2023

ICD-10-CM
FOR PHYSICIANS

Jackie L. Koesterman, CPC
Coding and Reimbursement Specialist
JDK Medical Coding EDU, LLC
Grand Forks, North Dakota

BUCK'S

INCLUDES
NETTER'S
ANATOMY
ART

ELSEVIER

Elsevier
3251 Riverport Lane
St. Louis, Missouri 63043

BUCK'S 2023 ICD-10-CM FOR PHYSICIANS   ISBN: 978-0-323-87417-5
Copyright © 2023, Elsevier Inc. All rights reserved.

Notice

Practitioners and researchers must always rely on their own experience and knowledge in evaluating
and using any information, methods, compounds or experiments described herein. Because of
rapid advances in the medical sciences, in particular, independent verification of diagnoses and
drug dosages should be made. To the fullest extent of the law, no responsibility is assumed by
Elsevier, authors, editors or contributors for any injury and/or damage to persons or property as a
matter of products liability, negligence or otherwise, or from any use or operation of any methods,
products, instructions, or ideas contained in the material herein.

Previous editions copyrighted 2022, 2021, 2020, 2019, 2018, 2017, 2016, 2015, 2014, 2013, 2010

International Standard Book Number: 978-0-323-87417-5

Content Strategist: Laura Klein
Senior Content Development Manager: Luke E. Held
Senior Content Development Specialist: Joshua S. Rapplean
Publishing Services Manager: Deepthi Unni
Project Manager: Aparna Venkatachalam
Senior Book Designer: Maggie Reid

Printed in Canada

 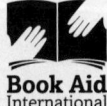

Working together
to grow libraries in
developing countries

www.elsevier.com • www.bookaid.org

Last digit is the print number: 9   8   7   6   5   4   3   2   1

DEDICATION

To all the brave medical coders who transitioned the nation into a new coding system.
Decades of waiting finally concluded with the implementation of I-10,
and you have been the pioneers leading the way.

With greatest appreciations for your efforts!

Carol J. Buck, MS

DEVELOPMENT OF THIS EDITION

Lead Technical Collaborator

Jackie L. Koesterman, CPC
Coding and Reimbursement Specialist
JDK Medical Coding EDU
Grand Forks, North Dakota

Query Team

Patricia Cordy Henricksen, MS, CHCA, CPC-I, CPC, CCP-P, ASC-PM
AAPC-Approved Instructor
Auditing, Coding, and Education Specialist
Soterion Medical Services
Lexington, Kentucky

CONTENTS

GUIDE TO USING THE 2023 ICD-10-CM FOR PHYSICIANS

Medical coding has long been a part of the health care profession. Through the years medical coding systems have become more complex and extensive. Today, medical coding is an intricate and immense process that is present in every health care setting. The increased use of electronic submissions for health care services only increases the need for coders who understand the coding process.

2023 ICD-10-CM for Physicians, Professional Edition was developed to help meet the needs of coding professionals at all levels by offering a comprehensive coding text at a reasonable price.

All material strictly adheres to the latest government versions available at the time of printing. Updates from the *Definitions of Medicare Code Edits* (MCE) will be posted to the companion website (www. codingupdates.com) when available.

Illustrations and Items

The ICD-10-CM Tabular List contains illustrations, pictures, and items to assist you in understanding difficult terminology, diseases/conditions, or coding in a specific category. Items are always printed in ███████ ink so that the added material is not mistaken for official notations or instructions. ███████ ink is used for other annotations in the text. Your ideas on what other descriptions or illustrations should be in future editions of this text are always appreciated.

Instructional Notations

Includes Notes

Includes

The word "Includes" appears immediately under certain categories to further define, or give examples of, the content of the category.

Excludes Notes

The ICD-10-CM has two types of excludes notes. Each note has a different definition for use, but they are both similar in that they indicate that codes excluded from each other are independent of each other.

Excludes1

A type 1 Excludes note is a pure excludes. It means "NOT CODED HERE!" An Excludes1 note indicates that the code excluded should never be used at the same time as the code above the Excludes1 note. An Excludes1 is for use when two conditions cannot occur together, such as a congenital form versus an acquired form of the same condition.

Excludes2

A type 2 Excludes note represents "NOT INCLUDED HERE." An Excludes2 note indicates that the condition excluded is not part of the condition it is excluded from, but a patient may have both conditions at the same time. When an Excludes2 note appears under a code, it is acceptable to use both the code and the excluded code together.

Code First/Use Additional Code notes (etiology/manifestation paired codes)

Certain conditions have both an underlying etiology and multiple body system manifestations due to the underlying etiology. For such conditions the ICD-10-CM has a coding convention that requires the underlying condition be sequenced first, followed by the manifestation. Wherever such a combination exists, there is a "use additional code" note at the etiology code, and a "code first" note at the manifestation code. These instructional notes indicate the proper sequencing order of the codes, etiology followed by manifestation.

In most cases the manifestation codes will have in the code title, "in diseases classified elsewhere." Codes with this title are a component of the etiology/manifestation convention. The code title indicates that it is a manifestation code. "In diseases classified elsewhere" codes are never permitted to be used as first-listed or principal diagnosis codes. They must be used in conjunction with an underlying condition code, and they must be listed following the underlying condition.

Use additional

The words indicate an instructional note that another code may be needed.

Code first

The words indicate an instructional note that directs the coder to sequence the underlying condition before the manifestation.

Code also

A "code also" note instructs that two codes may be required to fully describe a condition, but the sequencing of the two codes is discretionary, depending on the severity of the conditions and the reason for the encounter.

7th characters and placeholder X

For codes less than 6 characters that require a 7th character, a placeholder X should be assigned for all characters less than 6. The 7th character must always be the 7th character of a code.

Annotated

Throughout the manual, revisions, additions, and deleted codes or words are indicated by the following symbols:

⇛ **Revised:** Revisions within the line or code from the previous edition are indicated by the arrow.

▶ **New:** Additions to the previous edition are indicated by the triangle.

~~deleted~~ **Deleted:** Deletions from the previous edition are struck through.

ICD-10-CM Tabular List Symbols

⬤ **Use Additional Character(s):** The red stop sign cautions that the code requires additional character(s) to ensure the greatest specificity.

X For codes less than 6 characters that require a 7th character, a placeholder X should be assigned for all characters less than 6. The 7th character must always be the 7th character of a code.

OGCR The *Official Guidelines for Coding and Reporting* symbol includes the placement of a portion of a guideline as that guideline pertains to the code by which it is located. The complete OGCR are located in Part I.

🏵 The **Hierarchical condition category (HCC)** was initiated in 2004 for the reimbursement for patients with Medicare Advantage plans (Medicare Part C). HCC is based on a list of chronic or severity of illness diagnosis codes that CMS uses to determine reimbursements to Medicare Advantage plans. The HCC risk adjustment factor data is calculated for an entire year for encounters of the patient's care.

▷ **Manifestation Code:** Describes the manifestation of an underlying disease, not the disease itself, and therefore should not be assigned as a principal diagnosis, according to the *Definitions of Medicare Code Edits* (MCE).

Age conflict: The *Definitions of Medicare Code Edits* (MCE) detects inconsistencies between a patient's age and diagnosis. For example, a 5-year-old patient with benign prostatic hypertrophy or a 78-year-old pregnant female.

The diagnosis is clinically and virtually impossible in a patient of the stated age. Therefore, either the diagnosis or the age is presumed to be incorrect. There are four age categories for diagnoses in the *Definitions of Medicare Code Edits* (MCE):

N • Newborn. Age of 0 years; a subset of diagnoses intended only for newborns and neonates (e.g., fetal distress, perinatal jaundice).

P • Pediatric. Age range is 0-17 years inclusive (e.g., Reye's syndrome, routine child health exam).

M • Maternity. Age range is 9-64 years inclusive (e.g., diabetes in pregnancy, antepartum pulmonary complication).

A • Adult. Age range is 15-124 years inclusive (e.g., senile delirium, mature cataract).

♀♂ **Sex conflict:** *Definitions of Medicare Code Edits* (MCE) detects inconsistencies between a patient's sex and any diagnosis or procedure on the patient's record. For example, a male patient with cervical cancer (diagnosis) or a female patient with a prostatectomy (procedure). In both instances, the indicated diagnosis or the procedure conflicts with the stated sex of the patient. Therefore, either the patient's diagnosis, procedure, or sex is presumed to be incorrect.

Key words

Highlight identifies key words within similar code descriptions in a particular category.

Coding Clinic Identifies the year, quarter, and page number that presents information about an ICD-10-CM code in the American Hospital Association's *Coding Clinic*® for ICD-10-CM.

Visit codingupdates.com for the full list of 2022 Present on Admission codes.

SYMBOLS AND CONVENTIONS

ICD-10-CM Tabular

Use Additional Character(s): The red stop sign cautions you that the code requires additional character(s) to ensure greatest specificity.

Placeholder X: The red X reminds you that for codes less than 6 characters that require a 7th character, a placeholder X should be assigned to all characters less than 6.

Volume 1, Tabular List

● **K22   Other diseases of esophagus**

   Excludes2   esophageal varices (I85.-)

X● **V00.01   Pedestrian on foot injured in collision with roller-skater**

A02.20   Localized salmonella infection, unspecified

Unspecified: These codes are for use when the information in the medical record is insufficient to assign a more specific code. For those categories for which an unspecified code is not provided, the "other specified" code may represent both other and unspecified.

Use additional code: Located at the etiology code and directs you to assign a manifestation code.

A48.3   Toxic shock syndrome

   Use additional code to identify the organism (B95, B96)

Code first indicates the etiology code is to be first-listed before the manifestation code.

B39   Histoplasmosis

   Code first associated AIDS (B20)

Notes define terms or give coding instructions.

E34.0   Carcinoid syndrome

   Note: May be used as an additional code to identify functional activity associated with a carcinoid tumor.

Codes or index entries are for purposes of illustration only and may not be current.

OGCR Section I.C.6.B.5. ◀──────────────

Neoplasm Related Pain Code G89.3 is assigned to pain documented as being related, associated or due to cancer, primary or secondary malignancy, or tumor. This code is assigned regardless of whether the pain is acute or chronic.

OGCR: The *Official Guidelines for Coding and Reporting* are placed near the codes to which they refer and are highlighted.

I70.2   **Atherosclerosis of native arteries of the extremities**
Mönckeberg's (medial) sclerosis ◀──────

Use additional code, if applicable, to identify chronic total occlusion of artery of extremity (I70.92)

code, if applicable, directs the coder to other conditions that may be appropriate to report.

I74   **Arterial embolism and thrombosis**
Includes   embolic infarction
embolic occlusion
thrombotic infarction
thrombotic occlusion

The word "and" should be interpreted to mean either "and" or "or" when it appears in a statement.

Bold typeface is used on all codes and titles.

I83.001   **Varicose veins of unspecified lower extremity with ulcer of thigh**

"with" should be interpreted to mean "associated with" or "due to."

K73.2   **Chronic active hepatitis, not elsewhere classified**

"not elsewhere classified" or **NEC** identifies a code that is assigned only when the information at hand specifies a condition for which no more specific code is available.

"not otherwise specified" or **NOS** is equivalent to unspecified.

W13.9   **Fall from, out of or through building, not otherwise specified**

Codes or index entries are for purposes of illustration only and may not be current.

Excludes1 means "NOT CODED HERE!" An Excludes1 note indicates that the code excluded should never be assigned at the same time as the code above the Excludes1 note.

M19 **Other and unspecified osteoarthritis**
  Excludes1   polyarthritis (M15.-)
  Excludes2   arthrosis of spine (M47.-)
             hallux rigidus (M20.2)
             osteoarthritis of spine (M47.-)

Excludes2 represents "NOT INCLUDED HERE." An Excludes2 note indicates that the condition excluded is not part of the condition represented by the code, but a patient may have both conditions at the same time and it is acceptable to use both the code and the excluded code together, when appropriate.

Includes: This note appears immediately under a three-character code title to further define, or give examples of, the content.

A06 **Amebiasis**
  Includes   infection due to Entamoeba histolytica

E26.01 **Conn's syndrome**
          Code also adrenal adenoma (D35.0)

Code also instructs that two codes may be required to fully describe a condition, but this note does not provide sequencing direction.

Codes titled "other" or "other specified" are for use when the information in the medical record provides detail for which a specific code does not exist.

E25.8 **Other adrenogenital disorders**

O00.2 **Ovarian pregnancy**   M

Maternity DX (Diagnosis) for ages 9-64 according to the *Definitions of Medicare Code Edits* (MCE).

P02.20 **Newborn (suspected to be) affected by unspecified morphological and functional abnormalities of placenta**   N

Newborn, Age 0, according to the *Definitions of Medicare Code Edits* (MCE).

L21.0 **Seborrhea capitis**   P
          Cradle cap

Pediatric Age, 0-17, according to the *Definitions of Medicare Code Edits* (MCE).

G30.1 **Alzheimer's disease with late onset**   A

Adult Age, 15-124, according to the *Definitions of Medicare Code Edits* (MCE).

Females Only according to the *Definitions of Medicare Code Edits* (MCE).

B37.3 **Candidiasis of vulva and vagina** ♀

C60.1 **Malignant neoplasm of glans penis** ♂

Males Only according to the *Definitions of Medicare Code Edits* (MCE).

Codes or index entries are for purposes of illustration only and may not be current.

Manifestation according to the *Definitions of Medicare Code Edits* (MCE).

▶ H22 *Disorders of iris and ciliary body in diseases classified elsewhere*

   Code first *underlying disease, such as:*
      gout (M1A-, M10.-)

Key Term Highlight identifies key words within similar code descriptions in a particular category.

F10.21   Alcohol dependence, **in remission** ◀

Coding Clinic identifies the year, quarter, and page number that presents information about an ICD-10-PCS code in the American Hospital Association's *Coding Clinic®*.

B96.5   Pseudomonas (aeruginosa) (mallei) (pseudomallei) as the cause of diseases classified elsewhere
      ▶ Coding Clinic: 2015, Q1, P18

Codes or index entries are for purposes of illustration only and may not be current.

Alphabetic Index

Main terms are in **bold** typeface.

Aberrant (congenital) —*see also* Malposition, congenital
adrenal gland Q89.1

Etiology code first followed by the manifestation code in **brackets**. The code in brackets is always to be sequenced second.

Amyloid heart (disease) E85.4 *[I43]*

Amylophagia —*see* Pica

"see" indicates another term should be referenced.

Angiofibroma —*see also* Neoplasm, benign, by site

"see also" follows a main term and instructs that there is another main term that may also be referenced.

Appendicitis (pneumococcal) (retrocecal) K37
   with
      perforation NOS K35.32
      peritoneal abscess K35.33

A default code is listed next to the main term and represents that condition most commonly associated with the main term. If a condition is documented in a medical record without any additional information, such as acute or chronic, the default code should be assigned.

Use Additional Character(s): The red stop sign cautions you that the code requires additional character(s) to ensure greatest specificity.

Abrasion T14.8
   ankle S90.51-•

Codes or index entries are for purposes of illustration only and may not be current.

GUIDE TO THE 2023 ICD-10-CM UPDATES

No Change	**CHAPTER 1**	
No Change	**CERTAIN INFECTIOUS AND PARASITIC DISEASES (A00-B99)**	
No Change	**VIRAL AND PRION INFECTIONS OF THE CENTRAL NERVOUS SYSTEM (A80-A89)**	

No Change **A81** **Atypical virus infections of central nervous system**
No Change   Use additional
Revise from   code to identify:
Revise to   code, if applicable, to identify:
Revise from   dementia with behavioral disturbance (F02.81)
Revise to   dementia with anxiety (F02.84, F02.A4, F02.B4, F02.C4)
Delete   dementia without behavioral disturbance (F02.80)
Add   dementia with behavioral disturbance (F02.81-, F02.A1-, F02.B1-, F02.C1-)
Add   dementia with mood disturbance (F02.83, F02.A3, F02.B3, F02.C3)
Add   dementia with psychotic disturbance (F02.82, F02.A2, F02.B2, F02.C2)
Add   dementia without behavioral disturbance (F02.80, F02.A0, F02.B0, F02.C0)
Add   mild neurocognitive disorder due to known physiological condition (F06.7-)

No Change **A85** **Other viral encephalitis, not elsewhere classified**
No Change   **Excludes1**
Delete   benign myalgic encephalomyelitis (G93.3)
Add   myalgic encephalomyelitis (G93.32)

No Change **MYCOSES (B35-B49)**

No Change **B37** **Candidiasis**
No Change   **B37.3** **Candidiasis of vulva and vagina**
Add   **B37.31** **Acute candidiasis of vulva and vagina**
Add   Candidiasis of vulva and vagina NOS
Add   **B37.32** **Chronic candidiasis of vulva and vagina**
Add   Recurrent candidiasis of vulva and vagina

No Change **CHAPTER 2**

No Change **NEOPLASMS (C00-D49)**

No Change **MALIGNANT NEOPLASMS OF MALE GENITAL ORGANS (C60-C63)**

No Change **C61** **Malignant neoplasm of prostate**
No Change   Use additional
Revise from   code to identify:
Revise to   code, if applicable, to identify:

No Change **MALIGNANT NEOPLASMS OF LYMPHOID, HEMATOPOIETIC AND RELATED TISSUE (C81-C96)**

No Change **C84** **Mature T/NK-cell lymphomas**
No Change   **C84.0** **Mycosis fungoides**
No Change   **Excludes1**
Revise from   peripheral T-cell lymphoma, not classified (C84.4-)
Revise to   peripheral T-cell lymphoma, not elsewhere classified (C84.4-)
Revise from   **C84.4** **Peripheral T-cell lymphoma, not classified**
Revise to   **C84.4** **Peripheral T-cell lymphoma, not elsewhere classified**

Revise from **C84.40** Peripheral T-cell lymphoma, not classified, unspecified site
Revise to **C84.40** Peripheral T-cell lymphoma, not elsewhere classified, unspecified site
Revise from **C84.41** Peripheral T-cell lymphoma, not classified, lymph nodes of head, face, and neck
Revise to **C84.41** Peripheral T-cell lymphoma, not elsewhere classified, lymph nodes of head, face, and neck
Revise from **C84.42** Peripheral T-cell lymphoma, not classified, intrathoracic lymph nodes
Revise to **C84.42** Peripheral T-cell lymphoma, not elsewhere classified, intrathoracic lymph nodes
Revise from **C84.43** Peripheral T-cell lymphoma, not classified, intra-abdominal lymph nodes
Revise to **C84.43** Peripheral T-cell lymphoma, not elsewhere classified, intra-abdominal lymph nodes
Revise from **C84.44** Peripheral T-cell lymphoma, not classified, lymph nodes of axilla and upper limb
Revise to **C84.44** Peripheral T-cell lymphoma, not elsewhere classified, lymph nodes of axilla and upper limb
Revise from **C84.45** Peripheral T-cell lymphoma, not classified, lymph nodes of inguinal region and lower limb
Revise to **C84.45** Peripheral T-cell lymphoma, not elsewhere classified, lymph nodes of inguinal region and lower limb
Revise from **C84.46** Peripheral T-cell lymphoma, not classified, intrapelvic lymph nodes
Revise to **C84.46** Peripheral T-cell lymphoma, not elsewhere classified, intrapelvic lymph nodes
Revise from **C84.47** Peripheral T-cell lymphoma, not classified, spleen
Revise to **C84.47** Peripheral T-cell lymphoma, not elsewhere classified, spleen
Revise from **C84.48** Peripheral T-cell lymphoma, not classified, lymph nodes of multiple sites
Revise to **C84.48** Peripheral T-cell lymphoma, not elsewhere classified, lymph nodes of multiple sites
Revise from **C84.49** Peripheral T-cell lymphoma, not classified, extranodal and solid organ sites
Revise to **C84.49** Peripheral T-cell lymphoma, not elsewhere classified, extranodal and solid organ sites

No Change **C94** **Other leukemias of specified cell type**
Revise from **C94.6** **Myelodysplastic disease, not classified**
Revise to **C94.6** **Myelodysplastic disease, not elsewhere classified**
Delete   Myeloproliferative disease, not classified
Add   Myelodysplastic/myeloproliferative neoplasm, unclassifiable
Add   Myeloproliferative disease, not elsewhere classified

No Change		**BENIGN NEOPLASMS, EXCEPT BENIGN NEUROENDOCRINE TUMORS (D10-D36)**

No Change	D27	Benign neoplasm of ovary	
No Change		**Excludes2**	
Revise from			endometrial cyst (N80.1)
Revise to			endometrial cyst (N80.1-)

No Change	**CHAPTER 3**
No Change	**DISEASES OF THE BLOOD AND BLOOD-FORMING ORGANS AND CERTAIN DISORDERS INVOLVING THE IMMUNE MECHANISM (D50-D89)**

No Change		**HEMOLYTIC ANEMIAS (D55-D59)**	
No Change	D59	Acquired hemolytic anemia	
No Change		D59.3	Hemolytic-uremic syndrome
Delete			Use Additional code to identify associated:
Delete			E. coli infection (B96.2-)
Delete			Pneumococcal pneumonia (J13)
Delete			Shigella dysenteriae (A03.9)
Add			Code also, if applicable, any associated:
Add			acute kidney failure (N17.-)
Add			chronic kidney disease (N18.-)
Add		D59.30	**Hemolytic-uremic syndrome, unspecified**
			Hemolytic-uremic syndrome NOS
Add		D59.31	**Infection-associated hemolytic-uremic syndrome**
Add			Shiga toxin-producing E. coli [STEC] related hemolytic uremic syndrome
Add			Typical hemolytic uremic syndrome
Add			Use Additional code to identify associated infection, such as:
Add			E. coli infection (B96.2-)
Add			Human immunodeficiency virus [HIV] disease (B20)
Add			Pneumococcal meningitis (G00.1)
Add			Pneumococcal pneumonia (J13)
Add			Sepsis due to Streptococcus pneumoniae (A40.3)
Add			Shigella dysenteriae (A03.9)
Add			Streptococcus pneumoniae as the cause of diseases classified elsewhere (B95.3)
Add		D59.32	**Hereditary hemolytic-uremic syndrome**
Add			Atypical hemolytic uremic syndrome with an identified genetic cause
Add			Code also, if applicable:
Add			defects in the complement system (D84.1)
Add			methylmalonic acidemia (E71.120)
Add		D59.39	**Other hemolytic-uremic syndrome**
Add			Atypical (nongenetic) hemolytic uremic syndrome
Add			Secondary hemolytic-uremic syndrome
Add			*Code first, if applicable, any associated:*
Add			COVID-19 (U07.1)
Add			complications of kidney transplant (T86.1-)
Add			complications of heart transplant (T86.2-)
Add			complications of liver transplant (T86.4-)
Add			Code also, if applicable, any associated condition, such as:
Add			hypertensive emergency (I16.1)
Add			malignant neoplasm (C00-C96)
Add			systemic lupus erythematosus (M32.-)
Add			Use Additional code, if applicable, for adverse effect to identify drug (T36-T50 with fifth or sixth character 5)

No Change			**COAGULATION DEFECTS, PURPURA AND OTHER HEMORRHAGIC CONDITIONS (D65-D69)**
No Change	D66	Hereditary factor VIII deficiency	
No Change		**Excludes1**	
Revise from			factor VIII deficiency with vascular defect (D68.0)
Revise to			factor VIII deficiency with vascular defect (D68.0-)
No Change	D68	Other coagulation defects	
No Change		**Excludes1**	
Revise from			abnormal coagulation profile (R79.1)
Revise to			abnormal coagulation profile NOS (R79.1)
Delete			coagulation defects complicating abortion or ectopic or molar pregnancy (O00-O07, O08.1)
Delete			coagulation defects complicating pregnancy, childbirth and the puerperium (O45.0, O46.0, O67.0, O72.3)
Add		**Excludes2**	coagulation defects complicating abortion or ectopic or molar pregnancy (O00-O07, O08.1)
Add			coagulation defects complicating pregnancy, childbirth and the puerperium (O45.0, O46.0, O67.0, O72.3)
Revise from	D68.0	Von Willebrand's disease	
Revise to	D68.0	Von Willebrand disease	
Delete			Angiohemophilia
Delete			Factor VIII deficiency with vascular defect
Delete			Vascular hemophilia
Add		D68.00	**Von Willebrand disease, unspecified**
Add		D68.01	**Von Willebrand disease, type 1**
Add			Partial quantitative deficiency of von Willebrand factor
Add			Type 1C von Willebrand disease
Add		D68.02	**Von Willebrand disease, type 2**
Add			Qualitative defects of von Willebrand factor
Add			D68.020	**Von Willebrand disease, type 2A**
Add				Qualitative defects of von Willebrand factor with decreased platelet adhesion and selective deficiency of high-molecular-weight multimers
Add			D68.021	**Von Willebrand disease, type 2B**
Add				Qualitative defects of von Willebrand factor with high-molecular-weight von Willebrand factor loss
Add				Qualitative defects of von Willebrand factor with hyper-adhesive forms
Add				Qualitative defects of von Willebrand factor with increased affinity for platelet glycoprotein lb
Add			D68.022	**Von Willebrand disease, type 2M**
Add				Qualitative defects of von Willebrand factor with defective platelet adhesion with a normal size distribution of von Willebrand factor multimers

Add		D68.023	Von Willebrand disease, type 2N
Add			Qualitative defects of von Willebrand factor with defective von Willebrand factor to factor VIII binding
Add			Qualitative defects of von Willebrand factor with markedly decreased affinity for factor VIII
Add		D68.029	Von Willebrand disease, type 2, unspecified
Add			Qualitative defect in von Willebrand factor function, with no further subtyping
Add	D68.03	Von Willebrand disease, type 3	
Add			(Near) complete absence of von Willebrand factor
Add			Total quantitative deficiency of von Willebrand factor
Add	D68.04	Acquired von Willebrand disease	
Add			Acquired von Willebrand syndrome
Add	D68.09	Other von Willebrand disease	
Add			Platelet-type von Willebrand disease
Add			Pseudo-von Willebrand disease
Add			Code also, if applicable, qualitative platelet defects (D69.1)
No Change	D68.6	Other thrombophilia	
No Change		Excludes1	
Revise from			heparin induced thrombocytopenia (HIT) (D75.82)
Revise to			heparin induced thrombocytopenia (HIT) (D75.82-)
No Change	D69	Purpura and other hemorrhagic conditions	
No Change	D69.1	Qualitative platelet defects	
No Change		Excludes1	
Delete			von Willebrand's disease (D68.0)
Add			hemolytic-uremic syndrome (D59.3-)
Add		Excludes2	von Willebrand disease (D68.0-)
No Change	D69.5	Secondary thrombocytopenia	
No Change		Excludes1	
Revise from			heparin induced thrombocytopenia (HIT) (D75.82)
Revise to			heparin induced thrombocytopenia (HIT) (D75.82-)

No Change   **OTHER DISORDERS OF BLOOD AND BLOOD-FORMING ORGANS (D70-D77)**

No Change	D75	Other and unspecified diseases of blood and blood-forming organs	
No Change	D75.8	Other specified diseases of blood and blood-forming organs	
No Change	D75.82	Heparin induced thrombocytopenia (HIT)	
Add			Use Additional code, if applicable, for adverse effect of heparin (T45.515-)
Add		D75.821	Non-immune heparin-induced thrombocytopenia
Add			Non-immune HIT
Add			Type 1 heparin-induced thrombocytopenia
Add		D75.822	Immune-mediated heparin-induced thrombocytopenia
Add			Immune-mediated HIT
Add			Type 2 heparin-induced thrombocytopenia

Add		D75.828	Other heparin-induced thrombocytopenia syndrome
Add			Autoimmune heparin-induced thrombocytopenia syndrome
Add			Delayed-onset heparin-induced thrombocytopenia
Add			Persisting heparin-induced thrombocytopenia
Add		D75.829	Heparin-induced thrombocytopenia, unspecified
Add		D75.84	Other platelet-activating anti-PF4 disorders
Add			Spontaneous heparin-induced thrombocytopenia syndrome (without heparin exposure)
Add			Thrombosis with thrombocytopenia syndrome
Add			Vaccine-induced thrombotic thrombocytopenia
Add			Use Additional code, if applicable, for adverse effect of other viral vaccine (T50.B95-)

No Change   **CERTAIN DISORDERS INVOLVING THE IMMUNE MECHANISM (D80-D89)**

No Change	D81	Combined immunodeficiencies	
No Change	D81.8	Other combined immunodeficiencies	
Add		D81.82	Activated Phosphoinositide 3-kinase Delta Syndrome [APDS]
Add			p110d-activating mutation causing senescent T cells, lymphadenopathy, and immunodeficiency [PASLI] disease
Add			Code also, if applicable, any associated manifestations, such as:
Add			bronchiectasis (J47.-)
Add			herpes virus infections (B00.-)
Add			other acute respiratory tract infections (J00-J06; J20-J22)
Add			other infections (A00-B99)
Add			pneumonia (J12-J18)

No Change   # CHAPTER 4

No Change   # ENDOCRINE, NUTRITIONAL AND METABOLIC DISEASES (E00-E89)

No Change   **DISORDERS OF OTHER ENDOCRINE GLANDS (E20-E35)**

No Change	E23	Hypofunction and other disorders of the pituitary gland	
Add		Excludes1	short stature due to endocrine disorder (E34.3-)
No Change	E34	Other endocrine disorders	
No Change	E34.3	Short stature due to endocrine disorder	
Delete			Constitutional short stature
Delete			Laron-type short stature
Add		Excludes1	short stature (child) (R62.52)
Add		E34.30	Short stature due to endocrine disorder, unspecified
Add		E34.31	Constitutional short stature
			Constitutional delay of growth, puberty, or maturation
Add		E34.32	Genetic causes of short stature

Add		E34.321	**Primary insulin-like growth factor-1 (IGF-1) deficiency**
Add			Acid-labile subunit gene (IGFALS) defect
Add			Growth hormone gene 1 (GH1) defect with growth hormone neutralizing antibodies
Add			Growth hormone insensitivity syndrome (GHIS)
Add			Insulin-like growth factor 1 gene (IGF1) defect
Add			Laron type short stature
Add			Severe primary insulin-like growth factor-1 deficiency (SPIGFD)
Add			Signal transducer and activator of transcription 5B gene (STAT5b) defect
Add		E34.322	**Insulin-like growth factor-1 (IGF-1) resistance**
Add			Genetic syndrome with resistance to insulin-like growth factor-1
Add			Insulin-like growth factor-1 receptor (IGF-1R) defect
Add			Post-insulin-like growth factor-1 receptor signaling defect
Add		E34.328	**Other genetic causes of short stature**
Add			Short stature due to ACAN gene variant
Add			Short stature due to aggrecan deficiency
Add			Short stature due to NPR-2 gene variant
Add		E34.329	**Unspecified genetic causes of short stature**
Add		E34.39	**Other short stature due to endocrine disorder**

METABOLIC DISORDERS (E70-E88)

No Change			
No Change E87			**Other disorders of fluid, electrolyte and acid-base balance**
No Change	E87.2		**Acidosis**
Delete			Acidosis NOS
Delete			Lactic acidosis
Delete			Metabolic acidosis
Delete			Respiratory acidosis
Add		E87.20	**Acidosis, unspecified**
Add			Lactic acidosis NOS
Add			Metabolic acidosis NOS
Add			Code also, if applicable, respiratory failure with hypercapnia (J96. with 5th character 2)
Add		E87.21	**Acute metabolic acidosis**
Add			Acute lactic acidosis
Add		E87.22	**Chronic metabolic acidosis**
Add			Chronic lactic acidosis
Add			*Code first* underlying etiology, if applicable
Add		E87.29	**Other acidosis**
Add			Respiratory acidosis NOS
Add			**Excludes2** acute respiratory acidosis (J96.02)
Add			chronic respiratory acidosis (J96.12)

CHAPTER 5

MENTAL, BEHAVIORAL AND NEURODEVELOPMENTAL DISORDERS (F01-F99)

MENTAL DISORDERS DUE TO KNOWN PHYSIOLOGICAL CONDITIONS (F01-F09)

No Change			
No Change			
No Change			
No Change **F01**			**Vascular dementia**
Add		**Includes**	major neurocognitive disorder due to vascular disease
Add			multi-infarct dementia
Revise from	F01.5		Vascular dementia
Revise to	F01.5		Vascular dementia, unspecified severity
Revise from		F01.50	**Vascular dementia without behavioral disturbance**
Revise to		F01.50	**Vascular dementia, unspecified severity, without behavioral disturbance, psychotic disturbance, mood disturbance, and anxiety**
Revise from			Major neurocognitive disorder without behavioral disturbance
Revise to			Major neurocognitive disorder due to vascular disease NOS
Add			Vascular dementia NOS
Revise from		F01.51	**Vascular dementia with behavioral disturbance**
Revise to		F01.51	**Vascular dementia, unspecified severity, with behavioral disturbance**
Delete			Major neurocognitive disorder due to vascular disease, with behavioral disturbance
Delete			Major neurocognitive disorder with aggressive behavior
Delete			Major neurocognitive disorder with combative behavior
Delete			Major neurocognitive disorder with violent behavior
Delete			Vascular dementia with aggressive behavior
Delete			Vascular dementia with combative behavior
Delete			Vascular dementia with violent behavior
Delete			Use Additional code, if applicable, to identify wandering in vascular dementia (Z91.83)
Add		F01.511	**Vascular dementia, unspecified severity, with agitation**
Add			Major neurocognitive disorder due to vascular disease, unspecified severity, with aberrant motor behavior such as restlessness, rocking, pacing, or exit-seeking
Add			Major neurocognitive disorder due to vascular disease, unspecified severity, with verbal or physical behaviors such as profanity, shouting, threatening, anger, aggression, combativeness, or violence
Add			Vascular dementia, unspecified severity, with aberrant motor behavior such as restlessness, rocking, pacing, or exit-seeking
Add			Vascular dementia, unspecified severity, with verbal or physical behaviors such as profanity, shouting, threatening, anger, aggression, combativeness, or violence

Add		F01.518	**Vascular dementia, unspecified severity, with other behavioral disturbance**
Add			Major neurocognitive disorder due to vascular disease, unspecified severity, with behavioral disturbances such as sleep disturbance, social disinhibition, or sexual disinhibition
Add			Vascular dementia, unspecified severity, with behavioral disturbances such as sleep disturbance, social disinhibition, or sexual disinhibition
Add			Use Additional code, if applicable, to identify wandering in vascular dementia (Z91.83)
Add	F01.52		**Vascular dementia, unspecified severity, with psychotic disturbance**
Add			Major neurocognitive disorder due to vascular disease, unspecified severity, with psychotic disturbance such as hallucinations, paranoia, suspiciousness, or delusional state
Add			Vascular dementia, unspecified severity, with psychotic disturbance such as hallucinations, paranoia, suspiciousness, or delusional state
Add	F01.53		**Vascular dementia, unspecified severity, with mood disturbance**
Add			Major neurocognitive disorder due to vascular disease, unspecified severity, with mood disturbance such as depression, apathy, or anhedonia
Add			Vascular dementia, unspecified severity, with mood disturbance such as depression, apathy, or anhedonia
Add	F01.54		**Vascular dementia, unspecified severity, with anxiety**
Add			Major neurocognitive disorder due to vascular disease, unspecified severity, with anxiety
Add	F01.A		**Vascular dementia, mild**
Add		**Excludes1**	mild neurocognitive disorder due to known physiological condition with or without behavioral disturbance (F06.7-)
Add	F01.A0		**Vascular dementia, mild, without behavioral disturbance, psychotic disturbance, mood disturbance, and anxiety**
Add			Major neurocognitive disorder due to vascular disease, mild, NOS
Add			Vascular dementia, mild, NOS

Add		F01.A1	**Vascular dementia, mild, with behavioral disturbance**
Add		F01.A11	**Vascular dementia, mild, with agitation**
Add			Major neurocognitive disorder due to vascular disease, mild, with aberrant motor behavior such as restlessness, rocking, pacing, or exit-seeking
Add			Major neurocognitive disorder due to vascular disease, mild, with verbal or physical behaviors such as profanity, shouting, threatening, anger, aggression, combativeness, or violence
Add			Vascular dementia, mild, with aberrant motor behavior such as restlessness, rocking, pacing, or exit-seeking
Add			Vascular dementia, mild, with verbal or physical behaviors such as profanity, shouting, threatening, anger, aggression, combativeness, or violence
Add		F01.A18	**Vascular dementia, mild, with other behavioral disturbance**
Add			Major neurocognitive disorder due to vascular disease, mild, with behavioral disturbances such as sleep disturbance, social disinhibition, or sexual disinhibition
Add			Vascular dementia, mild, with behavioral disturbances such as sleep disturbance, social disinhibition, or sexual disinhibition
Add			Use Additional code, if applicable, to identify wandering in vascular dementia (Z91.83)
Add	F01.A2		**Vascular dementia, mild, with psychotic disturbance**
Add			Major neurocognitive disorder due to vascular disease, mild, with psychotic disturbance such as hallucinations, paranoia, suspiciousness, or delusional state
Add			Vascular dementia, mild, with psychotic disturbance such as hallucinations, paranoia, suspiciousness, or delusional state
Add	F01.A3		**Vascular dementia, mild, with mood disturbance**
Add			Major neurocognitive disorder due to vascular disease, mild, with mood disturbance such as depression, apathy, or anhedonia
Add			Vascular dementia, mild, with mood disturbance such as depression, apathy, or anhedonia
Add	F01.A4		**Vascular dementia, mild, with anxiety**
Add			Major neurocognitive disorder due to vascular disease, mild, with anxiety

Add	**F01.B Vascular dementia, moderate**
Add	**F01.B0 Vascular dementia, moderate, without behavioral disturbance, psychotic disturbance, mood disturbance, and anxiety**
Add	Major neurocognitive disorder due to vascular disease, moderate, NOS
Add	Vascular dementia, moderate, NOS
Add	**F01.B1 Vascular dementia, moderate, with behavioral disturbance**
Add	**F01.B11 Vascular dementia, moderate, with agitation**
Add	Major neurocognitive disorder due to vascular disease, moderate, with aberrant motor behavior such as restlessness, rocking, pacing, or exit-seeking
Add	Major neurocognitive disorder due to vascular disease, moderate, with verbal or physical behaviors such as profanity, shouting, threatening, anger, aggression, combativeness, or violence
Add	Vascular dementia, moderate, with aberrant motor behavior such as restlessness, rocking, pacing, or exit-seeking
Add	Vascular dementia, moderate, with verbal or physical behaviors such as profanity, shouting, threatening, anger, aggression, combativeness, or violence
Add	**F01.B18 Vascular dementia, moderate, with other behavioral disturbance**
Add	Major neurocognitive disorder due to vascular disease, moderate, with behavioral disturbances such as sleep disturbance, social disinhibition, or sexual disinhibition
Add	Vascular dementia, moderate, with behavioral disturbances such as sleep disturbance, social disinhibition, or sexual disinhibition
Add	Use Additional code, if applicable, to identify wandering in vascular dementia (Z91.83)
Add	**F01.B2 Vascular dementia, moderate, with psychotic disturbance**
Add	Major neurocognitive disorder due to vascular disease, moderate, with psychotic disturbance such as hallucinations, paranoia, suspiciousness, or delusional state
Add	Vascular dementia, moderate, with psychotic disturbance such as hallucinations, paranoia, suspiciousness, or delusional state

Add	**F01.B3 Vascular dementia, moderate, with mood disturbance**
Add	Major neurocognitive disorder due to vascular disease, moderate, with mood disturbance such as depression, apathy, or anhedonia
Add	Vascular dementia, moderate, with mood disturbance such as depression, apathy, or anhedonia
Add	**F01.B4 Vascular dementia, moderate, with anxiety**
Add	Major neurocognitive disorder due to vascular disease, moderate, with anxiety
Add	**F01.C Vascular dementia, severe**
Add	**F01.C0 Vascular dementia, severe, without behavioral disturbance, psychotic disturbance, mood disturbance, and anxiety**
Add	Major neurocognitive disorder due to vascular disease, severe, NOS
Add	Vascular dementia, severe, NOS
Add	**F01.C1 Vascular dementia, severe, with behavioral disturbance**
Add	**F01.C11 Vascular dementia, severe, with agitation**
Add	Major neurocognitive disorder due to vascular disease, severe, with aberrant motor behavior such as restlessness, rocking, pacing, or exit-seeking
Add	Major neurocognitive disorder due to vascular disease, severe, with verbal or physical behaviors such as profanity, shouting, threatening, anger, aggression, combativeness, or violence
Add	Vascular dementia, severe, with aberrant motor behavior such as restlessness, rocking, pacing, or exit-seeking
Add	Vascular dementia, severe, with verbal or physical behaviors such as profanity, shouting, threatening, anger, aggression, combativeness, or violence
Add	**F01.C18 Vascular dementia, severe, with other behavioral disturbance**
Add	Major neurocognitive disorder due to vascular disease, severe, with behavioral disturbances such as sleep disturbance, social disinhibition, or sexual disinhibition
Add	Vascular dementia, severe, with behavioral disturbances such as sleep disturbance, social disinhibition, or sexual disinhibition
Add	Use Additional code, if applicable, to identify wandering in vascular dementia (Z91.83)

Add		F01.C2	**Vascular dementia, severe, with psychotic disturbance**
Add			Major neurocognitive disorder due to vascular disease, severe, with psychotic disturbance such as hallucinations, paranoia, suspiciousness, or delusional state
Add			Vascular dementia, severe, with psychotic disturbance such as hallucinations, paranoia, suspiciousness, or delusional state
Add		F01.C3	**Vascular dementia, severe, with mood disturbance**
Add			Major neurocognitive disorder due to vascular disease, severe, with mood disturbance such as depression, apathy, or anhedonia
Add			Vascular dementia, severe, with mood disturbance such as depression, apathy, or anhedonia
Add		F01.C4	**Vascular dementia, severe, with anxiety**
Add			Major neurocognitive disorder due to vascular disease, severe, with anxiety
No Change	**F02**	**Dementia in other diseases classified elsewhere**	
Add		**Excludes1**	mild neurocognitive disorder due to known physiological condition with or without behavioral disturbance (F06.7-)
No Change		**Excludes2**	
Revise from			vascular dementia (F01.5-)
Revise to			vascular dementia (F01.5-, F01.A-, F01.B-, F01.C-)
Revise from	F02.8	**Dementia in other diseases classified elsewhere**	
Revise to	F02.8	**Dementia in other diseases classified elsewhere, unspecified severity**	
Revise from		F02.80	**Dementia in other diseases classified elsewhere without behavioral disturbance**
Revise to		F02.80	**Dementia in other diseases classified elsewhere, unspecified severity, without behavioral disturbance, psychotic disturbance, mood disturbance, and anxiety**
Revise from			Major neurocognitive disorder in other diseases classified elsewhere
Revise to			Major neurocognitive disorder in other diseases classified elsewhere NOS
Revise from		F02.81	**Dementia in other diseases classified elsewhere with behavioral disturbance**
Revise to		F02.81	**Dementia in other diseases classified elsewhere, unspecified severity, with behavioral disturbance**
Delete			Dementia in other diseases classified elsewhere with aggressive behavior
Delete			Dementia in other diseases classified elsewhere with combative behavior
Delete			Dementia in other diseases classified elsewhere with violent behavior
Delete			Major neurocognitive disorder in other diseases classified elsewhere with aggressive behavior
Delete			Major neurocognitive disorder in other diseases classified elsewhere with combative behavior
Delete			Major neurocognitive disorder in other diseases classified elsewhere with violent behavior
Delete			Use Additional code, if applicable, to identify wandering in dementia in conditions classified elsewhere (Z91.83)

Add		F02.811	**Dementia in other diseases classified elsewhere, unspecified severity, with agitation**
Add			Dementia in other diseases classified elsewhere, unspecified severity, with aberrant motor behavior such as restlessness, rocking, pacing, or exit-seeking
			Dementia in other diseases classified elsewhere, unspecified severity, with verbal or physical behaviors such as profanity, shouting, threatening, anger, aggression, combativeness, or violence
Add			Major neurocognitive disorder in other diseases classified elsewhere, unspecified severity, with aberrant motor behavior such as restlessness, rocking, pacing, or exit-seeking
Add			Major neurocognitive disorder in other diseases classified elsewhere, unspecified severity, with verbal or physical behaviors such as profanity, shouting, threatening, anger, aggression, combativeness, or violence
Add		F02.818	**Dementia in other diseases classified elsewhere, unspecified severity, with other behavioral disturbance**
Add			Dementia in other diseases classified elsewhere with sleep disturbance, social disinhibition, or sexual disinhibition
Add			Major neurocognitive disorder in other diseases classified elsewhere with sleep disturbance, social disinhibition, or sexual disinhibition
Add			Use Additional code, if applicable, to identify wandering in dementia in conditions classified elsewhere (Z91.83)
Add		F02.82	**Dementia in other diseases classified elsewhere, unspecified severity, with psychotic disturbance**
Add			Dementia in other diseases classified elsewhere, unspecified severity, with psychotic disturbance such as hallucinations, paranoia, suspiciousness, or delusional state
Add			Major neurocognitive disorder in other diseases classified elsewhere, unspecified, with psychotic disturbance such as hallucinations, paranoia, suspiciousness, or delusional state

Add		F02.83	**Dementia in other diseases classified elsewhere, unspecified severity, with mood disturbance**
Add			Dementia in other diseases classified elsewhere, unspecified severity, with mood disturbance such as depression, apathy, or anhedonia
Add			Major neurocognitive disorder in other diseases classified elsewhere unspecified severity, with mood disturbance such as with depression, apathy, or anhedonia
Add		F02.84	**Dementia in other diseases classified elsewhere, unspecified severity, with anxiety**
Add			Major neurocognitive disorder in other diseases classified elsewhere unspecified severity, with anxiety

Add   F02.A   **Dementia in other diseases classified elsewhere, mild**

Add   **Excludes1**   mild neurocognitive disorder due to known physiological condition with or without behavioral disturbance (F06.7-)

Add		F02.A0	**Dementia in other diseases classified elsewhere, mild, without behavioral disturbance, psychotic disturbance, mood disturbance, and anxiety**
Add			Dementia in other diseases classified elsewhere, mild, NOS
Add			Major neurocognitive disorder in other diseases classified elsewhere, mild, NOS
Add		F02.A1	**Dementia in other diseases classified elsewhere, mild, with behavioral disturbance**
Add		F02.A11	**Dementia in other diseases classified elsewhere, mild, with agitation**
Add			Dementia in other diseases classified elsewhere, mild, with aberrant motor behavior such as restlessness, rocking, pacing, or exit-seeking
Add			Dementia in other diseases classified elsewhere, mild, with verbal or physical behaviors such as profanity, shouting, threatening, anger, aggression, combativeness, or violence
Add			Major neurocognitive disorder in other diseases classified elsewhere, mild, with aberrant motor behavior such as restlessness, rocking, pacing, or exit-seeking
Add			Major neurocognitive disorder in other diseases classified elsewhere, mild, with verbal or physical behaviors such as profanity, shouting, threatening, anger, aggression, combativeness, or violence

Add		F02.A18	**Dementia in other diseases classified elsewhere, mild, with other behavioral disturbance**
Add			Dementia in other diseases classified elsewhere, mild, with behavioral disturbances such as sleep disturbance, social disinhibition, or sexual disinhibition
Add			Major neurocognitive disorder in other diseases classified elsewhere, mild, with behavioral disturbances such as sleep disturbance, social disinhibition, or sexual disinhibition
Add			Use Additional code, if applicable, to identify wandering in dementia in conditions classified elsewhere (Z91.83)
Add		F02.A2	**Dementia in other diseases classified elsewhere, mild, with psychotic disturbance**
Add			Dementia in other diseases classified elsewhere, mild, with psychotic disturbance such as hallucinations, paranoia, suspiciousness, or delusional state
Add			Major neurocognitive disorder in other diseases classified elsewhere, mild, with psychotic disturbance such as hallucinations, paranoia, suspiciousness, or delusional state
Add		F02.A3	**Dementia in other diseases classified elsewhere, mild, with mood disturbance**
Add			Dementia in other diseases classified elsewhere, mild, with mood disturbance such as depression, apathy, or anhedonia
Add			Major neurocognitive disorder in other diseases classified elsewhere, mild, with mood disturbance such as depression, apathy, or anhedonia
Add		F02.A4	**Dementia in other diseases classified elsewhere, mild, with anxiety**
Add			Major neurocognitive disorder in other diseases classified elsewhere, mild, with anxiety

Add   F02.B   **Dementia in other diseases classified elsewhere, moderate**

Add		F02.B0	**Dementia in other diseases classified elsewhere, moderate, without behavioral disturbance, psychotic disturbance, mood disturbance, and anxiety**
Add			Dementia in other diseases classified elsewhere, moderate, NOS
Add			Major neurocognitive disorder in other diseases classified elsewhere, moderate, NOS
Add		F02.B1	**Dementia in other diseases classified elsewhere, moderate, with behavioral disturbance**

Add		F02.B11	**Dementia in other diseases classified elsewhere, moderate, with agitation**
Add			Dementia in other diseases classified elsewhere, moderate, with aberrant motor behavior such as restlessness, rocking, pacing, or exit-seeking
Add			Dementia in other diseases classified elsewhere, moderate, with verbal or physical behaviors such as profanity, shouting, threatening, anger, aggression, combativeness, or violence
Add			Major neurocognitive disorder in other diseases classified elsewhere, moderate, with aberrant motor behavior such as restlessness, rocking, pacing, or exitseeking
Add			Major neurocognitive disorder in other diseases classified elsewhere, moderate, with verbal or physical behaviors such as profanity, shouting, threatening, anger, aggression, combativeness, or violence
Add		F02.B18	**Dementia in other diseases classified elsewhere, moderate, with other behavioral disturbance**
Add			Dementia in other diseases classified elsewhere, moderate, with behavioral disturbances such as sleep disturbance, social disinhibition, or sexual disinhibition
Add			Major neurocognitive disorder in other diseases classified elsewhere, moderate, with behavioral disturbance such as sleep disturbance, social disinhibition, or sexual disinhibition
Add			Use Additional code, if applicable, to identify wandering in dementia in conditions classified elsewhere (Z91.83)
Add	F02.B2		**Dementia in other diseases classified elsewhere, moderate, with psychotic disturbance**
Add			Dementia in other diseases classified elsewhere, moderate, with psychotic disturbance such as hallucinations, paranoia, suspiciousness, or delusional state
Add			Major neurocognitive disorder in other diseases classified elsewhere, moderate, with psychotic disturbance such as hallucinations, paranoia, suspiciousness, or delusional state

Add		F02.B3	**Dementia in other diseases classified elsewhere, moderate, with mood disturbance**
Add			Dementia in other diseases classified elsewhere, moderate, with mood disturbance such as depression, apathy, or anhedonia
Add			Major neurocognitive disorder in other diseases classified elsewhere, moderate, with mood disturbance such as depression, apathy, or anhedonia
Add		F02.B4	**Dementia in other diseases classified elsewhere, moderate, with anxiety**
Add			Major neurocognitive disorder in other diseases classified elsewhere, moderate, with anxiety
Add	F02.C		**Dementia in other diseases classified elsewhere, severe**
Add		F02.C0	**Dementia in other diseases classified elsewhere, severe, without behavioral disturbance, psychotic disturbance, mood disturbance, and anxiety**
Add			Dementia in other diseases classified elsewhere, severe, NOS
Add			Major neurocognitive disorder in other diseases classified elsewhere, severe, NOS
Add		F02.C1	**Dementia in other diseases classified elsewhere, severe, with behavioral disturbance**
Add		F02.C11	**Dementia in other diseases classified elsewhere, severe, with agitation**
Add			Dementia in other diseases classified elsewhere, severe, with aberrant motor behavior such as restlessness, rocking, pacing, or exit-seeking
Add			Dementia in other diseases classified elsewhere, severe, with verbal or physical behaviors such as profanity, shouting, threatening, anger, aggression, combativeness, or violence
Add			Major neurocognitive disorder in other diseases classified elsewhere, severe, with aberrant motor behavior such as restlessness, rocking, pacing, or exit-seeking
Add			Major neurocognitive disorder in other diseases classified elsewhere, severe, with verbal or physical behaviors such as profanity, shouting, threatening, anger, aggression, combativeness, or violence

Add　　F02.C18　**Dementia in other diseases classified elsewhere, severe, with other behavioral disturbance**

Add　　　　Dementia in other diseases classified elsewhere, severe, with behavioral disturbances such as sleep disturbance, social disinhibition, or sexual disinhibition

Add　　　　Major neurocognitive disorder in other diseases classified elsewhere, severe, with behavioral disturbances such as sleep disturbance, social disinhibition, or sexual disinhibition

Add　　　　Use Additional code, if applicable, to identify wandering in dementia in conditions classified elsewhere (Z91.83)

Add　　F02.C2　**Dementia in other diseases classified elsewhere, severe, with psychotic disturbance**

Add　　　　Dementia in other diseases classified elsewhere, severe, with psychotic disturbance such as hallucinations, paranoia, suspiciousness, or delusional state

Add　　　　Major neurocognitive disorder in other diseases classified elsewhere, severe, with psychotic disturbance such as hallucinations, paranoia, suspiciousness, or delusional state

Add　　F02.C3　**Dementia in other diseases classified elsewhere, severe, with mood disturbance**

Add　　　　Dementia in other diseases classified elsewhere, severe, with mood disturbance such as depression, apathy, or anhedonia

Add　　　　Major neurocognitive disorder in other diseases classified elsewhere, severe, with mood disturbance such as depression, apathy, or anhedonia

Add　　F02.C4　**Dementia in other diseases classified elsewhere, severe, with anxiety**

Add　　　　Major neurocognitive disorder in other diseases classified elsewhere, severe, with anxiety

No Change **F03**　**Unspecified dementia**

Add　　　　Major neurocognitive disorder NOS

Revise from　　F03.9　**Unspecified dementia**

Revise to　　F03.9　**Unspecified dementia, unspecified severity**

Revise from　　F03.90　**Unspecified dementia without behavioral disturbance**

Revise to　　F03.90　**Unspecified dementia, unspecified severity, without behavioral disturbance, psychotic disturbance, mood disturbance, and anxiety**

Revise from　　F03.91　**Unspecified dementia with behavioral disturbance**

Revise to　　F03.91　**Unspecified dementia, unspecified severity, with behavioral disturbance**

Delete　　　　Unspecified dementia with aggressive behavior

Delete　　　　Unspecified dementia with combative behavior

Delete　　　　Unspecified dementia with violent behavior

Delete　　　　Use Additional code, if applicable, to identify wandering in unspecified dementia (Z91.83)

Add　　F03.911　**Unspecified dementia, unspecified severity, with agitation**

Add　　　　Unspecified dementia, unspecified severity, with aberrant motor behavior such as restlessness, rocking, pacing, or exit-seeking

Add　　　　Unspecified dementia, unspecified severity, with verbal or physical behaviors such as profanity, shouting, threatening, anger, aggression, combativeness, or violence

Add　　F03.918　**Unspecified dementia, unspecified severity, with other behavioral disturbance**

Add　　　　Unspecified dementia, unspecified severity, with behavioral disturbances such as sleep disturbance, social disinhibition, or sexual disinhibition

Add　　　　Use Additional code, if applicable, to identify wandering in unspecified dementia (Z91.83)

Add　　F03.92　**Unspecified dementia, unspecified severity, with psychotic disturbance**

Add　　　　Unspecified dementia, unspecified severity, with psychotic disturbance such as hallucinations, paranoia, suspiciousness, or delusional state

Add　　F03.93　**Unspecified dementia, unspecified severity, with mood disturbance**

Add　　　　Unspecified dementia, unspecified severity, with mood disturbance such as depression, apathy, or anhedonia

Add　　F03.94　**Unspecified dementia, unspecified severity, with anxiety**

Add　　**F03.A Unspecified dementia, mild**

Add　　　　Excludes1　mild neurocognitive disorder due to known physiological condition with or without behavioral disturbance (F06.7-)

Add　　F03.A0　**Unspecified dementia, mild, without behavioral disturbance, psychotic disturbance, mood disturbance, and anxiety**

Add　　　　Dementia, mild, NOS

Add　　F03.A1　**Unspecified dementia, mild, with behavioral disturbance**

Add　　F03.A11　**Unspecified dementia, mild, with agitation**

Add　　　　Unspecified dementia, mild, with aberrant motor behavior such as restlessness, rocking, pacing, or exit-seeking

Add　　　　Unspecified dementia, mild, with verbal or physical behaviors such as profanity, shouting, threatening, anger, aggression, combativeness, or violence

Add		**F03.A18**	**Unspecified dementia, mild, with other behavioral disturbance**
Add			Unspecified dementia, mild, with behavioral disturbances such as sleep disturbance, social disinhibition, or sexual disinhibition
Add			Use Additional code, if applicable, to identify wandering in unspecified dementia (Z91.83)
Add		**F03.A2**	**Unspecified dementia, mild, with psychotic disturbance**
Add			Unspecified dementia, mild, with psychotic disturbance such as hallucinations, paranoia, suspiciousness, or delusional state
Add		**F03.A3**	**Unspecified dementia, mild, with mood disturbance**
Add			Unspecified dementia, mild, with mood disturbance such as depression, apathy, or anhedonia
Add		**F03.A4**	**Unspecified dementia, mild, with anxiety**
Add	**F03.B**	**Unspecified dementia, moderate**	
Add		**F03.B0**	**Unspecified dementia, moderate, without behavioral disturbance, psychotic disturbance, mood disturbance, and anxiety**
Add			Dementia, moderate, NOS
Add		**F03.B1**	**Unspecified dementia, moderate, with behavioral disturbance**
Add		**F03.B11**	**Unspecified dementia, moderate, with agitation**
Add			Unspecified dementia, moderate, with aberrant motor behavior such as restlessness, rocking, pacing, or exit-seeking
Add			Unspecified dementia, moderate, with verbal or physical behaviors such as profanity, shouting, threatening, anger, aggression, combativeness, or violence
Add		**F03.B18**	**Unspecified dementia, moderate, with other behavioral disturbance**
Add			Unspecified dementia, moderate, with behavioral disturbances such as sleep disturbance, social disinhibition, or sexual disinhibition
Add			Use Additional code, if applicable, to identify wandering in unspecified dementia (Z91.83)
Add		**F03.B2**	**Unspecified dementia, moderate, with psychotic disturbance**
Add			Unspecified dementia, moderate, with psychotic disturbance such as hallucinations, paranoia, suspiciousness, or delusional state

Add		**F03.B3**	**Unspecified dementia, moderate, with mood disturbance**
Add			Unspecified dementia, moderate, with mood disturbance such as depression, apathy, or anhedonia
Add		**F03.B4**	**Unspecified dementia, moderate, with anxiety**
Add	**F03.C**	**Unspecified dementia, severe**	
Add		**F03.C0**	**Unspecified dementia, severe, without behavioral disturbance, psychotic disturbance, mood disturbance, and anxiety**
Add			Dementia, severe, NOS
Add		**F03.C1**	**Unspecified dementia, severe, with behavioral disturbance**
Add		**F03.C11**	**Unspecified dementia, severe, with agitation**
Add			Unspecified dementia, severe, with aberrant motor behavior such as restlessness, rocking, pacing, or exit-seeking
Add			Unspecified dementia, severe, with verbal or physical behaviors such as profanity, shouting, threatening, anger, aggression, combativeness, or violence
Add		**F03.C18**	**Unspecified dementia, severe, with other behavioral disturbance**
Add			Unspecified dementia, severe, with behavioral disturbances such as sleep disturbance, social disinhibition, or sexual disinhibition
Add			Use Additional code, if applicable, to identify wandering in unspecified dementia (Z91.83)
Add		**F03.C2**	**Unspecified dementia, severe, with psychotic disturbance**
Add			Unspecified dementia, severe, with psychotic disturbance such as hallucinations, paranoia, suspiciousness, or delusional state
Add		**F03.C3**	**Unspecified dementia, severe, with mood disturbance**
Add			Unspecified dementia, severe, with mood disturbance such as depression, apathy, or anhedonia
Add		**F03.C4**	**Unspecified dementia, severe, with anxiety**

No Change	**F06**	**Other mental disorders due to known physiological condition**	
Add		**F06.7**	**Mild neurocognitive disorder due to known physiological condition**
Add			Mild neurocognitive impairment due to a known physiological condition
Add			*Code first the underlying physiological condition, such as:*
Add			Alzheimer's disease (G30.-)
Add			frontotemporal neurocognitive disorder (G31.09)
Add			human immunodeficiency virus [HIV] disease(B20)
Add			Huntington's disease (G10)
Add			Neurocognitive disorder with Lewy bodies (G31.83)
Add			Parkinson's disease (G20)
Add			systemic lupus erythematosus (M32.-)
Add			traumatic brain injury (S06.-)
Add			vitamin B deficiency (E53-)
Add			**Excludes1** age related cognitive decline (R41.81)
Add			altered mental status (R41.82)
Add			cerebral degeneration (G31.9)
Add			change in mental status (R41.82)
Add			cognitive deficits following (sequelae of) cerebral hemorrhage or infarction (I69.01I69.11-, I69.21-I69.31-, I69.81- I69.91-)
Add			dementia (F01.-, F02.-, F03)
Add			mild cognitive impairment due to unknown or unspecified etiology (G31.84)
Add			neurologic neglect syndrome (R41.4)
Add			personality change, nonpsychotic (F68.8)
Add		**F06.70**	**Mild neurocognitive disorder due to known physiological condition without behavioral disturbance**
Add			Mild neurocognitive disorder due to known physiological condition, NOS
Add		**F06.71**	**Mild neurocognitive disorder due to known physiological condition with behavioral disturbance**
No Change	**F07**	**Personality and behavioral disorders due to known physiological condition**	
No Change		**F07.0**	**Personality change due to known physiological condition**
Delete			*Code first underlying physiological condition*
No Change	**F09**	**Unspecified mental disorder due to known physiological condition**	
Add			**Excludes1** mild neurocognitive disorder due to known physiological condition (F06.7-)

MENTAL AND BEHAVIORAL DISORDERS DUE TO PSYCHOACTIVE SUBSTANCE USE (F10-F19)

No Change	**F10**	Alcohol related disorders	
No Change		F10.9	Alcohol use, unspecified
Add			F10.90 Alcohol use, unspecified, uncomplicated
Add			F10.91 Alcohol use, unspecified, in remission
No Change	**F11**	Opioid related disorders	
No Change		F11.9	Opioid use, unspecified
Add			F11.91 Opioid use, unspecified, in remission

No Change	**F12**	Cannabis related disorders	
No Change		F12.9	Cannabis use, unspecified
Add			F12.91 Cannabis use, unspecified, in remission
No Change	**F13**	Sedative, hypnotic, or anxiolytic related disorders	
No Change		F13.9	Sedative, hypnotic or anxiolytic-related use, unspecified
Add			F13.91 Sedative, hypnotic or anxiolytic use, unspecified, in remission
No Change	**F14**	Cocaine related disorders	
No Change		F14.9	Cocaine use, unspecified
Add			F14.91 Cocaine use, unspecified, in remission
No Change	**F15**	Other stimulant related disorders	
No Change		F15.9	Other stimulant use, unspecified
Add			F15.91 Other stimulant use, unspecified, in remission
No Change	**F16**	Hallucinogen related disorders	
No Change		F16.9	Hallucinogen use, unspecified
Add			F16.91 Hallucinogen use, unspecified, in remission
No Change	**F18**	Inhalant related disorders	
No Change		F18.9	Inhalant use, unspecified
Add			F18.91 Inhalant use, unspecified, in remission
No Change	**F19**	Other psychoactive substance related disorders	
No Change		F19.9	Other psychoactive substance use, unspecified
Add			F19.91 Other psychoactive substance use, unspecified, in remission

No Change **MOOD [AFFECTIVE] DISORDERS (F30-F39)**

No Change	**F31**	Bipolar disorder	
Add		**Includes** seasonal bipolar disorder	
No Change	**F33**	Major depressive disorder, recurrent	
Add		**Includes** recurrent episodes of seasonal affective disorder	

No Change **ANXIETY, DISSOCIATIVE, STRESS-RELATED, SOMATOFORM AND OTHER NONPSYCHOTIC MENTAL DISORDERS (F40-F48)**

No Change	**F43**	Reaction to severe stress, and adjustment disorders	
No Change		F43.8	Other reactions to severe stress
Add			F43.81 Prolonged grief disorder
Add			Complicated grief
Add			Complicated grief disorder
Add			Persistent complex bereavement disorder
Add			F43.89 Other reactions to severe stress
No Change		F43.9	Reaction to severe stress, unspecified
Add			Unspecified trauma and stressor-related disorder

No Change **CHAPTER 6**

No Change **DISEASES OF THE NERVOUS SYSTEM (G00-G99)**

No Change **INFLAMMATORY DISEASES OF THE CENTRAL NERVOUS SYSTEM (G00-G09)**

No Change	**G04**	Encephalitis, myelitis and encephalomyelitis	
No Change		**Excludes2**	
			benign myalgic encephalomyelitis (G93.3)
			myalgic encephalomyelitis (G93.32)

No Change — **SYSTEMIC ATROPHIES PRIMARILY AFFECTING THE CENTRAL NERVOUS SYSTEM (G10-G14)**

No Change **G10** Huntington's disease

Delete — Code also dementia in other diseases classified elsewhere without behavioral disturbance (F02.80)

Add — Use Additional code, if applicable, to identify:

Add — dementia with anxiety (F02.84, F02.A4, F02.B4, F02.C4)

Add — dementia with behavioral disturbance (F02.81-, F02.A1-, F02.B1-, F02.C1-)

Add — dementia with mood disturbance (F02.83, F02.A3, F02.B3, F02.C3)

Add — dementia with psychotic disturbance (F02.82, F02.A2, F02.B2, F02.C2)

Add — dementia without behavioral disturbance (F02.80, F02.A0, F02.B0, F02.C0)

Add — mild neurocognitive disorder due to known physiological condition (F06.7-)

No Change — **EXTRAPYRAMIDAL AND MOVEMENT DISORDERS (G20-G26)**

No Change **G20** Parkinson's disease

No Change — Use Additional
Revise from — code to identify:
Revise to — code, if applicable, to identify:
Revise from — dementia with behavioral disturbance (F02.81)
Revise to — dementia with anxiety (F02.84, F02.A4, F02.B4, F02.C4)

Delete — dementia without behavioral disturbance (F02.80)

Add — dementia with behavioral disturbance (F02.81-, F02.A1-, F02.B1-, F02.C1-)

Add — dementia with mood disturbance (F02.83, F02.A3, F02.B3, F02.C3)

Add — dementia with psychotic disturbance (F02.82, F02.A2, F02.B2, F02.C2)

Add — dementia without behavioral disturbance (F02.80, F02.A0, F02.B0, F02.C0)

Add — mild neurocognitive disorder due to known physiological condition (F06.7-)

Delete — **Excludes1** dementia with Parkinsonism (G31.83)

No Change — **OTHER DEGENERATIVE DISEASES OF THE NERVOUS SYSTEM (G30-G32)**

No Change **G30** Alzheimer's disease

No Change — Use Additional
Revise from — code to identify:
Revise to — code, if applicable, to identify:
Revise from — dementia with behavioral disturbance (F02.81)
Revise to — dementia with anxiety (F02.84, F02.A4, F02.B4, F02.C4)
Delete — dementia without behavioral disturbance (F02.80)
Add — dementia with behavioral disturbance (F02.81-, F02.A1-, F02.B1-, F02.C1-)

Add — dementia with mood disturbance (F02.83, F02.A3, F02.B3, F02.C3)

Add — dementia with psychotic disturbance (F02.82, F02.A2, F02.B2, F02.C2)

Add — dementia without behavioral disturbance (F02.80, F02.A0, F02.B0, F02.C0)

Add — mild neurocognitive disorder due to known physiological condition (F06.7-)

No Change **G31** Other degenerative diseases of nervous system, not elsewhere classified

No Change — **Use Additional**
Delete — For codes G31.0-G31.83, G31.85-G31.9, use additional code to identify:
Delete — dementia with behavioral disturbance (F02.81)
Delete — dementia without behavioral disturbance (F02.80)
Add — dementia with behavioral disturbance (F02.81-, F02.A1-, F02.B1-, F02.C1-)

Add — dementia with mood disturbance (F02.83, F02.A3, F02.B3, F02.C3)

Add — dementia with psychotic disturbance (F02.82, F02.A2, F02.B2, F02.C2)

Add — dementia without behavioral disturbance (F02.80, F02.A0, F02.B0, F02.C0)

Add — mild neurocognitive disorder due to known physiological condition (F06.7-)

No Change **G31.0** Frontotemporal dementia

Revise from — **G31.09** Other frontotemporal dementia
Revise to — **G31.09** Other frontotemporal neurocognitive disorder

Add — Use Additional code, if applicable, to identify mild neurocognitive disorders due to known physiological condition (F06.7-)

No Change **G31.8** Other specified degenerative diseases of nervous system

Revise from — **G31.83** Dementia with Lewy bodies
Revise to — **G31.83** Neurocognitive disorder with Lewy bodies

Delete — Dementia with Parkinsonism

Add — Use Additional code, if applicable, to identify mild neurocognitive disorders due to known physiological condition (F06.7-)

Revise from — **G31.84** Mild cognitive impairment, so stated
Revise to — **G31.84** Mild cognitive impairment of uncertain or unknown etiology

Delete — Mild neurocognitive disorder
Add — Mild cognitive disorder NOS
Add — Mild neurocognitive disorder of uncertain or unknown etiology

Add — Use Additional code to identify presence of:
Add — alcohol abuse and dependence (F10.-)
Add — exposure to environmental tobacco smoke (Z77.22)
Add — history of tobacco dependence (Z87.891)
Add — hypertension (I10-I16)
Add — occupational exposure to environmental tobacco smoke (Z57.31)
Add — tobacco dependence (F17.-)
Add — tobacco use (Z72.0)
No Change — **Excludes1**
Add — cerebrovascular diseases (I60-I69)
Delete — mild memory disturbance (F06.8)
Add — mild neurocognitive disorder due to a known physiological condition (F06.7-)

No Change — **EPISODIC AND PAROXYSMAL DISORDERS (G40-G47)**

No Change **G47** Sleep disorders
No Change **G47.3** Sleep apnea
No Change — **Excludes1**
Revise from — sleep apnea of newborn (P28.3)
Revise to — sleep apnea of newborn (P28.3-)

No Change **G47.33** Obstructive sleep apnea (adult) (pediatric)
No Change — **Excludes1**
Revise from — obstructive sleep apnea of newborn (P28.3)
Revise to — obstructive sleep apnea of newborn (P28.3-)

No Change	**DISEASES OF MYONEURAL JUNCTION AND MUSCLE (G70-G73)**		
No Change **G71**	**Primary disorders of muscles**		
No Change	**G71.0**	**Muscular dystrophy**	
Add		**G71.03**	**Limb girdle muscular dystrophies**
Add			**G71.031** **Autosomal dominant limb girdle muscular dystrophy**
Add			LGMD D4 calpain-3-related
Add			LGMD D5 collagen 6-related
Add			Limb girdle muscular dystrophy type 1
Add			**G71.032** **Autosomal recessive limb girdle muscular dystrophy due to calpain-3 dysfunction**
Add			Limb girdle muscular dystrophy type 2A
Add			LGMD R1 calpain-3-related
Add			Primary calpainopathy
Add			**G71.033** **Limb girdle muscular dystrophy due to dysferlin dysfunction**
Add			Dysferlinopathy
Add			LGMD R2 dysferlin-related
Add			Limb girdle muscular dystrophy type 2B
Add			Miyoshi Myopathy type 1
Add			**G71.034** **Limb girdle muscular dystrophy due to sarcoglycan dysfunction**
Add			**G71.0340** **Limb girdle muscular dystrophy due to sarcoglycan dysfunction, unspecified**
Add			Sarcoglycanopathy, NOS
Add			**G71.0341** **Limb girdle muscular dystrophy due to alpha sarcoglycan dysfunction**
Add			Alpha sarcoglycanopathy
Add			Limb-girdle muscular dystrophy due to alpha-sarcoglycan deficiency
Add			Limb girdle muscular dystrophy type 2D
Add			**G71.0342** **Limb girdle muscular dystrophy due to beta sarcoglycan dysfunction**
Add			Beta sarcoglycanopathy
Add			Limb girdle muscular dystrophy due to beta-sarcoglycan deficiency
Add			Limb girdle muscular dystrophy type 2E

Add			**G71.0349** **Limb girdle muscular dystrophy due to other sarcoglycan dysfunction**
Add			Delta sarcoglycanopathy
Add			Delta-sarcoglycan-related LGMD R6
Add			Gamma sarcoglycanopathy
Add			Gamma-sarcoglycan-related LGMD R5
Add			Limb girdle muscular dystrophy type 2C
Add			Limb girdle muscular dystrophy type 2F
Add			**G71.035** **Limb girdle muscular dystrophy due to anoctamin-5 dysfunction**
Add			Anoctamin-5-related LGMD R12
Add			Anoctaminopathy
Add			Autosomal recessive limb girdle muscular dystrophy type 2L
Add			Miyoshi myopathy type 3
Add			**G71.038** **Other limb girdle muscular dystrophy**
Add			LGMD R9 FKRP-related
Add			LGMD R22 collagen 6-related
Add			Limb girdle muscular dystrophy due to fukutin related protein dysfunction
Add			Limb girdle muscular dystrophy type 2I
Add			Other autosomal recessive limb girdle muscular dystrophy
Add			**G71.039** **Limb girdle muscular dystrophy, unspecified**
No Change		**G71.09** **Other specified muscular dystrophies**	
Delete		Limb-girdle muscular dystrophy	

No Change	**OTHER DISORDERS OF THE NERVOUS SYSTEM (G89-G99)**		
No Change **G90**	**Disorders of autonomic nervous system**		
Add	**G90.A** **Postural orthostatic tachycardia syndrome [POTS]**		
Add	Chronic orthostatic intolerance		
Add	Postural tachycardia syndrome		
No Change **G93**	**Other disorders of brain**		
Revise from	**G93.3** **Postviral fatigue syndrome**		
Revise to	**G93.3** **Postviral and related fatigue syndromes**		
Delete	Benign myalgic encephalomyelitis		
Add	Use Additional code, if applicable, for post COVID-19 condition, unspecified (U09.9)		
Add	**Excludes1** neurasthenia (F48.8)		
Add	**G93.31** **Postviral fatigue syndrome**		
Add	**G93.32** **Myalgic encephalomyelitis/chronic fatigue syndrome**		
Add	Chronic fatigue syndrome		
Add	ME/CFS		
Add	Myalgic encephalomyelitis		
Add	**G93.39** **Other post infection and related fatigue syndromes**		

No Change	G96	Other disorders of central nervous system
No Change	G96.0	Cerebrospinal fluid leak
No Change		G96.00 Cerebrospinal fluid leak, unspecified
No Change		Code also
Revise from		head injury (S00.- to S09.-)
Revise to		head injury (S00-S09)

No Change

CHAPTER 9

No Change

DISEASES OF THE CIRCULATORY SYSTEM (I00-I99)

No Change

ISCHEMIC HEART DISEASES (I20-I25)

No Change	I20	Angina pectoris
Add	I20.2	Refractory angina pectoris
No Change	I25	Chronic ischemic heart disease
No Change	I25.1	Atherosclerotic heart disease of native coronary artery
No Change		I25.11 Atherosclerotic heart disease of native coronary artery with angina pectoris
Add		I25.112 Atherosclerosic heart disease of native coronary artery with refractory angina pectoris
No Change	I25.7	Atherosclerosis of coronary artery bypass graft(s) and coronary artery of transplanted heart with angina pectoris
No Change		I25.70 Atherosclerosis of coronary artery bypass graft(s), unspecified, with angina pectoris
Add		I25.702 Atherosclerosis of coronary artery bypass graft(s), unspecified, with refractory angina pectoris
No Change		I25.71 Atherosclerosis of autologous vein coronary artery bypass graft(s) with angina pectoris
Add		I25.712 Atherosclerosis of autologous vein coronary artery bypass graft(s) with refractory angina pectoris
No Change		I25.72 Atherosclerosis of autologous artery coronary artery bypass graft(s) with angina pectoris
Add		I25.722 Atherosclerosis of autologous artery coronary artery bypass graft(s) with refractory angina pectoris
No Change		I25.73 Atherosclerosis of nonautologous biological coronary artery bypass graft(s) with angina pectoris
Add		I25.732 Atherosclerosis of nonautologous biological coronary artery bypass graft(s) with refractory angina pectoris
No Change		I25.75 Atherosclerosis of native coronary artery of transplanted heart with angina pectoris
Add		I25.752 Atherosclerosis of native coronary artery of transplanted heart with refractory angina pectoris
No Change		I25.76 Atherosclerosis of bypass graft of coronary artery of transplanted heart with angina pectoris
Add		I25.762 Atherosclerosis of bypass graft of coronary artery of transplanted heart with refractory angina pectoris
No Change		I25.79 Atherosclerosis of other coronary artery bypass graft(s) with angina pectoris
Add		I25.792 Atherosclerosis of other coronary artery bypass graft(s) with refractory angina pectoris

No Change

PULMONARY HEART DISEASE AND DISEASES OF PULMONARY CIRCULATION (I26-I28)

No Change	I27	Other pulmonary heart diseases
No Change	I27.8	Other specified pulmonary heart diseases
No Change		I27.83 Eisenmenger's syndrome
No Change		Code also
Revise from		atrial septal defect (Q21.1)
Revise to		atrial septal defect (Q21.1-)

No Change

OTHER FORMS OF HEART DISEASE (I30-I5A)

No Change	I31	Other diseases of pericardium
No Change	I31.2	Hemopericardium, not elsewhere classified
Add		**Excludes1** malignant pericardial effusion (I31.31)
No Change	I31.3	Pericardial effusion (noninflammatory)
Delete		Chylopericardium
Add		I31.31 Malignant pericardial effusion in diseases classified elsewhere
Add		Code first underlying neoplasm (C00-D49)
Add		I31.39 Other pericardial effusion (noninflammatory)
Add		Chylopericardium
No Change	I34	Nonrheumatic mitral valve disorders
		I34.0 Nonrheumatic mitral (valve) insufficiency
Add		Code also, if applicable:
Add		nonrheumatic mitral (valve) annulus calcification (I34.81)
No Change		I34.2 Nonrheumatic mitral (valve) stenosis
Add		Code also, if applicable:
Add		nonrheumatic mitral (valve) annulus calcification (I34.81)
No Change		I34.8 Other nonrheumatic mitral valve disorders
Add		I34.81 Nonrheumatic mitral (valve) annulus calcification
Add		Nonrheumatic mitral (valve) annular calcification
Add		Mitral (valve) annulus calcification NOS
Add		Code also, if applicable:
Add		nonrheumatic mitral (valve) insufficiency (I34.0)
Add		nonrheumatic mitral (valve) stenosis (I34.2)
Add		I34.89 Other nonrheumatic mitral valve disorders
No Change	I47	Paroxysmal tachycardia
No Change	I47.2	Ventricular tachycardia
Add		I47.20 Ventricular tachycardia, unspecified
Add		I47.21 Torsades de pointes
Add		Code also, if applicable, long QT syndrome (I45.81)
Add		Use Additional code for adverse effect, if applicable, to identify drug (T36-T50 with fifth or sixth character 5)
Add		I47.29 Other ventricular tachycardia

No Change		**CEREBROVASCULAR DISEASES (I60–I69)**	
No Change	I69	Sequelae of cerebrovascular disease	
No Change	I69.0	Sequelae of nontraumatic subarachnoid hemorrhage	
No Change		I69.09	Other sequelae of nontraumatic subarachnoid hemorrhage
No Change			I69.091 Dysphagia following nontraumatic subarachnoid hemorrhage
No Change			Use Additional
Revise from			code to identify the type of dysphagia, if known (R13.1-)
Revise to			code to identify the type of dysphagia, if known (R13.11-R13.19)
No Change	I69.1	Sequelae of nontraumatic intracerebral hemorrhage	
No Change		I69.19	Other sequelae of nontraumatic intracerebral hemorrhage
No Change			I69.191 Dysphagia following nontraumatic intracerebral hemorrhage
No Change			Use Additional
Revise from			code to identify the type of dysphagia, if known (R13.1-)
Revise to			code to identify the type of dysphagia, if known (R13.11-R13.19)
No Change	I69.2	Sequelae of other nontraumatic intracranial hemorrhage	
No Change		I69.29	Other sequelae of other nontraumatic intracranial hemorrhage
No Change			I69.291 Dysphagia following other nontraumatic intracranial hemorrhage
No Change			Use Additional
Revise from			code to identify the type of dysphagia, if known (R13.1-)
Revise to			code to identify the type of dysphagia, if known (R13.11-R13.19)
No Change	I69.3	Sequelae of cerebral infarction	
No Change		I69.39	Other sequelae of cerebral infarction
No Change			I69.391 Dysphagia following cerebral infarction
No Change			Use Additional
Revise from			code to identify the type of dysphagia, if known (R13.1-)
Revise to			code to identify the type of dysphagia, if known (R13.11-R13.19)
No Change	I69.8	Sequelae of other cerebrovascular diseases	
No Change		I69.89	Other sequelae of other cerebrovascular disease
No Change			I69.891 Dysphagia following other cerebrovascular disease
No Change			Use Additional
Revise from			code to identify the type of dysphagia, if known (R13.1-)
Revise to			code to identify the type of dysphagia, if known (R13.11-R13.19)

No Change	I69.9	Sequelae of unspecified cerebrovascular diseases	
No Change		I69.99	Other sequelae of unspecified cerebrovascular disease
No Change			I69.991 Dysphagia following unspecified cerebrovascular disease
No Change			Use Additional
Revise from			code to identify the type of dysphagia, if known (R13.1-)
Revise to			code to identify the type of dysphagia, if known (R13.11-R13.19)
No Change		**DISEASES OF ARTERIES, ARTERIOLES AND CAPILLARIES (I70–I79)**	
No Change	I71	Aortic aneurysm and dissection	
Delete		**Excludes1** aortic ectasia (I77.81-)	
Delete		syphilitic aortic aneurysm (A52.01)	
Delete		traumatic aortic aneurysm (S25.09, S35.09)	
Add		*Code first, if applicable:*	
Add		syphilitic aortic aneurysm (A52.01)	
Add		traumatic aortic aneurysm (S25.09, S35.09)	
No Change	I71.0	Dissection of aorta	
No Change		I71.01	Dissection of thoracic aorta
Add			I71.010 Dissection of ascending aorta
Add			I71.011 Dissection of aortic arch
Add			I71.012 Dissection of descending thoracic aorta
Add			I71.019 Dissection of thoracic aorta, unspecified
No Change	I71.1	Thoracic aortic aneurysm, ruptured	
Add		I71.10	Thoracic aortic aneurysm, ruptured, unspecified
Add		I71.11	Aneurysm of the ascending aorta, ruptured
Add		I71.12	Aneurysm of the aortic arch, ruptured
Add		I71.13	Aneurysm of the descending thoracic aorta, ruptured
No Change	I71.2	Thoracic aortic aneurysm, without rupture	
Add		I71.20	Thoracic aortic aneurysm, without rupture, unspecified
Add		I71.21	Aneurysm of the ascending aorta, without rupture
Add		I71.22	Aneurysm of the aortic arch, without rupture
Add		I71.23	Aneurysm of the descending thoracic aorta, without rupture
No Change	I71.3	Abdominal aortic aneurysm, ruptured	
Add		I71.30	Abdominal aortic aneurysm, ruptured, unspecified
Add		I71.31	Pararenal abdominal aortic aneurysm, ruptured
Add		I71.32	Juxtarenal abdominal aortic aneurysm, ruptured
Add		I71.33	Infrarenal abdominal aortic aneurysm, ruptured
No Change	I71.4	Abdominal aortic aneurysm, without rupture	
Add		I71.40	Abdominal aortic aneurysm, without rupture, unspecified
Add		I71.41	Pararenal abdominal aortic aneurysm, without rupture
Add		I71.42	Juxtarenal abdominal aortic aneurysm, without rupture
Add		I71.43	Infrarenal abdominal aortic aneurysm, without rupture
No Change	I71.5	Thoracoabdominal aortic aneurysm, ruptured	
Add		I71.50	Thoracoabdominal aortic aneurysm, ruptured, unspecified
Add		I71.51	Supraceliac aneurysm of the abdominal aorta, ruptured

Add		I71.52	Paravisceral aneurysm of the abdominal aorta, ruptured
No Change	I71.6		Thoracoabdominal aortic aneurysm, without rupture
Add		I71.60	Thoracoabdominal aortic aneurysm, without rupture, unspecified
Add		I71.61	Supraceliac aneurysm of the abdominal aorta, without rupture
Add		I71.62	Paravisceral aneurysm of the abdominal aorta, without rupture

No Change	I77	Other disorders of arteries and arterioles	
No Change		I77.8	Other specified disorders of arteries and arterioles
No Change		I77.81	Aortic ectasia
No Change			**Excludes1**
Revise from			aortic aneurysm and dissection (I71.0-)
Revise to			aortic aneurysm and dissection (I71.-)
Add		I77.82	Antineutrophilic cytoplasmic antibody [ANCA] vasculitis
Add			ANCA associated vasculitis
Add			ANCA positive vasculitis
Add			**Excludes2** eosinophilic granulomatosis with polyangiitis (M30.1)
Add			granulomatosis with polyangiitis (M31.3-)
Add			microscopic polyangiitis (M31.7)

No Change

CHAPTER 10

No Change

DISEASES OF THE RESPIRATORY SYSTEM (J00-J99)

No Change

OTHER DISEASES OF THE PLEURA (J90-J94)

No Change	J91	Pleural effusion in conditions classified elsewhere	
No Change		J91.0	Malignant pleural effusion
No Change			*Code first*
Revise from			underlying neoplasm
Revise to			underlying neoplasm (C00-D49)

No Change	J93	Pneumothorax and air leak	
No Change		J93.1	Other spontaneous pneumothorax
No Change		J93.12	Secondary spontaneous pneumothorax
No Change			*Code first*
Revise from			catamenial pneumothorax due to endometriosis (N80.8)
Revise to			catamenial pneumothorax due to endometriosis (N80.B-)

INTRAOPERATIVE AND POSTPROCEDURAL COMPLICATIONS AND DISORDERS OF RESPIRATORY SYSTEM, NOT ELSEWHERE CLASSIFIED (J95)

No Change	J95	Intraoperative and postprocedural complications and disorders of respiratory system, not elsewhere classified	
No Change		J95.8	Other intraoperative and postprocedural complications and disorders of respiratory system, not elsewhere classified
Add		J95.87	Transfusion-associated dyspnea (TAD)
Add			**Excludes1** transfusion associated circulatory overload (TACO) (E87.71)
Add			transfusion-related acute lung injury (TRALI) (J95.84)

No Change

OTHER DISEASES OF THE RESPIRATORY SYSTEM (J96-J99)

	J96	Respiratory failure, not elsewhere classified	
No Change		J96.0	Acute respiratory failure
No Change		J96.02	Acute respiratory failure with hypercapnia
Add			Acute respiratory acidosis

No Change		J96.1	Chronic respiratory failure
No Change		J96.12	Chronic respiratory failure with hypercapnia
Add			Chronic respiratory acidosis
No Change	J98	Other respiratory disorders	
No Change			**Excludes1**
Revise from			newborn apnea (P28.4)
Revise to			newborn apnea (P28.4-)
Revise from			newborn sleep apnea (P28.3)
Revise to			newborn sleep apnea (P28.3-)

No Change

CHAPTER 11

No Change

DISEASES OF THE DIGESTIVE SYSTEM (K00-K95)

No Change

DISEASES OF APPENDIX (K35-K38)

No Change	K35	Acute appendicitis	
No Change		K35.3	Acute appendicitis with localized peritonitis
Revise from		K35.32	Acute appendicitis with perforation and localized peritonitis, without abscess
Revise to		K35.32	Acute appendicitis with perforation, localized peritonitis, and gangrene, without abscess
Revise from		K35.33	Acute appendicitis with perforation and localized peritonitis, with abscess
Revise to		K35.33	Acute appendicitis with perforation, localized peritonitis, and gangrene, with abscess

No Change

DISEASES OF LIVER (K70-K77)

No Change	K72	Hepatic failure, not elsewhere classified	
Delete			**Includes** hepatic encephalopathy NOS
No Change	K76	Other diseases of liver	
No Change		K76.8	Other specified diseases of liver
Add		K76.82	Hepatic encephalopathy
Add			Hepatic encephalopathy, NOS
Add			Hepatic encephalopathy without coma
Add			Hepatocerebral intoxication
Add			Portal-systemic encephalopathy
Add			Code also underlying liver disease, such as:
Add			acute and subacute hepatic failure without coma (K72.00)
Add			alcoholic hepatic failure without coma (K70.40)
Add			chronic hepatic failure without coma (K72.10)
Add			hepatic failure with toxic liver disease without coma (K71.10)
Add			hepatic failure without coma (K72.90)
Add			icterus of newborn (P55-P59)
Add			postprocedural hepatic failure (K91.82)
Add			viral hepatitis without hepatic coma (B15.9, B16.1, B16.9, B17.10, B19.10, B19.20, B19.9)
Add			**Excludes1** acute and subacute hepatic failure with coma (K72.01)
Add			alcoholic hepatic failure with coma (K70.41)
Add			chronic hepatic failure with coma (K72.11)
Add			hepatic failure with coma (K72.91)
No Change	K77	Liver disorders in diseases classified elsewhere	
No Change			*Code first*
Revise from			infectious mononucleosis with liver disease (B27.0-B27.9 with .9)
Revise to			infectious mononucleosis with liver disease (B27.0-B27.9 with fifth character 9)

No Change	**DISORDERS OF GALLBLADDER, BILIARY TRACT AND PANCREAS (K80–K87)**
No Change **K80**	**Cholelithiasis**
No Change	**K80.4** **Calculus of bile duct with cholecystitis**
Delete	Codes also fistula of bile duct (K83.3)
Add	Code also fistula of bile duct (K83.3)

No Change

CHAPTER 12

No Change

DISEASES OF THE SKIN AND SUBCUTANEOUS TISSUE (L00–L99)

No Change **OTHER DISORDERS OF THE SKIN AND SUBCUTANEOUS TISSUE (L80–L99)**

No Change **L81**	**Other disorders of pigmentation**
No Change	Excludes1
Revise from	Peutz-Jeghers syndrome (Q85.8)
Revise to	Peutz-Jeghers syndrome (Q85.89)

No Change

CHAPTER 13

No Change

DISEASES OF THE MUSCULOSKELETAL SYSTEM AND CONNECTIVE TISSUE (M00–M99)

No Change **SYSTEMIC CONNECTIVE TISSUE DISORDERS (M30–M36)**

No Change **M31**	**Other necrotizing vasculopathies**
No Change	**M31.1** **Thrombotic microangiopathy**
No Change	**M31.11** **Hematopoietic stem cell transplantation-associated thrombotic microangiopathy [HSCT-TMA]**
No Change	Use Additional
Revise from	hemolytic uremic syndrome (D59.3)
Revise to	hemolytic uremic syndrome (D59.3-)
No Change **M36**	**Systemic disorders of connective tissue in diseases classified elsewhere**
No Change	**M36.2** **Hemophilic arthropathy**
No Change	*Code first*
Revise from	with vascular defect (D68.0)
Revise to	with vascular defect (D68.0-)

No Change **OTHER DORSOPATHIES (M50–M54)**

No Change **M50**	**Cervical disc disorders**
Delete	**Note:** code to the most superior level of disorder
No Change **M51**	**Thoracic, thoracolumbar, and lumbosacral intervertebral disc disorders**
Add	**M51.A Other lumbar and lumbosacral annulus fibrosus disc defects**
Add	**M51.A0** **Intervertebral annulus fibrosus defect, lumbar region, unspecified size**
Add	*Code first, if applicable, lumbar disc herniation (M51.06, M51.16, M51.26)*
Add	**M51.A1** **Intervertebral annulus fibrosus defect, small, lumbar region**
Add	*Code first, if applicable, lumbar disc herniation (M51.06, M51.16, M51.26)*
Add	**M51.A2** **Intervertebral annulus fibrosus defect, large, lumbar region**
Add	*Code first, if applicable, lumbar disc herniation (M51.06, M51.16, M51.26)*
Add	**M51.A3** **Intervertebral annulus fibrosus defect, lumbosacral region, unspecified size**
Add	*Code first, if applicable, lumbosacral disc herniation (M51.17, M51.27)*

Add	**M51.A4** **Intervertebral annulus fibrosus defect, small, lumbosacral region**
Add	*Code first, if applicable, lumbosacral disc herniation (M51.17, M51.27)*
Add	**M51.A5** **Intervertebral annulus fibrosus defect, large, lumbosacral region**
Add	*Code first, if applicable, lumbosacral disc herniation (M51.17, M51.27)*

No Change **DISORDERS OF MUSCLES (M60–M63)**

No Change **M62**	**Other disorders of muscle**
No Change	**M62.5** **Muscle wasting and atrophy, not elsewhere classified**
Add	**M62.5A Muscle wasting and atrophy, not elsewhere classified, back**
Add	**M62.5A0** **Muscle wasting and atrophy, not elsewhere classified, back, cervical**
Add	**M62.5A1** **Muscle wasting and atrophy, not elsewhere classified, back, thoracic**
Add	**M62.5A2** **Muscle wasting and atrophy, not elsewhere classified, back, lumbosacral**
Add	**M62.5A9** **Muscle wasting and atrophy, not elsewhere classified, back, unspecified level**

No Change **CHONDROPATHIES (M91–M94)**

No Change **M91**	**Juvenile osteochondrosis of hip and pelvis**
No Change	Excludes1
Revise from	slipped upper femoral epiphysis (nontraumatic) (M93.0)
Revise to	slipped upper femoral epiphysis (nontraumatic) (M93.0-)
No Change **M93**	**Other osteochondropathies**
No Change	**M93.0** **Slipped upper femoral epiphysis (nontraumatic)**
Add	Slipped capital femoral epiphysis (SCFE)
Add	Slipped upper femoral epiphysis (SUFE)
No Change	**M93.00** **Unspecified slipped upper femoral epiphysis (nontraumatic)**
Add	**M93.004** **Unspecified slipped upper femoral epiphysis (nontraumatic), bilateral hips**
Revise from	**M93.01** **Acute slipped upper femoral epiphysis (nontraumatic)**
Revise to	**M93.01** **Acute slipped upper femoral epiphysis, stable (nontraumatic)**
Revise from	**M93.011** **Acute slipped upper femoral epiphysis (nontraumatic), right hip**
Revise to	**M93.011** **Acute slipped upper femoral epiphysis, stable (nontraumatic), right hip**
Revise from	**M93.012** **Acute slipped upper femoral epiphysis (nontraumatic), left hip**
Revise to	**M93.012** **Acute slipped upper femoral epiphysis, stable (nontraumatic), left hip**
Revise from	**M93.013** **Acute slipped upper femoral epiphysis (nontraumatic), unspecified hip**
Revise to	**M93.013** **Acute slipped upper femoral epiphysis, stable (nontraumatic), unspecified hip**
Add	**M93.014** **Acute slipped upper femoral epiphysis, stable (nontraumatic), bilateral hips**

Revise from	M93.02	Chronic slipped upper femoral epiphysis (nontraumatic)
Revise to	M93.02	Chronic slipped upper femoral epiphysis, stable (nontraumatic)
Revise from	M93.021	Chronic slipped upper femoral epiphysis (nontraumatic), right hip
Revise to	M93.021	Chronic slipped upper femoral epiphysis, stable (nontraumatic), right hip
Revise from	M93.022	Chronic slipped upper femoral epiphysis (nontraumatic), left hip
Revise to	M93.022	Chronic slipped upper femoral epiphysis, stable (nontraumatic), left hip
Revise from	M93.023	Chronic slipped upper femoral epiphysis (nontraumatic), unspecified hip
Revise to	M93.023	Chronic slipped upper femoral epiphysis, stable (nontraumatic), unspecified hip
Add	M93.024	Chronic slipped upper femoral epiphysis, stable (nontraumatic), bilateral hips
Revise from	M93.03	Acute on chronic slipped upper femoral epiphysis (nontraumatic)
Revise to	M93.03	Acute on chronic slipped upper femoral epiphysis, stable (nontraumatic)
Revise from	M93.031	Acute on chronic slipped upper femoral epiphysis (nontraumatic), right hip
Revise to	M93.031	Acute on chronic slipped upper femoral epiphysis, stable (nontraumatic), right hip
Revise from	M93.032	Acute on chronic slipped upper femoral epiphysis (nontraumatic), left hip
Revise to	M93.032	Acute on chronic slipped upper femoral epiphysis, stable (nontraumatic), left hip
Revise from	M93.033	Acute on chronic slipped upper femoral epiphysis (nontraumatic), unspecified hip
Revise to	M93.033	Acute on chronic slipped upper femoral epiphysis, stable (nontraumatic), unspecified hip
Add	M93.034	Acute on chronic slipped upper femoral epiphysis, stable (nontraumatic), bilateral hips
Add	M93.04	Acute slipped upper femoral epiphysis, unstable (nontraumatic)
Add	M93.041	Acute slipped upper femoral epiphysis, unstable (nontraumatic), right hip
Add	M93.042	Acute slipped upper femoral epiphysis, unstable (nontraumatic), left hip
Add	M93.043	Acute slipped upper femoral epiphysis, unstable (nontraumatic), unspecified hip
Add	M93.044	Acute slipped upper femoral epiphysis, unstable (nontraumatic), bilateral hips
Add	M93.05	Acute on chronic slipped upper femoral epiphysis, unstable (nontraumatic)
Add	M93.051	Acute on chronic slipped upper femoral epiphysis, unstable (nontraumatic), right hip
Add	M93.052	Acute on chronic slipped upper femoral epiphysis, unstable (nontraumatic), left hip
Add	M93.053	Acute on chronic slipped upper femoral epiphysis, unstable (nontraumatic), unspecified hip
Add	M93.054	Acute on chronic slipped upper femoral epiphysis, unstable (nontraumatic), bilateral hips
Add	M93.06	Acute slipped upper femoral epiphysis, unspecified stability (nontraumatic)
Add	M93.061	Acute slipped upper femoral epiphysis, unspecified stability (nontraumatic), right hip
Add	M93.062	Acute slipped upper femoral epiphysis, unspecified stability (nontraumatic), left hip
Add	M93.063	Acute slipped upper femoral epiphysis, unspecified stability (nontraumatic), unspecified hip
Add	M93.064	Acute slipped upper femoral epiphysis, unspecified stability (nontraumatic), bilateral hips
Add	M93.07	Acute on chronic slipped upper femoral epiphysis, unspecified stability (nontraumatic)
Add	M93.071	Acute on chronic slipped upper femoral epiphysis, unspecified stability (nontraumatic), right hip
Add	M93.072	Acute on chronic slipped upper femoral epiphysis, unspecified stability (nontraumatic), left hip
Add	M93.073	Acute on chronic slipped upper femoral epiphysis, unspecified stability (nontraumatic), unspecified hip
Add	M93.074	Acute on chronic slipped upper femoral epiphysis, unspecified stability (nontraumatic), bilateral hips

No Change

INTRAOPERATIVE AND POSTPROCEDURAL COMPLICATIONS AND DISORDERS OF MUSCULOSKELETAL SYSTEM, NOT ELSEWHERE CLASSIFIED (M96)

No Change	M96	Intraoperative and postprocedural complications and disorders of musculoskeletal system, not elsewhere classified
Add	M96.A	Fracture of ribs, sternum and thorax associated with compression of the chest and cardiopulmonary resuscitation
Add	M96.A1	Fracture of sternum associated with chest compression and cardiopulmonary resuscitation
Add		Fracture of xiphoid process associated with chest compression and cardiopulmonary resuscitation
Add	M96.A2	Fracture of one rib associated with chest compression and cardiopulmonary resuscitation

Add	M96.A3	Multiple fractures of ribs associated with chest compression and cardiopulmonary resuscitation
Add	M96.A4	Flail chest associated with chest compression and cardiopulmonary resuscitation
Add	M96.A9	Other fracture associated with chest compression and cardiopulmonary resuscitation

No Change

CHAPTER 14

No Change

DISEASES OF THE GENITOURINARY SYSTEM (N00-N99)

No Change   **GLOMERULAR DISEASES (N00-N08)**

No Change **N08** Glomerular disorders in diseases classified elsewhere

No Change   **Excludes1**

Revise from   hemolytic-uremic syndrome (D59.3)
Revise to   hemolytic-uremic syndrome (D59.3-)

No Change   **RENAL TUBULO-INTERSTITIAL DISEASES (N10-N16)**

No Change **N14** Drug- and heavy-metal-induced tubulo-interstitial and tubular conditions

No Change   **N14.1** Nephropathy induced by other drugs, medicaments and biological substances

Add   **N14.11** Contrast-induced nephropathy
Add   Contrast medium, radiography nephropathy
Add   **Excludes2** acute kidney failure (N17.-)
Add   **N14.19** Nephropathy induced by other drugs, medicaments and biological substances

No Change   **ACUTE KIDNEY FAILURE AND CHRONIC KIDNEY DISEASE (N17-N19)**

No Change   **Excludes2**
Revise from   hemolytic-uremic syndrome (D59.3)
Revise to   hemolytic-uremic syndrome (D59.3-)

No Change   **INFLAMMATORY DISEASES OF FEMALE PELVIC ORGANS (N70-N77)**

No Change **N76** Other inflammation of vagina and vulva

No Change   **N76.8** Other specified inflammation of vagina and vulva
Add   **N76.82** Fournier disease of vagina and vulva
Add   Fournier gangrene of vagina and vulva
Add   Code also, if applicable, diabetes mellitus (E08-E13 with .9)
Add   **Excludes1** gangrene in diabetes mellitus (E08-E13 with .52)

No Change **N77** Vulvovaginal ulceration and inflammation in diseases classified elsewhere

No Change   **N77.1** Vaginitis, vulvitis and vulvovaginitis in diseases classified elsewhere
No Change   **Excludes1**
Revise from   candidal vulvovaginitis (B37.3)
Revise to   candidal vulvovaginitis (B37.3-)

No Change   **NONINFLAMMATORY DISORDERS OF FEMALE GENITAL TRACT (N80-N98)**

No Change **N80** Endometriosis

No Change   **N80.0** Endometriosis of uterus
Delete   Adenomyosis
Add   Endometriosis of the cervix
Add   **N80.00** Endometriosis of the uterus, unspecified
Add   **N80.01** Superficial endometriosis of the uterus
Add   **N80.02** Deep endometriosis of the uterus
Add   Deep retrocervical endometriosis
Add   **N80.03** Adenomyosis of the uterus
Add   Adenomyosis NOS

No Change **N80.1** Endometriosis of ovary
Add   **N80.10** Endometriosis of ovary, unspecified depth
Add   **N80.101** Endometriosis of right ovary, unspecified depth
Add   **N80.102** Endometriosis of left ovary, unspecified depth
Add   **N80.103** Endometriosis of bilateral ovaries, unspecified depth
Add   **N80.109** Endometriosis of ovary, unspecified side, unspecified depth
Add   Endometriosis of ovary NOS
Add   **N80.11** Superficial endometriosis of the ovary
Add   **N80.111** Superficial endometriosis of right ovary
Add   **N80.112** Superficial endometriosis of left ovary
Add   **N80.113** Superficial endometriosis of bilateral ovaries
Add   **N80.119** Superficial endometriosis of ovary, unspecified ovary
Add   **N80.12** Deep endometriosis of ovary
Add   Deep ovarian endometriosis
Add   Endometrioma
Add   **N80.121** Deep endometriosis of right ovary
Add   **N80.122** Deep endometriosis of left ovary
Add   **N80.123** Deep endometriosis of bilateral ovaries
Add   **N80.129** Deep endometriosis of ovary, unspecified ovary

No Change **N80.2** Endometriosis of fallopian tube
Add   **N80.20** Endometriosis of fallopian tube, unspecified depth
Add   **N80.201** Endometriosis of right fallopian tube, unspecified depth
Add   **N80.202** Endometriosis of left fallopian tube, unspecified depth
Add   **N80.203** Endometriosis of bilateral fallopian tubes, unspecified depth
Add   **N80.209** Endometriosis of unspecified fallopian tube, unspecified depth
Add   Endometriosis fallopian tube NOS
Add   **N80.21** Superficial endometriosis of fallopian tube
Add   **N80.211** Superficial endometriosis of right fallopian tube
Add   **N80.212** Superficial endometriosis of left fallopian tube
Add   **N80.213** Superficial endometriosis of bilateral fallopian tubes
Add   **N80.219** Superficial endometriosis of unspecified fallopian tube
Add   **N80.22** Deep endometriosis of the fallopian tube
Add   Deep endometriosis involving muscular wall of fallopian tube
Add   **N80.221** Deep endometriosis of right fallopian tube
Add   **N80.222** Deep endometriosis of left fallopian tube
Add   **N80.223** Deep endometriosis of bilateral fallopian tubes
Add   **N80.229** Deep endometriosis of unspecified fallopian tube

No Change	N80.3	Endometriosis of pelvic peritoneum	
Add	N80.30		Endometriosis of pelvic peritoneum, unspecified
Add			Endometriosis of the retroperitoneum NOS
Add	N80.31		Endometriosis of the anterior cul-de-sac
Add		N80.311	Superficial endometriosis of the anterior cul-de-sac
Add		N80.312	Deep endometriosis of the anterior cul-de-sac
Add		N80.319	Endometriosis of the anterior cul-de-sac, unspecified depth
Add			Endometriosis of the anterior cul-de-sac NOS
Add	N80.32		Endometriosis of the posterior cul-de-sac
Add		N80.321	Superficial endometriosis of the posterior cul-de-sac
Add		N80.322	Deep endometriosis of the posterior cul-de-sac
Add		N80.329	Endometriosis of the posterior cul-de-sac, unspecified depth
Add			Endometriosis of the posterior cul-de-sac NOS
Add	N80.33		Superficial endometriosis of the pelvic sidewall
Add		N80.331	Superficial endometriosis of the right pelvic sidewall
Add		N80.332	Superficial endometriosis of the left pelvic sidewall
Add		N80.333	Superficial endometriosis of bilateral pelvic sidewall
Add		N80.339	Superficial endometriosis of pelvic sidewall, unspecified side
Add	N80.34		Deep endometriosis of the pelvic sidewall
Add		N80.341	Deep endometriosis of the right pelvic sidewall
Add		N80.342	Deep endometriosis of the left pelvic sidewall
Add		N80.343	Deep endometriosis of the bilateral pelvic sidewall
Add		N80.349	Deep endometriosis of the pelvic sidewall, unspecified side
Add	N80.35		Endometriosis of the pelvic sidewall, unspecified depth
Add		N80.351	Endometriosis of the right pelvic sidewall, unspecified depth
Add		N80.352	Endometriosis of the left pelvic sidewall, unspecified depth
Add		N80.353	Endometriosis of bilateral pelvic sidewall, unspecified depth
Add		N80.359	Endometriosis of pelvic sidewall, unspecified side, unspecified depth
Add			Endometriosis of the pelvic sidewall NOS
Add	N80.36		Superficial endometriosis of the pelvic brim
Add		N80.361	Superficial endometriosis of the right pelvic brim
Add		N80.362	Superficial endometriosis of the left pelvic brim
Add		N80.363	Superficial endometriosis of bilateral pelvic brim
Add		N80.369	Superficial endometriosis of the pelvic brim, unspecified side
Add	N80.37		Deep endometriosis of the pelvic brim
Add		N80.371	Deep endometriosis of the right pelvic brim
Add		N80.372	Deep endometriosis of the left pelvic brim
Add		N80.373	Deep endometriosis of bilateral pelvic brim
Add		N80.379	Deep endometriosis of the pelvic brim, unspecified side
Add	N80.38		Endometriosis of the pelvic brim, unspecified depth
Add		N80.381	Endometriosis of the right pelvic brim, unspecified depth
Add		N80.382	Endometriosis of the left pelvic brim, unspecified depth
Add		N80.383	Endometriosis of bilateral pelvic brim, unspecified depth
Add		N80.389	Endometriosis of the pelvic brim, unspecified side, unspecified depth
Add			Endometriosis of the pelvic brim NOS
Add	N80.3A		Superficial endometriosis of the uterosacral ligament(s)
Add		N80.3A1	Superficial endometriosis of the right uterosacral ligament
Add		N80.3A2	Superficial endometriosis of the left uterosacral ligament
Add		N80.3A3	Superficial endometriosis of the bilateral uterosacral ligament(s)
Add		N80.3A9	Superficial endometriosis of the uterosacral ligament(s), unspecified side
Add	N80.3B		Deep endometriosis of the uterosacral ligament(s)
Add		N80.3B1	Deep endometriosis of the right uterosacral ligament
Add		N80.3B2	Deep endometriosis of the left uterosacral ligament
Add		N80.3B3	Deep endometriosis of bilateral uterosacral ligament(s)
Add		N80.3B9	Deep endometriosis of the uterosacral ligament(s), unspecified side
Add	N80.3C		Endometriosis of the uterosacral ligament(s), unspecified depth
Add		N80.3C1	Endometriosis of the right uterosacral ligament, unspecified depth
Add		N80.3C2	Endometriosis of the left uterosacral ligament, unspecified depth
Add		N80.3C3	Endometriosis of bilateral uterosacral ligament(s), unspecified depth
Add		N80.3C9	Endometriosis of the uterosacral ligament(s), unspecified side, unspecified depth
Add			Endometriosis of the uterosacral ligament(s) NOS
Add	N80.39		Endometriosis of other pelvic peritoneum
Add		N80.391	Superficial endometriosis of the pelvic peritoneum, other specified sites
Add		N80.392	Deep endometriosis of the pelvic peritoneum, other specified sites
Add		N80.399	Endometriosis of the pelvic peritoneum, other specified sites, unspecified depth

No Change	**N80.4**	**Endometriosis of rectovaginal septum and vagina**
Add	**N80.40**	**Endometriosis of rectovaginal septum, unspecified involvement of vagina**
Add		Endometriosis of the rectovaginal septum, NOS
Add	**N80.41**	**Endometriosis of rectovaginal septum without involvement of vagina**
Add	**N80.42**	**Endometriosis of rectovaginal septum with involvement of vagina**
No Change	**N80.5**	**Endometriosis of intestine**
Add	**N80.50**	**Endometriosis of intestine, unspecified**
Add	**N80.51**	**Endometriosis of the rectum**
Add	**N80.511**	**Superficial endometriosis of the rectum**
Add	**N80.512**	**Deep endometriosis of the rectum**
Add		Deep endometriosis of the rectum, multifocal
Add	**N80.519**	**Endometriosis of the rectum, unspecified depth**
Add		Endometriosis of the rectum NOS
Add	**N80.52**	**Endometriosis of the sigmoid colon**
Add	**N80.521**	**Superficial endometriosis of the sigmoid colon**
Add	**N80.522**	**Deep endometriosis of the sigmoid colon**
Add	**N80.529**	**Endometriosis of the sigmoid colon, unspecified depth**
Add		Endometriosis of the sigmoid colon NOS
Add	**N80.53**	**Endometriosis of the cecum**
Add	**N80.531**	**Superficial endometriosis of the cecum**
Add	**N80.532**	**Deep endometriosis of the cecum**
Add	**N80.539**	**Endometriosis of the cecum, unspecified depth**
Add		Endometriosis of the cecum NOS
Add	**N80.54**	**Endometriosis of the appendix**
Add	**N80.541**	**Superficial endometriosis of the appendix**
Add	**N80.542**	**Deep endometriosis of the appendix**
Add	**N80.549**	**Endometriosis of the appendix, unspecified depth**
Add		Endometriosis of the appendix NOS
Add	**N80.55**	**Endometriosis of other parts of the colon**
Add		Endometriosis of descending colon
Add		Endometriosis of transverse colon
Add	**N80.551**	**Superficial endometriosis of other parts of the colon**
Add	**N80.552**	**Deep endometriosis of other parts of the colon**
Add	**N80.559**	**Endometriosis of other parts of the colon, unspecified depth**
		Endometriosis of colon NOS
Add	**N80.56**	**Endometriosis of the small intestine**
Add	**N80.561**	**Superficial endometriosis of the small intestine**
Add	**N80.562**	**Deep endometriosis of the small intestine**
Add		Deep endometriosis of the small intestine, multifocal
Add	**N80.569**	**Endometriosis of the small intestine, unspecified depth**
Add		Endometriosis of the small intestine NOS

Add	**N80.A**	**Endometriosis of bladder and ureters**
Add	**N80.A0**	**Endometriosis of bladder, unspecified depth**
Add		Endometriosis of bladder NOS
Add	**N80.A1**	**Superficial endometriosis of bladder**
Add	**N80.A2**	**Deep endometriosis of bladder**
Add	**N80.A4**	**Superficial endometriosis of ureter**
Add		Extrinsic endometriosis of ureter
Add		Code also, if applicable, obstructive and reflux uropathy (N13.-)
Add	**N80.A41**	**Superficial endometriosis of right ureter**
Add	**N80.A42**	**Superficial endometriosis of left ureter**
Add	**N80.A43**	**Superficial endometriosis of bilateral ureters**
Add	**N80.A49**	**Superficial endometriosis of unspecified ureter**
Add	**N80.A5**	**Deep endometriosis of ureter**
Add		Intrinsic endometriosis of ureter
Add		Code also, if applicable, obstructive and reflux uropathy (N13.-)
Add	**N80.A51**	**Deep endometriosis of right ureter**
Add	**N80.A52**	**Deep endometriosis of left ureter**
Add	**N80.A53**	**Deep endometriosis of bilateral ureters**
Add	**N80.A59**	**Deep endometriosis of unspecified ureter**
Add	**N80.A6**	**Endometriosis of ureter, unspecified depth**
Add		Code also, if applicable, obstructive and reflux uropathy (N13.-)
Add	**N80.A61**	**Endometriosis of right ureter, unspecified depth**
Add	**N80.A62**	**Endometriosis of left ureter, unspecified depth**
Add	**N80.A63**	**Endometriosis of bilateral ureters, unspecified depth**
Add	**N80.A69**	**Endometriosis of unspecified ureter, unspecified depth**
Add	**N80.B**	**Endometriosis of cardiothoracic space**
Add		Endometriosis of thorax
Add		Code also, if applicable:
Add		catamenial hemothorax (J94.2)
Add		catamenial pneumothorax (J93.12)
Add	**N80.B1**	**Endometriosis of pleura**
Add	**N80.B2**	**Endometriosis of lung**
Add	**N80.B3**	**Endometriosis of diaphragm**
Add	**N80.B31**	**Superficial endometriosis of diaphragm**
Add	**N80.B32**	**Deep endometriosis of diaphragm**
Add	**N80.B39**	**Endometriosis of diaphragm, unspecified depth**
Add		Endometriosis of the diaphragm NOS
Add	**N80.B4**	**Endometriosis of the pericardial space**
Add	**N80.B5**	**Endometriosis of the mediastinal space**
Add	**N80.B6**	**Endometriosis of cardiothoracic space**
Add	**N80.C**	**Endometriosis of the abdomen**
Add	**N80.C0**	**Endometriosis of the abdomen, unspecified**
Add		Endometriosis of the abdomen NOS
Add	**N80.C1**	**Endometriosis of the anterior abdominal wall**
Add	**N80.C10**	**Endometriosis of the anterior abdominal wall, subcutaneous tissue**

Add		N80.C11	Endometriosis of the anterior abdominal wall, fascia and muscular layers
Add		N80.C19	Endometriosis of the anterior abdominal wall, unspecified depth
Add			Endometriosis of the anterior abdominal wall NOS
Add		N80.C2	Endometriosis of the umbilicus
Add		N80.C3	Endometriosis of the inguinal canal
Add		N80.C4	Endometriosis of extra-pelvic abdominal peritoneum
Add		N80.C9	Endometriosis of other site of abdomen
Add	N80.D		Endometriosis of the pelvic nerves
Add			Endometriosis of the nerves of the retroperitoneum
Add		N80.D0	Endometriosis of the pelvic nerves, unspecified
Add			Endometriosis of nerve of the retroperitoneum, NOS
Add		N80.D1	Endometriosis of the sacral splanchnic nerves
Add			Endometriosis of the pelvic splanchnic nerves
Add		N80.D2	Endometriosis of the sacral nerve roots
Add		N80.D3	Endometriosis of the obturator nerve
Add		N80.D4	Endometriosis of the sciatic nerve
Add		N80.D5	Endometriosis of the pudendal nerve
Add		N80.D6	Endometriosis of the femoral nerve
Add		N80.D9	Endometriosis of other pelvic nerve
Add			Endometriosis of the other nerves of the retroperitoneum
No Change	N80.8		Other endometriosis
Revise from			Endometriosis of thorax
Revise to			Endometriosis of other site
No Change	N85		Other noninflammatory disorders of uterus, except cervix
Add	N85.A		Isthmocele
Add			Isthmocele (non-pregnant state)
Add			Code also any associated conditions such as:
Add			abnormal uterine and vaginal bleeding, unspecified (N93.9)
Add			female infertility of uterine origin (N97.2)
Add			pelvic and perineal pain (R10.2)
Add		**Excludes1**	maternal care for cesarean scar defect (isthmocele) (O34.22)

No Change CHAPTER 15

No Change PREGNANCY, CHILDBIRTH AND THE PUERPERIUM (O00-O9A)

No Change **MATERNAL CARE RELATED TO THE FETUS AND AMNIOTIC CAVITY AND POSSIBLE DELIVERY PROBLEMS (O30-O48)**

No Change	O35		Maternal care for known or suspected fetal abnormality and damage
No Change		O35.0	Maternal care for (suspected) central nervous system malformation in fetus
Delete			Maternal care for fetal anencephaly
Delete			Maternal care for fetal hydrocephalus
Delete			Maternal care for fetal spina bifida
No Change		**Excludes2**	
Revise from			chromosomal abnormality in fetus (O35.1)
Revise to			chromosomal abnormality in fetus (O35.1-)
Add		O35.00	Maternal care for (suspected) central nervous system malformation or damage in fetus, unspecified
Add		O35.01	Maternal care for (suspected) central nervous system malformation or damage in fetus, agenesis of the corpus callosum

Add		O35.02	Maternal care for (suspected) central nervous system malformation or damage in fetus, anencephaly
Add		O35.03	Maternal care for (suspected) central nervous system malformation or damage in fetus, choroid plexus cysts
Add		O35.04	Maternal care for (suspected) central nervous system malformation or damage in fetus, encephalocele
Add		O35.05	Maternal care for (suspected) central nervous system malformation or damage in fetus, holoprosencephaly
Add		O35.06	Maternal care for (suspected) central nervous system malformation or damage in fetus, hydrocephaly
Add			Maternal care for fetal hydrocephalus
Add		O35.07	Maternal care for (suspected) central nervous system malformation or damage in fetus, microcephaly
Add		O35.08	Maternal care for (suspected) central nervous system malformation or damage in fetus, spina bifida
Add		O35.09	Maternal care for (suspected) other central nervous system malformation or damage in fetus
No Change		O35.1	Maternal care for (suspected) chromosomal abnormality in fetus
Add		O35.10	Maternal care for (suspected) chromosomal abnormality in fetus, unspecified
Add		O35.11	Maternal care for (suspected) chromosomal abnormality in fetus, Trisomy 13
Add		O35.12	Maternal care for (suspected) chromosomal abnormality in fetus, Trisomy 18
Add		O35.13	Maternal care for (suspected) chromosomal abnormality in fetus, Trisomy 21
Add		O35.14	Maternal care for (suspected) chromosomal abnormality in fetus, Turner Syndrome
Add		O35.15	Maternal care for (suspected) chromosomal abnormality in fetus, sex chromosome abnormality
Add		O35.19	Maternal care for (suspected) chromosomal abnormality in fetus, other chromosomal abnormality
Add		O35.A	Maternal care for other (suspected) fetal abnormality and damage, fetal facial anomalies
Add		O35.B	Maternal care for other (suspected) fetal abnormality and damage, fetal cardiac anomalies
Add		O35.C	Maternal care for other (suspected) fetal abnormality and damage, fetal pulmonary anomalies
Add		O35.D	Maternal care for other (suspected) fetal abnormality and damage, fetal gastrointestinal anomalies
Add		O35.E	Maternal care for other (suspected) fetal abnormality and damage, fetal genitourinary anomalies
Add		O35.F	Maternal care for other (suspected) fetal abnormality and damage, fetal musculoskeletal anomalies of trunk
Add		**Excludes2**	maternal care for other (suspected) fetal abnormality and damage, fetal lower extremities anomalies (O35.H)
Add			maternal care for other (suspected) fetal abnormality and damage, fetal upper extremities anomalies (O35.G)

Add	O35.G	Maternal care for other (suspected) fetal abnormality and damage, fetal upper extremities anomalies
Add	O35.H	Maternal care for other (suspected) fetal abnormality and damage, fetal lower extremities anomalies
No Change	O35.2	Maternal care for (suspected) hereditary disease in fetus
No Change		Excludes2
Revise from		chromosomal abnormality in fetus (O35.1)
Revise to		chromosomal abnormality in fetus (O35.1-)

No Change

CHAPTER 16

No Change

CERTAIN CONDITIONS ORIGINATING IN THE PERINATAL PERIOD (P00-P96)

No Change

RESPIRATORY AND CARDIOVASCULAR DISORDERS SPECIFIC TO THE PERINATAL PERIOD (P19-P29)

No Change P28		Other respiratory conditions originating in the perinatal period
Delete		Excludes1 congenital malformations of the respiratory system (Q30-Q34)
Add		Code also, if applicable, congenital malformations of the respiratory system (Q30-Q34)
No Change	P28.2	Cyanotic attacks of newborn
No Change		Excludes1
Revise from		apnea of newborn (P28.3-P28.4)
Revise to		apnea of newborn (P28.3- - P28.4-)
No Change	P28.3	Primary sleep apnea of newborn
Delete		Central sleep apnea of newborn
Delete		Obstructive sleep apnea of newborn
Add		Excludes2 other apnea of newborn (P28.4-)
Add	P28.30	Primary sleep apnea of newborn, unspecified
Add		Transient oxygen desaturation spells of newborn during sleep
Add	P28.31	Primary central sleep apnea of newborn
Add	P28.32	Primary obstructive sleep apnea of newborn
Add	P28.33	Primary mixed sleep apnea of newborn
Add	P28.39	Other primary sleep apnea of newborn
No Change	P28.4	Other apnea of newborn
Delete		Apnea of prematurity
Delete		Obstructive apnea of newborn
Delete		Excludes1 obstructive sleep apnea of newborn (P28.3)
Add		Excludes2 primary sleep apnea of newborn (P28.3-)
Add	P28.40	Unspecified apnea of newborn
Add		Apnea of newborn, NOS
Add		Transient oxygen desaturation spells of newborn
Add	P28.41	Central neonatal apnea of newborn
Add	P28.42	Obstructive apnea of newborn
Add	P28.43	Mixed neonatal apnea of newborn
Add	P28.49	Other apnea of newborn
Add		Apnea of prematurity

No Change

CHAPTER 17

No Change

CONGENITAL MALFORMATIONS, DEFORMATIONS AND CHROMOSOMAL ABNORMALITIES (Q00-Q99)

No Change

CONGENITAL MALFORMATIONS OF THE CIRCULATORY SYSTEM (Q20-Q28)

No Change Q21		Congenital malformations of cardiac septa
No Change	Q21.1	Atrial septal defect
Delete		Coronary sinus defect
Delete		Patent or persistent foramen ovale
Delete		Patent or persistent ostium secundum defect (type II)
Delete		Patent or persistent sinus venosus defect
Add		Excludes 2 ostium primum atrial septal defect (type I) (Q21.20)
Add	Q21.10	Atrial septal defect, unspecified
Add	Q21.11	Secundum atrial septal defect
Add		Fenestrated atrial septum
Add		Patent or persistent ostium secundum defect (type II)
Add	Q21.12	Patent foramen ovale
Add		Persistent foramen ovale
Add	Q21.13	Coronary sinus atrial septal defect
Add		Coronary sinus defect
Add		Unroofed coronary sinus
Add	Q21.14	Superior sinus venosus atrial septal defect
Add		Superior vena cava type atrial septal defect
Add	Q21.15	Inferior sinus venosus atrial septal defect
Add		Inferior vena cava type atrial septal defect
Add	Q21.16	Sinus venosus atrial septal defect, unspecified
Add		Sinus venosus defect, NOS
Add	Q21.19	Other specified atrial septal defect
Add		Common atrium
Add		Other specified atrial septal abnormality
No Change	Q21.2	Atrioventricular septal defect
Delete		Common atrioventricular canal
Add		Atrioventricular canal defect
Add	Q21.20	Atrioventricular septal defect, unspecified as to partial or complete
Add		Atrioventricular canal, NOS
Add		Endocardial cushion defect NOS
Add		Ostium primum atrial septal defect (type I) NOS
Add	Q21.21	Partial atrioventricular septal defect
Add		Incomplete atrioventricular canal
Add		Incomplete atrioventricular septal defect
Add		Incomplete endocardial cushion defect
Add		Ostium primum atrial septal defect (type I) with separate atrioventricular valves
Add		Partial atrioventricular canal
Add		Partial endocardial cushion defect
Add	Q21.22	Transitional atrioventricular septal defect
Add		Intermediate atrioventricular canal
Add		Intermediate atrioventricular septal defect
Add		Intermediate endocardial cushion defect
Add		Ostium primum atrial septal defect (type I) with separate atrioventricular valves and a small or restrictive inlet VSD
Add		Transitional atrioventricular canal
Add		Transitional endocardial cushion defect

Add   Q21.23   **Complete atrioventricular septal defect**
Add   Common atrioventricular canal
Add   Common atrioventricular septal defect
Add   Common endocardial cushion defect
Add   Ostium primum atrial septal defect (type I) with common atrioventricular valve and a moderate or larger inlet VSD

No Change   **OTHER CONGENITAL MALFORMATIONS (Q80-Q89)**

No Change **Q82**   **Other congenital malformations of skin**
No Change   **Excludes1**
Revise from   Sturge-Weber (-Dimitri) syndrome (Q85.8)
Revise to   Sturge-Weber (-Dimitri) syndrome (Q85.89)

No Change **Q85**   **Phakomatoses, not elsewhere classified**

No Change   **Q85.8**   **Other phakomatoses, not elsewhere classified**
Delete   Peutz-Jeghers Syndrome
Delete   Sturge-Weber(-Dimitri) syndrome
Delete   von Hippel-Lindau syndrome
Add   **Q85.81**   **PTEN tumor syndrome**
Add   PHTS
Add   PTEN hamartoma tumor syndrome
Add   PTEN related Cowden syndrome
Add   Code also, if applicable, genetic susceptibility to malignant neoplasm (Z15.0-)
Add   **Q85.82**   **Other Cowden syndrome**
Add   **Q85.83**   **Von Hippel-Lindau syndrome**
Add   Code also manifestations
Add   **Q85.89**   **Other phakomatoses, not elsewhere classified**
Add   Peutz-Jeghers syndrome
Add   Sturge-Weber(-Dimitri) syndrome

No Change **CHAPTER 18**

No Change **SYMPTOMS, SIGNS AND ABNORMAL CLINICAL AND LABORATORY FINDINGS, NOT ELSEWHERE CLASSIFIED (R00-R99)**

No Change   **SYMPTOMS AND SIGNS INVOLVING THE CIRCULATORY AND RESPIRATORY SYSTEMS (R00-R09)**

No Change **R04**   **Hemorrhage from respiratory passages**
No Change   **R04.8**   **Hemorrhage from other sites in respiratory passages**
No Change   **R04.81**   **Acute idiopathic pulmonary hemorrhage in infants**
No Change   **Excludes1**
Revise from   von Willebrand's disease (D68.0)
Revise to   von Willebrand disease (D68.0-)

No Change **R06**   **Abnormalities of breathing**
No Change   **R06.8**   **Other abnormalities of breathing**
No Change   **R06.81**   **Apnea, not elsewhere classified**
No Change   **Excludes1**
Revise from   apnea (of) newborn (P28.4)
Revise to   apnea (of) newborn (P28.4-)
Revise from   sleep apnea of newborn (primary) (P28.3)
Revise to   sleep apnea of newborn (primary) (P28.3-)

No Change   **GENERAL SYMPTOMS AND SIGNS (R50-R69)**

No Change **R53**   **Malaise and fatigue**
No Change   **R53.8**   **Other malaise and fatigue**
No Change   **R53.82**   **Chronic fatigue, unspecified**
Delete   Chronic fatigue syndrome NOS
No Change   **Excludes1**
Delete   postviral fatigue syndrome (G93.3)
Add   chronic fatigue syndrome (G93.32)
Add   myalgic encephalomyelitis (G93.32)
Add   post infection and related fatigue syndromes (G93.39)
Add   postviral fatigue syndrome (G93.31)

No Change **R62**   **Lack of expected normal physiological development in childhood and adults**
No Change   **R62.5**   **Other and unspecified lack of expected normal physiological development in childhood**
No Change   **R62.52**   **Short stature (child)**
No Change   **Excludes1**
Revise from   short stature due to endocrine disorder (E34.3)
Revise to   short stature due to endocrine disorder (E34.3-)

No Change   **ABNORMAL FINDINGS ON EXAMINATION OF BLOOD, WITHOUT DIAGNOSIS (R70-R79)**

No Change **R79**   **Other abnormal findings of blood chemistry**
No Change   **R79.1**   **Abnormal coagulation profile**
Add   Low von Willebrand factor

No Change **CHAPTER 19**

No Change **INJURY, POISONING AND CERTAIN OTHER CONSEQUENCES OF EXTERNAL CAUSES (S00-T88)**

No Change   **INJURIES TO THE HEAD (S00-S09)**

No Change **S06**   **Intracranial injury**
Add   **Use Additional** code, if applicable, to identify mild neurocognitive disorders due to known physiological condition (F06.7-)
No Change   **S06.0**   **Concussion**
No Change   **Excludes1**
Revise from   concussion with other intracranial injuries classified in subcategories S06.1- to S06.6-, S06.81- and S06.82- code to specified intracranial injury
Revise to   concussion with other intracranial injuries classified in subcategories S06.1- to S06.6-, and S06.81- to S06.89-, code to specified intracranial injury
No Change   **S06.0X Concussion**
No Change   **S06.0X1**   **Concussion with loss of consciousness of 30 minutes or less**
Add   Concussion with brief loss of consciousness
Add   **S06.0XA**   **Concussion with loss of consciousness status unknown**
Add   Concussion NOS
No Change   **S06.0X9**   **Concussion with loss of consciousness of unspecified duration**
Delete   Concussion NOS

No Change	S06.1	Traumatic cerebral edema
No Change		S06.1X Traumatic cerebral edema
No Change		S06.1X1 Traumatic cerebral edema with loss of consciousness of 30 minutes or less
Add		Traumatic cerebral edema with brief loss of consciousness
Add		S06.1XA Traumatic cerebral edema with loss of consciousness status unknown
Add		Traumatic cerebral edema NOS
No Change		S06.1X9 Traumatic cerebral edema with loss of consciousness of unspecified duration
Delete		Traumatic cerebral edema NOS
No Change	S06.2	Diffuse traumatic brain injury
No Change		S06.2X Diffuse traumatic brain injury
No Change		S06.2X1 Diffuse traumatic brain injury with loss of consciousness of 30 minutes or less
Add		Diffuse traumatic brain injury with brief loss of consciousness
Add		S06.2XA Diffuse traumatic brain injury with loss of consciousness status unknown
Add		Diffuse traumatic brain injury NOS
No Change		S06.2X9 Diffuse traumatic brain injury with loss of consciousness of unspecified duration
Delete		Diffuse traumatic brain injury NOS
No Change	S06.3	Focal traumatic brain injury
No Change		S06.30 Unspecified focal traumatic brain injury
		S06.301 Unspecified focal traumatic brain injury with loss of consciousness of 30 minutes or less
Add		Unspecified focal traumatic brain injury with brief loss of consciousness
Add		S06.30A Unspecified focal traumatic brain injury with loss of consciousness status unknown
Add		Unspecified focal traumatic brain injury NOS
No Change		S06.309 Unspecified focal traumatic brain injury with loss of consciousness of unspecified duration
Delete		Unspecified focal traumatic brain injury NOS
No Change		S06.31 Contusion and laceration of right cerebrum
No Change		S06.311 Contusion and laceration of right cerebrum with loss of consciousness of 30 minutes or less
Add		Contusion and laceration of right cerebrum with brief loss of consciousness
Add		S06.31A Contusion and laceration of right cerebrum with loss of consciousness status unknown
Add		Contusion and laceration of right cerebrum NOS
No Change		S06.319 Contusion and laceration of right cerebrum with loss of consciousness of unspecified duration
Delete		Contusion and laceration of right cerebrum NOS

No Change	S06.32	Contusion and laceration of left cerebrum
No Change		S06.321 Contusion and laceration of left cerebrum with loss of consciousness of 30 minutes or less
Add		Contusion and laceration of left cerebrum with brief loss of consciousness
Add		S06.32A Contusion and laceration of left cerebrum with loss of consciousness status unknown
Add		Contusion and laceration of left cerebrum NOS
No Change		S06.329 Contusion and laceration of left cerebrum with loss of consciousness of unspecified duration
Delete		Contusion and laceration of left cerebrum NOS
No Change	S06.33	Contusion and laceration of cerebrum, unspecified
No Change		S06.331 Contusion and laceration of cerebrum, unspecified, with loss of consciousness of 30 minutes or less
Add		Contusion and laceration of cerebrum, unspecified, with brief loss of consciousness
Add		S06.33A Contusion and laceration of cerebrum, unspecified, with loss of consciousness status unknown
Add		Contusion and laceration of cerebrum NOS
No Change		S06.339 Contusion and laceration of cerebrum, unspecified, with loss of consciousness of unspecified duration
Delete		Contusion and laceration of cerebrum NOS
No Change	S06.34	Traumatic hemorrhage of right cerebrum
No Change		S06.341 Traumatic hemorrhage of right cerebrum with loss of consciousness of 30 minutes or less
Add		Traumatic hemorrhage of right cerebrum with loss of consciousness
Add		S06.34A Traumatic hemorrhage of right cerebrum with loss of consciousness status unknown
Add		Traumatic hemorrhage of right cerebrum NOS
No Change		S06.349 Traumatic hemorrhage of right cerebrum with loss of consciousness of unspecified duration
Delete		Traumatic hemorrhage of right cerebrum NOS
No Change	S06.35	Traumatic hemorrhage of left cerebrum
No Change		S06.351 Traumatic hemorrhage of left cerebrum with loss of consciousness of 30 minutes or less
Add		Traumatic hemorrhage of left cerebrum with brief loss of consciousness
Add		S06.35A Traumatic hemorrhage of left cerebrum with loss of consciousness status unknown
Add		Traumatic hemorrhage of left cerebrum NOS

No Change		S06.359	Traumatic hemorrhage of left cerebrum with loss of consciousness of unspecified duration
Delete			Traumatic hemorrhage of left cerebrum NOS
No Change	S06.36		Traumatic hemorrhage of cerebrum, unspecified
No Change		S06.361	Traumatic hemorrhage of cerebrum, unspecified, with loss of consciousness of 30 minutes or less
Add			Traumatic hemorrhage of cerebrum, unspecified, with brief loss of consciousness
Add		S06.36A	Traumatic hemorrhage of cerebrum, unspecified, with loss of consciousness status unknown
Add			Traumatic hemorrhage of cerebrum NOS
No Change		S06.369	Traumatic hemorrhage of cerebrum, unspecified, with loss of consciousness of unspecified duration
Delete			Traumatic hemorrhage of cerebrum NOS
No Change	S06.37		Contusion, laceration, and hemorrhage of cerebellum
No Change		S06.371	Contusion, laceration, and hemorrhage of cerebellum with loss of consciousness of 30 minutes or less
Add			Contusion, laceration, and hemorrhage of cerebellum with brief loss of consciousness
Add		S06.37A	Contusion, laceration, and hemorrhage of cerebellum with loss of consciousness status unknown
Add			Contusion, laceration, and hemorrhage of cerebellum NOS
No Change		S06.379	Contusion, laceration, and hemorrhage of cerebellum with loss of consciousness of unspecified duration
Delete			Contusion, laceration, and hemorrhage of cerebellum NOS
No Change	S06.38		Contusion, laceration, and hemorrhage of brainstem
No Change		S06.381	Contusion, laceration, and hemorrhage of brainstem with loss of consciousness of 30 minutes or less
Add			Contusion, laceration, and hemorrhage of brainstem with brief loss of consciousness
Add		S06.38A	Contusion, laceration, and hemorrhage of brainstem with loss of consciousness status unknown
Add			Contusion, laceration, and hemorrhage of brainstem NOS
No Change		S06.389	Contusion, laceration, and hemorrhage of brainstem with loss of consciousness of unspecified duration
Delete			Contusion, laceration, and hemorrhage of brainstem NOS

No Change	S06.4			Epidural hemorrhage
No Change		S06.4X		Epidural hemorrhage
No Change			S06.4X1	Epidural hemorrhage with loss of consciousness of 30 minutes or less
Add				Epidural hemorrhage with brief loss of consciousness
Add			S06.4XA	Epidural hemorrhage with loss of consciousness status unknown
Add				Epidural hemorrhage NOS
No Change			S06.4X9	Epidural hemorrhage with loss of consciousness of unspecified duration
Delete				Epidural hemorrhage NOS
No Change	S06.5			Traumatic subdural hemorrhage
No Change		S06.5X		Traumatic subdural hemorrhage
No Change			S06.5X1	Traumatic subdural hemorrhage with loss of consciousness of 30 minutes or less
Add				Traumatic subdural hemorrhage with brief loss of consciousness
Add			S06.5XA	Traumatic subdural hemorrhage with loss of consciousness status unknown
Add				Traumatic subdural hemorrhage NOS
No Change			S06.5X9	Traumatic subdural hemorrhage with loss of consciousness of unspecified duration
Delete				Traumatic subdural hemorrhage NOS
No Change	S06.6			Traumatic subarachnoid hemorrhage
No Change		S06.6X		Traumatic subarachnoid hemorrhage
No Change			S06.6X1	Traumatic subarachnoid hemorrhage with loss of consciousness of 30 minutes or less
Add				Traumatic subarachnoid hemorrhage with brief loss of consciousness
Add			S06.6XA	Traumatic subarachnoid hemorrhage with loss of consciousness status unknown
Add				Traumatic subarachnoid hemorrhage NOS
No Change			S06.6X9	Traumatic subarachnoid hemorrhage with loss of consciousness of unspecified duration
Delete				Traumatic subarachnoid hemorrhage NOS
No Change	S06.8			Other specified intracranial injuries
No Change		S06.81		Injury of right internal carotid artery, intracranial portion, not elsewhere classified
No Change			S06.811	Injury of right internal carotid artery, intracranial portion, not elsewhere classified with loss of consciousness of 30 minutes or less
Add				Injury of right internal carotid artery, intracranial portion, not elsewhere classified with brief loss of consciousness

Add	S06.81A	**Injury of right internal carotid artery, intracranial portion, not elsewhere classified with loss of consciousness status unknown**
Add		Injury of right internal carotid artery, intracranial portion, not elsewhere classified NOS
No Change	S06.819	**Injury of right internal carotid artery, intracranial portion, not elsewhere classified with loss of consciousness of unspecified duration**
Delete		Injury of right internal carotid artery, intracranial portion, not elsewhere classified NOS
No Change	S06.82	**Injury of left internal carotid artery, intracranial portion, not elsewhere classified**
No Change	S06.821	**Injury of left internal carotid artery, intracranial portion, not elsewhere classified with loss of consciousness of 30 minutes or less**
Add		Injury of left internal carotid artery, intracranial portion, not elsewhere classified with brief loss of consciousness
Add	S06.82A	**Injury of left internal carotid artery, intracranial portion, not elsewhere classified with loss of consciousness status unknown**
Add		Injury of left internal carotid artery, intracranial portion, not elsewhere classified NOS
No Change	S06.829	**Injury of left internal carotid artery, intracranial portion, not elsewhere classified with loss of consciousness of unspecified duration**
Delete		Injury of left internal carotid artery, intracranial portion, not elsewhere classified NOS
Add	S06.8A	**Primary blast injury of brain, not elsewhere classified**
Add		Code also, if applicable, focal traumatic brain injury (S06.3-)
Add		**Excludes2** traumatic cerebral edema (S06.1)
Add	S06.8A0	**Primary blast injury of brain, not elsewhere classified without loss of consciousness**
Add	S06.8A1	**Primary blast injury of brain, not elsewhere classified with loss of consciousness of 30 minutes or less**
Add		Primary blast injury of brain, not elsewhere classified with brief loss of consciousness
Add	S06.8A2	**Primary blast injury of brain, not elsewhere classified with loss of consciousness of 31 minutes to 59 minutes**

Add	S06.8A3	**Primary blast injury of brain, not elsewhere classified with loss of consciousness of 1 hour to 5 hours 59 minutes**
Add	S06.8A4	**Primary blast injury of brain, not elsewhere classified with loss of consciousness of 6 hours to 24 hours**
Add	S06.8A5	**Primary blast injury of brain, not elsewhere classified with loss of consciousness greater than 24 hours with return to pre-existing conscious level**
Add	S06.8A6	**Primary blast injury of brain, not elsewhere classified with loss of consciousness greater than 24 hours without return to pre-existing conscious level with patient surviving**
Add	S06.8A7	**Primary blast injury of brain, not elsewhere classified with loss of consciousness of any duration with death due to brain injury prior to regaining consciousness**
Add	S06.8A8	**Primary blast injury of brain, not elsewhere classified with loss of consciousness of any duration with death due to other cause prior to regaining consciousness**
Add	S06.8AA	**Primary blast injury of brain, not elsewhere classified with loss of consciousness status unknown**
Add		Primary blast injury of brain NOS
Add	S06.8A9	**Primary blast injury of brain, not elsewhere classified with loss of consciousness of unspecified duration**
No Change	S06.89	**Other specified intracranial injury**
No Change	S06.891	**Other specified intracranial injury with loss of consciousness of 30 minutes or less**
Add		Other specified intracranial injury with brief loss of consciousness
Add	S06.89A	**Other specified intracranial injury with loss of consciousness status unknown**
No Change	S06.9	**Unspecified intracranial injury**
No Change	S06.9X	**Unspecified intracranial injury**
No Change	S06.9X1	**Unspecified intracranial injury with loss of consciousness of 30 minutes or less**
Add		Unspecified intracranial injury with brief loss of consciousness
Add	S06.9XA	**Unspecified intracranial injury with loss of consciousness status unknown**

No Change	**POISONING BY, ADVERSE EFFECTS OF AND UNDERDOSING OF DRUGS MEDICAMENTS AND BIOLOGICAL SUBSTANCES (T36-T50)**	

No Change T43 Poisoning by, adverse effect of and underdosing of psychotropic drugs, not elsewhere classified

No Change   T43.6 Poisoning by, adverse effect of and underdosing of psychostimulants

No Change   T43.62 Poisoning by, adverse effect of and underdosing of amphetamines

Delete   Poisoning by, adverse effect of and underdosing of methamphetamines

Add   T43.65 Poisoning by, adverse effect of and underdosing of methamphetamines

Add   T43.651 Poisoning by methamphetamines accidental (unintentional)
                         Poisoning by methamphetamines NOS

Add   T43.652 Poisoning by methamphetamines intentional self-harm

Add   T43.653 Poisoning by methamphetamines, assault

Add   T43.654 Poisoning by methamphetamines, undetermined

Add   T43.655 Adverse effect of methamphetamines

Add   T43.656 Underdosing of methamphetamines

No Change # CHAPTER 20

No Change # EXTERNAL CAUSES OF MORBIDITY (V00-Y99)

No Change **MOTORCYCLE RIDER INJURED IN TRANSPORT ACCIDENT (V20-V29)**

Add   **Includes**   electric bicycle
Add   e-bike
Add   e-bicycle

No Change V20 Motorcycle rider injured in collision with pedestrian or animal

No Change   V20.0 Motorcycle driver injured in collision with pedestrian or animal in nontraffic accident

Add   V20.01 Electric (assisted) bicycle driver injured in collision with pedestrian or animal in nontraffic accident

Add   V20.09 Other motorcycle driver injured in collision with pedestrian or animal in nontraffic accident

No Change   V20.1 Motorcycle passenger injured in collision with pedestrian or animal in nontraffic accident

Add   V20.11 Electric (assisted) bicycle passenger injured in collision with pedestrian or animal in nontraffic accident

Add   V20.19 Other motorcycle passenger injured in collision with pedestrian or animal in nontraffic accident

No Change   V20.2 Unspecified motorcycle rider injured in collision with pedestrian or animal in nontraffic accident

Add   V20.21 Unspecified electric (assisted) bicycle rider injured in collision with pedestrian or animal in nontraffic accident

Add   V20.29 Unspecified rider of other motorcycle injured in collision with pedestrian or animal in nontraffic accident

No Change   V20.3 Person boarding or alighting a motorcycle injured in collision with pedestrian or animal

Add   V20.31 Person boarding or alighting an electric (assisted) bicycle injured in collision with pedestrian or animal

Add   V20.39 Person boarding or alighting other motorcycle injured in collision with pedestrian or animal

No Change   V20.4 Motorcycle driver injured in collision with pedestrian or animal in traffic accident

Add   V20.41 Electric (assisted) bicycle driver injured in collision with pedestrian or animal in traffic accident

Add   V20.49 Other motorcycle driver injured in collision with pedestrian or animal in traffic accident

No Change   V20.5 Motorcycle passenger injured in collision with pedestrian or animal in traffic accident

Add   V20.51 Electric (assisted) bicycle passenger injured in collision with pedestrian or animal in traffic accident

Add   V20.59 Other motorcycle passenger injured in collision with pedestrian or animal in traffic accident

No Change   V20.9 Unspecified motorcycle rider injured in collision with pedestrian or animal in traffic accident

Add   V20.91 Unspecified electric (assisted) bicycle rider injured in collision with pedestrian or animal in traffic accident

Add   V20.99 Unspecified rider of other motorcycle injured in collision with pedestrian or animal in traffic accident

No Change V21 Motorcycle rider injured in collision with pedal cycle

No Change   V21.0 Motorcycle driver injured in collision with pedal cycle in nontraffic accident

Add   V21.01 Electric (assisted) bicycle driver injured in collision with pedal cycle in nontraffic accident

Add   V21.09 Other motorcycle driver injured in collision with pedal cycle in nontraffic accident

No Change   V21.1 Motorcycle passenger injured in collision with pedal cycle in nontraffic accident

Add   V21.11 Electric (assisted) bicycle passenger injured in collision with pedal cycle in nontraffic accident

Add   V21.19 Other motorcycle passenger injured in collision with pedal cycle in nontraffic accident

No Change   V21.2 Unspecified motorcycle rider injured in collision with pedal cycle in nontraffic accident

Add   V21.21 Unspecified electric (assisted) bicycle rider injured in collision with pedal cycle in nontraffic accident

Add   V21.29 Unspecified rider of other motorcycle injured in collision with pedal cycle in nontraffic accident

No Change   V21.3 Person boarding or alighting a motorcycle injured in collision with pedal cycle

Add   V21.31 Person boarding or alighting an electric (assisted) bicycle injured in collision with pedal cycle

Add   V21.39 Person boarding or alighting other motorcycle injured in collision with pedal cycle

No Change   V21.4 Motorcycle driver injured in collision with pedal cycle in traffic accident

Add   V21.41 Electric (assisted) bicycle driver injured in collision with pedal cycle in traffic accident

Add   V21.49 Other motorcycle driver injured in collision with pedal cycle in traffic accident

No Change	V21.5	Motorcycle passenger injured in collision with pedal cycle in traffic accident
Add	V21.51	Electric (assisted) bicycle passenger injured in collision with pedal cycle in traffic accident
Add	V21.59	Other motorcycle passenger injured in collision with pedal cycle in traffic accident
No Change	V21.9	Unspecified motorcycle rider injured in collision with pedal cycle in traffic accident
Add	V21.91	Unspecified electric (assisted) bicycle rider injured in collision with pedal cycle in traffic accident
Add	V21.99	Unspecified rider of other motorcycle injured in collision with pedal cycle in traffic accident
No Change	V22	Motorcycle rider injured in collision with two- or three-wheeled motor vehicle
No Change	V22.0	Motorcycle driver injured in collision with two- or three-wheeled motor vehicle in nontraffic accident
Add	V22.01	Electric (assisted) bicycle driver injured in collision with two- or three-wheeled motor vehicle in nontraffic accident
Add	V22.09	Other motorcycle driver injured in collision with two- or three-wheeled motor vehicle in nontraffic accident
No Change	V22.1	Motorcycle passenger injured in collision with two- or three-wheeled motor vehicle in nontraffic accident
Add	V22.11	Electric (assisted) bicycle passenger injured in collision with two- or three-wheeled motor vehicle in nontraffic accident
Add	V22.19	Other motorcycle passenger injured in collision with two- or three-wheeled motor vehicle in nontraffic accident
No Change	V22.2	Unspecified motorcycle rider injured in collision with two- or three-wheeled motor vehicle in nontraffic accident
Add	V22.21	Unspecified electric (assisted) bicycle rider injured in collision with two- or threewheeled motor vehicle in nontraffic accident
Add	V22.29	Unspecified rider of other motorcycle injured in collision with two- or three-wheeled motor vehicle in nontraffic accident
No Change	V22.3	Person boarding or alighting a motorcycle injured in collision with two- or three-wheeled motor vehicle
Add	V22.31	Person boarding or alighting an electric (assisted) bicycle injured in collision with two- or three-wheeled motor vehicle
Add	V22.39	Person boarding or alighting other motorcycle injured in collision with two- or threewheeled motor vehicle
No Change	V22.4	Motorcycle driver injured in collision with two- or three-wheeled motor vehicle in traffic accident
Add	V22.41	Electric (assisted) bicycle driver injured in collision with two- or three-wheeled motor vehicle in traffic accident
Add	V22.49	Other motorcycle driver injured in collision with two- or three-wheeled motor vehicle in traffic accident
No Change	V22.5	Motorcycle passenger injured in collision with two- or three-wheeled motor vehicle in traffic accident
Add	V22.51	Electric (assisted) bicycle passenger injured in collision with two- or three-wheeled motor vehicle in traffic accident
Add	V22.59	Other motorcycle passenger injured in collision with two- or three-wheeled motor vehicle in traffic accident
No Change	V22.9	Unspecified motorcycle rider injured in collision with two- or three-wheeled motor vehicle in traffic accident
Add	V22.91	Unspecified electric (assisted) bicycle rider injured in collision with two- or threewheeled motor vehicle in traffic accident
Add	V22.99	Unspecified rider of other motorcycle injured in collision with two- or three-wheeled motor vehicle in traffic accident
No Change	V23	Motorcycle rider injured in collision with car, pick-up truck or van
No Change	V23.0	Motorcycle driver injured in collision with car, pick-up truck or van in nontraffic accident
Add	V23.01	Electric (assisted) bicycle driver injured in collision with car, pick-up truck or van in nontraffic accident
Add	V23.09	Other motorcycle driver injured in collision with car, pick-up truck or van in nontraffic accident
No Change	V23.1	Motorcycle passenger injured in collision with car, pick-up truck or van in nontraffic accident
Add	V23.11	Electric (assisted) bicycle passenger injured in collision with car, pick-up truck or van in nontraffic accident
Add	V23.19	Other motorcycle passenger injured in collision with car, pick-up truck or van in nontraffic accident
No Change	V23.2	Unspecified motorcycle rider injured in collision with car, pick-up truck or van in nontraffic accident
Add	V23.21	Unspecified electric (assisted) bicycle rider injured in collision with car, pick-up truck or van in nontraffic accident
Add	V23.29	Unspecified rider of other motorcycle injured in collision with car, pick-up truck or van in nontraffic accident
No Change	V23.3	Person boarding or alighting a motorcycle injured in collision with car, pick-up truck or van
Add	V23.31	Person boarding or alighting an electric (assisted) bicycle injured in collision with car, pick-up truck or van
Add	V23.39	Person boarding or alighting other motorcycle injured in collision with car, pick-up truck or van
No Change	V23.4	Motorcycle driver injured in collision with car, pick-up truck or van in traffic accident
Add	V23.41	Electric (assisted) bicycle driver injured in collision with car, pick-up truck or van in traffic accident
Add	V23.49	Other motorcycle driver injured in collision with car, pick-up truck or van in traffic accident
No Change	V23.5	Motorcycle passenger injured in collision with car, pick-up truck or van in traffic accident
Add	V23.51	Electric (assisted) bicycle passenger injured in collision with car, pick-up truck or van in traffic accident
Add	V23.59	Other motorcycle passenger injured in collision with car, pick-up truck or van in traffic accident
No Change	V23.9	Unspecified motorcycle rider injured in collision with car, pick-up truck or van in traffic accident
Add	V23.91	Unspecified electric (assisted) bicycle rider injured in collision with car, pick-up truck or van in traffic accident
Add	V23.99	Unspecified rider of other motorcycle injured in collision with car, pick-up truck or van in traffic accident

No Change **V24**	Motorcycle rider injured in collision with heavy transport vehicle or bus	
No Change	**Excludes1:**	
Revise from		motorcycle rider injured in collision with military vehicle (V29.81)
Revise to		motorcycle rider injured in collision with military vehicle (V29.818)
No Change	**V24.0**	Motorcycle driver injured in collision with heavy transport vehicle or bus in nontraffic accident
Add	**V24.01**	Electric (assisted) bicycle driver injured in collision with heavy transport vehicle or bus in nontraffic accident
Add	**V24.09**	Other motorcycle driver injured in collision with heavy transport vehicle or bus in nontraffic accident
No Change	**V24.1**	Motorcycle passenger injured in collision with heavy transport vehicle or bus in nontraffic accident
Add	**V24.11**	Electric (assisted) bicycle passenger injured in collision with heavy transport vehicle or bus in nontraffic accident
Add	**V24.19**	Other motorcycle passenger injured in collision with heavy transport vehicle or bus in nontraffic accident
No Change	**V24.2**	Unspecified motorcycle rider injured in collision with heavy transport vehicle or bus in nontraffic accident
Add	**V24.21**	Unspecified electric (assisted) bicycle rider injured in collision with heavy transport vehicle or bus in nontraffic accident
Add	**V24.29**	Unspecified rider of other motorcycle injured in collision with heavy transport vehicle or bus in nontraffic accident
No Change	**V24.3**	Person boarding or alighting a motorcycle injured in collision with heavy transport vehicle or bus
Add	**V24.31**	Person boarding or alighting an electric (assisted) bicycle injured in collision with heavy transport vehicle or bus
Add	**V24.39**	Person boarding or alighting other motorcycle injured in collision with heavy transport vehicle or bus
No Change	**V24.4**	Motorcycle driver injured in collision with heavy transport vehicle or bus in traffic accident
Add	**V24.41**	Electric (assisted) bicycle driver injured in collision with heavy transport vehicle or bus in traffic accident
Add	**V24.49**	Other motorcycle driver injured in collision with heavy transport vehicle or bus in traffic accident
No Change	**V24.5**	Motorcycle passenger injured in collision with heavy transport vehicle or bus in traffic accident
Add	**V24.51**	Electric (assisted) bicycle passenger injured in collision with heavy transport vehicle or bus in traffic accident
Add	**V24.59**	Other motorcycle passenger injured in collision with heavy transport vehicle or bus in traffic accident
No Change	**V24.9**	Unspecified motorcycle rider injured in collision with heavy transport vehicle or bus in traffic accident
Add	**V24.91**	Unspecified electric (assisted) bicycle rider injured in collision with heavy transport vehicle or bus in traffic accident
Add	**V24.99**	Unspecified rider of other motorcycle injured in collision with heavy transport vehicle or bus in traffic accident

No Change **V25**	Motorcycle rider injured in collision with railway train or railway vehicle	
No Change	**V25.0**	Motorcycle driver injured in collision with railway train or railway vehicle in nontraffic accident
Add	**V25.01**	Electric (assisted) bicycle driver injured in collision with railway train or railway vehicle in nontraffic accident
Add	**V25.09**	Other motorcycle driver injured in collision with railway train or railway vehicle in nontraffic accident
No Change	**V25.1**	Motorcycle passenger injured in collision with railway train or railway vehicle in nontraffic accident
Add	**V25.11**	Electric (assisted) bicycle passenger injured in collision with railway train or railway vehicle in nontraffic accident
Add	**V25.19**	Other motorcycle passenger injured in collision with railway train or railway vehicle in nontraffic accident
No Change	**V25.2**	Unspecified motorcycle rider injured in collision with railway train or railway vehicle in nontraffic accident
Add	**V25.21**	Unspecified electric (assisted) bicycle rider injured in collision with railway train or railway vehicle in nontraffic accident
Add	**V25.29**	Unspecified rider of other motorcycle injured in collision with railway train or railway vehicle in nontraffic accident
No Change	**V25.3**	Person boarding or alighting a motorcycle injured in collision with railway train or railway vehicle
Add	**V25.31**	Person boarding or alighting an electric (assisted) bicycle injured in collision with railway train or railway vehicle
Add	**V25.39**	Person boarding or alighting other motorcycle injured in collision with railway train or railway vehicle
No Change	**V25.4**	Motorcycle driver injured in collision with railway train or railway vehicle in traffic accident
Add	**V25.41**	Electric (assisted) bicycle driver injured in collision with railway train or railway vehicle in traffic accident
Add	**V25.49**	Other motorcycle driver injured in collision with railway train or railway vehicle in traffic accident
No Change	**V25.5**	Motorcycle passenger injured in collision with railway train or railway vehicle in traffic accident
Add	**V25.51**	Electric (assisted) bicycle passenger injured in collision with railway train or railway vehicle in traffic accident
Add	**V25.59**	Other motorcycle passenger injured in collision with railway train or railway vehicle in traffic accident
No Change	**V25.9**	Unspecified motorcycle rider injured in collision with railway train or railway vehicle in traffic accident
Add	**V25.91**	Unspecified electric (assisted) bicycle rider injured in collision with railway train or railway vehicle in traffic accident
Add	**V25.99**	Unspecified rider of other motorcycle injured in collision with railway train or railway vehicle in traffic accident

No Change **V26**	Motorcycle rider injured in collision with other nonmotor vehicle	
No Change	**V26.0**	Motorcycle driver injured in collision with other nonmotor vehicle in nontraffic accident
Add	**V26.01**	Electric (assisted) bicycle driver injured in collision with other nonmotor vehicle in nontraffic accident
Add	**V26.09**	Other motorcycle driver injured in collision with other nonmotor vehicle in nontraffic accident

No Change	V26.1		Motorcycle passenger injured in collision with other nonmotor vehicle in nontraffic accident
Add		V26.11	Electric (assisted) bicycle passenger injured in collision with other nonmotor vehicle in nontraffic accident
Add		V26.19	Other motorcycle passenger injured in collision with other nonmotor vehicle in nontraffic accident
No Change	V26.2		Unspecified motorcycle rider injured in collision with other nonmotor vehicle in nontraffic accident
Add		V26.21	Unspecified electric (assisted) bicycle rider injured in collision with other nonmotor vehicle in nontraffic accident
Add		V26.29	Unspecified rider of other motorcycle injured in collision with other nonmotor vehicle in nontraffic accident
No Change	V26.3		Person boarding or alighting a motorcycle injured in collision with other nonmotor vehicle
Add		V26.31	Person boarding or alighting an electric (assisted) bicycle injured in collision with other nonmotor vehicle
Add		V26.39	Person boarding or alighting other motorcycle injured in collision with other nonmotor vehicle
No Change	V26.4		Motorcycle driver injured in collision with other nonmotor vehicle in traffic accident
Add		V26.41	Electric (assisted) bicycle driver injured in collision with other nonmotor vehicle in traffic accident
Add		V26.49	Other motorcycle driver injured in collision with other nonmotor vehicle in traffic accident
No Change	V26.5		Motorcycle passenger injured in collision with other nonmotor vehicle in traffic accident
Add		V26.51	Electric (assisted) bicycle passenger injured in collision with other nonmotor vehicle in traffic accident
Add		V26.59	Other motorcycle passenger injured in collision with other nonmotor vehicle in traffic accident
No Change	V26.9		Unspecified motorcycle rider injured in collision with other nonmotor vehicle in traffic accident
Add		V26.91	Unspecified electric (assisted) bicycle rider injured in collision with other nonmotor vehicle in traffic accident
Add		V26.99	Unspecified rider of other motorcycle injured in collision with other nonmotor vehicle in traffic accident
No Change	**V27**		Motorcycle rider injured in collision with fixed or stationary object
No Change	V27.0		Motorcycle driver injured in collision with fixed or stationary object in nontraffic accident
Add		V27.01	Electric (assisted) bicycle driver injured in collision with fixed or stationary object in nontraffic accident
Add		V27.09	Other motorcycle driver injured in collision with fixed or stationary object in nontraffic accident
No Change	V27.1		Motorcycle passenger injured in collision with fixed or stationary object in nontraffic accident
Add		V27.11	Electric (assisted) bicycle passenger injured in collision with fixed or stationary object in nontraffic accident
Add		V27.19	Other motorcycle passenger injured in collision with fixed or stationary object in nontraffic accident

No Change	V27.2		Unspecified motorcycle rider injured in collision with fixed or stationary object in nontraffic accident
Add		V27.21	Unspecified electric (assisted) bicycle rider injured in collision with fixed or stationary object in nontraffic accident
Add		V27.29	Unspecified rider of other motorcycle injured in collision with fixed or stationary object in nontraffic accident
No Change	V27.3		Person boarding or alighting a motorcycle injured in collision with fixed or stationary object
Add		V27.31	Person boarding or alighting an electric (assisted) bicycle injured in collision with fixed or stationary object
Add		V27.39	Person boarding or alighting other motorcycle injured in collision with fixed or stationary object
No Change	V27.4		Motorcycle driver injured in collision with fixed or stationary object in traffic accident
Add		V27.41	Electric (assisted) bicycle driver injured in collision with fixed or stationary object in traffic accident
Add		V27.49	Other motorcycle driver injured in collision with fixed or stationary object in traffic accident
No Change	V27.5		Motorcycle passenger injured in collision with fixed or stationary object in traffic accident
Add		V27.51	Electric (assisted) bicycle passenger injured in collision with fixed or stationary object in traffic accident
Add		V27.59	Other motorcycle passenger injured in collision with fixed or stationary object in traffic accident
No Change	V27.9		Unspecified motorcycle rider injured in collision with fixed or stationary object in traffic accident
Add		V27.91	Unspecified electric (assisted) bicycle rider injured in collision with fixed or stationary object in traffic accident
Add		V27.99	Unspecified rider of other motorcycle injured in collision with fixed or stationary object in traffic accident
No Change	**V28**		Motorcycle rider injured in noncollision transport accident
No Change	V28.0		Motorcycle driver injured in noncollision transport accident in nontraffic accident
Add		V28.01	Electric (assisted) bicycle driver injured in noncollision transport accident in nontraffic accident
Add		V28.09	Other motorcycle driver injured in noncollision transport accident in nontraffic accident
No Change	V28.1		Motorcycle passenger injured in noncollision transport accident in nontraffic accident
Add		V28.11	Electric (assisted) bicycle passenger injured in noncollision transport accident in nontraffic accident
Add		V28.19	Other motorcycle passenger injured in noncollision transport accident in nontraffic accident
No Change	V28.2		Unspecified motorcycle rider injured in noncollision transport accident in nontraffic accident
Add		V28.21	Unspecified electric (assisted) bicycle rider injured in noncollision transport accident in nontraffic accident
Add		V28.29	Unspecified rider of other motorcycle injured in noncollision transport accident in nontraffic accident

No Change	V28.3	Person boarding or alighting a motorcycle injured in noncollision transport accident
Add	V28.31	Person boarding or alighting an electric (assisted) bicycle injured in noncollision transport accident
Add	V28.39	Person boarding or alighting other motorcycle injured in noncollision transport accident
No Change	V28.4	Motorcycle driver injured in noncollision transport accident in traffic accident
Add	V28.41	Electric (assisted) bicycle driver injured in noncollision transport accident in traffic accident
Add	V28.49	Other motorcycle driver injured in noncollision transport accident in traffic accident
No Change	V28.5	Motorcycle passenger injured in noncollision transport accident in traffic accident
Add	V28.51	Electric (assisted) bicycle passenger injured in noncollision transport accident in traffic accident
Add	V28.59	Other motorcycle passenger injured in noncollision transport accident in traffic accident
No Change	V28.9	Unspecified motorcycle rider injured in noncollision transport accident in traffic accident
Add	V28.91	Unspecified electric (assisted) bicycle rider injured in noncollision transport accident in traffic accident
Add	V28.99	Unspecified rider of other motorcycle injured in noncollision transport accident in traffic accident

No Change V29	Motorcycle rider injured in other and unspecified transport accidents	
No Change	V29.0	Motorcycle driver injured in collision with other and unspecified motor vehicles in nontraffic accident
No Change	V29.00	Motorcycle driver injured in collision with unspecified motor vehicles in nontraffic accident
Add	V29.001	Electric (assisted) bicycle driver injured in collision with unspecified motor vehicles in nontraffic accident
Add	V29.008	Other motorcycle driver injured in collision with unspecified motor vehicles in nontraffic accident
No Change	V29.09	Motorcycle driver injured in collision with other motor vehicles in nontraffic accident
Add	V29.091	Electric (assisted) bicycle driver injured in collision with other motor vehicles in nontraffic accident
Add	V29.098	Other motorcycle driver injured in collision with other motor vehicles in nontraffic accident
No Change	V29.1	Motorcycle passenger injured in collision with other and unspecified motor vehicles in nontraffic accident
No Change	V29.10	Motorcycle passenger injured in collision with unspecified motor vehicles in nontraffic accident
Add	V29.101	Electric (assisted) bicycle passenger injured in collision with unspecified motor vehicles in nontraffic accident
Add	V29.108	Other motorcycle passenger injured in collision with unspecified motor vehicles in nontraffic accident

No Change	V29.19	Motorcycle passenger injured in collision with other motor vehicles in nontraffic accident
Add	V29.191	Electric (assisted) bicycle passenger injured in collision with other motor vehicles in nontraffic accident
Add	V29.198	Other motorcycle passenger injured in collision with other motor vehicles in nontraffic accident
No Change	V29.2	Unspecified motorcycle rider injured in collision with other and unspecified motor vehicles in nontraffic accident
No Change	V29.20	Unspecified motorcycle rider injured in collision with unspecified motor vehicles in nontraffic accident
Delete		Motorcycle collision NOS, nontraffic
Add	V29.201	Unspecified electric (assisted) bicycle rider injured in collision with unspecified motor vehicles in nontraffic accident
Add	V29.208	Unspecified rider of other motorcycle injured in collision with unspecified motor vehicles in nontraffic accident
Add		Motorcycle collision NOS, nontraffic
No Change	V29.29	Unspecified motorcycle rider injured in collision with other motor vehicles in nontraffic accident
Add	V29.291	Unspecified electric (assisted) bicycle rider injured in collision with other motor vehicles in nontraffic accident
Add	V29.298	Unspecified rider of other motorcycle injured in collision with other motor vehicles in nontraffic accident
No Change	V29.3	Motorcycle rider (driver) (passenger) injured in unspecified nontraffic accident
Delete		Motorcycle accident NOS, nontraffic
Delete		Motorcycle rider injured in nontraffic accident NOS
Add	V29.31	Electric (assisted) bicycle (driver) (passenger) injured in unspecified nontraffic accident
Add	V29.39	Other motorcycle (driver) (passenger) injured in unspecified nontraffic accident
Add		Motorcycle accident NOS, nontraffic
Add		Motorcycle rider injured in nontraffic accident NOS
No Change	V29.4	Motorcycle driver injured in collision with other and unspecified motor vehicles in traffic accident
No Change	V29.40	Motorcycle driver injured in collision with unspecified motor vehicles in traffic accident
Add	V29.401	Electric (assisted) bicycle driver injured in collision with unspecified motor vehicles in traffic accident
Add	V29.408	Other motorcycle driver injured in collision with unspecified motor vehicles in traffic accident

No Change   **V29.49**   Motorcycle driver injured in collision with other motor vehicles in traffic accident

Add   **V29.491**   Electric (assisted) bicycle driver injured in collision with other motor vehicles in traffic accident

Add   **V29.498**   Other motorcycle driver injured in collision with other motor vehicles in traffic accident

No Change   **V29.5**   Motorcycle passenger injured in collision with other and unspecified motor vehicles in traffic accident

No Change   **V29.50**   Motorcycle passenger injured in collision with unspecified motor vehicles in traffic accident

Add   **V29.501**   Electric (assisted) bicycle passenger injured in collision with unspecified motor vehicles in traffic accident

Add   **V29.508**   Other motorcycle passenger injured in collision with unspecified motor vehicles in traffic accident

No Change   **V29.59**   Motorcycle passenger injured in collision with other motor vehicles in traffic accident

Add   **V29.591**   Electric (assisted) bicycle passenger injured in collision with other motor vehicles in traffic accident

Add   **V29.598**   Other motorcycle passenger injured in collision with other motor vehicles in traffic accident

No Change   **V29.6**   Unspecified motorcycle rider injured in collision with other and unspecified motor vehicles in traffic accident

No Change   **V29.60**   Unspecified motorcycle rider injured in collision with unspecified motor vehicles in traffic accident

Delete   Motorcycle collision NOS (traffic)

Add   **V29.601**   Unspecified electric (assisted) bicycle rider injured in collision with unspecified motor vehicles in traffic accident

Add   **V29.608**   Unspecified rider of other motorcycle injured in collision with unspecified motor vehicles in traffic accident

   Motorcycle collision NOS (traffic)

No Change   **V29.69**   Unspecified motorcycle rider injured in collision with other motor vehicles in traffic accident

Add   **V29.691**   Unspecified electric (assisted) bicycle rider injured in collision with other motor vehicles in traffic accident

Add   **V29.698**   Unspecified rider of other motorcycle injured in collision with other motor vehicles in traffic accident

No Change   **V29.8**   Motorcycle rider (driver) (passenger) injured in other specified transport accidents

No Change   **V29.81**   Motorcycle rider (driver) (passenger) injured in transport accident with military vehicle

Add   **V29.811**   Electric (assisted) bicycle rider (driver) (passenger) injured in transport accident with military vehicle

Add   **V29.818**   Rider (driver) (passenger) of other motorcycle injured in transport accident with military vehicle

No Change   **V29.88**   Motorcycle rider (driver) (passenger) injured in other specified transport accidents

Add   **V29.881**   Electric (assisted) bicycle rider (driver) (passenger) injured in other specified transport accidents

Add   **V29.888**   Rider (driver) (passenger) of other motorcycle injured in other specified transport accidents

No Change   **V29.9**   Motorcycle rider (driver) (passenger) injured in unspecified traffic accident

Delete   Motorcycle accident NOS

Add   **V29.91**   Electric (assisted) bicycle rider (driver) (passenger) injured in unspecified traffic accident

Add   **V29.99**   Rider (driver) (passenger) of other motorcycle injured in unspecified traffic accident

Add   Motorcycle accident NOS

No Change   **SLIPPING, TRIPPING, STUMBLING AND FALLS (W00-W19)**

No Change **W08**   Fall from other furniture
Add   Fall from stool

No Change   **EXPOSURE TO INANIMATE MECHANICAL FORCES (W20-W49)**

No Change **W23**   Caught, crushed, jammed or pinched in or between objects

Add   **W23.2**   Caught, crushed, jammed or pinched between a moving and stationary object

---

No Change   **CONTACT WITH HEAT AND HOT SUBSTANCES (X10-X19)**

No Change **X15**   Contact with hot household appliances
No Change   **X15.3**   Contact with hot saucepan or skillet
Add   Contact with hot cooking pan
Add   Contact with hot cooking pot

No Change   **LEGAL INTERVENTION, OPERATIONS OF WAR, MILITARY OPERATIONS, AND TERRORISM (Y35-Y38)**

No Change **Y36**   Operations of war
No Change   **Excludes1**
Revise from   military vehicles involved in transport accidents with non-military vehicle during peacetime (V09.01, V09.21, V19.81, V29.81, V39.81, V49.81, V59.81, V69.81, V79.81)
Revise to   military vehicles involved in transport accidents with non-military vehicle during peacetime (V09.01, V09.21, V19.81, V29.818, V39.81, V49.81, V59.81, V69.81, V79.81)

No Change **Y37**   Military operations
No Change   **Excludes1**
Revise from   military vehicles involved in transport accident with civilian vehicle (V09.01, V09.21, V19.81, V29.81, V39.81, V49.81, V59.81, V69.81, V79.81)
Revise to   military vehicles involved in transport accident with civilian vehicle (V09.01, V09.21, V19.81, V29.818, V39.81, V49.81, V59.81, V69.81, V79.81)

No Change **CHAPTER 21**

No Change **FACTORS INFLUENCING HEALTH STATUS AND CONTACT WITH HEALTH SERVICES (Z00-Z99)**

No Change **PERSONS ENCOUNTERING HEALTH SERVICES FOR EXAMINATIONS (Z00-Z13)**

No Change **Z03** Encounter for medical observation for suspected diseases and conditions ruled out

No Change **Z03.8** Encounter for observation for other suspected diseases and conditions ruled out

Add **Z03.83** Encounter for observation for suspected conditions related to home physiologic monitoring device ruled out

Add Encounter for observation for apnea alarm without findings

Add Encounter for observation for bradycardia alarm without findings

Add Encounter for observation for malfunction of home cardiorespiratory monitor

Add Encounter for observation for non-specific findings home physiologic monitoring device

Add Encounter for observation for pulse oximeter alarm without findings

Add **Excludes1** apnea NOS (R06.81)
Add neonatal bradycardia (P29.12)
Add newborn apnea (P28.4-)
Add primary sleep apnea of newborn (P28.3-)
Add sleep apnea (G47.3-)

No Change **PERSONS WITH POTENTIAL HEALTH HAZARDS RELATED TO SOCIOECONOMIC AND PSYCHOSOCIAL CIRCUMSTANCES (Z55-Z65)**

No Change **Z59** Problems related to housing and economic circumstances

No Change **Z59.8** Other problems related to housing and economic circumstances

Add **Z59.82** **Transportation insecurity**
Add Excessive transportation time
Add Inaccessible transportation
Add Inadequate transportation
Add Lack of transportation
Add Unaffordable transportation
Add Unreliable transportation
Add Unsafe transportation

Add **Z59.86** **Financial insecurity**
Add Bankruptcy
Add Burdensome debt
Add Economic strain
Add Financial strain
Add Money problems
Add Running out of money
Add Unable to make ends meet
Add **Excludes2** extreme poverty (Z59.5)
Add low income (Z59.6)
Add material hardship, not elsewhere classified (Z59.87)

Add **Z59.87** **Material hardship**
Add Material deprivation
Add Unable to obtain adequate childcare
Add Unable to obtain adequate clothing
Add Unable to obtain adequate utilities
Add Unable to obtain basic needs
Add **Excludes2** extreme poverty (Z59.5)
Add financial insecurity, not elsewhere classified (Z59.86)
Add low income (Z59.6)

No Change **PERSONS ENCOUNTERING HEALTH SERVICES IN OTHER CIRCUMSTANCES (Z69-Z76)**

No Change **Z71** Persons encountering health services for other counseling and medical advice, not elsewhere classified

No Change **Z71.8** Other specified counseling

Add **Z71.87** Encounter for pediatric-to-adult transition counseling
Add Code also chronic condition, if applicable, such as:
Add autism spectrum disorder (F84.0)
Add congenital malformations of the circulatory system (Q20-Q28)
Add cystic fibrosis (E84-)
Add sickle-cell disorder (D57-)

Add **Z71.88** Encounter for counseling for socioeconomic factors

No Change **Z72** Problems related to lifestyle
No Change **Z72.8** Other problems related to lifestyle
No Change **Z72.82** Problems related to sleep
Add **Z72.823** **Risk of suffocation (smothering) under another while sleeping**
Add Child-caregiver co-sleeping
Add Infant bed-sharing

No Change **PERSONS WITH POTENTIAL HEALTH HAZARDS RELATED TO FAMILY AND PERSONAL HISTORY AND CERTAIN CONDITIONS INFLUENCING HEALTH STATUS (Z77-Z99)**

No Change **Z79** Long term (current) drug therapy
No Change **Z79.4** Long term (current) use of insulin
Add **Excludes2** long-term (current) use of injectable non-insulin antidiabetic drugs (Z79.85)

Add **Z79.6** Long term (current) use of immunomodulators and immunosuppressants
Add **Excludes2** long term (current) use of steroids (Z79.5-)
Add long term (current) use of agents affecting estrogen receptors and estrogen levels (Z79.81-)

Add **Z79.60** **Long term (current) use of unspecified immunomodulators and immunosuppressants**

Add **Z79.61** **Long term (current) use of immunomodulator**
Add Long term (current) use of apremilast
Add Long term (current) use of immunomodulatory imide drug
Add Long term (current) use of lenalidomide
Add Long term (current) use of pomalidomide

Add **Z79.62** **Long term (current) use of immunosuppressant**
Add **Z79.620** Long term (current) use of immunosuppressive biologic
Add Long term (current) use of adalimumab
Add Long term (current) use of etanercept
Add Long term (current) use of infliximab
Add Long term (current) use of monoclonal antibodies

Add **Z79.621** **Long term (current) use of calcineurin inhibitor**
Add Long term (current) use of cyclosporine
Add Long term (current) use of tacrolimus

Add	Z79.622	Long term (current) use of Janus kinase inhibitor
Add		Long term (current) use of tofacitinib
Add	Z79.623	Long term (current) use of mammalian target of rapamycin (mTOR) inhibitor
Add		Long term (current) use of sirolimus
Add	Z79.624	Long term (current) use of inhibitors of nucleotide synthesis
Add		Long term (current) use of azathioprine
Add		Long term (current) use omycophenolate
Add		Long term (current) use of purine synthesis (IMDH) inhibitors
Add	Z79.63	Long term (current) use of chemotherapeutic agent
Add	Z79.630	Long term (current) use of alkylating agent
Add		Long term (current) use of chlorambucil
Add		Long term (current) use of cisplatin
Add		Long term (current) use of cyclophosphamide
Add	Z79.631	Long term (current) use of antimetabolite agent
Add		Long term (current) use of 5-fluorouracil
Add		Long term (current) use of 6-mercaptopurine
Add		Long term (current) use of cytarabine
Add		Long term (current) use of methotrexate
Add	Z79.632	Long term (current) use of antitumor antibiotic
Add		Long term (current) use of bleomycin
Add		Long term (current) use of doxorubicin
Add		Long term (current) use of mitomycin C
Add	Z79.633	Long term (current) use of mitotic inhibitor
Add		Long term (current) use of paclitaxel
Add		Long term (current) use of plant alkaloids
Add		Long term (current) use of vinblastine
Add		Long term (current) use of vincristine
Add	Z79.634	Long term (current) use of topoisomerase inhibitor
Add		Long term (current) use of etoposide
Add		Long term (current) use of irinotecan
Add		Long term (current) use of topotecan
Add	Z79.64	Long term (current) use of myelosuppressive agent
Add		Long term (current) use of hydroxyurea
Add	Z79.69	Long term (current) use of other immunomodulators and immunosuppressants

No Change	Z79.8	Other long term (current) drug therapy
No Change	Z79.84	Long term (current) use of oral hypoglycemic drugs
Add		**Excludes2** long-term (current) use of injectable non-insulin antidiabetic drugs (Z79.85)
Add	Z79.85	Long-term (current) use of injectable non-insulin antidiabetic drugs
Add		**Excludes2** long term (current) use of insulin (Z79.4)
Add		long term (current) use of oral hypoglycemic drugs (Z79.84)
No Change Z87		Personal history of other diseases and conditions
Add	Z87.6	Personal history of certain (corrected) conditions arising in the perinatal period
		Conditions classifiable to P00-P96
Add		**Excludes1** personal history of (corrected) congenital malformations (Z87.7-)
Add	Z87.61	Personal history of (corrected) necrotizing enterocolitis of newborn
Add	Z87.68	Personal history of other (corrected) conditions arising in the perinatal period
No Change	Z87.7	Personal history of (corrected) congenital malformations
No Change	Z87.73	Personal history of (corrected) congenital malformations of digestive system
Add	Z87.731	Personal history of (corrected) tracheoesophageal fistula or atresia
Add	Z87.732	Personal history of (corrected) persistent cloaca or cloacal malformations
No Change	Z87.76	Personal history of (corrected) congenital malformations of integument, limbs and musculoskeletal system
Add	Z87.760	Personal history of (corrected) congenital diaphragmatic hernia or other congenital diaphragm malformations
Add	Z87.761	Personal history of (corrected) gastroschisis
Add	Z87.762	Personal history of (corrected) prune belly malformation
Add	Z87.763	Personal history of other (corrected) congenital abdominal wall malformations
Add	Z87.768	Personal history of other specified (corrected) congenital malformations of integument, limbs and musculoskeletal system
No Change Z91		Personal risk factors, not elsewhere classified
No Change		**Excludes2**
No Change	Z91.1	Patient's noncompliance with medical treatment and regimen
Add		**Excludes 2** caregiver noncompliance with patient's medical treatment and regimen (Z91.A-)
No Change	Z91.11	Patient's noncompliance with dietary regimen
Add		Code also, if applicable, food insecurity (Z59.4-)
Add	Z91.110	Patient's noncompliance with dietary regimen due to financial hardship

Add		Z91.118	Patient's noncompliance with dietary regimen for other reason
Add			Inability to comply with dietary regimen
Add		Z91.119	Patient's noncompliance with dietary regimen due to unspecified reason
No Change	Z91.19		Patient's noncompliance with other medical treatment and regimen
Revise from			Nonadherence to medical treatment
Revise to			Patient's nonadherence to medical treatment
Add		Z91.190	Patient's noncompliance with other medical treatment and regimen due to financial hardship
Add		Z91.198	Patient's noncompliance with other medical treatment and regimen for other reason
Add		Z91.199	Patient's noncompliance with other medical treatment and regimen due to unspecified reason
Add	Z91.A		Caregiver's noncompliance with patient's medical treatment and regimen
Add	Z91.A1		Caregiver's noncompliance with patient's dietary regimen
Add			Caregiver's inability to comply with patient's dietary regimen
Add			Code also, if applicable, food insecurity (Z59.4-)
Add		Z91.A10	Caregiver's noncompliance with patient's dietary regimen due to financial hardship
Add		Z91.A18	Caregiver's noncompliance with patient's dietary regimen for other reason

Add		Z91.A2	Caregiver's intentional underdosing of patient's medication regimen
Add			Code first underdosing of medication (T36-T50) with fifth or sixth character 6
Add		Z91.A20	Caregiver's intentional underdosing of patient's medication regimen due to financial hardship
Add		Z91.A28	Caregiver's intentional underdosing of medication regimen for other reason
Add		Z91.A3	Caregiver's unintentional underdosing of patient's medication regimen
Add			Code first underdosing of medication (T36-T50) with fifth or sixth character 6
Add		Z91.A4	Caregiver's other noncompliance with patient's medication regimen
Add			Caregiver's underdosing of patient's medication NOS
Add		Z91.A5	Caregiver's noncompliance with patient's renal dialysis
Add		Z91.A9	Caregiver's noncompliance with patient's other medical treatment and regimen
Add			Caregiver's nonadherence to patient's medical treatment
No Change	Z91.8		Other specified personal risk factors, not elsewhere classified
No Change		Z91.83	Wandering in diseases classified elsewhere
No Change			Code first
Revise from			unspecified dementia with behavioral disturbance (F03.9-)
Revise to			unspecified dementia with behavioral disturbance (F03.9-, F03.A-, F03.B-, F03.C-)

PART I

Introduction

ICD-10-CM Official Guidelines for Coding and Reporting FY2023
(October 1, 2022 - September 30, 2023)
Narrative changes appear in **bold** text
Items <u>underlined</u> have been moved within the guidelines since the 2022 version
Italics are used to indicate revisions to heading changes

The Centers for Medicare and Medicaid Services (CMS) and the National Center for Health Statistics (NCHS), two departments within the U.S. Federal Government's Department of Health and Human Services (DHHS), provide the following guidelines for coding and reporting using the International Classification of Diseases, 10th Revision, Clinical Modification (ICD-10-CM). These guidelines should be used as a companion document to the official version of the ICD-10-CM as published on the NCHS website. The ICD-10-CM is a morbidity classification published by the United States for classifying diagnoses and reason for visits in all health care settings. The ICD-10-CM is based on the ICD-10, the statistical classification of disease published by the World Health Organization (WHO).

These guidelines have been approved by the four organizations that make up the Cooperating Parties for the ICD-10-CM: the American Hospital Association (AHA), the American Health Information Management Association (AHIMA), CMS, and NCHS.

These guidelines are a set of rules that have been developed to accompany and complement the official conventions and instructions provided within the ICD-10-CM itself. The instructions and conventions of the classification take precedence over guidelines. These guidelines are based on the coding and sequencing instructions in the Tabular List and Alphabetic Index of ICD-10-CM, but provide additional instruction. Adherence to these guidelines when assigning ICD-10-CM diagnosis codes is required under the Health Insurance Portability and Accountability Act (HIPAA). The diagnosis codes (Tabular List and Alphabetic Index) have been adopted under HIPAA for all health care settings. A joint effort between the health care provider and the coder is essential to achieve complete and accurate documentation, code assignment, and reporting of diagnoses and procedures. These guidelines have been developed to assist both the health care provider and the coder in identifying those diagnoses that are to be reported. The importance of consistent, complete documentation in the medical record cannot be overemphasized. Without such documentation accurate coding cannot be achieved. The entire record should be reviewed to determine the specific reason for the encounter and the conditions treated.

The term "encounter" is used for all settings, including hospital admissions. In the context of these guidelines, the term "provider" is used throughout the guidelines to mean physician or any qualified health care practitioner who is legally accountable for establishing the patient's diagnosis. Only this set of guidelines, approved by the Cooperating Parties, is official.

The guidelines are organized into sections. Section I includes the structure and conventions of the classification and general guidelines that apply to the entire classification, and chapter-specific guidelines that correspond to the chapters as they are arranged in the classification. Section II includes guidelines for selection of principal diagnosis for non-outpatient settings. Section III includes guidelines for reporting additional diagnoses in non-outpatient settings. Section IV is for outpatient coding and reporting. It is necessary to review all sections of the guidelines to fully understand all of the rules and instructions needed to code properly.

ICD-10-CM Official Guidelines for Coding and Reporting

Section I. Conventions, General Coding Guidelines and Chapter Specific Guidelines

A. Conventions for the ICD-10-CM
1. The Alphabetic Index and Tabular List
2. Format and Structure:
3. Use of codes for reporting purposes
4. Placeholder character
5. 7th Characters
6. Abbreviations
   a. Alphabetic Index abbreviations
   b. Tabular List abbreviations
7. Punctuation
8. Use of "and"
9. Other and Unspecified codes
   a. "Other" codes
   b. "Unspecified" codes
10. Includes Notes
11. Inclusion terms
12. Excludes Notes
    a. Excludes1
    b. Excludes2
13. Etiology/manifestation convention ("code first", "use additional code" and "in diseases classified elsewhere" notes)
14. "And"
15. "With"
16. "See" and "See Also"
17. "Code also note"
18. Default codes
19. Code assignment and Clinical Criteria

B. General Coding Guidelines
1. Locating a code in the ICD-10-CM
2. Level of Detail in Coding
3. Code or codes from A00.0 through T88.9, Z00-Z99.8, U00-U85
4. Signs and symptoms
5. Conditions that are an integral part of a disease process
6. Conditions that are not an integral part of a disease process
7. Multiple coding for a single condition
8. Acute and Chronic Conditions
9. Combination Code
10. Sequela (Late Effects)
11. Impending or Threatened Condition
12. Reporting Same Diagnosis Code More than Once
13. Laterality
14. Documentation by Clinicians Other than the Patient's Provider
15. Syndromes
16. Documentation of Complications of Care
17. Borderline Diagnosis
18. Use of Sign/Symptom/Unspecified Codes
19. Coding for Healthcare Encounters in Hurricane Aftermath
    a. Use of External Cause of Morbidity Codes
    b. Sequencing of External Causes of Morbidity Codes
    c. Other External Causes of Morbidity Code Issues
    d. Use of Z codes

C. Chapter-Specific Coding Guidelines
1. Chapter 1: Certain Infectious and Parasitic Diseases (A00-B99, U07.1, U09.9)
   a. Human Immunodeficiency Virus (HIV) Infections
   b. Infectious agents as the cause of diseases classified to other chapters
   c. Infections resistant to antibiotics
   d. Sepsis, Severe Sepsis, and Septic Shock infection resistant to antibiotics
   e. Methicillin Resistant Staphylococcus aureus (MRSA) Conditions
   f. Zika virus infection
   g. Coronavirus infections
2. Chapter 2: Neoplasms (C00-D49)
   a. *Admission/Encounter for treatment of primary site*
   b. *Admission/Encounter for treatment of secondary site*
   c. Coding and sequencing of complications
   d. Primary malignancy previously excised
   e. Admissions/Encounters involving chemotherapy, immunotherapy and radiation therapy
   f. Admission/encounter to determine extent of malignancy
   g. Symptoms, signs, and abnormal findings listed in Chapter 18 associated with neoplasms
   h. Admission/encounter for pain control/management
   i. Malignancy in two or more noncontiguous sites
   j. Disseminated malignant neoplasm, unspecified
   k. Malignant neoplasm without specification of site
   l. Sequencing of neoplasm codes
   m. Current malignancy versus personal history of malignancy
   n. Leukemia, Multiple Myeloma, and Malignant Plasma Cell Neoplasms in remission versus personal history
   o. Aftercare following surgery for neoplasm
   p. Follow-up care for completed treatment of a malignancy
   q. Prophylactic organ removal for prevention of malignancy
   r. Malignant neoplasm associated with transplanted organ
   s. Breast Implant Associated Anaplastic Large Cell Lymphoma
   t. **Secondary malignant neoplasm of lymphoid tissue**
3. Chapter 3: Disease of the Blood and Blood-Forming Organs and Certain Disorders Involving the Immune Mechanism (D50-D89)
4. Chapter 4: Endocrine, Nutritional, and Metabolic Diseases (E00-E89)
   a. Diabetes mellitus
5. Chapter 5: Mental, Behavioral, and Neurodevelopmental disorders (F01 – F99)
   a. Pain disorders related to psychological factors
   b. Mental and behavioral disorders due to psychoactive substance use
   c. Factitious Disorder
6. Chapter 6: Diseases of the Nervous System (G00-G99)
   a. Dominant/nondominant side
   b. Pain - Category G89

GUIDELINES (ICD-10-CM)

Section I. Conventions, General Coding Guidelines, and Chapter Specific Guidelines

The conventions, general guidelines, and chapter-specific guidelines are applicable to all health care settings unless otherwise indicated. The conventions and instructions of the classification take precedence over guidelines.

A. Conventions for the ICD-10-CM

The conventions for the ICD-10-CM are the general rules for use of the classification independent of the guidelines. These conventions are incorporated within the Alphabetic Index and Tabular List of the ICD-10-CM as instructional notes.

  1. The Alphabetic Index and Tabular List

The ICD-10-CM is divided into the Alphabetic Index, an alphabetical list of terms and their corresponding code, and the Tabular List, a structured list of codes divided into chapters based on body system or condition. The Alphabetic Index consists of the following parts: the Index of Diseases and Injury, the Index of External Causes of Injury, the Table of Neoplasms, and the Table of Drugs and Chemicals.

See Section I.C.2. **Neoplasms**
See Section I.C.19. Adverse effects, poisoning, underdosing and toxic effects

  2. Format and Structure:

The ICD-10-CM Tabular List contains categories, subcategories and codes. Characters for categories, subcategories and codes may be either a letter or a number. All categories are 3 characters. A 3-character category that has no further subdivision is equivalent to a code. Subcategories are either 4 or 5 characters. Codes may be 3, 4, 5, 6 or 7 characters. That is, each level of subdivision after a category is a subcategory. The final level of subdivision is a code. Codes that have applicable 7th characters are still referred to as codes, not subcategories. A code that has an applicable 7th character is considered invalid without the 7th character.

The ICD-10-CM uses an indented format for ease in reference

  3. Use of codes for reporting purposes

For reporting purposes only codes are permissible, not categories or subcategories, and any applicable 7th character is required.

  4. Placeholder character

The ICD-10-CM utilizes a placeholder character "X". The "X" is used as a placeholder at certain codes to allow for future expansion. An example of this is at the poisoning, adverse effect and underdosing codes, categories T36-T50. Where a placeholder exists, the X must be used in order for the code to be considered a valid code.

  5. 7th Characters

Certain ICD-10-CM categories have applicable 7th characters. The applicable 7th character is required for all codes within the category, or as the notes in the Tabular List instruct. The 7th character must always be the 7th character in the data field. If a code that requires a 7th character is not 6 characters, a placeholder X must be used to fill in the empty characters.

6. Abbreviations

a. Alphabetic Index abbreviations

NEC "Not elsewhere classifiable"
This abbreviation in the Alphabetic Index represents "other specified". When a specific code is not available for a condition the Alphabetic Index directs the coder to the "other specified" code in the Tabular List.

NOS "Not otherwise specified"
This abbreviation is the equivalent of unspecified.

b. Tabular List abbreviations

NEC "Not elsewhere classifiable"
This abbreviation in the Tabular List represents "other specified". When a specific code is not available for a condition, the Tabular List includes an NEC entry under a code to identify the code as the "other specified" code.

NOS "Not otherwise specified"
This abbreviation is the equivalent of unspecified.

7. Punctuation

[ ] Brackets are used in the Tabular List to enclose synonyms, alternative wording or explanatory phrases. Brackets are used in the Alphabetic Index to identify manifestation codes.

( ) Parentheses are used in both the Alphabetic Index and Tabular List to enclose supplementary words that may be present or absent in the statement of a disease or procedure without affecting the code number to which it is assigned. The terms within the parentheses are referred to as nonessential modifiers. The nonessential modifiers in the Alphabetic Index to Diseases apply to subterms following a main term except when a nonessential modifier and a subentry are mutually exclusive, the subentry takes precedence. For example, in the ICD-10-CM Alphabetic Index under the main term Enteritis, "acute" is a nonessential modifier and "chronic" is a subentry. In this case, the nonessential modifier "acute" does not apply to the subentry "chronic".

: Colons are used in the Tabular List after an incomplete term which needs one or more of the modifiers following the colon to make it assignable to a given category.

8. Use of "and".
See Section I.A.14. Use of the term "And"

9. Other and Unspecified codes

a. "Other" codes

Codes titled "other" or "other specified" are for use when the information in the medical record provides detail for which a specific code does not exist. Alphabetic Index entries with NEC in the line designate "other" codes in the Tabular List.

These Alphabetic Index entries represent specific disease entities for which no specific code exists so the term is included within an "other" code.

b. "Unspecified" codes

Codes titled "unspecified" are for use when the information in the medical record is insufficient to assign a more specific code. For those categories for which an unspecified code is not provided, the "other specified" code may represent both other and unspecified.
See Section I.B.18 Use of signs/symptoms/unspecified codes

10. Includes Notes

This note appears immediately under a 3-character code title to further define, or give examples of, the content of the category.

11. Inclusion terms

List of terms is included under some codes. These terms are the conditions for which that code is to be used. The terms may be synonyms of the code title, or, in the case of "other specified" codes, the terms are a list of the various conditions assigned to that code. The inclusion terms are not necessarily exhaustive. Additional terms found only in the Alphabetic Index may also be assigned to a code.

12. Excludes Notes

The ICD-10-CM has two types of excludes notes. Each type of note has a different definition for use, but they are all similar in that they indicate that codes excluded from each other are independent of each other.

a. Excludes1

A type 1 Excludes note is a pure excludes note. It means "NOT CODED HERE!" An Excludes1 note indicates that the code excluded should never be used at the same time as the code above the Excludes1 note. An Excludes1 is used when two conditions cannot occur together, such as a congenital form versus an acquired form of the same condition.

An exception to the Excludes1 definition is the circumstance when the two conditions are unrelated to each other. If it is not clear whether the two conditions involving an Excludes1 note are related or not, query the provider. For example, code F45.8, Other somatoform disorders, has an Excludes1 note for "sleep related teeth grinding (G47.63)" because "teeth grinding" is an inclusion term under F45.8. Only one of these two codes should be assigned for teeth grinding. However, psychogenic dysmenorrhea is also an inclusion term under F45.8, and a patient could have both this condition and sleep-related teeth grinding. In this case, the two conditions are clearly unrelated to each other, and so it would be appropriate to report F45.8 and G47.63 together.

b. Excludes2

A Type 2 Excludes note represents "Not included here." An excludes2 note indicates that the condition excluded is not part of the condition represented by the code, but a patient may have both conditions at the same time. When

5

an Excludes2 note appears under a code, it is acceptable to use both the code and the excluded code together, when appropriate.

13. **Etiology/manifestation convention ("code first", "use additional code" and "in diseases classified elsewhere" notes)**

Certain conditions have both an underlying etiology and multiple body system manifestations due to the underlying etiology. For such conditions, the ICD-10-CM has a coding convention that requires the underlying condition be sequenced first, if applicable, followed by the manifestation. Wherever such a combination exists, there is a "use additional code" note at the etiology code, and a "code first" note at the manifestation code. These instructional notes indicate the proper sequencing order of the codes, etiology followed by manifestation.

In most cases the manifestation codes will have in the code title, "in diseases classified elsewhere." Codes with this title are a component of the etiology/manifestation convention. The code title indicates that it is a manifestation code. "In diseases classified elsewhere" codes are never permitted to be used as first-listed or principal diagnosis codes. They must be used in conjunction with an underlying condition code and they must be listed following the underlying condition. See category F02, Dementia in other diseases classified elsewhere, for an example of this convention.

There are manifestation codes that do not have "in diseases classified elsewhere" in the title. For such codes, there is a "use additional code" note at the etiology code and a "code first" note at the manifestation code and the rules for sequencing apply.

In addition to the notes in the Tabular List, these conditions also have a specific Alphabetic Index entry structure. In the Alphabetic Index both conditions are listed together with the etiology code first followed by the manifestation codes in brackets. The code in brackets is always to be sequenced second.

An example of the etiology/manifestation convention is dementia with Parkinson's disease. In the Alphabetic Index, code G20 is listed first, followed by code F02.80 or F02.81 in brackets. Code G20 represents the underlying etiology, Parkinson's disease, and must be sequenced first, whereas *codes* F02.80 and F02.81 represent the manifestation of dementia in diseases classified elsewhere, with or without behavioral disturbance.

"Code first" and "Use additional code" notes are also used as sequencing rules in the classification for certain codes that are not part of an etiology/manifestation combination.

See Section I.B.7. Multiple coding for a single condition.

14. **"And"**

The word "and" should be interpreted to mean either "and" or "or" when it appears in a title.

For example, cases of "tuberculosis of bones", "tuberculosis of joints" and "tuberculosis of bones and joints" are classified to subcategory A18.0, Tuberculosis of bones and joints.

15. **"With"**

The word "with" or "in" should be interpreted to mean "associated with" or "due to" when it appears in a code title, the Alphabetic Index, (either under a main term or subterm) or an instructional note in the Tabular List. The classification presumes a causal relationship between the two conditions linked by these terms in the Alphabetic Index or Tabular List. These conditions should be coded as related even in the absence of provider documentation explicitly linking them, unless the documentation clearly states the conditions are unrelated or when another guideline exists that specifically requires a documented linkage between two conditions (e.g., sepsis guideline for "acute organ dysfunction that is not clearly associated with the sepsis").

For conditions not specifically linked by these relational terms in the classification or when a guideline requires that a linkage between two conditions be explicitly documented provider documentation must link the conditions in order to code them as related.

The word "with" in the Alphabetic Index is sequenced immediately following the main term or subterm, not in alphabetical order.

16. **"See" and "See Also"**

The "see" instruction following a main term in the Alphabetic Index indicates that another term should be referenced. It is necessary to go to the main term referenced with the "see" note to locate the correct code.

A "see also" instruction following a main term in the Alphabetic Index instructs that there is another main term that may also be referenced that may provide additional Alphabetic Index entries that may be useful. It is not necessary to follow the "see also" note when the original main term provides the necessary code.

17. **"Code also" note**

A "code also" note instructs that two codes may be required to fully describe a condition, but this note does not provide sequencing direction. The sequencing depends on the circumstances of the encounter.

18. **Default codes**

A code listed next to a main term in the ICD-10-CM Alphabetic Index is referred to as a default code. The default code represents that condition that is most commonly associated with the main term, or is the unspecified code for the condition. If a condition is documented in a medical record (for example, appendicitis) without any additional information, such as acute or chronic, the default code should be assigned.

19. **Code assignment and Clinical Criteria**

The assignment of a diagnosis code is based on the provider's diagnostic statement that the condition exists. The provider's statement that the patient has a particular condition is sufficient. Code assignment is not based on clinical criteria used by the provider to establish the diagnosis. **If there is** conflicting medical record documentation, query the provider.

B. General Coding Guidelines

1. Locating a code in the ICD-10-CM

To select a code in the classification that corresponds to a diagnosis or reason for visit documented in a medical record, first locate the term in the Alphabetic Index, and then verify the code in the Tabular List. Read and be guided by instructional notations that appear in both the Alphabetic Index and the Tabular List.

It is essential to use both the Alphabetic Index and Tabular List when locating and assigning a code. The Alphabetic Index does not always provide the full code. Selection of the full code, including laterality and any applicable 7th character can only be done in the Tabular List. A dash (-) at the end of an Alphabetic Index entry indicates that additional characters are required. Even if a dash is not included at the Alphabetic Index entry, it is necessary to refer to the Tabular List to verify that no 7th character is required.

2. Level of Detail in Coding

Diagnosis codes are to be used and reported at their highest number of characters available and to the highest level of specificity documented in the medical record.

ICD-10-CM diagnosis codes are composed of codes with 3, 4, 5, 6, or 7 characters. Codes with three characters are included in ICD-10-CM as the heading of a category of codes that may be further subdivided by the use of 4th and/or 5th characters and/or 6th characters, which provide greater detail.

A 3-character code is to be used only if it is not further subdivided. A code is invalid if it has not been coded to the full number of characters required for that code, including the 7th character, if applicable.

3. Code or codes from A00.0 through T88.9, Z00-Z99.8, U00-U85

The appropriate code or codes from A00.0 through T88.9, Z00-Z99.8 and U00-U85 must be used to identify diagnoses, symptoms, conditions, problems, complaints or other reason(s) for the encounter/visit.

4. Signs and symptoms

Codes that describe symptoms and signs, as opposed to diagnoses, are acceptable for reporting purposes when a related definitive diagnosis has not been established (confirmed) by the provider. Chapter 18 of ICD-10-CM, Symptoms, Signs, and Abnormal Clinical and Laboratory Findings, Not Elsewhere Classified (codes R00.0 - R99) contains many, but not all codes for symptoms.

See Section I.B.18 Use of signs/symptoms/ unspecified codes

5. Conditions that are an integral part of a disease process

Signs and symptoms that are associated routinely with a disease process should not be assigned as additional codes, unless otherwise instructed by the classification.

6. Conditions that are not an integral part of a disease process

Additional signs and symptoms that may not be associated routinely with a disease process should be coded when present.

7. Multiple coding for a single condition

In addition to the etiology/manifestation convention that requires two codes to fully describe a single condition that affects multiple body systems, there are other single conditions that also require more than one code. "Use additional code" notes are found in the Tabular List at codes that are not part of an etiology/manifestation pair where a secondary code is useful to fully describe a condition. The sequencing rule is the same as the etiology/manifestation pair, "use additional code" indicates that a secondary code should be added, if known.

For example, for bacterial infections that are not included in Chapter 1, a secondary code from category B95, Streptococcus, Staphylococcus, and Enterococcus, as the cause of diseases classified elsewhere, or B96, Other bacterial agents as the cause of diseases classified elsewhere, may be required to identify the bacterial organism causing the infection. A "use additional code" note will normally be found at the infectious disease code, indicating a need for the organism code to be added as a secondary code.

"Code first" notes are also under certain codes that are not specifically manifestation codes but may be due to an underlying cause. When there is a "code first" note and an underlying condition is present, the underlying condition should be sequenced first, if known.

"Code, if applicable, any causal condition first," notes indicate that this code may be assigned as a principal diagnosis when the causal condition is unknown or not applicable. If a causal condition is known, then the code for that condition should be sequenced as the principal or first-listed diagnosis.

Multiple codes may be needed for sequela, complication codes and obstetric codes to more fully describe a condition. See the specific guidelines for these conditions for further instruction.

8. Acute and Chronic Conditions

If the same condition is described as both acute (subacute) and chronic, and separate subentries exist in the Alphabetic Index at the same indentation level, code both and sequence the acute (subacute) code first.

9. Combination Code

A combination code is a single code used to classify:
Two diagnoses, or
A diagnosis with an associated secondary process (manifestation)
A diagnosis with an associated complication
Combination codes are identified by referring to subterm entries in the Alphabetic Index and by reading the inclusion and exclusion notes in the Tabular List.

Assign only the combination code when that code fully identifies the diagnostic conditions involved or when the Alphabetic Index so directs. Multiple coding should not be used when the classification provides a combination code that clearly identifies all of the elements documented in the diagnosis. When the combination code lacks necessary specificity in describing the manifestation or complication, an additional code should be used as a secondary code.

10. **Sequela (Late Effects)**
A sequela is the residual effect (condition produced) after the acute phase of an illness or injury has terminated. There is no time limit on when a sequela code can be used. The residual may be apparent early, such as in cerebral infarction, or it may occur months or years later, such as that due to a previous injury. Examples of sequela include: scar formation resulting from a burn, deviated septum due to a nasal fracture, and infertility due to tubal occlusion from old tuberculosis. Coding of sequela generally requires two codes sequenced in the following order: the condition or nature of the sequela is sequenced first. The sequela code is sequenced second.

An exception to the above guidelines are those instances where the code for the sequela is followed by a manifestation code identified in the Tabular List and title, or the sequela code has been expanded (at the 4th, 5th, or 6th character levels) to include the manifestation(s). The code for the acute phase of an illness or injury that led to the sequela is never used with a code for the late effect.

See Section I.C.9. Sequelae of cerebrovascular disease
See Section I.C.15. Sequelae of complication of pregnancy, childbirth and the puerperium
See Section I.C.19. Application of 7th characters for Chapter 19

11. **Impending or Threatened Condition**
Code any condition described at the time of discharge as "impending" or "threatened" as follows:

If it did occur, code as confirmed diagnosis.

If it did not occur, reference the Alphabetic Index to determine if the condition has a subentry term for "impending" or "threatened" and also reference main term entries for "Impending" and for "Threatened."

If the subterms are listed, assign the given code.

If the subterms are not listed, code the existing underlying condition(s) and not the condition described as impending or threatened.

12. **Reporting Same Diagnosis Code More Than Once**
Each unique ICD-10-CM diagnosis code may be reported only once for an encounter. This applies to bilateral conditions when there are no distinct codes identifying laterality or two different conditions classified to the same ICD-10-CM diagnosis code.

13. **Laterality**
Some ICD-10-CM codes indicate laterality, specifying whether the condition occurs on the left, right or is bilateral. If no bilateral code is provided and the condition is bilateral, assign separate codes for both the left and right side. If the side is not identified in the medical record, assign the code for the unspecified side.

When a patient has a bilateral condition and each side is treated during separate encounters, assign the "bilateral" code (as the condition still exists on both sides), including for the encounter to treat the first side. For the second encounter for treatment after one side has previously been treated and the condition no longer exists on that side, assign the appropriate unilateral code for the side where the condition still exists (e.g., cataract surgery performed on each eye in separate encounters). The bilateral code would not be assigned for the subsequent encounter, as the patient no longer has the condition in the previously-treated site. If the treatment on the first side did not completely resolve the condition, then the bilateral code would still be appropriate.

When laterality is not documented by the patient's provider, code assignment for the affected side may be based on medical record documentation from other clinicians. If there is conflicting medical record documentation regarding the affected side, the patient's attending provider should be queried for clarification. Codes for "unspecified" side should rarely be used, such as when the documentation in the record is insufficient to determine the affected side and it is not possible to obtain clarification.

14. **Documentation by Clinicians Other than the Patient's Provider**
Code assignment is based on the documentation by the patient's provider (i.e., physician or other qualified healthcare practitioner legally accountable for establishing the patient's diagnosis). There are a few exceptions when code assignment may be based on medical record documentation from clinicians who are not the patient's provider (i.e., physician or other qualified healthcare practitioner legally accountable for establishing the patient's diagnosis).

In this context, "clinicians" other than the patient's provider refer to healthcare professionals permitted, based on regulatory or accreditation requirements or internal hospital policies, to document in a patient's official medical record.

These exceptions include codes for:
- Body Mass Index (BMI)
- Depth of non-pressure chronic ulcers
- Pressure ulcer stage
- Coma scale
- NIH stroke scale (NIHSS)
- Social determinants of health (SDOH)
- Laterality
- Blood alcohol level

This information is typically, **or may be,** documented by other clinicians involved in the care of the patient (e.g., a dietitian often documents the BMI, a nurse often documents the pressure ulcer stages, and an emergency medical technician often documents the coma scale). However, the associated diagnosis (such as overweight, obesity, acute stroke, pressure ulcer, or a condition classifiable to category F10, Alcohol related disorders) must be documented by the patient's provider. If there is conflicting medical record documentation, either from the same clinician or different clinicians, the patient's attending provider should be queried for clarification.

The BMI, coma scale, and NIHSS blood alcohol level codes, codes for social determinants of health **and underimmunization status** should only be reported as secondary diagnoses.

See Section I.C.21.c.17 for additional information regarding coding social determinants of health.

15. **Syndromes**
Follow the Alphabetic Index guidance when coding syndromes. In the absence of Alphabetic Index guidance, assign codes for the documented manifestations of the syndrome. Additional codes for manifestations that are not an integral part of the disease process may also be assigned when the condition does not have a unique code.

16. **Documentation of Complications of Care**
Code assignment is based on the provider's documentation of the relationship between the condition and the care or procedure, unless otherwise instructed by the classification. The guideline extends to any complications of care, regardless of the chapter the code is located in. It is important to note that not all conditions that occur during or following medical care or surgery are classified as complications. There must be a cause-and-effect relationship between the care provided and the condition, and **the documentation must support that the condition is clinically significant. It is not necessary for the provider to explicitly document the term "complication." For example, if the condition alters the course of the surgery as documented in the operative report, then it is would be appropriate to report a complication code.** Query the provider for clarification **if the documentation is not clear as to the relationship between the condition and the care or procedure.**

17. **Borderline Diagnosis**
If the provider documents a "borderline" diagnosis at the time of discharge, the diagnosis is coded as confirmed, unless the classification provides a specific entry (e.g., borderline diabetes). If a borderline condition has a specific index entry in ICD-10-CM, it should be coded as such. Since borderline conditions are not uncertain diagnoses, no distinction is made between the care setting (inpatient versus outpatient). Whenever the documentation is unclear regarding a borderline condition, coders are encouraged to query for clarification.

18. **Use of Sign/Symptom/Unspecified Codes**
Sign/symptom and "unspecified" codes have acceptable, even necessary, uses. While specific diagnosis codes should be reported when they are supported by the available medical record documentation and clinical knowledge of the patient's health condition, there are instances when signs/symptoms or unspecified codes are the best choices for accurately reflecting the healthcare encounter. Each healthcare encounter should be coded to the level of certainty known for that encounter.

As stated in the introductory section of these official coding guidelines, a joint effort between the healthcare provider and the coder is essential to achieve complete and accurate documentation, code assignment, and reporting of diagnoses and procedures. The importance of consistent, complete documentation in the medical record cannot be overemphasized. Without such documentation accurate coding cannot be achieved. The entire record should be reviewed to determine the specific reason for the encounter and the conditions treated.

If a definitive diagnosis has not been established by the end of the encounter, it is appropriate to report codes for sign(s) and/or symptom(s) in lieu of a definitive diagnosis. When sufficient clinical information isn't known or available about a particular health condition to assign a more specific code, it is acceptable to report the appropriate "unspecified" code (e.g., a diagnosis of pneumonia has been determined, but not the specific type). Unspecified codes should be reported when they are the codes that most accurately reflect what is known about the patient's condition at the time of that particular encounter. It would be inappropriate to select a specific code that is not supported by the medical record documentation or conduct medically unnecessary diagnostic testing in order to determine a more specific code.

19. **Coding for Healthcare Encounters in Hurricane Aftermath**

a. **Use of External Cause of Morbidity Codes**
An external cause of morbidity code should be assigned to identify the cause of the injury(ies) incurred as a result of the hurricane. The use of external cause of morbidity codes is supplemental to the application of ICD-10-CM codes. External cause of morbidity codes are never to be recorded as a principal diagnosis (first-listed in non-inpatient settings). The appropriate injury code should be sequenced before any external cause codes. The external cause of morbidity codes capture how the injury or health condition happened (cause), the intent (unintentional or accidental; or intentional, such as suicide or assault), the place where the event occurred, the activity of the patient at the time of the event, and the person's status (e.g., civilian, military). They should not be assigned for encounters to treat hurricane victims' medical conditions when no injury, adverse effect or poisoning is involved. External cause of morbidity codes should be assigned for each encounter for care and treatment of the injury. External cause of morbidity codes may be assigned in all health care settings. For

the purpose of capturing complete and accurate ICD-10-CM data in the aftermath of the hurricane, a healthcare setting should be considered as any location where medical care is provided by licensed healthcare professionals.

b. Sequencing of External Causes of Morbidity Codes

Codes for cataclysmic events, such as a hurricane, take priority over all other external cause codes except child and adult abuse and terrorism and should be sequenced before other external cause of injury codes. Assign as many external cause of morbidity codes as necessary to fully explain each cause. For example, if an injury occurs as a result of a building collapse during the hurricane, external cause codes for both the hurricane and the building collapse should be assigned, with the external causes code for hurricane being sequenced as the first external cause code. For injuries incurred as a direct result of the hurricane, assign the appropriate code(s) for the injuries, followed by the code X37.0-, Hurricane (with the appropriate 7th character), and any other applicable external cause of injury codes. Code X37.0- also should be assigned when an injury is incurred as a result of flooding caused by a levee breaking related to the hurricane. Code X38.-, Flood (with the appropriate 7th character), should be assigned when an injury is from flooding resulting directly from the storm. Code X36.0.-, Collapse of dam or man-made structure, should not be assigned when the cause of the collapse is due to the hurricane. Use of code X36.0- is limited to collapses of man-made structures due to earth surface movements, not due to storm surges directly from a hurricane.

c. Other External Causes of Morbidity Code Issues

For injuries that are not a direct result of the hurricane, such as an evacuee that has incurred an injury as a result of a motor vehicle accident, assign the appropriate external cause of morbidity code(s) to describe the cause of the injury, but do not assign code X37.0-, Hurricane. If it is not clear whether the injury was a direct result of the hurricane, assume the injury is due to the hurricane and assign code X37.0-, Hurricane, as well as any other applicable external cause of morbidity codes. In addition to code X37.0-, Hurricane, other possible applicable external cause of morbidity codes include:

X30-	Exposure to excessive natural heat
X31-	Exposure to excessive natural cold
X38-	Flood

d. Use of Z codes

Z codes (other reasons for healthcare encounters) may be assigned as appropriate to further explain the reasons for presenting for healthcare services, including transfers between healthcare facilities or provide additional information relevant to a patient encounter. The ICD-10-CM Official Guidelines for Coding and Reporting identify which codes maybe assigned as principal or first-listed diagnosis only, secondary diagnosis only, or principal/first-listed or secondary (depending on the circumstances). Possible applicable Z codes include:

Z59.0-	Homelessness
Z59.1	Inadequate housing
Z59.5	Extreme poverty
Z75.1	Person awaiting admission to adequate facility elsewhere
Z75.3	Unavailability and inaccessibility of health-care facilities
Z75.4	Unavailability and inaccessibility of other helping agencies
Z76.2	Encounter for health supervision and care of other healthy infant and child
Z99.12	Encounter for respirator [ventilator] dependence during power failure

The external cause of morbidity codes and the Z codes listed above are not an all-inclusive list. Other codes may be applicable to the encounter based upon the documentation. Assign as many codes as necessary to fully explain each healthcare encounter. Since patient history information may be very limited, use any available documentation to assign the appropriate external cause of morbidity and Z codes.

C. Chapter-Specific Coding Guidelines

In addition to general coding guidelines, there are guidelines for specific diagnoses and/or conditions in the classification. Unless otherwise indicated, these guidelines apply to all health care settings. Please refer to Section II for guidelines on the selection of principal diagnosis.

1. Chapter 1: Certain Infectious and Parasitic Diseases (A00-B99, U07.1, U09.9)

a. Human Immunodeficiency Virus (HIV) Infections

1) Code only confirmed cases

Code only confirmed cases of HIV infection/illness. This is an exception to the hospital inpatient guideline Section II, H.

In this context, "confirmation" does not require documentation of positive serology or culture for HIV; the provider's diagnostic statement that the patient is HIV positive, or has an HIV-related illness is sufficient.

2) Selection and sequencing of HIV codes

(a) Patient admitted for HIV-related condition

If a patient is admitted for an HIV-related condition, the principal diagnosis should be B20, Human immunodeficiency virus [HIV] disease followed by additional diagnosis codes for all reported HIV-related conditions.

An exception to this guideline is if the reason for admission is hemolytic-uremic syndrome associated with HIV disease. Assign code D59.31, Infection-associated hemolytic-uremic syndrome, followed by code B20, Human immunodeficiency virus [HIV] disease.

(b) Patient with HIV disease admitted for unrelated condition

If a patient with HIV disease is admitted for an unrelated condition (such as a traumatic injury), the code for the unrelated condition (e.g., the nature of injury code) should be the principal diagnosis. Other diagnoses would be B20 followed by additional diagnosis codes for all reported HIV-related conditions.

(c) Whether the patient is newly diagnosed

Whether the patient is newly diagnosed or has had previous admissions/encounters for HIV conditions is irrelevant to the sequencing decision.

(d) Asymptomatic human immunodeficiency virus

Z21, Asymptomatic human immunodeficiency virus [HIV] infection status, is to be applied when the patient without any documentation of symptoms is listed as being "HIV positive," "known HIV," "HIV test positive," or similar terminology. Do not use this code if the term "AIDS" **or** "HIV disease" is used or if the patient is treated for any HIV-related illness or is described as having any condition(s) resulting from his/her HIV positive status; use B20 in these cases.

(e) Patients with inconclusive HIV serology

Patients with inconclusive HIV serology, but no definitive diagnosis or manifestations of the illness, may be assigned code R75, Inconclusive laboratory evidence of human immunodeficiency virus [HIV].

(f) Previously diagnosed HIV-related illness

Patients with any known prior diagnosis of an HIV-related illness should be coded to B20. Once a patient has developed an HIV-related illness, the patient should always be assigned code B20 on every subsequent admission/encounter. Patients previously diagnosed with any HIV illness (B20) should never be assigned to R75 or Z21, Asymptomatic human immunodeficiency virus [HIV] infection status.

(g) HIV Infection in Pregnancy, Childbirth and the Puerperium

During pregnancy, childbirth or the puerperium, a patient admitted (or presenting for a health care encounter) because of an HIV-related illness should receive a principal diagnosis code of O98.7-, Human immunodeficiency [HIV] disease complicating pregnancy, childbirth and the puerperium, followed by B20 and the code(s) for the HIV-related illness(es). Codes from Chapter 15 always take sequencing priority.

Patients with asymptomatic HIV infection status admitted (or presenting for a health care encounter) during pregnancy, childbirth, or the puerperium should receive codes of O98.7- and Z21.

(h) Encounters for testing for HIV

If a patient is being seen to determine his/her HIV status, use code Z11.4, Encounter for screening for human immunodeficiency virus [HIV]. Use additional codes for any associated high-risk behavior, if applicable.

If a patient with signs or symptoms is being seen for HIV testing, code the signs and symptoms. An additional counseling code Z71.7, Human immunodeficiency virus [HIV] counseling, may be used if counseling is provided during the encounter for the test.

When a patient returns to be informed of his/her HIV test results and the test result is negative, use code Z71.7, Human immunodeficiency virus [HIV] counseling.

If the results are positive, see previous guidelines and assign codes as appropriate.

(i) HIV managed by **antiretroviral** medication

If a patient with documented HIV disease, **HIV-related illness or AIDS** is currently managed on antiretroviral medications, assign code B20, Human immunodeficiency virus [HIV] disease. Code Z79.899, Other long term (current) drug therapy, may be assigned as an additional code to identify the long-term (current) use of antiretroviral medications.

b. Infectious agents as the cause of diseases classified to other chapters

Certain infections are classified in chapters other than Chapter 1 and no organism is identified as part of the infection code. In these instances, it is necessary to use an additional code from Chapter 1 to identify the organism. A code from category B95, Streptococcus, Staphylococcus, and Enterococcus as the cause of diseases classified to other chapters, B96, Other bacterial agents as the cause of diseases classified to other chapters, or B97, Viral agents as the cause of diseases classified to other chapters, is to be used as an additional code to identify the organism. An instructional note will be found at the infection code advising that an additional organism code is required.

c. Infections resistant to antibiotics

Many bacterial infections are resistant to current antibiotics. It is necessary to identify all infections documented as antibiotic resistant. Assign a code from category Z16, Resistance to antimicrobial drugs, following the infection code only if the infection code does not identify drug resistance.

d. Sepsis, Severe Sepsis, and Septic Shock

1) Coding of Sepsis and Severe Sepsis

(a) Sepsis

For a diagnosis of sepsis, assign the appropriate code for the underlying systemic infection. If the type of infection or causal organism is not further specified, assign code A41.9, Sepsis, unspecified organism.

A code from subcategory R65.2, Severe sepsis, should not be assigned unless severe sepsis or an associated acute organ dysfunction is documented.

11

(i) Negative or inconclusive blood cultures and sepsis
Negative or inconclusive blood cultures do not preclude a diagnosis of sepsis in patients with clinical evidence of the condition, however, the provider should be queried.

(ii) Urosepsis
The term urosepsis is a nonspecific term. It is not to be considered synonymous with sepsis. It has no default code in the Alphabetic Index. Should a provider use this term, he/she must be queried for clarification.

(iii) Sepsis with organ dysfunction
If a patient has sepsis and associated acute organ dysfunction or multiple organ dysfunction (MOD), follow the instructions for coding severe sepsis.

(iv) Acute organ dysfunction that is not clearly associated with the sepsis
If a patient has sepsis and an acute organ dysfunction, but the medical record documentation indicates that the acute organ dysfunction is related to a medical condition other than the sepsis, do not assign a code from subcategory R65.2, Severe sepsis. An acute organ dysfunction must be associated with the sepsis in order to assign the severe sepsis code. If the documentation is not clear as to whether an acute organ dysfunction is related to the sepsis or another medical condition, query the provider.

(b) Severe sepsis
The coding of severe sepsis requires a minimum of 2 codes: first a code for the underlying systemic infection, followed by a code from subcategory R65.2, Severe sepsis. If the causal organism is not documented, assign code A41.9, Sepsis, unspecified organism, for the infection. Additional code(s) for the associated acute organ dysfunction are also required.

Due to the complex nature of severe sepsis, some cases may require querying the provider prior to assignment of the codes.

2) Septic shock
(a) Septic shock generally refers to circulatory failure associated with severe sepsis, and therefore, it represents a type of acute organ dysfunction.
For all cases of septic shock, the code for the systemic infection should be sequenced first, followed by code R65.21, Severe sepsis with septic shock or code T81.12, Postprocedural septic shock. Any additional codes for the other acute organ dysfunctions should also be assigned. As noted

in the sequencing instructions in the Tabular List, the code for septic shock cannot be assigned as a principal diagnosis.

3) Sequencing of severe sepsis
If severe sepsis is present on admission, and meets the definition of principal diagnosis, the underlying systemic infection should be assigned as principal diagnosis followed by the appropriate code from subcategory R65.2 as required by the sequencing rules in the Tabular List. A code from subcategory R65.2 can never be assigned as a principal diagnosis.

When severe sepsis develops during an encounter (it was not present on admission) the underlying systemic infection and the appropriate code from subcategory R65.2 should be assigned as secondary diagnoses.

Severe sepsis may be present on admission but the diagnosis may not be confirmed until sometime after admission. If the documentation is not clear whether severe sepsis was present on admission, the provider should be queried.

For infection-associated hemolytic-uremic syndrome with severe sepsis, see guideline I.C.1.d.9.

4) Sepsis or severe sepsis with a localized infection
If the reason for admission is sepsis or severe sepsis and a localized infection, such as pneumonia or cellulitis, a code(s) for the underlying systemic infection should be assigned first and the code for the localized infection should be assigned as a secondary diagnosis. If the patient has severe sepsis, a code from subcategory R65.2 should also be assigned as a secondary diagnosis. If the patient is admitted with a localized infection, such as pneumonia, and sepsis/severe sepsis doesn't develop until after admission, the localized infection should be assigned first, followed by the appropriate sepsis/severe sepsis codes.

For hemolytic-uremic syndrome associated with sepsis, see guideline I.C.1.d.9.

5) Sepsis due to a postprocedural infection
(a) Documentation of causal relationship
As with all postprocedural complications, code assignment is based on the provider's documentation of the relationship between the infection and the procedure.

(b) Sepsis due to a postprocedural infection
For infections following a procedure, a code from T81.40, to T81.43. Infection following a procedure, or a code from O86.00 to O86.03, Infection of obstetric surgical wound, that identifies the site of the infection should be coded first, if known. Assign an additional code for sepsis following a procedure (T81.44) or sepsis following an obstetrical procedure (O86.04). Use an additional code to identify the infectious agent. If the patient has severe sepsis the appropriate code from subcategory R65.2 should also be assigned with the additional code(s) for any acute organ dysfunction.

For infections following infusion, transfusion, therapeutic injection, or immunization, a code from subcategory T80.2, Infections following infusion, transfusion, and therapeutic injection, or code T88.0-, Infection following immunization, should be coded first, followed by the code for the specific infection. If the patient has severe sepsis, the appropriate code from subcategory R65.2 should also be assigned, with the additional codes(s) for any acute organ dysfunction.

(c) Postprocedural infection and postprocedural septic shock

If a postprocedural infection has resulted in postprocedural septic shock, assign the codes indicated above for sepsis due to a postprocedural infection, followed by code T81.12-, Postprocedural septic shock. Do not assign code R65.21, Severe sepsis with septic shock. Additional code(s) should be assigned
for any acute organ dysfunction.

6) Sepsis and severe sepsis associated with a noninfectious process (condition)

In some cases a noninfectious process (condition), such as trauma, may lead to an infection which can result in sepsis or severe sepsis. If sepsis or severe sepsis is documented as associated with a noninfectious condition, such as a burn or serious injury, and this condition meets the definition for principal diagnosis, the code for the noninfectious condition should be sequenced first, followed by the code for the resulting infection. If severe sepsis is present, a code from subcategory R65.2 should also be assigned with any associated organ dysfunction(s) codes. It is not necessary to assign a code from subcategory R65.1, Systemic inflammatory response syndrome (SIRS) of non-infectious origin, for these cases.

If the infection meets the definition of principal diagnosis it should be sequenced before the non-infectious condition. When both the associated non-infectious condition and the infection meet the definition of principal diagnosis either may be assigned as principal diagnosis.

Only one code from category R65, Symptoms and signs specifically associated with systemic inflammation and infection, should be assigned. Therefore, when a non-infectious condition leads to an infection resulting in severe sepsis, assign the appropriate code from subcategory R65.2, Severe sepsis. Do not additionally assign a code from subcategory R65.1, Systemic inflammatory response syndrome (SIRS) of non-infectious origin.

See Section I.C.18. SIRS due to non-infectious process

7) Sepsis and septic shock complicating abortion, pregnancy, childbirth, and the puerperium

See Section I.C.15. Sepsis and septic shock complicating abortion, pregnancy, childbirth and the puerperium

8) Newborn sepsis

See Section I.C.16. f. Bacterial sepsis of Newborn

9) Hemolytic-uremic syndrome associated with sepsis

If the reason for admission is hemolytic-uremic syndrome that is associated with sepsis, assign code D59.31, Infection-associated hemolytic-uremic syndrome, as the principal diagnosis. Codes for the underlying systemic infection and any other conditions (such as severe sepsis) should be assigned as secondary diagnoses.

e. Methicillin Resistant Staphylococcus aureus (MRSA) Conditions

1) Selection and sequencing of MRSA codes

(a) Combination codes for MRSA infection

When a patient is diagnosed with an infection that is due to methicillin resistant Staphylococcus aureus (MRSA), and that infection has a combination code that includes the causal organism (e.g., sepsis, pneumonia) assign the appropriate combination code for the condition (e.g., code A41.02, Sepsis due to Methicillin resistant Staphylococcus aureus or code J15.212, Pneumonia due to Methicillin resistant Staphylococcus aureus). Do not assign code B95.62, Methicillin resistant Staphylococcus aureus infection as the cause of diseases classified elsewhere, as an additional code because the combination code includes the type of infection and the MRSA organism. Do not assign a code from subcategory Z16.11, Resistance to penicillins, as an additional diagnosis.

See Section C.1. for instructions on coding and sequencing of sepsis and severe sepsis.

(b) Other codes for MRSA infection

When there is documentation of a current infection (e.g., wound infection, stitch abscess, urinary tract infection) due to MRSA, and that infection does not have a combination code that includes the causal organism, assign the appropriate code to identify the condition along with code B95.62, Methicillin resistant Staphylococcus aureus infection as the cause of diseases classified elsewhere for the MRSA infection. Do not assign a code from subcategory Z16.11, Resistance to penicillins.

(c) Methicillin susceptible Staphylococcus aureus (MSSA) and MRSA colonization

The condition or state of being colonized or carrying MSSA or MRSA is called colonization or carriage, while an individual person is described as being colonized or being a carrier. Colonization means that MSSA or MSRA is present on or in the body without necessarily causing illness. A positive MRSA colonization test might be documented by the provider as "MRSA screen positive" or "MRSA nasal swab positive".

Assign code Z22.322, Carrier or suspected carrier of Methicillin resistant Staphylococcus aureus, for patients documented as having MRSA colonization. Assign code Z22.321, Carrier or suspected carrier of Methicillin susceptible Staphylococcus aureus, for patients documented as having MSSA colonization. Colonization is not necessarily indicative of a disease process or as the cause of a specific condition the patient may have unless documented as such by the provider.

(d) MRSA colonization and infection

If a patient is documented as having both MRSA colonization and infection during a hospital admission, code Z22.322, Carrier or suspected carrier of Methicillin resistant Staphylococcus aureus, and a code for the MRSA infection may both be assigned.

f. Zika virus infections

1) Code only confirmed cases

Code only a confirmed diagnosis of Zika virus (A92.5, Zika virus disease) as documented by the provider. This is an exception to the hospital inpatient guideline Section II, H.

In this context, "confirmation" does not require documentation of the type of test performed; the provider's diagnostic statement that the condition is confirmed is sufficient. This code should be assigned regardless of the stated mode of transmission.

If the provider documents "suspected", "possible" or "probable" Zika, do not assign code A92.5. Assign a code(s) explaining the reason for encounter (such as fever, rash, or joint pain) or Z20.821, Contact with and (suspected) exposure to Zika virus.

g. Coronavirus infections

1) COVID-19 infection (infection due to SARS-CoV-2)

(a) Code only confirmed cases

Code only a confirmed diagnosis of the 2019 novel coronavirus disease (COVID-19) as documented by the provider, or documentation of a positive COVID-19 test result. For a confirmed diagnosis, assign code U07.1, COVID-19. This is an exception to the hospital inpatient guideline Section II, H. In this context, "confirmation" does not require documentation of a positive test result for COVID-19; the provider's documentation that the individual has COVID-19 is sufficient.

If the provider documents "suspected," "possible," "probable," or "inconclusive" COVID-19, do not assign code U07.1. Instead, code the signs and symptoms reported. *See guideline I.C.1.g.1.g.*

(b) Sequencing of codes

When COVID-19 meets the definition of principal diagnosis, code U07.1, COVID-19, should be sequenced first, followed by the appropriate codes for associated manifestations, except when another guideline requires that certain codes be sequenced first, such as obstetrics, sepsis, or transplant complications.

For a COVID-19 infection that progresses to sepsis, see Section I.C.1.d. Sepsis, Severe Sepsis, and Septic Shock

See Section I.C.15.s. for COVID-19 infection in pregnancy, childbirth, and the puerperium

See Section I.C.16.h. for COVID-19 infection in newborn

For a COVID-19 infection in a lung transplant patient, see Section I.C.19.g.3.a. Transplant complications other than kidney.

(c) Acute respiratory manifestations of COVID-19

When the reason for the encounter/admission is a respiratory manifestation of COVID-19, assign code U07.1, COVID-19, as the principal/first-listed diagnosis and assign code(s) for the respiratory manifestation(s) as additional diagnoses.

The following conditions are examples of common respiratory manifestations of COVID-19.

(i) Pneumonia
For a patient with pneumonia confirmed as due to COVID-19, assign codes U07.1, COVID-19, and J12.89, Other viral pneumonia.

(ii) Acute bronchitis
For a patient with acute bronchitis confirmed as due to COVID-19, assign codes U07.1, and J20.8, Acute bronchitis due to other specified organisms.
Bronchitis not otherwise specified (NOS) due to COVID-19 should be coded using code U07.1 and J40, Bronchitis, not specified as acute or chronic.

(iii) Lower respiratory infection
If the COVID-19 is documented as being associated with a lower respiratory infection, not otherwise specified (NOS), or an acute respiratory infection, NOS, codes U07.1 and J22, Unspecified acute lower respiratory infection, should be assigned.
If the COVID-19 is documented as being associated with a respiratory infection, NOS, codes U07.1 and J98.8, Other specified respiratory disorders, should be assigned.

(iv) Acute respiratory distress syndrome
For acute respiratory distress syndrome (ARDS) due to COVID-19, assign codes U07.1, and J80, Acute respiratory distress syndrome.

(v) Acute respiratory failure
For acute respiratory failure due to COVID-19, assign code U07.1, and code J96.0-, Acute respiratory failure.

(d) Non-respiratory manifestations of COVID-19

When the reason for the encounter/admission is a non-respiratory manifestation (e.g., viral enteritis) of COVID-19, assign code U07.1, COVID-19, as the principal/first-listed diagnosis and assign code(s) for the manifestation(s) as additional diagnoses.

(e) Exposure to COVID-19

For asymptomatic individuals with actual or suspected exposure to COVID-19, assign code Z20.828, Contact with and (suspected) exposure to other viral communicable diseases.

For symptomatic individuals with actual or suspected exposure to COVID-19 and the infection has been ruled out, or test results are inconclusive or unknown, assign code Z20.828, Contact with and (suspected) exposure to other viral communicable diseases. See guideline I.C.21.c.1, Contact/Exposure, for additional guidance regarding the use of category Z20 codes.

If COVID-19 is confirmed, see guideline I.C.1.g.1.a.

(f) Screening for COVID-19

During the COVID-19 pandemic, a screening code is generally not appropriate. For encounters for COVID-19 testing, including preoperative testing, code as exposure to COVID-19 (guideline I.C.1.g.1.e).

Coding guidance will be updated as new information concerning any changes in the pandemic status becomes available.

(g) Signs and symptoms without definitive diagnosis of COVID-19

For patients presenting with any signs/symptoms associated with COVID-19 (such as fever, etc.) but a definitive diagnosis has not been established, assign the appropriate code(s) for each of the presenting signs and symptoms such as:
- R05.1, Acute cough, or R05.9, Cough, unspecified
- R06.02 Shortness of breath
- R50.9 Fever, unspecified

If a patient with signs/symptoms associated with COVID-19 also has an actual or suspected contact with or exposure to COVID-19, assign Z20.828, Contact with and (suspected) exposure to other viral communicable diseases, as an additional code.

(h) Asymptomatic individuals who test positive for COVID-19

For asymptomatic individuals who test positive for COVID-19, see guideline I.C.1.g.1.a. Although the individual is asymptomatic, the individual has tested positive and is considered to have the COVID-19 infection.

(i) Personal history of COVID-19

For patients with a history of COVID-19, assign code Z86.19, Personal history of other infectious and parasitic diseases.

(j) Follow-up visits after COVID-19 infection has resolved

For individuals who previously had COVID-19 without residual symptom(s) or condition(s), and are being seen for follow-up evaluation, and COVID-19 test results are negative, assign codes Z09, Encounter for follow-up examination after completed treatment for conditions other than malignant neoplasm, and Z86.19, Personal history of other infectious and parasitic diseases.

For follow-up visits for individuals with symptom(s) or condition(s) related to a previous COVID-19 infection, see guideline I.C.1.g.1.m.

See Section I.C.21.c.8, Factors influencing health states and contact with health services, Follow-up

(k) Encounter for antibody testing

For an encounter for antibody testing that is not being performed to confirm a current COVID-19 infection, nor is a follow-up test after resolution of COVID-19, assign Z01.84, Encounter for antibody response examination.

Follow the applicable guidelines above if the individual is being tested to confirm a current COVID-19 infection.

For follow-up testing after a COVID-19 infection, see guideline I.C.1.g.1.j.

(l) Multisystem Inflammatory Syndrome

For individuals with multisystem inflammatory syndrome (MIS) and COVID-19, assign code U07.1, COVID-19, as the principal/first-listed diagnosis and assign code M35.81, Multisystem inflammatory syndrome, as an additional diagnosis.

If an individual with a history of COVID-19 develops MIS, assign codes M35.81, Multisystem inflammatory syndrome, and U09.9, Post COVID-19 condition, unspecified.

If an individual with a known or suspected exposure to COVID-19, and no current COVID-19 infection or history of COVID-19, develops MIS, assign codes M35.81, Multisystem inflammatory syndrome, and Z20.822, Contact with and (suspected) exposure to COVID-19.

Additional codes should be assigned for any associated complications of MIS.

(m) Post COVID-19 Condition

For sequela of COVID-19, or associated symptoms or conditions that develop following a previous COVID-19 infection, assign a code(s) for the specific symptom(s) or condition(s) related to the previous COVID-19 infection, if known, and code U09.9, Post COVID-19 condition, unspecified.

Code U09.9 should not be assigned for manifestations of an active (current) COVID-19 infection.

If a patient has a condition(s) associated with a previous COVID-19 infection and develops a new active (current) COVID-19 infection, code U09.9 may be assigned in conjunction with code U07.1, COVID-19, to identify that the patient also has a condition(s) associated with a previous COVID-19 infection. Code(s) for the specific condition(s) associated with the previous COVID-19 infection and code(s) for manifestation(s) of the new active (current) COVID-19 infection should also be assigned.

(n) Underimmunization for COVID-19 Status Code Z28.310, Unvaccinated for COVID-19, may be assigned when the patient has not received a COVID-19 vaccine of any type. Code Z28.311, Partially vaccinated for COVID-19, may be assigned when the patient has been partially

vaccinated for COVID-19 as per the recommendations of the Centers for Disease Control and Prevention (CDC) in place at the time of the encounter. For information, visit the CDC's website https://www.cdc.gov/coronavirus/2019-ncov/vaccines/.

See Section I.B.14. for underimmunization documentation by clinicians other than patient's provider.

2. **Chapter 2: Neoplasms (C00-D49)**
General guidelines
Chapter 2 of the ICD-10-CM contains the codes for most benign and all malignant neoplasms. Certain benign neoplasms, such as prostatic adenomas, may be found in the specific body system chapters. To properly code a neoplasm it is necessary to determine from the record if the neoplasm is benign, in-situ, malignant, or of uncertain histologic behavior. If malignant, any secondary (metastatic) sites should also be determined.

Primary malignant neoplasms overlapping site boundaries
A primary malignant neoplasm that overlaps two or more contiguous (next to each other) sites should be classified to the subcategory/code .8 ("overlapping lesion"), unless the combination is specifically indexed elsewhere. For multiple neoplasms of the same site that are not contiguous such as tumors in different quadrants of the same breast, codes for each site should be assigned.

Malignant neoplasm of ectopic tissue
Malignant neoplasms of ectopic tissue are to be coded to the site of origin mentioned (e.g., ectopic pancreatic malignant neoplasms involving the stomach are coded to malignant neoplasm of pancreas, unspecified) (C25.9).

The neoplasm table in the Alphabetic Index should be referenced first. However, if the histological term is documented, that term should be referenced first, rather than going immediately to the Neoplasm Table, in order to determine which column in the Neoplasm Table is appropriate. For example, if the documentation indicates "adenoma," refer to the term in the Alphabetic Index to review the entries under this term and the instructional note to "see also neoplasm, by site, benign." The table provides the proper code based on the type of neoplasm and the site. It is important to select the proper column in the table that corresponds to the type of neoplasm. The Tabular List should then be referenced to verify that the correct code has been selected from the table and that a more specific site code does not exist.

See Section I.C.21. Factors influencing health status and contact with health services, Status, for information regarding Z15.0, codes for genetic susceptibility to cancer.

a. *Admission/Encounter for treatment of primary site*
If the **malignancy is chiefly responsible for occasioning the patient admission/encounter and treatment is directed at the primary site,** designate the **primary** malignancy as the principal **/first-listed** diagnosis.

The only exception to this guideline is if the administration of chemotherapy, immunotherapy or external beam radiation therapy **is chiefly responsible for occasioning the admission/encounter. In that case,** assign the appropriate Z51.— code as the first-listed or principal diagnosis, and the **underlying** diagnosis or problem for which the service is being performed as a secondary diagnosis.

b. *Admission/Encounter for treatment of secondary site*
When a patient is admitted because of a primary neoplasm with metastasis and treatment is directed toward the secondary site only, the secondary neoplasm is designated as the principal diagnosis even though the primary malignancy is still present.

c. **Coding and sequencing of complications**
Coding and sequencing of complications associated with the malignancies or with the therapy thereof are subject to the following guidelines:

1) **Anemia associated with malignancy**
When admission/encounter is for management of an anemia associated with the malignancy, and the treatment is only for anemia, the appropriate code for the malignancy is sequenced as the principal or first-listed diagnosis followed by the appropriate code for the anemia (such as code D63.0, Anemia in neoplastic disease).

2) **Anemia associated with chemotherapy, immunotherapy and radiation therapy**
When the admission/encounter is for management of an anemia associated with an adverse effect of the administration of chemotherapy or immunotherapy and the only treatment is for the anemia, the anemia code is sequenced first followed by the appropriate codes for the neoplasm and the adverse effect (T45.1X5, Adverse effect of antineoplastic and immunosuppressive drugs).

When the admission/encounter is for management of an anemia associated with an adverse effect of radiotherapy, the anemia code should be sequenced first, followed by the appropriate neoplasm code and code Y84.2, Radiological procedure and radiotherapy as the cause of abnormal reaction of the patient, or of later complication, without mention of misadventure at the time of the procedure.

3) **Management of dehydration due to the malignancy**
When the admission/encounter is for management of dehydration due to the malignancy and only the dehydration is being treated (intravenous rehydration), the dehydration is sequenced first, followed by the code(s) for the malignancy.

4) Treatment of a complication resulting from a surgical procedure

When the admission/encounter is for treatment of a complication resulting from a surgical procedure, designate the complication as the principal or first-listed diagnosis if treatment is directed at resolving the complication.

d. Primary malignancy previously excised

When a primary malignancy has been previously excised or eradicated from its site and there is no further treatment directed to that site and there is no evidence of any existing primary malignancy, at that site a code from category Z85, Personal history of malignant neoplasm, should be used to indicate the former site of the malignancy. Any mention of extension, invasion, or metastasis to another site is coded as a secondary malignant neoplasm to that site. The secondary site may be the principal or first-listed diagnosis with the Z85 code used as a secondary code.

See section I.C.2.t. Secondary malignant neoplasm of lymphoid tissue.

e. Admissions/Encounters involving chemotherapy, immunotherapy and radiation therapy

1) Episode of care involves surgical removal of neoplasm

When an episode of care involves the surgical removal of a neoplasm, primary or secondary site, followed by adjunct chemotherapy or radiation treatment during the same episode of care, the code for the neoplasm should be assigned as principal or first-listed diagnosis.

2) Patient admission/encounter solely for administration of chemotherapy, immunotherapy and radiation therapy

If a patient admission/encounter is solely for the administration of chemotherapy, immunotherapy or external beam radiation therapy assign code Z51.0, Encounter for antineoplastic radiation therapy, or Z51.11, Encounter for antineoplastic chemotherapy, or Z51.12, Encounter for antineoplastic immunotherapy as the first-listed or principal diagnosis. If a patient receives more than one of these therapies during the same admission more than one of these codes may be assigned, in any sequence.

The malignancy for which the therapy is being administered should be assigned as a secondary diagnosis.

If a patient admission/encounter is for the insertion or implantation of radioactive elements (e.g., brachytherapy) the appropriate code for the malignancy is sequenced as the principal or first-listed diagnosis. Code Z51.0 should not be assigned.

3) Patient admitted for radiation therapy, chemotherapy or immunotherapy and develops complications

When a patient is admitted for the purpose of external beam radiotherapy, immunotherapy or chemotherapy and develops complications such as uncontrolled nausea and vomiting or dehydration, the principal or first-listed diagnosis is Z51.0, Encounter for antineoplastic radiation therapy, or Z51.11, Encounter for antineoplastic chemotherapy, or Z51.12, Encounter for antineoplastic immunotherapy followed by any codes for the complications.

When a patient is admitted for the purpose of insertion or implantation of radioactive elements (e.g., brachytherapy) and develops complications such as uncontrolled nausea and vomiting or dehydration, the principal or first-listed diagnosis is the appropriate code for the malignancy followed by any codes for the complications.

f. Admission/encounter to determine extent of malignancy

When the reason for admission/encounter is to determine the extent of the malignancy, or for a procedure such as paracentesis or thoracentesis, the primary malignancy or appropriate metastatic site is designated as the principal or first-listed diagnosis, even though chemotherapy or radiotherapy is administered.

g. Symptoms, signs, and abnormal findings listed in Chapter 18 associated with neoplasms

Symptoms, signs, and ill-defined conditions listed in Chapter 18 characteristic of, or associated with, an existing primary or secondary site malignancy cannot be used to replace the malignancy as principal or first-listed diagnosis, regardless of the number of admissions or encounters for treatment and care of the neoplasm.

See Section I.C.21. Factors influencing health status and contact with health services, Encounter for prophylactic organ removal.

h. Admission/encounter for pain control/management

See Section I.C.6. for information on coding admission/encounter for pain control/management.

i. Malignancy in two or more noncontiguous sites

A patient may have more than one malignant tumor in the same organ. These tumors may represent different primaries or metastatic disease, depending on the site. Should the documentation be unclear, the provider should be queried as to the status of each tumor so that the correct codes can be assigned.

j. Disseminated malignant neoplasm, unspecified

Code C80.0, Disseminated malignant neoplasm, unspecified, is for use only in those cases where the patient has advanced metastatic disease and no known primary or secondary sites are specified. It should not be used in place of assigning codes for the primary site and all known secondary sites.

k. Malignant neoplasm without specification of site

Code C80.1, Malignant (primary) neoplasm, unspecified, equates to Cancer, unspecified. This code should only be used when no determination can be made as to the primary site of a malignancy. This code should rarely be used in the inpatient setting.

l. **Sequencing of neoplasm codes**

   1) **Encounter for treatment of primary malignancy**

   If the reason for the encounter is for treatment of a primary malignancy, assign the malignancy as the principal/first-listed diagnosis. The primary site is to be sequenced first, followed by any metastatic sites.

   2) **Encounter for treatment of secondary malignancy**

   When an encounter is for a primary malignancy with metastasis and treatment is directed toward the metastatic (secondary) site(s) only, the metastatic site(s) is designated as the principal/first-listed diagnosis. The primary malignancy is coded as an additional code.

   3) **Malignant neoplasm in a pregnant patient**

   When a pregnant patient has a malignant neoplasm, a code from subcategory O9A.1-, Malignant neoplasm complicating pregnancy, childbirth, and the puerperium, should be sequenced first, followed by the appropriate code from Chapter 2 to indicate the type of neoplasm.

   4) **Encounter for complication associated with a neoplasm**

   When an encounter is for management of a complication associated with a neoplasm, such as dehydration, and the treatment is only for the complication, the complication is coded first, followed by the appropriate code(s) for the neoplasm.

   The exception to this guideline is anemia. When the admission/encounter is for management of an anemia associated with the malignancy, and the treatment is only for anemia, the appropriate code for the malignancy is sequenced as the principal or first-listed diagnosis followed by code D63.0, Anemia in neoplastic disease.

   5) **Complication from surgical procedure for treatment of a neoplasm**

   When an encounter is for treatment of a complication resulting from a surgical procedure performed for the treatment of the neoplasm, designate the complication as the principal/first-listed diagnosis. See the guideline regarding the coding of a current malignancy versus personal history to determine if the code for the neoplasm should also be assigned.

   6) **Pathologic fracture due to a neoplasm**

   When an encounter is for a pathological fracture due to a neoplasm, and the focus of treatment is the fracture, a code from subcategory M84.5, Pathological fracture in neoplastic disease, should be sequenced first, followed by the code for the neoplasm.

   If the focus of treatment is the neoplasm with an associated pathological fracture, the neoplasm code should be sequenced first, followed by a code from M84.5 for the pathological fracture.

m. **Current malignancy versus personal history of malignancy**

When a primary malignancy has been excised but further treatment, such as an additional surgery for the malignancy, radiation therapy or chemotherapy is directed to that site, the primary malignancy code should be used until treatment is completed.

When a primary malignancy has been previously excised or eradicated from its site, there is no further treatment (of the malignancy) directed to that site, and there is no evidence of any existing primary malignancy at that site, a code from category Z85, Personal history of malignant neoplasm, should be used to indicate the former site of the malignancy.

Codes from subcategories Z85.0 – Z85.85 should only be assigned for the former site of a primary malignancy, not the site of a secondary malignancy. Code Z85.89, may be assigned for the former site(s) of either a primary or secondary malignancy.

See Section I.C.21. Factors influencing health status and contact with health services, History (of)

n. **Leukemia, Multiple Myeloma, and Malignant Plasma Cell Neoplasms in remission versus personal history**

The categories for leukemia, and category C90, Multiple myeloma and malignant plasma cell neoplasms, have codes indicating whether or not the leukemia has achieved remission. There are also codes Z85.6, Personal history of leukemia, and Z85.79, Personal history of other malignant neoplasms of lymphoid, hematopoietic and related tissues. If the documentation is unclear, as to whether the leukemia has achieved remission, the provider should be queried.

See Section I.C.21. Factors influencing health status and contact with health services, History (of)

o. **Aftercare following surgery for neoplasm**

See Section I.C.21. Factors influencing health status and contact with health services, Aftercare

p. **Follow-up care for completed treatment of a malignancy**

See Section I.C.21. Factors influencing health status and contact with health services, Follow-up

q. **Prophylactic organ removal for prevention of malignancy**

See Section I.C. 21, Factors influencing health status and contact with health services, Prophylactic organ removal

r. **Malignant neoplasm associated with transplanted organ**

A malignant neoplasm of a transplanted organ should be coded as a transplant complication. Assign first the appropriate code from category T86.-, Complications of transplanted organs and tissue, followed by code C80.2, Malignant neoplasm associated with transplanted organ. Use an additional code for the specific malignancy.

s. **Breast Implant Associated Anaplastic Large Cell Lymphoma**

Breast implant associated anaplastic large cell lymphoma (BIA-ALCL) is a type of lymphoma that can develop around breast implants. Assign code C84.7A, Anaplastic large cell lymphoma, ALK-negative, breast, for BIA-ALCL. Do not assign a complication code from chapter 19.

t. Secondary malignant neoplasm of lymphoid tissue

When a malignant neoplasm of lymphoid tissue metastasizes beyond the lymph nodes, a code from categories C81-C85 with a final character "9" should be assigned identifying "extranodal and solid organ sites" rather than a code for the secondary neoplasm of the affected solid organ. For example, for metastasis of B-cell lymphoma to the lung, brain and left adrenal gland, assign code C83.39, Diffuse large B-cell lymphoma, extranodal and solid organ sites.

3. **Chapter 3: Disease of the blood and blood-forming organs and certain disorders involving the immune mechanism (D50-D89)**
Reserved for future guideline expansion

4. **Chapter 4: Endocrine, Nutritional, and Metabolic Diseases (E00-E89)**

a. **Diabetes mellitus**
The diabetes mellitus codes are combination codes that include the type of diabetes mellitus, the body system affected, and the complications affecting that body system. As many codes within a particular category as are necessary to describe all of the complications of the disease may be used. They should be sequenced based on the reason for a particular encounter. Assign as many codes from categories E08 – E13 as needed to identify all of the associated conditions that the patient has.

1) **Type of diabetes**
The age of a patient is not the sole determining factor, though most type 1 diabetics develop the condition before reaching puberty. For this reason type 1 diabetes mellitus is also referred to as juvenile diabetes.

2) **Type of diabetes mellitus not documented**
If the type of diabetes mellitus is not documented in the medical record the default is E11.-, Type 2 diabetes mellitus.

3) **Diabetes mellitus and the use of insulin, oral hypoglycemics, and injectable non-insulin drugs**
If the documentation in a medical record does not indicate the type of diabetes but does indicate that the patient uses insulin, code E11, Type 2 diabetes mellitus, should be assigned. Additional code(s) should be assigned from category Z79 to identify the long-term (current) use of insulin or oral hypoglycemic drugs, or injectable non-insulin antidiabetic, as follows: If the patient is treated with both oral **hypoglycemic drugs** and insulin, both code Z79.4, Long term (current) use of insulin, and code Z79.84, Long term (current) use of oral hypoglycemic drugs, should be assigned. If the patient is treated with both insulin and an injectable non-insulin antidiabetic drug, assign codes Z79.4, Long-term (current) use of insulin, and **Z79.85, Long-term (current) use of injectable non-insulin antidiabetic drugs.** If the patient is treated with both oral hypoglycemic drugs and an injectable non-insulin antidiabetic drug, assign codes Z79.84, Long-term (current) use of oral hypoglycemic drugs, and **Z79.85, Long-term (current) use of injectable non-insulin antidiabetic drugs.** Code Z79.4 should not be assigned if insulin is given temporarily to bring a type 2 patient's blood sugar under control during an encounter.

4) **Diabetes mellitus in pregnancy and gestational diabetes**
See Section I.C.15. Diabetes mellitus in pregnancy.
See Section I.C.15. Gestational (pregnancy induced)
diabetes

5) **Complications due to insulin pump malfunction**

(a) **Underdose of insulin due to insulin pump failure**
An underdose of insulin due to an insulin pump failure should be assigned to a code from subcategory T85.6, Mechanical complication of other specified internal and external prosthetic devices, implants and grafts, that specifies the type of pump malfunction, as the principal or first-listed code, followed by code T38.3X6-, Underdosing of insulin and oral hypoglycemic [antidiabetic] drugs. Additional codes for the type of diabetes mellitus and any associated complications due to the underdosing should also be assigned.

(b) **Overdose of insulin due to insulin pump failure**
The principal or first-listed code for an encounter due to an insulin pump malfunction resulting in an overdose of insulin, should also be T85.6-, Mechanical complication of other specified internal and external prosthetic devices, implants and grafts, followed by code T38.3X1-, Poisoning by insulin and oral hypoglycemic [antidiabetic] drugs, accidental (unintentional).

6) **Secondary diabetes mellitus**
Codes under categories E08, Diabetes mellitus due to underlying condition, E09, Drug or chemical induced diabetes mellitus and E13, Other specified diabetes mellitus, identify complications/manifestations associated with secondary diabetes mellitus. Secondary diabetes is always caused by another condition or event (e.g., cystic fibrosis, malignant neoplasm of pancreas, pancreatectomy, adverse effect of drug, or poisoning).

(a) **Secondary diabetes mellitus and the use of insulin or hypoglycemic drugs**
For patients with secondary diabetes mellitus who routinely use insulin or oral hypoglycemic drugs, or injectable non-insulin drugs, an additional code(s) from category Z79 should be assigned to identify the long-term (current) use of insulin or oral hypoglycemic drugs, or non-injectable non-insulin drugs as follows: If the patient is treated with both oral **hypoglycemic drugs** and insulin, both code Z79.4, Long term (current) use of insulin, and code Z79.84, Long term (current) use of oral hypoglycemic drugs, should be assigned. If the patient is treated with both insulin and an injectable non- insulin antidiabetic drug, assign

codes Z79.4, Long- term (current) use of insulin, and **Z79.85, Long-term (current) use of injectable non-insulin antidiabetic drugs.** If the patient is treated with both oral hypoglycemic drugs and an injectable non-insulin antidiabetic drug, assign codes Z79.84, Long-term (current) use of oral hypoglycemic drugs, and **Z79.85, Long-term (current) use of injectable non-insulin antidiabetic drugs.** Code Z79.4 should not be assigned if insulin is given temporarily to bring a type 2 patient's blood sugar under control during an encounter.

(b) Assigning and sequencing secondary diabetes codes and its causes

The sequencing of the secondary diabetes codes in relationship to codes for the cause of the diabetes is based on the Tabular List instructions for categories E08, E09 and E13.

(i) Secondary diabetes mellitus due to pancreatectomy
For postpancreatectomy diabetes mellitus (lack of insulin due to the surgical removal of all or part of the pancreas), assign code E89.1, Postprocedural hypoinsulinemia. Assign a code from category E13 and a code from subcategory Z90.41-, Acquired absence of pancreas, as additional codes.

(ii) Secondary diabetes due to drugs
Secondary diabetes may be caused by an adverse effect of correctly administered medications, poisoning or sequela of poisoning.

See Section I.C.19.e for coding of adverse effects and poisoning, and Section I.C.20 for external cause code reporting.

5. Chapter 5: Mental, Behavioral and Neurodevelopmental disorders (F01 – F99)

a. Pain disorders related to psychological factors
Assign code F45.41, for pain that is exclusively related to psychological disorders. As indicated by the Excludes1 note under category G89, a code from category G89 should not be assigned with code F45.41

Code F45.42, Pain disorders with related psychological factors, should be used with a code from category G89, Pain, not elsewhere classified, if there is documentation of a psychological component for a patient with acute or chronic pain.

See Section I.C.6. Pain

b. Mental and behavioral disorders due to psychoactive substance use

1) In Remission
Selection of codes **describing** "in remission" for categories F10-F19, Mental and behavioral disorders due to psychoactive substance use (categories F10-F19 with -11, -.21, **-91**) requires the provider's clinical judgment **and** are assigned only on the basis of provider documentation (as defined in the Official Guidelines for Coding and Reporting), unless otherwise instructed by the classification.

Mild substance use disorders in early or sustained remission are classified to the appropriate codes for substance abuse in remission, and moderate or severe substance use disorders in early or sustained remission are classified to the appropriate codes for substance dependence in remission.

2) Psychoactive Substance Use, Abuse and Dependence
When the provider documentation refers to use, abuse and dependence of the same substance (e.g., alcohol, opioid, cannabis, etc.), only one code should be assigned to identify the pattern of use based on the following hierarchy:

- If both use and abuse are documented, assign only the code for abuse
- If both abuse and dependence are documented, assign only the code for dependence
- If use, abuse and dependence are all documented, assign only the code for dependence
- If both use and dependence are documented, assign only the code for dependence.

3) Psychoactive Substance Use, Unspecified
As with all other unspecified diagnoses, the codes for unspecified psychoactive substance use disorders (F10.9-, F11.9-, F12.9-, F13.9-, F14.9-, F15.9-, F16.9-, F18.9-, F19.9-) should only be assigned based on provider documentation and when they meet the definition of a reportable diagnosis (see Section III, Reporting Additional Diagnoses). These codes are to be used only when the psychoactive substance use is associated 1with a substance related disorder (chapter 5 such as sexual dysfunction and sleep disorder, or a mental or behavioral disorder) or medical condition, and such a relationship is documented by the provider.

4) Medical Conditions Due to Psychoactive Substance Use, Abuse and Dependence
Medical conditions due to substance use, abuse, and dependence are not classified as substance-induced disorders. Assign the diagnosis code for the medical condition as directed by the Alphabetical Index along with the appropriate psychoactive substance use, abuse or dependence code. For example, for alcoholic pancreatitis due to alcohol dependence, assign the appropriate code from subcategory K85.2, Alcohol induced acute pancreatitis, and the appropriate code from subcategory F10.2, such as code F10.20, Alcohol dependence, uncomplicated. It would not be appropriate to assign code F10.288, Alcohol dependence with other alcohol-induced disorder.

5) Blood Alcohol Level
A code from category Y90, Evidence of alcohol involvement determined by blood alcohol level, may be assigned when this information is documented and the patient's provider has documented a condition classifiable to category

F10, Alcohol related disorders. The blood alcohol level does not need to be documented by the patient's provider in order for it to be coded.

See Section I.B.14. for blood alcohol level documentation by clinicians other than patient's provider.

c. Factitious Disorder
Factitious disorder imposed on self or Munchausen's syndrome is a disorder in which a person falsely reports or causes his or her own physical or psychological signs or symptoms. For patients with documented factitious disorder on self or Munchausen's syndrome, assign the appropriate code from subcategory F68.1-, Factitious disorder imposed on self.

Munchausen's syndrome by proxy (MSBP) is a disorder in which a caregiver (perpetrator) falsely reports or causes an illness or injury in another person (victim) under his or her care, such as a child, an elderly adult, or a person who has a disability. The condition is also referred to as "factitious disorder imposed on another" or "factitious disorder by proxy." The perpetrator, not the victim, receives this diagnosis. Assign code F68.A, Factitious disorder imposed on another, to the perpetrator's record. For the victim of a patient suffering from MSBP, assign the appropriate code from categories T74, Adult and child abuse, neglect and other maltreatment, confirmed, or T76, Adult and child abuse, neglect and other maltreatment, suspected.

See Section I.C.19.f. Adult and child abuse, neglect and other maltreatment

d. Dementia
The ICD-10-CM classifies dementia (categories F01, F02, and F03) on the basis of the etiology and severity (unspecified, mild, moderate or severe). Selection of the appropriate severity level requires the provider's clinical judgment and codes should be assigned only on the basis of provider documentation (as defined in the *Official Guidelines for Coding and Reporting*), unless otherwise instructed by the classification. If the documentation does not provide information about the severity of the dementia, assign the appropriate code for unspecified severity.

If a patient is admitted to an inpatient acute care hospital or other inpatient facility setting with dementia at one severity level and it progresses to a higher severity level, assign one code for the highest severity level reported during the stay.

6. Chapter 6: Diseases of the Nervous System (G00-G99)
a. Dominant/nondominant side
Codes from category G81, Hemiplegia and hemiparesis, and subcategories, G83.1, Monoplegia of lower limb, G83.2, Monoplegia of upper limb, and G83.3, Monoplegia, unspecified, identify whether the dominant or nondominant side is affected. Should the affected side be documented, but not specified as dominant or nondominant,

and the classification system does not indicate a default, code selection is as follows:
- For ambidextrous patients, the default should be dominant.
- If the left side is affected, the default is non-dominant.
- If the right side is affected, the default is dominant.

b. Pain - Category G89
1) General coding information
Codes in category G89, Pain, not elsewhere classified, may be used in conjunction with codes from other categories and chapters to provide more detail about acute or chronic pain and neoplasm-related pain, unless otherwise indicated below.

If the pain is not specified as acute or chronic, post-thoracotomy, postprocedural, or neoplasm-related, do not assign codes from category G89.

A code from category G89 should not be assigned if the underlying (definitive) diagnosis is known, unless the reason for the encounter is pain control/management and not management of the underlying condition.

When an admission or encounter is for a procedure aimed at treating the underlying condition (e.g., spinal fusion, kyphoplasty), a code for the underlying condition (e.g., vertebral fracture, spinal stenosis) should be assigned as the principal diagnosis. No code from category G89 should be assigned.

(a) Category G89 Codes as Principal or First-Listed Diagnosis
Category G89 codes are acceptable as principal diagnosis or the first-listed code:
- When pain control or pain management is the reason for the admission/encounter (e.g., a patient with displaced intervertebral disc, nerve impingement and severe back pain presents for injection of steroid into the spinal canal). The underlying cause of the pain should be reported as an additional diagnosis, if known.
- When a patient is admitted for the insertion of a neurostimulator for pain control, assign the appropriate pain code as the principal or first-listed diagnosis. When an admission or encounter is for a procedure aimed at treating the underlying condition and a neurostimulator is inserted for pain control during the same admission/encounter, a code for the underlying condition should be assigned as the principal diagnosis and the appropriate pain code should be assigned as a secondary diagnosis.

(b) Use of Category G89 Codes in Conjunction with Site-Specific Pain Codes
(i) Assigning Category G89 and Site-Specific Pain Codes
Codes from category G89 may be used in conjunction with codes that identify the site of pain

(including codes from Chapter 18) if the category G89 code provides additional information. For example, if the code describes the site of the pain, but does not fully describe whether the pain is acute or chronic, then both codes should be assigned.

(ii) Sequencing of Category G89 Codes with Site-Specific Pain Codes

The sequencing of category G89 codes with site-specific pain codes (including Chapter 18 codes), is dependent on the circumstances of the encounter/admission as follows:

- If the encounter is for pain control or pain management, assign the code from category G89 followed by the code identifying the specific site of pain (e.g., encounter for pain management for acute neck pain from trauma is assigned code G89.11, Acute pain due to trauma, followed by code M54.2, Cervicalgia, to identify the site of pain).
- If the encounter is for any other reason except pain control or pain management, and a related definitive diagnosis has not been established (confirmed) by the provider, assign the code for the specific site of pain first, followed by the appropriate code from category G89.

2) Pain due to devices, implants and grafts

See Section I.C.19. Pain due to medical devices

3) Postoperative Pain

The provider's documentation should be used to guide the coding of postoperative pain, as well as Section III. Reporting Additional Diagnoses and Section IV. Diagnostic Coding and Reporting in the Outpatient Setting.

The default for post-thoracotomy and other postoperative pain not specified as acute or chronic is the code for the acute form.

Routine or expected postoperative pain immediately after surgery should not be coded.

(a) Postoperative pain not associated with specific postoperative complication

Postoperative pain not associated with a specific postoperative complication is assigned to the appropriate postoperative pain code in category G89.

(b) Postoperative pain associated with specific postoperative complication

Postoperative pain associated with a specific postoperative complication (such as painful wire sutures) is assigned to the appropriate code(s) found in Chapter 19, Injury, poisoning, and certain other consequences of external causes. If appropriate, use additional code(s) from category G89 to identify acute or chronic pain (G89.18 or G89.28).

4) Chronic pain

Chronic pain is classified to subcategory G89.2. There is no time frame defining when pain becomes chronic pain. The provider's documentation should be used to guide use of these codes.

5) Neoplasm Related Pain

Code G89.3 is assigned to pain documented as being related, associated or due to cancer, primary or secondary malignancy, or tumor. This code is assigned regardless of whether the pain is acute or chronic.

This code may be assigned as the principal or first-listed code when the stated reason for the admission/encounter is documented as pain control/pain management. The underlying neoplasm should be reported as an additional diagnosis.

When the reason for the admission/encounter is management of the neoplasm and the pain associated with the neoplasm is also documented, code G89.3 may be assigned as an additional diagnosis. It is not necessary to assign an additional code for the site of the pain.

See Section I.C.2 for instructions on the sequencing of neoplasms for all other stated reasons for the admission/encounter (except for pain control/pain management).

6) Chronic pain syndrome

Central pain syndrome (G89.0) and chronic pain syndrome (G89.4) are different than the term "chronic pain," and therefore codes should only be used when the provider has specifically documented this condition.

See Section I.C.5. Pain disorders related to psychological factors

7. Chapter 7: Diseases of the Eye and Adnexa (H00-H59)

a. Glaucoma

1) Assigning Glaucoma Codes

Assign as many codes from category H40, Glaucoma, as needed to identify the type of glaucoma, the affected eye, and the glaucoma stage.

2) Bilateral glaucoma with same type and stage

When a patient has bilateral glaucoma and both eyes are documented as being the same type and stage, and there is a code for bilateral glaucoma, report only the code for the type of glaucoma, bilateral, with the seventh character for the stage.

When a patient has bilateral glaucoma and both eyes are documented as being the same type and stage, and the classification does not provide a code for bilateral glaucoma (i.e., subcategories H40.10, H40.11 and H40.20) report only one code for the type of glaucoma with the appropriate seventh character for the stage.

3) Bilateral glaucoma stage with different types or stages

When a patient has bilateral glaucoma and each eye is documented as having a different type or stage, and the classification distinguishes laterality, assign the appropriate code for each eye rather than the code for bilateral glaucoma.

When a patient has bilateral glaucoma and each eye is documented as having a different type, and the classification does not distinguish laterality (i.e., subcategories H40.10, H40.11 and H40.20), assign one code for each type of glaucoma with the appropriate 7th character for the stage.

When a patient has bilateral glaucoma and each eye is documented as having the same type, but different stage, and the classification does not distinguish laterality (i.e., subcategories H40.10, H40.11 and H40.20), assign a code for the type of glaucoma for each eye with the 7th character for the specific glaucoma stage documented for each eye.

4) Patient admitted with glaucoma and stage evolves during the admission

If a patient is admitted with glaucoma and the stage progresses during the admission, assign the code for highest stage documented.

5) Indeterminate stage glaucoma

Assignment of the 7th character "4" for "indeterminate stage" should be based on the clinical documentation. The 7th character "4" is used for glaucomas whose stage cannot be clinically determined. This 7th character should not be confused with the 7th character "0", unspecified, which should be assigned when there is no documentation regarding the stage of the glaucoma.

b. Blindness

If "blindness" or "low vision" of both eyes is documented but the visual impairment category is not documented, assign code H54.3, Unqualified visual loss, both eyes. If "blindness" or "low vision" in one eye is documented but the visual impairment category is not documented, assign a code from H54.6-, Unqualified visual loss, one eye. If "blindness" or "visual loss" is documented without any information about whether one or both eyes are affected, assign code H54.7, Unspecified visual loss.

8. Chapter 8: Diseases of the Ear and Mastoid Process (H60-H95)

Reserved for future guideline expansion

9. Chapter 9: Diseases of the Circulatory System (I00-I99)

a. Hypertension

The classification presumes a causal relationship between hypertension and heart involvement and between hypertension and kidney involvement, as the two conditions are linked by the term "with" in the Alphabetic Index. These conditions should be coded as related even in the absence of provider documentation explicitly linking them, unless the documentation clearly states the conditions are unrelated.

For hypertension and conditions not specifically linked by relational terms such as "with," "associated with" or "due to" in the classification, provider documentation must link the conditions in order to code them as related.

1) Hypertension with Heart Disease

Hypertension with heart conditions classified to I50.- or I51.4-I51.7, I51.89, I51.9, are assigned to, a code from category I11, Hypertensive heart disease. Use additional code(s) from category I50, Heart failure, to identify the type(s) of heart failure in those patients with heart failure.

The same heart conditions (I50.-, I51.4-I51.7, I51.89, I51.9) with hypertension are coded separately if the provider has documented they are unrelated to the hypertension. Sequence according to the circumstances of the admission/encounter.

2) Hypertensive Chronic Kidney Disease

Assign codes from category I12, Hypertensive chronic kidney disease, when both hypertension and a condition classifiable to category N18, Chronic kidney disease (CKD), are present. CKD should not be coded as hypertensive if the provider indicates the CKD is not related to the hypertension.

The appropriate code from category N18 should be used as a secondary code with a code from category I12 to identify the stage of chronic kidney disease.

See Section I.C.14. Chronic kidney disease.

If a patient has hypertensive chronic kidney disease and acute renal failure, the acute renal failure should also be coded. Sequence according to the circumstances of the admission/encounter.

3) Hypertensive Heart and Chronic Kidney Disease

Assign codes from combination category I13, Hypertensive heart and chronic kidney disease, when there is hypertension with both heart and kidney involvement. If heart failure is present, assign an additional code from category I50 to identify the type of heart failure.

The appropriate code from category N18, Chronic kidney disease, should be used as a secondary code with a code from category I13 to identify the stage of chronic kidney disease.

See Section I.C.14. Chronic kidney disease.

The codes in category I13, Hypertensive heart and chronic kidney disease, are combination codes that include hypertension, heart disease and chronic kidney disease. The Includes note at I13 specifies that the conditions included at I11 and I12 are included together in I13. If a patient has hypertension, heart disease and chronic kidney disease then a code from I13 should be used, not individual codes for hypertension, heart disease and chronic kidney disease, or codes from I11 or I12.

For patients with both acute renal failure and chronic kidney disease the acute renal failure should also be coded. Sequence according to the circumstances of the admission/encounter.

4) Hypertensive Cerebrovascular Disease

For hypertensive cerebrovascular disease, first assign the appropriate code from categories I60-I69, followed by the appropriate hypertension code.

5) Hypertensive Retinopathy

Subcategory H35.0, Background retinopathy and retinal vascular changes, should be used with a code from category I10 – I15, Hypertensive disease to include the systemic hypertension. The sequencing is based on the reason for the encounter.

6) Hypertension, Secondary

Secondary hypertension is due to an underlying condition. Two codes are required: one to identify the underlying etiology and one from category I15 to identify the hypertension. Sequencing of codes is determined by the reason for admission/encounter.

7) Hypertension, Transient

Assign code R03.0, Elevated blood pressure reading without diagnosis of hypertension, unless patient has an established diagnosis of hypertension. Assign code O13.-, Gestational [pregnancy-induced] hypertension without significant proteinuria, or O14.-, Pre-eclampsia, for transient hypertension of pregnancy.

8) Hypertension, Controlled

This diagnostic statement usually refers to an existing state of hypertension under control by therapy. Assign the appropriate code from categories I10-I15, Hypertensive diseases.

9) Hypertension, Uncontrolled

Uncontrolled hypertension may refer to untreated hypertension or hypertension not responding to current therapeutic regimen. In either case, assign the appropriate code from categories I10-I15, Hypertensive diseases.

10) Hypertensive Crisis

Assign a code from category I16, Hypertensive crisis, for documented hypertensive urgency, hypertensive emergency or unspecified hypertensive crisis. Code also any identified hypertensive disease (I10-I15). The sequencing is based on the reason for the encounter.

11) Pulmonary Hypertension

Pulmonary hypertension is classified to category I27, Other pulmonary heart diseases. For secondary pulmonary hypertension (I27.1, I27.2-), code also any associated conditions or adverse effects of drugs or toxins. The sequencing is based on the reason for the encounter, except for adverse effects of drugs.

See Section I.C.19.e

b. Atherosclerotic Coronary Artery Disease and Angina

ICD-10-CM has combination codes for atherosclerotic heart disease with angina pectoris. The subcategories for these codes are I25.11, Atherosclerotic heart disease of native coronary artery with angina pectoris and I25.7, Atherosclerosis of coronary artery bypass graft(s) and coronary artery of transplanted heart with angina pectoris.

When using one of these combination codes it is not necessary to use an additional code for angina pectoris. A causal relationship can be assumed in a patient with both atherosclerosis and angina pectoris, unless the documentation indicates the angina is due to something other than the atherosclerosis.

If a patient with coronary artery disease is admitted due to an acute myocardial infarction (AMI), the AMI should be sequenced before the coronary artery disease.

See Section I.C.9. Acute myocardial infarction (AMI)

c. Intraoperative and Postprocedural Cerebrovascular Accident

Medical record documentation should clearly specify the cause-and-effect relationship between the medical intervention and the cerebrovascular accident in order to assign a code for intraoperative or postprocedural cerebrovascular accident.

Proper code assignment depends on whether it was an infarction or hemorrhage and whether it occurred intraoperatively or postoperatively. If it was a cerebral hemorrhage, code assignment depends on the type of procedure performed.

d. Sequelae of Cerebrovascular Disease

1) Category I69, Sequelae of Cerebrovascular disease

Category I69 is used to indicate conditions classifiable to categories I60-I67 as the causes of sequela (neurologic deficits), themselves classified elsewhere. These "late effects" include neurologic deficits that persist after initial onset of conditions classifiable to categories I60-I67. The neurologic deficits caused by cerebrovascular disease may be present from the onset or may arise at any time after the onset of the condition classifiable to categories I60-I67.

Codes from category I69, Sequelae of cerebrovascular disease, that specify hemiplegia, hemiparesis and monoplegia identify whether the dominant or nondominant side is affected. Should the affected side be documented, but not specified as dominant or nondominant, and the classification system does not indicate a default, code selection is as follows:

- For ambidextrous patients, the default should be dominant.
- If the left side is affected, the default is non-dominant.
- If the right side is affected, the default is dominant.

2) Codes from category I69 with codes from I60-I67

Codes from category I69 may be assigned on a health care record with codes from I60-I67, if the patient has a current cerebrovascular disease and deficits from an old cerebrovascular disease.

3) Codes from category I69 and Personal history of transient ischemic attack (TIA) and cerebral infarction (Z86.73)

Codes from category I69 should not be assigned if the patient does not have neurologic deficits.

See Section I.C.21. 4. History (of) for use of personal history codes

e. Acute myocardial infarction (AMI)

1) Type 1 ST elevation myocardial infarction (STEMI) and non ST elevation myocardial infarction (NSTEMI)

The ICD-10-CM codes for type 1 acute myocardial infarction (AMI) identify the site, such as anterolateral wall or true posterior wall. Subcategories I21.0-I21.2 and code I21.3 are used for type 1 ST elevation myocardial infarction (STEMI). Code I21.4, Non-ST elevation (NSTEMI) myocardial infarction, is used for type 1 non ST elevation myocardial infarction (NSTEMI) and nontransmural MIs.

If a type 1 NSTEMI evolves to STEMI, assign the STEMI code. If a type 1 STEMI converts to NSTEMI due to thrombolytic therapy, it is still coded as STEMI.

For encounters occurring while the myocardial infarction is equal to, or less than, 4 weeks old, including transfers to another acute setting or a postacute setting, and the myocardial infarction meets the definition for "other diagnoses" (see Section III, Reporting Additional Diagnoses), codes from category I21 may continue to be reported. For encounters after the 4 week time frame and the patient is still receiving care related to the myocardial infarction, the appropriate aftercare code should be assigned, rather than a code from category I21. For old or healed myocardial infarctions not requiring further care, code I25.2, Old myocardial infarction, may be assigned.

2) Acute myocardial infarction, unspecified
Code I21.9, Acute myocardial infarction, unspecified, is the default for unspecified acute myocardial infarction or unspecified type. If only type 1 STEMI or transmural MI without the site is documented, assign code I21.3, ST elevation (STEMI) myocardial infarction of unspecified site.

3) AMI documented as nontransmural or subendocardial but site provided
If an AMI is documented as nontransmural or subendocardial, but the site is provided, it is still coded as a subendocardial AMI.

See Section I.C.21.3 for information on coding status post administration of tPA in a different facility within the last 24 hours.

4) Subsequent acute myocardial infarction
A code from category I22, Subsequent ST elevation (STEMI) and non ST elevation (NSTEMI) myocardial infarction, is to be used when a patient who has suffered a type 1 or unspecified AMI has a new AMI within the 4 week time frame of the initial AMI. A code from category I22 must be used in conjunction with a code from category I21. The sequencing of the I22 and I21 codes depends on the circumstances of the encounter.

Do not assign code I22 for subsequent myocardial infarctions other than type 1 or unspecified. For subsequent type 2 AMI assign only code I21.A1. For subsequent type 4 or type 5 AMI, assign only code I21.A9.

If a subsequent myocardial infarction of one type occurs within 4 weeks of a myocardial infarction of a different type, assign the appropriate codes from category I21 to identify each type. Do not assign a code from I22. Codes from category I22 should only be assigned if both the initial and subsequent myocardial infarctions are type 1 or unspecified.

5) Other Types of Myocardial Infarction
The ICD-10-CM provides codes for different types of myocardial infarction. Type 1 myocardial infarctions are assigned to codes I21.0-I21.4.

Type 2 myocardial infarction (myocardial infarction due to demand ischemia or secondary to ischemic imbalance) is assigned to code I21.A1, Myocardial infarction type 2 with the underlying cause coded first. Do not assign code I24.8, Other forms of acute ischemic heart disease, for the demand ischemia. If a type 2 AMI is described as NSTEMI or STEMI, only assign code I21.A1. Codes I21.01-I21.4 should only be assigned for type 1 AMIs.

Acute myocardial infarctions type 3, 4a, 4b, 4c, and 5 are assigned to code I21.A9, Other myocardial infarction type.

The "Code also" and "Code first" notes should be followed related to complications, and for coding of postprocedural myocardial infarctions during or following cardiac surgery.

10. Chapter 10: Diseases of the Respiratory System (J00-J99, U07.1)

a. Chronic Obstructive Pulmonary Disease [COPD] and Asthma

1) Acute exacerbation of chronic obstructive bronchitis and asthma
The codes in categories J44 and J45 distinguish between uncomplicated cases and those in acute exacerbation. An acute exacerbation is a worsening or a decompensation of a chronic condition. An acute exacerbation is not equivalent to an infection superimposed on a chronic condition, though an exacerbation may be triggered by an infection.

b. Acute Respiratory Failure

1) Acute respiratory failure as principal diagnosis
A code from subcategory J96.0, Acute respiratory failure, or subcategory J96.2, Acute and chronic respiratory failure, may be assigned as a principal diagnosis when it is the condition established after study to be chiefly responsible for occasioning the admission to the hospital, and the selection is supported by the Alphabetic Index and Tabular List. However, chapter-specific coding guidelines (such as obstetrics, poisoning, HIV, newborn) that provide sequencing direction take precedence.

2) Acute respiratory failure as secondary diagnosis
Respiratory failure may be listed as a secondary diagnosis if it occurs after admission, or if it is present on admission, but does not meet the definition of principal diagnosis.

3) Sequencing of acute respiratory failure and another acute condition
When a patient is admitted with respiratory failure and another acute condition (e.g., myocardial infarction, cerebrovascular accident, aspiration pneumonia), the principal diagnosis will not be the same in every situation. This applies whether the other acute condition is a respiratory or nonrespiratory condition. Selection of the principal diagnosis will be dependent on the circumstances of admission. If both the respiratory failure and the other acute condition are equally responsible for occasioning the admission to the hospital, and there are no chapter-specific sequencing rules, the guideline regarding two or more diagnoses that

equally meet the definition for principal diagnosis (Section II, C.) may be applied in these situations.

If the documentation is not clear as to whether acute respiratory failure and another condition are equally responsible for occasioning the admission, query the provider for clarification.

c. Influenza due to certain identified influenza viruses

Code only confirmed cases of influenza due to certain identified influenza viruses (category J09), and due to other identified influenza virus (category J10). This is an exception to the hospital inpatient guideline Section II, H. (Uncertain Diagnosis).

In this context, "confirmation" does not require documentation of positive laboratory testing specific for avian or other novel influenza A or other identified influenza virus. However, coding should be based on the provider's diagnostic statement that the patient has avian influenza, or other novel influenza A, for category J09, or has another particular identified strain of influenza, such as H1N1 or H3N2, but not identified as novel or variant, for category J10.

If the provider records "suspected" or "possible" or "probable" avian influenza, or novel influenza, or other identified influenza, then the appropriate influenza code from category J11, Influenza due to unidentified influenza virus, should be assigned. A code from category J09, Influenza due to certain identified influenza viruses, should not be assigned nor should a code from category J10, Influenza due to other identified influenza virus.

d. Ventilator associated Pneumonia

1) Documentation of Ventilator associated Pneumonia

As with all procedural or postprocedural complications, code assignment is based on the provider's documentation of the relationship between the condition and the procedure.

Code J95.851, Ventilator associated pneumonia, should be assigned only when the provider has documented ventilator associated pneumonia (VAP). An additional code to identify the organism (e.g., Pseudomonas aeruginosa, code B96.5) should also be assigned. Do not assign an additional code from categories J12-J18 to identify the type of pneumonia.

Code J95.851 should not be assigned for cases where the patient has pneumonia and is on a mechanical ventilator and the provider has not specifically stated that the pneumonia is ventilator-associated pneumonia. If the documentation is unclear as to whether the patient has a pneumonia that is a complication attributable to the mechanical ventilator, query the provider.

2) Ventilator associated Pneumonia Develops after Admission

A patient may be admitted with one type of pneumonia (e.g., code J13, Pneumonia due to Streptococcus pneumonia) and subsequently develop VAP. In this instance, the principal diagnosis would be the appropriate code from categories J12-J18 for the pneumonia diagnosed at the time of admission. Code J95.851, Ventilator associated pneumonia, would be assigned as an additional diagnosis when the provider has also documented the presence of ventilator associated pneumonia.

e. Vaping-related disorders

For patients presenting with condition(s) related to vaping, assign code U07.0, Vaping-related disorder, as the principal diagnosis. For lung injury due to vaping, assign only code U07.0. Assign additional codes for other manifestations, such as acute respiratory failure (subcategory J96.0-) or pneumonitis (code J68.0).

Associated respiratory signs and symptoms due to vaping, such as cough, shortness of breath, etc., are not coded separately, when a definitive diagnosis has been established. However, it would be appropriate to code separately any gastrointestinal symptoms, such as diarrhea and abdominal pain.

11. Chapter 11: Diseases of the Digestive System (K00-K95)

Reserved for future guideline expansion

12. Chapter 12: Diseases of the Skin and Subcutaneous Tissue (L00-L99)

a. Pressure ulcer stage codes

1) Pressure ulcer stages

Codes in category L89, Pressure ulcer, identify the site and stage of the pressure ulcer.

The ICD-10-CM classifies pressure ulcer stages based on severity, which is designated by stages 1-4, deep tissue pressure injury, unspecified stage, and unstageable.

Assign as many codes from category L89 as needed to identify all the pressure ulcers the patient has, if applicable.

See Section I.B.14 for pressure ulcer stage documentation by clinicians other than patient's provider

2) Unstageable pressure ulcers

Assignment of the code for unstageable pressure ulcer (L89.--0) should be based on the clinical documentation. These codes are used for pressure ulcers whose stage cannot be clinically determined (e.g., the ulcer is covered by eschar or has been treated with a skin or muscle graft). This code should not be confused with the codes for unspecified stage (L89.--9). When there is no documentation regarding the stage of the pressure ulcer, assign the appropriate code for unspecified stage (L89.9).

If during an encounter, the stage of an unstageable pressure ulcer is revealed after debridement, assign only the code for the stage revealed following debridement.

3) Documented pressure ulcer stage

Assignment of the pressure ulcer stage code should be guided by clinical documentation of the stage or documentation of the terms found in the Alphabetic Index. For clinical terms describing the stage that are not found in the Alphabetic Index, and there is no documentation of the stage, the provider should be queried.

4) Patients admitted with pressure ulcers documented as healed

No code is assigned if the documentation states that the pressure ulcer is completely healed at the time of admission.

5) Pressure ulcers documented as healing

Pressure ulcers described as healing should be assigned the appropriate pressure ulcer stage code based on the documentation in the medical record. If the documentation does not provide information about the stage of the healing pressure ulcer, assign the appropriate code for unspecified stage.

If the documentation is unclear as to whether the patient has a current (new) pressure ulcer or if the patient is being treated for a healing pressure ulcer, query the provider.

For ulcers that were present on admission but healed at the time of discharge, assign the code for the site and stage of the pressure ulcer at the time of admission.

6) Patient admitted with pressure ulcer evolving into another stage during the admission

If a patient is admitted to an inpatient hospital with a pressure ulcer at one stage and it progresses to a higher stage, two separate codes should be assigned: one code for the site and stage of the ulcer on admission and a second code for the same ulcer site and the highest stage reported during the stay.

7) Pressure-induced deep tissue damage

For pressure-induced deep tissue damage or deep tissue pressure injury, assign only the appropriate code for pressure-induced deep tissue damage (L89.--6).

b. Non-Pressure Chronic Ulcers

1) Patients admitted with non-pressure ulcers documented as healed

No code is assigned if the documentation states that the non-pressure ulcer is completely healed at the time of admission.

2) Non-pressure ulcers documented as healing

Non-pressure ulcers described as healing should be assigned the appropriate non-pressure ulcer code based on the documentation in the medical record. If the documentation does not provide information about the severity of the healing non-pressure ulcer, assign the appropriate code for unspecified severity.

If the documentation is unclear as to whether the patient has a current (new) non-pressure ulcer or if the patient is being treated for a healing non-pressure ulcer, query the provider.

For ulcers that were present on admission but healed at the time of discharge, assign the code for the site and severity of the non-pressure ulcer at the time of admission.

3) Patient admitted with non-pressure ulcer that progresses to another severity level during the admission

If a patient is admitted to an inpatient hospital with a non-pressure ulcer at one severity level and it progresses to a higher severity level, two separate codes should be assigned: one code for the site and severity level of the ulcer on admission and a second code for the same ulcer site and the highest severity level reported during the stay.

See Section I.B.14 for pressure ulcer stage documentation by clinicians other than patient's provider

13. Chapter 13: Diseases of the Musculoskeletal System and Connective Tissue (M00-M99)

a. Site and laterality

Most of the codes within Chapter 13 have site and laterality designations. The site represents the bone, joint or the muscle involved. For some conditions where more than one bone, joint or muscle is usually involved, such as osteoarthritis, there is a "multiple sites" code available. For categories where no multiple site code is provided and more than one bone, joint or muscle is involved, multiple codes should be used to indicate the different sites involved.

1) Bone versus joint

For certain conditions, the bone may be affected at the upper or lower end (e.g., avascular necrosis of bone, M87, Osteoporosis, M80, M81). Though the portion of the bone affected may be at the joint, the site designation will be the bone, not the joint.

b. Acute traumatic versus chronic or recurrent musculoskeletal conditions

Many musculoskeletal conditions are a result of previous injury or trauma to a site, or are recurrent conditions. Bone, joint or muscle conditions that are the result of a healed injury are usually found in Chapter 13. Recurrent bone, joint or muscle conditions are also usually found in Chapter 13. Any current, acute injury should be coded to the appropriate injury code from Chapter 19. Chronic or recurrent conditions should generally be coded with a code from Chapter 13. If it is difficult to determine from the documentation in the record which code is best to describe a condition, query the provider.

c. Coding of Pathologic Fractures

Seventh character A is for use as long as the patient is receiving active treatment for the fracture. While the patient may be seen by a new or different provider over the course of treatment for a pathological fracture, assignment of the 7th character is based on whether the patient is undergoing active treatment and not whether the provider is seeing the patient for the first time.

Seventh character, D is to be used for encounters after the patient has completed active treatment for the fracture and is receiving routine care for the fracture during the healing or recovery phase. The other 7th characters, listed under each subcategory in the Tabular List, are to be used for subsequent encounters for treatment of problems associated with the healing, such as malunions, nonunions, and sequelae.

Care for complications of surgical treatment for fracture repairs during the healing or recovery phase should be coded with the appropriate complication codes.

See Section I.C.19. Coding of traumatic fractures

d. Osteoporosis

Osteoporosis is a systemic condition, meaning that all bones of the musculoskeletal system are affected. Therefore, site is not a component of the codes under category M81, Osteoporosis without current pathological fracture. The site codes under category M80, Osteoporosis with current pathological fracture, identify the site of the fracture, not the osteoporosis.

1) Osteoporosis without pathological fracture

Category M81, Osteoporosis without current pathological fracture, is for use for patients with osteoporosis who do not currently have a pathologic fracture due to the osteoporosis, even if they have had a fracture in the past. For patients with a history of osteoporosis fractures, status code Z87.310, Personal history of (healed) osteoporosis fracture, should follow the code from M81.

2) Osteoporosis with current pathological fracture

Category M80, Osteoporosis with current pathological fracture, is for patients who have a current pathologic fracture at the time of an encounter. The codes under M80 identify the site of the fracture. A code from category M80, not a traumatic fracture code, should be used for any patient with known osteoporosis who suffers a fracture, even if the patient had a minor fall or trauma, if that fall or trauma would not usually break a normal, healthy bone.

e. Multisystem Inflammatory Syndrome

See Section I.C.1.g.1.l for Multisystem Inflammatory Syndrome

14. Chapter 14: Diseases of Genitourinary System (N00-N99)

a. Chronic kidney disease

1) Stages of chronic kidney disease (CKD)

The ICD-10-CM classifies CKD based on severity. The severity of CKD is designated by stages 1-5. Stage 2, code N18.2, equates to mild CKD; stage 3, codes N18.30-N18.32, equate to moderate CKD; and stage 4, code N18.4, equates to severe CKD. Code N18.6, End stage renal disease (ESRD), is assigned when the provider has documented end-stage-renal disease (ESRD).

If both a stage of CKD and ESRD are documented, assign code N18.6 only.

2) Chronic kidney disease and kidney transplant status

Patients who have undergone kidney transplant may still have some form of chronic kidney disease (CKD) because the kidney transplant may not fully restore kidney function. Therefore, the presence of CKD alone does not constitute a transplant complication. Assign the appropriate N18 code for the patient's stage of CKD and code Z94.0, Kidney transplant status. If a transplant complication such as failure or rejection or other transplant complication is documented, see Section I.C.19.g for information on coding complications of a kidney transplant. If the documentation is unclear as to whether the patient has a complication of the transplant, query the provider.

3) Chronic kidney disease with other conditions

Patients with CKD may also suffer from other serious conditions, most commonly diabetes mellitus and hypertension. The sequencing of the CKD code in relationship to codes for other contributing conditions is based on the conventions in the Tabular List.

See I.C.9. Hypertensive chronic kidney disease.
See I.C.19. Chronic kidney disease and kidney transplant complications.

15. Chapter 15: Pregnancy, Childbirth, and the Puerperium (O00-O9A)

a. General Rules for Obstetric Cases

1) Codes from chapter 15 and sequencing priority

Obstetric cases require codes from chapter 15, codes in the range O00-O9A, Pregnancy, Childbirth, and the Puerperium. Chapter 15 codes have sequencing priority over codes from other chapters. Additional codes from other chapters may be used in conjunction with chapter 15 codes to further specify conditions. Should the provider document that the pregnancy is incidental to the encounter, then code Z33.1, Pregnant state, incidental, should be used in place of any chapter 15 codes. It is the provider's responsibility to state that the condition being treated is not affecting the pregnancy.

2) Chapter 15 codes used only on the maternal record

Chapter 15 codes are to be used only on the maternal record, never on the record of the newborn.

3) Final character for trimester

The majority of codes in Chapter 15 have a final character indicating the trimester of pregnancy. The timeframes for the trimesters are indicated at the beginning of the chapter. If trimester is not a component of a code it is because the condition always occurs in a specific trimester, or the concept of trimester of pregnancy is not applicable. Certain codes have characters for only certain trimesters because the condition does not occur in all trimesters, but it may occur in more than just one.

Assignment of the final character for trimester should be based on the provider's documentation of the trimester (or number of weeks) for the current admission/encounter. This applies to the assignment of trimester for pre-existing conditions as well as those that develop during or are due to the pregnancy. The provider's documentation of the number of weeks may be used to assign the appropriate code identifying the trimester.

Whenever delivery occurs during the current admission, and there is an "in childbirth" option for the obstetric complication being coded, the "in childbirth" code should be assigned.

When the classification does not provide an obstetric code with an "in childbirth" option, it is appropriate to assign a code describing the current trimester.

4) Selection of trimester for inpatient admissions that encompass more than one trimester

In instances when a patient is admitted to a hospital for complications of pregnancy during one trimester and remains in the hospital into a subsequent trimester, the trimester character for the antepartum complication code should be assigned on the basis of the trimester when the complication developed, not the trimester of the discharge. If the condition developed prior to the current admission/encounter or represents a pre-existing condition, the trimester character for the trimester at the time of the admission/encounter should be assigned.

5) Unspecified trimester

Each category that includes codes for trimester has a code for "unspecified trimester." The "unspecified trimester" code should rarely be used, such as when the documentation in the record is insufficient to determine the trimester and it is not possible to obtain clarification.

6) 7th character for fetus identification

Where applicable, a 7th character is to be assigned for certain categories (O31, O32, O33.3 - O33.6, O35, O36, O40, O41, O60.1, O60.2, O64, and O69) to identify the fetus for which the complication code applies.

Assign 7th character "0":
- For single gestations
- When the documentation in the record is insufficient to determine the fetus affected and it is not possible to obtain clarification.
- When it is not possible to clinically determine which fetus is affected.

7) Completed weeks of gestation

In ICD-10-CM, "completed" weeks of gestation refers to full weeks. For example, if the provider documents gestation at 39 weeks and 6 days, the code for 39 weeks of gestation should be assigned, as the patient has not yet reached 40 completed weeks.

b. Selection of OB Principal or First-listed Diagnosis

1) Routine outpatient prenatal visits

For routine outpatient prenatal visits when no complications are present, a code from category Z34, Encounter for supervision of normal pregnancy, should be used as the first-listed diagnosis. These codes should not be used in conjunction with chapter 15 codes.

2) Supervision of High-Risk Pregnancy

Codes from category O09, Supervision of high-risk pregnancy, are intended for use only during the prenatal period. For complications during the labor or delivery episode as a result of a high-risk pregnancy, assign the applicable complication codes from chapter 15. If there are no complications during the labor or delivery episode, assign code O80, Encounter for full-term uncomplicated delivery.

For routine prenatal outpatient visits for patients with high-risk pregnancies, a code from category O09, Supervision of high-risk pregnancy, should be used as the first-listed diagnosis. Secondary Chapter 15 codes may be used in conjunction with these codes if appropriate.

3) Episodes when no delivery occurs

In episodes when no delivery occurs, the principal diagnosis should correspond to the principal complication of the pregnancy which necessitated the encounter. Should more than one complication exist, all of which are treated or monitored, any of the complication codes may be sequenced first.

4) When a delivery occurs

When an obstetric patient is admitted and delivers during that admission, the condition that prompted the admission should be sequenced as the principal diagnosis. If multiple conditions prompted the admission, sequence the one most related to the delivery as the principal diagnosis. A code for any complication of the delivery should be assigned as an additional diagnosis. In cases of cesarean delivery, if the patient was admitted with a condition that resulted in the performance of a cesarean procedure, that condition should be selected as the principal diagnosis. If the reason for the admission was unrelated to the condition resulting in the cesarean delivery, the condition related to the reason for the admission should be selected as the principal diagnosis.

5) Outcome of delivery

A code from category Z37, Outcome of delivery, should be included on every maternal record when a delivery has occurred. These codes are not to be used on subsequent records or on the newborn record.

c. Pre-existing conditions versus conditions due to the pregnancy

Certain categories in Chapter 15 distinguish between conditions of the mother that existed prior to pregnancy (pre-existing) and those that are a direct result of pregnancy. When assigning codes from Chapter 15, it is important to assess if a condition was pre-existing prior to pregnancy or developed during or due to the pregnancy in order to assign the correct code.

Categories that do not distinguish between pre-existing and pregnancy-related conditions may be used for either. It is acceptable to use codes specifically for the puerperium with codes complicating pregnancy and childbirth if a condition arises postpartum during the delivery encounter.

d. Pre-existing hypertension in pregnancy

Category O10, Pre-existing hypertension complicating pregnancy, childbirth and the puerperium, includes codes for hypertensive heart and hypertensive chronic kidney disease. When assigning one of the O10 codes that includes hypertensive heart disease or hypertensive chronic kidney disease, it is necessary to add a secondary code from the appropriate hypertension category to specify the type of heart failure or chronic kidney disease.

See Section I.C.9. Hypertension.

e. Fetal Conditions Affecting the Management of the Mother

1) Codes from categories O35 and O36

Codes from categories O35, Maternal care for known or suspected fetal abnormality and damage, and O36, Maternal care for other fetal problems, are assigned only when the fetal condition is actually responsible for modifying the management of the mother, i.e., by requiring diagnostic studies, additional observation, special care, or termination of pregnancy. The fact that the fetal condition exists does not justify assigning a code from this series to the mother's record.

2) In utero surgery

In cases when surgery is performed on the fetus, a diagnosis code from category O35, Maternal care for known or suspected fetal abnormality and damage, should be assigned identifying the fetal condition. Assign the appropriate procedure code for the procedure performed.

No code from Chapter 16, the perinatal codes, should be used on the mother's record to identify fetal conditions. Surgery performed in utero on a fetus is still to be coded as an obstetric encounter.

f. HIV Infection in Pregnancy, Childbirth and the Puerperium

During pregnancy, childbirth or the puerperium, a patient admitted because of an HIV-related illness should receive a principal diagnosis from subcategory O98.7-, Human immunodeficiency [HIV] disease complicating pregnancy, childbirth and the puerperium, followed by the code(s) for the HIV-related illness(es).

Patients with asymptomatic HIV infection status admitted during pregnancy, childbirth, or the puerperium should receive codes of O98.7- and Z21, Asymptomatic human immunodeficiency virus [HIV] infection status.

g. Diabetes mellitus in pregnancy

Diabetes mellitus is a significant complicating factor in pregnancy. Pregnant patients who are diabetic should be assigned a code from category O24, Diabetes mellitus in pregnancy, childbirth, and the puerperium, first, followed by the appropriate diabetes code(s) (E08-E13) from Chapter 4.

h. Longterm use of insulin and oral hypoglycemics

See section I.C.4.a.3 for information on the longterm use of insulin and oral hypoglycemics.

i. Gestational (pregnancy induced) diabetes

Gestational (pregnancy induced) diabetes can occur during the second and third trimester of pregnancy in patients who were not diabetic prior to pregnancy. Gestational diabetes can cause complications in the pregnancy similar to those of pre-existing diabetes mellitus. It also puts the patient at greater risk of developing diabetes after the pregnancy. Codes for gestational diabetes are in subcategory O24.4, Gestational diabetes mellitus. No other code from category O24, Diabetes mellitus in pregnancy, childbirth, and the puerperium, should be used with a code from O24.4.

The codes under subcategory O24.4 include diet controlled, insulin controlled, and controlled by oral hypoglycemic drugs. If a patient with gestational diabetes is treated with both diet and insulin, only the code for insulin-controlled is required. If a patient with gestational diabetes is treated with both diet and oral hypoglycemic medications, only the code for "controlled by oral hypoglycemic drugs" is required. Codes Z79.4, Long-term (current) use of insulin, Z79.84, Long-term (current) use of oral hypoglycemic drugs, **and Z79.85, Long-term (current) use of injectable non-insulin antidiabetic drugs,** should not be assigned with codes from subcategory O24.4.

An abnormal glucose tolerance in pregnancy is assigned a code from subcategory O99.81, Abnormal glucose complicating pregnancy, childbirth, and the puerperium.

j. Sepsis and septic shock complicating abortion, pregnancy, childbirth and the puerperium

When assigning a chapter 15 code for sepsis complicating abortion, pregnancy, childbirth, and the puerperium, a code for the specific type of infection should be assigned as an additional diagnosis. If severe sepsis is present, a code from subcategory R65.2, Severe sepsis, and code(s) for associated organ dysfunction(s) should also be assigned as additional diagnoses.

k. Puerperal sepsis

Code O85, Puerperal sepsis, should be assigned with a secondary code to identify the causal organism (e.g., for a bacterial infection, assign a code from category B95-B96, Bacterial infections in conditions classified elsewhere). A code from category A40, Streptococcal sepsis, or A41, Other sepsis, should not be used for puerperal sepsis. If applicable, use additional codes to identify severe sepsis (R65.2-) and any associated acute organ dysfunction.

Code O85 should not be assigned for sepsis following an obstetrical procedure (See Section I.C.1.d.5.b., Sepsis due to a postprocedural infection).

l. Alcohol, tobacco and drug use during pregnancy, childbirth and the puerperium

1) Alcohol use during pregnancy, childbirth and the puerperium

Codes under subcategory O99.31, Alcohol use complicating pregnancy, childbirth, and the puerperium, should be assigned for any pregnancy case when a patient uses alcohol during the pregnancy or postpartum. A secondary code from category F10, Alcohol related disorders, should also be assigned to identify manifestations of the alcohol use.

2) Tobacco use during pregnancy, childbirth and the puerperium

Codes under subcategory O99.33, Smoking (tobacco) complicating pregnancy, childbirth, and the puerperium, should be assigned for any pregnancy case when a patient uses any type of tobacco product during the pregnancy or postpartum. A secondary code from category F17, Nicotine dependence, should also be assigned to identify the type of nicotine dependence.

3) Drug use during pregnancy, childbirth and the puerperium

Codes under subcategory O99.32, Drug use complicating pregnancy, childbirth, and the puerperium, should be assigned for any pregnancy case when a patient uses drugs during the pregnancy or postpartum. This can involve illegal drugs, or inappropriate use or abuse of prescription drugs. Secondary code(s) from categories F11-F16 and F18-F19 should also be assigned to identify manifestations of the drug use.

m. Poisoning, toxic effects, adverse effects and underdosing in a pregnant patient

A code from subcategory O9A.2, Injury, poisoning and certain other consequences of external causes complicating pregnancy, childbirth, and the puerperium, should be sequenced first, followed by the appropriate injury, poisoning, toxic effect, adverse effect or underdosing code, and then the additional code(s) that specifies the condition caused by the poisoning, toxic effect, adverse effect or underdosing.

See Section I.C.19. Adverse effects, poisoning, underdosing and toxic effects.

n. Normal Delivery, Code O80

1) Encounter for full term uncomplicated delivery

Code O80 should be assigned when a patient is admitted for a full-term normal delivery and delivers a single, healthy infant without any complications antepartum, during the delivery, or postpartum during the delivery episode. Code O80 is always a principal diagnosis. It is not to be used if any other code from chapter 15 is needed to describe a current complication of the antenatal, delivery, or postnatal period. Additional codes from other chapters may be used with code O80 if they are not related to or are in any way complicating the pregnancy.

2) Uncomplicated delivery with resolved antepartum complication

Code O80 may be used if the patient had a complication at some point during the pregnancy, but the complication is not present at the time of the admission for delivery.

3) Outcome of delivery for O80

Z37.0, Single live birth, is the only outcome of delivery code appropriate for use with O80.

o. The Peripartum and Postpartum Periods

1) Peripartum and Postpartum periods

The postpartum period begins immediately after delivery and continues for six weeks following delivery. The peripartum period is defined as the last month of pregnancy to five months postpartum.

2) Peripartum and postpartum complication

A postpartum complication is any complication occurring within the six week period.

3) Pregnancy-related complications after 6-week period

Chapter 15 codes may also be used to describe pregnancy-related complications after the peripartum or postpartum period if the provider documents that a condition is pregnancy related.

4) Admission for routine postpartum care following delivery outside hospital

When the mother delivers outside the hospital prior to admission and is admitted for routine postpartum care and no complications are noted, code Z39.0, Encounter for care and examination of mother immediately after delivery, should be assigned as the principal diagnosis.

5) Pregnancy associated cardiomyopathy

Pregnancy associated cardiomyopathy, code O90.3, is unique in that it may be diagnosed in the third trimester of pregnancy but may continue to progress months after delivery. For this reason, it is referred to as peripartum cardiomyopathy. Code O90.3 is only for use when the cardiomyopathy develops as a result of pregnancy in a patient who did not have pre-existing heart disease.

p. Code O94, Sequelae of complication of pregnancy, childbirth, and the puerperium

1) Code O94

Code O94, Sequelae of complication of pregnancy, childbirth, and the puerperium, is for use in those cases when an initial complication of a pregnancy develops a sequela or sequelae requiring care or treatment at a future date.

2) After the initial postpartum period

This code may be used at any time after the initial postpartum period.

3) Sequencing of Code O94

This code, like all sequela codes, is to be sequenced following the code describing the sequelae of the complication.

q. Termination of Pregnancy and Spontaneous abortions

1) Abortion with Liveborn Fetus

When an attempted termination of pregnancy results in a liveborn fetus assign code Z33.2, Encounter for elective termination of pregnancy and a code from category Z37, Outcome of Delivery.

2) Retained Products of Conception following an abortion

Subsequent encounters for retained products of conception following a spontaneous abortion or elective termination of pregnancy, without complications are assigned O03.4, Incomplete spontaneous abortion without complication or code O07.4, Failed attempted termination of pregnancy without complication. This advice is appropriate even when the patient was discharged previously with a discharge diagnosis of complete abortion. If the patient has a specific complication associated with the spontaneous abortion or elective termination of pregnancy in addition to retained products of conception, assign the appropriate complication code (e.g., O03.-, O04.-, O07.-) instead of code O03.4 or O07.4

3) Complications leading to abortion

Codes from chapter 15 may be used as additional codes to identify any documented complications of the pregnancy in conjunction with codes in categories in O04, O07 and O08.

4) Hemorrhage following elective abortion

For hemorrhage post elective abortion, assign code O04.6, Delayed or excessive hemorrhage following (induced) termination of pregnancy. Do not assign code O72.1, Other immediate postpartum hemorrhage, as this code should not be assigned for post abortion conditions. Do not assign code Z33.2, Encounter for elective termination of pregnancy, when the patient experiences a complication post elective abortion.

r. Abuse in a pregnant patient

For suspected or confirmed cases of abuse of a pregnant patient, a code(s) from subcategories O9A.3, Physical abuse complicating pregnancy, childbirth, and the puerperium, O9A.4, Sexual abuse complicating pregnancy, childbirth, and the puerperium, and O9A.5, Psychological abuse complicating pregnancy, childbirth, and the puerperium, should be sequenced first, followed by the appropriate codes (if applicable) to identify any associated current injury due to physical abuse, sexual abuse, and the perpetrator of abuse.

See Section I.C.19. Adult and child abuse, neglect and other maltreatment.

s. COVID-19 infection in pregnancy, childbirth, and the puerperium

During pregnancy, childbirth or the puerperium, when COVID-19 is the reason for admission/ encounter, code O98.5-, Other viral diseases complicating pregnancy, childbirth and the puerperium, should be sequenced as the principal/ first-listed diagnosis, and code U07.1, COVID-19, and the appropriate codes for associated manifestation(s) should be assigned as additional diagnoses. Codes from Chapter 15 always take sequencing priority.

If the reason for admission/encounter is unrelated to COVID-19 but the patient tests positive for COVID-19 during the admission/ encounter, the appropriate code for the reason for admission/encounter should be sequenced as the principal/first-listed diagnosis, and codes O98.5- and U07.1, as well as the appropriate codes for associated COVID-19 manifestations, should be assigned as additional diagnoses.

16. Chapter 16: Certain Conditions Originating in the Perinatal Period (P00-P96)

For coding and reporting purposes the perinatal period is defined as before birth through the 28th day following birth. The following guidelines are provided for reporting purposes

a. General Perinatal Rules

1) Use of Chapter 16 Codes

Codes in this chapter are never for use on the maternal record. Codes from Chapter 15, the obstetric chapter, are never permitted on the newborn record.

Chapter 16 codes may be used throughout the life of the patient if the condition is still present.

2) Principal Diagnosis for Birth Record

When coding the birth episode in a newborn record, assign a code from category Z38, Liveborn infants according to place of birth and type of delivery, as the principal diagnosis. A code from category Z38 is assigned only once, to a newborn at the time of birth. If a newborn is transferred to another institution, a code from category Z38 should not be used at the receiving hospital.

A code from category Z38 is used only on the newborn record, not on the mother's record.

3) Use of Codes from other Chapters with Codes from Chapter 16

Codes from other chapters may be used with codes from chapter 16 if the codes from the other chapters provide more specific detail. Codes for signs and symptoms may be assigned when a definitive diagnosis has not been established. If the reason for the encounter is a perinatal condition, the code from chapter 16 should be sequenced first.

4) Use of Chapter 16 Codes after the Perinatal Period

Should a condition originate in the perinatal period, and continue throughout the life of the patient, the perinatal code should continue to be used regardless of the patient's age.

5) Birth process or community acquired conditions

If a newborn has a condition that may be either due to the birth process or community acquired and the documentation does not indicate which it is, the default is due to the birth process and the code from Chapter 16 should be used. If the condition is community-acquired, a code from Chapter 16 should not be assigned.

For COVID-19 infection in a newborn, see guideline I.C.16.h.

6) Code all clinically significant conditions

All clinically significant conditions noted on routine newborn examination should be coded. A condition is clinically significant if it requires:

- clinical evaluation; or
- therapeutic treatment; or
- diagnostic procedures; or
- extended length of hospital stay; or
- increased nursing care and/or monitoring; or
- has implications for future health care needs

Note: The perinatal guidelines listed above are the same as the general coding guidelines for "additional diagnoses," except for the final point regarding implications for future health care needs. Codes should be assigned for conditions that have been specified by the provider as having implications for future health care needs.

b. Observation and Evaluation of Newborns for Suspected Conditions not Found

1) Use of Z05 codes

Assign a code from category Z05, Observation and evaluation of newborn for suspected **diseases and** conditions ruled out, to identify those instances when a healthy newborn is evaluated for a suspected condition/**disease** that is determined after study not to be present. Do not use a code from category Z05 when the patient **is documented to have** signs or symptoms of a suspected problem; in such cases code the sign or symptom.

2) Z05 on other than the birth record
A code from category Z05 may also be assigned as a principal or firstlisted code for readmissions or encounters when the code from category Z38 code no longer applies. Codes from category Z05 are for use only for healthy newborns and infants for which no condition after study is found to be present.

3) Z05 on a birth record
A code from category Z05 is to be used as a secondary code after the code from category Z38, Liveborn infants according to place of birth and type of delivery.

c. Coding Additional Perinatal Diagnoses
1) Assigning codes for conditions that require treatment
Assign codes for conditions that require treatment or further investigation, prolong the length of stay, or require resource utilization.

2) Codes for conditions specified as having implications for future health care needs
Assign codes for conditions that have been specified by the provider as having implications for future health care needs.

Note: This guideline should not be used for adult patients.

d. Prematurity and Fetal Growth Retardation
Providers utilize different criteria in determining prematurity. A code for prematurity should not be assigned unless it is documented. Assignment of codes in categories P05, Disorders of newborn related to slow fetal growth and fetal malnutrition, and P07, Disorders of newborn related to short gestation and low birth weight, not elsewhere classified, should be based on the recorded birth weight and estimated gestational age.

When both birth weight and gestational age are available, two codes from category P07 should be assigned, with the code for birth weight sequenced before the code for gestational age.

e. Low birth weight and immaturity status
Codes from category P07, Disorders of newborn related to short gestation and low birth weight, not elsewhere classified, are for use for a child or adult who was premature or had a low birth weight as a newborn and this is affecting the patient's current health status.

See Section I.C.21. Factors influencing health status and contact with health services, Status.

f. Bacterial Sepsis of Newborn
Category P36, Bacterial sepsis of newborn, includes congenital sepsis. If a perinate is documented as having sepsis without documentation of congenital or community acquired, the default is congenital and a code from category P36 should

be assigned. If the P36 code includes the causal organism, an additional code from category B95, Streptococcus, Staphylococcus, and Enterococcus as the cause of diseases classified elsewhere, or B96, Other bacterial agents as the cause of diseases classified elsewhere, should not be assigned. If the P36 code does not include the causal organism, assign an additional code from category B96. If applicable, use additional codes to identify severe sepsis (R65.2-) and any associated acute organ dysfunction.

g. Stillbirth
Code P95, Stillbirth, is only for use in institutions that maintain separate records for stillbirths. No other code should be used with P95. Code P95 should not be used on the mother's record.

h. COVID-19 Infection in Newborn
For a newborn that tests positive for COVID-19, assign code U07.1, COVID-19, and the appropriate codes for associated manifestation(s) in neonates/newborns in the absence of documentation indicating a specific type of transmission. For a newborn that tests positive for COVID-19 and the provider documents the condition was contracted in utero or during the birth process, assign codes P35.8, Other congenital viral diseases, and U07.1, COVID-19. When coding the birth episode in a newborn record, the appropriate code from category Z38, Liveborn infants according to place of birth and type of delivery, should be assigned as the principal diagnosis.

17. **Chapter 17: Congenital malformations, deformations, and chromosomal abnormalities (Q00-Q99)**
Assign an appropriate code(s) from categories Q00-Q99, Congenital malformations, deformations, and chromosomal abnormalities when a malformation/deformation or chromosomal abnormality is documented. A malformation/deformation/or chromosomal abnormality may be the principal/first-listed diagnosis on a record or a secondary diagnosis.

When a malformation/deformation/or chromosomal abnormality does not have a unique code assignment, assign additional code(s) for any manifestations that may be present.

When the code assignment specifically identifies the malformation/deformation/or chromosomal abnormality, manifestations that are an inherent component of the anomaly should not be coded separately. Additional codes should be assigned for manifestations that are not an inherent component.

Codes from Chapter 17 may be used throughout the life of the patient. If a congenital malformation or deformity has been corrected, a personal history code should be used to identify the history of the malformation or deformity. Although present at birth, a malformation/deformation/or chromosomal abnormality may not be identified until later in life. Whenever the condition is diagnosed by the provider, it is appropriate to assign a code from codes Q00-Q99.

For the birth admission, the appropriate code from category Z38, Liveborn infants, according to place of birth and type of delivery, should be sequenced as the principal diagnosis, followed by any congenital anomaly codes, Q00-Q99.

18. **Chapter 18: Symptoms, signs, and abnormal clinical and laboratory findings, not elsewhere classified (R00-R99)**

Chapter 18 includes symptoms, signs, abnormal results of clinical or other investigative procedures, and ill-defined conditions regarding which no diagnosis classifiable elsewhere is recorded. Signs and symptoms that point to a specific diagnosis have been assigned to a category in other chapters of the classification.

a. Use of symptom codes

Codes that describe symptoms and signs are acceptable for reporting purposes when a related definitive diagnosis has not been established (confirmed) by the provider.

b. Use of a symptom code with a definitive diagnosis code

Codes for signs and symptoms may be reported in addition to a related definitive diagnosis when the sign or symptom is not routinely associated with that diagnosis, such as the various signs and symptoms associated with complex syndromes. The definitive diagnosis code should be sequenced before the symptom code.

Signs or symptoms that are associated routinely with a disease process should not be assigned as additional codes, unless otherwise instructed by the classification.

c. Combination codes that include symptoms

ICD-10-CM contains a number of combination codes that identify both the definitive diagnosis and common symptoms of that diagnosis. When using one of these combination codes, an additional code should not be assigned for the symptom.

d. Repeated falls

Code R29.6, Repeated falls, is for use for encounters when a patient has recently fallen and the reason for the fall is being investigated.

Code Z91.81, History of falling, is for use when a patient has fallen in the past and is at risk for future falls. When appropriate, both codes R29.6 and Z91.81 may be assigned together.

e. Coma

Code R40.20, Unspecified coma, may be assigned in conjunction with codes for any medical condition.

Do not report codes for unspecified coma, individual or total Glasgow coma scale scores for a patient with a medically induced coma or a sedated patient.

1) Coma Scale

The coma scale codes (R40.21- to R40.24-) can be used in conjunction with traumatic brain injury codes. These codes are primarily for use by trauma registries, but they may be used in any setting where this information is collected. The coma scale codes should be sequenced after the diagnosis code(s).

These codes, one from each subcategory, are needed to complete the scale. The 7th character indicates when the scale was recorded. The 7th character should match for all three codes.

At a minimum, report the initial score documented on presentation at your facility. This may be a score from the emergency medicine technician (EMT) or in the emergency department. If desired, a facility may choose to capture multiple coma scale scores.

Assign code R40.24-, Glasgow coma scale, total score, when only the total score is documented in the medical record and not the individual score(s).

If multiple coma scores are captured within the first 24 hours after hospital admission, assign only the code for the score at the time of admission. ICD-10-CM does not classify coma scores that are reported after admission but less than 24 hours later.

See Section I.B.14. for coma scale documentation by clinicians other than patient's provider

f. Functional quadriplegia

GUIDELINE HAS BEEN DELETED EFFECTIVE OCTOBER 1, 2017

g. SIRS due to Non-Infectious Process

The systemic inflammatory response syndrome (SIRS) can develop as a result of certain non-infectious disease processes, such as trauma, malignant neoplasm, or pancreatitis. When SIRS is documented with a noninfectious condition, and no subsequent infection is documented, the code for the underlying condition, such as an injury, should be assigned, followed by code R65.10, Systemic inflammatory response syndrome (SIRS) of non-infectious origin without acute organ dysfunction, or code R65.11, Systemic inflammatory response syndrome (SIRS) of non-infectious origin with acute organ dysfunction. If an associated acute organ dysfunction is documented, the appropriate code(s) for the specific type of organ dysfunction(s) should be assigned in addition to code R65.11. If acute organ dysfunction is documented, but it cannot be determined if the acute organ dysfunction is associated with SIRS or due to another condition (e.g., directly due to the trauma), the provider should be queried.

h. Death NOS

Code R99, Ill-defined and unknown cause of mortality, is only for use in the very limited circumstance when a patient who has already died is brought into an emergency department or other healthcare facility and is pronounced dead upon arrival. It does not represent the discharge disposition of death.

i. NIHSS Stroke Scale

The NIH stroke scale (NIHSS) codes (R29.7- -) can be used in conjunction with acute stroke codes (I63) to identify the patient's neurological status and the severity of the stroke. The stroke scale codes should be sequenced after the acute stroke diagnosis code(s).

At a minimum, report the initial score documented. If desired, a facility may choose to capture multiple stroke scale scores.

See Section I.B.14 for NIHSS stroke scale documentation by clinicians other than patient's provider

19. **Chapter 19: Injury, poisoning, and certain other consequences of external causes (S00-T88)**

   a. **Application of 7th Characters in Chapter 19**
   Most categories in chapter 19 have a 7th character requirement for each applicable code. Most categories in this chapter have three 7th character values (with the exception of fractures): A, initial encounter, D, subsequent encounter and S, sequela. Categories for traumatic fractures have additional 7th character values. While the patient may be seen by a new or different provider over the course of treatment for an injury, assignment of the 7th character is based on whether the patient is undergoing active treatment and not whether the provider is seeing the patient for the first time.

   For complication codes, active treatment refers to treatment for the condition described by the code, even though it may be related to an earlier precipitating problem. For example, code T84.50XA, Infection and inflammatory reaction due to unspecified internal joint prosthesis, initial encounter, is used when active treatment is provided for the infection, even though the condition relates to the prosthetic device, implant or graft that was placed at a previous encounter.

   7th character "A", initial encounter is used for each encounter where the patient is receiving active treatment for the condition.

   7th character "D" subsequent encounter is used for encounters after the patient has completed active treatment of the condition and is receiving routine care for the condition during the healing or recovery phase.

   The aftercare Z codes should not be used for aftercare for conditions such as injuries or poisonings, where 7th characters are provided to identify subsequent care. For example, for aftercare of an injury, assign the acute injury code with the 7th character "D" (subsequent encounter).

   7th character "S", sequela, is for use for complications or conditions that arise as a direct result of a condition, such as scar formation after a burn. The scars are sequelae of the burn. When using 7th character "S", it is necessary to use both the injury code that precipitated the sequela and the code for the sequela itself. The "S" is added only to the injury code, not the sequela code. The 7th character "S" identifies the injury responsible for the sequela. The specific type of sequela (e.g., scar) is sequenced first, followed by the injury code.
   See Section I.B.10. Sequelae, (Late Effects)

   b. **Coding of Injuries**
   When coding injuries, assign separate codes for each injury unless a combination code is provided, in which case the combination code is assigned. Codes from category T07, Unspecified multiple injuries should not be assigned in the inpatient setting unless information for a more specific code is not available. Traumatic injury codes (S00-T14.9) are not to be used for normal, healing surgical wounds or to identify complications of surgical wounds.

   The code for the most serious injury, as determined by the provider and the focus of treatment, is sequenced first.

   1) **Superficial injuries**
   Superficial injuries such as abrasions or contusions are not coded when associated with more severe injuries of the same site.

   2) **Primary injury with damage to nerves/ blood vessels**
   When a primary injury results in minor damage to peripheral nerves or blood vessels, the primary injury is sequenced first with additional code(s) for injuries to nerves and spinal cord (such as category S04), and/or injury to blood vessels (such as category S15). When the primary injury is to the blood vessels or nerves, that injury should be sequenced first.

   3) **Iatrogenic injuries**
   Injury codes from Chapter 19 should not be assigned for injuries that occur during, or as a result of, a medical intervention. Assign the appropriate complication code(s).

   c. **Coding of Traumatic Fractures**
   The principles of multiple coding of injuries should be followed in coding fractures. Fractures of specified sites are coded individually by site in accordance with both the provisions within categories S02, S12, S22, S32, S42, S49, S52, S59, S62, S72, S79, S82, S89, S92 and the level of detail furnished by medical record content.

   A fracture not indicated as open or closed should be coded to closed. A fracture not indicated whether displaced or not displaced should be coded to displaced.

   More specific guidelines are as follows:

   1) **Initial vs. subsequent encounter for fractures**
   Traumatic fractures are coded using the appropriate 7th character for initial encounter (A, B, C) for each encounter where the patient is receiving active treatment for the fracture. The appropriate 7th character for initial encounter should also be assigned for a patient who delayed seeking treatment for the fracture or nonunion.

   Fractures are coded using the appropriate 7th character for subsequent care for encounters after the patient has completed active treatment of the fracture and is receiving routine care for the fracture during the healing or recovery phase.

   Care for complications of surgical treatment for fracture repairs during the healing or recovery phase should be coded with the appropriate complication codes.

   Care of complications of fractures, such as malunion and nonunion, should be reported with the appropriate 7th character for subsequent care with nonunion (K, M, N,) or subsequent care with malunion (P, Q, R).

   Malunion/nonunion: The appropriate 7th character for initial encounter should also be assigned for a patient who delayed seeking treatment for the fracture or nonunion.

The open fracture designations in the assignment of the 7th character for fractures of the forearm, femur and lower leg, including ankle are based on the Gustilo open fracture classification. When the Gustilo classification type is not specified for an open fracture, the 7th character for open fracture type I or II should be assigned (B, E, H, M, Q).

A code from category M80, not a traumatic fracture code, should be used for any patient with known osteoporosis who suffers a fracture, even if the patient had a minor fall or trauma, if that fall or trauma would not usually break a normal, healthy bone.

See Section I.C.13. Osteoporosis.

The aftercare Z codes should not be used for aftercare for traumatic fractures. For aftercare of a traumatic fracture, assign the acute fracture code with the appropriate 7th character.

2) Multiple fractures sequencing
Multiple fractures are sequenced in accordance with the severity of the fracture.

3) Physeal fractures
For physeal fractures, assign only the code identifying the type of physeal fracture. Do not assign a separate code to identify the specific bone that is fractured.

d. Coding of Burns and Corrosions
The ICD-10-CM makes a distinction between burns and corrosions. The burn codes are for thermal burns, except sunburns, that come from a heat source, such as a fire or hot appliance. The burn codes are also for burns resulting from electricity and radiation. Corrosions are burns due to chemicals. The guidelines are the same for burns and corrosions.

Current burns (T20-T25) are classified by depth, extent and by agent (X code). Burns are classified by depth as first degree (erythema), second degree (blistering), and third degree (full-thickness involvement). Burns of the eye and internal organs (T26-T28) are classified by site, but not by degree.

1) Sequencing of burn and related condition codes
Sequence first the code that reflects the highest degree of burn when more than one burn is present.

a. When the reason for the admission or encounter is for treatment of external multiple burns, sequence first the code that reflects the burn of the highest degree.

b. When a patient has both internal and external burns, the circumstances of admission govern the selection of the principal diagnosis or first-listed diagnosis.

c. When a patient is admitted for burn injuries and other related conditions such as smoke inhalation and/or respiratory failure, the circumstances of admission govern the selection of the principal or first-listed diagnosis.

2) Burns of the same anatomic site
Classify burns of the same anatomic site and on the same side but of different degrees to the subcategory identifying the highest degree recorded in the diagnosis (e.g., for second and third degree burns of right thigh, assign only code T24.311-).

3) Non-healing burns
Non-healing burns are coded as acute burns.

Necrosis of burned skin should be coded as a non-healed burn.

4) Infected burn
For any documented infected burn site, use an additional code for the infection.

5) Assign separate codes for each burn site
When coding burns, assign separate codes for each burn site. Category T30, Burn and corrosion, body region unspecified is extremely vague and should rarely be used.

Codes for burns of "multiple sites" should only be assigned when the medical record documentation does not specify the individual sites.

6) Burns and corrosions classified according to extent of body surface involved
Assign codes from category T31, Burns classified according to extent of body surface involved, or T32, Corrosions classified according to extent of body surface involved, for acute burns or corrosions when the site of the burn or corrosion is not specified or when there is a need for additional data. It is advisable to use category T31 as additional coding when needed to provide data for evaluating burn mortality, such as that needed by burn units. It is also advisable to use category T31 as an additional code for reporting purposes when there is mention of a thirddegree burn involving 20 percent or more of the body surface. Codes from categories T31 and T32 should not be used for sequelae of burns or corrosions.

Categories T31 and T32 are based on the classic "rule of nines" in estimating body surface involved: head and neck are assigned nine percent, each arm nine percent, each leg 18 percent, the anterior trunk 18 percent, posterior trunk 18 percent, and genitalia one percent. Providers may change these percentage assignments where necessary to accommodate infants and children who have proportionately larger heads than adults, and patients who have large buttocks, thighs, or abdomen that involve burns.

7) Encounters for treatment of sequela of burns
Encounters for the treatment of the late effects of burns or corrosions (i.e., scars or joint contractures) should be coded with a burn or corrosion code with the 7th character "S" for sequela.

8) Sequelae with a late effect code and current burn
When appropriate, both a code for a current burn or corrosion with 7th character "A" or "D" and a burn or corrosion code with 7th character "S" may be assigned on the same record (when both a current burn and sequelae of an old burn exist). Burns and corrosions do not heal at the same rate and a current healing wound may still exist with sequela of a healed burn or corrosion.

See Section I.B.10. Sequela, (Late Effects)

9) Use of an external cause code with burns and corrosions

An external cause code should be used with burns and corrosions to identify the source and intent of the burn, as well as the place where it occurred.

e. Adverse Effects, Poisoning, Underdosing and Toxic Effects

Codes in categories T36-T65 are combination codes that include the substance that was taken as well as the intent. No additional external cause code is required for poisonings, toxic effects, adverse effects and underdosing codes.

1) Do not code directly from the Table of Drugs

Do not code directly from the Table of Drugs and Chemicals. Always refer back to the Tabular List.

2) Use as many codes as necessary to describe

Use as many codes as necessary to describe completely all drugs, medicinal or biological substances.

3) If the same code would describe the causative agent

If the same code would describe the causative agent for more than one adverse reaction, poisoning, toxic effect or underdosing, assign the code only once.

4) If two or more drugs, medicinal or biological substances

If two or more drugs, medicinal or biological substances are taken, code each individually unless a combination code is listed in the Table of Drugs and Chemicals.

If multiple unspecified drugs, medicinal or biological substances were taken, assign the appropriate code from subcategory T50.91, Poisoning by, adverse effect of and underdosing of multiple unspecified drugs, medicaments and biological substances.

5) The occurrence of drug toxicity is classified in ICD-10-CM as follows:

(a) Adverse Effect

When coding an adverse effect of a drug that has been correctly prescribed and properly administered, assign the appropriate code for the nature of the adverse effect followed by the appropriate code for the adverse effect of the drug (T36-T50). The code for the drug should have a 5th or 6th character "5" (for example T36.0X5-) Examples of the nature of an adverse effect are tachycardia, delirium, gastrointestinal hemorrhaging, vomiting, hypokalemia, hepatitis, renal failure, or respiratory failure.

(b) Poisoning

When coding a poisoning or reaction to the improper use of a medication (e.g., overdose, wrong substance given or taken in error, wrong route of administration), first assign the appropriate code from categories T36-T50. The poisoning codes have an associated intent as their 5th or 6th character (accidental, intentional self-harm, assault and undetermined). If the intent of the poisoning is unknown or unspecified, code the intent as accidental intent. The undetermined intent is only for use if the documentation in the record specifies that the intent cannot be determined. Use additional code(s) for all manifestations of poisonings.

If there is also a diagnosis of abuse or dependence of the substance, the abuse or dependence is assigned as an additional code.

Examples of poisoning include:

    (i) Error was made in drug prescription Errors made in drug prescription or in the administration of the drug by provider, nurse, patient, or other person.

    (ii) Overdose of a drug intentionally taken If an overdose of a drug was intentionally taken or administered and resulted in drug toxicity, it would be coded as a poisoning.

    (iii) Nonprescribed drug taken with correctly prescribed and properly administered drug.
If a nonprescribed drug or medicinal agent was taken in combination with a correctly prescribed and properly administered drug, any drug toxicity or other reaction resulting from the interaction of the two drugs would be classified as a poisoning.

    (iv) Interaction of drug(s) and alcohol. When a reaction results from the interaction of a drug(s) and alcohol, this would be classified as poisoning.

See Section I.C.4. if poisoning is the result of insulin pump malfunctions.

(c) Underdosing

Underdosing refers to taking less of a medication than is prescribed by a provider or a manufacturer's instruction. Discontinuing the use of a prescribed medication on the patient's own initiative (not directed by the patient's provider) is also classified as an underdosing. For underdosing, assign the code from categories T36-T50 (fifth or sixth character "6").

Documentation of a change in the patient's condition is not required in order to assign an underdosing code.

Documentation that the patient is taking less of a medication than is prescribed or discontinued the prescribed medication is sufficient for code assignment.

Codes for underdosing should never be assigned as principal or first-listed codes. If a patient has a relapse or exacerbation of the medical condition for which the drug is prescribed because of the reduction in dose, then the medical condition itself should be coded.

Noncompliance (Z91.12-, Z91.13- and Z91.14-) or complication of care (Y63.6-Y63.9) codes are to be used with an underdosing code to indicate intent, if known.

(d) Toxic Effects

When a harmful substance is ingested or comes in contact with a person, this is classified as a toxic effect. The toxic effect codes are in categories T51-T65.

Toxic effect codes have an associated intent: accidental, intentional self-harm, assault and undetermined.

f. Adult and child abuse, neglect and other maltreatment

Sequence first the appropriate code from categories T74, Adult and child abuse, neglect and other maltreatment, confirmed, or T76, Adult and child abuse, neglect and other maltreatment, suspected, for abuse, neglect and other maltreatment, followed by any accompanying mental health or injury code(s).

If the documentation in the medical record states abuse or neglect it is coded as confirmed (T74.-). It is coded as suspected if it is documented as suspected (T76.-).

For cases of confirmed abuse or neglect an external cause code from the assault section (X92-Y09) should be added to identify the cause of any physical injuries. A perpetrator code (Y07) should be added when the perpetrator of the abuse is known. For suspected cases of abuse or neglect, do not report external cause or perpetrator code.

If a suspected case of abuse, neglect or mistreatment is ruled out during an encounter code Z04.71, Encounter for examination and observation following alleged physical adult abuse, ruled out, or code Z04.72, Encounter for examination and observation following alleged child physical abuse, ruled out, should be used, not a code from T76.

If a suspected case of alleged rape or sexual abuse is ruled out during an encounter code Z04.41, Encounter for examination and observation following alleged adult rape or code Z04.42, Encounter for examination and observation following alleged child rape, should be used, not a code from T76.

If a suspected case of forced sexual exploitation or forced labor exploitation is ruled out during an encounter, code Z04.81, Encounter for examination and observation of victim following forced sexual exploitation, or code Z04.82, Encounter for examination and observation of victim following forced labor exploitation, should be used, not a code from T76.

See Section I.C.15. Abuse in a pregnant patient.

g. Complications of care

1) General guidelines for complications of care

(a) Documentation of complications of care

See Section I.B.16. for information on documentation of complications of care.

2) Pain due to medical devices

Pain associated with devices, implants or grafts left in a surgical site (for example painful hip prosthesis) is assigned to the appropriate code(s) found in Chapter 19, Injury, poisoning, and certain other consequences of external causes. Specific codes for pain due to medical devices are found in the T code section of the ICD-10-CM. Use additional code(s) from category G89 to identify acute or chronic pain due to presence of the device, implant or graft (G89.18 or G89.28).

3) Transplant complications

(a) Transplant complications other than kidney

Codes under category T86, Complications of transplanted organs and tissues, are for use for both complications and rejection of transplanted organs. A transplant complication code is only assigned if the complication affects the function of the transplanted organ. Two codes are required to fully describe a transplant complication: the appropriate code from category T86 and a secondary code that identifies the complication.

Pre-existing conditions or conditions that develop after the transplant are not coded as complications unless they affect the function of the transplanted organs.

See Section I.C.21. for transplant organ removal status
See Section I.C.2. for malignant neoplasm associated with transplanted organ.

(b) Kidney transplant complications

Patients who have undergone kidney transplant may still have some form of chronic kidney disease (CKD) because the kidney transplant may not fully restore kidney function. Code T86.1- should be assigned for documented complications of a kidney transplant, such as transplant failure or rejection or other transplant complication. Code T86.1- should not be assigned for post kidney transplant patients who have chronic kidney (CKD) unless a transplant complication such as transplant failure or rejection is documented. If the documentation is unclear as to whether the patient has a complication of the transplant, query the provider.

Conditions that affect the function of the transplanted kidney, other than CKD, should be assigned a code from subcategory T86.1, Complications of transplanted organ, Kidney, and a secondary code that identifies the complication.

For patients with CKD following a kidney transplant, but who do not have a complication such as failure or rejection, *see Section I.C.14. Chronic kidney disease and kidney transplant status.*

4) Complication codes that include the external cause

As with certain other T codes, some of the complications of care codes have the external cause included in the code. The code includes the nature of the complication as well as the type of procedure that caused the complication. No external cause code indicating the type of procedure is necessary for these codes.

5) Complications of care codes within the body system chapters

Intraoperative and postprocedural complication codes are found within the body system chapters with codes specific to the organs and structures of that body system. These codes should be sequenced first, followed by a code(s) for the specific complication, if applicable.

Complication codes from the body system chapters should be assigned for intraoperative and postprocedural complications (e.g., the appropriate complication code from chapter 9 would be assigned for a vascular intraoperative or postprocedural complication) unless the complication is specifically indexed to a T code in chapter 19.

20. **Chapter 20: External Causes of Morbidity (V00-Y99)**
The external causes of morbidity codes should never be sequenced as the first-listed or principal diagnosis.

External cause codes are intended to provide data for injury research and evaluation of injury prevention strategies. These codes capture how the injury or health condition happened (cause), the intent (unintentional or accidental; or intentional, such as suicide or assault), the place where the event occurred the activity of the patient at the time of the event, and the person's status (e.g., civilian, military).

There is no national requirement for mandatory ICD-10-CM external cause code reporting. Unless a provider is subject to a state-based external cause code reporting mandate or these codes are required by a particular payer, reporting of ICD-10-CM codes in Chapter 20, External Causes of Morbidity, is not required. In the absence of a mandatory reporting requirement, providers are encouraged to voluntarily report external cause codes, as they provide valuable data for injury research and evaluation of injury prevention strategies.

a. **General External Cause Coding Guidelines**

1) **Used with any code in the range of A00.0-T88.9, Z00-Z99**
An external cause code may be used with any code in the range of A00.0-T88.9, Z00-Z99, classification that represents a health condition due to an external cause. Though they are most applicable to injuries, they are also valid for use with such things as infections or diseases due to an external source, and other health conditions, such as a heart attack that occurs during strenuous physical activity.

2) **External cause code used for length of treatment**
Assign the external cause code, with the appropriate 7th character (initial encounter, subsequent encounter or sequela) for each encounter for which the injury or condition is being treated.

Most categories in Chapter 20 have a 7th character requirement for each applicable code. Most categories in this chapter have three 7th character values: A, initial encounter, D, subsequent encounter and S, sequela. While the patient may be seen by a new or different provider over the course of treatment for an injury or condition, assignment of the 7th character for external cause should match the 7th character of the code assigned for the associated injury or condition for the encounter.

3) **Use the full range of external cause codes**
Use the full range of external cause codes to completely describe the cause, the intent, the place of occurrence, and if applicable, the activity of the patient at the time of the event, and the patient's status, for all injuries, and other health conditions due to an external cause.

4) **Assign as many external cause codes as necessary**
Assign as many external cause codes as necessary to fully explain each cause. If only one external code can be recorded, assign the code most related to the principal diagnosis.

5) **The selection of the appropriate external cause code**
The selection of the appropriate external cause code is guided by the Alphabetic Index of External Causes and by Inclusion and Exclusion notes in the Tabular List.

6) **External cause code can never be a principal diagnosis**
An external cause code can never be a principal (first-listed) diagnosis.

7) **Combination external cause codes**
Certain of the external cause codes are combination codes that identify sequential events that result in an injury, such as a fall which results in striking against an object. The injury may be due to either event or both. The combination external cause code used should correspond to the sequence of events regardless of which caused the most serious injury.

8) **No external cause code needed in certain circumstances**
No external cause code from Chapter 20 is needed if the external cause and intent are included in a code from another chapter (e.g., T36.0X1- Poisoning by penicillins, accidental (unintentional)).

b. **Place of Occurrence Guideline**
Codes from category Y92, Place of occurrence of the external cause, are secondary codes for use after other external cause codes to identify the location of the patient at the time of injury or other condition.

Generally, a place of occurrence code is assigned only once, at the initial encounter for treatment. However, in the rare instance that a new injury occurs during hospitalization, an additional place of occurrence code may be assigned. No 7th characters are used for Y92.

Do not use place of occurrence code Y92.9 if the place is not stated or is not applicable.

c. **Activity Code**
Assign a code from category Y93, Activity code, to describe the activity of the patient at the time the injury or other health condition occurred.

An activity code is used only once, at the initial encounter for treatment. Only one code from Y93 should be recorded on a medical record.

The activity codes are not applicable to poisonings, adverse effects, misadventures or sequela.

Do not assign Y93.9, Unspecified activity, if the activity is not stated.

A code from category Y93 is appropriate for use with external cause and intent codes if identifying the activity provides additional information about the event.

d. Place of Occurrence, Activity, and Status Codes Used with other External Cause Code

When applicable, place of occurrence, activity, and external cause status codes are sequenced after the main external cause code(s). Regardless of the number of external cause codes assigned, generally there should be only one place of occurrence code, one activity code, and one external cause status code assigned to an encounter. However, in the rare instance that a new injury occurs during hospitalization, an additional place of occurrence code may be assigned.

e. If the Reporting Format Limits the Number of External Cause Codes

If the reporting format limits the number of external cause codes that can be used in reporting clinical data, report the code for the cause/intent most related to the principal diagnosis. If the format permits capture of additional external cause codes, the cause/intent, including medical misadventures, of the additional events should be reported rather than the codes for place, activity, or external status.

f. Multiple External Cause Coding Guidelines

More than one external cause code is required to fully describe the external cause of an illness or injury. The assignment of external cause codes should be sequenced in the following priority:

If two or more events cause separate injuries, an external cause code should be assigned for each cause. The first-listed external cause code will be selected in the following order:

External codes for child and adult abuse take priority over all other external cause codes.

See Section I.C.19., Child and Adult abuse guidelines.

External cause codes for terrorism events take priority over all other external cause codes except child and adult abuse.

External cause codes for cataclysmic events take priority over all other external cause codes except child and adult abuse and terrorism.

External cause codes for transport accidents take priority over all other external cause codes except cataclysmic events, child and adult abuse and terrorism.

Activity and external cause status codes are assigned following all causal (intent) external cause codes.

The first-listed external cause code should correspond to the cause of the most serious diagnosis due to an assault, accident, or self-harm, following the order of hierarchy listed above.

g. Child and Adult Abuse Guideline

Adult and child abuse, neglect and maltreatment are classified as assault. Any of the assault codes may be used to indicate the external cause of any injury resulting from the confirmed abuse.

For confirmed cases of abuse, neglect and maltreatment, when the perpetrator is known, a code from Y07, Perpetrator of maltreatment and neglect, should accompany any other assault codes.

See Section I.C.19. Adult and child abuse, neglect and other maltreatment

h. Unknown or Undetermined Intent Guideline

If the intent (accident, self-harm, assault) of the cause of an injury or other condition is unknown or unspecified, code the intent as accidental intent. All transport accident categories assume accidental intent.

1) Use of undetermined intent

External cause codes for events of undetermined intent are only for use if the documentation in the record specifies that the intent cannot be determined.

i. Sequelae (Late Effects) of External Cause Guidelines

1) Sequelae external cause codes

Sequela are reported using the external cause code with the 7th character "S" for sequela. These codes should be used with any report of a late effect or sequela resulting from a previous injury.

See Section I.B.10. Sequela (Late Effects)

2) Sequela external cause code with a related current injury

A sequela external cause code should never be used with a related current nature of injury code.

3) Use of sequela external cause codes for subsequent visits

Use a late effect external cause code for subsequent visits when a late effect of the initial injury is being treated. Do not use a late effect external cause code for subsequent visits for follow-up care (e.g., to assess healing, to receive rehabilitative therapy) of the injury when no late effect of the injury has been documented.

j. Terrorism Guidelines

1) Cause of injury identified by the Federal Government (FBI) as terrorism

When the cause of an injury is identified by the Federal Government (FBI) as terrorism, the first-listed external cause code should be a code from category Y38, Terrorism. The definition of terrorism employed by the FBI is found at the inclusion note at the beginning of category Y38. Use additional code for place of occurrence (Y92.-). More than one Y38 code may be assigned if the injury is the result of more than one mechanism of terrorism.

2) Cause of an injury is suspected to be the result of terrorism

When the cause of an injury is suspected to be the result of terrorism a code from category Y38 should not be assigned. Suspected cases should be classified as assault.

3) Code Y38.9, Terrorism, secondary effects

Assign code Y38.9, Terrorism, secondary effects, for conditions occurring subsequent to the terrorist event. This code should not be assigned for conditions that are due to the initial terrorist act.

It is acceptable to assign code Y38.9 with another code from Y38 if there is an injury due to the initial terrorist event and an injury that is a subsequent result of the terrorist event.

k. External Cause Status

A code from category Y99, External cause status, should be assigned whenever any other external cause code is assigned for an encounter, including an Activity code, except for the events noted below. Assign a code from category Y99, External cause status, to indicate the work status of the person at the time the event occurred. The status code indicates whether the event occurred during military activity, whether a non-military person was at work, whether an individual including a student or volunteer was involved in a non-work activity at the time of the causal event.

A code from Y99, External cause status, should be assigned, when applicable, with other external cause codes, such as transport accidents and falls. The external cause status codes are not applicable to poisonings, adverse effects, misadventures or late effects.

Do not assign a code from category Y99 if no other external cause codes (cause, activity) are applicable for the encounter.

An external cause status code is used only once, at the initial encounter for treatment. Only one code from Y99 should be recorded on a medical record.

Do not assign code Y99.9, Unspecified external cause status, if the status is not stated.

21. Chapter 21: Factors influencing health status and contact with health services (Z00-Z99)

Note: The chapter-specific guidelines provide additional information about the use of Z codes for specified encounters.

a. Use of Z Codes in Any Healthcare Setting

Z codes are for use in any healthcare setting. Z codes may be used as either a first-listed (principal diagnosis code in the inpatient setting) or secondary code, depending on the circumstances of the encounter. Certain Z codes may only be used as first-listed or principal diagnosis.

b. Z Codes Indicate a Reason for an Encounter *or Provide Additional Information about a Patient Encounter*

Z codes are not procedure codes. A corresponding procedure code must accompany a Z code to describe any procedure performed.

c. Categories of Z Codes

1) Contact/Exposure

Category Z20 indicates contact with, and suspected exposure to, communicable diseases. These codes are for patients who are suspected to have been exposed to a disease by close personal contact with an infected individual or are in an area where a disease is epidemic.

Category Z77, Other contact with and (suspected) exposures hazardous to health, indicates contact with and suspected exposures hazardous to health.

Contact/exposure codes may be used as a first-listed code to explain an encounter for testing, or, more commonly, as a secondary code to identify a potential risk.

2) Inoculations and vaccinations

Code Z23 is for encounters for inoculations and vaccinations. It indicates that a patient is being seen to receive a prophylactic inoculation against a disease. Procedure codes are required to identify the actual administration of the injection and the type(s) of immunizations given. Code Z23 may be used as a secondary code if the inoculation is given as a routine part of preventive health care, such as a well-baby visit.

3) Status

Status codes indicate that a patient is either a carrier of a disease or has the sequelae or residual of a past disease or condition. This includes such things as the presence of prosthetic or mechanical devices resulting from past treatment. A status code is informative, because the status may affect the course of treatment and its outcome. A status code is distinct from a history code. The history code indicates that the patient no longer has the condition.

A status code should not be used with a diagnosis code from one of the body system chapters, if the diagnosis code includes the information provided by the status code. For example, code Z94.1, Heart transplant status, should not be used with a code from subcategory T86.2, Complications of heart transplant. The status code does not provide additional information. The complication code indicates that the patient is a heart transplant patient.

For encounters for weaning from a mechanical ventilator, assign a code from subcategory J96.1, Chronic respiratory failure, followed by code Z99.11, Dependence on respirator [ventilator] status.

The status Z codes/categories are:

Z14	Genetic carrier
	Genetic carrier status indicates that a person carries a gene, associated with a particular disease, which may be passed to offspring who may develop that disease. The person does not have the disease and is not at risk of developing the disease.
Z15	Genetic susceptibility to disease Genetic susceptibility indicates that a person has a gene that increases the risk of that person developing the disease.

Codes from category Z15 should not be used as principal or first-listed codes. If the patient has the condition to which he/she is susceptible, and that condition is the reason for the encounter, the code for the current condition should be sequenced first. If the patient is being seen for follow-up after completed treatment for this condition, and the condition no longer exists, a follow-up code should be sequenced first, followed by the appropriate personal history and genetic susceptibility codes. If the purpose of the encounter is genetic counseling associated with procreative management, code Z31.5, Encounter for genetic counseling, should be assigned as the first-listed code, followed by a code from category Z15. Additional codes should be assigned for any applicable family or personal history.

Z16   Resistance to antimicrobial drugs
This code indicates that a patient has a condition that is resistant to antimicrobial drug treatment. Sequence the infection code first.

Z17   Estrogen receptor status

Z18   Retained foreign body fragments

Z19   Hormone sensitivity malignancy status

Z21   Asymptomatic HIV infection status This code indicates that a patient has tested positive for HIV but has manifested no signs or symptoms of the disease.

Z22   Carrier of infectious disease Carrier status indicates that a person harbors the specific organisms of a disease without manifest symptoms and is capable of transmitting the infection.

Z28.3   Underimmunization status
See Section I.B.14. for underimmunization documentation by clinicians other than the patient's provider.

Z33.1   Pregnant state, incidental This code is a secondary code only for use when the pregnancy is in no way complicating the reason for visit. Otherwise, a code from the obstetric chapter is required.

Z66   Do not resuscitate
This code may be used when it is documented by the provider that a patient is on do not resuscitate status at any time during the stay.

Z67   Blood type

Z68   Body mass index (BMI)
BMI codes should only be assigned when there is an associated reportable diagnosis (such as obesity). Do not assign BMI codes during pregnancy.
See Section I.B.14 for BMI documentation by clinicians other than the patient's provider.

Z74.01   Bed confinement status

Z76.82   Awaiting organ transplant status

Z78   Other specified health status
Code Z78.1, Physical restraint status, may be used when it is documented by the provider that a patient has been put in restraints during the current encounter. Please note that this code should not be reported when it is documented by the provider that a patient is temporarily restrained during a procedure.

Z79   Long-term (current) drug therapy
Codes from this category indicate a patient's continuous use of a prescribed drug (including such things as aspirin therapy) for the long-term treatment of a condition or for prophylactic use. It is not for use for patients who have addictions to drugs. This subcategory is not for use of medications for detoxification or maintenance programs to prevent withdrawal symptoms (e.g., methadone maintenance for opiate dependence).

Assign the appropriate code for the drug use, abuse, or dependence instead.

Assign a code from Z79 if the patient is receiving a medication for an extended period as a prophylactic measure (such as for the prevention of deep vein thrombosis) or as treatment of a chronic condition (such as arthritis) or a disease requiring a lengthy course of treatment (such as cancer). Do not assign a code from category Z79 for medication being administered for a brief period of time to treat an acute illness or injury (such as a course of antibiotics to treat acute bronchitis).

Z88   Allergy status to drugs, medicaments and biological substances Except: Z88.9, Allergy status to unspecified drugs, medicaments and biological substances status

Z89   Acquired absence of limb

Z90   Acquired absence of organs, not elsewhere classified

Z91.0-   Allergy status, other than to drugs and biological substances

Z92.82   Status post administration of tPA (rtPA) in a different facility within the last 24 hours prior to admission to a current facility Assign code Z92.82, Status post administration of tPA (rtPA) in a different facility within the last 24 hours prior to admission to current facility, as a secondary diagnosis when a patient is received by transfer into a facility and documentation indicates they were administered tissue plasminogen activator (tPA) within the last 24 hours prior to admission to the current facility. This guideline applies even if the patient is still receiving the tPA at the time they are received into the current facility. The appropriate code for the condition for which the tPA was administered (such as cerebrovascular disease or myocardial infarction) should be assigned first. Code Z92.82 is only applicable to the receiving facility record and not to the transferring facility record.

Z93   Artificial opening status

Z94   Transplanted organ and tissue status

Z95   Presence of cardiac and vascular implants and grafts

Z96   Presence of other functional implants

Z97   Presence of other devices

Z98   Other postprocedural states
Assign code Z98.85, Transplanted organ removal status, to indicate that a transplanted organ has been previously removed. This code should not be assigned for the encounter in which the transplanted organ is removed. The complication necessitating removal of the transplant organ should be assigned for that encounter.
See Section I.C.19. for information on the coding of organ transplant complications.

Z99   Dependence on enabling machines and devices, not elsewhere classified

Note: Categories Z89-Z90 and Z93-Z99 are for use only if there are no complications or malfunctions of the organ or tissue replaced, the amputation site or the equipment on which the patient is dependent.

4) History (of)

There are two types of history Z codes, personal and family. Personal history codes explain a patient's past medical condition that no longer exists and is not receiving any treatment, but that has the potential for recurrence, and therefore may require continued monitoring.

Family history codes are for use when a patient has a family member(s) who has had a particular disease that causes the patient to be at higher risk of also contracting the disease.

Personal history codes may be used in conjunction with follow-up codes and family history codes may be used in conjunction with screening codes to explain the need for a test or procedure. History codes are also acceptable on any medical record regardless of the reason for visit. A history of an illness, even if no longer present, is important information that may alter the type of treatment ordered.

The reason for the encounter (for example, screening or counseling) should be sequenced first and the appropriate personal and/or family history code(s) should be assigned as additional diagnos(es).

The history Z code categories are:

Z80	Family history of primary malignant neoplasm
Z81	Family history of mental and behavioral disorders
Z82	Family history of certain disabilities and chronic diseases (leading to disablement)
Z83	Family history of other specific disorders
Z84	Family history of other conditions
Z85	Personal history of malignant neoplasm
Z86	Personal history of certain other diseases
Z87	Personal history of other diseases and conditions
Z91.4-	Personal history of psychological trauma, not elsewhere classified
Z91.5	Personal history of self-harm
Z91.81	History of falling
Z91.82	Personal history of military deployment
Z92	Personal history of medical treatment Except: Z92.0, Personal history of contraception Except: Z92.82, Status post administration of tPA (rtPA) in a different facility within the last 24 hours prior to admission to a current facility

5) Screening

Screening is the testing for disease or disease precursors in seemingly well individuals so that early detection and treatment can be provided for those who test positive for the disease (e.g., screening mammogram).

The testing of a person to rule out or confirm a suspected diagnosis because the patient has some sign or symptom is a diagnostic examination, not a screening. In these cases, the sign or symptom is used to explain the reason for the test.

A screening code may be a first-listed code if the reason for the visit is specifically the screening exam. It may also be used as an additional code if the screening is done during an office visit for other health problems. A screening code is not necessary if the screening is inherent to a routine examination, such as a pap smear done during a routine pelvic examination.

Should a condition be discovered during the screening then the code for the condition may be assigned as an additional diagnosis.

The Z code indicates that a screening exam is planned. A procedure code is required to confirm that the screening was performed.

The screening Z codes/categories:

Z11	Encounter for screening for infectious and parasitic diseases
Z12	Encounter for screening for malignant neoplasms
Z13	Encounter for screening for other diseases and disorders Except: Z13.9, Encounter for screening, unspecified
Z36	Encounter for antenatal screening for mother

6) Observation

There are three observation Z code categories. They are for use in very limited circumstances when a person is being observed for a suspected condition that is ruled out. The observation codes are not for use if an injury or illness or any signs or symptoms related to the suspected condition are present. In such cases the diagnosis/symptom code is used with the corresponding external cause code.

The observation codes are primarily to be used as a principal/first-listed diagnosis. An observation code may be assigned as a secondary diagnosis code when the patient is being observed for a condition that is ruled out and is unrelated to the principal/first-listed diagnosis. Also, when the principal diagnosis is required to be a code from category Z38, Liveborn infants according to place of birth and type of delivery, then a code from category Z05, Encounter for observation and evaluation of newborn for suspected diseases and conditions ruled out, is sequenced after the Z38 code. Additional codes may be used in addition to the observation code, but only if they are unrelated to the suspected condition being observed.

Codes from subcategory Z03.7, Encounter for suspected maternal and fetal conditions ruled out, may either be used as a first-listed or as an additional code assignment depending on the case. They are for use in very limited circumstances on a maternal record when an encounter is for a suspected maternal or fetal condition that is ruled out during that encounter (for example, a maternal or fetal condition may be suspected due to an abnormal test result). These codes should not be used when the condition is confirmed. In those cases, the confirmed condition should be coded. In addition, these codes are not for use if an illness or any signs or symptoms related to the suspected condition or problem are present. In such cases the diagnosis/symptom code is used.

Additional codes may be used in addition to the code from subcategory Z03.7, but only if they are unrelated to the suspected condition being evaluated.

Codes from subcategory Z03.7, may not be used for encounters for antenatal screening of mother. *See Section I.C.21. Screening.*

For encounters for suspected fetal condition that are inconclusive following testing and evaluation, assign the appropriate code from category O35, O36, O40 or O41.

The observation Z code categories:

Z03   Encounter for medical observation for suspected diseases and conditions ruled out

Z04   Encounter for examination and observation for other reasons Except: Z04.9, Encounter for examination and observation for unspecified reason

Z05   Encounter for observation and evaluation of newborn for suspected diseases and conditions ruled out

7) Aftercare

Aftercare visit codes cover situations when the initial treatment of a disease has been performed and the patient requires continued care during the healing or recovery phase, or for the long-term consequences of the disease. The aftercare Z code should not be used if treatment is directed at a current, acute disease. The diagnosis code is to be used in these cases.

Exceptions to this rule are codes Z51.0, Encounter for antineoplastic radiation therapy, and codes from subcategory Z51.1, Encounter for antineoplastic chemotherapy and immunotherapy. These codes are to be first-listed, followed by the diagnosis code when a patient's encounter is solely to receive radiation therapy, chemotherapy, or immunotherapy for the treatment of a neoplasm. If the reason for the encounter is more than one type of antineoplastic therapy, code Z51.0 and a code from subcategory Z51.1 may be assigned together, in which case one of these codes would be reported as a secondary diagnosis.

The aftercare Z codes should also not be used for aftercare for injuries. For aftercare of an injury, assign the acute injury code with the appropriate 7th character (for subsequent encounter).

The aftercare codes are generally first-listed to explain the specific reason for the encounter. An aftercare code may be used as an additional code when some type of aftercare is provided in addition to the reason for admission and no diagnosis code is applicable. An example of this

would be the closure of a colostomy during an encounter for treatment of another condition.

Aftercare codes should be used in conjunction with other aftercare codes or diagnosis codes to provide better detail on the specifics of an aftercare encounter visit, unless otherwise directed by the classification. The sequencing of multiple aftercare codes depends on the circumstances of the encounter.

Certain aftercare Z code categories need a secondary diagnosis code to describe the resolving condition or sequelae. For others, the condition is included in the code title.

Additional Z code aftercare category terms include fitting and adjustment, and attention to artificial openings.

Status Z codes may be used with aftercare Z codes to indicate the nature of the aftercare. For example code Z95.1, Presence of aortocoronary bypass graft, may be used with code Z48.812, Encounter for surgical aftercare following surgery on the circulatory system, to indicate the surgery for which the aftercare is being performed. A status code should not be used when the aftercare code indicates the type of status, such as using Z43.0, Encounter for attention to tracheostomy, with Z93.0, Tracheostomy status.

The aftercare Z category/codes:

Z42   Encounter for plastic and reconstructive surgery following medical procedure or healed injury

Z43   Encounter for attention to artificial openings

Z44   Encounter for fitting and adjustment of external prosthetic device

Z45   Encounter for adjustment and management of implanted device

Z46   Encounter for fitting and adjustment of other devices

Z47   Orthopedic aftercare

Z48   Encounter for other postprocedural aftercare

Z49   Encounter for care involving renal dialysis

Z51   Encounter for other aftercare and medical care

8) Follow-up

The follow-up codes are used to explain continuing surveillance following completed treatment of a disease, condition, or injury. They imply that the condition has been fully treated and no longer exists. They should not be confused with aftercare codes, or injury codes with a 7th character for subsequent encounter, that explain ongoing care of a healing condition or its sequelae. Follow-up codes may be used in conjunction with history codes to provide the full picture of the healed condition and its treatment. The follow-up code is sequenced first, followed by the history code.

A follow-up code may be used to explain multiple visits. Should a condition be found to have recurred on the follow-up visit, then the diagnosis code for the condition should be assigned in place of the follow-up code.

The follow-up Z code categories:

Z08	Encounter for follow-up examination after completed treatment for malignant neoplasm
Z09	Encounter for follow-up examination after completed treatment for conditions other than malignant neoplasm
Z39	Encounter for maternal postpartum care and examination

9) Donor

Codes in category Z52, Donors of organs and tissues, are used for living individuals who are donating blood or other body tissue. These codes are for individuals donating for others, as well as for self-donations. They are not used to identify cadaveric donations.

10) Counseling

Counseling Z codes are used when a patient or family member receives assistance in the aftermath of an illness or injury, or when support is required in coping with family or social problems.

The counseling Z codes/categories:

Z30.0-	Encounter for general counseling and advice on contraception
Z31.5	Encounter for procreative genetic counseling
Z31.6-	Encounter for general counseling and advice on procreation
Z32.2	Encounter for childbirth instruction
Z32.3	Encounter for childcare instruction
Z69	Encounter for mental health services for victim and perpetrator of abuse
Z70	Counseling related to sexual attitude, behavior and orientation
Z71	Persons encountering health services for other counseling and medical advice, not elsewhere classified

Note: Code Z71.84, Encounter for health counseling related to travel, is to be used for health risk and safety counseling for future travel purposes. Code Z71.85, Encounter for immunization safety counseling, is to be used for counseling of the patient or caregiver regarding the safety of a vaccine. This code should not be used for the provision of general information regarding risks and potential side effects during routine encounters for the administration of vaccines.

Code Z71.87, Encounter for pediatric-to-adult transition counseling, should be assigned when pediatric-to-adult transition counseling is the sole reason for the encounter or when this counseling is provided in addition to other services, such as treatment of a chronic condition. If both transition counseling and treatment of a medical condition are provided during the **same encounter, the code(s) for the medical condition(s) treated and code Z71.87 should be assigned, with sequencing depending on the circumstances of the encounter.**

Z76.81	Expectant mother prebirth pediatrician visit

11) Encounters for Obstetrical and Reproductive Services

See Section I.C.15. Pregnancy, Childbirth, and the Puerperium, for further instruction on the use of these codes.

Z codes for pregnancy are for use in those circumstances when none of the problems or complications included in the codes from the Obstetrics chapter exist (a routine prenatal visit or postpartum care). Codes in category Z34, Encounter for supervision of normal pregnancy, are always first listed and are not to be used with any other code from the OB chapter.

Codes in category Z3A, Weeks of gestation, may be assigned to provide additional information about the pregnancy. Category Z3A codes should not be assigned for pregnancies with abortive outcomes (categories O00-O08), elective termination of pregnancy (code Z33.2), nor for postpartum conditions, as category Z3A is not applicable to these conditions. The date of the admission should be used to determine weeks of gestation for inpatient admissions that encompass more than one gestational week.

The outcome of delivery, category Z37, should be included on all maternal delivery records. It is always a secondary code. Codes in category Z37 should not be used on the newborn record.

Z codes for family planning (contraceptive) or procreative management and counseling should be included on an obstetric record either during the pregnancy or the postpartum stage, if applicable.

Z codes/categories for obstetrical and reproductive services:

Z30	Encounter for contraceptive management
Z31	Encounter for procreative management
Z32.2	Encounter for childbirth instruction
Z32.3	Encounter for childcare instruction
Z33	Pregnant state
Z34	Encounter for supervision of normal pregnancy
Z36	Encounter for antenatal screening of mother
Z3A	Weeks of gestation
Z37	Outcome of delivery
Z39	Encounter for maternal postpartum care and examination
Z76.81	Expectant mother prebirth pediatrician visit

12) Newborns and Infants

See Section I.C.16. Newborn (Perinatal) Guidelines, for further instruction on the use of these codes.

Newborn Z codes/categories:

Z76.1	Encounter for health supervision and care of foundling

Z00.1- Encounter for routine child health examination

Z38 Liveborn infants according to place of birth and type of delivery

13) Routine and Administrative Examinations

The Z codes allow for the description of encounters for routine examinations, such as, a general check-up, or, examinations for administrative purposes, such as, a pre-employment physical. The codes are not to be used if the examination is for diagnosis of a suspected condition or for treatment purposes. In such cases the diagnosis code is used. During a routine exam, should a diagnosis or condition be discovered, it should be coded as an additional code. Pre-existing and chronic conditions and history codes may also be included as additional codes as long as the examination is for administrative purposes and not focused on any particular condition.

Some of the codes for routine health examinations distinguish between "with" and "without" abnormal findings. Code assignment depends on the information that is known at the time the encounter is being coded. For example, if no abnormal findings were found during the examination, but the encounter is being coded before test results are back, it is acceptable to assign the code for "without abnormal findings." When assigning a code for "with abnormal findings," additional code(s) should be assigned to identify the specific abnormal finding(s).

Pre-operative examination and pre-procedural laboratory examination Z codes are for use only in those situations when a patient is being cleared for a procedure or surgery and no treatment is given.

The Z codes/categories for routine and administrative examinations:

Z00 Encounter for general examination without complaint, suspected or reported diagnosis

Z01 Encounter for other special examination without complaint, suspected or reported diagnosis

Z02 Encounter for administrative examination
Except: Z02.9, Encounter for administrative examinations, unspecified

Z32.0- Encounter for pregnancy test

14) Miscellaneous Z Codes

The miscellaneous Z codes capture a number of other health care encounters that do not fall into one of the other categories. Some of these codes identify the reason for the encounter; others are for use as additional codes that provide useful information on circumstances that may affect a patient's care and treatment.

Prophylactic Organ Removal

For encounters specifically for prophylactic removal of an organ (such as prophylactic removal of breasts due to a genetic susceptibility to cancer or a family history of cancer), the principal or first-listed code should be a code from category Z40, Encounter for prophylactic surgery, followed by the appropriate codes to identify the associated risk factor (such as genetic susceptibility or family history).

If the patient has a malignancy of one site and is having prophylactic removal at another site to prevent either a new primary malignancy or metastatic disease, a code for the malignancy should also be assigned in addition to a code from subcategory Z40.0, Encounter for prophylactic surgery for risk factors related to malignant neoplasms. A Z40.0 code should not be assigned if the patient is having organ removal for treatment of a malignancy, such as the removal of the testes for the treatment of prostate cancer.

Miscellaneous Z codes/categories:

Z28 Immunization not carried out
Except: Z28.3, Underimmunization status

Z29 Encounter for other prophylactic measures

Z40 Encounter for prophylactic surgery

Z41 Encounter for procedures for purposes other than remedying health state
Except: Z41.9, Encounter for procedure for purposes other than remedying health state, unspecified

Z72 Problems related to lifestyle
Note: These codes should be assigned only when the documentation specifies that the patient has an associated problem

Z73 Problems related to life management difficulty
Note: These codes should be assigned only when the documentation specifies that the patient has an associated problem.

Z74 Problems related to care provider dependency Except: Z74.01, Bed confinement status

Z75 Problems related to medical facilities and other health care

Z76.0 Encounter for issue of repeat prescription

Z76.3 Healthy person accompanying sick person

Z76.4 Other boarder to healthcare facility

Z76.5 Malingerer [conscious simulation]

Z91.1- Patient's noncompliance with medical treatment and regimen

Z91.83 Wandering in diseases classified elsewhere

Z91.84- Oral health risk factors

Z91.89 Other specified personal risk factors, not elsewhere classified

See Section I.B.14 for Z55-Z65 Persons with potential health hazards related to socioeconomic and psychosocial circumstances, documentation by clinicians other than the patient's provider

15) Nonspecific Z Codes

Certain Z codes are so non-specific, or potentially redundant with other codes in the classification, that there can be little justification for their use in the inpatient setting. Their use in the outpatient setting should be limited to those instances when there is no further documentation to permit more precise coding. Otherwise, any sign or symptom or any other reason for visit that is captured in another code should be used.

Nonspecific Z codes/categories:

Z02.9	Encounter for administrative examinations, unspecified
Z04.9	Encounter for examination and observation for unspecified reason
Z13.9	Encounter for screening, unspecified
Z41.9	Encounter for procedure for purposes other than remedying health state, unspecified
Z52.9	Donor of unspecified organ or tissue
Z86.59	Personal history of other mental and behavioral disorders
Z88.9	Allergy status to unspecified drugs, medicaments and biological substances status
Z92.0	Personal history of contraception

16) Z Codes That May Only be Principal/ First-Listed Diagnosis

The following Z codes/categories may only be reported as the principal/first-listed diagnosis, except when there are multiple encounters on the same day and the medical records for the encounters are combined:

Z00	Encounter for general examination without complaint, suspected or reported diagnosis Except: Z00.6
Z01	Encounter for other special examination without complaint, suspected or reported diagnosis
Z02	Encounter for administrative examination
Z04	Encounter for examination and observation for other reasons
Z33.2	Encounter for elective termination of pregnancy
Z31.81	Encounter for male factor infertility in female patient
Z31.83	Encounter for assisted reproductive fertility procedure cycle
Z31.84	Encounter for fertility preservation procedure
Z34	Encounter for supervision of normal pregnancy
Z39	Encounter for maternal postpartum care and examination
Z38	Liveborn infants according to place of birth and type of delivery
Z40	Encounter for prophylactic surgery
Z42	Encounter for plastic and reconstructive surgery following medical procedure or healed injury
Z51.0	Encounter for antineoplastic radiation therapy
Z51.1-	Encounter for antineoplastic chemotherapy and immunotherapy

Z52	Donors of organs and tissues Except: Z52.9, Donor of unspecified organ or tissue
Z76.1	Encounter for health supervision and care of foundling
Z76.2	Encounter for health supervision and care of other healthy infant and child
Z99.12	Encounter for respirator [ventilator] dependence during power failure

17) Social Determinants of Health

Codes describing **problems or risk factors related to** social determinants of health (SDOH) should be assigned when this information is documented. **Assign as many SDOH codes as are necessary to describe all of the problems or risk factors. These codes should be assigned only when the documentation specifies that the patient has an associated problem or risk factor. For example, not every individual living alone would be assigned code Z60.2, Problems related to living alone.**

For social determinants of health, such as information found in categories Z55-Z65, Persons with potential health hazards related to socioeconomic and psychosocial circumstances, code assignment may be based on medical record documentation from clinicians involved in the care of the patient who are not the patient's provider since this information represents social information, rather than medical diagnoses.

For example, coding professionals may utilize documentation of social information from social workers, community health workers, case managers, or nurses, if their documentation is included in the official medical record.

Patient self-reported documentation may be used to assign codes for social determinants of health, as long as the patient self-reported information is signed-off by and incorporated into the medical record by either a clinician or provider.

Social determinants of health codes are located primarily in these Z code categories:

Z55	Problems related to education and literacy
Z56	Problems related to employment and unemployment
Z57	Occupational exposure to risk factors
Z58	Problems related to physical environment
Z59	Problems related to housing and economic circumstances
Z60	Problems related to social environment
Z62	Problems related to upbringing
Z63	Other problems related to primary support group, including family circumstances
Z64	Problems related to certain psychosocial circumstances
Z65	Problems related to other psychosocial circumstances

See Section I.B.14. Documentation by Clinicians Other than the Patient's Provider.

22. **Chapter 22: Codes for Special Purposes (U00-U85)**
    U07.0 Vaping-related disorder (see Section
           I.C.10.e., Vaping-related disorders)
    U07.1 COVID-19 (see Section I.C.1.g.1.,
           COVID-19 infection)
    U09.9 Post COVID-19 condition, unspecified
           (see Section I.C.1.g.1.m)

Section II. Selection of Principal Diagnosis

The circumstances of inpatient admission always govern the selection of principal diagnosis. The principal diagnosis is defined in the Uniform Hospital Discharge Data Set (UHDDS) as "that condition established after study to be chiefly responsible for occasioning the admission of the patient to the hospital for care."

The UHDDS definitions are used by hospitals to report inpatient data elements in a standardized manner. These data elements and their definitions can be found in the July 31, 1985, Federal Register (Vol. 50, No, 147), pp. 31038-40.

Since that time, the application of the UHDDS definitions has been expanded to include all nonoutpatient settings (acute care, short term, long-term care and psychiatric hospitals; home health agencies; rehab facilities; nursing homes, etc. . .). The UHDDS definitions also apply to hospice services (all levels of care).

In determining principal diagnosis, coding conventions in the ICD-10-CM, the Tabular List and Alphabetic Index take precedence over these official coding guidelines.

(See Section I.A., Conventions for the ICD-10-CM)

The importance of consistent, complete documentation in the medical record cannot be overemphasized. Without such documentation the application of all coding guidelines is a difficult, if not impossible, task.

A. **Codes for symptoms, signs, and ill-defined conditions**
   Codes for symptoms, signs, and ill-defined conditions from Chapter 18 are not to be used as principal diagnosis when a related definitive diagnosis has been established.

B. **Two or more interrelated conditions, each potentially meeting the definition for principal diagnosis**
   When there are two or more interrelated conditions (such as diseases in the same ICD-10-CM chapter or manifestations characteristically associated with a certain disease) potentially meeting the definition of principal diagnosis, either condition may be sequenced first, unless the circumstances of the admission, the therapy provided, the Tabular List, or the Alphabetic Index indicate otherwise.

C. **Two or more diagnoses that equally meet the definition for principal diagnosis**
   In the unusual instance when two or more diagnoses equally meet the criteria for principal diagnosis as determined by the circumstances of admission, diagnostic workup and/or therapy provided, and the Alphabetic Index, Tabular List, or another coding guidelines does not provide sequencing direction, any one of the diagnoses may be sequenced first.

D. **Two or more comparative or contrasting conditions.**
   In those rare instances when two or more contrasting or comparative diagnoses are documented as "either/or" (or similar terminology), they are coded as if the diagnoses were confirmed and the diagnoses are sequenced according to the circumstances of the admission. If no further determination can be made as to which diagnosis should be principal, either diagnosis may be sequenced first

E. **A symptom(s) followed by contrasting/ comparative diagnoses**
   GUIDELINE HAS BEEN DELETED EFFECTIVE OCTOBER 1, 2014

F. **Original treatment plan not carried out**
   Sequence as the principal diagnosis the condition, which after study occasioned the admission to the hospital, even though treatment may not have been carried out due to unforeseen circumstances.

G. **Complications of surgery and other medical care**
   When the admission is for treatment of a complication resulting from surgery or other medical care, the complication code is sequenced as the principal diagnosis. If the complication is classified to the T80-T88 series and the code lacks the necessary specificity in describing the complication, an additional code for the specific complication should be assigned.

H. **Uncertain Diagnosis**
   If the diagnosis documented at the time of discharge is qualified as "probable," "suspected," "likely," "questionable," "possible," or "still to be ruled out," "compatible with," "consistent with," or other similar terms indicating uncertainty, code the condition as if it existed or was established. The bases for these guidelines are the diagnostic workup, arrangements for further workup or observation, and initial therapeutic approach that correspond most closely with the established diagnosis.
   Note: This guideline is applicable only to inpatient admissions to short-term, acute, long-term care and psychiatric hospitals.

I. **Admission from Observation Unit**
   1. **Admission Following Medical Observation**
   When a patient is admitted to an observation unit for a medical condition, which either worsens or does not improve, and is subsequently admitted as an inpatient of the same hospital for this same medical condition, the principal diagnosis would be the medical condition which led to the hospital admission.

   2. **Admission Following Post-Operative Observation**
   When a patient is admitted to an observation unit to monitor a condition (or complication) that develops following outpatient surgery, and then is subsequently admitted as an inpatient of the same hospital, hospitals should apply the Uniform Hospital Discharge Data Set (UHDDS) definition of principal diagnosis as "that condition established

after study to be chiefly responsible for occasioning the admission of the patient to the hospital for care."

J. Admission from Outpatient Surgery

When a patient receives surgery in the hospital's outpatient surgery department and is subsequently admitted for continuing inpatient care at the same hospital, the following guidelines should be followed in selecting the principal diagnosis for the inpatient admission:

- If the reason for the inpatient admission is a complication, assign the complication as the principal diagnosis.
- If no complication, or other condition, is documented as the reason for the inpatient admission, assign the reason for the outpatient surgery as the principal diagnosis.
- If the reason for the inpatient admission is another condition unrelated to the surgery, assign the unrelated condition as the principal diagnosis.

K. Admissions/Encounters for Rehabilitation

When the purpose for the admission/encounter is rehabilitation, sequence first the code for the condition for which the service is being performed. For example, for an admission/encounter for rehabilitation for right-sided dominant hemiplegia following a cerebrovascular infarction, report code I69.351, Hemiplegia and hemiparesis following cerebral infarction affecting right dominant side, as the first-listed or principal diagnosis.

If the condition for which the rehabilitation service is being provided is no longer present, report the appropriate aftercare code as the first-listed or principal diagnosis, unless the rehabilitation service is being provided following an injury. For rehabilitation services following active treatment of an injury, assign the injury code with the appropriate seventh character for subsequent encounter as the first-listed or principal diagnosis. For example, if a patient with severe degenerative osteoarthritis of the hip, underwent hip replacement and the current encounter/admission is for rehabilitation, report code Z47.1, Aftercare following joint replacement surgery, as the first-listed or principal diagnosis. If the patient requires rehabilitation post hip replacement for right intertrochanteric femur fracture, report code S72.141D, Displaced intertrochanteric fracture of right femur, subsequent encounter for closed fracture with routine healing, as the first-listed or principal diagnosis.

See Section I.C.21.c.7., Factors influencing health states and contact with health services, Aftercare.

See Section I.C.19.a., for additional information about the use of 7th characters for injury codes.

Section III. Reporting Additional Diagnoses

GENERAL RULES FOR OTHER (ADDITIONAL) DIAGNOSES
For reporting purposes the definition for "other diagnoses" is interpreted as additional conditions that affect patient care in terms of requiring:

clinical evaluation; or
therapeutic treatment; or
diagnostic procedures; or
extended length of hospital stay; or
increased nursing care and/or monitoring.

The UHDDS item #11-b defines Other Diagnoses as "all conditions that coexist at the time of admission, that develop subsequently, or that affect the treatment received and/or the length of stay. Diagnoses that relate to an earlier episode which have no bearing on the current hospital stay are to be excluded." UHDDS definitions apply to inpatients in acute care, short-term, long term care and psychiatric hospital setting. The UHDDS definitions are used by acute care short-term hospitals to report inpatient data elements in a standardized manner. These data elements and their definitions can be found in the July 31, 1985, Federal Register (Vol. 50, No, 147), pp. 31038-40.

Since that time, the application of the UHDDS definitions has been expanded to include all non-outpatient settings (acute care, short term, long term care and psychiatric hospitals; home health agencies; rehab facilities; nursing homes, etc. . .). The UHDDS definitions also apply to hospice services (all levels of care).

The following guidelines are to be applied in designating "other diagnoses" when neither the Alphabetic Index nor the Tabular List in ICD-10-CM provide direction. The listing of the diagnoses in the patient record is the responsibility of the attending provider.

A. Previous conditions

If the provider has included a diagnosis in the final diagnostic statement, such as the discharge summary or the face sheet, it should ordinarily be coded. Some providers include in the diagnostic statement resolved conditions or diagnoses and status-post procedures from previous admissions that have no bearing on the current stay. Such conditions are not to be reported and are coded only if required by hospital policy.

However, history codes (categories Z80-Z87) may be used as secondary codes if the historical condition or family history has an impact on current care or influences treatment.

B. Abnormal findings

Abnormal findings (laboratory, x-ray, pathologic, and other diagnostic results) are not coded and reported unless the provider indicates their clinical significance. If the findings are outside the normal range and the attending provider has ordered other tests to evaluate the condition or prescribed treatment, it is appropriate to ask the provider whether the abnormal finding should be added.

Please note: This differs from the coding practices in the outpatient setting for coding encounters for diagnostic tests that have been interpreted by a provider.

C. Uncertain Diagnosis

If the diagnosis documented at the time of discharge is qualified as "probable," "suspected," "likely," "questionable," "possible," or "still to be ruled out," "compatible with," "consistent with," or other similar terms indicating uncertainty, code the condition as if it existed or was established. The bases for these guidelines are the diagnostic workup, arrangements for further workup or observation, and initial therapeutic approach that correspond most closely with the established diagnosis.

Note: This guideline is applicable only to inpatient admissions to short-term, acute, long-term care and psychiatric hospitals.

Section IV. Diagnostic Coding and Reporting Guidelines for Outpatient Services

These coding guidelines for outpatient diagnoses have been approved for use by hospitals/ providers in coding and reporting hospital-based outpatient services and provider-based office visits. Guidelines in Section I, Conventions, general coding guidelines and chapter-specific guidelines, should also be applied for outpatient services and office visits.

Information about the use of certain abbreviations, punctuation, symbols, and other conventions used in the ICD-10-CM Tabular List (code numbers and titles), can be found in Section IA of these guidelines, under "Conventions Used in the Tabular List." Section I.B. contains general guidelines that apply to the entire classification. Section I.C. contains chapter-specific guidelines that correspond to the chapters as they are arranged in the classification. Information about the correct sequence to use in finding a code is also described in Section I.

The terms encounter and visit are often used interchangeably in describing outpatient service contacts and, therefore, appear together in these guidelines without distinguishing one from the other.

Though the conventions and general guidelines apply to all settings, coding guidelines for outpatient and provider reporting of diagnoses will vary in a number of instances from those for inpatient diagnoses, recognizing that:

The Uniform Hospital Discharge Data Set (UHDDS) definition of principal diagnosis does not apply to hospital-based outpatient services and provider-based office visits.

Coding guidelines for inconclusive diagnoses (probable, suspected, rule out, etc.) were developed for inpatient reporting and do not apply to outpatients.

A. Selection of first-listed condition

In the outpatient setting, the term first-listed diagnosis is used in lieu of principal diagnosis.

In determining the first-listed diagnosis the coding conventions of ICD-10-CM, as well as the general and disease specific guidelines take precedence over the outpatient guidelines.

Diagnoses often are not established at the time of the initial encounter/visit. It may take two or more visits before the diagnosis is confirmed.

The most critical rule involves beginning the search for the correct code assignment through the Alphabetic Index. Never begin searching initially in the Tabular List as this will lead to coding errors.

1. Outpatient Surgery

When a patient presents for outpatient surgery (same day surgery), code the reason for the surgery as the first-listed diagnosis (reason for the encounter), even if the surgery is not performed due to a contraindication.

2. Observation Stay

When a patient is admitted for observation for a medical condition, assign a code for the medical condition as the first-listed diagnosis.

When a patient presents for outpatient surgery and develops complications requiring admission to observation, code the reason for the surgery as the first reported diagnosis (reason for the encounter), followed by codes for the complications as secondary diagnoses.

B. Codes from A00.0 through T88.9, Z00-Z99, U00-U85

The appropriate code(s) from A00.0 through T88.9, Z00-Z99, and U00-U85 must be used to identify diagnoses, symptoms, conditions, problems, complaints, or other reason(s) for the encounter/ visit.

C. Accurate reporting of ICD-10-CM diagnosis codes

For accurate reporting of ICD-10-CM diagnosis codes, the documentation should describe the patient's condition, using terminology which includes specific diagnoses as well as symptoms, problems, or reasons for the encounter. There are ICD-10-CM codes to describe all of these.

D. Codes that describe symptoms and signs

Codes that describe symptoms and signs, as opposed to diagnoses, are acceptable for reporting purposes when a diagnosis has not been established (confirmed) by the provider. Chapter 18 of ICD-10-CM, Symptoms, Signs, and Abnormal Clinical and Laboratory Findings Not Elsewhere Classified (codes R00-R99) contains many, but not all codes for symptoms.

E. Encounters for circumstances other than a disease or injury

ICD-10-CM provides codes to deal with encounters for circumstances other than a disease or injury. The Factors Influencing Health Status and Contact with Health Services codes (Z00-Z99) are provided to deal with occasions when circumstances other than a disease or injury are recorded as diagnosis or problems.

See Section I.C.21., Factors influencing health status and contact with health services.

F. Level of Detail in Coding

1. ICD-10-CM codes with 3, 4, 5, 6 or 7 characters

ICD-10-CM is composed of codes with 3, 4, 5, 6 or 7 characters. Codes with three characters are included in ICD-10-CM as the heading of a category of codes that may be further subdivided by the use of fourth, fifth, sixth or seventh characters to provide greater specificity.

2. Use of full number of characters required for a code

A 3-character code is to be used only if it is not further subdivided. A code is invalid if it has not been coded to the full number of characters required for that code, including the 7th character, if applicable.

3. Highest level of specificity

Code to the highest level of specificity when supported by the medical record documentation.

G. ICD-10-CM code for the diagnosis, condition, problem, or other reason for encounter/visit

List first the ICD-10-CM code for the diagnosis, condition, problem, or other reason for encounter/visit shown in the medical record to be chiefly responsible for the services provided. List additional codes that describe any coexisting conditions. In some cases the first-listed diagnosis may be a symptom when a diagnosis has not been established (confirmed) by the provider.

H. Uncertain diagnosis

Do not code diagnoses documented as "probable," "suspected," "questionable," "rule out," "compatible with," "consistent with," or "working diagnosis" or other similar terms indicating uncertainty. Rather, code the condition(s) to the highest degree of certainty for that encounter/visit, such as symptoms, signs, abnormal test results, or other reason for the visit.

Please note: This differs from the coding practices used by short-term, acute care, long-term care and psychiatric hospitals.

I. Chronic diseases

Chronic diseases treated on an ongoing basis may be coded and reported as many times as the patient receives treatment and care for the condition(s)

J. Code all documented conditions that coexist

Code all documented conditions that coexist at the time of the encounter/visit, and that require or affect patient care treatment or management. Do not code conditions that were previously treated and no longer exist. However, history codes (categories Z80-Z87) may be used as secondary codes if the historical condition or family history has an impact on current care or influences treatment.

K. Patients receiving diagnostic services only

For patients receiving diagnostic services only during an encounter/visit, sequence first the diagnosis, condition, problem, or other reason for encounter/visit shown in the medical record to be chiefly responsible for the outpatient services provided during the encounter/visit. Codes for other diagnoses (e.g., chronic conditions) may be sequenced as additional diagnoses.

For encounters for routine laboratory/radiology testing in the absence of any signs, symptoms, or associated diagnosis, assign Z01.89, Encounter for other specified special examinations. If routine testing is performed during the same encounter as a test to evaluate a sign, symptom, or diagnosis, it is appropriate to assign both the Z code and the code describing the reason for the non-routine test.

For outpatient encounters for diagnostic tests that have been interpreted by a physician, and the final report is available at the time of coding, code any confirmed or definitive diagnosis(es) documented in the interpretation. Do not code related signs and symptoms as additional diagnoses.

Please note: This differs from the coding practice in the hospital inpatient setting regarding abnormal findings on test results.

L. Patients receiving therapeutic services only

For patients receiving therapeutic services only during an encounter/visit, sequence first the diagnosis, condition, problem, or other reason for encounter/visit shown in the medical record to be chiefly responsible for the outpatient services provided during the encounter/visit. Codes for other diagnoses (e.g., chronic conditions) may be sequenced as additional diagnoses.

The only exception to this rule is that when the primary reason for the admission/encounter is chemotherapy or radiation therapy, the appropriate Z code for the service is listed first, and the diagnosis or problem for which the service is being performed listed second.

M. Patients receiving preoperative evaluations only

For patients receiving preoperative evaluations only, sequence first a code from subcategory Z01.81, Encounter for pre-procedural examinations, to describe the pre-op consultations. Assign a code for the condition to describe the reason for the surgery as an additional diagnosis. Code also any findings related to the pre-op evaluation.

N. Ambulatory surgery

For ambulatory surgery, code the diagnosis for which the surgery was performed. If the postoperative diagnosis is known to be different from the preoperative diagnosis at the time the diagnosis is confirmed, select the postoperative diagnosis for coding, since it is the most definitive.

O. Routine outpatient prenatal visits

See Section I.C.15., Routine outpatient prenatal visits.

P. Encounters for general medical examinations with abnormal findings

The subcategories for encounters for general medical examinations, Z00.0- and encounter for routine child health examination, Z00.12-, provide codes for with and without abnormal findings. Should a general medical examination result in an abnormal finding, the code for general medical examination with abnormal finding should be assigned as the first-listed diagnosis. An examination with abnormal findings refers to a condition/diagnosis that is newly identified or a change in severity of a chronic condition (such as uncontrolled hypertension, or an acute exacerbation of chronic obstructive pulmonary disease) during a routine physical examination. A secondary code for the abnormal finding should also be coded.

Q. Encounters for routine health screenings

See Section I.C.21., Factors influencing health status and contact with health services, Screening

Appendix I
Present on Admission Reporting Guidelines

Introduction

These guidelines are to be used as a supplement to the ICD-10-CM Official Guidelines for Coding and Reporting to facilitate the assignment of the Present on Admission (POA) indicator for each diagnosis and external cause of injury code reported on claim forms (UB-04 and 837 Institutional).

These guidelines are not intended to replace any guidelines in the main body of the ICD-10-CM Official Guidelines for Coding and Reporting. The POA guidelines are not intended to provide guidance on when a condition should be coded, but rather, how to apply the POA indicator to the final set of diagnosis codes that have been assigned in accordance with Sections I, II, and III of the official coding guidelines. Subsequent to the assignment of the ICD-10-CM codes, the POA indicator should then be assigned to those conditions that have been coded.

As stated in the Introduction to the ICD-10-CM Official Guidelines for Coding and Reporting, a joint effort between the healthcare provider and the coder is essential to achieve complete and accurate documentation, code assignment, and reporting of diagnoses and procedures. The importance of consistent, complete documentation in the medical record cannot be overemphasized. Medical record documentation from any provider involved in the care and treatment of the patient may be used to support the determination of whether a condition was present on admission or not. In the context of the official coding guidelines, the term "provider" means a physician or any qualified healthcare practitioner who is legally accountable for establishing the patient's diagnosis.

These guidelines are not a substitute for the provider's clinical judgment as to the determination of whether a condition was/was not present on admission. The provider should be queried regarding issues related to the linking of signs/symptoms, timing of test results, and the timing of findings.

Please see the CDC website for the detailed list of ICD-10-CM codes that do not require the use of a POA indicator (https://www.cdc.gov/nchs/icd/icd10cm.htm). The codes and categories on this exempt list are for circumstances regarding the healthcare encounter or factors influencing health status that do not represent a current disease or injury or that describe conditions that are always present on admission.

General Reporting Requirements

All claims involving inpatient admissions to general acute care hospitals or other facilities that are subject to a law or regulation mandating collection of present on admission information.

Present on admission is defined as present at the time the order for inpatient admission occurs—conditions that develop during an outpatient encounter, including emergency department, observation, or outpatient surgery, are considered as present on admission.

POA indicator is assigned to principal and secondary diagnoses (as defined in Section II of the Official Guidelines for Coding and Reporting) and the external cause of injury codes.

Issues related to inconsistent, missing, conflicting or unclear documentation must still be resolved by the provider.

If a condition would not be coded and reported based on UHDDS definitions and current official coding guidelines, then the POA indicator would not be reported.

Reporting Options

Y - Yes

N - No

U - Unknown

W - Clinically undetermined

Unreported/Not used - (Exempt from POA reporting)

Reporting Definitions

Y = present at the time of inpatient admission

N = not present at the time of inpatient admission

U = documentation is insufficient to determine if condition is present on admission

W = provider is unable to clinically determine whether condition was present on admission or not

Timeframe for POA Identification and Documentation

There is no required timeframe as to when a provider (per the definition of "provider" used in these guidelines) must identify or document a condition to be present on admission. In some clinical situations, it may not be possible for a provider to make a definitive diagnosis (or a condition may not be recognized or reported by the patient) for a period of time after admission. In some cases it may be several days before the provider arrives at a definitive diagnosis. This does not mean that the condition was not present on admission. Determination of whether the condition was present on admission or not will be based on the applicable POA guideline as identified in this document, or on the provider's best clinical judgment.

If at the time of code assignment the documentation is unclear as to whether a condition was present on admission or not, it is appropriate to query the provider for clarification.

Assigning the POA Indicator

Condition is on the "Exempt from Reporting" list

Leave the "present on admission" field blank if the condition is on the list of ICD-10-CM codes for which this field is not applicable. This is the only circumstance in which the field may be left blank.

POA Explicitly Documented

Assign "Y" for any condition the provider explicitly documents as being present on admission.

Assign "N" for any condition the provider explicitly documents as not present at the time of admission.

Conditions diagnosed prior to inpatient admission

Assign "Y" for conditions that were diagnosed prior to admission (example: hypertension, diabetes mellitus, asthma)

Conditions diagnosed during the admission but clearly present before admission

Assign "Y" for conditions diagnosed during the admission that were clearly present but not diagnosed until after admission occurred.

Diagnoses subsequently confirmed after admission are considered present on admission if at the time of admission they are documented as suspected, possible, rule out, differential diagnosis, or constitute an underlying cause of a symptom that is present at the time of admission.

Condition develops during outpatient encounter prior to inpatient admission

Assign "Y" for any condition that develops during an outpatient encounter prior to a written order for inpatient admission.

Documentation does not indicate whether condition was present on admission

Assign "U" when the medical record documentation is unclear as to whether the condition was present on admission. "U" should not be routinely assigned and used only in very limited circumstances. Coders are encouraged to query the providers when the documentation is unclear.

Documentation states that it cannot be determined whether the condition was or was not present on admission

Assign "W" when the medical record documentation indicates that it cannot be clinically determined whether or not the condition was present on admission.

Chronic condition with acute exacerbation during the admission

If a single code identifies both the chronic condition and the acute exacerbation, see POA guidelines pertaining to codes that contain multiple clinical concepts.

If a single code only identifies the chronic condition and not the acute exacerbation (e.g., acute exacerbation of chronic leukemia), assign "Y."

Conditions documented as possible, probable, suspected, or rule out at the time of discharge

If the final diagnosis contains a possible, probable, suspected, or rule out diagnosis, and this diagnosis was based on signs, symptoms or clinical findings suspected at the time of inpatient admission, assign "Y."

If the final diagnosis contains a possible, probable, suspected, or rule out diagnosis, and this diagnosis was based on signs, symptoms or clinical findings that were not present on admission, assign "N".

Conditions documented as impending or threatened at the time of discharge

If the final diagnosis contains an impending or threatened diagnosis, and this diagnosis is based on symptoms or clinical findings that were present on admission, assign "Y".

If the final diagnosis contains an impending or threatened diagnosis, and this diagnosis is based on symptoms or clinical findings that were not present on admission, assign "N".

Acute and Chronic Conditions

Assign "Y" for acute conditions that are present at time of admission and "N" for acute conditions that are not present at time of admission.

Assign "Y" for chronic conditions, even though the condition may not be diagnosed until after admission.

If a single code identifies both an acute and chronic condition, see the POA guidelines for codes that contain multiple clinical concepts.

Codes That Contain Multiple Clinical Concepts

Assign "N" if at least one of the clinical concepts included in the code was not present on admission (e.g., COPD with acute exacerbation and the exacerbation was not present on admission; gastric ulcer that does not start bleeding until after admission; asthma patient develops status asthmaticus after admission).

Assign "Y" if all of the clinical concepts included in the code were present on admission (e.g., duodenal ulcer that perforates prior to admission).

For infection codes that include the causal organism, assign "Y" if the infection (or signs of the infection) were present on admission, even though the culture results may not be known until after admission (e.g., patient is admitted with pneumonia and the provider documents Pseudomonas as the causal organism a few days later).

Same Diagnosis Code for Two or More Conditions

When the same ICD-10-CM diagnosis code applies to two or more conditions during the same encounter (e.g., two separate conditions classified to the same ICD-10-CM diagnosis code):

Assign "Y" if all conditions represented by the single ICD-10-CM code were present on admission (e.g., bilateral unspecified age-related cataracts).

Assign "N" if any of the conditions represented by the single ICD-10-CM code was not present on admission (e.g., traumatic secondary and recurrent hemorrhage and seroma is assigned to a single code T79.2, but only one of the conditions was present on admission).

Obstetrical conditions

Whether or not the patient delivers during the current hospitalization does not affect assignment of the POA indicator. The determining factor for POA assignment is whether the pregnancy complication or obstetrical condition described by the code was present at the time of admission or not.

If the pregnancy complication or obstetrical condition was present on admission (e.g., patient admitted in preterm labor), assign "Y".

If the pregnancy complication or obstetrical condition was not present on admission (e.g., 2nd degree laceration during delivery, postpartum hemorrhage that occurred during current hospitalization, fetal distress develops after admission), assign "N".

If the obstetrical code includes more than one diagnosis and any of the diagnoses identified by the code were not present on admission assign "N".

(e.g., Category O11, Pre-existing hypertension with pre-eclampsia)

Perinatal conditions

Newborns are not considered to be admitted until after birth. Therefore, any condition present at birth or that developed in utero is considered present at admission and should be assigned "Y". This includes conditions that occur during delivery (e.g., injury during delivery, meconium aspiration, exposure to streptococcus B in the vaginal canal).

Congenital conditions and anomalies

Assign "Y" for congenital conditions and anomalies except for categories Q00-Q99, Congenital anomalies, which are on the exempt list. Congenital conditions are always considered present on admission.

External cause of injury codes

Assign "Y" for any external cause code representing an external cause of morbidity that occurred prior to inpatient admission (e.g., patient fell out of bed at home, patient fell out of bed in emergency room prior to admission).

Assign "N" for any external cause code representing an external cause of morbidity that occurred during inpatient hospitalization (e.g., patient fell out of hospital bed during hospital stay, patient experienced an adverse reaction to a medication administered after inpatient admission).

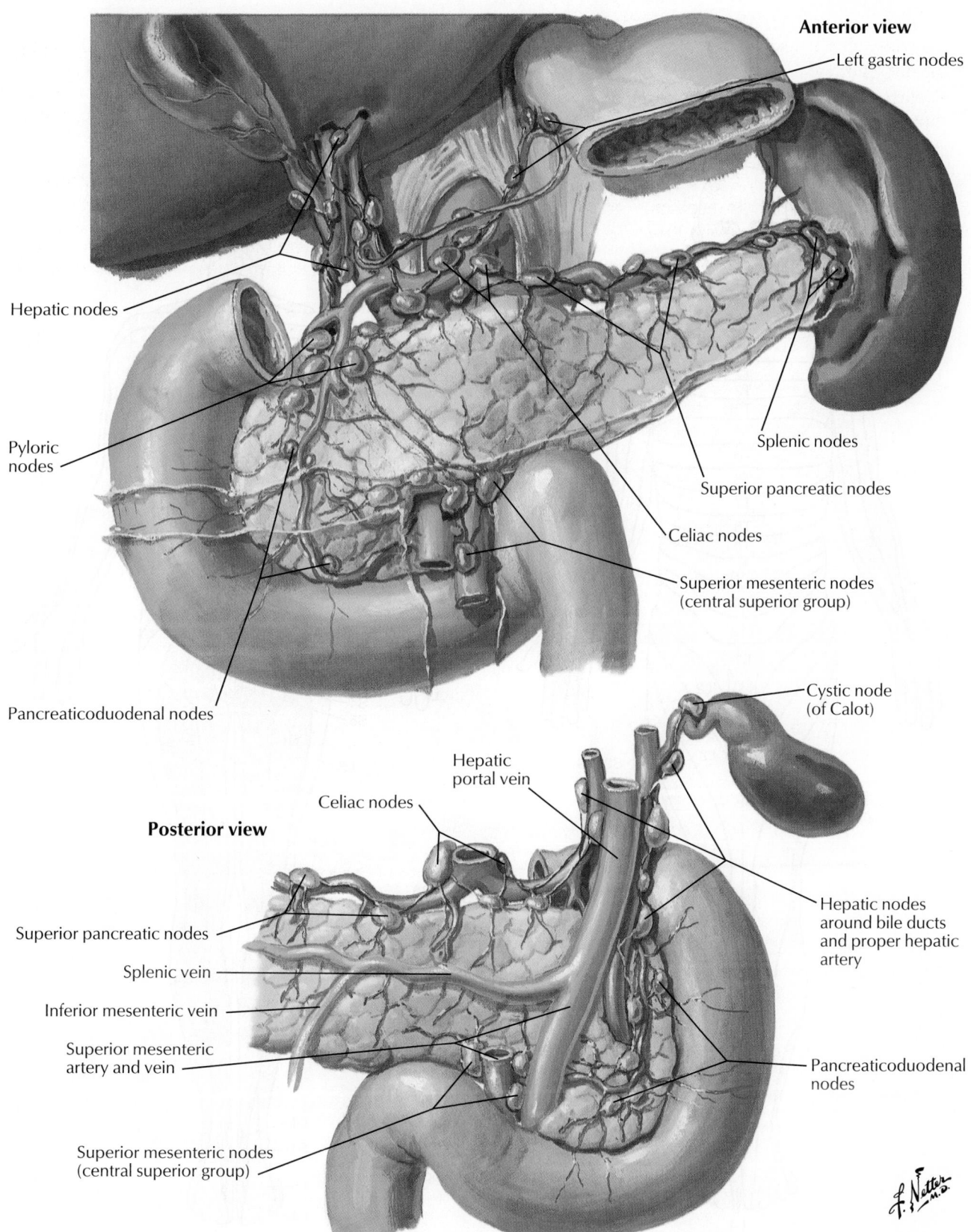

Anterior view

Left gastric nodes

Hepatic nodes

Pyloric nodes

Splenic nodes

Superior pancreatic nodes

Celiac nodes

Superior mesenteric nodes (central superior group)

Pancreaticoduodenal nodes

Cystic node (of Calot)

Hepatic portal vein

Celiac nodes

Posterior view

Superior pancreatic nodes

Splenic vein

Inferior mesenteric vein

Superior mesenteric artery and vein

Hepatic nodes around bile ducts and proper hepatic artery

Pancreaticoduodenal nodes

Superior mesenteric nodes (central superior group)

Plate 1 Lymph Vessels and Nodes of Pancreas. (Copyright 2022 Elsevier Inc. All rights reserved. www.netterimages.com. Image ID: 4420)

Levels of principal dermatomes

C5	Clavicles
C5, 6, 7	Lateral parts of upper limbs
C8, T1	Medial sides of upper limbs
C6	Thumb
C6, 7, 8	Hand
C8	Ring and little fingers
T4	Level of nipples
T10	Level of umbilicus
L1	Inguinal or groin regions
L1, 2, 3, 4	Anterior and inner surfaces of lower limbs
L4, 5, S1	Foot
L4	Medial side of great toe
S1, 2, L5	Posterior and other surfaces of lower limbs
S1	Lateral margin of foot and little toe
S2, 3, 4	Perineum

Plate 2 Schematic demarcation of Dermatomes. (Miller MD, Hart JA, MacKnight JM: Essential Orthopaedics, ed 2, Philadelphia, 2020, Elsevier.)

Female: frontal section

- Peritoneum
- Body of bladder
- Fundus of bladder
- Interureteric crest
- Left ureteric orifice
- Trigone of bladder
- Neck of bladder
- Paravesical endopelvic fascia and vesical venous plexus
- Vesical fascia
- Tendinous arch of levator ani muscle
- Obturator internus muscle
- Levator ani muscle
- Tendinous arch of pelvic fascia
- Urethra
- Sphincter urethrae muscle
- Perineal membrane
- Inferior pubic ramus
- Crus of clitoris and ischiocavernosus muscle
- Bulb of vestibule and bulbospongiosus muscle
- Deep perineal (investing or Gallaudet's) fascia
- Superficial perineal (Colles') fascia

Round ligament of uterus

Vagina

Male: frontal section

- Peritoneum
- Body of bladder
- Fundus of bladder
- Ductus (vas) deferens
- Interureteric crest
- Right ureteric orifice
- Trigone of bladder
- Neck of bladder
- Paravesical endopelvic fascia and vesical venous plexus
- Tendinous arch of levator ani muscle
- Uvula of bladder
- Obturator internus muscle
- Levator ani muscle
- Capsule of prostate
- Prostate and prostatic urethra
- Seminal colliculus
- Bulbourethral (Cowper's) gland
- Perineal membrane and sphincter urethrae muscle
- Bulbous portion of spongy urethra
- Corpus spongiosum and bulbospongiosus muscle
- Deep perineal (investing or Gallaudet's) fascia
- Internal urethral sphincter
- Tendinous arch of pelvic fascia
- Anterior recess of ischio-anal fossa
- Inferior pubic ramus
- Crus of penis and ischiocavernosus muscle
- Superficial perineal (Colles') fascia

ANATOMY ILLUSTRATIONS

Sites of ectopic implantation

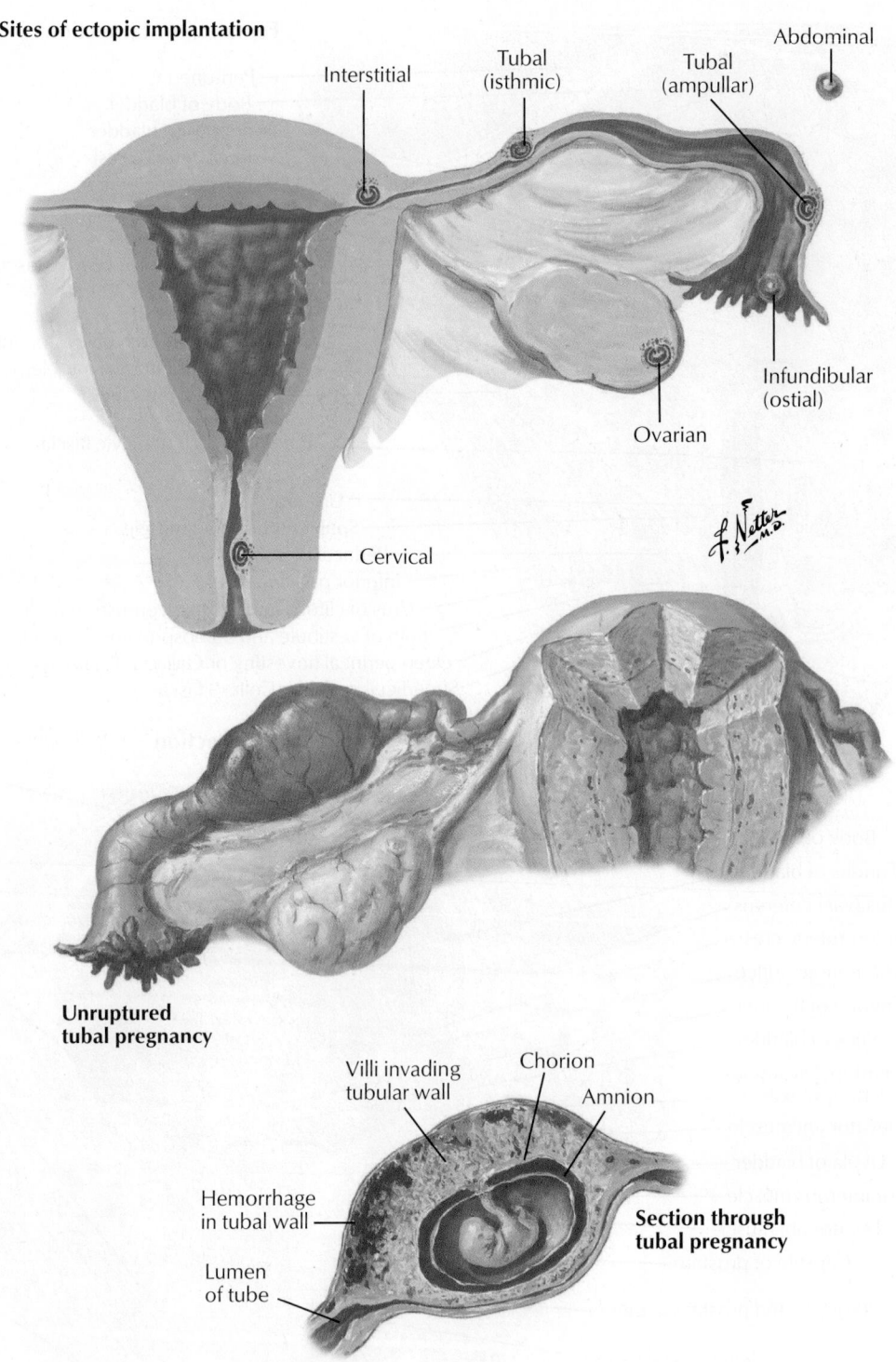

Interstitial

Tubal (isthmic)

Tubal (ampullar)

Abdominal

Infundibular (ostial)

Ovarian

Cervical

Unruptured tubal pregnancy

Villi invading tubular wall

Chorion

Amnion

Hemorrhage in tubal wall

Section through tubal pregnancy

Lumen of tube

Plate 4   Ectopic Pregnancy. (Copyright 2022 Elsevier Inc. All rights reserved. www.netterimages.com. Image ID: 5148)

Skin of penis

Superficial fascia
of penis (Colles' fascia)

Deep (Buck's)
fascia of penis

Testicular artery

Ductus deferens

Artery to ductus deferens

Genital branch of
genitofemoral nerve

Pampiniform (venous) plexus

Epididymis

Appendix of epididymis

Appendix of testis

Testis (covered by visceral
layer of tunica vaginalis)

Parietal layer of tunica vaginalis

Superficial
inguinal ring

External
spermatic fascia

Cremaster muscle
and fascia

Septum of scrotum
(formed by
dartos fascia)

Superficial
(dartos) fascia
of scrotum

Skin of scrotum

Superficial (dartos) fascia of scrotum

External spermatic fascia

Cremaster muscle and fascia

Internal spermatic fascia

Parietal layer of tunica vaginalis

Epididymis

Testis (covered by visceral layer of tunica vaginalis)

Skin of scrotum

Plate 5 Scrotum and Contents. (Copyright 2022 Elsevier Inc. All rights reserved. www.netterimages.com. Image ID: 4686)

Plate 6 Cranial Nerves (12 pairs) are known by their numbers (Roman numerals) and names. (Herlihy BL: The Human Body in Health and Illness, ed 6, St. Louis, 2018, Elsevier.)

Superior view

Supratrochlear nerve
Medial rectus muscle
Superior oblique muscle
Infratrochlear nerve
Nasociliary nerve
Trochlear nerve (IV)
Common tendinous ring
Ophthalmic nerve (V_1)
Optic nerve (II)
Internal carotid artery and nerve plexus
Oculomotor nerve (III)
Trochlear nerve (IV)
Abducent nerve (VI)
Tentorium cerebelli

Medial branch } Lateral branch } Supraorbital nerve
Levator palpebrae superioris muscle
Superior rectus muscle
Lacrimal gland
Lacrimal nerve
Lateral rectus muscle
Frontal nerve
Maxillary nerve (V_2)
Meningeal branch of maxillary nerve
Mandibular nerve (V_3)
Lesser petrosal nerve
Meningeal branch of mandibular nerve
Greater petrosal nerve
Trigeminal (semilunar) ganglion
Tentorial (meningeal) branch of ophthalmic nerve

Superior view:
levator palpebrae superioris, superior rectus, and superior oblique muscles partially cut away

Supratrochlear nerve *(cut)*
Supraorbital nerve branches *(cut)*
Infratrochlear nerve
Anterior ethmoidal nerve
Optic nerve (II)
Posterior ethmoidal nerve
Superior branch of oculomotor nerve (III) *(cut)*
Nasociliary nerve
Internal carotid plexus
Trochlear nerve (IV) *(cut)*
Oculomotor nerve (III)
Abducent nerve (VI)

Long ciliary nerves
Short ciliary nerves
Lacrimal nerve
Ciliary ganglion
Parasympathetic root of ciliary ganglion (from inferior branch of oculomotor nerve)
Sympathetic root of ciliary ganglion (from internal carotid plexus)
Sensory root of ciliary ganglion (from nasociliary nerve)
Branches to inferior and medial rectus muscles
Abducent nerve (VI)
Inferior branch of oculomotor nerve (III)
Lacrimal nerve
Frontal nerve *(cut)*
Ophthalmic nerve (V_1)

Proper palmar digital nerves (median nerve)

Medial two lumbricals innervated by ulnar nerve

Cutaneous innervation of the median nerve in the hand

Cutaneous innervation of the dorsal branch of the ulnar nerve

Cutaneous innervation of the palmar branch of the median nerve

Palmar view

Lateral two lumbricals innervated by median nerve

Dorsal view

Proper palmar digital nerve (ulnar nerve)

Intrinsic muscles innervated by ulnar nerve except the thenar muscles and the two lateral lumbricals

Common palmar digital nerve

Hypothenar muscles innervated by ulnar nerve

Palmaris brevis

Deep branch of the ulnar nerve

Superficial branch of the ulnar nerve

Palmar branch of the ulnar nerve

Ulnar nerve

Ulna

Common palmar digital nerves (median nerve)

Cutaneous innervation of the superficial branch of the ulnar nerve in the hand

Thenar muscles innervated by median nerve

Recurrent branch of median nerve

Cutaneous innervation of the palmar branch of the ulnar nerve

Palmar view

Palmar branch of the median nerve

Median nerve

Radius

Cutaneous innervation of the median nerve in the hand

Innervation of the hand, median and ulnar nerves (palmar view)

Dorsal view

Plate 8 Innervation of the Hand: Median and Ulnar Nerves (From Drake RL, Vogl AW, Mitchell AWM, Tibbitts RM, Richardson PE: Gray's Atlas of Anatomy, ed 2, Philadelphia, 2015, Churchill Livingstone.)

Biceps brachii

Posterior cutaneous nerve of forearm (cut) (from radial nerve)

Lateral cutaneous nerve of forearm (cut) (from musculocutaneous nerve)

Biceps brachii tendon

Radial artery

Brachioradialis

Radial artery

Palmaris longus tendon

Median nerve

Thenar muscles

Palmar branch of median nerve

Palmar aponeurosis

Ulnar nerve

Medial cutaneous nerve of forearm (from medial cord of brachial plexus)

Median nerve

Brachial artery

Medial epicondyle

Bicipital aponeurosis

Radial nerve

Brachial artery

Lateral epicondyle

Radial recurrent artery

Deep branch radial nerve

Radial artery

Supinator

Superficial branch radial nerve

Common interosseous artery

Posterior interosseous artery

Interosseous membrane

Pronator teres (cut)

Perforating branches of anterior interosseous artery

Ulnar artery

Brachioradialis tendon (cut)

Palmar branch of ulnar nerve

Hypothenar muscles

Median nerve

Flexor carpi radialis tendon (cut)

Flexor retinaculum

Superficial palmar branch of radial artery

Palmar branch of median nerve

Median nerve

Recurrent interosseous artery

Ulnar nerve

Humeral head of pronator teres (cut)

Posterior interosseous artery

Anterior ulnar recurrent artery

Humeral head of flexor carpi ulnaris

Posterior ulnar recurrent artery

Ulnar head of pronator teres

Ulnar artery

Anterior interosseous nerve

Anterior interosseous artery

Radial artery

Interosseous membrane

Flexor digitorum superficialis (cut)

Flexor digitorum profundus

Dorsal branch of ulnar nerve

Flexor carpi ulnaris tendon (cut)

Ulnar nerve

Palmar branch of ulnar nerve

Deep palmar branch of ulnar artery

Deep palmar arch

Superficial palmar arch

Superior ulnar collateral artery

Inferior ulnar collateral artery

Radial collateral artery

Brachial artery

Radial recurrent artery

Anterior ulnar recurrent artery

Posterior ulnar recurrent artery

Common interosseous artery

Anterior interosseous artery

Ulnar artery

Radius

Ulna

Superficial palmar branch of radial artery

Pisiform

Superficial palmar arch

Deep palmar arch

Arteries and nerves of forearm (anterior view)

Plate 9   Arteries and Nerves of the Forearm (Anterior View) (From Drake RL, Vogl AW, Mitchell AWM, Tibbitts RM, Richardson PE: Gray's Atlas of Anatomy, ed 2, Philadelphia, 2015, Churchill Livingstone.)

Lateral cutaneous branch of subcostal nerve

Inguinal ligament (Poupart's)

Superficial circumflex iliac vein

Femoral branches of genitofemoral nerve

Lateral femoral cutaneous nerve

Saphenous opening (fossa ovalis)

Fascia lata

Anterior cutaneous branches of femoral nerve

Patellar nerve plexus

Branches of lateral sural cutaneous nerve (from common fibular [peroneal] nerve)

Deep fascia of leg (crural fascia)

Superficial fibular (peroneal) nerve
Medial dorsal cutaneous branch

Intermediate dorsal cutaneous branch

Small saphenous vein and lateral dorsal cutaneous nerve (from sural nerve)

Lateral dorsal digital nerve and vein of 5th toe

Dorsal metatarsal veins

Dorsal digital nerves and veins

Superficial epigastric vein

Ilioinguinal nerve (scrotal branch) (usually passes through superficial inguinal ring)

Genital branch of genitofemoral nerve

Femoral vein

Superficial external pudendal vein

Accessory saphenous vein

Great saphenous vein

Cutaneous branches of obturator nerve

Infrapatellar branch of saphenous nerve

Saphenous nerve (terminal branch of femoral nerve)

Great saphenous vein

Dorsal digital nerves

Dorsal venous arch

Dorsal digital nerve and vein of medial side of great toe

Dorsal digital branch of deep fibular (peroneal) nerve

Plate 10 Superficial Nerves and Veins of Lower Limb: Anterior View. (Copyright 2022 Elsevier Inc. All rights reserved. www.netterimages.com. Image ID: 4846)

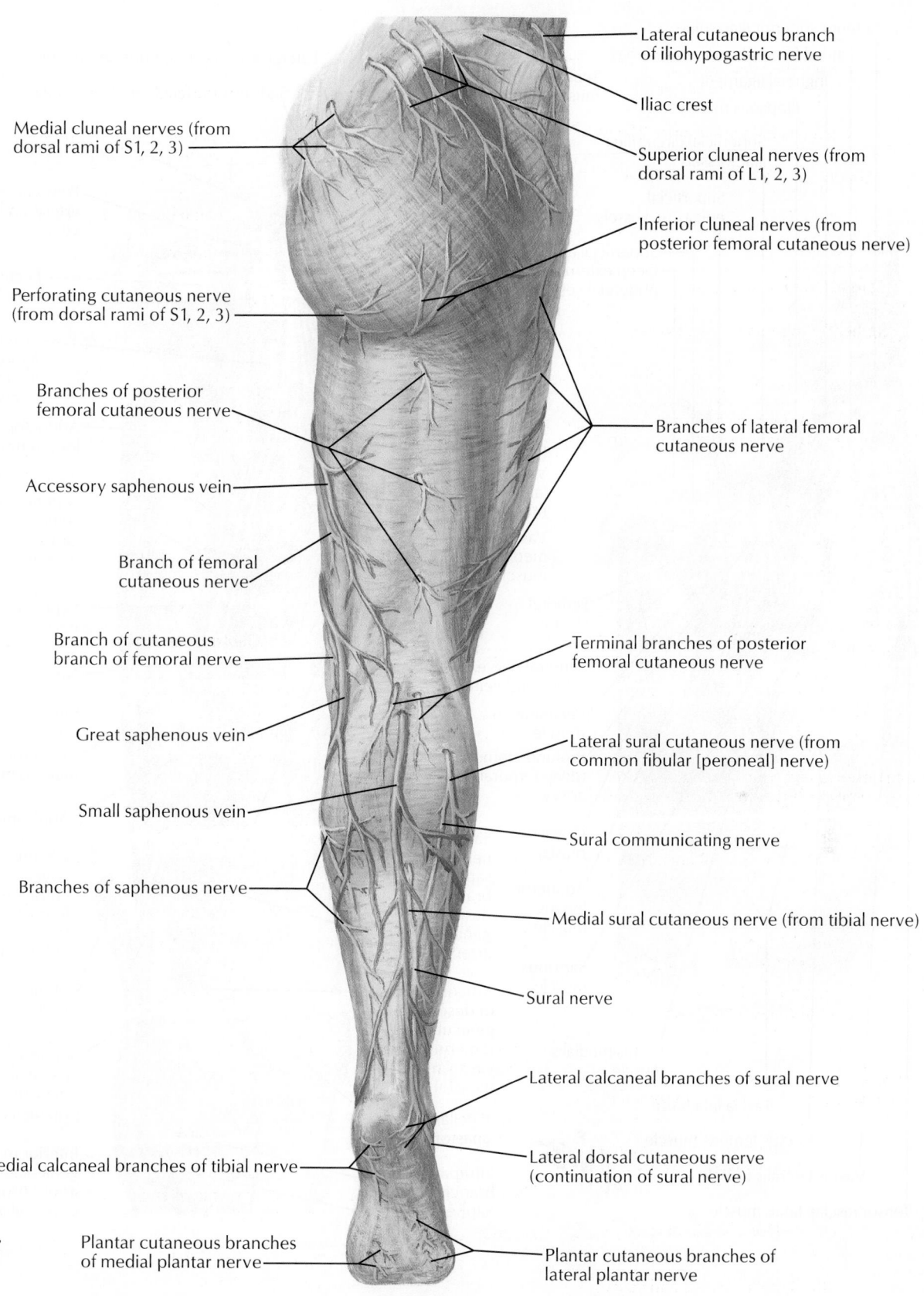

Lateral cutaneous branch of iliohypogastric nerve

Iliac crest

Medial cluneal nerves (from dorsal rami of S1, 2, 3)

Superior cluneal nerves (from dorsal rami of L1, 2, 3)

Inferior cluneal nerves (from posterior femoral cutaneous nerve)

Perforating cutaneous nerve (from dorsal rami of S1, 2, 3)

Branches of posterior femoral cutaneous nerve

Branches of lateral femoral cutaneous nerve

Accessory saphenous vein

Branch of femoral cutaneous nerve

Branch of cutaneous branch of femoral nerve

Terminal branches of posterior femoral cutaneous nerve

Great saphenous vein

Lateral sural cutaneous nerve (from common fibular [peroneal] nerve)

Small saphenous vein

Sural communicating nerve

Branches of saphenous nerve

Medial sural cutaneous nerve (from tibial nerve)

Sural nerve

Lateral calcaneal branches of sural nerve

Medial calcaneal branches of tibial nerve

Lateral dorsal cutaneous nerve (continuation of sural nerve)

Plantar cutaneous branches of medial plantar nerve

Plantar cutaneous branches of lateral plantar nerve

ANATOMY ILLUSTRATIONS

Plate 11 Superficial Nerves and Veins of Lower Limb: Posterior View. (Copyright 2022 Elsevier Inc. All rights reserved. www.netterimages.com. Image ID: 4669)

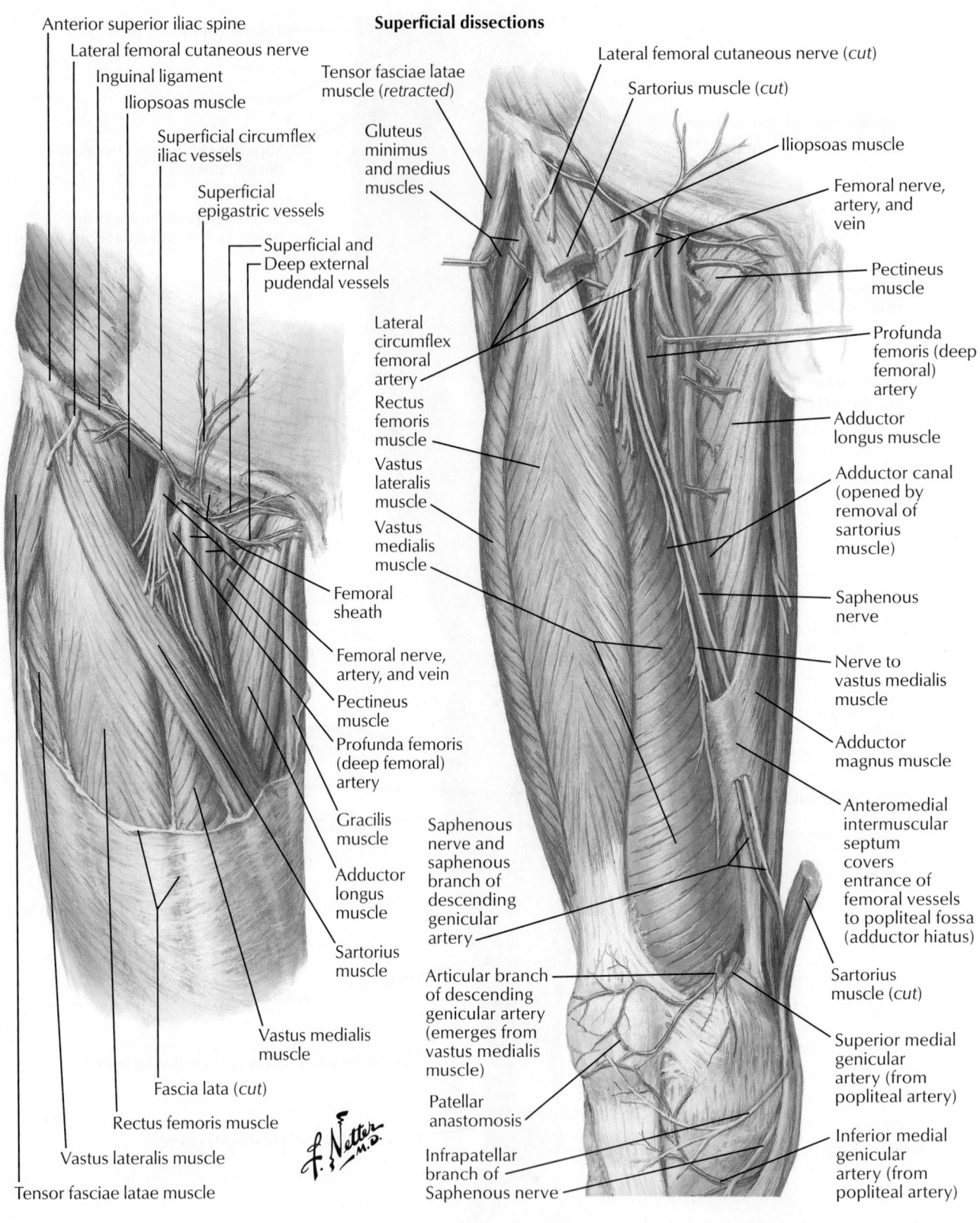

Anterior superior iliac spine

Lateral femoral cutaneous nerve

Inguinal ligament

Iliopsoas muscle

Superficial circumflex iliac vessels

Superficial epigastric vessels

Superficial and Deep external pudendal vessels

Superficial dissections

Tensor fasciae latae muscle (*retracted*)

Gluteus minimus and medius muscles

Lateral circumflex femoral artery

Rectus femoris muscle

Vastus lateralis muscle

Vastus medialis muscle

Femoral sheath

Femoral nerve, artery, and vein

Pectineus muscle

Profunda femoris (deep femoral) artery

Gracilis muscle

Adductor longus muscle

Sartorius muscle

Vastus medialis muscle

Fascia lata (*cut*)

Rectus femoris muscle

Vastus lateralis muscle

Tensor fasciae latae muscle

Saphenous nerve and saphenous branch of descending genicular artery

Articular branch of descending genicular artery (emerges from vastus medialis muscle)

Patellar anastomosis

Infrapatellar branch of Saphenous nerve

Lateral femoral cutaneous nerve (*cut*)

Sartorius muscle (*cut*)

Iliopsoas muscle

Femoral nerve, artery, and vein

Pectineus muscle

Profunda femoris (deep femoral) artery

Adductor longus muscle

Adductor canal (opened by removal of sartorius muscle)

Saphenous nerve

Nerve to vastus medialis muscle

Adductor magnus muscle

Anteromedial intermuscular septum covers entrance of femoral vessels to popliteal fossa (adductor hiatus)

Sartorius muscle (*cut*)

Superior medial genicular artery (from popliteal artery)

Inferior medial genicular artery (from popliteal artery)

ANATOMY ILLUSTRATIONS

Plate 12 Arteries and Nerves of Thigh: Anterior Views. (Copyright 2022 Elsevier Inc. All rights reserved. www.netterimages.com. Image ID: 4475)

Deep dissection

Deep circumflex iliac artery

Lateral femoral cutaneous nerve

Sartorius muscle (cut)

Iliopsoas muscle

Tensor fasciae latae muscle (retracted)

Gluteus medius and minimus muscles

Femoral nerve

Rectus femoris muscle (cut)

Ascending, transverse and descending branches of Lateral circumflex femoral artery

Medial circumflex femoral artery

Pectineus muscle (cut)

Profunda femoris (deep femoral) artery

Perforating branches

Adductor longus muscle (cut)

Vastus lateralis muscle

Vastus intermedius muscle

Rectus femoris muscle (cut)

Saphenous nerve

Anteromedial intermuscular septum (opened)

Vastus medialis muscle

Quadriceps femoris tendon

Patella and patellar anastomosis

Medial patellar retinaculum

Patellar ligament

External iliac artery and vein

Inguinal ligament (Poupart's)

Femoral artery and vein (cut)

Pectineus muscle (cut)

Obturator canal

Obturator externus muscle

Adductor longus muscle (cut)

Anterior branch and Posterior branch of obturator nerve

Quadratus femoris muscle

Adductor brevis muscle

Branches of posterior branch of obturator nerve

Adductor magnus muscle

Gracilis muscle

Cutaneous branch of obturator nerve

Femoral artery and vein (cut)

Descending genicular artery
Articular branch
Saphenous branch

Adductor hiatus

Sartorius muscle (cut)

Adductor magnus tendon

Adductor tubercle on medial epicondyle of femur

Superior medial genicular artery (from popliteal artery)

Infrapatellar branch of Saphenous nerve

Inferior medial genicular artery (from popliteal artery)

ANATOMY ILLUSTRATIONS

Deep dissection

Superior cluneal nerves

Gluteus maximus muscle (*cut*)

Medial cluneal nerves

Inferior gluteal artery and nerve

Pudendal nerve

Nerve to obturator internus (and superior gemellus)

Posterior femoral cutaneous nerve

Sacrotuberous ligament

Ischial tuberosity

Inferior cluneal nerves (*cut*)

Adductor magnus muscle

Gracilis muscle

Sciatic nerve

Muscular branches of sciatic nerve

Semitendinosus muscle (*retracted*)

Semimembranosus muscle

Sciatic nerve

Articular branch

Adductor hiatus

Popliteal vein and artery

Superior medial genicular artery

Medial epicondyle of femur

Tibial nerve

Gastrocnemius muscle (medial head)

Medial sural cutaneous nerve

Small saphenous vein

Iliac crest

Gluteal aponeurosis and gluteus medius muscle (*cut*)

Superior gluteal artery and nerve

Gluteus minimus muscle

Tensor fasciae latae muscle

Piriformis muscle

Gluteus medius muscle (*cut*)

Superior gemellus muscle

Greater trochanter of femur

Obturator internus muscle

Inferior gemellus muscle

Gluteus maximus muscle (*cut*)

Quadratus femoris muscle

Medial circumflex femoral artery

Vastus lateralis muscle and iliotibial tract

Adductor minimus part of adductor magnus muscle

1st perforating artery (from profunda femoris artery)

Adductor magnus muscle

2nd and 3rd perforating arteries (from profunda femoris artery)

4th perforating artery (from profunda femoris artery)

Long head (*retracted*)
Short head
Biceps femoris muscle

Superior lateral genicular artery

Common fibular (peroneal) nerve

Plantaris muscle

Gastrocnemius muscle (lateral head)

Lateral sural cutaneous nerve

ANATOMY ILLUSTRATIONS

Plate 14 Arteries and Nerves of Thigh: Posterior View. (Copyright 2022 Elsevier Inc. All rights reserved. www.netterimages.com. Image ID: 49317)

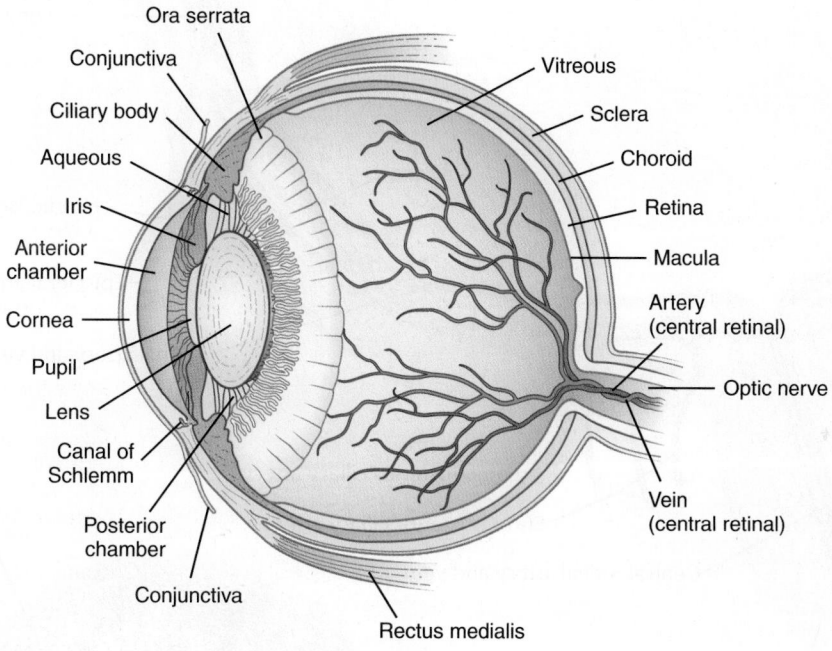

Ora serrata

Conjunctiva

Ciliary body

Aqueous

Iris

Anterior chamber

Cornea

Pupil

Lens

Canal of Schlemm

Posterior chamber

Conjunctiva

Rectus medialis

Vitreous

Sclera

Choroid

Retina

Macula

Artery (central retinal)

Optic nerve

Vein (central retinal)

Plate 15   Anatomy of the eye. (Dehn RW, Asprey DP: Essential Clinical Procedures, ed 3, Philadelphia, 2013, Saunders.)

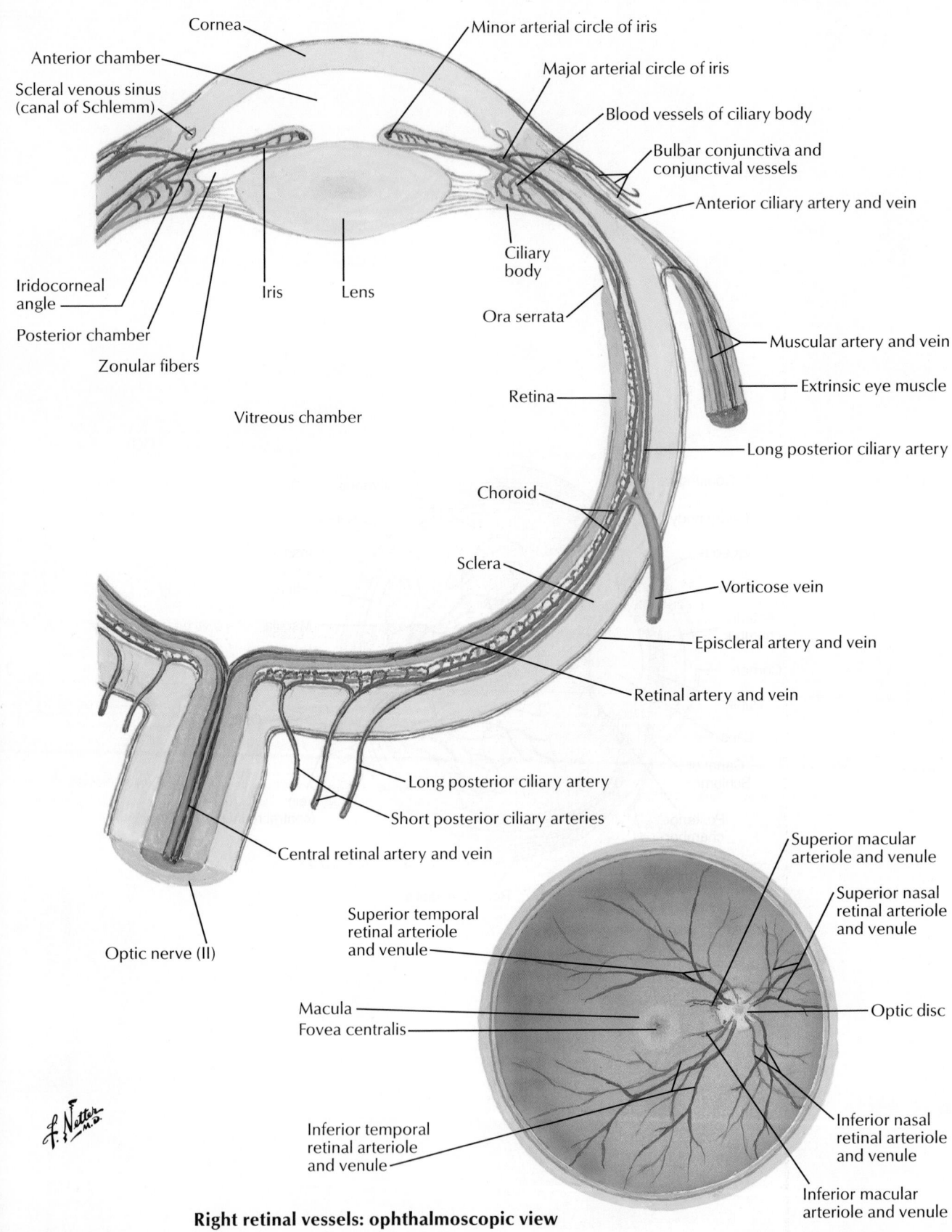

Cornea

Minor arterial circle of iris

Anterior chamber

Major arterial circle of iris

Scleral venous sinus
(canal of Schlemm)

Blood vessels of ciliary body

Bulbar conjunctiva and
conjunctival vessels

Anterior ciliary artery and vein

Iridocorneal
angle

Ciliary
body

Posterior chamber

Ora serrata

Iris

Lens

Muscular artery and vein

Zonular fibers

Extrinsic eye muscle

Vitreous chamber

Retina

Long posterior ciliary artery

Choroid

Sclera

Vorticose vein

Episcleral artery and vein

Retinal artery and vein

Long posterior ciliary artery

Short posterior ciliary arteries

Central retinal artery and vein

Optic nerve (II)

Superior macular
arteriole and venule

Superior nasal
retinal arteriole
and venule

Superior temporal
retinal arteriole
and venule

Macula

Optic disc

Fovea centralis

Inferior nasal
retinal arteriole
and venule

Inferior temporal
retinal arteriole
and venule

Inferior macular
arteriole and venule

Right retinal vessels: ophthalmoscopic view

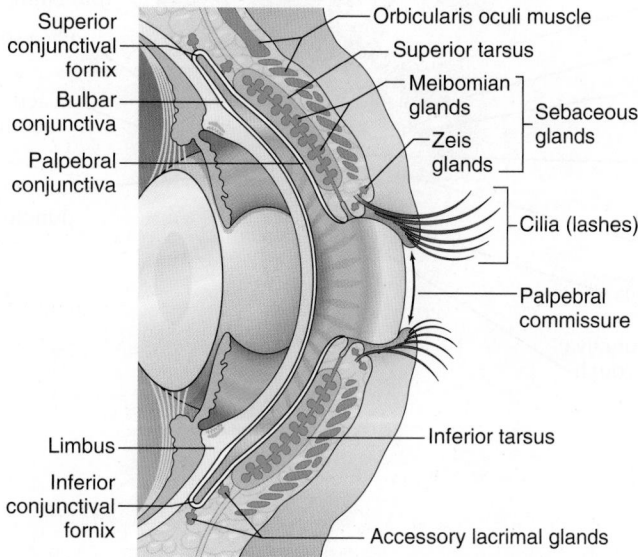

Superior conjunctival fornix

Bulbar conjunctiva

Palpebral conjunctiva

Orbicularis oculi muscle

Superior tarsus

Meibomian glands

Sebaceous glands

Zeis glands

Cilia (lashes)

Palpebral commissure

Limbus

Inferior conjunctival fornix

Inferior tarsus

Accessory lacrimal glands

Plate 17   Anatomy of the conjunctiva and eyelids. (Kumar V, Abbas AK, Aster JC: Robbins and Cotran Pathologic Basis of Disease, ed 9, Philadelphia, 2015, Saunders.)

Superior palpebral conjunctiva: tarsal (meibomian) glands shining through

Seen through cornea { Pupil / Iris

Corneoscleral junction (corneal limbus)

Bulbar conjunctiva over sclera

Inferior conjunctival fornix

Inferior palpebral conjunctiva: tarsal glands shining through

Superior lacrimal papilla and punctum

Plica semilunaris

Lacrimal caruncle in lacrimal lake (lacus lacrimalis)

Inferior lacrimal papilla and punctum

Plate 18 Eyelid. (Copyright 2022 Elsevier Inc. All rights reserved. www.netterimages.com. Image ID: 4557)

Orbital part of lacrimal gland

Palpebral part of lacrimal gland

Excretory ducts of lacrimal gland

Plica semilunaris

Lacrimal caruncle

Inferior lacrimal papilla and punctum

Superior lacrimal papilla and punctum

Lacrimal canaliculi

Lacrimal sac

Nasolacrimal duct

Opening of nasolacrimal duct

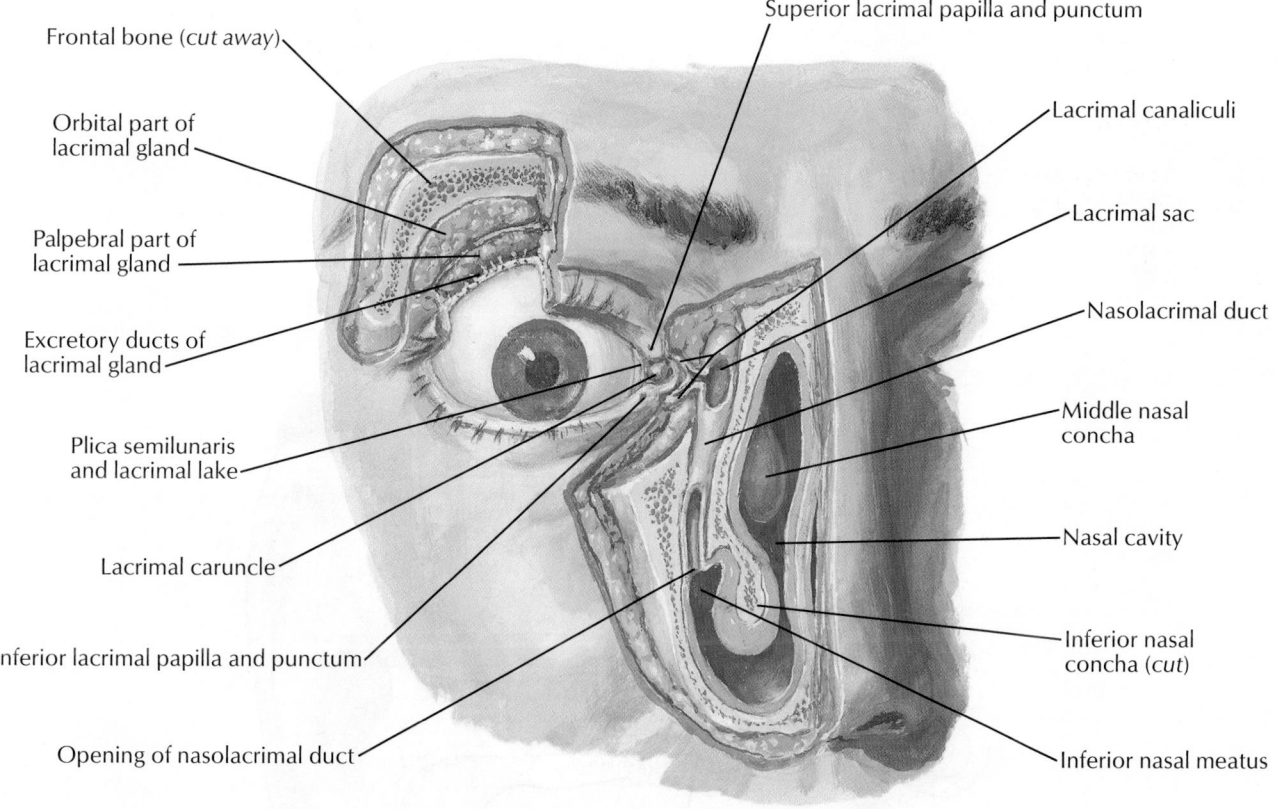

Frontal bone (*cut away*)

Orbital part of lacrimal gland

Palpebral part of lacrimal gland

Excretory ducts of lacrimal gland

Plica semilunaris and lacrimal lake

Lacrimal caruncle

Inferior lacrimal papilla and punctum

Opening of nasolacrimal duct

Superior lacrimal papilla and punctum

Lacrimal canaliculi

Lacrimal sac

Nasolacrimal duct

Middle nasal concha

Nasal cavity

Inferior nasal concha (*cut*)

Inferior nasal meatus

ANATOMY ILLUSTRATIONS

ANATOMY ILLUSTRATIONS

Plate 20 Pathway of Sound. (LaFleur Brooks D, LaFleur Brooks M: Basic Medical Language, ed 4, St. Louis, 2013, Mosby.)

Plate 21 Middle ear structures. (©Elsevier Collection.)

74

RIGHT TYMPANIC MEMBRANE

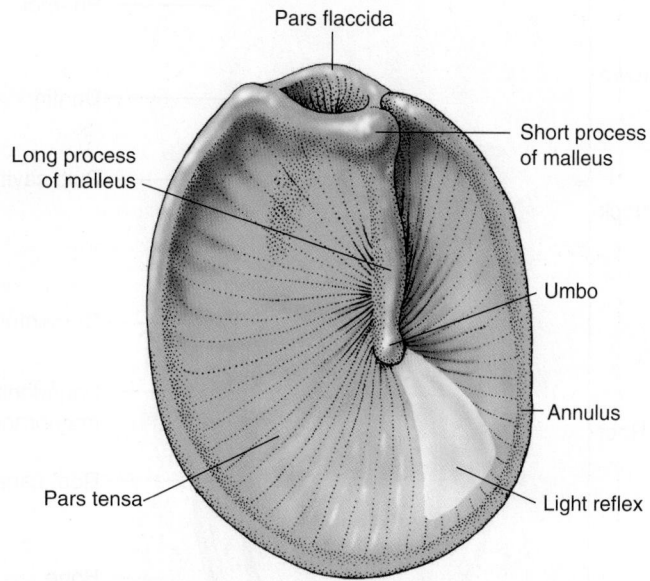

Pars flaccida

Short process
of malleus

Long process
of malleus

Umbo

Annulus

Pars tensa

Light reflex

Plate 22 Structural landmarks of tympanic membrane. (Ignatavicius DD, Workman ML: Medical-Surgical Nursing: Patient-Centered Collaborative Care, ed 7, St. Louis, 2013, Saunders.)

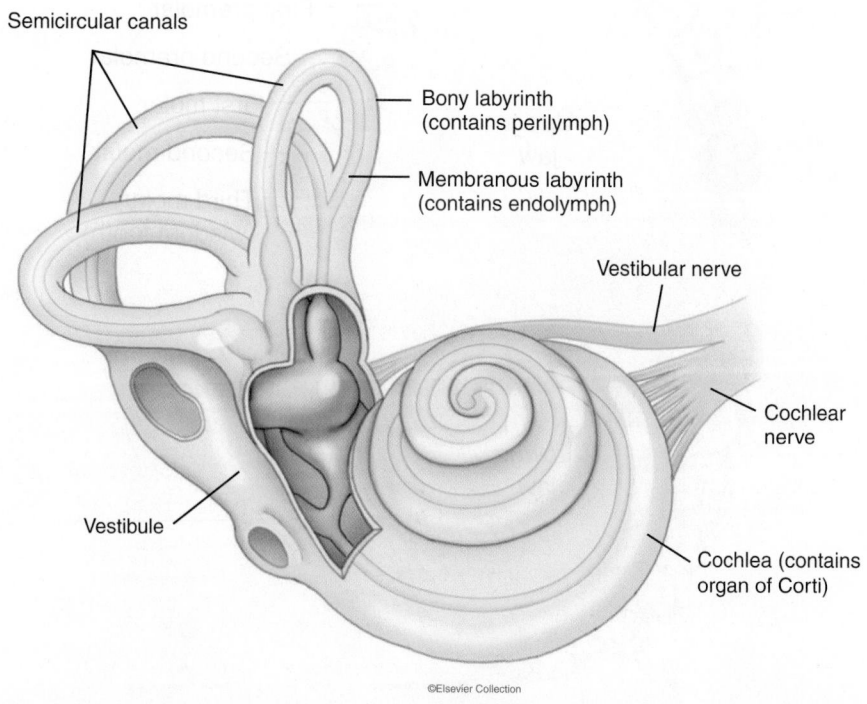

Semicircular canals

Bony labyrinth
(contains perilymph)

Membranous labyrinth
(contains endolymph)

Vestibular nerve

Cochlear
nerve

Vestibule

Cochlea (contains
organ of Corti)

©Elsevier Collection

Plate 23 Inner ear structures. (©Elsevier Collection.)

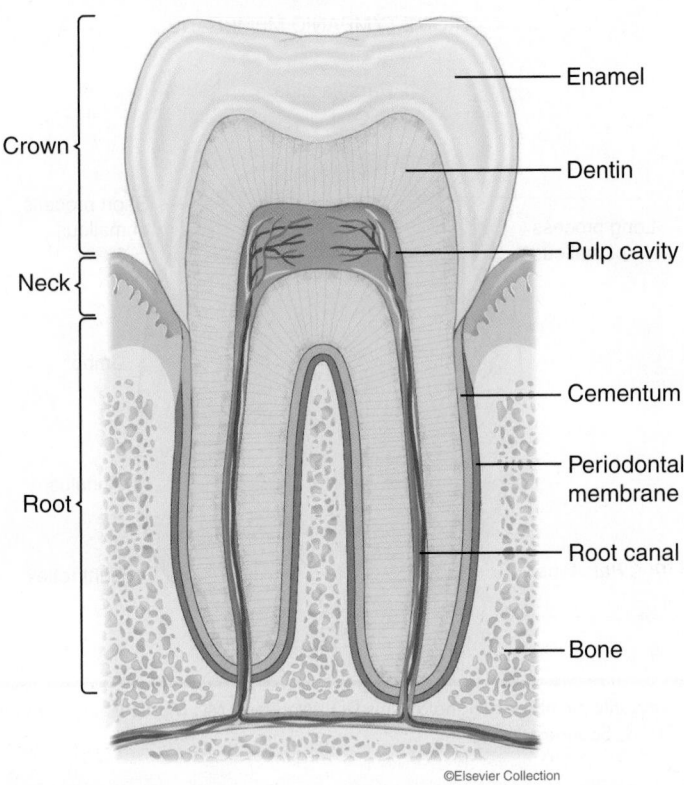

Crown {
Enamel

Dentin

Pulp cavity

Neck {

Cementum

Periodontal
membrane

Root {
Root canal

Bone

©Elsevier Collection

Plate 24 The Tooth. (©Elsevier Collection).

Central incisor

Lateral incisor

Canine

First premolar

Second premolar

First molar

Upper
jaw

Second molar

Third molar
(wisdom tooth)

Lower
jaw

©Elsevier Collection

Plate 25 Adult Teeth. (©Elsevier Collection).

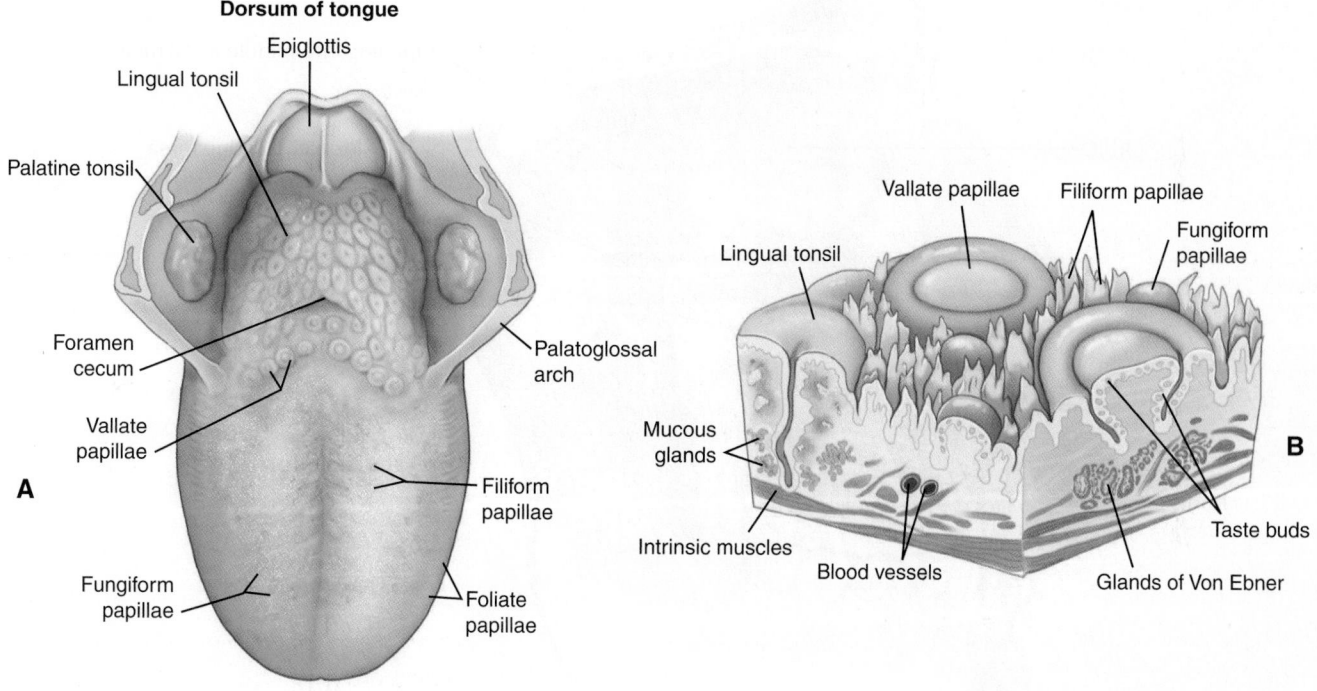

Dorsum of tongue

A

- Epiglottis
- Lingual tonsil
- Palatine tonsil
- Foramen cecum
- Vallate papillae
- Fungiform papillae
- Palatoglossal arch
- Filiform papillae
- Foliate papillae

B

- Vallate papillae
- Filiform papillae
- Fungiform papillae
- Lingual tonsil
- Mucous glands
- Intrinsic muscles
- Blood vessels
- Taste buds
- Glands of Von Ebner

© Elsevier Collection

Plate 26 A, Dorsal view of tongue showing the roughened large lingual tonsils on the posterior of the tongue and the foliate papillae on the side. B, Section of dorsal of the tongue showing a cutaway through lingual papillae and showing von Ebner's glands at the base of the vallate papilla. (Brand RW, Isselhard DE: Anatomy of Orofacial Structures: A Comprehensive Approach, ed 8, St. Louis, 2019, Elsevier.)

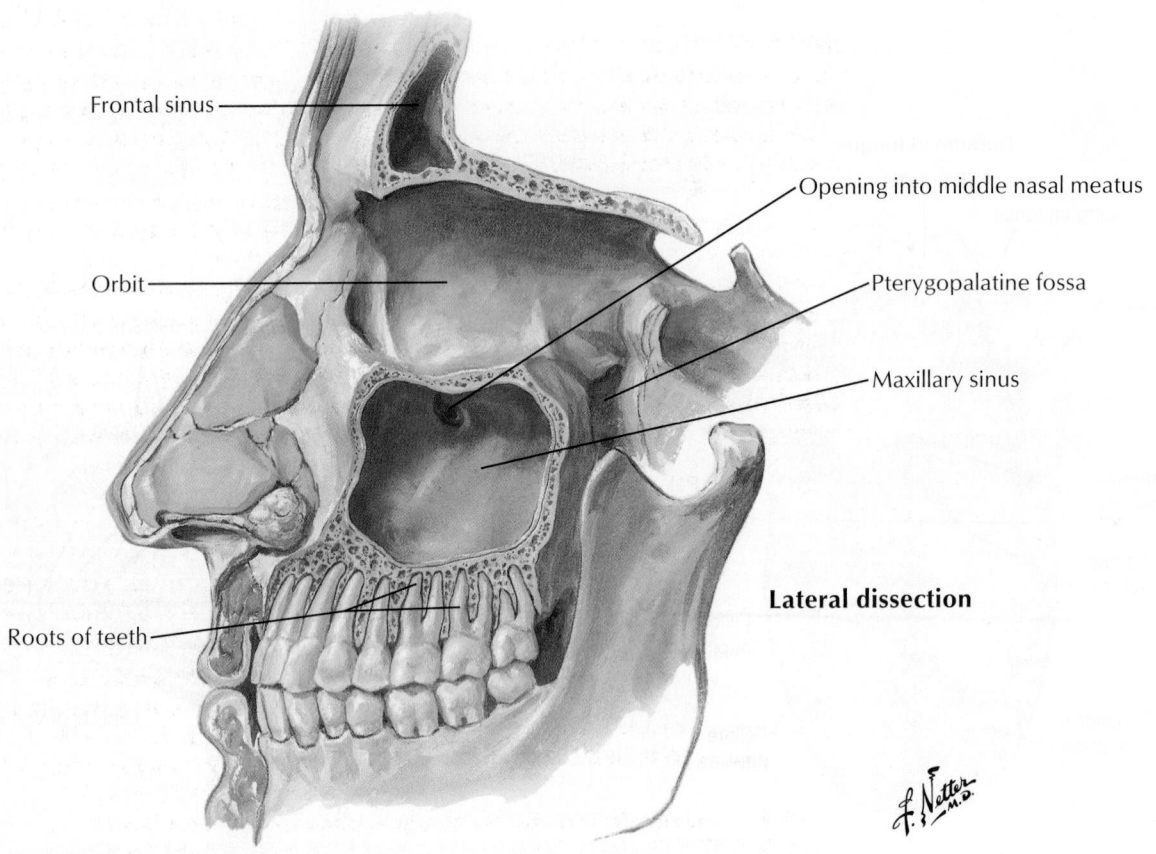

Frontal sinus

Opening into middle nasal meatus

Orbit

Pterygopalatine fossa

Maxillary sinus

Lateral dissection

Roots of teeth

Plate 27 Paranasal Sinuses. (Copyright 2022 Elsevier Inc. All rights reserved. www.netterimages.com. Image ID: 8427)

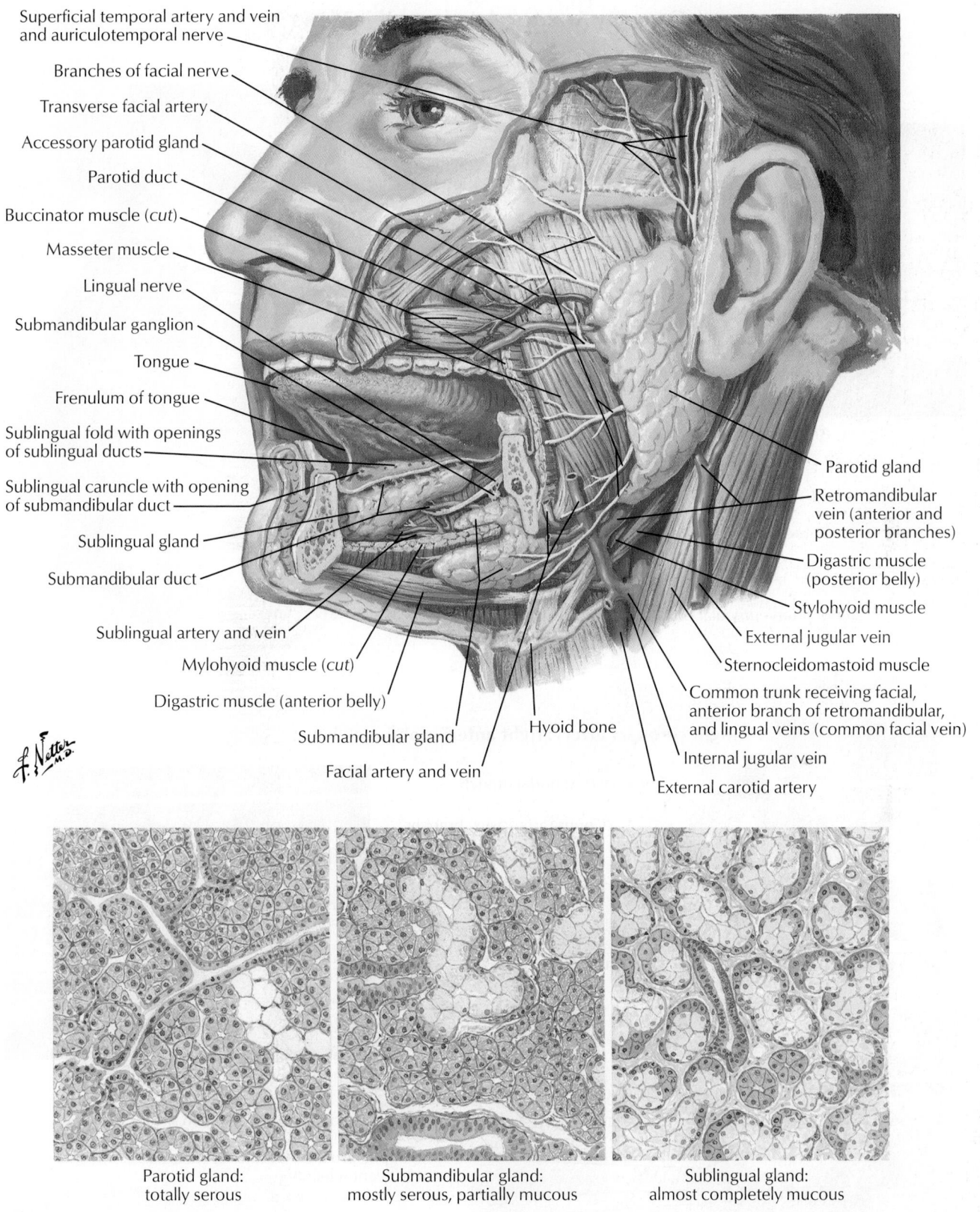

Superficial temporal artery and vein and auriculotemporal nerve

Branches of facial nerve

Transverse facial artery

Accessory parotid gland

Parotid duct

Buccinator muscle (*cut*)

Masseter muscle

Lingual nerve

Submandibular ganglion

Tongue

Frenulum of tongue

Sublingual fold with openings of sublingual ducts

Sublingual caruncle with opening of submandibular duct

Sublingual gland

Submandibular duct

Sublingual artery and vein

Mylohyoid muscle (*cut*)

Digastric muscle (anterior belly)

Submandibular gland

Facial artery and vein

Hyoid bone

Parotid gland

Retromandibular vein (anterior and posterior branches)

Digastric muscle (posterior belly)

Stylohyoid muscle

External jugular vein

Sternocleidomastoid muscle

Common trunk receiving facial, anterior branch of retromandibular, and lingual veins (common facial vein)

Internal jugular vein

External carotid artery

Parotid gland: totally serous

Submandibular gland: mostly serous, partially mucous

Sublingual gland: almost completely mucous

ANATOMY ILLUSTRATIONS

Coronary Arteries: Arteriographic Views

Right coronary artery: left anterior oblique view

Arteriogram

Sinuatrial (SA) nodal branch

Right coronary artery

Atrioventricular (AV) nodal branch

Branches to back of left ventricle

Right marginal branch

Posterior interventricular branch (posterior descending artery)

Right coronary artery: right anterior oblique view

Sinuatrial (SA) nodal branch

Conus (arteriosus) branch

Right coronary artery

Right marginal branch

Arteriogram

Atrioventricular (AV) nodal branch

Right posterolateral branches (to back of left ventricle)

Posterior interventricular branch (posterior descending artery)

ANATOMY ILLUSTRATIONS

Left coronary artery: left anterior oblique view

Left coronary artery

Circumflex branch

Arteriogram

Anterior interventricular branch (left anterior descending)

Diagonal branches of anterior interventricular branch

Atrioventricular branch of circumflex branch

Left (obtuse) marginal branch

Posterolateral branches

(Perforating) interventricular septal branches

Left coronary artery: right anterior oblique view

Left coronary artery

Anterior interventricular branch (left anterior descending)

Circumflex branch

(Perforating) interventricular septal branches

Arteriogram

Left (obtuse) marginal branch

Posterolateral branches

Diagonal branch of Anterior interventricular branch

Atrioventricular branch of circumflex branch

ANATOMY ILLUSTRATIONS

Corpus callosum

Anterolateral central (lenticulostriate) arteries

Lateral frontobasal (orbitofrontal) artery

Prefrontal artery

Precentral (pre-Rolandic) and central (Rolandic) sulcal arteries

Anterior parietal (postcentral sulcal) artery

Posterior parietal artery

Branch to angular gyrus

Temporal branches (anterior, middle, and posterior)

Middle cerebral artery and branches (deep in lateral cerebral [Sylvian] sulcus)

Anterior communicating artery

Posterior communicating artery

Anterior inferior cerebellar artery (AICA)

Posterior spinal artery

Paracentral artery

Medial frontal branches

Pericallosal artery

Callosomarginal artery

Polar frontal artery

Anterior cerebral arteries

Medial frontobasal (orbitofrontal) artery

Distal medial striate artery (recurrent artery of Heubner)

Internal carotid artery

Anterior choroidal artery

Posterior cerebral artery

Superior cerebellar artery

Basilar and pontine arteries

Labyrinthine (internal acoustic) artery

Vertebral artery

Posterior inferior cerebellar artery (PICA)

Anterior spinal artery

Corpus striatum (caudate and lentiform nuclei)

Anterolateral central (lenticulostriate) arteries

Insula (island of Reil)

Limen of insula

Precentral (pre-Rolandic), central (Rolandic) sulcal, and parietal arteries

Lateral cerebral (Sylvian) sulcus

Temporal branches of middle cerebral artery

Temporal lobe

Middle cerebral artery

Internal carotid artery

Falx cerebri

Callosomarginal arteries and Pericallosal arteries (branches of anterior cerebral arteries)

Trunk of corpus callosum

Internal capsule

Septum pellucidum

Rostrum of corpus callosum

Anterior cerebral arteries

Distal medial striate artery (recurrent artery of Heubner)

Anterior communicating artery

Optic chiasm

Plate 31   Arteries of Brain: Frontal View and Section. (Copyright 2022 Elsevier Inc. All rights reserved. www.netterimages.com. Image ID: 4588)

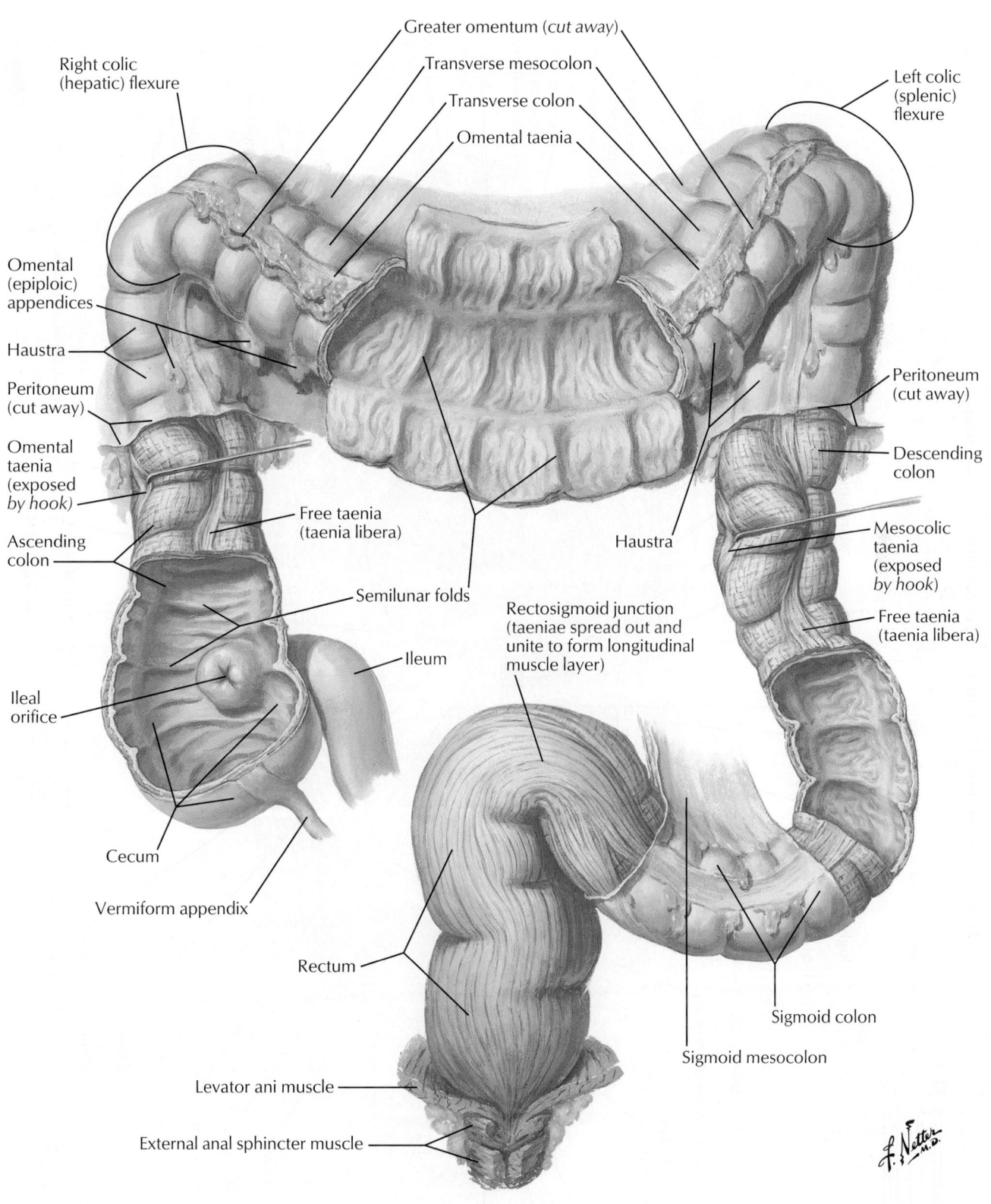

Right colic (hepatic) flexure

Greater omentum (*cut away*)

Transverse mesocolon

Transverse colon

Omental taenia

Left colic (splenic) flexure

Omental (epiploic) appendices

Haustra

Peritoneum (cut away)

Omental taenia (exposed *by hook)*

Ascending colon

Free taenia (taenia libera)

Semilunar folds

Ileum

Ileal orifice

Cecum

Vermiform appendix

Rectum

Haustra

Peritoneum (cut away)

Descending colon

Mesocolic taenia (exposed *by hook)*

Free taenia (taenia libera)

Rectosigmoid junction (taeniae spread out and unite to form longitudinal muscle layer)

Sigmoid colon

Sigmoid mesocolon

Levator ani muscle

External anal sphincter muscle

f. Netter m.d.

Plate 32 Mucosa and Musculature of Large Intestine. (Copyright 2022 Elsevier Inc. All rights reserved. www.netterimages.com. Image ID: 4778)

ANATOMY ILLUSTRATIONS

Transverse Section: T3–4 Intervertebral Disc, Manubrium

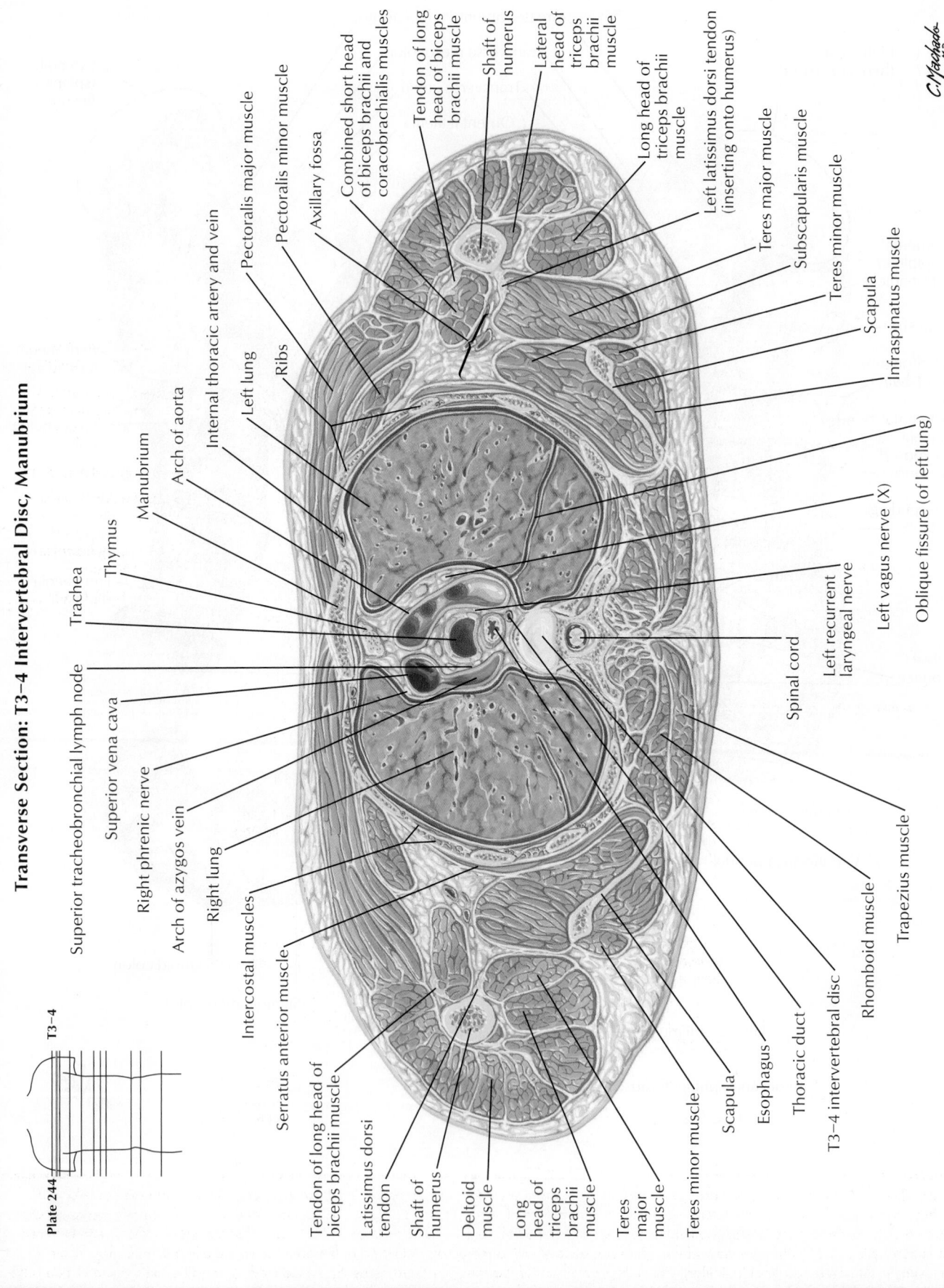

Plate 33 Cross Section of Thorax at T3-4 Disc Level. (Copyright 2022 Elsevier Inc. All rights reserved. www.netterimages.com. Image ID: 4880)

Anterior cruciate ligament

Fibular (lateral) collateral ligament

Tendon of popliteus m.

Lateral meniscus

Transverse ligament

Fibular head

Patellar tendon

A

Posterior cruciate ligament

Medial condyle

Tibial (medial) collateral ligament

Medial meniscus

Patellar ligament

Patella

Anterior cruciate ligament

Posterior menisco-femoral ligament

Fibular (lateral) collateral ligament

Lateral condyle

Lateral meniscus

Popliteus tendon

Oblique popliteal ligament

Fibular head

Semimembranous tendon

Popliteus m.

Tibia

B

Tibial tuberosity

Anterior cruciate ligament

Medial collateral ligament

Medial meniscus

Transverse ligament

Lateral meniscus

Posterior cruciate ligament

C

Plate 34 Knee joint opened; anterior, posterior, and proximal views. A, Anterior view of the knee joint, opened by folding the patella and patellar ligament inferiorly. On the lateral side is the fibular collateral ligament, separated by the popliteal tendon from the lateral meniscus. On the medial side, the tibial collateral ligament is attached to the medial meniscus. The anterior and posterior cruciate ligaments are seen between the femoral condyles. B, Posterior view of the opened knee joint with a more complete view of the posterior cruciate ligament. C, The femur is removed, showing the proximal (articular) end of the right tibia. On the medial side is the gently curved medial meniscus; on the lateral side is the more tightly curved lateral meniscus. The anterior end of the medial meniscus is anchored to the surface of the tibia by the transverse ligament. The cut ends of the anterior and posterior cruciate ligaments are shown, as well as the meniscofemoral ligament. (Fritz S: Mosby's Essential Sciences for Therapeutic Massage: Anatomy, Physiology, Biomechanics, and Pathology, ed 5, St. Louis, 2017, Elsevier.)

Paramedian (sagittal) dissection

Ureter

Uterine (fallopian) tube

Ovary

Ligament of ovary

Round ligament of uterus

Broad ligament (*cut*)

Superior pubic ramus (*cut*)

Inferior pubic ramus (*cut*)

Ischiocavernosus muscle

Body of clitoris

Labia minora

Labium majus

Rectouterine pouch (of Douglas)

Peritoneum (*cut edge*)

Vesicouterine pouch

Rectum

Ureter

Urinary bladder

Vagina

Pelvic diaphragm (levator ani muscle)

Deep transverse perineal muscle (*cut*)

External anal sphincter muscle

Median (sagittal) section

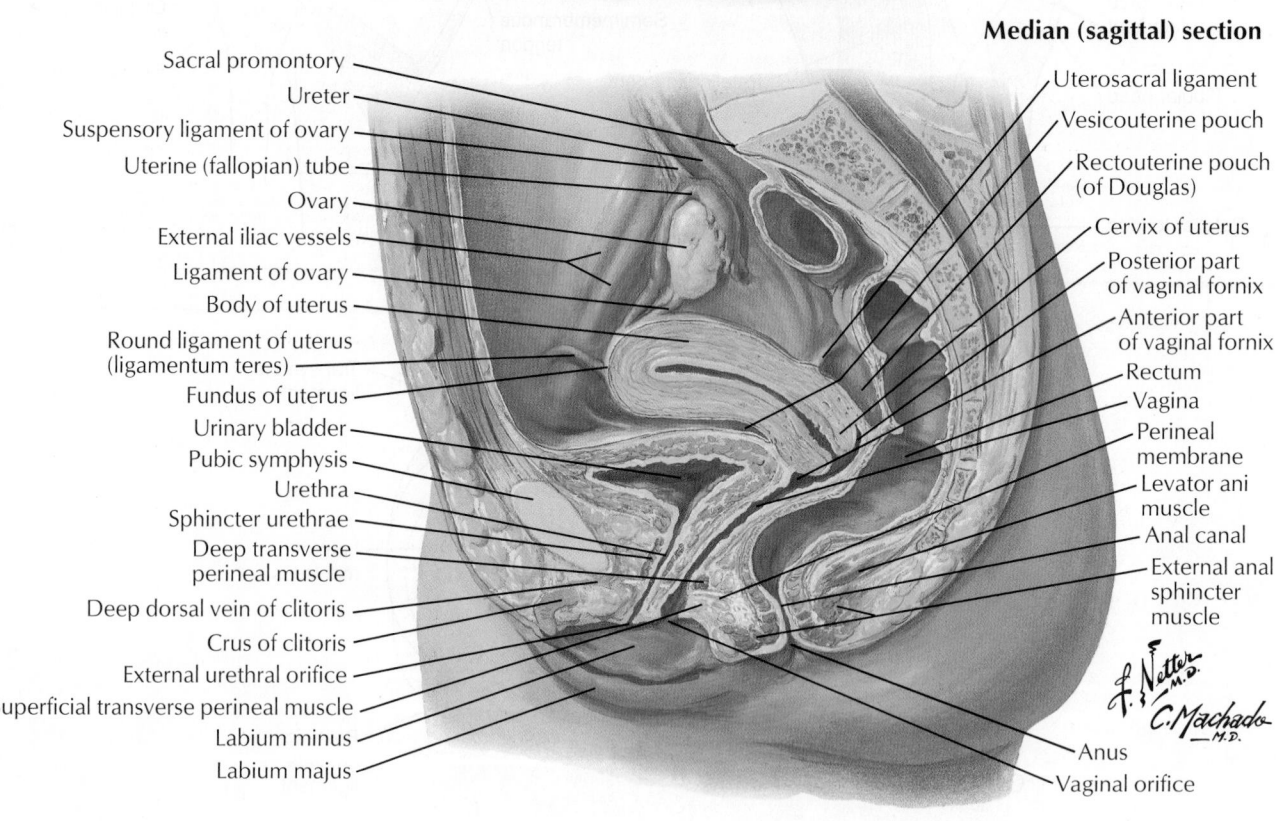

Sacral promontory

Ureter

Suspensory ligament of ovary

Uterine (fallopian) tube

Ovary

External iliac vessels

Ligament of ovary

Body of uterus

Round ligament of uterus (ligamentum teres)

Fundus of uterus

Urinary bladder

Pubic symphysis

Urethra

Sphincter urethrae

Deep transverse perineal muscle

Deep dorsal vein of clitoris

Crus of clitoris

External urethral orifice

Superficial transverse perineal muscle

Labium minus

Labium majus

Uterosacral ligament

Vesicouterine pouch

Rectouterine pouch (of Douglas)

Cervix of uterus

Posterior part of vaginal fornix

Anterior part of vaginal fornix

Rectum

Vagina

Perineal membrane

Levator ani muscle

Anal canal

External anal sphincter muscle

Anus

Vaginal orifice

F. Netter M.D.

C. Machado M.D.

PART II

Alphabetic Index

A

Aarskog's syndrome Q87.19
Abandonment —*see* Maltreatment
Abasia (-astasia) (hysterical) F44.4
Abderhalden-Kaufmann-Lignac syndrome
    (cystinosis) E72.04
Abdomen, abdominal —*see also* condition
  acute R10.0
  angina K55.1
  muscle deficiency syndrome Q79.4
Abdominalgia —*see* Pain, abdominal
Abduction contracture, hip or other joint —*see*
    Contraction, joint
Aberrant (congenital) —*see also* Malposition,
    congenital
  adrenal gland Q89.1
  artery (peripheral) Q27.8
    basilar NEC Q28.1
    cerebral Q28.3
    coronary Q24.5
    digestive system Q27.8
    eye Q15.8
    lower limb Q27.8
    precerebral Q28.1
    pulmonary Q25.79
    renal Q27.2
    retina Q14.1
    specified site NEC Q27.8
    subclavian Q27.8
    upper limb Q27.8
    vertebral Q28.1
  breast Q83.8
  endocrine gland NEC Q89.2
  hepatic duct Q44.5
  pancreas Q45.3
  parathyroid gland Q89.2
  pituitary gland Q89.2
  sebaceous glands, mucous membrane,
      mouth, congenital Q38.6
  spleen Q89.09
  subclavian artery Q27.8
  thymus (gland) Q89.2
  thyroid gland Q89.2
  vein (peripheral) NEC Q27.8
    cerebral Q28.3
    digestive system Q27.8
    lower limb Q27.8
    precerebral Q28.1
    specified site NEC Q27.8
    upper limb Q27.8
Aberration
  distantial —*see* Disturbance, visual
  mental F99
Abetalipoproteinemia E78.6
Abiotrophy R68.89
Ablatio, ablation
  retinae —*see* Detachment, retina
Ablepharia, ablepharon Q10.3
Abnormal, abnormality, abnormalities —*see*
    also Anomaly
  acid-base balance (mixed) E87.4
  albumin R77.0
  alphafetoprotein R77.2
  alveolar ridge K08.9
  anatomical relationship Q89.9
  apertures, congenital, diaphragm Q79.1
▶ atrial septal, specified NEC Q21.19
  auditory perception H93.29-●
    diplacusis —*see* Diplacusis
    hyperacusis —*see* Hyperacusis
    recruitment —*see* Recruitment, auditory
    threshold shift —*see* Shift, auditory
        threshold
  autosomes Q99.9
    fragile site Q95.5
  basal metabolic rate R94.8
  biosynthesis, testicular androgen E29.1
  bleeding time R79.1
  blood amino-acid level R79.83

Abnormal, abnormality, abnormalities —
    (*Continued*)
  blood level (of)
    cobalt R79.0
    copper R79.0
    iron R79.0
    lithium R78.89
    magnesium R79.0
    mineral NEC R79.0
    zinc R79.0
  blood pressure
    elevated R03.0
    low reading (nonspecific) R03.1
  blood sugar R73.09
  blood-gas level R79.81
  bowel sounds R19.15
    absent R19.11
    hyperactive R19.12
  brain scan R94.02
  breathing R06.9
  caloric test R94.138
  cerebrospinal fluid R83.9
    cytology R83.6
    drug level R83.2
    enzyme level R83.0
    hormones R83.1
    immunology R83.4
    microbiology R83.5
    nonmedicinal level R83.3
    specified type NEC R83.8
  chemistry, blood R79.9
    C-reactive protein R79.82
    drugs —*see* Findings, abnormal, in blood
    gas level R79.81
    minerals R79.0
    pancytopenia D61.818
    PTT R79.1
    specified NEC R79.89
    toxins —*see* Findings, abnormal, in
        blood
  chest sounds (friction) (rales) R09.89
  chromosome, chromosomal Q99.9
    with more than three X chromosomes,
        female Q97.1
    analysis result R89.8
      bronchial washings R84.8
      cerebrospinal fluid R83.8
      cervix uteri NEC R87.89
      nasal secretions R84.8
      nipple discharge R89.8
      peritoneal fluid R85.89
      pleural fluid R84.8
      prostatic secretions R86.8
      saliva R85.89
      seminal fluid R86.8
      sputum R84.8
      synovial fluid R89.8
      throat scrapings R84.8
      vagina R87.89
      vulva R87.89
      wound secretions R89.8
    dicentric replacement Q93.2
    ring replacement Q93.2
    sex Q99.8
      female phenotype Q97.9
        specified NEC Q97.8
      male phenotype Q98.9
        specified NEC Q98.8
      structural male Q98.6
    specified NEC Q99.8
  clinical findings NEC R68.89
  coagulation D68.9
    newborn, transient P61.6
    profile R79.1
    time R79.1
  communication —*see* Fistula
  conjunctiva, vascular H11.41-●
  coronary artery Q24.5
  cortisol-binding globulin E27.8
  course, eustachian tube Q17.8

Abnormal, abnormality, abnormalities —
    (*Continued*)
  creatinine clearance R94.4
  cytology
    anus R85.619
      atypical squamous cells cannot
          exclude high grade squamous
          intraepithelial lesion (ASC-H)
          R85.611
      atypical squamous cells of undetermined
          significance (ASC-US) R85.610
      cytologic evidence of malignancy
          R85.614
      high grade squamous intraepithelial
          lesion (HGSIL) R85.613
      human papillomavirus (HPV) DNA test
        high risk positive R85.81
        low risk postive R85.82
      inadequate smear R85.615
      low grade squamous intraepithelial
          lesion (LGSIL) R85.612
      satisfactory anal smear but lacking
          transformation zone R85.616
      specified NEC R85.618
      unsatisfactory smear R85.615
    female genital organs —*see* Abnormal,
        Papanicolaou (smear)
  dark adaptation curve H53.61
  dentofacial NEC —*see* Anomaly, dentofacial
  development, developmental Q89.9
    central nervous system Q07.9
  diagnostic imaging
    abdomen, abdominal region NEC R93.5
    biliary tract R93.2
    bladder R93.41
    breast R92.8
    central nervous system NEC R90.89
    cerebrovascular NEC R90.89
    coronary circulation R93.1
    digestive tract NEC R93.3
    gastrointestinal (tract) R93.3
    genitourinary organs R93.89
    head R93.0
    heart R93.1
    intrathoracic organ NEC R93.89
    kidney R93.42-●
    limbs R93.6
    liver R93.2
    lung (field) R91.8
    musculoskeletal system NEC R93.7
    renal pelvis R93.41
    retroperitoneum R93.5
    site specified NEC R93.89
    skin and subcutaneous tissue R93.89
    skull R93.0
    testis R93.81-●
    urinary organs specified NEC R93.49
    ureter R93.41
  direction, teeth, fully erupted M26.30
  ear ossicles, acquired NEC H74.39-●
    ankylosis —*see* Ankylosis, ear ossicles
    discontinuity —*see* Discontinuity, ossicles,
        ear
    partial loss —*see* Loss, ossicles, ear (partial)
  Ebstein Q22.5
  echocardiogram R93.1
  echoencephalogram R90.81
  echogram —*see* Abnormal, diagnostic
      imaging
  electrocardiogram [ECG] [EKG] R94.31
  electroencephalogram [EEG] R94.01
  electrolyte —*see* Imbalance, electrolyte
  electromyogram [EMG] R94.131
  electro-oculogram [EOG] R94.110
  electrophysiological intracardiac studies
      R94.39
  electroretinogram [ERG] R94.111
  erythrocytes
    congenital, with perinatal jaundice D58.9
  feces (color) (contents) (mucus) R19.5

▶ New   ⇒ Revised   ~~deleted~~ Deleted   ● Use Additional Character(s)

Abnormal, abnormality, abnormalities —
(Continued)
finding —see Findings, abnormal, without
diagnosis
fluid
amniotic —see Abnormal, specimen,
specified
cerebrospinal —see Abnormal,
cerebrospinal fluid
peritoneal —see Abnormal, specimen,
digestive organs
pleural —see Abnormal, specimen,
respiratory organs
synovial —see Abnormal, specimen,
specified
thorax (bronchial washings) (pleural
fluid) —see Abnormal, specimen,
respiratory organs
vaginal —see Abnormal, specimen, female
genital organs
form
teeth K00.2
uterus —see Anomaly, uterus
function studies
auditory R94.120
bladder R94.8
brain R94.09
cardiovascular R94.30
ear R94.128
endocrine NEC R94.7
eye NEC R94.118
kidney R94.4
liver R94.5
nervous system
central NEC R94.09
peripheral NEC R94.138
pancreas R94.8
placenta R94.8
pulmonary R94.2
special senses NEC R94.128
spleen R94.8
thyroid R94.6
vestibular R94.121
gait —see Gait
hysterical F44.4
gastrin secretion E16.4
globulin R77.1
cortisol-binding E27.8
thyroid-binding E07.89
glomerular, minor —see also N00-N07 with
fourth character .0 N05.0
glucagon secretion E16.3
glucose tolerance (test) (non-fasting)
R73.09
gravitational (G) forces or states (effect of)
T75.81
hair (color) (shaft) L67.9
specified NEC L67.8
hard tissue formation in pulp (dental)
K04.3
head movement R25.0
heart
rate R00.9
specified NEC R00.8
shadow R93.1
sounds NEC R01.2
hemoglobin (disease) —see also Disease,
hemoglobin D58.2
trait —see Trait, hemoglobin, abnormal
histology NEC R89.7
immunological findings R89.4
in serum R76.9
specified NEC R76.8
increase in appetite R63.2
involuntary movement —see Abnormal,
movement, involuntary
jaw closure M26.51
karyotype R89.8
kidney function test R94.4
knee jerk R29.2
leukocyte (cell) (differential) NEC D72.9

Abnormal, abnormality, abnormalities —
(Continued)
liver function test (see also Elevated, liver
function, test) R79.89
loss of
height R29.890
weight R63.4
mammogram NEC R92.8
calcification (calculus) R92.1
microcalcification R92.0
Mantoux test R76.11
movement (disorder) —see also Disorder,
movement
head R25.0
involuntary R25.9
fasciculation R25.3
of head R25.0
spasm R25.2
specified type NEC R25.8
tremor R25.1
myoglobin (Aberdeen) (Annapolis) R89.7
neonatal screening P09.9
for
congenital adrenal hyperplasia P09.2
congenital endocrine disease P09.2
congenital hematologic disorders P09.3
critical congenital heart disease P09.5
cystic fibrosis P09.4
hemoglobinothies P09.3
hypothyroidism P09.2
inborn errors of metabolism P09.1
neonatal hearing loss P09.6
red cell membrane defects P09.3
sickle cell P09.3
specified NEC P09.8
oculomotor study R94.113
palmar creases Q82.8
Papanicolaou (smear)
anus R85.619
atypical squamous cells cannot
exclude high grade squamous
intraepithelial lesion (ASC-H)
R85.611
atypical squamous cells of undetermined
significance (ASC-US) R85.610
cytologic evidence of malignancy
R85.614
high grade squamous intraepithelial
lesion (HGSIL) R85.613
human papillomavirus (HPV) DNA test
high risk positive R85.81
low risk postive R85.82
inadequate smear R85.615
low grade squamous intraepithelial
lesion (LGSIL) R85.612
satisfactory anal smear but lacking
transformation zone R85.616
specified NEC R85.618
unsatisfactory smear R85.615
bronchial washings R84.6
cerebrospinal fluid R83.6
cervix R87.619
atypical squamous cells cannot
exclude high grade squamous
intraepithelial lesion (ASC-H)
R87.611
atypical squamous cells of undetermined
significance (ASC-US) R87.610
cytologic evidence of malignancy
R87.614
high grade squamous intraepithelial
lesion (HGSIL) R87.613
inadequate smear R87.615
low grade squamous intraepithelial
lesion (LGSIL) R87.612
non-atypical endometrial cells R87.618
satisfactory cervical smear but lacking
transformation zone R87.616
specified NEC R87.618
thin preparaton R87.619
unsatisfactory smear R87.615

Abnormal, abnormality, abnormalities —
(Continued)
Papanicolaou (smear) (Continued)
nasal secretions R84.6
nipple discharge R89.6
peritoneal fluid R85.69
pleural fluid R84.6
prostatic secretions R86.6
saliva R85.69
seminal fluid R86.6
sites NEC R89.6
sputum R84.6
synovial fluid R89.6
throat scrapings R84.6
vagina R87.629
atypical squamous cells cannot
exclude high grade squamous
intraepithelial lesion (ASC-H)
R87.621
atypical squamous cells of undetermined
significance (ASC-US) R87.620
cytologic evidence of malignancy
R87.624
high grade squamous intraepithelial
lesion (HGSIL) R87.623
inadequate smear R87.625
low grade squamous intraepithelial
lesion (LGSIL) R87.622
specified NEC R87.628
thin preparation R87.629
unsatisfactory smear R87.625
vulva R87.69
wound secretions R89.6
partial thromboplastin time (PTT) R79.1
pelvis (bony) —see Deformity, pelvis
percussion, chest (tympany) R09.89
periods (grossly) —see Menstruation
phonocardiogram R94.39
plantar reflex R29.2
plasma
protein R77.9
specified NEC R77.8
viscosity R70.1
pleural (folds) Q34.0
posture R29.3
product of conception O02.9
specified type NEC O02.89
prothrombin time (PT) R79.1
pulmonary
artery, congenital Q25.79
function, newborn P28.89
test results R94.2
pulsations in neck R00.2
pupillary H21.56-●
function (reaction) (reflex) —see Anomaly,
pupil, function
radiological examination —see Abnormal,
diagnostic imaging
red blood cell(s) (morphology) (volume)
R71.8
reflex —see Reflex
renal function test R94.4
response to nerve stimulation R94.130
retinal correspondence H53.31
retinal function study R94.111
rhythm, heart —see also Arrhythmia
saliva —see Abnormal, specimen, digestive
organs
scan
kidney R94.4
liver R93.2
thyroid R94.6
secretion
gastrin E16.4
glucagon E16.3
semen, seminal fluid —see Abnormal,
specimen, male genital organs
serum level (of)
acid phosphatase R74.8
alkaline phosphatase R74.8
amylase R74.8

Abnormal, abnormality, abnormalities —
  (Continued)
  serum level (of) *(Continued)*
    enzymes R74.9
      specified NEC R74.8
    lipase R74.8
    triacylglycerol lipase R74.8
  shape
    gravid uterus —*see* Anomaly, uterus
  sinus venosus Q21.06
  size, tooth, teeth K00.2
  spacing, tooth, teeth, fully erupted M26.30
  specimen
    digestive organs (peritoneal fluid) (saliva)
      R85.9
      cytology R85.69
      drug level R85.2
      enzyme level R85.0
      histology R85.7
      hormones R85.1
      immunology R85.4
      microbiology R85.5
      nonmedicinal level R85.3
      specified type NEC R85.89
    female genital organs (secretions) (smears)
      R87.9
      cytology R87.69
        cervix R87.619
          human papillomavirus (HPV) DNA
            test
            high risk positive R87.810
            low risk positive R87.820
          inadequate (unsatisfactory) smear
            R87.615
          non-atypical endometrial cells
            R87.618
          specified NEC R87.618
        vagina R87.629
          human papillomavirus (HPV) DNA
            test
            high risk positive R87.811
            low risk positive R87.821
          inadequate (unsatisfactory) smear
            R87.625
        vulva R87.69
      drug level R87.2
      enzyme level R87.0
      histological R87.7
      hormones R87.1
      immunology R87.4
      microbiology R87.5
      nonmedicinal level R87.3
      specified type NEC R87.89
    male genital organs (prostatic secretions)
      (semen) R86.9
      cytology R86.6
      drug level R86.2
      enzyme level R86.0
      histological R86.7
      hormones R86.1
      immunology R86.4
      microbiology R86.5
      nonmedicinal level R86.3
      specified type NEC R86.8
    nipple discharge —*see* Abnormal,
      specimen, specified
    respiratory organs (bronchial washings)
      (nasal secretions) (pleural fluid)
      (sputum) R84.9
      cytology R84.6
      drug level R84.2
      enzyme level R84.0
      histology R84.7
      hormones R84.1
      immunology R84.4
      microbiology R84.5
      nonmedicinal level R84.3
      specified type NEC R84.8
    specified organ, system and tissue NOS
      R89.9
      cytology R89.6

Abnormal, abnormality, abnormalities —
  (Continued)
  specimen *(Continued)*
    specified organ, system and tissue NOS
      (Continued)
      drug level R89.2
      enzyme level R89.0
      histology R89.7
      hormones R89.1
      immunology R89.4
      microbiology R89.5
      nonmedicinal level R89.3
      specified type NEC R89.8
    synovial fluid —*see* Abnormal, specimen,
      specified
    thorax (bronchial washings) (pleural
      fluids) —*see* Abnormal, specimen,
      respiratory organs
    vagina (secretion) (smear) R87.629
    vulva (secretion) (smear) R87.69
    wound secretion —*see* Abnormal,
      specimen, specified
  spermatozoa —*see* Abnormal, specimen, male
    genital organs
  sputum (amount) (color) (odor) R09.3
  stool (color) (contents) (mucus) R19.5
    bloody K92.1
    guaiac positive R19.5
  synchondrosis Q78.8
  thermography —*see also* Abnormal,
    diagnostic imaging R93.89
  thyroid-binding globulin E07.89
  tooth, teeth (form) (size) K00.2
  toxicology (findings) R78.9
  transport protein E88.09
  tumor marker NEC R97.8
  ultrasound results —*see* Abnormal, diagnostic
    imaging
  umbilical cord complicating delivery O69.9
  urination NEC R39.198
  urine (constituents) R82.90
    bile R82.2
    cytological examination R82.89
    drugs R82.5
    fat R82.0
    glucose R81
    heavy metals R82.6
    hemoglobin R82.3
    histological examination R82.89
    ketones R82.4
    microbiological examination (culture) R82.79
    myoglobin R82.1
    positive culture R82.79
    protein —*see* Proteinuria
    specified substance NEC R82.998
      chromoabnormality NEC R82.91
    substances nonmedical R82.6
  uterine hemorrhage —*see* Hemorrhage, uterus
  vectorcardiogram R94.39
  visually evoked potential (VEP) R94.112
  white blood cells D72.9
    specified NEC D72.89
  X-ray examination —*see* Abnormal,
    diagnostic imaging
Abnormity (any organ or part) —*see* Anomaly
Abocclusion M26.29
  hemolytic disease (newborn) P55.1
  incompatibility reaction ABO —*see*
    Complication(s), transfusion,
    incompatibility reaction, ABO
Abolition, language R48.8
Aborter, habitual or recurrent —*see* Loss (of),
  pregnancy, recurrent
Abortion (complete) (spontaneous) O03.9
  with
    retained products of conception —*see*
      Abortion, incomplete
  attempted (elective) (failed) O07.4
    complicated by O07.30
      afibrinogenemia O07.1
      cardiac arrest O07.36

Abortion *(Continued)*
  attempted *(Continued)*
    complicated by *(Continued)*
      chemical damage of pelvic organ(s) O07.34
      circulatory collapse O07.31
      cystitis O07.38
      defibrination syndrome O07.1
      electrolyte imbalance O07.33
      embolism (air) (amniotic fluid) (blood
        clot) (fat) (pulmonary) (septic)
        (soap) O07.2
      endometritis O07.0
      genital tract and pelvic infection O07.0
      hemolysis O07.1
      hemorrhage (delayed) (excessive) O07.1
      infection
        genital tract or pelvic O07.0
        urinary tract tract O07.38
      intravascular coagulation O07.1
      laceration of pelvic organ(s) O07.34
      metabolic disorder O07.33
      oliguria O07.32
      oophoritis O07.0
      parametritis O07.0
      pelvic peritonitis O07.0
      perforation of pelvic organ(s) O07.34
      renal failure or shutdown O07.32
      salpingitis or salpingo-oophoritis O07.0
      sepsis O07.37
      shock O07.31
      specified condition NEC O07.39
      tubular necrosis (renal) O07.32
      uremia O07.32
      urinary tract infection O07.38
      venous complication NEC O07.35
        embolism (air) (amniotic fluid) (blood
          clot) (fat) (pulmonary) (septic)
          (soap) O07.2
  complicated (by) (following) O03.80
    afibrinogenemia O03.6
    cardiac arrest O03.86
    chemical damage of pelvic organ(s) O03.84
    circulatory collapse O03.81
    cystitis O03.88
    defibrination syndrome O03.6
    electrolyte imbalance O03.83
    embolism (air) (amniotic fluid) (blood clot)
      (fat) (pulmonary) (septic) (soap) O03.7
    endometritis O03.5
    genital tract and pelvic infection O03.5
    hemolysis O03.6
    hemorrhage (delayed) (excessive) O03.6
    infection
      genital tract or pelvic O03.5
      urinary tract O03.88
    intravascular coagulation O03.6
    laceration of pelvic organ(s) O03.84
    metabolic disorder O03.83
    oliguria O03.82
    oophoritis O03.5
    parametritis O03.5
    pelvic peritonitis O03.5
    perforation of pelvic organ(s) O03.84
    renal failure or shutdown O03.82
    salpingitis or salpingo-oophoritis O03.5
    sepsis O03.87
    shock O03.81
    specified condition NEC O03.89
    tubular necrosis (renal) O03.82
    uremia O03.82
    urinary tract infection O03.88
    venous complication NEC O03.85
      embolism (air) (amniotic fluid) (blood
        clot) (fat) (pulmonary) (septic)
        (soap) O03.7
  failed —*see* Abortion, attempted
  habitual or recurrent N96
    with current abortion —*see* categories
      O03-O04
    without current pregnancy N96
    care in current pregnancy O26.2-●

▶ New   ⇒ Revised   ~~deleted~~ Deleted   ● Use Additional Character(s)

Abortion *(Continued)*
  incomplete (spontaneous) O03.4
    complicated (by) (following) O03.30
      afibrinogenemia O03.1
      cardiac arrest O03.36
      chemical damage of pelvic organ(s) O03.34
      circulatory collapse O03.31
      cystitis O03.38
      defibrination syndrome O03.1
      electrolyte imbalance O03.33
      embolism (air) (amniotic fluid) (blood
          clot) (fat) (pulmonary) (septic)
          (soap) O03.2
      endometritis O03.0
      genital tract and pelvic infection O03.0
      hemolysis O03.1
      hemorrhage (delayed) (excessive) O03.1
      infection
          genital tract or pelvic O03.0
          urinary tract O03.38
      intravascular coagulation O03.1
      laceration of pelvic organ(s) O03.34
      metabolic disorder O03.33
      oliguria O03.32
      oophoritis O03.0
      parametritis O03.0
      pelvic peritonitis O03.0
      perforation of pelvic organ(s) O03.34
      renal failure or shutdown O03.32
      salpingitis or salpingo-oophoritis O03.0
      sepsis O03.37
      shock O03.31
      specified condition NEC O03.39
      tubular necrosis (renal) O03.32
      uremia O03.32
      urinary infection O03.38
      venous complication NEC O03.35
        embolism (air) (amniotic fluid) (blood
            clot) (fat) (pulmonary) (septic)
            (soap) O03.2
  induced (encounter for) Z33.2
    complicated by O04.80
      afibrinogenemia O04.6
      cardiac arrest O04.86
      chemical damage of pelvic organ(s) O04.84
      circulatory collapse O04.81
      cystitis O04.88
      defibrination syndrome O04.6
      electrolyte imbalance O04.83
      embolism (air) (amniotic fluid) (blood
          clot) (fat) (pulmonary) (septic)
          (soap) O04.7
      endometritis O04.5
      genital tract and pelvic infection O04.5
      hemolysis O04.6
      hemorrhage (delayed) (excessive) O04.6
      infection
          genital tract or pelvic O04.5
          urinary tract O04.88
      intravascular coagulation O04.6
      laceration of pelvic organ(s) O04.84
      metabolic disorder O04.83
      oliguria O04.82
      oophoritis O04.5
      parametritis O04.5
      pelvic peritonitis O04.5
      perforation of pelvic organ(s) O04.84
      renal failure or shutdown O04.82
      salpingitis or salpingo-oophoritis O04.5
      sepsis O04.87
      shock O04.81
      specified condition NEC O04.89
      tubular necrosis (renal) O04.82
      uremia O04.82
      urinary tract infection O04.88
      venous complication NEC O04.85
        embolism (air) (amniotic fluid) (blood
            clot) (fat) (pulmonary) (septic)
            (soap) O04.7
  inevitable O03.4
  missed O02.1

Abortion *(Continued)*
  spontaneous —*see* Abortion (complete)
      (spontaneous)
    threatened O20.0
  threatened (spontaneous) O20.0
  tubal O00.10-●
    with intrauterine pregnancy O00.11-
Abortus fever A23.1
Aboulomania F60.7
Abrami's disease D59.8
Abramov-Fiedler myocarditis (acute isolated
      myocarditis) I40.1
Abrasion T14.8
  abdomen, abdominal (wall) S30.811
  alveolar process S00.512
  ankle S90.51-●
  antecubital space —*see* Abrasion, elbow
  anus S30.817
  arm (upper) S40.81-●
  auditory canal —*see* Abrasion, ear
  auricle —*see* Abrasion, ear
  axilla —*see* Abrasion, arm
  back, lower S30.810
  breast S20.11-●
  brow S00.81
  buttock S30.810
  calf —*see* Abrasion, leg
  canthus —*see* Abrasion, eyelid
  cheek S00.81
    internal S00.512
  chest wall —*see* Abrasion, thorax
  chin S00.81
  clitoris S30.814
  cornea S05.0-●
  costal region —*see* Abrasion, thorax
  dental K03.1
  digit(s)
    foot —*see* Abrasion, toe
    hand —*see* Abrasion, finger
  ear S00.41-●
  elbow S50.31-●
  epididymis S30.813
  epigastric region S30.811
  epiglottis S10.11
  esophagus (thoracic) S27.818
    cervical S10.11
  eyebrow —*see* Abrasion, eyelid
  eyelid S00.21-●
  face S00.81
  finger(s) S60.41-●
    index S60.41-●
    little S60.41-●
    middle S60.41-●
    ring S60.41-●
  flank S30.811
  foot (except toe(s) alone) S90.81-●
    toe —*see* Abrasion, toe
  forearm S50.81-●
    elbow only —*see* Abrasion, elbow
  forehead S00.81
  genital organs, external
    female S30.816
    male S30.815
  groin S30.811
  gum S00.512
  hand S60.51-●
  head S00.91
    ear —*see* Abrasion, ear
    eyelid —*see* Abrasion, eyelid
    lip S00.511
    nose S00.31
    oral cavity S00.512
    scalp S00.01
    specified site NEC S00.81
  heel —*see* Abrasion, foot
  hip S70.21-●
  inguinal region S30.811
  interscapular region S20.419
  jaw S00.81
  knee S80.21-●
  labium (majus) (minus) S30.814

Abrasion *(Continued)*
  larynx S10.11
  leg (lower) S80.81-●
    knee —*see* Abrasion, knee
    upper —*see* Abrasion, thigh
  lip S00.511
  lower back S30.810
  lumbar region S30.810
  malar region S00.81
  mammary —*see* Abrasion, breast
  mastoid region S00.81
  mouth S00.512
  nail
    finger —*see* Abrasion, finger
    toe —*see* Abrasion, toe
  nape S10.81
  nasal S00.31
  neck S10.91
    specified site NEC S10.81
    throat S10.11
  nose S00.31
  occipital region S00.01
  oral cavity S00.512
  orbital region —*see* Abrasion, eyelid
  palate S00.512
  palm —*see* Abrasion, hand
  parietal region S00.01
  pelvis S30.810
  penis S30.812
  perineum
    female S30.814
    male S30.810
  periocular area —*see* Abrasion, eyelid
  phalanges
    finger —*see* Abrasion, finger
    toe —*see* Abrasion, toe
  pharynx S10.11
  pinna —*see* Abrasion, ear
  popliteal space —*see* Abrasion, knee
  prepuce S30.812
  pubic region S30.810
  pudendum
    female S30.816
    male S30.815
  sacral region S30.810
  scalp S00.01
  scapular region —*see* Abrasion, shoulder
  scrotum S30.813
  shin —*see* Abrasion, leg
  shoulder S40.21-●
  skin NEC T14.8
  sternal region S20.319
  submaxillary region S00.81
  submental region S00.81
  subungual
    finger(s) —*see* Abrasion, finger
    toe(s) —*see* Abrasion, toe
  supraclavicular fossa S10.81
  supraorbital S00.81
  temple S00.81
  temporal region S00.81
  testis S30.813
  thigh S70.31-●
  thorax, thoracic (wall) S20.91
    back S20.41-●
    front S20.31-●
  throat S10.11
  thumb S60.31-●
  toe(s) (lesser) S90.416
    great S90.41-●
  tongue S00.512
  tooth, teeth (dentifrice) (habitual) (hard
      tissues) (occupational) (ritual)
      (traditional) K03.1
  trachea S10.11
  tunica vaginalis S30.813
  tympanum, tympanic membrane —*see*
      Abrasion, ear
  uvula S00.512
  vagina S30.814
  vocal cords S10.11

Abrasion (*Continued*)
  vulva S30.814
  wrist S60.81-●
Abrism —*see* Poisoning, food, noxious, plant
Abruptio placentae O45.9-●
  with
    afibrinogenemia O45.01-●
    coagulation defect O45.00-●
      specified NEC O45.09-●
    disseminated intravascular coagulation
      O45.02-●
    hypofibrinogenemia O45.01-●
  specified NEC O45.8-●
Abruption, placenta —*see* Abruptio placentae
Abscess (connective tissue) (embolic) (fistulous)
    (infective) (metastatic) (multiple)
    (pernicious) (pyogenic) (septic) L02.91
  with
    diverticular disease (intestine) K57.80
      with bleeding K57.81
      large intestine K57.20
        with
          bleeding K57.21
          small intestine K57.40
            with bleeding K57.41
      small intestine K57.00
        with
          bleeding K57.01
          large intestine K57.40
            with bleeding K57.41
    lymphangitis - code by site under Abscess
  abdomen, abdominal
    cavity K65.1
    wall L02.211
  abdominopelvic K65.1
  accessory sinus —*see* Sinusitis
  adrenal (capsule) (gland) E27.8
  alveolar K04.7
    with sinus K04.6
  amebic A06.4
    brain (and liver or lung abscess) A06.6
    genitourinary tract A06.82
    liver (without mention of brain or lung
      abscess) A06.4
    lung (and liver) (without mention of brain
      abscess) A06.5
    specified site NEC A06.89
    spleen A06.89
  anerobic A48.0
  ankle —*see* Abscess, lower limb
  anorectal K61.2
  antecubital space —*see* Abscess, upper limb
  antrum (chronic) (Highmore) —*see* Sinusitis,
    maxillary
  anus K61.0
  apical (tooth) K04.7
    with sinus (alveolar) K04.6
  appendix K35.33
  areola (acute) (chronic) (nonpuerperal)
      N61.1
    puerperal, postpartum or gestational —*see*
      Infection, nipple
  arm (any part) —*see* Abscess, upper limb
  artery (wall) I77.89
  atheromatous I77.2
  auricle, ear —*see* Abscess, ear, external
  axilla (region) L02.41-●
    lymph gland or node L04.2
  back (any part, except buttock) L02.212
  Bartholin's gland N75.1
    with
      abortion —*see* Abortion, by type
        complicated by, sepsis
      ectopic or molar pregnancy O08.0
    following ectopic or molar pregnancy O08.0
  Bezold's —*see* Mastoiditis, acute
  bilharziasis B65.1
  bladder (wall) —*see* Cystitis, specified type
    NEC
  bone (subperiosteal) —*see also* Osteomyelitis,
    specified type NEC

Abscess (*Continued*)
  bone (*Continued*)
    accessory sinus (chronic) —*see* Sinusitis
    chronic or old —*see* Osteomyelitis, chronic
    jaw (lower) (upper) M27.2
    mastoid —*see* Mastoiditis, acute,
      subperiosteal
    petrous —*see* Petrositis
    spinal (tuberculous) A18.01
      nontuberculous —*see* Osteomyelitis,
        vertebra
  bowel K63.0
  brain (any part) (cystic) (otogenic) G06.0
    amebic (with abscess of any other site) A06.6
    gonococcal A54.82
    pheomycotic (chromomycotic) B43.1
    tuberculous A17.81
  breast (acute) (chronic) (nonpuerperal) N61.1
    newborn P39.0
    puerperal, postpartum, gestational —*see*
      Mastitis, obstetric, purulent
  broad ligament N73.2
    acute N73.0
    chronic N73.1
  Brodie's (localized) (chronic) M86.8X-●
  bronchi J98.09
  buccal cavity K12.2
  bulbourethral gland N34.0
  bursa M71.00
    ankle M71.07-●
    elbow M71.02-●
    foot M71.07-●
    hand M71.04-●
    hip M71.05-●
    knee M71.06-●
    multiple sites M71.09
    pharyngeal J39.1
    shoulder M71.01-●
    specified site NEC M71.08
    wrist M71.03-●
  buttock L02.31
  canthus —*see* Blepharoconjunctivitis
  cartilage —*see* Disorder, cartilage, specified
    type NEC
  cecum K35.33
  cerebellum, cerebellar G06.0
    sequelae G09
  cerebral (embolic) G06.0
    sequelae G09
  cervical (meaning neck) L02.11
    lymph gland or node L04.0
  cervix (stump) (uteri) —*see* Cervicitis
  cheek (external) L02.01
    inner K12.2
  chest J86.9
    with fistula J86.0
    wall L02.213
  chin L02.01
  choroid —*see* Inflammation, chorioretinal
  circumtonsillar J36
  cold (lung) (tuberculous) —*see also*
      Tuberculosis, abscess, lung
    articular —*see* Tuberculosis, joint
  colon (wall) K63.0
  colostomy K94.02
  conjunctiva —*see* Conjunctivitis, acute
  cornea H16.31-●
  corpus
    cavernosum N48.21
    luteum —*see* Oophoritis
  Cowper's gland N34.0
  cranium G06.0
  cul-de-sac (Douglas') (posterior) —*see*
      Peritonitis, pelvic, female
  cutaneous —*see* Abscess, by site
  dental K04.7
    with sinus (alveolar) K04.6
  dentoalveolar K04.7
    with sinus K04.6
  diaphragm, diaphragmatic K65.1
  Douglas' cul-de-sac or pouch —*see*
      Peritonitis, pelvic, female

Abscess (*Continued*)
  Dubois A50.59
  ear (middle) —*see also* Otitis, media,
      suppurative
    acute —*see* Otitis, media, suppurative,
      acute
    external H60.0-●
  entamebic —*see* Abscess, amebic
  enterostomy K94.12
  epididymis N45.4
  epidural G06.2
    brain G06.0
    spinal cord G06.1
  epiglottis J38.7
  epiploon, epiploic K65.1
  erysipelatous —*see* Erysipelas
  esophagus K20.80
  ethmoid (bone) (chronic) (sinus) J32.2
  external auditory canal —*see* Abscess, ear,
    external
  extradural G06.2
    brain G06.0
      sequelae G09
    spinal cord G06.1
  extraperitoneal K68.19
  eye —*see* Endophthalmitis, purulent
  eyelid H00.03-●
  face (any part, except ear, eye and nose) L02.01
  fallopian tube —*see* Salpingitis
  fascia M72.8
  fauces J39.1
  fecal K63.0
  femoral (region) —*see* Abscess, lower limb
  filaria, filarial —*see* Infestation, filarial
  finger (any) —*see also* Abscess, hand
    nail —*see* Cellulitis, finger
  foot L02.61-●
  forehead L02.01
  frontal sinus (chronic) J32.1
  gallbladder K81.0
  genital organ or tract
    female (external) N76.4
    male N49.9
      multiple sites N49.8
      specified NEC N49.8
  gestational mammary O91.11-●
  gestational subareolar O91.11-●
  gingival
    ▶aggressive K05.20
      ▶generalized K05.229
        ▶moderate K05.222
        ▶severe K05.223
        ▶slight K05.221
      ▶localized K05.219
        ▶moderate K05.212
        ▶severe K05.213
        ▶slight K05.211
  gland, glandular (lymph) (acute) —*see*
      Lymphadenitis, acute
  gluteal (region) L02.31
  gonorrheal —*see* Gonococcus
  groin L02.214
  gum
    ▶aggressive K05.20
      ▶generalized K05.229
        ▶moderate K05.222
        ▶severe K05.223
        ▶slight K05.221
      ▶localized K05.219
        ▶moderate K05.212
        ▶severe K05.213
        ▶slight K05.211
  hand L02.51-●
  head NEC L02.811
    face (any part, except ear, eye and nose)
      L02.01
  heart —*see* Carditis
  heel —*see* Abscess, foot
  helminthic —*see* Infestation, helminth
  hepatic (cholangitic) (hematogenic)
      (lymphogenic) (pylephlebitic) K75.0
    amebic A06.4

▶ New   ⇒ Revised   ~~deleted~~ Deleted   ● Use Additional Character(s)

Abscess (Continued)

hip (region) —see Abscess, lower limb
horseshoe K61.31
ileocecal K35.33
ileostomy (bud) K94.12
iliac (region) L02.214
  fossa K35.33
infraclavicular (fossa) —see Abscess, upper
  limb
inguinal (region) L02.214
  lymph gland or node L04.1
intersphincteric K61.4
intestine, intestinal NEC K63.0
  rectal K61.1
intra-abdominal —see also Abscess,
  peritoneum K65.1
  following procedure T81.43
    obstetrical O86.03
  postprocedural T81.43
    retroperitoneal K68.11
intracranial G06.0
intramammary —see Abscess, breast
intramuscular, following procedure T81.44
  obstetrical O86.02
intraorbital —see Abscess, orbit
intraperitoneal K65.1
intrasphincteric (anus) K61.4
intraspinal G06.1
intratonsillar J36
ischiorectal (fossa) (specified NEC) K61.39
jaw (bone) (lower) (upper) M27.2
joint —see Arthritis, pyogenic or pyemic
  spine (tuberculous) A18.01
    nontuberculous —see Spondylopathy,
      infective
kidney N15.1
  with calculus N20.0
    with hydronephrosis N13.6
  puerperal (postpartum) O86.21
knee —see also Abscess, lower limb
  joint M00.9
labium (majus) (minus) N76.4
lacrimal
  caruncle —see Inflammation, lacrimal,
    passages, acute
  gland —see Dacryoadenitis
  passages (duct) (sac) —see Inflammation,
    lacrimal, passages, acute
lacunar N34.0
larynx J38.7
lateral (alveolar) K04.7
  with sinus K04.6
leg (any part) —see Abscess, lower limb
lens H27.8
lingual K14.0
  tonsil J36
lip K13.0
Littre's gland N34.0
liver (cholangitic) (hematogenic) (lymphogenic)
  (pylephlebitic) (pyogenic) K75.0
  amebic (due to Entamoeba histolytica)
    (dysenteric) (tropical) A06.4
    with
      brain abscess (and liver or lung
        abscess) A06.6
      lung abscess A06.5
loin (region) L02.211
lower limb L02.41-●
lumbar (tuberculous) A18.01
  nontuberculous L02.212
lung (miliary) (putrid) J85.2
  with pneumonia J85.1
    due to specified organism (see
      Pneumonia, in (due to))
  amebic (with liver abscess) A06.5
    with
      brain abscess A06.6
      pneumonia A06.5
lymph, lymphatic, gland or node (acute) —see
  also Lymphadenitis, acute
  mesentery I88.0
malar M27.2
mammary gland —see Abscess, breast

Abscess (Continued)

marginal, anus K61.0
mastoid —see Mastoiditis, acute
maxilla, maxillary M27.2
  molar (tooth) K04.7
    with sinus K04.6
  premolar K04.7
  sinus (chronic) J32.0
mediastinum J85.3
meibomian gland —see Hordeolum
meninges G06.2
mesentery, mesenteric K65.1
mesosalpinx —see Salpingitis
mons pubis L02.215
mouth (floor) K12.2
muscle —see Myositis, infective
myocardium I40.0
nabothian (follicle) —see Cervicitis
nasal J32.9
nasopharyngeal J39.1
navel L02.216
  newborn P38.9
    with mild hemorrhage P38.1
    without hemorrhage P38.9
neck (region) L02.11
  lymph gland or node L04.0
nephritic —see Abscess, kidney
nipple N61.1
  associated with
    lactation —see Pregnancy, complicated by
    pregnancy —see Pregnancy, complicated
      by
nose (external) (fossa) (septum) J34.0
  sinus (chronic) —see Sinusitis
omentum K65.1
operative wound T81.49
orbit, orbital —see Cellulitis, orbit
otogenic G06.0
ovary, ovarian (corpus luteum) —see Oophoritis
oviduct —see Oophoritis
palate (soft) K12.2
  hard M27.2
palmar (space) —see Abscess, hand
pancreas (duct) —see Pancreatitis, acute
parafrenal N48.21
parametric, parametrium N73.2
  acute N73.0
  chronic N73.1
paranephric N15.1
parapancreatic —see Pancreatitis, acute
parapharyngeal J39.0
pararectal K61.1
parasinus —see Sinusitis
parauterine (see also Disease, pelvis,
  inflammatory) N73.2
paravaginal —see Vaginitis
parietal region (scalp) L02.811
parodontal —see Periodontitis, aggressive,
  localized
parotid (duct) (gland) K11.3
  region K12.2
pectoral (region) L02.213
pelvis, pelvic
  female —see Disease, pelvis, inflammatory
  male, peritoneal K65.1
penis N48.21
  gonococcal (accessory gland) (periurethral)
    A54.1
perianal K61.0
periapical K04.7
  with sinus (alveolar) K04.6
periappendicular K35.33
pericardial I30.1
pericecal K35.33
pericemental —see Periodontitis, aggressive,
  localized
pericholecystic —see Cholecystitis, acute
pericoronal —see Periodontitis, aggressive,
  localized
peridental —see Periodontitis, aggressive,
  localized
perimetric —see also Disease, pelvis,
  inflammatory N73.2

Abscess (Continued)

perinephric, perinephritic —see Abscess,
  kidney
perineum, perineal (superficial) L02.215
  urethra N34.0
periodontal (parietal) —see Periodontitis,
  aggressive, localized
  apical K04.7
periosteum, periosteal —see also
  Osteomyelitis, specified type NEC
  with osteomyelitis —see also Osteomyelitis,
    specified type NEC
  acute —see Osteomyelitis, acute
  chronic —see Osteomyelitis, chronic
peripharyngeal J39.0
peripleuritic J86.9
  with fistula J86.0
periprostatic N41.2
perirectal K61.1
perirenal (tissue) —see Abscess, kidney
perisinuous (nose) —see Sinusitis
peritoneum, peritoneal (perforated)
  (ruptured) K65.1
  with appendicitis (see also Appendicitis)
    K35.33
  pelvic
    female —see Peritonitis, pelvic, female
    male K65.1
  ➡postoperative T81.43
  puerperal, postpartum, childbirth O85
  tuberculous A18.31
peritonsillar J36
perityphlic K35.33
periureteral N28.89
periurethral N34.0
  gonococcal (accessory gland) (periurethral)
    A54.1
periuterine —see also Disease, pelvis,
  inflammatory N73.2
perivesical —see Cystitis, specified type NEC
petrous bone —see Petrositis
phagedenic NOS L02.91
  chancroid A57
pharynx, pharyngeal (lateral) J39.1
pilonidal L05.01
pituitary (gland) E23.6
pleura J86.9
  with fistula J86.0
popliteal —see Abscess, lower limb
postcecal K35.33
postlaryngeal J38.7
postnasal J34.0
postoperative (any site) (see also Infection,
  postoperative wound) T81.49
  retroperitoneal K68.11
postpharyngeal J39.0
posttonsillar J36
post-typhoid A01.09
pouch of Douglas —see Peritonitis, pelvic,
  female
premammary —see Abscess, breast
prepatellar —see Abscess, lower limb
presacral K68.19
prostate N41.2
  gonococcal (acute) (chronic) A54.22
psoas muscle K68.12
puerperal - code by site under Puerperal,
  abscess
pulmonary —see Abscess, lung
pulp, pulpal (dental) K04.01
  irreversible K04.02
  reversible K04.01
rectovaginal septum K63.0
rectovesical —see Cystitis, specified type NEC
rectum K61.1
renal —see Abscess, kidney
retina —see Inflammation, chorioretinal
retrobulbar —see Abscess, orbit
retrocecal K65.1
retrolaryngeal J38.7
retromammary —see Abscess, breast
retroperitoneal NEC K68.19
  postprocedural K68.11

Abscess (Continued)
retropharyngeal J39.0
retrouterine —see Peritonitis, pelvic, female
retrovesical —see Cystitis, specified type NEC
root, tooth K04.7
    with sinus (alveolar) K04.6
round ligament —see also Disease, pelvis,
    inflammatory N73.2
rupture (spontaneous) NOS L02.91
sacrum (tuberculous)
    nontuberculous M46.28
salivary (duct) (gland) K11.3
scalp (any part) L02.811
scapular —see Osteomyelitis, specified type
    NEC
sclera —see Scleritis
scrofulous (tuberculous) A18.2
scrotum N49.2
seminal vesicle N49.0
septal, dental K04.7
    with sinus (alveolar) K04.6
serous —see Periostitis
shoulder (region) —see Abscess, upper limb
sigmoid K63.0
sinus (accessory) (chronic) (nasal) —see also
    Sinusitis
    intracranial venous (any) G06.0
Skene's duct or gland N34.0
skin —see Abscess, by site
specified site NEC L02.818
spermatic cord N49.1
sphenoidal (sinus) (chronic) J32.3
spinal cord (any part) (staphylococcal) G06.1
    tuberculous A17.81
spine (column) (tuberculous) A18.01
    epidural G06.1
    nontuberculous —see Osteomyelitis, vertebra
spleen D73.3
    amebic A06.89
stitch T81.41
    following an obstetrical procedure O86.01
subarachnoid G06.2
    brain G06.0
    spinal cord G06.1
subareolar —see Abscess, breast
subcecal K35.33
subcutaneous —see also Abscess, by site
    following procedure T81.41
        obstetrical O86.01
    pheomycotic (chromomycotic) B43.2
subdiaphragmatic K65.1
subdural G06.2
    brain G06.0
        sequelae G09
    spinal cord G06.1
sub-fascial, following an obstetrical
    procedure O86.02
subgaleal L02.811
subhepatic K65.1
sublingual K12.2
    gland K11.3
submammary —see Abscess, breast
submandibular (region) (space) (triangle) K12.2
    gland K11.3
submaxillary (region) L02.01
    gland K11.3
submental L02.01
    gland K11.3
subperiosteal —see Osteomyelitis, specified
    type NEC
subphrenic K65.1
    following an obstetrical procedure O86.03
    postoperative T81.43
suburethral N34.0
sudoriparous L75.8
supraclavicular (fossa) —see Abscess, upper
    limb
supralevator K61.5
suprapelvic, acute N73.0
suprarenal (capsule) (gland) E27.8
sweat gland L74.8
tear duct —see Inflammation, lacrimal,
    passages, acute

Abscess (Continued)
temple L02.01
temporal region L02.01
temporosphenoidal G06.0
tendon (sheath) M65.00
    ankle M65.07-•
    foot M65.07-•
    forearm M65.03-•
    hand M65.04-•
    lower leg M65.06-•
    pelvic region M65.05-•
    shoulder region M65.01-•
    specified site NEC M65.08
    thigh M65.05-•
    upper arm M65.02-•
testis N45.4
thigh —see Abscess, lower limb
thorax J86.9
    with fistula J86.0
throat J39.1
thumb —see also Abscess, hand
    nail —see Cellulitis, finger
thymus (gland) E32.1
thyroid (gland) E06.0
toe (any) —see also Abscess, foot
    nail —see Cellulitis, toe
tongue (staphylococcal) K14.0
tonsil(s) (lingual) J36
tonsillopharyngeal J36
tooth, teeth (root) K04.7
    with sinus (alveolar) K04.6
    supporting structures NEC —see
        Periodontitis, aggressive, localized
trachea J39.8
trunk L02.219
    abdominal wall L02.211
    back L02.212
    chest wall L02.213
    groin L02.214
    perineum L02.215
    umbilicus L02.216
tubal —see Salpingitis
tuberculous —see Tuberculosis, abscess
tubo-ovarian —see Salpingo-oophoritis
tunica vaginalis N49.1
umbilicus L02.216
upper
    limb L02.41-•
    respiratory J39.8
urethral (gland) N34.0
urinary N34.0
uterus, uterine (wall) —see also Endometritis
    ligament —see also Disease, pelvis,
        inflammatory N73.2
    neck —see Cervicitis
uvula K12.2
vagina (wall) —see Vaginitis
vaginorectal —see Vaginitis
vas deferens N49.1
vermiform appendix K35.33
vertebra (column) (tuberculous) A18.01
    nontuberculous —see Osteomyelitis,
        vertebra
vesical —see Cystitis, specified type NEC
vesico-uterine pouch —see Peritonitis, pelvic,
    female
vitreous (humor) —see Endophthalmitis,
    purulent
vocal cord J38.3
von Bezold's —see Mastoiditis, acute
vulva N76.4
vulvovaginal gland N75.1
web space —see Abscess, hand
wound T81.49
wrist —see Abscess, upper limb
Absence (of) (organ or part) (complete or partial)
adrenal (gland) (congenital) Q89.1
    acquired E89.6
albumin in blood E88.09
alimentary tract (congenital) Q45.8
    upper Q40.8
alveolar process (acquired) —see Anomaly,
    alveolar

Absence (Continued)
ankle (acquired) Z89.44-•
anus (congenital) Q42.3
    with fistula Q42.2
aorta (congenital) Q25.41
appendix, congenital Q42.8
arm (acquired) Z89.20-•
    above elbow Z89.22-•
        congenital (with hand present) —see
            Agenesis, arm, with hand present
            and hand —see Agenesis, forearm,
                and hand
    below elbow Z89.21-•
        congenital (with hand present) —see
            Agenesis, arm, with hand present
            and hand —see Agenesis, forearm,
                and hand
    congenital —see Defect, reduction, upper
        limb
    shoulder (following explantation of
        shoulder joint prosthesis) (joint) (with
        or without presence of antibiotic-
        impregnated cement spacer) Z89.23-•
        congenital (with hand present) —see
            Agenesis, arm, with hand present
artery (congenital) (peripheral) Q27.8
    brain Q28.3
    coronary Q24.5
    pulmonary Q25.79
    specified NEC Q27.8
    umbilical Q27.0
atrial septum (congenital) Q21.19
auditory canal (congenital) (external) Q16.1
auricle (ear), congenital Q16.0
bile, biliary duct, congenital Q44.5
bladder (acquired) Z90.6
    congenital Q64.5
bowel sounds R19.11
brain Q00.0
    part of Q04.3
breast(s) (and nipple(s)) (acquired) Z90.1-•
    congenital Q83.8
broad ligament Q50.6
bronchus (congenital) Q32.4
canaliculus lacrimalis, congenital Q10.4
cerebellum (vermis) Q04.3
cervix (acquired) (with uterus) Z90.710
    with remaining uterus Z90.712
    congenital Q51.5
chin, congenital Q18.8
cilia (congenital) Q10.3
    acquired —see Madarosis
clitoris (congenital) Q52.6
coccyx, congenital Q76.49
cold sense R20.8
congenital
    lumen —see Atresia
    organ or site NEC —see Agenesis
    septum —see Imperfect, closure
corpus callosum Q04.0
cricoid cartilage, congenital Q31.8
diaphragm (with hernia), congenital Q79.1
digestive organ(s) or tract, congenital Q45.8
    acquired NEC Z90.49
    upper Q40.8
ductus arteriosus Q28.8
duodenum (acquired) Z90.49
    congenital Q41.0
ear, congenital Q16.9
    acquired H93.8-•
    auricle Q16.0
    external Q16.0
    inner Q16.5
    lobe, lobule Q17.8
    middle, except ossicles Q16.4
        ossicles Q16.3
    ossicles Q16.3
ejaculatory duct (congenital) Q55.4
endocrine gland (congenital) NEC Q89.2
    acquired E89.89
epididymis (congenital) Q55.4
    acquired Z90.79
epiglottis, congenital Q31.8

Absence *(Continued)*
esophagus (congenital) Q39.8
　acquired (partial) Z90.49
eustachian tube (congenital) Q16.2
extremity (acquired) Z89.9
　congenital Q73.0
　knee (following explantation of knee joint
　　prosthesis) (joint) (with or without
　　presence of antibiotic-impregnated
　　cement spacer) Z89.52-●
　lower (above knee) Z89.619
　　below knee Z89.51-●
　upper —*see* Absence, arm
eye (acquired) Z90.01
　congenital Q11.1
　muscle (congenital) Q10.3
eyeball (acquired) Z90.01
eyelid (fold) (congenital) Q10.3
　acquired Z90.01
face, specified part NEC Q18.8
fallopian tube(s) (acquired) Z90.79
　congenital Q50.6
family member (causing problem in home)
　NEC —*see also* Disruption, family Z63.32
femur, congenital —*see* Defect, reduction,
　lower limb, longitudinal, femur
fibrinogen (congenital) D68.2
　acquired D65
finger(s) (acquired) Z89.02-●
　congenital —*see* Agenesis, hand
foot (acquired) Z89.43-●
　congenital —*see* Agenesis, foot
forearm (acquired) —*see* Absence, arm, below
　elbow
gallbladder (acquired) Z90.49
　congenital Q44.0
gamma globulin in blood D80.1
　hereditary D80.0
genital organs
　acquired (female) (male) Z90.79
　female, congenital Q52.8
　　external Q52.71
　　internal NEC Q52.8
　male, congenital Q55.8
genitourinary organs, congenital NEC
　female Q52.8
　male Q55.8
globe (acquired) Z90.01
　congenital Q11.1
glottis, congenital Q31.8
hand and wrist (acquired) Z89.11-●
　congenital —*see* Agenesis, hand
head, part (acquired) NEC Z90.09
heat sense R20.8
hip (following explantation of hip joint
　　prosthesis) (joint) (with or without
　　presence of antibiotic-impregnated
　　cement spacer) Z89.62-●
hymen (congenital) Q52.4
ileum (acquired) Z90.49
　congenital Q41.2
immunoglobulin, isolated NEC D80.3
　IgA D80.2
　IgG D80.3
　IgM D80.4
incus (acquired) —*see* Loss, ossicles, ear
　congenital Q16.3
inner ear, congenital Q16.5
intestine (acquired) (small) Z90.49
　congenital Q41.9
　　specified NEC Q41.8
　large Z90.49
　　congenital Q42.9
　　　specified NEC Q42.8
iris, congenital Q13.1
jejunum (acquired) Z90.49
　congenital Q41.1
joint
　acquired
　　hip (following explantation of hip joint
　　　prosthesis) (with or without
　　　presence of antibiotic-impregnated
　　　cement spacer) Z89.62-●

Absence *(Continued)*
joint *(Continued)*
　acquired *(Continued)*
　　knee (following explantation of knee
　　　joint prosthesis) (with or without
　　　presence of antibiotic-impregnated
　　　cement spacer) Z89.52-●
　　shoulder (following explantation of
　　　shoulder joint prosthesis) (with or
　　　without presence of antibiotic-
　　　impregnated cement spacer) Z89.23-●
　　congenital NEC Q74.8
kidney(s) (acquired) Z90.5
　congenital Q60.2
　　bilateral Q60.1
　　unilateral Q60.0
knee (following explantation of knee joint
　　prosthesis) (joint) (with or without
　　presence of antibiotic-impregnated
　　cement spacer) Z89.52-●
labyrinth, membranous Q16.5
larynx (congenital) Q31.8
　acquired Z90.02
leg (acquired) (above knee) Z89.61-●
　below knee (acquired) Z89.51-●
　congenital —*see* Defect, reduction, lower
　　limb
lens (acquired) —*see also* Aphakia
　congenital Q12.3
　post cataract extraction Z98.4-●
limb (acquired) —*see* Absence, extremity
lip Q38.6
liver (congenital) Q44.7
lung (fissure) (lobe) (bilateral) (unilateral)
　(congenital) Q33.3
　acquired (any part) Z90.2
menstruation —*see* Amenorrhea
muscle (congenital) (pectoral) Q79.8
　ocular Q10.3
neck, part Q18.8
neutrophil —*see* Agranulocytosis
nipple(s) (with breast(s)) (acquired) Z90.1-●
　congenital Q83.2
nose (congenital) Q30.1
　acquired Z90.09
organ
　of Corti, congenital Q16.5
　or site, congenital NEC Q89.8
　　acquired NEC Z90.89
osseous meatus (ear) Q16.4
ovary (acquired)
　bilateral Z90.722
　congenital
　　bilateral Q50.02
　　unilateral Q50.01
　unilateral Z90.721
oviduct (acquired)
　bilateral Z90.722
　congenital Q50.6
　unilateral Z90.721
pancreas (congenital) Q45.0
　acquired Z90.410
　　complete Z90.410
　　partial Z90.411
　　total Z90.410
parathyroid gland (acquired) E89.2
　congenital Q89.2
patella, congenital Q74.1
penis (congenital) Q55.5
　acquired Z90.79
pericardium (congenital) Q24.8
pituitary gland (congenital) Q89.2
　acquired E89.3
prostate (acquired) Z90.79
　congenital Q55.4
pulmonary valve Q22.0
punctum lacrimale (congenital) Q10.4
radius, congenital —*see* Defect, reduction,
　upper limb, longitudinal, radius
rectum (congenital) Q42.1
　with fistula Q42.0
　acquired Z90.49
respiratory organ NOS Q34.9

Absence *(Continued)*
rib (acquired) Z90.89
　congenital Q76.6
sacrum, congenital Q76.49
salivary gland(s), congenital Q38.4
scrotum, congenital Q55.29
seminal vesicles (congenital) Q55.4
　acquired Z90.79
septum
▌atrial (congenital) Q21.19
　between aorta and pulmonary artery Q21.4
　ventricular (congenital) Q20.4
sex chromosome
　female phenotype Q97.8
　male phenotype Q98.8
skull bone (congenital) Q75.8
　with
　　anencephaly Q00.0
　　encephalocele —*see* Encephalocele
　　hydrocephalus Q03.9
　　　with spina bifida —*see* Spina bifida, by
　　　　site, with hydrocephalus
　　microcephaly Q02
spermatic cord, congenital Q55.4
spine, congenital Q76.49
spleen (congenital) Q89.01
　acquired Z90.81
sternum, congenital Q76.7
stomach (acquired) (partial) Z90.3
　congenital Q40.2
superior vena cava, congenital Q26.8
teeth, tooth (congenital) K00.0
　acquired (complete) K08.109
　　class I K08.101
　　class II K08.102
　　class III K08.103
　　class IV K08.104
　　due to
　　　caries K08.139
　　　　class I K08.131
　　　　class II K08.132
　　　　class III K08.133
　　　　class IV K08.134
　　　periodontal disease K08.129
　　　　class I K08.121
　　　　class II K08.122
　　　　class III K08.123
　　　　class IV K08.124
　　　specified NEC K08.199
　　　　class I K08.191
　　　　class II K08.192
　　　　class III K08.193
　　　　class IV K08.194
　　　trauma K08.119
　　　　class I K08.111
　　　　class II K08.112
　　　　class III K08.113
　　　　class IV K08.114
　　partial K08.409
　　　class I K08.401
　　　class II K08.402
　　　class III K08.403
　　　class IV K08.404
　　　due to
　　　　caries K08.439
　　　　　class I K08.431
　　　　　class II K08.432
　　　　　class III K08.433
　　　　　class IV K08.434
　　　　periodontal disease K08.429
　　　　　class I K08.421
　　　　　class II K08.422
　　　　　class III K08.423
　　　　　class IV K08.424
　　　　specified NEC K08.499
　　　　　class I K08.491
　　　　　class II K08.492
　　　　　class III K08.493
　　　　　class IV K08.494
　　　　trauma K08.419
　　　　　class I K08.411
　　　　　class II K08.412
　　　　　class III K08.413
　　　　　class IV K08.414

Absence (Continued)
  tendon (congenital) Q79.8
  testis (congenital) Q55.0
    acquired Z90.79
  thumb (acquired) Z89.01-●
    congenital —see Agenesis, hand
  thymus gland Q89.2
  thyroid (gland) (acquired) E89.0
    cartilage, congenital Q31.8
    congenital E03.1
  toe(s) (acquired) Z89.42-●
    with foot —see Absence, foot and ankle
    congenital —see Agenesis, foot
    great Z89.41-●
  tongue, congenital Q38.3
  trachea (cartilage), congenital Q32.1
  transverse aortic arch, congenital Q25.49
  tricuspid valve Q22.4
  umbilical artery, congenital Q27.0
  upper arm and forearm with hand present,
    congenital —see Agenesis, arm, with
    hand present
  ureter (congenital) Q62.4
    acquired Z90.6
  urethra, congenital Q64.5
  uterus (acquired) Z90.710
    with cervix Z90.710
    with remaining cervical stump Z90.711
    congenital Q51.0
  uvula, congenital Q38.5
  vagina, congenital Q52.0
  vas deferens (congenital) Q55.4
    acquired Z90.79
  vein (peripheral) congenital NEC Q27.8
    cerebral Q28.3
    digestive system Q27.8
    great Q26.8
    lower limb Q27.8
    portal Q26.5
    precerebral Q28.1
    specified site NEC Q27.8
    upper limb Q27.8
  vena cava (inferior) (superior), congenital Q26.8
  ventricular septum Q20.4
  vertebra, congenital Q76.49
▶von Willebrand factor, complete (near) (see
    also Disease, von Willebrand) D68.03
  vulva, congenital Q52.71
  wrist (acquired) Z89.12-●
Absorbent system disease I87.8
Absorption
  carbohydrate, disturbance K90.49
  chemical —see Table of Drugs and Chemicals
    through placenta (newborn) P04.9
      environmental substance P04.6
      nutritional substance P04.5
      obstetric anesthetic or analgesic drug P04.0
  drug NEC —see Table of Drugs and Chemicals
    addictive
      through placenta (newborn) (see also
        Newborn, affected by, maternal,
        use of) P04.40
        cocaine P04.41
        hallucinogens P04.42
        specified drug NEC P04.49
    medicinal
      through placenta (newborn) P04.19
    through placenta (newborn) P04.19
      obstetric anesthetic or analgesic drug P04.0
  fat, disturbance K90.49
    pancreatic K90.3
  noxious substance —see Table of Drugs and
    Chemicals
  protein, disturbance K90.49
  starch, disturbance K90.49
  toxic substance —see Table of Drugs and
    Chemicals
  uremic —see Uremia
Abstinence symptoms, syndrome
  alcohol F10.239
    with delirium F10.231
  cocaine F14.23
  neonatal P96.1

Abstinence symptoms, syndrome (Continued)
  nicotine —see Dependence, drug, nicotine,
    with, withdrawal
  opioid F11.93
    with dependence F11.23
  psychoactive NEC F19.939
    with
      delirium F19.931
      dependence F19.239
        with
          delirium F19.231
          perceptual disturbance F19.232
        uncomplicated F19.230
      perceptual disturbance F19.932
      uncomplicated F19.930
  sedative F13.939
    with
      delirium F13.931
      dependence F13.239
        with
          delirium F13.231
          perceptual disturbance F13.232
        uncomplicated F13.230
      perceptual disturbance F13.932
      uncomplicated F13.930
  stimulant NEC F15.93
    with dependence F15.23
Abulia R68.89
Abulomania F60.7
Abuse
  adult —see Maltreatment, adult
    as reason for
      couple seeking advice (including
        offender) Z63.0
  alcohol (non-dependent) F10.10
    with
      anxiety disorder F10.180
      intoxication F10.129
        with delirium F10.121
        uncomplicated F10.120
      mood disorder F10.14
      other specified disorder F10.188
      psychosis F10.159
        delusions F10.150
        hallucinations F10.151
      sexual dysfunction F10.181
      sleep disorder F10.182
      unspecified disorder F10.19
      withdrawal F10.139
        with
          perceptual disturbance F10.132
        delirium F10.131
        uncomplicated F10.130
    counseling and surveillance Z71.41
    in remission (early) (sustained) F10.11
  amphetamine (or related substance) —see also
    Abuse, drug, stimulant NEC
    stimulant NEC F15.10
      with
        anxiety disorder F15.180
        intoxication F15.129
          with
            delirium F15.121
            perceptual disturbance F15.122
        withdrawal F15.13
  analgesics (non-prescribed) (over the counter)
    F55.8
  antacids F55.0
  antidepressants —see Abuse, drug,
    psychoactive NEC
  anxiolytic —see Abuse, drug, sedative
  barbiturates —see Abuse, drug, sedative
  caffeine —see Abuse, drug, stimulant NEC
  cannabis, cannabinoids —see Abuse, drug,
    cannabis
  child —see Maltreatment, child
  cocaine —see Abuse, drug, cocaine
  drug NEC (non-dependent) F19.10
    with sleep disorder F19.182
    amphetamine type —see Abuse, drug,
      stimulant NEC
    analgesics (non-prescribed) (over the
      counter) F55.8

Abuse (Continued)
  drug NEC (Continued)
    antacids F55.0
    antidepressants —see Abuse, drug,
      psychoactive NEC
    anxiolytics —see Abuse, drug, sedative
    barbiturates —see Abuse, drug, sedative
    caffeine —see Abuse, drug, stimulant NEC
    cannabis F12.10
      with
        anxiety disorder F12.180
        intoxication F12.129
          with
            delirium F12.121
            perceptual disturbance F12.122
          uncomplicated F12.120
        other specified disorder F12.188
        psychosis F12.159
          delusions F12.150
          hallucinations F12.151
        unspecified disorder F12.19
        withdrawal F12.13
      in remission (early) (sustained) F12.11
    cocaine F14.10
      with
        anxiety disorder F14.180
        intoxication F14.129
          with
            delirium F14.121
            perceptual disturbance F14.122
          uncomplicated F14.120
        mood disorder F14.14
        other specified disorder F14.188
        psychosis F14.159
          delusions F14.150
          hallucinations F14.151
        sexual dysfunction F14.181
        sleep disorder F14.182
        unspecified disorder F14.19
        withdrawal F14.13
      in remission (early) (sustained) F14.11
    counseling and surveillance Z71.51
    hallucinogen F16.10
      with
        anxiety disorder F16.180
        flashbacks F16.183
        intoxication F16.129
          with
            delirium F16.121
            perceptual disturbance F16.122
          uncomplicated F16.120
        mood disorder F16.14
        other specified disorder F16.188
        perception disorder, persisting F16.183
        psychosis F16.159
          delusions F16.150
          hallucinations F16.151
        unspecified disorder F16.19
      in remission (early) (sustained) F16.11
    hashish —see Abuse, drug, cannabis
    herbal or folk remedies F55.1
    hormones F55.3
    hypnotics —see Abuse, drug, sedative
    inhalant F18.10
      with
        anxiety disorder F18.180
        dementia, persisting F18.17
        intoxication F18.129
          with delirium F18.121
          uncomplicated F18.120
        mood disorder F18.14
        other specified disorder F18.188
        psychosis F18.159
          delusions F18.150
          hallucinations F18.151
        unspecified disorder F18.19
      in remission (early) (sustained) F18.11
    in remission (early) (sustained) F19.11
    laxatives F55.2
    LSD —see Abuse, drug, hallucinogen
    marihuana —see Abuse, drug, cannabis
    morphine type (opioids) —see Abuse, drug,
      opioid

  ▶ New   ⇒ Revised   ~~deleted~~ Deleted   ● Use Additional Character(s)

Abuse *(Continued)*
  drug NEC *(Continued)*
    opioid F11.10
      with
        intoxication F11.129
          with
            delirium F11.121
            perceptual disturbance F11.122
          uncomplicated F11.120
        mood disorder F11.14
        other specified disorder F11.188
        psychosis F11.159
          delusions F11.150
          hallucinations F11.151
        sexual dysfunction F11.181
        sleep disorder F11.182
        unspecified disorder F11.19
        withdrawal F11.13
      in remission (early) (sustained) F11.11
    PCP (phencyclidine) (or related substance) —
        see Abuse, drug, hallucinogen
    psychoactive NEC F19.10
      with
        amnestic disorder F19.16
        anxiety disorder F19.180
        dementia F19.17
        intoxication F19.129
          with
            delirium F19.121
            perceptual disturbance F19.122
          uncomplicated F19.120
        mood disorder F19.14
        other specified disorder F19.188
        psychosis F19.159
          delusions F19.150
          hallucinations F19.151
        sexual dysfunction F19.181
        sleep disorder F19.182
        unspecified disorder F19.19
        withdrawal F19.139
          with
            perceptual disturbance F19.132
            delirium F19.131
          uncomplicated F19.130
    sedative, hypnotic or anxiolytic F13.10
      with
        anxiety disorder F13.180
        intoxication F13.129
          with delirium F13.121
          uncomplicated F13.120
        mood disorder F13.14
        other specified disorder F13.188
        psychosis F13.159
          delusions F13.150
          hallucinations F13.151
        sexual dysfunction F13.181
        sleep disorder F13.182
        unspecified disorder F13.19
        withdrawal F13.139
          with
            perceptual disturbance F13.132
            delirium F13.131
          uncomplicated F13.130
      in remission (early) (sustained) F13.11
    solvent —*see* Abuse, drug, inhalant
    steroids F55.3
    stimulant NEC F15.10
      with
        anxiety disorder F15.180
        intoxication F15.129
          with
            delirium F15.121
            perceptual disturbance F15.122
          uncomplicated F15.120
        mood disorder F15.14
        other specified disorder F15.188
        psychosis F15.159
          delusions F15.150
          hallucinations F15.151
        sexual dysfunction F15.181
        sleep disorder F15.182
        unspecified disorder F15.19
        withdrawal F15.13
      in remission (early) (sustained) F15.11

Abuse *(Continued)*
  drug NEC *(Continued)*
    tranquilizers —*see* Abuse, drug, sedative
    vitamins F55.4
    hallucinogens —*see* Abuse, drug, hallucinogen
    hashish —*see* Abuse, drug, cannabis
    herbal or folk remedies F55.1
    hormones F55.3
    hypnotic —*see* Abuse, drug, sedative
    inhalant —*see* Abuse, drug, inhalant
    laxatives F55.2
    LSD —*see* Abuse, drug, hallucinogen
    marihuana —*see* Abuse, drug, cannabis
    morphine type (opioids) —*see* Abuse, drug,
        opioid
    non-psychoactive substance NEC F55.8
      antacids F55.0
      folk remedies F55.1
      herbal remedies F55.1
      hormones F55.3
      laxatives F55.2
      steroids F55.3
      vitamins F55.4
    opioids —*see* Abuse, drug, opioid
    PCP (phencyclidine) (or related substance) —
        see Abuse, drug, hallucinogen
    physical (adult) (child) —*see* Maltreatment
    psychoactive substance —*see* Abuse, drug,
        psychoactive NEC
    psychological (adult) (child) —*see* Maltreatment
    sedative —*see* Abuse, drug, sedative
    sexual —*see* Maltreatment
    solvent —*see* Abuse, drug, inhalant
    steroids F55.3
    vitamins F55.4
Acalculia R48.8
  developmental F81.2
Acanthamebiasis (with) B60.10
  conjunctiva B60.12
  keratoconjunctivitis B60.13
  meningoencephalitis B60.11
  other specified B60.19
Acanthocephaliasis B83.8
Acanthocheilonemiasis B74.4
Acanthocytosis E78.6
Acantholysis L11.9
Acanthosis (acquired) (nigricans) L83
  benign Q82.8
  congenital Q82.8
  seborrheic L82.1
    inflamed L82.0
  tongue K14.3
Acapnia E87.3
▶Acarbia E87.29
Acardia, acardius Q89.8
Acardiacus amorphus Q89.8
Acardiotrophia I51.4
Acariasis B88.0
  scabies B86
Acarodermatitis (urticarioides) B88.0
Acarophobia F40.218
Acatalasemia, acatalasia E80.3
Acathisia (drug induced) G25.71
Accelerated atrioventricular conduction I45.6
Accentuation of personality traits (type A) Z73.1
Accessory (congenital)
  adrenal gland Q89.1
  anus Q43.4
  appendix Q43.4
  atrioventricular conduction I45.6
  auditory ossicles Q16.3
  auricle (ear) Q17.0
  biliary duct or passage Q44.5
  bladder Q64.79
  blood vessels NEC Q27.9
    coronary Q24.5
  bone NEC Q79.8
  breast tissue, axilla Q83.1
  carpal bones Q74.0
  cecum Q43.4
  chromosome(s) NEC (nonsex) Q92.9

Accessory *(Continued)*
  chromosome(s) NEC (nonsex) *(Continued)*
    with complex rearrangements NEC Q92.5
      seen only at prometaphase Q92.8
    13 —*see* Trisomy, 13
    18 —*see* Trisomy, 18
    21 —*see* Trisomy, 21
    partial Q92.9
    sex
      female phenotype Q97.8
  coronary artery Q24.5
  cusp(s), heart valve NEC Q24.8
    pulmonary Q22.3
  cystic duct Q44.5
  digit(s) Q69.9
  ear (auricle) (lobe) Q17.0
  endocrine gland NEC Q89.2
  eye muscle Q10.3
  eyelid Q10.3
  face bone(s) Q75.8
  fallopian tube (fimbria) (ostium) Q50.6
  finger(s) Q69.0
  foreskin N47.8
  frontonasal process Q75.8
  gallbladder Q44.1
  genital organ(s)
    female Q52.8
      external Q52.79
      internal NEC Q52.8
    male Q55.8
  genitourinary organs NEC Q89.8
    female Q52.8
    male Q55.8
  hallux Q69.2
  heart Q24.8
    valve NEC Q24.8
      pulmonary Q22.3
  hepatic ducts Q44.5
  hymen Q52.4
  intestine (large) (small) Q43.4
  kidney Q63.0
  lacrimal canal Q10.6
  leaflet, heart valve NEC Q24.8
  ligament, broad Q50.6
  liver Q44.7
    duct Q44.5
  lobule (ear) Q17.0
  lung (lobe) Q33.1
  muscle Q79.8
  navicular of carpus Q74.0
  nervous system, part NEC Q07.8
  nipple Q83.3
  nose Q30.8
  organ or site not listed —*see* Anomaly, by site
  ovary Q50.31
  oviduct Q50.6
  pancreas Q45.3
  parathyroid gland Q89.2
  parotid gland (and duct) Q38.4
  pituitary gland Q89.2
  preauricular appendage Q17.0
  prepuce N47.8
  renal arteries (multiple) Q27.2
  rib Q76.6
    cervical Q76.5
  roots (teeth) K00.2
  salivary gland Q38.4
  sesamoid bones Q74.8
    foot Q74.2
    hand Q74.0
  skin tags Q82.8
  spleen Q89.09
  sternum Q76.7
  submaxillary gland Q38.4
  tarsal bones Q74.2
  teeth, tooth K00.1
  tendon Q79.8
  thumb Q69.1
  thymus gland Q89.2
  thyroid gland Q89.2
  toes Q69.2

Accessory *(Continued)*
  tongue Q38.3
  tooth, teeth K00.1
  tragus Q17.0
  ureter Q62.5
  urethra Q64.79
  urinary organ or tract NEC Q64.8
  uterus Q51.28
  vagina Q52.10
  valve, heart NEC Q24.8
    pulmonary Q22.3
  vertebra Q76.49
  vocal cords Q31.8
  vulva Q52.79
Accident
  birth —*see* Birth, injury
  cardiac —*see* Infarct, myocardium
  cerebral I63.9
  cerebrovascular (embolic) (ischemic)
      (thrombotic) I63.9
    aborted I63.9
    hemorrhagic —*see* Hemorrhage,
        intracranial, intracerebral
    old (without sequelae) Z86.73
      with sequelae (of) —*see* Sequelae,
        infarction, cerebral
  coronary —*see* Infarct, myocardium
  craniovascular I63.9
  vascular, brain I63.9
Accidental —*see* condition
Accommodation (disorder) —*see also* condition
  hysterical paralysis of F44.89
  insufficiency of H52.4
  paresis —*see* Paresis, of accommodation
  spasm —*see* Spasm, of accommodation
Accouchement —*see* Delivery
Accreta placenta O43.21-•
Accretio cordis (nonrheumatic) I31.0
Accretions, tooth, teeth K03.6
Acculturation difficulty Z60.3
Accumulation secretion, prostate N42.89
Acephalia, acephalism, acephalus, acephaly
    Q00.0
Acephalobrachia monster Q89.8
Acephalochirus monster Q89.8
Acephalogaster Q89.8
Acephalostomus monster Q89.8
Acephalothorax Q89.8
Acerophobia F40.298
Acetonemia R79.89
  in Type 1 diabetes E10.10
    with coma E10.11
Acetonuria R82.4
Achalasia (cardia) (esophagus) K22.0
  congenital Q39.5
  pylorus Q40.0
  sphincteral NEC K59.89
Ache(s) —*see* Pain
Acheilia Q38.6
Achillobursitis —*see* Tendinitis, Achilles
Achillodynia —*see* Tendinitis, Achilles
Achlorhydria, achlorhydric (neurogenic) K31.83
  anemia D50.8
  diarrhea K31.83
  psychogenic F45.8
  secondary to vagotomy K91.1
Achluophobia F40.228
Acholia K82.8
Acholuric jaundice (familial)
    (splenomegalic) —*see also* Spherocytosis
  acquired D59.8
Achondrogenesis Q77.0
Achondroplasia (osteosclerosis congenita)
    Q77.4
Achroma, cutis L80
Achromat (ism), achromatopsia (acquired)
    (congenital) H53.51
Achromia, congenital —*see* Albinism
Achromia parasitica B36.0
Achylia gastrica K31.89
  psychogenic F45.8

Acid
  burn —*see* Corrosion
  deficiency
    amide nicotinic E52
    ascorbic E54
    folic E53.8
    nicotinic E52
    pantothenic E53.8
  intoxication (*see also* Acidosis) E87.29
  peptic disease K30
  phosphatase deficiency E83.39
  stomach K30
    psychogenic F45.8
Acidemia (*see also* Acidosis) E87.20
  argininosuccinic E72.22
  isovaleric E71.110
  metabolic (newborn) P19.9
    first noted before onset of labor P19.0
    first noted during labor P19.1
    noted at birth P19.2
  methylmalonic E71.120
  pipecolic E72.3
  propionic E71.121
Acidity, gastric (high) K30
  psychogenic F45.8
Acidocytopenia —*see* Agranulocytosis
Acidocytosis D72.10
Acidopenia —*see* Agranulocytosis
Acidosis (lactic) E87.20
  in Type 1 diabetes E10.10
    with coma E10.11
  kidney, tubular N25.89
  lactic E87.20
    acute E87.21
    chronic E87.22
  metabolic NEC E87.20
    acute E87.21
    chronic E87.22
    hyperchloremic, of newborn P74.421
    with respiratory acidosis E87.4
    late, of newborn P74.0
  mixed metabolic and respiratory, newborn P84
  newborn P84
  renal (hyperchloremic) (tubular) N25.89
  respiratory E87.29
    acute J96.02
    chronic J96.12
    complicated by
      metabolic
        acidosis E87.4
        alkalosis E87.4
    specified NEC E87.29
Aciduria
  4-hydroxybutyric E72.81
  argininosuccinic E72.22
  gamma-hydroxybutyric E72.81
  glutaric (type I) E72.3
    type II E71.313
    type III E71.5-•
  orotic (congenital) (hereditary) (pyrimidine
      deficiency) E79.8
    anemia D53.0
Acladiosis (skin) B36.0
Aclasis, diaphyseal Q78.6
Acleistocardia Q21.19
Aclusion —*see* Anomaly, dentofacial,
    malocclusion
Acne L70.9
  artificialis L70.8
  atrophica L70.2
  cachecticorum (Hebra) L70.8
  conglobata L70.1
  cystic L70.0
  decalvans L66.2
  excoriée (des jeunes filles) L70.5
  frontalis L70.2
  indurata L70.0
  infantile L70.4
  keloid L73.0
  lupoid L70.2
  necrotic, necrotica (miliaris) L70.2

Acne *(Continued)*
  neonatal L70.4
  nodular L70.0
  occupational L70.8
  picker's L70.5
  pustular L70.0
  rodens L70.2
  rosacea L71.9
  specified NEC L70.8
  tropica L70.3
  varioliformis L70.2
  vulgaris L70.0
Acnitis (primary) A18.4
Acosta's disease T70.29
Acoustic —*see* condition
Acousticophobia F40.298
ACPO (acute colonic pseudo-obstruction) K59.81
Acquired —*see also* condition
  immunodeficiency syndrome (AIDS) B20
Acrania Q00.0
Acroangiodermatitis I78.9
Acroasphyxia, chronic I73.89
Acrobystitis N47.7
Acrocephalopolysyndactyly Q87.0
Acrocephalosyndactyly Q87.0
Acrocephaly Q75.0
Acrochondrohyperplasia —*see* Syndrome,
    Marfan's
Acrocyanosis I73.89
  newborn P28.2
    meaning transient blue hands and feet -
      omit code
Acrodermatitis L30.8
  atrophicans (chronica) L90.4
  continua (Hallopeau) L40.2
  enteropathica (hereditary) E83.2
  Hallopeau's L40.2
  infantile papular L44.4
  perstans L40.2
  pustulosa continua L40.2
  recalcitrant pustular L40.2
Acrodynia —*see* Poisoning, mercury
Acromegaly, acromegalia E22.0
Acromelalgia I73.81
Acromicria, acromikria Q79.8
Acronyx L60.0
Acropachy, thyroid —*see* Thyrotoxicosis
Acroparesthesia (simple) (vasomotor) I73.89
Acropathy, thyroid —*see* Thyrotoxicosis
Acrophobia F40.241
Acroposthitis N47.7
Acroscleriasis, acroscleroderma,
    acrosclerosis —*see* Sclerosis, systemic
Acrosphacelus I96
Acrospiroma, eccrine —*see* Neoplasm, skin,
    benign
Acrostealgia —*see* Osteochondropathy
Acrotrophodynia —*see* Immersion
ACTH ectopic syndrome E24.3
Actinic —*see* condition
Actinobacillosis, actinobacillus A28.8
  mallei A24.0
  muris A25.1
Actinomyces israelii (infection) —*see*
    Actinomycosis
Actinomycetoma (foot) B47.1
Actinomycosis, actinomycotic A42.9
  with pneumonia A42.0
  abdominal A42.1
  cervicofacial A42.2
  cutaneous A42.89
  gastrointestinal A42.1
  pulmonary A42.0
  sepsis A42.7
  specified site NEC A42.89
Actinoneuritis G62.82
Action, heart
  disorder I49.9
  irregular I49.9
    psychogenic F45.8
Activated protein C resistance D68.51

Activation
  mast cell (disorder) (syndrome) D89.40
    idiopathic D89.42
    monoclonal D89.41
    secondary D89.43
    specified type NEC D89.49
Active —see condition
Acute —see also condition
  abdomen R10.0
  gallbladder —see Cholecystitis, acute
Acyanotic heart disease (congenital) Q24.9
Acystia Q64.5
Adair-Dighton syndrome (brittle bones and
    blue sclera, deafness) Q78.0
Adamantinoblastoma —see Ameloblastoma
Adamantinoma —see also Cyst, calcifying
    odontogenic
  long bones C40.90
    lower limb C40.2-●
    upper limb C40.0-●
  malignant C41.1
    jaw (bone) (lower) C41.1
      upper C41.0
  tibial C40.2-●
Adamantoblastoma —see Ameloblastoma
Adams-Stokes (-Morgagni) disease or
    syndrome I45.9
Adaption reaction —see Disorder, adjustment
Addiction —see also Dependence F19.20
  alcohol, alcoholic (ethyl) (methyl) (wood)
      (without remission) F10.20
    with remission F10.21
  drug —see Dependence, drug
  ethyl alcohol (without remission) F10.20
    with remission F10.21
  heroin —see Dependence, drug, opioid
  methyl alcohol (without remission) F10.20
    with remission F10.21
  methylated spirit (without remission) F10.20
    with remission F10.21
  morphine(-like substances) —see
      Dependence, drug, opioid
  nicotine —see Dependence, drug, nicotine
  opium and opioids —see Dependence, drug,
      opioid
  tobacco —see Dependence, drug, nicotine
Addisonian crisis E27.2
Addison's
  anemia (pernicious) D51.0
  disease (bronze) or syndrome E27.1
    tuberculous A18.7
  keloid L94.0
Addison-Biermer anemia (pernicious) D51.0
Addison-Schilder complex E71.528
Additional —see also Accessory
  chromosome(s) Q99.8
    21 —see Trisomy, 21
    sex —see Abnormal, chromosome, sex
Adduction contracture, hip or other joint —see
    Contraction, joint
Adenitis —see also Lymphadenitis
  acute, unspecified site L04.9
  axillary I88.9
    acute L04.2
    chronic or subacute I88.1
  Bartholin's gland N75.8
  bulbourethral gland —see Urethritis
  cervical I88.9
    acute L04.0
    chronic or subacute I88.1
  chancroid (Hemophilus ducreyi) A57
  chronic, unspecified site I88.1
  Cowper's gland —see Urethritis
  due to Pasteurella multocida (P. septica) A28.0
  epidemic, acute B27.09
  gangrenous L04.9
  gonorrheal NEC A54.89
  groin I88.9
    acute L04.1
    chronic or subacute I88.1
  infectious (acute) (epidemic) B27.09

Adenitis (Continued)
  inguinal I88.9
    acute L04.1
    chronic or subacute I88.1
  lymph gland or node, except mesenteric I88.9
    acute —see Lymphadenitis, acute
    chronic or subacute I88.1
  mesenteric (acute) (chronic) (nonspecific)
      (subacute) I88.0
  parotid gland (suppurative) —see Sialoadenitis
  salivary gland (any) (suppurative) —see
      Sialoadenitis
  scrofulous (tuberculous) A18.2
  Skene's duct or gland —see Urethritis
  strumous, tuberculous A18.2
  subacute, unspecified site I88.1
  sublingual gland (suppurative) —see
      Sialoadenitis
  submandibular gland (suppurative) —see
      Sialoadenitis
  submaxillary gland (suppurative) —see
      Sialoadenitis
  tuberculous —see Tuberculosis, lymph gland
  urethral gland —see Urethritis
  Wharton's duct (suppurative) —see
      Sialoadenitis
Adenoacanthoma —see Neoplasm, malignant,
    by site
Adenoameloblastoma —see Cyst, calcifying
    odontogenic
Adenocarcinoid (tumor) —see Neoplasm,
    malignant, by site
Adenocarcinoma —see also Neoplasm,
    malignant, by site
  acidophil
    specified site —see Neoplasm, malignant,
        by site
    unspecified site C75.1
  adrenal cortical C74.0-●
  alveolar —see Neoplasm, lung, malignant
  apocrine
    breast —see Neoplasm, breast, malignant
    in situ
      breast D05.8-●
      specified site NEC —see Neoplasm, skin,
          in situ
      unspecified site D04.9
    specified site NEC —see Neoplasm, skin,
        malignant
    unspecified site C44.99
  basal cell
    specified site —see Neoplasm, skin,
        malignant
    unspecified site C08.9
  basophil
    specified site —see Neoplasm, malignant,
        by site
    unspecified site C75.1
  bile duct type C22.1
    liver C22.1
    specified site NEC —see Neoplasm,
        malignant, by site
    unspecified site C22.1
  bronchiolar —see Neoplasm, lung, malignant
  bronchioloalveolar —see Neoplasm, lung,
      malignant
  ceruminous C44.29-●
  cervix, in situ (see also Carcinoma, cervix
      uteri, in situ) D06.9
  chromophobe
    specified site —see Neoplasm, malignant,
        by site
    unspecified site C75.1
  diffuse type
    specified site —see Neoplasm, malignant,
        by site
    unspecified site C16.9
  duct
    infiltrating
      with Paget's disease —see Neoplasm,
          breast, malignant
      specified site —see Neoplasm,
          malignant, by site

Adenocarcinoma (Continued)
  duct (Continued)
    infiltrating (Continued)
      unspecified site (female) C50.91-●
        male C50.92-●
      specified site —see Neoplasm, malignant,
          by site
      unspecified site
        female C56.9
        male C61
  eosinophil
    specified site —see Neoplasm, malignant,
        by site
    unspecified site C75.1
  follicular
    with papillary C73
    moderately differentiated C73
    specified site —see Neoplasm, malignant,
        by site
    trabecular C73
    unspecified site C73
    well differentiated C73
  Hurthle cell C73
  in
    adenomatous
      polyposis coli C18.9
  infiltrating duct
    with Paget's disease —see Neoplasm,
        breast, malignant
    specified site —see Neoplasm,
        malignant, by site
    unspecified site (female) C50.91-●
      male C50.92-●
  inflammatory
    specified site —see Neoplasm,
        malignant, by site
    unspecified site (female) C50.91-●
      male C50.92-●
  intestinal type
    specified site —see Neoplasm,
        malignant, by site
    unspecified site C16.9
  intracystic papillary
  intraductal
    breast D05.1-●
    noninfiltrating
      breast D05.1-●
      papillary
        with invasion
          specified site —see Neoplasm,
              malignant, by site
          unspecified site (female) C50.91-●
            male C50.92-●
        breast D05.1-●
        specified site NEC —see Neoplasm, in
            situ, by site
        unspecified site D05.1-●
      specified site NEC —see Neoplasm, in
          situ, by site
      unspecified site D05.1-●
    papillary
      with invasion
        specified site —see Neoplasm,
            malignant, by site
        unspecified site (female) C50.91-●
          male C50.92-●
      breast D05.1-●
      specified site —see Neoplasm, in situ,
          by site
      unspecified site D05.1-●
    specified site NEC —see Neoplasm, in situ,
        by site
    unspecified site D05.1-●
  islet cell
    with exocrine, mixed
      specified site —see Neoplasm,
          malignant, by site
      unspecified site C25.9
    pancreas C25.4
    specified site NEC —see Neoplasm,
        malignant, by site
    unspecified site C25.4

Adenocarcinoma (*Continued*)
lobular
in situ
breast D05.0-●
specified site NEC —*see* Neoplasm, in situ, by site
unspecified site D05.0-●
specified site —*see* Neoplasm, malignant, by site
unspecified site (female) C50.91-●
male C50.92-●
mucoid —*see also* Neoplasm, malignant, by site
cell
specified site —*see* Neoplasm, malignant, by site
unspecified site C75.1
nonencapsulated sclerosing C73
papillary
with follicular C73
follicular variant C73
intraductal (noninfiltrating)
with invasion
specified site —*see* Neoplasm, malignant, by site
unspecified site (female) C50.91-●
male C50.92-●
breast D05.1-●
specified site NEC —*see* Neoplasm, in situ, by site
unspecified site D05.1-●
serous
specified site —*see* Neoplasm, malignant, by site
unspecified site C56.9
papillocystic
specified site —*see* Neoplasm, malignant, by site
unspecified site C56.9
pseudomucinous
specified site —*see* Neoplasm, malignant, by site
unspecified site C56.9
renal cell C64-●
sebaceous —*see* Neoplasm, skin, malignant, by site
serous —*see also* Neoplasm, malignant, by site
papillary
specified site —*see* Neoplasm, malignant, by site
unspecified site C56.9
sweat gland —*see* Neoplasm, skin, malignant
water-clear cell C75.0
Adenocarcinoma-in-situ —*see also* Neoplasm, in situ, by site
breast D05.9-●
Adenofibroma
clear cell —*see* Neoplasm, benign, by site
endometrioid D27.9
borderline malignancy D39.10
malignant C56-●
mucinous
specified site —*see* Neoplasm, benign, by site
unspecified site D27.9
papillary
specified site —*see* Neoplasm, benign, by site
unspecified site D27.9
prostate —*see* Enlargement, enlarged, prostate
serous
specified site —*see* Neoplasm, benign, by site
unspecified site D27.9
specified site —*see* Neoplasm, benign, by site
unspecified site D27.9
Adenofibrosis
breast —*see* Fibroadenosis, breast
➠endometrioid N80.00

Adenoiditis (chronic) J35.02
with tonsillitis J35.03
acute J03.90
recurrent J03.91
specified organism NEC J03.80
recurrent J03.81
staphylococcal J03.80
recurrent J03.81
streptococcal J03.00
recurrent J03.01
Adenoids —*see* condition
Adenolipoma —*see* Neoplasm, benign, by site
Adenolipomatosis, Launois-Bensaude E88.89
Adenolymphoma
specified site —*see* Neoplasm, benign, by site
unspecified site D11.9
Adenoma —*see also* Neoplasm, benign, by site
acidophil
specified site —*see* Neoplasm, benign, by site
unspecified site D35.2
acidophil-basophil, mixed
specified site —*see* Neoplasm, benign, by site
unspecified site D35.2
adrenal (cortical) D35.00
clear cell D35.00
compact cell D35.00
glomerulosa cell D35.00
heavily pigmented variant D35.00
mixed cell D35.00
alpha-cell
pancreas D13.7
specified site NEC —*see* Neoplasm, benign, by site
unspecified site D13.7
alveolar D14.30
apocrine
breast D24-●
specified site NEC —*see* Neoplasm, skin, benign, by site
unspecified site D23.9
basal cell D11.9
basophil
specified site —*see* Neoplasm, benign, by site
unspecified site D35.2
basophil-acidophil, mixed
specified site —*see* Neoplasm, benign, by site
unspecified site D35.2
beta-cell
pancreas D13.7
specified site NEC —*see* Neoplasm, benign, by site
unspecified site D13.7
bile duct D13.4
common D13.5
extrahepatic D13.5
intrahepatic D13.4
specified site NEC —*see* Neoplasm, benign, by site
unspecified site D13.4
black D35.00
bronchial D38.1
cylindroid type —*see* Neoplasm, lung, malignant
ceruminous D23.2-●
chief cell D35.1
chromophobe
specified site —*see* Neoplasm, benign, by site
unspecified site D35.2
colloid
specified site —*see* Neoplasm, benign, by site
unspecified site D34
eccrine, papillary —*see* Neoplasm, skin, benign

Adenoma (*Continued*)
endocrine, multiple
single specified site —*see* Neoplasm, uncertain behavior, by site
two or more specified sites D44-●
unspecified site D44.9
endometrioid —*see also* Neoplasm, benign
borderline malignancy —*see* Neoplasm, uncertain behavior, by site
eosinophil
specified site —*see* Neoplasm, malignant, by site
unspecified site D35.2
fetal
specified site —*see* Neoplasm, benign, by site
unspecified site D34
follicular
specified site —*see* Neoplasm, benign, by site
unspecified site D34
hepatocellular D13.4
Hurthle cell D34
islet cell
pancreas D13.7
specified site NEC —*see* Neoplasm, benign, by site
unspecified site D13.7
liver cell D13.4
macrofollicular
specified site —*see* Neoplasm, benign, by site
unspecified site D34
malignant, malignum —*see* Neoplasm, malignant, by site
microcystic
pancreas D13.6
specified site NEC —*see* Neoplasm, benign, by site
unspecified site D13.6
microfollicular
specified site —*see* Neoplasm, benign, by site
unspecified site D34
mucoid cell
specified site —*see* Neoplasm, benign, by site
unspecified site D35.2
multiple endocrine
single specified site —*see* Neoplasm, uncertain behavior, by site
two or more specified sites D44-●
unspecified site D44.9
nipple D24-●
papillary —*see also* Neoplasm, benign, by site
eccrine —*see* Neoplasm, skin, benign, by site
Pick's tubular
specified site —*see* Neoplasm, benign, by site
unspecified site
female D27.9
male D29.20
pleomorphic
carcinoma in —*see* Neoplasm, salivary gland, malignant
specified site —*see* Neoplasm, malignant, by site
unspecified site C08.9
polypoid —*see also* Neoplasm, benign
adenocarcinoma in —*see* Neoplasm, malignant, by site
adenocarcinoma in situ —*see* Neoplasm, in situ, by site
prostate —*see* Neoplasm, benign, prostate
rete cell D29.20
sebaceous —*see* Neoplasm, skin, benign
Sertoli cell
specified site —*see* Neoplasm, benign, by site
unspecified site
female D27.9
male D29.20

▶ New   ➠ Revised   ~~deleted~~ Deleted   ● Use Additional Character(s)

Adenoma *(Continued)*
 skin appendage —*see* Neoplasm, skin, benign
 sudoriferous gland —*see* Neoplasm, skin, benign
 sweat gland —*see* Neoplasm, skin, benign
 testicular
  specified site —*see* Neoplasm, benign, by site
  unspecified site
   female D27.9
   male D29.20
 tubular —*see also* Neoplasm, benign, by site
  adenocarcinoma in —*see* Neoplasm, malignant, by site
  adenocarcinoma in situ —*see* Neoplasm, in situ, by site
  Pick's
   specified site —*see* Neoplasm, benign
   unspecified site
    female D27.9
    male D29.20
 tubulovillous —*see also* Neoplasm, benign, by site
  adenocarcinoma in —*see* Neoplasm, malignant, by site
  adenocarcinoma in situ —*see* Neoplasm, in situ, by site
 villous —*see* Neoplasm, uncertain behavior, by site
  adenocarcinoma in —*see* Neoplasm, malignant, by site
  adenocarcinoma in situ —*see* Neoplasm, in situ, by site
 water-clear cell D35.1
Adenomatosis
 endocrine (multiple) E31.20
  single specified site —*see* Neoplasm, uncertain behavior, by site
 erosive of nipple D24-●
 pluriendocrine —*see* Adenomatosis, endocrine
 pulmonary D38.1
  malignant —*see* Neoplasm, lung, malignant
 specified site —*see* Neoplasm, benign, by site
 unspecified site D12.6
Adenomatous
 goiter (nontoxic) E04.9
  with hyperthyroidism —*see* Hyperthyroidism, with, goiter, nodular
  toxic —*see* Hyperthyroidism, with, goiter, nodular
Adenomyoma —*see also* Neoplasm, benign, by site
 prostate —*see* Enlarged, prostate
➡**Adenomyometritis** N80.00
➡**Adenomyosis** (uterus) N80.03
Adenopathy (lymph gland) R59.9
 generalized R59.1
 inguinal R59.0
 localized R59.0
 mediastinal R59.0
 mesentery R59.0
 syphilitic (secondary) A51.49
 tracheobronchial R59.0
  tuberculous A15.4
   primary (progressive) A15.7
 tuberculous —*see also* Tuberculosis, lymph gland
  tracheobronchial A15.4
   primary (progressive) A15.7
Adenosalpingitis —*see* Salpingitis
Adenosarcoma —*see* Neoplasm, malignant, by site
Adenosclerosis I88.8
Adenosis (sclerosing) breast —*see* Fibroadenosis, breast
Adenovirus, as cause of disease classified elsewhere B97.0
Adentia (complete) (partial) —*see* Absence, teeth

Adherent —*see also* Adhesions
 labia (minora) N90.89
 pericardium (nonrheumatic) I31.0
  rheumatic I09.2
 placenta (with hemorrhage) O72.0
  without hemorrhage O73.0
 prepuce, newborn N47.0
 scar (skin) L90.5
 tendon in scar L90.5
Adhesions, adhesive (postinfective) K66.0
 with intestinal obstruction K56.50
  complete K56.52
  incomplete K56.51
  partial K56.51
 abdominal (wall) —*see* Adhesions, peritoneum
 appendix K38.8
 bile duct (common) (hepatic) K83.8
 bladder (sphincter) N32.89
 bowel —*see* Adhesions, peritoneum
 cardiac I31.0
  rheumatic I09.2
 cecum —*see* Adhesions, peritoneum
 cervicovaginal N88.1
  congenital Q52.8
  postpartal O90.89
   old N88.1
 cervix N88.1
 ciliary body NEC —*see* Adhesions, iris
 clitoris N90.89
 colon —*see* Adhesions, peritoneum
 common duct K83.8
 congenital —*see also* Anomaly, by site
  fingers —*see* Syndactylism, complex, fingers
  omental, anomalous Q43.3
  peritoneal Q43.3
  tongue (to gum or roof of mouth) Q38.3
 conjunctiva (acquired) H11.21-●
  congenital Q15.8
 cystic duct K82.8
 diaphragm —*see* Adhesions, peritoneum
 due to foreign body —*see* Foreign body
 duodenum —*see* Adhesions, peritoneum
 ear
  middle H74.1-●
 epididymis N50.89
 epidural —*see* Adhesions, meninges
 epiglottis J38.7
 eyelid H02.59
 female pelvis N73.6
 gallbladder K82.8
 globe H44.89
 heart I31.0
  rheumatic I09.2
 ileocecal (coil) —*see* Adhesions, peritoneum
 ileum —*see* Adhesions, peritoneum
 intestine —*see also* Adhesions, peritoneum
  with obstruction K56.50
   complete K56.52
   incomplete K56.51
   partial K56.51
 intra-abdominal —*see* Adhesions, peritoneum
 iris H21.50-●
  anterior H21.51-●
  goniosynechiae H21.52-●
  posterior H21.54-●
  to corneal graft T85.898
 joint —*see* Ankylosis
  knee M23.8X
  temporomandibular M26.61-●
 labium (majus) (minus), congenital Q52.5
 liver —*see* Adhesions, peritoneum
 lung J98.4
 mediastinum J98.59
 meninges (cerebral) (spinal) G96.12
  congenital Q07.8
  tuberculous (cerebral) (spinal) A17.0
 mesenteric —*see* Adhesions, peritoneum
 nasal (septum) (to turbinates) J34.89
 ocular muscle —*see* Strabismus, mechanical
 omentum —*see* Adhesions, peritoneum

Adhesions, adhesive *(Continued)*
 ovary N73.6
  congenital (to cecum, kidney or omentum) Q50.39
 paraovarian N73.6
 pelvic (peritoneal)
  female N73.6
   postprocedural N99.4
  male —*see* Adhesions, peritoneum
  postpartal (old) N73.6
  tuberculous A18.17
 penis to scrotum (congenital) Q55.8
 periappendiceal —*see also* Adhesions, peritoneum
 pericardium (nonrheumatic) I31.0
  focal I31.8
  rheumatic I09.2
  tuberculous A18.84
 pericholecystic K82.8
 perigastric —*see* Adhesions, peritoneum
 periovarian N73.6
 periprostatic N42.89
 perirectal —*see* Adhesions, peritoneum
 perirenal N28.89
 peritoneum, peritoneal (postinfective) K66.0
  with obstruction (intestinal) K56.50
   complete K56.52
   incomplete K56.51
   partial K56.51
  congenital Q43.3
  pelvic, female N73.6
   postprocedural N99.4
  postpartal, pelvic N73.6
  postprocedural K66.0
  to uterus N73.6
 peritubal N73.6
 periureteral N28.89
 periuterine N73.6
 perivesical N32.89
 perivesicular (seminal vesicle) N50.89
 pleura, pleuritic J94.8
  tuberculous NEC A15.6
 pleuropericardial J94.8
 postoperative (gastrointestinal tract) K66.0
  with obstruction —*see also* Obstruction, intestine, postoperative K91.30
  due to foreign body accidentally left in wound —*see* Foreign body, accidentally left during a procedure
  pelvic peritoneal N99.4
  urethra —*see* Stricture, urethra, postprocedural
  vagina N99.2
 postpartal, old (vulva or perineum) N90.89
 preputial, prepuce N47.5
 pulmonary J98.4
 pylorus —*see* Adhesions, peritoneum
 sciatic nerve —*see* Lesion, nerve, sciatic
 seminal vesicle N50.89
 shoulder (joint) —*see* Capsulitis, adhesive
 sigmoid flexure —*see* Adhesions, peritoneum
 spermatic cord (acquired) N50.89
  congenital Q55.4
 spinal canal G96.12
 stomach —*see* Adhesions, peritoneum
 subscapular —*see* Capsulitis, adhesive
 temporomandibular M26.61-●
 tendinitis —*see also* Tenosynovitis, specified type NEC
  shoulder —*see* Capsulitis, adhesive
 testis N44.8
 tongue, congenital (to gum or roof of mouth) Q38.3
  acquired K14.8
 trachea J39.8
 tubo-ovarian N73.6
 tunica vaginalis N44.8
 uterus N73.6
  internal N85.6
  to abdominal wall N73.6

Adhesions, adhesive (*Continued*)
  vagina (chronic) N89.5
    postoperative N99.2
  vitreomacular H43.82-●
  vitreous H43.89
  vulva N90.89
Adiaspiromycosis B48.8
Adie (-Holmes) pupil or syndrome —*see*
    Anomaly, pupil, function, tonic pupil
Adiponecrosis neonatorum P83.88
Adiposis —*see also* Obesity
  cerebralis E23.6
  dolorosa E88.2
Adiposity —*see also* Obesity
  heart —*see* Degeneration, myocardial
  localized E65
Adiposogenital dystrophy E23.6
Adjustment
  disorder —*see* Disorder, adjustment
  implanted device —*see* Encounter (for),
    adjustment (of)
  prosthesis, external —*see* Fitting
  reaction —*see* Disorder, adjustment
Administration of tPA (rtPA) in a different
    facility within the last 24 hours prior to
    admission to current facility Z92.82
Admission (for) —*see also* Encounter (for)
  adjustment (of)
    artificial
      arm Z44.00-●
        complete Z44.01-●
        partial Z44.02-●
      eye Z44.2
      leg Z44.10-●
        complete Z44.11-●
        partial Z44.12-●
    brain neuropacemaker Z46.2
      implanted Z45.42
    breast
      implant Z45.81
      prosthesis (external) Z44.3
    colostomy belt Z46.89
    contact lenses Z46.0
    cystostomy device Z46.6
    dental prosthesis Z46.3
    device NEC
      abdominal Z46.89
      implanted Z45.89
        cardiac Z45.09
          defibrillator (with synchronous
              cardiac pacemaker) Z45.02
          pacemaker (cardiac
              resynchronization therapy
              (CRT-P)) Z45.018
            pulse generator Z45.010
          resynchronization therapy
              defibrillator (CRT-D) Z45.02
        hearing device Z45.328
          bone conduction Z45.320
          cochlear Z45.321
        infusion pump Z45.1
        nervous system Z45.49
          CSF drainage Z45.41
          hearing device —*see* Admission,
              adjustment, device, implanted,
              hearing device
          neuropacemaker Z45.42
          visual substitution Z45.31
        specified NEC Z45.89
        vascular access Z45.2
        visual substitution Z45.31
      nervous system Z46.2
        implanted —*see* Admission,
            adjustment, device, implanted,
            nervous system
      orthodontic Z46.4
      prosthetic Z44.9
        arm —*see* Admission, adjustment,
            artificial, arm
        breast Z44.3
        dental Z46.3

Admission (*Continued*)
  adjustment (*Continued*)
    device NEC (*Continued*)
      prosthetic (*Continued*)
        eye Z44.2
        leg —*see* Admission, adjustment,
            artificial, leg
        specified type NEC Z44.8
      substitution
        auditory Z46.2
          implanted —*see* Admission,
              adjustment, device, implanted,
              hearing device
        nervous system Z46.2
          implanted —*see* Admission,
              adjustment, device, implanted,
              nervous system
        visual Z46.2
          implanted Z45.31
      urinary Z46.6
    hearing aid Z46.1
      implanted —*see* Admission, adjustment,
          device, implanted, hearing device
    ileostomy device Z46.89
    intestinal appliance or device NEC Z46.89
    neuropacemaker (brain) (peripheral nerve)
        (spinal cord) Z46.2
      implanted Z45.42
    orthodontic device Z46.4
    orthopedic (brace) (cast) (device) (shoes)
        Z46.89
    pacemaker (cardiac resynchronization
        therapy (CRT-P))
      cardiac Z45.018
        pulse generator Z45.010
      nervous system Z46.2
        implanted Z45.42
    portacath (port-a-cath) Z45.2
    prosthesis Z44.9
      arm —*see* Admission, adjustment,
          artificial, arm
      breast Z44.3
      dental Z46.3
      eye Z44.2
      leg —*see* Admission, adjustment,
          artificial, leg
      specified NEC Z44.8
    spectacles Z46.0
  aftercare (*see also* Aftercare) Z51.89
    postpartum
      immediately after delivery Z39.0
      routine follow-up Z39.2
    radiation therapy (antineoplastic) Z51.0
  attention to artificial opening (of) Z43.9
    artificial vagina Z43.7
    colostomy Z43.3
    cystostomy Z43.5
    enterostomy Z43.4
    gastrostomy Z43.1
    ileostomy Z43.2
    jejunostomy Z43.4
    nephrostomy Z43.6
    specified site NEC Z43.8
      intestinal tract Z43.4
      urinary tract Z43.6
    tracheostomy Z43.0
    ureterostomy Z43.6
    urethrostomy Z43.6
  breast augmentation or reduction Z41.1
  breast reconstruction following mastectomy
      Z42.1
  change of
    dressing (nonsurgical) Z48.00
    neuropacemaker device (brain) (peripheral
        nerve) (spinal cord) Z46.2
      implanted Z45.42
    surgical dressing Z48.01
  circumcision, ritual or routine (in absence of
      diagnosis) Z41.2
  clinical research investigation (control)
      (normal comparison) (participant) Z00.6

Admission (*Continued*)
  contraceptive management Z30.9
  cosmetic surgery NEC Z41.1
  counseling (*see also* Counseling)
    dietary Z71.3
    gestational carrier Z31.7
    HIV Z71.7
    human immunodeficiency virus Z71.7
    nonattending third party Z71.0
    procreative management NEC Z31.69
  delivery, full-term, uncomplicated O80
    cesarean, without indication O82
  desensitization to allergens Z51.6
  dietary surveillance and counseling Z71.3
  ear piercing Z41.3
  examination at health care facility (adult) —
      see also Examination Z00.00
    with abnormal findings Z00.01
    clinical research investigation (control)
        (normal comparison) (participant)
        Z00.6
    dental Z01.20
      with abnormal findings Z01.21
    donor (potential) Z00.5
    ear Z01.10
      with abnormal findings NEC Z01.118
        following failed vision screening
            Z01.020
          with abnormal findings Z01.021
    eye Z01.00
      with abnormal findings Z01.01
    general, specified reason NEC Z00.8
    hearing Z01.10
      with abnormal findings NEC Z01.118
      infant or child (over 28 days old) Z00.129
        with abnormal findings Z00.121
    postpartum checkup Z39.2
    psychiatric (general) Z00.8
      requested by authority Z04.6
    vision Z01.00
      with abnormal findings Z01.01
        following failed vision screening
            Z01.020
          with abnormal findings Z01.021
      infant or child (over 28 days old) Z00.129
        with abnormal findings Z00.121
  fitting (of)
    artificial
      arm —*see* Admission, adjustment,
          artificial, arm
      eye Z44.2
      leg —*see* Admission, adjustment,
          artificial, leg
    brain neuropacemaker Z46.2
      implanted Z45.42
    breast prosthesis (external) Z44.3
    colostomy belt Z46.89
    contact lenses Z46.0
    cystostomy device Z46.6
    dental prosthesis Z46.3
    dentures Z46.3
    device NEC
      abdominal Z46.89
      nervous system Z46.2
        implanted —*see* Admission,
            adjustment, device, implanted,
            nervous system
      orthodontic Z46.4
      prosthetic Z44.9
        breast Z44.3
        dental Z46.3
        eye Z44.2
      substitution
        auditory Z46.2
          implanted —*see* Admission,
              adjustment, device, implanted,
              hearing device
        nervous system Z46.2
          implanted —*see* Admission,
              adjustment, device, implanted,
              nervous system

Admission *(Continued)*
  fitting (of) *(Continued)*
    device NEC *(Continued)*
      substitution *(Continued)*
        visual Z46.2
          implanted Z45.31
    hearing aid Z46.1
    ileostomy device Z46.89
    intestinal appliance or device NEC
        Z46.89
    neuropacemaker (brain) (peripheral nerve)
        (spinal cord) Z46.2
      implanted Z45.42
    orthodontic device Z46.4
    orthopedic device (brace) (cast) (shoes)
        Z46.89
    prosthesis Z44.9
      arm —*see* Admission, adjustment,
          artificial, arm
      breast Z44.3
      dental Z46.3
      eye Z44.2
      leg —*see* Admission, adjustment,
          artificial, leg
      specified type NEC Z44.8
    spectacles Z46.0
  follow-up examination Z09
  intrauterine device management Z30.431
    initial prescription Z30.014
  mental health evaluation Z00.8
    requested by authority Z04.6
  observation —*see* Observation
  Papanicolaou smear, cervix Z12.4
    for suspected malignant neoplasm
        Z12.4
  plastic and reconstructive surgery following
      medical procedure or healed injury NEC
      Z42.8
  plastic surgery, cosmetic NEC Z41.1
  postpartum observation
    immediately after delivery Z39.0
    routine follow-up Z39.2
  poststerilization (for restoration) Z31.0
    aftercare Z31.42
  procreative management Z31.9
  prophylactic (measure) —*see also* Encounter,
      prophylactic measures
    organ removal Z40.00
      breast Z40.01
      fallopian tube(s) Z40.03
        with ovary(s) Z40.02
      ovary(s) Z40.02
      specified organ NEC Z40.09
      testes Z40.09
    vaccination Z23
  psychiatric examination (general) Z00.8
    requested by authority Z04.6
  radiation therapy (antineoplastic) Z51.0
  reconstructive surgery following medical
      procedure or healed injury NEC Z42.8
  removal of
    cystostomy catheter Z43.5
    drains Z48.03
    dressing (nonsurgical) Z48.00
    implantable subdermal contraceptive Z30.46
    intrauterine contraceptive device Z30.432
    neuropacemaker (brain) (peripheral nerve)
        (spinal cord) Z46.2
      implanted Z45.42
    staples Z48.02
    surgical dressing Z48.01
    sutures Z48.02
    ureteral stent Z46.6
  respirator [ventilator] use during power
      failure Z99.12
  restoration of organ continuity
      (poststerilization) Z31.0
    aftercare Z31.42
  sensitivity test —*see also* Test, skin
    allergy NEC Z01.82
    Mantoux Z11.1

Admission *(Continued)*
  tuboplasty following previous sterilization
      Z31.0
    aftercare Z31.42
  vasoplasty following previous sterilization
      Z31.0
    aftercare Z31.42
  vision examination Z01.00
    with abnormal findings Z01.01
      following failed vision screening
          Z01.020
        with abnormal findings Z01.021
    infant or child (over 28 days old) Z00.129
      with abnormal findings Z00.121
  waiting period for admission to other facility
      Z75.1
Adnexitis (suppurative) —*see*
    Salpingo-oophoritis
Adolescent X-linked adrenoleukodystrophy
    E71.521
Adrenal (gland) —*see* condition
Adrenalism, tuberculous A18.7
Adrenalitis, adrenitis E27.8
  autoimmune E27.1
  meningococcal, hemorrhagic A39.1
Adrenarche, premature E27.0
Adrenocortical syndrome —*see* Cushing's,
    syndrome
Adrenogenital syndrome E25.9
  acquired E25.8
  congenital E25.0
  salt loss E25.0
Adrenogenitalism, congenital E25.0
Adrenoleukodystrophy E71.529
  neonatal E71.511
  X-linked E71.529
    Addison only phenotype E71.528
    Addison-Schilder E71.528
    adolescent E71.521
    adrenomyeloneuropathy E71.522
    childhood cerebral E71.520
    other specified E71.528
Adrenomyeloneuropathy E71.522
Adventitious bursa —*see* Bursopathy, specified
    type NEC
Adverse effect —*see* Table of Drugs and
    Chemicals, categories T36-T50, with 6th
    character 5
Advice —*see* Counseling
Adynamia (episodica) (hereditary) (periodic)
    G72.3
Aeration lung imperfect, newborn —*see*
    Atelectasis
Aerobullosis T70.3
Aerocele —*see* Embolism, air
Aerodermectasia
  subcutaneous (traumatic) T79.7
Aerodontalgia T70.29
Aeroembolism T70.3
Aerogenes capsulatus infection A48.0
Aero-otitis media T70.0
Aerophagy, aerophagia (psychogenic) F45.8
Aerophobia F40.228
Aerosinusitis T70.1
Aerotitis T70.0
Affection —*see* Disease
Afibrinogenemia —*see also* Defect, coagulation
    D68.8
  acquired D65
  congenital D68.2
  following ectopic or molar pregnancy
      O08.1
  in abortion —*see* Abortion, by type,
      complicated by, afibrinogenemia
  puerperal O72.3
African
  sleeping sickness B56.9
  tick fever A68.1
  trypanosomiasis B56.9
    gambian B56.0
    rhodesian B56.1

Aftercare —*see also* Care Z51.89
  following surgery (for) (on)
    amputation Z47.81
    attention to
      drains Z48.03
      dressings (nonsurgical) Z48.00
        surgical Z48.01
      sutures Z48.02
    circulatory system Z48.812
    delayed (planned) wound closure Z48.1
    digestive system Z48.815
    explantation of joint prosthesis (staged
        procedure)
      hip Z47.32
      knee Z47.33
      shoulder Z47.31
    genitourinary system Z48.816
    joint replacement Z47.1
    neoplasm Z48.3
    nervous system Z48.811
    oral cavity Z48.814
    organ transplant
      bone marrow Z48.290
      heart Z48.21
      heart-lung Z48.280
      kidney Z48.22
      liver Z48.23
      lung Z48.24
      multiple organs NEC Z48.288
      specified NEC Z48.298
    orthopedic NEC Z47.89
    planned wound closure Z48.1
    removal of internal fixation device Z47.2
    respiratory system Z48.813
    scoliosis Z47.82
    sense organs Z48.810
    skin and subcutaneous tissue Z48.817
    specified body system
      circulatory Z48.812
      digestive Z48.815
      genitourinary Z48.816
      nervous Z48.811
      oral cavity Z48.814
      respiratory Z48.813
      sense organs Z48.810
      skin and subcutaneous tissue Z48.817
      teeth Z48.814
    specified NEC Z48.89
    spinal Z47.89
    teeth Z48.814
  fracture — code to fracture with seventh
      character D
  involving
    removal of
      drains Z48.03
      dressings (nonsurgical) Z48.00
      staples Z48.02
      surgical dressings Z48.01
      sutures Z48.02
  neuropacemaker (brain) (peripheral nerve)
      (spinal cord) Z46.2
    implanted Z45.42
  orthopedic NEC Z47.89
  postprocedural —*see* Aftercare, following
      surgery
After-cataract —*see* Cataract, secondary
Agalactia (primary) O92.3
  elective, secondary or therapeutic O92.5
Agammaglobulinemia (acquired (secondary))
    (nonfamilial) D80.1
  with
    immunoglobulin-bearing B-lymphocytes
        D80.1
    lymphopenia D81.9
  autosomal recessive (Swiss type) D80.0
  Bruton's X-linked D80.0
  common variable (CVAgamma) D80.1
  congenital sex-linked D80.0
  hereditary D80.0
  lymphopenic D81.9
  Swiss type (autosomal recessive) D80.0

Agammaglobulinemia (Continued)
  X-linked (with growth hormone deficiency)
      (Bruton) D80.0
Aganglionosis (bowel) (colon) Q43.1
Age (old) —see Senility
Agenesis
  adrenal (gland) Q89.1
  alimentary tract (complete) (partial) NEC
      Q45.8
    upper Q40.8
  anus, anal (canal) Q42.3
    with fistula Q42.2
  aorta Q25.41
  appendix Q42.8
  arm (complete) Q71.0-●
    with hand present Q71.1-●
  artery (peripheral) Q27.9
    brain Q28.3
    coronary Q24.5
    pulmonary Q25.79
    specified NEC Q27.8
    umbilical Q27.0
  auditory (canal) (external) Q16.1
  auricle (ear) Q16.0
  bile duct or passage Q44.5
  bladder Q64.5
  bone Q79.9
  brain Q00.0
    part of Q04.3
  breast (with nipple present) Q83.8
    with absent nipple Q83.0
  bronchus Q32.4
  canaliculus lacrimalis Q10.4
  carpus —see Agenesis, hand
  cartilage Q79.9
  cecum Q42.8
  cerebellum Q04.3
  cervix Q51.5
  chin Q18.8
  cilia Q10.3
  circulatory system, part NOS Q28.9
  clavicle Q74.0
  clitoris Q52.6
  coccyx Q76.49
  colon Q42.9
    specified NEC Q42.8
  corpus callosum Q04.0
  cricoid cartilage Q31.8
  diaphragm (with hernia) Q79.1
  digestive organ(s) or tract (complete) (partial)
      NEC Q45.8
    upper Q40.8
  ductus arteriosus Q28.8
  duodenum Q41.0
  ear Q16.9
    auricle Q16.0
    lobe Q17.8
  ejaculatory duct Q55.4
  endocrine (gland) NEC Q89.2
  epiglottis Q31.8
  esophagus Q39.8
  eustachian tube Q16.2
  eye Q11.1
    adnexa Q15.8
  eyelid (fold) Q10.3
  face
    bones NEC Q75.8
    specified part NEC Q18.8
  fallopian tube Q50.6
  femur —see Defect, reduction, lower limb,
      longitudinal, femur
  fibula —see Defect, reduction, lower limb,
      longitudinal, fibula
  finger (complete) (partial) —see Agenesis,
      hand
  foot (and toes) (complete) (partial) Q72.3-●
  forearm (with hand present) —see Agenesis,
      arm, with hand present
    and hand Q71.2-●
  gallbladder Q44.0
  gastric Q40.2

Agenesis (Continued)
  genitalia, genital (organ(s))
    female Q52.8
      external Q52.71
      internal NEC Q52.8
    male Q55.8
  glottis Q31.8
  hair Q84.0
  hand (and fingers) (complete) (partial) Q71.3-●
  heart Q24.8
    valve NEC Q24.8
      pulmonary Q22.0
  hepatic Q44.7
  humerus —see Defect, reduction, upper limb
  hymen Q52.4
  ileum Q41.2
  incus Q16.3
  intestine (small) Q41.9
    large Q42.9
      specified NEC Q42.8
  iris (dilator fibers) Q13.1
  jaw M26.09
  jejunum Q41.1
  kidney(s) (partial) Q60.2
    bilateral Q60.1
    unilateral Q60.0
  labium (majus) (minus) Q52.71
  labyrinth, membranous Q16.5
  lacrimal apparatus Q10.4
  larynx Q31.8
  leg (complete) Q72.0-●
    with foot present Q72.1-●
    lower leg (with foot present) —see
        Agenesis, leg, with foot present
      and foot Q72.2-●
  lens Q12.3
  limb (complete) Q73.0
    lower —see Agenesis, leg
    upper —see Agenesis, arm
  lip Q38.0
  liver Q44.7
  lung (fissure) (lobe) (bilateral) (unilateral)
      Q33.3
  mandible, maxilla M26.09
  metacarpus —see Agenesis, hand
  metatarsus —see Agenesis, foot
  muscle Q79.8
    eyelid Q10.3
    ocular Q15.8
  musculoskeletal system NEC Q79.8
  nail(s) Q84.3
  neck, part Q18.8
  nerve Q07.8
  nervous system, part NEC Q07.8
  nipple Q83.2
  nose Q30.1
  nuclear Q07.8
  organ
    of Corti Q16.5
    or site not listed —see Anomaly, by site
  osseous meatus (ear) Q16.1
  ovary
    bilateral Q50.02
    unilateral Q50.01
  oviduct Q50.6
  pancreas Q45.0
  parathyroid (gland) Q89.2
  parotid gland(s) Q38.4
  patella Q74.1
  pelvic girdle (complete) (partial) Q74.2
  penis Q55.5
  pericardium Q24.8
  pituitary (gland) Q89.2
  prostate Q55.4
  punctum lacrimale Q10.4
  radioulnar —see Defect, reduction, upper
      limb
  radius —see Defect, reduction, upper limb,
      longitudinal, radius
  rectum Q42.1
    with fistula Q42.0

Agenesis (Continued)
  renal Q60.2
    bilateral Q60.1
    unilateral Q60.0
  respiratory organ NEC Q34.8
  rib Q76.6
  roof of orbit Q75.8
  round ligament Q52.8
  sacrum Q76.49
  salivary gland Q38.4
  scapula Q74.0
  scrotum Q55.29
  seminal vesicles Q55.4
  septum
    atrial Q21.19
      between aorta and pulmonary artery
          Q21.4
    ventricular Q20.4
  shoulder girdle (complete) (partial)
      Q74.0
  skull (bone) Q75.8
    with
      anencephaly Q00.0
      encephalocele —see Encephalocele
      hydrocephalus Q03.9
        with spina bifida —see Spina bifida, by
            site, with hydrocephalus
      microcephaly Q02
  spermatic cord Q55.4
  spinal cord Q06.0
  spine Q76.49
  spleen Q89.01
  sternum Q76.7
  stomach Q40.2
  submaxillary gland(s) (congenital) Q38.4
  tarsus —see Agenesis, foot
  tendon Q79.8
  testicle Q55.0
  thymus (gland) Q89.2
  thyroid (gland) E03.1
    cartilage Q31.8
  tibia —see Defect, reduction, lower limb,
      longitudinal, tibia
  tibiofibular —see Defect, reduction, lower
      limb, specified type NEC
  toe (and foot) (complete) (partial) —see
      Agenesis, foot
  tongue Q38.3
  trachea (cartilage) Q32.1
  ulna —see Defect, reduction, upper limb,
      longitudinal, ulna
  upper limb —see Agenesis, arm
  ureter Q62.4
  urethra Q64.5
  urinary tract NEC Q64.8
  uterus Q51.0
  uvula Q38.5
  vagina Q52.0
  vas deferens Q55.4
  vein(s) (peripheral) Q27.9
    brain Q28.3
    great NEC Q26.8
    portal Q26.5
  vena cava (inferior) (superior) Q26.8
  vermis of cerebellum Q04.3
  vertebra Q76.49
  vulva Q52.71
Ageusia R43.2
Agitated —see condition
Agitation R45.1
Aglossia (congenital) Q38.3
Aglossia-adactylia syndrome Q87.0
Aglycogenosis E74.00
Agnosia (body image) (other senses) (tactile)
    R48.1
  developmental F88
  verbal R48.1
    auditory R48.1
      developmental F80.2
  developmental F80.2
  visual (object) R48.3

▶ New   ⇒ Revised   ~~deleted~~ Deleted   ● Use Additional Character(s)

Agoraphobia F40.00
  with panic disorder F40.01
  without panic disorder F40.02
Agrammatism R48.8
Agranulocytopenia —see Agranulocytosis
Agranulocytosis (chronic) (cyclical) (genetic)
    (infantile) (periodic) (pernicious) (see also
    Neutropenia) D70.9
  congenital D70.0
  cytoreductive cancer chemotherapy sequela
    D70.1
  drug-induced D70.2
    due to cytoreductive cancer chemotherapy
      D70.1
  due to infection D70.3
  secondary D70.4
    drug-induced D70.2
      due to cytoreductive cancer
        chemotherapy D70.1
Agraphia (absolute) R48.8
  with alexia R48.0
  developmental F81.81
Ague (dumb) —see Malaria
Agyria Q04.3
Ahumada-del Castillo syndrome E23.0
Aichmophobia F40.298
AIDS (related complex) B20
Ailment heart —see Disease, heart
Ailurophobia F40.218
Ainhum (disease) L94.6
AIN —see Neoplasia, intraepithelial, anal
AIPHI (acute idiopathic pulmonary hemorrhage
    in infants (over 28 days old)) R04.81
Air
  anterior mediastinum J98.2
  compressed, disease T70.3
  conditioner lung or pneumonitis J67.7
  embolism (artery) (cerebral) (any site)
    T79.0
    with ectopic or molar pregnancy O08.2
    due to implanted device NEC —see
      Complications, by site and type,
      specified NEC
    following
      abortion —see Abortion by type,
        complicated by, embolism
      ectopic or molar pregnancy O08.2
    infusion, therapeutic injection or
      transfusion T80.0
    in pregnancy, childbirth or puerperium —
      see Embolism, obstetric
    traumatic T79.0
  hunger, psychogenic F45.8
  rarefied, effects of —see Effect, adverse, high
    altitude
  sickness T75.3
Airplane sickness T75.3
Akathisia (drug-induced) (treatment- induced)
    G25.71
  neuroleptic induced (acute) G25.71
  tardive G25.71
Akinesia R29.898
Akinetic mutism R41.89
Akureyri's disease G93.39
Alactasia, congenital E73.0
Alagille's syndrome Q44.7
Alastrim B03
Albers-Schönberg syndrome Q78.2
Albert's syndrome —see Tendinitis,
    Achilles
Albinism, albino E70.30
  with hematologic abnormality E70.339
    Chédiak-Higashi syndrome E70.330
    Hermansky-Pudlak syndrome E70.331
    other specified E70.338
    I E70.320
    II E70.321
  ocular E70.319
    autosomal recessive E70.311
    other specified E70.318
    X-linked E70.310

Albinism, albino (Continued)
  oculocutaneous E70.329
    other specified E70.328
    tyrosinase (ty) negative E70.320
    tyrosinase (ty) positive E70.321
  other specified E70.39
Albinismus E70.30
Albright (-McCune)(-Sternberg) syndrome
    Q78.1
Albuminous —see condition
Albuminuria, albuminuric (acute) (chronic)
    (subacute) —see also Proteinuria R80.9
  complicating pregnancy —see Proteinuria,
    gestational
    with
      gestational hypertension —see
        Pre-eclampsia
      pre-existing hypertension —see
        Hypertension, complicating
        pregnancy, pre-existing, with,
        pre-eclampsia
  gestational —see Proteinuria, gestational
    with
      gestational hypertension —see
        Pre-eclampsia
      pre-existing hypertension —see
        Hypertension, complicating
        pregnancy, pre-existing, with,
        pre-eclampsia
  orthostatic R80.2
  postural R80.2
  pre-eclamptic —see Pre-eclampsia
  scarlatinal A38.8
Albuminurophobia F40.298
Alcaptonuria E70.29
Alcohol, alcoholic, alcohol-induced
  addiction (without remission) F10.20
    with remission F10.21
  amnestic disorder, persisting F10.96
    with dependence F10.26
  anxiety disorder F10.980
  bipolar and related disorder F10.94
  brain syndrome, chronic F10.97
    with dependence F10.27
  cardiopathy I42.6
  counseling and surveillance Z71.41
    family member Z71.42
  delirium (acute) (tremens) (withdrawal)
    F10.921
    with intoxication F10.921
    in
      abuse F10.121
      dependence F10.221
  dementia F10.97
    with dependence F10.27
  dependence (acute) (tremens) (withdrawal)
    F10.231
  depressive disorder F10.94
  deterioration F10.97
    with dependence F10.27
  hallucinosis (acute) F10.951
    in
      abuse F10.151
      dependence F10.251
  insanity F10.959
  intoxication (acute) (without dependence)
    F10.129
    with
      delirium F10.121
      dependence F10.229
        with delirium F10.221
        uncomplicated F10.220
      uncomplicated F10.120
  jealousy F10.988
  Korsakoff's, Korsakov's, Korsakow's F10.26
  liver K70.9
    acute —see Disease, liver, alcoholic,
      hepatitis
  major neurocognitive disorder, amnestic-
    confabulatory type F10.96
  major neurocognitive disorder, nonamnestic-
    confabulatory type F10.97

Alcohol, alcoholic, alcohol-induced (Continued)
  mania (acute) (chronic) F10.959
  mild neurocognitive disorder F10.988
  paranoia, paranoid (type) psychosis F10.950
  pellagra E52
  poisoning, accidental (acute) NEC —see
      Table of Drugs and Chemicals, alcohol,
      poisoning
  psychosis —see Psychosis, alcoholic
  psychotic disorder F10.959
  sexual dysfunction F10.981
  sleep disorder F10.982
  withdrawal (without convulsions) F10.239
    with delirium F10.231
Alcoholism (chronic) (without remission) F10.20
  with
    psychosis —see Psychosis, alcoholic
    remission F10.21
  Korsakov's F10.96
    with dependence F10.26
Alder (-Reilly) anomaly or syndrome
    (leukocyte granulation) D72.0
Aldosteronism E26.9
  familial (type I) E26.02
  glucocorticoid-remediable E26.02
  primary (due to (bilateral) adrenal
    hyperplasia) E26.09
  primary NEC E26.09
  secondary E26.1
  specified NEC E26.89
Aldosteronoma D44.10
Aldrich(-Wiskott) syndrome (eczema-
    thrombocytopenia) D82.0
Alektorophobia F40.218
Aleppo boil B55.1
Aleukemic —see condition Aleukia
  congenital D70.0
  hemorrhagica D61.9
    congenital D61.09
  splenica D73.1
Alexia R48.0
  developmental F81.0
  secondary to organic lesion R48.0
Algoneurodystrophy M89.00
  ankle M89.07-●
  foot M89.07-●
  forearm M89.03-●
  hand M89.04-●
  lower leg M89.06-●
  multiple sites M89.0-●
  shoulder M89.01-●
  specified site NEC M89.08
  thigh M89.05-●
  upper arm M89.02-●
Algophobia F40.298
Alienation, mental —see Psychosis
Alkalemia E87.3
Alkalosis E87.3
  metabolic E87.3
    with respiratory acidosis E87.4
  of newborn P74.41
  respiratory E87.3
Alkaptonuria E70.29
Allen-Masters syndrome N83.8
Allergy, allergic (reaction) (to) T78.40
  air-borne substance NEC (rhinitis) J30.89
  alveolitis (extrinsic) J67.9
    due to
      Aspergillus clavatus J67.4
      Cryptostroma corticale J67.6
      organisms (fungal, thermophilic
        actinomycete) growing in
        ventilation (air conditioning)
        systems J67.7
    specified type NEC J67.8
  anaphylactic reaction or shock T78.2
  angioneurotic edema T78.3
  animal (dander) (epidermal) (hair) (rhinitis)
    J30.81
  bee sting (anaphylactic shock) —see Toxicity,
    venom, arthropod, bee

Allergy, allergic *(Continued)*
  biological —*see* Allergy, drug
  colitis —*see also* Colitis, allergic K52.29
  dander (animal) (rhinitis) J30.81
  dandruff (rhinitis) J30.81
  dental restorative material (existing) K08.55
  dermatitis —*see* Dermatitis, contact, allergic
  diathesis —*see* History, allergy
  drug, medicament & biological (any)
    (external) (internal) T78.40
    correct substance properly administered —
      see Table of Drugs and Chemicals, by
      drug, adverse effect
    wrong substance given or taken NEC (by
      accident) —*see* Table of Drugs and
      Chemicals, by drug, poisoning
  due to pollen J30.1
  dust (house) (stock) (rhinitis) J30.89
    with asthma —*see* Asthma, allergic extrinsic
  eczema —*see* Dermatitis, contact, allergic
  epidermal (animal) (rhinitis) J30.81
  feathers (rhinitis) J30.89
  food (any) (ingested) NEC T78.1
    anaphylactic shock —*see* Shock,
      anaphylactic, due to food
    dermatitis —*see* Dermatitis, due to, food
    dietary counseling and surveillance Z71.3
    in contact with skin L23.6
    rhinitis J30.5
    status (without reaction) Z91.018
      beef Z91.014
      eggs Z91.012
      lamb Z91.014
      mammalian meats Z91.014
      milk products Z91.011
      peanuts Z91.010
      pork Z91.014
      red meats Z91.014
      seafood Z91.013
      specified NEC Z91.018
  gastrointestinal —*see also* specific type of
    allergic reaction
    meaning colitis —*see also* Colitis, allergic)
      K52.29
    meaning gastroenteritis —*see also*
      Gastroenteritis, allergic) K52.29
    meaning other adverse food reaction not
      elsewhere classified T78.1
  grain J30.1
  grass (hay fever) (pollen) J30.1
    asthma —*see* Asthma, allergic extrinsic
  hair (animal) (rhinitis) J30.81
  history (of) —*see* History, allergy
  horse serum —*see* Allergy, serum
  inhalant (rhinitis) J30.89
    pollen J30.1
  kapok (rhinitis) J30.89
  medicine —*see* Allergy, drug
  milk protein —*see also* Allergy, food Z91.011
    anaphylactic reaction T78.07
    dermatitis L27.2
    enterocolitis syndrome K52.21
    enteropathy K52.22
    gastroenteritis K52.29
    gastroesophageal reflux —*see also* Reaction,
      adverse, food) K21.9
      with esophagitis without bleeding K21.00
        with bleeding K21.01
    proctocolitis K52.29
  nasal, seasonal due to pollen J30.1
  pneumonia J82.89
  pollen (any) (hay fever) J30.1
    asthma —*see* Asthma, allergic extrinsic
  primrose J30.1
  primula J30.1
  proctocolitis K52.29
  purpura D69.0
  ragweed (hay fever) (pollen) J30.1
    asthma —*see* Asthma, allergic extrinsic
  rose (pollen) J30.1
  seasonal NEC J30.2

Allergy, allergic *(Continued)*
  Senecio jacobae (pollen) J30.1
  serum —*see also* Reaction, serum T80.69
    anaphylactic shock T80.59
  shock (anaphylactic) T78.2
    due to
      administration of blood and blood
        products T80.51
      adverse effect of correct medicinal
        substance properly administered
        T88.6
      immunization T80.52
      serum NEC T80.59
      vaccination T80.52
    specific NEC T78.49
  tree (any) (hay fever) (pollen) J30.1
    asthma —*see* Asthma, allergic extrinsic
  upper respiratory J30.9
  urticaria L50.0
  vaccine —*see* Allergy, serum
  wheat —*see* Allergy, food
Allescheriasis B48.2
Alligator skin disease Q80.9
Allocheiria, allochiria R20.8
Almeida's disease —*see*
    Paracoccidioidomycosis
Alopecia (hereditaria) (seborrheica) L65.9
  androgenic L64.9
    drug-induced L64.0
    specified NEC L64.8
  areata L63.9
    ophiasis L63.2
    specified NEC L63.8
    totalis L63.0
    universalis L63.1
  cicatricial L66.9
    specified NEC L66.8
  circumscripta L63.9
  congenital, congenitalis Q84.0
  due to cytotoxic drugs NEC L65.8
  mucinosa L65.2
  postinfective NEC L65.8
  postpartum L65.0
  premature L64.8
  specific (syphilitic) A51.32
  specified NEC L65.8
  syphilitic (secondary) A51.32
  totalis (capitis) L63.0
  universalis (entire body) L63.1
  X-ray L58.1
Alpers' disease G31.81
Alpine sickness T70.29
Alport syndrome Q87.81
ALTE (apparent life threatening event) in
    newborn and infant R68.13
Alteration (of), Altered
  awareness
    transient R40.4
    unintended under general anesthesia,
      during procedure T88.53
  mental status R41.82
  pattern of family relationships affecting child
    Z62.898
  sensation
    following
      cerebrovascular disease I69.998
        cerebral infarction I69.398
        intracerebral hemorrhage I69.198
        nontraumatic intracranial hemorrhage
          NEC I69.298
        specified disease NEC I69.898
        subarachnoid hemorrhage I69.098
Alternating —*see* condition
Altitude, high (effects) —*see* Effect, adverse,
    high altitude
Aluminosis (of lung) J63.0
Alveolitis
  allergic (extrinsic) —*see* Pneumonitis,
    hypersensitivity
  due to
    Aspergillus clavatus J67.4
    Cryptostroma corticale J67.6

Alveolitis *(Continued)*
  fibrosing (cryptogenic) (idiopathic) J84.112
  jaw M27.3
  sicca dolorosa M27.3
Alveolus, alveolar —*see* condition
Alymphocytosis D72.810
  thymic (with immunodeficiency) D82.1
Alymphoplasia, thymic D82.1
Alzheimer's disease or sclerosis —*see* Disease,
    Alzheimer's
Amastia (with nipple present) Q83.8
  with absent nipple Q83.0
Amathophobia F40.228
Amaurosis (acquired) (congenital) —*see also*
    Blindness
  fugax G45.3
  hysterical F44.6
  Leber's congenital H35.50
  uremic —*see* Uremia
Amaurotic idiocy (infantile) (juvenile) (late)
    E75.4
Amaxophobia F40.248
Ambiguous genitalia Q56.4
Amblyopia (congenital) (ex anopsia) (partial)
    (suppression) H53.00-●
  anisometropic —*see* Amblyopia, refractive
  deprivation H53.01-●
  hysterical F44.6
  nocturnal —*see also* Blindness, night
    vitamin A deficiency E50.5
  refractive H53.02-●
  strabismic H53.03-●
  suspect H53.04-●
  tobacco H53.8
  toxic NEC H53.8
  uremic —*see* Uremia
Ameba, amebic (histolytica) —*see also* Amebiasis
  abscess (liver) A06.4
Amebiasis A06.9
  with abscess —*see* Abscess, amebic
  acute A06.0
  chronic (intestine) A06.1
    with abscess —*see* Abscess, amebic
  cutaneous A06.7
  cutis A06.7
  cystitis A06.81
  genitourinary tract NEC A06.82
  hepatic —*see* Abscess, liver, amebic
  intestine A06.0
  nondysenteric colitis A06.2
  skin A06.7
  specified site NEC A06.89
Ameboma (of intestine) A06.3
Amelia Q73.0
  lower limb —*see* Agenesis, leg
  upper limb —*see* Agenesis, arm
Ameloblastoma —*see also* Cyst, calcifying
    odontogenic
  long bones C40.9-●
    lower limb C40.2-●
    upper limb C40.0-●
  malignant C41.1
    jaw (bone) (lower) C41.1
      upper C41.0
  tibial C40.2-●
Amelogenesis imperfecta K00.5
  nonhereditaria (segmentalis) K00.4
Amenorrhea N91.2
  hyperhormonal E28.8
  primary N91.0
  secondary N91.1
Amentia —*see* Disability, intellectual
  Meynert's (nonalcoholic) F04
American
  leishmaniasis B55.2
  mountain tick fever A93.2
Ametropia —*see* Disorder, refraction
AMH (asymptomatic microscopic hematuria)
    R31.21
Amianthosis J61
Amimia R48.8

Amino-acid disorder E72.9
    anemia D53.0
Aminoacidopathy E72.9
Aminoaciduria E72.9
Amnes (t)ic syndrome (post-traumatic) F04
    induced by
        alcohol F10.96
            with dependence F10.26
        psychoactive NEC F19.96
            with
                abuse F19.16
                dependence F19.26
        sedative F13.96
            with dependence F13.26
Amnesia R41.3
    anterograde R41.1
    auditory R48.8
    dissociative F44.0
        with dissociative fugue F44.1
    hysterical F44.0
    postictal in epilepsy —see Epilepsy
    psychogenic F44.0
    retrograde R41.2
    transient global G45.4
Amnion, amniotic —see condition
Amnionitis —see Pregnancy, complicated by
Amok F68.8
Amoral traits F60.89
Amphetamine (or other stimulant) —
        induced
    anxiety disorder F15.980
    bipolar and related disorder F15.94
    delirium F15.921
    depressive disorder F15.94
    obsessive-compulsive and related disorder
        F15.988
    psychotic disorder F15.959
    sexual dysfunction F15.981
    sleep disorder F15.982
    stimulant withdrawal F15.23
Ampulla
    lower esophagus K22.89
    phrenic K22.89
Amputation —see also Absence, by site,
        acquired
    neuroma (postoperative) (traumatic) —see
            Complications, amputation stump,
            neuroma
    stump (surgical)
        abnormal, painful, or with complication
                (late) —see Complications, amputation
                stump
        healed or old NOS Z89.9
    traumatic (complete) (partial)
        arm (upper) (complete) S48.91-●
            at
                elbow S58.01-●
                    partial S58.02-●
                shoulder joint (complete) S48.01-●
                    partial S48.02-●
            between
                elbow and wrist (complete) S58.11-●
                    partial S58.12-●
                shoulder and elbow (complete)
                        S48.11-●
                    partial S48.12-●
            partial S48.92-●
        breast (complete) S28.21-●
            partial S28.22-●
        clitoris (complete) S38.211
            partial S38.212
        ear (complete) S08.11-●
            partial S08.12-●
        finger (complete) (metacarpophalangeal)
                S68.11-●
            index S68.11-●
            little S68.11-●
            middle S68.11-●
            partial S68.12-●
                index S68.12-●
                little S68.12-●

Amputation (Continued)
    traumatic (Continued)
        finger (Continued)
            partial (Continued)
                middle S68.12-●
                ring S68.12-●
            ring S68.11-●
            thumb —see Amputation, traumatic,
                thumb
            transphalangeal (complete) S68.61-●
                index S68.61-●
                little S68.61-●
                middle S68.61-●
                partial S68.62-●
                    index S68.62-●
                    little S68.62-●
                    middle S68.62-●
                    ring S68.62-●
                ring S68.61-●
        foot (complete) S98.91-●
            at ankle level S98.01-●
                partial S98.02-●
            midfoot S98.31-●
                partial S98.32-●
            partial S98.92-●
        forearm (complete) S58.91-●
            at elbow level (complete) S58.01-●
                partial S58.02-●
            between elbow and wrist (complete)
                    S58.11-●
                partial S58.12-●
            partial S58.92-●
        genital organ(s) (external)
            female (complete) S38.211
                partial S38.212
            male
                penis (complete) S38.221
                    partial S38.222
                scrotum (complete) S38.231
                    partial S38.232
                testes (complete) S38.231
                    partial S38.232
        hand (complete) (wrist level) S68.41-●
            finger(s) alone —see Amputation,
                    traumatic, finger
            partial S68.42-●
            thumb alone —see Amputation,
                    traumatic, thumb
            transmetacarpal (complete) S68.71-●
                partial S68.72-●
        head
            ear —see Amputation, traumatic, ear
            nose (partial) S08.812
                complete S08.811
            part S08.89
                scalp S08.0
        hip (and thigh) (complete) S78.91-●
            at hip joint (complete) S78.01-●
                partial S78.02-●
            between hip and knee (complete)
                    S78.11-●
                partial S78.12-●
            partial S78.92-●
        labium (majus) (minus) (complete)
                S38.21-●
            partial S38.21-●
        leg (lower) S88.91-●
            at knee level S88.01-●
                partial S88.02-●
            between knee and ankle S88.11-●
                partial S88.12-●
            partial S88.92-●
        nose (partial) S08.812
            complete S08.811
        penis (complete) S38.221
            partial S38.222
        scrotum (complete) S38.231
            partial S38.232
        shoulder —see Amputation, traumatic, arm
            at shoulder joint —see Amputation,
                    traumatic, arm, at shoulder joint

Amputation (Continued)
    traumatic (Continued)
        testes (complete) S38.231
            partial S38.232
        thigh —see Amputation, traumatic, hip
        thorax, part of S28.1
            breast —see Amputation, traumatic, breast
        thumb (complete) (metacarpophalangeal)
                S68.01-●
            partial S68.02-●
            transphalangeal (complete) S68.51-●
                partial S68.52-●
        toe (lesser) S98.13-●
            great S98.11-●
                partial S98.12-●
            more than one S98.21-●
                partial S98.22-●
            partial S98.14-●
        vulva (complete) S38.211
            partial S38.212
Amputee (bilateral) (old) Z89.9
Amsterdam dwarfism Q87.19
Amusia R48.8
    developmental F80.89
Amyelencephalus, amyelencephaly Q00.0
Amyelia Q06.0
Amygdalitis —see Tonsillitis
Amygdalolith J35.8
Amyloid heart (disease) E85.4 [I43]
Amyloidosis (generalized) (primary) E85.9
    with lung involvement E85.4 [J99]
    familial E85.2
    genetic E85.2
    heart E85.4 [I43]
    hemodialysis-associated E85.3
    light chain (AL) E85.81
    liver E85.4 [K77]
    localized E85.4
    neuropathic heredofamilial E85.1
    non-neuropathic heredofamilial E85.0
    organ limited E85.4
    Portuguese E85.1
    pulmonary E85.4 [J99]
    secondary systemic E85.3
    senile systemic (SSA) E85.82
    skin (lichen) (macular) E85.4 [L99]
    specified NEC E85.89
    subglottic E85.4 [J99]
    wild-type transthyretin-related (ATTR)
            E85.82
Amylopectinosis (brancher enzyme deficiency)
        E74.03
Amylophagia —see Pica
Amyoplasia congenita Q79.8
Amyotonia M62.89
    congenita G70.2
Amyotrophia, amyotrophy, amyotrophic G71.8
    congenita Q79.8
    diabetic —see Diabetes, amyotrophy
    lateral sclerosis G12.21
    neuralgic G54.5
    spinal progressive G12.25
Anacidity, gastric K31.83
    psychogenic F45.8
Anaerosis of newborn P28.89
Analbuminemia E88.09
Analgesia —see Anesthesia
Analphalipoproteinemia E78.6
Anaphylactic
    purpura D69.0
    shock or reaction —see Shock, anaphylactic
Anaphylactoid shock or reaction —see Shock,
        anaphylactic
Anaphylactoid syndrome of pregnancy
        O88.01-●
Anaphylaxis —see Shock, anaphylactic
Anaplasia cervix —see also Dysplasia, cervix
        N87.9
Anaplasmosis [A. phagocytophilum]
        (transfusion transmitted) A79.82
    human A77.49

Anarthria R47.1
Anasarca R60.1
　　cardiac —*see* Failure, heart, congestive
　　lung J18.2
　　newborn P83.2
　　nutritional E43
　　pulmonary J18.2
　　renal N04.9
Anastomosis
　　aneurysmal —*see* Aneurysm
　　arteriovenous ruptured brain I60.8
　　intestinal K63.89
　　　　complicated NEC K91.89
　　　　　　involving urinary tract N99.89
　　intracerebral I61.8
　　intraparenchymal I61.8
　　intraventricular I61.5
　　retinal and choroidal vessels (congenital) Q14.8
　　subarachnoid I60.8
Anatomical narrow angle H40.03-●
Ancylostoma, ancylostomiasis (braziliense)
　　　　(caninum) (ceylanicum) (duodenale) B76.0
　　Necator americanus B76.1
Andersen's disease (glycogen storage) E74.09
Anderson-Fabry disease E75.21
Andes disease T70.29
Andrews' disease (bacterid) L08.89
Androblastoma
　　benign
　　　　specified site —*see* Neoplasm, benign, by
　　　　　　site
　　　　unspecified site
　　　　　　female D27.9
　　　　　　male D29.20
　　malignant
　　　　specified site —*see* Neoplasm, malignant,
　　　　　　by site
　　　　unspecified site
　　　　　　female C56.9
　　　　　　male C62.90
　　specified site —*see* Neoplasm, uncertain
　　　　behavior, by site
　　tubular
　　　　with lipid storage
　　　　　　specified site —*see* Neoplasm, benign,
　　　　　　　　by site
　　　　　　unspecified site
　　　　　　　　female D27.9
　　　　　　　　male D29.20
　　　　specified site —*see* Neoplasm, benign, by site
　　　　unspecified site
　　　　　　female D27.9
　　　　　　male D29.20
　　unspecified site
　　　　female D39.10
　　　　male D40.10
Androgen insensitivity syndrome —*see also*
　　Syndrome, androgen insensitivity E34.50
Androgen resistance syndrome —*see also*
　　Syndrome, androgen insensitivity E34.50
Android pelvis Q74.2
　　with disproportion (fetopelvic) O33.3
　　　　causing obstructed labor O65.3
Androphobia F40.290
Anectasis, pulmonary (newborn) —*see* Atelectasis
Anemia (essential) (general) (hemoglobin
　　deficiency) (infantile) (primary) (profound)
　　D64.9
　　with (due to) (in)
　　　　disorder of
　　　　　　anaerobic glycolysis D55.29
　　　　　　pentose phosphate pathway D55.1
　　　　koilonychia D50.9
　　achlorhydric D50.8
　　achrestic D53.1
　　Addison (-Biermer) (pernicious) D51.0
　　agranulocytic —*see* Agranulocytosis
　　amino-acid-deficiency D53.0
　　aplastic D61.9
　　　　congenital D61.09
　　　　drug-induced D61.1

Anemia *(Continued)*
　　aplastic *(Continued)*
　　　　due to
　　　　　　drugs D61.1
　　　　　　external agents NEC D61.2
　　　　　　infection D61.2
　　　　　　radiation D61.2
　　　　idiopathic D61.3
　　　　red cell (pure) D60.9
　　　　　　chronic D60.0
　　　　　　congenital D61.01
　　　　　　specified type NEC D60.8
　　　　　　transient D60.1
　　　　specified type NEC D61.89
　　　　toxic D61.2
　　aregenerative
　　　　congenital D61.09
　　asiderotic D50.9
　　atypical (primary) D64.9
　　Baghdad spring D55.0
　　Balantidium coli A07.0
　　Biermer's (pernicious) D51.0
　　blood loss (chronic) D50.0
　　　　acute D62
　　bothriocephalus B70.0 *[D63.8]*
　　brickmaker's B76.9 *[D63.8]*
　　cerebral I67.89
　　childhood D58.9
　　chlorotic D50.8
　　chronic
　　　　blood loss D50.0
　　　　hemolytic D58.9
　　　　　　idiopathic D59.9
　　　　simple D53.9
　　chronica congenita aregenerativa D61.09
　　combined system disease NEC D51.0 *[G32.0]*
　　　　due to dietary vitamin B12 deficiency
　　　　　　D51.3 *[G32.0]*
　　complicating pregnancy, childbirth
　　　　or puerperium —*see* Pregnancy,
　　　　complicated by (management affected
　　　　by), anemia
　　congenital P61.4
　　　　aplastic D61.09
　　　　due to isoimmunization NOS P55.9
　　　　dyserythropoietic, dyshematopoietic D64.4
　　　　following fetal blood loss P61.3
　　　　Heinz body D58.2
　　　　hereditary hemolytic NOS D58.9
　　　　pernicious D51.0
　　　　spherocytic D58.0
　　Cooley's (erythroblastic) D56.1
　　cytogenic D51.0
　　deficiency D53.9
　　　　2, 3 diphosphoglycurate mutase D55.29
　　　　2, 3 PG D55.29
　　　　6 phosphogluconate dehydrogenase D55.1
　　　　6-PGD D55.1
　　　　amino-acid D53.0
　　　　combined B12 and folate D53.1
　　　　enzyme D55.9
　　　　　　drug-induced (hemolytic) D59.2
　　　　　　glucose-6-phosphate dehydrogenase
　　　　　　　　(G6PD) D55.0
　　　　　　glycolytic D55.29
　　　　　　nucleotide metabolism D55.3
　　　　　　related to hexose monophosphate
　　　　　　　　(HMP) shunt pathway NEC D55.1
　　　　　　specified type NEC D55.8
　　　　erythrocytic glutathione D55.1
　　　　folate D52.9
　　　　　　dietary D52.0
　　　　　　drug-induced D52.1
　　　　folic acid D52.9
　　　　　　dietary D52.0
　　　　　　drug-induced D52.1
　　　　G SH D55.1
　　　　G6PD D55.0
　　　　GGS-R D55.1
　　　　glucose-6-phosphate dehydrogenase D55.0
　　　　glutathione reductase D55.1

Anemia *(Continued)*
　　deficiency *(Continued)*
　　　　glyceraldehyde phosphate dehydrogenase
　　　　　　D55.29
　　　　hexokinase D55.29
　　　　iron D50.9
　　　　　　secondary to blood loss (chronic) D50.0
　　　　nutritional D53.9
　　　　　　with
　　　　　　　　poor iron absorption D50.8
　　　　　　　　specified deficiency NEC D53.8
　　　　phosphofructo-aldolase D55.29
　　　　phosphoglycerate kinase D55.29
　　　　PK D55.21
　　　　protein D53.0
　　　　pyruvate kinase D55.21
　　　　transcobalamin II D55.22
　　　　triose-phosphate isomerase D55.29
　　　　vitamin B12 NOS D51.9
　　　　　　dietary D51.3
　　　　　　due to
　　　　　　　　intrinsic factor deficiency D51.0
　　　　　　　　selective vitamin B12 malabsorption
　　　　　　　　　　with proteinuria D51.1
　　　　　　pernicious D51.0
　　　　　　specified type NEC D51.8
　　Diamond-Blackfan (congenital hypoplastic)
　　　　D61.01
　　dibothriocephalus B70.0 *[D63.8]*
　　dimorphic D53.1
　　diphasic D53.1
　　Diphyllobothrium (Dibothriocephalus) B70.0
　　　　[D63.8]
　　due to (in) (with)
　　　　antineoplastic chemotherapy D64.81
　　　　blood loss (chronic) D50.0
　　　　　　acute D62
　　　　chemotherapy, antineoplastic D64.81
　　　　chronic disease classified elsewhere NEC
　　　　　　D63.8
　　　　chronic kidney disease D63.1
　　　　deficiency
　　　　　　amino-acid D53.0
　　　　　　copper D53.8
　　　　　　folate (folic acid) D52.9
　　　　　　　　dietary D52.0
　　　　　　　　drug-induced D52.1
　　　　　　molybdenum D53.8
　　　　　　protein D53.0
　　　　　　zinc D53.8
　　　　dietary vitamin B12 deficiency D51.3
　　　　disorder of
　　　　　　glutathione metabolism D55.1
　　　　　　nucleotide metabolism D55.3
　　　　drug —*see* Anemia, by type —*see also* Table
　　　　　　of Drugs and Chemicals
　　　　end stage renal disease D63.1
　　　　enzyme disorder D55.9
　　　　fetal blood loss P61.3
　　　　fish tapeworm (D latum) infestation B70.0
　　　　　　[D63.8]
　　　　hemorrhage (chronic) D50.0
　　　　　　acute D62
　　　　impaired absorption D50.9
　　　　loss of blood (chronic) D50.0
　　　　　　acute D62
　　　　myxedema E03.9 *[D63.8]*
　　　　Necator americanus B76.1 *[D63.8]*
　　　　prematurity P61.2
　　　　selective vitamin B12 malabsorption with
　　　　　　proteinuria D51.1
　　　　transcobalamin II deficiency D51.2
　　Dyke-Young type (secondary) (symptomatic)
　　　　D59.19
　　dyserythropoietic (congenital) D64.4
　　dyshematopoietic (congenital) D64.4
　　Egyptian B76.9 *[D63.8]*
　　elliptocytosis —*see* Elliptocytosis
　　enzyme-deficiency, drug-induced D59.2
　　epidemic —*see also* Ancylostomiasis B76.9
　　　　[D63.8]

▶ New　　⏩ Revised　　~~deleted~~ Deleted　　● Use Additional Character(s)

Anemia (Continued)
  erythroblastic
    familial D56.1
    newborn —see also Disease, hemolytic
        P55.9
    of childhood D56.1
  erythrocytic glutathione deficiency D55.1
  erythropoietin-resistant anemia (EPO
      resistant anemia) D63.1
  Faber's (achlorhydric anemia) D50.9
  factitious (self-induced blood letting) D50.0
  familial erythroblastic D56.1
  Fanconi's (congenital pancytopenia) D61.09
  favism D55.0
  fish tapeworm (D. latum) infestation B70.0
      [D63.8]
  folate (folic acid) deficiency D52.9
  glucose-6-phosphate dehydrogenase (G6PD)
      deficiency D55.0
  glutathione-reductase deficiency D55.1
  goat's milk D52.0
  granulocytic —see Agranulocytosis
  Heinz body, congenital D58.2
  hemolytic D58.9
    acquired D59.9
      with hemoglobinuria NEC D59.6
      autoimmune NEC D59.19
      infectious D59.4
      specified type NEC D59.8
      toxic D59.4
    acute D59.9
      due to enzyme deficiency specified type
          NEC D55.8
      Lederer's D59.19
    autoimmune D59.10
      cold D59.12
      drug-induced D59.0
      mixed D59.13
      warm D59.11
    chronic D58.9
      idiopathic D59.9
    cold type (secondary) (symptomatic)
        D59.12
    congenital (spherocytic) —see
        Spherocytosis
    due to
      cardiac conditions D59.4
      drugs (nonautoimmune) D59.2
        autoimmune D59.0
      enzyme disorder D55.9
        drug-induced D59.2
      presence of shunt or other internal
          prosthetic device D59.4
    familial D58.9
    hereditary D58.9
      due to enzyme disorder D55.9
        specified type NEC D55.8
      specified type NEC D58.8
    idiopathic (chronic) D59.9
    mechanical D59.4
    microangiopathic D59.4
    mixed type (primary) (secondary)
        (symptomatic) D59.13
    nonautoimmune D59.4
      drug-induced D59.2
    nonspherocytic
      congenital or hereditary NEC D55.8
        glucose-6-phosphate dehydrogenase
            deficiency D55.0
        pyruvate kinase deficiency D55.21
        type
          I D55.1
          II D55.29
      type
        I D55.1
        II D55.29
    primary
      autoimmune
        cold type D59.12
        mixed type D59.13
        warm type D59.11

Anemia (Continued)
  hemolytic (Continued)
    secondary D59.4
      autoimmune
        cold type D59.12
        mixed type D59.13
        warm type D59.11
      specified (hereditary) type NEC D58.8
      Stransky-Regala type —see also
          Hemoglobinopathy D58.8
    symptomatic D59.4
      autoimmune
        cold type D59.12
        mixed type D59.13
        warm type D59.11
    toxic D59.4
    warm type (primary) (secondary)
        (symptomatic) D59.11
  hemorrhagic (chronic) D50.0
    acute D62
  Herrick's D57.1
  hexokinase deficiency D55.29
  hookworm B76.9 [D63.8]
  hypochromic (idiopathic) (microcytic)
      (normoblastic) D50.9
    due to blood loss (chronic) D50.0
      acute D62
    familial sex-linked D64.0
    pyridoxine-responsive D64.3
    sideroblastic, sex-linked D64.0
  hypoplasia, red blood cells D61.9
    congenital or familial D61.01
  hypoplastic (idiopathic) D61.9
    congenital or familial (of childhood)
        D61.01
  hypoproliferative (refractive) D61.9
  idiopathic D64.9
    aplastic D61.3
    hemolytic, chronic D59.9
  in (due to) (with)
    chronic kidney disease D63.1
    end stage renal disease D63.1
    failure, kidney (renal) D63.1
    neoplastic disease —see also Neoplasm
        D63.0
  intertropical —see also Ancylostomiasis
      D63.8
  iron deficiency D50.9
    secondary to blood loss (chronic) D50.0
      acute D62
    specified type NEC D50.8
  Joseph-Diamond-Blackfan (congenital
      hypoplastic) D61.01
  Lederer's (hemolytic) D59.19
  leukoerythroblastic D61.82
  macrocytic D53.9
    nutritional D52.0
    tropical D52.8
  malarial (see also Malaria) B54 [D63.8]
  malignant (progressive) D51.0
  malnutrition D53.9
  marsh (see also Malaria) B54 [D63.8]
  Mediterranean (with other
      hemoglobinopathy) D56.9
  megaloblastic D53.1
    combined B12 and folate deficiency
        D53.1
    hereditary D51.1
    nutritional D52.0
    orotic aciduria D53.0
    refractory D53.1
    specified type NEC D53.1
  megalocytic D53.1
  microcytic (hypochromic) D50.9
    due to blood loss (chronic) D50.0
      acute D62
    familial D56.8
  microdrepanocytosis D57.40
  microelliptopoikilocytic (Rietti-Greppi-
      Micheli) D56.9
  miner's B76.9 [D63.8]

Anemia (Continued)
  myelodysplastic D46.9
  myelofibrosis D75.81
  myelogenous D64.89
  myelopathic D64.89
  myelophthisic D61.82
  myeloproliferative D47.Z9
  newborn P61.4
    due to
      ABO (antibodies, isoimmunization,
          maternal/fetal incompatibility)
          P55.1
      Rh (antibodies, isoimmunization,
          maternal/fetal incompatibility)
          P55.0
    following fetal blood loss P61.3
    posthemorrhagic (fetal) P61.3
  nonspherocytic hemolytic —see Anemia,
      hemolytic, nonspherocytic
  normocytic (infectional) D64.9
    due to blood loss (chronic) D50.0
      acute D62
    myelophthisic D61.82
  nutritional (deficiency) D53.9
    with
      poor iron absorption D50.8
      specified deficiency NEC D53.8
    megaloblastic D52.0
  of prematurity P61.2
  orotaciduric (congenital) (hereditary)
      D53.0
  osteosclerotic D64.89
  ovalocytosis (hereditary) —see Elliptocytosis
  paludal —see also Malaria B54 [D63.8]
  pernicious (congenital) (malignant)
      (progressive) D51.0
  pleochromic D64.89
    of sprue D52.8
  posthemorrhagic (chronic) D50.0
    acute D62
    newborn P61.3
  postoperative (postprocedural)
    due to (acute) blood loss D62
      chronic blood loss D50.0
    specified NEC D64.89
  postpartum O90.81
  pressure D64.89
  progressive D64.9
    malignant D51.0
    pernicious D51.0
  protein-deficiency D53.0
  pseudoleukemica infantum D64.89
  pure red cell D60.9
    congenital D61.01
  pyridoxine-responsive D64.3
  pyruvate kinase deficiency D55.21
  refractory D46.4
    with
      excess of blasts D46.20
        1 (RAEB 1) D46.21
        2 (RAEB 2) D46.22
        in transformation (RAEB T) —see
            Leukemia, acute myeloblastic
      hemochromatosis D46.1
      sideroblasts (ring) (RARS) D46.1
    without ring sideroblasts, so stated
        D46.0
    without sideroblasts without excess of
        blasts D46.0
    megaloblastic D53.1
    sideroblastic D46.1
    sideropenic D50.9
  Rietti-Greppi-Micheli D56.9
  scorbutic D53.2
  secondary to
    blood loss (chronic) D50.0
      acute D62
    hemorrhage (chronic) D50.0
      acute D62
  semiplastic D61.89
  sickle-cell —see Disease, sickle-cell

Anemia (Continued)
  sideroblastic D64.3
    hereditary D64.0
    hypochromic, sex-linked D64.0
    pyridoxine-responsive NEC D64.3
    refractory D46.1
    secondary (due to)
      disease D64.1
      drugs and toxins D64.2
    specified type NEC D64.3
  sideropenic (refractory) D50.9
    due to blood loss (chronic) D50.0
      acute D62
  simple chronic D53.9
  specified type NEC D64.89
  spherocytic (hereditary) —see Spherocytosis
  splenic D64.89
  splenomegalic D64.89
  stomatocytosis D58.8
  syphilitic (acquired) (late) A52.79 [D63.8]
  target cell D64.89
  thalassemia D56.9
  thrombocytopenic —see Thrombocytopenia
  toxic D61.2
  tropical B76.9 [D63.8]
    macrocytic D52.8
  tuberculous A18.89 [D63.8]
  vegan D51.3
  vitamin
    B6-responsive D64.3
    B12 deficiency (dietary) pernicious D51.0
  von Jaksch's D64.89
  Witts' (achlorhydric anemia) D50.8
Anemophobia F40.228
Anencephalus, anencephaly Q00.0
Anergasia —see Psychosis, organic
Anesthesia, anesthetic R20.0
  complication or reaction NEC —see also
      Complications, anesthesia T88.59
    due to
      correct substance properly
        administered —see Table of Drugs
        and Chemicals, by drug, adverse
        effect
      overdose or wrong substance given —see
        Table of Drugs and Chemicals, by
        drug, poisoning
      unintended awareness under general
        anesthesia during procedure T88.53
        personal history of Z92.84
  cornea H18.81-●
  dissociative F44.6
  functional (hysterical) F44.6
  hyperesthetic, thalamic G89.0
  hysterical F44.6
  local skin lesion R20.0
  sexual (psychogenic) F52.1
  shock (due to) T88.2
  skin R20.0
  testicular N50.9
Anetoderma (maculosum) (of) L90.8
  Jadassohn-Pellizzari L90.2
  Schweninger-Buzzi L90.1
Aneurin deficiency E51.9
Aneurysm (anastomotic) (artery) (cirsoid)
    (diffuse) (false) (fusiform) (multiple)
    (saccular) I72.9
  abdominal (aorta) I71.40
    infrarenal I71.43
      ruptured I71.33
    juxtarenal I71.42
      ruptured I71.32
    pararenal I71.41
      ruptured I71.31
    ruptured I71.30
    syphilitic A52.01
  aorta, aortic (nonsyphilitic) I71.9
    abdominal I71.40
      dissecting —see Dissection, aorta,
        abdominal
      ruptured I71.30

Aneurysm (Continued)
  aorta, aortic (nonsyphilitic) (Continued)
    arch I71.22
      ruptured I71.12
      arteriosclerotic I71.9
        ruptured I71.8
    ascending I71.21
      ruptured I71.11
    congenital Q25.43
    descending I71.9
      abdominal I71.40
        ruptured I71.30
      ruptured I71.8
      thoracic I71.23
        ruptured I71.13
    dissecting —see Dissection, aorta
    root Q25.43
    ruptured I71.8
    sinus, congenital Q25.43
    syphilitic A52.01
    thoracic I71.20
      ruptured I71.10
    thoracoabdominal I71.60
      paravisceral I71.62
        ruptured I71.52
      ruptured I71.50
      supraceliac I71.61
        ruptured I71.51
    thorax, thoracic I71.20
      arch I71.22
        ruptured I71.12
      ascending I71.21
        ruptured I71.11
      descending I71.23
        ruptured I71.13
      ruptured I71.10
        arch I71.12
        ascending I71.11
        descending I71.13
    transverse I71.22
      ruptured I71.12
    valve (heart) —see also Endocarditis, aortic
      I35.8
  arteriosclerotic I72.9
    cerebral I67.1
      ruptured —see Hemorrhage, intracranial,
        subarachnoid
  arteriovenous (congenital) —see also
      Malformation, arteriovenous
    acquired I77.0
      brain I67.1
        ruptured —see Aneurysm,
          arteriorvenous, brain, ruptured
      coronary I25.41
      pulmonary I28.0
    brain Q28.2
      ruptured I60.8
        intracerebral I61.8
        intraparenchymal I61.8
        intraventricular I61.5
        subarachnoid I60.8
    peripheral —see Malformation,
        arteriovenous, peripheral
    precerebral vessels Q28.0
    specified site NEC —see also Malformation,
        arteriovenous
      acquired I77.0
  basal —see Aneurysm, brain
  basilar (trunk) I72.5
  berry (congenital) (nonruptured) I67.1
    ruptured I60.7
  brain I67.1
    arteriosclerotic I67.1
      ruptured —see Hemorrhage, intracranial,
        subarachnoid
    arteriovenous (congenital) (nonruptured)
        Q28.2
      acquired I67.1
        ruptured —see Aneurysm,
          arteriorvenous, brain, ruptured
          I60.8-
      ruptured —see Aneurysm,
        arteriorvenous, brain, ruptured I60.8-

Aneurysm (Continued)
  brain (Continued)
    berry (congenital) (nonruptured) I67.1
      ruptured —see also Hemorrhage,
        intracranial, subarachnoid I60.7
    congenital Q28.3
      aorta (root) (sinus) Q25.43
      ruptured I60.7
    meninges I67.1
      ruptured I60.8
    miliary (congenital) (nonruptured) I67.1
      ruptured —see also Hemorrhage,
        intracranial, subarachnoid I60.7
    mycotic I33.0
    ruptured —see Hemorrhage, intracranial,
      subarachnoid
    syphilitic (hemorrhage) A52.05
  cardiac (false) —see also Aneurysm, heart I25.3
  carotid artery (common) (external) I72.0
    internal (intracranial) I67.1
      extracranial portion I72.0
    ruptured into brain I60.0-●
    syphilitic A52.09
      intracranial A52.05
  cavernous sinus I67.1
    arteriovenous (congenital) (nonruptured)
        Q28.3
      ruptured I60.8
  celiac I72.8
  central nervous system, syphilitic A52.05
  cerebral —see Aneurysm, brain
  chest —see Aneurysm, thorax
  circle of Willis I67.1
    congenital Q28.3
      ruptured I60.6
    ruptured I60.6
  common iliac artery I72.3
  congenital (peripheral) Q27.8
    aorta (root) (sinus) Q25.43
    brain Q28.3
      ruptured I60.7
    coronary Q24.5
    digestive system Q27.8
    lower limb Q27.8
    pulmonary Q25.79
    retina Q14.1
    specified site NEC Q27.8
    upper limb Q27.8
  conjunctiva —see Abnormality, conjunctiva,
      vascular
  conus arteriosus —see Aneurysm, heart
  coronary (arteriosclerotic) (artery) I25.41
    arteriovenous, congenital Q24.5
    congenital Q24.5
    ruptured —see Infarct, myocardium
    syphilitic A52.06
    vein I25.89
  cylindroid (aorta) I71.9
    ruptured I71.8
    syphilitic A52.01
  ductus arteriosus Q25.0
  endocardial, infective (any valve) I33.0
  femoral (artery) (ruptured) I72.4
  gastroduodenal I72.8
  gastroepiploic I72.8
  heart (wall) (chronic or with a stated duration
      of over 4 weeks) I25.3
    valve —see Endocarditis
  hepatic I72.8
  iliac (common) (artery) (ruptured) I72.3
  infective I72.9
    endocardial (any valve) I33.0
  innominate (nonsyphilitic) I72.8
    syphilitic A52.09
  interauricular septum —see Aneurysm, heart
  interventricular septum —see Aneurysm,
      heart
  intrathoracic (nonsyphilitic) (see also
      Aneurysm, aorta, thorax) I71.20
    ruptured (see also Aneurysm, aorta, thorax,
      ruptured) I71.10
    syphilitic A52.01

Aneurysm *(Continued)*
lower limb I72.4
lung (pulmonary artery) I28.1
mediastinal (nonsyphilitic) I72.8
syphilitic A52.09
miliary (congenital) I67.1
ruptured —*see* Hemorrhage, intracerebral, subarachnoid, intracranial
mitral (heart) (valve) I34.89
mural —*see* Aneurysm, heart
mycotic I72.9
endocardial (any valve) I33.0
ruptured, brain —*see* Hemorrhage, intracerebral, subarachnoid
myocardium —*see* Aneurysm, heart
neck I72.0
pancreaticoduodenal I72.8
patent ductus arteriosus Q25.0
peripheral NEC I72.8
congenital Q27.8
digestive system Q27.8
lower limb Q27.8
specified site NEC Q27.8
upper limb Q27.8
popliteal (artery) (ruptured) I72.4
precerebral
congenital (nonruptured) Q28.1
specified site, NEC I72.5
pulmonary I28.1
arteriovenous Q25.72
acquired I28.0
syphilitic A52.09
valve (heart) —*see* Endocarditis, pulmonary
racemose (peripheral) I72.9
congenital —*see* Aneurysm, congenital
radial I72.1
Rasmussen NEC A15.0
renal (artery) I72.2
retina —*see also* Disorder, retina, microaneurysms
congenital Q14.1
diabetic —*see* E08-E13 with .3- •
sinus of Valsalva Q25.49
specified NEC I72.8
spinal (cord) I72.8
syphilitic (hemorrhage) A52.09
splenic I72.8
subclavian (artery) (ruptured) I72.8
syphilitic A52.09
superior mesenteric I72.8
syphilitic (aorta) A52.01
central nervous system A52.05
congenital (late) A50.54 *[I79.0]*
spine, spinal A52.09
thoracoabdominal (aorta) I71.60
ruptured I71.50
syphilitic A52.01
thorax, thoracic (aorta) (arch) (nonsyphilitic) — *see* Aneurysm, aorta, thorax
ruptured —*see* Aneurysm, aorta, thorax, ruptured
syphilitic A52.01
traumatic (complication) (early), specified site —*see* Injury, blood vessel
tricuspid (heart) (valve) I07.8
ulnar I72.1
upper limb (ruptured) I72.1
valve, valvular —*see* Endocarditis
visceral NEC I72.8
venous —*see also* Varix I86.8
congenital Q27.8
digestive system Q27.8
lower limb Q27.8
specified site NEC Q27.8
upper limb Q27.8
ventricle —*see* Aneurysm, heart
vertebral artery I72.6
visceral NEC I72.8
Angelman syndrome Q93.51
Anger R45.4
Angiectasis, angiectopia I99.8

Angiitis I77.6
allergic granulomatous M30.1
hypersensitivity M31.0
necrotizing M31.9
specified NEC M31.8
nervous system, granulomatous I67.7
Angina (attack) (cardiac) (chest) (heart) (pectoris) (syndrome) (vasomotor) I20.9
with
atherosclerotic heart disease —*see* Arteriosclerosis, coronary (artery)
documented spasm I20.1
abdominal K55.1
accelerated —*see* Angina, unstable
agranulocytic —*see* Agranulocytosis
angiospastic —*see* Angina, with documented spasm
aphthous B08.5
crescendo —*see* Angina, unstable
croupous J05.0
cruris I73.9
de novo effort —*see* Angina, unstable
diphtheritic, membranous A36.0
equivalent I20.8
exudative, chronic J37.0
following acute myocardial infarction I23.7
gangrenous diphtheritic A36.0
intestinal K55.1
Ludovici K12.2
Ludwig's K12.2
malignant diphtheritic A36.0
membranous J05.0
diphtheritic A36.0
Vincent's A69.1
mesenteric K55.1
monocytic —*see* Mononucleosis, infectious
of effort —*see* Angina, specified NEC
phlegmonous J36
diphtheritic A36.0
post-infarctional I23.7
pre-infarctional —*see* Angina, unstable
Prinzmetal —*see* Angina, with documented spasm
progressive —*see* Angina, unstable
pseudomembranous A69.1
pultaceous, diphtheritic A36.0
▶ refractory I20.2
spasm-induced —*see* Angina, with documented spasm
specified NEC I20.8
stable I20.8
stenocardia —*see* Angina, specified NEC
stridulous, diphtheritic A36.2
tonsil J36
trachealis J05.0
unstable I20.0
variant —*see* Angina, with documented spasm
Vincent's A69.1
worsening effort —*see* Angina, unstable
Angioblastoma —*see* Neoplasm, connective tissue, uncertain behavior
Angiocholecystitis —*see* Cholecystitis, acute
Angiocholitis —*see also* Cholecystitis, acute K83.09
Angiodysgenesis spinalis G95.19
Angiodysplasia (cecum) (colon) K55.20
with bleeding K55.21
duodenum (and stomach) K31.819
with bleeding K31.811
stomach (and duodenum) K31.819
with bleeding K31.811
Angioedema (allergic) (any site) (with urticaria) T78.3
episodic, with eosinophilia D72.118
hereditary D84.1
Angioendothelioma —*see* Neoplasm, uncertain behavior, by site
benign D18.00
intra-abdominal D18.03
intracranial D18.02
skin D18.01
specified site NEC D18.09
bone —*see* Neoplasm, bone, malignant
Ewing's —*see* Neoplasm, bone, malignant

Angioendotheliomatosis C85.8- •
Angiofibroma —*see also* Neoplasm, benign, by site
juvenile
specified site —*see* Neoplasm, benign, by site
unspecified site D10.6
Angiohemophilia (A) (B) —*see* Disease, von Willebrand
Angioid streaks (choroid) (macula) (retina) H35.33
Angiokeratoma —*see* Neoplasm, skin, benign
corporis diffusum E75.21
Angioleiomyoma —*see* Neoplasm, connective tissue, benign
Angiolipoma —*see also* Lipoma
infiltrating —*see* Lipoma
Angioma —*see also* Hemangioma, by site
capillary I78.1
hemorrhagicum hereditaria I78.0
intra-abdominal D18.03
intracranial D18.02
malignant —*see* Neoplasm, connective tissue, malignant
plexiform D18.00
intra-abdominal D18.03
intracranial D18.02
skin D18.01
specified site NEC D18.09
senile I78.1
serpiginosum L81.7
skin D18.01
specified site NEC D18.09
spider I78.1
stellate I78.1
venous Q28.3
Angiomatosis Q82.8
bacillary A79.89
encephalotrigeminal Q85.89
hemorrhagic familial I78.0
hereditary familial I78.0
liver K76.4
Angiomyolipoma —*see* Lipoma
Angiomyoliposarcoma —*see* Neoplasm, connective tissue, malignant
Angiomyoma —*see* Neoplasm, connective tissue, benign
Angiomyosarcoma —*see* Neoplasm, connective tissue, malignant
Angiomyxoma —*see* Neoplasm, connective tissue, uncertain behavior
Angioneurosis F45.8
Angioneurotic edema (allergic) (any site) (with urticaria) T78.3
hereditary D84.1
Angiopathia, angiopathy I99.9
cerebral I67.9
amyloid E85.4 *[I68.0]*
diabetic (peripheral) —*see* Diabetes, angiopathy
peripheral I73.9
diabetic —*see* Diabetes, angiopathy
specified type NEC I73.89
retinae syphilitica A52.05
retinalis (juvenilis)
diabetic —*see* Diabetes, retinopathy
proliferative —*see* Retinopathy, proliferative
Angiosarcoma —*see also* Neoplasm, connective tissue, malignant
liver C22.3
Angiosclerosis —*see* Arteriosclerosis
Angiospasm (peripheral) (traumatic) (vessel) I73.9
brachial plexus G54.0
cerebral G45.9
cervical plexus G54.2
nerve
arm —*see* Mononeuropathy, upper limb
axillary G54.0
median —*see* Lesion, nerve, median
ulnar —*see* Lesion, nerve, ulnar

Angiospasm *(Continued)*
  nerve *(Continued)*
    axillary G54.0
    leg —*see* Mononeuropathy, lower limb
    median —*see* Lesion, nerve, median
    plantar —*see* Lesion, nerve, plantar
    ulnar —*see* Lesion, nerve, ulnar
Angiospastic disease or edema I73.9
Angiostrongyliasis
  due to
    Parastrongylus
      cantonensis B83.2
      costaricensis B81.3
    intestinal B81.3
Anguillulosis —*see* Strongyloidiasis
Angulation
  cecum —*see* Obstruction, intestine
  coccyx (acquired) —*see also* subcategory M43.8
    congenital NEC Q76.49
  femur (acquired) —*see also* Deformity, limb,
    specified type NEC, thigh
    congenital Q74.2
  intestine (large) (small) —*see* Obstruction,
    intestine
  sacrum (acquired) —*see also* subcategory
    M43.8
    congenital NEC Q76.49
  sigmoid (flexure) —*see* Obstruction, intestine
  spine —*see* Dorsopathy, deforming,
    specified NEC
  tibia (acquired) —*see also* Deformity, limb,
    specified type NEC, lower leg
    congenital Q74.2
  ureter N13.5
    with infection N13.6
  wrist (acquired) —*see also* Deformity,
    limb, specified type NEC, forearm
    congenital Q74.0
Angulus infectiosus (lips) K13.0
Anhedonia R45.84
  sexual F52.0
Anhidrosis L74.4
Anhydration E86.0
Anhydremia E86.0
Anidrosis L74.4
Aniridia (congenital) Q13.1
Anisakiasis (infection) (infestation) B81.0
Anisakis larvae infestation B81.0
Aniseikonia H52.32
Anisocoria (pupil) H57.02
  congenital Q13.2
Anisocytosis R71.8
Anisometropia (congenital) H52.31
Ankle —*see* condition
Ankyloblepharon (eyelid) (acquired) —*see also*
    Blepharophimosis
  filiforme (adnatum) (congenital) Q10.3
  total Q10.3
Ankyloglossia Q38.1
Ankylosis (fibrous) (osseous) (joint) M24.60
  ankle M24.67-●
  arthrodesis status Z98.1
  cricoarytenoid (cartilage) (joint) (larynx) J38.7
  dental K03.5
  ear ossicles H74.31-●
  elbow M24.62-●
  foot M24.67-●
  hand M24.64-●
  hip M24.65-●
  incostapedial joint (infectional) —*see*
    Ankylosis, ear ossicles
  jaw (temporomandibular) M26.61-●
  knee M24.66-●
  lumbosacral (joint) M43.27
  postoperative (status) Z98.1
  produced by surgical fusion, status Z98.1
  sacro-iliac (joint) M43.28
  shoulder M24.61-●
  specified site NEC M24.69
  spine (joint) —*see also* Fusion, spine
    spondylitic —*see* Spondylitis, ankylosing

Ankylosis *(Continued)*
  surgical Z98.1
  temporomandibular M26.61-●
  tooth, teeth (hard tissues) K03.5
  wrist M24.63-●
Ankylostoma —*see* Ancylostoma
Ankylostomiasis —*see* Ancylostomiasis
Ankylurethria —*see* Stricture, urethra
Annular —*see also* condition
  detachment, cervix N88.8
  organ or site, congenital NEC —*see* Distortion
  pancreas (congenital) Q45.1
▶**Anoctaminopathy** G71.035
Anodontia (complete) (partial) (vera) K00.0
  acquired K08.10
Anomaly, anomalous (congenital) (unspecified
    type) Q89.9
  abdominal wall NEC Q79.59
  acoustic nerve Q07.8
  adrenal (gland) Q89.1
  Alder (-Reilly) (leukocyte granulation) D72.0
  alimentary tract Q45.9
    upper Q40.9
  alveolar M26.70
    hyperplasia M26.79
      mandibular M26.72
      maxillary M26.71
    hypoplasia M26.79
      mandibular M26.74
      maxillary M26.73
    ridge (process) M26.79
    specified NEC M26.79
  ankle (joint) Q74.2
  anus Q43.9
  aorta (arch) NEC Q25.40
    coarctation (preductal) (postductal) Q25.1
  aortic cusp or valve Q23.9
  appendix Q43.8
  apple peel syndrome Q41.1
  aqueduct of Sylvius Q03.0
    with spina bifida —*see* Spina bifida, with
      hydrocephalus
  arm Q74.0
  arteriovenous NEC
    coronary Q24.5
    gastrointestinal Q27.33
      acquired —*see* Angiodysplasia
  artery (peripheral) Q27.9
    basilar NEC Q28.1
    cerebral Q28.3
    coronary Q24.5
    digestive system Q27.8
    eye Q15.8
    great Q25.9
      specified NEC Q25.8
    lower limb Q27.8
    peripheral Q27.9
      specified NEC Q27.8
    pulmonary NEC Q25.79
    renal Q27.2
    retina Q14.1
    specified site NEC Q27.8
    subclavian Q27.8
      origin Q25.48
    umbilical Q27.0
    upper limb Q27.8
    vertebral NEC Q28.1
  aryteno-epiglottic folds Q31.8
  atrial
    bands or folds Q20.8
    septa Q21.10
  atrioventricular
    excitation I45.6
    septum Q21.0
  auditory canal Q17.8
  auricle
    ear Q17.8
      causing impairment of hearing Q16.9
    heart Q20.8
  Axenfeld's Q15.0
  back Q89.9

Anomaly, anomalous *(Continued)*
  band
    atrial Q20.8
    heart Q24.8
    ventricular Q24.8
  Bartholin's duct Q38.4
  biliary duct or passage Q44.5
  bladder Q64.70
    absence Q64.5
    diverticulum Q64.6
    exstrophy Q64.10
      cloacal Q64.12
      extroversion Q64.19
      specified type NEC Q64.19
      supravesical fissure Q64.11
    neck obstruction Q64.31
    specified type NEC Q64.79
  bone Q79.9
    arm Q74.0
    face Q75.9
    leg Q74.2
    pelvic girdle Q74.2
    shoulder girdle Q74.0
    skull Q75.9
      with
        anencephaly Q00.0
        encephalocele —*see* Encephalocele
        hydrocephalus Q03.9
          with spina bifida —*see* Spina bifida,
            by site, with hydrocephalus
        microcephaly Q02
  brain (multiple) Q04.9
    vessel Q28.3
  breast Q83.9
  broad ligament Q50.6
  bronchus Q32.4
  bulbus cordis Q21.9
  bursa Q79.9
  canal of Nuck Q52.4
  canthus Q10.3
  capillary Q27.9
  cardiac Q24.9
    chambers Q20.9
      specified NEC Q20.8
    septal closure Q21.9
      specified NEC Q21.8
    valve NEC Q24.8
      pulmonary Q22.3
  cardiovascular system Q28.8
  carpus Q74.0
  caruncle, lacrimal Q10.6
  cascade stomach Q40.2
  cauda equina Q06.3
  cecum Q43.9
  cerebral Q04.9
    vessels Q28.3
  cervix Q51.9
  Chédiak-Higashi(-Steinbrinck) (congenital
      gigantism of peroxidase granules)
      E70.330
  cheek Q18.9
  chest wall Q67.8
    bones Q76.9
  chin Q18.9
  chordae tendineae Q24.8
  choroid Q14.3
    plexus Q07.8
  chromosomes, chromosomal Q99.9
    D (1) —*see* condition, chromosome 13
    E (3) —*see* condition, chromosome 18
    G —*see* condition, chromosome 21
    sex
      female phenotype Q97.8
      gonadal dysgenesis (pure) Q99.1
      Klinefelter's Q98.4
      male phenotype Q98.9
      Turner's Q96.9
    specified NEC Q99.8
  cilia Q10.3
  circulatory system Q28.9
  clavicle Q74.0
  clitoris Q52.6

Anomaly, anomalous *(Continued)*
  coccyx Q76.49
  colon Q43.9
  common duct Q44.5
  communication
    coronary artery Q24.5
    left ventricle with right atrium Q21.0
  concha (ear) Q17.3
  connection
    portal vein Q26.5
    pulmonary venous Q26.4
      partial Q26.3
      total Q26.2
    renal artery with kidney Q27.2
  cornea (shape) Q13.4
  coronary artery or vein Q24.5
  cranium —*see* Anomaly, skull
  cricoid cartilage Q31.8
  cystic duct Q44.5
  dental
    alveolar —*see* Anomaly, alveolar
    arch relationship M26.20
      specified NEC M26.29
  dentofacial M26.9
    alveolar —*see* Anomaly, alveolar
    dental arch relationship M26.20
      specified NEC M26.29
    functional M26.50
      specified NEC M26.59
    jaw-cranial base relationship M26.10
      asymmetry M26.12
        maxillary M26.11
      specified type NEC M26.19
    jaw size M26.00
      macrogenia M26.05
      mandibular
        hyperplasia M26.03
        hypoplasia M26.04
      maxillary
        hyperplasia M26.01
        hypoplasia M26.02
      microgenia M26.06
      specified type NEC M26.09
    malocclusion M26.4
      dental arch relationship NEC M26.29
      jaw-cranial base relationship —*see*
        Anomaly, dentofacial, jaw-cranial
        base relationship
      jaw size —*see* Anomaly, dentofacial, jaw
        size
      specified type NEC M26.89
    temporomandibular joint M26.60-●
      adhesions M26.61-●
      ankylosis M26.61-●
      arthralgia M26.62-●
      articular disc M26.63-●
      specified type NEC M26.69
    tooth position, fully erupted M26.30
      specified NEC M26.39
  dermatoglyphic Q82.8
  diaphragm (apertures) NEC Q79.1
  digestive organ(s) or tract Q45.9
    lower Q43.9
    upper Q40.9
  distance, interarch (excessive) (inadequate)
    M26.25
  distribution, coronary artery Q24.5
  ductus
    arteriosus Q25.0
    botalli Q25.0
  duodenum Q43.9
  dura (brain) Q04.9
    spinal cord Q06.9
  ear (external) Q17.9
    causing impairment of hearing Q16.9
    inner Q16.5
    middle (causing impairment of hearing)
      Q16.4
      ossicles Q16.3
  Ebstein's (heart) (tricuspid valve) Q22.5
  ectodermal Q82.9

Anomaly, anomalous *(Continued)*
  Eisenmenger's (ventricular septal defect) Q21.8
  ejaculatory duct Q55.4
  elbow Q74.0
  endocrine gland NEC Q89.2
  epididymis Q55.4
  epiglottis Q31.8
  esophagus Q39.9
  eustachian tube Q17.8
  eye Q15.9
    anterior segment Q13.9
      specified NEC Q13.89
    posterior segment Q14.9
      specified NEC Q14.8
    ptosis (eyelid) Q10.0
    specified NEC Q15.8
  eyebrow Q18.8
  eyelid Q10.3
    ptosis Q10.0
  face Q18.9
    bone(s) Q75.9
  fallopian tube Q50.6
  fascia Q79.9
  femur NEC Q74.2
  fibula NEC Q74.2
  finger Q74.0
  fixation, intestine Q43.3
  flexion (joint) NOS Q74.9
    hip or thigh Q65.89
  foot NEC Q74.2
    varus (congenital) Q66.3-●
  foramen
    ⇒Botalli Q21.12
    ⇒ovale Q21.12
  forearm Q74.0
  forehead Q75.8
  form, teeth K00.2
  fovea centralis Q14.1
  frontal bone —*see* Anomaly, skull
  gallbladder (position) (shape) (size) Q44.1
  Gartner's duct Q52.4
  gastrointestinal tract Q45.9
  genitalia, genital organ(s) or system
    female Q52.9
      external Q52.70
      internal NOS Q52.9
    male Q55.9
      hydrocele P83.5
      specified NEC Q55.8
  genitourinary NEC
    female Q52.9
    male Q55.9
  Gerbode Q21.0
  glottis Q31.8
  granulation or granulocyte, genetic
    (constitutional) (leukocyte) D72.0
  gum Q38.6
  gyri Q07.9
  hair Q84.2
  hand Q74.0
  hard tissue formation in pulp K04.3
  head —*see* Anomaly, skull
  heart Q24.9
    auricle Q20.8
    bands or folds Q24.8
    fibroelastosis cordis I42.4
    obstructive NEC Q22.6
    patent ductus arteriosus (Botalli) Q25.0
    septum Q21.9
      ⇒auricular Q21.19
      ⇒interatrial Q21.19
      interventricular Q21.0
        with pulmonary stenosis or atresia,
          dextraposition of aorta and
          hypertrophy of right ventricle
          Q21.3
      specified NEC Q21.8
      ventricular Q21.0
        with pulmonary stenosis or atresia,
          dextraposition of aorta and
          hypertrophy of right ventricle
          Q21.3

Anomaly, anomalous *(Continued)*
  heart *(Continued)*
    tetralogy of Fallot Q21.3
    valve NEC Q24.8
      aortic
        bicuspid valve Q23.1
        insufficiency Q23.1
        stenosis Q23.0
          subaortic Q24.4
      mitral
        insufficiency Q23.3
        stenosis Q23.2
      pulmonary Q22.3
        atresia Q22.0
        insufficiency Q22.2
        stenosis Q22.1
          infundibular Q24.3
          subvalvular Q24.3
      tricuspid
        atresia Q22.4
        stenosis Q22.4
    ventricle Q20.8
  heel NEC Q74.2
  Hegglin's D72.0
  hemianencephaly Q00.0
  hemicephaly Q00.0
  hemicrania Q00.0
  hepatic duct Q44.5
  hip NEC Q74.2
  hourglass stomach Q40.2
  humerus NEC Q74.2
  hydatid of Morgagni
    female Q50.5
    male (epididymal) Q55.4
      testicular Q55.29
  hymen Q52.4
  hypersegmentation of neutrophils, hereditary
    D72.0
  hypophyseal Q89.2
  ileocecal (coil) (valve) Q43.9
  ileum Q43.9
  ilium NEC Q74.2
  integument Q84.9
    specified NEC Q84.8
  interarch distance (excessive) (inadequate)
    M26.25
  intervertebral cartilage or disc Q76.49
  intestine (large) (small) Q43.9
    with anomalous adhesions, fixation or
      malrotation Q43.3
  iris Q13.2
  ischium NEC Q74.2
  jaw —*see* Anomaly, dentofacial
    alveolar —*see* Anomaly, alveolar
    jaw-cranial base relationship —*see* Anomaly,
      dentofacial, jaw-cranial base relationship
  jejunum Q43.8
  joint Q74.9
    specified NEC Q74.8
  Jordan's D72.0
  kidney(s) (calyx) (pelvis) Q63.9
    artery Q27.2
    specified NEC Q63.8
  Klippel-Feil (brevicollis) Q76.1
  knee Q74.1
  labium (majus) (minus) Q52.70
  labyrinth, membranous Q16.5
  lacrimal apparatus or duct Q10.6
  larynx, laryngeal (muscle) Q31.9
    web (bed) Q31.0
  lens Q12.9
  leukocytes, genetic D72.0
    granulation (constitutional) D72.0
  lid (fold) Q10.3
  ligament Q79.9
    broad Q50.6
    round Q52.8
  limb Q74.9
    lower NEC Q74.2
      reduction deformity —*see* Defect,
        reduction, lower limb
    upper Q74.0

Anomaly, anomalous (Continued)
lip Q38.0
liver Q44.7
    duct Q44.5
lower limb NEC Q74.2
lumbosacral (joint) (region) Q76.49
    kyphosis —see Kyphosis, congenital
    lordosis —see Lordosis, congenital
lung (fissure) (lobe) Q33.9
mandible —see Anomaly, dentofacial
maxilla —see Anomaly, dentofacial
May (-Hegglin) D72.0
meatus urinarius NEC Q64.79
meningeal bands or folds Q07.9
    constriction of Q07.8
    spinal Q06.9
meninges Q07.9
    cerebral Q04.8
    spinal Q06.9
meningocele Q05.9
mesentery Q45.9
metacarpus Q74.0
metatarsus NEC Q74.2
middle ear Q16.4
    ossicles Q16.3
mitral (leaflets) (valve) Q23.9
    insufficiency Q23.3
    specified NEC Q23.8
    stenosis Q23.2
mouth Q38.6
Müllerian —see also Anomaly, by site
    uterus NEC Q51.818
multiple NEC Q89.7
muscle Q79.9
    eyelid Q10.3
musculoskeletal system, except limbs Q79.9
myocardium Q24.8
nail Q84.6
narrowness, eyelid Q10.3
nasal sinus (wall) Q30.8
neck (any part) Q18.9
nerve Q07.9
    acoustic Q07.8
    optic Q07.8
nervous system (central) Q07.9
nipple Q83.9
nose, nasal (bones) (cartilage) (septum)
        (sinus) Q30.9
    specified NEC Q30.8
ocular muscle Q15.8
omphalomesenteric duct Q43.0
opening, pulmonary veins Q26.4
optic
    disc Q14.2
    nerve Q07.8
opticociliary vessels Q13.2
orbit (eye) Q10.7
organ Q89.9
    of Corti Q16.5
origin
    artery
        innominate Q25.8
        pulmonary Q25.79
        renal Q27.2
        subclavian Q25.48
osseous meatus (ear) Q16.1
ovary Q50.39
oviduct Q50.6
palate (hard) (soft) NEC Q38.5
pancreas or pancreatic duct Q45.3
papillary muscles Q24.8
parathyroid gland Q89.2
paraurethral ducts Q64.79
parotid (gland) Q38.4
patella Q74.1
Pelger-Huët (hereditary hyposegmentation)
        D72.0
pelvic girdle NEC Q74.2
pelvis (bony) NEC Q74.2
    rachitic E64.3
penis (glans) Q55.69
pericardium Q24.8

Anomaly, anomalous (Continued)
peripheral vascular system Q27.9
Peter's Q13.4
pharynx Q38.8
pigmentation L81.9
    congenital Q82.8
pituitary (gland) Q89.2
pleural (folds) Q34.0
portal vein Q26.5
    connection Q26.5
position, tooth, teeth, fully erupted M26.30
    specified NEC M26.39
precerebral vessel Q28.1
prepuce Q55.69
prostate Q55.4
pulmonary Q33.9
    artery NEC Q25.79
    valve Q22.3
        atresia Q22.0
        insufficiency Q22.2
        specified type NEC Q22.3
        stenosis Q22.1
            infundibular Q24.3
            subvalvular Q24.3
    venous connection Q26.4
        partial Q26.3
        total Q26.2
pupil Q13.2
    function H57.00
        anisocoria H57.02
        Argyll Robertson pupil H57.01
        miosis H57.03
        mydriasis H57.04
        specified type NEC H57.09
        tonic pupil H57.05-●
pylorus Q40.3
radius Q74.0
rectum Q43.9
reduction (extremity) (limb)
    femur (longitudinal) —see Defect,
        reduction, lower limb, longitudinal,
        femur
    fibula (longitudinal) —see Defect,
        reduction, lower limb, longitudinal,
        fibula
    lower limb —see Defect, reduction, lower
        limb
    radius (longitudinal) —see Defect,
        reduction, upper limb, longitudinal,
        radius
    tibia (longitudinal) —see Defect, reduction,
        lower limb, longitudinal, tibia
    ulna (longitudinal) —see Defect, reduction,
        upper limb, longitudinal, ulna
    upper limb —see Defect, reduction, upper
        limb
refraction —see Disorder, refraction
renal Q63.9
    artery Q27.2
    pelvis Q63.9
        specified NEC Q63.8
respiratory system Q34.9
    specified NEC Q34.8
retina Q14.1
rib Q76.6
    cervical Q76.5
Rieger's Q13.81
rotation —see Malrotation
    hip or thigh Q65.89
round ligament Q52.8
sacroiliac (joint) NEC Q74.2
sacrum NEC Q76.49
    kyphosis —see Kyphosis, congenital
    lordosis —see Lordosis, congenital
saddle nose, syphilitic A50.57
salivary duct or gland Q38.4
scapula Q74.0
scrotum —see Malformation, testis and
        scrotum
sebaceous gland Q82.9
seminal vesicles Q55.4
sense organs NEC Q07.8

Anomaly, anomalous (Continued)
sex chromosomes NEC —see also Anomaly,
        chromosomes
    female phenotype Q97.8
    male phenotype Q98.9
shoulder (girdle) (joint) Q74.0
sigmoid (flexure) Q43.9
simian crease Q82.8
sinus of Valsalva Q25.49
skeleton generalized Q78.9
skin (appendage) Q82.9
skull Q75.9
    with
        anencephaly Q00.0
        encephalocele —see Encephalocele
        hydrocephalus Q03.9
            with spina bifida —see Spina bifida, by
                site, with hydrocephalus
        microcephaly Q02
specified organ or site NEC Q89.8
spermatic cord Q55.4
spine, spinal NEC Q76.49
    column NEC Q76.49
        kyphosis —see Kyphosis, congenital
        lordosis —see Lordosis, congenital
    cord Q06.9
    nerve root Q07.8
spleen Q89.09
    agenesis Q89.01
stenonian duct Q38.4
sternum NEC Q76.7
stomach Q40.3
submaxillary gland Q38.4
tarsus NEC Q74.2
tendon Q79.9
testis —see Malformation, testis and scrotum
thigh NEC Q74.2
thorax (wall) Q67.8
    bony Q76.9
throat Q38.8
thumb Q74.0
thymus gland Q89.2
thyroid (gland) Q89.2
    cartilage Q31.8
tibia NEC Q74.2
    saber A50.56
toe Q74.2
tongue Q38.3
tooth, teeth K00.9
    eruption K00.6
    position, fully erupted M26.30
    spacing, fully erupted M26.30
trachea (cartilage) Q32.1
tragus Q17.9
tricuspid (leaflet) (valve) Q22.9
    atresia or stenosis Q22.4
    Ebstein's Q22.5
Uhl's (hypoplasia of myocardium, right
        ventricle) Q24.8
ulna Q74.0
umbilical artery Q27.0
union
    cricoid cartilage and thyroid cartilage
        Q31.8
    thyroid cartilage and hyoid bone Q31.8
    trachea with larynx Q31.8
upper limb Q74.0
urachus Q64.4
ureter Q62.8
    obstructive NEC Q62.39
        cecoureterocele Q62.32
        orthotopic ureterocele Q62.31
urethra Q64.70
    absence Q64.5
    double Q64.74
    fistula to rectum Q64.73
    obstructive Q64.39
        stricture Q64.32
    prolapse Q64.71
    specified type NEC Q64.79
urinary tract Q64.9
uterus Q51.9
    with only one functioning horn Q51.4

▶ New   ⇒ Revised   ~~deleted~~ Deleted   ● Use Additional Character(s)

Anomaly, anomalous (Continued)
  uvula Q38.5
  vagina Q52.4
  valleculae Q31.8
  valve (heart) NEC Q24.8
    coronary sinus Q24.5
    inferior vena cava Q24.8
    pulmonary Q22.3
    sinus coronario Q24.5
    venae cavae inferioris Q24.8
  vas deferens Q55.4
  vascular Q27.9
    brain Q28.3
    ring Q25.45
  vein(s) (peripheral) Q27.9
    brain Q28.3
    cerebral Q28.3
    coronary Q24.5
    developmental Q28.3
    great Q26.9
      specified NEC Q26.8
  vena cava (inferior) (superior) Q26.9
  venous —see Anomaly, vein(s)
  venous return Q26.8
  ventricular
    bands or folds Q24.8
    septa Q21.0
  vertebra Q76.49
    kyphosis —see Kyphosis, congenital
    lordosis —see Lordosis, congenital
  vesicourethral orifice Q64.79
  vessel(s) Q27.9
    optic papilla Q14.2
    precerebral Q28.1
  vitelline duct Q43.0
  vitreous body or humor Q14.0
  vulva Q52.70
  wrist (joint) Q74.0
Anomia R48.8
Anonychia (congenital) Q84.3
  acquired L60.8
Anophthalmos, anophthalmus (congenital)
    (globe) Q11.1
  acquired Z90.01
Anopia, anopsia H53.46-●
  quadrant H53.46-●
Anorchia, anorchism, anorchidism Q55.0
Anorexia R63.0
  hysterical F44.89
  nervosa F50.00
    atypical F50.9
    binge-eating type F50.2
      with purging F50.02
    restricting type F50.01
Anorgasmy, psychogenic (female) F52.31
  male F52.32
Anosmia R43.0
  hysterical F44.6
  postinfectional J39.8
Anosognosia R41.89
Anosteoplasia Q78.9
Anovulatory cycle N97.0
Anoxemia R09.02
  newborn P84
Anoxia (pathological) R09.02
  altitude T70.29
  cerebral G93.1
    complicating
      anesthesia (general) (local) or other
        sedation T88.59
      in labor and delivery O74.3
      in pregnancy O29.21-●
      postpartum, puerperal O89.2
    delivery (cesarean) (instrumental) O75.4
    during a procedure G97.81
    newborn P84
    resulting from a procedure G97.82
  due to
    drowning T75.1
    high altitude T70.29
  heart —see Insufficiency, coronary
  intrauterine P84

Anoxia (Continued)
  myocardial —see Insufficiency, coronary
  newborn P84
  spinal cord G95.11
  systemic (by suffocation) (low content in
    atmosphere) —see Asphyxia, traumatic
Anteflexion —see Anteversion
Antenatal
  care (normal pregnancy) Z34.90
  screening (encounter for) of mother —see also
    Encounter, antenatal screening Z36.9
Antepartum —see condition
Anterior —see condition
Antero-occlusion M26.220
Anteversion
  cervix —see Anteversion, uterus
  femur (neck), congenital Q65.89
  uterus, uterine (cervix) (postinfectional)
      (postpartal, old) N85.4
    congenital Q51.818
    in pregnancy or childbirth —see Pregnancy,
      complicated by
Anthophobia F40.228
Anthracosilicosis J60
Anthracosis (lung) (occupational) J60
  lingua K14.3
Anthrax A22.9
  with pneumonia A22.1
  cerebral A22.8
  colitis A22.2
  cutaneous A22.0
  gastrointestinal A22.2
  inhalation A22.1
  intestinal A22.2
  meningitis A22.8
  pulmonary A22.1
  respiratory A22.1
  sepsis A22.7
  specified manifestation NEC A22.8
Anthropoid pelvis Q74.2
  with disproportion (fetopelvic) O33.0
Anthropophobia F40.10
  generalized F40.11
Antibodies, maternal (blood group) —see
    Isoimmunization, affecting management of
    pregnancy
  anti-D —see Isoimmunization, affecting
    management of pregnancy, Rh
  newborn P55.0
Antibody
  anticardiolipin R76.0
    with
      hemorrhagic disorder D68.312
      hypercoagulable state D68.61
  antiphosphatidylglycerol R76.0
    with
      hemorrhagic disorder D68.312
      hypercoagulable state D68.61
  antiphosphatidylinositol R76.0
    with
      hemorrhagic disorder D68.312
      hypercoagulable state D68.61
  antiphosphatidylserine R76.0
    with
      hemorrhagic disorder D68.312
      hypercoagulable state D68.61
  antiphospholipid R76.0
    with
      hemorrhagic disorder D68.312
      hypercoagulable state D68.61
Anticardiolipin syndrome D68.61
Anticoagulant, circulating (intrinsic) —see also -
    Disorder, hemorrhagic D68.318
  drug-induced (extrinsic) —see also - Disorder,
    hemorrhagic D68.32
  iatrogenic D68.32
Antidiuretic hormone syndrome E22.2
Antimonial cholera —see Poisoning, antimony
Antiphospholipid
  antibody
    with hemorrhagic disorder D68.312
    syndrome D68.61

Antisocial personality F60.2
Antithrombinemia —see Circulating
    anticoagulants
Antithromboplastinemia D68.318
Antithromboplastinogenemia D68.318
Antitoxin complication or reaction —see
    Complications, vaccination
Antlophobia F40.228
Antritis J32.0
  maxilla J32.0
    acute J01.00
      recurrent J01.01
  stomach K29.50
    with bleeding K29.51
Antrum, antral —see condition
Anuria R34
  calculous (impacted) (recurrent) —see also
    Calculus, urinary N20.9
  following
    abortion —see Abortion by type
      complicated by, renal failure
    ectopic or molar pregnancy O08.4
  newborn P96.0
  postprocedural N99.0
  postrenal N13.8
  traumatic (following crushing) T79.5
Anus, anal —see condition
Anusitis K62.89
Anxiety F41.9
  depression F41.8
  episodic paroxysmal F41.0
  generalized F41.1
  hysteria F41.8
  neurosis F41.1
  panic type F41.0
  reaction F41.1
  separation, abnormal (of childhood) F93.0
  specified NEC F41.8
  state F41.1
Aorta, aortic —see condition
Aortectasia —see Ectasia, aorta
  with aneurysm —see Aneurysm, aorta
Aortitis (nonsyphilitic) (calcific) I77.6
  arteriosclerotic I70.0
  Doehle-Heller A52.02
  luetic A52.02
  rheumatic —see Endocarditis, acute,
    rheumatic
  specific (syphilitic) A52.02
  syphilitic A52.02
    congenital A50.54 [I79.1]
Apathetic thyroid storm —see Thyrotoxicosis
Apathy R45.3
Apeirophobia F40.228
Apepsia K30
  psychogenic F45.8
Aperistalsis, esophagus K22.0
Apertognathia M26.29
Apert's syndrome Q87.0
Aphagia R13.0
  psychogenic F50.9
Aphakia (acquired) (postoperative) H27.0-●
  congenital Q12.3
Aphasia (amnestic) (global) (nominal)
    (semantic) (syntactic) R47.01
  acquired, with epilepsy (Landau-Kleffner
    syndrome) —see Epilepsy,
    specified NEC
  auditory (developmental) F80.2
  developmental (receptive type) F80.2
    expressive type F80.1
    Wernicke's F80.2
  following
    cerebrovascular disease I69.920
      cerebral infarction I69.320
      intracerebral hemorrhage I69.120
      nontraumatic intracranial hemorrhage
        NEC I69.220
      specified disease NEC I69.820
      subarachnoid hemorrhage I69.020

Aphasia (Continued)
➠primary progressive (see also Dementia, in, diseases specified elsewhere) G31.01 [F02.80]
　➠with behavioral disturbance (see also Dementia, in, diseases specified elsewhere) G31.01 [F02.81-●]
➠progressive isolated (see also Dementia, in, diseases specified elsewhere) G31.01 [F02.80]
　➠with behavioral disturbance (see also Dementia, in, diseases specified elsewhere) G31.01 [F02.81-●]
sensory F80.2
syphilis, tertiary A52.19
Wernicke's (developmental) F80.2
Aphonia (organic) R49.1
hysterical F44.4
psychogenic F44.4
Aphthae, aphthous —see also condition
Bednar's K12.0
cachectic K14.0
epizootic B08.8
fever B08.8
oral (recurrent) K12.0
stomatitis (major) (minor) K12.0
thrush B37.0
ulcer (oral) (recurrent) K12.0
genital organ(s) NEC
female N76.6
male N50.89
larynx J38.7
Apical —see condition
Apiphobia F40.218
Aplasia —see also Agenesis
abdominal muscle syndrome Q79.4
alveolar process (acquired) —see Anomaly, alveolar
congenital Q38.6
aorta (congenital) Q25.41
axialis extracorticalis (congenita) E75.29
bone marrow (myeloid) D61.9
congenital D61.01
brain Q00.0
part of Q04.3
bronchus Q32.4
cementum K00.4
cerebellum Q04.3
cervix (congenital) Q51.5
congenital pure red cell D61.01
corpus callosum Q04.0
cutis congenita Q84.8
erythrocyte congenital D61.01
extracortical axial E75.29
eye Q11.1
fovea centralis (congenital) Q14.1
gallbladder, congenital Q44.0
iris Q13.1
labyrinth, membranous Q16.5
limb (congenital) Q73.8
lower —see Defect, reduction, lower limb
upper —see Agenesis, arm
lung, congenital (bilateral) (unilateral) Q33.3
pancreas Q45.0
parathyroid-thymic D82.1
Pelizaeus-Merzbacher E75.29
penis Q55.5
prostate Q55.4
red cell (with thymoma) D60.9
acquired D60.9
due to drugs D60.9
adult D60.9
chronic D60.0
congenital D61.01
constitutional D61.01
due to drugs D60.9
hereditary D61.01
of infants D61.01
primary D61.01
pure D61.01
due to drugs D60.9
specified type NEC D60.8
transient D60.1

Aplasia (Continued)
round ligament Q52.8
skin Q84.8
spermatic cord Q55.4
spleen Q89.01
testicle Q55.0
thymic, with immunodeficiency D82.1
thyroid (congenital) (with myxedema) E03.1
uterus Q51.0
ventral horn cell Q06.1
Apnea, apneic (of) (spells) R06.81
newborn NEC P28.4
obstructive P28.4
sleep (central) (obstructive) (primary) P28.3
▶newborn P28.40
▶central P28.41
▶mixed P28.43
▶obstructive P28.42
▶sleep
▶primary P28.30
▶central P28.31
▶mixed P28.33
▶obstructive P28.32
▶specified NEC P28.39
▶specified NEC P28.49
➠prematurity P28.49
sleep G47.30
central (primary) G47.31
idiopathic G47.31
in conditions classified elsewhere G47.37
obstructive (adult) (pediatric) G47.33
hypopnea G47.33
primary central G47.31
specified NEC G47.39
Apneumatosis, newborn P28.0
Apocrine metaplasia (breast) —see Dysplasia, mammary, specified type NEC
Apophysitis (bone) —see also Osteochondropathy
calcaneus M92.8
juvenile M92.9
Apoplectiform convulsions (cerebral ischemia) I67.82
Apoplexia, apoplexy, apoplectic
adrenal A39.1
heart (auricle) (ventricle) —see Infarct, myocardium
heat T67.01
hemorrhagic (stroke) —see Hemorrhage, intracranial
meninges, hemorrhagic —see Hemorrhage, intracranial, subarachnoid
uremic N18.9 [I68.8]
Appearance
bizarre R46.1
specified NEC R46.89
very low level of personal hygiene R46.0
Appendage
epididymal (organ of Morgagni) Q55.4
intestine (epiploic) Q43.8
preauricular Q17.0
testicular (organ of Morgagni) Q55.29
Appendicitis (pneumococcal) (retrocecal) K37
with
gangrene K35.891
▶with localized peritonitis K35.31
perforation NOS K35.32
peritoneal abscess K35.33
peritonitis NEC K35.33
generalized (with perforation or rupture) K35.20
with abscess K35.21
localized K35.30
with
gangrene K35.32
perforation K35.32
and abscess K35.33
ruptured NOS (with localized peritonitis) K35.32

Appendicitis (Continued)
➠acute (catarrhal) (fulminating) (obstructive) (retrocecal) (suppurative) K35.80
with
gangrene K35.891
peritoneal abscess K35.33
peritonitis NEC K35.33
generalized (with perforation or rupture) K35.20
with abscess K35.21
localized K35.30
with
gangrene K35.32
perforation K35.32
and abscess K35.33
specified NEC K35.890
with gangrene K35.891
▶with localized peritonitis K35.31
amebic A06.89
chronic (recurrent) K36
➠exacerbation —see Appendicitis, with, gangrene
gangrenous —see Appendicitis, acute
healed (obliterative) K36
interval K36
neurogenic K36
obstructive K36
recurrent K36
relapsing K36
ruptured NOS (with localized peritonitis) K35.32
subacute (adhesive) K36
subsiding K36
suppurative —see Appendicitis, acute
tuberculous A18.32
Appendicopathia oxyurica B80
Appendix, appendicular —see also condition
epididymis Q55.4
Morgagni
female Q50.5
male (epididymal) Q55.4
testicular Q55.29
testis Q55.29
Appetite
depraved —see Pica
excessive R63.2
lack or loss —see also Anorexia R63.0
nonorganic origin F50.89
psychogenic F50.89
perverted (hysterical) —see Pica
Apple peel syndrome Q41.1
Apprehension state F41.1
Apprehensiveness, abnormal F41.9
Approximal wear K03.0
Apraxia (classic) (ideational) (ideokinetic) (ideomotor) (motor) (verbal) R48.2
following
cerebrovascular disease I69.990
cerebral infarction I69.390
intracerebral hemorrhage I69.190
nontraumatic intracranial hemorrhage NEC I69.290
specified disease NEC I69.890
subarachnoid hemorrhage I69.090
oculomotor, congenital H51.8
Aptyalism K11.7
Apudoma —see Neoplasm, uncertain behavior, by site
Aqueous misdirection H40.83-●
Arabicum elephantiasis —see Infestation, filarial
Arachnitis —see Meningitis
Arachnodactyly —see Syndrome, Marfan's
Arachnoiditis (acute) (adhesive) (basal) (brain) (cerebrospinal) —see Meningitis
Arachnophobia F40.210
Arboencephalitis, Australian A83.4
Arborization block (heart) I45.5
ARC (AIDS-related complex) B20
Arch
aortic Q25.49
bovine Q25.49

▶ New　➠ Revised　deleted Deleted　● Use Additional Character(s)

Arches —*see* condition
Arcuate uterus Q51.810
Arcuatus uterus Q51.810
Arcus (cornea) senilis —*see* Degeneration, cornea, senile
Arc-welder's lung J63.4
Areflexia R29.2
Areola —*see* condition
Argentaffinoma —*see also* Neoplasm, uncertain behavior, by site
  malignant —*see* Neoplasm, malignant, by site
  syndrome E34.0
Argininemia E72.21
Arginosuccinic aciduria E72.22
Argyll Robertson phenomenon, pupil or syndrome (syphilitic) A52.19
  atypical H57.09
  nonsyphilitic H57.09
Argyria, argyriasis
  conjunctival H11.13-●
  from drug or medicament —*see* Table of Drugs and Chemicals, by substance
Argyrosis, conjunctival H11.13-●
Arhinencephaly Q04.1
Ariboflavinosis E53.0
Arm —*see* condition
Arnold-Chiari disease, obstruction or syndrome (type II) Q07.00
  with
    hydrocephalus Q07.02
      with spina bifida Q07.03
    spina bifida Q07.01
      with hydrocephalus Q07.03
  type III —*see* Encephalocele
  type IV Q04.8
Aromatic amino-acid metabolism disorder E70.9
  specified NEC E70.89
Arousals, confusional G47.51
Arrest, arrested
  cardiac I46.9
    complicating
      abortion —*see* Abortion, by type, complicated by, cardiac arrest
      anesthesia (general) (local) or other sedation —*see* Table of Drugs and Chemicals, by drug
        in labor and delivery O74.2
        in pregnancy O29.11-●
        postpartum, puerperal O89.1
      delivery (cesarean) (instrumental) O75.4
    due to
      cardiac condition I46.2
      specified condition NEC I46.8
    intraoperative I97.71-●
    newborn P29.81
    personal history, successfully resuscitated Z86.74
    postprocedural I97.12-●
      obstetric procedure O75.4
  cardiorespiratory —*see* Arrest, cardiac
  circulatory —*see* Arrest, cardiac
  deep transverse O64.0
  development or growth
    bone —*see* Disorder, bone, development or growth
    child R62.50
    tracheal rings Q32.1
  epiphyseal
    complete
      femur M89.15-●
      humerus M89.12-●
      tibia M89.16-●
      ulna M89.13-●
      forearm M89.13-●
        specified NEC M89.13-●
      ulna —*see* Arrest, epiphyseal, by type, ulna
      lower leg M89.16-●
        specified NEC M89.168
      tibia —*see* Arrest, epiphyseal, by type, tibia

Arrest, arrested (*Continued*)
  epiphyseal (*Continued*)
    partial
      femur M89.15-●
      humerus M89.12-●
      tibia M89.16-●
      ulna M89.13-●
      specified NEC M89.18
    granulopoiesis —*see* Agranulocytosis
    growth plate —*see* Arrest, epiphyseal
  heart —*see* Arrest, cardiac
  legal, anxiety concerning Z65.3
  physeal —*see* Arrest, epiphyseal
  respiratory R09.2
    newborn P28.81
  sinus I45.5
  spermatogenesis (complete) —*see* Azoospermia
    incomplete —*see* Oligospermia
  transverse (deep) O64.0
Arrhenoblastoma
  benign
    specified site —*see* Neoplasm, benign, by site
    unspecified site
      female D27.9
      male D29.20
  malignant
    specified site —*see* Neoplasm, malignant, by site
    unspecified site
      female C56.9
      male C62.90
  specified site —*see* Neoplasm, uncertain behavior, by site
  unspecified site
    female D39.10
    male D40.10
Arrhythmia (auricle)(cardiac) (juvenile)(nodal) (reflex)(supraventricular)(transitory) (ventricle) I49.9
  block I45.9
  extrasystolic I49.49
  newborn
    bradycardia P29.12
      occurring before birth P03.819
        before onset of labor P03.810
        during labor P03.811
    tachycardia P29.11
  psychogenic F45.8
  sinus I49.8
  specified NEC I49.8
  vagal R55
  ventricular re-entry I47.0
Arrillaga-Ayerza syndrome (pulmonary sclerosis with pulmonary hypertension) I27.0
Arsenical pigmentation L81.8
  from drug or medicament —*see* Table of Drugs and Chemicals
Arsenism —*see* Poisoning, arsenic
Arterial —*see* condition
Arteriofibrosis —*see* Arteriosclerosis
Arteriolar sclerosis —*see* Arteriosclerosis
Arteriolith —*see* Arteriosclerosis
Arteriolitis I77.6
  necrotizing, kidney I77.5
  renal —*see* Hypertension, kidney
Arteriolosclerosis —*see* Arteriosclerosis
Arterionephrosclerosis —*see* Hypertension, kidney
Arteriopathy I77.9
  cerebral autosomal dominant, with subcortical infarcts and leukoencephalopathy (CADASIL) I67.850
Arteriosclerosis, arteriosclerotic (diffuse) (obliterans) (of) (senile) (with calcification) I70.90
  with
    chronic limb-threatening ischemia —*see* Arteriosclerosis, with critical limb ischemia

Arteriosclerosis, arteriosclerotic (*Continued*)
  with (*Continued*)
    critical limb ischemia
      bypass graft I70.329
        autologous vein graft I70.429
          leg I70.429
            with
              gangrene (and intermittent claudication, rest pain, and ulcer) I70.469
              rest pain (and intermittent claudication) I70.429
      bilateral I70.423
        with
          gangrene (and intermittent claudication, rest pain, and ulcer) I70.463
          rest pain (and intermittent claudication) I70.423
      left I70.422
        with
          gangrene (and intermittent claudication, rest pain, and ulcer) I70.462
          rest pain (and intermittent claudication) I70.422
          ulceration (and intermittent claudication and rest pain) I70.449
          ankle I70.443
          calf I70.442
          foot site NEC I70.445
          heel I70.444
          lower leg NEC I70.448
          mid foot I70.444
          thigh I70.441
      right I70.421
        with
          gangrene (and intermittent claudication, rest pain, and ulcer) I70.461
          rest pain (and intermittent claudication) I70.421
          ulceration (and intermittent claudication and rest pain) I70.439
          ankle I70.433
          calf I70.432
          foot site NEC I70.435
          heel I70.434
          lower leg NEC I70.438
          midfoot I70.434
          thigh I70.431
    leg I70.329
      with
        gangrene (and intermittent claudication, rest pain, and ulcer) I70.369
        rest pain (and intermittent claudication) I70.329
      bilateral I70.323
        with
          gangrene (and intermittent claudication, rest pain, and ulcer) I70.363
          rest pain (and intermittent claudication) I70.323
      left I70.322
        with
          rest pain (and intermittent claudication) I70.322
          ulceration (and intermittent claudication and rest pain) I70.349
          ankle I70.343
          calf I70.342
          foot site NEC I70.345
          heel I70.344
          lower leg NEC I70.348
          midfoot I70.344
          thigh I70.341

Arteriosclerosis, arteriosclerotic (Continued)
  with (Continued)
    critical limb ischemia (Continued)
      bypass graft (Continued)
        leg (Continued)
          right I70.321
            with
              gangrene (and intermittent
                claudication, rest pain,
                and ulcer) I70.361
              rest pain (and intermittent
                claudication) I70.321
              ulceration (and intermittent
                claudication and rest
                pain) I70.339
                ankle I70.333
                calf I70.332
                foot site NEC I70.335
                heel I70.334
                lower leg NEC I70.338
                midfoot I70.334
                thigh I70.331
        nonautologous biological graft
          I70.529
          leg I70.529
            with
              gangrene (and intermittent
                claudication, rest pain,
                and ulcer) I70.569
              rest pain (and intermittent
                claudication) I70.529
          bilateral I70.523
            with
              gangrene (and intermittent
                claudication, rest pain,
                and ulcer) I70.563
              rest pain (and intermittent
                claudication) I70.523
          left I70.522
            with
              gangrene (and intermittent
                claudication, rest pain,
                and ulcer) I70.562
              rest pain (and intermittent
                claudication) I70.522
              ulceration (and intermittent
                claudication and rest
                pain) I70.549
                ankle I70.543
                calf I70.542
                foot site NEC I70.545
                heel I70.544
                lower leg NEC I70.548
                midfoot I70.544
                thigh I70.541
          right I70.521
            with
              gangrene (and intermittent
                claudication, rest pain,
                and ulcer) I70.561
              rest pain (and intermittent
                claudication) I70.521
              ulceration (and intermittent
                claudication and rest
                pain) I70.539
                ankle I70.533
                calf I70.532
                foot site NEC I70.535
                heel I70.534
                lower leg NEC I70.538
                midfoot I70.534
                thigh I70.531
        nonbiological graft I70.629
          leg I70.629
            with
              gangrene (and intermittent
                claudication, rest pain,
                and ulcer) I70.669
              rest pain (and intermittent
                claudication) I70.629

Arteriosclerosis, arteriosclerotic (Continued)
  with (Continued)
    critical limb ischemia (Continued)
      bypass graft (Continued)
        nonbiological graft (Continued)
          leg (Continued)
            bilateral I70.623
              with
                gangrene (and intermittent
                  claudication, rest pain,
                  and ulcer) I70.663
                rest pain (and intermittent
                  claudication)
                  I70.623
            left I70.622
              with
                gangrene (and intermittent
                  claudication, rest pain,
                  and ulcer) I70.662
                rest pain (and intermittent
                  claudication) I70.622
              ulceration (and intermittent
                claudication and rest
                pain) I70.649
                ankle I70.643
                calf I70.642
                foot site NEC I70.645
                heel I70.644
                lower leg NEC I70.648
                midfoot I70.644
                thigh I70.641
          right I70.621
            with
              gangrene (and intermittent
                claudication, rest pain,
                and ulcer) I70.661
              rest pain (and intermittent
                claudication) I70.621
              ulceration (and intermittent
                claudication and rest
                pain) I70.639
                ankle I70.633
                calf I70.632
                foot site NEC I70.635
                heel I70.634
                lower leg NEC I70.638
                midfoot I70.634
                thigh I70.631
        specified graft NEC I70.729
          leg I70.729
            with
              gangrene (and intermittent
                claudication, rest pain,
                and ulcer) I70.769
              rest pain (and intermittent
                claudication) I70.729
          bilateral I70.723
            with
              gangrene (and intermittent
                claudication, rest pain,
                and ulcer) I70.763
              rest pain (and intermittent
                claudication)
                I70.723
          left I70.722
            with
              gangrene (and intermittent
                claudication, rest pain,
                and ulcer) I70.762
              rest pain (and intermittent
                claudication) I70.722
              ulceration (and intermittent
                claudication and rest
                pain) I70.749
                ankle I70.743
                calf I70.742
                foot site NEC I70.745
                heel I70.744
                lower leg NEC I70.748
                midfoot I70.744
                thigh I70.741

Arteriosclerosis, arteriosclerotic (Continued)
  with (Continued)
    critical limb ischemia (Continued)
      bypass graft (Continued)
        specified graft (Continued)
          leg (Continued)
            right I70.721
              with
                gangrene (and intermittent
                  claudication, rest pain,
                  and ulcer) I70.761
                rest pain (and intermittent
                  claudication) I70.721
              ulceration (and intermittent
                claudication and rest
                pain) I70.739
                ankle I70.733
                calf I70.732
                foot site NEC I70.735
                heel I70.734
                lower leg NEC I70.738
                midfoot I70.734
                thigh I70.731
        leg I70.229
          with
            gangrene (and intermittent
              claudication, rest pain, and
              ulcer) I70.269
            rest pain (and intermittent
              claudication) I70.229
        bilateral I70.223
          with
            gangrene (and intermittent
              claudication, rest pain, and
              ulcer) I70.263
            rest pain (and intermittent
              claudication) I70.223
        left I70.222
          with
            gangrene (and intermittent
              claudication, rest pain, and
              ulcer) I70.262
            rest pain (and intermittent
              claudication) I70.222
            ulceration (and intermittent
              claudication and rest pain)
              I70.249
              ankle I70.243
              calf I70.242
              foot site NEC I70.245
              heel I70.244
              lower leg NEC I70.248
              midfoot I70.244
              thigh I70.241
        right I70.221
          with
            gangrene (and intermittent
              claudication, rest pain, and
              ulcer) I70.261
            rest pain (and intermittent
              claudication) I70.221
            ulceration (and intermittent
              claudication and rest pain)
              I70.239
              ankle I70.233
              calf I70.232
              foot site NEC I70.235
              heel I70.234
              lower leg NEC I70.238
              midfoot I70.234
              thigh I70.231
  aorta I70.0
  arteries of extremities —see Arteriosclerosis,
    extremities
  with
    chronic limb-threatening ischemia —see
      Arteriosclerosis, with critical limb
      ischemia
    critical limb ischemia —see
      Arteriosclerosis, with critical limb
      ischemia

▶ New   ⇒ Revised   ~~deleted~~ Deleted   ● Use Additional Character(s)

Arteriosclerosis, arteriosclerotic *(Continued)*
  brain I67.2
  bypass graft
    with
      chronic limb-threatening ischemia —*see*
        Arteriosclerosis, with critical limb
        ischemia
      critical limb ischemia —*see*
        Arteriosclerosis, with critical limb
        ischemia
      coronary —*see* Arteriosclerosis, coronary,
        bypass graft
      extremities —*see* Arteriosclerosis,
        extremities, bypass graft
  cardiac —*see* Disease, heart, ischemic,
    atherosclerotic
  cardiopathy —*see* Disease, heart, ischemic,
    atherosclerotic
  cardiorenal —*see* Hypertension, cardiorenal
  cardiovascular —*see* Disease, heart, ischemic,
    atherosclerotic
  carotid —*see also* Occlusion, artery, carotid
    I65.2-•
  central nervous system I67.2
  cerebral I67.2
  cerebrovascular I67.2
  coronary (artery) I25.10
    bypass graft I25.810
      with
        angina pectoris I25.709
          with documented spasm
            I25.701
          ▶refractory I25.702
          specified type NEC I25.708
          unstable I25.700
        ischemic chest pain I25.709
      autologous artery I25.810
        with
          angina pectoris I25.729
            with documented spasm
              I25.721
            ▶refractory I25.722
            specified type I25.728
            unstable I25.720
          ischemic chest pain I25.729
      autologous vein I25.810
        with
          angina pectoris I25.719
            with documented spasm I25.711
            ▶refractory I25.712
            specified type I25.718
            unstable I25.710
          ischemic chest pain I25.719
      nonautologous biological I25.810
        with
          angina pectoris I25.739
            with documented spasm I25.731
            ▶refractory I25.732
            specified type I25.738
            unstable I25.730
          ischemic chest pain I25.739
      specified type NEC I25.810
        with
          angina pectoris I25.799
            with documented spasm I25.791
            ▶refractory I25.792
            specified type I25.798
            unstable I25.790
          ischemic chest pain I25.799
    due to
      calcified coronary lesion (severely)
        I25.84
      lipid rich plaque I25.83
    native vessel
      with
        angina pectoris I25.119
          with documented spasm I25.111
          ▶refractory I25.112
          specified type NEC I25.118
          unstable I25.110
        ischemic chest pain I25.119

Arteriosclerosis, arteriosclerotic *(Continued)*
  coronary (artery) *(Continued)*
    transplanted heart I25.811
      bypass graft I25.812
        with
          angina pectoris I25.769
            with documented spasm I25.761
            ▶refractory I25.762
            specified type I25.768
            unstable I25.760
          ischemic chest pain I25.769
    native coronary artery I25.811
      with
        angina pectoris I25.759
          with documented spasm I25.751
          ▶refractory I25.752
          specified type I25.758
          unstable I25.750
        ischemic chest pain I25.759
  extremities (native arteries) I70.209
    with
      chronic limb-threatening ischemia —*see*
        Arteriosclerosis, with critical limb
        ischemia
      critical limb ischemia —*see*
        Arteriosclerosis, with critical limb
        ischemia
    bypass graft I70.309
      with
        chronic limb-threatening ischemia —
          see Arteriosclerosis, with critical
          limb ischemia
        critical limb ischemia —*see*
          Arteriosclerosis, with critical limb
          ischemia
      autologous vein graft I70.409
        leg I70.409
          with
            gangrene (and intermittent
              claudication, rest pain and
              ulcer) I70.469
            intermittent claudication I70.419
            rest pain (and intermittent
              claudication) I70.429
          bilateral I70.403
            with
              gangrene (and intermittent
                claudication, rest pain and
                ulcer) I70.463
              intermittent claudication
                I70.413
              rest pain (and intermittent
                claudication) I70.423
              specified type NEC I70.493
          left I70.402
            with
              gangrene (and intermittent
                claudication, rest pain and
                ulcer) I70.462
              intermittent claudication
                I70.412
              rest pain (and intermittent
                claudication) I70.422
              ulceration (and intermittent
                claudication and rest
                pain) I70.449
              ankle I70.443
              calf I70.442
              foot site NEC I70.445
              heel I70.444
              lower leg NEC I70.448
              midfoot I70.444
              thigh I70.441
              specified type NEC I70.492
          right I70.401
            with
              gangrene (and intermittent
                claudication, rest pain and
                ulcer) I70.461
              intermittent claudication
                I70.411

Arteriosclerosis, arteriosclerotic *(Continued)*
  extremities *(Continued)*
    bypass graft *(Continued)*
      autologous vein graft *(Continued)*
        leg *(Continued)*
          right *(Continued)*
            with
              rest pain (and intermittent
                claudication) I70.421
              ulceration (and intermittent
                claudication and rest
                pain) I70.439
              ankle I70.433
              calf I70.432
              foot site NEC I70.435
              heel I70.434
              lower leg NEC I70.438
              midfoot I70.434
              thigh I70.431
              specified type NEC I70.491
          specified type NEC I70.499
        specified NEC I70.408
          with
            gangrene (and intermittent
              claudication, rest pain and
              ulcer) I70.468
            intermittent claudication
              I70.418
            rest pain (and intermittent
              claudication) I70.428
            ulceration (and intermittent
              claudication and rest pain)
              I70.45
            specified type NEC I70.498
      leg I70.309
        with
          gangrene (and intermittent
            claudication, rest pain and
            ulcer) I70.369
          intermittent claudication I70.319
          rest pain (and intermittent
            claudication) I70.329
        bilateral I70.303
          with
            gangrene (and intermittent
              claudication, rest pain and
              ulcer) I70.363
            intermittent claudication
              I70.313
            rest pain (and intermittent
              claudication) I70.323
            specified type NEC I70.393
        left I70.302
          with
            gangrene (and intermittent
              claudication, rest pain and
              ulcer) I70.362
            intermittent claudication
              I70.312
            rest pain (and intermittent
              claudication) I70.322
            ulceration (and intermittent
              claudication and rest pain)
              I70.349
            ankle I70.343
            calf I70.342
            foot site NEC I70.345
            heel I70.344
            lower leg NEC I70.348
            midfoot I70.344
            thigh I70.341
            specified type NEC I70.392
        right I70.301
          with
            gangrene (and intermittent
              claudication, rest pain and
              ulcer) I70.361
            intermittent claudication
              I70.311
            rest pain (and intermittent
              claudication) I70.321

A

Arteriosclerosis, arteriosclerotic (Continued)
  extremities (Continued)
    bypass graft (Continued)
      leg (Continued)
        right (Continued)
          with (Continued)
            ulceration (and intermittent claudication and rest pain) I70.339
              ankle I70.333
              calf I70.332
              foot site NEC I70.335
              heel I70.334
              lower leg NEC I70.338
              midfoot I70.334
              thigh I70.331
            specified type NEC I70.391
          specified type NEC I70.399
      nonautologous biological graft I70.509
        leg I70.509
          with
            gangrene (and intermittent claudication, rest pain and ulcer) I70.569
            intermittent claudication I70.519
            rest pain (and intermittent claudication) I70.529
          bilateral I70.503
            with
              gangrene (and intermittent claudication, rest pain and ulcer) I70.563
              intermittent claudication I70.513
              rest pain (and intermittent claudication) I70.523
              specified type NEC I70.593
          left I70.502
            with
              gangrene (and intermittent claudication, rest pain and ulcer) I70.562
              intermittent claudication I70.512
              rest pain (and intermittent claudication) I70.522
              ulceration (and intermittent claudication and rest pain) I70.549
                ankle I70.543
                calf I70.542
                foot site NEC I70.545
                heel I70.544
                lower leg NEC I70.548
                midfoot I70.544
                thigh I70.541
            specified type NEC I70.592
          right I70.501
            with
              gangrene (and intermittent claudication, rest pain and ulcer) I70.561
              intermittent claudication I70.511
              rest pain (and intermittent claudication) I70.521
              ulceration (and intermittent claudication and rest pain) I70.539
                ankle I70.533
                calf I70.532
                foot site NEC I70.535
                heel I70.534
                lower leg NEC I70.538
                midfoot I70.534
                thigh I70.531
            specified type NEC I70.591
          specified type NEC I70.599

Arteriosclerosis, arteriosclerotic (Continued)
  extremities (Continued)
    bypass graft (Continued)
      nonautologous biological graft (Continued)
        specified NEC I70.508
          with
            gangrene (and intermittent claudication, rest pain and ulcer) I70.568
            intermittent claudication I70.518
            rest pain (and intermittent claudication) I70.528
            ulceration (and intermittent claudication and rest pain) I70.55
          specified NEC I70.598
      nonbiological graft I70.609
        leg I70.609
          with
            gangrene (and intermittent claudication, rest pain and ulcer) I70.669
            intermittent claudication I70.619
            rest pain (and intermittent claudication) I70.629
          bilateral I70.603
            with
              gangrene (and intermittent claudication, rest pain and ulcer) I70.663
              intermittent claudication I70.613
              rest pain (and intermittent claudication) I70.623
              specified type NEC I70.693
          left I70.602
            with
              gangrene (and intermittent claudication, rest pain and ulcer) I70.662
              intermittent claudication I70.612
              rest pain (and intermittent claudication) I70.622
              ulceration (and intermittent claudication and rest pain) I70.649
                ankle I70.643
                calf I70.642
                foot site NEC I70.645
                heel I70.644
                lower leg NEC I70.648
                midfoot I70.644
                thigh I70.641
            specified type NEC I70.692
          right I70.601
            with
              gangrene (and intermittent claudication, rest pain and ulcer) I70.661
              intermittent claudication I70.611
              rest pain (and intermittent claudication) I70.621
              ulceration (and intermittent claudication and rest pain) I70.639
                ankle I70.633
                calf I70.632
                foot site NEC I70.635
                heel I70.634
                lower leg NEC I70.638
                midfoot I70.634
                thigh I70.631
            specified type NEC I70.691
          specified type NEC I70.699

Arteriosclerosis, arteriosclerotic (Continued)
  extremities (Continued)
    bypass graft (Continued)
      nonbiological graft (Continued)
        specified NEC I70.608
          with
            gangrene (and intermittent claudication, rest pain and ulcer) I70.668
            intermittent claudication I70.618
            rest pain (and intermittent claudication) I70.628
            ulceration (and intermittent claudication and rest pain) I70.65
          specified type NEC I70.698
      specified graft NEC I70.709
        leg I70.709
          with
            gangrene (and intermittent claudication, rest pain and ulcer) I70.769
            intermittent claudication I70.719
            rest pain (and intermittent claudication) I70.729
          bilateral I70.703
            with
              gangrene (and intermittent claudication, rest pain and ulcer) I70.763
              intermittent claudication I70.713
              rest pain (and intermittent claudication) I70.723
              specified type NEC I70.793
          left I70.702
            with
              gangrene (and intermittent claudication, rest pain and ulcer) I70.762
              intermittent claudication I70.712
              rest pain (and intermittent claudication) I70.722
              ulceration (and intermittent claudication and rest pain) I70.749
                ankle I70.743
                calf I70.742
                foot site NEC I70.745
                heel I70.744
                lower leg NEC I70.748
                midfoot I70.744
                thigh I70.741
            specified type NEC I70.792
          right I70.701
            with
              gangrene (and intermittent claudication, rest pain and ulcer) I70.761
              intermittent claudication I70.711
              rest pain (and intermittent claudication) I70.721
              ulceration (and intermittent claudication and rest pain) I70.739
                ankle I70.733
                calf I70.732
                foot site NEC I70.735
                heel I70.734
                lower leg NEC I70.738
                midfoot I70.734
                thigh I70.731
            specified type NEC I70.791
          specified type NEC I70.799
        specified NEC I70.708
          with
            gangrene (and intermittent claudication, rest pain and ulcer) I70.768
            intermittent claudication I70.718

▶ New   ⇒ Revised   ~~deleted~~ Deleted   ● Use Additional Character(s)

Arteriosclerosis, arteriosclerotic *(Continued)*
  extremities *(Continued)*
    bypass graft *(Continued)*
      specified graft NEC *(Continued)*
        leg *(Continued)*
          with *(Continued)*
            rest pain (and intermittent
              claudication) I70.728
            ulceration (and intermittent
              claudication and rest pain)
              I70.75
            specified type NEC I70.798
      specified NEC I70.308
        with
          gangrene (and intermittent
            claudication, rest pain and
            ulcer) I70.368
          intermittent claudication I70.318
          rest pain (and intermittent
            claudication) I70.328
          ulceration (and intermittent
            claudication and rest pain)
            I70.35
        specified type NEC I70.398
    leg I70.209
      with
        gangrene (and intermittent
          claudication, rest pain and ulcer)
          I70.269
        intermittent claudication I70.219
        rest pain (and intermittent
          claudication) I70.229
      bilateral I70.203
        with
          gangrene (and intermittent
            claudication, rest pain and
            ulcer) I70.263
          intermittent claudication I70.213
          rest pain (and intermittent
            claudication) I70.223
        specified type NEC I70.293
      left I70.202
        with
          gangrene (and intermittent
            claudication, rest pain and
            ulcer) I70.262
          intermittent claudication I70.212
          rest pain (and intermittent
            claudication) I70.222
          ulceration (and intermittent
            claudication and rest pain)
            I70.249
            ankle I70.243
            calf I70.242
            foot site NEC I70.245
            heel I70.244
            lower leg NEC I70.248
            midfoot I70.244
            thigh I70.241
        specified type NEC I70.292
      right I70.201
        with
          gangrene (and intermittent
            claudication, rest pain and
            ulcer) I70.261
          intermittent claudication
            I70.211
          rest pain (and intermittent
            claudication) I70.221
          ulceration (and intermittent
            claudication and rest pain)
            I70.239
            ankle I70.233
            calf I70.232
            foot site NEC I70.235
            heel I70.234
            lower leg NEC I70.238
            midfoot I70.234
            thigh I70.231
        specified type NEC I70.291
    specified type NEC I70.299

Arteriosclerosis, arteriosclerotic *(Continued)*
  extremities *(Continued)*
    specified site NEC I70.208
      with
        gangrene (and intermittent claudication,
          rest pain and ulcer) I70.268
        intermittent claudication I70.218
        rest pain (and intermittent
          claudication) I70.228
        ulceration (and intermittent
          claudication and rest pain) I70.25
      specified type NEC I70.298
    generalized I70.91
    heart (disease) —see Arteriosclerosis,
      coronary (artery)
    kidney —see Hypertension, kidney
    medial —see Arteriosclerosis, extremities
    mesenteric (artery) K55.1
    Mönckeberg's —see Arteriosclerosis,
      extremities
    myocarditis I51.4
    peripheral (of extremities) —see
      Arteriosclerosis, extremities
    pulmonary (idiopathic) I27.0
    renal (arterioles) —see also Hypertension,
      kidney
      artery I70.1
    retina (vascular) I70.8 *[H35.0-●]*
    specified artery NEC I70.8
    spinal (cord) G95.19
    vertebral (artery) I67.2
Arteriospasm I73.9
Arteriovenous —see condition
Arteritis I77.6
  allergic M31.0
  aorta (nonsyphilitic) I77.6
    syphilitic A52.02
  aortic arch M31.4
  brachiocephalic M31.4
  brain I67.7
    syphilitic A52.04
  cerebral I67.7
    in
      diseases classified elsewhere I68.2
      systemic lupus erythematosus M32.19
    listerial A32.89
    syphilitic A52.04
    tuberculous A18.89
  coronary (artery) I25.89
    rheumatic I01.8
      chronic I09.89
    syphilitic A52.06
  cranial (left) (right), giant cell M31.6
  deformans —see Arteriosclerosis
  giant cell NEC M31.6
    with polymyalgia rheumatica M31.5
  necrosing or necrotizing M31.9
    specified NEC M31.8
  nodosa M30.0
  obliterans —see Arteriosclerosis
  pulmonary I28.8
  rheumatic —see Fever, rheumatic
  senile —see Arteriosclerosis
  suppurative I77.2
  syphilitic (general) A52.09
    brain A52.04
    coronary A52.06
    spinal A52.09
  temporal, giant cell M31.6
  young female aortic arch syndrome M31.4
Artery, arterial —see also condition
  abscess I77.89
  single umbilical Q27.0
Arthralgia (allergic) —see also Pain, joint
  in caisson disease T70.3
  temporomandibular M26.62
Arthritis, arthritic (acute) (chronic)
  (nonpyogenic) (subacute) M19.90
  allergic —see Arthritis, specified form NEC
  ankylosing (crippling) (spine) —see also
    Spondylitis, ankylosing
    sites other than spine —see Arthritis,
      specified form NEC

Arthritis, arthritic *(Continued)*
  atrophic —see Osteoarthritis
    spine —see Spondylitis, ankylosing
  back —see Spondylopathy, inflammatory
  blennorrhagic (gonococcal) A54.42
  Charcot's —see Arthropathy, neuropathic
    diabetic —see Diabetes, arthropathy,
      neuropathic
    syringomyelic G95.0
  chylous (filarial) —see also category M01 B74.9
  climacteric (any site) NEC —see Arthritis,
    specified form NEC
  crystal (-induced) —see Arthritis, in, crystals
  deformans —see Osteoarthritis
  degenerative —see Osteoarthritis
  due to or associated with
    acromegaly E22.0
    brucellosis —see Brucellosis
    caisson disease T70.3
    diabetes —see Diabetes, arthropathy
    dracontiasis —see also category M01 B72
    enteritis NEC
      regional —see Enteritis, regional
    erysipelas —see also category M01 A46
    erythema
      epidemic A25.1
      nodosum L52
    filariasis NOS B74.9
    glanders A24.0
    helminthiasis —see also category M01 B83.9
    hemophilia D66 *[M36.2]*
    Henoch-(Schönlein) purpura D69.0 *[M36.4]*
    human parvovirus —see also category M01
      B97.6
    infectious disease NEC —see category M01
    leprosy (see also category M01) —see also
      Leprosy A30.9
    Lyme disease A69.23
    mycobacteria —see also category M01 A31.8
    parasitic disease NEC —see also category
      M01 B89
    paratyphoid fever (see also category M01)
      —see also Fever, paratyphoid A01.4
    rat bite fever —see also category M01 A25.1
    regional enteritis —see Enteritis, regional
    respiratory disorder NOS J98.9
    serum sickness —see also Reaction, serum
      T80.69
    syringomyelia G95.0
    typhoid fever A01.04
  epidemic erythema A25.1
  facet joint (see also Spondylosis) M47.819
  febrile —see Fever, rheumatic
  gonococcal A54.42
  gouty (acute) —see Gout
  in (due to)
    acromegaly —see also subcategory
      M14.8-● E22.0
    amyloidosis —see also subcategory
      M14.8-● E85.4
    bacterial disease —see also subcategory
      M01 A49.9
    Behçet's syndrome M35.2
    caisson disease —see also subcategory
      M14.8-● T70.3
    coliform bacilli (Escherichia coli) —see
      Arthritis, in, pyogenic organism NEC
    crystals M11.9
      dicalcium phosphate —see Arthritis, in,
        crystals, specified type NEC
      hydroxyapatite M11.0-●
      pyrophosphate —see Arthritis, in,
        crystals, specified type NEC
      specified type NEC M11.80
        ankle M11.87-●
        elbow M11.82-●
        foot joint M11.87-●
        hand joint M11.84-●
        hip M11.85-●
        knee M11.86-●
        multiple sites M11.8-●

Arthritis, arthritic *(Continued)*
  in *(Continued)*
    crystals *(Continued)*
      specified type *(Continued)*
        shoulder M11.81-•
        vertebrae M11.88
        wrist M11.83-•
    dermatoarthritis, lipoid E78.81
    dracontiasis (dracunculiasis) —*see also*
      category M01 B72
    endocrine disorder NEC —*see also*
      subcategory M14.8-• E34.9
    enteritis, infectious NEC —*see also* category
      M01 A09
      specified organism NEC —*see also*
        category M01 A08.8
    erythema
      multiforme —*see also* subcategory
        M14.8-• L51.9
      nodosum —*see also* subcategory M14.8-•
        L52
    gout —*see* Gout
    helminthiasis NEC —*see also* category M01
      B83.9
    hemochromatosis —*see also* subcategory
      M14.8-• E83.118
    hemoglobinopathy NEC D58.2 *[M36.3]*
    hemophilia NEC D66 *[M36.2]*
    Hemophilus influenzae M00.8-• *[B96.3]*
    Henoch(-Schönlein) purpura D69.0 *[M36.4]*
    hyperparathyroidism NEC —*see also*
      subcategory M14.8-• E21.3
    hypersensitivity reaction NEC T78.49
      [M36.4]
    hypogammaglobulinemia —*see also*
      subcategory M14.8-• D80.1
    hypothyroidism NEC —*see also*
      subcategory M14.8-• E03.9
    infection —*see* Arthritis, pyogenic or
      pyemic
      spine —*see* Spondylopathy, infective
    infectious disease NEC —*see* category M01
    leprosy —*see also* category M01 A30.9
    leukemia NEC C95.9-• *[M36.1]*
    lipoid dermatoarthritis E78.81
    Lyme disease A69.23
    Mediterranean fever, familial —*see also*
      subcategory M14.8-• M04.1
    Meningococcus A39.83
    metabolic disorder NEC —*see also*
      subcategory M14.8-• E88.9
    multiple myelomatosis C90.0-• *[M36.1]*
    mumps B26.85
    mycosis NEC —*see also* category M01 B49
    myelomatosis (multiple) C90.0-• *[M36.1]*
    neurological disorder NEC G98.0
    ochronosis —*see also* subcategory M14.8-•
      E70.29
    O'nyong-nyong —*see also* category M01
      A92.1
    parasitic disease NEC —*see also* category
      M01 B89
    paratyphoid fever —*see also* category M01
      A01.4
    Pseudomonas —*see* Arthritis, pyogenic,
      bacterial NEC
    psoriasis L40.50
    pyogenic organism NEC —*see* Arthritis,
      pyogenic, bacterial NEC
    Reiter's disease —*see* Reiter's disease
    respiratory disorder NEC —*see also*
      subcategory M14.8-• J98.9
    reticulosis, malignant —*see also*
      subcategory M14.8-• C86.0
    rubella B06.82
    Salmonella (arizonae) (cholerae-suis)
      (enteritidis) (typhimurium) A02.23
    sarcoidosis D86.86
    specified bacteria NEC —*see* Arthritis,
      pyogenic, bacterial NEC
    sporotrichosis B42.82

Arthritis, arthritic *(Continued)*
  in *(Continued)*
    syringomyelia G95.0
    thalassemia NEC D56.9 *[M36.3]*
    tuberculosis —*see* Tuberculosis, arthritis
    typhoid fever A01.04
    urethritis, Reiter's —*see* Reiter's disease
    viral disease NEC —*see also* category M01
      B34.9
  infectious or infective —*see also* Arthritis,
    pyogenic or pyemic
    spine —*see* Spondylopathy, infective
  juvenile M08.90
    with systemic onset —*see* Still's disease
    ankle M08.97-•
    elbow M08.92-•
    foot joint M08.97-•
    hand joint M08.94-•
    hip M08.95-•
    knee M08.96-•
    multiple site M08.99
    pauciarticular M08.40
      ankle M08.47-•
      elbow M08.42-•
      foot joint M08.47-•
      hand joint M08.44-•
      hip M08.45-•
      knee M08.46-•
      shoulder M08.41-•
      specified site NEC M08.4A
      vertebrae M08.48
      wrist M08.43-•
    psoriatic L40.54
    rheumatoid —*see* Arthritis, rheumatoid,
      juvenile
    shoulder M08.91-•
    specified site NEC M08.9A
    specified type NEC M08.80
      ankle M08.87-•
      elbow M08.82-•
      foot joint M08.87-•
      hand joint M08.84-•
      hip M08.85-•
      knee M08.86-•
      multiple site M08.89
      shoulder M08.81-•
      specified joint NEC M08.88
      vertebrae M08.88
      wrist M08.83-•
    vertebra M08.98
    wrist M08.93-•
  meaning osteoarthritis —*see* Osteoarthritis
  meningococcal A39.83
  menopausal (any age) NEC —*see* Arthritis,
    specified form NEC
  mutilans (psoriatic) L40.52
  mycotic NEC —*see also* category M01 B49
  neuropathic (Charcot) —*see* Arthropathy,
    neuropathic
    diabetic —*see* Diabetes, arthropathy,
      neuropathic
    nonsyphilitic NEC G98.0
    syringomyelic G95.0
  ochronotic —*see also* subcategory M14.8-•
    E70.29
  palindromic (any site) —*see* Rheumatism,
    palindromic
  pneumococcal M00.10
    ankle M00.17-•
    elbow M00.12-•
    foot joint —*see* Arthritis, pneumococcal,
      ankle
    hand joint M00.14-•
    hip M00.15-•
    knee M00.16-•
    multiple site M00.19
    shoulder M00.11-•
    vertebra M00.18
    wrist M00.13-•
  postdysenteric —*see* Arthropathy,
    postdysenteric

Arthritis, arthritic *(Continued)*
  postmeningococcal A39.84
  postrheumatic, chronic —*see* Arthropathy,
    postrheumatic, chronic
  primary progressive —*see also* Arthritis,
    specified form NEC
    spine —*see* Spondylitis, ankylosing
  psoriatic L40.50
  purulent (any site except spine) —*see*
    Arthritis, pyogenic or pyemic
    spine —*see* Spondylopathy, infective
  pyogenic or pyemic (any site except spine)
    M00.9
    bacterial NEC M00.80
      ankle M00.87-•
      elbow M00.82-•
      foot joint —*see* Arthritis, pyogenic,
        bacterial NEC, ankle
      hand joint M00.84-•
      hip M00.85-•
      knee M00.86-•
      multiple site M00.89
      shoulder M00.81-•
      vertebra M00.88
      wrist M00.83-•
    pneumococcal —*see* Arthritis,
      pneumococcal
    spine —*see* Spondylopathy, infective
    staphylococcal —*see* Arthritis,
      staphylococcal
    streptococcal —*see* Arthritis, streptococcal
      NEC
      pneumococcal —*see* Arthritis,
        pneumococcal
  reactive —*see* Reiter's disease
  rheumatic —*see also* Arthritis, rheumatoid
    acute or subacute —*see* Fever, rheumatic
  rheumatoid M06.9
    with
      carditis —*see* Rheumatoid, carditis
      endocarditis —*see* Rheumatoid, carditis
      heart involvement NEC —*see*
        Rheumatoid, carditis
      lung involvement —*see* Rheumatoid, lung
      myocarditis —*see* Rheumatoid, carditis
      myopathy —*see* Rheumatoid, myopathy
      pericarditis —*see* Rheumatoid, carditis
      polyneuropathy —*see* Rheumatoid,
        polyneuropathy
      rheumatoid factor —*see* Arthritis,
        rheumatoid, seropositive
      splenoadenomegaly and leukopenia —
        see Felty's syndrome
      vasculitis —*see* Rheumatoid, vasculitis
      visceral involvement NEC —*see*
        Rheumatoid, arthritis, with
        involvement of organs NEC
    juvenile (with or without rheumatoid
      factor) M08.00
      with systemic onset —*see* Still's disease
      ankle M08.07-•
      elbow M08.02-•
      foot joint M08.07-•
      hand joint M08.04-•
      hip M08.05-•
      knee M08.06-•
      multiple site M08.09
      shoulder M08.01-•
      specified site NEC M08.0A
      vertebra M08.08
      wrist M08.03-•
    seronegative M06.00
      ankle M06.07-•
      elbow M06.02-•
      foot joint M06.07-•
      hand joint M06.04-•
      hip M06.05-•
      knee M06.06-•
      multiple sites M06.09
      shoulder M06.01-•
      specified site NEC M06.0A
      vertebra M06.08
      wrist M06.03-•

▶ New   ⇒ Revised   ~~deleted~~ Deleted   • Use Additional Character(s)

Arthritis, arthritic (Continued)
  rheumatoid (Continued)
    seropositive M05.9
      without organ involvement M05.70
        ankle M05.77- ●
        elbow M05.72- ●
        foot joint M05.77- ●
        hand joint M05.74- ●
        hip M05.75- ●
        knee M05.76- ●
        multiple sites M05.79
        shoulder M05.71- ●
        specified site NEC M05.7A
        vertebra —see Spondylitis, ankylosing
        wrist M05.73- ●
    specified NEC M05.80
      ankle M05.87- ●
      elbow M05.82- ●
      foot joint M05.87- ●
      hand joint M05.84- ●
      hip M05.85- ●
      knee M05.86- ●
      multiple sites M05.89
      specified site NEC M05.8A
      shoulder M05.81- ●
      vertebra —see Spondylitis, ankylosing
      wrist M05.83- ●
    specified type NEC M06.80
      ankle M06.87- ●
      elbow M06.82- ●
      foot joint M06.87- ●
      hand joint M06.84- ●
      hip M06.85- ●
      knee M06.86- ●
      multiple site M06.89
      shoulder M06.81- ●
      specified site NEC M06.8A
      vertebra M06.88
      wrist M06.83- ●
    spine —see Spondylitis, ankylosing
  rubella B06.82
  scorbutic —see also subcategory M14.8- ● E54
  senile or senescent —see Osteoarthritis
  septic (any site except spine) —see Arthritis,
      pyogenic or pyemic
    spine —see Spondylopathy, infective
  serum (nontherapeutic) (therapeutic) —see
      Arthropathy, postimmunization
  specified form NEC M13.80
    ankle M13.87- ●
    elbow M13.82- ●
    foot joint M13.87- ●
    hand joint M13.84- ●
    hip M13.85- ●
    knee M13.86- ●
    multiple site M13.89
    shoulder M13.81- ●
    specified joint NEC M13.88
    wrist M13.83- ●
  spine —see also Spondylosis
    infectious or infective NEC —see
        Spondylopathy, infective
    Marie-Strümpell —see Spondylitis,
        ankylosing
    pyogenic —see Spondylopathy, infective
    rheumatoid —see Spondylitis, ankylosing
    traumatic (old) —see Spondylopathy,
        traumatic
    tuberculous A18.01
  staphylococcal M00.00
    ankle M00.07- ●
    elbow M00.02- ●
    foot joint —see Arthritis, staphylococcal,
        ankle
    hand joint M00.04- ●
    hip M00.05- ●
    knee M00.06- ●
    multiple site M00.09
    shoulder M00.01- ●
    vertebra M00.08
    wrist M00.03- ●

Arthritis, arthritic (Continued)
  streptococcal NEC M00.20
    ankle M00.27- ●
    elbow M00.22- ●
    foot joint —see Arthritis, streptococcal,
        ankle
    hand joint M00.24- ●
    hip M00.25- ●
    knee M00.26- ●
    multiple site M00.29
    shoulder M00.21- ●
    vertebra M00.28
    wrist M00.23- ●
  suppurative —see Arthritis, pyogenic or
      pyemic
  syphilitic (late) A52.16
    congenital A50.55 [M12.80]
  syphilitica deformans (Charcot) A52.16
  temporomandibular joint M26.65- ●
  toxic of menopause (any site) —see Arthritis,
      specified form NEC
  transient —see Arthropathy, specified form
      NEC
  traumatic (chronic) —see Arthropathy,
      traumatic
  tuberculous A18.02
    spine A18.01
  uratic —see Gout
  urethritica (Reiter's) —see Reiter's disease
  vertebral —see Spondylopathy, inflammatory
  villous (any site) —see Arthropathy, specified
      form NEC
Arthrocele —see Effusion, joint
Arthrodesis status Z98.1
Arthrodynia —see also Pain, joint
Arthrodysplasia Q74.9
Arthrofibrosis, joint —see Ankylosis
Arthrogryposis (congenital) Q68.8
  multiplex congenita Q74.3
Arthrokatadysis M24.7
Arthropathy (see also Arthritis) M12.9
  Charcot's —see Arthropathy, neuropathic
    diabetic —see Diabetes, arthropathy,
        neuropathic
    syringomyelic G95.0
  cricoarytenoid J38.7
  crystal(-induced) —see Arthritis, in, crystals
  diabetic NEC —see Diabetes, arthropathy
  distal interphalangeal, psoriatic L40.51
  enteropathic M07.60
    ankle M07.67- ●
    elbow M07.62- ●
    foot joint M07.67- ●
    hand joint M07.64- ●
    hip M07.65- ●
    knee M07.66- ●
    multiple site M07.69
    shoulder M07.61- ●
    vertebra M07.68
    wrist M07.63- ●
  facet joint (see also Spondylosis) M47.819
  following intestinal bypass M02.00
    ankle M02.07- ●
    elbow M02.02- ●
    foot joint M02.07- ●
    hand joint M02.04- ●
    hip M02.05- ●
    knee M02.06- ●
    multiple site M02.09
    shoulder M02.01- ●
    vertebra M02.08
    wrist M02.03- ●
  gouty —see also Gout
    in (due to)
      Lesch-Nyhan syndrome E79.1 [M14.8-●]
      sickle-cell disorders D57- ● [M14.8-●]
  hemophilic NEC D66 [M36.2]
    in (due to)
      hyperparathyroidism NEC E21.3
          [M14.8-●]
      metabolic disease NOS E88.9 [M14.8-●]

Arthropathy (Continued)
  in (due to)
    acromegaly E22.0 [M14.8-●]
    amyloidosis E85.4 [M14.8-●]
    blood disorder NOS D75.9 [M36.3]
    diabetes —see Diabetes, arthropathy
    endocrine disease NOS E34.9 [M14.8-●]
    erythema
      multiforme L51.9 [M14.8-●]
      nodosum L52 [M14.8-●]
    hemochromatosis E83.118 [M14.8-●]
    hemoglobinopathy NEC D58.2 [M36.3]
    hemophilia NEC D66 [M36.2]
    Henoch-Schönlein purpura D69.0 [M36.4]
    hyperthyroidism E05.90 [M14.8-●]
    hypothyroidism E03.9 [M14.8-●]
    infective endocarditis I33.0 [M12.80]
    leukemia NEC C95.9- ● [M36.1]
    malignant histiocytosis C96.A [M36.1]
    metabolic disease NOS E88.9 [M14.8-●]
    multiple myeloma C90.0- ● [M36.1]
    neoplastic disease NOS (see also Neoplasm)
        D49.9 [M36.1]
    nutritional deficiency —see also
        subcategory M14.8- ● E63.9
    psoriasis NOS L40.50
    sarcoidosis D86.86
    syphilis (late) A52.77
      congenital A50.55 [M12.80]
    thyrotoxicosis —see also subcategory
        M14.8- ● E05.90
    ulcerative colitis K51.90 [M07.60]
    viral hepatitis (postinfectious) NEC B19.9
        [M12.80]
    Whipple's disease —see also subcategory
        M14.8- ● K90.81
  Jaccoud —see Arthropathy, postrheumatic,
      chronic
  juvenile —see Arthritis, juvenile
    psoriatic L40.54
  mutilans (psoriatic) L40.52
  neuropathic (Charcot) M14.60
    ankle M14.67- ●
    diabetic —see Diabetes, arthropathy,
        neuropathic
    elbow M14.62- ●
    foot joint M14.67- ●
    hand joint M14.64- ●
    hip M14.65- ●
    knee M14.66- ●
    multiple site M14.69
    nonsyphilitic NEC G98.0
    shoulder M14.61- ●
    syringomyelic G95.0
    vertebra M14.68
    wrist M14.63- ●
  osteopulmonary —see Osteoarthropathy,
      hypertrophic, specified NEC
  postdysenteric M02.10
    ankle M02.17- ●
    elbow M02.12- ●
    foot joint M02.17- ●
    hand joint M02.14- ●
    hip M02.15- ●
    knee M02.16- ●
    multiple site M02.19
    shoulder M02.11- ●
    vertebra M02.18
    wrist M02.13- ●
  postimmunization M02.20
    ankle M02.27- ●
    elbow M02.22- ●
    foot joint M02.27- ●
    hand joint M02.24- ●
    hip M02.25- ●
    knee M02.26- ●
    multiple site M02.29
    shoulder M02.21- ●
    vertebra M02.28
    wrist M02.23- ●

Arthropathy (Continued)
  postinfectious NEC B99 [M12.80]
    in (due to)
      enteritis due to Yersinia enterocolitica
        A04.6 [M12.80]
      syphilis A52.77
      viral hepatitis NEC B19.9 [M12.80]
  postrheumatic, chronic (Jaccoud) M12.00
    ankle M12.07-●
    elbow M12.02-●
    foot joint M12.07-●
    hand joint M12.04-●
    hip M12.05-●
    knee M12.06-●
    multiple site M12.09
    shoulder M12.01-●
    specified joint NEC M12.08
    vertebrae M12.08
    wrist M12.03-●
  psoriatic NEC L40.59
    interphalangeal, distal L40.51
  reactive M02.9
    in (due to)
      infective endocarditis I33.0 [M02.9]
    specified type NEC M02.80
      ankle M02.87-●
      elbow M02.82-●
      foot joint M02.87-●
      hand joint M02.84-●
      hip M02.85-●
      knee M02.86-●
      multiple site M02.89
      shoulder M02.81-●
      vertebra M02.88
      wrist M02.83-●
  specified form NEC M12.80
    ankle M12.87-●
    elbow M12.82-●
    foot joint M12.87-●
    hand joint M12.84-●
    hip M12.85-●
    knee M12.86-●
    multiple site M12.89
    shoulder M12.81-●
    specified joint NEC M12.88
    vertebrae M12.88
    wrist M12.83-●
  syringomyelic G95.0
  tabes dorsalis A52.16
  tabetic A52.16
  temporomandibular joint M26.65-●
  transient —see Arthropathy, specified form
    NEC
  traumatic M12.50
    ankle M12.57-●
    elbow M12.52-●
    foot joint M12.57-●
    hand joint M12.54-●
    hip M12.55-●
    knee M12.56-●
    multiple site M12.59
    shoulder M12.51-●
    specified joint NEC M12.58
    vertebrae M12.58
    wrist M12.53-●
Arthropyosis —see Arthritis, pyogenic or
  pyemic
Arthrosis (deformans) (degenerative)
  (localized) —see also Osteoarthritis M19.90
  spine —see Spondylosis
Arthus' phenomenon or reaction T78.41
  due to
    drug —see Table of Drugs and Chemicals,
      by drug
Articular —see condition
Articulation, reverse (teeth) M26.24
Artificial
  insemination complication —see
    Complications, artificial, fertilization
  opening status (functioning) (without
    complication) Z93.9

Artificial (Continued)
  opening status (functioning) (without
    complication) (Continued)
    anus (colostomy) Z93.3
    colostomy Z93.3
    cystostomy Z93.50
      appendico-vesicostomy Z93.52
      cutaneous Z93.51
      specified NEC Z93.59
    enterostomy Z93.4
    gastrostomy Z93.1
    ileostomy Z93.2
    intestinal tract NEC Z93.4
    jejunostomy Z93.4
    nephrostomy Z93.6
    specified site NEC Z93.8
    tracheostomy Z93.0
    ureterostomy Z93.6
    urethrostomy Z93.6
    urinary tract NEC Z93.6
    vagina Z93.8
  vagina status Z93.8
Arytenoid —see condition
Asbestosis (occupational) J61
ASC-H (atypical squamous cells cannot exclude
    high grade squamous intraepithelial lesion
    on cytologic smear)
  anus R85.611
  cervix R87.611
  vagina R87.621
ASC-US (atypical squamous cells of
    undetermined significance on cytologic
    smear)
  anus R85.610
  cervix R87.610
  vagina R87.620
Ascariasis B77.9
  with
    complications NEC B77.89
    intestinal complications B77.0
    pneumonia, pneumonitis B77.81
Ascaridosis, ascaridiasis —see Ascariasis
Ascaris (infection) (infestation)
    (lumbricoides) —see Ascariasis
Ascending —see condition
Aschoff's bodies —see Myocarditis, rheumatic
Ascites (abdominal) R18.8
  cardiac —see also Failure, heart, right I50.810
  chylous (nonfilarial) I89.8
    filarial —see Infestation, filarial
  due to
    cirrhosis, alcoholic K70.31
    hepatitis
      alcoholic K70.11
      chronic active K71.51
    S. japonicum B65.2
  heart —see also Failure, heart, right I50.810
  malignant R18.0
  pseudochylous R18.8
  syphilitic A52.74
  tuberculous A18.31
Aseptic —see condition
Asherman's syndrome N85.6
Asialia K11.7
Asiatic cholera —see Cholera
Asimultagnosia (simultanagnosia) R48.3
Askin's tumor —see Neoplasm, connective
    tissue, malignant
Asocial personality F60.2
Asomatognosia R41.4
Aspartylglucosaminuria E77.1
Asperger's disease or syndrome F84.5
Aspergilloma —see Aspergillosis
Aspergillosis (with pneumonia) B44.9
  bronchopulmonary, allergic B44.81
  disseminated B44.7
  generalized B44.7
  pulmonary NEC B44.1
    allergic B44.81
    invasive B44.0
  specified NEC B44.89
  tonsillar B44.2

Aspergillus (flavus) (fumigatus) (infection)
    (terreus) —see Aspergillosis
Aspermatogenesis —see Azoospermia
Aspermia (testis) —see Azoospermia
Asphyxia, asphyxiation (by) R09.01
  antenatal P84
  birth P84
  bunny bag —see Asphyxia, due to,
    mechanical threat to breathing, trapped
    in bed clothes
  crushing S28.0
  drowning T75.1
  gas, fumes, or vapor —see Table of Drugs and
    Chemicals
  inhalation —see Inhalation
  intrauterine P84
  local I73.00
    with gangrene I73.01
  mucus —see also Foreign body, respiratory
    tract, causing asphyxia
  newborn P84
  pathological R09.01
  postnatal P84
    mechanical —see Asphyxia, due to,
      mechanical threat to breathing
  prenatal P84
  reticularis R23.1
  strangulation —see Asphyxia, due to,
    mechanical threat to breathing
  submersion T75.1
  traumatic T71.9
    due to
      crushed chest S28.0
      foreign body (in) —see Foreign body,
        respiratory tract, causing asphyxia
      low oxygen content of ambient air
        T71.20
        due to
          being trapped in
            low oxygen environment
              T71.29
            in car trunk T71.221
              circumstances undetermined
                T71.224
              done with intent to harm by
                another person T71.223
              self T71.222
            in refrigerator T71.231
              circumstances undetermined
                T71.234
              done with intent to
                harm by
                another person T71.233
              self T71.232
          cave-in T71.21
      mechanical threat to breathing
        (accidental) T71.191
        circumstances undetermined T71.194
        done with intent to harm by
          another person T71.193
        self T71.192
        hanging T71.161
          circumstances undetermined
            T71.164
          done with intent to harm by
            another person T71.163
          self T71.162
        plastic bag T71.121
          circumstances undetermined
            T71.124
          done with intent to harm by
            another person T71.123
          self T71.122
        smothering
          in furniture T71.151
            circumstances undetermined
              T71.154
            done with intent to harm by
              another person T71.153
            self T71.152

▶ New   ⇒ Revised   ~~deleted~~ Deleted   ● Use Additional Character(s)

Asphyxia, asphyxiation (by) (Continued)
  traumatic (Continued)
    due to (Continued)
      mechanical threat to breathing
          (Continued)
        smothering (Continued)
          under
            another person's body T71.141
              circumstances undetermined
                  T71.144
              done with intent to harm
                  T71.143
            pillow T71.111
              circumstances undetermined
                  T71.114
              done with intent to harm by
                  another person T71.113
              self T71.112
          trapped in bed clothes T71.131
            circumstances undetermined
                T71.134
            done with intent to harm by
                another person T71.133
            self T71.132
  vomiting, vomitus —see Foreign body,
      respiratory tract, causing asphyxia
Aspiration
  amniotic (clear) fluid (newborn) P24.10
    with
      pneumonia (pneumonitis) P24.11
      respiratory symptoms P24.11
  blood
    newborn (without respiratory symptoms)
        P24.20
      with
        pneumonia (pneumonitis) P24.21
        respiratory symptoms P24.21
    specified age NEC —see Foreign body,
        respiratory tract
  bronchitis J69.0
  food or foreign body —see Foreign body,
      by site
  liquor (amnii) (newborn) P24.10
    with
      pneumonia (pneumonitis) P24.11
      respiratory symptoms P24.11
  meconium (newborn) (without respiratory
      symptoms) P24.00
    with
      pneumonitis (pneumonitis) P24.01
      respiratory symptoms P24.01
  milk (newborn) (without respiratory
      symptoms) P24.30
    with
      pneumonia (pneumonitis) P24.31
      respiratory symptoms P24.31
    specified age NEC —see Foreign body,
        respiratory tract
  mucus —see also Foreign body, by site,
      causing asphyxia
    newborn P24.10
      with
        pneumonia (pneumonitis) P24.11
        respiratory symptoms P24.11
  neonatal P24.9
    specific NEC (without respiratory
        symptoms) P24.80
      with
        pneumonia (pneumonitis) P24.81
        respiratory symptoms P24.81
  newborn P24.9
    specific NEC (without respiratory
        symptoms) P24.80
      with
        pneumonia (pneumonitis) P24.81
        respiratory symptoms P24.81
  pneumonia J69.0
  pneumonitis J69.0
  syndrome of newborn —see Aspiration, by
      substance, with pneumonia

Aspiration (Continued)
  vernix caseosa (newborn) P24.80
    with
      pneumonia (pneumonitis) P24.81
      respiratory symptoms P24.81
  vomitus —see also Foreign body, respiratory
      tract
    newborn (without respiratory symptoms)
        P24.30
      with
        pneumonia (pneumonitis) P24.31
        respiratory symptoms P24.31
Asplenia (congenital) Q89.01
  postsurgical Z90.81
Assam fever B55.0
Assault, sexual —see Maltreatment
Assmann's focus NEC A15.0
Astasia (-abasia) (hysterical) F44.4
Asteatosis cutis L85.3
Astereognosia, astereognosis R48.1
Asterixis R27.8
  in liver disease K71.3
Asteroid hyalitis —see Deposit, crystalline
Asthenia, asthenic R53.1
  cardiac —see also Failure, heart I50.9
    psychogenic F45.8
  cardiovascular —see also Failure, heart I50.9
    psychogenic F45.8
  heart —see also Failure, heart I50.9
    psychogenic F45.8
  hysterical F44.4
  myocardial —see also Failure, heart I50.9
    psychogenic F45.8
  nervous F48.8
  neurocirculatory F45.8
  neurotic F48.8
  psychogenic F48.8
  psychoneurotic F48.8
  psychophysiologic F48.8
  reaction (psychophysiologic) F48.8
  senile R54
Asthenopia —see also Discomfort, visual
  hysterical F44.6
  psychogenic F44.6
Asthenospermia —see Abnormal, specimen,
    male genital organs
Asthma, asthmatic (bronchial) (catarrh)
    (spasmodic) J45.909
  with
    chronic obstructive bronchitis J44.9
      with
        acute lower respiratory infection
            J44.0
        exacerbation (acute) J44.1
    chronic obstructive pulmonary disease
        J44.9
      with
        acute lower respiratory infection
            J44.0
        exacerbation (acute) J44.1
    exacerbation (acute) J45.901
    hay fever —see Asthma, allergic extrinsic
    rhinitis, allergic —see Asthma, allergic
        extrinsic
    status asthmaticus J45.902
  allergic extrinsic J45.909
    with
      exacerbation (acute) J45.901
      status asthmaticus J45.902
  atopic —see Asthma, allergic extrinsic
  cardiac —see Failure, ventricular, left
  cardiobronchial I50.1
  childhood J45.909
    with
      exacerbation (acute) J45.901
      status asthmaticus J45.902
  chronic obstructive J44.9
    with
      acute lower respiratory infection J44.0
      exacerbation (acute) J44.1
  collier's J60

Asthma, asthmatic (Continued)
  cough variant J45.991
  detergent J69.8
  due to
    detergent J69.8
    inhalation of fumes J68.3
  eosinophilic J82.83
  extrinsic, allergic —see Asthma, allergic
      extrinsic
  grinder's J62.8
  hay —see Asthma, allergic extrinsic
  heart I50.1
  idiosyncratic —see Asthma, nonallergic
  intermittent (mild) J45.20
    with
      exacerbation (acute) J45.21
      status asthmaticus J45.22
  intrinsic, nonallergic —see Asthma,
      nonallergic
  Kopp's E32.8
  late-onset J45.909
    with
      exacerbation (acute) J45.901
      status asthmaticus J45.902
  mild intermittent J45.20
    with
      exacerbation (acute) J45.21
      status asthmaticus J45.22
  mild persistent J45.30
    with
      exacerbation (acute) J45.31
      status asthmaticus J45.32
  Millar's (laryngismus stridulus) J38.5
  miner's J60
  mixed J45.909
    with
      exacerbation (acute) J45.901
      status asthmaticus J45.902
  moderate persistent J45.40
    with
      exacerbation (acute) J45.41
      status asthmaticus J45.42
  nervous —see Asthma, nonallergic
  nonallergic (intrinsic) J45.909
    with
      exacerbation (acute) J45.901
      status asthmaticus J45.902
  persistent
    mild J45.30
      with
        exacerbation (acute) J45.31
        status asthmaticus J45.32
    moderate J45.40
      with
        exacerbation (acute) J45.41
        status asthmaticus J45.42
    severe J45.50
      with
        exacerbation (acute) J45.51
        status asthmaticus J45.52
  platinum J45.998
  pneumoconiotic NEC J64
  potter's J62.8
  predominantly allergic J45.909
  psychogenic F54
  pulmonary eosinophilic J82.83
  red cedar J67.8
  Rostan's I50.1
  sandblaster's J62.8
  sequoiosis J67.8
  severe persistent J45.50
    with
      exacerbation (acute) J45.51
      status asthmaticus J45.52
  specified NEC J45.998
  stonemason's J62.8
  thymic E32.8
  tuberculous —see Tuberculosis, pulmonary
  Wichmann's (laryngismus stridulus) J38.5
  wood J67.8

Astigmatism (compound) (congenital)
H52.20-●
irregular H52.21-●
regular H52.22-●
Astraphobia F40.220
Astroblastoma
specified site —see Neoplasm, malignant, by
site
unspecified site C71.9
Astrocytoma (cystic)
anaplastic
specified site —see Neoplasm, malignant,
by site
unspecified site C71.9
fibrillary
specified site —see Neoplasm, malignant,
by site
unspecified site C71.9
fibrous
specified site —see Neoplasm, malignant,
by site
unspecified site C71.9
gemistocytic
specified site —see Neoplasm, malignant,
by site
unspecified site C71.9
juvenile
specified site —see Neoplasm, malignant,
by site
unspecified site C71.9
pilocytic
specified site —see Neoplasm, malignant,
by site
unspecified site C71.9
piloid
specified site —see Neoplasm, malignant,
by site
unspecified site C71.9
protoplasmic
specified site —see Neoplasm, malignant,
by site
unspecified site C71.9
specified site NEC —see Neoplasm,
malignant, by site
subependymal D43.2
giant cell
specified site —see Neoplasm, uncertain
behavior, by site
unspecified site D43.2
specified site —see Neoplasm, uncertain
behavior, by site
unspecified site D43.2
unspecified site C71.9
Astroglioma
specified site —see Neoplasm, malignant, by
site
unspecified site C71.9
Asymbolia R48.8
Asymmetry —see also Distortion
between native and reconstructed breast N65.1
face Q67.0

jaw (lower) —see Anomaly, dentofacial, jaw-
cranial base relationship, asymmetry
Asynergia, asynergy R27.8
ventricular I51.89
Asystole (heart) —see Arrest, cardiac
At risk
for
dental caries Z91.849
high Z91.843
low Z91.841
moderate Z91.842
falling Z91.81
Ataxia, ataxy, ataxic R27.0
acute R27.8
autosomal recessive Friedreich G11.11
brain (hereditary) G11.9
cerebellar (hereditary) G11.9
with defective DNA repair G11.3
alcoholic G31.2

Ataxia, ataxy, ataxic (Continued)
cerebellar (hereditary) (Continued)
early-onset G11.10
with
essential tremor G11.19
myoclonus [Hunt's ataxia] G11.19
retained tendon reflexes G11.19
in
alcoholism G31.2
myxedema E03.9 [G13.2]
neoplastic disease —see also Neoplasm
D49.9 [G32.81]
specified disease NEC G32.81
late-onset (Marie's) G11.2
cerebral (hereditary) G11.9
congenital nonprogressive G11.0
family, familial —see Ataxia, hereditary
following
cerebrovascular disease I69.993
cerebral infarction I69.393
intracerebral hemorrhage I69.193
nontraumatic intracranial hemorrhage
NEC I69.293
specified disease NEC I69.893
subarachnoid hemorrhage I69.093
Friedreich's (heredofamilial) (cerebellar)
(spinal) G11.11
gait R26.0
hysterical F44.4
general R27.8
gluten M35.9 [G32.81]
with celiac disease K90.0 [G32.81]
hereditary G11.9
with neuropathy G60.2
cerebellar —see Ataxia, cerebellar
spastic G11.4
specified NEC G11.8
spinal (Friedreich's) G11.11
heredofamilial —see Ataxia, hereditary
Hunt's G11.19
hysterical F44.4
locomotor (progressive) (syphilitic) (partial)
(spastic) A52.11
diabetic —see Diabetes, ataxia
Ataxia, ataxy, ataxic (Continued)
Marie's (cerebellar) (heredofamilial)
(late- onset) G11.2
nonorganic origin F44.4
nonprogressive, congenital G11.0
psychogenic F44.4
Roussy-Lévy G60.0
Sanger-Brown's (hereditary) G11.2
spastic hereditary G11.4
spinal
hereditary (Friedreich's) G11.11
progressive (syphilitic) A52.11
spinocerebellar, X-linked recessive G11.19
telangiectasia (Louis-Bar) G11.3
Ataxia-telangiectasia (Louis-Bar) G11.3
Atelectasis (massive) (partial) (pressure)
(pulmonary) J98.11
newborn P28.10
due to resorption P28.11
partial P28.19
primary P28.0
secondary P28.19
primary (newborn) P28.0
tuberculous —see Tuberculosis, pulmonary
Atelocardia Q24.9
Atelomyelia Q06.1
Atheroembolism
of
extremities
lower I75.02-●
upper I75.01-●
kidney I75.81
specified NEC I75.89
Atheroma, atheromatous —see also
Arteriosclerosis I70.90
aorta, aortic I70.0
valve —see also Endocarditis, aortic I35.8

Atheroma, atheromatous (Continued)
aorto-iliac I70.0
artery —see Arteriosclerosis
basilar (artery) I67.2
carotid (artery) (common) (internal) I67.2
cerebral (arteries) I67.2
coronary (artery) I25.10
with angina pectoris —see Arteriosclerosis,
coronary (artery)
degeneration —see Arteriosclerosis
heart, cardiac —see Disease, heart, ischemic,
atherosclerotic
mitral (valve) I34.89
myocardium, myocardial —see Disease, heart,
ischemic, atherosclerotic
pulmonary valve (heart) —see also
Endocarditis, pulmonary I37.8
tricuspid (heart) (valve) I36.8
valve, valvular —see Endocarditis
vertebral (artery) I67.2
Atheromatosis —see Arteriosclerosis
Atherosclerosis —see also Arteriosclerosis
coronary
artery I25.10
with angina pectoris —see
Arteriosclerosis, coronary (artery),
due to
calcified coronary lesion (severely)
I25.84
lipid rich plaque I25.83
transplanted heart I25.811
bypass graft I25.812
with angina pectoris —see
Arteriosclerosis, coronary (artery)
native coronary artery I25.811
with angina pectoris —see
Arteriosclerosis, coronary (artery)
Athetosis (acquired) R25.8
bilateral (congenital) G80.3
congenital (bilateral) (double) G80.3
double (congenital) G80.3
unilateral R25.8
Athlete's
foot B35.3
heart I51.7
Athrepsia E41
Athyrea (acquired) —see also Hypothyroidism
congenital E03.1
Atonia, atony, atonic
bladder (sphincter) (neurogenic) N31.2
capillary I78.8
cecum K59.89
psychogenic F45.8
colon —see Atony, intestine
congenital P94.2
esophagus K22.89
intestine K59.89
psychogenic F45.8
stomach K31.89
neurotic or psychogenic F45.8
uterus (during labor) O62.2
with hemorrhage (postpartum) O72.1
postpartum (with hemorrhage) O72.1
without hemorrhage O75.89
Atopy —see History, allergy
Atransferrinemia, congenital E88.09
Atresia, atretic
alimentary organ or tract NEC Q45.8
upper Q40.8
ani, anus, anal (canal) Q42.3
with fistula Q42.2
aorta (ring) Q25.29
aortic (orifice) (valve) Q23.0
arch Q25.21
congenital with hypoplasia of ascending
aorta and defective development of
left ventricle (with mitral stenosis)
Q23.4
in hypoplastic left heart syndrome Q23.4
aqueduct of Sylvius Q03.0
with spina bifida —see Spina bifida, with
hydrocephalus

▶ New   ⇒ Revised   ~~deleted~~ Deleted   ● Use Additional Character(s)

Atresia, atretic *(Continued)*
  artery NEC Q27.8
    cerebral Q28.3
    coronary Q24.5
    digestive system Q27.8
    eye Q15.8
    lower limb Q27.8
    pulmonary Q25.5
    specified site NEC Q27.8
    umbilical Q27.0
    upper limb Q27.8
  auditory canal (external) Q16.1
  bile duct (common) (congenital) (hepatic) Q44.2
    acquired —*see* Obstruction, bile duct
  bladder (neck) Q64.39
    obstruction Q64.31
  bronchus Q32.4
  cecum Q42.8
  cervix (acquired) N88.2
    congenital Q51.828
    in pregnancy or childbirth —*see* Anomaly, cervix, in pregnancy or childbirth
      causing obstructed labor O65.5
  choana Q30.0
  colon Q42.9
    specified NEC Q42.8
  common duct Q44.2
  cricoid cartilage Q31.8
  cystic duct Q44.2
    acquired K82.8
      with obstruction K82.0
  digestive organs NEC Q45.8
  duodenum Q41.0
  ear canal Q16.1
  ejaculatory duct Q55.4
  epiglottis Q31.8
  esophagus Q39.0
    with tracheoesophageal fistula Q39.1
  eustachian tube Q17.8
  fallopian tube (congenital) Q50.6
    acquired N97.1
  follicular cyst N83.0-●
  foramen of
    Luschka Q03.1
      with spina bifida —*see* Spina bifida, with hydrocephalus
    Magendie Q03.1
      with spina bifida —*see* Spina bifida, with hydrocephalus
  gallbladder Q44.1
  genital organ
    external
      female Q52.79
      male Q55.8
    internal
      female Q52.8
      male Q55.8
  glottis Q31.8
  gullet Q39.0
    with tracheoesophageal fistula Q39.1
  heart valve NEC Q24.8
    pulmonary Q22.0
    tricuspid Q22.4
  hymen Q52.3
    acquired (postinfective) N89.6
  ileum Q41.2
  intestine (small) Q41.9
    large Q42.9
      specified NEC Q42.8
  iris, filtration angle Q15.0
  jejunum Q41.1
  lacrimal apparatus Q10.4
  larynx Q31.8
  meatus urinarius Q64.33
  mitral valve Q23.2
    in hypoplastic left heart syndrome Q23.4
  nares (anterior) (posterior) Q30.0
  nasopharynx Q34.8
  nose, nostril Q30.0
    acquired J34.89

Atresia, atretic *(Continued)*
  organ or site NEC Q89.8
  osseous meatus (ear) Q16.1
  oviduct (congenital) Q50.6
    acquired N97.1
  parotid duct Q38.4
    acquired K11.8
  pulmonary (artery) Q25.5
    valve Q22.0
  pulmonic Q22.0
  pupil Q13.2
  rectum Q42.1
    with fistula Q42.0
  salivary duct Q38.4
    acquired K11.8
  sublingual duct Q38.4
    acquired K11.8
  submandibular duct Q38.4
    acquired K11.8
  submaxillary duct Q38.4
    acquired K11.8
  thyroid cartilage Q31.8
  trachea Q32.1
  tricuspid valve Q22.4
  ureter Q62.10
    pelvic junction Q62.11
    vesical orifice Q62.12
  ureteropelvic junction Q62.11
  ureterovesical orifice Q62.12
  urethra (valvular) Q64.39
    stricture Q64.32
  urinary tract NEC Q64.8
  uterus Q51.818
    acquired N85.8
  vagina (congenital) Q52.4
    acquired (postinfectional) (senile) N89.5
  vas deferens Q55.3
  vascular NEC Q27.8
    cerebral Q28.3
    digestive system Q27.8
    lower limb Q27.8
    specified site NEC Q27.8
    upper limb Q27.8
  vein NEC Q27.8
    digestive system Q27.8
    great Q26.8
    lower limb Q27.8
    portal Q26.5
    pulmonary Q26.4
      partial Q26.3
      total Q26.2
    specified site NEC Q27.8
    upper limb Q27.8
  vena cava (inferior) (superior) Q26.8
  vesicourethral orifice Q64.31
  vulva Q52.79
    acquired N90.5
Atrichia, atrichosis —*see* Alopecia
Atrophia —*see also* Atrophy
  cutis senilis L90.8
    due to radiation L57.8
  gyrata of choroid and retina H31.23
  senilis R54
    dermatological L90.8
      due to radiation (nonionizing) (solar) L57.8
  unguium L60.3
    congenita Q84.6
Atrophie blanche (en plaque) (de Milian) L95.0
Atrophoderma, atrophodermia (of) L90.9
  diffusum (idiopathic) L90.4
  maculatum L90.8
    et striatum L90.8
      due to syphilis A52.79
    syphilitic A51.39
  neuriticum L90.8
  Pasini and Pierini L90.3
  pigmentosum Q82.1
  reticulatum symmetricum faciei L66.4
  senile L90.8
    due to radiation (nonionizing) (solar) L57.8
  vermiculata (cheeks) L66.4

Atrophy, atrophic (of)
  adrenal (capsule) (gland) E27.49
    primary (autoimmune) E27.1
  alveolar process or ridge (edentulous) K08.20
  anal sphincter (disuse) N81.84
  appendix K38.8
  arteriosclerotic —*see* Arteriosclerosis
  bile duct (common) (hepatic) K83.8
  bladder N32.89
    neurogenic N31.8
  blanche (en plaque) (of Milian) L95.0
  bone (senile) NEC —*see also* Disorder, bone, specified type NEC
    due to
      tabes dorsalis (neurogenic) A52.11
  brain (cortex) (progressive) G31.9
  ➠frontotemporal circumscribed (see also Dementia, in, diseases specified elsewhere) G31.01 *[F02.80]*
    ➠with behavioral disturbance (see also Dementia, in, diseases specified elsewhere) G31.01 *[F02.81-●]*
    senile NEC G31.1
  breast N64.2
    obstetric —*see* Disorder, breast, specified type NEC
  buccal cavity K13.79
  cardiac —*see* Degeneration, myocardial
  cartilage (infectional) (joint) —*see* Disorder, cartilage, specified NEC
  cerebellar —*see* Atrophy, brain
  cerebral —*see* Atrophy, brain
  cervix (mucosa) (senile) (uteri) N88.8
    menopausal N95.8
  Charcot-Marie-Tooth G60.0
  choroid (central) (macular) (myopic) (retina) H31.10-●
    diffuse secondary H31.12-●
    gyrate H31.23
    senile H31.11-●
  ciliary body —*see* Atrophy, iris
  conjunctiva (senile) H11.89
  corpus cavernosum N48.89
  cortical —*see* Atrophy, brain
  cystic duct K82.8
  Déjérine-Thomas G23.8
  disuse NEC —*see* Atrophy, muscle
  Duchenne-Aran G12.21
  ear H93.8-●
  edentulous alveolar ridge K08.20
  endometrium (senile) N85.8
    cervix N88.8
  enteric K63.89
  epididymis N50.89
  eyeball —*see* Disorder, globe, degenerated condition, atrophy
  eyelid (senile) —*see* Disorder, eyelid, degenerative
  facial (skin) L90.9
  fallopian tube (senile) N83.32-●
    with ovary N83.33-●
  fascioscapulohumeral (Landouzy-Déjérine) G71.02
  fatty, thymus (gland) E32.8
  gallbladder K82.8
  gastric K29.40
    with bleeding K29.41
  gastrointestinal K63.89
  glandular I89.8
  globe H44.52-●
  gum —*see* Recession, gingival
  hair L67.8
  heart (brown) —*see* Degeneration, myocardial
  hemifacial Q67.4
    Romberg G51.8
  infantile E41
    paralysis, acute —*see* Poliomyelitis, paralytic
  intestine K63.89
  iris (essential) (progressive) H21.26-●
    specified NEC H21.29

Atrophy, atrophic *(Continued)*
  kidney (senile) (terminal) —*see also* Sclerosis,
    renal N26.1
    congenital or infantile Q60.5
      bilateral Q60.4
      unilateral Q60.3
    hydronephrotic —*see* Hydronephrosis
  lacrimal gland (primary) H04.14-●
    secondary H04.15-●
  Landouzy-Déjérine G71.02
  laryngitis, infective J37.0
  larynx J38.7
  Leber's optic (hereditary) H47.22
  lip K13.0
  liver (yellow) K72.90
    with coma K72.91
    acute, subacute K72.00
      with coma K72.01
    chronic K72.10
      with coma K72.11
  lung (senile) J98.4
  macular (dermatological) L90.8
    syphilitic, skin A51.39
      striated A52.79
  mandible (edentulous) K08.20
    minimal K08.21
    moderate K08.22
    severe K08.23
  maxilla K08.20
    minimal K08.24
    moderate K08.25
    severe K08.26
  muscle, muscular (diffuse) (general)
    (idiopathic) (primary) M62.50
    ankle M62.57-●
  ▶back M62.5A9
    ▶cervical M62.5A0
    ▶lumbosacral M62.5A2
    ▶thoracic M62.5A1
    Duchenne-Aran G12.21
    foot M62.57-●
    forearm M62.53-●
    hand M62.54-●
    infantile spinal G12.0
    lower leg M62.56-●
    multiple sites M62.59
    myelopathic —*see* Atrophy, muscle, spinal
    myotonic G71.11
    neuritic G58.9
    neuropathic (peroneal) (progressive) G60.0
    pelvic (disuse) N81.84
    peroneal G60.0
    progressive (bulbar) G12.21
      adult G12.1
      infantile (spinal) G12.0
      spinal G12.25
        adult G12.1
        infantile G12.0
    pseudohypertrophic G71.02
    shoulder region M62.51-●
    specified site NEC M62.58
    spinal G12.9
      adult form G12.1
      Aran-Duchenne G12.21
      childhood form, type II G12.1
      distal G12.1
      hereditary NEC G12.1
      infantile, type I (Werdnig-Hoffmann)
        G12.0
      juvenile form, type III (Kugelberg-
        Welander) G12.1
      progressive G12.25
      scapuloperoneal form G12.1
      specified NEC G12.8
    syphilitic A52.78
    thigh M62.55-●
    upper arm M62.52-●
  myocardium —*see* Degeneration, myocardial
  myometrium (senile) N85.8
    cervix N88.8
  myopathic NEC —*see* Atrophy, muscle

Atrophy, atrophic *(Continued)*
  myotonia G71.11
  nail L60.3
  nasopharynx J31.1
  nerve —*see also* Disorder, nerve
    abducens —*see* Strabismus, paralytic, sixth
      nerve
    accessory G52.8
    acoustic or auditory —*see* subcategory
      H93.3
    cranial G52.9
      eighth (auditory) —*see* subcategory
        H93.3
      eleventh (accessory) G52.8
      fifth (trigeminal) G50.8
      first (olfactory) G52.0
      fourth (trochlear) —*see* Strabismus,
        paralytic, fourth nerve
      second (optic) H47.20
      sixth (abducens) —*see* Strabismus,
        paralytic, sixth nerve
      tenth (pneumogastric) (vagus) G52.2
      third (oculomotor) —*see* Strabismus,
        paralytic, third nerve
      twelfth (hypoglossal) G52.3
    hypoglossal G52.3
    oculomotor —*see* Strabismus, paralytic,
      third nerve
    olfactory G52.0
    optic (papillomacular bundle)
      syphilitic (late) A52.15
        congenital A50.44
    pneumogastric G52.2
    trigeminal G50.8
    trochlear —*see* Strabismus, paralytic, fourth
      nerve
    vagus (pneumogastric) G52.2
  neurogenic, bone, tabetic A52.11
  nutritional E43
    with marasmus E41
  old age R54
  olivopontocerebellar G23.8
  optic (nerve) H47.20
    glaucomatous H47.23-●
    hereditary H47.22
    primary H47.21-●
    specified type NEC H47.29-●
    syphilitic (late) A52.15
      congenital A50.44
  orbit H05.31-●
  ovary (senile) N83.31-●
    with fallopian tube N83.33-●
  oviduct (senile) —*see* Atrophy, fallopian
    tube
  palsy, diffuse (progressive) G12.22
  pancreas (duct) (senile) K86.89
  parotid gland K11.0
  pelvic muscle N81.84
  penis N48.89
  pharynx J39.2
  pluriglandular E31.8
    autoimmune E31.0
  polyarthritis M15.9
  prostate N42.89
  pseudohypertrophic (muscle) G71.02
  renal —*see also* Sclerosis, renal N26.1
  retina, retinal (postinfectional) H35.89
  rhinitis J31.0
  salivary gland K11.0
  scar L90.5
 ⇒sclerosis, lobar (of brain) (*see also* Dementia,
    in, diseases specified elsewhere) G31.09
    [F02.80]
    ⇒with behavioral disturbance (*see also*
      Dementia, in, diseases specified
      elsewhere) G31.09 *[F02.81-●]*
  scrotum N50.89
  seminal vesicle N50.89
  senile R54
    due to radiation (nonionizing) (solar) L57.8

Atrophy, atrophic *(Continued)*
  skin (patches) (spots) L90.9
    degenerative (senile) L90.8
    due to radiation (nonionizing) (solar) L57.8
    senile L90.8
  spermatic cord N50.89
  spinal (acute) (cord) G95.89
    muscular —*see* Atrophy, muscle, spinal
    paralysis G12.20
      acute —*see* Poliomyelitis, paralytic
      meaning progressive muscular atrophy
        G12.25
  spine (column) —*see* Spondylopathy,
    specified NEC
  spleen (senile) D73.0
  stomach K29.40
    with bleeding K29.41
  striate (skin) L90.6
    syphilitic A52.79
  subcutaneous L90.9
  sublingual gland K11.0
  submandibular gland K11.0
  submaxillary gland K11.0
  Sudeck's —*see* Algoneurodystrophy
  suprarenal (capsule) (gland) E27.49
    primary E27.1
  systemic affecting central nervous system
    in
      myxedema E03.9 *[G13.2]*
      neoplastic disease —*see also* Neoplasm
        D49.9 *[G13.1]*
      specified disease NEC G13.8
  tarso-orbital fascia, congenital Q10.3
  testis N50.0
  thenar, partial —*see* Syndrome, carpal tunnel
  thymus (fatty) E32.8
  thyroid (gland) (acquired) E03.4
    with cretinism E03.1
    congenital (with myxedema) E03.1
  tongue (senile) K14.8
    papillae K14.4
  trachea J39.8
  tunica vaginalis N50.89
  turbinate J34.89
  tympanic membrane (nonflaccid) H73.82-●
    flaccid H73.81-●
  upper respiratory tract J39.8
  uterus, uterine (senile) N85.8
    cervix N88.8
    due to radiation (intended effect) N85.8
      adverse effect or misadventure N99.89
  vagina (senile) N95.2
  vas deferens N50.89
  vascular I99.8
  vertebra (senile) —*see* Spondylopathy,
    specified NEC
  vulva (senile) N90.5
  Werdnig-Hoffmann G12.0
  yellow —*see* Failure, hepatic
Attack, attacks
  with alteration of consciousness (with
    automatisms) —*see* Epilepsy,
    localization-related, symptomatic, with
    complex partial seizures
  without alteration of consciousness —
    see Epilepsy, localization-related,
    symptomatic, with simple partial
    seizures
  Adams-Stokes I45.9
  akinetic —*see* Epilepsy, generalized, specified
    NEC
  angina —*see* Angina
  atonic —*see* Epilepsy, generalized, specified
    NEC
  benign shuddering G25.83
  cataleptic —*see* Catalepsy
  coronary —*see* Infarct, myocardium
  cyanotic, newborn P28.2
  drop NEC R55
  epileptic —*see* Epilepsy
  heart —*see* infarct, myocardium

Attack, attacks *(Continued)*
  hysterical F44.9
  jacksonian —*see* Epilepsy, localization-
      related, symptomatic, with simple
      partial seizures
  myocardium, myocardial —*see* Infarct,
      myocardium
  myoclonic —*see* Epilepsy, generalized,
      specified NEC
  panic F41.0
  psychomotor —*see* Epilepsy, localization-
      related, symptomatic, with complex
      partial seizures
  salaam —*see* Epilepsy, spasms
  schizophreniform, brief F23
  shuddering, benign G25.83
  Stokes-Adams I45.9
  syncope R55
  transient ischemic (TIA) G45.9
    specified NEC G45.8
  unconsciousness R55
    hysterical F44.89
  vasomotor R55
  vasovagal (paroxysmal) (idiopathic) R55
Attention (to)
  artificial
    opening (of) Z43.9
      digestive tract NEC Z43.4
        colon Z43.3
        ilium Z43.2
        stomach Z43.1
      specified NEC Z43.8
      trachea Z43.0
      urinary tract NEC Z43.6
        cystostomy Z43.5
        nephrostomy Z43.6
        ureterostomy Z43.6
        urethrostomy Z43.6
      vagina Z43.7
  colostomy Z43.3
  cystostomy Z43.5
  deficit disorder or syndrome F98.8
    with hyperactivity —*see* Disorder,
        attention-deficit hyperactivity
  gastrostomy Z43.1
  ileostomy Z43.2
  jejunostomy Z43.4
  nephrostomy Z43.6
  surgical dressings Z48.01
  sutures Z48.02
  tracheostomy Z43.0
  ureterostomy Z43.6
  urethrostomy Z43.6
Attrition
  gum —*see* Recession, gingival
  tooth, teeth (excessive) (hard tissues) K03.0
Atypical, atypism —*see also* condition
  cells (on cytolgocial smear) (endocervical)
      (endometrial) (glandular)
    cervix R87.619
    vagina R87.629
  cervical N87.9
  endometrium N85.9
    hyperplasia N85.00
  parenting situation Z62.9

Auditory —*see* condition
Aujeszky's disease B33.8
Aurantiasis, cutis E67.1
Auricle, auricular —*see also* condition
  cervical Q18.2
Auriculotemporal syndrome G50.8
Austin Flint murmur (aortic insufficiency) I35.1
Australian
  Q fever A78
  X disease A83.4
Autism, autistic (childhood) (infantile) F84.0
  atypical F84.9
  spectrum disorder F84.0
Autodigestion R68.89
Autoerythrocyte sensitization (syndrome)
    D69.2
Autographism L50.3
Autoimmune
  disease (systemic) M35.9
  inhibitors to clotting factors D68.311
  lymphoproliferative syndrome [ALPS]
      D89.82
  thyroiditis E06.3
Autointoxication R68.89
Automatism G93.89
  with temporal sclerosis G93.81
  epileptic —*see* Epilepsy, localization- related,
      symptomatic, with complex partial
      seizures
  paroxysmal, idiopathic —*see* Epilepsy,
      localization-related, symptomatic, with
      complex partial seizures
Autonomic, autonomous
  bladder (neurogenic) N31.2
  hysteria seizure F44.5
Autosensitivity, erythrocyte D69.2
Autosensitization, cutaneous L30.2
Autosome —*see* condition by chromosome
    involved
Autotopagnosia R48.1
Autotoxemia R68.89
Autumn —*see* condition
Avellis' syndrome G46.8
Aversion
  oral R63.39
    newborn P92.- •
    nonorganic origin F98.2
  sexual F52.1
Aviator's
  disease or sickness —*see* Effect, adverse, high
      altitude
  ear T70.0
Avitaminosis (multiple) —*see also* Deficiency,
      vitamin E56.9
  B E53.9
    with
      beriberi E51.11
      pellagra E52
  B2 E53.0
  B6 E53.1
  B12 E53.8
  D E55.9
    with rickets E55.0
  G E53.0
  K E56.1
  nicotinic acid E52

AVNRT (atrioventricular nodal re-entrant
    tachycardia) I47.1
AVRT (atrioventricular nodal re-entrant
    tachycardia) I47.1
Avulsion (traumatic)
  blood vessel —*see* Injury, blood vessel
  bone —*see* Fracture, by site
  cartilage —*see also* Dislocation, by site
    symphyseal (inner), complicating delivery
        O71.6
  external site other than limb —*see* Wound,
      open, by site
  eye S05.7- •
  head (intracranial)
    external site NEC S08.89
    scalp S08.0
  internal organ or site —*see* Injury, by site
  joint —*see also* Dislocation, by site
    capsule —*see* Sprain, by site
  kidney S37.06- •
  ligament —*see* Sprain, by site
  limb —*see also* Amputation, traumatic, by site
    skin and subcutaneous tissue —*see* Wound,
        open, by site
  muscle —*see* Injury, muscle
  nerve (root) —*see* Injury, nerve
  scalp S08.0
  skin and subcutaneous tissue —*see* Wound,
      open, by site
  spleen S36.032
  symphyseal cartilage (inner), complicating
      delivery O71.6
  tendon —*see* Injury, muscle
  tooth S03.2
Awareness of heart beat R00.2
Axenfeld's
  anomaly or syndrome Q15.0
  degeneration (calcareous) Q13.4
Axilla, axillary —*see also* condition
  breast Q83.1
Axonotmesis —*see* Injury, nerve
Ayerza's disease or syndrome (pulmonary
    artery sclerosis with pulmonary
    hypertension) I27.0
Azoospermia (organic) N46.01
  due to
    drug therapy N46.021
    efferent duct obstruction N46.023
    infection N46.022
    radiation N46.024
    specified cause NEC N46.029
    systemic disease N46.025
Azotemia R79.89
  meaning uremia N19
Aztec ear Q17.3
Azygos
  continuation inferior vena cava Q26.8
  lobe (lung) Q33.1

A

B

Baastrup's disease —see Kissing spine
Babesiosis B60.00
  due to
    Babesia
      divergens B60.03
      duncani B60.02
      KO-1 B60.09
      microti B60.01
      MO-1 B60.03
      species
        unspecified B60.00
      venatorum B60.09
    specified NEC B60.09
Babington's disease (familial hemorrhagic
    telangiectasia) I78.0
Babinski's syndrome A52.79
Baby
  crying constantly R68.11
  floppy (syndrome) P94.2
Bacillary —see condition
Bacilluria R82.71
Bacillus —see also Infection, bacillus
  abortus infection A23.1
  anthracis infection A22.9
  coli infection —see also Escherichia coli B96.20
  Flexner's A03.1
  mallei infection A24.0
  Shiga's A03.0
  suipestifer infection —see Infection, salmonella
Back —see condition
Backache (postural) M54.9
  sacroiliac M53.3
  specified NEC M54.89
Backflow —see Reflux
Backward reading (dyslexia) F81.0
Bacteremia R78.81
  with sepsis —see Sepsis
Bactericholia —see Cholecystitis, acute
Bacterid, bacteride (pustular) L40.3
Bacterium, bacteria, bacterial
  agent NEC, as cause of disease classified
    elsewhere B96.89
  in blood —see Bacteremia
  in urine —see Bacteriuria
Bacteriuria, bacteruria R82.71
  asymptomatic R82.71
Bacteroides
  fragilis, as cause of disease classified
    elsewhere B96.6
Bad
  heart —see Disease, heart
  trip
    due to drug abuse —see Abuse, drug,
      hallucinogen
    due to drug dependence —see Dependence,
      drug, hallucinogen
Baelz's disease (cheilitis glandularis
    apostematosa) K13.0
Baerensprung's disease (eczema marginatum)
    B35.6
Bagasse disease or pneumonitis J67.1
Bagassosis J67.1
Baker's cyst —see Cyst, Baker's
Bakwin-Krida syndrome (metaphyseal
    dysplasia) Q78.5
Balancing side interference M26.56
Balanitis (circinata) (erosiva) (gangrenosa)
    (phagedenic) (vulgaris) N48.1
  amebic A06.82
  candidal B37.42
  due to Haemophilus ducreyi A57
  gonococcal (acute) (chronic) A54.23
  xerotica obliterans N48.0
Balanoposthitis N47.6
  gonococcal (acute) (chronic) A54.23
  ulcerative (specific) A63.8
Balanorrhagia —see Balanitis
Balantidiasis, balantidiosis A07.0
Bald tongue K14.4

Baldness —see also Alopecia
  male-pattern —see Alopecia, androgenic
Balkan grippe A78
Balloon disease —see Effect, adverse, high
    altitude
Balo's disease (concentric sclerosis) G37.5
Bamberger-Marie disease —see Osteoarthropathy,
    hypertrophic, specified type NEC
Bancroft's filariasis B74.0
Band(s)
  adhesive —see Adhesions, peritoneum
  anomalous or congenital —see also Anomaly,
      by site
    heart (atrial) (ventricular) Q24.8
    intestine Q43.3
    omentum Q43.3
  cervix N88.1
  constricting, congenital Q79.8
  gallbladder (congenital) Q44.1
  intestinal (adhesive) —see Adhesions,
      peritoneum
  obstructive
    intestine K56.50
      complete K56.52
      incomplete K56.51
      partial K56.51
    peritoneum K56.50
      complete K56.52
      incomplete K56.51
      partial K56.51
  periappendiceal, congenital Q43.3
  peritoneal (adhesive) —see Adhesions,
      peritoneum
  uterus N73.6
    internal N85.6
  vagina N89.5
Bandemia D72.825
Bandl's ring (contraction), complicating
    delivery O62.4
Bangkok hemorrhagic fever A91
Bang's disease (brucella abortus) A23.1
Bankruptcy, anxiety concerning Z59.89
▶Bankruptcy (anxiety concerning) Z59.86
Bannister's disease T78.3
  hereditary D84.1
Banti's disease or syndrome (with cirrhosis)
    (with portal hypertension) K76.6
Bar, median, prostate —see Enlargement,
    enlarged, prostate
Barcoo disease or rot —see Ulcer, skin
Barlow's disease E54
Barodontalgia T70.29
Baron Münchausen syndrome —see Disorder,
    factitious
Barosinusitis T70.1
Barotitis T70.0
Barotrauma T70.29
  odontalgia T70.29
  otitic T70.0
  sinus T70.1
Barraquer (-Simons) disease or syndrome
    (progressive lipodystrophy) E88.1
Barré-Guillain disease or syndrome G61.0
Barré-Liéou syndrome (posterior cervical
    sympathetic) M53.0
Barrel chest M95.4
Barrett's
  disease —see Barrett's, esophagus
  esophagus K22.70
    with dysplasia K22.719
      high grade K22.711
      low grade K22.710
    without dysplasia K22.70
  syndrome —see Barrett's, esophagus
  ulcer K22.10
    with bleeding K22.11
    without bleeding K22.10
Barth syndrome E78.71
Bársony (-Polgár) (-Teschendorf) syndrome
    (corkscrew esophagus) K22.4
Bartholinitis (suppurating) N75.5
  gonococcal (acute) (chronic) (with abscess)
    A54.1

Bartonellosis A44.9
  cutaneous A44.1
  mucocutaneous A44.1
  specified NEC A44.8
  systemic A44.0
Barton's fracture S52.56-●
Bartter's syndrome E26.81
Basal —see condition
Basan's (hidrotic) ectodermal dysplasia Q82.4
Baseball finger —see Dislocation, finger
Basedow's disease (exophthalmic goiter) —see
    Hyperthyroidism, with, goiter
Basic —see condition
Basilar —see condition
Bason's (hidrotic) ectodermal dysplasia Q82.4
Basopenia —see Agranulocytosis
Basophilia D72.824
Basophilism (cortico-adrenal) (Cushing's)
    (pituitary) E24.0
Bassen-Kornzweig disease or syndrome E78.6
Bat ear Q17.5
Bateman's
  disease B08.1
  purpura (senile) D69.2
Bathing cramp T75.1
Bathophobia F40.248
Batten (-Mayou) disease E75.4
  retina E75.4 [H36]
Batten-Steinert syndrome G71.11
Battered —see Maltreatment
Battey Mycobacterium infection A31.0
Battle exhaustion F43.0
Battledore placenta O43.19-●
Baumgarten-Cruveilhier cirrhosis, disease or
    syndrome K74.69
Bauxite fibrosis (of lung) J63.1
Bayle's disease (general paresis) A52.17
Bazin's disease (primary) (tuberculous) A18.4
Beach ear —see Swimmer's, ear
Beaded hair (congenital) Q84.1
Béal conjunctivitis or syndrome B30.2
Beard's disease (neurasthenia) F48.8
Beat(s)
  atrial, premature I49.1
  ectopic I49.49
  elbow —see Bursitis, elbow
  escaped, heart I49.49
  hand —see Bursitis, hand
  knee —see Bursitis, knee
  premature I49.40
    atrial I49.1
    auricular I49.1
    supraventricular I49.1
Beau's
  disease or syndrome —see Degeneration,
    myocardial
  lines (transverse furrows on fingernails) L60.4
Bechterev's syndrome —see Spondylitis,
    ankylosing
Beck's syndrome (anterior spinal artery
    occlusion) I65.8
Becker's
  cardiomyopathy I42.8
  disease
    idiopathic mural endomyocardial disease
      I42.3
    myotonia congenita, recessive form G71.12
  dystrophy G71.01
  pigmented hairy nevus D22.5
Beckwith-Wiedemann syndrome Q87.3
Bed confinement status Z74.01
▶Bed-sharing, infant Z72.823
Bed sore —see Ulcer, pressure, by site
Bedbug bite(s) —see Bite(s), by site, superficial,
    insect
Bedclothes, asphyxiation or suffocation
    by —see Asphyxia, traumatic, due to,
      mechanical, trapped
Bednar's
  aphthae K12.0
  tumor —see Neoplasm, malignant, by site
Bedridden Z74.01

▶ New   ⇒ Revised   ~~deleted~~ Deleted   ● Use Additional Character(s)

Bedsore —*see* Ulcer, pressure, by site
Bedwetting —*see* Enuresis
Bee sting (with allergic or anaphylactic shock) —
 see Toxicity, venom, arthropod, bee
Beer drinker's heart (disease) I42.6
Begbie's disease (exophthalmic goiter) —*see*
 Hyperthyroidism, with, goiter
Behavior
 antisocial
  adult Z72.811
  child or adolescent Z72.810
 disorder, disturbance —*see* Disorder, conduct
 disruptive —*see* Disorder, conduct
 drug seeking Z76.5
 inexplicable R46.2
 marked evasiveness R46.5
 obsessive-compulsive R46.81
 overactivity R46.3
 poor responsiveness R46.4
 self-damaging (life-style) Z72.89
 sleep-incompatible Z72.821
 slowness R46.4
 specified NEC R46.89
 strange (and inexplicable) R46.2
 suspiciousness R46.5
 type A pattern Z73.1
 undue concern or preoccupation with
  stressful events R46.6
 verbosity and circumstantial detail obscuring
  reason for contact R46.7
Behcet's disease or syndrome M35.2
Behr's disease —*see* Degeneration, macula
Beigel's disease or morbus (white piedra)
 B36.2
Bejel A65
Bekhterev's syndrome —*see* Spondylitis,
 ankylosing
Belching —*see* Eructation
Bell's
 mania F30.8
 palsy, paralysis G51.0
  infant or newborn P11.3
 spasm G51.3-●
Bence Jones albuminuria or proteinuria NEC
 R80.3
Bends T70.3
Benedikt's paralysis or syndrome G46.3
Benign (*see also* condition)
 prostatic hyperplasia —*see* Hyperplasia,
  prostate
Bennett's fracture (displaced) S62.21-●
Benson's disease —*see* Deposit, crystalline
Bent
 back (hysterical) F44.4
 nose M95.0
  congenital Q67.4
Bereavement (uncomplicated) Z63.4
Bergeron's disease (hysterical chorea) F44.4
Berger's disease —*see* Nephropathy, IgA
Beriberi (dry) E51.11
 heart (disease) E51.12
 polyneuropathy E51.11
 wet E51.12
 involving circulatory system E51.11
Berlin's disease or edema (traumatic) S05.8X-●
Berlock (berloque) dermatitis L56.2
Bernard-Horner syndrome G90.2
Bernard-Soulier disease or thrombopathia D69.1
Bernhardt (-Roth) disease —*see*
 Mononeuropathy, lower limb, meralgia
 paresthetica
Bernheim's syndrome —*see* Failure, heart,
 right
Bertielliasis B71.8
Berylliosis (lung) J63.2
Besnier-Boeck (-Schaumann) disease —*see*
 Sarcoidosis
Besnier's
 lupus pernio D86.3
 prurigo L20.0
Bestiality F65.89
Best's disease H35.50

Beta-mercaptolactate-cysteine disulfiduria
 E72.09
Betalipoproteinemia, broad or floating E78.2
Betting and gambling Z72.6
 pathological (compulsive) F63.0
Bezoar T18.9
 intestine T18.3
 stomach T18.2
Bezold's abscess —*see* Mastoiditis, acute
Bianchi's syndrome R48.8
Bicornate or bicornis uterus Q51.3
 in pregnancy or childbirth O34.00
  causing obstructed labor O65.5
Bicuspid aortic valve Q23.1
Biedl-Bardet syndrome Q87.89
Bielschowsky (-Jansky) disease E75.4
Biermer's (pernicious) anemia or disease D51.0
Biett's disease L93.0
Bifid (congenital)
 apex, heart Q24.8
 clitoris Q52.6
 kidney Q63.8
 nose Q30.2
 patella Q74.1
 scrotum Q55.29
 toe NEC Q74.2
 tongue Q38.3
 ureter Q62.8
 uterus Q51.3
 uvula Q35.7
Biforis uterus (suprasimplex) Q51.3
Bifurcation (congenital)
 gallbladder Q44.1
 kidney pelvis Q63.8
 renal pelvis Q63.8
 rib Q76.6
 tongue, congenital Q38.3
 trachea Q32.1
 ureter Q62.8
 urethra Q64.74
 vertebra Q76.49
Big spleen syndrome D73.1
Bigeminal pulse R00.8
Bilateral —*see* condition
Bile
 duct —*see* condition
 pigments in urine R82.2
Bilharziasis —*see also* Schistosomiasis
 chyluria B65.0
 cutaneous B65.3
 galacturia B65.0
 hematochyluria B65.0
 intestinal B65.1
 lipemia B65.9
 lipuria B65.0
 oriental B65.2
 piarhemia B65.9
 pulmonary NOS B65.9 [J99]
  pneumonia B65.9 [J17]
 tropical hematuria B65.0
 vesical B65.0
Biliary —*see* condition
Bilirubin metabolism disorder E80.7
 specified NEC E80.6
Bilirubinemia, familial nonhemolytic E80.4
Bilirubinuria R82.2
Biliuria R82.2
Bilocular stomach K31.2
Binswanger's disease I67.3
Biparta, bipartite
 carpal scaphoid Q74.0
 patella Q74.1
 vagina Q52.10
Bird
 face Q75.8
 fancier's disease or lung J67.2
Birt-Hogg-Dube syndrome Q87.89
Birth
 complications in mother —*see* Delivery,
  complicated
 compression during NOS P15.9

Birth (*Continued*)
 defect —*see* Anomaly
 immature (less than 37 completed weeks) —
  see Preterm, newborn
  extremely (less than 28 completed
   weeks) —*see* Immaturity, extreme
 inattention, at or after —*see* Maltreatment,
  child, neglect
 injury NOS P15.9
  basal ganglia P11.1
  brachial plexus NEC P14.3
  brain (compression) (pressure) P11.2
  central nervous system NOS P11.9
  cerebellum P11.1
  cerebral hemorrhage P10.1
  external genitalia P15.5
  eye P15.3
  face P15.4
  fracture
   bone P13.9
    specified NEC P13.8
   clavicle P13.4
   femur P13.2
   humerus P13.3
   long bone, except femur P13.3
   radius and ulna P13.3
   skull P13.0
   spine P11.5
   tibia and fibula P13.3
  intracranial P11.2
   laceration or hemorrhage P10.9
    specified NEC P10.8
  intraventricular hemorrhage P10.2
  laceration
   brain P10.1
   by scalpel P15.8
   peripheral nerve P14.9
  liver P15.0
  meninges
   brain P11.1
   spinal cord P11.5
  nerve
   brachial plexus P14.3
   cranial NEC (except facial) P11.4
   facial P11.3
   peripheral P14.9
   phrenic (paralysis) P14.2
  paralysis
   facial nerve P11.3
   spinal P11.5
  penis P15.5
  rupture
   spinal cord P11.5
  scalp P12.9
  scalpel wound P15.8
  scrotum P15.5
  skull NEC P13.1
   fracture P13.0
  specified type NEC P15.8
  spinal cord P11.5
  spine P11.5
  spleen P15.1
  sternomastoid (hematoma) P15.2
  subarachnoid hemorrhage P10.3
  subcutaneous fat necrosis P15.6
  subdural hemorrhage P10.0
  tentorial tear P10.4
  testes P15.5
  vulva P15.5
 lack of care, at or after —*see* Maltreatment,
  child, neglect
 neglect, at or after —*see* Maltreatment, child,
  neglect
 palsy or paralysis, newborn, NOS (birth
  injury) P14.9
 premature (infant) —*see* Preterm, newborn
 shock, newborn P96.89
 trauma —*see* Birth, injury
 weight
  4000 grams to 4499 grams P08.1
  4500 grams or more P08.0

Birth *(Continued)*
 weight *(Continued)*
  low (2499 grams or less) —*see* Low,
    birthweight
   extremely (999 grams or less) —*see* Low,
     birthweight, extreme
Birthmark Q82.5
Bisalbuminemia E88.09
Biskra's button B55.1
Bite(s) (animal) (human)
 abdomen, abdominal
  wall S31.159
   with penetration into peritoneal cavity
     S31.659
    epigastric region S31.152
     with penetration into peritoneal cavity
       S31.652
    left
     lower quadrant S31.154
      with penetration into peritoneal
        cavity S31.654
     upper quadrant S31.151
      with penetration into peritoneal
        cavity S31.651
    periumbilic region S31.155
     with penetration into peritoneal cavity
       S31.655
    right
     lower quadrant S31.153
      with penetration into peritoneal
        cavity S31.653
     upper quadrant S31.150
      with penetration into peritoneal
        cavity S31.650
   superficial NEC S30.871
    insect S30.861
 alveolar (process) —*see* Bite, oral cavity
 amphibian (venomous) —*see* Venom, bite,
   amphibian
 animal —*see also* Bite, by site
  venomous —*see* Venom
 ankle S91.05-●
  superficial NEC S90.57-●
   insect S90.56-●
 antecubital space —*see* Bite, elbow
 anus S31.835
  superficial NEC S30.877
   insect S30.867
 arm (upper) S41.15-●
  lower —*see* Bite, forearm
  superficial NEC S40.87-●
   insect S40.86-●
 arthropod NEC —*see* Venom, bite, arthropod
 auditory canal (external) (meatus) —
   see Bite, ear
 auricle, ear —*see* Bite, ear
 axilla —*see* Bite, arm
 back —*see also* Bite, thorax, back
  lower S31.050
   with penetration into retroperitoneal
     space S31.051
   superficial NEC S30.870
    insect S30.860
 bedbug —*see* Bite(s), by site, superficial,
   insect
 breast S21.05-●
  superficial NEC S20.17-●
   insect S20.16-●
 brow —*see* Bite, head, specified site NEC
 buttock S31.805
  left S31.825
  right S31.815
  superficial NEC S30.870
   insect S30.860
 calf —*see* Bite, leg
 canaliculus lacrimalis —*see* Bite, eyelid
 canthus, eye —*see* Bite, eyelid
 centipede —*see* Toxicity, venom, arthropod,
   centipede
 cheek (external) S01.45-●
  internal —*see* Bite, oral cavity
  superficial NEC S00.87
   insect S00.86

Bite *(Continued)*
 chest wall —*see* Bite, thorax
 chigger B88.0
 chin —*see* Bite, head, specified site NEC
 clitoris —*see* Bite, vulva
 costal region —*see* Bite, thorax
 digit(s)
  hand —*see* Bite, finger
  toe —*see* Bite, toe
 ear (canal) (external) S01.35-●
  superficial NEC S00.47-●
   insect S00.46-●
 elbow S51.05-●
  superficial NEC S50.37-●
   insect S50.36-●
 epididymis —*see* Bite, testis
 epigastric region —*see* Bite, abdomen
 epiglottis —*see* Bite, neck, specified site NEC
 esophagus, cervical S11.25
  superficial NEC S10.17
   insect S10.16
 eyebrow —*see* Bite, eyelid
 eyelid S01.15-●
  superficial NEC S00.27-●
   insect S00.26-●
 face NEC —*see* Bite, head, specified site NEC
 finger(s) S61.259
  with
   damage to nail S61.359
  index S61.258
   with
    damage to nail S61.358
   left S61.251
    with
     damage to nail S61.351
   right S61.250
    with
     damage to nail S61.350
   superficial NEC S60.478
    insect S60.46-●
  little S61.25-●
   with
    damage to nail S61.35-●
   superficial NEC S60.47-●
    insect S60.46-●
  middle S61.25-●
   with
    damage to nail S61.35-●
   superficial NEC S60.47-●
    insect S60.46-●
  ring S61.25-●
   with
    damage to nail S61.35-●
   superficial NEC S60.47-●
    insect S60.46-●
  superficial NEC S60.479
   insect S60.469
  thumb —*see* Bite, thumb
 flank —*see* Bite, abdomen, wall
 flea —*see* Bite, by site, superficial,
   insect
 foot (except toe(s) alone) S91.35-●
  superficial NEC S90.87-●
   insect S90.86-●
  toe —*see* Bite, toe
 forearm S51.85-●
  elbow only —*see* Bite, elbow
  superficial NEC S50.87-●
   insect S50.86-●
 forehead —*see* Bite, head, specified site
   NEC
 genital organs, external
  female S31.552
   superficial NEC S30.876
    insect S30.866
   vagina and vulva —*see* Bite, vulva
  male S31.551
   penis —*see* Bite, penis
   scrotum —*see* Bite, scrotum
   superficial NEC S30.875
    insect S30.865
   testes —*see* Bite, testis
 groin —*see* Bite, abdomen, wall

Bite *(Continued)*
 gum —*see* Bite, oral cavity
 hand S61.45-●
  finger —*see* Bite, finger
  superficial NEC S60.57-●
   insect S60.56-●
  thumb —*see* Bite, thumb
 head S01.95
  cheek —*see* Bite, cheek
  ear —*see* Bite, ear
  eyelid —*see* Bite, eyelid
  lip —*see* Bite, lip
  nose —*see* Bite, nose
  oral cavity —*see* Bite, oral cavity
  scalp —*see* Bite, scalp
  specified site NEC S01.85
   superficial NEC S00.87
    insect S00.86
  superficial NEC S00.97
   insect S00.96
  temporomandibular area —*see* Bite, cheek
 heel —*see* Bite, foot
 hip S71.05-●
  superficial NEC S70.27-●
   insect S70.26-●
 hymen S31.45
 hypochondrium —*see* Bite, abdomen, wall
 hypogastric region —*see* Bite, abdomen, wall
 inguinal region —*see* Bite, abdomen, wall
 insect —*see* Bite, by site, superficial, insect
 instep —*see* Bite, foot
 interscapular region —*see* Bite, thorax, back
 jaw —*see* Bite, head, specified site NEC
 knee S81.05-●
  superficial NEC S80.27-●
   insect S80.26-●
 labium (majus) (minus) —*see* Bite, vulva
 lacrimal duct —*see* Bite, eyelid
 larynx S11.015
  superficial NEC S10.17
   insect S10.16
 leg (lower) S81.85-●
  ankle —*see* Bite, ankle
  foot —*see* Bite, foot
  knee —*see* Bite, knee
  superficial NEC S80.87-●
   insect S80.86-●
  toe —*see* Bite, toe
  upper —*see* Bite, thigh
 lip S01.551
  superficial NEC S00.571
   insect S00.561
 lizard (venomous) —*see* Venom, bite, reptile
 loin —*see* Bite, abdomen, wall
 lower back —*see* Bite, back, lower
 lumbar region —*see* Bite, back, lower
 malar region —*see* Bite, head, specified site
   NEC
 mammary —*see* Bite, breast
 marine animals (venomous) —*see* Toxicity,
   venom, marine animal
 mastoid region —*see* Bite, head, specified site
   NEC
 mouth —*see* Bite, oral cavity
 nail
  finger —*see* Bite, finger
  toe —*see* Bite, toe
 nape —*see* Bite, neck, specified site NEC
 nasal (septum) (sinus) —*see* Bite, nose
 nasopharynx —*see* Bite, head, specified site
   NEC
 neck S11.95
  involving
   cervical esophagus —*see* Bite,
     esophagus, cervical
   larynx —*see* Bite, larynx
   pharynx —*see* Bite, pharynx
   thyroid gland S11.15
   trachea —*see* Bite, trachea
  specified site NEC S11.85
   superficial NEC S10.87
    insect S10.86

▶ New   ⇒ Revised   ~~deleted~~ Deleted   ● Use Additional Character(s)

Bite *(Continued)*
  neck *(Continued)*
    superficial NEC S10.97
      insect S10.96
    throat S11.85
      superficial NEC S10.17
        insect S10.16
  nose (septum) (sinus) S01.25
    superficial NEC S00.37
      insect S00.36
  occipital region —*see* Bite, scalp
  oral cavity S01.552
    superficial NEC S00.572
      insect S00.562
  orbital region —*see* Bite, eyelid
  palate —*see* Bite, oral cavity
  palm —*see* Bite, hand
  parietal region —*see* Bite, scalp
  pelvis S31.050
    with penetration into retroperitoneal space S31.051
    superficial NEC S30.870
      insect S30.860
  penis S31.25
    superficial NEC S30.872
      insect S30.862
  perineum
    female —*see* Bite, vulva
    male —*see* Bite, pelvis
  periocular area (with or without lacrimal passages) —*see* Bite, eyelid
  phalanges
    finger —*see* Bite, finger
    toe —*see* Bite, toe
  pharynx S11.25
    superficial NEC S10.17
      insect S10.16
  pinna —*see* Bite, ear
  poisonous —*see* Venom
  popliteal space —*see* Bite, knee
  prepuce —*see* Bite, penis
  pubic region —*see* Bite, abdomen, wall
  rectovaginal septum —*see* Bite, vulva
  red bug B88.0
  reptile NEC —*see also* Venom, bite, reptile
    nonvenomous —*see* Bite, by site
    snake —*see* Venom, bite, snake
  sacral region —*see* Bite, back, lower
  sacroiliac region —*see* Bite, back, lower
  salivary gland —*see* Bite, oral cavity
  scalp S01.05
    superficial NEC S00.07
      insect S00.06
  scapular region —*see* Bite, shoulder
  scrotum S31.35
    superficial NEC S30.873
      insect S30.863
  sea-snake (venomous) —*see* Toxicity, venom, snake, sea snake
  shin —*see* Bite, leg
  shoulder S41.05-●
    superficial NEC S40.27-●
      insect S40.26-●
  snake —*see also* Venom, bite, snake
    nonvenomous —*see* Bite, by site
  spermatic cord —*see* Bite, testis
  spider (venomous) —*see* Toxicity, venom, spider
    nonvenomous —*see* Bite, by site, superficial, insect
  sternal region —*see* Bite, thorax, front
  submaxillary region —*see* Bite, head, specified site NEC
  submental region —*see* Bite, head, specified site NEC
  subungual
    finger(s) —*see* Bite, finger
    toe —*see* Bite, toe
  superficial —*see* Bite, by site, superficial
  supraclavicular fossa S11.85

Bite *(Continued)*
  supraorbital —*see* Bite, head, specified site NEC
  temple, temporal region —*see* Bite, head, specified site NEC
  temporomandibular area —*see* Bite, cheek
  testis S31.35
    superficial NEC S30.873
      insect S30.863
  thigh S71.15-●
    superficial NEC S70.37-●
      insect S70.36-●
  thorax, thoracic (wall) S21.95
    back S21.25-●
      with penetration into thoracic cavity S21.45-●
    breast —*see* Bite, breast
    front S21.15-●
      with penetration into thoracic cavity S21.35-●
    superficial NEC S20.97
      back S20.47-●
      front S20.37-●
      insect S20.96
        back S20.46-●
        front S20.36-●
  throat —*see* Bite, neck, throat
  thumb S61.05-●
    with
      damage to nail S61.15-●
    superficial NEC S60.37-●
      insect S60.36-●
  thyroid S11.15
    superficial NEC S10.87
      insect S10.86
  toe(s) S91.15-●
    with
      damage to nail S91.25-●
    great S91.15-●
      with
        damage to nail S91.25-●
    lesser S91.15-●
      with
        damage to nail S91.25-●
    superficial NEC S90.47-●
      great S90.47-●
      insect S90.46-●
        great S90.46-●
  tongue S01.552
  trachea S11.025
    superficial NEC S10.17
      insect S10.16
  tunica vaginalis —*see* Bite, testis
  tympanum, tympanic membrane —*see* Bite, ear
  umbilical region S31.155
  uvula —*see* Bite, oral cavity
  vagina —*see* Bite, vulva
  venomous —*see* Venom
  vocal cords S11.035
    superficial NEC S10.17
      insect S10.16
  vulva S31.45
    superficial NEC S30.874
      insect S30.864
  wrist S61.55-●
    superficial NEC S60.87-●
      insect S60.86-●
Biting, cheek or lip K13.1
Biventricular failure (heart) I50.82
Björck (-Thorson) syndrome (malignant carcinoid) E34.0
Black
  death A20.9
  eye S00.1-●
  hairy tongue K14.3
  heel (foot) S90.3-●
  lung (disease) J60
  palm (hand) S60.22-●
Blackfan-Diamond anemia or syndrome (congenital hypoplastic anemia) D61.01

Blackhead L70.0
Blackout R55
Bladder —*see* condition
Blast (air) (hydraulic) (immersion) (underwater)
  blindness S05.8X-●
  injury
    abdomen or thorax —*see* Injury, by site
    ear (acoustic nerve trauma) —*see* Injury, nerve, acoustic, specified type NEC
    syndrome NEC T70.8
Blastoma —*see* Neoplasm, malignant, by site
  pulmonary —*see* Neoplasm, lung, malignant
Blastomycosis, blastomycotic B40.9
  Brazilian —*see* Paracoccidioidomycosis
  cutaneous B40.3
  disseminated B40.7
  European —*see* Cryptococcosis
  generalized B40.7
  keloidal B48.0
  North American B40.9
  primary pulmonary B40.0
  pulmonary B40.2
    acute B40.0
    chronic B40.1
  skin B40.3
  South American —*see* Paracoccidioidomycosis
  specified NEC B40.89
Bleb(s) R23.8
  emphysematous (lung) (solitary) J43.9
  endophthalmitis H59.43
  filtering (vitreous), after glaucoma surgery Z98.83
  inflamed (infected), postprocedural H59.40
    stage 1 H59.41
    stage 2 H59.42
    stage 3 H59.43
  lung (ruptured) J43.9
    congenital —*see* Atelectasis
    newborn P25.8
  subpleural (emphysematous) J43.9
Blebitis, postprocedural H59.40
  stage 1 H59.41
  stage 2 H59.42
  stage 3 H59.43
Bleeder (familial) (hereditary) —*see* Hemophilia
Bleeding —*see also* Hemorrhage
  anal K62.5
  anovulatory N97.0
  atonic, following delivery O72.1
  capillary I78.8
    puerperal O72.2
  contact (postcoital) N93.0
  due to uterine subinvolution N85.3
  ear —*see* Otorrhagia
  excessive, associated with menopausal onset N92.4
  familial —*see* Defect, coagulation
  following intercourse N93.0
  gastrointestinal K92.2
  hemorrhoids —*see* Hemorrhoids
  intermenstrual (regular) N92.3
    irregular N92.1
  intraoperative —*see* Complication, intraoperative, hemorrhage
  irregular N92.6
  menopausal N92.4
  newborn, intraventricular —*see* Newborn, affected by, hemorrhage, intraventricular
  nipple N64.59
  nose R04.0
  ovulation N92.3
  perimenopausal N92.4
  postclimacteric N95.0
  postcoital N93.0
  postmenopausal N95.0
  postoperative —*see* Complication, postprocedural, hemorrhage
  preclimacteric N92.4
  pre-pubertal vaginal N93.1
  puberty (excessive, with onset of menstrual periods) N92.2

Bleeding (Continued)
rectum, rectal K62.5
newborn P54.2
tendencies —see Defect, coagulation
throat R04.1
tooth socket (post-extraction) K91.840
umbilical stump P51.9
uterus, uterine NEC N93.9
climacteric N92.4
dysfunctional or functional N93.8
menopausal N92.4
preclimacteric or premenopausal N92.4
unrelated to menstrual cycle N93.9
vagina, vaginal (abnormal) N93.9
dysfunctional or functional N93.8
newborn P54.6
pre-pubertal N93.1
vicarious N94.89
Blennorrhagia, blennorrhagic —see Gonorrhea
Blennorrhea (acute) (chronic) —see also
Gonorrhea
inclusion (neonatal) (newborn) P39.1
lower genitourinary tract (gonococcal) A54.00
neonatorum (gonococcal ophthalmia) A54.31
Blepharelosis —see Entropion
Blepharitis (angularis) (ciliaris) (eyelid)
(marginal) (nonulcerative) H01.009
herpes zoster B02.39
left H01.006
lower H01.005
upper H01.004
upper and lower H01.00B
right H01.003
lower H01.002
upper H01.001
upper and lower H01.00A
squamous H01.029
left H01.026
lower H01.025
upper H01.024
upper and lower H01.02B
right H01.023
lower H01.022
upper H01.021
upper and lower H01.02A
ulcerative H01.019
left H01.016
lower H01.015
upper H01.014
upper and lower H01.01B
right H01.013
lower H01.012
upper H01.011
upper and lower H01.01B
Blepharochalasis H02.30
congenital Q10.0
left H02.36
lower H02.35
upper H02.34
right H02.33
lower H02.32
upper H02.31
Blepharoclonus H02.59
Blepharoconjunctivitis H10.50-●
angular H10.52-●
contact H10.53-●
ligneous H10.51-●
Blepharophimosis (eyelid) H02.529
congenital Q10.3
left H02.526
lower H02.525
upper H02.524
right H02.523
lower H02.522
upper H02.521
Blepharoptosis H02.40-●
congenital Q10.0
mechanical H02.41-●
myogenic H02.42-●
neurogenic H02.43-●
paralytic H02.43-●
Blepharopyorrhea, gonococcal A54.39

Blepharospasm G24.5
drug induced G24.01
Blighted ovum O02.0
Blind —see also Blindness
bronchus (congenital) Q32.4
loop syndrome K90.2
congenital Q43.8
sac, fallopian tube (congenital) Q50.6
spot, enlarged —see Defect, visual field,
localized, scotoma, blind spot area
tract or tube, congenital NEC —see Atresia,
by site
Blindness (acquired) (congenital) (both eyes)
H54.0X-●
blast S05.8X-●
color —see Deficiency, color vision
concussion S05.8X-●
cortical H47.619
left brain H47.612
right brain H47.611
day H53.11
due to injury (current episode) S05.9-●
sequelae — code to injury with seventh
character S
eclipse (total) —see Retinopathy, solar
emotional (hysterical) F44.6
face H53.16
hysterical F44.6
legal (both eyes) (USA definition) H54.8
mind R48.8
night H53.60
abnormal dark adaptation curve H53.61
acquired H53.62
congenital H53.63
specified type NEC H53.69
vitamin A deficiency E50.5
one eye (other eye normal) H54.40
left (normal vision on right) H54.42-●
low vision on right H54.12-●
low vision, other eye H54.10
right (normal vision on left) H54.41-●
low vision on left H54.11-●
psychic R48.8
river B73.01
snow —see Photokeratitis
sun, solar —see Retinopathy, solar
transient —see Disturbance, vision, subjective,
loss, transient
traumatic (current episode) S05.9-●
word (developmental) F81.0
acquired R48.0
secondary to organic lesion R48.0
Blister (nonthermal)
abdominal wall S30.821
alveolar process S00.522
ankle S90.52-●
antecubital space —see Blister, elbow
anus S30.827
arm (upper) S40.82-●
auditory canal —see Blister, ear
auricle —see Blister, ear
axilla —see Blister, arm
back, lower S30.820
beetle dermatitis L24.89
breast S20.12-●
brow S00.82
calf —see Blister, leg
canthus —see Blister, eyelid
cheek S00.82
internal S00.522
chest wall —see Blister, thorax
chin S00.82
costal region —see Blister, thorax
digit(s)
foot —see Blister, toe
hand —see Blister, finger
due to burn —see Burn, by site, second degree
ear S00.42-●
elbow S50.32-●
epiglottis S10.12
esophagus, cervical S10.12
eyebrow —see Blister, eyelid

Blister (Continued)
eyelid S00.22-●
face S00.82
fever B00.1
finger(s) S60.429
index S60.42-●
little S60.42-●
middle S60.42-●
ring S60.42-●
foot (except toe(s) alone) S90.82-●
toe —see Blister, toe
forearm S50.82-●
elbow only —see Blister, elbow
forehead S00.82
fracture - omit code
genital organ
female S30.826
male S30.825
gum S00.522
hand S60.52-●
head S00.92
ear —see Blister, ear
eyelid —see Blister, eyelid
lip S00.521
nose S00.32
oral cavity S00.522
scalp S00.02
specified site NEC S00.82
heel —see Blister, foot
hip S70.22-●
interscapular region S20.429
jaw S00.82
knee S80.22-●
larynx S10.12
leg (lower) S80.82-●
knee —see Blister, knee
upper —see Blister, thigh
lip S00.521
malar region S00.82
mammary —see Blister, breast
mastoid region S00.82
mouth S00.522
multiple, skin, nontraumatic R23.8
nail
finger —see Blister, finger
toe —see Blister, toe
nasal S00.32
neck S10.92
specified site NEC S10.82
throat S10.12
nose S00.32
occipital region S00.02
oral cavity S00.522
orbital region —see Blister, eyelid
palate S00.522
palm —see Blister, hand
parietal region S00.02
pelvis S30.820
penis S30.822
periocular area —see Blister, eyelid
phalanges
finger —see Blister, finger
toe —see Blister, toe
pharynx S10.12
pinna —see Blister, ear
popliteal space —see Blister, knee
scalp S00.02
scapular region —see Blister, shoulder
scrotum S30.823
shin —see Blister, leg
shoulder S40.22-●
sternal region S20.329
submaxillary region S00.82
submental region S00.82
subungual
finger(s) —see Blister, finger
toe(s) —see Blister, toe
supraclavicular fossa S10.82
supraorbital S00.82
temple S00.82
temporal region S00.82
testis S30.823

▶ New   ⇒ Revised   ~~deleted~~ Deleted   ● Use Additional Character(s)

Blister *(Continued)*
thermal —*see* Burn, second degree, by site
thigh S70.32-●
thorax, thoracic (wall) S20.92
back S20.42-●
front S20.32-●
throat S10.12
thumb S60.32-●
toe(s) S90.42-●
great S90.42-●
tongue S00.522
trachea S10.12
tympanum, tympanic membrane —*see* Blister, ear
upper arm —*see* Blister, arm (upper)
uvula S00.522
vagina S30.824
vocal cords S10.12
vulva S30.824
wrist S60.82-●
Bloating R14.0
Bloch-Sulzberger disease or syndrome Q82.3
Block, blocked
alveolocapillary J84.10
arborization (heart) I45.5
arrhythmic I45.9
atrioventricular (incomplete) (partial) I44.30
with atrioventricular dissociation I44.2
complete I44.2
congenital Q24.6
congenital Q24.6
first degree I44.0
second degree (types I and II) I44.1
specified NEC I44.39
third degree I44.2
types I and II I44.1
auriculoventricular —*see* Block, atrioventricular
bifascicular (cardiac) I45.2
bundle-branch (complete) (false) (incomplete) I45.4
bilateral I45.2
left I44.7
with right bundle branch block I45.2
hemiblock I44.60
anterior I44.4
posterior I44.5
incomplete I44.7
with right bundle branch block I45.2
right I45.10
with
left bundle branch block I45.2
left fascicular block I45.2
specified NEC I45.19
Wilson's type I45.19
cardiac I45.9
conduction I45.9
complete I44.2
fascicular (left) I44.60
anterior I44.4
posterior I44.5
right I45.0
specified NEC I44.69
foramen Magendie (acquired) G91.1
congenital Q03.1
with spina bifida —*see* Spina bifida, by site, with hydrocephalus
heart I45.9
bundle branch I45.4
bilateral I45.2
complete (atrioventricular) I44.2
congenital Q24.6
first degree (atrioventricular) I44.0
second degree (atrioventricular) I44.1
specified type NEC I45.5
third degree (atrioventricular) I44.2
hepatic vein I82.0
intraventricular (nonspecific) I45.4
bundle branch
bilateral I45.2
kidney N28.9
postcystoscopic or postprocedural N99.0

Block, blocked *(Continued)*
Mobitz (types I and II) I44.1
myocardial —*see* Block, heart
nodal I45.5
organ or site, congenital NEC —*see* Atresia, by site
portal (vein) I81
second degree (types I and II) I44.1
sinoatrial I45.5
sinoauricular I45.5
third degree I44.2
trifascicular I45.3
tubal N97.1
vein NOS I82.90
Wenckebach (types I and II) I44.1
Blockage —*see* Obstruction
Blocq's disease F44.4
Blood
constituents, abnormal R78.9
disease D75.9
donor —*see* Donor, blood
dyscrasia D75.9
with
abortion —*see* Abortion, by type, complicated by, hemorrhage
ectopic pregnancy O08.1
molar pregnancy O08.1
following ectopic or molar pregnancy O08.1
newborn P61.9
puerperal, postpartum O72.3
flukes NEC —*see* Schistosomiasis
in
feces K92.1
occult R19.5
urine —*see* Hematuria
mole O02.0
occult in feces R19.5
pressure
decreased, due to shock following injury T79.4
examination only Z01.30
fluctuating I99.8
high —*see* Hypertension
borderline R03.0
incidental reading, without diagnosis of hypertension R03.0
low —*see also* Hypotension
incidental reading, without diagnosis of hypotension R03.1
spitting —*see* Hemoptysis
staining cornea —*see* Pigmentation, cornea, stromal
transfusion
reaction or complication —*see* Complications, transfusion
type
A (Rh positive) Z67.10
Rh negative Z67.11
AB (Rh positive) Z67.30
Rh negative Z67.31
B (Rh positive) Z67.20
Rh negative Z67.21
O (Rh positive) Z67.40
Rh negative Z67.41
Rh (positive) Z67.90
negative Z67.91
vessel rupture —*see* Hemorrhage
vomiting —*see* Hematemesis
Blood-forming organs, disease D75.9
Bloodgood's disease —*see* Mastopathy, cystic
Bloom (-Machacek)(-Torre) **syndrome** Q82.8
Blount disease or osteochondrosis M92.51-●
Blue
baby Q24.9
diaper syndrome E72.09
dome cyst (breast) —*see* Cyst, breast
dot cataract Q12.0
nevus D22.9

Blue *(Continued)*
sclera Q13.5
with fragility of bone and deafness Q78.0
toe syndrome I75.02-●
Blueness —*see* Cyanosis
Blues, postpartal O90.6
baby O90.6
Blurring, visual H53.8
Blushing (abnormal) (excessive) R23.2
BMI —*see* Body, mass index
Boarder, hospital NEC Z76.4
accompanying sick person Z76.3
healthy infant or child Z76.2
foundling Z76.1
Bockhart's impetigo L01.02
Bodechtel-Guttman disease (subacute sclerosing panencephalitis) A81.1
Boder-Sedgwick syndrome (ataxia-telangiectasia) G11.3
Body, bodies
Aschoff's —*see* Myocarditis, rheumatic
asteroid, vitreous —*see* Deposit, crystalline
cytoid (retina) —*see* Occlusion, artery, retina
drusen (degenerative) (macula) (retinal) —*see also* Degeneration, macula, drusen
optic disc —*see* Drusen, optic disc
foreign —*see* Foreign body
loose
joint, except knee —*see* Loose, body, joint
knee M23.4-●
sheath, tendon —*see* Disorder, tendon, specified type NEC
mass index (BMI)
adult
19.9 or less Z68.1
20.0-20.9 Z68.20
21.0-21.9 Z68.21
22.0-22.9 Z68.22
23.0-23.9 Z68.23
24.0-24.9 Z68.24
25.0-25.9 Z68.25
26.0-26.9 Z68.26
27.0-27.9 Z68.27
28.0-28.9 Z68.28
29.0-29.9 Z68.29
30.0-30.9 Z68.30
31.0-31.9 Z68.31
32.0-32.9 Z68.32
33.0-33.9 Z68.33
34.0-34.9 Z68.34
35.0-35.9 Z68.35
36.0-36.9 Z68.36
37.0-37.9 Z68.37
38.0-38.9 Z68.38
39.0-39.9 Z68.39
40.0-44.9 Z68.41
45.0-49.9 Z68.42
50.0-59.9 Z68.43
60.0-69.9 Z68.44
70 and over Z68.45
pediatric
5th percentile to less than 85th percentile for age Z68.52
85th percentile to less than 95th percentile for age Z68.53
greater than or equal to ninety-fifth percentile for age Z68.54
less than fifth percentile for age Z68.51
Mooser's A75.2
rice —*see also* Loose, body, joint
knee M23.4-●
rocking F98.4
Boeck's
disease or sarcoid —*see* Sarcoidosis
lupoid (miliary) D86.3
Boerhaave's syndrome (spontaneous esophageal rupture) K22.3
Boggy
cervix N88.8
uterus N85.8

Boil —*see also* Furuncle, by site
  Aleppo B55.1
  Baghdad B55.1
  Delhi B55.1
  lacrimal
    gland —*see* Dacryoadenitis
    passages (duct) (sac) —*see* Inflammation,
      lacrimal, passages, acute
  Natal B55.1
  orbit, orbital —*see* Abscess, orbit
  tropical B55.1
Bold hives —*see* Urticaria
Bombé, iris —*see* Membrane, pupillary
Bone —*see* condition
Bonnevie-Ullrich syndrome —*see also* Turner's
  syndrome Q87.19
Bonnier's syndrome —*see* subcategory H81.8
Bonvale dam fever T73.3
Bony block of joint —*see* Ankylosis
BOOP (bronchiolitis obliterans organized
  pneumonia) J84.89
Borderline
  diabetes mellitus R73.03
  hypertension R03.0
  osteopenia M85.8-●
  pelvis, with obstruction during labor O65.1
  personality F60.3
Borna disease A83.9
Bornholm disease B33.0
Boston exanthem A88.0
Botalli, ductus (patent) (persistent) Q25.0
Bothriocephalus latus infestation B70.0
Botulism (foodborne intoxication) A05.1
  infant A48.51
  non-foodborne A48.52
  wound A48.52
Bouba —*see* Yaws
Bouchard's nodes (with arthropathy) M15.2
Bouffée délirante F23
Bouillaud's disease or syndrome (rheumatic
  heart disease) I01.9
Bourneville's disease Q85.1
Boutonniere deformity (finger) —*see*
  Deformity, finger, boutonniere
Bouveret (-Hoffmann) syndrome (paroxysmal
  tachycardia) I47.9
Bovine heart —*see* Hypertrophy, cardiac
Bowel —*see* condition
Bowen's
  dermatosis (precancerous) —*see* Neoplasm,
    skin, in situ
  disease —*see* Neoplasm, skin, in situ
  epithelioma —*see* Neoplasm, skin, in situ
  type
    epidermoid carcinoma-in-situ —*see*
      Neoplasm, skin, in situ
    intraepidermal squamous cell carcinoma —
      see Neoplasm, skin, in situ
Bowing
  femur —*see also* Deformity, limb, specified
    type NEC, thigh
    congenital Q68.3
  fibula —*see also* Deformity, limb, specified
    type NEC, lower leg
    congenital Q68.4
  forearm —*see* Deformity, limb, specified type
    NEC, forearm
  leg(s), long bones, congenital Q68.5
  radius —*see* Deformity, limb, specified type
    NEC, forearm
  tibia —*see also* Deformity, limb, specified type
    NEC, lower leg
    congenital Q68.4
Bowleg(s) (acquired) M21.16-●
  congenital Q68.5
  rachitic E64.3
Boyd's dysentery A03.2
Brachial —*see* condition
Brachycardia R00.1
Brachycephaly Q75.0
Bradley's disease A08.19

Bradyarrhythmia, cardiac I49.8
Bradycardia (sinoatrial) (sinus) (vagal) R00.1
  neonatal P29.12
  reflex G90.09
  tachycardia syndrome I49.5
Bradykinesia R25.8
Bradypnea R06.89
Bradytachycardia I49.5
Brailsford's disease or osteochondrosis —*see*
  Osteochondrosis, juvenile, radius
Brain —*see also* condition
  death G93.82
  syndrome —*see* Syndrome, brain
Branched-chain amino-acid disorder E71.2
Branchial —*see* condition
  cartilage, congenital Q18.2
Branchiogenic remnant (in neck) Q18.0
Brandt's syndrome (acrodermatitis
  enteropathica) E83.2
Brash (water) R12
Bravais-Jacksonian epilepsy —*see* Epilepsy,
  localization-related, symptomatic, with
  simple partial seizures
Braxton Hicks contractions —*see* False, labor
Brazilian leishmaniasis B55.2
BRBPR K62.5
Break, retina (without detachment) H33.30-●
  with retinal detachment —*see* Detachment,
    retina
  horseshoe tear H33.31-●
  multiple H33.33-●
  round hole H33.32-●
Breakdown
  device, graft or implant —*see also*
    Complications, by site and type,
    mechanical T85.618
    arterial graft NEC —*see* Complication,
      cardiovascular device, mechanical,
      vascular
    breast (implant) T85.41
    catheter NEC T85.618
      cystostomy T83.010
      dialysis (renal) T82.41
        intraperitoneal T85.611
      Hopkins T83.018
      ileostomy T83.018
      infusion NEC T82.514
        cranial T85.610
        epidural T85.610
        intrathecal T85.610
        spinal T85.610
        subarachnoid T85.610
        subdural T85.610
      nephrostomy T83.012
      urethral indwelling T83.011
      urinary NEC T83.018
      urostomy T83.018
    electronic (electrode) (pulse generator)
      (stimulator)
      bone T84.310
      cardiac T82.119
        electrode T82.110
        pulse generator T82.111
        specified type NEC T82.118
      nervous system —*see* Complication,
        prosthetic device, mechanical,
        electronic nervous system stimulator
      urinary —*see* Complication,
        genitourinary, device, urinary,
        mechanical
    fixation, internal (orthopedic) NEC —
      see Complication, fixation device,
      mechanical
    gastrointestinal —*see* Complications,
      prosthetic device, mechanical,
      gastrointestinal device
    genital NEC T83.418
      intrauterine contraceptive device T83.31
      penile prosthesis (cylinder) (implanted)
        (pump) (reservoir) T83.410
      testicular prosthesis T83.411

Breakdown (Continued)
  device, graft or implant (Continued)
    heart NEC —*see* Complication,
      cardiovascular device, mechanical
    intrathecal infusion pump T85.615
    joint prosthesis —*see* Complications..., joint
      prosthesis,internal, mechanical, by site
    nervous system, specified device NEC
      T85.615
    ocular NEC —*see* Complications, prosthetic
      device, mechanical, ocular device
    orthopedic NEC —*see* Complication,
      orthopedic, device, mechanical
    specified NEC T85.618
    subcutaneous device pocket
      nervous system prosthetic device,
        implant, or graft T85.890
      other internal prosthetic device, implant,
        or graft T85.898
    sutures, permanent T85.612
      used in bone repair —*see* Complications,
        fixation device, internal
        (orthopedic), mechanical
    urinary NEC T83.118
      graft T83.21
      sphincter, implanted T83.111
      stent (ileal conduit) (nephroureteral)
        T83.113
        ureteral indwelling T83.112
    vascular NEC —*see* Complication,
      cardiovascular device, mechanical
    ventricular intracranial shunt T85.01
  nervous F48.8
  perineum O90.1
  respirator J95.850
    specified NEC J95.859
  ventilator J95.850
    specified NEC J95.859
Breast —*see also* condition
  buds E30.1
    in newborn P96.89
  dense R92.2
  nodule —*see also* Lump, breast N63.0
Breath
  foul R19.6
  holder, child R06.89
  holding spell R06.89
  shortness R06.02
Breathing
  labored —*see* Hyperventilation
  mouth R06.5
    causing malocclusion M26.5
  periodic R06.3
    high altitude G47.32
Breathlessness R06.81
Breda's disease —*see* Yaws
Breech presentation (mother) O32.1
  causing obstructed labor O64.1
  footling O32.8
    causing obstructed labor O64.8
  incomplete O32.8
    causing obstructed labor O64.8
Breisky's disease N90.4
Brennemann's syndrome I88.0
Brenner
  tumor (benign) D27.9
    borderline malignancy D39.1-●
    malignant C56
    proliferating D39.1
Bretonneau's disease or angina A36.0
Breus' mole O02.0
Brevicollis Q76.49
Brickmakers' anemia B76.9 [D63.8]
Bridge, myocardial Q24.5
Bright red blood per rectum (BRBPR)
  K62.5
Bright's disease —*see also* Nephritis
  arteriosclerotic —*see* Hypertension, kidney
Brill (-Zinsser) disease (recrudescent typhus)
  A75.1
Brill-Symmers' disease C82.90

▶ New   ⇒ Revised   ~~deleted~~ Deleted   ● Use Additional Character(s)

Brion-Kayser disease —*see* Fever, parathyroid
Briquet's disorder or syndrome F45.0
Brissaud's
  infantilism or dwarfism E23.0
  motor-verbal tic F95.2
Brittle
  bones disease Q78.0
  nails L60.3
    congenital Q84.6
Broad —*see also* condition
  beta disease E78.2
  ligament laceration syndrome N83.8
Broad- or floating-betalipoproteinemia E78.2
Brock's syndrome (atelectasis due to enlarged
    lymph nodes) J98.19
Brocq-Duhring disease (dermatitis
    herpetiformis) L13.0
Brodie's abscess or disease M86.8X- ●
Broken
  arches —*see also* Deformity, limb, flat foot
  arm (meaning upper limb) —*see* Fracture, arm
  back —*see* Fracture, vertebra
  bone —*see* Fracture
  implant or internal device —*see*
    Complications, by site and type,
    mechanical
  leg (meaning lower limb) —*see* Fracture, leg
  nose S02.2
  tooth, teeth —*see* Fracture, tooth
Bromhidrosis, bromidrosis L75.0
Bromidism, bromism G92.8
  chronic (dependence) F13.20
  due to
    correct substance properly administered —
      see Table of Drugs and Chemicals, by
      drug, adverse effect
    overdose or wrong substance given
      or taken —*see* Table of Drugs and
      Chemicals, by drug, poisoning
Bromidrosiphobia F40.298
Bronchi, bronchial —*see* condition
Bronchiectasis (cylindrical) (diffuse) (fusiform)
    (localized) (saccular) J47.9
  with
    acute
      bronchitis J47.0
      lower respiratory infection J47.0
    exacerbation (acute) J47.1
  congenital Q33.4
  tuberculous NEC —*see* Tuberculosis,
    pulmonary
Bronchiolectasis —*see* Bronchiectasis
Bronchiolitis (acute) (infective) (subacute) J21.9
  with
    bronchospasm or obstruction J21.9
    influenza, flu or grippe —*see* Influenza,
      with, respiratory manifestations NEC
    chemical (chronic) J68.4
      acute J68.0
    chronic (fibrosing) (obliterative) J44.9
    due to
      external agent —*see* Bronchitis, acute,
        due to
      human metapneumovirus J21.1
      respiratory syncytial virus (RSV) J21.0
      specified organism NEC J21.8
    fibrosa obliterans J44.9
    influenzal —*see* Influenza, with, respiratory
      manifestations NEC
    obliterans J42
      with organizing pneumonia (BOOP) J84.89
    obliterative (chronic) (subacute) J44.9
      due to chemicals, gases, fumes or vapors
        (inhalation) J68.4
      due to fumes or vapors J68.4
    respiratory, interstitial lung disease J84.115
Bronchitis (diffuse) (fibrinous) (hypostatic)
    (infective) (membranous) J40
  with
    influenza, flu or grippe —*see* Influenza,
      with, respiratory manifestations NEC

Bronchitis (*Continued*)
  with (*Continued*)
    obstruction (airway) (lung) J44.9
    tracheitis (15 years of age and above) J40
      acute or subacute J20.9
      chronic J42
      under 15 years of age J20.9
  acute or subacute (with bronchospasm or
    obstruction) J20.9
    with
      bronchiectasis J47.0
      chronic obstructive pulmonary disease
        J44.0
      chemical (due to gases, fumes or vapors)
        J68.0
    due to
      fumes or vapors J68.0
      Haemophilus influenzae J20.1
      Mycoplasma pneumoniae J20.0
      radiation J70.0
      specified organism NEC J20.8
      Streptococcus J20.2
      virus
        coxsackie J20.3
        echovirus J20.7
        parainfluenzae J20.4
        respiratory syncytial (RSV) J20.5
        rhinovirus J20.6
    viral NEC J20.8
  allergic (acute) J45.909
    with
      exacerbation (acute) J45.901
      status asthmaticus J45.902
  arachidic T17.528
  aspiration (due to food and vomit) J69.0
  asthmatic J45.9
    chronic J44.9
      with
        acute lower respiratory infection J44.0
        exacerbation (acute) J44.1
  capillary —*see* Pneumonia, broncho
  caseous (tuberculous) A15.5
  Castellani's A69.8
  catarrhal (15 years of age and above) J40
    acute —*see* Bronchitis, acute
    chronic J41.0
    under 15 years of age J20.9
  chemical (acute) (subacute) J68.0
    chronic J68.4
    due to fumes or vapors J68.0
      chronic J68.4
  chronic J42
    with
      airways obstruction J44.9
      tracheitis (chronic) J42
    asthmatic (obstructive) J44.9
    catarrhal J41.0
    chemical (due to fumes or vapors) J68.4
    due to
      chemicals, gases, fumes or vapors
        (inhalation) J68.4
      radiation J70.1
      tobacco smoking J41.0
    emphysematous J44.9
    mucopurulent J41.1
    non-obstructive J41.0
    obliterans J44.9
    obstructive J44.9
    purulent J41.1
    simple J41.0
  croupous —*see* Bronchitis, acute
  due to gases, fumes or vapors (chemical)
    J68.0
  emphysematous (obstructive) J44.9
  exudative —*see* Bronchitis, acute
  fetid J41.1
  grippal —*see* Influenza, with, respiratory
    manifestations NEC
  in those under 15 years age —*see* Bronchitis,
    acute
    chronic —*see* Bronchitis, chronic

Bronchitis (*Continued*)
  influenzal —*see* Influenza, with, respiratory
    manifestations NEC
  mixed simple and mucopurulent J41.8
  moulder's J62.8
  mucopurulent (chronic) (recurrent) J41.1
    acute or subacute J20.9
    simple (mixed) J41.8
  obliterans (chronic) J44.9
  obstructive (chronic) (diffuse) J44.9
  pituitous J41.1
  pneumococcal, acute or subacute J20.2
  pseudomembranous, acute or subacute —*see*
    Bronchitis, acute
  purulent (chronic) (recurrent) J41.1
    acute or subacute —*see* Bronchitis, acute
  putrid J41.1
  senile (chronic) J42
  simple and mucopurulent (mixed) J41.8
  smokers' J41.0
  spirochetal NEC A69.8
  subacute —*see* Bronchitis, acute
  suppurative (chronic) J41.1
    acute or subacute —*see* Bronchitis, acute
  tuberculous A15.5
  under 15 years of age —*see* Bronchitis, acute
    chronic —*see* Bronchitis, chronic
  viral NEC, acute or subacute —*see also*
    Bronchitis, acute J20.8
Bronchoalveolitis J18.0
Bronchoaspergillosis B44.1
Bronchocele meaning goiter E04.0
Broncholithiasis J98.09
  tuberculous NEC A15.5
Bronchomalacia J98.09
  congenital Q32.2
Bronchomycosis NOS B49 [*J99*]
  candidal B37.1
Bronchopleuropneumonia —*see* Pneumonia,
  broncho
Bronchopneumonia —*see* Pneumonia, broncho
Bronchopneumonitis —*see* Pneumonia,
  broncho
Bronchopulmonary —*see* condition
Bronchopulmonitis —*see* Pneumonia, broncho
Bronchorrhagia (*see* Hemoptysis)
Bronchorrhea J98.09
  acute J20.9
  chronic (infective) (purulent) J42
Bronchospasm (acute) J98.01
  with
    bronchiolitis, acute J21.9
    bronchitis, acute (conditions in J20) —*see*
      Bronchitis, acute
  due to external agent —*see* condition,
    respiratory, acute, due to
  exercise induced J45.990
Bronchospirochetosis A69.8
  Castellani A69.8
Bronchostenosis J98.09
Bronchus —*see* condition
Brontophobia F40.220
Bronze baby syndrome P83.88
Brooke's tumor —*see* Neoplasm, skin, benign
Brown enamel of teeth (hereditary) K00.5
Brown's sheath syndrome H50.61- ●
Brown-Séquard disease, paralysis or
  syndrome G83.81
Bruce sepsis A23.0
Brucellosis (infection) A23.9
  abortus A23.1
  canis A23.3
  dermatitis A23.9
  melitensis A23.0
  mixed A23.8
  sepsis A23.9
    melitensis A23.0
    specified NEC A23.8
  suis A23.2
Bruck-de Lange disease Q87.19
Bruck's disease —*see* Deformity, limb

BRUE (brief resolved unexplained event) R68.13
Brugsch's syndrome Q82.8
Bruise (skin surface intact) —see also Contusion
    with
        open wound —see Wound, open
    internal organ —see Injury, by site
    newborn P54.5
    scalp, due to birth injury, newborn P12.3
    umbilical cord O69.5
Bruit (arterial) R09.89
    cardiac R01.1
Brush burn —see Abrasion, by site
Bruton's X-linked agammaglobulinemia D80.0
Bruxism
    psychogenic F45.8
    sleep related G47.63
Bubbly lung syndrome P27.0
Bubo I88.8
    blennorrhagic (gonococcal) A54.89
    chancroidal A57
    climatic A55
    due to Haemophilus ducreyi A57
    gonococcal A54.89
    indolent (nonspecific) I88.8
    inguinal (nonspecific) I88.8
        chancroidal A57
        climatic A55
        due to H. ducreyi A57
        infective I88.8
    scrofulous (tuberculous) A18.2
    soft chancre A57
    suppurating —see Lymphadenitis, acute
    syphilitic (primary) A51.0
        congenital A50.07
    tropical A55
    virulent (chancroidal) A57
Bubonic plague A20.0
Bubonocele —see Hernia, inguinal
Buccal —see condition
Buchanan's disease or osteochondrosis M91.0
Buchem's syndrome (hyperostosis corticalis)
    M85.2
Bucket-handle fracture or tear (semilunar
    cartilage) —see Tear, meniscus
Budd-Chiari syndrome (hepatic vein
    thrombosis) I82.0
Budgerigar fancier's disease or lung
    J67.2
Buds
    breast E30.1
        in newborn P96.89
Buerger's disease (thromboangiitis obliterans)
    I73.1
Bulbar —see condition
Bulbus cordis (left ventricle) (persistent) Q21.8
Bulimia (nervosa) F50.2
    atypical F50.9
    normal weight F50.9
Bulky
    stools R19.5
    uterus N85.2
Bulla (e) R23.8
    lung (emphysematous) (solitary) J43.9
        newborn P25.8
▸Bullet wound —see also Puncture
    fracture - code as Fracture, by site
    internal organ —see Injury, by site
Bundle
    branch block (complete) (false)
        (incomplete) —see Block, bundle-branch
    of His —see condition
Bunion M21.61-●
    tailor's M21.62-●
Bunionette M21.62-●
Buphthalmia, buphthalmos (congenital) Q15.0
Burdwan fever B55.0
Bürger-Grütz disease or syndrome E78.3
Buried
    penis (congenital) Q55.64
        acquired N48.83
    roots K08.3

Burke's syndrome K86.89
Burkitt
    cell leukemia C91.0-●
    lymphoma (malignant) C83.7-●
        small noncleaved, diffuse C83.7-●
        spleen C83.77
        undifferentiated C83.7-●
    tumor C83.7-●
    type
        acute lymphoblastic leukemia C91.0-●
        undifferentiated C83.7-●
Burn (electricity) (flame) (hot gas, liquid or hot
    object) (radiation) (steam) (thermal) T30.0
    abdomen, abdominal (muscle) (wall)
        T21.02
        first degree T21.12
        second degree T21.22
        third degree T21.32
    above elbow T22.039
        first degree T22.139
        left T22.032
            first degree T22.132
            second degree T22.232
            third degree T22.332
        right T22.031
            first degree T22.131
            second degree T22.231
            third degree T22.331
        second degree T22.239
        third degree T22.339
    acid (caustic) (external) (internal) —see
        Corrosion, by site
    alimentary tract NEC T28.2
        esophagus T28.1
        mouth T28.0
        pharynx T28.0
    alkaline (caustic) (external) (internal) —see
        Corrosion, by site
    ankle T25.019
        first degree T25.119
        left T25.012
            first degree T25.112
            second degree T25.212
            third degree T25.312
        multiple with foot —see Burn, lower, limb,
            multiple, ankle and foot
        right T25.011
            first degree T25.111
            second degree T25.211
            third degree T25.311
        second degree T25.219
        third degree T25.319
    anus —see Burn, buttock
    arm (lower) (upper) —see Burn, upper,
        limb
    axilla T22.049
        first degree T22.149
        left T22.042
            first degree T22.142
            second degree T22.242
            third degree T22.342
        right T22.041
            first degree T22.141
            second degree T22.241
            third degree T22.341
        second degree T22.249
        third degree T22.349
    back (lower) T21.04
        first degree T21.14
        second degree T21.24
        third degree T21.34
        upper T21.03
            first degree T21.13
            second degree T21.23
            third degree T21.33
    blisters - code as Burn, second degree, by site
    breast(s) —see Burn, chest wall
    buttock(s) T21.05
        first degree T21.15
        second degree T21.25
        third degree T21.35

Burn (Continued)
    calf T24.039
        first degree T24.139
        left T24.032
            first degree T24.132
            second degree T24.232
            third degree T24.332
        right T24.031
            first degree T24.131
            second degree T24.231
            third degree T24.331
        second degree T24.239
        third degree T24.339
    canthus (eye) —see Burn, eyelid
    caustic acid or alkaline —see Corrosion, by
        site
    cervix T28.3
    cheek T20.06
        first degree T20.16
        second degree T20.26
        third degree T20.36
    chemical (acids) (alkalines) (caustics) (external)
        (internal) —see Corrosion, by site
    chest wall T21.01
        first degree T21.11
        second degree T21.21
        third degree T21.31
    chin T20.03
        first degree T20.13
        second degree T20.23
        third degree T20.33
    colon T28.2
    conjunctiva (and cornea) —see Burn, cornea
    cornea (and conjunctiva) T26.1-●
        chemical —see Corrosion, cornea
    corrosion (external) (internal) —see
        Corrosion, by site
    deep necrosis of underlying tissue - code as
        Burn, third degree, by site
    dorsum of hand T23.069
        first degree T23.169
        left T23.062
            first degree T23.162
            second degree T23.262
            third degree T23.362
        right T23.061
            first degree T23.161
            second degree T23.261
            third degree T23.361
        second degree T23.269
        third degree T23.369
    due to ingested chemical agent —see
        Corrosion, by site
    ear (auricle) (external) (canal) T20.01
        first degree T20.11
        second degree T20.21
        third degree T20.31
    elbow T22.029
        first degree T22.129
        left T22.022
            first degree T22.122
            second degree T22.222
            third degree T22.322
        right T22.021
            first degree T22.121
            second degree T22.221
            third degree T22.321
        second degree T22.229
        third degree T22.329
    epidermal loss - code as Burn, second degree,
        by site
    erythema, erythematous - code as Burn, first
        degree, by site
    esophagus T28.1
    extent (percentage of body surface)
        less than 10 percent T31.0
        10-19 percent T31.10
            with 0-9 percent third degree burns
                T31.10
            with 10-19 percent third degree burns
                T31.11

▶ New   ▥ Revised   ~~deleted~~ Deleted   ● Use Additional Character(s)

Burn *(Continued)*
  extent *(Continued)*
    20-29 percent T31.20
      with 0-9 percent third degree burns T31.20
      with 10-19 percent third degree burns T31.21
      with 20-29 percent third degree burns T31.22
    30-39 percent T31.30
      with 0-9 percent third degree burns T31.30
      with 10-19 percent third degree burns T31.31
      with 20-29 percent third degree burns T31.32
      with 30-39 percent third degree burns T31.33
    40-49 percent T31.40
      with 0-9 percent third degree burns T31.40
      with 10-19 percent third degree burns T31.41
      with 20-29 percent third degree burns T31.42
      with 30-39 percent third degree burns T31.43
      with 40-49 percent third degree burns T31.44
    50-59 percent T31.50
      with 0-9 percent third degree burns T31.50
      with 10-19 percent third degree burns T31.51
      with 20-29 percent third degree burns T31.52
      with 30-39 percent third degree burns T31.53
      with 40-49 percent third degree burns T31.54
      with 50-59 percent third degree burns T31.55
    60-69 percent T31.60
      with 0-9 percent third degree burns T31.60
      with 10-19 percent third degree burns T31.61
      with 20-29 percent third degree burns T31.62
      with 30-39 percent third degree burns T31.63
      with 40-49 percent third degree burns T31.64
      with 50-59 percent third degree burns T31.65
      with 60-69 percent third degree burns T31.66
    70-79 percent T31.70
      with 0-9 percent third degree burns T31.70
      with 10-19 percent third degree burns T31.71
      with 20-29 percent third degree burns T31.72
      with 30-39 percent third degree burns T31.73
      with 40-49 percent third degree burns T31.74
      with 50-59 percent third degree burns T31.75
      with 60-69 percent third degree burns T31.76
      with 70-79 percent third degree burns T31.77
    80-89 percent T31.80
      with 0-9 percent third degree burns T31.80
      with 10-19 percent third degree burns T31.81
      with 20-29 percent third degree burns T31.82
      with 30-39 percent third degree burns T31.83
      with 40-49 percent third degree burns T31.84

Burn *(Continued)*
  extent *(Continued)*
    80-89 percent T31.80 *(Continued)*
      with 50-59 percent third degree burns T31.85
      with 60-69 percent third degree burns T31.86
      with 70-79 percent third degree burns T31.87
      with 80-89 percent third degree burns T31.88
    90 percent or more T31.90
      with 0-9 percent third degree burns T31.90
      with 10-19 percent third degree burns T31.91
      with 20-29 percent third degree burns T31.92
      with 30-39 percent third degree burns T31.93
      with 40-49 percent third degree burns T31.94
      with 50-59 percent third degree burns T31.95
      with 60-69 percent third degree burns T31.96
      with 70-79 percent third degree burns T31.97
      with 80-89 percent third degree burns T31.98
      with 90 percent or more third degree burns T31.99
  extremity —*see* Burn, limb
  eye(s) and adnexa T26.4-●
    with resulting rupture and destruction of eyeball T26.2-●
    conjunctival sac —*see* Burn, cornea
    cornea —*see* Burn, cornea
    lid —*see* Burn, eyelid
    periocular area —*see* Burn, eyelid
    specified site NEC T26.3-●
  eyeball —*see* Burn, eye
  eyelid(s) T26.0-●
    chemical —*see* Corrosion, eyelid
  face —*see* Burn, head
  finger T23.029
    first degree T23.129
    left T23.022
      first degree T23.122
      second degree T23.222
      third degree T23.322
    multiple sites (without thumb) T23.039
      with thumb T23.049
        first degree T23.149
        left T23.042
          first degree T23.142
          second degree T23.242
          third degree T23.342
        right T23.041
          first degree T23.141
          second degree T23.241
          third degree T23.341
        second degree T23.249
        third degree T23.349
      first degree T23.139
      left T23.032
        first degree T23.132
        second degree T23.232
        third degree T23.332
      right T23.031
        first degree T23.131
        second degree T23.231
        third degree T23.331
      second degree T23.239
      third degree T23.339
    right T23.021
      first degree T23.121
      second degree T23.221
      third degree T23.321
    second degree T23.229
    third degree T23.329
  flank —*see* Burn, abdominal wall

Burn *(Continued)*
  foot T25.029
    first degree T25.129
    left T25.022
      first degree T25.122
      second degree T25.222
      third degree T25.322
    multiple with ankle —*see* Burn, lower, limb, multiple, ankle and foot
    right T25.021
      first degree T25.121
      second degree T25.221
      third degree T25.321
    second degree T25.229
    third degree T25.329
  forearm T22.019
    first degree T22.119
    left T22.012
      first degree T22.112
      second degree T22.212
      third degree T22.312
    right T22.011
      first degree T22.111
      second degree T22.211
      third degree T22.311
    second degree T22.219
    third degree T22.319
  forehead T20.06
    first degree T20.16
    second degree T20.26
    third degree T20.36
  fourth degree - code as Burn, third degree, by site
  friction —*see* Burn, by site
  from swallowing caustic or corrosive substance NEC —*see* Corrosion, by site
  full thickness skin loss - code as Burn, third degree, by site
  gastrointestinal tract NEC T28.2
    from swallowing caustic or corrosive substance T28.7
  genital organs
    external
      female T21.07
        first degree T21.17
        second degree T21.27
        third degree T21.37
      male T21.06
        first degree T21.16
        second degree T21.26
        third degree T21.36
    internal T28.3
      from caustic or corrosive substance T28.8
  groin —*see* Burn, abdominal wall
  hand(s) T23.009
    back —*see* Burn, dorsum of hand
    finger —*see* Burn, finger
    first degree T23.109
    left T23.002
      first degree T23.102
      second degree T23.202
      third degree T23.302
    multiple sites with wrist T23.099
      first degree T23.199
      left T23.092
        first degree T23.192
        second degree T23.292
        third degree T23.392
      right T23.091
        first degree T23.191
        second degree T23.291
        third degree T23.391
      second degree T23.299
      third degree T23.399
    palm —*see* Burn, palm
    right T23.001
      first degree T23.101
      second degree T23.201
      third degree T23.301

Burn *(Continued)*
  hand *(Continued)*
    second degree T23.209
    third degree T23.309
    thumb —*see* Burn, thumb
  head (and face) (and neck) T20.00
    cheek —*see* Burn, cheek
    chin —*see* Burn, chin
    ear —*see* Burn, ear
    eye(s) only —*see* Burn, eye
    first degree T20.10
    forehead —*see* Burn, forehead
    lip —*see* Burn, lip
    multiple sites T20.09
      first degree T20.19
      second degree T20.29
      third degree T20.39
    neck —*see* Burn, neck
    nose —*see* Burn, nose
    scalp —*see* Burn, scalp
    second degree T20.20
    third degree T20.30
  hip(s) —*see* Burn, thigh
  inhalation —*see* Burn, respiratory tract
    caustic or corrosive substance (fumes) —*see* Corrosion, respiratory tract
  internal organ(s) T28.40
    alimentary tract T28.2
      esophagus T28.1
    eardrum T28.41
    esophagus T28.1
    from caustic or corrosive substance (swallowing) NEC —*see* Corrosion, by site
    genitourinary T28.3
    mouth T28.0
    pharynx T28.0
    respiratory tract —*see* Burn, respiratory tract
    specified organ NEC T28.49
  interscapular region —*see* Burn, back, upper
  intestine (large) (small) T28.2
  knee T24.029
    first degree T24.129
    left T24.022
      first degree T24.122
      second degree T24.222
      third degree T24.322
    right T24.021
      first degree T24.121
      second degree T24.221
      third degree T24.321
    second degree T24.229
    third degree T24.329
  labium (majus) (minus) —*see* Burn, genital organs, external, female
  lacrimal apparatus, duct, gland or sac —*see* Burn, eye, specified site NEC
  larynx T27.0
    with lung T27.1
  leg(s) (lower) (upper) —*see* Burn, lower, limb
  lightning —*see* Burn, by site
  limb(s)
    lower (except ankle or foot alone) —*see* Burn, lower, limb
    upper —*see* Burn, upper limb
  lip(s) T20.02
    first degree T20.12
    second degree T20.22
    third degree T20.32
  lower
    back —*see* Burn, back
    limb T24.009
      ankle —*see* Burn, ankle
      calf —*see* Burn, calf
      first degree T24.109
      foot —*see* Burn, foot
      hip —*see* Burn, thigh
      knee —*see* Burn, knee

Burn *(Continued)*
  lower *(Continued)*
    limb *(Continued)*
      left T24.002
        first degree T24.102
        second degree T24.202
        third degree T24.302
      multiple sites, except ankle and foot T24.099
      ankle and foot T25.099
        first degree T25.199
        left T25.092
          first degree T25.192
          second degree T25.292
          third degree T25.392
        right T25.091
          first degree T25.191
          second degree T25.291
          third degree T25.391
        second degree T25.299
        third degree T25.399
      first degree T24.199
      left T24.092
        first degree T24.192
        second degree T24.292
        third degree T24.392
      right T24.091
        first degree T24.191
        second degree T24.291
        third degree T24.391
      second degree T24.299
      third degree T24.399
      right T24.001
        first degree T24.101
        second degree T24.201
        third degree T24.301
      second degree T24.209
      thigh —*see* Burn, thigh
      third degree T24.309
      toe —*see* Burn, toe
  lung (with larynx and trachea) T27.1
  mouth T28.0
  neck T20.07
    first degree T20.17
    second degree T20.27
    third degree T20.37
  nose (septum) T20.04
    first degree T20.14
    second degree T20.24
    third degree T20.34
  ocular adnexa —*see* Burn, eye
  orbit region —*see* Burn, eyelid
  palm T23.059
    first degree T23.159
    left T23.052
      first degree T23.152
      second degree T23.252
      third degree T23.352
    right T23.051
      first degree T23.151
      second degree T23.251
      third degree T23.351
    second degree T23.259
    third degree T23.359
  partial thickness - code as Burn, by site, second degree
  pelvis —*see* Burn, trunk
  penis —*see* Burn, genital organs, external, male
  perineum
    female —*see* Burn, genital organs, external, female
    male —*see* Burn, genital organs, external, male
  periocular area —*see* Burn, eyelid
  pharynx T28.0
  rectum T28.2
  respiratory tract T27.3
    larynx —*see* Burn, larynx
    specified part NEC T27.2
    trachea —*see* Burn, trachea

Burn *(Continued)*
  sac, lacrimal —*see* Burn, eye, specified site NEC
  scalp T20.05
    first degree T20.15
    second degree T20.25
    third degree T20.35
  scapular region T22.069
    first degree T22.169
    left T22.062
      first degree T22.162
      second degree T22.262
      third degree T22.362
    right T22.061
      first degree T22.161
      second degree T22.261
      third degree T22.361
    second degree T22.269
    third degree T22.369
  sclera —*see* Burn, eye, specified site NEC
  scrotum —*see* Burn, genital organs, external, male
  shoulder T22.059
    first degree T22.159
    left T22.052
      first degree T22.152
      second degree T22.252
      third degree T22.352
    right T22.051
      first degree T22.151
      second degree T22.251
      third degree T22.351
    second degree T22.259
    third degree T22.359
  stomach T28.2
  temple —*see* Burn, head
  testis —*see* Burn, genital organs, external, male
  thigh T24.019
    first degree T24.119
    left T24.012
      first degree T24.112
      second degree T24.212
      third degree T24.312
    right T24.011
      first degree T24.111
      second degree T24.211
      third degree T24.311
    second degree T24.219
    third degree T24.319
  thorax (external) —*see* Burn, trunk
  throat (meaning pharynx) T28.0
  thumb(s) T23.019
    first degree T23.119
    left T23.012
      first degree T23.112
      second degree T23.212
      third degree T23.312
    multiple sites with fingers T23.049
      first degree T23.149
      left T23.042
        first degree T23.142
        second degree T23.242
        third degree T23.342
      right T23.041
        first degree T23.141
        second degree T23.241
        third degree T23.341
      second degree T23.249
      third degree T23.349
    right T23.011
      first degree T23.111
      second degree T23.211
      third degree T23.311
    second degree T23.219
    third degree T23.319
  toe T25.039
    first degree T25.139
    left T25.032
      first degree T25.132
      second degree T25.232
      third degree T25.332

▶ New   ⇒ Revised   ~~deleted~~ Deleted   ● Use Additional Character(s)

Burn (Continued)
  toe (Continued)
    right T25.031
      first degree T25.131
      second degree T25.231
      third degree T25.331
    second degree T25.239
    third degree T25.339
  tongue T28.0
  tonsil(s) T28.0
  trachea T27.0
    with lung T27.1
  trunk T21.00
    abdominal wall —see Burn, abdominal
      wall
    anus —see Burn, buttock
    axilla —see Burn, upper limb
    back —see Burn, back
    breast —see Burn, chest wall
    buttock —see Burn, buttock
    chest wall —see Burn, chest wall
    first degree T21.10
    flank —see Burn, abdominal wall
    genital
      female —see Burn, genital organs,
        external, female
      male —see Burn, genital organs, external,
        male
    groin —see Burn, abdominal wall
    interscapular region —see Burn, back,
      upper
    labia —see Burn, genital organs, external,
      female
    lower back —see Burn, back
    penis —see Burn, genital organs, external,
      male
    perineum
      female —see Burn, genital organs,
        external, female
      male —see Burn, genital organs, external,
        male
    scapula region —see Burn, scapular
      region
    scrotum —see Burn, genital organs,
      external, male
    second degree T21.20
    specified site NEC T21.09
      first degree T21.19
      second degree T21.29
      third degree T21.39
    testes —see Burn, genital organs, external,
      male
    third degree T21.30
    upper back —see Burn, back, upper
    vulva —see Burn, genital organs, external,
      female
  unspecified site with extent of body surface
    involved specified
    less than 10 percent T31.0
    10-19 percent (0-9 percent third degree)
      T31.10
      with 10-19 percent third degree
        T31.11
    20-29 percent (0-9 percent third degree)
      T31.20
      with
        10-19 percent third degree T31.21
        20-29 percent third degree T31.22
    30-39 percent (0-9 percent third degree)
      T31.30
      with
        10-19 percent third degree T31.31
        20-29 percent third degree T31.32
        30-39 percent third degree T31.33
    40-49 percent (0-9 percent third degree)
      T31.40
      with
        10-19 percent third degree T31.41
        20-29 percent third degree T31.42
        30-39 percent third degree T31.43
        40-49 percent third degree T31.44

Burn (Continued)
  unspecified site with extent of body surface
    involved specified (Continued)
    50-59 percent (0-9 percent third degree)
      T31.50
      with
        10-19 percent third degree T31.51
        20-29 percent third degree T31.52
        30-39 percent third degree T31.53
        40-49 percent third degree T31.54
        50-59 percent third degree T31.55
    60-69 percent (0-9 percent third degree)
      T31.60
      with
        10-19 percent third degree T31.61
        20-29 percent third degree T31.62
        30-39 percent third degree T31.63
        40-49 percent third degree T31.64
        50-59 percent third degree T31.65
        60-69 percent third degree T31.66
    70-79 percent (0-9 percent third degree)
      T31.70
      with
        10-19 percent third degree T31.71
        20-29 percent third degree T31.72
        30-39 percent third degree T31.73
        40-49 percent third degree T31.74
        50-59 percent third degree T31.75
        60-69 percent third degree T31.76
        70-79 percent third degree T31.77
    80-89 percent (0-9 percent third degree)
      T31.80
      with
        10-19 percent third degree T31.81
        20-29 percent third degree T31.82
        30-39 percent third degree T31.83
        40-49 percent third degree T31.84
        50-59 percent third degree T31.85
        60-69 percent third degree T31.86
        70-79 percent third degree T31.87
        80-89 percent third degree T31.88
    90 percent or more (0-9 percent third
      degree) T31.90
      with
        10-19 percent third degree T31.91
        20-29 percent third degree T31.92
        30-39 percent third degree T31.93
        40-49 percent third degree T31.94
        50-59 percent third degree T31.95
        60-69 percent third degree T31.96
        70-79 percent third degree T31.97
        80-89 percent third degree T31.98
        90-99 percent third degree T31.99
  upper limb T22.00
    above elbow —see Burn, above elbow
    axilla —see Burn, axilla
    elbow —see Burn, elbow
    first degree T22.10
    forearm —see Burn, forearm
    hand —see Burn, hand
    interscapular region —see Burn, back,
      upper
    multiple sites T22.099
      first degree T22.199
      left T22.092
        first degree T22.192
        second degree T22.292
        third degree T22.392
      right T22.091
        first degree T22.191
        second degree T22.291
        third degree T22.391
      second degree T22.299
      third degree T22.399
    scapular region —see Burn, scapular region
    second degree T22.20
    shoulder —see Burn, shoulder
    third degree T22.30
    wrist —see Burn, wrist
  uterus T28.3
  vagina T28.3

Burn (Continued)
  vulva —see Burn, genital organs, external,
    female
  wrist T23.079
    first degree T23.179
    left T23.072
      first degree T23.172
      second degree T23.272
      third degree T23.372
    multiple sites with hand T23.099
      first degree T23.199
      left T23.092
        first degree T23.192
        second degree T23.292
        third degree T23.392
      right T23.091
        first degree T23.191
        second degree T23.291
        third degree T23.391
      second degree T23.299
      third degree T23.399
    right T23.071
      first degree T23.171
      second degree T23.271
      third degree T23.371
    second degree T23.279
    third degree T23.379
Burnett's syndrome E83.52
Burning
  feet syndrome E53.9
  sensation R20.8
  tongue K14.6
Burn-out (state) Z73.0
Burns' disease or osteochondrosis —see
  Osteochondrosis, juvenile, ulna
Bursa —see condition
Bursitis M71.9
  Achilles —see Tendinitis, Achilles
  adhesive —see Bursitis, specified NEC
  ankle —see Enthesopathy, lower limb, ankle,
    specified type NEC
  calcaneal —see Enthesopathy, foot, specified
    type NEC
  collateral ligament, tibial —see Bursitis, tibial
    collateral
  due to use, overuse, pressure —see also
    Disorder, soft tissue, due to use,
    specified type NEC
    specified NEC —see Disorder, soft tissue,
      due to use, specified NEC
  Duplay's M75.0
  elbow NEC M70.3-•
    olecranon M70.2-•
  finger —see Disorder, soft tissue, due to use,
    specified type NEC, hand
  foot —see Enthesopathy, foot, specified type
    NEC
  gonococcal A54.49
  gouty —see Gout
  hand M70.1-•
  hip NEC M70.7-•
    trochanteric M70.6-•
  infective NEC M71.10
    abscess —see Abscess, bursa
    ankle M71.17-•
    elbow M71.12-•
    foot M71.17-•
    hand M71.14-•
    hip M71.15-•
    knee M71.16-•
    multiple sites M71.19
    shoulder M71.11-•
    specified site NEC M71.18
    wrist M71.13-•
  ischial —see Bursitis, hip
  knee NEC M70.5-•
    prepatellar M70.4-•
  occupational NEC —see also Disorder, soft
    tissue, due to, use
  olecranon —see Bursitis, elbow, olecranon
  pharyngeal J39.1

Bursitis *(Continued)*
  popliteal —*see* Bursitis, knee
  prepatellar M70.4-●
  radiohumeral M70.3-●
  rheumatoid M06.20
    ankle M06.27-●
    elbow M06.22-●
    foot joint M06.27-●
    hand joint M06.24-●
    hip M06.25-●
    knee M06.26-●
    multiple site M06.29
    shoulder M06.21-●
    vertebra M06.28
    wrist M06.23-●
  scapulohumeral —*see* Bursitis, shoulder
  semimembranous muscle (knee) —*see*
      Bursitis, knee
  shoulder M75.5-●
    adhesive —*see* Capsulitis, adhesive
  specified NEC M71.50
    ankle M71.57-●
    due to use, overuse or pressure —*see*
        Disorder, soft tissue, due to, use
    elbow M71.52-●
    foot M71.57-●
    hand M71.54-●

Bursitis *(Continued)*
  specified NEC *(Continued)*
    hip M71.55-●
    knee M71.56-●
    shoulder —*see* Bursitis, shoulder
    specified site NEC M71.58
    tibial collateral M76.4-●
    wrist M71.53-●
  subacromial —*see* Bursitis, shoulder
  subcoracoid —*see* Bursitis, shoulder
  subdeltoid —*see* Bursitis, shoulder
  syphilitic A52.78
  Thornwaldt, Tornwaldt J39.2
  tibial collateral M76.4-●
  toe —*see* Enthesopathy, foot, specified type
      NEC
  trochanteric (area) —*see* Bursitis, hip,
      trochanteric
  wrist —*see* Bursitis, hand
Bursopathy M71.9
  specified type NEC M71.80
    ankle M71.87-●
    elbow M71.82-●
    foot M71.87-●
    hand M71.84-●
    hip M71.85-●
    knee M71.86-●

Bursopathy *(Continued)*
  specified type NEC *(Continued)*
    multiple sites M71.89
    shoulder M71.81-●
    specified site NEC M71.88
    wrist M71.83-●
Burst stitches or sutures (complication of
    surgery) T81.31
  external operation wound T81.31
  internal operation wound T81.32
Buruli ulcer A31.1
Bury's disease L95.1
Buschke's
  disease —*see* Cryptococcosis by site
  scleredema —*see* Sclerosis, systemic
Busse-Buschke disease —*see* Cryptococcosis
    by site
Buttock —*see* condition
Button
  Biskra B55.1
  Delhi B55.1
  oriental B55.1
Buttonhole deformity (finger) —*see* Deformity,
    finger, boutonniere
Bwamba fever A92.8
Byssinosis J66.0
Bywaters' syndrome T79.5

▶ New ➡ Revised ~~deleted~~ Deleted ● Use Additional Character(s)

C

Cachexia R64
  cancerous R64
  cardiac —see Disease, heart
  dehydration E86.0
  due to malnutrition R64
  exophthalmic —see Hyperthyroidism
  heart —see Disease, heart
  hypophyseal E23.0
  hypopituitary E23.0
  lead —see Poisoning, lead
  malignant R64
  marsh —see Malaria
  nervous F48.8
  old age R54
  paludal —see Malaria
  pituitary E23.0
  pulmonary R64
  renal N28.9
  saturnine —see Poisoning, lead
  senile R54
  Simmonds' E23.0
  splenica D73.0
  strumipriva E03.4
  tuberculous NEC —see Tuberculosis
CADASIL (cerebral autosomal dominant
    arteriopathy with subcortical infarcts
    and leukoencephalopathy) I67.850
Café au lait spots L81.3
Caffeine-induced
  anxiety disorder F15.980
  sleep disorder F15.982
Caffey's syndrome Q78.8
Caisson disease T70.3
Cake kidney Q63.1
Caked breast (puerperal, postpartum) O92.79
Calabar swelling B74.3
Calcaneal spur —see Spur, bone, calcaneal
Calcaneo-apophysitis M92.8
Calcareous —see condition
Calcicosis J62.8
Calciferol (vitamin D) deficiency E55.9
  with rickets E55.0
Calcification
  adrenal (capsule) (gland) E27.49
    tuberculous E35 [B90.8]
  aorta I70.0
  artery (annular) —see Arteriosclerosis
  auricle (ear) —see Disorder, pinna, specified
      type NEC
  basal ganglia G23.8
  bladder N32.89
    due to Schistosoma hematobium B65.0
  brain (cortex) —see Calcification, cerebral
  bronchus J98.09
  bursa M71.40
    ankle M71.47-•
    elbow M71.42-•
    foot M71.47-•
    hand M71.44-•
    hip M71.45-•
    knee M71.46-•
    multiple sites M71.49
    shoulder M75.3-•
    specified site NEC M71.48
    wrist M71.43-•
  cardiac —see Degeneration, myocardial
  cerebral (cortex) G93.89
    artery I67.2
  cervix (uteri) N88.8
  choroid plexus G93.89
  conjunctiva —see Concretion, conjunctiva
  corpora cavernosa (penis) N48.89
  cortex (brain) —see Calcification, cerebral
  dental pulp (nodular) K04.2
  dentinal papilla K00.4
  fallopian tube N83.8
  falx cerebri G96.198
  gallbladder K82.8
  general E83.59
  heart —see also Degeneration, myocardial
    ▶valve —see also Endocarditis
    ▶mitral —see Calcification, mitral

Calcification (Continued)
  idiopathic infantile arterial (IIAC) Q28.8
  intervertebral cartilage or disc (postinfective) —
      see Disorder, disc, specified NEC
  intracranial —see Calcification, cerebral
  joint —see Disorder, joint, specified type NEC
  kidney N28.89
    tuberculous N29 [B90.1]
  larynx (senile) J38.7
  lens —see Cataract, specified NEC
  lung (active) (postinfectional) J98.4
    tuberculous B90.9
  lymph gland or node (postinfectional) I89.8
    tuberculous —see also Tuberculosis, lymph
        gland B90.8
  mammographic R92.1
  massive (paraplegic) —see Myositis,
      ossificans, in, quadriplegia
  medial —see Arteriosclerosis, extremities
  meninges (cerebral) (spinal) G96.198
  metastatic E83.59
  ▶mitral (valve)
    ▶annular I34.81
      ▶nonrheumatic I34.81
      ▶rheumatic I05.8
    ▶annulus I34.81
      ▶nonrheumatic I34.81
      ▶rheumatic I05.8
  Mönckeberg's —see Arteriosclerosis,
      extremities
  muscle M61.9
    due to burns —see Myositis, ossificans, in,
        burns
    paralytic —see Myositis, ossificans, in,
        quadriplegia
    specified type NEC M61.40
      ankle M61.47-•
      foot M61.47-•
      forearm M61.43-•
      hand M61.44-•
      lower leg M61.46-•
      multiple sites M61.49
      pelvic region M61.45-•
      shoulder region M61.41-•
      specified site NEC M61.48
      thigh M61.45-•
      upper arm M61.42-•
  myocardium, myocardial —see Degeneration,
      myocardial
  ovary N83.8
  pancreas K86.89
  penis N48.89
  periarticular —see Disorder, joint, specified
      type NEC
  pericardium —see also Pericarditis I31.1
  pineal gland E34.8
  pleura J94.8
    postinfectional J94.8
    tuberculous NEC B90.9
  pulpal (dental) (nodular) K04.2
  sclera H15.89
  spleen D73.89
  subcutaneous L94.2
  suprarenal (capsule) (gland) E27.49
  tendon (sheath) —see also Tenosynovitis,
      specified type NEC
    with bursitis, synovitis or tenosynovitis —
        see Tendinitis, calcific
  trachea J39.8
  ureter N28.89
  vitreous —see Deposit, crystalline
Calcified —see Calcification
Calcinosis (interstitial) (tumoral) (universalis)
    E83.59
  with Raynaud's phenomenon, esophageal
      dysfunction, sclerodactyly, telangiectasia
      (CREST syndrome) M34.1
  circumscripta (skin) L94.2
  cutis L94.2
Calciphylaxis —see also Calcification, by site
    E83.59

Calcium
  deposits —see Calcification, by site
  metabolism disorder E83.50
  salts or soaps in vitreous —see Deposit,
      crystalline
Calciuria R82.994
Calculi —see Calculus
Calculosis, intrahepatic —see Calculus, bile duct
Calculus, calculi, calculous
  ampulla of Vater —see Calculus, bile duct
  anuria (impacted) (recurrent) —see also
      Calculus, urinary N20.9
  appendix K38.1
  bile duct (common) (hepatic) K80.50
    with
      calculus of gallbladder —see Calculus,
          gallbladder and bile duct
      cholangitis K80.30
        with
          cholecystitis —see Calculus, bile
              duct, with cholecystitis
          obstruction K80.31
        acute K80.32
          with
            chronic cholangitis K80.36
              with obstruction K80.37
            obstruction K80.33
        chronic K80.34
          with
            acute cholangitis K80.36
              with obstruction K80.37
            obstruction K80.35
      cholecystitis (with cholangitis) K80.40
        with obstruction K80.41
        acute K80.42
          with
            chronic cholecystitis K80.46
              with obstruction K80.47
            obstruction K80.43
        chronic K80.44
          with
            acute cholecystitis K80.46
              with obstruction K80.47
            obstruction K80.45
      obstruction K80.51
  biliary —see also Calculus, gallbladder
    specified NEC K80.80
      with obstruction K80.81
  bilirubin, multiple —see Calculus, gallbladder
  bladder (encysted) (impacted) (urinary)
      (diverticulum) N21.0
  bronchus J98.09
  calyx (kidney) (renal) —see Calculus, kidney
  cholesterol (pure) (solitary) —see Calculus,
      gallbladder
  common duct (bile) —see Calculus, bile duct
  conjunctiva —see Concretion, conjunctiva
  cystic N21.0
    duct —see Calculus, gallbladder
  dental (subgingival) (supragingival) K03.6
  diverticulum
    bladder N21.0
    kidney N20.0
  epididymis N50.89
  gallbladder K80.20
    with
      bile duct calculus —see Calculus,
          gallbladder and bile duct
      cholecystitis K80.10
        with obstruction K80.11
        acute K80.00
          with
            chronic cholecystitis K80.12
              with obstruction K80.13
            obstruction K80.01
        chronic K80.10
          with
            acute cholecystitis K80.12
              with obstruction K80.13
            obstruction K80.11
      specified NEC K80.18
        with obstruction K80.19
    obstruction K80.21

Calculus, calculi, calculous (Continued)
  gallbladder and bile duct K80.70
    with
      cholecystitis K80.60
        with obstruction K80.61
        acute K80.62
          with
            chronic cholecystitis K80.66
              with obstruction K80.67
              obstruction K80.63
            obstruction K80.63
        chronic K80.64
          with
            acute cholecystitis K80.66
              with obstruction K80.67
            obstruction K80.65
      obstruction K80.71
  hepatic (duct) —see Calculus, bile duct
  hepatobiliary K80.80
    with obstruction K80.81
  ileal conduit N21.8
  intestinal (impaction) (obstruction) K56.49
  kidney (impacted) (multiple) (pelvis)
    (recurrent) (staghorn) N20.0
    with calculus, ureter N20.2
    congenital Q63.8
  lacrimal passages —see Dacryolith
  liver (impacted) —see Calculus, bile duct
  lung J98.4
  mammographic R92.1
  nephritic (impacted) (recurrent) —see
    Calculus, kidney
  nose J34.89
  pancreas (duct) K86.89
  parotid duct or gland K11.5
  pelvis, encysted —see Calculus, kidney
  prostate N42.0
  pulmonary J98.4
  pyelitis (impacted) (recurrent) N20.0
    with hydronephrosis N13.6
  pyelonephritis (impacted) (recurrent) —see
    category N20
    with hydronephrosis N13.6
  renal (impacted) (recurrent) —see Calculus,
    kidney
  salivary (duct) (gland) K11.5
  seminal vesicle N50.89
  staghorn —see Calculus, kidney
  Stensen's duct K11.5
  stomach K31.89
  sublingual duct or gland K11.5
    congenital Q38.4
  submandibular duct, gland or region K11.5
  submaxillary duct, gland or region K11.5
  suburethral N21.8
  tonsil J35.8
  tooth, teeth (subgingival) (supragingival) K03.6
  tunica vaginalis N50.89
  ureter (impacted) (recurrent) N20.1
    with calculus, kidney N20.2
      with hydronephrosis N13.2
        with infection N13.6
  ureteropelvic junction N20.1
  urethra (impacted) N21.1
  urinary (duct) (impacted) (passage) (tract)
    N20.9
    with hydronephrosis N13.2
      with infection N13.6
    in (due to)
    lower N21.9
      specified NEC N21.8
  vagina N89.8
  vesical (impacted) N21.0
  Wharton's duct K11.5
  xanthine E79.8 [N22]
Calicectasis N28.89
Caliectasis N28.89
California
  disease B38.9
  encephalitis A83.5
Caligo cornea —see Opacity, cornea, central
Callositas, callosity (infected) L84

Callus (infected) L84
  bone —see Osteophyte
    excessive, following fracture - code as
      Sequelae of fracture
CALME (childhood asymmetric labium majus
  enlargement) N90.61
Calorie deficiency or malnutrition —see also
  Malnutrition E46
Calpainopathy (primary) G71.032
  autosomal dominant G71.031
  autosomal recessive G71.032
Calvé-Perthes disease —see Legg-Calve-Perthes
  disease
Calvé's disease —see Osteochondrosis, juvenile,
  spine
Calvities —see Alopecia, androgenic
Cameroon fever —see Malaria
Camptocormia (hysterical) F44.4
Camurati-Engelmann syndrome Q78.3
Canal —see also condition
  atrioventricular common Q21.2
  atrioventricular Q21.20
    common Q21.23
    incomplete Q21.21
    intermediate Q21.22
    partial Q21.21
    transitional Q21.22
Canaliculitis (lacrimal) (acute) (subacute)
  H04.33-●
  Actinomyces A42.89
  chronic H04.42-●
Canavan's disease E75.29
Canceled procedure (surgical) Z53.9
  because of
    contraindication Z53.09
      smoking Z53.01
    left against medical advice (AMA) Z53.29
    patient's decision Z53.20
      for reasons of belief or group pressure
        Z53.1
      specified reason NEC Z53.29
    specified reason NEC Z53.8
Cancer —see also Neoplasm, by site, malignant
  bile duct type, liver C22.1
  blood —see Leukemia
  breast —see also Neoplasm, breast, malignant
    C50.91-●
  hepatocellular C22.0
  lung —see also Neoplasm, lung, malignant
    C34.90-●
  ovarian —see also Neoplasm, ovary,
    malignant C56.9-●
  unspecified site (primary) C80.1
Cancer (o)phobia F45.29
Cancerous —see Neoplasm, malignant, by site
Cancrum oris A69.0
Candidiasis, candidal B37.9
  balanitis B37.42
  bronchitis B37.1
  cheilitis B37.83
  congenital P37.5
  cystitis B37.41
  disseminated B37.7
  endocarditis B37.6
  enteritis B37.82
  esophagitis B37.81
  intertrigo B37.2
  lung B37.1
  meningitis B37.5
  mouth B37.0
  nails B37.2
  neonatal P37.5
  onychia B37.2
  oral B37.0
  osteomyelitis B37.89
  otitis externa B37.84
  paronychia B37.2
  perionyxis B37.2
  pneumonia B37.1
  proctitis B37.82
  pulmonary B37.1
  pyelonephritis B37.49
  sepsis B37.7

Candidiasis, candidal (Continued)
  skin B37.2
  specified site NEC B37.89
  stomatitis B37.0
  systemic B37.7
  urethritis B37.41
  urogenital site NEC B37.49
  vagina (acute) B37.31
    chronic (recurrent) B37.32
  vulva (acute) B37.31
    chronic (recurrent) B37.32
  vulvovaginitis (acute) B37.31
    chronic (recurrent) B37.32
Candidid L30.2
Candidosis —see Candidiasis
Candiru infection or infestation B88.8
Canities (premature) L67.1
  congenital Q84.2
Canker (mouth) (sore) K12.0
  rash A38.9
Cannabinosis J66.2
Cannabis induced
  anxiety disorder F12.980
  psychotic disorder F12.959
  sleep disorder F12.988
Canton fever A75.9
Cantrell's syndrome Q87.89
Capillariasis (intestinal) B81.1
  hepatic B83.8
Capillary —see condition
Caplan's syndrome —see Rheumatoid, lung
Capsule —see condition
Capsulitis (joint) —see also Enthesopathy
  adhesive (shoulder) M75.0-●
  hepatic K65.8
  labyrinthine —see Otosclerosis, specified NEC
  thyroid E06.9
Caput
  crepitus Q75.8
  medusae I86.8
  succedaneum P12.81
Car sickness T75.3
Carapata (disease) A68.0
Carate —see Pinta
Carbon lung J60
Carbuncle L02.93
  abdominal wall L02.231
  anus K61.0
  auditory canal, external —see Abscess, ear,
    external
  auricle ear —see Abscess, ear, external
  axilla L02.43-●
  back (any part) L02.232
  breast N61.1
  buttock L02.33
  cheek (external) L02.03
  chest wall L02.233
  chin L02.03
  corpus cavernosum N48.21
  ear (any part) (external) (middle) —see
    Abscess, ear, external
  external auditory canal —see Abscess, ear,
    external
  eyelid —see Abscess, eyelid
  face NEC L02.03
  femoral (region) —see Carbuncle, lower limb
  finger —see Carbuncle, hand
  flank L02.231
  foot L02.63-●
  forehead L02.03
  genital —see Abscess, genital
  gluteal (region) L02.33
  groin L02.234
  hand L02.53-●
  head NEC L02.831
  heel —see Carbuncle, foot
  hip —see Carbuncle, lower limb
  kidney —see Abscess, kidney
  knee —see Carbuncle, lower limb
  labium (majus) (minus) N76.4
  lacrimal
    gland —see Dacryoadenitis
    passages (duct) (sac) —see Inflammation,
      lacrimal, passages, acute

Carbuncle *(Continued)*
  leg —*see* Carbuncle, lower limb
  lower limb L02.43-●
  malignant A22.0
  navel L02.236
  neck L02.13
  nose (external) (septum) J34.0
  orbit, orbital —*see* Abscess, orbit
  palmar (space) —*see* Carbuncle, hand
  partes posteriores L02.33
  pectoral region L02.233
  penis N48.21
  perineum L02.235
  pinna —*see* Abscess, ear, external
  popliteal —*see* Carbuncle, lower limb
  scalp L02.831
  seminal vesicle N49.0
  shoulder —*see* Carbuncle, upper limb
  specified site NEC L02.838
  temple (region) L02.03
  thumb —*see* Carbuncle, hand
  toe —*see* Carbuncle, foot
  trunk L02.239
    abdominal wall L02.231
    back L02.232
    chest wall L02.233
    groin L02.234
    perineum L02.235
    umbilicus L02.236
  umbilicus L02.236
  upper limb L02.43-●
  urethra N34.0
  vulva N76.4
Carbunculus —*see* Carbuncle
Carcinoid (tumor) —*see* Tumor, carcinoid
Carcinoidosis E34.0
Carcinoma (malignant) —*see also* Neoplasm,
  by site, malignant
  acidophil
    specified site —*see* Neoplasm, malignant,
      by site
    unspecified site C75.1
  acidophil-basophil, mixed
    specified site —*see* Neoplasm, malignant,
      by site
    unspecified site C75.1
  adnexal (skin) —*see* Neoplasm, skin, malignant
  adrenal cortical C74.0-●
  alveolar —*see* Neoplasm, lung, malignant
    cell —*see* Neoplasm, lung, malignant
  ameloblastic C41.1
    upper jaw (bone) C41.0
  apocrine
    breast —*see* Neoplasm, breast, malignant
    specified site NEC —*see* Neoplasm, skin,
      malignant
    unspecified site C44.99
  basal cell (pigmented) (*see also* Neoplasm,
    skin, malignant) C44.91
    fibro-epithelial —*see* Neoplasm, skin,
      malignant
    morphea —*see* Neoplasm, skin, malignant
    multicentric —*see* Neoplasm, skin,
      malignant
  basaloid
  basal-squamous cell, mixed —*see* Neoplasm,
    skin, malignant
  basophil
    specified site —*see* Neoplasm, malignant,
      by site
    unspecified site C75.1
  basophil-acidophil, mixed
    specified site —*see* Neoplasm, malignant,
      by site
    unspecified site C75.1
  basosquamous —*see* Neoplasm, skin, malignant
  bile duct
    with hepatocellular, mixed C22.0
    liver C22.1
    specified site NEC —*see* Neoplasm,
      malignant, by site
    unspecified site C22.1

Carcinoma *(Continued)*
  branchial or branchiogenic C10.4
  bronchial or bronchogenic —*see* Neoplasm,
    lung, malignant
  bronchiolar —*see* Neoplasm, lung, malignant
  bronchioloalveolar —*see* Neoplasm, lung,
    malignant
  C cell
    specified site —*see* Neoplasm, malignant,
      by site
    unspecified site C73
  ceruminous C44.29-●
  cervix uteri
    in situ D06.9
      endocervix D06.0
      exocervix D06.1
      specified site NEC D06.7
  chorionic
    specified site —*see* Neoplasm, malignant,
      by site
    unspecified site
      female C58
      male C62.90
  chromophobe
    specified site —*see* Neoplasm, malignant,
      by site
    unspecified site C75.1
  cloacogenic
    specified site —*see* Neoplasm, malignant,
      by site
    unspecified site C21.2
  diffuse type
    specified site —*see* Neoplasm, malignant,
      by site
    unspecified site C16.9
  duct (cell)
    with Paget's disease —*see* Neoplasm,
      breast, malignant
    infiltrating
      with lobular carcinoma (in situ)
        specified site —*see* Neoplasm,
          malignant, by site
        unspecified site (female) C50.91-●
          male C50.92-●
      specified site —*see* Neoplasm,
        malignant, by site
      unspecified site (female) C50.91-●
        male C50.92-●
  ductal
    with lobular
      specified site —*see* Neoplasm,
        malignant, by site
      unspecified site (female) C50.91-●
        male C50.92-●
  ductular, infiltrating
    specified site —*see* Neoplasm, malignant,
      by site
    unspecified site (female) C50.91-●
      male C50.92-●
  embryonal
    liver C22.7
  endometrioid
    specified site —*see* Neoplasm, malignant,
      by site
    unspecified site
      female C56.9
      male C61
  eosinophil
    specified site —*see* Neoplasm, malignant,
      by site
    unspecified site C75.1
  epidermoid —*see also* Neoplasm, skin
    malignant
    in situ, Bowen's type —*see* Neoplasm, skin,
      in situ
  fibroepithelial, basal cell —*see* Neoplasm,
    skin, malignant
  follicular
    with papillary (mixed) C73
    moderately differentiated C73
    pure follicle C73
    specified site —*see* Neoplasm, malignant,
      by site

Carcinoma *(Continued)*
  follicular *(Continued)*
    trabecular C73
    unspecified site C73
    well differentiated C73
  generalized, with unspecified primary site C80.0
  glycogen-rich —*see* Neoplasm, breast,
    malignant
  granulosa cell C56-●
  hepatic cell C22.0
  hepatocellular C22.0
    with bile duct, mixed C22.0
    fibrolamellar C22.0
  hepatocholangiolitic C22.0
  Hurthle cell C73
  in
    adenomatous
      polyposis coli C18.9
    pleomorphic adenoma —*see* Neoplasm,
      salivary glands, malignant
    situ —*see* Carcinoma-in-situ
  infiltrating
    duct
      with lobular
        specified site —*see* Neoplasm,
          malignant, by site
        unspecified site (female) C50.91-●
          male C50.92-●
      with Paget's disease —*see* Neoplasm,
        breast, malignant
      specified site —*see* Neoplasm, malignant
      unspecified site (female) C50.91-●
        male C50.92-●
    ductular
      specified site —*see* Neoplasm, malignant
      unspecified site (female) C50.91-●
        male C50.92-●
    lobular
      specified site —*see* Neoplasm, malignant
      unspecified site (female) C50.91-●
        male C50.92-●
  inflammatory
    specified site —*see* Neoplasm, malignant
    unspecified site (female) C50.91-●
      male C50.92-●
  intestinal type
    specified site —*see* Neoplasm, malignant,
      by site
    unspecified site C16.9
  intracystic
    noninfiltrating —*see* Neoplasm, in situ,
      by site
  intraductal (noninfiltrating)
    with Paget's disease —*see* Neoplasm,
      breast, malignant
    breast D05.1-●
    papillary
      with invasion
        specified site —*see* Neoplasm,
          malignant, by site
        unspecified site (female) C50.91-●
          male C50.92-●
      breast D05.1-●
      specified site NEC —*see* Neoplasm,
        in situ, by site
      unspecified site (female) D05.1-●
    specified site NEC —*see* Neoplasm,
      in situ, by site
    unspecified site (female) D05.1-●
  intraepidermal —*see* Neoplasm, in situ
    squamous cell, Bowen's type —*see*
      Neoplasm, skin, in situ
  intraepithelial —*see* Neoplasm, in situ, by site
    squamous cell —*see* Neoplasm, in situ, by
      site
  intraosseous C41.1
    upper jaw (bone) C41.0
  islet cell
    with exocrine, mixed
      specified site —*see* Neoplasm,
        malignant, by site
      unspecified site C25.9
    pancreas C25.4

Carcinoma *(Continued)*
  islet cell *(Continued)*
    specified site NEC —*see* Neoplasm,
      malignant, by site
    unspecified site C25.4
  juvenile, breast —*see* Neoplasm, breast,
    malignant
  large cell
    small cell
      specified site —*see* Neoplasm,
        malignant, by site
      unspecified site C34.90
  Leydig cell (testis)
    specified site —*see* Neoplasm, malignant,
      by site
    unspecified site
      female C56.9
      male C62.90
  lipid-rich (female) C50.91-●
    male C50.92-●
  liver cell C22.0
  liver NEC C22.7
  lobular (infiltrating)
    with intraductal
      specified site —*see* Neoplasm,
        malignant, by site
      unspecified site (female) C50.91-●
        male C50.92-●
    noninfiltrating
      breast D05.0-●
      specified site NEC —*see* Neoplasm, in
        situ, by site
      unspecified site D05.0-●
    specified site —*see* Neoplasm, malignant,
      by site
    unspecified site (female) C50.91-●
      male C50.92-●
  medullary
    with
      amyloid stroma
        specified site —*see* Neoplasm,
          malignant, by site
        unspecified site C73
      lymphoid stroma
        specified site —*see* Neoplasm,
          malignant, by site
        unspecified site (female) C50.91-●
          male C50.92-●
  Merkel cell C4A.9
    anal margin C4A.51
    anal skin C4A.51
    canthus C4A.1-●
    ear and external auricular canal C4A.2-●
    external auricular canal C4A.2-●
    eyelid, including canthus C4A.1-●
    face C4A.30
      specified NEC C4A.39
    hip C4A.7-●
    lip C4A.0
    lower limb, including hip C4A.7-●
    neck C4A.4
    nodal presentation C7B.1
    nose C4A.31
    overlapping sites C4A.8
    perianal skin C4A.51
    scalp C4A.4
    secondary C7B.1
    shoulder C4A.6-●
    skin of breast C4A.52
    trunk NEC C4A.59
    upper limb, including shoulder C4A.6-●
    visceral metastatic C7B.1
  metastatic —*see* Neoplasm, secondary
  metatypical —*see* Neoplasm, skin, malignant
  morphea, basal cell —*see* Neoplasm, skin,
    malignant
  mucoid
    cell
      specified site —*see* Neoplasm,
        malignant, by site
      unspecified site C75.1

Carcinoma *(Continued)*
  neuroendocrine —*see also* Tumor,
    neuroendocrine
    high grade, any site C7A.1
    poorly differentiated, any site C7A.1
  nonencapsulated sclerosing C73
  noninfiltrating
    intracystic —*see* Neoplasm, in situ, by site
    intraductal
      breast D05.1-●
      papillary
        breast D05.1-●
        specified site NEC —*see* Neoplasm, in
          situ, by site
        unspecified site D05.1-●
      specified site —*see* Neoplasm, in situ,
        by site
      unspecified site D05.1-●
    lobular
      breast D05.0-●
      specified site NEC —*see* Neoplasm, in
        situ, by site
      unspecified site (female) D05.0-●
  oat cell
    specified site —*see* Neoplasm, malignant,
      by site
    unspecified site C34.90
  odontogenic C41.1
    upper jaw (bone) C41.0
  papillary
    with follicular (mixed) C73
    follicular variant C73
    intraductal (noninfiltrating)
      with invasion
        specified site —*see* Neoplasm,
          malignant, by site
        unspecified site (female) C50.91-●
          male C50.92-●
      breast D05.1-●
      specified site NEC —*see* Neoplasm, in
        situ, by site
      unspecified site D05.1-●
    serous
      specified site —*see* Neoplasm,
        malignant, by site
      surface
        specified site —*see* Neoplasm,
          malignant, by site
        unspecified site C56.9
      unspecified site C56.9
  papillocystic
    specified site —*see* Neoplasm, malignant,
      by site
    unspecified site C56.9
  parafollicular cell
    specified site —*see* Neoplasm, malignant,
      by site
    unspecified site C73
  pilomatrix —*see* Neoplasm, skin, malignant
  pseudomucinous
    specified site —*see* Neoplasm, malignant,
      by site
    unspecified site C56.9
  renal cell C64-●
  Schmincke —*see* Neoplasm, nasopharynx,
    malignant
  Schneiderian
    specified site —*see* Neoplasm, malignant,
      by site
    unspecified site C30.0
  sebaceous —*see* Neoplasm, skin, malignant
  secondary —*see also* Neoplasm, secondary,
    by site
    Merkel cell C7B.1
  secretory, breast —*see* Neoplasm, breast,
    malignant
  serous
    papillary
      specified site —*see* Neoplasm,
        malignant, by site
      unspecified site C56.9

Carcinoma *(Continued)*
  serous *(Continued)*
    surface, papillary
      specified site —*see* Neoplasm,
        malignant, by site
      unspecified site C56.9
  Sertoli cell
    specified site —*see* Neoplasm, malignant,
      by site
    unspecified site C62.90
      female C56.9
      male C62.90
  skin appendage —*see* Neoplasm, skin,
    malignant
  small cell
    fusiform cell
      specified site —*see* Neoplasm,
        malignant, by site
      unspecified site C34.90
    intermediate cell
      specified site —*see* Neoplasm,
        malignant, by site
      unspecified site C34.90
    large cell
      specified site —*see* Neoplasm,
        malignant, by site
      unspecified site C34.90
  solid
    with amyloid stroma
      specified site —*see* Neoplasm,
        malignant, by site
      unspecified site C73
    microinvasive
      specified site —*see* Neoplasm,
        malignant, by site
      unspecified site C53.9
  sweat gland —*see* Neoplasm, skin, malignant
  theca cell C56.-●
  thymic C37
  unspecified site (primary) C80.1
  water-clear cell C75.0
Carcinoma-in-situ —*see also* Neoplasm, in situ,
  by site
  breast NOS D05.9-●
    specified type NEC D05.8-●
  epidermoid —*see also* Neoplasm, in situ, by site
    with questionable stromal invasion
      cervix D06.9
      specified site NEC —*see* Neoplasm, in
        situ, by site
      unspecified site D06.9
    Bowen's type —*see* Neoplasm, skin, in situ
  intraductal
    breast D05.1-●
    specified site NEC —*see* Neoplasm, in situ,
      by site
    unspecified site D05.1-●
  lobular
    with
      infiltrating duct
        breast (female) C50.91-●
          male C50.92-●
        specified site NEC —*see* Neoplasm,
          malignant
        unspecified site (female) C50.91-●
          male C50.92-●
    intraductal
      breast D05.8-●
      specified site NEC —*see* Neoplasm, in
        situ, by site
      unspecified site (female) D05.8-●
    breast D05.0-●
    specified site NEC —*see* Neoplasm, in situ,
      by site
    unspecified site D05.0-●
  squamous cell —*see also* Neoplasm, in situ,
    by site
    with questionable stromal invasion
      cervix D06.9
      specified site NEC —*see* Neoplasm, in
        situ, by site
      unspecified site D06.9

Carcinomaphobia F45.29
Carcinomatosis C80.0
  peritonei C78.6
  unspecified site (primary) (secondary) C80.0
Carcinosarcoma —*see* Neoplasm, malignant,
  by site
  embryonal —*see* Neoplasm, malignant, by site
Cardia, cardial —*see* condition
Cardiac —*see also* condition
  death, sudden —*see* Arrest, cardiac
  pacemaker
    in situ Z95.0
    management or adjustment Z45.018
  tamponade I31.4
Cardialgia —*see* Pain, precordial
Cardiectasis —*see* Hypertrophy, cardiac
Cardiochalasia K21.9
Cardiomalacia I51.5
Cardiomegalia glycogenica diffusa E74.02 [143]
Cardiomegaly —*see also* Hypertrophy, cardiac
  congenital Q24.8
  glycogen E74.02 [143]
  idiopathic I51.7
Cardiomyoliposis I51.5
Cardiomyopathy (familial) (idiopathic) I42.9
  alcoholic I42.6
  amyloid E85.4 [143]
    transthyretin-related (ATTR) familial E85.4
      [143]
  arteriosclerotic —*see* Disease, heart, ischemic,
    atherosclerotic
  beriberi E51.12
  cobalt-beer I42.6
  congenital I42.4
  congestive I42.0
  constrictive NOS I42.5
  dilated I42.0
  due to
    alcohol I42.6
    beriberi E51.12
    cardiac glycogenosis E74.02 [143]
    drugs I42.7
    external agents NEC I42.7
    Friedreich's ataxia G11.11
    myotonia atrophica G71.11 [143]
    progressive muscular dystrophy (*see also*
      Dystrophy, muscular, by type) G71.09
      [143]
  glycogen storage E74.02 [143]
  hypertensive —*see* Hypertension, heart
  hypertrophic (nonobstructive) I42.2
    obstructive I42.1
      congenital Q24.8
  in
    Chagas' disease (chronic) B57.2
      acute B57.0
    sarcoidosis D86.85
  ischemic I25.5
  metabolic E88.9 [143]
    thyrotoxic E05.90 [143]
      with thyroid storm E05.91 [143]
  newborn I42.8
    congenital I42.4
  non-ischemic (*see also* by cause) I42.8
  nutritional E63.9 [143]
    beriberi E51.12
  obscure of Africa I42.8
  peripartum O90.3
  postpartum O90.3
  restrictive NEC I42.5
  rheumatic I09.0
  secondary I42.9
  specified NEC I42.8
  stress induced I51.81
  takotsubo I51.81
  thyrotoxic E05.90 [143]
    with thyroid storm E05.91 [143]
  toxic NEC I42.7
  transthyretin-related (ATTR) familial amyloid
    E85.4
  tuberculous A18.84
  viral B33.24

Cardionephritis —*see* Hypertension, cardiorenal
Cardionephropathy —*see* Hypertension,
  cardiorenal
Cardionephrosis —*see* Hypertension, cardiorenal
Cardiopathia nigra I27.0
Cardiopathy —*see also* Disease, heart I51.9
  idiopathic I42.9
  mucopolysaccharidosis E76.3 [152]
Cardiopericarditis —*see* Pericarditis
Cardiophobia F45.29
Cardiorenal —*see* condition
Cardiorrhexis —*see* Infarct, myocardium
Cardiosclerosis —*see* Disease, heart, ischemic,
  atherosclerotic
Cardiosis —*see* Disease, heart
Cardiospasm (esophagus) (reflex) (stomach)
  K22.0
  congenital Q39.5
  with megaesophagus Q39.5
Cardiostenosis —*see* Disease, heart
Cardiosymphysis I31.0
Cardiovascular —*see* condition
Carditis (acute) (bacterial) (chronic) (subacute)
  I51.89
  meningococcal A39.50
  rheumatic —*see* Disease, heart, rheumatic
  rheumatoid —*see* Rheumatoid, carditis
  viral B33.20
Care (of) (for) (following)
  child (routine) Z76.2
  family member (handicapped) (sick)
    creating problem for family Z63.6
    provided away from home for holiday
      relief Z75.5
    unavailable, due to
      absence (person rendering care)
        (sufferer) Z74.2
      inability (any reason) of person
        rendering care Z74.2
  foundling Z76.1
  holiday relief Z75.5
  improper —*see* Maltreatment
  lack of (at or after birth) (infant) —*see*
    Maltreatment, child, neglect
  lactating mother Z39.1
  palliative Z51.5
  postpartum
    immediately after delivery Z39.0
    routine follow-up Z39.2
  respite Z75.5
  unavailable, due to
    absence of person rendering care Z74.2
    inability (any reason) of person rendering
      care Z74.2
  well-baby Z76.2
Caries
  bone NEC A18.03
  dental (dentino enamel junction) (early
    childhood) (of dentine) (pre-eruptive)
    (recurrent) (to the pulp) K02.9
    arrested (coronal) (root) K02.3
    chewing surface
      limited to enamel K02.51
      penetrating into dentin K02.52
      penetrating into pulp K02.53
    coronal surface
      chewing surface
        limited to enamel K02.51
        penetrating into dentin K02.52
        penetrating into pulp K02.53
      pit and fissure surface
        limited to enamel K02.51
        penetrating into dentin K02.52
        penetrating into pulp K02.53
      smooth surface
        limited to enamel K02.61
        penetrating into dentin K02.62
        penetrating into pulp K02.63
    pit and fissure surface
      limited to enamel K02.51
      penetrating into dentin K02.52
      penetrating into pulp K02.53

Caries (Continued)
  dental (Continued)
    primary, cervical origin K02.52
    root K02.7
    smooth surface
      limited to enamel K02.61
      penetrating into dentin K02.62
      penetrating into pulp K02.63
  external meatus —*see* Disorder, ear, external,
    specified type NEC
  hip (tuberculous) A18.02
  initial (tooth)
    chewing surface K02.51
    pit and fissure surface K02.51
    smooth surface K02.61
  knee (tuberculous) A18.02
  labyrinth —*see* subcategory H83.8
  limb NEC (tuberculous) A18.03
  mastoid process (chronic) —*see* Mastoiditis,
    chronic
    tuberculous A18.03
  middle ear —*see* subcategory H74.8
  nose (tuberculous) A18.03
  orbit (tuberculous) A18.03
  ossicles, ear —*see* Abnormal, ear ossicles
  petrous bone —*see* Petrositis
  root (dental) (tooth) K02.7
  sacrum (tuberculous) A18.01
  spine, spinal (column) (tuberculous) A18.01
  syphilitic A52.77
    congenital (early) A50.02 [M90.80]
  tooth, teeth —*see* Caries, dental
  tuberculous A18.03
  vertebra (column) (tuberculous) A18.01
Carious teeth —*see* Caries, dental
Carneous mole O02.0
Carnitine insufficiency E71.40
Carotenemia (dietary) E67.1
Carotenosis (cutis) (skin) E67.1
Carotid body or sinus syndrome G90.01
Carotidynia G90.01
Carpal tunnel syndrome —*see* Syndrome,
  carpal tunnel
Carpenter's syndrome Q87.0
Carpopedal spasm —*see* Tetany
Carr-Barr-Plunkett syndrome Q97.1
Carrier (suspected) of
  amebiasis Z22.1
  bacterial disease NEC Z22.39
    diphtheria Z22.2
    intestinal infectious NEC Z22.1
      typhoid Z22.0
    meningococcal Z22.31
    sexually transmitted Z22.4
    specified NEC Z22.39
    staphylococcal (Methicillin susceptible)
      Z22.321
      Methicillin resistant Z22.322
    streptococcal Z22.338
      group B Z22.330
        complicating pregnancy or delivery
          O99.82-●
    typhoid Z22.0
  cholera Z22.1
  diphtheria Z22.2
  gastrointestinal pathogens NEC Z22.1
  genetic Z14.8
    cystic fibrosis Z14.1
    hemophilia A (asymptomatic) Z14.01
      symptomatic Z14.02
  gestational, pregnant Z33.1
  gonorrhea Z22.4
  HAA (hepatitis Australian-antigen) B18.8
  HB (c)(s)-AG B18.1
  hepatitis (viral) B18.9
    Australia-antigen (HAA) B18.8
    B surface antigen (HBsAg) B18.1
      with acute delta- (super)infection B17.0
    C B18.2
    specified NEC B18.8
  human T-cell lymphotropic virus type-1
    (HTLV-1) infection Z22.6

Carrier of *(Continued)*
  infectious organism Z22.9
    specified NEC Z22.8
  meningococci Z22.31
  Salmonella typhosa Z22.0
  serum hepatitis —*see* Carrier, hepatitis
  staphylococci (Methicillin susceptible) Z22.321
    Methicillin resistant Z22.322
  streptococci Z22.338
    group B Z22.330
      complicating pregnancy or delivery
        O99.82-●
  syphilis Z22.4
  typhoid Z22.0
  venereal disease NEC Z22.4
Carrion's disease A44.0
Carter's relapsing fever (Asiatic) A68.1
Cartilage —*see* condition
Caruncle (inflamed)
  conjunctiva (acute) —*see* Conjunctivitis, acute
  labium (majus) (minus) N90.89
  lacrimal —*see* Inflammation, lacrimal,
    passages
  myrtiform N89.8
  urethral (benign) N36.2
Cascade stomach K31.2
Caseation lymphatic gland (tuberculous) A18.2
Cassidy (-Scholte) syndrome (malignant
  carcinoid) E34.0
Castellani's disease A69.8
Castration, traumatic, male S38.231
Casts in urine R82.998
Cat
  cry syndrome Q93.4
  ear Q17.3
  eye syndrome Q92.8
Catabolism, senile R54
Catalepsy (hysterical) F44.2
  schizophrenic F20.2
Cataplexy (idiopathic) —*see* Narcolepsy
Cataract (cortical) (immature) (incipient) H26.9
  with
    neovascularization —*see* Cataract,
      complicated
  age-related —*see* Cataract, senile
  anterior
    and posterior axial embryonal Q12.0
    pyramidal Q12.0
  associated with
    galactosemia E74.21 *[H28]*
    myotonic disorders G71.19 *[H28]*
  blue Q12.0
  central Q12.0
  cerulean Q12.0
  complicated H26.20
    with
      neovascularization H26.21-●
      ocular disorder H26.22-●
      glaucomatous flecks H26.23-●
  congenital Q12.0
  coraliform Q12.0
  coronary Q12.0
  crystalline Q12.0
  diabetic —*see* Diabetes, cataract
  drug-induced H26.3-●
  due to
    ocular disorder —*see* Cataract, complicated
    radiation H26.8
  electric H26.8
  extraction status Z98.4-●
  glass-blower's H26.8
  heat ray H26.8
  heterochromic —*see* Cataract, complicated
  hypermature —*see* Cataract, senile,
    morgagnian type
  in (due to)
    chronic iridocyclitis —*see* Cataract,
      complicated
    diabetes —*see* Diabetes, cataract
    endocrine disease E34.9 *[H28]*
    eye disease —*see* Cataract, complicated

Cataract *(Continued)*
  in (due to) *(Continued)*
    hypoparathyroidism E20.9 *[H28]*
    malnutrition-dehydration E46 *[H28]*
    metabolic disease E88.9 *[H28]*
    myotonic disorders G71.19 *[H28]*
    nutritional disease E63.9 *[H28]*
  infantile —*see* Cataract, presenile
  irradiational —*see* Cataract, specified NEC
  juvenile —*see* Cataract, presenile
  malnutrition-dehydration E46 *[H28]*
  morgagnian —*see* Cataract, senile,
    morgagnian type
  myotonic G71.19 *[H28]*
  myxedema E03.9 *[H28]*
  nuclear
    embryonal Q12.0
    sclerosis —*see* Cataract, senile, nuclear
  presenile H26.00-●
    combined forms H26.06-●
    cortical H26.01-●
    lamellar —*see* Cataract, presenile, cortical
    nuclear H26.03-●
    specified NEC H26.09
    subcapsular polar (anterior) H26.04-●
      posterior H26.05-●
    zonular —*see* Cataract, presenile, cortical
  secondary H26.40
    Soemmering's ring H26.41-●
    specified NEC H26.49-●
    to eye disease —*see* Cataract, complicated
  senile H25.9
    brunescens —*see* Cataract, senile, nuclear
    combined forms H25.81-●
    coronary —*see* Cataract, senile, incipient
    cortical H25.01-●
    hypermature —*see* Cataract, senile,
      morgagnian type
    incipient (mature) (total) H25.09-●
      cortical —*see* Cataract, senile, cortical
      subcapsular —*see* Cataract, senile,
        subcapsular
    morgagnian type (hypermature) H25.2-●
    nuclear (sclerosis) H25.1-●
    polar subcapsular (anterior) (posterior) —
      see Cataract, senile, incipient
    punctate —*see* Cataract, senile, incipient
    specified NEC H25.89
    subcapsular polar (anterior) H25.03-●
      posterior H25.04-●
  snowflake —*see* Diabetes, cataract
  specified NEC H26.8
  toxic —*see* Cataract, drug-induced
  traumatic H26.10-●
    localized H26.11-●
    partially resolved H26.12-●
    total H26.13-●
  zonular (perinuclear) Q12.0
Cataracta —*see also* Cataract
  brunescens —*see* Cataract, senile, nuclear
  centralis pulverulenta Q12.0
  cerulea Q12.0
  complicata —*see* Cataract, complicated
  congenita Q12.0
  coralliformis Q12.0
  coronaria Q12.0
  diabetic —*see* Diabetes, cataract
  membranacea
    accreta —*see* Cataract, secondary
    congenita Q12.0
  nigra —*see* Cataract, senile, nuclear
  sunflower —*see* Cataract, complicated
Catarrh, catarrhal (acute) (febrile) (infectious)
  (inflammation) (*see also* condition) J00
  bronchial —*see* Bronchitis
  chest —*see* Bronchitis
  chronic J31.0
  due to congenital syphilis A50.03
  enteric —*see* Enteritis
  eustachian H68.009
  fauces —*see* Pharyngitis

Catarrh, catarrhal *(Continued)*
  gastrointestinal —*see* Enteritis
  gingivitis K05.00
    nonplaque induced K05.01
    plaque induced K05.00
  hay —*see* Fever, hay
  intestinal —*see* Enteritis
  larynx, chronic J37.0
  liver B15.9
    with hepatic coma B15.0
  lung —*see* Bronchitis
  middle ear, chronic —*see* Otitis, media,
    nonsuppurative, chronic, serous
  mouth K12.1
  nasal (chronic) —*see* Rhinitis
  nasobronchial J31.1
  nasopharyngeal (chronic) J31.1
    acute J00
  pulmonary —*see* Bronchitis
  spring (eye) (vernal) —*see* Conjunctivitis,
    acute, atopic
  summer (hay) —*see* Fever, hay
  throat J31.2
  tubotympanal —*see also* Otitis, media,
    nonsuppurative
    chronic —*see* Otitis, media,
      nonsuppurative, chronic, serous
Catatonia (schizophrenic) F20.2
Catatonic
  disorder due to known physiologic condition
    F06.1
  schizophrenia F20.2
  stupor R40.1
Cat-scratch —*see also* Abrasion
  disease or fever A28.1
Cauda equina —*see* condition
Cauliflower ear M95.1-●
Causalgia (upper limb) G56.4-●
  lower limb G57.7-●
Cause
  external, general effects T75.89
Caustic burn —*see* Corrosion, by site
Cavare's disease (familial periodic paralysis)
  G72.3
Cave-in, injury
  crushing (severe) —*see* Crush
  suffocation —*see* Asphyxia, traumatic, due to
    low oxygen, due to cave-in
Cavernitis (penis) N48.29
Cavernositis N48.29
Cavernous —*see* condition
Cavitation of lung —*see also* Tuberculosis,
  pulmonary
  nontuberculous J98.4
Cavities, dental —*see* Caries, dental
Cavity
  lung —*see* Cavitation of lung
  optic papilla Q14.2
  pulmonary —*see* Cavitation of lung
Cavovarus foot, congenital Q66.1-●
Cavus foot (congenital) Q66.7-●
  acquired —*see* Deformity, limb, foot, specified
    NEC
Cazenave's disease L10.2
CDKL5 (Cyclin-Dependent Kinase-Like 5
  Deficiency Disorder) G40.42
Cecitis K52.9
  with perforation, peritonitis, or rupture K65.8
Cecoureterocele Q62.32
Cecum —*see* condition
Celiac
  artery compression syndrome I77.4
  disease (with steatorrhea) K90.0
  infantilism K90.0
Cell(s), cellular —*see also* condition
  in urine R82.998
Cellulitis (diffuse) (phlegmonous) (septic)
  (suppurative) L03.90
  abdominal wall L03.311
  anaerobic A48.0
  ankle —*see* Cellulitis, lower limb
  anus K61.0

Cellulitis *(Continued)*
  arm —*see* Cellulitis, upper limb
  auricle (ear) —*see* Cellulitis, ear
  axilla L03.11-●
  back (any part) L03.312
  breast (acute) (nonpuerperal) (subacute)
    N61.0
    nipple N61.0
  broad ligament
    acute N73.0
  buttock L03.317
  cervical (meaning neck) L03.221
  cervix (uteri) —*see* Cervicitis
  cheek (external) L03.211
    internal K12.2
  chest wall L03.313
  chronic L03.90
  clostridial A48.0
  corpus cavernosum N48.22
  digit
    finger —*see* Cellulitis, finger
    toe —*see* Cellulitis, toe
  Douglas' cul-de-sac or pouch
    acute N73.0
  drainage site (following operation) T81.49
  ear (external) H60.1-●
  eosinophilic (granulomatous) L98.3
  erysipelatous —*see* Erysipelas
  external auditory canal —*see* Cellulitis, ear
  eyelid —*see* Abscess, eyelid
  face NEC L03.211
  finger (intrathecal) (periosteal)
    (subcutaneous) (subcuticular) L03.01-●
  foot —*see* Cellulitis, lower limb
  gangrenous —*see* Gangrene
  genital organ NEC
    female (external) N76.4
    male N49.9
      multiple sites N49.8
      specified NEC N49.8
  gluteal (region) L03.317
  gonococcal A54.89
  groin L03.314
  hand —*see* Cellulitis, upper limb
  head NEC L03.811
    face (any part, except ear, eye and nose)
      L03.211
  heel —*see* Cellulitis, lower limb
  hip —*see* Cellulitis, lower limb
  jaw (region) L03.211
  knee —*see* Cellulitis, lower limb
  labium (majus) (minus) —*see* Vulvitis
  lacrimal passages —*see* Inflammation,
    lacrimal, passages
  larynx J38.7
  leg —*see* Cellulitis, lower limb
  lip K13.0
  lower limb L03.11-●
    toe —*see* Cellulitis, toe
  mouth (floor) K12.2
  multiple sites, so stated L03.90
  nasopharynx J39.1
  navel L03.316
    newborn P38.9
      with mild hemorrhage P38.1
      without hemorrhage P38.9
  neck (region) L03.221
  nipple (acute) (nonpuerperal) (subacute) N61.0
  nose (septum) (external) J34.0
  orbit, orbital H05.01-●
  palate (soft) K12.2
  pectoral (region) L03.313
  pelvis, pelvic (chronic)
    female —*see also* Disease, pelvis,
      inflammatory N73.2
      acute N73.0
      following ectopic or molar pregnancy O08.0
    male K65.0
  penis N48.22
  perineal, perineum L03.315
  periorbital L03.213

Cellulitis *(Continued)*
  perirectal K61.1
  peritonsillar J36
  periurethral N34.0
  periuterine —*see also* Disease, pelvis,
    inflammatory N73.2
    acute N73.0
  pharynx J39.1
  preseptal L03.213
  rectum K61.1
  retroperitoneal K68.9
  round ligament
    acute N73.0
  scalp (any part) L03.811
  scrotum N49.2
  seminal vesicle N49.0
  shoulder —*see* Cellulitis, upper limb
  specified site NEC L03.818
  submandibular (region) (space) (triangle) K12.2
    gland K11.3
  submaxillary (region) K12.2
    gland K11.3
  thigh —*see* Cellulitis, lower limb
  thumb (intrathecal) (periosteal)
    (subcutaneous) (subcuticular) —*see*
    Cellulitis, finger
  toe (intrathecal) (periosteal) (subcutaneous)
    (subcuticular) L03.03-●
  tonsil J36
  trunk L03.319
    abdominal wall L03.311
    back (any part) L03.312
    buttock L03.317
    chest wall L03.313
    groin L03.314
    perineal, perineum L03.315
    umbilicus L03.316
  tuberculous (primary) A18.4
  umbilicus L03.316
  upper limb L03.11-●
    axilla —*see* Cellulitis, axilla
    finger —*see* Cellulitis, finger
    thumb —*see* Cellulitis, finger
  vaccinal T88.0
  vocal cord J38.3
  vulva —*see* Vulvitis
  wrist —*see* Cellulitis, upper limb
Cementoblastoma, benign —*see* Cyst,
  calcifying odontogenic
Cementoma —*see* Cyst, calcifying odontogenic
Cementoperiostitis —*see* Periodontitis
Cementosis K03.4
Central auditory processing disorder H93.25
Central pain syndrome G89.0
Cephalematocele, cephal (o)hematocele
  newborn P52.8
    birth injury P10.8
  traumatic —*see* Hematoma, brain
Cephalematoma, cephalhematoma (calcified)
  newborn (birth injury) P12.0
  traumatic —*see* Hematoma, brain
Cephalgia, cephalalgia —*see also* Headache
  histamine G44.009
    intractable G44.001
    not intractable G44.009
  trigeminal autonomic (TAC) NEC G44.099
    intractable G44.091
    not intractable G44.099
Cephalic —*see* condition
Cephalitis —*see* Encephalitis
Cephalocele —*see* Encephalocele
Cephalomenia N94.89
Cephalopelvic —*see* condition
Cerclage (with cervical incompetence) in
  pregnancy —*see* Incompetence, cervix, in
  pregnancy
Cerebellitis —*see* Encephalitis
Cerebellum, cerebellar —*see* condition
Cerebral —*see* condition
Cerebritis —*see* Encephalitis
Cerebro-hepato-renal syndrome Q87.89

Cerebromalacia —*see* Softening, brain
  sequelae of cerebrovascular disease I69.398
Cerebroside lipidosis E75.22
Cerebrospasticity (congenital) G80.1
Cerebrospinal —*see* condition
Cerebrum —*see* condition
Ceroid-lipofuscinosis, neuronal E75.4
Cerumen (accumulation) (impacted) H61.2-●
Cervical —*see also* condition
  auricle Q18.2
  dysplasia in pregnancy —*see* Abnormal,
    cervix, in pregnancy or childbirth
  erosion in pregnancy —*see* Abnormal, cervix,
    in pregnancy or childbirth
  fibrosis in pregnancy —*see* Abnormal, cervix,
    in pregnancy or childbirth
  fusion syndrome Q76.1
  rib Q76.5
  shortening (complicating pregnancy) O26.87-●
Cervicalgia M54.2
➠Cervicitis (acute) (atrophic) (chronic)
    (nonvenereal) (senile) (subacute) (with
    ulceration) N72
  with
    abortion —*see* Abortion, by type complicated
      by genital tract and pelvic infection
    ectopic pregnancy O08.0
    molar pregnancy O08.0
  chlamydial A56.09
  gonococcal A54.03
  herpesviral A60.03
  puerperal (postpartum) O86.11
  syphilitic A52.76
  trichomonal A59.09
  tuberculous A18.16
Cervicocolpitis (emphysematosa) (*see also*
  Cervicitis) N72
Cervix —*see* condition
Cesarean delivery, previous, affecting
  management of pregnancy O34.219
  classical (vertical) scar O34.212
➠isthmocele (non-pregnant state) N85.A
▶maternal care for O34.22
  low transverse scar O34.211
  mid-transverse T incision O34.218
  scar
    ➠defect (non-pregnant state) N85.A
    ▶maternal care for O34.22
    specified type NEC O34.218
Céstan (-Chenais) paralysis or syndrome G46.3
Céstan-Raymond syndrome I65.8
Cestode infestation B71.9
  specified type NEC B71.8
Cestodiasis B71.9
Chabert's disease A22.9
Chacaleh E53.8
Chafing L30.4
Chagas' (-Mazza) disease (chronic) B57.2
  with
    cardiovascular involvement NEC B57.2
    digestive system involvement B57.30
      megacolon B57.32
      megaesophagus B57.31
      other specified B57.39
    megacolon B57.32
    megaesophagus B57.31
    myocarditis B57.2
    nervous system involvement B57.40
      meningitis B57.41
      meningoencephalitis B57.42
      other specified B57.49
    specified organ involvement NEC B57.5
  acute (with) B57.1
    cardiovascular NEC B57.0
    myocarditis B57.0
Chagres fever B50.9
Chairridden Z74.09
Chalasia (cardiac sphincter) K21.9
Chalazion H00.19
  left H00.16
    lower H00.15
    upper H00.14

Chalazion *(Continued)*
  right H00.13
    lower H00.12
    upper H00.11
Chalcosis *—see also* Disorder, globe,
    degenerative, chalcosis
  cornea *—see* Deposit, cornea
  crystalline lens *—see* Cataract, complicated
  retina H35.89
Chalicosis (pulmonum) J62.8
Chancre (any genital site) (hard) (hunterian)
    (mixed) (primary) (seronegative)
    (seropositive) (syphilitic) A51.0
  congenital A50.07
  conjunctiva NEC A51.2
  Ducrey's A57
  extragenital A51.2
  eyelid A51.2
  lip A51.2
  nipple A51.2
  Nisbet's A57
  of
    carate A67.0
    pinta A67.0
    yaws A66.0
  palate, soft A51.2
  phagedenic A57
  simple A57
  soft A57
    bubo A57
    palate A51.2
  urethra A51.0
  yaws A66.0
Chancroid (anus) (genital) (penis) (perineum)
    (rectum) (urethra) (vulva) A57
Chandler's disease (osteochondritis dissecans,
    hip) *—see* Osteochondritis, dissecans, hip
Change(s) (in) (of) *—see also* Removal
  arteriosclerotic *—see* Arteriosclerosis
  bone *—see also* Disorder, bone
    diabetic *—see* Diabetes, bone change
  bowel habit R19.4
  cardiorenal (vascular) *—see* Hypertension,
    cardiorenal
  cardiovascular *—see* Disease, cardiovascular
  circulatory I99.9
  cognitive (mild) (organic) R41.89
  color, tooth, teeth
    during formation K00.8
    posteruptive K03.7
  contraceptive device Z30.433
  corneal membrane H18.30
    Bowman's membrane fold or rupture
      H18.31-●
    Descemet's membrane
      fold H18.32-●
      rupture H18.33-●
  coronary *—see* Disease, heart, ischemic
  degenerative, spine or vertebra *—see*
    Spondylosis
  dental pulp, regressive K04.2
  dressing (nonsurgical) Z48.00
    surgical Z48.01
  heart *—see* Disease, heart
  hip joint *—see* Derangement, joint, hip
  hyperplastic larynx J38.7
  hypertrophic
    nasal sinus J34.89
    turbinate, nasal J34.3
    upper respiratory tract J39.8
  indwelling catheter Z46.6
  inflammatory *—see also* Inflammation
    sacroiliac M46.1
  job, anxiety concerning Z56.1
  joint *—see* Derangement, joint
  life *—see* Menopause
  mental status R41.82
  minimal (glomerular) *—see also* N00-N07
    with fourth character .0 N05.0
  myocardium, myocardial *—see* Degeneration,
    myocardial - of life *—see* Menopause
  pacemaker Z45.018
    pulse generator Z45.010

Change *(Continued)*
  personality (enduring) F68.8
    due to (secondary to)
      general medical condition F07.0
    secondary (nonspecific) F60.89
  regressive, dental pulp K04.2
  renal *—see* Disease, renal
  retina H35.9
    myopic *—see also* Myopia, degenerative
      H44.2-●
  sacroiliac joint M53.3
  senile *—see also* condition R54
  sensory R20.8
  skin R23.9
    acute, due to ultraviolet radiation L56.9
      specified NEC L56.8
    chronic, due to nonionizing radiation L57.9
      specified NEC L57.8
    cyanosis R23.0
    flushing R23.2
    pallor R23.1
    petechiae R23.3
    specified change NEC R23.8
    swelling *—see* Mass, localized
    texture R23.4
  trophic
    arm *—see* Mononeuropathy, upper limb
    leg *—see* Mononeuropathy, lower limb
  vascular I99.9
  vasomotor I73.9
  voice R49.9
    psychogenic F44.4
    specified NEC R49.8
Changing sleep-work schedule, affecting sleep
    G47.26
Changuinola fever A93.1
Chapping skin T69.8
Charcot-Marie-Tooth disease, paralysis or
    syndrome G60.0
Charcot's
  arthropathy *—see* Arthropathy, neuropathic
  cirrhosis K74.3
  disease (tabetic arthropathy) A52.16
  joint (disease) (tabetic) A52.16
    diabetic *—see* Diabetes, with, arthropathy
    syringomyelic G95.0
  syndrome (intermittent claudication) I73.9
CHARGE association Q89.8
Charley-horse (quadriceps) M62.831
  traumatic (quadriceps) S76.11-●
Charlouis' disease *—see* Yaws
Cheadle's disease E54
Checking (of)
  cardiac pacemaker (battery) (electrode(s))
    Z45.018
    pulse generator Z45.010
  implantable subdermal contraceptive Z30.46
  intrauterine contraceptive device Z30.431
  wound Z48.0-●
    due to injury - code to Injury, by site, using
      appropriate seventh character for
      subsequent encounter
Check-up *—see* Examination
Chédiak-Higashi (-Steinbrinck) syndrome
    (congenital gigantism of peroxidase
    granules) E70.330
Cheek *—see* condition
Cheese itch B88.0
Cheese-washer's lung J67.8
Cheese-worker's lung J67.8
Cheilitis (acute) (angular) (catarrhal) (chronic)
    (exfoliative) (gangrenous) (glandular)
    (infectional) (suppurative) (ulcerative)
    (vesicular) K13.0
  actinic (due to sun) L56.8
    other than from sun L59.8
  candidal B37.83
Cheilodynia K13.0
Cheiloschisis *—see* Cleft, lip
Cheilosis (angular) K13.0
  with pellagra E52
  due to
    vitamin B2 (riboflavin) deficiency E53.0

Cheiromegaly M79.89
Cheiropompholyx L30.1
Cheloid *—see* Keloid
Chemical burn *—see* Corrosion, by site
Chemodectoma *—see* Paraganglioma,
    nonchromaffin
Chemosis, conjunctiva *—see* Edema,
    conjunctiva
Chemotherapy (session) (for)
  cancer Z51.11
  neoplasm Z51.11
Cherubism M27.8
Chest *—see* condition
Cheyne-Stokes breathing (respiration) R06.3
Chiari's
  disease or syndrome (hepatic vein
    thrombosis) I82.0
  malformation
    type I G93.5
    type II *—see* Spina bifida
  net Q24.8
Chicago disease B40.9
Chickenpox *—see* Varicella
Chiclero ulcer or sore B55.1
Chigger (infestation) B88.0
Chignon (disease) B36.8
  newborn (from vacuum extraction) (birth
    injury) P12.1
Chilaiditi's syndrome (subphrenic
    displacement, colon) Q43.3
Chilblain(s) (lupus) T69.1
Child
  custody dispute Z65.3
Childbirth *—see* Delivery
Childhood
  cerebral X-linked adrenoleukodystrophy
    E71.520
  period of rapid growth Z00.2
Chill(s) R68.83
  with fever R50.9
  without fever R68.83
  congestive in malarial regions B54
Chilomastigiasis A07.8
Chimera 46,XX/46,XY Q99.0
Chin *—see* condition
Chinese dysentery A03.9
Chionophobia F40.228
Chitral fever A93.1
Chlamydia, chlamydial A74.9
  cervicitis A56.09
  conjunctivitis A74.0
  cystitis A56.01
  endometritis A56.11
  epididymitis A56.19
  female
    pelvic inflammatory disease A56.11
    pelviperitonitis A56.11
  orchitis A56.19
  peritonitis A74.81
  pharyngitis A56.4
  proctitis A56.3
  psittaci (infection) A70
  salpingitis A56.11
  sexually-transmitted infection NEC A56.8
  specified NEC A74.89
  urethritis A56.01
  vulvovaginitis A56.02
Chlamydiosis *—see* Chlamydia
Chloasma (skin) (idiopathic) (symptomatic)
    L81.1
  eyelid H02.719
    hyperthyroid E05.90 *[H02.719]*
      with thyroid storm E05.91 *[H02.719]*
    left H02.716
      lower H02.715
      upper H02.714
    right H02.713
      lower H02.712
      upper H02.711
Chloroma C92.3-●
Chlorosis D50.9
  Egyptian B76.9 *[D63.8]*
  miner's B76.9 *[D63.8]*

Chlorotic anemia D50.8
Chocolate cyst (ovary) N80.10-●
Choked
  disc or disk —see Papilledema
  on food, phlegm, or vomitus NOS —see
      Foreign body, by site
  while vomiting NOS —see Foreign body, by
      site
Chokes (resulting from bends) T70.3
Choking sensation R09.89
Cholangiectasis K83.8
Cholangiocarcinoma
  with hepatocellular carcinoma, combined
      C22.0
  liver C22.1
  specified site NEC —see Neoplasm,
      malignant, by site
  unspecified site C22.1
Cholangiohepatitis K83.8
  due to fluke infestation B66.1
Cholangiohepatoma C22.0
Cholangiolitis (acute) (chronic) (extrahepatic)
      (gangrenous) (intrahepatic) K83.09
  paratyphoidal —see Fever, paratyphoid
  typhoidal A01.09
Cholangioma D13.4
  malignant —see Cholangiocarcinoma
Cholangitis (ascending) (primary) (recurrent)
      (sclerosing) (secondary) (stenosing)
      (suppurative) K83.09
  with calculus, bile duct —see Calculus, bile
      duct, with cholangitis
  chronic nonsuppurative destructive K74.3
  primary K83.09
    sclerosing K83.01
  sclerosing K83.09
Cholecystectasia K82.8
Cholecystitis K81.9
  with
    calculus, stones in
      bile duct (common) (hepatic) —
          see Calculus, bile duct, with
          cholecystitis
      cystic duct —see Calculus, gallbladder,
          with cholecystitis
      gallbladder —see Calculus, gallbladder,
          with cholecystitis
      choledocholithiasis —see Calculus, bile
          duct, with cholecystitis
      cholelithiasis —see Calculus, gallbladder,
          with cholecystitis
    gangrene of gallbladder K82.A1
    perforation of gallbladder K82.A2
  acute (emphysematous) (gangrenous)
      (suppurative) K81.0
    with
      calculus, stones in
        cystic duct —see Calculus, gallbladder,
            with cholecystitis, acute
        gallbladder —see Calculus, gallbladder,
            with cholecystitis, acute
        choledocholithiasis —see Calculus, bile
            duct, with cholecystitis, acute
        cholelithiasis —see Calculus, gallbladder,
            with cholecystitis, acute
      chronic cholecystitis K81.2
        with gallbladder calculus K80.12
          with obstruction K80.13
  chronic K81.1
    with acute cholecystitis K81.2
      with gallbladder calculus K80.12
        with obstruction K80.13
    emphysematous (acute) —see Cholecystitis,
        acute
    gangrenous —see Cholecystitis, acute
    paratyphoidal, current A01.4
    suppurative —see Cholecystitis, acute
    typhoidal A01.09
Cholecystolithiasis —see Calculus, gallbladder
Choledochitis (suppurative) K83.09
Choledocholith —see Calculus, bile duct

Choledocholithiasis (common duct) (hepatic
      duct) —see Calculus, bile duct
  cystic —see Calculus, gallbladder
  typhoidal A01.09
Cholelithiasis (cystic duct) (gallbladder)
      (impacted) (multiple) —see Calculus,
      gallbladder
  bile duct (common) (hepatic) —see Calculus,
      bile duct
  hepatic duct —see Calculus, bile duct
  specified NEC K80.80
    with obstruction K80.81
Cholemia —see also Jaundice
  familial (simple) (congenital) E80.4
  Gilbert's E80.4
Choleperitoneum, choleperitonitis K65.3
Cholera (Asiatic) (epidemic) (malignant) A00.9
  antimonial —see Poisoning, antimony
  classical A00.0
  due to Vibrio cholerae 01 A00.9
    biovar cholerae A00.0
    biovar eltor A00.1
    el tor A00.1
  el tor A00.1
Cholerine —see Cholera
Cholestasis NEC K83.1
  with hepatocyte injury K71.0
  due to total parenteral nutrition (TPN) K76.89
  pure K71.0
Cholesteatoma (ear) (middle) (with reaction)
      H71.9-●
  attic H71.0-●
  external ear (canal) H60.4-●
  mastoid H71.2-●
  postmastoidectomy cavity (recurrent) —see
      Complications, postmastoidectomy,
      recurrent cholesteatoma
  recurrent (postmastoidectomy) —see
      Complications, postmastoidectomy,
      recurrent cholesteatoma
  tympanum H71.1-●
Cholesteatosis, diffuse H71.3-●
Cholesteremia E78.00
Cholesterin in vitreous —see Deposit, crystalline
Cholesterol
  deposit
    retina H35.89
    vitreous —see Deposit, crystalline
  elevated (high) E78.00
    with elevated (high) triglycerides E78.2
    screening for Z13.220
  imbibition of gallbladder K82.4
Cholesterolemia (essential) (pure) E78.00
  familial E78.01
  hereditary E78.01
Cholesterolosis, cholesterosis (gallbladder)
      K82.4
  cerebrotendinous E75.5
Cholocolic fistula K82.3
Choluria R82.2
Chondritis M94.8X9
  auricular H61.03-●
  costal (Tietze's) M94.0
  external ear H61.03-●
  patella, posttraumatic —see Chondromalacia,
      patella
  pinna H61.03-●
  purulent M94.8X-●
  tuberculous NEC A18.02
    intervertebral A18.01
Chondroblastoma —see also Neoplasm, bone,
      benign
  malignant —see Neoplasm, bone, malignant
Chondrocalcinosis M11.20
  ankle M11.27-●
  elbow M11.22-●
  familial M11.10
    ankle M11.17-●
    elbow M11.12-●
    foot joint M11.17-●
    hand joint M11.14-●

Chondrocalcinosis (Continued)
  familial (Continued)
    hip M11.15-●
    knee M11.16-●
    multiple site M11.19
    shoulder M11.11-●
    vertebrae M11.18
    wrist M11.13-●
  foot joint M11.27-●
  hand joint M11.24-●
  hip M11.25-●
  knee M11.26-●
  multiple site M11.29
  shoulder M11.21-●
  specified type NEC M11.20
    ankle M11.27-●
    elbow M11.22-●
    foot joint M11.27-●
    hand joint M11.24-●
    hip M11.25-●
    knee M11.26-●
    multiple site M11.29
    shoulder M11.21-●
    vertebrae M11.28
    wrist M11.23-●
  vertebrae M11.28
  wrist M11.23-●
Chondrodermatitis nodularis helicis or
      anthelicis —see Perichondritis, ear
Chondrodysplasia Q78.9
  with hemangioma Q78.4
  calcificans congenita Q77.3
  fetalis Q77.4
  metaphyseal (Jansen's) (McKusick's)
      (Schmid's) Q78.8
  punctata Q77.3
Chondrodystrophy, chondrodystrophia
      (familial) (fetalis) (hypoplastic) Q78.9
  calcificans congenita Q77.3
  myotonic (congenital) G71.13
  punctata Q77.3
Chondroectodermal dysplasia Q77.6
Chondrogenesis imperfecta Q77.4
Chondrolysis M94.35-●
Chondroma —see also Neoplasm, cartilage,
      benign
  juxtacortical —see Neoplasm, bone, benign
  periosteal —see Neoplasm, bone, benign
Chondromalacia (systemic) M94.20
  acromioclavicular joint M94.21-●
  ankle M94.27-●
  elbow M94.22-●
  foot joint M94.27-●
  glenohumeral joint M94.21-●
  hand joint M94.24-●
  hip M94.25-●
  knee M94.26-●
    patella M22.4-●
  multiple sites M94.29
  patella M22.4-●
  rib M94.28
  sacroiliac joint M94.259
  shoulder M94.21-●
  sternoclavicular joint M94.21-●
  vertebral joint M94.28
  wrist M94.23-●
Chondromatosis —see also Neoplasm, cartilage,
      uncertain behavior
  internal Q78.4
Chondromyxosarcoma —see Neoplasm,
      cartilage, malignant
Chondro-osteodysplasia (Morquio-Brailsford
      type) E76.219
Chondro-osteodystrophy E76.29
Chondro-osteoma —see Neoplasm, bone, benign
Chondropathia tuberosa M94.0
Chondrosarcoma —see Neoplasm, cartilage,
      malignant
  juxtacortical —see Neoplasm, bone, malignant
  mesenchymal —see Neoplasm, connective
      tissue, malignant
  myxoid —see Neoplasm, cartilage, malignant

Chordee (nonvenereal) N48.89
  congenital Q54.4
  gonococcal A54.09
Chorditis (fibrinous) (nodosa) (tuberosa) J38.2
Chordoma —see Neoplasm, vertebral (column),
  malignant
Chorea (chronic) (gravis) (posthemiplegic)
  (senile) (spasmodic) G25.5
  with
    heart involvement I02.0
      active or acute (conditions in I01-●) I02.0
        rheumatic I02.9
          with valvular disorder I02.0
      rheumatic heart disease (chronic) (inactive)
        (quiescent) — code to rheumatic heart
        condition involved
  drug-induced G25.4
  habit F95.8
  hereditary G10
  Huntington's G10
  hysterical F44.4
  minor I02.9
    with heart involvement I02.0
  progressive G25.5
    hereditary G10
  rheumatic (chronic) I02.9
    with heart involvement I02.0
  Sydenham's I02.9
    with heart involvement —see Chorea, with
      rheumatic heart disease
    nonrheumatic G25.5
Choreoathetosis (paroxysmal) G25.5
Chorioadenoma (destruens) D39.2
Chorioamnionitis O41.12-●
Chorioangioma D26.7
Choriocarcinoma —see Neoplasm, malignant,
  by site
  combined with
    embryonal carcinoma —see Neoplasm,
      malignant, by site
    other germ cell elements —see Neoplasm,
      malignant, by site
    teratoma —see Neoplasm, malignant, by site
  specified site —see Neoplasm, malignant, by
    site
  unspecified site
    female C58
    male C62.90
Chorioencephalitis (acute) (lymphocytic)
  (serous) A87.2
Chorioepithelioma —see Choriocarcinoma
Choriomeningitis (acute) (lymphocytic)
  (serous) A87.2
Chorionepithelioma —see Choriocarcinoma
Chorioretinitis —see also Inflammation,
  chorioretinal
  disseminated —see also Inflammation,
    chorioretinal, disseminated
    in neurosyphilis A52.19
  Egyptian B76.9 [D63.8]
  focal —see also Inflammation, chorioretinal,
    focal
    histoplasmic B39.9 [H32]
  in (due to)
    histoplasmosis B39.9 [H32]
    syphilis (secondary) A51.43
      late A52.71
    toxoplasmosis (acquired) B58.01
      congenital (active) P37.1 [H32]
    tuberculosis A18.53
  juxtapapillary, juxtapapillaris —see
    Inflammation, chorioretinal, focal,
    juxtapapillary
  leprous A30.9 [H32]
  miner's B76.9 [D63.8]
  progressive myopia (degeneration) —see also
    Myopia, degenerative H44.2-●
  syphilitic (secondary) A51.43
    congenital (early) A50.01 [H32]
      late A50.32
    late A52.71
  tuberculous A18.53

Chorioretinopathy, central serous H35.71-●
Choroid —see condition
Choroideremia H31.21
Choroiditis —see Chorioretinitis
Choroidopathy —see Disorder, choroid
Choroidoretinitis —see Chorioretinitis
Choroidoretinopathy, central serous —see
  Chorioretinopathy, central serous
Christian-Weber disease M35.6
Christmas disease D67
Chromaffinoma —see also Neoplasm, benign,
  by site
  malignant —see Neoplasm, malignant, by site
Chromatopsia —see Deficiency, color vision
Chromhidrosis, chromidrosis L75.1
Chromoblastomycosis —see Chromomycosis
Chromoconversion R82.91
Chromomycosis B43.9
  brain abscess B43.1
  cerebral B43.1
  cutaneous B43.0
  skin B43.0
  specified NEC B43.8
  subcutaneous abscess or cyst B43.2
Chromophytosis B36.0
Chromosome —see condition by chromosome
  involved
  D (1) —see condition, chromosome 13
  E (3) —see condition, chromosome 18
  G —see condition, chromosome 21
Chromotrichomycosis B36.8
Chronic —see condition
  fracture —see Fracture, pathological
Churg-Strauss syndrome M30.1
Chyle cyst, mesentery I89.8
Chylocele (nonfilarial) I89.8
  filarial —see also Infestation, filarial B74.9
    [N51]
  tunica vaginalis N50.89
    filarial —see also Infestation, filarial B74.9
      [N51]
Chylomicronemia (fasting) (with
  hyperprebetalipoproteinemia) E78.3
⇒Chylopericardium I31.39
  acute I30.9
Chylothorax (nonfilarial) J94.0
  filarial —see also Infestation, filarial B74.9 [J91.8]
Chylous —see condition
Chyluria (nonfilarial) R82.0
  due to
    bilharziasis B65.0
    Brugia (malayi) B74.1
      timori B74.2
    schistosomiasis (bilharziasis) B65.0
    Wuchereria (bancrofti) B74.0
  filarial —see Infestation, filarial
Cicatricial (deformity) —see Cicatrix
Cicatrix (adherent) (contracted) (painful)
  (vicious) —see also Scar L90.5
  adenoid (and tonsil) J35.8
  alveolar process M26.79
  anus K62.89
  auricle —see Disorder, pinna, specified type
    NEC
  bile duct (common) (hepatic) K83.8
  bladder N32.89
  bone —see Disorder, bone, specified type NEC
  brain G93.89
  cervix (postoperative) (postpartal) N88.1
  common duct K83.8
  cornea H17.9
    tuberculous A18.59
  duodenum (bulb), obstructive K31.5
  esophagus K22.2
  eyelid —see Disorder, eyelid function
  hypopharynx J39.2
  lacrimal passages —see Obstruction, lacrimal
  larynx J38.7
  lung J98.4
  middle ear —see subcategory H74.8
  mouth K13.79

Cicatrix (Continued)
  muscle M62.89
    with contracture —see Contraction, muscle
      NEC
  nasopharynx J39.2
  palate (soft) K13.79
  penis N48.89
  pharynx J39.2
  prostate N42.89
  rectum K62.89
  retina —see Scar, chorioretinal
  semilunar cartilage —see Derangement,
    meniscus
  seminal vesicle N50.89
  skin L90.5
    infected L08.89
    postinfective L90.5
    tuberculous B90.8
  specified site NEC L90.5
  throat J39.2
  tongue K14.8
  tonsil (and adenoid) J35.8
  trachea J39.8
  tuberculous NEC B90.9
  urethra N36.8
  uterus N85.8
  vagina N89.8
    postoperative N99.2
  vocal cord J38.3
  wrist, constricting (annular) L90.5
CIDP (chronic inflammatory demyelinating
  polyneuropathy) G61.81
CIN —see Neoplasia, intraepithelial, cervix
CINCA (chronic infantile neurological,
  cutaneous and articular syndrome)
  M04.1
Cinchonism —see Deafness, ototoxic
  correct substance properly administered —see
    Table of Drugs and Chemicals, by drug,
    adverse effect
  overdose or wrong substance given
    or taken —see Table of Drugs and
    Chemicals, by drug, poisoning
Circle of Willis —see condition
Circular —see condition
Circulating anticoagulants —see also - Disorder,
  hemorrhagic D68.318
  due to drugs —see also - Disorder,
    hemorrhagic D68.32
  following childbirth O72.3
Circulation
  collateral, any site I99.8
  defective (lower extremity) I99.9
    congenital Q28.9
  embryonic Q28.9
  failure (peripheral) R57.9
    newborn P29.89
  fetal, persistent P29.38
  heart, incomplete Q28.9
Circulatory system —see condition
Circulus senilis (cornea) —see Degeneration,
  cornea, senile
Circumcision (in absence of medical indication)
  (ritual) (routine) Z41.2
Circumscribed —see condition
Circumvallate placenta O43.11-●
Cirrhosis, cirrhotic (hepatic) (liver) K74.60
  alcoholic K70.30
    with ascites K70.31
  atrophic —see Cirrhosis, liver
  Baumgarten-Cruveilhier K74.69
  biliary (cholangiolitic) (cholangitic)
    (hypertrophic) (obstructive)
    (pericholangiolitic) K74.5
  due to
    Clonorchiasis B66.1
    flukes B66.3
  primary K74.3
  secondary K74.4
  cardiac (of liver) K76.1
  Charcot's K74.3

Cirrhosis, cirrhotic (Continued)
  cholangiolitic, cholangitic, cholostatic
    (primary) K74.3
  congestive K76.1
  Cruveilhier-Baumgarten K74.69
  cryptogenic (liver) K74.69
  due to
    hepatolenticular degeneration E83.01
    Wilson's disease E83.01
    xanthomatosis E78.2
  fatty K76.0
    alcoholic K70.0
  Hanot's (hypertrophic) K74.3
  hepatic —see Cirrhosis, liver
  hypertrophic K74.3
  Indian childhood K74.69
  kidney —see Sclerosis, renal
  Laennec's K70.30
    with ascites K70.31
    alcoholic K70.30
      with ascites K70.31
    nonalcoholic K74.69
  liver K74.60
    alcoholic K70.30
      with ascites K70.31
      fatty K70.0
    congenital P78.81
    syphilitic A52.74
  lung (chronic) J84.10
  macronodular K74.69
    alcoholic K70.30
      with ascites K70.31
  micronodular K74.69
    alcoholic K70.30
      with ascites K70.31
  mixed type K74.69
  monolobular K74.3
  nephritis —see Sclerosis, renal
  nutritional K74.69
    alcoholic K70.30
      with ascites K70.31
  obstructive —see Cirrhosis, biliary
  ovarian N83.8
  pancreas (duct) K86.89
  pigmentary E83.110
  portal K74.69
    alcoholic K70.30
      with ascites K70.31
  postnecrotic K74.69
    alcoholic K70.30
      with ascites K70.31
  pulmonary J84.10
  renal —see Sclerosis, renal
  spleen D73.2
  stasis K76.1
  Todd's K74.3
  unilobar K74.3
  xanthomatous (biliary) K74.5
    due to xanthomatosis (familial) (metabolic)
      (primary) E78.2
Cistern, subarachnoid R93.0
Citrullinemia E72.23
Citrullinuria E72.23
Civatte's disease or poikiloderma L57.3
Clam digger's itch B65.3
Clammy skin R23.1
Clap —see Gonorrhea
Clarke-Hadfield syndrome (pancreatic
  infantilism) K86.89
Clark's paralysis G80.9
Clastothrix L67.8
Claude Bernard-Horner syndrome G90.2
  traumatic —see Injury, nerve, cervical
    sympathetic
Claude's disease or syndrome G46.3
Claudicatio venosa intermittens I87.8
Claudication (intermittent) I73.9
  cerebral (artery) G45.9
  spinal cord (arteriosclerotic) G95.19
    syphilitic A52.09
  venous (axillary) I87.8

Claustrophobia F40.240
Clavus (infected) L84
Clawfoot (congenital) Q66.89
  acquired —see Deformity, limb, clawfoot
Clawhand (acquired) —see also Deformity, limb,
  clawhand
  congenital Q68.1
Clawtoe (congenital) Q66.89
  acquired —see Deformity, toe, specified NEC
Clay eating —see Pica
Cleansing of artificial opening —see Attention
  to, artificial, opening
Cleft (congenital) —see also Imperfect, closure
  alveolar process M26.79
  branchial (persistent) Q18.2
  cyst Q18.0
    fistula Q18.0
    sinus Q18.0
  cricoid cartilage, posterior Q31.8
  foot Q72.7
  hand Q71.6
  lip (unilateral) Q36.9
    with cleft palate Q37.9
      hard Q37.1
        with soft Q37.5
      soft Q37.3
        with hard Q37.5
    bilateral Q36.0
      with cleft palate Q37.8
        hard Q37.0
          with soft Q37.4
        soft Q37.2
          with hard Q37.4
    median Q36.1
  nose Q30.2
  palate Q35.9
    with cleft lip (unilateral) Q37.9
      bilateral Q37.8
    hard Q35.1
      with
        cleft lip (unilateral) Q37.1
          bilateral Q37.0
        soft Q35.5
          with cleft lip (unilateral) Q37.5
            bilateral Q37.4
    medial Q35.5
    soft Q35.3
      with
        cleft lip (unilateral) Q37.3
          bilateral Q37.2
        hard Q35.5
          with cleft lip (unilateral) Q37.5
            bilateral Q37.4
  penis Q55.69
  scrotum Q55.29
  thyroid cartilage Q31.8
  uvula Q35.7
Cleidocranial dysostosis Q74.0
Cleptomania F63.2
Clicking hip (newborn) R29.4
Climacteric (female) —see also Menopause
  arthritis (any site) NEC —see Arthritis,
    specified form NEC
  depression (single episode) F32.89
    recurrent episode F33.8
  male (symptoms) (syndrome) NEC N50.89
  melancholia (single episode) F32.89
    recurrent episode F33.8
  paranoid state F22
  polyarthritis NEC —see Arthritis, specified
    form NEC
  symptoms (female) N95.1
Clinical research investigation (clinical trial)
  (control subject) (normal comparison)
  (participant) Z00.6
Clitoris —see condition Cloaca (persistent)
  Q43.7
Clonorchiasis, clonorchis infection (liver)
  B66.1
Clonus R25.8
Closed bite M26.29

Clostridium (C.) perfringens, as cause of
  disease classified elsewhere B96.7
Closure
  congenital, nose Q30.0
  cranial sutures, premature Q75.0
  defective or imperfect NEC —see Imperfect,
    closure
  fistula, delayed —see Fistula
  foramen ovale, imperfect Q21.12
  hymen N89.6
  interauricular septum, defective Q21.19
  interventricular septum, defective Q21.0
  lacrimal duct —see also Stenosis, lacrimal,
    duct
    congenital Q10.5
  nose (congenital) Q30.0
    acquired M95.0
  of artificial opening —see Attention to,
    artificial, opening
  primary angle, without glaucoma damage
    H40.06-●
  vagina N89.5
  valve —see Endocarditis
  vulva N90.5
Clot (blood) —see also Embolism
  artery (obstruction) (occlusion) —see
    Embolism
  bladder N32.89
  brain (intradural or extradural) —see
    Occlusion, artery, cerebral
  circulation I74.9
  heart —see also Infarct, myocardium
    not resulting in infarction I51.3
  vein —see Thrombosis
Clouded state R40.1
  epileptic —see Epilepsy, specified NEC
  paroxysmal —see Epilepsy, specified NEC
Cloudy antrum, antra J32.0
Clouston's (hidrotic) ectodermal dysplasia
  Q82.4
Clubbed nail pachydermoperiostosis M89.40
  [L62]
Clubbing of finger(s) (nails) R68.3
Clubfinger R68.3
  congenital Q68.1
Clubfoot (congenital) Q66.89
  acquired —see Deformity, limb, clubfoot
  equinovarus Q66.0-●
  paralytic —see Deformity, limb, clubfoot
Clubhand (congenital) (radial) Q71.4-●
  acquired —see Deformity, limb, clubhand
Clubnail R68.3
  congenital Q84.6
Clump, kidney Q63.1
Clumsiness, clumsy child syndrome F82
Cluttering F98.81
Clutton's joints A50.51 [M12.80]
Coagulation, intravascular (diffuse)
  (disseminated) —see also Defibrination
    syndrome
  complicating abortion —see Abortion, by
    type, complicated by, intravascular
    coagulation
  following ectopic or molar pregnancy
    O08.1
Coagulopathy —see also Defect, coagulation
  consumption D65
  intravascular D65
    newborn P60
Coalition
  calcaneo-scaphoid Q66.89
  tarsal Q66.89
Coalminer's
  elbow —see Bursitis, elbow, olecranon
  lung or pneumoconiosis J60
Coalworker's lung or pneumoconiosis
  J60
Coarctation
  aorta (preductal) (postductal) Q25.1
  pulmonary artery Q25.71
Coated tongue K14.3

Coats' disease (exudative retinopathy) —*see*
  Retinopathy, exudative
Cocaine-induced
  anxiety disorder F14.980
  bipolar and related disorder F14.94
  depressive disorder F14.94
  obsessive-compulsive and related disorder
    F14.988
  psychotic disorder F14.959
  sleep disorder F14.982
  sexual dysfunction F14.981
Cocainism —*see* Disorder, cocaine use
Coccidioidomycosis B38.9
  cutaneous B38.3
  disseminated B38.7
  generalized B38.7
  meninges B38.4
  prostate B38.81
  pulmonary B38.2
    acute B38.0
    chronic B38.1
  skin B38.3
  specified NEC B38.89
Coccidioidosis —*see* Coccidioidomycosis
Coccidiosis (intestinal) A07.3
Coccydynia, coccygodynia M53.3
Coccyx —*see* condition
Cochin-China diarrhea K90.1
Cockayne's syndrome Q87.19
Cocked up toe —*see* Deformity, toe, specified
  NEC
Cock's peculiar tumor L72.3
Codman's tumor —*see* Neoplasm, bone, benign
Coenurosis B71.8
Coffee-worker's lung J67.8
Cogan's syndrome H16.32-•
  oculomotor apraxia H51.8
Coitus, painful (female) N94.10
  male N53.12
  psychogenic F52.6
Cold J00
  with influenza, flu, or grippe —*see* Influenza,
    with, respiratory manifestations NEC
  agglutinin disease or hemoglobinuria
    (chronic) D59.12
  bronchial —*see* Bronchitis
  chest —*see* Bronchitis
  common (head) J00
  effects of T69.9
    specified effect NEC T69.8
  excessive, effects of T69.9
    specified effect NEC T69.8
  exhaustion from T69.8
  exposure to T69.9
    specified effect NEC T69.8
  head J00
  injury syndrome (newborn) P80.0
  on lung —*see* Bronchitis
  rose J30.1
  sensitivity, auto-immune D59.12
  symptoms J00
  virus J00
Coldsore B00.1
Colibacillosis A49.8
  as the cause of other disease (see also
    Escherichia coli) B96.20
  generalized A41.50
Colic (bilious) (infantile) (intestinal) (recurrent)
    (spasmodic) R10.83
  abdomen R10.83
    psychogenic F45.8
  appendix, appendicular K38.8
  bile duct —*see* Calculus, bile duct
  biliary —*see* Calculus, bile duct
  common duct —*see* Calculus, bile duct
  cystic duct —*see* Calculus, gallbladder
  Devonshire NEC —*see* Poisoning, lead
  gallbladder —*see* Calculus, gallbladder
  gallstone —*see* Calculus, gallbladder
    gallbladder or cystic duct —*see* Calculus,
      gallbladder

Colic (Continued)
  hepatic (duct) —*see* Calculus, bile duct
  hysterical F45.8
  kidney N23
  lead NEC —*see* Poisoning, lead
  mucous K58.9
    with diarrhea K58.0
    psychogenic F54
  nephritic N23
  painter's NEC —*see* Poisoning, lead
  pancreas K86.89
  psychogenic F45.8
  renal N23
  saturnine NEC —*see* Poisoning, lead
  ureter N23
  urethral N36.8
    due to calculus N21.1
  uterus NEC N94.89
    menstrual —*see* Dysmenorrhea
  worm NOS B83.9
Colicystitis —*see* Cystitis
Colitis (acute) (catarrhal) (chronic)
    (noninfective) (hemorrhagic) (see also
    Enteritis) K52.9
  allergic K52.29
    with
      food protein-induced enterocolitis
        syndrome K52.21
      proctocolitis K52.29
  amebic (acute) —*see also* Amebiasis A06.0
    nondysenteric A06.2
  anthrax A22.2
  bacillary —*see* Infection, Shigella
  balantidial A07.0
  Clostridium difficile
    not specified as recurrent A04.72
    recurrent A04.71
  coccidial A07.3
  collagenous K52.831
  cystica superficialis K52.89
  dietary counseling and surveillance (for) Z71.3
  dietetic —*see also* Colitis, allergic K52.29
  drug-induced K52.1
  due to radiation K52.0
  eosinophilic K52.82
  food hypersensitivity —*see also* Colitis,
    allergic K52.29
  giardial A07.1
  granulomatous —*see* Enteritis, regional, large
    intestine
  infectious —*see* Enteritis, infectious
  indeterminate, so stated K52.3
  ischemic K55.9
    acute (subacute) —*see also* Ischemia,
      intestine, acute K55.039
    chronic K55.1
    due to mesenteric artery insufficiency K55.1
    fulminant (acute) —*see also* Ischemia,
      intestine, acute K55.039
  left sided K51.50
    with
      abscess K51.514
      complication K51.519
        specified NEC K51.518
      fistula K51.513
      obstruction K51.512
      rectal bleeding K51.511
  lymphocytic K52.832
  membranous
    psychogenic F54
  microscopic K52.839
    specified NEC K52.838
  mucous —*see* Syndrome, irritable, bowel
    psychogenic F54
  noninfective K52.9
    specified NEC K52.89
  polyposa —*see* Polyp, colon, inflammatory
  protozoal A07.9
  pseudomembranous
    not specified as recurrent A04.72
    recurrent A04.71

Colitis (Continued)
  pseudomucinous —*see* Syndrome, irritable,
    bowel
  regional —*see* Enteritis, regional, large intestine
    infectious A09
  segmental —*see* Enteritis, regional, large
    intestine
  septic —*see* Enteritis, infectious
  spastic K58.9
    with diarrhea K58.0
    psychogenic F54
  staphylococcal A04.8
    foodborne A05.0
  subacute ischemic —*see also* Ischemia,
    intestine, acute K55.039
  thromboulcerative —*see also* Ischemia,
    intestine, acute K55.039
  toxic NEC K52.1
    due to Clostridium difficile
      not specified as recurrent A04.72
      recurrent A04.71
  transmural —*see* Enteritis, regional, large
    intestine
  trichomonal A07.8
  tuberculous (ulcerative) A18.32
  ulcerative (chronic) K51.90
    with
      complication K51.919
        abscess K51.914
        fistula K51.913
        obstruction K51.912
        rectal bleeding K51.911
        specified complication NEC K51.918
    enterocolitis —*see* Enterocolitis, ulcerative
    ileocolitis —*see* Ileocolitis, ulcerative
    mucosal proctocolitis —*see* Proctocolitis,
      mucosal
    proctitis —*see* Proctitis, ulcerative
    pseudopolyposis —*see* Polyp, colon,
      inflammatory
    psychogenic F54
    rectosigmoiditis —*see* Rectosigmoiditis,
      ulcerative
    specified type NEC K51.80
      with
        complication K51.819
          abscess K51.814
          fistula K51.813
          obstruction K51.812
          rectal bleeding K51.811
          specified complication NEC K51.818
Collagenosis, collagen disease (nonvascular)
    (vascular) M35.9
  cardiovascular I42.8
  reactive perforating L87.1
  specified NEC M35.89
Collapse R55
  adrenal E27.2
  cardiorespiratory R57.0
  cardiovascular R57.0
    newborn P29.89
  circulatory (peripheral) R57.9
    during or after labor and delivery O75.1
    following ectopic or molar pregnancy O08.3
    newborn P29.89
  during or
    after labor and delivery O75.1
    resulting from a procedure, not elsewhere
      classified T81.10
  external ear canal —*see* Stenosis, external ear
    canal
  general R55
  heart —*see* Disease, heart
  heat T67.1
  hysterical F44.89
  labyrinth, membranous (congenital) Q16.5
  lung (massive) —*see also* Atelectasis J98.19
    pressure due to anesthesia (general) (local)
      or other sedation T88.2
    during labor and delivery O74.1
    in pregnancy O29.02-•
    postpartum, puerperal O89.09

▶ New   ⇒ Revised   ~~deleted~~ Deleted   • Use Additional Character(s)

Collapse *(Continued)*
   myocardial —*see* Disease, heart
   nervous F48.8
   neurocirculatory F45.8
   nose M95.0
   postoperative T81.10
   pulmonary —*see also* Atelectasis J98.19
      newborn —*see* Atelectasis
   trachea J39.8
   tracheobronchial J98.09
   valvular —*see* Endocarditis
   vascular (peripheral) R57.9
      during or after labor and delivery O75.1
      following ectopic or molar pregnancy O08.3
      newborn P29.89
   vertebra M48.50-●
      cervical region M48.52-●
      cervicothoracic region M48.53-●
      in (due to)
         metastasis —*see* Collapse, vertebra, in,
            specified disease NEC
      ▶neoplasm (metastasis) M84.58-●
         osteoporosis —*see also* Osteoporosis
            M80.88
            cervical region M80.88
            cervicothoracic region M80.88
            lumbar region M80.88
            lumbosacral region M80.88
            multiple sites M80.88
            occipito-atlanto-axial region M80.88
            sacrococcygeal region M80.88
            thoracic region M80.88
            thoracolumbar region M80.88
         specified disease NEC M48.50-●
            cervical region M48.52-●
            cervicothoracic region M48.53-●
            lumbar region M48.56-●
            lumbosacral region M48.57-●
            occipito-atlanto-axial region M48.51-●
            sacrococcygeal region M48.58-●
            thoracic region M48.54-●
            thoracolumbar region M48.55-●
      lumbar region M48.56-●
      lumbosacral region M48.57-●
      occipito-atlanto-axial region M48.51-●
      sacrococcygeal region M48.58-●
      thoracic region M48.54-●
      thoracolumbar region M48.55-●
Collateral —*see also* condition
   circulation (venous) I87.8
   dilation, veins I87.8
Colles' fracture S52.53-●
Collet (-Sicard) syndrome G52.7
Collier's asthma or lung J60
Collodion baby Q80.2
Colloid nodule (of thyroid) (cystic) E04.1
Coloboma (iris) Q13.0
   eyelid Q10.3
   fundus Q14.8
   lens Q12.2
   optic disc (congenital) Q14.2
      acquired H47.31-●
Coloenteritis —*see* Enteritis
Colon —*see* condition
Colonization
   MRSA (Methicillin resistant Staphylococcus
      aureus) Z22.322
   MSSA (Methicillin susceptible
      Staphylococcus aureus) Z22.321
   status —*see* Carrier (suspected) of
Coloptosis K63.4
Color blindness —*see* Deficiency, color vision
Colostomy
   attention to Z43.3
   fitting or adjustment Z46.89
   malfunctioning K94.03
   status Z93.3
Colpitis (acute) —*see* Vaginitis
Colpocele N81.5
Colpocystitis —*see* Vaginitis
Colpospasm N94.2

Column, spinal, vertebral —*see* condition
Coma R40.20
   with
      motor response (none) R40.231
         abnormal R40.233
         abnormal extensor posturing to pain or
            noxious stimuli (<2 years of age)
            R40.232
         abnormal flexure posturing to pain or
            noxious stimuli (0-5 years of age)
            R40.233
         extension R40.232
         extensor posturing to pain or noxious
            stimuli (2-5 years of age) R40.232
         flexion/decorticate posturing
            (<2 years of age) R40.233
         flexion withdrawal R40.234
         localizes pain (2-5 years of age) R40.235
         normal or spontaneous movement
            (<2 years of age) R40.236
         obeys commands (2-5 years of age)
            R40.236
         score of
            1 R40.231
            2 R40.232
            3 R40.233
            4 R40.234
            5 R40.235
            6 R40.236
         withdraws from pain or noxious stimuli
            (0-5 years of age) R40.234
         withdraws to touch (<2 years of age)
            R40.235
      opening of eyes (never) R40.211
         in response to
            pain R40.212
            sound R40.213
         score of
            1 R40.211
            2 R40.212
            3 R40.213
            4 R40.214
         spontaneous R40.214
      verbal response (none) R40.221
         confused conversation R40.224
         cooing or babbling or crying
            appropriately (<2 years of age)
            R40.225
         inappropriate crying or screaming
            (<2 years of age) R40.223
         inappropriate words R40.223
         inappropriate words (2-5 years of age)
            R40.224
         incomprehensible sounds (2-5 years of
            age) R40.222
         incomprehensible words R40.222
         irritable cries (<2 years of age) R40.224
      ▶moans/grunts to pain; restless
            (<2 years old) R40.222
         oriented R40.225
         score of
            1 R40.221
            2 R40.222
            3 R40.223
            4 R40.224
            5 R40.225
         screaming (2-5 years of age) R40.223
         uses appropriate words (2-5 years of
            age) R40.225
   eclamptic —*see* Eclampsia
   epileptic —*see* Epilepsy
   Glasgow, scale score —*see* Glasgow coma
      scale
   hepatic —*see* Failure, hepatic, by type, with
      coma
   hyperglycemic (diabetic) —*see* Diabetes, by
      type, with hyperosmolarity, with coma
   hyperosmolar (diabetic) —*see* Diabetes, by
      type, with hyperosmolarity, with coma
   hypoglycemic (diabetic) —*see* Diabetes, by
      type, with hypoglycemia, with coma
      nondiabetic E15

Coma *(Continued)*
   in diabetes —*see* Diabetes, coma
   insulin-induced —*see* Coma, hypoglycemic
   ketoacidotic (diabetic) —*see* Diabetes, by
      type, with ketoacidosis, with coma
   myxedematous E03.5
   newborn P91.5
   persistent vegetative state R40.3
   specified NEC, without documented
      Glasgow coma scale score, or with
      partial Glasgow coma scale score
      reported R40.244
Comatose —*see* Coma
Combat fatigue F43.0
Combined —*see* condition
Comedo, comedones (giant) L70.0
Comedocarcinoma —*see also* Neoplasm, breast,
   malignant
   noninfiltrating
      breast D05.8-●
      specified site —*see* Neoplasm, in situ, by site
      unspecified site D05.8-●
Comedomastitis —*see* Ectasia, mammary duct
Comminuted fracture - code as Fracture, closed
Common
   arterial trunk Q20.0
  ▶atrioventricular canal Q21.23
  ▶atrium Q21.19
   cold (head) J00
   truncus (arteriosus) Q20.0
   variable immunodeficiency —*see*
      Immunodeficiency, common variable
   ventricle Q20.4
Commotio, commotion (current)
   brain —*see* Injury, intracranial, concussion
   cerebri —*see* Injury, intracranial, concussion
   retinae S05.8X-●
   spinal cord —*see* Injury, spinal cord, by region
   spinalis —*see* Injury, spinal cord, by region
Communication
   between
      base of aorta and pulmonary artery Q21.4
      left ventricle and right atrium Q20.5
      pericardial sac and pleural sac Q34.8
      pulmonary artery and pulmonary vein,
         congenital Q25.72
   congenital between uterus and digestive or
      urinary tract Q51.7
Compartment syndrome (deep) (posterior)
   (traumatic) T79.A0
   abdomen T79.A3
   lower extremity (hip, buttock, thigh, leg, foot,
      toes) T79.A2
   nontraumatic
      abdomen M79.A3
      lower extremity (hip, buttock, thigh, leg,
         foot, toes) M79.A2-●
      specified site NEC M79.A9
      upper extremity (shoulder, arm, forearm,
         wrist, hand, fingers) M79.A1-●
   specified site NEC T79.A9
   upper extremity (shoulder, arm, forearm,
      wrist, hand, fingers) T79.A1
Compensation
   failure —*see* Disease, heart
   neurosis, psychoneurosis —*see* Disorder,
      factitious
Complaint —*see also* Disease
   bowel, functional K59.9
      psychogenic F45.8
   intestine, functional K59.9
      psychogenic F45.8
   kidney —*see* Disease, renal
   miners' J60
Complete —*see* condition
Complex
   Addison-Schilder E71.528
   cardiorenal —*see* Hypertension, cardiorenal
   Costen's M26.69
   disseminated mycobacterium avium-
      intracellulare (DMAC) A31.2

Complex *(Continued)*
Eisenmenger's (ventricular septal defect) I27.83
hypersexual F52.8
jumped process, spine —*see* Dislocation, vertebra
primary, tuberculous A15.7
Schilder-Addison E71.528
subluxation (vertebral) M99.19
  abdomen M99.19
  acromioclavicular M99.17
  cervical region M99.11
  cervicothoracic M99.11
  costochondral M99.18
  costovertebral M99.18
  head region M99.10
  hip M99.15
  lower extremity M99.16
  lumbar region M99.13
  lumbosacral M99.13
  occipitocervical M99.10
  pelvic region M99.15
  pubic M99.15
  rib cage M99.18
  sacral region M99.14
  sacrococcygeal M99.14
  sacroiliac M99.14
  specified NEC M99.19
  sternochondral M99.18
  sternoclavicular M99.17
  thoracic region M99.12
  thoracolumbar M99.12
  upper extremity M99.17
Taussig-Bing (transposition, aorta and overriding pulmonary artery) Q20.1
Complication(s) (from) (of)
accidental puncture or laceration during a procedure (of) —*see* Complications, intraoperative (intraprocedural), puncture or laceration
amputation stump (surgical) (late) NEC T87.9
  dehiscence T87.81
  infection or inflammation T87.40
    lower limb T87.4-•
    upper limb T87.4-•
  necrosis T87.50
    lower limb T87.5-•
    upper limb T87.5-•
  neuroma T87.30
    lower limb T87.3-•
    upper limb T87.3-•
  specified type NEC T87.89
anastomosis (and bypass) —*see also* Complications, prosthetic device or implant
  intestinal (internal) NEC K91.89
    involving urinary tract N99.89
  urinary tract (involving intestinal tract) N99.89
  vascular —*see* Complications, cardiovascular device or implant
anesthesia, anesthetic —*see also* Anesthesia, complication T88.59
  brain, postpartum, puerperal O89.2
  cardiac
    in
      labor and delivery O74.2
      pregnancy O29.19-•
    postpartum, puerperal O89.1
  central nervous system
    in
      labor and delivery O74.3
      pregnancy O29.29-•
    postpartum, puerperal O89.2
  difficult or failed intubation T88.4
    in pregnancy O29.6-•
  failed sedation (conscious) (moderate) during procedure T88.52
  general, unintended awareness during procedure T88.53
  hyperthermia, malignant T88.3
  hypothermia T88.51
  intubation failure T88.4

Complication *(Continued)*
anesthesia, anesthetic *(Continued)*
  malignant hyperthermia T88.3
  pulmonary
    in
      labor and delivery O74.1
      pregnancy NEC O29.09-•
    postpartum, puerperal O89.09
  shock T88.2
  spinal and epidural
    in
      labor and delivery NEC O74.6
        headache O74.5
      pregnancy NEC O29.5X-•
    postpartum, puerperal NEC O89.5
      headache O89.4
  unintended awareness under general anesthesia during procedure T88.53
anti-reflux device —*see* Complications, esophageal anti-reflux device
aortic (bifurcation) graft —*see* Complications, graft, vascular
aortocoronary (bypass) graft —*see* Complications, coronary artery (bypass) graft
aortofemoral (bypass) graft —*see* Complications, extremity artery (bypass) graft
arteriovenous
  fistula, surgically created T82.9
    embolism T82.818
    fibrosis T82.828
    hemorrhage T82.838
    infection or inflammation T82.7
    mechanical
      breakdown T82.510
      displacement T82.520
      leakage T82.530
      malposition T82.520
      obstruction T82.590
      perforation T82.590
      protrusion T82.590
    pain T82.848
    specified type NEC T82.898
    stenosis T82.858
    thrombosis T82.868
  shunt, surgically created T82.9
    embolism T82.818
    fibrosis T82.828
    hemorrhage T82.838
    infection or inflammation T82.7
    mechanical
      breakdown T82.511
      displacement T82.521
      leakage T82.531
      malposition T82.521
      obstruction T82.591
      perforation T82.591
      protrusion T82.591
    pain T82.848
    specified type NEC T82.898
    stenosis T82.858
    thrombosis T82.868
arthroplasty —*see* Complications, joint prosthesis
artificial
  fertilization or insemination N98.9
    attempted introduction (of)
      embryo in embryo transfer N98.3
      ovum following in vitro fertilization N98.2
    hyperstimulation of ovaries N98.1
    infection N98.0
    specified NEC N98.8
  heart T82.9
    embolism T82.817
    fibrosis T82.827
    hemorrhage T82.837
    infection or inflammation T82.7
    mechanical
      breakdown T82.512
      displacement T82.522
      leakage T82.532

Complication *(Continued)*
artificial *(Continued)*
  heart *(Continued)*
    mechanical *(Continued)*
      malposition T82.522
      obstruction T82.592
      perforation T82.592
      protrusion T82.592
    pain T82.847
    specified type NEC T82.897
    stenosis T82.857
    thrombosis T82.867
  opening
    cecostomy —*see* Complications, colostomy
    colostomy —*see* Complications, colostomy
    cystostomy —*see* Complications, cystostomy
    enterostomy —*see* Complications, enterostomy
    gastrostomy —*see* Complications, gastrostomy
    ileostomy —*see* Complications, enterostomy
    jejunostomy —*see* Complications, enterostomy
    nephrostomy —*see* Complications, stoma, urinary tract
    tracheostomy —*see* Complications, tracheostomy
    ureterostomy —*see* Complications, stoma, urinary tract
    urethrostomy —*see* Complications, stoma, urinary tract
balloon implant or device
  gastrointestinal T85.9
    embolism T85.818
    fibrosis T85.828
    hemorrhage T85.838
    infection and inflammation T85.79
    pain T85.848
    specified type NEC T85.898
    stenosis T85.858
    thrombosis T85.868
  vascular (counterpulsation) T82.9
    embolism T82.818
    fibrosis T82.828
    hemorrhage T82.838
    infection or inflammation T82.7
    mechanical
      breakdown T82.513
      displacement T82.523
      leakage T82.533
      malposition T82.523
      obstruction T82.593
      perforation T82.593
      protrusion T82.593
    pain T82.848
    specified type NEC T82.898
    stenosis T82.858
    thrombosis T82.868
bariatric procedure
  gastric band procedure K95.09
    infection K95.01
  specified procedure NEC K95.89
    infection K95.81
bile duct implant (prosthetic) T85.9
  embolism T85.818
  fibrosis T85.828
  hemorrhage T85.838
  infection and inflammation T85.79
  mechanical
    breakdown T85.510
    displacement T85.520
    malfunction T85.510
    malposition T85.520
    obstruction T85.590
    perforation T85.590
    protrusion T85.590
    specified NEC T85.590
  pain T85.848
  specified type NEC T85.898

▶ New   ⇒ Revised   ~~deleted~~ Deleted   • Use Additional Character(s)

Complication *(Continued)*
  bile duct implant *(Continued)*
    stenosis T85.858
    thrombosis T85.868
  bladder device (auxiliary) —*see*
    Complications, genitourinary, device or
    implant, urinary system
  bleeding (postoperative) —*see* Complication,
    postoperative, hemorrhage
    intraoperative —*see* Complication,
      intraoperative, hemorrhage
  blood vessel graft —*see* Complications, graft,
    vascular
  bone
    device NEC T84.9
      embolism T84.81
      fibrosis T84.82
      hemorrhage T84.83
      infection or inflammation T84.7
      mechanical
        breakdown T84.318
        displacement T84.328
        malposition T84.328
        obstruction T84.398
        perforation T84.398
        protrusion T84.398
      pain T84.84
      specified type NEC T84.89
      stenosis T84.85
      thrombosis T84.86
    graft —*see* Complications, graft, bone
    growth stimulator (electrode) —*see*
      Complications, electronic stimulator
      device, bone
    marrow transplant —*see* Complications,
      transplant, bone, marrow
  brain neurostimulator (electrode) —*see*
    Complications, electronic stimulator
    device, brain
  breast implant (prosthetic) T85.9
    capsular contracture T85.44
    embolism T85.818
    fibrosis T85.828
    hemorrhage T85.838
    infection and inflammation T85.79
    mechanical
      breakdown T85.41
      displacement T85.42
      leakage T85.43
      malposition T85.42
      obstruction T85.49
      perforation T85.49
      protrusion T85.49
      specified NEC T85.49
    pain T85.848
    specified type NEC T85.898
    stenosis T85.858
    thrombosis T85.868
  bypass —*see also* Complications, prosthetic
    device or implant
    aortocoronary —*see* Complications,
      coronary artery (bypass) graft
    arterial —*see also* Complications, graft,
      vascular
      extremity —*see* Complications, extremity
        artery (bypass) graft
  cardiac —*see also* Disease, heart
    device, implant or graft T82.9
      embolism T82.817
      fibrosis T82.827
      hemorrhage T82.837
      infection or inflammation T82.7
        valve prosthesis T82.6
      mechanical
        breakdown T82.519
          specified device NEC T82.518
        displacement T82.529
          specified device NEC T82.528
        leakage T82.539
          specified device NEC T82.538
        malposition T82.529
          specified device NEC T82.528

Complication *(Continued)*
  cardiac *(Continued)*
    device, implant or graft *(Continued)*
      mechanical *(Continued)*
        obstruction T82.599
          specified device NEC T82.598
        perforation T82.599
          specified device NEC T82.598
        protrusion T82.599
          specified device NEC T82.598
      pain T82.847
      specified type NEC T82.897
      stenosis T82.857
      thrombosis T82.867
  cardiovascular device, graft or implant T82.9
    aortic graft —*see* Complications, graft,
      vascular
    arteriovenous
      fistula, artificial —*see* Complication,
        arteriovenous, fistula, surgically
        created
      shunt —*see* Complication, arteriovenous,
        shunt, surgically created
    artificial heart —*see* Complication,
      artificial, heart
    balloon (counterpulsation) device —*see*
      Complication, balloon implant,
      vascular
    carotid artery graft —*see* Complications,
      graft, vascular
    coronary bypass graft —*see* Complication,
      coronary artery (bypass) graft
    dialysis catheter (vascular) —*see*
      Complication, catheter, dialysis
    electronic T82.9
      electrode T82.9
        embolism T82.817
        fibrosis T82.827
        hemorrhage T82.837
        infection T82.7
        mechanical
          breakdown T82.110
          displacement T82.120
          leakage T82.190
          obstruction T82.190
          perforation T82.190
          protrusion T82.190
          specified type NEC T82.190
        pain T82.847
        specified NEC T82.897
        stenosis T82.857
        thrombosis T82.867
      embolism T82.817
      fibrosis T82.827
      hemorrhage T82.837
      infection T82.7
      mechanical
        breakdown T82.119
        displacement T82.129
        leakage T82.199
        obstruction T82.199
        perforation T82.199
        protrusion T82.199
        specified type NEC T82.199
      pain T82.847
      pulse generator T82.9
        embolism T82.817
        fibrosis T82.827
        hemorrhage T82.837
        infection T82.7
        mechanical
          breakdown T82.111
          displacement T82.121
          leakage T82.191
          obstruction T82.191
          perforation T82.191
          protrusion T82.191
          specified type NEC T82.191
        pain T82.847
        specified NEC T82.897
        stenosis T82.857
        thrombosis T82.867

Complication *(Continued)*
  cardiovascular device, graft or implant
    (Continued)
    electronic *(Continued)*
      specified condition NEC T82.897
      specified device NEC T82.9
        embolism T82.817
        fibrosis T82.827
        hemorrhage T82.837
        infection T82.7
        mechanical
          breakdown T82.118
          displacement T82.128
          leakage T82.198
          obstruction T82.198
          perforation T82.198
          protrusion T82.198
          specified type NEC T82.198
        pain T82.847
        specified NEC T82.897
        stenosis T82.857
        thrombosis T82.867
      stenosis T82.857
      thrombosis T82.867
    extremity artery graft —*see* Complication,
      extremity artery (bypass) graft
    femoral artery graft —*see* Complication,
      extremity artery (bypass) graft
    heart
      transplant —*see* Complication,
        transplant, heart
      valve —*see* Complication, prosthetic
        device, heart valve
        graft —*see* Complication, heart, valve,
          graft
    heart-lung transplant —*see* Complication,
      transplant, heart, with lung
    infection or inflammation T82.7
    umbrella device —*see* Complication,
      umbrella device, vascular
    vascular graft (or anastomosis) —*see*
      Complication, graft, vascular
  carotid artery (bypass) graft —*see*
    Complications, graft, vascular
  catheter (device) NEC —*see also*
    Complications, prosthetic device or
    implant
    cranial infusion
      infection and inflammation T85.735
      mechanical
        breakdown T85.610
        displacement T85.620
        leakage T85.630
        malfunction T85.690
        malposition T85.620
        obstruction T85.690
        perforation T85.690
        protrusion T85.690
        specified NEC T85.690
    cystostomy T83.9
      embolism T83.81
      fibrosis T83.82
      hemorrhage T83.83
      infection and inflammation T83.510
      mechanical
        breakdown T83.010
        displacement T83.020
        leakage T83.030
        malposition T83.020
        obstruction T83.090
        perforation T83.090
        protrusion T83.090
        specified NEC T83.090
      pain T83.84
      specified type NEC T83.89
      stenosis T83.85
      thrombosis T83.86
    dialysis (vascular) T82.9
      embolism T82.818
      fibrosis T82.828
      hemorrhage T82.838

Complication *(Continued)*
  catheter NEC *(Continued)*
    dialysis *(Continued)*
      infection and inflammation T82.7
      intraperitoneal —*see* Complications, catheter, intraperitoneal
      mechanical
        breakdown T82.41
        displacement T82.42
        leakage T82.43
        malposition T82.42
        obstruction T82.49
        perforation T82.49
        protrusion T82.49
      pain T82.848
      specified type NEC T82.898
      stenosis T82.858
      thrombosis T82.868
    epidural infusion T85.9
      embolism T85.810
      fibrosis T85.820
      hemorrhage T85.830
      infection and inflammation T85.735
      mechanical
        breakdown T85.610
        displacement T85.620
        leakage T85.630
        malfunction T85.610
        malposition T85.620
        obstruction T85.690
        perforation T85.690
        protrusion T85.690
        specified NEC T85.690
      pain T85.840
      specified type NEC T85.890
      stenosis T85.850
      thrombosis T85.860
    intraperitoneal dialysis T85.9
      embolism T85.818
      fibrosis T85.828
      hemorrhage T85.838
      infection and inflammation T85.71
      mechanical
        breakdown T85.611
        displacement T85.621
        leakage T85.631
        malfunction T85.611
        malposition T85.621
        obstruction T85.691
        perforation T85.691
        protrusion T85.691
        specified NEC T85.691
      pain T85.848
      specified type NEC T85.898
      stenosis T85.858
      thrombosis T85.868
    intrathecal infusion
      infection and inflammation T85.735
      mechanical
        breakdown T85.610
        displacement T85.620
        leakage T85.630
        malfunction T85.690
        malposition T85.620
        obstruction T85.690
        perforation T85.690
        protrusion T85.690
        specified NEC T85.690
    intravenous infusion T82.9
      embolism T82.818
      fibrosis T82.828
      hemorrhage T82.838
      infection or inflammation T82.7
      mechanical
        breakdown T82.514
        displacement T82.524
        leakage T82.534
        malposition T82.524
        obstruction T82.594
        perforation T82.594
        protrusion T82.594
      pain T82.848

Complication *(Continued)*
  catheter NEC *(Continued)*
    intravenous infusion *(Continued)*
      specified type NEC T82.898
      stenosis T82.858
      thrombosis T82.868
    spinal infusion
      infection and inflammation T85.735
      mechanical
        breakdown T85.610
        displacement T85.620
        leakage T85.630
        malfunction T85.690
        malposition T85.620
        obstruction T85.690
        perforation T85.690
        protrusion T85.690
        specified NEC T85.690
    subarachnoid infusion
      infection and inflammation T85.735
      mechanical
        breakdown T85.610
        displacement T85.620
        leakage T85.630
        malfunction T85.690
        malposition T85.620
        obstruction T85.690
        perforation T85.690
        protrusion T85.690
        specified NEC T85.690
    subdural infusion T85.9
      embolism T85.810
      fibrosis T85.820
      hemorrhage T85.830
      infection and inflammation T85.735
      mechanical
        breakdown T85.610
        displacement T85.620
        leakage T85.630
        malfunction T85.610
        malposition T85.620
        obstruction T85.690
        perforation T85.690
        protrusion T85.690
        specified NEC T85.690
      pain T85.840
      specified type NEC T85.890
      stenosis T85.850
      thrombosis T85.860
    urethral T83.9
      displacement T83.028
      embolism T83.81
      fibrosis T83.82
      hemorrhage T83.83
      indwelling
        breakdown T83.011
        displacement T83.021
        infection and inflammation T83.511
        leakage T83.031
        specified complication NEC T83.091
      infection and inflammation T83.511
      leakage T83.038
      malposition T83.028
      mechanical
        breakdown T83.011
      obstruction (mechanical) T83.091
      pain T83.84
      perforation T83.091
      protrusion T83.091
      specified type NEC T83.091
      stenosis T83.85
      thrombosis T83.86
    urinary NEC
      breakdown T83.018
      displacement T83.028
      infection and inflammation T83.518
      leakage T83.038
      specified complication NEC T83.098
  cecostomy (stoma) —*see* Complications, colostomy

Complication *(Continued)*
  cesarean delivery wound NEC O90.89
    disruption O90.0
    hematoma O90.2
    infection (following delivery) O86.00
  chemotherapy (antineoplastic) NEC T88.7
  chimeric antigen receptor (CAR-T) cell therapy T80.82
  chin implant (prosthetic) —*see* Complication, prosthetic device or implant, specified NEC
  circulatory system I99.8
    intraoperative I97.88
    postprocedural I97.89
      following cardiac surgery —*see also* Infarct, myocardium, associated with revascularization procedure I97.19-●
      postcardiotomy syndrome I97.0
      hypertension I97.3
      lymphedema after mastectomy I97.2
      postcardiotomy syndrome I97.0
      specified NEC I97.89
  colostomy (stoma) K94.00
    hemorrhage K94.01
    infection K94.02
    malfunction K94.03
    mechanical K94.03
    specified complication NEC K94.09
  contraceptive device, intrauterine — *see* Complications, intrauterine, contraceptive device
  cord (umbilical) —*see* Complications, umbilical cord
  corneal graft —*see* Complications, graft, cornea
  coronary artery (bypass) graft T82.9
    atherosclerosis —*see* Arteriosclerosis, coronary (artery)
    ⇒embolism T82.817
    ⇒fibrosis T82.827
    ⇒hemorrhage T82.837
    infection and inflammation T82.7
    mechanical
      breakdown T82.211
      displacement T82.212
      leakage T82.213
      malposition T82.212
      obstruction T82.218
      perforation T82.218
      protrusion T82.218
      specified NEC T82.218
    ⇒pain T82.847
    specified type NEC T82.898
    ⇒stenosis T82.857
    ⇒thrombosis T82.867
  counterpulsation device (balloon), intra-aortic —*see* Complications, balloon implant, vascular
  cystostomy (stoma) N99.518
    catheter —*see* Complications, catheter, cystostomy
    hemorrhage N99.510
    infection N99.511
    malfunction N99.512
    specified type NEC N99.518
  delivery —*see also* Complications, obstetric O75.9
    procedure (instrumental) (manual) (surgical) O75.4
    specified NEC O75.89
  dialysis (peritoneal) (renal) —*see also* Complications, infusion
    catheter (vascular) —*see* Complication, catheter, dialysis
      peritoneal, intraperitoneal —*see* Complications, catheter, intraperitoneal
  dorsal column (spinal) neurostimulator —*see* Complications, electronic stimulator device, spinal cord
  drug NEC T88.7
  ear procedure —*see also* Disorder, ear
    intraoperative H95.88-●

▶ New   ⇒ Revised   ~~deleted~~ Deleted   ● Use Additional Character(s)

Complication *(Continued)*
  ear procedure *(Continued)*
    intraoperative *(Continued)*
      hematoma —*see* Complications,
        intraoperative, hematoma (of), ear
      hemorrhage —*see* Complications,
        intraoperative, hemorrhage (of), ear
      laceration —*see* Complications,
        intraoperative, puncture or
        laceration..., ear
      seroma —*see* Complications,
        postprocedural, seroma (of),
        mastoid process
      specified NEC H95.88-•
    postoperative H95.89-•
      external ear canal stenosis H95.81-•
      hematoma —*see* Complications,
        postprocedural, hemorrhage
        (hematoma) (of), ear
      hemorrhage —*see* Complications,
        postprocedural, hemorrhage
        (hematoma) (of), ear
      postmastoidectomy —*see* Complications,
        postmastoidectomy
      specified NEC H95.89-•
  ectopic pregnancy O08.9
    damage to pelvic organs O08.6
    embolism O08.2
    genital infection O08.0
    hemorrhage (delayed) (excessive) O08.1
    metabolic disorder O08.5
    renal failure O08.4
    shock O08.3
    specified type NEC O08.0
    venous complication NEC O08.7
  electronic stimulator device
    bladder (urinary) —*see* Complications,
      electronic stimulator device, urinary
    bone T84.9
      breakdown T84.310
      displacement T84.320
      embolism T84.81
      fibrosis T84.82
      hemorrhage T84.83
      infection or inflammation T84.7
      malfunction T84.310
      malposition T84.320
      mechanical NEC T84.390
      obstruction T84.390
      pain T84.84
      perforation T84.390
      protrusion T84.390
      specified type NEC T84.89
      stenosis T84.85
      thrombosis T84.86
    brain T85.9
      embolism T85.810
      fibrosis T85.820
      hemorrhage T85.830
      infection and inflammation T85.731
      mechanical
        breakdown T85.110
        displacement T85.120
        leakage T85.190
        malposition T85.120
        obstruction T85.190
        perforation T85.190
        protrusion T85.190
        specified NEC T85.190
      pain T85.840
      specified type NEC T85.890
      stenosis T85.850
      thrombosis T85.860
    cardiac (defibrillator) (pacemaker) —*see*
      Complications, cardiovascular device
      or implant, electronic
    generator (brain) (gastric) (peripheral)
      (sacral) (spinal)
      breakdown T85.113
      displacement T85.123
      leakage T85.193

Complication *(Continued)*
  electronic stimulator device *(Continued)*
    generator *(Continued)*
      malposition T85.123
      obstruction T85.193
      perforation T85.193
      protrusion T85.193
      specified type NEC T85.193
    muscle T84.9
      breakdown T84.418
      displacement T84.428
      embolism T84.81
      fibrosis T84.82
      hemorrhage T84.83
      infection or inflammation T84.7
      mechanical NEC T84.498
      pain T84.84
      specified type NEC T84.89
      stenosis T84.85
      thrombosis T84.86
    nervous system T85.9
      brain —*see* Complications, electronic
        stimulator device, brain
      cranial nerve —*see* Complications,
        electronic stimulator device,
        peripheral nerve
      embolism T85.810
      fibrosis T85.820
      gastric nerve —*see* Complications,
        electronic stimulator device,
        peripheral nerve
      hemorrhage T85.830
      infection and inflammation T85.738
      mechanical
        breakdown T85.118
        displacement T85.128
        leakage T85.199
        malposition T85.128
        obstruction T85.199
        perforation T85.199
        protrusion T85.199
        specified NEC T85.199
      pain T85.840
      peripheral nerve —*see* Complications,
        electronic stimulator device,
        peripheral nerve
      sacral nerve —*see* Complications, electronic
        stimulator device, peripheral nerve
      specified type NEC T85.890
      spinal cord —*see* Complications, electronic
        stimulator device, spinal cord
      stenosis T85.850
      thrombosis T85.860
      vagal nerve —*see* Complications, electronic
        stimulator device, peripheral nerve
    peripheral nerve T85.9
      embolism T85.810
      fibrosis T85.820
      hemorrhage T85.830
      infection and inflammation T85.732
      mechanical
        breakdown T85.111
        displacement T85.121
        leakage T85.191
        malposition T85.121
        obstruction T85.191
        perforation T85.191
        protrusion T85.191
        specified NEC T85.191
      pain T85.840
      specified type NEC T85.890
      stenosis T85.850
      thrombosis T85.860
    spinal cord T85.9
      embolism T85.810
      fibrosis T85.820
      hemorrhage T85.830
      infection and inflammation T85.733
      mechanical
        breakdown T85.112
        displacement T85.122

Complication *(Continued)*
  electronic stimulator device *(Continued)*
    spinal cord *(Continued)*
      mechanical *(Continued)*
        leakage T85.192
        malposition T85.122
        obstruction T85.192
        perforation T85.192
        protrusion T85.192
        specified NEC T85.192
      pain T85.840
      specified type NEC T85.890
      stenosis T85.850
      thrombosis T85.860
    urinary T83.9
      embolism T83.81
      fibrosis T83.82
      hemorrhage T83.83
      infection and inflammation T83.598
      mechanical
        breakdown T83.110
        displacement T83.120
        malposition T83.120
        perforation T83.190
        protrusion T83.190
        specified NEC T83.190
      pain T83.84
      specified type NEC T83.89
      stenosis T83.85
      thrombosis T83.86
  electroshock therapy T88.9
    specified NEC T88.8
  endocrine E34.9
    postprocedural
      adrenal hypofunction E89.6
      hypoinsulinemia E89.1
      hypoparathyroidism E89.2
      hypopituitarism E89.3
      hypothyroidism E89.0
      ovarian failure E89.40
        asymptomatic E89.40
        symptomatic E89.41
      specified NEC E89.89
      testicular hypofunction E89.5
  endodontic treatment NEC M27.59
  enterostomy (stoma) K94.10
    hemorrhage K94.11
    infection K94.12
    malfunction K94.13
    mechanical K94.13
    specified complication NEC K94.19
  episiotomy, disruption O90.1
  esophageal anti-reflux device T85.9
    embolism T85.818
    fibrosis T85.828
    hemorrhage T85.838
    infection and inflammation T85.79
    mechanical
      breakdown T85.511
      displacement T85.521
      malfunction T85.511
      malposition T85.521
      obstruction T85.591
      perforation T85.591
      protrusion T85.591
      specified NEC T85.591
    pain T85.848
    specified type NEC T85.898
    stenosis T85.858
    thrombosis T85.868
  esophagostomy K94.30
    hemorrhage K94.31
    infection K94.32
    malfunction K94.33
    mechanical K94.33
    specified complication NEC K94.39
  extracorporeal circulation T80.90
  extremity artery (bypass) graft T82.9
    arteriosclerosis —*see* Arteriosclerosis,
      extremities, bypass graft
    embolism T82.818
    fibrosis T82.828

Complication *(Continued)*
  extremity artery (bypass) graft *(Continued)*
    hemorrhage T82.838
    infection and inflammation T82.7
    mechanical
      breakdown T82.318
        femoral artery T82.312
      displacement T82.328
        femoral artery T82.322
      leakage T82.338
        femoral artery T82.332
      malposition T82.328
        femoral artery T82.322
      obstruction T82.398
        femoral artery T82.392
      perforation T82.398
        femoral artery T82.392
      protrusion T82.398
        femoral artery T82.392
    pain T82.848
    specified type NEC T82.898
    stenosis T82.858
    thrombosis T82.868
  eye H57.9
    corneal graft —*see* Complications, graft,
      cornea
    implant (prosthetic) T85.9
      embolism T85.818
      fibrosis T85.828
      hemorrhage T85.838
      infection and inflammation T85.79
      mechanical
        breakdown T85.318
        displacement T85.328
        leakage T85.398
        malposition T85.328
        obstruction T85.398
        perforation T85.398
        protrusion T85.398
        specified NEC T85.398
      pain T85.848
      specified type NEC T85.898
      stenosis T85.858
      thrombosis T85.868
    intraocular lens —*see* Complications,
      intraocular lens
    orbital prosthesis —*see* Complications,
      orbital prosthesis
  female genital N94.9
    device, implant or graft NEC —*see*
      Complications, genitourinary, device
      or implant, genital tract
  femoral artery (bypass) graft —*see*
    Complication, extremity artery (bypass)
    graft
  fixation device, internal (orthopedic) T84.9
    infection and inflammation T84.60
      arm T84.61-●
        humerus T84.61-●
        radius T84.61-●
        ulna T84.61-●
      leg T84.629
        femur T84.62-●
        fibula T84.62-●
        tibia T84.62-●
      specified site NEC T84.69
      spine T84.63
    mechanical
      breakdown
        limb T84.119
          carpal T84.210
          femur T84.11-●
          fibula T84.11-●
          humerus T84.11-●
          metacarpal T84.210
          metatarsal T84.213
          phalanx
            foot T84.213
            hand T84.210
          radius T84.11-●
          tarsal T84.213

Complication *(Continued)*
  fixation device, internal *(Continued)*
    mechanical *(Continued)*
      breakdown *(Continued)*
        limb *(Continued)*
          tibia T84.11-●
          ulna T84.11-●
        specified bone NEC T84.218
        spine T84.216
      displacement
        limb T84.129
          carpal T84.220
          femur T84.12-●
          fibula T84.12-●
          humerus T84.12-●
          metacarpal T84.220
          metatarsal T84.223
          phalanx
            foot T84.223
            hand T84.220
          radius T84.12-●
          tarsal T84.223
          tibia T84.12-●
          ulna T84.12-●
        specified bone NEC T84.228
        spine T84.226
      malposition —*see* Complications,
        fixation device, internal,
        mechanical, displacement
      obstruction —*see* Complications, fixation
        device, internal, mechanical,
        specified type NEC
      perforation —*see* Complications, fixation
        device, internal, mechanical,
        specified type NEC
      protrusion —*see* Complications, fixation
        device, internal, mechanical,
        specified type NEC
      specified type NEC
        limb T84.199
          carpal T84.290
          femur T84.19-●
          fibula T84.19-●
          humerus T84.19-●
          metacarpal T84.290
          metatarsal T84.293
          phalanx
            foot T84.293
            hand T84.290
          radius T84.19-●
          tarsal T84.293
          tibia T84.19-●
          ulna T84.19-●
        specified bone NEC T84.298
        vertebra T84.296
    specified type NEC T84.89
      embolism T84.81
      fibrosis T84.82
      hemorrhage T84.83
      pain T84.84
      specified complication NEC T84.89
      stenosis T84.85
      thrombosis T84.86
  following
    acute myocardial infarction NEC I23.8
    aneurysm (false) (of cardiac wall)
      (of heart wall) (ruptured) I23.3
    angina I23.7
    atrial
      septal defect I23.1
      thrombosis I23.6
    cardiac wall rupture I23.3
    chordae tendinae rupture I23.4
    defect
      septal
        atrial (heart) I23.1
        ventricular (heart) I23.2
    hemopericardium I23.0
    papillary muscle rupture I23.5
    rupture
      cardiac wall I23.3
        with hemopericardium I23.0

Complication *(Continued)*
  following *(Continued)*
    acute myocardial infarction NEC
      (Continued)
      rupture *(Continued)*
        chordae tendineae I23.4
        papillary muscle I23.5
      specified NEC I23.8
      thrombosis
        atrium I23.6
        auricular appendage I23.6
        ventricle (heart) I23.6
      ventricular
        septal defect I23.2
        thrombosis I23.6
    ectopic or molar pregnancy O08.9
      cardiac arrest O08.81
      sepsis O08.82
      specified type NEC O08.89
      urinary tract infection O08.83
    termination of pregnancy —*see* Abortion
  gastrointestinal K92.9
    bile duct prosthesis —*see* Complications,
      bile duct implant
    esophageal anti-reflux device —*see*
      Complications, esophageal
      anti-reflux device
    postoperative
      colostomy —*see* Complications, colostomy
      dumping syndrome K91.1
      enterostomy —*see* Complications,
        enterostomy
      gastrostomy —*see* Complications,
        gastrostomy
      malabsorption NEC K91.2
      obstruction —*see also* Obstruction,
        intestine, postoperative K91.30
      postcholecystectomy syndrome K91.5
      specified NEC K91.89
      vomiting after GI surgery K91.0
    prosthetic device or implant
      bile duct prosthesis —*see* Complications,
        bile duct implant
      esophageal anti-reflux device —*see*
        Complications, esophageal
        anti-reflux device
      specified type NEC
        embolism T85.818
        fibrosis T85.828
        hemorrhage T85.838
        mechanical
          breakdown T85.518
          displacement T85.528
          malfunction T85.518
          malposition T85.528
          obstruction T85.598
          perforation T85.598
          protrusion T85.598
          specified NEC T85.598
        pain T85.848
        specified complication NEC T85.898
        stenosis T85.858
        thrombosis T85.868
  gastrostomy (stoma) K94.20
    hemorrhage K94.21
    infection K94.22
    malfunction K94.23
    mechanical K94.23
    specified complication NEC K94.29
  genitourinary
    device or implant T83.9
      genital tract T83.9
        infection or inflammation T83.69
        intrauterine contraceptive device —*see*
          Complications, intrauterine,
          contraceptive device
        mechanical —*see* Complications, by
          device, mechanical
        mesh —*see* Complications, prosthetic
          device or implant, mesh
        penile prosthesis —*see* Complications,
          prosthetic device, penile

▶ New   ⇨ Revised   ~~deleted~~ Deleted   ● Use Additional Character(s)

Complication *(Continued)*
  genitourinary *(Continued)*
    device or implant *(Continued)*
      genital tract *(Continued)*
        specified type NEC T83.89
          embolism T83.81
          fibrosis T83.82
          hemorrhage T83.83
          pain T83.84
          specified complication NEC T83.89
          stenosis T83.85
          thrombosis T83.86
        vaginal mesh —*see* Complications, prosthetic device or implant, mesh
    urinary system T83.9
      cystostomy catheter —*see* Complication, catheter, cystostomy
      electronic stimulator —*see* Complications, electronic stimulator device, urinary
      indwelling urethral catheter —*see* Complications, catheter, urethral, indwelling
      infection or inflammation T83.598
        indwelling urethral catheter T83.511
      kidney transplant —*see* Complication, transplant, kidney
      organ graft —*see* Complication, graft, urinary organ
      specified type NEC T83.89
        embolism T83.81
        fibrosis T83.82
        hemorrhage T83.83
        mechanical T83.198
          breakdown T83.118
          displacement T83.128
          malfunction T83.118
          malposition T83.128
          obstruction T83.198
          perforation T83.198
          protrusion T83.198
          specified NEC T83.198
      sphincter, implanted T83.191
      stent (ileal conduit) (nephroureteral) T83.193
        ureteral indwelling T83.192
      pain T83.84
      specified complication NEC T83.89
      stenosis T83.85
      thrombosis T83.86
      sphincter implant —*see* Complications, implant, urinary sphincter
  postprocedural
    pelvic peritoneal adhesions N99.4
    renal failure N99.0
    specified NEC N99.89
    stoma —*see* Complications, stoma, urinary tract
    urethral stricture —*see* Stricture, urethra, postprocedural
    vaginal
      adhesions N99.2
      vault prolapse N99.3
  graft (bypass) (patch) —*see also* Complications, prosthetic device or implant
    aorta —*see* Complications, graft, vascular
    arterial —*see* Complication, graft, vascular
    bone T86.839
      failure T86.831
      infection T86.832
      mechanical T84.318
        breakdown T84.318
        displacement T84.328
        protrusion T84.398
        specified type NEC T84.398
      rejection T86.830
      specified type NEC T86.838
    carotid artery —*see* Complications, graft, vascular

Complication *(Continued)*
  graft *(Continued)*
    cornea T86.849-
      failure T86.841-
      infection T86.842-
      mechanical T85.398
        breakdown T85.318
        displacement T85.328
        protrusion T85.398
        specified type NEC T85.398
      rejection T86.840-
      retroprosthetic membrane T85.398
      specified type NEC T86.848-
    femoral artery (bypass) —*see* Complication, extremity artery (bypass) graft
    genital organ or tract —*see* Complications, genitourinary, device or implant, genital tract
    muscle T84.9
      breakdown T84.410
      displacement T84.420
      embolism T84.81
      fibrosis T84.82
      hemorrhage T84.83
      infection and inflammation T84.7
      mechanical NEC T84.490
      pain T84.84
      specified type NEC T84.89
      stenosis T84.85
      thrombosis T84.86
    nerve —*see* Complication, prosthetic device or implant, specified NEC
    skin —*see* Complications, prosthetic device or implant, skin graft
    tendon T84.9
      breakdown T84.410
      displacement T84.420
      embolism T84.81
      fibrosis T84.82
      hemorrhage T84.83
      infection and inflammation T84.7
      mechanical NEC T84.490
      pain T84.84
      specified type NEC T84.89
      stenosis T84.85
      thrombosis T84.86
    urinary organ T83.9
      embolism T83.81
      fibrosis T83.82
      hemorrhage T83.83
      infection and inflammation T83.598
        indwelling urethral catheter T83.511
      mechanical
        breakdown T83.21
        displacement T83.22
        erosion T83.24
        exposure T83.25
        leakage T83.23
        malposition T83.22
        obstruction T83.29
        perforation T83.29
        protrusion T83.29
        specified NEC T83.29
      pain T83.84
      specified type NEC T83.89
      stenosis T83.85
      thrombosis T83.86
    vascular T82.9
      embolism T82.818
      femoral artery —*see* Complication, extremity artery (bypass) graft
      fibrosis T82.828
      hemorrhage T82.838
      mechanical
        breakdown T82.319
          aorta (bifurcation) T82.310
          carotid artery T82.311
          specified vessel NEC T82.318
        displacement T82.329
          aorta (bifurcation) T82.320
          carotid artery T82.321
          specified vessel NEC T82.328

Complication *(Continued)*
  graft *(Continued)*
    vascular *(Continued)*
      mechanical *(Continued)*
        leakage T82.339
          aorta (bifurcation) T82.330
          carotid artery T82.331
          specified vessel NEC T82.338
        malposition T82.329
          aorta (bifurcation) T82.320
          carotid artery T82.321
          specified vessel NEC T82.328
        obstruction T82.399
          aorta (bifurcation) T82.390
          carotid artery T82.391
          specified vessel NEC T82.398
        perforation T82.399
          aorta (bifurcation) T82.390
          carotid artery T82.391
          specified vessel NEC T82.398
        protrusion T82.399
          aorta (bifurcation) T82.390
          carotid artery T82.391
          specified vessel NEC T82.398
      pain T82.848
      specified complication NEC T82.898
      stenosis T82.858
      thrombosis T82.868
  heart I51.9
    assist device
      infection and inflammation T82.7
    following acute myocardial infarction — *see* Complications, following, acute myocardial infarction
    postoperative —*see* Complications, circulatory system
    transplant —*see* Complication, transplant, heart
    and lung(s) —*see* Complications, transplant, heart, with lung
    valve
      graft (biological) T82.9
        embolism T82.817
        fibrosis T82.827
        hemorrhage T82.837
        infection and inflammation T82.7
        mechanical T82.228
          breakdown T82.221
          displacement T82.222
          leakage T82.223
          malposition T82.222
          obstruction T82.228
          perforation T82.228
          protrusion T82.228
        pain T82.847
        specified type NEC T82.897
        stenosis T82.857
        thrombosis T82.867
      prosthesis T82.9
        embolism T82.817
        fibrosis T82.827
        hemorrhage T82.837
        infection or inflammation T82.6
        mechanical T82.09
          breakdown T82.01
          displacement T82.02
          leakage T82.03
          malposition T82.02
          obstruction T82.09
          perforation T82.09
          protrusion T82.09
        pain T82.847
        specified type NEC T82.897
          mechanical T82.09
        stenosis T82.857
        thrombosis T82.867
  hematoma
    intraoperative —*see* Complication, intraoperative, hemorrhage
    postprocedural —*see* Complication, postprocedural, hematoma
  hemodialysis —*see* Complications, dialysis

Complication (*Continued*)
- hemorrhage
  - intraoperative —*see* Complication, intraoperative, hemorrhage
  - postprocedural —*see* Complication, postprocedural, hemorrhage
- IEC (immune effector cellular) therapy T80.82
- ileostomy (stoma) —*see* Complications, enterostomy
- immune effector cellular (IEC) therapy T80.82
- immunization (procedure) —*see* Complications, vaccination
- implant —*see also* Complications, by site and type
  - urinary sphincter T83.9
    - embolism T83.81
    - fibrosis T83.82
    - hemorrhage T83.83
    - infection and inflammation T83.591
    - mechanical
      - breakdown T83.111
      - displacement T83.121
      - leakage T83.191
      - malposition T83.121
      - obstruction T83.191
      - perforation T83.191
      - protrusion T83.191
      - specified NEC T83.191
    - pain T83.84
    - specified type NEC T83.89
    - stenosis T83.85
    - thrombosis T83.86
- infusion (procedure) T80.90
  - air embolism T80.0
  - blood —*see* Complications, transfusion
  - catheter —*see* Complications, catheter
  - infection T80.29
  - pump —*see* Complications, cardiovascular, device or implant
  - sepsis T80.29
  - serum reaction —*see also* Reaction, serum T80.69
    - anaphylactic shock —*see also* Shock, anaphylactic T80.59
  - specified type NEC T80.89
- inhalation therapy NEC T81.81
- injection (procedure) T80.90
  - drug reaction —*see* Reaction, drug
  - infection T80.29
  - sepsis T80.29
  - serum (prophylactic) (therapeutic) —*see* Complications, vaccination
  - specified type NEC T80.89
  - vaccine (any) —*see* Complications, vaccination
- inoculation (any) —*see* Complications, vaccination
- insulin pump
  - infection and inflammation T85.72
  - mechanical
    - breakdown T85.614
    - displacement T85.624
    - leakage T85.633
    - malposition T85.624
    - obstruction T85.694
    - perforation T85.694
    - protrusion T85.694
    - specified NEC T85.694
- intestinal pouch NEC K91.858
- intraocular lens (prosthetic) T85.9
  - embolism T85.818
  - fibrosis T85.828
  - hemorrhage T85.838
  - infection and inflammation T85.79
  - mechanical
    - breakdown T85.21
    - displacement T85.22
    - malposition T85.22
    - obstruction T85.29
    - perforation T85.29
    - protrusion T85.29
    - specified NEC T85.29

Complication (*Continued*)
- intraocular lens (*Continued*)
  - pain T85.848
  - specified type NEC T85.898
  - stenosis T85.858
  - thrombosis T85.868
- intraoperative (intraprocedural)
  - cardiac arrest —*see also* Infarct, myocardium, associated with revascularization procedure
    - during cardiac surgery I97.710
    - during other surgery I97.711
  - cardiac functional disturbance NEC —*see also* Infarct, myocardium, associated with revascularization procedure
    - during cardiac surgery I97.790
    - during other surgery I97.791
  - hemorrhage (hematoma) (of)
    - circulatory system organ or structure
      - during cardiac bypass I97.411
      - during cardiac catheterization I97.410
      - during other circulatory system procedure I97.418
      - during other procedure I97.42
    - digestive system organ
      - during procedure on digestive system K91.61
      - during procedure on other organ K91.62
    - ear
      - during procedure on ear and mastoid process H95.21
      - during procedure on other organ H95.22
    - endocrine system organ or structure
      - during procedure on endocrine system organ or structure E36.01
      - during procedure on other organ E36.02
    - eye and adnexa
      - during ophthalmic procedure H59.11-●
      - during other procedure H59.12-●
    - genitourinary organ or structure
      - during procedure on genitourinary organ or structure N99.61
      - during procedure on other organ N99.62
    - mastoid process
      - during procedure on ear and mastoid process H95.21
      - during procedure on other organ H95.22
    - musculoskeletal structure
      - during musculoskeletal surgery M96.810
      - during non-orthopedic surgery M96.811
      - during orthopedic surgery M96.810
    - nervous system
      - during a nervous system procedure G97.31
      - during other procedure G97.32
    - respiratory system
      - during other procedure J95.62
      - during procedure on respiratory system organ or structure J95.61
    - skin and subcutaneous tissue
      - during a dermatologic procedure L76.01
      - during a procedure on other organ L76.02
    - spleen
      - during a procedure on other organ D78.02
      - during a procedure on the spleen D78.01
  - puncture or laceration (accidental) (unintentional) (of)
    - brain
      - during a nervous system procedure G97.48
      - during other procedure G97.49

Complication (*Continued*)
- intraoperative (*Continued*)
  - puncture or laceration (*Continued*)
    - circulatory system organ or structure
      - during circulatory system procedure I97.51
      - during other procedure I97.52
    - digestive system
      - during procedure on digestive system K91.71
      - during procedure on other organ K91.72
    - ear
      - during procedure on ear and mastoid process H95.31
      - during procedure on other organ H95.32
    - endocrine system organ or structure
      - during procedure on endocrine system organ or structure E36.11
      - during procedure on other organ E36.12
    - eye and adnexa
      - during ophthalmic procedure H59.21-●
      - during other procedure H59.22-●
    - genitourinary organ or structure
      - during procedure on genitourinary organ or structure N99.71
      - during procedure on other organ N99.72
    - mastoid process
      - during procedure on ear and mastoid process H95.31
      - during procedure on other organ H95.32
    - musculoskeletal structure
      - during musculoskeletal surgery M96.820
      - during non-orthopedic surgery M96.821
      - during orthopedic surgery M96.820
    - nervous system
      - during a nervous system procedure G97.48
      - during other procedure G97.49
    - respiratory system
      - during other procedure J95.72
      - during procedure on respiratory system organ or structure J95.71
    - skin and subcutaneous tissue
      - during a dermatologic procedure L76.11
      - during a procedure on other organ L76.12
    - spleen
      - during a procedure on other organ D78.12
      - during a procedure on the spleen D78.11
  - specified NEC
    - circulatory system I97.88
    - digestive system K91.81
    - ear H95.88
    - endocrine system E36.8
    - eye and adnexa H59.88
    - genitourinary system N99.81
    - mastoid process H95.88
    - musculoskeletal structure M96.89
    - nervous system G97.81
    - respiratory system J95.88
    - skin and subcutaneous tissue L76.81
    - spleen D78.81
- intraperitoneal catheter (dialysis) (infusion) —*see* Complication(s), catheter, intraperitoneal dialysis
- intrathecal infusion pump
  - infection and inflammation T85.738
  - mechanical
    - breakdown T85.615
    - displacement T85.625
    - leakage T85.635
    - malfunction T85.695
    - malposition T85.625
    - obstruction T85.695

▶ New   ⇒ Revised   ~~deleted~~ Deleted   ● Use Additional Character(s)

Complication *(Continued)*
  intrathecal infusion pump *(Continued)*
    mechanical *(Continued)*
      perforation T85.695
      protrusion T85.695
      specified NEC T85.695
  intrauterine
    contraceptive device
      embolism T83.81
      fibrosis T83.82
      hemorrhage T83.83
      infection and inflammation T83.69
      mechanical
        breakdown T83.31
        displacement T83.32
        malposition T83.32
        obstruction T83.39
        perforation T83.39
        protrusion T83.39
        specified NEC T83.39
      pain T83.84
      specified type NEC T83.89
      stenosis T83.85
      thrombosis T83.86
    procedure (fetal), to newborn P96.5
  jejunostomy (stoma) —*see* Complications,
    enterostomy
  joint prosthesis, internal T84.9
    breakage (fracture) T84.01-●
    dislocation T84.02-●
    fracture T84.01-●
    infection or inflammation T84.50
      hip T84.5-●
      knee T84.5-●
      specified joint NEC T84.59
    instability T84.02-●
    malposition —*see* Complications, joint
      prosthesis, mechanical, displacement
    mechanical
      breakage, broken T84.01-●
      dislocation T84.02-●
      fracture T84.01-●
      instability T84.02-●
      leakage —*see* Complications, joint
        prosthesis, mechanical, specified
        NEC
      loosening T84.039
        hip T84.03-●
        knee T84.03-●
        specified joint NEC T84.038
      obstruction —*see* Complications, joint
        prosthesis, mechanical, specified
        NEC
      perforation —*see* Complications, joint
        prosthesis, mechanical, specified
        NEC
      osteolysis T84.059
        hip T84.05-●
        knee T84.05-●
        other specified joint T84.058
      ~~periprosthetic osteolysis T84.059~~
    ▶ periprosthetic osteolysis, by site T84.05-●
      protrusion —*see* Complications, joint
        prosthesis, mechanical, specified
        NEC
      specified complication NEC T84.099
        hip T84.09-●
        knee T84.09-●
        other specified joint T84.098
      subluxation T84.02-●
      wear of articular bearing surface T84.069
        hip T84.06-●
        knee T84.06-●
        other specified joint T84.068
    specified joint NEC T84.89
      embolism T84.81
      fibrosis T84.82
      hemorrhage T84.83
      pain T84.84
      specified complication NEC T84.89
      stenosis T84.85
      thrombosis T84.86
    subluxation T84.02-●

Complication *(Continued)*
  kidney transplant —*see* Complications,
    transplant, kidney
  labor O75.9
    specified NEC O75.89
  liver transplant (immune or nonimmune) —
    see Complications, transplant,
    liver
  lumbar puncture G97.1
    cerebrospinal fluid leak G97.0
    headache or reaction G97.1
  lung transplant —*see* Complications,
    transplant, lung
    and heart —*see* Complications, transplant,
      lung, with heart
  male genital N50.9
    device, implant or graft —*see*
      Complications, genitourinary,
      device or implant, genital tract
    postprocedural or postoperative —*see*
      Complications, genitourinary,
      postprocedural
      specified NEC N99.89
  mastoid (process) procedure
    intraoperative H95.88-●
      hematoma —*see* Complications,
        intraoperative, hemorrhage
        (hematoma) (of), mastoid process
      hemorrhage —*see* Complications,
        intraoperative, hemorrhage
        (hematoma) (of), mastoid process
      laceration —*see* Complications,
        intraoperative, puncture or
        laceration..., mastoid process
      specified NEC H95.88-●
    postmastoidectomy —*see* Complications,
      postmastoidectomy
    postoperative H95.89-●
      external ear canal stenosis H95.81-●
      hematoma —*see* Complications...,
        postprocedural, hematoma (of),
        mastoid process
      hemorrhage —*see* Complications...,
        postprocedural, hemorrhage (of),
        mastoid process
      postmastoidectomy —*see* Complications,
        postmastoidectomy
      seroma —*see* Complications,
        postprocedural, seroma (of),
        mastoid process
      specified NEC H95.89-●
  mastoidectomy cavity —*see* Complications,
    postmastoidectomy
  mechanical —*see* Complications, by site and
    type, mechanical
  medical procedures *(see also* Complication(s),
    intraoperative) T88.9
  metabolic E88.9
    postoperative E89.89
    specified NEC E89.89
  molar pregnancy NOS O08.9
    damage to pelvic organs O08.6
    embolism O08.2
    genital infection O08.0
    hemorrhage (delayed) (excessive) O08.1
    metabolic disorder O08.5
    renal failure O08.4
    shock O08.3
    specified type NEC O08.0
    venous complication NEC O08.7
  musculoskeletal system —*see also*
    Complication, intraoperative
    (intraprocedural), by site
    device, implant or graft NEC —*see*
      Complications, orthopedic, device or
      implant
    internal fixation (nail) (plate) (rod) —*see*
      Complications, fixation device,
      internal
    joint prosthesis —*see* Complications, joint
      prosthesis

Complication *(Continued)*
  musculoskeletal system *(Continued)*
    postoperative (postprocedural) M96.89
      with osteoporosis —*see* Osteoporosis
      fracture following insertion of device —
        see Fracture, following insertion of
        orthopedic implant, joint prosthesis
        or bone plate
      joint instability after prosthesis removal
        M96.89
      lordosis M96.4
      postlaminectomy syndrome NEC M96.1
        kyphosis M96.2
      pseudarthrosis M96.0
      specified complication NEC M96.89
    post radiation M96.89
      kyphosis M96.3
      scoliosis M96.5
      specified complication NEC M96.89
  nephrostomy (stoma) —*see* Complications,
    stoma, urinary tract, external NEC
  nervous system G98.8
    central G96.9
    device, implant or graft —*see also*
      Complication, prosthetic device or
      implant, specified NEC
      electronic stimulator (electrode(s)) —*see*
        Complications, electronic stimulator
        device
      specified NEC
        infection and inflammation T85.738
        mechanical T85.695
          breakdown T85.615
          displacement T85.625
          leakage T85.635
          malfunction T85.695
          malposition T85.625
          obstruction T85.695
          perforation T85.695
          protrusion T85.695
          specified NEC T85.695
      ventricular shunt —*see* Complications,
        ventricular shunt
    electronic stimulator (electrode(s)) —*see*
      Complications, electronic stimulator
      device
    postprocedural G97.82
      intracranial hypotension G97.2
      specified NEC G97.82
      spinal fluid leak G97.0
  newborn, due to intrauterine (fetal)
    procedure P96.5
  nonabsorbable (permanent) sutures —*see*
    Complication, sutures, permanent
  obstetric O75.9
    procedure (instrumental) (manual)
      (surgical) specified NEC O75.4
    specified NEC O75.89
    surgical wound NEC O90.89
      hematoma O90.2
      infection O86.00
  ocular lens implant —*see* Complications,
    intraocular lens
  ophthalmologic
    postprocedural bleb —*see* Blebitis
  orbital prosthesis T85.9
    embolism T85.818
    fibrosis T85.828
    hemorrhage T85.838
    infection and inflammation T85.79
    mechanical
      breakdown T85.31-●
      displacement T85.32-●
      malposition T85.32-●
      obstruction T85.39-●
      perforation T85.39-●
      protrusion T85.39-●
      specified NEC T85.39-●
    pain T85.848
    specified type NEC T85.898
    stenosis T85.858
    thrombosis T85.868

Complication (Continued)

organ or tissue transplant (partial) (total) —
see Complications, transplant
orthopedic —see also Disorder, soft tissue
  device or implant T84.9
    bone
      device or implant —see Complication,
        bone, device NEC
      graft —see Complication, graft, bone
    breakdown T84.418
    displacement T84.428
    electronic bone stimulator —see
      Complications, electronic stimulator
      device, bone
    embolism T84.81
    fibrosis T84.82
    fixation device —see Complication,
      fixation device, internal
    hemorrhage T84.83
    infection or inflammation T84.7
    joint prosthesis —see Complication, joint
      prosthesis, internal
    malfunction T84.418
    malposition T84.428
    mechanical NEC T84.498
    muscle graft —see Complications, graft,
      muscle
    obstruction T84.498
    pain T84.84
    perforation T84.498
    protrusion T84.498
    specified complication NEC T84.89
    stenosis T84.85
    tendon graft —see Complications, graft,
      tendon
    thrombosis T84.86
  fracture (following insertion of device) —
    see Fracture, following insertion of
    orthopedic implant, joint prosthesis or
    bone plate
  postprocedural M96.89
    fracture —see Fracture, following
      insertion of orthopedic implant,
      joint prosthesis or bone plate
    postlaminectomy syndrome NEC M96.1
      kyphosis M96.3
      lordosis M96.4
    postradiation
      kyphosis M96.2
      scoliosis M96.5
    pseudarthrosis post-fusion M96.0
    specified type NEC M96.89
pacemaker (cardiac) —see Complications,
  cardiovascular device or implant,
  electronic
pancreas transplant —see Complications,
  transplant, pancreas
penile prosthesis (implant) —see
  Complications, prosthetic device, penile
perfusion NEC T80.90
perineal repair (obstetrical) NEC O90.89
  disruption O90.1
  hematoma O90.2
  infection (following delivery) O86.09
phototherapy T88.9
  specified NEC T88.8
postmastoidectomy NEC H95.19-●
  cyst, mucosal H95.13-●
  granulation H95.12-●
  inflammation, chronic H95.11-●
  recurrent cholesteatoma H95.0-●
postoperative —see Complications,
  postprocedural
  circulatory —see Complications, circulatory
    system
  ear —see Complications, ear
  endocrine —see Complications,
    endocrine
  eye —see Complications, eye
  lumbar puncture G97.1
    cerebrospinal fluid leak G97.0

Complication (Continued)

postoperative (Continued)
  nervous system (central) (peripheral) —see
    Complications, nervous system
  respiratory system —see Complications,
    respiratory system
postprocedural —see also Complications,
  surgical procedure
  cardiac arrest —see also Infarct,
    myocardium, associated with
    revascularization procedure
    following cardiac surgery I97.120
    following other surgery I97.121
  cardiac functional disturbance NEC —see
    also Infarct, myocardium, associated
    with revascularization procedure
    following cardiac surgery I97.190
    following other surgery I97.191
  cardiac insufficiency
    following cardiac surgery I97.110
    following other surgery I97.111
  chorioretinal scars following retinal
    surgery H59.81-●
  following cataract surgery
    cataract (lens) fragments H59.02-●
    cystoid macular edema H59.03-●
    specified NEC H59.09-●
    vitreous (touch) syndrome H59.01-●
  heart failure
    following cardiac surgery I97.130
    following other surgery I97.131
  hematoma (of)
    circulatory system organ or structure
      following cardiac bypass I97.631
      following cardiac catheterization
        I97.630
      following other circulatory system
        procedure I97.638
      following other procedure I97.621
    digestive system
      following procedure on digestive
        system K91.870
      following procedure on other organ
        K91.871
    ear
      following other procedure H95.52
      following procedure on ear and
        mastoid process H95.51
    endocrine system
      following endocrine system procedure
        E89.820
      following other procedure E89.821
    eye and adnexa
      following ophthalmic procedure
        H59.33-●
      following other procedure H59.34-●
    genitourinary organ or structure
      following procedure on genitourinary
        organ or structure N99.840
      following procedure on other organ
        N99.841
    mastoid process
      following other procedure H95.52
      following procedure on ear and
        mastoid process H95.51
    musculoskeletal structure
      following musculoskeletal surgery
        M96.840
      following non-orthopedic surgery
        M96.841
      following orthopedic surgery M96.840
    nervous system
      following nervous system procedure
        G97.61
      following other procedure G97.62
    respiratory system
      following other procedure J95.861
      following procedure on respiratory
        system organ or structure J95.860
    skin and subcutaneous tissue
      following dermatologic procedure
        L76.31

Complication (Continued)

postprocedural (Continued)
  hematoma (Continued)
    skin and subcutaneous tissue (Continued)
      following procedure on other organ
        L76.32
    spleen
      following procedure on other organ
        D78.32
      following procedure on the spleen
        D78.31
  hemorrhage (of)
    circulatory system organ or structure
      following cardiac bypass I97.611
      following cardiac catheterization
        I97.610
      following other circulatory system
        procedure I97.618
      following other procedure I97.620
    digestive system
      following procedure on digestive
        system K91.840
      following procedure on other organ
        K91.841
    ear
      following other procedure H95.42
      following procedure on ear and
        mastoid process H95.41
    endocrine system
      following endocrine system procedure
        E89.810
      following other procedure E89.811
    eye and adnexa
      following ophthalmic procedure
        H59.31-●
      following other procedure H59.32-●
    genitourinary organ or structure
      following procedure on genitourinary
        organ or structure N99.820
      following procedure on other organ
        N99.821
    mastoid process
      following other procedure H95.42
      following procedure on ear and
        mastoid process H95.41
    musculoskeletal structure
      following musculoskeletal surgery
        M96.830
      following non-orthopedic surgery
        M96.831
      following orthopedic surgery M96.830
    nervous system
      following nervous system procedure
        G97.51
      following other procedure G97.52
    respiratory system
      following other procedure J95.831
      following procedure on respiratory
        system organ or structure J95.830
    skin and subcutaneous tissue
      following dermatologic procedure
        L76.21
      following a procedure on other organ
        L76.22
    spleen
      following procedure on other organ
        D78.22
      following procedure on the spleen
        D78.21
  seroma (of)
    circulatory system organ or structure
      following cardiac bypass I97.641
      following cardiac catheterization
        I97.640
      following other circulatory system
        procedure I97.648
      following other procedure I97.622
    digestive system
      following procedure on digestive
        system K91.872
      following procedure on other organ
        K91.873

▶ New   ⇒ Revised   ~~deleted~~ Deleted   ● Use Additional Character(s)

Complication *(Continued)*
  postprocedural *(Continued)*
    seroma *(Continued)*
      ear
        following other procedure H95.54
        following procedure on ear and
          mastoid process H95.53
      endocrine system
        following endocrine system procedure
          E89.822
        following other procedure E89.823
      eye and adnexa
        following ophthalmic procedure
          H59.35-•
        following other procedure H59.36-•
      genitourinary organ or structure
        following procedure on genitourinary
          organ or structure N99.842
        following procedure on other organ
          N99.843
      mastoid process
        following other procedure H95.54
        following procedure on ear and
          mastoid process H95.53
      musculoskeletal structure
        following musculoskeletal surgery
          M96.842
        following non-orthopedic surgery
          M96.843
        following orthopedic surgery M96.842
      nervous system
        following nervous system procedure
          G97.63
        following other procedure G97.64
      respiratory system
        following other procedure J95.863
        following procedure on respiratory
          system organ or structure J95.862
      skin and subcutaneous tissue
        following dermatologic procedure
          L76.33
        following procedure on other organ
          L76.34
      spleen
        following procedure on other organ
          D78.34
        following procedure on the spleen
          D78.33
    specified NEC
      circulatory system I97.89
      digestive K91.89
      ear H95.89
      endocrine E89.89
      eye and adnexa H59.89
      genitourinary N99.89
      mastoid process H95.89
      metabolic E89.89
      musculoskeletal structure M96.89
      nervous system G97.82
      respiratory system J95.89
      skin and subcutaneous tissue L76.82
      spleen D78.89
  pregnancy NEC —*see* Pregnancy,
    complicated by
  prosthetic device or implant T85.9
    bile duct —*see* Complications, bile duct
      implant
    breast —*see* Complications, breast
      implant
    bulking agent
      ureteral
        erosion T83.714
        exposure T83.724
      urethral
        erosion T83.713
        exposure T83.723
    cardiac and vascular NEC —*see*
      Complications, cardiovascular device
      or implant
    corneal transplant —*see* Complications,
      graft, cornea

Complication *(Continued)*
  prosthetic device or implant *(Continued)*
    electronic nervous system stimulator —*see*
      Complications, electronic stimulator
      device
    epidural infusion catheter —*see*
      Complications, catheter, epidural
    esophageal anti-reflux device —*see*
      Complications, esophageal anti-reflux
      device
    genital organ or tract —*see* Complications,
      genitourinary, device or implant,
      genital tract
      specified NEC T83.79
    heart valve —*see* Complications, heart,
      valve, prosthesis
    infection or inflammation T85.79
    ➠intestine transplant T86.852
    liver transplant T86.43
    lung transplant T86.812
    pancreas transplant T86.892
    skin graft T86.822
    intraocular lens —*see* Complications,
      intraocular lens
    intraperitoneal (dialysis) catheter —
      see Complication(s), catheter,
      intraperitoneal dialysis
    joint —*see* Complications, joint prosthesis,
      internal
    mechanical NEC T85.698
      dialysis catheter (vascular) —*see also*
        Complication, catheter, dialysis,
        mechanical
        peritoneal —*see* Complication(s),
          catheter, intraperitoneal dialysis
      gastrointestinal device T85.598
      ocular device T85.398
      subdural (infusion) catheter T85.690
      suture, permanent T85.692
        that for bone repair —*see*
          Complications, fixation device,
          internal (orthopedic), mechanical
      ventricular shunt
        breakdown T85.01
        displacement T85.02
        leakage T85.03
        malposition T85.02
        obstruction T85.09
        perforation T85.09
        protrusion T85.09
        specified NEC T85.09
    mesh
      erosion (to surrounding organ or tissue)
        T83.718
        urethral (into pelvic floor muscles)
          T83.712
        vaginal (into pelvic floor muscles)
          T83.711
      exposure (into surrounding organ or
        tissue) T83.728
        urethral (through urethral wall)
          T83.722
        vaginal (into vagina) (through vaginal
          wall) T83.721
    orbital —*see* Complications, orbital
      prosthesis
    penile T83.9
      embolism T83.81
      fibrosis T83.82
      hemorrhage T83.83
      infection and inflammation T83.61
      mechanical
        breakdown T83.410
        displacement T83.420
        leakage T83.490
        malposition T83.420
        obstruction T83.490
        perforation T83.490
        protrusion T83.490
        specified NEC T83.490
      pain T83.84

Complication *(Continued)*
  prosthetic device or implant *(Continued)*
    penile *(Continued)*
      specified type NEC T83.89
      stenosis T83.85
      thrombosis T83.86
    prosthetic materials NEC
      erosion (to surrounding organ or tissue)
        T83.718
      exposure (into surrounding organ or
        tissue) T83.728
    skin graft T86.829
      artificial skin or decellularized
        allodermis
        embolism T85.818
        fibrosis T85.828
        hemorrhage T85.838
        infection and inflammation T85.79
        mechanical
          breakdown T85.613
          displacement T85.623
          malfunction T85.613
          malposition T85.623
          obstruction T85.693
          perforation T85.693
          protrusion T85.693
          specified NEC T85.693
        pain T85.848
        specified type NEC T85.898
        stenosis T85.858
        thrombosis T85.868
      failure T86.821
      infection T86.822
      rejection T86.820
      specified NEC T86.828
    sling
      urethral (female) (male)
        erosion T83.712
        exposure T83.722
    specified NEC T85.9
      embolism T85.818
      fibrosis T85.828
      hemorrhage T85.838
      infection and inflammation T85.79
      mechanical
        breakdown T85.618
        displacement T85.628
        leakage T85.638
        malfunction T85.618
        malposition T85.628
        obstruction T85.698
        perforation T85.698
        protrusion T85.698
        specified NEC T85.698
      pain T85.848
      specified type NEC T85.898
      stenosis T85.858
      thrombosis T85.868
    subdural infusion catheter —*see*
      Complications, catheter, subdural
    sutures —*see* Complications, sutures
    urinary organ or tract NEC —*see*
      Complications, genitourinary, device
      or implant, urinary system
    vascular —*see* Complications,
      cardiovascular device or implant
    ventricular shunt —*see* Complications,
      ventricular shunt (device)
  puerperium —*see* Puerperal
  puncture, spinal G97.1
    cerebrospinal fluid leak G97.0
    headache or reaction G97.1
  pyelogram N99.89
  radiation
    kyphosis M96.2
    scoliosis M96.5
  reattached
    extremity (infection) (rejection)
      lower T87.1X-•
      upper T87.0X-•
    specified body part NEC T87.2

Complication *(Continued)*
  reconstructed breast
    asymmetry between native and
      reconstructed breast N65.1
    deformity N65.0
    disproportion between native and
      reconstructed breast N65.1
    excess tissue N65.0
    misshappen N65.0
  reimplant NEC —*see also* Complications,
    prosthetic device or implant
    limb (infection) (rejection) —*see*
      Complications, reattached,
      extremity
    organ (partial) (total) —*see* Complications,
      transplant
    prosthetic device NEC —*see* Complications,
      prosthetic device
  renal N28.9
    allograft —*see* Complications, transplant,
      kidney
    dialysis —*see* Complications, dialysis
  respirator
    mechancial J95.850
      specified NEC J95.859
  respiratory system J98.9
    device, implant or graft —*see*
      Complication, prosthetic device or
      implant, specified NEC
    lung transplant —*see* Complications,
      prosthetic device or implant, lung
      transplant
    postoperative J95.89
      air leak J95.812
      Mendelson's syndrome (chemical
        pneumonitis) J95.4
      pneumothorax J95.811
      pulmonary insufficiency (acute) (after
        nonthoracic surgery) J95.2
        chronic J95.3
        following thoracic surgery J95.1
      respiratory failure (acute) J95.821
        acute and chronic J95.822
      specified NEC J95.89
      subglottic stenosis J95.5
      tracheostomy complication —*see*
        Complications, tracheostomy
    therapy T81.89
  sedation during labor and delivery O74.9
    cardiac O74.2
    central nervous system O74.3
    pulmonary NEC O74.1
  shunt —*see also* Complications, prosthetic
    device or implant
    arteriovenous —*see* Complications,
      arteriovenous, shunt
    ventricular (communicating) —*see*
      Complications, ventricular shunt
  skin
    graft T86.829
      failure T86.821
      infection T86.822
      rejection T86.820
      specified type NEC T86.828
  spinal
    anesthesia —*see* Complications, anesthesia,
      spinal
    catheter (epidural) (subdural) —*see*
      Complications, catheter
    puncture or tap G97.1
      cerebrospinal fluid leak G97.0
      headache or reaction G97.1
  stent
    bile duct —*see* Complications, bile duct
      prosthesis
    ureteral indwelling
      breakdown T83.112
      displacement T83.122
      leakage T83.192
      malposition T83.122

Complication *(Continued)*
  stent *(Continued)*
    ureteral indwelling *(Continued)*
      obstruction T83.192
      perforation T83.192
      protrusion T83.192
      specified NEC T83.192
    urinary (ileal conduit) (nephroureteral)
      T83.193
      embolism T83.81
      fibrosis T83.82
      hemorrhage T83.83
      infection and inflammation T83.593
      mechanical
        breakdown T83.113
        displacement T83.123
        leakage T83.193
        malposition T83.123
        obstruction T83.193
        perforation T83.193
        protrusion T83.193
        specified NEC T83.193
      pain T83.84
      specified type NEC T83.89
      stenosis T83.85
      thrombosis T83.86
    vascular
      end stent stenosis —*see* Restenosis,
        stent
      in stent stenosis —*see* Restenosis, stent
  stoma
    digestive tract
      colostomy —*see* Complications,
        colostomy
      enterostomy —*see* Complications,
        enterostomy
      esophagostomy —*see* Complications,
        esophagostomy
      gastrostomy —*see* Complications,
        gastrostomy
    urinary tract N99.528
      continent N99.538
        hemorrhage N99.530
        herniation N99.533
        infection N99.531
        malfunction N99.532
        specified type NEC N99.538
        stenosis N99.534
      cystostomy —*see* Complications,
        cystostomy
      external NOS N99.528
      hemorrhage N99.520
      herniation N99.523
      incontinent N99.528
        hemorrhage N99.520
        herniation N99.523
        infection N99.521
        malfunction N99.522
        specified type NEC N99.528
        stenosis N99.524
      infection N99.521
      malfunction N99.522
      specified type NEC N99.528
      stenosis N99.524
  stomach banding —*see* Complication(s),
    bariatric procedure
  stomach stapling —*see* Complication(s),
    bariatric procedure
  surgical material, nonabsorbable —*see*
    Complication, suture, permanent
  surgical procedure (on) T81.9
    amputation stump (late) —*see*
      Complications, amputation stump
    cardiac —*see* Complications, circulatory
      system
    cholesteatoma, recurrent —*see*
      Complications, postmastoidectomy,
      recurrent cholesteatoma
    circulatory (early) —*see* Complications,
      circulatory system

Complication *(Continued)*
  surgical procedure *(Continued)*
    digestive system —*see* Complications,
      gastrointestinal
    dumping syndrome (postgastrectomy)
      K91.1
    ear —*see* Complications, ear
    elephantiasis or lymphedema I97.89
      postmastectomy I97.2
    emphysema (surgical) T81.82
    endocrine —*see* Complications, endocrine
    eye —*see* Complications, eye
    fistula (persistent postoperative) T81.83
    foreign body inadvertently left in wound
      (sponge) (suture) (swab) —*see* Foreign
      body, accidentally left during a
      procedure
    gastrointestinal —*see* Complications,
      gastrointestinal
    genitourinary NEC N99.89
    hematoma
      intraoperative —*see* Complication,
        intraoperative, hemorrhage
      postprocedural —*see* Complication,
        postprocedural, hematoma
    hemorrhage
      intraoperative —*see* Complication,
        intraoperative, hemorrhage
      postprocedural —*see* Complication,
        postprocedural, hemorrhage
    hepatic failure K91.82
    hyperglycemia (postpancreatectomy) E89.1
    hypoinsulinemia (postpancreatectomy)
      E89.1
    hypoparathyroidism
      (postparathyroidectomy) E89.2
    hypopituitarism (posthypophysectomy)
      E89.3
    hypothyroidism (post-thyroidectomy)
      E89.0
    intestinal obstruction —*see also*
      Obstruction, intestine, postoperative
      K91.30
    intracranial hypotension following
      ventricular shunting
      (ventriculostomy) G97.2
    lymphedema I97.89
      postmastectomy I97.2
    malabsorption (postsurgical) NEC K91.2
      osteoporosis —*see* Osteoporosis,
        postsurgical malabsorption
    mastoidectomy cavity NEC —*see*
      Complications, postmastoidectomy
    metabolic E89.89
      specified NEC E89.89
    musculoskeletal —*see* Complications,
      musculoskeletal system
    nervous system (central) (peripheral) —*see*
      Complications, nervous system
    ovarian failure E89.40
      asymptomatic E89.40
      symptomatic E89.41
    peripheral vascular —*see* Complications,
      surgical procedure, vascular
    postcardiotomy syndrome I97.0
    postcholecystectomy syndrome K91.5
    postcommissurotomy syndrome I97.0
    postgastrectomy dumping syndrome K91.1
    postlaminectomy syndrome NEC M96.1
      kyphosis M96.3
    postmastectomy lymphedema syndrome
      I97.2
    postmastoidectomy cholesteatoma —*see*
      Complications, postmastoidectomy,
      recurrent cholesteatoma
    postvagotomy syndrome K91.1
    postvalvulotomy syndrome I97.0
    pulmonary insufficiency (acute) J95.2
      chronic J95.3
      following thoracic surgery J95.1

► New   ⇒ Revised   ~~deleted~~ Deleted   ● Use Additional Character(s)

Complication *(Continued)*
    surgical procedure *(Continued)*
        reattached body part —*see* Complications,
            reattached
        respiratory —*see* Complications,
            respiratory system
        shock (hypovolemic) T81.19
        spleen (postoperative) D78.89
            intraoperative D78.81
        stitch abscess T81.41
        subglottic stenosis (postsurgical) J95.5
        testicular hypofunction E89.5
        transplant —*see* Complications, organ or
            tissue transplant
        urinary NEC N99.89
        vaginal vault prolapse (posthysterectomy)
            N99.3
        vascular (peripheral)
            artery T81.719
                mesenteric T81.710
                renal T81.711
                specified NEC T81.718
            vein T81.72
        wound infection T81.49
    suture, permanent (wire) NEC T85.9
        with repair of bone —*see* Complications,
            fixation device, internal
        embolism T85.818
        fibrosis T85.828
        hemorrhage T85.838
        infection and inflammation T85.79
        mechanical
            breakdown T85.612
            displacement T85.622
            malfunction T85.612
            malposition T85.622
            obstruction T85.692
            perforation T85.692
            protrusion T85.692
            specified NEC T85.692
        pain T85.848
        specified type NEC T85.898
        stenosis T85.858
        thrombosis T85.868
    tracheostomy J95.00
        granuloma J95.09
        hemorrhage J95.01
        infection J95.02
        malfunction J95.03
        mechanical J95.03
        obstruction J95.03
        specified type NEC J95.09
        tracheo-esophageal fistula J95.04
    transfusion (blood) (lymphocytes) (plasma)
        T80.92
        air embolism T80.0
        circulatory overload E87.71
        febrile nonhemolytic transfusion reaction
            R50.84
        hemochromatosis E83.111
        hemolysis T80.89
        hemolytic reaction (antigen unspecified)
            T80.919
        incompatibility reaction (antigen
            unspecified) T80.919
            ABO T80.30
                delayed serologic (DSTR) T80.39
                hemolytic transfusion reaction
                    (HTR) (unspecified time after
                    transfusion) T80.319
                    acute (AHTR) (less than 24 hours
                        after transfusion) T80.310
                    delayed (DHTR) (24 hours or
                        more after transfusion)
                        T80.311
                specified NEC T80.39
                acute (antigen unspecified) T80.910
                delayed (antigen unspecified)
                    T80.911
                delayed serologic (DSTR) T80.89

Complication *(Continued)*
    transfusion *(Continued)*
        incompatibility reaction *(Continued)*
            Non-ABO (minor antigens (Duffy)
                (K) (Kell) (Kidd) (Lewis) (M) (N)
                (P) (S)) T80.A0
                delayed serologic (DSTR) T80.A9
                hemolytic transfusion reaction
                    (HTR) (unspecified time after
                    transfusion) T80.A19
                    acute (AHTR) (less than 24 hours
                        after transfusion) T80.A10
                    delayed (DHTR) (24 hours or more
                        after transfusion) T80.A11
                specified NEC T80.A9
            Rh (antigens (C) (c) (D) (E) (e)) (factor)
                T80.40
                delayed serologic (DSTR) T80.49
                hemolytic transfusion reaction
                    (HTR) (unspecified time after
                    transfusion) T80.419
                    acute (AHTR) (less than 24 hours
                        after transfusion) T80.410
                    delayed (DHTR) (24 hours or more
                        after transfusion) T80.411
                specified NEC T80.49
        infection T80.29
            acute T80.22
        reaction NEC T80.89
        sepsis T80.29
        shock T80.89
    transplant T86.90
        bone T86.839
            failure T86.831
            infection T86.832
            rejection T86.830
            specified type NEC T86.838
        bone marrow T86.00
            failure T86.02
            infection T86.03
            rejection T86.01
            specified type NEC T86.09
        cornea T86.849-
            failure T86.841-
            infection T86.842-
            rejection T86.840-
            specified type NEC T86.848-
        failure T86.92
        heart T86.20
            with lung T86.30
                cardiac allograft vasculopathy T86.290
                    failure T86.32
                    infection T86.33
                    rejection T86.31
                    specified type NEC T86.39
                failure T86.22
                infection T86.23
                rejection T86.21
                specified type NEC T86.298
            infection T86.93
        intestine T86.859
            failure T86.851
            infection T86.852
            rejection T86.850
            specified type NEC T86.858
        kidney T86.10
            failure T86.12
            infection T86.13
            rejection T86.11
            specified type NEC T86.19
        liver T86.40
            failure T86.42
            infection T86.43
            rejection T86.41
            specified type NEC T86.49
        lung T86.819
            with heart T86.30
                failure T86.32
                infection T86.33
                rejection T86.31
                specified type NEC T86.39

Complication *(Continued)*
    transplant *(Continued)*
        lung *(Continued)*
            failure T86.811
            infection T86.812
            rejection T86.810
            specified type NEC T86.818
        malignant neoplasm C80.2
        pancreas T86.899
            failure T86.891
            infection T86.892
            rejection T86.890
            specified type NEC T86.898
        peripheral blood stem cells T86.5
        post-transplant lymphoproliferative
            disorder (PTLD) D47.Z1
        rejection T86.91
        skin T86.829
            failure T86.821
            infection T86.822
            rejection T86.820
            specified type NEC T86.828
        specified
            tissue T86.899
                failure T86.891
                infection T86.892
                rejection T86.890
                specified type NEC T86.898
            type NEC T86.99
        stem cell (from peripheral blood) (from
            umbilical cord) T86.5
        umbilical cord stem cells T86.5
    trauma (early) T79.9
        specified NEC T79.8
    ultrasound therapy NEC T88.9
    umbilical cord NEC
        complicating delivery O69.9
            specified NEC O69.89
    umbrella device, vascular T82.9
        embolism T82.818
        fibrosis T82.828
        hemorrhage T82.838
        infection or inflammation T82.7
        mechanical
            breakdown T82.515
            displacement T82.525
            leakage T82.535
            malposition T82.525
            obstruction T82.595
            perforation T82.595
            protrusion T82.595
        pain T82.848
        specified type NEC T82.898
        stenosis T82.858
        thrombosis T82.868
    urethral catheter —*see* Complications,
        catheter, urethral, indwelling
    vaccination T88.1
        anaphylaxis NEC T80.52
        arthropathy —*see* Arthropathy,
            postimmunization
        cellulitis T88.0
        encephalitis or encephalomyelitis
            G04.02
        infection (general) (local) NEC T88.0
        meningitis G03.8
        myelitis G04.02
        protein sickness T80.62
        rash T88.1
        reaction (allergic) T88.1
            serum T80.62
        sepsis T88.0
        serum intoxication, sickness, rash, or other
            serum reaction NEC T80.62
            anaphylactic shock T80.52
        shock (allergic) (anaphylactic) T80.52
        vaccinia (generalized) (localized) T88.1
    vas deferens device or implant —*see*
        Complications, genitourinary, device or
        implant, genital tract

Complication *(Continued)*
  vascular I99.9
    device or implant T82.9
      embolism T82.818
      fibrosis T82.828
      hemorrhage T82.838
      infection or inflammation T82.7
      mechanical
        breakdown T82.519
          specified device NEC T82.518
        displacement T82.529
          specified device NEC T82.528
        leakage T82.539
          specified device NEC T82.538
        malposition T82.529
          specified device NEC T82.528
        obstruction T82.599
          specified device NEC T82.598
        perforation T82.599
          specified device NEC T82.598
        protrusion T82.599
          specified device NEC T82.598
      pain T82.848
      specified type NEC T82.898
      stenosis T82.858
      thrombosis T82.868
    dialysis catheter —*see* Complication,
        catheter, dialysis
    following infusion, therapeutic injection or
        transfusion T80.1
    graft T82.9
      embolism T82.818
      fibrosis T82.828
      hemorrhage T82.838
      mechanical
        breakdown T82.319
          aorta (bifurcation) T82.310
          carotid artery T82.311
          specified vessel NEC T82.318
        displacement T82.329
          aorta (bifurcation) T82.320
          carotid artery T82.321
          specified vessel NEC T82.328
        leakage T82.339
          aorta (bifurcation) T82.330
          carotid artery T82.331
          ▶femoral artery T82.332
          specified vessel NEC T82.338
        malposition T82.329
          aorta (bifurcation) T82.320
          carotid artery T82.321
          specified vessel NEC T82.328
        obstruction T82.399
          aorta (bifurcation) T82.390
          carotid artery T82.391
          specified vessel NEC T82.398
        perforation T82.399
          aorta (bifurcation) T82.390
          carotid artery T82.391
          specified vessel NEC T82.398
        protrusion T82.399
          aorta (bifurcation) T82.390
          carotid artery T82.391
          specified vessel NEC T82.398
      pain T82.848
      specified complication NEC T82.898
      stenosis T82.858
      thrombosis T82.868
    postoperative —*see* Complications,
        postoperative, circulatory
  vena cava device (filter) (sieve) (umbrella) —
      see Complications, umbrella device,
      vascular
  ventilation therapy NEC T81.81
  ventilator
    mechanical J95.850
      specified NEC J95.859
  ventricular (communicating) shunt (device)
      T85.9
    embolism T85.810
    fibrosis T85.820
    hemorrhage T85.830
    infection and inflammation T85.730

Complication *(Continued)*
  ventricular shunt *(Continued)*
    mechanical
      breakdown T85.01
      displacement T85.02
      leakage T85.03
      malposition T85.02
      obstruction T85.09
      perforation T85.09
      protrusion T85.09
      specified NEC T85.09
    pain T85.840
    specified type NEC T85.890
    stenosis T85.850
    thrombosis T85.860
  wire suture, permanent (implanted) —*see*
      Complications, suture, permanent
Compressed air disease T70.3
Compression
  with injury - code by Nature of injury
  artery I77.1
    celiac, syndrome I77.4
  brachial plexus G54.0
  brain (stem) G93.5
    due to
      contusion (diffuse) (*see also* Injury,
          intracranial, diffuse) S06.A0
        with herniation S06.A1
      focal (*see also* Injury, intracranial, focal)
          S06.A0
        with herniation S06.A1
      injury NEC (*see also* Injury, intracranial,
          diffuse) S06.A0
    nontraumatic G93.5
    traumatic (*see also* Injury, intracranial,
        diffuse) S06.A0
      with herniation S06.A1
  bronchus J98.09
  cauda equina G83.4
  celiac (artery) (axis) I77.4
  cerebral —*see* Compression, brain
  cervical plexus G54.2
  cord
    spinal —*see* Compression, spinal
    umbilical —*see* Compression, umbilical cord
  cranial nerve G52.9
    eighth —*see* subcategory H93.3
    eleventh G52.8
    fifth G50.8
    first G52.0
    fourth —*see* Strabismus, paralytic, fourth
        nerve
    ninth G52.1
    second —*see* Disorder, nerve, optic
    seventh G51.8
    sixth —*see* Strabismus, paralytic, sixth nerve
    tenth G52.2
    third —*see* Strabismus, paralytic, third nerve
    twelfth G52.3
  diver's squeeze T70.3
  during birth (newborn) P15.9
  esophagus K22.2
  eustachian tube —*see* Obstruction, eustachian
      tube, cartilaginous
  facies Q67.1
  fracture
    nontraumatic NOS —*see* Collapse, vertebra
    pathological —*see* Fracture, pathological
    traumatic —*see* Fracture, traumatic
  heart —*see* Disease, heart
  intestine —*see* Obstruction, intestine
  laryngeal nerve, recurrent G52.2
    with paralysis of vocal cords and larynx
        J38.00
      bilateral J38.02
      unilateral J38.01
  lumbosacral plexus G54.1
  lung J98.4
  lymphatic vessel I89.0
  medulla —*see* Compression, brain
  nerve —*see also* Disorder, nerve G58.9
    arm NEC —*see* Mononeuropathy, upper limb

Compression *(Continued)*
  nerve *(Continued)*
    axillary G54.0
    cranial —*see* Compression, cranial nerve
    leg NEC —*see* Mononeuropathy, lower
        limb
    median (in carpal tunnel) —*see* Syndrome,
        carpal tunnel
    optic —*see* Disorder, nerve, optic
    plantar —*see* Lesion, nerve, plantar
    posterior tibial (in tarsal tunnel) —*see*
        Syndrome, tarsal tunnel
    root or plexus NOS (in) G54.9
      intervertebral disc disorder NEC —
          see Disorder, disc, with,
          radiculopathy
        with myelopathy —*see* Disorder, disc,
            with, myelopathy
      neoplastic disease —*see also* Neoplasm
          D49.9 [G55]
      spondylosis —*see* Spondylosis, with
          radiculopathy
    sciatic (acute) —*see* Lesion, nerve, sciatic
    sympathetic G90.8
    traumatic —*see* Injury, nerve
    ulnar —*see* Lesion, nerve, ulnar
    upper extremity NEC —*see*
        Mononeuropathy, upper limb
  spinal (cord) G95.20
    by displacement of intervertebral disc
        NEC —*see also* Disorder, disc, with,
        myelopathy
    nerve root NOS G54.9
      due to displacement of intervertebral
          disc NEC —*see* Disorder, disc, with,
          radiculopathy
        with myelopathy —*see* Disorder, disc,
            with, myelopathy
    specified NEC G95.29
    spondylogenic (cervical) (lumbar,
        lumbosacral) (thoracic) —*see*
        Spondylosis, with myelopathy NEC
    anterior —*see* Syndrome, anterior, spinal
        artery, compression
    traumatic —*see* Injury, spinal cord, by
        region
  subcostal nerve (syndrome) —*see*
      Mononeuropathy, upper limb, specified
      NEC
  sympathetic nerve NEC G90.8
  syndrome T79.5
  trachea J39.8
  ulnar nerve (by scar tissue) —*see* Lesion,
      nerve, ulnar
  umbilical cord
    complicating delivery O69.2
      cord around neck O69.1
      prolapse O69.0
      specified NEC O69.2
  ureter N13.5
  vein I87.1
  vena cava (inferior) (superior) I87.1
Compulsion, compulsive
  gambling F63.0
  neurosis F42.8
  personality F60.5
  states F42.8
  swearing F42.8
    in Gilles de la Tourette's syndrome F95.2
  tics and spasms F95.9
Concato's disease (pericardial polyserositis)
    A19.9
  nontubercular I31.1
  pleural —*see* Pleurisy, with effusion
Concavity chest wall M95.4
Concealed penis Q55.64
Concern (normal) about sick person in family
    Z63.6
Concrescence (teeth) K00.2
Concretio cordis I31.1
  rheumatic I09.2

▶ New   ⇒ Revised   ~~deleted~~ Deleted   ● Use Additional Character(s)

Concretion —*see also* Calculus
  appendicular K38.1
  canaliculus —*see* Dacryolith
  clitoris N90.89
  conjunctiva H11.12-●
  eyelid —*see* Disorder, eyelid, specified type NEC
  lacrimal passages —*see* Dacryolith
  prepuce (male) N47.8
  salivary gland (any) K11.5
  seminal vesicle N50.89
  tonsil J35.8
Concussion (brain) (cerebral) (current) S06.0X9
  with
    ~~loss of consciousness of 30 minutes or less~~
      ~~S06.0X1~~
    ~~loss of consciousness of unspecified~~
      ~~duration S06.0X9~~
  ▶loss of consciousness
    ▶30 minutes or less S06.0X1
    ▶brief S06.0X1
    ▶status unknown S06.0XA
    ▶unspecified duration S06.0X9
  ▶no loss of consciousness S06.0X0
  blast (air) (hydraulic) (immersion)
      (underwater)
    abdomen or thorax —*see* Injury, blast, by
      site
    ear with acoustic nerve injury —*see* Injury,
      nerve, acoustic, specified type NEC
  cauda equina S34.3
  conus medullaris S34.02
  ocular S05.8X-●
  spinal (cord)
    cervical S14.0
    lumbar S34.01
    sacral S34.02
    thoracic S24.0
  syndrome F07.81
  without loss of consciousness S06.0X0
Condition —*see also* Disease
  post COVID-19 U09.9
Conditions arising in the perinatal period —
  see Newborn, affected by
Conduct disorder —*see* Disorder, conduct
Condyloma A63.0
  acuminatum A63.0
  gonorrheal A54.09
  latum A51.31
  syphilitic A51.31
    congenital A50.07
  venereal, syphilitic A51.31
Conflagration —*see also* Burn
  asphyxia (by inhalation of gases, fumes or
      vapors) —*see also* Table of Drugs and
      Chemicals T59.9-●
Conflict (with) —*see also* Discord
  family Z73.9
  marital Z63.0
    involving divorce or estrangement Z63.5
  parent-child Z62.820
    parent-adopted child Z62.821
    parent-biological child Z62.820
    parent-foster child Z62.822
  social role NEC Z73.5
Confluent —*see* condition
Confusion, confused R41.0
  epileptic F05
  mental state (psychogenic) F44.89
  psychogenic F44.89
  reactive (from emotional stress, psychological
      trauma) F44.89
Confusional arousals G47.51
Congelation T69.9
Congenital —*see also* condition
  aortic septum Q25.49
  intrinsic factor deficiency D51.0
  malformation —*see* Anomaly
Congestion, congestive
  bladder N32.89
  bowel K63.89
  brain G93.89
  breast N64.59
  bronchial J98.09

Congestion, congestive *(Continued)*
  catarrhal J31.0
  chest R09.89
  chill, malarial —*see* Malaria
  circulatory NEC I99.8
  duodenum K31.89
  eye —*see* Hyperemia, conjunctiva
  facial, due to birth injury P15.4
  general R68.89
  glottis J37.0
  heart —*see* Failure, heart, congestive
  hepatic K76.1
  hypostatic (lung) —*see* Edema, lung
  intestine K63.89
  kidney N28.89
  labyrinth —*see* subcategory H83.8
  larynx J37.0
  liver K76.1
  lung R09.89
    active or acute —*see* Pneumonia
  malaria, malarial —*see* Malaria
  nasal R09.81
  nose R09.81
  orbit, orbital —*see also* Exophthalmos
    inflammatory (chronic) —*see* Inflammation,
      orbit
  ovary N83.8
  pancreas K86.89
  pelvic, female N94.89
  pleural J94.8
  prostate (active) N42.1
  pulmonary —*see* Congestion, lung
  renal N28.89
  retina H35.81
  seminal vesicle N50.1
  spinal cord G95.19
  spleen (chronic) D73.2
  stomach K31.89
  trachea —*see* Tracheitis
  urethra N36.8
  uterus N85.8
    with subinvolution N85.3
  venous (passive) I87.8
  viscera R68.89
Congestive —*see* Congestion
Conical
  cervix (hypertrophic elongation) N88.4
  cornea —*see* Keratoconus
  teeth K00.2
Conjoined twins Q89.4
Conjugal maladjustment Z63.0
  involving divorce or estrangement Z63.5
Conjunctiva —*see* condition
Conjunctivitis (staphylococcal) (streptococcal)
      NOS H10.9
  Acanthamoeba B60.12
  acute H10.3-●
    atopic H10.1-●
    chemical —*see also* Corrosion, cornea
      H10.21-●
    mucopurulent H10.02-●
      follicular H10.01-●
    pseudomembranous H10.22-●
    serous except viral H10.23-●
      viral —*see* Conjunctivitis, viral
    toxic H10.21-●
  adenoviral (acute) (follicular) B30.1
  allergic (acute) —*see* Conjunctivitis, acute,
      atopic
    chronic H10.45
      vernal H10.44
  anaphylactic —*see* Conjunctivitis, acute, atopic
  Apollo B30.3
  atopic (acute) —*see* Conjunctivitis, acute, atopic
  Béal's B30.2
  blennorrhagic (gonococcal) (neonatorum)
      A54.31
  chemical (acute) —*see also* Corrosion, cornea
      H10.21-●
  chlamydial A74.0
    due to trachoma A71.1
    neonatal P39.1

Conjunctivitis *(Continued)*
  chronic (nodosa) (petrificans) (phlyctenular)
      H10.40-●
    allergic H10.45
      vernal H10.44
    follicular H10.43-●
    giant papillary H10.41-●
    simple H10.42-●
    vernal H10.44
  coxsackievirus 24 B30.3
  diphtheritic A36.86
  due to
    dust —*see* Conjunctivitis, acute, atopic
    filariasis B74.9
    mucocutaneous leishmaniasis B55.2
  enterovirus type 70 (hemorrhagic) B30.3
  epidemic (viral) B30.9
    hemorrhagic B30.3
  gonococcal (neonatorum) A54.31
  granular (trachomatous) A71.1
    sequelae (late effect) B94.0
  hemorrhagic (acute) (epidemic) B30.3
  herpes zoster B02.31
  in (due to)
    Acanthamoeba B60.12
    adenovirus (acute) (follicular) B30.1
    Chlamydia A74.0
    coxsackievirus 24 B30.3
    diphtheria A36.86
    enterovirus type 70 (hemorrhagic) B30.3
    filariasis B74.9
    gonococci A54.31
    herpes (simplex) virus B00.53
      zoster B02.31
    infectious disease NEC B99
    meningococci A39.89
    mucocutaneous leishmaniasis B55.2
    rosacea H10.82-●
    syphilis (late) A52.71
    zoster B02.31
  inclusion A74.0
  infantile P39.1
    gonococcal A54.31
  Koch-Weeks' —*see* Conjunctivitis, acute,
      mucopurulent
  light —*see* Conjunctivitis, acute, atopic
  ligneous —*see* Blepharoconjunctivitis,
      ligneous
  meningococcal A39.89
  mucopurulent —*see* Conjunctivitis, acute,
      mucopurulent
  neonatal P39.1
    gonococcal A54.31
  Newcastle B30.8
  of Béal B30.2
  parasitic
    filariasis B74.9
    mucocutaneous leishmaniasis B55.2
  Parinaud's H10.89
  petrificans H10.89
  rosacea H10.82-●
  specified NEC H10.89
  swimming-pool B30.1
  trachomatous A71.1
    acute A71.0
    sequelae (late effect) B94.0
  traumatic NEC H10.89
  tuberculous A18.59
  tularemic A21.1
  tularensis A21.1
  viral B30.9
    due to
      adenovirus B30.1
      enterovirus B30.3
    specified NEC B30.8
Conjunctivochalasis H11.82-●
Connective tissue —*see* condition
Conn's syndrome E26.01
Conradi (-Hunermann) disease Q77.3
Consanguinity Z84.3
  counseling Z71.89

Conscious simulation (of illness) Z76.5
Consecutive —see condition
Consolidation lung (base) —see Pneumonia, lobar
Constipation (atonic) (neurogenic) (simple) (spastic) K59.00
  chronic K59.09
    idiopathic K59.04
  drug-induced K59.03
  functional K59.04
  outlet dysfunction K59.02
  psychogenic F45.8
  slow transit K59.01
  specified NEC K59.09
Constitutional —see also condition
  substandard F60.7
Constitutionally substandard F60.7
Constriction —see also Stricture
  auditory canal —see Stenosis, external ear canal
  bronchial J98.09
  duodenum K31.5
  esophagus K22.2
  external
    abdomen, abdominal (wall) S30.841
    alveolar process S00.542
    ankle S90.54-●
    antecubital space —see Constriction, external, forearm
    arm (upper) S40.84-●
    auricle —see Constriction, external, ear
    axilla —see Constriction, external, arm
    back, lower S30.840
    breast S20.14-●
    brow S00.84
    buttock S30.840
    calf —see Constriction, external, leg
    canthus —see Constriction, external, eyelid
    cheek S00.84
      internal S00.542
    chest wall —see Constriction, external, thorax
    chin S00.84
    clitoris S30.844
    costal region —see Constriction, external, thorax
    digit(s)
      foot —see Constriction, external, toe
      hand —see Constriction, external, finger
    ear S00.44-●
    elbow S50.34-●
    epididymis S30.843
    epigastric region S30.841
    esophagus, cervical S10.14
    eyebrow —see Constriction, external, eyelid
    eyelid S00.24-●
    face S00.84
    finger(s) S60.44-●
      index S60.44-●
      little S60.44-●
      middle S60.44-●
      ring S60.44-●
    flank S30.841
    foot (except toe(s) alone) S90.84-●
      toe —see Constriction, external, toe
    forearm S50.84-●
      elbow only —see Constriction, external, elbow
    forehead S00.84
    genital organs, external
      female S30.846
      male S30.845
    groin S30.841
    gum S00.542
    hand S60.54-●
    head S00.94
      ear —see Constriction, external, ear
      eyelid —see Constriction, external, eyelid
      lip S00.541
      nose S00.34
      oral cavity S00.542

Constriction (Continued)
  external (Continued)
    head (Continued)
      scalp S00.04
      specified site NEC S00.84
    heel —see Constriction, external, foot
    hip S70.24-●
    inguinal region S30.841
    interscapular region S20.449
    jaw S00.84
    knee S80.24-●
    labium (majus) (minus) S30.844
    larynx S10.14
    leg (lower) S80.84-●
      knee —see Constriction, external, knee
      upper —see Constriction, external, thigh
    lip S00.541
    lower back S30.840
    lumbar region S30.840
    malar region S00.84
    mammary —see Constriction, external, breast
    mastoid region S00.84
    mouth S00.542
    nail
      finger —see Constriction, external, finger
      toe —see Constriction, external, toe
    nasal S00.34
    neck S10.94
      specified site NEC S10.84
      throat S10.14
    nose S00.34
    occipital region S00.04
    oral cavity S00.542
    orbital region —see Constriction, external, eyelid
    palate S00.542
    palm —see Constriction, external, hand
    parietal region S00.04
    pelvis S30.840
    penis S30.842
    perineum
      female S30.844
      male S30.840
    periocular area —see Constriction, external, eyelid
    phalanges
      finger —see Constriction, external, finger
      toe —see Constriction, external, toe
    pharynx S10.14
    pinna —see Constriction, external, ear
    popliteal space —see Constriction, external, knee
    prepuce S30.842
    pubic region S30.840
    pudendum
      female S30.846
      male S30.845
    sacral region S30.840
    scalp S00.04
    scapular region —see Constriction, external, shoulder
    scrotum S30.843
    shin —see Constriction, external, leg
    shoulder S40.24-●
    sternal region S20.349
    submaxillary region S00.84
    submental region S00.84
    subungual
      finger(s) —see Constriction, external, finger
      toe(s) —see Constriction, external, toe
    supraclavicular fossa S10.84
    supraorbital S00.84
    temple S00.84
    temporal region S00.84
    testis S30.843
    thigh S70.34-●
    thorax, thoracic (wall) S20.94
      back S20.44-●
      front S20.34-●
    throat S10.14

Constriction (Continued)
  external (Continued)
    thumb S60.34-●
    toe(s) (lesser) S90.44-●
      great S90.44-●
    tongue S00.542
    trachea S10.14
    tunica vaginalis S30.843
    uvula S00.542
    vagina S30.844
    vulva S30.844
    wrist S60.84-●
  gallbladder —see Obstruction, gallbladder
  intestine —see Obstruction, intestine
  larynx J38.6
    congenital Q31.8
      specified NEC Q31.8
      subglottic Q31.1
  organ or site, congenital NEC —see Atresia, by site
  prepuce (acquired) (congenital) N47.1
  pylorus (adult hypertrophic) K31.1
    congenital or infantile Q40.0
    newborn Q40.0
  ring dystocia (uterus) O62.4
  spastic —see also Spasm
    ureter N13.5
  ureter N13.5
    with infection N13.6
  urethra —see Stricture, urethra
  visual field (peripheral) (functional) —see Defect, visual field
Constrictive —see condition
Consultation
  without complaint or sickness Z71.9
    feared complaint unfounded Z71.1
    specified reason NEC Z71.89
  medical —see Counseling, medical
  religious Z71.81
  specified reason NEC Z71.89
  spiritual Z71.81
Consumption —see Tuberculosis
Contact (with) —see also Exposure (to)
  acariasis Z20.7
  AIDS virus Z20.6
  air pollution Z77.110
  algae and algae toxins Z77.121
  algae bloom Z77.121
  anthrax Z20.810
  aromatic (hazardous) compounds NEC Z77.028
  aromatic amines Z77.020
  aromatic dyes NOS Z77.028
  arsenic Z77.010
  asbestos Z77.090
  bacterial disease NEC Z20.818
  benzene Z77.021
  blue-green algae bloom Z77.121
  body fluids (potentially hazardous) Z77.21
  brown tide Z77.121
  chemicals (chiefly nonmedicinal) (hazardous) NEC Z77.098
  cholera Z20.09
  chromium compounds Z77.018
  communicable disease Z20.9
    bacterial NEC Z20.818
    specified NEC Z20.89
    viral NEC Z20.828
    Zika virus Z20.821
  coronavirus (disease) (novel) 2019 Z20.822
  COVID-19 Z20.822
  cyanobacteria bloom Z77.121
  dyes Z77.098
  Escherichia coli (E. coli) Z20.01
  fiberglass —see Table of Drugs and Chemicals, fiberglass
  German measles Z20.4
  gonorrhea Z20.2
  hazardous metals NEC Z77.018
  hazardous substances NEC Z77.29
  hazards in the physical environment NEC Z77.128
  hazards to health NEC Z77.9

▶ New   ⇒ Revised   ~~deleted~~ Deleted   ● Use Additional Character(s)

Contact *(Continued)*
HIV Z20.6
HTLV-III/LAV Z20.6
human immunodeficiency virus (HIV) Z20.6
infection Z20.9
  specified NEC Z20.89
infestation (parasitic) NEC Z20.7
intestinal infectious disease NEC Z20.09
  Escherichia coli (E. coli) Z20.01
lead Z77.011
meningococcus Z20.811
mold (toxic) Z77.120
nickel dust Z77.018
noise Z77.122
parasitic disease Z20.7
pediculosis Z20.7
pfiesteria piscicida Z77.121
poliomyelitis Z20.89
pollution
  air Z77.110
  environmental NEC Z77.118
  soil Z77.112
  water Z77.111
polycyclic aromatic hydrocarbons Z77.028
positive maternal group B streptococcus P00.82
rabies Z20.3
radiation, naturally occurring NEC Z77.123
radon Z77.123
red tide (Florida) Z77.121
rubella Z20.4
SARS-CoV-2 Z20.822
sexually-transmitted disease Z20.2
smallpox (laboratory) Z20.89
syphilis Z20.2
tuberculosis Z20.1
uranium Z77.012
varicella Z20.820
venereal disease Z20.2
viral disease NEC Z20.828
viral hepatitis Z20.5
water pollution Z77.111
Zika virus Z20.821
Contamination, food —*see* Intoxication, foodborne
Contraception, contraceptive
advice Z30.09
counseling Z30.09
device (intrauterine) (in situ) Z97.5
  causing menorrhagia T83.83
  checking Z30.431
  complications —*see* Complications, intrauterine, contraceptive device
  in place Z97.5
  initial prescription Z30.014
  reinsertion Z30.433
  removal Z30.432
  replacement Z30.433
emergency (postcoital) Z30.012
initial prescription Z30.019
  barrier Z30.018
  diaphragm Z30.018
  injectable Z30.013
  intrauterine device Z30.014
  pills Z30.011
  postcoital (emergency) Z30.012
  specified type NEC Z30.018
  subdermal implantable Z30.017
  transdermal patch hormonal Z30.016
  vaginal ring hormonal Z30.015
maintenance Z30.40
  barrier Z30.49
  diaphragm Z30.49
  examination Z30.8
  injectable Z30.42
  intrauterine device Z30.431
  pills Z30.41
  specified type NEC Z30.49
  subdermal implantable Z30.46
  transdermal patch hormonal Z30.45
  vaginal ring hormonal Z30.44
management Z30.9
  specified NEC Z30.8
postcoital (emergency) Z30.012

Contraception, contraceptive *(Continued)*
prescription Z30.019
  repeat Z30.40
sterilization Z30.2
surveillance (drug) —*see* Contraception, maintenance
Contraction(s), contracture, contracted
Achilles tendon —*see also* Short, tendon, Achilles
  congenital Q66.89
amputation stump (surgical) (flexion) (late) next proximal joint T87.89
anus K59.89
bile duct (common) (hepatic) K83.8
bladder N32.89
  neck or sphincter N32.0
bowel, cecum, colon or intestine, any part —*see* Obstruction, intestine
Braxton Hicks —*see* False, labor
breast implant, capsular T85.44
bronchial J98.09
burn (old) —*see* Cicatrix
cervix —*see* Stricture, cervix
cicatricial —*see* Cicatrix
conjunctiva, trachomatous, active A71.1
  sequelae (late effect) B94.0
Dupuytren's M72.0
eyelid —*see* Disorder, eyelid function
fascia (lata) (postural) M72.8
  Dupuytren's M72.0
  palmar M72.0
  plantar M72.2
finger NEC —*see also* Deformity, finger
  congenital Q68.1
  joint —*see* Contraction, joint, hand
flaccid —*see* Contraction, paralytic
gallbladder K82.0
heart valve —*see* Endocarditis
hip —*see* Contraction, joint, hip
hourglass
  bladder N32.89
    congenital Q64.79
  gallbladder K82.0
    congenital Q44.1
  stomach K31.89
    congenital Q40.2
    psychogenic F45.8
  uterus (complicating delivery) O62.4
hysterical F44.4
internal os —*see* Stricture, cervix
joint (abduction) (acquired) (adduction) (flexion) (rotation) M24.50
  ankle M24.57-●
  congenital NEC Q68.8
    hip Q65.89
  elbow M24.52-●
  foot joint M24.57-●
  hand joint M24.54-●
  hip M24.55-●
    congenital Q65.89
  hysterical F44.4
  knee M24.56-●
  shoulder M24.51-●
  specified site NEC M24.59
  wrist M24.53-●
kidney (granular) (secondary) N26.9
  congenital Q63.8
  hydronephritic —*see* Hydronephrosis Page N26.2
  pyelonephritic —*see* Pyelitis, chronic
  tuberculous A18.11
ligament —*see also* Disorder, ligament
  congenital Q79.8
muscle (postinfective) (postural) NEC M62.40
  with contracture of joint —*see* Contraction, joint
  ankle M62.47-●
  congenital Q79.8
    sternocleidomastoid Q68.0
  extraocular —*see* Strabismus
  eye (extrinsic) —*see* Strabismus
  foot M62.47-●

Contraction, contracture, contracted *(Continued)*
muscle *(Continued)* forearm M62.43-●
  hand M62.44-●
  hysterical F44.4
  ischemic (Volkmann's) T79.6
  lower leg M62.46-●
  multiple sites M62.49
  pelvic region M62.45-●
  posttraumatic —*see* Strabismus, paralytic
  psychogenic F45.8
    conversion reaction F44.4
  shoulder region M62.41-●
  specified site NEC M62.48
  thigh M62.45-●
  upper arm M62.42-●
neck —*see* Torticollis
ocular muscle —*see* Strabismus
organ or site, congenital NEC —*see* Atresia, by site
outlet (pelvis) —*see* Contraction, pelvis
palmar fascia M72.0
paralytic
  joint —*see* Contraction, joint
  muscle —*see also* Contraction, muscle NEC
    ocular —*see* Strabismus, paralytic
pelvis (acquired) (general) M95.5
  with disproportion (fetopelvic) O33.1
    causing obstructed labor O65.1
    inlet O33.2
    mid-cavity O33.3
    outlet O33.3
plantar fascia M72.2
premature
  atrium I49.1
  auriculoventricular I49.49
  heart I49.49
  junctional I49.2
  supraventricular I49.1
  ventricular I49.3
prostate N42.89
pylorus NEC —*see also* Pylorospasm
  psychogenic F45.8
rectum, rectal (sphincter) K59.89
ring (Bandl's) (complicating delivery) O62.4
scar —*see* Cicatrix
spine —*see* Dorsopathy, deforming
sternocleidomastoid (muscle), congenital Q68.0
stomach K31.89
  hourglass K31.89
    congenital Q40.2
    psychogenic F45.8
  psychogenic F45.8
tendon (sheath) M62.40
  with contracture of joint —*see* Contraction, joint
  Achilles —*see* Short, tendon, Achilles
  ankle M62.47-●
    Achilles —*see* Short, tendon, Achilles
  foot M62.47-●
  forearm M62.43-●
  hand M62.44-●
  lower leg M62.46-●
  multiple sites M62.49
  neck M62.48
  pelvic region M62.45-●
  shoulder region M62.41-●
  specified site NEC M62.48
  thigh M62.45-●
  thorax M62.48
  trunk M62.48
  upper arm M62.42-●
toe —*see* Deformity, toe, specified NEC
ureterovesical orifice (postinfectional) N13.5
  with infection N13.6
urethra —*see also* Stricture, urethra
  orifice N32.0
uterus N85.8
  abnormal NEC O62.9
  clonic (complicating delivery) O62.4
  dyscoordinate (complicating delivery) O62.4

Contraction, contracture, contracted
    (Continued)
  uterus (Continued)
    hourglass (complicating delivery) O62.4
    hypertonic O62.4
    hypotonic NEC O62.2
    inadequate
      primary O62.0
      secondary O62.1
    incoordinate (complicating delivery) O62.4
    poor O62.2
    tetanic (complicating delivery) O62.4
  vagina (outlet) N89.5
  vesical N32.89
    neck or urethral orifice N32.0
  visual field —see Defect, visual field,
      generalized
  Volkmann's (ischemic) T79.6
Contusion (skin surface intact) T14.8
  abdomen, abdominal (muscle) (wall) S30.1
  adnexa, eye NEC S05.8X-•
  adrenal gland S37.812
  alveolar process S00.532
  ankle S90.0-•
  antecubital space —see Contusion, forearm
  anus S30.3
  arm (upper) S40.02-•
    lower (with elbow) —see Contusion,
        forearm
  auditory canal —see Contusion, ear
  auricle —see Contusion, ear
  axilla —see Contusion, arm, upper
  back —see also Contusion, thorax, back
    lower S30.0
  bile duct S36.13
  bladder S37.22
  bone NEC T14.8
  brain (diffuse) —see Injury, intracranial, diffuse
    focal —see Injury, intracranial, focal
  brainstem S06.38-•
  breast S20.0-•
  broad ligament S37.892
  brow S00.83
  buttock S30.0
  canthus, eye S00.1-•
  cauda equina S34.3
  cerebellar, traumatic S06.37-•
  cerebral S06.33-•
    left side S06.32-•
    right side S06.31-•
  cheek S00.83
    internal S00.532
  chest (wall) —see Contusion, thorax
  chin S00.83
  clitoris S30.23
  colon —see Injury, intestine, large, contusion
  common bile duct S36.13
  conjunctiva S05.1-•
    with foreign body (in conjunctival sac) —
        see Foreign body, conjunctival sac
  conus medullaris (spine) S34.139
  cornea —see Contusion, eyeball
    with foreign body —see Foreign body,
        cornea
  corpus cavernosum S30.21
  cortex (brain) (cerebral) —see Injury,
      intracranial, diffuse
    focal —see Injury, intracranial, focal
  costal region —see Contusion, thorax
  cystic duct S36.13
  diaphragm S27.802
  duodenum S36.420
  ear S00.43-•
  elbow S50.0-•
    with forearm —see Contusion, forearm
  epididymis S30.22
  epigastric region S30.1
  epiglottis S10.0
  esophagus (thoracic) S27.812
    cervical S10.0
  eyeball S05.1-•

Contusion (Continued)
  eyebrow S00.1-•
  eyelid (and periocular area) S00.1-•
  face NEC S00.83
  fallopian tube S37.529
    bilateral S37.522
    unilateral S37.521
  femoral triangle S30.1
  finger(s) S60.00
    with damage to nail (matrix) S60.10
    index S60.02-•
      with damage to nail S60.12-•
    little S60.05-•
      with damage to nail S60.15-•
    middle S60.03-•
      with damage to nail S60.13-•
    ring S60.04-•
      with damage to nail S60.14-•
    thumb —see Contusion, thumb
  flank S30.1
  foot (except toe(s) alone) S90.3-•
    toe —see Contusion, toe
  forearm S50.1-•
    elbow only —see Contusion, elbow
  forehead S00.83
  gallbladder S36.122
  genital organs, external
    female S30.202
    male S30.201
  globe (eye) —see Contusion, eyeball
  groin S30.1
  gum S00.532
  hand S60.22-•
    finger(s) —see Contusion, finger
    wrist —see Contusion, wrist
  head S00.93
    ear —see Contusion, ear
    eyelid —see Contusion, eyelid
    lip S00.531
    nose S00.33
    oral cavity S00.532
    scalp S00.03
    specified part NEC S00.83
  heart —see also Injury, heart S26.91
  heel —see Contusion, foot
  hepatic duct S36.13
  hip S70.0-•
  ileum S36.428
  iliac region S30.1
  inguinal region S30.1
  interscapular region S20.229
  intra-abdominal organ S36.92
    colon —see Injury, intestine, large, contusion
    liver S36.112
    pancreas —see Contusion, pancreas
    rectum S36.62
    small intestine —see Injury, intestine, small,
        contusion
    specified organ NEC S36.892
    spleen —see Contusion, spleen
    stomach S36.32
  iris (eye) —see Contusion, eyeball
  jaw S00.83
  jejunum S36.428
  kidney S37.01-•
    major (greater than 2 cm) S37.02-•
    minor (less than 2 cm) S37.01-•
  knee S80.0-•
  labium (majus) (minus) S30.23
  lacrimal apparatus, gland or sac S05.8X-•
  larynx S10.0
  leg (lower) S80.1-•
    knee —see Contusion, knee
  lens —see Contusion, eyeball
  lip S00.531
  liver S36.112
  lower back S30.0
  lumbar region S30.0
  lung S27.329
    bilateral S27.322
    unilateral S27.321

Contusion (Continued)
  malar region S00.83
  mastoid region S00.83
  membrane, brain —see Injury, intracranial,
      diffuse
    focal —see Injury, intracranial, focal
  mesentery S36.892
  mesosalpinx S37.892
  mouth S00.532
  muscle —see Contusion, by site
  nail
    finger —see Contusion, finger, with
        damage to nail
    toe —see Contusion, toe, with damage to
        nail
  nasal S00.33
  neck S10.93
    specified site NEC S10.83
    throat S10.0
  nerve —see Injury, nerve
  newborn P54.5
  nose S00.33
  occipital
    lobe (brain) —see Injury, intracranial,
        diffuse
    focal —see Injury, intracranial,
        focal
    region (scalp) S00.03
  orbit (region) (tissues) S05.1-•
  ovary S37.429
    bilateral S37.422
    unilateral S37.421
  palate S00.532
  pancreas S36.229
    body S36.221
    head S36.220
    tail S36.222
  parietal
    lobe (brain) —see Injury, intracranial,
        diffuse
    focal —see Injury, intracranial, focal
    region (scalp) S00.03
  pelvic organ S37.92
    adrenal gland S37.812
    bladder S37.22
    fallopian tube —see Contusion, fallopian
        tube
    kidney —see Contusion, kidney
    ovary —see Contusion, ovary
    prostate S37.822
    specified organ NEC S37.892
    ureter S37.12
    urethra S37.32
    uterus S37.62
  pelvis S30.0
  penis S30.21
  perineum
    female S30.23
    male S30.0
  periocular area S00.1-•
  peritoneum S36.81
  periurethral tissue —see Contusion,
      urethra
  pharynx S10.0
  pinna —see Contusion, ear
  popliteal space —see Contusion, knee
  prepuce S30.21
  prostate S37.822
  pubic region S30.1
  pudendum
    female S30.202
    male S30.201
  quadriceps femoris —see Contusion, thigh
  rectum S36.62
  retroperitoneum S36.892
  round ligament S37.892
  sacral region S30.0
  scalp S00.03
    due to birth injury P12.3
  scapular region —see Contusion, shoulder
  sclera —see Contusion, eyeball

▶ New   ⇒ Revised   ~~deleted~~ Deleted   • Use Additional Character(s)

▶ New   ⇒ Revised   ~~deleted~~ Deleted   ● Use Additional Character(s)

Corrosion (Continued)
  hand(s) (Continued)
    multiple sites with wrist T23.499
      first degree T23.599
      left T23.492
        first degree T23.592
        second degree T23.692
        third degree T23.792
      right T23.491
        first degree T23.591
        second degree T23.691
        third degree T23.791
      second degree T23.699
      third degree T23.799
    palm —see Corrosion, palm
    right T23.401
      first degree T23.501
      second degree T23.601
      third degree T23.701
    second degree T23.609
    third degree T23.709
    thumb —see Corrosion, thumb
  head (and face) (and neck) T20.40
    cheek —see Corrosion, cheek
    chin —see Corrosion, chin
    ear —see Corrosion, ear
    eye(s) only —see Corrosion, eye
    first degree T20.50
    forehead —see Corrosion, forehead
    lip —see Corrosion, lip
    multiple sites T20.49
      first degree T20.59
      second degree T20.69
      third degree T20.79
    neck —see Corrosion, neck
    nose —see Corrosion, nose
    scalp —see Corrosion, scalp
    second degree T20.60
    third degree T20.70
  hip(s) —see Corrosion, lower, limb
  inhalation —see Corrosion, respiratory
      tract
  internal organ(s) (see also Corrosion, by site)
      T28.90
    alimentary tract T28.7
      esophagus T28.6
    esophagus T28.6
    genitourinary T28.8
    mouth T28.5
    pharynx T28.5
    specified organ NEC T28.99
  interscapular region —see Corrosion, back,
      upper
  intestine (large) (small) T28.7
  knee T24.429
    first degree T24.529
    left T24.422
      first degree T24.522
      second degree T24.622
      third degree T24.722
    right T24.421
      first degree T24.521
      second degree T24.621
      third degree T24.721
    second degree T24.629
    third degree T24.729
  labium (majus) (minus) —see Corrosion,
      genital organs, external, female
  lacrimal apparatus, duct, gland or sac —see
      Corrosion, eye, specified site NEC
  larynx T27.4
    with lung T27.5
  leg(s) (meaning lower limb(s)) —see
      Corrosion, lower limb
  limb(s)
    lower —see Corrosion, lower, limb
    upper —see Corrosion, upper limb
  lip(s) T20.42
    first degree T20.52
    second degree T20.62
    third degree T20.72

Corrosion (Continued)
  lower
    back —see Corrosion, back
    limb T24.409
      ankle —see Corrosion, ankle
      calf —see Corrosion, calf
      first degree T24.509
      foot —see Corrosion, foot
      hip —see Corrosion, thigh
      knee —see Corrosion, knee
      left T24.402
        first degree T24.502
        second degree T24.602
        third degree T24.702
      multiple sites, except ankle and foot
          T24.499
        ankle and foot T25.499
          first degree T25.599
          left T25.492
            first degree T25.592
            second degree T25.692
            third degree T25.792
          right T25.491
            first degree T25.591
            second degree T25.691
            third degree T25.791
          second degree T25.699
          third degree T25.799
        first degree T24.599
        left T24.492
          first degree T24.592
          second degree T24.692
          third degree T24.792
        right T24.491
          first degree T24.591
          second degree T24.691
          third degree T24.791
        second degree T24.699
        third degree T24.799
      right T24.401
        first degree T24.501
        second degree T24.601
        third degree T24.701
      second degree T24.609
      thigh —see Corrosion, thigh
      third degree T24.709
  lung (with larynx and trachea) T27.5
  mouth T28.5
  neck T20.47
    first degree T20.57
    second degree T20.67
    third degree T20.77
  nose (septum) T20.44
    first degree T20.54
    second degree T20.64
    third degree T20.74
  ocular adnexa —see Corrosion, eye
  orbit region —see Corrosion, eyelid
  palm T23.459
    first degree T23.559
    left T23.452
      first degree T23.552
      second degree T23.652
      third degree T23.752
    right T23.451
      first degree T23.551
      second degree T23.651
      third degree T23.751
    second degree T23.659
    third degree T23.759
  partial thickness - code as Corrosion,
      unspecified degree, by site
  pelvis —see Corrosion, trunk
  penis —see Corrosion, genital organs,
      external, male
  perineum
    female —see Corrosion, genital organs,
        external, female
    male —see Corrosion, genital organs,
        external, male
  periocular area —see Corrosion, eyelid

Corrosion (Continued)
  pharynx T28.5
  rectum T28.7
  respiratory tract T27.7
    larynx —see Corrosion, larynx
    specified part NEC T27.6
    trachea —see Corrosion, larynx
  sac, lacrimal —see Corrosion, eye,
      specified site NEC
  scalp T20.45
    first degree T20.55
    second degree T20.65
    third degree T20.75
  scapular region T22.469
    first degree T22.569
    left T22.462
      first degree T22.562
      second degree T22.662
      third degree T22.762
    right T22.461
      first degree T22.561
      second degree T22.661
      third degree T22.761
    second degree T22.669
    third degree T22.769
  sclera —see Corrosion, eye, specified site NEC
  scrotum —see Corrosion, genital organs,
      external, male
  shoulder T22.459
    first degree T22.559
    left T22.452
      first degree T22.552
      second degree T22.652
      third degree T22.752
    right T22.451
      first degree T22.551
      second degree T22.651
      third degree T22.751
    second degree T22.659
    third degree T22.759
  stomach T28.7
  temple —see Corrosion, head
  testis —see Corrosion, genital organs,
      external, male
  thigh T24.419
    first degree T24.519
    left T24.412
      first degree T24.512
      second degree T24.612
      third degree T24.712
    right T24.411
      first degree T24.511
      second degree T24.611
      third degree T24.711
    second degree T24.619
    third degree T24.719
  thorax (external) —see Corrosion, trunk
  throat (meaning pharynx) T28.5
  thumb(s) T23.419
    first degree T23.519
    left T23.412
      first degree T23.512
      second degree T23.612
      third degree T23.712
    multiple sites with fingers T23.449
      first degree T23.549
      left T23.442
        first degree T23.542
        second degree T23.642
        third degree T23.742
      right T23.441
        first degree T23.541
        second degree T23.641
        third degree T23.741
      second degree T23.649
      third degree T23.749
    right T23.411
      first degree T23.511
      second degree T23.611
      third degree T23.711
    second degree T23.619
    third degree T23.719

Corrosion (Continued)
- toe T25.439
  - first degree T25.539
  - left T25.432
    - first degree T25.532
    - second degree T25.632
    - third degree T25.732
  - right T25.431
    - first degree T25.531
    - second degree T25.631
    - third degree T25.731
  - second degree T25.639
  - third degree T25.739
- tongue T28.5
- tonsil(s) T28.5
- total body —see Corrosion, multiple body regions
- trachea T27.4
  - with lung T27.5
- trunk T21.40
  - abdominal wall —see Corrosion, abdominal wall
  - anus —see Corrosion, buttock
  - axilla —see Corrosion, upper limb
  - back —see Corrosion, back
  - breast —see Corrosion, chest wall
  - buttock —see Corrosion, buttock
  - chest wall —see Corrosion, chest wall
  - first degree T21.50
  - flank —see Corrosion, abdominal wall
  - genital
    - female —see Corrosion, genital organs, external, female
    - male —see Corrosion, genital organs, external, male
  - groin —see Corrosion, abdominal wall
  - interscapular region —see Corrosion, back, upper
  - labia —see Corrosion, genital organs, external, female
  - lower back —see Corrosion, back
  - penis —see Corrosion, genital organs, external, male
  - perineum
    - female —see Corrosion, genital organs, external, female
    - male —see Corrosion, genital organs, external, male
  - scapular region —see Corrosion, upper limb
  - scrotum —see Corrosion, genital organs, external, male
  - second degree T21.60
  - shoulder —see Corrosion, upper limb
  - specified site NEC T21.49
    - first degree T21.59
    - second degree T21.69
    - third degree T21.79
  - testes —see Corrosion, genital organs, external, male
  - third degree T21.70
  - upper back —see Corrosion, back, upper
  - vagina T28.8
  - vulva —see Corrosion, genital organs, external, female
- unspecified site with extent of body surface involved specified
  - less than 10 percent T32.0
  - 10-19 percent (0-9 percent third degree) T32.10
    - with 10-19 percent third degree T32.11
  - 20-29 percent (0-9 percent third degree) T32.20
    - with
      - 10-19 percent third degree T32.21
      - 20-29 percent third degree T32.22
  - 30-39 percent (0-9 percent third degree) T32.30
    - with
      - 10-19 percent third degree T32.31
      - 20-29 percent third degree T32.32
      - 30-39 percent third degree T32.33

Corrosion (Continued)
- unspecified site with extent of body surface involved specified (Continued)
  - 40-49 percent (0-9 percent third degree) T32.40
    - with
      - 10-19 percent third degree T32.41
      - 20-29 percent third degree T32.42
      - 30-39 percent third degree T32.43
      - 40-49 percent third degree T32.44
  - 50-59 percent (0-9 percent third degree) T32.50
    - with
      - 10-19 percent third degree T32.51
      - 20-29 percent third degree T32.52
      - 30-39 percent third degree T32.53
      - 40-49 percent third degree T32.54
      - 50-59 percent third degree T32.55
  - 60-69 percent (0-9 percent third degree) T32.60
    - with
      - 10-19 percent third degree T32.61
      - 20-29 percent third degree T32.62
      - 30-39 percent third degree T32.63
      - 40-49 percent third degree T32.64
      - 50-59 percent third degree T32.65
      - 60-69 percent third degree T32.66
  - 70-79 percent (0-9 percent third degree) T32.70
    - with
      - 10-19 percent third degree T32.71
      - 20-29 percent third degree T32.72
      - 30-39 percent third degree T32.73
      - 40-49 percent third degree T32.74
      - 50-59 percent third degree T32.75
      - 60-69 percent third degree T32.76
      - 70-79 percent third degree T32.77
  - 80-89 percent (0-9 percent third degree) T32.80
    - with
      - 10-19 percent third degree T32.81
      - 20-29 percent third degree T32.82
      - 30-39 percent third degree T32.83
      - 40-49 percent third degree T32.84
      - 50-59 percent third degree T32.85
      - 60-69 percent third degree T32.86
      - 70-79 percent third degree T32.87
      - 80-89 percent third degree T32.88
  - 90 percent or more (0-9 percent third degree) T32.90
    - with
      - 10-19 percent third degree T32.91
      - 20-29 percent third degree T32.92
      - 30-39 percent third degree T32.93
      - 40-49 percent third degree T32.94
      - 50-59 percent third degree T32.95
      - 60-69 percent third degree T32.96
      - 70-79 percent third degree T32.97
      - 80-89 percent third degree T32.98
      - 90-99 percent third degree T32.99
- upper limb (axilla) (scapular region) T22.40
  - above elbow —see Corrosion, above elbow
  - axilla —see Corrosion, axilla
  - elbow —see Corrosion, elbow
  - first degree T22.50
  - forearm —see Corrosion, forearm
  - hand —see Corrosion, hand
  - interscapular region —see Corrosion, back, upper
  - multiple sites T22.499
    - first degree T22.599
    - left T22.492
      - first degree T22.592
      - second degree T22.692
      - third degree T22.792
    - right T22.491
      - first degree T22.591
      - second degree T22.691
      - third degree T22.791
    - second degree T22.699
    - third degree T22.799
  - scapular region —see Corrosion, scapular region

Corrosion (Continued)
- upper limb (axilla) (scapular region) (Continued)
  - second degree T22.60
  - shoulder —see Corrosion, shoulder
  - third degree T22.70
  - wrist —see Corrosion, hand
- uterus T28.8
- vagina T28.8
- vulva —see Corrosion, genital organs, external, female
- wrist T23.479
  - first degree T23.579
  - left T23.472
    - first degree T23.572
    - second degree T23.672
    - third degree T23.772
  - multiple sites with hand T23.499
    - first degree T23.599
    - left T23.492
      - first degree T23.592
      - second degree T23.692
      - third degree T23.792
    - right T23.491
      - first degree T23.591
      - second degree T23.691
      - third degree T23.791
    - second degree T23.699
    - third degree T23.799
  - right T23.471
    - first degree T23.571
    - second degree T23.671
    - third degree T23.771
  - second degree T23.679
  - third degree T23.779
Corrosive burn —see Corrosion
Corsican fever —see Malaria
Cortical —see condition
Cortico-adrenal —see condition
Coryza (acute) J00
- with grippe or influenza —see Influenza, with, respiratory manifestations NEC
- syphilitic
  - congenital (chronic) A50.05
▶ Co-sleeping, child-caregiver Z72.823
Costen's syndrome or complex M26.69
Costiveness —see Constipation
Costochondritis M94.0
Cot death R99
Cotard's syndrome F22
Cotia virus B08.8
Cotton wool spots (retinal) H35.81
Cotungo's disease —see Sciatica
Cough (affected) (epidemic) (nervous) R05.9
- with hemorrhage —see Hemoptysis
- acute R05.1
- bronchial R05.8
  - with grippe or influenza —see Influenza, with, respiratory manifestations NEC
- chronic R05.3
- functional F45.8
- hysterical F45.8
- laryngeal, spasmodic R05.8
- paroxysmal, due to Bordetella pertussis (without pneumonia) A37.00
  - with pneumonia A37.01
- persistent R05.3
- refractory R05.3
- psychogenic F45.8
- smokers' J41.0
- specified NEC R05.8
- subacute R05.2
- syncope R05.4
- tea taster's B49
- unexplained R05.3
Counseling (for) Z71.9
- abuse NEC
  - perpetrator Z69.82
  - victim Z69.81
- alcohol abuser Z71.41
  - family Z71.42
- child abuse
  - nonparental
    - perpetrator Z69.021
    - victim Z69.020

Counseling (Continued)
parental
perpetrator Z69.011
victim Z69.010
consanguinity Z71.89
contraceptive Z30.09
dietary Z71.3
drug abuser Z71.51
family member Z71.52
exercise Z71.82
family Z71.89
fertility preservation (prior to cancer therapy)
(prior to removal of gonads) Z31.62
for non-attending third party Z71.0
related to sexual behavior or orientation Z70.2
genetic
nonprocreative Z71.83
procreative NEC Z31.5
gestational carrier Z31.7
health (advice) (education) (instruction) —see
Counseling, medical
risk for travel (international) Z71.84
human immunodeficiency virus (HIV) Z71.7
immunization safety Z71.85
impotence Z70.1
insulin pump use Z46.81
medical (for) Z71.9
boarding school resident Z59.3
consanguinity Z71.89
feared complaint and no disease found Z71.1
human immunodeficiency virus (HIV) Z71.7
institutional resident Z59.3
on behalf of another Z71.0
related to sexual behavior or orientation
Z70.2
person living alone Z60.2
specified reason NEC Z71.89
natural family planning
procreative Z31.61
to avoid pregnancy Z30.02
▶ pediatric-to-adult transition Z71.87
perpetrator (of)
abuse NEC Z69.82
child abuse
non-parental Z69.021
parental Z69.011
rape NEC Z69.82
spousal abuse Z69.12
procreative NEC Z31.69
fertility preservation (prior to cancer therapy)
(prior to removal of gonads) Z31.62
using natural family planning Z31.61
promiscuity Z70.1
rape victim Z69.81
religious Z71.81
safety for travel (international) Z71.84
sex, sexual (related to) Z70.9
attitude(s) Z70.0
behavior or orientation Z70.1
combined concerns Z70.3
non-responsiveness Z70.1
on behalf of third party Z70.2
specified reason NEC Z70.8
▶ socioeconomic factors Z71.88
specified reason NEC Z71.89
spiritual Z71.81
spousal abuse (perpetrator) Z69.12
victim Z69.11
substance abuse Z71.89
alcohol Z71.41
drug Z71.51
tobacco Z71.6
travel (international) Z71.84
tobacco use Z71.6
use (of)
insulin pump Z46.81
vaccine product safety Z71.85
victim (of)
abuse Z69.81
child abuse
by parent Z69.010
non-parental Z69.020
rape NEC Z69.81
Coupled rhythm R00.8

Couvelaire syndrome or uterus (complicating
delivery) O45.8X-●
COVID-19 U07.1
condition post U09.9
contact (with) Z20.822
exposure (to) Z20.822
history of (personal) Z86.16
long (haul) U09.9
pneumonia J12.82
screening Z11.52
sequelae (post acute) U09.9
Cowperitis —see Urethritis
Cowper's gland —see condition
Cowpox B08.010
due to vaccination T88.1
Coxa
magna M91.4-●
plana M91.2-●
valga (acquired) —see also Deformity, limb,
specified type NEC, thigh
congenital Q65.81
sequelae (late effect) of rickets E64.3
vara (acquired) —see also Deformity, limb,
specified type NEC, thigh
congenital Q65.82
sequelae (late effect) of rickets E64.3
Coxalgia, coxalgic (nontuberculous) —see also
Pain, joint, hip
tuberculous A18.02
Coxitis —see Monoarthritis, hip
Coxsackie (virus) (infection) B34.1
as cause of disease classified elsewhere B97.11
carditis B33.20
central nervous system NEC A88.8
endocarditis B33.21
enteritis A08.39
meningitis (aseptic) A87.0
myocarditis B33.22
pericarditis B33.23
pharyngitis B08.5
pleurodynia B33.0
specific disease NEC B33.8
Crabs, meaning pubic lice B85.3
Crack baby P04.41
Cracked nipple N64.0
associated with
lactation O92.13
pregnancy O92.11-●
puerperium O92.12
Cracked tooth K03.81
Cradle cap L21.0
Craft neurosis F48.8
Cramp(s) R25.2
abdominal —see Pain, abdominal
bathing T75.1
colic R10.83
psychogenic F45.8
due to immersion T75.1
fireman T67.2
heat T67.2
immersion T75.1
intestinal —see Pain, abdominal
psychogenic F45.8
leg, sleep related G47.62
limb (lower) (upper) NEC R25.2
sleep related G47.62
linotypist's F48.8
organic G25.89
muscle (limb) (general) R25.2
due to immersion T75.1
psychogenic F45.8
occupational (hand) F48.8
organic G25.89
salt-depletion E87.1
sleep related, leg G47.62
stoker's T67.2
swimmer's T75.1
telegrapher's F48.8
organic G25.89
typist's F48.8
organic G25.89
uterus N94.89
menstrual —see Dysmenorrhea

Cramp(s) (Continued)
writer's F48.8
organic G25.89
Cranial —see condition
Craniocleidodysostosis Q74.0
Craniofenestria (skull) Q75.8
Craniolacunia (skull) Q75.8
Craniopagus Q89.4
Craniopathy, metabolic M85.2
Craniopharyngeal —see condition
Craniopharyngioma D44.4
Craniorachischisis (totalis) Q00.1
Cranioschisis Q75.8
Craniostenosis Q75.0
Craniosynostosis Q75.0
Craniotabes (cause unknown) M83.8
neonatal P96.3
rachitic E64.3
syphilitic A50.56
Cranium —see condition
Craw-craw —see Onchocerciasis
Creaking joint —see Derangement, joint,
specified type NEC
Creeping
eruption B76.9
palsy or paralysis G12.22
Crenated tongue K14.8
Creotoxism A05.9
Crepitus
caput Q75.8
joint —see Derangement, joint, specified type
NEC
Crescent or conus choroid, congenital Q14.3
CREST syndrome M34.1
Cretin, cretinism (congenital) (endemic)
(nongoitrous) (sporadic) E00.9
pelvis
with disproportion (fetopelvic) O33.0
causing obstructed labor O65.0
type
hypothyroid E00.1
mixed E00.2
myxedematous E00.1
neurological E00.0
Creutzfeldt-Jakob disease or syndrome (with
dementia) A81.00
familial A81.09
iatrogenic A81.09
specified NEC A81.09
sporadic A81.09
variant (vCJD) A81.01
Crib death R99
Cribriform hymen Q52.3
Cri-du-chat syndrome Q93.4
Crigler-Najjar disease or syndrome E80.5
Crime, victim of Z65.4
Crimean hemorrhagic fever A98.0
Criminalism F60.2
Crisis
abdomen R10.0
acute reaction F43.0
addisonian E27.2
adrenal (cortical) E27.2
celiac K90.0
Dietl's N13.8
emotional —see also Disorder, adjustment
acute reaction to stress F43.0
specific to childhood and adolescence F93.8
glaucomatocyclitic —see Glaucoma,
secondary, inflammation
heart —see Failure, heart
nitritoid I95.2
correct substance properly administered —
see Table of Drugs and Chemicals, by
drug, adverse effect
overdose or wrong substance given
or taken —see Table of Drugs and
Chemicals, by drug, poisoning
oculogyric H51.8
psychogenic F45.8
Pel's (tabetic) A52.11
psychosexual identity F64.2
renal N28.0

Crisis (Continued)
▶ sickle-cell (see also Disease, sickle-cell, by type, with crisis) D57.00
  with
    acute chest syndrome D57.01
    cerebral vascular involvement D57.03
    crisis (painful) D57.00
      with complication specified NEC D57.09
    ▶complication specified NEC D57.09
    splenic sequestration D57.02
    vasoocclusive pain D57.00
  state (acute reaction) F43.0
  tabetic A52.11
  thyroid —see Thyrotoxicosis with thyroid storm
  thyrotoxic —see Thyrotoxicosis with thyroid storm
Crocq's disease (acrocyanosis) I73.89
Crohn's disease —see Enteritis, regional
Crooked septum, nasal J34.2
Cross syndrome E70.328
Crossbite (anterior) (posterior) M26.24
Cross-eye —see Strabismus, convergent concomitant
Croup, croupous (catarrhal) (infectious) (inflammatory) (nondiphtheritic) J05.0
  bronchial J20.9
  diphtheritic A36.2
  false J38.5
  spasmodic J38.5
    diphtheritic A36.2
  stridulous J38.5
    diphtheritic A36.2
Crouzon's disease Q75.1
Crowding, tooth, teeth, fully erupted M26.31
CRST syndrome M34.1
Cruchet's disease A85.8
Cruelty in children —see also Disorder, conduct
Crural ulcer —see Ulcer, lower limb
Crush, crushed, crushing T14.8
  abdomen S38.1
  ankle S97.0-●
  arm (upper) (and shoulder) S47.-●
  axilla —see Crush, arm
  back, lower S38.1
  buttock S38.1
  cheek S07.0
  chest S28.0
  cranium S07.1
  ear S07.0
  elbow S57.0-●
  extremity
    lower
      ankle —see Crush, ankle
      below knee —see Crush, leg
      foot —see Crush, foot
      hip —see Crush, hip
      knee —see Crush, knee
      thigh —see Crush, thigh
      toe —see Crush, toe
    upper
      below elbow S67.9-●
      elbow —see Crush, elbow
      finger —see Crush, finger
      forearm —see Crush, forearm
      hand —see Crush, hand
      thumb —see Crush, thumb
      upper arm —see Crush, arm
      wrist —see Crush, wrist
  face S07.0
  finger(s) S67.1-●
    with hand (and wrist) —see Crush, hand, specified site NEC
    index S67.19-●
    little S67.19-●
    middle S67.19-●
    ring S67.19-●
    thumb —see Crush, thumb
  foot S97.8-●
    toe —see Crush, toe
  forearm S57.8-●
  genitalia, external
    female S38.002
      vagina S38.03
      vulva S38.03

Crush, crushed, crushing (Continued)
  genitalia, external (Continued)
    male S38.001
      penis S38.01
      scrotum S38.02
      testis S38.02
  hand (except fingers alone) S67.2-●
    with wrist S67.4-●
  head S07.9
    specified NEC S07.8
  heel —see Crush, foot
  hip S77.0-●
    with thigh S77.2-●
  internal organ (abdomen, chest, or pelvis) NEC T14.8
  knee S87.0-●
  labium (majus) (minus) S38.03
  larynx S17.0
  leg (lower) S87.8-●
    knee —see Crush, knee
  lip S07.0
  lower
    back S38.1
    leg —see Crush, leg
  neck S17.9
  nerve —see Injury, nerve
  nose S07.0
  pelvis S38.1
  penis S38.01
  scalp S07.8
  scapular region —see Crush, arm
  scrotum S38.02
  severe, unspecified site T14.8
  shoulder (and upper arm) —see Crush, arm
  skull S07.1
  syndrome (complication of trauma) T79.5
  testis S38.02
  thigh S77.1-●
    with hip S77.2-●
  throat S17.8
  thumb S67.0-●
    with hand (and wrist) —see Crush, hand, specified site NEC
  toe(s) S97.10-●
    great S97.11-●
    lesser S97.12-●
  trachea S17.0
  vagina S38.03
  vulva S38.03
  wrist S67.3-●
    with hand S67.4-●
Crusta lactea L21.0
Crusts R23.4
Crutch paralysis —see Injury, brachial plexus
Cruveilhier-Baumgarten cirrhosis, disease or syndrome K74.69
Cruveilhier's atrophy or disease G12.8
Crying (constant) (continuous) (excessive)
  child, adolescent, or adult R45.83
  infant (baby) (newborn) R68.11
Cryofibrinogenemia D89.2
Cryoglobulinemia (essential) (idiopathic) (mixed) (primary) (purpura) (secondary) (vasculitis) D89.1
  with lung involvement D89.1 [J99]
Cryptitis (anal) (rectal) K62.89
Cryptococcosis, cryptococcus (infection) (neoformans) B45.9
  bone B45.3
  cerebral B45.1
  cutaneous B45.2
  disseminated B45.7
  generalized B45.7
  meningitis B45.1
  meningocerebralis B45.1
  osseous B45.3
  pulmonary B45.0
  skin B45.2
  specified NEC B45.8
Cryptopapillitis (anus) K62.89
Cryptophthalmos Q11.2
  syndrome Q87.0

Cryptorchid, cryptorchism, cryptorchidism Q53.9
  bilateral Q53.20
    abdominal Q53.211
    perineal Q53.22
  unilateral Q53.10
    abdominal Q53.111
    perineal Q53.12
Cryptosporidiosis A07.2
  hepatobiliary B88.8
  respiratory B88.8
Cryptostromosis J67.6
Crystalluria R82.998
Cubitus
  congenital Q68.8
  valgus (acquired) M21.0-●
    congenital Q68.8
    sequelae (late effect) of rickets E64.3
  varus (acquired) M21.1-●
    congenital Q68.8
    sequelae (late effect) of rickets E64.3
Cultural deprivation or shock Z60.3
Curling esophagus K22.4
Curling's ulcer —see Ulcer, peptic, acute
Curschmann (-Batten) (-Steinert) disease or syndrome G71.11
Curse, Ondine's —see Apnea, sleep
Curvature
  organ or site, congenital NEC —see Distortion
  penis (lateral) Q55.61
  Pott's (spinal) A18.01
  radius, idiopathic, progressive (congenital) Q74.0
  spine (acquired) (angular) (idiopathic) (incorrect) (postural) —see Dorsopathy, deforming
    congenital Q67.5
    due to or associated with
      Charcot-Marie-Tooth disease —see also subcategory M49.8 G60.0
      osteitis
        deformans M88.88
        fibrosa cystica —see also subcategory M49.8 E21.0
      tuberculosis (Pott's curvature) A18.01
    sequelae (late effect) of rickets E64.3
    tuberculous A18.01
Cushingoid due to steroid therapy E24.2
  correct substance properly administered —see Table of Drugs and Chemicals, by drug, adverse effect
  overdose or wrong substance given or taken —see Table of Drugs and Chemicals, by drug, poisoning
Cushing's
  syndrome or disease E24.9
    drug-induced E24.2
    iatrogenic E24.2
    pituitary-dependent E24.0
    specified NEC E24.8
  ulcer —see Ulcer, peptic, acute
Cusp, Carabelli - omit code
Cut (external) —see also Laceration
  muscle —see Injury, muscle
Cutaneous —see also condition
  hemorrhage R23.3
  larva migrans B76.9
Cutis —see also condition
  hyperelastica Q82.8
    acquired L57.4
  laxa (hyperelastica) —see Dermatolysis
  marmorata R23.8
  osteosis L94.2
  pendula —see Dermatolysis
  rhomboidalis nuchae L57.2
  verticis gyrata Q82.8
    acquired L91.8
Cyanosis R23.0
  due to
    ⇨patent foramen botalli Q21.12
    ⇨persistent foramen ovale Q21.12
  enterogenous D74.8
  paroxysmal digital —see Raynaud's disease
    with gangrene I73.01
  retina, retinal H35.89

Cyanotic heart disease I24.9
  congenital Q24.9
Cycle
  anovulatory N97.0
  menstrual, irregular N92.6
Cyclencephaly Q04.9
Cyclical vomiting, in migraine (see also
    Vomiting, cyclical) G43.A0
  psychogenic F50.89
Cyclitis —see also Iridocyclitis H20.9
  chronic —see Iridocyclitis, chronic
  Fuchs' heterochromic H20.81-●
  granulomatous —see Iridocyclitis, chronic
  lens-induced —see Iridocyclitis,
      lens-induced
  posterior H30.2-●
Cycloid personality F34.0
Cyclophoria H50.54
Cyclopia, cyclops Q87.0
Cyclopism Q87.0
Cyclosporiasis A07.4
Cyclothymia F34.0
Cyclothymic personality F34.0
Cyclotropia H50.41-●
Cylindroma —see also Neoplasm, malignant,
    by site
  eccrine dermal —see Neoplasm, skin, benign
  skin —see Neoplasm, skin, benign
Cylindruria R82.998
Cynanche
  diphtheritic A36.2
  tonsillaris J36
Cynophobia F40.218
Cynorexia R63.2
Cyphosis —see Kyphosis
Cyprus fever —see Brucellosis
Cyst (colloid) (mucous) (simple) (retention)
  adenoid (infected) J35.8
  adrenal gland E27.8
    congenital Q89.1
  air, lung J98.4
  allantoic Q64.4
  alveolar process (jaw bone) M27.40
  amnion, amniotic O41.8X-●
  aneurysmal M27.49
  anterior
    chamber (eye) —see Cyst, iris
    nasopalatine K09.1
  antrum J34.1
  anus K62.89
  apical (tooth) (periodontal) K04.8
  appendix K38.8
  arachnoid, brain (acquired) G93.0
    congenital Q04.6
  arytenoid J38.7
  Baker's M71.2-●
    ruptured M66.0
    tuberculous A18.02
  Bartholin's gland N75.0
  bile duct (common) (hepatic) K83.5
  bladder (multiple) (trigone) N32.89
  blue dome (breast) —see Cyst, breast
  bone (local) NEC M85.60
    aneurysmal M85.50
      ankle M85.57-●
      foot M85.57-●
      forearm M85.53-●
      hand M85.54-●
      jaw M27.49
      lower leg M85.56-●
      multiple site M85.59
      neck M85.58
      rib M85.58
      shoulder M85.51-●
      skull M85.58
      specified site NEC M85.58
      thigh M85.55-●
      toe M85.57-●
      upper arm M85.52-●
      vertebra M85.58
    solitary M85.40
      ankle M85.47-●
      fibula M85.46-●

Cyst (Continued)
  bone NEC (Continued)
    solitary (Continued)
      foot M85.47-●
      hand M85.44-●
      humerus M85.42-●
      jaw M27.49
      neck M85.48
      pelvis M85.45-●
      radius M85.43-●
      rib M85.48
      shoulder M85.41-●
      skull M85.48
      specified site NEC M85.48
      tibia M85.46-●
      toe M85.47-●
      ulna M85.43-●
      vertebra M85.48
    specified type NEC M85.60
      ankle M85.67-●
      foot M85.67-●
      forearm M85.63-●
      hand M85.64-●
      jaw M27.40
        developmental (nonodontogenic) K09.1
          odontogenic K09.0
        latent M27.0
      lower leg M85.66-●
      multiple site M85.69
      neck M85.68
      rib M85.68
      shoulder M85.61-●
      skull M85.68
      specified site NEC M85.68
      thigh M85.65-●
      toe M85.67-●
      upper arm M85.62-●
      vertebra M85.68
  brain (acquired) G93.0
    congenital Q04.6
    hydatid B67.99 [G94]
    third ventricle (colloid), congenital Q04.6
  branchial (cleft) Q18.0
  branchiogenic Q18.0
  breast (benign) (blue dome) (pedunculated)
      (solitary) N60.0-●
    involution —see Dysplasia, mammary,
        specified type NEC
    sebaceous —see Dysplasia, mammary,
        specified type NEC
  broad ligament (benign) N83.8
  bronchogenic (mediastinal) (sequestration)
      J98.4
    congenital Q33.0
  buccal K09.8
  bulbourethral gland N36.8
  bursa, bursal NEC M71.30
    with rupture —see Rupture, synovium
    ankle M71.37-●
    elbow M71.32-●
    foot M71.37-●
    hand M71.34-●
    hip M71.35-●
    multiple sites M71.39
    pharyngeal J39.2
    popliteal space —see Cyst, Baker's
    shoulder M71.31-●
    specified site NEC M71.38
    wrist M71.33-●
  calcifying odontogenic D16.5
    upper jaw (bone) (maxilla) D16.4
  canal of Nuck (female) N94.89
    congenital Q52.4
  canthus —see Cyst, conjunctiva
  carcinomatous —see Neoplasm, malignant,
    by site
  cauda equina G95.89
  cavum septi pellucidi —see Cyst, brain
  celomic (pericardium) Q24.8
  cerebellopontine (angle) —see Cyst, brain
  cerebellum —see Cyst, brain
  cerebral —see Cyst, brain
  cervical lateral Q18.0

Cyst (Continued)
  cervix NEC N88.8
    embryonic Q51.6
    nabothian N88.8
  chiasmal optic NEC —see Disorder, optic,
      chiasm
  chocolate (ovary) N80.10-●
  choledochus, congenital Q44.4
  chorion O41.8X-●
  choroid plexus G93.0
    congenital Q04.6
  ciliary body —see Cyst, iris
  clitoris N90.7
  colon K63.89
  common (bile) duct K83.5
  congenital NEC Q89.8
    adrenal gland Q89.1
    epiglottis Q31.8
    esophagus Q39.8
    fallopian tube Q50.4
    kidney Q61.00
      more than one (multiple) Q61.02
        specified as polycystic Q61.3
          adult type Q61.2
          infantile type NEC Q61.19
            collecting duct dilation Q61.11
      solitary Q61.01
    larynx Q31.8
    liver Q44.6
    lung Q33.0
    mediastinum Q34.1
    ovary Q50.1
    oviduct Q50.4
    periurethral (tissue) Q64.79
    prepuce Q55.69
    salivary gland (any) Q38.4
    sublingual Q38.6
    submaxillary gland Q38.6
    thymus (gland) Q89.2
    tongue Q38.3
    ureterovesical orifice Q62.8
    vulva Q52.79
  conjunctiva H11.44-●
  cornea H18.89-●
  corpora quadrigemina G93.0
  corpus
    albicans N83.29-●
    luteum (hemorrhagic) (ruptured) N83.1-●
  Cowper's gland (benign) (infected) N36.8
  cranial meninges G93.0
  craniobuccal pouch E23.6
  craniopharyngeal pouch E23.6
  cystic duct K82.8
  Cysticercus —see Cysticercosis
  Dandy-Walker Q03.1
    with spina bifida —see Spina bifida
  dental (root) K04.8
    developmental K09.0
    eruption K09.0
    primordial K09.0
  dentigerous (mandible) (maxilla) K09.0
  dermoid —see Neoplasm, benign, by site
    with malignant transformation C56.-●
    implantation
      external area or site (skin) NEC L72.0
      iris —see Cyst, iris, implantation
      vagina N89.8
      vulva N90.7
    mouth K09.8
    oral soft tissue K09.8
    sacrococcygeal —see Cyst, pilonidal
  developmental K09.1
    odontogenic K09.0
    oral region (nonodontogenic) K09.1
    ovary, ovarian Q50.1
  dura (cerebral) G93.0
    spinal G96.198
  ear (external) Q18.1
  echinococcal —see Echinococcus
  embryonic
    cervix uteri Q51.6
    fallopian tube Q50.4
    vagina Q52.4

Cyst (Continued)
   endometrium, endometrial (uterus) N85.8
     ectopic —see Endometriosis
   enterogenous Q43.8
   epidermal, epidermoid (inclusion) (see also
     Cyst, skin) L72.0
     mouth K09.8
     oral soft tissue K09.8
   epididymis N50.3
   epiglottis J38.7
   epiphysis cerebri E34.8
   epithelial (inclusion) L72.0
   epoophoron Q50.5
   eruption K09.0
   esophagus K22.89
   ethmoid sinus J34.1
   external female genital organs NEC N90.7
   eye NEC H57.89
     congenital Q15.8
   eyelid (sebaceous) H02.829
     infected —see Hordeolum
     left H02.826
       lower H02.825
       upper H02.824
     right H02.823
       lower H02.822
       upper H02.821
   fallopian tube N83.8
     congenital Q50.4
   fimbrial (twisted) Q50.4
   fissural (oral region) K09.1
   follicle (graafian) (hemorrhagic) N83.0-•
     nabothian N88.8
   follicular (atretic) (hemorrhagic) (ovarian)
     N83.0-•
     dentigerous K09.0
     odontogenic K09.0
     skin L72.9
     specified NEC L72.8
   frontal sinus J34.1
   gallbladder K82.8
   ganglion —see Ganglion
   Gartner's duct Q52.4
   gingiva K09.0
   gland of Moll —see Cyst, eyelid
   globulomaxillary K09.1
   graafian follicle (hemorrhagic) N83.0-•
   granulosal lutein (hemorrhagic) N83.1-•
   hemangiomatous D18.00
     intra-abdominal D18.03
     intracranial D18.02
     skin D18.01
     specified site NEC D18.09
   hemorrhagic M27.49
   hydatid —see also Echinococcus B67.90
     brain B67.99 [G94]
     liver —see also Cyst, liver, hydatid B67.8
     lung NEC B67.99 [J99]
     Morgagni
       female Q50.5
       male (epididymal) Q55.4
         testicular Q55.29
     specified site NEC B67.99
   hymen N89.8
     embryonic Q52.4
   hypopharynx J39.2
   hypophysis, hypophyseal (duct) (recurrent)
     E23.6
     cerebri E23.6
   implantation (dermoid)
     external area or site (skin) NEC L72.0
     iris —see Cyst, iris, implantation
     vagina N89.8
     vulva N90.7
   incisive canal K09.1
   inclusion (epidermal) (epithelial)
     (epidermoid) (squamous) L72.0
     not of skin - code under Cyst, by site
   intestine (large) (small) K63.89
   intracranial —see Cyst, brain
   intraligamentous —see also Disorder, ligament
     knee —see Derangement, knee

Cyst (Continued)
   intrasellar E23.6
   iris H21.309
     exudative H21.31-•
     idiopathic H21.30-•
     implantation H21.32-•
     parasitic H21.33-•
     pars plana (primary) H21.34-•
       exudative H21.35-•
   jaw (bone) M27.40
     aneurysmal M27.49
     developmental (odontogenic) K09.0
     fissural K09.1
     hemorrhagic M27.49
     traumatic M27.49
   joint NEC —see Disorder, joint, specified type
     NEC
▸kidney N28.1
   ▸acquired N28.1
     calyceal —see Hydronephrosis
     congenital Q61.00
     more than one (multiple) Q61.02
       specified as polycystic Q61.3
         adult type (autosomal dominant)
           Q61.2
         infantile type (autosomal recessive)
           NEC Q61.19
             collecting duct dilation Q61.11
     pyelogenic —see Hydronephrosis
     simple N28.1
   ▸solitary (single) N28.1
     acquired N28.1
▸congenital Q61.01
   labium (majus) (minus) N90.7
     sebaceous N90.7
   lacrimal —see also Disorder, lacrimal system,
     specified NEC
     gland H04.13-•
     passages or sac —see Disorder, lacrimal
       system, specified NEC
   larynx J38.7
   lateral periodontal K09.0
   lens H27.8
     congenital Q12.8
   lip (gland) K13.0
   liver (idiopathic) (simple) K76.89
     congenital Q44.6
     hydatid B67.8
       granulosus B67.0
       multilocularis B67.5
   lung J98.4
     congenital Q33.0
     giant bullous J43.9
   lutein N83.1-•
   lymphangiomatous D18.1
   lymphoepithelial, oral soft tissue K09.8
   macula —see Degeneration, macula, hole
   malignant —see Neoplasm, malignant, by site
   mammary gland —see Cyst, breast
   mandible M27.40
     dentigerous K09.0
     radicular K04.8
   maxilla M27.40
     dentigerous K09.0
     radicular K04.8
   medial, face and neck Q18.8
   median
     anterior maxillary K09.1
     palatal K09.1
   mediastinum, congenital Q34.1
   meibomian (gland) —see Chalazion
     infected —see Hordeolum
   membrane, brain G93.0
   meninges (cerebral) G93.0
     spinal G96.198
   meniscus, knee —see Derangement, knee,
     meniscus, cystic
   mesentery, mesenteric K66.8
     chyle I89.8
   mesonephric duct
     female Q50.5
     male Q55.4
   milk N64.89

Cyst (Continued)
   Morgagni (hydatid)
     female Q50.5
     male (epididymal) Q55.4
       testicular Q55.29
   mouth K09.8
   Müllerian duct Q50.4
     appendix testis Q55.29
     cervix Q51.6
     fallopian tube Q50.4
     female Q50.4
     male Q55.29
     prostatic utricle Q55.4
     vagina (embryonal) Q52.4
   multilocular (ovary) D39.10
     benign —see Neoplasm, benign, by site
   myometrium N85.8
   nabothian (follicle) (ruptured) N88.8
   nasoalveolar K09.1
   nasolabial K09.1
   nasopalatine (anterior) (duct) K09.1
   nasopharynx J39.2
   neoplastic —see Neoplasm, uncertain
     behavior, by site
     benign —see Neoplasm, benign, by site
   nerve root
     cervical G96.191
     lumbar G96.191
     sacral G96.191
     thoracic G96.191
   nervous system NEC G96.89
   neuroenteric (congenital) Q06.8
   nipple —see Cyst, breast
   nose (turbinates) J34.1
     sinus J34.1
   odontogenic, developmental K09.0
   omentum (lesser) K66.8
     congenital Q45.8
   ora serrata —see Cyst, retina, ora serrata
   oral
     region K09.9
       developmental (nonodontogenic) K09.1
       specified NEC K09.8
     soft tissue K09.9
       specified NEC K09.8
   orbit H05.81-•
   ovary, ovarian (twisted) N83.20-•
     adherent N83.20-•
   ▸chocolate N80.10-•
     corpus
       albicans N83.29-•
       luteum (hemorrhagic) N83.1-•
     dermoid D27.9
     developmental Q50.1
     due to failure of involution NEC N83.20-•
   ▸endometrial N80.10-•
     follicular (graafian) (hemorrhagic) N83.0-•
     hemorrhagic N83.20-•
     in pregnancy or childbirth O34.8-•
       with obstructed labor O65.5
     multilocular D39.10
     pseudomucinous D27.9
     retention N83.29-•
     serous N83.20-•
     specified NEC N83.29-•
     theca lutein (hemorrhagic) N83.1-•
     tuberculous A18.18
   oviduct N83.8
   palate (median) (fissural) K09.1
   palatine papilla (jaw) K09.1
   pancreas, pancreatic (hemorrhagic) (true) K86.2
     congenital Q45.2
     false K86.3
   paralabral
     hip M24.85-•
     shoulder S43.43-•
   paramesonephric duct Q50.4
     female Q50.4
     male Q55.29
   paranephric N28.1
   paraphysis, cerebri, congenital Q04.6
   parasitic B89
   parathyroid (gland) E21.4

▶ New   ⇛ Revised   deleted Deleted   • Use Additional Character(s)

Cyst (Continued)
  paratubal N83.8
  paraurethral duct N36.8
  paroophoron Q50.5
  parotid gland K11.6
  parovarian Q50.5
  pelvis, female N94.89
    in pregnancy or childbirth O34.8-•
      causing obstructed labor O65.5
  penis (sebaceous) N48.89
  periapical K04.8
  pericardial (congenital) Q24.8
    acquired (secondary) I31.8
  pericoronal K09.0
  perineural G96.191
  periodontal K04.8
    lateral K09.0
  peripelvic (lymphatic) N28.1
  peritoneum K66.8
    chylous I89.8
  periventricular, acquired, newborn P91.1
  pharynx (wall) J39.2
  pilar L72.11
  pilonidal (infected) (rectum) L05.91
    with abscess L05.01
    malignant C44.59-•
  pituitary (duct) (gland) E23.6
  placenta O43.19-•
  pleura J94.8
  popliteal —see Cyst, Baker's
  porencephalic Q04.6
    acquired G93.0
  postanal (infected) —see Cyst, pilonidal
  postmastoidectomy cavity (mucosal) —see
    Complications, postmastoidectomy, cyst
  preauricular Q18.1
  prepuce N47.4
    congenital Q55.69
  primordial (jaw) K09.0
  prostate N42.83
  pseudomucinous (ovary) D27.9
  pupillary, miotic H21.27-•
  radicular (residual) K04.8
  radiculodental K04.8
  ranular K11.8
  Rathke's pouch E23.6
  rectum (epithelium) (mucous) K62.89
  renal —see Cyst, kidney
  residual (radicular) K04.8
  retention (ovary) N83.29-•
    salivary gland K11.6
  retina H33.19-•
    ora serrata H33.11-•
    parasitic H33.12-•
  retroperitoneal K68.9
  sacrococcygeal (dermoid) —see Cyst,
    pilonidal
  salivary gland or duct (mucous extravasation
    or retention) K11.6
  Sampson's N80.10-•
  sclera H15.89
  scrotum L72.9
    sebaceous L72.3
  sebaceous (duct) (gland) L72.3
    breast —see Dysplasia, mammary, specified
      type NEC
    eyelid —see Cyst, eyelid
    genital organ NEC
      female N94.89
      male N50.89
    scrotum L72.3
  semilunar cartilage (knee) (multiple) —see
    Derangement, knee, meniscus, cystic
  seminal vesicle N50.89
  serous (ovary) N83.20-•
  sinus (accessory) (nasal) J34.1
  Skene's gland N36.8
  skin L72.9
    breast —see Dysplasia, mammary, specified
      type NEC
    epidermal, epidermoid L72.0
    epithelial L72.0
    eyelid —see Cyst, eyelid

Cyst (Continued)
  skin (Continued)
    genital organ NEC
      female N90.7
      male N50.89
    inclusion L72.0
    scrotum L72.9
    sebaceous L72.3
    sweat gland or duct L74.8
  solitary
    bone —see Cyst, bone, solitary
    jaw M27.40
    kidney N28.1
  spermatic cord N50.89
  sphenoid sinus J34.1
  spinal meninges G96.198
  spleen NEC D73.4
    congenital Q89.09
    hydatid —see also Echinococcus B67.99 [D77]
  Stafne's M27.0
  subarachnoid intrasellar R93.0
  subcutaneous, pheomycotic (chromomycotic)
    B43.2
  subdural (cerebral) G93.0
    spinal cord G96.198
  sublingual gland K11.6
  submandibular gland K11.6
  submaxillary gland K11.6
  suburethral N36.8
  suprarenal gland E27.8
  suprasellar —see Cyst, brain
  sweat gland or duct L74.8
  synovial —see also Cyst, bursa
    ruptured —see Rupture, synovium
  Tarlov G96.191
  tarsal —see Chalazion
  tendon (sheath) —see Disorder, tendon,
    specified type NEC
  testis N44.2
    tunica albuginea N44.1
  theca lutein (ovary) N83.1-•
  Thornwaldt's J39.2
  thymus (gland) E32.8
  thyroglossal duct (infected) (persistent) Q89.2
  thyroid (gland) E04.1
  thyrolingual duct (infected) (persistent) Q89.2
  tongue K14.8
  tonsil J35.8
  tooth —see Cyst, dental
  Tornwaldt's J39.2
  trichilemmal (proliferating) L72.12
  trichodermal L72.12
  tubal (fallopian) N83.8
    inflammatory —see Salpingitis, chronic
  tubo-ovarian N83.8
    inflammatory N70.13
  tunica
    albuginea testis N44.1
    vaginalis N50.89
  turbinate (nose) J34.1
  Tyson's gland N48.89
  urachus, congenital Q64.4
  ureter N28.89
  ureterovesical orifice N28.89
  urethra, urethral (gland) N36.8
  uterine ligament N83.8
  uterus (body) (corpus) (recurrent)
    N85.8
    embryonic Q51.818
    cervix Q51.6
  vagina, vaginal (implantation) (inclusion)
    (squamous cell) (wall) N89.8
    embryonic Q52.4
  vallecula, vallecular (epiglottis) J38.7
  vesical (orifice) N32.89
  vitreous body H43.89
  vulva (implantation) (inclusion) N90.7
    congenital Q52.79
    sebaceous gland N90.7
  vulvovaginal gland N90.7
  wolffian
    female Q50.5
    male Q55.4

Cystadenocarcinoma —see Neoplasm,
    malignant, by site
  bile duct C22.1
  endometrioid —see Neoplasm, malignant,
    by site
    specified site —see Neoplasm, malignant,
      by site
    unspecified site
      female C56.9
      male C61
  mucinous
    papillary
      specified site —see Neoplasm,
        malignant, by site
      unspecified site C56.9
    specified site —see Neoplasm, malignant,
      by site
    unspecified site C56.9
  papillary
    mucinous
      specified site —see Neoplasm,
        malignant, by site
      unspecified site C56.9
    pseudomucinous
      specified site —see Neoplasm,
        malignant, by site
      unspecified site C56.9
    serous
      specified site —see Neoplasm,
        malignant, by site
      unspecified site C56.9
    specified site —see Neoplasm, malignant,
      by site
    unspecified site C56.9
  pseudomucinous
    papillary
      specified site —see Neoplasm,
        malignant, by site
      unspecified site C56.9
    specified site —see Neoplasm, malignant,
      by site
    unspecified site C56.9
  serous
    papillary
      specified site —see Neoplasm,
        malignant, by site
      unspecified site C56.9
    specified site —see Neoplasm, malignant,
      by site
    unspecified site C56.9
Cystadenofibroma
  clear cell —see Neoplasm, benign, by site
  endometrioid D27.9
    borderline malignancy D39.1-•
    malignant C56.-•
  mucinous
    specified site —see Neoplasm, benign, by site
    unspecified site D27.9
  serous
    specified site —see Neoplasm, benign, by site
    unspecified site D27.9
  specified site —see Neoplasm, benign, by site
  unspecified site D27.9
Cystadenoma —see also Neoplasm, benign, by
    site
  bile duct D13.4
  endometrioid —see Neoplasm, benign, by site
    borderline malignancy —see Neoplasm,
      uncertain behavior, by site
  malignant —see Neoplasm, malignant, by site
  mucinous
    borderline malignancy
      ovary C56.-•
      specified site NEC —see Neoplasm,
        uncertain behavior, by site
      unspecified site C56.9
    papillary
      borderline malignancy
        ovary C56.-•
        specified site NEC —see Neoplasm,
          uncertain behavior, by site
        unspecified site C56.9

Cystadenoma (Continued)
 mucinous (Continued)
  papillary (Continued)
   specified site —see Neoplasm, benign,
    by site
   unspecified site D27.9
  specified site —see Neoplasm, benign, by site
  unspecified site D27.9
 papillary
  borderline malignancy
   ovary C56.-●
   specified site NEC —see Neoplasm,
    uncertain behavior, by site
   unspecified site C56.9
  lymphomatosum
   specified site —see Neoplasm, benign,
    by site
   unspecified site D11.9
  mucinous
   borderline malignancy
    ovary C56.-●
    specified site NEC —see Neoplasm,
     uncertain behavior, by site
    unspecified site C56.9
   specified site —see Neoplasm, benign,
    by site
   unspecified site D27.9
  pseudomucinous
   borderline malignancy
    ovary C56.-●
    specified site NEC —see Neoplasm,
     uncertain behavior, by site
    unspecified site C56.9
   specified site —see Neoplasm, benign,
    by site
   unspecified site D27.9
  serous
   borderline malignancy
    ovary C56.-●
    specified site NEC —see Neoplasm,
     uncertain behavior, by site
    unspecified site C56.9
   specified site —see Neoplasm, benign,
    by site
   unspecified site D27.9
  specified site —see Neoplasm, benign, by site
  unspecified site D27.9
 pseudomucinous
  borderline malignancy
   ovary C56.-●
   specified site NEC —see Neoplasm,
    uncertain behavior, by site
   unspecified site C56.9
  papillary
   borderline malignancy
    ovary C56.-●
    specified site NEC —see Neoplasm,
     uncertain behavior, by site
    unspecified site C56.9
   specified site —see Neoplasm, benign,
    by site
   unspecified site D27.9
  specified site —see Neoplasm, benign, by site
  unspecified site D27.9
 serous
  borderline malignancy
   ovary C56.-●
   specified site NEC —see Neoplasm,
    uncertain behavior, by site
   unspecified site C56.9
  papillary
   borderline malignancy
    ovary C56.-●
    specified site NEC —see Neoplasm,
     uncertain behavior, by site
    unspecified site C56.9
   specified site —see Neoplasm, benign,
    by site
   unspecified site D27.9
  specified site —see Neoplasm, benign, by site
  unspecified site D27.9

Cystathionine synthase deficiency E72.11
Cystathioninemia E72.19
Cystathioninuria E72.19
Cystic —see also condition
 breast (chronic) —see Mastopathy, cystic
 corpora lutea (hemorrhagic) N83.1-●
 duct —see condition
 eyeball (congenital) Q11.0
 fibrosis —see Fibrosis, cystic
 kidney (congenital) Q61.9
  adult type Q61.2
  infantile type NEC Q61.19
   collecting duct dilatation Q61.11
  medullary Q61.5
 liver, congenital Q44.6
 lung disease J98.4
  congenital Q33.0
 mastitis, chronic —see Mastopathy, cystic
 medullary, kidney Q61.5
 meniscus —see Derangement, knee,
  meniscus, cystic
 ovary N83.20-●
Cysticercosis, cysticerciasis B69.9
 with
  epileptiform fits B69.0
  myositis B69.81
 brain B69.0
 central nervous system B69.0
 cerebral B69.0
 ocular B69.1
 specified NEC B69.89
Cysticercus cellulose infestation —see
  Cysticercosis
Cystinosis (malignant) E72.04
Cystinuria E72.01
Cystitis (exudative) (hemorrhagic) (septic)
  (suppurative) N30.90
 with
  fibrosis —see Cystitis, chronic, interstitial
  hematuria N30.91
  leukoplakia —see Cystitis, chronic,
   interstitial
  malakoplakia —see Cystitis, chronic,
   interstitial
  metaplasia —see Cystitis, chronic, interstitial
  prostatitis N41.3
 acute N30.00
  with hematuria N30.01
  of trigone N30.30
   with hematuria N30.31
 allergic —see Cystitis, specified type NEC
 amebic A06.81
 bilharzial B65.9 [N33]
 blennorrhagic (gonococcal) A54.01
 bullous —see Cystitis, specified type NEC
 calculous N21.0
 chlamydial A56.01
 chronic N30.20
  with hematuria N30.21
  interstitial N30.10
   with hematuria N30.11
  of trigone N30.30
   with hematuria N30.31
  specified NEC N30.20
   with hematuria N30.21
 cystic (a) —see Cystitis, specified type NEC
 diphtheritic A36.85
 echinococcal
  granulosus B67.39
  multilocularis B67.69
 emphysematous —see Cystitis, specified type
  NEC
 encysted —see Cystitis, specified type NEC
 eosinophilic —see Cystitis, specified type
  NEC
 follicular —see Cystitis, of trigone
 gangrenous —see Cystitis, specified type
  NEC
 glandularis —see Cystitis, specified type
  NEC

Cystitis (Continued)
 gonococcal A54.01
 incrusted —see Cystitis, specified type
  NEC
 interstitial (chronic) —see Cystitis, chronic,
  interstitial
 irradiation N30.40
  with hematuria N30.41
 irritation —see Cystitis, specified type
  NEC
 malignant —see Cystitis, specified type
  NEC
 of trigone N30.30
  with hematuria N30.31
 panmural —see Cystitis, chronic, interstitial
 polyposa —see Cystitis, specified type NEC
 prostatic N41.3
 puerperal (postpartum) O86.22
 radiation —see Cystitis, irradiation
 specified type NEC N30.80
  with hematuria N30.81
 subacute —see Cystitis, chronic
 submucous —see Cystitis, chronic, interstitial
 syphilitic (late) A52.76
 trichomonal A59.03
 tuberculous A18.12
 ulcerative —see Cystitis, chronic, interstitial
Cystocele (-urethrocele)
 female N81.10
  with prolapse of uterus —see Prolapse,
   uterus
  lateral N81.12
  midline N81.11
  paravaginal N81.12
 in pregnancy or childbirth O34.8-●
  causing obstructed labor O65.5
 male N32.89
Cystolithiasis N21.0
Cystoma —see also Neoplasm, benign, by site
 endometrial, ovary N80.10-●
 mucinous
  specified site —see Neoplasm, benign, by site
  unspecified site D27.9
 serous
  specified site —see Neoplasm, benign, by site
  unspecified site D27.9
 simple (ovary) N83.29-●
Cystoplegia N31.2
Cystoptosis N32.89
Cystopyelitis —see Pyelonephritis
Cystorrhagia N32.89
Cystosarcoma phyllodes D48.6-●
 benign D24-●
 malignant —see Neoplasm, breast, malignant
Cystostomy
 attention to Z43.5
 complication —see Complications, cystostomy
 status Z93.50
  appendico-vesicostomy Z93.52
  cutaneous Z93.51
  specified NEC Z93.59
Cystourethritis —see Urethritis
Cystourethrocele —see also Cystocele
 female N81.10
  with uterine prolapse —see Prolapse,
   uterus
  lateral N81.12
  midline N81.11
  paravaginal N81.12
 male N32.89
Cytomegalic inclusion disease
 congenital P35.1
Cytomegalovirus infection B25.9
Cytomycosis (reticuloendothelial) B39.4
Cytopenia D75.9
 refractory
  with multilineage dysplasia D46.A
   and ring sideroblasts (RCMD RS) D46.B
Czerny's disease (periodic hydrarthrosis of the
 knee) —see Effusion, joint, knee

► New   ⇒ Revised   ~~deleted~~ Deleted   ● Use Additional Character(s)

D

Daae (-Finsen) disease (epidemic pleurodynia) B33.0
Dabney's grip B33.0
Da Costa's syndrome F45.8
Dacryoadenitis, dacryadenitis H04.00-•
  acute H04.01-•
  chronic H04.02-•
Dacryocystitis H04.30-•
  acute H04.32-•
  chronic H04.41-•
  neonatal P39.1
  phlegmonous H04.31-•
  syphilitic A52.71
    congenital (early) A50.01
  trachomatous, active A71.1
    sequelae (late effect) B94.0
Dacryocystoblenorrhea —see Inflammation, lacrimal, passages, chronic
Dacryocystocele —see Disorder, lacrimal system, changes
Dacryolith, dacryolithiasis H04.51-•
Dacryoma —see Disorder, lacrimal system, changes
Dacryopericystitis —see Dacryocystitis
Dacryops H04.11-•
Dacryostenosis —see also Stenosis, lacrimal
  congenital Q10.5
Dactylitis
  bone —see Osteomyelitis
  sickle-cell D57.00
    Hb C D57.219
    Hb SS D57.00
    specified NEC D57.819
  skin L08.9
  syphilitic A52.77
  tuberculous A18.03
Dactylolysis spontanea (ainhum) L94.6
Dactylosymphysis Q70.9
  fingers —see Syndactylism, complex, fingers
  toes —see Syndactylism, complex, toes
Damage
  arteriosclerotic —see Arteriosclerosis
  brain (nontraumatic) G93.9
    anoxic, hypoxic G93.1
      resulting from a procedure G97.82
    child NEC G80.9
    due to birth injury P11.2
  cardiorenal (vascular) —see Hypertension, cardiorenal
  cerebral NEC —see Damage, brain
  coccyx, complicating delivery O71.6
  coronary —see Disease, heart, ischemic
  deep tissue, pressure-induced —see also L89
    with final character .6
  eye, birth injury P15.3
  liver (nontraumatic) K76.9
    alcoholic K70.9
    due to drugs —see Disease, liver, toxic
    toxic —see Disease, liver, toxic
  lung
    dabbing (related) U07.0
    electronic cigarette (related) U07.0
    vaping (associated) (device) (product) (use) U07.0
  medication T88.7
  organ
    dabbing (related) U07.0
    electronic cigarette (related) U07.0
    vaping (associated) (device) (product) (use) U07.0
  pelvic
    joint or ligament, during delivery O71.6
    organ NEC
      during delivery O71.5
      following ectopic or molar pregnancy O08.6
  renal —see Disease, renal
  subendocardium, subendocardial —see Degeneration, myocardial
  vascular I99.9

Dana-Putnam syndrome (subacute combined sclerosis with pernicious anemia) —see Degeneration, combined
Danbolt (-Cross) syndrome (acrodermatitis enteropathica) E83.2
Dandruff L21.0
Dandy-Walker syndrome Q03.1
  with spina bifida —see Spina bifida
Danlos' syndrome (see also Syndrome, Ehler-Danlos) Q79.60
Darier (-White) disease (congenital) Q82.8
  meaning erythema annulare centrifugum L53.1
Darier-Roussy sarcoid D86.3
Darling's disease or histoplasmosis B39.4
Darwin's tubercle Q17.8
Dawson's (inclusion body) encephalitis A81.1
De Beurmann (-Gougerot) disease B42.1
De la Tourette's syndrome F95.2
De Lange's syndrome Q87.19
De Morgan's spots (senile angiomas) I78.1
De Quervain's
  disease (tendon sheath) M65.4
  syndrome E34.51
  thyroiditis (subacute granulomatous thyroiditis) E06.1
De Toni-Fanconi (-Debré) syndrome E72.09
  with cystinosis E72.04
Dead
  fetus, retained (mother) O36.4
    early pregnancy O02.1
  labyrinth —see subcategory H83.2
  ovum, retained O02.0
Deaf nonspeaking NEC H91.3
Deafmutism (acquired) (congenital) NEC H91.3
  hysterical F44.6
  syphilitic, congenital —see also subcategory H94.8 A50.09
Deafness (acquired) (complete) (hereditary) (partial) H91.9-•
  with blue sclera and fragility of bone Q78.0
  auditory fatigue —see Deafness, specified type NEC
  aviation T70.0
    nerve injury —see Injury, nerve, acoustic, specified type NEC
  boilermaker's —see subcategory H83.3
  central —see Deafness, sensorineural
  conductive H90.2
    and sensorineural
      mixed H90.8
        bilateral H90.6
    bilateral H90.0
    unilateral H90.1-•
      with restricted hearing on the contralateral side H90.A-•
  congenital H90.5
    with blue sclera and fragility of bone Q78.0
  due to toxic agents —see Deafness, ototoxic
  emotional (hysterical) F44.6
  functional (hysterical) F44.6
  high frequency H91.9-•
  hysterical F44.6
  low frequency H91.9-•
  mental R48.8
  mixed conductive and sensorineural H90.8
    bilateral H90.6
    unilateral H90.7-•
  nerve —see Deafness, sensorineural
  neural —see Deafness, sensorineural
  noise-induced —see also subcategory H83.3
    nerve injury —see Injury, nerve, acoustic, specified type NEC
  nonspeaking H91.3
  ototoxic —see subcategory H91.0
  perceptive —see Deafness, sensorineural
  psychogenic (hysterical) F44.6
  sensorineural H90.5
    and conductive
      mixed H90.8
        bilateral H90.6
    bilateral H90.3

Deafness (Continued)
  sensorineural (Continued)
    unilateral H90.4-•
      with restricted hearing on the contralateral side H90.A-•
  sensory —see Deafness, sensorineural
  specified type NEC —see subcategory H91.8
  sudden (idiopathic) H91.2-•
  syphilitic A52.15
  transient ischemic H93.01-•
  traumatic —see Injury, nerve, acoustic, specified type NEC
  word (developmental) H93.25
Death (cause unknown) (of) (unexplained) (unspecified cause) R99
  brain G93.82
  cardiac (sudden) (with successful resuscitation) —see Arrest, cardiac
    family history of Z82.41
    personal history of Z86.74
  family member (assumed) Z63.4
Debt, burdensome Z59.86
Debility (chronic) (general) (nervous) R53.81
  congenital or neonatal NOS P96.9
  nervous R53.81
  old age R54
  senile R54
Débove's disease (splenomegaly) R16.1
Decalcification
  bone —see Osteoporosis
  teeth K03.89
Decapsulation, kidney N28.89
Decay
  dental —see Caries, dental
  senile R54
  tooth, teeth —see Caries, dental
Deciduitis (acute)
  following ectopic or molar pregnancy O08.0
Decline (general) —see Debility
  cognitive, age-associated R41.81
Decompensation
  cardiac (acute) (chronic) —see Disease, heart
  cardiovascular —see Disease, cardiovascular
  heart —see Disease, heart
  hepatic —see Failure, hepatic
  myocardial (acute) (chronic) —see Disease, heart
  respiratory J98.8
Decompression sickness T70.3
Decrease (d)
  absolute neutrophile count —see Neutropenia
  blood
    platelets —see Thrombocytopenia
    pressure R03.1
      due to shock following
        injury T79.4
        operation T81.19
  estrogen E28.39
    postablative E89.40
      asymptomatic E89.40
      symptomatic E89.41
  fragility of erythrocytes D58.8
  function
    lipase (pancreatic) K90.3
    ovary in hypopituitarism E23.0
    parenchyma of pancreas K86.89
    pituitary (gland) (anterior) (lobe) E23.0
      posterior (lobe) E23.0
  functional activity R68.89
  glucose R73.09
  hematocrit R71.0
  hemoglobin R71.0
  leukocytes D72.819
    specified NEC D72.818
  libido R68.82
  lymphocytes D72.810
  platelets D69.6
  respiration, due to shock following injury T79.4
  sexual desire R68.82
  tear secretion NEC —see Syndrome, dry eye

Decrease *(Continued)*
  tolerance
    fat K90.49
    glucose R73.09
    pancreatic K90.3
    salt and water E87.8
  vision NEC H54.7
  white blood cell count D72.819
    specified NEC D72.818
Decubitus (ulcer) *—see* Ulcer, pressure, by site
  cervix N86
Deepening acetabulum *—see* Derangement,
    joint, specified type NEC, hip
Defect, defective Q89.9
  3-beta-hydroxysteroid dehydrogenase E25.0
  11-hydroxylase E25.0
  21-hydroxylase E25.0
  abdominal wall, congenital Q79.59
  antibody immunodeficiency D80.9
  aorticopulmonary septum Q21.4
  atrial septal Q21.1
    coronary sinus Q21.13
    following acute myocardial infarction
      (current complication) I23.1
    ostium primum type (type I) Q21.20
      with
        common atrioventricular valves and
          moderate or larger inlet VSD
          Q21.23
        separate atrioventricular valves
          Q21.21
          and small or restrictive inlet VSD
            Q21.22
    ostium secundum type (patent persistent)
      (type II) Q21.11
    sinus venosus Q21.16
      inferior Q21.15
      superior Q21.14
    specified NEC Q21.19
    vena cava type
      inferior Q21.15
      superior Q21.14
  atrioventricular
    canal Q21.20
    septal
      common Q21.23
      complete Q21.23
      incomplete Q21.21
      intermediate Q21.22
      partial Q21.21
      transitional Q21.22
      unspecified as to partial or complete
        Q21.20
    septum Q21.20
  auricular septal Q21.10
  bilirubin excretion NEC E80.6
  biosynthesis, androgen (testicular) E29.1
  bulbar septum Q21.0
  catalase E80.3
  cell membrane receptor complex (CR3) D71
  circulation I99.9
    congenital Q28.9
    newborn Q28.9
  coagulation (factor) *—see also* Deficiency,
    factor D68.9
    with
      ectopic pregnancy O08.1
      molar pregnancy O08.1
    acquired D68.4
    antepartum with hemorrhage *—see*
      Hemorrhage, antepartum, with
      coagulation defect
    due to
      liver disease D68.4
      vitamin K deficiency D68.4
    hereditary NEC D68.2
    intrapartum O67.0
    newborn, transient P61.6
    postpartum O99.13
      with hemorrhage O72.3
    specified type NEC D68.8

Defect, defective *(Continued)*
  complement system D84.1
  conduction (heart) I45.9
    bone *—see* Deafness, conductive
  congenital, organ or site not listed *—see*
    Anomaly, by site
  coronary sinus Q21.13
  cushion, endocardial Q21.20
    common Q21.23
    incomplete Q21.21
    intermediate Q21.22
    transitional Q21.22
  degradation, glycoprotein E77.1
  dental bridge, crown, fillings *—see* Defect,
    dental restoration
  dental restoration K08.50
    specified NEC K08.59
  dentin (hereditary) K00.5
  Descemet's membrane, congenital Q13.89
  developmental *—see also* Anomaly
    cauda equina Q06.3
  diaphragm
    with elevation, eventration or hernia *—see*
      Hernia, diaphragm
    congenital Q79.1
      with hernia Q79.0
      gross (with hernia) Q79.0
  ectodermal, congenital Q82.9
  Eisenmenger's Q21.8
  enzyme
    catalase E80.3
    peroxidase E80.3
  esophagus, congenital Q39.9
  extensor retinaculum M62.89
  fibrin polymerization D68.2
  filling
    bladder R93.41
    kidney R93.42-●
    renal pelvis R93.41
    stomach R93.3
    ureter R93.41
    urinary organs, specified NEC R93.49
  GABA (gamma aminobutyric acid) metabolic
    E72.81
  Gerbode Q21.0
  glucose transport, blood-brain barrier E74.810
  glycoprotein degradation E77.1
  Hageman (factor) D68.2
  hearing *—see* Deafness
  high grade F70
  interatrial septal Q21.19
  interauricular septal Q21.19
  interventricular septal Q21.0
    with dextroposition of aorta, pulmonary
      stenosis and hypertrophy of right
      ventricle Q21.3
    in tetralogy of Fallot Q21.3
  intervertebral annular fibrosis *(see also*
    Disease, intervertebral disc, by site)* M51.9
    lumbar M51.A0
      large M51.A2
      small M51.A1
    lumbosacral M51.A3
      large M51.A5
      small M51.A4
  learning (specific) *—see* Disorder, learning
  lymphocyte function antigen-1 (LFA-1) D84.0
  lysosomal enzyme, post-translational
    modification E77.0
  major osseous M89.70
    ankle M89.77-●
    carpus M89.74-●
    clavicle M89.71-●
    femur M89.75-●
    fibula M89.76-●
    fingers M89.74-●
    foot M89.77-●
    forearm M89.73-●
    hand M89.74-●
    humerus M89.72-●
    lower leg M89.76-●
    metacarpus M89.74-●

Defect, defective *(Continued)*
  major osseous *(Continued)*
    metatarsus M89.77-●
    multiple sites M89.79
    pelvic region M89.75-●
    pelvis M89.75-●
    radius M89.73-●
    scapula M89.71-●
    shoulder region M89.71-●
    specified NEC M89.78
    tarsus M89.77-●
    thigh M89.75-●
    tibia M89.76-●
    toes M89.77-●
    ulna M89.73-●
  mental *—see* Disability, intellectual
  modification, lysosomal enzymes, post-
    translational E77.0
  obstructive, congenital
    renal pelvis Q62.39
    ureter Q62.39
      atresia *—see* Atresia, ureter
      cecoureterocele Q62.32
      megaureter Q62.2
      orthotopic ureterocele Q62.31
  osseous, major M89.70
    ankle M89.77-●
    carpus M89.74-●
    clavicle M89.71-●
    femur M89.75-●
    fibula M89.76-●
    fingers M89.74-●
    foot M89.77-●
    forearm M89.73-●
    hand M89.74-●
    humerus M89.72-●
    lower leg M89.76-●
    metacarpus M89.74-●
    metatarsus M89.77-●
    multiple sites M89.9
    pelvic region M89.75-●
    pelvis M89.75-●
    radius M89.73-●
    scapula M89.71-●
    shoulder region M89.71-●
    specified NEC M89.78
    tarsus M89.77-●
    thigh M89.75-●
    tibia M89.76-●
    toes M89.77-●
    ulna M89.73-●
  osteochondral NEC *—see also* Deformity
    M95.8-●
  ostium
    primum Q21.20
    secundum Q21.11
  peroxidase E80.3
  placental blood supply *—see* Insufficiency,
    placental
  platelets, qualitative D69.1
  constitutional *—see* Disease, von
    Willebrand
  postural NEC, spine *—see* Dorsopathy,
    deforming
  qualitative, of von Willebrand factor
    with
      decreased platelet adhesion and
        selective deficiency of high-
        molecular-weight multimers *(see*
        also Disease, von Willebrand)*
        D68.020
      defective platelet adhesion with a
        normal size distribution of von
        Willebrand factor multimers *(see*
        also Disease, von Willebrand)*
        D68.022
      defective von Willebrand factor to factor
        VIII binding *(see also* Disease, von
        Willebrand)* D68.023
      high-molecular-weight von Willebrand
        factor loss *(see also* Disease, von
        Willebrand)* D68.021

  ▶ New   ⇨ Revised   ~~deleted~~ Deleted   ● Use Additional Character(s)

Defect, defective *(Continued)*
qualitative, of von Willebrand factor *(Continued)*
  with *(Continued)*
  ▶hyper-adhesive forms (*see also* Disease, von Willebrand) D68.021
  ▶increased affinity for platelet glycoprotein lb (*see also* Disease, von Willebrand) D68.021
  ▶markedly decreased affinity for factor VIII (*see also* Disease, von Willebrand) D68.023
  ▶in von Willebrand factor function, with no further subtyping (*see also* Disease, von Willebrand) D68.029
reduction
  limb Q73.8
    lower Q72.9-●
      absence —*see* Agenesis, leg
      foot —*see* Agenesis, foot
      longitudinal
        femur Q72.4-●
        fibula Q72.6-●
        tibia Q72.5-●
      specified type NEC Q72.89-●
      split foot Q72.7-●
    specified type NEC Q73.8
    upper Q71.9-●
      absence —*see* Agenesis, arm
        forearm —*see* Agenesis, forearm
        hand —*see* Agenesis, hand
      lobster-claw hand Q71.6-●
      longitudinal
        radius Q71.4-●
        ulna Q71.5-●
      specified type NEC Q71.89-●
  renal pelvis Q63.8
    obstructive Q62.39
  respiratory system, congenital Q34.9
  restoration, dental K08.50
    specified NEC K08.59
  retinal nerve bundle fibers H35.89
  septal (heart) NOS Q21.9
    acquired (atrial) (auricular) (ventricular) (old) I51.0
    atrial (*see also* Defect, atrial septal) Q21.10
      concurrent with acute myocardial infarction —*see* Infarct, myocardium
      following acute myocardial infarction (current complication) I23.1
    ventricular —*see also* Defect, ventricular septal Q21.0
  sinus venosus (*see also* Defect, atrial septal, sinus venosus) Q21.16
  speech —*see* Disorder, speech
    developmental F80.9
    specified NEC R47.89
  Taussig-Bing (aortic transposition and overriding pulmonary artery) Q20.1
  teeth, wedge K03.1
  vascular (local) I99.9
    congenital Q27.9
  ventricular septal Q21.0
    concurrent with acute myocardial infarction —*see* Infarct, myocardium
    following acute myocardial infarction (current complication) I23.2
    in tetralogy of Fallot Q21.3
  vision NEC H54.7
  visual field H53.40
    bilateral
      heteronymous H53.47
      homonymous H53.46-●
    generalized contraction H53.48-●
    localized
      arcuate H53.43-●
      scotoma (central area) H53.41-●
        blind spot area H53.42-●
      sector H53.43-●
    specified type NEC H53.45-●
  voice R49.9
    specified NEC R49.8
  wedge, tooth, teeth (abrasion) K03.1

Deferentitis N49.1
  gonorrheal (acute) (chronic) A54.23
Defibrination (syndrome) D65
  antepartum —*see* Hemorrhage, antepartum, with coagulation defect, disseminated intravascular coagulation
  following ectopic or molar pregnancy O08.1
  intrapartum O67.0
  newborn P60
  postpartum O72.3
Deficiency, deficient
  3-beta hydroxysteroid dehydrogenase E25.0
  11-hydroxylase E25.0
  21-hydroxylase E25.0
  5-alpha reductase (with male pseudohermaphroditism) E29.1
  AADC (aromatic L-amino acid decarboxylase) E70.81
  abdominal muscle syndrome Q79.4
  AC globulin (congenital) (hereditary) D68.2
    acquired D68.4
  accelerator globulin (Ac G) (blood) D68.2
  acid phosphatase E83.39
  acid sphingomyelinase (ASMD) E75.249
    type
      A E75.240
      A/B E75.244
      B E75.241
  activating factor (blood) D68.2
  ADA2 (adenosine deaminase 2) D81.32
  adenosine deaminase (ADA) D81.30
    with severe combined immunodeficiency (SCID) D81.31
    partial (type 1) D81.39
    specified NEC D81.39
    type 1 (without SCID) (without severe combined immunodeficiency) D81.39
    type 2 D81.32
  aldolase (hereditary) E74.19
  alpha-1-antitrypsin E88.01
  amino-acids E72.9
  anemia —*see* Anemia
  aneurin E51.9
  antibody with
    hyperimmunoglobulinemia D80.6
    near-normal immunoglobins D80.6
  antidiuretic hormone E23.2
  anti-hemophilic
    factor (A) D66
      B D67
      C D68.1
    globulin (AHG) NEC D66
  antithrombin (antithrombin III) D68.59
  aromatic L-amino acid decarboxylase (AADC) E70.81
  ascorbic acid E54
  attention (disorder) (syndrome) F98.8
    with hyperactivity —*see* Disorder, attention-deficit hyperactivity
  autoprothrombin
    I D68.2
    II D67
    C D68.2
  beta-glucuronidase E76.29
  biotin E53.8
  biotin-dependent carboxylase D81.819
  biotinidase D81.810
  brancher enzyme (amylopectinosis) E74.03
  C1 esterase inhibitor (C1-INH) D84.1
  calciferol E55.9
    with
      adult osteomalacia M83.8
      rickets —*see* Rickets
  calcium (dietary) E58
  calorie, severe E43
    with marasmus E41
      and kwashiorkor E42
  cardiac —*see* Insufficiency, myocardial
  carnitine E71.40
    due to
      hemodialysis E71.43
      inborn errors of metabolism E71.42
      Valproic acid therapy E71.43

Deficiency, deficient *(Continued)*
  carnitine *(Continued)*
    iatrogenic E71.43
    muscle palmityltransferase E71.314
    primary E71.41
    secondary E71.448
  carotene E50.9
  central nervous system G96.89
  ceruloplasmin (Wilson) E83.01
  choline E53.8
  Christmas factor D67
  chromium E61.4
  chronic neurovisceral acid sphingomyelinase E75.244
  chronic visceral acid sphingomyelinase E75.241
  clotting (blood) —*see also* Deficiency, coagulation factor D68.9
  clotting factor NEC (hereditary) —*see also* Deficiency, factor D68.2
  coagulation NOS D68.9
    with
      ectopic pregnancy O08.1
      molar pregnancy O08.1
    acquired (any) D68.4
    antepartum hemorrhage —*see* Hemorrhage, antepartum, with coagulation defect
    clotting factor NEC —*see also* Deficiency, factor D68.2
    due to
      hyperprothrombinemia D68.4
      liver disease D68.4
      vitamin K deficiency D68.4
    newborn, transient P61.6
    postpartum O72.3
    specified NEC D68.8
  cognitive F09
  color vision H53.50
    achromatopsia H53.51
    acquired H53.52
    deuteranomaly H53.53
    protanomaly H53.54
    specified type NEC H53.59
    tritanomaly H53.55
  combined glucocorticoid and mineralocorticoid E27.49
  contact factor D68.2
  copper (nutritional) E61.0
  corticoadrenal E27.40
    primary E27.1
  craniofacial axis Q75.0
  cyanocobalamin E53.8
  debrancher enzyme (limit dextrinosis) E74.03
  dehydrogenase
    long chain/very long chain acyl CoA E71.310
    medium chain acyl CoA E71.311
    short chain acyl CoA E71.312
  diet E63.9
  dihydropyrimidine dehydrogenase (DPD) E88.89
  disaccharidase E73.9
  edema —*see* Malnutrition, severe
  endocrine E34.9
  energy-supply —*see* Malnutrition
  enzymes, circulating NEC E88.09
  ergosterol E55.9
    with
      adult osteomalacia M83.8
      rickets —*see* Rickets
  essential fatty acid (EFA) E63.0
  eye movements
    saccadic H55.81
    smooth pursuit H55.82
  factor —*see also* Deficiency, coagulation
    Hageman D68.2
    I (congenital) (hereditary) D68.2
    II (congenital) (hereditary) D68.2
    IX (congenital) (functional) (hereditary) (with functional defect) D67
    multiple (congenital) D68.8
      acquired D68.4

Deficiency, deficient (Continued)
  factor (Continued)
    V (congenital) (hereditary) D68.2
    Hageman D68.2
    VII (congenital) (hereditary) D68.2
    VIII (congenital) (functional) (hereditary)
        (with functional defect) D66
      ⬧with vascular defect —see Disease, von
        Willebrand
    X (congenital) (hereditary) D68.2
    XI (congenital) (hereditary) D68.1
    XII (congenital) (hereditary) D68.2
    XIII (congenital) (hereditary) D68.2
  femoral, proximal focal (congenital) —
      see Defect, reduction, lower limb,
      longitudinal, femur
  fibrin-stabilizing factor (congenital)
      (hereditary) D68.2
    acquired D68.4
  fibrinase D68.2
  fibrinogen (congenital) (hereditary) D68.2
    acquired D65
  folate E53.8
  folic acid E53.8
  foreskin N47.3
  fructokinase E74.11
  fructose 1,6-diphosphatase E74.19
  fructose-1-phosphate aldolase E74.19
  GABA (gamma aminobutyric acid)
      transaminase E72.81
  GABA-T (gamma aminobutyric acid
      transaminase) E72.81
  galactokinase E74.29
  galactose-1-phosphate uridyl transferase E74.29
  gammaglobulin in blood D80.1
    hereditary D80.0
  glass factor D68.2
  glucocorticoid E27.49
    mineralocorticoid E27.49
  glucose-6-phosphatase E74.01
  glucose-6-phosphate dehydrogenase anemia
      anemia D55.0
    without anemia D75.A
  glucose transporter protein type 1 E74.810
  glucuronyl transferase E80.5
  Glut1 E74.810
  glycogen synthetase E74.09
  gonadotropin (isolated) E23.0
  growth hormone (idiopathic) (isolated) E23.0
  Hageman factor D68.2
  hemoglobin D64.9
  hepatophosphorylase E74.09
  homogentisate 1,2-dioxygenase E70.29
  hormone
    anterior pituitary (partial) NEC E23.0
      growth E23.0
    growth (isolated) E23.0
    pituitary E23.0
    testicular E29.1
  hypoxanthine-(guanine)-
      phosphoribosyltransferase (HG-PRT)
      (total HG-PRT) E79.1
  immunity D84.9
    cell-mediated D84.89
      with thrombocytopenia and eczema D82.0
    combined D81.9
    humoral D80.9
    IgA (secretory) D80.2
    IgG D80.3
    IgM D80.4
  immuno —see Immunodeficiency
  immunoglobulin, selective
    A (IgA) D80.2
    G (IgG) (subclasses) D80.3
    M (IgM) D80.4
  infantile neurovisceral acid sphingomyelinase
      E75.240
  inositol (B complex) E53.8
  intrinsic
    factor (congenital) D51.0
    sphincter N36.42
      with urethral hypermobility N36.43

Deficiency, deficient (Continued)
  iodine E61.8
    congenital syndrome —see Syndrome,
      iodine-deficiency, congenital
  iron E61.1
    anemia D50.9
  kalium E87.6
  kappa-light chain D80.8
  labile factor (congenital) (hereditary) D68.2
    acquired D68.4
  lacrimal fluid (acquired) —see also Syndrome,
      dry eye
    congenital Q10.6
  lactase
    congenital E73.0
    secondary E73.1
  Laki-Lorand factor D68.2
  lecithin cholesterol acyltransferase E78.6
  lipocaic K86.89
  lipoprotein (familial) (high density) E78.6
  liver phosphorylase E74.09
  lysosomal alpha-1, 4 glucosidase E74.02
  magnesium E61.2
  major histocompatibility complex
    class I D81.6
    class II D81.7
  manganese E61.3
  menadione (vitamin K) E56.1
    newborn P53
  mental (familial) (hereditary) —see Disability,
      intellectual
  methylenetetrahydrofolate reductase
      (MTHFR) E72.12
  mevalonate kinase M04.1
  mineral NEC E61.8
  mineralocorticoid E27.49
    with glucocorticoid E27.49
  molybdenum (nutritional) E61.5
  moral F60.2
  multiple nutrient elements E61.7
  multiple sulfatase (MSD) E75.26
  muscle
    carnitine (palmityltransferase) E71.314
    phosphofructokinase E74.09
  myoadenylate deaminase E79.2
  myocardial —see Insufficiency, myocardial
  myophosphorylase E74.04
  NADH diaphorase or reductase (congenital)
      D74.0
  NADH-methemoglobin reductase
      (congenital) D74.0
  natrium E87.1
  niacin (amide) (-tryptophan) E52
  nicotinamide E52
  nicotinic acid E52
  number of teeth —see Anodontia
  nutrient element E61.9
    multiple E61.7
    specified NEC E61.8
  ⬧nutrition, nutritional (see also Nutrition
      deficient) E63.9
    sequelae —see Sequelae, nutritional
      deficiency
    specified NEC E63.8
  of interleukin 1 receptor antagonist [DIRA]
      M04.8
  ornithine transcarbamylase E72.4
  ovarian E28.39
  oxygen —see Anoxia
  pantothenic acid E53.8
  parathyroid (gland) E20.9
  perineum (female) N81.89
  phenylalanine hydroxylase E70.1
  phosphoenolpyruvate carboxykinase E74.4
  phosphofructokinase E74.19
  phosphomannomutase E74.818
  phosphomannose isomerase E74.818
  phosphomannosyl mutase E74.818
  phosphorylase kinase, liver E74.09
  pituitary hormone (isolated) E23.0
  plasma thromboplastin
    antecedent (PTA) D68.1
    component (PTC) D67

Deficiency, deficient (Continued)
  plasminogen (type 1) (type 2) E88.02
  platelet NEC D69.1
    ⬧constitutional —see Disease, von Willebrand
  polyglandular E31.8
    autoimmune E31.0
  potassium (K) E87.6
  prepuce N47.3
  proaccelerin (congenital) (hereditary) D68.2
    acquired D68.4
  proconvertin factor (congenital) (hereditary)
      D68.2
    acquired D68.4
  protein —see also Malnutrition E46
    anemia D53.0
    C D68.59
    S D68.59
  prothrombin (congenital) (hereditary) D68.2
    acquired D68.4
  Prower factor D68.2
  pseudocholinesterase E88.09
  PTA (plasma thromboplastin antecedent)
      D68.1
  PTC (plasma thromboplastin component) D67
  purine nucleoside phosphorylase (PNP) D81.5
  pyracin (alpha) (beta) E53.1
  pyridoxal E53.1
  pyridoxamine E53.1
  pyridoxine (derivatives) E53.1
  pyruvate
    carboxylase E74.4
    dehydrogenase E74.4
  riboflavin (vitamin B2) E53.0
  salt E87.1
  secretion
    ovary E28.39
    salivary gland (any) K11.7
    urine R34
  selenium (dietary) E59
  serum antitrypsin, familial E88.01
  short stature homeobox gene (SHOX)
    with
      dyschondrosteosis Q78.8
      ⬧short stature (idiopathic) E34.328
      Turner's syndrome Q96.9
  sodium (Na) E87.1
  SPCA (factor VII) D68.2
  sphincter, intrinsic N36.42
    with urethral hypermobility N36.43
  stable factor (congenital) (hereditary) D68.2
    acquired D68.4
  Stuart-Prower (factor X) D68.2
  succinic semialdehyde dehydrogenase E72.81
  sucrase E74.39
  sulfatase E75.26
  sulfite oxidase E72.19
  thiamin, thiaminic (chloride) E51.9
    beriberi (dry) E51.11
      wet E51.12
  thrombokinase D68.2
    newborn P53
  thyroid (gland) —see Hypothyroidism
  tocopherol E56.0
  tooth bud K00.0
  transcobalamine II (anemia) D51.2
  vanadium E61.6
  vascular I99.9
  vasopressin E23.2
  vertical ridge K06.8
  viosterol —see Deficiency, calciferol
  vitamin (multiple) NOS E56.9
    A E50.9
      with
        Bitot's spot (corneal) E50.1
        follicular keratosis E50.8
        keratomalacia E50.4
        manifestations NEC E50.8
        night blindness E50.5
        scar of cornea, xerophthalmic E50.6
        xeroderma E50.8
        xerophthalmia E50.7

▶ New   ⬧ Revised   ~~deleted~~ Deleted   ● Use Additional Character(s)

Deficiency, deficient *(Continued)*
  vitamin (multiple) NOS *(Continued)*
    A *(Continued)*
      with *(Continued)*
        xerosis
          conjunctival E50.0
            and Bitot's spot E50.1
          cornea E50.2
            and ulceration E50.3
      sequelae E64.1
    B (complex) NOS E53.9
      with
        beriberi (dry) E51.11
          wet E51.12
        pellagra E52
    B1 NOS E51.9
      beriberi (dry) E51.11
        with circulatory system
          manifestations E51.11
        wet E51.12
    B12 E53.8
    B2 (riboflavin) E53.0
    B6 E53.1
    C E54
      sequelae E64.2
    D E55.9
      with
        adult osteomalacia M83.8
        rickets —*see* Rickets
      25-hydroxylase E83.32
    E E56.0
    folic acid E53.8
    G E53.0
    group B E53.9
      specified NEC E53.8
    H (biotin) E53.8
    K E56.1
      of newborn P53
    nicotinic E52
    P E56.8
    PP (pellagra-preventing) E52
    specified NEC E56.8
    thiamin E51.9
      beriberi —*see* Beriberi
▶ von Willebrand factor
  ▶ partial quantitative *(see also* Disease, von
      Willebrand) D68.01
  ▶ total quantitative *(see also* Disease, von
      Willebrand) D68.03
  zinc, dietary E60
Deficit —*see also* Deficiency
  attention and concentration R41.840
    following
      cerebral infarction I69.310
      cerebrovascular disease I69.910
        specified disease NEC I69.810
      nontraumatic
        intracerebral hemorrhage I69.110
        specified intracranial hemorrhage
          NEC I69.210
        subarachnoid hemorrhage I69.010
    disorder —*see* Attention, deficit
  cognitive
    communication R41.841
    emotional
      following
        cerebral infarction I69.315
        cerebrovascular disease I69.915
          specified disease NEC I69.815
        nontraumatic
          intracerebral hemorrhage I69.115
          specified intracranial hemorrhage
            NEC I69.215
          subarachnoid hemorrhage I69.015
    following
      cerebral infarction I69.319
      cerebrovascular disease I69.919
        specified disease NEC I69.819
      nontraumatic
        intracerebral hemorrhage I69.119
        specified intracranial hemorrhage
          NEC I69.219
        subarachnoid hemorrhage I69.019

Deficit *(Continued)*
  cognitive *(Continued)*
    social
      following
        cerebral infarction I69.315
        cerebrovascular disease I69.915
          specified disease NEC I69.815
        nontraumatic
          intracerebral hemorrhage I69.115
          specified intracranial hemorrhage
            NEC I69.215
          subarachnoid hemorrhage I69.015
  cognitive NEC R41.89
    following
      cerebral infarction I69.318
      cerebrovascular disease I69.918
        specified disease NEC I69.818
      nontraumatic
        intracerebral hemorrhage I69.118
        specified intracranial hemorrhage
          NEC I69.218
        subarachnoid hemorrhage I69.018
  concentration R41.840
  executive function R41.844
    following
      cerebral infarction I69.314
      cerebrovascular disease I69.914
        specified disease NEC I69.814
      nontraumatic
        intracerebral hemorrhage I69.114
        specified intracranial hemorrhage
          NEC I69.214
        subarachnoid hemorrhage I69.014
  frontal lobe R41.844
    following
      cerebral infarction I69.314
      cerebrovascular disease I69.914
        specified disease NEC I69.814
      nontraumatic
        intracerebral hemorrhage I69.114
        specified intracranial hemorrhage
          NEC I69.214
        subarachnoid hemorrhage I69.014
  memory
    following
      cerebral infarction I69.311
      cerebrovascular disease I69.911
        specified disease NEC I69.811
      nontraumatic
        intracerebral hemorrhage I69.111
        specified intracranial hemorrhage
          NEC I69.211
        subarachnoid hemorrhage I69.011
  neurologic NEC R29.818
    ischemic
      reversible (RIND) I63.9
        prolonged (PRIND) I63.9
  oxygen R09.02
  prolonged reversible ischemic neurologic
    (PRIND) I63.9
  psychomotor R41.843
    following
      cerebral infarction I69.313
      cerebrovascular disease I69.913
        specified disease NEC I69.813
      nontraumatic
        intracerebral hemorrhage I69.113
        specified intracranial hemorrhage
          NEC I69.213
        subarachnoid hemorrhage I69.013
  visuospatial R41.842
    following
      cerebral infarction I69.312
      cerebrovascular disease I69.912
        specified disease NEC I69.812
      nontraumatic
        intracerebral hemorrhage I69.112
        specified intracranial hemorrhage
          NEC I69.212
        subarachnoid hemorrhage I69.012

Deflection
  radius —*see* Deformity, limb, specified type
    NEC, forearm
  septum (acquired) (nasal) (nose) J34.2
  spine —*see* Curvature, spine
  turbinate (nose) J34.2
Defluvium
  capillorum —*see* Alopecia
  ciliorum —*see* Madarosis
  unguium L60.8
Deformity Q89.9
  abdomen, congenital Q89.9
  abdominal wall
    acquired M95.8
    congenital Q79.59
  acquired (unspecified site) M95.9
  adrenal gland Q89.1
  alimentary tract, congenital Q45.9
    upper Q40.9
  ankle (joint) (acquired) —*see also* Deformity,
    limb, lower leg
    abduction —*see* Contraction, joint, ankle
    congenital Q68.8
    contraction —*see* Contraction, joint, ankle
    specified type NEC —*see* Deformity, limb,
      foot, specified NEC
  anus (acquired) K62.89
    congenital Q43.9
  aorta (arch) (congenital) Q25.40
    acquired I77.89
  aortic
    arch, acquired I77.89
    cusp or valve (congenital) Q23.8
      acquired —*see also* Endocarditis, aortic
        I35.8
  arm (acquired) (upper) —*see also* Deformity,
    limb, upper arm
    congenital Q68.8
    forearm —*see* Deformity, limb, forearm
  artery (congenital) (peripheral) NOS Q27.9
    acquired I77.89
    coronary (acquired) I25.9
      congenital Q24.5
    umbilical Q27.0
⇛ atrial septal *(see also* Defect, atrial septal) Q21.10
  auditory canal (external) (congenital) —*see*
    also Malformation, ear, external
    acquired —*see* Disorder, ear, external,
      specified type NEC
  auricle
    ear (congenital) —*see also* Malformation,
      ear, external
    acquired —*see* Disorder, pinna,
      deformity
  back —*see* Dorsopathy, deforming
  bile duct (common) (congenital) (hepatic)
    Q44.5
    acquired K83.8
  biliary duct or passage (congenital) Q44.5
    acquired K83.8
  bladder (neck) (trigone) (sphincter)
    (acquired) N32.89
    congenital Q64.79
  bone (acquired) NOS M95.9
    congenital Q79.9
    turbinate M95.0
  brain (congenital) Q04.9
    acquired G93.89
    reduction Q04.3
  breast (acquired) N64.89
    congenital Q83.9
    reconstructed N65.0
  bronchus (congenital) Q32.4
    acquired NEC J98.09
  bursa, congenital Q79.9
  canaliculi (lacrimalis) (acquired) —*see also*
    Disorder, lacrimal system, changes
    congenital Q10.6
  canthus, acquired —*see* Disorder, eyelid,
    specified type NEC
  capillary (acquired) I78.8

Deformity *(Continued)*
    cardiovascular system, congenital Q28.9
    caruncle, lacrimal (acquired) —*see also*
        Disorder, lacrimal system, changes
        congenital Q10.6
    cascade, stomach K31.2
    cecum (congenital) Q43.9
        acquired K63.89
    cerebral, acquired G93.89
        congenital Q04.9
    cervix (uterus) (acquired) NEC N88.8
        congenital Q51.9
    cheek (acquired) M95.2
        congenital Q18.9
    chest (acquired) (wall) M95.4
        congenital Q67.8
        sequelae (late effect) of rickets E64.3
    chin (acquired) M95.2
        congenital Q18.9
    choroid (congenital) Q14.3
        acquired H31.8
        plexus Q07.8
            acquired G96.198
    cicatricial —*see* Cicatrix
    cilia, acquired —*see* Disorder, eyelid,
        specified type NEC
    clavicle (acquired) M95.8
        congenital Q68.8
    clitoris (congenital) Q52.6
        acquired N90.89
    clubfoot —*see* Clubfoot
    coccyx (acquired) —*see* subcategory M43.8
    colon (congenital) Q43.9
        acquired K63.89
    concha (ear), congenital —*see also*
        Malformation, ear, external
        acquired —*see* Disorder, pinna, deformity
    cornea (acquired) H18.70
        congenital Q13.4
        descemetocele —*see* Descemetocele
        ectasia —*see* Ectasia, cornea
        specified NEC H18.79-●
        staphyloma —*see* Staphyloma, cornea
    coronary artery (acquired) I25.9
        congenital Q24.5
    cranium (acquired) —*see* Deformity, skull
    cricoid cartilage (congenital) Q31.8
        acquired J38.7
    cystic duct (congenital) Q44.5
        acquired K82.8
    Dandy-Walker Q03.1
        with spina bifida —*see* Spina bifida
    diaphragm (congenital) Q79.1
        acquired J98.6
    digestive organ NOS Q45.9
    ductus arteriosus Q25.0
    duodenal bulb K31.89
    duodenum (congenital) Q43.9
        acquired K31.89
    dura —*see* Deformity, meninges
    ear (acquired) —*see also* Disorder, pinna,
        deformity
        congenital (external) Q17.9
            internal Q16.5
            middle Q16.4
                ossicles Q16.3
            ossicles Q16.3
    ectodermal (congenital) NEC Q84.9
    ejaculatory duct (congenital) Q55.4
        acquired N50.89
    elbow (joint) (acquired) —*see also* Deformity,
        limb, upper arm
        congenital Q68.8
        contraction —*see* Contraction, joint, elbow
    endocrine gland NEC Q89.2
    epididymis (congenital) Q55.4
        acquired N50.89
    epiglottis (congenital) Q31.8
        acquired J38.7
    esophagus (congenital) Q39.9
        acquired K22.89
    eustachian tube (congenital) NEC Q17.8

Deformity *(Continued)*
    eye, congenital Q15.9
    eyebrow (congenital) Q18.8
    eyelid (acquired) —*see also* Disorder, eyelid,
        specified type NEC
        congenital Q10.3
    face (acquired) M95.2
        congenital Q18.9
    fallopian tube, acquired N83.8
    femur (acquired) —*see* Deformity, limb,
        specified type NEC, thigh
    fetal
        with fetopelvic disproportion O33.7
        causing obstructed labor O66.3
    finger (acquired) M20.00-●
        boutonniere M20.02-●
        congenital Q68.1
        flexion contracture —*see* Contraction, joint,
            hand
        mallet finger M20.01-●
        specified NEC M20.09-●
        swan-neck M20.03-●
    flexion (joint) (acquired) —*see also* Deformity,
        limb, flexion M21.20
        congenital NOS Q74.9
        hip Q65.89
    foot (acquired) —*see also* Deformity, limb,
        lower leg
        cavovarus (congenital) Q66.1-●
        congenital NOS Q66.9-●
            specified type NEC Q66.89
        specified type NEC —*see* Deformity, limb,
            foot, specified NEC
        valgus (congenital) Q66.6
            acquired —*see* Deformity, valgus, ankle
        varus (congenital) NEC Q66.3-●
            acquired —*see* Deformity, varus, ankle
    forearm (acquired) —*see also* Deformity, limb,
        forearm
        congenital Q68.8
    forehead (acquired) M95.2
        congenital Q75.8
    frontal bone (acquired) M95.2
        congenital Q75.8
    gallbladder (congenital) Q44.1
        acquired K82.8
    gastrointestinal tract (congenital) NOS Q45.9
        acquired K63.89
    genitalia, genital organ(s) or system NEC
        female (congenital) Q52.9
            acquired N94.89
            external Q52.70
        male (congenital) Q55.9
            acquired N50.89
    globe (eye) (congenital) Q15.8
        acquired H44.89
    gum, acquired NEC K06.8
    hand (acquired) —*see also* Deformity, limb, hand
        congenital Q68.1
    head (acquired) M95.2
        congenital Q75.8
    heart (congenital) Q24.9
        septum Q21.9
            auricular (*see also* Defect, atrial septal)
                Q21.10
            ventricular Q21.0
        valve (congenital) NEC Q24.8
            acquired —*see* Endocarditis
    heel (acquired) —*see* Deformity, foot
    hepatic duct (congenital) Q44.5
        acquired K83.8
    hip (joint) (acquired) —*see also* Deformity,
        limb, thigh
        congenital Q65.9
        due to (previous) juvenile
            osteochondrosis —*see* Coxa, plana
        flexion —*see* Contraction, joint, hip
    hourglass —*see* Contraction, hourglass
    humerus (acquired) M21.82-●
        congenital Q74.0
    hypophyseal (congenital) Q89.2

Deformity *(Continued)*
    ileocecal (coil) (valve) (acquired) K63.89
        congenital Q43.9
    ileum (congenital) Q43.9
        acquired K63.89
    ilium (acquired) M95.5
        congenital Q74.2
    integument (congenital) Q84.9
    intervertebral cartilage or disc (acquired) —
        see Disorder, disc, specified NEC
    intestine (large) (small) (congenital) NOS
        Q43.9
        acquired K63.89
    intrinsic minus or plus (hand) —*see*
        Deformity, limb, specified type NEC,
        forearm
    iris (acquired) H21.89
        congenital Q13.2
    ischium (acquired) M95.5
        congenital Q74.2
    jaw (acquired) (congenital) M26.9
    joint (acquired) NEC M21.90
        congenital Q68.8
        elbow M21.92-●
        hand M21.94-●
        hip M21.95-●
        knee M21.96-●
        shoulder M21.92-●
        wrist M21.93-●
    kidney(s) (calyx) (pelvis) (congenital) Q63.9
        acquired N28.89
        artery (congenital) Q27.2
            acquired I77.89
    Klippel-Feil (brevicollis) Q76.1
    knee (acquired) NEC —*see also* Deformity,
        limb, lower leg
        congenital Q68.2
    labium (majus) (minus) (congenital) Q52.79
        acquired N90.89
    lacrimal passages or duct (congenital) NEC
        Q10.6
        acquired —*see* Disorder, lacrimal system,
            changes
    larynx (muscle) (congenital) Q31.8
        acquired J38.7
        web (glottic) Q31.0
    leg (upper) (acquired) NEC —*see also*
        Deformity, limb, thigh
        congenital Q68.8
        lower leg —*see* Deformity, limb, lower leg
    lens (acquired) H27.8
        congenital Q12.9
    lid (fold) (acquired) —*see also* Disorder,
        eyelid, specified type NEC
        congenital Q10.3
    ligament (acquired) —*see* Disorder, ligament
        congenital Q79.9
    limb (acquired) M21.90
        clawfoot M21.53-●
        clawhand M21.51-●
        ▶congenital Q68.1
        clubfoot M21.54-●
        clubhand M21.52-●
        congenital, except reduction deformity
            Q74.9
        flat foot M21.4-●
        flexion M21.20
            ankle M21.27-●
            elbow M21.22-●
            finger M21.24-●
            hip M21.25-●
            knee M21.26-●
            shoulder M21.21-●
            toe M21.27-●
            wrist M21.23-●
        foot
            claw —*see* Deformity, limb, clawfoot
            club —*see* Deformity, limb, clubfoot
            drop M21.37-●
            flat —*see* Deformity, limb, flat foot
            specified NEC M21.6X-●

▶ New   ⇒ Revised   ~~deleted~~ Deleted   ● Use Additional Character(s)

Deformity (Continued)

limb (Continued)

forearm M21.93-•

hand M21.94-•

lower leg M21.96-•

specified type NEC M21.80

   forearm M21.83-•

   lower leg M21.86-•

   thigh M21.85-•

   upper arm M21.82-•

thigh M21.95-•

unequal length M21.70

   short site is

      femur M21.75-•

      fibula M21.76-•

      humerus M21.72-•

      radius M21.73-•

      tibia M21.76-•

      ulna M21.73-•

upper arm M21.92-•

valgus —see Deformity, valgus

varus —see Deformity, varus

wrist drop M21.33-•

lip (acquired) NEC K13.0

congenital Q38.0

liver (congenital) Q44.7

acquired K76.89

lumbosacral (congenital) (joint) (region) Q76.49

acquired —see subcategory M43.8

kyphosis —see Kyphosis, congenital

lordosis —see Lordosis, congenital

lung (congenital) Q33.9

acquired J98.4

lymphatic system, congenital Q89.9

Madelung's (radius) Q74.0

mandible (acquired) (congenital) M26.9

maxilla (acquired) (congenital) M26.9

meninges or membrane (congenital) Q07.9

cerebral Q04.8

   acquired G96.198

spinal cord (congenital) Q06.-•

   acquired G96.198

metacarpus (acquired) —see Deformity, limb, forearm

congenital Q74.0

metatarsus (acquired) —see Deformity, foot

congenital Q66.9-•

middle ear (congenital) Q16.4

ossicles Q16.3

mitral (leaflets) (valve) I05.8

parachute Q23.2

stenosis, congenital Q23.2

mouth (acquired) K13.79

congenital Q38.6

multiple, congenital NEC Q89.7

muscle (acquired) M62.89

congenital Q79.9

   sternocleidomastoid Q68.0

musculoskeletal system (acquired) M95.9

congenital Q79.9

specified NEC M95.8

nail (acquired) L60.8

congenital Q84.6

nasal —see Deformity, nose

neck (acquired) M95.3

congenital Q18.9

   sternocleidomastoid Q68.0

nervous system (congenital) Q07.9

nipple (congenital) Q83.9

acquired N64.89

nose (acquired) (cartilage) M95.0

bone (turbinate) M95.0

congenital Q30.9

   bent or squashed Q67.4

saddle M95.0

   syphilitic A50.57

septum (acquired) J34.2

   congenital Q30.8

sinus (wall) (congenital) Q30.8

   acquired M95.0

syphilitic (congenital) A50.57

   late A52.73

Deformity (Continued)

ocular muscle (congenital) Q10.3

acquired —see Strabismus, mechanical

opticociliary vessels (congenital) Q13.2

orbit (eye) (acquired) H05.30

atrophy —see Atrophy, orbit

congenital Q10.7

due to

   bone disease NEC H05.32-•

   trauma or surgery H05.33-•

enlargement —see Enlargement, orbit

exostosis —see Exostosis, orbit

organ of Corti (congenital) Q16.5

ovary (congenital) Q50.39

acquired N83.8

oviduct, acquired N83.8

palate (congenital) Q38.5

acquired M27.8

cleft (congenital) —see Cleft, palate

pancreas (congenital) Q45.3

acquired K86.89

parathyroid (gland) Q89.2

parotid (gland) (congenital) Q38.4

acquired K11.8

patella (acquired) —see Disorder, patella, specified NEC

pelvis, pelvic (acquired) (bony) M95.5

with disproportion (fetopelvic) O33.0

   causing obstructed labor O65.0

congenital Q74.2

rachitic sequelae (late effect) E64.3

penis (glans) (congenital) Q55.69

acquired N48.89

pericardium (congenital) Q24.8

acquired —see Pericarditis

pharynx (congenital) Q38.8

acquired J39.2

pinna, acquired —see also Disorder, pinna, deformity

congenital Q17.9

pituitary (congenital) Q89.2

posture —see Dorsopathy, deforming

prepuce (congenital) Q55.69

acquired N47.8

prostate (congenital) Q55.4

acquired N42.89

pupil (congenital) Q13.2

acquired —see Abnormality, pupillary

pylorus (congenital) Q40.3

acquired K31.89

rachitic (acquired), old or healed E64.3

radius (acquired) —see also Deformity, limb, forearm

congenital Q68.8

rectum (congenital) Q43.9

acquired K62.89

reduction (extremity) (limb), congenital (see also condition and site) Q73.8

brain Q04.3

lower —see Defect, reduction, lower limb

upper —see Defect, reduction, upper limb

renal —see Deformity, kidney

respiratory system (congenital) Q34.9

rib (acquired) M95.4

congenital Q76.6

   cervical Q76.5

rotation (joint) (acquired) —see Deformity, limb, specified site NEC

congenital Q74.9

hip —see Deformity, limb, specified type NEC, thigh

   congenital Q65.89

sacroiliac joint (congenital) Q74.2

acquired —see subcategory M43.8

sacrum (acquired) —see subcategory M43.8

saddle

back —see Lordosis

nose M95.0

   syphilitic A50.57

salivary gland or duct (congenital) Q38.4

acquired K11.8

scapula (acquired) M95.8

congenital Q68.8

Deformity (Continued)

scrotum (congenital) —see also Malformation, testis and scrotum

acquired N50.89

seminal vesicles (congenital) Q55.4

acquired N50.89

septum, nasal (acquired) J34.2

shoulder (joint) (acquired) —see Deformity, limb, upper arm

congenital Q74.0

contraction —see Contraction, joint, shoulder

sigmoid (flexure) (congenital) Q43.9

acquired K63.89

skin (congenital) Q82.9

skull (acquired) M95.2

congenital Q75.8

with

   anencephaly Q00.0

   encephalocele —see Encephalocele

   hydrocephalus Q03.9

      with spina bifida —see Spina bifida, by site, with hydrocephalus

   microcephaly Q02

soft parts, organs or tissues (of pelvis)

in pregnancy or childbirth NEC O34.8-•

   causing obstructed labor O65.5

spermatic cord (congenital) Q55.4

acquired N50.89

torsion —see Torsion, spermatic cord

spinal —see Dorsopathy, deforming

column (acquired) —see Dorsopathy, deforming

congenital Q67.5

cord (congenital) Q06.9

   acquired G95.89

nerve root (congenital) Q07.9

spine (acquired) —see also Dorsopathy, deforming

congenital Q67.5

rachitic E64.3

specified NEC —see Dorsopathy, deforming, specified NEC

spleen

acquired D73.89

congenital Q89.09

Sprengel's (congenital) Q74.0

sternocleidomastoid (muscle), congenital Q68.0

sternum (acquired) M95.4

congenital NEC Q76.7

stomach (congenital) Q40.3

acquired K31.89

submandibular gland (congenital) Q38.4

submaxillary gland (congenital) Q38.4

acquired K11.8

talipes —see Talipes

testis (congenital) —see also Malformation, testis and scrotum

acquired N44.8

torsion —see Torsion, testis

thigh (acquired) —see also Deformity, limb, thigh

congenital NEC Q68.8

thorax (acquired) (wall) M95.4

congenital Q67.8

sequelae of rickets E64.3

thumb (acquired) —see also Deformity, finger

congenital NEC Q68.1

thymus (tissue) (congenital) Q89.2

thyroid (gland) (congenital) Q89.2

cartilage Q31.8

   acquired J38.7

tibia (acquired) —see also Deformity, limb, specified type NEC, lower leg

congenital NEC Q68.8

saber (syphilitic) A50.56

toe (acquired) M20.6-•

congenital Q66.9-•

hallux rigidus M20.2-•

hallux valgus M20.1-•

hallux varus M20.3-•

hammer toe M20.4-•

specified NEC M20.5X-•

Deformity (Continued)
  tongue (congenital) Q38.3
    acquired K14.8
  tooth, teeth K00.2
  trachea (rings) (congenital) Q32.1
    acquired J39.8
  transverse aortic arch (congenital) Q25.49
  tricuspid (leaflets) (valve) I07.8
    atresia or stenosis Q22.4
    Ebstein's Q22.5
  trunk (acquired) M95.8
    congenital Q89.9
  ulna (acquired) —*see also* Deformity, limb, forearm
    congenital NEC Q68.8
  urachus, congenital Q64.4
  ureter (opening) (congenital) Q62.8
    acquired N28.89
  urethra (congenital) Q64.79
    acquired N36.8
  urinary tract (congenital) Q64.9
    urachus Q64.4
  uterus (congenital) Q51.9
    acquired N85.8
  uvula (congenital) Q38.5
  vagina (acquired) N89.8
    congenital Q52.4
  valgus NEC M21.00
    ankle M21.07-●
    elbow M21.02-●
    hip M21.05-●
    knee M21.06-●
  valve, valvular (congenital) (heart) Q24.8
    acquired —*see* Endocarditis
  varus NEC M21.10
    ankle M21.17-●
    elbow M21.12-●
    hip M21.15
    knee M21.16-●
    tibia —*see* Osteochondrosis, juvenile, tibia
  vas deferens (congenital) Q55.4
    acquired N50.89
  vein (congenital) Q27.9
    great Q26.9
  vertebra —*see* Dorsopathy, deforming
  vertical talus (congenital) Q66.80
    left foot Q66.82
    right foot Q66.81
  vesicourethral orifice (acquired) N32.89
    congenital NEC Q64.79
  vessels of optic papilla (congenital) Q14.2
  visual field (contraction) —*see* Defect, visual field
  vitreous body, acquired H43.89
  vulva (congenital) Q52.79
    acquired N90.89
  wrist (joint) (acquired) —*see also* Deformity, limb, forearm
    congenital Q68.8
    contraction —*see* Contraction, joint, wrist
Degeneration, degenerative
  adrenal (capsule) (fatty) (gland) (hyaline) (infectional) E27.8
  amyloid —*see also* Amyloidosis E85.9
  anterior cornua, spinal cord G12.29
  anterior labral S43.49-●
  aorta, aortic I70.0
    fatty I77.89
  aortic valve (heart) —*see* Endocarditis, aortic
  arteriovascular —*see* Arteriosclerosis
  artery, arterial (atheromatous) (calcareous) — *see also* Arteriosclerosis
    cerebral, amyloid E85.4 [I68.0]
    medial —*see* Arteriosclerosis, extremities
  articular cartilage NEC —*see* Derangement, joint, articular cartilage, by site
  atheromatous —*see* Arteriosclerosis
  basal nuclei or ganglia G23.9
    specified NEC G23.8
  bone NEC —*see* Disorder, bone, specified type NEC
  brachial plexus G54.0

Degeneration, degenerative (Continued)
  brain (cortical) (progressive) G31.9
    alcoholic G31.2
    arteriosclerotic I67.2
    childhood G31.9
      specified NEC G31.89
    cystic G31.89
      congenital Q04.6
    in
      alcoholism G31.2
      beriberi E51.2
      cerebrovascular disease I67.9
      congenital hydrocephalus Q03.9
        with spina bifida —*see also* Spina bifida
      Fabry-Anderson disease E75.21
      Gaucher's disease E75.22
      Hunter's syndrome E76.1
      lipidosis
        cerebral E75.4
        generalized E75.6
      mucopolysaccharidosis —*see* Mucopolysaccharidosis
      myxedema E03.9 [G32.89]
      neoplastic disease —*see also* Neoplasm D49.6 [G32.89]
      Niemann-Pick disease E75.249 [G32.89]
      sphingolipidosis E75.3 [G32.89]
      vitamin B12 deficiency E53.8 [G32.89]
    senile NEC G31.1
  breast N64.89
  Bruch's membrane —*see* Degeneration, choroid
  capillaries (fatty) I78.8
    amyloid E85.89 [I79.8]
  cardiac —*see also* Degeneration, myocardial
    valve, valvular —*see* Endocarditis
  cardiorenal —*see* Hypertension, cardiorenal
  cardiovascular —*see also* Disease, cardiovascular
    renal —*see* Hypertension, cardiorenal
  cerebellar NOS G31.9
    alcoholic G31.2
    primary (hereditary) (sporadic) G11.9
  cerebral —*see* Degeneration, brain
  cerebrovascular I67.9
    due to hypertension I67.4
  cervical plexus G54.2
  cervix N88.8
    due to radiation (intended effect) N88.8
      adverse effect or misadventure N99.89
  chamber angle H21.21-●
  changes, spine or vertebra —*see* Spondylosis
  chorioretinal —*see also* Degeneration, choroid
    hereditary H31.20
  choroid (colloid) (drusen) H31.10-●
    atrophy —*see* Atrophy, choroidal
    hereditary —*see* Dystrophy, choroidal, hereditary
  ciliary body H21.22-●
  cochlear —*see* subcategory H83.8
  combined (spinal cord) (subacute) E53.8 [G32.0]
    with anemia (pernicious) D51.0 [G32.0]
      due to dietary vitamin B12 deficiency D51.3 [G32.0]
    in (due to)
      vitamin B12 deficiency E53.8 [G32.0]
        anemia D51.9 [G32.0]
  conjunctiva H11.10
    concretions —*see* Concretion, conjunctiva
    deposits —*see* Deposit, conjunctiva
    pigmentations —*see* Pigmentation, conjunctiva
    pinguecula —*see* Pinguecula
    xerosis —*see* Xerosis, conjunctiva
  cornea H18.40
    calcerous H18.43
      band keratopathy H18.42-●
    familial, hereditary —*see* Dystrophy, cornea
    hyaline (of old scars) H18.49
    keratomalacia —*see* Keratomalacia
    nodular H18.45-●
    peripheral H18.46-●

Degeneration, degenerative (Continued)
  cornea (Continued)
    senile H18.41-●
    specified type NEC H18.49
  cortical (cerebellar) (parenchymatous) G31.89
    alcoholic G31.2
    diffuse, due to arteriopathy I67.2
  corticobasal G31.85
  cutis L98.8
    amyloid E85.4 [L99]
  dental pulp K04.2
  disc disease —*see* Degeneration, intervertebral disc, by site
  dorsolateral (spinal cord) —*see* Degeneration, combined
  extrapyramidal G25.9
  eye, macular —*see also* Degeneration, macula
    congenital or hereditary —*see* Dystrophy, retina
  facet joints —*see* Spondylosis
  fatty
    liver NEC K76.0
      alcoholic K70.0
  grey matter (brain) (Alpers') G31.81
  heart —*see also* Degeneration, myocardial
    amyloid E85.4 [I43]
    atheromatous —*see* Disease, heart, ischemic, atherosclerotic
    ischemic —*see* Disease, heart, ischemic
  hepatolenticular (Wilson's) E83.01
  hepatorenal K76.7
  hyaline (diffuse) (generalized)
    localized —*see* Degeneration, by site
  infrapatellar fat pad M79.4
  intervertebral disc NOS
    with
      myelopathy —*see* Disorder, disc, with, myelopathy
      radiculitis or radiculopathy —*see* Disorder, disc, with, radiculopathy
    cervical, cervicothoracic —*see* Disorder, disc, cervical, degeneration
    with
      myelopathy —*see* Disorder, disc, cervical, with myelopathy
      neuritis, radiculitis or radiculopathy —*see* Disorder, disc, cervical, with neuritis
    lumbar region M51.36
      with
        myelopathy M51.06
        neuritis, radiculitis, radiculopathy or sciatica M51.16
    lumbosacral region M51.37
      with
        neuritis, radiculitis, radiculopathy or sciatica M51.17
    sacrococcygeal region M53.3
    thoracic region M51.34
      with
        myelopathy M51.04
        neuritis, radiculitis, radiculopathy M51.14
    thoracolumbar region M51.35
      with
        myelopathy M51.05
        neuritis, radiculitis, radiculopathy M51.15
  intestine, amyloid E85.4
  iris (pigmentary) H21.23-●
  ischemic —*see* Ischemia
  joint disease —*see* Osteoarthritis
  kidney N28.89
    amyloid E85.4 [N29]
    cystic, congenital Q61.9
    fatty N28.89
    polycystic Q61.3
      adult type (autosomal dominant) Q61.2
      infantile type (autosomal recessive) NEC Q61.19
        collecting duct dilatation Q61.11

▶ New   ⇒ Revised   ~~deleted~~ Deleted   ● Use Additional Character(s)

Degeneration, degenerative (Continued)
Kuhnt-Junius —see also Degeneration, macula
    H35.32-●
lens —see Cataract
lenticular (familial) (progressive) (Wilson's)
    (with cirrhosis of liver) E83.01
liver (diffuse) NEC K76.89
    amyloid E85.4 [K77]
    cystic K76.89
        congenital Q44.6
    fatty NEC K76.0
        alcoholic K70.0
    hypertrophic K76.89
    parenchymatous, acute or subacute K72.00
        with coma K72.01
    pigmentary K76.89
    toxic (acute) K71.9
lung J98.4
lymph gland I89.8
    hyaline I89.8
macula, macular (acquired) (age-related)
    (senile) H35.30
    angioid streaks H35.33
    atrophic age-related H35.31-●
    congenital or hereditary —see Dystrophy,
        retina
    cystoid H35.35-●
    drusen H35.36-●
    dry age-related H35.31-●
    exudative H35.32-●
    hole H35.34-●
    nonexudative H35.31-●
    puckering H35.37-●
    toxic H35.38-●
    wet age-related H35.32-●
membranous labyrinth, congenital (causing
    impairment of hearing) Q16.5
meniscus —see Derangement, meniscus
mitral —see Insufficiency, mitral
Mönckeberg's —see Arteriosclerosis,
    extremities
motor centers, senile G31.1
multi-system G90.3
mural —see Degeneration, myocardial
muscle (fatty) (fibrous) (hyaline)
    (progressive) M62.89
    heart —see Degeneration, myocardial
myelin, central nervous system G37.9
myocardial, myocardium (fatty) (hyaline)
    (senile) I51.5
    with rheumatic fever (conditions in I00) I09.0
        active, acute or subacute I01.2
            with chorea I02.0
        inactive or quiescent (with chorea) I09.0
    hypertensive —see Hypertension, heart
    rheumatic —see Degeneration, myocardial,
        with rheumatic fever
    syphilitic A52.06
nasal sinus (mucosa) J32.9
    frontal J32.1
    maxillary J32.0
nerve —see Disorder, nerve
nervous system G31.9
    alcoholic G31.2
    amyloid E85.4 [G99.8]
    autonomic G90.9
    fatty G31.89
    specified NEC G31.89
nipple N64.89
olivopontocerebellar (hereditary) (familial)
    G23.8
osseous labyrinth —see subcategory H83.8
ovary N83.8
    cystic N83.20-●
    microcystic N83.20-●
pallidal pigmentary (progressive) G23.0
pancreas K86.89
    tuberculous A18.83
penis N48.89
pigmentary (diffuse) (general)
    localized —see Degeneration, by site
    pallidal (progressive) G23.0

Degeneration, degenerative (Continued)
pineal gland E34.8
pituitary (gland) E23.6
popliteal fat pad M79.4
posterolateral (spinal cord) —see
    Degeneration, combined
pulmonary valve (heart) I37.8
pulp (tooth) K04.2
pupillary margin H21.24-●
renal —see Degeneration, kidney
retina H35.9
    hereditary (cerebroretinal) (congenital)
        (juvenile) (macula) (peripheral)
        (pigmentary) —see Dystrophy, retina
    Kuhnt-Junius —see also Degeneration,
        macula H35.32-●
    macula (cystic) (exudative) (hole)
        (nonexudative) (pseudohole) (senile)
        (toxic) —see Degeneration, macula
    peripheral H35.40
        lattice H35.41-●
        microcystoid H35.42-●
        paving stone H35.43-●
        secondary
            pigmentary H35.45-●
            vitreoretinal H35.46-●
        senile reticular H35.44-●
    pigmentary (primary) —see also Dystrophy,
        retina
        secondary —see Degeneration, retina,
            peripheral, secondary
    posterior pole —see Degeneration, macula
saccule, congenital (causing impairment of
    hearing) Q16.5
senile R54
    brain G31.1
    cardiac, heart or myocardium —see
        Degeneration, myocardial
    motor centers G31.1
    vascular —see Arteriosclerosis
sinus (cystic) —see also Sinusitis
    polypoid J33.1
skin L98.8
    amyloid E85.4 [L99]
    colloid L98.8
spinal (cord) G31.89
    amyloid E85.4 [G32.89]
    combined (subacute) —see Degeneration,
        combined
    dorsolateral —see Degeneration, combined
    familial NEC G31.89
    fatty G31.89
    funicular —see Degeneration, combined
    posterolateral —see Degeneration,
        combined
    subacute combined —see Degeneration,
        combined
    tuberculous A17.81
spleen D73.0
    amyloid E85.4 [D77]
stomach K31.89
striatonigral G23.2
suprarenal (capsule) (gland) E27.8
synovial membrane (pulpy) —see Disorder,
    synovium, specified type NEC
tapetoretinal —see Dystrophy, retina
thymus (gland) E32.8
    fatty E32.8
thyroid (gland) E07.89
tricuspid (heart) (valve) I07.9
tuberculous NEC —see Tuberculosis
turbinate J34.89
uterus (cystic) N85.8
vascular (senile) —see Arteriosclerosis
    hypertensive —see Hypertension
vitreoretinal, secondary —see Degeneration,
    retina, peripheral, secondary,
    vitreoretinal
vitreous (body) H43.81-●
Wallerian —see Disorder, nerve
Wilson's hepatolenticular E83.01

Deglutition
paralysis R13.0
    hysterical F44.4
pneumonia J69.0
Degos' disease I77.89
Dehiscence (of)
amputation stump T87.81
cesarean wound O90.0
closure of
    cornea T81.31
    craniotomy T81.32
    fascia (muscular) (superficial) T81.32
    internal organ or tissue T81.32
    laceration (external) (internal) T81.33
    ligament T81.32
    mucosa T81.31
    muscle or muscle flap T81.32
    ribs or rib cage T81.32
    skin and subcutaneous tissue (full-
        thickness) (superficial) T81.31
    skull T81.32
    sternum (sternotomy) T81.32
    tendon T81.32
    traumatic laceration (external) (internal)
        T81.33
episiotomy O90.1
operation wound NEC T81.31
    external operation wound (superficial) T81.31
    internal operation wound (deep) T81.32
perineal wound (postpartum) O90.1
traumatic injury wound repair T81.33
wound T81.30
    traumatic repair T81.33
Dehydration E86.0
newborn P74.1
Déjérine-Roussy syndrome G93.89
Déjérine-Sottas disease or neuropathy
    (hypertrophic) G60.0
Déjérine-Thomas atrophy G23.8
Delay, delayed
any plane in pelvis
    complicating delivery O66.9
birth or delivery NOS O63.9
closure, ductus arteriosus (Botalli) P29.38
coagulation —see Defect, coagulation
conduction (cardiac) (ventricular) I45.9
delivery, second twin, triplet, etc O63.2
development R62.50
    global F88
    intellectual (specific) F81.9
    language F80.9
        due to hearing loss F80.4
    learning F81.9
    ▶milestone R62.0
    pervasive F84.9
    physiological R62.50
        specified stage NEC R62.0
    reading F81.0
    sexual E30.0
    speech F80.9
        due to hearing loss F80.4
    spelling F81.81
ejaculation F52.32
gastric emptying K30
menarche E30.0
menstruation (cause unknown) N91.0
milestone R62.0
passage of meconium (newborn) P76.0
primary respiration P28.9
puberty (constitutional) E30.0
separation of umbilical cord P96.82
sexual maturation, female E30.0
sleep phase syndrome G47.21
union, fracture —see Fracture, by site
vaccination Z28.9
Deletion(s)
autosome Q93.9
    identified by fluorescence in situ
        hybridization (FISH) Q93.89
    identified by in situ hybridization (ISH)
        Q93.89

Deletion *(Continued)*
  chromosome
    with complex rearrangements NEC Q93.7
    part of NEC Q93.59
    seen only at prometaphase Q93.89
    short arm
      4 Q93.3
      5p Q93.4
      22q11.2 Q93.81
    specified NEC Q93.89
    long arm chromosome 18 or 21 Q93.89
      with complex rearrangements NEC
        Q93.7
  microdeletions NEC Q93.88
Delhi boil or button B55.1
Delinquency (juvenile) (neurotic) F91.8
  group Z72.810
Delinquent immunization status Z28.3
Delirious (acute or subacute) (not alcohol or
    drug-induced) (with dementia) R41.0
  alcoholic (acute) (tremens) (withdrawal)
      F10.921
    with intoxication F10.921
      in
        abuse F10.121
        dependence F10.221
  due to (secondary to)
    alcohol
      intoxication F10.921
        in
          abuse F10.121
          dependence F10.221
      withdrawal F10.231
    amphetamine intoxication F15.921
      in
        abuse F15.121
        dependence F15.221
    anxiolytic
      intoxication F13.921
        in
          abuse F13.121
          dependence F13.221
      withdrawal F13.231
    cannabis intoxication (acute) F12.921
      in
        abuse F12.121
        dependence F12.221
    cocaine intoxication (acute) F14.921
      in
        abuse F14.121
        dependence F14.221
    general medical condition F05
    hallucinogen intoxication F16.921
      in
        abuse F16.121
        dependence F16.221
    hypnotic
      intoxication F13.921
        in
          abuse F13.121
          dependence F13.221
      withdrawal F13.231
    inhalant intoxication (acute) F18.921
      in
        abuse F18.121
        dependence F18.221
    multiple etiologies F05
    opioid intoxication (acute) F11.921
      in
        abuse F11.121
        dependence F11.221
    other (or unknown) substance F19.921
    phencyclidine intoxication (acute) F16.921
      in
        abuse F16.121
        dependence F16.221
    psychoactive substance NEC intoxication
        (acute) F19.921
      in
        abuse F19.121
        dependence F19.221

Delirious *(Continued)*
  due to *(Continued)*
    sedative
      intoxication F13.921
        in
          abuse F13.121
          dependence F13.221
      withdrawal F13.231
    unknown etiology R41.0
  exhaustion F43.0
  hysterical F44.89
  postprocedural (postoperative) F05
  puerperal F05
  thyroid —*see* Thyrotoxicosis with thyroid
    storm
  traumatic —*see* Injury, intracranial
  tremens (alcohol-induced) F10.231
    sedative-induced F13.231
Delivery (childbirth) (labor)
  arrested active phase O62.1
  cesarean (for)
    without indication O82
    abnormal
      pelvis (bony) (deformity) (major) NEC
        with disproportion (fetopelvic) O33.0
        with obstructed labor O65.0
      presentation or position O32.9
    abruptio placentae —*see also* Abruptio
        placentae O45.9-●
    acromion presentation O32.2
    atony, uterus O62.2
    breech presentation O32.1
      incomplete O32.8
    brow presentation O32.3
    cephalopelvic disproportion O33.9
    cerclage O34.3-●
    chin presentation O32.3
    cicatrix of cervix O34.4-●
    contracted pelvis (general)
      inlet O33.2
      outlet O33.3
    cord presentation or prolapse O69.0
    cystocele O34.8-●
    deformity (acquired) (congenital)
      pelvic organs or tissues NEC O34.8-●
      pelvis (bony) NEC O33.0
    disproportion NOS O33.9
    eclampsia —*see* Eclampsia
    face presentation O32.3
    failed
      forceps O66.5
      induction of labor O61.9
        instrumental O61.1
        mechanical O61.1
        medical O61.0
        specified NEC O61.8
        surgical O61.1
      trial of labor NOS O66.40
        following previous cesarean delivery
          O66.41
      vacuum extraction O66.5
      ventouse O66.5
    fetal-maternal hemorrhage O43.01-●
    hemorrhage (intrapartum) O67.9
      with coagulation defect O67.0
      specified cause NEC O67.8
    high head at term O32.4
    hydrocephalic fetus O33.6
    incarceration of uterus O34.51-●
    incoordinate uterine action O62.4
    increased size, fetus O33.5
    inertia, uterus O62.2
      primary O62.0
      secondary O62.1
    isthmocele O34.22
    lateroversion, uterus O34.59-●
    mal lie O32.9
    malposition
      fetus O32.9
      pelvic organs or tissues NEC O34.8-●
      uterus NEC O34.59-●

Delivery *(Continued)*
  cesarean *(Continued)*
    malpresentation NOS O32.9
    oblique presentation O32.2
    occurring after 37 completed weeks of
      gestation but before 39 completed
      weeks gestation due to (spontaneous)
      onset of labor O75.82
    oversize fetus O33.5
    pelvic tumor NEC O34.8-●
    placenta previa O44.0-●
      complete O44.0-●
        with hemorrhage O44.1-●
    placental insufficiency O36.51-●
    planned, occurring after 37 completed
      weeks of gestation but before 39
      completed weeks gestation due to
      (spontaneous) onset of labor O75.82
    polyp, cervix O34.4-●
      causing obstructed labor O65.5
    poor dilatation, cervix O62.0
    pre-eclampsia O14.94
      mild O14.04
      moderate O14.04
      severe O14.14
        with hemolysis, elevated liver
          enzymes and low platelet count
          (HELLP) O14.24
    previous
      cesarean delivery O34.219
        classical (vertical) scar O34.212
        isthmocele O34.22
        low transverse scar O34.211
        mid-transverse T incision O34.218
        scar
          defect (isthmocele) O34.22
          specified type NEC O34.218
      surgery (to)
        cervix O34.4-●
        gynecological NEC O34.8-●
        rectum O34.7-●
        uterus O34.29
        vagina O34.6-●
    prolapse
      arm or hand O32.2
      uterus O34.52-●
    prolonged labor NOS O63.9
    rectocele O34.8-●
    retroversion
      uterus O34.53-●
    rigid
      cervix O34.4-●
      pelvic floor O34.8-●
      perineum O34.7-●
      vagina O34.6-●
      vulva O34.7-●
    sacculation, pregnant uterus O34.59-●
    scar(s)
      cervix O34.4-●
      cesarean delivery O34.219
        classical (vertical) O34.212
        isthmocele O34.22
        low transverse O34.211
        mid-transverse T incision O34.218
        scar
          defect (isthmocele) O34.22
          specified type NEC O34.218
      defect (isthmocele) O34.22
      transmural uterine O34.29
      uterus O34.29
    Shirodkar suture in situ O34.3-●
    shoulder presentation O32.2
    stenosis or stricture, cervix O34.4-●
    streptococcus group B (GBS) carrier state
      O99.824
    transmural uterine scar O34.29
    transverse presentation or lie O32.2
    tumor, pelvic organs or tissues NEC O34.8-●
      cervix O34.4-●
    umbilical cord presentation or prolapse O69.0
  completely normal case O80

Delivery (Continued)
  complicated O75.9
    by
      abnormal, abnormality (of)
        forces of labor O62.9
          specified type NEC O62.8
        glucose O99.814
        uterine contractions NOS O62.9
      abruptio placentae —see also Abruptio
          placentae O45.9-●
      abuse
        physical O9A.32
        psychological O9A.52
        sexual O9A.42
      adherent placenta O72.0
        without hemorrhage O73.0
      alcohol use O99.314
      anemia (pre-existing) O99.02
      anesthetic death O74.8
      annular detachment of cervix O71.3
      atony, uterus O62.2
      attempted vacuum extraction and
          forceps O66.5
      Bandl's ring O62.4
      bariatric surgery status O99.844
      biliary tract disorder O26.62
      bleeding —see Delivery, complicated by,
          hemorrhage
      blood disorder NEC O99.12
      cervical dystocia (hypotonic) O62.2
        primary O62.0
        secondary O62.1
      circulatory system disorder O99.42
      compression of cord (umbilical) NEC
          O69.2
      condition NEC O99.892
      contraction, contracted ring O62.4
      cord (umbilical)
        around neck
          with compression O69.1
          without compression O69.81
        bruising O69.5
        complication O69.9
          specified NEC O69.89
        compression NEC O69.2
        entanglement O69.2
          without compression O69.82
        hematoma O69.5
        presentation O69.0
        prolapse O69.0
        short O69.3
        thrombosis (vessels) O69.5
        vascular lesion O69.5
      Couvelaire uterus O45.8X-●
      damage to (injury to) NEC
        perineum O71.82
        periurethral tissue O71.82
        vulva O71.82
      delay following rupture of membranes
          (spontaneous) —see Pregnancy,
          complicated by, premature rupture
          of membranes
      depressed fetal heart tones O76
      diabetes O24.92
        gestational O24.429
          diet controlled O24.420
          insulin controlled O24.424
          oral drug controlled (antidiabetic)
              (hypoglycemic) O24.425
        pre-existing O24.32
          specified NEC O24.82
          type 1 O24.02
          type 2 O24.12
      diastasis recti (abdominis) O71.89
      dilatation
        bladder O66.8
        cervix incomplete, poor or slow O62.0
      disease NEC O99.892
      disruptio uteri —see Delivery,
          complicated by, rupture, uterus
      drug use O99.324

Delivery (Continued)
  complicated (Continued)
    by (Continued)
      dysfunction, uterus NOS O62.9
        hypertonic O62.4
        hypotonic O62.2
          primary O62.0
          secondary O62.1
        incoordinate O62.4
      eclampsia O15.1
      embolism (pulmonary) —see Embolism,
          obstetric
      endocrine, nutritional or metabolic
          disease NEC O99.284
      failed
        attempted vaginal birth after previous
            cesarean delivery O66.41
        induction of labor O61.9
          instrumental O61.1
          mechanical O61.1
          medical O61.0
          specified NEC O61.8
          surgical O61.1
        trial of labor O66.40
      female genital mutilation O65.5
      fetal
        abnormal acid-base balance O68
        acidemia O68
        acidosis O68
        alkalosis O68
        death, early O02.1
        deformity O66.3
        heart rate or rhythm (abnormal) (non-
            reassuring) O76
        hypoxia O77.8
        stress O77.9
          due to drug administration O77.1
          electrocardiographic evidence of
              O77.8
          specified NEC O77.8
          ultrasound evidence of O77.8
      fever during labor O75.2
      gastric banding status O99.844
      gastric bypass status O99.844
      gastrointestinal disease NEC O99.62
      gestational
        diabetes O24.429
          diet controlled O24.420
          insulin (and diet) controlled O24.424
          oral drug controlled (antidiabetic)
              (hypoglycemic) O24.425
        edema O12.04
          with proteinuria O12.24
        proteinuria O12.14
      gonorrhea O98.22
      hematoma O71.7
        ischial spine O71.7
        pelvic O71.7
        vagina O71.7
        vulva or perineum O71.7
      hemorrhage (uterine) O67.9
        associated with
          afibrinogenemia O67.0
          coagulation defect O67.0
          hyperfibrinolysis O67.0
          hypofibrinogenemia O67.0
        due to
          low implantation of placenta O44.5-●
          low-lying placenta O44.5-●
          placenta previa O44.1-●
            marginal O44.3-●
            partial O44.3-●
          premature separation of placenta
              (normally implanted) (see also
              Abruptio placentae) O45.9-●
          retained placenta O72.0
          uterine leiomyoma O67.8
        placenta NEC O67.8
        postpartum NEC (atonic) (immediate)
            O72.1
          with retained or trapped placenta
              O72.0

Delivery (Continued)
  complicated (Continued)
    by (Continued)
      hemorrhage (uterine) (Continued)
        postpartum NEC (Continued)
          delayed O72.2
          secondary O72.2
          third stage O72.0
      hourglass contraction, uterus O62.4
      hypertension, hypertensive (pre-
          existing) —see Hypertension,
          complicated by, childbirth (labor)
      hypotension O26.5-●
      incomplete dilatation (cervix) O62.0
      incoordinate uterus contractions
          O62.4
      inertia, uterus O62.2
        during latent phase of labor O62.0
        primary O62.0
        secondary O62.1
      infection (maternal) O98.92
        carrier state NEC O99.834
        gonorrhea O98.22
        human immunodeficiency virus (HIV)
            O98.72
        sexually transmitted NEC O98.32
        specified NEC O98.82
        syphilis O98.12
        tuberculosis O98.02
        viral hepatitis O98.42
        viral NEC O98.52
      injury (to mother) (see also Delivery,
          complicated, by, damage to) O71.9
        nonobstetric O9A.22
          caused by abuse —see Delivery,
              complicated by, abuse
      intrauterine fetal death, early O02.1
      inversion, uterus O71.2
      laceration (perineal) O70.9
        anus (sphincter) O70.4
          with third degree laceration —see
              also Delivery, complicated, by,
              laceration, perineum, third
              degree O70.20
          with mucosa O70.3
          without third degree laceration
              O70.4
        bladder (urinary) O71.5
        bowel O71.5
        cervix (uteri) O71.3
        fourchette O70.0
        hymen O70.0
        labia O70.0
        pelvic
          floor O70.1
          organ NEC O71.5
        perineum, perineal O70.9
          first degree O70.0
          fourth degree O70.3
          muscles O70.1
          second degree O70.1
          skin O70.0
          slight O70.0
          third degree O70.20
            with
              both external anal sphincter
                  (EAS) and internal anal
                  sphincter (IAS) torn (IIIc)
                  O70.23
              less than 50% of external anal
                  sphincter (EAS) thickness
                  torn (IIIa) O70.21
              more than 50% external anal
                  sphincter (EAS) thickness
                  torn (IIIb) O70.22
            IIIa O70.21
            IIIb O70.22
            IIIc O70.23
        peritoneum (pelvic) O71.5
        rectovaginal (septum) (without
            perineal laceration) O71.4

Delivery *(Continued)*
　complicated *(Continued)*
　　by *(Continued)*
　　　laceration *(Continued)*
　　　　rectovaginal *(Continued)*
　　　　　with perineum —*see also* Delivery,
　　　　　　complicated, by, laceration,
　　　　　　perineum, third degree O70.20
　　　　　　with anal or rectal mucosa
　　　　　　　O70.3
　　　　specified NEC O71.89
　　　　sphincter ani —*see* Delivery,
　　　　　complicated, by, laceration, anus
　　　　　(sphincter)
　　　　urethra O71.5
　　　　uterus O71.81
　　　　　before labor O71.81
　　　　vagina, vaginal (deep) (high)
　　　　　(without perineal laceration)
　　　　　O71.4
　　　　　with perineum O70.0
　　　　　　muscles, with perineum O70.1
　　　　vulva O70.0
　　　liver disorder O26.62
　　　malignancy O9A.12
　　　malnutrition O25.2
　　　malposition, malpresentation
　　　　without obstruction O32.9 —*see
　　　　　also* Delivery, complicated by,
　　　　　obstruction
　　　　breech O32.1
　　　　compound O32.6
　　　　face (brow) (chin) O32.3
　　　　footling O38.8
　　　　high head O32.4
　　　　oblique O32.2
　　　　specified NEC O32.8
　　　　transverse O32.2
　　　　unstable lie O32.0
　　　　placenta O44.0-•
　　　　　with hemorrhage O44.1-•
　　　　uterus or cervix O65.5
　　　meconium in amniotic fluid O77.0
　　　mental disorder NEC O99.344
　　　metrorrhexis —*see* Delivery, complicated
　　　　by, rupture, uterus
　　　nervous system disorder O99.354
　　　obesity (pre-existing) O99.214
　　　obesity surgery status O99.844
　　　obstetric trauma O71.9
　　　　specified NEC O71.89
　　　obstructed labor
　　　　due to
　　　　　breech (complete) (frank)
　　　　　　presentation O64.1
　　　　　　incomplete O64.8
　　　　　brow presenation O64.3
　　　　　buttock presentation O64.1
　　　　　chin presentation O64.2
　　　　　compound presentation O64.5
　　　　　contracted pelvis O65.1
　　　　　deep transverse arrest O64.0
　　　　　deformed pelvis O65.0
　　　　　dystocia (fetal) O66.9
　　　　　　due to
　　　　　　　conjoined twins O66.3
　　　　　　　fetal
　　　　　　　　abnormality NEC O66.3
　　　　　　　　ascites O66.3
　　　　　　　　hydrops O66.3
　　　　　　　　meningomyelocele O66.3
　　　　　　　　sacral teratoma O66.3
　　　　　　　　tumor O66.3
　　　　　　　hydrocephalic fetus O66.3
　　　　　　　shoulder O66.0
　　　　　face presentation O64.2
　　　　　fetopelvic disproportion O65.4
　　　　　footling presentation O64.8
　　　　　impacted shoulders O66.0
　　　　　incomplete rotation of fetal head
　　　　　　O64.0

Delivery *(Continued)*
　complicated *(Continued)*
　　by *(Continued)*
　　　obstructed labor *(Continued)*
　　　　due to *(Continued)*
　　　　　large fetus O66.2
　　　　　locked twins O66.1
　　　　　malposition O64.9
　　　　　　specified NEC O64.8
　　　　　malpresentation O64.9
　　　　　　specified NEC O64.8
　　　　　multiple fetuses NEC O66.6
　　　　　pelvic
　　　　　　abnormality (maternal) O65.9
　　　　　　　organ O65.5
　　　　　　　specified NEC O65.8
　　　　　　contraction
　　　　　　　inlet O65.2
　　　　　　　mid-cavity O65.3
　　　　　　　outlet O65.3
　　　　　persistent (position)
　　　　　　occipitoiliac O64.0
　　　　　　occipitoposterior O64.0
　　　　　　occipitosacral O64.0
　　　　　　occipitotransverse O64.0
　　　　　prolapsed arm O64.4
　　　　　shoulder presentation O64.4
　　　　specified NEC O66.8
　　　pathological retraction ring, uterus
　　　　O62.4
　　　penetration, pregnant uterus by
　　　　instrument O71.1
　　　perforation —*see* Delivery, complicated
　　　　by, laceration
　　　placenta, placental
　　　　ablatio —*see also* Abruptio placentae
　　　　　O45.9-•
　　　　abnormality O43.9-•
　　　　　specified NEC O43.89-•
　　　　abruptio —*see also* Abruptio placentae
　　　　　O45.9-•
　　　　accreta O43.21-•
　　　　adherent (with hemorrhage) O72.0
　　　　　without hemorrhage O73.0
　　　　detachment (premature) —*see also*
　　　　　Abruptio placentae O45.9-•
　　　　disorder O43.9-•
　　　　　specified NEC O43.89-•
　　　　hemorrhage NEC O67.8
　　　　increta O43.22-•
　　　　low (implantation) (lying) O44.4-•
　　　　　with hemorrhage O44.5-•
　　　　malformation O43.10-•
　　　　malposition O44.0-•
　　　　　without hemorrhage O44.1-•
　　　　percreta O43.23-•
　　　　previa (central) (complete) (lateral)
　　　　　(total) O44.0-•
　　　　　with hemorrhage O44.1-•
　　　　　　marginal O44.2-•
　　　　　　　with hemorrhage O44.3-•
　　　　　　partial O44.2-•
　　　　　　　with hemorrhage O44.3-•
　　　　retained (with hemorrhage) O72.0
　　　　　without hemorrhage O73.0
　　　　separation (premature) O45.9-•
　　　　　specified NEC O45.8X-•
　　　　vicious insertion O44.1-•
　　　precipitate labor O62.3
　　　premature rupture, membranes (see
　　　　also Pregnancy, complicated by,
　　　　premature rupture of membranes)
　　　　O42.90
　　　prolapse
　　　　arm or hand O32.2
　　　　cord (umbilical) O69.0
　　　　foot or leg O32.8
　　　　uterus O34.52-•
　　　prolonged labor O63.9
　　　　first stage O63.0
　　　　second stage O63.1

Delivery *(Continued)*
　complicated *(Continued)*
　　by *(Continued)*
　　　protozoal disease (maternal) O98.62
　　　respiratory disease NEC O99.52
　　　retained membranes or portions of
　　　　placenta O72.2
　　　　without hemorrhage O73.1
　　　retarded birth O63.9
　　　retention of secundines (with
　　　　hemorrhage) O72.0
　　　　without hemorrhage O73.0
　　　　partial O72.2
　　　　　without hemorrhage O73.1
　　　rupture
　　　　bladder (urinary) O71.5
　　　　cervix O71.3
　　　　pelvic organ NEC O71.5
　　　　urethra O71.5
　　　　uterus (during or after labor) O71.1
　　　　　before labor O71.0-•
　　　separation, pubic bone (symphysis
　　　　pubis) O71.6
　　　shock O75.1
　　　shoulder presentation O64.4
　　　skin disorder NEC O99.72
　　　spasm, cervix O62.4
　　　stenosis or stricture, cervix O65.5
　　　streptococcus group B (GBS) carrier state
　　　　O99.824
　　　subluxation of symphysis (pubis)
　　　　O26.72
　　　syphilis (maternal) O98.12
　　　tear —*see* Delivery, complicated by,
　　　　laceration
　　　tetanic uterus O62.4
　　　trauma (obstetrical) —*see also* Delivery,
　　　　complicated, by, damage to O71.9
　　　　non-obstetric O9A.22
　　　　periurethral O71.82
　　　　specified NEC O71.89
　　　tuberculosis (maternal) O98.02
　　　tumor, pelvic organs or tissues NEC
　　　　O65.5
　　　umbilical cord around neck
　　　　with compression O69.1
　　　　without compression O69.81
　　　uterine inertia O62.2
　　　　during latent phase of labor O62.0
　　　　primary O62.0
　　　　secondary O62.1
　　　vasa previa O69.4
　　　velamentous insertion of cord
　　　　O43.12-•
　　specified complication NEC O75.89
　delayed NOS O63.9
　　following rupture of membranes
　　　artificial O75.5
　　second twin, triplet, etc. O63.2
　forceps, low following failed vacuum
　　extraction O66.5
　missed (at or near term) O36.4
　normal O80
　obstructed —*see* Delivery, complicated by,
　　obstructed labor
　precipitate O62.3
　preterm —*see also* Pregnancy, complicated by,
　　preterm labor O60.10
　spontaneous O80
　term pregnancy NOS O80
　uncomplicated O80
　vaginal, following previous cesarean delivery
　　O34.219
　　classical (vertical) scar O34.212
　　low transverse scar O34.211
　　mid-transverse T incision O34.218
　　scar
　　　defect (isthmocele) O34.22
　　　specified type NEC O34.218]
Delusions (paranoid) —*see* Disorder, delusional

▶ New　⇒ Revised　~~deleted~~ Deleted　• Use Additional Character(s)

Dementia (degenerative (primary)) (old age)
(persisting) (unspecified severity) (without
behavioral disturbance, psychotic
disturbance, mood disturbance, and
anxiety) F03.90
  with
    aggressive behavior F03.91
    behavioral disturbance F03.91
    combative behavior F03.91
    aberrant motor behavior (exit-seeking)
      (pacing) (restlessness) (rocking) F03.911
    agitation F03.911
    anxiety F03.94
    behavioral disturbances (sexual
      disinhibition) (sleep disturbance)
      (social disinhibition) F03.918
      specified NEC F03.918
  Lewy bodies (see also Dementia, in,
    diseases specified elsewhere) G31.83
    [F02.80]
    with behavioral disturbance (see also
      Dementia, in, diseases specified
      elsewhere) G31.83 [F02.81-•]
    mood disturbance (anhedonia) (apathy)
      (depression) F03.93
  Parkinson's disease (see also Dementia, in,
    diseases specified elsewhere) G20
    [F02.80]
    with behavioral disturbance G20
      [F02.81-•]
  Parkinsonism (see also Dementia, in,
    diseases specified elsewhere) G31.83
    [F02.80]
    with behavioral disturbance (see also
      Dementia, in, diseases specified
      elsewhere) G31.83 [F02.81-•]
    violent behavior F03.91
    psychotic disturbance (delusional state)
      (hallucinations) (paranoia)
      (suspiciousness) F03.92
    verbal or physical behaviors (anger)
      (aggression) (combativeness)
      (profanity) (shouting) (threatening)
      (violence) F03.911
  alcoholic F10.97
    with dependence F10.27
  Alzheimer's type —see Disease, Alzheimer's
  arteriosclerotic —see Dementia, vascular
  atypical, Alzheimer's type —see Disease,
    Alzheimer's, specified NEC
  congenital —see Disability, intellectual
  frontal (lobe) (see also Dementia, in, diseases
    specified elsewhere) G31.09 [F02.80]
    with behavioral disturbance (see also
      Dementia, in, diseases specified
      elsewhere) G31.09 [F02.81-•]
  frontotemporal (see also Dementia, in,
    diseases specified elsewhere) G31.09
    [F02.80]
    with behavioral disturbance (see also
      Dementia, in, diseases specified
      elsewhere) G31.09 [F02.81-•]
    specified NEC (see also Dementia, in,
      diseases specified elsewhere) G31.09
      [F02.80]
      with behavioral disturbance (see also
        Dementia, in, diseases specified
        elsewhere) G31.09 [F02.81-•]
  in (due to)
    alcohol F10.97
      with dependence F10.27
    Alzheimer's disease —see Disease,
      Alzheimer's
    arteriosclerotic brain disease —see
      Dementia, vascular
    cerebral lipidoses (see also Dementia, in,
      diseases specified elsewhere)
      E75.-• [F02.80]
      with behavioral disturbance (see also
        Dementia, in, diseases specified
        elsewhere) E75.-• [F02.81-•]

Dementia (Continued)
  in (Continued)
    Creutzfeldt-Jakob disease —see also
      Creutzfeldt-Jakob disease or
      syndrome (with dementia) A81.00
    diseases specified elsewhere (unspecified
      severity) (without behavioral
      disturbance, psychotic disturbance,
      mood disturbance, and anxiety) F02.80
      with
        aberrant motor behavior (exit-seeking)
          (pacing) (restlessness) (rocking)
          F02.811
        agitation F02.811
        anxiety F02.84
        behavioral disturbances (sexual
          disinhibition) (sleep disturbance)
          (social disinhibition) F02.818
          specified NEC F02.818
        mood disturbance (anhedonia)
          (apathy) (depression) F02.83
        psychotic disturbance (delusional
          state) (hallucinations) (paranoia)
          (suspiciousness) F02.82
        verbal or physical behaviors (anger)
          (aggression) (combativeness)
          (profanity) (shouting)
          (threatening)(violence) F02.811
      mild F02.A0
      with
        aberrant motor behavior (exit-
          seeking) (pacing) (restlessness)
          (rocking) F02.A11
        agitation F02.A11
        anxiety F02.A4
        behavioral disturbances (sexual
          disinhibition) (sleep
          disturbance) (social
          disinhibition) F02.A18
          specified NEC F02.A18
        mood disturbance (anhedonia)
          (apathy) (depression) F02.A3
        psychotic disturbance (delusional
          state) (hallucinations) (paranoia)
          (suspiciousness) F02.A2
        verbal or physical behaviors (anger)
          (aggression) (combativeness)
          (profanity) (shouting)
          (threatening)(violence) F02.A11
      moderate F02.B0
      with
        aberrant motor behavior (exit-
          seeking) (pacing) (restlessness)
          (rocking) F02.B11
        agitation F02.B11
        anxiety F02.B4
        behavioral disturbances (sexual
          disinhibition) (sleep
          disturbance) (social
          disinhibition) F02.B18
          specified NEC F02.B18
        mood disturbance (anhedonia)
          (apathy) (depression) F02.B3
        psychotic disturbance (delusional
          state) (hallucinations) (paranoia)
          (suspiciousness) F02.B2
        verbal or physical behaviors (anger)
          (aggression) (combativeness)
          (profanity) (shouting)
          (threatening)(violence) F02.B11
      severe F02.C0
      with
        aberrant motor behavior (exit-
          seeking) (pacing) (restlessness)
          (rocking) F02.C11
        agitation F02.C11
        anxiety F02.C4
        behavioral disturbances (sexual
          disinhibition) (sleep
          disturbance) (social
          disinhibition) F02.C18
          specified NEC F02.C18

Dementia (Continued)
  in (Continued)
    diseases specified elsewhere (Continued)
      severe (Continued)
        with (Continued)
          mood disturbance (anhedonia)
            (apathy) (depression) F02.C3
          psychotic disturbance (delusional
            state) (hallucinations)
            (paranoia) (suspiciousness)
            F02.C2
          verbal or physical behaviors (anger)
            (aggression) (combativeness)
            (profanity) (shouting)
            (threatening)(violence) F02.C11
    epilepsy (see also Dementia, in, diseases
      specified elsewhere) G40.-• [F02.80]
    with behavioral disturbance (see also
      Dementia, in, diseases specified
      elsewhere) G40.-• [F02.81-•]
    hepatolenticular degeneration (see also
      Dementia, in, diseases specified
      elsewhere) E83.01 [F02.80]
    with behavioral disturbance (see also
      Dementia, in, diseases specified
      elsewhere) E83.01 [F02.81-•]
    human immunodeficiency virus (HIV)
      disease (see also Dementia, in, diseases
      specified elsewhere) B20 [F02.80]
    with behavioral disturbance (see also
      Dementia, in, diseases specified
      elsewhere) B20 [F02.81-•]
    Huntington's disease or chorea (see also
      Dementia, in, diseases specified
      elsewhere) G10 [F02.80]
    with behavioral disturbance (see also
      Dementia, in, diseases specified
      elsewhere) G10 [F02.81-•]
    hypercalcemia (see also Dementia, in,
      diseases specified elsewhere) E83.52
      [F02.80]
    with behavioral disturbance (see also
      Dementia, in, diseases specified
      elsewhere) E83.52 [F02.81-•]
    hypothyroidism, acquired (see also
      Dementia, in, diseases specified
      elsewhere) E03.9 [F02.80]
    with behavioral disturbance (see also
      Dementia, in, diseases specified
      elsewhere) E03.9 [F02.81-•]
    due to iodine deficiency (see also
      Dementia, in, diseases specified
      elsewhere) E01.8 [F02.80]
      with behavioral disturbance (see also
        Dementia, in, diseases specified
        elsewhere) E01.8 [F02.81-•]
    inhalants F18.97
      with dependence F18.27
    multiple
      etiologies F03
    sclerosis (see also Dementia, in, diseases
      specified elsewhere) G35 [F02.80]
    with behavioral disturbance (see also
      Dementia, in, diseases specified
      elsewhere) G35 [F02.81-•]
    neurosyphilis (see also Dementia, in,
      diseases specified elsewhere) A52.17
      [F02.80]
    with behavioral disturbance (see also
      Dementia, in, diseases specified
      elsewhere) A52.17 [F02.81-•]
    juvenile (see also Dementia, in, diseases
      specified elsewhere) A50.49 [F02.80]
    with behavioral disturbance (see also
      Dementia, in, diseases specified
      elsewhere) A50.49 [F02.81-•]
    niacin deficiency (see also Dementia, in,
      diseases specified elsewhere) E52
      [F02.80]
    with behavioral disturbance (see also
      Dementia, in, diseases specified
      elsewhere) E52 [F02.81-•]

Dementia *(Continued)*
  in *(Continued)*
    ➠paralysis agitans *(see also* Dementia, in, diseases specified elsewhere) G20 *[F02.80]*
      ➠with behavioral disturbance *(see also* Dementia, in, diseases specified elsewhere) G20 *[F02.81-●]*
    ➠Parkinson's disease *(see also* Dementia, in, diseases specified elsewhere) G20 *[F02.80]*
    ➠pellagra *(see also* Dementia, in, diseases specified elsewhere) E52 *[F02.80]*
      ➠with behavioral disturbance *(see also* Dementia, in, diseases specified elsewhere) E52 *[F02.81-●]*
    ➠Pick's G31.01 *(see also* Dementia, in, diseases specified elsewhere) *[F02.80]*
      ➠with behavioral disturbance *(see also* Dementia, in, diseases specified elsewhere) G31.01 *[F02.81-●]*
    ➠polyarteritis nodosa *(see also* Dementia, in, diseases specified elsewhere) M30.0 *[F02.80]*
      ➠with behavioral disturbance *(see also* Dementia, in, diseases specified elsewhere) M30.0 *[F02.81-●]*
    psychoactive drug F19.97
      with dependence F19.27
      inhalants F18.97
        with dependence F18.27
      sedatives, hypnotics or anxiolytics F13.97
        with dependence F13.27
    sedatives, hypnotics or anxiolytics F13.97
      with dependence F13.27
    ➠systemic lupus erythematosus *(see also* Dementia, in, diseases specified elsewhere) M32.-● *[F02.80]*
      ➠with behavioral disturbance *(see also* Dementia, in, diseases specified elsewhere) M32.-● *[F02.81-●]*
    trypanosomiasis
      ➠African *(see also* Dementia, in, diseases specified elsewhere) B56.9 *[F02.80]*
        ➠with behavioral disturbance *(see also* Dementia, in, diseases specified elsewhere) B56.9 *[F02.81-●]*
    ➠unknown etiology *(see also* Dementia, in, diseases specified elsewhere) F03.-●
    ➠vitamin B12 deficiency *(see also* Dementia, in, diseases specified elsewhere) E53.8 *[F02.80]*
      ➠with behavioral disturbance *(see also* Dementia, in, diseases specified elsewhere) E53.8 *[F02.81-●]*
    volatile solvents F18.97
      with dependence F18.27
  infantile, infantilis F84.3
  ➠Lewy body *(see also* Dementia, in, diseases specified elsewhere) G31.83 *[F02.80]*
    ➠with behavioral disturbance *(see also* Dementia, in, diseases specified elsewhere) G31.83 *[F02.81-●]*
  ▶mild F02.A0
    ▶with
      ▶aberrant motor behavior (exit-seeking) (pacing) (restlessness) (rocking) F02.A11
      ▶agitation F02.A11
      ▶anxiety F02.A4
      ▶behavioral disturbances (sexual disinhibition) (sleep disturbance) (social disinhibition) F02.A18
        ▶specified NEC F02.A18
      ▶mood disturbance (anhedonia) (apathy) (depression) F02.A3
      ▶psychotic disturbance (delusional state) (hallucinations) (paranoia) (suspiciousness) F02.A2
      ▶verbal or physical behaviors (anger) (aggression) (combativeness) (profanity) (shouting) (threatening) (violence) F02.A11

Dementia *(Continued)*
  in *(Continued)*
    ▶moderate F02.B0
      ▶with
        ▶aberrant motor behavior (exit-seeking) (pacing) (restlessness) (rocking) F02.B11
        ▶agitation F02.B11
        ▶anxiety F02.B4
        ▶behavioral disturbances (sexual disinhibition) (sleep disturbance) (social disinhibition) F02.B18
          ▶specified NEC F02.B18
        ▶mood disturbance (anhedonia) (apathy) (depression) F02.B3
        ▶psychotic disturbance (delusional state) (hallucinations) (paranoia) (suspiciousness) F02.B2
        ▶verbal or physical behaviors (anger) (aggression) (combativeness) (profanity) (shouting) (threatening)(violence) F02.B11
    multi-infarct —*see* Dementia, vascular
  ➠paralytica, paralytic (syphilitic) *(see also* Dementia, in, diseases specified elsewhere) A52.17 *[F02.80]*
    ➠with behavioral disturbance *(see also* Dementia, in, diseases specified elsewhere) A52.17 *[F02.81-●]*
    juvenilis A50.45
  paretic A52.17
  praecox —*see* Schizophrenia
  presenile F03
    Alzheimer's type —*see* Disease, Alzheimer's, early onset
  primary degenerative F03
  progressive, syphilitic A52.17
  senile F03
    with acute confusional state F05
    Alzheimer's type —*see* Disease, Alzheimer's, late onset
    depressed or paranoid type F03
  ▶severe F02.C0
    ▶with
      ▶aberrant motor behavior (exit-seeking) (pacing) (restlessness) (rocking) F02.C11
      ▶agitation F02.C11
      ▶anxiety F02.C4
      ▶behavioral disturbances (sexual disinhibition) (sleep disturbance) (social disinhibition) F02.C18
        ▶specified NEC F02.C18
      ▶mood disturbance (anhedonia) (apathy) (depression) F02.C3
      ▶psychotic disturbance (delusional state) (hallucinations) (paranoia) (suspiciousness) F02.C2
      ▶verbal or physical behaviors (anger) (aggression) (combativeness) (profanity) (shouting) (threatening) (violence) F02.C11
  ➠vascular (acute onset) (mixed) (multi-infarct) (subcortical) (unspecified severity) (without behavioral disturbance, psychotic disturbance, mood disturbance, and anxiety) F01.50
    ~~with behavioral disturbance F01.51~~
    ▶with
      ▶aberrant motor behavior (exit-seeking) (pacing) (restlessness) (rocking) F01.511
      ▶agitation F01.511
      ▶anxiety F01.54
      ▶behavioral disturbances (sleep disturbance) (sexual disinhibition) (social disinhibition) F01.518
        ▶specified NEC F01.518
      ▶mood disturbance (anhedonia) (apathy) (depression) F01.53

Dementia *(Continued)*
  vascular *(Continued)*
    with *(Continued)*
      ▶psychotic disturbance (delusional state) (hallucinations) (paranoia) (suspiciousness) F01.52
      ▶verbal or physical behaviors (anger) (aggression) (combativeness) (profanity) (shouting) (threatening) (violence) F01.511
    ▶mild F01.A0
      ▶with
        ▶aberrant motor behavior (exit-seeking) (pacing) (restlessness) (rocking) F01.A11
        ▶agitation F01.A11
        ▶anxiety F01.A4
        ▶behavioral disturbances (sleep disturbance) (sexual disinhibition) (social disinhibition) F01.A18
          ▶specified NEC F01.A18
        ▶mood disturbance (anhedonia) (apathy) (depression) F01.A3
        ▶psychotic disturbance (delusional state) (hallucinations) (paranoia) (suspiciousness) F01.A2
        ▶verbal or physical behaviors (anger) (aggression) (combativeness) (profanity) (shouting) (threatening)(violence) F01.A11
    ▶moderate F01.B0
      ▶with
        ▶aberrant motor behavior (exit-seeking) (pacing) (restlessness) (rocking) F01.B11
        ▶agitation F01.B11
        ▶anxiety F01.B4
        ▶behavioral disturbances (sleep disturbance) (sexual disinhibition) (social disinhibition) F01.B18
          ▶specified NEC F01.B18
        ▶mood disturbance (anhedonia) (apathy) (depression) F01.B3
        ▶psychotic disturbance (delusional state) (hallucinations) (paranoia) (suspiciousness) F01.B2
        ▶verbal or physical behaviors (anger) (aggression) (combativeness) (profanity) (shouting) (threatening)(violence) F01.B11
    ▶severe F01.C0
      ▶with
        ▶aberrant motor behavior (exit-seeking) (pacing) (restlessness) (rocking) F01.C11
        ▶agitation F01.C11
        ▶anxiety F01.C4
        ▶behavioral disturbances (sleep disturbance) (sexual disinhibition) (social disinhibition) F01.C18
          ▶specified NEC F01.C18
        ▶mood disturbance (anhedonia) (apathy) (depression) F01.C3
        ▶psychotic disturbance (delusional state) (hallucinations) (paranoia) (suspiciousness) F01.C2
        ▶verbal or physical behaviors (anger) (aggression) (combativeness) (profanity) (shouting) (threatening)(violence) F01.C11
Demineralization, bone —*see* Osteoporosis
Demodex folliculorum (infestation) B88.0
Demophobia F40.248
Demoralization R45.3
Demyelination, demyelinization
  central nervous system G37.9
    specified NEC G37.8
  corpus callosum (central) G37.1

Demyelination, demyelinization *(Continued)*
  disseminated, acute G36.9
    specified NEC G36.8
  global G35
  in optic neuritis G36.0
Dengue (classical) (fever) A90
  hemorrhagic A91
  sandfly A93.1
Dennie-Marfan syphilitic syndrome A50.45
Dens evaginatus, in dente or invaginatus
    K00.2
Dense breasts R92.2
Density
  increased, bone (disseminated) (generalized)
      (spotted) —*see* Disorder, bone, density
      and structure, specified type NEC
  lung (nodular) J98.4
Dental —*see also* condition
  examination Z01.20
    with abnormal findings Z01.21
  restoration
    aesthetically inadequate or displeasing
        K08.56
    defective K08.50
      specified NEC K08.59
    failure of marginal integrity K08.51
    failure of periodontal anatomical integrity
        K08.54
Dentia praecox K00.6
Denticles (pulp) K04.2
Dentigerous cyst K09.0
Dentin
  irregular (in pulp) K04.3
  opalescent K00.5
  secondary (in pulp) K04.3
  sensitive K03.89
Dentinogenesis imperfecta K00.5
Dentinoma —*see* Cyst, calcifying odontogenic
Dentition (syndrome) K00.7
  delayed K00.6
  difficult K00.7
  precocious K00.6
  premature K00.6
  retarded K00.6
Dependence (on) (syndrome) F19.20
  with remission F19.21
  alcohol (ethyl) (methyl) (without remission)
      F10.20
    with
      amnestic disorder, persisting F10.26
      anxiety disorder F10.280
      dementia, persisting F10.27
      intoxication F10.229
        with delirium F10.221
        uncomplicated F10.220
      mood disorder F10.24
      psychotic disorder F10.259
        with
          delusions F10.250
          hallucinations F10.251
      remission F10.21
      sexual dysfunction F10.281
      sleep disorder F10.282
      specified disorder NEC F10.288
      withdrawal F10.239
        with
          delirium F10.231
          perceptual disturbance F10.232
        uncomplicated F10.230
    counseling and surveillance Z71.41
    in remission F10.21
  amobarbital —*see* Dependence, drug,
      sedative
  amphetamine(s) (type) —*see* Dependence,
      drug, stimulant NEC
  amytal (sodium) —*see* Dependence, drug,
      sedative
  analgesic NEC F55.8
  anesthetic (agent) (gas) (general) (local)
      NEC —*see* Dependence, drug,
      psychoactive NEC

Dependence *(Continued)*
  anxiolytic NEC —*see* Dependence, drug,
      sedative
  barbital(s) —*see* Dependence, drug, sedative
  barbiturate(s) (compounds) (drugs
      classifiable to T42) —*see* Dependence,
      drug, sedative
  benzedrine —*see* Dependence, drug,
      stimulant NEC
  bhang —*see* Dependence, drug, cannabis
  bromide(s) NEC —*see* Dependence, drug,
      sedative
  caffeine —*see* Dependence, drug, stimulant
      NEC
  cannabis (sativa) (indica) (resin) (derivatives)
      (type) —*see* Dependence, drug, cannabis
  chloral (betaine) (hydrate) —*see* Dependence,
      drug, sedative
  chlordiazepoxide —*see* Dependence, drug,
      sedative
  coca (leaf) (derivatives) —*see* Dependence,
      drug, cocaine
  cocaine —*see* Dependence, drug, cocaine
  codeine —*see* Dependence, drug, opioid
  combinations of drugs F19.20
  dagga —*see* Dependence, drug, cannabis
  demerol —*see* Dependence, drug, opioid
  dexamphetamine —*see* Dependence, drug,
      stimulant NEC
  dexedrine —*see* Dependence, drug, stimulant
      NEC
  dextromethorphan —*see* Dependence, drug,
      opioid
  dextromoramide —*see* Dependence, drug,
      opioid
  dextro-nor-pseudo-ephedrine —*see*
      Dependence, drug, stimulant NEC
  dextrorphan —*see* Dependence, drug, opioid
  diazepam —*see* Dependence, drug,
  sedative
  dilaudid —*see* Dependence, drug, opioid
  D-lysergic acid diethylamide —*see*
      Dependence, drug, hallucinogen
  drug NEC F19.20
    with sleep disorder F19.282
    cannabis F12.20
      with
        anxiety disorder F12.280
        intoxication F12.229
          with
            delirium F12.221
            perceptual disturbance F12.222
          uncomplicated F12.220
        other specified disorder F12.288
        psychosis F12.259
          delusions F12.250
          hallucinations F12.251
        unspecified disorder F12.29
        withdrawal F12.23
      in remission F12.21
    cocaine F14.20
      with
        anxiety disorder F14.280
        intoxication F14.229
          with
            delirium F14.221
            perceptual disturbance F14.222
          uncomplicated F14.220
        mood disorder F14.24
        other specified disorder F14.288
        psychosis F14.259
          delusions F14.250
          hallucinations F14.251
        sexual dysfunction F14.281
        sleep disorder F14.282
        unspecified disorder F14.29
        withdrawal F14.23
      in remission F14.21
      withdrawal symptoms in newborn
          P96.1
    counseling and surveillance Z71.51

Dependence *(Continued)*
  drug NEC *(Continued)*
    hallucinogen F16.20
      with
        anxiety disorder F16.280
        flashbacks F16.283
        intoxication F16.229
          with delirium F16.221
          uncomplicated F16.220
        mood disorder F16.24
        other specified disorder F16.288
        perception disorder, persisting F16.283
        psychosis F16.259
          delusions F16.250
          hallucinations F16.251
        unspecified disorder F16.29
      in remission F16.21
    in remission F19.21
    inhalant F18.20
      with
        anxiety disorder F18.280
        dementia, persisting F18.27
        intoxication F18.229
          with delirium F18.221
          uncomplicated F18.220
        mood disorder F18.24
        other specified disorder F18.288
        psychosis F18.259
          delusions F18.250
          hallucinations F18.251
        unspecified disorder F18.29
      in remission F18.21
    nicotine F17.200
      with disorder F17.209
        in remission F17.201
        specified disorder NEC F17.208
        withdrawal F17.203
      chewing tobacco F17.220
        with disorder F17.229
          in remission F17.221
          specified disorder NEC F17.228
          withdrawal F17.223
      cigarettes F17.210
        with disorder F17.219
          in remission F17.211
          specified disorder NEC F17.218
          withdrawal F17.213
      specified product NEC F17.290
        with disorder F17.299
          remission F17.291
          specified disorder NEC F17.298
          withdrawal F17.293
    opioid F11.20
      with
        intoxication F11.229
          with
            delirium F11.221
            perceptual disturbance F11.222
          uncomplicated F11.220
        mood disorder F11.24
        other specified disorder F11.288
        psychosis F11.259
          delusions F11.250
          hallucinations F11.251
        sexual dysfunction F11.281
        sleep disorder F11.282
        unspecified disorder F11.29
        withdrawal F11.23
      in remission F11.21
    psychoactive NEC F19.20
      with
        amnestic disorder F19.26
        anxiety disorder F19.280
        dementia F19.27
        intoxication F19.229
          with
            delirium F19.221
            perceptual disturbance F19.222
          uncomplicated F19.220
        mood disorder F19.24
        other specified disorder F19.288
        psychosis F19.259
          delusions F19.250
          hallucinations F19.251

Dependence (Continued)
  hallucinogen (Continued)
    psychoactive NEC (Continued)
      with (Continued)
        sexual dysfunction F19.281
        sleep disorder F19.282
        unspecified disorder F19.29
        withdrawal F19.239
          with
            delirium F19.231
            perceptual disturbance F19.232
          uncomplicated F19.230
    sedative, hypnotic or anxiolytic F13.20
      with
        amnestic disorder F13.26
        anxiety disorder F13.280
        dementia, persisting F13.27
        intoxication F13.229
          with delirium F13.221
          uncomplicated F13.220
        mood disorder F13.24
        other specified disorder F13.288
        psychosis F13.259
          delusions F13.250
          hallucinations F13.251
        sexual dysfunction F13.281
        sleep disorder F13.282
        unspecified disorder F13.29
        withdrawal F13.239
          with
            delirium F13.231
            perceptual disturbance F13.232
          uncomplicated F13.230
      in remission F13.21
    stimulant NEC F15.20
      with
        anxiety disorder F15.280
        intoxication F15.229
          with
            delirium F15.221
            perceptual disturbance F15.222
          uncomplicated F15.220
        mood disorder F15.24
        other specified disorder F15.288
        psychosis F15.259
          delusions F15.250
          hallucinations F15.251
        sexual dysfunction F15.281
        sleep disorder F15.282
        unspecified disorder F15.29
        withdrawal F15.23
      in remission F15.21
  ethyl
    alcohol (without remission) F10.20
      with remission F10.21
    bromide —see Dependence, drug, sedative
    carbamate F19.20
    chloride F19.20
    morphine —see Dependence, drug, opioid
  ganja —see Dependence, drug, cannabis
  glue (airplane) (sniffing) —see Dependence, drug, inhalant
  glutethimide —see Dependence, drug, sedative
  hallucinogenics —see Dependence, drug, hallucinogen
  hashish —see Dependence, drug, cannabis
  hemp —see Dependence, drug, cannabis
  heroin (salt) (any) —see Dependence, drug, opioid
  hypnotic NEC —see Dependence, drug, sedative
  Indian hemp —see Dependence, drug, cannabis
  inhalants —see Dependence, drug, inhalant
  khat —see Dependence, drug, stimulant NEC
  laudanum —see Dependence, drug, opioid
  LSD (-25) (derivatives) —see Dependence, drug, hallucinogen
  luminal —see Dependence, drug, sedative
  lysergic acid —see Dependence, drug, hallucinogen

Dependence (Continued)
  maconha —see Dependence, drug, cannabis
  marihuana —see Dependence, drug, cannabis
  meprobamate —see Dependence, drug, sedative
  mescaline —see Dependence, drug, hallucinogen
  methadone —see Dependence, drug, opioid
  methamphetamine(s) —see Dependence, drug, stimulant NEC
  methaqualone —see Dependence, drug, sedative
  methyl
    alcohol (without remission) F10.20
      with remission F10.21
    bromide —see Dependence, drug, sedative
    morphine —see Dependence, drug, opioid
    phenidate —see Dependence, drug, stimulant NEC
    sulfonal —see Dependence, drug, sedative
  morphine (sulfate) (sulfite) (type) —see Dependence, drug, opioid
  narcotic (drug) NEC —see Dependence, drug, opioid
  nembutal —see Dependence, drug, sedative
  neraval —see Dependence, drug, sedative
  neravan —see Dependence, drug, sedative
  neurobarb —see Dependence, drug, sedative
  nicotine —see Dependence, drug, nicotine
  nitrous oxide F19.20
  nonbarbiturate sedatives and tranquilizers with similar effect —see Dependence, drug, sedative
  on
    artificial heart (fully implantable) (mechanical) Z95.812
    aspirator Z99.0
    care provider (because of) Z74.9
      impaired mobility Z74.09
      need for
        assistance with personal care Z74.1
        continuous supervision Z74.3
      no other household member able to render care Z74.2
      specified reason NEC Z74.8
    machine Z99.89
      enabling NEC Z99.89
      specified type NEC Z99.89
    renal dialysis (hemodialysis) (peritoneal) Z99.2
    respirator Z99.11
    ventilator Z99.11
    wheelchair Z99.3
  opiate —see Dependence, drug, opioid
  opioids —see Dependence, drug, opioid
  opium (alkaloids) (derivatives) (tincture) —see Dependence, drug, opioid
  oxygen (long-term) (supplemental) Z99.81
  paraldehyde —see Dependence, drug, sedative
  paregoric —see Dependence, drug, opioid
  PCP (phencyclidine) (or related substance) —see Dependence, drug, hallucinogen
  pentobarbital —see Dependence, drug, sedative
  pentobarbitone (sodium) —see Dependence, drug, sedative
  pentothal —see Dependence, drug, sedative
  peyote —see Dependence, drug, hallucinogen
  phencyclidine (PCP) (or related substance) —see Dependence, drug, hallucinogen
  phenmetrazine —see Dependence, drug, stimulant NEC
  phenobarbital —see Dependence, drug, sedative
  polysubstance F19.20
  psilocibin, psilocin, psilocyn, psilocyline —see Dependence, drug, hallucinogen
  psychostimulant NEC —see Dependence, drug, stimulant NEC
  secobarbital —see Dependence, drug, sedative

Dependence (Continued)
  seconal —see Dependence, drug, sedative
  sedative NEC —see Dependence, drug, sedative
  specified drug NEC —see Dependence, drug
  stimulant NEC —see Dependence, drug, stimulant NEC
  substance NEC —see Dependence, drug
  supplemental oxygen Z99.81
  tobacco —see Dependence, drug, nicotine
    counseling and surveillance Z71.6
  tranquilizer NEC —see Dependence, drug, sedative
  vitamin B6 E53.1
  volatile solvents —see Dependence, drug, inhalant
Dependency
  care-provider Z74.9
  passive F60.7
  reactions (persistent) F60.7
Depersonalization (in neurotic state) (neurotic) (syndrome) F48.1
Depletion
  extracellular fluid E86.9
  plasma E86.1
  potassium E87.6
    nephropathy N25.89
  salt or sodium E87.1
    causing heat exhaustion or prostration T67.4
    nephropathy N28.9
  volume NOS E86.9
Deployment (current) (military) status Z56.82
  in theater or in support of military war, peacekeeping and humanitarian operations Z56.82
  personal history of Z91.82
    military war, peacekeeping and humanitarian deployment (current or past conflict) Z91.82
  returned from Z91.82
Depolarization, premature I49.40
  atrial I49.1
  junctional I49.2
  specified NEC I49.49
  ventricular I49.3
Deposit
  bone in Boeck's sarcoid D86.89
  calcareous, calcium —see Calcification
  cholesterol
    retina H35.89
    vitreous (body) (humor) —see Deposit, crystalline
  conjunctiva H11.11-●
  cornea H18.00-●
    argentous H18.02-●
    due to metabolic disorder H18.03-●
    Kayser-Fleischer ring H18.04-●
    pigmentation —see Pigmentation, cornea
  crystalline, vitreous (body) (humor) H43.2-●
  hemosiderin in old scars of cornea —see Pigmentation, cornea, stromal
  metallic in lens —see Cataract, specified NEC
  skin R23.8
  tooth, teeth (betel) (black) (green) (materia alba) (orange) (tobacco) K03.6
  urate, kidney —see Calculus, kidney
Depraved appetite —see Pica
Depressed
  HDL cholesterol E78.6
Depression (acute) (mental) F32.A
  agitated (single episode) F32.2
  anaclitic —see Disorder, adjustment
  anxiety F41.8
    persistent F34.1
  arches —see also Deformity, limb, flat foot
  atypical (single episode) F32.89
    recurrent episode F33.8
  basal metabolic rate R94.8
  bone marrow D75.89
  central nervous system R09.2

▶ New   ⇒ Revised   ~~deleted~~ Deleted   ● Use Additional Character(s)

Depression (Continued)
cerebral R29.818
newborn P91.4
cerebrovascular I67.9
chest wall M95.4
climacteric (single episode) F32.89
recurrent episode F33.8
endogenous (without psychotic symptoms)
F33.2
with psychotic symptoms F33.3
functional activity R68.89
hysterical F44.89
involutional (single episode) F32.89
recurrent episode F33.8
major F32.9
with psychotic symptoms F32.3
recurrent —see Disorder, depressive,
recurrent
manic-depressive —see Disorder, depressive,
recurrent
masked (single episode) F32.89
medullary G93.89
menopausal (single episode) F32.89
recurrent episode F33.8
metatarsus —see Depression, arches
monopolar F33.9
nervous F34.1
neurotic F34.1
nose M95.0
postnatal (NOS) F53.0
postpartum (NOS) F53.0
post-psychotic of schizophrenia F32.89
post-schizophrenic F32.89
psychogenic (reactive) (single episode) F32.9
psychoneurotic F34.1
psychotic (single episode) F32.3
recurrent F33.3
reactive (psychogenic) (single episode) F32.9
psychotic (single episode) F32.3
recurrent —see Disorder, depressive, recurrent
respiratory center G93.89
seasonal —see Disorder, depressive, recurrent
senile F03
severe, single episode F32.2
situational F43.21
skull Q67.4
specified NEC (single episode) F32.89
sternum M95.4
visual field —see Defect, visual field
vital (recurrent) (without psychotic
symptoms) F33.2
with psychotic symptoms F33.3
single episode F32.2
Deprivation
cultural Z60.3
effects NOS T73.9
specified NEC T73.8
emotional NEC Z65.8
affecting infant or child —see
Maltreatment, child, psychological
food T73.0
▶material Z59.87
protein —see Malnutrition
sleep Z72.820
social Z60.4
affecting infant or child —see
Maltreatment, child, psychological
specified NEC T73.8
vitamins —see Deficiency, vitamin
water T73.1
Derangement
⇒ankle (internal) —see Derangement, joint,
articular cartilage, ankle
cartilage (articular) NEC —see Derangement,
joint, articular cartilage, by site
recurrent —see Dislocation, recurrent
cruciate ligament, anterior, current injury —
see Sprain, knee, cruciate, anterior
⇒elbow (internal) —see Derangement, joint,
articular cartilage, elbow
⇒hip (joint) (internal) (old) —see Derangement,
joint, articular cartilage, hip

Derangement (Continued)
joint (internal) M24.9
ankylosis —see Ankylosis
articular cartilage M24.10
ankle M24.17-•
elbow M24.12-•
foot M24.17-•
hand M24.14-•
hip M24.15-•
knee NEC M23.9-•
loose body —see Loose, body
shoulder M24.11-•
specified site NEC M24.19
wrist M24.13-•
contracture —see Contraction, joint
current injury —see also Dislocation
knee, meniscus or cartilage —see Tear,
meniscus
dislocation
pathological —see Dislocation, pathological
recurrent —see Dislocation, recurrent
knee —see Derangement, knee
ligament —see Disorder, ligament
loose body —see Loose, body
recurrent —see Dislocation, recurrent
specified type NEC M24.80
ankle M24.87-•
elbow M24.82-•
foot joint M24.87-•
hand joint M24.84-•
hip M24.85-•
shoulder M24.81-•
specified site NEC M24.89
wrist M24.83-•
temporomandibular M26.69
knee (recurrent) M23.9-•
ligament disruption, spontaneous M23.60-•
anterior cruciate M23.61-•
capsular M23.67-•
instability, chronic M23.5-•
lateral collateral M23.64-•
medial collateral M23.63-•
posterior cruciate M23.62-•
loose body M23.4-•
meniscus M23.30-•
cystic M23.00-•
lateral M23.002
anterior horn M23.04-•
posterior horn M23.05-•
specified NEC M23.06-•
medial M23.005
anterior horn M23.01-•
posterior horn M23.02-•
specified NEC M23.03-•
degenerate —see Derangement, knee,
meniscus, specified NEC
detached —see Derangement, knee,
meniscus, specified NEC
due to old tear or injury M23.20-•
lateral M23.20-•
anterior horn M23.24-•
posterior horn M23.25-•
specified NEC M23.26-•
medial M23.20-•
anterior horn M23.21-•
posterior horn M23.22-•
specified NEC M23.23-•
retained —see Derangement, knee,
meniscus, specified NEC
specified NEC M23.30-•
lateral M23.30-•
anterior horn M23.34-•
posterior horn M23.35-•
specified NEC M23.36-•
medial M23.30-•
anterior horn M23.31-•
posterior horn M23.32-•
specified NEC M23.33-•
old M23.8X-•
specified NEC —see subcategory M23.8
low back NEC —see Dorsopathy, specified NEC
meniscus —see Derangement, knee, meniscus

Derangement (Continued)
mental —see Psychosis
patella, specified NEC —see Disorder,
patella, derangement NEC
semilunar cartilage (knee) —see
Derangement, knee, meniscus,
specified NEC
shoulder (internal) —see Derangement,
joint, shoulder
Dercum's disease E88.2
Derealization (neurotic) F48.1
Dermal —see condition
Dermaphytid —see Dermatophytosis
Dermatitis (eczematous) L30.9
ab igne L59.0
acarine B88.0
actinic (due to sun) L57.8
other than from sun L59.8
allergic —see Dermatitis, contact, allergic
ambustionis, due to burn or scald —see Burn
amebic A06.7
ammonia L22
arsenical (ingested) L27.8
artefacta L98.1
psychogenic F54
atopic L20.9
psychogenic F54
specified NEC L20.89
autoimmune progesterone L30.8
berlock, berloque L56.2
blastomycotic B40.3
blister beetle L24.89
bullous, bullosa L13.9
mucosynechial, atrophic L12.1
seasonal L30.8
specified NEC L13.8
calorica L59.0
due to burn or scald —see Burn
caterpillar L24.89
cercarial B65.3
combustionis L59.0
due to burn or scald —see Burn
congelationis T69.1
contact (occupational) L25.9
allergic L23.9
due to
adhesives L23.1
cement L23.5
chemical products NEC L23.5
chromium L23.0
cosmetics L23.2
dander (cat) (dog) L23.81
drugs in contact with skin L23.3
dyes L23.4
food in contact with skin L23.6
hair (cat) (dog) L23.81
insecticide L23.5
metals L23.0
nickel L23.0
plants, non-food L23.7
plastic L23.5
rubber L23.5
specified agent NEC L23.89
due to
cement L25.3
chemical products NEC L25.3
cosmetics L25.0
dander (cat) (dog) L23.81
drugs in contact with skin L25.1
dyes L25.2
food in contact with skin L25.4
hair (cat) (dog) L23.81
plants, non-food L25.5
specified agent NEC L25.8
irritant L24.9
due to
body fluids L24.A0
incontinence (dual) (fecal) (urinary)
24.A2
saliva L24.A1
specified NEC L24.A9
cement L24.5

Dermatitis (Continued)
  contact (Continued)
    irritant (Continued)
      due to (Continued)
        chemical products NEC L24.5
        cosmetics L24.3
        detergents L24.0
        drugs in contact with skin L24.4
        food in contact with skin L24.6
        oils and greases L24.1
        plants, non-food L24.7
        related to
          colostomy L24.B3
          endotracheal tube L24.A9
          enterocutaneous
            fistula L24.B3
          gastrostomy L24.B1
          ileostomy L24.B3
          jejunostomy L24.B1
          saliva or spit fistula L24.B1
          stoma or fistula L24.B0
            digestive L24.B1
            fecal or urinary L24.B3
            respiratory L24.B2
          tracheostomy L24.B2
        solvents L24.2
        specified agent NEC L24.89
  contusiformis L52
  desquamative L30.8
  diabetic —see E08-E13 with .620
  diaper L22
  diphtheritica A36.3
  dry skin L85.3
  due to
    acetone (contact) (irritant) L24.2
    acids (contact) (irritant) L24.5
    adhesive(s) (allergic) (contact) (plaster) L23.1
      irritant L24.5
    alcohol (irritant) (skin contact) (substances
      in category T51) L24.2
      taken internally L27.8
    alkalis (contact) (irritant) L24.5
    arsenic (ingested) L27.8
    carbon disulfide (contact) (irritant) L24.2
    caustics (contact) (irritant) L24.5
    cement (contact) L25.3
    cereal (ingested) L27.2
    chemical(s) NEC L25.3
      taken internally L27.8
    chlorocompounds L24.2
    chromium (contact) (irritant) L24.81
    coffee (ingested) L27.2
    cold weather L30.8
    cosmetics (contact) L25.0
      allergic L23.2
      irritant L24.3
    cyclohexanes L24.2
    dander (cat) (dog) L23.81
    Demodex species B88.0
    Dermanyssus gallinae B88.0
    detergents (contact) (irritant) L24.0
    dichromate L24.81
    drugs and medicaments (generalized)
      (internal use) L27.0
      external —see Dermatitis, due to, drugs,
        in contact with skin
      in contact with skin L25.1
        allergic L23.3
        irritant L24.4
      localized skin eruption L27.1
      specified substance —see Table of Drugs
        and Chemicals
    dyes (contact) L25.2
      allergic L23.4
      irritant L24.89
    epidermophytosis —see Dermatophytosis
    esters L24.2
    external irritant NEC L24.9
    fish (ingested) L27.2
    flour (ingested) L27.2
    food (ingested) L27.2
      in contact with skin L25.4

Dermatitis (Continued)
  due to (Continued)
    fruit (ingested) L27.2
    furs (allergic) (contact) L23.81
    glues —see Dermatitis, due to, adhesives
    glycols L24.2
    greases NEC (contact) (irritant) L24.1
    hair (cat) (dog) L23.81
    hot
      objects and materials —see Burn
      weather or places L59.0
    hydrocarbons L24.2
    infrared rays L59.8
    ingestion, ingested substance L27.9
      chemical NEC L27.8
      drugs and medicaments —see
        Dermatitis, due to, drugs
      food L27.2
      specified NEC L27.8
    insecticide in contact with skin L24.5
    internal agent L27.9
      drugs and medicaments (generalized) —
        see Dermatitis, due to, drugs
      food L27.2
    irradiation —see Dermatitis, due to,
      radioactive substance
    ketones L24.2
    lacquer tree (allergic) (contact) L23.7
    light (sun) NEC L57.8
      acute L56.8
      other L59.8
    Liponyssoides sanguineus B88.0
    low temperature L30.8
    meat (ingested) L27.2
    metals, metal salts (contact) (irritant) L24.81
    milk (ingested) L27.2
    nickel (contact) (irritant) L24.81
    nylon (contact) (irritant) L24.5
    oils NEC (contact) (irritant) L24.1
    paint solvent (contact) (irritant) L24.2
    petroleum products (contact) (irritant)
      (substances in T52) L24.2
    plants NEC (contact) L25.5
      allergic L23.7
      irritant L24.7
    plasters (adhesive) (any) (allergic) (contact)
      L23.1
      irritant L24.5
    plastic (contact) L25.3
    preservatives (contact) —see Dermatitis,
      due to, chemical, in contact with skin
    primrose (allergic) (contact) L23.7
    primula (allergic) (contact) L23.7
    radiation L59.8
      nonionizing (chronic exposure) L57.8
      sun NEC L57.8
        acute L56.8
    radioactive substance L58.9
      acute L58.0
      chronic L58.1
    radium L58.9
      acute L58.0
      chronic L58.1
    ragweed (allergic) (contact) L23.7
    Rhus (allergic) (contact) (diversiloba)
      (radicans) (toxicodendron) (venenata)
      (verniciflua) L23.7
    rubber (contact) L24.5
    Senecio jacobaea (allergic) (contact) L23.7
    solvents (contact) (irritant) (substances in
      categories T52) L24.2
    specified agent NEC (contact) L25.8
      allergic L23.89
      irritant L24.89
    sunshine NEC L57.8
      acute L56.8
    tetrachlorethylene (contact) (irritant) L24.2
    toluene (contact) (irritant) L24.2
    turpentine (contact) L24.2
    ultraviolet rays (sun NEC) (chronic
      exposure) L57.8
      acute L56.8

Dermatitis (Continued)
  due to (Continued)
    vaccine or vaccination L27.0
      specified substance —see Table of Drugs
        and Chemicals
    varicose veins —see Varix, leg, with,
      inflammation
    X-rays L58.9
      acute L58.0
      chronic L58.1
  dyshydrotic L30.1
  dysmenorrheica N94.6
  escharotica —see Burn
  exfoliative, exfoliativa (generalized) L26
    neonatorum L00
  eyelid —(see also Dermatosis, eyelid) H01.9
    allergic H01.119
      left H01.116
        lower H01.115
        upper H01.114
      right H01.113
        lower H01.112
        upper H01.111
    contact —see Dermatitis, eyelid, allergic
    due to
      Demodex species B88.0
      herpes (zoster) B02.39
        simplex B00.59
    eczematous H01.139
      left H01.136
        lower H01.135
        upper H01.134
      right H01.133
        lower H01.132
        upper H01.131
    specified NEC H01.8
  facta, factitia, factitial L98.1
    psychogenic F54
  flexural NEC L20.82
  friction L30.4
  fungus B36.9
    specified type NEC B36.8
  gangrenosa, gangrenous infantum L08.0
  harvest mite B88.0
  heat L59.0
  herpesviral, vesicular (ear) (lip) B00.1
  herpetiformis (bullous) (erythematous)
    (pustular) (vesicular) L13.0
    juvenile L12.2
    senile L12.0
  hiemalis L30.8
  hypostatic, hypostatica —see Varix, leg, with,
    inflammation
  infectious eczematoid L30.3
  infective L30.3
  irritant —see Dermatitis, contact, irritant
  Jacquet's (diaper dermatitis) L22
  Leptus B88.0
  lichenified NEC L28.0
  medicamentosa (generalized) (internal
    use) —see Dermatitis, due to drugs
  mite B88.0
  multiformis L13.0
    juvenile L12.2
  napkin L22
  neurotica L13.0
  nummular L30.0
  papillaris capillitii L73.0
  pellagrous E52
  perioral L71.0
  photocontact L56.2
  polymorpha dolorosa L13.0
  pruriginosa L13.0
  pruritic NEC L30.8
  psychogenic F54
  purulent L08.0
  pustular
    contagious B08.02
    subcorneal L13.1
  pyococcal L08.0
  pyogenica L08.0
  repens L40.2
  Ritter's (exfoliativa) L00

▶ New   ⟹ Revised   ~~deleted~~ Deleted   ● Use Additional Character(s)

Dermatitis *(Continued)*
 Schamberg's L81.7
 schistosome B65.3
 seasonal bullous L30.8
 seborrheic L21.9
  infantile L21.1
  specified NEC L21.8
 sensitization NOS L23.9
 septic L08.0
 solare L57.8
 specified NEC L30.8
 stasis I87.2
  with
   varicose ulcer —*see* Varix, leg, with
    ulcer, with inflammation
   varicose veins —*see* Varix, leg, with,
    inflammation
  due to postthrombotic syndrome —*see*
   Syndrome, postthrombotic
 suppurative L08.0
 traumatic NEC L30.4
 trophoneurotica L13.0
 ultraviolet (sun) (chronic exposure) L57.8
  acute L56.8
 varicose —*see* Varix, leg, with, inflammation
 vegetans L10.1
 verrucosa B43.0
 vesicular, herpesviral B00.1
Dermatoarthritis, lipoid E78.81
Dermatochalasis, eyelid H02.839
 left H02.836
  lower H02.835
  upper H02.834
 right H02.833
  lower H02.832
  upper H02.831
Dermatofibroma (lenticulare) —*see* Neoplasm,
 skin, benign
 protuberans —*see* Neoplasm, skin, uncertain
  behavior
Dermatofibrosarcoma (pigmented)
 (protuberans) —*see* Neoplasm, skin,
 malignant
Dermatographia L50.3
Dermatolysis (exfoliativa) (congenital) Q82.8
 acquired L57.4
 eyelids —*see* Blepharochalasis
 palpebrarum —*see* Blepharochalasis
 senile L57.4
Dermatomegaly NEC Q82.8
Dermatomucosomyositis *(see also*
 Dermatomyositis) M33.10
 with
  myopathy M33.12
  respiratory involvement M33.11
  specified organ involvement NEC M33.19
Dermatomycosis B36.9
 furfuracea B36.0
 specified type NEC B36.8
Dermatomyositis (acute) (chronic) —*see also*
 Dermatopolymyositis
 adult —*see also* Dermatomyositis, specified
  NEC M33.10
 in (due to) neoplastic disease —*see also*
  Neoplasm D49.9 *[M36.0]*
 juvenile M33.00
  with
   myopathy M33.02
   respiratory involvement M33.01
   specified organ involvement NEC M33.09
   ▶amyopathic M33.03
  without myopathy M33.03
 specified NEC M33.10
  with
   myopathy M33.12
   respiratory involvement M33.11
   specified organ involvement NEC M33.19
   ▶amyopathic M33.13
  without myopathy M33.13
Dermatoneuritis of children —*see* Poisoning,
 mercury
Dermatophilosis A48.8
Dermatophytid L30.2

Dermatophytide —*see* Dermatophytosis
Dermatophytosis (epidermophyton) (infection)
 (Microsporum) (tinea) (Trichophyton) B35.9
 beard B35.0
 body B35.4
 capitis B35.0
 corporis B35.4
 deep-seated B35.8
 disseminated B35.8
 foot B35.3
 granulomatous B35.8
 groin B35.6
 hand B35.2
 nail B35.1
 perianal (area) B35.6
 scalp B35.0
 specified NEC B35.8
Dermatopolymyositis M33.90
 with
  myopathy M33.92
  respiratory involvement M33.91
  specified organ involvement NEC M33.99
  ▶amyopathic M33.93
 in neoplastic disease —*see also* Neoplasm
  D49.9 *[M36.0]*
 juvenile M33.00
  with
   myopathy M33.02
   respiratory involvement M33.01
   specified organ involvement NEC M33.09
   ▶amyopathic M33.03
   ▶without myopathy M33.03
 specified NEC M33.10
  myopathy M33.12
  respiratory involvement M33.11
  specified organ involvement NEC M33.19
  ▶amyopathic M33.13
  ▶without myopathy M33.13
 without myopathy M33.93
Dermatopolyneuritis —*see* Poisoning, mercury
Dermatorrhexis (*see also* Syndrome, Ehlers-
 Danlos) Q79.60
 acquired L57.4
Dermatosclerosis —*see also* Scleroderma
 localized L94.0
Dermatosis L98.9
 Andrews' L08.89
 Bowen's —*see* Neoplasm, skin, in situ
 bullous L13.9
  specified NEC L13.8
 exfoliativa L26
 eyelid (noninfectious) (*see also* Dermatitis,
  eyelid) H01.9
  discoid lupus erythematosus —*see* Lupus,
   erythematosus, eyelid
  xeroderma —*see* Xeroderma, acquired,
   eyelid
 factitial L98.1
 febrile neutrophilic L98.2
 gonococcal A54.89
 herpetiformis L13.0
  juvenile L12.2
 linear IgA L13.8
 menstrual NEC L98.8
 neutrophilic, febrile L98.2
 occupational —*see* Dermatitis, contact
 papulosa nigra L82.1
 pigmentary L81.9
  progressive L81.7
  Schamberg's L81.7
 psychogenic F54
 purpuric, pigmented L81.7
 pustular, subcorneal L13.1
 transient acantholytic L11.1
Dermographia, dermographism L50.3
Dermoid (cyst) —*see also* Neoplasm, benign,
 by site
 with malignant transformation C56-●
 due to radiation (nonionizing) L57.8
Dermopathy
 infiltrative with thyrotoxicosis —*see*
  Thyrotoxicosis
 nephrogenic fibrosing L90.8

Dermophytosis —*see* Dermatophytosis
Descemetocele H18.73-●
Descemet's membrane —*see* condition
Descending —*see* condition
Descensus uteri —*see* Prolapse, uterus
Desert
 rheumatism B38.0
 sore —*see* Ulcer, skin
Desertion (newborn) —*see* Maltreatment
Desmoid (extra-abdominal) (tumor) —*see*
 Neoplasm, connective tissue, uncertain
 behavior
 abdominal D48.1
Despondency F32.A
Desquamation, skin R23.4
Destruction, destructive —*see also* Damage
 articular facet —*see also* Derangement, joint,
  specified type NEC
  knee M23.8X-●
  vertebra —*see* Spondylosis
 bone —*see also* Disorder, bone, specified type
  NEC
  syphilitic A52.77
 joint —*see also* Derangement, joint, specified
  type NEC
  sacroiliac M53.3
 rectal sphincter K62.89
 septum (nasal) J34.89
 tuberculous NEC —*see* Tuberculosis
 tympanum, tympanic membrane
  (nontraumatic) —*see* Disorder, tympanic
  membrane, specified NEC
 vertebral disc —*see* Degeneration,
  intervertebral disc
Destructiveness —*see also* Disorder, conduct
 adjustment reaction —*see* Disorder,
  adjustment
Desultory labor O62.2
Detachment
 cartilage —*see* Sprain
 cervix, annular N88.8
  complicating delivery O71.3
 choroid (old) (postinfectional) (simple)
  (spontaneous) H31.40-●
  hemorrhagic H31.41-●
  serous H31.42-●
 ligament —*see* Sprain
 meniscus (knee) —*see also* Derangement,
  knee, meniscus, specified NEC
  current injury —*see* Tear, meniscus
  due to old tear or injury —*see*
   Derangement, knee, meniscus, due to
   old tear
 retina (without retinal break) (serous)
  H33.2-●
  with retinal:
   break H33.00-●
    giant H33.03-●
    multiple H33.02-●
    single H33.01-●
   dialysis H33.04-●
  pigment epithelium —*see* Degeneration,
   retina, separation of layers, pigment
   epithelium detachment
  rhegmatogenous —*see* Detachment, retina,
   with retinal, break
  specified NEC H33.8
  total H33.05-●
  traction H33.4-●
 vitreous (body) H43.81
Detergent asthma J69.8
Deterioration
 epileptic F06.8
 general physical R53.81
 heart, cardiac —*see* Degeneration, myocardial
 mental —*see* Psychosis
 myocardial, myocardium —*see* Degeneration,
  myocardial
 senile (simple) R54
Deuteranomaly (anomalous trichromat) H53.53
Deuteranopia (complete) (incomplete) H53.53

Development
- abnormal, bone Q79.9
- arrested R62.50
  - bone —*see* Arrest, development or growth, bone
  - child R62.50
    - due to malnutrition E45
- defective, congenital —*see also* Anomaly, by site
  - cauda equina Q06.3
  - left ventricle Q24.8
    - in hypoplastic left heart syndrome Q23.4
  - valve Q24.8
    - pulmonary Q22.3
- delayed (*see also* Delay, development) R62.50
  - arithmetical skills F81.2
  - language (skills) (expressive) F80.1
  - learning skill F81.9
  - mixed skills F88
  - motor coordination F82
  - reading F81.0
  - specified learning skill NEC F81.89
  - speech F80.9
  - spelling F81.81
  - written expression F81.81
- imperfect, congenital —*see also* Anomaly, by site
  - heart Q24.9
  - lungs Q33.6
- incomplete
  - bronchial tree Q32.4
  - organ or site not listed —*see* Hypoplasia, by site
  - respiratory system Q34.9
- sexual, precocious NEC E30.1
- tardy, mental (*see also* Disability, intellectual) F79

Developmental —*see* condition
- testing, infant or child —*see* Examination, child

Devergie's disease (pityriasis rubra pilaris) L44.0

Deviation (in)
- conjugate palsy (eye) (spastic) H51.0
- esophagus (acquired) K22.89
- eye, skew H51.8
- midline (jaw) (teeth) (dental arch) M26.29
  - specified site NEC —*see* Malposition
- nasal septum J34.2
  - congenital Q67.4
- opening and closing of the mandible M26.53
- organ or site, congenital NEC —*see* Malposition, congenital
- septum (nasal) (acquired) J34.2
  - congenital Q67.4
- sexual F65.9
  - bestiality F65.89
  - erotomania F52.8
  - exhibitionism F65.2
  - fetishism, fetishistic F65.0
    - transvestism F65.1
  - frotteurism F65.81
  - masochism F65.51
  - multiple F65.89
  - necrophilia F65.89
  - nymphomania F52.8
  - pederosis F65.4
  - pedophilia F65.4
  - sadism, sadomasochism F65.52
  - satyriasis F52.8
  - specified type NEC F65.89
  - transvestism F64.1
  - voyeurism F65.3
- teeth, midline M26.29
- trachea J39.8
- ureter, congenital Q62.61

Device
- cerebral ventricle (communicating) in situ Z98.2
- contraceptive —*see* Contraceptive, device
- drainage, cerebrospinal fluid, in situ Z98.2

Devic's disease G36.0

Devil's
- grip B33.0
- pinches (purpura simplex) D69.2

Devitalized tooth K04.99

Devonshire colic —*see* Poisoning, lead

Dextraposition, aorta Q20.3
- in tetralogy of Fallot Q21.3

Dextrinosis, limit (debrancher enzyme deficiency) E74.03

Dextrocardia (true) Q24.0
- with
  - complete transposition of viscera Q89.3
  - situs inversus Q89.3

Dextrotransposition, aorta Q20.3

d-glycericacidemia E72.59

Dhat syndrome F48.8

Dhobi itch B35.6

Di George's syndrome D82.1

Di Guglielmo's disease C94.0-•

Diabetes, diabetic (mellitus) (sugar) E11.9
- with
  - amyotrophy E11.44
  - arthropathy NEC E11.618
  - autonomic (poly)neuropathy E11.43
  - cataract E11.36
  - Charcot's joints E11.610
  - chronic kidney disease E11.22
  - circulatory complication NEC E11.59
  - coma due to
    - hyperosmolarity E11.01
    - hypoglycemia E11.641
    - ketoacidosis E11.11
  - complication E11.8
    - specified NEC E11.69
  - dermatitis E11.620
  - foot ulcer E11.621
  - gangrene E11.52
  - gastroparalysis E11.43
  - gastroparesis E11.43
  - glomerulonephrosis, intracapillary E11.21
  - glomerulosclerosis, intercapillary E11.21
  - hyperglycemia E11.65
  - hyperosmolarity E11.00
    - with coma E11.01
  - hypoglycemia E11.649
    - with coma E11.641
  - ketoacidosis E11.10
    - with coma E11.11
  - kidney complications NEC E11.29
  - Kimmelsteil-Wilson disease E11.21
  - loss of protective sensation (LOPS) —*see* Diabetes, by type, with neuropathy
  - mononeuropathy E11.41
  - myasthenia E11.44
  - necrobiosis lipoidica E11.620
  - nephropathy E11.21
  - neuralgia E11.42
  - neurologic complication NEC E11.49
  - neuropathic arthropathy E11.610
  - neuropathy E11.40
  - ophthalmic complication NEC E11.39
  - oral complication NEC E11.638
  - osteomyelitis E11.69
  - periodontal disease E11.630
  - peripheral angiopathy E11.51
    - with gangrene E11.52
  - polyneuropathy E11.42
  - renal complication NEC E11.29
  - renal tubular degeneration E11.29
  - retinopathy E11.319
    - with macular edema E11.311
      - resolved following treatment E11.37
    - nonproliferative E11.329
      - with macular edema E11.321
      - mild E11.329
        - with macular edema E11.321
      - moderate E11.339
        - with macular edema E11.331
      - severe E11.349
        - with macular edema E11.341

Diabetes, diabetic (*Continued*)
- with (*Continued*)
  - retinopathy (*Continued*)
    - proliferative E11.359
      - with
        - combined traction retinal detachment and rhegmatogenous retinal detachment E11.354
        - macular edema E11.351
        - stable proliferative diabetic retinopathy E11.355
        - traction retinal detachment involving the macula E11.352
        - traction retinal detachment not involving the macula E11.353
  - skin complication NEC E11.628
  - skin ulcer NEC E11.622
- brittle —*see* Diabetes, type 1
- bronzed E83.110
- complicating pregnancy —*see* Pregnancy, complicated by, diabetes
- dietary counseling and surveillance Z71.3
- due to
  - autoimmune process —*see* Diabetes, type 1
  - immune mediated pancreatic islet beta-cell destruction —*see* Diabetes, type 1
- due to drug or chemical E09.9
  - with
    - amyotrophy E09.44
    - arthropathy NEC E09.618
    - autonomic (poly)neuropathy E09.43
    - cataract E09.36
    - Charcot's joints E09.610
    - chronic kidney disease E09.22
    - circulatory complication NEC E09.59
    - complication E09.8
      - specified NEC E09.69
    - dermatitis E09.620
    - foot ulcer E09.621
    - gangrene E09.52
    - gastroparalysis E09.43
    - gastroparesis E09.43
    - glomerulonephrosis, intracapillary E09.21
    - glomerulosclerosis, intercapillary E09.21
    - hyperglycemia E09.65
    - hyperosmolarity E09.00
      - with coma E09.01
    - hypoglycemia E09.649
      - with coma E09.641
    - ketoacidosis E09.10
      - with coma E09.11
    - kidney complications NEC E09.29
    - Kimmelsteil-Wilson disease E09.21
    - mononeuropathy E09.41
    - myasthenia E09.44
    - necrobiosis lipoidica E09.620
    - nephropathy E09.21
    - neuralgia E09.42
    - neurologic complication NEC E09.49
    - neuropathic arthropathy E09.610
    - neuropathy E09.40
    - ophthalmic complication NEC E09.39
    - oral complication NEC E09.638
    - periodontal disease E09.630
    - peripheral angiopathy E09.51
      - with gangrene E09.52
    - polyneuropathy E09.42
    - renal complication NEC E09.29
    - renal tubular degeneration E09.29
    - retinopathy E09.319
      - with macular edema E09.311
        - resolved following treatment E09.37
      - nonproliferative E09.329
        - with macular edema E09.321
        - mild E09.329
          - with macular edema E09.321
        - moderate E09.339
          - with macular edema E09.331
        - severe E09.349
          - with macular edema E09.341

▶ New   ⟹ Revised   ~~deleted~~ Deleted   • Use Additional Character(s)

Diabetes, diabetic *(Continued)*
  due to drug or chemical *(Continued)*
    with *(Continued)*
      retinopathy *(Continued)*
        proliferative E09.359
          with
            combined traction retinal
              detachment and
              rhegmatogenous retinal
              detachment E09.354
            macular edema E09.351
            stable proliferative diabetic
              retinopathy E09.355
            traction retinal detachment
              involving the macula
              E09.352
            traction retinal detachment not
              involving the macula
              E09.353
      skin complication NEC E09.628
      skin ulcer NEC E09.622
  due to underlying condition E08.9
    with
      amyotrophy E08.44
      arthropathy NEC E08.618
      autonomic (poly)neuropathy E08.43
      cataract E08.36
      Charcot's joints E08.610
      chronic kidney disease E08.22
      circulatory complication NEC E08.59
      complication E08.8
        specified NEC E08.69
      dermatitis E08.620
      foot ulcer E08.621
      gangrene E08.52
      gastroparalysis E08.43
      gastroparesis E08.43
      glomerulonephrosis, intracapillary E08.21
      glomerulosclerosis, intercapillary E08.21
      hyperglycemia E08.69
      hyperosmolarity E08.00
        with coma E08.01
      hypoglycemia E08.649
        with coma E08.641
      ketoacidosis E08.10
        with coma E08.11
      kidney complications NEC E08.29
      Kimmelsteil-WIlson disease E08.21
      mononeuropathy E08.41
      myasthenia E08.44
      necrobiosis lipoidica E08.620
      nephropathy E08.21
      neuralgia E08.42
      neurologic complication NEC E08.49
      neuropathic arthropathy E08.610
      neuropathy E08.40
      ophthalmic complication NEC E08.39
      oral complication NEC E08.638
      periodontal disease E08.630
      peripheral angiopathy E08.51
        with gangrene E08.52
      polyneuropathy E08.42
      renal complication NEC E08.29
      renal tubular degeneration E08.29
      retinopathy E08.319
        with macular edema E08.311
          resolved following treatment E08.37
        nonproliferative E08.329
          with macular edema E08.321
          mild E08.329
            with macular edema E08.321
          moderate E08.339
            with macular edema E08.331
          severe E08.349
            with macular edema E08.341
        proliferative E08.359
          with
            combined traction retinal
              detachment and
              rhegmatogenous retinal
              detachment E08.354

Diabetes, diabetic *(Continued)*
  due to underlying condition *(Continued)*
    with *(Continued)*
      retinopathy *(Continued)*
        proliferative *(Continued)*
          with *(Continued)*
            macular edema E08.351
            stable proliferative diabetic
              retinopathy E08.355
            traction retinal detachment
              involving the macula
              E08.352
            traction retinal detachment not
              involving the macula
              E08.353
      skin complication NEC E08.628
      skin ulcer NEC E08.622
  gestational (in pregnancy) O24.419
    affecting newborn P70.0
    diet-controlled O24.410
    in childbirth O24.429
      diet-controlled O24.420
      insulin (and diet) controlled O24.424
      oral drug controlled (antidiabetic)
        (hypoglycemic) O24.425
    insulin (and diet) controlled O24.414
    oral drug controlled (antidiabetic)
      (hypoglycemic) O24.415
    puerperal O24.439
      diet-controlled O24.430
      insulin (and diet) controlled O24.434
      oral drug controlled (antidiabetic)
        (hypoglycemic) O24.435
  hepatogenous E13.9
  idiopathic —*see* Diabetes, type 1
  ~~inadequately controlled — code to Diabetes,~~
    ~~by type, with hyperglycemia~~
  ▶inadequately controlled —*see* Diabetes, by
    type, with hyperglycemia
  insipidus E23.2
    nephrogenic N25.1
    pituitary E23.2
    vasopressin resistant N25.1
  insulin dependent — code to type of diabetes
  juvenile-onset —*see* Diabetes, type 1
  ketosis-prone —*see* Diabetes, type 1
  latent R73.03
  neonatal (transient) P70.2
  non-insulin dependent — code to type of
    diabetes
  ~~out of control — code to Diabetes, by type,~~
    ~~with hyperglycemia~~
  ▶out of control —*see* Diabetes, by type, with
    hyperglycemia
  phosphate E83.39
  ▶poorly controlled —*see* Diabetes, by type,
    with hyperglycemia
  ~~poorly controlled — code to Diabetes, by~~
    ~~type, with hyperglycemia~~
  postpancreatectomy —*see* Diabetes, specified
    type NEC
  postprocedural —*see* Diabetes, specified type
    NEC
  ▶retina, hemorrhage E13.39
  secondary diabetes mellitus NEC —*see*
    Diabetes, specified type NEC
  specified type NEC E13.9
    with
      amyotrophy E13.44
      arthropathy NEC E13.618
      autonomic (poly)neuropathy E13.43
      cataract E13.36
      Charcot's joints E13.610
      chronic kidney disease E13.22
      circulatory complication NEC E13.59
      complication E13.8
        specified NEC E13.69
      dermatitis E13.620
      foot ulcer E13.621
      gangrene E13.52
      gastroparalysis E13.43

Diabetes, diabetic *(Continued)*
  specified type NEC *(Continued)*
    with *(Continued)*
      gastroparesis E13.43
      glomerulonephrosis, intracapillary
        E13.21
      glomerulosclerosis, intercapillary E13.21
      hyperglycemia E13.65
      hyperosmolarity E13.00
        with coma E13.01
      hypoglycemia E13.649
        with coma E13.641
      ketoacidosis E13.10
        with coma E13.11
      kidney complications NEC E13.29
      Kimmelsteil-Wilson disease E13.21
      mononeuropathy E13.41
      myasthenia E13.44
      necrobiosis lipoidica E13.620
      nephropathy E13.21
      neuralgia E13.42
      neurologic complication NEC E13.49
      neuropathic arthropathy E13.610
      neuropathy E13.40
      ophthalmic complication NEC E13.39
      oral complication NEC E13.638
      periodontal disease E13.630
      peripheral angiopathy E13.51
        with gangrene E13.52
      polyneuropathy E13.42
      renal complication NEC E13.29
      renal tubular degeneration E13.29
      retinopathy E13.319
        with macular edema E13.311
          resolved following treatment
            E13.37
        nonproliferative E13.329
          with macular edema E13.321
          mild E13.329
            with macular edema E13.321
          moderate E13.339
            with macular edema E13.331
          severe E13.349
            with macular edema E13.341
        proliferative E13.359
          with
            combined traction retinal
              detachment and
              rhegmatogenous retinal
              detachment E13.354
            macular edema E13.351
            stable proliferative diabetic
              retinopathy E13.355
            traction retinal detachment
              involving the macula
              E13.352
            traction retinal detachment not
              involving the macula
              E13.353
      skin complication NEC E13.628
      skin ulcer NEC E13.622
  steroid-induced —*see* Diabetes, due to, drug
    or chemical
  type 1 E10.9
    with
      amyotrophy E10.44
      arthropathy NEC E10.618
      autonomic (poly)neuropathy E10.43
      cataract E10.36
      Charcot's joints E10.610
      chronic kidney disease E10.22
      circulatory complication NEC E10.59
      coma due to
        hypoglycemia E11.641
        ketoacidosis E11.11
      complication E10.8
        specified NEC E10.69
      dermatitis E10.620
      foot ulcer E10.621
      gangrene E10.52
      gastroparalysis E10.43

Diabetes, diabetic *(Continued)*
  type 1 *(Continued)*
    with *(Continued)*
      gastroparesis E10.43
      glomerulonephrosis, intracapillary E10.21
      glomerulosclerosis, intercapillary E10.21
      hyperglycemia E10.65
      hypoglycemia E10.649
        with coma E10.641
      ketoacidosis E10.10
        with coma E10.11
      kidney complications NEC E10.29
      Kimmelsteil-Wilson disease E10.21
      mononeuropathy E10.41
      myasthenia E10.44
      necrobiosis lipoidica E10.620
      nephropathy E10.21
      neuralgia E10.42
      neurologic complication NEC E10.49
      neuropathic arthropathy E10.610
      neuropathy E10.40
      ophthalmic complication NEC E10.39
      oral complication NEC E10.638
      osteomyelitis E10.69
      periodontal disease E10.630
      peripheral angiopathy E10.51
        with gangrene E10.52
      polyneuropathy E10.42
      renal complication NEC E10.29
      renal tubular degeneration E10.29
      retinopathy E10.319
        with macular edema E10.311
          resolved following treatment E10.37
        nonproliferative E10.329
          with macular edema E10.321
          mild E10.329
            with macular edema E10.321
          moderate E10.339
            with macular edema E10.331
          severe E10.349
            with macular edema E10.341
        proliferative E10.359
          with
            combined traction retinal
              detachment and
              rhegmatogenous retinal
              detachment E13.354
            macular edema E13.351
            stable proliferative diabetic
              retinopathy E13.355
            traction retinal detachment
              involving the macula E13.352
            traction retinal detachment not
              involving the macula E13.353
      skin complication NEC E10.628
      skin ulcer NEC E10.622
  type 2 E11.9
    with
      amyotrophy E11.44
      arthropathy NEC E11.618
      autonomic (poly)neuropathy E11.43
      cataract E11.36
      Charcot's joints E11.610
      chronic kidney disease E11.22
      circulatory complication NEC E11.59
      coma due to
        hyperosmolarity E11.01
        hypoglycemia E11.641
        ketoacidosis E11.1-●
      complication E11.8
        specified NEC E11.69
      dermatitis E11.620
      foot ulcer E11.621
      gangrene E11.52
      gastroparalysis E11.43
      gastroparesis E11.43
      glomerulonephrosis, intracapillary E11.21
      glomerulosclerosis, intercapillary E11.21
      hyperglycemia E11.65
      hyperosmolarity E11.00
        with coma E11.01
      hypoglycemia E11.649
        with coma E11.641

Diabetes, diabetic *(Continued)*
  type 2 *(Continued)*
    with *(Continued)*
      ketoacidosis E11.10
        with coma E11.11
      kidney complications NEC E11.29
      Kimmelsteil-Wilson disease E11.21
      mononeuropathy E11.41
      myasthenia E11.44
      necrobiosis lipoidica E11.620
      nephropathy E11.21
      neuralgia E11.42
      neurologic complication NEC E11.49
      neuropathic arthropathy E11.610
      neuropathy E11.40
      ophthalmic complication NEC E11.39
      oral complication NEC E11.638
      osteomyelitis E11.69
      periodontal disease E11.630
      peripheral angiopathy E11.51
        with gangrene E11.52
      polyneuropathy E11.42
      renal complication NEC E11.29
      renal tubular degeneration E11.29
      retinopathy E11.319
        with macular edema E11.311
          resolved following treatment E11.37
        nonproliferative E11.329
          with macular edema E11.321
          mild E11.329
            with macular edema E11.321
          moderate E11.339
            with macular edema E11.331
          severe E11.349
            with macular edema E11.341
        proliferative E11.359
          with
            combined traction retinal
              detachment and
              rhegmatogenous retinal
              detachment E11.354
            macular edema E11.351
            stable proliferative diabetic
              retinopathy E11.355
            traction retinal detachment
              involving the macula E11.352
            traction retinal detachment not
              involving the macula E11.353
      skin complication NEC E11.628
      skin ulcer NEC E11.622
  uncontrolled
    meaning
      hyperglycemia —*see* Diabetes, by type,
        with, hyperglycemia
      hypoglycemia —*see* Diabetes, by type,
        with, hypoglycemia
Diacyclothrombopathia D69.1
Diagnosis deferred R69
Dialysis (intermittent) (treatment)
  noncompliance (with) Z91.15
  renal (hemodialysis) (peritoneal), status Z99.2
  retina, retinal —*see* Detachment, retina, with
    retinal, dialysis
Diamond-Blackfan anemia (congenital
  hypoplastic) D61.01
Diamond-Gardener syndrome
  (autoerythrocyte sensitization) D69.2
Diaper rash L22
Diaphoresis (excessive) R61
Diaphragm —*see* condition
Diaphragmalgia R07.1
Diaphragmatitis, diaphragmitis J98.6
Diaphysial aclasis Q78.6
Diaphysitis —*see* Osteomyelitis, specified type
  NEC
Diarrhea, diarrheal (disease) (infantile)
  (inflammatory) R19.7
  achlorhydric K31.83
  allergic K52.29
    due to
      colitis —*see* Colitis, allergic
      enteritis —*see* Enteritis, allergic

Diarrhea, diarrheal *(Continued)*
  amebic —*see also* Amebiasis A06.0
    with abscess —*see* Abscess, amebic
    acute A06.0
    chronic A06.1
    nondysenteric A06.2
  bacillary —*see* Dysentery, bacillary
  balantidial A07.0
  cachectic NEC K52.89
  Chilomastix A07.8
  choleriformis A00.1
  chronic (noninfectious) K52.9
  coccidial A07.3
  Cochin-China K90.1
    strongyloidiasis B78.0
  Dientamoeba A07.8
  dietetic —*see also* Diarrhea, allergic K52.29
  drug-induced K52.1
  due to
    bacteria A04.9
      specified NEC A04.8
    Campylobacter A04.5
    Capillaria philippinensis B81.1
    Clostridium difficile
      not specified as recurrent A04.72
      recurrent A04.71
    Clostridium perfringens (C) (F) A04.8
    Cryptosporidium A07.2
    drugs K52.1
    Escherichia coli A04.4
      enteroaggregative A04.4
      enterohemorrhagic A04.3
      enteroinvasive A04.2
      enteropathogenic A04.0
      enterotoxigenic A04.1
      specified NEC A04.4
    food hypersensitivity —*see also* Diarrhea,
      allergic K52.29
    Necator americanus B76.1
    S. japonicum B65.2
    specified organism NEC A08.8
      bacterial A04.8
      viral A08.39
    Staphylococcus A04.8
    Trichuris trichiuria B79
    virus —*see* Enteritis, viral
    Yersinia enterocolitica A04.6
  dysenteric A09
  endemic A09
  epidemic A09
  flagellate A07.9
  Flexner's (ulcerative) A03.1
  functional K59.1
    following gastrointestinal surgery K91.89
    psychogenic F45.8
  Giardia lamblia A07.1
  giardial A07.1
  hill K90.1
  infectious A09
  malarial —*see* Malaria
  mite B88.0
  mycotic NEC B49
  neonatal (noninfectious) P78.3
  nervous F45.8
  neurogenic K59.1
  noninfectious K52.9
  postgastrectomy K91.1
  postvagotomy K91.1
  protozoal A07.9
    specified NEC A07.8
  psychogenic F45.8
  specified
    bacterium NEC A04.8
    virus NEC A08.39
  strongyloidiasis B78.0
  toxic K52.1
  trichomonal A07.8
  tropical K90.1
  tuberculous A18.32
  viral —*see* Enteritis, viral

▶ New   ⇒ Revised   ~~deleted~~ Deleted   ● Use Additional Character(s)

Diastasis
  cranial bones M84.88
    congenital NEC Q75.8
  joint (traumatic) —see Dislocation
  muscle M62.00
    ankle M62.07-●
    congenital Q79.8
    foot M62.07-●
    forearm M62.03-●
    hand M62.04-●
    lower leg M62.06-●
    pelvic region M62.05-●
    shoulder region M62.01-●
    specified site NEC M62.08
    thigh M62.05-●
    upper arm M62.02-●
  recti (abdomen)
    complicating delivery O71.89
    congenital Q79.59
Diastema, tooth, teeth, fully erupted M26.32
Diastematomyelia Q06.2
Diataxia, cerebral G80.4
Diathesis
  allergic —see History, allergy
  bleeding (familial) D69.9
  cystine (familial) E72.00
  gouty —see Gout
  hemorrhagic (familial) D69.9
    newborn NEC P53
  spasmophilic R29.0
Diaz's disease or osteochondrosis (juvenile)
    (talus) —see Osteochondrosis, juvenile,
    tarsus
Dibothriocephalus, dibothriocephaliasis
    (latus) (infection) (infestation) B70.0
  larval B70.1
Dicephalus, dicephaly Q89.4
Dichotomy, teeth K00.2
Dichromat, dichromatopsia (congenital) —see
    Deficiency, color vision
Dichuchwa A65
Dicroceliasis B66.2
Didelphia, didelphys —see Double uterus
Didymytis N45.1
  with orchitis N45.3
Dietary
  inadequacy or deficiency E63.9
  surveillance and counseling Z71.3
Dietl's crisis N13.8
Dieulafoy lesion (hemorrhagic)
  duodenum K31.82
  esophagus K22.89
  intestine (colon) K63.81
  stomach K31.82
Difficult, difficulty (in)
  acculturation Z60.3
  feeding R63.30
    newborn P92.9
      breast P92.5
      specified NEC P92.8
    nonorganic (infant or child) F98.29
    specified NEC R63.39
  intubation, in anesthesia T88.4
  mechanical, gastroduodenal stoma K91.89
    causing obstruction —see also Obstruction,
      intestine, postoperative K91.30
  micturition
    need to immediately re-void R39.191
    position dependent R39.192
    specified NEC R39.198
  reading (developmental) F81.0
    secondary to emotional disorders F93.9
  spelling (specific) F81.81
    with reading disorder F81.89
    due to inadequate teaching Z55.8
  swallowing —see Dysphagia
  walking R26.2
  work
    conditions NEC Z56.5
    schedule Z56.3
Diffuse —see condition
DiGeorge's syndrome (thymic hypoplasia) D82.1

Digestive —see condition
Dihydropyrimidine dehydrogenase disease
    (DPD) E88.89
Diktyoma —see Neoplasm, malignant, by site
Dilaceration, tooth K00.4
Dilatation
  anus K59.89
    venule —see Hemorrhoids
  aorta (focal) (general) —see Ectasia, aorta
    with aneurysm —see Aneurysm, aorta
    congenital Q25.44
  artery —see Aneurysm
  bladder (sphincter) N32.89
    congenital Q64.79
  blood vessel I99.8
  bronchial J47.9
    with
      exacerbation (acute) J47.1
      lower respiratory infection J47.0
  calyx N28.89
    due to obstruction —see Hydronephosis
  capillaries I78.8
  cardiac (acute) (chronic) —see also
      Hypertrophy, cardiac
    congenital Q24.8
      valve NEC Q24.8
        pulmonary Q22.3
    valve —see Endocarditis
  cavum septi pellucidi Q06.8
  cervix (uteri) —see also Incompetency, cervix
    incomplete, poor, slow complicating
      delivery O62.0
  colon K59.39
    congenital Q43.1
    psychogenic F45.8
    toxic K59.31
  common duct (acquired) K83.8
    congenital Q44.5
  cystic duct (acquired) K82.8
    congenital Q44.5
  duct, mammary —see Ectasia, mammary duct
  duodenum K59.89
  esophagus K22.89
    congenital Q39.5
    due to achalasia K22.0
  eustachian tube, congenital Q17.8
  gallbladder K82.8
  gastric —see Dilatation, stomach
  heart (acute) (chronic) —see also Hypertrophy,
      cardiac
    congenital Q24.8
    valve —see Endocarditis
  ileum K59.89
    psychogenic F45.8
  jejunum K59.89
    psychogenic F45.8
  kidney (calyx) (collecting structures) (cystic)
      (parenchyma) (pelvis) (idiopathic) N28.89
    due to obstruction —see Hydronephrosis
  lacrimal passages or duct —see Disorder,
      lacrimal system, changes
  lymphatic vessel I89.0
  mammary duct —see Ectasia, mammary duct
  Meckel's diverticulum (congenital) Q43.0
    malignant —see Table of Neoplasms, small
      intestine, malignant
  myocardium (acute) (chronic) —see
      Hypertrophy, cardiac organ or site,
      congenital NEC —see Distortion
  pancreatic duct K86.89
  pericardium —see Pericarditis
  pharynx J39.2
  prostate N42.89
  pulmonary
    artery (idiopathic) I28.8
    valve, congenital Q22.3
  pupil H57.04
  rectum K59.39
  saccule, congenital Q16.5
  salivary gland (duct) K11.8
  sphincter ani K62.89

Dilatation (Continued)
  stomach K31.89
    acute K31.0
    psychogenic F45.8
  submaxillary duct K11.8
  trachea, congenital Q32.1
  ureter (idiopathic) N28.82
    congenital Q62.2
    due to obstruction N13.4
  urethra (acquired) N36.8
  vasomotor I73.9
  vein I86.8
  ventricular, ventricle (acute) (chronic) —see
      also Hypertrophy, cardiac
    cerebral, congenital Q04.8
  venule NEC I86.8
  vesical orifice N32.89
Dilated, dilation —see Dilatation
Diminished, diminution
  hearing (acuity) —see Deafness
  sense or sensation (cold) (heat) (tactile)
      (vibratory) R20.8
  vision NEC H54.7
  vital capacity R94.2
Diminuta taenia B71.0
Dimitri-Sturge-Weber disease Q85.89
Dimple
  congenital sacral Q82.6
  parasacral Q82.6
  pilonidal or postanal —see Cyst, pilonidal
Dioctophyme renalis (infection) (infestation)
    B83.8
Dipetalonemiasis B74.4
Diphallus Q55.69
Diphtheria, diphtheritic (gangrenous)
    (hemorrhagic) A36.9
  carrier (suspected) Z22.2
  cutaneous A36.3
  faucial A36.0
  infection of wound A36.3
  laryngeal A36.2
  myocarditis A36.81
  nasal, anterior A36.89
  nasopharyngeal A36.1
  neurological complication A36.89
  pharyngeal A36.0
  specified site NEC A36.89
  tonsillar A36.0
Diphyllobothriasis (intestine) B70.0
  larval B70.1
Diplacusis H93.22-●
Diplegia (upper limbs) G83.0
  congenital (cerebral) G80.8
  facial G51.0
  lower limbs G82.20
  spastic G80.1
Diplococcus, diplococcal —see condition
Diplopia H53.2
Dipsomania F10.20
  with
    psychosis —see Psychosis, alcoholic
    remission F10.21
Dipylidiasis B71.1
DIRA (deficiency of interleukin 1 receptor
    antagonist) M04.8
Direction, teeth, abnormal, fully erupted M26.30
Dirofilariasis B74.8
Dirt-eating child F98.3
Disability, disabilities
  heart —see Disease, heart
  intellectual F79
    with
      autistic features F84.9
        pathogenic CHAMP1 (genetic)
          (variant) F78.A9
        pathogenic HNRNPH2 (genetic)
          (variant) F78.A9
        pathogenic SATB2 (genetic) (variant)
          F78.A9
        pathogenic SETBP1 (genetic) (variant)
          F78.A9

Disability, disabilities (Continued)
  heart (Continued)
    with (Continued)
      autistic features (Continued)
        pathogenic STXBP1 (genetic) (variant)
            F78.A9
        pathogenic SYNGAP1 (genetic)
            (variant) F78.A1
      autosomal dominant F78.A9
      autosomal recessive F78.A9
      genetic related F78.A9
        with
          pathogenic CHAMP1 (variant) F78.
              A9
          pathogenic HNRNPH2 (variant)
              F78.A9
          pathogenic SATB2 (variant) F78.A9
          pathogenic SETBP1 (variant) F78.A9
          pathogenic STXBP1 (variant) F78.A9
          pathogenic SYNGAP1 (variant)
              F78.A1
          specified NEC F78.A9
          SYNGAP1-related F78.A1
      in
        autosomal dominant mental
            retardation F78.A9
        autosomal recessive mental
            retardation F78.A9
        SATB2-associated syndrome F78.A9
        SETBP1 disorder F78.A9
        STXBP1 encephalopathy with epilepsy
            (see also Encephalopathy; and see
            also Epilepsy) F78.A9
        X-linked mental retardation
            (syndromic) (Bain type) F78.A9
      mild (I.Q. 50-69) F70
      moderate (I.Q. 35-49) F71
      profound (I.Q. under 20) F73
      severe (I.Q. 20-34) F72
      specified level NEC F78.A9
      SYNGAP1-related F78.A1
      X-linked (syndromic) (Bain type) F78.A9
  knowledge acquisition F81.9
  learning F81.9
  limiting activities Z73.6
  spelling, specific F81.81
Disappearance of family member Z63.4
Disarticulation —see Amputation
  meaning traumatic amputation —see
      Amputation, traumatic
Discharge (from)
  abnormal finding in —see Abnormal, specimen
  breast (female) (male) N64.52
  diencephalic autonomic idiopathic —
      see Epilepsy, specified NEC
  ear —see also Otorrhea
    blood —see Otorrhagia
  excessive urine R35.89
  nipple N64.52
  penile R36.9
  postnasal R09.82
  prison, anxiety concerning Z65.2
  urethral R36.9
    without blood R36.0
    hematospermia R36.1
  vaginal N89.8
Discitis, diskitis M46.40
  cervical region M46.42
  cervicothoracic region M46.43
  lumbar region M46.46
  lumbosacral region M46.47
  multiple sites M46.49
  occipito-atlanto-axial region M46.41
  pyogenic —see Infection, intervertebral
      disc, pyogenic
  sacrococcygeal region M46.48
  thoracic region M46.44
  thoracolumbar region M46.45
Discoid
  meniscus (congenital) Q68.6
  semilunar cartilage (congenital) —see
      Derangement, knee, meniscus,
      specified NEC

Discoloration
  nails L60.8
  teeth (posteruptive) K03.7
    during formation K00.8
Discomfort
  chest R07.89
  visual H53.14-●
Discontinuity, ossicles, ear H74.2-●
Discord (with)
  boss Z56.4
  classmates Z55.4
  counselor Z64.4
  employer Z56.4
  family Z63.8
  fellow employees Z56.4
  in-laws Z63.1
  landlord Z59.2
  lodgers Z59.2
  neighbors Z59.2
  probation officer Z64.4
  social worker Z64.4
  teachers Z55.4
  workmates Z56.4
Discordant connection
  atrioventricular (congenital) Q20.5
  ventriculoarterial Q20.3
Discrepancy
  centric occlusion maximum intercuspation
      M26.55
  leg length (acquired) —see Deformity, limb,
      unequal length
    congenital —see Defect, reduction, lower
        limb
  uterine size date O26.84-●
Discrimination
  ethnic Z60.5
  political Z60.5
  racial Z60.5
  religious Z60.5
  sex Z60.5
Disease, diseased —see also Syndrome
  absorbent system I87.8
  acid-peptic K30
  Acosta's T70.29
  Adams-Stokes (-Morgagni) (syncope with
      heart block) I45.9
  Addison's anemia (pernicious) D51.0
  adenoids (and tonsils) J35.9
  adrenal (capsule) (cortex) (gland) (medullary)
      E27.9
    hyperfunction E27.0
    specified NEC E27.8
  ainhum L94.6
  airway
    obstructive, chronic J44.9
      due to
        cotton dust J66.0
        specific organic dusts NEC J66.8
      reactive —see Asthma
  akamushi (scrub typhus) A75.3
  Albers-Schönberg (marble bones) Q78.2
  Albert's —see Tendinitis, Achilles
  alimentary canal K63.9
  alligator-skin Q80.9
    acquired L85.0
  alpha heavy chain C88.3
  alpine T70.29
  altitude T70.20
  alveolar ridge
    edentulous K06.9
      specified NEC K06.8
  alveoli, teeth K08.9
  ⮕Alzheimer's (see also Dementia, in, diseases
      specified elsewhere) G30.9 [F02.80]
    ⮕with behavioral disturbance (see also
        Dementia, in, diseases specified
        elsewhere) G30.9 [F02.81-●]
    ⮕early onset (see also Dementia, in, diseases
        specified elsewhere) G30.0 [F02.80]
      ⮕with behavioral disturbance (see also
          Dementia, in, diseases specified
          elsewhere) G30.0 [F02.81-●]

Disease, diseased (Continued)
  Alzheimer's (Continued)
    ⮕late onset (see also Dementia, in, diseases
        specified elsewhere) G30.1 [F02.80]
      ⮕with behavioral disturbance (see also
          Dementia, in, diseases specified
          elsewhere) G30.1 [F02.81-●]
    ⮕specified NEC (see also Dementia, in,
        diseases specified elsewhere) G30.8
        [F02.80]
      ⮕with behavioral disturbance (see also
          Dementia, in, diseases specified
          elsewhere) G30.8 [F02.81-●]
  amyloid —see Amyloidosis
  Andersen's (glycogenosis IV) E74.09
  Andes T70.29
  Andrews' (bacterid) L08.89
  angiospastic I73.9
    cerebral G45.9
    vein I87.8
  anterior
    chamber H21.9
    horn cell G12.29
  antiglomerular basement membrane
      (anti-GBM) antibody M31.0
    tubulo-interstitial nephritis N12
  antral —see Sinusitis, maxillary
  anus K62.9
    specified NEC K62.89
  aorta (nonsyphilitic) I77.9
    syphilitic NEC A52.02
  aortic (heart) (valve) I35.9
    rheumatic I06.9
  Apollo B30.3
  aponeuroses —see Enthesopathy
  appendix K38.9
    specified NEC K38.8
  aqueous (chamber) H21.9
  Arnold-Chiari —see Arnold-Chiari disease
  arterial I77.9
    occlusive —see Occlusion, by site
      due to stricture or stenosis I77.1
    peripheral I73.9
  arteriocardiorenal —see Hypertension,
      cardiorenal
  arteriolar (generalized) (obliterative) I77.9
  arteriorenal —see Hypertension, kidney
  arteriosclerotic —see also Arteriosclerosis
    cardiovascular —see Disease, heart,
        ischemic, atherosclerotic
    coronary (artery) —see Disease, heart,
        ischemic, atherosclerotic
    heart —see Disease, heart, ischemic,
        atherosclerotic
  artery I77.9
    cerebral I67.9
    coronary I25.10
      with angina pectoris —see
          Arteriosclerosis, coronary (artery)
    peripheral I73.9
  arthropod-borne NOS (viral) A94
    specified type NEC A93.8
  atticoantral, chronic H66.20
    left H66.22
      with right H66.23
    right H66.21
      with left H66.23
  auditory canal —see Disorder, ear, external
  auricle, ear NEC —see Disorder, pinna
  Australian X A83.4
  autoimmune (systemic) NOS M35.9
    hemolytic D59.10
      cold type (primary) (secondary)
          (symptomatic) D59.12
      drug-induced D59.0
      mixed type (primary) (secondary)
          (symptomatic) D59.13
      warm type (primary) (secondary)
          (symptomatic) D59.11
    thyroid E06.3
  autoinflammatory M04.9
    NOD2-associated M04.8
    specified type NEC M04.8

▶ New   ⮕ Revised   ~~deleted~~ Deleted   ● Use Additional Character(s)

Disease, diseased *(Continued)*
  aviator's —*see* Effect, adverse, high altitude
  Ayerza's (pulmonary artery sclerosis with
    pulmonary hypertension) I27.0
  Babington's (familial hemorrhagic
    telangiectasia) I78.0
  bacterial A49.9
    specified NEC A48.8
    zoonotic A28.9
      specified type NEC A28.8
  Baelz's (cheilitis glandularis apostematosa)
    K13.0
  bagasse J67.1
  balloon —*see* Effect, adverse, high altitude
  Bang's (brucella abortus) A23.1
  Bannister's T78.3
  barometer makers' —*see* Poisoning, mercury
  Barraquer (-Simons') (progressive
    lipodystrophy) E88.1
  Barrett's —*see* Barrett's, esophagus
  Bartholin's gland N75.9
  basal ganglia G25.9
    degenerative G23.9
      specified NEC G23.8
    specified NEC G25.89
  Basedow's (exophthalmic goiter) —*see*
    Hyperthyroidism, with, goiter (diffuse)
  Bateman's B08.1
  Batten-Steinert G71.11
  Battey A31.0
  Beard's (neurasthenia) F48.8
  Becker
    idiopathic mural endomyocardial I42.3
    myotonia congenita G71.12
  Begbie's (exophthalmic goiter) —*see*
    Hyperthyroidism, with, goiter (diffuse)
  behavioral, organic F07.9
  Beigel's (white piedra) B36.2
  Benson's —*see* Deposit, crystalline
  Bernard-Soulier (thrombopathy) D69.1
  Bernhardt (-Roth) —*see* Mononeuropathy,
    lower limb, meralgia paresthetica
  Biermer's (pernicious anemia) D51.0
  bile duct (common) (hepatic) K83.9
    with calculus, stones —*see* Calculus, bile duct
    specified NEC K83.8
  biliary (tract) K83.9
    specified NEC K83.8
  Billroth's —*see* Spina bifida
  bird fancier's J67.2
  black lung J60
  bladder N32.9
    in (due to)
      schistosomiasis (bilharziasis) B65.0 [N33]
    specified NEC N32.89
  bleeder's D66
  blood D75.9
    forming organs D75.9
    vessel I99.9
  Bloodgood's —*see* Mastopathy, cystic
  Blount M92.51-●
  Bodechtel-Guttmann (subacute sclerosing
    panencephalitis) A81.1
  bone —*see also* Disorder, bone
    aluminum M83.4
    fibrocystic NEC
      jaw M27.49
  bone-marrow D75.9
  Borna A83.9
  Bornholm (epidemic pleurodynia) B33.0
  Bouchard's (myopathic dilatation of the
    stomach) K31.0
  Bouillaud's (rheumatic heart disease) I01.9
  Bourneville (-Brissaud) (tuberous sclerosis)
    Q85.1
  Bouveret (-Hoffmann) (paroxysmal
    tachycardia) I47.9
  bowel K63.9
    functional K59.9
      psychogenic F45.8
  brain G93.9
    arterial, artery I67.9
    arteriosclerotic I67.2

Disease, diseased *(Continued)*
  brain *(Continued)*
    congenital Q04.9
    degenerative —*see* Degeneration, brain
    inflammatory —*see* Encephalitis
    organic G93.9
      arteriosclerotic I67.2
    parasitic NEC B71.9 [G94]
    senile NEC G31.1
    specified NEC G93.89
  breast (see also Disorder, breast) N64.9
    cystic (chronic) —*see* Mastopathy, cystic
    fibrocystic —*see* Mastopathy, cystic
    Paget's
      female, unspecified side C50.91-●
      male, unspecified side C50.92-●
    specified NEC N64.89
  Breda's —*see* Yaws
  Bretonneau's (diphtheritic malignant angina)
    A36.0
  Bright's —*see* Nephritis
    arteriosclerotic —*see* Hypertension, kidney
  Brill's (recrudescent typhus) A75.1
  Brill-Zinsser (recrudescent typhus) A75.1
  Brion-Kayser —*see* Fever, paratyphoid
  broad
    beta E78.2
    ligament (noninflammatory) N83.9
      inflammatory —*see* Disease, pelvis,
        inflammatory
      specified NEC N83.8
  Brocq-Duhring (dermatitis herpetiformis) L13.0
  Brocq's
    meaning
      dermatitis herpetiformis L13.0
      prurigo L28.2
  bronchopulmonary J98.4
  bronchus NEC J98.09
  bronze Addison's E27.1
    tuberculous A18.7
  budgerigar fancier's J67.2
  Buerger's (thromboangiitis obliterans) I73.1
  bullous L13.9
    chronic of childhood L12.2
    specified NEC L13.8
  Bürger-Grütz (essential familial
    hyperlipemia) E78.3
  bursa —*see* Bursopathy
  caisson T70.3
  California —*see* Coccidioidomycosis
  capillaries I78.9
    specified NEC I78.8
  Carapata A68.0
  cardiac —*see* Disease, heart
  cardiopulmonary, chronic I27.9
  cardiorenal (hepatic) (hypertensive)
    (vascular) —*see* Hypertension,
    cardiorenal
  cardiovascular (atherosclerotic) I25.10
    with angina pectoris —*see* Arteriosclerosis,
      coronary (artery),
    congenital Q28.9
    hypertensive —*see* Hypertension, heart
    newborn P29.9
      specified NEC P29.89
    renal (hypertensive) —*see* Hypertension,
      cardiorenal
    syphilitic (asymptomatic) A52.00
  cartilage —*see* Disorder, cartilage
  Castellani's A69.8
  Castleman (unicentric) (multicentric) D47.Z2
    HHV-8-associated —*see also* Herpesvirus,
      human, 8 D47.Z2
  cat-scratch A28.1
  Cavare's (familial periodic paralysis) G72.3
  cecum K63.9
  celiac (adult) (infantile) (with steatorrhea)
    K90.0
  cellular tissue L98.9
  central core G71.29
  cerebellar, cerebellum —*see* Disease, brain
  cerebral —*see also* Disease, brain
    degenerative —*see* Degeneration, brain

Disease, diseased *(Continued)*
  cerebrospinal G96.9
  cerebrovascular I67.9
    acute I67.89
      embolic I63.4-●
      thrombotic I63.3-●
    arteriosclerotic I67.2
    hereditary NEC I67.858
    specified NEC I67.89
  cervix (uteri) (noninflammatory) N88.9
    inflammatory —*see* Cervicitis
    specified NEC N88.8
  Chabert's A22.9
  Chandler's (osteochondritis dissecans, hip) —
    see Osteochondritis, dissecans, hip
  Charlouis —*see* Yaws
  Chédiak-Steinbrinck (-Higashi) (congenital
    gigantism of peroxidase granules) E70.330
  chest J98.9
  Chiari's (hepatic vein thrombosis) I82.0
  Chicago B40.9
  Chignon B36.8
  chigo, chigoe B88.1
  childhood granulomatous D71
  Chinese liver fluke B66.1
  chlamydial A74.9
    specified NEC A74.89
  cholecystic K82.9
  choroid H31.9
    specified NEC H31.8
  Christmas D67
  chronic bullous of childhood L12.2
  chylomicron retention E78.3
  ciliary body H21.9
    specified NEC H21.89
  circulatory (system) NEC I99.8
    newborn P29.9
    syphilitic A52.00
      congenital A50.54
  coagulation factor deficiency (congenital) —
    see Defect, coagulation
  coccidioidal —*see* Coccidioidomycosis
  cold
    agglutinin or hemoglobinuria D59.12
      paroxysmal D59.6
    hemagglutinin (chronic) D59.12
  collagen NOS (nonvascular) (vascular) M35.9
    specified NEC M35.89
  colon K63.9
    functional K59.9
      congenital Q43.2
    ischemic —*see also* Ischemia, intestine,
      acute K55.039
  colonic inflammatory bowel, unclassified
    (IBDU) K52.3
  combined system —*see* Degeneration,
    combined
  compressed air T70.3
  Concato's (pericardial polyserositis) A19.9
    nontubercular I31.1
    pleural —*see* Pleurisy, with effusion
  conjunctiva H11.9
    chlamydial A74.0
    specified NEC H11.89
    viral B30.9
      specified NEC B30.8
  connective tissue, systemic (diffuse) M35.9
    in (due to)
      hypogammaglobulinemia D80.1 [M36.8]
      ochronosis E70.29 [M36.8]
    specified NEC M35.89
  Conor and Bruch's (boutonneuse fever) A77.1
  Cooper's —*see* Mastopathy, cystic
  Cori's (glycogenosis III) E74.03
  corkhandler's or corkworker's J67.3
  cornea H18.9
    specified NEC H18.89-●
  coronary (artery) —*see* Disease, heart,
    ischemic, atherosclerotic
    congenital Q24.5
    ostial, syphilitic (aortic) (mitral)
      (pulmonary) A52.03

Disease, diseased *(Continued)*
- corpus cavernosum N48.9
  - specified NEC N48.89
- Cotugno's —*see* Sciatica
- COVID-19 U07.1
- coxsackie (virus) NEC B34.1
- cranial nerve NOS G52.9
- Creutzfeldt-Jakob —*see* Creutzfeldt-Jakob disease or syndrome
- Crocq's (acrocyanosis) I73.89
- Crohn's —*see* Enteritis, regional
- Curschmann G71.11
- cystic
  - breast (chronic) —*see* Mastopathy, cystic
  - kidney, congenital Q61.9
  - liver, congenital Q44.6
  - lung J98.4
    - congenital Q33.0
- cytomegalic inclusion (generalized) B25.9
  - with pneumonia B25.0
  - congenital P35.1
- cytomegaloviral B25.9
  - specified NEC B25.8
- Czerny's (periodic hydrarthrosis of the knee) —*see* Effusion, joint, knee
- Daae (-Finsen) (epidemic pleurodynia) B33.0
- Darling's —*see* Histoplasmosis capsulati
- deer fly —*see* Tularemia
- Degos' I77.8
- demyelinating, demyelinizating (nervous system) G37.9
  - multiple sclerosis G35
  - specified NEC G37.8
- dense deposit —*see also* N00-N07 with fourth character .6 N05.6
- deposition, hydroxyapatite —*see* Disease, hydroxyapatite deposition
- de Quervain's (tendon sheath) M65.4
  - thyroid (subacute granulomatous thyroiditis) E06.1
- Devergie's (pityriasis rubra pilaris) L44.0
- Devic's G36.0
- diaphorase deficiency D74.0
- diaphragm J98.6
- diarrheal, infectious NEC A09
- digestive system K92.9
  - specified NEC K92.89
- disc, degenerative —*see* Degeneration, intervertebral disc
- discogenic —*see also* Displacement, intervertebral disc NEC
  - with myelopathy —*see* Disorder, disc, with, myelopathy
- diverticular —*see* Diverticula
- Dubois (thymus) A50.59 *[E35]*
- Duchenne-Griesinger G71.01
- Duchenne's
  - muscular dystrophy G71.01
  - pseudohypertrophy, muscles G71.01
- ductless glands E34.9
- Duhring's (dermatitis herpetiformis) L13.0
- duodenum K31.9
  - specified NEC K31.89
- Dupré's (meningism) R29.1
- Dupuytren's (muscle contracture) M72.0
- Durand-Nicholas-Favre (climatic bubo) A55
- Duroziez's (congenital mitral stenosis) Q23.2
- ear —*see* Disorder, ear
- Eberth's —*see* Fever, typhoid
- Ebola (virus) A98.4
- Ebstein's heart Q22.5
- Echinococcus —*see* Echinococcus
- echovirus NEC B34.1
- Eddowes' (brittle bones and blue sclera) Q78.0
- edentulous (alveolar) ridge K06.9
  - specified NEC K06.8
- Edsall's T67.2
- Eichstedt's (pityriasis versicolor) B36.0
- Eisenmenger's (irreversible) I27.83
- Ellis-van Creveld (chondroectodermal dysplasia) Q77.6

Disease, diseased *(Continued)*
- end stage renal (ESRD) N18.6
  - due to hypertension I12.0
- endocrine glands or system NEC E34.9
- endomyocardial (eosinophilic) I42.3
- English (rickets) E55.0
- enteroviral, enterovirus NEC B34.1
  - central nervous system NEC A88.8
- epidemic B99.9
  - specified NEC B99.8
- epididymis N50.9
- Erb (-Landouzy) G71.02
- Erdheim-Chester (ECD) E88.89
- esophagus K22.9
  - functional K22.4
  - psychogenic F45.8
  - specified NEC K22.89
- Eulenburg's (congenital paramyotonia) G71.19
- eustachian tube —*see* Disorder, eustachian tube
- external
  - auditory canal —*see* Disorder, ear, external
  - ear —*see* Disorder, ear, external
- extrapyramidal G25.9
  - specified NEC G25.89
- eye H57.9
  - anterior chamber H21.9
  - inflammatory NEC H57.89
  - muscle (external) —*see* Strabismus
  - specified NEC H57.89
  - syphilitic —*see* Oculopathy, syphilitic
- eyeball H44.9
  - specified NEC H44.89
- eyelid —*see* Disorder, eyelid
  - specified NEC —*see* Disorder, eyelid, specified type NEC
- eyeworm of Africa B74.3
- facial nerve (seventh) G51.9
  - newborn (birth injury) P11.3
- Fahr (of brain) G23.8
- Fahr Volhard (of kidney) I12.-●
- fallopian tube (noninflammatory) N83.9
  - inflammatory —*see* Salpingo-oophoritis
  - specified NEC N83.8
- familial periodic paralysis G72.3
- Fanconi's (congenital pancytopenia) D61.09
- fascia NEC —*see also* Disorder, muscle
  - inflammatory —*see* Myositis
  - specified NEC M62.89
- Fauchard's (periodontitis) —*see* Periodontitis
- Favre-Durand-Nicolas (climatic bubo) A55
- Fede's K14.0
- Feer's —*see* Poisoning, mercury
- female pelvic inflammatory —*see also* Disease, pelvis, inflammatory N73.9
  - syphilitic (secondary) A51.42
  - tuberculous A18.17
- Fernels' (aortic aneurysm) I71.9
- fibrocaseous of lung —*see* Tuberculosis, pulmonary
- fibrocystic —*see* Fibrocystic disease
- Fiedler's (leptospiral jaundice) A27.0
- fifth B08.3
- file-cutter's —*see* Poisoning, lead
- fish-skin Q80.9
  - acquired L85.0
- Flajani (-Basedow) (exophthalmic goiter) —*see* Hyperthyroidism, with, goiter (diffuse)
- flax-dresser's J66.1
- fluke —*see* Infestation, fluke
- foot and mouth B08.8
- foot process N04.9
- Forbes' (glycogenosis III) E74.03
- Fordyce-Fox (apocrine miliaria) L75.2
- Fordyce's (ectopic sebaceous glands) (mouth) Q38.6
- Forestier's (rhizomelic pseudopolyarthritis) M35.3
  - meaning ankylosing hyperostosis —*see* Hyperostosis, ankylosing
- Fothergill's
  - neuralgia —*see* Neuralgia, trigeminal
  - scarlatina anginosa A38.9

Disease, diseased *(Continued)*
- Fournier (gangrene) N49.3
- ▶▶female N76.82
  - ▶vagina and vulva N76.82
- fourth B08.8
- Fox (-Fordyce) (apocrine miliaria) L75.2
- Francis' —*see* Tularemia
- Franklin C88.2
- Frei's (climatic bubo) A55
- Friedreich's
  - combined systemic or ataxia G11.11
  - myoclonia G25.3
- frontal sinus —*see* Sinusitis, frontal
- fungus NEC B49
- Gaisböck's (polycythemia hypertonica) D75.1
- gallbladder K82.9
  - calculus —*see* Calculus, gallbladder
  - cholecystitis —*see* Cholecystitis
  - cholesterolosis K82.4
  - fistula —*see* Fistula, gallbladder
  - hydrops K82.1
  - obstruction —*see* Obstruction, gallbladder
  - perforation K82.2
  - specified NEC K82.8
- gamma heavy chain C88.2
- Gamna's (siderotic splenomegaly) D73.2
- Gamstorp's (adynamia episodica hereditaria) G72.3
- Gandy-Nanta (siderotic splenomegaly) D73.2
- ganister J62.8
- gastric —*see* Disease, stomach
- gastroesophageal reflux (GERD) K21.9
  - with esophagitis (without bleeding) K21.00
  - with bleeding K21.01
- gastrointestinal (tract) K92.9
  - amyloid E85.4
  - functional K59.9
    - psychogenic F45.8
  - specified NEC K92.89
- Gee (-Herter) (-Heubner) (-Thaysen) (nontropical sprue) K90.0
- genital organs
  - female N94.9
  - male N50.9
- Gerhardt's (erythromelalgia) I73.81
- Gibert's (pityriasis rosea) L42
- Gierke's (glycogenosis I) E74.01
- Gilles de la Tourette's (motor-verbal tic) F95.2
- gingiva K06.9
  - plaque induced K05.00
  - specified NEC K06.8
- gland (lymph) I89.9
- Glanzmann's (hereditary hemorrhagic thrombasthenia) D69.1
- glass-blower's (cataract) —*see* Cataract, specified NEC
  - salivary gland hypertrophy K11.1
- Glisson's —*see* Rickets
- globe H44.9
  - specified NEC H44.89
- glomerular —*see also* Glomerulonephritis
  - with edema —*see* Nephrosis
  - acute —*see* Nephritis, acute
  - chronic —*see* Nephritis, chronic
  - minimal change N05.0
  - rapidly progressive N01.9
- glycogen storage E74.00
  - Andersen's E74.09
  - Cori's E74.03
  - Forbes' E74.03
  - generalized E74.00
  - glucose-6-phosphatase deficiency E74.01
  - heart E74.02 *[I43]*
  - hepatorenal E74.09
  - Hers' E74.09
  - liver and kidney E74.09
  - McArdle's E74.04
  - muscle phosphofructokinase E74.09
  - myocardium E74.02 *[I43]*
  - Pompe's E74.02
  - Tauri's E74.09
  - type 0 E74.09

Disease, diseased *(Continued)*
  glycogen storage *(Continued)*
    type I E74.01
    type II E74.02
    type III E74.03
    type IV E74.09
    type V E74.04
    type VI-XI E74.09
    Von Gierke's E74.01
  Goldstein's (familial hemorrhagic
      telangiectasia) I78.0
  gonococcal NOS A54.9
  graft-versus-host (GVH) D89.813
    acute D89.810
    acute on chronic D89.812
    chronic D89.811
  grainhandler's J67.8
  granulomatous (childhood) (chronic) D71
  Graves' (exophthalmic goiter) —*see*
      Hyperthyroidism, with, goiter (diffuse)
  Griesinger's —*see* Ancylostomiasis
  Grisel's M43.6
  Gruby's (tinea tonsurans) B35.0
  Guillain-Barré G61.0
  Guinon's (motor-verbal tic) F95.2
  gum K06.9
  gynecological N94.9
  H (Hartnup's) E72.02
  Haff —*see* Poisoning, mercury
  Hageman (congenital factor XII deficiency)
      D68.2
  hair (color) (shaft) L67.9
    follicles L73.9
      specified NEC L73.8
  Hamman's (spontaneous mediastinal
      emphysema) J98.2
  hand, foot and mouth B08.4
  Hansen's —*see* Leprosy
  Hantavirus, with pulmonary manifestations
      B33.4
    with renal manifestations A98.5
  Harada's H30.81-●
  Hartnup (pellagra-cerebellar ataxia-renal
      aminoaciduria) E72.02
  Hart's (pellagra-cerebellar ataxia-renal
      aminoaciduria) E72.02
  Hashimoto's (struma lymphomatosa) E06.3
  Hb —*see* Disease, hemoglobin
  heart (organic) I51.9
    with
      pulmonary edema (acute) —*see also*
          Failure, ventricular, left I50.1
      rheumatic fever (conditions in I00)
          active I01.9
            with chorea I02.0
            specified NEC I01.8
          inactive or quiescent (with chorea) I09.9
            specified NEC I09.89
    amyloid E85.4 *[I43]*
    aortic (valve) I35.9
    arteriosclerotic or sclerotic (senile) —*see*
        Disease, heart, ischemic, atherosclerotic
    artery, arterial —*see* Disease, heart,
        ischemic, atherosclerotic
    beer drinkers' I42.6
    beriberi (wet) E51.12
    black I27.0
    congenital Q24.9
      cyanotic Q24.9
      specified NEC Q24.8
    coronary —*see* Disease, heart, ischemic
    cryptogenic I51.9
    fibroid —*see* Myocarditis
    functional I51.89
      psychogenic F45.8
    glycogen storage E74.02 *[I43]*
    gonococcal A54.83
    hypertensive —*see* Hypertension, heart
    hyperthyroid —*see also* Hyperthyroidism
        E05.90 *[I43]*
      with thyroid storm E05.91 *[I43]*

Disease, diseased *(Continued)*
  heart *(Continued)*
    ischemic (chronic or with a stated duration
        of over 4 weeks) I25.9
      atherosclerotic (of) I25.10
        with angina pectoris —*see*
            Arteriosclerosis, coronary
            (artery)
        coronary artery bypass graft —*see*
            Arteriosclerosis, coronary
            (artery),
      cardiomyopathy I25.5
      diagnosed on ECG or other special
          investigation, but currently
          presenting no symptoms I25.6
      silent I25.6
      specified form NEC I25.89
    kyphoscoliotic I27.1
    meningococcal A39.50
      endocarditis A39.51
      myocarditis A39.52
      pericarditis A39.53
    mitral I05.9
      specified NEC I05.8
    muscular —*see* Degeneration, myocardial
    psychogenic (functional) F45.8
    pulmonary (chronic) I27.9
      in schistosomiasis B65.9 *[I52]*
      specified NEC I27.89
    rheumatic (chronic) (inactive) (old)
        (quiescent) (with chorea) I09.9
      active or acute I01.9
        with chorea (acute) (rheumatic)
            (Sydenham's) I02.0
      specified NEC I09.89
    senile —*see* Myocarditis
    syphilitic A52.06
      aortic A52.03
        aneurysm A52.01
      congenital A50.54 *[I52]*
    thyrotoxic —*see also* Thyrotoxicosis E05.90
        [I43]
      with thyroid storm E05.91 *[I43]*
    valve, valvular (obstructive)
        (regurgitant) —*see also* Endocarditis
      congenital NEC Q24.8
        pulmonary Q22.3
    vascular —*see* Disease, cardiovascular
  heavy chain NEC C88.2
    alpha C88.3
    gamma C88.2
    mu C88.2
  Hebra's
    pityriasis
      maculata et circinata L42
      rubra pilaris L44.0
    prurigo L28.2
  hematopoietic organs D75.9
  hemoglobin or Hb
    abnormal (mixed) NEC D58.2
      with thalassemia D56.9
    AS genotype D57.3
    Bart's D56.0
    C (Hb-C) D58.2
      with other abnormal hemoglobin NEC
          D58.2
      elliptocytosis D58.1
      Hb-S D57.2-●
      sickle-cell D57.2-●
      thalassemia D56.8
    Constant Spring D58.2
    D (Hb-D) D58.2
    E (Hb-E) D58.2
    E-beta thalassemia D56.5
    elliptocytosis D58.1
    H (Hb-H) (thalassemia) D56.0
      with other abnormal hemoglobin NEC
          D56.9
      Constant Spring D56.0
    I thalassemia D56.9
    M D74.0

Disease, diseased *(Continued)*
  hemoglobin or Hb *(Continued)*
    S or SS D57.1
      with
        acute chest syndrome D57.01
        cerebral vascular involvement D57.03
        crisis (painful) D57.00
          with complication specified NEC
              D57.09
        splenic sequestration D57.02
        vasoocclusive pain D57.00
      beta plus D57.44
        with
          acute chest syndrome D57.451
          cerebral vascular involvement
              D57.453
          crisis D57.459
            with specified complication NEC
                D57.458
          splenic sequestration D57.452
          vasoocclusive pain D57.459
        without crisis D57.44
      beta zero D57.42
        with
          acute chest syndrome D57.431
          cerebral vascular involvement
              D57.433
          crisis D57.439
            with specified complication NEC
                D57.438
          splenic sequestration D57.432
          vasoocclusive pain D57.439
        without crisis D57.42
    SC D57.2-●
    SD D57.8-●
    SE D57.8-●
    spherocytosis D58.0
    unstable, hemolytic D58.2
  hemolytic (newborn) P55.9
    autoimmune D59.10
      cold type (primary) (secondary)
          (symptomatic) D59.12
      mixed type (primary) (secondary)
          (symptomatic) D59.13
      warm type (primary) (secondary)
          (symptomatic) D59.11
    drug-induced D59.0
    due to or with
      incompatibility
        ABO (blood group) P55.1
        blood (group) (Duffy) (K) (Kell)
            (Kidd) (Lewis) (M) (S) NEC P55.8
        Rh (blood group) (factor) P55.0
        Rh negative mother P55.0
    specified type NEC P55.8
    unstable hemoglobin D58.2
  hemorrhagic D69.9
    newborn P53
  Henoch (-Schönlein) (purpura nervosa) D69.0
  hepatic —*see* Disease, liver
  hepatobiliary K83.9
    toxic K71.9
  hepatolenticular E83.01
  heredodegenerative NEC
    spinal cord G95.89
  herpesviral, disseminated B00.7
  Hers' (glycogenosis VI) E74.09
  Herter (-Gee) (-Heubner) (nontropical sprue)
      K90.0
  Heubner-Herter (nontropical sprue) K90.0
  high fetal gene or hemoglobin thalassemia
      D56.9
  Hildenbrand's —*see* Typhus
  hip (joint) M25.9
    congenital Q65.89
    suppurative M00.9
    tuberculous A18.02
  His (-Werner) (trench fever) A79.0
  ⮞ Hodgson's *(see also* Aneurysm, aorta, thorax)
      I71.20
  ⮞ ruptured *(see also* Aneurysm, aorta, thorax,
      ruptured) I71.10
  Holla —*see* Spherocytosis

Disease, diseased *(Continued)*
  hookworm B76.9
    specified NEC B76.8
  host-versus-graft D89.813
    acute D89.810
    acute on chronic D89.812
    chronic D89.811
  human immunodeficiency virus (HIV) B20
  Huntington's G10
  ➡with dementia *(see also* Dementia, in, diseases specified elsewhere) G10 *[F02.80]*
  Hutchinson's (cheiropompholyx) —*see* Hutchinson's disease
  hyaline (diffuse) (generalized)
    membrane (lung) (newborn) P22.0
      adult J80
  hydatid —*see* Echinococcus
  hydroxyapatite deposition M11.00
    ankle M11.07-●
    elbow M11.02-●
    foot joint M11.07-●
    hand joint M11.04-●
    hip M11.05-●
    knee M11.06-●
    multiple site M11.09
    shoulder M11.01-●
    vertebra M11.08
    wrist M11.03-●
  hyperkinetic —*see* Hyperkinesia
  hypertensive —*see* Hypertension
  hypophysis E23.7
  ➡Iceland G93.39
  I-cell E77.0
  immune D89.9
  immunoproliferative (malignant) C88.9
    small intestinal C88.3
    specified NEC C88.8
  inclusion B25.9
    salivary gland B25.9
  infectious, infective B99.9
    congenital P37.9
      specified NEC P37.8
      viral P35.9
        specified type NEC P35.8
    specified NEC B99.8
  inflammatory
    penis N48.29
      abscess N48.21
      cellulitis N48.22
    prepuce N47.7
      balanoposthitis N47.6
    tubo-ovarian —*see* Salpingo-oophoritis
  intervertebral disc —*see also* Disorder, disc
    with myelopathy —*see* Disorder, disc, with, myelopathy
    cervical, cervicothoracic —*see* Disorder, disc, cervical
    with
      myelopathy —*see* Disorder, disc, cervical, with myelopathy
      neuritis, radiculitis or radiculopathy —*see* Disorder, disc, cervical, with neuritis
      specified NEC —*see* Disorder, disc, cervical, specified type NEC
    lumbar (with)
      myelopathy M51.06
      neuritis, radiculitis, radiculopathy or sciatica M51.16
      specified NEC M51.86
    lumbosacral (with)
      neuritis, radiculitis, radiculopathy or sciatica M51.17
      specified NEC M51.87
    specified NEC —*see* Disorder, disc, specified NEC
    thoracic (with)
      myelopathy M51.04
      neuritis, radiculitis or radiculopathy M51.14
      specified NEC M51.84

Disease, diseased *(Continued)*
  intervertebral disc *(Continued)*
    thoracolumbar (with)
      myelopathy M51.05
      neuritis, radiculitis or radiculopathy M51.15
      specified NEC M51.85
  intestine K63.9
    functional K59.9
      psychogenic F45.8
      specified NEC K59.89
    organic K63.9
    protozoal A07.9
    specified NEC K63.89
  iris H21.9
    specified NEC H21.89
  iron metabolism or storage E83.10
  island (scrub typhus) A75.3
  itai-itai —*see* Poisoning, cadmium
  Jakob-Creutzfeldt —*see* Creutzfeldt-Jakob disease or syndrome
  jaw M27.9
    fibrocystic M27.49
    specified NEC M27.8
  jigger B88.1
  joint —*see also* Disorder, joint
    Charcot's —*see* Arthropathy, neuropathic (Charcot)
    degenerative —*see* Osteoarthritis
      multiple M15.9
      spine —*see* Spondylosis
    facet joint *(see also* Spondylosis) M47.819
    hypertrophic —*see* Osteoarthritis
    sacroiliac M53.3
    specified NEC —*see* Disorder, joint, specified type NEC
    spine NEC —*see* Dorsopathy
    suppurative —*see* Arthritis, pyogenic or pyemic
  Jourdain's (acute gingivitis) K05.00
    nonplaque induced K05.01
    plaque induced K05.00
  Kaschin-Beck (endemic polyarthritis) M12.10
    ankle M12.17-●
    elbow M12.12-●
    foot joint M12.17-●
    hand joint M12.14-●
    hip M12.15-●
    knee M12.16-●
    multiple site M12.19
    shoulder M12.11-●
    vertebra M12.18
    wrist M12.13-●
  Katayama B65.2
  Kedani (scrub typhus) A75.3
  Keshan E59
  kidney (functional) (pelvis) N28.9
    chronic N18.9
      hypertensive —*see* Hypertension, kidney
      stage 1 N18.1
      stage 2 (mild) N18.2
      stage 3 (moderate) N18.30
        stage 3a N18.31
        stage 3b N18.32
      stage 4 (severe) N18.4
      stage 5 N18.5
    complicating pregnancy —*see* Pregnancy, complicated by, renal disease
    cystic (congenital) Q61.9
    diabetic —*see* E08-E13 with .22
    fibrocystic (congenital) Q61.8
    hypertensive —*see* Hypertension, kidney
    in (due to)
      schistosomiasis (bilharziasis) B65.9 *[N29]*
    multicystic Q61.4
    polycystic Q61.3
      adult type Q61.2
      childhood type NEC Q61.19
        collecting duct dilatation Q61.11
  Kimmelstiel (-Wilson) (intercapillary polycystic (congenital) glomerulosclerosis) —*see* E08-E13 with .21

Disease, diseased *(Continued)*
  Kimura D21.9
    specified site *(see* Neoplasm, connective tissue benign)
  Kinnier Wilson's (hepatolenticular degeneration) E83.01
  kissing —*see* Mononucleosis, infectious
  Klebs' —*see also* Glomerulonephritis N05.-●
  Klippel-Feil (brevicollis) Q76.1
  Köhler-Pellegrini-Stieda (calcification, knee joint) —*see* Bursitis, tibial collateral
  Kok Q89.8
  König's (osteochondritis dissecans) —*see* Osteochondritis, dissecans
  Korsakoff's (nonalcoholic) F04
    alcoholic F10.96
      with dependence F10.26
  Kostmann's (infantile genetic agranulocytosis) D70.0
  kuru A81.81
  Kyasanur Forest A98.2
  labyrinth, ear —*see* Disorder, ear, inner
  lacrimal system —*see* Disorder, lacrimal system
  Lafora's —*see* Epilepsy, generalized, idiopathic
  Lancereaux-Mathieu (leptospiral jaundice) A27.0
  Landry's G61.0
  Larrey-Weil (leptospiral jaundice) A27.0
  larynx J38.7
  legionnaires' A48.1
    nonpneumonic A48.2
  Lenegre's I44.2
  lens H27.9
    specified NEC H27.8
  Lev's (acquired complete heart block) I44.2
  ➡Lewy body (dementia) *(see also* Dementia, in, diseases specified elsewhere) G31.83 *[F02.80]*
    with behavioral disturbance *(see also* Dementia, in, diseases specified elsewhere) G31.83 *[F02.81-●]*
  Lichtheim's (subacute combined sclerosis with pernicious anemia) D51.0
  Lightwood's (renal tubular acidosis) N25.89
  Lignac's (cystinosis) E72.04
  lip K13.0
  lipid-storage E75.6
    specified NEC E75.5
  Lipschütz's N76.6
  liver (chronic) (organic) K76.9
    alcoholic (chronic) K70.9
      acute —*see* Disease, liver, alcoholic, hepatitis
      cirrhosis K70.30
        with ascites K70.31
      failure K70.40
        with coma K70.41
      fatty liver K70.0
      fibrosis K70.2
      hepatitis K70.10
        with ascites K70.11
      sclerosis K70.2
    cystic, congenital Q44.6
    drug-induced (idiosyncratic) (toxic) (predictable) (unpredictable) —*see* Disease, liver, toxic
  ➡end stage K72.1-●
      due to hepatitis —*see* Hepatitis
      with coma K72.11
    fatty, nonalcoholic (NAFLD) K76.0
      alcoholic K70.0
    fibrocystic (congenital) Q44.6
    fluke
      Chinese B66.1
      oriental B66.1
      sheep B66.3
    gestational alloimmune (GALD) P78.84
    glycogen storage E74.09 *[K77]*
    in (due to)
      schistosomiasis (bilharziasis) B65.9 *[K77]*

▶ New　⟹ Revised　~~deleted~~ Deleted　● Use Additional Character(s)

Disease, diseased (Continued)
liver (Continued)
  inflammatory K75.9
    alcoholic K70.1
    specified NEC K75.89
  polycystic (congenital) Q44.6
  toxic K71.9
    with
      cholestasis K71.0
      cirrhosis (liver) K71.7
      fibrosis (liver) K71.7
      focal nodular hyperplasia K71.8
      hepatic granuloma K71.8
      hepatic necrosis K71.10
        with coma K71.11
      hepatitis NEC K71.6
        acute K71.2
        chronic
          active K71.50
            with ascites K71.51
          lobular K71.4
          persistent K71.3
        lupoid K71.50
          with ascites K71.51
      peliosis hepatis K71.8
      veno-occlusive disease (VOD) of liver K71.8
  veno-occlusive K76.5
Lobo's (keloid blastomycosis) B48.0
Lobstein's (brittle bones and blue sclera) Q78.0
Ludwig's (submaxillary cellulitis) K12.2
lumbosacral region M53.87
lung J98.4
  black J60
  congenital Q33.9
  cystic J98.4
    congenital Q33.0
  dabbing (related) U07.0
  electronic cigarette (related) U07.0
  fibroid (chronic) —see Fibrosis, lung
  fluke B66.4
    oriental B66.4
  in
    amyloidosis E85.4 [J99]
    sarcoidosis D86.0
    Sjögren's syndrome M35.02
    systemic
      lupus erythematosus M32.13
      sclerosis M34.81
  interstitial J84.9
    of childhood, specified NEC J84.848
    respiratory bronchiolitis J84.115
    specified NEC J84.89
    with progressive fibrotic phenotype, in diseases classified elsewhere J84.170
  obstructive (chronic) J44.9
    with
      acute
        bronchitis J44.0
        exacerbation NEC J44.1
        lower respiratory infection J44.0
      alveolitis, allergic J67.9
      asthma J44.9
      bronchiectasis J47.9
        with
          exacerbation (acute) J47.1
          lower respiratory infection J47.0
      bronchitis J44.9
        with
          exacerbation (acute) J44.1
          lower respiratory infection J44.0
      emphysema J43.9
      hypersensitivity pneumonitis J67.9
    decompensated J44.1
      with
        exacerbation (acute) J44.1
  polycystic J98.4
    congenital Q33.0
  rheumatoid (diffuse) (interstitial) —see Rheumatoid, lung
  vaping (associated) (device) (product) (use) U07.0

➠Lutembacher's (atrial septal defect with mitral stenosis) Q21.19
Lyme A69.20
lymphatic (gland) (system) (channel) (vessel) I89.9
lymphoproliferative D47.9
  specified NEC D47.Z9
  T-gamma D47.Z9
  X-linked D82.3
Magitot's M27.2
malarial —see Malaria
malignant —see also Neoplasm, malignant, by site
Manson's B65.1
maple bark J67.6
maple-syrup-urine E71.0
Marburg (virus) A98.3
Marion's (bladder neck obstruction) N32.0
Marsh's (exophthalmic goiter) —see Hyperthyroidism, with, goiter (diffuse)
mastoid (process) —see Disorder, ear, middle
Mathieu's (leptospiral jaundice) A27.0
Maxcy's A75.2
McArdle (-Schmid-Pearson) (glycogenosis V) E74.04
mediastinum J98.59
medullary center (idiopathic) (respiratory) G93.89
Meige's (chronic hereditary edema) Q82.0
meningococcal —see Infection, meningococcal
mental F99
  organic F09
mesenchymal M35.9
mesenteric embolic —see also Ischemia, intestine, acute K55.039
metabolic, metabolism E88.9
  bilirubin E80.7
metal-polisher's J62.8
metastatic —see also Neoplasm, secondary, by site C79.9
microvascular — code to condition
microvillus
  atrophy Q43.8
  inclusion (MVD) Q43.8
middle ear —see Disorder, ear, middle
Mikulicz' (dryness of mouth, absent or decreased lacrimation) K11.8
Milroy's (chronic hereditary edema) Q82.0
Minamata —see Poisoning, mercury
minicore G71.29
Minor's G95.19
Minot's (hemorrhagic disease, newborn) P53
➠Minot-von Willebrand-Jürgens (angiohemophilia) —see Disease, von Willebrand
Mitchell's (erythromelalgia) I73.81
mitral (valve) I05.9
  nonrheumatic I34.9
mixed connective tissue M35.1
moldy hay J67.0
Monge's T70.29
Morgagni-Adams-Stokes (syncope with heart block) I45.9
Morgagni's (syndrome) (hyperostosis frontalis interna) M85.2
Morton's (with metatarsalgia) —see Lesion, nerve, plantar
Morvan's G60.8
motor neuron (bulbar) (mixed type) (spinal) G12.20
  amyotrophic lateral sclerosis G12.21
  familial G12.24
  progressive bulbar palsy G12.22
  specified NEC G12.29
moyamoya I67.5
mu heavy chain disease C88.2
multicore G71.29
multiminicore G71.29
muscle —see also Disorder, muscle
  inflammatory —see Myositis
  ocular (external) —see Strabismus

Disease, diseased (Continued)
musculoskeletal system, soft tissue —see also Disorder, soft tissue
  specified NEC —see Disorder, soft tissue, specified type NEC
mushroom workers' J67.5
mycotic B49
~~myelodysplastic, not classified (see also Syndrome, myelodysplasia) C94.6~~
~~myeloproliferative, not classified C94.6 chronic D47.1~~
▶myelodysplastic (see also Syndrome, myelodysplasia) C94.6
▶myelodysplastic/myeloproliferative neoplasm, unclassifiable C94.6
▶myeloproliferative D47.1
  ▶chronic D47.1
  ▶not classified C94.6
  ▶specified NEC C94.6
  ▶unclassifiable C94.6
myocardium, myocardial —see also Degeneration, myocardial I51.5
  primary (idiopathic) I42.9
myoneural G70.9
Naegeli's D69.1
nails L60.9
  specified NEC L60.8
Nairobi (sheep virus) A93.8
nasal J34.9
nemaline body G71.21
nerve —see Disorder, nerve
nervous system G98.8
  autonomic G90.9
  central G96.9
    specified NEC G96.89
  congenital Q07.9
  parasympathetic G90.9
  specified NEC G98.8
  sympathetic G90.9
  vegetative G90.9
neuromuscular system G70.9
Newcastle B30.8
Nicolas (-Durand)-Favre (climatic bubo) A55
nipple N64.9
  Paget's C50.01-●
    female C50.01-●
    male C50.02-●
Nishimoto (-Takeuchi) I67.5
nonarthropod-borne NOS (viral) B34.9
  enterovirus NEC B34.1
nonautoimmune hemolytic D59.4
  drug-induced D59.2
Nonne-Milroy-Meige (chronic hereditary edema) Q82.0
nose J34.9
nucleus pulposus —see Disorder, disc
nutritional E63.9
oast-house-urine E72.19
ocular
  herpesviral B00.50
  zoster B02.30
obliterative vascular I77.1
Ohara's —see Tularemia
Opitz's (congestive splenomegaly) D73.2
Oppenheim-Urbach (necrobiosis lipoidica diabeticorum) —see E08-E13 with .620
optic nerve NEC —see Disorder, nerve, optic
orbit —see Disorder, orbit
organ
  dabbing (related) U07.0
  electronic cigarette (related) U07.0
  vaping (associated) (device) (product) (use) U07.0
Oriental liver fluke B66.1
Oriental lung fluke B66.4
Ormond's N13.5
Oropouche virus A93.0
Osler-Rendu (familial hemorrhagic telangiectasia) I78.0
osteofibrocystic E21.0
Otto's M24.7

Disease, diseased (Continued)
  outer ear —see Disorder, ear, external
  ovary (noninflammatory) N83.9
    cystic N83.20-●
    inflammatory —see Salpingo-oophoritis
    polycystic E28.2
    specified NEC N83.8
  Owren's (congenital) —see Defect,
    coagulation
▶ p110d-activating mutation causing senescent
    T cells, lymphadenopathy, and
    immunodeficiency [PASLI] D81.82
  pancreas K86.9
    cystic K86.2
    fibrocystic E84.9
    specified NEC K86.89
  panvalvular I08.9
    specified NEC I08.8
  parametrium (noninflammatory) N83.9
  parasitic B89
    cerebral NEC B71.9 [G94]
    intestinal NOS B82.9
    mouth B37.0
    skin NOS B88.9
    specified type —see Infestation
    tongue B37.0
  parathyroid (gland) E21.5
    specified NEC E21.4
  Parkinson's G20
  parodontal K05.6
  Parrot's (syphilitic osteochondritis) A50.02
  Parry's (exophthalmic goiter) —see
    Hyperthyroidism, with, goiter (diffuse)
  Parson's (exophthalmic goiter) —see
    Hyperthyroidism, with, goiter (diffuse)
  Paxton's (white piedra) B36.2
  pearl-worker's —see Osteomyelitis, specified
    type NEC
  Pellegrini-Stieda (calcification, knee joint) —
    see Bursitis, tibial collateral
  pelvis, pelvic
    female NOS N94.9
      specified NEC N94.89
    gonococcal (acute) (chronic) A54.24
    inflammatory (female) N73.9
      acute N73.0
      chlamydial A56.11
      chronic N73.1
      specified NEC N73.8
      syphilitic (secondary) A51.42
        late A52.76
      tuberculous A18.17
    organ, female N94.9
    peritoneum, female NEC N94.89
  penis N48.9
    inflammatory N48.29
      abscess N48.21
      cellulitis N48.22
    specified NEC N48.89
  periapical tissues NOS K04.90
  periodontal K05.6
    specified NEC K05.5
  periosteum —see Disorder, bone, specified
    type NEC
  peripheral
    arterial I73.9
    autonomic nervous system G90.9
    nerves —see Polyneuropathy
    vascular NOS I73.9
  peritoneum K66.9
    pelvic, female NEC N94.89
    specified NEC K66.8
  persistent mucosal (middle ear) H66.20
    left H66.22
      with right H66.23
    right H66.21
      with left H66.23
  Petit's —see Hernia, abdomen, specified site
    NEC
  pharynx J39.2
    specified NEC J39.2
  Phocas' —see Mastopathy, cystic

Disease, diseased (Continued)
  photochromogenic (acid-fast bacilli)
    (pulmonary) A31.0
    nonpulmonary A31.9
▶ Pick's (see also Dementia, in, diseases
    specified elsewhere) G31.01 [F02.80]
▶ with behavioral disturbance (see also
    Dementia, in, diseases specified
    elsewhere) G31.01 [F02.81-●]
▶ brain (see also Dementia, in, diseases
    specified elsewhere) G31.01 [F02.80]
▶ with behavioral disturbance (see also
    Dementia, in, diseases specified
    elsewhere) G31.01 [F02.81-●]
    of pericardium (pericardial pseudocirrhosis
    of liver) I31.1
  pigeon fancier's J67.2
  pineal gland E34.8
  pink —see Poisoning, mercury
  Pinkus' (lichen nitidus) L44.1
  pinworm B80
  Piry virus A93.8
  pituitary (gland) E23.7
  pituitary-snuff-taker's J67.8
  pleura (cavity) J94.9
    specified NEC J94.8
  pneumatic drill (hammer) T75.21
  Pollitzer's (hidradenitis suppurativa)
    L73.2
  polycystic
    kidney or renal Q61.3
      adult type Q61.2
      childhood type NEC Q61.19
        collecting duct dilatation Q61.11
    liver or hepatic Q44.6
    lung or pulmonary J98.4
      congenital Q33.0
    ovary, ovaries E28.2
    spleen Q89.09
  polyethylene T84.05-●
  Pompe's (glycogenosis II) E74.02
  Posadas-Wernicke B38.9
  Potain's (pulmonary edema) —see Edema,
    lung
  prepuce N47.8
    inflammatory N47.7
      balanoposthitis N47.6
  Pringle's (tuberous sclerosis) Q85.1
  prion, central nervous system A81.9
    specified NEC A81.89
  prostate N42.9
    specified NEC N42.89
  protozoal B64
    acanthamebiasis —see Acanthamebiasis
    African trypanosomiasis —see African
      trypanosomiasis
    babesiosis —(see also Babesiosis) B60.00
    Chagas disease —see Chagas disease
    intestine, intestinal A07.9
    leishmaniasis —see Leishmaniasis
    malaria —see Malaria
    naegleriasis B60.2
    pneumocystosis B59
    specified organism NEC B60.8
    toxoplasmosis —see Toxoplasmosis
  pseudo-Hurler's E77.0
  psychiatric F99
  psychotic —see Psychosis
  Puente's (simple glandular cheilitis) K13.0
  puerperal —see also Puerperal O90.89
  pulmonary —see also Disease, lung
    artery I28.9
    chronic obstructive J44.9
      with
        acute bronchitis J44.0
        exacerbation (acute) J44.1
        lower respiratory infection (acute)
          J44.0
      decompensated J44.1
        with
          exacerbation (acute) J44.1

Disease, diseased (Continued)
  pulmonary (Continued)
    heart I27.9
      specified NEC I27.89
    hypertensive (vascular) —see also
      Hypertension, pulmonary I27.20
      primary (idiopathic) I27.0
    valve I37.9
      rheumatic I09.89
  pulp (dental) NOS K04.90
  pulseless M31.4
  Putnam's (subacute combined sclerosis with
    pernicious anemia) D51.0
  Pyle (-Cohn) (metaphyseal dysplasia)
    Q78.5
  ragpicker's or ragsorter's A22.1
  Raynaud's —see Raynaud's disease
  reactive airway —see Asthma
  Reclus' (cystic) —see Mastopathy, cystic
  rectum K62.9
    specified NEC K62.89
  Refsum's (heredopathia atactica
    polyneuritiformis) G60.1
  renal (functional) (pelvis) —see also Disease,
    kidney N28.9
    with
      edema —see Nephrosis
      glomerular lesion —see
        Glomerulonephritis
        with edema —see Nephrosis
      interstitial nephritis N12
    acute N28.9
    chronic —see also Disease, kidney, chronic
      N18.9
    cystic, congenital Q61.9
    diabetic —see E08-E13 with .22
    end-stage (failure) N18.6
      due to hypertension I12.0
    fibrocystic (congenital) Q61.8
    hypertensive —see Hypertension, kidney
    lupus M32.14
    phosphate-losing (tubular) N25.0
    polycystic (congenital) Q61.3
      adult type Q61.2
      childhood type NEC Q61.19
        collecting duct dilatation Q61.11
    rapidly progressive N01.9
    subacute N01.9
  Rendu-Osler-Weber (familial hemorrhagic
    telangiectasia) I78.0
  renovascular (arteriosclerotic) —see
    Hypertension, kidney
  respiratory (tract) J98.9
    acute or subacute NOS J06.9
      due to
        chemicals, gases, fumes or vapors
          (inhalation) J68.3
        external agent J70.9
          specified NEC J70.8
        radiation J70.0
        smoke inhalation J70.5
      noninfectious J39.8
    chronic NOS J98.9
      due to
        chemicals, gases, fumes or vapors
          J68.4
        external agent J70.9
          specified NEC J70.8
        radiation J70.1
    newborn P27.9
      specified NEC P27.8
    due to
      chemicals, gases, fumes or vapors
        J68.9
      acute or subacute NEC J68.3
      chronic J68.4
    external agent J70.9
      specified NEC J70.8
    newborn P28.9
      specified type NEC P28.89

▶ New   ⇒ Revised   ~~deleted~~ Deleted   ● Use Additional Character(s)

Disease, diseased *(Continued)*
  respiratory (tract) *(Continued)*
    upper J39.9
      acute or subacute J06.9
      noninfectious NEC J39.8
      specified NEC J39.8
      streptococcal J06.9
  retina, retinal H35.9
    Batten's or Batten-Mayou E75.4 *[H36]*
    specified NEC H35.89
  rheumatoid —*see* Arthritis, rheumatoid
  rickettsial NOS A79.9
    specified type NEC A79.89
  Riga (-Fede) (cachectic aphthae) K14.0
  Riggs' (compound periodontitis) —*see*
    Periodontitis
  Ritter's L00
  Rivalta's (cervicofacial actinomycosis) A42.2
  rod body G71.21
  Robles' (onchocerciasis) B73.01
  Roger's (congenital interventricular septal
    defect) Q21.0
  Rosenthal's (factor XI deficiency) D68.1
  Ross River B33.1
  Rossbach's (hyperchlorhydria) K31.89
    psychogenic F45.8
  Rotes Quérol —*see* Hyperostosis, ankylosing
  Roth (-Bernhardt) —*see* Mononeuropathy,
    lower limb, meralgia paresthetica
  Runeberg's (progressive pernicious anemia)
    D51.0
  sacroiliac NEC M53.3
  salivary gland or duct K11.9
    inclusion B25.9
    specified NEC K11.8
    virus B25.9
  sandworm B76.9
  Schimmelbusch's —*see* Mastopathy, cystic
  Schmorl's —*see* Schmorl's disease or nodes
  Schönlein (-Henoch) (purpura rheumatica)
    D69.0
  Schottmüller's —*see* Fever, paratyphoid
  Schultz's (agranulocytosis) —*see*
    Agranulocytosis
  Schwalbe-Ziehen-Oppenheim G24.1
  Schwartz-Jampel G71.13
  sclera H15.9
    specified NEC H15.89
  scrofulous (tuberculous) A18.2
  scrotum N50.9
  sebaceous glands L73.9
  semilunar cartilage, cystic —*see also*
    Derangement, knee, meniscus, cystic
  seminal vesicle N50.9
  serum NEC —*see also* Reaction, serum
    T80.69
  sexually transmitted A64
    anogenital
      herpesviral infection —*see* Herpes,
        anogenital
      warts A63.0
    chancroid A57
    chlamydial infection —*see* Chlamydia
    gonorrhea —*see* Gonorrhea
    granuloma inguinale A58
    specified organism NEC A63.8
    syphilis —*see* Syphilis
    trichomoniasis —*see* Trichomoniasis
  Sézary C84.1-•
  shimamushi (scrub typhus) A75.3
  shipyard B30.0
  sickle-cell D57.1
    with
      acute chest syndrome D57.01
      cerebral vascular involvement D57.03
      crisis (painful) D57.00
        with complication specified NEC
          D57.09
      splenic sequestration D57.02
      vasoocclusive pain D57.00
    elliptocytosis D57.8-•

Disease, diseased *(Continued)*
  sickle-cell *(Continued)*
    Hb-C D57.20
      with
        acute chest syndrome D57.211
        cerebral vascular involvement D57.213
        crisis (painful) D57.219
          with specified complication NEC
            D57.218
        splenic sequestration D57.212
        vasoocclusive pain D57.219
      without crisis D57.20
    Hb-SD D57.80
      with
        acute chest syndrome D57.811
        cerebral vascular involvement D57.813
        crisis (painful) D57.819
          with complication specified NEC
            D57.818
        splenic sequestration D57.812
        vasoocclusive pain D57.819
      without crisis D57.80
    Hb-SE D57.80
      with
        acute chest syndrome D57.811
        cerebral vascular involvement D57.813
        crisis (painful) D57.819
          with complication specified NEC
            D57.818
        splenic sequestration D57.812
        vasoocclusive pain D57.819
      without crisis D57.80
    specified NEC D57.80
      with
        acute chest syndrome D57.811
        cerebral vascular involvement D57.813
        crisis (painful) D57.819
          with complication specified NEC
            D57.818
        splenic sequestration D57.812
        vasoocclusive pain D57.819
      without crisis D57.80
    spherocytosis D57.80
      with
        acute chest syndrome D57.811
        cerebral vascular involvement D57.813
        crisis (painful) D57.819
          with complication specified NEC
            D57.818
        splenic sequestration D57.812
        vasoocclusive pain D57.819
      without crisis D57.80
    thalassemia D57.40
      with
        acute chest syndrome D57.411
        cerebral vascular involvement D57.413
        crisis (painful) D57.419
          with specified complication NEC
            D57.418
        splenic sequestration D57.412
        vasoocclusive pain D57.419
    beta plus D57.44
      with
        acute chest syndrome D57.451
        cerebral vascular involvement
          D57.453
        crisis D57.459
          with specified complication NEC
            D57.458
        splenic sequestration D57.452
        vasoocclusive pain D57.459
      without crisis D57.44
    beta zero D57.42
      with
        acute chest syndrome D57.431
        cerebral vascular involvement
          D57.433
        crisis D57.439
          with specified complication NEC
            D57.438
        splenic sequestration D57.432
        vasoocclusive pain D57.439
      without crisis D57.42

Disease, diseased *(Continued)*
  silo-filler's J68.8
    bronchitis J68.0
    pneumonitis J68.0
    pulmonary edema J68.1
  simian B B00.4
  Simons' (progressive lipodystrophy) E88.1
  sin nombre virus B33.4
  sinus —*see* Sinusitis
  Sirkari's B55.0
  sixth B08.20
    due to human herpesvirus 6 B08.21
    due to human herpesvirus 7 B08.22
  skin L98.9
    due to metabolic disorder NEC
      E88.9 *[L99]*
    specified NEC L98.8
  slim (HIV) B20
  small vessel I73.9
  Sneddon-Wilkinson (subcorneal pustular
    dermatosis) L13.1
  South African creeping B88.0
  spinal (cord) G95.9
    congenital Q06.9
    specified NEC G95.89
  spine —*see also* Spondylopathy
    joint —*see* Dorsopathy
    tuberculous A18.01
  spinocerebellar (hereditary) G11.9
    specified NEC G11.8
  spleen D73.9
    amyloid E85.4 *[D77]*
    organic D73.9
    polycystic Q89.09
    postinfectional D73.89
  sponge-diver's —*see* Toxicity, venom, marine
    animal, sea anemone
  Startle Q89.8
  Steinert's G71.11
  Sticker's (erythema infectiosum) B08.3
  Stieda's (calcification, knee joint) —*see*
    Bursitis, tibial collateral
  Stokes' (exophthalmic goiter) —*see*
    Hyperthyroidism, with, goiter
    (diffuse)
  Stokes-Adams (syncope with heart block)
    I45.9
  stomach K31.9
    functional, psychogenic F45.8
    specified NEC K31.89
  stonemason's J62.8
  storage
    glycogen —*see* Disease, glycogen storage
    mucopolysaccharide —*see*
      Mucopolysaccharidosis
  striatopallidal system NEC G25.89
  Stuart-Prower (congenital factor X deficiency)
    D68.2
  Stuart's (congenital factor X deficiency)
    D68.2
  subcutaneous tissue —*see* Disease, skin
  supporting structures of teeth K08.9
    specified NEC K08.89
  suprarenal (capsule) (gland) E27.9
    hyperfunction E27.0
    specified NEC E27.8
  sweat glands L74.9
    specified NEC L74.8
  Sweeley-Klionsky E75.21
  Swift (-Feer) —*see* Poisoning, mercury
  swimming-pool granuloma A31.1
  Sylvest's (epidemic pleurodynia) B33.0
  sympathetic nervous system G90.9
  synovium —*see* Disorder, synovium
  syphilitic —*see* Syphilis
  systemic tissue mast cell D47.02
  tanapox (virus) B08.71
  Tangier E78.6
  Tarral-Besnier (pityriasis rubra pilaris) L44.0
  Tauri's E74.09
  tear duct —*see* Disorder, lacrimal system

▶ New   ⇒ Revised   ~~deleted~~ Deleted   • Use Additional Character(s)

Disease, diseased *(Continued)*
tendon, tendinous —*see also* Disorder, tendon
   nodular —*see* Trigger finger
terminal vessel I73.9
testis N50.9
thalassemia Hb-S —*see* Disease, sickle-cell,
   thalassemia
Thaysen-Gee (nontropical sprue) K90.0
Thomsen G71.12
throat J39.2
   septic J02.0
thromboembolic —*see* Embolism
thymus (gland) E32.9
   specified NEC E32.8
thyroid (gland) E07.9
   heart —*see also* Hyperthyroidism
     E05.90 *[I43]*
      with thyroid storm E05.91 *[I43]*
   specified NEC E07.8
Tietze's M94.0
tongue K14.9
   specified NEC K14.89
tonsils, tonsillar (and adenoids) J35.9
tooth, teeth K08.9
   hard tissues K03.9
     specified NEC K03.89
   pulp NEC K04.99
   specified NEC K08.89
Tourette's F95.2
trachea NEC J39.8
tricuspid I07.9
   nonrheumatic I36.9
triglyceride-storage E75.5
trophoblastic —*see* Mole, hydatidiform
tsutsugamushi A75.3
tube (fallopian) (noninflammatory) N83.9
   inflammatory —*see* Salpingitis
   specified NEC N83.8
tuberculous NEC —*see* Tuberculosis
tubo-ovarian (noninflammatory) N83.9
   inflammatory —*see* Salpingo-oophoritis
   specified NEC N83.8
tubotympanic, chronic —*see* Otitis, media,
   suppurative, chronic, tubotympanic
tubulo-interstitial N15.9
   specified NEC N15.8
tympanum —*see* Disorder, tympanic
   membrane
Uhl's Q24.8
Underwood's (sclerema neonatorum)
   P83.0
Unverricht (-Lundborg) —*see* Epilepsy,
   generalized, idiopathic
Urbach-Oppenheim (necrobiosis lipoidica
   diabeticorum) —*see* E08-E13 with .620
ureter N28.9
   in (due to)
     schistosomiasis (bilharziasis)
      B65.0 *[N29]*
urethra N36.9
   specified NEC N36.8
urinary (tract) N39.9
   bladder N32.9
     specified NEC N32.89
   specified NEC N39.8
uterus (noninflammatory) N85.9
   infective —*see* Endometritis
   inflammatory —*see* Endometritis
   specified NEC N85.8
uveal tract (anterior) H21.9
   posterior H31.9
vagabond's B85.1
vagina, vaginal (noninflammatory) N89.9
   inflammatory NEC N76.89
   specified NEC N89.8
valve, valvular I38
   multiple I08.9
     specified NEC I08.8
van Creveld-von Gierke (glycogenosis I)
   E74.01
vas deferens N50.9

Disease, diseased *(Continued)*
vascular *(Continued)*
   arteriosclerotic —*see* Arteriosclerosis
   ciliary body NEC —*see* Disorder, iris,
     vascular
   hypertensive —*see* Hypertension
   iris NEC —*see* Disorder, iris, vascular
   obliterative I77.1
     peripheral I73.9
   occlusive I99.8
   peripheral (occlusive) I73.9
     in diabetes mellitus —*see* E08-E13 with .51
vasomotor I73.9
vasospastic I73.9
vein I87.9
venereal —*see also* Disease, sexually
   transmitted A64
   chlamydial NEC A56.8
     anus A56.3
     genitourinary NOS A56.2
     pharynx A56.4
     rectum A56.3
   fifth A55
   sixth A55
   specified nature or type NEC A63.8
vertebra, vertebral —*see also* Spondylopathy
   disc —*see* Disorder, disc
vibration —*see* Vibration, adverse effects
viral, virus —*see also* Disease, by type of virus
   B34.9
   arbovirus NOS A94
   arthropod-borne NOS A94
   congenital P35.9
     specified NEC P35.8
   Hanta (with renal manifestations)
     (Dobrava) (Puumala) (Seoul) A98.5
     with pulmonary manifestations (Andes)
      (Bayou) (Bermejo) (Black Creek
      Canal) (Choclo) (Juquitiba) (Laguna
      negra) (Lechiguanas) (New York)
      (Oran) (Sin nombre) B33.4
   Hantaan (Korean hemorrhagic fever) A98.5
   human immunodeficiency (HIV) B20
   Kunjin A83.4
   nonarthropod-borne NOS B34.9
   Powassan A84.81
   Rocio (encephalitis) A83.6
   Sin nombre (Hantavirus) (cardio)-
     pulmonary syndrome B33.4
   Tahyna B33.8
   vesicular stomatitis A93.8
vitreous H43.9
   specified NEC H43.89
vocal cord J38.3
Volkmann's, acquired T79.6
von Eulenburg's (congenital paramyotonia)
   G71.19
von Gierke's (glycogenosis I) E74.01
von Graefe's —*see* Strabismus, paralytic,
   ophthalmoplegia, progressive
⇢von Willebrand (-Jürgens) (angiohemophilia)
   D68.00
  ▶acquired D68.04
  ▶platelet-type D68.09
  ▶pseudo D68.09
  ▶specified NEC D68.09
  ▶type 1 D68.01
  ▶type 1C D68.01
  ▶type 2 D68.029
    ▶type 2A D68.020
    ▶type 2B D68.021
    ▶type 2M D68.022
    ▶type 2N D68.023
  ▶type 3 D68.03
Vrolik's (osteogenesis imperfecta) Q78.0
vulva (noninflammatory) N90.9
   inflammatory NEC N76.89
   specified NEC N90.89
Wallgren's (obstruction of splenic vein with
   collateral circulation) I87.8
Wassilieff's (leptospiral jaundice) A27.0

Disease, diseased *(Continued)*
wasting NEC R64
   due to malnutrition E43
     with marasmus E41
Waterhouse-Friderichsen A39.1
Wegner's (syphilitic osteochondritis) A50.02
Weil's (leptospiral jaundice of lung) A27.0
Weir Mitchell's (erythromelalgia) I73.81
Werdnig-Hoffmann G12.0
Werner's E31.21
Werner-His (trench fever) A79.0
Werner-Schultz (neutropenic splenomegaly)
   D73.81
Wernicke-Posadas B38.9
whipworm B79
white blood cells D72.9
   specified NEC D72.89
white matter R90.82
white-spot, meaning lichen sclerosus et
   atrophicus L90.0
   penis N48.0
   vulva N90.4
Wilkie's K55.1
Wilkinson-Sneddon (subcorneal pustular
   dermatosis) L13.1
Willis' —*see* Diabetes
Wilson's (hepatolenticular degeneration) E83.01
woolsorter's A22.1
yaba monkey tumor B08.72
yaba pox (virus) B08.72
Zika virus A92.5
zoonotic, bacterial A28.9
   congenital P35.4
   specified type NEC A28.8
Disfigurement (due to scar) L90.5
Disgerminoma —*see* Dysgerminoma
DISH (diffuse idiopathic skeletal
   hyperostosis) —*see* Hyperostosis, ankylosing
Disinsertion, retina —*see* Detachment, retina
Dislocatable hip, congenital Q65.6
Dislocation (articular)
   with fracture —*see* Fracture
   acromioclavicular (joint) S43.10-●
     with displacement
      100%-200% S43.12-●
      more than 200% S43.13-●
     inferior S43.14-●
     posterior S43.15-●
   ankle S93.0-●
   astragalus —*see* Dislocation, ankle
   atlantoaxial S13.121
   atlantooccipital S13.111
   atloidooccipital S13.111
   breast bone S23.29
   capsule, joint code by site under Dislocation
   carpal (bone) —*see* Dislocation, wrist
   carpometacarpal (joint) NEC S63.05-●
     thumb S63.04-●
   cartilage (joint) - code by site under
     Dislocation
   cervical spine (vertebra) —*see* Dislocation,
     vertebra, cervical
   chronic —*see* Dislocation, recurrent
   clavicle —*see* Dislocation, acromioclavicular
     joint
   coccyx S33.2
   congenital NEC Q68.8
   coracoid —*see* Dislocation, shoulder
   costal cartilage S23.29
   costochondral S23.29
   cricoarytenoid articulation S13.29
   cricothyroid articulation S13.29
   dorsal vertebra —*see* Dislocation, vertebra,
     thoracic
   ear ossicle —*see* Discontinuity, ossicles, ear
   elbow S53.10-●
     congenital Q68.8
     pathological —*see* Dislocation, pathological
      NEC, elbow
     radial head alone —*see* Dislocation, radial
      head

▶ New   ⇢ Revised   ~~deleted~~ Deleted   ● Use Additional Character(s)

Dislocation *(Continued)*
  elbow *(Continued)*
    recurrent —*see* Dislocation, recurrent, elbow
    traumatic S53.10-•
      anterior S53.11-•
      lateral S53.14-•
      medial S53.13-•
      posterior S53.12-•
      specified type NEC S53.19-•
  eye, nontraumatic —*see* Luxation, globe
  eyeball, nontraumatic —*see* Luxation, globe
  femur
    distal end —*see* Dislocation, knee
    proximal end —*see* Dislocation, hip
  fibula
    distal end —*see* Dislocation, ankle
    proximal end —*see* Dislocation, knee
  finger S63.25-•
    index S63.25-•
    interphalangeal S63.27-•
      distal S63.29-•
        index S63.29-•
        little S63.29-•
        middle S63.29-•
        ring S63.29-•
      index S63.27-•
      little S63.27-•
      middle S63.27-•
      proximal S63.28-•
        index S63.28-•
        little S63.28-•
        middle S63.28-•
        ring S63.28-•
      ring S63.27-•
    little S63.25-•
    metacarpophalangeal S63.26-•
      index S63.26-•
      little S63.26-•
      middle S63.26-•
      ring S63.26-•
    middle S63.25-•
    recurrent —*see* Dislocation, recurrent, finger
    ring S63.25-•
    thumb —*see* Dislocation, thumb
  foot S93.30-•
    recurrent —*see* Dislocation, recurrent, foot
    specified site NEC S93.33-•
    tarsal joint S93.31-•
    tarsometatarsal joint S93.32-•
    toe —*see* Dislocation, toe
  fracture —*see* Fracture
  glenohumeral (joint) —*see* Dislocation, shoulder
  glenoid —*see* Dislocation, shoulder
  habitual —*see* Dislocation, recurrent
  hip S73.00-•
    anterior S73.03-•
      obturator S73.02-•
    central S73.04-•
    congenital (total) Q65.2
      bilateral Q65.1
      partial Q65.5
        bilateral Q65.4
        unilateral Q65.3-•
      unilateral Q65.0-•
    developmental M24.85-•
    pathological —*see* Dislocation, pathological NEC, hip
    posterior S73.01-•
    recurrent —*see* Dislocation, recurrent, hip
  humerus, proximal end —*see* Dislocation, shoulder
  incomplete —*see* Subluxation, by site
  incus —*see* Discontinuity, ossicles, ear
  infracoracoid —*see* Dislocation, shoulder

Dislocation *(Continued)*
  innominate (pubic junction) (sacral junction) S33.39
    acetabulum —*see* Dislocation, hip
  interphalangeal (joint(s))
    finger S63.279
      distal S63.29-•
        index S63.29-•
        little S63.29-•
        middle S63.29-•
        ring S63.29-•
      index S63.27-•
      little S63.27-•
      middle S63.27-•
      proximal S63.28-•
        index S63.28-•
        little S63.28-•
        middle S63.28-•
        ring S63.28-•
      ring S63.27-•
    foot or toe —*see* Dislocation, toe
    thumb S63.12-•
  jaw (cartilage) (meniscus) S03.0-•
  joint prosthesis —*see* Complications, joint prosthesis, mechanical, displacement, by site
  knee S83.106
    cap —*see* Dislocation, patella
    congenital Q68.2
    old M23.8X-•
    patella —*see* Dislocation, patella
    pathological —*see* Dislocation, pathological NEC, knee
    proximal tibia
      anteriorly S83.11-•
      laterally S83.14-•
      medially S83.13-•
      posteriorly S83.12-•
    recurrent —*see also* Derangement, knee, specified NEC
    specified type NEC S83.19-•
  lacrimal gland H04.16-•
  lens (complete) H27.10-•
    anterior H27.12-•
    congenital Q12.1
    ocular implant —*see* Complications, intraocular lens
    partial H27.11-•
    posterior H27.13-•
    traumatic S05.8X-•
  ligament code by site under Dislocation
  lumbar (vertebra) —*see* Dislocation, vertebra, lumbar
  lumbosacral (vertebra) —*see also* Dislocation, vertebra, lumbar
    congenital Q76.49
  mandible S03.0-•
  meniscus (knee) —*see* Tear, meniscus
    other sites code by site under Dislocation
  metacarpal (bone)
    distal end —*see* Dislocation, finger
    proximal end S63.06-•
  metacarpophalangeal (joint)
    finger S63.26-•
      index S63.26-•
      little S63.26-•
      middle S63.26-•
      ring S63.26-•
    thumb S63.11-•
  metatarsal (bone) —*see* Dislocation, foot
  metatarsophalangeal (joint(s)) —*see* Dislocation, toe
  midcarpal (joint) S63.03-•
  midtarsal (joint) —*see* Dislocation, foot
  neck S13.20
    specified site NEC S13.29
    vertebra —*see* Dislocation, vertebra, cervical
  nose (septal cartilage) S03.1
  occipitoatloid S13.111

Dislocation *(Continued)*
  old —*see* Derangement, joint, specified type NEC
  ossicles, ear —*see* Discontinuity, ossicles, ear
  partial —*see* Subluxation, by site
  patella S83.006
    congenital Q74.1
    lateral S83.01-•
    recurrent (nontraumatic) M22.0-•
      incomplete M22.1-•
    specified type NEC S83.09-•
  pathological NEC M24.30
    ankle M24.37-•
    elbow M24.32-•
    foot joint M24.37-•
    hand joint M24.34-•
    hip M24.35-•
    knee M24.36-•
    lumbosacral joint —*see* subcategory M53.2
    pelvic region —*see* Dislocation, pathological, hip
    sacroiliac —*see* subcategory M53.2
    shoulder M24.31-•
    specified site NEC M24.39
    wrist M24.33-•
  pelvis NEC S33.30
    specified NEC S33.39
  phalanx
    finger or hand —*see* Dislocation, finger
    foot or toe —*see* Dislocation, toe
  prosthesis, internal —*see* Complications, prosthetic device, by site, mechanical
  radial head S53.006
    anterior S53.01-•
    posterior S53.02-•
    specified type NEC S53.09-•
  radiocarpal (joint) S63.02-•
  radiohumeral (joint) —*see* Dislocation, radial head
  radioulnar (joint)
    distal S63.01-•
    proximal —*see* Dislocation, elbow
  radius
    distal end —*see* Dislocation, wrist
    proximal end —*see* Dislocation, radial head
  recurrent M24.40
    ankle M24.47-•
    elbow M24.42-•
    finger M24.44-•
    foot joint M24.47-•
    hand joint M24.44-•
    hip M24.45-•
    knee M24.46-•
      patella —*see* Dislocation, patella, recurrent
    patella —*see* Dislocation, patella, recurrent
    sacroiliac —*see* subcategory M53.2
    shoulder M24.41-•
    specified site NEC M24.49
    toe M24.47-•
    vertebra —*see also* subcategory M43.5
      atlantoaxial M43.4
        with myelopathy M43.3
    wrist M24.43-•
  rib (cartilage) S23.29
  sacrococcygeal S33.2
  sacroiliac (joint) (ligament) S33.2
    congenital Q74.2
    recurrent —*see* subcategory M53.2
  sacrum S33.2
  scaphoid (bone) (hand) (wrist) —*see* Dislocation, wrist
    foot —*see* Dislocation, foot
  scapula —*see* Dislocation, shoulder, girdle, scapula
  semilunar cartilage, knee —*see* Tear, meniscus
  septal cartilage (nose) S03.1
  septum (nasal) (old) J34.2
  sesamoid bone code by site under Dislocation

Dislocation *(Continued)*
  shoulder (blade) (ligament) (joint) (traumatic) S43.006
    acromioclavicular —*see* Dislocation, acromioclavicular
    chronic —*see* Dislocation, recurrent, shoulder
    congenital Q68.8
    girdle S43.30-●
      scapula S43.31-●
      specified site NEC S43.39-●
    humerus S43.00-●
      anterior S43.01-●
      inferior S43.03-●
      posterior S43.02-●
    pathological —*see* Dislocation, pathological NEC, shoulder
    recurrent —*see* Dislocation, recurrent, shoulder
    specified type NEC S43.08-●
  spine
    cervical —*see* Dislocation, vertebra, cervical
    congenital Q76.49
    due to birth trauma P11.5
    lumbar —*see* Dislocation, vertebra, lumbar
    thoracic —*see* Dislocation, vertebra, thoracic
  spontaneous —*see* Dislocation, pathological
  sternoclavicular (joint) S43.206
    anterior S43.21-●
    posterior S43.22-●
  sternum S23.29
  subglenoid —*see* Dislocation, shoulder
  symphysis pubis S33.4
  talus —*see* Dislocation, ankle
  tarsal (bone(s)) (joint(s)) —*see* Dislocation, foot
  tarsometatarsal (joint(s)) —*see* Dislocation, foot
  temporomandibular (joint) S03.0-●
  thigh, proximal end —*see* Dislocation, hip
  thorax S23.20
    specified site NEC S23.29
    vertebra —*see* Dislocation, vertebra
  thumb S63.10-●
    interphalangeal joint —*see* Dislocation, interphalangeal (joint), thumb
    metacarpophalangeal joint —*see* Dislocation, metacarpophalangeal (joint), thumb
  thyroid cartilage S13.29
  tibia
    distal end —*see* Dislocation, ankle
    proximal end —*see* Dislocation, knee
  tibiofibular (joint)
    distal —*see* Dislocation, ankle
    superior —*see* Dislocation, knee
  toe(s) S93.106
    great S93.10-●
      interphalangeal joint S93.11-●
      metatarsophalangeal joint S93.12-●
    interphalangeal joint S93.119
    lesser S93.106
      interphalangeal joint S93.11-●
      metatarsophalangeal joint S93.12-●
    metatarsophalangeal joint S93.12-●
  tooth S03.2
  trachea S23.29
  ulna
    distal end S63.07-●
    proximal end —*see* Dislocation, elbow
  ulnohumeral (joint) —*see* Dislocation, elbow
  vertebra (articular process) (body) (traumatic)
    cervical S13.101
      atlantoaxial joint S13.121
      atlantooccipital joint S13.111
      atloidooccipital joint S13.111
      joint between
        C0 and C1 S13.111
        C1 and C2 S13.121

Dislocation *(Continued)*
  vertebra *(Continued)*
    cervical *(Continued)*
      joint between *(Continued)*
        C2 and C3 S13.131
        C3 and C4 S13.141
        C4 and C5 S13.151
        C5 and C6 S13.161
        C6 and C7 S13.171
        C7 and T1 S13.181
      occipitoatloid joint S13.111
    congenital Q76.49
    lumbar S33.101
      joint between
        L1 and L2 S33.111
        L2 and L3 S33.121
        L3 and L4 S33.131
        L4 and L5 S33.141
    nontraumatic —*see* Displacement, intervertebral disc
    partial —*see* Subluxation, by site
    recurrent NEC —*see* subcategory M43.5
    thoracic S23.101
      joint between
        T1 and T2 S23.111
        T2 and T3 S23.121
        T3 and T4 S23.123
        T4 and T5 S23.131
        T5 and T6 S23.133
        T6 and T7 S23.141
        T7 and T8 S23.143
        T8 and T9 S23.151
        T9 and T10 S23.153
        T10 and T11 S23.161
        T11 and T12 S23.163
        T12 and L1 S23.171
  wrist (carpal bone) S63.006
    carpometacarpal joint —*see* Dislocation, carpometacarpal (joint)
    distal radioulnar joint —*see* Dislocation, radioulnar (joint), distal
    metacarpal bone, proximal —*see* Dislocation, metacarpal (bone), proximal end
    midcarpal —*see* Dislocation, midcarpal (joint)
    radiocarpal joint —*see* Dislocation, radiocarpal (joint)
    recurrent —*see* Dislocation, recurrent, wrist
    specified site NEC S63.09-●
    ulna —*see* Dislocation, ulna, distal end
  xiphoid cartilage S23.29
Disorder (of) —*see also* Disease
  acantholytic L11.9
    specified NEC L11.8
  acute
    psychotic —*see* Psychosis, acute
    stress F43.0
  adjustment (grief) F43.20
    with
      anxiety F43.22
        with depressed mood F43.23
      conduct disturbance F43.24
        with emotional disturbance F43.25
      depressed mood F43.21
        with anxiety F43.23
      other specified symptom F43.29
  adrenal (capsule) (gland) (medullary) E27.9
    specified NEC E27.8
  ▥adrenogenital (*see also* Adrenogenital syndrome) E25.9
    drug-induced E25.8
    iatrogenic E25.8
    idiopathic E25.8
  adult personality (and behavior) F69
    specified NEC F68.8
  affective (mood) —*see* Disorder, mood
  aggressive, unsocialized F91.1

Disorder *(Continued)*
  alcohol-related F10.99
    with
      amnestic disorder, persisting F10.96
      anxiety disorder F10.980
      dementia, persisting F10.97
      intoxication F10.929
        with delirium F10.921
        uncomplicated F10.920
      mood disorder F10.94
      other specified F10.988
      psychotic disorder F10.959
        with
          delusions F10.950
          hallucinations F10.951
      sexual dysfunction F10.981
      sleep disorder F10.982
  alcohol use
    mild F10.10
      with
        alcohol-induced
          anxiety disorder F10.180
          bipolar and related disorder F10.14
          depressive disorder F10.14
          psychotic disorder F10.159
          sexual dysfunction F10.181
          sleep disorder F10.182
        alcohol intoxication F10.129
          delirium F10.121
      in remission (early) (sustained) F10.11
    moderate or severe F10.20
      with
        alcohol-induced
          anxiety disorder F10.280
          bipolar and related disorder F10.24
          depressive disorder F10.24
          major neurocognitive disorder, amnestic-confabulatory type F10.26
          major neurocognitive disorder, nonamnestic-confabulatory type F10.27
          mild neurocognitive disorder F10.288
          psychotic disorder F10.259
          sexual dysfunction F10.281
          sleep disorder F10.282
        alcohol intoxication F10.229
          delirium F10.221
      in remission (early) (sustained) F10.21
  allergic —*see* Allergy
  alveolar NEC J84.09
  amino-acid
    cystathioninuria E72.19
    cystinosis E72.04
    cystinuria E72.01
    glycinuria E72.09
    homocystinuria E72.11
    metabolism —*see* Disturbance, metabolism, amino-acid
    specified NEC E72.89
    neonatal, transitory P74.8
    renal transport NEC E72.09
    transport NEC E72.09
  amnesic, amnestic
    alcohol-induced F10.96
      with dependence F10.26
    due to (secondary to) general medical condition F04
    psychoactive NEC-induced F19.96
      with
        abuse F19.16
        dependence F19.26
    sedative, hypnotic or anxiolytic-● induced F13.96
      with dependence F13.26

▶ New   ⇒ Revised   ~~deleted~~ Deleted   ● Use Additional Character(s)

Disorder (Continued)
  amphetamine-type substance use
    mild F15.10
      in remission (early) (sustained) F15.11
    moderate F15.20
      in remission (early) (sustained) F15.21
    severe F15.20
      in remission (early) (sustained) F15.21
  amphetamine (or other stimulant) use
    mild
      with
        amphetamine (or other stimulant)
          -induced
          anxiety disorder F15.180
          bipolar and related disorder F15.14
          depressive disorder F15.14
          obsessive-compulsive and related
            disorder F15.188
          psychotic disorder F15.159
          sexual dysfunction F15.181
        amphetamine, cocaine, or other
          stimulant intoxication
          with perceptual disturbances
            F15.122
          without perceptual disturbances
            F15.129
        intoxication delirium F15.121
    moderate or severe
      with
        amphetamine (or other stimulant)
          -induced
          anxiety disorder F15.280
          obsessive-compulsive and related
            disorder F15.288
          sexual dysfunction F15.281
          bipolar and related disorder F15.24
          depressive disorder F15.24
          psychotic disorder F15.259
        amphetamine, cocaine, or other
          stimulant intoxication
           with perceptual disturbances
            F15.222
          without perceptual disturbances
            F15.229
        intoxication delirium F15.221
  anaerobic glycolysis with anemia D55.29
  anxiety F41.9
    due to (secondary to)
      alcohol F10.980
        in
          abuse F10.180
          dependence F10.280
      amphetamine F15.980
        in
          abuse F15.180
          dependence F15.280
      anxiolytic F13.980
        in
          abuse F13.180
          dependence F13.280
      caffeine F15.980
        in
          abuse F15.180
          dependence F15.280
      cannabis F12.980
        in
          abuse F12.180
          dependence F12.280
      cocaine F14.980
        in
          abuse F14.180
          dependence F14.180
      general medical condition F06.4
      hallucinogen F16.980
        in
          abuse F16.180
          dependence F16.280
      hypnotic F13.980
        in
          abuse F13.180
          dependence F13.280

Disorder (Continued)
  anxiety (Continued)
    due to (Continued)
      inhalant F18.980
        in
          abuse F18.180
          dependence F18.280
      phencyclidine F16.980
        in
          abuse F16.180
          dependence F16.280
      psychoactive substance NEC
        F19.980
        in
          abuse F19.180
          dependence F19.280
      sedative F13.980
        in
          abuse F13.180
          dependence F13.280
      volatile solvents F18.980
        in
          abuse F18.180
          dependence F18.280
    generalized F41.1
    illness F45.21
    mixed
      with depression (mild) F41.8
      specified NEC F41.3
    organic F06.4
    phobic F40.9
      of childhood F40.8
    specified NEC F41.8
  aortic valve —see Endocarditis, aortic
  aromatic amino-acid metabolism E70.9
    specified NEC E70.89
  arteriole NEC I77.89
  artery NEC I77.89
  articulation —see Disorder, joint
  attachment (childhood)
    disinhibited F94.2
    reactive F94.1
  attention-deficit hyperactivity (adolescent)
    (adult) (child) F98.8
    combined
      presentation F90.2
      type F90.2
    hyperactive
      impulsive presentation F90.1
      type F90.1
    inattentive
      presentation F90.0
      type F90.0
    specified type NEC F90.8
  attention-deficit without hyperactivity
    (adolescent) (adult) (child) F90.0
  auditory processing (central) H93.25
  autism spectrum F84.0
  autistic F84.0
  autoimmune D89.89
  autonomic nervous system G90.9
    specified NEC G90.8
  avoidant
    child or adolescent F40.10
    restrictive food intake F50.82
  balance
    acid-base E87.8
      mixed E87.4
    electrolyte E87.8
    fluid NEC E87.8
  behavioral (disruptive) —see Disorder,
    conduct
▸ bereavement, persistent complex F43.81
  beta-amino-acid metabolism E72.89
  bile acid and cholesterol metabolism E78.70
    Barth syndrome E78.71
    other specified E78.79
    Smith-Lemli-Opitz syndrome
      E78.72
  bilirubin excretion E80.6
  binge eating F50.81

Disorder (Continued)
  binocular
    movement H51.9
      convergence
        excess H51.12
        insufficiency H51.11
      internuclear ophthalmoplegia —see
        Ophthalmoplegia, internuclear
      palsy of conjugate gaze H51.0
      specified type NEC H51.8
    vision NEC —see Disorder, vision, binocular
▸ bipolar (I) (seasonal) (type 1) F31.9
    and related due to a known physiological
      condition
      with
        manic features F06.33
        manic- or hypomanic-like episodes
          F06.33
        mixed features F06.34
    current (or most recent) episode
      depressed F31.9
        with psychotic features F31.5
        without psychotic features
          F31.30
          mild F31.31
          moderate F31.32
          severe (without psychotic features)
            F31.4
            with psychotic features
              F31.5
      hypomanic F31.0
      manic F31.9
        with psychotic features F31.2
        without psychotic features
          F31.10
          mild F31.11
          moderate F31.12
          severe (without psychotic features)
            F31.13
            with psychotic features
              F31.2
      mixed F31.60
        mild F31.61
        moderate F31.62
        severe (without psychotic features)
          F31.63
          with psychotic features F31.64
        severe depression (without psychotic
          features) F31.4
          with psychotic features F31.5
    II (type 2) F31.81
    in remission (currently) F31.70
      in full remission
        most recent episode
          depressed F31.76
          hypomanic F31.72
          manic F31.74
          mixed F31.78
      in partial remission
        most recent episode
          depressed F31.75
          hypomanic F31.71
          manic F31.73
          mixed F31.77
    organic F06.30
    single manic episode F30.9
      mild F30.11
      moderate F30.12
      hhsevere (without psychotic symptoms)
        F30.13
      with psychotic symptoms F30.2
    specified NEC F31.89
  bladder N32.9
    functional NEC N31.9
    in schistosomiasis B65.0 [N33]
    specified NEC N32.89
  bleeding D68.9
  blood D75.9
    in congenital early syphilis A50.09
      [D77]
  body dysmorphic F45.22

Disorder (*Continued*)
  bone M89.9
    continuity M84.9
      specified type NEC M84.80
        ankle M84.87-●
        fibula M84.86-●
        foot M84.87-●
        hand M84.84-●
        humerus M84.82-●
        neck M84.88
        pelvis M84.859
        radius M84.83-●
        rib M84.88
        shoulder M84.81-●
        skull M84.88
        thigh M84.85-●
        tibia M84.86-●
        ulna M84.83-●
        vertebra M84.88
    density and structure M85.9
      cyst —*see also* Cyst, bone, specified type NEC
        aneurysmal —*see* Cyst, bone, aneurysmal
        solitary —*see* Cyst, bone, solitary
      diffuse idiopathic skeletal hyperostosis —*see* Hyperostosis, ankylosing
      fibrous dysplasia (monostotic) —*see* Dysplasia, fibrous, bone
      fluorosis —*see* Fluorosis, skeletal
      hyperostosis of skull M85.2
      osteitis condensans —*see* Osteitis, condensans
      specified type NEC M85.8-●
        ankle M85.87-●
        foot M85.87-●
        forearm M85.83-●
        hand M85.84-●
        lower leg M85.86-●
        multiple sites M85.89
        neck M85.88
        rib M85.88
        shoulder M85.81-●
        skull M85.88
        thigh M85.85-●
        upper arm M85.82-●
        vertebra M85.88
    development and growth NEC M89.20
      carpus M89.24-●
      clavicle M89.21-●
      femur M89.25-●
      fibula M89.26-●
      finger M89.24-●
      humerus M89.22-●
      ilium M89.259
      ischium M89.259
      metacarpus M89.24-●
      metatarsus M89.27-●
      multiple sites M89.29
      neck M89.28
      radius M89.23-●
      rib M89.28
      scapula M89.21-●
      skull M89.28
      tarsus M89.27-●
      tibia M89.26-●
      toe M89.27-●
      ulna M89.23-●
      vertebra M89.28
    specified type NEC M89.8X-●
  brachial plexus G54.0
  branched-chain amino-acid metabolism E71.2
    specified NEC E71.19
  breast N64.9
    agalactia —*see* Agalactia
    associated with
      lactation O92.70
        specified NEC O92.79
      pregnancy O92.20
        specified NEC O92.29

Disorder (*Continued*)
  breast (*Continued*)
    associated with (*Continued*)
      puerperium O92.20
        specified NEC O92.29
    cracked nipple —*see* Cracked nipple
    galactorrhea —*see* Galactorrhea
    hypogalactia O92.4
    lactation disorder NEC O92.79
    mastitis —*see* Mastitis
    nipple infection —*see* Infection, nipple
    retracted nipple —*see* Retraction, nipple
    specified type NEC N64.89
  Briquet's F45.0
  bullous, in diseases classified elsewhere L14
  caffeine use
    mild
      with
        caffeine-induced
          anxiety disorder F15.180
          sleep disorder F15.182
    moderate or severe
      with
        caffeine-induced
          anxiety disorder F15.280
          sleep disorder F15.282
  cannabis use
    mild F12.10
      with
        cannabis-induced
          anxiety disorder F12.180
          psychotic disorder F12.159
          sleep disorder F12.188
        cannabis intoxication delirium F12.121
          with perceptual disturbances F12.122
          without perceptual disturbances F12.129
    in remission (early) (sustained) F12.11
    moderate or severe F12.20
      with
        cannabis-induced
          anxiety disorder F12.280
          psychotic disorder F12.259
          sleep disorder F12.288
        cannabis intoxication
          with perceptual disturbances F12.222
          without perceptual disturbances F12.229
        delirium F12.221
    in remission (early) (sustained) F12.21
  carbohydrate
    absorption, intestinal NEC E74.39
    metabolism (congenital) E74.9
      specified NEC E74.89
  cardiac, functional I51.89
  carnitine metabolism E71.40
  cartilage M94.9
    articular NEC —*see* Derangement, joint, articular cartilage
    chondrocalcinosis —*see* Chondrocalcinosis
    specified type NEC M94.8X-●
      articular —*see* Derangement, joint, articular cartilage
      multiple sites M94.8X0
  catatonia (due to known physiological condition) (with another mental disorder) F06.1
  catatonic
    due to (secondary to) known physiological condition F06.1
    organic F06.1
  central auditory processing H93.25
  cervical
    region NEC M53.82
    root (nerve) NEC G54.2
  character NOS F60.9
  childhood disintegrative NEC F84.3

Disorder (*Continued*)
  cholesterol and bile acid metabolism E78.70
    Barth syndrome E78.71
    other specified E78.79
    Smith-Lemli-Opitz syndrome E78.72
  choroid H31.9
    atrophy —*see* Atrophy, choroid
    degeneration —*see* Degeneration, choroid
    detachment —*see* Detachment, choroid
    dystrophy —*see* Dystrophy, choroid
    hemorrhage —*see* Hemorrhage, choroid
    rupture —*see* Rupture, choroid
    scar —*see* Scar, chorioretinal
    solar retinopathy —*see* Retinopathy, solar
    specified type NEC H31.8
  ciliary body —*see* Disorder, iris
    degeneration —*see* Degeneration, ciliary body
  coagulation (factor) (*see also* Defect, coagulation) D68.9
    newborn, transient P61.6
  cocaine use
    mild F14.10
      with
        amphetamine, cocaine, or other stimulant intoxication
          with perceptual disturbances F14.122
          without perceptual disturbances F14.129
        cocaine-induced
          anxiety disorder F14.180
          bipolar and related disorder F14.14
          depressive disorder F14.14
          obsessive-compulsive and related disorder F14.188
          psychotic disorder F14.159
          sexual dysfunction F14.181
          sleep disorder F14.182
        cocaine intoxication delirium F14.121
    in remission (early) (sustained) F14.11
    moderate or severe F14.20
      with
        amphetamine, cocaine, or other stimulant intoxication
          with perceptual disturbances F14.222
          without perceptual disturbances F14.229
        cocaine-induced
          anxiety disorder F14.280
          bipolar and related disorder F14.24
          depressive disorder F14.24
          obsessive-compulsive and related disorder F14.288
          psychotic disorder F14.259
          sexual dysfunction F14.281
          sleep disorder F14.282
        cocaine intoxication delirium F14.221
    in remission (early) (sustained) F14.21
  coccyx NEC M53.3
  cognitive F09
    due to (secondary to) general medical condition F09
    persisting R41.89
      due to
        alcohol F10.97
          with dependence F10.27
        anxiolytics F13.97
          with dependence F13.27
        hypnotics F13.97
          with dependence F13.27
        sedatives F13.97
          with dependence F13.27
        specified substance NEC F19.97
          with
            abuse F19.17
            dependence F19.27

▶ New ⇒ Revised ~~deleted~~ Deleted ● Use Additional Character(s)

Disorder *(Continued)*
　communication F80.9
　　social pragmatic F80.82
　conduct (childhood) F91.9
　　adjustment reaction —*see* Disorder,
　　　adjustment
　　adolescent onset type F91.2
　　childhood onset type F91.1
　　compulsive F63.9
　　confined to family context F91.0
　　depressive F91.8
　　group type F91.2
　　hyperkinetic —*see* Disorder, attention-
　　　deficit hyperactivity
　　oppositional defiance F91.3
　　socialized F91.2
　　solitary aggressive type F91.1
　　specified NEC F91.8
　　unsocialized (aggressive) F91.1
　conduction, heart I45.9
　congenital glycosylation (CDG) E74.89
　conjunctiva H11.9
　　infection —*see* Conjunctivitis
　connective tissue, localized L94.9
　　specified NEC L94.8
　conversion (functional neurological symptom
　　disorder)
　　with
　　　abnormal movement F44.4
　　　anesthesia or sensory loss F44.6
　　　attacks or seizures F44.5
　　　mixed symptoms F44.7
　　　special sensory symptoms F44.6
　　　speech symptoms F44.4
　　　swallowing symptoms F44.4
　　　weakness or paralysis F44.4
　convulsive (secondary) —*see* Convulsions
　cornea H18.9
　　deformity —*see* Deformity, cornea
　　degeneration —*see* Degeneration, cornea
　　deposits —*see* Deposit, cornea
　　due to contact lens H18.82-●
　　　specified as edema —*see* Edema, cornea
　　edema —*see* Edema, cornea
　　keratitis —*see* Keratitis
　　keratoconjunctivitis —*see*
　　　Keratoconjunctivitis
　　membrane change —*see* Change, corneal
　　　membrane
　　neovascularization —*see*
　　　Neovascularization, cornea
　　scar —*see* Opacity, cornea
　　specified type NEC H18.89-●
　　ulcer —*see* Ulcer, cornea
　corpus cavernosum N48.9
　cranial nerve —*see* Disorder, nerve, cranial
　Cyclin-Dependent Kinase-Like 5 Deficiency
　　(CDKL5) G40.42
　cyclothymic F34.0
　defiant oppositional F91.3
　delusional (persistent) (systematized) F22
　　induced F24
　depersonalization F48.1
　depressive F32.A
　　due to known physiological condition
　　　with
　　　　depressive features F06.31
　　　　major depressive-like episode F06.32
　　　　mixed features F06.34
　　major F32.9
　　　with psychotic symptoms F32.3
　　　in remission (full) F32.5
　　　　partial F32.4
　　　recurrent F33.9
　　　　with psychotic features F33.3
　　　single episode F32.9
　　　　mild F32.0
　　　　moderate F32.1
　　　　severe (without psychotic symptoms)
　　　　　F32.2
　　　　　with psychotic symptoms F32.3

Disorder *(Continued)*
　depressive *(Continued)*
　　organic F06.31
　　persistent F34.1
　　recurrent F33.9
　　　current episode
　　　　mild F33.0
　　　　moderate F33.1
　　　　severe (without psychotic symptoms)
　　　　　F33.2
　　　　　with psychotic symptoms F33.3
　　　in remission F33.40
　　　　full F33.42
　　　　partial F33.41
　　　specified NEC F33.8
　　single episode —*see* Episode, depressive
　　specified NEC F32.89
　developmental F89
　　arithmetical skills F81.2
　　coordination (motor) F82
　　expressive writing F81.81
　　language F80.9
　　　expressive F80.1
　　　mixed receptive and expressive
　　　　F80.2
　　　receptive type F80.2
　　　specified NEC F80.89
　　learning F81.9
　　　arithmetical F81.2
　　　reading F81.0
　　mixed F88
　　motor coordination or function F82
　　pervasive F84.9
　　　specified NEC F84.8
　　phonological F80.0
　　reading F81.0
　　scholastic skills —*see also* Disorder,
　　　learning
　　　mixed F81.89
　　specified NEC F88
　　speech F80.9
　　　articulation F80.0
　　　specified NEC F80.89
　　written expression F81.81
　diaphragm J98.6
　digestive (system) K92.9
　　newborn P78.9
　　　specified NEC P78.89
　　postprocedural —*see* Complication,
　　　gastrointestinal
　　psychogenic F45.8
　disc (intervertebral) M51.9
　　with
　　　myelopathy
　　　　cervical region M50.00
　　　　cervicothoracic region M50.03
　　　　high cervical region M50.01
　　　　lumbar region M51.06
　　　　mid-cervical region M50.020
　　　　sacrococcygeal region M53.3
　　　　thoracic region M51.04
　　　　thoracolumbar region M51.05
　　　radiculopathy
　　　　cervical region M50.10
　　　　cervicothoracic region M50.13
　　　　high cervical region M50.11
　　　　lumbar region M51.16
　　　　lumbosacral region M51.17
　　　　mid-cervical region M50.120
　　　　sacrococcygeal region M53.3
　　　　thoracic region M51.14
　　　　thoracolumbar region M51.15
　　cervical M50.90
　　　with
　　　　myelopathy M50.00
　　　　　C2-C3 M50.01
　　　　　C3-C4 M50.01
　　　　　C4-C5 M50.021
　　　　　C5-C6 M50.022
　　　　　C6-C7 M50.023
　　　　　C7-T1 M50.03

Disorder *(Continued)*
　disc *(Continued)*
　　cervical *(Continued)*
　　　with *(Continued)*
　　　　myelopathy *(Continued)*
　　　　　cervicothoracic region M50.03
　　　　　high cervical region M50.01
　　　　　mid-cervical region M50.020
　　　　　neuritis, radiculitis or radiculopathy
　　　　　　M50.10
　　　　　　C2-C3 M50.11
　　　　　　C3-C4 M50.11
　　　　　　C4-C5 M50.121
　　　　　　C5-C6 M50.122
　　　　　　C6-C7 M50.123
　　　　　　C7-T1 M50.13
　　　　　　cervicothoracic region M50.13
　　　　　　high cervical region M50.11
　　　　　　mid-cervical region M50.120
　　　　C2-C3 M50.91
　　　　C3-C4 M50.91
　　　　C4-C5 M50.921
　　　　C5-C6 M50.922
　　　　C6-C7 M50.923
　　　　C7-T1 M50.93
　　　　cervicothoracic region M50.93
　　　　degeneration M50.30
　　　　　C2-C3 M50.31
　　　　　C3-C4 M50.31
　　　　　C4-C5 M50.321
　　　　　C5-C6 M50.322
　　　　　C6-C7 M50.323
　　　　　C7-T1 M50.33
　　　　　cervicothoracic region M50.33
　　　　　high cervical region M50.31
　　　　　mid-cervical region M50.320
　　　　displacement M50.20
　　　　　C2-C3 M50.21
　　　　　C3-C4 M50.21
　　　　　C4-C5 M50.221
　　　　　C5-C6 M50.222
　　　　　C6-C7 M50.223
　　　　　C7-T1 M50.23
　　　　　cervicothoracic region M50.23
　　　　　high cervical region M50.21
　　　　　mid-cervical region M50.220
　　　　high cervical region M50.91
　　　　mid-cervical region M50.920
　　　　specified type NEC M50.80
　　　　　C2-C3 M50.81
　　　　　C3-C4 M50.81
　　　　　C4-C5 M50.821
　　　　　C5-C6 M50.822
　　　　　C6-C7 M50.823
　　　　　C7-T1 M50.83
　　　　　cervicothoracic region M50.83
　　　　　high cervical region M50.81
　　　　　mid-cervical region M50.820
　　　specified NEC
　　　　lumbar region M51.86
　　　　lumbosacral region M51.87
　　　　sacrococcygeal region M53.3
　　　　thoracic region M51.84
　　　　thoracolumbar region M51.85
　　disinhibited attachment (childhood) F94.2
　　disintegrative, childhood NEC F84.3
　　disruptive F91.9
　　　mood dysregulation F34.81
　　　specified NEC F91.8
　　disruptive behavior —*see* Disorder, conduct
　　dissocial personality F60.2
　　dissociative F44.9
　　　affecting
　　　　motor function F44.4
　　　　　and sensation F44.7
　　　　sensation F44.6
　　　　　and motor function F44.7
　　　brief reactive F43.0
　　　due to (secondary to) general medical
　　　　condition F06.8
　　　mixed F44.7

Disorder *(Continued)*
  dissociative *(Continued)*
    organic F06.8
    other specified NEC F44.89
  double heterozygous sickling —*see* Disease, sickle-cell
  dream anxiety F51.5
  drug induced hemorrhagic D68.32
  drug related F19.99
    abuse —*see* Abuse, drug
    dependence —*see* Dependence, drug
  dysmorphic body F45.22
  dysthymic F34.1
  ear H93.9-●
    bleeding —*see* Otorrhagia
    deafness —*see* Deafness
    degenerative H93.09-●
    discharge —*see* Otorrhea
    external H61.9-●
      auditory canal stenosis —*see* Stenosis, external ear canal
      exostosis —*see* Exostosis, external ear canal
      impacted cerumen —*see* Impaction, cerumen
      otitis —*see* Otitis, externa
      perichondritis —*see* Perichondritis, ear
      pinna —*see* Disorder, pinna
      specified type NEC H61.89-●
        in diseases classified elsewhere H62.8X-●
    inner H83.9-●
      vestibular dysfunction —*see* Disorder, vestibular function
    middle H74.9-●
      adhesive H74.1-●
      ossicle —*see* Abnormal, ear ossicles
      polyp —*see* Polyp, ear (middle)
      specified NEC, in diseases classified elsewhere H75.8-●
    postprocedural —*see* Complications, ear, procedure
    specified NEC, in diseases classified elsewhere H94.8-●
  eating (adult) (psychogenic) F50.9
    anorexia —*see* Anorexia
    binge F50.81
    bulimia F50.2
    child F98.29
      pica F98.3
      rumination disorder F98.21
    pica F50.89
      childhood F98.3
  electrolyte (balance) NEC E87.8
    with
      abortion —*see* Abortion by type complicated by specified condition NEC
      ectopic pregnancy O08.5
      molar pregnancy O08.5
    acidosis (metabolic) (respiratory) E87.2
    alkalosis (lactic) (metabolic) E87.20
      ▶acute E87.21
      ▶chronic E87.22
      ▶respiratory E87.29
      ▶specified NEC E87.29
  elimination, transepidermal L87.9
    specified NEC L87.8
  emotional (persistent) F34.9
    of childhood F93.9
      specified NEC F93.8
  endocrine E34.9
    postprocedural E89.89
    specified NEC E89.89
  erectile (male) (organic) —*see also* Dysfunction, sexual, male, erectile N52.9
    nonorganic F52.21
  erythematous —*see* Erythema
  esophagus K22.9
    functional K22.4
    psychogenic F45.8

Disorder *(Continued)*
  eustachian tube H69.9-●
    infection —*see* Salpingitis, eustachian
    obstruction —*see* Obstruction, eustachian tube
    patulous —*see* Patulous, eustachian tube
    specified NEC H69.8-●
  exhibitionistic F65.2
  extrapyramidal G25.9
    in diseases classified elsewhere —*see* category G26
    specified type NEC G25.89
  eye H57.9
    postprocedural —*see* Complication, postprocedural, eye
  eyelid H02.9
    cyst —*see* Cyst, eyelid
    degenerative H02.70
      chloasma —*see* Chloasma, eyelid
      madarosis —*see* Madarosis
      specified type NEC H02.79
      vitiligo —*see* Vitiligo, eyelid
      xanthelasma —*see* Xanthelasma
    dermatochalasis —*see* Dermato-chalasis
    edema —*see* Edema, eyelid
    elephantiasis —*see* Elephantiasis, eyelid
    foreign body, retained —*see* Foreign body, retained, eyelid
    function H02.59
      abnormal innervation syndrome —*see* Syndrome, abnormal innervation
      blepharochalasis —*see* Blepharochalasis
      blepharoclonus —*see* Blepharoclonus
      blepharophimosis —*see* Blepharophimosis
      blepharoptosis —*see* Blepharoptosis
      lagophthalmos —*see* Lagophthalmos
      lid retraction —*see* Retraction, lid
    hypertrichosis —*see* Hypertrichosis, eyelid
    specified type NEC H02.89
    vascular H02.879
      left H02.876
        lower H02.875
        upper H02.874
      right H02.873
        lower H02.872
        upper H02.871
  factitious
    by proxy F68.A
    imposed on another F68.A
    imposed on self F68.10
      with predominantly
        psychological symptoms F68.11
          with physical symptoms F68.13
        physical symptoms F68.12
          with psychological symptoms F68.13
  factor, coagulation —*see* Defect, coagulation
  fatty acid
    metabolism E71.30
      specified NEC E71.39
    oxidation
      LCAD E71.310
      MCAD E71.311
      SCAD E71.312
      specified deficiency NEC E71.318
  feeding (infant or child) —*see also* Disorder, eating R63.30
    or eating disorder F50.9
    pediatric
      acute R63.31
      chronic R63.32
    specified NEC F50.9
  feigned (with obvious motivation) Z76.5
    without obvious motivation —*see* Disorder, factitious
  female
    hypoactive sexual desire F52.0
    orgasmic F52.31
    sexual interest/arousal F52.22
  fetishistic F65.0
  fibroblastic M72.9
    specified NEC M72.8

Disorder *(Continued)*
  fluency
    adult onset F98.5
    childhood onset F80.81
    following
      cerebral infarction I69.323
      cerebrovascular disease I69.923
        specified disease NEC I69.823
      intracerebral hemorrhage I69.123
      nontraumatic intracranial hemorrhage NEC I69.223
      subarachnoid hemorrhage I69.023
    in conditions classified elsewhere R47.82
  fluid balance E87.8
  follicular (skin) L73.9
    specified NEC L73.8
  frotteuristic F65.81
  fructose metabolism E74.10
    essential fructosuria E74.11
    fructokinase deficiency E74.11
    fructose-1, 6-diphosphatase deficiency E74.19
    hereditary fructose intolerance E74.12
    other specified E74.19
  functional polymorphonuclear neutrophils D71
  gallbladder, biliary tract and pancreas in diseases classified elsewhere K87
  gambling F63.0
  gamma aminobutyric acid (GABA) metabolism E72.81
  gamma-glutamyl cycle E72.89
  gastric (functional) K31.9
    motility K30
    psychogenic F45.8
    secretion K30
  gastrointestinal (functional) NOS K92.9
    newborn P78.9
    psychogenic F45.8
  gender-identity or -role F64.9
    childhood F64.2
    effect on relationship F66
    of adolescence or adulthood F64.0
      nontranssexual F64.8
    specified NEC F64.8
    uncertainty F66
  genito-pelvic pain penetration F52.6
  genitourinary system
    female N94.9
    male N50.9
    psychogenic F45.8
  globe H44.9
    degenerated condition H44.50
      absolute glaucoma H44.51-●
      atrophy H44.52-●
      leucocoria H44.53-●
    degenerative H44.30
      chalcosis H44.31-●
      myopia —*see also* Myopia, degenerative H44.2-●
      siderosis H44.32-●
      specified type NEC H44.39-●
    endophthalmitis —*see* Endophthalmitis
    foreign body, retained —*see* Foreign body, intraocular, old, retained
    hemophthalmos —*see* Hemophthalmos
    hypotony H44.40
      due to
        ocular fistula H44.42-●
        specified disorder NEC H44.43-●
      flat anterior chamber H44.41-●
      primary H44.44-●
    luxation —*see* Luxation, globe
    specified type NEC H44.89
  glomerular (in) N05.9
    amyloidosis E85.4 *[N08]*
    cryoglobulinemia D89.1 *[N08]*
    disseminated intravascular coagulation D65 *[N08]*
    Fabry's disease E75.21 *[N08]*

Disorder *(Continued)*
  glomerular *(Continued)*
    familial lecithin cholesterol acyltransferase deficiency E78.6 *[N08]*
    Goodpasture's syndrome M31.0
    hemolytic-uremic syndrome —*see* Syndrome, hemolytic-uremic
    Henoch (-Schönlein) purpura D69.0 *[N08]*
    malariae malaria B52.0
    microscopic polyangiitis M31.7 *[N08]*
    multiple myeloma C90.0-• *[N08]*
    mumps B26.83
    schistosomiasis B65.9 *[N08]*
    sepsis NEC A41.-• *[N08]*
      streptococcal A40.-• *[N08]*
    sickle-cell disorders D57.-• *[N08]*
    strongyloidiasis B78.9 *[N08]*
    subacute bacterial endocarditis I33.0 *[N08]*
    syphilis A52.75
    systemic lupus erythematosus M32.14
    thrombotic thrombocytopenic purpura M31.19 *[N08]*
    Waldenström macroglobulinemia C88.0 *[N08]*
    Wegener's granulomatosis M31.31
  gluconeogenesis E74.4
  glucosaminoglycan metabolism —*see* Disorder, metabolism, glucosaminoglycan
  glucose transport E74.819
    specified NEC E74.818
  glycine metabolism E72.50
    d-glycericacidemia E72.59
    hyperhydroxyprolinemia E72.59
    hyperoxaluria R82.992
      primary E72.53
    hyperprolinemia E72.59
    non-ketotic hyperglycinemia E72.51
    oxalosis E72.53
    oxaluria E72.53
    sarcosinemia E72.59
    trimethylaminuria E72.52
  glycoprotein metabolism E77.9
    specified NEC E77.8
  grief
    complicated F43.81
    prolonged F43.81
  habit (and impulse) F63.9
    involving sexual behavior NEC F65.9
    specified NEC F63.89
  hallucinogen use
    mild F16.10
      with
        hallucinogen-induced
          anxiety disorder F16.180
          bipolar and related disorder F16.14
          depressive disorder F16.14
          psychotic disorder F16.159
        hallucinogen intoxication delirium F16.121
        other hallucinogen intoxication F16.129
      in remission (early) (sustained) F16.11
    moderate or severe F16.20
      with
        hallucinogen-induced
          anxiety disorder F16.280
          bipolar and related disorder F16.24
          depressive disorder F16.24
          psychotic disorder F16.259
        hallucinogen intoxication delirium F16.221
        other hallucinogen intoxication F16.229
      in remission (early) (sustained) F16.21
  heart action I49.9
  hematological D75.9
    newborn (transient) P61.9
      specified NEC P61.8
  hematopoietic organs D75.9

  hemorrhagic NEC D69.9
    drug-induced D68.32
    due to
      extrinsic circulating anticoagulants D68.32
      increase in
        anti-IIa D68.32
        anti-Xa D68.32
      intrinsic
        circulating anticoagulants D68.318
        increase in
          antithrombin D68.318
          anti-VIIIa D68.318
          anti-IXa D68.318
          anti-XIa D68.318
    following childbirth O72.3
  hemostasis —*see* Defect, coagulation
  histidine metabolism E70.40
    histidinemia E70.41
    other specified E70.49
  hoarding F42.3
  hyperkinetic —*see* Disorder, attention-deficit hyperactivity
  hyperleucine-isoleucinemia E71.19
  hypervalinemia E71.19
  hypoactive sexual desire F52.0
  hypochondriacal F45.20
    body dysmorphic F45.22
    neurosis F45.21
    other specified F45.29
  identity
    dissociative F44.81
    illness anxiety F45.21
    of childhood F93.8
  immune mechanism (immunity) D89.9
    specified type NEC D89.89
  impaired renal tubular function N25.9
    specified NEC N25.89
  impulse (control) F63.9
  inflammatory
    pelvic, in diseases classified elsewhere —*see* category N74
    penis N48.29
      abscess N48.21
      cellulitis N48.22
  inhalant use
    mild F18.10
      with
        inhalant-induced
          anxiety disorder F18.180
          depressive disorder F18.14
          major neurocognitive disorder F18.17
          mild neurocognitive disorder F18.188
          psychotic disorder F18.159
        inhalant intoxication F18.129
        inhalant intoxication delirium F18.121
      in remission (early) (sustained) F18.11
    moderate or severe F18.20
      with
        inhalant-induced
          anxiety disorder F18.280
          depressive disorder F18.24
          major neurocognitive disorder F18.27
          mild neurocognitive disorder F18.288
          psychotic disorder F18.259
        inhalant intoxication F18.229
        inhalant intoxication delirium F18.221
      in remission (early) (sustained) F18.21
  integument, newborn P83.9
    specified NEC P83.88
  intermittent explosive F63.81
  internal secretion pancreas —*see* Increased, secretion, pancreas, endocrine
  intestine, intestinal
    carbohydrate absorption NEC E74.39
      postoperative K91.2

  intestine, intestinal *(Continued)*
    functional NEC K59.9
      postoperative K91.89
    psychogenic F45.8
    vascular K55.9
      chronic K55.1
      specified NEC K55.8
  intraoperative (intraprocedural) —*see* Complications, intraoperative
  involuntary emotional expression (IEED) F48.2
  iris H21.9
    adhesions —*see* Adhesions, iris
    atrophy —*see* Atrophy, iris
    chamber angle recession —*see* Recession, chamber angle
    cyst —*see* Cyst, iris
    degeneration —*see* Degeneration, iris
    in diseases classified elsewhere H22
    iridodialysis —*see* Iridodialysis
    iridoschisis —*see* Iridoschisis
    miotic pupillary cyst —*see* Cyst, pupillary
    pupillary
      abnormality —*see* Abnormality, pupillary
      membrane —*see* Membrane, pupillary
    specified type NEC H21.89
    vascular NEC H21.1X-•
  iron metabolism E83.10
    specified NEC E83.19
  isovaleric acidemia E71.110
  jaw, developmental M27.0
    temporomandibular —*see also* Anomaly, dentofacial, temporomandibular joint M26.60-•
  joint M25.9
    derangement —*see* Derangement, joint
    effusion —*see* Effusion, joint
    fistula —*see* Fistula, joint
    hemarthrosis —*see* Hemarthrosis
    instability —*see* Instability, joint
    osteophyte —*see* Osteophyte
    pain —*see* Pain, joint
    psychogenic F45.8
    specified type NEC M25.80
      ankle M25.87-•
      elbow M25.82-•
      foot joint M25.87-•
      hand joint M25.84-•
      hip M25.85-•
      knee M25.86-•
      shoulder M25.81-•
      wrist M25.83-•
    stiffness —*see* Stiffness, joint
  ketone metabolism E71.32
  kidney N28.9
    functional (tubular) N25.9
    in
      schistosomiasis B65.9 *[N29]*
    tubular function N25.9
      specified NEC N25.89
  lacrimal system H04.9
    changes H04.69
      fistula —*see* Fistula, lacrimal
    gland H04.19
      atrophy —*see* Atrophy, lacrimal gland
      cyst —*see* Cyst, lacrimal, gland
      dacryops —*see* Dacryops
      dislocation —*see* Dislocation, lacrimal gland
      dry eye syndrome —*see* Syndrome, dry eye
      infection —*see* Dacryoadenitis
      granuloma —*see* Granuloma, lacrimal
      inflammation —*see* Inflammation, lacrimal
      obstruction —*see* Obstruction, lacrimal
      specified NEC H04.89
  lactation NEC O92.79
  language (developmental) F80.9
    expressive F80.1
    mixed receptive and expressive F80.2
    receptive F80.2

Disorder *(Continued)*
　late luteal phase dysphoric N94.89
　learning (specific) F81.9
　　acalculia R48.8
　　alexia R48.0
　　mathematics F81.2
　　reading F81.0
　　specified
　　　with impairment in
　　　　mathematics F81.2
　　　　reading F81.0
　　　　written expression F81.81
　　specified NEC F81.89
　　spelling F81.81
　　written expression F81.81
　lens H27.9
　　aphakia —*see* Aphakia
　　cataract —*see* Cataract
　　dislocation —*see* Dislocation, lens
　　specified type NEC H27.8
　ligament M24.20
　　ankle M24.27-●
　　attachment, spine —*see* Enthesopathy,
　　　spinal
　　elbow M24.22-●
　　foot joint M24.27-●
　　hand joint M24.24-●
　　hip M24.25-●
　　knee —*see* Derangement, knee, specified
　　　NEC
　　shoulder M24.21-●
　　specified site NEC M24.29
　　vertebra M24.28
　　wrist M24.23-●
　ligamentous attachments —*see also*
　　　Enthesopathy
　　spine —*see* Enthesopathy, spinal
　lipid
　　metabolism, congenital E78.9
　　storage E75.6
　　　specified NEC E75.5
　lipoprotein
　　deficiency (familial) E78.6
　　metabolism E78.9
　　　specified NEC E78.89
　liver K76.9
　　malarial B54 *[K77]*
　low back —*see also* Dorsopathy, specified NEC
　lumbosacral
　　plexus G54.1
　　root (nerve) NEC G54.4
　lung, interstitial, drug-induced J70.4
　　acute J70.2
　　chronic J70.3
　　dabbing (related) U07.0
　　e-cigarette (related) U07.0
　　electronic cigarette (related) U07.0
　　vaping (associated) (device) (product)
　　　(related) (use) U07.0
　lymphoproliferative, post-transplant (PTLD)
　　　D47.Z1
　lysine and hydroxylysine metabolism E72.3
　major neurocognitive *(see also* Dementia, in
　　(due to)) F03-●
　male
　　erectile (organic) —*see also* Dysfunction,
　　　sexual, male, erectile N52.9
　　　nonorganic F52.21
　　hypoactive sexual desire F52.0
　　orgasmic F52.32
　manic F30.9
　　organic F06.33
　mast cell activation —*see* Activation, mast cell
　mastoid —*see also* Disorder, ear, middle
　　postprocedural —*see* Complications, ear,
　　　procedure
　meninges, specified type NEC G96.198
　meniscus —*see* Derangement, knee,
　　　meniscus
　menopausal N95.9
　　specified NEC N95.8

Disorder *(Continued)*
　menstrual N92.6
　　psychogenic F45.8
　　specified NEC N92.5
　mental (or behavioral) (nonpsychotic) F99
　　due to (secondary to)
　　　amphetamine
　　　　due to drug abuse —*see* Abuse, drug,
　　　　　stimulant
　　　　due to drug dependence —*see*
　　　　　Dependence, drug, stimulant
　　　brain disease, damage and dysfunction
　　　　F09
　　　caffeine use
　　　　due to drug abuse —*see* Abuse, drug,
　　　　　stimulant
　　　　due to drug dependence —*see*
　　　　　Dependence, drug, stimulant
　　　cannabis use
　　　　due to drug abuse —*see* Abuse, drug,
　　　　　cannabis
　　　　due to drug dependence —*see*
　　　　　Dependence, drug, cannabis
　　　general medical condition F09
　　　sedative or hypnotic use
　　　　due to drug abuse —*see* Abuse, drug,
　　　　　sedative
　　　　due to drug dependence —*see*
　　　　　Dependence, drug, sedative
　　　tobacco (nicotine) use —*see* Dependence,
　　　　drug, nicotine
　　following organic brain damage F07.9
　　　frontal lobe syndrome F07.0
　　　personality change F07.0
　　　postconcussional syndrome F07.81
　　　specified NEC F07.89
　　infancy, childhood or adolescence F98.9
　　neurotic —*see* Neurosis
　　organic or symptomatic F09
　　presenile, psychotic F03
　　problem NEC
　　psychoneurotic —*see* Neurosis
　　psychotic —*see* Psychosis
　　puerperal F53.0
　　senile, psychotic NEC F03
　metabolic, amino acid, transitory, newborn
　　　P74.8
　metabolism NOS E88.9
　　amino-acid E72.9
　　　aromatic E70.9
　　　　albinism —*see* Albinism
　　　　histidine E70.40
　　　　　histidinemia E70.41
　　　　　other specified E70.49
　　　　hyperphenylalaninemia E70.1
　　　　　classical phenylketonuria E70.0
　　　　other specified E70.89
　　　　tryptophan E70.5
　　　　tyrosine E70.20
　　　　　hypertyrosinemia E70.21
　　　　　other specified E70.29
　　　branched chain E71.2
　　　　3-methylglutaconic aciduria E71.111
　　　　hyperleucine-isoleucinemia E71.19
　　　　hypervalinemia E71.19
　　　　isovaleric acidemia E71.110
　　　　maple syrup urine disease E71.0
　　　　methylmalonic acidemia E71.120
　　　　organic aciduria NEC E71.118
　　　　other specified E71.19
　　　　proprionate NEC E71.128
　　　　proprionic acidemia E71.121
　　　glycine E72.50
　　　　d-glycericacidemia E72.59
　　　　hyperhydroxyprolinemia E72.59
　　　　hyperoxaluria R82.992
　　　　　primary E72.53
　　　　hyperprolinemia E72.59
　　　　non-ketotic hyperglycinemia
　　　　　E72.51
　　　　other specified E72.59

Disorder *(Continued)*
　metabolism *(Continued)*
　　amino-acid *(Continued)*
　　　glycine *(Continued)*
　　　　sarcosinemia E72.59
　　　　trimethylaminuria E72.52
　　　hydroxylysine E72.3
　　　lysine E72.3
　　　ornithine E72.4
　　　other specified E72.89
　　　　beta-amino acid E72.89
　　　　gamma-glutamyl cycle E72.89
　　　straight-chain E72.89
　　　sulfur-bearing E72.10
　　　　homocystinuria E72.11
　　　　methylenetetrahydrofolate reductase
　　　　　deficiency E72.12
　　　other specified E72.19
　　bile acid and cholesterol metabolism E78.70
　　bilirubin E80.7
　　　specified NEC E80.6
　　calcium E83.50
　　　hypercalcemia E83.52
　　　hypocalcemia E83.51
　　　other specified E83.59
　　carbohydrate E74.9
　　　specified NEC E74.89
　　cholesterol and bile acid metabolism E78.70
　　congenital E88.9
　　copper E83.00
　　　specified type NEC E83.09
　　　Wilson's disease E83.01
　　cystinuria E72.01
　　fructose E74.10
　　galactose E74.20
　　glucosaminoglycan E76.9
　　　mucopolysaccharidosis —*see*
　　　　Mucopolysaccharidosis
　　　specified NEC E76.8
　　glutamine E72.89
　　glycine E72.50
　　glycogen storage (hepatorenal) E74.09
　　glycoprotein E77.9
　　　specified NEC E77.8
　　glycosaminoglycan E76.9
　　　specified NEC E76.8
　　in labor and delivery O75.89
　　iron E83.10
　　isoleucine E71.19
　　leucine E71.19
　　lipoid E78.9
　　lipoprotein E78.9
　　　specified NEC E78.89
　　magnesium E83.40
　　　hypermagnesemia E83.41
　　　hypomagnesemia E83.42
　　　other specified E83.49
　　mineral E83.9
　　　specified NEC E83.89
　　mitochondrial E88.40
　　　MELAS syndrome E88.41
　　　MERRF syndrome (myoclonic epilepsy
　　　　associated with ragged-red fibers)
　　　　E88.42
　　　other specified E88.49
　　ornithine E72.4
　　phosphatases E83.30
　　phosphorus E83.30
　　　acid phosphatase deficiency E83.39
　　　hypophosphatasia E83.39
　　　hypophosphatemia E83.39
　　　　familial E83.31
　　　other specified E83.39
　　　pseudovitamin D deficiency E83.32
　　plasma protein NEC E88.09
　　porphyrin —*see* Porphyria
　　postprocedural E89.89
　　　specified NEC E89.89
　　purine E79.9
　　　specified NEC E79.8
　　pyrimidine E79.9
　　　specified NEC E79.8

Disorder (Continued)

  metabolism (Continued)

    pyruvate E74.4

    serine E72.89

    sodium E87.8

    specified NEC E88.89

    threonine E72.89

    valine E71.19

    zinc E83.2

  methylmalonic acidemia E71.120

  micturition NEC —see also Difficulty,
    micturition R39.198

    feeling of incomplete emptying R39.14

    hesitancy R39.11

    poor stream R39.12

    psychogenic F45.8

    split stream R39.13

    straining R39.16

    urgency R39.15

  mild neurocognitive G31.84

  ▶due to known physiological condition
    (without behavioral disturbance)
    F06.70

    ▶with behavioral disturbance F06.71

  mitochondrial metabolism E88.40

  mitral (valve) —see Endocarditis, mitral

  mixed

    anxiety and depressive F41.8

    of scholastic skills (developmental) F81.89

    receptive expressive language F80.2

  mood F39

    bipolar —see Disorder, bipolar

    depressive —see Disorder, depressive

    due to (secondary to)

      alcohol F10.94

      amphetamine F15.94

        in

          abuse F15.14

          dependence F15.24

      anxiolytic F13.94

        in

          abuse F13.14

          dependence F13.24

      cocaine F14.94

        in

          abuse F14.14

          dependence F14.24

      general medical condition F06.30

      hallucinogen F16.94

        in

          abuse F16.14

          dependence F16.24

      hypnotic F13.94

        in

          abuse F13.14

          dependence F13.24

      inhalant F18.94

        in

          abuse F18.14

          dependence F18.24

      opioid F11.94

        in

          abuse F11.14

          dependence F11.24

      phencyclidine (PCP) F16.94

        in

          abuse F16.14

          dependence F16.24

      physiological condition F06.30

        with

          depressive features F06.31

          major depressive-like episode
            F06.32

          manic features F06.33

          mixed features F06.34

      psychoactive substance NEC F19.94

        in

          abuse F19.14

          dependence F19.24

      sedative F13.94

        in

          abuse F13.14

          dependence F13.24

Disorder (Continued)

  mood (Continued)

    due to (Continued)

      volatile solvents F18.94

        in

          abuse F18.14

          dependence F18.24

    manic episode F30.9

      with psychotic symptoms F30.2

      without psychotic symptoms F30.10

        mild F30.11

        moderate F30.12

        severe F30.13

      in remission (full) F30.4

        partial F30.3

      specified type NEC F30.8

    organic F06.30

      right hemisphere F07.89

    persistent F34.9

      cyclothymia F34.0

      dysthymia F34.1

      specified type NEC F34.89

    recurrent F39

    right hemisphere organic F07.89

  movement G25.9

    drug-induced G25.70

      akathisia G25.71

      specified NEC G25.79

    hysterical F44.4

    in diseases classified elsewhere —see
      category G26

    periodic limb G47.61

      sleep related G47.61

    sleep related NEC G47.69

    specified NEC G25.89

    stereotyped F98.4

    treatment-induced G25.9

  multiple personality F44.81

  muscle M62.9

    attachment, spine —see Enthesopathy,
      spinal

    in trichinellosis —see Trichinellosis, with
      muscle disorder

    psychogenic F45.8

    specified type NEC M62.89

    tone, newborn P94.9

      specified NEC P94.8

  muscular

    attachments —see also Enthesopathy

      spine —see Enthesopathy, spinal

    urethra N36.44

  musculoskeletal system, soft tissue —see
    Disorder, soft tissue

    postprocedural M96.89

    psychogenic F45.8

  myoneural G70.9

    due to lead G70.1

    specified NEC G70.89

    toxic G70.1

  myotonic NEC G71.19

  nail, in diseases classified elsewhere L62

  neck region NEC —see Dorsopathy, specified
    NEC

  neonatal onset multisystemic inflammatory
    (NOMID) M04.2

  nerve G58.9

    abducent NEC —see Strabismus, paralytic,
      sixth nerve

    accessory G52.8

    acoustic —see subcategory H93.3

    auditory —see subcategory H93.3

    auriculotemporal G50.8

    axillary G54.0

    cerebral —see Disorder, nerve, cranial

    cranial G52.9

      eighth —see subcategory H93.3

      eleventh G52.8

      fifth G50.9

      first G52.0

      fourth NEC —see Strabismus, paralytic,
        fourth nerve

Disorder (Continued)

  nerve (Continued)

    cranial (Continued)

      multiple G52.7

      ninth G52.1

      second NEC —see Disorder, nerve,
        optic

      seventh NEC G51.8

      sixth NEC —see Strabismus, paralytic,
        sixth nerve

      specified NEC G52.8

      tenth G52.2

      third NEC —see Strabismus, paralytic,
        third nerve

      twelfth G52.3

    entrapment —see Neuropathy,
      entrapment

    facial G51.9

      specified NEC G51.8

    femoral —see Lesion, nerve, femoral

    glossopharyngeal NEC G52.1

    hypoglossal G52.3

    intercostal G58.0

    lateral

      cutaneous of thigh —see
        Mononeuropathy, lower limb,
        meralgia paresthetica

      popliteal —see Lesion, nerve, popliteal

    lower limb —see Mononeuropathy, lower
      limb

    medial popliteal —see Lesion, nerve,
      popliteal, medial

    median NEC —see Lesion, nerve,
      median

    multiple G58.7

    oculomotor NEC —see Strabismus,
      paralytic, third nerve

    olfactory G52.0

    optic NEC H47.09-●

      hemorrhage into sheath —see
        Hemorrhage, optic nerve

      ischemic H47.01-●

    peroneal —see Lesion, nerve, popliteal

    phrenic G58.8

    plantar —see Lesion, nerve, plantar

    pneumogastric G52.2

    posterior tibial —see Syndrome, tarsal
      tunnel

    radial —see Lesion, nerve, radial

    recurrent laryngeal G52.2

    root G54.9

      cervical G54.2

      lumbosacral G54.1

      specified NEC G54.8

      thoracic G54.3

    sciatic NEC —see Lesion, nerve, sciatic

    specified NEC G58.8

      lower limb —see Mononeuropathy,
        lower limb, specified NEC

      upper limb —see Mononeuropathy,
        upper limb, specified NEC

    sympathetic G90.9

    tibial —see Lesion, nerve, popliteal,
      medial

    trigeminal G50.9

      specified NEC G50.8

    trochlear NEC —see Strabismus, paralytic,
      fourth nerve

    ulnar —see Lesion, nerve, ulnar

    upper limb —see Mononeuropathy, upper
      limb

    vagus G52.2

  nervous system G98.8

    autonomic (peripheral) G90.9

      specified NEC G90.8

    central G96.9

      specified NEC G96.89

    parasympathetic G90.9

    specified NEC G98.8

    sympathetic G90.9

    vegetative G90.9

Disorder (Continued)
  neurocognitive R41.9
    ▶with Lewy bodies (see also Dementia, in, diseases specified elsewhere) G31.83 [F02.-]
    ▶frontotemporal, specified NEC (see also Dementia, in, diseases specified elsewhere) G31.09 [F02.-●]
    ⫸major (see also Dementia) F03.-●
      with
        aggressive behavior F01.51
        combative behavior F01.51
        violent behavior F01.51
      due to vascular disease, with behavioral disturbance F01.51
      ▶due to vascular disease —see Dementia, vascular
      ▶mild —see Dementia, vascular, mild
      ▶moderate —see Dementia, vascular, moderate
      ▶severe —see Dementia, vascular, severe
      in (due to) (other diseases classified elsewhere) —see also Dementia, in (due to) F02.80
        with
          ⫸aggressive behavior (see also Dementia, in (due to)) F02.81-●
          combative behavior (see also Dementia, in (due to)) F02.81-●
          violent behavior (see also Dementia, in (due to)) F02.81-●
        without behavioral disturbance F01.50
    ⫸mild (of uncertain or unknown etiology) (see also Disorder, mild neurocognitive) G31.84
  neurodevelopmental F89
    specified NEC F88
  neurohypophysis NEC E23.3
  neurological NEC R29.818
  neuromuscular G70.9
    hereditary NEC G71.9
    specified NEC G70.89
    toxic G70.1
  neurotic F48.9
    specified NEC F48.8
  neutrophil, polymorphonuclear D71
  nicotine use —see Dependence, drug, nicotine
  nightmare F51.5
  non-rapid eye movement sleep arousal
    sleep terror type F51.4
    sleepwalking type F51.3
  nose J34.9
    specified NEC J34.89
  obsessive-compulsive F42.9
    and related disorder due to a known physiological condition F06.8
  odontogenesis NOS K00.9
  opioid use
    with
      opioid-induced psychotic disorder F11.959
        with
          delusions F11.950
          hallucinations F11.951
    due to drug abuse —see Abuse, drug, opioid
    due to drug dependence —see Dependence, drug, opioid
    mild F11.10
      with
        opioid-induced
          anxiety disorder F11.188
          depressive disorder F11.14
          sexual dysfunction F11.181
        opioid intoxication
          with perceptual disturbances F11.122
          delirium F11.121
          without perceptual disturbances F11.129
      in remission (early) (sustained) F11.11

Disorder (Continued)
  opioid use (Continued)
    moderate or severe F11.20
      with
        opioid-induced
          anxiety disorder F11.288
          anxiety disorder F11.988
          depressive disorder F11.24
          depressive disorder F11.94
          sexual dysfunction F11.281
          sexual dysfunction F11.981
        opioid intoxication
          with perceptual disturbances F11.222
          delirium F11.221
          without perceptual disturbances F11.229
      in remission (early) (sustained) F11.21
  oppositional defiant F91.3
  optic
    chiasm H47.49
      due to
        inflammatory disorder H47.41
        neoplasm H47.42
        vascular disorder H47.43
    disc H47.39-●
      coloboma —see Coloboma, optic disc
      drusen —see Drusen, optic disc
      pseudopapilledema —see Pseudopapilledema
    radiations —see Disorder, visual, pathway
    tracts —see Disorder, visual, pathway
  orbit H05.9
    cyst —see Cyst, orbit
    deformity —see Deformity, orbit
    edema —see Edema, orbit
    enophthalmos —see Enophthalmos
    exophthalmos —see Exophthalmos
    hemorrhage —see Hemorrhage, orbit
    inflammation —see Inflammation, orbit
    myopathy —see Myopathy, extraocular muscles
    retained foreign body —see Foreign body, orbit, old
    specified type NEC H05.89
  organic
    anxiety F06.4
    catatonic F06.1
    delusional F06.2
    dissociative F06.8
    emotionally labile (asthenic) F06.8
    mood (affective) F06.30
    schizophrenia-like F06.2
  orgasmic (female) F52.31
    male F52.32
  ornithine metabolism E72.4
  overanxious F41.1
    of childhood F93.8
  pain
    with related psychological factors F45.42
    exclusively related to psychological factors F45.41
    genito-pelvic penetration disorder F52.6
  pancreatic internal secretion E16.9
    specified NEC E16.8
  panic F41.0
    with agoraphobia F40.01
  papulosquamous L44.9
    in diseases classified elsewhere L45
    specified NEC L44.8
  paranoid F22
    induced F24
    shared F24
  paraphilic F65.9
    specified NEC F65.89
  parathyroid (gland) E21.5
    specified NEC E21.4
  parietoalveolar NEC J84.09
  paroxysmal, mixed R56.9
  patella M22.9-●
    chondromalacia —see Chondromalacia, patella

Disorder (Continued)
  patella (Continued)
    derangement NEC M22.3X-●
    recurrent
      dislocation —see Dislocation, patella, recurrent
      subluxation —see Dislocation, patella, recurrent, incomplete
    specified NEC M22.8X-●
  patellofemoral M22.2X-●
  pedophilic F65.4
  pentose phosphate pathway with anemia D55.1
  perception, due to hallucinogens F16.983
    in
      abuse F16.183
      dependence F16.283
  peripheral nervous system NEC G64
  peroxisomal E71.50
    biogenesis
      neonatal adrenoleukodystrophy E71.511
      specified disorder NEC E71.518
      Zellweger syndrome E71.510
    rhizomelic chondrodysplasia punctata E71.540
    specified form NEC E71.548
      group 1 E71.518
      group 2 E71.53
      group 3 E71.542
    X-linked adrenoleukodystrophy E71.529
      adolescent E71.521
      adrenomyeloneuropathy E71.522
      childhood E71.520
      specified form NEC E71.528
    Zellweger-like syndrome E71.541
  persistent
    (somatoform) pain F45.41
    affective (mood) F34.9
  personality —see also Personality F60.9
    affective F34.0
    aggressive F60.3
    amoral F60.2
    anankastic F60.5
    antisocial F60.2
    anxious F60.6
    asocial F60.2
    asthenic F60.7
    avoidant F60.6
    borderline F60.3
    change (secondary) due to general medical condition F07.0
    compulsive F60.5
    cyclothymic F34.0
    dependent (passive) F60.7
    depressive F34.1
    dissocial F60.2
    emotional instability F60.3
    expansive paranoid F60.0
    explosive F60.3
    following organic brain damage F07.9
    histrionic F60.4
    hyperthymic F34.0
    hypothymic F34.1
    hysterical F60.4
    immature F60.89
    inadequate F60.7
    labile F60.3
    mixed (nonspecific) F60.89
    moral deficiency F60.2
    narcissistic F60.81
    negativistic F60.89
    obsessional F60.5
    obsessive (-compulsive) F60.5
    organic F07.9
    overconscientious F60.5
    paranoid F60.0
    passive (-dependent) F60.7
    passive-aggressive F60.89
    pathological NEC F60.9
    pseudosocial F60.2
    psychopathic F60.2

▶ New   ⫸ Revised   deleted Deleted   ● Use Additional Character(s)

Disorder *(Continued)*
  personality *(Continued)*
    schizoid F60.1
    schizotypal F21
    self-defeating F60.7
    specified NEC F60.89
    type A F60.5
    unstable (emotional) F60.3
  pervasive, developmental F84.9
  phencyclidine use
    mild F16.10
      with
        phencyclidine-induced
          anxiety disorder F16.180
          bipolar and related disorder F16.14
          depressive disorder F16.14
          psychotic disorder F16.159
        phencyclidine intoxication F16.129
        phencyclidine intoxication delirium F16.121
      in remission (early) (sustained) F16.11
    moderate or severe F16.20
      with
        phencyclidine-induced
          anxiety disorder F16.280
          bipolar and related disorder F16.24
          depressive disorder F16.24
          psychotic disorder F16.259
        phencyclidine intoxication F16.229
        phencyclidine intoxication delirium F16.221
      in remission (early) (sustained) F16.21
  phobic anxiety, childhood F40.8
  phosphate-losing tubular N25.0
  pigmentation L81.9
    choroid, congenital Q14.3
    diminished melanin formation L81.6
    iron L81.8
    specified NEC L81.8
  pinna (noninfective) H61.10-•
    deformity, acquired H61.11-•
    hematoma H61.12-•
    perichondritis —*see* Perichondritis, ear
    specified type NEC H61.19-•
  pituitary gland E23.7
    iatrogenic (postprocedural) E89.3
    specified NEC E23.6
 ▶ platelet-activating anti-PF4, specified NEC D75.84
  platelets D69.1
  plexus G54.9
    specified NEC G54.8
  polymorphonuclear neutrophils D71
  porphyrin metabolism —*see* Porphyria
  postconcussional F07.81
  posthallucinogen perception F16.983
    in
      abuse F16.183
      dependence F16.283
  postmenopausal N95.9
    specified NEC N95.8
  postprocedural (postoperative) —*see* Complications, postprocedural
  post-transplant lymphoproliferative D47.z1
  post-traumatic stress (PTSD) F43.10
    acute F43.11
    chronic F43.12
  premenstrual dysphoric (PMDD) F32.81
  prepuce N47.8
  propionic acidemia E71.121
  prostate N42.9
    specified NEC N42.89
  psychogenic NOS —*see also* condition F45.9
    anxiety F41.8
    appetite F50.9
    asthenic F48.8
    cardiovascular (system) F45.8
    compulsive F42.8
    cutaneous F54
    depressive F32.9
    digestive (system) F45.8

Disorder *(Continued)*
  psychogenic NOS *(Continued)*
    dysmenorrheic F45.8
    dyspneic F45.8
    endocrine (system) F54
    eye NEC F45.8
    feeding —*see* Disorder, eating
    functional NEC F45.8
    gastric F45.8
    gastrointestinal (system) F45.8
    genitourinary (system) F45.8
    heart (function) (rhythm) F45.8
    hyperventilatory F45.8
    hypochondriacal —*see* Disorder, hypochondriacal
    intestinal F45.8
    joint F45.8
    learning F81.9
    limb F45.8
    lymphatic (system) F45.8
    menstrual F45.8
    micturition F45.8
    monoplegic NEC F44.4
    motor F44.4
    muscle F45.8
    musculoskeletal F45.8
    neurocirculatory F45.8
    obsessive F42.8
    occupational F48.8
    organ or part of body NEC F45.8
    paralytic NEC F44.4
    phobic F40.9
    physical NEC F45.8
    rectal F45.8
    respiratory (system) F45.8
    rheumatic F45.8
    sexual (function) F52.9
    skin (allergic) (eczematous) F54
    sleep F51.9
    specified part of body NEC F45.8
    stomach F45.8
  psychological F99
    associated with
      disease classified elsewhere F54
      sexual
        development F66
        relationship F66
      uncertainty about gender identity F64.9
  psychomotor NEC F44.4
    hysterical F44.4
  psychoneurotic —*see also* Neurosis
    mixed NEC F48.8
  psychophysiologic —*see* Disorder, somatoform
  psychosexual F65.9
    development F66
    identity of childhood F64.2
  psychosomatic NOS —*see* Disorder, somatoform
    multiple F45.0
    undifferentiated F45.1
  psychotic —*see* Psychosis
    transient (acute) F23
  puberty E30.9
    specified NEC E30.8
  pulmonary (valve) —*see* Endocarditis, pulmonary
  purine metabolism E79.9
  pyrimidine metabolism E79.9
  pyruvate metabolism E74.4
  reactive attachment (childhood) F94.1
  reading R48.0
    developmental (specific) F81.0
  receptive language F80.2
  receptor, hormonal, peripheral —*see also* Syndrome, androgen insensitivity E34.50
  recurrent brief depressive F33.8
  reflex R29.2
  refraction H52.7
    aniseikonia H52.32
    anisometropia H52.31
    astigmatism —*see* Astigmatism

Disorder *(Continued)*
  refraction *(Continued)*
    hypermetropia —*see* Hypermetropia
    myopia —*see* Myopia
    presbyopia H52.4
    specified NEC H52.6
  relationship F68.8
    due to sexual orientation F66
  REM sleep behavior G47.52
  renal function, impaired (tubular) N25.9
  resonance R49.9
    specified NEC R49.8
  respiratory function, impaired —*see also* Failure, respiration
    postprocedural —*see* Complication, postoperative, respiratory system
    psychogenic F45.8
  retina H35.9
    angioid streaks H35.33
    changes in vascular appearance H35.01-•
    degeneration —*see* Degeneration, retina
    dystrophy (hereditary) —*see* Dystrophy, retina
    edema H35.81
    hemorrhage —*see* Hemorrhage, retina
    ischemia H35.82
    macular degeneration —*see* Degeneration, macula
    microaneurysms H35.04-•
    microvascular abnormality NEC H35.09
    neovascularization —*see* Neovascularization, retina
    retinopathy —*see* Retinopathy
    separation of layers H35.70
      central serous chorioretinopathy H35.71-•
      pigment epithelium detachment (serous) H35.72-•
        hemorrhagic H35.73-•
    specified type NEC H35.89
    telangiectasis —*see* Telangiectasis, retina
    vasculitis —*see* Vasculitis, retina
  retroperitoneal K68.9
  right hemisphere organic affective F07.89
  rumination (infant or child) F98.21
  sacrum, sacrococcygeal NEC M53.3
  schizoaffective F25.9
    bipolar type F25.0
    depressive type F25.1
    manic type F25.0
    mixed type F25.0
    specified NEC F25.8
  schizoid of childhood F84.5
  schizophrenia spectrum and other psychotic disorder F29
    specified NEC F28
  schizophreniform F20.81
    brief F23
  schizotypal (personality) F21
 ▶ seasonal affective, recurrent episodes F33.-•
  secretion, thyrocalcitonin E07.0
  sedative, hypnotic, or anxiolytic use
    mild F13.10
      with
        sedative, hypnotic, or anxiolytic-induced
          anxiety disorder F13.180
          bipolar and related disorder F13.14
          depressive disorder F13.14
          psychotic disorder F13.159
          sexual dysfunction F13.181
        sedative, hypnotic, or anxiolytic intoxication F13.129
        sedative, hypnotic, or anxiolytic intoxication delirium F13.121
      in remission (early) (sustained) F13.11
    moderate or severe F13.20
      with
        sedative, hypnotic, or anxiolytic-induced
          anxiety disorder F13.280
          bipolar and related disorder F13.24

Disorder (Continued)
  sedative, hypnotic, or anxiolytic use
      (Continued)
    moderate or severe (Continued)
      with (Continued)
        sedative, hypnotic, or anxiolytic-
            induced (Continued)
          anxiety disorder depressive
              disorder F13.24
          major neurocognitive disorder
              F13.27
          mild neurocognitive disorder
              F13.288
          psychotic disorder F13.259
          sexual dysfunction F13.281
          sedative, hypnotic, or anxiolytic
              intoxication F13.229
          sedative, hypnotic, or anxiolytic
              intoxication delirium F13.221
        in remission (early) (sustained) F13.21
  seizure —see also Epilepsy G40.909
    intractable G40.919
      with status epilepticus G40.911
  semantic pragmatic F80.89
    with autism F84.0
  sense of smell R43.1
    psychogenic F45.8
  separation anxiety, of childhood F93.0
  sexual
    arousal, female F52.22
    aversion F52.1
    function, psychogenic F52.9
    interest/arousal, female F52.22
    masochism F65.51
    maturation F66
    nonorganic F52.9
    preference —see also Deviation, sexual
        F65.9
      fetishistic transvestism F65.1
    relationship F66
    sadism F65.52
  shyness, of childhood and adolescence
      F40.10
  sibling rivalry F93.8
  sickle-cell (sickling) (homozygous) —see
        Disease, sickle-cell
    heterozygous D57.3
    specified type NEC D57.8-●
    trait D57.3
  sinus (nasal) J34.9
    specified NEC J34.89
  skin L98.9
    atrophic L90.9
      specified NEC L90.8
    granulomatous L92.9
      specified NEC L92.8
    hypertrophic L91.9
      specified NEC L91.8
    infiltrative NEC L98.6
    newborn P83.9
      specified NEC P83.88
    picking F42.4
    psychogenic (allergic) (eczematous) F54
  sleep G47.9
    breathing-related —see Apnea, sleep
    circadian rhythm G47.20
      advance sleep phase type G47.22
      delayed sleep phase type G47.21
      due to
        alcohol
          abuse F10.182
          dependence F10.282
          use F10.982
        amphetamines
          abuse F15.182
          dependence F15.282
          use F15.982
        caffeine
          abuse F15.182
          dependence F15.282
          use F15.982

Disorder (Continued)
  sleep (Continued)
    circadian rhythm (Continued)
      due to (Continued)
        cocaine
          abuse F14.182
          dependence F14.282
          use F14.982
        drug NEC
          abuse F19.182
          dependence F19.282
          use F19.982
        opioid
          abuse F11.182
          dependence F11.282
          use F11.982
        psychoactive substance NEC
          abuse F19.182
          dependence F19.282
          use F19.982
        sedative, hypnotic, or anxiolytic
          abuse F13.182
          dependence F13.282
          use F13.982
        stimulant NEC
          abuse F15.182
          dependence F15.282
          use F15.982
      free running type G47.24
      in conditions classified elsewhere
          G47.27
      irregular sleep wake type G47.23
      jet lag type G47.25
      non-24-hour sleep-wake type G47.24
      shift work type G47.26
      specified NEC G47.29
    due to
      alcohol
        abuse F10.182
        dependence F10.282
        use F10.982
      amphetamine
        abuse F15.182
        dependence F15.282
        use F15.982
      anxiolytic
        abuse F13.182
        dependence F13.282
        use F13.982
      caffeine
        abuse F15.182
        dependence F15.282
        use F15.982
      cocaine
        abuse F14.182
        dependence F14.282
        use F14.982
      drug NEC
        abuse F19.182
        dependence F19.282
        use F19.982
      hypnotic
        abuse F13.182
        dependence F13.282
        use F13.982
      opioid
        abuse F11.182
        dependence F11.282
        use F11.982
      psychoactive substance NEC
        abuse F19.182
        dependence F19.282
        use F19.982
      sedative
        abuse F13.182
        dependence F13.282
        use F13.982
      stimulant NEC
        abuse F15.182
        dependence F15.282
        use F15.982

Disorder (Continued)
  sleep (Continued)
    emotional F51.9
    excessive somnolence —see Hypersomnia
    hypersomnia type —see Hypersomnia
    initiating or maintaining —see Insomnia
    nightmares F51.5
    nonorganic F51.9
      specified NEC F51.8
    parasomnia type G47.50
    specified NEC G47.8
    terrors F51.4
    walking F51.3
  sleep-wake pattern or schedule —see also
        Disorder, sleep, circadian rhythm G47.9
    specified NEC G47.8
  social
    anxiety (of childhood) F40.10
      generalized F40.11
    functioning in childhood F94.9
      specified NEC F94.8
    pragmatic F80.82
  soft tissue M79.9
    ankle M79.9
    due to use, overuse and pressure M70.90
      ankle M70.97-●
      bursitis —see Bursitis
      foot M70.97-●
      forearm M70.93-●
      hand M70.94-●
      lower leg M70.96-●
      multiple sites M70.99
      pelvic region M70.95-●
      shoulder region M70.91-●
      specified site NEC M70.98
      specified type NEC M70.80
        ankle M70.87-●
        foot M70.87-●
        forearm M70.83-●
        hand M70.84-●
        lower leg M70.86-●
        multiple sites M70.89
        pelvic region M70.85-●
        shoulder region M70.81-●
        specified site NEC M70.88
        thigh M70.85-●
        upper arm M70.82-●
      thigh M70.95-●
      upper arm M70.92-●
    foot M79.9
    forearm M79.9
    hand M79.9
    lower leg M79.9
    multiple sites M79.9
    occupational —see Disorder, soft tissue,
        due to use, overuse and pressure
    pelvic region M79.9
    shoulder region M79.9
    specified type NEC M79.89
    thigh M79.9
    upper arm M79.9
  somatic symptom F45.1
  somatization F45.0
  somatoform F45.9
    pain (persistent) F45.41
    somatization (multiple) (long-lasting) F45.0
    specified NEC F45.8
    undifferentiated F45.1
  somnolence, excessive —see Hypersomnia
  specific
    arithmetical F81.2
    developmental, of motor F82
    reading F81.0
    speech and language F80.9
    spelling F81.81
    written expression F81.81
  speech R47.9
    articulation (functional) (specific) F80.0
    developmental F80.9
    specified NEC R47.89
  speech-sound F80.0

▶ New   ➡ Revised   ~~deleted~~ Deleted   ● Use Additional Character(s)

Disorder *(Continued)*
  spelling (specific) F81.81
  spine —*see also* Dorsopathy
    ligamentous or muscular attachments,
        peripheral —*see* Enthesopathy, spinal
    specified NEC —*see* Dorsopathy, specified
        NEC
  stereotyped, habit or movement F98.4
  stimulant use (other) (unspecified)
    mild F15.10
      in remission (early) (sustained) F15.11
    moderate or severe F15.20
      in remission (early) (sustained) F15.21
  stomach (functional) —*see* Disorder, gastric
  stress F43.9
    acute F43.0
    post-traumatic F43.10
      acute F43.11
      chronic F43.12
  substance use (other) (unknown)
    mild F19.10
      with substance-induced
        anxiety disorder F19.180
        bipolar and related disorder F19.14
        depressive disorder F19.14
        major neurocognitive disorder
            F19.17
        mild neurocognitive disorder F19.188
        obsessive-compulsive and related
            disorder F19.188
        sexual dysfunction F19.181
      substance intoxication F19.129
      substance intoxication delirium F19.121
    moderate or severe F19.20
      with substance-induced
        anxiety disorder F19.280
        bipolar and related disorder F19.24
        depressive disorder F19.24
        major neurocognitive disorder
            F19.27
        mild neurocognitive disorder F19.288
        obsessive-compulsive and related
            disorder F19.288
        sexual dysfunction F19.281
      in remission (early) (sustained) F19.21
      substance intoxication F19.229
      substance intoxication delirium F19.221
  sulfur-bearing amino-acid metabolism
      E72.10
  sweat gland (eccrine) L74.9
    apocrine L75.9
      specified NEC L75.8
    specified NEC L74.8
  synovium M67.90
    acromioclavicular M67.91-●
    ankle M67.97-●
    elbow M67.92-●
    foot M67.97-●
    forearm M67.93-●
    hand M67.94-●
    hip M67.95-●
    knee M67.96-●
    multiple sites M67.99
    rupture —*see* Rupture, synovium
    shoulder M67.91-●
    specified type NEC M67.80
      acromioclavicular M67.81-●
      ankle M67.87-●
      elbow M67.82-●
      foot M67.87-●
      hand M67.84-●
      hip M67.85-●
      knee M67.86-●
      multiple sites M67.89
      wrist M67.83-●
    synovitis —*see* Synovitis
    upper arm M67.92-●
    wrist M67.93-●
  temperature regulation, newborn P81.9
    specified NEC P81.8
  temporomandibular joint M26.60-●

Disorder *(Continued)*
  tendon M67.90
    acromioclavicular M67.91-●
    ankle M67.97-●
    contracture —*see* Contracture, tendon
    elbow M67.92-●
    foot M67.97-●
    forearm M67.93-●
    hand M67.94-●
    hip M67.95-●
    knee M67.96-●
    multiple sites M67.99
    rupture —*see* Rupture, tendon
    shoulder M67.91-●
    specified type NEC M67.80
      acromioclavicular M67.81-●
      ankle M67.87-●
      elbow M67.82-●
      foot M67.87-●
      hand M67.84-●
      hip M67.85-●
      knee M67.86-●
      multiple sites M67.89
      trunk M67.88
      wrist M67.83-●
    synovitis —*see* Synovitis
    tendinitis —*see* Tendinitis
    tenosynovitis —*see* Tenosynovitis
    trunk M67.98
    upper arm M67.92-●
    wrist M67.93-●
  thoracic root (nerve) NEC G54.3
  thyrocalcitonin hypersecretion E07.0
  thyroid (gland) E07.9
    function NEC, neonatal, transitory P72.2
    iodine-deficiency related E01.8
    specified NEC E07.89
  tic —*see* Tic
  tobacco use
    chewing tobacco (mild) (moderate) (severe)
      in remission (early) (sustained) F17.221
    cigarettes (mild) (moderate) (severe)
      in remission (early) (sustained) F17.211
    mild F17.200
      in remission (early) (sustained) F17.201
    moderate F17.200
      in remission (early) (sustained) F17.201
    severe F17.200
      in remission (early) (sustained) F17.201
    specified product NEC (mild) (moderate)
        (severe)
      in remission (early) (sustained) F17.291
  tooth K08.9
    development K00.9
      specified NEC K00.8
    eruption K00.6
  Tourette's F95.2
  trance and possession F44.89
  transvestic F65.1
  ~~trauma and stressor-related F43.9~~
    ~~other specified F43.8~~
  ▶trauma and stressor-related NOS F43.9
    ▶other specified F43.89
    ▶unspecified F43.9
  tricuspid (valve) —*see* Endocarditis, tricuspid
  tryptophan metabolism E70.5
  tubular, phosphate-losing N25.0
  tubulo-interstitial (in)
    brucellosis A23.9 *[N16]*
    cystinosis E72.04
    diphtheria A36.84
    glycogen storage disease E74.00 *[N16]*
    leukemia NEC C95.9-● *[N16]*
    lymphoma NEC C85.9-● *[N16]*
    mixed cryoglobulinemia D89.1 *[N16]*
    multiple myeloma C90.0-● *[N16]*
    Salmonella infection A02.25
    sarcoidosis D86.84
    sepsis A41.9 *[N16]*
      streptococcal A40.9 *[N16]*
    systemic lupus erythematosus M32.15

Disorder *(Continued)*
  tubulo-interstitial *(Continued)*
    toxoplasmosis B58.83
    transplant rejection T86.91 *[N16]*
    Wilson's disease E83.01 *[N16]*
  tubulo-renal function, impaired N25.9
    specified NEC N25.89
  tympanic membrane H73.9-●
    atrophy —*see* Atrophy, tympanic membrane
    infection —*see* Myringitis
    perforation —*see* Perforation, tympanum
    specified NEC H73.89-●
  unsocialized aggressive F91.1
  urea cycle metabolism E72.20
    argininemia E72.21
    argininosuccinic aciduria E72.22
    citrullinemia E72.23
    ornithine transcarbamylase deficiency
        E72.4
    other specified E72.29
  ureter (in) N28.9
    schistosomiasis B65.0 *[N29]*
    tuberculosis A18.11
  urethra N36.9
    specified NEC N36.8
  urinary system N39.9
    specified NEC N39.8
  valve, heart
    aortic —*see* Endocarditis, aortic
    mitral —*see* Endocarditis, mitral
    pulmonary —*see* Endocarditis, pulmonary
    rheumatic
      aortic —*see* Endocarditis, aortic,
          rheumatic
      mitral —*see* Endocarditis, mitral
      pulmonary —*see* Endocarditis,
          pulmonary, rheumatic
      tricuspid —*see* Endocarditis, tricuspid
    tricuspid —*see* Endocarditis, tricuspid
  vestibular function H81.9-●
    specified NEC —*see* subcategory H81.8
    in diseases classified elsewhere H82.-●
  vertigo —*see* Vertigo
  vision, binocular H53.30
    abnormal retinal correspondence H53.31
    diplopia H53.2
    fusion with defective stereopsis H53.32
    simultaneous perception H53.33
    suppression H53.34
  visual
    cortex
      blindness H47.619
        left brain H47.612
        right brain H47.611
      due to
        inflammatory disorder H47.629
          left brain H47.622
          right brain H47.621
        neoplasm H47.639
          left brain H47.632
          right brain H47.631
        vascular disorder H47.649
          left brain H47.642
          right brain H47.641
    pathway H47.9
      due to
        inflammatory disorder H47.51-●
        neoplasm H47.52-●
        vascular disorder H47.53-●
      optic chiasm —*see* Disorder, optic,
          chiasm
  vitreous body H43.9
    crystalline deposits —*see* Deposit,
        crystalline
    degeneration —*see* Degeneration, vitreous
    hemorrhage —*see* Hemorrhage, vitreous
    opacities —*see* Opacity, vitreous
    prolapse —*see* Prolapse, vitreous
    specified NEC H43.89
  voice R49.9
    specified type NEC R49.8

Disorder *(Continued)*
volatile solvent use
due to drug abuse —*see* Abuse, drug,
inhalant
due to drug dependence —*see* Dependence,
drug, inhalant
voyeuristic F65.3
white blood cells D72.9
specified NEC D72.89
withdrawing, child or adolescent F40.10
Disorientation R41.0
Displacement, displaced
acquired traumatic of bone, cartilage, joint,
tendon NEC —*see* Dislocation
adrenal gland (congenital) Q89.1
appendix, retrocecal (congenital) Q43.8
auricle (congenital) Q17.4
bladder (acquired) N32.89
congenital Q64.19
brachial plexus (congenital) Q07.8
brain stem, caudal (congenital) Q04.8
canaliculus (lacrimalis), congenital Q10.6
cardia through esophageal hiatus (congenital)
Q40.1
cerebellum, caudal (congenital) Q04.8
cervix —*see* Malposition, uterus
colon (congenital) Q43.3
device, implant or graft —*see also*
Complications, by site and type,
mechanical T85.628
arterial graft NEC —*see* Complication,
cardiovascular device, mechanical,
vascular
breast (implant) T85.42
catheter NEC T85.628
dialysis (renal) T82.42
intraperitoneal T85.621
infusion NEC T82.524
spinal (epidural) (subdural) T85.620
urinary
cystostomy T83.020
Hopkins T83.028
ileostomy T83.028
indwelling T83.021
nephrostomy T83.022
specified NEC T83.028
urostomy T83.028
electronic (electrode) (pulse generator)
(stimulator) —*see* Complication,
electronic stimulator
fixation, internal (orthopedic) NEC —
see Complication, fixation device,
mechanical
gastrointestinal —*see* Complications,
prosthetic device, mechanical,
gastrointestinal device
genital NEC T83.428
intrauterine contraceptive device (string)
T83.32
penile prosthesis (cylinder) (implanted)
(pump) (resevoir) T83.420
testicular prosthesis T83.421
heart NEC —*see* Complication,
cardiovascular device, mechanical
joint prosthesis —*see* Complications, joint
prosthesis, mechanical
ocular —*see* Complications, prosthetic
device, mechanical, ocular device
orthopedic NEC —*see* Complication,
orthopedic, device or graft,
mechanical
specified NEC T85.628
urinary NEC T83.128
graft T83.22
sphincter, implanted T83.121
stent (ileal conduit) (nephroureteral)
T83.123
ureteral indwelling T83.122
vascular NEC —*see* Complication,
cardiovascular device, mechanical
ventricular intracranial shunt T85.02

Displacement, displaced *(Continued)*
electronic stimulator
bone T84.320
cardiac —*see* Complications, cardiac
device, electronic
nervous system —*see* Complication,
prosthetic device, mechanical,
electronic nervous system stimulator
urinary —*see* Complications, electronic
stimulator, urinary
esophageal mucosa into cardia of stomach,
congenital Q39.8
esophagus (acquired) K22.89
congenital Q39.8
eyeball (acquired) (lateral) (old) —*see*
Displacement, globe
congenital Q15.8
current —*see* Avulsion, eye
fallopian tube (acquired) N83.4-●
congenital Q50.6
opening (congenital) Q50.6
gallbladder (congenital) Q44.1
gastric mucosa (congenital) Q40.2
globe (acquired) (old) (lateral) H05.21-●
current —*see* Avulsion, eye
heart (congenital) Q24.8
acquired I51.89
hymen (upward) (congenital) Q52.4
intervertebral disc NEC
with myelopathy —*see* Disorder, disc, with,
myelopathy
cervical, cervicothoracic (with) M50.20
myelopathy —*see* Disorder, disc,
cervical, with myelopathy
neuritis, radiculitis or radiculopathy —
see Disorder, disc, cervical, with
neuritis
due to trauma —*see* Dislocation, vertebra
lumbar region M51.26
with
neuritis, radiculitis, radiculopathy or
sciatica M51.16
lumbosacral region M51.27
with
myelopathy M51.07
neuritis, radiculitis, radiculopathy or
sciatica M51.17
sacrococcygeal region M53.3
thoracic region M51.24
with
myelopathy M51.04
neuritis, radiculitis, radiculopathy
M51.14
thoracolumbar region M51.25
with
myelopathy M51.05
neuritis, radiculitis, radiculopathy
M51.15
intrauterine device (string) T83.32
kidney (acquired) N28.83
congenital Q63.2
lachrymal, lacrimal apparatus or duct
(congenital) Q10.6
lens, congenital Q12.1
macula (congenital) Q14.1
Meckel's diverticulum Q43.0
malignant —*see* Table of Neoplasms, small
intestine, malignant
nail (congenital) Q84.6
acquired L60.8
opening of Wharton's duct in mouth
Q38.4
organ or site, congenital NEC —*see*
Malposition, congenital
ovary (acquired) N83.4-●
congenital Q50.39
free in peritoneal cavity (congenital)
Q50.39
into hernial sac N83.4-●
oviduct (acquired) N83.4-●
congenital Q50.6

Displacement, displaced *(Continued)*
parathyroid (gland) E21.4
parotid gland (congenital) Q38.4
punctum lacrimale (congenital) Q10.6
sacro-iliac (joint) (congenital) Q74.2
current injury S33.2
old —*see* subcategory M53.2
salivary gland (any) (congenital) Q38.4
spleen (congenital) Q89.09
stomach, congenital Q40.2
sublingual duct Q38.4
tongue (downward) (congenital) Q38.3
tooth, teeth, fully erupted M26.30
horizontal M26.33
vertical M26.34
trachea (congenital) Q32.1
ureter or ureteric opening or orifice
(congenital) Q62.62
uterine opening of oviducts or fallopian tubes
Q50.6
uterus, uterine —*see* Malposition, uterus
ventricular septum Q21.0
with rudimentary ventricle Q20.4
Disproportion
between native and reconstructed breast
N65.1
fiber-type G71.20
congenital G71.29
Disruptio uteri —*see* Rupture, uterus
Disruption (of)
ciliary body NEC H21.89
closure of
cornea T81.31
craniotomy T81.32
fascia (muscular) (superficial)
T81.32
internal organ or tissue T81.32
laceration (external) (internal)
T81.33
ligament T81.32
mucosa T81.31
muscle or muscle flap T81.32
ribs or rib cage T81.32
skin and subcutaneous tissue (full-
thickness) (superficial) T81.31
skull T81.32
sternum (sternotomy) T81.32
tendon T81.32
traumatic laceration (external) (internal)
T81.33
family Z63.8
due to
absence of family member due to
military deployment Z63.31
absence of family member NEC
Z63.32
alcoholism and drug addiction in
family Z63.72
bereavement Z63.4
death (assumed) or disappearance of
family member Z63.4
divorce or separation Z63.5
drug addiction in family Z63.72
return of family member from military
deployment (current or past
conflict) Z63.71
stressful life events NEC Z63.79
iris NEC H21.89
ligament(s) —*see also* Sprain
knee
current injury —*see* Dislocation, knee
old (chronic) —*see* Derangement, knee,
ligament, instability, chronic
spontaneous NEC —*see* Derangement,
knee, disruption ligament
ossicular chain —*see* Discontinuity, ossicles,
ear
pelvic ring (stable) S32.810
unstable S32.811
traumatic injury wound repair T81.33

▶ New   ⇒ Revised   ~~deleted~~ Deleted   ● Use Additional Character(s)

Disruption *(Continued)*
wound T81.30
episiotomy O90.1
operation T81.31
cesarean O90.0
external operation wound (superficial)
T81.31
internal operation wound (deep)
T81.32
perineal (obstetric) O90.1
traumatic injury repair T81.33
Dissatisfaction with
employment Z56.9
school environment Z55.4
Dissecting —*see* condition
Dissection
aorta I71.00
abdominal I71.02
thoracic I71.019
▶ aortic arch I71.011
▶ ascending aorta I71.010
▶ descending thoracic aorta I71.012
thoracoabdominal I71.03
artery I77.70
basilar (trunk) I77.75
carotid I77.71
cerebral (nonruptured) I67.0
ruptured —*see* Hemorrhage, intracranial,
subarachnoid
coronary I25.42
extremity
lower I77.77
upper I77.76
iliac I77.72
precerebral
congenital (nonruptured) Q28.1
specified site NEC I77.75
renal I77.73
specified NEC I77.79
vertebral I77.74
precerebral artery, congenital (nonruptured)
Q28.1
Heartland A93.8
traumatic —*see* Wound, open, by site
vascular I99.8
wound —*see* Wound, open
Disseminated —*see* condition
Dissociation
auriculoventricular or atrioventricular (AV)
(any degree) (isorhythmic) I45.89
with heart block I44.2
interference I45.89
Dissociative reaction, state F44.9
Dissolution, vertebra —*see* Osteoporosis
Distension, distention
abdomen R14.0
bladder N32.89
cecum K63.89
colon K63.89
gallbladder K82.8
intestine K63.89
kidney N28.89
liver K76.89
seminal vesicle N50.89
stomach K31.89
acute K31.0
psychogenic F45.8
ureter —*see* Dilatation, ureter
uterus N85.8
Distoma hepaticum infestation B66.3
Distomiasis B66.9
bile passages B66.3
hemic B65.9
hepatic B66.3
due to Clonorchis sinensis B66.1
intestinal B66.5
liver B66.3
due to Clonorchis sinensis B66.1
lung B66.4
pulmonary B66.4

Distomolar (fourth molar) K00.1
Disto-occlusion (Division I) (Division II)
M26.212
Distortion(s) (congenital)
adrenal (gland) Q89.1
arm NEC Q68.8
bile duct or passage Q44.5
bladder Q64.79
brain Q04.9
cervix (uteri) Q51.9
chest (wall) Q67.8
bones Q76.8
clavicle Q74.0
clitoris Q52.6
coccyx Q76.49
common duct Q44.5
coronary Q24.5
cystic duct Q44.5
ear (auricle) (external) Q17.3
inner Q16.5
middle Q16.4
ossicles Q16.3
endocrine NEC Q89.2
eustachian tube Q17.8
eye (adnexa) Q15.8
face bone(s) NEC Q75.8
fallopian tube Q50.6
femur NEC Q68.8
fibula NEC Q68.8
finger(s) Q68.1
foot Q66.9-●
genitalia, genital organ(s)
female Q52.8
external Q52.79
internal NEC Q52.8
gyri Q04.8
hand bone(s) Q68.1
heart (auricle) (ventricle) Q24.8
valve (cusp) Q24.8
hepatic duct Q44.5
humerus NEC Q68.8
hymen Q52.4
intrafamilial communications Z63.8
jaw NEC M26.89
labium (majus) (minus) Q52.79
leg NEC Q68.8
lens Q12.8
liver Q44.7
lumbar spine Q76.49
with disproportion O33.8
causing obstructed labor O65.0
lumbosacral (joint) (region) Q76.49
kyphosis —*see* Kyphosis, congenital
lordosis —*see* Lordosis, congenital
nerve Q07.8
nose Q30.8
organ
of Corti Q16.5
or site not listed —*see* Anomaly, by site
ossicles, ear Q16.3
oviduct Q50.6
pancreas Q45.3
parathyroid (gland) Q89.2
pituitary (gland) Q89.2
radius NEC Q68.8
sacroiliac joint Q74.2
sacrum Q76.49
scapula Q74.0
shoulder girdle Q74.0
skull bone(s) NEC Q75.8
with
anencephalus Q00.0
encephalocele —*see* Encephalocele
hydrocephalus Q03.9
with spina bifida —*see* Spina bifida,
with hydrocephalus
microcephaly Q02
spinal cord Q06.8
spine Q76.49
kyphosis —*see* Kyphosis, congenital
lordosis —*see* Lordosis, congenital

Distortion *(Continued)*
spleen Q89.09
sternum NEC Q76.7
thorax (wall) Q67.8
bony Q76.8
thymus (gland) Q89.2
thyroid (gland) Q89.2
tibia NEC Q68.8
toe(s) Q66.9-●
tongue Q38.3
trachea (cartilage) Q32.1
ulna NEC Q68.8
ureter Q62.8
urethra Q64.79
causing obstruction Q64.39
uterus Q51.9
vagina Q52.4
vertebra Q76.49
kyphosis —*see* Kyphosis, congenital
lordosis —*see* Lordosis, congenital
visual —*see also* Disturbance, vision
shape and size H53.15
vulva Q52.79
wrist (bones) (joint) Q68.8
Distress
abdomen —*see* Pain, abdominal
acute respiratory R06.03
syndrome (adult) (child) J80
epigastric R10.13
fetal P84
complicating pregnancy —*see* Stress, fetal
gastrointestinal (functional) K30
psychogenic F45.8
intestinal (functional) NOS K59.9
psychogenic F45.8
maternal, during labor and delivery O75.0
relationship, with spouse or intimate partner
Z63.0
respiratory (adult) (child) R06.03
newborn P22.9
specified NEC P22.8
orthopnea R06.01
psychogenic F45.8
shortness of breath R06.02
specified type NEC R06.09
Distribution vessel, atypical Q27.9
coronary artery Q24.5
precerebral Q28.1
Districhiasis L68.8
Disturbance(s) —*see also* Disease
absorption K90.9
calcium E58
carbohydrate K90.49
fat K90.49
pancreatic K90.3
protein K90.49
starch K90.49
vitamin —*see* Deficiency, vitamin
acid-base equilibrium E87.8
mixed E87.4
activity and attention (with hyperkinesis) —
see Disorder, attention-deficit
hyperactivity
amino acid transport E72.00
assimilation, food K90.9
auditory nerve, except deafness —*see*
subcategory H93.3
behavior —*see* Disorder, conduct
blood clotting (mechanism) —*see also* Defect,
coagulation D68.9
cerebral
nerve —*see* Disorder, nerve, cranial
status, newborn P91.9
specified NEC P91.88
circulatory I99.9
conduct —*see also* Disorder, conduct F91.9
adjustment reaction —*see* Disorder,
adjustment
compulsive F63.9
disruptive F91.9

Disturbance *(Continued)*

conduct *(Continued)*
hyperkinetic —*see* Disorder, attention-deficit hyperactivity
socialized F91.2
specified NEC F91.8
unsocialized F91.1
coordination R27.8
cranial nerve —*see* Disorder, nerve, cranial
deep sensibility —*see* Disturbance, sensation
digestive K30
psychogenic F45.8
electrolyte —*see also* Imbalance, electrolyte
newborn, transitory P74.49
hyperammonemia P74.6
hyperchloremia P74.421
hyperchloremic metabolic acidosis P74.421
hypochloremia P74.422
potassium balance
hyperkalemia P74.31
hypokalemia P74.32
sodium balance
hypernatremia P74.21
hyponatremia P74.22
specified type NEC P74.49
emotions specific to childhood and adolescence F93.9
with
anxiety and fearfulness NEC F93.8
elective mutism F94.0
oppositional disorder F91.3
sensitivity (withdrawal) F40.10
shyness F40.10
social withdrawal F40.10
involving relationship problems F93.8
mixed F93.8
specified NEC F93.8
endocrine (gland) E34.9
neonatal, transitory P72.9
specified NEC P72.8
equilibrium R42
fructose metabolism E74.10
gait —*see* Gait
hysterical F44.4
psychogenic F44.4
gastrointestinal (functional) K30
psychogenic F45.8
habit, child F98.9
hearing, except deafness and tinnitus —*see* Abnormal, auditory perception
heart, functional (conditions in I44-I50)
due to presence of (cardiac) prosthesis I97.19-●
postoperative I97.89
cardiac surgery —*see also* Infarct, myocardium, associated with revascularization procedure I97.19-●
hormones E34.9
innervation uterus (parasympathetic) (sympathetic) N85.8
keratinization NEC
gingiva K05.10
nonplaque induced K05.11
plaque induced K05.10
lip K13.0
oral (mucosa) (soft tissue) K13.29
tongue K13.29
learning (specific) —*see* Disorder, learning
memory —*see* Amnesia
mild, following organic brain damage F06.8
mental F99
associated with diseases classified elsewhere F54
metabolism E88.9
with
abortion —*see* Abortion, by type with other specified complication
ectopic pregnancy O08.5
molar pregnancy O08.5

Disturbance *(Continued)*

metabolism *(Continued)*
amino-acid E72.9
aromatic E70.9
branched-chain E71.2
straight-chain E72.89
sulfur-bearing E72.10
ammonia E72.20
arginine E72.21
arginosuccinic acid E72.22
carbohydrate E74.9
cholesterol E78.9
citrulline E72.23
cystathionine E72.19
general E88.9
glutamine E72.89
histidine E70.40
homocystine E72.19
hydroxylysine E72.3
in labor or delivery O75.89
iron E83.10
lipoid E78.9
lysine E72.3
methionine E72.19
neonatal, transitory P74.9
calcium and magnesium P71.9
specified type NEC P71.8
carbohydrate metabolism P70.9
specified type NEC P70.8
specified NEC P74.8
ornithine E72.4
phosphate E83.39
sodium NEC E87.8
threonine E72.89
tryptophan E70.5
tyrosine E70.20
urea cycle E72.20
motor R29.2
nervous, functional R45.0
neuromuscular mechanism (eye), due to syphilis A52.15
nutritional E63.9
nail L60.3
ocular motion H51.9
psychogenic F45.8
oculogyric H51.8
psychogenic F45.8
oculomotor H51.9
psychogenic F45.8
olfactory nerve R43.1
optic nerve NEC —*see* Disorder, nerve, optic
oral epithelium, including tongue NEC K13.29
perceptual due to
alcohol withdrawal F10.232
amphetamine intoxication F15.922
in
abuse F15.122
dependence F15.222
anxiolytic withdrawal F13.232
cannabis intoxication (acute) F12.922
in
abuse F12.122
dependence F12.222
cocaine intoxication (acute) F14.922
in
abuse F14.122
dependence F14.222
hypnotic withdrawal F13.232
opioid intoxication (acute) F11.922
in
abuse F11.122
dependence F11.222
phencyclidine intoxication (acute) F16.122
sedative withdrawal F13.232
personality (pattern) (trait) —*see also* Disorder, personality F60.9
following organic brain damage F07.9
polyglandular E31.9
specified NEC E31.8

Disturbance *(Continued)*

potassium balance, newborn
hyperkalemia P74.31
hypokalemia P74.32
psychogenic F45.9
psychomotor F44.4
psychophysical visual H53.16
pupillary —*see* Anomaly, pupil, function
reflex R29.2
rhythm, heart I49.9
salivary secretion K11.7
sensation (cold) (heat) (localization) (tactile discrimination) (texture) (vibratory) NEC R20.9
hysterical F44.6
skin R20.9
anesthesia R20.0
hyperesthesia R20.3
hypoesthesia R20.1
paresthesia R20.2
specified type NEC R20.8
smell R43.9
and taste (mixed) R43.8
anosmia R43.0
parosmia R43.1
specified NEC R43.8
taste R43.9
and smell (mixed) R43.8
parageusia R43.2
specified NEC R43.8
sensory —*see* Disturbance, sensation
situational (transient) —*see also* Disorder, adjustment
acute F43.0
sleep G47.9
nonorganic origin F51.9
smell —*see* Disturbance, sensation, smell
sociopathic F60.2
sodium balance, newborn
hypernatremia P74.21
hyponatremia P74.22
speech R47.9
developmental F80.9
specified NEC R47.89
stomach (functional) K31.9
sympathetic (nerve) G90.9
taste —*see* Disturbance, sensation, taste
temperature
regulation, newborn P81.9
specified NEC P81.8
sense R20.8
hysterical F44.6
tooth
eruption K00.6
formation K00.4
structure, hereditary NEC K00.5
touch —*see* Disturbance, sensation
vascular I99.9
arteriosclerotic —*see* Arteriosclerosis
vasomotor I73.9
vasospastic I73.9
vision, visual H53.9
following
cerebral infarction I69.398
cerebrovascular disease I69.998
specified NEC I69.898
intracerebral hemorrhage I69.198
nontraumatic intracranial hemorrhage NEC I69.298
specified disease NEC I69.898
subarachnoid hemorrhage I69.098
psychophysical H53.16
specified NEC H53.8
subjective H53.10
day blindness H53.11
discomfort H53.14-●
distortions of shape and size H53.15
loss
sudden H53.13-●
transient H53.12-●
specified type NEC H53.19

► New   ⇒ Revised   ~~deleted~~ Deleted   ● Use Additional Character(s)

Disturbance *(Continued)*
  voice R49.9
    psychogenic F44.4
    specified NEC R49.8
Diuresis R35.89
Diver's palsy, paralysis or squeeze T70.3
Diverticulitis (acute) K57.92
  bladder —*see* Cystitis
  ileum —*see* Diverticulitis, intestine, small
  intestine K57.92
    with
      abscess, perforation K57.80
        with bleeding K57.81
      bleeding K57.93
    congenital Q43.8
    large K57.32
      with
        abscess, perforation K57.20
          with bleeding K57.21
        bleeding K57.33
        small intestine K57.52
          with
            abscess, perforation K57.40
              with bleeding K57.41
            bleeding K57.53
    small K57.12
      with
        abscess, perforation K57.00
          with bleeding K57.01
        bleeding K57.13
        large intestine K57.52
          with
            abscess, perforation K57.40
              with bleeding K57.41
            bleeding K57.53
Diverticulosis K57.90
  with bleeding K57.91
  large intestine K57.30
    with
      bleeding K57.31
      small intestine K57.50
        with bleeding K57.51
  small intestine K57.10
    with
      bleeding K57.11
      large intestine K57.50
        with bleeding K57.51
Diverticulum, diverticula (multiple) K57.90
  appendix (noninflammatory) K38.2
  bladder (sphincter) N32.3
    congenital Q64.6
  bronchus (congenital) Q32.4
    acquired J98.09
  calyx, calyceal (kidney) N28.89
  cardia (stomach) K31.4
  cecum —*see* Diverticulosis, intestine, large
    congenital Q43.8
  colon —*see* Diverticulosis, intestine, large
    congenital Q43.8
  duodenum —*see* Diverticulosis, intestine,
      small
    congenital Q43.8
  epiphrenic (esophagus) K22.5
  esophagus (congenital) Q39.6
    acquired (epiphrenic) (pulsion) (traction)
        K22.5
  eustachian tube —*see* Disorder, eustachian
      tube, specified NEC
  fallopian tube N83.8
  gastric K31.4
  heart (congenital) Q24.8
  ileum —*see* Diverticulosis, intestine, small
  jejunum —*see* Diverticulosis, intestine, small
  kidney (pelvis) (calyces) N28.89
    with calculus —*see* Calculus, kidney
  Meckel's (displaced) (hypertrophic) Q43.0
    malignant —*see* Table of Neoplasms, small
        intestine, malignant
  midthoracic K22.5
  organ or site, congenital NEC —*see* Distortion

Diverticulum, diverticula *(Continued)*
  pericardium (congenital) (cyst) Q24.8
    acquired I31.8
  pharyngoesophageal (congenital) Q39.6
    acquired K22.5
  pharynx (congenital) Q38.7
  rectosigmoid —*see* Diverticulosis, intestine,
      large
    congenital Q43.8
  rectum —*see* Diverticulosis, intestine, large
  Rokitansky's K22.5
  seminal vesicle N50.89
  sigmoid —*see* Diverticulosis, intestine, large
    congenital Q43.8
  stomach (acquired) K31.4
    congenital Q40.2
  trachea (acquired) J39.8
  ureter (acquired) N28.89
    congenital Q62.8
  ureterovesical orifice N28.89
  urethra (acquired) N36.1
    congenital Q64.79
  ventricle, left (congenital) Q24.8
  vesical N32.3
    congenital Q64.6
  Zenker's (esophagus) K22.5
Division
  cervix uteri (acquired) N88.8
  glans penis Q55.69
  labia minora (congenital) Q52.79
  ligament (partial or complete) (current) —*see
      also* Sprain
    with open wound —*see* Wound, open
  muscle (partial or complete) (current) —*see
      also* Injury, muscle
    with open wound —*see* Wound, open
  nerve (traumatic) —*see* Injury, nerve
  spinal cord —*see* Injury, spinal cord,
      by region
  vein I87.8
Divorce, causing family disruption Z63.5
Dix-Hallpike neurolabyrinthitis —*see*
      Neuronitis, vestibular
Dizziness R42
  hysterical F44.89
  psychogenic F45.8
DMAC (disseminated mycobacterium avium-
      intracellulare complex) A31.2
DNR (do not resuscitate) Z66
Doan-Wiseman syndrome (primary splenic
      neutropenia) —*see* Agranulocytosis
Doehle-Heller aortitis A52.02
Dog bite —*see* Bite
Dohle body panmyelopathic syndrome D72.0
Dolichocephaly Q67.2
Dolichocolon Q43.8
Dolichostenomelia —*see* Syndrome, Marfan's
Donohue's syndrome E34.8
Donor (organ or tissue) Z52.9
  blood (whole) Z52.000
    autologous Z52.010
    specified component (lymphocytes)
        (platelets) NEC Z52.008
      autologous Z52.018
      specified donor NEC Z52.098
    specified donor NEC Z52.090
    stem cells Z52.001
      autologous Z52.011
      specified donor NEC Z52.091
  bone Z52.20
    autologous Z52.21
    marrow Z52.3
    specified type NEC Z52.29
  cornea Z52.5
  egg (Oocyte) Z52.819
    age 35 and over Z52.812
      anonymous recipient Z52.812
      designated recipient Z52.813
    under age 35 Z52.810
      anonymous recipient Z52.810
      designated recipient Z52.811

Donor *(Continued)*
  kidney Z52.4
  liver Z52.6
  lung Z52.89
  lymphocyte —*see* Donor, blood, specified
      components NEC
  Oocyte —*see* Donor, egg
  platelets Z52.008
  potential, examination of Z00.5
  semen Z52.89
  skin Z52.10
    autologous Z52.11
    specified type NEC Z52.19
  specified organ or tissue NEC Z52.89
  sperm Z52.89
Donovanosis A58
Dorsalgia M54.9
  psychogenic F45.41
  specified NEC M54.89
Dorsopathy M53.9
  deforming M43.9
    specified NEC —*see* subcategory M43.8
  specified NEC M53.80
    cervical region M53.82
    cervicothoracic region M53.83
    lumbar region M53.86
    lumbosacral region M53.87
    occipito-atlanto-axial region M53.81
    sacrococcygeal region M53.88
    thoracic region M53.84
    thoracolumbar region M53.85
Double
  albumin E88.09
  aortic arch Q25.45
  auditory canal Q17.8
  auricle (heart) Q20.8
  bladder Q64.79
  cervix Q51.820
    with doubling of uterus (and vagina)
        Q51.10
      with obstruction Q51.11
  inlet ventricle Q20.4
  kidney with double pelvis (renal) Q63.0
  meatus urinarius Q64.75
  monster Q89.4
  outlet
    left ventricle Q20.2
    right ventricle Q20.1
  pelvis (renal) with double ureter Q62.5
  tongue Q38.3
  ureter (one or both sides) Q62.5
    with double pelvis (renal) Q62.5
  urethra Q64.74
  urinary meatus Q64.75
  uterus Q51.28
    with
      doubling of cervix (and vagina) Q51.10
        with obstruction Q51.11
      complete Q51.21
      in pregnancy or childbirth O34.0-●
        causing obstructed labor O65.5
      partial Q51.22
    specified NEC Q51.28
  vagina Q52.10
    with doubling of uterus (and cervix)
        Q51.10
      with obstruction Q51.11
  vision H53.2
  vulva Q52.79
Doubled up Z59.01
Douglas' pouch, cul-de-sac —*see* condition
Down syndrome Q90.9
  meiotic nondisjunction Q90.0
  mitotic nondisjunction Q90.1
  mosaicism Q90.1
  translocation Q90.2
DPD (dihydropyrimidine dehydrogenase
      deficiency) E88.89
Dracontiasis B72
Dracunculiasis, dracunculosis B72
Dream state, hysterical F44.89

Drepanocytic anemia —see Disease, sickle-cell
Dresbach's syndrome (elliptocytosis) D58.1
Dreschlera (hawaiiensis) (infection)
B43.8
Dressler's syndrome I24.1
Drift, ulnar —see Deformity, limb, specified
type NEC, forearm
Drinking (alcohol)
excessive, to excess NEC (without
dependence) F10.10
habitual (continual) (without remission)
F10.20
with remission F10.21
Drip, postnasal (chronic) R09.82
due to
allergic rhinitis —see Rhinitis, allergic
common cold J00
gastroesophageal reflux —see Reflux,
gastroesophageal
nasopharyngitis —see Nasopharyngitis
other known condition — code to
condition
sinusitis —see Sinusitis
Droop
facial R29.810
cerebrovascular disease I69.992
cerebral infarction I69.392
intracerebral hemorrhage I69.192
nontraumatic intracranial hemorrhage
NEC I69.292
specified disease NEC I69.892
subarachnoid hemorrhage I69.092
Drop (in)
attack NEC R55
finger —see Deformity, finger
foot —see Deformity, limb, foot, drop
hematocrit (precipitous) R71.0
hemoglobin R71.0
toe —see Deformity, toe, specified NEC
wrist —see Deformity, limb, wrist drop
Dropped heart beats I45.9
Dropsy, dropsical —see also Hydrops
abdomen R18.8
brain —see Hydrocephalus
cardiac, heart —see Failure, heart, congestive
gangrenous —see Gangrene
heart —see Failure, heart, congestive
kidney —see Nephrosis
lung —see Edema, lung
newborn due to isoimmunization P56.0
pericardium —see Pericarditis
Drowned, drowning (near) T75.1
Drowsiness R40.0
Drug
abuse counseling and surveillance Z71.51
addiction —see Dependence
dependence —see Dependence
habit —see Dependence
harmful use —see Abuse, drug
induced fever R50.2
overdose —see Table of Drugs and Chemicals,
by drug, poisoning
poisoning —see Table of Drugs and
Chemicals, by drug, poisoning
resistant organism infection —see also
Resistant, organism, to, drug Z16.30
therapy
long term (current) (prophylactic) —see
Therapy, drug long-term (current)
(prophylactic)
short term - omit code
wrong substance given or taken in error —see
Table of Drugs and Chemicals, by drug,
poisoning
Drunkenness (without dependence) F10.129
acute in alcoholism F10.229
chronic (without remission) F10.20
with remission F10.21
pathological (without dependence) F10.129
with dependence F10.229
sleep F51.9

Drusen
macula (degenerative) (retina) —see
Degeneration, macula, drusen
optic disc H47.32-●
Dry, dryness —see also condition
larynx J38.7
mouth R68.2
due to dehydration E86.0
nose J34.89
socket (teeth) M27.3
throat J39.2
DSAP L56.5
Duane's syndrome H50.81-●
Dubin-Johnson disease or syndrome E80.6
Dubois' disease (thymus gland) A50.59 [E35]
Dubowitz' syndrome Q87.19
Duchenne-Aran muscular atrophy G12.21
Duchenne-Griesinger disease G71.01
Duchenne's
disease or syndrome
motor neuron disease G12.22
muscular dystrophy G71.01
locomotor ataxia (syphilitic) A52.11
paralysis
birth injury P14.0
due to or associated with
motor neuron disease G12.22
muscular dystrophy G71.01
Ducrey's chancre A57
Duct, ductus —see condition
Duhring's disease (dermatitis herpetiformis)
L13.0
Dullness, cardiac (decreased) (increased) R01.2
Dumb ague —see Malaria
Dumbness —see Aphasia
Dumdum fever B55.0
Dumping syndrome (postgastrectomy) K91.1
Duodenitis (nonspecific) (peptic) K29.80
with bleeding K29.81
Duodenocholangitis —see Cholangitis
Duodenum, duodenal —see condition
Duplay's bursitis or periarthritis M75.0
Duplication, duplex —see also Accessory
alimentary tract Q45.8
anus Q43.4
appendix (and cecum) Q43.4
biliary duct (any) Q44.5
bladder Q64.79
cecum (and appendix) Q43.4
cervix Q51.820
chromosome NEC
with complex rearrangements NEC Q92.5
seen only at prometaphase Q92.8
cystic duct Q44.5
digestive organs Q45.8
esophagus Q39.8
frontonasal process Q75.8
intestine (large) (small) Q43.4
kidney Q63.0
liver Q44.7
pancreas Q45.3
penis Q55.69
respiratory organs NEC Q34.8
salivary duct Q38.4
spinal cord (incomplete) Q06.2
stomach Q40.2
Dupré's disease (meningism) R29.1
Dupuytren's contraction or disease M72.0
Durand-Nicolas-Favre disease A55
Durotomy (inadvertent) (incidental) G97.41
Duroziez's disease (congenital mitral stenosis)
Q23.2
Dutton's relapsing fever (West African)
A68.1
➡Dwarfism (see also Stature, short) E34.328
achondroplastic Q77.4
➡congenital (see also Stature, short) E34.328
➡constitutional E34.31
hypochondroplastic Q77.4
hypophyseal E23.0
➡infantile (see also Stature, short) E34.328

Dwarfism (Continued)
➡Laron-type (see also Stature, short) E34.321
Lorain (-Levi) type E23.0
metatropic Q77.8
nephrotic-glycosuric (with
hypophosphatemic rickets) E72.09
nutritional E45
pancreatic K86.89
pituitary E23.0
renal N25.0
thanatophoric Q77.1
Dyke-Young anemia (secondary)
(symptomatic) D59.19
Dysacusis —see Abnormal, auditory
perception
Dysadrenocortism E27.9
hyperfunction E27.0
Dysarthria R47.1
following
cerebral infarction I69.322
cerebrovascular disease I69.922
specified disease NEC I69.822
intracerebral hemorrhage I69.122
nontraumatic intracranial hemorrhage
NEC I69.222
subarachnoid hemorrhage I69.022
Dysautonomia (familial) G90.1
Dysbarism T70.3
Dysbasia R26.2
angiosclerotica intermittens I73.9
hysterical F44.4
lordotica (progressiva) G24.1
nonorganic origin F44.4
psychogenic F44.4
Dysbetalipoproteinemia (familial) E78.2
Dyscalculia R48.8
developmental F81.2
Dyschezia K59.00
Dyschondroplasia (with hemangiomata) Q78.4
Dyschromia (skin) L81.9
Dyscollagenosis M35.9
Dyscranio-pygo-phalangy Q87.0
Dyscrasia
blood (with) D75.9
antepartum hemorrhage —see Hemorrhage,
antepartum, with coagulation defect
intrapartum hemorrhage O67.0
newborn P61.9
specified type NEC P61.8
puerperal, postpartum O72.3
polyglandular, pluriglandular E31.9
Dysendocrinism E34.9
Dysentery, dysenteric (catarrhal) (diarrhea)
(epidemic) (hemorrhagic) (infectious)
(sporadic) (tropical) A09
abscess, liver A06.4
amebic —see also Amebiasis A06.0
with abscess —see Abscess, amebic
acute A06.0
chronic A06.1
arthritis —see also category M01 A09
bacillary —see also category M01 A03.9
bacillary A03.9
arthritis —see also category M01 A03.9
Boyd A03.2
Flexner A03.1
Schmitz (-Stutzer) A03.0
Shiga (-Kruse) A03.0
Shigella A03.9
boydii A03.2
dysenteriae A03.0
flexneri A03.1
group A A03.0
group B A03.1
group C A03.2
group D A03.3
sonnei A03.3
specified type NEC A03.8
Sonne A03.3
specified type NEC A03.8
balantidial A07.0

Dysentery, dysenteric *(Continued)*
  Balantidium coli A07.0
  Boyd's A03.2
  candidal B37.82
  Chilomastix A07.8
  Chinese A03.9
  coccidial A07.3
  Dientamoeba (fragilis) A07.8
  Embadomonas A07.8
  Entamoeba, entamebic —*see* Dysentery, amebic
  Flexner-Boyd A03.2
  Flexner's A03.1
  Giardia lamblia A07.1
  Hiss-Russell A03.1
  Lamblia A07.1
  leishmanial B55.0
  malarial —*see* Malaria
  metazoal B82.0
  monilial B37.82
  protozoal A07.9
  Salmonella A02.0
  schistosomal B65.1
  Schmitz (-Stutzer) A03.0
  Shiga (-Kruse) A03.0
  Shigella NOS —*see* Dysentery, bacillary
  Sonne A03.3
  strongyloidiasis B78.0
  trichomonal A07.8
  viral —*see also* Enteritis, viral A08.4
Dysequilibrium R42
Dysesthesia R20.8
  hysterical F44.6
▶**Dysferlinopathy** G71.033
Dysfibrinogenemia (congenital) D68.2
Dysfunction
  adrenal E27.9
    hyperfunction E27.0
  autonomic
    due to alcohol G31.2
    somatoform F45.8
  bladder N31.9
    neurogenic NOS —*see* Dysfunction, bladder, neuromuscular
    neuromuscular NOS N31.9
      atonic (motor) (sensory) N31.2
      autonomous N31.2
      flaccid N31.2
      nonreflex N31.2
      reflex N31.1
      specified NEC N31.8
      uninhibited N31.0
  bleeding, uterus N93.8
  cerebral G93.89
  colon K59.9
    psychogenic F45.8
  colostomy K94.03
  cystic duct K82.8
  cystostomy (stoma) —*see* Complications, cystostomy
  ejaculatory N53.19
    anejaculatory orgasm N53.13
    painful N53.12
    premature F52.4
    retarded N53.11
  endocrine NOS E34.9
  endometrium N85.8
  enterostomy K94.13
  erectile —*see* Dysfunction, sexual, male, erectile
  feeding, pediatric
    acute R63.31
    chronic R63.32
  gallbladder K82.8
  gastrostomy (stoma) K94.23
  gland, glandular NOS E34.9
    meibomian, of eyelid —*see* Dysfunction, meibomian gland
  heart I51.89
  hemoglobin D75.89
  hepatic K76.89
  hypophysis E23.7

Dysfunction *(Continued)*
  hypothalamic NEC E23.3
  ileostomy (stoma) K94.13
  jejunostomy (stoma) K94.13
  kidney —*see* Disease, renal
  labyrinthine —*see* subcategory H83.2
  left ventricular, following sudden emotional stress I51.81
  liver K76.89
  male —*see* Dysfunction, sexual, male
  meibomian gland, of eyelid H02.889
    left H02.886
      lower H02.885
      upper H02.884
      upper and lower eyelids H02.88B
    right H02.883
      lower H02.882
      upper H02.881
      upper and lower eyelids H02.88A
  orgasmic (female) F52.31
    male F52.32
  ovary E28.9
    specified NEC E28.8
  papillary muscle I51.89
  parathyroid E21.4
  physiological NEC R68.89
    psychogenic F59
  pineal gland E34.8
  pituitary (gland) E23.3
  platelets D69.1
  polyglandular E31.9
    specified NEC E31.8
  psychophysiologic F59
  psychosexual F52.9
    with
      dyspareunia F52.6
      premature ejaculation F52.4
      vaginismus F52.5
  pylorus K31.9
  rectum K59.9
    psychogenic F45.8
  reflex (sympathetic) —*see* Syndrome, pain, complex regional I
  segmental —*see* Dysfunction, somatic
  senile R54
  sexual (due to) R37
    alcohol F10.981
    amphetamine F15.981
      in
        abuse F15.181
        dependence F15.281
    anxiolytic F13.981
      in
        abuse F13.181
        dependence F13.281
    cocaine F14.981
      in
        abuse F14.181
        dependence F14.281
    excessive sexual drive F52.8
    failure of genital response (male) F52.21
      female F52.22
    female N94.9
      aversion F52.1
      dyspareunia N94.10
        psychogenic F52.6
      frigidity F52.22
      nymphomania F52.8
      orgasmic F52.31
      psychogenic F52.9
        aversion F52.1
        dyspareunia F52.6
        frigidity F52.22
        nymphomania F52.8
        orgasmic F52.31
        vaginismus F52.5
      vaginismus N94.2
        psychogenic F52.5
    hypnotic F13.981
      in
        abuse F13.181
        dependence F13.281

Dysfunction *(Continued)*
  sexual *(Continued)*
    inhibited orgasm (female) F52.31
      male F52.32
    lack
      of sexual enjoyment F52.1
      or loss of sexual desire F52.0
    male N53.9
      anejaculatory orgasm N53.13
      ejaculatory N53.19
        painful N53.12
        premature F52.4
        retarded N53.11
      erectile N52.9
        drug induced N52.2
        due to
          disease classified elsewhere N52.1
          drug N52.2
        postoperative (postprocedural) N52.39
          following
            cryotherapy N52.37
            interstitial seed therapy N52.36
            prostate ablative therapy N52.37
            prostatectomy N52.34
              radical N52.31
            radiation therapy N52.35
            radical cystectomy N52.32
            ultrasound ablative therapy N52.37
            urethral surgery N52.33
        psychogenic F52.21
        specified cause NEC N52.8
        vasculogenic
          arterial insufficiency N52.01
            with corporo-venous occlusive N52.03
          corporo-venous occlusive N52.02
            with arterial insufficiency N52.03
      impotence —*see* Dysfunction, sexual, male, erectile
      psychogenic F52.9
        aversion F52.1
        erectile F52.21
        orgasmic F52.32
        premature ejaculation F52.4
        satyriasis F52.8
        specified type NEC F52.8
      specified type NEC N53.8
    nonorganic F52.9
      specified NEC F52.8
    opioid F11.981
      in
        abuse F11.181
        dependence F11.281
    orgasmic dysfunction (female) F52.31
      male F52.32
    premature ejaculation F52.4
    psychoactive substances NEC F19.981
      in
        abuse F19.181
        dependence F19.281
    psychogenic F52.9
    sedative F13.981
      in
        abuse F13.181
        dependence F13.281
    sexual aversion F52.1
    vaginismus (nonorganic) (psychogenic) F52.5
  sinoatrial node I49.5
  somatic M99.09
    abdomen M99.09
    acromioclavicular M99.07
    cervical region M99.01
    cervicothoracic M99.01
    costochondral M99.08
    costovertebral M99.08
    head region M99.00
    hip M99.05
    lower extremity M99.06
    lumbar region M99.03

Dysfunction (Continued)
  somatic (Continued)
    lumbosacral M99.03
    occipitocervical M99.00
    pelvic region M99.05
    pubic M99.05
    rib cage M99.08
    sacral region M99.04
    sacrococcygeal M99.04
    sacroiliac M99.04
    specified NEC M99.09
    sternochondral M99.08
    sternoclavicular M99.07
    thoracic region M99.02
    thoracolumbar M99.02
    upper extremity M99.07
  somatoform autonomic F45.8
  stomach K31.89
    psychogenic F45.8
  suprarenal E27.9
    hyperfunction E27.0
  symbolic R48.9
    specified type NEC R48.8
  temporomandibular (joint) M26.69
    joint-pain syndrome M26.62-●
  testicular (endocrine) E29.9
    specified NEC E29.8
  thymus E32.9
  thyroid E07.9
  ureterostomy (stoma) —see Complications,
    stoma, urinary tract
  urethrostomy (stoma) —see Complications,
    stoma, urinary tract
  uterus, complicating delivery O62.9
    hypertonic O62.4
    hypotonic O62.2
      primary O62.0
      secondary O62.1
  ventricular I51.9
    with congestive heart failure —see also
      Failure, heart I50.9
    left, reversible, following sudden
      emotional stress I51.81
Dysgenesis
  gonadal (due to chromosomal anomaly) Q96.9
    pure Q99.1
  renal Q60.5
    bilateral Q60.4
    unilateral Q60.3
  reticular D72.0
  tidal platelet D69.3
Dysgerminoma
  specified site —see Neoplasm, malignant,
    by site
  unspecified site
    female C56.9
    male C62.90
Dysgeusia R43.2
Dysgraphia R27.8
Dyshidrosis, dysidrosis L30.1
Dyskaryotic cervical smear R87.619
Dyskeratosis L85.8
  cervix —see Dysplasia, cervix
  congenital Q82.8
  uterus NEC N85.8
Dyskinesia G24.9
  biliary (cystic duct or gallbladder) K82.8
  drug induced
    orofacial G24.01
  esophagus K22.4
  hysterical F44.4
  intestinal K59.89
  nonorganic origin F44.4
  orofacial (idiopathic) G24.4
    drug induced G24.01
  psychogenic F44.4
  subacute, drug induced G24.01
  tardive G24.01
    neuroleptic induced G24.01
  trachea J39.8
  tracheobronchial J98.09

Dyslalia (developmental) F80.0
Dyslexia R48.0
  developmental F81.0
Dyslipidemia E78.5
  depressed HDL cholesterol E78.6
  elevated fasting triglycerides E78.1
Dysmaturity —see also Light for dates
  pulmonary (newborn) (Wilson-Mikity)
    P27.0
Dysmenorrhea (essential) (exfoliative)
    N94.6
  congestive (syndrome) N94.6
  primary N94.4
  psychogenic F45.8
  secondary N94.5
Dysmetabolic syndrome X E88.81
Dysmetria R27.8
Dysmorphism (due to)
  alcohol Q86.0
  exogenous cause NEC Q86.8
  hydantoin Q86.1
  warfarin Q86.2
Dysmorphophobia (nondelusional)
    F45.22
  delusional F22
Dysnomia R47.01
Dysorexia R63.0
  psychogenic F50.89
Dysostosis
  cleidocranial, cleidocranialis Q74.0
  craniofacial Q75.1
  Fairbank's (idiopathic familial generalized
    osteophytosis) Q78.9
  mandibulofacial (incomplete) Q75.4
  multiplex E76.01
  oculomandibular Q75.5
Dyspareunia (female) N94.10
  deep N94.12
  male N53.12
  nonorganic F52.6
  psychogenic F52.6
  secondary N94.19
  specified NEC N94.19
  superficial (introital) N94.11
Dyspepsia R10.13
  atonic K30
  functional (allergic) (congenital)
    (gastrointestinal) (occupational)
    (reflex) K30
  intestinal K59.89
  nervous F45.8
  neurotic F45.8
  psychogenic F45.8
Dysphagia R13.10
  cervical R13.19
  following
    cerebral infarction I69.391
    cerebrovascular disease I69.991
      specified NEC I69.891
    intracerebral hemorrhage I69.191
    nontraumatic intracranial hemorrhage
      NEC I69.291
    specified disease NEC I69.891
    subarachnoid hemorrhage I69.091
  functional (hysterical) F45.8
  hysterical F45.8
  nervous (hysterical) F45.8
  neurogenic R13.19
  oral phase R13.11
  oropharyngeal phase R13.12
  pharyngeal phase R13.13
  pharyngoesophageal phase R13.14
  psychogenic F45.8
  sideropenic D50.1
  spastica K22.4
  specified NEC R13.19
Dysphagocytosis, congenital D71
Dysphasia R47.02
  developmental
    expressive type F80.1
    receptive type F80.2

Dysphasia (Continued)
  following
    cerebrovascular disease I69.921
      cerebral infarction I69.321
      intracerebral hemorrhage I69.121
    nontraumatic intracranial hemorrhage NEC
      I69.221
      specified disease NEC I69.821
      subarachnoid hemorrhage I69.021
Dysphonia R49.0
  functional F44.4
  hysterical F44.4
  psychogenic F44.4
  spastica J38.3
Dysphoria
  gender F64.9
    in
      adolescence and adulthood
        F64.0
      children F64.2
    specified NEC F64.8
    postpartal O90.6
Dyspituitarism E23.3
Dysplasia —see also Anomaly
  acetabular, congenital Q65.89
  alveolar capillary, with vein misalignment
    J84.843
  anus (histologically confirmed) (mild)
    (moderate) K62.82
    severe D01.3
  arrhythmogenic right ventricular I42.8
  arterial, fibromuscular I77.3
  asphyxiating thoracic (congenital) Q77.2
  brain Q07.9
  bronchopulmonary, perinatal P27.1
  cervix (uteri) N87.9
    mild N87.0
    moderate N87.1
    severe D06.9
  chondroectodermal Q77.6
  colon D12.6
  craniometaphyseal Q78.58
  dentinal K00.5
  diaphyseal, progressive Q78.3
  dystrophic Q77.5
  ectodermal (anhidrotic) (congenital)
    (hereditary) Q82.4
    hydrotic Q82.8
  epithelial, uterine cervix —see Dysplasia,
    cervix
  eye (congenital) Q11.2
  fibrous
    bone NEC (monostotic) M85.00
      ankle M85.07-●
      foot M85.07-●
      forearm M85.03-●
      hand M85.04-●
      lower leg M85.06-●
      multiple site M85.09
      neck M85.08
      rib M85.08
      shoulder M85.01-●
      skull M85.08
      specified site NEC M85.08
      thigh M85.05-●
      toe M85.07-●
      upper arm M85.02-●
      vertebra M85.08
    diaphyseal, progressive Q78.3
    jaw M27.8
    polyostotic Q78.1
  florid osseous —see also Cyst, calcifying
    odontogenic
  high grade, focal D12.6
  hip, congenital Q65.89
  joint, congenital Q74.8
  kidney Q61.4
    multicystic Q61.4
  leg Q74.2
  lung, congenital (not associated with short
    gestation) Q33.6

▶ New ⇒ Revised ~~deleted~~ Deleted ● Use Additional Character(s)

▶ New　⇒ Revised　deleted Deleted　● Use Additional Character(s)

Dystrophy, dystrophia *(Continued)*
  muscular *(Continued)*
    limb-girdle *(Continued)*
      ▶ type 2 (autosomal recessive) G71.038
        ▶ specified NEC G71.038
      ▶ type 2A (autosomal recessive) G71.032
      ▶ type 2B (autosomal recessive) G71.033
      ▶ type 2C (autosomal recessive) G71.0349
      ▶ type 2D (autosomal recessive) G71.0341
      ▶ type 2E (autosomal recessive) G71.0342
      ▶ type 2F (autosomal recessive) G71.0349
      ▶ type 2I (autosomal recessive) G71.038
      ▶ type 2L (autosomal recessive) G71.035
    myotonic G71.11
    progressive (hereditary) G71.09
      Charcot-Marie (-Tooth) type G60.0
    pseudohypertrophic (infantile) G71.01
    scapulohumeral G71.02
    scapuloperoneal G71.09
    severe (Duchenne type) G71.01
    specified type NEC G71.09

Dystrophy, dystrophia *(Continued)*
  myocardium, myocardial —*see*
    Degeneration, myocardial
  nail L60.3
    congenital Q84.6
  nutritional E45
  ocular G71.09
  oculocerebrorenal E72.03
  oculopharyngeal G71.09
  ovarian N83.8
  polyglandular E31.8
  reflex (neuromuscular) (sympathetic) —
    see Syndrome, pain, complex regional I
  retinal (hereditary) H35.50
    in
      lipid storage disorders E75.6 *[H36]*
      systemic lipidoses E75.6 *[H36]*
    involving
      pigment epithelium H35.54
      sensory area H35.53

Dystrophy, dystrophia *(Continued)*
  retinal *(Continued)*
    pigmentary H35.52
    vitreoretinal H35.51
  Salzmann's nodular —*see* Degeneration,
    cornea, nodular
  scapuloperoneal G71.09
  skin NEC L98.8
  sympathetic (reflex) —*see* Syndrome, pain,
    complex regional I
    cervical G90.2
  tapetoretinal H35.54
  thoracic, asphyxiating Q77.2
  unguium L60.3
    congenital Q84.6
  vitreoretinal H35.51
  vulva N90.4
  yellow (liver) —*see* Failure, hepatic
Dysuria R30.0
  psychogenic F45.8

▶ New   ⇒ Revised   ~~deleted~~ Deleted   ● Use Additional Character(s)

Edema, edematous *(Continued)*
  cardiovascular —*see* Failure, heart, congestive
  cerebral —*see* Edema, brain
  cerebrospinal —*see* Edema, brain
  cervix (uteri) (acute) N88.8
    puerperal, postpartum O90.89
  chronic hereditary Q82.0
  circumscribed, acute T78.3
    hereditary D84.1
  conjunctiva H11.42-●
  cornea H18.2-●
    idiopathic H18.22-●
    secondary H18.23-●
      due to contact lens H18.21-●
  due to
    lymphatic obstruction I89.0
    salt retention E87.0
  epiglottis —*see* Edema, glottis
  essential, acute T78.3
    hereditary D84.1
  extremities, lower —*see* Edema, legs
  eyelid NEC H02.849
    left H02.846
      lower H02.845
      upper H02.844
    right H02.843
      lower H02.842
      upper H02.841
  familial, hereditary Q82.0
  famine —*see* Malnutrition, severe
  generalized R60.1
  glottis, glottic, glottidis (obstructive) (passive)
      J38.4
    allergic T78.3
      hereditary D84.1
  heart —*see* Failure, heart, congestive
  heat T67.7
  hereditary Q82.0
  inanition —*see* Malnutrition, severe
  intracranial G93.6
  iris H21.89
  joint —*see* Effusion, joint
  larynx —*see* Edema, glottis
  legs R60.0
    due to venous obstruction I87.1
    hereditary Q82.0
  localized R60.0
    due to venous obstruction I87.1
  lower limbs —*see* Edema, legs
  lung J81.1
    with heart condition or failure —*see*
        Failure, ventricular, left
    acute J81.0
    chemical (acute) J68.1
      chronic J68.1
    chronic J81.1
      due to
        chemicals, gases, fumes or vapors
            (inhalation) J68.1
        external agent J70.9
          specified NEC J70.8
        radiation J70.1
    due to
      chemicals, fumes or vapors (inhalation)
          J68.1
      external agent J70.9
        specified NEC J70.8
      high altitude T70.29
      near drowning T75.1
      radiation J70.0
    meaning failure, left ventricle I50.1
  lymphatic I89.0
    due to mastectomy I97.2
  macula H35.81
    cystoid, following cataract surgery —*see*
        Complications, postprocedural,
        following cataract surgery
    diabetic —*see* Diabetes, by type, with,
        retinopathy, with macular edema
  malignant —*see* Gangrene, gas
  Milroy's Q82.0

Edema, edematous *(Continued)*
  nasopharynx J39.2
  newborn P83.30
    hydrops fetalis —*see* Hydrops, fetalis
    specified NEC P83.39
  nutritional —*see also* Malnutrition, severe
    with dyspigmentation, skin and hair E40
  optic disc or nerve —*see* Papilledema
  orbit H05.22-●
  pancreas K86.89
  papilla, optic —*see* Papilledema
  penis N48.89
  periodic T78.3
    hereditary D84.1
  pharynx J39.2
  pulmonary —*see* Edema, lung
  Quincke's T78.3
    hereditary D84.1
  renal —*see* Nephrosis
  retina H35.81
    diabetic —*see* Diabetes, by type, with,
        retinopathy, with macular edema
  salt E87.0
  scrotum N50.89
  seminal vesicle N50.89
  spermatic cord N50.89
  spinal (cord) (vascular) (nontraumatic) G95.19
  starvation —*see* Malnutrition, severe
  stasis —*see* Hypertension, venous, (chronic)
  subglottic —*see* Edema, glottis
  supraglottic —*see* Edema, glottis
  testis N44.8
  tunica vaginalis N50.89
  vas deferens N50.89
  vulva (acute) N90.89
Edentulism —*see* Absence, teeth, acquired
Edsall's disease T67.2
Educational handicap Z55.9
  less than a high school diploma Z55.5
  no general equivalence degree (GED) Z55.5
  specified NEC Z55.8
Edward's syndrome —*see* Trisomy, 18
Effect, adverse
  abnormal gravitational (G) forces or states
      T75.81
  abuse —*see* Maltreatment
  air pressure T70.9
    specified NEC T70.8
  altitude (high) —*see* Effect, adverse, high
      altitude
  anesthesia —*see also* Anesthesia T88.59
    in labor and delivery O74.9
    local, toxic
      in labor and delivery O74.4-●
      in pregnancy NEC O29.3-●
      postpartum, puerperal O89.3
    postpartum, puerperal O89.9
    specified NEC T88.59
      in labor and delivery O74.8
      postpartum, puerperal O89.8
    spinal and epidural T88.59
      headache T88.59
        in labor and delivery O74.5
        postpartum, puerperal O89.4
      specified NEC
        in labor and delivery O74.6
        postpartum, puerperal O89.5
  antitoxin —*see* Complications, vaccination
  atmospheric pressure T70.9
    due to explosion T70.8
    high T70.3
    low —*see* Effect, adverse, high altitude
    specified effect NEC T70.8
  biological, correct substance properly
      administered —*see* Effect, adverse, drug
  blood (derivatives) (serum) (transfusion) —
      see Complications, transfusion
  chemical substance —*see* Table of Drugs and
      Chemicals
  cold (temperature) (weather) T69.9
    chilblains T69.1
    frostbite —*see* Frostbite
    specified effect NEC T69.8

Effect, adverse *(Continued)*
  drugs and medicaments T88.7
    specified drug —*see* Table of Drugs and
        Chemicals, by drug, adverse effect
    specified effect — code to condition
  electric current, electricity (shock) T75.4
    burn —*see* Burn
  exertion (excessive) T73.3
  exposure —*see* Exposure
  external cause NEC T75.89
  foodstuffs T78.1
    allergic reaction —*see* Allergy, food
      causing anaphylaxis —*see* Shock,
          anaphylactic, due to food
    noxious —*see* Poisoning, food, noxious
  gases, fumes, or vapors T59.9-●
    specified agent —*see* Table of Drugs and
        Chemicals
  glue (airplane) sniffing
    due to drug abuse —*see* Abuse, drug,
        inhalant
    due to drug dependence —*see* Dependence,
        drug, inhalant
  heat —*see* Heat
  high altitude NEC T70.29
    anoxia T70.29
    on
      ears T70.0
      sinuses T70.1
    polycythemia D75.1
  high pressure fluids T70.4
  hot weather —*see* Heat
  hunger T73.0
  immersion, foot —*see* Immersion
  immunization —*see* Complications,
      vaccination
  immunological agents —*see* Complications,
      vaccination
  infrared (radiation) (rays) NOS T66
    dermatitis or eczema L59.8
  infusion —*see* Complications, infusion
  lack of care of infants —*see* Maltreatment,
      child
  lightning —*see* Lightning
  medical care T88.9
    specified NEC T88.8
  medicinal substance, correct, properly
      administered —*see* Effect, adverse, drug
  motion T75.3
  noise, on inner ear —*see* subcategory H83.3
  overheated places —*see* Heat
  psychosocial, of work environment Z56.5
  radiation (diagnostic) (infrared) (natural
      source) (therapeutic) (ultraviolet) (X-ray)
      NOS T66
    dermatitis or eczema —*see* Dermatitis, due
        to, radiation
    fibrosis of lung J70.1
    pneumonitis J70.0
    pulmonary manifestations
      acute J70.0
      chronic J70.1
    skin L59.9
  radioactive substance NOS
    dermatitis or eczema —*see* Radiodermatitis
  reduced temperature T69.9
    immersion foot or hand —*see* Immersion
    specified effect NEC T69.8
  serum NEC (*see also* Reaction, serum) T80.69
  specified NEC T78.8
    external cause NEC T75.89
  strangulation —*see* Asphyxia, traumatic
  submersion T75.1
  thirst T73.1
  toxic —*see* Toxicity
  transfusion —*see* Complications, transfusion
  ultraviolet (radiation) (rays) NOS T66
    burn —*see* Burn
    dermatitis or eczema —*see* Dermatitis, due
        to, ultraviolet rays
      acute L56.8

▶ New   ⇒ Revised   ~~deleted~~ Deleted   ● Use Additional Character(s)

Effect, adverse *(Continued)*
  vaccine (any) —*see* Complications, vaccination
  vibration —*see* Vibration, adverse effects
  water pressure NEC T70.9
    specified NEC T70.8
  weightlessness T75.82
  whole blood —*see* Complications, transfusion
  work environment Z56.5
Effect(s) (of) (from) —*see* Effect, adverse NEC
Effects, late —*see* Sequelae
Effluvium
  anagen L65.1
  telogen L65.0
Effort syndrome (psychogenic) F45.8
Effusion
  amniotic fluid —*see* Pregnancy, complicated
    by, premature rupture of membranes
  brain (serous) G93.6
  bronchial —*see* Bronchitis
  cerebral G93.6
  cerebrospinal —*see also* Meningitis
    vessel G93.6
  chest —*see* Effusion, pleura
  chylous, chyliform (pleura) J94.0
  intracranial G93.6
  joint M25.40
    ankle M25.47-●
    elbow M25.42-●
    foot joint M25.47-●
    hand joint M25.44-●
    hip M25.45-●
    knee M25.46-●
    shoulder M25.41-●
    specified joint NEC M25.48
    wrist M25.43-●
  malignant pleural J91.0
  meninges —*see* Meningitis
  pericardium, pericardial (noninflammatory)
    I31.39
    acute —*see* Pericarditis, acute
    ▶malignant, in disease classified elsewhere
      I31.31
    ▶specified type, NEC I31.39
  peritoneal (chronic) R18.8
  pleura, pleurisy, pleuritic, pleuropericardial
    J90
    chylous, chyliform J94.0
    due to systemic lupus erythematosis M32.13
    in conditions classified elsewhere J91.8
    influenzal —*see* Influenza, with, respiratory
      manifestations NEC
    malignant J91.0
    newborn P28.89
    tuberculous NEC A15.6
      primary (progressive) A15.7
  spinal —*see* Meningitis
  thorax, thoracic —*see* Effusion, pleura
Egg shell nails L60.3
  congenital Q84.6
EGPA (eosinophilic granulomatosis with
    polyangiitis) M30.1
Egyptian splenomegaly B65.1
Ehlers-Danlos syndrome (*see also* Syndrome,
    Ehlers-Danlos) Q79.60
Ehrlichiosis A77.40
  due to
    E. chafeensis A77.41
    E. ewingii A77.49
    E. muris euclairensis A77.49
    E. sennetsu A79.81
    specified organism NEC A77.49
Eichstedt's disease B36.0
Eisenmenger's
  complex or syndrome I27.83
  defect Q21.8
Ejaculation
  delayed F52.32
  painful N53.12
  premature F52.4
  retarded N53.11
  retrograde N53.14
  semen, painful N53.12
    psychogenic F52.6

Ekbom's syndrome (restless legs) G25.81
Ekman's syndrome (brittle bones and blue
    sclera) Q78.0
Elastic skin Q82.8
  acquired L57.4
Elastofibroma —*see* Neoplasm, connective
    tissue, benign
Elastoma (juvenile) Q82.8
  Miescher's L87.2
Elastomyofibrosis I42.4
Elastosis
  actinic, solar L57.8
  atrophicans (senile) L57.4
  perforans serpiginosa L87.2
  senilis L57.4
Elbow —*see* condition
Electric current, electricity, effects (concussion)
    (fatal) (nonfatal) (shock) T75.4
  burn —*see* Burn
Electric feet syndrome E53.8
Electrocution T75.4
  from electroshock gun (taser) T75.4
Electrolyte imbalance E87.8
  with
    abortion —*see* Abortion by type,
      complicated by, electrolyte imbalance
    ectopic pregnancy O08.5
    molar pregnancy O08.5
Elephantiasis (nonfilarial) I89.0
  arabicum —*see* Infestation, filarial
  bancroftian B74.0
  congenital (any site) (hereditary) Q82.0
  due to
    Brugia (malayi) B74.1
      timori B74.2
    mastectomy I97.2
    Wuchereria (bancrofti) B74.0
  eyelid H02.859
    left H02.856
      lower H02.855
      upper H02.854
    right H02.853
      lower H02.852
      upper H02.851
  filarial, filariensis —*see* Infestation, filarial
  glandular I89.0
  graecorum A30.9
  lymphangiectatic I89.0
  lymphatic vessel I89.0
    due to mastectomy I97.2
  scrotum (nonfilarial) I89.0
  streptococcal I89.0
  surgical I97.89
    postmastectomy I97.2
  telangiectodes I89.0
  vulva (nonfilarial) N90.89
Elevated, elevation
  alanine transaminase (ALT) R74.01
  ALT (alanine transaminase) R74.01
  antibody titer R76.0
  aspartate transaminase (AST) R74.01
  AST (aspartate transaminase) R74.01
  basal metabolic rate R94.8
  blood pressure —*see also* Hypertension
    reading (incidental) (isolated) (nonspecific),
      no diagnosis of hypertension R03.0
  blood sugar R73.9
  body temperature (of unknown origin) R50.9
  C-reactive protein (CRP) R79.82
  cancer antigen 125 [CA 125] R97.1
  carcinoembryonic antigen [CEA] R97.0
  cholesterol E78.00
    with high triglycerides E78.2
  conjugate, eye H51.0
  diaphragm, congenital Q79.1
  erythrocyte sedimentation rate R70.0
  fasting glucose R73.01
  fasting triglycerides E78.1
  finding on laboratory examination —*see*
    Findings, abnormal, inconclusive,
    without diagnosis, by type of exam

Elevated, elevation *(Continued)*
  GFR (glomerular filtration rate) —*see*
    Findings, abnormal, inconclusive,
    without diagnosis, by type of exam
  glucose tolerance (oral) R73.02
  immunoglobulin level R76.8
  indoleacetic acid R82.5
  lactic acid dehydrogenase (LDH) level R74.02
  leukocytes D72.829
  lipoprotein a (Lp(a)) level E78.41
  liver function
    study R94.5
    test R79.89
      alkaline phosphatase R74.8
      aminotransferase R74.01
      bilirubin R17
      hepatic enzyme R74.8
      lactate dehydrogenase R74.02
  (Lp(a)) (lipoprotein(a)) E78.41
  lymphocytes D72.820
  prostate specific antigen [PSA] R97.20
  Rh titer —*see* Complication(s), transfusion,
    incompatibility reaction, Rh (factor)
  scapula, congenital Q74.0
  sedimentation rate R70.0
  SGOT R74.01
  SGPT R74.01
  transaminase level R74.01
  triglycerides E78.1
    with high cholesterol E78.2
  troponin R77.8
  tumor associated antigens [TAA] NEC R97.8
  tumor specific antigens [TSA] NEC R97.8
  urine level of
    17-ketosteroids R82.5
    catecholamine R82.5
    indoleacetic acid R82.5
    steroids R82.5
    vanillylmandelic acid (VMA) R82.5
  venous pressure I87.8
  white blood cell count D72.829
    specified NEC D72.828
Elliptocytosis (congenital) (hereditary) D58.1
  Hb C (disease) D58.1
  hemoglobin disease D58.1
  sickle-cell (disease) D57.8-●
    trait D57.3
Ellison-Zollinger syndrome E16.4
Ellis-van Creveld syndrome
    (chondroectodermal dysplasia) Q77.6
Elongated, elongation (congenital) —*see also*
    Distortion
  bone Q79.9
  cervix (uteri) Q51.828
    acquired N88.4
    hypertrophic N88.4
  colon Q43.8
  common bile duct Q44.5
  cystic duct Q44.5
  frenulum, penis Q55.69
  labia minora (acquired) N90.69
  ligamentum patellae Q74.1
  petiolus (epiglottidis) Q31.8
  tooth, teeth K00.2
  uvula Q38.6
Eltor cholera A00.1
Emaciation R64
  due to manutrition E43
Embadomoniasis A07.8
Embedded tooth, teeth K01.0
  root only K08.3
Embolic —*see* condition
Embolism (multiple) (paradoxical) I74.9
  air (any site) (traumatic) T79.0
    following
      abortion —*see* Abortion by type
        complicated by embolism
      ectopic pregnancy O08.2
      infusion, therapeutic injection or
        transfusion T80.0
      molar pregnancy O08.2

Embolism (Continued)
  air (Continued)
    following (Continued)
      procedure NEC
        artery T81.719
          mesenteric T81.710
          renal T81.711
          specified NEC T81.718
        vein T81.72
    in pregnancy, childbirth or puerperium —
      see Embolism, obstetric
  amniotic fluid (pulmonary) —see also
    Embolism, obstetric
    following
      abortion —see Abortion by type
        complicated by embolism
      ectopic pregnancy O08.2
      molar pregnancy O08.2
  aorta, aortic I74.10
    abdominal I74.09
      saddle I74.01
    bifurcation I74.09
    saddle I74.01
    thoracic I74.11
  artery I74.9
    auditory, internal I65.8
    basilar —see Occlusion, artery, basilar
    carotid (common) (internal) —see
      Occlusion, artery, carotid
    cerebellar (anterior inferior) (posterior
      inferior) (superior) I66.3
    cerebral —see Occlusion, artery, cerebral
    choroidal (anterior) I65.8
    communicating posterior I65.8
    coronary —see also Infarct, myocardium
      not resulting in infarction I24.0
    extremity I74.4
      lower I74.3
      upper I74.2
    hypophyseal I65.8
    iliac I74.5
    limb I74.4
      lower I74.3
      upper I74.2
    mesenteric (with gangrene) —see also
      Ischemia, intestine, acute K55.09
    ophthalmic —see Occlusion, artery, retina
    peripheral I74.4
    pontine I65.8
    precerebral —see Occlusion, artery,
      precerebral
    pulmonary —see Embolism, pulmonary
    renal N28.0
    retinal —see Occlusion, artery, retina
    septic I76
    specified NEC I74.8
    vertebral —see Occlusion, artery, vertebral
  basilar (artery) I65.1
  blood clot
    following
      abortion —see Abortion by type
        complicated by embolism
      ectopic or molar pregnancy O08.2
    in pregnancy, childbirth or puerperium —
      see Embolism, obstetric
  brain —see also Occlusion, artery, cerebral
    following
      abortion —see Abortion by type
        complicated by embolism
      ectopic or molar pregnancy O08.2
    puerperal, postpartum, childbirth —see
      Embolism, obstetric
  capillary I78.8
  cardiac —see also Infarct, myocardium
    not resulting in infarction I51.3
  carotid (artery) (common) (internal) —see
    Occlusion, artery, carotid
  cavernous sinus (venous) —see Embolism,
    intracranial venous sinus
  cerebral —see Occlusion, artery, cerebral
  cholesterol —see Atheroembolism

Embolism (Continued)
  coronary (artery or vein) (systemic) —see
    Occlusion, coronary
  due to device, implant or graft —see also
    Complications, by site and type,
    specified NEC
    arterial graft NEC T82.818
    breast (implant) T85.818
    catheter NEC T85.818
      dialysis (renal) T82.818
        intraperitoneal T85.818
      infusion NEC T82.818
        spinal (epidural) (subdural) T85.810
      urinary (indwelling) T83.81
    electronic (electrode) (pulse generator)
      (stimulator)
      bone T84.81
      cardiac T82.817
      nervous system (brain) (peripheral
        nerve) (spinal) T85.810
      urinary T83.81
    fixation, internal (orthopedic) NEC T84.81
    gastrointestinal (bile duct) (esophagus)
      T85.818
    genital NEC T83.81
    heart (graft) (valve) T82.817
    joint prosthesis T84.81
    ocular (corneal graft) (orbital implant)
      T85.818
    orthopedic (bone graft) NEC T86.838
    specified NEC T85.818
    urinary (graft) NEC T83.81
    vascular NEC T82.818
    ventricular intracranial shunt T85.810
  extremities
    lower —see Embolism, vein, lower
      extremity
      arterial I74.3
    upper I74.2
  eye H34.9
  fat (cerebral) (pulmonary) (systemic) T79.1
    complicating delivery —see Embolism,
      obstetric
    following
      abortion —see Abortion by type
        complicated by embolism
      ectopic or molar pregnancy O08.2
  following
    abortion —see Abortion by type
      complicated by embolism
    ectopic or molar pregnancy O08.2
    infusion, therapeutic injection or transfusion
      air T80.0
  heart (fatty) —see also Infarct, myocardium
    not resulting in infarction I51.3
  hepatic (vein) I82.0
  in pregnancy, childbirth or puerperium —see
    Embolism, obstetric
  intestine (artery) (vein) (with gangrene) —see
    also Ischemia, intestine, acute K55.039
  intracranial —see also Occlusion, artery,
    cerebral
    venous sinus (any) G08
      nonpyogenic I67.6
  intraspinal venous sinuses or veins G08
    nonpyogenic G95.19
  kidney (artery) N28.0
  lateral sinus (venous) —see Embolism,
    intracranial, venous sinus
  leg —see Embolism, vein, lower extremity
    arterial I74.3
  longitudinal sinus (venous) —see Embolism,
    intracranial, venous sinus
  lung (massive) —see Embolism, pulmonary
  meninges I66.8
  mesenteric (artery) (vein) (with gangrene) —
    see also Ischemia, intestine, acute K55.059
  obstetric (in) (pulmonary)
    childbirth O88.22
      air O88.02
      amniotic fluid O88.12
      blood clot O88.22

Embolism (Continued)
  obstetric (Continued)
    childbirth (Continued)
      fat O88.82
      pyemic O88.32
      septic O88.32
      specified type NEC O88.82
    pregnancy O88.21-•
      air O88.01-•
      amniotic fluid O88.11-•
      blood clot O88.21-•
      fat O88.81-•
      pyemic O88.31-•
      septic O88.31-•
      specified type NEC O88.81-•
    puerperal O88.23
      air O88.03
      amniotic fluid O88.13
      blood clot O88.23
      fat O88.83
      pyemic O88.33
      septic O88.33
      specified type NEC O88.83
  ophthalmic —see Occlusion, artery, retina
  penis N48.81
  peripheral artery NOS I74.4
  pituitary E23.6
  popliteal (artery) I74.3
  portal (vein) I81
  postoperative, postprocedural
    artery T81.719
      mesenteric T81.710
      renal T81.711
      specified NEC T81.718
    vein T81.72
  precerebral artery —see Occlusion, artery,
    precerebral
  puerperal —see Embolism, obstetric
  pulmonary (acute) (artery) (vein) I26.99
    with acute cor pulmonale I26.09
    chronic I27.82
    following
      abortion —see Abortion by type
        complicated by embolism
      ectopic or molar pregnancy O08.2
    healed or old Z86.711
    in pregnancy, childbirth or puerperium —
      see Embolism, obstetric
    multiple subsegmental without acute cor
      pulmonale I26.94
    personal history of Z86.711
    saddle I26.92
      with acute cor pulmonale I26.02
    septic I26.90
      with acute cor pulmonale I26.01
    single subsegmental without acute cor
      pulmonale I26.93
    subsegmental NOS I26.93
  pyemic (multiple) I76
    following
      abortion —see Abortion by type
        complicated by embolism
      ectopic or molar pregnancy O08.2
    Hemophilus influenzae A41.3
    pneumococcal A40.3
      with pneumonia J13
    puerperal, postpartum, childbirth (any
      organism) —see Embolism, obstetric
    specified organism NEC A41.89
    staphylococcal A41.2
    streptococcal A40.9
  renal (artery) N28.0
    vein I82.3
  retina, retinal —see Occlusion, artery,
    retina
  saddle
    abdominal aorta I74.01
    pulmonary artery I26.92
      with acute cor pulmonale I26.02
  septic (arterial) I76
    complicating abortion —see Abortion, by
      type, complicated by, embolism

▶ New   ⇒ Revised   ~~deleted~~ Deleted   • Use Additional Character(s)

Embolism (Continued)
sinus —see Embolism, intracranial, venous
    sinus
soap complicating abortion —see Abortion,
    by type, complicated by, embolism
spinal cord G95.19
    pyogenic origin G06.1
spleen, splenic (artery) I74.8
upper extremity I74.2
vein (acute) I82.90
    antecubital I82.61-●
        chronic I82.71-●
    axillary I82.A1-●
        chronic I82.A2-●
    basilic I82.61-●
        chronic I82.71-●
    brachial I82.62-●
        chronic I82.72-●
    brachiocephalic (innominate) I82.290
        chronic I82.291
  ▶calf, muscle I82.46-●
      ▶chronic I82.56-●
    cephalic I82.61-●
        chronic I82.71-●
    chronic I82.91
    deep (DVT) I82.40-●
        calf I82.4Z-●
            chronic I82.5Z-●
        lower leg I82.4Z-●
            chronic I82.5Z-●
        thigh I82.4Y-●
            chronic I82.5Y-●
        upper leg I82.4Y
            chronic I82.5y-●
    femoral I82.41-●
        chronic I82.51-●
  ▶gastrocnemial I82.46-●
      ▶chronic I82.56-●
    iliac (iliofemoral) I82.42-●
        chronic I82.52-●
    innominate I82.290
        chronic I82.291
    internal jugular I82.C1-●
        chronic I82.C2-●
    lower extremity
        deep I82.40-●
            chronic I82.50-●
            specified NEC I82.49-●
                chronic NEC I82.59-●
        distal
            deep I82.4Z-●
        proximal
            deep I82.4Y-●
                chronic I82.5Y-●
        superficial I82.81-●
  ▶peroneal I82.45-●
      ▶chronic I82.55-●
    popliteal I82.43-●
        chronic I82.53-●
    radial I82.62-●
        chronic I82.72-●
    renal I82.3
    saphenous (greater) (lesser) I82.81-●
  ▶soleal I82.46-●
      ▶chronic I82.56-●
    specified NEC I82.890
        chronic NEC I82.891
    subclavian I82.B1-●
        chronic I82.B2-●
    thoracic NEC I82.290
        chronic I82.291
    tibial I82.44-●
        chronic I82.54-●
    ulnar I82.62-●
        chronic I82.72-●
    upper extremity I82.60-●
        chronic I82.70-●
        deep I82.62-●
            chronic I82.72-●
        superficial I82.61-●
            chronic I82.71-●

Embolism (Continued)
vena cava
    inferior (acute) I82.220
        chronic I82.221
    superior (acute) I82.210
        chronic I82.211
venous sinus G08
vessels of brain —see Occlusion, artery, cerebral
Embolus —see Embolism
Embryoma —see also Neoplasm, uncertain
        behavior, by site
    benign —see Neoplasm, benign, by site
    kidney C64.-●
    liver C22.0
    malignant —see also Neoplasm, malignant,
        by site
        kidney C64.-●
        liver C22.0
        testis C62.9-●
            descended (scrotal) C62.1-●
            undescended C62.0-●
    testis C62.9-●
        descended (scrotal) C62.1-●
        undescended C62.0-●
Embryonic
    circulation Q28.9
    heart Q28.9
    vas deferens Q55.4
Embryopathia NOS Q89.9
Embryotoxon Q13.4
Emesis —see Vomiting
Emotional lability R45.86
Emotionality, pathological F60.3
Emotogenic disease —see Disorder,
        psychogenic
Emphysema (atrophic) (bullous) (chronic)
        (interlobular) (lung) (obstructive)
        (pulmonary) (senile) (vesicular) J43.9
    cellular tissue (traumatic) T79.7
        surgical T81.82
    centrilobular J43.2
    compensatory J98.3
    congenital (interstitial) P25.0
    conjunctiva H11.89
    connective tissue (traumatic) T79.7
        surgical T81.82
    due to chemicals, gases, fumes or vapors J68.4
    eyelid(s) —see Disorder, eyelid, specified type
            NEC
        surgical T81.82
        traumatic T79.7
    interstitial J98.2
        congenital P25.0
        perinatal period P25.0
    laminated tissue T79.7
        surgical T81.82
    mediastinal J98.2
        newborn P25.2
    orbit, orbital —see Disorder, orbit, specified
            type NEC
    panacinar J43.1
    panlobular J43.1
    specified NEC J43.8
    subcutaneous (traumatic) T79.7
        nontraumatic J98.2
        postprocedural T81.82
        surgical T81.82
    surgical T81.82
    thymus (gland) (congenital) E32.8
    traumatic (subcutaneous) T79.7
    unilateral J43.0
Empty nest syndrome Z60.0
Empyema (acute) (chest) (double) (pleura)
        (supradiaphragmatic) (thorax) J86.9
    with fistula J86.0
    accessory sinus (chronic) —see Sinusitis
    antrum (chronic) —see Sinusitis, maxillary
    brain (any part) —see Abscess, brain
    ethmoidal (chronic) (sinus) —see Sinusitis,
            ethmoidal
    extradural —see Abscess, extradural
    frontal (chronic) (sinus) —see Sinusitis, frontal
    gallbladder K81.0

Empyema (Continued)
mastoid (process) (acute) —see Mastoiditis,
        acute
maxilla, maxillary M27.2
    sinus (chronic) —see Sinusitis, maxillary
nasal sinus (chronic) —see Sinusitis
sinus (accessory) (chronic) (nasal) —see
        Sinusitis
sphenoidal (sinus) (chronic) —see Sinusitis,
        sphenoidal
subarachnoid —see Abscess, extradural
subdural —see Abscess, subdural
tuberculous A15.6
ureter —see Ureteritis
ventricular —see Abscess, brain
En coup de sabre lesion L94.1
Enamel pearls K00.2
Enameloma K00.2
Enanthema, viral B09
Encephalitis (chronic) (hemorrhagic)
        (idiopathic) (nonepidemic) (spurious)
        (subacute) G04.90
    acute —see also Encephalitis, viral A86
        disseminated G04.00
            infectious G04.01
            noninfectious G04.81
            postimmunization (postvaccination)
                    G04.02
            postinfectious G04.01
        inclusion body A85.8
        necrotizing hemorrhagic G04.30
            postimmunization G04.32
            postinfectious G04.31
            specified NEC G04.39
    arboviral, arbovirus NEC A85.2
    arthropod-borne NEC (viral) A85.2
    Australian A83.4
    California (virus) A83.5
    Central European (tick-borne) A84.1
    Czechoslovakian A84.1
    Dawson's (inclusion body) A81.1
    diffuse sclerosing A81.1
    disseminated, acute G04.00
    due to
        cat scratch disease A28.1
        human immunodeficiency virus (HIV)
                disease B20 [G05.3]
        malaria —see Malaria
        rickettsiosis —see Rickettsiosis
        smallpox inoculation G04.02
        typhus —see Typhus
    Eastern equine A83.2
    endemic (viral) A86
    epidemic NEC (viral) A86
    equine (acute) (infectious) (viral) A83.9
        Eastern A83.2
        Venezuelan A92.2
        Western A83.1
    Far Eastern (tick-borne) A84.0
    following vaccination or other immunization
            procedure G04.02
    herpes zoster B02.0
    herpesviral B00.4
        due to herpesvirus 6 B10.01
        due to herpesvirus 7 B10.09
        specified NEC B10.09
    Ilheus (virus) A83.8
    in (due to)
        actinomycosis A42.82
        adenovirus A85.1
        African trypanosomiasis B56.9 [G05.3]
        Chagas' disease (chronic) B57.42
        cytomegalovirus B25.8
        enterovirus A85.0
        herpes (simplex) virus B00.4
            due to herpesvirus 6 B10.01
            due to herpesvirus 7 B10.09
            specified NEC B10.09
        infectious disease NEC B99 [G05.3]
        influenza —see Influenza, with,
                encephalopathy
        listeriosis A32.12
        measles B05.0

Encephalitis (Continued)
in (Continued)
mumps B26.2
naegleriasis B60.2
parasitic disease NEC B89 [G05.3]
poliovirus A80.9 [G05.3]
rubella B06.01
syphilis
congenital A50.42
late A52.14
systemic lupus erythematosus M32.19
toxoplasmosis (acquired) B58.2
congenital P37.1
tuberculosis A17.82
zoster B02.0
inclusion body A81.1
infectious (acute) (virus) NEC A86
Japanese (B type) A83.0
La Crosse A83.5
lead —see Poisoning, lead
lethargica (acute) (infectious) A85.8
louping ill A84.89
lupus erythematosus, systemic M32.19
lymphatica A87.2
Mengo A85.8
meningococcal A39.81
Murray Valley A83.4
otitic NEC H66.40 [G05.3]
parasitic NOS B71.9
periaxial G37.0
periaxialis (concentrica) (diffuse) G37.5
postchickenpox B01.11
postexanthematous NEC B09
postimmunization G04.02
postinfectious NEC G04.01
postmeasles B05.0
postvaccinal G04.02
postvaricella B01.11
postviral NEC A86
Powassan A84.81
Rasmussen G04.81
Rio Bravo A85.8
Russian
autumnal A83.0
spring-summer (taiga) A84.0
saturnine —see Poisoning, lead
specified NEC G04.81
St. Louis A83.3
subacute sclerosing A81.1
summer A83.0
suppurative G04.81
tick-borne A84.9
Torula, torular (cryptococcal) B45.1
toxic NEC G92.8
trichinosis B75 [G05.3]
type
B A83.0
C A83.3
van Bogaert's A81.1
Venezuelan equine A92.2
Vienna A85.8
viral, virus A86
arthropod-borne NEC A85.2
mosquito-borne A83.9
Australian X disease A83.4
California virus A83.5
Eastern equine A83.2
Japanese (B type) A83.0
Murray Valley A83.4
specified NEC A83.8
St. Louis A83.3
type B A83.0
type C A83.3
Western equine A83.1
tick-borne A84.9
biundulant A84.1
central European A84.1
Czechoslovakian A84.1
diphasic meningoencephalitis A84.1
Far Eastern A84.0
Russian spring-summer (taiga) A84.0
specified NEC A84.89

Encephalitis (Continued)
in (Continued)
specified type NEC A85.8
tick-borne, specified NEC A84.89
Western equine A83.1
Encephalocele Q01.9
frontal Q01.0
nasofrontal Q01.1
occipital Q01.2
specified NEC Q01.8
Encephalocystocele —see Encephalocele
Encephaloduroarteriomyosynangiosis
(EDAMS) I67.5
Encephalomalacia (brain) (cerebellar)
(cerebral) —see Softening, brain
Encephalomeningitis —see
Meningoencephalitis
Encephalomeningocele —see Encephalocele
Encephalomeningomyelitis —see
Meningoencephalitis
Encephalomyelitis —see also Encephalitis G04.90
acute disseminated G04.00
infectious G04.01
noninfectious G04.81
postimmunization G04.02
postinfectious G04.01
acute necrotizing hemorrhagic G04.30
postimmunization G04.32
postinfectious G04.31
specified NEC G04.39
benign myalgic G93.3
equine A83.9
Eastern A83.2
Venezuelan A92.2
Western A83.1
in diseases classified elsewhere G05.3
myalgic, benign G93.3
▶myalgic G93.32
▶chronic fatigue syndrome [ME/CFS] G93.32
postchickenpox B01.11
postinfectious NEC G04.01
postmeasles B05.0
postvaccinal G04.02
postvaricella B01.11
rubella B06.01
specified NEC G04.81
Venezuelan equine A92.2
Encephalomyelocele —see Encephalocele
Encephalomyelomeningitis —see
Meningoencephalitis
Encephalomyelopathy G96.9
Encephalomyeloradiculitis (acute) G61.0
Encephalomyeloradiculoneuritis (acute)
(Guillain-Barré) G61.0
Encephalomyeloradiculopathy G96.9
Encephalopathia hyperbilirubinemica,
newborn P57.9
due to isoimmunization (conditions in P55)
P57.0
Encephalopathy (acute) G93.40
acute necrotizing hemorrhagic G04.30
postimmunization G04.32
postinfectious G04.31
specified NEC G04.39
alcoholic G31.2
anoxic —see Damage, brain, anoxic
arteriosclerotic I67.2
centrolobar progressive (Schilder) G37.0
congenital Q07.9
degenerative, in specified disease NEC G32.89
due to
drugs (see also Table of Drugs and
Chemicals) G92.8
demyelinating callosal G37.1
▶hepatic (without coma) K76.82
hyperbilirubinemic, newborn P57.9
due to isoimmunization (conditions in P55)
P57.0
hypertensive I67.4
hypoglycemic E16.2
hypoxic —see Damage, brain, anoxic

Encephalopathy (Continued)
hypoxic ischemic (Continued)
mild P91.61
moderate P91.62
severe P91.63
in (due to) (with)
birth injury P11.1
hyperinsulinism E16.1 [G94]
influenza —see Influenza, with,
encephalopathy
lack of vitamin (see also Deficiency, vitamin)
E56.9 [G32.89]
neoplastic disease (see also Neoplasm)
D49.9 [G13.1]
serum (see also Reaction, serum) T80.69
syphilis A52.17
trauma (postconcussional) F07.81
current injury —see Injury, intracranial
vaccination G04.02
lead —see Poisoning, lead
metabolic G93.41
drug induced G92.8
toxic G92.8
myoclonic, early, symptomatic —see Epilepsy,
generalized, specified NEC
necrotizing, subacute (Leigh) G31.82
neonatal P91.819
in diseases classified elsewhere P91.811
pellagrous E52 [G32.89]
portosystemic —see Failure, hepatic
▶portal-systemic K76.82
postcontusional F07.81
current injury —see Injury, intracranial,
diffuse
posthypoglycemic (coma) E16.1 [G94]
postradiation G93.89
saturnine —see Poisoning, lead
septic G93.41
specified NEC G93.49
spongiform, subacute (viral) A81.09
toxic G92.8
metabolic G92.8
traumatic (postconcussional) F07.81
current injury —see Injury, intracranial
vitamin B deficiency NEC E53.9 [G32.89]
vitamin B1 E51.2
Wernicke's E51.2
Encephalorrhagia —see Hemorrhage,
intracranial, intracerebral
Encephalosis, posttraumatic F07.81
Enchondroma —see also Neoplasm, bone,
benign
Enchondromatosis (cartilaginous) (multiple)
Q78.4
Encopresis R15.9
functional F98.1
nonorganic origin F98.1
psychogenic F98.1
Encounter (with health service) (for) Z76.89
adjustment and management (of)
breast implant Z45.81
implanted device NEC Z45.89
myringotomy device (stent) (tube) Z45.82
neurostimulator (brain) (gastric)
(peripheral nerve) (sacral nerve)
(spinal cord) (vagus nerve) Z45.42
administrative purpose only Z02.9
examination for
adoption Z02.82
armed forces Z02.3
disability determination Z02.71
driving license Z02.4
employment Z02.1
insurance Z02.6
medical certificate NEC Z02.79
paternity testing Z02.81
residential institution admission Z02.2
school admission Z02.0
sports Z02.5
specified reason NEC Z02.89
aftercare —see Aftercare

▶ New   ⇒ Revised   ~~deleted~~ Deleted   ● Use Additional Character(s)

Encounter (Continued)
antenatal screening Z36.9
cervical length Z36.86
chromosomal anomalies Z36.0
congenital cardiac abnormalities Z36.83
elevated maternal serum alphafetoprotein level Z36.1
fetal growth retardation Z36.4
fetal lung maturity Z36.84
fetal macrosomia Z36.88
hydrops fetalis Z36.81
intrauterine growth restriction (IUGR)/ small-for-dates Z36.4
isoimmunization Z36.5
large-for-dates Z36.88
malformations Z36.3
non-visualized anatomy on a previous scan Z36.2
nuchal translucency Z36.82
raised alphafetoprotein level Z36.1
risk of pre-term labor Z36.86
specified type NEC Z36.89
specified follow-up NEC Z36.2
specified genetic defects NEC Z36.8A
Streptococcus B Z36.85
suspected anomaly Z36.3
uncertain dates Z36.87
assisted reproductive fertility procedure cycle Z31.83
blood typing Z01.83
Rh typing Z01.83
breast augmentation or reduction Z41.1
breast implant exchange (different material) (different size) Z45.81
breast reconstruction following mastectomy Z42.1
check-up —see Examination
chemotherapy for neoplasm Z51.11
colonoscopy, screening Z12.11
counseling —see Counseling
delivery, full-term, uncomplicated O80
cesarean, without indication O82
desensitization to allergens Z51.6
ear piercing Z41.3
examination —see Examination
expectant parent(s) (adoptive) pre-birth pediatrician visit Z76.81
fertility preservation procedure (prior to cancer therapy) (prior to removal of gonads) Z31.84
fitting (of) —see Fitting (and adjustment) (of)
genetic
counseling
nonprocreative Z71.83
procreative Z31.5
testing —see Test, genetic
hearing conservation and treatment Z01.12
immunotherapy for neoplasm Z51.12
in vitro fertilization cycle Z31.83
instruction (in)
child care (postpartal) (prenatal) Z32.3
childbirth Z32.2
natural family planning
procreative Z31.61
to avoid pregnancy Z30.02
insulin pump titration Z46.81
joint prosthesis insertion following prior explantation of joint prosthesis (staged procedure)
hip Z47.32
knee Z47.33
shoulder Z47.31
laboratory (as part of a general medical examination) Z00.00
with abnormal findings Z00.01
mental health services (for)
abuse NEC
perpetrator Z69.82
victim Z69.81
child abuse
nonparental
perpetrator Z69.021
victim Z69.020

Encounter (Continued)
mental health services (for) (Continued)
abuse NEC (Continued)
parental
perpetrator Z69.011
victim Z69.010
child neglect
nonparental
perpetrator Z69.021
victim Z69.020
parental
perpetrator Z69.011
victim Z69.010
child psychological abuse
nonparental
perpetrator Z69.021
victim Z69.020
parental
perpetrator Z69.011
victim Z69.010
child sexual abuse
nonparental
perpetrator Z69.021
victim Z69.020
parental
perpetrator Z69.011
victim Z69.010
non-spousal adult abuse
perpetrator Z69.82
victim Z69.81
spousal or partner
abuse
perpetrator Z69.12
victim Z69.11
neglect
perpetrator Z69.12
victim Z69.11
psychological abuse
perpetrator Z69.12
victim Z69.11
violence
perpetrator (physical) (sexual) Z69.12
victim (physical) Z69.11
sexual Z69.81
observation (for) (ruled out)
▶ alarm, without findings
▶ apnea Z03.83
▶ bradycardia Z03.83
▶ oximeter Z03.83
▶ condition suspected related to home physiologic monitoring device Z03.83
exposure to (suspected)
anthrax Z03.810
biological agent NEC Z03.818
▶ malfunction of home cardiorespiratory monitor Z03.83
▶ non-specific findings home physiologic monitoring device Z03.83
pediatrician visit, by expectant parent(s) (adoptive) Z76.81
placental sample (taken vaginally) —see also Encounter, antenatal screening Z36.9
plastic and reconstructive surgery following medical procedure or healed injury NEC Z42.8
pregnancy
supervision of —see Pregnancy, supervision of
test Z32.00
result negative Z32.02
result positive Z32.01
procreative management and counseling for gestational carrier Z31.7
prophylactic measures Z29.9
antivenin Z29.12
fluoride administration Z29.3
immunotherapy for respiratory syncytial virus (RSV) Z29.11
rabies immune globin Z29.14
Rho (D) immune globulin Z29.13
specified NEC Z29.8
radiation therapy (antineoplastic) Z51.0

Encounter (Continued)
radiological (as part of a general medical examination) Z00.00
with abnormal findings Z00.01
reconstructive surgery following medical procedure or healed injury NEC Z42.8
removal (of) —see also Removal
artificial
arm Z44.00-●
complete Z44.01-●
partial Z44.02-●
eye Z44.2-●
leg Z44.10-●
complete Z44.11-●
partial Z44.12-●
breast implant Z45.81
tissue expander (with or without synchronous insertion of permanent implant) Z45.81
device Z46.9
specified NEC Z46.89
external
fixation device — code to fracture with seventh character D
prosthesis, prosthetic device Z44.9
breast Z44.3-●
specified NEC Z44.8
implanted device NEC Z45.89
insulin pump Z46.81
internal fixation device Z47.2
myringotomy device (stent) (tube) Z45.82
nervous system device NEC Z46.2
brain neuropacemaker Z46.2
visual substitution device Z46.2
implanted Z45.31
non-vascular catheter Z46.82
orthodontic device Z46.4
stent
ureteral Z46.6
urinary device Z46.6
repeat cervical smear to confirm findings of recent normal smear following initial abnormal smear Z01.42
respirator [ventilator] use during power failure (Z99.12)
Rh typing Z01.83
screening —see Screening
specified NEC Z76.89
sterilization Z30.2
suspected condition, ruled out
amniotic cavity and membrane Z03.71
cervical shortening Z03.75
fetal anomaly Z03.73
fetal growth Z03.74
maternal and fetal conditions NEC Z03.79
oligohydramnios Z03.71
placental problem Z03.72
polyhydramnios Z03.71
suspected exposure (to), ruled out
anthrax Z03.810
biological agents NEC Z03.818
termination of pregnancy, elective Z33.2
testing —see Test
therapeutic drug level monitoring Z51.81
titration, insulin pump Z46.81
to determine fetal viability of pregnancy O36.80
training
insulin pump Z46.81
X-ray of chest (as part of a general medical examination) Z00.00
with abnormal findings Z00.01
Encystment —see Cyst
Endarteritis (bacterial, subacute) (infective) I77.6
brain I67.7
cerebral or cerebrospinal I67.7
deformans —see Arteriosclerosis
embolic —see Embolism
obliterans —see also Arteriosclerosis
pulmonary I28.8
pulmonary I28.8

Endarteritis (Continued)
retina —see Vasculitis, retina
senile —see Arteriosclerosis
syphilitic A52.09
brain or cerebral A52.04
congenital A50.54 [I79.8]
tuberculous A18.89
Endemic —see condition
Endocarditis (chronic) (marantic) (nonbacterial)
(thrombotic) (valvular) I38
with rheumatic fever (conditions in I00)
active —see Endocarditis, acute, rheumatic
inactive or quiescent (with chorea) I09.1
acute or subacute I33.9
infective I33.0
rheumatic (aortic) (mitral) (pulmonary)
(tricuspid) I01.1
with chorea (acute) (rheumatic)
(Sydenham's) I02.0
aortic (heart) (nonrheumatic) (valve) I35.8
with
mitral disease I08.0
with tricuspid (valve) disease I08.3
active or acute I01.1
with chorea (acute) (rheumatic)
(Sydenham's) I02.0
rheumatic fever (conditions in I00)
active —see Endocarditis, acute,
rheumatic
inactive or quiescent (with chorea) I06.9
tricuspid (valve) disease I08.2
with mitral (valve) disease I08.3
acute or subacute I33.9
arteriosclerotic I35.8
rheumatic I06.9
with mitral disease I08.0
with tricuspid (valve) disease I08.3
active or acute I01.1
with chorea (acute) (rheumatic)
(Sydenham's) I02.0
active or acute I01.1
with chorea (acute) (rheumatic)
(Sydenham's) I02.0
specified NEC I06.8
specified cause NEC I35.8
syphilitic A52.03
arteriosclerotic I38
atypical verrucous (Libman-Sacks) M32.11
bacterial (acute) (any valve) (subacute) I33.0
candidal B37.6
congenital Q24.8
constrictive I33.0
Coxiella burnetii A78 [I39]
Coxsackie B33.21
due to
prosthetic cardiac valve T82.6
Q fever A78 [I39]
Serratia marcescens I33.0
typhoid (fever) A01.02
gonococcal A54.83
infectious or infective (acute) (any valve)
(subacute) I33.0
lenta (acute) (any valve) (subacute) I33.0
Libman-Sacks M32.11
listerial A32.82
Löffler's I42.3
malignant (acute) (any valve) (subacute) I33.0
meningococcal A39.51
mitral (chronic) (double) (fibroid) (heart)
(inactive) (valve) (with chorea) I05.9
with
aortic (valve) disease I08.0
with tricuspid (valve) disease I08.3
active or acute I01.1
with chorea (acute) (rheumatic)
(Sydenham's) I02.0
rheumatic fever (conditions in I00)
active —see Endocarditis, acute,
rheumatic
inactive or quiescent (with chorea) I05.9
tricuspid (valve) disease I08.1
with aortic (valve) disease I08.3

Endocarditis (Continued)
mitral (Continued)
active or acute I01.1
with chorea (acute) (rheumatic)
(Sydenham's) I02.0
bacterial I33.0
arteriosclerotic I34.89
nonrheumatic I34.89
acute or subacute I33.9
specified NEC I05.8
monilial B37.6
multiple valves I08.9
specified disorders I08.8
mycotic (acute) (any valve) (subacute) I33.0
pneumococcal (acute) (any valve) (subacute)
I33.0
pulmonary (chronic) (heart) (valve) I37.8
with rheumatic fever (conditions in I00)
active —see Endocarditis, acute, rheumatic
inactive or quiescent (with chorea) I09.89
with aortic, mitral or tricuspid disease
I08.8
acute or subacute I33.9
rheumatic I01.1
with chorea (acute) (rheumatic)
(Sydenham's) I02.0
arteriosclerotic I37.8
congenital Q22.2
rheumatic (chronic) (inactive) (with chorea)
I09.89
active or acute I01.1
with chorea (acute) (rheumatic)
(Sydenham's) I02.0
syphilitic A52.03
purulent (acute) (any valve) (subacute) I33.0
Q fever A78 [I39]
rheumatic (chronic) (inactive) (with chorea)
I09.1
active or acute (aortic) (mitral)
(pulmonary) (tricuspid) I01.1
with chorea (acute) (rheumatic)
(Sydenham's) I02.0
rheumatoid —see Rheumatoid, carditis
septic (acute) (any valve) (subacute) I33.0
streptococcal (acute) (any valve) (subacute)
I33.0
subacute —see Endocarditis, acute
suppurative (acute) (any valve) (subacute) I33.0
syphilitic A52.03
toxic I33.9
tricuspid (chronic) (heart) (inactive)
(rheumatic) (valve) (with chorea) I07.9
with
aortic (valve) disease I08.2
mitral (valve) disease I08.3
mitral (valve) disease I08.1
aortic (valve) disease I08.3
rheumatic fever (conditions in I00)
active —see Endocarditis, acute,
rheumatic
inactive or quiescent (with chorea) I07.8
active or acute I01.1
with chorea (acute) (rheumatic)
(Sydenham's) I02.0
arteriosclerotic I36.8
nonrheumatic I36.8
acute or subacute I33.9
specified cause, except rheumatic I36.8
tuberculous —see Tuberculosis, endocarditis
typhoid A01.02
ulcerative (acute) (any valve) (subacute) I33.0
vegetative (acute) (any valve) (subacute) I33.0
verrucous (atypical) (nonbacterial)
(nonrheumatic) M32.11
Endocardium, endocardial —see also condition
cushion defect Q21.20
Endocervicitis —see also Cervicitis
due to intrauterine (contraceptive) device
T83.69
hyperplastic N72
Endocrine —see condition

Endocrinopathy, pluriglandular E31.9
Endodontic
overfill M27.52
underfill M27.53
Endodontitis K04.01
irreversible K04.02
reversible K04.01
Endomastoiditis —see Mastoiditis
Endometrioma N80.12-●
Endometriosis N80.9
abdomen, abdominal N80.C0
specified site, NEC N80.C9
wall N80.C19
fascia and muscular layers N80.C11
subcutaneous tissue N80.C10
unspecified depth N80.C19
appendix N80.549
deep N80.542
superficial N80.541
bladder (unspecified depth) N80.A0
deep N80.A2
superficial N80.A1
bowel N80.50
broad ligament N80.3C
cardiothoracic space N80.B6
cecum N80.539
N80.532
superficial N80.531
cervix N80.0-●
colon N80.559
descending N80.559
deep N80.552
superficial N80.551
sigmoid N80.529
deep N80.522
superficial N80.521
transverse N80.559
deep N80.552
superficial N80.551
cul-de-sac (Douglas')
anterior (unspecified depth) N80.319
deep N80.312
superficial N80.311
posterior (unspecified depth) N80.329
deep N80.322
superficial N80.321
deep
involving muscular wall of fallopian tube
N80.22
retrocervical N80.02
diaphragm N80.B39
deep N80.B32
superficial N80.B31
unspecified depth N80.B39
exocervix N80.01
extra-pelvic abdominal peritoneum N80.C4
fallopian tube (unspecified depth) N80.20-●
deep N80.22-●
superficial N80.21-●
female genital organ NEC N80.8
gallbladder N80.8
inguinal canal N80.C3
in scar of skin N80.6
internal N80.02
intestine N80.50
small N80.569
deep (multifocal) N80.562
superficial N80.561
lung N80.B2
mediastinal space N80.B5
myometrium N80.03
nerve
femoral N80.D6
obturator N80.D3
pelvic N80.D0
splanchnic N80.D1
pudendal N80.D5
retroperitoneum, NEC N80.D9
sacral splanchnic N80.D1
sciatic N80.D4
specified, NEC N80.D9

▶ New   ⇒ Revised   ~~deleted~~ Deleted   ● Use Additional Character(s)

Endometriosis *(Continued)*
⫸ovary (unspecified depth) N80.10-●
　▶deep N80.12-●
　▶superficial N80.11-●
⫸parametrium N80.399
　~~pelvic peritoneum N80.3~~
▶pelvic
　▶brim N80.38-●
　　▶deep N80.37-●
　　▶superficial N80.36-●
　▶peritoneum N80.30
　　▶specified sites, NEC N80.399
　　　▶deep N80.392
　　　▶superficial N80.391
　▶sidewall N80.35-●
　　▶deep N80.34-●
　　▶superficial N80.33-●
▶pericardial space N80.B4
⫸peritoneal (pelvic) N80.30
▶pleura N80.B1
⫸rectovaginal septum N80.40
　▶with involvement of vagina N80.42
　▶without involvement of vagina N80.41
▶rectum N80.519
　▶deep (multifocal) N80.512
　▶superficial N80.511
▶retroperitoneum N80.30
⫸round ligament N80.3C9
▶sacral nerve roots N80.D2
　skin (scar) N80.6
　specified site NEC N80.8
　stromal D39.0
⫸thorax N80.B-●
⫸umbilicus N80.C2
▶ureter N80.A69
　▶deep N80.A5-●
　▶extrinsic N80.A4-●
　▶intrinsic N80.A5-●
　▶unspecified depth N80.A6-●
⫸uterosacral ligament(s) N80.3C-●
　▶deep N80.3B-●
　▶superficial N80.3A-●
⫸uterus N80.00
　▶deep N80.02
　▶internal N80.02
　▶superficial N80.01
⫸vagina N80.42
　vulva N80.8
Endometritis (decidual) (nonspecific) (purulent)
　　(senile (atrophic) (suppurative) N71.9
　with ectopic pregnancy O08.0
　acute N71.0
　blenorrhagic (gonococcal) (acute) (chronic)
　　　A54.24
　cervix, cervical (with erosion or ectropion) —
　　　see also Cervicitis
　　hyperplastic N72
　chlamydial A56.11
　chronic N71.1
　following
　　abortion —*see* Abortion by type
　　　complicated by genital infection
　　ectopic or molar pregnancy O08.0
・ gonococcal, gonorrheal (acute) (chronic)
　　　A54.24
　hyperplastic —*see also* Hyperplasia,
　　　endometrial N85.00-●
　　cervix N72
　puerperal, postpartum, childbirth
　　　O86.12
　subacute N71.0
　tuberculous A18.17
Endometrium —*see* condition
Endomyocardiopathy, South African I42.3
Endomyocarditis —*see* Endocarditis
Endomyofibrosis I42.3
Endomyometritis —*see* Endometritis
Endopericarditis —*see* Endocarditis
Endoperineuritis —*see* Disorder, nerve
Endophlebitis —*see* Phlebitis

Endophthalmia —*see* Endophthalmitis,
　　purulent
Endophthalmitis (acute) (infective) (metastatic)
　　(subacute) H44.009
　bleb associated H59.4 —*see also* Bleb,
　　　inflammed (infected), postprocedural
　gonorrheal A54.39
　in (due to)
　　cysticercosis B69.1
　　onchocerciasis B73.01
　　toxocariasis B83.0
　panuveitis —*see* Panuveitis
　parasitic H44.12-●
　purulent H44.00-●
　　panophthalmitis —*see* Panophthalmitis
　　vitreous abscess H44.02-●
　specified NEC H44.19
　sympathetic —*see* Uveitis, sympathetic
Endosalpingioma D28.2
Endosalpingiosis N94.89
Endosteitis —*see* Osteomyelitis
Endothelioma, bone —*see* Neoplasm, bone,
　　malignant
Endotheliosis (hemorrhagic infectional)
　　D69.8
Endotoxemia — code to condition
Endotrachelitis —*see* Cervicitis
Engelmann (-Camurati) syndrome Q78.3
English disease —*see* Rickets
Engman's disease L30.3
Engorgement
　breast N64.59
　　newborn P83.4
　　puerperal, postpartum O92.79
　lung (passive) —*see* Edema, lung
　pulmonary (passive) —*see* Edema, lung
　stomach K31.89
　venous, retina —*see* Occlusion, retina, vein,
　　　engorgement
Enlargement, enlarged —*see also* Hypertrophy
　adenoids J35.2
　　with tonsils J35.3
　alveolar ridge K08.89
　　congenital —*see* Anomaly, alveolar
　apertures of diaphragm (congenital)
　　　Q79.1
　gingival K06.1
　heart, cardiac —*see* Hypertrophy, cardiac
　labium majus, childhood asymmetric
　　　(CALME) N90.61
　lacrimal gland, chronic H04.03-●
　liver —*see* Hypertrophy, liver
　lymph gland or node R59.9
　　generalized R59.1
　　localized R59.0
　orbit H05.34-●
　organ or site, congenital NEC —*see* Anomaly,
　　　by site
　parathyroid (gland) E21.0
　pituitary fossa R93.0
　prostate N40.0
　　with lower urinary tract symptoms (LUTS)
　　　N40.1
　　without lower urinary tract symptoms
　　　(LUTS) N40.0
　sella turcica R93.0
　spleen —*see* Splenomegaly
　thymus (gland) (congenital) E32.0
　thyroid (gland) —*see* Goiter
　tongue K14.8
　tonsils J35.1
　　with adenoids J35.3
　uterus N85.2
　vestibular aqueduct Q16.5
Enophthalmos H05.40-●
　due to
　　orbital tissue atrophy H05.41-●
　　trauma or surgery H05.42-●
Enostosis M27.8
Entamebic, entamebiasis —*see* Amebiasis

Entanglement
　umbilical cord(s) O69.82
　　with compression O69.2
　　around neck (with compression)
　　　O69.81
　　　with compression O69.1
　　　without compression O69.81
　　of twins in monoamniotic sac O69.2
　　without compression O69.82
Enteralgia —*see* Pain, abdominal
Enteric —*see* condition
Enteritis (acute) (diarrheal) (hemorrhagic)
　　(noninfective) K52.9
　adenovirus A08.2
　aertrycke infection A02.0
　allergic K52.29
　　with
　　　eosinophilic gastritis or gastroenteritis
　　　　K52.81
　　　food protein-induced enterocolitis
　　　　　syndrome K52.21
　　　food protein-induced enteropathy K52.22
　　　FPIES K52.21
　amebic (acute) A06.0
　　with abscess —*see* Abscess, amebic
　　chronic A06.1
　　　with abscess —*see* Abscess, amebic
　　　nondysenteric A06.2
　　nondysenteric A06.2
　astrovirus A08.32
　bacillary NOS A03.9
　bacterial A04.9
　　specified NEC A04.8
　calicivirus A08.31
　candidal B37.82
　Chilomastix A07.8
　choleriformis A00.1
　chronic (noninfectious) K52.9
　　ulcerative —*see* Colitis, ulcerative
　cicatrizing (chronic) —*see* Enteritis, regional,
　　　small intestine
　Clostridium
　　botulinum (food poisoning) A05.1
　　difficile
　　　not specified as recurrent A04.72
　　　recurrent A04.71
　coccidial A07.3
　coxsackie virus A08.39
　dietetic —*see also* Enteritis, allergic K52.29
　drug-induced K52.1
　due to
　　astrovirus A08.32
　　calicivirus A08.31
　　coxsackie virus A08.39
　　drugs K52.1
　　echovirus A08.39
　　enterovirus NEC A08.39
　　food hypersensitivity —*see also* Enteritis,
　　　　allergic K52.29
　　infectious organism (bacterial) (viral) —*see*
　　　　Enteritis, infectious
　　torovirus A08.39
　　Yersinia enterocolitica A04.6
　echovirus A08.39
　eltor A00.1
　enterovirus NEC A08.39
　eosinophilic K52.81
　epidemic (infectious) A09
　fulminant —*see also* Ischemia, intestine, acute
　　　K55.019
　gangrenous —*see* Enteritis, infectious
　giardial A07.1
　infectious NOS A09
　　due to
　　　adenovirus A08.2
　　　Aerobacter aerogenes A04.8
　　　Arizona (bacillus) A02.0
　　　bacteria NOS A04.9
　　　　specified NEC A04.8
　　　Campylobacter A04.5
　　　Clostridium difficile
　　　　not specified as recurrent A04.72
　　　　recurrent A04.71

Enteritis *(Continued)*
  infectious NOS *(Continued)*
    due to *(Continued)*
      Clostridium perfringens A04.8
      Enterobacter aerogenes A04.8
      enterovirus A08.39
      Escherichia coli A04.4
        enteroaggregative A04.4
        enterohemorrhagic A04.3
        enteroinvasive A04.2
        enteropathogenic A04.0
        enterotoxigenic A04.1
        specified NEC A04.4
      specified
        bacteria NEC A04.8
        virus NEC A08.39
      Staphylococcus A04.8
      virus NEC A08.4
        specified type NEC A08.39
      Yersinia enterocolitica A04.6
    specified organism NEC A08.8
  influenzal —*see* Influenza, with, digestive
    manifestations
  ischemic K55.9
    acute —*see also* Ischemia, intestine, acute
      K55.019
    chronic K55.1
  microsporidial A07.8
  mucomembranous, myxomembranous —*see*
    Syndrome, irritable bowel
  mucous —*see* Syndrome, irritable bowel
  necroticans A05.2
  necrotizing of newborn —*see* Enterocolitis,
    necrotizing, in newborn
  neurogenic —*see* Syndrome, irritable bowel
  newborn necrotizing —*see* Enterocolitis,
    necrotizing, in newborn
  noninfectious K52.9
  norovirus A08.11
  parasitic NEC B82.9
  paratyphoid (fever) —*see* Fever, paratyphoid
  protozoal A07.9
    specified NEC A07.8
  radiation K52.0
  regional (of) K50.90
    with
      complication K50.919
        abscess K50.914
        fistula K50.913
        intestinal obstruction K50.912
        rectal bleeding K50.911
        specified complication NEC K50.918
    colon —*see* Enteritis, regional, large
      intestine
    duodenum —*see* Enteritis, regional, small
      intestine
    ileum —*see* Enteritis, regional, small
      intestine
    jejunum —*see* Enteritis, regional, small
      intestine
    large bowel —*see* Enteritis, regional, large
      intestine
    large intestine (colon) (rectum) K50.10
      with
        complication K50.119
          abscess K50.114
          fistula K50.113
          intestinal obstruction K50.112
          rectal bleeding K50.111
          small intestine (duodenum) (ileum)
            (jejunum) involvement K50.80
            with
              complication K50.819
                abscess K50.814
                fistula K50.813
                intestinal obstruction
                  K50.812
                rectal bleeding K50.811
                specified complication NEC
                  K50.818
          specified complication NEC K50.118

Enteritis *(Continued)*
  regional *(Continued)*
    rectum —*see* Enteritis, regional, large
      intestine
    small intestine (duodenum) (ileum)
      (jejunum) K50.00
      with
        complication K50.019
          abscess K50.014
          fistula K50.013
          intestinal obstruction K50.012
          large intestine (colon) (rectum)
            involvement K50.80
            with
              complication K50.819
                abscess K50.814
                fistula K50.813
                intestinal obstruction
                  K50.812
                rectal bleeding K50.811
                specified complication NEC
                  K50.818
          rectal bleeding K50.011
          specified complication NEC K50.018
  rotaviral A08.0
  Salmonella, salmonellosis (arizonae)
    (cholerae-suis) (enteritidis)
    (typhimurium) A02.0
  segmental —*see* Enteritis, regional
  septic A09
  Shigella —*see* Infection, Shigella
  small round structured NEC A08.19
  spasmodic, spastic —*see* Syndrome, irritable
    bowel
  staphylococcal A04.8
    due to food A05.0
  torovirus A08.39
  toxic NEC K52.1
    due to Clostridium difficile
      not specified as recurrent A04.72
      recurrent A04.71
  trichomonal A07.8
  tuberculous A18.32
  typhosa A01.00
  ulcerative (chronic) —*see* Colitis, ulcerative
  viral A08.4
    adenovirus A08.2
    enterovirus A08.39
    Rotavirus A08.0
    small round structured NEC A08.19
    specified NEC A08.39
    virus specified NEC A08.39
Enterobiasis B80
Enterobius vermicularis (infection) (infestation)
  B80
Enterocele —*see also* Hernia, abdomen
  pelvic, pelvis (acquired) (congenital) N81.5
  vagina, vaginal (acquired) (congenital)
    NEC N81.5
Enterocolitis —*see also* Enteritis K52.9
  due to Clostridium difficile
    not specified as recurrent A04.72
    recurrent A04.71
  fulminant ischemic —*see also* Ischemia,
    intestine, acute K55.059
  granulomatous —*see* Enteritis, regional
  hemorrhagic (acute) —*see also* Ischemia,
    intestine, acute K55.059
    chronic K55.1
  infectious NEC A09
  ischemic K55.9
  necrotizing K55.30
    with
      perforation K55.33
      pneumatosis K55.32
      and perforation K55.33
    due to Clostridium difficile
      not specified as recurrent A04.72
      recurrent A04.71
    in non-newborn K55.30
      stage 1 (without pneumatosis, without
        perforation) K55.31

Enterocolitis *(Continued)*
  necrotizing *(Continued)*
    in non-newborn *(Continued)*
      stage 2 (with pneumatosis, without
        perforation) K55.32
      stage 3 (with pneumatosis, with
        perforation) K55.33
    in newborn P77.9
      stage 1 (without pneumatosis, without
        perforation) P77.1
      stage 2 (with pneumatosis, without
        perforation) P77.2
      stage 3 (with pneumatosis, with
        perforation) P77.3
    without pneumatosis or perforation K55.31
  noninfectious K52.9
    newborn —*see* Enterocolitis, necrotizing, in
      newborn
  pseudomembranous (newborn)
    not specified as recurrent A04.72
    recurrent A04.71
  radiation K52.0
    newborn —*see* Enterocolitis, necrotizing, in
      newborn
  ulcerative (chronic) —*see* Pancolitis,
    ulcerative (chronic)
Enterogastritis —*see* Enteritis
Enteropathy K63.9
  celiac-gluten-sensitive K90.0
    non-celiac K90.41
  food protein-induced K52.22
  hemorrhagic, terminal —*see also* Ischemia,
    intestine, acute K55.059
  protein-losing K90.49
Enteroperitonitis —*see* Peritonitis
Enteroptosis K63.4
Enterorrhagia K92.2
Enterospasm —*see also* Syndrome, irritable,
  bowel
  psychogenic F45.8
Enterostenosis —*see also* Obstruction, intestine,
  specified NEC K56.699
Enterostomy
  complication —*see* Complication, enterostomy
  status Z93.4
Enterovirus, as cause of disease classified
  elsewhere B97.10
  coxsackievirus B97.11
  echovirus B97.12
  other specified B97.19
Enthesopathy (peripheral) M77.5-●
  Achilles tendinitis —*see* Tendinitis, Achilles
  ankle and tarsus M77.9
    specified type NEC —*see* Enthesopathy,
      foot, specified type NEC
  anterior tibial syndrome M76.81-●
  calcaneal spur —*see* Spur, bone, calcaneal
  elbow region M77.8
    lateral epicondylitis —*see* Epicondylitis,
      lateral
    medial epicondylitis —*see* Epicondylitis,
      medial
  foot NEC M77.8
    metatarsalgia —*see* Metatarsalgia
    specified type NEC M77.5-●
  forearm M77.8
  gluteal tendinitis —*see* Tendinitis, gluteal
  hand M77.8
  hip —*see* Enthesopathy, lower limb, specified
    type NEC
  iliac crest spur —*see* Spur, bone, iliac crest
  iliotibial band syndrome —*see* Syndrome,
    iliotibial band
  knee —*see* Enthesopathy, lower limb, lower
    leg, specified type NEC
  lateral epicondylitis —*see* Epicondylitis,
    lateral
  lower limb (excluding foot) M76.9
    Achilles tendinitis —*see* Tendinitis, Achilles
    ankle and tarsus M77.5-
      specified type NEC - *see* Enthesopathy,
        foot, specified type NEC

▶ New   ⇒ Revised   ~~deleted~~ Deleted   ● Use Additional Character(s)

Enthesopathy *(Continued)*
  lower limb *(Continued)*
    anterior tibial syndrome M76.81- •
    gluteal tendinitis —*see* Tendinitis, gluteal
    iliac crest spur —*see* Spur, bone, iliac crest
    iliotibial band syndrome —*see* Syndrome,
      iliotibial band
    patellar tendinitis —*see* Tendinitis, patellar
    pelvic region —*see* Enthesopathy, lower
      limb, specified type NEC
    peroneal tendinitis —*see* Tendinitis, peroneal
    posterior tibial syndrome M76.82- •
    psoas tendinitis —*see* Tendinitis, psoas
    specified type NEC M76.89- •
    tibial collateral bursitis —*see* Bursitis, tibial
      collateral
  medial epicondylitis —*see* Epicondylitis, medial
  multiple sites M77.8
  patellar tendinitis —*see* Tendinitis, patellar
  pelvis M77.8
  periarthritis of wrist —*see* Periarthritis, wrist
  peroneal tendinitis —*see* Tendinitis, peroneal
  posterior tibial syndrome M76.82- •
  psoas tendinitis —*see* Tendinitis, psoas
  shoulder M77.8
  shoulder region —*see* Lesion, shoulder
  specified type NEC M77.8
  spinal M46.00
    cervical region M46.02
    cervicothoracic region M46.03
    lumbar region M46.06
    lumbosacral region M46.07
    multiple sites M46.09
    occipito-atlanto-axial region M46.01
    sacrococcygeal region M46.08
    thoracic region M46.04
    thoracolumbar region M46.05
  tibial collateral bursitis —*see* Bursitis, tibial
    collateral
  upper arm M77.8
  wrist and carpus NEC M77.8
    calcaneal spur —*see* Spur, bone, calcaneal
    periarthritis of wrist —*see* Periarthritis, wrist
Entomophobia F40.218
Entomophthoromycosis B46.8
Entrance, air into vein —*see* Embolism, air
Entrapment, nerve —*see* Neuropathy,
  entrapment
Entropion (eyelid) (paralytic) H02.009
  cicatricial H02.019
    left H02.016
      lower H02.015
      upper H02.014
    right H02.013
      lower H02.012
      upper H02.011
  congenital Q10.2
  left H02.006
    lower H02.005
    upper H02.004
  mechanical H02.029
    left H02.026
      lower H02.025
      upper H02.024
    right H02.023
      lower H02.022
      upper H02.021
  right H02.003
    lower H02.002
    upper H02.001
  senile H02.039
    left H02.036
      lower H02.035
      upper H02.034
    right H02.033
      lower H02.032
      upper H02.031
  spastic H02.049
    left H02.046
      lower H02.045
      upper H02.044

Entropion *(Continued)*
  spastic *(Continued)*
    right H02.043
      lower H02.042
      upper H02.041
Enucleated eye (traumatic, current) S05.7- •
Enuresis R32
  functional F98.0
  habit disturbance F98.0
  nocturnal N39.44
    psychogenic F98.0
  nonorganic origin F98.0
  psychogenic F98.0
Eosinopenia —*see* Agranulocytosis
Eosinophilia (allergic) (idiopathic) (secondary)
  D72.10
  with
    angiolymphoid hyperplasia (ALHE)
      D18.01
  familial D72.19
  hereditary D72.19
  in disease classified elsewhere D72.18
  infiltrative —*see* Eosinophilia, pulmonary
  Löffler's J82.89
  peritoneal —*see* Peritonitis, eosinophilic
  pulmonary NEC J82.89
    acute J82.82
    asthmatic J82.83
    chronic J82.81
  specified NEC D72.19
  tropical (pulmonary) J82.89
Eosinophilia-myalgia syndrome M35.89
Ependymitis (acute) (cerebral) (chronic)
  (granular) —*see* Encephalomyelitis
Ependymoblastoma
  specified site —*see* Neoplasm, malignant, by
    site
  unspecified site C71.9
Ependymoma (epithelial) (malignant)
  anaplastic
    specified site —*see* Neoplasm, malignant,
      by site
    unspecified site C71.9
  benign
    specified site —*see* Neoplasm, benign, by
      site
    unspecified site D33.2
  myxopapillary D43.2
    specified site —*see* Neoplasm, uncertain
      behavior, by site
    unspecified site D43.2
  papillary D43.2
    specified site —*see* Neoplasm, uncertain
      behavior, by site
    unspecified site D43.2
  specified site —*see* Neoplasm, malignant, by
    site
  unspecified site C71.9
Ependymopathy G93.89
Ephelis, ephelides L81.2
Epiblepharon (congenital) Q10.3
Epicanthus, epicanthic fold (eyelid)
  (congenital) Q10.3
Epicondylitis (elbow)
  lateral M77.1- •
  medial M77.0- •
Epicystitis —*see* Cystitis
Epidemic —*see* condition
Epidermidalization, cervix —*see* Dysplasia,
  cervix
Epidermis, epidermal —*see* condition
Epidermodysplasia verruciformis B07.8
Epidermolysis
  bullosa (congenital) Q81.9
    acquired L12.30
      drug-induced L12.31
      specified cause NEC L12.35
    dystrophica Q81.2
    letalis Q81.1
    simplex Q81.0
    specified NEC Q81.8

Epidermolysis *(Continued)*
  necroticans combustiformis L51.2
    due to drug —*see* Table of Drugs and
      Chemicals, by drug
Epidermophytid —*see* Dermatophytosis
Epidermophytosis (infected) —*see*
  Dermatophytosis
Epididymis —*see* condition
Epididymitis (acute) (nonvenereal) (recurrent)
  (residual) N45.1
  with orchitis N45.3
  blennorrhagic (gonococcal) A54.23
  caseous (tuberculous) A18.15
  chlamydial A56.19
  filarial —*see also* Infestation, filarial B74.9
    [N51]
  gonococcal A54.23
  syphilitic A52.76
  tuberculous A18.15
Epididymo-orchitis —*see also* Epididymitis
  N45.3
Epidural —*see* condition
Epigastrium, epigastric —*see* condition
Epigastrocele —*see* Hernia, ventral
Epiglottis —*see* condition
Epiglottitis, epiglottiditis (acute) J05.10
  with obstruction J05.11
  chronic J37.0
Epignathus Q89.4
Epilepsia partialis continua —*see also*
  Kozhevnikof's epilepsy G40.1- •
Epilepsy, epileptic, epilepsia (attack) (cerebral)
  (convulsion) (fit) (seizure) G40.909

Note: the following terms are to be
considered equivalent to intractable:
pharmacoresistant (pharmacologically
resistant), treatment resistant, refractory
(medically) and poorly controlled

with
  complex partial seizures —*see* Epilepsy,
    localization-related, symptomatic,
    with complex partial seizures
  grand mal seizures on awakening —
    see Epilepsy, generalized, specified
    NEC
  myoclonic absences —*see* Epilepsy,
    generalized, specified NEC
  myoclonic-astatic seizures —*see* Epilepsy,
    generalized, specified NEC
  simple partial seizures —*see* Epilepsy,
    localization-related, symptomatic,
    with simple partial seizures
akinetic —*see* Epilepsy, generalized, specified
  NEC
benign childhood with centrotemporal EEG
  spikes —*see* Epilepsy, localization-
    related, idiopathic
benign myoclonic in infancy G40.80- •
Bravais-jacksonian —*see* Epilepsy,
  localization-related, symptomatic,
  with simple partial seizures
childhood
  with occipital EEG paroxysms —*see*
    Epilepsy, localization-related,
    idiopathic
  absence G40.A09
    intractable G40.A19
      with status epilepticus G40.A11
      without status epilepticus G40.A19
    not intractable G40.A09
      with status epilepticus G40.A01
      without status epilepticus G40.A09
climacteric —*see* Epilepsy, specified NEC
cysticercosis B69.0
deterioration (mental) F06.8
due to syphilis A52.19
focal —*see* Epilepsy, localization-related,
  symptomatic, with simple partial
  seizures

Epilepsy, epileptic, epilepsia (Continued)
  generalized
    idiopathic G40.309
      intractable G40.319
        with status epilepticus G40.311
        without status epilepticus G40.319
      not intractable G40.309
        with status epilepticus G40.301
        without status epilepticus G40.309
    specified NEC G40.409
      intractable G40.419
        with status epilepticus G40.411
        without status epilepticus G40.419
      not intractable G40.409
        with status epilepticus G40.401
        without status epilepticus G40.409
  impulsive petit mal —see Epilepsy, juvenile
      myoclonic
  intractable G40.919
    with status epilepticus G40.911
    without status epilepticus G40.919
  juvenile absence G40.A09
    intractable G40.A19
      with status epilepticus G40.A11
      without status epilepticus G40.A19
    not intractable G40.A09
      with status epilepticus G40.A01
      without status epilepticus G40.A09
  juvenile myoclonic G40.B11
    intractable G40.B19
      with status epilepticus G40.B11
      without status epilepticus G40.B19
    not intractable G40.B09
      with status epilepticus G40.B01
      without status epilepticus G40.B09
  localization-related (focal) (partial)
    idiopathic G40.009
      with seizures of localized onset G40.009
        intractable G40.019
          with status epilepticus G40.011
          without status epilepticus G40.019
        not intractable G40.009
          with status epilepticus G40.001
          without status epilepticus G40.009
    symptomatic
      with complex partial seizures G40.209
        intractable G40.219
          with status epilepticus G40.211
          without status epilepticus G40.219
        not intractable G40.209
          with status epilepticus G40.201
          without status epilepticus
            G40.209
      with simple partial seizures G40.109
        intractable G40.119
          with status epilepticus G40.111
          without status epilepticus
            G40.119
        not intractable G40.109
          with status epilepticus G40.101
          without status epilepticus G40.109
  myoclonus, myoclonic —see also Epilepsy,
      generalized, specified NEC
    progressive —see Epilepsy, generalized,
        idiopathic
    severe, in infancy (SMEI) G40.83-•
  not intractable G40.909
    with status epilepticus G40.901
    without status epilepticus G40.909
  on awakening —see Epilepsy, generalized,
      specified NEC
  parasitic NOS B71.9 [G94]
  partialis continua —see also Kozhevnikof's
      epilepsy G40.1-•
  peripheral —see Epilepsy, specified NEC
  polymorphic, in infancy (PMEI) G40.83-•
  procursiva —see Epilepsy, localization-
      related, symptomatic, with simple
      partial seizures
  progressive (familial) myoclonic —see
      Epilepsy, generalized, idiopathic

Epilepsy, epileptic, epilepsia (Continued)
  reflex —see Epilepsy, specified NEC
  related to
    alcohol G40.509
      not intractable G40.509
        with status epilepticus G40.501
        without status epilepticus G40.509
    drugs G40.509
      not intractable G40.509
        with status epilepticus G40.501
        without status epilepticus G40.509
    external causes G40.509
      not intractable G40.509
        with status epilepticus G40.501
        without status epilepticus G40.509
    hormonal changes G40.509
      not intractable G40.509
        with status epilepticus G40.501
        without status epilepticus G40.509
    sleep deprivation G40.509
      not intractable G40.509
        with status epilepticus G40.501
        without status epilepticus G40.509
    stress G40.509
      not intractable G40.509
        with status epilepticus G40.501
        without status epilepticus G40.509
  somatomotor —see Epilepsy, localization-
      related, symptomatic, with simple
      partial seizures
  somatosensory —see Epilepsy, localization-
      related, symptomatic, with simple
      partial seizures
  spasms G40.822
    intractable G40.824
      with status epilepticus G40.823
      without status epilepticus G40.824
    not intractable G40.822
      with status epilepticus G40.821
      without status epilepticus G40.822
  specified NEC G40.802
    intractable G40.804
      with status epilepticus G40.803
      without status epilepticus G40.804
    not intractable G40.802
      with status epilepticus G40.801
      without status epilepticus G40.802
  syndromes
    generalized
      idiopathic G40.309
        intractable G40.319
          with status epilepticus G40.311
          without status epilepticus G40.319
        not intractable G40.309
          with status epilepticus G40.301
          without status epilepticus G40.309
      specified NEC G40.409
        intractable G40.419
          with status epilepticus G40.411
          without status epilepticus G40.419
        not intractable G40.409
          with status epilepticus G40.401
          without status epilepticus G40.409
    localization-related (focal) (partial)
      idiopathic G40.009
        with seizures of localized onset
            G40.009
          intractable G40.019
            with status epilepticus G40.011
            without status epilepticus
              G40.019
          not intractable G40.009
            with status epilepticus G40.001
            without status epilepticus
              G40.009
      symptomatic
        with complex partial seizures
            G40.209
          intractable G40.219
            with status epilepticus G40.211
            without status epilepticus G40.219

Epilepsy, epileptic, epilepsia (Continued)
  syndromes (Continued)
    localization-related (Continued)
      symptomatic (Continued)
        with complex partial seizures
            (Continued)
          not intractable G40.209
            with status epilepticus G40.201
            without status epilepticus
              G40.209
        with simple partial seizures G40.109
          intractable G40.119
            with status epilepticus G40.111
            without status epilepticus
              G40.119
          not intractable G40.109
            with status epilepticus G40.101
            without status epilepticus
              G40.109
    specified NEC G40.802
      intractable G40.804
        with status epilepticus G40.803
        without status epilepticus G40.804
      not intractable G40.802
        with status epilepticus G40.801
        without status epilepticus G40.802
  tonic (-clonic) —see Epilepsy, generalized,
      specified NEC
  twilight F05
  uncinate (gyrus) —see Epilepsy, localization-
      related, symptomatic, with complex
      partial seizures
  Unverricht (-Lundborg) (familial myoclonic) —
      see Epilepsy, generalized, idiopathic
  visceral —see Epilepsy, specified NEC
  visual —see Epilepsy, specified NEC
Epiloia Q85.1
Epimenorrhea N92.0
Epipharyngitis —see Nasopharyngitis
Epiphora H04.20-•
  due to
    excess lacrimation H04.21-•
    insufficient drainage H04.22-•
Epiphyseal arrest —see Arrest, epiphyseal
Epiphyseolysis, epiphysiolysis —see
    Osteochondropathy
Epiphysitis —see also Osteochondropathy
  juvenile M92.9
  syphilitic (congenital) A50.02
Epiplocele —see Hernia, abdomen
Epiploitis —see Peritonitis
Epiplosarcomphalocele —see Hernia,
    umbilicus
Episcleritis (suppurative) H15.10-•
  in (due to)
    syphilis A52.71
    tuberculosis A18.51
  nodular H15.12-•
  periodica fugax H15.11-•
    angioneurotic —see Edema, angioneurotic
  syphilitic (late) A52.71
  tuberculous A18.51
Episode
  affective, mixed F39
  depersonalization (in neurotic state) F48.1
  depressive F32.A
    major F32.9
      mild F32.0
      moderate F32.1
      severe (without psychotic symptoms)
        F32.2
        with psychotic symptoms F32.3
    recurrent F33.9
      brief F33.8
    specified NEC F32.89
  hypomanic F30.8
  manic F30.9
    with
      psychotic symptoms F30.2
      remission (full) F30.4
        partial F30.3

Episode *(Continued)*
  manic *(Continued)*
    without psychotic symptoms F30.10
      mild F30.11
      moderate F30.12
      severe (without psychotic symptoms)
        F30.13
        with psychotic symptoms F30.2
    other specified F30.8
    recurrent F31.89
  psychotic F23
    organic F06.8
  schizophrenic (acute) NEC, brief F23
Epispadias (female) (male) Q64.0
Episplenitis D73.89
Epistaxis (multiple) R04.0
  hereditary I78.0
  vicarious menstruation N94.89
Epithelioma (malignant) —*see also* Neoplasm,
    malignant, by site
  adenoides cysticum —*see* Neoplasm, skin,
    benign
  basal cell —*see* Neoplasm, skin, malignant
  benign —*see* Neoplasm, benign, by site
  Bowen's —*see* Neoplasm, skin, in situ
  calcifying, of Malherbe —*see* Neoplasm, skin,
    benign
  external site —*see* Neoplasm, skin, malignant
  intraepidermal, Jadassohn —*see* Neoplasm,
    skin, benign
  squamous cell —*see* Neoplasm, malignant,
    by site
Epitheliomatosis pigmented Q82.1
Epitheliopathy, multifocal placoid pigment
    H30.14-●
Epithelium, epithelial —*see* condition
Epituberculosis (with atelectasis) (allergic)
    A15.7
Eponychia Q84.6
Epstein's
  nephrosis or syndrome —*see* Nephrosis
  pearl K09.8
Epulis (gingiva) (fibrous) (giant cell) K06.8
Equinia A24.0
Equinovarus (congenital) (talipes) Q66.0-●
  acquired —*see* Deformity, limb, clubfoot
Equivalent
  convulsive (abdominal) —*see* Epilepsy,
    specified NEC
  epileptic (psychic) —*see* Epilepsy,
    localization-related, symptomatic, with
    complex partial seizures
Erb (-Duchenne) **paralysis** (birth injury)
    (newborn) P14.0
Erb's
  disease G71.02
  palsy, paralysis (brachial) (birth) (newborn)
    P14.0
    spinal (spastic) syphilitic A52.17
  pseudohypertrophic muscular dystrophy
    G71.02
Erb-Goldflam disease or syndrome G70.00
  with exacerbation (acute) G70.01
  in crisis G70.01
Erdheim's syndrome (acromegalic
    macrospondylitis) E22.0
Erection, painful (persistent) —*see* Priapism
Ergosterol deficiency (vitamin D) E55.9
  with
    adult osteomalacia M83.8
    rickets —*see* Rickets
Ergotism —*see also* Poisoning, food, noxious,
    plant
  from ergot used as drug (migraine therapy) —
    see Table of Drugs and Chemicals
Erosio interdigitalis blastomycetica B37.2
Erosion
  artery I77.2
    without rupture I77.89
  bone —*see* Disorder, bone, density and
    structure, specified NEC

Erosion *(Continued)*
  bronchus J98.09
  cartilage (joint) —*see* Disorder, cartilage,
    specified type NEC
  cervix (uteri) (acquired) (chronic) (congenital)
    N86
    with cervicitis N72
  cornea (nontraumatic) —*see* Ulcer, cornea
    recurrent H18.83-●
    traumatic —*see* Abrasion, cornea
  dental (idiopathic) (occupational) (due to
    diet, drugs or vomiting) K03.2
  duodenum, postpyloric —*see* Ulcer,
    duodenum
  esophagus K22.10
    with bleeding K22.11
  gastric —*see* Ulcer, stomach
  gastrojejunal —*see* Ulcer, gastrojejunal
  implanted mesh —*see* Complications,
    prosthetic device or implant, mesh
  intestine K63.3
  lymphatic vessel I89.8
  pylorus, pyloric (ulcer) —*see* Ulcer, stomach
  spine, aneurysmal A52.09
  stomach —*see* Ulcer, stomach
  subcutaneous device pocket
    nervous system prosthetic device, implant,
      or graft T85.890
    other internal prosthetic device, implant, or
      graft T85.898
  teeth (idiopathic) (occupational) (due to diet,
    drugs or vomiting) K03.2
  urethra N36.8
  uterus N85.8
Erotomania F52.8
Error
  metabolism, inborn —*see* Disorder,
    metabolism
  refractive —*see* Disorder, refraction
Eructation R14.2
  nervous or psychogenic F45.8
Eruption
  creeping B76.9
  drug (generalized) (taken internally) L27.0
    fixed L27.1
    in contact with skin —*see* Dermatitis, due
      to drugs
    localized L27.1
  Hutchinson, summer L56.4
  Kaposi's varicelliform B00.0
  napkin L22
  polymorphous light (sun) L56.4
  recalcitrant pustular L13.8
  ringed R23.8
  skin (nonspecific) R21
    creeping (meaning hookworm) B76.9
    due to inoculation/vaccination
      (generalized) —*see also* Dermatitis,
      due to, vaccine L27.0
      localized L27.1
    erysipeloid A26.0
    feigned L98.1
    Kaposi's varicelliform B00.0
    lichenoid L28.0
    meaning dermatitis —*see* Dermatitis
    toxic NEC L53.0
  tooth, teeth, abnormal (incomplete) (late)
    (premature) (sequence) K00.6
  vesicular R23.8
Erysipelas (gangrenous) (infantile) (newborn)
    (phlegmonous) (suppurative) A46
  external ear A46 [H62.40]
  puerperal, postpartum O86.89
Erysipeloid A26.9
  cutaneous (Rosenbach's) A26.0
  disseminated A26.8
  sepsis A26.7
  specified NEC A26.8
Erythema, erythematous (infectional)
    (inflammation) L53.9
  ab igne L59.0

Erythema, erythematous *(Continued)*
  annulare (centrifugum) (rheumaticum)
    L53.1
  arthriticum epidemicum A25.1
  brucellum —*see* Brucellosis
  chronic figurate NEC L53.3
  chronicum migrans (Borrelia burgdorferi)
    A69.20
  diaper L22
  due to
    chemical NEC L53.0
      in contact with skin L24.5
    drug (internal use) —*see* Dermatitis, due
      to, drugs
  elevatum diutinum L95.1
  endemic E52
  epidemic, arthritic A25.1
  figuratum perstans L53.3
  gluteal L22
  heat - code by site under Burn, first degree
  ichthyosiforme congenitum bullous
    Q80.3
  in diseases classified elsewhere L54
  induratum (nontuberculous) L52
    tuberculous A18.4
  infectiosum B08.3
  intertrigo L30.4
  iris L51.9
  marginatum L53.2
    in (due to) acute rheumatic fever I00
  medicamentosum —*see* Dermatitis, due to,
    drugs
  migrans A26.0
    chronicum A69.20
    tongue K14.1
  multiforme (major) (minor) L51.9
    bullous, bullosum L51.1
    conjunctiva L51.1
    nonbullous L51.0
    pemphigoides L12.0
    specified NEC L51.8
  napkin L22
  neonatorum P83.88
    toxic P83.1
  nodosum L52
    tuberculous A18.4
  palmar L53.8
  pernio T69.1
  rash, newborn P83.88
  scarlatiniform (recurrent) (exfoliative)
    L53.8
  solare L55.0
  specified NEC L53.8
  toxic, toxicum NEC L53.0
    newborn P83.1
  tuberculous (primary) A18.4
Erythematous, erythematosus —*see* condition
Erythermalgia (primary) I73.81
Erythralgia I73.81
Erythrasma L08.1
Erythredema (polyneuropathy) —*see* Poisoning,
    mercury
Erythremia (acute) C94.0-●
  chronic D45
  secondary D75.1
Erythroblastopenia —*see also* Aplasia, red cell
    D60.9
  congenital D61.01
Erythroblastophthisis D61.09
Erythroblastosis (fetalis) (newborn) P55.9
  due to
    ABO (antibodies) (incompatibility)
      (isoimmunization) P55.1
    Rh (antibodies) (incompatibility)
      (isoimmunization) P55.0
Erythrocyanosis (crurum) I73.89
Erythrocythemia —*see* Erythremia
Erythrocytosis (megalosplenic) (secondary)
    D75.1
  familial D75.0
  oval, hereditary —*see* Elliptocytosis

Erythrocytosis *(Continued)*
  secondary D75.1
  stress D75.1
Erythroderma (secondary) —*see also* Erythema
  L53.9
  bullous ichthyosiform, congenital Q80.3
  desquamativum L21.1
  ichthyosiform, congenital (bullous) Q80.3
  neonatorum P83.88
  psoriaticum L40.8
Erythrodysesthesia, palmar plantar (PPE)
  L27.1
Erythrogenesis imperfecta D61.09
Erythroleukemia C94.0-•
Erythromelalgia I73.81
Erythrophagocytosis D75.89
Erythrophobia F40.298
Erythroplakia, oral epithelium, and tongue
  K13.29
Erythroplasia (Queyrat) D07.4
  specified site —*see* Neoplasm, skin, in situ
  unspecified site D07.4
Escherichia coli (E. coli), as cause of disease
  classified elsewhere B96.20
  non-O157 Shiga toxin-producing (with
    known O group) B96.22
  non-Shiga toxin-producing B96.29
  O157 with confirmation of Shiga toxin when
    H antigen is unknown, or is not H7
    B96.21
  O157:H- (nonmotile) with confirmation of
    Shiga toxin B96.21
  Shiga toxin-producing (with unspecified O
    group) (STEC) B96.23
  O157 B96.21
  O157:H7 with or without confirmation of
    Shiga toxin-production B96.21
  specified NEC B96.29
Esophagismus K22.4
Esophagitis (acute) (alkaline) (chemical)
  (chronic) (infectional) (necrotic) (peptic)
  (postoperative) (without bleeding)
  K20.90
  with bleeding K20.91
  candidal B37.81
  due to gastrointestinal reflux disease (without
    bleeding) K21.00
    with bleeding K21.01
  eosinophilic K20.0
  reflux K21.00
  specified NEC (without bleeding) K20.80
    with bleeding K21.81
  tuberculous A18.83
  ulcerative K22.10
    with bleeding K22.11
Esophagocele K22.5
Esophagomalacia K22.89
Esophagospasm K22.4
Esophagostenosis K22.2
Esophagostomiasis B81.8
Esophagotracheal —*see* condition
Esophagus —*see* condition
Esophoria H50.51
  convergence, excess H51.12
  divergence, insufficiency H51.8
Esotropia —*see* Strabismus, convergent
  concomitant
Espundia B55.2
Essential —*see* condition
Esthesioneuroblastoma C30.0
Esthesioneurocytoma C30.0
Esthesioneuroepithelioma C30.0
Esthiomene A55
Estivo-autumnal malaria (fever) B50.9
Estrangement (marital) Z63.5
  parent-child NEC Z62.890
Estriasis —*see* Myiasis
Ethanolism —*see* Alcoholism
Etherism —*see* Dependence, drug, inhalant
Ethmoid, ethmoidal —*see* condition

Ethmoiditis (chronic) (nonpurulent)
  (purulent) —*see also* Sinusitis, ethmoidal
  influenzal —*see* Influenza, with, respiratory
    manifestations NEC
  Woakes' J33.1
Ethylism —*see* Alcoholism
Eulenburg's disease (congenital paramyotonia)
  G71.19
Eumycetoma B47.0
Eunuchoidism E29.1
  hypogonadotropic E23.0
European blastomycosis —*see* Cryptococcosis
Eustachian —*see* condition
Evaluation (for) (of)
  development state
    adolescent Z00.3
    period of
      delayed growth in childhood Z00.70
        with abnormal findings Z00.71
      rapid growth in childhood Z00.2
    puberty Z00.3
  growth and developmental state (period of
    rapid growth) Z00.2
    delayed growth Z00.70
      with abnormal findings Z00.71
  mental health (status) Z00.8
    requested by authority Z04.6
  period of
    delayed growth in childhood Z00.70
      with abnormal findings Z00.71
    rapid growth in childhood Z00.2
  suspected condition —*see* Observation
Evans syndrome D69.41
Event
  apparent life threatening in newborn and
    infant (ALTE) R68.13
  brief resolved unexplained event (BRUE)
    R68.13
Eventration —*see also* Hernia, ventral
  colon into chest —*see* Hernia, diaphragm
  diaphragm (congenital) Q79.1
Eversion
  bladder N32.89
  cervix (uteri) N86
    with cervicitis N72
  foot NEC —*see also* Deformity, valgus, ankle
    congenital Q66.6
  punctum lacrimale (postinfectional) (senile)
    H04.52-•
  ureter (meatus) N28.89
  urethra (meatus) N36.8
  uterus N81.4
Evidence
  cytologic
    of malignancy on anal smear R85.614
    of malignancy on cervical smear R87.614
    of malignancy on vaginal smear R87.624
Evisceration
  birth injury P15.8
  traumatic NEC
    eye —*see* Enucleated eye
Evulsion —*see* Avulsion
Ewing's sarcoma or tumor —*see* Neoplasm,
  bone, malignant
Examination (for) (following) (general) (of)
  (routine) Z00.00
  with abnormal findings Z00.01
  abuse, physical (alleged), ruled out
    adult Z04.71
    child Z04.72
  adolescent (development state) Z00.3
  alleged rape or sexual assault (victim), ruled
    out
    adult Z04.41
    child Z04.42
  allergy Z01.82
  annual (adult) (periodic) (physical) Z00.00
    with abnormal findings Z00.01
    gynecological Z01.419
      with abnormal findings Z01.411
  antibody response Z01.84

Examination *(Continued)*
  blood —*see* Examination, laboratory
  blood pressure Z01.30
    with abnormal findings Z01.31
  cancer staging —*see* Neoplasm, malignant,
    by site
  cervical Papanicolaou smear Z12.4
    as part of routine gynecological
      examination Z01.419
      with abnormal findings Z01.411
  child (over 28 days old) Z00.129
    with abnormal findings Z00.121
    under 28 days old —*see* Newborn,
      examination
  clinical research control or normal
    comparison (control) (participant)
    Z00.6
  contraceptive (drug) maintenance (routine)
    Z30.8
    device (intrauterine) Z30.431
  dental Z01.20
    with abnormal findings Z01.21
  developmental —*see* Examination, child
  donor (potential) Z00.5
  ear Z01.10
    with abnormal findings NEC Z01.118
  eye Z01.00
    with abnormal findings Z01.01
    following failed vision screening Z01.020
      with abnormal findings Z01.021
  following
    accident NEC Z04.3
      transport Z04.1
      work Z04.2
    assault, alleged, ruled out
      adult Z04.71
      child Z04.72
    motor vehicle accident Z04.1
    treatment (for) Z09
      combined NEC Z09
        fracture Z09
        malignant neoplasm Z08
      malignant neoplasm Z08
      mental disorder Z09
      specified condition NEC Z09
  follow-up (routine) (following) Z09
    chemotherapy NEC Z09
      malignant neoplasm Z08
    fracture Z09
    malignant neoplasm Z08
    postpartum Z39.2
    psychotherapy Z09
    radiotherapy NEC Z09
      malignant neoplasm Z08
    surgery NEC Z09
      malignant neoplasm Z08
  forced sexual exploitation Z04.81
  forced labor exploitation Z04.82
  gynecological Z01.419
    with abnormal findings Z01.411
    for contraceptive maintenance Z30.8
  health —*see* Examination, medical
  hearing Z01.10
    with abnormal findings NEC Z01.118
    infant or child (over 28 days old) Z00.129
      with abnormal findings Z00.121
    following failed hearing screening
      Z01.110
  immunity status testing Z01.84
  laboratory (as part of a general medical
    examination) Z00.00
    with abnormal findings Z00.01
    preprocedural Z01.812
  lactating mother Z39.1
  medical (adult) (for) (of) Z00.00
    with abnormal findings Z00.01
    administrative purpose only Z02.9
      specified NEC Z02.89
    admission to
      armed forces Z02.3
      old age home Z02.2

  ▶ New   ⇛ Revised   ~~deleted~~ Deleted   • Use Additional Character(s)

Examination *(Continued)*
  medical *(Continued)*
    admission to *(Continued)*
      prison Z02.89
      residential institution Z02.2
      school Z02.0
        following illness or medical treatment Z02.0
      summer camp Z02.89
    adoption Z02.82
    blood alcohol or drug level Z02.83
    camp (summer) Z02.89
    clinical research, normal subject (control) (participant) Z00.6
    control subject in clinical research (normal comparison) (participant) Z00.6
    donor (potential) Z00.5
    driving license Z02.4
    general (adult) Z00.00
      with abnormal findings Z00.01
    immigration Z02.89
    insurance purposes Z02.6
    marriage Z02.89
    medicolegal reasons NEC Z04.89
    naturalization Z02.89
    participation in sport Z02.5
    paternity testing Z02.81
    population survey Z00.8
    pre-employment Z02.1
    pre-operative —*see* Examination, pre-procedural
    pre-procedural
      cardiovascular Z01.810
      respiratory Z01.811
      specified NEC Z01.818
    preschool children
      for admission to school Z02.0
    prisoners
      for entrance into prison Z02.89
    recruitment for armed forces Z02.3
    specified NEC Z00.8
    sport competition Z02.5
  medicolegal reason NEC Z04.89
    forced sexual exploitation Z04.81
    forced labor exploitation Z04.82
  newborn —*see* Newborn, examination
  pelvic (annual) (periodic) Z01.419
    with abnormal findings Z01.411
  period of rapid growth in childhood Z00.2
  periodic (adult) (annual) (routine) Z00.00
    with abnormal findings Z00.01
  physical (adult) —*see also* Examination, medical Z00.00
    sports Z02.5
  postpartum
    immediately after delivery Z39.0
    routine follow-up Z39.2
  pre-chemotherapy (antineoplastic) Z01.818
  prenatal (normal pregnancy) —*see also* Pregnancy, normal Z34.9-●
  pre-procedural (pre-operative)
    cardiovascular Z01.810
    laboratory Z01.812
    respiratory Z01.811
    specified NEC Z01.818
  prior to chemotherapy (antineoplastic) Z01.818
  psychiatric NEC Z00.8
    follow-up not needing further care Z09
    requested by authority Z04.6
  radiological (as part of a general medical examination) Z00.00
    with abnormal findings Z00.01
  repeat cervical smear to confirm findings of recent normal smear following initial abnormal smear Z01.42
  skin (hypersensitivity) Z01.82
  special —*see also* Examination, by type Z01.89
    specified type NEC Z01.89
  specified type or reason NEC Z04.89
  teeth Z01.20
    with abnormal findings Z01.21

Examination *(Continued)*
  urine —*see* Examination, laboratory
  vision Z01.00
    with abnormal findings Z01.01
    following failed vision screening Z01.020
      with abnormal findings Z01.021
    infant or child (over 28 days old) Z00.129
      with abnormal findings Z00.121
Exanthem, exanthema —*see also* Rash
  with enteroviral vesicular stomatitis B08.4
  Boston A88.0
  epidemic with meningitis A88.0 [G02]
  subitum B08.20
    due to human herpesvirus 6 B08.21
    due to human herpesvirus 7 B08.22
  viral, virus B09
    specified type NEC B08.8
Excess, excessive, excessively
  alcohol level in blood R78.0
  androgen (ovarian) E28.1
  attrition, tooth, teeth K03.0
  carotene, carotin (dietary) E67.1
  cold, effects of T69.9
    specified effect NEC T69.8
  convergence H51.12
  crying
    in child, adolescent, or adult R45.83
    in infant R68.11
  development, breast N62
  divergence H51.8
  drinking (alcohol) NEC (without dependence) F10.10
    habitual (continual) (without remission) F10.20
  eating R63.2
  estrogen E28.0
  fat —*see also* Obesity
    in heart —*see* Degeneration, myocardial
    localized E65
  foreskin N47.8
  gas R14.0
  glucagon E16.3
  heat —*see* Heat
  intermaxillary vertical dimension of fully erupted teeth M26.37
  interocclusal distance of fully erupted teeth M26.37
  kalium E87.5
  large
    colon K59.39
      congenital Q43.8
    infant P08.0
    organ or site, congenital NEC —*see* Anomaly, by site
  long
    organ or site, congenital NEC —*see* Anomaly, by site
  menstruation (with regular cycle) N92.0
    with irregular cycle N92.1
  napping Z72.821
  natrium E87.0
  number of teeth K00.1
  nutrient (dietary) NEC R63.2
  potassium (K) E87.5
  salivation K11.7
  secretion —*see also* Hypersecretion
    milk O92.6
    sputum R09.3
    sweat R61
  sexual drive F52.8
  short
    organ or site, congenital NEC —*see* Anomaly, by site
    umbilical cord in labor or delivery O69.3
  skin L98.7
    and subcutaneous tissue L98.7
    eyelid (acquired) —*see* Blepharochalasis
      congenital Q10.3
  sodium (Na) E87.0
  spacing of fully erupted teeth M26.32
  sputum R09.3

Excess, excessive, excessively *(Continued)*
  sweating R61
  thirst R63.1
    due to deprivation of water T73.1
  ▶transportation time Z59.82
  tuberosity of jaw M26.07
  vitamin
    A (dietary) E67.0
      administered as drug (prolonged intake) —*see* Table of Drugs and Chemicals, vitamins, adverse effect
      overdose or wrong substance given or taken —*see* Table of Drugs and Chemicals, vitamins, poisoning
    D (dietary) E67.3
      administered as drug (prolonged intake) —*see* Table of Drugs and Chemicals, vitamins, adverse effect
      overdose or wrong substance given or taken —*see* Table of Drugs and Chemicals, vitamins, poisoning
  weight
    gain R63.5
    loss R63.4
Excitability, abnormal, under minor stress (personality disorder) F60.3
Excitation
  anomalous atrioventricular I45.6
  psychogenic F30.8
  reactive (from emotional stress, psychological trauma) F30.8
Excitement
  hypomanic F30.8
  manic F30.9
  mental, reactive (from emotional stress, psychological trauma) F30.8
  state, reactive (from emotional stress, psychological trauma) F30.8
Excoriation (traumatic) —*see also* Abrasion
  neurotic L98.1
  skin picking disorder F42.4
Exfoliation
  due to erythematous conditions according to extent of body surface involved L49.0
    10-19 percent of body surface L49.1
    20-29 percent of body surface L49.2
    30-39 percent of body surface L49.3
    40-49 percent of body surface L49.4
    50-59 percent of body surface L49.5
    60-69 percent of body surface L49.6
    70-79 percent of body surface L49.7
    80-89 percent of body surface L49.8
    90-99 percent of body surface L49.9
    less than 10 percent of body surface L49.0
  teeth, due to systemic causes K08.0
Exfoliative —*see* condition
Exhaustion, exhaustive (physical NEC) R53.83
  battle F43.0
  cardiac —*see* Failure, heart
  delirium F43.0
  due to
    cold T69.8
    excessive exertion T73.3
    exposure T73.2
    neurasthenia F48.8
  heart —*see* Failure, heart
  heat —*see also* Heat, exhaustion T67.5
    due to
      salt depletion T67.4
      water depletion T67.3
  maternal, complicating delivery O75.81
  mental F48.8
  myocardium, myocardial —*see* Failure, heart
  nervous F48.8
  old age R54
  psychogenic F48.8
  psychosis F43.0
  senile R54
  vital NEC T73.0
Exhibitionism F65.2

Exocervicitis —see Cervicitis
Exomphalos Q79.2
    meaning hernia —see Hernia, umbilicus
Exophoria H50.52
    convergence, insufficiency H51.11
    divergence, excess H51.8
Exophthalmos H05.2-●
    congenital Q15.8
    constant NEC H05.24-●
    displacement, globe —see Displacement,
        globe
    due to thyrotoxicosis (hyperthyroidism) —see
        Hyperthyroidism, with, goiter (diffuse)
    dysthyroid —see Hyperthyroidism, with,
        goiter (diffuse)
    goiter —see Hyperthyroidism, with, goiter
        (diffuse)
    intermittent NEC H05.25-●
    malignant —see Hyperthyroidism, with,
        goiter (diffuse)
    orbital
        edema —see Edema, orbit
        hemorrhage —see Hemorrhage, orbit
    pulsating NEC H05.26-●
    thyrotoxic, thyrotropic —see
        Hyperthyroidism, with, goiter (diffuse)
Exostosis —see also Disorder, bone
    cartilaginous —see Neoplasm, bone, benign
    congenital (multiple) Q78.6
    external ear canal H61.81-●
    gonococcal A54.49
    jaw (bone) M27.8
    multiple, congenital Q78.6
    orbit H05.35-●
    osteocartilaginous —see Neoplasm, bone,
        benign
    syphilitic A52.77
Exotropia —see Strabismus, divergent
    concomitant
Explanation of
    investigation finding Z71.2
    medication Z71.89
Exploitation
    labor
        confirmed
            adult forced T74.61
            child forced T74.62
        suspected
            adult forced T76.61
            child forced T76.62
    sexual
        confirmed
            adult forced T74.51
            child T74.52
        suspected
            adult forced T76.51
            child T76.52
Exposure (to) —see also Contact, with
    T75.89
    acariasis Z20.7
    AIDS virus Z20.6
    air pollution Z77.110
    algae and algae toxins Z77.121
    algae bloom Z77.121
    anthrax Z20.810
    aromatic amines Z77.020
    aromatic (hazardous) compounds NEC
        Z77.028
    aromatic dyes NOS Z77.028
    arsenic Z77.010
    asbestos Z77.090
    bacterial disease NEC Z20.818
    benzene Z77.021
    blue-green algae bloom Z77.121
    body fluids (potentially hazardous)
        Z77.21
    brown tide Z77.121

Exposure (Continued)
    chemicals (chiefly nonmedicinal) (hazardous)
        NEC Z77.098
    cholera Z20.09
    chromium compounds Z77.018
    cold, effects of T69.9
        specified effect NEC T69.8
    communicable disease Z20.9
        bacterial NEC Z20.818
        specified NEC Z20.89
        viral NEC Z20.828
        Zika virus Z20.821
        coronavirus (disease) (novel) 2019 Z20.822
    cyanobacteria bloom Z77.121
    disaster Z65.5
    discrimination Z60.5
    dyes Z77.098
    effects of T73.9
    environmental tobacco smoke (acute)
        (chronic) Z77.22
    Escherichia coli (E. coli) Z20.01
    exhaustion due to T73.2
    fiberglass —see Table of Drugs and
        Chemicals, fiberglass
    German measles Z20.4
    gonorrhea Z20.2
    hazardous metals NEC Z77.018
    hazardous substances NEC Z77.29
    hazards in the physical environment NEC
        Z77.128
    hazards to health NEC Z77.9
    human immunodeficiency virus (HIV)
        Z20.6
    human T-lymphotropic virus type-1 (HTLV-1)
        Z20.89
    implanted
        mesh —see Complications, prosthetic
            device or implant, mesh
        prosthetic materials NEC —see
            Complications, prosthetic materials
            NEC
    infestation (parasitic) NEC Z20.7
    intestinal infectious disease NEC Z20.09
        Escherichia coli (E. coli) Z20.01
    lead Z77.011
    meningococcus Z20.811
    mold (toxic) Z77.120
    nickel dust Z77.018
    noise Z77.122
    occupational
        air contaminants NEC Z57.39
        dust Z57.2
        environmental tobacco smoke Z57.31
        extreme temperature Z57.6
        noise Z57.0
        radiation Z57.1
        risk factors Z57.9
            specified NEC Z57.8
        toxic agents (gases) (liquids) (solids)
            (vapors) in agriculture Z57.4
        toxic agents (gases) (liquids) (solids)
            (vapors) in industry NEC Z57.5
        vibration Z57.7
    parasitic disease NEC Z20.7
    pediculosis Z20.7
    persecution Z60.5
    pfiesteria piscicida Z77.121
    poliomyelitis Z20.89
    pollution
        air Z77.110
        environmental NEC Z77.118
        soil Z77.112
        water Z77.111
    polycyclic aromatic hydrocarbons Z77.028
    prenatal (drugs) (toxic chemicals) —see
        Newborn, affected by, noxious substances
        transmitted via placenta or breast milk

Exposure (Continued)
    rabies Z20.3
    radiation, naturally occurring NEC Z77.123
    radon Z77.123
    red tide (Florida) Z77.121
    rubella Z20.4
    second hand tobacco smoke (acute) (chronic)
        Z77.22
        in the perinatal period P96.81
    sexually-transmitted disease Z20.2
    smallpox (laboratory) Z20.89
    syphilis Z20.2
    terrorism Z65.4
    torture Z65.4
    tuberculosis Z20.1
    uranium Z77.012
    varicella Z20.820
    venereal disease Z20.2
    viral disease NEC Z20.828
    war Z65.5
    water pollution Z77.111
    Zika virus Z20.821
Exsanguination —see Hemorrhage
Exstrophy
    abdominal contents Q45.8
    bladder Q64.10
        cloacal Q64.12
        specified type NEC Q64.19
        supravesical fissure Q64.11
Extensive —see condition
Extra —see also Accessory
    marker chromosomes (normal individual)
        Q92.61
        in abnormal individual Q92.62
    rib Q76.6
        cervical Q76.5
Extrasystoles (supraventricular) I49.49
    atrial I49.1
    auricular I49.1
    junctional I49.2
    ventricular I49.3
Extrauterine gestation or pregnancy —see
    Pregnancy, by site
Extravasation
    blood R58
    chyle into mesentery I89.8
    pelvicalyceal N13.8
    pyelosinus N13.8
    urine (from ureter) R39.0
    vesicant agent
        antineoplastic chemotherapy T80.810
        other agent NEC T80.818
Extremity —see condition, limb
Extrophy —see Exstrophy
Extroversion
    bladder Q64.19
    uterus N81.4
        complicating delivery O71.2
        postpartal (old) N81.4
Extruded tooth (teeth) M26.34
Extrusion
    breast implant (prosthetic) T85.42
    eye implant (globe) (ball) T85.328
    intervertebral disc —see Displacement,
        intervertebral disc
    ocular lens implant (prosthetic) —see
        Complications, intraocular lens
    vitreous —see Prolapse, vitreous
Exudate
    pleural —see Effusion, pleura
    retina H35.89
    wound fluids L24.A9
Exudative —see condition
Eye, eyeball, eyelid —see condition
Eyestrain —see Disturbance, vision, subjective
Eyeworm disease of Africa B74.3

▶ New   ⇒ Revised   ~~deleted~~ Deleted   ● Use Additional Character(s)

F

Faber's syndrome (achlorhydric anemia) D50.9
Fabry (-Anderson) disease E75.21
Facet syndrome M47.89-●
Faciocephalalgia, autonomic —see also
    Neuropathy, peripheral, autonomic G90.09
Factor(s)
    psychic, associated with diseases classified
        elsewhere F54
    psychological
        affecting physical conditions F54
        or behavioral
            affecting general medical condition F54
            associated with disorders or diseases
                classified elsewhere F54
Fahr disease (of brain) G23.8
Fahr Volhard disease (of kidney) I12.-●
Failure, failed
    abortion —see Abortion, attempted
    aortic (valve) I35.8
        rheumatic I06.8
    attempted abortion —see Abortion, attempted
    biventricular I50.82
        due to left heart failure I50.814
    bone marrow —see Anemia, aplastic
    cardiac —see Failure, heart
    cardiorenal (chronic) —see also Failure, renal,
        and Failure, heart I50.9
        hypertensive I13.2
    cardiorespiratory (see also Failure, heart) R09.2
    cardiovascular (chronic) —see Failure, heart
    cerebrovascular I67.9
    cervical dilatation in labor O62.0
    circulation, circulatory (peripheral) R57.9
        newborn P29.89
    compensation —see Disease, heart
    compliance with medical treatment or
        regimen —see Noncompliance
    congestive —see Failure, heart, congestive
    dental implant (endosseous) M27.69
        due to
            failure of dental prosthesis M27.63
            lack of attached gingiva M27.62
            occlusal trauma (poor prosthetic design)
                M27.62
            parafunctional habits M27.62
            periodontal infection (peri-implantitis)
                M27.62
            poor oral hygiene M27.62
        osseointegration M27.61
            due to
                complications of systemic disease
                    M27.61
                poor bone quality M27.61
            iatrogenic M27.61
        post-osseointegration
            biological M27.62
            due to complications of systemic disease
                M27.62
            iatrogenic M27.62
            mechanical M27.63
        pre-integration M27.61
        pre-osseointegration M27.61
        specified NEC M27.69
    descent of head (at term) of pregnancy
        (mother) O32.4
    endosseous dental implant —see Failure,
        dental implant
    engagement of head (term of pregnancy)
        (mother) O32.4
    erection (penile) —see also Dysfunction,
        sexual, male, erectile N52.9
        nonorganic F52.21
    examination(s), anxiety concerning Z55.2
    expansion terminal respiratory units
        (newborn) (primary) P28.0
    forceps NOS (with subsequent cesarean
        delivery) O66.5
    gain weight (child over 28 days old) R62.51
        adult R62.7
        newborn P92.6

Failure, failed (Continued)
    genital response (male) F52.21
        female F52.22
    heart (acute) (senile) (sudden) I50.9
        with
            acute pulmonary edema —see Failure,
                ventricular, left
            decompensation I50.9
                with
                    normal ejection fraction I50.33
                    preserved ejection fraction I50.33
                    reduced ejection fraction I50.23
                        with diastolic dysfunction I50.43
                    combined systolic and diastolic
                        I50.43
                    diastolic I50.33
                    right I50.813
                    systolic I50.23
            dilatation —see Disease, heart
            hypertension —see Hypertension, heart
            normal ejection fraction —see Failure,
                heart, diastolic
            preserved ejection fraction —see Failure,
                heart, diastolic
            reduced ejection fraction —see Failure,
                heart, systolic
        arteriosclerotic I70.90
        biventricular I50.82
            due to left heart failure I50.814
        combined left-right sided I50.82
            due to left heart failure I50.814
        compensated —see also Failure, heart, by
            type as diastolic or systolic, chronic
            I50.9
        complicating
            anesthesia (general) (local) or other
                sedation
                in labor and delivery O74.2
                in pregnancy O29.12-●
                postpartum, puerperal O89.1
            delivery (cesarean) (instrumental) O75.4
        congestive I50.9
            with rheumatic fever (conditions in I00)
                active I01.8
                inactive or quiescent (with chorea)
                    I09.81
            newborn P29.0
            rheumatic (chronic) (inactive) (with
                chorea) I09.81
                active or acute I01.8
                with chorea I02.0
        decompensated —see also Failure, heart, by
            type as diastolic or systolic, acute and
            chronic I50.9
        degenerative —see Degeneration, myocardial
        diastolic (congestive) (left ventricular) I50.30
            acute (congestive) I50.31
                and (on) chronic (congestive) I50.33
            chronic (congestive) I50.32
                and (on) acute (congestive) I50.33
            combined with systolic (congestive)
                I50.40
                acute (congestive) I50.41
                    and (on) chronic (congestive) I50.43
                chronic (congestive) I50.42
                    and (on) acute (congestive) I50.43
        due to presence of cardiac prosthesis I97.13-●
        end stage —see also Failure, heart, by type
            as diastolic or systolic, chronic I50.84
        following cardiac surgery I97.13-●
        high output NOS I50.83
        hypertensive —see Hypertension, heart
        left (ventricular) —see also Failure,
            ventricular, left
            combined diastolic and systolic —see
                Failure, heart, diastolic, combined
                with systolic
            diastolic —see Failure, heart, diastolic
            systolic —see Failure, heart, systolic
        low output (syndrome) NOS I50.9
        newborn P29.0
        organic —see Disease, heart
        peripartum O90.3

Failure, failed (Continued)
    heart (Continued)
        postprocedural I97.13-●
        rheumatic (chronic) (inactive) I09.9
        right (isolated) (ventricular) I50.810
            acute I50.811
                and (on) chronic I50.813
            chronic I50.812
                and acute I50.813
            secondary to left heart failure I50.814
        specified NEC I50.89

> Note: heart failure stages A, B, C, and
> D are based on the American College of
> Cardiology and American Heart Association
> stages of heart failure, which complement
> and should not be confused with the New
> York Heart Association Classification of
> Heart Failure, into Class I, Class II, Class III,
> and Class IV

        stage A Z91.89
        stage B (see also Failure, heart, by type as
            diastolic or systolic) I50.9
        stage C (see also Failure, heart, by type as
            diastolic or systolic) I50.9
        stage D (see also Failure, heart, by type
            as diastolic or systolic, chronic)
            I50.84
        systolic (congestive) (left ventricular)
            I50.20
            acute (congestive) I50.21
                and (on) chronic (congestive) I50.23
            chronic (congestive) I50.22
                and (on) acute (congestive) I50.23
            combined with diastolic (congestive)
                I50.40
                acute (congestive) I50.41
                    and (on) chronic (congestive)
                        I50.43
                chronic (congestive) I50.42
                    and (on) acute (congestive) I50.43
        thyrotoxic (see also Thyrotoxicosis) E05.90
            [I43]
            with
                high output (see also Thyrotoxicosis)
                    I50.83
                thyroid storm E05.91 [I43]
                    high output (see also
                        Thyrotoxicosis) I50.83
        valvular —see Endocarditis
    hepatic K72.90
        with coma K72.91
        acute or subacute K72.00
            with coma K72.01
            due to drugs K71.10
                with coma K71.11
        alcoholic (acute) (chronic) (subacute)
            K70.40
            with coma K70.41
        chronic K72.10
            with coma K72.11
            due to drugs (acute) (subacute) (chronic)
                K71.10
                with coma K71.11
        due to drugs (acute) (subacute) (chronic)
            K71.10
            with coma K71.11
        postprocedural K91.82
    hepatorenal K76.7
    induction (of labor) O61.9
        abortion —see Abortion, attempted
        by
            oxytocic drugs O61.0
            prostaglandins O61.0
        instrumental O61.1
        mechanical O61.1
        medical O61.0
        specified NEC O61.8
        surgical O61.1

Failure, failed *(Continued)*
- intubation during anesthesia T88.4
  - in pregnancy O29.6-●
  - labor and delivery O74.7
  - postpartum, puerperal O89.6
- involution, thymus (gland) E32.0
- kidney —*see also* Disease, kidney, chronic N19
  - acute —*see also* Failure, renal, acute N17.9-●
  - diabetic —*see* E08-E13 with .22
- lactation (complete) O92.3
  - partial O92.4
- Leydig's cell, adult E29.1
- liver —*see* Failure, hepatic
- menstruation at puberty N91.0
- mitral I05.8
- myocardial, myocardium —*see also* Failure, heart I50.9
  - chronic —*see also* Failure, heart, congestive I50.9
  - congestive —*see also* Failure, heart, congestive I50.9
- newborn screening —*see* Abnormal, neonatal screening
  - neonatal congenital heart disease P09.5
- orgasm (female) (psychogenic) F52.31
  - male F52.32
- ovarian (primary) E28.39
  - iatrogenic E89.40
    - asymptomatic E89.40
    - symptomatic E89.41
  - postprocedural (postablative) (postirradiation) (postsurgical) E89.40
    - asymptomatic E89.40
    - symptomatic E89.41
- ovulation causing infertility N97.0
- polyglandular, autoimmune E31.0
- prosthetic joint implant —*see* Complications, joint prosthesis, mechanical, breakdown, by site
- renal N19
  - with
    - tubular necrosis (acute) N17.0
  - acute N17.9
    - with
      - cortical necrosis N17.1
      - medullary necrosis N17.2
      - tubular necrosis N17.0
    - specified NEC N17.8
  - chronic N18.9
    - hypertensive —*see* Hypertension, kidney
  - congenital P96.0
  - end stage (chronic) N18.6
    - due to hypertension I12.0
  - following
    - abortion —*see* Abortion by type
      - complicated by specified condition NEC
    - crushing T79.5
    - ectopic or molar pregnancy O08.4
    - labor and delivery (acute) O90.4
  - hypertensive —*see* Hypertension, kidney
  - postprocedural N99.0
- respiration, respiratory J96.90
  - with
    - hypercapnia J96.92
    - hypercarbia J96.02
    - hypoxia J96.91
  - acute J96.00
    - with
      - hypercapnia J96.02
      - hypercarbia J96.92
      - hypoxia J96.01
  - acute and (on) chronic J96.20
    - with
      - hypercapnia J96.22
      - hypercarbia J96.22
      - hypoxia J96.21
  - center G93.89
  - chronic J96.10
    - with
      - hypercapnia J96.12
      - hypercarbia J96.12
      - hypoxia J96.11

Failure, failed *(Continued)*
- respiration, respiratory *(Continued)*
  - newborn P28.5
  - postprocedural (acute) J95.821
    - acute and chronic J95.822
- rotation
  - cecum Q43.3
  - colon Q43.3
  - intestine Q43.3
  - kidney Q63.2
- sedation (conscious) (moderate) during procedure T88.52
  - history of Z92.83
- segmentation —*see also* Fusion
  - fingers —*see* Syndactylism, complex, fingers
  - vertebra Q76.49
    - with scoliosis Q76.3
- seminiferous tubule, adult E29.1
- senile (general) R54
- sexual arousal (male) F52.21
  - female F52.22
- testicular endocrine function E29.1
- to thrive (child over 28 days old) R62.51
  - adult R62.7
  - newborn P92.6
- transplant T86.92
  - bone T86.831
    - marrow T86.02
  - cornea T86.841-●
  - heart T86.22
    - with lung(s) T86.32
  - intestine T86.851
  - kidney T86.12
  - liver T86.42
  - lung(s) T86.811
    - with heart T86.32
  - pancreas T86.891
  - skin (allograft) (autograft) T86.821
  - specified organ or tissue NEC T86.891
  - stem cell (peripheral blood) (umbilical cord) T86.5
- trial of labor (with subsequent cesarean delivery) O66.40
  - following previous cesarean delivery O66.41
- tubal ligation N99.89
- urinary —*see* Disease, kidney, chronic
- vacuum extraction NOS (with subsequent cesarean delivery) O66.5
- vasectomy N99.89
- ventouse NOS (with subsequent cesarean delivery) O66.5
- ventricular —*see also* Failure, heart I50.9
  - left —*see also* Failure, heart, left I50.1
    - with rheumatic fever (conditions in I00)
      - active I01.8
        - with chorea I02.0
      - inactive or quiescent (with chorea) I09.81
    - rheumatic (chronic) (inactive) (with chorea) I09.81
      - active or acute I01.8
        - with chorea I02.0
  - right —*see* Failure, heart, right
- vital centers, newborn P91.88

Fainting (fit) R55
Fallen arches —*see* Deformity, limb, flat foot
Falling, falls (repeated) R29.6
- any organ or part —*see* Prolapse
Fallopian
- insufflation Z31.41
- tube —*see* condition
Fallot's
- pentalogy Q21.8
- tetrad or tetralogy Q21.3
- triad or trilogy Q22.3
False —*see also* condition
- croup J38.5
- joint —*see* Nonunion, fracture

False *(Continued)*
- labor (pains) O47.9
  - at or after 37 completed weeks of gestation O47.1
  - before 37 completed weeks of gestation O47.0-●
- passage, urethra (prostatic) N36.5
- pregnancy F45.8
Family, familial —*see also* condition
- disruption Z63.8
  - involving divorce or separation Z63.5
- Li-Fraumeni (syndrome) Z15.01
- planning advice Z30.09
- problem Z63.9
  - specified NEC Z63.8
- retinoblastoma C69.2-●
Famine (effects of) T73.0
- edema —*see* Malnutrition, severe
Fanconi (-de Toni)(-Debré) **syndrome** E72.09
- with cystinosis E72.04
Fanconi's anemia (congenital pancytopenia) D61.09
Farber's disease or syndrome E75.29
Farcy A24.0
Farmer's
- lung J67.0
- skin L57.8
Farsightedness —*see* Hypermetropia
Fascia —*see* condition
Fasciculation R25.3
Fasciitis M72.9
- diffuse (eosinophilic) M35.4
- infective M72.8
  - necrotizing M72.6
- necrotizing M72.6
- nodular M72.4
- perirenal (with ureteral obstruction) N13.5
  - with infection N13.6
- plantar M72.2
- specified NEC M72.8
- traumatic (old) M72.8
  - current - code by site under Sprain
Fascioliasis B66.3
Fasciolopsis, fasciolopsiasis (intestinal) B66.5
Fascioscapulohumeral myopathy G71.02
Fast pulse R00.0
Fat
- embolism —*see* Embolism, fat
- excessive —*see also* Obesity
  - in heart —*see* Degeneration, myocardial
- in stool R19.5
- localized (pad) E65
  - heart —*see* Degeneration, myocardial
  - knee M79.4
  - retropatellar M79.4
- necrosis
  - breast N64.1
  - mesentery K65.4
  - omentum K65.4
- pad E65
  - knee M79.4
Fatigue R53.83
- auditory deafness —*see* Deafness
- chronic R53.82
- combat F43.0
- general R53.83
  - psychogenic F48.8
- heat (transient) T67.6
- muscle M62.89
- myocardium —*see* Failure, heart
- neoplasm-related R53.0
- nervous, neurosis F48.8
- operational F48.8
- psychogenic (general) F48.8
- senile R54
- voice R49.8
Fatness —*see* Obesity

▶ New   ➡ Revised   ~~deleted~~ Deleted   ● Use Additional Character(s)

Fatty —see also condition
  apron E65
  degeneration —see Degeneration, fatty
  heart (enlarged) —see Degeneration,
    myocardial
  liver NEC K76.0
    alcoholic K70.0
    nonalcoholic K76.0
  necrosis —see Degeneration, fatty
Fauces —see condition
Fauchard's disease (periodontitis) —see
  Periodontitis
Faucitis J02.9
Favism (anemia) D55.0
Favus —see Dermatophytosis
Fazio-Londe disease or syndrome
  G12.1
Fear complex or reaction F40.9
Fear of —see Phobia
Feared complaint unfounded Z71.1
Febris, febrile —see also Fever
  flava —see also Fever, yellow A95.9
  melitensis A23.0
  pestis —see Plague
  recurrens —see Fever, relapsing
  rubra A38.9
Fecal
  incontinence R15.9
  smearing R15.1
  soiling R15.1
  urgency R15.2
Fecalith (impaction) K56.41
  appendix K38.1
  congenital P76.8
Fede's disease K14.0
Feeble rapid pulse due to shock following
  injury T79.4
Feeble-minded F70
Feeding
  difficulties R63.30
  problem (elderly) (infant) R63.39
    newborn P92.9
      specified NEC P92.8
    nonorganic (adult) —see Disorder,
      eating
Feeling (of)
  foreign body in throat R09.89
Feer's disease —see Poisoning, mercury
Feet —see condition
Feigned illness Z76.5
Feil-Klippel syndrome (brevicollis) Q76.1
Feinmesser's (hidrotic) ectodermal dysplasia
  Q82.4
Felinophobia F40.218
Felon —see also Cellulitis, digit
  with lymphangitis —see Lymphangitis,
    acute, digit
Felty's syndrome M05.00
  ankle M05.07-●
  elbow M05.02-●
  foot joint M05.07-●
  hand joint M05.04-●
  hip M05.05-●
  knee M05.06-●
  multiple site M05.09
  shoulder M05.01-●
  vertebra —see Spondylitis, ankylosing
  wrist M05.03-●
Female genital cutting status —see Female
  genital mutilation status (FGM)
Female genital mutilation status (FGM)
  N90.810
  specified NEC N90.818
  type I (clitorectomy status) N90.811
  type II (clitorectomy with excision
    of labia minora status)
    N90.812
  type III (infibulation status)
    N90.813
  type IV N90.818
Femur, femoral —see condition

Fenestration, fenestrated —see also Imperfect,
  closure
  aortico-pulmonary Q21.4
  ▶ atrial septum Q21.11
  cusps, heart valve NEC Q24.8
    pulmonary Q22.3
  pulmonic cusps Q22.3
Fernell's disease (aortic aneurysm) I71.9
Fertile eunuch syndrome E23.0
Fetid
  breath R19.6
  sweat L75.0
Fetishism F65.0
  transvestic F65.1
Fetus, fetal —see also condition
  alcohol syndrome (dysmorphic) Q86.0
  compressus O31.0-●
  hydantoin syndrome Q86.1
  lung tissue P28.0
  papyraceous O31.0-●
Fever (inanition) (of unknown origin)
  (persistent) (with chills) (with rigor) R50.9
  abortus A23.1
  Aden (dengue) A90
  African tick bite A77.8
  African tick-borne A68.1
  American
    mountain (tick) A93.2
      spotted A77.0
  aphthous B08.8
  arbovirus, arboviral A94
    hemorrhagic A94
    specified NEC A93.8
  Argentinian hemorrhagic A96.0
  Assam B55.0
  Australian Q A78
  Bangkok hemorrhagic A91
  Barmah forest A92.8
  Bartonella A44.0
  bilious, hemoglobinuric B50.8
  blackwater B50.8
  blister B00.1
  Bolivian hemorrhagic A96.1
  Bonvale dam T73.3
  boutonneuse A77.1
  brain —see Encephalitis
  Brazilian purpuric A48.4
  breakbone A90
  Bullis A77.0
  Bunyamwera A92.8
  Burdwan B55.0
  Bwamba A92.8
  Cameroon —see Malaria
  Canton A75.9
  catarrhal (acute) J00
    chronic J31.0
  cat-scratch A28.1
  Central Asian hemorrhagic A98.0
  cerebral —see Encephalitis
  cerebrospinal meningococcal A39.0
  Chagres B50.9
  Chandipura A92.8
  Changuinola A93.1
  Charcot's (biliary) (hepatic) (intermittent) —
    see Calculus, bile duct
  Chikungunya (viral) (hemorrhagic) A92.0
  Chitral A93.1
  Colombo —see Fever, paratyphoid
  Colorado tick (virus) A93.2
  congestive (remittent) —see Malaria
  Congo virus A98.0
  continued malarial B50.9
  Corsican —see Malaria
  Crimean-Congo hemorrhagic A98.0
  Cyprus —see Brucellosis
  dandy A90
  deer fly —see Tularemia
  dengue (virus) A90
    hemorrhagic A91
    sandfly A93.1
  desert B38.0
  drug induced R50.2

Fever (Continued)
  due to
    conditions classified elsewhere R50.81
    heat T67.01
  enteric A01.00
  enteroviral exanthematous (Boston
    exanthem) A88.0
  ephemeral (of unknown origin) R50.9
  epidemic hemorrhagic A98.5
  erysipelatous —see Erysipelas
  estivo-autumnal (malarial) B50.9
  famine A75.0
  five day A79.0
  following delivery O86.4
  Fort Bragg A27.89
  gastroenteric A01.00
  gastromalarial —see Malaria
  Gibraltar —see Brucellosis
  glandular —see Mononucleosis, infectious
  Guama (viral) A92.8
  Haverhill A25.1
  hay (allergic) J30.1
    with asthma (bronchial) J45.909
      with
        exacerbation (acute) J45.901
        status asthmaticus J45.902
      due to
        allergen other than pollen J30.89
        pollen, any plant or tree J30.1
  heat (effects) T67.01
  hematuric, bilious B50.8
  hemoglobinuric (malarial) (bilious) B50.8
  hemorrhagic (arthropod-borne) NOS A94
    with renal syndrome A98.5
    arenaviral A96.9
      specified NEC A96.8
    Argentinian A96.0
    Bangkok A91
    Bolivian A96.1
    Central Asian A98.0
    Chikungunya A92.0
    Crimean-Congo A98.0
    dengue (virus) A91
    epidemic A98.5
    Junin (virus) A96.0
    Korean A98.5
    Kyasanur forest A98.2
    Machupo (virus) A96.1
    mite-borne A93.8
    mosquito-borne A92.8
    Omsk A98.1
    Philippine A91
    Russian A98.5
    Singapore A91
    Southeast Asia A91
    Thailand A91
    tick-borne NEC A93.8
    viral A99
      specified NEC A98.8
  hepatic —see Cholecystitis
  herpetic —see Herpes
  icterohemorrhagic A27.0
  Indiana A93.8
  infective B99.9
    specified NEC B99.8
  intermittent (bilious) —see also Malaria
    of unknown origin R50.9
    pernicious B50.9
  iodide R50.2
  Japanese river A75.3
  jungle —see also Malaria
    yellow A95.0
  Junin (virus) hemorrhagic A96.0
  Katayama B65.2
  kedani A75.3
  Kenya (tick) A77.1
  Kew Garden A79.1
  Korean hemorrhagic A98.5
  Lassa A96.2
  Lone Star A77.0
  Machupo (virus) hemorrhagic A96.1

Fever (Continued)
  malaria, malarial —see Malaria
  Malta A23.9
  Marseilles A77.1
  marsh —see Malaria
  Mayaro (viral) A92.8
  Mediterranean —see also Brucellosis A23.9
    familial M04.1
    tick A77.1
  meningeal —see Meningitis
  Meuse A79.0
  Mexican A75.2
  mianeh A68.1
  miasmatic —see Malaria
  mosquito-borne (viral) A92.9
    hemorrhagic A92.8
  mountain —see also Brucellosis
    meaning Rocky Mountain spotted fever
      A77.0
    tick (American) (Colorado) (viral) A93.2
  Mucambo (viral) A92.8
  mud A27.9
  Neapolitan —see Brucellosis
  neutropenic D70.9
  newborn P81.9
    environmental P81.0
  Nine-Mile A78
  non-exanthematous tick A93.2
  North Asian tick-borne A77.2
  Omsk hemorrhagic A98.1
  O'nyong-nyong (viral) A92.1
  Oropouche (viral) A93.0
  Oroya A44.0
  pacific coast tick A77.8
  paludal —see Malaria
  Panama (malarial) B50.9
  Pappataci A93.1
  paratyphoid A01.4
    A A01.1
    B A01.2
    C A01.3
  parrot A70
  periodic (Mediterranean) M04.1
  persistent (of unknown origin) R50.9
  petechial A39.0
  pharyngoconjunctival B30.2
  Philippine hemorrhagic A91
  phlebotomus A93.1
  Piry (virus) A93.8
  Pixuna (viral) A92.8
  Plasmodium ovale B53.0
  polioviral (nonparalytic) A80.4
  Pontiac A48.2
  postimmunization R50.83
  postoperative R50.82
    due to infection T81.40
  posttransfusion R50.84
  postvaccination R50.83
  presenting with conditions classified
    elsewhere R50.81
  pretibial A27.89
  puerperal O86.4
  Q A78
  quadrilateral A78
  quartan (malaria) B52.9
  Queensland (coastal) (tick) A77.3
  quintan A79.0
  rabbit —see Tularemia
  rat-bite A25.9
    due to
      Spirillum A25.0
      Streptobacillus moniliformis A25.1
  recurrent —see Fever, relapsing
  relapsing (Borrelia) A68.9
    Carter's (Asiatic) A68.1
    Dutton's (West African) A68.1
    Koch's A68.9
    louse-borne A68.0
    Novy's
      louse-borne A68.0
      tick-borne A68.1

Fever (Continued)
  relapsing (Borrelia) (Continued)
    Obermeyer's (European) A68.0
    tick-borne A68.1
  remittent (bilious) (congestive) (gastric) —see
    Malaria
  rheumatic (active) (acute) (chronic) (subacute)
    I00
    with central nervous system involvement
      I02.9
    active with heart involvement —see
      category I01
    inactive or quiescent with
      cardiac hypertrophy I09.89
      carditis I09.9
      endocarditis I09.1
        aortic (valve) I06.9
          with mitral (valve) disease I08.0
        mitral (valve) I05.9
          with aortic (valve) disease I08.0
        pulmonary (valve) I09.89
        tricuspid (valve) I07.8
      heart disease NEC I09.89
      heart failure (congestive) (conditions in
        category I50.) I09.81
      left ventricular failure (conditions in
        I50.1-I50.4-) I09.81
      myocarditis, myocardial degeneration
        (conditions in I51.4) I09.0
      pancarditis I09.9
      pericarditis I09.2
  Rift Valley (viral) A92.4
  Rocky Mountain spotted A77.0
  rose J30.1
  Ross River B33.1
  Russian hemorrhagic A98.5
  San Joaquin (Valley) B38.0
  sandfly A93.1
  Sao Paulo A77.0
  scarlet A38.9
  seven day (leptospirosis) (autumnal)
    (Japanese) A27.89
  dengue A90
  shin-bone A79.0
  Singapore hemorrhagic A91
  solar A90
  Songo A98.5
  sore B00.1
  South African tick-bite A68.1
  Southeast Asia hemorrhagic A91
  spinal —see Meningitis
  spirillary A25.0
  splenic —see Anthrax
  spotted A77.9
    American A77.0
    Brazilian A77.0
    cerebrospinal meningitis A39.0
    Colombian A77.0
    due to Rickettsia
      africae (African tick bite fever) A77.8
      australis A77.3
      conorii A77.1
      parkeri A77.8
      rickettsii A77.0
      sibirica A77.2
      specified type NEC A77.8
    Ehrlichiosis A77.40
      due to
        E. chafeensis A77.41
        specified organism NEC A77.49
    Rocky Mountain A77.0
  steroid R50.2
  streptobacillary A25.1
  subtertian B50.9
  Sumatran mite A75.3
  sun A90
  swamp A27.9
  swine A02.8
  sylvatic, yellow A95.0
  Tahyna B33.8
  tertian —see Malaria, tertian

Fever (Continued)
  Thailand hemorrhagic A91
  thermic T67.01
  three-day A93.1
  tick
    American mountain A93.2
    Colorado A93.2
    Kemerovo A93.8
    Mediterranean A77.1
    mountain A93.2
    nonexanthematous A93.2
    Quaranfil A93.8
  tick-bite NEC A93.8
  tick-borne (hemorrhagic) NEC A93.8
  trench A79.0
  tsutsugamushi A75.3
  typhogastric A01.00
  typhoid (abortive) (hemorrhagic)
    (intermittent) (malignant) A01.00
    complicated by
      arthritis A01.04
      heart involvement A01.02
      meningitis A01.01
      osteomyelitis A01.05
      pneumonia A01.03
      specified NEC A01.09
  typhomalarial —see Malaria
  typhus —see Typhus (fever)
  undulant —see Brucellosis
  unknown origin R50.9
  uveoparotid D86.89
  valley B38.0
  Venezuelan equine A92.2
  vesicular stomatitis A93.8
  viral hemorrhagic —see Fever, hemorrhagic,
    by type of virus
  Volhynian A79.0
  Wesselsbron (viral) A92.8
  West
    African B50.8
    Nile (viral) A92.30
      with
        complications NEC A92.39
        cranial nerve disorders A92.32
        encephalitis A92.31
        encephalomyelitis A92.31
        neurologic manifestation NEC
          A92.32
        optic neuritis A92.32
        polyradiculitis A92.32
  Whitmore's —see Melioidosis
  Wolhynian A79.0
  worm B83.9
  yellow A95.9
    jungle A95.0
    sylvatic A95.0
    urban A95.1
  Zika virus A92.5
Fibrillation
  atrial or auricular (established) I48.91
    chronic I48.20
    persistent I48.19
    paroxysmal I48.0
    permanent I48.21
    persistent (chronic) (NOS) (other) I48.19
    longstanding I48.11
  cardiac I49.8
  heart I49.8
  muscular M62.89
  ventricular I49.01
Fibrin
  ball or bodies, pleural (sac) J94.1
  chamber, anterior (eye) (gelatinous
    exudate) —see Iridocyclitis, acute
Fibrinogenolysis —see Fibrinolysis
Fibrinogenopenia D68.8
  acquired D65
  congenital D68.2
Fibrinolysis (hemorrhagic) (acquired) D65
  antepartum hemorrhage —see Hemorrhage,
    antepartum, with coagulation defect

▶ New   ⇒ Revised   ~~deleted~~ Deleted   ● Use Additional Character(s)

Fibrinolysis (Continued)
  following
    abortion —see Abortion by type
      complicated by hemorrhage
    ectopic or molar pregnancy O08.1
  intrapartum O67.0
  newborn, transient P60
  postpartum O72.3
Fibrinopenia (hereditary) D68.2
  acquired D68.4
Fibrinopurulent —see condition
Fibrinous —see condition
Fibroadenoma
  cellular intracanalicular D24-•
  giant D24-•
  intracanalicular
    cellular D24-•
    giant D24-•
    specified site —see Neoplasm, benign, by
      site
    unspecified site D24-•
  juvenile D24-•
  pericanalicular
    specified site —see Neoplasm, benign, by
      site
    unspecified site D24-•
  phyllodes D24-•
  prostate D29.1
  specified site NEC —see Neoplasm, benign,
    by site
  unspecified site D24-•
Fibroadenosis, breast (chronic) (cystic) (diffuse)
  (periodic) (segmental) N60.2-•
Fibroangioma —see also Neoplasm, benign, by
  site
  juvenile
    specified site —see Neoplasm, benign, by
      site
    unspecified site D10.6
Fibrochondrosarcoma —see Neoplasm,
  cartilage, malignant
Fibrocystic
  disease —see also Fibrosis, cystic
    breast —see Mastopathy, cystic
    jaw M27.49
    kidney (congenital) Q61.8
    liver Q44.6
    pancreas E84.9
  kidney (congenital) Q61.8
Fibrodysplasia ossificans progressiva —see
  Myositis, ossificans, progressiva
Fibroelastosis (cordis) (endocardial)
  (endomyocardial) I42.4
Fibroid (tumor) —see also Neoplasm, connective
  tissue, benign
  disease, lung (chronic) —see Fibrosis, lung
  heart (disease) —see Myocarditis
  in pregnancy or childbirth O34.1-•
    causing obstructed labor O65.5
  induration, lung (chronic) —see Fibrosis, lung
  lung —see Fibrosis, lung
  pneumonia (chronic) —see Fibrosis, lung
  uterus —see also Leiomyoma, uterus D25.9
Fibrolipoma —see Lipoma
Fibroliposarcoma —see Neoplasm, connective
  tissue, malignant
Fibroma —see also Neoplasm, connective tissue,
  benign
  ameloblastic —see Cyst, calcifying odontogenic
  bone (nonossifying) —see Disorder, bone,
    specified type NEC
    ossifying —see Neoplasm, bone, benign
  cementifying —see Neoplasm, bone, benign
  chondromyxoid —see Neoplasm, bone,
    benign
  desmoplastic —see Neoplasm, connective
    tissue, uncertain behavior
  durum —see Neoplasm, connective tissue,
    benign
  fascial —see Neoplasm, connective tissue,
    benign

Fibroma (Continued)
  invasive —see Neoplasm, connective tissue,
    uncertain behavior
  molle —see Lipoma
  myxoid —see Neoplasm, connective tissue,
    benign
  nasopharynx, nasopharyngeal (juvenile)
    D10.6
  nonosteogenic (nonossifying) —see Dysplasia,
    fibrous
  odontogenic (central) —see Cyst, calcifying
    odontogenic
  ossifying —see Neoplasm, bone, benign
  periosteal —see Neoplasm, bone, benign
  soft —see Lipoma
Fibromatosis M72.9
  abdominal —see Neoplasm, connective tissue,
    uncertain behavior
  aggressive —see Neoplasm, connective tissue,
    uncertain behavior
  congenital generalized —see Neoplasm,
    connective tissue, uncertain behavior
  Dupuytren's M72.0
  gingival K06.1
  palmar (fascial) M72.0
  plantar (fascial) M72.2
  pseudosarcomatous (proliferative)
    (subcutaneous) M72.4
  retroperitoneal D48.3
  specified NEC M72.8
Fibromyalgia M79.7
Fibromyoma —see also Neoplasm, connective
  tissue, benign
  uterus (corpus) —see also Leiomyoma, uterus
    in pregnancy or childbirth —see Fibroid, in
      pregnancy or childbirth
      causing obstructed labor O65.5
Fibromyositis M79.7
Fibromyxolipoma D17.9
Fibromyxoma —see Neoplasm, connective
  tissue, benign
Fibromyxosarcoma —see Neoplasm, connective
  tissue, malignant
Fibro-odontoma, ameloblastic —see Cyst,
  calcifying odontogenic
Fibro-osteoma —see Neoplasm, bone, benign
Fibroplasia, retrolental H35.17
Fibropurulent —see condition
Fibrosarcoma —see also Neoplasm, connective
  tissue, malignant
  ameloblastic C41.1
    upper jaw (bone) C41.0
  congenital —see Neoplasm, connective tissue,
    malignant
  fascial —see Neoplasm, connective tissue,
    malignant
  infantile —see Neoplasm, connective tissue,
    malignant
  odontogenic C41.1
    upper jaw (bone) C41.0
  periosteal —see Neoplasm, bone, malignant
Fibrosclerosis
  breast N60.3-•
  multifocal M35.5
  penis (corpora cavernosa) N48.6
Fibrosis, fibrotic
  adrenal (gland) E27.8
  amnion O41.8X-•
  anal papillae K62.89
  arteriocapillary —see Arteriosclerosis
  bladder N32.89
    interstitial —see Cystitis, chronic,
      interstitial
    localized submucosal —see Cystitis,
      chronic, interstitial
    panmural —see Cystitis, chronic, interstitial
  breast —see Fibrosclerosis, breast
  capillary —see also Arteriosclerosis I70.90
    lung (chronic) —see Fibrosis, lung
  cardiac —see Myocarditis
  cervix N88.8

Fibrosis, fibrotic (Continued)
  chorion O41.8X-•
  corpus cavernosum (sclerosing) N48.6
  cystic (of pancreas) E84.9
    with
      distal intestinal obstruction syndrome
        E84.19
      fecal impaction E84.19
      intestinal manifestations NEC E84.19
      pulmonary manifestations E84.0
      specified manifestations NEC E84.8
  due to device, implant or graft —see also
    Complications, by site and type,
    specified NEC T85.828
    arterial graft NEC T82.828
    breast (implant) T85.828
    catheter NEC T85.828
      dialysis (renal) T82.828
        intraperitoneal T85.828
      infusion NEC T82.828
        spinal (epidural) (subdural)
          T85.820
      urinary (indwelling) T83.82
    electronic (electrode) (pulse generator)
      (stimulator)
      bone T84.82
      cardiac T82.827
      nervous system (brain) (peripheral
        nerve) (spinal) T85.820
      urinary T83.82
    fixation, internal (orthopedic) NEC T84.82
    gastrointestinal (bile duct) (esophagus)
      T85.828
    genital NEC T83.82
    heart NEC T82.827
    joint prosthesis T84.82
    ocular (corneal graft) (orbital implant)
      NEC T85.828
    orthopedic NEC T84.82
    specified NEC T85.828
    urinary NEC T83.82
    vascular NEC T82.828
    ventricular intracranial shunt T85.820
  ejaculatory duct N50.89
  endocardium —see Endocarditis
  endomyocardial (tropical) I42.3
  epididymis N50.89
  eye muscle —see Strabismus, mechanical
  heart —see Myocarditis
  hepatic —see Fibrosis, liver
  hepatolienal (portal hypertension) K76.6
  hepatosplenic (portal hypertension) K76.6
  infrapatellar fat pad M79.4
  intrascrotal N50.89
  kidney N26.9
  liver K74.00
    with sclerosis K74.2
    advanced K74.02
    alcoholic K70.2
    early K74.01
    stage
      F1 or F2 K74.01
      F3 K74.02
  lung (atrophic) (chronic) (confluent)
    (massive) (perialveolar) (peribronchial)
    J84.10
    with
      anthracosilicosis J60
      anthracosis J60
      asbestosis J61
      bagassosis J67.1
      bauxite J63.1
      berylliosis J63.2
      byssinosis J66.0
      calcicosis J62.8
      chalicosis J62.8
      dust reticulation J64
      farmer's lung J67.0
      ganister disease J62.8
      graphite J63.3
      pneumoconiosis NOS J64

Fibrosis, fibrotic *(Continued)*
  lung *(Continued)*
    with *(Continued)*
      siderosis J63.4
      silicosis J62.8
    capillary J84.10
    congenital P27.8
    diffuse (idiopathic) J84.10
      chemicals, gases, fumes or vapors
        (inhalation) J68.4
      interstitial J84.10
        acute J84.114
      talc J62.0
    following radiation J70.1
    idiopathic J84.112
    postinflammatory J84.10
    silicotic J62.8
    tuberculous —*see* Tuberculosis, pulmonary
  lymphatic gland I89.8
  median bar —*see* Hyperplasia, prostate
  mediastinum (idiopathic) J98.59
  meninges G96.198
  myocardium, myocardial —*see* Myocarditis
  ovary N83.8
  oviduct N83.8
  pancreas K86.89
  penis NEC N48.6
  pericardium I31.0
  perineum, in pregnancy or childbirth O34.7-•
    causing obstructed labor O65.5
  pleura J94.1
  popliteal fat pad M79.4
  prostate (chronic) —*see* Hyperplasia, prostate
  pulmonary —*see also* Fibrosis, lung J84.10
    congenital P27.8
    idiopathic J84.112
  rectal sphincter K62.89
  retroperitoneal, idiopathic (with ureteral
    obstruction) N13.5
    with infection N13.6
  sclerosing mesenteric (idiopathic) K65.4
  scrotum N50.89
  seminal vesicle N50.89
  senile R54
  skin L90.5
  spermatic cord N50.89
  spleen D73.89
    in schistosomiasis (bilharziasis) B65.9 [D77]
  subepidermal nodular —*see* Neoplasm, skin,
    benign
  submucous (oral) (tongue) K13.5
  testis N44.8
    chronic, due to syphilis A52.76
  thymus (gland) E32.8
  tongue, submucous K13.5
  tunica vaginalis N50.89
  uterus (non-neoplastic) N85.8
  vagina N89.8
  valve, heart —*see* Endocarditis
  vas deferens N50.89
  vein I87.8
Fibrositis (periarticular) M79.7
  nodular, chronic (Jaccoud's) (rheumatoid) —
    see Arthropathy, postrheumatic, chronic
Fibrothorax J94.1
Fibrotic —*see* Fibrosis
Fibrous —*see* condition
Fibroxanthoma —*see also* Neoplasm, connective
  tissue, benign
  atypical —*see* Neoplasm, connective tissue,
    uncertain behavior
  malignant —*see* Neoplasm, connective tissue,
    malignant
Fibroxanthosarcoma —*see* Neoplasm,
  connective tissue, malignant
Fiedler's
  disease (icterohemorrhagic leptospirosis) A27.0
  myocarditis (acute) I40.1
Fifth disease B08.3
  venereal A55
Filaria, filarial, filariasis —*see* Infestation, filarial

Filatov's disease —*see* Mononucleosis, infectious
File-cutter's disease —*see* Poisoning, lead
Filling defect
  biliary tract R93.2
  bladder R93.41
  duodenum R93.3
  gallbladder R93.2
  gastrointestinal tract R93.3
  intestine R93.3
  kidney R93.42-•
  stomach R93.3
  ureter R93.41
  urinary organs, specified NEC R93.49
Fimbrial cyst Q50.4
Financial problem affecting care NOS Z59.9
  bankruptcy Z59.89
  foreclosure on loan Z59.89
  home loan Z59.81-•
  ▶strain Z59.86
Findings, abnormal, inconclusive, without
  diagnosis —*see also* Abnormal
  17-ketosteroids, elevated R82.5
  acetonuria R82.4
  alcohol in blood R78.0
  anisocytosis R71.8
  antenatal screening of mother O28.9
    biochemical O28.1
    chromosomal O28.5
    cytological O28.2
    genetic O28.5
    hematological O28.0
    radiological O28.4
    specified NEC O28.8
    ultrasonic O28.3
  antibody titer, elevated R76.0
  anticardiolipin antibody R76.0
  antiphosphatidylglycerol antibody R76.0
  antiphosphatidylinositol antibody R76.0
  antiphosphatidylserine antibody R76.0
  antiphospholipid antibody R76.0
  bacteriuria R82.71
  bicarbonate E87.8
  bile in urine R82.2
  blood sugar R73.09
    high R73.9
    low (transient) E16.2
  body fluid or substance, specified NEC
    R88.8
  casts, urine R82.998
  catecholamines R82.5
  cells, urine R82.998
  chloride E87.8
  cholesterol E78.9
    high E78.00
      with high triglycerides E78.2
  chyluria R82.0
  cloudy
    dialysis effluent R88.0
    urine R82.90
  creatinine clearance R94.4
  crystals, urine R82.998
  culture
    blood R78.81
    positive —*see* Positive, culture
  echocardiogram R93.1
  electrolyte level, urinary R82.998
  function study NEC R94.8
    bladder R94.8
    endocrine NEC R94.7
      thyroid R94.6
    kidney R94.4
    liver R94.5
    pancreas R94.8
    placenta R94.8
    pulmonary R94.2
    spleen R94.8
  gallbladder, nonvisualization R93.2
  glucose (tolerance test) (non-fasting) R73.09
  glycosuria R81
  heart
    shadow R93.1
    sounds R01.2
  hematinuria R82.3

Findings, abnormal, inconclusive, without
  diagnosis *(Continued)*
  hematocrit drop (precipitous) R71.0
  hemoglobinuria R82.3
  human papillomavirus (HPV) DNA test
    positive
    cervix
      high risk R87.810
      low risk R87.820
    vagina
      high risk R87.811
      low risk R87.821
  in blood (of substance not normally found in
    blood) R78.9
    addictive drug NEC R78.4
    alcohol (excessive level) R78.0
    cocaine R78.2
    hallucinogen R78.3
    heavy metals (abnormal level) R78.79
    lead R78.71
    lithium (abnormal level) R78.89
    opiate drug R78.1
    psychotropic drug R78.5
    specified substance NEC R78.89
    steroid agent R78.6
  indoleacetic acid, elevated R82.5
  ketonuria R82.4
  lactic acid dehydrogenase (LDH) R74.02
  liver function test (*see also* Elevated, liver
    function, test) R79.89
  mammogram NEC R92.8
    calcification (calculus) R92.1
    inconclusive result (due to dense breasts)
      R92.2
    microcalcification R92.0
  mediastinal shift R93.89
  melanin, urine R82.998
  myoglobinuria R82.1
  neonatal screening —*see* Abnormal, neonatal
    screening
  newborn screens, state mandated —*see*
    Abnormal, neonatal screening
  nonvisualization of gallbladder R93.2
  odor of urine NOS R82.90
  Papanicolaou cervix R87.619
    non-atypical endometrial cells R87.618
  pneumoencephalogram R93.0
  poikilocytosis R71.8
  potassium (deficiency) E87.6
    excess E87.5
  PPD R76.11
  radiologic (X-ray) R93.89
    abdomen R93.5
    biliary tract R93.2
    breast R92.8
    gastrointestinal tract R93.3
    genitourinary organs R93.89
    head R93.0
    inconclusive due to excess body fat of
      patient R93.9
    intrathoracic organs NEC R93.1
    musculoskeletal
      limbs R93.6
      other than limb R93.7
    placenta R93.89
    retroperitoneum R93.5
    skin R93.89
    skull R93.0
    subcutaneous tissue R93.89
    testis R93.81-•
  red blood cell (count) (morphology) (sickling)
    (volume) R71.8
  scan NEC R94.8
    bladder R94.8
    bone R94.8
    kidney R94.4
    liver R93.2
    lung R94.2
    pancreas R94.8
    placental R94.8
    spleen R94.8
    thyroid R94.6
  sedimentation rate, elevated R70.0

▶ New   ⇒ Revised   ~~deleted~~ Deleted   • Use Additional Character(s)

Findings, abnormal, inconclusive, without diagnosis *(Continued)*
SGOT R74.01
SGPT R74.01
sodium (deficiency) E87.1
  excess E87.0
specified body fluid NEC R88.8
stress test R94.39
thyroid (function) (metabolic rate) (scan) (uptake) R94.6
transaminase (level) R74.01
triglycerides E78.9
  high E78.1
    with high cholesterol E78.2
tuberculin skin test (without active tuberculosis) R76.11
urine R82.90
  acetone R82.4
  bacteria R82.71
  bile R82.2
  casts or cells R82.998
  chyle R82.0
  culture positive R82.79
  glucose R81
  hemoglobin R82.3
  ketone R82.4
  sugar R81
vanillylmandelic acid (VMA), elevated R82.5
vectorcardiogram (VCG) R94.39
ventriculogram R93.0
white blood cell (count) (differential) (morphology) D72.9
xerography R92.8
Finger —*see* condition
Fire, Saint Anthony's —*see* Erysipelas
Fire-setting
  pathological (compulsive) F63.1
Fish hook stomach K31.89
Fishmeal-worker's lung J67.8
Fissure, fissured
anus, anal K60.2
  acute K60.0
  chronic K60.1
  congenital Q43.8
ear, lobule, congenital Q17.8
epiglottis (congenital) Q31.8
larynx J38.7
  congenital Q31.8
lip K13.0
  congenital —*see* Cleft, lip
nipple N64.0
  associated with
    lactation O92.13
    pregnancy O92.11- •
    puerperium O92.12
nose Q30.2
palate (congenital) —*see* Cleft, palate
skin R23.4
spine (congenital) —*see also* Spina bifida
  with hydrocephalus —*see* Spina bifida, by site, with hydrocephalus
tongue (acquired) K14.5
  congenital Q38.3
Fistula (cutaneous) L98.8
abdomen (wall) K63.2
  bladder N32.2
  intestine NEC K63.2
  ureter N28.89
  uterus N82.5
abdominorectal K63.2
abdominosigmoidal K63.2
abdominothoracic J86.0
abdominouterine N82.5
  congenital Q51.7
abdominovesical N32.2
accessory sinuses —*see* Sinusitis
actinomycotic —*see* Actinomycosis
alveolar antrum —*see* Sinusitis, maxillary
alveolar process K04.6
anorectal K60.5
antrobuccal —*see* Sinusitis, maxillary
antrum —*see* Sinusitis, maxillary

Fistula *(Continued)*
anus, anal (recurrent) (infectional) K60.3
  congenital Q43.6
    with absence, atresia and stenosis Q42.2
  tuberculous A18.32
aorta-duodenal I77.2
appendix, appendicular K38.3
arteriovenous (acquired) (nonruptured) I77.0
  brain I67.1
    congenital Q28.2
      ruptured —*see* Fistula, arteriovenous, brain, ruptured
    ruptured I60.8
      intracerebral I61.8
      intraparenchymal I61.8
      intraventricular I61.5
      subarachnoid I60.8
  cerebral —*see* Fistula, arteriovenous, brain
  congenital (peripheral) —*see also* Malformation, arteriovenous
    brain Q28.2
      ruptured —*see* Fistula, arteriovenous, brain, ruptured
    coronary Q24.5
    pulmonary Q25.72
  coronary I25.41
    congenital Q24.5
  pulmonary I28.0
    congenital Q25.72
  surgically created (for dialysis) Z99.2
    complication —*see* Complication, arteriovenous, fistula, surgically created
  traumatic —*see* Injury, blood vessel
artery I77.2
aural (mastoid) —*see* Mastoiditis, chronic
auricle —*see also* Disorder, pinna, specified type NEC
  congenital Q18.1
Bartholin's gland N82.8
bile duct (common) (hepatic) K83.3
  with calculus, stones —*see also* Calculus, bile duct K83.3
biliary (tract) —*see* Fistula, bile duct
bladder (sphincter) NEC —*see also* Fistula, vesico- N32.2
  into seminal vesicle N32.2
bone —*see also* Disorder, bone, specified type NEC
  with osteomyelitis, chronic —*see* Osteomyelitis, chronic, with draining sinus
brain G93.89
  arteriovenous (acquired) (see Fistula, arteriovenous, brain) I67.1
  congenital Q28.2
branchial (cleft) Q18.0
branchiogenous Q18.0
breast N61.0
  puerperal, postpartum or gestational, due to mastitis (purulent) —*see* Mastitis, obstetric, purulent
bronchial J86.0
bronchocutaneous, bronchomediastinal, bronchopleural, bronchopleuromediastinal (infective) J86.0
  tuberculous NEC A15.5
bronchoesophageal J86.0
  congenital Q39.2
    with atresia of esophagus Q39.1
bronchovisceral J86.0
buccal cavity (infective) K12.2
cecosigmoidal K63.2
cecum K63.2
cerebrospinal (fluid) G96.08
cervical, lateral Q18.1
cervicoaural Q18.1
cervicosigmoidal N82.4
cervicovesical N82.1
cervix N82.8
chest (wall) J86.0

Fistula *(Continued)*
cholecystenteric —*see* Fistula, gallbladder
cholecystocolic —*see* Fistula, gallbladder
cholecystocolonic —*see* Fistula, gallbladder
cholecystoduodenal —*see* Fistula, gallbladder
cholecystogastric —*see* Fistula, gallbladder
cholecystointestinal —*see* Fistula, gallbladder
choledochoduodenal —*see* Fistula, bile duct
cholocolic K82.3
coccyx —*see* Sinus, pilonidal
colon K63.2
colostomy K94.09
colovesical N32.1
common duct —*see* Fistula, bile duct
congenital, site not listed —*see* Anomaly, by site
coronary, arteriovenous I25.41
  congenital Q24.5
costal region J86.0
cul-de-sac, Douglas' N82.8
cystic duct —*see also* Fistula, gallbladder
  congenital Q44.5
dental K04.6
diaphragm J86.0
duodenum K31.6
ear (external) (canal) —*see* Disorder, ear, external, specified type NEC
enterocolic K63.2
enterocutaneous K63.2
enterouterine N82.4
  congenital Q51.7
enterovaginal N82.4
  congenital Q52.2
  large intestine N82.3
  small intestine N82.2
enterovesical N32.1
epididymis N50.89
  tuberculous A18.15
esophagobronchial J86.0
  congenital Q39.2
    with atresia of esophagus Q39.1
esophagocutaneous K22.89
esophagopleural-cutaneous J86.0
esophagotracheal J86.0
  congenital Q39.2
    with atresia of esophagus Q39.1
esophagus K22.89
  congenital Q39.2
    with atresia of esophagus Q39.1
ethmoid —*see* Sinusitis, ethmoidal
eyeball (cornea) (sclera) —*see* Disorder, globe, hypotony
eyelid H01.8
fallopian tube, external N82.5
fecal K63.2
  congenital Q43.6
from periapical abscess K04.6
frontal sinus —*see* Sinusitis, frontal
gallbladder K82.3
  with calculus, cholelithiasis, stones —*see* Calculus, gallbladder
gastric K31.6
gastrocolic K31.6
  congenital Q40.2
  tuberculous A18.32
gastroenterocolic K31.6
gastroesophageal K31.6
gastrojejunal K31.6
gastrojejunocolic K31.6
genital tract (female) N82.9
  specified NEC N82.8
  to intestine NEC N82.4
  to skin N82.5
hepatic artery-portal vein, congenital Q26.6
hepatopleural J86.0
hepatopulmonary J86.0
ileorectal or ileosigmoidal K63.2
ileovaginal N82.2
ileovesical N32.1
ileum K63.2
in ano K60.3
  tuberculous A18.32

Fistula *(Continued)*
  inner ear (labyrinth) —*see* subcategory H83.1
  intestine NEC K63.2
  intestinocolonic (abdominal) K63.2
  intestinoureteral N28.89
  intestinouterine N82.4
  intestinovaginal N82.4
    large intestine N82.3
    small intestine N82.2
  intestinovesical N32.1
  ischiorectal (fossa) K61.39
  jejunum K63.2
  joint M25.10
    ankle M25.17-●
    elbow M25.12-●
    foot joint M25.17-●
    hand joint M25.14-●
    hip M25.15-●
    knee M25.16-●
    shoulder M25.11-●
    specified joint NEC M25.18
    tuberculous —*see* Tuberculosis, joint
    vertebrae M25.18
    wrist M25.13-●
  kidney N28.89
  labium (majus) (minus) N82.8
  labyrinth —*see* subcategory H83.1
  lacrimal (gland) (sac) H04.61-●
  lacrimonasal duct —*see* Fistula, lacrimal
  laryngotracheal, congenital Q34.8
  larynx J38.7
  lip K13.0
    congenital Q38.0
  lumbar, tuberculous A18.01
  lung J86.0
  lymphatic I89.8
  mammary (gland) N61.0
  mastoid (process) (region) —*see* Mastoiditis, chronic
  maxillary J32.0
  medial, face and neck Q18.8
  mediastinal J86.0
  mediastinobronchial J86.0
  mediastinocutaneous J86.0
  middle ear —*see* subcategory H74.8
  mouth K12.2
  nasal J34.89
    sinus —*see* Sinusitis
  nasopharynx J39.2
  nipple N64.0
  nose J34.89
  oral (cutaneous) K12.2
    maxillary J32.0
    nasal (with cleft palate) —*see* Cleft, palate
  orbit, orbital —*see* Disorder, orbit, specified type NEC
  oroantral J32.0
  oviduct, external N82.5
  palate (hard) M27.8
  pancreatic K86.89
  pancreaticoduodenal K86.89
  parotid (gland) K11.4
    region K12.2
  penis N48.89
  perianal K60.3
  pericardium (pleura) (sac) —*see* Pericarditis
  pericecal K63.2
  perineorectal K60.4 perineosigmoidal K63.2
  perineosigmoidal K63.2
  perineum, perineal (with urethral involvement) NEC N36.0
    tuberculous A18.13
    ureter N28.89
  perirectal K60.4
    tuberculous A18.32
  peritoneum K65.9
  pharyngoesophageal J39.2
  pharynx J39.2
    branchial cleft (congenital) Q18.0
  pilonidal (infected) (rectum) —*see* Sinus, pilonidal

Fistula *(Continued)*
  pleura, pleural, pleurocutaneous, pleuroperitoneal J86.0
    tuberculous NEC A15.6
  pleuropericardial I31.8
  portal vein-hepatic artery, congenital Q26.6
  postauricular H70.81-●
  postoperative, persistent T81.83
    specified site —*see* Fistula, by site
  preauricular (congenital) Q18.1
  prostate N42.89
  pulmonary J86.0
    arteriovenous I28.0
      congenital Q25.72
    tuberculous —*see* Tuberculosis, pulmonary
  pulmonoperitoneal J86.0
  rectolabial N82.4
  rectosigmoid (intercommunicating) K63.2
  rectoureteral N28.89
  rectourethral N36.0
    congenital Q64.73
  rectouterine N82.4
    congenital Q51.7
  rectovaginal N82.3
    congenital Q52.2
    tuberculous A18.18
  rectovesical N32.1
    congenital Q64.79
  rectovesicovaginal N82.3
  rectovulval N82.4
    congenital Q52.79
  rectum (to skin) K60.4
    congenital Q43.6
      with absence, atresia and stenosis Q42.0
    tuberculous A18.32
  renal N28.89
  retroauricular —*see* Fistula, postauricular
  salivary duct or gland (any) K11.4
    congenital Q38.4
  scrotum (urinary) N50.89
    tuberculous A18.15
  semicircular canals —*see* subcategory H83.1
  sigmoid K63.2
    to bladder N32.1
  sinus —*see* Sinusitis
  skin L98.8
    to genital tract (female) N82.5
  splenocolic D73.89
  stercoral K63.2
  stomach K31.6
  sublingual gland K11.4
  submandibular gland K11.4
  submaxillary (gland) K11.4
    region K12.2
  thoracic J86.0
    duct I89.8
  thoracoabdominal J86.0
  thoracogastric J86.0
  thoracointestinal J86.0
  thorax J86.0
  thyroglossal duct Q89.2
  thyroid E07.89
  trachea, congenital (external) (internal) Q32.1
  tracheoesophageal J86.0
    congenital Q39.2
      with atresia of esophagus Q39.1
    following tracheostomy J95.04
  traumatic arteriovenous —*see* Injury, blood vessel, by site
  tuberculous - code by site under Tuberculosis
  typhoid A01.09
  umbilicourinary Q64.8
  urachus, congenital Q64.4
  ureter (persistent) N28.89
  ureteroabdominal N28.89
  ureterorectal N28.89
  ureterosigmoido-abdominal N28.89
  ureterovaginal N82.1
  ureterovesical N32.2
  urethra N36.0
    congenital Q64.79
    tuberculous A18.13

Fistula *(Continued)*
  urethroperineal N36.0
  urethroperineovesical N32.2
  urethrorectal N36.0
    congenital Q64.73
  urethroscrotal N50.89
  urethrovaginal N82.1
  urethrovesical N32.2
  urinary (tract) (persistent) (recurrent) N36.0
  uteroabdominal N82.5
    congenital Q51.7
  uteroenteric, uterointestinal N82.4
    congenital Q51.7
  uterorectal N82.4
    congenital Q51.7
  uteroureteric N82.1
  uterourethral Q51.7
  uterovaginal N82.8
  uterovesical N82.1
    congenital Q51.7
  uterus N82.8
  vagina (postpartal) (wall) N82.8
  vaginocutaneous (postpartal) N82.5
  vaginointestinal NEC N82.4
    large intestine N82.3
    small intestine N82.2
  vaginoperineal N82.5
  vasocutaneous, congenital Q55.7
  vesical NEC N32.2
  vesicoabdominal N32.2
  vesicocervicovaginal N82.1
  vesicocolic N32.1
  vesicocutaneous N32.2
  vesicoenteric N32.1
  vesicointestinal N32.1
  vesicometrorectal N82.4
  vesicoperineal N32.2
  vesicorectal N32.1
    congenital Q64.79
  vesicosigmoidal N32.1
  vesicosigmoidovaginal N82.3
  vesicoureteral N32.2
  vesicoureterovaginal N82.1
  vesicourethral N32.2
  vesicourethrorectal N32.1
  vesicouterine N82.1
    congenital Q51.7
  vesicovaginal N82.0
  vulvorectal N82.4
    congenital Q52.79
Fit R56.9
  epileptic —*see* Epilepsy
  fainting R55
  hysterical F44.5
  newborn P90
Fitting (and adjustment) (of)
  artificial
    arm —*see* Admission, adjustment, artificial, arm
    breast Z44.3
    eye Z44.2
    leg —*see* Admission, adjustment, artificial, leg
  automatic implantable cardiac defibrillator (with synchronous cardiac pacemaker) Z45.02
  brain neuropacemaker Z46.2
    implanted Z45.42
  cardiac defibrillator —*see* Fitting (and adjustment) (of), automatic implantable cardiac defibrillator
  catheter, non-vascular Z46.82
  colostomy belt Z46.89
  contact lenses Z46.0
  CRT-D (resynchronization therapy defibrillator) Z45.02
  CRT-P (cardiac resynchronization therapy pacemaker) Z45.018
    pulse generator Z45.010
  cystostomy device Z46.6

▶ New   ➡ Revised   ~~deleted~~ Deleted   ● Use Additional Character(s)

Fitting *(Continued)*
defibrillator, cardiac —*see* Fitting (and adjustment) (of), automatic implantable cardiac defibrillator
dentures Z46.3
device NOS Z46.9
abdominal Z46.89
gastrointestinal NEC Z46.59
implanted NEC Z45.89
nervous system Z46.2
implanted —*see* Admission, adjustment, device, implanted, nervous system
orthodontic Z46.4
orthoptic Z46.0
orthotic Z46.89
prosthetic (external) Z44.9
breast Z44.3
dental Z46.3
eye Z44.2
specified NEC Z44.8
specified NEC Z46.89
substitution
auditory Z46.2
implanted —*see* Admission, adjustment, device, implanted, hearing device
nervous system Z46.2
implanted —*see* Admission, adjustment, device, implanted, nervous system
visual Z46.2
implanted Z45.31
urinary Z46.6
gastric lap band Z46.51
gastrointestinal appliance NEC Z46.59
glasses (reading) Z46.0
hearing aid Z46.1
ileostomy device Z46.89
insulin pump Z46.81
intestinal appliance NEC Z46.89
myringotomy device (stent) (tube) Z45.82
neuropacemaker Z46.2
implanted Z45.42
non-vascular catheter Z46.82
orthodontic device Z46.4
orthopedic device (brace) (cast) (corset) (shoes) Z46.89
pacemaker (cardiac) (cardiac resynchronization therapy (CRT-P)) Z45.018
nervous system (brain) (peripheral nerve) (spinal cord) Z46.2
implanted Z45.42
pulse generator Z45.010
portacath (port-a-cath) Z45.2
prosthesis (external) Z44.9
arm —*see* Admission, adjustment, artificial, arm
breast Z44.3
dental Z46.3
eye Z44.2
leg —*see* Admission, adjustment, artificial, leg
specified NEC Z44.8
spectacles Z46.0
wheelchair Z46.89
Fitzhugh-Curtis syndrome
due to
Chlamydia trachomatis A74.81
Neisseria gonorrhorea (gonococcal peritonitis) A54.85
Fitz's syndrome (acute hemorrhagic pancreatitis) —*see also* Pancreatitis, acute K85.80
Fixation
joint —*see* Ankylosis
larynx J38.7
stapes —*see* Ankylosis, ear ossicles
deafness —*see* Deafness, conductive
uterus (acquired) —*see* Malposition, uterus
vocal cord J38.3

Flabby ridge K06.8
Flaccid —*see also* condition
palate, congenital Q38.5
Flail
chest S22.5-•
►associated with chest compression and cardiopulmonary resuscitation M96.A4
newborn (birth injury) P13.8
joint (paralytic) M25.20
ankle M25.27-•
elbow M25.22-•
foot joint M25.27-•
hand joint M25.24-•
hip M25.25-•
knee M25.26-•
shoulder M25.21-•
specified joint NEC M25.28
wrist M25.23-•
Flajani's disease —*see* Hyperthyroidism, with, goiter (diffuse)
Flap, liver K71.3
Flashbacks (residual to hallucinogen use) F16.283
Flat
chamber (eye) —*see* Disorder, globe, hypotony, flat anterior chamber
chest, congenital Q67.8
foot (acquired) (fixed type) (painful) (postural) —*see also* Deformity, limb, flat foot
congenital (rigid) (spastic (everted)) Q66.5-•
rachitic sequelae (late effect) E64.3
organ or site, congenital NEC —*see* Anomaly, by site
pelvis M95.5
with disproportion (fetopelvic) O33.0
causing obstructed labor O65.0
congenital Q74.2
Flatau-Schilder disease G37.0
Flatback syndrome M40.30
lumbar region M40.36
lumbosacral region M40.37
thoracolumbar region M40.35
Flattening
head, femur M89.8X5
hip —*see* Coxa, plana
lip (congenital) Q18.8
nose (congenital) Q67.4
acquired M95.0
Flatulence R14.3
psychogenic F45.8
Flatus R14.3
vaginalis N89.8
Flax-dresser's disease J66.1
Flea bite —*see* Injury, bite, by site, superficial, insect
Flecks, glaucomatous (subcapsular) —*see* Cataract, complicated
Fleischer (-Kayser) ring (cornea) H18.04-•
Fleshy mole O02.0
Flexibilitas cerea —*see* Catalepsy
Flexion
amputation stump (surgical) T87.89
cervix —*see* Malposition, uterus
contracture, joint —*see* Contraction, joint
deformity, joint —*see also* Deformity, limb, flexion M21.20
hip, congenital Q65.89
uterus —*see also* Malposition, uterus
lateral —*see* Lateroversion, uterus
Flexner-Boyd dysentery A03.2
Flexner's dysentery A03.1
Flexure —*see* Flexion
Flint murmur (aortic insufficiency) I35.1
Floater, vitreous —*see* Opacity, vitreous
Floating
cartilage (joint) —*see also* Loose, body, joint
knee —*see* Derangement, knee, loose body
gallbladder, congenital Q44.1
kidney N28.89
congenital Q63.8
spleen D73.89

Flooding N92.0
Floor —*see* condition
Floppy
baby syndrome (nonspecific) P94.2
iris syndrome (intraoperative) (IFIS) H21.81
nonrheumatic mitral valve syndrome I34.1
Flu —*see also* Influenza
avian —*see also* Influenza, due to, identified novel influenza A virus J09.X2
bird —*see also* Influenza, due to, identified novel influenza A virus J09.X2
intestinal NEC A08.4
swine (viruses that normally cause infections in pigs) —*see also* Influenza, due to, identified novel influenza A virus J09.X2
Fluctuating blood pressure I99.8
Fluid
abdomen R18.8
chest J94.8
heart —*see* Failure, heart, congestive
joint —*see* Effusion, joint
loss (acute) E86.9
lung —*see* Edema, lung
overload E87.70
specified NEC E87.79
peritoneal cavity R18.8
pleural cavity J94.8
retention R60.9
Flukes NEC —*see also* Infestation, fluke
blood NEC —*see* Schistosomiasis
liver B66.3
Fluor (vaginalis) N89.8
trichomonal or due to Trichomonas (vaginalis) A59.00
Fluorosis
dental K00.3
skeletal M85.10
ankle M85.17-•
foot M85.17-•
forearm M85.13-•
hand M85.14-•
lower leg M85.16-•
multiple site M85.19
neck M85.18
rib M85.18
shoulder M85.11-•
skull M85.18
specified site NEC M85.18
thigh M85.15-•
toe M85.17-•
upper arm M85.12-•
vertebra M85.18
Flush syndrome E34.0
Flushing R23.2
menopausal N95.1
Flutter
atrial or auricular I48.92
atypical I48.4
type I I48.3
type II I48.4
typical I48.3
heart I49.8
atrial or auricular I48.92
atypical I48.4
type I I48.3
type II I48.4
typical I48.3
ventricular I49.02
ventricular I49.02
FNHTR (febrile nonhemolytic transfusion reaction) R50.84
Fochier's abscess - code by site under Abscess
Focus, Assmann's —*see* Tuberculosis, pulmonary
Fogo selvagem L10.3
Foix-Alajouanine syndrome G95.19
Fold, folds (anomalous) —*see also* Anomaly, by site
Descemet's membrane —*see* Change, corneal membrane, Descemet's, fold
epicanthic Q10.3
heart Q24.8

Folie à deux F24
Follicle
  cervix (nabothian) (ruptured) N88.8
  graafian, ruptured, with hemorrhage N83.0-●
  nabothian N88.8
Follicular —see condition
Folliculitis (superficial) L73.9
  abscedens et suffodiens L66.3
  cyst N83.0-●
  decalvans L66.2
  deep —see Furuncle, by site
  gonococcal (acute) (chronic) A54.01
  keloid, keloidalis L73.0
  pustular L01.02
  ulerythematosa reticulata L66.4
Folliculome lipidique
  specified site —see Neoplasm, benign, by site
  unspecified site
    female D27.9
    male D29.20
Folling's disease E70.0
Follow-up —see Examination, follow-up
Fong's syndrome (hereditary osteo-
  onychodysplasia) Q87.2
Food
  allergy L27.2
  asphyxia (from aspiration or inhalation) —see
    Foreign body, by site
  choked on —see Foreign body, by site
  deprivation T73.0
    specified kind of food NEC E63.8
  insecurity Z59.41
  intoxication —see Poisoning, food
  lack of T73.0
  poisoning —see Poisoning, food
  rejection NEC —see Disorder, eating
  strangulation or suffocation —see Foreign
    body, by site
  toxemia —see Poisoning, food
Foot —see condition
Foramen ovale (nonclosure) (patent)
  (persistent) Q21.12
Forbes' glycogen storage disease E74.03
Fordyce-Fox disease L75.2
Fordyce's disease (mouth) Q38.6
Forearm —see condition
Foreclosure on loan Z59.89
Foreign body
  with
    laceration —see Laceration, by site, with
      foreign body
    puncture wound —see Puncture, by site,
      with foreign body
  accidentally left following a procedure
    T81.509
    aspiration T81.506
      resulting in
        adhesions T81.516
        obstruction T81.526
        perforation T81.536
        specified complication NEC
          T81.596
    cardiac catheterization T81.505
      resulting in
        acute reaction T81.60
          aseptic peritonitis T81.61
          specified NEC T81.69
        adhesions T81.515
        obstruction T81.525
        perforation T81.535
        specified complication NEC
          T81.595
    causing
      acute reaction T81.60
        aseptic peritonitis T81.61
        specified complication NEC T81.69
      adhesions T81.519
      aseptic peritonitis T81.61
      obstruction T81.529
      perforation T81.539
      specified complication NEC T81.599

Foreign body (Continued)
  accidentally left following a procedure
    (Continued)
    endoscopy T81.504
      resulting in
        adhesions T81.514
        obstruction T81.524
        perforation T81.534
        specified complication NEC T81.594
    immunization T81.503
      resulting in
        adhesions T81.513
        obstruction T81.523
        perforation T81.533
        specified complication NEC T81.593
    infusion T81.501
      resulting in
        adhesions T81.511
        obstruction T81.521
        perforation T81.531
        specified complication NEC T81.591
    injection T81.503
      resulting in
        adhesions T81.513
        obstruction T81.523
        perforation T81.533
        specified complication NEC T81.593
    kidney dialysis T81.502
      resulting in
        adhesions T81.512
        obstruction T81.522
        perforation T81.532
        specified complication NEC T81.592
    packing removal T81.507
      resulting in
        acute reaction T81.60
          aseptic peritonitis T81.61
          specified NEC T81.69
        adhesions T81.517
        obstruction T81.527
        perforation T81.537
        specified complication NEC T81.597
    puncture T81.506
      resulting in
        adhesions T81.516
        obstruction T81.526
        perforation T81.536
        specified complication NEC T81.596
    specified procedure NEC T81.508
      resulting in
        acute reaction T81.60
          aseptic peritonitis T81.61
          specified NEC T81.69
        adhesions T81.518
        obstruction T81.528
        perforation T81.538
        specified complication NEC T81.598
    surgical operation T81.500
      resulting in
        acute reaction T81.60
          aseptic peritonitis T81.61
          specified NEC T81.69
        adhesions T81.510
        obstruction T81.520
        perforation T81.530
        specified complication NEC T81.590
    transfusion T81.501
      resulting in
        adhesions T81.511
        obstruction T81.521
        perforation T81.531
        specified complication NEC T81.591
  alimentary tract T18.9
    anus T18.5
    colon T18.4
    esophagus —see Foreign body, esophagus
    mouth T18.0
    multiple sites T18.8
    rectosigmoid (junction) T18.5
    rectum T18.5
    small intestine T18.3

Foreign body (Continued)
  alimentary tract (Continued)
    specified site NEC T18.8
    stomach T18.2
  anterior chamber (eye) S05.5-●
  auditory canal —see Foreign body, entering
    through orifice, ear
  bronchus T17.508
    causing
      asphyxiation T17.500
        food (bone) (seed) T17.520
        gastric contents (vomitus) T17.510
        specified type NEC T17.590
      injury NEC T17.508
        food (bone) (seed) T17.528
        gastric contents (vomitus) T17.518
        specified type NEC T17.598
  canthus —see Foreign body, conjunctival sac
  ciliary body (eye) S05.5-●
  conjunctival sac T15.1-●
  cornea T15.0-●
  entering through orifice
    accessory sinus T17.0
    alimentary canal T18.9
      multiple parts T18.8
      specified part NEC T18.8
    alveolar process T18.0
    antrum (Highmore's) T17.0
    anus T18.5
    appendix T18.4
    auditory canal —see Foreign body, entering
      through orifice, ear
    auricle —see Foreign body, entering
      through orifice, ear
    bladder T19.1
    bronchioles —see Foreign body, respiratory
      tract, specified site NEC
    bronchus (main) —see Foreign body,
      bronchus
    buccal cavity T18.0
    canthus (inner) —see Foreign body,
      conjunctival sac
    cecum T18.4
    cervix (canal) (uteri) T19.3
    colon T18.4
    conjunctival sac —see Foreign body,
      conjunctival sac
    cornea —see Foreign body, cornea
    digestive organ or tract NOS T18.9
      multiple parts T18.8
      specified part NEC T18.8
    duodenum T18.3
    ear (external) T16.-●
    esophagus —see Foreign body, esophagus
    eye (external) NOS T15.9-●
      conjunctival sac —see Foreign body,
        conjunctival sac
      cornea —see Foreign body, cornea
      specified part NEC T15.8-●
    eyeball —see also Foreign body, entering
      through orifice, eye, specified part
      NEC
      with penetrating wound —see Puncture,
        eyeball
    eyelid —see also Foreign body, conjunctival
      sac
      with
        laceration —see Laceration, eyelid,
          with foreign body
        puncture —see Puncture, eyelid, with
          foreign body
        superficial injury —see Foreign body,
          superficial, eyelid
    gastrointestinal tract T18.9
      multiple parts T18.8
      specified part NEC T18.8
    genitourinary tract T19.9
      multiple parts T19.8
      specified part NEC T19.8
    globe —see Foreign body, entering through
      orifice, eyeball

▶ New   ⟹ Revised   ~~deleted~~ Deleted   ● Use Additional Character(s)

Foreign body (Continued)
  entering through orifice (Continued)
    gum T18.0
    Highmore's antrum T17.0
    hypopharynx —see Foreign body, pharynx
    ileum T18.3
    intestine (small) T18.3
      large T18.4
    lacrimal apparatus (punctum) —see
        Foreign body, entering through orifice,
        eye, specified part NEC
    large intestine T18.4
    larynx —see Foreign body, larynx
    lung —see Foreign body, respiratory tract,
        specified site NEC
    maxillary sinus T17.0
    mouth T18.0
    nasal sinus T17.0
    nasopharynx —see Foreign body, pharynx
    nose (passage) T17.1
    nostril T17.1
    oral cavity T18.0
    palate T18.0
    penis T19.4
    pharynx —see Foreign body, pharynx
    piriform sinus —see Foreign body, pharynx
    rectosigmoid (junction) T18.5
    rectum T18.5
    respiratory tract —see Foreign body,
        respiratory tract
    sinus (accessory) (frontal) (maxillary)
        (nasal) T17.0
      piriform —see Foreign body, pharynx
    small intestine T18.3
    stomach T18.2
    suffocation by —see Foreign body, by site
    tear ducts or glands —see Foreign body,
        entering through orifice, eye, specified
        part NEC
    throat —see Foreign body, pharynx
    tongue T18.0
    tonsil, tonsillar (fossa) —see Foreign body,
        pharynx
    trachea —see Foreign body, trachea
    ureter T19.8
    urethra T19.0
    uterus (any part) T19.3
    vagina T19.2
    vulva T19.2
  esophagus T18.108
    causing
      injury NEC T18.108
        food (bone) (seed) T18.128
        gastric contents (vomitus) T18.118
        specified type NEC T18.198
      tracheal compression T18.100
        food (bone) (seed) T18.120
        gastric contents (vomitus) T18.110
        specified type NEC T18.190
  feeling of, in throat R09.89
  fragment —see Retained, foreign body
      fragments (type of)
  genitourinary tract T19.9
    bladder T19.1
    multiple parts T19.8
    penis T19.4
    specified site NEC T19.8
    urethra T19.0
    uterus T19.3
      IUD Z97.5
    vagina T19.2
      contraceptive device Z97.5
    vulva T19.2
  granuloma (old) (soft tissue) —see also
      Granuloma, foreign body
    skin L92.3
  in
    laceration —see Laceration, by site, with
        foreign body
    puncture wound —see Puncture, by site,
        with foreign body
    soft tissue (residual) M79.5

Foreign body (Continued)
  inadvertently left in operation wound —see
      Foreign body, accidentally left during a
      procedure
  ingestion, ingested NOS T18.9
  inhalation or inspiration —see Foreign body,
      by site
  internal organ, not entering through a natural
      orifice - code as specific injury with
      foreign body
  intraocular S05.5-●
    old, retained (nonmagnetic) H44.70-●
      anterior chamber H44.71-●
      ciliary body H44.72-●
      iris H44.72-●
      lens H44.73-●
      magnetic H44.60-●
        anterior chamber H44.61-●
        ciliary body H44.62-●
        iris H44.62-●
        lens H44.63-●
        posterior wall H44.64-●
        specified site NEC H44.69-●
        vitreous body H44.65-●
      posterior wall H44.74-●
      specified site NEC H44.79-●
      vitreous body H44.75-●
    iris —see Foreign body, intraocular
  lacrimal punctum —see Foreign body,
      entering through orifice, eye, specified
      part NEC
  larynx T17.308
    causing
      asphyxiation T17.300
        food (bone) (seed) T17.320
        gastric contents (vomitus) T17.310
        specified type NEC T17.390
      injury NEC T17.308
        food (bone) (seed) T17.328
        gastric contents (vomitus) T17.318
        specified type NEC T17.398
  lens —see Foreign body, intraocular
  ocular muscle S05.4-●
    old, retained —see Foreign body, orbit, old
  old or residual
    soft tissue (residual) M79.5
  operation wound, left accidentally —see
      Foreign body, accidentally left during a
      procedure
  orbit S05.4-●
    old, retained H05.5-●
  pharynx T17.208
    causing
      asphyxiation T17.200
        food (bone) (seed) T17.220
        gastric contents (vomitus)
            T17.210
        specified type NEC T17.290
      injury NEC T17.208
        food (bone) (seed) T17.228
        gastric contents (vomitus)
            T17.218
        specified type NEC T17.298
  respiratory tract T17.908
    bronchioles —see Foreign body, respiratory
        tract, specified site NEC
    bronchus —see Foreign body, bronchus
    causing
      asphyxiation T17.900
        food (bone) (seed) T17.920
        gastric contents (vomitus) T17.910
        specified type NEC T17.990
      injury NEC T17.908
        food (bone) (seed) T17.928
        gastric contents (vomitus) T17.918
        specified type NEC T17.998
    larynx —see Foreign body, larynx
    lung —see Foreign body, respiratory tract,
        specified site NEC
    multiple parts —see Foreign body,
        respiratory tract, specified site NEC

Foreign body (Continued)
  respiratory tract (Continued)
    nasal sinus T17.0
    nasopharynx —see Foreign body,
        pharynx
    nose T17.1
    nostril T17.1
    pharynx —see Foreign body, pharynx
    specified site NEC T17.808
      causing
        asphyxiation T17.800
          food (bone) (seed) T17.820
          gastric contents (vomitus) T17.810
          specified type NEC T17.890
        injury NEC T17.808
          food (bone) (seed) T17.828
          gastric contents (vomitus) T17.818
          specified type NEC T17.898
    throat —see Foreign body, pharynx
    trachea —see Foreign body, trachea
  retained (old) (nonmagnetic) (in)
    anterior chamber (eye) —see Foreign body,
        intraocular, old, retained, anterior
        chamber
      magnetic —see Foreign body, intraocular,
          old, retained, magnetic, anterior
          chamber
    ciliary body —see Foreign body,
        intraocular, old, retained, ciliary body
      magnetic —see Foreign body, intraocular,
          old, retained, magnetic, ciliary body
    eyelid H02.819
      left H02.816
        lower H02.815
        upper H02.814
      right H02.813
        lower H02.812
        upper H02.811
    fragments —see Retained, foreign body
        fragments (type of)
    globe —see Foreign body, intraocular, old,
        retained
      magnetic —see Foreign body, intraocular,
          old, retained, magnetic
    intraocular —see Foreign body, intraocular,
        old, retained
      magnetic —see Foreign body, intraocular,
          old, retained, magnetic
    iris —see Foreign body, intraocular, old,
        retained, iris
      magnetic —see Foreign body, intraocular,
          old, retained, magnetic, iris
    lens —see Foreign body, intraocular, old,
        retained, lens
      magnetic —see Foreign body, intraocular,
          old, retained, magnetic, lens
    muscle —see Foreign body, retained, soft
        tissue
    orbit —see Foreign body, orbit, old
    posterior wall of globe —see Foreign body,
        intraocular, old, retained, posterior
        wall
      magnetic —see Foreign body, intraocular,
          old, retained, magnetic, posterior
          wall
    retrobulbar —see Foreign body, orbit, old,
        retrobulbar
    soft tissue M79.5
    vitreous —see Foreign body, intraocular,
        old, retained, vitreous body
      magnetic —see Foreign body, intraocular,
          old, retained, magnetic, vitreous
          body
  retina S05.5-●
  superficial, without open wound
    abdomen, abdominal (wall) S30.851
    alveolar process S00.552
    ankle S90.55-●
    antecubital space —see Foreign body,
        superficial, forearm
    anus S30.857

Foreign body *(Continued)*
  superficial, without open wound *(Continued)*
    arm (upper) S40.85-●
    auditory canal —*see* Foreign body,
      superficial, ear
    auricle —*see* Foreign body, superficial, ear
    axilla —*see* Foreign body, superficial, arm
    back, lower S30.850
    breast S20.15-●
    brow S00.85
    buttock S30.850
    calf —*see* Foreign body, superficial, leg
    canthus —*see* Foreign body, superficial,
      eyelid
    cheek S00.85
      internal S00.552
    chest wall —*see* Foreign body, superficial,
      thorax
    chin S00.85
    clitoris S30.854
    costal region —*see* Foreign body,
      superficial, thorax
    digit(s)
      foot —*see* Foreign body, superficial, toe
      hand —*see* Foreign body, superficial,
        finger
    ear S00.45-●
    elbow S50.35-●
    epididymis S30.853
    epigastric region S30.851
    epiglottis S10.15
    esophagus, cervical S10.15
    eyebrow —*see* Foreign body, superficial,
      eyelid
    eyelid S00.25-●
    face S00.85
    finger(s) S60.459
      index S60.45-●
      little S60.45-●
      middle S60.45-●
      ring S60.45-●
    flank S30.851
    foot (except toe(s) alone) S90.85-●
      toe —*see* Foreign body, superficial, toe
    forearm S50.85-●
      elbow only —*see* Foreign body,
        superficial, elbow
    forehead S00.85
    genital organs, external
      female S30.856
      male S30.855
    groin S30.851
    gum S00.552
    hand S60.55-●
    head S00.95
      ear —*see* Foreign body, superficial, ear
      eyelid —*see* Foreign body, superficial,
        eyelid
      lip S00.551
      nose S00.35
      oral cavity S00.552
      scalp S00.05
      specified site NEC S00.85
    heel —*see* Foreign body, superficial, foot
    hip S70.25-●
    inguinal region S30.851
    interscapular region S20.459
    jaw S00.85
    knee S80.25-●
    labium (majus) (minus) S30.854
    larynx S10.15
    leg (lower) S80.85-●
      knee —*see* Foreign body, superficial, knee
      upper —*see* Foreign body, superficial,
        thigh
    lip S00.551
    lower back S30.850
    lumbar region S30.850
    malar region S00.85
    mammary —*see* Foreign body, superficial,
      breast

Foreign body *(Continued)*
  superficial, without open wound *(Continued)*
    mastoid region S00.85
    mouth S00.552
    nail
      finger —*see* Foreign body, superficial,
        finger
      toe —*see* Foreign body, superficial, toe
    nape S10.85
    nasal S00.35
    neck S10.95
      specified site NEC S10.85
      throat S10.15
    nose S00.35
    occipital region S00.05
    oral cavity S00.552
    orbital region —*see* Foreign body,
      superficial, eyelid
    palate S00.552
    palm —*see* Foreign body, superficial,
      hand
    parietal region S00.05
    pelvis S30.850
    penis S30.852
    perineum
      female S30.854
      male S30.850
    periocular area —*see* Foreign body,
      superficial, eyelid
    phalanges
      finger —*see* Foreign body, superficial,
        finger
      toe —*see* Foreign body, superficial, toe
    pharynx S10.15
    pinna —*see* Foreign body, superficial, ear
    popliteal space —*see* Foreign body,
      superficial, knee
    prepuce S30.852
    pubic region S30.850
    pudendum
      female S30.856
      male S30.855
    sacral region S30.850
    scalp S00.05
    scapular region —*see* Foreign body,
      superficial, shoulder
    scrotum S30.853
    shin —*see* Foreign body, superficial, leg
    shoulder S40.25-●
    sternal region S20.359
    submaxillary region S00.85
    submental region S00.85
    subungual
      finger(s) —*see* Foreign body, superficial,
        finger
      toe(s) —*see* Foreign body, superficial,
        toe
    supraclavicular fossa S10.85
    supraorbital S00.85
    temple S00.85
    temporal region S00.85
    testis S30.853
    thigh S70.35-●
    thorax, thoracic (wall) S20.95
      back S20.45-●
      front S20.35-●
    throat S10.15
    thumb S60.35-●
    toe(s) (lesser) S90.456
      great S90.45-●
    tongue S00.552
    trachea S10.15
    tunica vaginalis S30.853
    tympanum, tympanic membrane —*see*
      Foreign body, superficial, ear
    uvula S00.552
    vagina S30.854
    vocal cords S10.15
    vulva S30.854
    wrist S60.85-●
  swallowed T18.9

Foreign body *(Continued)*
  trachea T17.408
    causing
      asphyxiation T17.400
        food (bone) (seed) T17.420
        gastric contents (vomitus) T17.410
        specified type NEC T17.490
      injury NEC T17.408
        food (bone) (seed) T17.428
        gastric contents (vomitus) T17.418
        specified type NEC T17.498
    type of fragment —*see* Retained, foreign body
      fragments (type of)
    vitreous (humor) S05.5-●
Forestier's disease (rhizomelic
  pseudopolyarthritis) M35.3-●
  meaning ankylosing hyperostosis —*see*
    Hyperostosis, ankylosing
Formation
  hyalin in cornea —*see* Degeneration, cornea
  sequestrum in bone (due to infection) —*see*
    Osteomyelitis, chronic
  valve
    colon, congenital Q43.8
    ureter (congenital) Q62.39
Formication R20.2
Fort Bragg fever A27.89
Fossa —*see also* condition
  pyriform —*see* condition
Foster-Kennedy syndrome H47.14-●
Fothergill's
  disease (trigeminal neuralgia) —*see also*
    Neuralgia, trigeminal
  scarlatina anginosa A38.9
Foul breath R19.6
Foundling Z76.1
Fournier disease or gangrene N49.3
  ▦female N76.82
  ▶vagina and vulva N76.82
Fourth
  cranial nerve —*see* condition
  molar K00.1
Foville's (peduncular) **disease or syndrome** G46.3
Fox (-Fordyce) **disease** (apocrine miliaria) L75.2
FPIES (food protein-induced enterocolitis
  syndrome) K52.21
Fracture, burst —*see* Fracture, traumatic, by site
Fracture, chronic —*see* Fracture, pathological,
  by site
Fracture, insufficiency —*see* Fracture,
  pathological, by site
Fracture, nontraumatic, NEC
  atypical
    femur M84.750-●
      complete
        oblique M84.759
          left side M84.758
          right side M84.757
        transverse M84.756
          left side M84.755
          right side M84.754
      incomplete M84.753
        left side M84.752
        right side M84.751
Fracture, pathological (pathologic) —*see also*
  Fracture, traumatic M84.40
  ankle M84.47-●
  carpus M84.44-●
  clavicle M84.41-●
  compression (not due to trauma) —*see also*
    Collapse, vertebra M48.50-●
  dental implant M27.63
  dental restorative material K08.539
    with loss of material K08.531
    without loss of material K08.530
  due to
    neoplastic disease NEC —*see also*
      Neoplasm M84.50
      ankle M84.57-●
      carpus M84.54-●
      clavicle M84.51-●
      femur M84.55-●

Fracture, pathological *(Continued)*
  due to *(Continued)*
    neoplastic disease NEC *(Continued)*
      fibula M84.56-●
      finger M84.54-●
      hip M84.559
      humerus M84.52-●
      ilium M84.550
      ischium M84.550
      metacarpus M84.54-●
      metatarsus M84.57-●
      neck M84.58
      pelvis M84.550
      radius M84.53-●
      rib M84.58
      scapula M84.51-●
      skull M84.58
      specified site NEC M84.58
      tarsus M84.57-●
      tibia M84.56-●
      toe M84.57-●
      ulna M84.53-●
      vertebra M84.58
    osteoporosis M80.00
      disuse —*see* Osteoporosis, specified type
        NEC, with pathological fracture
      drug-induced —*see* Osteoporosis, drug
        induced, with pathological fracture
      idiopathic —*see* Osteoporosis, specified
        type NEC, with pathological
        fracture
      postmenopausal —*see* Osteoporosis,
        postmenopausal, with pathological
        fracture
      postoophorectomy —*see* Osteo-
        porosis, postoophorectomy, with
        pathological fracture
      postsurgical malabsorption —*see*
        Osteoporosis, specified type NEC,
        with pathological fracture
      specified cause NEC —*see* Osteoporosis,
        specified type NEC, with
        pathological fracture
    specified disease NEC M84.60
      ankle M84.67-●
      carpus M84.64-●
      clavicle M84.61-●
      femur M84.65-●
      fibula M84.66-●
      finger M84.64-●
      hip M84.65-●
      humerus M84.62-●
      ilium M84.650
      ischium M84.650
      metacarpus M84.64-●
      metatarsus M84.67-●
      neck M84.68
      radius M84.63-●
      rib M84.68
      scapula M84.61-●
      skull M84.68
      tarsus M84.67-●
      tibia M84.66-●
      toe M84.67-●
      ulna M84.63-●
      vertebra M84.68
  femur M84.45-●
  fibula M84.46-●
  finger M84.44-●
  hip M84.459
  humerus M84.42-●
  ilium M84.454
  ischium M84.454
  joint prosthesis —*see* Complications, joint
    prosthesis, mechanical, breakdown, by
    site
    periprosthetic —*see* Fracture, pathological,
      periprosthetic
  metacarpus M84.44-●
  metatarsus M84.47-●
  neck M84.48

Fracture, pathological *(Continued)*
  pelvis M84.454
  periprosthetic M97.9
    ankle M97.2-●
    elbow M97.4-●
    finger M97.8
    hip M97.0-●
    knee M97.1-●
    other specified joint M97.8
    shoulder M97.3-●
    spinal joint M97.8
    toe joint M97.8
    wrist joint M97.8
  radius M84.43-●
  restorative material (dental) K08.539
    with loss of material K08.531
    without loss of material K08.530
  rib M84.48
  scapula M84.41-●
  skull M84.48
  tarsus M84.47-●
  tibia M84.46-●
  toe M84.47-●
  ulna M84.43-●
  vertebra M84.48
Fracture, traumatic (abduction) (adduction)
    (separation) —*see also* Fracture,
    pathological T14.8
▶associated with chest compression and
    cardiopulmonary resuscitation M96.A9
  acetabulum S32.40-●
    column
      anterior (displaced) (iliopubic) S32.43-●
        nondisplaced S32.436
      posterior (displaced) (ilioischial) S32.443
        nondisplaced S32.44-●
    dome (displaced) S32.48-●
      nondisplaced S32.48
    specified NEC S32.49-●
    transverse (displaced) S32.45-●
      with associated posterior wall fracture
        (displaced) S32.46-●
        nondisplaced S32.46-●
      nondisplaced S32.45-●
    wall
      anterior (displaced) S32.41-●
        nondisplaced S32.41-●
      medial (displaced) S32.47-●
        nondisplaced S32.47-●
      posterior (displaced) S32.42-●
        with associated transverse fracture
          (displaced) S32.46-●
          nondisplaced S32.46-●
        nondisplaced S32.42-●
  acromion —*see* Fracture, scapula, acromial
    process
  ankle S82.899
    bimalleolar (displaced) S82.84-●
      nondisplaced S82.84-●
    lateral malleolus only (displaced) S82.6-●
      nondisplaced S82.6-●
    medial malleolus (displaced) S82.5-●
      associated with Maisonneuve's
        fracture —*see* Fracture,
        Maisonneuve's
      nondisplaced S82.5-●
    talus —*see* Fracture, tarsal, talus
    trimalleolar (displaced) S82.85-●
      nondisplaced S82.85-●
  arm (upper) —*see also* Fracture, humerus, shaft
    humerus —*see* Fracture, humerus
    radius —*see* Fracture, radius
    ulna —*see* Fracture, ulna
  astragalus —*see* Fracture, tarsal, talus
  atlas —*see* Fracture, neck, cervical vertebra,
    first
  axis —*see* Fracture, neck, cervical vertebra,
    second
  back —*see* Fracture, vertebra
  Barton's —*see* Barton's fracture
  base of skull —*see* Fracture, skull, base

Fracture, traumatic *(Continued)*
  basicervical (basal) (femoral) S72.0
  Bennett's —*see* Bennett's fracture
  bimalleolar —*see* Fracture, ankle,
    bimalleolar
  blow-out S02.3-●
  bone NEC T14.8
    birth injury P13.9
    following insertion of orthopedic implant,
      joint prosthesis or bone plate —*see*
      Fracture, following insertion of
      orthopedic implant, joint prosthesis or
      bone plate
    in (due to) neoplastic disease NEC —
      see Fracture, pathological, due to,
      neoplastic disease
    pathological (cause unknown) —*see*
      Fracture, pathological
  breast bone —*see* Fracture, sternum
  buckle —*see* Fracture, by site, torus
  bucket handle (semilunar cartilage) —*see*
    Tear, meniscus
  burst —*see* Fracture, traumatic, by site
  calcaneus —*see* Fracture, tarsal, calcaneus
  carpal bone(s) S62.10-●
    capitate (displaced) S62.13-●
      nondisplaced S62.13-●
    cuneiform —*see* Fracture, carpal bone,
      triquetrum
    hamate (body) (displaced) S62.143
      hook process (displaced) S62.15-●
        nondisplaced S62.15-●
      nondisplaced S62.14-●
    larger multangular —*see* Fracture, carpal
      bones, trapezium
    lunate (displaced) S62.12-●
      nondisplaced S62.12-●
    navicular S62.00-●
      distal pole (displaced) S62.01-●
        nondisplaced S62.01-●
      middle third (displaced) S62.02-●
        nondisplaced S62.02-●
      proximal third (displaced) S62.03-●
        nondisplaced S62.03-●
      volar tuberosity —*see* Fracture, carpal
        bones, navicular, distal pole
    os magnum —*see* Fracture, carpal bones,
      capitate
    pisiform (displaced) S62.16-●
      nondisplaced S62.16-●
    semilunar —*see* Fracture, carpal bones,
      lunate
    smaller multangular —*see* Fracture, carpal
      bones, trapezoid
    trapezium (displaced) S62.17-●
      nondisplaced S62.17-●
    trapezoid (displaced) S62.18-●
      nondisplaced S62.18-●
    triquetrum (displaced) S62.11-●
      nondisplaced S62.11-●
    unciform —*see* Fracture, carpal bones,
      hamate
  cervical —*see* Fracture, vertebra, cervical
  clavicle S42.00-●
    acromial end (displaced) S42.03-●
      nondisplaced S42.03-●
    birth injury P13.4
    lateral end —*see* Fracture, clavicle, acromial
      end
    shaft (displaced) S42.02-●
      nondisplaced S42.02-●
    sternal end (anterior) (displaced) S42.01-●
      nondisplaced S42.01-●
      posterior S42.01-●
  coccyx S32.2
  collapsed —*see* Collapse, vertebra
  collar bone —*see* Fracture, clavicle
  Colles' —*see* Colles' fracture
  coronoid process —*see* Fracture, ulna, upper
    end, coronoid process
  corpus cavernosum penis S39.840

Fracture, traumatic *(Continued)*
  costochondral cartilage S23.41
  costochondral, costosternal junction —*see*
    Fracture, rib
  cranium —*see* Fracture, skull
  cricoid cartilage S12.8
  cuboid (ankle) —*see* Fracture, tarsal, cuboid
  cuneiform
    foot —*see* Fracture, tarsal, cuneiform
    wrist —*see* Fracture, carpal, triquetrum
  delayed union —*see* Delay, union, fracture
  dental restorative material K08.539
    with loss of material K08.531
    without loss of material K08.530
  due to
    birth injury —*see* Birth, injury, fracture
    osteoporosis —*see* Osteoporosis, with
      fracture
  Dupuytren's —*see* Fracture, ankle, lateral
    malleolus
  elbow S42.40-●
  ethmoid (bone) (sinus) —*see* Fracture, skull,
    base
  face bone S02.92
  fatigue —*see also* Fracture, stress
    vertebra M48.40
      cervical region M48.42
      cervicothoracic region M48.43
      lumbar region M48.46
      lumbosacral region M48.47
      occipito-atlanto-axial region M48.41
      sacrococcygeal region M48.48
      thoracic region M48.44
      thoracolumbar region M48.45
  femur, femoral S72.9-●
    basicervical (basal) S72.0
    birth injury P13.2
    capital epiphyseal S79.01-●
    condyles, epicondyles —*see* Fracture,
      femur, lower end
    distal end —*see* Fracture, femur, lower end
    epiphysis
      head —*see* Fracture, femur, upper end,
        epiphysis
      lower —*see* Fracture, femur, lower end,
        epiphysis
      upper —*see* Fracture, femur, upper end,
        epiphysis
    following insertion of implant, prosthesis
      or plate M96.66-●
    head —*see* Fracture, femur, upper end,
      head
    intertrochanteric —*see* Fracture, femur,
      trochanteric
    intratrochanteric —*see* Fracture, femur,
      trochanteric
    lower end S72.40-●
      condyle (displaced) S72.41-●
        lateral (displaced) S72.42-●
          nondisplaced S72.42-●
        medial (displaced) S72.43-●
          nondisplaced S72.43-●
        nondisplaced S72.41-●
      epiphysis (displaced) S72.44-●
        nondisplaced S72.44-●
      physeal S79.10-●
        Salter-Harris
          Type I S79.11-●
          Type II S79.12-●
          Type III S79.13-●
          Type IV S79.14-●
        specified NEC S79.19-●
      specified NEC S72.49-●
      supracondylar (displaced) S72.45-●
        with intracondylar extension
          (displaced) S72.46-●
          nondisplaced S72.46-●
        nondisplaced S72.45-●
      torus S72.47-●
    neck —*see* Fracture, femur, upper end,
      neck

femur, femoral *(Continued)*
  pertrochanteric —*see* Fracture, femur,
    trochanteric
  shaft (lower third) (middle third) (upper
    third) S72.30-●
    comminuted (displaced) S72.35-●
      nondisplaced S72.35-●
    oblique (displaced) S72.33-●
      nondisplaced S72.33-●
    segmental (displaced) S72.36-●
      nondisplaced S72.36-●
    specified NEC S72.39-●
    spiral (displaced) S72.34-●
      nondisplaced S72.34-●
    transverse (displaced) S72.32-●
      nondisplaced S72.32-●
  specified site NEC —*see* subcategory
    S72.8
  subcapital (displaced) S72.01-●
  subtrochanteric (region) (section)
    (displaced) S72.2-●
    nondisplaced S72.2-●
  transcervical —*see* Fracture, femur,
    midcervical
  transtrochanteric —*see* Fracture, femur,
    trochanteric
  trochanteric S72.10-●
    apophyseal (displaced) S72.13-●
      nondisplaced S72.13-●
    greater trochanter (displaced) S72.11-●
      nondisplaced S72.11-●
    intertrochanteric (displaced) S72.14-●
      nondisplaced S72.14-●
    lesser trochanter (displaced) S72.12-●
      nondisplaced S72.12-●
  upper end S72.00-●
    apophyseal (displaced) S72.13-●
      nondisplaced S72.13-●
    cervicotrochanteric —*see* Fracture,
      femur, upper end, neck, base
    epiphysis (displaced) S72.02-●
      nondisplaced S72.02-●
    head S72.05-●
      articular (displaced) S72.06-●
        nondisplaced S72.06-●
      specified NEC S72.09-●
    intertrochanteric (displaced)
      S72.14-●
      nondisplaced S72.14-●
    intracapsular S72.01-●
    midcervical (displaced) S72.03-●
      nondisplaced S72.03-●
    neck S72.00-●
      base (displaced) S72.04-●
        nondisplaced S72.04-●
      specified NEC S72.09-●
    pertrochanteric —*see* Fracture, femur,
      upper end, trochanteric
    physeal S79.00-●
      Salter-Harris type I S79.01-●
      specified NEC S79.09-●
    subcapital (displaced) S72.01-●
    subtrochanteric (displaced) S72.2-●
      nondisplaced S72.2-●
    transcervical —*see* Fracture, femur,
      upper end, midcervical
    trochanteric S72.10-●
      greater (displaced) S72.11-●
        nondisplaced S72.11-●
      lesser (displaced) S72.12-●
        nondisplaced S72.12-●
fibula (shaft) (styloid) S82.40-●
  comminuted (displaced) S82.45-●
    nondisplaced S82.45-●
  following insertion of implant, prosthesis
    or plate M96.67-●
  involving ankle or malleolus —*see*
    Fracture, fibula, lateral malleolus
  lateral malleolus (displaced) S82.6-●
    nondisplaced S82.6-●

fibula (shaft) (styloid) *(Continued)*
  lower end
    physeal S89.30-●
      Salter-Harris
        Type I S89.31-●
        Type II S89.32-●
      specified NEC S89.39-●
    specified NEC S82.83-●
    torus S82.82-●
  oblique (displaced) S82.43-●
    nondisplaced S82.43-●
  segmental (displaced) S82.46-●
    nondisplaced S82.46-●
  specified NEC S82.49-●
  spiral (displaced) S82.44-●
    nondisplaced S82.44-●
  transverse (displaced) S82.42-●
    nondisplaced S82.42-●
  upper end
    physeal S89.20-●
      Salter-Harris
        Type I S89.21-●
        Type II S89.22-●
      specified NEC S89.29-●
    specified NEC S82.83-●
    torus S82.81-●
finger (except thumb) S62.60-●
  distal phalanx (displaced) S62.63-●
    nondisplaced S62.66-●
  index S62.60-●
    distal phalanx (displaced) S62.63-●
      nondisplaced S62.66-●
    middle phalanx (displaced) S62.62-●
      nondisplaced S62.65-●
    proximal phalanx (displaced) S62.61-●
      nondisplaced S62.64-●
  little S62.60-●
    distal phalanx (displaced) S62.63-●
      nondisplaced S62.66-●
    middle phalanx (displaced) S62.62-●
      nondisplaced S62.65-●
    proximal phalanx (displaced) S62.61-●
      nondisplaced S62.64-●
  middle phalanx (displaced) S62.62-●
    nondisplaced S62.65-●
  middle S62.60-●
    distal phalanx (displaced) S62.63-●
      nondisplaced S62.66-●
    middle phalanx (displaced) S62.62-●
      nondisplaced S62.65-●
    proximal phalanx (displaced) S62.61-●
      nondisplaced S62.64-●
  proximal phalanx (displaced) S62.61-●
    nondisplaced S62.64-●
  ring S62.60-●
    distal phalanx (displaced) S62.63-●
      nondisplaced S62.66-●
    middle phalanx (displaced) S62.62-●
      nondisplaced S62.65-●
    proximal phalanx (displaced) S62.61-●
      nondisplaced S62.64-●
  thumb —*see* Fracture, thumb
following insertion (intraoperative)
  (postoperative) of orthopedic implant,
  joint prosthesis or bone plate M96.69
  femur M96.66-●
  fibula M96.67-●
  humerus M96.62-●
  pelvis M96.65
  radius M96.63-●
  specified bone NEC M96.69
  tibia M96.67-●
  ulna M96.63-●
foot S92.90-●
  astragalus —*see* Fracture, tarsal, talus
  calcaneus —*see* Fracture, tarsal, calcaneus
  cuboid —*see* Fracture, tarsal, cuboid
  cuneiform —*see* Fracture, tarsal, cuneiform
  metatarsal —*see* Fracture, metatarsal
  navicular —*see* Fracture, tarsal, navicular

▶ New   ⇒ Revised   ~~deleted~~ Deleted   ● Use Additional Character(s)

Fracture, traumatic *(Continued)*
  foot *(Continued)*
    sesamoid S92.81-●
    specified NEC S92.81-●
    talus —*see* Fracture, tarsal, talus
    tarsal —*see* Fracture, tarsal
    toe —*see* Fracture, toe
  forearm S52.9-●
    radius —*see* Fracture, radius
    ulna —*see* Fracture, ulna
  fossa (anterior) (middle) (posterior) S02.19
  fragility —*see* Fracture, pathological, due to
    osteoporosis
  frontal (bone) (skull) S02.0
    sinus S02.19
  glenoid (cavity) (scapula) —*see* Fracture,
    scapula, glenoid cavity
  greenstick —*see* Fracture, by site
  hallux —*see* Fracture, toe, great
  hand S62.9-●
    carpal —*see* Fracture, carpal bone
    finger (except thumb) —*see* Fracture,
      finger
    metacarpal —*see* Fracture, metacarpal
    navicular (scaphoid) (hand) —*see* Fracture,
      carpal bone, navicular
    thumb —*see* Fracture, thumb
  healed or old
    with complications - code by Nature of the
      complication
  heel bone —*see* Fracture, tarsal, calcaneus
  Hill-Sachs S42.29-●
  hip —*see* Fracture, femur, neck
  humerus S42.30-●
    anatomical neck —*see* Fracture, humerus,
      upper end
    articular process —*see* Fracture, humerus,
      lower end
    capitellum —*see* Fracture, humerus, lower
      end, condyle, lateral
    distal end —*see* Fracture, humerus, lower
      end
    epiphysis
      lower —*see* Fracture, humerus, lower
        end, physeal
      upper —*see* Fracture, humerus, upper
        end, physeal
    external condyle —*see* Fracture, humerus,
      lower end, condyle, lateral
    following insertion of implant, prosthesis
      or plate M96.62-●
    great tuberosity —*see* Fracture, humerus,
      upper end, greater tuberosity
    intercondylar —*see* Fracture, humerus,
      lower end
    internal epicondyle —*see* Fracture, humerus,
      lower end, epicondyle, medial
    lesser tuberosity —*see* Fracture, humerus,
      upper end, lesser tuberosity
    lower end S42.40-●
      condyle
        lateral (displaced) S42.45-●
          nondisplaced S42.45-●
        medial (displaced) S42.46-●
          nondisplaced S42.46-●
      epicondyle
        lateral (displaced) S42.43-●
          nondisplaced S42.43-●
        medial (displaced) S42.44-●
          incarcerated S42.44-●
          nondisplaced S42.44-●
      physeal S49.10-●
        Salter-Harris
          Type I S49.11-●
          Type II S49.12-●
          Type III S49.13-●
          Type IV S49.14-●
        specified NEC S49.19-●
      specified NEC (displaced)
        S42.49-●
      nondisplaced S42.49-●

humerus *(Continued)*
  lower end *(Continued)*
    supracondylar (simple) (displaced)
      S42.41-●
      with intercondylar fracture —*see*
        Fracture, humerus, lower end
      comminuted (displaced) S42.42-●
        nondisplaced S42.42-●
      nondisplaced S42.41-●
      torus S42.48-●
      transcondylar (displaced) S42.47-●
        nondisplaced S42.47-●
    proximal end —*see* Fracture, humerus,
      upper end
    shaft S42.30-●
      comminuted (displaced) S42.35-●
        nondisplaced S42.35-●
      greenstick S42.31-●
      oblique (displaced) S42.33-●
        nondisplaced S42.33-●
      segmental (displaced) S42.36-●
        nondisplaced S42.36-●
      specified NEC S42.39-●
      spiral (displaced) S42.34-●
        nondisplaced S42.34-●
      transverse (displaced) S42.32-●
        nondisplaced S42.32-●
    supracondylar —*see* Fracture, humerus,
      lower end
    surgical neck —*see* Fracture, humerus,
      upper end, surgical neck
    trochlea —*see* Fracture, humerus, lower
      end, condyle, medial
    tuberosity —*see* Fracture, humerus, upper
      end
    upper end S42.20-●
      anatomical neck —*see* Fracture,
        humerus, upper end, specified NEC
      articular head —*see* Fracture, humerus,
        upper end, specified NEC
      epiphysis —*see* Fracture, humerus,
        upper end, physeal
      greater tuberosity (displaced) S42.25-●
        nondisplaced S42.25-●
      lesser tuberosity (displaced) S42.26-●
        nondisplaced S42.26-●
      physeal S49.00-●
        Salter-Harris
          Type I S49.01-●
          Type II S49.02-●
          Type III S49.03-●
          Type IV S49.04-●
        specified NEC S49.09-●
      specified NEC (displaced) S42.29-●
        nondisplaced S42.29-●
      surgical neck (displaced) S42.21-●
        four-part S42.24-●
        nondisplaced S42.21-●
        three-part S42.23-●
        two-part (displaced) S42.22-●
          nondisplaced S42.22-●
      torus S42.27-●
      transepiphyseal —*see* Fracture, humerus,
        upper end, physeal
  hyoid bone S12.8
  ilium S32.30-●
    with disruption of pelvic ring —*see*
      Disruption, pelvic ring
    avulsion (displaced) S32.31-●
      nondisplaced S32.31-●
    specified NEC S32.39-●
  impaction, impacted - code as Fracture, by
    site
  innominate bone —*see* Fracture, ilium
  instep —*see* Fracture, foot
  ischium S32.60-●
    with disruption of pelvic ring —*see*
      Disruption, pelvic ring
    avulsion (displaced) S32.61-●
      nondisplaced S32.61-●
    specified NEC S32.69-●

jaw (bone) (lower) —*see* Fracture, mandible
  upper —*see* Fracture, maxilla
joint prosthesis —*see* Complications, joint
  prosthesis, mechanical, breakdown,
  by site
  periprosthetic —*see* Fracture, traumatic,
    periprosthetic
knee cap —*see* Fracture, patella
larynx S12.8
late effects —*see* Sequelae, fracture
leg (lower) S82.9-●
  ankle —*see* Fracture, ankle
  femur —*see* Fracture, femur
  fibula —*see* Fracture, fibula
  malleolus —*see* Fracture, ankle
  patella —*see* Fracture, patella
  specified site NEC S82.89-●
  tibia —*see* Fracture, tibia
lumbar spine —*see* Fracture, vertebra, lumbar
lumbosacral spine S32.9
Maisonneuve's (displaced) S82.86-●
  nondisplaced S82.86-●
malar bone —*see also* Fracture, maxilla
  S02.400
  left side S02.40B
  right side S02.40A
malleolus —*see* Fracture, ankle
malunion —*see* Fracture, by site
mandible (lower jawbone) S02.609
  alveolus S02.67-●
  angle (of jaw) S02.65-●
  body, unspecified S02.600-●
    left side S02.602
    right side S02.601
  condylar process S02.61-●
  coronoid process S02.63-●
  ramus, unspecified S02.64-●
  specified site NEC S02.69
  subcondylar process S02.62-●
  symphysis S02.66
manubrium (sterni) S22.21
  dissociation from sternum S22.23
march —*see* Fracture, traumatic, stress, by site
maxilla, maxillary (bone) (sinus) (superior)
  (upper jaw) S02.401
  alveolus S02.42
  inferior —*see* Fracture, mandible
  LeFort I S02.411
  LeFort II S02.412
  LeFort III S02.413
  left side S02.40D
  right side S02.40C
metacarpal S62.309
  base (displaced) S62.319
    nondisplaced S62.349
  fifth S62.30-●
    base (displaced) S62.31-●
      nondisplaced S62.34-●
    neck (displaced) S62.33-●
      nondisplaced S62.36-●
    shaft (displaced) S62.32-●
      nondisplaced S62.35-●
    specified NEC S62.398
  first S62.20-●
    base NEC (displaced) S62.23-●
      nondisplaced S62.23-●
    Bennett's —*see* Bennett's fracture
    neck (displaced) S62.25-●
      nondisplaced S62.25-●
    shaft (displaced) S62.24-●
      nondisplaced S62.24-●
    specified NEC S62.29-●
  fourth S62.30-●
    base (displaced) S62.31-●
      nondisplaced S62.34-●
    neck (displaced) S62.33-●
      nondisplaced S62.36-●
    shaft (displaced) S62.32-●
      nondisplaced S62.35-●
    specified NEC S62.39-●

Fracture, traumatic *(Continued)*
  metacarpal *(Continued)*
    neck (displaced) S62.33-●
      nondisplaced S62.36-●
    Rolando's —*see* Rolando's fracture
    second S62.30-●
      base (displaced) S62.31-●
        nondisplaced S62.34-●
      neck (displaced) S62.33-●
        nondisplaced S62.36-●
      shaft (displaced) S62.32-●
        nondisplaced S62.35-●
      specified NEC S62.39-●
    shaft (displaced) S62.32-●
      nondisplaced S62.35-●
    specified NEC S62.399
    third S62.30-●
      base (displaced) S62.31-●
        nondisplaced S62.34-●
      neck (displaced) S62.33-●
        nondisplaced S62.36-●
      shaft (displaced) S62.32-●
        nondisplaced S62.35-●
      specified NEC S62.39-●
  metaphyseal —*see* Fracture, traumatic, by
    site, shaft
  metastatic —*see* Fracture, pathological,
    due to, neoplastic disease —*see also*
    Neoplasm
  metatarsal bone S92.30-●
    fifth (displaced) S92.35-●
      nondisplaced S92.35-●
    first (displaced) S92.31-●
      nondisplaced S92.31-●
    fourth (displaced) S92.34-●
      nondisplaced S92.34-●
    physeal S99.10-●
      Salter-Harris
        Type I S99.11-●
        Type II S99.12-●
        Type III S99.13-●
        Type IV S99.14-●
      specified NEC S99.19-●
    second (displaced) S92.32-●
      nondisplaced S92.32-●
    third (displaced) S92.33-●
      nondisplaced S92.33-●
  Monteggia's —*see* Monteggia's fracture
  multiple
    hand (and wrist) NEC —*see* Fracture,
      by site
    ribs —*see* Fracture, rib, multiple
  nasal (bone(s)) S02.2
  navicular (scaphoid) (foot) —*see also* Fracture,
    tarsal, navicular
    hand —*see* Fracture, carpal, navicular
  neck S12.9
    cervical vertebra S12.9
      fifth (displaced) S12.400
        nondisplaced S12.401
        specified type NEC (displaced)
          S12.490
          nondisplaced S12.491
      first (displaced) S12.000
        burst (stable) S12.01
          unstable S12.02
        lateral mass (displaced)
          S12.040
          nondisplaced S12.041
        nondisplaced S12.001
        posterior arch (displaced)
          S12.030
          nondisplaced S12.031
        specified type NEC (displaced)
          S12.090
          nondisplaced S12.091
      fourth (displaced) S12.300
        nondisplaced S12.301
        specified type NEC (displaced)
          S12.390
          nondisplaced S12.391

Fracture, traumatic *(Continued)*
  neck *(Continued)*
    cervical vertebra *(Continued)*
      second (displaced) S12.100
        dens (anterior) (displaced) (type II)
          S12.110
          nondisplaced S12.112
          posterior S12.111
          specified type NEC (displaced)
            S12.120
            nondisplaced S12.121
        nondisplaced S12.101
        specified type NEC (displaced)
          S12.190
          nondisplaced S12.191
      seventh (displaced) S12.600
        nondisplaced S12.601
        specified type NEC (displaced)
          S12.690
          nondisplaced S12.691
      sixth (displaced) S12.500
        nondisplaced S12.501
        specified type NEC (displaced)
          S12.590
          nondisplaced S12.591
      third (displaced) S12.200
        nondisplaced S12.201
        specified type NEC (displaced)
          S12.290
          nondisplaced S12.291
    hyoid bone S12.8
    larynx S12.8
    specified site NEC S12.8
    thyroid cartilage S12.8
    trachea S12.8
  neoplastic NEC —*see* Fracture, pathological,
    due to, neoplastic disease
  neural arch —*see* Fracture, vertebra
  newborn —*see* Birth, injury, fracture
  nontraumatic —*see* Fracture, pathological
  nonunion —*see* Nonunion, fracture
  nose, nasal (bone) (septum) S02.2
  occiput —*see* Fracture, skull, base,
    occiput
  odontoid process —*see* Fracture, neck,
    cervical vertebra, second
  olecranon (process) (ulna) —*see* Fracture,
    ulna, upper end, olecranon process
  orbit, orbital (bone) (region) S02.85
    floor (blow-out) S02.3-●
    roof S02.12-●
    wall S02.85
      lateral S02.84-●
      medial S02.83-●
  os
    calcis —*see* Fracture, tarsal,
      calcaneus
    magnum —*see* Fracture, carpal,
      capitate
    pubis —*see* Fracture, pubis
  palate S02.8-●
  parietal bone (skull) S02.0
  patella S82.00-●
    comminuted (displaced) S82.04-●
      nondisplaced S82.04-●
    longitudinal (displaced) S82.02-●
      nondisplaced S82.02-●
    osteochondral (displaced) S82.01-●
      nondisplaced S82.01-●
    specified NEC S82.09-●
    transverse (displaced) S82.03-●
      nondisplaced S82.03-●
  pedicle (of vertebral arch) —*see* Fracture,
    vertebra
  pelvis, pelvic (bone) S32.9
    acetabulum —*see* Fracture, acetabulum
    circle —*see* Disruption, pelvic ring
    following insertion of implant, prosthesis
      or plate M96.65
    ilium —*see* Fracture, ilium
    ischium —*see* Fracture, ischium

Fracture, traumatic *(Continued)*
  pelvis, pelvic *(Continued)*
    multiple
      with disruption of pelvic ring (circle) —
        see Disruption, pelvic ring
      without disruption of pelvic ring (circle)
        S32.82
    pubis —*see* Fracture, pubis
    sacrum —*see* Fracture, sacrum
    specified site NEC S32.89
  periprosthetic, around internal prosthetic
    joint M97.9
    ankle M97.2-●
    elbow M97.4-●
    finger M97.8
    hip M97.0-●
    knee M97.1-●
    shoulder M97.3-●
    specified joint NEC M97.8
    spine M97.8
    toe M97.8
    wrist M97.8
  phalanx
    foot —*see* Fracture, toe
    hand —*see* Fracture, finger
  pisiform —*see* Fracture, carpal, pisiform
  pond —*see* Fracture, skull
  prosthetic device, internal —*see*
    Complications, prosthetic device, by site,
    mechanical
  pubis S32.50-●
    with disruption of pelvic ring —*see*
      Disruption, pelvic ring
    specified site NEC S32.59-●
    superior rim S32.59-●
  radius S52.9-●
    distal end —*see* Fracture, radius, lower end
    following insertion of implant, prosthesis
      or plate M96.63-●
    head —*see* Fracture, radius, upper end,
      head
    lower end S52.50-●
      Barton's —*see* Barton's fracture
      Colles' —*see* Colles' fracture
      extraarticular NEC S52.55-●
      intraarticular NEC S52.57-●
      physeal S59.20-●
        Salter-Harris
          Type I S59.21-●
          Type II S59.22-●
          Type III S59.23-●
          Type IV S59.24-●
        specified NEC S59.29-●
      Smith's —*see* Smith's fracture
      specified NEC S52.59-●
      styloid process (displaced) S52.51-●
        nondisplaced S52.51-●
      torus S52.52-●
    neck —*see* Fracture, radius, upper end
    proximal end —*see* Fracture, radius, upper
      end
    shaft S52.30-●
      bent bone S52.38-●
      comminuted (displaced) S52.35-●
        nondisplaced S52.35-●
      Galeazzi's —*see* Galeazzi's fracture
      greenstick S52.31-●
      oblique (displaced) S52.33-●
        nondisplaced S52.33-●
      segmental (displaced) S52.36-●
        nondisplaced S52.36-●
      specified NEC S52.39-●
      spiral (displaced) S52.34-●
        nondisplaced S52.34-●
      transverse (displaced) S52.32-●
        nondisplaced S52.32-●
    upper end S52.10-●
      head (displaced) S52.12-●
        nondisplaced S52.12-●
      neck (displaced) S52.13-●
        nondisplaced S52.13-●

▶ New   ⇒ Revised   ~~deleted~~ Deleted   ● Use Additional Character(s)

Fracture, traumatic *(Continued)*
  radius *(Continued)*
    upper end *(Continued)*
      physeal S59.10- ●
        Salter-Harris
          Type I S59.11- ●
          Type II S59.12- ●
          Type III S59.13- ●
          Type IV S59.14- ●
        specified NEC S59.19- ●
      specified NEC S52.18- ●
      torus S52.11- ●
  ramus
    inferior or superior, pubis —*see* Fracture, pubis
    mandible —*see* Fracture, mandible
  restorative material (dental) K08.539
    with loss of material K08.531
    without loss of material K08.530
  rib S22.3- ●
    with flail chest —*see* Flail, chest
    ▶associated with chest compression and cardiopulmonary resuscitation M96.A2
    multiple S22.4- ●
      with flail chest —*see* Flail, chest
      ▶associated with chest compression and cardiopulmonary resuscitation M96.A3
  root, tooth —*see* Fracture, tooth
  sacrum S32.10
    specified NEC S32.19
    Type
      1 S32.14
      2 S32.15
      3 S32.16
      4 S32.17
    Zone
      I S32.119
        displaced (minimally) S32.111
          severely S32.112
        nondisplaced S32.110
      II S32.129
        displaced (minimally) S32.121
          severely S32.122
        nondisplaced S32.120
      III S32.139
        displaced (minimally) S32.131
          severely S32.132
        nondisplaced S32.130
  scaphoid (hand) —*see also* Fracture, carpal, navicular
    foot —*see* Fracture, tarsal, navicular
  scapula S42.10- ●
    acromial process (displaced) S42.12- ●
      nondisplaced S42.12- ●
    body (displaced) S42.11- ●
      nondisplaced S42.11- ●
    coracoid process (displaced) S42.13- ●
      nondisplaced S42.13- ●
    glenoid cavity (displaced) S42.14- ●
      nondisplaced S42.14- ●
    neck (displaced) S42.15- ●
      nondisplaced S42.15- ●
    specified NEC S42.19- ●
  semilunar bone, wrist —*see* Fracture, carpal, lunate
  sequelae —*see* Sequelae, fracture
  sesamoid bone
    foot S92.81- ●
    hand —*see* Fracture, carpal
    other —*see* Fracture, traumatic, by site
  shepherd's —*see* Fracture, tarsal, talus
  shoulder (girdle) S42.9- ●
    blade —*see* Fracture, scapula
  sinus (ethmoid) (frontal) S02.19
  skull S02.91
    base S02.10- ●
      occiput S02.119
        condyle S02.113

Fracture, traumatic *(Continued)*
  skull *(Continued)*
    base *(Continued)*
      occiput *(Continued)*
        condyle *(Continued)*
          type I S02.110
            left side S02.11B
            right side S02.11A
          type II S02.111
            left side S02.11D
            right side S02.11C
          type III S02.112
            left side S02.11F
            right side S02.11E
          specified NEC S02.118
            left side S02.11H
            right side S02.11G
        specified NEC S02.19- ●
    birth injury P13.0
    frontal bone S02.0
    parietal bone S02.0
    specified site NEC S02.8
    temporal bone S02.19
    vault S02.0
  Smith's —*see* Smith's fracture
  sphenoid (bone) (sinus) S02.19
  spine —*see* Fracture, vertebra
  spinous process —*see* Fracture, vertebra
  spontaneous (cause unknown) —*see* Fracture, pathological
  stave (of thumb) —*see* Fracture, metacarpal, first
  sternum S22.20
    with flail chest —*see* Flail, chest
    ▶associated with chest compression and cardiopulmonary resuscitation M96.A1
    body S22.22
    manubrium S22.21
    xiphoid (process) S22.24
    ▶associated with chest compression and cardiopulmonary resuscitation M96.A1
  stress M84.30
    ankle M84.37- ●
    carpus M84.34- ●
    clavicle M84.31- ●
    femoral neck M84.359
    femur M84.35- ●
    fibula M84.36- ●
    finger M84.34- ●
    hip M84.359
    humerus M84.32- ●
    ilium M84.350
    ischium M84.350
    metacarpus M84.34- ●
    metatarsus M84.37- ●
    neck —*see* Fracture, fatigue, vertebra
    pelvis M84.350
    radius M84.33- ●
    rib M84.38
    scapula M84.31- ●
    skull M84.38
    tarsus M84.37- ●
    tibia M84.36- ●
    toe M84.37- ●
    ulna M84.33- ●
    vertebra —*see* Fracture, fatigue, vertebra
  supracondylar, elbow —*see* Fracture, humerus, lower end, supracondylar
  symphysis pubis —*see* Fracture, pubis
  talus (ankle bone) —*see* Fracture, tarsal, talus
  tarsal bone(s) S92.20- ●
    astragalus —*see* Fracture, tarsal, talus
    calcaneus S92.00- ●
      anterior process (displaced) S92.02- ●
        nondisplaced S92.02- ●
      body (displaced) S92.01- ●
        nondisplaced S92.01- ●
      extraarticular NEC (displaced) S92.05- ●
        nondisplaced S92.05- ●

Fracture, traumatic *(Continued)*
  tarsal bone(s) *(Continued)*
    calcaneus *(Continued)*
      intraarticular (displaced) S92.06- ●
        nondisplaced S92.06- ●
      physeal S99.00- ●
        Salter-Harris
          Type I S99.01- ●
          Type II S99.02- ●
          Type III S99.03- ●
          Type IV S99.04- ●
        specified NEC S99.09- ●
      tuberosity (displaced) S92.04- ●
        avulsion (displaced) S92.03- ●
          nondisplaced S92.03- ●
        nondisplaced S92.04- ●
    cuboid (displaced) S92.21- ●
      nondisplaced S92.21- ●
    cuneiform
      intermediate (displaced) S92.23- ●
        nondisplaced S92.23- ●
      lateral (displaced) S92.22- ●
        nondisplaced S92.22- ●
      medial (displaced) S92.24- ●
        nondisplaced S92.24- ●
    navicular (displaced) S92.25- ●
      nondisplaced S92.25- ●
    scaphoid —*see* Fracture, tarsal, navicular
    talus S92.10- ●
      avulsion (displaced) S92.15- ●
        nondisplaced S92.15- ●
      body (displaced) S92.12- ●
        nondisplaced S92.12- ●
      dome (displaced) S92.14- ●
        nondisplaced S92.14- ●
      head (displaced) S92.12- ●
        nondisplaced S92.12- ●
      lateral process (displaced) S92.14- ●
        nondisplaced S92.14- ●
      neck (displaced) S92.11- ●
        nondisplaced S92.11- ●
      posterior process (displaced) S92.13- ●
        nondisplaced S92.13- ●
      specified NEC S92.19- ●
  temporal bone (styloid) S02.19
  thorax (bony) S22.9
    with flail chest —*see* Flail, chest
    rib S22.3- ●
      multiple S22.4- ●
        with flail chest —*see* Flail, chest
    sternum S22.20
      body S22.22
      manubrium S22.21
      xiphoid process S22.24
      ▶associated with chest compression and cardiopulmonary resuscitation M96.A1
    vertebra (displaced) S22.009
      burst (stable) S22.001
        unstable S22.002
      eighth S22.069
        burst (stable) S22.061
          unstable S22.062
        specified type NEC S22.068
        wedge compression S22.060
      eleventh S22.089
        burst (stable) S22.081
          unstable S22.082
        specified type NEC S22.088
        wedge compression S22.080
      fifth S22.059
        burst (stable) S22.051
          unstable S22.052
        specified type NEC S22.058
        wedge compression S22.050
      first S22.019
        burst (stable) S22.011
          unstable S22.012
        specified type NEC S22.018
        wedge compression S22.010

Fracture, traumatic (Continued)
  thorax (Continued)
    vertebra (Continued)
      fourth S22.049
        burst (stable) S22.041
          unstable S22.042
        specified type NEC S22.048
        wedge compression S22.040
      ninth S22.079
        burst (stable) S22.071
          unstable S22.072
        specified type NEC S22.078
        wedge compression S22.070
      nondisplaced S22.001
      second S22.029
        burst (stable) S22.021
          unstable S22.022
        specified type NEC S22.028
        wedge compression S22.020
      seventh S22.069
        burst (stable) S22.061
          unstable S22.062
        specified type NEC S22.068
        wedge compression S22.060
      sixth S22.059
        burst (stable) S22.051
          unstable S22.052
        specified type NEC S22.058
        wedge compression S22.050
      specified type NEC S22.008
      tenth S22.079
        burst (stable) S22.071
          unstable S22.072
        specified type NEC S22.078
        wedge compression S22.070
      third S22.039
        burst (stable) S22.031
          unstable S22.032
        specified type NEC S22.038
        wedge compression S22.030
      twelfth S22.089
        burst (stable) S22.081
          unstable S22.082
        specified type NEC S22.088
        wedge compression S22.080
      wedge compression S22.000
  thumb S62.50-●
    distal phalanx (displaced) S62.52-●
      nondisplaced S62.52-●
    proximal phalanx (displaced) S62.51-●
      nondisplaced S62.51-●
  thyroid cartilage S12.8
  tibia (shaft) S82.20-●
    comminuted (displaced) S82.25-●
      nondisplaced S82.25-●
    condyles —see Fracture, tibia, upper end
    distal end —see Fracture, tibia, lower end
    epiphysis
      lower —see Fracture, tibia, lower end
      upper —see Fracture, tibia, upper end
    following insertion of implant, prosthesis
      or plate M96.67-●
    head (involving knee joint) —see Fracture,
      tibia, upper end
    intercondyloid eminence —see Fracture,
      tibia, upper end
    involving ankle or malleolus —see
      Fracture, ankle, medial malleolus
    lower end S82.30-●
      physeal S89.10-●
        Salter-Harris
          Type I S89.11-●
          Type II S89.12-●
          Type III S89.13-●
          Type IV S89.14-●
        specified NEC S89.19-●
      pilon (displaced) S82.87-●
        nondisplaced S82.87-●
      specified NEC S82.39-●
      torus S82.31-●
    malleolus —see Fracture, ankle, medial
      malleolus

Fracture, traumatic (Continued)
  tibia (Continued)
    oblique (displaced) S82.23-●
      nondisplaced S82.23-●
    pilon —see Fracture, tibia, lower end, pilon
    proximal end —see Fracture, tibia, upper end
    segmental (displaced) S82.26-●
      nondisplaced S82.26-●
    specified NEC S82.29-●
    spine —see Fracture, tibia, upper end, spine
    spiral (displaced) S82.24-●
      nondisplaced S82.24-●
    transverse (displaced) S82.22-●
      nondisplaced S82.22-●
    tuberosity —see Fracture, tibia, upper end,
      tuberosity
    upper end S82.10-●
      bicondylar (displaced) S82.14-●
        nondisplaced S82.14-●
      lateral condyle (displaced) S82.12-●
        nondisplaced S82.12-●
      medial condyle (displaced) S82.13-●
        nondisplaced S82.13-●
      physeal S89.00-●
        Salter-Harris
          Type I S89.01-●
          Type II S89.02-●
          Type III S89.03-●
          Type IV S89.04-●
        specified NEC S89.09-●
      plateau —see Fracture, tibia, upper end,
        bicondylar
      specified NEC S82.19-●
      spine (displaced) S82.11-●
        nondisplaced S82.11-●
      torus S82.16-●
      tuberosity (displaced) S82.15-●
        nondisplaced S82.15-●
  toe S92.91-●
    great (displaced) S92.40-●
      distal phalanx (displaced) S92.42-●
        nondisplaced S92.42-●
      nondisplaced S92.40-●
      proximal phalanx (displaced) S92.41-●
        nondisplaced S92.41-●
      specified NEC S92.49-●
    lesser (displaced) S92.50-●
      distal phalanx (displaced) S92.53-●
        nondisplaced S92.53-●
      middle phalanx (displaced) S92.52-●
        nondisplaced S92.52-●
      nondisplaced S92.50-●
      proximal phalanx (displaced) S92.51-●
        nondisplaced S92.51-●
      specified NEC S92.59-●
    physeal
      phalanx S99.20-●
        Salter-Harris
          Type I S99.21-●
          Type II S99.22-●
          Type III S99.23-●
          Type IV S99.24-●
        specified NEC S99.29-●
  tooth (root) S02.5
  trachea (cartilage) S12.8
  transverse process —see Fracture, vertebra
  trapezium or trapezoid bone —see Fracture,
    carpal
  trimalleolar —see Fracture, ankle, trimalleolar
  triquetrum (cuneiform of carpus) —see
    Fracture, carpal, triquetrum
  trochanter —see Fracture, femur, trochanteric
  tuberosity (external) —see Fracture,
    traumatic, by site
  ulna (shaft) S52.20-●
    bent bone S52.28-●
    coronoid process —see Fracture, ulna,
      upper end, coronoid process
    distal end —see Fracture, ulna, lower end
    following insertion of implant, prosthesis
      or plate M96.63-●
    head S52.60-●

Fracture, traumatic (Continued)
  ulna (Continued)
    lower end S52.60-●
      physeal S59.00-●
        Salter-Harris
          Type I S59.01-●
          Type II S59.02-●
          Type III S59.03-●
          Type IV S59.04-●
        specified NEC S59.09-●
      specified NEC S52.69-●
      styloid process (displaced) S52.61-●
        nondisplaced S52.61-●
      torus S52.62-●
    proximal end —see Fracture, ulna, upper end
    shaft S52.20-●
      comminuted (displaced) S52.25-●
        nondisplaced S52.25-●
      greenstick S52.21-●
      Monteggia's —see Monteggia's fracture
      oblique (displaced) S52.23-●
        nondisplaced S52.23-●
      segmental (displaced) S52.26-●
        nondisplaced S52.26-●
      specified NEC S52.29-●
      spiral (displaced) S52.24-●
        nondisplaced S52.24-●
      transverse (displaced) S52.22-●
        nondisplaced S52.22-●
    upper end S52.00-●
      coronoid process (displaced) S52.04-●
        nondisplaced S52.04-●
      olecranon process (displaced) S52.02-●
        with intraarticular extension S52.03-●
        nondisplaced S52.02-●
          with intraarticular extension S52.03-●
      specified NEC S52.09-●
      torus S52.01-●
  unciform —see Fracture, carpal, hamate
  vault of skull S02.0
  vertebra, vertebral (arch) (body) (column)
    (neural arch) (pedicle) (spinous process)
    (transverse process)
    atlas —see Fracture, neck, cervical vertebra,
      first
    axis —see Fracture, neck, cervical vertebra,
      second
    cervical (teardrop) S12.9
      axis —see Fracture, neck, cervical
        vertebra, second
      first (atlas) —see Fracture, neck, cervical
        vertebra, first
      second (axis) —see Fracture, neck,
        cervical vertebra, second
    chronic M84.48
    coccyx S32.2
    dorsal —see Fracture, thorax, vertebra
    lumbar S32.009
      burst (stable) S32.001
        unstable S32.002
      fifth S32.059
        burst (stable) S32.051
          unstable S32.052
        specified type NEC S32.058
        wedge compression S32.050
      first S32.019
        burst (stable) S32.011
          unstable S32.012
        specified type NEC S32.018
        wedge compression S32.010
      fourth S32.049
        burst (stable) S32.041
          unstable S32.042
        specified type NEC S32.048
        wedge compression S32.040
      second S32.029
        burst (stable) S32.021
          unstable S32.022
        specified type NEC S32.028
        wedge compression S32.020
      specified type NEC S32.008

▶ New   ⇒ Revised   ~~deleted~~ Deleted   ● Use Additional Character(s)

Fracture, traumatic *(Continued)*
  vertebra, vertebral *(Continued)*
    lumbar *(Continued)*
      third S32.039
        burst (stable) S32.031
          unstable S32.032
        specified type NEC S32.038
        wedge compression S32.030
      wedge compression S32.000
    metastatic —*see* Collapse, vertebra, in,
      specified disease NEC —*see also*
      Neoplasm
    newborn (birth injury) P11.5
    sacrum S32.10
      specified NEC S32.19
      Type
        1 S32.14
        2 S32.15
        3 S32.16
        4 S32.17
      Zone
        I S32.119
          displaced (minimally) S32.111
            severely S32.112
          nondisplaced S32.110
        II S32.129
          displaced (minimally) S32.121
            severely S32.122
          nondisplaced S32.120
        III S32.139
          displaced (minimally) S32.131
            severely S32.132
          nondisplaced S32.130
    thoracic —*see* Fracture, thorax, vertebra
  vertex S02.0
  vomer (bone) S02.2
  wrist S62.10-•
    carpal —*see* Fracture, carpal bone
    navicular (scaphoid) (hand) —*see* Fracture,
      carpal, navicular
  xiphisternum, xiphoid (process) S22.24
  ▶associated with chest compression and
    cardiopulmonary resuscitation
    M96.A1
  zygoma S02.442
    left side S02.40F
    right side S02.40E
Fragile, fragility
  autosomal site Q95.5
  bone, congenital (with blue sclera) Q78.0
  capillary (hereditary) D69.8
  hair L67.8
  nails L60.3
  non-sex chromosome site Q95.5
  X chromosome Q99.2
Fragilitas
  crinium L67.8
  ossium (with blue sclerae) (hereditary)
    Q78.0
  unguium L60.3
    congenital Q84.6
Fragments, cataract (lens), following cataract
    surgery H59.02-•
  retained foreign body —*see* Retained, foreign
    body fragments (type of)
Frailty (frail) R54
  mental R41.81
Frambesia, frambesial (tropica) —*see also* Yaws
  initial lesion or ulcer A66.0
  primary A66.0
Frambeside
  gummatous A66.4
  of early yaws A66.2
Frambesioma A66.1
Franceschetti-Klein (-Wildervanck) disease or
    syndrome Q75.4
Francis' disease —*see* Tularemia
Franklin disease C88.2
Frank's essential thrombocytopenia D69.3
Fraser's syndrome Q87.0

Freckle(s) L81.2
  malignant melanoma in —*see* Melanoma
  melanotic (Hutchinson's) —*see* Melanoma,
    in situ
  retinal D49.81
Frederickson's hyperlipoproteinemia, type
  I and V E78.3
  IIA E78.00
  IIB and III E78.2
  IV E78.1
Freeman Sheldon syndrome Q87.0
Freezing —*see also* Effect, adverse, cold T69.9
Freiberg's disease (infraction of metatarsal head
    or osteochondrosis) —*see* Osteochondrosis,
    juvenile, metatarsus
Frei's disease A55
Fremitus, friction, cardiac R01.2
Frenum, frenulum
  external os Q51.828
  tongue (shortening) (congenital) Q38.1
Frequency micturition (nocturnal) R35.0
  psychogenic F45.8
Frey's syndrome
  auriculotemporal G50.8
  hyperhidrosis L74.52
Friction
  burn —*see* Burn, by site
  fremitus, cardiac R01.2
  precordial R01.2
  sounds, chest R09.89
Friderichsen-Waterhouse syndrome or disease
    A39.1
Friedländer's B (bacillus) NEC —*see also*
    condition A49.8
Friedreich's
  ataxia G11.11
  combined systemic disease G11.11
  facial hemihypertrophy Q67.4
  sclerosis (cerebellum) (spinal cord) G11.11
Frigidity F52.22
Fröhlich's syndrome E23.6
Frontal —*see also* condition
  lobe syndrome F07.0
Frostbite (superficial) T33.90
  with
    partial thickness skin loss —*see* Frostbite
      (superficial), by site
    tissue necrosis T34.90
  abdominal wall T33.3
    with tissue necrosis T34.3
  ankle T33.81-•
    with tissue necrosis T34.81-•
  arm T33.4-•
    with tissue necrosis T34.4-•
      finger(s) —*see* Frostbite, finger
      hand —*see* Frostbite, hand
      wrist —*see* Frostbite, wrist
  ear T33.01-•
    with tissue necrosis T34.01-•
  face T33.09
    with tissue necrosis T34.09
  finger T33.53-•
    with tissue necrosis T34.53-•
  foot T33.82-•
    with tissue necrosis T34.82-•
  hand T33.52-•
    with tissue necrosis T34.52-•
  head T33.09
    with tissue necrosis T34.09
      ear —*see* Frostbite, ear
      nose —*see* Frostbite, nose
  hip (and thigh) T33.6-•
    with tissue necrosis T34.6-•
  knee T33.7-•
    with tissue necrosis T34.7-•
  leg T33.9-•
    with tissue necrosis T34.9-•
      ankle —*see* Frostbite, ankle
      foot —*see* Frostbite, foot
      knee —*see* Frostbite, knee
      lower T33.7-•
        with tissue necrosis T34.7-•

Frostbite *(Continued)*
  leg *(Continued)*
    thigh —*see* Frostbite, hip
    toe —*see* Frostbite, toe
  limb
    lower T33.99
      with tissue necrosis T34.99
    upper —*see* Frostbite, arm
  neck T33.1
    with tissue necrosis T34.1
  nose T33.02
    with tissue necrosis T34.02
  pelvis T33.3
    with tissue necrosis T34.3
  specified site NEC T33.99
    with tissue necrosis T34.99
  thigh —*see* Frostbite, hip
  thorax T33.2
    with tissue necrosis T34.2
  toes T33.83-•
    with tissue necrosis T34.83-•
  trunk T33.99
    with tissue necrosis T34.99
  wrist T33.51-•
    with tissue necrosis T34.51-•
Frotteurism F65.81
Frozen —*see also* Effect, adverse, cold T69.9
  pelvis (female) N94.89
    male K66.8
  shoulder —*see* Capsulitis, adhesive
Fructokinase deficiency E74.11
Fructose 1,6 diphosphatase deficiency E74.19
Fructosemia (benign) (essential) E74.12
Fructosuria (benign) (essential) E74.11
Fuchs'
  black spot (myopic) —*see also* Myopia,
    degenerative H44.2-•
  dystrophy (corneal endothelium) H18.51-•
  heterochromic cyclitis —*see* Cyclitis, Fuchs'
    heterochromic
Fucosidosis E77.1
Fugue R68.89
  dissociative F44.1
  hysterical (dissociative) F44.1
  postictal in epilepsy —*see* Epilepsy
  reaction to exceptional stress (transient)
    F43.0
Fulminant, fulminating —*see* condition
Functional —*see also* condition
  bleeding (uterus) N93.8
Functioning, intellectual, borderline R41.83
Fundus —*see* condition
Fungemia NOS B49
Fungus, fungous
  cerebral G93.89
  disease NOS B49
  infection —*see* Infection, fungus
Funiculitis (acute) (chronic) (endemic)
    N49.1
  gonococcal (acute) (chronic) A54.23
  tuberculous A18.15
Funnel
  breast (acquired) M95.4
    congenital Q67.6
    sequelae (late effect) of rickets E64.3
  chest (acquired) M95.4
    congenital Q67.6
    sequelae (late effect) of rickets E64.3
  pelvis (acquired) M95.5
    with disproportion (fetopelvic) O33.3
      causing obstructed labor O65.3
    congenital Q74.2
FUO (fever of unknown origin) R50.9
Furfur L21.0
  microsporon B36.0
Furrier's lung J67.8
Furrowed K14.5
  nail(s) (transverse) L60.4
    congenital Q84.6
  tongue K14.5
    congenital Q38.3

Furuncle L02.92
  abdominal wall L02.221
  ankle —see Furuncle, lower limb
  antecubital space —see Furuncle, upper limb
  anus K61.0
  arm —see Furuncle, upper limb
  auditory canal, external —see Abscess, ear, external
  auricle (ear) —see Abscess, ear, external
  axilla (region) L02.42-•
Furuncle (Continued)
  back (any part) L02.222
  breast N61.1
  buttock L02.32
  cheek (external) L02.02
  chest wall L02.223
  chin L02.02
  corpus cavernosum N48.21
  ear, external —see Abscess, ear, external
  external auditory canal —see Abscess, ear, external
  eyelid —see Abscess, eyelid
  face L02.02
  femoral (region) —see Furuncle, lower limb
  finger —see Furuncle, hand
  flank L02.221
  foot L02.62-•
  forehead L02.02
  gluteal (region) L02.32
  groin L02.224
  hand L02.52-•
  head L02.821
    face L02.02
  hip —see Furuncle, lower limb
  kidney —see Abscess, kidney
  knee —see Furuncle, lower limb
  labium (majus) (minus) N76.4
  lacrimal
    gland —see Dacryoadenitis
    passages (duct) (sac) —see Inflammation, lacrimal, passages, acute
  leg (any part) —see Furuncle, lower limb
  lower limb L02.42-•
  malignant A22.0
  mouth K12.2
  navel L02.226
  neck L02.12

Furuncle (Continued)
  nose J34.0
  orbit, orbital —see Abscess, orbit
  palmar (space) —see Furuncle, hand
  partes posteriores L02.32
  pectoral region L02.223
  penis N48.21
  perineum L02.225
  pinna —see Abscess, ear, external
  popliteal —see Furuncle, lower limb
  prepatellar —see Furuncle, lower limb
  scalp L02.821
  seminal vesicle N49.0
  shoulder —see Furuncle, upper limb
  specified site NEC L02.828
  submandibular K12.2
  temple (region) L02.02
  thumb —see Furuncle, hand
  toe —see Furuncle, foot
  trunk L02.229
    abdominal wall L02.221
    back L02.222
    chest wall L02.223
    groin L02.224
    perineum L02.225
    umbilicus L02.226
  umbilicus L02.226
  upper limb L02.42-•
  vulva N76.4
Furunculosis —see Furuncle
Fused —see Fusion, fused
Fusion, fused (congenital)
  astragaloscaphoid Q74.2
  ➡atria Q21.19
  auditory canal Q16.1
  ➡auricles, heart Q21.19
  binocular with defective stereopsis H53.32
  bone Q79.8
  cervical spine M43.22
  choanal Q30.0
  commissure, mitral valve Q23.2
  cusps, heart valve NEC Q24.8
    mitral Q23.2
    pulmonary Q22.1
    tricuspid Q22.4
  ear ossicles Q16.3
  fingers Q70.0-•
  hymen Q52.3
  joint (acquired) —see also Ankylosis
    congenital Q74.8

Fusion, fused (Continued)
  kidneys (incomplete) Q63.1
  labium (majus) (minus) Q52.5
  larynx and trachea Q34.8
  limb, congenital Q74.8
    lower Q74.2
    upper Q74.0
  lobes, lung Q33.8
  lumbosacral (acquired) M43.27
    arthrodesis status Z98.1
    congenital Q76.49
    postprocedural status Z98.1
  nares, nose, nasal, nostril(s) Q30.0
  organ or site not listed —see Anomaly, by site
  ossicles Q79.9
    auditory Q16.3
  pulmonic cusps Q22.1
  ribs Q76.6
  sacroiliac (joint) (acquired) M43.28
    arthrodesis status Z98.1
    congenital Q74.2
    postprocedural status Z98.1
  spine (acquired) NEC M43.20
    arthrodesis status Z98.1
    cervical region M43.22
    cervicothoracic region M43.23
    congenital Q76.49
    lumbar M43.26
    lumbosacral region M43.27
    occipito-atlanto-axial region M43.21
    postoperative status Z98.1
    sacrococcygeal region M43.28
    thoracic region M43.24
    thoracolumbar region M43.25
  sublingual duct with submaxillary duct at opening in mouth Q38.4
  testes Q55.1
  toes Q70.2
  tooth, teeth K00.2
  trachea and esophagus Q39.8
  twins Q89.4
  vagina Q52.4
  ventricles, heart Q21.0
  vertebra (arch) —see Fusion, spine
  vulva Q52.5
Fusospirillosis (mouth) (tongue) (tonsil) A69.1
Fussy baby R68.12

▶ New   ➡ Revised   ~~deleted~~ Deleted   • Use Additional Character(s)

G

Gain in weight (abnormal) (excessive) —see also
    Weight, gain
Gaisböck's disease (polycythemia hypertonica)
    D75.1
Gait abnormality R26.9
    ataxic R26.0
    falling R29.6
    hysterical (ataxic) (staggering) F44.4
    paralytic R26.1
    spastic R26.1
    specified type NEC R26.89
    staggering R26.0
    unsteadiness R26.81
    walking difficulty NEC R26.2
Galactocele (breast) N64.89
    puerperal, postpartum O92.79
Galactokinase deficiency E74.29
Galactophoritis N61.0
    gestational, puerperal, postpartum O91.2-•
Galactorrhea O92.6
    not associated with childbirth N64.3
Galactosemia (classic) (congenital) E74.21
Galactosuria E74.29
Galacturia R82.0
    schistosomiasis (bilharziasis) B65.0
GALD (gestational alloimmune liver disease)
    P78.84
Galeazzi's fracture S52.37-•
Galen's vein —see condition
Galeophobia F40.218
Gall duct —see condition
Gallbladder —see also condition
    acute K81.0
Gallop rhythm R00.8
Gallstone (colic) (cystic duct) (gallbladder)
    (impacted) (multiple) —see also Calculus,
    gallbladder
    with
        cholecystitis —see Calculus, gallbladder,
            with cholecystitis
        bile duct (common) (hepatic) —see Calculus,
            bile duct
        causing intestinal obstruction K56.3
        specified NEC K80.80
            with obstruction K80.81
Gambling Z72.6
    pathological (compulsive) F63.0
Gammopathy (of undetermined significance
    [MGUS]) D47.2
    associated with lymphoplasmacytic dyscrasia
        D47.2
    monoclonal D47.2
    polyclonal D89.0
Gamna's disease (siderotic splenomegaly)
    D73.1
Gamophobia F40.298
Gampsodactylia (congenital) Q66.7-•
Gamstorp's disease (adynamia episodica
    hereditaria) G72.3
Gandy-Nanta disease (siderotic splenomegaly)
    D73.1
Gang
    membership offenses Z72.810
Gangliocytoma D36.10
Ganglioglioma —see Neoplasm, uncertain
    behavior, by site
Ganglion (compound) (diffuse) (joint) (tendon
    (sheath)) M67.40
    ankle M67.47-•
    foot M67.47-•
    forearm M67.43-•
    hand M67.44-•
    lower leg M67.46-•
    multiple sites M67.49
    of yaws (early) (late) A66.6
    pelvic region M67.45-•
    periosteal —see Periostitis
    shoulder region M67.41-•
    specified site NEC M67.48

Ganglion (Continued)
    thigh region M67.45-•
    tuberculous A18.09
    upper arm M67.42-•
    wrist M67.43-•
Ganglioneuroblastoma —see Neoplasm, nerve,
    malignant
Ganglioneuroma D36.10
    malignant —see Neoplasm, nerve, malignant
Ganglioneuromatosis D36.10
Ganglionitis
    fifth nerve —see Neuralgia, trigeminal
    gasserian (postherpetic) (postzoster) B02.21
    geniculate G51.1
        newborn (birth injury) P11.3
        postherpetic, postzoster B02.21
    herpes zoster B02.21
    postherpetic geniculate B02.21
Gangliosidosis E75.10
    GM1 E75.19
    GM2 E75.00
        other specified E75.09
        Sandhoff disease E75.01
        Tay-Sachs disease E75.02
    GM3 E75.19
    mucolipidosis IV E75.11
Gangosa A66.5
Gangrene, gangrenous (connective tissue)
    (dropsical) (dry) (moist) (skin) (ulcer) —see
    also Necrosis I96
    with diabetes (mellitus) —see Diabetes, with
        gangrene
    abdomen (wall) I96
    alveolar M27.3
    appendix K35.80
        with
            peritonitis, localized (see also
                Appendicitis) K35.31
    arteriosclerotic (general) (senile) —see
        Arteriosclerosis, extremities, with,
        gangrene
    auricle I96
    Bacillus welchii A48.0
    bladder (infectious) —see Cystitis, specified
        type NEC
    bowel, cecum, or colon —see Gangrene,
        intestine
    Clostridium perfringens or welchii A48.0
    cornea H18.89-•
    corpora cavernosa N48.29
        noninfective N48.89
    cutaneous, spreading I96
    decubital —see Ulcer, pressure, by site
    diabetic (any site) —see Diabetes, with gangrene
    emphysematous —see Gangrene, gas
    epidemic —see Poisoning, food, noxious,
        plant
    epididymis (infectional) N45.1
    erysipelas —see Erysipelas
    extremity (lower) (upper) I96
    Fournier N49.3
    ▥female N76.82
    ▶vagina and vulva N76.82
    fusospirochetal A69.0
    gallbladder —see Cholecystitis, acute
    gas (bacillus) A48.0
        following
            abortion —see Abortion by type
                complicated by infection
            ectopic or molar pregnancy O08.0
    glossitis K14.0
    hernia —see Hernia, by site, with gangrene
    intestine, intestinal (hemorrhagic)
        (massive) —see also Infarct, intestine
        K55.069
        with
            mesenteric embolism —see also Infarct,
                intestine K55.069
            obstruction —see Obstruction, intestine
    laryngitis J04.0
    limb (lower) (upper) I96

Gangrene, gangrenous (Continued)
    lung J85.0
        spirochetal A69.8
    lymphangitis I89.1
    Meleney's (synergistic) —see Ulcer, skin
    mesentery —see also Infarct, intestine
        K55.069
        with
            embolism —see also Infarct, intestine
                K55.069
            intestinal obstruction —see Obstruction,
                intestine
    mouth A69.0
    ovary —see Oophoritis
    pancreas —see Pancreatitis, acute
    penis N48.29
        noninfective N48.89
    perineum I96
    pharynx —see also Pharyngitis
        Vincent's A69.1
    presenile I73.1
    progressive synergistic —see Ulcer, skin
    pulmonary J85.0
    pulpal (dental) K04.1
    quinsy J36
    Raynaud's (symmetric gangrene) I73.01
    retropharyngeal J39.2
    scrotum N49.3
        noninfective N50.89
    senile (atherosclerotic) —see Arteriosclerosis,
        extremities, with, gangrene
    spermatic cord N49.1
        noninfective N50.89
    spine I96
    spirochetal NEC A69.8
    spreading cutaneous I96
    stomatitis A69.0
    symmetrical I73.01
    testis (infectional) N45.2
        noninfective N44.8
    throat —see also Pharyngitis
        diphtheritic A36.0
        Vincent's A69.1
    thyroid (gland) E07.89
    tooth (pulp) K04.1
    tuberculous NEC —see Tuberculosis
    tunica vaginalis N49.1
        noninfective N50.89
    umbilicus I96
    uterus —see Endometritis
    uvulitis K12.2
    vas deferens N49.1
        noninfective N50.89
    ▥vulva N76.82
Ganister disease J62.8
Ganser's syndrome (hysterical) F44.89
Gardner-Diamond syndrome (autoerythrocyte
    sensitization) D69.2
Gargoylism E76.01
Garré's disease, osteitis (sclerosing),
    osteomyelitis —see Osteomyelitis,
    specified type NEC
Garrod's pad, knuckle M72.1
Gartner's duct
    cyst Q52.4
    persistent Q50.6
Gas R14.3
    asphyxiation, inhalation, poisoning,
        suffocation NEC —see Table of Drugs
        and Chemicals
    excessive R14.0
    gangrene A48.0
        following
            abortion —see Abortion by type
                complicated by infection
            ectopic or molar pregnancy O08.0
    on stomach R14.0
    pains R14.1
Gastralgia —see also Pain, abdominal
Gastrectasis K31.0
    psychogenic F45.8

Gastric —*see* condition
Gastrinoma
  malignant
    pancreas C25.4
    specified site NEC —*see* Neoplasm,
      malignant, by site
    unspecified site C25.4
  specified site —*see* Neoplasm, uncertain
    behavior
  unspecified site D37.9
Gastritis (simple) K29.70
  with bleeding K29.71
  acute (erosive) K29.00
    with bleeding K29.01
  alcoholic K29.20
    with bleeding K29.21
  allergic K29.60
    with bleeding K29.61
  atrophic (chronic) K29.40
    with bleeding K29.41
  chronic (antral) (fundal) K29.50
    with bleeding K29.51
    atrophic K29.40
      with bleeding K29.41
    superficial K29.30
      with bleeding K29.31
  dietary counseling and surveillance Z71.3
  due to diet deficiency E63.9
  eosinophilic K52.81
  giant hypertrophic K29.60
    with bleeding K29.61
  granulomatous K29.60
    with bleeding K29.61
  hypertrophic (mucosa) K29.60
    with bleeding K29.61
  nervous F54
  spastic K29.60
    with bleeding K29.61
  specified NEC K29.60
    with bleeding K29.61
  superficial chronic K29.30
    with bleeding K29.31
  tuberculous A18.83
  viral NEC A08.4
Gastrocarcinoma —*see* Neoplasm, malignant,
  stomach
Gastrocolic —*see* condition
Gastrodisciasis, gastrodiscoidiasis B66.8
Gastroduodenitis K29.90
  with bleeding K29.91
  virus, viral A08.4
    specified type NEC A08.39
Gastrodynia —*see* Pain, abdominal
Gastroenteritis (acute) (chronic) (noninfectious)
  (*see also* Enteritis) K52.9
  allergic K52.29
  with
    eosinophilic gastritis or gastroenteritis
      K52.81
    food protein-induced enterocolitis
      syndrome K52.21
    food protein-induced enteropathy K52.22
  dietetic —*see also* Gastroenteritis, allergic
    K52.29
  drug-induced K52.1
  due to
    Cryptosporidium A07.2
    drugs K52.1
    food poisoning —*see* Intoxication,
      foodborne
    radiation K52.0
  eosinophilic K52.81
  epidemic (infectious) A09
  food hypersensitivity —*see also*
    Gastroenteritis, allergic K52.29
  infectious —*see* Enteritis, infectious
  influenzal —*see* Influenza, with
    gastroenteritis
  noninfectious K52.9
    specified NEC K52.89
  rotaviral A08.0

Gastroenteritis (Continued)
  Salmonella A02.0
  toxic K52.1
  viral NEC A08.4
    acute infectious A08.39
      type Norwalk A08.11
    infantile (acute) A08.39
    Norwalk agent A08.11
    rotaviral A08.0
    severe of infants A08.39
    specified type NEC A08.39
Gastroenteropathy —*see also* Gastroenteritis K52.9
  acute, due to Norovirus A08.11
  acute, due to Norwalk agent A08.11
  infectious A09
Gastroenteroptosis K63.4
Gastroesophageal laceration-hemorrhage
  syndrome K22.6
Gastrointestinal —*see* condition
Gastrojejunal —*see* condition
Gastrojejunitis —*see also* Enteritis K52.9
Gastrojejunocolic —*see* condition
Gastroliths K31.89
Gastromalacia K31.89
Gastroparalysis K31.84
  diabetic —*see* Diabetes, gastroparalysis
Gastroparesis K31.84
  diabetic —*see* Diabetes, by type, with
    gastroparesis
Gastropathy K31.9
  congestive portal (*see also*, Hypertension,
    portal) K31.89
  erythematous K29.70
  exudative K90.89
  portal hypertensive (*see also*, Hypertension,
    portal) K31.89
Gastroptosis K31.89
Gastrorrhagia K92.2
  psychogenic F45.8
Gastroschisis (congenital) Q79.3
Gastrospasm (neurogenic) (reflex) K31.89
  neurotic F45.8
  psychogenic F45.8
Gastrostaxis —*see* Gastritis, with bleeding
Gastrostenosis K31.89
Gastrostomy
  attention to Z43.1
  status Z93.1
Gastrosuccorrhea (continuous) (intermittent)
  K31.89
  neurotic F45.8
  psychogenic F45.8
Gatophobia F40.218
Gaucher's disease or splenomegaly (adult)
  (infantile) E75.22
Gee (-Herter)(-Thaysen) disease (nontropical
  sprue) K90.0
Gélineau's syndrome G47.419
  with cataplexy G47.411
Gemination, tooth, teeth K00.2
Gemistocytoma
  specified site —*see* Neoplasm, malignant, by
    site
  unspecified site C71.9
General, generalized —*see* condition
Genetic
  carrier (status)
    cystic fibrosis Z14.1
    hemophilia A (asymptomatic) Z14.01
      symptomatic Z14.02
    specified NEC Z14.8
  susceptibility to disease NEC Z15.89
    malignant neoplasm Z15.09
      breast Z15.01
      endometrium Z15.04
      ovary Z15.02
      prostate Z15.03
      specified NEC Z15.09
    multiple endocrine neoplasia Z15.81
Genital —*see* condition
Genito-anorectal syndrome A55

Genitourinary system —*see* condition
Genu
  congenital Q74.1
  extrorsum (acquired) —*see also* Deformity,
    varus, knee
    congenital Q74.1
    sequelae (late effect) of rickets E64.3
  introrsum (acquired) —*see also* Deformity,
    valgus, knee
    congenital Q74.1
    sequelae (late effect) of rickets E64.3
  rachitic (old) E64.3
  recurvatum (acquired) —*see also* Deformity,
    limb, specified type NEC, lower leg
    congenital Q68.2
    sequelae (late effect) of rickets E64.3
  valgum (acquired) (knock-knee) M21.06-●
    congenital Q74.1
    sequelae (late effect) of rickets E64.3
  varum (acquired) (bowleg) M21.16-●
    congenital Q74.1
    sequelae (late effect) of rickets E64.3
Geographic tongue K14.1
Geophagia —*see* Pica
Geotrichosis B48.3
  stomatitis B48.3
Gephyrophobia F40.242
Gerbode defect Q21.0
GERD (gastroesophageal reflux disease) K21.9
Gerhardt's
  disease (erythromelalgia) I73.81
  syndrome (vocal cord paralysis) J38.00
    bilateral J38.02
    unilateral J38.01
German measles —*see also* Rubella
  exposure to Z20.4
Germinoblastoma (diffuse) C85.9-●
  follicular C82.9-●
Germinoma —*see* Neoplasm, malignant, by site
Gerontoxon —*see* Degeneration, cornea, senile
Gerstmann-Sträussler-Scheinker syndrome
  (GSS) A81.82
Gerstmann's syndrome R48.8
  developmental F81.2
Gestation (period) —*see also* Pregnancy
  ectopic —*see* Pregnancy, by site
  multiple O30.9-●
    greater than quadruplets —*see* Pregnancy,
      multiple (gestation), specified NEC
    specified NEC —*see* Pregnancy, multiple
      (gestation), specified NEC
Gestational
  mammary abscess O91.11-●
  purulent mastitis O91.11-●
  subareolar abscess O91.11-●
Ghon tubercle, primary infection A15.7
Ghost
  teeth K00.4
  vessels (cornea) H16.41-●
Ghoul hand A66.3
Gianotti-Crosti disease L44.4
Giant
  cell
    epulis K06.8
    peripheral granuloma K06.8
  esophagus, congenital Q39.5
  kidney, congenital Q63.3
  urticaria T78.3
    hereditary D84.1
Giardiasis A07.1
Gibert's disease or pityriasis L42
Giddiness R42
  hysterical F44.89
  psychogenic F45.8
Gierke's disease (glycogenosis I) E74.01
Gigantism (cerebral) (hypophyseal) (pituitary)
  E22.0
  constitutional E34.4
Gilbert's disease or syndrome E80.4
Gilchrist's disease B40.9
Gilford-Hutchinson disease E34.8

▶ New   ⇒ Revised   ~~deleted~~ Deleted   ● Use Additional Character(s)

Gilles de la Tourette's disease or syndrome
(motor-verbal tic) F95.2
Gingivitis K05.10
acute (catarrhal) K05.00
necrotizing A69.1
nonplaque induced K05.01
plaque induced K05.00
chronic (desquamative) (hyperplastic)
(simple marginal) (pregnancy
associated) (ulcerative) K05.10
nonplaque induced K05.11
plaque induced K05.10
expulsiva —see Periodontitis
necrotizing ulcerative (acute) A69.1
pellagrous E52
acute necrotizing A69.1
Vincent's A69.1
Gingivoglossitis K14.0
Gingivopericementitis —see Periodontitis
Gingivosis —see Gingivitis, chronic
Gingivostomatitis K05.10
herpesviral B00.2
necrotizing ulcerative (acute) A69.1
Gland, glandular —see condition
Glanders A24.0
Glanzmann (-Naegeli) disease or
thrombasthenia D69.1
Glasgow coma scale
total score
3-8 R40.243
9-12 R40.242
13-15 R40.241
Glass-blower's disease (cataract) —see
Cataract, specified NEC
Glaucoma H40.9
with
increased episcleral venous pressure
H40.81-●
pseudoexfoliation of lens —see Glaucoma,
open angle, primary, capsular
absolute H44.51-●
angle-closure (primary) H40.20-●
acute (attack) (crisis) H40.21-●
chronic H40.22-●
intermittent H40.23-●
residual stage H40.24-●
borderline H40.00-●
capsular (with pseudoexfoliation of lens) —
see Glaucoma, open angle, primary,
capsular
childhood Q15.0
closed angle —see Glaucoma, angle-closure
congenital Q15.0
corticosteroid-induced —see Glaucoma,
secondary, drugs
hypersecretion H40.82-●
in (due to)
amyloidosis E85.4 [H42]
aniridia Q13.1 [H42]
concussion of globe —see Glaucoma,
secondary, trauma
dislocation of lens —see Glaucoma,
secondary
disorder of lens NEC —see Glaucoma,
secondary
drugs —see Glaucoma, secondary, drugs
endocrine disease NOS E34.9 [H42]
eye
inflammation —see Glaucoma,
secondary, inflammation
trauma —see Glaucoma, secondary,
trauma
hypermature cataract —see Glaucoma,
secondary
iridocyclitis —see Glaucoma, secondary,
inflammation
lens disorder —see Glaucoma, secondary,
Lowe's syndrome E72.03 [H42]
metabolic disease NOS E88.9 [H42]
ocular disorders NEC —see Glaucoma,
secondary

Glaucoma (Continued)
in (due to) (Continued)
onchocerciasis B73.02
pupillary block —see Glaucoma, secondary
retinal vein occlusion —see Glaucoma,
secondary
Rieger's anomaly Q13.81 [H42]
rubeosis of iris —see Glaucoma, secondary
tumor of globe —see Glaucoma, secondary
infantile Q15.0
low tension —see Glaucoma, open angle,
primary, low-tension
malignant H40.83-●
narrow angle —see Glaucoma, angle-closure
newborn Q15.0
noncongestive (chronic) —see Glaucoma,
open angle
nonobstructive —see Glaucoma, open angle
obstructive —see also Glaucoma,
angle-closure
due to lens changes —see Glaucoma,
secondary
open angle H40.10-●
primary H40.11-●
capsular (with pseudoexfoliation of lens)
H40.14-●
low-tension H40.12-●
pigmentary H40.13-●
residual stage H40.15-●
phacolytic —see Glaucoma, secondary
pigmentary —see Glaucoma, open angle,
primary, pigmentary
postinfectious —see Glaucoma, secondary,
inflammation
secondary (to) H40.5-●
drugs H40.6-●
inflammation H40.4-●
trauma H40.3-●
simple (chronic) H40.11-●
simplex H40.11-●
specified type NEC H40.89
suspect H40.00-●
syphilitic A52.71
traumatic —see also Glaucoma, secondary,
trauma
newborn (birth injury) P15.3
tuberculous A18.59
Glaucomatous flecks (subcapsular) —see
Cataract, complicated
Glazed tongue K14.4
Gleet (gonococcal) A54.01
Glénard's disease K63.4
Glioblastoma (multiforme)
with sarcomatous component
specified site —see Neoplasm, malignant,
by site
unspecified site C71.9
giant cell
specified site —see Neoplasm, malignant,
by site
unspecified site C71.9
specified site —see Neoplasm, malignant, by
site
unspecified site C71.9
Glioma (malignant)
astrocytic
specified site —see Neoplasm, malignant,
by site
unspecified site C71.9
mixed
specified site —see Neoplasm, malignant,
by site
unspecified site C71.9
nose Q30.8
specified site NEC —see Neoplasm,
malignant, by site
subependymal D43.2
specified site —see Neoplasm, uncertain
behavior, by site
unspecified site D43.2
unspecified site C71.9
Gliomatosis cerebri C71.0

Glioneuroma —see Neoplasm, uncertain
behavior, by site
Gliosarcoma
specified site —see Neoplasm, malignant, by
site
unspecified site C71.9
Gliosis (cerebral) G93.89
spinal G95.89
Glisson's disease —see Rickets
Globinuria R82.3
Globus (hystericus) F45.8
Glomangioma D18.00
intra-abdominal D18.03
intracranial D18.02
skin D18.01
specified site NEC D18.09
Glomangiomyoma D18.00
intra-abdominal D18.03
intracranial D18.02
skin D18.01
specified site NEC D18.09
Glomangiosarcoma —see Neoplasm, connective
tissue, malignant
Glomerular
disease in syphilis A52.75
nephritis —see Glomerulonephritis
Glomerulitis —see Glomerulonephritis
Glomerulonephritis —see also Nephritis N05.9
with
C3
glomerulonephritis N05.A
glomerulopathy N05.A
with dense deposit disease N05.6
edema —see Nephrosis
minimal change N05.0
minor glomerular abnormality N05.0
acute N00.9
chronic N03.9
crescentic (diffuse) NEC —see also N00-N07
with fourth character .7 N05.7
dense deposit —see also N00-N07 with fourth
character .6 N05.6
diffuse
crescentic —see also N00-N07 with fourth
character .7 N05.7
endocapillary proliferative —see also
N00N07 with fourth character .4 N05.4
membranous —see also N00-N07 with
fourth character .2 N05.2
mesangial proliferative —see also N00-N07
with fourth character .3 N05.3
mesangiocapillary —see also N00-N07 with
fourth character .5 N05.5
sclerosing N18.9
endocapillary proliferative (diffuse) NEC —
see also N00-N07 with fourth character
.4 N05.4
extracapillary NEC —see also N00-N07 with
fourth character .7 N05.7
focal (and segmental) —see also N00-N07 with
fourth character .1 N05.1
hypocomplementemic —
see Glomerulonephritis,
membranoproliferative
IgA —see Nephropathy, IgA
immune complex (circulating) NEC N05.8
in (due to)
amyloidosis E85.4 [N08]
bilharziasis B65.9 [N08]
cryoglobulinemia D89.1 [N08]
defibrination syndrome D65 [N08]
diabetes mellitus —see Diabetes,
glomerulosclerosis
disseminated intravascular coagulation
D65 [N08]
Fabry (-Anderson) disease E75.21 [N08]
Goodpasture's syndrome M31.0
hemolytic-uremic syndrome —see
Syndrome, hemolytic-uremic
Henoch (-Schönlein) purpura D69.0 [N08]
lecithin cholesterol acyltransferase
deficiency E78.6 [N08]

Glomerulonephritis (Continued)
in (Continued)
microscopic polyangiitis M31.7 [N08]
multiple myeloma C90.0-● [N08]
Plasmodium malariae B52.0
schistosomiasis B65.9 [N08]
sepsis A41.9-● [N08]
streptococcal A40-● [N08]
sickle-cell disorders D57.-● [N08]
strongyloidiasis B78.9 [N08]
subacute bacterial endocarditis I33.0
[N08]
syphilis (late) congenital A50.59 [N08]
systemic lupus erythematosus M32.14
thrombotic thrombocytopenic purpura
M31.19 [N08]
typhoid fever A01.09
Waldenström macroglobulinemia C88.0
[N08]
Wegener's granulomatosis M31.31
latent or quiescent N03.9
lobular, lobulonodular —
see Glomerulonephritis,
membranoproliferative
membranoproliferative (diffuse) (type 1
or 3) —see also N00-N07 with fourth
character .5 N05.5
dense deposit (type 2) NEC —see also
N00-N07 with fourth character .6
N05.6
membranous (diffuse) NEC —see also
N00-N07 with fourth character .2 N05.2
mesangial
IgA/IgG —see Nephropathy, IgA
proliferative (diffuse) NEC —see also
N00-N07 with fourth character .3
N05.3
mesangiocapillary (diffuse) NEC —see also
N00-N07 with fourth character .5 N05.5
necrotic, necrotizing NEC —see also N00-N07
with fourth character .8 N05.8
nodular —see Glomerulonephritis,
membranoproliferative
poststreptococcal NEC N05.9
acute N00.9
chronic N03.9
rapidly progressive N01.9
proliferative NEC —see also N00-N07 with
fourth character .8 N05.8
diffuse (lupus) M32.14
rapidly progressive N01.9
sclerosing, diffuse N18.9
specified pathology NEC —see also N00-N07
with fourth character .8 N05.8
subacute N01.9
Glomerulopathy —see Glomerulonephritis
Glomerulosclerosis —see also Sclerosis, renal
intercapillary (nodular) (with diabetes) —see
Diabetes, glomerulosclerosis
intracapillary —see Diabetes, glomerulosclerosis
Glossagra K14.6
Glossalgia K14.6
Glossitis (chronic superficial) (gangrenous)
(Moeller's) K14.0
areata exfoliativa K14.1
atrophic K14.4
benign migratory K14.1
cortical superficial, sclerotic K14.0
Hunter's D51.0
interstitial, sclerous K14.0
median rhomboid K14.2
pellagrous E52
superficial, chronic K14.0
Glossocele K14.8
Glossodynia K14.6
exfoliativa K14.4
Glossoncus K14.8
Glossopathy K14.9
Glossophytia K14.3
Glossoplegia K14.8
Glossoptosis K14.8

Glossopyrosis K14.6
Glossotrichia K14.3
Glossy skin L90.8
Glottis —see condition
Glottitis —see also Laryngitis J04.0
Glucagonoma
pancreas
benign D13.7
malignant C25.4
uncertain behavior D37.8
specified site NEC
benign —see Neoplasm, benign, by site
malignant —see Neoplasm, malignant, by
site
uncertain behavior —see Neoplasm,
uncertain behavior, by site
unspecified site
benign D13.7
malignant C25.4
uncertain behavior D37.8
Glucoglycinuria E72.51
Glucose-galactose malabsorption E74.39
Glue
ear —see Otitis, media, nonsuppurative,
chronic, mucoid
sniffing (airplane) —see Abuse, drug, inhalant
dependence —see Dependence, drug,
inhalant
GLUT1 deficiency syndrome 1, infantile onset
E74.810
GLUT1 deficiency syndrome or 2, childhood
onset E74.810
Glutaric aciduria E72.3
Glycinemia E72.51
Glycinuria (renal) (with ketosis) E72.09
Glycogen
infiltration —see Disease, glycogen storage
storage disease —see Disease, glycogen storage
Glycogenosis (diffuse) (generalized) —see also
Disease, glycogen storage
cardiac E74.02 [I43]
diabetic, secondary —see Diabetes,
glycogenosis, secondary
pulmonary interstitial J84.842
Glycopenia E16.2
Glycosuria R81
renal (familial) E74.818
Gnathostoma spinigerum (infection)
(infestation), gnathostomiasis (wandering
swelling) B83.1
Goiter (plunging) (substernal) E04.9
with
hyperthyroidism (recurrent) —see
Hyperthyroidism, with, goiter
thyrotoxicosis —see Hyperthyroidism,
with, goiter
adenomatous —see Goiter, nodular
cancerous C73
congenital (nontoxic) E03.0
diffuse E03.0
parenchymatous E03.0
transitory, with normal functioning P72.0
cystic E04.2
due to iodine-deficiency E01.1
due to
enzyme defect in synthesis of thyroid
hormone E07.1
iodine-deficiency (endemic) E01.2
dyshormonogenetic (familial) E07.1
endemic (iodine-deficiency) E01.2
diffuse E01.0
multinodular E01.1
exophthalmic —see Hyperthyroidism, with,
goiter
iodine-deficiency (endemic) E01.2
diffuse E01.0
multinodular E01.1
nodular E01.1
lingual Q89.2
lymphadenoid E06.3
malignant C73

Goiter (Continued)
multinodular (cystic) (nontoxic) E04.2
toxic or with hyperthyroidism E05.20
with thyroid storm E05.21
neonatal NEC P72.0
nodular (nontoxic) (due to) E04.9
with
hyperthyroidism E05.20
with thyroid storm E05.21
thyrotoxicosis E05.20
with thyroid storm E05.21
endemic E01.1
iodine-deficiency E01.1
sporadic E04.9
toxic E05.20
with thyroid storm E05.21
nontoxic E04.9
diffuse (colloid) E04.0
multinodular E04.2
simple E04.0
specified NEC E04.8
uninodular E04.1
simple E04.0
toxic —see Hyperthyroidism, with, goiter
uninodular (nontoxic) E04.1
toxic or with hyperthyroidism E05.10
with thyroid storm E05.11
Goiter-deafness syndrome E07.1
Goldberg syndrome Q89.8
Goldberg-Maxwell syndrome E34.51
Goldblatt's hypertension or kidney I70.1
Goldenhar (-Gorlin) syndrome Q87.0
Goldflam-Erb disease or syndrome G70.00
with exacerbation (acute) G70.01
in crisis G70.01
Goldscheider's disease Q81.8
Goldstein's disease (familial hemorrhagic
telangiectasia) I78.0
Golfer's elbow —see Epicondylitis, medial
Gonadoblastoma
specified site —see Neoplasm, uncertain
behavior, by site
unspecified site
female D39.10
male D40.10
Gonecystitis —see Vesiculitis
Gongylonemiasis B83.8
Goniosynechiae —see Adhesions, iris,
goniosynechiae
Gonococcemia A54.86
Gonococcus, gonococcal (disease) (infection)
—see also condition A54.9
anus A54.6
bursa, bursitis A54.49
conjunctiva, conjunctivitis (neonatorum)
A54.31
endocardium A54.83
eye A54.30
conjunctivitis A54.31
iridocyclitis A54.32
keratitis A54.33
newborn A54.31
other specified A54.39
fallopian tubes (acute) (chronic) A54.24
genitourinary (organ) (system) (tract) (acute)
lower A54.00
with abscess (accessory gland)
(periurethral) A54.1
upper —see also condition A54.29
heart A54.83
iridocyclitis A54.32
joint A54.42
lymphatic (gland) (node) A54.89
meninges, meningitis A54.81
musculoskeletal A54.40
arthritis A54.42
osteomyelitis A54.43
other specified A54.49
spondylopathy A54.41
pelviperitonitis A54.24
pelvis (acute) (chronic) A54.24

▶ New   ⇒ Revised   ~~deleted~~ Deleted   ● Use Additional Character(s)

Gonococcus, gonococcal (Continued)
  pharynx A54.5
  proctitis A54.6
  pyosalpinx (acute) (chronic) A54.24
  rectum A54.6
  skin A54.89
  specified site NEC A54.89
  tendon sheath A54.49
  throat A54.5
  urethra (acute) (chronic) A54.01
    with abscess (accessory gland)
      (periurethral) A54.1
  vulva (acute) (chronic) A54.02
Gonocytoma
  specified site —see Neoplasm, uncertain
    behavior, by site
  unspecified site
    female D39.10
    male D40.10
Gonorrhea (acute) (chronic) A54.9
  Bartholin's gland (acute) (chronic) (purulent)
    A54.02
    with abscess (accessory gland)
      (periurethral) A54.1
  bladder A54.01
  cervix A54.03
  conjunctiva, conjunctivitis (neonatorum)
    A54.31
  contact Z20.2
  Cowper's gland (with abscess) A54.1
  exposure to Z20.2
  fallopian tube (acute) (chronic) A54.24
  kidney (acute) (chronic) A54.21
  lower genitourinary tract A54.00
    with abscess (accessory gland)
      (periurethral) A54.1
  ovary (acute) (chronic) A54.24
  pelvis (acute) (chronic) A54.24
    female pelvic inflammatory disease A54.24
  penis A54.09
  prostate (acute) (chronic) A54.22
  seminal vesicle (acute) (chronic) A54.23
  specified site not listed —see also Gonococcus
    A54.89
  spermatic cord (acute) (chronic) A54.23
  urethra A54.01
    with abscess (accessory gland)
      (periurethral) A54.1
  vagina A54.02
  vas deferens (acute) (chronic) A54.23
  vulva A54.02
Goodall's disease A08.19
Goodpasture's syndrome M31.0
Gopalan's syndrome (burning feet) E53.0
Gorlin-Chaudry-Moss syndrome Q87.0
Gottron's papules L94.4
Gougerot's syndrome (trisymptomatic) L81.7
Gougerot-Blum syndrome (pigmented
  purpuric lichenoid dermatitis) L81.7
Gougerot-Carteaud disease or syndrome
  (confluent reticulate papillomatosis) L83
Gouley's syndrome (constrictive pericarditis)
  I31.1
Goundou A66.6
Gout, chronic (see also Gout, gouty) M1A.9-●
  drug-induced M1A.20
    ankle M1A.27-●
    elbow M1A.22-●
    foot joint M1A.27-●
    hand joint M1A.24-●
    hip M1A.25-●
    knee M1A.26-●
    multiple site M1A.29-●
    shoulder M1A.21-●
    vertebrae M1A.28
    wrist M1A.23-●
  idiopathic M1A.00
    ankle M1A.07-●
    elbow M1A.02-●
    foot joint M1A.07-●
    hand joint M1A.04-●

Gout, chronic (Continued)
  idiopathic (Continued)
    hip M1A.05-●
    knee M1A.06-●
    multiple site M1A.09
    shoulder M1A.01-●
    vertebrae M1A.08
    wrist M1A.03-●
  in (due to) renal impairment M1A.30
    ankle M1A.37-●
    elbow M1A.32-●
    foot joint M1A.37-●
    hand joint M1A.34-●
    hip M1A.35-●
    knee M1A.36-●
    multiple site M1A.39
    shoulder M1A.31-●
    vertebrae M1A.38
    wrist M1A.33-●
  lead-induced M1A.10
    ankle M1A.17-●
    elbow M1A.12-●
    foot joint M1A.17-●
    hand joint M1A.14-●
    hip M1A.15-●
    knee M1A.16-●
    multiple site M1A.19
    shoulder M1A.11-●
    vertebrae M1A.18
    wrist M1A.13-●
  primary —see Gout, chronic, idiopathic
  saturnine —see Gout, chronic, lead-induced
  secondary NEC M1A.40
    ankle M1A.47-●
    elbow M1A.42-●
    foot joint M1A.47-●
    hand joint M1A.44-●
    hip M1A.45-●
    knee M1A.46-●
    multiple site M1A.49
    shoulder M1A.41-●
    vertebrae M1A.48
    wrist M1A.43-●
  syphilitic —see also subcategory M14.8-●
    A52.77
  tophi M1A.9
Gout, gouty (acute) (attack) (flare) —see also
  Gout, chronic M10.9-●
  drug-induced M10.20
    ankle M10.27-●
    elbow M10.22-●
    foot joint M10.27-●
    hand joint M10.24-●
    hip M10.25-●
    knee M10.26-●
    multiple site M10.29
    shoulder M10.21-●
    vertebrae M10.28
    wrist M10.23-●
  idiopathic M10.00
    ankle M10.07-●
    elbow M10.02-●
    foot joint M10.07-●
    hand joint M10.04-●
    hip M10.05-●
    knee M10.06-●
    multiple site M10.09
    shoulder M10.01-●
    vertebrae M10.08
    wrist M10.03-●
  in (due to) renal impairment M10.30
    ankle M10.37-●
    elbow M10.32-●
    foot joint M10.37-●
    hand joint M10.34-●
    hip M10.35-●
    knee M10.36-●
    multiple site M10.39
    shoulder M10.31-●
    vertebrae M10.38
    wrist M10.33-●

Gout, gouty (Continued)
  lead-induced M10.10
    ankle M10.17-●
    elbow M10.12-●
    foot joint M10.17-●
    hand joint M10.14-●
    hip M10.15-●
    knee M10.16-●
    multiple site M10.19
    shoulder M10.11-●
    vertebrae M10.18
    wrist M10.13-●
  primary —see Gout, idiopathic
  saturnine —see Gout, lead-induced
  secondary NEC M10.40
    ankle M10.47-●
    elbow M10.42-●
    foot joint M10.47-●
    hand joint M10.44-●
    hip M10.45-●
    knee M10.46-●
    multiple site M10.49
    shoulder M10.41-●
    vertebrae M10.48
    wrist M10.43-●
  syphilitic —see also subcategory M14.8-●
    A52.77
  tophi NEC —see Gout, chronic
Gower's
  muscular dystrophy G71.01
  syndrome (vasovagal attack) R55
Gradenigo's syndrome —see Otitis, media,
  suppurative, acute
Graefe's disease —see Strabismus, paralytic,
  ophthalmoplegia, progressive
Graft-versus-host disease D89.813
  acute D89.810
  acute on chronic D89.812
  chronic D89.811
Grain mite (itch) B88.0
Grainhandler's disease or lung J67.8
Grand mal —see Epilepsy, generalized,
  specified NEC
Grand multipara status only (not pregnant)
  Z64.1
  pregnant —see Pregnancy, complicated by,
    grand multiparity
Granite worker's lung J62.8
Granular —see also condition
  inflammation, pharynx J31.2
  kidney (contracting) —see Sclerosis, renal
  liver K74.69
Granulation tissue (abnormal) (excessive) L92.9
  postmastoidectomy cavity —see
    Complications, postmastoidectomy,
    granulation
Granulocytopenia (primary) (malignant) —see
  Agranulocytosis
Granuloma L92.9
  abdomen K66.8
    from residual foreign body L92.3
    pyogenicum L98.0
  actinic L57.5
  annulare (perforating) L92.0
  apical K04.5
  aural —see Otitis, externa, specified NEC
  beryllium (skin) L92.3
  bone
    eosinophilic C96.6
    from residual foreign body —see
      Osteomyelitis, specified type NEC
    lung C96.6
  brain (any site) G06.0
    schistosomiasis B65.9 [G07]
  canaliculus lacrimalis —see Granuloma,
    lacrimal
  candidal (cutaneous) B37.2
  cerebral (any site) G06.0
  coccidioidal (primary) (progressive) B38.7
    lung B38.1
    meninges B38.4

Granuloma (Continued)
  colon K63.89
  conjunctiva H11.22-•
  dental K04.5
  ear, middle —see Cholesteatoma
  eosinophilic C96.6
    bone C96.6
    lung C96.6
    oral mucosa K13.4
    skin L92.2
  eyelid H01.8
  facial (e) L92.2
  foreign body (in soft tissue) NEC M60.20
    ankle M60.27-•
    foot M60.27-•
    forearm M60.23-•
    hand M60.24-•
    in operation wound —see Foreign body,
        accidentally left during a procedure
    lower leg M60.26-•
    pelvic region M60.25-•
    shoulder region M60.21-•
    skin L92.3
    specified site NEC M60.28
    subcutaneous tissue L92.3
    thigh M60.25-•
    upper arm M60.22-•
  gangraenescens M31.2
  genito-inguinale A58
  giant cell (central) (reparative) (jaw) M27.1
    gingiva (peripheral) K06.8
  gland (lymph) I88.8
  hepatic NEC K75.3
    in (due to)
      berylliosis J63.2 [K77]
      sarcoidosis D86.89
  Hodgkin C81.9
  ileum K63.89
  infectious B99.9
    specified NEC B99.8
  inguinale (Donovan) (venereal) A58
  intestine NEC K63.89
  intracranial (any site) G06.0
  intraspinal (any part) G06.1
  iridocyclitis —see Iridocyclitis, chronic
  jaw (bone) (central) M27.1
    reparative giant cell M27.1
  kidney —see also Infection, kidney N15.8
  lacrimal H04.81-•
  larynx J38.7
  lethal midline (faciale (e)) M31.2
  liver NEC —see Granuloma, hepatic
  lung (infectious) —see also Fibrosis, lung
    coccidioidal B38.1
    eosinophilic C96.6
  Majocchi's B35.8
  malignant (facial (e)) M31.2
  mandible (central) M27.1
  midline (lethal) M31.2
  monilial (cutaneous) B37.2
  nasal sinus —see Sinusitis
  operation wound T81.89
    foreign body —see Foreign body,
        accidentally left during a procedure
    stitch T81.89
    talc —see Foreign body, accidentally left
        during a procedure
  oral mucosa K13.4
  orbit, orbital H05.11-•
  paracoccidioidal B41.8
  penis, venereal A58
  periapical K04.5
  peritoneum K66.8
    due to ova of helminths NOS —see also
        Helminthiasis B83.9 [K67]
  postmastoidectomy cavity —see
        Complications, postmastoidectomy,
        recurrent cholesteatoma
  prostate N42.89
  pudendi (ulcerating) A58
  pulp, internal (tooth) K03.3

Granuloma (Continued)
  pyogenic, pyogenicum (of) (skin) L98.0
    gingiva K06.8
    maxillary alveolar ridge K04.5
    oral mucosa K13.4
  rectum K62.89
  reticulohistiocytic D76.3
  rubrum nasi L74.8
  Schistosoma —see Schistosomiasis
  septic (skin) L98.0
  silica (skin) L92.3
  sinus (accessory) (infective) (nasal) —see
        Sinusitis
  skin L92.9
    from residual foreign body L92.3
    pyogenicum L98.0
  spine
    syphilitic (epidural) A52.19
    tuberculous A18.01
  stitch (postoperative) T81.89
  suppurative (skin) L98.0
  swimming pool A31.1
  talc —see also Granuloma, foreign body
    in operation wound —see Foreign body,
        accidentally left during a procedure
  telangiectaticum (skin) L98.0
  tracheostomy J95.09
  trichophyticum B35.8
  tropicum A66.4
  umbilical P83.81
  umbilicus P83.81
  urethra N36.8
  uveitis —see Iridocyclitis, chronic
  vagina A58
  venereum A58
  vocal cord J38.3
Granulomatosis L92.9
  with polyangiitis M31.3-•
  eosinophilic, with polyangiitis [EGPA] M30.1
  lymphoid C83.8-•
  miliary (listerial) A32.89
  necrotizing, respiratory M31.30
  progressive septic D71
  specified NEC L92.8
  Wegener's M31.30
    with renal involvement M31.31
Granulomatous tissue (abnormal) (excessive)
    L92.9
Granulosis rubra nasi L74.8
Graphite fibrosis (of lung) J63.3
Graphospasm F48.8
  organic G25.89
Grating scapula M89.8X1
Gravel (urinary) —see Calculus, urinary
Graves' disease —see Hyperthyroidism, with,
    goiter
Gravis —see condition
Grawitz tumor C64.-•
Gray syndrome (newborn) P93.0
Grayness, hair (premature) L67.1
  congenital Q84.2
Green sickness D50.8
Greenfield's disease
  meaning
    concentric sclerosis (encephalitis periaxialis
        concentrica) G37.5
    metachromatic leukodystrophy E75.25
Greenstick fracture - code as Fracture, by site
Grey syndrome (newborn) P93.0
Grief F43.21
  complicated F43.81
  prolonged F43.29
  reaction —see also Disorder, adjustment F43.20
Griesinger's disease B76.0
Grinder's lung or pneumoconiosis J62.8
Grinding, teeth
  psychogenic F45.8
  sleep related G47.63
Grip
  Dabney's B33.0
  devil's B33.0
Grippe, grippal —see also Influenza
  Balkan A78
  summer, of Italy A93.1

Grisel's disease M43.6
Groin —see condition
Grooved tongue K14.5
Ground itch B76.9
Grover's disease or syndrome L11.1
Growing pains, children R29.898
Growth (fungoid) (neoplastic) (new) —see also
    Neoplasm
  adenoid (vegetative) J35.8
  benign —see Neoplasm, benign, by site
  malignant —see Neoplasm, malignant, by site
  rapid, childhood Z00.2
  secondary —see Neoplasm, secondary, by site
Gruby's disease B35.0
Gubler-Millard paralysis or syndrome G46.3
Guerin-Stern syndrome Q74.3
Guidance, insufficient anterior (occlusal) M26.54
Guillain-Barré disease or syndrome G61.0
  sequelae G65.0
Guinea worms (infection) (infestation) B72
Guinon's disease (motor-verbal tic) F95.2
Gull's disease E03.4
Gum —see condition
Gumboil K04.7
  with sinus K04.6
Gumma (syphilitic) A52.79
  artery A52.09
    cerebral A52.04
  bone A52.77
    of yaws (late) A66.6
  brain A52.19
  cauda equina A52.19
  central nervous system A52.3
  ciliary body A52.71
  congenital A50.59
  eyelid A52.71
  heart A52.06
  intracranial A52.19
  iris A52.71
  kidney A52.75
  larynx A52.73
  leptomeninges A52.19
  liver A52.74
  meninges A52.19
  myocardium A52.06
  nasopharynx A52.73
  neurosyphilitic A52.3
  nose A52.73
  orbit A52.71
  palate (soft) A52.79
  penis A52.76
  pericardium A52.06
  pharynx A52.73
  pituitary A52.79
  scrofulous (tuberculous) A18.4
  skin A52.79
  specified site NEC A52.79
  spinal cord A52.19
  tongue A52.79
  tonsil A52.73
  trachea A52.73
  tuberculous A18.4
  ulcerative due to yaws A66.4
  ureter A52.75
  yaws A66.4
    bone A66.6
Gunn's syndrome Q07.8
Gunshot wound —see also Puncture, open
  fracture - code as Fracture, by site
  internal organs —see Injury, by site
Gynandrism Q56.0
Gynandroblastoma
  specified site —see Neoplasm, uncertain
      behavior, by site
  unspecified site
    female D39.10
    male D40.10
Gynecological examination (periodic) (routine)
    Z01.419
  with abnormal findings Z01.411
Gynecomastia N62
Gynephobia F40.291
Gyrate scalp Q82.8

▶ New ⇒ Revised deleted Deleted • Use Additional Character(s)

H

H (Hartnup's) disease E72.02
Haas' disease or osteochondrosis (juvenile) (head of humerus) —*see* Osteochondrosis, juvenile, humerus
Habit, habituation
  bad sleep Z72.821
  chorea F95.8
  disturbance, child F98.9
  drug —*see* Dependence, drug
  irregular sleep Z72.821
  laxative F55.2
  spasm —*see* Tic
  tic —*see* Tic
Haemophilus (H.) influenzae, as cause of disease classified elsewhere B96.3
Haff disease —*see* Poisoning, mercury
Hageman's factor defect, deficiency or disease D68.2
Haglund's disease or osteochondrosis (juvenile) (os tibiale externum) —*see* Osteochondrosis, juvenile, tarsus
Hailey-Hailey disease Q82.8
Hair —*see also* condition
  plucking F63.3
    in stereotyped movement disorder F98.4
  tourniquet syndrome —*see also* Constriction, external, by site
    finger S60.44-●
    penis S30.842
    thumb S60.34-●
    toe S90.44-●
Hairball in stomach T18.2
Hair-pulling, pathological (compulsive) F63.3
Hairy black tongue K14.3
Half vertebra Q76.49
Halitosis R19.6
Hallerman-Streiff syndrome Q87.0
Hallervorden-Spatz disease G23.0
Hallopeau's acrodermatitis or disease L40.2
Hallucination R44.3
  auditory R44.0
  gustatory R44.2
  olfactory R44.2
  specified NEC R44.2
  tactile R44.2
  visual R44.1
Hallucinosis (chronic) F28
  alcoholic (acute) F10.951
    in
      abuse F10.151
      dependence F10.251
  drug-induced F19.951
    cannabis F12.951
    cocaine F14.951
    hallucinogen F16.151
    in
      abuse F19.151
        cannabis F12.151
        cocaine F14.151
        hallucinogen F16.151
        inhalant F18.151
        opioid F11.151
        sedative, anxiolytic or hypnotic F13.151
        stimulant NEC F15.151
      dependence F19.251
        cannabis F12.251
        cocaine F14.251
        hallucinogen F16.251
        inhalant F18.251
        opioid F11.251
        sedative, anxiolytic or hypnotic F13.251
        stimulant NEC F15.251
    inhalant F18.951
    opioid F11.951
    sedative, anxiolytic or hypnotic F13.951
    stimulant NEC F15.951
  organic F06.0

Hallux
  deformity (acquired) NEC M20.5X-●
  limitus M20.5X-●
  malleus (acquired) NEC M20.3-●
  rigidus (acquired) M20.2-●
    congenital Q74.2
    sequelae (late effect) of rickets E64.3
  valgus (acquired) M20.1-●
    congenital Q66.6
  varus (acquired) M20.3-●
    congenital Q66.3-●
Halo, visual H53.19
Hamartoma, hamartoblastoma Q85.9
  epithelial (gingival), odontogenic, central or peripheral —*see* Cyst, calcifying odontogenic
Hamartosis Q85.9
Hamman-Rich syndrome J84.114
Hammer toe (acquired) NEC —*see also* Deformity, toe, hammer toe
  congenital Q66.89
  sequelae (late effect) of rickets E64.3
Hand —*see* condition
Hand-foot syndrome L27.1
Handicap, handicapped
  educational Z55.9
    specified NEC Z55.8
Hand-Schüller-Christian disease or syndrome C96.5
Hanging (asphyxia) (strangulation) (suffocation) —*see* Asphyxia, traumatic, due to mechanical threat
Hangnail —*see also* Cellulitis, digit
  with lymphangitis —*see* Lymphangitis, acute, digit
Hangover (alcohol) F10.129
Hanhart's syndrome Q87.0
Hanot-Chauffard (-Troisier) syndrome E83.19
Hanot's cirrhosis or disease K74.3
Hansen's disease —*see* Leprosy
Hantaan virus disease (Korean hemorrhagic fever) A98.5
Hantavirus disease (with renal manifestations) (Dobrava) (Puumala) (Seoul) A98.5
  with pulmonary manifestations (Andes) (Bayou) (Bermejo) (Black Creek Canal) (Choclo) (Juquitiba) (Laguna negra) (Lechiguanas) (New York) (Oran) (Sin nombre) B33.4
Happy puppet syndrome Q93.59
Harada's disease or syndrome H30.81-●
Hardening
  artery —*see* Arteriosclerosis
  brain G93.89
Harelip (complete) (incomplete) —*see* Cleft, lip
Harlequin (newborn) Q80.4
Harley's disease D59.6
Harmful use (of)
  alcohol F10.10
  anxiolytics —*see* Abuse, drug, sedative
  cannabinoids —*see* Abuse, drug, cannabis
  cocaine —*see* Abuse, drug, cocaine
  drug —*see* Abuse, drug
  hallucinogens —*see* Abuse, drug, hallucinogen
  hypnotics —*see* Abuse, drug, sedative -
    opioids —*see* Abuse, drug, opioid
  PCP (phencyclidine) —*see* Abuse, drug, hallucinogen
  sedatives —*see* Abuse, drug, sedative
  stimulants NEC —*see* Abuse, drug, stimulant
Harris' lines —*see* Arrest, epiphyseal
▶ Hardship, material Z59.87
Hartnup's disease E72.02
Harvester's lung J67.0
Harvesting ovum for in vitro fertilization Z31.83
Hashimoto's disease or thyroiditis E06.3
Hashitoxicosis (transient) E06.3
Hassal-Henle bodies or warts (cornea) H18.49
Haut mal —*see* Epilepsy, generalized, specified NEC
Haverhill fever A25.1

Hay fever —*see also* Fever, hay J30.1
Hayem-Widal syndrome D59.8
Haygarth's nodes M15.8
Haymaker's lung J67.0
Hb (abnormal)
  Bart's disease D56.0
  disease —*see* Disease, hemoglobin
  trait —*see* Trait
Head —*see* condition
Headache R51.9
  with
    orthostatic component NEC R51.0
    positional component NEC R51.0
  allergic NEC G44.89
  associated with sexual activity G44.82
  cervicogenic G44.86
  chronic daily R51.9
  cluster G44.009
    chronic G44.029
      intractable G44.021
      not intractable G44.029
    episodic G44.019
      intractable G44.011
      not intractable G44.019
    intractable G44.001
    not intractable G44.009
  cough (primary) G44.83
  daily chronic R51.9
  drug-induced NEC G44.40
    intractable G44.41
    not intractable G44.40
  exertional (primary) G44.84
  histamine G44.009
    intractable G44.001
    not intractable G44.009
  hypnic G44.81
  lumbar puncture G97.1
  medication overuse G44.40
    intractable G44.41
    not intractable G44.40
  menstrual —*see* Migraine, menstrual
  migraine (type) —*see also* Migraine G43.909
  nasal septum R51.9
  neuralgiform, short lasting unilateral, with conjunctival injection and tearing (SUNCT) G44.059
    intractable G44.051
    not intractable G44.059
  new daily persistent (NDPH) G44.52
  orgasmic G44.82
  periodic syndromes in adults and children G43.C0
    with refractory migraine G43.C1
    intractable G43.C1
    not intractable G43.C0
    without refractory migraine G43.C0
  postspinal puncture G97.1
  post-traumatic G44.309
    acute G44.319
      intractable G44.311
      not intractable G44.319
    chronic G44.329
      intractable G44.321
      not intractable G44.329
    intractable G44.301
    not intractable G44.309
  pre-menstrual —*see* Migraine, menstrual
  preorgasmic G44.82
  primary
    cough G44.83
    exertional G44.84
    stabbing G44.85
    thunderclap G44.53
  rebound G44.40
    intractable G44.41
    not intractable G44.40
  short lasting unilateral neuralgiform, with conjunctival injection and tearing (SUNCT) G44.059
    intractable G44.051
    not intractable G44.059
  specified syndrome NEC G44.89

▶ New   ⇒ Revised   ~~deleted~~ Deleted   ● Use Additional Character(s)

Headache (Continued)
spinal and epidural anesthesia - induced T88.59
in labor and delivery O74.5
in pregnancy O29.4-●
postpartum, puerperal O89.4
spinal fluid loss (from puncture) G97.1
stabbing (primary) G44.85
tension (-type) G44.209
chronic G44.229
intractable G44.221
not intractable G44.229
episodic G44.219
intractable G44.211
not intractable G44.219
intractable G44.201
not intractable G44.209
thunderclap (primary) G44.53
vascular NEC G44.1
Healthy
infant
accompanying sick mother Z76.3
receiving care Z76.2
person accompanying sick person Z76.3
Hearing examination Z01.10
with abnormal findings NEC Z01.118
infant or child (over 28 days old) Z00.129
with abnormal findings Z00.121
following failed hearing screening Z01.110
for hearing conservation and treatment Z01.12
Heart —see condition
Heart beat
abnormality R00.9
specified NEC R00.8
awareness R00.2
rapid R00.0
slow R00.1
Heartburn R12
psychogenic F45.8
Heartland virus disease A93.8
Heat (effects) T67.9
apoplexy T67.01
burn —see also Burn L55.9
collapse T67.1
cramps T67.2
dermatitis or eczema L59.0
edema T67.7
erythema - code by site under Burn, first degree
excessive T67.9
specified effect NEC T67.8
exhaustion T67.5
anhydrotic T67.3
due to
salt (and water) depletion T67.4
water depletion T67.3
with salt depletion T67.4
fatigue (transient) T67.6
fever T67.01
hyperpyrexia T67.01
prickly L74.0
prostration —see Heat, exhaustion
pyrexia T67.01
rash L74.0
specified effect NEC T67.8
stroke T67.01
exertional T67.02
specified NEC T67.09
sunburn —see Sunburn
syncope T67.1
Heavy-for-dates NEC (infant) (4000g to 4499g) P08.1
exceptionally (4500g or more) P08.0
Hebephrenia, hebephrenic (schizophrenia) F20.1
Heberden's disease or nodes (with arthropathy) M15.1
Hebra's
pityriasis L26
prurigo L28.2
Heel —see condition
Heerfordt's disease D86.89
Hegglin's anomaly or syndrome D72.0
Heilmeyer-Schoner disease D45

Heine-Medin disease A80.9
Heinz body anemia, congenital D58.2
Heliophobia F40.228
Heller's disease or syndrome F84.3
HELLP syndrome (hemolysis, elevated liver enzymes and low platelet count) O14.2-●
complicating
childbirth O14.24
puerperium O14.25
Helminthiasis —see also Infestation, helminth
Ancylostoma B76.0
intestinal B82.0
mixed types (types classifiable to more than one of the titles B65.0-B81.3 and B81.8) B81.4
specified type NEC B81.8
mixed types (intestinal) (types classifiable to more than one of the titles B65.0-B81.3 and B81.8) B81.4
Necator (americanus) B76.1
specified type NEC B83.8
Heloma L84
Hemangioblastoma —see Neoplasm, connective tissue, uncertain behavior
malignant —see Neoplasm, connective tissue, malignant
Hemangioendothelioma —see also Neoplasm, uncertain behavior, by site
benign D18.00
intra-abdominal D18.03
intracranial D18.02
skin D18.01
specified site NEC D18.09
bone (diffuse) —see Neoplasm, bone, malignant
epithelioid —see also Neoplasm, uncertain behavior, by site
malignant —see Neoplasm, malignant, by site
malignant —see Neoplasm, connective tissue, malignant
Hemangiofibroma —see Neoplasm, benign, by site
Hemangiolipoma —see Lipoma
Hemangioma D18.00
arteriovenous D18.00
intra-abdominal D18.03
intracranial D18.02
skin D18.01
specified site NEC D18.09
capillary I78.1
intra-abdominal D18.03
intracranial D18.02
skin D18.01
specified site NEC D18.09
cavernous D18.00
intra-abdominal D18.03
intracranial D18.02
skin D18.01
specified site NEC D18.09
epithelioid D18.00
intra-abdominal D18.03
intracranial D18.02
skin D18.01
specified site NEC D18.09
histiocytoid D18.00
intra-abdominal D18.03
intracranial D18.02
skin D18.01
specified site NEC D18.09
infantile D18.00
intra-abdominal D18.03
intracranial D18.02
skin D18.01
specified site NEC D18.09
intra-abdominal D18.03
intracranial D18.02
intramuscular D18.00
intra-abdominal D18.03
intracranial D18.02
skin D18.01
specified site NEC D18.09

Hemangioma (Continued)
intrathoracic structures D18.09
juvenile D18.00
malignant —see Neoplasm, connective tissue, malignant
plexiform D18.00
intra-abdominal D18.03
intracranial D18.02
skin D18.01
specified site NEC D18.09
racemose D18.00
intra-abdominal D18.03
intracranial D18.02
skin D18.01
specified site NEC D18.09
sclerosing —see Neoplasm, skin, benign
simplex D18.00
intra-abdominal D18.03
intracranial D18.02
skin D18.01
specified site NEC D18.09
skin D18.01
specified site NEC D18.09
venous D18.00
intra-abdominal D18.03
intracranial D18.02
skin D18.01
specified site NEC D18.09
verrucous keratotic D18.00
intra-abdominal D18.03
intracranial D18.02
skin D18.01
specified site NEC D18.09
Hemangiomatosis (systemic) I78.8
involving single site —see Hemangioma
Hemangiopericytoma —see also Neoplasm, connective tissue, uncertain behavior
benign —see Neoplasm, connective tissue, benign
malignant —see Neoplasm, connective tissue, malignant
Hemangiosarcoma —see Neoplasm, connective tissue, malignant
Hemarthrosis (nontraumatic) M25.00
ankle M25.07-●
elbow M25.02-●
foot joint M25.07-●
hand joint M25.04-●
hip M25.05-●
in hemophilic arthropathy —see Arthropathy, hemophilic
knee M25.06-●
shoulder M25.01-●
specified joint NEC M25.08
traumatic —see Sprain, by site
vertebrae M25.08
wrist M25.03-●
Hematemesis K92.0
with ulcer - code by site under Ulcer, with hemorrhage K27.4
newborn, neonatal P54.0
due to swallowed maternal blood P78.2
Hematidrosis L74.8
Hematinuria —see also Hemoglobinuria
malarial B50.8
Hematobilia K83.8
Hematocele
female NEC N94.89
with ectopic pregnancy O00.90
with intrauterine pregnancy O00.91
ovary N83.8
male N50.1
Hematochezia —see also Melena K92.1
Hematochyluria —see also Infestation, filarial
schistosomiasis (bilharziasis) B65.0
Hematocolpos (with hematometra or hematosalpinx) N89.7
Hematocornea —see Pigmentation, cornea, stromal
Hematogenous —see condition

Hematoma (traumatic) (skin surface intact) —
see also Contusion
with
    injury of internal organs —see Injury, by site
    open wound —see Wound, open
amputation stump (surgical) (late) T87.89
aorta, dissecting I71.00
    abdominal I71.02
➡ thoracic (see also Dissection, aorta, thoracic)
        I71.019
    thoracoabdominal I71.03
aortic intramural —see Dissection, aorta
arterial (complicating trauma) —see Injury,
    blood vessel, by site
auricle —see Contusion, ear
    nontraumatic —see Disorder, pinna,
        hematoma
birth injury NEC P15.8
brain (traumatic)
    with
        cerebral laceration or contusion
            (diffuse) —see Injury, intracranial,
            diffuse
            focal —see Injury, intracranial, focal
    cerebellar, traumatic S06.37-●
    intracerebral, traumatic —see Injury,
        intracranial, intracerebral hemorrhage
    newborn NEC P52.4
        birth injury P10.1
    nontraumatic —see Hemorrhage,
        intracranial
    subarachnoid, arachnoid, traumatic —see
        Injury, intracranial, subarachnoid
        hemorrhage
    subdural, traumatic —see Injury,
        intracranial, subdural hemorrhage
breast (nontraumatic) N64.89
broad ligament (nontraumatic) N83.7
    traumatic S37.892
cerebellar, traumatic S06.37-●
cerebral —see Hematoma, brain
cerebrum S06.36-●
    left S06.35-●
    right S06.34-●
cesarean delivery wound O90.2
complicating delivery (perineal) (pelvic)
    (vagina) (vulva) O71.7
corpus cavernosum (nontraumatic) N48.89
epididymis (nontraumatic) N50.1
epidural (traumatic) —see Injury, intracranial,
    epidural hemorrhage
    spinal —see Injury, spinal cord, by region
episiotomy O90.2
face, birth injury P15.4
genital organ NEC (nontraumatic)
    female (nonobstetric) N94.89
        traumatic S30.202
    male N50.1
        traumatic S30.201
internal organs —see Injury, by site
intracerebral, traumatic —see Injury,
    intracranial, intracerebral hemorrhage
intraoperative —see Complications,
    intraoperative, hemorrhage
labia (nontraumatic) (nonobstetric) N90.8
liver (subcapsular) (nontraumatic) K76.89
    birth injury P15.0
mediastinum —see Injury, intrathoracic
mesosalpinx (nontraumatic) N83.7
    traumatic S37.898
muscle - code by site under Contusion
nontraumatic
    muscle M79.81
    soft tissue M79.81
obstetrical surgical wound O90.2
orbit, orbital (nontraumatic) —see also
        Hemorrhage, orbit
    traumatic —see Contusion, orbit
pelvis (female) (nontraumatic) (nonobstetric)
    N94.89
    obstetric O71.7
    traumatic —see Injury, by site

Hematoma (Continued)
penis (nontraumatic) N48.89
    birth injury P15.5
perianal (nontraumatic) K64.5
perineal S30.23
    complicating delivery O71.7
perirenal —see Injury, kidney
pinna —see Contusion, ear
    nontraumatic —see Disorder, pinna,
        hematoma
placenta O43.89-●
postoperative (postprocedural) —see
        Complication, postprocedural,
        hematoma
retroperitoneal (nontraumatic) K66.1
    traumatic S36.892
scrotum, superficial S30.22
    birth injury P15.5
seminal vesicle (nontraumatic) N50.1
    traumatic S37.892
spermatic cord (traumatic) S37.892
    nontraumatic N50.1
spinal (cord) (meninges) —see also Injury,
    spinal cord, by region
    newborn (birth injury) P11.5
spleen D73.5
    intraoperative —see Complications,
        intraoperative, hemorrhage, spleen
    postprocedural (postoperative) —see
        Complications, postprocedural,
        hemorrhage, spleen
sternocleidomastoid, birth injury P15.2
sternomastoid, birth injury P15.2
subarachnoid (traumatic) —see Injury,
    intracranial, subarachnoid hemorrhage
    newborn (nontraumatic) P52.5
        due to birth injury P10.3
    nontraumatic —see Hemorrhage,
        intracranial, subarachnoid
subdural (traumatic) —see Injury, intracranial,
    subdural hemorrhage
    newborn (localized) P52.8
        birth injury P10.0
    nontraumatic —see Hemorrhage,
        intracranial, subdural
superficial, newborn P54.5
testis (nontraumatic) N50.1
    birth injury P15.5
tunica vaginalis (nontraumatic) N50.1
umbilical cord, complicating delivery O69.5
uterine ligament (broad) (nontraumatic) N83.7
    traumatic S37.892
vagina (ruptured) (nontraumatic) N89.8
    complicating delivery O71.7
vas deferens (nontraumatic) N50.1
    traumatic S37.892
vitreous —see Hemorrhage, vitreous
vulva (nontraumatic) (nonobstetric) N90.89
    complicating delivery O71.7
    newborn (birth injury) P15.5
Hematometra N85.7
    with hematocolpos N89.7
Hematomyelia (central) G95.19
    newborn (birth injury) P11.5
    traumatic T14.8
Hematomyelitis G04.90
Hematoperitoneum —see Hemoperitoneum
Hematophobia F40.230
Hematopneumothorax (see Hemothorax)
Hematopoiesis, cyclic D70.4
Hematoporphyria —see Porphyria
Hematorachis, hematorrhachis G95.19
    newborn (birth injury) P11.5
Hematosalpinx N83.6
    with
        hematocolpos N89.7
        hematometra N85.7
            with hematocolpos N89.7
        infectional —see Salpingitis
Hematospermia R36.1
Hematothorax (see Hemothorax)

Hematuria R31.9
benign (familial) (of childhood) —see also
        Hematuria, idiopathic
    essential microscopic R31.1
due to sulphonamide, sulfonamide —see Table
    of Drugs and Chemicals, by drug
endemic —see also Schistosomiasis B65.0
gross R31.0
idiopathic N02.9
    with glomerular lesion
        C3
            glomerulonephritis N02.A
            glomerulopathy N02.A
                with dense deposit disease N02.6
        crescentic (diffuse) glomerulonephritis
            N02.7
        dense deposit disease N02.6
        endocapillary proliferative
            glomerulonephritis N02.4
        focal and segmental hyalinosis or
            sclerosis N02.1
        membranoproliferative (diffuse) N02.5
        membranous (diffuse) N02.2
        mesangial proliferative (diffuse) N02.3
        mesangiocapillary (diffuse) N02.5
        minor abnormality N02.0
        proliferative NEC N02.8
        specified pathology NEC N02.8
intermittent —see Hematuria, idiopathic
malarial B50.8
microscopic NEC (with symptoms) R31.29
    asymptomatic R31.21
    benign essential R31.1
paroxysmal —see also Hematuria, idiopathic
    nocturnal D59.5
persistent —see Hematuria, idiopathic
recurrent —see Hematuria, idiopathic
tropical —see also Schistosomiasis B65.0
tuberculous A18.13
Hemeralopia (day blindness) H53.11
    vitamin A deficiency E50.5
Hemi-akinesia R41.4
Hemianalgesia R20.0
Hemianencephaly Q00.0
Hemianesthesia R20.0
Hemianopia, hemianopsia (heteronymous)
    H53.47
    homonymous H53.46-●
    syphilitic A52.71
Hemiathetosis R25.8
Hemiatrophy R68.89
    cerebellar G31.9
    face, facial, progressive (Romberg) G51.8
    tongue K14.8
Hemiballism (us) G25.5
Hemicardia Q24.8
Hemicephalus, hemicephaly Q00.0
Hemichorea G25.5
Hemicolitis, left —see Colitis, left sided
Hemicrania
    congenital malformation Q00.0
    continua G44.51
    meaning migraine —see also Migraine G43.909
    paroxysmal G44.039
        chronic G44.049
            intractable G44.041
            not intractable G44.049
        episodic G44.039
            intractable G44.031
            not intractable G44.039
        intractable G44.031
        not intractable G44.039
Hemidystrophy —see Hemiatrophy
Hemiectromelia Q73.8
Hemihypalgesia R20.8
Hemihypesthesia R20.1
Hemi-inattention R41.4
Hemimelia Q73.8
    lower limb —see Defect, reduction, lower
        limb, specified type NEC
    upper limb —see Defect, reduction, upper
        limb, specified type NEC

Hemiparalysis —*see* Hemiplegia
Hemiparesis —*see* Hemiplegia
Hemiparesthesia R20.2
Hemiparkinsonism G20
Hemiplegia G81.9-●
  alternans facialis G83.89
  ascending NEC G81.90
    spinal G95.89
  congenital (cerebral) G80.8
    spastic G80.2
  embolic (current episode) I63.4-●
  flaccid G81.0-●
  following
    cerebrovascular disease I69.959
      cerebral infarction I69.35-●
      intracerebral hemorrhage I69.15-●
      nontraumatic intracranial hemorrhage
        NEC I69.25-●
      specified disease NEC I69.85-●
      stroke NOS I69.35-●
      subarachnoid hemorrhage I69.05-●
  hysterical F44.4
  newborn NEC P91.88
    birth injury P11.9
  spastic G81.1-●
    congenital G80.2
  thrombotic (current episode) I63.3-●
Hemisection, spinal cord —*see* Injury, spinal
    cord, by region
Hemispasm (facial) R25.2
Hemisporosis B48.8
Hemitremor R25.1
Hemivertebra Q76.49
  failure of segmentation with scoliosis Q76.3
  fusion with scoliosis Q76.3
Hemochromatosis E83.119
  with refractory anemia D46.1
  due to repeated red blood cell transfusion
    E83.111
  hereditary (primary) E83.110
  neonatal P78.84
  primary E83.110
  specified NEC E83.118
Hemoglobin —*see also* condition
  abnormal (disease) —*see* Disease, hemoglobin
  AS genotype D57.3
  Constant Spring D58.2
  E-beta thalassemia D56.5
  fetal, hereditary persistence (HPFH) D56.4
  H Constant Spring D56.0
  low NOS D64.9
  S (Hb S), heterozygous D57.3
Hemoglobinemia D59.9
  due to blood transfusion T80.89
  paroxysmal D59.6
    nocturnal D59.5
Hemoglobinopathy (mixed) D58.2
  with thalassemia D56.8
  sickle-cell D57.1
    with thalassemia D57.40
      with
        acute chest syndrome D57.411
        cerebral vascular involvement
          D57.413
        crisis (painful) D57.419
          with specified complication NEC
            D57.418
        splenic sequestration D57.412
        vasoocclusive pain D57.419
      without crisis D57.40
Hemoglobinuria R82.3
  with anemia, hemolytic, acquired (chronic)
    NEC D59.6
  cold (paroxysmal) (with Raynaud's
    syndrome) D59.6
    agglutinin D59.12
  due to exertion or hemolysis NEC D59.6
  intermittent D59.6
  malarial B50.8
  march D59.6

Hemoglobinuria (Continued)
  nocturnal (paroxysmal) D59.5
  paroxysmal (cold) D59.6
    nocturnal D59.5
Hemolymphangioma D18.1
Hemolysis
  intravascular
    with
      abortion —*see* Abortion, by type,
        complicated by, hemorrhage
      ectopic or molar pregnancy O08.1
      hemorrhage
        antepartum —*see* Hemorrhage,
          antepartum, with coagulation
          defect
        intrapartum —*see also* Hemorrhage,
          complicating, delivery O67.0
      postpartum O72.3
  neonatal (excessive) P58.9
    specified NEC P58.8
Hemolytic —*see* condition
Hemopericardium I31.2
  following acute myocardial infarction
    (current complication) I23.0
  newborn P54.8
  traumatic —*see* Injury, heart, with
    hemopericardium
Hemoperitoneum K66.1
  infectional K65.9
  traumatic S36.899
    with open wound —*see* Wound, open,
      with penetration into peritoneal
      cavity
Hemophilia (classical) (familial) (hereditary)
    D66
  A D66
  B D67
  C D68.1
  acquired D68.311
  autoimmune D68.311
  calcipriva —*see also* Defect, coagulation
    D68.4
  nonfamilial —*see also* Defect, coagulation
    D68.4
  secondary D68.311
  vascular —*see* Disease, von Willebrand
Hemophthalmos H44.81-●
Hemopneumothorax —*see also* Hemothorax
  traumatic S27.2
Hemoptysis R04.2
  newborn P26.9
  tuberculous —*see* Tuberculosis, pulmonary
Hemorrhage, hemorrhagic (concealed) R58
  abdomen R58
  accidental antepartum —*see* Hemorrhage,
    antepartum
  acute idiopathic pulmonary, in infants
    R04.81
  adenoid J35.8
  adrenal (capsule) (gland) E27.49
    medulla E27.8
    newborn P54.4
  after delivery —*see* Hemorrhage,
    postpartum
  alveolar
    lung, newborn P26.8
    process K08.89
  alveolus K08.89
  amputation stump (surgical) T87.89
  anemia (chronic) D50.0
    acute D62
  antepartum (with) O46.90
    with coagulation defect O46.00-●
      afibrinogenemia O46.01-●
      disseminated intravascular coagulation
        O46.02-●
      hypofibrinogenemia O46.01-●
      specified defect NEC O46.09-●
    before 20 weeks gestation O20.9
      specified type NEC O20.8
      threatened abortion O20.0

Hemorrhage, hemorrhagic (Continued)
  antepartum (Continued)
    due to
      abruptio placenta —*see also* Abruptio
        placentae O45.9-●
      leiomyoma, uterus —*see* Hemorrhage,
        antepartum, specified cause NEC
      placenta previa O44.1-●
      specified cause NEC —*see* subcategory
        O46.8X-●
  anus (sphincter) K62.5
  apoplexy (stroke) —*see* Hemorrhage,
    intracranial, intracerebral
  arachnoid —*see* Hemorrhage, intracranial,
    subarachnoid
  artery R58
    brain —*see* Hemorrhage, intracranial,
      intracerebral
  basilar (ganglion) I61.0
  bladder N32.89
  bowel K92.2
    newborn P54.3
  brain (miliary) (nontraumatic) —*see*
      Hemorrhage, intracranial, intracerebral
    due to
      birth injury P10.1
      syphilis A52.05
    epidural or extradural (traumatic) —
      see Injury, intracranial, epidural
      hemorrhage
    newborn P52.4
      birth injury P10.1
    subarachnoid —*see* Hemorrhage,
      intracranial, subarachnoid
    subdural —*see* Hemorrhage, intracranial,
      subdural
  brainstem (nontraumatic) I61.3
    traumatic S06.38-●
  breast N64.59
  bronchial tube —*see* Hemorrhage, lung
  bronchopulmonary —*see* Hemorrhage, lung
  bronchus —*see* Hemorrhage, lung
  bulbar I61.5
  capillary I78.8
    primary D69.8
  cecum K92.2
  cerebellar, cerebellum (nontraumatic) I61.4
    newborn P52.6
    traumatic S06.37-●
  cerebral, cerebrum —*see also* Hemorrhage,
      intracranial, intracerebral
    lobe I61.1
    newborn (anoxic) P52.4
      birth injury P10.1
  cerebromeningeal I61.8
  cerebrospinal —*see* Hemorrhage, intracranial,
    intracerebral
  cervix (uteri) (stump) NEC N88.8
  chamber, anterior (eye) —*see* Hyphema
  childbirth —*see* Hemorrhage, complicating,
    delivery
  choroid H31.30-●
    expulsive H31.31-●
  ciliary body —*see* Hyphema
  cochlea —*see* subcategory H83.8
  colon K92.2
  complicating
    abortion —*see* Abortion, by type,
      complicated by, hemorrhage
    delivery O67.9
      associated with coagulation defect
        (afibrinogenemia) (DIC)
        (hyperfibrinolysis) O67.0
      specified cause NEC O67.8
    surgical procedure —*see* Hemorrhage,
      intraoperative
  conjunctiva H11.3-●
    newborn P54.8
  cord, newborn (stump) P51.9
  corpus luteum (ruptured) cyst N83.1-●
  cortical (brain) I61.1

▶ New   ⇒ Revised   ~~deleted~~ Deleted   ● Use Additional Character(s)

Hemorrhage, hemorrhagic *(Continued)*
cranial —*see* Hemorrhage, intracranial
cutaneous R23.3
    due to autosensitivity, erythrocyte D69.2
    newborn P54.5
delayed
    following ectopic or molar pregnancy
        O08.1
    postpartum O72.2
diathesis (familial) D69.9
disease D69.9
    newborn P53
    specified type NEC D69.8
due to or associated with
    afibrinogenemia or other coagulation defect
        (conditions in categories D65-D69)
        antepartum —*see* Hemorrhage,
            antepartum, with coagulation
            defect
        intrapartum O67.0
    dental implant M27.61
    device, implant or graft —*see also*
        Complications, by site and type,
        specified NEC T85.838
        arterial graft NEC T82.838
        breast T85.838
        catheter NEC T85.838
            dialysis (renal) T82.838
                intraperitoneal T85.838
            infusion NEC T82.838
                spinal (epidural) (subdural)
                    T85.830
            urinary (indwelling) T83.83
        electronic (electrode) (pulse generator)
            (stimulator)
            bone T84.83
            cardiac T82.837
            nervous system (brain) (peripheral
                nerve) (spinal) T85.830
            urinary T83.83
        fixation, internal (orthopedic) NEC
            T84.83
        gastrointestinal (bile duct) (esophagus)
            T85.838
        genital NEC T83.83
        heart NEC T82.837
        joint prosthesis T84.83
        ocular (corneal graft) (orbital implant)
            NEC T85.838
        orthopedic NEC T84.83
            bone graft T86.838
        specified NEC T85.838
        urinary NEC T83.83
        vascular NEC T82.838
        ventricular intracranial shunt T85.838
duodenum, duodenal K92.2
    ulcer —*see* Ulcer, duodenum, with
        hemorrhage
dura mater —*see* Hemorrhage, intracranial,
    subdural
endotracheal —*see* Hemorrhage, lung
epicranial subaponeurotic (massive), birth
    injury P12.2
epidural (traumatic) —*see also* Injury,
    intracranial, epidural hemorrhage
    nontraumatic I62.1
esophagus K22.89
    varix I85.01
        secondary I85.11
excessive, following ectopic gestation
    (subsequent episode) O08.1
extradural (traumatic) —*see* Injury,
    intracranial, epidural hemorrhage
    birth injury P10.8
    newborn (anoxic) (nontraumatic) P52.8
    nontraumatic I62.1
eye NEC H57.89
    fundus —*see* Hemorrhage, retina
    lid —*see* Disorder, eyelid, specified type
        NEC
fallopian tube N83.6

Hemorrhage, hemorrhagic *(Continued)*
fibrinogenolysis —*see* Fibrinolysis
fibrinolytic (acquired) —*see* Fibrinolysis
from
    ear (nontraumatic) —*see* Otorrhagia
    tracheostomy stoma J95.01
fundus, eye —*see* Hemorrhage, retina
funis —*see* Hemorrhage, umbilicus, cord
gastric —*see* Hemorrhage, stomach
gastroenteric K92.2
    newborn P54.3
gastrointestinal (tract) K92.2
    newborn P54.3
genital organ, male N50.1
genitourinary (tract) NOS R31.9
gingiva K06.8
globe (eye) —*see* Hemophthalmos
graafian follicle cyst (ruptured) N83.0-•
gum K06.8
heart I51.89
hypopharyngeal (throat) R04.1
intermenstrual (regular) N92.3
    irregular N92.1
internal (organs) NEC R58
    capsule I61.0
    ear —*see* subcategory H83.8
    newborn P54.8
intestine K92.2
    newborn P54.3
intra-abdominal R58
intra-alveolar (lung), newborn P26.8
intracerebral (nontraumatic) —*see*
    Hemorrhage, intracranial,
    intracerebral
intracranial (nontraumatic) I62.9
    birth injury P10.9
    epidural, nontraumatic I62.1
    extradural, nontraumatic I62.1
    intracerebral (nontraumatic) (in) I61.9
        brain stem I61.3
        cerebellum I61.4
        hemisphere I61.2
            cortical (superficial) I61.1
            subcortical (deep) I61.0
        intraoperative
            during a nervous system procedure
                G97.31
            during other procedure G97.32
        intraventricular I61.5
        multiple localized I61.6
        newborn P52.4
            birth injury P10.1
        postprocedural
            following a nervous system procedure
                G97.51
            following other procedure
                G97.52
        specified NEC I61.8
        superficial I61.1
        traumatic (diffuse) —*see* Injury,
            intracranial, diffuse
        focal —*see* Injury, intracranial, focal
    newborn P52.9
        specified NEC P52.8
    subarachnoid (nontraumatic) (from) I60.9
        intracranial (cerebral) artery I60.7
            anterior communicating I60.2
            basilar I60.4
            carotid siphon and bifurcation
                I60.0-•
            communicating I60.7
                anterior I60.2
                posterior I60.3-•
            middle cerebral I60.1-•
            posterior communicating I60.3-•
            specified artery NEC I60.6
            vertebral I60.5-•
        newborn P52.5
            birth injury P10.3
        specified NEC I60.8
        traumatic S06.6X-•

Hemorrhage, hemorrhagic *(Continued)*
intracranial *(Continued)*
    subdural (nontraumatic) I62.00
        acute I62.01
        birth injury P10.0
        chronic I62.03
        newborn (anoxic) (hypoxic) P52.8
            birth injury P10.0
        spinal G95.19
        subacute I62.02
        traumatic —*see* Injury, intracranial,
            subdural hemorrhage
    traumatic —*see* Injury, intracranial, focal
        brain injury
intramedullary NEC G95.19
intraocular —*see* Hemophthalmos
intraoperative, intraprocedural —*see*
    Complication, hemorrhage (hematoma),
    intraoperative (intraprocedural), by site
intrapartum —*see* Hemorrhage, complicating,
    delivery
intrapelvic
    female N94.89
    male K66.1
intraperitoneal K66.1
intrapontine I61.3
intraprocedural —*see* Complication,
    hemorrhage (hematoma), intraoperative
    (intraprocedural), by site
intrauterine N85.7
    complicating delivery —*see also* Hemorrhage,
        complicating, delivery O67.9
    postpartum —*see* Hemorrhage, postpartum
intraventricular I61.5
    newborn (nontraumatic) —*see also* Newborn,
        affected by, hemorrhage P52.3
    due to birth injury P10.2
    grade
        1 P52.0
        2 P52.1
        3 P52.21
        4 P52.22
intravesical N32.89
iris (postinfectional) (postinflammatory)
    (toxic) —*see* Hyphema
joint (nontraumatic) —*see* Hemarthrosis
kidney N28.89
knee (joint) (nontraumatic) —*see*
    Hemarthrosis, knee
labyrinth —*see* subcategory H83.8
lenticular striate artery I61.0
ligature, vessel —*see* Hemorrhage,
    postoperative
liver K76.89
lung R04.89
    newborn P26.9
        massive P26.1
        specified NEC P26.8
    tuberculous —*see* Tuberculosis, pulmonary
massive umbilical, newborn P51.0
mediastinum —*see* Hemorrhage, lung
medulla I61.3
membrane (brain) I60.8
    spinal cord —*see* Hemorrhage, spinal cord
meninges, meningeal (brain) (middle) I60.8
    spinal cord —*see* Hemorrhage, spinal cord
mesentery K66.1
metritis —*see* Endometritis
mouth K13.79
mucous membrane NEC R58
    newborn P54.8
muscle M62.89
nail (subungual) L60.8
nasal turbinate R04.0
    newborn P54.8
navel, newborn P51.9
newborn P54.9
    specified NEC P54.8
nipple N64.59
nose R04.0
    newborn P54.8

Hemorrhage, hemorrhagic (Continued)
- omentum K66.1
- optic nerve (sheath) H47.02-•
- orbit, orbital H05.23-•
- ovary NEC N83.8
- oviduct N83.6
- pancreas K86.89
- parathyroid (gland) (spontaneous) E21.4
- parturition —see Hemorrhage, complicating, delivery
- penis N48.89
- pericardium, pericarditis I31.2
- peritoneum, peritoneal K66.1
- peritonsillar tissue J35.8
  - due to infection J36
- petechial R23.3
  - due to autosensitivity, erythrocyte D69.2
- pituitary (gland) E23.6
- pleura —see Hemorrhage, lung
- polioencephalitis, superior E51.2
- polymyositis —see Polymyositis
- pons, pontine I61.3
- posterior fossa (nontraumatic) I61.8
  - newborn P52.6
- postmenopausal N95.0
- postnasal R04.0
- postoperative —see Complications, postprocedural, hemorrhage, by site
- postpartum NEC (following delivery of placenta) O72.1
  - delayed or secondary O72.2
  - retained placenta O72.0
  - third stage O72.0
- pregnancy —see Hemorrhage, antepartum
- preretinal —see Hemorrhage, retina
- prostate N42.1
- puerperal —see Hemorrhage, postpartum
  - delayed or secondary O72.2
- pulmonary R04.89
  - newborn P26.9
    - massive P26.1
    - specified NEC P26.8
  - tuberculous —see Tuberculosis, pulmonary
- purpura (primary) D69.3
- rectum (sphincter) K62.5
  - newborn P54.2
- recurring, following initial hemorrhage at time of injury T79.2
- renal N28.89
- respiratory passage or tract R04.9
  - specified NEC R04.89
- retina, retinal (vessels) H35.6-•
  - ▥diabetic —see Microaneurysm, retinal, diabetic
- retroperitoneal R58
- scalp R58
- scrotum N50.1
- secondary (nontraumatic) R58
  - following initial hemorrhage at time of injury T79.2
- seminal vesicle N50.1
- skin R23.3
  - newborn P54.5
- slipped umbilical ligature P51.8
- spermatic cord N50.1
- spinal (cord) G95.19
  - newborn (birth injury) P11.5
- spleen D73.5
  - intraoperative —see Complications, intraoperative, hemorrhage, spleen
  - postprocedural —see Complications, postprocedural, hemorrhage, spleen
- stomach K92.2
  - newborn P54.3
  - ulcer —see Ulcer, stomach, with hemorrhage
- subarachnoid (nontraumatic) —see Hemorrhage, intracranial, subarachnoid
- subconjunctival —see also Hemorrhage, conjunctiva
  - birth injury P15.3
- subcortical (brain) I61.0

Hemorrhage, hemorrhagic (Continued)
- subcutaneous R23.3
- subdiaphragmatic R58
- subdural (acute) (nontraumatic) —see Hemorrhage, intracranial, subdural
- subependymal
  - newborn P52.0
    - with intraventricular extension P52.1
      - and intracerebral extension P52.22
- subgaleal P12.2
- subhyaloid —see Hemorrhage, retina
- subperiosteal —see Disorder, bone, specified type NEC
- subretinal —see Hemorrhage, retina
- subtentorial —see Hemorrhage, intracranial, subdural
- subungual L60.8
- suprarenal (capsule) (gland) E27.49
  - newborn P54.4
- tentorium (traumatic) NEC —see Hemorrhage, brain
  - newborn (birth injury) P10.4
- testis N50.1
- third stage (postpartum) O72.0
- thorax —see Hemorrhage, lung
- throat R04.1
- thymus (gland) E32.8
- thyroid (cyst) (gland) E07.89
- tongue K14.8
- tonsil J35.8
- trachea —see Hemorrhage, lung
- tracheobronchial R04.89
  - newborn P26.0
- traumatic — code to specific injury
  - cerebellar —see Hemorrhage, brain
  - intracranial —see Hemorrhage, brain
  - recurring or secondary (following initial hemorrhage at time of injury) T79.2
- tuberculous NEC —see also Tuberculosis, pulmonary A15.0
- tunica vaginalis N50.1
- ulcer - code by site under Ulcer, with hemorrhage K27.4
- umbilicus, umbilical
  - cord
    - after birth, newborn P51.9
    - complicating delivery O69.5
  - newborn P51.9
    - massive P51.0
    - slipped ligature P51.8
  - stump P51.9
- urethra (idiopathic) N36.8
- uterus, uterine (abnormal) N93.9
  - climacteric N92.4
  - complicating delivery —see Hemorrhage, complicating, delivery
  - dysfunctional or functional N93.8
  - intermenstrual (regular) N92.3
    - irregular N92.1
  - postmenopausal N95.0
  - postpartum —see Hemorrhage, postpartum
  - preclimacteric or premenopausal N92.4
  - prepubertal N93.8
  - pubertal N92.2
- vagina (abnormal) N93.9
  - newborn P54.6
- vas deferens N50.1
- vasa previa O69.4
- ventricular I61.5
- vesical N32.89
- viscera NEC R58
  - newborn P54.8
- vitreous (humor) (intraocular) H43.1-•
- vulva N90.89

Hemorrhoids (bleeding) (without mention of degree) K64.9
- 1st degree (grade/stage I) (without prolapse outside of anal canal) K64.0
- 2nd degree (grade/stage II) (that prolapse with straining but retract spontaneously) K64.1

Hemorrhoids (Continued)
- 3rd degree (grade/stage III) (that prolapse with straining and require manual replacement back inside anal canal) K64.2
- 4th degree (grade/stage IV) (with prolapsed tissue that cannot be manually replaced) K64.3
- complicating
  - pregnancy O22.4
  - puerperium O87.2
- external K64.4
  - with
    - thrombosis K64.5
- internal (without mention of degree) K64.8
- prolapsed K64.8
- skin tags
  - anus K64.4
  - residual K64.4
- specified NEC K64.8
- strangulated —see also Hemorrhoids, by degree K64.8
- thrombosed —see also Hemorrhoids, by degree K64.5
- ulcerated —see also Hemorrhoids, by degree K64.8
Hemosalpinx N83.6
- with
  - hematocolpos N89.7
  - hematometra N85.7
    - with hematocolpos N89.7
Hemosiderosis (dietary) E83.19
- pulmonary, idiopathic E83.1 [J84.03]
- transfusion T80.89
Hemothorax (bacterial) (nontuberculous) J94.2
- newborn P54.8
- traumatic S27.1
  - with pneumothorax S27.2
- tuberculous NEC A15.6
Henoch (-Schönlein) **disease or syndrome** (purpura) D69.0
Henpue, henpuye A66.6
Hepar lobatum (syphilitic) A52.74
Hepatalgia K76.89
Hepatitis K75.9
- acute B17.9
  - with coma K72.01
  - with hepatic failure —see Failure, hepatic
  - alcoholic —see Hepatitis, alcoholic
  - infectious B15.9
  - non-viral K72.0
  - viral B17.9
- alcoholic (acute) (chronic) K70.10
  - with ascites K70.11
- amebic —see Abscess, liver, amebic
- anicteric (viral) —see Hepatitis, viral
- antigen-associated (HAA) —see Hepatitis, B
- Australia-antigen (positive) —see Hepatitis, B
- autoimmune K75.4
- B B19.10
  - with hepatic coma B19.11
  - acute B16.9
    - with
      - delta-agent (coinfection) (without hepatic coma) B16.1
        - with hepatic coma B16.0
      - hepatic coma (without delta-agent coinfection) B16.2
  - chronic B18.1
    - with delta-agent B18.0
- bacterial NEC K75.89
- C (viral) B19.20
  - with hepatic coma B19.21
  - acute B17.10
    - with hepatic coma B17.11
  - chronic B18.2
- catarrhal (acute) B15.9
  - with hepatic coma B15.0
- cholangiolitic K75.89
- cholestatic K75.89

▶ New   ⇨ Revised   ~~deleted~~ Deleted   • Use Additional Character(s)

Hepatitis (Continued)
  chronic K73.9
    active NEC K73.2
    lobular NEC K73.1
    persistent NEC K73.0
    specified NEC K73.8
  cytomegaloviral B25.1
  due to ethanol (acute) (chronic) —see
      Hepatitis, alcoholic
  epidemic B15.9
    with hepatic coma B15.0
  fulminant NEC (viral) —see Hepatitis, viral
  granulomatous NEC K75.3
  herpesviral B00.81
  history of
    B Z86.19
    C Z86.19
  homologous serum —see Hepatitis, viral,
      type B
  in (due to)
    mumps B26.81
    toxoplasmosis (acquired) B58.1
      congenital (active) P37.1 [K77]
  infectious, infective B15.9
    acute (subacute) B17.9
    chronic B18.9
  inoculation —see Hepatitis, viral, type B
  interstitial (chronic) K74.69
  ischemia, ischemic K72.00
  lupoid NEC K75.2
  malignant NEC (with hepatic failure)
      K72.90
    with coma K72.91
  neonatal giant cell P59.29
  neonatal (idiopathic) (toxic) P59.29
  newborn P59.29
  postimmunization —see Hepatitis, viral,
      type B
  post-transfusion —see Hepatitis, viral, type B
  reactive, nonspecific K75.2
  serum —see Hepatitis, viral, type B
  shock K72.00
  specified type NEC
    with hepatic failure —see Failure, hepatic
  syphilitic (late) A52.74
    congenital (early) A50.08 [K77]
      late A50.59 [K77]
    secondary A51.45
  toxic —see also Disease, liver, toxic K71.6
  tuberculous A18.83
  viral, virus B19.9
    with hepatic coma B19.0
    acute B17.9
    chronic B18.9
      specified NEC B18.8
      type
        B B18.1
          with delta-agent B18.0
        C B18.2
    congenital P35.3
    coxsackie B33.8 [K77]
    cytomegalic inclusion B25.1
    in remission, any type — code to Hepatitis,
        chronic, by type
    non-A, non-B B17.8
    specified type NEC (with or without coma)
        B17.8
    type
      A B15.9
        with hepatic coma B15.0
      B B19.10
        with hepatic coma B19.11
        acute B16.9
          with
            delta-agent (coinfection) (without
                hepatic coma) B16.1
              with hepatic coma B16.0
            hepatic coma (without delta-
                agent coinfection) B16.2
        chronic B18.1
          with delta-agent B18.0

Hepatitis (Continued)
  viral, virus (Continued)
    type (Continued)
      C B19.20
        with hepatic coma B19.21
        acute B17.10
          with hepatic coma B17.11
        chronic B18.2
      E B17.2
      non-A, non-B B17.8
Hepatization lung (acute) —see Pneumonia, lobar
Hepatoblastoma C22.2
Hepatocarcinoma C22.0
Hepatocholangiocarcinoma C22.0
Hepatocholangioma, benign D13.4
Hepatocholangitis K75.89
Hepatolenticular degeneration E83.01
Hepatoma (malignant) C22.0
  benign D13.4
  embryonal C22.0
Hepatomegaly —see also Hypertrophy, liver
  with splenomegaly R16.2
  congenital Q44.7
  in mononucleosis
    gammaherpesviral B27.09
    infectious specified NEC B27.89
Hepatoptosis K76.89
Hepatorenal syndrome following labor and
    delivery O90.4
Hepatosis K76.89
Hepatosplenomegaly R16.2
  hyperlipemic (Bürger-Grütz type) E78.3 [K77]
Hereditary —see condition
Hereditary alpha tryptasemia (syndrome) D89.44
Heredodegeneration, macular —see Dystrophy,
    retina
Heredopathia atactica polyneuritiformis G60.1
Heredosyphilis —see Syphilis, congenital
Herlitz' syndrome Q81.1
Hermansky-Pudlak syndrome E70.331
Hermaphrodite, hermaphroditism (true) Q56.0
  46,XX with streak gonads Q99.1
  46,XX/46,XY Q99.0
  46,XY with streak gonads Q99.1
  chimera 46,XX/46,XY Q99.0
Hernia, hernial (acquired) (recurrent) K46.9
  with
    gangrene —see Hernia, by site, with,
        gangrene
    incarceration —see Hernia, by site, with,
        obstruction
    irreducible —see Hernia, by site, with,
        obstruction
    obstruction —see Hernia, by site, with,
        obstruction
    strangulation —see Hernia, by site, with,
        obstruction
  abdomen, abdominal K46.9
    with
      gangrene (and obstruction) K46.1
      obstruction K46.0
    femoral —see Hernia, femoral
    incisional —see Hernia, incisional
    inguinal —see Hernia, inguinal
    specified site NEC K45.8
      with
        gangrene (and obstruction) K45.1
        obstruction K45.0
    umbilical —see Hernia, umbilical
    wall —see Hernia, ventral
  appendix —see Hernia, abdomen
  bladder (mucosa) (sphincter)
    congenital (female) (male) Q79.51
    female —see Cystocele
    male N32.89
  brain, congenital —see Encephalocele
  cartilage, vertebra —see Displacement,
      intervertebral disc
  cerebral, congenital —see also Encephalocele
    endaural Q01.8
  ciliary body (traumatic) S05.2-●

Hernia, hernial (Continued)
  colon —see Hernia, abdomen
  Cooper's —see Hernia, abdomen, specified
      site NEC
  crural —see Hernia, femoral
  diaphragm, diaphragmatic K44.9
    with
      gangrene (and obstruction) K44.1
      obstruction K44.0
    congenital Q79.0
  direct (inguinal) —see Hernia, inguinal
  diverticulum, intestine —see Hernia,
      abdomen
  double (inguinal) —see Hernia, inguinal,
      bilateral
  due to adhesions (with obstruction) K56.50
  epigastric —see also Hernia, ventral K43.9
  esophageal hiatus —see Hernia, hiatal
  external (inguinal) —see Hernia, inguinal
  fallopian tube N83.4-●
  fascia M62.89
  femoral K41.90
    with
      gangrene (and obstruction) K41.40
        not specified as recurrent K41.40
        recurrent K41.41
      obstruction K41.30
        not specified as recurrent K41.30
        recurrent K41.31
    bilateral K41.20
      with
        gangrene (and obstruction) K41.10
          not specified as recurrent K41.10
          recurrent K41.11
        obstruction K41.00
          not specified as recurrent K41.00
          recurrent K41.01
      not specified as recurrent K41.20
      recurrent K41.21
    not specified as recurrent K41.90
    recurrent K41.91
    unilateral K41.90
      with
        gangrene (and obstruction) K41.40
          not specified as recurrent K41.40
          recurrent K41.41
        obstruction K41.30
          not specified as recurrent K41.30
          recurrent K41.31
      not specified as recurrent K41.90
      recurrent K41.91
  foramen magnum G93.5
    congenital Q01.8
  funicular (umbilical) —see also Hernia,
      umbilicus
    spermatic (cord) —see Hernia, inguinal
  gastrointestinal tract —see Hernia, abdomen
  Hesselbach's —see Hernia, femoral, specified
      site NEC
  hiatal (esophageal) (sliding) K44.9
    with
      gangrene (and obstruction) K44.1
      obstruction K44.0
    congenital Q40.1
  hypogastric —see Hernia, ventral
  incarcerated —see also Hernia, by site, with
      obstruction
    with gangrene —see Hernia, by site, with
        gangrene
  incisional K43.2
    with
      gangrene (and obstruction) K43.1
      obstruction K43.0
  indirect (inguinal) —see Hernia, inguinal
  inguinal (direct) (external) (funicular)
      (indirect) (internal) (oblique) (scrotal)
      (sliding) K40.90
    with
      gangrene (and obstruction) K40.40
        not specified as recurrent K40.40
        recurrent K40.41

▶ New   ⇒ Revised   deleted Deleted   ● Use Additional Character(s)

Hernia, hernial *(Continued)*
  inguinal *(Continued)*
    with *(Continued)*
      obstruction K40.30
        not specified as recurrent K40.30
        recurrent K40.31
      bilateral K40.20
        with
          gangrene (and obstruction) K40.10
            not specified as recurrent K40.10
            recurrent K40.11
          obstruction K40.00
            not specified as recurrent K40.00
            recurrent K40.01
        not specified as recurrent K40.20
        recurrent K40.21
      not specified as recurrent K40.90
      recurrent K40.91
      unilateral K40.90
        with
          gangrene (and obstruction) K40.40
            not specified as recurrent K40.40
            recurrent K40.41
          obstruction K40.30
            not specified as recurrent K40.30
            recurrent K40.31
        not specified as recurrent K40.90
        recurrent K40.91
  internal —*see also* Hernia, abdomen
    inguinal —*see* Hernia, inguinal
  interstitial —*see* Hernia, abdomen
  intervertebral cartilage or disc —*see* Displacement, intervertebral disc
  intestine, intestinal —*see* Hernia, by site
  intra-abdominal —*see* Hernia, abdomen
  iris (traumatic) S05.2-●
  irreducible —*see also* Hernia, by site, with obstruction
    with gangrene —*see* Hernia, by site, with gangrene
  ischiatic —*see* Hernia, abdomen, specified site NEC
  ischiorectal —*see* Hernia, abdomen, specified site NEC
  lens (traumatic) S05.2-●
  linea (alba) (semilunaris) —*see* Hernia, ventral
  Littre's —*see* Hernia, abdomen
  lumbar —*see* Hernia, abdomen, specified site NEC
  lung (subcutaneous) J98.4
  mediastinum J98.59
  mesenteric (internal) —*see* Hernia, abdomen
  midline —*see* Hernia, ventral
  muscle (sheath) M62.89
  nucleus pulposus —*see* Displacement, intervertebral disc
  oblique (inguinal) —*see* Hernia, inguinal
  obstructive —*see also* Hernia, by site, with obstruction
    with gangrene —*see* Hernia, by site, with gangrene
  obturator —*see* Hernia, abdomen, specified site NEC
  omental —*see* Hernia, abdomen
  ovary N83.4-●
  oviduct N83.4-●
  paraesophageal —*see also* Hernia, diaphragm
    congenital Q40.1
  parastomal K43.5
    with
      gangrene (and obstruction) K43.4
      obstruction K43.3
  paraumbilical —*see* Hernia, umbilicus
  perineal —*see* Hernia, abdomen, specified site NEC
  Petit's —*see* Hernia, abdomen, specified site NEC
  postoperative —*see* Hernia, incisional
  pregnant uterus —*see* Abnormal, uterus in pregnancy or childbirth
  prevesical N32.89

Hernia, hernial *(Continued)*
  properitoneal —*see* Hernia, abdomen, specified site NEC
  pudendal —*see* Hernia, abdomen, specified site NEC
  rectovaginal N81.6
  retroperitoneal —*see* Hernia, abdomen, specified site NEC
  Richter's —*see* Hernia, abdomen, with obstruction
  Rieux's, Riex's —*see* Hernia, abdomen, specified site NEC
  sac condition (adhesion) (dropsy) (inflammation) (laceration) (suppuration) - code by site under Hernia
  sciatic —*see* Hernia, abdomen, specified site NEC
  scrotum, scrotal —*see* Hernia, inguinal
  sliding (inguinal) —*see also* Hernia, inguinal
    hiatus —*see* Hernia, hiatal
  spigelian —*see* Hernia, ventral
  spinal —*see* Spina bifida
  strangulated —*see also* Hernia, by site, with obstruction
    with gangrene —*see* Hernia, by site, with gangrene
  subxiphoid —*see* Hernia, ventral
  supra-umbilicus —*see* Hernia, ventral
  tendon —*see* Disorder, tendon, specified type NEC
  Treitz's (fossa) —*see* Hernia, abdomen, specified site NEC
  tunica vaginalis Q55.29
  umbilicus, umbilical K42.9
    with
      gangrene (and obstruction) K42.1
      obstruction K42.0
  ureter N28.89
  urethra, congenital Q64.79
  urinary meatus, congenital Q64.79
  uterus N81.4
    pregnant —*see* Abnormal, uterus in pregnancy or childbirth
  vaginal (anterior) (wall) —*see* Cystocele
  Velpeau's —*see* Hernia, femoral
  ventral K43.9
    with
      gangrene (and obstruction) K43.7
      obstruction K43.6
    incisional K43.2
      with
        gangrene (and obstruction) K43.1
        obstruction K43.0
      recurrent —*see* Hernia, incisional
    specified NEC K43.9
      with
        gangrene (and obstruction) K43.7
        obstruction K43.6
  vesical
    congenital (female) (male) Q79.51
    female —*see* Cystocele
    male N32.89
  vitreous (into wound) S05.2-●
    into anterior chamber —*see* Prolapse, vitreous
Herniation —*see also* Hernia
  brain (stem) G93.5
    nontraumatic G93.5
    traumatic S06.A1
      cerebellar S06.A1
      subfalcine (cingulate) S06.A1
      tonsillar S06.A1
      transtentorial (central) (upward cerebellar) S06.A1
      uncal S06.A1
  cerebral G93.5
    nontraumatic G93.5
    traumatic S06.A1
  mediastinum J98.59
  nucleus pulposus —*see* Displacement, intervertebral disc
Herpangina B08.5

Herpes, herpesvirus, herpetic B00.9
  anogenital A60.9
    perianal skin A60.1
    rectum A60.1
    urogenital tract A60.00
      cervix A60.03
      male genital organ NEC A60.02
      penis A60.01
      specified site NEC A60.09
      vagina A60.04
      vulva A60.04
  blepharitis (zoster) B02.39
    simplex B00.59
  circinatus B35.4
    bullosus L12.0
  conjunctivitis (simplex) B00.53
    zoster B02.31
  cornea B02.33
  encephalitis B00.4
    due to herpesvirus 6 B10.01
    due to herpesvirus 7 B10.09
    specified NEC B10.09
  eye (zoster) B02.30
    simplex B00.50
  eyelid (zoster) B02.39
    simplex B00.59
  facialis B00.1
  febrilis B00.1
  geniculate ganglionitis B02.21
  genital, genitalis A60.00
    female A60.09
    male A60.02
  gestational, gestationis O26.4-●
  gingivostomatitis B00.2
  human B00.9
    1 —*see* Herpes, simplex
    2 —*see* Herpes, simplex
    3 —*see* Varicella
    4 —*see* Mononucleosis, Epstein-Barr (virus)
    5 —*see* Disease, cytomegalic inclusion (generalized)
    6
      encephalitis B10.01
      specified NEC B10.81
    7
      encephalitis B10.09
      specified NEC B10.82
    8 B10.89
  infection NEC B10.89
    Kaposi's sarcoma associated B10.89
  iridocyclitis (simplex) B00.51
    zoster B02.32
  iris (vesicular erythema multiforme) L51.9
  iritis (simplex) B00.51
  Kaposi's sarcoma associated B10.89
  keratitis (simplex) (dendritic) (disciform) (interstitial) B00.52
    zoster (interstitial) B02.33
  keratoconjunctivitis (simplex) B00.52
    zoster B02.33
  labialis B00.1
  lip B00.1
  meningitis (simplex) B00.3
    zoster B02.1
  ophthalmicus (zoster) NEC B02.30
    simplex B00.50
  penis A60.01
  perianal skin A60.1
  pharyngitis, pharyngotonsillitis B00.2
  rectum A60.1
  scrotum A60.02
  sepsis B00.7
  simplex B00.9
    complicated NEC B00.89
    congenital P35.2
    conjunctivitis B00.53
    external ear B00.1
    eyelid B00.59
    hepatitis B00.81
    keratitis (interstitial) B00.52
    myeitis B00.82
    specified complication NEC B00.89
    visceral B00.89

Herpes, herpesvirus, herpetic *(Continued)*
 stomatitis B00.2
 tonsurans B35.0
 visceral B00.89
 vulva A60.04
 whitlow B00.89
 zoster —*see also* condition B02.9
  auricularis B02.21
  complicated NEC B02.8
  conjunctivitis B02.31
  disseminated B02.7
  encephalitis B02.0
  eye(lid) B02.39
  geniculate ganglionitis B02.21
  keratitis (interstitial) B02.33
  meningitis B02.1
  myelitis B02.24
  neuritis, neuralgia B02.29
  ophthalmicus NEC B02.30
  oticus B02.21
  polyneuropathy B02.23
  specified complication NEC B02.8
  trigeminal neuralgia B02.22
Herpesvirus (human) —*see* Herpes
Herpetophobia F40.218
Herrick's anemia —*see* Disease, sickle-cell
Hers' disease E74.09
Herter-Gee syndrome K90.0
Herxheimer's reaction R68.89
Hesitancy
 of micturition R39.11
 urinary R39.11
Hesselbach's hernia —*see* Hernia, femoral,
   specified site NEC
Heterochromia (congenital) Q13.2
 cataract —*see* Cataract, complicated
 cyclitis (Fuchs) —*see* Cyclitis, Fuchs'
   heterochromic
 hair L67.1
 iritis —*see* Cyclitis, Fuchs' heterochromic
 retained metallic foreign body
    (nonmagnetic) —*see* Foreign body,
    intraocular, old, retained
   magnetic —*see* Foreign body, intraocular,
    old, retained, magnetic
 uveitis —*see* Cyclitis, Fuchs' heterochromic
Heterophoria —*see* Strabismus, heterophoria
Heterophyes, heterophyiasis (small intestine)
  B66.8
Heterotopia, heterotopic —*see also* Malposition,
  congenital
 cerebralis Q04.8
Heterotropia —*see* Strabismus
Heubner-Herter disease K90.0
Hexadactylism Q69.9
HGSIL (cytology finding) (high grade
  squamous intraepithelial lesion on
  cytologic smear) (Pap smear finding)
 anus R85.613
 cervix R87.613
  biopsy (histology) finding — *see* Neoplasia,
    intraepithelial, cervix, grade II or
    grade III
 vagina R87.623
  biopsy (histology) finding — *see* Neoplasia,
    intraepithelial, vagina, grade II or
    grade III
Hibernoma —*see* Lipoma
Hiccup, hiccough R06.6
 epidemic B33.0
 psychogenic F45.8
Hidden penis (congenital) Q55.64
 acquired N48.83
Hidradenitis (axillaris) (suppurative)
  L73.2
Hidradenoma (nodular) —*see also* Neoplasm,
  skin, benign
 clear cell —*see* Neoplasm, skin, benign
 papillary —*see* Neoplasm, skin, benign
Hidrocystoma —*see* Neoplasm, skin,
  benign

High
 altitude effects T70.20
  anoxia T70.29
  on
   ears T70.0
   sinuses T70.1
  polycythemia D75.1
 arch
  foot Q66.7-●
  palate, congenital Q38.5
 arterial tension —*see* Hypertension
 basal metabolic rate R94.8
 blood pressure —*see also* Hypertension
  borderline R03.0
  reading (incidental) (isolated)
    (nonspecific), without diagnosis of
    hypertension R03.0
 cholesterol E78.00
  with high triglycerides E78.2
 diaphragm (congenital) Q79.1
 expressed emotional level within family Z63.8
 head at term O32.4
 palate, congenital Q38.5
 risk
  infant NEC Z76.2
  sexual behavior (heterosexual) Z72.51
   bisexual Z72.53
   homosexual Z72.52
 scrotal testis, testes
  bilateral Q53.23
  unilateral Q53.13
 temperature (of unknown origin) R50.9
 thoracic rib Q76.6
 triglycerides E78.1
  with high cholesterol E78.2
Hildenbrand's disease A75.0
Hilum —*see* condition
Hip —*see* condition
➡Hippel's disease Q85.83
Hippophobia F40.218
Hippus H57.09
Hirschsprung's disease or megacolon Q43.1
Hirsutism, hirsuties L68.0
Hirudiniasis
 external B88.3
 internal B83.4
Hiss-Russell dysentery A03.1
Histidinemia, histidinuria E70.41
Histiocytoma —*see also* Neoplasm, skin, benign
 fibrous —*see also* Neoplasm, skin, benign
  atypical —*see* Neoplasm, connective tissue,
    uncertain behavior
  malignant —*see* Neoplasm, connective
    tissue, malignant
Histiocytosis D76.3
 acute differentiated progressive C96.0
 Langerhans' cell NEC C96.6
  multifocal X
   multisystemic (disseminated) C96.0
   unisystemic C96.5
  pulmonary, adult (adult PLCH) J84.82
  unifocal (X) C96.6
 lipid, lipoid D76.3
  essential E75.29
 malignant C96.A
 mononuclear phagocytes NEC D76.1
  Langerhans' cells C96.6
 non-Langerhans' cell D76.3
 polyostotic sclerosing D76.3
 sinus, with massive lymphadenopathy D76.3
 syndrome NEC D76.3
 X NEC C96.6
  acute (progressive) C96.0
  chronic C96.6
  multifocal C96.5
  multisystemic C96.0
  unifocal C96.6
Histoplasmosis B39.9
 with pneumonia NEC B39.2
 African B39.5
 American —*see* Histoplasmosis, capsulati

Histoplasmosis *(Continued)*
 capsulati B39.4
  disseminated B39.3
  generalized B39.3
  pulmonary B39.2
   acute B39.0
   chronic B39.1
 Darling's B39.4
 duboisii B39.5
 lung NEC B39.2
History
 family (of) —*see also* History, personal (of)
  alcohol abuse Z81.1
  allergy NEC Z84.89
  anemia Z83.2
  arthritis Z82.61
  asthma Z82.5
  blindness Z82.1
  cardiac death (sudden) Z82.41
  carrier of genetic disease Z84.81
  chromosomal anomaly Z82.79
  chronic
   disabling disease NEC Z82.8
   lower respiratory disease Z82.5
  colonic polyps Z83.71
  congenital malformations and
    deformations Z82.79
   polycystic kidney Z82.71
  consanguinity Z84.3
  deafness Z82.2
  diabetes mellitus Z83.3
  disability NEC Z82.8
  disease or disorder (of)
   allergic NEC Z84.89
   behavioral NEC Z81.8
   blood and blood-forming organs Z83.2
   cardiovascular NEC Z82.49
   chronic disabling NEC Z82.8
   digestive Z83.79
   ear NEC Z83.52
   elevated lipoprotein (a) (Lp(a)) Z83.430
   endocrine NEC Z83.49
   eye NEC Z83.518
    glaucoma Z83.511
   familial hypercholesterolemia Z83.42
   genitourinary NEC Z84.2
   glaucoma Z83.511
   hematological Z83.2
   immune mechanism Z83.2
   infectious NEC Z83.1
   ischemic heart Z82.49
   kidney Z84.1
   lipoprotein metabolism Z83.438
   mental NEC Z81.8
   metabolic Z83.49
   musculoskeletal NEC Z82.69
   neurological NEC Z82.0
   nutritional Z83.49
   parasitic NEC Z83.1
   psychiatric NEC Z81.8
   respiratory NEC Z83.6
   skin and subcutaneous tissue NEC Z84.0
   specified NEC Z84.89
  drug abuse NEC Z81.3
  elevated lipoprotein(a) (Lp (a)) Z83.430
  epilepsy Z82.0
  familial hypercholesterolemia Z83.42
  genetic disease carrier Z84.81
  glaucoma Z83.511
  hearing loss Z82.2
  human immunodeficiency virus (HIV)
    infection Z83.0
  Huntington's chorea Z82.0
  hyperlipidemia, familial combined Z83.438
  intellectual disability Z81.0
  leukemia Z80.6
  lipidemia NEC Z83.438
  malignant neoplasm (of) NOS Z80.9
   bladder Z80.52
   breast Z80.3
   bronchus Z80.1

History *(Continued)*
  family *(Continued)*
    malignant neoplasm *(Continued)*
      digestive organ Z80.0
      gastrointestinal tract Z80.0
      genital organ Z80.49
        ovary Z80.41
        prostate Z80.42
        specified organ NEC Z80.49
        testis Z80.43
      hematopoietic NEC Z80.7
      intrathoracic organ NEC Z80.2
      kidney Z80.51
      lung Z80.1
      lymphatic NEC Z80.7
      ovary Z80.41
      prostate Z80.42
      respiratory organ NEC Z80.2
      specified site NEC Z80.8
      testis Z80.43
      trachea Z80.1
      urinary organ or tract Z80.59
        bladder Z80.52
        kidney Z80.51
    mental
      disorder NEC Z81.8
    multiple endocrine neoplasia (MEN)
      syndrome Z83.41
    osteoporosis Z82.62
    polycystic kidney Z82.71
    polyps (colon) Z83.71
    psychiatric disorder Z81.8
    psychoactive substance abuse NEC Z81.3
    respiratory condition NEC Z83.6
      asthma and other lower respiratory
        conditions Z82.5
    self-harmful behavior Z81.8
    SIDS (sudden infant death syndrome) Z84.82
    skin condition Z84.0
    specified condition NEC Z84.89
    stroke (cerebrovascular) Z82.3
    substance abuse NEC Z81.4
      alcohol Z81.1
      drug NEC Z81.3
      psychoactive NEC Z81.3
      tobacco Z81.2
    sudden
      cardiac death Z82.41
      infant death syndrome (SIDS) Z84.82
    tobacco abuse Z81.2
    violence, violent behavior Z81.8
    visual loss Z82.1
  personal (of) —*see also* History, family (of)
    abuse
      adult Z91.419
        forced labor or sexual exploitation
          Z91.42
        physical and sexual Z91.410
        psychological Z91.411
      childhood Z62.819
        forced labor or sexual exploitation in
          childhood Z62.813
        physical Z62.810
        psychological Z62.811
        sexual Z62.810
    alcohol dependence F10.21
    allergy (to) Z88.9
      analgesic agent NEC Z88.6
      anesthetic Z88.4
      antibiotic agent NEC Z88.1
      anti-infective agent NEC Z88.3
      contrast media Z91.041
      drugs, medicaments and biological
        substances Z88.9
        specified NEC Z88.8
      food Z91.018
        additives Z91.02
        beef Z91.014
        eggs Z91.012
        lamb Z91.014
        mammalian meats Z91.014
        milk products Z91.011
        peanuts Z91.010

History *(Continued)*
  personal *(Continued)*
    allergy *(Continued)*
      food *(Continued)*
        pork Z91.014
        red meats Z91.014
        seafood Z91.013
        specified food NEC Z91.018
      insect Z91.038
        bee Z91.030
      latex Z91.040
      medicinal agents Z88.9
        specified NEC Z88.8
      narcotic agent NEC Z88.5
      nonmedicinal agents Z91.048
      penicillin Z88.0
      serum Z88.7
      specified NEC Z91.09
      sulfonamides Z88.2
      vaccine Z88.7
    anaphylactic shock Z87.892
    anaphylaxis Z87.892
    behavioral disorders Z86.59
    benign carcinoid tumor Z86.012
    benign neoplasm Z86.018
      brain Z86.011
      carcinoid Z86.012
      colonic polyps Z86.010
    brain injury (traumatic) Z87.820
    breast implant removal Z98.86
    calculi, renal Z87.442
    cancer —*see* History, personal (of),
      malignant neoplasm (of)
    cardiac arrest (death), successfully
      resuscitated Z86.74
    CAR-T (Chimeric Antigen Receptor T-cell)
      therapy Z92.850
    cellular therapy Z92.859
      specified NEC Z92.858
    cerebral infarction without residual deficit
      Z86.73
    ▶certain (corrected) conditions arising in the
      perinatal period, specified NEC
      Z87.68
    cervical dysplasia Z87.410
    chemotherapy for neoplastic condition
      Z92.21
    childhood abuse —*see* History, personal
      (of), abuse
    Chimeric Antigen Receptor T-cell (CAR-T)
      therapy Z92.850
    cleft lip (corrected) Z87.730
    cleft palate (corrected) Z87.730
    ▶cloaca, persistent Z87.732
    ▶cloacal malformations Z87.732
    collapsed vertebra (healed) Z87.311
      due to osteoporosis Z87.310
    combat and operational stress reaction
      Z86.51
    congenital malformation (corrected)
      Z87.798
      circulatory system (corrected) Z87.74
      ▶diaphragmatic hernia Z87.760
      digestive system (corrected) NEC
        Z87.738
      ear (corrected) Z87.721
      eye (corrected) Z87.720
      face and neck (corrected) Z87.790
      ▶gastroschisis Z87.761
      genitourinary system (corrected) NEC
        Z87.718
      heart (corrected) Z87.74
      ⫸integument (corrected) Z87.768
      ⫸limb(s) (corrected) Z87.768
      ▶malformations
        ▶abdominal wall Z87.763
        ▶diaphragm NEC Z87.760
        ▶integument Z87.768
        ▶limbs Z87.768
        ▶musculoskeletal system Z87.768
        ▶prune belly Z87.762

History *(Continued)*
  personal *(Continued)*
    congenital malformation *(Continued)*
      ⫸musculoskeletal system (corrected)
        Z87.768
      neck (corrected) Z87.790
      ▶necrotizing enterocolitis of newborn
        (corrected) Z87.61
      nervous system (corrected) NEC
        Z87.728
      respiratory system (corrected) Z87.75
      sense organs (corrected) NEC Z87.728
      specified NEC Z87.798
      ▶tracheoesophageal
        ▶atresia Z87.731
        ▶fistula Z87.731
    contraception Z92.0
    coronavirus (disease) (novel) 2019 Z86.16
    COVID-19 Z86.16
    deployment (military) Z91.82
    diabetic foot ulcer Z86.31
    disease or disorder (of) Z87.898
      blood and blood-forming organs Z86.2
      circulatory system Z86.79
        specified condition NEC Z86.79
      connective tissue NEC Z87.39
      digestive system Z87.19
        colonic polyp Z86.010
        peptic ulcer disease Z87.11
        specified condition NEC Z87.19
      ear Z86.69
      endocrine Z86.39
        diabetic foot ulcer Z86.31
        gestational diabetes Z86.32
        specified type NEC Z86.39
      eye Z86.69
      genital (track) system NEC
        female Z87.42
        male Z87.438
      hematological Z86.2
      Hodgkin Z85.71
      immune mechanism Z86.2
      infectious Z86.19
        coronavirus (disease) (novel) 2019
          Z86.16
        COVID-19 Z86.16
        malaria Z86.13
        Methicillin resistant Staphylococcus
          aureus (MRSA) Z86.14
        poliomyelitis Z86.12
        SARS-CoV-2   Z86.16
        specified NEC Z86.19
        tuberculosis Z86.11
      mental NEC Z86.59
      metabolic Z86.39
        diabetic foot ulcer Z86.31
        gestational diabetes Z86.32
        specified type NEC Z86.39
      musculoskeletal NEC Z87.39
      nervous system Z86.69
      nutritional Z86.39
      parasitic Z86.19
      respiratory system NEC Z87.09
      sense organs Z86.69
      skin Z87.2
      specified site or type NEC Z87.898
      subcutaneous tissue Z87.2
      trophoblastic Z87.59
      urinary system NEC Z87.448
    drug dependence —*see* Dependence, drug,
      by type, in remission
    drug therapy
      antineoplastic chemotherapy Z92.21
      estrogen Z92.23
      immunosuppression Z92.25
      inhaled steroids Z92.240
      monoclonal drug Z92.22
      specified NEC Z92.29
      steroid Z92.241
      systemic steroids Z92.241

▶ New   ⫸ Revised   ~~deleted~~ Deleted   • Use Additional Character(s)

History *(Continued)*
  personal *(Continued)*
    dysplasia
      cervical (mild) (moderate) Z87.410
        severe (grade III) Z86.001
      prostatic Z87.430
      vaginal (mild) (moderate) Z87.411
        severe (grade III) Z86.002
      vulvar (mild) (moderate) Z87.412
        severe (grade III) Z86.002
    embolism (venous) Z86.718
      pulmonary Z86.711
    encephalitis Z86.61
    estrogen therapy Z92.23
    extracorporeal membrane oxygenation
      (ECMO) Z92.81
    failed conscious sedation Z92.83
    failed moderate sedation Z92.83
    fall, falling Z91.81
    forced labor or sexual exploitation Z91.42
      in childhood Z62.813
    fracture (healed)
      fatigue Z87.312
      fragility Z87.310
      osteoporosis Z87.310
      pathological NEC Z87.311
      stress Z87.312
      traumatic Z87.81
    gene therapy Z92.86
    gestational diabetes Z86.32
    hepatitis
      B Z86.19
      C Z86.19
    Hodgkin disease Z85.71
    hyperthermia, malignant Z88.4
    hypospadias (corrected) Z87.710
    hysterectomy Z90.710
    immunosuppression therapy Z92.25
    in situ neoplasm
      breast Z86.000
      cervix uteri Z86.001
      digestive organs, specified NEC Z86.004
      esophagus Z86.003
      genital organs, specified NEC Z86.002
      melanoma Z86.006
      middle ear Z86.005
      oral cavity Z86.003
      respiratory system Z86.005
      skin Z86.007
      specified NEC Z86.008
      stomach Z86.003
    infection NEC Z86.19
      central nervous system Z86.61
      coronavirus (disease) (novel) 2019 Z86.16
      COVID-19 Z86.16
      latent tuberculosis Z86.15
      Methicillin resistant Staphylococcus
        aureus (MRSA) Z86.14
      SARS-CoV-2 Z86.16
      urinary (recurrent) (tract) Z87.41
    injury NEC Z87.828
    in utero procedure during pregnancy
      Z98.870
    in utero procedure while a fetus Z98.871
    irradiation Z92.3
    kidney stones Z87.442
    latent tuberculosis Z86.15
    leukemia Z85.6
    lymphoma (non-Hodgkin) Z85.72
    malignant melanoma (skin) Z85.820
    malignant neoplasm (of) Z85.9
      accessory sinuses Z85.22
      anus NEC Z85.048
        carcinoid Z85.040
      bladder Z85.51
      bone Z85.830
      brain Z85.841
      breast Z85.3
      bronchus NEC Z85.118
        carcinoid Z85.110
      carcinoid —*see* History, personal (of),
        malignant neoplasm, by site,
        carcinioid

History *(Continued)*
  personal *(Continued)*
    malignant neoplasm (of) *(Continued)*
      cervix Z85.41
      colon NEC Z85.038
        carcinoid Z85.030
      digestive organ Z85.00
        specified NEC Z85.09
      endocrine gland NEC Z85.858
      epididymis Z85.48
      esophagus Z85.01
      eye Z85.840
      gastrointestinal tract —*see* History,
        malignant neoplasm, digestive organ
      genital organ
        female Z85.40
          specified NEC Z85.44
        male Z85.45
          specified NEC Z85.49
      hematopoietic NEC Z85.79
      intrathoracic organ Z85.20-●
      kidney NEC Z85.528
        carcinoid Z85.520
      large intestine NEC Z85.038
        carcinoid Z85.030
      larynx Z85.21
      liver Z85.05
      lung NEC Z85.118
        carcinoid Z85.110
      mediastinum Z85.29
      Merkel cell Z85.821
      middle ear Z85.22
      nasal cavities Z85.22
      nervous system NEC Z85.848
        oral cavity Z85.819
        specified site NEC Z85.818
      ovary Z85.43
      pancreas Z85.07
      pelvis Z85.53
      pharynx Z85.819
        specified site NEC Z85.818
      pleura Z85.29
      prostate Z85.46
      rectosigmoid junction NEC Z85.048
        carcinoid Z85.040
      rectum NEC Z85.048
        carcinoid Z85.040
      respiratory organ Z85.20
      sinuses, accessory Z85.22
      skin NEC Z85.828
        melanoma Z85.820
        Merkel cell Z85.821
      small intestine NEC Z85.068
        carcinoid Z85.060
      soft tissue Z85.831
      specified site NEC Z85.89
      stomach NEC Z85.028
        carcinoid Z85.020
      testis Z85.47
      thymus NEC Z85.238
        carcinoid Z85.230
      thyroid Z85.850
      tongue Z85.810
      trachea Z85.12
      ureter Z85.54
      urinary organ or tract Z85.50
        specified NEC Z85.59
      uterus Z85.42
    maltreatment Z91.89
    medical treatment NEC Z92.89
    melanoma Z85.820
      in situ Z86.06
      malignant (skin) Z85.820
    meningitis Z86.61
    mental disorder Z86.59
    Merkel cell carcinoma (skin) Z85.821
    Methicillin resistant Staphylococcus aureus
      (MRSA) Z86.14
    military deployment Z91.82
    military war, peacekeeping and
      humanitarian deployment (current or
      past conflict) Z91.82
    myocardial infarction (old) I25.2

History *(Continued)*
  personal *(Continued)*
    neglect (in)
      adult Z91.412
      childhood Z62.812
    neoplasia
      anal intraepithelial, III [AIN III] Z86.004
      high-grade prostatic intraepithelial, III
        [HGPIN III] Z86.002
      vaginal intraepithelial, III [VAIN III]
        Z86.002
      vulvar intraepithelial, III [VIN III] Z86.002
    neoplasm
      benign Z86.018
        brain Z86.011
        colon polyp Z86.010
      in situ
        breast Z86.000
        cervix uteri Z86.001
        digestive organs, specified NEC Z86.004
        esophagus Z86.003
        genital organs, specified NEC Z86.002
        melanoma Z86.006
        middle ear Z86.005
        oral cavity Z86.003
        respiratory system Z86.005
        skin Z86.007
        specified NEC Z86.008
        stomach Z86.003
      malignant —*see* History of, malignant
        neoplasm
      uncertain behavior Z86.03
    nephrotic syndrome Z87.441
    nicotine dependence Z87.891
    noncompliance with medical treatment or
      regimen —*see* Noncompliance
    nutritional deficiency Z86.39
    obstetric complications Z87.59
      childbirth Z87.59
      pregnancy Z87.59
      pre-term labor Z87.51
      puerperium Z87.59
    osteoporosis fractures Z87.31
    parasuicide (attempt) Z91.51
    physical trauma NEC Z87.828
      self-harm or suicide attempt Z91.51
    pneumonia (recurrent) Z87.01
    poisoning NEC Z91.89
      self-harm or suicide attempt Z91.51
    poor personal hygiene Z91.89
    preterm labor Z87.51
    procedure during pregnancy Z98.870
    procedure while a fetus Z98.871
    prolonged reversible ischemic neurologic
      deficit (PRINO) Z86.73
    prostatic dysplasia Z87.430
    psychiatric disorder NEC Z87.89
    psychological
      abuse
        adult Z91.411
        child Z62.811
      trauma, specified NEC Z91.49
    radiation therapy Z92.3
    removal
      implant
        breast Z98.86
    renal calculi Z87.442
    respiratory condition NEC Z87.09
    retained foreign body fully removed
      Z87.821
    risk factors NEC Z91.89
    SARS-CoV-2 infection Z86.16
    self-harm
      nonsuicidal Z91.52
      suicidal Z91.51
    self-inflicted injury without suicidal intent
      Z91.52
    self-injury
      nonsuicidal Z91.52
    self-mutilation Z91.52
    self-poisoning attempt Z91.51
      suicidal behavior Z91.51
    sex reassignment Z87.890

History *(Continued)*
  personal *(Continued)*
    sleep-wake cycle problem Z72.821
    specified NEC Z87.898
    steroid therapy (systemic) Z92.241
      inhaled Z92.240
    stroke without residual deficits Z86.73
    substance abuse NEC F10-F19
    sudden cardiac arrest Z86.74
    sudden cardiac death successfully
      resuscitated Z86.74
    suicide attempt Z91.51
    surgery NEC Z98.890
      with uterine scar Z98.891
      sex reassignment Z87.890
      transplant —see Transplant
    thrombophlebitis Z86.72
    thrombosis (venous) Z86.718
      pulmonary Z86.711
    tobacco dependence Z87.891
    transient ischemic attack (TIA) without
      residual deficits Z86.73
    trauma (physical) NEC Z87.828
      psychological NEC Z91.49
      self-harm Z91.51
    traumatic brain injury Z87.820
    tuberculosis, latent infection Z86.15
    unhealthy sleep-wake cycle Z72.821
    unintended awareness under general
      anesthesia Z92.84
    urinary (recurrent) (tract) infection(s) Z87.440
    urinary calculi Z87.42
    uterine scar from previous surgery Z98.891
    vaginal dysplasia Z87.411
    venous thrombosis or embolism Z86.718
      pulmonary Z86.711
    vulvar dysplasia Z87.412
His-Werner disease A79.0
HIV —see also Human, immunodeficiency virus B20
  laboratory evidence (nonconclusive) R75
  nonconclusive test (in infants) R75
  positive, seropositive Z21
Hives (bold) —see Urticaria
Hoarseness R49.0
Hobo Z59.00
Hodgkin disease —see Lymphoma, Hodgkin
~~Hodgson's disease I71.2~~
~~ruptured I71.1~~
►Hodgson's (see also Aneurysm, aorta, thorax) I71.20
  ►ruptured (see also Aneurysm, aorta, thorax, ruptured) I71.10
Hoffa-Kastert disease E88.89
Hoffa's disease E88.89
Hoffmann-Bouveret syndrome I47.9
Hoffmann's syndrome E03.9 [G73.7]
Hole (round)
  macula H35.34-●
  retina (without detachment) —see Break, retina, round hole
    with detachment —see Detachment, retina, with retinal, break
Holiday relief care Z75.5
Hollenhorst's plaque —see Occlusion, artery, retina
Hollow foot (congenital) Q66.7-●
  acquired —see Deformity, limb, foot, specified NEC
Holoprosencephaly Q04.2
Holt-Oram syndrome Q87.2
Homelessness Z59.00
  sheltered Z59.01
  unsheltered Z59.02
Homesickness —see Disorder, adjustment
Homocysteinemia R79.83
Homocystinemia, homocystinuria E72.11
Homogentisate 1,2-dioxygenase deficiency E70.29
Homologous serum hepatitis (prophylactic) (therapeutic) —see Hepatitis, viral, type B
Honeycomb lung J98.4
  congenital Q33.0

Hooded
  clitoris Q52.6
  penis Q55.69
Hookworm (disease) (infection) (infestation) B76.9
  with anemia B76.9 [D63.8]
  specified NEC B76.8
Hordeolum (eyelid) (externum) (recurrent) H00.019
  internum H00.029
    left H00.026
      lower H00.025
      upper H00.024
    right H00.023
      lower H00.022
      upper H00.021
  left H00.016
    lower H00.015
    upper H00.014
  right H00.013
    lower H00.012
    upper H00.011
Horn
  cutaneous L85.8
  nail L60.2
    congenital Q84.6
Horner (-Claude Bernard) syndrome G90.2
  traumatic —see Injury, nerve, cervical sympathetic
Horseshoe kidney (congenital) Q63.1
Horton's headache or neuralgia G44.099
  intractable G44.091
  not intractable G44.099
Hospital hopper syndrome —see Disorder, factitious
Hospitalism in children —see Disorder, adjustment
Hostility R45.5
  towards child Z62.3
Hot flashes
  menopausal N95.1
Hourglass (contracture) —see also Contraction, hourglass
  stomach K31.89
    congenital Q40.2
    stricture K31.2
Household, housing circumstance affecting care Z59.9
  specified NEC Z59.89
Housemaid's knee —see Bursitis, prepatellar
HSCT-TMA (hematopoietic stem cell transplantation-associated thrombotic microangiopathy) M31.11
Hudson (-Stähli) line (cornea) —see Pigmentation, cornea, anterior
Human
  bite (open wound) —see also Bite
    intact skin surface —see Bite, superficial
  herpesvirus —see Herpes
  immunodeficiency virus (HIV) disease (infection) B20
    asymptomatic status Z21
    contact Z20.6
    counseling Z71.7
    ⇒dementia (see also Dementia, in, diseases specified elsewhere) B20 [F02.80]
      ⇒with behavioral disturbance (see also Dementia, in, diseases specified elsewhere) B20 [F02.81-●]
    exposure to Z20.6
    laboratory evidence R75
    type-2 (HIV 2) as cause of disease classified elsewhere B97.35
  papillomavirus (HPV)
    DNA test positive
      high risk
        cervix R87.810
        vagina R87.811
      low risk
        cervix R87.820
        vagina R87.821
    screening for Z11.51

Human *(Continued)*
  T-cell lymphotropic virus
    type-1 (HTLV-I) infection B33.3
      as cause of disease classified elsewhere B97.33
      carrier Z22.6
    type-2 (HTLV-II) as cause of disease classified elsewhere B97.34
Humidifier lung or pneumonitis J67.7
Humiliation (experience) in childhood Z62.898
Humpback (acquired) —see Kyphosis
Hunchback (acquired) —see Kyphosis
Hunger T73.0
  air, psychogenic F45.8
Hungry bone syndrome E83.81
Hunner's ulcer —see Cystitis, chronic, interstitial
Hunter's
  glossitis D51.0
  syndrome E76.1
Huntington's disease or chorea G10
⇒with dementia (see also Dementia, in, diseases specified elsewhere) G10 [F02.80]
  ⇒with behavioral disturbance (see also Dementia, in, diseases specified elsewhere) G10 [F02.81-●]
Hunt's
  disease or syndrome (herpetic geniculate ganglionitis) B02.21
  dyssynergia cerebellaris myoclonica G11.19
  neuralgia B02.21
Hurler (-Scheie) disease or syndrome E76.02
Hurst's disease G36.1
Hurthle cell
  adenocarcinoma C73
  adenoma D34
  carcinoma C73
  tumor D34
Hutchinson-Boeck disease or syndrome —see Sarcoidosis
Hutchinson-Gilford disease or syndrome E34.8
Hutchinson's
  disease, meaning
    angioma serpiginosum L81.7
    pompholyx (cheiropompholyx) L30.1
    prurigo estivalis L56.4
    summer eruption or summer prurigo L56.4
  melanotic freckle —see Melanoma, in situ
    malignant melanoma in —see Melanoma
  teeth or incisors (congenital syphilis) A50.52
  triad (congenital syphilis) A50.53
Hyalin plaque, sclera, senile H15.89
Hyaline membrane (disease) (lung) (pulmonary) (newborn) P22.0
Hyalinosis
  cutis (et mucosae) E78.89
  focal and segmental (glomerular) —see also N00-N07 with fourth character .1 N05.1
Hyalitis, hyalosis, asteroid —see also Deposit, crystalline
  syphilitic (late) A52.71
Hydatid
  cyst or tumor —see Echinococcus
  mole —see Hydatidiform mole
  Morgagni
    female Q50.5
    male (epididymal) Q55.4
    testicular Q55.29
Hydatidiform mole (benign) (complicating pregnancy) (delivered) (undelivered) O01.9
  classical O01.0
  complete O01.0
  incomplete O01.1
  invasive D39.2
  malignant D39.2
  partial O01.1
Hydatidosis —see Echinococcus
Hydradenitis (axillaris) (suppurative) L73.2
Hydradenoma —see Hidradenoma
Hydramnios O40.-●
Hydrancephaly, hydranencephaly Q04.3
  with spina bifida —see Spina bifida, with hydrocephalus
Hydrargyrism NEC —see Poisoning, mercury

► New   ⇒ Revised   ~~deleted~~ Deleted   ● Use Additional Character(s)

Hydrarthrosis —*see also* Effusion, joint
  gonococcal A54.42
  intermittent M12.40
    ankle M12.47-•
    elbow M12.42-•
    foot joint M12.47-•
    hand joint M12.44-•
    hip M12.45-•
    knee M12.46-•
    multiple site M12.49
    shoulder M12.41-•
    specified joint NEC M12.48
    wrist M12.43-•
  of yaws (early) (late) —*see also* subcategory
    M14.8-• A66.6
  syphilitic (late) A52.77
    congenital A50.55 [*M12.80*]
Hydremia D64.89
Hydrencephalocele (congenital) —*see*
  Encephalocele
Hydrencephalomeningocele (congenital) —*see*
  Encephalocele
Hydroa R23.8
  aestivale L56.4
  vacciniforme L56.4
Hydroadenitis (axillaris) (suppurative) L73.2
Hydrocalycosis —*see* Hydronephrosis
Hydrocele (spermatic cord) (testis) (tunica
    vaginalis) N43.3
  canal of Nuck N94.89
  communicating N43.2
    congenital P83.5
  congenital P83.5
  encysted N43.0
  female NEC N94.89
  infected N43.1
  newborn P83.5
  round ligament N94.89
  specified NEC N43.2
  spinalis —*see* Spina bifida
  vulva N90.89
Hydrocephalus (acquired) (external) (internal)
    (malignant) (recurrent) G91.9
  aqueduct Sylvius stricture Q03.0
  causing disproportion O33.6
    with obstructed labor O66.3
  communicating G91.0
  congenital (external) (internal) Q03.9
    with spina bifida Q05.4
      cervical Q05.0
      dorsal Q05.1
      lumbar Q05.2
      lumbosacral Q05.2
      sacral Q05.3
      thoracic Q05.1
      thoracolumbar Q05.1
    specified NEC Q03.8
  due to toxoplasmosis (congenital) P37.1
  foramen Magendie block (acquired) G91.1
    congenital —*see also* Hydrocephalus,
      congenital Q03.1
  in (due to)
    infectious disease NEC B89 [*G91.4*]
    neoplastic disease NEC (*see also* Neoplasm)
      G91.4
    parasitic disease B89 [*G91.4*]
  newborn Q03.9
    with spina bifida —*see* Spina bifida, with
      hydrocephalus
  noncommunicating G91.1
  normal pressure G91.2
    secondary G91.0
  obstructive G91.1
  otitic G93.2
  post-traumatic NEC G91.3
  secondary G91.4
    post-traumatic G91.3
  specified NEC G91.8
  syphilitic, congenital A50.49
Hydrocolpos (congenital) N89.8
Hydrocystoma —*see* Neoplasm, skin, benign
Hydroencephalocele (congenital) —*see*
  Encephalocele

Hydroencephalomeningocele (congenital) —
  see Encephalocele
Hydrohematopneumothorax —*see* Hemothorax
Hydromeningitis —*see* Meningitis
Hydromeningocele (spinal) —*see also* Spina bifida
  cranial —*see* Encephalocele
Hydrometra N85.8
Hydrometrocolpos N89.8
Hydromicrocephaly Q02
Hydromphalos (since birth) Q45.8
Hydromyelia Q06.4
Hydromyelocele —*see* Spina bifida
Hydronephrosis (atrophic) (early)
    (functionless) (intermittent) (primary)
    (secondary) NEC N13.30
  with
    infection N13.6
    obstruction (by) (of)
      renal calculus N13.2
        with infection N13.6
      ureteral NEC N13.1
        with infection N13.6
        calculus N13.2
          with infection N13.6
      ureteropelvic junction (congenital) Q62.11
        acquired N13.0
          with infection N13.6
      ureteral stricture NEC N13.1
        with infection N13.6
  congenital Q62.0
    due to acquired occlusion of ureteropelvic
      junction N13.0
  specified type NEC N13.39
  tuberculous A18.11
Hydropericarditis —*see* Pericarditis
Hydropericardium —*see* Pericarditis
Hydroperitoneum R18.8
Hydrophobia —*see* Rabies
Hydrophthalmos Q15.0
Hydropneumohemothorax —*see* Hemothorax
Hydropneumopericarditis —*see* Pericarditis
Hydropneumopericardium —*see* Pericarditis
Hydropneumothorax J94.8
  traumatic —*see* Injury, intrathoracic, lung
  tuberculous NEC A15.6
Hydrops R60.9
  abdominis R18.8
  articulorum intermittens —*see* Hydrarthrosis,
    intermittent
  cardiac —*see* Failure, heart, congestive
  causing obstructed labor (mother) O66.3
  endolymphatic H81.0-•
  fetal —*see* Pregnancy, complicated by,
    hydrops, fetalis
  fetalis P83.2
    due to
      ABO isoimmunization P56.0
      alpha thalassemia D56.0
      hemolytic disease P56.90
        specified NEC P56.99
      isoimmunization (ABO) (Rh) P56.0
      other specified nonhemolytic disease
        NEC P83.2
      Rh incompatibility P56.0
    during pregnancy —*see* Pregnancy,
      complicated by, hydrops, fetalis
  gallbladder K82.1
  joint —*see* Effusion, joint
  labyrinth H81.0
  newborn (idiopathic) P83.2
    due to
      ABO isoimmunization P56.0
      alpha thalassemia D56.0
      hemolytic disease P56.90
        specified NEC P56.99
      isoimmunization (ABO) (Rh) P56.0
      Rh incompatibility P56.0
  nutritional —*see* Malnutrition, severe
  pericardium —*see* Pericarditis
  pleura —*see* Hydrothorax
  spermatic cord —*see* Hydrocele
Hydropyonephrosis N13.6
Hydrorachis Q06.4

Hydrorrhea (nasal) J34.89
  pregnancy —*see* Rupture, membranes,
    premature
Hydrosadenitis (axillaris) (suppurative) L73.2
Hydrosalpinx (fallopian tube) (follicularis) N70.11
Hydrothorax (double) (pleura) J94.8
  chylous (nonfilarial) I89.8
    filarial —*see also* Infestation, filarial B74.9
      [*I91.8*]
  traumatic —*see* Injury, intrathoracic
  tuberculous NEC (non primary) A15.6
Hydroureter —*see also* Hydronephrosis N13.4
  with infection N13.6
  congenital Q62.39
Hydroureteronephrosis —*see* Hydronephrosis
Hydrourethra N36.8
Hydroxykynureninuria E70.89
Hydroxylysinemia E72.3
Hydroxyprolinemia E72.59
Hygiene, sleep
  abuse Z72.821
  inadequate Z72.821
  poor Z72.821
Hygroma (congenital) (cystic) D18.1
  praepatellare, prepatellar —*see* Bursitis,
    prepatellar
Hymen —*see* condition
Hymenolepis, hymenolepiasis (diminuta)
    (infection) (infestation) (nana) B71.0
Hypalgesia R20.8
Hyperacidity (gastric) K31.89
  psychogenic F45.8
Hyperactive, hyperactivity F90.9
  basal cell, uterine cervix —*see* Dysplasia, cervix
  bowel sounds R19.12
  cervix epithelial (basal) —*see* Dysplasia, cervix
  child F90.9
    attention deficit —*see* Disorder, attention-
      deficit hyperactivity
  detrusor muscle N32.81
  gastrointestinal K31.89
    psychogenic F45.8
  nasal mucous membrane J34.3
  stomach K31.89
  thyroid (gland) —*see* Hyperthyroidism
Hyperacusis H93.23-•
Hyperadrenalism E27.5
Hyperadrenocorticism E24.9
  congenital E25.0
  iatrogenic E24.2
    correct substance properly administered —
      see Table of Drugs and Chemicals, by
      drug, adverse effect
    overdose or wrong substance given
      or taken —*see* Table of Drugs and
      Chemicals, by drug, poisoning
  not associated with Cushing's syndrome
    E27.0
  pituitary-dependent E24.0
Hyperaldosteronism E26.9
  familial (type I) E26.02
  glucocorticoid-remediable E26.02
  primary (due to (bilateral) adrenal
    hyperplasia) E26.09
  primary NEC E26.09
  secondary E26.1
  specified NEC E26.89
Hyperalgesia R20.8
Hyperalimentation R63.2
  carotene, carotin E67.1
  specified NEC E67.8
  vitamin
    A E67.0
    D E67.3
Hyperaminoaciduria
  arginine E72.21
  cystine E72.01
  lysine E72.3
  ornithine E72.4
Hyperammonemia (congenital) E72.20
Hyperazotemia —*see* Uremia
Hyperbetalipoproteinemia (familial) E78.00
  with prebetalipoproteinemia E78.2

Hyperbilirubinemia
constitutional E80.6
familial conjugated E80.6
neonatal (transient) —*see* Jaundice, newborn
Hypercalcemia, hypocalciuric, familial E83.52
Hypercalciuria, idiopathic R82.994
Hypercapnia R06.89
newborn P84
Hypercarotenemia (dietary) E67.1
Hypercementosis K03.4
Hyperchloremia E87.8
Hyperchlorhydria K31.89
neurotic F45.8
psychogenic F45.8
Hypercholesterinemia —*see*
Hypercholesterolemia
Hypercholesterolemia (essential) (primary)
(pure) E78.00
with hyperglyceridemia, endogenous E78.2
dietary counseling and surveillance Z71.3
familial E78.01
hereditary E78.01
Hyperchylia gastrica, psychogenic F45.8
Hyperchylomicronemia (familial) (primary) E78.3
with hyperbetalipoproteinemia E78.3
Hypercoagulable (state) D68.59
activated protein C resistance D68.51
antithrombin (III) deficiency D68.59
factor V Leiden mutation D68.51
primary NEC D68.59
protein C deficiency D68.59
protein S deficiency D68.59
prothrombin gene mutation D68.52
secondary D68.69
specified NEC D68.69
Hypercoagulation (state) D68.59
Hypercorticalism, pituitary-dependent E24.0
Hypercorticosolism —*see* Cushing's, syndrome
Hypercorticosteronism E24.2
correct substance properly administered —*see*
Table of Drugs and Chemicals, by drug,
adverse effect
overdose or wrong substance given
or taken —*see* Table of Drugs and
Chemicals, by drug, poisoning
Hypercortisonism E24.2
correct substance properly administered —*see*
Table of Drugs and Chemicals, by drug,
adverse effect
overdose or wrong substance given
or taken —*see* Table of Drugs and
Chemicals, by drug, poisoning
Hyperekplexia Q89.8
Hyperelectrolytemia E87.8
Hyperemesis R11.10
with nausea R11.2
gravidarum (mild) O21.0
with
carbohydrate depletion O21.1
dehydration O21.1
electrolyte imbalance O21.1
metabolic disturbance O21.1
severe (with metabolic disturbance) O21.1
projectile R11.12
psychogenic F45.8
Hyperemia (acute) (passive) R68.89
anal mucosa K62.89
bladder N32.89
cerebral I67.89
conjunctiva H11.43-●
ear internal, acute —*see* subcategory H83.0
enteric K59.89
eye —*see* Hyperemia, conjunctiva
eyelid (active) (passive) —*see* Disorder,
eyelid, specified type NEC
intestine K59.89
iris —*see* Disorder, iris, vascular
kidney N28.89
labyrinth —*see* subcategory H83.0
liver (active) K76.89
lung (passive) —*see* Edema, lung
pulmonary (passive) —*see* Edema, lung
renal N28.89

Hyperemia (*Continued*)
retina H35.89
stomach K31.89
Hyperesthesia (body surface) R20.3
larynx (reflex) J38.7
hysterical F44.89
pharynx (reflex) J39.2
hysterical F44.89
Hyperestrogenism (drug-induced) (iatrogenic)
E28.0
Hyperexplexia Q89.8
Hyperfibrinolysis —*see* Fibrinolysis
Hyperfructosemia E74.19
Hyperfunction
adrenal cortex, not associated with Cushing's
syndrome E27.0
medulla E27.5
adrenomedullary E27.5
virilism E25.9
congenital E25.0
ovarian E28.8
pancreas K86.89
parathyroid (gland) E21.3
pituitary (gland) (anterior) E22.9
specified NEC E22.8
polyglandular E31.1
testicular E29.0
Hypergammaglobulinemia D89.2
polyclonal D89.0
Waldenström D89.0
Hypergastrinemia E16.4
Hyperglobulinemia R77.1
Hyperglycemia, hyperglycemic (transient)
R73.9
coma —*see* Diabetes, by type, with coma
postpancreatectomy E89.1
Hyperglyceridemia (endogenous) (essential)
(familial) (hereditary) (pure) E78.1
mixed E78.3
Hyperglycinemia (non-ketotic) E72.51
Hypergonadism
ovarian E28.8
testicular (primary) (infantile) E29.0
Hyperheparinemia D68.32
Hyperhidrosis, hyperidrosis R61
focal
primary L74.519
axilla L74.510
face L74.511
palms L74.512
soles L74.513
secondary L74.52
generalized R61
localized
primary L74.519
axilla L74.510
face L74.511
palms L74.512
soles L74.513
secondary L74.52
psychogenic F45.8
secondary R61
focal L74.52
Hyperhistidinemia E70.41
Hyperhomocysteinemia E72.11
Hyperhydroxyprolinemia E72.59
Hyperinsulinism (functional) E16.1
with
coma (hypoglycemic) E15
encephalopathy E16.1 [*G94*]
ectopic E16.1
therapeutic misadventure (from administration
of insulin) —*see* subcategory T38.3
Hyperkalemia E87.5
Hyperkeratosis —*see also* Keratosis L85.9
cervix N88.0
due to yaws (early) (late) (palmar or plantar)
A66.3
follicularis Q82.8
penetrans (in cutem) L87.0
palmoplantaris climacterica L85.1
pinta A67.1
senile (with pruritus) L57.0

Hyperkeratosis (*Continued*)
universalis congenita Q80.8
vocal cord J38.3
vulva N90.4
Hyperkinesia, hyperkinetic (disease) (reaction)
(syndrome) (childhood) (adolescence) —
see also Disorder, attention-deficit
hyperactivity
heart I51.89
Hyperleucine-isoleucinemia E71.19
Hyperlipemia, hyperlipidemia E78.5
combined E78.2
familial E78.49
group
A E78.00
B E78.1
C E78.2
D E78.3
mixed E78.2
specified NEC E78.49
Hyperlipidosis E75.6
hereditary NEC E75.5
Hyperlipoproteinemia E78.5
Fredrickson's type
I E78.3
IIa E78.00
IIb E78.2
III E78.2
IV E78.1
V E78.3
low-density-lipoprotein-type (LDL) E78.00
very-low-density-lipoprotein-type (VLDL)
E78.1
Hyperlucent lung, unilateral J43.0
Hyperlysinemia E72.3
Hypermagnesemia E83.41
neonatal P71.8
Hypermenorrhea N92.0
Hypermethioninemia E72.19
Hypermetropia (congenital) H52.0-●
Hypermobility, hypermotility
cecum —*see* Syndrome, irritable bowel
coccyx —*see* subcategory M53.2
colon —*see* Syndrome, irritable bowel
psychogenic F45.8
ileum K58.9
intestine —*see also* Syndrome, irritable bowel
K58.9
psychogenic F45.8
meniscus (knee) —*see* Derangement, knee,
meniscus
scapula —*see* Instability, joint, shoulder
stomach K31.89
psychogenic F45.8
syndrome M35.7
urethra N36.41
with intrinsic sphincter deficiency N36.43
Hypernasality R49.21
Hypernatremia E87.0
Hypernephroma C64.-●
Hyperopia —*see* Hypermetropia
Hyperorexia nervosa F50.2
Hyperornithinemia E72.4
Hyperosmia R43.1
Hyperosmolality E87.0
Hyperostosis (monomelic) —*see also* Disorder,
bone, density and structure, specified NEC
ankylosing (spine) M48.10
cervical region M48.12
cervicothoracic region M48.13
lumbar region M48.16
lumbosacral region M48.17
multiple sites M48.19
occipito-atlanto-axial region M48.11
sacrococcygeal region M48.18
thoracic region M48.14
thoracolumbar region M48.15
cortical (skull) M85.2
infantile M89.8X-●
frontal, internal of skull M85.2
interna frontalis M85.2

▶ New   ⇒ Revised   ~~deleted~~ Deleted   ● Use Additional Character(s)

Hyperostosis (Continued)
- skeletal, diffuse idiopathic —see Hyperostosis, ankylosing
- skull M85.2
  - congenital Q75.8
- vertebral, ankylosing —see Hyperostosis, ankylosing

Hyperovarism E28.8
Hyperoxaluria (primary) R82.992
Hyperparathyroidism E21.3
- primary E21.0
- secondary (renal) N25.81
  - non-renal E21.1
- specified NEC E21.2
- tertiary E21.2

Hyperpathia R20.8
Hyperperistalsis R19.2
- psychogenic F45.8

Hyperpermeability, capillary I78.8
Hyperphagia R63.2
Hyperphenylalaninemia NEC E70.1
Hyperphoria (alternating) H50.53
Hyperphosphatemia E83.39
Hyperpiesis, hyperpiesia —see Hypertension
Hyperpigmentation —see also Pigmentation
- melanin NEC L81.4
- postinflammatory L81.0

Hyperpinealism E34.8
Hyperpituitarism E22.9
Hyperplasia, hyperplastic
- adenoids J35.2
- adrenal (capsule) (cortex) (gland) E27.8
  - with
    - sexual precocity (male) E25.9
      - congenital E25.0
    - virilism, adrenal E25.9
      - congenital E25.0
    - virilization (female) E25.9
      - congenital E25.0
  - congenital E25.0
  - salt-losing E25.0
- adrenomedullary E27.5
- angiolymphoid, eosinophilia (ALHE) D18.01
- appendix (lymphoid) K38.0
- artery, fibromuscular I77.3
- bone —see also Hypertrophy, bone
  - marrow D75.89
- breast —see also Hypertrophy, breast
  - atypical, atypia N60.9-●
    - ductal N60.9-●
    - lobular N60.9-●
- C-cell, thyroid E07.0
- cementation (tooth) (teeth) K03.4
- cervical gland R59.0
- cervix (uteri) (basal cell) (endometrium) (polypoid) —see also Dysplasia, cervix
  - congenital Q51.828
- clitoris, congenital Q52.6
- denture K06.2
- endocervicitis N72
- endometrium, endometrial (adenomatous) (cystic) (glandular) (glandular-cystic) (polypoid) N85.00
  - with atypia N85.02
  - benign N85.01
  - cervix —see Dysplasia, cervix
  - complex (without atypia) N85.01
  - simple (without atypia) N85.01
- epithelial L85.9
  - focal, oral, including tongue K13.29
  - nipple N62
  - skin L85.9
  - tongue K13.29
  - vaginal wall N89.3
- erythroid D75.89
- fibromuscular of artery (carotid) (renal) I77.3
- genital
  - female NEC N94.89
  - male N50.89
- gingiva K06.1

Hyperplasia, hyperplastic
- glandularis cystica uteri (interstitialis) —see also Hyperplasia, endometrial N85.00-●
- gum K06.1
- hymen, congenital Q52.4
- irritative, edentulous (alveolar) K06.2
- jaw M26.09
  - alveolar M26.79
  - lower M26.03
    - alveolar M26.72
  - upper M26.01
    - alveolar M26.71
- kidney (congenital) Q63.3
- labia N90.69
  - epithelial N90.3
- liver (congenital) Q44.7
  - nodular, focal K76.89
- lymph gland or node R59.9
- mandible, mandibular M26.03
  - alveolar M26.72
  - unilateral condylar M27.8
- maxilla, maxillary M26.01
  - alveolar M26.71
- myometrium, myometrial N85.2
- neuroendocrine cell, of infancy J84.841
- nose
  - lymphoid J34.89
  - polypoid J33.9
- oral mucosa (irritative) K13.6
- organ or site, congenital NEC —see Anomaly, by site
- ovary N83.8
- palate, papillary (irritative) K13.6
- pancreatic islet cells E16.9
  - alpha E16.8
    - with excess
      - gastrin E16.4
      - glucagon E16.3
  - beta E16.1
- parathyroid (gland) E21.0
- pharynx (lymphoid) J39.2
- prostate (adenofibromatous) (nodular) N40.0
  - with lower urinary tract symptoms (LUTS) N40.1
  - without lower urinary tract symptoms (LUTS) N40.0
- renal artery I77.89
- reticulo-endothelial (cell) D75.89
- salivary gland (any) K11.1
- Schimmelbusch's —see Mastopathy, cystic
- suprarenal capsule (gland) E27.8
- thymus (gland) (persistent) E32.0
- thyroid (gland) —see Goiter
- tonsils (faucial) (infective) (lingual) (lymphoid) J35.1
  - with adenoids J35.3
- unilateral condylar M27.8
- uterus, uterine N85.2
  - endometrium (glandular) —see also Hyperplasia, endometrial N85.00-●
- vulva N90.69
  - epithelial N90.3

Hyperpnea —see Hyperventilation
Hyperpotassemia E87.5
Hyperprebetalipoproteinemia (familial) E78.1
Hyperprolactinemia E22.1
Hyperprolinemia (type I) (type II) E72.59
Hyperproteinemia E88.09
Hyperprothrombinemia, causing coagulation factor deficiency D68.4
Hyperpyrexia R50.9
- heat (effects) T67.01
- malignant, due to anesthetic T88.3
- rheumatic —see Fever, rheumatic
- unknown origin R50.9

Hyper-reflexia R29.2
Hypersalivation K11.7

Hypersecretion
- ACTH (not associated with Cushing's syndrome) E27.0
  - pituitary E24.0
- adrenaline E27.5
- adrenomedullary E27.5
- androgen (testicular) E29.0
  - ovarian (drug-induced) (iatrogenic) E28.1
- calcitonin E07.0
- catecholamine E27.5
- corticoadrenal E24.9
- cortisol E24.9
- epinephrine E27.5
- estrogen E28.0
- gastric K31.89
  - psychogenic F45.8
- gastrin E16.4
- glucagon E16.3
- hormone(s)
  - ACTH (not associated with Cushing's syndrome) E27.0
    - pituitary E24.0
  - antidiuretic E22.2
  - growth E22.0
  - intestinal NEC E34.1
  - ovarian androgen E28.1
  - pituitary E22.9
  - testicular E29.0
  - thyroid stimulating E05.80
    - with thyroid storm E05.81
- insulin —see Hyperinsulinism
- lacrimal glands —see Epiphora
- medulloadrenal E27.5
- milk O92.6
- ovarian androgens E28.1
- salivary gland (any) K11.7
- thyrocalcitonin E07.0
- upper respiratory J39.8

Hypersegmentation, leukocytic, hereditary D72.0
Hypersensitive, hypersensitiveness, hypersensitivity —see also Allergy
- carotid sinus G90.01
- colon —see Irritable, colon
- drug T88.7
- gastrointestinal K52.29
  - immediate K52.29
  - psychogenic F45.8
- labyrinth —see subcategory H83.2
- pain R20.8
- pneumonitis —see Pneumonitis, allergic
- reaction T78.40
  - upper respiratory tract NEC J39.3

Hypersomnia (organic) G47.10
- due to
  - alcohol
    - abuse F10.182
    - dependence F10.282
    - use F10.982
  - amphetamines
    - abuse F15.182
    - dependence F15.282
    - use F15.982
  - caffeine
    - abuse F15.182
    - dependence F15.282
    - use F15.982
  - cocaine
    - abuse F14.182
    - dependence F14.282
    - use F14.982
  - drug NEC
    - abuse F19.182
    - dependence F19.282
    - use F19.982
  - medical condition G47.14
  - mental disorder F51.13
  - opioid
    - abuse F11.182
    - dependence F11.282
    - use F11.982

▶ New   ⇒ Revised   ~~deleted~~ Deleted   ● Use Additional Character(s)

Hypersomnia *(Continued)*
 due to *(Continued)*
  psychoactive substance NEC
   abuse F19.182
   dependence F19.282
   use F19.982
  sedative, hypnotic, or anxiolytic
   abuse F13.182
   dependence F13.282
   use F13.982
  stimulant NEC
   abuse F15.182
   dependence F15.282
   use F15.982
 idiopathic G47.11
  with long sleep time G47.11
  without long sleep time G47.12
 menstrual related G47.13
 nonorganic origin F51.11
  specified NEC F51.19
 not due to a substance or known
   physiological condition F51.11
  specified NEC F51.19
 primary F51.11
 recurrent G47.13
 specified NEC G47.19
Hypersplenia, hypersplenism D73.1
Hyperstimulation, ovaries (associated with
  induced ovulation) N98.1
Hypersusceptibility —*see* Allergy
Hypertelorism (ocular) (orbital) Q75.2
Hypertension, hypertensive (accelerated)
  (benign) (essential) (idiopathic)
  (malignant) (systemic) I10
 with
  heart failure (congestive) I11.0
  heart involvement (conditions in I50.-
   or I51.4-I51.7, I51.89, I51.9, due to
   hypertension) —*see* Hypertension,
   heart
  kidney involvement —*see* Hypertension,
   kidney
 benign, intracranial G93.2
 borderline R03.0
 cardiorenal (disease) I13.10
  with heart failure I13.0
   with stage 1 through stage 4 chronic
    kidney disease I13.0
   with stage 5 or end stage renal disease
    I13.2
  without heart failure I13.10
   with stage 1 through stage 4 chronic
    kidney disease I13.10
   with stage 5 or end stage renal disease
    I13.11
 cardiovascular
  disease (arteriosclerotic) (sclerotic) —*see*
   Hypertension, heart
  renal (disease) —*see* Hypertension,
   cardiorenal
 chronic venous —*see* Hypertension, venous
  (chronic)
 complicating
  childbirth (labor) O16.4
   pre-existing O10.92
    with
     heart disease O10.12
      with renal disease O10.32
     pre-eclampsia O11.4
     renal disease O10.22
      with heart disease O10.32
     essential O10.02
    secondary O10.42
   pregnancy O16.-●
    with edema —*see also* Pre-eclampsia
     O14.9-●
    gestational (pregnancy induced)
     (without proteinuria) O13.-●
     with proteinuria O14.9-●
      mild pre-eclampsia O14.0-●
      moderate pre-eclampsia O14.0-●

Hypertension, hypertensive *(Continued)*
 complicating *(Continued)*
  pregnancy *(Continued)*
   gestational (pregnancy induced)
    (Continued)
    with proteinuria *(Continued)*
     severe pre-eclampsia O14.1-●
      with hemolysis, elevated liver
       enzymes and low platelet
       count (HELLP) O14.2-●
   pre-existing O10.91-●
    with
     heart disease O10.11-●
      with renal disease O10.31-●
     pre-eclampsia —*see* category O11
     renal disease O10.21-●
      with heart disease O10.31-●
    essential O10.01-●
    secondary O10.41-●
   transient O13.-●
  puerperium pre-existing O16.5
   pre-existing
    with
     heart disease O10.13
      with renal disease O10.33
     pre-eclampsia O11.5
     renal disease O10.23
      with heart disease O10.33
    essential O10.03
   pregnancy-induced O13.9
   secondary O10.43
 crisis I16.9
 due to
  endocrine disorders I15.2
  pheochromocytoma I15.2
  renal disorders NEC I15.1
   arterial I15.0
  renovascular disorders I15.0
  specified disease NEC I15.8
 emergency I16.1
 encephalopathy I67.4
 gestational (without significant proteinuria)
   (pregnancy-induced) (transient)
   O13.-●
  with significant proteinuria —*see*
   Pre-eclampsia
  complicating
   delivery O13.4
   puerperium O13.5
 Goldblatt's I70.1
 heart (disease) (conditions in I51.4-I51.9 due
   to hypertension) I11.9
  with
   heart failure (congestive) I11.0
   kidney disease (chronic) —*see*
    Hypertension, cardiorenal
 intracranial, benign G93.2
 kidney I12.9
  with
   heart disease —*see* Hypertension,
    cardiorenal
   stage 1 through stage 4 chronic kidney
    disease I12.9
   stage 5 chronic kidney disease (CKD) or
    end stage renal disease (ESRD) I12.0
 lesser circulation I27.0

 maternal O16.-●
 newborn P29.2
  pulmonary (persistent) P29.30
 ocular H40.05-●
 pancreatic duct — code to underlying
   condition
  with chronic pancreatitis K86.1
 portal (due to chronic liver disease)
   (idiopathic) K76.6
  gastropathy K31.89
  in (due to) schistosomiasis (bilharziasis)
   B65.9 *[K77]*
 postoperative I97.3
 psychogenic F45.8

Hypertension, hypertensive *(Continued)*
 pulmonary NEC I27.20
  with
   cor pulmonale (chronic) I27.29
    acute I26.09
   right heart ventricular strain/failure
    I27.29
    acute I26.09
   right to left shunt related to congenital
    heart disease I27.83
   unclear multifactorial mechanisms
    I27.29
  arterial (associated) (drug-induced) (toxin-
   induced) I27.21
  chronic thromboembolic I27.24
  due to
   hematologic disorders I27.29
   kyphoscoliotic heart disease I27.1
   left heart disease I27.22
   lung diseases and hypoxia I27.23
   metabolic disorders I27.29
   specified systemic disorders NEC I27.29
  group 1 (associated) (drug-induced) (toxin-
   induced) I27.21
  group 2 I27.22
  group 3 I27.23
  group 4 I27.24
  group 5 I27.29
  of newborn (persistent) P29.30
  secondary
   arterial I27.21
   specified NEC I27.29
  primary (idiopathic) I27.0
 renal —*see* Hypertension, kidney
 renovascular I15.0
 secondary NEC I15.9
  due to
   endocrine disorders I15.2
   pheochromocytoma I15.2
   renal disorders NEC I15.1
    arterial I15.0
   renovascular disorders I15.0
  specified NEC I15.8
 transient R03.0
  of pregnancy O13.●
 urgency I16.0
 venous (chronic)
  due to
   deep vein thrombosis —*see* Syndrome,
    postthrombotic
  idiopathic I87.309
   with
    inflammation I87.32-●
     with ulcer I87.33-●
    specified complication NEC I87.39-●
    ulcer I87.31-●
     with inflammation I87.33-●
   asymptomatic I87.30-●
Hypertensive urgency —*see* Hypertension
Hyperthecosis ovary E28.8
Hyperthermia (of unknown origin) —*see also*
  Hyperpyrexia
 malignant, due to anesthesia T88.3
 newborn P81.9
  environmental P81.0
Hyperthyroid (recurrent) —*see* Hyperthyroidism
Hyperthyroidism (latent) (pre-adult) (recurrent)
  E05.90
 with
  goiter (diffuse) E05.00
   with thyroid storm E05.01
   nodular (multinodular) E05.20
    with thyroid storm E05.21
    uninodular E05.10
     with thyroid storm E05.11
  storm E05.91
 due to ectopic thyroid tissue E05.30
  with thyroid storm E05.31
 neonatal, transitory P72.1
 specified NEC E05.80
  with thyroid storm E05.81

▶ New   ⇒ Revised   ~~deleted~~ Deleted   ● Use Additional Character(s)

Hypertony, hypertonia, hypertonicity
bladder N31.8
congenital P94.1
stomach K31.89
psychogenic F45.8
uterus, uterine (contractions) (complicating
delivery) O62.4
Hypertrichosis L68.9
congenital Q84.2
eyelid H02.869
left H02.866
lower H02.865
upper H02.864
right H02.863
lower H02.862
upper H02.861
lanuginosa Q84.2
acquired L68.1
localized L68.2
specified NEC L68.8
Hypertriglyceridemia, essential E78.1
Hypertrophy, hypertrophic
adenofibromatous, prostate —*see*
Enlargement, enlarged, prostate
adenoids (infective) J35.2
with tonsils J35.3
adrenal cortex E27.8
alveolar process or ridge —*see* Anomaly,
alveolar
anal papillae K62.89
artery I77.89
congenital NEC Q27.8
digestive system Q27.8
lower limb Q27.8
specified site NEC Q27.8
upper limb Q27.8
auricular —*see* Hypertrophy, cardiac
Bartholin's gland N75.8
bile duct (common) (hepatic) K83.8
bladder (sphincter) (trigone) N32.89
bone M89.30
carpus M89.34-●
clavicle M89.31-●
femur M89.35-●
fibula M89.36-●
finger M89.34-●
humerus M89.32-●
ilium M89.359
ischium M89.359
metacarpus M89.34-●
metatarsus M89.37-●
multiple sites M89.39
neck M89.38
radius M89.33-●
rib M89.38
scapula M89.31-●
skull M89.38
tarsus M89.37-●
tibia M89.36-●
toe M89.37-●
ulna M89.33-●
vertebra M89.38
brain G93.89
breast N62
cystic —*see* Mastopathy, cystic
newborn P83.4
pubertal, massive N62
puerperal, postpartum —*see* Disorder,
breast, specified type NEC
senile (parenchymatous) N62
cardiac (chronic) (idiopathic) I51.7
with rheumatic fever (conditions in I00)
active I01.8
inactive or quiescent (with chorea) I09.89
congenital NEC Q24.8
fatty —*see* Degeneration, myocardial
hypertensive —*see* Hypertension, heart
rheumatic (with chorea) I09.89
active or acute I01.8
with chorea I02.0
valve —*see* Endocarditis

Hypertrophy, hypertrophic *(Continued)*
cartilage —*see* Disorder, cartilage, specified
type NEC
cecum —*see* Megacolon
cervix (uteri) N88.8
congenital Q51.828
elongation N88.4
clitoris (cirrhotic) N90.89
congenital Q52.6
colon —*see also* Megacolon
congenital Q43.2
conjunctiva, lymphoid H11.89
corpora cavernosa N48.89
cystic duct K82.8
duodenum K31.89
endometrium (glandular) —*see also*
Hyperplasia, endometrial N85.00-●
cervix N88.8
epididymis N50.89
esophageal hiatus (congenital) Q79.1
with hernia —*see* Hernia, hiatal
eyelid —*see* Disorder, eyelid, specified type
NEC
facet joint (see also Spondylosis) M47.819
fat pad E65
knee (infrapatellar) (popliteal) (prepatellar)
(retropatellar) M79.4
foot (congenital) Q74.2
frenulum, frenum (tongue) K14.8
lip K13.0
gallbladder K82.8
gastric mucosa K29.60
with bleeding K29.61
gland, glandular R59.9
generalized R59.1
localized R59.0
gum (mucous membrane) K06.1
heart (idiopathic) —*see also* Hypertrophy,
cardiac
valve —*see also* Endocarditis I38
hemifacial Q67.4
hepatic —*see* Hypertrophy, liver
hiatus (esophageal) Q79.1
hilus gland R59.0
hymen, congenital Q52.4
ileum K63.89
intestine NEC K63.89
jejunum K63.89
kidney (compensatory) N28.81
congenital Q63.3
labium (majus) (minus) N90.60
ligament —*see* Disorder, ligament
lingual tonsil (infective) J35.1
with adenoids J35.3
lip K13.0
congenital Q18.6
liver R16.0
acute K76.89
cirrhotic —*see* Cirrhosis, liver
congenital Q44.7
fatty —*see* Fatty, liver
lymph, lymphatic gland R59.9
generalized R59.1
localized R59.0
tuberculous —*see* Tuberculosis, lymph
gland
mammary gland —*see* Hypertrophy, breast
Meckel's diverticulum (congenital) Q43.0
malignant —*see* Table of Neoplasms, small
intestine, malignant
median bar —*see* Hyperplasia, prostate
meibomian gland —*see* Chalazion
meniscus, knee, congenital Q74.1
metatarsal head —*see* Hypertrophy, bone,
metatarsus
metatarsus —*see* Hypertrophy, bone,
metatarsus
mucous membrane
alveolar ridge K06.2
gum K06.1
nose (turbinate) J34.3

Hypertrophy, hypertrophic *(Continued)*
muscle M62.89
muscular coat, artery I77.89
myocardium —*see also* Hypertrophy, cardiac
idiopathic I42.2
myometrium N85.2
nail L60.2
congenital Q84.5
nasal J34.89
alae J34.89
bone J34.89
cartilage J34.89
mucous membrane (septum) J34.3
sinus J34.89
turbinate J34.3
nasopharynx, lymphoid (infectional) (tissue)
(wall) J35.2
nipple N62
organ or site, congenital NEC —*see* Anomaly,
by site - ovary N83.8
palate (hard) M27.8
soft K13.79
pancreas, congenital Q45.3
parathyroid (gland) E21.0
parotid gland K11.1
penis N48.89
pharyngeal tonsil J35.2
pharynx J39.2
lymphoid (infectional) (tissue) (wall)
J35.2
pituitary (anterior) (fossa) (gland) E23.6
prepuce (congenital) N47.8
female N90.89
prostate —*see* Enlargement, enlarged,
prostate
congenital Q55.4
pseudomuscular (*see also* Dystrophy,
muscular, by type, if applicable)
pylorus (adult) (muscle) (sphincter) K31.1
congenital or infantile Q40.0
rectal, rectum (sphincter) K62.89
rhinitis (turbinate) J31.0
salivary gland (any) K11.1
congenital Q38.4
scaphoid (tarsal) —*see* Hypertrophy, bone,
tarsus
scar L91.0
scrotum N50.89
seminal vesicle N50.89
sigmoid —*see* Megacolon
skin L91.9
specified NEC L91.8
spermatic cord N50.89
spleen —*see* Splenomegaly
spondylitis —*see* Spondylosis
stomach K31.89
sublingual gland K11.1
submandibular gland K11.1
suprarenal cortex (gland) E27.8
synovial NEC M67.20
acromioclavicular M67.21-●
ankle M67.27-●
elbow M67.22-●
foot M67.27-●
hand M67.24-●
hip M67.25-●
knee M67.26-●
multiple sites M67.29
specified site NEC M67.28
wrist M67.23-●
tendon —*see* Disorder, tendon, specified type
NEC
testis N44.8
congenital Q55.29
thymic, thymus (gland) (congenital)
E32.0
thyroid (gland) —*see* Goiter
toe (congenital) Q74.2
acquired —*see also* Deformity, toe, specified
NEC

Hypertrophy, hypertrophic *(Continued)*
  tongue *(Continued)*
    congenital Q38.2
    papillae (foliate) K14.3
  tonsils (faucial) (infective) (lingual) (lymphoid) J35.1
    with adenoids J35.3
  tunica vaginalis N50.89
  ureter N28.89
  urethra N36.8
  uterus N85.2
    neck (with elongation) N88.4
    puerperal O90.89
  uvula K13.79
  vagina N89.8
  vas deferens N50.89
  vein I87.8
  ventricle, ventricular (heart) —*see also* Hypertrophy, cardiac
    congenital Q24.8
    in tetralogy of Fallot Q21.3
  verumontanum N36.8
  vocal cord J38.3
  vulva N90.60
    stasis (nonfilarial) N90.69
Hypertropia H50.2-●
Hypertyrosinemia E70.21
Hyperuricemia (asymptomatic) E79.0
Hyperuricosuria R82.993
Hypervalinemia E71.19
Hyperventilation (tetany) R06.4
  hysterical F45.8
  psychogenic F45.8
  syndrome F45.8
Hypervitaminosis (dietary) NEC E67.8
  A E67.0
    administered as drug (prolonged intake) — *see* Table of Drugs and Chemicals, vitamins, adverse effect
    overdose or wrong substance given or taken —*see* Table of Drugs and Chemicals, vitamins, poisoning
  B6 E67.2
  D E67.3
    administered as drug (prolonged intake) — *see* Table of Drugs and Chemicals, vitamins, adverse effect
    overdose or wrong substance given or taken —*see* Table of Drugs and Chemicals, vitamins, poisoning
  K E67.8
    administered as drug (prolonged intake) — *see* Table of Drugs and Chemicals, vitamins, adverse effect
    overdose or wrong substance given or taken —*see* Table of Drugs and Chemicals, vitamins, poisoning
Hypervolemia E87.70
  specified NEC E87.79
Hypesthesia R20.1
  cornea —*see* Anesthesia, cornea
Hyphema H21.0-●
  traumatic S05.1-●
Hypoacidity, gastric K31.89
  psychogenic F45.8
Hypoadrenalism, hypoadrenia E27.40
  primary E27.1
  tuberculous A18.7
Hypoadrenocorticism E27.40
  pituitary E23.0
  primary E27.1
Hypoalbuminemia E88.09
Hypoaldosteronism E27.40
Hypoalphalipoproteinemia E78.6
Hypobarism T70.29
Hypobaropathy T70.29
Hypobetalipoproteinemia (familial) E78.6
Hypocalcemia E83.51
  dietary E58
  neonatal P71.1
    due to cow's milk P71.0
  phosphate-loading (newborn) P71.1

Hypochloremia E87.8
Hypochlorhydria K31.89
  neurotic F45.8
  psychogenic F45.8
Hypochondria, hypochondriac, hypochondriasis (reaction) F45.21
  sleep F51.03
Hypochondrogenesis Q77.0
Hypochondroplasia Q77.4
Hypochromasia, blood cells D50.8
Hypodontia —*see* Anodontia
Hypocitraturia R82.991
Hypoeosinophilia D72.89
Hypoesthesia R20.1
Hypofibrinogenemia D68.8
  acquired D65
  congenital (hereditary) D68.2
Hypofunction
  adrenocortical E27.40
    drug-induced E27.3
    postprocedural E89.6
    primary E27.1
  adrenomedullary, postprocedural E89.6
  cerebral R29.818
  corticoadrenal NEC E27.40
  intestinal K59.89
  labyrinth —*see* subcategory H83.2
  ovary E28.39
  pituitary (gland) (anterior) E23.0
  testicular E29.1
    postprocedural (postsurgical) (postirradiation) (iatrogenic) E89.5
Hypogalactia O92.4
Hypogammaglobulinemia —*see also* Agammaglobulinemia D80.1
  hereditary D80.0
  nonfamilial D80.1
  transient, of infancy D80.7
Hypogenitalism (congenital) —*see* Hypogonadism
Hypoglossia Q38.3
Hypoglycemia (spontaneous) E16.2
  coma E15
    diabetic —*see* Diabetes, by type, with hypoglycemia, with coma
  diabetic —*see* Diabetes, hypoglycemia
  dietary counseling and surveillance Z71.3
  drug-induced E16.0
    with coma (nondiabetic) E15
  due to insulin E16.0
    with coma (nondiabetic) E15
    therapeutic misadventure —*see* subcategory T38.3
  functional, nonhyperinsulinemic E16.1
  iatrogenic E16.0
    with coma (nondiabetic) E15
  in infant of diabetic mother P70.1
    gestational diabetes P70.0
  infantile E16.1
  leucine-induced E71.19
  neonatal (transitory) P70.4
    iatrogenic P70.3
  reactive (not drug-induced) E16.1
  transitory neonatal P70.4
Hypogonadism
  female E28.39
  hypogonadotropic E23.0
  male E29.1
  ovarian (primary) E28.39
  pituitary E23.0
  testicular (primary) E29.1
Hypohidrosis, hypoidrosis L74.4
Hypoinsulinemia, postprocedural E89.1
Hypokalemia E87.6
Hypoleukocytosis —*see* Agranulocytosis
Hypolipoproteinemia (alpha) (beta) E78.6
Hypomagnesemia E83.42
  neonatal P71.2
Hypomania, hypomanic reaction F30.8
Hypomenorrhea —*see* Oligomenorrhea

Hypometabolism R63.8
Hypomotility
  gastrointestinal (tract) K31.89
    psychogenic F45.8
  intestine K59.89
    psychogenic F45.8
  stomach K31.89
    psychogenic F45.8
Hyponasality R49.22
Hyponatremia E87.1
Hypo-osmolality E87.1
Hypo-ovarianism, hypo-ovarism E28.39
Hypoparathyroidism E20.9
  familial E20.8
  idiopathic E20.0
  neonatal, transitory P71.4
  postprocedural E89.2
  specified NEC E20.8
Hypoperfusion (in)
  newborn P96.89
Hypopharyngitis —*see* Laryngopharyngitis
Hypophoria H50.53
Hypophosphatemia, hypophosphatasia (acquired) (congenital) (renal) E83.39
  familial E83.31
Hypophyseal, hypophysis —*see also* condition
  dwarfism E23.0
  gigantism E22.0
Hypopiesis —*see* Hypotension
Hypopinealism E34.8
Hypopituitarism (juvenile) E23.0
  drug-induced E23.1
  due to
    hypophysectomy E89.3
    radiotherapy E89.3
  iatrogenic NEC E23.1
  postirradiation E89.3
  postpartum O99.285
  postprocedural E89.3
Hypoplasia, hypoplastic
  adrenal (gland), congenital Q89.1
  alimentary tract, congenital Q45.8
    upper Q40.8
  anus, anal (canal) Q42.3
    with fistula Q42.2
  aorta, aortic Q25.42
    ascending, in hypoplastic left heart syndrome Q23.4
    valve Q23.1
      in hypoplastic left heart syndrome Q23.4
  areola, congenital Q83.8
  arm (congenital) —*see* Defect, reduction, upper limb
  artery (peripheral) Q27.8
    brain (congenital) Q28.3
    coronary Q24.5
    digestive system Q27.8
    lower limb Q27.8
    pulmonary Q25.79
      functional, unilateral J43.0
    retinal (congenital) Q14.1
    specified site NEC Q27.8
    umbilical Q27.0
    upper limb Q27.8
  auditory canal Q17.8
    causing impairment of hearing Q16.9
  biliary duct or passage Q44.5
  bone NOS Q79.9
    face Q75.8
    marrow D61.9
      megakaryocytic D69.49
    skull —*see* Hypoplasia, skull
  brain Q02
    gyri Q04.3
    part of Q04.3
  breast (areola) N64.82
  bronchus Q32.4
  cardiac Q24.8

▶ New   ⇒ Revised   ~~deleted~~ Deleted   ● Use Additional Character(s)

Hypoplasia, hypoplastic *(Continued)*
carpus —*see* Defect, reduction, upper limb,
    specified type NEC
cartilage hair Q78.8
cecum Q42.8
cementum K00.4
cephalic Q02
cerebellum Q04.3
cervix (uteri), congenital Q51.821
clavicle (congenital) Q74.0
coccyx Q76.49
colon Q42.9
    specified NEC Q42.8
corpus callosum Q04.0
cricoid cartilage Q31.2
digestive organ(s) or tract NEC Q45.8
    upper (congenital) Q40.8
ear (auricle) (lobe) Q17.2
    middle Q16.4
enamel of teeth (neonatal) (postnatal)
    (prenatal) K00.4
endocrine (gland) NEC Q89.2
endometrium N85.8
epididymis (congenital) Q55.4
epiglottis Q31.2
erythroid, congenital D61.01
esophagus (congenital) Q39.8
eustachian tube Q17.8
eye Q11.2
eyelid (congenital) Q10.3
face Q18.8
    bone(s) Q75.8
femur (congenital) —*see* Defect, reduction,
    lower limb, specified type NEC
fibula (congenital) —*see* Defect, reduction,
    lower limb, specified type NEC
finger (congenital) —*see* Defect, reduction,
    upper limb, specified type NEC
focal dermal Q82.8
foot —*see* Defect, reduction, lower limb,
    specified type NEC
gallbladder Q44.0
genitalia, genital organ(s)
    female, congenital Q52.8
        external Q52.79
        internal NEC Q52.8
    in adiposogenital dystrophy E23.6
glottis Q31.2
hair Q84.2
hand (congenital) —*see* Defect, reduction,
    upper limb, specified type NEC
heart Q24.8
humerus (congenital) —*see* Defect, reduction,
    upper limb, specified type NEC
intestine (small) Q41.9
    large Q42.9
        specified NEC Q42.8
jaw M26.09
    alveolar M26.79
    lower M26.04
        alveolar M26.74
    upper M26.02
        alveolar M26.73
kidney(s) Q60.5
    bilateral Q60.4
    unilateral Q60.3
labium (majus) (minus), congenital Q52.79
larynx Q31.2
left heart syndrome Q23.4
leg (congenital) —*see* Defect, reduction, lower
    limb
limb Q73.8
    lower (congenital) —*see* Defect, reduction,
        lower limb
    upper (congenital) —*see* Defect, reduction,
        upper limb
liver Q44.7
lung (lobe) (not associated with short
    gestation) Q33.6
    associated with immaturity, low birth
        weight, prematurity, or short gestation
        P28.0

Hypoplasia, hypoplastic *(Continued)*
mammary (areola), congenital Q83.8
mandible, mandibular M26.04
    alveolar M26.74
    unilateral condylar M27.8
maxillary M26.02
    alveolar M26.73
medullary D61.9
megakaryocytic D69.49
metacarpus —*see* Defect, reduction, upper
    limb, specified type NEC
metatarsus —*see* Defect, reduction, lower
    limb, specified type NEC
muscle Q79.8
nail(s) Q84.6
nose, nasal Q30.1
optic nerve H47.03-•
osseous meatus (ear) Q17.8
ovary, congenital Q50.39
pancreas Q45.0
parathyroid (gland) Q89.2
parotid gland Q38.4
patella Q74.1
pelvis, pelvic girdle Q74.2
penis (congenital) Q55.62
peripheral vascular system Q27.8
    digestive system Q27.8
    lower limb Q27.8
    specified site NEC Q27.8
    upper limb Q27.8
pituitary (gland) (congenital) Q89.2
pulmonary (not associated with short
    gestation) Q33.6
    artery, functional J43.0
    associated with short gestation P28.0
radioulnar —*see* Defect, reduction, upper
    limb, specified type NEC
radius —*see* Defect, reduction, upper limb
rectum Q42.1
    with fistula Q42.0
respiratory system NEC Q34.8
rib Q76.6
right heart syndrome Q22.6
sacrum Q76.49
scapula Q74.0
scrotum Q55.1
shoulder girdle Q74.0
skin Q82.8
skull (bone) Q75.8
    with
        anencephaly Q00.0
        encephalocele —*see* Encephalocele
        hydrocephalus Q03.9
            with spina bifida —*see* Spina bifida, by
                site, with hydrocephalus
        microcephaly Q02
spinal (cord) (ventral horn cell) Q06.1
spine Q76.49
sternum Q76.7
tarsus —*see* Defect, reduction, lower limb,
    specified type NEC
testis Q55.1
thymic, with immunodeficiency D82.1
thymus (gland) Q89.2
    with immunodeficiency D82.1
thyroid (gland) E03.1
    cartilage Q31.2
tibiofibular (congenital) —*see* Defect,
    reduction, lower limb, specified type
    NEC
toe —*see* Defect, reduction, lower limb,
    specified type NEC
tongue Q38.3
Turner's K00.4
ulna (congenital) —*see* Defect, reduction,
    upper limb
umbilical artery Q27.0
unilateral condylar M27.8
ureter Q62.8
uterus, congenital Q51.811
vagina Q52.4

Hypoplasia, hypoplastic *(Continued)*
vascular NEC peripheral Q27.8
    brain Q28.3
    digestive system Q27.8
    lower limb Q27.8
    specified site NEC Q27.8
    upper limb Q27.8
vein(s) (peripheral) Q27.8
    brain Q28.3
    digestive system Q27.8
    great Q26.8
    lower limb Q27.8
    specified site NEC Q27.8
    upper limb Q27.8
vena cava (inferior) (superior) Q26.8
vertebra Q76.49
vulva, congenital Q52.79
zonule (ciliary) Q12.8
Hypoplasminogenemia E88.02
Hypopnea, obstructive sleep apnea G47.33
Hypopotassemia E87.6
Hypoproconvertinemia, congenital
    (hereditary) D68.2
Hypoproteinemia E77.8
Hypoprothrombinemia (congenital)
    (hereditary) (idiopathic) D68.2
    acquired D68.4
    newborn, transient P61.6
Hypoptyalism K11.7
Hypopyon (eye) (anterior chamber) —*see*
    Iridocyclitis, acute, hypopyon
Hypopyrexia R68.0
Hyporeflexia R29.2
Hyposecretion
    ACTH E23.0
    antidiuretic hormone E23.2
    ovary E28.39
    salivary gland (any) K11.7
    vasopressin E23.2
Hyposegmentation, leukocytic, hereditary
    D72.0
Hyposiderinemia D50.9
Hyposplenism D73.0
Hypospadias Q54.9
    balanic Q54.0
    coronal Q54.0
    glandular Q54.0
    penile Q54.1
    penoscrotal Q54.2
    perineal Q54.3
    specified NEC Q54.8
Hypospermatogenesis —*see* Oligospermia
Hyposplenism D73.0
Hypostasis pulmonary, passive —*see* Edema,
    lung
Hypostatic —*see* condition
Hyposthenuria N28.89
Hypotension (arterial) (constitutional) I95.9
    chronic I95.89
    drug-induced I95.2
    due to (of) hemodialysis I95.3
    iatrogenic I95.89
    idiopathic (permanent) I95.0
    intracranial G96.810
        following
            lumbar cerebrospinal fluid shunting
                G97.83
            specified procedure NEC G97.84
            ventricular shunting (ventriculostomy)
                G97.2
        specified NEC G96.819
        spontaneous G96.811
    intra-dialytic I95.3
    maternal, syndrome (following labor and
        delivery) O26.5-•
    neurogenic, orthostatic G90.3
    orthostatic (chronic) I95.1
        due to drugs I95.2
        neurogenic G90.3
    postoperative I95.81
    postural I95.1
    specified NEC I95.89

Hypothermia (accidental) T68
  due to anesthesia, anesthetic T88.51
  low environmental temperature T68
  neonatal P80.9
    environmental (mild) NEC P80.8
    mild P80.8
    severe (chronic) (cold injury syndrome)
      P80.0
    specified NEC P80.8
  not associated with low environmental
    temperature R68.0
Hypothyroidism (acquired) E03.9
  autoimmune —see Thyroiditis, autoimmune
  congenital (without goiter) E03.1
    with goiter (diffuse) E03.0
  due to
    exogenous substance NEC E03.2
    iodine-deficiency, acquired E01.8
      subclinical E02
    irradiation therapy E89.0
    medicament NEC E03.2
    P-aminosalicylic acid (PAS) E03.2
    phenylbutazone E03.2
    resorcinol E03.2
    sulfonamide E03.2
    surgery E89.0
    thiourea group drugs E03.2

Hypothyroidism (Continued)
  iatrogenic NEC E03.2
  iodine-deficiency (acquired) E01.8
    congenital —see Syndrome, iodine-
      deficiency, congenital
    subclinical E02
  neonatal, transitory P72.2
  postinfectious E03.3
  postirradiation E89.0
  postprocedural E89.0
  postsurgical E89.0
  specified NEC E03.8
  subclinical, iodine-deficiency related E02
Hypotonia, hypotonicity, hypotony
  bladder N31.2
  congenital (benign) P94.2
  eye —see Disorder, globe, hypotony
Hypotrichosis —see Alopecia
Hypotropia H50.2-●
Hypoventilation R06.89
  congenital central alveolar G47.35
  sleep related
    idiopathic nonobstructive alveolar
      G47.34
    in conditions classified elsewhere G47.36

Hypovitaminosis —see Deficiency, vitamin
Hypovolemia E86.1
  surgical shock T81.19
  traumatic (shock) T79.4
Hypoxemia R09.02
  newborn P84
  sleep related, in conditions classified
    elsewhere G47.36
Hypoxia —see also Anoxia R09.02
  cerebral, during a procedure NEC G97.81
    postprocedural NEC G97.82
  intrauterine P84
  myocardial —see Insufficiency, coronary
  newborn P84
  sleep-related G47.34
Hypsarhythmia —see Epilepsy, generalized,
    specified NEC
Hysteralgia, pregnant uterus O26.89-●
Hysteria, hysterical (conversion) (dissociative
    state) F44.9
  anxiety F41.8
  convulsions F44.5
  psychosis, acute F44.9
Hysteroepilepsy F44.5

▶ New   ⇒ Revised   ~~deleted~~ Deleted   ● Use Additional Character(s)

I

IBDU (colonic inflammatory bowel disease unclassified) K52.3
ICANS (immune effector cell-associated neurotoxicity syndrome) —see Syndrome, immune effector cell-associated neurotoxicity
Ichthyoparasitism due to Vandellia cirrhosa B88.8
Ichthyosis (congenital) Q80.9
  acquired L85.0
  fetalis Q80.4
  hystrix Q80.8
  lamellar Q80.2
  lingual K13.29
  palmaris and plantaris Q82.8
  simplex Q80.0
  vera Q80.8
  vulgaris Q80.0
  X-linked Q80.1
Ichthyotoxism —see Poisoning, fish
  bacterial —see Intoxication, foodborne
Icteroanemia, hemolytic (acquired) D59.9
  congenital —see Spherocytosis
Icterus —see also Jaundice
  conjunctiva R17
  gravis, newborn P55.0
  hematogenous (acquired) D59.9
  hemolytic (acquired) D59.9
    congenital —see Spherocytosis
  hemorrhagic (acute) (leptospiral) (spirochetal) A27.0
    newborn P53
  infectious B15.9
    with hepatic coma B15.0
    leptospiral A27.0
    spirochetal A27.0
  neonatorum —see Jaundice, newborn
  newborn P59.9
  spirochetal A27.0
Ictus solaris, solis T67.01
Ideation
  homicidal R45.850
  suicidal R45.851
Identity disorder (child) F64.9
  gender role F64.2
  psychosexual F64.2
Idioglossia F80.0
Idiopathic —see condition
Idiot, idiocy (congenital) F73
  amaurotic (Bielschowsky(-Jansky)) (family) (infantile (late)) (juvenile (late)) (Vogt-Spielmeyer) E75.4
  microcephalic Q02
Id reaction (due to bacteria) L30.2
IgE asthma J45.909
IIAC (idiopathic infantile arterial calcification) Q28.8
Ileitis (chronic) (noninfectious) —see also Enteritis K52.9
  backwash —see Pancolitis, ulcerative (chronic)
  infectious A09
  regional (ulcerative) —see Enteritis, regional, small intestine
  segmental —see Enteritis, regional
  terminal (ulcerative) —see Enteritis, regional, small intestine
Ileocolitis —see also Enteritis K52.9
  infectious A09
  regional —see Enteritis, regional
  ulcerative K51.0-●
Ileostomy
  attention to Z43.2
  malfunctioning K94.13
  status Z93.2
  with complication —see Complications, enterostomy
Ileotyphus —see Typhoid
Ileum —see condition
Ileus (bowel) (colon) (inhibitory) (intestine) K56.7
  adynamic K56.0

Ileus (Continued)
  due to gallstone (in intestine) K56.3
  duodenal (chronic) K31.5
  gallstone K56.3
  mechanical NEC —see also Obstruction, intestine, specified K56.699
  meconium P76.0
    in cystic fibrosis E84.11
    meaning meconium plug (without cystic fibrosis) P76.0
  myxedema K59.89
  neurogenic K56.0
    Hirschsprung's disease or megacolon Q43.1
  newborn
    due to meconium P76.0
      in cystic fibrosis E84.11
      meaning meconium plug (without cystic fibrosis) P76.0
    transitory P76.1
  obstructive —see also Obstruction, intestine, specified K56.699
  paralytic K56.0
  postoperative K91.89
Iliac —see condition
Iliotibial band syndrome M76.3-●
Illiteracy Z55.0
Illness—see also Disease R69
  manic-depressive —see Disorder, bipolar
Imbalance R26.89
  autonomic G90.8
  constituents of food intake E63.1
  electrolyte E87.8
    with
      abortion —see Abortion by type, complicated by, electrolyte imbalance
      molar pregnancy O08.5
    due to hyperemesis gravidarum O21.1
    following ectopic or molar pregnancy O08.5
    neonatal, transitory NEC P74.49
      potassium
        hyperkalemia P74.31
        hypokalemia P74.32
      sodium
        hypernatremia P74.21
        hyponatremia P74.22
  endocrine E34.9
  eye muscle NOS H50.9
  hormone E34.9
  hysterical F44.4
  labyrinth —see subcategory H83.2
  posture R29.3
  protein-energy —see Malnutrition
  sympathetic G90.8
Imbecile, imbecility (I.Q. 35-49) F71
Imbedding, intrauterine device T83.39
Imbibition, cholesterol (gallbladder) K82.4
Imbrication, teeth, fully erupted M26.30
Imerslund (-Gräsbeck) syndrome D51.1
Immature —see also Immaturity
  birth (less than 37 completed weeks) —see Preterm, newborn
    extremely (less than 28 completed weeks) —see Immaturity, extreme
  personality F60.89
Immaturity (less than 37 completed weeks) —see also Preterm, newborn
  extreme of newborn (less than 28 completed weeks of gestation) (less than 196 completed days of gestation) (unspecified weeks of gestation) P07.20
    gestational age
      23 completed weeks (23 weeks, 0 days through 23 weeks, 6 days) P07.22
      24 completed weeks (24 weeks, 0 days through 24 weeks, 6 days) P07.23
      25 completed weeks (25 weeks, 0 days through 25 weeks, 6 days) P07.24
      26 completed weeks (26 weeks, 0 days through 26 weeks, 6 days) P07.25
      27 completed weeks (27 weeks, 0 days through 27 weeks, 6 days) P07.26
      less than 23 completed weeks P07.21

Immaturity (Continued)
  fetus or infant light-for-dates —see Light-for-dates
  lung, newborn P28.0
  organ or site NEC —see Hypoplasia
  pulmonary, newborn P28.0
  reaction F60.89
  sexual (female) (male), after puberty E30.0
Immersion T75.1
  foot T69.02-●
  hand T69.01-●
Immobile, immobility
  complete, due to severe physical disability or frailty R53.2
  intestine K59.89
  syndrome (paraplegic) M62.3
Immune reconstitution (inflammatory) syndrome [IRIS] D89.3
Immunization —see also Vaccination
  ABO —see Incompatibility, ABO
    in newborn P55.1
  appropriate for age
    child (over 28 days old) Z00.129
      with abnormal findings Z00.121
  complication —see Complications, vaccination
  encounter for Z23
  not done (not carried out) Z28.9
    because (of)
      acute illness of patient Z28.01
      allergy to vaccine (or component) Z28.04
      caregiver refusal Z28.82
      chronic illness of patient Z28.02
      contraindication NEC Z28.09
      delay in delivery of vaccine Z28.83
      group pressure Z28.1
      guardian refusal Z28.82
      immune compromised state of patient Z28.03
      lack of availability of vaccine Z28.83
      manufacturer delay of vaccine Z28.83
      parent refusal Z28.82
      patient's belief Z28.1
      patient had disease being vaccinated against Z28.81
      patient refusal Z28.21
      religious beliefs of patient Z28.1
      specified reason NEC Z28.89
        of patient Z28.29
      unavailability of vaccine Z28.83
      unspecified patient reason Z28.20
  Rh factor
    affecting management of pregnancy NEC O36.09-●
    anti-D antibody O36.01-●
    from transfusion —see Complication(s), transfusion, incompatibility reaction, Rh (factor)
Immunocompromised NOS D84.9
Immunocytoma C83.0-●
Immunodeficiency D84.9
  with
    adenosine-deaminase deficiency (see also Deficiency, adenosine deaminase) D81.30
    antibody defects D80.9
      specified type NEC D80.8
    hyperimmunoglobulinemia D80.6
    increased immunoglobulin M (IgM) D80.5
    major defect D82.9
      specified type NEC D82.8
    partial albinism D82.8
    short-limbed stature D82.2
    thrombocytopenia and eczema D82.0
  antibody with
    hyperimmunoglobulinemia D80.6
    near-normal immunoglobulins D80.6
  autosomal recessive, Swiss type D80.0

Immunodeficiency (Continued)
  combined D81.9
    biotin-dependent carboxylase D81.819
      biotinidase D81.810
      holocarboxylase synthetase D81.818
      specified type NEC D81.818
    severe (SCID) D81.9
      with
        low or normal B-cell numbers D81.2
        low T- and B-cell numbers D81.1
        reticular dysgenesis D81.0
      specified type NEC D81.89
  common variable D83.9
    with
      abnormalities of B-cell numbers and
        function D83.0
      autoantibodies to B- or T-cells D83.2
      immunoregulatory T-cell disorders
        D83.1
    specified type NEC D83.8
  due to
    conditions classified elsewhere D84.81
    drugs D84.821
    external causes D84.822
    medication (current or past) D84.821
  following hereditary defective response to
    Epstein-Barr virus (EBV) D82.3
  selective, immunoglobulin
    A (IgA) D80.2
    G (IgG) (subclasses) D80.3
    M (IgM) D80.4
  severe combined (SCID) D81.9
    due to adenosine deaminase deficiency
      D81.31
  specified type NEC D84.89
  X-linked, with increased IgM D80.5
Immunodeficient NOS D84.9
Immunosuppressed NOS D84.9
Immunotherapy (encounter for)
  antineoplastic Z51.12
Impaction, impacted
  bowel, colon, rectum —see also Impaction,
    fecal K56.49
    by gallstone K56.3
  calculus —see Calculus
  cerumen (ear) (external) H61.2-●
  cuspid —see Impaction, tooth
  dental (same or adjacent tooth) K01.1
  fecal, feces K56.41
  fracture —see Fracture, by site
  gallbladder —see Calculus, gallbladder
  gallstone(s) —see Calculus, gallbladder
    bile duct (common) (hepatic) —see
      Calculus, bile duct
    cystic duct —see Calculus, gallbladder
    in intestine, with obstruction (any part)
      K56.3
  intestine (calculous) NEC —see also
    Impaction, fecal K56.49
    gallstone, with ileus K56.3
  intrauterine device (IUD) T83.39
  molar —see Impaction, tooth
  shoulder, causing obstructed labor O66.0
  tooth, teeth K01.1
  turbinate J34.89
Impaired, impairment (function)
  auditory discrimination —see Abnormal,
    auditory perception
  cognitive, mild, so stated G31.84
  ▶cognitive, mild, of uncertain or unknown
    etiology G31.84
  dual sensory Z73.82
  fasting glucose R73.01
  glucose tolerance (oral) R73.02
  hearing —see Deafness
  heart —see Disease, heart
  kidney N28.9
    disorder resulting from N25.9
      specified NEC N25.89
  liver K72.90
    with coma K72.91

Impaired, impairment (Continued)
  mastication K08.89
  mild cognitive, so stated G31.84
  ▶mild cognitive G31.84
    ▶of uncertain or unknown etiology G31.84
  ▶mild neurocognitive
    ▶due to known physiological condition
      (without behavioral disturbance) F06.70
    ▶with behavioral disturbance F06.71
  mobility
    ear ossicles —see Ankylosis, ear ossicles
    requiring care provider Z74.09
  myocardium, myocardial —see Insufficiency,
    myocardial
  rectal sphincter R19.8
  renal (acute) (chronic) N28.9
    disorder resulting from N25.9
      specified NEC N25.89
  vision NEC H54.7
    both eyes H54.3
Impediment, speech (see also Disorder, speech)
  R47.9
  psychogenic (childhood) F98.8
  slurring R47.81
  specified NEC R47.89
Impending
  coronary syndrome I20.0
  delirium tremens F10.239
  myocardial infarction I20.0
Imperception auditory (acquired) —see also
  Deafness
  congenital H93.25
Imperfect
  aeration, lung (newborn) NEC —see
    Atelectasis
  closure (congenital)
    alimentary tract NEC Q45.8
      lower Q43.8
      upper Q40.8
    ⇒atrioventricular ostium NEC Q21.20
    ⇒atrium (secundum) Q21.11
    branchial cleft NOS Q18.2
      cyst Q18.0
      fistula Q18.0
      sinus Q18.0
    choroid Q14.3
    cricoid cartilage Q31.8
    cusps, heart valve NEC Q24.8
      pulmonary Q22.3
    ductus
      arteriosus Q25.0
      Botalli Q25.0
    ear drum (causing impairment of hearing)
      Q16.4
    esophagus with communication to
      bronchus or trachea Q39.1
    eyelid Q10.3
    foramen
      ⇒botalli Q21.12
      ⇒ovale Q21.12
    genitalia, genital organ(s) or system
      female Q52.8
        external Q52.79
        internal NEC Q52.8
      male Q55.8
    glottis Q31.8
    ⇒interatrial ostium or septum Q21.19
    ⇒interauricular ostium or septum Q21.19
    interventricular ostium or septum Q21.0
    larynx Q31.8
    lip —see Cleft, lip
    nasal septum Q30.3
    nose Q30.2
    omphalomesenteric duct Q43.0
    optic nerve entry Q14.2
    organ or site not listed —see Anomaly,
      by site
    ostium
      ⇒interatrial Q21.19
      ⇒interauricular Q21.19
      interventricular Q21.0

Imperfect (Continued)
  closure (Continued)
    palate —see Cleft, palate
    preauricular sinus Q18.1
    retina Q14.1
    roof of orbit Q75.8
    sclera Q13.5
    septum
      aorticopulmonary Q21.4
      ⇒atrial (secundum) Q21.19
      between aorta and pulmonary artery
        Q21.4
      heart Q21.9
      ⇒interatrial (secundum) Q21.19
      ⇒interauricular (secundum) Q21.19
      interventricular Q21.0
        in tetralogy of Fallot Q21.3
      nasal Q30.3
      ventricular Q21.0
        with pulmonary stenosis or atresia,
          dextraposition of aorta, and
          hypertrophy of right ventricle
          Q21.3
        in tetralogy of Fallot Q21.3
    skull Q75.0
      with
        anencephaly Q00.0
        encephalocele —see Encephalocele
        hydrocephalus Q03.9
          with spina bifida —see Spina bifida,
            by site, with hydrocephalus
        microcephaly Q02
    spine (with meningocele) —see Spina bifida
    trachea Q32.1
    tympanic membrane (causing impairment
      of hearing) Q16.4
    uterus Q51.818
    vitelline duct Q43.0
  erection —see Dysfunction, sexual, male,
    erectile
  fusion —see Imperfect, closure
  inflation, lung (newborn) —see Atelectasis
  posture R29.3
  rotation, intestine Q43.3
  septum, ventricular Q21.0
Imperfectly descended testis —see Cryptorchid
Imperforate (congenital) —see also Atresia
  anus Q42.3
    with fistula Q42.2
  cervix (uteri) Q51.828
  esophagus Q39.0
    with tracheoesophageal fistula Q39.1
  hymen Q52.3
  jejunum Q41.1
  pharynx Q38.8
  rectum Q42.1
    with fistula Q42.0
  urethra Q64.39
  vagina Q52.4
Impervious (congenital) —see also Atresia
  anus Q42.3
    with fistula Q42.2
  bile duct Q44.2
  esophagus Q39.0
    with tracheoesophageal fistula Q39.1
  intestine (small) Q41.9
    large Q42.9
      specified NEC Q42.8
  rectum Q42.1
    with fistula Q42.0
  ureter —see Atresia, ureter
  urethra Q64.39
Impetiginization of dermatoses L01.1
Impetigo (any organism) (any site) (circinate)
  (contagiosa) (simplex) (vulgaris) L01.00
  Bockhart's L01.02
  bullous, bullosa L01.03
  external ear L01.00 [H62.40]
  follicularis L01.02
  furfuracea L30.5
  herpetiformis L40.1
    nonobstetrical L40.1

▶ New   ⇒ Revised   ~~deleted~~ Deleted   ● Use Additional Character(s)

Impetigo *(Continued)*
  neonatorum L01.03
  nonbullous L01.01
  specified type NEC L01.09
  ulcerative L01.09
Impingement (on teeth)
  joint —*see* Disorder, joint, specified type NEC
  soft tissue
    anterior M26.81
    posterior M26.82
Implant, endometrial N80.9
Implantation
  anomalous —*see* Anomaly, by site
    ureter Q62.63
  cyst
    external area or site (skin) NEC L72.0
    iris —*see* Cyst, iris, implantation
    vagina N89.8
    vulva N90.7
  dermoid (cyst) —*see* Implantation, cyst
Impotence (sexual) N52.9
  counseling Z70.1
  organic origin —*see also* Dysfunction, sexual, male, erectile N52.9
  psychogenic F52.21
Impression, basilar Q75.8
Imprisonment, anxiety concerning Z65.1
Improper care (child) (newborn) —*see* Maltreatment
Improperly tied umbilical cord (causing hemorrhage) P51.8
Impulsiveness (impulsive) R45.87
Inability to swallow —*see* Aphagia
▶ comply with dietary regimen Z91.118
▶ swallow - *see* Aphagia
Inaccessible, inaccessibility
  health care NEC Z75.3
    due to
      waiting period Z75.2
        for admission to facility elsewhere Z75.1
    other helping agencies Z75.4
▶ transportation Z59.82
Inactive —*see* condition
Inadequate, inadequacy
  aesthetics of dental restoration K08.56
  biologic, constitutional, functional, or social F60.7
  development
    child R62.50
    genitalia
      after puberty NEC E30.0
      congenital
        female Q52.8
          external Q52.79
          internal Q52.8
        male Q55.8
    lungs Q33.6
      associated with short gestation P28.0
    organ or site not listed —*see* Anomaly, by site
  diet (causing nutritional deficiency) E63.9
  drinking-water supply Z58.6
  eating habits Z72.4
  environment, household Z59.1
  family support Z63.8
  food (supply) NEC Z59.48
    hunger effects T73.0
  functional F60.7
  household care, due to
    family member
      handicapped or ill Z74.2
      on vacation Z75.5
      temporarily away from home Z74.2
    technical defects in home Z59.1
    temporary absence from home of person rendering care Z74.2
  housing (heating) (space) Z59.1
  income (financial) Z59.6
  intrafamilial communication Z63.8
⇒ material resources Z59.87
  mental —*see* Disability, intellectual

Inadequate, inadequacy *(Continued)*
  parental supervision or control of child Z62.0
  personality F60.7
  pulmonary
    function R06.89
      newborn P28.5
    ventilation, newborn P28.5
  sample of cytologic smear
    anus R85.615
    cervix R87.615
    vagina R87.625
  social F60.7
    insurance Z59.7
    skills NEC Z73.4
  supervision of child by parent Z62.0
  teaching affecting education Z55.8
▶ transportation Z59.82
  welfare support Z59.7
Inanition R64
  with edema —*see* Malnutrition, severe
  due to
    deprivation of food T73.0
    malnutrition —*see* Malnutrition
  fever R50.9
Inappropriate
  change in quantitative human chorionic gonadotropin (hCG) in early pregnancy O02.81
  diet or eating habits Z72.4
  level of quantitative human chorionic gonadotropin (hCG) for gestational age in early pregnancy O02.81
  secretion
    antidiuretic hormone (ADH) (excessive) E22.2
      deficiency E23.2
    pituitary (posterior) E22.2
Inattention at or after birth —*see* Neglect
Incarceration, incarcerated
  enterocele K46.0
    gangrenous K46.1
  epiplocele K46.0
    gangrenous K46.1
  exomphalos K42.0
    gangrenous K42.1
  hernia —*see also* Hernia, by site, with obstruction
    with gangrene —*see* Hernia, by site, with gangrene
  iris, in wound —*see* Injury, eye, laceration, with prolapse
  lens, in wound —*see* Injury, eye, laceration, with prolapse
  omphalocele K42.0
  prison, anxiety concerning Z65.1
  rupture —*see* Hernia, by site
  sarcoepiplocele K46.0
    gangrenous K46.1
  sarcoepiplomphalocele K42.0
    with gangrene K42.1
  uterus N85.8
    gravid O34.51-●
      causing obstructed labor O65.5
Incised wound
  external —*see* Laceration
  internal organs —*see* Injury, by site
Incision, incisional
  hernia K43.2
    with
      gangrene (and obstruction) K43.1
      obstruction K43.0
    surgical, complication —*see* Complications, surgical procedure
    traumatic
      external —*see* Laceration
      internal organs —*see* Injury, by site
Inclusion
  azurophilic leukocytic D72.0
  blennorrhea (neonatal) (newborn) P39.1
  gallbladder in liver (congenital) Q44.1

Incompatibility
  ABO
    affecting management of pregnancy O36.11-●
      anti-A sensitization O36.11-●
      anti-B sensitization O36.19-●
      specified NEC O36.19-●
    infusion or transfusion reaction —*see* Complication(s), transfusion, incompatibility reaction, ABO
    newborn P55.1
  blood (group) (Duffy) (K) (Kell) (Kidd) (Lewis) (M) (S) NEC
    affecting management of pregnancy O36.11-●
      anti-A sensitization O36.11-●
      anti-B sensitization O36.19-●
    infusion or transfusion reaction T80.89
    newborn P55.8
  divorce or estrangement Z63.5
  Rh (blood group) (factor) Z31.82
    affecting management of pregnancy NEC O36.09-●
      anti-D antibody O36.01-●
    infusion or transfusion reaction —*see* Complication(s), transfusion, incompatibility reaction, Rh (factor)
    newborn P55.0
  rhesus —*see* Incompatibility, Rh
Incompetency, incompetent, incompetence
  annular
    aortic (valve) —*see* Insufficiency, aortic
    mitral (valve) I34.0
    pulmonary valve (heart) I37.1
  aortic (valve) —*see* Insufficiency, aortic
  cardiac valve —*see* Endocarditis
  cervix, cervical (os) N88.3
    in pregnancy O34.3-●
  chronotropic I45.89
    with
      autonomic dysfunction G90.8
      ischemic heart disease I25.89
      left ventricular dysfunction I51.89
      sinus node dysfunction I49.8
  esophagogastric (junction) (sphincter) K22.0
  mitral (valve) —*see* Insufficiency, mitral
  pelvic fundus N81.89
  pubocervical tissue N81.82
  pulmonary valve (heart) I37.1
    congenital Q22.3
  rectovaginal tissue N81.83
  tricuspid (annular) (valve) —*see* Insufficiency, tricuspid
  valvular —*see* Endocarditis
    congenital Q24.8
  vein, venous (saphenous) (varicose) —*see* Varix, leg
Incomplete —*see also* condition
▶ atrioventricular
  ▶ canal Q21.21
  ▶ septal defect Q21.21
  bladder, emptying R33.9
  defecation R15.0
▶ endocardial cushion defect Q21.21
  expansion lungs (newborn) NEC —*see* Atelectasis
  rotation, intestine Q43.3
Inconclusive
  diagnostic imaging due to excess body fat of patient R93.9
  findings on diagnostic imaging of breast NEC R92.8
  mammogram (due to dense breasts) R92.2
Incontinence R32
  anal sphincter R15.9
  coital N39.491
  feces R15.9
    nonorganic origin F98.1
  insensible (urinary) N39.42
  overflow N39.490

Incontinence (*Continued*)
 postural (urinary) N39.492
 psychogenic F45.8
 rectal R15.9
 reflex N39.498
 stress (female) (male) N39.3
  and urge N39.46
 urethral sphincter R32
 urge N39.41
  and stress (female) (male) N39.46
 urine (urinary) R32
  continuous N39.45
  due to cognitive impairment, or severe
    physical disability or immobility
    R39.81
  functional R39.81
  insensible N39.42
  mixed (stress and urge) N39.46
  nocturnal N39.44
  nonorganic origin F98.0
  overflow N39.490
  post dribbling N39.43
  postural N39.492
  reflex N39.498
  specified NEC N39.498
  stress (female) (male) N39.3
   and urge N39.46
  total N39.498
  unaware N39.42
  urge N39.41
   and stress (female) (male) N39.46
Incontinentia pigmenti Q82.3
Incoordinate, incoordination
 esophageal-pharyngeal (newborn) —*see*
   Dysphagia
 muscular R27.8
 uterus (action) (contractions) (complicating
   delivery) O62.4
Increase, increased
 abnormal, in development R63.8
 androgens (ovarian) E28.1
 anticoagulants (antithrombin) (anti-VIIIa)
   (anti-IXa) (anti-Xa) (anti-XIa) —*see*
   Circulating anticoagulants
 cold sense R20.8
 estrogen E28.0
 function
  adrenal
   cortex —*see* Cushing's, syndrome
   medulla E27.5
  pituitary (gland) (anterior) (lobe) E22.9
   posterior E22.2
 heat sense R20.8
 intracranial pressure (benign) G93.2
 permeability, capillaries I78.8
 pressure, intracranial G93.2
 secretion
  gastrin E16.4
  glucagon E16.3
  pancreas, endocrine E16.9
   growth hormone-releasing hormone
    E16.8
   pancreatic polypeptide E16.8
   somatostatin E16.8
   vasoactive-intestinal polypeptide E16.8
 sphericity, lens Q12.4
 splenic activity D73.1
 venous pressure I87.8
  portal K76.6
Increta placenta O43.22-●
Incrustation, cornea, foreign body (lead)
   (zinc) —*see* Foreign body, cornea
Incyclophoria H50.54
Incyclotropia —*see* Cyclotropia
Indeterminate sex Q56.4
India rubber skin Q82.8
Indigestion (acid) (bilious) (functional) K30
 catarrhal K31.89
 due to decomposed food NOS A05.9
 nervous F45.8
 psychogenic F45.8

Indirect —*see* condition
Induratio penis plastica N48.6
Induration, indurated
 brain G93.89
 breast (fibrous) N64.51
  puerperal, postpartum O92.29
 broad ligament N83.8
 chancre
  anus A51.1
  congenital A50.07
  extragenital NEC A51.2
 corpora cavernosa (penis) (plastic) N48.6
 liver (chronic) K76.89
 lung (black) (chronic) (fibroid) —*see also*
   Fibrosis, lung J84.10
  essential brown J84.03
 penile (plastic) N48.6
 phlebitic —*see* Phlebitis
 skin R23.4
Inebriety (without dependence) —*see* Alcohol,
   intoxication
Inefficiency, kidney N28.9
Inelasticity, skin R23.4
Inequality, leg (length) (acquired) —*see also*
   Deformity, limb, unequal length
 congenital —*see* Defect, reduction, lower limb
 lower leg —*see* Deformity, limb, unequal
   length
Inertia
 bladder (neurogenic) N31.2
 stomach K31.89
  psychogenic F45.8
 uterus, uterine during labor O62.2
  during latent phase of labor O62.0
  primary O62.0
  secondary O62.1
 vesical (neurogenic) N31.2
Infancy, infantile, infantilism —*see also*
   condition
 celiac K90.0
 genitalia, genitals (after puberty) E30.0
 Herter's (nontropical sprue) K90.0
 intestinal K90.0
 Lorain E23.0
 pancreatic K86.89
 pelvis M95.5
  with disproportion (fetopelvic) O33.1
   causing obstructed labor O65.1
 pituitary E23.0
 renal N25.0
 uterus —*see* Infantile, genitalia
Infant(s) —*see also* Infancy
 excessive crying R68.11
 irritable child R68.12
 lack of care —*see* Neglect
 liveborn (singleton) Z38.2
  born in hospital Z38.00
   by cesarean Z38.01
  born outside hospital Z38.1
  multiple NEC Z38.8
   born in hospital Z38.68
    by cesarean Z38.69
   born outside hospital Z38.7
  quadruplet Z38.8
   born in hospital Z38.63
    by cesarean Z38.64
   born outside hospital Z38.7
  quintuplet Z38.8
   born in hospital Z38.65
    by cesarean Z38.66
   born outside hospital Z38.7
  triplet Z38.8
   born in hospital Z38.61
    by cesarean Z38.62
   born outside hospital Z38.7
  twin Z38.5
   born in hospital Z38.30
    by cesarean Z38.31
   born outside hospital Z38.4
 of diabetic mother (syndrome of) P70.1
  gestational diabetes P70.0

Infantile —*see also* condition
 genitalia, genitals E30.0
 os, uterine E30.0
 penis E30.0
 testis E29.1
 uterus E30.0
Infantilism —*see* Infancy
Infarct, infarction
 adrenal (capsule) (gland) E27.49
 appendices epiploicae —*see also* Infarct,
   intestine K55.069
 bowel —*see also* Infarct, intestine K55.069
 brain (stem) —*see* Infarct, cerebral
 breast N64.89
 brewer's (kidney) N28.0
 cardiac —*see* Infarct, myocardium
 cerebellar —*see* Infarct, cerebral
 cerebral (acute) (chronic) (*see also* Occlusion,
   artery cerebral or precerebral, with
   infarction) I63.9-●
  aborted I63.9
  cortical I63.9
  due to
   cerebral venous thrombosis,
     nonpyogenic I63.6
   embolism
    cerebral arteries I63.4-●
    precerebral arteries I63.1-●
   occlusion NEC
    cerebral arteries I63.5-●
    precerebral arteries I63.2-●
    small artery I63.81
   stenosis NEC
    cerebral arteries I63.5-●
    precerebral arteries I63.2-●
    small artery I63.81
   thrombosis
    cerebral artery I63.3-●
    precerebral artery I63.0-●
  intraoperative
   during cardiac surgery I97.810
   during other surgery I97.811
  neonatal P91.82-●
  perinatal (arterial ischemic) P91.82-●
  postprocedural
   following cardiac surgery I97.820
   following other surgery I97.821
  specified NEC I63.89
 colon (acute) (agnogenic) (embolic)
   (hemorrhagic) (nonocclusive)
   (nonthrombotic) (occlusive) (segmental)
   (thrombotic) (with gangrene) —*see also*
   Infarct, intestine K55.049
 coronary artery —*see* Infarct, myocardium
 embolic —*see* Embolism
 fallopian tube N83.8
 gallbladder K82.8
 heart —*see* Infarct, myocardium
 hepatic K76.3
 hypophysis (anterior lobe) E23.6
 impending (myocardium) I20.0
 intestine (acute) (agnogenic) (embolic)
   (hemorrhagic) (nonocclusive)
   (nonthrombotic) (occlusive) (thrombotic)
   (with gangrene) K55.069
  diffuse K55.062
  focal K55.061
  large K55.049
   diffuse K55.042
   focal K55.041
  small K55.029
   diffuse K55.022
   focal K55.021
 kidney N28.0
 lacunar I63.81
 liver K76.3
 lung (embolic) (thrombotic) —*see* Embolism,
   pulmonary
 lymph node I89.8
 mesentery, mesenteric (embolic) (thrombotic)
   (with gangrene) —*see also* Infarct,
   intestine K55.069

Infarct, infarction *(Continued)*
  muscle (ischemic) M62.20
    ankle M62.27-●
    foot M62.27-●
    forearm M62.23-●
    hand M62.24-●
    lower leg M62.26-●
    pelvic region M62.25-●
    shoulder region M62.21-●
    specified site NEC M62.28
    thigh M62.25-●
    upper arm M62.22-●
  myocardium, myocardial (acute) (with stated duration of 4 weeks or less) I21.9
    associated with revascularization procedure I21.A9
    diagnosed on ECG, but presenting no symptoms I25.2
    due to
      demand ischemia I21.A1
      ischemic imbalance I21.A1
    healed or old I25.2
    intraoperative —*see also* Infarct, myocardium, associated with revascularization procedure
      during cardiac surgery I97.790
      during other surgery I97.791
    non-Q wave I21.4
    non-ST elevation (NSTEMI) I21.4
      subsequent I22.2
    nontransmural I21.4
    past (diagnosed on ECG or other investigation, but currently presenting no symptoms) I25.2
    postprocedural —*see also* Infarct, myocardium, associated with revascularization procedure
      following cardiac surgery —*see also* Infarct, myocardium, type 4 or type 5 I97.190
      following other surgery I97.191
    Q wave —*see also* Infarct, myocardium, by site I21.3
    secondary to
      demand ischemia I21.A1
      ischemic imbalance I21.A1
    ST elevation (STEMI) I21.3
      anterior (anteroapical) (anterolateral) (anteroseptal) (Q wave) (wall) I21.09
        subsequent I22.0
      inferior (diaphragmatic) (inferolateral) (inferoposterior) (wall) NEC I21.19
        subsequent I22.1
      inferoposterior transmural (Q wave) I21.11
      involving
        coronary artery of anterior wall NEC I21.09
        coronary artery of inferior wall NEC I21.19
        diagonal coronary artery I21.02
        left anterior descending coronary artery I21.02
        left circumflex coronary artery I21.21
        left main coronary artery I21.01
        oblique marginal coronary artery I21.21
        right coronary artery I21.11
      lateral (apical-lateral) (basal-lateral) (high) I21.29
        subsequent I22.8
      posterior (posterobasal) (posterolateral) (posteroseptal) (true) I21.29
        subsequent I22.8
      septal I21.29
        subsequent I22.8
      specified NEC I21.29
        subsequent I22.8
    subsequent I22.9
    subsequent (recurrent) (reinfarction) I22.9
      anterior (anteroapical) (anterolateral) (anteroseptal) (wall) I22.0
      diaphragmatic (wall) I22.1
      inferior (diaphragmatic) (inferolateral) (inferoposterior) (wall) I22.1

Infarct, infarction *(Continued)*
  myocardium, myocardial *(Continued)*
    subsequent *(Continued)*
      lateral (apical-lateral) (basal-lateral) (high) I22.8
      non-ST elevation (NSTEMI) I22.2
      posterior (posterobasal) (posterolateral) (posteroseptal) (true) I22.8
      septal I22.8
      specified NEC I22.8
      ST elevation I22.9
        anterior (anteroapical) (anterolateral) (anteroseptal) (wall) I22.0
        inferior (diaphragmatic) (inferolateral) (inferoposterior) (wall) I22.1
        specified NEC I22.8
      subendocardial I22.2
      ⟹transmural I22.9
        anterior (anteroapical) (anterolateral) (anteroseptal) (wall) I22.0
        diaphragmatic (wall) I22.1
        inferior (diaphragmatic) (inferolateral) (inferoposterior) (wall) I22.1
        lateral (apical-lateral) (basal-lateral) (high) I22.8
        posterior (posterobasal) (posterolateral) (posteroseptal) (true) I22.8
        specified NEC I22.8
    type 1 —*see also* Infarction, myocardial, subsequent, by site, or by ST elevation or non-ST elevation I22.9
    type 2 I21.A1
    type 3 I21.A9
    type 4 I21.A9
    type 5 I21.A9
    syphilitic A52.06
    transmural I21.9
      anterior (anteroapical) (anterolateral) (anteroseptal) (Q wave) (wall) NEC I21.09
      inferior (diaphragmatic) (inferolateral) (inferoposterior) (Q wave) (wall) NEC I21.19
      inferoposterior (Q wave) I21.11
      lateral (apical-lateral) (basal-lateral) (high) NEC I21.29
      posterior (posterobasal) (posterolateral) (posteroseptal) (true) NEC I21.29
      septal NEC I21.29
      specified NEC I21.29
    type 1 —*see also* Infarction, myocardial, by site, or by ST elevation or non-ST elevation I21.9
    type 2 I21.A1
    type 3 I21.A9
    type 4 (a) (b) (c) I21.A9
    type 5 I21.A9
  nontransmural I21.4
  omentum —*see also* Infarct, intestine K55.069
  ovary N83.8
  pancreas K86.89
  papillary muscle —*see* Infarct, myocardium
  parathyroid gland E21.4
  pituitary (gland) E23.6
  placenta O43.81-●
  prostate N42.89
  pulmonary (artery) (vein) (hemorrhagic) —*see* Embolism, pulmonary
  renal (embolic) (thrombotic) N28.0
  retina, retinal (artery) —*see* Occlusion, artery, retina
  spinal (cord) (acute) (embolic) (nonembolic) G95.11
  spleen D73.5
    embolic or thrombotic I74.8
  subendocardial (acute) (nontransmural) I21.4
  suprarenal (capsule) (gland) E27.49
  testis N50.1
  thrombotic —*see also* Thrombosis
    artery, arterial —*see* Embolism
  thyroid (gland) E07.89
  ventricle (heart) —*see* Infarct, myocardium

Infecting —*see* condition
Infection, infected, infective (opportunistic) B99.9
  with
    drug resistant organism —*see* Resistance (to), drug —*see also* specific organism
    lymphangitis —*see* Lymphangitis
    organ dysfunction (acute) R65.20
      with septic shock R65.21
  abscess (skin) - code by site under Abscess
  Absidia —*see* Mucormycosis
  Acanthamoeba —*see* Acanthamebiasis
  Acanthocheilonema (perstans) (streptocerca) B74.4
  accessory sinus (chronic) —*see* Sinusitis
  achorion —*see* Dermatophytosis
  Acremonium falciforme B47.0
  acromioclavicular M00.9
  Actinobacillus (actinomycetem-comitans) A28.8
    mallei A24.0
    muris A25.1
  Actinomadura B47.1
  Actinomyces (israelii) —*see also* Actinomycosis A42.9
  Actinomycetales —*see* Actinomycosis
  actinomycotic NOS —*see* Actinomycosis
  adenoid (and tonsil) J03.90
    chronic J35.02
  adenovirus NEC
    as cause of disease classified elsewhere B97.0
    unspecified nature or site B34.0
  aerogenes capsulatus A48.0
  aertrycke —*see* Infection, salmonella
  alimentary canal NOS —*see* Enteritis, infectious
  Allescheria boydii B48.2
  Alternaria B48.8
  alveolus, alveolar (process) K04.7
  Ameba, amebic (histolytica) —*see* Amebiasis
  amniotic fluid, sac or cavity O41.10-●
    chorioamnionitis O41.12-●
    placentitis O41.14-●
  amputation stump (surgical) —*see* Complication, amputation stump, infection
  Ancylostoma (duodenalis) B76.0
  Anisakiasis, Anisakis larvae B81.0
  anthrax —*see* Anthrax
  antrum (chronic) —*see* Sinusitis, maxillary
  anus, anal (papillae) (sphincter) K62.89
  arbovirus (arbor virus) A94
    specified type NEC A93.8
  artificial insemination N98.0
  Ascaris lumbricoides —*see* Ascariasis
  Ascomycetes B47.0
  Aspergillus (flavus) (fumigatus) (terreus) —*see* Aspergillosis
  atypical
    acid-fast (bacilli) —*see* Mycobacterium, atypical
    mycobacteria —*see* Mycobacterium, atypical
    virus A81.9
      specified type NEC A81.89
  auditory meatus (external) —*see* Otitis, externa, infective
  auricle (ear) —*see* Otitis, externa, infective
  axillary gland (lymph) L04.2
  Bacillus A49.9
    abortus A23.1
    anthracis —*see* Anthrax
    Ducrey's (any location) A57
    Flexner's A03.1
    Friedländer's NEC A49.8
    gas (gangrene) A48.0
    mallei A24.0
    melitensis A23.0
    paratyphoid, paratyphosus A01.4
      A A01.1
      B A01.2
      C A01.3

Infection, infected, infective (Continued)
  Bacillus (Continued)
    Shiga (-Kruse) A03.0
    suipestifer —see Infection, salmonella
    swimming pool A31.1
    typhosa A01.00
    welchii —see Gangrene, gas
  bacterial NOS A49.9
    as cause of disease classified elsewhere
        B96.89
      Bacteroides fragilis [B. fragilis] B96.6
      Clostridium perfringens [C. perfringens]
          B96.7
      Enterobacter sakazakii B96.89
      Enterococcus B95.2
      Escherichia coli [E. coli] (see also
          Escherichia coli) B96.20
      Helicobacter pylori [H.pylori] B96.81
      Hemophilus influenzae [H. influenzae]
          B96.3
      Klebsiella pneumoniae [K. pneumoniae]
          B96.1
      Mycoplasma pneumoniae [M.
          pneumoniae] B96.0
      Proteus (mirabilis) (morganii) B96.4
      Pseudomonas (aeruginosa) (mallei)
          (pseudomallei) B96.5
      Staphylococcus B95.8
        aureus (methicillin susceptible)
            (MSSA) B95.61
          methicillin resistant (MRSA) B95.62
        specified NEC B95.7
      Streptococcus B95.5
        group A B95.0
        group B B95.1
        pneumoniae B95.3
        specified NEC B95.4
      Vibrio vulnificus B96.82
    specified NEC A48.8
  Bacterium
    paratyphosum A01.4
      A A01.1
      B A01.2
      C A01.3
    typhosum A01.00
  Bacteroides NEC A49.8
    fragilis, as cause of disease classified
        elsewhere B96.6
  Balantidium coli A07.0
  Bartholin's gland N75.8
  Basidiobolus B46.8
  bile duct (common) (hepatic) —see
      Cholangitis
  bladder —see Cystitis
  Blastomyces, blastomycotic —see also
      Blastomycosis
    brasiliensis —see Paracoccidioidomycosis
    dermatitidis —see Blastomycosis
    European —see Cryptococcosis
    Loboi B48.0
    North American B40.9
    South American —see
        Paracoccidioidomycosis
  bleb, postprocedure —see Blebitis
  bone —see Osteomyelitis
  Bordetella —see Whooping cough
  Borrelia bergdorfi A69.20
  brain —see also Encephalitis G04.90
    membranes —see Meningitis
    septic G06.0
      meninges —see Meningitis, bacterial
  branchial cyst Q18.0
  breast —see Mastitis
  bronchus —see Bronchitis
  Brucella A23.9
    abortus A23.1
    canis A23.3
    melitensis A23.0
    mixed A23.8
    specified NEC A23.8
    suis A23.2

Infection, infected, infective (Continued)
  Brugia (malayi) B74.1
    timori B74.2
  bursa —see Bursitis, infective
  buttocks (skin) L08.9
  Campylobacter, intestinal A04.5
    as cause of disease classified elsewhere
        B96.81
  Candida (albicans) (tropicalis) —see
      Candidiasis
  candiru B88.8
  Capillaria (intestinal) B81.1
    hepatica B83.8
    philippinensis B81.1
  cartilage —see Disorder, cartilage, specified
      type NEC
  catheter-related bloodstream (CRBSI)
      T80.211
  cat liver fluke B66.0
  cellulitis - code by site under Cellulitis
  central line-associated T80.219
    bloodstream (CLABSI) T80.211
    specified NEC T80.218
  Cephalosporium falciforme B47.0
  cerebrospinal —see Meningitis
  cervical gland (lymph) L04.0
  cervix —see Cervicitis
  cesarean delivery wound (puerperal)
      O86.00
  cestodes —see Infestation, cestodes
  chest J22
  Chilomastix (intestinal) A07.8
  Chlamydia, chlamydial A74.9
    anus A56.3
    genitourinary tract A56.2
      lower A56.00
      specified NEC A56.19
    lymphogranuloma A55
    pharynx A56.4
    psittaci A70
    rectum A56.3
    sexually transmitted NEC A56.8
  cholera —see Cholera
  Cladosporium
    bantianum (brain abscess) B43.1
    carrionii B43.0
    castellanii B36.1
    trichoides (brain abscess) B43.1
    werneckii B36.1
  Clonorchis (sinensis) (liver) B66.1
  Clostridium NEC
    bifermentans A48.0
    botulinum (food poisoning) A05.1
      infant A48.51
      wound A48.52
    difficile
      as cause of disease classified elsewhere
          B96.89
      foodborne (disease)
        not specified as recurrent A04.72
        recurrent A04.71
      gas gangrene A48.0
      necrotizing enterocolitis
        not specified as recurrent A04.72
        recurrent A04.71
      sepsis A41.4
    gas-forming NEC A48.0
    histolyticum A48.0
    novyi, causing gas gangrene A48.0
    oedematiens A48.0
    perfringens
      as cause of disease classified elsewhere
          B96.7
      due to food A05.2
      foodborne (disease) A05.2
      gas gangrene A48.0
      sepsis A41.4
    septicum, causing gas gangrene
        A48.0
    sordellii, causing gas gangrene
        A48.0

Infection, infected, infective (Continued)
  Clostridium NEC (Continued)
    welchii
      as cause of disease classified elsewhere
          B96.7
      foodborne (disease) A05.2
      gas gangrene A48.0
      necrotizing enteritis A05.2
      sepsis A41.4
  Coccidioides (immitis) —see
      Coccidioidomycosis
  colon —see Enteritis, infectious
  colostomy K94.02
  common duct —see Cholangitis
  congenital P39.9
    Candida (albicans) P37.5
    cytomegalovirus P35.1
    hepatitis, viral P35.3
    herpes simplex P35.2
    infectious or parasitic disease P37.9
      specified NEC P37.8
    listeriosis (disseminated) P37.2
    malaria NEC P37.4
      falciparum P37.3
    Plasmodium falciparum P37.3
    poliomyelitis P35.8
    rubella P35.0
    skin P39.4
    toxoplasmosis (acute) (subacute) (chronic)
        P37.1
    tuberculosis P37.0
    urinary (tract) P39.3
    vaccinia P35.8
    virus P35.9
      specified type NEC P35.8
  Conidiobolus B46.8
  coronavirus-2019 U07.1
  coronavirus NEC B34.2
    as cause of disease classified elsewhere
        B97.29
    severe acute respiratory syndrome (SARS
        associated) B97.21
  corpus luteum —see Salpingo-oophoritis
  Corynebacterium diphtheriae —see
      Diphtheria
  cotia virus B08.8
  COVID-19 U07.1
  Coxiella burnetii A78
  coxsackie —see Coxsackie
  Cryptococcus neoformans —see
      Cryptococcosis
  Cryptosporidium A07.2
  Cunninghamella —see Mucormycosis
  cyst —see Cyst
  cystic duct —see also Cholecystitis K81.9
  Cysticercus cellulosae —see Cysticercosis
  cytomegalovirus, cytomegaloviral B25.9
    congenital P35.1
    maternal, maternal care for (suspected)
        damage to fetus O35.3
    mononucleosis B27.10
      with
        complication NEC B27.19
        meningitis B27.12
        polyneuropathy B27.11
  delta-agent (acute), in hepatitis B carrier
      B17.0
  dental (pulpal origin) K04.7
  Deuteromycetes B47.0
  Dicrocoelium dendriticum B66.2
  Dipetalonema (perstans) (streptocerca) B74.4
  diphtherial —see Diphtheria
  Diphyllobothrium (adult) (latum) (pacificum)
      B70.0
    larval B70.1
  Diplogonoporus (grandis) B71.8
  Dipylidium caninum B67.4
  Dirofilaria B74.8
  Dracunculus medinensis B72
  Drechslera (hawaiiensis) B43.8
  Ducrey Haemophilus (any location) A57

▶ New   ⇒ Revised   ~~deleted~~ Deleted   ● Use Additional Character(s)

Infection, infected, infective *(Continued)*
 due to or resulting from
  artificial insemination N98.0
  Babesia
   divergens (-like) strain B60.03
   duncani (-type) species B60.02
   microti B60.01
   species
    specified NEC B60.09
  central venous catheter T80.219
   bloodstream T80.211
   exit or insertion site T80.212
   localized T80.212
   port or reservoir T80.212
   specified NEC T80.218
   tunnel T80.212
  device, implant or graft —*see also*
    Complications, by site and type,
    infection or inflammation T85.79
   arterial graft NEC T82.7
   breast (implant) T85.79
   catheter NEC T85.79
    dialysis (renal) T82.7
     central line T80.211
     intraperitoneal T85.71
    infusion NEC T82.7
     cranial T85.735
     intrathecal T85.735
     spinal (epidural) (subdural) T85.735
     subarachnoid T85.735
    urinary T83.518
     cystostomy T83.510
     Hopkins T83.518
     ileostomy T83.518
     nephrostomy T83.512
     specified NEC T83.518
     urethral indwelling T83.511
     urostomy T83.518
   electronic (electrode) (pulse generator)
     (stimulator)
    bone T84.7
    cardiac T82.7
    nervous system T85.738
     brain T85.731
     cranial nerve T85.732
     gastric nerve T85.732
     generator pocket T85.734
     neurostimulator generator
       T85.734
     peripheral nerve T85.732
     sacral nerve T85.732
     spinal cord T85.733
     vagal nerve T85.732
    urinary T83.590
   fixation, internal (orthopedic) NEC —
     see Complication, fixation device,
     infection
   gastrointestinal (bile duct) (esophagus)
     T85.79
    neurostimulator electrode (lead)
      T85.732
   genital NEC T83.69
   heart NEC T82.7
    valve (prosthesis) T82.6
     graft T82.7
   joint prosthesis —*see* Complication, joint
     prosthesis, infection
   ocular (corneal graft) (orbital implant)
     NEC T85.79
   orthopedic NEC T84.7
   penile (cylinder) (pump) (resevoir)
     T83.61
   specified NEC T85.79
   testicular T83.62
   urinary NEC T83.598
    ileal conduit stent T83.593
    implanted neurostimulation T83.590
    implanted sphincter T83.591
    indwelling ureteral stent T83.592
    nephroureteral stent T83.593
    specified stent NEC T83.593

Infection, infected, infective *(Continued)*
 due to or resulting from *(Continued)*
  device, implant or graft *(Continued)*
   vascular NEC T82.7
   ventricular intracranial (communicating)
     shunt T85.730
  Hickman catheter T80.219
   bloodstream T80.211
   localized T80.212
   specified NEC T80.218
  immunization or vaccination
    T88.0
  infusion, injection or transfusion
    NEC T80.29
   acute T80.22
  injury NEC - code by site under Wound,
    open
  peripherally inserted central catheter
    (PICC) T80.219
   bloodstream T80.211
   localized T80.212
   specified NEC T80.218
  portacath (port-a-cath) T80.219
   bloodstream T80.211
   localized T80.212
   specified NEC T80.218
  protozoa of the order Piroplasmida NEC
    B60.09
  pulmonary artery catheter —*see* Infection,
    due to or resulting from, central
    venous catheter
  surgery T81.40
  Swan Ganz catheter —*see* Infection, due
    to or resulting from, central venous
    catheter
  triple lumen catheter T80.219
   bloodstream T80.211
   localized T80.212
   specified NEC T80.218
  umbilical venous catheter T80.219
   bloodstream T80.211
   localized T80.212
   specified NEC T80.218
 during labor NEC O75.3
 ear (middle) —*see also* Otitis media
  external —*see* Otitis, externa, infective
  inner —*see* subcategory H83.0
 Eberthella typhosa A01.00
 Echinococcus —*see* Echinococcus
 echovirus
  as cause of disease classified elsewhere
    B97.12
  unspecified nature or site B34.1
 endocardium I33.0
 endocervix —*see* Cervicitis
 Entamoeba —*see* Amebiasis
 enteric —*see* Enteritis, infectious
 Enterobacter sakazakii B96.89
 Enterobius vermicularis B80
 enterostomy K94.12
 enterovirus B34.1
  as cause of disease classified elsewhere
    B97.10
   coxsackievirus B97.11
   echovirus B97.12
   specified NEC B97.19
 Entomophthora B46.8
 Epidermophyton —*see* Dermatophytosis
 epididymis —*see* Epididymitis
 episiotomy (puerperal) O86.09
 Erysipelothrix (insidiosa) (rhusiopathiae) —
    see Erysipeloid
 erythema infectiosum B08.3
 Escherichia (E.) coli NEC A49.8
  as cause of disease classified elsewhere —
    see also Escherichia coli B96.20
   congenital P39.8
    sepsis P36.4
   generalized A41.51
   intestinal —*see* Enteritis, infectious, due to,
     Escherichia coli

Infection, infected, infective *(Continued)*
 ethmoidal (chronic) (sinus) —*see* Sinusitis,
   ethmoidal
 eustachian tube (ear) —*see* Salpingitis,
   eustachian
 external auditory canal (meatus) NEC —*see*
   Otitis, externa, infective
 eye (purulent) —*see* Endophthalmitis, purulent
 eyelid —*see* Inflammation, eyelid
 fallopian tube —*see* Salpingo-oophoritis
 Fasciola (gigantica) (hepatica) (indica) B66.3
 Fasciolopsis (buski) B66.5
 filarial —*see* Infestation, filarial
 finger (skin) L08.9
  nail L03.01-●
   fungus B35.1
 fish tapeworm B70.0
  larval B70.1
 flagellate, intestinal A07.9
 fluke —*see* Infestation, fluke
 focal
  teeth (pulpal origin) K04.7
  tonsils J35.01
 Fonsecaea (compactum) (pedrosoi) B43.0
 food —*see* Intoxication, foodborne
 foot (skin) L08.9
  dermatophytic fungus B35.3
 Francisella tularensis —*see* Tularemia
 frontal (sinus) (chronic) —*see* Sinusitis, frontal
 fungus NOS B49
  beard B35.0
  dermatophytic —*see* Dermatophytosis
  foot B35.3
  groin B35.6
  hand B35.2
  nail B35.1
  pathogenic to compromised host only B48.8
  perianal (area) B35.6
  scalp B35.0
  skin B36.9
   foot B35.3
   hand B35.2
   toenails B35.1
 Fusarium B48.8
 gallbladder —*see* Cholecystitis
 gas bacillus —*see* Gangrene, gas
 gastrointestinal —*see* Enteritis, infectious
 generalized NEC —*see* Sepsis
 generator pocket, implanted electronic
   neurostimulator T85.734
 genital organ or tract
  female —*see* Disease, pelvis, inflammatory
  male N49.9
   multiple sites N49.8
   specified NEC N49.8
 Ghon tubercle, primary A15.7
 Giardia lamblia A07.1
 gingiva (chronic) K05.10
  acute K05.00
   nonplaque induced K05.01
   plaque induced K05.00
  nonplaque induced K05.11
  plaque induced K05.10
 glanders A24.0
 glenosporopsis B48.0
 Gnathostoma (spinigerum) B83.1
 Gongylonema B83.8
 gonococcal —*see* Gonococcus
 gram-negative bacilli NOS A49.9
 guinea worm B72
 gum (chronic) K05.10
  acute K05.00
   nonplaque induced K05.01
   plaque induced K05.00
  nonplaque induced K05.11
  plaque induced K05.10
 Haemophilus —*see* Infection, Hemophilus
 heart —*see* Carditis
 Helicobacter pylori A04.8
  as cause of disease classified elsewhere
    B96.81

Infection, infected, infective *(Continued)*
  helminths B83.9
    intestinal B82.0
      mixed (types classifiable to more than one of the titles B65.0-B81.3 and B81.8) B81.4
      specified type NEC B81.8
    specified type NEC B83.8
  Hemophilus
    aegyptius, systemic A48.4
    ducrey (any location) A57
    generalized A41.3
    influenzae NEC A49.2
      as cause of disease classified elsewhere B96.3
  herpes (simplex) —*see also* Herpes
    congenital P35.2
    disseminated B00.7
    zoster B02.9
  herpesvirus, herpesviral —*see* Herpes
  Heterophyes (heterophyes) B66.8
  hip (joint) NEC M00.9
    due to internal joint prosthesis
      left T84.52
      right T84.51
    skin NEC L08.9
  Histoplasma —*see* Histoplasmosis
    American B39.4
    capsulatum B39.4
  hookworm B76.9
  human
    papilloma virus A63.0
    T-cell lymphotropic virus type-1 (HTLV-1) B33.3
  hydrocele N43.0
  Hymenolepis B71.0
  hypopharynx —*see* Pharyngitis
  inguinal (lymph) glands L04.1
    due to soft chancre A57
  intervertebral disc, pyogenic M46.30
    cervical region M46.32
    cervicothoracic region M46.33
    lumbar region M46.36
    lumbosacral region M46.37
    multiple sites M46.39
    occipito-atlanto-axial region M46.31
    sacrococcygeal region M46.38
    thoracic region M46.34
    thoracolumbar region M46.35
  intestine, intestinal —*see* Enteritis, infectious
    specified NEC A08.8
  intra-amniotic affecting newborn NEC P39.2
  intrauterine inflammation O41.12-•
  Isospora belli or hominis A07.3
  Japanese B encephalitis A83.0
  jaw (bone) (lower) (upper) M27.2
  joint NEC M00.9
    due to internal joint prosthesis T84.50
  kidney (cortex) (hematogenous) N15.9
    with calculus N20.0
      with hydronephrosis N13.6
    following ectopic gestation O08.83
    pelvis and ureter (cystic) N28.85
    puerperal (postpartum) O86.21
    specified NEC N15.8
  Klebsiella (K.) pneumoniae NEC A49.8
    as cause of disease classified elsewhere B96.1
  knee (joint) NEC M00.9
    due to internal joint prosthesis
      left T84.54
      right T84.53
    joint M00.9
    skin L08.9
  Koch's —*see* Tuberculosis
  labia (majora) (minora) (acute) —*see* Vulvitis
  lacrimal
    gland —*see* Dacryoadenitis
    passages (duct) (sac) —*see* Inflammation, lacrimal, passages
  lancet fluke B66.2

Infection, infected, infective *(Continued)*
  larynx NEC J38.7
  leg (skin) NOS L08.9
  Legionella pneumophila A48.1
    nonpneumonic A48.2
  Leishmania —*see also* Leishmaniasis
    aethiopica B55.1
    braziliensis B55.2
    chagasi B55.0
    donovani B55.0
    infantum B55.0
    major B55.1
    mexicana B55.1
    tropica B55.1
  lentivirus, as cause of disease classified elsewhere B97.31
  Leptosphaeria senegalensis B47.0
  Leptospira interrogans A27.9
    autumnalis A27.89
    canicola A27.89
    hebdomadis A27.89
    icterohaemorrhagiae A27.0
    pomona A27.89
    specified type NEC A27.89
  leptospirochetal NEC —*see* Leptospirosis
  Listeria monocytogenes —*see also* Listeriosis
    congenital P37.2
  Loa loa B74.3
    with conjunctival infestation B74.3
    eyelid B74.3
  Loboa loboi B48.0
  local, skin (staphylococcal) (streptococcal) L08.9
    abscess - code by site under Abscess
    cellulitis - code by site under Cellulitis
    specified NEC L08.89
    ulcer —*see* Ulcer, skin
  Loefflerella mallei A24.0
  lung —*see also* Pneumonia J18.9
    atypical Mycobacterium A31.0
    spirochetal A69.8
    tuberculous —*see* Tuberculosis, pulmonary
    virus —*see* Pneumonia, viral
  lymph gland —*see also* Lymphadenitis, acute
    mesenteric I88.0
  lymphoid tissue, base of tongue or posterior pharynx, NEC (chronic) J35.03
  Madurella (grisea) (mycetomii) B47.0
  major
    following ectopic or molar pregnancy O08.0
    puerperal, postpartum, childbirth O85
  Malassezia furfur B36.0
  Malleomyces
    mallei A24.0
    pseudomallei (whitmori) —*see* Melioidosis
  mammary gland N61.0
  Mansonella (ozzardi) (perstans) (streptocerca) B74.4
  mastoid —*see* Mastoiditis
  maxilla, maxillary M27.2
    sinus (chronic) —*see* Sinusitis, maxillary
  mediastinum J98.51
  Medina (worm) B72
  meibomian cyst or gland —*see* Hordeolum
  meninges —*see* Meningitis, bacterial
  meningococcal —*see also* condition A39.9
    adrenals A39.1
    brain A39.81
    cerebrospinal A39.0
    conjunctiva A39.89
    endocardium A39.51
    heart A39.50
      endocardium A39.51
      myocardium A39.52
      pericardium A39.53
    joint A39.83
    meninges A39.0
    meningococcemia A39.4
      acute A39.2
      chronic A39.3

Infection, infected, infective *(Continued)*
  meningococcal *(Continued)*
    myocardium A39.52
    pericardium A39.53
    retrobulbar neuritis A39.82
    specified site NEC A39.89
  mesenteric lymph nodes or glands NEC I88.0
  Metagonimus B66.8
  metatarsophalangeal M00.9
  methicillin
    resistant Staphylococcus aureus (MRSA) A49.02
    susceptible Staphylococcus aureus (MSSA) A49.01
  Microsporum, microsporic —*see* Dermatophytosis
  mixed flora (bacterial) NEC A49.8
  Monilia —*see* Candidiasis
  Monosporium apiospermum B48.2
  mouth, parasitic B37.0
  Mucor —*see* Mucormycosis
  muscle NEC —*see* Myositis, infective
  mycelium NOS B49
  mycetoma B47.9
    actinomycotic NEC B47.1
    mycotic NEC B47.0
  Mycobacterium, mycobacterial —*see* Mycobacterium
  Mycoplasma NEC A49.3
    pneumoniae, as cause of disease classified elsewhere B96.0
  mycotic NOS B49
    pathogenic to compromised host only B48.8
    skin NOS B36.9
  myocardium NEC I40.0
  nail (chronic)
    with lymphangitis —*see* Lymphangitis, acute, digit
    finger L03.01-•
      fungus B35.1
    ingrowing L60.0
    toe L03.03-•
      fungus B35.1
  nasal sinus (chronic) —*see* Sinusitis
  nasopharynx —*see* Nasopharyngitis
  navel L08.82
  Necator americanus B76.1
  Neisseria —*see* Gonococcus
  Neotestudina rosatii B47.0
  newborn P39.9
    intra-amniotic NEC P39.2
    skin P39.4
    specified type NEC P39.8
  nipple N61.0
    associated with
      lactation O91.03
        pregnancy O91.01-•
        puerperium O91.02
  Nocardia —*see* Nocardiosis
  obstetrical surgical wound (puerperal) O86.00
    incisional site
      deep O86.02
      superficial O86.01
    organ and space site O86.03
    surgical site specified NEC O86.09
  Oesophagostomum (apiostomum) B81.8
  Oestrus ovis —*see* Myiasis
  Oidium albicans B37.9
  Onchocerca (volvulus) —*see* Onchocerciasis - oncovirus, as cause of disease classified elsewhere B97.32
  operation wound T81.49
  Opisthorchis (felineus) (viverrini) B66.0
  orbit, orbital —*see* Inflammation, orbit
  orthopoxvirus NEC B08.09
  ovary —*see* Salpingo-oophoritis
  Oxyuris vermicularis B80

Infection, infected, infective (Continued)
  pancreas (acute) —see Pancreatitis, acute
    abscess —see Pancreatitis, acute
    specified NEC —see also Pancreatitis, acute
      K85.80
  papillomavirus, as cause of disease classified
    elsewhere B97.7
  papovavirus NEC B34.4
  Paracoccidioides brasiliensis —see
    Paracoccidioidomycosis
  Paragonimus (westermani) B66.4
  parainfluenza virus B34.8
  parameningococcus NOS A39.9
  parapoxvirus B08.60
    specified NEC B08.69
  parasitic B89
  Parastrongylus
    cantonensis B83.2
    costaricensis B81.3
    paratyphoid A01.4
      Type A A01.1
      Type B A01.2
      Type C A01.3
  paraurethral ducts N34.2
  parotid gland —see Sialoadenitis
  parvovirus NEC B34.3
    as cause of disease classified elsewhere
      B97.6
  Pasteurella NEC A28.0
    multocida A28.0
    pestis —see Plague
    pseudotuberculosis A28.0
    septica (cat bite) (dog bite) A28.0
    tularensis —see Tularemia
  pelvic, female —see Disease, pelvis,
    inflammatory
  Penicillium (marneffei) B48.4
  penis (glans) (retention) NEC N48.29
  periapical K04.5
  peridental, periodontal K05.20
    generalized —see Periodontitis, aggressive,
      generalized
    localized —see Periodontitis, aggressive,
      localized
  perinatal period P39.9
    specified type NEC P39.8
  perineal repair (puerperal) O86.09
  periorbital —see Inflammation, orbit
  perirectal K62.89
  perirenal —see Infection, kidney
  peritoneal —see Peritonitis
  periureteral N28.89
  Petriellidium boydii B48.2
  pharynx —see also Pharyngitis
    coxsackievirus B08.5
    posterior, lymphoid (chronic) J35.03
  Phialophora
    gougerotii (subcutaneous abscess or cyst)
      B43.2
    jeanselmei (subcutaneous abscess or cyst)
      B43.2
    verrucosa (skin) B43.0
  Piedraia hortae B36.3
  pinta A67.9
    intermediate A67.1
    late A67.2
    mixed A67.3
    primary A67.0
  pinworm B80
  pityrosporum furfur B36.0
  pleuro-pneumonia-like organism (PPLO)
    NEC A49.3
    as cause of disease classified elsewhere
      B96.0
  pneumococcus, pneumococcal NEC A49.1
    as cause of disease classified elsewhere
      B95.3
    generalized (purulent) A40.3
      with pneumonia J13
  Pneumocystis carinii (pneumonia) B59
  Pneumocystis jiroveci (pneumonia) B59

Infection, infected, infective (Continued)
  port or reservoir T80.212
  postoperative T81.40
  postoperative wound T81.49
  postprocedural T81.40
    surgical site
      deep incisional T81.42
      organ and space T81.43
      specified NEC T81.49
      superficial incisional T81.41
  postvaccinal T88.0
  prepuce NEC N47.7
    with penile inflammation N47.6
  prion —see Disease, prion, central nervous
    system
  prostate (capsule) —see Prostatitis
  Proteus (mirabilis) (morganii) (vulgaris) NEC
    A49.8
    as cause of disease classified elsewhere
      B96.4
  protozoal NEC B64
    intestinal A07.9
      specified NEC A07.8
    specified NEC B60.8
  Pseudoallescheria boydii B48.2
  Pseudomonas NEC A49.8
    as cause of disease classified elsewhere
      B96.5
    mallei A24.0
    pneumonia J15.1
    pseudomallei —see Melioidosis
  puerperal O86.4
    genitourinary tract NEC O86.89
    major or generalized O85
    minor O86.4
    specified NEC O86.89
  pulmonary —see Infection, lung
  purulent —see Abscess
  Pyrenochaeta romeroi B47.0
  Q fever A78
  rectum (sphincter) K62.89
  renal —see also Infection, kidney
    pelvis and ureter (cystic) N28.85
  reovirus, as cause of disease classified
    elsewhere B97.5
  respiratory (tract) NEC J98.8
    acute J22
    chronic J98.8
    influenzal (upper) (acute) —see Influenza,
      with, respiratory manifestations
      NEC
    lower (acute) J22
      chronic —see Bronchitis, chronic
    rhinovirus J00
    syncytial virus (RSV) —see Infection, virus,
      respiratory syncytial (RSV)
    upper (acute) NOS J06.9
      chronic J39.8
      streptococcal J06.9
      viral NOS J06.9
        due to respiratory syncytial virus
          (RSV) J06.9 [B97.1]
  resulting from
    presence of internal prosthesis, implant,
      graft —see Complications, by site and
      type, infection
  retortamoniasis A07.8
  retroperitoneal NEC K68.9
  retrovirus B33.3
    as cause of disease classified elsewhere
      B97.30
    human
      immunodeficiency, type 2 (HIV 2)
        B97.35
      T-cell lymphotropic
        type I (HTLV-I) B97.33
        type II (HTLV-II) B97.34
    lentivirus B97.31
    oncovirus B97.32
    specified NEC B97.39
  Rhinosporidium (seeberi) B48.1

Infection, infected, infective (Continued)
  rhinovirus
    as cause of disease classified elsewhere
      B97.89
    unspecified nature or site B34.8
  Rhizopus —see Mucormycosis
  rickettsial NOS A79.9
  roundworm (large) NEC B82.0
    Ascariasis —see also Ascariasis B77.9
  rubella —see Rubella
  Saccharomyces —see Candidiasis
  salivary duct or gland (any) —see
    Sialoadenitis
  Salmonella (aertrycke) (arizonae)
    (callinarum) (cholerae-suis) (enteritidis)
    (suipestifer) (typhimurium) A02.9
    with
      (gastro) enteritis A02.0
      sepsis A02.1
      specified manifestation NEC
        A02.8
    due to food (poisoning) A02.9
    hirschfeldii A01.3
    localized A02.20
      arthritis A02.23
      meningitis A02.21
      osteomyelitis A02.24
      pneumonia A02.22
      pyelonephritis A02.25
      specified NEC A02.29
    paratyphi A01.4
      A A01.1
      B A01.2
      C A01.3
    schottmuelleri A01.2
    typhi, typhosa —see Typhoid
  Sarcocystis A07.8
  scabies B86
  Schistosoma —see Infestation, Schistosoma
  scrotum (acute) NEC N49.2
  seminal vesicle —see Vesiculitis
  septic
    localized, skin —see Abscess
  sheep liver fluke B66.3
  Shigella A03.9
    boydii A03.2
    dysenteriae A03.0
    flexneri A03.1
    group
      A A03.0
      B A03.1
      C A03.2
      D A03.3
    Schmitz (-Stutzer) A03.0
    schmitzii A03.0
    shigae A03.0
    sonnei A03.3
    specified NEC A03.8
  shoulder (joint) NEC M00.9
    due to internal joint prosthesis
      T84.59
    skin NEC L08.9
  sinus (accessory) (chronic) (nasal) —see also
    Sinusitis
    pilonidal —see Sinus, pilonidal
    skin NEC L08.89
  Skene's duct or gland —see Urethritis
  skin (local) (staphylococcal) (streptococcal)
    L08.9
    abscess - code by site under Abscess
    cellulitis - code by site under Cellulitis
    due to fungus B36.9
      specified NEC B36.8
    mycotic B36.9
      specified type NEC B36.8
    newborn P39.4
    ulcer —see Ulcer, skin
  slow virus A81.9
    specified NEC A81.89
  Sparganum (mansoni) (proliferum) (baxteri)
    B70.1

Infection, infected, infective (Continued)
specific —see also Syphilis
  to perinatal period —see Infection,
    congenital
specified NEC B99.8
spermatic cord NEC N49.1
sphenoidal (sinus) —see Sinusitis,
  sphenoidal
spinal cord NOS —see also Myelitis G04.91
  abscess G06.1
  meninges —see Meningitis
  streptococcal G04.89
Spirillum A25.0
spirochetal NOS A69.9
  lung A69.8
  specified NEC A69.8
Spirometra larvae B70.1
spleen D73.89
Sporotrichum, Sporothrix (schenckii) —see
  Sporotrichosis
staphylococcal, unspecified site
  aureus (methicillin susceptible) (MSSA)
    A49.01
    methicillin resistant (MRSA) A49.02
  as cause of disease classified elsewhere
    B95.8
    aureus (methicillin susceptible) (MSSA)
      B95.61
      methicillin resistant (MRSA)
        B95.62
    specified NEC B95.7
  food poisoning A05.0
  generalized (purulent) A41.2
  pneumonia —see Pneumonia,
    staphylococcal
Stellantchasmus falcatus B66.8
streptobacillus moniliformis A25.1
streptococcal NEC A49.1
  as cause of disease classified elsewhere
    B95.5
  B genitourinary complicating
    childbirth O98.82
    pregnancy O98.81-•
    puerperium O98.83
  congenital
    sepsis P36.10
      group B P36.0
      specified NEC P36.19
  generalized (purulent) A40.9
Streptomyces B47.1
Strongyloides (stercoralis) —see
  Strongyloidiasis
stump (amputation) (surgical) —see
  Complication, amputation stump,
  infection
subcutaneous tissue, local L08.9
suipestifer —see Infection, salmonella
swimming pool bacillus A31.1
Taenia —see Infestation, Taenia
Taeniarhynchus saginatus B68.1
tapeworm —see Infestation,
  tapeworm
tendon (sheath) —see Tenosynovitis, infective
  NEC
Ternidens diminutus B81.8
testis —see Orchitis
threadworm B80
throat —see Pharyngitis
thyroglossal duct K14.8
toe (skin) L08.9
  cellulitis L03.03-•
    fungus B35.1
  nail L03.03-•
    fungus B35.1
tongue NEC K14.0
  parasitic B37.0
tonsil (and adenoid) (faucial) (lingual)
  (pharyngeal) —see Tonsillitis
tooth, teeth K04.7
  irreversible K04.02
  periapical K04.7

Infection, infected, infective (Continued)
tooth, teeth (Continued)
  peridental, periodontal K05.20
    generalized —see Periodontitis,
      aggressive, generalized
    localized —see Periodontitis, aggressive,
      localized
  pulp K04.01
    irreversible K04.02
    reversible K04.01
TORCH —see Infection, congenital
  without active infection P00.2
Torula histolytica —see Cryptococcosis
Toxocara (canis) (cati) (felis) B83.0
Toxoplasma gondii —see Toxoplasma
trachea, chronic J42
trematode NEC —see Infestation, fluke
trench fever A79.0
Treponema pallidum —see Syphilis
Trichinella (spiralis) B75
Trichomonas A59.9
  cervix A59.09
  intestine A07.8
  prostate A59.02
  specified site NEC A59.8
  urethra A59.03
  urogenitalis A59.00
  vagina A59.01
  vulva A59.01
Trichophyton, trichophytic —see
  Dermatophytosis
Trichosporon (beigelii) cutaneum B36.2
Trichostrongylus B81.2
Trichuris (trichiura) B79
Trombicula (irritans) B88.0
Trypanosoma
  brucei
    gambiense B56.0
    rhodesiense B56.1
  cruzi —see Chagas' disease
tubal —see Salpingo-oophoritis
tuberculous
  latent (LTBI) Z22.7
  NEC —see Tuberculosis
tubo-ovarian —see Salpingo-oophoritis
tunica vaginalis N49.1
tunnel T80.212
tympanic membrane NEC —see Myringitis
typhoid (abortive) (ambulant) (bacillus) —see
  Typhoid
typhus A75.9
  flea-borne A75.2
  mite-borne A75.3
  recrudescent A75.1
  tick-borne A77.9
    African A77.1
    North Asian A77.2
umbilicus L08.82
ureter —see Ureteritis
urethra —see Urethritis
urinary (tract) N39.0
  bladder —see Cystitis
  complicating
    pregnancy O23.4-•
      specified type NEC O23.3-•
  kidney —see Infection, kidney
  newborn P39.3
  puerperal (postpartum) O86.20
  tuberculous A18.13
  urethra —see Urethritis
uterus, uterine —see Endometritis
vaccination T88.0
vaccinia not from vaccination B08.011
vagina (acute) —see Vaginitis
varicella B01.9
varicose veins —see Varix
vas deferens NEC N49.1
vesical —see Cystitis
Vibrio
  cholerae A00.0
    El Tor A00.1

Infection, infected, infective (Continued)
Vibrio (Continued)
  parahaemolyticus (food poisoning)
    A05.3
  vulnificus
    as cause of disease classified elsewhere
      B96.82
    foodborne intoxication A05.5
Vincent's (gum) (mouth) (tonsil) A69.1
virus, viral NOS B34.9
  adenovirus
    as cause of disease classified elsewhere
      B97.0
    unspecified nature or site B34.0
  arborvirus, arbovirus arthropod-borne
    A94
  as cause of disease classified elsewhere
    B97.89
    adenovirus B97.0
    coronavirus B97.29
      SARS-associated B97.21
    coxsackievirus B97.11
    echovirus B97.12
    enterovirus B97.10
      coxsackievirus B97.11
      echovirus B97.12
      specified NEC B97.19
    human
      immunodeficiency, type 2 (HIV 2)
        B97.35
      metapneumovirus B97.81
      T-cell lymphotropic,
        type I (HTLV-I) B97.33
        type II (HTLV-II) B97.34
    papillomavirus B97.7
    parvovirus B97.6
    reovirus B97.5
    respiratory syncytial (RSV) —see
      Infection virus, respiratory
      syncytial (RSV)
    retrovirus B97.30
      human
        immunodeficiency, type 2 (HIV 2)
          B97.35
        T-cell lymphotropic,
          type I (HTLV-I) B97.33
          type II (HTLV-II) B97.34
      lentivirus B97.31
      oncovirus B97.32
      specified NEC B97.39
    specified NEC B97.89
  central nervous system A89
    atypical A81.9
      specified NEC A81.89
    enterovirus NEC A88.8
      meningitis A87.0
    slow virus A81.9
      specified NEC A81.89
    specified NEC A88.8
  chest J98.8
  cotia B08.8
  COVID-19 U07.1
  coxsackie —see also Infection, coxsackie
    B34.1
    as cause of disease classified elsewhere
      B97.11
  ECHO
    as cause of disease classified elsewhere
      B97.12
    unspecified nature or site B34.1
  encephalitis, tick-borne A84.9
  enterovirus, as cause of disease classified
    elsewhere B97.10
    coxsackievirus B97.11
    echovirus B97.12
    specified NEC B97.19
  exanthem NOS B09
  human metapneumovirus as cause of
    disease classified elsewhere B97.81
  human papilloma as cause of disease
    classified elsewhere B97.7

▶ New   ⇒ Revised   ~~deleted~~ Deleted   • Use Additional Character(s)

Infection, infected, infective *(Continued)*
  virus, viral NOS *(Continued)*
    intestine —*see* Enteritis, viral
    respiratory syncytial (RSV) —*see* Infection
        virus, respiratory syncytial (RSV)
      bronchiolitis J21.0
      bronchitis J20.5
      bronchopneumonia J12.1
      otitis media H65.-● *[B97.4]*
      pneumonia J12.1
      upper respiratory infection J06.9
          [B97.4]
    rhinovirus
      as cause of disease classified elsewhere
          B97.89
      unspecified nature or site B34.8
    slow A81.9
      specified NEC A81.89
    specified type NEC B33.8
      as cause of disease classified elsewhere
          B97.89
      unspecified nature or site B34.9
    West Nile —*see* Virus, West Nile
  vulva (acute) —*see* Vulvitis
  West Nile —*see* Virus, West Nile
  whipworm B79
  worms B83.9
    specified type NEC B83.8
  Wuchereria (bancrofti) B74.0
    malayi B74.1
    yatapoxvirus B08.70
      specified NEC B08.79
  yeast *(see also* Candidiasis) B37.9
  yellow fever —*see* Fever, yellow
  Yersinia
    enterocolitica (intestinal) A04.6
    pestis —*see* Plague
    pseudotuberculosis A28.2
  Zeis' gland —*see* Hordeolum
  Zika virus A92.5
    congenital P35.4
  zoonotic bacterial NOS A28.9
  Zopfia senegalensis B47.0
Infective, infectious —*see* condition
Infertility
  female N97.9
    age-related N97.8
    associated with
      anovulation N97.0
      cervical (mucus) disease or anomaly
          N88.3
      congenital anomaly
        cervix N88.3
        fallopian tube N97.1
        uterus N97.2
        vagina N97.8
      dysmucorrhea N88.3
      fallopian tube disease or anomaly
          N97.1
      pituitary-hypothalamic origin
          E23.0
      specified origin NEC N97.8
      Stein-Leventhal syndrome E28.2
      uterine disease or anomaly N97.2
      vaginal disease or anomaly N97.8
    due to
      cervical anomaly N88.3
      fallopian tube anomaly N97.1
      ovarian failure E28.39
      Stein-Leventhal syndrome
          E28.2
      uterine anomaly N97.2
      vaginal anomaly N97.8
    nonimplantation N97.2
    origin
      cervical N88.3
      tubal (block) (occlusion) (stenosis)
          N97.1
      uterine N97.2
      vaginal N97.8

Infertility *(Continued)*
  male N46.9
    azoospermia N46.01
      extratesticular cause N46.029
        drug therapy N46.021
        efferent duct obstruction N46.023
        infection N46.022
        radiation N46.024
        specified cause NEC N46.029
        systemic disease N46.025
    oligospermia N46.11
      extratesticular cause N46.129
        drug therapy N46.121
        efferent duct obstruction N46.123
        infection N46.122
        radiation N46.124
        specified cause NEC N46.129
        systemic disease N46.125
    specified type NEC N46.8
Infestation B88.9
  Acanthocheilonema (perstans) (streptocerca)
      B74.4
  Acariasis B88.0
    demodex folliculorum B88.0
    sarcoptes scabiei B86
    trombiculae B88.0
  Agamofilaria streptocerca B74.4
  Ancylostoma, ankylostoma (braziliense)
      (caninum) (ceylanicum) (duodenale)
      B76.0
    americanum B76.1
    new world B76.1
  Anisakis larvae, anisakiasis B81.0
  arthropod NEC B88.2
  Ascaris lumbricoides —*see* Ascariasis
  Balantidium coli A07.0
  beef tapeworm B68.1
  Bothriocephalus (latus) B70.0
    larval B70.1
  broad tapeworm B70.0
    larval B70.1
  Brugia (malayi) B74.1
    timori B74.2
  candiru B88.8
  Capillaria
    hepatica B83.8
    philippinensis B81.1
  cat liver fluke B66.0
  cestodes B71.9
    diphyllobothrium —*see* Infestation,
        diphyllobothrium
    dipylidiasis B71.1
    hymenolepiasis B71.0
    specified type NEC B71.8
  chigger B88.0
  chigo, chigoe B88.1
  Clonorchis (sinensis) (liver) B66.1
  coccidial A07.3
  crab-lice B85.3
  Cysticercus cellulosae —*see* Cysticercosis
  Demodex (folliculorum) B88.0
  Dermanyssus gallinae B88.0
  Dermatobia (hominis) —*see* Myiasis
  Dibothriocephalus (latus) B70.0
    larval B70.1
  Dicrocoelium dendriticum B66.2
  Diphyllobothrium (adult) (latum) (intestinal)
      (pacificum) B70.0
    larval B70.1
  Diplogonoporus (grandis) B71.8
  Dipylidium caninum B67.4
  Distoma hepaticum B66.3
  dog tapeworm B67.4
  Dracunculus medinensis B72
  dragon worm B72
  dwarf tapeworm B71.0
  Echinococcus —*see* Echinococcus
  Echinostomum ilocanum B66.8
  Entamoeba (histolytica) —*see* Infection,
      Ameba
  Enterobius vermicularis B80

Infestation *(Continued)*
  eyelid
    in (due to)
      leishmaniasis B55.1
      loiasis B74.3
      onchocerciasis B73.09
      phthiriasis B85.3
    parasitic NOS B89
  eyeworm B74.3
  Fasciola (gigantica) (hepatica) (indica) B66.3
  Fasciolopsis (buski) (intestine) B66.5
  filarial B74.9
    bancroftian B74.0
    conjunctiva B74.9
    due to
      Acanthocheilonema (perstans)
          (streptocerca) B74.4
      Brugia (malayi) B74.1
        timori B74.2
      Dracunculus medinensis B72
      guinea worm B72
      loa loa B74.3
      Mansonella (ozzardi) (perstans)
          (streptocerca) B74.4
      Onchocerca volvulus B73.00
        eye B73.00
        eyelid B73.09
      Wuchereria (bancrofti) B74.0
    Malayan B74.1
    ozzardi B74.4
    specified type NEC B74.8
  fish tapeworm B70.0
    larval B70.1
  fluke B66.9
    blood NOS —*see* Schistosomiasis
    cat liver B66.0
    intestinal B66.5
    lancet B66.2
    liver (sheep) B66.3
      cat B66.0
      Chinese B66.1
      due to clonorchiasis B66.1
      oriental B66.1
    lung (oriental) B66.4
    sheep liver B66.3
    specified type NEC B66.8
  fly larvae —*see* Myiasis
  Gasterophilus (intestinalis) —*see* Myiasis
  Gastrodiscoides hominis B66.8
  Giardia lamblia A07.1
  Gnathostoma (spinigerum) B83.1
  Gongylonema B83.8
  guinea worm B72
  helminth B83.9
    angiostrongyliasis B83.2
      intestinal B81.3
    gnathostomiasis B83.1
    hirudiniasis, internal B83.4
    intestinal B82.0
      angiostrongyliasis B81.3
      anisakiasis B81.0
      ascariasis —*see* Ascariasis
      capillariasis B81.1
      cysticercosis —*see* Cysticercosis
      diphyllobothriasis —*see* Infestation,
          diphyllobothriasis
      dracunculiasis B72
      echinococcus —*see* Echinococcosis
      enterobiasis B80
      filariasis —*see* Infestation, filarial
      fluke —*see* Infestation, fluke
      hookworm —*see* Infestation, hookworm
      mixed (types classifiable to more than
          one of the titles B65.0-B81.3 and
          B81.8) B81.4
      onchocerciasis —*see* Onchocerciasis
      schistosomiasis —*see* Infestation,
          schistosoma
    specified
      cestode NEC —*see* Infestation, cestode
      type NEC B81.8

Infestation *(Continued)*
  helminth *(Continued)*
    intestinal *(Continued)*
      strongyloidiasis —*see* Strongyloidiasis
      taenia —*see* Infestation, taenia
      trichinellosis B75
      trichostrongyliasis B81.2
      trichuriasis B79
     specified type NEC B83.8
     syngamiasis B83.3
     visceral larva migrans B83.0
   Heterophyes (heterophyes) B66.8
   hookworm B76.9
    ancylostomiasis B76.0
    necatoriasis B76.1
    specified type NEC B76.8
   Hymenolepis (diminuta) (nana) B71.0
   intestinal NEC B82.9
   leeches (aquatic) (land) —*see* Hirudiniasis
   Leishmania —*see* Leishmaniasis
   lice, louse —*see* Infestation, Pediculus
   Linguatula B88.8
   Liponyssoides sanguineus B88.0
   Loa loa B74.3
    conjunctival B74.3
    eyelid B74.3
   louse —*see* Infestation, Pediculus
   maggots —*see* Myiasis
   Mansonella (ozzardi) (perstans) (streptocerca) B74.4
   Medina (worm) B72
   Metagonimus (yokogawai) B66.8
   microfilaria streptocerca —*see* Onchocerciasis
    eye B73.00
    eyelid B73.09
   mites B88.9
    scabic B86
   Monilia (albicans) —*see* Candidiasis
   mouth B37.0
   Necator americanus B76.1
   nematode NEC (intestinal) B82.0
    Ancylostoma B76.0
    conjunctiva NEC B83.9
    Enterobius vermicularis B80
    Gnathostoma spinigerum B83.1
    physaloptera B80
    specified NEC B81.8
    trichostrongylus B81.2
    trichuris (trichuria) B79
   Oesophagostomum (apiostomum) B81.8
   Oestrus ovis —*see also* Myiasis B87.9
   Onchocerca (volvulus) —*see* Onchocerciasis
   Opisthorchis (felineus) (viverrini) B66.0
   orbit, parasitic NOS B89
   Oxyuris vermicularis B80
   Paragonimus (westermani) B66.4
   parasite, parasitic B89
    eyelid B89
    intestinal NOS B82.9
    mouth B37.0
    skin B88.9
    tongue B37.0
   Parastrongylus
    cantonensis B83.2
    costaricensis B81.3
   Pediculus B85.2
    body B85.1
    capitis (humanus) (any site) B85.0
    corporis (humanus) (any site) B85.1
    head B85.0
    mixed (classifiable to more than one of the titles B85.0-B85.3) B85.4
    pubis (any site) B85.3
   Pentastoma B88.8
   Phthirus (pubis) (any site) B85.3
    with any infestation classifiable to B85.0-B85.2 B85.4
   pinworm B80
   pork tapeworm (adult) B68.0

Infestation *(Continued)*
  protozoal NEC B64
   intestinal A07.9
    specified NEC A07.8
   specified NEC B60.8
  pubic, louse B85.3
  rat tapeworm B71.0
  red bug B88.0
  roundworm (large) NEC B82.0
   Ascariasis —*see also* Ascariasis B77.9
  sandflea B88.1
  Sarcoptes scabiei B86
  scabies B86
  Schistosoma B65.9
   bovis B65.8
   cercariae B65.3
   haematobium B65.0
   intercalatum B65.8
   japonicum B65.2
   mansoni B65.1
   mattheei B65.8
   mekongi B65.8
   specified type NEC B65.8
   spindale B65.8
  screw worms —*see* Myiasis
  skin NOS B88.9
  Sparganum (mansoni) (proliferum) (baxteri) B70.1
   larval B70.1
  specified type NEC B88.8
  Spirometra larvae B70.1
  Stellantchasmus falcatus B66.8
  Strongyloides stercoralis —*see* Strongyloidiasis
  Taenia B68.9
   diminuta B71.0
   echinococcus —*see* Echinococcus
   mediocanellata B68.1
   nana B71.0
   saginata B68.1
   solium (intestinal form) B68.0
    larval form —*see* Cysticercosis
  Taeniarhynchus saginatus B68.1
  tapeworm B71.9
   beef B68.1
   broad B70.0
    larval B70.1
   dog B67.4
   dwarf B71.0
   fish B70.0
    larval B70.1
   pork B68.0
   rat B71.0
  Ternidens diminutus B81.8
  Tetranychus molestissimus B88.0
  threadworm B80
  tongue B37.0
  Toxocara (canis) (cati) (felis) B83.0
  trematode(s) NEC —*see* Infestation, fluke
  Trichinella (spiralis) B75
  Trichocephalus B79
  Trichomonas —*see* Trichomoniasis
  Trichostrongylus B81.2
  Trichuris (trichiura) B79
  Trombicula (irritans) B88.0
  Tunga penetrans B88.1
  Uncinaria americana B76.1
  Vandellia cirrhosa B88.8
  whipworm B79
  worms B83.9
   intestinal B82.0
  Wuchereria (bancrofti) B74.0

Infiltrate, infiltration
  amyloid (generalized) (localized) —*see* Amyloidosis
  calcareous NEC R89.7
   localized —*see* Degeneration, by site
  calcium salt R89.7
  cardiac
   fatty —*see* Degeneration, myocardial
   glycogenic E74.02 *[143]*

Infiltrate, infiltration *(Continued)*
  corneal —*see* Edema, cornea
  eyelid —*see* Inflammation, eyelid
  glycogen, glycogenic —*see* Disease, glycogen storage
  heart, cardiac
   fatty —*see* Degeneration, myocardial
   glycogenic E74.02 *[143]*
  inflammatory in vitreous H43.89
  kidney N28.89
  leukemic —*see* Leukemia
  liver K76.89
   fatty —*see* Fatty, liver NEC
   glycogen —*see also* Disease, glycogen storage E74.03 *[K77]*
  lung R91.8
   eosinophilic —*see* Eosinophilia, pulmonary
  lymphatic —*see also* Leukemia, lymphatic C91.9-•
   gland I88.9
  muscle, fatty M62.89
  myocardium, myocardial
   fatty —*see* Degeneration, myocardial
   glycogenic E74.02 *[143]*
  on chest x-ray R91.8
  pulmonary R91.8
   with eosinophilia —*see* Eosinophilia, pulmonary
  skin (lymphocytic) L98.6
  thymus (gland) (fatty) E32.8
  urine R39.0
  vesicant agent
   antineoplastic chemotherapy T80.810
   other agent NEC T80.818
  vitreous body H43.89
Infirmity R68.89
  senile R54
Inflammation, inflamed, inflammatory (with exudation)
  abducent (nerve) —*see* Strabismus, paralytic, sixth nerve
  accessory sinus (chronic) —*see* Sinusitis
  adrenal (gland) E27.8
  alveoli, teeth M27.3
   scorbutic E54
  anal canal, anus K62.89
  antrum (chronic) —*see* Sinusitis, maxillary
  appendix —*see* Appendicitis
  arachnoid —*see* Meningitis
  areola N61.0
   puerperal, postpartum or gestational —*see* Infection, nipple
  areolar tissue NOS L08.9
  artery —*see* Arteritis
  auditory meatus (external) —*see* Otitis, externa
  Bartholin's gland N75.8
  bile duct (common) (hepatic) or passage —*see* Cholangitis
  bladder —*see* Cystitis
  bone —*see* Osteomyelitis
  brain —*see also* Encephalitis
   membrane —*see* Meningitis
  breast N61.0
   puerperal, postpartum, gestational —*see* Mastitis, obstetric
  broad ligament —*see* Disease, pelvis, inflammatory
  bronchi —*see* Bronchitis
  catarrhal J00
  cecum —*see* Appendicitis
  cerebral —*see also* Encephalitis
   membrane —*see* Meningitis
  cerebrospinal
   meningococcal A39.0
  cervix (uteri) —*see* Cervicitis
  chest J98.8
  chorioretinal H30.9-•
   cyclitis —*see* Cyclitis
   disseminated H30.10-•
    generalized H30.13-•
    peripheral H30.12-•
    posterior pole H30.11-•

Inflammation, inflamed, inflammatory
  (Continued)
  chorioretinal (Continued)
    epitheliopathy —see Epitheliopathy
    focal H30.00-●
      juxtapapillary H30.01-●
      macular H30.04-●
      paramacular —see Inflammation,
          chorioretinal, focal, macular
      peripheral H30.03-●
      posterior pole H30.02-●
      specified type NEC H30.89-●
  choroid —see Inflammation, chorioretinal
  chronic, postmastoidectomy cavity —see
      Complications, postmastoidectomy,
      inflammation
  colon —see Enteritis
  connective tissue (diffuse) NEC —see
      Disorder, soft tissue, specified type NEC
  cornea —see Keratitis
  corpora cavernosa N48.29
  cranial nerve —see Disorder, nerve, cranial
  Douglas' cul-de-sac or pouch (chronic) N73.0
  due to device, implant or graft —see also
      Complications, by site and type,
      infection or inflammation
    arterial graft T82.7
    breast (implant) T85.79
    catheter T85.79
      dialysis (renal) T82.7
        intraperitoneal T85.71
      infusion T82.7
        cranial T85.735
        intrathecal T85.735
        spinal (epidural) (subdural) T85.735
        subarachnoid T85.735
      urinary T83.518
        cystostomy T83.510
        Hopkins T83.518
        ileostomy T83.518
        nephrostomy T83.512
        specified NEC T83.518
        urethral indwelling T83.511
        urostomy T83.518
    electronic (electrode) (pulse generator)
        (stimulator)
      bone T84.7
      cardiac T82.7
      nervous system T85.738
        brain T85.731
        cranial nerve T85.732
        gastric nerve T85.732
        neurostimulator generator T85.734
        peripheral nerve T85.732
        sacral nerve T85.732
        spinal cord T85.733
        vagal nerve T85.732
      urinary T83.590
    fixation, internal (orthopedic) NEC —
        see Complication, fixation device,
        infection
    gastrointestinal (bile duct) (esophagus)
        T85.79
    neurostimulator electrode (lead) T85.732
    genital NEC T83.69
    heart NEC T82.7
      valve (prosthesis) T82.6
        graft T82.7
    joint prosthesis —see Complication, joint
        prosthesis, infection
    ocular (corneal graft) (orbital implant)
        NEC T85.79
    orthopedic NEC T84.7
    penile (cylinder) (pump) (resevoir) T83.61
    specified NEC T85.79
    testicular T83.62
    urinary NEC T83.598
      ileal conduit stent T83.593
      implanted neurostimulation T83.590
      implanted sphincter T83.591
      indwelling ureteral stent T83.592

Inflammation, inflamed, inflammatory
  (Continued)
  due to device, implant or graft (Continued)
    (Continued)
    urinary NEC (Continued)
      nephroureteral stent T83.593
      specified stent NEC T83.593
    vascular NEC T82.7
    ventricular intracranial (communicating)
        shunt T85.730
  duodenum K29.80
    with bleeding K29.81
  dura mater —see Meningitis
  ear (middle) —see also Otitis, media
    external —see Otitis, externa
    inner —see subcategory H83.0
  epididymis —see Epididymitis
  esophagus —see Esophagitis
  ethmoidal (sinus) (chronic) —see Sinusitis,
      ethmoidal
  eustachian tube (catarrhal) —see Salpingitis,
      eustachian
  eyelid H01.9
    abscess —see Abscess, eyelid
    blepharitis —see Blepharitis
    chalazion —see Chalazion
    dermatosis (noninfectious) —see
        Dermatosis, eyelid
    hordeolum —see Hordeolum
    specified NEC H01.8
  fallopian tube —see Salpingo-oophoritis
  fascia —see Myositis
  follicular, pharynx J31.2
  frontal (sinus) (chronic) —see Sinusitis, frontal
  gallbladder —see Cholecystitis
  gastric —see Gastritis
  gastrointestinal —see Enteritis
  genital organ (internal) (diffuse)
    female —see Disease, pelvis, inflammatory
    male N49.9
      multiple sites N49.8
      specified NEC N49.8
  gland (lymph) —see Lymphadenitis
  glottis —see Laryngitis
  granular, pharynx J31.2
  gum K05.10
    nonplaque induced K05.11
    plaque induced K05.10
  heart —see Carditis
  hepatic duct —see Cholangitis
  ileoanal (internal) pouch K91.850
  ileum —see also Enteritis
    regional or terminal —see Enteritis, regional
  intestinal pouch K91.850
  intestine (any part) —see Enteritis
  jaw (acute) (bone) (chronic) (lower)
      (suppurative) (upper) M27.2
  joint NEC —see Arthritis
    sacroiliac M46.1
  kidney —see Nephritis
  knee (joint) M13.169
    tuberculous A18.02
  labium (majus) (minus) —see Vulvitis
  lacrimal
    gland —see Dacryoadenitis
    passages (duct) (sac) —see also Dacryocystitis
      canaliculitis —see Canaliculitis, lacrimal
  larynx —see Laryngitis
  leg NOS L08.9
  lip K13.0
  liver (capsule) —see also Hepatitis
    chronic K73.9
    suppurative K75.0
  lung (acute) —see also Pneumonia
    chronic J98.4
  lymphatic vessel —see Lymphangitis
  lymph gland or node —see Lymphadenitis
  maxilla, maxillary M27.2
    sinus (chronic) —see Sinusitis, maxillary
  membranes of brain or spinal cord —see
      Meningitis

Inflammation, inflamed, inflammatory
  (Continued)
  meninges —see Meningitis
  mouth K12.1
  muscle —see Myositis
  myocardium —see Myocarditis
  nasal sinus (chronic) —see Sinusitis
  nasopharynx —see Nasopharyngitis
  navel L08.82
  nerve NEC —see Neuritis
  nipple N61.0
    puerperal, postpartum or gestational —see
        Infection, nipple
  nose —see Rhinitis
  oculomotor (nerve) —see Strabismus,
      paralytic, third nerve
  optic nerve —see Neuritis, optic
  orbit (chronic) H05.10
    acute H05.00
      abscess —see Abscess, orbit
      cellulitis —see Cellulitis, orbit
      osteomyelitis —see Osteomyelitis, orbit
      periostitis —see Periostitis, orbital
      tenonitis —see Tenonitis, eye
    granuloma —see Granuloma, orbit
    myositis —see Myositis, orbital
  ovary —see Salpingo-oophoritis
  oviduct —see Salpingo-oophoritis
  pancreas (acute) —see Pancreatitis
  parametrium N73.0
  parotid region L08.9
  pelvis, female —see Disease, pelvis,
      inflammatory
  penis (corpora cavernosa) N48.29
  perianal K62.89
  pericardium —see Pericarditis
  perineum (female) (male) L08.9
  perirectal K62.89
  peritoneum —see Peritonitis
  periuterine —see Disease, pelvis, inflammatory
  perivesical —see Cystitis
  petrous bone (acute) (chronic) —see Petrositis
  pharynx (acute) —see Pharyngitis
  pia mater —see Meningitis
  pleura —see Pleurisy
  polyp, colon —see also Polyp, colon,
      inflammatory K51.40
  prostate —see also Prostatitis
    specified type NEC N41.8
  rectosigmoid —see Rectosigmoiditis
  rectum —see also Proctitis K62.89
  respiratory, upper —see also Infection,
      respiratory, upper J06.9
    acute, due to radiation J70.0
    chronic, due to external agent —see
        condition, respiratory, chronic, due to
    due to
      chemicals, gases, fumes or vapors
          (inhalation) J68.2
      radiation J70.1
  retina —see Chorioretinitis
  retrocecal —see Appendicitis
  retroperitoneal —see Peritonitis
  salivary duct or gland (any) (suppurative) —
      see Sialoadenitis
  scorbutic, alveoli, teeth E54
  scrotum N49.2
  seminal vesicle —see Vesiculitis
  sigmoid —see Enteritis
  sinus —see Sinusitis
  Skene's duct or gland —see Urethritis
  skin L08.9
  spermatic cord N49.1
  sphenoidal (sinus) —see Sinusitis, sphenoidal
  spinal
    cord —see Encephalitis
    membrane —see Meningitis
    nerve —see Disorder, nerve
  spine —see Spondylopathy, inflammatory
  spleen (capsule) D73.89
  stomach —see Gastritis

Inflammation, inflamed, inflammatory
(Continued)
subcutaneous tissue L08.9
suprarenal (gland) E27.8
synovial —*see* Tenosynovitis
tendon (sheath) NEC —*see* Tenosynovitis
testis —*see* Orchitis
throat (acute) —*see* Pharyngitis
thymus (gland) E32.8
thyroid (gland) —*see* Thyroiditis
tongue K14.0
tonsil —*see* Tonsillitis
trachea —*see* Tracheitis
trochlear (nerve) —*see* Strabismus, paralytic,
fourth nerve
tubal —*see* Salpingo-oophoritis
tuberculous NEC —*see* Tuberculosis
tubo-ovarian —*see* Salpingo-oophoritis
tunica vaginalis N49.1
tympanic membrane —*see* Tympanitis
umbilicus, umbilical L08.82
uterine ligament —*see* Disease, pelvis,
inflammatory
uterus (catarrhal) —*see* Endometritis
uveal tract (anterior) NOS —*see also*
Iridocyclitis
posterior —*see* Chorioretinitis
vagina —*see* Vaginitis
vas deferens N49.1
vein —*see also* Phlebitis
intracranial or intraspinal (septic) G08
thrombotic I80.9
leg —*see* Phlebitis, leg
lower extremity —*see* Phlebitis, leg
vocal cord J38.3
vulva —*see* Vulvitis
Wharton's duct (suppurative) —*see*
Sialoadenitis
Inflation, lung, imperfect (newborn) —*see*
Atelectasis
Influenza (bronchial) (epidemic) (respiratory
(upper)) (unidentified influenza virus) J11.1
with
digestive manifestations J11.2
encephalopathy J11.81
enteritis J11.2
gastroenteritis J11.2
gastrointestinal manifestations J11.2
laryngitis J11.1
myocarditis J11.82
otitis media J11.83
pharyngitis J11.1
pneumonia J11.00
specified type J11.08
respiratory manifestations NEC J11.1
specified manifestation NEC J11.89
A (non-novel) J10-●
A/H5N1 —*see also* Influenza, due to,
identified novel influenza A virus J09.X2
avian —*see also* Influenza, due to, identified
novel influenza A virus J09.X2
B J10-●
bird —*see also* Influenza, due to, identified
novel influenza A virus J09.X2
C J10-●
novel (2009) H1N1 influenza —*see also*
Influenza, due to, identified influenza
virus NEC J10.1
novel influenza A/H1N1 —*see also* Influenza,
due to, identified influenza virus NEC
J10.1
due to
avian (*see also* Influenza, due to, identified
novel influenza A virus) J09.X2
identified influenza virus NEC J10.1
with
digestive manifestations J10.2
encephalopathy J10.81
enteritis J10.2
gastroenteritis J10.2
gastrointestinal manifestations J10.2

Influenza *(Continued)*
due to *(Continued)*
identified influenza virus NEC *(Continued)*
with *(Continued)*
laryngitis J10.1
myocarditis J10.82
otitis media J10.83
pharyngitis J10.1
pneumonia (unspecified type) J10.00
with same identified influenza virus
J10.01
specified type NEC J10.08
respiratory manifestations NEC J10.1
specified manifestation NEC J10.89
identified novel influenza A virus J09.X2
with
digestive manifestations J09.X3
encephalopathy J09.X9
enteritis J09.X3
gastroenteritis J09.X3
gastrointestinal manifestations J09.X3
laryngitis J09.X2
myocarditis J09.X9
otitis media J09.X9
pharyngitis J09.X2
pneumonia J09.X1
respiratory manifestations NEC
J09.X2
specified manifestation NEC J09.X9
upper respiratory symptoms J09.X2
of other animal origin, not bird or swine (*see
also* Influenza, due to, identified novel
influenza A virus) J09.X2
swine (viruses that normally cause infections
in pigs) —*see also* Influenza, due to,
identified novel influenza A virus
J09.X2
Influenza-like disease —*see* Influenza
Influenzal —*see* Influenza
Infraction, Freiberg's (metatarsal head) —*see*
Osteochondrosis, juvenile, metatarsus
Infraeruption of tooth (teeth) M26.34
**Infusion complication, misadventure, or
reaction** —*see* Complications, infusion
Ingestion
chemical —*see* Table of Drugs and Chemicals,
by substance, poisoning
drug or medicament
correct substance properly administered —
see Table of Drugs and Chemicals, by
drug, adverse effect
overdose or wrong substance given
or taken —*see* Table of Drugs and
Chemicals, by drug, poisoning
foreign body —*see* Foreign body, alimentary
tract
multiple drug —*see* Table of Drugs and
Chemicals, multiple
tularemia A21.3
Ingrowing
hair (beard) L73.1
nail (finger) (toe) L60.0
Inguinal —*see also* condition
testicle Q53.9
bilateral Q53.212
unilateral Q53.112
Inhalant-induced
anxiety disorder F18.980
depressive disorder F18.94
major neurocognitive disorder F18.97
mild neurocognitive disorder F18.988
psychotic disorder F18.959
Inhalation
anthrax A22.1
flame T27.3
food or foreign body —*see* Foreign body, by
site
gases, fumes, or vapors T59.9-●
specified agent NEC —*see* Table of Drugs
and Chemicals, by substance
T59.89-●

Inhalation *(Continued)*
liquid or vomitus —*see* Asphyxia
meconium (newborn) P24.00
with
with respiratory symptoms P24.01
pneumonia (pneumonitis) P24.01
mucus —*see* Asphyxia, mucus
oil or gasoline (causing suffocation) —*see*
Foreign body, by site
smoke T59.81-●
with respiratory conditions J70.5
due to chemicals, gases, fumes and
vapors J68.9
steam (*see also* Burn, respiratory tract) T59.9-●
stomach contents or secretions —*see* Foreign
body, by site
due to anesthesia (general) (local) or other
sedation T88.59
in labor and delivery O74.0
in pregnancy O29.01-●
postpartum, puerperal O89.01
Inhibition, orgasm
female F52.31
male F52.32
Inhibitor, systemic lupus erythematosus
(presence of) D68.62
Iniencephalus, iniencephaly Q00.2
Injection, traumatic jet (air) (industrial) (water)
(paint or dye) T70.4
Injury —*see also* specified injury type T14.90
abdomen, abdominal S39.91
blood vessel —*see* Injury, blood vessel,
abdomen
cavity —*see* Injury, intra-abdominal
contusion S30.1
internal —*see* Injury, intra-abdominal
intra-abdominal organ —*see* Injury,
intra-abdominal
nerve —*see* Injury, nerve, abdomen
open —*see* Wound, open, abdomen
specified NEC S39.81
superficial —*see* Injury, superficial,
abdomen
Achilles tendon S86.00-●
laceration S86.02-●
specified type NEC S86.09-●
strain S86.01-●
acoustic, resulting in deafness —*see* Injury,
nerve, acoustic
adrenal (gland) S37.819
contusion S37.812
laceration S37.813
specified type NEC S37.818
alveolar (process) S09.93
ankle S99.91-●
contusion —*see* Contusion, ankle
dislocation —*see* Dislocation, ankle
fracture —*see* Fracture, ankle
nerve —*see* Injury, nerve, ankle
open —*see* Wound, open, ankle
specified type NEC S99.81-●
sprain —*see* Sprain, ankle
superficial —*see* Injury, superficial, ankle
anterior chamber, eye —*see* Injury, eye,
specified site NEC
anus —*see* Injury, abdomen
aorta (thoracic) S25.00
abdominal S35.00
laceration (minor) (superficial) S35.01
major S35.02
specified type NEC S35.09
laceration (minor) (superficial) S25.01
major S25.02
specified type NEC S25.09
arm (upper) S49.9-●
blood vessel —*see* Injury, blood vessel,
arm
contusion —*see* Contusion, arm, upper
fracture —*see* Fracture, humerus
lower —*see* Injury, forearm
muscle —*see* Injury, muscle, shoulder

▶ New ⇒ Revised ~~deleted~~ Deleted ● Use Additional Character(s)

Injury *(Continued)*
  arm *(Continued)*
    nerve —*see* Injury, nerve, arm
    open —*see* Wound, open, arm
    specified type NEC S49.8-●
    superficial —*see* Injury, superficial, arm
  artery (complicating trauma) —*see also* Injury, blood vessel, by site
    cerebral or meningeal —*see* Injury, intracranial
  auditory canal (external) (meatus) S09.91
  auricle, auris, ear S09.91
  axilla —*see* Injury, shoulder
  back —*see* Injury, back, lower
  bile duct S36.13
  birth —*see also* Birth, injury P15.9
  bladder (sphincter) S37.20
    at delivery O71.5
    contusion S37.22
    laceration S37.23
    obstetrical trauma O71.5
    specified type NEC S37.29
  blast (air) (hydraulic) (immersion) (underwater) NEC T14.8
    acoustic nerve trauma —*see* Injury, nerve, acoustic
    bladder —*see* Injury, bladder
    brain —*see* Concussion
    ▶ primary, specified NEC S06.8A-●
    colon —*see* Injury, intestine, large, blast injury
    ear (primary) S09.31-●
      secondary S09.39-●
    generalized T70.8
    lung —*see* Injury, intrathoracic, lung, blast injury
    multiple body organs T70.8
    peritoneum S36.81
    rectum S36.61
    retroperitoneum S36.898
    small intestine S36.419
      duodenum S36.410
      specified site NEC S36.418
    specified
      intra-abdominal organ NEC S36.898
      pelvic organ NEC S37.899
  blood vessel NEC T14.8
    abdomen S35.9-●
      aorta —*see* Injury, aorta, abdominal
      celiac artery —*see* Injury, blood vessel, celiac artery
      iliac vessel —*see* Injury, blood vessel, iliac
      laceration S35.91
      mesenteric vessel —*see* Injury, mesenteric
      portal vein —*see* Injury, blood vessel, portal vein
      renal vessel —*see* Injury, blood vessel, renal
      specified vessel NEC S35.8X-●
      splenic vessel —*see* Injury, blood vessel, splenic
      vena cava —*see* Injury, vena cava, inferior
    ankle —*see* Injury, blood vessel, foot
    aorta (abdominal) (thoracic) —*see* Injury, aorta
    arm (upper) NEC S45.90-●
      forearm —*see* Injury, blood vessel, forearm
      laceration S45.91-●
      specified
        site NEC S45.80-●
          laceration S45.81-●
          specified type NEC S45.89-●
        type NEC S45.99-●
      superficial vein S45.30-●
        laceration S45.31-●
        specified type NEC S45.39-●
    axillary
      artery S45.00-●
        laceration S45.01-●
        specified type NEC S45.09-●

Injury *(Continued)*
  blood vessel NEC *(Continued)*
    axillary *(Continued)*
      vein S45.20-●
        laceration S45.21-●
        specified type NEC S45.29-●
    azygos vein —*see* Injury, blood vessel, thoracic, specified site NEC
    brachial
      artery S45.10-●
        laceration S45.11-●
        specified type NEC S45.19-●
      vein S45.20-●
        laceration S45.219
        specified type NEC S45.29-●
    carotid artery (common) (external) (internal, extracranial) S15.00-●
      internal, intracranial S06.8-●
      laceration (minor) (superficial) S15.01-●
        major S15.02-●
      specified type NEC S15.09-●
    celiac artery S35.219
      branch S35.299
        laceration (minor) (superficial) S35.291
          major S35.292
        specified NEC S35.298
      laceration (minor) (superficial) S35.211
        major S35.212
      specified type NEC S35.218
    cerebral —*see* Injury, intracranial
    deep plantar —*see* Injury, blood vessel, plantar artery
    digital (hand) —*see* Injury, blood vessel, finger
    dorsal
      artery (foot) S95.00-●
        laceration S95.01-●
        specified type NEC S95.09-●
      vein (foot) S95.20-●
        laceration S95.21-●
        specified type NEC S95.29-●
    due to accidental laceration during procedure —*see* Laceration, accidental complicating surgery
    extremity —*see* Injury, blood vessel, limb
    femoral
      artery (common) (superficial) S75.00-●
        laceration (minor) (superficial) S75.01-●
          major S75.02-●
        specified type NEC S75.09-●
      vein (hip level) (thigh level) S75.10-●
        laceration (minor) (superficial) S75.11-●
          major S75.12-●
        specified type NEC S75.19-●
    finger S65.50-●
      index S65.50-●
        laceration S65.51-●
        specified type NEC S65.59-●
      laceration S65.51-●
      little S65.50-●
        laceration S65.51-●
        specified type NEC S65.59-●
      middle S65.50-●
        laceration S65.51-●
        specified type NEC S65.59-●
      specified type NEC S65.59-●
      thumb —*see* Injury, blood vessel, thumb
    foot S95.90-●
      dorsal
        artery —*see* Injury, blood vessel, dorsal, artery
        vein —*see* Injury, blood vessel, dorsal, vein
      laceration S95.91-●
      plantar artery —*see* Injury, blood vessel, plantar artery
      specified
        site NEC S95.80-●
          laceration S95.81-●
          specified type NEC S95.89-●
        specified type NEC S95.99-●

Injury *(Continued)*
  blood vessel NEC *(Continued)*
    forearm S55.90-●
      laceration S55.91-●
      radial artery —*see* Injury, blood vessel, radial artery
      specified
        site NEC S55.80-●
          laceration S55.81-●
          specified type NEC S55.89-●
        type NEC S55.99-●
      ulnar artery —*see* Injury, blood vessel, ulnar artery
      vein S55.20-●
        laceration S55.21-●
        specified type NEC S55.29-●
    gastric
      artery —*see* Injury, mesenteric, artery, branch
      vein —*see* Injury, blood vessel, abdomen
    gastroduodenal artery —*see* Injury, mesenteric, artery, branch
    greater saphenous vein (lower leg level) S85.30-●
      hip (and thigh) level S75.20-●
        laceration (minor) (superficial) S75.21-●
          major S75.22-●
        specified type NEC S75.29-●
      laceration S85.31-●
      specified type NEC S85.39-●
    hand (level) S65.90-●
      finger —*see* Injury, blood vessel, finger
      laceration S65.91-●
      palmar arch —*see* Injury, blood vessel, palmar arch
      radial artery —*see* Injury, blood vessel, radial artery, hand
      specified
        site NEC S65.80-●
          laceration S65.81-●
          specified type NEC S65.89-●
        type NEC S65.99-●
      thumb —*see* Injury, blood vessel, thumb
      ulnar artery —*see* Injury, blood vessel, ulnar artery, hand
    head S09.0
      intracranial —*see* Injury, intracranial
      multiple S09.0
    hepatic
      artery —*see* Injury, mesenteric, artery
      vein —*see* Injury, vena cava, inferior
    hip S75.90-●
      femoral artery —*see* Injury, blood vessel, femoral, artery
      femoral vein —*see* Injury, blood vessel, femoral, vein
      greater saphenous vein —*see* Injury, blood vessel, greater saphenous, hip level
      laceration S75.91-●
      specified
        site NEC S75.80-●
          laceration S75.81-●
          specified type NEC S75.89-●
        type NEC S75.99-●
    hypogastric (artery) (vein) —*see* Injury, blood vessel, iliac
    iliac S35.5-●
      artery S35.51-●
      specified vessel NEC S35.5-●
      uterine vessel —*see* Injury, blood vessel, uterine
      vein S35.51-●
    innominate —*see* Injury, blood vessel, thoracic, innominate
    intercostal (artery) (vein) —*see* Injury, blood vessel, thoracic, intercostal
    jugular vein (external) S15.20-●
      internal S15.30-●
        laceration (minor) (superficial) S15.31-●
          major S15.32-●
        specified type NEC S15.39-●

Injury (Continued)
  blood vessel NEC (Continued)
    jugular vein (Continued)
      laceration (minor) (superficial) S15.21-●
        major S15.22-●
      specified type NEC S15.29-●
    leg (level) (lower) S85.90-●
      greater saphenous —see Injury, blood
          vessel, greater saphenous
      laceration S85.91-●
      lesser saphenous —see Injury, blood
          vessel, lesser saphenous
      peroneal artery —see Injury, blood
          vessel, peroneal artery
      popliteal
        artery —see Injury, blood vessel,
            popliteal, artery
        vein —see Injury, blood vessel,
            popliteal, vein
      specified
        site NEC S85.80-●
          laceration S85.81-●
          specified type NEC S85.89-●
        type NEC S85.99-●
      thigh —see Injury, blood vessel, hip
      tibial artery —see Injury, blood vessel,
          tibial artery
    lesser saphenous vein (lower leg level)
        S85.40-●
      laceration S85.41-●
      specified type NEC S85.49-●
    limb
      lower —see Injury, blood vessel, leg
      upper —see Injury, blood vessel, arm
    lower back —see Injury, blood vessel,
        abdomen
      specified NEC —see Injury, blood vessel,
          abdomen, specified, site NEC
    mammary (artery) (vein) —see Injury, blood
        vessel, thoracic, specified site NEC
    mesenteric (inferior) (superior)
      artery —see Injury, mesenteric, artery
      vein —see Injury, mesenteric, vein
    neck S15.9
      specified site NEC S15.8
    ovarian (artery) (vein) —see subcategory
        S35.8
    palmar arch (superficial) S65.20-●
      deep S65.30-●
        laceration S65.31-●
        specified type NEC S65.39-●
      laceration S65.21-●
      specified type NEC S65.29-●
    pelvis —see Injury, blood vessel, abdomen
      specified NEC —see Injury, blood vessel,
          abdomen, specified, site NEC
    peroneal artery S85.20-●
      laceration S85.21-●
      specified type NEC S85.29-●
    plantar artery (deep) (foot) S95.10-●
      laceration S95.11-●
      specified type NEC S95.19-●
    popliteal
      artery S85.00-●
        laceration S85.01-●
        specified type NEC S85.09-●
      vein S85.50-●
        laceration S85.51-●
        specified type NEC S85.59-●
    portal vein S35.319
      laceration S35.311
      specified type NEC S35.318
    precerebral —see Injury, blood vessel, neck
    pulmonary (artery) (vein) —see Injury,
        blood vessel, thoracic, pulmonary
    radial artery (forearm level) S55.10-●
      hand and wrist (level) S65.10-●
        laceration S65.11-●
        specified type NEC S65.19-●
      laceration S55.11-●
      specified type NEC S55.19-●

Injury (Continued)
  blood vessel NEC (Continued)
    renal
      artery S35.40-●
        laceration S35.41-●
        specified NEC S35.49-●
      vein S35.40-●
        laceration S35.41-●
        specified NEC S35.49-●
    saphenous vein (greater) (lower leg
        level) —see Injury, blood vessel,
        greater saphenous
      hip and thigh level —see Injury, blood
          vessel, greater saphenous, hip level
      lesser —see Injury, blood vessel, lesser
          saphenous
    shoulder
      specified NEC —see Injury, blood vessel,
          arm, specified site NEC
      superficial vein —see Injury, blood
          vessel, arm, superficial vein
    specified NEC T14.8
    splenic
      artery —see Injury, blood vessel, celiac
          artery, branch
      vein S35.329
        laceration S35.321
        specified NEC S35.328
    subclavian —see Injury, blood vessel,
        thoracic, innominate
    thigh —see Injury, blood vessel, hip
    thoracic S25.90
      aorta S25.00
        laceration (minor) (superficial)
            S25.01
          major S25.02
        specified type NEC S25.09
      azygos vein —see Injury, blood vessel,
          thoracic, specified, site NEC
      innominate
        artery S25.10-●
          laceration (minor) (superficial)
              S25.11-●
            major S25.12-●
          specified type NEC S25.19-●
        vein S25.30-●
          laceration (minor) (superficial)
              S25.31-●
            major S25.32-●
          specified type NEC S25.39-●
      intercostal S25.50-●
        laceration S25.51-●
        specified type NEC S25.59-●
      laceration S25.91
      mammary vessel —see Injury, blood
          vessel, thoracic, specified, site NEC
      pulmonary S25.40-●
        laceration (minor) (superficial)
            S25.41-●
          major S25.42-●
        specified type NEC S25.49-●
      specified
        site NEC S25.80-●
          laceration S25.81-●
          specified type NEC S25.89-●
        type NEC S25.99
      subclavian —see Injury, blood vessel,
          thoracic, innominate
      vena cava (superior) S25.20
        laceration (minor) (superficial)
            S25.21
          major S25.22
        specified type NEC S25.29
    thumb S65.40-●
      laceration S65.41-●
      specified type NEC S65.49-●
    tibial artery S85.10-●
      anterior S85.13-●
        laceration S85.14-●
        specified injury NEC S85.15-●
      laceration S85.11-●

Injury (Continued)
  blood vessel NEC (Continued)
    tibial artery (Continued)
      posterior S85.16-●
        laceration S85.17-●
        specified injury NEC S85.18-●
      specified injury NEC S85.12-●
    ulnar artery (forearm level) S55.00-●
      hand and wrist (level) S65.00-●
        laceration S65.01-●
        specified type NEC S65.09-●
      laceration S55.01-●
      specified type NEC S55.09-●
    upper arm (level) —see Injury, blood vessel,
        arm
    superficial vein —see Injury, blood
        vessel, arm, superficial vein
    uterine S35.5-●
      artery S35.53-●
      vein S35.53-●
    vena cava —see Injury, vena cava
    vertebral artery S15.10-●
      laceration (minor) (superficial)
          S15.11-●
        major S15.12-●
      specified type NEC S15.19-●
    wrist (level) —see Injury, blood vessel,
        hand
  brachial plexus S14.3
    newborn P14.3
  brain (traumatic) S06.9-●
    diffuse (axonal) S06.2X-●
    focal S06.30-●
  brainstem S06.38-●
  breast NOS S29.9
  broad ligament —see Injury, pelvic organ,
      specified site NEC
  bronchus, bronchi —see Injury, intrathoracic,
      bronchus
  brow S09.90
  buttock S39.92
  canthus, eye S05.90
  cardiac plexus —see Injury, nerve, thorax,
      sympathetic
  cauda equina S34.3
  cavernous sinus —see Injury, intracranial
  cecum —see Injury, colon
  celiac ganglion or plexus —see Injury, nerve,
      lumbosacral, sympathetic
  cerebellum —see Injury, intracranial
  cerebral —see Injury, intracranial
  cervix (uteri) —see Injury, uterus
  cheek (wall) S09.93
  chest —see Injury, thorax
  childbirth (newborn) —see also Birth, injury
    maternal NEC O71.9
  chin S09.93
  choroid (eye) —see Injury, eye, specified site
      NEC
  clitoris S39.94
  coccyx —see also Injury, back, lower
    complicating delivery O71.6
  colon —see Injury, intestine, large
  common bile duct —see Injury, liver
  conjunctiva (superficial) —see Injury, eye,
      conjunctiva
  conus medullaris —see Injury, spinal, sacral
      cord
    spermatic (pelvic region) S37.898
      scrotal region S39.848
    spinal —see Injury, spinal cord, by region
  cornea —see Injury, eye, specified site NEC
    abrasion —see Injury, eye, cornea,
        abrasion
  cortex (cerebral) —see also Injury, intracranial
    visual —see Injury, nerve, optic
  costal region NEC S29.9
  costochondral NEC S29.9
  cranial
    cavity —see Injury, intracranial
    nerve —see Injury, nerve, cranial

▶ New   ⇒ Revised   ~~deleted~~ Deleted   ● Use Additional Character(s)

Injury *(Continued)*
crushing —*see* Crush
cutaneous sensory nerve
cystic duct —*see* Injury, liver
deep tissue —*see* Contusion, by site
  meaning pressure ulcer —*see* Ulcer,
    pressure L89 with final character .6
delivery (newborn) P15.9
  maternal NEC O71.9
Descemet's membrane —*see* Injury, eyeball,
  penetrating
diaphragm —*see* Injury, intrathoracic,
  diaphragm
duodenum —*see* Injury, intestine, small,
  duodenum
ear (auricle) (external) (canal) S09.91
  abrasion —*see* Abrasion, ear
  bite —*see* Bite, ear
  blister —*see* Blister, ear
  bruise —*see* Contusion, ear
  contusion —*see* Contusion, ear
  external constriction —*see* Constriction,
    external, ear
  hematoma —*see* Hematoma, ear
  inner —*see* Injury, ear, middle
  laceration —*see* Laceration, ear
  middle S09.30-•
    blast —*see* Injury, blast, ear
    specified NEC S09.39-•
  puncture —*see* Puncture, ear
  superficial —*see* Injury, superficial, ear
eighth cranial nerve (acoustic or auditory) —
  see Injury, nerve, acoustic
elbow S59.90-•
  contusion —*see* Contusion, elbow
  dislocation —*see* Dislocation, elbow
  fracture —*see* Fracture, ulna, upper
    end
  open —*see* Wound, open, elbow
  specified NEC S59.80-•
  sprain —*see* Sprain, elbow
  superficial —*see* Injury, superficial,
    elbow
eleventh cranial nerve (accessory) —*see*
  Injury, nerve, accessory
epididymis S39.94
epigastric region S39.91
epiglottis NEC S19.89
esophageal plexus —*see* Injury, nerve, thorax,
  sympathetic
esophagus (thoracic part) —*see also* Injury,
  intrathoracic, esophagus
  cervical NEC S19.85
eustachian tube S09.30-•
eye S05.9-•
  avulsion S05.7-•
  ball —*see* Injury, eyeball
  conjunctiva S05.0-•
  cornea
    abrasion S05.0-•
  laceration S05.3-•
    with prolapse S05.2-•
  lacrimal apparatus S05.8X-•
  orbit penetration S05.4-•
  specified site NEC S05.8X-•
eyeball S05.8X-•
  contusion S05.1-•
  penetrating S05.6-•
    with
      foreign body S05.5-•
      prolapse or loss of intraocular tissue
        S05.2-•
      without prolapse or loss of intraocular
        tissue S05.3-•
  specified type NEC S05.8-•
eyebrow S09.93
eyelid S09.93
  abrasion —*see* Abrasion, eyelid
  contusion —*see* Contusion, eyelid
  open —*see* Wound, open, eyelid
face S09.93

Injury *(Continued)*
fallopian tube S37.509
  bilateral S37.502
    blast injury S37.512
    contusion S37.522
    laceration S37.532
    specified type NEC S37.592
  blast injury (primary) S37.519
    bilateral S37.512
    secondary —*see* Injury, fallopian tube,
      specified type NEC
    unilateral S37.511
  contusion S37.529
    bilateral S37.522
    unilateral S37.521
  laceration S37.539
    bilateral S37.532
    unilateral S37.531
  specified type NEC S37.599
    bilateral S37.592
    unilateral S37.591
  unilateral S37.501
    blast injury S37.511
    contusion S37.521
    laceration S37.531
    specified type NEC S37.591
fascia —*see* Injury, muscle
fifth cranial nerve (trigeminal) —*see* Injury,
  nerve, trigeminal
finger (nail) S69.9-•
  blood vessel —*see* Injury, blood vessel,
    finger
  contusion —*see* Contusion, finger
  dislocation —*see* Dislocation, finger
  fracture —*see* Fracture, finger
  muscle —*see* Injury, muscle, finger
  nerve —*see* Injury, nerve, digital, finger
  open —*see* Wound, open, finger
  specified NEC S69.8-•
  sprain —*see* Sprain, finger
  superficial —*see* Injury, superficial, finger
first cranial nerve (olfactory) —*see* Injury,
  nerve, olfactory
flank —*see* Injury, abdomen
foot S99.92-•
  blood vessel —*see* Injury, blood vessel,
    foot
  contusion —*see* Contusion, foot
  dislocation —*see* Dislocation, foot
  fracture —*see* Fracture, foot
  muscle —*see* Injury, muscle, foot
  open —*see* Wound, open, foot
  specified type NEC S99.82-•
  sprain —*see* Sprain, foot
  superficial —*see* Injury, superficial, foot
forceps NOS P15.9
forearm S59.91-•
  blood vessel —*see* Injury, blood vessel,
    forearm
  contusion —*see* Contusion, forearm
  fracture —*see* Fracture, forearm
  muscle —*see* Injury, muscle, forearm
  nerve —*see* Injury, nerve, forearm
  open —*see* Wound, open, forearm
  specified NEC S59.81-•
  superficial —*see* Injury, superficial, forearm
forehead S09.90
fourth cranial nerve (trochlear) —*see* Injury,
  nerve, trochlear
gallbladder S36.129
  contusion S36.122
  laceration S36.123
  specified NEC S36.128
ganglion
  celiac, coeliac —*see* Injury, nerve,
    lumbosacral, sympathetic
  gasserian —*see* Injury, nerve, trigeminal
  stellate —*see* Injury, nerve, thorax,
    sympathetic
  thoracic sympathetic —*see* Injury, nerve,
    thorax, sympathetic

Injury *(Continued)*
gasserian ganglion —*see* Injury, nerve,
  trigeminal
gastric artery —*see* Injury, blood vessel, celiac
  artery, branch
gastroduodenal artery —*see* Injury, blood
  vessel, celiac artery, branch
gastrointestinal tract —*see* Injury,
  intra-abdominal
  with open wound into abdominal cavity —
    see Wound, open, with penetration
    into peritoneal cavity
  colon —*see* Injury, intestine, large
  rectum —*see* Injury, intestine, large, rectum
    with open wound into abdominal cavity
    S36.61
  small intestine —*see* Injury, intestine, small
  specified site NEC —*see* Injury, intra-
    abdominal, specified, site NEC
  stomach —*see* Injury, stomach
genital organ(s)
  external S39.94
    specified NEC S39.848
  internal S37.90
    fallopian tube —*see* Injury, fallopian tube
    ovary —*see* Injury, ovary
    prostate —*see* Injury, prostate
    seminal vesicle —*see* Injury, pelvis,
      organ, specified site NEC
    uterus —*see* Injury, uterus
    vas deferens —*see* Injury, pelvis, organ,
      specified site NEC
  obstetrical trauma O71.9
gland
  lacrimal laceration —*see* Injury, eye,
    specified site NEC
  salivary S09.93
  thyroid NEC S19.84
globe (eye) S05.90
  specified NEC S05.8X-•
groin —*see* Injury, abdomen
gum S09.90
hand S69.9-•
  blood vessel —*see* Injury, blood vessel,
    hand
  contusion —*see* Contusion, hand
  fracture —*see* Fracture, hand
  muscle —*see* Injury, muscle, hand
  nerve —*see* Injury, nerve, hand
  open —*see* Wound, open, hand
  specified NEC S69.8-•
  sprain —*see* Sprain, hand
  superficial —*see* Injury, superficial, hand
head S09.90
  with loss of consciousness S06.9-•
  specified NEC S09.8-•
heart (traumatic) S26.90
  with hemopericardium S26.00
    contusion S26.01
    laceration (mild) S26.020
      major S26.022
      moderate S26.021
    specified type NEC S26.09
  without hemopericardium S26.10
    contusion S26.11
    laceration S26.12
    specified type NEC S26.19
  contusion S26.91
  laceration S26.92
  non-traumatic (acute) (chronic) (non-
    ischemic) I5A
  specified type NEC S26.99
heel —*see* Injury, foot
hepatic
  artery —*see* Injury, blood vessel, celiac
    artery, branch
  duct —*see* Injury, liver
  vein —*see* Injury, vena cava, inferior
hip S79.91-•
  blood vessel —*see* Injury, blood vessel, hip
  contusion —*see* Contusion, hip
  dislocation —*see* Dislocation, hip

Injury *(Continued)*
  hip *(Continued)*
    fracture —*see* Fracture, femur, neck
    muscle —*see* Injury, muscle, hip
    nerve —*see* Injury, nerve, hip
    open —*see* Wound, open, hip
    specified NEC S79.81-●
    sprain —*see* Sprain, hip
    superficial —*see* Injury, superficial, hip
  hymen S39.94
  hypogastric
    blood vessel —*see* Injury, blood vessel, iliac
    plexus —*see* Injury, nerve, lumbosacral,
        sympathetic
  ileum —*see* Injury, intestine, small
  iliac region S39.91
  instrumental (during surgery) —*see*
        Laceration, accidental complicating
        surgery
    birth injury —*see* Birth, injury
    nonsurgical —*see* Injury, by site
    obstetrical O71.9
      bladder O71.5
      cervix O71.3
      high vaginal O71.4
      perineal NOS O70.9
      urethra O71.5
      uterus O71.5
        with rupture or perforation O71.1
  internal T14.8
    aorta —*see* Injury, aorta
    bladder (sphincter) —*see* Injury, bladder
      with
        ectopic or molar pregnancy O08.6
        following ectopic or molar pregnancy
          O08.6
        obstetrical trauma O71.5
    bronchus, bronchi —*see* Injury,
        intrathoracic, bronchus
    cecum —*see* Injury, intestine, large
    cervix (uteri) —*see also* Injury, uterus
      with ectopic or molar pregnancy O08.6
      following ectopic or molar pregnancy
          O08.6
      obstetrical trauma O71.3
    chest —*see* Injury, intrathoracic
    gastrointestinal tract —*see* Injury,
        intra-abdominal
    heart —*see* Injury, heart
    intestine NEC —*see* Injury, intestine
    intrauterine —*see* Injury, uterus
    mesentery —*see* Injury, intra-abdominal,
        specified, site NEC
    pelvis, pelvic (organ) S37.90
      following ectopic or molar pregnancy
          (subsequent episode) O08.6
      obstetrical trauma NEC O71.5
        rupture or perforation O71.1
      specified NEC S39.83
    rectum —*see* Injury, intestine, large, rectum
    stomach —*see* Injury, stomach
    ureter —*see* Injury, ureter
    urethra (sphincter) following ectopic or
        molar pregnancy O08.6
    uterus —*see* Injury, uterus
  interscapular area —*see* Injury, thorax
  intestine
    large S36.509
      ascending (right) S36.500
        blast injury (primary) S36.510
          secondary S36.590
        contusion S36.520
        laceration S36.530
        specified type NEC S36.590
      blast injury (primary) S36.519
        ascending (right) S36.510
        descending (left) S36.512
        rectum S36.61
        sigmoid S36.513
        specified site NEC S36.518
        transverse S36.511

Injury *(Continued)*
  intestine *(Continued)*
    large *(Continued)*
      contusion S36.529
        ascending (right) S36.520
        descending (left) S36.522
        rectum S36.62
        sigmoid S36.523
        specified site NEC S36.528
        transverse S36.521
      descending (left) S36.502
        blast injury (primary) S36.512
          secondary S36.592
        contusion S36.522
        laceration S36.532
        specified type NEC S36.592
      laceration S36.539
        ascending (right) S36.530
        descending (left) S36.532
        rectum S36.63
        sigmoid S36.533
        specified site NEC S36.538
        transverse S36.531
      rectum S36.60
        blast injury (primary) S36.61
          secondary S36.69
        contusion S36.62
        laceration S36.63
        specified type NEC S36.69
      sigmoid S36.503
        blast injury (primary) S36.513
          secondary S36.593
        contusion S36.523
        laceration S36.533
        specified type NEC S36.593
      specified
        site NEC S36.508
          blast injury (primary)
            S36.518
            secondary S36.598
          contusion S36.528
          laceration S36.538
          specified type NEC S36.598
        type NEC S36.599
          ascending (right) S36.590
          descending (left) S36.592
          rectum S36.69
          sigmoid S36.593
          specified site NEC S36.598
          transverse S36.591
      transverse S36.501
        blast injury (primary) S36.511
          secondary S36.591
        contusion S36.521
        laceration S36.531
        specified type NEC S36.591
    small S36.409
      blast injury (primary) S36.419
        duodenum S36.410
        secondary S36.499
          duodenum S36.490
          specified site NEC S36.498
        specified site NEC S36.418
      contusion S36.429
        duodenum S36.420
        specified site NEC S36.428
      duodenum S36.400
        blast injury (primary) S36.410
          secondary S36.490
        contusion S36.420
        laceration S36.430
        specified NEC S36.490
      laceration S36.439
        duodenum S36.430
        specified site NEC S36.438
      specified
        site NEC S36.408
        type NEC S36.499
          duodenum S36.490
          specified site NEC
            S36.498

Injury *(Continued)*
  intra-abdominal S36.90
    adrenal gland —*see* Injury, adrenal gland
    bladder —*see* Injury, bladder
    colon —*see* Injury, intestine, large
    contusion S36.92
    fallopian tube —*see* Injury, fallopian tube
    gallbladder —*see* Injury, gallbladder
    intestine —*see* Injury, intestine
    kidney —*see* Injury, kidney
    laceration S36.93
    liver —*see* Injury, liver
    ovary —*see* Injury, ovary
    pancreas —*see* Injury, pancreas
    pelvic NOS S37.90
    peritoneum —*see* Injury, intra-abdominal,
        specified, site NEC
    prostate —*see* Injury, prostate
    rectum —*see* Injury, intestine, large, rectum
    retroperitoneum —*see* Injury, intra-
        abdominal, specified, site NEC
    seminal vesicle —*see* Injury, pelvis, organ,
        specified site NEC
    small intestine —*see* Injury, intestine, small
    specified
      pelvic S37.90
        specified
          site NEC S37.899
            specified type NEC S37.898
          type NEC S37.99
      site NEC S36.899
        contusion S36.892
        laceration S36.893
        specified type NEC S36.898
      type NEC S36.99
    spleen —*see* Injury, spleen
    stomach —*see* Injury, stomach
    ureter —*see* Injury, ureter
    urethra —*see* Injury, urethra
    uterus —*see* Injury, uterus
    vas deferens —*see* Injury, pelvis, organ,
        specified site NEC
  intracranial (traumatic) *(see also*, if applicable,
      Compression, brain, traumatic) S06.9-●
    cerebellar hemorrhage, traumatic —*see*
        Injury, intracranial, focal
    cerebral edema, traumatic S06.1X-●
      diffuse S06.1X-●
      focal S06.1X-●
    diffuse (axonal) S06.2X-●
    epidural hemorrhage (traumatic) S06.4X-●
    focal brain injury S06.30-●
      contusion —*see* Contusion, cerebral
      laceration —*see* Laceration, cerebral
    intracerebral hemorrhage, traumatic
        S06.36-●
      left side S06.35-●
      right side S06.34-●
    ▶specified NEC S06.89-●
    subarachnoid hemorrhage, traumatic
        S06.6X-●
    subdural hemorrhage, traumatic S06.5X-●
  intraocular —*see* Injury, eyeball, penetrating
  intrathoracic S27.9
    bronchus S27.409
      bilateral S27.402
      blast injury (primary) S27.419
        bilateral S27.412
        secondary —*see* Injury, intrathoracic,
            bronchus, specified type NEC
        unilateral S27.411
      contusion S27.429
        bilateral S27.422
        unilateral S27.421
      laceration S27.439
        bilateral S27.432
        unilateral S27.431
      specified type NEC S27.499
        bilateral S27.492
        unilateral S27.491
      unilateral S27.401

▶ New   ⇒ Revised   ~~deleted~~ Deleted   ● Use Additional Character(s)

Injury *(Continued)*
  intrathoracic *(Continued)*
    diaphragm S27.809
      contusion S27.802
      laceration S27.803
      specified type NEC S27.808
    esophagus (thoracic) S27.819
      contusion S27.812
      laceration S27.813
      specified type NEC S27.818
    heart —*see* Injury, heart
    hemopneumothorax S27.2
    hemothorax S27.1
    lung S27.309
      aspiration J69.0
      bilateral S27.302
      blast injury (primary) S27.319
        bilateral S27.312
        secondary —*see* Injury, intrathoracic,
          lung, specified type NEC
        unilateral S27.311
      contusion S27.329
        bilateral S27.322
        unilateral S27.321
      laceration S27.339
        bilateral S27.332
        unilateral S27.331
      specified type NEC S27.399
        bilateral S27.392
        unilateral S27.391
      unilateral S27.301
    pleura S27.60
      laceration S27.63
      specified type NEC S27.69
    pneumothorax S27.0
    specified organ NEC S27.899
      contusion S27.892
      laceration S27.893
      specified type NEC S27.898
    thoracic duct —*see* Injury, intrathoracic,
      specified organ NEC
    thymus gland —*see* Injury, intrathoracic,
      specified organ NEC
    trachea, thoracic S27.50
      blast (primary) S27.51
      contusion S27.52
      laceration S27.53
      specified type NEC S27.59
  iris —*see* Injury, eye, specified site NEC
    penetrating —*see* Injury, eyeball,
      penetrating
  jaw S09.93
  jejunum —*see* Injury, intestine, small
  joint NOS T14.8
    old or residual —*see* Disorder, joint,
      specified type NEC
  kidney S37.00-●
    acute (nontraumatic) N17.9
    contusion —*see* Contusion, kidney
    laceration —*see* Laceration, kidney
    specified NEC S37.09-●
  knee S89.9-●
    contusion —*see* Contusion, knee
    dislocation —*see* Dislocation, knee
    meniscus (lateral) (medial) —*see* Sprain,
      knee, specified site NEC
      old injury or tear —*see* Derangement,
        knee, meniscus, due to old injury
    open —*see* Wound, open, knee
    specified NEC S89.8-●
    sprain —*see* Sprain, knee
    superficial —*see* Injury, superficial, knee
  labium (majus) (minus) S39.94
  labyrinth, ear S09.30-●
  lacrimal apparatus, duct, gland, or sac —*see*
    Injury, eye, specified site NEC
  larynx NEC S19.81
  leg (lower) S89.9-●
    blood vessel —*see* Injury, blood vessel, leg
    contusion —*see* Contusion, leg
    fracture —*see* Fracture, leg

Injury *(Continued)*
  leg *(Continued)*
    muscle —*see* Injury, muscle, leg
    nerve —*see* Injury, nerve, leg
    open —*see* Wound, open, leg
    specified NEC S89.8-●
    superficial —*see* Injury, superficial, leg
  lens, eye —*see* Injury, eye, specified site
    NEC
    penetrating —*see* Injury, eyeball,
      penetrating
  limb NEC T14.8
  lip S09.93
  liver S36.119
    contusion S36.112
    laceration S36.113
      major (stellate) S36.116
      minor S36.114
      moderate S36.115
    specified NEC S36.118
  lower back S39.92
    specified NEC S39.82
  lumbar, lumbosacral (region) S39.92
    plexus —*see* Injury, lumbosacral plexus
  lumbosacral plexus S34.4
  lung —*see also* Injury, intrathoracic, lung
    aspiration J69.0
    dabbing (related) U07.0
    electronic cigarette (related) U07.0
    EVALI - [e-cigarette, or vaping, product
      use associated] U07.0
    transfusion-related (TRALI) J95.84
    vaping (associated) (device) (product) (use)
      U07.0
  lymphatic thoracic duct —*see* Injury,
    intrathoracic, specified organ NEC
  malar region S09.93
  mastoid region S09.90
  maxilla S09.93
  mediastinum —*see* Injury, intrathoracic,
    specified organ NEC
  membrane, brain —*see* Injury, intracranial
  meningeal artery —*see* Injury, intracranial,
    subdural hemorrhage
  meninges (cerebral) —*see* Injury, intracranial
  mesenteric
    artery
      branch S35.299
        laceration (minor) (superficial) S35.291
          major S35.292
        specified NEC S35.298
      inferior S35.239
        laceration (minor) (superficial) S35.231
          major S35.232
        specified NEC S35.238
      superior S35.229
        laceration (minor) (superficial) S35.221
          major S35.222
        specified NEC S35.228
    plexus (inferior) (superior) —*see* Injury,
      nerve, lumbosacral, sympathetic
    vein
      inferior S35.349
        laceration S35.341
        specified NEC S35.348
      superior S35.339
        laceration S35.331
        specified NEC S35.338
  mesentery —*see* Injury, intra-abdominal,
    specified site NEC
  mesosalpinx —*see* Injury, pelvic organ,
    specified site NEC
  middle ear S09.30-●
  midthoracic region NOS S29.9
  mouth S09.93
  multiple NOS T07
  muscle (and fascia) (and tendon)
    abdomen S39.001
      laceration S39.021
      specified type NEC S39.091
      strain S39.011

Injury *(Continued)*
  muscle *(Continued)*
    abductor
      thumb, forearm level —*see* Injury,
        muscle, thumb, abductor
    adductor
      thigh S76.20-●
        laceration S76.22-●
        specified type NEC S76.29-●
        strain S76.21-●
    ankle —*see* Injury, muscle, foot
    anterior muscle group, at leg level (lower)
      S86.20-●
      laceration S86.22-●
      specified type NEC S86.29-●
      strain S86.21-●
    arm (upper) —*see* Injury, muscle,
      shoulder
    biceps (parts NEC) S46.20-●
      laceration S46.22-●
      long head S46.10-●
        laceration S46.12-●
        specified type NEC S46.19-●
        strain S46.11-●
      specified type NEC S46.29-●
      strain S46.21-●
    extensor
      finger(s) (other than thumb) —*see* Injury,
        muscle, finger by site, extensor
      forearm level, specified NEC —*see*
        Injury, muscle, forearm, extensor
      thumb —*see* Injury, muscle, thumb,
        extensor
      toe (large) (ankle level) (foot level) —*see*
        Injury, muscle, toe, extensor
    finger
      extensor (forearm level) S56.40-●
        hand level S66.309
          laceration S66.329
          specified type NEC S66.399
          strain S66.319
        laceration S56.429
        specified type NEC S56.499
        strain S56.419
      flexor (forearm level) S56.10-●
        hand level S66.109
          laceration S66.129
          specified type NEC S66.199
          strain S66.119
        laceration S56.129
        specified type NEC S56.199
        strain S56.119
      index
        extensor (forearm level)
          hand level S66.308
            laceration S66.32-●
            specified type NEC S66.39-●
            strain S66.31-●
          specified type NEC S56.492-●
        flexor (forearm level)
          hand level S66.108
            laceration S66.12-●
            specified type NEC
              S66.19-●
            strain S66.11-●
          specified type NEC S56.19-●
          strain S56.11-●
        intrinsic S66.50-●
          laceration S66.52-●
          specified type NEC S66.59-●
          strain S66.51-●
      intrinsic S66.509
        laceration S66.529
        specified type NEC S66.599
        strain S66.519
      little
        extensor (forearm level)
          hand level S66.30-●
            laceration S66.32-●
            specified type NEC S66.39-●
            strain S66.31-●

Injury *(Continued)*
  muscle *(Continued)*
    finger *(Continued)*
      little *(Continued)*
        extensor *(Continued)*
          laceration S56.42-●
          specified type NEC S56.49-●
          strain S56.41-●
        flexor (forearm level)
          hand level S66.10-●
            laceration S66.12-●
            specified type NEC S66.19-●
            strain S66.11-●
          laceration S56.12-●
          specified type NEC S56.19-●
          strain S56.11-●
        intrinsic S66.50-●
          laceration S66.52-●
          specified type NEC S66.59-●
          strain S66.51-●
      middle
        extensor (forearm level)
          hand level S66.30-●
            laceration S66.32-●
            specified type NEC
              S66.39-●
            strain S66.31-●
          laceration S56.42-●
          specified type NEC
            S56.49-●
          strain S56.41-●
        flexor (forearm level)
          hand level S66.10-●
            laceration S66.12-●
            specified type NEC
              S66.19-●
            strain S66.11-●
          laceration S56.12-●
          specified type NEC S56.19-●
          strain S56.11-●
        intrinsic S66.50-●
          laceration S66.52-●
          specified type NEC S66.59-●
          strain S66.51-●
      ring
        extensor (forearm level)
          hand level S66.30-●
           laceration S66.32-●
           specified type NEC S66.39-●
           strain S66.31-●
          laceration S56.42-●
          specified type NEC S56.49-●
          strain S56.41-●
        flexor (forearm level)
          hand level S66.10-●
           laceration S66.12-●
           specified type NEC S66.19-●
           strain S66.11-●
          laceration S56.12-●
          specified type NEC S56.19-●
          strain S56.11-●
        intrinsic S66.50-●
          laceration S66.52-●
          specified type NEC S66.59-●
          strain S66.51-●
    flexor
      finger(s) (other than thumb) — *see* Injury,
        muscle, finger
      forearm level, specified NEC —
        see Injury, muscle, forearm,
        flexor
      thumb —*see* Injury, muscle, thumb,
        flexor
      toe (long) (ankle level) (foot level) —*see*
        Injury, muscle, toe, flexor
    foot S96.90-●
      intrinsic S96.20-●
        laceration S96.22-●
        specified type NEC S96.29-●
        strain S96.21-●
      laceration S96.92-●

Injury *(Continued)*
  muscle *(Continued)*
    foot *(Continued)*
      long extensor, toe —*see* Injury, muscle,
        toe, extensor
      long flexor, toe —*see* Injury, muscle, toe,
        flexor
      specified
        site NEC S96.80-●
          laceration S96.82-●
          specified type NEC S96.89-●
          strain S96.81-●
        type NEC S96.99-●
      strain S96.91-●
    forearm (level) S56.90-●
      extensor S56.50-●
        laceration S56.52-●
        specified type NEC S56.59-●
        strain S56.51-●
      flexor S56.20-●
        laceration S56.22-●
        specified type NEC S56.29-●
        strain S56.21-●
      laceration S56.92-●
      specified S56.99-●
        site NEC S56.80-●
          laceration S56.82-●
          strain S56.81-●
        type NEC S56.89-●
      strain S56.91-●
    hand (level) S66.90-●
      laceration S66.92-●
      specified
        site NEC S66.80-●
          laceration S66.82-●
          specified type NEC S66.89-●
          strain S66.81-●
        type NEC S66.99-●
      strain S66.91-●
    head S09.10
      laceration S09.12
      specified type NEC S09.19
      strain S09.11
    hip NEC S76.00-●
      laceration S76.02-●
      specified type NEC S76.09-●
      strain S76.01-●
    intrinsic
      ankle and foot level —*see* Injury, muscle,
        foot, intrinsic
      finger (other than thumb) —*see* Injury,
        muscle, finger by site, intrinsic
      foot (level) —*see* Injury, muscle, foot,
        intrinsic
      thumb —*see* Injury, muscle, thumb,
        intrinsic
    leg (level) (lower) S86.90-●
      Achilles tendon —*see* Injury, Achilles
        tendon
      anterior muscle group —*see* Injury,
        muscle, anterior muscle group
      laceration S86.92-●
      peroneal muscle group —*see* Injury,
        muscle, peroneal muscle group
      posterior muscle group —*see* Injury,
        muscle, posterior muscle group,
        leg level
      specified
        site NEC S86.80-●
          laceration S86.82-●
          specified type NEC S86.89-●
          strain S86.81-●
        type NEC S86.99-●
      strain S86.91-●
    long
      extensor toe, at ankle and foot level —*see*
        Injury, muscle, toe, extensor
      flexor, toe, at ankle and foot level —*see*
        Injury, muscle, toe, flexor
      head, biceps —*see* Injury, muscle, biceps,
        long head

Injury *(Continued)*
  muscle *(Continued)*
    lower back S39.002
      laceration S39.022
      specified type NEC S39.092
      strain S39.012
    neck (level) S16.9
      laceration S16.2
      specified type NEC S16.8
      strain S16.1
    pelvis S39.003
      laceration S39.023
      specified type NEC S39.093
      strain S39.013
    peroneal muscle group, at leg level (lower)
      S86.30-●
      laceration S86.32-●
      specified type NEC S86.39-●
      strain S86.31-●
    posterior muscle (group)
      leg level (lower) S86.10-●
        laceration S86.12-●
        specified type NEC S86.19-●
        strain S86.11-●
      thigh level S76.30-●
        laceration S76.32-●
        specified type NEC S76.39-●
        strain S76.31-●
    quadriceps (thigh) S76.10-●
      laceration S76.12-●
      specified type NEC S76.19-●
      strain S76.11-●
    shoulder S46.90-●
      laceration S46.92-●
      rotator cuff —*see* Injury, rotator cuff
      specified site NEC S46.80-●
        laceration S46.82-●
        specified type NEC S46.89-●
        strain S46.81-●
      specified type NEC S46.99-●
      strain S46.91-●
    thigh NEC (level) S76.90-●
      adductor —*see* Injury, muscle, adductor,
        thigh
      laceration S76.92-●
      posterior muscle (group) —*see* Injury,
        muscle, posterior muscle, thigh level
      quadriceps —*see* Injury, muscle,
        quadriceps
      specified
        site NEC S76.80-●
          laceration S76.82-●
          specified type NEC S76.89-●
          strain S76.81-●
        type NEC S76.99-●
      strain S76.91-●
    thorax (level) S29.009
      back wall S29.002
      front wall S29.001
      laceration S29.029
        back wall S29.022
        front wall S29.021
      specified type NEC S29.099
        back wall S29.092
        front wall S29.091
      strain S29.019
        back wall S29.012
        front wall S29.011
    thumb
      abductor (forearm level) S56.30-●
        laceration S56.32-●
        specified type NEC S56.39-●
        strain S56.31-●
      extensor (forearm level) S56.30-●
        hand level S66.20-●
          laceration S66.22-●
          specified type NEC S66.29-●
          strain S66.21-●
        laceration S56.32-●
        specified type NEC S56.39-●
        strain S56.31-●

▶ New   ⇒ Revised   ~~deleted~~ Deleted   ● Use Additional Character(s)

Injury *(Continued)*
  muscle *(Continued)*
    thumb *(Continued)*
      flexor (forearm level) S56.00-●
        hand level S66.00-●
          laceration S66.02-●
          specified type NEC S66.09-●
          strain S66.01-●
        laceration S56.02-●
        specified type NEC S56.09-●
        strain S56.01-●
        wrist level —*see* Injury, muscle, thumb, flexor, hand level
      intrinsic S66.40-●
        laceration S66.42-●
        specified type NEC S66.49-●
        strain S66.41-●
    toe —*see also* Injury, muscle, foot
      extensor, long S96.10-●
        laceration S96.12-●
        specified type NEC S96.19-●
        strain S96.11-●
      flexor, long S96.00-●
        laceration S96.02-●
        specified type NEC S96.09-●
        strain S96.01-●
    triceps S46.30-●
      laceration S46.32-●
      specified type NEC S46.39-●
      strain S46.31-●
    wrist (and hand) level —*see* Injury, muscle, hand
  musculocutaneous nerve —*see* Injury, nerve, musculocutaneous
  myocardial (acute) (chronic) (non-ischemic) (non-traumatic) I5A
    traumatic —*see* Injury, heart
  myocardium —*see also* Injury, heart
    non-traumatic —*see* Injury, myocardial
  nape —*see* Injury, neck
  nasal (septum) (sinus) S09.92
  nasopharynx S09.92
  neck S19.9
    specified NEC S19.80
      specified site NEC S19.89
  nerve NEC T14.8
    abdomen S34.9
      peripheral S34.6
      specified site NEC S34.8
    abducens S04.4-●
      contusion S04.4-●
      laceration S04.4-●
      specified type NEC S04.4-●
    abducent —*see* Injury, nerve, abducens
    accessory S04.7-●
      contusion S04.7-●
      laceration S04.7-●
      specified type NEC S04.7-●
    acoustic S04.6-●
      contusion S04.6-●
      laceration S04.6-●
      specified type NEC S04.6-●
    ankle S94.9-●
      cutaneous sensory S94.3-●
      specified site NEC —*see* subcategory S94.8
    anterior crural, femoral —*see* Injury, nerve, femoral
    arm (upper) S44.9-●
      axillary —*see* Injury, nerve, axillary
      cutaneous —*see* Injury, nerve, cutaneous, arm
      median —*see* Injury, nerve, median, upper arm
      musculocutaneous —*see* Injury, nerve, musculocutaneous
      radial —*see* Injury, nerve, radial, upper arm
      specified site NEC —*see* subcategory S44.8
      ulnar —*see* Injury, nerve, ulnar, arm
    auditory —*see* Injury, nerve, acoustic

Injury *(Continued)*
  nerve NEC *(Continued)*
    axillary S44.3-●
    brachial plexus —*see* Injury, brachial plexus
    cervical sympathetic S14.5
    cranial S04.9
      contusion S04.9
      eighth (acoustic or auditory) —*see* Injury, nerve, acoustic
      eleventh (accessory) —*see* Injury, nerve, accessory
      fifth (trigeminal) —*see* Injury, nerve, trigeminal
      first (olfactory) —*see* Injury, nerve, olfactory
      fourth (trochlear) —*see* Injury, nerve, trochlear
      laceration S04.9
      ninth (glossopharyngeal) —*see* Injury, nerve, glossopharyngeal
      second (optic) —*see* Injury, nerve, optic
      seventh (facial) —*see* Injury, nerve, facial
      sixth (abducent) —*see* Injury, nerve, abducens
      specified
        nerve NEC S04.89-●
          contusion S04.89-●
          laceration S04.89-●
          specified type NEC S04.89-●
        type NEC S04.9
      tenth (pneumogastric or vagus) —*see* Injury, nerve, vagus
      third (oculomotor) —*see* Injury, nerve, oculomotor
      twelfth (hypoglossal) —*see* Injury, nerve, hypoglossal
    cutaneous sensory
      ankle (level) S94.3-●
      arm (upper) (level) S44.5-●
      foot (level) —*see* Injury, nerve, cutaneous sensory, ankle
      forearm (level) S54.3-●
      hip (level) S74.2-●
      leg (lower level) S84.2-●
      shoulder (level) —*see* Injury, nerve, cutaneous sensory, arm
      thigh (level) —*see* Injury, nerve, cutaneous sensory, hip
    deep peroneal —*see* Injury, nerve, peroneal, foot
    digital
      finger S64.4-●
        index S64.49-●
        little S64.49-●
        middle S64.49-●
        ring S64.49-●
        thumb S64.3-●
      toe —*see* Injury, nerve, ankle, specified site NEC
    eighth cranial (acoustic or auditory) —*see* Injury, nerve, acoustic
    eleventh cranial (accessory) —*see* Injury, nerve, accessory
    facial S04.5-●
      contusion S04.5-●
      laceration S04.5-●
      newborn P11.3
      specified type NEC S04.5-●
    femoral (hip level) (thigh level) S74.1-●
    fifth cranial (trigeminal) —*see* Injury, nerve, trigeminal
    finger (digital) —*see* Injury, nerve, digital, finger
    first cranial (olfactory) —*see* Injury, nerve, olfactory
    foot S94.9-●
      cutaneous sensory S94.3-●
      deep peroneal S94.2-●
      lateral plantar S94.0-●

Injury *(Continued)*
  nerve NEC *(Continued)*
    foot *(Continued)*
      medial plantar S94.1-●
      specified site NEC —*see* subcategory S94.8
    forearm (level) S54.9-●
      cutaneous sensory —*see* Injury, nerve, cutaneous sensory, forearm
      median —*see* Injury, nerve, median
      radial —*see* Injury, nerve, radial
      specified site NEC —*see* subcategory S54.8
      ulnar —*see* Injury, nerve, ulnar
    fourth cranial (trochlear) —*see* Injury, nerve, trochlear
    glossopharyngeal S04.89-●
      specified type NEC S04.89-●
    hand S64.9-●
      median —*see* Injury, nerve, median, hand
      radial —*see* Injury, nerve, radial, hand
      specified NEC —*see* subcategory S64.8
      ulnar —*see* Injury, nerve, ulnar, hand
    hip (level) S74.9-●
      cutaneous sensory —*see* Injury, nerve, cutaneous sensory, hip
      femoral —*see* Injury, nerve, femoral
      sciatic —*see* Injury, nerve, sciatic
      specified site NEC —*see* subcategory S74.8
    hypoglossal S04.89-●
      specified type NEC S04.89-●
    lateral plantar S94.0-●
    leg (lower) S84.9-●
      cutaneous sensory —*see* Injury, nerve, cutaneous sensory, leg
      peroneal —*see* Injury, nerve, peroneal
      specified site NEC —*see* subcategory S84.8
      tibial —*see* Injury, nerve, tibial
      upper —*see* Injury, nerve, thigh
    lower
      back —*see* Injury, nerve, abdomen, specified site NEC
        peripheral —*see* Injury, nerve, abdomen, peripheral
      limb —*see* Injury, nerve, leg
    lumbar plexus —*see* Injury, nerve, lumbosacral, sympathetic
    ➠lumbar spinal —*see* Injury, spinal, lumbar
    peripheral S34.6
      root S34.21
      sympathetic S34.5
    lumbosacral
      plexus —*see* Injury, nerve, lumbosacral, sympathetic
      sympathetic S34.5
    medial plantar S94.1-●
    median (forearm level) S54.1-●
      hand (level) S64.1-●
      upper arm (level) S44.1-●
      wrist (level) —*see* Injury, nerve, median, hand
    musculocutaneous S44.4-●
    musculospiral (upper arm level) —*see* Injury, nerve, radial, upper arm
    neck S14.9
      peripheral S14.4
      specified site NEC S14.8
      sympathetic S14.5
    ninth cranial (glossopharyngeal) —*see* Injury, nerve, glossopharyngeal
    oculomotor S04.1-●
      contusion S04.1-●
      laceration S04.1-●
      specified type NEC S04.1-●
    olfactory S04.81-●
      specified type NEC S04.81-●
    optic S04.01-●
      contusion S04.01-●
      laceration S04.01-●
      specified type NEC S04.01-●

Injury *(Continued)*
 nerve NEC *(Continued)*
  pelvic girdle —*see* Injury, nerve, hip
  pelvis —*see* Injury, nerve, abdomen, specified site NEC
  peripheral —*see* Injury, nerve, abdomen, peripheral
  peripheral NEC T14.8
   abdomen —*see* Injury, nerve, abdomen, peripheral
   lower back —*see* Injury, nerve, abdomen, peripheral
   neck —*see* Injury, nerve, neck, peripheral
   pelvis —*see* Injury, nerve, abdomen, peripheral
   specified NEC T14.8
  peroneal (lower leg level) S84.1-●
   foot S94.2-●
  plexus
   brachial —*see* Injury, brachial plexus
   celiac, coeliac —*see* Injury, nerve, lumbosacral, sympathetic
   mesenteric, inferior —*see* Injury, nerve, lumbosacral, sympathetic
   sacral —*see* Injury, lumbosacral plexus
   spinal
    brachial —*see* Injury, brachial plexus
    lumbosacral —*see* Injury, lumbosacral plexus
   pneumogastric —*see* Injury, nerve, vagus
  radial (forearm level) S54.2-●
   hand (level) S64.2-●
   upper arm (level) S44.2-●
   wrist (level) —*see* Injury, nerve, radial, hand
  root —*see* Injury, nerve, spinal, root
  sacral plexus —*see* Injury, lumbosacral plexus
  ▶sacral spinal —*see* Injury, spinal, sacral
  peripheral S34.6
   root S34.22
   sympathetic S34.5
  sciatic (hip level) (thigh level) S74.0-●
  second cranial (optic) —*see* Injury, nerve, optic
  self-inflicted, without suicidal intent R45.88
  seventh cranial (facial) —*see* Injury, nerve, facial
  shoulder —*see* Injury, nerve, arm
  sixth cranial (abducent) —*see* Injury, nerve, abducens
  spinal
   plexus —*see* Injury, nerve, plexus, spinal
   root
    cervical S14.2
    dorsal S24.2
    lumbar S34.21
    sacral S34.22
    thoracic —*see* Injury, nerve, spinal, root, dorsal
  splanchnic —*see* Injury, nerve, lumbosacral, sympathetic
  sympathetic NEC —*see* Injury, nerve, lumbosacral, sympathetic
   cervical —*see* Injury, nerve, cervical sympathetic
  tenth cranial (pneumogastric or vagus) —*see* Injury, nerve, vagus
  thigh (level) —*see* Injury, nerve, hip
   cutaneous sensory —*see* Injury, nerve, cutaneous sensory, hip
   femoral —*see* Injury, nerve, femoral
   sciatic —*see* Injury, nerve, sciatic
   specified NEC —*see* Injury, nerve, hip
  third cranial (oculomotor) —*see* Injury, nerve, oculomotor
  thorax S24.9
   peripheral S24.3
   specified site NEC S24.8
   sympathetic S24.4

Injury *(Continued)*
 nerve NEC *(Continued)*
  thumb, digital —*see* Injury, nerve, digital, thumb
  tibial (lower leg level) (posterior) S84.0-●
  toe —*see* Injury, nerve, ankle
  trigeminal S04.3-●
   contusion S04.3-●
   laceration S04.3-●
   specified type NEC S04.3-●
  trochlear S04.2-●
   contusion S04.2-●
   laceration S04.2-●
   specified type NEC S04.2-●
  twelfth cranial (hypoglossal) —*see* Injury, nerve, hypoglossal
  ulnar (forearm level) S54.0-●
   arm (upper) (level) S44.0-●
   hand (level) S64.0-●
   wrist (level) —*see* Injury, nerve, ulnar, hand
  vagus S04.89-●
   specified type NEC S04.89-●
  wrist (level) —*see* Injury, nerve, hand
 ninth cranial nerve (glossopharyngeal) —*see* Injury, nerve, glossopharyngeal
 nose (septum) S09.92
 obstetrical O71.9
  specified NEC O71.89
 occipital (region) (scalp) S09.90
  lobe —*see* Injury, intracranial
 optic chiasm S04.02
 optic radiation S04.03-●
 optic tract and pathways S04.03-●
 orbit, orbital (region) —*see* Injury, eye
  penetrating (with foreign body) —*see* Injury, eye, orbit, penetrating
  specified NEC —*see* Injury, eye, specified site NEC
 ovary, ovarian S37.409
  bilateral S37.402
   contusion S37.422
   laceration S37.432
   specified type NEC S37.492
  blood vessel —*see* Injury, blood vessel, ovarian
  contusion S37.429
   bilateral S37.422
   unilateral S37.421
  laceration S37.439
   bilateral S37.432
   unilateral S37.431
  specified type NEC S37.499
   bilateral S37.492
   unilateral S37.491
  unilateral S37.401
   contusion S37.421
   laceration S37.431
   specified type NEC S37.491
 palate (hard) (soft) S09.93
 pancreas S36.209
  body S36.201
   contusion S36.221
   laceration S36.231
    major S36.261
    minor S36.241
    moderate S36.251
   specified type NEC S36.291
  contusion S36.229
  head S36.200
   contusion S36.220
   laceration S36.230
    major S36.260
    minor S36.240
    moderate S36.250
   specified type NEC S36.290
  laceration S36.239
   major S36.269
   minor S36.249
   moderate S36.259
  specified type NEC S36.299
  tail S36.202
   contusion S36.222

Injury *(Continued)*
 pancreas *(Continued)*
  tail *(Continued)*
   laceration S36.232
    major S36.262
    minor S36.242
    moderate S36.252
   specified type NEC S36.292
 parietal (region) (scalp) S09.90
  lobe —*see* Injury, intracranial
 patellar ligament (tendon) S76.10-●
  laceration S76.12-●
  specified NEC S76.19-●
  strain S76.11-●
 pelvis, pelvic (floor) S39.93
  complicating delivery O70.1
  joint or ligament, complicating delivery O71.6
  organ S37.90
   with ectopic or molar pregnancy O08.6
   complication of abortion —*see* Abortion
   contusion S37.92
   following ectopic or molar pregnancy O08.6
   laceration S37.93
   obstetrical trauma NEC O71.5
   specified
    site NEC S37.899
     contusion S37.892
     laceration S37.893
     specified type NEC S37.898
    type NEC S37.99
  specified NEC S39.83
 penis S39.94
 perineum S39.94
 peritoneum S36.81
  laceration S36.893
 periurethral tissue —*see* Injury, urethra
  complicating delivery O71.82
 phalanges
  foot —*see* Injury, foot
  hand —*see* Injury, hand
 pharynx NEC S19.85
 pleura —*see* Injury, intrathoracic, pleura
 plexus
  brachial —*see* Injury, brachial plexus
  cardiac —*see* Injury, nerve, thorax, sympathetic
  celiac, coeliac —*see* Injury, nerve, lumbosacral, sympathetic
  esophageal —*see* Injury, nerve, thorax, sympathetic
  hypogastric —*see* Injury, nerve, lumbosacral, sympathetic
  lumbar, lumbosacral —*see* Injury, lumbosacral plexus
  mesenteric —*see* Injury, nerve, lumbosacral, sympathetic
  pulmonary —*see* Injury, nerve, thorax, sympathetic
 postcardiac surgery (syndrome) I97.0
 prepuce S39.94
 pressure
  injury —*see* Ulcer, pressure, by site
 prostate S37.829
  contusion S37.822
  laceration S37.823
  specified type NEC S37.828
 pubic region S39.94
 pudendum S39.94
 pulmonary plexus —*see* Injury, nerve, thorax, sympathetic
 rectovaginal septum NEC S39.83
 rectum —*see* Injury, intestine, large, rectum
 retina —*see* Injury, eye, specified site NEC
  penetrating —*see* Injury, eyeball, penetrating
 retroperitoneal —*see* Injury, intra-abdominal, specified site NEC

▶ New ⇒ Revised ~~deleted~~ Deleted ● Use Additional Character(s)

Injury *(Continued)*
  rotator cuff (muscle(s)) (tendon(s)) S46.00-●
    laceration S46.02-●
    specified type NEC S46.09-●
    strain S46.01-●
  round ligament —*see* Injury, pelvic organ, specified site NEC
  sacral plexus —*see* Injury, lumbosacral plexus
  salivary duct or gland S09.93
  scalp S09.90
    newborn (birth injury) P12.9
      due to monitoring (electrode) (sampling incision) P12.4
      specified NEC P12.89
        caput succedaneum P12.81
  scapular region —*see* Injury, shoulder
  sclera —*see* Injury, eye, specified site NEC
    penetrating —*see* Injury, eyeball, penetrating
  scrotum S39.94
  second cranial nerve (optic) —*see* Injury, nerve, optic
  seminal vesicle —*see* Injury, pelvic organ, specified site NEC
  seventh cranial nerve (facial) —*see* Injury, nerve, facial
  shoulder S49.9-●
    blood vessel —*see* Injury, blood vessel, arm
    contusion —*see* Contusion, shoulder
    dislocation —*see* Dislocation, shoulder
    fracture —*see* Fracture, shoulder
    muscle —*see* Injury, muscle, shoulder
    nerve —*see* Injury, nerve, shoulder
    open —*see* Wound, open, shoulder
    specified type NEC S49.8-●
    sprain —*see* Sprain, shoulder girdle
    superficial —*see* Injury, superficial, shoulder
  sinus
    cavernous —*see* Injury, intracranial
    nasal S09.92
  sixth cranial nerve (abducent) —*see* Injury, nerve, abducens
  skeleton, birth injury P13.9
    specified part NEC P13.8
  skin NEC T14.8
    surface intact —*see* Injury, superficial
  skull NEC S09.90
  specified NEC T14.8
  spermatic cord (pelvic region) S37.898
    scrotal region S39.848
  spinal (cord)
    cervical (neck) S14.109
      anterior cord syndrome S14.139
        C1 level S14.131
        C2 level S14.132
        C3 level S14.133
        C4 level S14.134
        C5 level S14.135
        C6 level S14.136
        C7 level S14.137
        C8 level S14.138
      Brown-Séquard syndrome S14.149
        C1 level S14.141
        C2 level S14.142
        C3 level S14.143
        C4 level S14.144
        C5 level S14.145
        C6 level S14.146
        C7 level S14.147
        C8 level S14.148
      C1 level S14.101
      C2 level S14.102
      C3 level S14.103
      C4 level S14.104
      C5 level S14.105
      C6 level S14.106
      C7 level S14.107
      C8 level S14.108

Injury *(Continued)*
  spinal *(Continued)*
    cervical *(Continued)*
      central cord syndrome S14.129
        C1 level S14.121
        C2 level S14.122
        C3 level S14.123
        C4 level S14.124
        C5 level S14.125
        C6 level S14.126
        C7 level S14.127
        C8 level S14.128
      complete lesion S14.119
        C1 level S14.111
        C2 level S14.112
        C3 level S14.113
        C4 level S14.114
        C5 level S14.115
        C6 level S14.116
        C7 level S14.117
        C8 level S14.118
      concussion S14.0
      edema S14.0
      incomplete lesion specified NEC S14.159
        C1 level S14.151
        C2 level S14.152
        C3 level S14.153
        C4 level S14.154
        C5 level S14.155
        C6 level S14.156
        C7 level S14.157
        C8 level S14.158
      posterior cord syndrome S14.159
        C1 level S14.151
        C2 level S14.152
        C3 level S14.153
        C4 level S14.154
        C5 level S14.155
        C6 level S14.156
        C7 level S14.157
        C8 level S14.158
    dorsal —*see* Injury, spinal, thoracic
    lumbar S34.109
      complete lesion S34.119
        L1 level S34.111
        L2 level S34.112
        L3 level S34.113
        L4 level S34.114
        L5 level S34.115
      concussion S34.01
      edema S34.01
      incomplete lesion S34.129
        L1 level S34.121
        L2 level S34.122
        L3 level S34.123
        L4 level S34.124
        L5 level S34.125
      L1 level S34.101
      L2 level S34.102
      L3 level S34.103
      L4 level S34.104
      L5 level S34.105
    nerve root NEC
      cervical —*see* Injury, nerve, spinal, root, cervical
      dorsal —*see* Injury, nerve, spinal, root, dorsal
      lumbar S34.21
      sacral S34.22
      thoracic —*see* Injury, nerve, spinal, root, dorsal
    plexus
      brachial —*see* Injury, brachial plexus
      lumbosacral —*see* Injury, lumbosacral plexus
    sacral S34.139
      complete lesion S34.131
      incomplete lesion S34.132

Injury *(Continued)*
  spinal *(Continued)*
    thoracic S24.109
      anterior cord syndrome S24.139
        T1 level S24.131
        T2-T6 level S24.132
        T7-T10 level S24.133
        T11-T12 level S24.134
      Brown-Séquard syndrome S24.149
        T1 level S24.141
        T2-T6 level S24.142
        T7-T10 level S24.143
        T11-T12 level S24.144
      complete lesion S24.119
        T1 level S24.111
        T2-T6 level S24.112
        T7-T10 level S24.113
        T11-T12 level S24.114
      concussion S24.0
      edema S24.0
      incomplete lesion specified NEC S24.159
        T1 level S24.151
        T2-T6 level S24.152
        T7-T10 level S24.153
        T11-T12 level S24.154
      posterior cord syndrome S24.159
        T1 level S24.151
        T2-T6 level S24.152
        T7-T10 level S24.153
        T11-T12 level S24.154
      T1 level S24.101
      T2-T6 level S24.102
      T7-T10 level S24.103
      T11-T12 level S24.104
  splanchnic nerve —*see* Injury, nerve, lumbosacral, sympathetic
  spleen S36.00
    contusion S36.029
      major S36.021
      minor S36.020
    laceration S36.039
      major (massive) (stellate) S36.032
      moderate S36.031
      superficial (capsular) (minor) S36.030
    specified type NEC S36.09
  splenic artery —*see* Injury, blood vessel, celiac artery, branch
  stellate ganglion —*see* Injury, nerve, thorax, sympathetic
  sternal region S29.9
  stomach S36.30
    contusion S36.32
    laceration S36.33
    specified type NEC S36.39
  subconjunctival —*see* Injury, eye, conjunctiva
  subcutaneous NEC T14.8
  submaxillary region S09.93
  submental region S09.93
  subungual
    fingers —*see* Injury, hand
    toes —*see* Injury, foot
  superficial NEC T14.8
    abdomen, abdominal (wall) S30.92
      abrasion S30.811
      bite S30.871
        insect S30.861
      contusion S30.1
      external constriction S30.841
      foreign body S30.851
    abrasion —*see* Abrasion, by site
    adnexa, eye NEC —*see* Injury, eye, specified site NEC
    alveolar process —*see* Injury, superficial, oral cavity
    ankle S90.91-●
      abrasion —*see* Abrasion, ankle
      bite —*see* Bite, ankle
      blister —*see* Blister, ankle
      contusion —*see* Contusion, ankle

Injury *(Continued)*
   superficial NEC *(Continued)*
      ankle *(Continued)*
         external constriction —*see* Constriction,
           external, ankle
         foreign body —*see* Foreign body,
           superficial, ankle
      anus S30.98
      arm (upper) S40.92-●
         abrasion —*see* Abrasion, arm
         bite —*see* Bite, superficial, arm
         blister —*see* Blister, arm (upper)
         contusion —*see* Contusion, arm
         external constriction —*see* Constriction,
           external, arm
         foreign body —*see* Foreign body,
           superficial, arm
      auditory canal (external) (meatus) —*see*
         Injury, superficial, ear
      auricle —*see* Injury, superficial, ear
      axilla —*see* Injury, superficial, arm
      back —*see also* Injury, superficial, thorax,
         back
        lower S30.91
           abrasion S30.810
           contusion S30.0
           external constriction S30.840
           superficial
              bite NEC S30.870
                 insect S30.860
              foreign body S30.850
      bite NEC —*see* Bite, superficial NEC, by
         site
      blister —*see* Blister, by site
      breast S20.10-●
         abrasion —*see* Abrasion, breast
         bite —*see* Bite, superficial, breast
         contusion —*see* Contusion, breast
         external constriction —*see* Constriction,
           external, breast
         foreign body —*see* Foreign body,
           superficial, breast
      brow —*see* Injury, superficial, head,
         specified NEC
      buttock S30.91
      calf —*see* Injury, superficial, leg
      canthus, eye —*see* Injury, superficial,
         periocular area
      cheek (external) —*see* Injury, superficial,
         head, specified NEC
         internal —*see* Injury, superficial, oral
           cavity
      chest wall —*see* Injury, superficial, thorax
      chin —*see* Injury, superficial, head NEC
      clitoris S30.95
      conjunctiva —*see* Injury, eye, conjunctiva
         with foreign body (in conjunctival
         sac) —*see* Foreign body,
         conjunctival sac
      contusion —*see* Contusion, by site
      costal region —*see* Injury, superficial,
         thorax
      digit(s)
        hand —*see* Injury, superficial, finger
      ear (auricle) (canal) (external) S00.40-●
         abrasion —*see* Abrasion, ear
         bite —*see* Bite, superficial, ear
         contusion —*see* Contusion, ear
         external constriction —*see* Constriction,
           external, ear
         foreign body —*see* Foreign body,
           superficial, ear
      elbow S50.90-●
         abrasion —*see* Abrasion, elbow
         bite —*see* Bite, superficial, elbow
         blister —*see* Blister, elbow
         contusion —*see* Contusion, elbow
         external constriction —*see* Constriction,
           external, elbow
         foreign body —*see* Foreign body,
           superficial, elbow

Injury *(Continued)*
   superficial NEC *(Continued)*
      epididymis S30.94
      epigastric region S30.92
      epiglottis —*see* Injury, superficial, throat
      esophagus
        cervical —*see* Injury, superficial,
         throat
      external constriction —*see* Constriction,
        external, by site
      extremity NEC T14.8
      eyeball NEC —*see* Injury, eye, specified
        site NEC
      eyebrow —*see* Injury, superficial,
        periocular area
      eyelid S00.20-●
        abrasion —*see* Abrasion, eyelid
        bite —*see* Bite, superficial, eyelid
        contusion —*see* Contusion, eyelid
        external constriction —*see* Constriction,
         external, eyelid
        foreign body —*see* Foreign body,
         superficial, eyelid
      face NEC —*see* Injury, superficial, head,
        specified NEC
      finger(s) S60.949
        abrasion —*see* Abrasion, finger
        bite —*see* Bite, superficial, finger
        blister —*see* Blister, finger
        contusion —*see* Contusion, finger
        external constriction —*see* Constriction,
         external, finger
        foreign body —*see* Foreign body,
         superficial, finger
        index S60.94-●
        insect bite —*see* Bite, by site, superficial,
         insect
        little S60.94-●
        middle S60.94-●
        ring S60.94-●
      flank S30.92
      foot S90.92-●
        abrasion —*see* Abrasion, foot
        bite —*see* Bite, foot
        blister —*see* Blister, foot
        contusion —*see* Contusion, foot
        external constriction —*see* Constriction,
         external, foot
        foreign body —*see* Foreign body,
         superficial, foot
      forearm S50.91-●
        abrasion —*see* Abrasion, forearm
        bite —*see* Bite, forearm, superficial
        blister —*see* Blister, forearm
        contusion —*see* Contusion, forearm
        elbow only —*see* Injury, superficial,
         elbow
        external constriction —*see* Constriction,
         external, forearm
        foreign body —*see* Foreign body,
         superficial, forearm
      forehead —*see* Injury, superficial, head
        NEC
      foreign body —*see* Foreign body,
        superficial
      genital organs, external
        female S30.97
        male S30.96
      globe (eye) —*see* Injury, eye, specified site
        NEC
      groin S30.92
      gum —*see* Injury, superficial, oral
        cavity
      hand S60.92-●
        abrasion —*see* Abrasion, hand
        bite —*see* Bite, superficial, hand
        contusion —*see* Contusion, hand
        external constriction —*see* Constriction,
         external, hand
        foreign body —*see* Foreign body,
         superficial, hand

Injury *(Continued)*
   superficial NEC *(Continued)*
      head S00.90
        ear —*see* Injury, superficial, ear
        eyelid —*see* Injury, superficial, eyelid
        nose S00.30
        oral cavity S00.502
        scalp S00.00
        specified site NEC S00.80
      heel —*see* Injury, superficial, foot
      hip S70.91-●
        abrasion —*see* Abrasion, hip
        bite —*see* Bite, superficial, hip
        blister —*see* Blister, hip
        contusion —*see* Contusion, hip
        external constriction —*see* Constriction,
         external, hip
        foreign body —*see* Foreign body,
         superficial, hip
      iliac region —*see* Injury, superficial,
        abdomen
      inguinal region —*see* Injury, superficial,
        abdomen
      insect bite —*see* Bite, by site, superficial,
        insect
      interscapular region —*see* Injury,
        superficial, thorax, back
      jaw —*see* Injury, superficial, head, specified
        NEC
      knee S80.91-●
        abrasion —*see* Abrasion, knee
        bite —*see* Bite, superficial, knee
        blister —*see* Blister, knee
        contusion —*see* Contusion, knee
        external constriction —*see* Constriction,
         external, knee
        foreign body —*see* Foreign body,
         superficial, knee
      labium (majus) (minus) S30.95
      lacrimal (apparatus) (gland) (sac) —*see*
        Injury, eye, specified site NEC
      larynx —*see* Injury, superficial, throat
      leg (lower) S80.92-●
        abrasion —*see* Abrasion, leg
        bite —*see* Bite, superficial, leg
        contusion —*see* Contusion, leg
        external constriction —*see* Constriction,
         external, leg
        foreign body —*see* Foreign body,
         superficial, leg
        knee —*see* Injury, superficial, knee
      limb NEC T14.8
      lip S00.501
      lower back S30.91
      lumbar region S30.91
      malar region —*see* Injury, superficial, head,
        specified NEC
      mammary —*see* Injury, superficial, breast
      mastoid region —*see* Injury, superficial,
        head, specified NEC
      mouth —*see* Injury, superficial, oral cavity
      muscle NEC T14.8
      nail NEC T14.8
        finger —*see* Injury, superficial, finger
        toe —*see* Injury, superficial, toe
      nasal (septum) —*see* Injury, superficial, nose
      neck S10.90
        specified site NEC S10.80
      nose (septum) S00.30
      occipital region —*see* Injury, superficial,
        scalp
      oral cavity S00.502
      orbital region —*see* Injury, superficial,
        periocular area
      palate —*see* Injury, superficial, oral
        cavity
      palm —*see* Injury, superficial, hand
      parietal region —*see* Injury, superficial,
        scalp
      pelvis S30.91
        girdle —*see* Injury, superficial, hip

▶ New   ⇒ Revised   ~~deleted~~ Deleted   ● Use Additional Character(s)

Injury (Continued)
    superficial NEC (Continued)
        penis S30.93
        perineum
            female S30.95
            male S30.91
        periocular area S00.20-●
            abrasion —see Abrasion, eyelid
            bite —see Bite, superficial, eyelid
            contusion —see Contusion, eyelid
            external constriction —see Constriction,
                external, eyelid
            foreign body —see Foreign body,
                superficial, eyelid
        phalanges
            finger —see Injury, superficial, finger
            toe —see Injury, superficial, toe
        pharynx —see Injury, superficial, throat
        pinna —see Injury, superficial, ear
        popliteal space —see Injury, superficial,
            knee
        prepuce S30.93
        pubic region S30.91
        pudendum
            female S30.97
            male S30.96
        sacral region S30.91
        scalp S00.00
        scapular region —see Injury, superficial,
            shoulder
        sclera —see Injury, eye, specified site NEC
        scrotum S30.94
        shin —see Injury, superficial, leg
        shoulder S40.91-●
            abrasion —see Abrasion, shoulder
            bite —see Bite, superficial, shoulder
            blister —see Blister, shoulder
            contusion —see Contusion, shoulder
            external constriction —see Constriction,
                external, shoulder
            foreign body —see Foreign body,
                superficial, shoulder
        skin NEC T14.8
        sternal region —see Injury, superficial,
            thorax, front
        subconjunctival —see Injury, eye, specified
            site NEC
        subcutaneous NEC T14.8
        submaxillary region —see Injury,
            superficial, head, specified NEC
        submental region —see Injury, superficial,
            head, specified NEC
        subungual
            finger(s) —see Injury, superficial, finger
            toe(s) —see Injury, superficial, toe
        supraclavicular fossa —see Injury,
            superficial, neck
        supraorbital —see Injury, superficial, head,
            specified NEC
        temple —see Injury, superficial, head,
            specified NEC
        temporal region —see Injury, superficial,
            head, specified NEC
        testis S30.94
        thigh S70.92-●
            abrasion —see Abrasion, thigh
            bite —see Bite, superficial, thigh
            blister —see Blister, thigh
            contusion —see Contusion, thigh
            external constriction —see Constriction,
                external, thigh
            foreign body —see Foreign body,
                superficial, thigh
        thorax, thoracic (wall) S20.90
            abrasion —see Abrasion, thorax
            back S20.40-●
            bite —see Bite, thorax, superficial
            blister —see Blister, thorax
            contusion —see Contusion, thorax
            external constriction —see Constriction,
                external, thorax

Injury (Continued)
    superficial NEC (Continued)
        thorax, thoracic (Continued)
            foreign body —see Foreign body,
                superficial, thorax
            front S20.30-●
        throat S10.10
            abrasion S10.11
            bite S10.17
                insect S10.16
            blister S10.12
            contusion S10.0
            external constriction S10.14
            foreign body S10.15
        thumb S60.93-●
            abrasion —see Abrasion, thumb
            bite —see Bite, superficial, thumb
            blister —see Blister, thumb
            contusion —see Contusion, thumb
            external constriction —see Constriction,
                external, thumb
            foreign body —see Foreign body,
                superficial, thumb
            insect bite —see Bite, by site, superficial,
                insect
            specified type NEC S60.39-●
        toe(s) S90.93-●
            abrasion —see Abrasion, toe
            bite —see Bite, toe
            blister —see Blister, toe
            contusion —see Contusion, toe
            external constriction —see Constriction,
                external, toe
            foreign body —see Foreign body,
                superficial, toe
            great S90.93-●
        tongue —see Injury, superficial, oral cavity
        tooth, teeth —see Injury, superficial, oral
            cavity
        trachea S10.10
        tunica vaginalis S30.94
        tympanum, tympanic membrane —see
            Injury, superficial, ear
        uvula —see Injury, superficial, oral cavity
        vagina S30.95
        vocal cords —see Injury, superficial, throat
        vulva S30.95
        wrist S60.91-●
    supraclavicular region —see Injury, neck
    supraorbital S09.93
    suprarenal gland (multiple) —see Injury,
        adrenal
    surgical complication (external or internal
        site) —see Laceration, accidental
        complicating surgery
    temple S09.90
    temporal region S09.90
    tendon —see also Injury, muscle, by site
        abdomen —see Injury, muscle, abdomen
        Achilles —see Injury, Achilles tendon
        lower back —see Injury, muscle, lower
            back
        pelvic organs —see Injury, muscle, pelvis
    tenth cranial nerve (pneumogastric or
        vagus) —see Injury, nerve, vagus
    testis S39.94
    thigh S79.92-●
        blood vessel —see Injury, blood vessel, hip
        contusion —see Contusion, thigh
        fracture —see Fracture, femur
        muscle —see Injury, muscle, thigh
        nerve —see Injury, nerve, thigh
        open —see Wound, open, thigh
        specified NEC S79.82-●
        superficial —see Injury, superficial, thigh
    third cranial nerve (oculomotor) —see Injury,
        nerve, oculomotor
    thorax, thoracic S29.9
        blood vessel —see Injury, blood vessel,
            thorax
        cavity —see Injury, intrathoracic

Injury (Continued)
    thorax, thoracic (Continued)
        dislocation —see Dislocation, thorax
        external (wall) S29.9
            contusion —see Contusion, thorax
            nerve —see Injury, nerve, thorax
            open —see Wound, open, thorax
            specified NEC S29.8
            sprain —see Sprain, thorax
            superficial —see Injury, superficial,
                thorax
        fracture —see Fracture, thorax
        internal —see Injury, intrathoracic
        intrathoracic organ —see Injury,
            intrathoracic
        sympathetic ganglion —see Injury, nerve,
            thorax, sympathetic
    throat —see also Injury, neck S19.9
    thumb S69.9-●
        blood vessel —see Injury, blood vessel,
            thumb
        contusion —see Contusion, thumb
        dislocation —see Dislocation, thumb
        fracture —see Fracture, thumb
        muscle —see Injury, muscle, thumb
        nerve —see Injury, nerve, digital, thumb
        open —see Wound, open, thumb
        specified NEC S69.8-●
        sprain —see Sprain, thumb
        superficial —see Injury, superficial, thumb
    thymus (gland) —see Injury, intrathoracic,
        specified organ NEC
    thyroid (gland) NEC S19.84
    toe S99.92-●
        contusion —see Contusion, toe
        dislocation —see Dislocation, toe
        fracture —see Fracture, toe
        muscle —see Injury, muscle, toe
        open —see Wound, open, toe
        specified type NEC S99.82-●
        sprain —see Sprain, toe
        superficial —see Injury, superficial, toe
    tongue S09.93
    tonsil S09.93
    tooth S09.93
    trachea (cervical) NEC S19.82
        thoracic —see Injury, intrathoracic, trachea,
            thoracic
    transfusion-related acute lung (TRALI)
        J95.84
    tunica vaginalis S39.94
    twelfth cranial nerve (hypoglossal) —see
        Injury, nerve, hypoglossal
    ureter S37.10
        contusion S37.12
        laceration S37.13
        specified type NEC S37.19
    urethra (sphincter) S37.30
        at delivery O71.5
        contusion S37.32
        laceration S37.33
        specified type NEC S37.38
    urinary organ S37.899
        contusion S37.92
        laceration S37.93
        specified
            site NEC S37.899
                contusion S37.892
                laceration S37.893
                specified type NEC S37.898
            type NEC S37.99
    uterus, uterine S37.60
        with ectopic or molar pregnancy O08.6
        blood vessel —see Injury, blood vessel, iliac
        contusion S37.62
        laceration S37.63
            cervix at delivery O71.3
        rupture associated with obstetrics —see
            Rupture, uterus
        specified type NEC S37.69
    uvula S09.93

Injury *(Continued)*
  vagina S39.93
    abrasion S30.814
    bite S31.45
      insect S30.864
      superficial NEC S30.874
    contusion S30.23
    crush S38.03
    during delivery —*see* Laceration, vagina,
        during delivery
    external constriction S30.844
    insect bite S30.864
    laceration S31.41
      with foreign body S31.42
    open wound S31.40
    puncture S31.43
      with foreign body S31.44
    superficial S30.95
      foreign body S30.854
  vas deferens —*see* Injury, pelvic organ,
      specified site NEC
  vascular NEC T14.8
  vein —*see* Injury, blood vessel
  vena cava (superior) S25.20
    inferior S35.10
      laceration (minor) (superficial) S35.11
        major S35.12
      specified type NEC S35.19
    laceration (minor) (superficial) S25.21
      major S25.22
    specified type NEC S25.29
  vesical (sphincter) —*see* Injury, bladder
  visual cortex S04.04-●
  vitreous (humor) S05.90
    specified NEC S05.8X-●
  vocal cord NEC S19.83
  vulva S39.94
    abrasion S30.814
    bite S31.45
      insect S30.864
      superficial NEC S30.874
    contusion S30.23
    crush S38.03
    during delivery —*see* Laceration,
        perineum, female, during delivery
    external constriction S30.844
    insect bite S30.864
    laceration S31.41
      with foreign body S31.42
    open wound S31.40
    puncture S31.43
      with foreign body S31.44
    superficial S30.95
      foreign body S30.854
  whiplash (cervical spine) S13.4
  wrist S69.9-●
    blood vessel —*see* Injury, blood vessel,
        hand
    contusion —*see* Contusion, wrist
    dislocation —*see* Dislocation, wrist
    fracture —*see* Fracture, wrist
    muscle —*see* Injury, muscle, hand
    nerve —*see* Injury, nerve, hand
    open —*see* Wound, open, wrist
    specified NEC S69.8-●
    sprain —*see* Sprain, wrist
    superficial —*see* Injury, superficial, wrist
Inoculation —*see also* Vaccination
  complication or reaction —*see* Complications,
      vaccination
Insanity, insane —*see also* Psychosis
  adolescent —*see* Schizophrenia
  confusional F28
    acute or subacute F05
  delusional F22
  senile F03
Insect
  bite —*see* Bite, by site, superficial, insect
  venomous, poisoning NEC (by) —*see* Venom,
      arthropod
  Insecurity, food Z59.41

► Insecurity
► financial Z59.86
► food Z59.41
► transportation Z59.82
Insensitivity
  adrenocorticotropin hormone (ACTH) E27.49
  androgen E34.50
    complete E34.51
    partial E34.52
Insertion
  cord (umbilical) lateral or velamentous
      O43.12-●
  intrauterine contraceptive device (encounter
      for) —*see* Intrauterine contraceptive
      device
Insolation (sunstroke) T67.01
Insomnia (organic) G47.00
  without objective findings F51.02
  adjustment F51.02
  adjustment disorder F51.02
  behavioral, of childhood Z73.819
    combined type Z73.812
    limit setting type Z73.811
    sleep-onset association type Z73.810
  childhood Z73.819
  chronic F51.04
    somatized tension F51.04
  conditioned F51.04
  due to
    alcohol
      abuse F10.182
      dependence F10.282
      use F10.982
    amphetamines
      abuse F15.182
      dependence F15.282
      use F15.982
    anxiety disorder F51.05
    caffeine
      abuse F15.182
      dependence F15.282
      use F15.982
    cocaine
      abuse F14.182
      dependence F14.282
      use F14.982
    depression F51.05
    drug NEC
      abuse F19.182
      dependence F19.282
      use F19.982
    medical condition G47.01
    mental disorder NEC F51.05
    opioid
      abuse F11.182
      dependence F11.282
      use F11.982
    psychoactive substance NEC
      abuse F19.182
      dependence F19.282
      use F19.982
    sedative, hypnotic, or anxiolytic
      abuse F13.182
      dependence F13.282
      use F13.982
    stimulant NEC
      abuse F15.182
      dependence F15.282
      use F15.982
  fatal familial (FFI) A81.83
  idiopathic F51.01
  learned F51.3
  nonorganic origin F51.01
  not due to a substance or known
      physiological condition F51.01
    specified NEC F51.09
  paradoxical F51.03
  primary F51.01
  psychiatric F51.05
  psychophysiologic F51.04
  related to psychopathology F51.05
  short-term F51.02

Insomnia *(Continued)*
  specified NEC G47.09
  stress-related F51.02
  transient F51.02
Inspiration
  food or foreign body —*see* Foreign body, by site
  mucus —*see* Asphyxia, mucus
Inspissated bile syndrome (newborn) P59.1
Instability
  emotional (excessive) F60.3
  housing
    housed Z59.819
      with risk of homelessness Z59.811
      homelessness in past 12 months Z59.812
  joint (post-traumatic) M25.30
    ankle M25.37-●
    due to old ligament injury —*see* Disorder,
        ligament
    elbow M25.32-●
    flail —*see* Flail, joint
    foot M25.37-●
    hand M25.34-●
    hip M25.35-●
    knee M25.36-●
    lumbosacral —*see* subcategory M53.2
    prosthesis —*see* Complications, joint
        prosthesis, mechanical, displacement,
        by site
    sacroiliac —*see* subcategory M53.2
    secondary to
        old ligament injury —*see* Disorder,
            ligament
        removal of joint prosthesis M96.89
    shoulder (region) M25.31-●
    specified site NEC M25.39
    spine —*see* subcategory M53.2
    wrist M25.33-●
  knee (chronic) M23.5-●
  lumbosacral —*see* subcategory M53.2
  nervous F48.8
  personality (emotional) F60.3
  spine —*see* Instability, joint, spine
  vasomotor R55
Institutional syndrome (childhood) F94.2
Institutionalization, affecting child Z62.22
  disinhibited attachment F94.2
Insufficiency, insufficient
  accommodation, old age H52.4
  adrenal (gland) E27.40
    primary E27.1
  adrenocortical E27.40
    drug-induced E27.3
    iatrogenic E27.3
    primary E27.1
  anatomic crown height K08.89
  anterior (occlusal) guidance M26.54
  anus K62.89
  aortic (valve) I35.1
    with
      mitral (valve) disease I08.0
        with tricuspid (valve) disease I08.3
      stenosis I35.2
      tricuspid (valve) disease I08.2
        with mitral (valve) disease I08.3
    congenital Q23.1
    rheumatic I06.1
      with
        mitral (valve) disease I08.0
          with tricuspid (valve) disease I08.3
        stenosis I06.2
          with mitral (valve) disease I08.0
            with tricuspid (valve) disease
                I08.3
        tricuspid (valve) disease I08.2
          with mitral (valve) disease I08.3
    specified cause NEC I35.1
    syphilitic A52.03
  arterial I77.1
    basilar G45.0
    carotid (hemispheric) G45.1
    cerebral I67.81
    coronary (acute or subacute) I24.8

► New   ⇒ Revised   ~~deleted~~ Deleted   ● Use Additional Character(s)

Insufficiency, insufficient *(Continued)*
  arterial *(Continued)*
    mesenteric K55.1
    peripheral I73.9
    precerebral (multiple) (bilateral) G45.2
    vertebral G45.0
  arteriovenous I99.8
  biliary K83.8
  cardiac —*see also* Insufficiency, myocardial
    due to presence of (cardiac) prosthesis
      I97.11-•
    postprocedural I97.11-•
  cardiorenal, hypertensive I13.2
  cardiovascular —*see* Disease, cardiovascular
  cerebrovascular (acute) I67.81
    with transient focal neurological signs and
      symptoms G45.8
  circulatory NEC I99.8
    newborn P29.89
  clinical crown length K08.89
  convergence H51.11
  coronary (acute or subacute) I24.8
    chronic or with a stated duration of over 4
      weeks I25.89
  corticoadrenal E27.40
    primary E27.1
  dietary E63.9
  divergence H51.8
  food T73.0
  gastroesophageal K22.89
  gonadal
    ovary E28.39
    testis E29.1
  heart —*see also* Insufficiency, myocardial
    newborn P29.0
    valve —*see* Endocarditis
  hepatic —*see* Failure, hepatic
  idiopathic autonomic G90.09
  interocclusal distance of fully erupted teeth
    (ridge) M26.36
  kidney N28.9
    acute N28.9
    chronic N18.9
  lacrimal (secretion) H04.12-•
    passages —*see* Stenosis, lacrimal
  liver —*see* Failure, hepatic
  lung —*see* Insufficiency, pulmonary
  mental (congenital) —*see* Disability, intellectual
  mesenteric K55.1
  mitral (valve) I34.0
    with
      aortic valve disease I08.0
        with tricuspid (valve) disease I08.3
      obstruction or stenosis I05.2
        with aortic valve disease I08.0
      tricuspid (valve) disease I08.1
        with aortic (valve) disease I08.3
    congenital Q23.3
    rheumatic I05.1
      with
        aortic valve disease I08.0
          with tricuspid (valve) disease I08.3
        obstruction or stenosis I05.2
          with aortic valve disease I08.0
            with tricuspid (valve) disease I08.3
        tricuspid (valve) disease I08.1
          with aortic (valve) disease I08.3
      active or acute I01.1
        with chorea, rheumatic (Sydenham's)
          I02.0
    specified cause, except rheumatic I34.0
  muscle —*see also* Disease, muscle
    heart —*see* Insufficiency, myocardial
  ocular NEC H50.9
  myocardial, myocardium (with
    arteriosclerosis) —*see also* Failure,
    heart I50.9
    with
      rheumatic fever (conditions in I00) I09.0
        active, acute or subacute I01.2
          with chorea I02.0
        inactive or quiescent (with chorea)
          I09.0
    congenital Q24.8

Insufficiency, insufficient *(Continued)*
  myocardial, myocardium *(Continued)*
    hypertensive —*see* Hypertension, heart
    newborn P29.0
    rheumatic I09.0
      active, acute, or subacute I01.2
    syphilitic A52.06
➡nourishment *(see also* Nutrition deficient) T73.0
  pancreatic K86.89
    exocrine K86.81
  parathyroid (gland) E20.9
  peripheral vascular (arterial) I73.9
  pituitary E23.0
  placental (mother) O36.51-•
  platelets D69.6
  prenatal care affecting management of
    pregnancy O09.3-•
  progressive pluriglandular E31.0
  pulmonary J98.4
    acute, following surgery (nonthoracic)
      J95.2
      thoracic J95.1
    chronic, following surgery J95.3
    following
      shock J98.4
      trauma J98.4
    newborn P28.89
    valve I37.1
      with stenosis I37.2
      congenital Q22.2
      rheumatic I09.89
        with aortic, mitral or tricuspid (valve)
          disease I08.8
  pyloric K31.89
  renal (acute) N28.9
    chronic N18.9
  respiratory R06.89
    newborn P28.5
  rotation —*see* Malrotation
  sleep syndrome F51.12
  social insurance Z59.7
  suprarenal E27.40
    primary E27.1
  tarso-orbital fascia, congenital Q10.3
  testis E29.1
  thyroid (gland) (acquired) E03.9
    congenital E03.1
  tricuspid (valve) (rheumatic) I07.1
    with
      aortic (valve) disease I08.2
        with mitral (valve) disease I08.3
      mitral (valve) disease I08.1
        with aortic (valve) disease I08.3
      obstruction or stenosis I07.2
        with aortic (valve) disease I08.2
          with mitral (valve) disease I08.3
    congenital Q22.8
    nonrheumatic I36.1
      with stenosis I36.2
  urethral sphincter R32
  valve, valvular (heart) I38
    aortic —*see* Insufficiency, aortic (valve)
    mitral —*see* Insufficiency, mitral (valve)
    pulmonary —*see* Insufficiency, pulmonary,
      valve
    tricuspid —*see* Insufficiency, tricuspid
      (valve)
    congenital Q24.8
  vascular I99.8
    intestine K55.9
      acute —*see also* Ischemia, intestine, acute
        K55.059
      mesenteric K55.1
      peripheral I73.9
      renal —*see* Hypertension, kidney
  velopharyngeal
    acquired K13.79
    congenital Q38.8
  venous (chronic) (peripheral) I87.2
  ventricular —*see* Insufficiency, myocardial
  welfare support Z59.7

Insufflation, fallopian Z31.41
Insular —*see* condition
Insulinoma
  pancreas
    benign D13.7
    malignant C25.4
    uncertain behavior D37.8
  specified site
    benign —*see* Neoplasm, by site, benign
    malignant —*see* Neoplasm, by site,
      malignant
    uncertain behavior —*see* Neoplasm, by site,
      uncertain behavior
  unspecified site
    benign D13.7
    malignant C25.4
    uncertain behavior D37.8
Insuloma —*see* Insulinoma
Interference
  balancing side M26.56
  non-working side M26.56
Intermenstrual —*see* condition
Intermittent —*see* condition
Internal —*see* condition
Interrogation
  cardiac defibrillator (automatic) (implantable)
    Z45.02
  cardiac pacemaker Z45.018
  cardiac (event) (loop) recorder Z45.09
  infusion pump (implanted) (intrathecal) Z45.1
  neurostimulator Z46.2
Interruption
  aortic arch Q25.21
  phase-shift, sleep cycle —*see* Disorder, sleep,
    circadian rhythm
  sleep phase-shift, or 24 hour sleep-wake
    cycle —*see* Disorder, sleep, circadian
    rhythm
Interstitial —*see* condition
Intertrigo L30.4
  labialis K13.0
Intervertebral disc —*see* condition
Intestine, intestinal —*see* condition
Intolerance
  carbohydrate K90.49
  disaccharide, hereditary E73.0
  fat NEC K90.49
    pancreatic K90.3
  food K90.49
    dietary counseling and surveillance Z71.3
  fructose E74.10
    hereditary E74.12
  glucose(-galactose) E74.39
  gluten K90.01
  lactose E73.9
    specified NEC E73.8
  lysine E72.3
  milk NEC K90.49
    lactose E73.9
▶orthostatic, chronic G90.A
  protein K90.49
  starch NEC K90.49
  sucrose (-isomaltose) E74.31
Intoxicated NEC (without dependence) —*see*
  Alcohol, intoxication
Intoxication
➡acid *(see also* Acidosis) E87.29
  alcoholic (acute) (without dependence) —*see*
    Alcohol, intoxication
  alimentary canal K52.1
  amphetamine (without dependence) —*see*
    also Abuse, drug, stimulant, with
    intoxication
    stimulant NEC F15.10
      with
        anxiety disorder F15.180
        intoxication F15.129
          with
            delirium F15.121
            perceptual disturbance F15.122
      with dependence —*see* Dependence, drug,
        stimulant, with intoxication

Intoxication *(Continued)*
  anxiolytic (acute) (without dependence) —*see*
      Abuse, drug, sedative, with intoxication
    with dependence —*see* Dependence, drug,
        sedative, with intoxication
  caffeine F15.929
    with dependence —*see* Dependence, drug,
        stimulant, with intoxication
  cannabinoids (acute) (without
      dependence) —*see* Use, cannabis, with
      intoxication
    with
      abuse —*see* Abuse, drug, cannabis, with
          intoxication
      dependence —*see* Dependence, drug,
          cannabis, with intoxication
  chemical —*see* Table of Drugs and
      Chemicals
    via placenta or breast milk —*see*
        Absorption, chemical, through
        placenta
  cocaine (acute) (without dependence) —*see*
      Abuse, drug, cocaine, with intoxication
    with dependence —*see* Dependence, drug,
        cocaine, with intoxication
  drug
    acute (without dependence) —*see* Abuse,
        drug, by type with intoxication
      with dependence —*see* Dependence,
          drug, by type with intoxication
    addictive
      via placenta or breast milk —*see*
          Absorption, drug, addictive,
          through placenta
    newborn P93.8
      gray baby syndrome P93.0
    overdose or wrong substance given
        or taken —*see* Table of Drugs and
        Chemicals, by drug, poisoning
  enteric K52.1
  foodborne A05.9
    bacterial A05.9
    classical (Clostridium botulinum)
        A05.1
    due to
      Bacillus cereus A05.4
      bacterium A05.9
        specified NEC A05.8
      Clostridium
        botulinum A05.1
        perfringens A05.2
        welchii A05.2
      Salmonella A02.9
        with
          (gastro) enteritis A02.0
          localized infection(s) A02.20
            arthritis A02.23
            meningitis A02.21
            osteomyelitis A02.24
            pneumonia A02.22
            pyelonephritis A02.25
            specified NEC A02.29
          sepsis A02.1
          specified manifestation NEC A02.8
      Staphylococcus A05.0
      Vibrio
        parahaemolyticus A05.3
        vulnificus A05.5
    enterotoxin, staphylococcal A05.0
    noxious —*see* Poisoning, food, noxious
  gastrointestinal K52.1
  hallucinogenic (without dependence) —
      see Abuse, drug, hallucinogen, with
      intoxication
    with dependence —*see* Dependence, drug,
        hallucinogen, with intoxication
▶ hepatocerebral intoxication K76.82
  hypnotic (acute) (without dependence) —*see*
      Abuse, drug, sedative, with intoxication
    with dependence —*see* Dependence, drug,
        sedative, with intoxication

Intoxication *(Continued)*
  inhalant (acute) (without dependence) —*see*
      Abuse, drug, inhalant, with intoxication
    with dependence —*see* Dependence, drug,
        inhalant, with intoxication
  meaning
    inebriation —*see* category F10
    poisoning —*see* Table of Drugs and
        Chemicals
  methyl alcohol (acute) (without
      dependence) —*see* Alcohol, intoxication
  opioid (acute) (without dependence) —*see*
      Abuse, drug, opioid, with intoxication
    with dependence —*see* Dependence, drug,
        opioid, with intoxication
  pathologic NEC (without dependence) —*see*
      Alcohol, intoxication
  phencyclidine (without dependence) —*see*
      Abuse, drug, hallucinogen, with
      intoxication
    with dependence —*see* Dependence, drug,
        hallucinogen, with intoxication
  potassium (K) E87.5
  psychoactive substance NEC (without
      dependence) —*see* Abuse, drug,
      psychoactive NEC, with intoxication
    with dependence —*see* Dependence, drug,
        psychoactive NEC, with intoxication
  sedative (acute) (without dependence) —*see*
      Abuse, drug, sedative, with intoxication
    with dependence —*see* Dependence, drug,
        sedative, with intoxication
  serum —*see also* Reaction, serum T80.69
  uremic —*see* Uremia
  volatile solvents (acute) (without
      dependence) —*see* Abuse, drug,
      inhalant, with intoxication
    with dependence —*see* Dependence, drug,
        inhalant, with intoxication
  water E87.79
Intraabdominal testis, testes
  bilateral Q53.211
  unilateral Q53.111
Intracranial —*see* condition
Intrahepatic gallbladder Q44.1
Intraligamentous —*see* condition
Intrathoracic —*see also* condition
  kidney Q63.2
Intrauterine contraceptive device
  checking Z30.431
  in situ Z97.5
  insertion Z30.430
    immediately following removal
        Z30.433
  management Z30.431
  reinsertion Z30.433
  removal Z30.432
  replacement Z30.433
  retention in pregnancy O26.3-●
Intraventricular —*see* condition
Intrinsic deformity —*see* Deformity
Intubation, difficult or failed T88.4
Intumescence, lens (eye) (cataract) —*see*
    Cataract
Intussusception (bowel) (colon) (enteric)
    (ileocecal) (ileocolic) (intestine) (rectum)
    K56.1
  appendix K38.8
  congenital Q43.8
  ureter (with obstruction) N13.5
Invagination (bowel, colon, intestine or rectum)
    K56.1
Inversion
  albumin-globulin (A-G) ratio E88.09
  bladder N32.89
  cecum —*see* Intussusception
  cervix N88.8
  chromosome in normal individual
      Q95.1
  circadian rhythm —*see* Disorder, sleep,
      circadian rhythm

Inversion *(Continued)*
  nipple N64.59
    congenital Q83.8
      gestational —*see* Retraction, nipple
      puerperal, postpartum —*see* Retraction,
          nipple
  nyctohemeral rhythm —*see* Disorder, sleep,
      circadian rhythm
  optic papilla Q14.2
  organ or site, congenital NEC —*see* Anomaly,
      by site
  sleep rhythm —*see* Disorder, sleep, circadian
      rhythm
  testis (congenital) Q55.29
  uterus (chronic) (postinfectional) (postpartal,
      old) N85.5
    postpartum O71.2
  vagina (posthysterectomy) N99.3
  ventricular Q20.5
Investigation —*see also* Examination Z04.9
  clinical research subject (control) (normal
      comparison) (participant) Z00.6
Involuntary movement, abnormal R25.9
Involution, involutional —*see also* condition
  breast, cystic —*see* Dysplasia, mammary,
      specified type NEC
  depression (single episode) F32.89
    recurrent episode F33.9
  melancholia (single episode) F32.89
    recurrent episode F33.8
  ovary, senile —*see* Atrophy, ovary
  thymus failure E32.8
I.Q.
  under 20 F73
  20-34 F72
  35-49 F71
  50-69 F70
IRDS (type I) P22.0
  type II P22.1
Irideremia Q13.1
Iridis rubeosis —*see* Disorder, iris, vascular
Iridochoroiditis (panuveitis) —*see* Panuveitis
Iridocyclitis H20.9-●
  acute H20.0-●
    hypopyon H20.05-●
    primary H20.01-●
    recurrent H20.02-●
    secondary (noninfectious) H20.04-●
      infectious H20.03-●
  chronic H20.1-●
  due to allergy —*see* Iridocyclitis, acute,
      secondary
  endogenous —*see* Iridocyclitis, acute,
      primary
  Fuchs' —*see* Cyclitis, Fuchs' heterochromic
  gonococcal A54.32
  granulomatous —*see* Iridocyclitis, chronic
  herpes, herpetic (simplex) B00.51
    zoster B02.32
  hypopyon —*see* Iridocyclitis, acute,
      hypopyon
  in (due to)
    ankylosing spondylitis M45.9
    gonococcal infection A54.32
    herpes (simplex) virus B00.51
      zoster B02.32
    infectious disease NOS B99
    parasitic disease NOS B89 *[H22]*
    sarcoidosis D86.83
    syphilis A51.43
    tuberculosis A18.54
    zoster B02.32
  lens-induced H20.2-●
  nongranulomatous —*see* Iridocyclitis, acute
  recurrent —*see* Iridocyclitis, acute, recurrent
  rheumatic —*see* Iridocyclitis, chronic
  subacute —*see* Iridocyclitis, acute
  sympathetic —*see* Uveitis, sympathetic
  syphilitic (secondary) A51.43
  tuberculous (chronic) A18.54
  Vogt-Koyanagi H20.82-●

Iridocyclochoroiditis (panuveitis) —see
   Panuveitis
Iridodialysis H21.53-●
Iridodonesis H21.89
Iridoplegia (complete) (partial) (reflex) H57.09
Iridoschisis H21.25-●
Iris —see also condition
   bombé —see Membrane, pupillary
Iritis —see also Iridocyclitis
   chronic —see Iridocyclitis, chronic
   diabetic —see E08-E13 with .39
   due to
      herpes simplex B00.51
      leprosy A30.9 [H22]
   gonococcal A54.32
   gouty —see also Gout, by type M10.9 [H22]
   granulomatous —see Iridocyclitis, chronic
   lens induced —see Iridocyclitis, lens-induced
   papulosa (syphilitic) A52.71
   rheumatic —see Iridocyclitis, chronic
   syphilitic (secondary) A51.43
      congenital (early) A50.01
      late A52.71
   tuberculous A18.54
Iron —see condition
Iron-miner's lung J63.4
Irradiated enamel (tooth, teeth) K03.89
Irradiation effects, adverse T66
Irreducible, irreducibility —see condition
Irregular, irregularity
   action, heart I49.9
   alveolar process K08.89
   bleeding N92.6
   breathing R06.89
   contour of cornea (acquired) —see Deformity,
      cornea
      congenital Q13.4
   contour, reconstructed breast N65.0
   dentin (in pulp) K04.3
   eye movements H55.89
      deficient
         saccadic H55.81
         smooth H55.82
      nystagmus —see Nystagmus
   labor O62.2
   menstruation (cause unknown) N92.6
   periods N92.6
   prostate N42.9
   pupil —see Abnormality, pupillary
   reconstructed breast N65.0
   respiratory R06.89
   septum (nasal) J34.2
   shape, organ or site, congenital NEC —see
      Distortion
   sleep-wake pattern (rhythm) G47.23
Irritable, irritability R45.4
   bladder N32.89
   bowel (syndrome) K58.9
      with
         constipation K58.1
         diarrhea K58.0
      mixed K58.2
      psychogenic F45.8
      specified NEC K58.8
   bronchial —see Bronchitis
   cerebral, in newborn P91.3
   colon —see also Irritable, bowel K58.9
      with diarrhea K58.0
      psychogenic F45.8
   duodenum K59.89
   heart (psychogenic) F45.8
   hip —see Derangement, joint, specified type
      NEC, hip
   ileum K59.89
   infant R68.12
   jejunum K59.89
   rectum K59.89
   stomach K31.89
      psychogenic F45.8
   sympathetic G90.8
   urethra N36.8

Irritation
   anus K62.89
   axillary nerve G54.0
   bladder N32.89
   brachial plexus G54.0
   bronchial —see Bronchitis
   cervical plexus G54.2
   cervix —see Cervicitis
   choroid, sympathetic —see Endophthalmitis
   cranial nerve —see Disorder, nerve, cranial
   gastric K31.89
      psychogenic F45.8
   globe, sympathetic —see Uveitis, sympathetic
   labyrinth —see subcategory H83.2
   lumbosacral plexus G54.1
   meninges (traumatic) —see Injury, intracranial
      nontraumatic —see Meningismus
   nerve —see Disorder, nerve
   nervous R45.0
   penis N48.89
   perineum NEC L29.3
   peripheral autonomic nervous system G90.8
   peritoneum —see Peritonitis
   pharynx J39.2
   plantar nerve —see Lesion, nerve, plantar
   spinal (cord) (traumatic) —see also Injury,
      spinal cord, by region
      nerve G58.9
         root NEC —see Radiculopathy
      nontraumatic —see Myelopathy
   stomach K31.89
      psychogenic F45.8
   sympathetic nerve NEC G90.8
   ulnar nerve —see Lesion, nerve, ulnar
   vagina N89.8
Ischemia, ischemic I99.8
   bowel (transient)
      acute —see also Ischemia, intestine, acute
         K55.059
      chronic K55.1
      due to mesenteric artery insufficiency
         K55.1
   brain —see Ischemia, cerebral
   cardiac (see Disease, heart, ischemic)
   cardiomyopathy I25.5
   cerebral (chronic) (generalized) I67.82
      arteriosclerotic I67.2
      intermittent G45.9
      newborn P91.0
      recurrent focal G45.8
      transient G45.9
   colon chronic (due to mesenteric artery
      insufficiency) K55.1
   coronary —see Disease, heart, ischemic
   demand (coronary) —see also Angina
      I24.8
      with myocardial infarction I21.A1
      resulting in myocardial infarction
         I21.A1
   heart (chronic or with a stated duration of
      over 4 weeks) I25.9
      acute or with a stated duration of 4 weeks
        or less I24.9
      subacute I24.9
   infarction, muscle —see Infarct, muscle
   intestine (large) (small) (transient) K55.9
      acute K55.059
         diffuse K55.052
         focal K55.051
         large K55.039
            diffuse K55.032
            focal K55.031
         small K55.019
            diffuse K55.012
            focal K55.011
      chronic K55.1
      due to mesenteric artery insufficiency
         K55.1
   kidney N28.0
   limb, critical —see Arteriosclerosis, with
      critical limb ischemia

Ischemia, ischemic (Continued)
   limb-threatening, chronic —see
      Arteriosclerosis, with critical limb
      ischemia
   mesenteric, acute —see also Ischemia,
      intestine, acute K55.059
   muscle, traumatic T79.6
   myocardium, myocardial (chronic or with
      a stated duration of over 4 weeks)
      I25.9
      acute, without myocardial infarction
         I51.3
      silent (asymptomatic) I25.6
      transient of newborn P29.4
   renal N28.0
   retina, retinal —see Occlusion, artery, retina
   small bowel
      acute K55.019
         diffuse K55.012
         focal K55.011
      chronic K55.1
      due to mesenteric artery insufficiency
         K55.1
   spinal cord G95.11
   subendocardial —see Insufficiency,
      coronary
   supply (coronary) —see also Angina
      I25.9
      due to vasospasm I20.1
Ischial spine —see condition
Ischialgia —see Sciatica
Ischiopagus Q89.4
Ischium, ischial —see condition
Ischuria R34
Iselin's disease or osteochondrosis —see
   Osteochondrosis, juvenile, metatarsus
Islands of
   parotid tissue in
      lymph nodes Q38.6
      neck structures Q38.6
   submaxillary glands in
      fascia Q38.6
      lymph nodes Q38.6
      neck muscles Q38.6
Islet cell tumor, pancreas D13.7
Isoimmunization NEC —see also
   Incompatibility
   affecting management of pregnancy (ABO)
      (with hydrops fetalis) O36.11-●
      anti-A sensitization O36.11-●
      anti-B sensitization O36.19-●
      anti-c sensitization O36.09-●
      anti-C sensitization O36.09-●
      anti-e sensitization O36.09-●
      anti-E sensitization O36.09-●
      Rh NEC O36.09-●
         anti-D antibody O36.01-●
      specified NEC O36.19-●
   newborn P55.9
      with
         hydrops fetalis P56.0
         kernicterus P57.0
      ABO (blood groups) P55.1
      Rhesus (Rh) factor P55.0
      specified type NEC P55.8
Isolation, isolated
   dwelling Z59.89
   family Z63.79
   social Z60.4
Isoleucinosis E71.19
Isomerism atrial appendages (with asplenia or
   polysplenia) Q20.6
Isosporiasis, isosporosis A07.3
Isovaleric acidemia E71.110
Issue of
   medical certificate Z02.79
      for disability determination Z02.71
   repeat prescription (appliance) (glasses)
      (medicinal substance, medicament,
      medicine) Z76.0
      contraception —see Contraception

Itch, itching —*see also* Pruritus
  baker's L23.6
  barber's B35.0
  bricklayer's L24.5
  cheese B88.0
  clam digger's B65.3
  coolie B76.9
  copra B88.0
  dew B76.9
  dhobi B35.6
  filarial —*see* Infestation, filarial
  grain B88.0
  grocer's B88.0

Itch, itching (Continued)
  ground B76.9
  harvest B88.0
  jock B35.6
  Malabar B35.5
    beard B35.0
    foot B35.3
    scalp B35.0
  meaning scabies B86
  Norwegian B86
  perianal L29.0
  poultrymen's B88.0

Itch, itching (Continued)
  sarcoptic B86
  scabies B86
  scrub B88.0
  straw B88.0
  swimmer's B65.3
  water B76.9
  winter L29.8
Ivemark's syndrome (asplenia with congenital heart disease) Q89.01
Ivory bones Q78.2
Ixodiasis NEC B88.8

▶ New   ⇒ Revised   ~~deleted~~ Deleted   • Use Additional Character(s)

J

Jaccoud's syndrome —*see* Arthropathy, postrheumatic, chronic
Jackson's
  membrane Q43.3
  paralysis or syndrome G83.89
  veil Q43.3
Jacquet's dermatitis (diaper dermatitis) L22
Jadassohn-Pellizari's disease or anetoderma L90.2
Jadassohn's
  blue nevus —*see* Nevus
  intraepidermal epithelioma —*see* Neoplasm, skin, benign
Jaffe-Lichtenstein (-Uehlinger) syndrome —*see* Dysplasia, fibrous, bone NEC
Jakob-Creutzfeldt disease or syndrome —*see* Creutzfeldt-Jakob disease or syndrome
Jaksch-Luzet disease D64.89
Jamaican
  neuropathy G92.8
  paraplegic tropical ataxic-spastic syndrome G92.8
Janet's disease F48.8
Janiceps Q89.4
Jansky-Bielschowsky amaurotic idiocy E75.4
Japanese
  B-type encephalitis A83.0
  river fever A75.3
Jaundice (yellow) R17
  acholuric (familial) (splenomegalic) —*see also* Spherocytosis
    acquired D59.8
  breast-milk (inhibitor) P59.3
  catarrhal (acute) B15.9
    with hepatic coma B15.0
  cholestatic (benign) R17
  due to or associated with
    delayed conjugation P59.8
      associated with (due to) preterm delivery P59.0
    preterm delivery P59.0
  epidemic (catarrhal) B15.9
    with hepatic coma B15.0
    leptospiral A27.0
    spirochetal A27.0
  familial nonhemolytic (congenital) (Gilbert) E80.4
    Crigler-Najjar E80.5
  febrile (acute) B15.9
    with hepatic coma B15.0
    leptospiral A27.0
    spirochetal A27.0
  hematogenous D59.9
  hemolytic (acquired) D59.9
    congenital —*see* Spherocytosis

Jaundice (Continued)
  hemorrhagic (acute) (leptospiral) (spirochetal) A27.0
  infectious (acute) (subacute) B15.9
    with hepatic coma B15.0
    leptospiral A27.0
    spirochetal A27.0
  leptospiral (hemorrhagic) A27.0
  malignant (without coma) K72.90
    with coma K72.91
  neonatal —*see* Jaundice, newborn
  newborn P59.9
    due to or associated with
      ABO
        antibodies P55.1
        incompatibility, maternal/fetal P55.1
        isoimmunization P55.1
      absence or deficiency of enzyme system for bilirubin conjugation (congenital) P59.8
      bleeding P58.1
      breast milk inhibitors to conjugation P59.3
        associated with preterm delivery P59.0
      bruising P58.0
      Crigler-Najjar syndrome E80.5
      delayed conjugation P59.8
        associated with preterm delivery P59.0
      drugs or toxins
        given to newborn P58.42
        transmitted from mother P58.41
      excessive hemolysis P58.9
        due to
          bleeding P58.1
          bruising P58.0
          drugs or toxins
            given to newborn P58.42
            transmitted from mother P58.41
          infection P58.2
          polycythemia P58.3
          swallowed maternal blood P58.5
        specified type NEC P58.8
      galactosemia E74.21
      Gilbert syndrome E80.4
      hemolytic disease P55.9
        ABO isoimmunization P55.1
        Rh isoimmunization P55.0
        specified NEC P55.8
      hepatocellular damage P59.20
        specified NEC P59.29
      hereditary hemolytic anemia P58.8
      hypothyroidism, congenital E03.1
      incompatibility, maternal/fetal NOS P55.9
      infection P58.2

Jaundice (Continued)
  newborn (Continued)
    due to or associated with (Continued)
      inspissated bile syndrome P59.1
      isoimmunization NOS P55.9
      mucoviscidosis E84.9
      polycythemia P58.3
      preterm delivery P59.0
      Rh
        antibodies P55.0
        incompatibility, maternal/fetal P55.0
        isoimmunization P55.0
      specified cause NEC P59.8
      swallowed maternal blood P58.5
    spherocytosis (congenital) D58.0
  nonhemolytic congenital familial (Gilbert) E80.4
  nuclear, newborn —*see also* Kernicterus of newborn P57.9
  obstructive —*see also* Obstruction, bile duct K83.1
  post-immunization —*see* Hepatitis, viral, type, B
  post-transfusion —*see* Hepatitis, viral, type, B
  regurgitation —*see also* Obstruction, bile duct K83.1
  serum (homologous) (prophylactic) (therapeutic) —*see* Hepatitis, viral, type, B
  spirochetal (hemorrhagic) A27.0
  symptomatic R17
    newborn P59.9
Jaw —*see* condition
Jaw-winking phenomenon or syndrome Q07.8
Jealousy
  alcoholic F10.988
  childhood F93.8
  sibling F93.8
Jejunitis —*see* Enteritis
Jejunostomy status Z93.4
Jejunum, jejunal —*see* condition
Jensen's disease —*see* Inflammation, chorioretinal, focal, juxtapapillary
Jerks, myoclonic G25.3
Jervell-Lange-Nielsen syndrome I45.81
Jeune's disease Q77.2
Jigger disease B88.1
Job's syndrome (chronic granulomatous disease) D71
Joint —*see also* condition
  mice —*see* Loose, body, joint
    knee M23.4-●
Jordan's anomaly or syndrome D72.0
Joseph-Diamond-Blackfan anemia (congenital hypoplastic) D61.01
Jungle yellow fever A95.0
Jüngling's disease —*see* Sarcoidosis
Juvenile —*see* condition

K

Kahler's disease C90.0-●
Kakke E51.11
Kala-azar B55.0
Kallmann's syndrome E23.0
Kanner's syndrome (autism) —see Psychosis, childhood
Kaposi's
  dermatosis (xeroderma pigmentosum) Q82.1
  lichen ruber L44.0
    acuminatus L44.0
  sarcoma
    colon C46.4
    connective tissue C46.1
    gastrointestinal organ C46.4
    lung C46.5-●
    lymph node (multiple) C46.3
    palate (hard) (soft) C46.2
    rectum C46.4
    skin (multiple sites) C46.0
    specified site NEC C46.7
    stomach C46.4
    unspecified site C46.9
  varicelliform eruption B00.0
  vaccinia T88.1
Kartagener's syndrome or triad (sinusitis, bronchiectasis, situs inversus) Q89.3
Karyotype
  with abnormality except iso (Xq) Q96.2
  45,X Q96.0
  46,X
    iso (Xq) Q96.1
  46,XX Q98.3
    with streak gonads Q50.32
    hermaphrodite (true) Q99.1
    male Q98.3
  46,XY
    with streak gonads Q56.1
    female Q97.3
    hermaphrodite (true) Q99.1
  47,XXX Q97.0
  47,XXY Q98.0
  47,XYY Q98.5
Kaschin-Beck disease —see Disease, Kaschin-Beck
Katayama's disease or fever B65.2
Kawasaki's syndrome M30.3
Kayser-Fleischer ring (cornea) (pseudosclerosis) H18.04-●
Kaznelson's syndrome (congenital hypoplastic anemia) D61.01
Kearns-Sayre syndrome H49.81-●
Kedani fever A75.3
Kelis L91.0
Kelly (-Patterson) syndrome (sideropenic dysphagia) D50.1
Keloid, cheloid L91.0
  acne L73.0
  Addison's L94.0
  cornea —see Opacity, cornea
  Hawkin's L91.0
  scar L91.0
Keloma L91.0
Kenya fever A77.1
Keratectasia —see also Ectasia, cornea
  congenital Q13.4
Keratinization of alveolar ridge mucosa
  excessive K13.23
  minimal K13.22
Keratinized residual ridge mucosa
  excessive K13.23
  minimal K13.22
Keratitis (nodular) (nonulcerative) (simple) (zonular) H16.9
  with ulceration (central) (marginal) (perforated) (ring) —see Ulcer, cornea
  actinic —see Photokeratitis
  arborescens (herpes simplex) B00.52
  areolar H16.11-●
  bullosa H16.8

Keratitis (Continued)
  deep H16.309
    specified type NEC H16.399
  dendritic (a) (herpes simplex) B00.52
  disciform (is) (herpes simplex) B00.52
    varicella B01.81
  filamentary H16.12-●
  gonococcal (congenital or prenatal) A54.33
  herpes, herpetic (simplex) B00.52
    zoster B02.33
  in (due to)
    acanthamebiasis B60.13
    adenovirus B30.0
    exanthema —see also Exanthem B09
    herpes (simplex) virus B00.52
    measles B05.81
    syphilis A50.31
    tuberculosis A18.52
    zoster B02.33
  interstitial (nonsyphilitic) H16.30-●
    diffuse H16.32-●
    herpes, herpetic (simplex) B00.52
      zoster B02.33
    sclerosing H16.33-●
    specified type NEC H16.39-●
    syphilitic (congenital) (late) A50.31
    tuberculous A18.52
  macular H16.11-●
  nummular H16.11-●
  oyster shuckers' H16.8
  parenchymatous —see Keratitis, interstitial
  petrificans H16.8
  postmeasles B05.81
  punctata
    leprosa A30.9 [H16.14-●]
    syphilitic (profunda) A50.31
  punctate H16.14-●
  purulent H16.8
  rosacea L71.8
  sclerosing H16.33-●
  specified type NEC H16.8
  stellate H16.11-●
  striate H16.11-●
  superficial H16.10-●
    with conjunctivitis —see Keratoconjunctivitis
    due to light —see Photokeratitis
  suppurative H16.8
  syphilitic (congenital) (prenatal) A50.31
  trachomatous A71.1
    sequelae B94.0
  tuberculous A18.52
  vesicular H16.8
  xerotic —see also Keratomalacia H16.8
    vitamin A deficiency E50.4
Keratoacanthoma L85.8
Keratocele —see Descemetocele
Keratoconjunctivitis H16.20-●
  Acanthamoeba B60.13
  adenoviral B30.0
  epidemic B30.0
  exposure H16.21-●
  herpes, herpetic (simplex) B00.52
    zoster B02.33
  in exanthema —see also Exanthem B09
  infectious B30.0
  lagophthalmic —see Keratoconjunctivitis, specified type NEC
  neurotrophic H16.23-●
  phlyctenular H16.25-●
  postmeasles B05.81
  shipyard B30.0
  sicca (Sjogren's) M35.0-●
    not Sjogren's H16.22-●
  specified type NEC H16.29-●
  tuberculous (phlyctenular) A18.52
  vernal H16.26-●
Keratoconus H18.60-●
  congenital Q13.4
  stable H18.61-●
  unstable H18.62-●

Keratocyst (dental) (odontogenic) —see Cyst, calcifying odontogenic
Keratoderma, keratodermia (congenital) (palmaris et plantaris) (symmetrical) Q82.8
  acquired L85.1
    in diseases classified elsewhere L86
  climactericum L85.1
  gonococcal A54.89
  gonorrheal A54.89
  punctata L85.2
  Reiter's —see Reiter's disease
Keratodermatocele —see Descemetocele
Keratoglobus H18.79
  congenital Q15.8
    with glaucoma Q15.0
Keratohemia —see Pigmentation, cornea, stromal
Keratoiritis —see also Iridocyclitis
  syphilitic A50.39
  tuberculous A18.54
Keratoma L57.0
  palmaris and plantaris hereditarium Q82.8
  senile L57.0
Keratomalacia H18.44-●
  vitamin A deficiency E50.4
Keratomegaly Q13.4
Keratomycosis B49
  nigrans, nigricans (palmaris) B36.1
Keratopathy H18.9
  band H18.42-●
  bullous H18.1-●
  bullous (aphakic), following cataract surgery H59.01-●
Keratoscleritis, tuberculous A18.52
Keratosis L57.0
  actinic L57.0
  arsenical L85.8
  congenital, specified NEC Q80.8
  female genital NEC N94.89
  follicularis Q82.8
    acquired L11.0
    congenita Q82.8
    et parafollicularis in cutem penetrans L87.0
    spinulosa (decalvans) Q82.8
    vitamin A deficiency E50.8
  gonococcal A54.89
  male genital (external) N50.89
  nigricans L83
  obturans, external ear (canal) —see Cholesteatoma, external ear
  palmaris et plantaris (inherited) (symmetrical) Q82.8
    acquired L85.1
  penile N48.89
  pharynx J39.2
  pilaris, acquired L85.8
  punctata (palmaris et plantaris) L85.2
  scrotal N50.89
  seborrheic L82.1
    inflamed L82.0
  senile L57.0
  solar L57.0
  tonsillaris J35.8
  vagina N89.4
  vegetans Q82.8
  vitamin A deficiency E50.8
  vocal cord J38.3
Kerato-uveitis —see Iridocyclitis
Kerion (celsi) B35.0
Kernicterus of newborn (not due to isoimmunization) P57.9
  due to isoimmunization (conditions in P55.0-P55.9) P57.0
  specified type NEC P57.8
Kerunoparalysis T75.09
Keshan disease E59
▶ Ketoacidosis E87.29
  diabetic —see Diabetes, by type, with ketoacidosis
Ketonuria R82.4

▶ New   ⇒ Revised   deleted Deleted   ● Use Additional Character(s)

Ketosis NEC E88.89
  diabetic —see Diabetes, by type, with
    ketoacidosis
Kew Garden fever A79.1
Kidney —see condition
Kienböck's disease —see also Osteochondrosis,
    juvenile, hand, carpal lunate
  adult M93.1
Kimmelstiel (-Wilson) disease —see Diabetes,
    Kimmelstiel (-Wilson) disease
Kimura disease D21.9
  specified site (see Neoplasm, connective
    tissue benign)
Kink, kinking
  artery I77.1
  hair (acquired) L67.8
  ileum or intestine —see Obstruction,
    intestine
  Lane's —see Obstruction, intestine
  organ or site, congenital NEC —see Anomaly,
    by site
  ureter (pelvic junction) N13.5
    with
      hydronephrosis N13.1
        with infection N13.6
      pyelonephritis (chronic) N11.1
    congenital Q62.39
  vein(s) I87.8
    caval I87.1
    peripheral I87.1
Kinnier Wilson's disease (hepatolenticular
    degeneration) E83.01
Kissing spine M48.20
  cervical region M48.22
  cervicothoracic region M48.23
  lumbar region M48.26
  lumbosacral region M48.27
  occipito-atlanto-axial region M48.21
  thoracic region M48.24
  thoracolumbar region M48.25
Klatskin's tumor C24.0
Klauder's disease A26.8
Klebs' disease —see also Glomerulonephritis
    N05.-●
Klebsiella (K.) pneumoniae, as cause of
    disease classified elsewhere B96.1
Klein (e)-Levin syndrome G47.13
Kleptomania F63.2
Klinefelter's syndrome Q98.4
  karyotype 47,XXY Q98.0
  male with more than two X chromosomes
    Q98.1
Klippel-Feil deficiency, disease, or syndrome
    (brevicollis) Q76.1
Klippel's disease I67.2
Klippel-Trenaunay (-Weber) syndrome
    Q87.2
Klumpke (-Déjerine) palsy, paralysis (birth)
    (newborn) P14.1
Knee —see condition
Knock knee (acquired) M21.06-●
  congenital Q74.1

Knot(s)
  intestinal, syndrome (volvulus) K56.2
  surfer S89.8-●
  umbilical cord (true) O69.2
Knotting (of)
  hair L67.8
  intestine K56.2
Knuckle pad (Garrod's) M72.1
Koch's
  infection —see Tuberculosis
  relapsing fever A68.9
Koch-Weeks' conjunctivitis —see
    Conjunctivitis, acute, mucopurulent
Köebner's syndrome Q81.8
Köenig's disease (osteochondritis dissecans) —
    see Osteochondritis, dissecans
Köhler-Pellegrini-Steida disease or syndrome
    (calcification, knee joint) —see Bursitis,
    tibial collateral
Köhler's disease
  patellar —see Osteochondrosis, juvenile,
    patella
  tarsal navicular —see Osteochondrosis,
    juvenile, tarsus
Koilonychia L60.3
  congenital Q84.6
Kojevnikov's, epilepsy —see Kozhevnikof's
    epilepsy
Koplik's spots B05.9
Kopp's asthma E32.8
Korsakoff's (Wernicke) disease, psychosis or
    syndrome (alcoholic) F10.96
  with dependence F10.26
  drug-induced
    due to drug abuse —see Abuse, drug, by
      type, with amnestic disorder
    due to drug dependence —see Dependence,
      drug, by type, with amnestic disorder
  nonalcoholic F04
Korsakov's disease, psychosis or syndrome —
    see Korsakoff's disease
Korsakow's disease, psychosis or syndrome —
    see Korsakoff's disease
Kostmann's disease or syndrome (infantile
    genetic agranulocytosis) —see
    Agranulocytosis
Kozhevnikof's epilepsy G40.109
  intractable G40.119
    with status epilepticus G40.111
    without status epilepticus G40.119
  not intractable G40.109
    with status epilepticus G40.101
    without status epilepticus G40.109
Krabbe's
  disease E75.23
  syndrome, congenital muscle hypoplasia
    Q79.8
Kraepelin-Morel disease —see Schizophrenia
Kraft-Weber-Dimitri disease Q85.89
Kraurosis
  ani K62.89
  penis N48.0

Kraurosis (Continued)
  vagina N89.8
  vulva N90.4
Kreotoxism A05.9
Krukenberg's
  spindle —see Pigmentation, cornea, posterior
  tumor C79.6-●
Kufs' disease E75.4
Kugelberg-Welander disease G12.1
Kuhnt-Junius degeneration —see also
    Degeneration, macula H35.32-●
Kümmell's disease or spondylitis —see
    Spondylopathy, traumatic
Kupffer cell sarcoma C22.3
Kuru A81.81
Kussmaul's
  disease M30.0
  respiration E87.29
    in diabetic acidosis —see Diabetes, by type,
      with ketoacidosis
Kwashiorkor E40
  marasmic, marasmus type E42
Kyasanur Forest disease A98.2
Kyphoscoliosis, kyphoscoliotic (acquired) —
    see also Scoliosis M41.9
  congenital Q67.5
  heart (disease) I27.1
  sequelae of rickets E64.3
  tuberculous A18.01
Kyphosis, kyphotic (acquired) M40.209
  cervical region M40.202
  cervicothoracic region M40.203
  congenital Q76.419
    cervical region Q76.412
    cervicothoracic region Q76.413
    occipito-atlanto-axial region Q76.411
    thoracic region Q76.414
    thoracolumbar region Q76.415
  Morquio-Brailsford type (spinal) —see also
    subcategory M49.8 E76.219
  postlaminectomy M96.3
  postradiation therapy M96.2
  postural (adolescent) M40.00
    cervicothoracic region M40.03
    thoracic region M40.04
    thoracolumbar region M40.05
  secondary NEC M40.10
    cervical region M40.12
    cervicothoracic region M40.13
    thoracic region M40.14
    thoracolumbar region M40.15
  sequelae of rickets E64.3
  specified type NEC M40.299
    cervical region M40.292
    cervicothoracic region M40.293
    thoracic region M40.294
    thoracolumbar region M40.295
  syphilitic, congenital A50.56
  thoracic region M40.204
  thoracolumbar region M40.205
  tuberculous A18.01
Kyrle disease L87.0

K

L

Labia, labium —*see* condition
Labile
  blood pressure R09.89
  vasomotor system I73.9
Labioglossal paralysis G12.29
Labium leporinum —*see* Cleft, lip
Labor —*see* Delivery
Labored breathing —*see* Hyperventilation
Labyrinthitis (circumscribed) (destructive)
  (diffuse) (inner ear) (latent) (purulent)
  (suppurative) (*see also* subcategory)
  H83.0
  syphilitic A52.79
Laceration
  with abortion —*see* Abortion, by type,
    complicated by laceration of pelvic
    organs
  abdomen, abdominal
    wall S31.119
      with
        foreign body S31.129
        penetration into peritoneal cavity
          S31.619
          with foreign body S31.629
      epigastric region S31.112
        with
          foreign body S31.122
          penetration into peritoneal cavity
            S31.612
            with foreign body S31.622
      left
        lower quadrant S31.114
          with
            foreign body S31.124
            penetration into peritoneal cavity
              S31.614
              with foreign body S31.624
        upper quadrant S31.111
          with
            foreign body S31.121
            penetration into peritoneal cavity
              S31.611
              with foreign body S31.621
      periumbilic region S31.115
        with
          foreign body S31.125
          penetration into peritoneal cavity
            S31.615
            with foreign body S31.625
      right
        lower quadrant S31.113
          with
            foreign body S31.123
            penetration into peritoneal cavity
              S31.613
              with foreign body S31.623
        upper quadrant S31.110
          with
            foreign body S31.120
            penetration into peritoneal cavity
              S31.610
              with foreign body S31.620
  accidental, complicating surgery —*see*
    Complications, surgical, accidental
    puncture or laceration
  Achilles tendon S86.02-●
  adrenal gland S37.813
  alveolar (process) —*see* Laceration, oral cavity
  ankle S91.01-●
    with
      foreign body S91.02-●
  antecubital space —*see* Laceration, elbow
  anus (sphincter) S31.831
    with
      ectopic or molar pregnancy O08.6
      foreign body S31.832
    complicating delivery —*see* Delivery,
      complicated, by, laceration, anus
      (sphincter)

Laceration (*Continued*)
  anus (*Continued*)
    following ectopic or molar pregnancy
      O08.6
    nontraumatic, nonpuerperal —*see* Fissure,
      anus
  arm (upper) S41.11-●
    with foreign body S41.12-●
    lower —*see* Laceration, forearm
  auditory canal (external) (meatus) —*see*
    Laceration, ear
  auricle, ear —*see* Laceration, ear
  axilla —*see* Laceration, arm
  back —*see also* Laceration, thorax, back
    lower S31.010
      with
        foreign body S31.020
          with penetration into
            retroperitoneal space S31.021
        penetration into retroperitoneal space
          S31.011
  bile duct S36.13
  bladder S37.23
    with ectopic or molar pregnancy O08.6
    following ectopic or molar pregnancy
      O08.6
    obstetrical trauma O71.5
  blood vessel —*see* Injury, blood vessel
  bowel —*see also* Laceration, intestine
    with ectopic or molar pregnancy O08.6
    complicating abortion —*see* Abortion,
      by type, complicated by, specified
      condition NEC
    following ectopic or molar pregnancy
      O08.6
    obstetrical trauma O71.5
  brain (any part) (cortex) (diffuse)
    (membrane) —*see also* Injury,
    intracranial, diffuse
    during birth P10.8
      with hemorrhage P10.1
    focal —*see* Injury, intracranial, focal brain
      injury
  brainstem S06.38-●
  breast S21.01-●
    with foreign body S21.02-●
  broad ligament S37.893
    with ectopic or molar pregnancy O08.6
    following ectopic or molar pregnancy
      O08.6
    laceration syndrome N83.8
    obstetrical trauma O71.6
    syndrome (laceration) N83.8
  buttock S31.801
    with foreign body S31.802
    left S31.821
      with foreign body S31.822
    right S31.811
      with foreign body S31.812
  calf —*see* Laceration, leg
  canaliculus lacrimalis —*see* Laceration,
    eyelid
  canthus, eye —*see* Laceration, eyelid
  capsule, joint —*see* Sprain
  causing eversion of cervix uteri (old) N86
  central (perineal), complicating delivery
    O70.9
  cerebellum, traumatic S06.37-●
  cerebral S06.33-●
    during birth P10.8
      with hemorrhage P10.1
    left side S06.32-●
    right side S06.31-●
  cervix (uteri)
    with ectopic or molar pregnancy O08.6
    following ectopic or molar pregnancy
      O08.6
    nonpuerperal, nontraumatic N88.1
    obstetrical trauma (current) O71.3
    old (postpartal) N88.1
    traumatic S37.63

Laceration (*Continued*)
  cheek (external) S01.41-●
    with foreign body S01.42-●
    internal —*see* Laceration, oral cavity
  chest wall —*see* Laceration, thorax
  chin —*see* Laceration, head, specified site
    NEC
  chordae tendinae NEC I51.1
    concurrent with acute myocardial
      infarction —*see* Infarct, myocardium
    following acute myocardial infarction
      (current complication) I23.4
  clitoris —*see* Laceration, vulva
  colon —*see* Laceration, intestine, large,
    colon
  common bile duct S36.13
  cortex (cerebral) —*see* Injury, intracranial,
    diffuse
  costal region —*see* Laceration, thorax
  cystic duct S36.13
  diaphragm S27.803
  digit(s)
    foot —*see* Laceration, toe
    hand —*see* Laceration, finger
  duodenum S36.430
  ear (canal) (external) S01.31-●
    with foreign body S01.32-●
    drum S09.2-●
  elbow S51.01-●
    with
      foreign body S51.02-●
  epididymis —*see* Laceration, testis
  epigastric region —*see* Laceration, abdomen,
    wall, epigastric region
  esophagus K22.89
    traumatic
      cervical S11.21
        with foreign body S11.22
      thoracic S27.813
  eye (ball) S05.3-●
    with prolapse or loss of intraocular tissue
      S05.2-●
    penetrating S05.6-●
  eyebrow —*see* Laceration, eyelid
  eyelid S01.11-●
    with foreign body S01.12-●
  face NEC —*see* Laceration, head, specified
    site NEC
  fallopian tube S37.539
    bilateral S37.532
    unilateral S37.531
  finger(s) S61.219
    with
      damage to nail S61.319
        with
          foreign body S61.329
      foreign body S61.229
    index S61.218
      with
        damage to nail S61.318
          with
            foreign body S61.328
        foreign body S61.228
    left S61.211
      with
        damage to nail S61.311
          with
            foreign body S61.321
        foreign body S61.221
    right S61.210
      with
        damage to nail S61.310
          with
            foreign body S61.320
        foreign body S61.220
    little S61.218
      with
        damage to nail S61.318
          with
            foreign body S61.328
        foreign body S61.228

▶ New   ⟹ Revised   ~~deleted~~ Deleted   ● Use Additional Character(s)

Laceration *(Continued)*
finger *(Continued)*
little *(Continued)*
left S61.217
with
damage to nail S61.317
with
foreign body S61.327
foreign body S61.227
right S61.216
with
damage to nail S61.316
with
foreign body S61.326
foreign body S61.226
middle S61.218
with
damage to nail S61.318
with
foreign body S61.328
foreign body S61.228
left S61.213
with
damage to nail S61.313
with
foreign body S61.323
foreign body S61.223
right S61.212
with
damage to nail S61.312
with
foreign body S61.322
foreign body S61.222
ring S61.218
with
damage to nail S61.318
with
foreign body S61.328
foreign body S61.228
left S61.215
with
damage to nail S61.315
with
foreign body S61.325
foreign body S61.225
right S61.214
with
damage to nail S61.314
with
foreign body S61.324
foreign body S61.224
flank S31.119
with foreign body S31.129
foot (except toe(s) alone) S91.319
with foreign body S91.329
left S91.312
with foreign body S91.322
right S91.311
with foreign body S91.321
toe —*see* Laceration, toe
forearm S51.819
with
foreign body S51.829
elbow only —*see* Laceration,
elbow
left S51.812
with
foreign body S51.822
right S51.811
with
foreign body S51.821
forehead S01.81
with foreign body S01.82
fourchette O70.0
with ectopic or molar pregnancy
O08.6
complicating delivery O70.0
following ectopic or molar pregnancy
O08.6
gallbladder S36.123

Laceration *(Continued)*
genital organs, external
female S31.512
with foreign body S31.522
vagina —*see* Laceration, vagina
vulva —*see* Laceration, vulva
male S31.511
with foreign body S31.521
penis —*see* Laceration, penis
scrotum —*see* Laceration, scrotum
testis —*see* Laceration, testis
groin —*see* Laceration, abdomen, wall
gum —*see* Laceration, oral cavity
hand S61.419
with
foreign body S61.429
finger —*see* Laceration, finger
left S61.412
with
foreign body S61.422
right S61.411
with
foreign body S61.421
thumb —*see* Laceration, thumb
head S01.91
with foreign body S01.92
cheek —*see* Laceration, cheek
ear —*see* Laceration, ear
eyelid —*see* Laceration, eyelid
lip —*see* Laceration, lip
nose —*see* Laceration, nose
oral cavity —*see* Laceration, oral
cavity
scalp S01.01
with foreign body S01.02
specified site NEC S01.81
with foreign body S01.82
temporomandibular area —*see* Laceration,
cheek
heart —*see* Injury, heart, laceration
heel —*see* Laceration, foot
hepatic duct S36.13
hip S71.019
with foreign body S71.029
left S71.012
with foreign body S71.022
right S71.011
with foreign body S71.021
hymen —*see* Laceration, vagina
hypochondrium —*see* Laceration, abdomen,
wall
hypogastric region —*see* Laceration,
abdomen, wall
ileum S36.438
inguinal region —*see* Laceration, abdomen,
wall
instep —*see* Laceration, foot
internal organ —*see* Injury, by site
interscapular region —*see* Laceration, thorax,
back
intestine
large
colon S36.539
ascending S36.530
descending S36.532
sigmoid S36.533
specified site NEC S36.538
rectum S36.63
transverse S36.531
small S36.439
duodenum S36.430
specified site NEC S36.438
intra-abdominal organ S36.93
intestine —*see* Laceration, intestine
liver —*see* Laceration, liver
pancreas —*see* Laceration, pancreas
peritoneum S36.81
specified site NEC S36.893
spleen —*see* Laceration, spleen
stomach —*see* Laceration, stomach

Laceration *(Continued)*
intracranial NEC —*see also* Injury,
intracranial, diffuse
birth injury P10.9
jaw —*see* Laceration, head, specified site NEC
jejunum S36.438
joint capsule —*see* Sprain, by site
kidney S37.03- ●
major (greater than 3 cm) (massive)
(stellate) S37.06- ●
minor (less than 1 cm) S37.04- ●
moderate (1 to 3 cm) S37.05- ●
multiple S37.06- ●
knee S81.01- ●
with foreign body S81.02- ●
labium (majus) (minus) —*see* Laceration,
vulva
lacrimal duct —*see* Laceration, eyelid
large intestine —*see* Laceration, intestine,
large
larynx S11.011
with foreign body S11.012
leg (lower) S81.819
with foreign body S81.829
foot —*see* Laceration, foot
knee —*see* Laceration, knee
left S81.812
with foreign body S81.822
right S81.811
with foreign body S81.821
upper —*see* Laceration, thigh
ligament —*see* Sprain
lip S01.511
with foreign body S01.521
liver S36.113
major (stellate) S36.116
minor S36.114
moderate S36.115
loin —*see* Laceration, abdomen, wall
lower back —*see* Laceration, back, lower
lumbar region —*see* Laceration, back, lower
lung S27.339
bilateral S27.332
unilateral S27.331
malar region —*see* Laceration, head, specified
site NEC
mammary —*see* Laceration, breast
mastoid region —*see* Laceration, head,
specified site NEC
meninges —*see* Injury, intracranial, diffuse
meniscus —*see* Tear, meniscus
mesentery S36.893
mesosalpinx S37.893
mouth —*see* Laceration, oral cavity
muscle —*see* Injury, muscle, by site,
laceration
nail
finger —*see* Laceration, finger, with
damage to nail
toe —*see* Laceration, toe, with damage to nail
nasal (septum) (sinus) —*see* Laceration, nose
nasopharynx —*see* Laceration, head, specified
site NEC
neck S11.91
with foreign body S11.92
involving
cervical esophagus S11.21
with foreign body S11.22
larynx —*see* Laceration, larynx
pharynx —*see* Laceration, pharynx
thyroid gland —*see* Laceration, thyroid
gland
trachea —*see* Laceration, trachea
specified site NEC S11.81
with foreign body S11.82
nerve —*see* Injury, nerve
nose (septum) (sinus) S01.21
with foreign body S01.22
ocular NOS S05.3- ●
adnexa NOS S01.11- ●

▶ New   ⇒ Revised   ~~deleted~~ Deleted   ● Use Additional Character(s)

Laceration (Continued)
  trachea S11.021
    with foreign body S11.022
  tunica vaginalis —see Laceration, testis
  tympanum, tympanic membrane —see
    Laceration, ear, drum
  umbilical region S31.115
    with foreign body S31.125
  ureter S37.13
  urethra S37.33
    with or following ectopic or molar
      pregnancy O08.6
    obstetrical trauma O71.5
  urinary organ NEC S37.893
  uterus S37.63
    with ectopic or molar pregnancy O08.6
    following ectopic or molar pregnancy O08.6
    nonpuerperal, nontraumatic N85.8
    obstetrical trauma NEC O71.81
    old (postpartal) N85.8
  uvula —see Laceration, oral cavity
  vagina S31.41
    with
      ectopic or molar pregnancy O08.6
      foreign body S31.42
    during delivery O71.4
      with perineal laceration —see Laceration,
        perineum, female, during delivery
    following ectopic or molar pregnancy
      O08.6
    nonpuerperal, nontraumatic N89.8
    old (postpartal) N89.8
  vas deferens S37.893
  vesical —see Laceration, bladder
  vocal cords S11.031
    with foreign body S11.032
  vulva S31.41
    with
      ectopic or molar pregnancy O08.6
      foreign body S31.42
    complicating delivery O70.0
    following ectopic or molar pregnancy
      O08.6
    nonpuerperal, nontraumatic N90.89
    old (postpartal) N90.89
  wrist S61.519
    with
      foreign body S61.529
    left S61.512
      with
        foreign body S61.522
    right S61.511
      with
        foreign body S61.521
Lack of
  achievement in school Z55.3
  adequate
    food Z59.48
    intermaxillary vertical dimension of fully
      erupted teeth M26.36
    sleep Z72.820
  appetite (see Anorexia) R63.0
  awareness R41.9
  care
    in home Z74.2
    of infant (at or after birth) T76.02
      confirmed T74.02
  cognitive functions R41.9
  coordination R27.9
    ataxia R27.0
    specified type NEC R27.8
  development (physiological) R62.50
    failure to thrive (child over 28 days old)
      R62.51
    adult R62.7
    newborn P92.6
    short stature R62.52
    specified type NEC R62.59
  energy R53.83
  financial resources Z59.6

Lack of (Continued)
  food Z59.48
  growth R62.52
  heating Z59.1
  housing (permanent) (temporary) Z59.00
    adequate Z59.1
  learning experiences in childhood Z62.898
  leisure time (affecting life-style) Z73.2
  material resources Z59.87
  memory —see also Amnesia
    mild, following organic brain damage F06.8
  ovulation N97.0
  parental supervision or control of child Z62.0
  person able to render necessary care Z74.2
  physical exercise Z72.3
  play experience in childhood Z62.898
  posterior occlusal support M26.57
  relaxation (affecting life-style) Z73.2
  safe drinking water Z58.6
  sexual
    desire F52.0
    enjoyment F52.1
  shelter Z59.02
  sleep (adequate) Z72.820
  supervision of child by parent Z62.0
  support, posterior occlusal M26.57
  transportation Z59.82
  water T73.1
    safe drinking Z58.6
Lacrimal —see condition
Lacrimation, abnormal —see Epiphora
Lacrimonasal duct —see condition
Lactation, lactating (breast) (puerperal,
  postpartum)
  associated
    cracked nipple O92.13
    retracted nipple O92.03
  defective O92.4
  disorder NEC O92.79
  excessive O92.6
  failed (complete) O92.3
    partial O92.4
  mastitis NEC —see Mastitis, obstetric
  mother (care and/or examination) Z39.1
  nonpuerperal N64.3
Lacticemia, excessive (see also Acidosis) E87.20
Lacunar skull Q75.8
Laennec's cirrhosis K70.30
  with ascites K70.31
  nonalcoholic K74.69
Lafora's disease —see Epilepsy, generalized,
  idiopathic
Lag, lid (nervous) —see Retraction, lid
Lagophthalmos (eyelid) (nervous) H02.209
  bilateral, upper and lower eyelids H02.20C
  cicatricial H02.219
    bilateral, upper and lower eyelids H02.21C
    left H02.216
      lower H02.215
      upper H02.214
      upper and lower eyelids H02.21B
    right H02.213
      lower H02.212
      upper H02.211
      upper and lower eyelids H02.21A
  keratoconjunctivitis —see Keratoconjunctivitis
  left H02.206
    lower H02.205
    upper H02.204
    upper and lower eyelids H02.20B
  mechanical H02.229
    bilateral, upper and lower eyelids H02.22C
    left H02.226
      lower H02.225
      upper H02.224
      upper and lower eyelids H02.22B
    right H02.223
      lower H02.222
      upper H02.221
      upper and lower eyelids H02.22A

Lagophthalmos (Continued)
  paralytic H02.239
    bilateral, upper and lower eyelids H02.23C
    left H02.236
      lower H02.235
      upper H02.234
      upper and lower eyelids H02.23B
    right H02.233
      lower H02.232
      upper H02.231
      upper and lower eyelids H02.23A
  right H02.203
    lower H02.202
    upper H02.201
    upper and lower eyelids H02.20A
Laki-Lorand factor deficiency —see Defect,
  coagulation, specified type NEC
Lalling F80.0
Lambert-Eaton syndrome —see Syndrome,
  Lambert-Eaton
Lambliasis, lambliosis A07.1
Landau-Kleffner syndrome —see Epilepsy,
  specified NEC
Landouzy-Déjérine dystrophy or
  facioscapulohumeral atrophy G71.02
Landouzy's disease (icterohemorrhagic
  leptospirosis) A27.0
Landry-Guillain-Barré, syndrome or paralysis
  G61.0
Landry's disease or paralysis G61.0
Lane's
  band Q43.3
  kink —see Obstruction, intestine
  syndrome K90.2
Langdon Down's syndrome —see Trisomy, 21
Lapsed immunization schedule status Z28.3
Large
  baby (regardless of gestational age) (4000g to
    4499g) P08.1
  ear, congenital Q17.1
  physiological cup Q14.2
  stature R68.89
Large-for-dates NEC (infant) (4000g to 4499g)
  P08.1
  affecting management of pregnancy O36.6-•
  exceptionally (4500g or more) P08.0
Larsen-Johansson disease
  orosteochondrosis —see Osteochondrosis,
    juvenile, patella
Larsen's syndrome (flattened facies and
  multiple congenital dislocations) Q74.8
Larva migrans
  cutaneous B76.9
    Ancylostoma B76.0
  visceral B83.0
Laryngeal —see condition
Laryngismus (stridulus) J38.5
  congenital P28.89
  diphtheritic A36.2
Laryngitis (acute) (edematous) (fibrinous)
  (infective) (infiltrative) (malignant)
  (membranous) (phlegmonous)
  (pneumococcal) (pseudomembranous)
  (septic) (subglottic) (suppurative)
  (ulcerative) J04.0
  with
    influenza, flu, or grippe —see Influenza,
      with, laryngitis
    tracheitis (acute) —see Laryngotracheitis
  atrophic J37.0
  catarrhal J37.0
  chronic J37.0
    with tracheitis (chronic) J37.1
  diphtheritic A36.2
  due to external agent —see Inflammation,
    respiratory, upper, due to
  Hemophilus influenzae J04.0
  H. influenzae J04.0
  hypertrophic J37.0
  influenzal —see Influenza, with, respiratory
    manifestations NEC

Laryngitis (Continued)
  obstructive J05.0
  sicca J37.0
  spasmodic J05.0
    acute J04.0
  streptococcal J04.0
  stridulous J05.0
  syphilitic (late) A52.73
    congenital A50.59 [J99]
      early A50.03 [J99]
  tuberculous A15.5
  Vincent's A69.1
Laryngocele (congenital) (ventricular) Q31.3
Laryngofissure J38.7
  congenital Q31.8
Laryngomalacia (congenital) Q31.5
Laryngopharyngitis (acute) J06.0
  chronic J37.0
  due to external agent —see Inflammation,
    respiratory, upper, due to
Laryngoplegia J38.00
  bilateral J38.02
  unilateral J38.01
Laryngoptosis J38.7
Laryngospasm J38.5
Laryngostenosis J38.6
Laryngotracheitis (acute) (Infectional)
    (infective) (viral) J04.2
  atrophic J37.1
  catarrhal J37.1
  chronic J37.1
  diphtheritic A36.2
  due to external agent —see Inflammation,
    respiratory, upper, due to
  Hemophilus influenzae J04.2
  hypertrophic J37.1
  influenzal —see Influenza, with, respiratory
    manifestations NEC
  pachydermic J38.7
  sicca J37.1
  spasmodic J38.5
    acute J05.0
  streptococcal J04.2
  stridulous J38.5
  syphilitic (late) A52.73
    congenital A50.59 [J99]
      early A50.03 [J99]
  tuberculous A15.5
  Vincent's A69.1
Laryngotracheobronchitis —see Bronchitis
Larynx, laryngeal —see condition
Lassa fever A96.2
Lassitude —see Weakness
Late
  talker R62.0
  walker R62.0
Late effect(s) —see Sequelae
Latent —see condition
Laterocession —see Lateroversion
Lateroflexion —see Lateroversion
Lateroversion
  cervix —see Lateroversion, uterus
  uterus, uterine (cervix) (postinfectional)
    (postpartal, old) N85.4
    congenital Q51.818
    in pregnancy or childbirth O34.59-•
Lathyrism —see Poisoning, food, noxious,
    plant
Launois' syndrome (pituitary gigantism) E22.0
Launois-Bensaude adenolipomatosis E88.89
Laurence-Moon (-Bardet)-Biedl syndrome
    Q87.89
Lax, laxity —see also Relaxation
  ligament (ous) —see also Disorder, ligament
    familial M35.7
    knee —see Derangement, knee
  skin (acquired) L57.4
    congenital Q82.8
Laxative habit F55.2
Lazy leukocyte syndrome D70.8
Lead miner's lung J63.6

Leak, leakage
  air NEC J93.82
    postprocedural J95.812
  amniotic fluid —see Rupture, membranes,
    premature
  blood (microscopic), fetal, into maternal
    circulation affecting management
    of pregnancy —see Pregnancy,
    complicated by
  cerebrospinal fluid G96.00
    cranial
      postoperative G96.08
      specified NEC G96.08
      spontaneous G96.01
      traumatic G96.08
    from spinal (lumbar) puncture G97.0
    spinal
      postoperative G96.09
      post-traumatic G96.09
      specified NEC G96.09
      spontaneous G96.02
    spontaneous
      from
        skull base G96.01
        spine G96.02
  CSF —see Leak, cerebrospinal fluid
  device, implant or graft —see also
    Complications, by site and type,
    mechanical
⇒ arterial graft NEC —see Complication,
      vascular, graft, mechanical, leakage
      T82.838
    breast (implant) T85.43
    catheter NEC T85.638
      dialysis (renal) T82.43
        intraperitoneal T85.631
      infusion NEC T82.534
        spinal (epidural) (subdural)
          T85.630
      urinary T83.038
        cystostomy T83.030
        Hopkins T83.038
        ileostomy T83.038
        indwelling T83.031
        nephrostomy T83.032
        specified NEC T83.038
        urostomy T83.038
    gastrointestinal —see Complications,
      prosthetic device, mechanical,
      gastrointestinal device
    genital NEC T83.498
      penile prosthesis (cylinder) (implanted)
        (pump) (resevoir) T83.490
      testicular prosthesis T83.491
    heart NEC —see Complication,
      cardiovascular device, mechanical
    joint prosthesis —see Complications, joint
      prosthesis, mechanical, specified NEC,
      by site
    ocular NEC —see Complications, prosthetic
      device, mechanical, ocular device
    orthopedic NEC —see Complication,
      orthopedic, device, mechanical
    persistent air J93.82
    specified NEC T85.638
    urinary NEC —see also Complication,
      genitourinary, device, urinary,
      mechanical
      graft T83.23
    vascular NEC —see Complication,
      cardiovascular device, mechanical
    ventricular intracranial shunt T85.03
  urine —see Incontinence
Leaky heart —see Endocarditis
Learning defect (specific) F81.9
Leather bottle stomach C16.9
Leber's
  congenital amaurosis H35.50
  optic atrophy (hereditary) H47.22
Lederer's anemia D59.19
Leeches (external) —see Hirudiniasis

Leg —see condition
Legg (-Calvé)-Perthes disease, syndrome or
    osteochondrosis M91.1-•
Legionellosis A48.1
  nonpneumonic A48.2
Legionnaires'
  disease A48.1
    nonpneumonic A48.2
  pneumonia A48.1
Leigh's disease G31.82
Leiner's disease L21.1
Leiofibromyoma —see Leiomyoma
Leiomyoblastoma —see Neoplasm, connective
    tissue, benign
Leiomyofibroma —see also Neoplasm,
    connective tissue, benign
  uterus (cervix) (corpus) D25.9
Leiomyoma —see also Neoplasm, connective
    tissue, benign
  bizarre —see Neoplasm, connective tissue,
    benign
  cellular —see Neoplasm, connective tissue,
    benign
  epithelioid —see Neoplasm, connective
    tissue, benign
  uterus (cervix) (corpus) D25.9
    intramural D25.1
    submucous D25.0
    subserosal D25.2
  vascular —see Neoplasm, connective tissue,
    benign
Leiomyoma, leiomyomatosis (intravascular) —
    see Neoplasm, connective tissue, uncertain
    behavior
Leiomyosarcoma —see also Neoplasm,
    connective tissue, malignant
  epithelioid —see Neoplasm, connective
    tissue, malignant
  myxoid —see Neoplasm, connective tissue,
    malignant
Leishmaniasis B55.9
  American (mucocutaneous) B55.2
    cutaneous B55.1
  Asian Desert B55.1
  Brazilian B55.2
  cutaneous (any type) B55.1
    dermal —see also Leishmaniasis, cutaneous
      post-kala-azar B55.0
  eyelid B55.1
  infantile B55.0
  Mediterranean B55.0
  mucocutaneous (American) (New World)
    B55.2
  naso-oral B55.2
  nasopharyngeal B55.2
  old world B55.1
  tegumentaria diffusa B55.1
  visceral B55.0
Leishmanoid, dermal —see also Leishmaniasis,
    cutaneous
  post-kala-azar B55.0
Lenegre's disease I44.2
Lengthening, leg —see Deformity, limb,
    unequal length
Lennert's lymphoma —see Lymphoma,
    Lennert's
Lennox-Gastaut syndrome G40.812
  intractable G40.814
    with status epilepticus G40.813
    without status epilepticus G40.814
  not intractable G40.812
    with status epilepticus G40.811
    without status epilepticus G40.812
Lens —see condition
Lenticonus (anterior) (posterior) (congenital)
    Q12.8
Lenticular degeneration, progressive E83.01
Lentiglobus (posterior) (congenital) Q12.8
Lentigo (congenital) L81.4
  maligna —see also Melanoma, in situ
    melanoma —see Melanoma

Lentivirus, as cause of disease classified
   elsewhere B97.31
Leontiasis
   ossium M85.2
   syphilitic (late) A52.78
      congenital A50.59
Lepothrix A48.8
Lepra —see Leprosy
Leprechaunism E34.8
Leprosy A30.-●
   with muscle disorder A30.9 [M63.80]
      ankle A30.9 [M63.87-●]
      foot A30.9 [M63.87-●]
      forearm A30.9 [M63.83-●]
      hand A30.9 [M63.84-●]
      lower leg A30.9 [M63.86-●]
      multiple sites A30.9 [M63.89]
      pelvic region A30.9 [M63.85-●]
      shoulder region A30.9 [M63.81-●]
      specified site NEC A30.9 [M63.88]
      thigh A30.9 [M63.85-●]
      upper arm A30.9 [M63.82-●]
   anesthetic A30.9
   BB A30.3
   BL A30.4
   borderline (infiltrated) (neuritic) A30.3
      lepromatous A30.4
      tuberculoid A30.2
   BT A30.2
   dimorphous (infiltrated) (neuritic) A30.3
   I A30.0
   indeterminate (macular) (neuritic) A30.0
   lepromatous (diffuse) (infiltrated) (macular)
      (neuritic) (nodular) A30.5
   LL A30.5
   macular (early) (neuritic) (simple) A30.9
   maculoanesthetic A30.9
   mixed A30.3
   neural A30.9
   nodular A30.5
   primary neuritic A30.3
   specified type NEC A30.8
   TT A30.1
   tuberculoid (major) (minor) A30.1
Leptocytosis, hereditary D56.9
Leptomeningitis (chronic) (circumscribed)
   (hemorrhagic) (nonsuppurative) —see
      Meningitis
Leptomeningopathy G96.198
Leptospiral —see condition
Leptospirochetal —see condition
Leptospirosis A27.9
   canicola A27.89
   due to Leptospira interrogans serovar
      icterohaemorrhagiae A27.0
   icterohemorrhagica A27.0
   pomona A27.89
   Weil's disease A27.0
Leptus dermatitis B88.0
Leriche's syndrome (aortic bifurcation
      occlusion) I74.09
Leri's pleonosteosis Q78.8
Leri-Weill syndrome Q77.8
Lermoyez' syndrome —see Vertigo, peripheral
      NEC
Lesch-Nyhan syndrome E79.1
Leser-Trélat disease L82.1
   inflamed L82.0
Lesion(s) (nontraumatic)
   abducens nerve —see Strabismus, paralytic,
      sixth nerve
   alveolar process K08.9
   angiocentric immunoproliferative
      D47.Z9
   anorectal K62.9
   aortic (valve) I35.9
   auditory nerve —see subcategory
      H93.3
   basal ganglion G25.9
   bile duct —see Disease, bile duct
   biomechanical M99.9

Lesion (Continued)
   biomechanical (Continued)
      specified type NEC M99.89
         abdomen M99.89
         acromioclavicular M99.87
         cervical region M99.81
         cervicothoracic M99.81
         costochondral M99.88
         costovertebral M99.88
         head region M99.80
         hip M99.85
         lower extremity M99.86
         lumbar region M99.83
         lumbosacral M99.83
         occipitocervical M99.80
         pelvic region M99.85
         pubic M99.85
         rib cage M99.88
         sacral region M99.84
         sacrococcygeal M99.84
         sacroiliac M99.84
         specified NEC M99.89
         sternochondral M99.88
         sternoclavicular M99.87
         thoracic region M99.82
         thoracolumbar M99.82
         upper extremity M99.87
   bladder N32.9
   bone —see Disorder, bone
   brachial plexus G54.0
   brain G93.9
      congenital Q04.9
      vascular I67.9
         degenerative I67.9
         hypertensive I67.4
   buccal cavity K13.79
   calcified —see Calcification
   canthus —see Disorder, eyelid
   carate —see Pinta, lesions
   cardia K31.9
   cardiac —see also Disease, heart I51.9
      congenital Q24.9
      valvular —see Endocarditis
   cauda equina G83.4
   cecum K63.9
   cerebral —see Lesion, brain
   cerebrovascular I67.9
      degenerative I67.9
      hypertensive I67.4
   cervical (nerve) root NEC G54.2
   chiasmal —see Disorder, optic, chiasm
   chorda tympani G51.8
   coin, lung R91.1
   colon K63.9
   combined periodontic - endodontic K05.5
   congenital —see Anomaly, by site
   conjunctiva H11.9
   conus medullaris —see Injury, conus
      medullaris
   coronary artery —see Ischemia, heart
   cranial nerve G52.9
      eighth —see Disorder, ear
      eleventh G52.9
      fifth G50.9
      first G52.0
      fourth —see Strabismus, paralytic, fourth
         nerve
      seventh G51.9
      sixth —see Strabismus, paralytic, sixth nerve
      tenth G52.2
      twelfth G52.3
   cystic —see Cyst
   degenerative —see Degeneration
   duodenum K31.9
   edentulous (alveolar) ridge, associated with
      trauma, due to traumatic occlusion K06.2
   en coup de sabre L94.1
   eyelid —see Disorder, eyelid
   gasserian ganglion G50.8
   gastric K31.9
   gastroduodenal K31.9

Lesion (Continued)
   gastrointestinal K63.9
   gingiva, associated with trauma K06.2
   glomerular
      focal and segmental —see also N00-N07
         with fourth character .1 N05.1
      minimal change —see also N00-N07 with
         fourth character .0 N05.0
   heart (organic) —see Disease, heart
   hyperchromic, due to pinta (carate) A67.1
   hyperkeratotic —see Hyperkeratosis
   hypothalamic E23.7
   ileocecal K63.9
   ileum K63.9
   iliohypogastric nerve G57.8-●
   inflammatory —see Inflammation
   intestine K63.9
   intracerebral —see Lesion, brain
   intrachiasmal (optic) —see Disorder, optic,
      chiasm
   intracranial, space-occupying R90.0
   joint —see Disorder, joint
      sacroiliac (old) M53.3
   keratotic —see Keratosis
   kidney —see Disease, renal
   laryngeal nerve (recurrent) G52.2
   lip K13.0
   liver K76.9
   lumbosacral
      plexus G54.1
      root (nerve) NEC G54.4
   lung (coin) R91.1
   maxillary sinus J32.0
   mitral I05.9
   Morel-Lavallée —see Hematoma,
      by site
   motor cortex NEC G93.89
   mouth K13.79
   nerve G58.9
      femoral G57.2-●
      median G56.1-●
         carpal tunnel syndrome —see Syndrome,
            carpal tunnel
      plantar G57.6-●
      popliteal (lateral) G57.3-●
         medial G57.4-●
      radial G56.3-●
      sciatic G57.0-●
      spinal —see Injury, nerve, spinal
      ulnar G56.2-●
   nervous system, congenital Q07.9
   nonallopathic —see Lesion, biomechanical
   nose (internal) J34.89
   obstructive —see Obstruction
   obturator nerve G57.8-●
   oral mucosa K13.70
   organ or site NEC —see Disease, by site
   osteolytic —see Osteolysis
   peptic K27.9
   periodontal, due to traumatic occlusion K05.5
   pharynx J39.2
   pigment, pigmented (skin) L81.9
   pinta —see Pinta, lesions
   polypoid —see Polyp
   prechiasmal (optic) —see Disorder, optic,
      chiasm
   primary —see also Syphilis, primary A51.0
      carate A67.0
      pinta A67.0
      yaws A66.0
   pulmonary J98.4
      valve I37.9
   pylorus K31.9
   rectosigmoid K63.9
   retina, retinal H35.9
   sacroiliac (joint) (old) M53.3
   salivary gland K11.9
      benign lymphoepithelial K11.8
   saphenous nerve G57.8-●
   sciatic nerve G57.0-●
   secondary —see Syphilis, secondary

Lesion *(Continued)*
　shoulder (region) M75.9-●
　　specified NEC M75.8-●
　sigmoid K63.9
　sinus (accessory) (nasal) J34.89
　skin L98.9
　　suppurative L08.0
　SLAP S43.43-●
　spinal cord G95.9
　　congenital Q06.9
　spleen D73.89
　stomach K31.9
　superior glenoid labrum S43.43-●
　syphilitic —*see* Syphilis
　tertiary —*see* Syphilis, tertiary
　thoracic root (nerve) NEC G54.3
　tonsillar fossa J35.9
　tooth, teeth K08.9
　　white spot
　　　chewing surface K02.51
　　　pit and fissure surface K02.51
　　　smooth surface K02.61
　traumatic —*see* specific type of injury by site
　tricuspid (valve) I07.9
　　nonrheumatic I36.9
　trigeminal nerve G50.9
　ulcerated or ulcerative —*see* Ulcer, skin
　uterus N85.9
　vagina N89.8
　vulva N90.89
　vagus nerve G52.2
　valvular —*see* Endocarditis
　vascular I99.9
　　affecting central nervous system I67.9
　　following trauma NEC T14.8
　　umbilical cord, complicating delivery O69.5
　warty —*see* Verruca
　white spot (tooth)
　　chewing surface K02.51
　　pit and fissure surface K02.51
　　smooth surface K02.61
Less than a high school diploma Z55.5
Lethargic —*see* condition
Lethargy R53.83
Letterer-Siwe's disease C96.0
Leukemia, leukemic C95.9-●
　acute basophilic C94.8-●
　acute bilineal C95.0-●
　acute erythroid C94.0-●
　acute lymphoblastic C91.0-●
　acute megakaryoblastic C94.2-●
　acute megakaryocytic C94.2-●
　acute mixed lineage C95.0-●
　acute monoblastic (monoblastic/monocytic)
　　C93.0-●
　acute monocytic (monoblastic/monocytic)
　　C93.0-●
　acute myeloblastic (minimal differentiation)
　　(with maturation) C92.0-●
　acute myeloid, NOS C92.0-●
　　with
　　　11q23-abnormality C92.6-●
　　　dysplasia of remaining hematopoesis
　　　　and/or myelodysplastic disease in
　　　　its history C92.A-●
　　　multilineage dysplasia C92.A-●
　　　variation of MLL-gene C92.6-●
　　M6 (a)(b) C94.0-●
　　M7 C94.2-●
　acute myelomonocytic C92.5-●
　acute promyelocytic C92.4-●
　adult T-cell (HTLV-1-associated) (acute
　　variant) (chronic variant)
　　(lymphomatoid variant) (smouldering
　　variant) C91.5-●
　aggressive NK-cell C94.8-●
　AML (1/ETO) (M0) (M1) (M2) (without a
　　FAB classification) C92.0-●
　AML M3 C92.4-●
　AML M4 (Eo with inv(16) or t(16;16)) C92.5-●
　AML M5 C93.0-●

Leukemia, leukemic *(Continued)*
　AML M5a C93.0-●
　AML M5b C93.0-●
　AML Me with t (15;17) and variants C92.4-●
　atypical chronic myeloid, BCR/ABL-negative
　　C92.2-●
　biphenotypic acute C95.0-●
　blast cell C95.0-●
　Burkitt-type, mature B-cell C91.A-●
　chronic eosinophilic (*see also* Syndrome,
　　hypereosinophilic, myeloid) C94.8-●
　chronic lymphocytic, of B-cell type C91.1-●
　chronic monocytic C93.1-●
　chronic myelogenous (Philadelphia
　　chromosome (Ph1) positive) (t(9;22))
　　(q34;q11) (with crisis of blast cells)
　　C92.1-●
　chronic myeloid, BCR/ABL-positive C92.1-●
　　atypical, BCR/ABL-negative C92.2-●
　chronic myelomonocytic C93.1-●
　chronic neutrophilic D47.1
　CMML (-1) (-2) (with eosinophilia) C93.1-●
　granulocytic —*see also* Category C92 C92.9-●
　hairy-cell C91.4-●
　juvenile myelomonocytic C93.3-●
　lymphoid C91.9-●
　　specified NEC C91.Z-●
　mast cell C94.3-●
　mature B-cell, Burkitt-type C91.A-●
　monocytic (subacute) C93.9-●
　　specified NEC C93.Z-●
　myelogenous —*see also* Category
　　C92 C92.9-●
　myeloid C92.9-●
　　specified NEC C92.Z-●
　plasma cell C90.1-●
　plasmacytic C90.1-●
　prolymphocytic
　　of B-cell type C91.3-●
　　of T-cell type C91.6-●
　specified NEC C94.8-●
　stem cell, of unclear lineage C95.0-●
　subacute lymphocytic C91.9-●
　T-cell large granular lymphocytic C91.Z-●
　unspecified cell type C95.9-●
　　acute C95.0-●
　　chronic C95.1-●
Leukemoid reaction —*see also* Reaction,
　　leukemoid D72.823-●
Leukoaraiosis (hypertensive) I67.81
Leukoariosis —*see* Leukoaraiosis
Leukocoria —*see* Disorder, globe, degenerated
　　condition, leucocoria
Leukocytopenia D72.819
Leukocytosis D72.829
　eosinophilic D72.19
Leukoderma, leukodermia NEC L81.5
　syphilitic A51.39
　　late A52.79
Leukodystrophy E75.29
Leukoedema, oral epithelium K13.29
Leukoencephalitis G04.81
　acute (subacute) hemorrhagic G36.1
　　postimmunization or postvaccinal
　　　G04.02
　postinfectious G04.01
　subacute sclerosing A81.1
　van Bogaert's (sclerosing) A81.1
Leukoencephalopathy —*see also*
　　Encephalopathy G93.49
　Binswanger's I67.3
　heroin vapor G92.8
　metachromatic E75.25
　multifocal (progressive) A81.2
　postimmunization and postvaccinal
　　G04.02
　progressive multifocal A81.2
　reversible, posterior G93.6
　van Bogaert's (sclerosing) A81.1
　vascular, progressive I67.3
Leukoerythroblastosis D75.9

Leukokeratosis —*see also* Leukoplakia
　mouth K13.21
　nicotina palati K13.24
　oral mucosa K13.21
　tongue K13.21
　vocal cord J38.3
Leukokraurosis vulva (e) N90.4
Leukoma (cornea) —*see also* Opacity, cornea
　adherent H17.0-●
　interfering with central vision —*see* Opacity,
　　cornea, central
Leukomalacia, cerebral, newborn P91.2
　periventricular P91.2
Leukomelanopathy, hereditary D72.0
Leukonychia (punctata) (striata) L60.8
　congenital Q84.4
Leukopathia unguium L60.8
　congenital Q84.4
Leukopenia D72.819
　basophilic D72.818
　chemotherapy (cancer) induced D70.1
　congenital D70.0
　cyclic D70.0
　drug induced NEC D70.2
　　due to cytoreductive cancer chemotherapy
　　　D70.1
　eosinophilic D72.818
　familial D70.0
　infantile genetic D70.0
　malignant D70.9
　periodic D70.0
　transitory neonatal P61.5
Leukopenic —*see* condition
Leukoplakia
　anus K62.89
　bladder (postinfectional) N32.89
　buccal K13.21
　cervix (uteri) N88.0
　esophagus K22.89
　gingiva K13.21
　hairy (oral mucosa) (tongue) K13.3
　kidney (pelvis) N28.89
　larynx J38.7
　lip K13.21
　mouth K13.21
　oral epithelium, including tongue (mucosa)
　　K13.21
　palate K13.21
　pelvis (kidney) N28.89
　penis (infectional) N48.0
　rectum K62.89
　syphilitic (late) A52.79
　tongue K13.21
　ureter (postinfectional) N28.89
　urethra (postinfectional) N36.8
　uterus N85.8
　vagina N89.4
　vocal cord J38.3
　vulva N90.4
Leukorrhea N89.8
　due to Trichomonas (vaginalis) A59.00
　trichomonal A59.00
Leukosarcoma C85.9
Levocardia (isolated) Q24.1
　with situs inversus Q89.3
Levotransposition Q20.5
Lev's disease or syndrome (acquired complete
　　heart block) I44.2
Levulosuria —*see* Fructosuria
Levurid L30.2
➥ Lewy body (ies) (disease) G31.83
~~Leyden-Moebius dystrophy G71.09~~
▶ Leyden-Möbius dystrophy —*see* Dystrophy,
　　Leyden-Möbius
Leydig cell
　carcinoma
　　specified site —*see* Neoplasm, malignant,
　　　by site
　　unspecified site
　　　female C56.9-●
　　　male C62.9-●

Leydig cell (Continued)
  tumor
    benign
      specified site —see Neoplasm, benign,
        by site
      unspecified site
        female D27.-●
        male D29.2-●
    malignant
      specified site —see Neoplasm,
        malignant, by site
      unspecified site
        female C56.-●
        male C62.9-●
    specified site —see Neoplasm, uncertain
      behavior, by site
    unspecified site
      female D39.1-●
      male D40.1-●
Leydig-Sertoli cell tumor
  specified site —see Neoplasm, benign,
    by site
  unspecified site
    female D27.-●
    male D29.2-●
▶LGMD —see Dystrophy, muscular, limb-girdle
LGSIL (Low grade squamous intraepithelial
  lesion on cytologic smear of)
  anus R85.612
  cervix R87.612
  vagina R87.622
Liar, pathologic F60.2
Libido
  decreased R68.82
Libman-Sacks disease M32.11
Lice (infestation) B85.2
  body (Pediculus corporis) B85.1
  crab B85.3
  head (Pediculus capitis) B85.0
  mixed (classifiable to more than one of the
    titles B85.0-B85.3) B85.4
  pubic (Phthirus pubis) B85.3
Lichen L28.0
  albus L90.0
    penis N48.0
    vulva N90.4
  amyloidosis E85.4 [L99]
  atrophicus L90.0
    penis N48.0
    vulva N90.4
  congenital Q82.8
  myxedematosus L98.5
  nitidus L44.1
  pilaris Q82.8
    acquired L85.8
  planopilaris L66.1
  planus (chronicus) L43.9
    annularis L43.8
    bullous L43.1
    follicular L66.1
    hypertrophic L43.0
    moniliformis L44.3
    of Wilson L43.9
    specified NEC L43.8
    subacute (active) L43.3
    tropicus L43.3
  ruber
    acuminatus L44.0
    moniliformis L44.3
    planus L43.9
  sclerosus (et atrophicus) L90.0
    penis N48.0
    vulva N90.4
  scrofulosus (primary) (tuberculous) A18.4
  simplex (chronicus) (circumscriptus)
    L28.0
  striatus L44.2
  urticatus L28.2
Lichenification L28.0
Lichenoides tuberculosis (primary) A18.4
Lichtheim's disease or syndrome D51.0

Lien migrans D73.89
Ligament —see condition
Light
  for gestational age —see Light for dates
  headedness R42
Light-for-dates (infant) P05.00
  with weight of
    499 grams or less P05.01
    500-749 grams P05.02
    750-999 grams P05.03
    1000-1249 grams P05.04
    1250-1499 grams P05.05
    1500-1749 grams P05.06
    1750-1999 grams P05.07
    2000-2499 grams P05.08
    2500 grams and over P05.09
  affecting management of pregnancy O36.59-●
  and small-for-dates —see Small for dates
  specified NEC P05.09
Lightning (effects) (stroke) (struck by) T75.00
  burn —see Burn
  foot E53.8
  shock T75.01
  specified effect NEC T75.09
Lightwood-Albright syndrome N25.89
Lightwood's disease or syndrome (renal
  tubular acidosis) N25.89
Lignac (-de Toni) (-Fanconi) (-Debré) disease or
  syndrome E72.09
  with cystinosis E72.04
Ligneous thyroiditis E06.5
Likoff's syndrome I20.8
Limb —see condition
Limbic epilepsy personality syndrome F07.0
Limitation, limited
  activities due to disability Z73.6
  cardiac reserve —see Disease, heart
  eye muscle duction, traumatic —see
    Strabismus, mechanical
  mandibular range of motion M26.52
⇒Lindau (-von Hippel) disease Q85.83
Line(s)
  Beau's L60.4
  Harris' —see Arrest, epiphyseal
  Hudson's (cornea) —see Pigmentation,
    cornea, anterior
  Stähli's (cornea) —see Pigmentation, cornea,
    anterior
Linea corneae senilis —see Change, cornea,
  senile
Lingua
  geographica K14.1
  nigra (villosa) K14.3
  plicata K14.5
  tylosis K13.29
Lingual —see condition
Linguatulosis B88.8
Linitis (gastric) plastica C16.9
Lip —see condition
Lipedema —see Edema
Lipemia —see also Hyperlipidemia
  retina, retinalis E78.3
Lipidosis E75.6
  cerebral (infantile) (juvenile) (late) E75.4
  cerebroretinal E75.4
  cerebroside E75.22
  cholesterol (cerebral) E75.5
  glycolipid E75.21
  hepatosplenomegalic E78.3
  sphingomyelin —see Niemann-Pick disease
    or syndrome
  sulfatide E75.29
Lipoadenoma —see Neoplasm, benign, by site
Lipoblastoma —see Lipoma
Lipoblastomatosis —see Lipoma
Lipochondrodystrophy E76.01
Lipochrome histiocytosis (familial) D71
Lipodermatosclerosis —see Varix, leg, with,
  inflammation
  ulcerated —see Varix, leg, with, ulcer, with
    inflammation by site

Lipodystrophia progressiva E88.1
Lipodystrophy (progressive) E88.1
  insulin E88.1
  intestinal K90.81
  mesenteric K65.4
Lipofibroma —see Lipoma
Lipofuscinosis, neuronal (with ceroidosis) E75.4
Lipogranuloma, sclerosing L92.8
Lipogranulomatosis E78.89
Lipoid —see also condition
  histiocytosis D76.3
    essential E75.29
  nephrosis N04.9
  proteinosis of Urbach E78.89
Lipoidemia —see Hyperlipidemia
Lipoidosis —see Lipidosis
Lipoma D17.9
  fetal D17.9
    fat cell D17.9
  infiltrating D17.9
  intramuscular D17.9
  pleomorphic D17.9
  site classification
    arms (skin) (subcutaneous) D17.2-●
    connective tissue D17.30
      intra-abdominal D17.5
      intrathoracic D17.4
      peritoneum D17.79
      retroperitoneum D17.79
      specified site NEC D17.39
      spermatic cord D17.6
    face (skin) (subcutaneous) D17.0
    genitourinary organ NEC D17.72
    head (skin) (subcutaneous) D17.0
    intra-abdominal D17.5
    intrathoracic D17.4
    kidney D17.71
    legs (skin) (subcutaneous) D17.2-●
    neck (skin) (subcutaneous) D17.0
    peritoneum D17.79
    retroperitoneum D17.79
    skin D17.30
      specified site NEC D17.39
    specified site NEC D17.79
    spermatic cord D17.6
    subcutaneous D17.30
      specified site NEC D17.39
    trunk (skin) (subcutaneous) D17.1
    unspecified D17.9
  spindle cell D17.9
Lipomatosis E88.2
  dolorosa (Dercum) E88.2
  fetal —see Lipoma
  Launois-Bensaude E88.89
Lipomyoma —see Lipoma
Lipomyxoma —see Lipoma
Lipomyxosarcoma —see Neoplasm, connective
  tissue, malignant
Lipoprotein metabolism disorder E78.9
Lipoproteinemia E78.5
  broad-beta E78.2
  floating-beta E78.2
  hyper-pre-beta E78.1
Liposarcoma —see also Neoplasm, connective
  tissue, malignant
  dedifferentiated —see Neoplasm, connective
    tissue, malignant
  differentiated type —see Neoplasm,
    connective tissue, malignant
  embryonal —see Neoplasm, connective tissue,
    malignant
  mixed type —see Neoplasm, connective
    tissue, malignant
  myxoid —see Neoplasm, connective tissue,
    malignant
  pleomorphic —see Neoplasm, connective
    tissue, malignant
  round cell —see Neoplasm, connective tissue,
    malignant
  well differentiated type —see Neoplasm,
    connective tissue, malignant

Liposynovitis prepatellaris E88.89
Lipping, cervix N86
Lipschütz disease or ulcer N76.6
Lipuria R82.0
  schistosomiasis (bilharziasis) B65.0
Lisping F80.0
Lissauer's paralysis A52.17
Lissencephalia, lissencephaly Q04.3
Listeriosis, listerellosis A32.9
  congenital (disseminated) P37.2
  cutaneous A32.0
  neonatal, newborn (disseminated) P37.2
  oculoglandular A32.81
  specified NEC A32.89
Lithemia E79.0
Lithiasis —see Calculus
Lithosis J62.8
Lithuria R82.998
Litigation, anxiety concerning Z65.3
Little leaguer's elbow —see Epicondylitis, medial
Little's disease G80.9
Littre's
  gland —see condition
  hernia —see Hernia, abdomen
Littritis —see Urethritis
Livedo (annularis) (racemosa) (reticularis) R23.1
Liver —see condition
Living alone (problems with) Z60.2
  with handicapped person Z74.2
Living in a shelter (motel) (scattered site
    housing) (temporary or transitional living
    situation) Z59.01
Lloyd's syndrome —see Adenomatosis, endocrine
Loa loa, loaiasis, loasis B74.3
Lobar —see condition
Lobomycosis B48.0
Lobo's disease B48.0
Lobotomy syndrome F07.0
Lobstein (-Ekman) disease or syndrome Q78.0
Lobster-claw hand Q71.6-•
Lobulation (congenital) —see also Anomaly,
    by site
  kidney, Q63.1
  liver, abnormal Q44.7
  spleen Q89.09
Lobule, lobular —see condition
Local, localized —see condition
Locked twins causing obstructed labor O66.1
Locked-in state G83.5
Locking
  joint —see Derangement, joint, specified type
    NEC
    knee —see Derangement, knee
Lockjaw —see Tetanus
Löffler's
  endocarditis I42.3
  eosinophilia J82.89
  pneumonia J82.89
  syndrome (eosinophilic pneumonitis)
    J82.89
Loiasis (with conjunctival infestation) (eyelid)
    B74.3
Lone Star fever A77.0
Long
  COVID (-19) (see also COVID-19) U09.9
  labor O63.9
    first stage O63.0
    second stage O63.1
  QT syndrome I45.81
Long-term (current) (prophylactic) drug
    therapy (use of)
▶ 5-fluorouracil Z79.631
▶ 6-mercaptopurine Z79.631
▶ adalimumab Z79.620
  agents affecting estrogen receptors and
    estrogen levels NEC Z79.818
▶ alkylating agent Z79.630
  anastrozole (Arimidex) Z79.811
  antibiotics Z79.2
    short-term use - omit code
  anticoagulants Z79.01
▶ antidiabetic drugs, injectable, non-insulin
    Z79.85

Long-term (Continued)
  anti-inflammatory, non-steroidal (NSAID)
    Z79.1
▶ antimetabolite agent Z79.631
  antiplatelet Z79.02
  antithrombotics Z79.02
▶ antitumor antibiotic Z79.632
▶ apremilast Z79.61
  aromatase inhibitors Z79.811
  aspirin Z79.82
▶ azathioprine Z79.624
  birth control pill or patch Z79.3
  bisphosphonates Z79.83
▶ bleomycin Z79.632
▶ calcineurin inhibitor Z79.621
▶ chlorambucil Z79.630
▶ cisplatin Z79.630
  contraceptive, oral Z79.3
▶ cyclophosphamide Z79.630
▶ cyclosporine Z79.621
▶ cytarabine Z79.631
▶ doxorubicin Z79.632
  drug, specified NEC Z79.899
  estrogen receptor downregulators Z79.818
▶ etanercept Z79.620
▶ etoposide Z79.634
  Evista Z79.810
  exemestane (Aromasin) Z79.811
  Fareston Z79.810
  fulvestrant (Faslodex) Z79.818
  gonadotropin-releasing hormone (GnRH)
    agonist Z79.818
  goserelin acetate (Zoladex) Z79.818
  hormone replacement Z79.890
▶ hydroxyurea Z79.64
▶ immunomodulators, unspecified Z79.60
▶ specified NEC Z79.69
▶ immunomodulatory imide drug Z79.61
▶ immunosuppressants, unspecified Z79.60
  ▶ specified NEC Z79.69
  immunosuppressive biologic Z79.620
▶ infliximab Z79.620
▶ inhibitors of nucleotide synthesis Z79.624
  insulin Z79.4
▶ irinotecan Z79.634
▶ Janus kinase inhibitor Z79.622
▶ lenalidomide Z79.61
  letrozole (Femara) Z79.811
  leuprolide acetate (leuprorelin) (Lupron)
    Z79.818
▶ mammalian target of rapamycin (mTOR)
    inhibitor Z79.623
  megestrol acetate (Megace) Z79.818
  methadone for pain management Z79.891
▶ mitomycin C Z79.632
▶ mitotic inhibitor Z79.633
▶ monoclonal antibodies Z79.620
▶ myelosuppressive agent Z79.64
  Nolvadex Z79.810
  non-insulin antidiabetic drug, injectable
    Z79.899
  non-steroidal anti-inflammatories (NSAID)
    Z79.1
▶ omycophenolate Z79.624
  opiate analgesic Z79.891
  oral
    antidiabetic Z79.84
    contraceptive Z79.3
    hypoglycemic Z79.84
▶ paclitaxel Z79.633
▶ plant alkaloids Z79.633
▶ pomalidomide Z79.61
▶ purine synthesis (IMDH) inhibitors
    Z79.624
  raloxifene (Evista) Z79.810
  selective estrogen receptor modulators
    (SERMs) Z79.810
▶ sirolimus Z79.623
  steroids
    inhaled Z79.51
    systemic Z79.52
▶ tacrolimus Z79.621

Long-term (Continued)
  tamoxifen (Nolvadex) Z79.810
▶ tofacitinib Z79.622
▶ topoisomerase inhibitor Z79.634
▶ topotecan Z79.634
  toremifene (Fareston) Z79.810
▶ vinblastine Z79.633
▶ vincristine Z79.633
Longitudinal stripes or grooves, nails L60.8
  congenital Q84.6
Loop
  intestine —see Volvulus
  vascular on papilla (optic) Q14.2
Loose —see also condition
  body
    joint M24.00
      ankle M24.07-•
      elbow M24.02-•
      hand M24.04-•
      hip M24.05-•
      knee M23.4-•
      shoulder (region) M24.01-•
      specified site NEC M24.08
      toe M24.07-•
      vertebra M24.08
      wrist M24.03-•
    knee M23.4-•
  sheath, tendon —see Disorder, tendon,
    specified type NEC
  cartilage —see Loose, body, joint
  skin and subcutaneous tissue (following
    bariatric surgery weight loss) (following
    dietary weight loss) L98.7
  tooth, teeth K08.89
Loosening
  aseptic
    joint prosthesis —see Complications, joint
      prosthesis, mechanical, loosening,
      by site
    epiphysis —see Osteochondropathy
  mechanical
    joint prosthesis —see Complications, joint
      prosthesis, mechanical, loosening,
      by site
Looser-Milkman (-Debray) syndrome M83.8
Lop ear (deformity) Q17.3
Lorain (-Levi) short stature syndrome E23.0
Lordosis M40.50
  acquired —see Lordosis, specified type NEC
  congenital Q76.429
    lumbar region Q76.426
    lumbosacral region Q76.427
    sacral region Q76.428
    sacrococcygeal region Q76.428
    thoracolumbar region Q76.425
  lumbar region M40.56
  lumbosacral region M40.57
  postsurgical M96.4
  postural —see Lordosis, specified type NEC
  rachitic (late effect) (sequelae) E64.3
  sequelae of rickets E64.3
  specified type NEC M40.40
    lumbar region M40.46
    lumbosacral region M40.47
    thoracolumbar region M40.45
  thoracolumbar region M40.55
  tuberculous A18.01
Loss (of)
  appetite (see Anorexia) R63.0
    hysterical F50.89
    nonorganic origin F50.89
    psychogenic F50.89
  blood —see Hemorrhage
  bone —see Loss, substance of, bone
  consciousness, transient R55
    traumatic —see Injury, intracranial
  control, sphincter, rectum R15.9
    nonorganic origin F98.1
  elasticity, skin R23.4
  family (member) in childhood Z62.898
  fluid (acute) E86.9
  function of labyrinth —see subcategory H83.2
  hair, nonscarring —see Alopecia

▶ New   ⇒ Revised   ~~deleted~~ Deleted   • Use Additional Character(s)

Loss *(Continued)*
  hearing —*see also* Deafness
    central NOS H90.5
    conductive H90.2
      bilateral H90.0
      unilateral
        with
          restricted hearing on the
            contralateral side H90.A1-•
          unrestricted hearing on the
            contralateral side H90.1-•
    mixed conductive and sensorineural
        hearing loss H90.8
      bilateral H90.6
      unilateral
        with
          restricted hearing on the
            contralateral side H90.A3-•
          unrestricted hearing on the
            contralateral side H90.7-•
    neural NOS H90.5
    perceptive NOS H90.5
    sensorineural NOS H90.5
      bilateral H90.3
      unilateral
        with
          restricted hearing on the
            contralateral side H90.A2-•
          unrestricted hearing on the
            contralateral side H90.4-•
    sensory NOS H90.5
  height R29.890
  limb or member, traumatic, current —*see*
    Amputation, traumatic
  love relationship in childhood Z62.898
  memory —*see also* Amnesia
    mild, following organic brain damage F06.8
  mind —*see* Psychosis
  occlusal vertical dimension of fully erupted
    teeth M26.37
  organ or part —*see* Absence, by site, acquired
  ossicles, ear (partial) H74.32-•
  parent in childhood Z63.4
  pregnancy, recurrent N96
    without current pregnancy N96
    care in current pregnancy O26.2-•
  recurrent pregnancy —*see* Loss, pregnancy,
    recurrent
  self-esteem, in childhood Z62.898
  sense of
    smell —*see* Disturbance, sensation, smell
    taste —*see* Disturbance, sensation, taste
    touch R20.8
  sensory R44.9
    dissociative F44.6
  sexual desire F52.0
  sight (acquired) (complete) (congenital) —*see*
    Blindness
  substance of
    bone —*see* Disorder, bone, density and
      structure, specified NEC
      horizontal alveolar K06.3
    cartilage —*see* Disorder, cartilage, specified
      type NEC
      auricle (ear) —*see* Disorder, pinna,
        specified type NEC
    vitreous (humor) H15.89
  tooth, teeth —*see* Absence, teeth, acquired
  vision, visual H54.7
    both eyes H54.3
    one eye H54.60
      left (normal vision on right) H54.62
      right (normal vision on left) H54.61
    specified as blindness —*see* Blindness
    subjective
      sudden H53.13-•
      transient H53.12-•
  vitreous —*see* Prolapse, vitreous
  voice —*see* Aphonia
  weight (abnormal) (cause unknown) R63.4
Louis-Bar syndrome (ataxia-telangiectasia)
  G11.3

Louping ill (encephalitis) A84.89
Louse, lousiness —*see* Lice
Low
  achiever, school Z55.3
  back syndrome M54.50
  basal metabolic rate R94.8
  birthweight (2499 grams or less) P07.10
    with weight of
      1000-1249 grams P07.14
      1250-1499 grams P07.15
      1500-1749 grams P07.16
      1750-1999 grams P07.17
      2000-2499 grams P07.18
    extreme (999 grams or less) P07.00
      with weight of
        499 grams or less P07.01
        500-749 grams P07.02
        750-999 grams P07.03
    for gestational age —*see* Light for dates
  blood pressure —*see also* Hypotension
    reading (incidental) (isolated) (nonspecific)
      R03.1
  cardiac reserve —*see* Disease, heart
  function —*see also* Hypofunction
    kidney N28.9
  hematocrit D64.9
  hemoglobin D64.9
  income Z59.6
  level of literacy Z55.0
  lying
    kidney N28.89
    organ or site, congenital —*see* Malposition,
      congenital
  output syndrome (cardiac) —*see* Failure,
    heart
  platelets (blood) —*see* Thrombocytopenia
  reserve, kidney N28.89
  salt syndrome E87.1
  self esteem R45.81
  set ears Q17.4
  vision H54.2X-
    one eye (other eye normal) H54.50
      left (normal vision on right)
        H54.52A-
      other eye blind —*see* Blindness
      right (normal vision on left) H54.511-
▶von Willebrand factor R79.1
Low-density-lipoprotein-type (LDL)
  hyperlipoproteinemia E78.00
Lowe's syndrome E72.03
Lown-Ganong-Levine syndrome I45.6
LSD reaction (acute) (without dependence)
  F16.90
  with dependence F16.20
L-shaped kidney Q63.8
LTBI (lantent tuberculosis infection) Z22.7
Ludwig's angina or disease K12.2
Lues (venerea), luetic —*see* Syphilis
Luetscher's syndrome (dehydration) E86.0
Lumbago, lumbalgia M54.50
  with sciatica M54.4-•
    due to intervertebral disc disorder
      M51.17
  due to displacement, intervertebral disc
    M51.27
    with sciatica M51.17
Lumbar —*see* condition
Lumbarization, vertebra, congenital Q76.49
Lumbermen's itch B88.0
Lump —*see also* Mass
  breast N63.0
    axillary tail
      left N63.32
      right N63.31
    left
      lower inner quadrant N63.24
      lower outer quadrant N63.23
      overlapping quadrants N63.25
      unspecified quadrant N63.20
      upper inner quadrant N63.22
      upper outer quadrant N63.21

Lump *(Continued)*
  breast *(Continued)*
    right
      lower inner quadrant N63.14
      lower outer quadrant N63.13
      overlapping quadrants N63.15
      unspecified quadrant N63.10
      upper inner quadrant N63.12
      upper outer quadrant N63.11
    subareolar
      left N63.42
      right N63.41
Lunacy —*see* Psychosis
Lung —*see* condition
Lupoid (miliary) of Boeck D86.3
Lupus
  anticoagulant D68.62
    with
      hemorrhagic disorder D68.312
      hypercoagulable state D68.62
    finding without diagnosis R76.0
  discoid (local) L93.0
  erythematosus (discoid) (local) L93.0
    disseminated —*see* Lupus, erythematosus,
      systemic
    eyelid H01.129
      left H01.126
        lower H01.125
        upper H01.124
      right H01.123
        lower H01.122
        upper H01.121
    profundus L93.2
    specified NEC L93.2
    subacute cutaneous L93.1
    systemic M32.9
      with organ or system involvement
        M32.10
        endocarditis M32.11
        lung M32.13
        pericarditis M32.12
        renal (glomerular) M32.14
          tubulo-interstitial M32.15
        specified organ or system NEC
          M32.19
      drug-induced M32.0
      inhibitor (presence of) D68.62
        with
          hemorrhagic disorder D68.312
          hypercoagulable state D68.62
        finding without diagnosis R76.0
      specified NEC M32.8
  exedens A18.4
  hydralazine M32.0
    correct substance properly administered —
      see Table of Drugs and Chemicals, by
      drug, adverse effect
    overdose or wrong substance given
      or taken —*see* Table of Drugs and
      Chemicals, by drug, poisoning
  nephritis (chronic) M32.14
  nontuberculous, not disseminated L93.0
  panniculitis L93.2
  pernio (Besnier) D86.3
  systemic —*see* Lupus, erythematosus,
    systemic
  tuberculous A18.4
    eyelid A18.4
  vulgaris A18.4
    eyelid A18.4
Luteinoma D27.-•
▶Lutembacher's disease or syndrome (atrial
  septal defect with mitral stenosis)
  Q21.19
Luteoma D27.-•
Lutz (-Splendore-de Almeida) disease —*see*
  Paracoccidioidomycosis
Luxation —*see also* Dislocation
  eyeball (nontraumatic) —*see* Luxation, globe
    birth injury P15.3
  globe, nontraumatic H44.82-•

Luxation (Continued)
  lacrimal gland —see Dislocation, lacrimal
    gland
  lens (old) (partial) (spontaneous)
    congenital Q12.1
    syphilitic A50.39
Lycanthropy F22
Lyell's syndrome L51.2
  due to drug L51.2
    correct substance properly administered —
      see Table of Drugs and Chemicals, by
      drug, adverse effect
    overdose or wrong substance given
      or taken —see Table of Drugs and
      Chemicals, by drug, poisoning
Lyme disease A69.20
Lymph
  gland or node —see condition
  scrotum —see Infestation, filarial
Lymphadenitis I88.9
  with ectopic or molar pregnancy O08.0
  acute L04.9
    axilla L04.2
    face L04.0
    head L04.0
    hip L04.3
    limb
      lower L04.3
      upper L04.2
    neck L04.0
    shoulder L04.2
    specified site NEC L04.8
    trunk L04.1
  anthracosis (occupational) J60
  any site, except mesenteric I88.9
    chronic I88.1
    subacute I88.1
  breast
    gestational —see Mastitis, obstetric
    puerperal, postpartum (nonpurulent) O91.22
  chancroidal (congenital) A57
  chronic I88.1
    mesenteric I88.0
  due to
    Brugia (malayi) B74.1
      timori B74.2
    chlamydial lymphogranuloma A55
    diphtheria (toxin) A36.89
    lymphogranuloma venereum A55
    Wuchereria bancrofti B74.0
  following ectopic or molar pregnancy O08.0
  gonorrheal A54.89
  infective —see Lymphadenitis, acute
  mesenteric (acute) (chronic) (nonspecific)
    (subacute) I88.0
    due to Salmonella typhi A01.09
    tuberculous A18.39
  mycobacterial A31.8
  purulent —see Lymphadenitis, acute
  pyogenic —see Lymphadenitis, acute
  regional, nonbacterial I88.8
  septic —see Lymphadenitis, acute
  subacute, unspecified site I88.1
  suppurative —see Lymphadenitis, acute
  syphilitic (early) (secondary) A51.49
    late A52.79
  tuberculous —see Tuberculosis, lymph gland
  venereal (chlamydial) A55
Lymphadenoid goiter E06.3
Lymphadenopathy (generalized) R59.1
  angioimmunoblastic, with dysproteinemia
    (AILD) C86.5
  due to toxoplasmosis (acquired) B58.89
    congenital (acute) (subacute) (chronic) P37.1
  localized R59.0
  syphilitic (early) (secondary) A51.49
Lymphadenosis R59.1
Lymphangiectasis I89.0
  conjunctiva H11.89
  postinfectional I89.0
  scrotum I89.0

Lymphangiectatic elephantiasis, nonfilarial I89.0
Lymphangioendothelioma D18.1
  malignant —see Neoplasm, connective tissue,
    malignant
Lymphangioleiomyomatosis J84.81
Lymphangioma D18.1
  capillary D18.1
  cavernous D18.1
  cystic D18.1
  malignant —see Neoplasm, connective tissue,
    malignant
Lymphangiomyoma D18.1
Lymphangiomyomatosis J84.81
Lymphangiosarcoma —see Neoplasm,
  connective tissue, malignant
Lymphangitis I89.1
  with
    abscess - code by site under Abscess
    cellulitis - code by site under Cellulitis
    ectopic or molar pregnancy O08.0
  acute L03.91
    abdominal wall L03.321
    ankle —see Lymphangitis, acute, lower
      limb
    arm —see Lymphangitis, acute, upper limb
    auricle (ear) —see Lymphangitis, acute, ear
    axilla L03.12-●
    back (any part) L03.322
    buttock L03.327
    cervical (meaning neck) L03.222
    cheek (external) L03.212
    chest wall L03.323
    digit
      finger —see Lymphangitis, acute, finger
      toe —see Lymphangitis, acute, toe
    ear (external) H60.1-●
    external auditory canal —see
      Lymphangitis, acute, ear
    eyelid —see Abscess, eyelid
    face NEC L03.212
    finger (intrathecal) (periosteal)
      (subcutaneous) (subcuticular)
      L03.02-●
    foot —see Lymphangitis, acute, lower limb
    gluteal (region) L03.327
    groin L03.324
    hand —see Lymphangitis, acute, upper
      limb
    head NEC L03.891
      face (any part, except ear, eye and nose)
        L03.212
    heel —see Lymphangitis, acute, lower limb
    hip —see Lymphangitis, acute, lower limb
    jaw (region) L03.212
    knee —see Lymphangitis, acute, lower limb
    leg —see Lymphangitis, acute, lower limb
    lower limb L03.12-●
      toe —see Lymphangitis, acute, toe
    navel L03.326
    neck (region) L03.222
    orbit, orbital —see Cellulitis, orbit
    pectoral (region) L03.323
    perineal, perineum L03.325
    scalp (any part) L03.891
    shoulder —see Lymphangitis, acute, upper
      limb
    specified site NEC L03.898
    thigh —see Lymphangitis, acute, lower limb
    thumb (intrathecal) (periosteal)
      (subcutaneous) (subcuticular) —see
      Lymphangitis, acute, finger
    toe (intrathecal) (periosteal) (subcutaneous)
      (subcuticular) L03.04-●
    trunk L03.329
      abdominal wall L03.321
      back (any part) L03.322
      buttock L03.327
      chest wall L03.323
      groin L03.324
      perineal, perineum L03.325
      umbilicus L03.326

Lymphangitis (Continued)
  with (Continued)
    umbilicus L03.326
    upper limb L03.12-●
      axilla —see Lymphangitis, acute, axilla
      finger —see Lymphangitis, acute, finger
      thumb —see Lymphangitis, acute, finger
      wrist —see Lymphangitis, acute, upper
        limb
  breast
    gestational —see Mastitis, obstetric
  chancroidal A57
  chronic (any site) I89.1
  due to
    Brugia (malayi) B74.1
      timori B74.2
    Wuchereria bancrofti B74.0
  following ectopic or molar pregnancy
    O08.89
  penis
    acute N48.29
    gonococcal (acute) (chronic) A54.09
  puerperal, postpartum, childbirth O86.89
  strumous, tuberculous A18.2
  subacute (any site) I89.1
  tuberculous —see Tuberculosis, lymph gland
Lymphatic (vessel) —see condition
Lymphatism E32.8
Lymphectasia I89.0
Lymphedema (acquired) —see also Elephantiasis
  congenital Q82.0
  hereditary (chronic) (idiopathic) Q82.0
  postmastectomy I97.2
  praecox I89.0
  secondary I89.0
  surgical NEC I97.89
    postmastectomy (syndrome) I97.2
Lymphoblastic —see condition
Lymphoblastoma (diffuse) —see Lymphoma,
  lymphoblastic (diffuse)
  giant follicular —see Lymphoma,
    lymphoblastic (diffuse)
  macrofollicular —see Lymphoma,
    lymphoblastic (diffuse)
Lymphocele I89.8
Lymphocytic
  chorioencephalitis (acute) (serous) A87.2
  choriomeningitis (acute) (serous) A87.2
  meningoencephalitis A87.2
Lymphocytoma, benign cutis L98.8
Lymphocytopenia D72.810
Lymphocytosis (symptomatic) D72.820
  infectious (acute) B33.8
Lymphoepithelioma —see Neoplasm,
  malignant, by site
Lymphogranuloma (malignant) —see also
  Lymphoma, Hodgkin
  chlamydial A55
  inguinale A55
  venereum (any site) (chlamydial) (with
    stricture of rectum) A55
Lymphogranulomatosis (malignant) —see also
  Lymphoma, Hodgkin
  benign (Boeck's sarcoid) (Schaumann's)
    D86.1
Lymphohistiocytosis, hemophagocytic
  (familial) D76.1
Lymphoid —see condition
Lymphoma (of) (malignant) C85.90
  adult T-cell (HTLV-1-associated) (acute
    variant) (chronic variant)
    (lymphomatoid variant) (smouldering
    variant) C91.5-●
  anaplastic large cell
    ALK-negative C84.7-●
    ALK-positive C84.6-●
    breast implant associated (BIA-ALCL)
      C84.7A
    CD30-positive C84.6-●
    primary cutaneous C86.6
  angioimmunoblastic T-cell C86.5

▶ New   ⇒ Revised   ~~deleted~~ Deleted   ● Use Additional Character(s)

Lymphoma *(Continued)*
  BALT C88.4
  B-cell C85.1-•
  B-precursor C83.5-•
  blastic NK-cell C86.4
  blastic plasmacytoid dendritic cell neoplasm
    (BPDCN) C86.4
  bronchial-associated lymphoid tissue
    [BALT-lymphoma] C88.4
  Burkitt (atypical) C83.7-•
  Burkitt-like C83.7-•
  centrocytic C83.1-•
  cutaneous follicle center C82.6-•
  cutaneous T-cell C84.A-•
  diffuse follicle center C82.5-•
  diffuse large cell C83.3-•
    anaplastic C83.3-•
    B-cell C83.3-•
    CD30-positive C83.3-•
    centroblastic C83.3-•
    immunoblastic C83.3-•
    plasmablastic C83.3-•
    subtype not specified C83.3-•
    T-cell rich C83.3-•
  enteropathy-type (associated) (intestinal)
    T-cell C86.2
  extranodal marginal zone B-cell lymphoma
    of mucosa-associated lymphoid tissue
    [MALT-lymphoma] C88.4
  extranodal NK/T-cell, nasal type C86.0
  follicular C82.9-•
    grade
      I C82.0-•
      II C82.1-•
      III C82.2-•
      IIIa C82.3-•
      IIIb C82.4-•
    specified NEC C82.8-•

Lymphoma *(Continued)*
  hepatosplenic T-cell (alpha-beta) (gamma-
    delta) C86.1
  histiocytic C85.9-•
    true C96.A
  Hodgkin C81.9
    lymphocyte-rich (classical) C81.4-•
    lymphocyte depleted (classical) C81.3-•
    mixed cellularity (classical) C81.2-•
    nodular sclerosis (classical) C81.1-•
    specified NEC (classical) C81.7-•
    lymphocyte-rich classical C81.4-•
    lymphocyte depleted classical C81.3-•
    mixed cellularity classical C81.2-•
    nodular
      lymphocyte predominant C81.0-•
      sclerosis (classical) C81.1-•
  intravascular large B-cell C83.8-•
  Lennert's C84.4-•
  lymphoblastic (diffuse) C83.5-•
  lymphoblastic B-cell C83.5-•
  lymphoblastic T-cell C83.5-•
  lymphoepithelioid C84.4-•
  lymphoplasmacytic C83.0-•
    with IgM-production C88.0
  MALT C88.4
  mantle cell C83.1-•
  mature T-cell NEC C84.4-•
  mature T/NK-cell C84.9-•
    specified NEC C84.Z-•
  mediastinal (thymic) large B-cell C85.2-•
  Mediterranean C88.3
  mucosa-associated lymphoid tissue
    [MALT-lymphoma] C88.4
  NK/T cell C84.9-•
  nodal marginal zone C83.0-•
  non-follicular (diffuse) C83.9-•
    specified NEC C83.8-•

Lymphoma *(Continued)*
  non-Hodgkin —*see also* Lymphoma, by type
    C85.9-•
    specified NEC C85.8-•
  non-leukemic variant of B-CLL C83.0-•
  ~~peripheral T-cell, not classified C84.4-~~•
  ▶peripheral T-cell NEC C84.4-•
  primary cutaneous
    anaplastic large cell C86.6
    CD30-positive large T-cell C86.6
  primary effusion B-cell C83.8-•
  SALT C88.4
  skin-associated lymphoid tissue
    [SALT-lymphoma] C88.4
  small cell B-cell C83.0-•
  splenic marginal zone C83.0-•
  subcutaneous panniculitis-like T-cell
    C86.3
  T-precursor C83.5-•
  true histiocytic C96.A
Lymphomatosis —*see* Lymphoma
Lymphopathia venereum, veneris A55
Lymphopenia D72.810
Lymphoplasmacytic leukemia —*see* Leukemia,
  chronic lymphocytic, B-cell type
Lymphoproliferation, X-linked disease D82.3
Lymphoreticulosis, benign (of inoculation)
  A28.1
Lymphorrhea I89.8
Lymphosarcoma (diffuse) —*see also* Lymphoma
  C85.9-•
Lymphostasis I89.8
Lypemania —*see* Melancholia
Lysine and hydroxylysine metabolism
  disorder E72.3
Lyssa —*see* Rabies

M

Macacus ear Q17.3
Maceration, wet feet, tropical (syndrome)
T69.02-●
MacLeod's syndrome J43.0
Macrocephalia, macrocephaly Q75.3
Macrocheilia, macrochilia (congenital)Q18.6
Macrocolon —see also Megacolon Q43.1
Macrocornea Q15.8
  with glaucoma Q15.0
Macrocytic —see condition
Macrocytosis D75.89
Macrodactylia, macrodactylism (fingers)
  (thumbs) Q74.0
  toes Q74.2
Macrodontia K00.2
Macrogenia M26.05
Macrogenitosomia (adrenal) (male) (praecox)
  E25.9
  congenital E25.0
Macroglobulinemia (idiopathic) (primary)
  C88.0
  monoclonal (essential) D47.2
  Waldenström C88.0
Macroglossia (congenital) Q38.2
  acquired K14.8
Macrognathia, macrognathism (congenital)
  (mandibular) (maxillary) M26.09
Macrogyria (congenital) Q04.8
Macrohydrocephalus —see Hydrocephalus
Macromastia —see Hypertrophy, breast
Macrophthalmos Q11.3
  in congenital glaucoma Q15.0
Macropsia H53.15
Macrosigmoid K59.39
  congenital Q43.2
Macrospondylitis, acromegalic E22.0
Macrostomia (congenital) Q18.4
Macrotia (external ear) (congenital) Q17.1
Macula
  cornea, corneal —see Opacity, cornea
  degeneration (atrophic) (exudative)
    (senile) —see also Degeneration, macula
  hereditary —see Dystrophy, retina
Maculae ceruleae — B85.1
Maculopathy, toxic —see Degeneration, macula,
  toxic
Madarosis (eyelid) H02.729
  left H02.726
    lower H02.725
    upper H02.724
  right H02.723
    lower H02.722
    upper H02.721
Madelung's
  deformity (radius) Q74.0
  disease
    radial deformity Q74.0
    symmetrical lipomas, neck E88.89
Madness —see Psychosis
Madura
  foot B47.9
    actinomycotic B47.1
    mycotic B47.0
Maduromycosis B47.0
Maffucci's syndrome Q78.4
Magnesium metabolism disorder —see
  Disorder, metabolism, magnesium
Main en griffe (acquired) —see also Deformity,
  limb, clawhand
▦congenital Q68.1
Maintenance (encounter for)
  antineoplastic chemotherapy Z51.11
  antineoplastic radiation therapy Z51.0
  methadone F11.20
Majocchi's
  disease L81.7
  granuloma B35.8
Major —see condition
Malabar itch (any site) B35.5

Malabsorption K90.9
  calcium K90.89
  carbohydrate K90.49
  disaccharide E73.9
  fat K90.49
  galactose E74.20
  glucose(-galactose) E74.39
  intestinal K90.9
    specified NEC K90.89
  isomaltose E74.31
  lactose E73.9
  methionine E72.19
  monosaccharide E74.39
  postgastrectomy K91.2
  postsurgical K91.2
  protein K90.49
  starch K90.49
  sucrose E74.39
  syndrome K90.9
    postsurgical K91.2
Malacia, bone (adult) M83.9
  juvenile —see Rickets
Malacoplakia
  bladder N32.89
  pelvis (kidney) N28.89
  ureter N28.89
  urethra N36.8
Malacosteon, juvenile —see Rickets
Maladaptation —see Maladjustment
Maladie de Roger Q21.0
Maladjustment
  conjugal Z63.0
    involving divorce or estrangement Z63.5
  educational Z55.4
  family Z63.9
  marital Z63.0
    involving divorce or estrangement Z63.5
  occupational NEC Z56.89
  simple, adult —see Disorder, adjustment
  situational —see Disorder, adjustment
  social Z60.9
    due to
      acculturation difficulty Z60.3
      discrimination and persecution
        (perceived) Z60.5
      exclusion and isolation Z60.4
      life-cycle (phase of life) transition Z60.0
      rejection Z60.4
      specified reason NEC Z60.8
Malaise R53.81
Malakoplakia —see Malacoplakia
Malaria, malarial (fever) B54
  with
    blackwater fever B50.8
      hemoglobinuric (bilious) B50.8
    hemoglobinuria B50.8
  accidentally induced (therapeutically) - code
    by type under Malaria
  algid B50.9
  cerebral B50.0 [G94]
  clinically diagnosed (without parasitological
    confirmation) B54
  congenital NEC P37.4
    falciparum P37.3
  congestion, congestive B54
  continued (fever) B50.9
  estivo-autumnal B50.9
  falciparum B50.9
    with complications NEC B50.8
      cerebral B50.0 [G94]
    severe B50.8
  hemorrhagic B54
  malariae B52.9
    with
      complications NEC B52.8
      glomerular disorder B52.0
  malignant (tertian) —see Malaria, falciparum
  mixed infections — code to first listed type
    in B50-B53
  ovale B53.0
  parasitologically confirmed NEC B53.8

Malaria, malarial (Continued)
  pernicious, acute —see Malaria, falciparum
  Plasmodium (P.)
    falciparum NEC —see Malaria, falciparum
    malariae NEC B52.9
      with Plasmodium
        falciparum (and or vivax) —see
          Malaria, falciparum
        vivax —see also Malaria, vivax
          and falciparum —see Malaria,
            falciparum
    ovale B53.0
      with Plasmodium malariae —see also
        Malaria, malariae
      and vivax —see also Malaria, vivax
        and falciparum —see Malaria,
          falciparum
    simian B53.1
      with Plasmodium malariae —see also
        Malaria, malariae
      and vivax —see also Malaria, vivax
        and falciparum —see Malaria,
          falciparum
    vivax NEC B51.9
      with Plasmodium falciparum —see
        Malaria, falciparum
  quartan —see Malaria, malariae
  quotidian —see Malaria, falciparum
  recurrent B54
  remittent B54
  specified type NEC (parasitologically
    confirmed) B53.8
  spleen B54
  subtertian (fever) —see Malaria, falciparum
  tertian (benign) —see also Malaria, vivax
    malignant B50.9
  tropical B50.9
  typhoid B54
  vivax B51.9
    with
      complications NEC B51.8
      ruptured spleen B51.0
Malassez's disease (cystic) N50.89
Malassimilation K90.9
Mal de los pintos —see Pinta
Mal de mer T75.3
Maldescent, testis Q53.9
  bilateral Q53.20
    abdominal Q53.211
    perineal Q53.22
  unilateral Q53.10
    abdominal Q53.111
    perineal Q53.12
Maldevelopment —see also Anomaly
  brain Q07.9
  colon Q43.9
  hip Q74.2
    congenital dislocation Q65.2
      bilateral Q65.1
      unilateral Q65.0-●
  mastoid process Q75.8
  middle ear Q16.4
    except ossicles Q16.4
    ossicles Q16.3
  ossicles Q16.3
  spine Q76.49
  toe Q74.2
Male type pelvis Q74.2
  with disproportion (fetopelvic) O33.3
    causing obstructed labor O65.3
Malformation (congenital) —see also Anomaly
  adrenal gland Q89.1
  affecting multiple systems with skeletal
    changes NEC Q87.5
  alimentary tract Q45.9
    specified type NEC Q45.8
    upper Q40.9
      specified type NEC Q40.8
  aorta Q25.40
    absence Q25.41
    aneurysm, congenital Q25.43

▶ New   ⇒ Revised   ~~deleted~~ Deleted   ● Use Additional Character(s)

Malformation *(Continued)*
  aorta *(Continued)*
    aplasia Q25.41
    atresia Q25.29
      aortic arch Q25.21
    coarctation (preductal) (postductal) Q25.1
    dilatation, congenital Q25.44
    hypoplasia Q25.42
    patent ductus arteriosus Q25.0
    specified type NEC Q25.49
    stenosis Q25.1
      supravalvular Q25.3
  aortic valve Q23.9
    specified NEC Q23.8
  arteriovenous, aneurysmatic (congenital) Q27.30
    brain Q28.2
      ruptured I60.8
        intracerebral I61.8
        intraparenchymal I61.8
        intraventricular I61.5
        subarachnoid I60.8
    cerebral *(see* Malformation, arteriovenous, brain) Q28.2
    peripheral Q27.30
      congenital Q27.33
      digestive system —*see* Angiodysplasia
      lower limb Q27.32
      other specified site Q27.39
      renal vessel Q27.34
      upper limb Q27.31
    precerebral vessels (nonruptured) Q28.0
  auricle
    ear (congenital) Q17.3
      acquired H61.119
        left H61.112
          with right H61.113
        right H61.111
          with left H61.113
  bile duct Q44.5
  bladder Q64.79
    aplasia Q64.5
    diverticulum Q64.6
    exstrophy —*see* Exstrophy, bladder
    neck obstruction Q64.31
  bone Q79.9
    face Q75.9
      specified type NEC Q75.8
    skull Q75.9
      specified type NEC Q75.8
  brain (multiple) Q04.9
    arteriovenous Q28.2
    specified type NEC Q04.8
  branchial cleft Q18.2
  breast Q83.9
    specified type NEC Q83.8
  broad ligament Q50.6
  bronchus Q32.4
  bursa Q79.9
  cardiac
    chambers Q20.9
      specified type NEC Q20.8
    septum Q21.9
      specified type NEC Q21.8
  cerebral Q04.9
    vessels Q28.3
  cervix uteri Q51.9
    specified type NEC Q51.828
  Chiari
    Type I G93.5
    Type II Q07.01
  choroid (congenital) Q14.3
    plexus Q07.8
  circulatory system Q28.9
  cochlea Q16.5
  cornea Q13.4
  coronary vessels Q24.5
  corpus callosum (congenital) Q04.0
  diaphragm Q79.1
  digestive system NEC, specified type NEC Q45.8

Malformation *(Continued)*
  dura Q07.9
    brain Q04.9
    spinal Q06.9
  ear Q17.9
    causing impairment of hearing Q16.9
    external Q17.9
      accessory auricle Q17.0
      causing impairment of hearing Q16.9
        absence of
          auditory canal Q16.1
          auricle Q16.0
      macrotia Q17.1
      microtia Q17.2
      misplacement Q17.4
      misshapen NEC Q17.3
      prominence Q17.5
      specified type NEC Q17.8
    inner Q16.5
    middle Q16.4
      absence of eustachian tube Q16.2
      ossicles (fusion) Q16.3
    ossicles Q16.3
    specified type NEC Q17.8
  epididymis Q55.4
  esophagus Q39.9
    specified type NEC Q39.8
  eye Q15.9
    lid Q10.3
    specified NEC Q15.8
  fallopian tube Q50.6
  genital organ —*see* Anomaly, genitalia
  great
    artery Q25.9
      aorta —*see* Malformation, aorta
      pulmonary artery —*see* Malformation, pulmonary, artery
      specified type NEC Q25.8
    vein Q26.9
      anomalous
        portal venous connection Q26.5
        pulmonary venous connection Q26.4
          partial Q26.3
          total Q26.2
      persistent left superior vena cava Q26.1
      portal vein-hepatic artery fistula Q26.6
      specified type NEC Q26.8
      vena cava stenosis, congenital Q26.0
  gum Q38.6
  hair Q84.2
  heart Q24.9
    specified type NEC Q24.8
  integument Q84.9
    specified type NEC Q84.8
  internal ear Q16.5
  intestine Q43.9
    specified type NEC Q43.8
  iris Q13.2
  joint Q74.9
    ankle Q74.2
    lumbosacral Q76.49
    sacroiliac Q74.2
    specified type NEC Q74.8
  kidney Q63.9
    accessory Q63.0
    giant Q63.3
    horseshoe Q63.1
    hydronephrosis Q62.0
    malposition Q63.2
    specified type NEC Q63.8
  lacrimal apparatus Q10.6
  lingual Q38.3
  lip Q38.0
  liver Q44.7
  lung Q33.9
  meninges or membrane (congenital) Q07.9
    cerebral Q04.8
    spinal (cord) Q06.9
  middle ear Q16.4
    ossicles Q16.3
  mitral valve Q23.9
    specified NEC Q23.8

Malformation *(Continued)*
  Mondini's (congenital) (malformation, cochlea) Q16.5
  mouth (congenital) Q38.6
  multiple types NEC Q89.7
  musculoskeletal system Q79.9
  myocardium Q24.8
  nail Q84.6
  nervous system (central) Q07.9
  nose Q30.9
    specified type NEC Q30.8
  optic disc Q14.2
  orbit Q10.7
  ovary Q50.39
  palate Q38.5
  parathyroid gland Q89.2
  pelvic organs or tissues NEC
    in pregnancy or childbirth O34.8-●
      causing obstructed labor O65.5
  penis Q55.69
    aplasia Q55.5
    curvature (lateral) Q55.61
    hypoplasia Q55.62
  pericardium Q24.8
  peripheral vascular system Q27.9
    specified type NEC Q27.8
  pharynx Q38.8
  precerebral vessels Q28.1
  prostate Q55.4
  pulmonary
    arteriovenous Q25.72
    artery Q25.9
      atresia Q25.5
      specified type NEC Q25.79
      stenosis Q25.6
    valve Q22.3
  renal artery Q27.2
  respiratory system Q34.9
  retina Q14.1
  scrotum —*see* Malformation, testis and scrotum
  seminal vesicles Q55.4
  sense organs NEC Q07.9
  skin Q82.9
  specified NEC Q89.8
  spinal
    cord Q06.9
    nerve root Q07.8
  spine Q76.49
    kyphosis —*see* Kyphosis, congenital
    lordosis —*see* Lordosis, congenital
  spleen Q89.09
  stomach Q40.3
    specified type NEC Q40.2
  teeth, tooth K00.9
  tendon Q79.9
  testis and scrotum Q55.20
    aplasia Q55.0
    hypoplasia Q55.1
    polyorchism Q55.21
    retractile testis Q55.22
    scrotal transposition Q55.23
    specified NEC Q55.29
  thorax, bony Q76.9
  throat Q38.8
  thyroid gland Q89.2
  tongue (congenital) Q38.3
    hypertrophy Q38.2
    tie Q38.1
  trachea Q32.1
  tricuspid valve Q22.9
    specified type NEC Q22.8
  umbilical cord NEC (complicating delivery) O69.89
  umbilicus Q89.9
  ureter Q62.8
    agenesis Q62.4
    duplication Q62.5
    malposition —*see* Malposition, congenital, ureter
    obstructive defect —*see* Defect, obstructive, ureter
    vesico-uretero-renal reflux Q62.7

Malformation *(Continued)*
    urethra Q64.79
      aplasia Q64.5
      duplication Q64.74
      posterior valves Q64.2
      prolapse Q64.71
      stricture Q64.32
    urinary system Q64.9
    uterus Q51.9
      specified type NEC Q51.818
    vagina Q52.4
    vascular system, peripheral Q27.9
    vas deferens Q55.4
      atresia Q55.3
    venous —*see* Anomaly, vein(s)
    vulva Q52.70
Malfunction —*see also* Dysfunction
    cardiac electronic device T82.119
      electrode T82.110
      pulse generator T82.111
      specified type NEC T82.118
    catheter device NEC T85.618
      cystostomy T83.010
      dialysis (renal) (vascular) T82.41
        intraperitoneal T85.611
      infusion NEC T82.514
        cranial T85.610
        epidural T85.610
        intrathecal T85.610
        spinal T85.610
        subarachnoid T85.610
        subdural T85.610
      urinary —*see also* Breakdown, device,
        catheter T83.018
    colostomy K94.03
      valve K94.03
    cystostomy (stoma) N99.512
      catheter T83.010
    enteric stoma K94.13
    enterostomy K94.13
    esophagostomy K94.33
    gastroenteric K31.89
    gastrostomy K94.23
    ileostomy K94.13
      valve K94.13
    intrathecal infusion pump T85.615
    jejunostomy K94.13
    nervous system device, implant or graft,
      specified NEC T85.615
    pacemaker —*see* Malfunction, cardiac
      electronic device
    prosthetic device, internal —*see*
      Complications, prosthetic device, by site,
      mechanical
    tracheostomy J95.03
    urinary device NEC —*see* Complication,
      genitourinary, device, urinary,
      mechanical
    valve
      colostomy K94.03
      heart T82.09
      ileostomy K94.13
    vascular graft or shunt NEC —*see*
      Complication, cardiovascular device,
      mechanical, vascular
    ventricular (communicating shunt) T85.01
Malherbe's tumor —*see* Neoplasm, skin,
    benign
Malibu disease L98.8-●
Malignancy —*see also* Neoplasm, malignant,
    by site
    unspecified site (primary) C80.1
Malignant —*see* condition
Malingerer, malingering Z76.5
Mallet finger (acquired) —*see* Deformity, finger,
    mallet finger
    congenital Q74.0
    sequelae of rickets E64.3
Malleus A24.0
Mallory's bodies R89.7
Mallory-Weiss syndrome K22.6

Malnutrition E46
    degree
      first E44.1
      mild (protein) E44.1
      moderate (protein) E44.0
      second E44.0
      severe (protein-energy) E43
        intermediate form E42
          with
          ➠kwashiorkor E42
            marasmus E41
      third E43
    following gastrointestinal surgery K91.2
    intrauterine
      light-for-dates —*see* Light for dates
      small-for-dates —*see* Small for dates
    lack of care, or neglect (child) (infant) T76.02
      confirmed T74.02
    malignant E40
    protein E46
      calorie E46
        mild E44.1
        moderate E44.0
        severe E43
          intermediate form E42
            with
              kwashiorkor (and marasmus)
                E42
              marasmus E41
      energy E46
        mild E44.1
        moderate E44.0
        severe E43
          intermediate form E42
            with
              kwashiorkor (and marasmus)
                E42
              marasmus E41
    severe (protein-energy) E43
      with
        kwashiorkor (and marasmus) E42
        marasmus E41
Malocclusion (teeth) M26.4
    Angle's M26.219
      class I M26.211
      class II M26.212
      class III M26.213
    due to
      abnormal swallowing M26.59
      mouth breathing M26.59
      tongue, lip or finger habits M26.59
    temporomandibular (joint) M26.69
Malposition
    cervix —*see* Malposition, uterus
    congenital
      adrenal (gland) Q89.1
      alimentary tract Q45.8
        lower Q43.8
        upper Q40.8
      aorta Q25.49
      appendix Q43.8
      arterial trunk Q20.0
      artery (peripheral) Q27.8
        coronary Q24.5
        digestive system Q27.8
        lower limb Q27.8
        pulmonary Q25.79
        specified site NEC Q27.8
        upper limb Q27.8
      auditory canal Q17.8
        causing impairment of hearing Q16.9
      auricle (ear) Q17.4
        causing impairment of hearing Q16.9
      cervical Q18.2
      biliary duct or passage Q44.5
      bladder (mucosa) —*see* Exstrophy,
        bladder
      brachial plexus Q07.8
      brain tissue Q04.8
      breast Q83.8
      bronchus Q32.4

Malposition *(Continued)*
    congenital *(Continued)*
      cecum Q43.8
      clavicle Q74.0
      colon Q43.8
      digestive organ or tract NEC Q45.8
        lower Q43.8
        upper Q40.8
      ear (auricle) (external) Q17.4
        ossicles Q16.3
      endocrine (gland) NEC Q89.2
      epiglottis Q31.8
      eustachian tube Q17.8
      eye Q15.8
      facial features Q18.8
      fallopian tube Q50.6
      finger(s) Q68.1
        supernumerary Q69.0
      foot Q66.9-●
      gallbladder Q44.1
      gastrointestinal tract Q45.8
      genitalia, genital organ(s) or tract
        female Q52.8
          external Q52.79
          internal NEC Q52.8
        male Q55.8
      glottis Q31.8
      hand Q68.1
      heart Q24.8
        dextrocardia Q24.0
          with complete transposition of viscera
            Q89.3
      hepatic duct Q44.5
      hip (joint) Q65.89
      intestine (large) (small) Q43.8
        with anomalous adhesions, fixation or
          malrotation Q43.3
      joint NEC Q68.8
      kidney Q63.2
      larynx Q31.8
      limb Q68.8
        lower Q68.8
        upper Q68.8
      liver Q44.7
      lung (lobe) Q33.8
      nail(s) Q84.6
      nerve Q07.8
      nervous system NEC Q07.8
      nose, nasal (septum) Q30.8
      organ or site not listed —*see* Anomaly,
        by site
      ovary Q50.39
      pancreas Q45.3
      parathyroid (gland) Q89.2
      patella Q74.1
      peripheral vascular system Q27.8
      pituitary (gland) Q89.2
      respiratory organ or system NEC
        Q34.8
      rib (cage) Q76.6
        supernumerary in cervical region
          Q76.5
      scapula Q74.0
      shoulder Q74.0
      spinal cord Q06.8
      spleen Q89.09
      sternum NEC Q76.7
      stomach Q40.2
      symphysis pubis Q74.2
      thymus (gland) Q89.2
      thyroid (gland) (tissue) Q89.2
        cartilage Q31.8
      toe(s) Q66.9-●
        supernumerary Q69.2
      tongue Q38.3
      trachea Q32.1
      ureter Q62.60
        deviation Q62.61
        displacement Q62.62
        ectopia Q62.63
        specified type NEC Q62.69

▶ New   ➠ Revised   ~~deleted~~ Deleted   ● Use Additional Character(s)

Malposition *(Continued)*
  congenital *(Continued)*
    uterus Q51.818
    vein(s) (peripheral) Q27.8
      great Q26.8
    vena cava (inferior) (superior) Q26.8
  device, implant or graft —*see also*
    Complications, by site and type,
    mechanical T85.628
    arterial graft NEC —*see* Complication,
      cardiovascular device, mechanical,
      vascular
    breast (implant) T85.42
    catheter NEC T85.628
      cystostomy T83.020
      dialysis (renal) T82.42
        intraperitoneal T85.621
      infusion NEC T82.524
        spinal (epidural) (subdural) T85.620
      urinary —*see also* Displacement, device,
        catheter, urinary T83.028
    electronic (electrode) (pulse generator)
      (stimulator)
      bone T84.320
      cardiac T82.129
        electrode T82.120
        pulse generator T82.121
        specified type NEC T82.128
      nervous system —*see* Complication,
        prosthetic device, mechanical,
        electronic nervous system
        stimulator
      urinary —*see* Complication,
        genitourinary, device, urinary,
        mechanical
    fixation, internal (orthopedic) NEC —
      see Complication, fixation device,
      mechanical
    gastrointestinal —*see* Complications,
      prosthetic device, mechanical,
      gastrointestinal device
    genital NEC T83.428
      intrauterine contraceptive device (string)
        T83.32
      penile prosthesis (cylinder) (implanted)
        (pump) (resevoir) T83.420
      testicular prosthesis T83.421
    heart NEC —*see* Complication,
      cardiovascular device, mechanical
    joint prosthesis —*see* Complication, joint
      prosthesis, mechanical
    ocular NEC —*see* Complications,
      prosthetic device, mechanical,
      ocular device
    orthopedic NEC —*see* Complication,
      orthopedic, device, mechanical
    specified NEC T85.628
    urinary NEC —*see also* Complication,
      genitourinary, device, urinary,
      mechanical
      graft T83.22
    vascular NEC —*see* Complication,
      cardiovascular device, mechanical
    ventricular intracranial shunt T85.02
  fetus —*see* Pregnancy, complicated by
    (management affected by), presentation,
    fetal
  gallbladder K82.8
  gastrointestinal tract, congenital Q45.8
  heart, congenital NEC Q24.8
  joint prosthesis —*see* Complications, joint
    prosthesis, mechanical, displacement,
    by site
  stomach K31.89
    congenital Q40.2
  tooth, teeth, fully erupted M26.30
  uterus (acute) (acquired) (adherent)
    (asymptomatic) (postinfectional)
    (postpartal, old) N85.4
    anteflexion or anteversion N85.4
      congenital Q51.818

Malposition *(Continued)*
  uterus *(Continued)*
    flexion N85.4
      lateral —*see* Lateroversion, uterus
    inversion N85.5
    lateral (flexion) (version) —*see*
      Lateroversion, uterus
    in pregnancy or childbirth —*see*
      subcategory O34.5
    retroflexion or retroversion —*see*
      Retroversion, uterus
Malposture R29.3
Malrotation
  cecum Q43.3
  colon Q43.3
  intestine Q43.3
  kidney Q63.2
Malta fever —*see* Brucellosis
Maltreatment
  adult
    abandonment
      confirmed T74.01
      suspected T76.01
    bullying
      confirmed T74.31
      suspected T76.31
    confirmed T74.91
    history of Z91.419
    intimidation (through social media)
      confirmed T74.31
      suspected T76.31
    neglect
      confirmed T74.01
      suspected T76.01
    physical abuse
      confirmed T74.11
      suspected T76.11
    psychological abuse
      confirmed T74.31
      history of Z91.411
      suspected T76.31
    sexual abuse
      confirmed T74.21
      suspected T76.21
    suspected T76.91
  child
    abandonment
      confirmed T74.02
      suspected T76.02
    bullying
      confirmed T74.32
      suspected T76.32
    confirmed T74.92
    history of —*see* History, personal (of),
      abuse
    intimidation (through social media)
      confirmed T74.32
      suspected T76.32
    neglect
      confirmed T74.02
      history of —*see* History, personal (of),
        abuse
      suspected T76.02
    physical abuse
      confirmed T74.12
      history of —*see* History, personal (of),
        abuse
      suspected T76.12
    psychological abuse
      confirmed T74.32
      history of —*see* History, personal (of),
        abuse
      suspected T76.32
    sexual abuse
      confirmed T74.22
      history of —*see* History, personal (of),
        abuse
      suspected T76.22
    suspected T76.92
  personal history of Z91.89
Maltworker's lung J67.4

Malunion, fracture —*see* Fracture, by site
Mammillitis N61.0
  puerperal, postpartum O91.02
Mammitis —*see* Mastitis
Mammogram (examination) Z12.39
  routine Z12.31
Mammoplasia N62
Management (of)
  bone conduction hearing device (implanted)
    Z45.320
  cardiac pacemaker NEC Z45.018
  cerebrospinal fluid drainage device Z45.41
  cochlear device (implanted) Z45.321
  contraceptive Z30.9
    specified NEC Z30.8
  implanted device Z45.9
    specified NEC Z45.89
  infusion pump Z45.1
  procreative Z31.9
    male factor infertility in female Z31.81
    specified NEC Z31.89
  prosthesis (external) —*see also* Fitting
    Z44.9
    implanted Z45.9
      specified NEC Z45.89
  renal dialysis catheter Z49.01
  vascular access device Z45.2
Mangled —*see* specified injury by site
Mania (monopolar) —*see also* Disorder, mood,
  manic episode
  with psychotic symptoms F30.2
  without psychotic symptoms F30.10
    mild F30.11
    moderate F30.12
    severe F30.13
  Bell's F30.8
  chronic (recurrent) F31.89
  hysterical F44.89
  puerperal F30.8
  recurrent F31.89
Manic depression F31.9
Manic-depressive insanity, psychosis, or
  syndrome —*see* Disorder, bipolar
Mannosidosis E77.1
Mansonelliasis, mansonellosis B74.4
Manson's
  disease B65.1
  schistosomiasis B65.1
Manual —*see* condition
Maple-bark-stripper's lung (disease) J67.6
Maple-syrup-urine disease E71.0
Marable's syndrome (celiac artery
  compression) I77.4
Marasmus E41
  due to malnutrition E41
  intestinal E41
  nutritional E41
  senile R54
  tuberculous NEC —*see* Tuberculosis
Marble
  bones Q78.2
  skin R23.8
Marburg virus disease A98.3
March
  fracture —*see* Fracture, traumatic, stress, by
    site
  hemoglobinuria D59.6
Marchesani (-Weill) syndrome Q87.0
Marchiafava (-Bignami) syndrome or disease
  G37.1
Marchiafava-Micheli syndrome D59.5
Marcus Gunn's syndrome Q07.8
Marfan's syndrome —*see* Syndrome, Marfan's
Marie-Bamberger disease —*see*
  Osteoarthropathy, hypertrophic, specified
  NEC
Marie-Charcot-Tooth neuropathic muscular
  atrophy G60.0
Marie's
  cerebellar ataxia (late-onset) G11.2
  disease or syndrome (acromegaly) E22.0

Marie-Strümpell arthritis, disease or
    spondylitis —*see* Spondylitis, ankylosing
Marion's disease (bladder neck obstruction)
    N32.0
Marital conflict Z63.0
Mark
    port wine Q82.5
    raspberry Q82.5
    strawberry Q82.5
    stretch L90.6
    tattoo L81.8
Marker heterochromatin —*see* Extra, marker
    chromosomes
Maroteaux-Lamy syndrome (mild) (severe)
    E76.29
Marrow (bone)
    arrest D61.9
    poor function D75.89
Marseilles fever A77.1
Marsh fever —*see* Malaria
Marshall's (hidrotic) ectodermal dysplasia
    Q82.4
Marsh's disease (exophthalmic goiter)
    E05.00
    with storm E05.01
Masculinization (female) with adrenal
    hyperplasia E25.9
    congenital E25.0
Masculinovoblastoma D27.-●
Masochism (sexual) F65.51
Mason's lung J62.8
Mass
    abdominal R19.00
        epigastric R19.06
        generalized R19.07
        left lower quadrant R19.04
        left upper quadrant R19.02
        periumbilic R19.05
        right lower quadrant R19.03
        right upper quadrant R19.01
        specified site NEC R19.09
    breast —*see also* Lump, breast N63.0
    chest R22.2
    cystic —*see* Cyst
    ear H93.8-●
    head R22.0
    intra-abdominal (diffuse) (generalized) —*see*
        Mass, abdominal
    kidney N28.89
    liver R16.0
    localized (skin) R22.9
        chest R22.2
        head R22.0
        limb
            lower R22.4-●
            upper R22.3-●
        neck R22.1
        trunk R22.2
    lung R91.8
    malignant —*see* Neoplasm, malignant,
        by site
    neck R22.1
    pelvic (diffuse) (generalized) —*see* Mass,
        abdominal
    specified organ NEC —*see* Disease, by site
    splenic R16.1
    substernal thyroid —*see* Goiter
    superficial (localized) R22.9
    umbilical (diffuse) (generalized) R19.09
Massive —*see* condition
Mast cell
    disease, systemic tissue D47.02
    leukemia C94.3-●
    neoplasm
        malignant C96.20
            specified type NEC C96.29
        of uncertain behavior NEC D47.09
    sarcoma C96.22
    tumor D47.09
Mastalgia N64.4
Masters-Allen syndrome N83.8

Mastitis (acute) (diffuse) (nonpuerperal)
    (subacute) N61.0
    with abscess N61.1
    chronic (cystic) —*see* Mastopathy, cystic
    cystic (Schimmelbusch's type) —*see*
        Mastopathy, cystic
    fibrocystic —*see* Mastopathy, cystic
    granulomatous N61.2-●
    infective N61.0
        newborn P39.0
    interstitial, gestational or puerperal —*see*
        Mastitis, obstetric
    neonatal (noninfective) P83.4
        infective P39.0
    obstetric (interstitial) (nonpurulent)
        associated with
            lactation O91.23
            pregnancy O91.21-●
            puerperium O91.22
        purulent
            associated with
                lactation O91.13
                pregnancy O91.11-●
                puerperium O91.12
    periductal —*see* Ectasia, mammary duct
    phlegmonous —*see* Mastopathy, cystic
    plasma cell —*see* Ectasia, mammary duct
    without abscess N61.0
Mastocytoma (extracutaneous) D47.09
    malignant C96.29
    solitary D47.01
Mastocytosis D47.09
    aggressive systemic C96.21
    cutaneous (diffuse) (maculopapular) D47.01
        congenital Q82.2
        of neonatal onset Q82.2
        of newborn onset Q82.2
    indolent systemic D47.02
    isolated bone marrow D47.02
    malignant C96.29
    systemic (indolent) (smoldering)
        with an associated hematological
            non-mast cell lineage disease (SM-
            AHNMD) D47.02
Mastodynia N64.4
Mastoid —*see* condition
Mastoidalgia —*see* subcategory H92.0
Mastoiditis (coalescent) (hemorrhagic)
    (suppurative) H70.9-●
    acute, subacute H70.00-●
        complicated NEC H70.09-●
        subperiosteal H70.01-●
    chronic (necrotic) (recurrent) H70.1-●
    in (due to)
        infectious disease NEC B99 [H75.0-●]
        parasitic disease NEC B89 [H75.0-●]
        tuberculosis A18.03
    petrositis —*see* Petrositis
    postauricular fistula —*see* Fistula, postauricular
    specified NEC H70.89-●
    tuberculous A18.03
Mastopathy, mastopathia N64.9
    chronica cystica —*see* Mastopathy, cystic
    cystic (chronic) (diffuse) N60.1
        with epithelial proliferation N60.3-●
    diffuse cystic —*see* Mastopathy, cystic
    estrogenic, oestrogenica N64.89
    ovarian origin N64.89
Mastoplasia, mastoplastia N62
Masturbation (excessive) F98.8
Maternal care (for) —*see* Pregnancy
    (complicated by) (management affected by)
Matheiu's disease (leptospiral jaundice) A27.0
Mauclaire's disease or osteochondrosis —*see*
    Osteochondrosis, juvenile, hand, metacarpal
Maxcy's disease A75.2
Maxilla, maxillary —*see* condition
May (-Hegglin) anomaly or syndrome D72.0
McArdle (-Schmid)(-Pearson) disease
    (glycogen storage) E74.04
McCune-Albright syndrome Q78.1

McQuarrie's syndrome (idiopathic familial
    hypoglycemia) E16.2
▶ME/CFS (myalgic encephalomyelitis/chronic
    fatigue syndrome) G93.32
Meadow's syndrome Q86.1
Measles (black) (hemorrhagic) (suppressed)
    B05.9
    with
        complications NEC B05.89
        encephalitis B05.0
        intestinal complications B05.4
        keratitis (keratoconjunctivitis) B05.81
        meningitis B05.1
        otitis media B05.3
        pneumonia B05.2
    French —*see* Rubella
    German —*see* Rubella
    Liberty —*see* Rubella
Meatitis, urethral —*see* Urethritis
Meatus, meatal —*see* condition
Meat-wrappers' asthma J68.9
Meckel-Gruber syndrome Q61.9
Meckel's diverticulitis, diverticulum
    (displaced) (hypertrophic) Q43.0
Meconium
    ileus, newborn P76.0
        in cystic fibrosis E84.11
        meaning meconium plug (without cystic
            fibrosis) P76.0
    obstruction, newborn P76.0
        due to fecaliths P76.0
        in mucoviscidosis E84.11
    peritonitis P78.0
    plug syndrome (newborn) NEC P76.0
Median —*see also* condition
    arcuate ligament syndrome I77.4
    bar (prostate) (vesical orifice) —*see*
        Hyperplasia, prostate
    rhomboid glossitis K14.2
Mediastinal shift R93.89
Mediastinitis (acute) (chronic) J98.51
    syphilitic A52.73
    tuberculous A15.8
Mediastinopericarditis —*see also* Pericarditis
    acute I30.9
    adhesive I31.0
    chronic I31.8
        rheumatic I09.2
Mediastinum, mediastinal —*see* condition
Medicine poisoning —*see* Table of Drugs and
    Chemicals, by drug, poisoning
Mediterranean
    fever —*see* Brucellosis
        familial M04.1
        tick A77.1
    kala-azar B55.0
    leishmaniasis B55.0
    tick fever A77.1
Medulla —*see* condition
Medullary cystic kidney Q61.5
Medullated fibers
    optic (nerve) Q14.8
    retina Q14.1
Medulloblastoma
    desmoplastic C71.6
    specified site —*see* Neoplasm, malignant, by
        site
    unspecified site C71.6
Medulloepithelioma —*see also* Neoplasm,
    malignant, by site
    teratoid —*see* Neoplasm, malignant, by site
Medullomyoblastoma
    specified site —*see* Neoplasm, malignant, by
        site
    unspecified site C71.6
Meekeren-Ehlers-Danlos syndrome —*see also*
    Syndrome, Ehlers-Danlos Q79.6
Megacolon (acquired) (functional) (not
    Hirschsprung's disease) (in) K59.39
    Chagas' disease B57.32
    congenital, congenitum (aganglionic) Q43.1

▶ New   ⇒ Revised   ~~deleted~~ Deleted   ● Use Additional Character(s)

Megacolon *(Continued)*
 Hirschsprung's (disease) Q43.1
 toxic NEC K59.31
  due to Clostridium difficile
   not specified as recurrent A04.72
   recurrent A04.71
Megaesophagus (functional) K22.0
 congenital Q39.5
 in (due to) Chagas' disease B57.31
Megalencephaly Q04.5
Megalerythema (epidemic) B08.3
Megaloappendix Q43.8
Megalocephalus, megalocephaly NEC Q75.3
Megalocornea Q15.8
 with glaucoma Q15.0
Megalocytic anemia D53.1
Megalodactylia (fingers) (thumbs) (congenital)
  Q74.0
 toes Q74.2
Megaloduodenum Q43.8
Megaloesophagus (functional) K22.0
 congenital Q39.5
Megalogastria (acquired) K31.89
 congenital Q40.2
Megalophthalmos Q11.3
Megalopsia H53.15
Megalosplenia —*see* Splenomegaly
Megaloureter N28.82
 congenital Q62.2
Megarectum K62.89
Megasigmoid K59.39
 congenital Q43.2
Megaureter N28.82
 congenital Q62.2
Megavitamin-B6 syndrome E67.2
Megrim —*see* Migraine
Meibomian
 cyst, infected —*see* Hordeolum
 gland —*see* condition
 sty, stye —*see* Hordeolum
Meibomitis —*see* Hordeolum
Meige-Milroy disease (chronic hereditary
  edema) Q82.0
Meige's syndrome Q82.0
Melalgia, nutritional E53.8
Melancholia F32.A
 climacteric (single episode) F32.89
  recurrent episode F33.8
 hypochondriac F45.29
 intermittent (single episode) F32.89
  recurrent episode F33.8
 involutional (single episode) F32.89
  recurrent episode F33.8
 menopausal (single episode) F32.89
  recurrent episode F33.8
 puerperal F32.89
 reactive (emotional stress or trauma) F32.3
 recurrent F33.9
 senile F03
 stuporous (single episode) F32.89
  recurrent episode F33.8
Melanemia R79.89
Melanoameloblastoma —*see* Neoplasm, bone,
  benign
Melanoblastoma —*see* Melanoma
Melanocarcinoma —*see* Melanoma
Melanocytoma, eyeball D31.9-●
Melanocytosis, neurocutaneous Q82.8
Melanoderma, melanodermia L81.4
Melanodontia, infantile K03.89
Melanodontoclasia K03.89
Melanoepithelioma —*see* Melanoma
Melanoma (malignant) C43.9
 acral lentiginous, malignant —*see* Melanoma,
  skin, by site
 amelanotic —*see* Melanoma, skin, by site
 balloon cell —*see* Melanoma, skin, by site
 benign —*see* Nevus
 desmoplastic, malignant —*see* Melanoma,
  skin, by site
 epithelioid cell —*see* Melanoma, skin, by site
  with spindle cell, mixed —*see* Melanoma,
   skin, by site

Melanoma *(Continued)*
 in
  giant pigmented nevus —*see* Melanoma,
   skin, by site
  Hutchinson's melanotic freckle —*see*
   Melanoma, skin, by site
  junctional nevus —*see* Melanoma, skin,
   by site
  precancerous melanosis —*see* Melanoma,
   skin, by site
 in situ D03.9
  abdominal wall D03.59
  ala nasi D03.39
  ankle D03.7-●
  anus, anal (margin) (skin) D03.51
  arm D03.6-●
  auditory canal D03.2-●
  auricle (ear) D03.2-●
  auricular canal (external) D03.2-●
  axilla, axillary fold D03.59
  back D03.59
  breast D03.52
  brow D03.39
  buttock D03.59
  canthus (eye) D03.1-●
  cheek (external) D03.39
  chest wall D03.59
  chin D03.39
  choroid D03.8
  conjunctiva D03.8
  ear (external) D03.2-●
  external meatus (ear) D03.2-●
  eye D03.8
  eyebrow D03.39
  eyelid (lower) (upper) D03.1-●
  face D03.30
   specified NEC D03.39
  female genital organ (external) NEC D03.8
  finger D03.6-●
  flank D03.59
  foot D03.7-●
  forearm D03.6-●
  forehead D03.39
  foreskin D03.8
  gluteal region D03.59
  groin D03.59
  hand D03.6-●
  heel D03.7-●
  helix D03.2-●
  hip D03.7-●
  interscapular region D03.59
  iris D03.8
  jaw D03.39
  knee D03.7-●
  labium (majus) (minus) D03.8
  lacrimal gland D03.8
  leg D03.7-●
  lip (lower) (upper) D03.0
  lower limb NEC D03.7-●
  male genital organ (external) NEC D03.8
  nail D03.9
   finger D03.6-●
   toe D03.7-●
  neck D03.4
  nose (external) D03.39
  orbit D03.8
  penis D03.8
  perianal skin D03.51
  perineum D03.51
  pinna D03.2-●
  popliteal fossa or space D03.7-●
  prepuce D03.8
  pudendum D03.8
  retina D03.8
  retrobulbar D03.8
  scalp D03.4
  scrotum D03.8
  shoulder D03.6-●
  specified site NEC D03.8
  submammary fold D03.52
  temple D03.39

Melanoma *(Continued)*
 in situ *(Continued)*
  thigh D03.7-●
  toe D03.7-●
  trunk NEC D03.59
  umbilicus D03.59
  upper limb NEC D03.6-●
  vulva D03.8
 juvenile —*see* Nevus
 malignant, of soft parts except skin —*see*
   Neoplasm, connective tissue, malignant
 metastatic
  breast C79.81
  genital organ C79.82
  specified site NEC C79.89
 neurotropic, malignant —*see* Melanoma, skin,
  by site
 nodular —*see* Melanoma, skin, by site
 regressing, malignant —*see* Melanoma, skin,
  by site
 skin C43.9
  abdominal wall C43.59
  ala nasi C43.31
  ankle C43.7-●
  anus, anal (skin) C43.51
  arm C43.6-●
  auditory canal (external) C43.2-●
  auricle (ear) C43.2-●
  auricular canal (external) C43.2-●
  axilla, axillary fold C43.59
  back C43.59
  breast (female) (male) C43.52
  brow C43.39
  buttock C43.59
  canthus (eye) C43.1-●
  cheek (external) C43.39
  chest wall C43.59
  chin C43.39
  ear (external) C43.2-●
  elbow C43.6-●
  external meatus (ear) C43.2-●
  eyebrow C43.39
  eyelid (lower) (upper) C43.1-●
  face C43.30
   specified NEC C43.39
  female genital organ (external) NEC C51.9
  finger C43.6-●
  flank C43.59
  foot C43.7-●
  forearm C43.6-●
  forehead C43.39
  foreskin C60.0
  glabella C43.39
  gluteal region C43.59
  groin C43.59
  hand C43.6-●
  heel C43.7-●
  helix C43.2-●
  hip C43.7-●
  interscapular region C43.59
  jaw (external) C43.39
  knee C43.7-●
  labium C51.9
   majus C51.0
   minus C51.1
  leg C43.7-●
  lip (lower) (upper) C43.0
  lower limb NEC C43.7-●
  male genital organ (external) NEC C63.9
  nail
   finger C43.6-●
   toe C43.7-●
  nasolabial groove C43.39
  nates C43.59
  neck C43.4
  nose (external) C43.31
  overlapping site C43.8
  palpebra C43.1-●
  penis C60.9
  perianal skin C43.51
  perineum C43.51

Melanoma *(Continued)*
  skin *(Continued)*
    pinna C43.2-●
    popliteal fossa or space C43.7-●
    prepuce C60.0
    pudendum C51.9
    scalp C43.4
    scrotum C63.2
    shoulder C43.6-●
    skin NEC C43.9
    submammary fold C43.52
    temple C43.39
    thigh C43.7-●
    toe C43.7-●
    trunk NEC C43.59
    umbilicus C43.59
    upper limb NEC C43.6-●
    vulva C51.9
      overlapping sites C51.8
  spindle cell
    with epithelioid, mixed —*see* Melanoma,
      skin, by site
    type A C69.4-●
    type B C69.4-●
  superficial spreading —*see* Melanoma, skin,
    by site
Melanosarcoma —*see also* Melanoma
  epithelioid cell —*see* Melanoma
Melanosis L81.4
  addisonian E27.1
    tuberculous A18.7
  adrenal E27.1
  colon K63.89
  conjunctiva —*see* Pigmentation, conjunctiva
    congenital Q13.89
  cornea (presenile) (senile) —*see also*
    Pigmentation, cornea
    congenital Q13.4
  eye NEC H57.89
    congenital Q15.8
  lenticularis progressiva Q82.1
  liver K76.89
  precancerous —*see also* Melanoma, in situ
    malignant melanoma in —*see* Melanoma
  Riehl's L81.4
  sclera H15.89
    congenital Q13.89
  suprarenal E27.1
  tar L81.4
  toxic L81.4
Melanuria R82.998
MELAS syndrome E88.41
Melasma L81.1
  adrenal (gland) E27.1
  suprarenal (gland) E27.1
Melena K92.1
  with ulcer - code by site under Ulcer, with
    hemorrhage K27.4
  due to swallowed maternal blood P78.2
  newborn, neonatal P54.1
    due to swallowed maternal blood P78.2
Meleney's
  gangrene (cutaneous) —*see* Ulcer, skin
  ulcer (chronic undermining) —*see* Ulcer, skin
Melioidosis A24.9
  acute A24.1
  chronic A24.2
  fulminating A24.1
  pneumonia A24.1
  pulmonary (chronic) A24.2
    acute A24.1
    subacute A24.2
  sepsis A24.1
  specified NEC A24.3
  subacute A24.2
Melitensis, febris A23.0
Melkersson (-Rosenthal) syndrome G51.2
Mellitus, diabetes —*see* Diabetes
Melorheostosis (bone) —*see* Disorder, bone,
  density and structure, specified NEC
Meloschisis Q18.4

Melotia Q17.4
Membrana
  capsularis lentis posterior Q13.89
  epipapillaris Q14.2
Membranacea placenta O43.19-●
Membranaceous uterus N85.8
Membrane(s), membranous —*see also* condition
  cyclitic —*see* Membrane, pupillary
  folds, congenital —*see* Web
  Jackson's Q43.3
  over face of newborn P28.9
  premature rupture —*see* Rupture,
    membranes, premature
  pupillary H21.4-●
    persistent Q13.89
  retained (with hemorrhage) (complicating
    delivery) O72.2
    without hemorrhage O73.1
  secondary cataract —*see* Cataract, secondary
  unruptured (causing asphyxia) —*see*
    Asphyxia, newborn
  vitreous —*see* Opacity, vitreous, membranes
    and strands
Membranitis —*see* Chorioamnionitis
Memory disturbance, lack or loss —*see also*
  Amnesia
  mild, following organic brain damage F06.8
Menadione deficiency E56.1
Menarche
  delayed E30.0
  precocious E30.1
Mendacity, pathologic F60.2
Mendelson's syndrome (due to anesthesia) J95.4
  in labor and delivery O74.0
  in pregnancy O29.01-●
  obstetric O74.0
  postpartum, puerperal O89.01
Ménétrier's disease or syndrome K29.60
  with bleeding K29.61
Ménière's disease, syndrome or vertigo H81.0-●
Meninges, meningeal —*see* condition
Meningioma —*see also* Neoplasm, meninges,
  benign
  angioblastic —*see* Neoplasm, meninges,
    benign
  angiomatous —*see* Neoplasm, meninges,
    benign
  atypical —*see* Neoplasm, meninges, uncertain
    behavior
  endotheliomatous —*see* Neoplasm, meninges,
    benign
  fibroblastic —*see* Neoplasm, meninges,
    benign
  fibrous —*see* Neoplasm, meninges, benign
  hemangioblastic —*see* Neoplasm, meninges,
    benign
  hemangiopericytic —*see* Neoplasm,
    meninges, benign
  malignant —*see* Neoplasm, meninges,
    malignant
  meningiothelial —*see* Neoplasm, meninges,
    benign
  meningotheliomatous —*see* Neoplasm,
    meninges, benign
  mixed —*see* Neoplasm, meninges, benign
  multiple —*see* Neoplasm, meninges,
    uncertain behavior
  papillary —*see* Neoplasm, meninges,
    uncertain behavior
  psammomatous —*see* Neoplasm, meninges,
    benign
  syncytial —*see* Neoplasm, meninges, benign
  transitional —*see* Neoplasm, meninges,
    benign
Meningiomatosis (diffuse) —*see* Neoplasm,
  meninges, uncertain behavior
Meningism —*see* Meningismus
Meningismus (infectional) (pneumococcal) R29.1
  due to serum or vaccine R29.1
  influenzal —*see* Influenza, with,
    manifestations NEC

Meningitis (basal) (basic) (brain) (cerebral)
  (cervical) (congestive) (diffuse)
  (hemorrhagic) infantile) (membranous)
  (metastatic) (nonspecific) (pontine)
  (progressive) (simple) (spinal) (subacute)
  (sympathetic) (toxic) G03.9
  abacterial G03.0
  actinomycotic A42.81
  adenoviral A87.1
  arbovirus A87.8
  aseptic (acute) G03.0
  bacterial G00.9
    Escherichia coli (E. coli) G00.8
    Friedländer (bacillus) G00.8
    gram-negative G00.9
    H. influenzae G00.0
    Klebsiella G00.8
    pneumococcal G00.1
    specified organism NEC G00.8
    staphylococcal G00.3
    streptococcal (acute) G00.2
  benign recurrent (Mollaret) G03.2
  candidal B37.5
  caseous (tuberculous) A17.0
  cerebrospinal A39.0
  chronic NEC G03.1
  clear cerebrospinal fluid NEC G03.0
  coxsackievirus A87.0
  cryptococcal B45.1
  diplococcal (gram positive) A39.0
  echovirus A87.0
  enteroviral A87.0
  eosinophilic B83.2
  epidemic NEC A39.0
  Escherichia coli (E. coli) G00.8
  fibrinopurulent G00.9
    specified organism NEC G00.8
  Friedländer (bacillus) G00.8
  gonococcal A54.81
  gram-negative cocci G00.9
  gram-positive cocci G00.9
  Haemophilus (influenzae) G00.0
  H. influenzae G00.0
  in (due to)
    adenovirus A87.1
    African trypanosomiasis B56.9 *[G02]*
    anthrax A22.8
    bacterial disease NEC A48.8 *[G01]*
    Chagas' disease (chronic) B57.41
    chickenpox B01.0
    coccidioidomycosis B38.4
    Diplococcus pneumoniae G00.1
    enterovirus A87.0
    herpes (simplex) virus B00.3
      zoster B02.1
    infectious mononucleosis B27.92
    leptospirosis A27.81
    Listeria monocytogenes A32.11
    Lyme disease A69.21
    measles B05.1
    mumps (virus) B26.1
    neurosyphilis (late) A52.13
    parasitic disease NEC B89 *[G02]*
    poliovirus A80.9 *[G02]*
    preventive immunization, inoculation or
      vaccination G03.8
    rubella B06.02
    Salmonella infection A02.21
    specified cause NEC G03.8
    Streptococcal pneumoniae G00.1
    typhoid fever A01.01
    varicella B01.0
    viral disease NEC A87.8
    whooping cough A37.90
    zoster B02.1
  infectious G00.9
  influenzal (H. influenzae) G00.0
  Klebsiella G00.8
  leptospiral (aseptic) A27.81
  lymphocytic (acute) (benign) (serous) A87.2
  meningococcal A39.0

▶ New   ⇒ Revised   ~~deleted~~ Deleted   ● Use Additional Character(s)

Meningitis (Continued)
Mima polymorpha G00.8
Mollaret (benign recurrent) G03.2
monilial B37.5
mycotic NEC B49 *[G02]*
Neisseria A39.0
nonbacterial G03.0
nonpyogenic NEC G03.0
ossificans G96.198
pneumococcal streptococcus pneumoniae
    G00.1
poliovirus A80.9 *[G02]*
postmeasles B05.1
purulent G00.9
    specified organism NEC G00.8
pyogenic G00.9
    specified organism NEC G00.8
Salmonella (arizonae) (Cholerae-Suis)
    (enteritidis) (typhimurium) A02.21
septic G00.9
    specified organism NEC G00.8
serosa circumscripta NEC G03.0
serous NEC G93.2
specified organism NEC G00.8
sporotrichosis B42.81
staphylococcal G00.3
sterile G03.0
Streptococcal (acute) G00.2
    pneumoniae G00.1
suppurative G00.9
    specified organism NEC G00.8
syphilitic (late) (tertiary) A52.13
    acute A51.41
    congenital A50.41
    secondary A51.41
Torula histolytica (cryptococcal) B45.1
traumatic (complication of injury) T79.8
tuberculous A17.0
typhoid A01.01
viral NEC A87.9
Yersinia pestis A20.3
Meningocele (spinal) —*see also* Spina bifida
with hydrocephalus —*see* Spina bifida, by
    site, with hydrocephalus
acquired (traumatic) G96.198
cerebral —*see* Encephalocele
Meningocerebritis —*see* Meningoencephalitis
Meningococcemia A39.4
acute A39.2
chronic A39.3
Meningococcus, meningococcal —*see also*
    condition A39.9
adrenalitis, hemorrhagic A39.1
carrier (suspected) of Z22.31
meningitis (cerebrospinal) A39.0
Meningoencephalitis —*see also* Encephalitis
    G04.90
acute NEC —*see also* Encephalitis, viral A86
bacterial NEC G04.2
California A83.5
diphasic A84.1
eosinophilic B83.2
epidemic A39.81
herpesviral, herpetic B00.4
    due to herpesvirus 6 B10.01
    due to herpesvirus 7 B10.09
    specified NEC B10.09
in (due to)
    blastomycosis NEC B40.81
    diseases classified elsewhere G05.3
    free-living amebae B60.2
    Hemophilus influenzae (H. influenzae)
        G00.0
    herpes B00.4
        due to herpesvirus 6 B10.01
        due to herpesvirus 7 B10.09
        specified NEC B10.09
    H. influenzae G00.0
    Lyme disease A69.22
    mercury —*see* subcategory T56.1
    mumps B26.2

Meningoencephalitis (Continued)
in (due to) (Continued)
    Naegleria (amebae) (organisms) (fowleri)
        B60.2
    Parastrongylus cantonensis B83.2
    toxoplasmosis (acquired) B58.2
        congenital P37.1
infectious (acute) (viral) A86
influenzal (H. influenzae) G00.0
Listeria monocytogenes A32.12
lymphocytic (serous) A87.2
mumps B26.2
parasitic NEC B89 *[G05.3]*
pneumococcal G04.2
primary amebic B60.2
specific (syphilitic) A52.14
specified organism NEC G04.81
staphylococcal G04.2
streptococcal G04.2
syphilitic A52.14
toxic NEC G92.8
    due to mercury —*see* subcategory T56.1
tuberculous A17.82
virus NEC A86
Meningoencephalocele —*see also* Encephalocele
syphilitic A52.19
    congenital A50.49
Meningoencephalomyelitis —*see also*
    Meningoencephalitis
acute NEC (viral) A86
    disseminated G04.00
        postimmunization or postvaccination
            G04.02
        postinfectious G04.01
    due to
        actinomycosis A42.82
        Torula B45.1
        Toxoplasma or toxoplasmosis (acquired)
            B58.2
            congenital P37.1
    postimmunization or postvaccination G04.02
Meningoencephalomyelopathy G96.9
Meningoencephalopathy G96.9
Meningomyelitis —*see also*
    Meningoencephalitis
bacterial NEC G04.2
blastomycotic NEC B40.81
cryptococcal B45.1
in diseases classified elsewhere G05.4
meningococcal A39.81
syphilitic A52.14
tuberculous A17.82
Meningomyelocele —*see also* Spina bifida
syphilitic A52.19
Meningomyeloneuritis —*see*
    Meningoencephalitis
Meningoradiculitis —*see* Meningitis
Meningovascular —*see* condition
Menkes' disease or syndrome E83.09
meaning maple-syrup-urine disease E71.0
Menometrorrhagia N92.1
Menopause, menopausal (asymptomatic)
    (state) Z78.0
arthritis (any site) NEC —*see* Arthritis,
    specified form NEC
bleeding N92.4
depression (single episode) F32.89
    agitated (single episode) F32.2
        recurrent episode F33.9
    psychotic (single episode) F32.89
        zrecurrent episode F33.8
    recurrent episode F33.9
melancholia (single episode) F32.89
    recurrent episode F33.8
paranoid state F22
▶postirradiation (postprocedural)
    ▶asymptomatic E89.40
    ▶symptomatic E89.41
premature E28.319
    asymptomatic E28.319
        postirradiation E89.40
        postsurgical E89.40

Menopause, menopausal (Continued)
premature (Continued)
    symptomatic E28.310
        postirradiation E89.41
        postsurgical E89.41
    psychosis NEC F28
    symptomatic N95.1
    toxic polyarthritis NEC —*see* Arthritis,
        specified form NEC
Menorrhagia (primary) N92.0
climacteric N92.4
    menopausal N92.4
menopausal N92.4
perimenopausal N92.4
postclimacteric N95.0
postmenopausal N95.0
preclimacteric or premenopausal N92.4
pubertal (menses retained) N92.2
Menostaxis N92.0
Menses, retention N94.89
Menstrual —*see* Menstruation
Menstruation
absent —*see* Amenorrhea
anovulatory N97.0
cycle, irregular N92.6
delayed N91.0
disorder N93.9
    psychogenic F45.8
during pregnancy O20.8
excessive (with regular cycle) N92.0
    with irregular cycle N92.1
    at puberty N92.2
frequent N92.0
infrequent —*see* Oligomenorrhea
irregular N92.6
    specified NEC N92.5
latent N92.5
membranous N92.5
painful —*see also* Dysmenorrhea N94.6
    primary N94.4
    psychogenic F45.8
    secondary N94.5
passage of clots N92.0
precocious E30.1
protracted N92.5
rare —*see* Oligomenorrhea
retained N94.89
retrograde N92.5
scanty —*see* Oligomenorrhea
suppression N94.89
vicarious (nasal) N94.89
Mental —*see also* condition
deficiency —*see* Disability, intellectual
deterioration —*see* Psychosis
disorder —*see* Disorder, mental
exhaustion F48.8
insufficiency (congenital) —*see* Disability,
    intellectual
observation without need for further medical
    care Z03.89
retardation —*see* Disability, intellectual
subnormality —*see* Disability, intellectual
upset —*see* Disorder, mental
Meralgia paresthetica G57.1-●
Mercurial —*see* condition
Mercurialism —*see* subcategory T56.1
MERRF syndrome (myoclonic epilepsy
    associated with ragged-red fiber) E88.42
Merkel cell tumor —*see* Carcinoma, Merkel cell
Merocele —*see* Hernia, femoral
Meromelia
lower limb —*see* Defect, reduction, lower
    limb
    intercalary
        femur —*see* Defect, reduction, lower
            limb, specified type NEC
        tibiofibular (complete) (incomplete) —
            see Defect, reduction, lower limb
upper limb —*see* Defect, reduction, upper
    limb
    intercalary, humeral, radioulnar —*see*
        Agenesis, arm, with hand present

M

Merzbacher-Pelizaeus disease E75.29
Mesaortitis —see Aortitis
Mesarteritis —see Arteritis
Mesencephalitis —see Encephalitis
Mesenchymoma —see also Neoplasm,
    connective tissue, uncertain behavior
  benign —see Neoplasm, connective tissue,
    benign
  malignant —see Neoplasm, connective tissue,
    malignant
Mesenteritis
  retractile K65.4
  sclerosing K65.4
Mesentery, mesenteric —see condition
Mesiodens, mesiodentes K00.1
Mesio-occlusion M26.213
Mesocolon —see condition
Mesonephroma (malignant) —see Neoplasm,
    malignant, by site
  benign —see Neoplasm, benign, by site
Mesophlebitis —see Phlebitis
Mesostromal dysgenesia Q13.89
Mesothelioma (malignant) C45.9
  benign
    mesentery D19.1
    mesocolon D19.1
    omentum D19.1
    peritoneum D19.1
    pleura D19.0
    specified site NEC D19.7
    unspecified site D19.9
  biphasic C45.9
    benign
      mesentery D19.1
      mesocolon D19.1
      omentum D19.1
      peritoneum D19.1
      pleura D19.0
      specified site NEC D19.7
      unspecified site D19.9
  cystic D48.4
  epithelioid C45.9
    benign
      mesentery D19.1
      mesocolon D19.1
      omentum D19.1
      peritoneum D19.1
      pleura D19.0
      specified site NEC D19.7
      unspecified site D19.9
  fibrous C45.9
    benign
      mesentery D19.1
      mesocolon D19.1
      omentum D19.1
      peritoneum D19.1
      pleura D19.0
      specified site NEC D19.7
      unspecified site D19.9
  site classification
    liver C45.7
    lung C45.7
    mediastinum C45.7
    mesentery C45.1
    mesocolon C45.1
    omentum C45.1
    pericardium C45.2
    peritoneum C45.1
    pleura C45.0
      parietal C45.0
    retroperitoneum C45.7
    specified site NEC C45.7
    unspecified site C45.9
Metabolic syndrome E88.81
Metagonimiasis B66.8
Metagonimus infestation (intestine)
    B66.8
Metal
  pigmentation L81.8
  polisher's disease J62.8
Metamorphopsia H53.15

Metaplasia
  apocrine (breast) —see Dysplasia, mammary,
    specified type NEC
  cervix (squamous) —see Dysplasia, cervix
  endometrium (squamous) (uterus) N85.8
  esophagus K22.7-●
  gastric intestinal K31.A0
    with dysplasia K31.A29
      high grade K31.A22
      low grade K31.A21
    indefinite for dysplasia K31.A0
    without dysplasia K31.A19
      involving
        antrum K31.A11
        body (corpus) K31.A12
        cardia K31.A14
        fundus K31.A13
        multiple sites K31.A15
  kidney (pelvis) (squamous) N28.89
  myelogenous D73.1
  myeloid (agnogenic) (megakaryocytic) D73.1
  spleen D73.1
  squamous cell, bladder N32.89
Metastasis, metastatic
  abscess —see Abscess
  calcification E83.59
  cancer
    from specified site —see Neoplasm,
      malignant, by site
    to specified site —see Neoplasm, secondary,
      by site
  deposits (in) —see Neoplasm, secondary, by site
  disease (see also Neoplasm, secondary, by site)
    C79.9
  spread (to) —see Neoplasm, secondary, by site
Metastrongyliasis B83.8
Metatarsalgia M77.4-●
  anterior G57.6-●
  Morton's G57.6-●
Metatarsus, metatarsal —see also condition
  adductus, congenital Q66.22-●
  valgus (abductus), congenital Q66.6
  varus (congenital) Q66.22-●
  primus Q66.21-●
Methadone use —see Use, opioid
Methemoglobinemia D74.9
  acquired (with sulfhemoglobinemia) D74.8
  congenital D74.0
  enzymatic (congenital) D74.0
  Hb M disease D74.0
  hereditary D74.0
  toxic D74.8
Methemoglobinuria —see Hemoglobinuria
Methioninemia E72.19
Methylmalonic acidemia E71.120
Metritis (catarrhal) (hemorrhagic) (septic)
    (suppurative) —see also Endometritis
  cervical —see Cervicitis
Metropathia hemorrhagica N93.8
Metroperitonitis —see Peritonitis, pelvic, female
Metrorrhagia N92.1
  climacteric N92.4
  menopausal N92.4
  perimenopausal N92.4
  postpartum NEC (atonic) (following delivery
    of placenta) O72.1
    delayed or secondary O72.2
  preclimacteric or premenopausal N92.4
  psychogenic F45.8
Metrorrhexis —see Rupture, uterus
Metrosalpingitis N70.91
Metrostaxis N93.8
Metrovaginitis —see Endometritis
Meyer-Schwickerath and Weyers syndrome
    Q87.0
Meynert's amentia (nonalcoholic) F04
  alcoholic F10.96
    with dependence F10.26
Mibelli's disease (porokeratosis) Q82.8
Mice, joint —see Loose, body, joint
  knee M23.4
Micrencephalon, micrencephaly Q02

Microalbuminuria R80.9
Microaneurysm, retinal —see also Disorder,
    retina, microaneurysms
  diabetic —see E08-E13 with .31
Microangiopathy (peripheral) I73.9
  thrombotic M31.10
    hematopoietic stem cell transplantation-
      associated [HSCT-TMA] M31.10
Microcalcifications, breast R92.0
Microcephalus, microcephalic, microcephaly
    Q02
  due to toxoplasmosis (congenital) P37.1
Microcheilia Q18.7
Microcolon (congenital) Q43.8
Microcornea (congenital) Q13.4
Microcytic —see condition D57.40
Microdeletions NEC Q93.88
Microdontia K00.2
Microdrepanocytosis D57.40
  with
    acute chest syndrome D57.411
    cerebral vascular involvement D57.413
    crisis (painful) D57.419
      with specified complication NEC D57.418
    splenic sequestration D57.412
    vasoocclusive pain D57.419
Microembolism
  atherothrombotic —see Atheroembolism
  retinal —see Occlusion, artery, retina
Microencephalon Q02
Microfilaria streptocerca infestation —see
    Onchocerciasis
Microgastria (congenital) Q40.2
Microgenia M26.06
Microgenitalia, congenital
  female Q52.8
  male Q55.8
Microglioma —see Lymphoma, non-Hodgkin,
    specified NEC
Microglossia (congenital) Q38.3
Micrognathia, micrognathism (congenital)
    (mandibular) (maxillary) M26.09
Microgyria (congenital) Q04.3
Microinfarct of heart —see Insufficiency, coronary
Microlentia (congenital) Q12.8
Microlithiasis, alveolar, pulmonary J84.02
Micromastia N64.82
Micromyelia (congenital) Q06.8
Micropenis Q55.62
Microphakia (congenital) Q12.8
Microphthalmos, microphthalmia (congenital)
    Q11.2
  due to toxoplasmosis P37.1
Micropsia H53.15
Microscopic polyangiitis (polyarteritis) M31.7
Microsporidiosis B60.8
  intestinal A07.8
Microsporon furfur infestation B36.0
Microsporosis —see also Dermatophytosis
  nigra B36.1
Microstomia (congenital) Q18.5
Microtia (congenital) (external ear) Q17.2
Microtropia H50.40
Microvillus inclusion disease (MVD) (MVID)
    Q43.8
Micturition
  disorder NEC —see also Difficulty, micturition
    R39.198
    psychogenic F45.8
  frequency R35.0
    psychogenic F45.8
  hesitancy R39.11
  incomplete emptying R39.14
  nocturnal R35.1
  painful R30.9
    dysuria R30.0
    psychogenic F45.8
    tenesmus R30.1
  poor stream R39.12
  position dependent R39.192
  split stream R39.13
  straining R39.16
  urgency R39.15

▶ New   ⇒ Revised   ~~deleted~~ Deleted   ● Use Additional Character(s)

Mid plane —*see* condition
Middle
　ear —*see* condition
　lobe (right) syndrome J98.19
Miescher's elastoma L87.2
Mietens' syndrome Q87.2
Migraine (idiopathic) G43.909
　with refractory migraine G43.919
　　with status migrainosus G43.911
　　without status migrainosus G43.919
　with aura (acute-onset) (prolonged) (typical)
　　　(without headache) G43.109
　　with refractory migraine G43.119
　　　with status migrainosus G43.111
　　　without status migrainosus G43.119
　　intractable G43.119
　　　with status migrainosus G43.111
　　　without status migrainosus G43.119
　　not intractable G43.109
　　　with status migrainosus G43.101
　　　without status migrainosus G43.109
　　persistent G43.509
　　　with cerebral infarction G43.609
　　　　with refractory migraine G43.619
　　　　　with status migrainosus G43.611
　　　　　without status migrainosus G43.619
　　　　intractable G43.619
　　　　　with status migrainosus G43.611
　　　　　without status migrainosus G43.619
　　　　not intractable G43.609
　　　　　with status migrainosus G43.601
　　　　　without status migrainosus G43.609
　　　　without refractory migraine G43.609
　　　　　with status migrainosus G43.601
　　　　　without status migrainosus G43.609
　　　without cerebral infarction G43.509
　　　　with refractory migraine G43.519
　　　　　with status migrainosus G43.511
　　　　　without status migrainosus G43.519
　　　　intractable G43.519
　　　　　with status migrainosus G43.511
　　　　　without status migrainosus G43.519
　　　　not intractable G43.509
　　　　　with status migrainosus G43.501
　　　　　without status migrainosus G43.509
　　　　without refractory migraine G43.509
　　　　　with status migrainosus G43.501
　　　　　without status migrainosus G43.509
　　without mention of refractory migraine
　　　　G43.109
　　　with status migrainosus G43.101
　　　without status migrainosus G43.109
　abdominal G43.D0
　　with refractory migraine G43.D1
　　intractable G43.D1
　　not intractable G43.D0
　　without refractory migraine G43.D0
　basilar —*see* Migraine, with aura
　classical —*see* Migraine, with aura
　common —*see* Migraine, without aura
　complicated G43.109
　equivalents —*see* Migraine, with aura
　familiar —*see* Migraine, hemiplegic
　hemiplegic G43.409
　　with refractory migraine G43.419
　　　with status migrainosus G43.411
　　　without status migrainosus G43.419
　　intractable G43.419
　　　with status migrainosus G43.411
　　　without status migrainosus G43.419
　　not intractable G43.409
　　　with status migrainosus G43.401
　　　without status migrainosus G43.409
　　without refractory migraine G43.409
　　　with status migrainosus G43.401
　　　without status migrainosus G43.409
　intractable G43.919
　　with status migrainosus G43.911
　　without status migrainosus G43.919
　menstrual G43.829
　　with refractory migraine G43.839
　　　with status migrainosus G43.831
　　　without status migrainosus G43.839

Migraine (*Continued*)
　menstrual (*Continued*)
　　intractable G43.839
　　　with status migrainosus G43.831
　　　without status migrainosus G43.839
　　not intractable G43.829
　　　with status migrainosus G43.821
　　　without status migrainosus G43.829
　　without refractory migraine G43.829
　　　with status migrainosus G43.821
　　　without status migrainosus G43.829
　menstrually related —*see* Migraine, menstrual
　not intractable G43.909
　　with status migrainosus G43.901
　　without status migrainosus G43.919
　ophthalmoplegic G43.B0
　　with refractory migraine G43.B1
　　intractable G43.B1
　　not intractable G43.B0
　　　without refractory migraine G43.B0
　persistent aura (with, without) cerebral
　　　infarction —*see* Migraine, with aura,
　　　persistent
　preceded or accompanied by transient focal
　　　neurological phenomena —*see* Migraine,
　　　with aura
　pre-menstrual —*see* Migraine, menstrual
　pure menstrual —*see* Migraine, menstrual
　retinal —*see* Migraine, with aura
　specified NEC G43.809
　　intractable G43.819
　　　with status migrainosus G43.811
　　　without status migrainosus G43.819
　　not intractable G43.809
　　　with status migrainosus G43.801
　　　without status migrainosus G43.809
　sporadic —*see* Migraine, hemiplegic
　transformed —*see* Migraine, without aura,
　　　chronic
　triggered seizures —*see* Migraine, with aura
　without aura G43.009
　　with refractory migraine G43.019
　　　with status migrainosus G43.011
　　　without status migrainosus G43.019
　　chronic G43.709
　　　with refractory migraine G43.719
　　　　with status migrainosus G43.711
　　　　without status migrainosus G43.719
　　　intractable
　　　　with status migrainosus G43.711
　　　　without status migrainosus G43.719
　　　not intractable
　　　　with status migrainosus G43.701
　　　　without status migrainosus G43.709
　　　without refractory migraine G43.709
　　　　with status migrainosus G43.701
　　　　without status migrainosus G43.709
　　intractable
　　　with status migrainosus G43.011
　　　without status migrainosus G43.019
　　not intractable
　　　with status migrainosus G43.001
　　　without status migrainosus G43.009
　　without mention of refractory migraine
　　　　G43.009
　　　with status migrainosus G43.001
　　　without status migrainosus G43.009
　　without refractory migraine G43.909
　　　with status migrainosus G43.901
➠　　　without status migrainosus G43.909
Migrant, social Z59.00
Migration, anxiety concerning Z60.3
Migratory, migrating —*see also* condition
　person Z59.00
　testis Q55.29
Mikity-Wilson disease or syndrome P27.0
Mikulicz' disease or syndrome K11.8
Miliaria L74.3
　alba L74.1
　apocrine L75.2
　crystallina L74.1
　profunda L74.2
　rubra L74.0

Miliaria (*Continued*)
　tropicalis L74.2
Miliary —*see* condition
Milium L72.0
　colloid L57.8
Milk
　crust L21.0
　excessive secretion O92.6
　poisoning —*see* Poisoning, food, noxious
　retention O92.79
　sickness —*see* Poisoning, food, noxious
　spots I31.0
Milk-alkali disease or syndrome E83.52
Milk-leg (deep vessels) (nonpuerperal) —*see*
　　Embolism, vein, lower extremity
　complicating pregnancy O22.3-●
　puerperal, postpartum, childbirth O87.1
Milkman's disease or syndrome M83.8
Milky urine —*see* Chyluria
Millard-Gubler (-Foville) paralysis or
　　syndrome G46.3
Millar's asthma J38.5
Miller-Fisher syndrome G61.0
Mills' disease —*see* Hemiplegia
Millstone maker's pneumoconiosis J62.8
Milroy's disease (chronic hereditary edema)
　　Q82.0
Minamata disease T56.1-●
Miners' asthma or lung J60
Minkowski-Chauffard syndrome —*see*
　　Spherocytosis
Minor —*see* condition
Minor's disease (hematomyelia) G95.19
Minot's disease (hemorrhagic disease),
　　newborn P53
➠Minot-von Willebrand-Jurgens disease or
　　syndrome (angiohemophilia) —*see* Disease,
　　von Willebrand
Minus (and plus) hand (intrinsic) —*see* Deformity,
　　limb, specified type NEC, forearm
Miosis (pupil) H57.03
Mirizzi's syndrome (hepatic duct stenosis) K83.1
Mirror writing F81.0
MIS-A M35.81
MIS-C M35.81
Misadventure (of) (prophylactic) (therapeutic) —
　　see also Complications T88.9
　administration of insulin (by accident) —*see*
　　　subcategory T38.3
　infusion —*see* Complications, infusion
　local applications (of fomentations, plasters,
　　　etc.) T88.9
　　burn or scald —*see* Burn
　　specified NEC T88.8
　medical care (early) (late) T88.9
　　adverse effect of drugs or chemicals —*see*
　　　Table of Drugs and Chemicals
　medical care (early) (late)
　　burn or scald —*see* Burn
　　specified NEC T88.8
　specified NEC T88.8
　surgical procedure (early) (late) —*see*
　　　Complications, surgical procedure
　transfusion —*see* Complications, transfusion
　vaccination or other immunological
　　　procedure —*see* Complications,
　　　vaccination
Miscarriage O03.9
Misdirection, aqueous H40.83-●
Misperception, sleep state F51.02
Misplaced, misplacement
　ear Q17.4
　kidney (acquired) N28.89
　　congenital Q63.2
　organ or site, congenital NEC —*see*
　　　Malposition, congenital
Missed
　abortion O02.1
　delivery O36.4
Missing —*see also* Absence
　string of intrauterine contraceptive device
　　　T83.32

Misuse of drugs F19.99
Mitchell's disease (erythromelalgia) I73.81
Mite(s) (infestation) B88.9
  diarrhea B88.0
  grain (itch) B88.0
  hair follicle (itch) B88.0
  in sputum B88.0
Mitral —see condition
Mittelschmerz N94.0
Mixed —see condition
MMN (multifocal motor neuropathy) G61.82
MNGIE (Mitochondrial Neurogastrointestinal
    Encephalopathy) syndrome E88.49
Mobile, mobility
  cecum Q43.3
  excessive —see Hypermobility
  gallbladder, congenital Q44.1
  kidney N28.89
  organ or site, congenital NEC —see
    Malposition, congenital
Mobitz heart block (atrioventricular) I44.1
Moebius, Möbius
  disease (ophthalmoplegic migraine) —see
    Migraine, ophthalmoplegic
  syndrome Q87.0
    congenital oculofacial paralysis (with other
      anomalies) Q87.0
    ophthalmoplegic migraine —see Migraine,
      ophthalmoplegic
Moeller's glossitis K14.0
Mohr's syndrome (Types I and II) Q87.0
Mola destruens D39.2
Molar pregnancy O02.0
Molarization of premolars K00.2
Molding, head (during birth) - omit code
Mole (pigmented) —see also Nevus
  blood O02.0
  Breus' O02.0
  cancerous —see Melanoma
  carneous O02.0
  destructive D39.2
  fleshy O02.0
  hydatid, hydatidiform (benign) (complicating
    pregnancy) (delivered) (undelivered)
    O01.9
    classical O01.0
    complete O01.0
    incomplete O01.1
    invasive D39.2
    malignant D39.2
    partial O01.1
  intrauterine O02.0
  invasive (hydatidiform) D39.2
  malignant
    meaning
      malignant hydatidiform mole D39.2
      melanoma —see Melanoma
  nonhydatidiform O02.0
  nonpigmented —see Nevus
  pregnancy NEC O02.0
  skin —see Nevus
  tubal O00.10-
    with intrauterine pregnancy O00.11-
  vesicular —see Mole, hydatidiform
Molimen, molimina (menstrual) N94.3
Molluscum contagiosum (epitheliale) B08.1
Mönckeberg's arteriosclerosis, disease, or
    sclerosis —see Arteriosclerosis, extremities
Mondini's malformation (cochlea) Q16.5
Mondor's disease I80.8
Monge's disease T70.29
Monilethrix (congenital) Q84.1
Moniliasis —see also Candidiasis B37.9
  neonatal P37.5
Monitoring (encounter for)
  therapeutic drug level Z51.81
Monkey malaria B53.1
Monkeypox B04
Monoarthritis M13.10
  ankle M13.17-•
  elbow M13.12-•

Monoarthritis (Continued)
  foot joint M13.17-•
  hand joint M13.14-•
  hip M13.15-•
  knee M13.16-•
  shoulder M13.11-•
  wrist M13.13-•
Monoblastic —see condition
Monochromat (ism), monochromatopsia
    (acquired) (congenital) H53.51
Monocytic —see condition
Monocytopenia D72.818
Monocytosis (symptomatic) D72.821
Monomania —see Psychosis
Mononeuritis G58.9
  cranial nerve —see Disorder, nerve,
    cranial
  femoral nerve G57.2-•
  lateral
    cutaneous nerve of thigh G57.1-•
    popliteal nerve G57.3-•
  lower limb G57.9-•
    specified nerve NEC G57.8-•
  medial popliteal nerve G57.4-•
  median nerve G56.1-•
  multiplex G58.7
  plantar nerve G57.6-•
  posterior tibial nerve G57.5-•
  radial nerve G56.3-•
  sciatic nerve G57.0-•
  specified NEC G58.8
  tibial nerve G57.4-•
  ulnar nerve G56.2-•
  upper limb G56.9-•
    specified nerve NEC G56.8-•
  vestibular —see subcategory H93.3
Mononeuropathy G58.9
  carpal tunnel syndrome —see Syndrome,
    carpal tunnel
  diabetic NEC —see E08-E13 with .41
  femoral nerve —see Lesion, nerve, femoral
  ilioinguinal nerve G57.8-•
  in diseases classified elsewhere —see category
    G59
  intercostal G58.0
  lower limb G57.9-•
    causalgia —see Causalgia, lower limb
    femoral nerve —see Lesion, nerve,
      femoral
    meralgia paresthetica G57.1-•
    plantar nerve —see Lesion, nerve, plantar
    popliteal nerve —see Lesion, nerve,
      popliteal
    sciatic nerve —see Lesion, nerve, sciatic
    specified NEC G57.8-•
    tarsal tunnel syndrome —see Syndrome,
      tarsal tunnel
  median nerve —see Lesion, nerve, median
  multiplex G58.7
  obturator nerve G57.8-•
  popliteal nerve —see Lesion, nerve, popliteal
  radial nerve —see Lesion, nerve, radial
  saphenous nerve G57.8-•
  specified NEC G58.8
  tarsal tunnel syndrome —see Syndrome,
    tarsal tunnel
  tuberculous A17.83
  ulnar nerve —see Lesion, nerve, ulnar
  upper limb G56.9-•
    carpal tunnel syndrome —see Syndrome,
      carpal tunnel
    causalgia —see Causalgia
    median nerve —see Lesion, nerve, median
    radial nerve —see Lesion, nerve, radial
    specified site NEC G56.8-•
    ulnar nerve —see Lesion, nerve, ulnar
Mononucleosis, infectious B27.90
  with
    complication NEC B27.99
    meningitis B27.92
    polyneuropathy B27.91

Mononucleosis, infectious (Continued)
  cytomegaloviral B27.10
    with
      complication NEC B27.19
      meningitis B27.12
      polyneuropathy B27.11
  Epstein-Barr (virus) B27.00
    with
      complication NEC B27.09
      meningitis B27.02
      polyneuropathy B27.01
  gammaherpesviral B27.00
    with
      complication NEC B27.09
      meningitis B27.02
      polyneuropathy B27.01
  specified NEC B27.80
    with
      complication NEC B27.89
      meningitis B27.82
      polyneuropathy B27.81
Monoplegia G83.3-•
  congenital (cerebral) G80.8
    spastic G80.1
  embolic (current episode) I63.4-•
  following
    cerebrovascular disease
      cerebral infarction
        lower limb I69.34-•
        upper limb I69.33-•
      intracerebral hemorrhage
        lower limb I69.14-•
        upper limb I69.13-•
      lower limb I69.94-•
      nontraumatic intracranial hemorrhage
        NEC
        lower limb I69.24-•
        upper limb I69.23-•
      specified disease NEC
        lower limb I69.84-•
        upper limb I69.83-•
      stroke NOS
        lower limb I69.34-•
        upper limb I69.33-•
      subarachnoid hemorrhage
        lower limb I69.04-•
        upper limb I69.03-•
      upper limb I69.93-•
  hysterical (transient) F44.4
  lower limb G83.1-•
  psychogenic (conversion reaction) F44.4
  thrombotic (current episode) I63.3-•
  transient R29.818
  upper limb G83.2-•
Monorchism, monorchidism Q55.0
Monosomy —see also Deletion, chromosome
    Q93.9
  specified NEC Q93.89
  whole chromosome
    meiotic nondisjunction Q93.0
    mitotic nondisjunction Q93.1
    mosaicism Q93.1
  X Q96.9
Monster, monstrosity (single) Q89.7
  acephalic Q00.0
  twin Q89.4
Monteggia's fracture (-dislocation) S52.27-•
Mooren's ulcer (cornea) —see Ulcer, cornea,
    Mooren's
Moore's syndrome —see Epilepsy, specified
    NEC
Mooser-Neill reaction A75.2
Mooser's bodies A75.2
Morbidity not stated or unknown R69
Morbilli —see Measles
Morbus —see also Disease
  angelicus, anglorum E55.0
  Beigel B36.2
  caducus —see Epilepsy
  celiacus K90.0
  comitialis —see Epilepsy

▶ New   ⇒ Revised   ~~deleted~~ Deleted   • Use Additional Character(s)

Morbus *(Continued)*
  cordis —*see also* Disease, heart I51.9
    valvulorum —*see* Endocarditis
  coxae senilis M16.9
    tuberculous A18.02
  hemorrhagicus neonatorum P53
  maculosus neonatorum P54.5
Morel (-Stewart)(-Morgagni) **syndrome**
  M85.2
Morel-Kraepelin disease —*see* Schizophrenia
Morel-Moore syndrome M85.2
Morgagni's
  cyst, organ, hydatid, or appendage
    female Q50.5
    male (epididymal) Q55.4
      testicular Q55.29
  syndrome M85.2
Morgagni-Stewart-Morel syndrome M85.2
Morgagni-Stokes-Adams syndrome I45.9
Morgagni-Turner (-Albright) syndrome
  Q96.9
Moria F07.0
Moron (I.Q. 50-69) F70
Morphea L94.0
Morphinism (without remission) F11.20
  with remission F11.21
Morphinomania (without remission) F11.20
  with remission F11.21
Morquio (-Ullrich)(-Brailsford) **disease or**
  syndrome —*see* Mucopolysaccharidosis
Mortification (dry) (moist) —*see* Gangrene
Morton's metatarsalgia (neuralgia)(neuroma)
  (syndrome) G57.6
Morvan's disease or syndrome G60.8
Mosaicism, mosaic (autosomal) (chromosomal)
  45,X/46,XX Q96.3
  45,X/other cell lines NEC with abnormal sex
    chromosome Q96.4
  sex chromosome
    female Q97.8
    lines with various numbers of
      X chromosomes Q97.2
    male Q98.7
  XY Q96.3
Moschowitz' disease M31.19
Mother yaw A66.0
Motion sickness (from travel, any vehicle)
  (from roundabouts or swings) T75.3
Mottled, mottling, teeth (enamel) (endemic)
  (nonendemic) K00.3
Mounier-Kuhn syndrome Q32.4
  with bronchiectasis J47.9
    exacerbation (acute) J47.1
    lower respiratory infection J47.0
  acquired J98.09
    with bronchiectasis J47.9
      with
        exacerbation (acute) J47.1
        lower respiratory infection J47.0
Mountain
  sickness T70.29
    with polycythemia , acquired (acute)
      D75.1
  tick fever A93.2
Mouse, joint —*see* Loose, body, joint
  knee M23.4-●
Mouth —*see* condition
Movable
  coccyx —*see* subcategory M53.2
  kidney N28.89
    congenital Q63.8
  spleen D73.89
Movements, dystonic R25.8
Moyamoya disease I67.5
MRSA (Methicillin resistant Staphylococcus
  aureus)
  infection A49.02
    as the cause of diseases classified
      elsewhere B95.62
  sepsis A41.02
MSD (multiple sulfatase deficiency) E75.26

MSSA (Methicillin susceptible Staphylococcus
  aureus)
  infection A49.01
    as the cause of diseases classified
      elsewhere B95.61
  sepsis A41.01
Mucha-Habermann disease L41.0
Mucinosis (cutaneous) (focal) (papular)
  (reticular erythematous) (skin) L98.5
  oral K13.79
Mucocele
  appendix K38.8
  buccal cavity K13.79
  gallbladder K82.1
  lacrimal sac, chronic H04.43-●
  nasal sinus J34.1
  nose J34.1
  salivary gland (any) K11.6
  sinus (accessory) (nasal) J34.1
  turbinate (bone) (middle) (nasal) J34.1
  uterus N85.8
Mucolipidosis
  I E77.1
  II, III E77.0
  IV E75.11
Mucopolysaccharidosis E76.3
  beta-gluduronidase deficiency E76.29
  cardiopathy E76.3 *[I52]*
  Hunter's syndrome E76.1
  Hurler's syndrome E76.01
  Hurler-Scheie syndrome E76.02
  Maroteaux-Lamy syndrome E76.29
  Morquio syndrome E76.219
    A E76.210
    B E76.211
    classic E76.210
  Sanfilippo syndrome E76.22
  Scheie's syndrome E76.03
  specified NEC E76.29
  type
    I
      Hurler's syndrome E76.01
      Hurler-Scheie syndrome E76.02
      Scheie's syndrome E76.03
    II E76.1
    III E76.22
    IV E76.219
    IVA E76.210
    IVB E76.211
    VI E76.29
    VII E76.29
Mucormycosis B46.5
  cutaneous B46.3
  disseminated B46.4
  gastrointestinal B46.2
  generalized B46.4
  pulmonary B46.0
  rhinocerebral B46.1
  skin B46.3
  subcutaneous B46.3
Mucositis (ulcerative) K12.30
  due to drugs NEC K12.32
  gastrointestinal K92.81
  mouth (oral) (oropharyngeal) K12.30
    due to antineoplastic therapy
      K12.31
    due to drugs NEC K12.32
    due to radiation K12.33
    specified NEC K12.39
    viral K12.39
  nasal J34.81
  oral cavity —*see* Mucositis, mouth
  oral soft tissues —*see* Mucositis, mouth
  vagina and vulva N76.81
Mucositis necroticans agranulocytica —*see*
  Agranulocytosis
Mucous —*see also* condition
  patches (syphilitic) A51.39
    congenital A50.07
Mucoviscidosis E84.9
  with meconium obstruction E84.11

Mucus
  asphyxia or suffocation —*see* Asphyxia, mucus
  in stool R19.5
  plug —*see* Asphyxia, mucus
Muguet B37.0
Mulberry molars (congenital syphilis) A50.52
Müllerian mixed tumor
  specified site —*see* Neoplasm, malignant, by
    site
  unspecified site C54.9
Multicystic kidney (development) Q61.4
Multiparity (grand) Z64.1
  affecting management of pregnancy, labor
    and delivery (supervision only)
    O09.4-●
  requiring contraceptive management —*see*
    Contraception
Multipartita placenta O43.19-●
Multiple, multiplex —*see also* condition
  digits (congenital) Q69.9
  endocrine neoplasia —*see* Neoplasia,
    endocrine, multiple [MEN}
  personality F44.81
Multisystem inflammatory syndrome (in
  adults) (in children) M35.81
Mumps B26.9
  arthritis B26.85
  complication NEC B26.89
  encephalitis B26.2
  hepatitis B26.81
  meningitis (aseptic) B26.1
  meningoencephalitis B26.2
  myocarditis B26.82
  oophoritis B26.89
  orchitis B26.0
  pancreatitis B26.3
  polyneuropathy B26.84
Mumu —*see also* Infestation, filarial B74.9 *[N51]*
Münchhausen's syndrome —*see* Disorder,
  factitious
Münchmeyer's syndrome —*see* Myositis,
  ossificans, progressiva
Mural —*see* condition
Murmur (cardiac) (heart) (organic) R01.1
  abdominal R19.15
  aortic (valve) —*see* Endocarditis, aortic
  benign R01.0
  diastolic —*see* Endocarditis
  Flint I35.1
  functional R01.0
  Graham Steell I37.1
  innocent R01.0
  mitral (valve) —*see* Insufficiency, mitral
  nonorganic R01.0
  presystolic, mitral —*see* Insufficiency, mitral
  pulmonic (valve) I37.8
  systolic R01.1
  tricuspid (valve) I07.9
  valvular —*see* Endocarditis
Murri's disease (intermittent hemoglobinuria)
  D59.6
Muscle, muscular —*see also* condition
  carnitine (palmityltransferase) deficiency
    E71.314
Musculoneuralgia —*see* Neuralgia
Mushroom-workers' (pickers') **disease or lung**
  J67.5
Mushrooming hip —*see* Derangement, joint,
  specified NEC, hip
Mutation(s)
  factor V Leiden D68.51
  surfactant, of lung J84.83
  prothrombin gene D68.52
Mutism —*see also* Aphasia
  deaf (acquired) (congenital) NEC H91.3
  elective (adjustment reaction) (childhood)
    F94.0
  hysterical F44.4
  selective (childhood) F94.0
MVD (microvillus inclusion disease) Q43.8
MVID (microvillus inclusion disease) Q43.8

M

Myalgia M79.10
  auxiliary muscles, head and neck M79.12
  epidemic (cervical) B33.0
  mastication muscle M79.11
  site specified NEC M79.18
  traumatic NEC T14.8
Myasthenia G70.9
  congenital G70.2
  cordis —see Failure, heart
  developmental G70.2
  gravis G70.00
    with exacerbation (acute) G70.01
    in crisis G70.01
    neonatal, transient P94.0
    pseudoparalytica G70.00
      with exacerbation (acute) G70.01
      in crisis G70.01
  stomach, psychogenic F45.8
  syndrome
    in
      diabetes mellitus —see E08-E13 with .44
      neoplastic disease —see also Neoplasm
        D49.9 [G73.3]
      pernicious anemia D51.0 [G73.3]
      thyrotoxicosis E05.90 [G73.3]
        with thyroid storm E05.91 [G73.3]
Myasthenic M62.81
Mycelium infection B49
Mycetismus —see Poisoning, food, noxious,
  mushroom
Mycetoma B47.9
  actinomycotic B47.1
  bone (mycotic) B47.9 [M90.80]
  eumycotic B47.0
  foot B47.9
    actinomycotic B47.1
    mycotic B47.0
  madurae NEC B47.9
    mycotic B47.0
  maduromycotic B47.0
  mycotic B47.0
  nocardial B47.1
Mycobacteriosis —see Mycobacterium
Mycobacterium, mycobacterial (infection)
    A31.9
  anonymous A31.9
  atypical A31.9
    cutaneous A31.1
    pulmonary A31.0
      tuberculous —see Tuberculosis,
        pulmonary
    specified site NEC A31.8
  avium (intracellulare complex) A31.0
  balnei A31.1
  Battey A31.0
  chelonei A31.8
  cutaneous A31.1
  extrapulmonary systemic A31.8
  fortuitum A31.8
  intracellulare (Battey bacillus) A31.0
  kakaferifu A31.8
  kansasii (yellow bacillus) A31.0
  kasongo A31.8
  leprae —see also Leprosy A30.9
  luciflavum A31.1
  marinum (M. balnei) A31.1
  nonspecific —see Mycobacterium, atypical
  pulmonary (atypical) A31.0
    tuberculous —see Tuberculosis, pulmonary
  scrofulaceum A31.8
  simiae A31.8
  systemic, extrapulmonary A31.8
  szulgai A31.8
  terrae A31.8
  triviale A31.8
  tuberculosis (human, bovine) —see
    Tuberculosis
  ulcerans A31.1
  xenopi A31.8
Mycoplasma (M.) pneumoniae, as cause of
  disease classified elsewhere B96.0

Mycosis, mycotic B49
  cutaneous NEC B36.9
  ear B36.9
    in
      aspergillosis B44.89
      candidiasis B37.84
      moniliasis B37.84
  fungoides (extranodal) (solid organ) C84.0-●
  mouth B37.0
  nails B35.1
  opportunistic B48.8
  skin NEC B36.9
  specified NEC B48.8
  stomatitis B37.0
▶vagina, vaginitis (candidal) (acute) B37.31
  ▶chronic (recurrent) B37.32
Mydriasis (pupil) H57.04
Myelatelia Q06.1
Myelinolysis, pontine, central G37.2
Myelitis (acute) (ascending) (childhood)
    (chronic) (descending) (diffuse)
    (disseminated) (idiopathic) (pressure)
    (progressive) (spinal cord) (subacute) —see
    also Encephalitis G04.91
  flaccid G04.82
  herpes simplex B00.82
  herpes zoster B02.24
  in diseases classified elsewhere G05.4
  necrotizing, subacute G37.4
  optic neuritis in G36.0
  postchickenpox B01.12
  postherpetic B02.24
  postimmunization G04.02
  postinfectious NEC G04.89
  postvaccinal G04.02
  specified NEC G04.89
  syphilitic (transverse) A52.14
  toxic G92.9
  transverse (in demyelinating diseases of
    central nervous system) G37.3
  tuberculous A17.82
  varicella B01.12
Myeloblastic —see condition
Myeloblastoma
  granular cell —see also Neoplasm, connective
    tissue
    malignant —see Neoplasm, connective
      tissue, malignant
    tongue D10.1
Myelocele —see Spina bifida
Myelocystocele —see Spina bifida
Myelocytic —see condition
Myelodysplasia D46.9
  specified NEC D46.Z
  spinal cord (congenital) Q06.1
Myelodysplastic syndrome (see also Syndrome,
  myelodysplastic) D46.9
  with
    5q deletion D46.C
    isolated del (5q) chromosomal abnormality
      C46.C
  specified NEC D46.Z
Myeloencephalitis —see Encephalitis
Myelofibrosis D75.81
  with myeloid metaplasia D47.4
  acute C94.4-●
  idiopathic (chronic) D47.4
  primary D47.1
  secondary D75.81
    in myeloproliferative disease D47.4
Myelogenous —see condition
Myeloid —see condition
Myelokathexis D70.9
Myeloleukodystrophy E75.29
Myelolipoma —see Lipoma
Myeloma (multiple) C90.0-●
  monostotic C90.3
    plasma cell C90.0-●
  plasma cell C90.0-●
  solitary —see also Plasmacytoma, solitary
    C90.3-●

Myelomalacia G95.89
Myelomatosis C90.0-●
Myelomeningitis —see Meningoencephalitis
Myelomeningocele (spinal cord) —see Spina
  bifida
Myelo-osteo-musculodysplasia hereditaria
  Q79.8
Myelopathic
  anemia D64.89
  muscle atrophy —see Atrophy, muscle,
    spinal
  pain syndrome G89.0
Myelopathy (spinal cord) G95.9
  drug-induced G95.89
  in (due to)
    degeneration or displacement,
      intervertebral disc NEC —see
      Disorder, disc, with, myelopathy
    infection —see Encephalitis
    intervertebral disc disorder —see also
      Disorder, disc, with, myelopathy
    mercury —see subcategory T56.1
    neoplastic disease —see also Neoplasm
      D49.9 [G99.2]
    pernicious anemia D51.0 [G99.2]
    spondylosis —see Spondylosis, with
      myelopathy NEC
  necrotic (subacute) (vascular) G95.19
  radiation-induced G95.89
  spondylogenic NEC —see Spondylosis, with
    myelopathy NEC
  toxic G95.89
  transverse, acute G37.3
  vascular G95.19
  vitamin B12 E53.8 [G32.0]
Myelophthisis D61.82
Myeloradiculitis G04.91
Myeloradiculodysplasia (spinal)
  Q06.1
Myelosarcoma C92.3-●
Myelosclerosis D75.89
  with myeloid metaplasia D47.4
  disseminated, of nervous system
    G35
  megakaryocytic D47.4
    with myeloid metaplasia
      D47.4
Myelosis
  acute C92.0-●
  aleukemic C92.9-●
  chronic D47.1
  erythremic (acute) C94.0-●
  megakaryocytic C94.2-●
  nonleukemic D72.828
  subacute C92.9-●
Myiasis (cavernous) B87.9
  aural B87.4
  creeping B87.0
  cutaneous B87.0
  dermal B87.0
  ear (external) (middle) B87.4
  eye B87.2
  genitourinary B87.81
  intestinal B87.82
  laryngeal B87.3
  nasopharyngeal B87.3
  ocular B87.2
  orbit B87.2
  skin B87.0
  specified site NEC B87.89
  traumatic B87.1
  wound B87.1
Myoadenoma, prostate —see Hyperplasia,
  prostate
Myoblastoma
  granular cell —see also Neoplasm, connective
    tissue, benign
    malignant —see Neoplasm, connective
      tissue, malignant
    tongue D10.1
Myocardial —see condition

▶ New   ▦ Revised   ~~deleted~~ Deleted   ● Use Additional Character(s)

Myocardiopathy (congestive) (constrictive)
(familial) (hypertrophic nonobstructive)
(idiopathic) (infiltrative) (obstructive)
(primary) (restrictive) (sporadic) —see also
Cardiomyopathy I42.9
alcoholic I42.6
cobalt-beer I42.6
glycogen storage E74.02 [I43]
hypertrophic obstructive I42.1
in (due to)
beriberi E51.12
cardiac glycogenosis E74.02 [I43]
Friedreich's ataxia G11.11 [I43]
myotonia atrophica G71.11 [I43]
➠progressive muscular dystrophy (see also
Dystrophy, muscular, by type)
G71.03 [I43]
obscure (African) I42.8
secondary I42.9
thyrotoxic E05.90 [I43]
with storm E05.91 [I43]
toxic NEC I42.7
Myocarditis (with arteriosclerosis) (chronic)
(fibroid) (interstitial) (old) (progressive)
(senile) I51.4
with
rheumatic fever (conditions in I00) I09.0
active —see Myocarditis, acute,
rheumatic
inactive or quiescent (with chorea) I09.0
active I40.9
rheumatic I01.2
with chorea (acute) (rheumatic)
(Sydenham's) I02.0
acute or subacute (interstitial) I40.9
due to
streptococcus (beta-hemolytic) I01.2
idiopathic I40.1
rheumatic I01.2
with chorea (acute) (rheumatic)
(Sydenham's) I02.0
specified NEC I40.8
aseptic of newborn B33.22
bacterial (acute) I40.0
Coxsackie (virus) B33.22
diphtheritic A36.81
eosinophilic I40.1
epidemic of newborn (Coxsackie) B33.22
Fiedler's (acute) (isolated) I40.1
giant cell (acute) (subacute) I40.1
gonococcal A54.83
granulomatous (idiopathic) (isolated)
(nonspecific) I40.1
hypertensive —see Hypertension, heart
idiopathic (granulomatous) I40.1
in (due to)
diphtheria A36.81
epidemic louse-borne typhus A75.0 [I41]
Lyme disease A69.29
sarcoidosis D86.85
scarlet fever A38.1
toxoplasmosis (acquired) B58.81
typhoid A01.02
typhus NEC A75.9 [I41]
infective I40.0
influenzal —see Influenza, with, myocarditis
isolated (acute) I40.1
meningococcal A39.52
mumps B26.82
nonrheumatic, active I40.9
parenchymatous I40.9
pneumococcal I40.0
rheumatic (chronic) (inactive) (with chorea)
I09.0
active or acute I01.2
with chorea (acute) (rheumatic)
(Sydenham's) I02.0
rheumatoid —see Rheumatoid, carditis
septic I40.0
staphylococcal I40.0
suppurative I40.0

Myocarditis (Continued)
syphilitic (chronic) A52.06
toxic I40.8
rheumatic —see Myocarditis, acute,
rheumatic
tuberculous A18.84
typhoid A01.02
valvular —see Endocarditis
virus, viral I40.0
of newborn (Coxsackie) B33.22
Myocardium, myocardial —see condition
Myocardosis —see Cardiomyopathy
Myoclonus, myoclonic, myoclonia (familial)
(essential) (multifocal) (simplex) G25.3
drug-induced G25.3
epilepsy —see also Epilepsy, generalized,
specified NEC G40.4-●
familial (progressive) G25.3
epileptica G40.409
with status epilepticus G40.401
facial G51.3-●
familial progressive G25.3
Friedreich's G25.3
jerks G25.3
massive G25.3
palatal G25.3
pharyngeal G25.3
Myocytolysis I51.5
Myodiastasis —see Diastasis, muscle
Myoendocarditis —see Endocarditis
Myoepithelioma —see Neoplasm, benign, by
site
Myofasciitis (acute) —see Myositis
Myofibroma —see also Neoplasm, connective
tissue, benign
uterus (cervix) (corpus) —see Leiomyoma
Myofibromatosis D48.1
infantile Q89.8
Myofibrosis M62.89
heart —see Myocarditis
scapulohumeral —see Lesion, shoulder,
specified NEC
Myofibrositis M79.7
scapulohumeral —see Lesion, shoulder,
specified NEC
Myoglobulinuria, myoglobinuria (primary)
R82.1
Myokymia, facial G51.4
Myolipoma —see Lipoma
Myoma —see also Neoplasm, connective tissue,
benign
malignant —see Neoplasm, connective tissue,
malignant
prostate D29.1
uterus (cervix) (corpus) —see Leiomyoma
Myomalacia M62.89
Myometritis —see Endometritis
Myometrium —see condition
Myonecrosis, clostridial A48.0
Myopathy G72.9
acute
necrotizing G72.81
quadriplegic G72.81
alcoholic G72.1
benign congenital G71.20
central core G71.29
centronuclear G71.228
autosomal (dominant) (recessive)
G71.228
other specified NEC G71.228
congenital (benign) G71.20
critical illness G72.81
distal G71.09
drug-induced G72.0
endocrine NEC E34.9 [G73.7]
extraocular muscles H05.82-●
facioscapulohumeral G71.02
hereditary G71.9
specified NEC G71.8
hyaline body G71.29
myosin storage G71.29

Myopathy (Continued)
immune NEC G72.49
in (due to)
Addison's disease E27.1 [G73.7]
alcohol G72.1
amyloidosis E85.0 [G73.7]
cretinism E00.9 [G73.7]
Cushing's syndrome E24.9 [G73.7]
drugs G72.0
endocrine disease NEC E34.9 [G73.7]
giant cell arteritis M31.6 [G73.7]
glycogen storage disease E74.00 [G73.7]
hyperadrenocorticism E24.9 [G73.7]
hyperparathyroidism NEC E21.3 [G73.7]
hypoparathyroidism E20.9 [G73.7]
hypopituitarism E23.0 [G73.7]
hypothyroidism E03.9 [G73.7]
infectious disease NEC B99 [G73.7]
lipid storage disease E75.6 [G73.7]
metabolic disease NEC E88.9 [G73.7]
myxedema E03.9 [G73.7]
parasitic disease NEC B89 [G73.7]
polyarteritis nodosa M30.0 [G73.7]
rheumatoid arthritis —see Rheumatoid,
myopathy
sarcoidosis D86.87
scleroderma M34.82
sicca syndrome M35.03
Sjögren's syndrome M35.03
systemic lupus erythematosus M32.19
thyrotoxicosis (hyperthyroidism) E05.90
[G73.7]
with thyroid storm E05.91 [G73.7]
toxic agent NEC G72.2
inflammatory NEC G72.49
intensive care (ICU) G72.81
➠limb-girdle —see Dystrophy, muscular,
limb-girdle
mitochondrial NEC G71.3
▶Miyoshi, type 3 G71.035
myosin storage G71.29
mytonic, proximal (PROMM) G71.11
myotubular (centronuclear) G71.220
X-linked G71.220
nemaline G71.21
ocular G71.09
oculopharyngeal G71.09
of critical illness G72.81
primary G71.9
specified NEC G71.8
progressive NEC G72.89
proximal myotonic (PROMM) G71.11
rod (body) G71.21
scapulohumeral G71.02
specified NEC G72.89
toxic G72.2
Myopericarditis —see also Pericarditis
chronic rheumatic I09.2
Myopia (axial) (congenital) H52.1-●
degenerative (malignant) H44.20
with
choroidal neovascularization
H44.2A-●
foveoschisis H44.2D-●
macular hole H44.2B-●
retinal detachment H44.2C-●
specified maculopathy NEC H44.2E-●
bilateral H44.23
left eye H44.22
right eye H44.21
malignant —see also Myopia, degenerative
H44.2-●
pernicious —see also Myopia, degenerative
H44.2-●
progressive high (degenerative) —see also
Myopia, degenerative H44.2-●
Myosarcoma —see Neoplasm, connective tissue,
malignant
Myosis (pupil) H57.03
stromal (endolymphatic) D39.0

M

Myositis M60.9
  clostridial A48.0
  due to posture —see Myositis, specified type
      NEC
  epidemic B33.0
  fibrosa or fibrous (chronic), Volkmann's T79.6
  foreign body granuloma —see Granuloma,
      foreign body
  in (due to)
    bilharziasis B65.9 [M63.8-●]
    cysticercosis B69.81
    leprosy A30.9 [M63.8-●]
    mycosis B49 [M63.8-●]
    sarcoidosis D86.87
    schistosomiasis B65.9 [M63.8-●]
    syphilis
      late A52.78
      secondary A51.49
    toxoplasmosis (acquired) B58.82
    trichinellosis B75 [M63.8-●]
    tuberculosis A18.09
  inclusion body [IBM] G72.41
  infective M60.009
    arm M60.002
      left M60.001
      right M60.000
    leg M60.005
      left M60.004
      right M60.003
    lower limb M60.005
      ankle M60.07-●
      foot M60.07-●
      lower leg M60.06-●
      thigh M60.05-●
      toe M60.07-●
    multiple sites M60.09
    specified site NEC M60.08
    upper limb M60.002
      finger M60.04-●
      forearm M60.03-●
      hand M60.04-●
      shoulder region M60.01-●
      upper arm M60.02-●
  interstitial M60.10
    ankle M60.17-●
    foot M60.17-●
    forearm M60.13-●
    hand M60.14-●
    lower leg M60.16-●
    multiple sites M60.19
    shoulder region M60.11-●
    specified site NEC M60.18
    thigh M60.15-●
    upper arm M60.12-●
  mycotic B49 [M63.8-●]
  ossificans or ossifying (circumscripta) —see
      also Ossification, muscle, specified NEC
    in (due to)
      burns M61.30
        ankle M61.37-●
        foot M61.37-●
        forearm M61.33-●
        hand M61.34-●

Myositis (Continued)
  ossificans or ossifying (Continued)
    in (due to) (Continued)
      burns (Continued)
        lower leg M61.36-●
        multiple sites M61.39
        pelvic region M61.35-●
        shoulder region M61.31-●
        specified site NEC M61.38
        thigh M61.35-●
        upper arm M61.32-●
      quadriplegia or paraplegia M61.20
        ankle M61.27-●
        foot M61.27-●
        forearm M61.23-●
        hand M61.24-●
        lower leg M61.26-●
        multiple sites M61.29
        pelvic region M61.25-●
        shoulder region M61.21-●
        specified site NEC M61.28
        thigh M61.25-●
        upper arm M61.22-●
    progressiva M61.10
      ankle M61.17-●
      finger M61.14-●
      foot M61.17-●
      forearm M61.13-●
      hand M61.14-●
      lower leg M61.16-●
      multiple sites M61.19
      pelvic region M61.15-●
      shoulder region M61.11-●
      specified site NEC M61.18
      thigh M61.15-●
      toe M61.17-●
      upper arm M61.12-●
    traumatica M61.00
      ankle M61.07-●
      foot M61.07-●
      forearm M61.03-●
      hand M61.04-●
      lower leg M61.06-●
      multiple sites M61.09
      pelvic region M61.05-●
      shoulder region M61.01-●
      specified site NEC M61.08
      thigh M61.05-●
      upper arm M61.02-●
  purulent —see Myositis, infective
  specified type NEC M60.80
    ankle M60.87-●
    foot M60.87-●
    forearm M60.83-●
    hand M60.84-●
    lower leg M60.86-●
    multiple sites M60.89
    pelvic region M60.85-●
    shoulder region M60.81-●
    specified site NEC M60.88
    thigh M60.85-●
    upper arm M60.82-●

Myositis (Continued)
  suppurative —see Myositis, infective
  traumatic (old) —see Myositis, specified type
      NEC
Myospasia impulsiva F95.2
Myotonia (acquisita) (intermittens) M62.89
  atrophica G71.11
  chondrodystrophic G71.13
  congenita (acetazolamide responsive)
      (dominant) (recessive) G71.12
  drug-induced G71.14
  dystrophica G71.11
  fluctuans G71.19
  levior G71.12
  permanens G71.19
  symptomatic G71.19
Myotonic pupil —see Anomaly, pupil, function,
      tonic pupil
Myriapodiasis B88.2
Myringitis H73.2-●
  with otitis media —see Otitis, media
  acute H73.00-●
    bullous H73.01-●
    specified NEC H73.09-●
  bullous —see Myringitis, acute, bullous
  chronic H73.1-●
Mysophobia F40.228
Mytilotoxism —see Poisoning, fish
Myxadenitis labialis K13.0
Myxedema (adult) (idiocy) (infantile)
      (juvenile) —see also Hypothyroidism
      E03.9
  circumscribed E05.90
    with storm E05.91
  coma E03.5
  congenital E00.1
  cutis L98.5
  localized (pretibial) E05.90
    with storm E05.91
  papular L98.5
Myxochondrosarcoma —see Neoplasm,
      cartilage, malignant
Myxofibroma —see Neoplasm, connective
      tissue, benign
  odontogenic —see Cyst, calcifying
      odontogenic
Myxofibrosarcoma —see Neoplasm, connective
      tissue, malignant
Myxolipoma D17.9
Myxoliposarcoma —see Neoplasm, connective
      tissue, malignant
Myxoma —see also Neoplasm, connective tissue,
      benign
  nerve sheath —see Neoplasm, nerve,
      benign
  odontogenic —see Cyst, calcifying
      odontogenic
Myxosarcoma —see Neoplasm, connective
      tissue, malignant

▶ New   ⇒ Revised   ~~deleted~~ Deleted   ● Use Additional Character(s)

N

Naegeli's
  disease Q82.8
  leukemia, monocytic C93.1-●
Naegleriasis (with meningoencephalitis)
  B60.2
Naffziger's syndrome G54.0
Naga sore —see Ulcer, skin
Nägele's pelvis M95.5
  with disproportion (fetopelvic) O33.0
    causing obstructed labor O65.0
Nail —see also condition
  biting F98.8
  patella syndrome Q87.2
Nanism, nanosomia —see Dwarfism
Nanophyetiasis B66.8
Nanukayami A27.89
Napkin rash L22
Narcolepsy G47.419
  with cataplexy G47.411
  in conditions classified elsewhere G47.429
    with cataplexy G47.421
Narcosis R06.89
Narcotism —see Dependence
NARP (Neuropathy, Ataxia and Retinitis
  pigmentosa) syndrome E88.49
Narrow
  anterior chamber angle H40.03-●
  gingival width (of periodontal soft tissue)
    K05.5
  pelvis —see Contraction, pelvis
Narrowing —see also Stenosis
  artery I77.1
    auditory, internal I65.8
    basilar —see Occlusion, artery, basilar
    carotid —see Occlusion, artery, carotid
    cerebellar —see Occlusion, artery, cerebellar
    cerebral —see Occlusion artery, cerebral
    choroidal —see Occlusion, artery,
      precerebral, specified NEC
    communicating posterior —see
      Occlusion, artery, precerebral,
      specified NEC
    coronary —see also Disease, heart, ischemic,
      atherosclerotic
      congenital Q24.5
        syphilitic A50.54 [152]
        due to syphilis NEC A52.06
    hypophyseal —see Occlusion, artery,
      precerebral, specified NEC
    pontine —see Occlusion, artery, precerebral,
      specified NEC
    precerebral —see Occlusion, artery,
      precerebral
    vertebral —see Occlusion, artery, vertebral
  auditory canal (external) —see Stenosis,
    external ear canal
  eustachian tube —see Obstruction, eustachian
    tube
  eyelid —see Disorder, eyelid function
  larynx J38.6
  mesenteric artery —see also Ischemia,
    intestine, acute K55.059
  palate M26.89
  palpebral fissure —see Disorder, eyelid
    function
  ureter N13.5
    with infection N13.6
  urethra —see Stricture, urethra
Narrowness, abnormal, eyelid Q10.3
Nasal —see condition
Nasolachrymal, nasolacrimal —see condition
Nasopharyngeal —see also condition
  pituitary gland Q89.2
  torticollis M43.6
Nasopharyngitis (acute) (infective)
  (streptococcal) (subacute) J00
  chronic (suppurative) (ulcerative) J31.1
Nasopharynx, nasopharyngeal —see condition
Natal tooth, teeth K00.6

Nausea (without vomiting) R11.0
  with vomiting R11.2
  gravidarum —see Hyperemesis, gravidarum
  marina T75.3
  navalis T75.3
Navel —see condition
Neapolitan fever —see Brucellosis
Near drowning T75.1
Nearsightedness —see Myopia
Near-syncope R55
Nebula, cornea —see Opacity, cornea
Necator americanus infestation B76.1
Necatoriasis B76.1
Neck —see condition
Necrobiosis R68.89
  lipoidica NEC L92.1
    with diabetes —see E08-E13 with .620
Necrolysis, toxic epidermal L51.2
  due to drug
    correct substance properly administered —
      see Table of Drugs and Chemicals, by
      drug, adverse effect
    overdose or wrong substance given
      or taken —see Table of Drugs and
      Chemicals, by drug, poisoning
Necrophilia F65.89
Necrosis, necrotic (ischemic) —see also
  Gangrene
  adrenal (capsule) (gland) E27.49
  amputation stump (surgical) (late) T87.50
    arm T87.5-●
    leg T87.5-●
  antrum J32.0
  aorta (hyaline) —see also Aneurysm, aorta
    cystic medial —see Dissection, aorta
  artery I77.5
  bladder (aseptic) (sphincter) N32.89
  bone —see also Osteonecrosis M87.9
    aseptic or avascular —see Osteonecrosis
      idiopathic M87.00
    ethmoid J32.2
    jaw M27.2
    tuberculous —see Tuberculosis, bone
  brain I67.89
  breast (aseptic) (fat) (segmental) N64.1
  bronchus J98.09
  central nervous system NEC I67.89
  cerebellar I67.89
  cerebral I67.89
  colon —see also Infarct, intestine K55.049
  cornea H18.89-●
  cortical (acute) (renal) N17.1
  cystic medial (aorta) —see Dissection, aorta
  dental pulp K04.1
  esophagus K22.89
  ethmoid (bone) J32.2
  eyelid —see Disorder, eyelid, degenerative
  fat, fatty (generalized) —see also Disorder, soft
    tissue, specified type NEC
    abdominal wall K65.4
    breast (aseptic) (segmental) N64.1
    localized —see Degeneration, by site, fatty
    mesentery K65.4
    omentum K65.4
    pancreas K86.89
    peritoneum K65.4
    skin (subcutaneous), newborn P83.0
    subcutaneous, due to birth injury P15.6
  gallbladder —see Cholecystitis, acute
  heart —see Infarct, myocardium
  hip, aseptic or avascular —see Osteonecrosis,
    by type, femur
  intestine (acute) (hemorrhagic) (massive) —
    see also Infarct, intestine K55.069
  jaw M27.2
  kidney (bilateral) N28.0
    acute N17.9
      cortical (acute) (bilateral) N17.1
        with ectopic or molar pregnancy O08.4
      medullary (bilateral) (in acute renal failure)
        (papillary) N17.2

Necrosis, necrotic (Continued)
  kidney (Continued)
    papillary (bilateral) (in acute renal
      failure) N17.2
    tubular N17.0
      with ectopic or molar pregnancy
        O08.4
      complicating
        abortion —see Abortion, by type,
          complicated by, tubular necrosis
        ectopic or molar pregnancy O08.4
        pregnancy —see Pregnancy,
          complicated by, diseases of,
          specified type or system NEC
      following ectopic or molar pregnancy
        O08.4
      traumatic T79.5
  larynx J38.7
  liver (with hepatic failure) (cell) —see Failure,
    hepatic
    hemorrhagic, central K76.2
  lung J85.0
  lymphatic gland —see Lymphadenitis, acute
  mammary gland (fat) (segmental) N64.1
  mastoid (chronic) —see Mastoiditis, chronic
  medullary (acute) (renal) N17.2
  mesentery —see also Infarct, intestine
    K55.069
    fat K65.4
  mitral valve —see Insufficiency, mitral
  myocardium, myocardial —see Infarct,
    myocardium
  nose J34.0
  omentum (with mesenteric infarction) —see
    also Infarct, intestine K55.069
    fat K65.4
  orbit, orbital —see Osteomyelitis, orbit
  ossicles, ear —see Abnormal, ear ossicles
  ovary N70.92
  pancreas (aseptic) (duct) (fat) K86.89
    acute (infective) —see Pancreatitis, acute
    infective —see Pancreatitis, acute
  papillary (acute) (renal) N17.2
  perineum N90.89
  peritoneum (with mesenteric infarction) —see
    also Infarct, intestine K55.069
    fat K65.4
  pharynx J02.9
    in granulocytopenia —see Neutropenia
      Vincent's A69.1
  phosphorus —see subcategory T54.2
  pituitary (gland) E23.0
    postpartum O99.285
    Sheehan O99.285
  pressure —see Ulcer, pressure, by site
  pulmonary J85.0
  pulp (dental) K04.1
  radiation —see Necrosis, by site
  radium —see Necrosis, by site
  renal —see Necrosis, kidney
  sclera H15.89
  scrotum N50.89
  skin or subcutaneous tissue NEC I96
  spine, spinal (column) —see also
    Osteonecrosis, by type, vertebra
    cord G95.19
  spleen D73.5
  stomach K31.89
  stomatitis (ulcerative) A69.0
  subcutaneous fat, newborn P83.88
  subendocardial (acute) I21.4
    chronic I25.89
  suprarenal (capsule) (gland) E27.49
  testis N50.89
  thymus (gland) E32.8
  tonsil J35.8
  trachea J39.8
  tuberculous NEC —see Tuberculosis
  tubular (acute) (anoxic) (renal) (toxic)
    N17.0
    postprocedural N99.0

Necrosis, necrotic *(Continued)*
  vagina N89.8
  vertebra —*see also* Osteonecrosis, by type,
    vertebra
    tuberculous A18.01
  vulva N90.89
  X-ray —*see* Necrosis, by site
Necrospermia —*see* Infertility, male
Need (for)
  care provider because (of)
    assistance with personal care Z74.1
    continuous supervision required Z74.3
    impaired mobility Z74.09
    no other household member able to render
      care Z74.2
    specified reason NEC Z74.8
  immunization —*see* Vaccination
  vaccination —*see* Vaccination
Neglect
  adult
    confirmed T74.01
    history of Z91.412
    suspected T76.01
  child (childhood)
    confirmed T74.02
    history of Z62.812
    suspected T76.02
  emotional, in childhood Z62.898
  hemispatial R41.4
  left-sided R41.4
  sensory R41.4
  visuospatial R41.4
Neisserian infection NEC —*see* Gonococcus
Nelaton's syndrome G60.8
Nelson's syndrome E24.1
Nematodiasis (intestinal) B82.0
  Ancylostoma B76.0
Neonatal —*see also* Newborn
  acne L70.4
  bradycardia P29.12
  screening, abnormal findings on —*see*
    Abnormal, neonatal screening
  tachycardia P29.11
  tooth, teeth K00.6
Neonatorum —*see* condition
Neoplasia
  endocrine, multiple (MEN) E31.20
    type I E31.21
    type IIA E31.22
    type IIB E31.23
  intraepithelial (histologically confirmed)
    anal (AIN) (histologically confirmed)
      K62.82
      grade I K62.82
      grade II K62.82
      severe D01.3
    cervical glandular (histologically
      confirmed) D06.9
    cervix (uteri) (CIN) (histologically
      confirmed) N87.9
      glandular D06.9
      grade I N87.0
      grade II N87.1
      grade III (severe dysplasia) —*see also*
        Carcinoma, cervix uteri, in situ
        D06.9
    prostate (histologically confirmed) (PIN)
      N42.31
      grade I N42.31
      grade II N42.31
      grade III (severe dysplasia) D07.5
    vagina (histologically confirmed) (VAIN)
      N89.3
      grade I N89.0
      grade II N89.1
      grade III (severe dysplasia) D07.2
    vulva (histologically confirmed) (VIN)
      N90.3
      grade I N90.0
      grade II N90.1
      grade III (severe dysplasia) D07.1

Neoplasm, neoplastic —*see also* Table of
  Neoplasms
  lipomatous, benign —*see* Lipoma
  malignant mast cell C96.20
    specified type NEC C96.29
  mast cell, of uncertain behavior NEC D47.09
▶myelodysplastic/myeloproliferative,
    unclassifiable C94.6
Neovascularization
  ciliary body —*see* Disorder, iris, vascular
  cornea H16.40-●
    deep H16.44-●
    ghost vessels —*see* Ghost, vessels
    localized H16.43-●
    pannus —*see* Pannus
  iris —*see* Disorder, iris, vascular
  retina H35.05-●
Nephralgia N23
Nephritis, nephritic (albuminuric) (azotemic)
  (congenital) (disseminated) (epithelial)
  (familial) (focal) (granulomatous)
  (hemorrhagic) (infantile) (nonsuppurative,
  excretory) (uremic) N05.9
  with
    C3
      glomerulonephritis N05.A
      glomerulopathy N05.A
        with dense deposit disease N05.6
      dense deposit disease N05.6
      diffuse
        crescentic glomerulonephritis N05.7
        endocapillary proliferative
          glomerulonephritis N05.4
        membranous glomerulonephritis N05.2
        mesangial proliferative
          glomerulonephritis N05.3
        mesangiocapillary glomerulonephritis
          N05.5
      edema —*see* Nephrosis
      focal and segmental glomerular lesions
        N05.1
      foot process disease N04.9
      glomerular lesion
        diffuse sclerosing N05.8
        hypocomplementemic —*see* Nephritis,
          membranoproliferative
        IgA —*see* Nephropathy, IgA
        lobular, lobulonodular —*see* Nephritis,
          membranoproliferative
        nodular —*see* Nephritis,
          membranoproliferative
      lesion of
        glomerulonephritis, proliferative N05.8
        renal necrosis N05.9
      minor glomerular abnormality N05.0
      specified morphological changes NEC N05.8
  acute N00.9
    with
      C3
        glomerulonephritis N00.A
        glomerulopathy N00.A
          with dense deposit disease N00.6
        dense deposit disease N00.6
        diffuse
          crescentic glomerulonephritis N00.7
          endocapillary proliferative
            glomerulonephritis N00.4
          membranous glomerulonephritis N00.2
          mesangial proliferative
            glomerulonephritis N00.3
          mesangiocapillary glomerulonephritis
            N00.5
        focal and segmental glomerular lesions
          N00.1
        minor glomerular abnormality N00.0
        specified morphological changes NEC
          N00.8
  amyloid E85.4 *[N08]*
  antiglomerular basement membrane (anti-
    GBM) antibody NEC
    in Goodpasture's syndrome M31.0

Nephritis, nephritic *(Continued)*
  antitubular basement membrane (tubulo-
    interstitial) NEC N12
    toxic —*see* Nephropathy, toxic
  arteriolar —*see* Hypertension, kidney
  arteriosclerotic —*see* Hypertension, kidney
  ascending —*see* Nephritis, tubulo-interstitial
  atrophic N03.9
  Balkan (endemic) N15.0
  calculous, calculus —*see* Calculus,
    kidney
  cardiac —*see* Hypertension, kidney
  cardiovascular —*see* Hypertension,
    kidney
  chronic N03.9
    with
      C3
        glomerulonephritis N03.A
        glomerulopathy N03.A
          with dense deposit disease N03.6
        dense deposit disease N03.6
        diffuse
          crescentic glomerulonephritis
            N03.7
          endocapillary proliferative
            glomerulonephritis N03.4
          membranous glomerulonephritis
            N03.2
          mesangial proliferative
            glomerulonephritis N03.3
          mesangiocapillary glomerulonephritis
            N03.5
        focal and segmental glomerular lesions
          N03.1
        minor glomerular abnormality
          N03.0
        specified morphological changes
          NEC N03.8
    arteriosclerotic —*see* Hypertension,
      kidney
  cirrhotic N26.9
  complicating pregnancy O26.83-●
  croupous N00.9
  degenerative —*see* Nephrosis
  diffuse sclerosing N05.8
  due to
    diabetes mellitus —*see* E08-E13 with .21
    subacute bacterial endocarditis I33.0
    systemic lupus erythematosus (chronic)
      M32.14
    typhoid fever A01.09
  gonococcal (acute) (chronic) A54.21
  hypocomplementemic —*see* Nephritis,
    membranoproliferative
  IgA —*see* Nephropathy, IgA
  immune complex (circulating) NEC N05.8
  infective —*see* Nephritis, tubulo-interstitial
  interstitial —*see* Nephritis, tubulo-interstitial
  lead N14.3
  membranoproliferative (diffuse) (type 1
    or 3) —*see also* N00-N07 with fourth
    character .5 N05.5
    type 2 —*see also* N00-N07 with fourth
      character .6 N05.6
  minimal change N05.0
  necrotic, necrotizing NEC —*see also* N00-N07
    with fourth character .8 N05.8
  nephrotic —*see* Nephrosis
  nodular —*see* Nephritis,
    membranoproliferative
  polycystic Q61.3
    adult type Q61.2
    autosomal
      dominant Q61.2
      recessive NEC Q61.19
    childhood type NEC Q61.19
    infantile type NEC Q61.19
  poststreptococcal N05.9
    acute N00.9
    chronic N03.9
    rapidly progressive N01.9

▶ New   ⇒ Revised   ~~deleted~~ Deleted   ● Use Additional Character(s)

Nephritis, nephritic (Continued)
  proliferative NEC —see also N00-N07 with
    fourth character .8 N05.8
  purulent —see Nephritis, tubulo-interstitial
  rapidly progressive N01.9
    with
      C3
        glomerulonephritis N01.A
        glomerulopathy N01.A
          with dense deposit disease N01.6
      dense deposit disease N01.6
      diffuse
        crescentic glomerulonephritis N01.7
        endocapillary proliferative
          glomerulonephritis N01.4
        membranous glomerulonephritis N01.2
        mesangial proliferative
          glomerulonephritis N01.3
        mesangiocapillary glomerulonephritis
          N01.5
      focal and segmental glomerular lesions
        N01.1
      minor glomerular abnormality N01.0
      specified morphological changes NEC
        N01.8
  salt losing or wasting NEC N28.89
  saturnine N14.3
  sclerosing, diffuse N05.8
  septic —see Nephritis, tubulo-interstitial
  specified pathology NEC —see also N00-N07
    with fourth character .8 N05.8
  subacute N01.9
  suppurative —see Nephritis,
    tubulo-interstitial
  syphilitic (late) A52.75
    congenital A50.59 [N08]
    early (secondary) A51.44
  toxic —see Nephropathy, toxic
  tubal, tubular —see Nephritis,
    tubulo-interstitial
  tuberculous A18.11
  tubulo-interstitial (in) N12
    acute (infectious) N10
    chronic (infectious) N11.9
      nonobstructive N11.8
        reflux-associated N11.0
      obstructive N11.1
      specified NEC N11.8
    due to
      brucellosis A23.9 [N16]
      cryoglobulinemia D89.1 [N16]
      glycogen storage disease E74.00 [N16]
      Sjögren's syndrome M35.04
  vascular —see Hypertension, kidney
  war N00.9
Nephroblastoma (epithelial) (mesenchymal)
  C64-●
Nephrocalcinosis E83.59 [N29]
Nephrocystitis, pustular —see Nephritis,
  tubulo-interstitial
Nephrolithiasis (congenital) (pelvis)
  (recurrent) —see also Calculus, kidney
Nephroma C64-●
  mesoblastic D41.0-●
Nephronephritis —see Nephrosis
Nephronophthisis Q61.5
Nephropathia epidemica A98.5
Nephropathy —see also Nephritis N28.9
  with
    edema —see Nephrosis
    glomerular lesion —see Glomerulonephritis
  amyloid, hereditary E85.0
  analgesic N14.0
    with medullary necrosis, acute N17.2
  Balkan (endemic) N15.0
  chemical —see Nephropathy, toxic
  ▶contrast-induced N14.11
  ▶contrast medium, radiography N14.11
  diabetic —see E08-E13 with .21
  drug-induced N14.2
    ▶contrast-induced N14.11
    ⇒specified NEC N14.19

Nephropathy (Continued)
  focal and segmental hyalinosis or sclerosis
    N02.1
  heavy metal-induced N14.3
  hereditary NEC N07.9
    with
      C3
        glomerulonephritis N07.A
        glomerulopathy N07.A
          with dense deposit disease N07.6
      dense deposit disease N07.6
      diffuse
        crescentic glomerulonephritis N07.7
        endocapillary proliferative
          glomerulonephritis N07.4
        membranous glomerulonephritis
          N07.2
        mesangial proliferative
          glomerulonephritis N07.3
        mesangiocapillary glomerulonephritis
          N07.5
      focal and segmental glomerular lesions
        N07.1
      minor glomerular abnormality N07.0
      specified morphological changes NEC
        N07.8
  hypercalcemic N25.89
  hypertensive —see Hypertension, kidney
  hypokalemic (vacuolar) N25.89
  IgA N02.8
    with glomerular lesion N02.9
      focal and segmental hyalinosis or
        sclerosis N02.1
      membranoproliferative (diffuse) N02.5
      membranous (diffuse) N02.2
      mesangial proliferative (diffuse) N02.3
      mesangiocapillary (diffuse) N02.5
      proliferative NEC N02.8
      specified pathology NEC N02.8
  lead N14.3
  membranoproliferative (diffuse) N02.5
  membranous (diffuse) N02.2
  mesangial (IgA/IgG) —see Nephropathy, IgA
    proliferative (diffuse) N02.3
  mesangiocapillary (diffuse) N02.5
  obstructive N13.8
  phenacetin N17.2
  phosphate-losing N25.0
  potassium depletion N25.89
  pregnancy-related O26.83-●
  proliferative NEC (see also N00-N07 with
    fourth character .8) N05.8
  protein-losing N25.89
  saturnine N14.3
  sickle-cell D57.-● [N08]
  toxic NEC N14.4
    due to
      drugs N14.2
        analgesic N14.0
      ⇒specified NEC N14.19
      heavy metals N14.3
  vasomotor N17.0
  water-losing N25.89
Nephroptosis N28.83
Nephropyosis —see Abscess, kidney
Nephrorrhagia N28.89
Nephrosclerosis (arteriolar) (arteriosclerotic)
  (chronic) (hyaline) —see also Hypertension,
  kidney
  hyperplastic —see Hypertension, kidney
  senile N26.9
Nephrosis, nephrotic (Epstein's) (syndrome)
  (congenital) N04.9
  with
    foot process disease N04.9
    glomerular lesion N04.1
    hypocomplementemic N04.5
  acute N04.9
  anoxic —see Nephrosis, tubular
  chemical —see Nephrosis, tubular
  cholemic K76.7

Nephrosis, nephrotic (Continued)
  diabetic —see E08-E13 with .21
  Finnish type (congenital) Q89.8
  hemoglobin N10
  hemoglobinuric —see Nephrosis, tubular
  in
    amyloidosis E85.4 [N08]
    diabetes mellitus —see E08-E13 with .21
    epidemic hemorrhagic fever A98.5
    malaria (malariae) B52.0
  ischemic —see Nephrosis, tubular
  lipoid N04.9
  lower nephron —see Nephrosis, tubular
  malarial (malariae) B52.0
  minimal change N04.0
  myoglobin N10
  necrotizing —see Nephrosis, tubular
  osmotic (sucrose) N25.89
  radiation N04.9
  syphilitic (late) A52.75
  toxic —see Nephrosis, tubular
  tubular (acute) N17.0
    postprocedural N99.0
    radiation N04.9
Nephrosonephritis, hemorrhagic (endemic)
  A98.5
Nephrostomy
  attention to Z43.6
  status Z93.6
Nerve —see also condition
  injury —see Injury, nerve, by body site
Nerves R45.0
Nervous —see also condition R45.0
  heart F45.8
  stomach F45.8
  tension R45.0
Nervousness R45.0
Nesidioblastoma
  pancreas D13.7
  specified site NEC —see Neoplasm, benign,
    by site
  unspecified site D13.7
Nettleship's syndrome —see Urticaria
  pigmentosa
Neumann's disease or syndrome L10.1
Neuralgia, neuralgic (acute) M79.2
  accessory (nerve) G52.8
  acoustic (nerve) —see subcategory H93.3
  auditory (nerve) —see subcategory H93.3
  ciliary G44.009
    intractable G44.001
    not intractable G44.009
  cranial
    nerve —see also Disorder, nerve, cranial
      fifth or trigeminal —see Neuralgia,
        trigeminal
    postherpetic, postzoster B02.29
  ear —see subcategory H92.0
  facialis vera G51.1
  Fothergill's —see Neuralgia, trigeminal
  glossopharyngeal (nerve) G52.1
  Horton's G44.099
    intractable G44.091
    not intractable G44.099
  Hunt's B02.21
  hypoglossal (nerve) G52.3
  infraorbital —see Neuralgia, trigeminal
  malarial —see Malaria
  migrainous G44.009
    intractable G44.001
    not intractable G44.009
  Morton's G57.6-●
  nerve, cranial —see Disorder, nerve, cranial
  nose G52.0
  occipital M54.81
  olfactory G52.0
  penis N48.9
  perineum R10.2
  postherpetic NEC B02.29
    trigeminal B02.22
  pubic region R10.2

Neuralgia, neuralgic *(Continued)*
  scrotum R10.2
  Sluder's G44.89
  specified nerve NEC G58.8
  spermatic cord R10.2
  sphenopalatine (ganglion) G90.09
  trifacial —*see* Neuralgia, trigeminal
  trigeminal G50.0
    postherpetic, postzoster B02.22
  vagus (nerve) G52.2
  writer's F48.8
    organic G25.89
Neurapraxia —*see* Injury, nerve
Neurasthenia F48.8
  cardiac F45.8
  gastric F45.8
  heart F45.8
Neurilemmoma —*see also* Neoplasm, nerve,
    benign
  acoustic (nerve) D33.3
  malignant —*see also* Neoplasm, nerve,
    malignant
    acoustic (nerve) C72.4
Neurilemmosarcoma —*see* Neoplasm, nerve,
    malignant
Neurinoma —*see* Neoplasm, nerve, benign
Neurinomatosis —*see* Neoplasm, nerve,
    uncertain behavior
Neuritis (rheumatoid) M79.2
  abducens (nerve) —*see* Strabismus, paralytic,
    sixth nerve
  accessory (nerve) G52.8
  acoustic (nerve) —*see also* subcategory H93.3
    in (due to)
      infectious disease NEC B99 *[H94.0-●]*
      parasitic disease NEC B89 *[H94.0-●]*
    syphilitic A52.15
  alcoholic G62.1
    with psychosis —*see* Psychosis, alcoholic
  amyloid, any site E85.4 *[G63]*
  auditory (nerve) —*see* subcategory H93.3
  brachial —*see* Radiculopathy
    due to displacement, intervertebral disc —
      see Disorder, disc, cervical, with neuritis
  cranial nerve
    due to Lyme disease A69.22
    eighth or acoustic or auditory —*see*
      subcategory H93.3
    eleventh or accessory G52.8
➡ fifth or trigeminal G50.-●
    first or olfactory G52.0
    fourth or trochlear —*see* Strabismus,
      paralytic, fourth nerve
    second or optic —*see* Neuritis, optic
    seventh or facial G51.8
      newborn (birth injury) P11.3
    sixth or abducent —*see* Strabismus,
      paralytic, sixth nerve
    tenth or vagus G52.2
    third or oculomotor —*see* Strabismus,
      paralytic, third nerve
    twelfth or hypoglossal G52.3
  Déjérine-Sottas G60.0
  diabetic (mononeuropathy) —*see* E08-E13
    with .41
    polyneuropathy —*see* E08-E13 with .42
  due to
    beriberi E51.11
    displacement, prolapse or rupture,
      intervertebral disc —*see* Disorder, disc,
      with, radiculopathy
    herniation, nucleus pulposus M51.9 *[G55]*
  endemic E51.11
  facial G51.8
    newborn (birth injury) P11.3
  general —*see* Polyneuropathy
  geniculate ganglion G51.1
    due to herpes (zoster) B02.21
  gouty —*see also* Gout, by type M10.9 *[G63]*
  hypoglossal (nerve) G52.3
  ilioinguinal (nerve) G57.9-●
  infectious (multiple) NEC G61.0

Neuritis *(Continued)*
  interstitial hypertrophic progressive G60.0
  lumbar M54.16
  lumbosacral M54.17
  multiple —*see also* Polyneuropathy
    endemic E51.11
    infective, acute G61.0
  multiplex endemica E51.11
  nerve root —*see* Radiculopathy
  oculomotor (nerve) —*see* Strabismus,
    paralytic, third nerve
  olfactory nerve G52.0
  optic (nerve) (hereditary) (sympathetic) H46.9
    with demyelination G36.0
    in myelitis G36.0
    nutritional H46.2
    papillitis —*see* Papillitis, optic
    retrobulbar H46.1-●
    specified type NEC H46.8
    toxic H46.3
  peripheral (nerve) G62.9
    multiple —*see* Polyneuropathy
    single —*see* Mononeuritis
  pneumogastric (nerve) G52.2
  postherpetic, postzoster B02.29
  progressive hypertrophic interstitial G60.0
  retrobulbar —*see also* Neuritis, optic,
      retrobulbar
    in (due to)
      late syphilis A52.15
      meningococcal infection A39.82
    meningococcal A39.82
    syphilitic A52.15
  sciatic (nerve) —*see also* Sciatica
    due to displacement of intervertebral
      disc —*see* Disorder, disc, with,
      radiculopathy
  serum —*see also* Reaction, serum T80.69
  shoulder-girdle G54.5
  specified nerve NEC G58.8
  spinal (nerve) root —*see* Radiculopathy
  syphilitic A52.15
  thenar (median) G56.1-●
  thoracic M54.14
  toxic NEC G62.2
  trochlear (nerve) —*see* Strabismus, paralytic,
      fourth nerve
  vagus (nerve) G52.2
Neuroastrocytoma —*see* Neoplasm, uncertain
    behavior, by site
Neuroavitaminosis E56.9 *[G99.8]*
Neuroblastoma
  olfactory C30.0
  specified site —*see* Neoplasm, malignant, by
    site
  unspecified site C74.90
Neurochorioretinitis —*see* Chorioretinitis
Neurocirculatory asthenia F45.8
Neurocysticercosis B69.0
Neurocytoma —*see* Neoplasm, benign, by site
Neurodermatitis (circumscribed)
    (circumscripta) (local) L28.0
  atopic L20.81
  diffuse (Brocq) L20.81
  disseminated L20.81
Neuroencephalomyelopathy, optic G36.0
Neuroepithelioma —*see also* Neoplasm,
    malignant, by site
  olfactory C30.0
Neurofibroma —*see also* Neoplasm, nerve,
    benign
  melanotic —*see* Neoplasm, nerve, benign
  multiple —*see* Neurofibromatosis
  plexiform —*see* Neoplasm, nerve, benign
Neurofibromatosis (multiple) (nonmalignant)
    Q85.00
  acoustic Q85.02
  malignant —*see* Neoplasm, nerve, malignant
  specified NEC Q85.09
  type 1 (von Recklinghausen) Q85.01
  type 2 Q85.02

Neurofibrosarcoma —*see* Neoplasm, nerve,
    malignant
Neurogenic —*see also* condition
  bladder —*see also* Dysfunction, bladder,
    neuromuscular N31.9
    cauda equina syndrome G83.4
  bowel NEC K59.2
  heart F45.8
Neuroglioma —*see* Neoplasm, uncertain
    behavior, by site
Neurolabyrinthitis (of Dix and Hallpike) —*see*
    Neuronitis, vestibular
Neurolathyrism —*see* Poisoning, food, noxious,
    plant
Neuroleprosy A30.9
Neuroma —*see also* Neoplasm, nerve, benign
  acoustic (nerve) D33.3
  amputation (stump) (traumatic) (surgical
      complication) (late) T87.3-●
    arm T87.3-●
    leg T87.3-●
  digital (toe) G57.6-●
  interdigital G58.8
    lower limb toe G57.8-●
    upper limb G56.8-●
  intermetatarsal G57.8-●
  Morton's G57.6-●
  nonneoplastic
    arm G56.9-●
    leg G57.9-●
    lower extremity G57.9-●
    upper extremity G56.9-●
  optic (nerve) D33.3
  plantar G57.6-●
  plexiform —*see* Neoplasm, nerve,
    benign
  surgical (nonneoplastic)
    arm G56.9-●
    leg G57.9-●
    lower extremity G57.9-●
    upper extremity G56.9-●
Neuromyalgia —*see* Neuralgia
➡**Neuromyasthenia** (epidemic) (postinfectious)
    G93.39
Neuromyelitis G36.9
  ascending G61.0
  optica G36.0
Neuromyopathy G70.9
  paraneoplastic D49.9 *[G13.0]*
Neuromyotonia (Isaacs) G71.19
Neuronevus —*see* Nevus
Neuronitis G58.9
  ascending (acute) G57.2-●
  vestibular H81.2-●
Neuroparalytic —*see* condition
Neuropathy, neuropathic G62.9
  acute motor G62.81
  alcoholic G62.1
    with psychosis —*see* Psychosis,
      alcoholic
  arm G56.9-●
  autonomic, peripheral —*see* Neuropathy,
    peripheral, autonomic
  axillary G56.9-●
  bladder N31.9
    atonic (motor) (sensory) N31.2
    autonomous N31.2
    flaccid N31.2
    nonreflex N31.2
    reflex N31.1
    uninhibited N31.0
  brachial plexus G54.0
  cervical plexus G54.2
  chronic
    progressive segmentally demyelinating
      G62.89
    relapsing demyelinating G62.89
  Déjérine-Sottas G60.0
  diabetic —*see* E08-E13 with .40
    mononeuropathy —*see* E08-E13 with .41
    polyneuropathy —*see* E08-E13 with .42

▶ New   ➡ Revised   ~~deleted~~ Deleted   ● Use Additional Character(s)

Neuropathy, neuropathic (Continued)
  entrapment G58.9
    iliohypogastric nerve G57.8-•
    ilioinguinal nerve G57.8-•
    lateral cutaneous nerve of thigh
      G57.1-•
    median nerve G56.0-•
    obturator nerve G57.8-•
    peroneal nerve G57.3-•
    posterior tibial nerve G57.5-•
    saphenous nerve G57.8-•
    ulnar nerve G56.2-•
  facial nerve G51.9
  hereditary G60.9
    motor and sensory (types I-IV) G60.0
    sensory G60.8
    specified NEC G60.8
  hypertrophic G60.0
    Charcot-Marie-Tooth G60.0
    Déjérine-Sottas G60.0
    interstitial progressive G60.0
    of infancy G60.0
    Refsum G60.1
  idiopathic G60.9
    progressive G60.3
    specified NEC G60.8
  in association with hereditary ataxia
    G60.2
  intercostal G58.0
  ischemic —see Disorder, nerve
  Jamaica (ginger) G62.2
  leg NEC G57.9-•
  lower extremity G57.9-•
  lumbar plexus G54.1
  median nerve G56.1-•
  motor and sensory —see also Polyneuropathy
    hereditary (types I-IV) G60.0
  multifocal motor (MMN) G61.82
  multiple (acute) (chronic) —see
    Polyneuropathy
  optic (nerve) —see also Neuritis, optic
    ischemic H47.01-•
  paraneoplastic (sensorial) (Denny Brown)
    D49.9 [G13.0]
  peripheral (nerve) —see also Polyneuropathy
    G62.9
    autonomic G90.9
      idiopathic G90.09
      in (due to)
        amyloidosis E85.4 [G99.0]
        diabetes mellitus —see E08-E13 with
          .43
        endocrine disease NEC E34.9 [G99.0]
        gout M10.00 [G99.0]
        hyperthyroidism E05.90 [G99.0]
          with thyroid storm E05.91 [G99.0]
        metabolic disease NEC E88.9 [G99.0]
    idiopathic G60.9
      progressive G60.3
    in (due to)
      antitetanus serum G62.0
      arsenic G62.2
      drugs NEC G62.0
      lead G62.2
      organophosphate compounds G62.2
      toxic agent NEC G62.2
  plantar nerves G57.6-•
  progressive
    hypertrophic interstitial G60.0
    inflammatory G62.81
  radicular NEC —see Radiculopathy
  sacral plexus G54.1
  sciatic G57.0-•
  serum G61.1
  toxic NEC G62.2
  trigeminal sensory G50.8
  ulnar nerve G56.2-•
  uremic N18.9 [G63]
  vitamin B12 E53.8 [G63]
    with anemia (pernicious) D51.0 [G63]
      due to dietary deficiency D51.3 [G63]

Neurophthisis —see also Disorder, nerve
  peripheral, diabetic —see E08-E13 with .42
Neuroretinitis —see Chorioretinitis
Neuroretinopathy, hereditary optic H47.22
Neurosarcoma —see Neoplasm, nerve, malignant
Neurosclerosis —see Disorder, nerve
Neurosis, neurotic F48.9
  anankastic F42.8
  anxiety (state) F41.1
    panic type F41.0
  asthenic F48.8
  bladder F45.8
  cardiac (reflex) F45.8
  cardiovascular F45.8
  character F60.9
  colon F45.8
  compensation F68.10
  compulsive, compulsion F42.8
  conversion F44.9
  craft F48.8
  cutaneous F45.8
  depersonalization F48.1
  depressive (reaction) (type) F34.1
  environmental F48.8
  excoriation L98.1
  fatigue F48.8
  functional —see Disorder, somatoform
  gastric F45.8
  gastrointestinal F45.8
  heart F45.8
  hypochondriacal F45.21
  hysterical F44.9
  incoordination F45.8
    larynx F45.8
    vocal cord F45.8
  intestine F45.8
  larynx (sensory) F45.8
    hysterical F44.4
  mixed NEC F48.8
  musculoskeletal F45.8
  obsessional F42.8
  obsessive-compulsive F42.8
  occupational F48.8
  ocular NEC F45.8
  organ —see Disorder, somatoform
  pharynx F45.8
  phobic F40.9
  posttraumatic (situational) F43.10
    acute F43.11
    chronic F43.12
  psychasthenic (type) F48.8
  railroad F48.8
  rectum F45.8
  respiratory F45.8
  rumination F45.8
  sexual F65.9
  situational F48.8
  social F40.10
    generalized F40.11
  specified type NEC F48.8
  state F48.9
    with depersonalization episode F48.1
  stomach F45.8
  traumatic F43.10
    acute F43.11
    chronic F43.12
  vasomotor F45.8
  visceral F45.8
  war F48.8
Neurospongioblastosis diffusa Q85.1
Neurosyphilis (arrested) (early) (gumma) (late)
  (latent) (recurrent) (relapse) A52.3
  with ataxia (cerebellar) (locomotor) (spastic)
    (spinal) A52.19
  aneurysm (cerebral) A52.05
  arachnoid (adhesive) A52.13
  arteritis (any artery) (cerebral) A52.04
  asymptomatic A52.2
  congenital A50.40
  dura (mater) A52.13
  general paresis A52.17

Neurosyphilis (Continued)
  hemorrhagic A52.05
  juvenile (asymptomatic) (meningeal)
    A50.40
  leptomeninges (aseptic) A52.13
  meningeal, meninges (adhesive) A52.13
  meningitis A52.13
  meningovascular (diffuse) A52.13
  optic atrophy A52.15
  parenchymatous (degenerative) A52.19
  paresis, paretic A52.17
    juvenile A50.45
  remission in (sustained) A52.3
  serological (without symptoms) A52.2
  specified nature or site NEC A52.19
  tabes, tabetic (dorsalis) A52.11
    juvenile A50.45
  taboparesis A52.17
    juvenile A50.45
  thrombosis (cerebral) A52.05
  vascular (cerebral) NEC A52.05
Neurothekeoma —see Neoplasm, nerve, benign
Neurotic —see Neurosis
Neurotoxemia —see Toxemia
Neutroclusion M26.211
Neutropenia, neutropenic (chronic) (genetic)
  (idiopathic) (immune) (infantile)
  (malignant) (pernicious) (splenic) D70.9
  congenital (primary) D70.0
  cyclic D70.4
  cytoreductive cancer chemotherapy sequela
    D70.1
  drug-induced D70.2
    due to cytoreductive cancer chemotherapy
      D70.1
  due to infection D70.3
  fever D70.9
  neonatal, transitory (isoimmune) (maternal
    transfer) P61.5
  periodic D70.4
  secondary (cyclic) (periodic) (splenic) D70.4
    drug-induced D70.2
      due to cytoreductive cancer
        chemotherapy D70.1
  toxic D70.8
Neutrophilia, hereditary giant D72.0
Nevocarcinoma —see Melanoma
Nevus D22.9
  achromic —see Neoplasm, skin, benign
  amelanotic —see Neoplasm, skin, benign
  angiomatous D18.00
    intra-abdominal D18.03
    intracranial D18.02
    skin D18.01
    specified site NEC D18.09
  araneus I78.1
  balloon cell —see Neoplasm, skin, benign
  bathing trunk D48.5
  blue —see Neoplasm, skin, benign
    cellular —see Neoplasm, skin, benign
    giant —see Neoplasm, skin, benign
    Jadassohn's —see Neoplasm, skin, benign
    malignant —see Melanoma
  capillary D18.00
    intra-abdominal D18.03
    intracranial D18.02
    skin D18.01
    specified site NEC D18.09
  cavernous D18.00
    intra-abdominal D18.03
    intracranial D18.02
    skin D18.01
    specified site NEC D18.09
  cellular —see Neoplasm, skin, benign
    blue —see Neoplasm, skin, benign
  choroid D31.3-•
  comedonicus Q82.5
  conjunctiva D31.0-•
  dermal —see Neoplasm, skin, benign
    with epidermal nevus —see Neoplasm,
      skin, benign

Nevus *(Continued)*
  dysplastic —*see* Neoplasm, skin, benign
  eye D31.9-●
  flammeus Q82.5
  hemangiomatous D18.00
    intra-abdominal D18.03
    intracranial D18.02
    skin D18.01
    specified site NEC D18.09
  iris D31.4-●
  lacrimal gland D31.5-●
  lymphatic D18.1
  magnocellular
    specified site —*see* Neoplasm, benign, by
      site
    unspecified site D31.40
  malignant —*see* Melanoma
  meaning hemangioma D18.00
    intra-abdominal D18.03
    intracranial D18.02
    skin D18.01
    specified site NEC D18.09
  mouth (mucosa) D10.30
    specified site NEC D10.39
    white sponge Q38.6
  multiplex Q85.1
  non-neoplastic I78.1
  oral mucosa D10.30
    specified site NEC D10.39
    white sponge Q38.6
  orbit D31.6-●
  pigmented
    giant —*see also* Neoplasm, skin, uncertain
      behavior D48.5
      malignant melanoma in —*see* Melanoma
  portwine Q82.5
  retina D31.2-●
  retrobulbar D31.6-●
  sanguineous Q82.5
  senile I78.1
  skin D22.9
    abdominal wall D22.5
    ala nasi D22.39
    ankle D22.7-●
    anus, anal D22.5
    arm D22.6-●
    auditory canal (external) D22.2-●
    auricle (ear) D22.2-●
    auricular canal (external) D22.2-●
    axilla, axillary fold D22.5
    back D22.5
    breast D22.5
    brow D22.39
    buttock D22.5
    canthus (eye) D22.1-●
    cheek (external) D22.39
    chest wall D22.5
    chin D22.39
    ear (external) D22.2-●
    external meatus (ear) D22.2-●
    eyebrow D22.39
    eyelid (lower) (upper) D22.1-●
    face D22.30
      specified NEC D22.39
    female genital organ (external) NEC D28.0
    finger D22.6-●
    flank D22.5
    foot D22.7-●
    forearm D22.6-●
    forehead D22.39
    foreskin D29.0
    genital organ (external) NEC
      female D28.0
      male D29.9
    gluteal region D22.5
    groin D22.5
    hand D22.6-●
    heel D22.7-●
    helix D22.2-●
    hip D22.7-●
    interscapular region D22.5

Nevus *(Continued)*
  skin *(Continued)*
    jaw D22.39
    knee D22.7-●
    labium (majus) (minus) D28.0
    leg D22.7-●
    lip (lower) (upper) D22.0
    lower limb D22.7-●
    male genital organ (external) D29.9
    nail D22.9
      finger D22.6-●
      toe D22.7-●
    nasolabial groove D22.39
    nates D22.5
    neck D22.4
    nose (external) D22.39
    palpebra D22.1-●
    penis D29.0
    perianal skin D22.5
    perineum D22.5
    pinna D22.2-●
    popliteal fossa or space D22.7-●
    prepuce D29.0
    pudendum D28.0
    scalp D22.4
    scrotum D29.4
    shoulder D22.6-●
    submammary fold D22.5
    temple D22.39
    thigh D22.7-●
    toe D22.7-●
    trunk NEC D22.5
    umbilicus D22.5
    upper limb D22.6-●
    vulva D28.0
  specified site NEC —*see* Neoplasm, benign,
    by site
  spider I78.1
  stellar I78.1
  strawberry Q82.5
  Sutton's benign D22.9
  unius lateris Q82.5
  Unna's Q82.5
  vascular Q82.5
  verrucous Q82.5
Newborn (infant) (liveborn) (singleton)
  Z38.2
  abstinence syndrome P96.1
  acne L70.4
  affected by
    abnormalities of membranes P02.9
      specified NEC P02.8
    abruptio placenta P02.1
    amino-acid metabolic disorder, transitory
      P74.8
    amniocentesis (while in utero) P00.6
    amnionitis P02.78
    apparent life threatening event (ALTE)
      R68.13
    bleeding (into)
      cerebral cortex P52.22
      germinal matrix P52.0
      ventricles P52.1
    breech delivery P03.0
    cardiac arrest P29.81
    cardiomyopathy I42.8
      congenital I42.4
    cerebral ischemia P91.0
    Cesarean delivery P03.4
    chemotherapy agents P04.11
    chorioamnionitis P02.78
    cocaine (crack) P04.41
    complications of labor and delivery P03.9
      specified NEC P03.89
    compression of umbilical cord NEC P02.5
    contracted pelvis P03.1
    cyanosis P28.2
    delivery P03.9
      Cesarean P03.4
      forceps P03.2
      vacuum extractor P03.3

Newborn *(Continued)*
  affected by *(Continued)*
    drugs of addiction P04.40
      cocaine P04.41
      hallucinogens P04.42
      specified drug NEC P04.49
    entanglement (knot) in umbilical cord P02.5
    environmental chemicals P04.6
    fetal (intrauterine)
      growth retardation P05.9
      inflammatory response syndrome (FIRS)
        P02.70
      malnutrition not light or small for
        gestational age P05.2
    FIRS (fetal inflammatory response
      syndrome) P02.70
    forceps delivery P03.2
    heart rate abnormalities
      bradycardia P29.12
      intrauterine P03.819
        before onset of labor P03.810
        during labor P03.811
      tachycardia P29.11
    hemorrhage (antepartum) P02.1
      cerebellar (nontraumatic) P52.6
      intracerebral (nontraumatic) P52.4
      intracranial (nontraumatic) P52.9
        specified NEC P52.8
      intraventricular (nontraumatic) P52.3
        grade 1 P52.0
        grade 2 P52.1
        grade 3 P52.21
        grade 4 P52.22
      posterior fossa (nontraumatic) P52.6
      subarachnoid (nontraumatic) P52.5
      subependymal P52.0
        with intracerebral extension P52.22
        with intraventricular extension P52.1
          with enlargment of ventricles P52.21
        without intraventricular extension
          P52.0
    hypoxic ischemic encephalopathy [HIE]
      P91.60
      mild P91.61
      moderate P91.62
      severe P91.63
    induction of labor P03.89
    intestinal perforation P78.0
    intrauterine (fetal) blood loss P50.9
      due to (from)
        cut end of co-twin cord P50.5
        hemorrhage into
          co-twin P50.3
          maternal circulation P50.4
        placenta P50.2
        ruptured cord blood P50.1
        vasa previa P50.0
      specified NEC P50.8
    intrauterine (fetal) hemorrhage P50.9
    intrauterine (in utero) procedure P96.5
    malpresentation (malposition) NEC P03.1
    maternal (complication of) (use of)
      alcohol P04.3
      amphetamines P04.16
      analgesia (maternal) P04.0
      anesthesia (maternal) P04.0
      anticonvulsants P04.13
      antidepressants P04.15
      antineoplastic chemotherapy P04.11
      anxiolytics P04.1A
      blood loss P02.1
      cannabis P04.81
      circulatory disease P00.3
      condition P00.9
        specified NEC P00.89
      cytotoxic drugs P04.12
      delivery P03.9
        Cesarean P03.4
        forceps P03.2
        vacuum extractor P03.3
      diabetes mellitus (pre-existing) P70.1

▶ New   ⇒ Revised   ~~deleted~~ Deleted   ● Use Additional Character(s)

Newborn *(Continued)*
  affected by *(Continued)*
    maternal *(Continued)*
      disorder P00.9
        specified NEC P00.89
      drugs (addictive) (illegal) NEC P04.49
      ectopic pregnancy P01.4
      gestational diabetes P70.0
      group B streptococcus (GBS)
        colonization (positive) P00.82
      hemorrhage P02.1
      hypertensive disorder P00.0
      incompetent cervix P01.0
      infectious disease P00.2
      injury P00.5
      labor and delivery P03.9
      malpresentation before labor P01.7
      maternal death P01.6
      medical procedure P00.7
      medication P04.19
        specified type NEC P04.18
      multiple pregnancy P01.5
      nutritional disorder P00.4
      oligohydramnios P01.2
      opiates P04.14
        administered for procedures during
          pregnancy or labor and delivery
          P04.0
      parasitic disease P00.2
      periodontal disease P00.81
      placenta previa P02.0
      polyhydramnios P01.3
      precipitate delivery P03.5
      pregnancy P01.9
        specified P01.8
      premature rupture of membranes P01.1
      renal disease P00.1
      respiratory disease P00.3
      sedative-hypnotics P04.17
      surgical procedure P00.6
      tranquilizers administered for
        procedures during pregnancy or
        labor and delivery P04.0
      urinary tract disease P00.1
      uterine contraction (abnormal) P03.6
  meconium peritonitis P78.0
  medication (legal) (maternal use)
    (prescribed) P04.19
  membrane abnormalities P02.9
    specified NEC P02.8
  membranitis P02.78
  methamphetamine(s) P04.49
  mixed metabolic and respiratory acidosis P84
  neonatal abstinence syndrome P96.1
  noxious substances transmitted via
    placenta or breast milk P04.9
    cannabis P04.81
    specified NEC P04.89
  nutritional supplements P04.5
  placenta previa P02.0
  placental
    abnormality (functional)
      (morphological) P02.20
      specified NEC P02.29
    dysfunction P02.29
    infarction P02.29
    insufficiency P02.29
    separation NEC P02.1
    transfusion syndromes P02.3
  placentitis P02.78
  precipitate delivery P03.5
  prolapsed cord P02.4
  respiratory arrest P28.81
  slow intrauterine growth P05.9
  tobacco P04.2
  twin to twin transplacental transfusion P02.3
  umbilical cord (tightly) around neck P02.5
  umbilical cord condition P02.60
    short cord P02.69
    specified NEC P02.69
  uterine contractions (abnormal) P03.6
  vasa previa P02.69
    from intrauterine blood loss P50.0

Newborn *(Continued)*
  apnea *(see also* Apnea, newborn) P28.40
    obstructive P28.42
    primary *(see also* Apnea, newborn, sleep,
      primary) P28.30
    sleep (central) (obstructive) (primary) *(see
      also* Apnea, newborn, sleep, primary)
      P28.30
  born in hospital Z38.00
    by cesarean Z38.01
  born outside hospital Z38.1
  breast buds P96.89
  breast engorgement P83.4
  check-up *—see* Newborn, examination
  convulsion P90
  dehydration P74.1
  examination
    8 to 28 days old Z00.111
    under 8 days old Z00.110
  fever P81.9
    environmentally-induced P81.0
  hyperbilirubinemia P59.9
    of prematurity P59.0
  hypernatremia P74.21
  hyponatremia P74.22
  infection P39.9
    candidal P37.5
    specified NEC P39.8
    urinary tract P39.3
  jaundice P59.9
    due to
      breast milk inhibitor P59.3
      hepatocellular damage P59.20
        specified NEC P59.29
      preterm delivery P59.0
    of prematurity P59.0
    specified NEC P59.8
  late metabolic acidosis P74.0
  mastitis P39.0
    infective P39.0
    noninfective P83.4
  multiple born NEC Z38.8
    born in hospital Z38.68
      by cesarean Z38.69
    born outside hospital Z38.7
  omphalitis P38.9
    with mild hemorrhage P38.1
    without hemorrhage P38.9
  post-term P08.21
  prolonged gestation (over 42 completed
    weeks) P08.22
  quadruplet Z38.8
    born in hospital Z38.63
      by cesarean Z38.64
    born outside hospital Z38.7
  quintuplet Z38.8
    born in hospital Z38.65
      by cesarean Z38.66
    born outside hospital Z38.7
  seizure P90
  sepsis (congenital) P36.9
    due to
      anaerobes NEC P36.5
      Escherichia coli P36.4
      Staphylococcus P36.30
        aureus P36.2
        specified NEC P36.39
      Streptococcus P36.10
        group B P36.0
        specified NEC P36.19
      specified NEC P36.8
  triplet Z38.8
    born in hospital Z38.61
      by cesarean Z38.62
    born outside hospital Z38.7
  twin Z38.5
    born in hospital Z38.30
      by cesarean Z38.31
    born outside hospital Z38.4
  vomiting P92.09
    bilious P92.01
  weight check Z00.111

Newcastle conjunctivitis or disease B30.8
Nezelof's syndrome (pure alymphocytosis) D81.4
Niacin (amide) deficiency E52
Nicolas (-Durand)-Favre disease A55
Nicotine *—see* Tobacco
Nicotinic acid deficiency E52
Niemann-Pick disease or syndrome E75.249
  specified NEC E75.248
  type
    A E75.240
    A/B E75.244
    B E75.241
    C E75.242
    D E75.243
Night
  blindness *—see* Blindness, night
  sweats R61
  terrors (child) F51.4
Nightmares (REM sleep type) F51.5
NIHSS (National Institutes of Health Stroke
  Scale) score R29.7-•
Nipple *—see* condition
Nisbet's chancre A57
Nishimoto (-Takeuchi) disease I67.5
Nitritoid crisis or reaction *—see* Crisis, nitritoid
Nitrosohemoglobinemia D74.8
Njovera A65
No general equivalence degree (GED) Z55.5
Nocardiosis, nocardiasis A43.9
  cutaneous A43.1
  lung A43.0
  pneumonia A43.0
  pulmonary A43.0
  specified site NEC A43.8
Nocturia R35.1
  psychogenic F45.8
Nocturnal *—see* condition
Nodal rhythm I49.8
Node(s) *—see also* Nodule
  Bouchard's (with arthropathy) M15.2
  Haygarth's M15.8
  Heberden's (with arthropathy) M15.1
  larynx J38.7
  lymph *—see* condition
  milker's B08.03
  Osler's I33.0
  Schmorl's *—see* Schmorl's disease
  singer's J38.2
  teacher's J38.2
  tuberculous *—see* Tuberculosis, lymph
    gland
  vocal cord J38.2
Nodule(s), nodular
  actinomycotic *—see* Actinomycosis
  breast NEC *—see also* Lump, breast N63.0
  colloid (cystic), thyroid E04.1
  cutaneous *—see* Swelling, localized
  endometrial (stromal) D26.1
  Haygarth's M15.8
  inflammatory *—see* Inflammation
  juxta-articular
    syphilitic A52.77
    yaws A66.7
  larynx J38.7
  lung, solitary (subsegmental branch of the
    bronchial tree) R91.1
    multiple R91.8
  milker's B08.03
  prostate N40.2
    with lower urinary tract symptoms (LUTS)
      N40.3
    without lower urinary tract symptoms
      (LUTS) N40.2
  pulmonary, solitary (subsegmental branch of
    the bronchial tree) R91.1
  retrocardiac R09.89
  rheumatoid M06.30
    ankle M06.37-•
    elbow M06.32-•
    foot joint M06.37-•
    hand joint M06.34-•

Nodule(s), nodular (Continued)
  rheumatoid (Continued)
    hip M06.35-●
    knee M06.36-●
    multiple site M06.39
    shoulder M06.31-●
    vertebra M06.38
    wrist M06.33-●
  scrotum (inflammatory) N49.2
  singer's J38.2
  solitary, lung (subsegmental branch of the
    bronchial tree) R91.1
    multiple R91.8
  subcutaneous —*see* Swelling, localized
  teacher's J38.2
  thyroid (cold) (gland) (nontoxic) E04.1
    with thyrotoxicosis E05.20
      with thyroid storm E05.21
    toxic or with hyperthyroidism E05.20
      with thyroid storm E05.21
  vocal cord J38.2
Noma (gangrenous) (hospital) (infective)
  A69.0
  auricle I96
  mouth A69.0
  pudendi N76.89
  vulvae N76.89
Nomad, nomadism Z59.00
NOMID (neonatal onset multisystemic
  inflammatory disorder) M04.2
~~Nonadherence to medical treatment Z91.19~~
►Nonadherence to medical treatment, specified
  NEC Z91.199
►due to
  ►financial hardship Z91.190
  ►specified reason NEC Z91.198
Nonautoimmune hemolytic anemia D59.4
  drug-induced D59.2
Nonclosure —*see also* Imperfect, closure
  ductus arteriosus (Botallo's) Q25.0
  foramen
    ⇒botalli Q21.12
    ⇒ovale Q21.12
⇒Noncompliance Z91.199
  with
    dialysis Z91.15
    ⇒dietary regimen Z91.119
    ►due to
      ►financial hardship Z91.110
      ►specified reason NEC Z91.118
    ~~medical treatment Z91.19~~
    ►medical treatment, specified NEC Z91.199
    ►due to
      ►financial hardship Z91.190
      ►specified reason NEC Z91.198
    medication regimen NEC Z91.14
      underdosing —*see also* Table of Drugs
        and Chemicals, categories T36-T50,
        with final character 6 Z91.14
      intentional NEC Z91.128
      ►by caregiver Z91.A4
      ►due to
        ►financial hardship Z91.A20
        ►specified reason NEC Z91.A28
        due to financial hardship of
          patient Z91.120
      unintentional NEC Z91.138
      ►by caregiver Z91.A3

Noncompliance (Continued)
  with (Continued)
    ►caregiver
      ►with patient's
      ►dietary regimen
      ►due to
        ►financial hardship Z91.A10
        ►specified reason NEC Z91.A18
      ►medical treatment and regimen Z91.
        A9
      ►medication regimen, specified NEC
        Z91.A4
      ►renal dialysis Z91.A5
Nondescent (congenital) —*see also* Malposition,
  congenital
  cecum Q43.3
  colon Q43.3
  testicle Q53.9
    bilateral Q53.20
      abdominal Q53.211
      perineal Q53.22
    unilateral Q53.10
      abdominal Q53.111
      perineal Q53.12
Nondevelopment
  brain Q02
    part of Q04.3
  heart Q24.8
  organ or site, congenital NEC —*see*
    Hypoplasia
Nonengagement
  head NEC O32.4
    in labor, causing obstructed labor
      O64.8
Nonexanthematous tick fever A93.2
Nonexpansion, lung (newborn) P28.0
Nonfunctioning
  cystic duct —*see also* Disease, gallbladder
    K82.8
  gallbladder —*see also* Disease, gallbladder
    K82.8
  kidney N28.9
  labyrinth —*see* subcategory H83.2
Non-Hodgkin lymphoma NEC —*see*
  Lymphoma, non-Hodgkin
Nonimplantation, ovum N97.2
Noninsufflation, fallopian tube N97.1
Non-ketotic hyperglycinemia E72.51
Nonne-Milroy syndrome Q82.0
Nonovulation N97.0
Non-palpable testicle(s)
  bilateral R39.84
  unilateral R39.83
Nonpatent fallopian tube N97.1
Nonpneumatization, lung NEC P28.0
Nonrotation —*see* Malrotation
Nonsecretion, urine —*see* Anuria
Nonunion
  fracture —*see* Fracture, by site
  joint, following fusion or arthrodesis M96.0
  organ or site, congenital NEC —*see*
    Imperfect, closure
  symphysis pubis, congenital Q74.2
Nonvisualization, gallbladder R93.2
Nonvital, nonvitalized tooth K04.99
Non-working side interference M26.56
Noonan's syndrome Q87.19

Normocytic anemia (infectional) due to
  blood loss (chronic) D50.0
  acute D62
Norrie's disease (congenital) Q15.8
North American blastomycosis B40.9
Norwegian itch B86
Nose, nasal —*see* condition
Nosebleed R04.0
Nose-picking F98.8
Nosomania F45.21
Nosophobia F45.22
Nostalgia F43.20
Notch of iris Q13.2
Notching nose, congenital (tip) Q30.2
Nothnagel's
  syndrome —*see* Strabismus, paralytic, third
    nerve
  vasomotor acroparesthesia I73.89
Novy's relapsing fever A68.9
  louse-borne A68.0
  tick-borne A68.1
Noxious
  foodstuffs, poisoning by —*see* Poisoning,
    food, noxious, plant
  substances transmitted through placenta or
    breast milk P04.9
Nucleus pulposus —*see* condition
Numbness R20.0
Nuns' knee —*see* Bursitis, prepatellar
Nursemaid's elbow S53.03-●
Nutcracker esophagus K22.4
Nutmeg liver K76.1
Nutrient element deficiency E61.9
  specified NEC E61.8
⇒Nutrition deficient or insufficient —*see also*
  Malnutrition E63.9
  due to
    insufficient food T73.0
    lack of
      care (child) T76.02
        adult T76.01
      food T73.0
  ►specific element deficiency —*see* Nutrient
    element deficiency, or by element
  ►sequelae —*see* Sequalae, nutritional
    deficiency
  ►specified NEC E63.8
Nutritional stunting E45
Nyctalopia (night blindness) —*see* Blindness,
  night
Nycturia R35.1
  psychogenic F45.8
Nymphomania F52.8
Nystagmus H55.00
  benign paroxysmal —*see* Vertigo, benign
    paroxysmal
  central positional H81.4
  congenital H55.01
  dissociated H55.04
  latent H55.02
  miners' H55.09
  positional
    benign paroxysmal H81.4
    central H81.4
  specified form NEC H55.09
  visual deprivation H55.03

O

Obermeyer's relapsing fever (European) A68.0
Obesity E66.9
  with alveolar hypoventilation E66.2
  adrenal E27.8
  complicating
    childbirth O99.214
    pregnancy O99.21-•
    puerperium O99.215
  constitutional E66.8
  dietary counseling and surveillance Z71.3
  drug-induced E66.1
  due to
    drug E66.1
    excess calories E66.09
      morbid E66.01
      severe E66.01
  endocrine E66.8
  endogenous E66.8
  exogenous E66.09
  familial E66.8
  glandular E66.8
  hypothyroid —see Hypothyroidism
  hypoventilation syndrome (OHS) E66.2
  morbid E66.01
    with
      alveolar hypoventilation E66.2
      obesity hypoventilation syndrome (OHS) E66.2
    due to excess calories E66.01
  nutritional E66.09
  pituitary E23.6
  severe E66.01
  specified type NEC E66.8
Oblique —see condition
Obliteration
  appendix (lumen) K38.8
  artery I77.1
  bile duct (noncalculous) K83.1
  common duct (noncalculous) K83.1
  cystic duct —see Obstruction, gallbladder
  disease, arteriolar I77.1
  endometrium N85.8
  eye, anterior chamber —see Disorder, globe, hypotony
  fallopian tube N97.1
  lymphatic vessel I89.0
    due to mastectomy I97.2
  organ or site, congenital NEC —see Atresia, by site
  ureter N13.5
    with infection N13.6
  urethra —see Stricture, urethra
  vein I87.8
  vestibule (oral) K08.89
Observation (following) (for) (without need for further medical care) Z04.9
  accident NEC Z04.3
    at work Z04.2
    transport Z04.1
  adverse effect of drug Z03.6
  alleged rape or sexual assault (victim), ruled out
    adult Z04.41
    child Z04.42
  criminal assault Z04.89
  development state
    adolescent Z00.3
    period of rapid growth in childhood Z00.2
    puberty Z00.3
  disease, specified NEC Z03.89
  following work accident Z04.2
  forced sexual exploitation Z04.81
  forced labor exploitation Z04.82
  growth and development state —see Observation, development state
  injuries (accidental) NEC —see also Observation, accident

Observation (Continued)
  newborn (for)
    suspected condition, related to exposure from the mother or birth process —see Newborn, affected by, maternal
    ruled out Z05.9
      cardiac Z05.0
      connective tissue Z05.73
      gastrointestinal Z05.5
      genetic Z05.41
      genitourinary Z05.6
      immunologic Z05.43
      infectious Z05.1
      metabolic Z05.42
      musculoskeletal Z05.72
      neurological Z05.2
      respiratory Z05.3
      skin and subcutaneous tissue Z05.71
      specified condition NEC Z05.8
  postpartum
    immediately after delivery Z39.0
    routine follow-up Z39.2
  pregnancy (normal) (without complication) Z34.9-•
    high risk O09.9-•
  suicide attempt, alleged NEC Z03.89
    self-poisoning Z03.6
  suspected, ruled out —see also Suspected condition, ruled out
    abuse, physical
      adult Z04.71
      child Z04.72
    accident at work Z04.2
    adult battering victim Z04.71
    child battering victim Z04.72
    condition NEC Z03.89
      newborn —see also Observation, newborn (for), suspected condition, ruled out Z05.9
    drug poisoning or adverse effect Z03.6
    exposure (to)
      anthrax Z03.810
      biological agent NEC Z03.818
      foreign body
        aspirated (inhaled) Z03.822
        ingested Z03.821
        inserted (injected), in (eye) (orifice) (skin) Z03.823
      inflicted injury NEC Z04.89
      suicide attempt, alleged Z03.89
        self-poisoning Z03.6
      toxic effects from ingested substance (drug) (poison) Z03.6
    toxic effects from ingested substance (drug) (poison) Z03.6
Obsession, obsessional state F42.8
  mixed thoughts and acts F42.2
Obsessive-compulsive neurosis or reaction F42.8
Obstetric embolism, septic —see Embolism, obstetric, septic
Obstetrical trauma (complicating delivery) O71.9
  with or following ectopic or molar pregnancy O08.6
  specified type NEC O71.89
Obstipation —see Constipation
Obstruction, obstructed, obstructive
  airway J98.8
    with
      allergic alveolitis J67.9
      asthma J45.909
        with
          exacerbation (acute) J45.901
          status asthmaticus J45.902
      bronchiectasis J47.9
        with
          exacerbation (acute) J47.1
          lower respiratory infection J47.0
      bronchitis (chronic) J44.9
      emphysema J43.9

Obstruction, obstructed, obstructive (Continued)
  airway (Continued)
    chronic J44.9
      with
        allergic alveolitis —see Pneumonitis, hypersensitivity
        bronchiectasis J47.9
          with
            exacerbation (acute) J47.1
            lower respiratory infection J47.0
      due to
        foreign body —see Foreign body, by site, causing asphyxia
        inhalation of fumes or vapors J68.9
        laryngospasm J38.5
  ampulla of Vater K83.1
  aortic (heart) (valve) —see Stenosis, aortic
  aortoiliac I74.09
  aqueduct of Sylvius G91.1
    congenital Q03.0
      with spina bifida —see Spina bifida, by site, with hydrocephalus
  Arnold-Chiari —see Arnold-Chiari disease
  artery (see also Atherosclerosis, artery) I70.9
    basilar (complete) (partial) —see Occlusion, artery, basilar
    carotid (complete) (partial) —see Occlusion, artery, carotid
    cerebellar —see Occlusion, artery, cerebellar
    cerebral (anterior) (middle) (posterior) —see Occlusion, artery, cerebral
    precerebral —see Occlusion, artery, precerebral
    renal N28.0
    retinal NEC —see Occlusion, artery, retina
    stent —see Restenosis, stent
    vertebral (complete) (partial) —see Occlusion, artery, vertebral
  band (intestinal) —see also Obstruction, intestine, specified NEC K56.699
  bile duct or passage (common) (hepatic) (noncalculous) K83.1
    with calculus K80.51
    congenital (causing jaundice) Q44.3
  biliary (duct) (tract) K83.1
    gallbladder K82.0
  bladder-neck (acquired) N32.0
    congenital Q64.31
    due to hyperplasia (hypertrophy) of prostate —see Hyperplasia, prostate
  bowel —see Obstruction, intestine
  bronchus J98.09
  canal, ear —see Stenosis, external ear canal
  cardia K22.2
  caval veins (inferior) (superior) I87.1
  cecum —see Obstruction, intestine
  circulatory I99.8
  colon —see Obstruction, intestine
  common duct (noncalculous) K83.1
  coronary (artery) —see Occlusion, coronary
  cystic duct —see also Obstruction, gallbladder
    with calculus K80.21
  device, implant or graft —see also Complications, by site and type, mechanical T85.698
    arterial graft NEC —see Complication, cardiovascular device, mechanical, vascular
    catheter NEC T85.628
      cystostomy T83.090
      dialysis (renal) T82.49
        intraperitoneal T85.691
      Hopkins T83.098
      ileostomy T83.098
      infusion NEC T82.594
        spinal (epidural) (subdural) T85.690
      nephrostomy T83.092
      urethral indwelling T83.091
      urinary T83.098
      urostomy T83.098

Obstruction, obstructed, obstructive
(Continued)
  device, implant or graft *(Continued)*
    due to infection T85.79
    gastrointestinal —*see* Complications,
      prosthetic device, mechanical,
      gastrointestinal device
    genital NEC T83.498
      intrauterine contraceptive device T83.39
      penile prosthesis (cylinder) (implanted)
        (pump) (resevoir) T83.490
      testicular prosthesis T83.491
    heart NEC —*see* Complication,
      cardiovascular device, mechanical
    joint prosthesis —*see* Complications, joint
      prosthesis, mechanical, specified NEC,
      by site
    orthopedic NEC —*see* Complication,
      orthopedic, device, mechanical
    specified NEC T85.628
    urinary NEC —*see also* Complication,
      genitourinary, device, urinary,
      mechanical
      graft T83.29
    vascular NEC —*see* Complication,
      cardiovascular device, mechanical
    ventricular intracranial shunt T85.09
  due to foreign body accidentally left in
    operative wound T81.529
  duodenum K31.5
  ejaculatory duct N50.89
  esophagus K22.2
  eustachian tube (complete) (partial) H68.10-●
    cartilagenous (extrinsic) H68.13-●
      intrinsic H68.12-●
      osseous H68.11-●
  fallopian tube (bilateral) N97.1
  fecal K56.41
    with hernia —*see* Hernia, by site, with
      obstruction
  foramen of Monro (congenital) Q03.8
    with spina bifida —*see* Spina bifida,
      by site, with hydrocephalus
  foreign body —*see* Foreign body
  gallbladder K82.0
    with calculus, stones K80.21
    congenital Q44.1
  gastric outlet K31.1
  gastrointestinal —*see* Obstruction, intestine
  hepatic K76.89
    duct (noncalculous) K83.1
  hepatobiliary K83.1
  ileum —*see* Obstruction, intestine
  iliofemoral (artery) I74.5
  intestine K56.609
    complete K56.601
    incomplete K56.600
    partial K56.600
    with
      adhesions (intestinal) (peritoneal) K56.50
        complete K56.52
        incomplete K56.51
        partial K56.51
    adynamic K56.0
    by gallstone K56.3
    congenital (small) Q41.9
      large Q42.9
        specified part NEC Q42.8
    neurogenic K56.0
      Hirschsprung's disease or megacolon
        Q43.1
    newborn P76.9
      due to
        fecaliths P76.8
        inspissated milk P76.2
        meconium (plug) P76.0
          in mucoviscidosis E84.11
      specified NEC P76.8
    postoperative K91.30
      complete K91.32
      incomplete K91.31
      partial K91.31

Obstruction, obstructed, obstructive
(Continued)
  intestine *(Continued)*
    reflex K56.0
    specified NEC K56.699
      complete K56.691
      incomplete K56.690
      partial K56.690
    volvulus K56.2
  intracardiac ball valve prosthesis T82.09
  jejunum —*see* Obstruction, intestine
  joint prosthesis —*see* Complications, joint
    prosthesis, mechanical, specified NEC,
    by site
  kidney (calices) (*see also* Hydronephrosis)
    N28.89
  labor —*see* Delivery
  lacrimal (passages) (duct)
    by
      dacryolith —*see* Dacryolith
      stenosis —*see* Stenosis, lacrimal
    congenital Q10.5
    neonatal H04.53-●
  lacrimonasal duct —*see* Obstruction, lacrimal
  lacteal, with steatorrhea K90.2
  laryngitis —*see* Laryngitis
  larynx NEC J38.6
    congenital Q31.8
  lung J98.4
    disease, chronic J44.9
  lymphatic I89.0
  meconium (plug)
    newborn P76.0
      due to fecaliths P76.0
      in mucoviscidosis E84.11
  mitral —*see* Stenosis, mitral
  nasal J34.89
  nasolacrimal duct —*see also* Obstruction,
    lacrimal
    congenital Q10.5
  nasopharynx J39.2
  nose J34.89
  organ or site, congenital NEC —*see* Atresia,
    by site
  pancreatic duct K86.89
  parotid duct or gland K11.8
  pelviureteral junction N13.5
    with hydronephrosis N13.0
    congenital Q62.39
  pharynx J39.2
  portal (circulation) (vein) I81
  prostate —*see also* Hyperplasia, prostate
    valve (urinary) N32.0
  pulmonary valve (heart) I37.0
  pyelonephritis (chronic) N11.1
  pylorus
    adult K31.1
    congenital or infantile Q40.0
  rectosigmoid —*see* Obstruction, intestine
  rectum K62.4
  renal (*see also* Hydronephrosis) N28.89
    outflow N13.8
    pelvis, congenital Q62.39
  respiratory J98.8
    chronic J44.9
  retinal (vessels) H34.9
  salivary duct (any) K11.8
    with calculus K11.5
  sigmoid —*see* Obstruction, intestine
  sinus (accessory) (nasal) J34.89
  Stensen's duct K11.8
  stomach NEC K31.89
    acute K31.0
    congenital Q40.2
    due to pylorospasm K31.3
  submandibular duct K11.8
  submaxillary gland K11.8
    with calculus K11.5
  thoracic duct I89.0
  thrombotic —*see* Thrombosis
  trachea J39.8

Obstruction, obstructed, obstructive
(Continued)
  tracheostomy airway J95.03
  tricuspid (valve) —*see* Stenosis, tricuspid
  upper respiratory, congenital Q34.8
  ureter (functional) (pelvic junction) NEC N13.5
    with
      hydronephrosis N13.1
        with infection N13.6
        congenital Q62.39
      pyelonephritis (chronic) N11.1
    congenital Q62.39
    due to calculus —*see* Calculus, ureter
  urethra NEC N36.8
    congenital Q64.39
  urinary (moderate) N13.9
    due to hyperplasia (hypertrophy) of
      prostate —*see* Hyperplasia, prostate
    organ or tract (lower) N13.9
    prostatic valve N32.0
    specified NEC N13.8
  uropathy N13.9
  uterus N85.8
  vagina N89.5
  valvular —*see* Endocarditis
  vein, venous I87.1
    caval (inferior) (superior) I87.1
      thrombotic —*see* Thrombosis
  vena cava (inferior) (superior) I87.1
  vesical NEC N32.0
  vesicourethral orifice N32.0
    congenital Q64.31
  vessel NEC I99.8
    stent —*see* Restenosis, stent
Obturator —*see* condition
Occlusal wear, teeth K03.0
Occlusio pupillae —*see* Membrane, pupillary
Occlusion, occluded
  anus K62.4
    congenital Q42.3
      with fistula Q42.2
  aortoiliac (chronic) I74.09
  aqueduct of Sylvius G91.1
    congenital Q03.0
      with spina bifida —*see* Spina bifida, by
        site, with hydrocephalus
  artery —*see also* Atherosclerosis, artery I70.9
    auditory, internal I65.8
    basilar I65.1
      with
        infarction I63.22
          due to
            embolism I63.12
            thrombosis I63.02
    brain or cerebral I66.9
      with infarction (due to) I63.5-●
        embolism I63.4-●
        thrombosis I63.3-●
    carotid I65.2-●
      with
        infarction I63.23-●
          due to
            embolism I63.13-●
            thrombosis I63.03-●
    cerebellar (anterior inferior) (posterior
      inferior) (superior) I66.3
      with infarction I63.54-●
        due to
          embolism I63.44-●
          thrombosis I63.34-●
    cerebral I66.9
      with infarction I63.50
        due to
          embolism I63.40
            specified NEC I63.49
          thrombosis I63.30
            specified NEC I63.39
      anterior I66.1-●
        with infarction I63.52-●
          due to
            embolism I63.42-●
            thrombosis I63.32-●

Occlusion, occluded *(Continued)*
artery *(Continued)*
  cerebral *(Continued)*
    middle I66.0-●
      with infarction I63.51-●
        due to
          embolism I63.41-●
          thrombosis I63.31-●
    posterior I66.2-●
      with infarction I63.53-●
        due to
          embolism I63.43-●
          thrombosis I63.33-●
    specified NEC I66.8
      with infarction I63.59
        due to
          embolism I63.4-●
          thrombosis I63.3-●
  choroidal (anterior) —*see* Occlusion,
    artery, cerebral, specified NEC
  communicating posterior —*see* Occlusion,
    artery, precerebral, specified NEC
  complete
    coronary I25.82
    extremities I70.92
  coronary (acute) (thrombotic) (without
    myocardial infarction) I24.0
    with myocardial infarction —*see*
      Infarction, myocardium
    chronic total I25.82
    complete I25.82
    healed or old I25.2
    total (chronic) I25.82
  hypophyseal —*see* Occlusion, artery,
    precerebral, specified NEC
  iliac I74.5
  lower extremities due to stenosis or
    stricture I77.1
  mesenteric (embolic) (thrombotic) —*see also*
    Infarct, intestine K55.069
  perforating —*see* Occlusion, artery,
    cerebral, specified NEC
  peripheral I77.9
    thrombotic or embolic I74.4
  pontine —*see* Occlusion, artery, precerebral,
    specified NEC
  precerebral I65.9
    with infarction I63.20
      due to
        embolism I63.10
          specified NEC I63.19
        thrombosis I63.00
          specified NEC I63.09
      specified NEC I63.29
    basilar —*see* Occlusion, artery, basilar
    carotid —*see* Occlusion, artery, carotid
    puerperal O88.23
    specified NEC I65.8
      with infarction I63.29
        due to
          embolism I63.19
          thrombosis I63.09
    vertebral —*see* Occlusion, artery,
      vertebral
  renal N28.0
  retinal
    branch H34.23-●
    central H34.1-●
    partial H34.21-●
    transient H34.0-●
  spinal —*see* Occlusion, artery, precerebral,
    vertebral
  total (chronic)
    coronary I25.82
    extremities I70.92
  vertebral I65.0-●
    with
      infarction I63.21-●
        due to
          embolism I63.11-●
          thrombosis I63.01-●

Occlusion, occluded *(Continued)*
  basilar artery —*see* Occlusion, artery, basilar
  bile duct (common) (hepatic) (noncalculous)
    K83.1
  bowel —*see* Obstruction, intestine
  carotid (artery) (common) (internal) —*see*
    Occlusion, artery, carotid
  centric (of teeth) M26.59
    maximum intercuspation discrepancy
      M26.55
  cerebellar (artery) —*see* Occlusion, artery,
    cerebellar
  cerebral (artery) —*see* Occlusion, artery,
    cerebral
  cerebrovascular —*see also* Occlusion, artery,
    cerebral
    with infarction I63.5-●
  cervical canal —*see* Stricture, cervix
  cervix (uteri) —*see* Stricture, cervix
  choanal Q30.0
  choroidal (artery) —*see* Occlusion, artery,
    precerebral, specified NEC
  colon —*see* Obstruction, intestine
  communicating posterior artery —*see*
    Occlusion, artery, precerebral, specified
    NEC
  coronary (artery) (vein) (thrombotic) —*see*
    also Infarct, myocardium
    chronic total I25.82
    healed or old I25.2
    not resulting in infarction I24.0
    total (chronic) I25.82
  cystic duct —*see* Obstruction, gallbladder
  embolic —*see* Embolism
  fallopian tube N97.1
    congenital Q50.6
  gallbladder —*see also* Obstruction,
    gallbladder
    congenital (causing jaundice) Q44.1
  gingiva, traumatic K06.2
  hymen N89.6
    congenital Q52.3
  hypophyseal (artery) —*see* Occlusion, artery,
    precerebral, specified NEC
  iliac artery I74.5
  intestine —*see* Obstruction, intestine
  lacrimal passages —*see* Obstruction, lacrimal
  lung J98.4
  lymph or lymphatic channel I89.0
  mammary duct N64.89
  mesenteric artery (embolic) (thrombotic) —
    see also Infarct, intestine K55.069
  nose J34.89
    congenital Q30.0
  organ or site, congenital NEC —*see* Atresia,
    by site
  oviduct N97.1
    congenital Q50.6
  peripheral arteries
    due to stricture or stenosis I77.1
    upper extremity I74.2
  pontine (artery) —*see* Occlusion, artery,
    precerebral, specified NEC
  posterior lingual, of mandibular teeth M26.29
  precerebral artery —*see* Occlusion, artery,
    precerebral
  punctum lacrimale —*see* Obstruction,
    lacrimal
  pupil —*see* Membrane, pupillary
  pylorus, adult —*see also* Stricture, pylorus
    K31.1
  renal artery N28.0
  retina, retinal
    artery —*see* Occlusion, artery, retinal
    vein (central) H34.81-●
      engorgement H34.82-●
      tributary H34.83-●
    vessels H34.9
  spinal artery —*see* Occlusion, artery,
    precerebral, vertebral
  teeth (mandibular) (posterior lingual) M26.29

Occlusion, occluded *(Continued)*
  thoracic duct I89.0
  thrombotic —*see* Thrombosis, artery
  traumatic
    edentulous (alveolar) ridge K06.2
    gingiva K06.2
    periodontal K05.5
  tubal N97.1
  ureter (complete) (partial) N13.5
    congenital Q62.10
  ureteropelvic junction N13.5
    congenital Q62.11
  ureterovesical orifice N13.5
    congenital Q62.12
  urethra —*see* Stricture, urethra
  uterus N85.8
  vagina N89.5
  vascular NEC I99.8
  vein —*see* Thrombosis
    retinal —*see* Occlusion, retinal, vein
  vena cava (inferior) (superior) —*see*
    Embolism, vena cava
  ventricle (brain) NEC G91.1
  vertebral (artery) —*see* Occlusion, artery,
    vertebral
  vessel (blood) I99.8
  vulva N90.5
Occult
  blood in feces (stools) R19.5
Occupational
  problems NEC Z56.89
Ochlophobia —*see* Agoraphobia
Ochronosis (endogenous) E70.29
Ocular muscle —*see* condition
Oculogyric crisis or disturbance H51.8
  psychogenic F45.8
Oculomotor syndrome H51.9
Oculopathy
  syphilitic NEC A52.71
    congenital
      early A50.01
      late A50.30
    early (secondary) A51.43
    late A52.71
Oddi's sphincter spasm K83.4
Odontalgia K08.89
Odontoameloblastoma —*see* Cyst, calcifying
  odontogenic
Odontoclasia K03.89
Odontodysplasia, regional K00.4
Odontogenesis imperfecta K00.5
Odontoma (ameloblastic) (complex)
  (compound) (fibroameloblastic) —*see* Cyst,
  calcifying odontogenic
Odontomyelitis (closed) (open) K04.01
  irreversible K04.02
  reversible K04.01
Odontorrhagia K08.89
Odontosarcoma, ameloblastic C41.1
  upper jaw (bone) C41.0
Oestriasis —*see* Myiasis
Oguchi's disease H53.63
Ohara's disease —*see* Tularemia
OHS (obesity hypoventilation syndrome) E66.2

Oidiomycosis —*see* Candidiasis
Oidium albicans infection —*see* Candidiasis
Old (previous) **myocardial infarction**
  I25.2
Old age (without mention of debility) R54-●
  dementia F03
Olfactory —*see* condition
Oligemia —*see* Anemia
Oligoastrocytoma
  specified site —*see* Neoplasm, malignant,
    by site
  unspecified site C71.9
Oligocythemia D64.9
Oligodendroblastoma
  specified site —*see* Neoplasm, malignant
  unspecified site C71.9

Oligodendroglioma
  anaplastic type
    specified site —see Neoplasm, malignant,
      by site
    unspecified site C71.9
  specified site —see Neoplasm, malignant,
    by site
  unspecified site C71.9
Oligodontia —see Anodontia
Oligoencephalon Q02
Oligohidrosis L74.4
Oligohydramnios O41.0-●
Oligohydrosis L74.4
Oligomenorrhea N91.5
  primary N91.3
  secondary N91.4
Oligophrenia —see also Disability, intellectual
  phenylpyruvic E70.0
Oligospermia N46.11
  due to
    drug therapy N46.121
    efferent duct obstruction N46.123
    infection N46.122
    radiation N46.124
    specified cause NEC N46.129
    systemic disease N46.125
Oligotrichia —see Alopecia
Oliguria R34
  with, complicating or following ectopic or
    molar pregnancy O08.4
  postprocedural N99.0
Ollier's disease Q78.4
Omenotocele —see Hernia, abdomen, specified
  site NEC
Omentitis —see Peritonitis
Omentum, omental —see condition
Omphalitis (congenital) (newborn) P38.9
  with mild hemorrhage P38.1
  without hemorrhage P38.9
  not of newborn L08.82
  tetanus A33
Omphalocele Q79.2
Omphalomesenteric duct, persistent Q43.0
Omphalorrhagia, newborn P51.9
Omsk hemorrhagic fever A98.1
Onanism (excessive) F98.8
Onchocerciasis, onchocercosis B73.1
  with
    eye disease B73.00
      endophthalmitis B73.01
      eyelid B73.09
      glaucoma B73.02
      specified NEC B73.09
    eye NEC B73.00
    eyelid B73.09
Oncocytoma —see Neoplasm, benign, by site
Oncovirus, as cause of disease classified
  elsewhere B97.32
Ondine's curse —see Apnea, sleep
Oneirophrenia F23
Onychauxis L60.2
  congenital Q84.5
Onychia —see also Cellulitis, digit
  with lymphangitis —see Lymphangitis, acute,
    digit
  candidal B37.2
  dermatophytic B35.1
Onychitis —see also Cellulitis, digit
  with lymphangitis —see Lymphangitis, acute,
    digit
Onychocryptosis L60.0
Onychodystrophy L60.3
  congenital Q84.6
Onychogryphosis, onychogryposis L60.2
Onycholysis L60.1
Onychomadesis L60.8
Onychomalacia L60.3
Onychomycosis (finger) (toe) B35.1
Onycho-osteodysplasia Q87.2
Onychophagia F98.8
Onychophosis L60.8

Onychoptosis L60.8
Onychorrhexis L60.3
  congenital Q84.6
Onychoschizia L60.3
Onyxis (finger) (toe) L60.0
Onyxitis —see also Cellulitis, digit
  with lymphangitis —see Lymphangitis, acute,
    digit
Oophoritis (cystic) (infectional) (interstitial)
    N70.92
  with salpingitis N70.93
  acute N70.02
    with salpingitis N70.03
  chronic N70.12
    with salpingitis N70.13
  complicating abortion —see Abortion, by
    type, complicated by, oophoritis
Oophorocele N83.4-●
Opacity, opacities
  cornea H17.-●
    central H17.1-●
    congenital Q13.3
    degenerative —see Degeneration, cornea
    hereditary —see Dystrophy, cornea
    inflammatory —see Keratitis
    minor H17.81-●
    peripheral H17.82-●
    sequelae of trachoma (healed) B94.0
    specified NEC H17.89
  enamel (teeth) (fluoride) (nonfluoride) K00.3
  lens —see Cataract
  snowball —see Deposit, crystalline
  vitreous (humor) NEC H43.39-●
    congenital Q14.0
    membranes and strands H43.31-●
Opalescent dentin (hereditary) K00.5
Open, opening
  abnormal, organ or site, congenital —see
    Imperfect, closure
  angle with
    borderline
      findings
        high risk H40.02-●
        low risk H40.01-●
      intraocular pressure H40.00-●
    cupping of discs H40.01-●
    glaucoma (primary) —see Glaucoma, open
      angle
  bite
    anterior M26.220
    posterior M26.221
  false —see Imperfect, closure
  margin on tooth restoration K08.51
  restoration margins of tooth K08.51
  wound —see Wound, open
Operational fatigue F48.8
Operative —see condition
Operculitis —see Periodontitis
Operculum —see Break, retina
Ophiasis L63.2
Ophthalmia —see also Conjunctivitis H10.9
  actinic rays —see Photokeratitis
  allergic (acute) —see Conjunctivitis, acute,
    atopic
  blennorrhagic (gonococcal) (neonatorum)
    A54.31
  diphtheritic A36.86
  Egyptian A71.1
  electrica —see Photokeratitis
  gonococcal (neonatorum) A54.31
  metastatic —see Endophthalmitis, purulent
  migraine —see Migraine, ophthalmoplegic
  neonatorum, newborn P39.1
    gonococcal A54.31
  nodosa H16.24-●
  purulent —see Conjunctivitis, acute,
    mucopurulent
  spring —see Conjunctivitis, acute, atopic
  sympathetic —see Uveitis, sympathetic
Ophthalmitis —see Ophthalmia
Ophthalmocele (congenital) Q15.8

Ophthalmoneuromyelitis G36.0
Ophthalmoplegia —see also Strabismus, paralytic
  anterior internuclear —see Ophthalmoplegia,
    internuclear
  ataxia-areflexia G61.0
  diabetic —see E08-E13 with .39
  exophthalmic E05.00
    with thyroid storm E05.01
  external H49.88-●
    progressive H49.4-●
      with pigmentary retinopathy —see
        Kearns-Sayre syndrome
    total H49.3-●
  internal (complete) (total) H52.51-●
  internuclear H51.2-●
  migraine —see Migraine, ophthalmoplegic
  Parinaud's H49.88-●
  progressive external —see Ophthalmoplegia,
    external, progressive
  supranuclear, progressive G23.1
  total (external) —see Ophthalmoplegia,
    external, total
Opioid(s)
  abuse —see Abuse, drug, opioids
  dependence —see Dependence, drug, opioids
  induced, without use disorder
    anxiety disorder F11.988
    delirium F11.921
    depressive disorder F11.94
    sexual dysfunction F11.981
    sleep disorder F11.982
Opisthognathism M26.09
Opisthorchiasis (felineus) (viverrini) B66.0
Opitz' disease D73.2
Opiumism —see Dependence, drug, opioid
Oppenheim's disease G70.2
Oppenheim-Urbach disease (necrobiosis
    lipoidica diabeticorum) —see E08-E13 with
    .620
Optic nerve —see condition
Orbit —see condition
Orchioblastoma C62.9-●
Orchitis (gangrenous) (nonspecific) (septic)
    (suppurative) N45.2
  blennorrhagic (gonococcal) (acute) (chronic)
    A54.23
  chlamydial A56.19
  filarial —see also Infestation, filarial B74.9
    [N51]
  gonococcal (acute) (chronic) A54.23
  mumps B26.0
  syphilitic A52.76
  tuberculous A18.15
Orf (virus disease) B08.02
Organic —see also condition
  brain syndrome F09
  heart —see Disease, heart
  mental disorder F09
  psychosis F09
Orgasm
  anejaculatory N53.13
Oriental
  bilharziasis B65.2
  schistosomiasis B65.2
Orifice —see condition
Origin of both great vessels from right
    ventricle Q20.1
Ormond's disease (with ureteral obstruction)
    N13.5
  with infection N13.6
Ornithine metabolism disorder E72.4
Ornithinemia (Type I) (Type II) E72.4
Ornithosis A70
Orotaciduria, oroticaciduria (congenital)
    (hereditary) (pyrimidine deficiency) E79.8
  anemia D53.0
Orthodontics
  adjustment Z46.4
  fitting Z46.4
Orthopnea R06.01
Orthopoxvirus B08.09

▶ New   ⇥ Revised   ~~deleted~~ Deleted   ● Use Additional Character(s)

Os, uterus —*see* condition
Osgood-Schlatter disease or osteochondrosis M92.52-●
Osler (-Weber)-Rendu disease I78.0
Osler's nodes I33.0
Osmidrosis L75.0
Osseous —*see* condition
Ossification
  artery —*see* Arteriosclerosis
  auricle (ear) —*see* Disorder, pinna, specified type NEC
  bronchial J98.09
  cardiac —*see* Degeneration, myocardial
  cartilage (senile) —*see* Disorder, cartilage, specified type NEC
  coronary (artery) —*see* Disease, heart, ischemic, atherosclerotic
  diaphragm J98.6
  ear, middle —*see* Otosclerosis
  falx cerebri G96.198
  fontanel, premature Q75.0
  heart —*see also* Degeneration, myocardial
    valve —*see* Endocarditis
  larynx J38.7
  ligament —*see* Disorder, tendon, specified type NEC
    posterior longitudinal —*see* Spondylopathy, specified NEC
  meninges (cerebral) (spinal) G96.198
  multiple, eccentric centers —*see* Disorder, bone, development or growth
  muscle —*see also* Calcification, muscle
    due to burns —*see* Myositis, ossificans, in, burns
    paralytic —*see* Myositis, ossificans, in, quadriplegia
    progressive —*see* Myositis, ossificans, progressiva
    specified NEC M61.50
      ankle M61.57-●
      foot M61.57-●
      forearm M61.53-●
      hand M61.54-●
      lower leg M61.56-●
      multiple sites M61.59
      pelvic region M61.55-●
      shoulder region M61.51-●
      specified site NEC M61.58
      thigh M61.55-●
      upper arm M61.52-●
    traumatic —*see* Myositis, ossificans, traumatica
  myocardium, myocardial —*see* Degeneration, myocardial
  penis N48.89
  periarticular —*see* Disorder, joint, specified type NEC
  pinna —*see* Disorder, pinna, specified type NEC
  rider's bone —*see* Ossification, muscle, specified NEC
  sclera H15.89
  subperiosteal, post-traumatic M89.8X-●
  tendon —*see* Disorder, tendon, specified type NEC
  trachea J39.8
  tympanic membrane —*see* Disorder, tympanic membrane, specified NEC
  vitreous (humor) —*see* Deposit, crystalline
Osteitis —*see also* Osteomyelitis
  alveolar M27.3
  condensans M85.30
    ankle M85.37-●
    foot M85.37-●
    forearm M85.33-●
    hand M85.34-●
    lower leg M85.36-●
    multiple site M85.39
    neck M85.38
    rib M85.38
    shoulder M85.31-●

Osteitis *(Continued)*
  condensans *(Continued)*
    skull M85.38
    specified site NEC M85.38
    thigh M85.35-●
    toe M85.37-●
    upper arm M85.32-●
    vertebra M85.38
  deformans M88.9
    in (due to)
      malignant neoplasm of bone C41.9 *[M90.60]*
      neoplastic disease —*see also* Neoplasm D49.9 *[M90.60]*
        carpus D49.9 *[M90.64-●]*
        clavicle D49.9 *[M90.61-●]*
        femur D49.9 *[M90.65-●]*
        fibula D49.9 *[M90.66-●]*
        finger D49.9 *[M90.64-●]*
        humerus D49.9 *[M90.62-●]*
        ilium D49.9 *[M90.65-●]*
        ischium D49.9 *[M90.65-●]*
        metacarpus D49.9 *[M90.64-●]*
        metatarsus D49.9 *[M90.67-●]*
        multiple sites D49.9 *[M90.69]*
        neck D49.9 *[M90.68]*
        radius D49.9 *[M90.63-●]*
        rib D49.9 *[M90.68]*
        scapula D49.9 *[M90.61-●]*
        skull D49.9 *[M90.68]*
        tarsus D49.9 *[M90.67-●]*
        tibia D49.9 *[M90.66-●]*
        toe D49.9 *[M90.67-●]*
        ulna D49.9 *[M90.63-●]*
        vertebra D49.9 *[M90.68]*
    skull M88.0
    specified NEC —*see* Paget's disease, bone, by site
    vertebra M88.1
  due to yaws A66.6
  fibrosa NEC —*see* Cyst, bone, by site
    circumscripta —*see* Dysplasia, fibrous, bone NEC
    cystica (generalisata) E21.0
    disseminata Q78.1
    osteoplastica E21.0
  fragilitans Q78.0
  Garr's (sclerosing) —*see* Osteomyelitis, specified type NEC
  jaw (acute) (chronic) (lower) (suppurative) (upper) M27.2
  parathyroid E21.0
  petrous bone (acute) (chronic) —*see* Petrositis
  sclerotic, nonsuppurative —*see* Osteomyelitis, specified type NEC
  tuberculosa A18.09
    cystica D86.89
    multiplex cystoides D86.89
Osteoarthritis M19.90
  ankle M19.07-●
  ▶post-traumatic M19.17-●
  ▶primary M19.07-●
  ▶secondary M19.27-●
  elbow M19.02-●
  ▶post-traumatic M19.12-●
  ▶primary M19.02-●
  ▶secondary M19.22-●
  foot joint M19.07-●
  ▶post-traumatic M19.17-●
  ▶primary M19.07-●
  ▶secondary M19.27-●
  generalized (multiple joints) M15.9
    erosive M15.4
    primary M15.0
    specified NEC M15.8
  hand joint M19.04-●
    first carpometacarpal joint M18.9-●
    ▶post-traumatic —*see* Osteoarthritis, post-traumatic NEC, hand joint, first carpometacarpal joint

Osteoarthritis *(Continued)*
  hand joint *(Continued)*
    first carpometacarpal joint *(Continued)*
    ▶primary —*see* Osteoarthritis, primary, hand joint, first carpometacarpal joint
    ▶secondary —*see* Osteoarthritis, secondary, hand joint, first carpometacarpal joint
  ▶post-traumatic M19.14-●
  ▶primary M19.04-●
  ▶secondary M19.24-●
  ⧯hip M16.9
    bilateral M16.0
    ▶due to hip dysplasia M16.2
    ▶post-traumatic M16.4
    ▶secondary M16.6
    due to hip dysplasia (unilateral) M16.3-●
      bilateral M16.2
    ▶post-traumatic —*see* Osteoarthritis, post-traumatic, hip
    ▶primary M16.1-●
      ▶bilateral M16.0
    ▶secondary —*see* Osteoarthritis, secondary, hip
    ▶unilateral M16.1-●
      ▶due to hip dysplasia M16.3-●
      ▶post-traumatic M16.5-●
      ▶primary M16.1-●
      ▶secondary NEC M16.7
  interphalangeal
    distal (Heberden) M15.1
    proximal (Bouchard) M15.2
  ⧯knee M17.9
    bilateral M17.0
    ▶post-traumatic M17.2
    ▶secondary M17.4
    ▶post-traumatic —*see* Osteoarthritis, post-traumatic, knee
    ▶primary M17.1-●
      ▶bilateral M17.0
    ▶secondary —*see* Osteoarthritis, secondary, knee
    ▶unilateral M17.1-●
      ▶post-traumatic M17.3-●
      ▶primary M17.1-●
      ▶secondary NEC M17.5
  post-traumatic NEC M19.92
    ankle M19.17-●
    elbow M19.12-●
    foot joint M19.17-●
    hand joint M19.14-●
      first carpometacarpal joint M18.3-●
        bilateral M18.2
    hip M16.5-●
      bilateral M16.4
    knee M17.3-●
      bilateral M17.2
    shoulder M19.11-●
    specified site NEC M19.19
    wrist M19.13-●
  primary M19.91
    ankle M19.07-●
    elbow M19.02-●
    foot joint M19.07-●
    hand joint M19.04-●
      first carpometacarpal joint M18.1-●
        bilateral M18.0
    hip M16.1-●
      bilateral M16.0
    knee M17.1-●
      bilateral M17.0
    multiple sites M15.9
    shoulder M19.01-●
    ▶specified site NEC M19.09
    spine —*see* Spondylosis
    wrist M19.03-●
  secondary M19.93
    ankle M19.27-●
    elbow M19.22-●

Osteoarthritis (Continued)
  secondary (Continued)
    foot joint M19.27-●
    hand joint M19.24-●
      first carpometacarpal joint M18.5-●
        bilateral M18.4
    ➠hip M16.7-●
      bilateral M16.6
    ➠knee M17.5-●
      bilateral M17.4
    multiple M15.3
    shoulder M19.21-●
    specified site NEC M19.29
    spine —see Spondylosis
    wrist M19.23-●
  shoulder M19.01-●
    ▶post-traumatic M19.11-●
    ▶primary M19.01-●
    ▶secondary M19.21-●
  specified site NEC M19.09
  spine —see Spondylosis
  wrist M19.03-●
    ▶first carpometacarpal joint —see
        Osteoarthritis, hand joint, first
        carpometacarpal joint
    ▶post-traumatic M19.13-●
    ▶primary M19.03-●
    ▶secondary M19.23-●
Osteoarthropathy (hypertrophic) M19.90
  ankle —see Osteoarthritis, primary, ankle
  elbow —see Osteoarthritis, primary, elbow
  foot joint —see Osteoarthritis, primary, foot
  hand joint —see Osteoarthritis, primary, hand
      joint
  knee joint —see Osteoarthritis, primary, knee
  multiple site —see Osteoarthritis, primary,
      multiple joint
  pulmonary —see also Osteoarthropathy,
      specified type NEC
    hypertrophic —see Osteoarthropathy,
        hypertrophic, specified type NEC
    secondary —see Osteoarthropathy, specified
        type NEC
  secondary hypertrophic —see
      Osteoarthropathy, specified type NEC
  shoulder —see Osteoarthritis, primary,
      shoulder
  specified joint NEC —see Osteoarthritis,
      primary, specified joint NEC
  specified type NEC M89.40
    carpus M89.44-●
    clavicle M89.41-●
    femur M89.45-●
    fibula M89.46-●
    finger M89.44-●
    humerus M89.42-●
    ilium M89.459
    ischium M89.459
    metacarpus M89.44-●
    metatarsus M89.47-●
    multiple sites M89.49
    neck M89.48
    radius M89.43-●
    rib M89.48
    scapula M89.41-●
    skull M89.48
    tarsus M89.47-●
    tibia M89.46-●
    toe M89.47-●
    ulna M89.43-●
    vertebra M89.48
  spine —see Spondylosis
  wrist —see Osteoarthritis, primary, wrist
Osteoarthrosis (degenerative) (hypertrophic)
    (joint) —see also Osteoarthritis
  deformans alkaptonurica E70.29 [M36.8]
  erosive M15.4
  generalized M15.9
    primary M15.0
  polyarticular M15.9
  spine —see Spondylosis

Osteoblastoma —see Neoplasm, bone, benign
  aggressive —see Neoplasm, bone, uncertain
      behavior
Osteochondroarthrosis deformans
    endemica —see Disease, Kaschin-Beck
Osteochondritis —see also Osteochondropathy,
    by site
  Brailsford's —see Osteochondrosis, juvenile,
      radius
  dissecans M93.20
    ankle M93.27-●
    elbow M93.22-●
    foot M93.27-●
    hand M93.24-●
    hip M93.25-●
    knee M93.26-●
    multiple sites M93.29
    shoulder joint M93.21-●
    specified site NEC M93.28
    wrist M93.23-●
  juvenile M92.9
    patellar —see Osteochondrosis, juvenile,
        patella
  syphilitic (congenital) (early) A50.02
      [M90.80]
    ankle A50.02 [M90.87-●]
    elbow A50.02 [M90.82-●]
    foot A50.02 [M90.87-●]
    forearm A50.02 [M90.83-●]
    hand A50.02 [M90.84-●]
    hip A50.02 [M90.85-●]
    knee A50.02 [M90.86●-]
    multiple sites A50.02 [M90.89]
    shoulder joint A50.02 [M90.81-●]
    specified site NEC A50.02 [M90.88]
Osteochondrodysplasia Q78.9
  with defects of growth of tubular bones and
      spine Q77.9
    specified NEC Q77.8
  specified NEC Q78.8
Osteochondrodystrophy E78.9
Osteochondrolysis —see Osteochondritis,
    dissecans
Osteochondroma —see Neoplasm, bone, benign
➠Osteochondromatosis D16.9
  syndrome Q78.4
Osteochondromyxosarcoma —see Neoplasm,
    bone, malignant
Osteochondropathy M93.90
  ankle M93.97-●
  elbow M93.92-●
  foot M93.97-●
  hand M93.94-●
  hip M93.95-●
  Kienböck's disease of adults M93.1
  knee M93.96-●
  multiple joints M93.99
  osteochondritis dissecans —see
      Osteochondritis, dissecans
  osteochondrosis —see Osteochondrosis
  shoulder region M93.91-●
  slipped upper femoral epiphysis —see
      Slipped, epiphysis, upper femoral
  specified joint NEC M93.98
  specified type NEC M93.80
    ankle M93.87-●
    elbow M93.82-●
    foot M93.87-●
    hand M93.84-●
    hip M93.85-●
    knee M93.86-●
    multiple joints M93.89
    shoulder region M93.81-●
    specified joint NEC M93.88
    wrist M93.83-●
  syphilitic, congenital
    early A50.02 [M90.80]
    late A50.56 [M90.80]
  wrist M93.93-●
Osteochondrosarcoma —see Neoplasm, bone,
    malignant

Osteochondrosis —see also Osteochondropathy,
    by site
  acetabulum (juvenile) M91.0
  adult —see Osteochondropathy, specified
      type NEC, by site
  astragalus (juvenile) —see Osteochondrosis,
      juvenile, tarsus
  Blount M92.51-●
  Buchanan's M91.0
  Burns' —see Osteochondrosis, juvenile, ulna
  calcaneus (juvenile) —see Osteochondrosis,
      juvenile, tarsus
  capitular epiphysis (femur) (juvenile) —see
      Legg-Calvé-Perthes disease
  carpal (juvenile) (lunate) (scaphoid) —see
      Osteochondrosis, juvenile, hand, carpal
      lunate
    adult M93.1
  coxae juvenilis —see Legg-Calvé-Perthes
      disease
  deformans juvenilis, coxae —see Legg-Calvé-
      Perthes disease
  Diaz's —see Osteochondrosis, juvenile, tarsus
  dissecans (knee) (shoulder) —see
      Osteochondritis, dissecans
  femoral capital epiphysis (juvenile) —see
      Legg-Calvé-Perthes disease
  femur (head), juvenile —see Legg-Calvé-
      Perthes disease
  fibula (juvenile) —see Osteochondrosis,
      juvenile, fibula
  foot NEC (juvenile) M92.8
  Freiberg's —see Osteochondrosis, juvenile,
      metatarsus
  Haas' (juvenile) —see Osteochondrosis,
      juvenile, humerus
  Haglund's —see Osteochondrosis, juvenile,
      tarsus
  hip (juvenile) —see Legg-Calvé-Perthes
      disease
  humerus (capitulum) (head) (juvenile) —see
      Osteochondrosis, juvenile, humerus
  ilium, iliac crest (juvenile) M91.0
  ischiopubic synchondrosis M91.0
  Iselin's —see Osteochondrosis, juvenile,
      metatarsus
  juvenile, juvenilis M92.9
    after congenital dislocation of hip
        reduction —see Osteochondrosis,
        juvenile, hip, specified NEC
    arm —see Osteochondrosis, juvenile, upper
        limb NEC
    capitular epiphysis (femur) —see Legg-
        Calvé-Perthes disease
    clavicle, sternal epiphysis —see
        Osteochondrosis, juvenile, upper limb
        NEC
    coxae —see Legg-Calvé-Perthes disease
    deformans M92.9
    fibula M92.50-●
    foot NEC M92.8
    hand M92.20-●
      carpal lunate M92.21-●
      metacarpal head M92.22-●
      specified site NEC M92.29-●
    head of femur —see Legg-Calvé-Perthes
        disease
    hip and pelvis M91.9-●
      coxa plana —see Coxa, plana
      femoral head —see Legg-Calvé-Perthes
          disease
      pelvis M91.0
      pseudocoxalgia —see Pseudocoxalgia
      specified NEC M91.8-●
    humerus M92.0-●
    limb
      lower NEC M92.8
      upper NEC —see Osteochondrosis,
          juvenile, upper limb NEC
    medial cuneiform bone —see
        Osteochondrosis, juvenile, tarsus

▶ New   ➠ Revised   ~~deleted~~ Deleted   ● Use Additional Character(s)

Osteochondrosis *(Continued)*
  juvenile, juvenilis *(Continued)*
    metatarsus M92.7-●
    patella M92.4-●
    radius M92.1-●
    specified
      site NEC M92.8
      type NEC M92.8
        tibia and fibula M92.59-●
    spine M42.00
      cervical region M42.02
      cervicothoracic region M42.03
      lumbar region M42.06
      lumbosacral region M42.07
      multiple sites M42.09
      occipito-atlanto-axial region M42.01
      sacrococcygeal region M42.08
      thoracic region M42.04
      thoracolumbar region M42.05
    tarsus M92.6-●
    tibia M92.50-●
      proximal M92.51-●
      tubercle M92.52-●
    ulna M92.1-●
    upper limb NEC M92.3-●
    vertebra (body) (epiphyseal plates) (Calvé's) (Scheuermann's) —*see* Osteochondrosis, juvenile, spine
  Kienböck's —*see* Osteochondrosis, juvenile, hand, carpal lunate
    adult M93.1
  Köhler's
    patellar —*see* Osteochondrosis, juvenile, patella
    tarsal navicular —*see* Osteochondrosis, juvenile, tarsus
  Legg-Perthes (-Calvé's) (-Waldenström) —*see* Legg-Calvé-Perthes disease
  limb
    lower NEC (juvenile) M92.8
      tibia and fibula M92.59-●
    upper NEC (juvenile) —*see* Osteochondrosis, juvenile, upper limb NEC
  lunate bone (carpal) (juvenile) —*see also* Osteochondrosis, juvenile, hand, carpal lunate
    adult M93.1
  Mauclaire's —*see* Osteochondrosis, juvenile, hand, metacarpal
  metacarpal (head) (juvenile) —*see* Osteochondrosis, juvenile, hand, metacarpal
  metatarsus (fifth) (head) (juvenile) (second) —*see* Osteochondrosis, juvenile, metatarsus
  navicular (juvenile) —*see* Osteochondrosis, juvenile, tarsus
  os
    calcis (juvenile) —*see* Osteochondrosis, juvenile, tarsus
    tibiale externum (juvenile) —*see* Osteochondrosis, juvenile, tarsus
  Osgood-Schlatter M92.52-●
  Panner's —*see* Osteochondrosis, juvenile, humerus
  patellar center (juvenile) (primary) (secondary) —*see* Osteochondrosis, juvenile, patella
  pelvis (juvenile) M91.0
  Pierson's M91.0
  radius (head) (juvenile) —*see* Osteochondrosis, juvenile, radius
  Scheuermann's —*see* Osteochondrosis, juvenile, spine
  Sever's —*see* Osteochondrosis, juvenile, tarsus
  Sinding-Larsen —*see* Osteochondrosis, juvenile, patella

Osteochondrosis *(Continued)*
  spine *(Continued)*
    adult M42.10
      cervical region M42.12
      cervicothoracic region M42.13
      lumbar region M42.16
      lumbosacral region M42.17
      multiple sites M42.19
      occipito-atlanto-axial region M42.11
      sacrococcygeal region M42.18
      thoracic region M42.14
      thoracolumbar region M42.15
    juvenile —*see* Osteochondrosis, juvenile, spine
  symphysis pubis (juvenile) M91.0
  syphilitic (congenital) A50.02
  talus (juvenile) —*see* Osteochondrosis, juvenile, tarsus
  tarsus (navicular) (juvenile) —*see* Osteochondrosis, juvenile, tarsus
  tibia (proximal) (tubercle) (juvenile) —*see* Osteochondrosis, juvenile, tibia
  tuberculous —*see* Tuberculosis, bone
  ulna (lower) (juvenile) —*see* Osteochondrosis, juvenile, ulna
  van Neck's M91.0
  vertebral —*see* Osteochondrosis, spine
Osteoclastoma D48.0
  malignant —*see* Neoplasm, bone, malignant
Osteodynia —*see* Disorder, bone, specified type NEC
Osteodystrophy Q78.9
  azotemic N25.0
  congenital Q78.9
  parathyroid, secondary E21.1
  renal N25.0
Osteofibroma —*see* Neoplasm, bone, benign
Osteofibrosarcoma —*see* Neoplasm, bone, malignant
Osteogenesis imperfecta Q78.0
Osteogenic —*see* condition
Osteolysis M89.50
  carpus M89.54-●
  clavicle M89.51-●
  femur M89.55-●
  fibula M89.56-●
  finger M89.54-●
  humerus M89.52-●
  ilium M89.559
  ischium M89.559
  joint prosthesis (periprosthetic) —*see* Complications, joint prosthesis, mechanical, periprosthetic, osteolysis, by site
  metacarpus M89.54-●
  metatarsus M89.57-●
  multiple sites M89.59
  neck M89.58
  periprosthetic —*see* Complications, joint prosthesis, mechanical, periprosthetic, osteolysis, by site
  radius M89.53-●
  rib M89.58
  scapula M89.51-●
  skull M89.58
  tarsus M89.57-●
  tibia M89.56-●
  toe M89.57-●
  ulna M89.53-●
  vertebra M89.58
Osteoma —*see also* Neoplasm, bone, benign
  osteoid —*see also* Neoplasm, bone, benign
    giant —*see* Neoplasm, bone, benign
Osteomalacia M83.9
  adult M83.9
    drug-induced NEC M83.5
    due to
      malabsorption (postsurgical) M83.2
      malnutrition M83.3
    specified NEC M83.8
  aluminium-induced M83.4
  infantile —*see* Rickets

Osteomalacia *(Continued)*
  juvenile —*see* Rickets
  oncogenic E83.89
  pelvis M83.8
  puerperal M83.0
  senile M83.1
  vitamin-D-resistant in adults E83.31 *[M90.8-●]*
    carpus E83.31 *[M90.84-●]*
    clavicle E83.31 *[M90.81-●]*
    femur E83.31 *[M90.85-●]*
    fibula E83.31 *[M90.86-●]*
    finger E83.31 *[M90.84-●]*
    humerus E83.31 *[M90.82-●]*
    ilium E83.31 *[M90.859]*
    ischium E83.31 *[M90.859]*
    metacarpus E83.31 *[M90.84-●]*
    metatarsus E83.31 *[M90.87-●]*
    multiple sites E83.31 *[M90.89]*
    neck E83.31 *[M90.88]*
    radius E83.31 *[M90.83-●]*
    rib E83.31 *[M90.88]*
    scapula E83.31 *[M90.819]*
    skull E83.31 *[M90.88]*
    tarsus E83.31 *[M90.879]*
    tibia E83.31 *[M90.869]*
    toe E83.31 *[M90.879]*
    ulna E83.31 *[M90.839]*
    vertebra E83.31 *[M90.88]*
Osteomyelitis (general) (infective) (localized) (neonatal) (septic) (staphylococcal) (streptococcal) (suppurative) (with periostitis) M86.9
  acute M86.10
    carpus M86.14-●
    clavicle M86.11-●
    femur M86.15-●
    fibula M86.16-●
    finger M86.14-●
    hematogenous M86.00
      carpus M86.04-●
      clavicle M86.01-●
      femur M86.05-●
      fibula M86.06-●
      finger M86.04-●
      humerus M86.02-●
      ilium M86.08
      ischium M86.08
      mandible M27.2
      metacarpus M86.04-●
      metatarsus M86.07-●
      multiple sites M86.09
      neck M86.08
      orbit H05.02-●
      petrous bone —*see* Petrositis
      radius M86.03-●
      rib M86.08
      scapula M86.01-●
      skull M86.08
      tarsus M86.07-●
      tibia M86.06-●
      toe M86.07-●
      ulna M86.03-●
      vertebra —*see* Osteomyelitis, vertebra
    humerus M86.12-●
    ilium M86.18
    ischium M86.18
    mandible M27.2
    metacarpus M86.14-●
    metatarsus M86.17-●
    multiple sites M86.19
    neck M86.18
    orbit H05.02-●
    petrous bone —*see* Petrositis
    radius M86.13-●
    rib M86.18
    scapula M86.11-●
    skull M86.18
    tarsus M86.17-●
    tibia M86.16-●
    toe M86.17-●
    ulna M86.13-●
    vertebra —*see* Osteomyelitis, vertebra

Osteomyelitis *(Continued)*
  chronic (or old) M86.60
    with draining sinus M86.40
      carpus M86.44-●
      clavicle M86.41-●
      femur M86.45-●
      fibula M86.46-●
      finger M86.44-●
      humerus M86.42-●
      ilium M86.459
      ischium M86.459
      mandible M27.2
      metacarpus M86.44-●
      metatarsus M86.47-●
      multiple sites M86.49
      neck M86.48
      orbit H05.02-●
      petrous bone —*see* Petrositis
      radius M86.43-●
      rib M86.48
      scapula M86.41-●
      skull M86.48
      tarsus M86.47-●
      tibia M86.46-●
      toe M86.47-●
      ulna M86.43-●
      vertebra —*see* Osteomyelitis, vertebra
    carpus M86.64-●
    clavicle M86.61-●
    femur M86.65-●
    fibula M86.66-●
    finger M86.64-●
    hematogenous NEC M86.50
      carpus M86.54-●
      clavicle M86.51-●
      femur M86.55-●
      fibula M86.56-●
      finger M86.54-●
      humerus M86.52-●
      ilium M86.559
      ischium M86.559
      mandible M27.2
      metacarpus M86.54-●
      metatarsus M86.57-●
      multifocal M86.30
        carpus M86.34-●
        clavicle M86.31-●
        femur M86.35-●
        fibula M86.36-●
        finger M86.34-●
        humerus M86.32-●
        ilium M86.359
        ischium M86.359
        metacarpus M86.34-●
        metatarsus M86.37-●
        multiple sites M86.39
        neck M86.38
        radius M86.33-●
        rib M86.38
        scapula M86.31-●
        skull M86.38
        tarsus M86.37-●
        tibia M86.36-●
        toe M86.37-●
        ulna M86.33-●
        vertebra —*see* Osteomyelitis, vertebra
      multiple sites M86.59
      neck M86.58
      orbit H05.02-●
      petrous bone —*see* Petrositis
      radius M86.53-●
      rib M86.58
      scapula M86.51-●
      skull M86.58
      tarsus M86.57-●
      tibia M86.56-●
      toe M86.57-●
      ulna M86.53-●
      vertebra —*see* Osteomyelitis, vertebra
    humerus M86.62-●
    ilium M86.659

Osteomyelitis *(Continued)*
  chronic *(Continued)*
    ischium M86.659
    mandible M27.2
    metacarpus M86.64-●
    metatarsus M86.67-●
    multifocal —*see* Osteomyelitis, chronic, hematogenous, multifocal
    multiple sites M86.69
    neck M86.68
    orbit H05.02-●
    petrous bone —*see* Petrositis
    radius M86.63-●
    rib M86.68
    scapula M86.61-●
    skull M86.68
    tarsus M86.67-●
    tibia M86.66-●
    toe M86.67-●
    ulna M86.63-●
    vertebra —*see* Osteomyelitis, vertebra
  echinococcal B67.2
  Garr's —*see* Osteomyelitis, specified type NEC
  in diabetes mellitus —*see* E08-E13 with .69
  jaw (acute) (chronic) (lower) (neonatal) (suppurative) (upper) M27.2
  nonsuppurating —*see* Osteomyelitis, specified type NEC
  orbit H05.02-●
  petrous bone —*see* Petrositis
  Salmonella (arizonae) (cholerae-suis) (enteritidis) (typhimurium) A02.24
  sclerosing, nonsuppurative —*see* Osteomyelitis, specified type NEC
  specified type NEC —*see also* subcategory M86.8X-●
    mandible M27.2
    orbit H05.02-●
    petrous bone —*see* Petrositis
    vertebra —*see* Osteomyelitis, vertebra
  subacute M86.20
    carpus M86.24-●
    clavicle M86.21-●
    femur M86.25-●
    fibula M86.26-●
    finger M86.24-●
    humerus M86.22-●
    mandible M27.2
    metacarpus M86.24-●
    metatarsus M86.27-●
    multiple sites M86.29
    neck M86.28
    orbit H05.02-●
    petrous bone —*see* Petrositis
    radius M86.23-●
    rib M86.28
    scapula M86.21-●
    skull M86.28
    tarsus M86.27-●
    tibia M86.26-●
    toe M86.27-●
    ulna M86.23-●
    vertebra —*see* Osteomyelitis, vertebra
  syphilitic A52.77
    congenital (early) A50.02 [M90.80]
  tuberculous —*see* Tuberculosis, bone
  typhoid A01.05
  vertebra M46.20
    cervical region M46.22
    cervicothoracic region M46.23
    lumbar region M46.26
    lumbosacral region M46.27
    occipito-atlanto-axial region M46.21
    sacrococcygeal region M46.28
    thoracic region M46.24
    thoracolumbar region M46.25
Osteomyelofibrosis D47.4
Osteomyelosclerosis D75.89

Osteonecrosis M87.9
  due to
    drugs —*see* Osteonecrosis, secondary, due to, drugs
    trauma —*see* Osteonecrosis, secondary, due to, trauma
  idiopathic aseptic M87.00
    ankle M87.07-●
    carpus M87.03-●
    clavicle M87.01-●
    femur M87.05-●
    fibula M87.06-●
    finger M87.04-●
    humerus M87.02-●
    ilium M87.050
    ischium M87.050
    metacarpus M87.04-●
    metatarsus M87.07-●
    multiple sites M87.09
    neck M87.08
    pelvis M87.050
    radius M87.03-●
    rib M87.08
    scapula M87.01-●
    skull M87.08
    tarsus M87.07-●
    tibia M87.06-●
    toe M87.07-●
    ulna M87.03-●
    vertebra M87.08
  secondary NEC M87.30
    carpus M87.33-●
    clavicle M87.31-●
    due to
      drugs M87.10
        carpus M87.13-●
        clavicle M87.11-●
        femur M87.15-●
        fibula M87.16-●
        finger M87.14-●
        humerus M87.12-●
        ilium M87.159
        ischium M87.159
        jaw M87.180
        metacarpus M87.14-●
        metatarsus M87.17-●
        multiple sites M87.19
        neck M87.18
        radius M87.13-●
        rib M87.18
        scapula M87.11-●
        skull M87.18
        tarsus M87.17-●
        tibia M87.16-●
        toe M87.17-●
        ulna M87.13-●
        vertebra M87.18
      hemoglobinopathy NEC D58.2 [M90.50]
        carpus D58.2 [M90.54-●]
        clavicle D58.2 [M90.51-●]
        femur D58.2 [M90.55-●]
        fibula D58.2 [M90.56-●]
        finger D58.2 [M90.54-●]
        humerus D58.2 [M90.52-●]
        ilium D58.2 [M90.55-●]
        ischium D58.2 [M90.55-●]
        metacarpus D58.2 [M90.54-●]
        metatarsus D58.2 [M90.57-●]
        multiple sites D58.2 [M90.58]
        neck D58.2 [M90.58]
        radius D58.2 [M90.53-●]
        rib D58.2 [M90.58]
        scapula D58.2 [M90.51-●]
        skull D58.2 [M90.58]
        tarsus D58.2 [M90.57-●]
        tibia D58.2 [M90.56-●]
        toe D58.2 [M90.57-●]
        ulna D58.2 [M90.53-●]
        vertebra D58.2 [M90.58]

▶ New   ⇒ Revised   ~~deleted~~ Deleted   ● Use Additional Character(s)

Osteonecrosis *(Continued)*
  secondary NEC *(Continued)*
    due to *(Continued)*
      trauma (previous) M87.20
        carpus M87.23-●
        clavicle M87.21-●
        femur M87.25-●
        fibula M87.26-●
        finger M87.24-●
        humerus M87.22-●
        ilium M87.25-●
        ischium M87.25-●
        metacarpus M87.24-●
        metatarsus M87.27-●
        multiple sites M87.29
        neck M87.28
        radius M87.23-●
        rib M87.28
        scapula M87.21-●
        skull M87.28
        tarsus M87.27-●
        tibia M87.26-●
        toe M87.27-●
        ulna M87.23-●
        vertebra M87.28
    femur M87.35-●
    fibula M87.36-●
    finger M87.34-●
    humerus M87.32
    ilium M87.350
    in
      caisson disease T70.3 *[M90.50]*
        carpus T70.3 *[M90.54-●]*
        clavicle T70.3 *[M90.51-●]*
        femur T70.3 *[M90.55-●]*
        fibula T70.3 *[M90.56-●]*
        finger T70.3 *[M90.54-●]*
        humerus T70.3 *[M90.52-●]*
        ilium T70.3 *[M90.55-●]*
        ischium T70.3 *[M90.55-●]*
        metacarpus T70.3 *[M90.54-●]*
        metatarsus T70.3 *[M90.57-●]*
        multiple sites T70.3 *[M90.59]*
        neck T70.3 *[M90.58]*
        radius T70.3 *[M90.53-●]*
        rib T70.3 *[M90.58]*
        scapula T70.3 *[M90.51-●]*
        skull T70.3 *[M90.58]*
        tarsus T70.3 *[M90.57-●]*
        tibia T70.3 *[M90.56-●]*
        toe T70.3 *[M90.57-●]*
        ulna T70.3 *[M90.53-●]*
        vertebra T70.3 *[M90.58]*
    ischium M87.350
    metacarpus M87.34-●
    metatarsus M87.37-●
    multiple site M87.39
    neck M87.38
    radius M87.33-●
    rib M87.38
    scapula M87.319
    skull M87.38
    tarsus M87.379
    tibia M87.366
    toe M87.379
    ulna M87.33-●
    vertebra M87.38
  specified type NEC M87.80
    carpus M87.83-●
    clavicle M87.81-●
    femur M87.85-●
    fibula M87.86-●
    finger M87.84-●
    humerus M87.82-●
    ilium M87.85-●
    ischium M87.85-●
    metacarpus M87.84-●
    metatarsus M87.87-●
    multiple sites M87.89
    neck M87.88
    radius M87.83-●

Osteonecrosis *(Continued)*
  specified type NEC *(Continued)*
    rib M87.88-●
    scapula M87.81-●
    skull M87.88
    tarsus M87.87-●
    tibia M87.86-●
    toe M87.87-●
    ulna M87.83-●
    vertebra M87.88
Osteo-onycho-arthro-dysplasia Q87.2
Osteo-onychodysplasia, hereditary Q87.2
Osteopathia condensans disseminata Q78.8
Osteopathy —*see also* Osteomyelitis,
  Osteonecrosis, Osteoporosis
  after poliomyelitis M89.60
    carpus M89.64-●
    clavicle M89.61-●
    femur M89.65-●
    fibula M89.66-●
    finger M89.64-●
    humerus M89.62-●
    ilium M89.659
    ischium M89.659
    metacarpus M89.64-●
    metatarsus M89.67-●
    multiple sites M89.69
    neck M89.68
    radius M89.63-●
    rib M89.68
    scapula M89.61-●
    skull M89.68
    tarsus M89.67-●
    tibia M89.66-●
    toe M89.67-●
    ulna M89.63-●
    vertebra M89.68
  in (due to)
    renal osteodystrophy N25.0
    specified diseases classified elsewhere —
      see subcategory M90.8
Osteopenia M85.8-●
  borderline M85.8-●
Osteoperiostitis —*see* Osteomyelitis, specified
  type NEC
Osteopetrosis (familial) Q78.2
Osteophyte M25.70
  ankle M25.77-●
  elbow M25.72-●
  foot joint M25.77-●
  hand joint M25.74-●
  hip M25.75-●
  knee M25.76-●
  shoulder M25.71-●
  spine M25.78
  vertebrae M25.78
  wrist M25.73-●
Osteopoikilosis Q78.8
Osteoporosis (female) (male) M81.0
  with current pathological fracture M80.00
  age-related M81.0
    with current pathologic fracture M80.00
      carpus M80.04-●
      clavicle M80.01-●
      fibula M80.06-●
      finger M80.04-●
      humerus M80.02-●
      ilium M80.05-●
      ischium M80.05-●
      metacarpus M80.04-●
      metatarsus M80.07-●
      pelvis M80.05-●
      radius M80.03-●
      ▶rib(s) —*see* Osteoporosis, specified site
        NEC
      scapula M80.01-●
      site specified NEC M80.0A
      ▶specified site NEC M80.0A
      tarsus M80.07-●
      tibia M80.06-●
      toe M80.07-●

Osteoporosis *(Continued)*
  age-related *(Continued)*
    with current pathologic fracture
      (Continued)
      ulna M80.03-●
      vertebra M80.08
  disuse M81.8
    with current pathological fracture M80.80
      carpus M80.84-●
      clavicle M80.81-●
      fibula M80.86-●
      finger M80.84-●
      humerus M80.82-●
      ilium M80.85-●
      ischium M80.85-●
      metacarpus M80.84-●
      metatarsus M80.87-●
      pelvis M80.85-●
      radius M80.83-●
      scapula M80.81-●
      site specified NEC M80.8A
      tarsus M80.87-●
      tibia M80.86-●
      toe M80.87-●
      ulna M80.83-●
      vertebra M80.88
  drug-induced —*see* Osteoporosis, specified
    type NEC
  idiopathic —*see* Osteoporosis, specified type
    NEC
  involutional —*see* Osteoporosis, age-related
  Lequesne M81.6
  localized M81.6
  postmenopausal M81.0
    with pathological fracture M80.00
      carpus M80.04-●
      clavicle M80.01-●
      fibula M80.06-●
      finger M80.04-●
      humerus M80.02-●
      ilium M80.05-●
      ischium M80.05-●
      metacarpus M80.04-●
      metatarsus M80.07-●
      pelvis M80.05-●
      radius M80.03-●
      scapula M80.01-●
      site specified NEC M80.0A
      tarsus M80.07-●
      tibia M80.06-●
      toe M80.07-●
      ulna M80.03-●
      vertebra M80.08
  postoophorectomy —*see* Osteoporosis,
    specified type NEC
  postsurgical malabsorption —*see*
    Osteoporosis, specified type NEC
  post-traumatic —*see* Osteoporosis, specified
    type NEC
  senile —*see* Osteoporosis, age-related
  specified type NEC M81.8
    with pathological fracture M80.80
      carpus M80.84-●
      clavicle M80.81-●
      fibula M80.86-●
      finger M80.84-●
      humerus M80.82-●
      ilium M80.85-●
      ischium M80.85-●
      metacarpus M80.84-●
      metatarsus M80.87-●
      pelvis M80.85-●
      radius M80.83-●
      scapula M80.81-●
      site specified NEC M80.8A
      tarsus M80.87-●
      tibia M80.86-●
      toe M80.87-●
      ulna M80.83-●
      vertebra M80.88
Osteopsathyrosis (idiopathica) Q78.0

Osteoradionecrosis, jaw (acute) (chronic) (lower) (suppurative) (upper) M27.2
Osteosarcoma (any form) —see Neoplasm, bone, malignant
Osteosclerosis Q78.2
  acquired M85.8-●
  congenita Q77.4
  fragilitas (generalisata) Q78.2
  myelofibrosis D75.81
Osteosclerotic anemia D64.89
Osteosis
  cutis L94.2
  renal fibrocystic N25.0
Österreicher-Turner syndrome Q87.2
Ostium
  atrioventriculare commune Q21.23
  primum (arteriosum) (defect) (persistent) Q21.20
  secundum (arteriosum) (defect) (patent) (persistent) Q21.11
Ostrum-Furst syndrome Q75.8
Otalgia —see subcategory H92.0
Otitis (acute) H66.90
  with effusion —see also Otitis, media, nonsuppurative
    purulent —see Otitis, media, suppurative
  adhesive —see subcategory H74.1
  chronic —see also Otitis, media, chronic
    with effusion —see also Otitis, media, nonsuppurative, chronic
  externa H60.9-●
    abscess —see Abscess, ear, external
    acute (noninfective) H60.50-●
      actinic H60.51-●
      chemical H60.52-●
      contact H60.53-●
      eczematoid H60.54-●
      infective —see Otitis, externa, infective
      reactive H60.55-●
      specified NEC H60.59-●
    cellulitis —see Cellulitis, ear
    chronic H60.6-●
    diffuse —see Otitis, externa, infective, diffuse
    hemorrhagic —see Otitis, externa, infective, hemorrhagic
    in (due to)
      aspergillosis B44.89
      candidiasis B37.84
      erysipelas A46 [H62.40]
      herpes (simplex) virus infection B00.1
        zoster B02.8
      impetigo L01.00 [H62.40]
      infectious disease NEC B99 [H62.4-●]
      mycosis NEC B36.9 [H62.40]
      parasitic disease NEC B89 [H62.40]
      viral disease NEC B34.9 [H62.40]
      zoster B02.8
    infective NEC H60.39-●
      abscess —see Abscess, ear, external
      cellulitis —see Cellulitis, ear
      diffuse H60.31-●
      hemorrhagic H60.32-●
      swimmer's ear —see Swimmer's, ear
    malignant H60.2-●
    mycotic NEC B36.9 [H62.40]
      in
        aspergillosis B44.89
        candidiasis B37.84
        moniliasis B37.84
    necrotizing —see Otitis, externa, malignant
    Pseudomonas aeruginosa —see Otitis, externa, malignant
    reactive —see Otitis, externa, acute, reactive
    specified NEC —see subcategory H60.8
    tropical NEC B36.9 [H62.40]
      in
        aspergillosis B44.89
        candidiasis B37.84
        moniliasis B37.84

Otitis (Continued)
  insidiosa —see Otosclerosis
  interna —see subcategory H83.0
  media (hemorrhagic) (staphylococcal) (streptococcal) H66.9-●
    with effusion (nonpurulent) —see Otitis, media, nonsuppurative
    acute, subacute H66.90
      allergic —see Otitis, media, nonsuppurative, acute, allergic
      exudative —see Otitis, media, suppurative, acute
      mucoid —see Otitis, media, nonsuppurative, acute
      necrotizing —see also Otitis, media, suppurative, acute
        in
          measles B05.3
          scarlet fever A38.0
      nonsuppurative NEC —see Otitis, media, nonsuppurative, acute
      purulent —see Otitis, media, suppurative, acute
      sanguinous —see Otitis, media, nonsuppurative, acute
      secretory —see Otitis, media, nonsuppurative, acute, serous
      seromucinous —see Otitis, media, nonsuppurative, acute
      serous —see Otitis, media, nonsuppurative, acute, serous
      suppurative —see Otitis, media, suppurative, acute
    allergic —see Otitis, media, nonsuppurative
    catarrhal —see Otitis, media, nonsuppurative
    chronic H66.90
      with effusion (nonpurulent) —see Otitis, media, nonsuppurative, chronic
      allergic —see Otitis, media, nonsuppurative, chronic, allergic
      benign suppurative —see Otitis, media, suppurative, chronic, tubotympanic
      catarrhal —see Otitis, media, nonsuppurative, chronic, serous
      exudative —see Otitis, media, suppurative, chronic
      mucinous —see Otitis, media, nonsuppurative, chronic, mucoid
      mucoid —see Otitis, media, nonsuppurative, chronic, mucoid
      nonsuppurative NEC —see Otitis, media, nonsuppurative, chronic
      purulent —see Otitis, media, suppurative, chronic
      secretory —see Otitis, media, nonsuppurative, chronic, mucoid
      seromucinous —see Otitis, media, nonsuppurative, chronic
      serous —see Otitis, media, nonsuppurative, chronic, serous
      suppurative —see Otitis, media, suppurative, chronic
      transudative —see Otitis, media, nonsuppurative, chronic, mucoid
    exudative —see Otitis, media, nonsuppurative
    in (due to) (with)
      influenza —see Influenza, with, otitis media
      measles B05.3
      scarlet fever A38.0
      tuberculosis A18.6
      viral disease NEC B34.-● [H67.-●]
    mucoid —see Otitis, media, nonsuppurative
    nonsuppurative H65.9-●
      acute or subacute NEC H65.19-●
        allergic H65.11-●
          recurrent H65.11-●
        recurrent H65.19-●

Otitis (Continued)
  media (Continued)
    nonsuppurative (Continued)
      acute or subacute (Continued)
        secretory —see Otitis, media, nonsuppurative, serous
        serous H65.0-●
          recurrent H65.0-●
      chronic H65.49-●
        allergic H65.41-●
        mucoid H65.3-●
        serous H65.2-●
      postmeasles B05.3
      purulent —see Otitis, media, suppurative
      secretory —see Otitis, media, nonsuppurative
      seromucinous —see Otitis, media, nonsuppurative
      serous —see Otitis, media, nonsuppurative
      suppurative H66.4-●
        acute H66.00-●
          with rupture of ear drum H66.01-●
          recurrent H66.00-●
            with rupture of ear drum H66.01-●
        chronic —see also subcategory H66.3
          atticoantral H66.2-●
          benign —see Otitis, media, suppurative, chronic, tubotympanic
          tubotympanic H66.1-●
      transudative —see Otitis, media, nonsuppurative
      tuberculous A18.6
Otocephaly Q18.2
Otolith syndrome —see subcategory H81.8
Otomycosis (diffuse) NEC B36.9 [H62.40]
  in
    aspergillosis B44.89
    candidiasis B37.84
    moniliasis B37.84
Otoporosis —see Otosclerosis
Otorrhagia (nontraumatic) H92.2-●
  traumatic - code by Type of injury
Otorrhea H92.1-●
  cerebrospinal (fluid) G96.01
    postoperative G96.08
    specified NEC G96.08
    spontaneous G96.01
    traumatic G96.08
Otosclerosis (general) H80.9-●
  cochlear (endosteal) H80.2-●
  involving
    otic capsule —see Otosclerosis, cochlear
    oval window
      nonobliterative H80.0-●
      obliterative H80.1-●
    round window —see Otosclerosis, cochlear
  nonobliterative —see Otosclerosis, involving, oval window, nonobliterative
  obliterative —see Otosclerosis, involving, oval window, obliterative
  specified NEC H80.8-●
Otospongiosis —see Otosclerosis
Otto's disease or pelvis M24.7
Outcome of delivery Z37.9
  multiple births Z37.9
    all liveborn Z37.50
      quadruplets Z37.52
      quintuplets Z37.53
      sextuplets Z37.54
      specified number NEC Z37.59
      triplets Z37.51
    all stillborn Z37.7
    some liveborn Z37.60
      quadruplets Z37.62
      quintuplets Z37.63
      sextuplets Z37.64
      specified number NEC Z37.69
      triplets Z37.61

▶ New   ➠ Revised   ~~deleted~~ Deleted   ● Use Additional Character(s)

Outcome of delivery *(Continued)*
  single NEC Z37.9
    liveborn Z37.0
    stillborn Z37.1
  twins NEC Z37.9
    both liveborn Z37.2
    both stillborn Z37.4
    one liveborn, one stillborn Z37.3
Outlet —*see* condition
Ovalocytosis (congenital) (hereditary) —*see*
    Elliptocytosis
Ovarian —*see* Condition
Ovariocele N83.4-●
Ovaritis (cystic) —*see* Oophoritis
Ovary, ovarian —*see also* condition
  resistant syndrome E28.39
  vein syndrome N13.8
Overactive —*see also* Hyperfunction
  adrenal cortex NEC E27.0
  bladder N32.81
  hypothalamus E23.3
  thyroid —*see* Hyperthyroidism
Overactivity R46.3
  child —*see* Disorder, attention-deficit
    hyperactivity
Overbite (deep) (excessive) (horizontal)
    (vertical) M26.29
Overbreathing —*see* Hyperventilation
Overconscientious personality F60.5
Overdevelopment —*see* Hypertrophy
Overdistension —*see* Distension
Overdose, overdosage (drug) —*see* Table of
    Drugs and Chemicals, by drug, poisoning

Overeating R63.2
  nonorganic origin F50.89
  psychogenic F50.89
Overexertion (effects) (exhaustion) T73.3
Overexposure (effects) T73.9
  exhaustion T73.2
Overfeeding —*see* Overeating
  newborn P92.4
Overfill, endodontic M27.52
Overgrowth, bone —*see* Hypertrophy, bone
Overhanging of dental restorative material
    (unrepairable) K08.52
Overheated (places) (effects) —*see* Heat
Overjet (excessive horizontal) M26.23
Overlaid, overlying (suffocation) —
    see Asphyxia, traumatic, due to mechanical
    threat
Overlap, excessive horizontal (teeth) M26.23
Overlapping toe (acquired) —*see also*
    Deformity, toe, specified NEC
  congenital (fifth toe) Q66.89
Overload
  circulatory, due to transfusion (blood) (blood
    components) (TACO) E87.71
  fluid E87.70
    due to transfusion (blood) (blood
      components) E87.71
    specified NEC E87.79
  iron, due to repeated red blood cell
    transfusions E83.111
  potassium (K) E87.5
  sodium (Na) E87.0
Overnutrition —*see* Hyperalimentation

Overproduction —*see also* Hypersecretion
  ACTH E27.0
  catecholamine E27.5
  growth hormone E22.0
Overprotection, child by parent Z62.1
Overriding
  aorta Q25.49
  finger (acquired) —*see* Deformity, finger
    congenital Q68.1
  toe (acquired) —*see also* Deformity, toe,
    specified NEC
    congenital Q66.89
Overstrained R53.83
  heart —*see* Hypertrophy, cardiac
Overuse, muscle NEC M70.8-●
Overweight E66.3
Overworked R53.83
Oviduct —*see* condition
Ovotestis Q56.0
Ovulation (cycle)
  failure or lack of N97.0
  pain N94.0
Ovum —*see* condition
Owren's disease or syndrome (parahemophilia)
    D68.2
Ox heart —*see* Hypertrophy, cardiac
Oxalosis E72.53
Oxaluria E72.53
Oxycephaly, oxycephalic Q75.0
  syphilitic, congenital A50.02
Oxyuriasis B80
Oxyuris vermicularis (infestation) B80
Ozena J31.0

P

Pachyderma, pachydermia L85.9
  larynx (verrucosa) J38.7
Pachydermatocele (congenital) Q82.8
Pachydermoperiostosis —see also
    Osteoarthropathy, hypertrophic, specified
    type NEC
  clubbed nail M89.40 [L62]
Pachygyria Q04.3
Pachymeningitis (adhesive) (basal) (brain)
    (cervical) (chronic) (circumscribed)
    (external) (fibrous) (hemorrhagic)
    (hypertrophic) (internal) (purulent) (spinal)
    (suppurative) —see Meningitis
Pachyonychia (congenital) Q84.5
Pacinian tumor —see Neoplasm, skin, benign
Pad, knuckle or Garrod's M72.1
Paget-Schroetter syndrome I82.890
Paget's disease
  with infiltrating duct carcinoma —see
      Neoplasm, breast, malignant
  bone M88.9
    carpus M88.84-●
    clavicle M88.81-●
    femur M88.85-●
    fibula M88.86-●
    finger M88.84-●
    humerus M88.82-●
    ilium M88.85-●
    in neoplastic disease —see Osteitis,
        deformans, in neoplastic disease
    ischium M88.85-●
    metacarpus M88.84-●
    metatarsus M88.87-●
    multiple sites M88.89
    neck M88.88
    radius M88.83-●
    rib M88.88
    scapula M88.81-●
    skull M88.0
    specified NEC M88.88
    tarsus M88.87-●
    tibia M88.86-●
    toe M88.87-●
    ulna M88.83-●
    vertebra M88.1
  breast (female) C50.01-●
    male C50.02-●
  extramammary —see also Neoplasm, skin,
      malignant
    anus C21.0
      margin C44.590
      skin C44.590
  intraductal carcinoma —see Neoplasm,
      breast, malignant
  malignant —see Neoplasm, skin, malignant
    breast (female) C50.01-●
      male C50.02-●
    unspecified site (female) C50.01-●
      male C50.02-●
  mammary —see Paget's disease, breast
  nipple —see Paget's disease, breast
  osteitis deformans —see Paget's disease, bone
Pain(s) —see also Painful R52
  abdominal R10.9
    colic R10.83
    generalized R10.84
      with acute abdomen R10.0
    lower R10.30
      left quadrant R10.32
      pelvic or perineal R10.2
      periumbilical R10.33
      right quadrant R10.31
    rebound —see Tenderness, abdominal,
        rebound
    severe with abdominal rigidity R10.0
    tenderness —see Tenderness, abdominal
    upper R10.10
      epigastric R10.13
      left quadrant R10.12
      right quadrant R10.11

Pain (Continued)
  acute R52
    due to trauma G89.11
    neoplasm related G89.3
    postprocedural NEC G89.18
    post-thoracotomy G89.12
    specified by site — code to Pain, by site
  adnexa (uteri) R10.2
  anginoid —see Pain, precordial
  anus K62.89
  arm —see Pain, limb, upper
  axillary (axilla) M79.62-●
  back (postural) M54.9
  bladder R39.89
    associated with micturition —see
        Micturition, painful
    chronic R39.82
  bone —see Disorder, bone, specified type NEC
  breast N64.4
  broad ligament R10.2
  cancer associated (acute) (chronic) G89.3
  cecum —see Pain, abdominal
  cervicobrachial M53.1
  chest (central) R07.9
    anterior wall R07.89
    atypical R07.89
    ischemic I20.9
    musculoskeletal R07.89
    non-cardiac R07.89
    on breathing R07.1
    pleurodynia R07.81
    precordial R07.2
    wall (anterior) R07.89
  chronic G89.29
    associated with significant psychosocial
        dysfunction G89.4
    due to trauma G89.21
    neoplasm related G89.3
    postoperative NEC G89.28
    postprocedural NEC G89.28
    post-thoracotomy G89.22
    specified NEC G89.29
  coccyx M53.3
  colon —see Pain, abdominal
  coronary —see Angina
  costochondral R07.1
  diaphragm R07.1
  due to cancer G89.3
  due to device, implant or graft —see also
      Complications, by site and type,
      specified NEC T85.848
    arterial graft NEC T82.848
    breast (implant) T85.848
    catheter NEC T85.848
      dialysis (renal) T82.848
        intraperitoneal T85.848
      infusion NEC T82.848
        spinal (epidural) (subdural) T85.840
      urinary (indwelling) T83.84
    electronic (electrode) (pulse generator)
        (stimulator)
      bone T84.84
      cardiac T82.847
      nervous system (brain) (peripheral
          nerve) (spinal) T85.840
      urinary T83.84
    fixation, internal (orthopedic) NEC T84.84
    gastrointestinal (bile duct) (esophagus)
        T85.848
    genital NEC T83.84
    heart NEC T82.847
    infusion NEC T85.848
    joint prosthesis T84.84
    ocular (corneal graft) (orbital implant)
        NEC T85.848
    orthopedic NEC T84.84
    specified NEC T85.848
    urinary NEC T83.84
    vascular NEC T82.848
    ventricular intracranial shunt T85.840
  due to malignancy (primary) (secondary) G89.3
  ear —see subcategory H92.0
  epigastric, epigastrium R10.13

Pain (Continued)
  eye —see Pain, ocular
  face, facial R51.9
    atypical G50.1
  female genital organs NEC N94.89
  finger —see Pain, limb, upper
  flank —see Pain, abdominal
  foot —see Pain, limb, lower
  gallbladder K82.9
  gas (intestinal) R14.1
  gastric —see Pain, abdominal
  generalized NOS R52
  genital organ
    female N94.89
    male N50.89
  groin —see Pain, abdominal, lower
  hand —see Pain, limb, upper
  head —see Headache
  heart —see Pain, precordial
  infra-orbital —see Neuralgia, trigeminal
  intercostal R07.82
  intermenstrual N94.0
  jaw R68.84
  joint M25.50
    ankle M25.57-●
    elbow M25.52-●
    finger M25.54-●
    foot M25.57-●
    hand M25.54-●
    hip M25.55-●
    knee M25.56-●
    shoulder M25.51-●
    specified site NEC M25.59
    toe M25.57-●
    wrist M25.53-●
  kidney N23
  laryngeal R07.0
  leg —see Pain, limb, lower
  limb M79.609
    lower M79.60-●
      foot M79.67-●
      lower leg M79.66-●
      thigh M79.65-●
      toe M79.67-●
    upper M79.60-●
      axilla M79.62-●
      finger M79.64-●
      forearm M79.63-●
      hand M79.64-●
      upper arm M79.62-●
  loin M54.50
  low back M54.50
    specified NEC M54.59
    vertebral end plate M54.51
    vertebrogenic M54.51
  lumbar region M54.50
    vertebral end plate M54.51
    vertebrogenic M54.51
  mandibular R68.84
  mastoid —see subcategory H92.0
  maxilla R68.84
  menstrual —see also Dysmenorrhea N94.6
  metacarpophalangeal (joint) —see Pain, joint,
      hand
  metatarsophalangeal (joint) —see Pain, joint,
      foot
  mouth K13.79
  muscle —see Myalgia
  musculoskeletal —see also Pain, by site M79.18
  myofascial M79.18
  nasal J34.89
  nasopharynx J39.2
  neck NEC M54.2
  nerve NEC —see Neuralgia
  neuromuscular —see Neuralgia
  nose J34.89
  ocular H57.1-●
  ophthalmic —see Pain, ocular
  orbital region —see Pain, ocular
  ovary N94.89
  over heart —see Pain, precordial
  ovulation N94.0

▶ New   ⟹ Revised   ~~deleted~~ Deleted   ● Use Additional Character(s)

Pain *(Continued)*
pelvic (female) R10.2
penis N48.89
pericardial —*see* Pain, precordial
perineal, perineum R10.2
pharynx J39.2
pleura, pleural, pleuritic R07.81
postoperative NOS G89.18
postprocedural NOS G89.18
post-thoracotomy G89.12
precordial (region) R07.2
premenstrual N94.3
psychogenic (persistent) (any site) F45.41
radicular (spinal) —*see* Radiculopathy
rectum K62.89
respiration R07.1
retrosternal R07.2
rheumatoid, muscular —*see* Myalgia
rib R07.81
root (spinal) —*see* Radiculopathy
round ligament (stretch) R10.2
sacroiliac M53.3
sciatic —*see* Sciatica
scrotum N50.82
seminal vesicle N50.89
shoulder M25.51-●
spermatic cord N50.89
spinal root —*see* Radiculopathy
spine M54.9
cervical M54.2
low back M54.50
with sciatica M54.4-●
vertebral end plate —*see* Pain, vertebrogenic
thoracic M54.6
stomach —*see* Pain, abdominal
substernal R07.2
temporomandibular (joint) M26.62-●
testis N50.81-●
thoracic spine M54.6
with radicular and visceral pain M54.14
throat R07.0
tibia —*see* Pain, limb, lower
toe —*see* Pain, limb, lower
tongue K14.6
tooth K08.89
trigeminal —*see* Neuralgia, trigeminal
tumor associated G89.3
ureter N23
urinary (organ) (system) N23
uterus NEC N94.89
vagina R10.2
vertebrogenic M54.89
low back M54.51
lumbar M54.51
syndrome M54.89
vesical R39.89
associated with micturition —*see* Micturition, painful
vulva R10.2
Painful —*see also* Pain
coitus
female N94.10
male N53.12
psychogenic F52.6
ejaculation (semen) N53.12
psychogenic F52.6
erection —*see* Priapism
feet syndrome E53.8
joint replacement (hip) (knee) T84.84
menstruation —*see* Dysmenorrhea
psychogenic F45.8
micturition —*see* Micturition, painful
respiration R07.1
scar NEC L90.5
wire sutures T81.89
Painter's colic —*see* subcategory T56.0
Palate —*see* condition
Palatoplegia K13.79
Palatoschisis —*see* Cleft, palate
Palilalia R48.8
Palliative care Z51.5

Pallor R23.1
optic disc, temporal —*see* Atrophy, optic
Palmar —*see also* condition
fascia —*see* condition
Palpable
cecum K63.89
kidney N28.89
ovary N83.8
prostate N42.9
spleen —*see* Splenomegaly
Palpitations (heart) R00.2
psychogenic F45.8
Palsy —*see also* Paralysis G83.9
atrophic diffuse (progressive) G12.22
Bell's —*see also* Palsy, facial
newborn P11.3
brachial plexus NEC G54.0
newborn (birth injury) P14.3
brain —*see* Palsy, cerebral
bulbar (progressive) (chronic) G12.22
of childhood (Fazio-Londe) G12.1
pseudo NEC G12.29
supranuclear (progressive) G23.1
cerebral (congenital) G80.9
ataxic G80.4
athetoid G80.3
choreathetoid G80.3
diplegic G80.8
spastic G80.1
dyskinetic G80.3
athetoid G80.3
choreathetoid G80.3
distonic G80.3
dystonic G80.3
hemiplegic G80.8
spastic G80.2
mixed G80.8
monoplegic G80.8
spastic G80.1
paraplegic G80.8
spastic G80.1
quadriplegic G80.8
spastic G80.0
spastic G80.1
diplegic G80.1
hemiplegic G80.2
monoplegic G80.1
quadriplegic G80.0
specified NEC G80.1
tetrapelgic G80.0
specified NEC G80.8
syphilitic A52.12
congenital A50.49
tetraplegic G80.8
spastic G80.0
cranial nerve —*see also* Disorder, nerve, cranial
multiple G52.7
in
infectious disease B99 [G53]
neoplastic disease —*see also* Neoplasm D49.9 [G53]
parasitic disease B89 [G53]
sarcoidosis D86.82
creeping G12.22
diver's T70.3
Erb's P14.0
facial G51.0
newborn (birth injury) P11.3
glossopharyngeal G52.1
Klumpke (-Déjérine) P14.1
lead —*see* subcategory T56.0
median nerve (tardy) G56.1-●
nerve G58.9
specified NEC G58.8
peroneal nerve (acute) (tardy) G57.3-●
progressive supranuclear G23.1
pseudobulbar NEC G12.29
radial nerve (acute) G56.3-●
seventh nerve —*see also* Palsy, facial
newborn P11.3
shaking —*see* Parkinsonism
spastic (cerebral) (spinal) G80.1

Palsy *(Continued)*
ulnar nerve (tardy) G56.2-●
wasting G12.29
Paludism —*see* Malaria
Panangiitis M30.0
Panaris, panaritium —*see also* Cellulitis, digit
with lymphangitis —*see* Lymphangitis, acute, digit
Panarteritis nodosa M30.0
brain or cerebral I67.7
Pancake heart R93.1
with cor pulmonale (chronic) I27.81
Pancarditis (acute) (chronic) I51.89
rheumatic I09.89
active or acute I01.8
Pancoast's syndrome or tumor C34.1-●
Pancolitis, ulcerative (chronic) K51.00
with
abscess K51.014
complication K51.019
fistula K51.013
obstruction K51.012
rectal bleeding K51.011
specified complication NEC K51.018
Pancreas, pancreatic —*see* condition
Pancreatitis (annular) (apoplectic) (calcareous) (edematous) (hemorrhagic) (malignant) (subacute) (suppurative) K85.90
with necrosis (uninfected) K85.91
infected K85.92
acute (without necrosis or infection) K85.90
with necrosis (uninfected) K85.91
infected K85.92
alcohol induced (without necrosis or infection) K85.20
with necrosis (uninfected) K85.21
infected K85.22
biliary (without necrosis or infection) K85.10
with necrosis (uninfected) K85.11
infected K85.12
drug induced (without necrosis or infection) K85.30
with necrosis (uninfected) K85.31
infected K85.32
gallstone (without necrosis or infection) K85.10
with necrosis (uninfected) K85.11
infected K85.12
idiopathic (without necrosis or infection) K85.00
with necrosis (uninfected) K85.01
infected K85.02
specified NEC (without necrosis or infection) K85.80
with necrosis (uninfected) K85.81
infected K85.82
chronic (infectious) K86.1
alcohol-induced K86.0
recurrent K86.1
relapsing K86.1
cystic (chronic) K86.1
cytomegaloviral B25.2
fibrous (chronic) K86.1
gallstone (without necrosis or infection) K85.10
with necrosis (uninfected) K85.11
infected K85.12
gangrenous —*see* Pancreatitis, acute
interstitial (chronic) K86.1
acute —*see also* Pancreatitis, acute K85.80
mumps B26.3
recurrent
acute —*see* Pancreatitis, acute by type
chronic
relapsing, chronic K86.1
syphilitic A52.74
Pancreatoblastoma —*see* Neoplasm, pancreas, malignant
Pancreolithiasis K86.89
Pancytolysis D75.89

Pancytopenia (acquired) D61.818
  with
    malformations D61.09
    myelodysplastic syndrome —*see*
        Syndrome, myelodysplastic
  antineoplastic chemotherapy induced
      D61.810
  congenital D61.09
  drug-induced NEC D61.811
PANDAS (pediatric autoimmune
    neuropsychiatric disorders associated with
    streptococcal infections syndrome) D89.89
Panencephalitis, subacute, sclerosing
    A81.1
Panhematopenia D61.9
  congenital D61.09
  constitutional D61.09
  splenic, primary D73.1
Panhemocytopenia D61.9
  congenital D61.09
  constitutional D61.09
Panhypogonadism E29.1
Panhypopituitarism E23.0
  prepubertal E23.0
Panic (attack) (state) F41.0
  reaction to exceptional stress (transient) F43.0
Panmyelopathy, familial, constitutional D61.09
Panmyelophthisis D61.82
  congenital D61.09
Panmyelosis (acute) (with myelofibrosis)
    C94.4-●
Panner's disease —*see* Osteochondrosis,
    juvenile, humerus
Panneuritis endemica E51.11
Panniculitis (nodular) (nonsuppurative) M79.3
  back M54.00
    cervical region M54.02
    cervicothoracic region M54.03
    lumbar region M54.06
    lumbosacral region M54.07
    multiple sites M54.09
    occipito-atlanto-axial region M54.01
    sacrococcygeal region M54.08
    thoracic region M54.04
    thoracolumbar region M54.05
  lupus L93.2
  mesenteric K65.4
  neck M54.02
    cervicothoracic region M54.03
    occipito-atlanto-axial region M54.01
  relapsing M35.6
Panniculus adiposus (abdominal) E65
Pannus (allergic) (cornea) (degenerativus)
    (keratic) H16.42-●
  abdominal (symptomatic) E65
  trachomatosus, trachomatous (active) A71.1
Panophthalmitis H44.01-●
Pansinusitis (chronic) (hyperplastic)
    (nonpurulent) (purulent) J32.4
  acute J01.40
    recurrent J01.41
  tuberculous A15.8
Panuveitis (sympathetic) H44.11-●
Panvalvular disease I08.9
  specified NEC I08.8
PAPA (pyogenic arthritis, pyoderma
    gangrenosum, and acne syndrome) M04.8
Papanicolaou smear, cervix Z12.4
  as part of routine gynecological examination
      Z01.419
    with abnormal findings Z01.411
  for suspected neoplasm Z12.4
  nonspecific abnormal finding R87.619
  routine Z01.419
    with abnormal findings Z01.411
Papilledema (choked disc) H47.10
  associated with
    decreased ocular pressure H47.12
    increased intracranial pressure H47.11
    retinal disorder H47.13
  Foster-Kennedy syndrome H47.14-●

Papillitis H46.00
  anus K62.89
  chronic lingual K14.4
  necrotizing, kidney N17.2
  optic H46.0-●
  rectum K62.89
  renal, necrotizing N17.2
  tongue K14.0
Papilloma —*see also* Neoplasm, benign,
    by site
  acuminatum (female) (male) (anogenital)
      A63.0
  basal cell L82.1
    inflamed L82.0
  benign pinta (primary) A67.0
  bladder (urinary) (transitional cell) D41.4
  choroid plexus (lateral ventricle) (third
      ventricle) D33.0
    anaplastic C71.5
    fourth ventricle D33.1
    malignant C71.5
  renal pelvis (transitional cell) D41.1-●
    benign D30.1-●
  Schneiderian
    specified site —*see* Neoplasm, benign, by
        site
    unspecified site D14.0
  serous surface
    borderline malignancy
      specified site —*see* Neoplasm, uncertain
          behavior, by site
      unspecified site D39.10
    specified site —*see* Neoplasm, benign, by
        site
    unspecified site D27.9
  transitional (cell)
    bladder (urinary) D41.4
    inverted type —*see* Neoplasm, uncertain
        behavior, by site
    renal pelvis D41.1-●
    ureter D41.2-●
  ureter (transitional cell) D41.2-●
    benign D30.2-●
  urothelial —*see* Neoplasm, uncertain
      behavior, by site
  villous —*see* Neoplasm, uncertain behavior,
      by site
    adenocarcinoma in —*see* Neoplasm,
        malignant, by site
    in situ —*see* Neoplasm, in situ
  yaws, plantar or palmar A66.1
Papillomata, multiple, of yaws A66.1
Papillomatosis —*see also* Neoplasm, benign,
    by site
  confluent and reticulated L83
  cystic, breast —*see* Mastopathy, cystic
  ductal, breast —*see* Mastopathy, cystic
  intraductal (diffuse) —*see* Neoplasm, benign,
      by site
  subareolar duct D24-●
Papillomavirus, as cause of disease classified
    elsewhere B97.7
Papillon-Léage and Psaume syndrome
    Q87.0
Papule(s) R23.8
  carate (primary) A67.0
  fibrous, of nose D22.39
  Gottron's L94.4
  pinta (primary) A67.0
Papulosis
  lymphomatoid C86.6
  malignant I77.89
Papyraceous fetus O31.0-●
Para-albuminemia E88.09
Paracephalus Q89.7
Parachute mitral valve Q23.2
Paracoccidioidomycosis B41.9
  disseminated B41.7
  generalized B41.7
  mucocutaneous-lymphangitic B41.8
  pulmonary B41.0

Paracoccidioidomycosis *(Continued)*
  specified NEC B41.8
  visceral B41.8
Paradentosis K05.4
Paraffinoma T88.8
Paraganglioma D44.7
  adrenal D35.0-●
    malignant C74.1-●
  aortic body D44.7
    malignant C75.5
  carotid body D44.6
    malignant C75.4
  chromaffin —*see also* Neoplasm, benign, by
      site
    malignant —*see* Neoplasm, malignant, by
        site
  extra-adrenal D44.7
    malignant C75.5
      specified site —*see* Neoplasm,
          malignant, by site
      unspecified site C75.5
    specified site —*see* Neoplasm, uncertain
        behavior, by site
    unspecified site D44.7
  gangliocytic D13.2
    specified site —*see* Neoplasm, benign, by
        site
    unspecified site D13.2
  glomus jugulare D44.7
    malignant C75.5
  jugular D44.7
  malignant C75.5
    specified site —*see* Neoplasm, malignant,
        by site
    unspecified site C75.5
  nonchromaffin D44.7
    malignant C75.5
      specified site —*see* Neoplasm,
          malignant, by site
      unspecified site C75.5
    specified site —*see* Neoplasm, uncertain
        behavior, by site
    unspecified site D44.7
  parasympathetic D44.7
    specified site —*see* Neoplasm, uncertain
        behavior, by site
    unspecified site D44.7
  specified site —*see* Neoplasm, uncertain
      behavior, by site
  sympathetic D44.7
    specified site —*see* Neoplasm, uncertain
        behavior, by site
    unspecified site D44.7
  unspecified site D44.7
Parageusia R43.2
  psychogenic F45.8
Paragonimiasis B66.4
Paragranuloma, Hodgkin —*see* Lymphoma,
    Hodgkin, specified NEC
Parahemophilia —*see also* Defect, coagulation
    D68.2
Parakeratosis R23.4
  variegata L41.0
Paralysis, paralytic (complete) (incomplete)
    G83.9
  with
    syphilis A52.17
  abducens, abducent (nerve) —*see* Strabismus,
      paralytic, sixth nerve
  abductor, lower extremity G57.9-●
  accessory nerve G52.8
  accommodation —*see also* Paresis, of
      accommodation
    hysterical F44.89
  acoustic nerve (except Deafness) —*see*
      subcategory H93.3
  agitans —*see also* Parkinsonism G20
    arteriosclerotic G21.4
  alternating (oculomotor) G83.89
  amyotrophic G12.21

Paralysis, paralytic *(Continued)*
  ankle G57.9-●
  anus (sphincter) K62.89
  arm —*see* Monoplegia, upper limb
  ascending (spinal), acute G61.0
  association G12.29
  asthenic bulbar G70.00
    with exacerbation (acute) G70.01
    in crisis G70.01
  ataxic (hereditary) G11.9
    general (syphilitic) A52.17
  atrophic G58.9
    infantile, acute —*see* Poliomyelitis, paralytic
    progressive G12.22
    spinal (acute) —*see* Poliomyelitis, paralytic
  axillary G54.0
  Babinski-Nageotte's G83.89
  Bell's G51.0
    newborn P11.3
  Benedikt's G46.3
  birth injury P14.9
    spinal cord P11.5
  bladder (neurogenic) (sphincter)
    N31.2
  bowel, colon or intestine K56.0
  brachial plexus G54.0
    birth injury P14.3
    newborn (birth injury) P14.3
  brain G83.9
    diplegia G83.0
    triplegia G83.89
  bronchial J98.09
  Brown-Séquard G83.81
  bulbar (chronic) (progressive) G12.22
    infantile —*see* Poliomyelitis, paralytic
    poliomyelitic —*see* Poliomyelitis, paralytic
    pseudo G12.29
  bulbospinal G70.00
    with exacerbation (acute) G70.01
    in crisis G70.01
  cardiac —*see also* Failure, heart I50.9
  cerebrocerebellar, diplegic G80.1
  cervical
    plexus G54.2
    sympathetic G90.09
  Céstan-Chenais G46.3
  Charcot-Marie-Tooth type G60.0
  Clark's G80.9
  colon K56.0
  compressed air T70.3
  compression
    arm G56.9-●
    leg G57.9-●
    lower extremity G57.9-●
    upper extremity G56.9-●
  congenital (cerebral) —*see* Palsy, cerebral
  conjugate movement (gaze) (of eye) H51.0
    cortical (nuclear) (supranuclear) H51.0
  cordis —*see* Failure, heart
  cranial or cerebral nerve G52.9
  creeping G12.22
  crossed leg G83.89
  crutch —*see* Injury, brachial plexus
  deglutition R13.0
    hysterical F44.4
  dementia A52.17
  descending (spinal) NEC G12.29
  diaphragm (flaccid) J98.6
    due to accidental dissection of phrenic
      nerve during procedure —*see*
      Puncture, accidental complicating
      surgery
  digestive organs NEC K59.89
  diplegic —*see* Diplegia
  divergence (nuclear) H51.8
  diver's T70.3
  Duchenne's
    birth injury P14.0
    due to or associated with
      motor neuron disease G12.22
      muscular dystrophy G71.01

Paralysis, paralytic *(Continued)*
  due to intracranial or spinal birth injury —*see*
    Palsy, cerebral
  embolic (current episode) I63.4-●
  Erb (-Duchenne) (birth) (newborn) P14.0
  Erb's syphilitic spastic spinal A52.17
  esophagus K22.89
  eye muscle (extrinsic) H49.9
    intrinsic —*see also* Paresis, of
      accommodation
  facial (nerve) G51.0
    birth injury P11.3
    congenital P11.3
    following operation NEC —*see* Puncture,
      accidental complicating surgery
    newborn (birth injury) P11.3
  familial (recurrent) (periodic) G72.3
    spastic G11.4
  fauces J39.2
  finger G56.9-●
  gait R26.1
  gastric nerve (nondiabetic) G52.2
  gaze, conjugate H51.0
  general (progressive) (syphilitic) A52.17
    juvenile A50.45
  glottis J38.00
    bilateral J38.02
    unilateral J38.01
  gluteal G54.1
  Gubler (-Millard) G46.3
  hand —*see* Monoplegia, upper limb
  heart —*see* Arrest, cardiac
  hemiplegic —*see* Hemiplegia
  hyperkalemic periodic (familial) G72.3
  hypoglossal (nerve) G52.3
  hypokalemic periodic G72.3
  hysterical F44.4
  ileus K56.0
  infantile —*see also* Poliomyelitis, paralytic
    A80.30
    bulbar —*see* Poliomyelitis, paralytic
    cerebral —*see* Palsy, cerebral
    spastic —*see* Palsy, cerebral, spastic
  infective —*see* Poliomyelitis, paralytic
  inferior nuclear G83.9
  internuclear —*see* Ophthalmoplegia,
    internuclear
  intestine K56.0
  iris H57.09
    due to diphtheria (toxin) A36.89
  ischemic, Volkmann's (complicating trauma)
    T79.6
  Jackson's G83.89
  jake —*see* Poisoning, food, noxious, plant
  Jamaica ginger (jake) G62.2
  juvenile general A50.45
  Klumpke (-Déjérine) (birth) (newborn) P14.1
  labioglossal (laryngeal) (pharyngeal) G12.29
  Landry's G61.0
  laryngeal nerve (recurrent) (superior)
    (unilateral) J38.00
    bilateral J38.02
    unilateral J38.01
  larynx J38.00
    bilateral J38.02
    due to diphtheria (toxin) A36.2
    unilateral J38.01
  lateral G12.23
  lead —*see* subcategory T56.0
  left side —*see* Hemiplegia
  leg G83.1-●
    both —*see* Paraplegia
    crossed G83.89
    hysterical F44.4
    psychogenic F44.4
    transient or transitory R29.818
      traumatic NEC —*see* Injury, nerve, leg
  levator palpebrae superioris —*see*
    Blepharoptosis, paralytic
  limb —*see* Monoplegia
  lip K13.0

Paralysis, paralytic *(Continued)*
  Lissauer's A52.17
  lower limb —*see* Monoplegia, lower limb
    both —*see* Paraplegia
  lung J98.4
  median nerve G56.1-●
  medullary (tegmental) G83.89
  mesencephalic NEC G83.89
    tegmental G83.89
  middle alternating G83.89
  Millard-Gubler-Foville G46.3
  monoplegic —*see* Monoplegia
  motor G83.9
  muscle, muscular NEC G72.89
    due to nerve lesion G58.9
    eye (extrinsic) H49.9
      intrinsic —*see* Paresis, of accommodation
      oblique —*see* Strabismus, paralytic,
        fourth nerve
    iris sphincter H21.9
    ischemic (Volkmann's) (complicating
      trauma) T79.6
    progressive G12.21
    progressive, spinal G12.25
    pseudohypertrophic G71.02
    spinal progressive G12.25
  musculocutaneous nerve G56.9-●
  musculospiral G56.9-●
  nerve —*see also* Disorder, nerve
    abducent —*see* Strabismus, paralytic, sixth
      nerve
    accessory G52.8
    auditory (except Deafness) —*see*
      subcategory H93.3
    birth injury P14.9
    cranial or cerebral G52.9
    facial G51.0
      birth injury P11.3
      congenital P11.3
      newborn (birth injury) P11.3
    fourth or trochlear —*see* Strabismus,
      paralytic, fourth nerve
    newborn (birth injury) P14.9
    oculomotor —*see* Strabismus, paralytic,
      third nerve
    phrenic (birth injury) P14.2
    radial G56.3-●
    seventh or facial G51.0
      newborn (birth injury) P11.3
    sixth or abducent —*see* Strabismus,
      paralytic, sixth nerve
    syphilitic A52.15
    third or oculomotor —*see* Strabismus,
      paralytic, third nerve
    trigeminal G50.9
    trochlear —*see* Strabismus, paralytic, fourth
      nerve
    ulnar G56.2-●
  normokalemic periodic G72.3
  ocular H49.9
    alternating G83.89
  oculofacial, congenital (Moebius) Q87.0
  oculomotor (external bilateral) (nerve) —*see*
    Strabismus, paralytic, third nerve
  palate (soft) K13.79
  paratrigeminal G50.9
  periodic (familial) (hyperkalemic)
    (hypokalemic) (myotonic)
    (normokalemic) (potassium sensitive)
    (secondary) G72.3
  peripheral autonomic nervous system —*see*
    Neuropathy, peripheral, autonomic
  peroneal (nerve) G57.3-●
  pharynx J39.2
  phrenic nerve G56.8-●
  plantar nerve(s) G57.6-●
  pneumogastric nerve G52.2
  poliomyelitis (current) —*see* Poliomyelitis,
    paralytic
  popliteal nerve G57.3-●
  postepileptic transitory G83.84

Paralysis, paralytic *(Continued)*
  progressive (atrophic) (bulbar) (spinal)
    G12.22
    general A52.17
    infantile acute —*see* Poliomyelitis, paralytic
    supranuclear G23.1
  pseudobulbar G12.29
  ➧pseudohypertrophic (muscle) (*see also*
    Dystrophy, muscular, by type, if
    applicable) G71.09
  psychogenic F44.4
  quadriceps G57.9-●
  quadriplegic —*see* Tetraplegia
  radial nerve G56.3-●
  rectus muscle (eye) H49.9
  recurrent isolated sleep G47.53
  respiratory (muscle) (system) (tract) R06.81
    center NEC G93.89
    congenital P28.89
    newborn P28.89
  right side —*see* Hemiplegia
  saturnine —*see* subcategory T56.0
  sciatic nerve G57.0-●
  senile G83.9
  shaking —*see* Parkinsonism
  shoulder G56.9-●
  sleep, recurrent isolated G47.53
  spastic G83.9
    cerebral —*see* Palsy, cerebral, spastic
    congenital (cerebral) —*see* Palsy, cerebral,
      spastic
    familial G11.4
    hereditary G11.4
    quadriplegic G80.0
    syphilitic (spinal) A52.17
  sphincter, bladder —*see* Paralysis, bladder
  spinal (cord) G83.9
    accessory nerve G52.8
    acute —*see* Poliomyelitis, paralytic
    ascending acute G61.0
    atrophic (acute) —*see also* Poliomyelitis,
      paralytic
      spastic, syphilitic A52.17
    congenital NEC —*see* Palsy, cerebral
    hereditary G95.89
    infantile —*see* Poliomyelitis, paralytic
    progressive G12.21
    muscle G12.25
    sequelae NEC G83.89
  sternomastoid G52.8
  stomach K31.84
    diabetic —*see* Diabetes, by type, with
      gastroparesis
    nerve G52.2
      diabetic —*see* Diabetes, by type, with
        gastroparesis
  stroke —*see* Infarct, brain
  subcapsularis G56.8-●
  supranuclear (progressive) G23.1
  sympathetic G90.8
    cervical G90.09
    nervous system —*see* Neuropathy,
      peripheral, autonomic
  syndrome G83.9
    specified NEC G83.89
  syphilitic spastic spinal (Erb's) A52.17
  thigh G57.9-●
  throat J39.2
    diphtheritic A36.0
    muscle J39.2
  thrombotic (current episode) I63.3-●
  thumb G56.9-●
  tick —*see* Toxicity, venom, arthropod,
    specified NEC
  Todd's (postepileptic transitory paralysis)
    G83.84
  toe G57.6-●
  tongue K14.8
  transient R29.5
    arm or leg NEC R29.818
    traumatic NEC —*see* Injury, nerve

Paralysis, paralytic *(Continued)*
  trapezius G52.8
  traumatic, transient NEC —*see* Injury, nerve
  trembling —*see* Parkinsonism
  triceps brachii G56.9-●
  trigeminal nerve G50.9
  trochlear (nerve) —*see* Strabismus, paralytic,
    fourth nerve
  ulnar nerve G56.2-●
  upper limb —*see* Monoplegia, upper limb
  uremic N18.9 *[G99.8]*
  uveoparotitic D86.89
  uvula K13.79
    postdiphtheritic A36.0
  vagus nerve G52.2
  vasomotor NEC G90.8
  velum palati K13.79
  vesical —*see* Paralysis, bladder
  vestibular nerve (except Vertigo) —*see*
    subcategory H93.3
  vocal cords J38.00
    bilateral J38.02
    unilateral J38.01
  Volkmann's (complicating trauma) T79.6
  wasting G12.29
  Weber's G46.3
  wrist G56.9-●
Paramedial urethrovesical orifice Q64.79
Paramenia N92.6
Parametritis —*see also* Disease, pelvis,
  inflammatory N73.2
  acute N73.0
  complicating abortion —*see* Abortion, by
    type, complicated by, parametritis
Parametrium, parametric —*see* condition
Paramnesia —*see* Amnesia
Paramolar K00.1
Paramyloidosis E85.89
Paramyoclonus multiplex G25.3
Paramyotonia (congenita) G71.19
Parangi —*see* Yaws
Paranoia (querulans) F22
  senile F03
Paranoid
  dementia (senile) F03
    praecox —*see* Schizophrenia
  personality F60.0
  psychosis (climacteric) (involutional)
    (menopausal) F22
    psychogenic (acute) F23
    senile F03
  reaction (acute) F23
    chronic F22
  schizophrenia F20.0
  state (climacteric) (involutional)
    (menopausal) (simple) F22
    senile F03
  tendencies F60.0
  traits F60.0
  trends F60.0
  type, psychopathic personality F60.0
Paraparesis —*see* Paraplegia
Paraphasia R47.02
Paraphilia F65.9
Paraphimosis (congenital) N47.2
  chancroidal A57
Paraphrenia, paraphrenic (late) F22
  schizophrenia F20.0
Paraplegia (lower) G82.20
  ataxic —*see* Degeneration, combined, spinal
    cord
  complete G82.21
  congenital (cerebral) G80.8
    spastic G80.1
  familial spastic G11.4
  functional (hysterical) F44.4
  hereditary, spastic G11.4
  hysterical F44.4
  incomplete G82.22
  Pott's A18.01
  psychogenic F44.4

Paraplegia *(Continued)*
  spastic
    Erb's spinal, syphilitic A52.17
    hereditary G11.4
    tropical G04.1
  syphilitic (spastic) A52.17
  traumatic
    current injury - code to injury with seventh
      character A
      sequela of previous injury - code to
        injury with seventh character S
  tropical spastic G04.1
Parapoxvirus B08.60
  specified NEC B08.69
Paraproteinemia D89.2
  benign (familial) D89.2
  monoclonal D47.2
  secondary to malignant disease D47.2
Parapsoriasis L41.9
  en plaques L41.4
  guttata L41.1
  large plaque L41.4
  retiform, retiformis L41.5
  small plaque L41.3
  specified NEC L41.8
  varioliformis (acuta) L41.0
Parasitic —*see also* condition
  disease NEC B89
  stomatitis B37.0
  sycosis (beard) (scalp) B35.0
  twin Q89.4
Parasitism B89
  intestinal B82.9
  skin B88.9
  specified —*see* Infestation
Parasitophobia F40.218
Parasomnia G47.50
  due to
    alcohol
      abuse F10.182
      dependence F10.282
      use F10.982
    amphetamines
      abuse F15.182
      dependence F15.282
      use F15.982
    caffeine
      abuse F15.182
      dependence F15.282
      use F15.982
    cocaine
      abuse F14.182
      dependence F14.282
      use F14.982
    drug NEC
      abuse F19.182
      dependence F19.282
      use F19.982
    opioid
      abuse F11.182
      dependence F11.282
      use F11.982
    psychoactive substance NEC
      abuse F19.182
      dependence F19.282
      use F19.982
    sedative, hypnotic, or anxiolytic
      abuse F13.182
      dependence F13.282
      use F13.982
    stimulant NEC
      abuse F15.182
      dependence F15.282
      use F15.982
  in conditions classified elsewhere
    G47.54
  nonorganic origin F51.8
  organic G47.50
  specified NEC G47.59
Paraspadias Q54.9
Paraspasmus facialis G51.8

▶ New   ➔ Revised   ~~deleted~~ Deleted   ● Use Additional Character(s)

Parasuicide (attempt)
  history of (personal) Z91.51
    in family Z81.8
Parathyroid gland —see condition
Parathyroid tetany E20.9
Paratrachoma A74.0
Paratyphilitis —see Appendicitis
Paratyphoid (fever) —see Fever, paratyphoid
Paratyphus —see Fever, paratyphoid
Paraurethral duct Q64.79
Paraurethritis —see also Urethritis
  gonococcal (acute) (chronic) (with abscess) A54.1
Paravaccinia NEC B08.04
Paravaginitis —see Vaginitis
Parencephalitis —see also Encephalitis
  sequelae G09
Parent-child conflict —see Conflict, parent-child
  estrangement NEC Z62.890
Paresis —see also Paralysis
  accommodation —see Paresis, of accommodation
  Bernhardt's G57.1-●
  bladder (sphincter) —see also Paralysis, bladder
    tabetic A52.17
  bowel, colon or intestine K56.0
  extrinsic muscle, eye H49.9
  general (progressive) (syphilitic) A52.17
    juvenile A50.45
  heart —see Failure, heart
  insane (syphilitic) A52.17
  juvenile (general) A50.45
  of accommodation H52.52-●
  peripheral progressive (idiopathic) G60.3
  ⇒pseudohypertrophic (see also Dystrophy, muscular, by type, if applicable) G71.09
  senile G83.9
  syphilitic (general) A52.17
    congenital A50.45
  vesical NEC N31.2
Paresthesia —see also Disturbance, sensation, skin R20.2
  Bernhardt G57.1-●
Paretic —see condition
Parinaud's
  conjunctivitis H10.89
  oculoglandular syndrome H10.89
  ophthalmoplegia H49.88
Parkinsonism (idiopathic) (primary) G20
  with neurogenic orthostatic hypotension (symptomatic) G90.3
  arteriosclerotic G21.4
  ⇒dementia (see also Dystrophy, muscular, by type, if applicable) G31.83 [F02.80]
    ⇒with behavioral disturbance (see also Dystrophy, muscular, by type, if applicable) G31.83 [F02.81-●]
  due to
    drugs NEC G21.19
      neuroleptic G21.11
    medication-induced NEC G21.19
  neuroleptic induced G21.11
  postencephalitic G21.3
  secondary G21.9
    due to
      arteriosclerosis G21.4
      drugs NEC G21.19
        neuroleptic G21.11
      encephalitis G21.3
      external agents NEC G21.2
      syphilis A52.19
    specified NEC G21.8
  syphilitic A52.19
  treatment-induced NEC G21.19
  vascular G21.4
Parkinson's disease, syndrome or tremor —see Parkinsonism
Parodontitis —see Periodontitis
Parodontosis K05.4

Paronychia —see also Cellulitis, digit
  with lymphangitis —see Lymphangitis, acute, digit
  candidal (chronic) B37.2
  tuberculous (primary) A18.4
Parorexia (psychogenic) F50.89
Parosmia R43.1
  psychogenic F45.8
Parotid gland —see condition
Parotitis, parotiditis (allergic) (nonspecific toxic) (purulent) (septic) (suppurative) — see also Sialoadenitis
  epidemic —see Mumps
  infectious —see Mumps
  postoperative K91.89
  surgical K91.89
Parrot fever A70
Parrot's disease (early congenital syphilitic pseudoparalysis) A50.02
Parry-Romberg syndrome G51.8
Parry's disease or syndrome E05.00
  with thyroid storm E05.01
Pars planitis —see Cyclitis
Parsonage (-Aldren)-Turner syndrome G54.5
Parson's disease (exophthalmic goiter) E05.00
  with thyroid storm E05.01
Particolored infant Q82.8
Parturition —see Delivery
Parulis K04.7
  with sinus K04.6
Parvovirus, as cause of disease classified elsewhere B97.6
Pasini and Pierini's atrophoderma L90.3
Passage
  false, urethra N36.5
  meconium (newborn) during delivery P03.82
  of sounds or bougies —see Attention to, artificial, opening
Passive —see condition
  smoking Z77.22
Past due on rent or mortgage Z59.81- ●
Pasteurella septica A28.0
Pasteurellosis —see Infection, Pasteurella
PAT (paroxysmal atrial tachycardia) I47.1
Patau's syndrome —see Trisomy, 13
Patches
  mucous (syphilitic) A51.39
    congenital A50.07
  smokers' (mouth) K13.24
Patellar —see condition
Patent —see also Imperfect, closure
  canal of Nuck Q52.4
  cervix N88.3
  ductus arteriosus or Botallo's Q25.0
  foramen
    ⇒botalli Q21.12
    ⇒ovale Q21.12
  ⇒interauricular septum Q21.19
  interventricular septum Q21.0
  omphalomesenteric duct Q43.0
  os (uteri) —see Patent, cervix
  ⇒ostium secundum (type II) Q21.11
  urachus Q64.4
  vitelline duct Q43.0
Paterson (-Brown)(-Kelly) syndrome or web D50.1
Pathologic, pathological —see also condition
  asphyxia R09.01
  fire-setting F63.1
  gambling F63.0
  ovum O02.0
  resorption, tooth K03.3
  stealing F63.2
Pathology (of) —see Disease
  periradicular, associated with previous endodontic treatment NEC M27.59
Pattern, sleep-wake, irregular G47.23
Patulous —see also Imperfect, closure (congenital)
  alimentary tract Q45.8
    lower Q43.8
    upper Q40.8
  eustachian tube H69.0-●

Pause, sinoatrial I49.5
Paxton's disease B36.2
Pearl(s)
  enamel K00.2
  Epstein's K09.8
Pearl-worker's disease —see Osteomyelitis, specified type NEC
Pectenosis K62.4
Pectoral —see condition
Pectus
  carinatum (congenital) Q67.7
    acquired M95.4
    rachitic sequelae (late effect) E64.3
  excavatum (congenital) Q67.6
    acquired M95.4
    rachitic sequelae (late effect) E64.3
  recurvatum (congenital) Q67.6
Pedatrophia E41
Pederosis F65.4
Pediatric inflammatory multisystem syndrome M35.81
Pediculosis (infestation) B85.2
  capitis (head-louse) (any site) B85.0
  corporis (body-louse) (any site) B85.1
  eyelid B85.0
  mixed (classifiable to more than one of the titles B85.0-B85.3) B85.4
  pubis (pubic louse) (any site) B85.3
  vestimenti B85.1
  vulvae B85.3
Pediculus (infestation) —see Pediculosis
Pedophilia F65.4
Peg-shaped teeth K00.2
Pelade —see Alopecia, areata
Pelger-Huët anomaly or syndrome D72.0
Peliosis (rheumatica) D69.0
  hepatis K76.4
    with toxic liver disease K71.8
Pelizaeus-Merzbacher disease E75.29
Pellagra (alcoholic) (with polyneuropathy) E52
Pellagra-cerebellar-ataxia-renal aminoaciduria syndrome E72.02
Pellegrini (-Stieda) disease or syndrome —see Bursitis, tibial collateral
Pellizzi's syndrome E34.8
Pel's crisis A52.11
Pelvic —see also condition
  examination (periodic) (routine) Z01.419
    with abnormal findings Z01.411
  kidney, congenital Q63.2
Pelviolithiasis —see Calculus, kidney
Pelviperitonitis —see also Peritonitis, pelvic
  gonococcal A54.24
  puerperal O85
Pelvis —see condition or type
Pemphigoid L12.9
  benign, mucous membrane L12.1
  bullous L12.0
  cicatricial L12.1
  juvenile L12.2
  ocular L12.1
  specified NEC L12.8
Pemphigus L10.9
  benign familial (chronic) Q82.8
  Brazilian L10.3
  circinatus L13.0
  conjunctiva L12.1
  drug-induced L10.5
  erythematosus L10.4
  foliaceus L10.2
  gangrenous —see Gangrene
  neonatorum L01.03
  ocular L12.1
  paraneoplastic L10.81
  specified NEC L10.89
  syphilitic (congenital) A50.06
  vegetans L10.1
  vulgaris L10.0
  wildfire L10.3
Pendred's syndrome E07.1

Pendulous
  abdomen, in pregnancy —*see* Pregnancy,
      complicated by, abnormal, pelvic organs
      or tissues NEC
  breast N64.89
Penetrating wound —*see also* Puncture
  with internal injury —*see* Injury, by site
  eyeball —*see* Puncture, eyeball
  orbit (with or without foreign body) —*see*
      Puncture, orbit
  uterus by instrument with or following
      ectopic or molar pregnancy O08.6
Penicillosis B48.4
Penis —*see* condition
Penitis N48.29
Pentalogy of Fallot Q21.8
Pentasomy X syndrome Q97.1
Pentosuria (essential) E74.89
Percreta placenta O43.23-●
Peregrinating patient —*see* Disorder, factitious
Perforation, perforated (nontraumatic) (of)
  accidental during procedure (blood vessel)
      (nerve) (organ) —*see* Complication,
      accidental puncture or laceration
  antrum —*see* Sinusitis, maxillary
  appendix K35.22
    with localized peritonitis K35.32
  atrial septum, multiple Q21.19
  attic, ear —*see* Perforation, tympanum, attic
  bile duct (common) (hepatic) K83.2
    cystic K82.2
  bladder (urinary)
    with or following ectopic or molar
        pregnancy O08.6
    obstetrical trauma O71.5
    traumatic S37.29
      at delivery O71.5
  bowel K63.1
    with or following ectopic or molar
        pregnancy O08.6
    newborn P78.0
    obstetrical trauma O71.5
    traumatic —*see* Laceration, intestine
  broad ligament N83.8
    with or following ectopic or molar
        pregnancy O08.6
    obstetrical trauma O71.6
  by
    device, implant or graft —*see also*
        Complications, by site and type,
        mechanical T85.628
      arterial graft NEC —*see* Complication,
          cardiovascular device, mechanical,
          vascular
      breast (implant) T85.49
      catheter NEC T85.698
        cystostomy T83.090
        dialysis (renal) T82.49
          intraperitoneal T85.691
        infusion NEC T82.594
          spinal (epidural) (subdural)
              T85.690
        urinary —*see also* Complications,
            catheter, urinary T83.098
      electronic (electrode) (pulse generator)
          (stimulator)
        bone T84.390
        cardiac T82.199
          electrode T82.190
          pulse generator T82.191
          specified type NEC T82.198
        nervous system —*see* Complication,
            prosthetic device, mechanical,
            electronic nervous system
            stimulator
        urinary —*see* Complication,
            genitourinary, device, urinary,
            mechanical
      fixation, internal (orthopedic) NEC —
          see Complication, fixation device,
          mechanical

Perforation, perforated (*Continued*)
  by (*Continued*)
    device, implant or graft (*Continued*)
      gastrointestinal —*see* Complications,
          prosthetic device, mechanical,
          gastrointestinal device
      genital NEC T83.498
        intrauterine contraceptive device T83.39
        penile prosthesis T83.490
      heart NEC —*see* Complication,
          cardiovascular device, mechanical
      joint prosthesis —*see* Complications,
          joint prosthesis, mechanical,
          specified NEC, by site
      ocular NEC —*see* Complications,
          prosthetic device, mechanical,
          ocular device
      orthopedic NEC —*see* Complication,
          orthopedic, device, mechanical
      specified NEC T85.628
      urinary NEC —*see also* Complication,
          genitourinary, device, urinary,
          mechanical
        graft T83.29
      vascular NEC —*see* Complication,
          cardiovascular device, mechanical
      ventricular intracranial shunt T85.09
    foreign body left accidentally in
        operative wound T81.539
    instrument (any) during a procedure,
        accidental —*see* Puncture, accidental
        complicating surgery
  cecum K35.22
    with localized peritonitis K35.32
  cervix (uteri) N88.8
    with or following ectopic or molar
        pregnancy O08.6
    obstetrical trauma O71.3
  colon K63.1
    newborn P78.0
    obstetrical trauma O71.5
    traumatic —*see* Laceration, intestine, large
  common duct (bile) K83.2
  cornea (due to ulceration) —*see* Ulcer,
      cornea, perforated
  cystic duct K82.2
  diverticulum (intestine) K57.80
    with bleeding K57.81
    large intestine K57.20
      with
        bleeding K57.21
        small intestine K57.40
          with bleeding K57.41
      small intestine K57.00
      with
        bleeding K57.01
        large intestine K57.40
          with bleeding K57.41
  ear drum —*see* Perforation, tympanum
  esophagus K22.3
  ethmoidal sinus —*see* Sinusitis, ethmoidal
  frontal sinus —*see* Sinusitis, frontal
  gallbladder K82.2
  heart valve —*see* Endocarditis
  ileum K63.1
    newborn P78.0
    obstetrical trauma O71.5
    traumatic —*see* Laceration, intestine, small
  instrumental, surgical (accidental) (blood
      vessel) (nerve) (organ) —*see* Puncture,
      accidental complicating surgery
  intestine NEC K63.1
    with ectopic or molar pregnancy O08.6
    newborn P78.0
    obstetrical trauma O71.5
    traumatic —*see* Laceration, intestine
    ulcerative NEC K63.1
      newborn P78.0
  jejunum, jejunal K63.1
    obstetrical trauma O71.5
    traumatic —*see* Laceration, intestine, small
    ulcer —*see* Ulcer, gastrojejunal, with
        perforation

Perforation, perforated (*Continued*)
  joint prosthesis —*see* Complications, joint
      prosthesis, mechanical, specified NEC,
      by site
  mastoid (antrum) (cell) —*see* Disorder,
      mastoid, specified NEC
  maxillary sinus —*see* Sinusitis, maxillary
  membrana tympani —*see* Perforation,
      tympanum
  nasal
    septum J34.89
      congenital Q30.3
      syphilitic A52.73
    sinus J34.89
      congenital Q30.8
      due to sinusitis —*see* Sinusitis
  palate —*see also* Cleft, palate Q35.9
    syphilitic A52.79
  palatine vault —*see also* Cleft, palate, hard
      Q35.1
    syphilitic A52.79
    congenital A50.59
  pars flaccida (ear drum) —*see* Perforation,
      tympanum, attic
  pelvic
    floor S31.030
      with
        ectopic or molar pregnancy O08.6
        penetration into retroperitoneal space
            S31.031
        retained foreign body S31.040
          with penetration into
              retroperitoneal space S31.041
      following ectopic or molar pregnancy
          O08.6
      obstetrical trauma O70.1
    organ S37.99
      adrenal gland S37.818
      bladder —*see* Perforation, bladder
      fallopian tube S37.599
        bilateral S37.592
        unilateral S37.591
      kidney S37.09-●
      obstetrical trauma O71.5
      ovary S37.499
        bilateral S37.492
        unilateral S37.491
      prostate S37.828
      specified organ NEC S37.898
      ureter —*see* Perforation, ureter
      urethra —*see* Perforation, urethra
      uterus —*see* Perforation, uterus
  perineum —*see* Laceration, perineum
  pharynx J39.2
  rectum K63.1
    newborn P78.0
    obstetrical trauma O71.5
    traumatic S36.63
  root canal space due to endodontic treatment
      M27.51
  sigmoid K63.1
    newborn P78.0
    obstetrical trauma O71.5
    traumatic S36.533
  sinus (accessory) (chronic) (nasal) J34.89
  sphenoidal sinus —*see* Sinusitis, sphenoidal
  surgical (accidental) (by instrument) (blood
      vessel) (nerve) (organ) —*see* Puncture,
      accidental complicating surgery
  traumatic
    external —*see* Puncture
    eye —*see* Puncture, eyeball
    internal organ —*see* Injury, by site
  tympanum, tympanic (membrane) (persistent
      post-traumatic) (postinflammatory)
      H72.9-●
    attic H72.1-●
      multiple —*see* Perforation, tympanum,
          multiple
      total —*see* Perforation, tympanum, total
    central H72.0-●
      multiple —*see* Perforation, tympanum,
          multiple
      total —*see* Perforation, tympanum, total

▶ New   ⇒ Revised   ~~deleted~~ Deleted   ● Use Additional Character(s)

Perforation, perforated *(Continued)*
  tympanum, tympanic *(Continued)*
    marginal NEC —*see* subcategory H72.2
    multiple H72.81-●
    pars flaccida —*see* Perforation, tympanum,
      attic
    total H72.82-●
    traumatic, current episode S09.2-●
  typhoid, gastrointestinal —*see* Typhoid
  ulcer —*see* Ulcer, by site, with perforation
  ureter N28.89
    traumatic S37.19
  urethra N36.8
    with ectopic or molar pregnancy O08.6
    following ectopic or molar pregnancy O08.6
    obstetrical trauma O71.5
    traumatic S37.39
      at delivery O71.5
  uterus
    with ectopic or molar pregnancy O08.6
    by intrauterine contraceptive device T83.39
    following ectopic or molar pregnancy O08.6
    obstetrical trauma O71.1
    traumatic S37.69
      obstetric O71.1
  uvula K13.79
    syphilitic A52.79
  vagina
    obstetrical trauma O71.4
    other trauma - *see* Puncture, vagina
Periadenitis mucosa necrotica recurrens K12.0
Periappendicitis (acute) —*see* Appendicitis
Periarteritis nodosa (disseminated) (infectious)
  (necrotizing) M30.0
Periarthritis (joint) —*see also* Enthesopathy
  Duplay's M75.0-●
  gonococcal A54.42
  humeroscapularis —*see* Capsulitis, adhesive
  scapulohumeral —*see* Capsulitis, adhesive
  shoulder —*see* Capsulitis, adhesive
  wrist M77.2-●
Periarthrosis (angioneural) —*see* Enthesopathy
Pericapsulitis, adhesive (shoulder) —*see*
  Capsulitis, adhesive
Pericarditis (with decompensation) (with
  effusion) I31.9
  with rheumatic fever (conditions in I00) I01.0
    active —*see* Pericarditis, rheumatic
    inactive or quiescent I09.2
  acute (hemorrhagic) (nonrheumatic) (Sicca)
    I30.9
    with chorea (acute) (rheumatic)
      (Sydenham's) I02.0
    benign I30.8
    nonspecific I30.0
    rheumatic I01.0
      with chorea (acute) (Sydenham's) I02.0
  adhesive or adherent (chronic) (external)
    (internal) I31.0
    acute —*see* Pericarditis, acute
    rheumatic I09.2
  bacterial (acute) (subacute) (with serous or
    seropurulent effusion) I30.1
  calcareous I31.1
  cholesterol (chronic) I31.8
    acute I30.9
  chronic (nonrheumatic) I31.9
    rheumatic I09.2
  constrictive (chronic) I31.1
  coxsackie B33.23
  fibrinocaseous (tuberculous) A18.84
  fibrinopurulent I30.1
  fibrinous I30.8
  fibrous I31.0
  gonococcal A54.83
  idiopathic I30.0
  in systemic lupus erythematosus M32.12
  infective I30.1
  meningococcal A39.53
  neoplastic (chronic) I31.8
    acute I30.9

Pericarditis *(Continued)*
  obliterans, obliterating I31.0
  plastic I31.0
  pneumococcal I30.1
  postinfarction I24.1
  purulent I30.1
  rheumatic (active) (acute) (with effusion)
    (with pneumonia) I01.0
    with chorea (acute) (rheumatic)
      (Sydenham's) I02.0
    chronic or inactive (with chorea) I09.2
  rheumatoid —*see* Rheumatoid, carditis
  septic I30.1
  serofibrinous I30.8
  staphylococcal I30.1
  streptococcal I30.1
  suppurative I30.1
  syphilitic A52.06
  tuberculous A18.84
  uremic N18.9 *[I32]*
  viral I30.1
Pericardium, pericardial —*see* condition
Pericellulitis —*see* Cellulitis
Pericementitis (chronic) (suppurative) —*see also*
  Periodontitis
  acute K05.20
    generalized —*see* Periodontitis, aggressive,
      generalized
    localized —*see* Periodontitis, aggressive,
      localized
Perichondritis
  auricle —*see* Perichondritis, ear
  bronchus J98.09
  ear (external) H61.00-●
    acute H61.01-●
    chronic H61.02-●
  external auditory canal —*see* Perichondritis, ear
  larynx J38.7
    syphilitic A52.73
    typhoid A01.09
  nose J34.89
  pinna —*see* Perichondritis, ear
  trachea J39.8
Periclasia K05.4
Pericoronitis —*see* Periodontitis
Pericystitis N30.90
  with hematuria N30.91
Peridiverticulitis (intestine) K57.92
  cecum —*see* Diverticulitis, intestine, large
  colon —*see* Diverticulitis, intestine, large
  duodenum —*see* Diverticulitis, intestine, small
  intestine —*see* Diverticulitis, intestine
  jejunum —*see* Diverticulitis, intestine, small
  rectosigmoid —*see* Diverticulitis, intestine,
    large
  rectum —*see* Diverticulitis, intestine, large
  sigmoid —*see* Diverticulitis, intestine, large
Periendocarditis —*see* Endocarditis
Periepididymitis N45.1
Perifolliculitis L01.02
  abscedens, caput, scalp L66.3
  capitis, abscedens (et suffodiens) L66.3
  superficial pustular L01.02
Perihepatitis K65.8
Perilabyrinthitis (acute) —*see* subcategory H83.0
Perimeningitis —*see* Meningitis
Perimetritis —*see* Endometritis
Perimetrosalpingitis —*see* Salpingo-oophoritis
Perineocele N81.81
Perinephric, perinephritic —*see* condition
Perinephritis —*see also* Infection, kidney
  purulent —*see* Abscess, kidney
Perineum, perineal —*see* condition
Perineuritis NEC —*see* Neuralgia
Periodic —*see* condition
Periodontitis (chronic) (complex) (compound)
  (local) (simplex) K05.30
  acute K05.20
    generalized K05.229
      moderate K05.222
      severe K05.223
      slight K05.221

Periodontitis *(Continued)*
  acute *(Continued)*
    localized K05.219
      moderate K05.212
      severe K05.213
      slight K05.211
  ▶aggressive K05.20
    ▶generalized K05.229
      ▶moderate K05.222
      ▶severe K05.223
      ▶slight K05.221
    ▶localized K05.219
      ▶moderate K05.212
      ▶severe K05.213
      ▶slight K05.211
  apical K04.5
    acute (pulpal origin) K04.4
  generalized K05.329
    moderate K05.322
    severe K05.323
    slight K05.321
  localized K05.319
    moderate K05.312
    severe K05.313
    slight K05.311
Periodontoclasia K05.4
Periodontosis (juvenile) K05.4
Periods —*see also* Menstruation
  heavy N92.0
  irregular N92.6
  shortened intervals (irregular) N92.1
Perionychia —*see also* Cellulitis, digit
  with lymphangitis —*see* Lymphangitis, acute,
    digit
Perioophoritis —*see* Salpingo-oophoritis
Periorchitis N45.2
Periosteum, periosteal —*see* condition
Periostitis (albuminosa) (circumscribed)
  (diffuse) (infective) (monomelic) —*see also*
  Osteomyelitis
  alveolar M27.3
  alveolodental M27.3
  dental M27.3
  gonorrheal A54.43
  jaw (lower) (upper) M27.2
  orbit H05.03-●
  syphilitic A52.77
    congenital (early) A50.02 *[M90.80]*
    secondary A51.46
  tuberculous —*see* Tuberculosis, bone
  yaws (hypertrophic) (early) (late) A66.6
    [M90.80]
Periostosis (hyperplastic) —*see also* Disorder,
  bone, specified type NEC
  with osteomyelitis —*see* Osteomyelitis,
    specified type NEC
Peripartum
  cardiomyopathy O90.3
Periphlebitis —*see* Phlebitis
Periproctitis K62.89
Periprostatitis —*see* Prostatitis
Perirectal —*see* condition
Perirenal —*see* condition
Perisalpingitis —*see* Salpingo-oophoritis
Perisplenitis (infectional) D73.89
Peristalsis, visible or reversed R19.2
Peritendinitis —*see* Enthesopathy
Peritoneum, peritoneal —*see* condition
Peritonitis (adhesive) (bacterial) (fibrinous)
  (hemorrhagic) (idiopathic) (localized)
  (perforative) (primary) (with adhesions)
  (with effusion) K65.9
  with or following
    abscess K65.1
    appendicitis
      with perforation or rupture K35.32
      generalized (*see also* Appendicitis) K35.20
      localized (*see also* Appendicitis) K35.30
    diverticular disease (intestine) K57.80
      with bleeding K57.81
    ectopic or molar pregnancy O08.0

▶ New ⟹ Revised ~~deleted~~ Deleted ● Use Additional Character(s)

Personality *(Continued)*
 passive-aggressive F60.89
 pathologic F60.9
 pattern defect or disturbance F60.9
 pseudopsychopathic (organic) F07.0
 pseudoretarded (organic) F07.0
 psychoinfantile F60.4
 psychoneurotic NEC F60.89
 psychopathic F60.2
 querulant F60.0
 sadistic F60.89
 schizoid F60.1
 self-defeating F60.89
 sensitive paranoid F60.0
 sociopathic (amoral) (antisocial) (asocial)
  (dissocial) F60.2
 specified NEC F60.89
 type A Z73.1
 unstable (emotional) F60.3
Perthes' disease —*see* Legg-Calvé-Perthes
 disease
Pertussis *(see also* Whooping cough) A37.90
Perversion, perverted
 appetite F50.89
  psychogenic F50.89
 function
  pituitary gland E23.2
   posterior lobe E22.2
 sense of smell and taste R43.8
  psychogenic F45.8
 sexual —*see* Deviation, sexual
Pervious, congenital —*see also* Imperfect,
 closure
 ductus arteriosus Q25.0
Pes (congenital) —*see also* Talipes
 acquired —*see also* Deformity, limb, foot,
  specified NEC
  planus —*see* Deformity, limb, flat foot
 adductus Q66.89
 cavus Q66.7-●
 deformity NEC, acquired —*see* Deformity,
  limb, foot, specified NEC
 planus (acquired) (any degree) —*see also*
  Deformity, limb, flat foot
  rachitic sequelae (late effect) E64.3
 valgus Q66.6
Pest, pestis —*see* Plague
Petechia, petechiae R23.3
 newborn P54.5
Petechial typhus A75.9
Peter's anomaly Q13.4
Petit mal seizure —*see* Epilepsy, childhood,
 absence
Petit's hernia —*see* Hernia, abdomen, specified
 site NEC
Petrellidosis B48.2
Petrositis H70.20-●
 acute H70.21-●
 chronic H70.22-●
Peutz-Jeghers disease or syndrome Q85.89
Peyronie's disease N48.6
PFAPA (periodic fever, aphthous stomatitis,
 pharyngitis, and adenopathy syndrome)
 M04.8
Pfeiffer's disease —*see* Mononucleosis,
 infectious
Phagedena (dry) (moist) (sloughing) —*see also*
 Gangrene
 geometric L88
 penis N48.29
 tropical —*see* Ulcer, skin
 vulva N76.6
Phagedenic —*see* condition
Phakoma H35.89
Phakomatosis —*see also* specific eponymous
 syndromes Q85.9
 Bourneville's Q85.1
 specified NEC Q85.89
Phantom limb syndrome (without pain)
 G54.7
 with pain G54.6

Pharyngeal pouch syndrome D82.1
Pharyngitis (acute) (catarrhal) (gangrenous)
 (infective) (malignant) (membranous)
 (phlegmonous) (pseudomembranous)
 (simple) (subacute) (suppurative)
 (ulcerative) (viral) J02.9
 with influenza, flu, or grippe —*see* Influenza,
  with, pharyngitis
 aphthous B08.5
 atrophic J31.2
 chlamydial A56.4
 chronic (atrophic) (granular) (hypertrophic)
  J31.2
 coxsackievirus B08.5
 diphtheritic A36.0
 enteroviral vesicular B08.5
 follicular (chronic) J31.2
 fusospirochetal A69.1
 gonococcal A54.5
 granular (chronic) J31.2
 herpesviral B00.2
 hypertrophic J31.2
 infectional, chronic J31.2
 influenzal —*see* Influenza, with, respiratory
  manifestations NEC
 lymphonodular, acute (enteroviral) B08.8
 pneumococcal J02.8
 purulent J02.9
 putrid J02.9
 septic J02.0
 sicca J31.2
 specified organism NEC J02.8
 staphylococcal J02.8
 streptococcal J02.0
 syphilitic, congenital (early) A50.03
 tuberculous A15.8
 vesicular, enteroviral B08.5
 viral NEC J02.8
Pharyngoconjunctivitis, viral B30.2
Pharyngolaryngitis (acute) J06.0
 chronic J37.0
Pharyngoplegia J39.2
Pharyngotonsillitis, herpesviral B00.2
Pharyngotracheitis, chronic J42
Pharynx, pharyngeal —*see* condition
Phencyclidine-induced
 anxiety disorder F16.980
 bipolar and related disorder F16.94
 depressive disorder F16.94
 psychotic disorder F16.959
Phenomenon
 Arthus' —*see* Arthus' phenomenon
 jaw-winking Q07.8
 lupus erythematosus (LE) cell M32.9
 Raynaud's (secondary) I73.00
  with gangrene I73.01
 vasomotor R55
 vasospastic I73.9
 vasovagal R55
 Wenckebach's I44.1
Phenylketonuria E70.1
 classical E70.0
 maternal E70.1
Pheochromoblastoma
 specified site —*see* Neoplasm, malignant, by
  site
 unspecified site C74.10
Pheochromocytoma
 malignant
  specified site —*see* Neoplasm, malignant,
   by site
  unspecified site C74.10
 specified site —*see* Neoplasm, benign, by site
 unspecified site D35.00
Pheohyphomycosis —*see* Chromomycosis
Pheomycosis —*see* Chromomycosis
Phimosis (congenital) (due to infection) N47.1
 chancroidal A57
Phlebectasia —*see also* Varix
 congenital Q27.4

Phlebitis (infective) (pyemic) (septic)
 (suppurative) I80.9
 antepartum —*see* Thrombophlebitis,
  antepartum
 blue —*see* Phlebitis, leg, deep
 breast, superficial I80.8
 calf muscular vein (NOS) I80.25-●
 cavernous (venous) sinus —*see* Phlebitis,
  intracranial (venous) sinus
 cerebral (venous) sinus —*see* Phlebitis,
  intracranial (venous) sinus
 chest wall, superficial I80.8
 cranial (venous) sinus —*see* Phlebitis,
  intracranial (venous) sinus
 deep (vessels) —*see* Phlebitis, leg, deep
 due to implanted device —*see* Complications,
  by site and type, specified NEC
 during or resulting from a procedure T81.72
 femoral vein (superficial) I80.1-●
 femoropopliteal vein I80.0-●
 gastrocnemial vein I80.25-●
 gestational —*see* Phlebopathy, gestational
 hepatic veins I80.8
 iliac vein (common) (external) (internal)
  I80.21-●
 iliofemoral —*see* Phlebitis, femoral vein
 intracranial (venous) sinus (any) G08
  nonpyogenic I67.6
 intraspinal venous sinuses and veins G08
  nonpyogenic G95.19
 lateral (venous) sinus —*see* Phlebitis,
  intracranial (venous) sinus
 leg I80.3
  antepartum —*see* Thrombophlebitis,
   antepartum
  deep (vessels) NEC I80.20-●
   iliac I80.21-●
   popliteal vein I80.22-●
   specified vessel NEC I80.29-●
   tibial vein (anterior) (posterior) I80.23-●
  femoral vein (superficial) I80.1-●
  superficial (vessels) I80.0-●
 longitudinal sinus —*see* Phlebitis, intracranial
  (venous) sinus
 lower limb —*see* Phlebitis, leg
 migrans, migrating (superficial) I82.1
 pelvic
  with ectopic or molar pregnancy O08.0
  following ectopic or molar pregnancy O08.0
  puerperal, postpartum O87.1
 peroneal vein I80.24-●
 popliteal vein —*see* Phlebitis, leg, deep,
  popliteal
 portal (vein) K75.1
 postoperative T81.72
 pregnancy —*see* Thrombophlebitis,
  antepartum
 puerperal, postpartum, childbirth O87.0
  deep O87.1
  pelvic O87.1
  superficial O87.0
 retina —*see* Vasculitis, retina
 saphenous (accessory) (great) (long)
  (small) —*see* Phlebitis, leg, superficial
 sinus (meninges) —*see* Phlebitis, intracranial
  (venous) sinus
 soleal vein I80.25-●
 specified site NEC I80.8
 syphilitic A52.09
 tibial vein —*see* Phlebitis, leg, deep, tibial
 ulcerative I80.9
  leg —*see* Phlebitis, leg
 umbilicus I80.8
 uterus (septic) —*see* Endometritis
 varicose (leg) (lower limb) —*see* Varix, leg,
  with, inflammation
Phlebofibrosis I87.8
Phleboliths I87.8
Phlebopathy
 gestational O22.9-●
 puerperal O87.9
Phlebosclerosis I87.8

Phlebothrombosis —*see also* Thrombosis
　antepartum —*see* Thrombophlebitis, antepartum
　pregnancy —*see* Thrombophlebitis, antepartum
　puerperal —*see* Thrombophlebitis, puerperal
Phlebotomus fever A93.1
Phlegmasia
　alba dolens O87.1
　　nonpuerperal —*see* Phlebitis, femoral vein
　cerulea dolens —*see* Phlebitis, leg, deep
Phlegmon —*see* Abscess
Phlegmonous —*see* condition
Phlyctenulosis (allergic) (keratoconjunctivitis) (nontuberculous) —*see also* Keratoconjunctivitis
　cornea —*see* Keratoconjunctivitis
　tuberculous A18.52
Phobia, phobic F40.9
　animal F40.218
　　spiders F40.210
　examination F40.298
　reaction F40.9
　simple F40.298
　social F40.10
　　generalized F40.11
　specific (isolated) F40.298
　　animal F40.218
　　　spiders F40.210
　　blood F40.230
　　injection F40.231
　　injury F40.233
　　men F40.290
　　natural environment F40.228
　　　thunderstorms F40.220
　　situational F40.248
　　　bridges F40.242
　　　closed in spaces F40.240
　　　flying F40.243
　　　heights F40.241
　　specified focus NEC F40.298
　　transfusion F40.231
　　women F40.291
　specified NEC F40.8
　　medical care NEC F40.232
　state F40.9
Phocas' disease —*see* Mastopathy, cystic
Phocomelia Q73.1
　lower limb —*see* Agenesis, leg, with foot present
　upper limb —*see* Agenesis, arm, with hand present
Phoria H50.50
Phosphate-losing tubular disorder N25.0
Phosphatemia E83.39
Phosphaturia E83.39
Photodermatitis (sun) L56.8
　chronic L57.8
　due to drug L56.8
　light other than sun L59.8
Photokeratitis H16.13-●
Photophobia H53.14-●
Photophthalmia —*see* Photokeratitis
Photopsia H53.19
Photoretinitis —*see* Retinopathy, solar
Photosensitivity, photosensitization (sun) skin L56.8
　light other than sun L59.8
Phrenitis —*see* Encephalitis
Phrynoderma (vitamin A deficiency) E50.8
Phthiriasis (pubis) B85.3
　with any infestation classifiable to B85.0-B85.2 B85.4
Phthirus infestation —*see* Phthiriasis
Phthisis —*see also* Tuberculosis
　bulbi (infectional) —*see* Disorder, globe, degenerated condition, atrophy
　eyeball (due to infection) —*see* Disorder, globe, degenerated condition, atrophy
▶PHTS Q85.81
Phycomycosis —*see* Zygomycosis

Physalopteriasis B81.8
Physical restraint status Z78.1
Phytobezoar T18.9
　intestine T18.3
　stomach T18.2
Pian —*see* Yaws
Pianoma A66.1
Pica F50.89
　in adults F50.89
　infant or child F98.3
Picking, nose F98.8
Pick-Niemann disease —*see* Niemann-Pick disease or syndrome
Pick's
➡cerebral atrophy (*see also* Dementia, in, diseases specified elsewhere) G31.01 [F02.80]
　➡with behavioral disturbance (*see also* Dementia, in, diseases specified elsewhere) G31.01 [F02.81-●]
➡disease or syndrome (brain) (*see also* Dementia, in, diseases specified elsewhere) G31.01 [F02.80]
　➡with behavioral disturbance (*see also* Dementia, in, diseases specified elsewhere) G31.01 [F02.81-●]
　➡brain (*see also* Dementia, in, diseases specified elsewhere) G31.01 [F02.80]
　　➡with behavioral disturbance (*see also* Dementia, in, diseases specified elsewhere) G31.01 [F02.81-●]
　pericardium (pericardial pseudocirrhosis of liver) I31.1
syndrome
➡brain (*see also* Dementia, in, diseases specified elsewhere) G31.01 [F02.80]
　➡with behavioral disturbance (*see also* Dementia, in, diseases specified elsewhere) G31.01 [F02.81-●]
　of heart (pericardial pseudocirrhosis of liver) I31.1
Pickwickian syndrome E66.2
Piebaldism E70.39
Piedra (beard) (scalp) B36.8
　black B36.3
　white B36.2
Pierre Robin deformity or syndrome Q87.0
Pierson's disease or osteochondrosis M91.0
Pig-bel A05.2
Pigeon
　breast or chest (acquired) M95.4
　　congenital Q67.7
　　rachitic sequelae (late effect) E64.3
　breeder's disease or lung J67.2
　fancier's disease or lung J67.2
　toe —*see* Deformity, toe, specified NEC
Pigmentation (abnormal) (anomaly) L81.9
　conjunctiva H11.13-●
　cornea (anterior) H18.01-●
　　posterior H18.05-●
　　stromal H18.06-●
　diminished melanin formation NEC L81.6
　iron L81.8
　lids, congenital Q82.8
　limbus corneae —*see* Pigmentation, cornea
　metals L81.8
　optic papilla, congenital Q14.2
　retina, congenital (grouped) (nevoid) Q14.1
　scrotum, congenital Q82.8
　tattoo L81.8
Piles —*see also* Hemorrhoids K64.9
Pili
　annulati or torti (congenital) Q84.1
　incarnati L73.1
Pill roller hand (intrinsic) —*see* Parkinsonism
Pilomatrixoma —*see* Neoplasm, skin, benign
　malignant —*see* Neoplasm, skin, malignant
Pilonidal —*see* condition
Pimple R23.8
PIMS M35.81
PIN —*see* Neoplasia, intraepithelial, prostate

Pinched nerve —*see* Neuropathy, entrapment
Pindborg tumor —*see* Cyst, calcifying odontogenic
Pineal body or gland —*see* condition
Pinealoblastoma C75.3
Pinealoma D44.5
　malignant C75.3
Pineoblastoma C75.3
Pineocytoma D44.5
Pinguecula H11.15-●
Pingueculitis H10.81-●
Pinhole meatus —*see also* Stricture, urethra N35.919
Pink
　disease —*see* subcategory T56.1
　eye —*see* Conjunctivitis, acute, mucopurulent
Pinkus' disease (lichen nitidus) L44.1
Pinpoint
　meatus —*see* Stricture, urethra
　os (uteri) —*see* Stricture, cervix
Pins and needles R20.2
Pinta A67.9
　cardiovascular lesions A67.2
　chancre (primary) A67.0
　erythematous plaques A67.1
　hyperchromic lesions A67.1
　hyperkeratosis A67.1
　lesions A67.9
　　cardiovascular A67.2
　　hyperchromic A67.1
　　intermediate A67.1
　　late A67.2
　　mixed A67.3
　　primary A67.0
　　skin (achromic) (cicatricial) (dyschromic) A67.2
　　　hyperchromic A67.1
　　　mixed (achromic and hyperchromic) A67.3
　papule (primary) A67.0
　skin lesions (achromic) (cicatricial) (dyschromic) A67.2
　　hyperchromic A67.1
　　mixed (achromic and hyperchromic) A67.3
　vitiligo A67.2
Pintids A67.1
Pinworm (disease) (infection) (infestation) B80
Piroplasmosis (*see also* Babesiosis) B60.00
　specified NEC B60.09
Pistol wound —*see* Gunshot wound
Pitchers' elbow —*see* Derangement, joint, specified type NEC, elbow
Pithecoid pelvis Q74.2
　with disproportion (fetopelvic) O33.0
　　causing obstructed labor O65.0
Pithiatism F48.8
Pitted —*see* Pitting
Pitting —*see also* Edema R60.9
　lip R60.0
　nail L60.8
　teeth K00.4
Pituitary gland —*see* condition
Pituitary-snuff-taker's disease J67.8
Pityriasis (capitis) L21.0
　alba L30.5
　circinata (et maculata) L42
　furfuracea L21.0
　Hebra's L26
　lichenoides L41.0
　　chronica L41.1
　　et varioliformis (acuta) L41.0
　maculata (et circinata) L30.5
　nigra B36.1
　pilaris, Hebra's L44.0
　rosea L42
　rotunda L44.8
　rubra (Hebra) pilaris L44.0
　simplex L30.5
　specified type NEC L30.5
　streptogenes L30.5
　versicolor (scrotal) B36.0

Placenta, placental —see Pregnancy,
    complicated by (care of) (management
    affected by), specified condition
Placentitis O41.14-●
Plagiocephaly Q67.3
Plague A20.9
    abortive A20.8
    ambulatory A20.8
    asymptomatic A20.8
    bubonic A20.0
    cellulocutaneous A20.1
    cutaneobubonic A20.1
    lymphatic gland A20.0
    meningitis A20.3
    pharyngeal A20.8
    pneumonic (primary) (secondary) A20.2
    pulmonary, pulmonic A20.2
    septicemic A20.7
    tonsillar A20.8
        septicemic A20.7
Planning, family
    contraception Z30.9
    procreation Z31.69
Plaque(s)
    artery, arterial —see Arteriosclerosis
    calcareous —see Calcification
    coronary, lipid rich I25.83
    epicardial I31.8
    erythematous, of pinta A67.1
    Hollenhorst's —see Occlusion, artery, retina
    lipid rich, coronary I25.83
    pleural (without asbestos) J92.9
        with asbestos J92.0
    tongue K13.29
Plasmacytoma C90.3-●
    extramedullary C90.2-●
    medullary C90.0-●
    solitary C90.3-●
Plasmacytopenia D72.818
Plasmacytosis D72.822
Plaster ulcer —see Ulcer, pressure, by site
Plateau iris syndrome (post-iridectomy)
    (postprocedural) (without glaucoma)H21.82
    with glaucoma H40.22-●
Platybasia Q75.8
Platyonychia (congenital) Q84.6
    acquired L60.8
Platypelloid pelvis M95.5
    with disproportion (fetopelvic) O33.0
        causing obstructed labor O65.0
    congenital Q74.2
Platyspondylisis Q76.49
Plaut (-Vincent) disease —see also Vincent's A69.1
Plethora R23.2
    newborn P61.1
Pleura, pleural —see condition
Pleuralgia R07.81
Pleurisy (acute) (adhesive) (chronic) (costal)
    (diaphragmatic) (double) (dry) (fibrinous)
    (fibrous) (interlobar) (latent) (plastic)
    (primary) (residual) (sicca) (sterile)
    (subacute) (unresolved) R09.1
    with
        adherent pleura J86.0
        effusion J90
            chylous, chyliform J94.0
            tuberculous (non primary) A15.6
                primary (progressive) A15.7
            tuberculosis —see Pleurisy, tuberculous
                (non primary)
    encysted —see Pleurisy, with effusion
    exudative —see Pleurisy, with effusion
    fibrinopurulent, fibropurulent —see Pyothorax
    hemorrhagic —see Hemothorax
    pneumococcal J90
    purulent —see Pyothorax
    septic —see Pyothorax
    serofibrinous —see Pleurisy, with effusion
    seropurulent —see Pyothorax
    serous —see Pleurisy, with effusion
    staphylococcal J86.9

Pleurisy (Continued)
    streptococcal J90
    suppurative —see Pyothorax
    traumatic (post) (current) —see Injury,
        intrathoracic, pleura
    tuberculous (with effusion) (non primary) A15.6
        primary (progressive) A15.7
Pleuritis sicca —see Pleurisy
Pleurobronchopneumonia —see Pneumonia,
    broncho
Pleurodynia R07.81
    epidemic B33.0
    viral B33.0
Pleuropericarditis —see also Pericarditis
    acute I30.9
Pleuropneumonia (acute) (bilateral) (double)
    (septic) —see also Pneumonia J18.8
    chronic —see Fibrosis, lung
Pleuro-pneumonia-like-organism (PPLO), as
    cause of disease classified elsewhere B96.0
Pleurorrhea —see Pleurisy, with effusion
Plexitis, brachial G54.0
Plica
    polonica B85.0
    syndrome, knee M67.5
    tonsil J35.8
Plicated tongue K14.5
Plug
    bronchus NEC J98.09
    meconium (newborn) NEC syndrome P76.0
    mucus —see Asphyxia, mucus
Plumbism —see subcategory T56.0
Plummer's disease E05.20
    with thyroid storm E05.21
Plummer-Vinson syndrome D50.1
Pluricarential syndrome of infancy E40
Plus (and minus) hand (intrinsic) —see
    Deformity, limb, specified type NEC,
    forearm
PMEI (polymorphic epilepsy in infancy)
    G40.83-●
Pneumathemia —see Air, embolism
Pneumatic hammer (drill) syndrome T75.21
Pneumatocele (lung) J98.4
    intracranial G93.89
    tension J44.9
Pneumatosis
    cystoides intestinalis K63.89
    intestinalis K63.89
    peritonei K66.8
Pneumaturia R39.89
Pneumoblastoma —see Neoplasm, lung,
    malignant
Pneumocephalus G93.89
Pneumococcemia A40.3
Pneumococcus, pneumococcal —see condition
Pneumoconiosis (due to) (inhalation of) J64
    with tuberculosis (any type in A15) J65
    aluminum J63.0
    asbestos J61
    bagasse, bagassosis J67.1
    bauxite J63.1
    beryllium J63.2
    coal miners' (simple) J60
    coalworkers' (simple) J60
    collier's J60
    cotton dust J66.0
    diatomite (diatomaceous earth) J62.8
    dust
        inorganic NEC J63.6
        lime J62.8
        marble J62.8
        organic NEC J66.8
    fumes or vapors (from silo) J68.9
    graphite J63.3
    grinder's J62.8
    kaolin J62.8
    mica J62.8
    millstone maker's J62.8
    mineral fibers NEC J61
    miner's J60

Pneumoconiosis (Continued)
    moldy hay J67.0
    potter's J62.8
    rheumatoid —see Rheumatoid, lung
    sandblaster's J62.8
    silica, silicate NEC J62.8
        with carbon J60
    stonemason's J62.8
    talc (dust) J62.0
Pneumocystis carinii pneumonia B59
Pneumocystis jiroveci (pneumonia) B59
Pneumocystosis (with pneumonia) B59
Pneumohemopericardium I31.2
Pneumohemothorax J94.2
    traumatic S27.2
Pneumohydropericardium —see Pericarditis
Pneumohydrothorax —see Hydrothorax
Pneumomediastinum J98.2
    congenital or perinatal P25.2
Pneumomycosis B49 [J99]
Pneumonia (acute) (double) (migratory)
    (purulent) (septic) (unresolved) J18.9
    with
        influenza —see Influenza, with, pneumonia
        lung abscess J85.1
        due to specified organism —see
            Pneumonia, in (due to)
    2019 (novel) coronavirus J12.82
    adenoviral J12.0
    adynamic J18.2
    alba A50.04
    allergic (see also Pneumonitis,
        hypersensitivity) J82.89
    alveolar —see Pneumonia, lobar
    anaerobes J15.8
    anthrax A22.1
    apex, apical —see Pneumonia, lobar
    Ascaris B77.81
    aspiration J69.0
        due to
            aspiration of microorganisms
                bacterial J15.9
                viral J12.9
            food (regurgitated) J69.0
            gastric secretions J69.0
            milk (regurgitated) J69.0
            oils, essences J69.1
            solids, liquids NEC J69.8
            vomitus J69.0
        newborn P24.81
            amniotic fluid (clear) P24.11
            blood P24.21
            food (regurgitated) P24.31
            liquor (amnii) P24.11
            meconium P24.01
            milk P24.31
            mucus P24.11
            specified NEC P24.81
            stomach contents P24.31
        postprocedural J95.4
    atypical NEC J18.9
    bacillus J15.9
        specified NEC J15.8
    bacterial J15.9
        specified NEC J15.8
    Bacteroides (fragilis) (oralis)
        (melaninogenicus) J15.8
    basal, basic, basilar —see Pneumonia, by type
    bronchiolitis obliterans organized (BOOP)
        J84.89
    broncho-, bronchial (confluent) (croupous)
        (diffuse) (disseminated) (hemorrhagic)
        (involving lobes) (lobar) (terminal) J18.0
        allergic (see also Pneumonitis,
            hypersensitivity) J82.89
        aspiration —see Pneumonia, aspiration
        bacterial J15.9
            specified NEC J15.8
        chronic —see Fibrosis, lung
        diplococcal J13
        Eaton's agent J15.7

Pneumonia (Continued)
  broncho-, bronchial (Continued)
    Escherichia coli (E. coli) J15.5
    Friedländer's bacillus J15.0
    Hemophilus influenzae J14
    hypostatic J18.2
    inhalation —see also Pneumonia, aspiration
      due to fumes or vapors (chemical) J68.0
      of oils or essences J69.1
    Klebsiella (pneumoniae) J15.0
    lipid, lipoid J69.1
      endogenous J84.89
    Mycoplasma (pneumoniae) J15.7
    pleuro-pneumonia-like-organisms (PPLO)
      J15.7
    pneumococcal J13
    Proteus J15.6
    Pseudomonas J15.1
    Serratia marcescens J15.6
    specified organism NEC J16.8
    staphylococcal —see Pneumonia,
      staphylococcal
    streptococcal NEC J15.4
      group B J15.3
      pneumoniae J13
    viral, virus —see Pneumonia, viral
  Butyrivibrio (fibriosolvens) J15.8
  Candida B37.1
  caseous —see Tuberculosis, pulmonary
  catarrhal —see Pneumonia, broncho
  chlamydial J16.0
    congenital P23.1
  cholesterol J84.89
  cirrhotic (chronic) —see Fibrosis, lung
  Clostridium (haemolyticum) (novyi) J15.8
  confluent —see Pneumonia, broncho
  congenital (infective) P23.9
    due to
      bacterium NEC P23.6
      Chlamydia P23.1
      Escherichia coli P23.4
      Haemophilus influenzae P23.6
      infective organism NEC P23.8
      Klebsiella pneumoniae P23.6
      Mycoplasma P23.6
      Pseudomonas P23.5
      Staphylococcus P23.2
      Streptococcus (except group B) P23.6
        group B P23.3
      viral agent P23.0
    specified NEC P23.8
  coronavirus (novel) (disease) 2019 J12.82
  COVID-19 J12.82
  croupous —see Pneumonia, lobar
  cryptogenic organizing J84.116
  cytomegalic inclusion B25.0
  cytomegaloviral B25.0
  deglutition —see Pneumonia, aspiration
  desquamative interstitial J84.117
  diffuse —see Pneumonia, broncho
  diplococcal, diplococcus (broncho-) (lobar) J13
  disseminated (focal) —see Pneumonia, broncho
  Eaton's agent J15.7
  embolic, embolism —see Embolism,
    pulmonary
  Enterobacter J15.6
  eosinophilic J82.81
    acute J82.82
    chronic J82.81
  Escherichia coli (E. coli) J15.5
  Eubacterium J15.8
  fibrinous —see Pneumonia, lobar
  fibroid, fibrous (chronic) —see Fibrosis, lung
  Friedländer's bacillus J15.0
  Fusobacterium (nucleatum) J15.8
  gangrenous J85.0
  giant cell (measles) B05.2
  gonococcal A54.84
  gram-negative bacteria NEC J15.6
    anaerobic J15.8
  Hemophilus influenzae (broncho) (lobar) J14
  human metapneumovirus J12.3

Pneumonia (Continued)
  hypostatic (broncho) (lobar) J18.2
  in (due to)
    actinomycosis A42.0
    adenovirus J12.0
    anthrax A22.1
    ascariasis B77.81
    aspergillosis B44.9
    Bacillus anthracis A22.1
    Bacterium anitratum J15.6
    candidiasis B37.1
    chickenpox B01.2
    Chlamydia J16.0
      neonatal P23.1
    coccidioidomycosis B38.2
      acute B38.0
      chronic B38.1
    cytomegalovirus disease B25.0
    Diplococcus (pneumoniae) J13
    Eaton's agent J15.7
    Enterobacter J15.6
    Escherichia coli (E. coli) J15.5
    Friedländer's bacillus J15.0
    fumes and vapors (chemical) (inhalation)
      J68.0
    gonorrhea A54.84
    Hemophilus influenzae (H. influenzae) J14
    Herellea J15.6
    histoplasmosis B39.2
      acute B39.0
      chronic B39.1
    human metapneumovirus J12.3
    Klebsiella (pneumoniae) J15.0
    measles B05.2
    Mycoplasma (pneumoniae) J15.7
    nocardiosis, nocardiasis A43.0
    ornithosis A70
    parainfluenza virus J12.2
    pleuro-pneumonia-like-organism (PPLO)
      J15.7
    pneumococcus J13
    pneumocystosis (Pneumocystis carinii)
      (Pneumocystis jiroveci) B59
    Proteus J15.6
    Pseudomonas NEC J15.1
      pseudomallei A24.1
    psittacosis A70
    Q fever A78
    respiratory syncytial virus (RSV) J12.1
    rheumatic fever I00 [J17]
    rubella B06.81
    Salmonella (infection) A02.22
      typhi A01.03
    schistosomiasis B65.9 [J17]
    Serratia marcescens J15.6
    specified
      bacterium NEC J15.8
      organism NEC J16.8
    spirochetal NEC A69.8
    Staphylococcus J15.20
      aureus (methicillin susceptible) (MSSA)
        J15.211
        methicillin resistant (MRSA) J15.212
      specified NEC J15.29
    Streptococcus J15.4
      group B J15.3
      pneumoniae J13
      specified NEC J15.4
    toxoplasmosis B58.3
    tularemia A21.2
    typhoid (fever) A01.03
    varicella B01.2
    virus —see Pneumonia, viral
    whooping cough A37.91
      due to
        Bordetella parapertussis A37.11
        Bordetella pertussis A37.01
        specified NEC A37.81
    Yersinia pestis A20.2
  inhalation of food or vomit —see Pneumonia,
    aspiration

Pneumonia (Continued)
  interstitial J84.9
    chronic J84.111
    desquamative J84.117
    due to
      collagen vascular disease J84.178
      known underlying cause J84.178
    idiopathic NOS J84.111
    in disease classified elsewhere J84.178
    lymphocytic (due to collagen vascular
      disease) (in diseases classified
      elsewhere) J84.178
    lymphoid J84.2
    non-specific J84.89
    due to
      collagen vascular disease J84.178
      known underlying cause J84.178
    idiopathic J84.113
    in diseases classified elsewhere J84.178
    plasma cell B59
    pseudomonas J15.1
    usual J84.112
      due to collagen vascular disease J84.178
      idiopathic J84.112
      in diseases classified elsewhere J84.178
  Klebsiella (pneumoniae) J15.0
  lipid, lipoid (exogenous) J69.1
    endogenous J84.89
  lobar (disseminated) (double) (interstitial) J18.1
    bacterial J15.9
      specified NEC J15.8
    chronic —see Fibrosis, lung
    Escherichia coli (E. coli) J15.5
    Friedländer's bacillus J15.0
    Hemophilus influenzae J14
    hypostatic J18.2
    Klebsiella (pneumoniae) J15.0
    pneumococcal J13
    Proteus J15.6
    Pseudomonas J15.1
    specified organism NEC J16.8
    staphylococcal —see Pneumonia,
      staphylococcal
    streptococcal NEC J15.4
    Streptococcus pneumoniae J13
    viral, virus —see Pneumonia, viral
  lobular —see Pneumonia, broncho
  Löffler's J82.89
  lymphoid interstitial J84.2
  massive —see Pneumonia, lobar
  meconium P24.01
  MRSA (Methicillin resistant Staphylococcus
    aureus) J15.212
  MSSA (methicillin susceptible Staphylococcus
    aureus) J15.211
  multilobar —see Pneumonia, by type
  Mycoplasma (pneumoniae) J15.7
  necrotic J85.0
  neonatal P23.9
    aspiration —see Aspiration, by substance,
      with pneumonia
  nitrogen dioxide J68.0
  organizing J84.89
    due to
      collagen vascular disease J84.178
      known underlying cause J84.178
    in diseases classified elsewhere J84.178
  orthostatic J18.2
  parainfluenza virus J12.2
  parenchymatous —see Fibrosis, lung
  passive J18.2
  patchy —see Pneumonia, broncho
  Peptococcus J15.8
  Peptostreptococcus J15.8
  plasma cell (of infants) B59
  pleurolobar —see Pneumonia, lobar
  pleuro-pneumonia-like organism (PPLO) J15.7
  pneumococcal (broncho) (lobar) J13
  Pneumocystis (carinii) (jiroveci) B59
  postinfectional NEC B99 [J17]
  postmeasles B05.2
  Proteus J15.6

▶ New   ⟹ Revised   ~~deleted~~ Deleted   ● Use Additional Character(s)

Pneumonia *(Continued)*
  Pseudomonas J15.1
  psittacosis A70
  radiation J70.0
    respiratory syncytial virus (RSV) J12.1
  resulting from a procedure J95.89
  rheumatic I00 *[J17]*
  Salmonella (arizonae) (cholerae-suis)
      (enteritidis) (typhimurium) A02.22
    typhi A01.03
    typhoid fever A01.03
  SARS-associated coronavirus J12.81
  SARS-CoV-2 J12.82
  segmented, segmental —*see* Pneumonia,
      broncho-●
  Serratia marcescens J15.6
  specified NEC J18.8
    bacterium NEC J15.8
    organism NEC J16.8
    virus NEC J12.89
  spirochetal NEC A69.8
  staphylococcal (broncho) (lobar) J15.20
    aureus (methicillin susceptible) (MSSA)
        J15.211
      methicillin resistant (MRSA) J15.212
    specified NEC J15.29
  static, stasis J18.2
  streptococcal NEC (broncho) (lobar) J15.4
    group
      A J15.4
      B J15.3
      specified NEC J15.4
  Streptococcus pneumoniae J13
  syphilitic, congenital (early) A50.04
  traumatic (complication) (early) (secondary)
      T79.8
  tuberculous (any) —*see* Tuberculosis,
      pulmonary
  tularemic A21.2
  varicella B01.2
  Veillonella J15.8
  ventilator associated J95.851
  viral, virus (broncho) (interstitial) (lobar) J12.9
    adenoviral J12.0
    congenital P23.0
    human metapneumovirus J12.3
    parainfluenza J12.2
    respiratory syncytial (RSV) J12.1
    SARS-associated coronavirus J12.81
    specified NEC J12.89
  white (congenital) A50.04
Pneumonic —*see* condition
Pneumonitis (acute) (primary) —*see also*
    Pneumonia
  air-conditioner J67.7
  allergic (due to) J67.9
    organic dust NEC J67.8
    red cedar dust J67.8
    sequoiosis J67.8
    wood dust J67.8
  aspiration J69.0
    due to
      anesthesia J95.4
        during
          labor and delivery O74.0
          pregnancy O29.01-●
          puerperium O89.01
        fumes or gases J68.0
      obstetric O74.0
  chemical (due to gases, fumes or vapors)
      (inhalation) J68.0
    due to anesthesia J95.4
  cholesterol J84.89
  chronic —*see* Fibrosis, lung
  congenital rubella P35.0
  crack (cocaine) J68.0
  due to
    beryllium J68.0
    cadmium J68.0
    crack (cocaine) J68.0
    detergent J69.8
    fluorocarbon-polymer J68.0

Pneumonitis *(Continued)*
  due to *(Continued)*
    food, vomit (aspiration) J69.0
    fumes or vapors J68.0
    gases, fumes or vapors (inhalation) J68.0
    inhalation
      blood J69.8
      essences J69.1
      food (regurgitated), milk, vomit J69.0
      oils, essences J69.1
      saliva J69.0
      solids, liquids NEC J69.8
    manganese J68.0
    nitrogen dioxide J68.0
    oils, essences J69.1
    solids, liquids NEC J69.8
    toxoplasmosis (acquired) B58.3
      congenital P37.1
    vanadium J68.0
    ventilator J95.851
  eosinophilic J82.81
    acute J82.82
    chronic J82.81
  hypersensitivity J67.9
    air conditioner lung J67.7
    bagassosis J67.1
    bird fancier's lung J67.2
    farmer's lung J67.0
    maltworker's lung J67.4
    maple bark-stripper's lung J67.6
    mushroom worker's lung J67.5
    specified organic dust NEC J67.8
    suberosis J67.3
  interstitial (chronic) J84.89
    acute J84.114
    lymphoid J84.2
    non-specific J84.89
      idiopathic J84.113
  lymphoid, interstitial J84.2
  meconium P24.01
  postanesthetic J95.4
    correct substance properly administered —
        see Table of Drugs and Chemcials, by
        drug, adverse effect
    in labor and delivery O74.0
    in pregnancy O29.01-●
    obstetric O74.0
    overdose or wrong substance given or taken
        (by accident) —*see* Table of Drugs and
        Chemicals, by drug, poisoning
    postpartum, puerperal O89.01
  postoperative J95.4
    obstetric O74.0
  radiation J70.0
  rubella, congenital P35.0
  ventilation (air-conditioning) J67.7
  ventilator associated J95.851
  wood-dust J67.8
Pneumonoconiosis —*see* Pneumoconiosis
Pneumoparotid K11.8
Pneumopathy NEC J98.4
  alveolar J84.09
  due to organic dust NEC J66.8
  parietoalveolar J84.09
Pneumopericarditis —*see also* Pericarditis
  acute I30.9
Pneumopericardium —*see also* Pericarditis
  congenital P25.3
  newborn P25.3
  traumatic (post) —*see* Injury, heart
Pneumophagia (psychogenic) F45.8
Pneumopleurisy, pneumopleuritis —*see also*
    Pneumonia J18.8
Pneumopyopericardium I30.1
Pneumopyothorax —*see* Pyopneumothorax
  with fistula J86.0
Pneumorrhagia —*see also* Hemorrhage, lung
  tuberculous —*see* Tuberculosis, pulmonary
Pneumothorax NOS J93.9
  acute J93.83
  chronic J93.81

Pneumothorax NOS *(Continued)*
  congenital P25.1
  perinatal period P25.1
  postprocedural J95.811
  specified NEC J93.83
  spontaneous NOS J93.83
    newborn P25.1
    primary J93.11
    secondary J93.12
    tension J93.0
  tense valvular, infectional J93.0
  tension (spontaneous) J93.0
  traumatic S27.0
    with hemothorax S27.2
  tuberculous —*see* Tuberculosis, pulmonary
Podagra —*see also* Gout M10.9
Podencephalus Q01.9
Poikilocytosis R71.8
Poikiloderma L81.6
  Civatte's L57.3
  congenital Q82.8
  vasculare atrophicans L94.5
Poikilodermatomyositis M33.10
  with
    myopathy M33.12
    respiratory involvement M33.11
    specified organ involvement NEC M33.19
    ▶amyopathic M33.13
    ▶without myopathy M33.13
Pointed ear (congenital) Q17.3
Poison ivy, oak, sumac or other plant
    dermatitis (allergic) (contact) L23.7
Poisoning (acute) —*see also* Table of Drugs and
    Chemicals
  algae and toxins T65.82-●
  Bacillus B (aertrycke) (cholerae (suis))
      (paratyphosus) (suipestifer) A02.9
  botulinus A05.1
  bacterial toxins A05.9
  berries, noxious —*see* Poisoning, food,
      noxious, berries
  botulism A05.1
  ciguatera fish T61.0-●
  Clostridium botulinum A05.1
  death-cap (Amanita phalloides) (Amanita
      verna) —*see* Poisoning, food, noxious,
      mushrooms
  drug —*see* Table of Drugs and Chemicals, by
      drug, poisoning
  epidemic, fish (noxious) —*see* Poisoning,
      seafood
    bacterial A05.9
  fava bean D55.0
  fish (noxious) T61.9-●
    bacterial —*see* Intoxication, foodborne, by
        agent
    ciguatera fish —*see* Poisoning, ciguatera
        fish
    scombroid fish —*see* Poisoning, scombroid
        fish
    specified type NEC T61.77-●
  food NEC A05.9
    bacterial —*see* Intoxication, foodborne, by
        agent
    due to
      Bacillus (aertrycke) (choleraesuis)
          (paratyphosus) (suipestifer)
          A02.9
      botulinus A05.1
      Clostridium (perfringens) (Welchii)
          A05.2
      salmonella (aertrycke) (callinarum)
          (choleraesuis) (enteritidis)
          (paratyphi) (suipestifer) A02.9
        with
          gastroenteritis A02.0
          sepsis A02.1
      staphylococcus A05.0
      Vibrio
        parahaemolyticus A05.3
        vulnificus A05.5

Poisoning (Continued)
 food NEC (Continued)
  noxious or naturally toxic T62.9-●
   berries —see subcategory T62.1-●
   fish —see Poisoning, seafood
   mushrooms —see subcategory T62.0X-●
   plants NEC —see subcategory T62.2X-●
   seafood —see Poisoning, seafood
   specified NEC —see subcategory
    T62.8X-●
  ichthyotoxism —see Poisoning, seafood
  kreotoxism, food A05.9
  latex T65.81-●
  lead T56.0-●
  mushroom —see Poisoning, food, noxious,
   mushroom
  mussels —see also Poisoning, shellfish
   bacterial —see Intoxication, foodborne, by
    agent
  nicotine (tobacco) T65.2-●
  noxious foodstuffs —see Poisoning, food,
   noxious
  plants, noxious —see Poisoning, food,
   noxious, plants NEC
  ptomaine —see Poisoning, food
  radiation J70.0
  Salmonella (arizonae) (cholerae-suis)
   (enteritidis) (typhimurium) A02.9
  scombroid fish T61.1-●
  seafood (noxious) T61.9-●
   bacterial —see Intoxication, foodborne, by
    agent
   fish —see Poisoning, fish
   shellfish —see Poisoning, shellfish
   specified NEC —see subcategory T61.8X-●
  shellfish (amnesic) (azaspiracid) (diarrheic)
   (neurotoxic) (noxious) (paralytic) T61.78-●
   bacterial —see Intoxication, foodborne, by
    agent
   ciguatera mollusk —see Poisoning,
    ciguatera fish
  specified substance NEC T65.891
  Staphylococcus, food A05.0
  tobacco (nicotine) T65.2-●
  water E87.79
Poker spine —see Spondylitis, ankylosing
Poland syndrome Q79.8
Polioencephalitis (acute) (bulbar) A80.9
 inferior G12.22
 influenzal —see Influenza, with,
  encephalopathy
 superior hemorrhagic (acute) (Wernicke's)
  E51.2
 Wernicke's E51.2
Polioencephalomyelitis (acute) (anterior) A80.9
 with beriberi E51.2
Polioencephalopathy, superior hemorrhagic
 E51.2
 with
  beriberi E51.11
  pellagra E52
Poliomeningoencephalitis —see
 Meningoencephalitis
Poliomyelitis (acute) (anterior) (epidemic) A80.9
 with paralysis (bulbar) —see Poliomyelitis,
  paralytic
 abortive A80.4
 ascending (progressive) —see Poliomyelitis,
  paralytic
 bulbar (paralytic) —see Poliomyelitis,
  paralytic
 congenital P35.8
 nonepidemic A80.9
 nonparalytic A80.4
 paralytic A80.30
  specified NEC A80.39
  vaccine-associated A80.0
  wild virus
   imported A80.1
   indigenous A80.2
 spinal, acute A80.9

Poliosis (eyebrow) (eyelashes) L67.1
 circumscripta, acquired L67.1
Pollakiuria R35.0
 psychogenic F45.8
Pollinosis J30.1
Pollitzer's disease L73.2
Polyadenitis —see also Lymphadenitis
 malignant A20.0
Polyalgia M79.89
Polyangiitis M30.0
 microscopic M31.7
 overlap syndrome M30.8
Polyarteritis
 microscopic M31.7
 nodosa M30.0
  with lung involvement M30.1
  juvenile M30.2
  related condition NEC M30.8
Polyarthralgia —see Pain, joint
Polyarthritis, polyarthropathy —see also
 Arthritis M13.0
 due to or associated with other specified
  conditions —see Arthritis
 epidemic (Australian) (with exanthema) B33.1
 infective —see Arthritis, pyogenic or pyemic
 inflammatory M06.4
 juvenile (chronic) (seronegative) M08.3
 migratory M13.8-●
 rheumatic, acute —see Fever, rheumatic
Polyarthrosis M15.9
 post-traumatic M15.3
 primary M15.0
 specified NEC M15.8
Polycarential syndrome of infancy E40
Polychondritis (atrophic) (chronic) —see also
 Disorder, cartilage, specified type NEC
 relapsing M94.1
Polycoria Q13.2
Polycystic (disease)
 degeneration, kidney Q61.3
  autosomal dominant (adult type) Q61.2
  autosomal recessive (infantile type) NEC
   Q61.19
 kidney Q61.3
  autosomal
   dominant Q61.2
   recessive NEC Q61.19
  autosomal dominant (adult type) Q61.2
  autosomal recessive (childhood type) NEC
   Q61.19
  infantile type NEC Q61.19
 liver Q44.6
 lung J98.4
  congenital Q33.0
 ovary, ovaries E28.2
 spleen Q89.09
Polycythemia (secondary) D75.1
 acquired D75.1
 benign (familial) D75.0
 due to
  donor twin P61.1
  erythropoietin D75.1
  fall in plasma volume D75.1
  high altitude D75.1
  maternal-fetal transfusion P61.1
  stress D75.1
 emotional D75.1
 erythropoietin D75.1
 familial (benign) D75.0
 Gaisböck's (hypertonica) D75.1
 high altitude D75.1
 hypertonica D75.1
 hypoxemic D75.1
 neonatorum P61.1
 nephrogenous D75.1
 relative D75.1
 secondary D75.1
 spurious D75.1
 stress D75.1
 vera D45
Polycytosis cryptogenica D75.1

Polydactylism, polydactyly Q69.9
 toes Q69.2
Polydipsia R63.1
Polydystrophy, pseudo-Hurler E77.0
Polyembryoma —see Neoplasm, malignant,
 by site
Polyglandular
 deficiency E31.0
 dyscrasia E31.9
 dysfunction E31.9
 syndrome E31.8
Polyhydramnios O40.-●
Polymastia Q83.1
Polymenorrhea N92.0
Polymyalgia M35.3
 arteritica, giant cell M31.5
 rheumatica M35.3
  with giant cell arteritis M31.5
Polymyositis (acute) (chronic) (hemorrhagic)
 M33.20
 with
  myopathy M33.22
  respiratory involvement M33.21
  skin involvement —see
   Dermatopolymyositis
  specified organ involvement NEC M33.29
 ossificans (generalisata) (progressiva) —see
  Myositis, ossificans, progressiva
Polyneuritis, polyneuritic —see also
 Polyneuropathy
 acute (post-)infective G61.0
 alcoholic G62.1
 cranialis G52.7
 demyelinating, chronic inflammatory (CIDP)
  G61.81
 diabetic —see Diabetes, polyneuropathy
 diphtheritic A36.83
 due to lack of vitamin NEC E56.9 [G63]
 endemic E51.11
 erythredema —see subcategory T56.1
 febrile, acute G61.0
 hereditary ataxic G60.1
 idiopathic, acute G61.0
 infective (acute) G61.0
 inflammatory, chronic demyelinating (CIDP)
  G61.81
 nutritional E63.9 [G63]
 postinfective (acute) G61.0
 specified NEC G62.89
Polyneuropathy (peripheral) G62.9
 alcoholic G62.1
 amyloid (Portuguese) E85.1 [G63]
  transthyretin-related (ATTR) familial
   E85.1
 arsenical E85.1 [G63]
 critical illness G62.81
 demyelinating, chronic inflammatory (CIDP)
  G61.81
 diabetic —see Diabetes, polyneuropathy
 drug-induced G62.0
 hereditary G60.9
  specified NEC G60.8
 idiopathic G60.9
  progressive G60.3
 in (due to)
  alcohol G62.1
   sequelae G65.2
  amyloidosis, familial (Portuguese) E85.1
   [G63]
  antitetanus serum G61.1
  arsenic G62.2
   sequelae G65.2
  avitaminosis NEC E56.9 [G63]
  beriberi E51.11
  collagen vascular disease NEC M35.9 [G63]
  deficiency (of)
   B (-complex) vitamins E53.9 [G63]
   vitamin B6 E53.1 [G63]
  diabetes —see Diabetes, polyneuropathy
  diphtheria A36.83

Polyneuropathy (Continued)
in (Continued)
drug or medicament G62.0
correct substance properly administered —see Table of Drugs and Chemicals, by drug, adverse effect
overdose or wrong substance given or taken —see Table of Drugs and Chemicals, by drug, poisoning
endocrine disease NEC E34.9 [G63]
herpes zoster B02.23
hypoglycemia E16.2 [G63]
infectious
disease NEC B99 [G63]
mononucleosis B27.91
lack of vitamin NEC E56.9 [G63]
lead G62.2
sequelae G65.2
leprosy A30.9 [G63]
Lyme disease A69.22
metabolic disease NEC E88.9 [G63]
microscopic polyangiitis M31.7 [G63]
mumps B26.84
neoplastic disease —see also Neoplasm D49.9 [G63]
nutritional deficiency NEC E63.9 [G63]
organophosphate compounds G62.2
sequelae G65.2
parasitic disease NEC B89 [G63]
pellagra E52 [G63]
polyarteritis nodosa M30.0
porphyria E80.20 [G63]
radiation G62.82
rheumatoid arthritis —see Rheumatoid, polyneuropathy
sarcoidosis D86.89
serum G61.1
syphilis (late) A52.15
congenital A50.43
systemic
connective tissue disorder M35.9 [G63]
lupus erythematosus M32.19
toxic agent NEC G62.2
sequelae G65.2
transthyretin-related (ATTR) familial amyloid E85.1
triorthocresyl phosphate G62.2
sequelae G65.2
tuberculosis A17.89
uremia N18.9 [G63]
vitamin B12 deficiency E53.8 [G63]
with anemia (pernicious) D51.0 [G63]
due to dietary deficiency D51.3 [G63]
zoster B02.23
inflammatory G61.9
chronic demyelinating (CIDP) G61.81
sequelae G65.1
specified NEC G61.89
lead G62.2
sequelae G65.2
nutritional NEC E63.9 [G63]
postherpetic (zoster) B02.23
progressive G60.3
radiation-induced G62.82
sensory (hereditary) (idiopathic) G60.8
specified NEC G62.89
syphilitic (late) A52.15
congenital A50.43
Polyopia H53.8
Polyorchism, polyorchidism Q55.21
Polyosteoarthritis —see also Osteoarthritis, generalized M15.9- •
post-traumatic M15.3
specified NEC M15.8
Polyostotic fibrous dysplasia Q78.1
Polyotia Q17.0
Polyp, polypus
accessory sinus J33.8
adenocarcinoma in —see Neoplasm, malignant, by site
adenocarcinoma in situ in —see Neoplasm, in situ, by site

Polyp, polypus (Continued)
adenoid tissue J33.0
adenomatous —see also Neoplasm, benign, by site
adenocarcinoma in —see Neoplasm, malignant, by site
adenocarcinoma in situ in —see Neoplasm, in situ, by site
carcinoma in —see Neoplasm, malignant, by site
carcinoma in situ in —see Neoplasm, in situ, by site
multiple —see Neoplasm, benign
adenocarcinoma in —see Neoplasm, malignant, by site
adenocarcinoma in situ in —see Neoplasm, in situ, by site
antrum J33.8
anus, anal (canal) K62.0
Bartholin's gland N84.3
bladder D41.4
carcinoma in —see Neoplasm, malignant, by site
carcinoma in situ in —see Neoplasm, in situ, by site
cecum D12.0
cervix (uteri) N84.1
in pregnancy or childbirth —see Pregnancy, complicated by, abnormal, cervix
mucous N84.1
nonneoplastic N84.1
choanal J33.0
cholesterol K82.4
clitoris N84.3
colon K63.5
adenomatous D12.6
ascending D12.6
cecum D12.0
descending D12.4
ascending K63.5
sigmoid D12.5
transverse D12.3
cecum K63.5
descending K63.5
inflammatory K51.40
with
abscess K51.414
complication K51.419
specified NEC K51.418
fistula K51.413
intestinal obstruction K51.412
rectal bleeding K51.411
sigmoid D12.5
transverse D12.3
corpus uteri N84.0
dental K04.01
irreversible K04.02
reversible K04.01
duodenum K31.7
ear (middle) H74.4- •
endometrium N84.0
esophageal K22.81
esophagogastric junction K22.82
ethmoidal (sinus) J33.8
fallopian tube N84.8
female genital tract N84.9
specified NEC N84.8
frontal (sinus) J33.8
gallbladder K82.4
gingiva, gum K06.8
hyperplastic, (any site) K63.5
labia, labium (majus) (minus) N84.3
larynx (mucous) J38.1
adenomatous D14.1
malignant —see Neoplasm, malignant, by site
maxillary (sinus) J33.8
middle ear —see Polyp, ear (middle)
myometrium N84.0
nares
anterior J33.9
posterior J33.0

Polyp, polypus (Continued)
nasal (mucous) J33.9
cavity J33.0
septum J33.0
nasopharyngeal J33.0
nose (mucous) J33.9
oviduct N84.8
pharynx J39.2
placenta O90.89
prostate —see Enlargement, enlarged, prostate
pudenda, pudendum N84.3
pulpal (dental) K04.01
irreversible K04.02
reversible K04.01
rectum (nonadenomatous) K62.1
adenomatous —see Polyp, adenomatous
septum (nasal) J33.0
sinus (accessory) (ethmoidal) (frontal) (maxillary) (sphenoidal) J33.8
sphenoidal (sinus) J33.8
stomach K31.7
adenomatous D13.1
tube, fallopian N84.8
turbinate, mucous membrane J33.8
umbilical, newborn P83.6
ureter N28.89
urethra N36.2
uterus (body) (corpus) (mucous) N84.0
cervix N84.1
in pregnancy or childbirth —see Pregnancy, complicated by, tumor, uterus
vagina N84.2
vocal cord (mucous) J38.1
vulva N84.3
Polyphagia R63.2
Polyploidy Q92.7
Polypoid —see condition
Polyposis —see also Polyp
coli (adenomatous) D12.6
adenocarcinoma in C18.9
adenocarcinoma in situ in —see Neoplasm, in situ, by site
carcinoma in C18.9
colon (adenomatous) D12.6
familial D12.6
adenocarcinoma in situ in —see Neoplasm, in situ, by site
intestinal (adenomatous) D12.6
malignant lymphomatous C83.1
multiple, adenomatous —see also Neoplasm, benign D36.9
Polyradiculitis —see Polyneuropathy
Polyradiculoneuropathy (acute) (postinfective) (segmentally demyelinating) G61.0
Polyserositis
due to pericarditis I31.1
pericardial I31.1
periodic, familial E85.0
tuberculous A19.9
acute A19.1
chronic A19.8
Polysplenia syndrome Q89.09
Polysyndactyly —see also Syndactylism, syndactyly Q70.4
Polytrichia L68.3
Polyunguia Q84.6
Polyuria R35.89
nocturnal R35.81
psychogenic F45.8
specified NEC R35.89
Pompe's disease (glycogen storage) E74.02
Pompholyx L30.1
Poncet's disease (tuberculous rheumatism) A18.09
Pond fracture —see Fracture, skull
Ponos B55.0
Pons, pontine —see condition
Poor
aesthetic of existing restoration of tooth K08.56
contractions, labor O62.2
gingival margin to tooth restoration K08.51

Poor *(Continued)*
  personal hygiene R46.0
  prenatal care, affecting management of
      pregnancy —see Pregnancy, complicated
      by, insufficient, prenatal care
  sucking reflex (newborn) R29.2
  urinary stream R39.12
  vision NEC H54.7
Poradenitis, nostras inguinalis or venerea A55
Porencephaly (congenital) (developmental)
      (true) Q04.6
  acquired G93.0
  nondevelopmental G93.0
  traumatic (post) F07.89
Porocephaliasis B88.8
Porokeratosis Q82.8
Poroma, eccrine —see Neoplasm, skin, benign
Porphyria (South African) E80.20
  acquired E80.20
  acute intermittent (hepatic) (Swedish) E80.21
  cutanea tarda (hereditary) (symptomatic) E80.1
  due to drugs E80.20
      correct substance properly administered —
          see Table of Drugs and Chemicals, by
          drug, adverse effect
      overdose or wrong substance given
          or taken —see Table of Drugs and
          Chemicals, by drug, poisoning
  erythropoietic (congenital) (hereditary) E80.0
  hepatocutaneous type E80.1
  secondary E80.20
  toxic NEC E80.20
  variegata E80.20
Porphyrinuria —see Porphyria
Porphyruria —see Porphyria
Portal —see condition
Port wine nevus, mark, or stain Q82.5
Posadas-Wernicke disease B38.9
Positive
  culture (nonspecific)
      blood R78.81
      bronchial washings R84.5
      cerebrospinal fluid R83.5
      cervix uteri R87.5
      nasal secretions R84.5
      nipple discharge R89.5
      nose R84.5
          staphylococcus (Methicillin susceptible)
              Z22.321
              Methicillin resistant Z22.322
      peritoneal fluid R85.5
      pleural fluid R84.5
      prostatic secretions R86.5
      saliva R85.5
      seminal fluid R86.5
      sputum R84.5
      synovial fluid R89.5
      throat scrapings R84.5
      urine R82.79
      vagina R87.5
      vulva R87.5
      wound secretions R89.5
  PPD (skin test) R76.11
  serology for syphilis A53.0
      with signs or symptoms - code as Syphilis,
          by site and stage
      false R76.8
  skin test, tuberculin (without active
      tuberculosis) R76.11
  test, human immunodeficiency virus (HIV)
      R75
  VDRL A53.0
      with signs or symptoms - code by site and
          stage under Syphilis A53.9
  Wassermann reaction A53.0
Post COVID-19 condition, unspecified U09.9
Postcardiotomy syndrome I97.0
Postcaval ureter Q62.62
Postcholecystectomy syndrome K91.5
Postclimacteric bleeding N95.0
Postcommissurotomy syndrome I97.0

Postconcussional syndrome F07.81
Postcontusional syndrome F07.81
Postcricoid region —see condition
Post-dates (40-42 weeks) (pregnancy) (mother)
      O48.0
  more than 42 weeks gestation O48.1
Postencephalitic syndrome F07.89
Posterior —see condition
Posterolateral sclerosis (spinal cord) —see
      Degeneration, combined
Postexanthematous —see condition
Postfebrile —see condition
Postgastrectomy dumping syndrome K91.1
Posthemiplegic chorea —see Monoplegia
Posthemorrhagic anemia (chronic) D50.0
  acute D62
  newborn P61.3
Postherpetic neuralgia (zoster) B02.29
  trigeminal B02.22
Posthitis N47.7
Postimmunization complication or reaction —
      see Complications, vaccination
Postinfectious —see condition
Postlaminectomy syndrome NEC M96.1
Postleukotomy syndrome F07.0
Postmastectomy lymphedema (syndrome)
      I97.2
Postmaturity, postmature (over 42 weeks)
  maternal (over 42 weeks gestation) O48.1
  newborn P08.22
Postmeasles complication NEC —see also
      condition B05.89
Postmenopausal
  endometrium (atrophic) N95.8
      suppurative —see also Endometritis N71.9
  osteoporosis —see Osteoporosis,
      postmenopausal
Postnasal drip R09.82
  due to
      allergic rhinitis —see Rhinitis, allergic
      common cold J00
      gastroesophageal reflux —see Reflux,
          gastroesophageal
      nasopharyngitis —see Nasopharyngitis
      other know condition — code to condition
      sinusitis —see Sinusitis
Postnatal —see condition
Postoperative (postprocedural) —see
      Complication, postoperative
  pneumothorax, therapeutic Z98.3
  state NEC Z98.890
Postpancreatectomy hyperglycemia E89.1
Postpartum —see Puerperal
Postphlebitic syndrome —see Syndrome,
      postthrombotic
Postpolio (myelitic) syndrome G14
Postpoliomyelitic —see also condition
  osteopathy —see Osteopathy, after
      poliomyelitis
Postprocedural —see also Postoperative
  hypoinsulinemia E89.1
Postschizophrenic depression F32.89
Postsurgery status —see also Status (post)
  pneumothorax, therapeutic Z98.3
Post-term (40-42 weeks) (pregnancy) (mother)
      O48.0
  infant P08.21
  more than 42 weeks gestation (mother)
      O48.1
Post-traumatic brain syndrome, nonpsychotic
      F07.81
Post-typhoid abscess A01.09
Postures, hysterical F44.2
Postvaccinal reaction or complication —see
      Complications, vaccination
Postvalvulotomy syndrome I97.0
Potain's
  disease (pulmonary edema) —see Edema, lung
  syndrome (gastrectasis with dyspepsia) K31.0
▶POTS (postural orthostatic tachycardia
      syndrome) G90.A

Potter's
  asthma J62.8
  facies Q60.6
  lung J62.8
  syndrome (with renal agenesis) Q60.6
Pott's
  curvature (spinal) A18.01
  disease or paraplegia A18.01
  spinal curvature A18.01
  tumor, puffy —see Osteomyelitis, specified
      type NEC
Pouch
  bronchus Q32.4
  Douglas' —see condition
  esophagus, esophageal, congenital Q39.6
      acquired K22.5
  gastric K31.4
  Hartmann's K82.8
  pharynx, pharyngeal (congenital) Q38.7
Pouchitis K91.850
Poultrymen's itch B88.0
Poverty NEC Z59.6
  extreme Z59.5
Poxvirus NEC B08.8
Prader-Willi syndrome Q87.11
Prader-Willi-like syndrome Q87.11
Preauricular appendage or tag Q17.0
Prebetalipoproteinemia (acquired) (essential)
      (familial) (hereditary) (primary)
      (secondary) E78.1
  with chylomicronemia E78.3
Precipitate labor or delivery O62.3
Preclimacteric bleeding (menorrhagia) N92.4
Precocious
  adrenarche E30.1
  menarche E30.1
  menstruation E30.1
  pubarche E30.1
  puberty E30.1
      central E22.8
  sexual development NEC E30.1
  thelarche E30.8
Precocity, sexual (constitutional) (cryptogenic)
      (female) (idiopathic) (male) E30.1
  with adrenal hyperplasia E25.9
      congenital E25.0
Precordial pain R07.2
Predeciduous teeth K00.2
Prediabetes, prediabetic R73.03
  complicating
      pregnancy —see Pregnancy, complicated
          by, diseases of, specified type or
          system NEC
      puerperium O99.893
Predislocation status of hip at birth Q65.6
Pre-eclampsia O14.9-●
  with pre-existing hypertension —see
      Hypertension, complicating pregnancy,
      pre-existing, with, pre-eclampsia
  complicating
      childbirth O14.94
      puerperium O14.95
  mild O14.0-●
      complicating
          childbirth O14.04
          puerperium O14.05
  moderate O14.0-●
      complicating
          childbirth O14.04
          puerperium O14.05
  severe O14.1-●
      with hemolysis, elevated liver enzymes
          and low platelet count (HELLP)
          O14.2-●
      complicating
          childbirth O14.24
          puerperium O14.25
      complicating
          childbirth O14.14
          puerperium O14.15
Pre-eruptive color change, teeth, tooth K00.8

▶ New   ⇒ Revised   ~~deleted~~ Deleted   ● Use Additional Character(s)

Pre-excitation atrioventricular conduction I45.6
Preglaucoma H40.00- ●
Pregnancy (single) (uterine) —*see also* Delivery
and Puerperal Z33.1

Note: The Tabular must be reviewed for
assignment of the appropriate character
indicating the trimester of the pregnancy

Note: The Tabular must be reviewed for
assignment of appropriate seventh character
for multiple gestation codes in Chapter 15

abdominal (ectopic) O00.00
  with intrauterine pregnancy O00.01
  with viable fetus O36.7- ●
ampullar O00.10- ●
  with intrauterine pregnancy O00.11- ●
biochemical O02.81
broad ligament O00.80
  with intrauterine pregnancy O00.81
cervical O00.80
  with intrauterine pregnancy O00.81
chemical O02.81
complicated NOS O26.9- ●
complicated by (care of) (management
  affected by)
  abnormal, abnormality
    cervix O34.4- ●
      causing obstructed labor O65.5
    cord (umbilical) O69.9
    fetal heart rate or rhythm O36.83- ●
    findings on antenatal screening of
      mother O28.9
      biochemical O28.1
      chromosomal O28.5
      cytological O28.2
      genetic O28.5
      hematological O28.0
      radiological O28.4
      specified NEC O28.8
      ultrasonic O28.3
    glucose (tolerance) NEC O99.810
    pelvic organs O34.9- ●
      specified NEC O34.8- ●
        causing obstructed labor O65.5
    pelvis (bony) (major) NEC O33.0
    perineum O34.7- ●
    position
      placenta O44.0- ●
        with hemorrhage O44.1- ●
      uterus O34.59- ●
    uterus O34.59- ●
      causing obstructed labor O65.5
      congenital O34.0- ●
    vagina O34.6- ●
      causing obstructed labor O65.5
    vulva O34.7- ●
      causing obstructed labor O65.5
  abruptio placentae —*see* Abruptio
    placentae
  abscess or cellulitis
    bladder O23.1- ●
    breast O91.11- ●
    genital organ or tract O23.9- ●
  abuse
    physical O9A.31- ●
    psychological O9A.51- ●
    sexual O9A.41- ●
  adverse effect anesthesia O29.9- ●
    aspiration pneumonitis O29.01- ●
    cardiac arrest O29.11- ●
    cardiac complication NEC O29.19- ●
    cardiac failure O29.12- ●
    central nervous system complication
      NEC O29.29- ●
    cerebral anoxia O29.21- ●
    failed or difficult intubation O29.6- ●
    inhalation of stomach contents or
      secretions NOS O29.01- ●
    local, toxic reaction O29.3X
    Mendelson's syndrome O29.01- ●

Pregnancy (*Continued*)
  complicated by (*Continued*)
    adverse effect anesthesia (*Continued*)
      pressure collapse of lung O29.02- ●
      pulmonary complications NEC O29.09- ●
      specified NEC O29.8X
      spinal and epidural type NEC O29.5X
        induced headache O29.4- ●
    albuminuria —*see also* Proteinuria,
      gestational O12.1- ●
    alcohol use O99.31- ●
    amnionitis O41.12- ●
    anaphylactoid syndrome of pregnancy
      O88.01- ●
    anemia (conditions in D50-D64) (pre-
      existing) O99.01- ●
      complicating the puerperium O99.03
    antepartum hemorrhage O46.9- ●
      with coagulation defect —*see*
        Hemorrhage, antepartum, with
        coagulation defect
      specified NEC O46.8X- ●
    appendicitis O99.61- ●
    atrophy (yellow) (acute) liver (subacute)
      O26.61- ●
    bariatric surgery status O99.84- ●
    bicornis or bicornuate uterus O34.0- ●
    biliary tract problems O26.61- ●
    breech presentation O32.1
    cardiovascular diseases (conditions in
      I00-I09, I20-I52, I70-I99) O99.41- ●
    cerebrovascular disorders (conditions in
      I60-I69) O99.41- ●
    cervical shortening O26.87- ●
    cervicitis O23.51- ●
    cesarean scar defect (isthmocele) O34.22
    chloasma (gravidarum) O26.89- ●
    cholecystitis O99.61- ●
    cholestasis (intrahepatic) O26.61- ●
    chorioamnionitis O41.12- ●
    circulatory system disorder (conditions in
      I00-I09, I20-I99, O99.41- ●)
    compound presentation O32.6
    conjoined twins O30.02- ●
    connective system disorders (conditions in
      M00-M99) O99.891
    contracted pelvis (general) O33.1
      inlet O33.2
      outlet O33.3
    convulsions (eclamptic) (uremic) —*see also*
      Eclampsia O15.9- ●
    cracked nipple O92.11- ●
    cystitis O23.1- ●
    cystocele O34.8- ●
    death of fetus (near term) O36.4
      early pregnancy O02.1
      of one fetus or more in multiple
        gestation O31.2- ●
    deciduitis O41.14- ●
    decreased fetal movement O36.81- ●
    dental problems O99.61- ●
    diabetes (mellitus) O24.91- ●
      gestational (pregnancy induced) —*see*
        Diabetes, gestational
      pre-existing O24.31- ●
        specified NEC O24.81- ●
        type 1 O24.01- ●
        type 2 O24.11- ●
    digestive system disorders (conditions in
      K00-K93) O99.61- ●
    diseases of —*see* Pregnancy, complicated
      by, specified body system disease
      biliary tract O26.61- ●
      blood NEC (conditions in D65-D77)
        O99.11- ●
      liver O26.61- ●
      specified NEC O99.891
    disorders of —*see* Pregnancy, complicated
      by, specified body system disorder
      amniotic fluid and membranes O41.9- ●
        specified NEC O41.8X- ●
      biliary tract O26.61- ●

Pregnancy (*Continued*)
  complicated by (*Continued*)
    diseases of (*Continued*)
      ear and mastoid process (conditions in
        H60-H95) O99.891
      eye and adnexa (conditions in H00-H59)
        O99.891
      liver O26.61- ●
      skin (conditions in L00-L99) O99.71- ●
      specified NEC O99.891
    displacement, uterus NEC O34.59- ●
      causing obstructed labor O65.5
    disproportion (due to) O33.9
      fetal (ascites) (hydrops)
        (meningomyelocele) (sacral
        teratoma) (tumor) deformities NEC
        O33.7
      generally contracted pelvis O33.1
      hydrocephalic fetus O33.6
      inlet contraction of pelvis O33.2
      mixed maternal and fetal origin O33.4
      specified NEC O33.8
    double uterus O34.0- ●
      causing obstructed labor O65.5
    drug use (conditions in F11-F19) O99.32- ●
    eclampsia, eclamptic (coma) (convulsions)
      (delirium) (nephritis) (uremia) (*see also*
      Eclampsia) O15- ●
    ectopic pregnancy —*see* Pregnancy, ectopic
    edema O12.0- ●
      with
        gestational hypertension, mild —*see*
          also Pre-eclampsia O14.0- ●
        proteinuria O12.2- ●
    effusion, amniotic fluid —*see* Pregnancy,
      complicated by, premature rupture of
      membranes
    elderly
      multigravida O09.52- ●
      primigravida O09.51- ●
    embolism —*see also* Embolism, obstetric,
      pregnancy O88.- ●
    endocrine diseases NEC O99.28- ●
    endometritis O86.12
    excessive weight gain O26.0- ●
    exhaustion O26.81- ●
      during labor and delivery O75.81
    face presentation O32.3
    failed induction of labor O61.9
    failed or difficult intubation for anesthesia
      O29.6- ●
      instrumental O61.1
      mechanical O61.1
      medical O61.0
      specified NEC O61.8
      surgical O61.1
    false labor (pains) O47.9
      at or after 37 completed weeks of
        pregnancy O47.1
      before 37 completed weeks of pregnancy
        O47.0- ●
    fatigue O26.81- ●
      during labor and delivery O75.81
    fatty metamorphosis of liver O26.61- ●
    female genital mutilation O34.8- ● [*N90.81- ●*]
    fetal (maternal care for)
      abnormality or damage O35.9
        acid-base balance O68
        specified type NEC O35.8
      acidemia O68
      acidosis O68
     ▶ agenesis of corpus callosum O35.01
      alkalosis O68
      anemia and thrombocytopenia O36.82- ●
     ⇒ anencephaly O35.02
      bradycardia O36.83- ●
     ▶ cardiac anomalies O35.B
     ▶ central nervous system malformation or
        damage O35.00
       ▶ specified type NEC O35.09
     ▶ choroid plexus cysts O35.03

Pregnancy *(Continued)*
  complicated by *(Continued)*
    fetal *(Continued)*
      ▶chromosomal abnormality (conditions in Q90-Q99) O35.10
        ▶sex chromosome O35.15
        ▶specified NEC O35.19
        ▶Trisomy 13 O35.11
        ▶Trisomy 18 O35.12
        ▶Trisomy 21 O35.13
        ▶Turner Syndrome O35.14
      conjoined twins O30.02-●
      damage from
        amniocentesis O35.7
        biopsy procedures O35.7
        drug addiction O35.5
        hematological investigation O35.7
        intrauterine contraceptive device O35.7
        maternal
          alcohol addiction O35.4
          cytomegalovirus infection O35.3
          disease NEC O35.8
          drug addiction O35.5
          listeriosis O35.8
          rubella O35.3
          toxoplasmosis O35.8
          viral infection O35.3
        medical procedure NEC O35.7
        radiation O35.6
      death (near term) O36.4
        early pregnancy O02.1
      decreased movement O36.81-●
      depressed heart rate tones O36.83-●
      disproportion due to deformity (fetal) O33.7
      ▶encephalocele O35.04
      excessive growth (large for dates) O36.6-●
      ▶facial anomalies O35.A
      ▶gastrointestinal anomalies O35.D
      ▶genitourinary anomalies O35.E
      growth retardation O36.59-●
        light for dates O36.59-●
        small for dates O36.59-●
      heart rate irregularity (abnormal variability) (bradycardia) (decelerations) (tachycardia) O36.83-●
      hereditary disease O35.2
      ▶holoprosencephaly O35.05
      ▶hydrocephalus O35.06
      ▶hydrocephaly O35.06
      intrauterine death O36.4
      ▶microcephaly O35.07
      ▶musculoskeletal anomalies
        ▶lower extremities O35.H
        ▶trunk O35.F
        ▶upper extremities O35.G
      non-reassuring heart rate or rhythm O36.83-●
      poor growth O36.59-●
        light for dates O36.59-●
        small for dates O36.59-●
      problem O36.9-●
        specified NEC O36.89-●
      ▶pulmonary anomalies O35.C
      reduction (elective) O31.3-●
      selective termination O31.3-●
      ▶spina bifida Q35.08
      thrombocytopenia O36.82-●
    fibroid (tumor) (uterus) O34.1-●
    fissure of nipple O92.11-●
    gallstones O99.61-●
    gastric banding status O99.84-●
    gastric bypass status O99.84-●
    genital herpes (asymptomatic) (history of) (inactive) O98.3-●
    genital tract infection O23.9-●
    glomerular diseases (conditions in N00-N07) O26.83-●
      with hypertension, pre-existing —*see* Hypertension, complicating, pregnancy, pre-existing, with, renal disease

Pregnancy *(Continued)*
  complicated by *(Continued)*
    gonorrhea O98.21-●
    grand multiparity O09.4
    habitual aborter —*see* Pregnancy, complicated by, recurrent pregnancy loss
    HELLP syndrome (hemolysis, elevated liver enzymes and low platelet count) O14.2-●
    hemorrhage
      antepartum —*see* Hemorrhage, antepartum
      before 20 completed weeks gestation O20.9
        specified NEC O20.8
      due to premature separation, placenta — *see also* Abruptio placentae O45.9-●
      early O20.9
        specified NEC O20.8
      threatened abortion O20.0
    hemorrhoids O22.4-●
    hepatitis (viral) O98.41-●
    herniation of uterus O34.59-●
    high
      head at term O32.4
      risk —*see* Supervision (of) (for), high-risk
    history of in utero procedure during previous pregnancy O09.82-●
    HIV O98.71-●
    human immunodeficiency virus (HIV) disease O98.71-●
    hydatidiform mole —*see also* Mole, hydatidiform O01.9-●
    hydramnios O40.-●
    hydrocephalic fetus (disproportion) O33.6
    hydrops
      amnii O40.-●
      fetalis O36.2-●
        associated with isoimmunization —*see also* Pregnancy, complicated by, isoimmunization O36.11-●
    hydrorrhea O42.90
    hyperemesis (gravidarum) (mild) —*see also* Hyperemesis, gravidarum O21.0-●
    hypertension —*see* Hypertension, complicating pregnancy
    hypertensive
      heart and renal disease, pre-existing — *see* Hypertension, complicating, pregnancy, pre-existing, with, heart disease, with renal disease
      heart disease, pre-existing —*see* Hypertension, complicating, pregnancy, pre-existing, with, heart disease
      renal disease, pre-existing —*see* Hypertension, complicating, pregnancy, pre-existing, with, renal disease
    hypotension O26.5-●
    immune disorders NEC (conditions in D80-D89) O99.11-●
    incarceration, uterus O34.51-●
    incompetent cervix O34.3-●
    inconclusive fetal viability O36.80
    infection(s) O98.91-●
      amniotic fluid or sac O41.10-●
      bladder O23.1-●
      carrier state NEC O99.830
        streptococcus B O99.820
      genital organ or tract O23.9-●
        specified NEC O23.59-●
      genitourinary tract O23.9-●
      gonorrhea O98.21-●
      hepatitis (viral) O98.41-●
      HIV O98.71-●
      human immunodeficiency virus (HIV) O98.71-●
      intrauterine O41.12
      kidney O23.0-●
      nipple O91.01-●

Pregnancy *(Continued)*
  complicated by *(Continued)*
    infection(s) *(Continued)*
      parasitic disease O98.91-●
        specified NEC O98.81-●
      protozoal disease O98.61-●
      sexually transmitted NEC O98.31-●
      specified type NEC O98.81-●
      syphilis O98.11-●
      tuberculosis O98.01-●
      urethra O23.2-●
      urinary (tract) O23.4-●
        specified NEC O23.3-●
      viral disease O98.51-●
    inflammation
      intrauterine O41.12
    injury or poisoning (conditions in S00-T88) O9A.21-●
      due to abuse
        physical O9A.31-●
        psychological O9A.51-●
        sexual O9A.41-●
    insufficient
      prenatal care O09.3-●
      weight gain O26.1-●
    insulin resistance O26.89
    intrauterine fetal death (near term) O36.4
      early pregnancy O02.1
      multiple gestation (one fetus or more) O31.2-●
    isoimmunization O36.11-●
      anti-A sensitization O36.11-●
      anti-B sensitization O36.19-●
      Rh O36.09-●
        anti-D antibody O36.01-●
      specified NEC O36.19-●
    laceration of uterus NEC O71.81
    malformation
      ▶central nervous system O35.00
        ▶specified type NEC O35.09
      placenta, placental (vessel) O43.10-●
        specified NEC O43.19-●
      uterus (congenital) O34.0-●
    malnutrition (conditions in E40-E46) O25.1-●
    maternal hypotension syndrome O26.5-●
    mental disorders (conditions in F01-F09, F20-F52 and F54-F99) O99.34-●
      alcohol use O99.31-●
      drug use O99.32-●
      smoking O99.33-●
    mentum presentation O32.3
    metabolic disorders O99.28-●
    missed
      abortion O02.1
      delivery O36.4
    multiple gestations O30.9-●
      conjoined twins O30.02-●
      quadruplet —*see* Pregnancy, quadruplet
      specified complication NEC O31.8X-●
      specified number of multiples NEC —*see* Pregnancy, multiple (gestation), specified NEC
      triplet —*see* Pregnancy, triplet
      twin —*see* Pregnancy, twin
    musculoskeletal condition (conditions is M00-M99) O99.891
    necrosis, liver (conditions in K72) O26.61-●
    neoplasm
      benign
        cervix O34.4-●
        corpus uteri O34.1-●
        uterus O34.1-●
      malignant O9A.11-●
    nephropathy NEC O26.83-●
    nervous system condition (conditions in G00-G99) O99.35-●
    nutritional diseases NEC O99.28-●
    obesity (pre-existing) O99.21-●
    obesity surgery status O99.84-●
    oblique lie or presentation O32.2
    older mother —*see* Pregnancy, complicated by, elderly

▶ New   ⇒ Revised   ~~deleted~~ Deleted   ● Use Additional Character(s)

▶ New   ⇒ Revised   ~~deleted~~ Deleted   • Use Additional Character(s)

Pregnancy (Continued)
  twin (Continued)
    unable to determine number of placenta
      and number of amniotic sacs O30.09-●
    unspecified number of placenta and
      unspecified number of amniotic sacs
      O30.00-●
  unwanted Z64.0
  weeks of gestation
    8 weeks Z3A.08
    9 weeks Z3A.09
    10 weeks Z3A.10
    11 weeks Z3A.11
    12 weeks Z3A.12
    13 weeks Z3A.13
    14 weeks Z3A.14
    15 weeks Z3A.15
    16 weeks Z3A.16
    17 weeks Z3A.17
    18 weeks Z3A.18
    19 weeks Z3A.19
    20 weeks Z3A.20
    21 weeks Z3A.21
    22 weeks Z3A.22
    23 weeks Z3A.23
    24 weeks Z3A.24
    25 weeks Z3A.25
    26 weeks Z3A.26
    27 weeks Z3A.27
    28 weeks Z3A.28
    29 weeks Z3A.29
    30 weeks Z3A.30
    31 weeks Z3A.31
    32 weeks Z3A.32
    33 weeks Z3A.33
    34 weeks Z3A.34
    35 weeks Z3A.35
    36 weeks Z3A.36
    37 weeks Z3A.37
    38 weeks Z3A.38
    39 weeks Z3A.39
    40 weeks Z3A.40
    41 weeks Z3A.41
    42 weeks Z3A.42
    greater than 42 weeks Z3A.49
    less than 8 weeks Z3A.01
    not specified Z3A.00
Preiser's disease —see Osteonecrosis,
  secondary, due to, trauma, metacarpus
Pre-kwashiorkor —see Malnutrition, severe
Preleukemia (syndrome) D46.9
Preluxation, hip, congenital Q65.6
Premature —see also condition
  adrenarche E27.0
  aging E34.8
  beats I49.40
    atrial I49.1
    auricular I49.1
    supraventricular I49.1
  birth NEC —see Preterm, newborn
  closure, foramen ovale Q21.8
  contraction
    atrial I49.1
    atrioventricular I49.49
    auricular I49.1
    auriculoventricular I49.2
    heart (extrasystole) I49.49
    junctional I49.2
    ventricular I49.3
  delivery —see also Pregnancy, complicated by,
    preterm labor O60.10
  ejaculation F52.4
  infant NEC —see Preterm, newborn
    light-for-dates —see Light for dates
  labor —see Pregnancy, complicated by,
    preterm labor
  lungs P28.0
  menopause E28.319
    asymptomatic E28.319
    symptomatic E28.310

Pregnancy (Continued)
  newborn
    extreme (less than 28 completed weeks) —
      see Immaturity, extreme
    less than 37 completed weeks —see
      Preterm, newborn
  puberty E30.1
  rupture membranes or amnion —see
    Pregnancy, complicated by, premature
    rupture of membranes
  senility E34.8
  thelarche E30.8
  ventricular systole I49.3
Prematurity NEC (less than 37 completed
  weeks) —see Preterm, newborn
  extreme (less than 28 completed weeks) —see
    Immaturity, extreme
Premenstrual
  dysphoric disorder (PMDD) F32.81
  tension (syndrome) N94.3
Premolarization, cuspids K00.2
Prenatal
  care, normal pregnancy —see Pregnancy,
    normal
  screening of mother —see also Encounter,
    antenatal Z36.9
  teeth K00.6
Preparatory care for subsequent treatment NEC
  for dialysis Z49.01
    peritoneal Z49.02
Prepartum —see condition
Preponderance, left or right ventricular I51.7
Prepuce —see condition
PRES (posterior reversible encephalopathy
  syndrome) I67.83
Presbycardia R54
Presbycusis, presbyacusia H91.1-●
Presbyesophagus K22.89
Presbyophrenia F03
Presbyopia H52.4
Prescription of contraceptives (initial)
  Z30.019
  barrier Z30.018
  diaphragm Z30.018
  emergency (postcoital) Z30.012
  implantable subdermal Z30.017
  injectable Z30.013
  intrauterine contraceptive device Z30.014
  pills Z30.011
  postcoital (emergency) Z30.012
  repeat Z30.40
    barrier Z30.49
    diaphragm Z30.49
    implantable subdermal Z30.46
    injectable Z30.42
    pills Z30.41
    specified type NEC Z30.49
    transdermal patch hormonal Z30.45
    vaginal ring hormonal Z30.44
  specified type NEC Z30.018
    transdermal patch hormonal Z30.016
    vaginal ring hormonal Z30.015
Presence (of)
  ankle-joint implant (functional) (prosthesis)
    Z96.66-●
  aortocoronary (bypass) graft Z95.1
  arterial-venous shunt (dialysis) Z99.2
  artificial
    eye (globe) Z97.0
    heart (fully implantable) (mechanical)
      Z95.812
      valve Z95.2
    larynx Z96.3
    lens (intraocular) Z96.1
    limb (complete) (partial) Z97.1-●
      arm Z97.1-●
        bilateral Z97.15
      leg Z97.1-●
        bilateral Z97.16
  audiological implant (functional) Z96.29
  bladder implant (functional) Z96.0

Presence (Continued)
  bone
    conduction hearing device Z96.29
    implant (functional) NEC Z96.7
    joint (prosthesis) —see Presence, joint
      implant
  cardiac
    defibrillator (functional) (with synchronous
      cardiac pacemaker)Z95.810
    implant or graft Z95.9
      specified type NEC Z95.818
    pacemaker Z95.0
    resynchronization therapy
      defibrillator Z95.810
      pacemaker Z95.0
  ► cardioverter-defibrillator (ICD) Z95.810
  cerebrospinal fluid drainage device Z98.2
  cochlear implant (functional) Z96.21
  contact lens (es) Z97.3
  coronary artery graft or prosthesis Z95.5
  CRT-D (cardiac resynchronization therapy
    defibrillator) Z95.810
  CRT-P (cardiac resynchronization therapy
    pacemaker) Z95.0
  cardioverter-defribillator (ICD) Z95.810
  CSF shunt Z98.2
  dental prosthesis device Z97.2
  dentures Z97.2
  device (external) NEC Z97.8
    cardiac NEC Z95.818
    heart assist Z95.811
    implanted (functional) Z96.9
      specified NEC Z96.89
    prosthetic Z97.8
  ear implant Z96.20
    cochlear implant Z96.21
    myringotomy tube Z96.22
    specified type NEC Z96.29
  elbow-joint implant (functional) (prosthesis)
    Z96.62-●
  endocrine implant (functional) NEC Z96.49
  eustachian tube stent or device (functional)
    Z96.29
  external hearing-aid or device Z97.4
  finger-joint implant (functional) (prosthetic)
    Z96.69-●
  functional implant Z96.9
    specified NEC Z96.89
  graft
    cardiac NEC Z95.818
    vascular NEC Z95.828
  hearing-aid or device (external) Z97.4
    implant (bone) (cochlear) (functional) Z96.21
  heart assist device Z95.811
  heart valve implant (functional) Z95.2
    prosthetic Z95.2
    specified type NEC Z95.4
    xenogenic Z95.3
  hip-joint implant (functional) (prosthesis)
    Z96.64-●
  ICD (cardioverter-defibrillator) Z95.810
  implanted device (artificial) (functional)
    (prosthetic) Z96.9
    automatic cardiac defibrillator (with
      synchronous cardiac pacemaker)
      Z95.810
    cardiac pacemaker Z95.0
    cochlear Z96.21
    dental Z96.5
    heart Z95.812
    heart valve Z95.2
      prosthetic Z95.2
      specified NEC Z95.4
      xenogenic Z95.3
    insulin pump Z96.41
    intraocular lens Z96.1
    joint Z96.60
      ankle Z96.66-●
      elbow Z96.62-●
      finger Z96.69-●
      hip Z96.64-●

Presence (Continued)
  implanted device (Continued)
    joint (Continued)
      knee Z96.65-●
      shoulder Z96.61-●
      specified NEC Z96.698
      wrist Z96.63-●
    larynx Z96.3
    myringotomy tube Z96.22
    otological Z96.20
      cochlear Z96.21
      eustachian stent Z96.29
      myringotomy Z96.22
      specified NEC Z96.29
      stapes Z96.29
    skin Z96.81
    skull plate Z96.7
    specified NEC Z96.89
    urogenital Z96.0
  insulin pump (functional) Z96.41
  intestinal bypass or anastomosis Z98.0
  intraocular lens (functional) Z96.1
  intrauterine contraceptive device (IUD) Z97.5
  intravascular implant (functional) (prosthetic) NEC Z95.9
    coronary artery Z95.5
    defibrillator (with synchronous cardiac pacemaker) Z95.810
    peripheral vessel (with angioplasty) Z95.820
  joint implant (prosthetic) (any) Z96.60
    ankle —see Presence, ankle joint implant
    elbow —see Presence, elbow joint implant
    finger —see Presence, finger joint implant
    hip —see Presence, hip joint implant
    knee —see Presence, knee joint implant
    shoulder —see Presence, shoulder joint implant
    specified joint NEC Z96.698
    wrist —see Presence, wrist joint implant
  knee-joint implant (functional) (prosthesis) Z96.65-●
  laryngeal implant (functional) Z96.3
  mandibular implant (dental) Z96.5
  myringotomy tube(s) Z96.22
  neurostimulator (brain) (gastric) (peripheral nerve) (sacral nerve) (spinal cord) (vagus nerve) Z96.82
  orthopedic-joint implant (prosthetic) (any) —see Presence, joint implant
  otological implant (functional) Z96.29
  shoulder-joint implant (functional) (prosthesis) Z96.61-●
  skull-plate implant Z96.7
  spectacles Z97.3
  stapes implant (functional) Z96.29
  systemic lupus erythematosus [SLE] inhibitor D68.62
  tendon implant (functional) (graft) Z96.7
  tooth root(s) implant Z96.5
  ureteral stent Z96.0
  urethral stent Z96.0
  urogenital implant (functional) Z96.0
  vascular implant or device Z95.9
    access port device Z95.828
    specified type NEC Z95.828
  wrist-joint implant (functional) (prosthesis) Z96.63-●
Presenile —see also condition
  dementia F03
  premature aging E34.8
Presentation, fetal —see Delivery, complicated by, malposition
Prespondylolisthesis (congenital) Q76.2
Pressure
  area, skin —see Ulcer, pressure, by site
  brachial plexus G54.0
  brain G93.5
    injury at birth NEC P11.1
  cerebral —see Pressure, brain
  chest R07.89
  cone, tentorial G93.5

Pressure (Continued)
  hyposystolic —see also Hypotension
    incidental reading, without diagnosis of hypotension R03.1
  increased
    intracranial, benign G93.2
      injury at birth P11.0
    intraocular H40.05-●
  injury —see Ulcer, pressure, by site
  lumbosacral plexus G54.1
  mediastinum J98.59
  necrosis (chronic) —see Ulcer, pressure, by site
  parental, inappropriate (excessive) Z62.6
  sore (chronic) —see Ulcer, pressure, by site
  spinal cord G95.20
  ulcer (chronic) —see Ulcer, pressure, by site
  venous, increased I87.8
Pre-syncope R55
Preterm
  delivery (see also Pregnancy, complicated by, preterm labor) O60.10
  labor —see Pregnancy, complicated by, preterm labor
  newborn (infant) P07.30
    gestational age
      28 completed weeks (28 weeks, 0 days through 28 weeks, 6 days) P07.31
      29 completed weeks (29 weeks, 0 days through 29 weeks, 6 days) P07.32
      30 completed weeks (30 weeks, 0 days through 30 weeks, 6 days) P07.33
      31 completed weeks (31 weeks, 0 days through 31 weeks, 6 days) P07.34
      32 completed weeks (32 weeks, 0 days through 32 weeks, 6 days) P07.35
      33 completed weeks (33 weeks, 0 days through 33 weeks, 6 days) P07.36
      34 completed weeks (34 weeks, 0 days through 34 weeks, 6 days) P07.37
      35 completed weeks (35 weeks, 0 days through 35 weeks, 6 days) P07.38
      36 completed weeks (36 weeks, 0 days through 36 weeks, 6 days) P07.39
Previa
  placenta (total) (without hemorrhage) O44.0-●
    with hemorrhage O44.1-●
    complete O44.0-●
      with hemorrhage O44.1-●
    low —see also Delivery, complicated, by, placenta, low O44.4-●
      with hemorrhage O44.5-●
    marginal O44.2-●
      with hemorrhage O44.3-●
    partial O44.2-●
      with hemorrhage O44.3-●
  vasa O69.4
Priapism N48.30
  due to
    disease classified elsewhere N48.32
    drug N48.33
    specified cause NEC N48.39
    trauma N48.31
Prickling sensation (skin) R20.2
Prickly heat L74.0
Primary —see condition
Primigravida
  elderly, affecting management of pregnancy, labor and delivery (supervision only) —see Pregnancy, complicated by, elderly, primigravida
  older, affecting management of pregnancy, labor and delivery (supervision only) —see Pregnancy, complicated by, elderly, primigravida
  very young, affecting management of pregnancy, labor and delivery (supervision only) —see Pregnancy, complicated by, young mother, primigravida

Primipara
  elderly, affecting management of pregnancy, labor and delivery (supervision only) —see Pregnancy, complicated by, elderly, primigravida
  older, affecting management of pregnancy, labor and delivery (supervision only) —see Pregnancy, complicated by, elderly, primigravida
  very young, affecting management of pregnancy, labor and delivery (supervision only) —see Pregnancy, complicated by, young mother, primigravida
Primus varus (bilateral) Q66.21-●
PRIND (Prolonged reversible ischemic neurologic deficit) I63.9
Pringle's disease (tuberous sclerosis) Q85.1
Prinzmetal angina I20.1
Prizefighter ear —see Cauliflower ear
Problem (with) (related to)
  academic Z55.8
  acculturation Z60.3
  adjustment (to)
    change of job Z56.1
    life-cycle transition Z60.0
    pension Z60.0
    retirement Z60.0
  adopted child Z62.821
  alcoholism in family Z63.72
  atypical parenting situation Z62.9
  bankruptcy Z59.89
  behavioral (adult) F69
    drug seeking Z76.5
  birth of sibling affecting child Z62.898
  care (of)
    provider dependency Z74.9
      specified NEC Z74.8
    sick or handicapped person in family or household Z63.6
  child
    abuse (affecting the child) —see Maltreatment, child
    custody or support proceedings Z65.3
    in care of non-parental family member Z62.21
    in foster care Z62.21
    in welfare custody Z62.21
    living in orphanage or group home Z62.22
  child-rearing Z62.9
    specified NEC Z62.898
  communication (developmental) F80.9
  conflict or discord (with)
    boss Z56.4
    classmates Z55.4
    counselor Z64.4
    employer Z56.4
    family Z63.9
      specified NEC Z63.8
    probation officer Z64.4
    social worker Z64.4
    teachers Z55.4
    workmates Z56.4
  conviction in legal proceedings Z65.0
    with imprisonment Z65.1
  counselor Z64.4
  creditors Z59.89
  digestive K92.9
  drug addict in family Z63.72
  ear —see Disorder, ear
  economic Z59.9
    affecting care Z59.9
    specified NEC Z59.89
  ▶strain Z59.86
  education Z55.9
    specified NEC Z55.8
  employment Z56.9
    change of job Z56.1
    discord Z56.4
    environment Z56.5
    sexual harassment Z56.81

▶ New   ⇒ Revised   ~~deleted~~ Deleted   ● Use Additional Character(s)

Problem *(Continued)*
  employment *(Continued)*
    specified NEC Z56.89
    stress NEC Z56.6
    stressful schedule Z56.3
    threat of job loss Z56.2
    unemployment Z56.0
  enuresis, child F98.0
  eye H57.9
  failed examinations (school) Z55.2
  falling Z91.81
  family —*see also* Disruption, family Z63.9-●
    specified NEC Z63.8
  feeding (elderly) (infant) R63.39
    newborn P92.9
      breast P92.5
      overfeeding P92.4
      slow P92.2
      specified NEC P92.8
      underfeeding P92.3
    nonorganic F50.89
  finance Z59.9
    specified NEC Z59.89
  foreclosure on loan Z59.89
  foster child Z62.822
  frightening experience(s) in childhood Z62.898
  genital NEC
    female N94.9
    male N50.9
  health care Z75.9
    specified NEC Z75.8
  hearing —*see* Deafness
  homelessness Z59.00
  housing Z59.9
    inadequate Z59.1
    isolated Z59.89
    specified NEC Z59.89
  identity (of childhood) F93.8
  illegitimate pregnancy (unwanted) Z64.0
  illiteracy Z55.0
  impaired mobility Z74.09
  imprisonment or incarceration Z65.1
  inadequate teaching affecting education Z55.8
  inappropriate (excessive) parental pressure Z62.6
  influencing health status NEC Z78.9
  in-law Z63.1
  institutionalization, affecting child Z62.22
  intrafamilial communication Z63.8
  jealousy, child F93.8
  landlord Z59.2
  language (developmental) F80.9
  learning (developmental) F81.9
  legal Z65.3
    conviction without imprisonment Z65.0
    imprisonment Z65.1
    release from prison Z65.2
  life-management Z73.9
    specified NEC Z73.89
  life-style Z72.9
    gambling Z72.6
    high-risk sexual behavior (heterosexual) Z72.51
      bisexual Z72.53
      homosexual Z72.52
    inappropriate eating habits Z72.4
    self-damaging behavior NEC Z72.89
    specified NEC Z72.89
    tobacco use Z72.0
  literacy Z55.9
    low level Z55.0
    specified NEC Z55.8
  living alone Z60.2
  lodgers Z59.2
  loss of love relationship in childhood Z62.898
  marital Z63.0
    involving
      divorce Z63.5
      estrangement Z63.5
      gender identity F66
  mastication K08.89

Problem *(Continued)*
  medical
    care, within family Z63.6
    facilities Z75.9
      specified NEC Z75.8
  mental F48.9
  ▶money Z59.86
  multiparity Z64.1
  negative life events in childhood Z62.9
    altered pattern of family relationships Z62.898
    frightening experience Z62.898
    loss of
      love relationship Z62.898
      self-esteem Z62.898
    physical abuse (alleged) —*see* Maltreatment, child
    removal from home Z62.29
    specified event NEC Z62.898
  neighbor Z59.2
  neurological NEC R29.818
  new step-parent affecting child Z62.898
  none (feared complaint unfounded) Z71.1
  occupational NEC Z56.89
  parent-child —*see* Conflict, parent-child
  personal hygiene Z91.89
  personality F69
  phase-of-life transition, adjustment Z60.0
  presence of sick or disabled person
    in family or household Z63.79
    needing care Z63.6
  primary support group (family) Z63.9
    specified NEC Z63.8
  probation officer Z64.4
  psychiatric F99
  psychosexual (development) F66
  psychosocial Z65.9
    religious or spiritual Z65.8
    specified NEC Z65.8
  relationship Z63.9
    childhood F93.8
  release from prison Z65.2
    religious or spiritual Z65.8
  removal from home affecting child Z62.29
  seeking and accepting known hazardous and harmful
    behavioral or psychological interventions Z65.8
    chemical, nutritional or physical interventions Z65.8
  sexual function (nonorganic) F52.9
  sight H54.7
  sleep disorder, child F51.9
  smell —*see* Disturbance, sensation, smell
  social
    environment Z60.9
      specified NEC Z60.8
    exclusion and rejection Z60.4
    worker Z64.4
  speech R47.9
    developmental F80.9
    specified NEC R47.89
  swallowing —*see* Dysphagia
  taste —*see* Disturbance, sensation, taste
  tic, child F95.0
  underachievement in school Z55.3
  unemployment Z56.0
    threatened Z56.2
  unwanted pregnancy Z64.0
  upbringing Z62.9
    specified NEC Z62.898
  urinary N39.9
  voice production R47.89
  work schedule (stressful) Z56.3
Procedure (surgical)
  converted
    arthroscopic to open Z53.33
    laparoscopic to open Z53.31
    specified procedure NEC to open Z53.39
    thoracoscopic to open Z53.32
  for purpose other than remedying health state Z41.9
    specified NEC Z41.8

Procedure *(Continued)*
  not done Z53.9
    because of
      administrative reasons Z53.8
      contraindication Z53.09
        smoking Z53.01
      patient's decision Z53.20
        for reasons of belief or group pressure Z53.1
        left against medical advice (AMA) Z53.29
        left without being seen Z53.21
        specified reason NEC Z53.29
      specified reason NEC Z53.8
Procidentia (uteri) N81.3
Proctalgia K62.89
  fugax K59.4
  spasmodic K59.4
Proctitis K62.89
  amebic (acute) A06.0
  chlamydial A56.3
  gonococcal A54.6
  granulomatous —*see* Enteritis, regional, large intestine
  herpetic A60.1
  radiation K62.7
  tuberculous A18.32
  ulcerative (chronic) K51.20
    with
      complication K51.219
        abscess K51.214
        fistula K51.213
        obstruction K51.212
        rectal bleeding K51.211
        specified NEC K51.218
Proctocele
  female (without uterine prolapse) N81.6
    with uterine prolapse N81.2
      complete N81.3
  male K62.3
Proctocolitis
  allergic K52.29
  food-induced eosinophilic K52.29
  food protein-induced K52.29
  milk protein-induced K52.29
  mucosal —*see* Rectosigmoiditis, ulcerative
Proctoptosis K62.3
Proctorrhagia K62.5
Proctosigmoiditis K63.89
  ulcerative (chronic) —*see* Rectosigmoiditis, ulcerative
Proctospasm K59.4
  psychogenic F45.8
Profichet's disease —*see* Disorder, soft tissue, specified type NEC
Progeria E34.8
Prognathism (mandibular) (maxillary) M26.19
Progonoma (melanotic) —*see* Neoplasm, benign, by site
Progressive —*see* condition
Prolactinoma
  specified site —*see* Neoplasm, benign, by site
  unspecified site D35.2
Prolapse, prolapsed
  anus, anal (canal) (sphincter) K62.2
  arm or hand O32.2
    causing obstructed labor O64.4
  bladder (mucosa) (sphincter) (acquired)
    congenital Q79.4
    female —*see* Cystocele
    male N32.89
  breast implant (prosthetic) T85.49
  cecostomy K94.09
  cecum K63.4
  cervix, cervical (hypertrophied) N81.2
    anterior lip, obstructing labor O65.5
    congenital Q51.828
    postpartal, old N81.2
    stump N81.85
  ciliary body (traumatic) —*see* Laceration, eye(ball), with prolapse or loss of interocular tissue

Prolapse, prolapsed (Continued)
- colon (pedunculated) K63.4
- colostomy K94.09
- disc (intervertebral) —see Displacement, intervertebral disc
- eye implant (orbital) T85.398
  - lens (ocular) —see Complications, intraocular lens
- fallopian tube N83.4-●
- gastric (mucosa) K31.89
- genital, female N81.9
  - specified NEC N81.89
- globe, nontraumatic —see Luxation, globe
- ileostomy bud K94.19
- intervertebral disc —see Displacement, intervertebral disc
- intestine (small) K63.4
- iris (traumatic) —see Laceration, eye(ball), with prolapse or loss of interocular tissue
  - nontraumatic H21.89
- kidney N28.83
  - congenital Q63.2
- laryngeal muscles or ventricle J38.7
- liver K76.89
- meatus urinarius N36.8
- mitral (valve) I34.1
- ocular lens implant —see Complications, intraocular lens
- organ or site, congenital NEC —see Malposition, congenital
- ovary N83.4-●
- pelvic floor, female N81.89
- perineum, female N81.89
- rectum (mucosa) (sphincter) K62.3
  - due to trichuris trichuria B79
- spleen D73.89
- stomach K31.89
- umbilical cord
  - complicating delivery O69.0
- urachus, congenital Q64.4
- ureter N28.89
  - with obstruction N13.5
    - with infection N13.6
- ureterovesical orifice N28.89
- urethra (acquired) (infected) (mucosa) N36.8
  - congenital Q64.71
- urinary meatus N36.8
  - congenital Q64.72
- uterovaginal N81.4
  - complete N81.3
  - incomplete N81.2
- uterus (with prolapse of vagina) N81.4
  - complete N81.3
  - congenital Q51.818
  - first degree N81.2
  - in pregnancy or childbirth —see Pregnancy, complicated by, abnormal, uterus
  - incomplete N81.2
  - postpartal (old) N81.4
  - second degree N81.2
  - third degree N81.3
- uveal (traumatic) —see Laceration, eye(ball), with prolapse or loss of interocular tissue
- vagina (anterior) (wall) —see Cystocele
  - with prolapse of uterus N81.4
    - complete N81.3
    - incomplete N81.2
  - posterior wall N81.6
  - posthysterectomy N99.3
- vitreous (humor) H43.0-●
  - in wound —see Laceration, eye(ball), with prolapse or loss of interocular tissue
- womb —see Prolapse, uterus

Prolapsus, female N81.9
- specified NEC N81.89

Proliferation(s)
- primary cutaneous CD30-positive large T-cell C86.6
- prostate, atypical small acinar N42.32

Proliferative —see condition

Prolonged, prolongation (of)
- bleeding (time) (idiopathic) R79.1
- coagulation (time) R79.1
- gestation (over 42 completed weeks)
  - mother O48.1
  - newborn P08.22
- interval I44.0
- labor O63.9
  - first stage O63.0
  - second stage O63.1
- partial thromboplastin time (PTT) R79.1
- pregnancy (more than 42 weeks gestation) O48.1
- prothrombin time R79.1
- QT interval R94.31
- uterine contractions in labor O62.4

Prominence, prominent
- ischial spine or sacral promontory with disproportion (fetopelvic) O33.0
  - causing obstructed labor O65.0
- auricle (congenital) (ear) Q17.5
- nose (congenital) acquired M95.0

Promiscuity —see High, risk, sexual behavior

Pronation
- ankle —see Deformity, limb, foot, specified NEC
- foot —see also Deformity, limb, foot, specified NEC
  - congenital Q74.2

Prophylactic
- administration of
  - antibiotics, long-term Z79.2
    - short-term use - omit code
  - drug —see also Long-term (current) drug therapy (use of) Z79.899-●
  - medication Z79.899
- organ removal (for neoplasia management) Z40.00
  - breast Z40.01
  - fallopian tube(s) Z40.03
    - with ovary(s) Z40.02
  - ovary(s) Z40.02
  - specified site NEC Z40.09
- surgery Z40.9
  - for risk factors related to malignant neoplasm —see Prophylactic, organ removal
  - specified NEC Z40.8
- vaccination Z23

Propionic acidemia E71.121

Proptosis (ocular) —see also Exophthalmos
- thyroid —see Hyperthyroidism, with goiter

Prosecution, anxiety concerning Z65.3

Prosopagnosia R48.3

Prostadynia N42.81

Prostate, prostatic —see condition

Prostatism —see Hyperplasia, prostate

Prostatitis (congestive) (suppurative) (with cystitis) N41.9
- acute N41.0
- cavitary N41.8
- chronic N41.1
- diverticular N41.8
- due to Trichomonas (vaginalis) A59.02
- fibrous N41.1
- gonococcal (acute) (chronic) A54.22
- granulomatous N41.4
- hypertrophic N41.1
- subacute N41.1
- trichomonal A59.02
- tuberculous A18.14

Prostatocystitis N41.3

Prostatorrhea N42.89

Prostatosis N42.82

Prostration R53.83
- heat —see also Heat, exhaustion
  - anhydrotic T67.3
  - due to
    - salt (and water) depletion T67.4
    - water depletion T67.3
- nervous F48.8
- senile R54

Protanomaly (anomalous trichromat) H53.54

Protanopia (complete) (incomplete) H53.54

Protection (against) (from) —see Prophylactic

Protein
- deficiency NEC —see Malnutrition
- malnutrition —see Malnutrition
- sickness —see also Reaction, serum T80.69

Proteinemia R77.9

Proteinosis
- alveolar (pulmonary) J84.01
- lipid or lipoid (of Urbach) E78.89

Proteinuria R80.9
- Bence Jones R80.3
- complicating pregnancy —see Proteinuria, gestational
- gestational
  - complicating
    - childbirth O12.14
    - pregnancy O12.1-●
      - with edema O12.2-●
    - puerperium O12.15
- idiopathic R80.0
- isolated R80.0
  - with glomerular lesion N06.9
    - C3
      - glomerulonephritis N06.A
      - glomerulopathy N06.A
        - with dense deposit disease N06.6
    - dense deposit disease N06.6
    - diffuse
      - crescentic glomerulonephritis N06.7
      - endocapillary proliferative glomerulonephritis N06.4
      - mesangiocapillary glomerulonephritis N06.5
    - focal and segmental hyalinosis or sclerosis N06.1
    - membranous (diffuse) N06.2
    - mesangial proliferative (diffuse) N06.3
    - minimal change N06.0
    - specified pathology NEC N06.8
- orthostatic R80.2
  - with glomerular lesion —see Proteinuria, isolated, with glomerular lesion
- persistent R80.1
  - with glomerular lesion —see Proteinuria, isolated, with glomerular lesion
- postural R80.2
  - with glomerular lesion —see Proteinuria, isolated, with glomerular lesion
- pre-eclamptic —see Pre-eclampsia
- puerperal O12.15
- specified type NEC R80.8

Proteolysis, pathologic D65

Proteus (mirabilis) (morganii), as cause of disease classified elsewhere B96.4

Prothrombin gene mutation D68.52

Protoporphyria, erythropoietic E80.0

Protozoal —see also condition
- disease B64
  - specified NEC B60.8

Protrusion, protrusio
- acetabuli M24.7
- acetabulum (into pelvis) M24.7
- device, implant or graft —see also Complications, by site and type, mechanical T85.698
  - arterial graft NEC —see Complication, cardiovascular device, mechanical, vascular
  - breast (implant) T85.49

▶ New ⇒ Revised ~~deleted~~ Deleted ● Use Additional Character(s)

Protrusion, protrusio (Continued)
  device, implant or graft (Continued)
    catheter NEC T85.698
      cystostomy T83.090
      dialysis (renal) T82.49
        intraperitoneal T85.691
      infusion NEC T82.594
        spinal (epidural) (subdural) T85.690
      urinary —see also Complications,
          catheter, urinary T83.098
    electronic (electrode) (pulse generator)
        (stimulator)
      bone T84.390
      nervous system —see Complication,
          prosthetic device, mechanical,
          electronic nervous system
          stimulator
    fixation, internal (orthopedic) NEC —
        see Complication, fixation device,
        mechanical
    gastrointestinal —see Complications,
        prosthetic device, mechanical,
        gastrointestinal device
    genital NEC T83.498
      intrauterine contraceptive device
          T83.39
      penile prosthesis (cylinder) (implanted)
          (pump) (resevoir) T83.490
      testicular prosthesis T83.491
    heart NEC —see Complication,
        cardiovascular device, mechanical
    joint prosthesis —see Complications, joint
        prosthesis, mechanical, specified NEC,
        by site
    ocular NEC —see Complications, prosthetic
        device, mechanical, ocular device
    orthopedic NEC —see Complication,
        orthopedic, device, mechanical
    specified NEC T85.628
    urinary NEC —see also Complication,
        genitourinary, device, urinary,
        mechanical
      graft T83.29
    vascular NEC —see Complication,
        cardiovascular device, mechanical
    ventricular intracranial shunt T85.09
  intervertebral disc —see Displacement,
      intervertebral disc
  joint prosthesis —see Complications, joint
      prosthesis, mechanical, specified NEC,
      by site
  nucleus pulposus —see Displacement,
      intervertebral disc
Prune belly (syndrome) Q79.4
Prurigo (ferox) (gravis) (Hebrae) (Hebra's)
    (mitis) (simplex) L28.2
  Besnier's L20.0
  estivalis L56.4
  nodularis L28.1
  psychogenic F45.8
Pruritus, pruritic (essential) L29.9
  ani, anus L29.0
    psychogenic F45.8
  anogenital L29.3
    psychogenic F45.8
  due to onchocerca volvulus B73.1
  gravidarum —see Pregnancy, complicated by,
      specified pregnancy-related condition
      NEC
  hiemalis L29.8
  neurogenic (any site) F45.8
  perianal L29.0
  psychogenic (any site) F45.8
  scroti, scrotum L29.1
    psychogenic F45.8
  senile, senilis L29.8
  specified NEC L29.8
    psychogenic F45.8
  Trichomonas A59.9
  vulva, vulvae L29.2
    psychogenic F45.8

Pseudarthrosis, pseudoarthrosis (bone) —see
    Nonunion, fracture
  clavicle, congenital Q74.0
  joint, following fusion or arthrodesis M96.0
Pseudoaneurysm —see Aneurysm
Pseudoangina (pectoris) —see Angina
Pseudoangioma I81
Pseudoarteriosus Q28.8
Pseudoarthrosis —see Pseudarthrosis
Pseudobulbar affect (PBA) F48.2
Pseudochromhidrosis L67.8
Pseudocirrhosis, liver, pericardial I31.1
Pseudocowpox B08.03
Pseudocoxalgia M91.3-●
Pseudocroup J38.5
Pseudo-Cushing's syndrome, alcohol-induced
    E24.4
Pseudocyesis F45.8
Pseudocyst
  lung J98.4
  pancreas K86.3
  retina —see Cyst, retina
Pseudoelephantiasis neuroarthritica Q82.0
Pseudoexfoliation, capsule (lens) —see
    Cataract, specified NEC
Pseudofolliculitis barbae L73.1
Pseudoglioma H44.89
Pseudohemophilia (Bernuth's) (hereditary)
    (type B) —see Disease, von Willebrand
  Type A D69.8
  vascular D69.8
Pseudohermaphroditism Q56.3
  adrenal E25.8
  female (see also Disorder, adrenogenital)
      Q56.2
    with adrenocortical disorder E25.8
    without adrenocortical disorder Q56.2
    adrenal (congenital) E25.0
    unspecified E25.9
  male (see also Disorder, adrenogenital) Q56.1
    with
      adrenocortical disorder E25.8
      androgen resistance E34.51
      cleft scrotum Q56.1
      feminizing testis E34.51
      5-alpha-reductase deficiency E29.1
    without gonadal disorder Q56.1
    adrenal E25.8
    unspecified E25.9
Pseudo-Hurler's polydystrophy E77.0
Pseudohydrocephalus G93.2
Pseudohypertrophic muscular dystrophy
    (Erb's) G71.02
Pseudohypertrophy, muscle (see also
    Dystrophy, muscular, by type, if
    applicable) G71.09
Pseudohypoparathyroidism E20.1
Pseudoinsomnia F51.03
Pseudoleukemia, infantile D64.89
Pseudomembranous —see condition
Pseudomeningocele (cerebral) (infective) (post-
    traumatic) G96.198
  postprocedural (spinal) G97.82
Pseudomenses (newborn) P54.6
Pseudomenstruation (newborn) P54.6
Pseudomonas
  aeruginosa, as cause of disease classified
      elsewhere B96.5
  mallei infection A24.0
    as cause of disease classified elsewhere
        B96.5
  pseudomallei, as cause of disease classified
      elsewhere B96.5
Pseudomyotonia G71.19
Pseudomyxoma peritonei C78.6
Pseudoneuritis, optic (nerve) (disc) (papilla),
    congenital Q14.2
Pseudo-obstruction intestine (acute) (chronic)
    (idiopathic) (intermittent secondary)
    (primary) K59.89
  colonic K59.81

Pseudopapilledema H47.33-●
  congenital Q14.2
Pseudoparalysis
  arm or leg R29.818
  atonic, congenital P94.2
Pseudopelade L66.0
Pseudophakia Z96.1
Pseudopolyarthritis, rhizomelic M35.3
Pseudopolycythemia D75.1
Pseudopseudohypoparathyroidism E20.1
Pseudopterygium H11.81-●
Pseudoptosis (eyelid) —see Blepharochalasis
Pseudopuberty, precocious
  female heterosexual E25.8
  male isosexual E25.8
Pseudorickets (renal) N25.0
Pseudorubella B08.20
Pseudosclerema, newborn P83.88
Pseudosclerosis (brain)
  Jakob's —see Creutzfeldt-Jakob disease or
      syndrome
  of Westphal (Strüümpell) E83.01
  spastic —see Creutzfeldt-Jakob disease or
      syndrome
Pseudotetanus —see Convulsions
Pseudotetany R29.0
  hysterical F44.5
Pseudotruncus arteriosus Q25.49
Pseudotuberculosis A28.2
  enterocolitis A04.8
  pasteurella (infection) A28.0
Pseudotumor G93.2
  cerebri G93.2
  orbital H05.11-●
Pseudoxanthoma elasticum Q82.8
Psilosis (sprue) (tropical) K90.1
  nontropical K90.0
Psittacosis A70
Psoitis M60.88
Psoriasis L40.9
  arthropathic L40.50
    arthritis mutilans L40.52
    distal interphalangeal L40.51
    juvenile L40.54
    other specified L40.59
    spondylitis L40.53
  buccal K13.29
  flexural L40.8
  guttate L40.4
  mouth K13.29
  nummular L40.0
  plaque L40.0
  psychogenic F54
  pustular (generalized) L40.1
    palmaris et plantaris L40.3
  specified NEC L40.8
  vulgaris L40.0
Psychasthenia F48.8
Psychiatric disorder or problem F99
Psychogenic —see also condition
  factors associated with physical conditions
      F54
Psychological and behavioral factors affecting
    medical condition F59
Psychoneurosis, psychoneurotic —see also
    Neurosis
  anxiety (state) F41.1
  depersonalization F48.1
  hypochondriacal F45.21
  hysteria F44.9
  neurasthenic F48.8
  personality NEC F60.89
Psychopathy, psychopathic
  affectionless F94.2
  autistic F84.5
  constitution, post-traumatic F07.81
  personality —see Disorder, personality
  sexual —see Deviation, sexual
  state F60.2
Psychosexual identity disorder of childhood
    F64.2

P

Psychosis, psychotic F29
  acute (transient) F23
    hysterical F44.9
  affective —see Disorder, mood
  alcoholic F10.959
    with
      abuse F10.159
      anxiety disorder F10.980
        with
          abuse F10.180
          dependence F10.280
      delirium tremens F10.231
      delusions F10.950
        with
          abuse F10.150
          dependence F10.250
      dementia F10.97
        with dependence F10.27
      dependence F10.259
      hallucinosis F10.951
        with
          abuse F10.151
          dependence F10.251
      mood disorder F10.94
        with
          abuse F10.14
          dependence F10.24
      paranoia F10.950
        with
          abuse F10.150
          dependence F10.250
      persisting amnesia F10.96
        with dependence F10.26
    amnestic confabulatory F10.96
      with dependence F10.26
    delirium tremens F10.231
    Korsakoff's, Korsakov's, Korsakow's F10.26
    paranoid type F10.950
      with
        abuse F10.150
        dependence F10.250
  anergastic —see Psychosis, organic
  ▪arteriosclerotic (simple type) (uncomplicated)
      (see also Dementia, vascular) F01.50
    ▪with behavioral disturbance —see
        Dementia, vascular
  childhood F84.0
    atypical F84.8
  climacteric —see Psychosis, involutional
  confusional F29
    acute or subacute F05
    reactive F23
  cycloid F23
  depressive —see Disorder, depressive
  disintegrative (childhood) F84.3
  drug-induced —see F11-F19 with .x59
    paranoid and hallucinatory states —see
        F11-F19 with .x50 or .x51
  due to or associated with
    addiction, drug —see F11-F19 with .X59
    dependence
      alcohol F10.259
      drug —see F11-F19 with .x59
    epilepsy F06.8
    Huntington's chorea F06.8
    ischemia, cerebrovascular (generalized)
        F06.8
    multiple sclerosis F06.8
    physical disease F06.8
    presenile dementia F03
    senile dementia F03
    ▪vascular disease (arteriosclerotic) (cerebral)
        (see also Dementia, vascular) F01.50
      ▪with behavioral disturbance —see
          Dementia, vascular
  epileptic F06.8
  episode F23
    due to or associated with physical
        condition F06.8
  exhaustive F43.0
  hallucinatory, chronic F28

Psychosis, psychotic F29
  hypomanic F30.8
  hysterical (acute) F44.9
  induced F24
  infantile F84.0
    atypical F84.8
  infective (acute) (subacute) F05
  involutional F28
    depressive —see Disorder, depressive
    melancholic —see Disorder, depressive
    paranoid (state) F22
  Korsakoff's, Korsakov's, Korsakow's
      (nonalcoholic) F04
    alcoholic F10.96
      in dependence F10.26
    induced by other psychoactive
        substance —see categories F11-F19
        with .x5x
  mania, manic (single episode) F30.2
    recurrent type F31.89
  manic-depressive —see Disorder, bipolar
  menopausal —see Psychosis, involutional
  mixed schizophrenic and affective F25.8
  ▪multi-infarct (cerebrovascular) (see also
      Dementia, vascular) F01.50
    ▪with behavioral disturbance —see
        Dementia, vascular
  nonorganic F29
    specified NEC F28
  organic F09
    due to or associated with
      arteriosclerosis (cerebral) —see
          Psychosis, arteriosclerotic
      cerebrovascular disease,
          arteriosclerotic —see Psychosis,
          arteriosclerotic
      childbirth —see Psychosis, puerperal
      Creutzfeldt-Jakob disease or
          syndrome —see Creutzfeldt-Jakob
          disease or syndrome
      dependence, alcohol F10.259
      disease
        alcoholic liver F10.259
        brain, arteriosclerotic —see Psychosis,
            arteriosclerotic
        ▪cerebrovascular (see also Dementia,
            vascular) F01.50
          ▪with behavioral disturbance —see
              Dementia, vascular
        Creutzfeldt-Jakob —see Creutzfeldt-
            Jakob disease or syndrome
        endocrine or metabolic F06.8
          acute or subacute F05
        liver, alcoholic F10.259
      epilepsy transient (acute) F05
      infection
        brain (intracranial) F06.8
          acute or subacute F05
      intoxication
        alcoholic (acute) F10.259
        drug F11-F19 with .x59
      ischemia, cerebrovascular
          (generalized) —see Psychosis,
          arteriosclerotic
      puerperium —see Psychosis, puerperal
      trauma, brain (birth) (from electric
          current) (surgical) F06.8
        acute or subacute F05
    infective F06.8
      acute or subacute F05
    post-traumatic F06.8
      acute or subacute F05
  paranoiac F22
  paranoid (climacteric) (involutional)
      (menopausal) F22
    psychogenic (acute) F23
    schizophrenic F20.0
    senile F03
  postpartum F53.1
  presbyophrenic (type) F03
  presenile F03

Psychosis, psychotic F29
  psychogenic (paranoid) F23
    depressive F32.3
  puerperal F53.1
    specified type —see Psychosis, by type
  reactive (brief) (transient) (emotional stress)
      (psychological trauma) F23
    depressive F32.3
      recurrent F33.3
    excitative type F30.8
  schizoaffective F25.9
    depressive type F25.1
    manic type F25.0
  schizophrenia, schizophrenic —see
      Schizophrenia
  schizophrenia-like, in epilepsy F06.2
  schizophreniform F20.81
    affective type F25.9
    brief F23
    confusional type F23
    mixed type F25.0
  senile NEC F03
    depressed or paranoid type F03
    simple deterioration F03
    specified type — code to condition
  shared F24
  situational (reactive) F23
  symbiotic (childhood) F84.3
  symptomatic F09
Psychosomatic —see Disorder, psychosomatic
Psychosyndrome, organic F07.9
Psychotic episode due to or associated with
      physical condition F06.8
Pterygium (eye) H11.00-●
  amyloid H11.01-●
  central H11.02-●
  colli Q18.3
  double H11.03-●
  peripheral
    progressive H11.05-●
    stationary H11.04-●
  recurrent H11.06-●
Ptilosis (eyelid) —see Madarosis
Ptomaine (poisoning) —see Poisoning, food
Ptosis —see also Blepharoptosis
  adiposa (false) —see Blepharoptosis
  breast N64.81
  brow H57.81-●
  cecum K63.4
  colon K63.4
  congenital (eyelid) Q10.0
    specified site NEC —see Anomaly, by site
  eyebrow H57.81-●
  eyelid —see Blepharoptosis
    congenital Q10.0
  gastric K31.89
  intestine K63.4
  kidney N28.83
  liver K76.89
  renal N28.83
  splanchnic K63.4
  spleen D73.89
  stomach K31.89
  viscera K63.4
PTP D69.51
Ptyalism (periodic) K11.7
  hysterical F45.8
  pregnancy —see Pregnancy, complicated by,
      specified pregnancy-related condition
      NEC
  psychogenic F45.8
Ptyalolithiasis K11.5
Pubarche, precocious E30.1
Pubertas praecox E30.1
Puberty (development state) Z00.3
  bleeding (excessive) N92.2
  delayed E30.0
  precocious (constitutional) (cryptogenic)
      (idiopathic) E30.1
    central E22.8

▶ New   ▪ Revised   ~~deleted~~ Deleted   ● Use Additional Character(s)

Puberty *(Continued)*
  precocious *(Continued)*
    due to
      ovarian hyperfunction E28.1
        estrogen E28.0
      testicular hyperfunction E29.0
    premature E30.1
    due to
      adrenal cortical hyperfunction E25.8
      pineal tumor E34.8
      pituitary (anterior) hyperfunction E22.8
Puckering, macula —*see* Degeneration, macula, puckering
Pudenda, pudendum —*see* condition
Puente's disease (simple glandular cheilitis) K13.0
Puerperal, puerperium (complicated by, complications)
  abnormal glucose (tolerance test) O99.815
  abscess
    areola O91.02
      associated with lactation O91.03
    Bartholin's gland O86.19
    breast O91.12
      associated with lactation O91.13
    cervix (uteri) O86.11
    genital organ NEC O86.19
    kidney O86.21
    mammary O91.12
      associated with lactation O91.13
    nipple O91.02
      associated with lactation O91.03
    peritoneum O85
    subareolar O91.12
      associated with lactation O91.13
    urinary tract —*see* Puerperal, infection, urinary
    uterus O86.12
    vagina (wall) O86.13
    vaginorectal O86.13
    vulvovaginal gland O86.13
  adnexitis O86.19
  afibrinogenemia, or other coagulation defect O72.3
  albuminuria (acute) (subacute) —*see* Proteinuria, gestational
  alcohol use O99.315
  anemia O90.81
    pre-existing (pre-pregnancy) O99.03
  anesthetic death O89.8
  apoplexy O99.43
  bariatric surgery status O99.845
  blood disorder NEC O99.13
  blood dyscrasia O72.3
  cardiomyopathy O90.3
  cerebrovascular disorder (conditions in I60-I69) O99.43
  cervicitis O86.11
  circulatory system disorder O99.43
  coagulopathy (any) O99.13
    with hemorrhage O72.3
  complications O90.9
    specified NEC O90.89
  convulsions —*see* Eclampsia
  cystitis O86.22
  cystopyelitis O86.29
  delirium NEC F05
  diabetes O24.93
    gestational —*see* Puerperal, gestational diabetes
    pre-existing O24.33
      specified NEC O24.83
      type 1 O24.03
      type 2 O24.13
  digestive system disorder O99.63
  disease O90.9
    breast NEC O92.29
    cerebrovascular (acute) O99.43
    nonobstetric NEC O99.893
    tubo-ovarian O86.19
    Valsuani's O99.03

Puerperal, puerperium *(Continued)*
  disorder O90.9
    biliary tract O26.63
    lactation O92.70
    liver O26.63
    nonobstetric NEC O99.893
  disruption
    cesarean wound O90.0
    episiotomy wound O90.1
    perineal laceration wound O90.1
  drug use O99.325
  eclampsia (with pre-existing hypertension) O15.2
  embolism (pulmonary) (blood clot) —*see* Embolism, obstetric, puerperal
  endocrine, nutritional or metabolic disease NEC O99.285
  endophlebitis —*see* Puerperal, phlebitis
  endotrachelitis O86.11
  failure
    lactation (complete) O92.3
      partial O92.4
    renal, acute O90.4
  fever (of unknown origin) O86.4
    septic O85
  fissure, nipple O92.12
    associated with lactation O92.13
  fistula
    breast (due to mastitis) O91.12
      associated with lactation O91.13
    nipple O91.02
      associated with lactation O91.03
  galactophoritis O91.22
    associated with lactation O91.23
  galactorrhea O92.6
  gastric banding status O99.845
  gastric bypass status O99.845
  gastrointestinal disease NEC O99.63
  gestational
    diabetes O24.439
      diet controlled O24.430
      insulin (and diet) controlled O24.434
      oral drug controlled (antidiabetic) (hypoglycemic) O24.435
    edema O12.05
      with proteinuria O12.25
    proteinuria O12.15
  gonorrhea O98.23
  hematoma, subdural O99.43
  hemiplegia, cerebral O99.355- •
    due to cerebrovascular disorder O99.43
  hemorrhage O72.1
    brain O99.43
    bulbar O99.43
    cerebellar O99.43
    cerebral O99.43
    cortical O99.43
    delayed or secondary O72.2
    extradural O99.43
    internal capsule O99.43
    intracranial O99.43
    intrapontine O99.43
    meningeal O99.43
    pontine O99.43
    retained placenta O72.0
    subarachnoid O99.43
    subcortical O99.43
    subdural O99.43
    third stage O72.0
    uterine, delayed O72.2
    ventricular O99.43
  hemorrhoids O87.2
  hepatorenal syndrome O90.4
  hypertension —*see* Hypertension, complicating, puerperium
  hypertrophy, breast O92.29
  induration breast (fibrous) O92.29
  infection O86.4
    cervix O86.11
    generalized O85
    genital tract NEC O86.19
      obstetric surgical wound O86.09

Puerperal, puerperium *(Continued)*
  infection *(Continued)*
    kidney (bacillus coli) O86.21
    maternal O98.93
      carrier state NEC O99.835
      gonorrhea O98.23
      human immunodeficiency virus (HIV) O98.73
      protozoal O98.63
      sexually transmitted NEC O98.33
      specified NEC O98.83
      streptococcus group B (GBS) carrier state O99.825
      syphilis O98.13
      tuberculosis O98.03
      viral hepatitis O98.43
      viral NEC O98.53
    nipple O91.02
      associated with lactation O91.03
    peritoneum O85
    renal O86.21
    specified NEC O86.89
    urinary (asymptomatic) (tract) NEC O86.20
      bladder O86.22
      kidney O86.21
      specified site NEC O86.29
      urethra O86.22
    vagina O86.13
    vein —*see* Puerperal, phlebitis
  ischemia, cerebral O99.43
  lymphangitis O86.89
    breast O91.22
      associated with lactation O91.23
  malignancy O9A.13
  malnutrition O25.3
  mammillitis O91.02
    associated with lactation O91.03
  mammitis O91.22
    associated with lactation O91.23
  mania F30.8
  mastitis O91.22
    associated with lactation O91.23
    purulent O91.12
      associated with lactation O91.13
  melancholia —*see* Disorder, depressive
  mental disorder NEC O99.345
  metroperitonitis O85
  metrorrhagia —*see* Hemorrhage, postpartum
  metrosalpingitis O86.19
  metrovaginitis O86.13
  milk leg O87.1
  monoplegia, cerebral O99.43
  mood disturbance O90.6
  necrosis, liver (acute) (subacute) (conditions in subcategory K72.0) O26.63
    with renal failure O90.4
  nervous system disorder O99.355
  neuritis O90.89
  obesity (pre-existing prior to pregnancy) O99.215
  obesity surgery status O99.845
  occlusion, precerebral artery O99.43
  paralysis
    bladder (sphincter) O90.89
    cerebral O99.43
  paralytic stroke O99.43
  parametritis O85
  paravaginitis O86.13
  pelviperitonitis O85
  perimetritis O86.12
  perimetrosalpingitis O86.19
  perinephritis O86.21
  periphlebitis —*see* Puerperal phlebitis
  peritoneal infection O85
  peritonitis (pelvic) O85
  perivaginitis O86.13
  phlebitis O87.0
    deep O87.1
    pelvic O87.1
    superficial O87.0

Puerperal, puerperium *(Continued)*
  phlebothrombosis, deep O87.1
  phlegmasia alba dolens O87.1
  placental polyp O90.89
  pneumonia, embolic —*see* Embolism,
    obstetric, puerperal
  pre-eclampsia —*see* Pre-eclampsia
  psychosis F53.1
  pyelitis O86.21
  pyelocystitis O86.29
  pyelonephritis O86.21
  pyelonephrosis O86.21
  pyemia O85
  pyocystitis O86.29
  pyohemia O85
  pyometra O86.12
  pyonephritis O86.21
  pyosalpingitis O86.19
  pyrexia (of unknown origin) O86.4
  renal
    disease NEC O90.89
    failure O90.4
  respiratory disease NEC O99.53
  retention
    decidua —*see* Retention, decidua
    placenta O72.0
    secundines —*see* Retention,
      secundines
  retrated nipple O92.02
  salpingo-ovaritis O86.19
  salpingoperitonitis O85
  secondary perineal tear O90.1
  sepsis O85
  sepsis (pelvic) O85
  septic thrombophlebitis O86.81
  skin disorder NEC O99.73
  specified condition NEC O99.893
  stroke O99.43
  subinvolution (uterus) O90.89
  subluxation of symphysis (pubis) O26.73
  suppuration —*see* Puerperal, abscess
  tetanus A34
  thelitis O91.02
    associated with lactation O91.03
  thrombocytopenia O72.3
  thrombophlebitis (superficial) O87.0
    deep O87.1
    pelvic O87.1
    septic O86.81
  thrombosis (venous) —*see* Thrombosis,
    puerperal
  thyroiditis O90.5
  toxemia (eclamptic) (pre-eclamptic)
    (with convulsions) O15.2
  trauma, non-obstetric O9A.23
    caused by abuse (physical) (suspected)
      O9A.33
      confirmed O9A.33
      psychological (suspected) O9A.53
        confirmed O9A.53
      sexual (suspected) O9A.43
        confirmed O9A.43
  uremia (due to renal failure) O90.4
  urethritis O86.22
  vaginitis O86.13
  varicose veins (legs) O87.4
    vulva or perineum O87.8
  venous O87.9
  vulvitis O86.19
  vulvovaginitis O86.13
  white leg O87.1
Puerperium —*see* Puerperal
Pulmolithiasis J98.4
Pulmonary —*see* condition
Pulpitis (acute) (anachoretic) (chronic)
  (hyperplastic) (putrescent) (suppurative)
  (ulcerative) K04.01
  irreversible K04.02
  reversible K04.01
Pulpless tooth K04.99

Pulse
  alternating R00.8
  bigeminal R00.8
  fast R00.0
  feeble, rapid due to shock following injury
    T79.4
  rapid R00.0
  weak R09.89
Pulsus alternans or trigeminus R00.8
Punch drunk F07.81
Punctum lacrimale occlusion —*see* Obstruction,
  lacrimal
Puncture
  abdomen, abdominal
    wall S31.139
      with
        foreign body S31.149
        penetration into peritoneal cavity
          S31.639
          with foreign body S31.649
      epigastric region S31.132
        with
          foreign body S31.142
          penetration into peritoneal cavity
            S31.632
            with foreign body S31.642
      left
        lower quadrant S31.134
          with
            foreign body S31.144
            penetration into peritoneal cavity
              S31.634
              with foreign body S31.644
        upper quadrant S31.131
          with
            foreign body S31.141
            penetration into peritoneal cavity
              S31.631
              with foreign body S31.641
      periumbilic region S31.135
        with
          foreign body S31.145
          penetration into peritoneal cavity
            S31.635
            with foreign body S31.645
      right
        lower quadrant S31.133
          with
            foreign body S31.143
            penetration into peritoneal cavity
              S31.633
              with foreign body S31.643
        upper quadrant S31.130
          with
            foreign body S31.140
            penetration into peritoneal cavity
              S31.630
              with foreign body S31.640
    accidental, complicating surgery —*see*
      Complication, accidental puncture or
      laceration
    alveolar (process) —*see* Puncture, oral cavity
    ankle S91.039
      with
        foreign body S91.049
      left S91.032
        with
          foreign body S91.042
      right S91.031
        with
          foreign body S91.041
    anus S31.833
      with foreign body S31.834
    arm (upper) S41.139
      with foreign body S41.149
      left S41.132
        with foreign body S41.142
      lower —*see* Puncture, forearm
      right S41.131
        with foreign body S41.141
    auditory canal (external) (meatus) —*see*
      Puncture, ear

Puncture *(Continued)*
  auricle, ear —*see* Puncture, ear
  axilla —*see* Puncture, arm
  back —*see also* Puncture, thorax, back
    lower S31.030
      with
        foreign body S31.040
          with penetration into
            retroperitoneal space S31.041
        penetration into retroperitoneal space
          S31.031
  bladder (traumatic) S37.29
    nontraumatic N32.89
  breast S21.039
    with foreign body S21.049
    left S21.032
      with foreign body S21.042
    right S21.031
      with foreign body S21.041
  buttock S31.803
    with foreign body S31.804
    left S31.823
      with foreign body S31.824
    right S31.813
      with foreign body S31.814
  by
    device, implant or graft —*see*
      Complications, by site and type,
      mechanical
    foreign body left accidentally in operative
      wound T81.539
    instrument (any) during a procedure,
      accidental —*see* Puncture, accidental
      complicating surgery
  calf —*see* Puncture, leg
  canaliculus lacrimalis —*see* Puncture, eyelid
  canthus, eye —*see* Puncture, eyelid
  cervical esophagus S11.23
    with foreign body S11.24
  cheek (external) S01.439
    with foreign body S01.449
    internal —*see* Puncture, oral cavity
    left S01.432
      with foreign body S01.442
    right S01.431
      with foreign body S01.441
  chest wall —*see* Puncture, thorax
  chin —*see* Puncture, head, specified site NEC
  clitoris —*see* Puncture, vulva
  costal region —*see* Puncture, thorax
  digit(s)
    foot —*see* Puncture, toe
    hand —*see* Puncture, finger
  ear (canal) (external) S01.339
    with foreign body S01.349
    drum S09.2-•
    left S01.332
      with foreign body S01.342
    right S01.331
      with foreign body S01.341
  elbow S51.039
    with
      foreign body S51.049
    left S51.032
      with
        foreign body S51.042
    right S51.031
      with
        foreign body S51.041
  epididymis —*see* Puncture, testis
  epigastric region —*see* Puncture, abdomen,
    wall, epigastric
  epiglottis S11.83
    with foreign body S11.84
  esophagus
    cervical S11.23
      with foreign body S11.24
    thoracic S27.818
  eyeball S05.6-•
    with foreign body S05.5-•

▶ New   ⇒ Revised   ~~deleted~~ Deleted   • Use Additional Character(s)

Puncture *(Continued)*
  ocular —*see* Puncture, eyeball - oral cavity
    S01.532
    with foreign body S01.542
  orbit S05.4-•
  palate —*see* Puncture, oral cavity
  palm —*see* Puncture, hand
  pancreas S36.299
    body S36.291
    head S36.290
    tail S36.292
  pelvis —*see* Puncture, back, lower
  penis S31.23
    with foreign body S31.24
  perineum
    female S31.43
      with foreign body S31.44
    male S31.139
      with foreign body S31.149
  periocular area (with or without lacrimal
    passages) —*see* Puncture, eyelid
  phalanges
    finger —*see* Puncture, finger
    toe —*see* Puncture, toe
  pharynx S11.23
    with foreign body S11.24
  pinna —*see* Puncture, ear
  popliteal space —*see* Puncture, knee
  prepuce —*see* Puncture, penis
  pubic region S31.139
    with foreign body S31.149
  pudendum —*see* Puncture, genital organs,
    external
  rectovaginal septum —*see* Puncture, vagina
  sacral region —*see* Puncture, back, lower
  sacroiliac region —*see* Puncture, back, lower
  salivary gland —*see* Puncture, oral cavity
  scalp S01.03
    with foreign body S01.04
  scapular region —*see* Puncture, shoulder
  scrotum S31.33
    with foreign body S31.34
  shin —*see* Puncture, leg
  shoulder S41.039
    with foreign body S41.049
    left S41.032
      with foreign body S41.042
    right S41.031
      with foreign body S41.041
  spermatic cord —*see* Puncture, testis
  sternal region —*see* Puncture, thorax, front
  submaxillary region —*see* Puncture, head,
    specified site NEC
  submental region —*see* Puncture, head,
    specified site NEC
  subungual
    finger(s) —*see* Puncture, finger, with
      damage to nail
    toe —*see* Puncture, toe, with damage to
      nail
  supraclavicular fossa —*see* Puncture, neck,
    specified site NEC
  temple, temporal region —*see* Puncture, head,
    specified site NEC
  temporomandibular area —*see* Puncture,
    cheek
  testis S31.33
    with foreign body S31.34
  thigh S71.139
    with foreign body S71.149
    left S71.132
      with foreign body S71.142
    right S71.131
      with foreign body S71.141
  thorax, thoracic (wall) S21.93
    with foreign body S21.94
    back S21.23-•
      with
        foreign body S21.24-•
          with penetration S21.44
        penetration S21.43

Puncture *(Continued)*
  thorax, thoracic *(Continued)*
    breast —*see* Puncture, breast
    front S21.13-•
      with
        foreign body S21.14-•
          with penetration S21.34
        penetration S21.33
  throat —*see* Puncture, neck
  thumb S61.039
    with
      damage to nail S61.139
        with
          foreign body S61.149
      foreign body S61.049
    left S61.032
      with
        damage to nail S61.132
          with
            foreign body S61.142
        foreign body S61.042
    right S61.031
      with
        damage to nail S61.131
          with
            foreign body S61.141
        foreign body S61.041
  thyroid gland S11.13
    with foreign body S11.14
  toe(s) S91.139
    with
      damage to nail S91.239
        with
          foreign body S91.249
      foreign body S91.149
    great S91.133
      with
        damage to nail S91.233
          with
            foreign body S91.243
        foreign body S91.143
      left S91.132
        with
          damage to nail S91.232
            with
              foreign body S91.242
          foreign body S91.142
      right S91.131
        with
          damage to nail S91.231
            with
              foreign body S91.241
          foreign body S91.141
    lesser S91.136
      with
        damage to nail S91.236
          with
            foreign body S91.246
        foreign body S91.146
      left S91.135
        with
          damage to nail S91.235
            with
              foreign body S91.245
          foreign body S91.145
      right S91.134
        with
          damage to nail S91.234
            with
              foreign body S91.244
          foreign body S91.144
  tongue —*see* Puncture, oral cavity
  trachea S11.023
    with foreign body S11.024
  tunica vaginalis —*see* Puncture, testis
  tympanum, tympanic membrane S09.2-•
  umbilical region S31.135
    with foreign body S31.145
  uvula —*see* Puncture, oral cavity
  vagina S31.43
    with foreign body S31.44

Puncture *(Continued)*
  vocal cords S11.033
    with foreign body S11.034
  vulva S31.43
    with foreign body S31.44
  wrist S61.539
    with
      foreign body S61.549
    left S61.532
      with
        foreign body S61.542
    right S61.531
      with
        foreign body S61.541
PUO (pyrexia of unknown origin) R50.9
Pupillary membrane (persistent) Q13.89
Pupillotonia —*see* Anomaly, pupil, function,
  tonic pupil
Purpura D69.2
  abdominal D69.0
  allergic D69.0
  anaphylactoid D69.0
  annularis telangiectodes L81.7
  arthritic D69.0
  autoerythrocyte sensitization D69.2
  autoimmune D69.0
  bacterial D69.0
  Bateman's (senile) D69.2
  capillary fragility (hereditary) (idiopathic)
    D69.8
  cryoglobulinemic D89.1
  Devil's pinches D69.2
  fibrinolytic —*see* Fibrinolysis
  fulminans, fulminous D65
  gangrenous D65
  hemorrhagic, hemorrhagica D69.3
    not due to thrombocytopenia D69.0
  Henoch (-Schönlein) (allergic) D69.0
  hypergammaglobulinemic (benign)
    (Waldenström's) D89.0
  idiopathic (thrombocytopenic) D69.3
    nonthrombocytopenic D69.0
  immune thrombocytopenic D69.3
  infectious D69.0
  malignant D69.0
  neonatorum P54.5
  nervosa D69.0
  newborn P54.5
  nonthrombocytopenic D69.2
    hemorrhagic D69.0
    idiopathic D69.0
  nonthrombopenic D69.2
  peliosis rheumatica D69.0
  posttransfusion (post-transfusion) (from
    (fresh) whole blood or blood products)
    D69.51
  primary D69.49
  red cell membrane sensitivity D69.2
  rheumatica D69.0
  Schönlein (-Henoch) (allergic) D69.0
  scorbutic E54 [D77]
  senile D69.2
  simplex D69.2
  symptomatica D69.0
  telangiectasia annularis L81.7
  thrombocytopenic D69.49
    congenital D69.42
    hemorrhagic D69.3
    hereditary D69.42
    idiopathic D69.3
    immune D69.3
    neonatal, transitory P61.0
    thrombotic M31.19
  thrombohemolytic —*see* Fibrinolysis
  thrombolytic —*see* Fibrinolysis
  thrombopenic D69.49
  thrombotic, thrombocytopenic
    M31.19
  toxic D69.0
  vascular D69.0
  visceral symptoms D69.0

Purpuric spots R23.3
Purulent —*see* condition
Pus
  in
    stool R19.5
    urine N39.0
  tube (rupture) —*see* Salpingo-oophoritis
Pustular rash L08.0
Pustule (nonmalignant) L08.9
  malignant A22.0
Pustulosis palmaris et plantaris
  L40.3
Putnam (-Dana) disease or syndrome —*see*
  Degeneration, combined
Putrescent pulp (dental) K04.1
Pyarthritis, pyarthrosis —*see* Arthritis,
  pyogenic or pyemic
  tuberculous —*see* Tuberculosis, joint
Pyelectasis —*see* Hydronephrosis
Pyelitis (congenital) (uremic) —*see also*
  Pyelonephritis
  with
    calculus —*see* category N20
      with hydronephrosis N13.6
    contracted kidney N11.9
  acute N10
  chronic N11.9
    with calculus —*see* category N20
      with hydronephrosis N13.6
  cystica N28.84
  puerperal (postpartum) O86.21
  tuberculous A18.11
Pyelocystitis —*see* Pyelonephritis
Pyelonephritis —*see also* Nephritis,
  tubulo-interstitial
  with
    calculus —*see* category N20
      with hydronephrosis N13.6
    contracted kidney N11.9
  acute N10
  calculus —*see* category N20
    with hydronephrosis N13.6
  chronic N11.9
    with calculus —*see* category N20
      with hydronephrosis N13.6
    associated with ureteral obstruction or
      stricture N11.1
    nonobstructive N11.8
      with reflux (vesicoureteral) N11.0
    obstructive N11.1
    specified NEC N11.8
  in (due to)
    brucellosis A23.9 *[N16]*
    cryoglobulinemia (mixed) D89.1 *[N16]*

Pyelonephritis *(Continued)*
  with *(Continued)*
    cystinosis E72.04
    diphtheria A36.84
    glycogen storage disease E74.09 *[N16]*
    leukemia NEC C95.9-● *[N16]*
    lymphoma NEC C85.90 *[N16]*
    multiple myeloma C90.0-● *[N16]*
    obstruction N11.1
    Salmonella infection A02.25
    sarcoidosis D86.84
    sepsis A41.9 *[N16]*
    Sjögren's disease M35.04
    toxoplasmosis B58.83
    transplant rejection T86.91 *[N16]*
    Wilson's disease E83.01 *[N16]*
  nonobstructive N12
    with reflux (vesicoureteral) N11.0
    chronic N11.8
  syphilitic A52.75
Pyelonephrosis (obstructive) N11.1
  chronic N11.9
Pyelophlebitis I80.8
Pyeloureteritis cystica N28.85
Pyemia, pyemic (fever) (infection) (purulent) —
  see also Sepsis
  joint —*see* Arthritis, pyogenic or pyemic
  liver K75.1
  pneumococcal A40.3
  portal K75.1
  postvaccinal T88.0
  puerperal, postpartum, childbirth O85
  specified organism NEC A41.89
  tuberculous —*see* Tuberculosis, miliary
Pygopagus Q89.4
Pyknoepilepsy (idiopathic) —*see* Pyknolepsy
Pyknolepsy G40.A09
  intractable G40.A19
    with status epilepticus G40.A11
    without status epilepticus G40.A19
  not intractable G40.A09
    with status epilepticus G40.A01
    without status epilepticus G40.A09
Pylephlebitis K75.1
Pyle's syndrome Q78.5
Pylethrombophlebitis K75.1
Pylethrombosis K75.1
Pyloritis K29.90
  with bleeding K29.91
Pylorospasm (reflex) NEC K31.3
  congenital or infantile Q40.0
  neurotic F45.8
  newborn Q40.0
  psychogenic F45.8

Pylorus, pyloric —*see* condition
Pyoarthrosis —*see* Arthritis, pyogenic or
  pyemic
Pyocele
  mastoid —*see* Mastoiditis, acute
  sinus (accessory) —*see* Sinusitis
  turbinate (bone) J32.9
  urethra —*see also* Urethritis N34.0
Pyocolpos —*see* Vaginitis
Pyocystitis N30.80
  with hematuria N30.81
Pyoderma, pyodermia L08.0
  gangrenosum L88
  newborn P39.4
  phagedenic L88
  vegetans L08.81
Pyodermatitis L08.0
  vegetans L08.81
Pyogenic —*see* condition
Pyohydronephrosis N13.6
Pyometra, pyometrium, pyometritis —*see*
  Endometritis
Pyomyositis (tropical) —*see* Myositis,
  infective
Pyonephritis N12
Pyonephrosis N13.6
  tuberculous A18.11
Pyo-oophoritis —*see* Salpingo-oophoritis
Pyo-ovarium —*see* Salpingo-oophoritis
Pyopericarditis, pyopericardium I30.1
Pyophlebitis —*see* Phlebitis
Pyopneumopericardium I30.1
Pyopneumothorax (infective) J86.9
  with fistula J86.0
  tuberculous NEC A15.6
Pyosalpinx, pyosalpingitis —*see also*
  Salpingo-oophoritis
Pyothorax J86.9
  with fistula J86.0
  tuberculous NEC A15.6
Pyoureter N28.89
  tuberculous A18.11
Pyramidopallidonigral syndrome G20
Pyrexia (of unknown origin) R50.9
  atmospheric T67.01
  during labor NEC O75.2
  heat T67.01
  newborn P81.9
    environmentally-induced P81.0
  persistent R50.9
  puerperal O86.4
Pyroglobulinemia NEC E88.09
Pyromania F63.1
Pyrosis R12
Pyuria (bacterial) R82.81

Q

Q fever A78
    with pneumonia A78
Quadricuspid aortic valve Q23.8
Quadrilateral fever A78
Quadriparesis —see Quadriplegia
    meaning muscle weakness M62.81
Quadriplegia G82.50-●
    complete
        C1-C4 level G82.51
        C5-C7 level G82.53
    congenital (cerebral) (spinal) G80.8
        spastic G80.0

Quadriplegia (Continued)
    embolic (current episode) I63.4-●
    functional R53.2
    incomplete
        C1-C4 level G82.52
        C5-C7 level G82.54
    thrombotic (current episode) I63.3-●
    traumatic — code to injury with seventh
        character S
        current episode —see Injury, spinal (cord),
            cervical
Quadruplet, pregnancy —see Pregnancy,
    quadruplet
Quarrelsomeness F60.3

Queensland fever A77.3
Quervain's disease M65.4
    thyroid E06.1
Queyrat's erythroplasia D07.4
    penis D07.4
    specified site —see Neoplasm, skin,
        in situ
    unspecified site D07.4
Quincke's disease or edema T78.3
    hereditary D84.1
Quinsy (gangrenous) J36
Quintan fever A79.0
Quintuplet, pregnancy —see Pregnancy,
    quintuplet

▶ New   ⇒ Revised   ~~deleted~~ Deleted   ● Use Additional Character(s)

R

Rabbit fever —*see* Tularemia
Rabies A82.9
  contact Z20.3
  exposure to Z20.3
  inoculation reaction —*see* Complications,
    vaccination
  sylvatic A82.0
  urban A82.1
Rachischisis —*see* Spina bifida
Rachitic —*see also* condition
  deformities of spine (late effect) (sequelae)
    E64.3
  pelvis (late effect) (sequelae) E64.3
    with disproportion (fetopelvic) O33.0
      causing obstructed labor O65.0
Rachitis, rachitism (acute) (tarda) —*see also*
    Rickets
  renalis N25.0
  sequelae E64.3
Radial nerve —*see* condition
Radiation
  burn —*see* Burn
  effects NOS T66
  sickness NOS T66
  therapy, encounter for Z51.0
Radiculitis (pressure) (vertebrogenic) —*see*
    Radiculopathy
Radiculomyelitis —*see also* Encephalitis
  toxic, due to
    Clostridium tetani A35
    Corynebacterium diphtheriae A36.82
Radiculopathy M54.10
  cervical region M54.12
  cervicothoracic region M54.13
  due to
    disc disorder
      C3 M50.11
      C4 M50.11
      C5 M50.121
      C6 M50.122
      C7 M50.123
      C8 M50.13
    displacement of intervertebral disc —*see*
      Disorder, disc, with, radiculopathy
  leg M54.1-•
  lumbar region M54.16
  lumbosacral region M54.17
  occipito-atlanto-axial region M54.11
  postherpetic B02.29
  sacrococcygeal region M54.18
  syphilitic A52.11
  thoracic region (with visceral pain)
    M54.14
  thoracolumbar region M54.15
Radiodermal burns (acute, chronic, or
    occupational) —*see* Burn
Radiodermatitis L58.9
  acute L58.0
  chronic L58.1
Radiotherapy session Z51.0
RAEB (refractory anemia with excess blasts)
    D46.2-•
Rage, meaning rabies —*see* Rabies
Ragpicker's disease A22.1
Ragsorter's disease A22.1
Raillietiniasis B71.8
Railroad neurosis F48.8
Railway spine F48.8
Raised —*see also* Elevated
  antibody titer R76.0
Rake teeth, tooth M26.39
Rales R09.89
Ramifying renal pelvis Q63.8
Ramsay-Hunt disease or syndrome —*see also*
    Hunt's disease B02.21
  meaning dyssynergia cerebellaris myoclonica
    G11.19
Ranula K11.6
  congenital Q38.4

Rape
  adult
    confirmed T74.21
    suspected T76.21
  alleged, observation or examination, ruled out
    adult Z04.41
    child Z04.42
  child
    confirmed T74.22
    suspected T76.22
Rapid
  feeble pulse, due to shock, following injury
    T79.4
  heart (beat) R00.0
    psychogenic F45.8
  second stage (delivery) O62.3
  time-zone change syndrome G47.25
Rarefaction, bone —*see* Disorder, bone, density
    and structure, specified NEC
Rash (toxic) R21
  canker A38.9
  diaper L22
  drug (internal use) L27.0
    contact —*see also* Dermatitis, due to, drugs,
      external L25.1
  following immunization T88.1
  food —*see* Dermatitis, due to, food
  heat L74.0
  napkin (psoriasiform) L22
  nettle —*see* Urticaria
  pustular L08.0
  rose R21
    epidemic B06.9
  scarlet A38.9
  serum —*see also* Reaction, serum T80.69
  wandering tongue K14.1
Rasmussen aneurysm —*see* Tuberculosis,
    pulmonary
Rasmussen encephalitis G04.81
Rat-bite fever A25.9
  due to Streptobacillus moniliformis A25.1
  spirochetal (morsus muris) A25.0
Rathke's pouch tumor D44.3
Raymond (-Céstan) syndrome I65.8
Raynaud's disease, phenomenon or syndrome
    (secondary) I73.00
  with gangrene (symmetric) I73.01
RDS (newborn) (type I) P22.0
  type II P22.1
Reaction —*see also* Disorder
  adaptation —*see* Disorder, adjustment
  adjustment (anxiety) (conduct disorder)
    (depressiveness) (distress) —*see*
      Disorder, adjustment
    with
      mutism, elective (child) (adolescent) F94.0
  adverse
    food (any) (ingested) NEC T78.1
      anaphylactic —*see* Shock, anaphylactic,
        due to food
  anaphylactoid —*see* Shock, anaphylactic
  affective —*see* Disorder, mood
  allergic —*see* Allergy
  anaphylactic —*see* Shock, anaphylactic
  anesthesia —*see* Anesthesia, complication
  antitoxin (prophylactic) (therapeutic) —*see*
    Complications, vaccination
  anxiety F41.1
  Arthus —*see* Arthus' phenomenon
  asthenic F48.8
  combat and operational stress F43.0
  compulsive F42.8
  conversion F44.9
  crisis, acute F43.0
  deoxyribonuclease (DNA) (DNase)
    hypersensitivity D69.2
  depressive (single episode) F32.9
    affective (single episode) F31.4
      recurrent episode F33.9
    neurotic F34.1
    psychoneurotic F34.1

Reaction *(Continued)*
  depressive *(Continued)*
    psychotic F32.3
    recurrent —*see* Disorder, depressive,
      recurrent
  dissociative F44.9
  drug NEC T88.7
    addictive —*see* Dependence, drug
      transmitted via placenta or breast
        milk —*see* Absorption, drug,
        addictive, through placenta
    allergic —*see* Allergy, drug
    lichenoid L43.2
    newborn P93.8
      gray baby syndrome P93.0
    overdose or poisoning (by accident) —*see*
      Table of Drugs and Chemicals, by
      drug, poisoning
    photoallergic L56.1
    phototoxic L56.0
    withdrawal —*see* Dependence, by drug,
      with, withdrawal
      infant of dependent mother P96.1
    newborn P96.1
    wrong substance given or taken (by
      accident) —*see* Table of Drugs and
      Chemicals, by drug, poisoning
  fear F40.9
    child (abnormal) F93.8
  febrile nonhemolytic transfusion (FNHTR)
    R50.84
  fluid loss, cerebrospinal G97.1
  foreign
    body NEC —*see* Granuloma, foreign body
      in operative wound (inadvertently
        left) —*see* Foreign body, accidentally
        left during a procedure
    substance accidentally left during a
      procedure (chemical) (powder) (talc)
      T81.60
        aseptic peritonitis T81.61
        body or object (instrument) (sponge)
          (swab) —*see* Foreign body,
          accidentally left during a
          procedure
        specified reaction NEC T81.69
  grief —*see* Disorder, adjustment
  Herxheimer's R68.89
  hyperkinetic —*see* Hyperkinesia
  hypochondriacal F45.20
  hypoglycemic, due to insulin E16.0
    with coma (diabetic) —*see* Diabetes, coma
    nondiabetic E15
    therapeutic misadventure —*see*
      subcategory T38.3
  hypomanic F30.8
  hysterical F44.9
  immunization —*see* Complications, vaccination
  incompatibility
    ABO blood group (infusion) (transfusion) —
      see Complication(s), transfusion,
      incompatibility reaction, ABO
        delayed serologic T80.39
    minor blood group (Duffy) (E) (K) (Kell)
      (Kidd) (Lewis) (M) (N) (P) (S)
      T80.89
    Rh (factor) (infusion) (transfusion) —
      see Complication(s), transfusion,
      incompatibility reaction, Rh (factor)
  inflammatory —*see* Infection
  infusion —*see* Complications, infusion
  inoculation (immune serum) —*see*
    Complications, vaccination
  insulin T38.3-•
  involutional psychotic —*see* Disorder,
    depressive
  leukemoid D72.823
    basophilic D72.823
    lymphocytic D72.823
    monocytic D72.823
    myelocytic D72.823
    neutrophilic D72.823

Reaction *(Continued)*
 LSD (acute)
  due to drug abuse —*see* Abuse, drug,
   hallucinogen
  due to drug dependence —*see* Dependence,
   drug, hallucinogen
 lumbar puncture G97.1
 manic-depressive —*see* Disorder, bipolar
 neurasthenic F48.8
 neurogenic —*see* Neurosis
 neurotic F48.9
 neurotic-depressive F34.1
 nitritoid —*see* Crisis, nitritoid - obsessive-
   compulsive F42
 nonspecific
  to
   cell mediated immunity measurement
    of gamma interferon antigen
    response without active
    tuberculosis R76.12
   QuantiFERON-TB test (QFT) without
    active tuberculosis R76.12
   tuberculin test —*see also* Reaction,
    tuberculin skin test R76.11
 obsessive-compulsive F42.8
 organic, acute or subacute —*see* Delirium
 paranoid (acute) F23
  chronic F22
  senile F03
 passive dependency F60.7
 phobic F40.9
 post-traumatic stress, uncomplicated Z73.3
 psychogenic F99
 psychoneurotic —*see also* Neurosis
  compulsive F42.8
  depersonalization F48.1
  depressive F34.1
  hypochondriacal F45.20
  neurasthenic F48.8
  obsessive F42.8
 psychophysiologic —*see* Disorder,
   somatoform
 psychosomatic —*see* Disorder, somatoform
 psychotic —*see* Psychosis
 scarlet fever toxin —*see* Complications,
   vaccination
 schizophrenic F23
  acute (brief) (undifferentiated) F23
  latent F21
  undifferentiated (acute) (brief) F23
 serological for syphilis —*see* Serology for
   syphilis
 serum T80.69
  anaphylactic (immediate) —*see also* Shock,
   anaphylactic T80.59
  specified reaction NEC
   due to
    administration of blood and blood
     products T80.61
    immunization T80.62
    serum specified NEC T80.69
    vaccination T80.62
 situational —*see* Disorder, adjustment
 somatization —*see* Disorder, somatoform
 spinal puncture G97.1
  dural G97.1
 stress (severe) F43.9
  acute (agitation) ("daze") (disorientation)
   (disturbance of consciousness) (flight
   reaction) (fugue) F43.0
  ⇒specified NEC F43.89
 surgical procedure —*see* Complications,
   surgical procedure
 tetanus antitoxin —*see* Complications,
   vaccination
 toxic, to local anesthesia T81.59
  in labor and delivery O74.4
  in pregnancy O29.3X-●
  postpartum, puerperal O89.3
 toxin-antitoxin —*see* Complications,
   vaccination

Reaction *(Continued)*
 transfusion (blood) (bone marrow)
   (lymphocytes) (allergic) —*see*
   Complications, transfusion
 tuberculin skin test, abnormal R76.11
 vaccination (any) —*see* Complications,
   vaccination
 withdrawing, child or adolescent F93.8
Reactive airway disease —*see* Asthma
Reactive depression —*see* Reaction, depressive
Rearrangement
 chromosomal
  balanced (in) Q95.9
   abnormal individual (autosomal) Q95.2
    non-sex (autosomal) chromosomes
     Q95.2
    sex/non-sex chromosomes Q95.3
    specified NEC Q95.8
Recalcitrant patient —*see* Noncompliance
Recanalization, thrombus —*see* Thrombosis
Recession, receding
 chamber angle (eye) H21.55-●
 chin M26.09
 gingival (postinfective) (postoperative)
  generalized K06.020
   minimal K06.021
   moderate K06.022
   severe K06.023
  localized K06.010
   minimal K06.011
   moderate K06.012
   severe K06.013
Recklinghausen's disease Q85.01
 bones E21.0
Reclus' disease (cystic) —*see* Mastopathy, cystic
Recrudescent typhus (fever) A75.1
Recruitment, auditory H93.21-●
Rectalgia K62.89
Rectitis K62.89
Rectocele
 female (without uterine prolapse) N81.6
  with uterine prolapse N81.4
   incomplete N81.2
 in pregnancy —*see* Pregnancy, complicated
   by, abnormal, pelvic organs or tissues
   NEC
 male K62.3
Rectosigmoid junction —*see* condition
Rectosigmoiditis K63.89
 ulcerative (chronic) K51.30
  with
   complication K51.319
    abscess K51.314
    fistula K51.313
    obstruction K51.312
    rectal bleeding K51.311
    specified NEC K51.318
Rectourethral —*see* condition
Rectovaginal —*see* condition
Rectovesical —*see* condition
Rectum, rectal —*see* condition
Recurrent —*see* condition
 pregnancy loss —*see* Loss (of), pregnancy,
   recurrent
Red bugs B88.0
Red-cedar lung or pneumonitis J67.8
Red tide —*see also* Table of Drugs and
   Chemicals T65.82-●
Reduced
 mobility Z74.09
 ventilatory or vital capacity R94.2
Redundant, redundancy
 anus (congenital) Q43.8
 clitoris N90.89
 colon (congenital) Q43.8
 foreskin (congenital) N47.8
 intestine (congenital) Q43.8
 labia N90.69
 organ or site, congenital NEC —*see* Accessory
 panniculus (abdominal) E65
 prepuce (congenital) N47.8

Redundant, redundancy *(Continued)*
 pylorus K31.89
 rectum (congenital) Q43.8
 scrotum N50.89
 sigmoid (congenital) Q43.8
 skin L98.7
  and subcutaneous tissue L98.7
  of face L57.4
  eyelids —*see* Blepharochalasis
 stomach K31.89
Reduplication —*see* Duplication
Reflex R29.2
 hyperactive gag J39.2
 pupillary, abnormal —*see* Anomaly, pupil,
   function
 vasoconstriction I73.9
 vasovagal R55
Reflux K21.9
 acid K21.9
 esophageal K21.9
  with esophagitis (without bleeding) K21.00
   with bleeding K21.01
  newborn P78.83
 gastroesophageal K21.9
  with esophagitis (without bleeding) K21.00
   with bleeding K21.01
 mitral —*see* Insufficiency, mitral
 ureteral —*see* Reflux, vesicoureteral
 vesicoureteral (with scarring) N13.70
  with
   nephropathy N13.729
    with hydroureter N13.739
     bilateral N13.732
     unilateral N13.731
    without hydroureter N13.729
     bilateral N13.722
     unilateral N13.721
    bilateral N13.722
    unilateral N13.721
   pyelonephritis (chronic) N11.0
  without nephropathy N13.71
  congenital Q62.7
Reforming, artificial openings —*see* Attention
   to, artificial, opening
Refractive error —*see* Disorder, refraction
Refsum's disease or syndrome G60.1
Refusal of
 food, psychogenic F50.89
 treatment (because of) Z53.20
  left against medical advice (AMA) Z53.29
  left without being seen Z53.21
  patient's decision NEC Z53.29
  reasons of belief or group pressure Z53.1
Regional —*see* condition
Regurgitation R11.10
 aortic (valve) —*see* Insufficiency, aortic
 food —*see also* Vomiting
  with reswallowing —*see* Rumination
  newborn P92.1
 gastric contents —*see* Vomiting
 heart —*see* Endocarditis
 mitral (valve) —*see* Insufficiency, mitral
  congenital Q23.3
 myocardial —*see* Endocarditis
 pulmonary (valve) (heart) I37.1
  congenital Q22.2
  syphilitic A52.03
 tricuspid —*see* Insufficiency, tricuspid
 valve, valvular —*see* Endocarditis
  congenital Q24.8
 vesicoureteral —*see* Reflux, vesicoureteral
Reichmann's disease or syndrome K31.89
Reifenstein syndrome E34.52
Reinsertion
 implantable subdermal contraceptive Z30.46
 intrauterine contraceptive device Z30.433
Reiter's disease, syndrome, or urethritis
   M02.30
 ankle M02.37-●
 elbow M02.32-●
 foot joint M02.37-●
 hand joint M02.34-●

Reiter's disease, syndrome, or urethritis
    (Continued)
  hip M02.35-●
  knee M02.36-●
  multiple site M02.39
  shoulder M02.31-●
  vertebra M02.38
  wrist M02.33-●
Rejection
  food, psychogenic F50.89
  transplant T86.91
    bone T86.830
      marrow T86.01
    cornea T86.840-●
    heart T86.21
      with lung(s) T86.31
    intestine T86.850
    kidney T86.11
    liver T86.41
    lung(s) T86.810
      with heart T86.31
    organ (immune or nonimmune cause)
      T86.91
    pancreas T86.890
    skin (allograft) (autograft) T86.820
    specified NEC T86.890
    stem cell (peripheral blood) (umbilical
      cord) T86.5
Relapsing fever A68.9
  Carter's (Asiatic) A68.1
  Dutton's (West African) A68.1
  Koch's A68.9
  louse-borne (epidemic) A68.0
  Novy's (American) A68.1
  Obermeyers's (European) A68.0
  Spirillum A68.9
  tick-borne (endemic) A68.1
Relationship
  occlusal
    open anterior M26.220
    open posterior M26.221
Relaxation
  anus (sphincter) K62.89
    psychogenic F45.8
  arch (foot) —*see also* Deformity, limb, flat foot
  back ligaments —*see* Instability, joint, spine
  bladder (sphincter) N31.2
  cardioesophageal K21.9
  cervix —*see* Incompetency, cervix
  diaphragm J98.6
  joint (capsule) (ligament) (paralytic) —*see*
    Flail, joint
    congenital NEC Q74.8
  lumbosacral (joint) —*see* subcategory M53.2
  pelvic floor N81.89
  perineum N81.89
  posture R29.3
  rectum (sphincter) K62.89
  sacroiliac (joint) —*see* subcategory M53.2
  scrotum N50.89
  urethra (sphincter) N36.44
  vesical N31.2
Release from prison, anxiety concerning Z65.2
Remains
  canal of Cloquet Q14.0
  capsule (opaque) Q14.8
Remittent fever (malarial) B54
Remnant
  canal of Cloquet Q14.0
  capsule (opaque) Q14.8
  cervix, cervical stump (acquired)
    (postoperative) N88.8
  cystic duct, postcholecystectomy K91.5
  fingernail L60.8
    congenital Q84.6
  meniscus, knee —*see* Derangement, knee,
    meniscus, specified NEC
  thyroglossal duct Q89.2
  tonsil J35.8
    infected (chronic) J35.01
  urachus Q64.4

Removal (from) (of)
  artificial
    arm Z44.00-●
      complete Z44.01-●
      partial Z44.02-●
    eye Z44.2-●
    leg Z44.10-●
      complete Z44.11-●
      partial Z44.12-●
  breast implant Z45.81
  cardiac pulse generator (battery) (end-of-life)
    Z45.010
  catheter (urinary) (indwelling) Z46.6
    from artificial opening —*see* Attention to,
      artificial, opening
    non-vascular Z46.82
    vascular NEC Z45.2
  device Z46.9
    contraceptive Z30.432
      implantable subdermal Z30.46
    implanted NEC Z45.89
    specified NEC Z46.89
  drains Z48.03
  dressing (nonsurgical) Z48.00
    surgical Z48.01
  external
    fixation device — code to fracture with
      seventh character D
    prosthesis, prosthetic device Z44.9
      breast Z44.3-●
      specified NEC Z44.8
  home in childhood (to foster home or
    institution) Z62.29
  ileostomy Z43.2
  insulin pump Z46.81
  myringotomy device (stent) (tube) Z45.82
  nervous system device NEC Z46.2
    brain neuropacemaker Z46.2
    visual substitution device Z46.2
      implanted Z45.31
  non-vascular catheter Z46.82
  organ, prophylactic (for neoplasia
    management) —*see* Prophylactic, organ
    removal
  orthodontic device Z46.4
  staples Z48.02
  stent
    ureteral Z46.6
  suture Z48.02
  urinary device Z46.6
  vascular access device or catheter Z45.2
Ren
  arcuatus Q63.1
  mobile, mobilis N28.89
    congenital Q63.8
  unguliformis Q63.1
Renal —*see* condition
Rendu-Osler-Weber disease or syndrome I78.0
Reninoma D41.0-●
Renon-Delille syndrome E23.3
Reovirus, as cause of disease classified
    elsewhere B97.5
Repeated falls NEC R29.6
Replaced chromosome by dicentric ring Q93.2
Replacement by artificial or mechanical device
    or prosthesis of
  bladder Z96.0
  blood vessel NEC Z95.828
  bone NEC Z96.7
  cochlea Z96.21
  coronary artery Z95.5
  eustachian tube Z96.29
  eye globe Z97.0
  heart Z95.812
    valve Z95.2
      prosthetic Z95.2
      specified NEC Z95.4
      xenogenic Z95.3
  intestine Z96.89
  joint Z96.60
    hip —*see* Presence, hip joint implant
    knee —*see* Presence, knee joint implant
    specified site NEC Z96.698

Replacement by artificial or mechanical device
    or prosthesis of *(Continued)*
  larynx Z96.3
  lens Z96.1
  limb(s) —*see* Presence, artificial, limb
  mandible NEC (for tooth root implant(s)) Z96.5
  organ NEC Z96.89
  peripheral vessel NEC Z95.828
  stapes Z96.29
  teeth Z97.2
  tendon Z96.7
  tissue NEC Z96.89
  tooth root(s) Z96.5
  vessel NEC Z95.828
    coronary (artery) Z95.5
Request for expert evidence Z04.89
Reserve, decreased or low
  cardiac —*see* Disease, heart
  kidney N28.89
Residing
  in place not meant for human habitation
    (abandoned building) (car) (park)
    (sidewalk) Z59.02
  on the street Z59.02
Residual —*see also* condition
  ovary syndrome N99.83
  state, schizophrenic F20.5
  urine R39.198
Resistance, resistant (to)
  activated protein C D68.51
  complicating pregnancy O26.89
  insulin E88.81
  organism(s)
    to
      drug Z16.30
        aminoglycosides Z16.29
        amoxicillin Z16.11
        ampicillin Z16.11
        antibiotic(s) Z16.20
          multiple Z16.24
          specified NEC Z16.29
        antifungal Z16.32
        antimicrobial (single) Z16.30
          multiple Z16.35
          specified NEC Z16.39
        antimycobacterial (single) Z16.341
          multiple Z16.342
        antiparasitic Z16.31
        antiviral Z16.33
        beta lactam antibiotics Z16.10
          specified NEC Z16.19
        cephalosporins Z16.19
        extended beta lactamase (ESBL) Z16.12
        fluoroquinolones Z16.23
        macrolides Z16.29
        methicillin —*see* MRSA
        multiple drugs (MDRO)
          antibiotics Z16.24
          antimicrobial Z16.35
          antimycobacterials Z16.342
        penicillins Z16.11
        quinine (and related compounds)
          Z16.31
        quinolones Z16.23
        sulfonamides Z16.29
        tetracyclines Z16.29
        tuberculostatics (single) Z16.341
          multiple Z16.342
        vancomycin Z16.21
          related antibiotics Z16.22
  thyroid hormone E07.89
Resorption
  dental (roots) K03.3
    alveoli M26.79
  teeth (external) (internal) (pathological)
    (roots) K03.3
Respiration
  Cheyne-Stokes R06.3
  decreased due to shock, following injury T79.4
  disorder of, psychogenic F45.8
  insufficient, or poor R06.89
    newborn P28.5

Respiration *(Continued)*
  painful R07.1
  sighing, psychogenic F45.8
Respiratory —*see also* condition
  distress syndrome (newborn) (type I) P22.0
    type II P22.1
  syncytial virus, as cause of disease classified
    elsewhere (*see also* Virus, respiratory
    syncytial (RSV)) B97.4
Respite care Z75.5
Response (drug)
  photoallergic L56.1
  phototoxic L56.0
Restenosis
  stent
    vascular
      end stent
        adjacent to stent —*see* Arteriosclerosis

        within the stent
          coronary T82.855
            peripheral T82.856
      in stent
        coronary vessel T82.855
        peripheral vessel T82.856
Restless legs (syndrome) G25.81
Restlessness R45.1
Restoration (of)
  dental
    aesthetically inadequate or displeasing
      K08.56
    defective K08.50
      specified NEC K08.59
    failure of marginal integrity K08.51
    failure of periodontal anatomical intergrity
      K08.54
  organ continuity from previous sterilization
    (tuboplasty) (vasoplasty) Z31.0
    aftercare Z31.42
  tooth (existing)
    contours biologically incompatible with
      oral health K08.54
    open margins K08.51
    overhanging K08.52
    poor aesthetic K08.56
    poor gingival margins K08.51
  unsatisfactory, of tooth K08.50
    specified NEC K08.59
Restorative material (dental)
  allergy to K08.55
  fractured K08.539
    with loss of material K08.531
    without loss of material K08.530
  unrepairable overhanging of K08.52
Restriction of housing space Z59.1
Rests, ovarian, in fallopian tube Q50.6
Restzustand (schizophrenic) F20.5
Retained —*see also* Retention
  cholelithiasis following cholecystectomy K91.86
  foreign body fragments (type of) Z18.9
    acrylics Z18.2
    animal quill(s) or spines Z18.31
    cement Z18.83
    concrete Z18.83
    crystalline Z18.83
    depleted isotope Z18.09
    depleted uranium Z18.01
    diethylhexyl phthalates Z18.2
    glass Z18.81
    isocyanate Z18.2
    magnetic metal Z18.11
    metal Z18.10
    nonmagnetic metal Z18.12
    nontherapeutic radioactive Z18.09
    organic NEC Z18.39
    plastic Z18.2
    quill(s) (animal) Z18.31
    radioactive (nontherapeutic) NEC Z18.09
    specified NEC Z18.89
    spine(s) (animal) Z18.31
    stone Z18.83
    tooth (teeth) Z18.32
    wood Z18.33

Retained *(Continued)*
  fragments (type of) Z18.9
    acrylics Z18.2
    animal quill(s) or spines Z18.31
    cement Z18.83
    concrete Z18.83
    crystalline Z18.83
    depleted isotope Z18.09
    depleted uranium Z18.01
    diethylhexyl phthalates Z18.2
    glass Z18.81
    isocyanate Z18.2
    magnetic metal Z18.11
    metal Z18.10
    nonmagnectic metal Z18.12
    nontherapeutic radioactive Z18.09
    organic NEC Z18.39
    plastic Z18.2
    quill(s) (animal) Z18.31
    radioactive (nontherapeutic) NEC Z18.09
    specified NEC Z18.89
    spine(s) (animal) Z18.31
    stone Z18.83
    tooth (teeth) Z18.32
    wood Z18.33
  gallstones, following cholecystectomy
    K91.86
Retardation
  development, developmental, specific —*see*
    Disorder, developmental
  endochondral bone growth —*see* Disorder,
    bone, development or growth
  growth R62.50
    due to malnutrition E45
  mental —*see* Disability, intellectual
  motor function, specific F82
  physical (child) R62.52
    due to malnutrition E45
  reading (specific) F81.0
  spelling (specific) (without reading disorder)
    F81.81
Retching —*see* Vomiting
Retention —*see also* Retained
  bladder —*see* Retention, urine
➤carbon dioxide E87.29
  cholelithiasis following cholecystectomy K91.86
  cyst —*see* Cyst
  dead
    fetus (at or near term) (mother) O36.4
      early fetal death O02.1
    ovum O02.0
  decidua (fragments) (following delivery)
    (with hemorrhage) O72.2
    without hemorrhage O73.1
  deciduous tooth K00.6
  dental root K08.3
  fecal —*see* Constipation
  fetus
    dead O36.4
      early O02.1
  fluid R60.9
  foreign body —*see also* Foreign body, retained
    current trauma - code as Foreign body, by
      site or type
  gallstones, following cholecystectomy K91.86
  gastric K31.89
  intrauterine contraceptive device, in
    pregnancy —*see* Pregnancy, complicated
    by, retention, intrauterine device
  membranes (complicating delivery) (with
    hemorrhage) O72.2
    with abortion —*see* Abortion, by type
    without hemorrhage O73.1
  meniscus —*see* Derangement, meniscus
  menses N94.89
  milk (puerperal, postpartum) O92.79
  nitrogen, extrarenal R39.2
  ovary syndrome N99.83
  placenta (total) (with hemorrhage) O72.0
    without hemorrhage O73.0
    portions or fragments (with hemorrhage)
      O72.2
      without hemorrhage O73.1

Retention *(Continued)*
  products of conception
    early pregnancy (dead fetus) O02.1
    following
      delivery (with hemorrhage) O72.2
        without hemorrhage O73.1
    secundines (following delivery) (with
      hemorrhage) O72.0
      without hemorrhage O73.0
    complicating puerperium (delayed
      hemorrhage) O72.2
    partial O72.2
      without hemorrhage O73.1
  smegma, clitoris N90.89
  urine R33.9
    drug-induced R33.0
    due to hyperplasia (hypertrophy) of
      prostate —*see* Hyperplasia, prostate
    organic R33.8
      drug-induced R33.0
    psychogenic F45.8
    specified NEC R33.8
  water (in tissues) —*see* Edema
Reticular erythematous mucinosis L98.5
Reticulation, dust —*see* Pneumoconiosis
Reticulocytosis R70.1
Reticuloendotheliosis
  acute infantile C96.0
  leukemic C91.4-●
  nonlipid C96.0
Reticulohistiocytoma (giant-cell) D76.3
Reticuloid, actinic L57.1
Reticulosis (skin)
  acute of infancy C96.0
  hemophagocytic, familial D76.1
  histiocytic medullary C96.A
  lipomelanotic I89.8
  malignant (midline) C86.0
  polymorphic C86.0
  Sézary —*see* Sézary disease
Retina, retinal —*see also* condition
  dark area D49.81
Retinitis —*see also* Inflammation, chorioretinal
  albuminurica N18.9 *[H32]*
  diabetic —*see* Diabetes, retinitis
  disciformis —*see* Degeneration, macula
  focal —*see* Inflammation, chorioretinal, focal
  gravidarum —*see* Pregnancy, complicated by,
    specified pregnancy-related condition
    NEC
  juxtapapillaris —*see* Inflammation,
    chorioretinal, focal, juxtapapillary
  luetic —*see* Retinitis, syphilitic
  pigmentosa H35.52
  proliferans —*see* Disorder, globe,
    degenerative, specified type NEC
  proliferating —*see* Disorder, globe,
    degenerative, specified type NEC
  renal N18.9 *[H32]*
  syphilitic (early) (secondary) A51.43
    central, recurrent A52.71
    congenital (early) A50.01 *[H32]*
    late A52.71
  tuberculous A18.53
Retinoblastoma C69.2-●
  differentiated C69.2-●
  undifferentiated C69.2-●
Retinochoroiditis —*see also* Inflammation,
    chorioretinal
  disseminated —*see* Inflammation,
    chorioretinal, disseminated
    syphilitic A52.71
  focal —*see* Inflammation, chorioretinal
  juxtapapillaris —*see* Inflammation,
    chorioretinal, focal, juxtapapillary
Retinopathy (background) H35.00
  arteriosclerotic I70.8 *[H35.0-●]*
  atherosclerotic I70.8 *[H35.0-●]*
  central serous —*see* Chorioretinopathy,
    central serous
  Coats H35.02-●

▶ New   ➡ Revised   ~~deleted~~ Deleted   ● Use Additional Character(s)

Retinopathy (Continued)
diabetic —see Diabetes, retinopathy
exudative H35.02-●
hypertensive H35.03-●
in (due to)
  diabetes —see Diabetes, retinopathy
sickle-cell disorders D57.-● [H36]
of prematurity H35.10-●
  stage 0 H35.11-●
  stage 1 H35.12-●
  stage 2 H35.13-●
  stage 3 H35.14-●
  stage 4 H35.15-●
  stage 5 H35.16-●
pigmentary, congenital —see Dystrophy,
  retina
proliferative NEC H35.2-●
  diabetic —see Diabetes, retinopathy,
    proliferative
  sickle-cell D57.-● [H36]
solar H31.02-●
Retinoschisis H33.10-●
congenital Q14.1
specified type NEC H33.19-●
Retortamoniasis A07.8
Retractile testis Q55.22
Retraction
cervix —see Retroversion, uterus
drum (membrane) —see Disorder, tympanic
  membrane, specified NEC
finger —see Deformity, finger
lid H02.539
  left H02.536
    lower H02.535
    upper H02.534
  right H02.533
    lower H02.532
    upper H02.531
lung J98.4
mediastinum J98.59
nipple N64.53
  associated with
    lactation O92.03
    pregnancy O92.01-●
    puerperium O92.02
  congenital Q83.8
palmar fascia M72.0
pleura —see Pleurisy
ring, uterus (Bandl's) (pathological)
  O62.4
sternum (congenital) Q76.7
  acquired M95.4
uterus —see Retroversion, uterus
valve (heart) —see Endocarditis
Retrobulbar —see condition
Retrocecal —see condition
Retrocession —see Retroversion
Retrodisplacement —see Retroversion
Retroflection, retroflexion —see Retroversion
Retrognathia, retrognathism (mandibular)
  (maxillary) M26.19
Retrograde menstruation N92.5
Retroperineal —see condition
Retroperitoneal —see condition
Retroperitonitis K68.9
Retropharyngeal —see condition
Retroplacental —see condition
Retroposition —see Retroversion
Retroprosthetic membrane T85.398
Retrosternal thyroid (congenital)
  Q89.2
Retroversion, retroverted
cervix —see Retroversion, uterus
female NEC —see Retroversion, uterus
iris H21.89
testis (congenital) Q55.29
uterus (acquired) (acute) (any degree)
  (asymptomatic) (cervix) (postinfectional)
  (postpartal, old) N85.4
  congenital Q51.818
  in pregnancy O34.53-●

Retrovirus, as cause of disease classified
  elsewhere B97.30
human
  immunodeficiency, type 2 (HIV 2) B97.35
  T-cell lymphotropic
    type I (HTLV-I) B97.33
    type II (HTLV-II) B97.34
lentivirus B97.31
oncovirus B97.32
specified NEC B97.39
Retrusion, premaxilla (developmental) M26.09
Rett's disease or syndrome F84.2
Reverse peristalsis R19.2
Reye's syndrome G93.7
Rh (factor)
hemolytic disease (newborn) P55.0
incompatibility, immunization or sensitization
  affecting management of pregnancy NEC
    O36.09-●
    anti-D antibody O36.01-●
  newborn P55.0
  transfusion reaction —see Complication(s),
    transfusion, incompatibility reaction,
    Rh (factor)
negative mother affecting newborn P55.0
titer elevated —see Complication(s),
  transfusion, incompatibility reaction, Rh
  (factor)
transfusion reaction —see Complication(s),
  transfusion, incompatibility reaction, Rh
  (factor)
Rhabdomyolysis (idiopathic) NEC M62.82
traumatic T79.6
Rhabdomyoma —see also Neoplasm, connective
  tissue, benign
adult —see Neoplasm, connective tissue, benign
fetal —see Neoplasm, connective tissue, benign
glycogenic —see Neoplasm, connective tissue,
  benign
Rhabdomyosarcoma (any type) —see
  Neoplasm, connective tissue, malignant
Rhabdosarcoma —see Rhabdomyosarcoma
Rhesus (factor) **incompatibility** —see Rh,
  incompatibility
Rheumatic (acute) (subacute)
adherent pericardium I09.2
chronic I09.89
coronary arteritis I01.8
degeneration, myocardium I09.0
fever (acute) —see Fever, rheumatic
heart —see Disease, heart, rheumatic
myocardial degeneration —see Degeneration,
  myocardium
myocarditis (chronic) (inactive) (with chorea)
  I09.0
  with chorea (acute) (rheumatic)
    (Sydenham's) I02.0
  active or acute I01.2
pancarditis, acute I01.8
  with chorea (acute (rheumatic)
    Sydenham's) I02.0
pericarditis (active) (acute) (with effusion)
  (with pneumonia) I01.0
  with chorea (acute) (rheumatic)
    (Sydenham's) I02.0
  chronic or inactive I09.2
pneumonia I00 [J17]
torticollis M43.6
typhoid fever A01.09
Rheumatism (articular) (neuralgic)
  (nonarticular) M79.0
gout —see Arthritis, rheumatoid
intercostal, meaning Tietze's disease M94.0
palindromic (any site) M12.30
  ankle M12.37-●
  elbow M12.32-●
  foot joint M12.37-●
  hand joint M12.34-●
  hip M12.35-●
  knee M12.36-●
  multiple site M12.39

Rheumatism (Continued)
palindromic (Continued)
  shoulder M12.31-●
  specified joint NEC M12.38
  vertebrae M12.38
  wrist M12.33-●
sciatic M54.4-●
Rheumatoid —see also condition
arthritis —see also Arthritis, rheumatoid
  with involvement of organs NEC M05.60
    ankle M05.67-●
    elbow M05.62-●
    foot joint M05.67-●
    hand joint M05.64-●
    hip M05.65-●
    knee M05.66-●
    multiple site M05.69
    shoulder M05.61-●
    vertebra —see Spondylitis, ankylosing
    wrist M05.63-●
  seronegative —see Arthritis, rheumatoid,
    seronegative
  seropositive —see Arthritis, rheumatoid,
    seropositive
carditis M05.30
  ankle M05.37-●
  elbow M05.32-●
  foot joint M05.37-●
  hand joint M05.34-●
  hip M05.35-●
  knee M05.36-●
  multiple site M05.39
  shoulder M05.31-●
  vertebra —see Spondylitis, ankylosing
  wrist M05.33-●
endocarditis —see Rheumatoid, carditis
lung (disease) M05.10
  ankle M05.17-●
  elbow M05.12-●
  foot joint M05.17-●
  hand joint M05.14-●
  hip M05.15-●
  knee M05.16-●
  multiple site M05.19
  shoulder M05.11-●
  vertebra —see Spondylitis, ankylosing
  wrist M05.13-●
myocarditis —see Rheumatoid, carditis
myopathy M05.40
  ankle M05.47-●
  elbow M05.42-●
  foot joint M05.47-●
  hand joint M05.44-●
  hip M05.45-●
  knee M05.46-●
  multiple site M05.49
  shoulder M05.41-●
  vertebra —see Spondylitis, ankylosing
  wrist M05.43-●
pericarditis —see Rheumatoid, carditis
polyarthritis —see Arthritis, rheumatoid
polyneuropathy M05.50
  ankle M05.57-●
  elbow M05.52-●
  foot joint M05.57-●
  hand joint M05.54-●
  hip M05.55-●
  knee M05.56-●
  multiple site M05.59
  shoulder M05.51-●
  vertebra —see Spondylitis, ankylosing
  wrist M05.53-●
vasculitis M05.20
  ankle M05.27-●
  elbow M05.22-●
  foot joint M05.27-●
  hand joint M05.24-●
  hip M05.25-●
  knee M05.26-●
  multiple site M05.29
  shoulder M05.21-●
  vertebra —see Spondylitis, ankylosing
  wrist M05.23-●

R

Rhinitis (atrophic) (catarrhal) (chronic)
(croupous) (fibrinous) (granulomatous)
(hyperplastic) (hypertrophic)
(membranous) (obstructive) (purulent)
(suppurative) (ulcerative) J31.0
  with
    sore throat —see Nasopharyngitis
  acute J00
  allergic J30.9
    with asthma J45.909
      with
        exacerbation (acute) J45.901
        status asthmaticus J45.902
      due to
        food J30.5
        pollen J30.1
      nonseasonal J30.89
      perennial J30.89
      seasonal NEC J30.2
      specified NEC J30.89
  infective J00
  pneumococcal J00
  syphilitic A52.73
    congenital A50.05 [J99]
  tuberculous A15.8
  vasomotor J30.0
Rhinoantritis (chronic) —see Sinusitis, maxillary
Rhinodacryolith —see Dacryolith
Rhinolith (nasal sinus) J34.89
Rhinomegaly J34.89
Rhinopharyngitis (acute) (subacute) —see also
    Nasopharyngitis
  chronic J31.1
  destructive ulcerating A66.5
  mutilans A66.5
Rhinophyma L71.1
Rhinorrhea J34.89
  cerebrospinal (fluid) G96.01
    postoperative G96.08
    specified NEC G96.08
    spontaneous G96.01
    traumatic G96.08
  paroxysmal —see Rhinitis, allergic
  spasmodic —see Rhinitis, allergic
Rhinosalpingitis —see Salpingitis, eustachian
Rhinoscleroma A48.8
Rhinosporidiosis B48.1
Rhinovirus infection NEC B34.8
Rhizomelic chondrodysplasia punctata E71.540
Rhythm
  atrioventricular nodal I49.8
  disorder I49.9
    coronary sinus I49.8
    ectopic I49.8
    nodal I49.8
  escape I49.9
  heart, abnormal I49.9
  idioventricular I44.2
  nodal I49.8
  sleep, inversion G47.2-●
    nonorganic origin —see Disorder, sleep,
      circadian rhythm, psychogenic
Rhytidosis facialis L98.8
Rib —see also condition
  cervical Q76.5
Riboflavin deficiency E53.0
Rice bodies —see also Loose, body, joint
  knee M23.4-●
Richter syndrome —see Leukemia, chronic
  lymphocytic, B-cell type
Richter's hernia —see Hernia, abdomen, with
  obstruction
Ricinism —see Poisoning, food, noxious, plant
Rickets (active) (acute) (adolescent) (chest wall)
  (congenital) (current) (infantile) (intestinal)
  E55.0
  adult —see Osteomalacia
  celiac K90.0
  hypophosphatemic with nephrotic-glycosuric
    dwarfism E72.09
  inactive E64.3
  kidney N25.0

Rickets (Continued)
  renal N25.0
  sequelae, any E64.3
  vitamin-D-resistant E83.31 [M90.80]
Rickettsia 364D/R. philipii (Pacific Coast tick
  fever) A77.8
Rickettsial disease A79.9
  specified type NEC A79.89
Rickettsialpox (Rickettsia akari) A79.1
Rickettsiosis A79.9
  due to
    Ehrlichia sennetsu A79.81
    Neorickettsia sennetsu A79.81
    Rickettsia akari (rickettsialpox) A79.1
  specified type NEC A79.89
  tick-borne A77.9
  vesicular A79.1
Rider's bone —see Ossification, muscle,
  specified NEC
Ridge, alveolus —see also condition
  flabby K06.8
Ridged ear, congenital Q17.3
Riedel's
  lobe, liver Q44.7
  struma, thyroiditis or disease E06.5
Rieger's anomaly or syndrome Q13.81
Riehl's melanosis L81.4
Rietti-Greppi-Micheli anemia D56.9
Rieux's hernia —see Hernia, abdomen, specified
  site NEC
Riga (-Fede) disease K14.0
Riggs' disease —see Periodontitis
Right aortic arch Q25.47
Right middle lobe syndrome J98.11
Rigid, rigidity —see also condition
  abdominal R19.30
    with severe abdominal pain R10.0
    epigastric R19.36
    generalized R19.37
    left lower quadrant R19.34
    left upper quadrant R19.32
    periumbilic R19.35
    right lower quadrant R19.33
    right upper quadrant R19.31
  articular, multiple, congenital Q68.8
  cervix (uteri) in pregnancy —see Pregnancy,
    complicated by, abnormal, cervix
  hymen (acquired) (congenital) N89.6
  nuchal R29.1
  pelvic floor in pregnancy —see Pregnancy,
    complicated by, abnormal, pelvic organs
    or tissues NEC
  perineum or vulva in pregnancy —see
    Pregnancy, complicated by, abnormal,
    vulva
  spine —see Dorsopathy, specified NEC
  vagina in pregnancy —see Pregnancy,
    complicated by, abnormal, vagina
Rigors R68.89
  with fever R50.9
Riley-Day syndrome G90.1
RIND (reversible ischemic neurologic deficit)
  I63.9
Ring(s)
  aorta (vascular) Q25.45
  Bandl's O62.4
  contraction, complicating delivery O62.4
  esophageal, lower (muscular) K22.2
  Fleischer's (cornea) H18.04-●
  hymenal, tight (acquired) (congenital) N89.6
  Kayser-Fleischer (cornea) H18.04-●
  retraction, uterus, pathological O62.4
  Schatzki's (esophagus) (lower) K22.2
    congenital Q39.3
  Soemmerring's —see Cataract, secondary
  vascular (congenital) Q25.8
    aorta Q25.45
Ringed hair (congenital) Q84.1
Ringworm B35.9
  beard B35.0
  black dot B35.0
  body B35.4

Ringworm (Continued)
  Burmese B35.5
  corporeal B35.4
  foot B35.3
  groin B35.6
  hand B35.2
  honeycomb B35.0
  nails B35.1
  perianal (area) B35.6
  scalp B35.0
  specified NEC B35.8
  Tokelau B35.5
Rise, venous pressure I87.8
Rising, PSA following treatment for malignant
  neoplasm of prostate R97.21
Risk
  for
    dental caries Z91.849
      high Z91.843
      low Z91.841
      moderate Z91.842
    homelessness, imminent Z59.811
  ▶suffocation (smothering) under another while
    sleeping Z72.823
  suicidal
    meaning personal history of attempted
      suicide Z91.51
    meaning suicidal ideation —see Ideation,
      suicidal
Ritter's disease L00
Rivalry, sibling Z62.891
Rivalta's disease A42.2
River blindness B73.01
Robert's pelvis Q74.2
  with disproportion (fetopelvic) O33.0
    causing obstructed labor O65.0
Robin (-Pierre) syndrome Q87.0
Robinow-Silvermann-Smith syndrome Q87.19
Robinson's (hidrotic) ectodermal dysplasia or
  syndrome Q82.4
Robles' disease B73.01
Rocky Mountain (spotted) fever A77.0
Roetheln —see Rubella
Roger's disease Q21.0
Rokitansky-Aschoff sinuses (gallbladder) K82.8
Rolando's fracture (displaced) S62.22-●
  nondisplaced S62.22-●
Romano-Ward (prolonged QT interval)
  syndrome I45.81
Romberg's disease or syndrome G51.8
Roof, mouth —see condition
Rosacea L71.9
  acne L71.9
  keratitis L71.8
  specified NEC L71.8
Rosary, rachitic E55.0
Rose
  cold J30.1
  fever J30.1
  rash R21
    epidemic B06.9
Rosenbach's erysipeloid A26.0
Rosenthal's disease or syndrome D68.1
Roseola B09
  infantum B08.20
    due to human herpesvirus 6 B08.21
    due to human herpesvirus 7 B08.22
Ross River disease or fever B33.1
Rossbach's disease K31.89
  psychogenic F45.8
Rostan's asthma (cardiac) —see Failure,
  ventricular, left
Rotation
  anomalous, incomplete or insufficient,
    intestine Q43.3
  cecum (congenital) Q43.3
  colon (congenital) Q43.3
  spine, incomplete or insufficient —see
    Dorsopathy, deforming, specified NEC
  tooth, teeth, fully erupted M26.35
  vertebra, incomplete or insufficient —see
    Dorsopathy, deforming, specified NEC

▶ New   ⇒ Revised   ~~deleted~~ Deleted   ● Use Additional Character(s)

Rotes Quérol disease or syndrome —see
Hyperostosis, ankylosing
Roth (-Bernhardt) disease or syndrome —see
Meralgia paraesthetica
Rothmund (-Thomson) syndrome Q82.8
Rotor's disease or syndrome E80.6
Round
back (with wedging of vertebrae) —see
Kyphosis
sequelae (late effect) of rickets E64.3
worms (large) (infestation) NEC B82.0
Ascariasis —see also Ascariasis B77.9
Roussy-Lévy syndrome G60.0
Rubella (German measles) B06.9
complication NEC B06.09
neurological B06.00
congenital P35.0
contact Z20.4
exposure to Z20.4
maternal
care for (suspected) damage to fetus O35.3
manifest rubella in infant P35.0
suspected damage to fetus affecting
management of pregnancy O35.3
specified complications NEC B06.89
Rubeola (meaning measles) —see Measles
meaning rubella —see Rubella
Rubeosis, iris —see Disorder, iris, vascular
Rubinstein-Taybi syndrome Q87.2
Rudimentary (congenital) —see also Agenesis
arm —see Defect, reduction, upper limb
bone Q79.9
cervix uteri Q51.828
eye Q11.2
lobule of ear Q17.3
patella Q74.1
respiratory organs in thoracopagus Q89.4
tracheal bronchus Q32.4
uterus Q51.818
in male Q56.1
vagina Q52.0
Ruled out condition —see Observation,
suspected
Rumination R11.10
with nausea R11.2
disorder of infancy F98.21
neurotic F42.8
newborn P92.1
obsessional F42.8
psychogenic F42.8
Runeberg's disease D51.0
Runny nose R09.89
▶Running out of money Z59.86
Rupia (syphilitic) A51.39
congenital A50.06
tertiary A52.79
Rupture, ruptured
abscess (spontaneous) - code by site under
Abscess
aneurysm —see Aneurysm
anus (sphincter) —see Laceration, anus
aorta, aortic I71.8
abdominal I71.30
infrarenal I71.33
juxtarenal I71.32
pararenal I71.31
arch I71.12
ascending I71.11
descending I71.8
abdominal I71.30
thoracic I71.13
syphilitic A52.01
thoracoabdominal I71.50
paravisceral I71.52
supraceliac I71.51
thorax, thoracic I71.10
transverse I71.12
traumatic —see Injury, aorta, laceration,
major
valve or cusp —see also Endocarditis, aortic
I35.8

Rupture, ruptured (Continued)
appendix (with peritonitis) (see also
Appendicitis) K35.32
with localized peritonitis (see also
Appendicitis) K35.32
arteriovenous fistula, brain —see Fistula,
arteriovenous, brain, ruptured
artery I77.2
brain —see Hemorrhage, intracranial,
intracerebral
coronary —see Infarct, myocardium
heart —see Infarct, myocardium
pulmonary I28.8
traumatic (complication) —see Injury,
blood vessel
bile duct (common) (hepatic) K83.2
cystic K82.2
bladder (sphincter) (nontraumatic)
(spontaneous) N32.89
following ectopic or molar pregnancy
O08.6
obstetrical trauma O71.5
traumatic S37.29
blood vessel —see also Hemorrhage
brain —see Hemorrhage, intracranial,
intracerebral
heart —see Infarct, myocardium
traumatic (complication) —see Injury,
blood vessel, laceration, major, by site
bone —see Fracture
bowel (nontraumatic) K63.1
brain
aneurysm (congenital) —see also
Hemorrhage, intracranial, subarachnoid
syphilitic A52.05
hemorrhagic —see Hemorrhage,
intracranial, intracerebral
capillaries I78.8
cardiac (auricle) (ventricle) (wall) I23.3
with hemopericardium I23.0
infectional I40.9
traumatic —see Injury, heart
cartilage (articular) (current) —
see also Sprain
knee S83.3-●
semilunar —see Tear, meniscus
cecum (with peritonitis) K65.0
with peritoneal abscess K35.33
traumatic S36.598
celiac artery, traumatic —see Injury, blood
vessel, celiac artery, laceration, major
cerebral aneurysm (congenital) (see
Hemorrhage, intracranial, subarachnoid)
cervix (uteri)
with ectopic or molar pregnancy O08.6
following ectopic or molar pregnancy
O08.6
obstetrical trauma O71.3
traumatic S37.69
chordae tendineae NEC I51.1
concurrent with acute myocardial
infarction —see Infarct, myocardium
following acute myocardial infarction
(current complication) I23.4
choroid (direct) (indirect) (traumatic)
H31.32-●
circle of Willis I60.6
colon (nontraumatic) K63.1
traumatic —see Injury, intestine, large
cornea (traumatic) —see Injury, eye, laceration
coronary (artery) (thrombotic) —see Infarct,
myocardium
corpus luteum (infected) (ovary) N83.1-●
cyst —see Cyst
cystic duct K82.2
Descemet's membrane —see Change, corneal
membrane, Descemet's, rupture
traumatic —see Injury, eye, laceration
diaphragm, traumatic —see Injury,
intrathoracic, diaphragm
disc —see Rupture, intervertebral disc

Rupture, ruptured (Continued)
diverticulum (intestine) K57.80
with bleeding K57.81
bladder N32.3
large intestine K57.20
with
bleeding K57.21
small intestine K57.40
with bleeding K57.41
small intestine K57.00
with
bleeding K57.01
large intestine K57.40
with bleeding K57.41
duodenal stump K31.89
ear drum (nontraumatic) —see also
Perforation, tympanum
traumatic S09.2-●
due to blast injury —see Injury,
blast, ear
esophagus K22.3
eye (without prolapse or loss of intraocular
tissue) —see Injury, eye, laceration
fallopian tube NEC (nonobstetric)
(nontraumatic) N83.8
due to pregnancy O00.10-●
with intrauterine pregnancy O00.11-●
fontanel P13.1
gallbladder K82.2
traumatic S36.128
gastric —see also Rupture, stomach
vessel K92.2
globe (eye) (traumatic) —see Injury, eye,
laceration
graafian follicle (hematoma) N83.0-●
heart —see Rupture, cardiac
hymen (nontraumatic) (nonintentional)
N89.8
internal organ, traumatic —see Injury,
by site
intervertebral disc —see Displacement,
intervertebral disc
traumatic —see Rupture, traumatic,
intervertebral disc
intestine NEC (nontraumatic) K63.1
traumatic —see Injury, intestine
iris —see also Abnormality, pupillary
traumatic —see Injury, eye, laceration
joint capsule, traumatic —see Sprain
kidney (traumatic) S37.06-●
birth injury P15.8
nontraumatic N28.89
lacrimal duct (traumatic) —see Injury, eye,
specified site NEC
lens (cataract) (traumatic) —see Cataract,
traumatic
ligament, traumatic —see Rupture, traumatic,
ligament, by site
liver S36.116
birth injury P15.0
lymphatic vessel I89.8
marginal sinus (placental) (with
hemorrhage) —see Hemorrhage,
antepartum, specified cause NEC
membrana tympani (nontraumatic) —see
Perforation, tympanum
membranes (spontaneous)
artificial
delayed delivery following O75.5
delayed delivery following —see
Pregnancy, complicated by, premature
rupture of membranes
meningeal artery I60.8
meniscus (knee) —see also Tear, meniscus
old —see Derangement, meniscus
site other than knee - code as Sprain
mesenteric artery, traumatic —see Injury,
mesenteric, artery, laceration, major
mesentery (nontraumatic) K66.8
traumatic —see Injury, intra-abdominal,
specified, site NEC

Rupture, ruptured *(Continued)*
mitral (valve) I34.89
muscle (traumatic) —*see also* Strain
diastasis —*see* Diastasis, muscle
nontraumatic M62.10
ankle M62.17-•
foot M62.17-•
forearm M62.13-•
hand M62.14-•
lower leg M62.16-•
pelvic region M62.15-•
shoulder region M62.11-•
specified site NEC M62.18
thigh M62.15-•
upper arm M62.12-•
traumatic —*see* Strain, by site
musculotendinous junction NEC,
nontraumatic —*see* Rupture, tendon,
spontaneous
mycotic aneurysm causing cerebral
hemorrhage —*see* Hemorrhage,
intracranial, subarachnoid
myocardium, myocardial —*see* Rupture,
cardiac
traumatic —*see* Injury, heart
nontraumatic, meaning hernia —*see* Hernia
obstructed —*see* Hernia, by site, obstructed
operation wound —*see* Disruption, wound,
operation
ovary, ovarian N83.8
corpus luteum cyst N83.1-•
follicle (graafian) N83.0-•
oviduct (nonobstetric) (nontraumatic) N83.8
due to pregnancy O00.10-•
with intrauterine pregnancy O00.11-•
pancreas (nontraumatic) K86.89
traumatic S36.299
papillary muscle NEC I51.2
following acute myocardial infarction
(current complication) I23.5
pelvic
floor, complicating delivery O70.1
organ NEC, obstetrical trauma O71.5
perineum (nonobstetric) (nontraumatic)
N90.89
complicating delivery —*see* Delivery,
complicated, by, laceration, anus
(sphincter)
postoperative wound —*see* Disruption,
wound, operation
prostate (traumatic) S37.828
pulmonary
artery I28.8
valve (heart) I37.8
vein I28.8
vessel I28.8
pus tube —*see* Salpingitis
pyosalpinx —*see* Salpingitis
rectum (nontraumatic) K63.1
traumatic S36.69
retina, retinal (traumatic) (without
detachment) —*see also* Break, retina
with detachment —*see* Detachment,
retina, with retinal, break
rotator cuff (nontraumatic) M75.10-•
complete M75.12-•
incomplete M75.11-•
sclera —*see* Injury, eye, laceration
sigmoid (nontraumatic) K63.1
traumatic S36.593
spinal cord —*see also* Injury, spinal cord, by
region
due to injury at birth P11.5
newborn (birth injury) P11.5
spleen (traumatic) S36.09
birth injury P15.1
congenital (birth injury) P15.1
due to P. vivax malaria B51.0
nontraumatic D73.5
spontaneous D73.5

Rupture, ruptured *(Continued)*
splenic vein R58
traumatic —*see* Injury, blood vessel,
splenic vein
stomach (nontraumatic) (spontaneous)
K31.89
traumatic S36.39
supraspinatus (complete) (incomplete)
(nontraumatic) —*see* Tear, rotator cuff
symphysis pubis
obstetric O71.6
traumatic S33.4
synovium (cyst) M66.10
ankle M66.17-•
elbow M66.12-•
finger M66.14-•
foot M66.17-•
forearm M66.13-•
hand M66.14-•
pelvic region M66.15-•
shoulder region M66.11-•
specified site NEC M66.18
thigh M66.15-•
toe M66.17-•
upper arm M66.12-•
wrist M66.13-•
tendon (traumatic) —*see* Strain
nontraumatic (spontaneous) M66.9
ankle M66.87-•
extensor M66.20
ankle M66.27-•
foot M66.27-•
forearm M66.23-•
hand M66.24-•
lower leg M66.26-•
multiple sites M66.29
pelvic region M66.25-•
shoulder region M66.21-•
specified site NEC M66.28
thigh M66.25-•
upper arm M66.22-•
flexor M66.30
ankle M66.37-•
foot M66.37-•
forearm M66.33-•
hand M66.34-•
lower leg M66.36-•
multiple sites M66.39
pelvic region M66.35-•
shoulder region M66.31-•
specified site NEC M66.38
thigh M66.35-•
upper arm M66.32-•
foot M66.87-•
forearm M66.83-•
hand M66.84-•
lower leg M66.86-•
multiple sites M66.89
pelvic region M66.85-•
shoulder region M66.81-•
specified
site NEC M66.88
tendon M66.80
thigh M66.85-•
upper arm M66.82-•
thoracic duct I89.8
tonsil J35.8
traumatic
aorta —*see* Injury, aorta, laceration, major
diaphragm —*see* Injury, intrathoracic,
diaphragm
external site —*see* Wound, open, by site
eye —*see* Injury, eye, laceration
internal organ —*see* Injury, by site
intervertebral disc
cervical S13.0
lumbar S33.0
thoracic S23.0
kidney S37.06-•

Rupture, ruptured *(Continued)*
traumatic *(Continued)*
ligament —*see also* Sprain
ankle —*see* Sprain, ankle
carpus —*see* Rupture, traumatic,
ligament, wrist
collateral (hand) —*see* Rupture,
traumatic, ligament, finger,
collateral
finger (metacarpophalangeal)
(interphalangeal) S63.40-•
collateral S63.41-•
index S63.41-•
little S63.41-•
middle S63.41-•
ring S63.41-•
index S63.40-•
little S63.40-•
middle S63.40-•
palmar S63.42-•
index S63.42-•
little S63.42-•
middle S63.42-•
ring S63.42-•
ring S63.40-•
specified site NEC S63.499
index S63.49-•
little S63.49-•
middle S63.49-•
ring S63.49-•
volar plate S63.43-•
index S63.43-•
little S63.43-•
middle S63.43-•
ring S63.43-•
foot —*see* Sprain, foot
radial collateral S53.2-•
radiocarpal —*see* Rupture, traumatic,
ligament, wrist, radiocarpal
ulnar collateral S53.3-•
ulnocarpal —*see* Rupture, traumatic,
ligament, wrist, ulnocarpal
wrist S63.30-•
collateral S63.31-•
radiocarpal S63.32-•
specified site NEC S63.39-•
ulnocarpal (palmar) S63.33-•
liver S36.116
membrana tympani —*see* Rupture, ear
drum, traumatic
muscle or tendon —*see* Strain
myocardium —*see* Injury, heart
pancreas S36.299
rectum S36.69
sigmoid S36.593
spleen S36.09
stomach S36.39
symphysis pubis S33.4
tympanum, tympanic (membrane) —*see*
Rupture, ear drum, traumatic
ureter S37.19
uterus S37.69
vagina —*see* Injury, vagina
vena cava —*see* Injury, vena cava,
laceration, major
tricuspid (heart) (valve) I07.8
tube, tubal (nonobstetric) (nontraumatic)
N83.8
abscess —*see* Salpingitis
due to pregnancy O00.10-•
with intrauterine pregnancy O00.11-•
tympanum, tympanic (membrane)
(nontraumatic) —*see also* Perforation,
tympanic membrane H72.9-•
traumatic —*see* Rupture, ear drum,
traumatic
umbilical cord, complicating delivery
O69.89
ureter (traumatic) S37.19
nontraumatic N28.89

▶ New   ⇒ Revised   ~~deleted~~ Deleted   • Use Additional Character(s)

Rupture, ruptured *(Continued)*
  urethra (nontraumatic) N36.8
    with ectopic or molar pregnancy O08.6
    following ectopic or molar pregnancy
        O08.6
    obstetrical trauma O71.5
    traumatic S37.39
  uterosacral ligament (nonobstetric)
        (nontraumatic) N83.8
  uterus (traumatic) S37.69
    before labor O71.0-●
    during or after labor O71.1

Rupture, ruptured *(Continued)*
  traumatic *(Continued)*
    nonpuerperal, nontraumatic N85.8
    pregnant (during labor) O71.1
      before labor O71.0-●
  vagina —*see* Injury, vagina
  valve, valvular (heart) —*see* Endocarditis
  varicose vein —*see* Varix
  varix —*see* Varix
  vena cava R58
    traumatic —*see* Injury, vena cava,
        laceration, major
  vesical (urinary) N32.89

Rupture, ruptured *(Continued)*
  vessel (blood) R58
    pulmonary I28.8
    traumatic —*see* Injury, blood vessel
  viscus R19.8
  vulva complicating delivery O70.0
Russell-Silver syndrome Q87.19
Russian spring-summer type encephalitis
    A84.0
Rust's disease (tuberculous cervical spondylitis)
    A18.01
Ruvalcaba-Myhre-Smith syndrome E71.440
Rytand-Lipsitch syndrome I44.2

R

S

Saber, sabre shin or tibia (syphilitic) A50.56
    [M90.8-●]
Sac lacrimal —see condition
Saccharomyces infection B37.9
Saccharopinuria E72.3
Saccular —see condition
Sacculation
    aorta (nonsyphilitic) —see Aneurysm, aorta
    bladder N32.3
    intralaryngeal (congenital) (ventricular) Q31.3
    larynx (congenital) (ventricular) Q31.3
    organ or site, congenital —see Distortion
    pregnant uterus —see Pregnancy, complicated
        by, abnormal, uterus
    ureter N28.89
    urethra N36.1
    vesical N32.3
Sachs' amaurotic familial idiocy or disease
    E75.02
Sachs-Tay disease E75.02
Sacks-Libman disease M32.11
Sacralgia M53.3
Sacralization Q76.49
Sacrodynia M53.3
Sacroiliac joint —see condition
Sacroiliitis NEC M46.1
Sacrum —see condition
Saddle
    back —see Lordosis
    embolus
        abdominal aorta I74.01
        pulmonary artery I26.92
            with acute cor pulmonale I26.02
    injury — code to condition
    nose M95.0
        due to syphilis A50.57
Sadism (sexual) F65.52
Sadness, postpartal O90.6
Sadomasochism F65.50
Saemisch's ulcer (cornea) —see Ulcer, cornea,
    central
Sagging
    skin and subcutaneous tissue (following
        bariatric surgery weight loss) (following
        dietary weight loss) L98.7
Sahib disease B55.0
Sailors' skin L57.8
Saint
    Anthony's fire —see Erysipelas
    triad —see Hernia, diaphragm
    Vitus' dance —see Chorea, Sydenham's
Salaam
    attack(s) —see Epilepsy, spasms
    tic R25.8
Salicylism
    abuse F55.8
    overdose or wrong substance given —see
        Table of Drugs and Chemicals, by drug,
        poisoning
Salivary duct or gland —see condition
Salivation, excessive K11.7
Salmonella —see Infection, Salmonella
Salmonellosis A02.0
Salpingitis (catarrhal) (fallopian tube) (nodular)
    (pseudofollicular) (purulent) (septic)
    N70.91
    with oophoritis N70.93
    acute N70.01
        with oophoritis N70.03
    chlamydial A56.11
    chronic N70.11
        with oophoritis N70.13
    complicating abortion —see Abortion, by
        type, complicated by, salpingitis
    ear —see Salpingitis, eustachian
    eustachian (tube) H68.00-●
        acute H68.01-●
        chronic H68.02-●
    follicularis N70.11
        with oophoritis N70.13

Salpingitis (Continued)
    gonococcal (acute) (chronic) A54.24
    interstitial, chronic N70.11
        with oophoritis N70.13
    isthmica nodosa N70.11
        with oophoritis N70.13
    specific (gonococcal) (acute) (chronic) A54.24
    tuberculous (acute) (chronic) A18.17
    venereal (gonococcal) (acute) (chronic) A54.24
Salpingocele N83.4-●
Salpingo-oophoritis (catarrhal) (purulent)
    (ruptured) (septic) (suppurative) N70.93
    acute N70.03
        with ectopic or molar pregnancy O08.0
        following ectopic or molar pregnancy O08.0
        gonococcal A54.24
    chronic N70.13
    following ectopic or molar pregnancy O08.0
    gonococcal (acute) (chronic) A54.24
    puerperal O86.19
    specific (gonococcal) (acute) (chronic) A54.24
    subacute N70.03
    tuberculous (acute) (chronic) A18.17
    venereal (gonococcal) (acute) (chronic) A54.24
Salpingo-ovaritis —see Salpingo-oophoritis
Salpingoperitonitis —see Salpingo-oophoritis
Salzmann's nodular dystrophy —see
    Degeneration, cornea, nodular
▶Sampson's cyst or tumor N80.10-●
San Joaquin (Valley) fever B38.0
Sandblaster's asthma, lung or pneumoconiosis
    J62.8
Sander's disease (paranoia) F22
Sandfly fever A93.1
Sandhoff's disease E75.01
Sanfilippo (Type B) (Type C) (Type D)
    syndrome E76.22
Sanger-Brown ataxia G11.2
Sao Paulo fever or typhus A77.0
Saponification, mesenteric K65.8
Sarcocele (benign)
    syphilitic A52.76
        congenital A50.59
Sarcocystosis A07.8
Sarcoepiplocele —see Hernia
Sarcoepiplomphalocele Q79.2
▶Sarcoglycanopathy G71.0340
    ▶alpha G71.0341
    ▶beta G71.0342
    ▶delta G71.0349
    ▶gamma G71.0349
Sarcoid —see also Sarcoidosis
    arthropathy D86.86
    Boeck's D86.9
    Darier-Roussy D86.3
    iridocyclitis D86.83
    meningitis D86.81
    myocarditis D86.85
    myositis D86.87
    pyelonephritis D86.84
    Spiegler-Fendt L08.89
Sarcoidosis D86.9
    with
        cranial nerve palsies D86.82
        hepatic granuloma D86.89
        polyarthritis D86.86
        tubulo-interstitial nephropathy D86.84
    combined sites NEC D86.89
    lung D86.0
        and lymph nodes D86.2
    lymph nodes D86.1
        and lung D86.2
    meninges D86.81
    skin D86.3
    specified type NEC D86.89
Sarcoma (of) —see also Neoplasm, connective
    tissue, malignant
    alveolar soft part —see Neoplasm, connective
        tissue, malignant
    ameloblastic C41.1
        upper jaw (bone) C41.0

Sarcoma (Continued)
    botryoid —see Neoplasm, connective tissue,
        malignant
    botryoides —see Neoplasm, connective tissue,
        malignant
    cerebellar C71.6
        circumscribed (arachnoidal) C71.6
    circumscribed (arachnoidal) cerebellar C71.6
    clear cell —see also Neoplasm, connective
        tissue, malignant
        kidney C64.-●
    dendritic cells (accessory cells) C96.4
    embryonal —see Neoplasm, connective tissue,
        malignant
    endometrial (stromal) C54.1
        isthmus C54.0
    epithelioid (cell) —see Neoplasm, connective
        tissue, malignant
    Ewing's —see Neoplasm, bone, malignant
    follicular dendritic cell C96.4
    germinoblastic (diffuse) —see Lymphoma,
        diffuse, large cell
        follicular —see Lymphoma, follicular,
            specified NEC
    giant cell (except of bone) —see also
        Neoplasm, connective tissue, malignant
        bone —see Neoplasm, bone, malignant
    glomoid —see Neoplasm, connective tissue,
        malignant
    granulocytic C92.3-●
    hemangioendothelial —see Neoplasm,
        connective tissue, malignant
    hemorrhagic, multiple —see Sarcoma,
        Kaposi's
    histiocytic C96.A
    Hodgkin —see Lymphoma, Hodgkin
    immunoblastic (diffuse) —see Lymphoma,
        diffuse large cell
    interdigitating dendritic cell C96.4
    Kaposi's
        colon C46.4
        connective tissue C46.1
        gastrointestinal organ C46.4
        lung C46.5-●
        lymph node(s) C46.3
        palate (hard) (soft) C46.2
        rectum C46.4
        skin C46.0
        specified site NEC C46.7
        stomach C46.4
        unspecified site C46.9
    Kupffer cell C22.3
    Langerhans cell C96.4
    leptomeningeal —see Neoplasm, meninges,
        malignant
    liver NEC C22.4
    lymphangioendothelial —see Neoplasm,
        connective tissue, malignant
    lymphoblastic —see Lymphoma,
        lymphoblastic (diffuse)
    lymphocytic —see Lymphoma, small cell
        B-cell
    mast cell C96.22
    melanotic —see Melanoma
    meningeal —see Neoplasm, meninges,
        malignant
    meningothelial —see Neoplasm, meninges,
        malignant
    mesenchymal —see also Neoplasm,
        connective tissue, malignant
        mixed —see Neoplasm, connective tissue,
            malignant
    mesothelial —see Mesothelioma
    monstrocellular
        specified site —see Neoplasm, malignant,
            by site
        unspecified site C71.9
    myeloid C92.3-●
    neurogenic —see Neoplasm, nerve, malignant
    odontogenic C41.1
        upper jaw (bone) C41.0

▶ New   ⇒ Revised   ~~deleted~~ Deleted   ● Use Additional Character(s)

Sarcoma *(Continued)*
  osteoblastic —*see* Neoplasm, bone, malignant
  osteogenic —*see also* Neoplasm, bone, malignant
    juxtacortical —*see* Neoplasm, bone, malignant
    periosteal —*see* Neoplasm, bone, malignant
  periosteal —*see also* Neoplasm, bone, malignant
    osteogenic —*see* Neoplasm, bone, malignant
  pleomorphic cell —*see* Neoplasm, connective tissue, malignant
  reticulum cell (diffuse) —*see* Lymphoma, diffuse large cell
    nodular —*see* Lymphoma, follicular
    pleomorphic cell type —*see* Lymphoma, diffuse large cell
  rhabdoid —*see* Neoplasm, malignant, by site
  round cell —*see* Neoplasm, connective tissue, malignant
  small cell —*see* Neoplasm, connective tissue, malignant
  soft tissue —*see* Neoplasm, connective tissue, malignant
  spindle cell —*see* Neoplasm, connective tissue, malignant
  stromal (endometrial) C54.1
    isthmus C54.0
  synovial —*see also* Neoplasm, connective tissue, malignant
    biphasic —*see* Neoplasm, connective tissue, malignant
    epithelioid cell —*see* Neoplasm, connective tissue, malignant
    spindle cell —*see* Neoplasm, connective tissue, malignant
Sarcomatosis
  meningeal —*see* Neoplasm, meninges, malignant
  specified site NEC —*see* Neoplasm, connective tissue, malignant
  unspecified site C80.1
Sarcopenia (age-related) M62.84
Sarcosinemia E72.59
Sarcosporidiosis (intestinal) A07.8
SARS-CoV-2 —*see also* COVID-19
  sequelae (post acute) U09.9
Satiety, early R68.81
Saturnine —*see* condition
Saturnism
  overdose or wrong substance given or taken —*see* Table of Drugs and Chemicals, by drug, poisoning
Satyriasis F52.8
Sauriasis —*see* Ichthyosis
SBE (subacute bacterial endocarditis) I33.0
Scabies (any site) B86
Scabs R23.4
Scaglietti-Dagnini syndrome E22.0
Scald —*see* Burn
Scalenus anticus (anterior) syndrome G54.0
Scales R23.4
Scaling, skin R23.4
Scalp —*see* condition
Scapegoating affecting child Z62.3
Scaphocephaly Q75.0
Scapulalgia M89.8X1
Scapulohumeral myopathy G71.02
Scar, scarring —*see also* Cicatrix L90.5
  adherent L90.5
  atrophic L90.5
  cervix
    in pregnancy or childbirth —*see* Pregnancy, complicated by, abnormal cervix
  cheloid L91.0
  chorioretinal H31.00-•
    posterior pole macula H31.01-•
    postsurgical H59.81-•
    solar retinopathy H31.02-•
    specified type NEC H31.09-•

Scar, scarring *(Continued)*
  choroid —*see* Scar, chorioretinal
  conjunctiva H11.24-•
  cornea H17.9
    xerophthalmic —*see also* Opacity, cornea
      vitamin A deficiency E50.6
  defect (isthmocele) O34.22
  duodenum, obstructive K31.5
  hypertrophic L91.0
  keloid L91.0
  labia N90.89
  lung (base) J98.4
  macula —*see* Scar, chorioretinal, posterior pole
  muscle M62.89
  myocardium, myocardial I25.2
  painful L90.5
  posterior pole (eye) —*see* Scar, chorioretinal, posterior pole
  retina —*see* Scar, chorioretinal
  trachea J39.8
  transmural uterine, in pregnancy O34.29
  uterus N85.8
    in pregnancy O34.29
  vagina N89.8
    postoperative N99.2
  vulva N90.89
Scarabiasis B88.2
Scarlatina (anginosa) (maligna) A38.9
  myocarditis (acute) A38.1
    old —*see* Myocarditis
  otitis media A38.0
  ulcerosa A38.8
Scarlet fever (albuminuria) (angina) A38.9
Schamberg's disease (progressive pigmentary dermatosis) L81.7
Schatzki's ring (acquired) (esophagus) (lower) K22.2
  congenital Q39.3
Schaufenster krankheit I20.8
Schaumann's
  benign lymphogranulomatosis D86.1
  disease or syndrome —*see* Sarcoidosis
Scheie's syndrome E76.03
Schenck's disease B42.1
Scheuermann's disease or osteochondrosis — *see* Osteochondrosis, juvenile, spine
Schilder (-Flatau) disease G37.0
Schilling-type monocytic leukemia C93.0-•
Schimmelbusch's disease, cystic mastitis, or hyperplasia —*see* Mastopathy, cystic
Schistosoma infestation —*see* Infestation, Schistosoma
Schistosomiasis B65.9
  with muscle disorder B65.9 *[M63.80]*
    ankle B65.9 *[M63.87-•]*
    foot B65.9 *[M63.87-•]*
    forearm B65.9 *[M63.83-•]*
    hand B65.9 *[M63.84-•]*
    lower leg B65.9 *[M63.86-•]*
    multiple sites B65.9 *[M63.89]*
    pelvic region B65.9 *[M63.85-•]*
    shoulder region B65.9 *[M63.81-•]*
    specified site NEC B65.9 *[M63.88]*
    thigh B65.9 *[M63.85-•]*
    upper arm B65.9 *[M63.82-•]*
  Asiatic B65.2
  bladder B65.0
  chestermani B65.8
  colon B65.1
  cutaneous B65.3
  due to
    S. haematobium B65.0
    S. japonicum B65.2
    S. mansoni B65.1
    S. mattheii B65.8
  Eastern B65.2
  genitourinary tract B65.0
  intestinal B65.1
  lung NEC B65.9 *[J99]*
    pneumonia B65.9 *[J17]*
  Manson's (intestinal) B65.1

Schistosomiasis *(Continued)*
  oriental B65.2
  pulmonary NEC B65.9 *[J99]*
    pneumonia B65.9
  Schistosoma
    haematobium B65.0
    japonicum B65.2
    mansoni B65.1
  specified type NEC B65.8
  urinary B65.0
  vesical B65.0
Schizencephaly Q04.6
Schizoaffective psychosis F25.9
Schizodontia K00.2
Schizoid personality F60.1
Schizophrenia, schizophrenic F20.9
  acute (brief) (undifferentiated) F23
  atypical (form) F20.3
  borderline F21
  catalepsy F20.2
  catatonic (type) (excited) (withdrawn) F20.2
  cenesthopathic, cenesthesiopathic F20.89
  childhood type F84.5
  chronic undifferentiated F20.9
  cyclic F25.0
  disorganized (type) F20.1
  flexibilitas cerea F20.2
  hebephrenic (type) F20.1
  incipient F21
  latent F21
  negative type F20.5
  paranoid (type) F20.0
  paraphrenic F20.0
  post-psychotic depression F32.89
  prepsychotic F21
  prodromal F21
  pseudoneurotic F21
  pseudopsychopathic F21
  reaction F23
  residual (state) (type) F20.5
  restzustand F20.5
  schizoaffective (type) —*see* Psychosis, schizoaffective
  simple (type) F20.89
  simplex F20.89
  specified type NEC F20.89
  spectrum and other psychotic disorder F29
    specified NEC F28
  stupor F20.2
  syndrome of childhood F84.5
  undifferentiated (type) F20.3
    ➡chronic F20.9
Schizothymia (persistent) F60.1
Schlatter-Osgood disease or osteochondrosis M92.52-•
Schlatter's tibia —*see* Osteochondrosis, juvenile, tibia
Schmidt's syndrome (polyglandular, autoimmune) E31.0
Schmincke's carcinoma or tumor —*see* Neoplasm, nasopharynx, malignant
Schmitz (-Stutzer) dysentery A03.0
Schmorl's disease or nodes
  lumbar region M51.46
  lumbosacral region M51.47
  sacrococcygeal region M53.3
  thoracic region M51.44
  thoracolumbar region M51.45
Schneiderian
  papilloma —*see* Neoplasm, nasopharynx benign
    specified site —*see* Neoplasm, benign, by site
    unspecified site D14.0
  specified site —*see* Neoplasm, malignant, by site
    unspecified site C30.0
Scholte's syndrome (malignant carcinoid) E34.0
Scholz (-Bielchowsky-Henneberg) disease or syndrome E75.25
Schönlein (-Henoch) disease or purpura (primary) (rheumatic) D69.0

Schottmuller's disease A01.4
Schroeder's syndrome (endocrine hypertensive) E27.0
Schüller-Christian disease or syndrome C96.5
Schultze's type acroparesthesia, simple I73.89
Schultz's disease or syndrome —see Agranulocytosis
Schwalbe-Ziehen-Oppenheim disease G24.1
Schwannoma —see also Neoplasm, nerve, benign
  malignant —see also Neoplasm, nerve, malignant
    with rhabdomyoblastic differentiation — see Neoplasm, nerve, malignant
  melanocytic —see Neoplasm, nerve, benign
  pigmented —see Neoplasm, nerve, benign
Schwannomatosis Q85.03
Schwartz (-Jampel) syndrome G71.13
Schwartz-Bartter syndrome E22.2
Schweniger-Buzzi anetoderma L90.1
Sciatic —see condition
Sciatica (infective) M54.3
  with lumbago M54.4-●
    due to intervertebral disc disorder —see Disorder, disc, with, radiculopathy
  due to displacement of intervertebral disc (with lumbago) —see Disorder, disc, with, radiculopathy
  wallet M54.3-●
Scimitar syndrome Q26.8
Sclera —see condition
Sclerectasia H15.84-●
Scleredema
  adultorum —see Sclerosis, systemic
  Buschke's —see Sclerosis, systemic
  newborn P83.0
Sclerema (adiposum) (edematosum) (neonatorum) (newborn) P83.0
  adultorum —see Sclerosis, systemic
Scleriasis —see Scleroderma
Scleritis H15.00-●
  with corneal involvement H15.04-●
  anterior H15.01-●
  brawny H15.02-●
  in (due to) zoster B02.34
  posterior H15.03-●
  specified type NEC H15.09-●
  syphilitic A52.71
  tuberculous (nodular) A18.51
Sclerochoroiditis H31.8
Scleroconjunctivitis —see Scleritis
Sclerocystic ovary syndrome E28.2
Sclerodactyly, sclerodactylia L94.3
Scleroderma, sclerodermia (acrosclerotic) (diffuse) (generalized) (progressive) (pulmonary) —see also Sclerosis, systemic M34.9-●
  circumscribed L94.0
  linear L94.1
  localized L94.0
  newborn P83.88
  systemic M34.9
Sclerokeratitis H16.8
  tuberculous A18.52
Scleroma nasi A48.8
Scleromalacia (perforans) H15.05-●
Scleromyxedema L98.5
Sclérose en plaques G35
Sclerosis, sclerotic
  adrenal (gland) E27.8
  Alzheimer's —see Disease, Alzheimer's
  amyotrophic (lateral) G12.21
  aorta, aortic I70.0
    valve —see Endocarditis, aortic
  artery, arterial, arteriolar, arteriovascular — see Arteriosclerosis
  ascending multiple G35
  brain (generalized) (lobular) G37.9
    artery, arterial I67.2
    diffuse G37.0
    disseminated G35

Sclerosis, sclerotic (Continued)
  brain (Continued)
    insular G35
    Krabbe's E75.23
    miliary G35
    multiple G35
    presenile (Alzheimer's) —see Disease, Alzheimer's, early onset
    senile (arteriosclerotic) I67.2
    stem, multiple G35
    tuberous Q85.1
  bulbar, multiple G35
  bundle of His I44.39
  cardiac —see Disease, heart, ischemic, atherosclerotic
  cardiorenal —see Hypertension, cardiorenal
  cardiovascular —see also Disease, cardiovascular
    renal —see Hypertension, cardiorenal
  cerebellar —see Sclerosis, brain
  cerebral —see Sclerosis, brain
  cerebrospinal (disseminated) (multiple) G35
  cerebrovascular I67.2
  choroid —see Degeneration, choroid
  combined (spinal cord) —see also Degeneration, combined
    multiple G35
  concentric (Balo) G37.5
  cornea —see Opacity, cornea
  coronary (artery) I25.10
    with angina pectoris —see Arteriosclerosis, coronary (artery),
  corpus cavernosum
    female N90.89
    male N48.6
  diffuse (brain) (spinal cord) G37.0
  disseminated G35
  dorsal G35
  dorsolateral (spinal cord) —see Degeneration, combined
  endometrium N85.5
  extrapyramidal G25.9
  eye, nuclear (senile) —see Cataract, senile, nuclear
  focal and segmental (glomerular) —see also N00-N07 with fourth character .1 N05.1
  Friedreich's (spinal cord) G11.11
  funicular (spermatic cord) N50.89
  general (vascular) —see Arteriosclerosis
  gland (lymphatic) I89.8
  hepatic K74.1
    alcoholic K70.2
  hereditary
    cerebellar G11.9
    spinal (Friedreich's ataxia) G11.11
  hippocampal G93.81
  insular G35
  kidney —see Sclerosis, renal
  larynx J38.7
  lateral (amyotrophic) (descending) (spinal) G12.21
    primary G12.23
  lens, senile nuclear —see Cataract, senile, nuclear
  liver K74.1
    with fibrosis K74.2
      alcoholic K70.2
    alcoholic K70.2
    cardiac K76.1
  lung —see Fibrosis, lung
  mastoid —see Mastoiditis, chronic
  mesial temporal G93.81
  mitral I05.8
  Mönckeberg's (medial) —see Arteriosclerosis, extremities
  multiple (brain stem) (cerebral) (generalized) (spinal cord) G35
  myocardium, myocardial —see Disease, heart, ischemic, atherosclerotic
  nuclear (senile), eye —see Cataract, senile, nuclear

Sclerosis, sclerotic (Continued)
  ovary N83.8
  pancreas K86.89
  penis N48.6
  peripheral arteries —see Arteriosclerosis, extremities
  plaques G35
  pluriglandular E31.8
  polyglandular E31.8
  posterolateral (spinal cord) —see Degeneration, combined
  presenile (Alzheimer's) —see Disease, Alzheimer's, early onset
  primary, lateral G12.23
  progressive, systemic M34.0
  pulmonary —see Fibrosis, lung
    artery I27.0
    valve (heart) —see Endocarditis, pulmonary
  renal N26.9
    with
      cystine storage disease E72.09
      hypertensive heart disease (conditions in I11) —see Hypertension, cardiorenal
    arteriolar (hyaline) (hyperplastic) —see Hypertension, kidney
  retina (senile) (vascular) H35.00
  senile (vascular) —see Arteriosclerosis
  spinal (cord) (progressive) G95.89
    ascending G61.0
    combined —see also Degeneration, combined
      multiple G35
      syphilitic A52.11
    disseminated G35
    dorsolateral —see Degeneration, combined
    hereditary (Friedreich's) (mixed form) G11.11
    lateral (amyotrophic) G12.21
      progressive G12.23
    multiple G35
    posterior (syphilitic) A52.11
  stomach K31.89
  subendocardial, congenital I42.4
  systemic M34.9
    with
      lung involvement M34.81
      myopathy M34.82
      polyneuropathy M34.83
    drug-induced M34.2
    due to chemicals NEC M34.2
    progressive M34.0
    specified NEC M34.89
  temporal (mesial) G93.81
  tricuspid (heart) (valve) I07.8
  tuberous (brain) Q85.1
  tympanic membrane —see Disorder, tympanic membrane, specified NEC
  valve, valvular (heart) —see Endocarditis
  vascular —see Arteriosclerosis
  vein I87.8
Scoliosis (acquired) (postural) M41.9
  adolescent (idiopathic) —see Scoliosis, idiopathic, adolescent
  congenital Q67.5
    due to bony malformation Q76.3
    failure of segmentation (hemivertebra) Q76.3
    hemivertebra fusion Q76.3
    postural Q67.5
  ▸▸degenerative M41.5-●
  idiopathic M41.20
    adolescent M41.129
      cervical region M41.122
      cervicothoracic region M41.123
      lumbar region M41.126
      lumbosacral region M41.127
      thoracic region M41.124
      thoracolumbar region M41.125
    cervical region M41.22
    cervicothoracic region M41.23

▶ New   ⇒ Revised   deleted Deleted   ● Use Additional Character(s)

Scoliosis *(Continued)*
  idiopathic *(Continued)*
    infantile M41.00
      cervical region M41.02
      cervicothoracic region M41.03
      lumbar region M41.06
      lumbosacral region M41.07
      sacrococcygeal region M41.08
      thoracic region M41.04
      thoracolumbar region M41.05
    juvenile M41.119
      cervical region M41.112
      cervicothoracic region M41.113
      lumbar region M41.116
      lumbosacral region M41.117
      thoracic region M41.114
      thoracolumbar region M41.115
    lumbar region M41.26
    lumbosacral region M41.27
    thoracic region M41.24
    thoracolumbar region M41.25
  infantile —*see* Scoliosis, idiopathic, infantile
  neuromuscular M41.40
    cervical region M41.42
    cervicothoracic region M41.43
    lumbar region M41.46
    lumbosacral region M41.47
    occipito-atlanto-axial region M41.41
    thoracic region M41.44
    thoracolumbar region M41.45
  paralytic —*see* Scoliosis, neuromuscular
  postradiation therapy M96.5
  rachitic (late effect or sequelae) E64.3 *[M49.80]*
    cervical region E64.3 *[M49.82]*
    cervicothoracic region E64.3 *[M49.83]*
    lumbar region E64.3 *[M49.86]*
    lumbosacral region E64.3 *[M49.87]*
    multiple sites E64.3 *[M49.89]*
    occipito-atlanto-axial region E64.3 *[M49.81]*
    sacrococcygeal region E64.3 *[M49.88]*
    thoracic region E64.3 *[M49.84]*
    thoracolumbar region E64.3 *[M49.85]*
  sciatic M54.4-•
  secondary (to) NEC M41.50
    cerebral palsy, Friedreich's ataxia,
      poliomyelitis, neuromuscular
      disorders —*see* Scoliosis,
      neuromuscular
    cervical region M41.52
    cervicothoracic region M41.53
    lumbar region M41.56
    lumbosacral region M41.57
    thoracic region M41.54
    thoracolumbar region M41.55
  specified form NEC M41.80
    cervical region M41.82
    cervicothoracic region M41.83
    lumbar region M41.86
    lumbosacral region M41.87
    thoracic region M41.84
    thoracolumbar region M41.85
  thoracogenic M41.30
    thoracic region M41.34
    thoracolumbar region M41.35
  tuberculous A18.01
Scoliotic pelvis
  with disproportion (fetopelvic) O33.0
    causing obstructed labor O65.0
Scorbutus, scorbutic —*see also* Scurvy
  anemia D53.2
Score, NIHSS (National Institutes of Health
    Stroke Scale) R29.7-•
Scotoma (arcuate) (Bjerrum) (central) (ring) —
    see also Defect, visual field, localized, scotoma
  scintillating H53.12-•
Scratch —*see* Abrasion
Scratchy throat R09.89
Screening (for) Z13.9
  alcoholism Z13.33
  anemia Z13.0
  anomaly, congenital Z13.89

Screening *(Continued)*
  antenatal, of mother —*see also* Encounter,
    antenatal Z36.9
  arterial hypertension Z13.6
  arthropod-borne viral disease NEC Z11.59
  autism Z13.41
  bacteriuria, asymptomatic Z13.89
    specified NEC Z13.39
  behavioral disorder Z13.30
  brain injury, traumatic Z13.850
  bronchitis, chronic Z13.83
  brucellosis Z11.2
  cardiovascular disorder Z13.6
  cataract Z13.5
  chlamydial diseases Z11.8
  cholera Z11.0
  chromosomal abnormalities (nonprocreative)
    NEC Z13.79
  colonoscopy Z12.11
  congenital
    dislocation of hip Z13.89
    eye disorder Z13.5
    malformation or deformation Z13.89
  contamination NEC Z13.88
  coronavirus (disease) (novel) 2019 Z11.52
  COVID-19 Z11.52
  cystic fibrosis Z13.228
  dengue fever Z11.59
  dental disorder Z13.84
  depression (adult) (adolescent) (child) Z13.31
    maternal Z13.32
    perinatal Z13.32
  developmental
    delays Z13.40
      global (milestones) Z13.42
      specified NEC Z13.49
    handicap Z13.42
      in early childhood Z13.42
  diabetes mellitus Z13.1
  diphtheria Z11.2
  disability, intellectual Z13.39
  disease or disorder Z13.9
    bacterial NEC Z11.2
      intestinal infectious Z11.0
      respiratory tuberculosis Z11.1
    behavioral Z13.30
      specified NEC Z13.39
    developmental delays Z13.40
      global (milestones) Z13.42
      specified NEC Z13.49
    mental health and behavioral Z13.30
      specified NEC Z13.39
    blood or blood-forming organ Z13.0
    cardiovascular Z13.6
    Chagas' Z11.6
    chlamydial Z11.8
    coronavirus (novel) 2019 Z11.52
    COVID-19 Z11.52
    dental Z13.89
    digestive tract NEC Z13.818
      lower GI Z13.811
      upper GI Z13.810
    ear Z13.5
    endocrine Z13.29
    eye Z13.5
    genitourinary Z13.89
    heart Z13.6
    human immunodeficiency virus (HIV)
      infection Z11.4
    immunity Z13.0
    infection
      intestinal Z11.0
        specified NEC Z11.6
    infectious Z11.9
    metabolic Z13.228
    neurological Z13.89
    nutritional Z13.21
      metabolic Z13.228
        lipoid disorders Z13.220
    protozoal Z11.6
      intestinal Z11.0

Screening *(Continued)*
  disease or disorder *(Continued)*
    respiratory Z13.83
    rheumatic Z13.828
    rickettsial Z11.8
    sexually-transmitted NEC Z11.3
      human immunodeficiency virus (HIV)
        Z11.4
    sickle-cell (trait) Z13.0
    skin Z13.89
    specified NEC Z13.89
    spirochetal Z11.8
    thyroid Z13.29
    vascular Z13.6
    venereal Z11.3
    viral NEC Z11.59
      coronavirus (disease) (novel) 2019
        Z11.52
      COVID-19 Z11.52
      human immunodeficiency virus (HIV)
        Z11.4
      intestinal Z11.0
      SARS-CoV-2 Z11.52
  elevated titer Z13.89
  emphysema Z13.83
  encephalitis, viral (mosquito- or tick-borne)
    Z11.59
  exposure to contaminants (toxic) Z13.88
  fever
    dengue Z11.59
    hemorrhagic Z11.59
    yellow Z11.59
  filariasis Z11.6
  galactosemia Z13.228
  gastrointestinal condition Z13.818
  genetic (nonprocreative)- for procreative
    management —*see* Testing, genetic, for
    procreative management
    disease carrier status (nonprocreative)
      Z13.71
    specified NEC (nonprocreative) Z13.79
  genitourinary condition Z13.89
  glaucoma Z13.5
  gonorrhea Z11.3
  gout Z13.89
  helminthiasis (intestinal) Z11.6
  hematopoietic malignancy Z12.89
  hemoglobinopathies NEC Z13.0
  hemorrhagic fever Z11.59
  Hodgkin disease Z12.89
  human immunodeficiency virus (HIV) Z11.4
  human papillomavirus Z11.51
  hypertension Z13.6
  infant or child (over 28 days old) Z00.129
    with abnormal findings Z00.121
  immunity disorders Z13.0
  infection
    mycotic Z11.8
    parasitic Z11.8
  ingestion of radioactive substance Z13.88
  intellectual disability Z13.39
  intestinal
    helminthiasis Z11.6
    infectious disease Z11.0
  leishmaniasis Z11.6
  leprosy Z11.2
  leptospirosis Z11.8
  leukemia Z12.89
  lymphoma Z12.89
  malaria Z11.6
  malnutrition Z13.29
    metabolic Z13.228
    nutritional Z13.21
  measles Z11.59
  mental health disorder Z13.30
    specified NEC Z13.39
  metabolic errors, inborn Z13.228
  multiphasic Z13.89
  musculoskeletal disorder Z13.828
    osteoporosis Z13.820
  mycoses Z11.8

S

▶ New   ⇒ Revised   ~~deleted~~ Deleted   ● Use Additional Character(s)

Senile, senility *(Continued)*
  debility R54
  endometrium (atrophic) N85.8
  fallopian tube (atrophic) —*see* Atrophy,
    fallopian tube
  heart (failure) R54
  ovary (atrophic) —*see* Atrophy, ovary
  premature E34.8
  vagina, vaginitis (atrophic) N95.2
  wart L82.1
Sensation
  burning (skin) R20.8
    tongue K14.6
  loss of R20.8
  prickling (skin) R20.2
  tingling (skin) R20.2
Sense loss
  smell —*see* Disturbance, sensation, smell
  taste —*see* Disturbance, sensation, taste
  touch R20.8
Sensibility disturbance (cortical) (deep)
  (vibratory) R20.9
Sensitive, sensitivity —*see also* Allergy
  carotid sinus G90.01
  child (excessive) F93.8
  cold, autoimmune D59.12
  dentin K03.89
  gluten (non-celiac) K90.41
  latex Z91.040
  methemoglobin D74.8
  tuberculin, without clinical or radiological
    symptoms R76.11
  visual
    glare H53.71
    impaired contrast H53.72
Sensitiver Beziehungswahn F22
Sensitization, auto-erythrocytic D69.2
Separation
  anxiety, abnormal (of childhood) F93.0
  apophysis, traumatic - code as Fracture, by site
  choroid —*see* Detachment, choroid
  epiphysis, epiphyseal
    nontraumatic —*see also* Osteochondropathy,
      specified type NEC
      upper femoral —*see* Slipped, epiphysis,
        upper femoral
    traumatic - code as Fracture, by site
  fracture —*see* Fracture
  infundibulum cardiac from right ventricle by
    a partition Q24.3
  joint (traumatic) (current) - code by site under
    Dislocation
  muscle (nontraumatic) —*see* Diastasis, muscle
  pubic bone, obstetrical trauma O71.6
  retina, retinal —*see* Detachment, retina
  symphysis pubis, obstetrical trauma O71.6
  tracheal ring, incomplete, congenital Q32.1
Sepsis (generalized) (unspecified organism)
  A41.9
  with
    organ dysfunction (acute) (multiple) R65.20
      with septic shock R65.21
  actinomycotic A42.7
  adrenal hemorrhage syndrome
    (meningococcal) A39.1
  anaerobic A41.4
  Bacillus anthracis A22.7
  Brucella —*see also* Brucellosis A23.9
  candidal B37.7
  cryptogenic A41.9
  due to device, implant or graft T85.79
    arterial graft NEC T82.7
    breast (implant) T85.79
    catheter NEC T85.79
      dialysis (renal) T82.7
        intraperitoneal T85.71
      infusion NEC T82.7
        spinal (cranial) (epidural) (intrathecal)
          (spinal) (subarachnoid)
          (subdural) T85.735
      urethral indwelling T83.511
      urinary T83.518
    ectopic or molar pregnancy O08.82

Sepsis *(Continued)*
  due to device, implant or graft*(Continued)*
    electronic (electrode) (pulse generator)
      (stimulator)
      bone T84.7
      cardiac T82.7
      nervous system T85.738
        brain T85.731
        neurostimulator generator T85.734
        peripheral nerve T85.732
        spinal cord T85.733
      urinary T83.590
    fixation, internal (orthopedic) —*see*
      Complication, fixation device,
      infection
    gastrointestinal (bile duct) (esophagus)
      T85.79
      neurostimulator electrode (lead) T85.732
    genital T83.69
    heart NEC T82.7
      valve (prosthesis) T82.6
        graft T82.7
    joint prosthesis —*see* Complication, joint
      prosthesis, infection
    ocular (corneal graft) (orbital implant) T85.79
    orthopedic NEC T84.7
      fixation device, internal —*see*
        Complication, fixation device,
        infection
    specified NEC T85.79
    vascular T82.7
    ventricular intracranial (communicating)
      shunt T85.730
  during labor O75.3
  Enterococcus A41.81
  Erysipelothrix (rhusiopathiae) (erysipeloid)
    A26.7
  Escherichia coli (E. coli) A41.5
  extraintestinal yersiniosis A28.2
  following
    abortion (subsequent episode) O08.0
      current episode —*see* Abortion
    ectopic or molar pregnancy O08.82
    immunization T88.0
    infusion, therapeutic injection or
      transfusion NEC T80.29
    obstetrical procedure O86.04
  gangrenous A41.9
  gonococcal A54.86
  Gram-negative (organism) A41.5
    anaerobic A41.4
  Haemophilus influenzae A41.3
  herpesviral B00.7
  intra-abdominal K65.1
  intraocular —*see* Endophthalmitis, purulent
  Listeria monocytogenes A32.7
  localized — code to specific localized infection
    in operation wound T81.49
    skin —*see* Abscess
  malleus A24.0
  melioidosis A24.1
  meningeal —*see* Meningitis
  meningococcal A39.4
    acute A39.2
    chronic A39.3
  MSSA (Methicillin susceptible
    Staphylococcus aureus) A41.01
  newborn P36.9
    due to
      anaerobes NEC P36.5
      Escherichia coli P36.4
      Staphylococcus P36.30
        aureus P36.2
        specified NEC P36.39
      Streptococcus P36.10
        group B P36.0
        specified NEC P36.19
    specified NEC P36.8
  Pasteurella multocida A28.0
  pelvic, puerperal, postpartum, childbirth O85
  pneumococcal A40.3
  postprocedural T81.44

Sepsis *(Continued)*
  puerperal, postpartum, childbirth (pelvic) O85
  Salmonella (arizonae) (cholerae-suis)
    (enteritidis) (typhimurium) A02.1
  severe R65.20
    with septic shock R65.21
  Shigella (*see also* Dysentery, bacillary) A03.9
  skin, localized —*see* Abscess
  specified organism NEC A41.89
  Staphylococcus, staphylococcal A41.2
    aureus (methicillin susceptible) (MSSA)
      A41.01
      methicillin resistant (MRSA) A41.02
    coagulase-negative A41.1
    specified NEC A41.1
  Streptococcus, streptococcal A40.9
    agalactiae A40.1
    group
      A A40.0
      B A40.1
      D A41.81
    neonatal P36.10
      group B P36.0
      specified NEC P36.19
    pneumoniae A40.3
    pyogenes A40.0
    specified NEC A40.8
  tracheostomy stoma J95.02
  tularemic A21.7
  umbilical, umbilical cord (newborn) —*see*
    Sepsis, newborn
  Yersinia pestis A20.7
Septate —*see* Septum
Septic —*see* condition
  arm —*see* Cellulitis, upper limb
    with lymphangitis —*see* Lymphangitis,
      acute, upper limb
  embolus —*see* Embolism
  finger —*see* Cellulitis, digit
    with lymphangitis —*see* Lymphangitis,
      acute, digit
  foot —*see* Cellulitis, lower limb
    with lymphangitis —*see* Lymphangitis,
      acute, lower limb
  gallbladder (acute) K81.0
  hand —*see* Cellulitis, upper limb
    with lymphangitis —*see* Lymphangitis,
      acute, upper limb
  joint —*see* Arthritis, pyogenic or pyemic
  leg —*see* Cellulitis, lower limb
    with lymphangitis —*see* Lymphangitis,
      acute, lower limb
  nail —*see also* Cellulitis, digit
    with lymphangitis —*see* Lymphangitis,
      acute, digit
  sore —*see also* Abscess
    throat J02.0
      streptococcal J02.0
  spleen (acute) D73.89
  teeth, tooth (pulpal origin) K04.4
  throat —*see* Pharyngitis
  thrombus —*see* Thrombosis
  toe —*see* Cellulitis, digit
    with lymphangitis —*see* Lymphangitis,
      acute, digit
  tonsils, chronic J35.01
    with adenoiditis J35.03
  uterus —*see* Endometritis
Septicemia A41.9
  meaning sepsis —*see* Sepsis
Septum, septate (congenital) —*see also*
  Anomaly, by site
  anal Q42.3
    with fistula Q42.2
  aqueduct of Sylvius Q03.0
    with spina bifida —*see* Spina bifida, by site,
      with hydrocephalus
  uterus (complete) (partial) Q51.28
    complete Q51.21
    partial Q51.22
    specified NEC Q51.28

▶ New   ⇒ Revised   ~~deleted~~ Deleted   ● Use Additional Character(s)

Septum, septate *(Continued)*
vagina Q52.10
in pregnancy —*see* Pregnancy, complicated
by, abnormal vagina
causing obstructed labor O65.5
longitudinal Q52.129
microperforate
left side Q52.124
right side Q52.123
nonobstruction Q52.120
obstructing Q52.129
left side Q52.122
right side Q52.121
transverse Q52.11
Sequelae (of) —*see also* condition
abscess, intracranial or intraspinal (conditions
in G06) G09
amputation — code to injury with seventh
character S
burn and corrosion — code to injury with
seventh character S
calcium deficiency E64.8
cerebrovascular disease —*see* Sequelae,
disease, cerebrovascular
childbirth O94
contusion — code to injury with seventh
character S
corrosion —*see* Sequelae, burn and corrosion
COVID-19 (post acute) U09.9
crushing injury — code to injury with
seventh character S
disease
cerebrovascular I69.90
alteration of sensation I69.998
aphasia I69.920
apraxia I69.990
ataxia I69.993
cognitive deficits I69.91
disturbance of vision I69.998
dysarthria I69.922
dysphagia I69.991
dysphasia I69.921
facial droop I69.992
facial weakness I69.992
fluency disorder I69.923
hemiplegia I69.95-●
hemorrhage
intracerebral —*see* Sequelae,
hemorrhage, intracerebral
intracranial, nontraumatic NEC —
see Sequelae, hemorrhage,
intracranial, nontraumatic
subarachnoid —*see* Sequelae,
hemorrhage, subarachnoid
language deficit I69.928
monoplegia
lower limb I69.94-●
upper limb I69.93-●
paralytic syndrome I69.96-●
specified effect NEC I69.998
specified type NEC I69.80
alteration of sensation I69.898
aphasia I69.820
apraxia I69.890
ataxia I69.893
cognitive deficits I69.81
disturbance of vision I69.898
dysarthria I69.822
dysphagia I69.891
dysphasia I69.821
facial droop I69.892
facial weakness I69.892
fluency disorder I69.823
hemiplegia I69.85-●
language deficit I69.828
monoplegia
lower limb I69.84-●
upper limb I69.83-●
paralytic syndrome I69.86-●
specified effect NEC I69.898
speech deficit I69.928
speech deficit I69.828
stroke NOS —*see* Sequelae, stroke NOS

Sequelae *(Continued)*
dislocation — code to injury with seventh
character S
encephalitis or encephalomyelitis (conditions
in G04) G09
in infectious disease NEC B94.8
viral B94.1
external cause — code to injury with seventh
character S
foreign body entering natural orifice — code
to injury with seventh character S
fracture — code to injury with seventh
character S
frostbite — code to injury with seventh
character S
Hansen's disease B92
hemorrhage
intracerebral I69.10
alteration of sensation I69.198
aphasia I69.120
apraxia I69.190
ataxia I69.193
cognitive deficits I69.11
disturbance of vision I69.198
dysarthria I69.122
dysphagia I69.191
dysphasia I69.121
facial droop I69.192
facial weakness I69.192
fluency disorder I69.123
hemiplegia I69.15-●
language deficit NEC I69.128
monoplegia
lower limb I69.14-●
upper limb I69.13-●
paralytic syndrome I69.16-●
specified effect NEC I69.198
speech deficit NEC I69.128
intracranial, nontraumatic NEC I69.20
alteration of sensation I69.298
aphasia I69.220
apraxia I69.290
ataxia I69.293
cognitive deficits I69.21
disturbance of vision I69.298
dysarthria I69.222
dysphagia I69.291
dysphasia I69.221
facial droop I69.292
facial weakness I69.292
fluency disorder I69.223
hemiplegia I69.25-●
language deficit NEC I69.228
monoplegia
lower limb I69.24-●
upper limb I69.23-●
paralytic syndrome I69.26-●
specified effect NEC I69.298
speech deficit NEC I69.228
subarachnoid I69.00
alteration of sensation I69.098
aphasia I69.020
apraxia I69.090
ataxia I69.093
cognitive deficits —*see* subcategory
I69.01-●
disturbance of vision I69.098
dysarthria I69.022
dysphagia I69.091
dysphasia I69.021
facial droop I69.092
facial weakness I69.092
fluency disorder I69.023
hemiplegia I69.05-●
language deficit NEC I69.028
monoplegia
lower limb I69.04-●
upper limb I69.03-●
paralytic syndrome I69.06-●
specified effect NEC I69.098
speech deficit NEC I69.028

Sequelae *(Continued)*
hepatitis, viral B94.2
hyperalimentation E68
infarction
cerebral I69.30
alteration of sensation I69.398
aphasia I69.320
apraxia I69.390
ataxia I69.393
cognitive deficits I69.31
disturbance of vision I69.398
dysarthria I69.322
dysphagia I69.391
dysphasia I69.321
facial droop I69.392
facial weakness I69.392
fluency disorder I69.323
hemiplegia I69.35-●
language deficit NEC I69.328
monoplegia
lower limb I69.34-●
upper limb I69.33-●
paralytic syndrome I69.36-●
specified effect NEC I69.398
speech deficit NEC I69.328
infection, pyogenic, intracranial or intraspinal
G09
infectious disease B94.9
specified NEC B94.8
injury — code to injury with seventh
character S
leprosy B92
meningitis
bacterial (conditions in G00) G09
other or unspecified cause (conditions in
G03) G09
muscle (and tendon) injury — code to injury
with seventh character S
myelitis —*see* Sequelae, encephalitis
niacin deficiency E64.8
nutritional deficiency E64.9
specified NEC E64.8
obstetrical condition O94
parasitic disease B94.9
phlebitis or thrombophlebitis of intracranial
or intraspinal venous sinuses and veins
(conditions in G08) G09
poisoning — code to poisoning with seventh
character S
nonmedicinal substance —*see* Sequelae,
toxic effect, nonmedicinal substance
poliomyelitis (acute) B91
pregnancy O94
protein-energy malnutrition E64.0
puerperium O94
rickets E64.3
SARS-CoV-2 (post acute) U09.9
selenium deficiency E64.8
sprain and strain — code to injury with
seventh character S
stroke NOS I69.30
alteration in sensation I69.398
aphasia I69.320
apraxia I69.390
ataxia I69.393
cognitive deficits I69.31
disturbance of vision I69.398
dysarthria I69.322
dysphagia I69.391
dysphasia I69.321
facial droop I69.392
facial weakness I69.392
hemiplegia I69.35-●
language deficit NEC I69.328
monoplegia
lower limb I69.34-●
upper limb I69.33-●
paralytic syndrome I69.36-●
specified effect NEC I69.398
speech deficit NEC I69.328
tendon and muscle injury — code to injury
with seventh character S

▶ New   ➡ Revised   ~~deleted~~ Deleted   ● Use Additional Character(s)

Sequelae (Continued)
thiamine deficiency E64.8
trachoma B94.0
tuberculosis B90.9
bones and joints B90.2
central nervous system B90.0
genitourinary B90.1
pulmonary (respiratory) B90.9
specified organs NEC B90.8
viral
encephalitis B94.1
hepatitis B94.2
vitamin deficiency NEC E64.8
A E64.1
B E64.8
C E64.2
wound, open — code to injury with seventh
character S
Sequestration —see also Sequestrum
disc —see Displacement, intervertebral
disc
lung, congenital Q33.2
Sequestrum
bone —see Osteomyelitis, chronic
dental M27.2
jaw bone M27.2
orbit —see Osteomyelitis, orbit
sinus (accessory) (nasal) —see Sinusitis
Sequoiosis lung or pneumonitis J67.8
Serology for syphilis
doubtful
with signs or symptoms - code by site and
stage under Syphilis
follow-up of latent syphilis —see Syphilis,
latent
negative, with signs or symptoms — code by
site and stage under Syphilis
positive A53.0
with signs or symptoms - code by site and
stage under Syphilis
reactivated A53.0
Seroma —see also Hematoma
postprocedural —see Complication,
postprocedural, seroma
traumatic, secondary and recurrent
T79.2
Seropurulent —see condition
Serositis, multiple K65.8
pericardial I31.1
peritoneal K65.8
Serous —see condition
Sertoli cell
adenoma
specified site —see Neoplasm, benign, by
site
unspecified site
female D27.9
male D29.20
carcinoma
specified site —see Neoplasm, malignant,
by site
unspecified site (male) C62.9-●
female C56.9
tumor
with lipid storage
specified site —see Neoplasm, benign,
by site
unspecified site
female D27.9
male D29.20
specified site —see Neoplasm, benign, by
site
unspecified site
female D27.9
male D29.20
Sertoli-Leydig cell tumor —see Neoplasm,
benign, by site
specified site —see Neoplasm, benign, by site
unspecified site
female D27.9
male D29.20

Serum
allergy, allergic reaction —see also Reaction,
serum T80.69
shock —see also Shock, anaphylactic T80.59
arthritis —see also Reaction, serum T80.69
complication or reaction NEC —see also
Reaction, serum T80.69
disease NEC —see also Reaction, serum T80.69
hepatitis —see also Hepatitis, viral, type B
carrier (suspected) of B18.1
intoxication —see also Reaction, serum T80.69
neuritis —see also Reaction, serum T80.69
neuropathy G61.1
poisoning NEC —see also Reaction, serum
T80.69
rash NEC —see also Reaction, serum T80.69
reaction NEC —see also Reaction, serum
T80.69
sickness NEC —see also Reaction, serum
T80.69
urticaria —see also Reaction, serum T80.69
Sesamoiditis M25.8-●
Sever's disease or osteochondrosis —see
Osteochondrosis, juvenile, tarsus
Severe sepsis R65.20
with septic shock R65.21
Sex
chromosome mosaics Q97.8
lines with various numbers of
X chromosomes Q97.2
education Z70.8
reassignment surgery status Z87.890
Sextuplet pregnancy —see Pregnancy,
sextuplet
Sexual
function, disorder of (psychogenic) F52.9
immaturity (female) (male) E30.0
impotence (psychogenic) organic origin
NEC —see Dysfunction, sexual, male
precocity (constitutional) (cryptogenic)
(female) (idiopathic) (male) E30.1
Sexuality, pathologic —see Deviation, sexual
Sézary disease C84.1-●
Shadow, lung R91.8
Shaking palsy or paralysis —see Parkinsonism
Shallowness, acetabulum —see Derangement,
joint, specified type NEC, hip
Shaver's disease J63.1
Sheath (tendon) —see condition
Sheathing, retinal vessels H35.01-●
Shedding
nail L60.8
premature, primary (deciduous) teeth
K00.6
Sheehan's disease or syndrome E23.0
Shelf, rectal K62.89
Shell teeth K00.5
Shellshock (current) F43.0
lasting state —see Disorder, post-traumatic
stress
Shield kidney Q63.1
Shift
auditory threshold (temporary) H93.24-●
mediastinal R93.89
Shifting sleep-work schedule (affecting sleep)
G47.26
Shiga (-Kruse) dysentery A03.0
Shiga's bacillus A03.0
Shigella (dysentery) —see Dysentery,
bacillary
Shigellosis A03.9
Group A A03.0
Group B A03.1
Group C A03.2
Group D A03.3
Shin splints S86.89
Shingles —see Herpes, zoster
Shipyard disease or eye B30.0
Shirodkar suture, in pregnancy —see
Pregnancy, complicated by, incompetent
cervix

Shock R57.9
with ectopic or molar pregnancy O08.3
adrenal (cortical) (Addisonian) E27.2
adverse food reaction (anaphylactic) —see
Shock, anaphylactic, due to food
allergic —see Shock, anaphylactic
anaphylactic T78.2
chemical —see Table of Drugs and
Chemicals
due to drug or medicinal substance
correct substance properly administered
T88.6
overdose or wrong substance given or
taken (by accident) —see Table of
Drugs and Chemicals, by drug,
poisoning
due to food (nonpoisonous) T78.00
additives T78.06
dairy products T78.07
eggs T78.08
fish T78.03
shellfish T78.02
fruit T78.04
milk T78.07
nuts T78.05
multiple types T78.05
peanuts T78.01
peanuts T78.01
seeds T78.05
specified type NEC T78.09
vegetable T78.04
following sting(s) —see Venom
immunization T80.52
serum T80.59
blood and blood products T80.51
immunization T80.52
specified NEC T80.59
vaccination T80.52
anaphylactoid —see Shock, anaphylactic
anesthetic
correct substance properly administered
T88.2
overdose or wrong substance given
or taken —see Table of Drugs and
Chemicals, by drug, poisoning
specified anesthetic —see Table of
Drugs and Chemicals, by drug,
poisoning
cardiogenic R57.0
chemical substance —see Table of Drugs and
Chemicals
complicating ectopic or molar pregnancy O08.3
culture —see Disorder, adjustment
drug
due to correct substance properly
administered T88.6
overdose or wrong substance given or
taken (by accident) —see Table of
Drugs and Chemicals, by drug,
poisoning
during or after labor and delivery O75.1
electric T75.4
(taser) T75.4
endotoxic R65.21
postprocedural (resulting from a procedure,
not elsewhere classified) T81.12
following
ectopic or molar pregnancy O08.3
injury (immediate) (delayed) T79.4
labor and delivery O75.1
food (anaphylactic) —see Shock, anaphylactic,
due to food
from electroshock gun (taser) T75.4
gram-negative R65.21
postprocedural (resulting from a procedure,
not elsewhere classified) T81.12
hematologic R57.8
hemorrhagic R57.8
surgery (intraoperative) (postoperative)
T81.19
trauma T79.4

Shock *(Continued)*
hypovolemic R57.1
surgical T81.19
traumatic T79.4
insulin E15
therapeutic misadventure —*see*
subcategory T38.3
kidney N17.0
traumatic (following crushing) T79.5
lightning T75.01
liver K72.00
lung J80
obstetric O75.1
with ectopic or molar pregnancy O08.3
following ectopic or molar pregnancy
O08.3
pleural (surgical) T81.19
due to trauma T79.4
postprocedural (postoperative) T81.10
with ectopic or molar pregnancy O08.3
cardiogenic T81.11
endotoxic T81.12
following ectopic or molar pregnancy
O08.3
gram-negative T81.12
hypovolemic T81.19
septic T81.12
specified type NEC T81.19
psychic F43.0
septic (due to severe sepsis) R65.21
specified NEC R57.8
surgical T81.10
taser gun (taser) T75.4
therapeutic misadventure NEC T81.10
thyroxin
overdose or wrong substance given
or taken —*see* Table of Drugs and
Chemicals, by drug, poisoning
toxic, syndrome A48.3
transfusion —*see* Complications, transfusion
traumatic (immediate) (delayed) T79.4
Shoemaker's chest M95.4
Short, shortening, shortness
arm (acquired) —*see also* Deformity, limb,
unequal length
congenital Q71.81-●
forearm —*see* Deformity, limb, unequal
length
bowel syndrome K91.2
breath R06.02
cervical (complicating pregnancy) O26.87-●
non-gravid uterus N88.3
common bile duct, congenital Q44.5
cord (umbilical), complicating delivery O69.3
cystic duct, congenital Q44.5
esophagus (congenital) Q39.8
femur (acquired) —*see* Deformity, limb,
unequal length, femur
congenital —*see* Defect, reduction, lower
limb, longitudinal, femur
frenum, frenulum, linguae (congenital) Q38.1
hip (acquired) —*see also* Deformity, limb,
unequal length
congenital Q65.89
leg (acquired) —*see also* Deformity, limb,
unequal length
congenital Q72.81-●
lower leg —*see also* Deformity, limb,
unequal length
congenital Q72.81-●
limbed stature, with immunodeficiency
D82.2
lower limb (acquired) —*see also* Deformity,
limb, unequal length
organ or site, congenital NEC —*see* Distortion
palate, congenital Q38.5
radius (acquired) —*see also* Deformity, limb,
unequal length
congenital —*see* Defect, reduction, upper
limb, longitudinal, radius
rib syndrome Q77.2

Short, shortening, shortness*(Continued)*
stature (child) (hereditary) (idiopathic) NEC
R62.52
➠constitutional E34.31
~~due to endocrine disorder E34.3~~
▶due to
▶endocrine disorder E34.30
▶specified type NEC, due to endocrine
disorder E34.39
▶genetic causes E34.329
▶ACAN gene variant E34.828
▶acid-labile subunit gene (IGFALS)
defect E34.321
▶aggrecan deficiency E34.828
▶genetic syndrome with resistance to
insulin-like growth factor-1
E34.322
▶growth hormone gene 1 (GH1) defect
with growth hormone
neutralizing antibodies E34.321
▶growth hormone insensitivity
syndrome (GHIS) E34.321
▶insulin-like growth factor 1 gene
(IGF1) defect E34.321
▶insulin-like growth factor-1 receptor
(IGF-1R) defect E34.322
▶insulin-like growth factor-1 (IGF-1)
resistance E34.322
▶NPR-2 gene variant E34.828
▶post-insulin-like growth factor-1
receptor signaling defect E34.322
▶primary insulin-like growth factor-1
(IGF-1) deficiency E34.321
▶severe primary insulin-like growth
factor-1 deficiency (SPIGFD)
E34.321
▶signal transducer and activator of
transcription 5B gene (STAT5b)
defect E34.321
▶specified genetic cause NEC E34.828
➠Laron-type E34.321
tendon —*see also* Contraction, tendon
with contracture of joint —*see* Contraction,
joint
Achilles (acquired) M67.0-●
congenital Q66.89
congenital Q79.8
thigh (acquired) —*see also* Deformity, limb,
unequal length, femur
congenital —*see* Defect, reduction, lower
limb, longitudinal, femur
tibialis anterior (tendon) —*see* Contraction,
tendon
umbilical cord
complicating delivery O69.3
upper limb, congenital —*see* Defect,
reduction, upper limb, specified type
NEC
urethra N36.8
uvula, congenital Q38.5
vagina (congenital) Q52.4
Shortsightedness —*see* Myopia
Shoshin (acute fulminating beriberi) E51.11
Shoulder —*see* condition
Shovel-shaped incisors K00.2
Shower, thromboembolic —*see* Embolism
Shunt
arterial-venous (dialysis) Z99.2
arteriovenous, pulmonary (acquired) I28.0
congenital Q25.72
cerebral ventricle (communicating) in situ
Z98.2
surgical, prosthetic, with complications —*see*
Complications, cardiovascular, device or
implant Shutdown, renal N28.9
Shutdown, renal N28.9
Shy-Drager syndrome G90.3
Sialadenitis, sialadenosis (any gland) (chronic)
(periodic) (suppurative) —*see* Sialoadenitis
Sialectasia K11.8
Sialidosis E77.1

Sialitis, silitis (any gland) (chronic)
(suppurative) —*see* Sialoadenitis
Sialoadenitis (any gland) (periodic)
(suppurative) K11.20
acute K11.21
recurrent K11.22
chronic K11.23
Sialoadenopathy K11.9
Sialoangitis —*see* Sialoadenitis
Sialodochitis (fibrinosa) —*see* Sialoadenitis
Sialodocholithiasis K11.5
Sialolithiasis K11.5
Sialometaplasia, necrotizing K11.8
Sialorrhea —*see also* Ptyalism
periodic —*see* Sialoadenitis
Sialosis K11.7
Siamese twin Q89.4
Sibling rivalry Z62.891
Sicard's syndrome G52.7
Sicca syndrome —*see* Syndrome, Sjogren
Sick R69
or handicapped person in family Z63.79
needing care at home Z63.6
sinus (syndrome) I49.5
Sick-euthyroid syndrome E07.81
Sickle-cell
anemia —*see* Disease, sickle-cell
beta plus —*see* Disease, sickle-cell,
thalassemia, beta plus
beta zero —*see* Disease, sickle-cell,
thalassemia, beta zero
trait D57.3
Sicklemia —*see also* Disease, sickle-cell
trait D57.3
Sickness
air (travel) T75.3
airplane T75.3
alpine T70.29
altitude T70.20
Andes T70.29
aviator's T70.29
balloon T70.29
car T75.3
compressed air T70.3
decompression T70.3
green D50.8
milk —*see* Poisoning, food, noxious
motion T75.3
mountain T70.29
acute D75.1
protein —*see also* Reaction, serum T80.69
radiation T66
roundabout (motion) T75.3
sea T75.3
serum NEC —*see also* Reaction, serum T80.69
sleeping (African) B56.9
by Trypanosoma B56.9
brucei
gambiense B56.0
rhodesiense B56.1
East African B56.1
Gambian B56.0
Rhodesian B56.1
West African B56.0
swing (motion) T75.3
train (railway) (travel) T75.3
travel (any vehicle) T75.3
Sideropenia —*see* Anemia, iron deficiency
Siderosilicosis J62.8
Siderosis (lung) J63.4
brain G93.89
eye (globe) —*see* Disorder, globe,
degenerative, siderosis
Siemens' syndrome (ectodermal dysplasia) Q82.8
Sighing R06.89
psychogenic F45.8
Sigmoid —*see also* condition
flexure —*see* condition
kidney Q63.1
Sigmoiditis —*see also* Enteritis K52.9
infectious A09
noninfectious K52.9

▶ New   ➠ Revised   ~~deleted~~ Deleted   ● Use Additional Character(s)

Silfverskiöld's syndrome Q78.9
Silicosiderosis J62.8
Silicosis, silicotic (simple) (complicated)
  J62.8
  with tuberculosis J65
Silicotuberculosis J65
Silo-fillers' disease J68.8
  bronchitis J68.0
  pneumonitis J68.0
  pulmonary edema J68.1
Silver's syndrome Q87.19
Simian malaria B53.1
Simmonds' cachexia or disease E23.0
Simons' disease or syndrome (progressive
  lipodystrophy) E88.1
Simple, simplex —see condition
Simulation, conscious (of illness) Z76.5
Simultanagnosia (asimultagnosia) R48.3
Sin Nombre virus disease (Hantavirus)
  (cardio)-pulmonary syndrome) B33.4
Sinding-Larsen disease or osteochondrosis —
  see Osteochondrosis, juvenile, patella
Singapore hemorrhagic fever A91
Singer's node or nodule J38.2
Single
  atrium Q21.20
  coronary artery Q24.5
  umbilical artery Q27.0
  ventricle Q20.4
Singultus R06.6
  epidemicus B33.0
Sinus —see also Fistula
  abdominal K63.89
  arrest I45.5
  arrhythmia I49.8
  bradycardia R00.1
  branchial cleft (internal) (external) Q18.0
  coccygeal —see Sinus, pilonidal
  dental K04.6
  dermal (congenital) Q06.8
    with abscess Q06.8
    coccygeal, pilonidal —see Sinus, coccygeal
  infected, skin NEC L08.89
  marginal, ruptured or bleeding —see
    Hemorrhage, antepartum, specified
    cause NEC
  medial, face and neck Q18.8
  pause I45.5
  pericranii Q01.9
  pilonidal (infected) (rectum) L05.92
    with abscess L05.02
  preauricular Q18.1
  rectovaginal N82.3
  Rokitansky-Aschoff (gallbladder) K82.8
  sacrococcygeal (dermoid) (infected) —see
    Sinus, pilonidal
  tachycardia R00.0
    paroxysmal I47.1
  tarsi syndrome M25.57-●
  testis N50.89
  tract (postinfective) —see Fistula
  urachus Q64.4
Sinusitis (accessory) (chronic) (hyperplastic)
  (nasal) (nonpurulent) (purulent) J32.9
  acute J01.90
    ethmoidal J01.20
      recurrent J01.21
    frontal J01.10
      recurrent J01.11
    involving more than one sinus, other than
      pansinusitis J01.80
      recurrent J01.81
    maxillary J01.00
      recurrent J01.01
    pansinusitis J01.40
      recurrent J01.41
    recurrent J01.91
    specified NEC J01.80
      recurrent J01.81
    sphenoidal J01.30
      recurrent J01.31

Sinus(Continued)
  allergic —see Rhinitis, allergic
  due to high altitude T70.1
  ethmoidal J32.2
    acute J01.20
      recurrent J01.21
  frontal J32.1
    acute J01.10
      recurrent J01.11
  influenzal —see Influenza, with, respiratory
    manifestations NEC
  involving more than one sinus but not
    pansinusitis J32.8
    acute J01.80
      recurrent J01.81
  maxillary J32.0
    acute J01.00
      recurrent J01.01
  sphenoidal J32.3
    acute J01.30
      recurrent J01.31
  tuberculous, any sinus A15.8
Sinusitis-bronchiectasis-situs inversus
  (syndrome) (triad) Q89.3
Sipple's syndrome E31.22
Sirenomelia (syndrome) Q87.2
Siriasis T67.01
Sirkari's disease B55.0
Siti A65
Situation, psychiatric F99
Situational
  disturbance (transient) —see Disorder,
    adjustment
    acute F43.0
  maladjustment —see Disorder, adjustment
  reaction —see Disorder, adjustment
    acute F43.0
Situs inversus or transversus (abdominalis)
  (thoracis) Q89.3
Sixth disease B08.20
  due to human herpesvirus 6 B08.21
  due to human herpesvirus 7 B08.22
Sjögren-Larsson syndrome Q87.19
Sjögren's syndrome or disease —see Syndrome,
  Sjogren
Skeletal —see condition
Skene's gland —see condition
Skenitis —see Urethritis
Skerljevo A65
Skevas-Zerfus disease —see Toxicity, venom,
  marine animal, sea anemone
Skin —see also condition
  clammy R23.1
  donor —see Donor, skin
  dry L85.3
  hidebound M35.9
Slate-dressers' or slate-miners' lung
  J62.8
Sleep
  apnea —see Apnea, sleep
  deprivation Z72.820
  disorder or disturbance G47.9
    child F51.9
    nonorganic origin F51.9
    specified NEC G47.8
  disturbance G47.9
    nonorganic origin F51.9
  drunkenness F51.9
  rhythm inversion G47.2-●
  terrors F51.4
  walking F51.3
    hysterical F44.89
Sleep hygiene
  abuse Z72.821
  inadequate Z72.821
  poor Z72.821
Sleeping sickness —see Sickness, sleeping
Sleeplessness —see Insomnia
  menopausal N95.11
Sleep-wake schedule disorder G47.20
Slim disease (in HIV infection) B20

Slipped, slipping
  epiphysis (traumatic) —see also
    Osteochondropathy, specified type NEC
    capital femoral (traumatic) [SCFE]
      acute (on chronic) S79.01-●
      ▶nontraumatic M93.00-●
    current traumatic - code as Fracture, by site
    upper femoral (nontraumatic) [SUFE]
      M93.00-●
      acute M93.01-●
      on chronic M93.03-●
      chronic M93.02-●
  intervertebral disc —see Displacement,
    intervertebral disc
  ligature, umbilical P51.8
  patella —see Disorder, patella, derangement
    NEC
  rib M89.8X8
  sacroiliac joint —see subcategory M53.2
  tendon —see Disorder, tendon
  ulnar nerve, nontraumatic —see Lesion,
    nerve, ulnar
  vertebra NEC —see Spondylolisthesis
Slocumb's syndrome E27.0
Sloughing (multiple) (phagedena) (skin) —see
  also Gangrene
  abscess —see Abscess
  appendix K38.8
  fascia —see Disorder, soft tissue, specified
    type NEC
  scrotum N50.89
  tendon —see Disorder, tendon
  transplanted organ —see Rejection, transplant
  ulcer —see Ulcer, skin
Slow
  feeding, newborn P92.2
  flow syndrome, coronary I20.8
  heart(beat) R00.1
Slowing, urinary stream R39.198
Sluder's neuralgia (syndrome) G44.89
Slurred, slurring speech R47.81
Small (ness)
  for gestational age —see Small for dates
  introitus, vagina N89.6
  kidney (unknown cause) N27.9
    bilateral N27.1
    unilateral N27.0
  ovary (congenital) Q50.39
  pelvis
    with disproportion (fetopelvic) O33.1
      causing obstructed labor O65.1
  uterus N85.8
  white kidney N03.9
Small-and-light-for-dates —see Small for dates
Small-for-dates (infant) P05.10
  with weight of
    499 grams or less P05.11
    500-749 grams P05.12
    750-999 grams P05.13
    1000-1249 grams P05.14
    1250-1499 grams P05.15
    1500-1749 grams P05.16
    1750-1999 grams P05.17
    2000-2499 grams P05.18
    2500 grams and over P05.19
  specified NEC P05.19
Smallpox B03
Smearing, fecal R15.1
SMEI (severe myoclonic epilepsy in infancy)
  G40.83-●
Smith-Lemli-Opitz syndrome E78.72
Smith's fracture S52.54-●
Smoker —see Dependence, drug, nicotine
Smoker's
  bronchitis J41.0
  cough J41.0
  palate K13.24
  throat J31.2
  tongue K13.24
Smoking
  passive Z77.22

S

Smothering spells R06.81
Snaggle teeth, tooth M26.39
Snapping
   finger —*see* Trigger finger
   hip —*see* Derangement, joint, specified type
      NEC, hip
      involving the iliotibial band M76.3-●
   knee —*see* Derangement, knee
      involving the iliotibial band M76.3-●
Sneddon-Wilkinson disease or syndrome
   (sub-corneal pustular dermatosis)
   L13.1
Sneezing (intractable) R06.7
Sniffing
   cocaine
      abuse —*see* Abuse, drug, cocaine
      dependence —*see* Dependence, drug,
         cocaine
   gasoline
      abuse —*see* Abuse, drug, inhalant
      dependence —*see* Dependence, drug,
         inhalant
   glue (airplane)
      abuse —*see* Abuse, drug, inhalant
      drug dependence —*see* Dependence, drug,
         inhalant
Sniffles
   newborn P28.89
Snoring R06.83
Snow blindness —*see* Photokeratitis
Snuffles (non-syphilitic) R06.5
   newborn P28.89
   syphilitic (infant) A50.05 *[J99]*
Social
   exclusion Z60.4
      due to discrimination or persecution
         (perceived) Z60.5
   migrant Z59.00
      acculturation difficulty Z60.3
   rejection Z60.4
      due to discrimination or persecution Z60.5
   role conflict NEC Z73.5
   skills inadequacy NEC Z73.4
   transplantation Z60.3
Sodoku A25.0
Soemmerring's ring —*see* Cataract, secondary
Soft —*see also* condition
   nails L60.3
Softening
   bone —*see* Osteomalacia
   brain (necrotic) (progressive) G93.89
      congenital Q04.8
      embolic I63.4-●
      hemorrhagic —*see* Hemorrhage,
         intracranial, intracerebral
      occlusive I63.5-●
      thrombotic I63.3-●
   cartilage M94.2-●
      patella M22.4-●
   cerebellar —*see* Softening, brain
   cerebral —*see* Softening, brain
   cerebrospinal —*see* Softening, brain
   myocardial, heart —*see* Degeneration,
      myocardial
   spinal cord G95.89
   stomach K31.89
Soldier's
   heart F45.8
   patches I31.0
Solitary
   cyst, kidney N28.1
   kidney, congenital Q60.0
Solvent abuse —*see* Abuse, drug, inhalant
   dependence —*see* Dependence, drug,
      inhalant
Somatization reaction, somatic reaction —*see*
   Disorder, somatoform
Somnambulism F51.3
   hysterical F44.89
Somnolence R40.0
   nonorganic origin F51.11

Sonne dysentery A03.3
Soor B37.0
Sore
   bed —*see* Ulcer, pressure, by site
   chiclero B55.1
   Delhi B55.1
   desert —*see* Ulcer, skin
   eye H57.1-●
   Lahore B55.1
   mouth K13.79
      canker K12.0
   muscle M79.10
   Naga —*see* Ulcer, skin
   of skin —*see* Ulcer, skin - oriental B55.1
   pressure —*see* Ulcer, pressure, by site
   skin L98.9
   soft A57
   throat (acute) —*see also* Pharyngitis
      with influenza, flu, or grippe —*see*
         Influenza, with, respiratory
         manifestations NEC
      chronic J31.2
      coxsackie (virus) B08.5
      diphtheritic A36.0
      herpesviral B00.2
      influenzal —*see* Influenza, with, respiratory
         manifestations NEC
      septic J02.0
      streptococcal (ulcerative) J02.0
      viral NEC J02.8
         coxsackie B08.5
   tropical —*see* Ulcer, skin
   veldt —*see* Ulcer, skin
Soto's syndrome (cerebral gigantism) Q87.3
South African cardiomyopathy syndrome I42.8
Southeast Asian hemorrhagic fever A91
Spacing
   abnormal, tooth, teeth, fully erupted M26.30
   excessive, tooth, fully erupted M26.32
Spade-like hand (congenital) Q68.1
Spading nail L60.8
   congenital Q84.6
Spanish collar N47.1
Sparganosis B70.1
Spasm(s), spastic, spasticity —*see also* condition
   R25.2
   accommodation —*see* Spasm, of
      accommodation
   ampulla of Vater K83.4
   anus, ani (sphincter) (reflex) K59.4
      psychogenic F45.8
   artery I73.9
      cerebral G45.9
   Bell's G51.3-●
   bladder (sphincter, external or internal)
      N32.89
      psychogenic F45.8
   bronchus, bronchiole J98.01
   cardia K22.0
   cardiac I20.1
   carpopedal —*see* Tetany
   cerebral (arteries) (vascular) G45.9
   cervix, complicating delivery O62.4
   ciliary body (of accommodation) —*see* Spasm,
      of accommodation
   colon —*see also* Irritable, bowel K58.9
      with diarrhea K58.0
      psychogenic F45.8
   common duct K83.8
   compulsive —*see* Tic
   conjugate H51.8
   coronary (artery) I20.1
   diaphragm (reflex) R06.6
      epidemic B33.0
      psychogenic F45.8
   duodenum K59.89
   epidemic diaphragmatic (transient) B33.0
   esophagus (diffuse) K22.4
      psychogenic F45.8
   facial G51.3-●
   fallopian tube N83.8

Spasm(s), spastic, spasticity *(Continued)*
   gastrointestinal (tract) K31.89
      psychogenic F45.8
   glottis J38.5
      hysterical F44.4
      psychogenic F45.8
         conversion reaction F44.4
      reflex through recurrent laryngeal nerve
         J38.5
   habit —*see* Tic
   heart I20.1
   hemifacial (clonic) G51.3-●
   hourglass —*see* Contraction, hourglass
   hysterical F44.4
   infantile —*see* Epilepsy, spasms
   inferior oblique, eye H51.8
   intestinal —*see also* Syndrome, irritable bowel
      K58.9
      psychogenic F45.8
   larynx, laryngeal J38.5
      hysterical F44.4
      psychogenic F45.8
         conversion reaction F44.4
   levator palpebrae superioris —*see* Disorder,
      eyelid function
   muscle NEC M62.838
      back M62.830
   nerve, trigeminal G51.0
   nervous F45.8
   nodding F98.4
   occupational F48.8
   oculogyric H51.8
      psychogenic F45.8
   of accommodation H52.53-●
   ophthalmic artery —*see* Occlusion, artery,
      retina
   perineal, female N94.89
   peroneo-extensor —*see also* Deformity, limb,
      flat foot
   pharynx (reflex) J39.2
      hysterical F45.8
      psychogenic F45.8
   psychogenic F45.8
   pylorus NEC K31.3
      adult hypertrophic K31.89
      congenital or infantile Q40.0
      psychogenic F45.8
   rectum (sphincter) K59.4
      psychogenic F45.8
   retinal (artery) —*see* Occlusion, artery, retina
   sigmoid —*see also* Syndrome, irritable bowel
      K58.9
      psychogenic F45.8
   sphincter of Oddi K83.4
   stomach K31.89
      neurotic F45.8
   throat J39.2
      hysterical F45.8
      psychogenic F45.8
   tic F95.9
      chronic F95.1
      transient of childhood F95.0
   tongue K14.8
   torsion (progressive) G24.1
   trigeminal nerve —*see* Neuralgia, trigeminal
   ureter N13.5
   urethra (sphincter) N35.919
   uterus N85.8
      complicating labor O62.4
   vagina N94.2
      psychogenic F52.5
   vascular I73.9
   vasomotor I73.9
   vein NEC I87.8
   viscera —*see* Pain, abdominal
Spasmodic —*see* condition
Spasmophilia —*see* Tetany
Spasmus nutans F98.4
Spastic, spasticity —*see also* Spasm
   child (cerebral) (congenital) (paralysis) G80.1
Speaker's throat R49.8

▶ New   ⇒ Revised   ~~deleted~~ Deleted   ● Use Additional Character(s)

Specific, specified —*see* condition
Speech
   defect, disorder, disturbance, impediment —
      see Disorder, speech R47.9
      psychogenic, in childhood and adolescence
         F98.8
      slurring R47.81
      specified NEC R47.89
▶Spells, transient oxygen desaturation of
      newborn (*see also* Apnea, newborn) P28.40
   ▶during sleep (*see also* Apnea, newborn, sleep,
      primary) P28.30
Spencer's disease A08.19
Spens' syndrome (syncope with heart block)
   I45.9
Sperm counts (fertility testing) Z31.41
   postvasectomy Z30.8
      reversal Z31.42
Spermatic cord —*see* condition
Spermatocele N43.40
   congenital Q55.4
   multiple N43.42
   single N43.41
Spermatocystitis N49.0
Spermatocytoma C62.9-●
   specified site —*see* Neoplasm, malignant, by
      site
Spermatorrhea N50.89
Sphacelus —*see* Gangrene
Sphenoidal —*see* condition
Sphenoiditis (chronic) —*see* Sinusitis,
   sphenoidal
Sphenopalatine ganglion neuralgia G90.09
Sphericity, increased, lens (congenital) Q12.4
Spherocytosis (congenital) (familial)
      (hereditary) D58.0
   hemoglobin disease D58.0
   sickle-cell (disease) D57.8-●
Spherophakia Q12.4
Sphincter —*see* condition
Sphincteritis, sphincter of Oddi —*see*
   Cholangitis
Sphingolipidosis E75.3
   specified NEC E75.29
Sphingomyelinosis E75.3
Spicule tooth K00.2
Spider
   bite —*see* Toxicity, venom, spider
      nonvenomous —*see* Bite, by site,
         superficial, insect
   fingers —*see* Syndrome, Marfan's
   nevus I78.1
   toes —*see* Syndrome, Marfan's
   vascular I78.1
Spiegler-Fendt
   benign lymphocytoma L98.8
   sarcoid L08.89
Spielmeyer-Vogt disease E75.4
Spina bifida (aperta) Q05.9
   with hydrocephalus NEC Q05.4
   cervical Q05.5
      with hydrocephalus Q05.0
   dorsal Q05.6
      with hydrocephalus Q05.1
   lumbar Q05.7
      with hydrocephalus Q05.2
   lumbosacral Q05.7
      with hydrocephalus Q05.2
   occulta Q76.0
   sacral Q05.8
      with hydrocephalus Q05.3
   thoracic Q05.6
      with hydrocephalus Q05.1
   thoracolumbar Q05.6
      with hydrocephalus Q05.1
Spindle, Krukenberg's —*see* Pigmentation,
   cornea, posterior
Spine, spinal —*see* condition
Spiradenoma (eccrine) —*see* Neoplasm, skin,
   benign
Spirillosis A25.0

Spirillum
   minus A25.0
   obermeieri infection A68.0
Spirochetal —*see* condition
Spirochetosis A69.9
   arthritic, arthritica A69.9
   bronchopulmonary A69.8
   icterohemorrhagic A27.0
   lung A69.8
Spirometrosis B70.1
Spitting blood —*see* Hemoptysis
Splanchnoptosis K63.4
Spleen, splenic —*see* condition
Splenectasis —*see* Splenomegaly
Splenitis (interstitial) (malignant) (nonspecific)
   D73.89
   malarial —*see also* Malaria B54 [*D77*]
   tuberculous A18.85
Splenocele D73.89
Splenomegaly, splenomegalia (Bengal)
      (cryptogenic) (idiopathic) (tropical) R16.1
   with hepatomegaly R16.2
   cirrhotic D73.2
   congenital Q89.09
   congestive, chronic D73.2
   Egyptian B65.1
   Gaucher's E75.22
   malarial —*see also* Malaria B54 [*D77*]
   neutropenic D73.81
   Niemann-Pick —*see* Niemann-Pick disease or
      syndrome
   siderotic D73.2
   syphilitic A52.79
      congenital (early) A50.08 [*D77*]
Splenopathy D73.9
Splenoptosis D73.89
Splenosis D73.89
Splinter —*see* Foreign body, superficial, by site
Split, splitting
   foot Q72.7-●
   hand Q71.6
   heart sounds R01.2
   lip, congenital —*see* Cleft, lip
   nails L60.3
   urinary stream R39.13
Spondylarthrosis —*see* Spondylosis
Spondylitis (chronic) —*see also* Spondylopathy,
      inflammatory
   ankylopoietica —*see* Spondylitis, ankylosing
   ankylosing (chronic) M45.9
      with lung involvement M45.9 [*J99*]
      cervical region M45.2
      cervicothoracic region M45.3
      juvenile M08.1
      lumbar region M45.6
      lumbosacral region M45.7
      multiple sites M45.0
      occipito-atlanto-axial region M45.1
      sacrococcygeal region M45.8
      thoracic region M45.4
      thoracolumbar region M45.5
   atrophic (ligamentous) —*see* Spondylitis,
      ankylosing
   deformans (chronic) —*see* Spondylosis
   gonococcal A54.41
   gouty —*see also* Gout, by type, vertebrae
      M10.08
   in (due to)
      brucellosis A23.9 [*M49.80*]
         cervical region A23.9 [*M49.82*]
         cervicothoracic region A23.9 [*M49.83*]
         lumbar region A23.9 [*M49.86*]
         lumbosacral region A23.9 [*M49.87*]
         multiple sites A23.9 [*M49.89*]
         occipito-atlanto-axial region A23.9
            [*M49.81*]
         sacrococcygeal region A23.9 [*M49.88*]
         thoracic region A23.9 [*M49.84*]
         thoracolumbar region A23.9 [*M49.85*]
      enterobacteria —*see also* subcategory M49.8
         A04.9
      tuberculosis A18.01

Spondylitis (Continued)
   infectious NEC —*see* Spondylopathy,
      infective
   juvenile ankylosing (chronic) M08.1
   Kümmell's —*see* Spondylopathy, traumatic
   Marie-Strümpell —*see* Spondylitis,
      ankylosing
   muscularis —*see* Spondylopathy, specified
      NEC
   psoriatic L40.53
   rheumatoid —*see* Spondylitis, ankylosing
   rhizomelica —*see* Spondylitis, ankylosing
   sacroiliac NEC M46.1
   senescent, senile —*see* Spondylosis
   traumatic (chronic) or post-traumatic —*see*
      Spondylopathy, traumatic
   tuberculous A18.01
   typhosa A01.05
Spondyloarthritis
   axial —*see also* Spondlyitis, ankylosing
      non-radiographic M45.A0
         cervical M45.A2
         cervicothoracic M45.A3
         lumbar M45.A6
         lumbosacral M45.A7
         multiple sites M45.AB
         occipito-atlanto-axial region M45.A1
         sacral and sacrococcygeal M45.A8
         thoracic M45.A4
         thoracolumbar M45.A5
Spondylolisthesis (acquired) (degenerative)
      M43.10
   with disproportion (fetopelvic) O33.0
      causing obstructed labor O65.0
   cervical region M43.12
   cervicothoracic region M43.13
   congenital Q76.2
   lumbar region M43.16
   lumbosacral region M43.17
   multiple sites M43.19
   occipito-atlanto-axial region M43.11
   sacrococcygeal region M43.18
   thoracic region M43.14
   thoracolumbar region M43.15
   traumatic (old) M43.10
      acute
         fifth cervical (displaced) S12.430
            nondisplaced S12.431
            specified type NEC (displaced)
               S12.450
               nondisplaced S12.451
            type III S12.44
         fourth cervical (displaced) S12.330
            nondisplaced S12.331
            specified type NEC (displaced)
               S12.350
               nondisplaced S12.351
            type III S12.34
         second cervical (displaced) S12.130
            nondisplaced S12.131
            specified type NEC (displaced)
               S12.150
               nondisplaced S12.151
            type III S12.14
         seventh cervical (displaced) S12.630
            nondisplaced S12.631
            specified type NEC (displaced)
               S12.650
               nondisplaced S12.651
            type III S12.64
         sixth cervical (displaced) S12.530
            nondisplaced S12.531
            specified type NEC (displaced)
               S12.550
               nondisplaced S12.551
            type III S12.54
         third cervical (displaced) S12.230
            nondisplaced S12.231
            specified type NEC (displaced)
               S12.250
               nondisplaced S12.251
            type III S12.24

Spondylolysis (acquired) M43.00
  cervical region M43.02
  cervicothoracic region M43.03
  congenital Q76.2
  lumbar region M43.06
  lumbosacral region M43.07
    with disproportion (fetopelvic) O33.0
      causing obstructed labor O65.8
  multiple sites M43.09
  occipito-atlanto-axial region M43.01
  sacrococcygeal region M43.08
  thoracic region M43.04
  thoracolumbar region M43.05
Spondylopathy M48.9
  infective NEC M46.50
    cervical region M46.52
    cervicothoracic region M46.53
    lumbar region M46.56
    lumbosacral region M46.57
    multiple sites M46.59
    occipito-atlanto-axial region M46.51
    sacrococcygeal region M46.58
    thoracic region M46.54
    thoracolumbar region M46.55
  inflammatory M46.90
    cervical region M46.92
    cervicothoracic region M46.93
    lumbar region M46.96
    lumbosacral region M46.97
    multiple sites M46.99
    occipito-atlanto-axial region M46.91
    sacrococcygeal region M46.98
    specified type NEC M46.80
      cervical region M46.82
      cervicothoracic region M46.83
      lumbar region M46.86
      lumbosacral region M46.87
      multiple sites M46.89
      occipito-atlanto-axial region M46.81
      sacrococcygeal region M46.88
      thoracic region M46.84
      thoracolumbar region M46.85
    thoracic region M46.94
    thoracolumbar region M46.95
  neuropathic, in
    syringomyelia and syringobulbia G95.0
    tabes dorsalis A52.11
  specified NEC —see subcategory M48.8
  traumatic M48.30
    cervical region M48.32
    cervicothoracic region M48.33
    lumbar region M48.36
    lumbosacral region M48.37
    occipito-atlanto-axial region M48.31
    sacrococcygeal region M48.38
    thoracic region M48.34
    thoracolumbar region M48.35
Spondylosis M47.9
  with
    disproportion (fetopelvic) O33.0
      causing obstructed labor O65.0
    myelopathy NEC M47.10
      cervical region M47.12
      cervicothoracic region M47.13
      lumbar region M47.16
      occipito-atlanto-axial region M47.11
      thoracic region M47.14
      thoracolumbar region M47.15
    radiculopathy M47.20
      cervical region M47.22
      cervicothoracic region M47.23
      lumbar region M47.26
      lumbosacral region M47.27
      occipito-atlanto-axial region M47.21
      sacrococcygeal region M47.28
      thoracic region M47.24
      thoracolumbar region M47.25
  without myelopathy or radiculopathy
      M47.819
    cervical region M47.812
    cervicothoracic region M47.813
    lumbar region M47.816

Spondylolysis (Continued)
  without myelopathy or radiculopathy
      (Continued)
    lumbosacral region M47.817
    occipito-atlanto-axial region M47.811
    sacrococcygeal region M47.818
    thoracic region M47.814
    thoracolumbar region M47.815
  specified NEC M47.899
    cervical region M47.892
    cervicothoracic region M47.893
    facet joint (see also Spondylosis) M47.819
    lumbar region M47.896
    lumbosacral region M47.897
    occipito-atlanto-axial region M47.891
    sacrococcygeal region M47.898
    thoracic region M47.894
    thoracolumbar region M47.895
  traumatic —see Spondylopathy, traumatic
Sponge
  inadvertently left in operation wound —see
      Foreign body, accidentally left during a
      procedure
  kidney (medullary) Q61.5
Sponge-diver's disease —see Toxicity, venom,
    marine animal, sea anemone
Spongioblastoma (any type) —see Neoplasm,
    malignant, by site
  specified site —see Neoplasm, malignant, by
    site
  unspecified site C71.9
Spongioneuroblastoma —see Neoplasm,
    malignant, by site
Spontaneous —see also condition
  fracture (cause unknown) —see Fracture,
    pathological
Spoon nail L60.3
  congenital Q84.6
Sporadic —see condition
Sporothrix schenckii infection —see
    Sporotrichosis
Sporotrichosis B42.9
  arthritis B42.82
  disseminated B42.7
  generalized B42.7
  lymphocutaneous (fixed) (progressive)
    B42.1
  pulmonary B42.0
  specified NEC B42.89
Spots, spotting (in) (of)
  Bitot's —see also Pigmentation, conjunctiva
    in the young child E50.1
    vitamin A deficiency E50.1
  café, au lait L81.3
  Cayenne pepper I78.1
  cotton wool, retina —see Occlusion, artery,
    retina
  de Morgan's (senile angiomas) I78.1
  Fuchs' black (myopic) —see also Myopia,
    degenerative H44.2-●
  intermenstrual (regular) N92.0
    irregular N92.1
  Koplik's B05.9
  liver L81.4
  pregnancy O26.85-●
  purpuric R23.3
  ruby I78.1
Spotted fever —see Fever, spotted A77.9
Sprain (joint) (ligament)
  acromioclavicular joint or ligament S43.5-●
  ankle S93.40-●
    calcaneofibular ligament S93.41-●
    deltoid ligament S93.42-●
    internal collateral ligament —see Sprain,
      ankle, specified ligament NEC
    specified ligament NEC S93.49-●
    talofibular ligament —see Sprain, ankle,
      specified ligament NEC
    tibiofibular ligament S93.43-●
  anterior longitudinal, cervical S13.4
  atlas, atlanto-axial, atlanto-occipital S13.4
  breast bone —see Sprain, sternum

Sprain (Continued)
  calcaneofibular —see Sprain, ankle
  carpal —see Sprain, wrist
  carpometacarpal —see Sprain, hand, specified
    site NEC
  cartilage
    costal S23.41
    semilunar (knee) —see Sprain, knee,
      specified site NEC
      with current tear —see Tear, meniscus
    thyroid region S13.5
    xiphoid —see Sprain, sternum
  cervical, cervicodorsal, cervicothoracic S13.4
  chondrosternal S23.421
  coracoclavicular S43.8-●
  coracohumeral S43.41-●
  coronary, knee —see Sprain, knee, specified
    site NEC
  costal cartilage S23.41
  cricoarytenoid articulation or ligament S13.5
  cricothyroid articulation S13.5
  cruciate, knee —see Sprain, knee, cruciate
  deltoid, ankle —see Sprain, ankle
  dorsal (spine) S23.3
  elbow S53.40-●
    radial collateral ligament S53.43-●
    radiohumeral S53.41-●
    rupture
      radial collateral ligament —see Rupture,
        traumatic, ligament, radial
        collateral
      ulnar collateral ligament —see Rupture,
        traumatic, ligament, ulnar collateral
    specified type NEC S53.49-●
    ulnar collateral ligament S53.44-●
    ulnohumeral S53.42-●
  femur, head —see Sprain, hip
  fibular collateral, knee —see Sprain, knee,
    collateral
  fibulocalcaneal —see Sprain, ankle
  finger(s) S63.61-●
    index S63.61-●
    interphalangeal (joint) S63.63-●
      index S63.63-●
      little S63.63-●
      middle S63.63-●
      ring S63.63-●
    little S63.61-●
    metacarpophalangeal (joint) S63.65-●
    middle S63.61-●
    ring S63.61-●
    specified site NEC S63.69-●
      index S63.69-●
      little S63.69-●
      middle S63.69-●
      ring S63.69-●
  foot S93.60-●
    specified ligament NEC S93.69-●
    tarsal ligament S93.61-●
    tarsometatarsal ligament S93.62-●
    toe —see Sprain, toe
  hand S63.9-●
    finger —see Sprain, finger
    specified site NEC —see subcategory S63.8
    thumb —see Sprain, thumb
  head S03.9
  hip S73.10-●
    iliofemoral ligament S73.11-●
    ischiocapsular (ligament) S73.12-●
    specified NEC S73.19-●
  iliofemoral —see Sprain, hip
  innominate
    acetabulum —see Sprain, hip
    sacral junction S33.6
  internal
    collateral, ankle —see Sprain, ankle
    semilunar cartilage —see Sprain, knee,
      specified site NEC
  interphalangeal
    finger —see Sprain, finger, interphalangeal
      (joint)
    toe —see Sprain, toe, interphalangeal joint

▶ New   ⇒ Revised   ~~deleted~~ Deleted   ● Use Additional Character(s)

Sprain *(Continued)*
 ischiocapsular —*see* Sprain, hip
 ischiofemoral —*see* Sprain, hip
 jaw (articular disc) (cartilage) (meniscus)
  S03.4-●
  old M26.69
 knee S83.9-●
  collateral ligament S83.40-●
   lateral (fibular) S83.42-●
   medial (tibial) S83.41-●
  cruciate ligament S83.50-●
   anterior S83.51-●
   posterior S83.52-●
  lateral (fibular) collateral ligament S83.42-●
  medial (tibial) collateral ligament S83.41-●
  patellar ligament S76.11-●
  specified site NEC S83.8X-●
  superior tibiofibular joint (ligament) S83.6-●
 lateral collateral, knee —*see* Sprain, knee, collateral
 lumbar (spine) S33.5
 lumbosacral S33.9
 mandible (articular disc) S03.4-●
  old M26.69
 medial collateral, knee —*see* Sprain, knee, collateral
 meniscus
  jaw S03.4-●
   old M26.69
  knee —*see* Sprain, knee, specified site NEC
   with current tear —*see* Tear, meniscus
    old —*see* Derangement, knee, meniscus, due to old tear
  mandible S03.4-●
   old M26.69
 metacarpal (distal) (proximal) —*see* Sprain, hand, specified site NEC
 metacarpophalangeal —*see* Sprain, finger, metacarpophalangeal (joint)
 metatarsophalangeal —*see* Sprain, toe, metatarsophalangeal joint
 midcarpal —*see* Sprain, hand, specified site NEC
 midtarsal —*see* Sprain, foot, specified site NEC
 neck S13.9
  anterior longitudinal cervical ligament S13.4
  atlanto-axial joint S13.4
  atlanto-occipital joint S13.4
  cervical spine S13.4
  cricoarytenoid ligament S13.5
  cricothyroid ligament S13.5
  specified site NEC S13.8
  thyroid region (cartilage) S13.5
 nose S03.8
 orbicular, hip —*see* Sprain, hip
 patella —*see* Sprain, knee, specified site NEC
 patellar ligament S76.11-●
 pelvis NEC S33.8
 phalanx
  finger —*see* Sprain, finger
  toe —*see* Sprain, toe
 pubofemoral —*see* Sprain, hip
 radiocarpal —*see* Sprain, wrist
 radiohumeral —*see* Sprain, elbow
 radius, collateral —*see* Rupture, traumatic, ligament, radial collateral
 rib (cage) S23.41
 rotator cuff (capsule) S43.42-●
 sacroiliac (region)
  chronic or old —*see* subcategory M53.2
  joint S33.6
 scaphoid (hand) —*see* Sprain, hand, specified site NEC
 scapula (r) —*see* Sprain, shoulder girdle, specified site NEC
 semilunar cartilage (knee) —*see* Sprain, knee, specified site NEC
  with current tear —*see* Tear, meniscus
   old —*see* Derangement, knee, meniscus, due to old tear

Sprain *(Continued)*
 shoulder joint S43.40-●
  acromioclavicular joint (ligament) —*see* Sprain, acromioclavicular joint
  blade —*see* Sprain, shoulder, girdle, specified site NEC
  coracoclavicular joint (ligament) —*see* Sprain, coracoclavicular joint
  coracohumeral ligament —*see* Sprain, coracohumeral joint
  girdle S43.9-●
   specified site NEC S43.8-●
  rotator cuff —*see* Sprain, rotator cuff
  specified site NEC S43.49-●
  sternoclavicular joint (ligament) —*see* Sprain, sternoclavicular joint
 spine
  cervical S13.4
  lumbar S33.5
  thoracic S23.3
 sternoclavicular joint S43.6-●
 sternum S23.429
  chondrosternal joint S23.421
  specified site NEC S23.428
  sternoclavicular (joint) (ligament) S23.420
 symphysis
  jaw S03.4-●
   old M26.69
  mandibular S03.4-●
   old M26.69
 talofibular —*see* Sprain, ankle
 tarsal —*see* Sprain, foot, specified site NEC
 tarsometatarsal —*see* Sprain, foot, specified site NEC
 temporomandibular S03.4-●
  old M26.69
 thorax S23.9
  ribs S23.41
  specified site NEC S23.8
  spine S23.3
  sternum —*see* Sprain, sternum
 thumb S63.60-●
  interphalangeal (joint) S63.62-●
  metacarpophalangeal (joint) S63.64-●
  specified site NEC S63.68-●
 thyroid cartilage or region S13.5
 tibia (proximal end) —*see* Sprain, knee, specified site NEC
 tibial collateral, knee —*see* Sprain, knee, collateral
 tibiofibular
  distal —*see* Sprain, ankle
  superior —*see* Sprain, knee, specified site NEC
 toe(s) S93.50-●
  great S93.50-●
  interphalangeal joint S93.51-●
   great S93.51-●
   lesser S93.51-●
  lesser S93.50-●
  metatarsophalangeal joint S93.52-●
   great S93.52-●
   lesser S93.52-●
 ulna, collateral —*see* Rupture, traumatic, ligament, ulnar collateral
 ulnohumeral —*see* Sprain, elbow
 wrist S63.50-●
  carpal S63.51-●
  radiocarpal S63.52-●
  specified site NEC S63.59-●
 xiphoid cartilage —*see* Sprain, sternum
Sprengel's deformity (congenital) Q74.0
Sprue (tropical) K90.1
 celiac K90.0
 idiopathic K90.49
 meaning thrush B37.0
 nontropical K90.0
Spur, bone —*see also* Enthesopathy
 calcaneal M77.3-●
 iliac crest M76.2-●
 nose (septum) J34.89

Spurway's syndrome Q78.0
Sputum
 abnormal (amount) (color) (odor) (purulent) R09.3
 blood-stained R04.2
 excessive (cause unknown) R09.3
Squamous —*see also* condition
 epithelium in
  cervical canal (congenital) Q51.828
  uterine mucosa (congenital) Q51.818
Squashed nose M95.0
 congenital Q67.4
Squeeze, diver's T70.3
Squint —*see also* Strabismus
 accommodative —*see* Strabismus, convergent concomitant
SSADHD (succinic semialdehyde dehydrogenase deficiency) E72.81
St. Hubert's disease A82.9
Stab —*see also* Laceration
 internal organs —*see* Injury, by site
Stafne's cyst or cavity M27.0
Staggering gait R26.0
 hysterical F44.4
Staghorn calculus —*see* Calculus, kidney
Stähli's line (cornea) (pigment) —*see* Pigmentation, cornea, anterior
Stain, staining
 meconium (newborn) P96.83
 port wine Q82.5
 tooth, teeth (hard tissues) (extrinsic) K03.6
  due to
   accretions K03.6
   deposits (betel) (black) (green) (materia alba) (orange) (soft) (tobacco) K03.6
   metals (copper) (silver) K03.7
   nicotine K03.6
   pulpal bleeding K03.7
   tobacco K03.6
  intrinsic K00.8
Stammering —*see also* Disorder, fluency F80.81
Standstill
 auricular I45.5
 cardiac —*see* Arrest, cardiac
 sinoatrial I45.5
 ventricular —*see* Arrest, cardiac
Stannosis J63.5
Stanton's disease —*see* Melioidosis
Staphylitis (acute) (catarrhal) (chronic) (gangrenous) (membranous) (suppurative) (ulcerative) K12.2
Staphylococcal scalded skin syndrome L00
Staphylococcemia A41.2
Staphylococcus, staphylococcal —*see also* condition
 as cause of disease classified elsewhere B95.8
  aureus (methicillin susceptible) (MSSA) B95.61
   methicillin resistant (MRSA) B95.62
  specified NEC, as cause of disease classified elsewhere B95.7
Staphyloma (sclera)
 cornea H18.72-●
 equatorial H15.81-●
 localized (anterior) H15.82-●
 posticum H15.83-●
 ring H15.85-●
Stargardt's disease —*see* Dystrophy, retina
Starvation (inanition) (due to lack of food) T73.0
 edema —*see* Malnutrition, severe
Stasis
 bile (noncalculous) K83.1
 bronchus J98.09
  with infection —*see* Bronchitis
 cardiac —*see* Failure, heart, congestive
 cecum K59.89
 colon K59.89

Stasis *(Continued)*
  dermatitis I87.2
    with
      varicose ulcer —*see* Varix, leg, with ulcer,
        with inflammation
      varicose veins —*see* Varix, leg, with,
        inflammation
      due to postthrombotic syndrome —*see*
        Syndrome, postthrombotic
    duodenal K31.5
    eczema —*see* Varix, leg, with, inflammation
    edema —*see* Hypertension, venous (chronic),
      idiopathic
    foot T69.0-●
    ileocecal coil K59.89
    ileum K59.89
    intestinal K59.89
    jejunum K59.89
    kidney N19
    liver (cirrhotic) K76.1
    lymphatic I89.8
    pneumonia J18.2
    pulmonary —*see* Edema, lung
    rectal K59.89
    renal N19
      tubular N17.0
    ulcer —*see* Varix, leg, with, ulcer
      without varicose veins I87.2
    urine —*see* Retention, urine
    venous I87.8
State (of)
  affective and paranoid, mixed, organic
      psychotic F06.8
  agitated R45.1
    acute reaction to stress F43.0
  anxiety (neurotic) F41.1
  apprehension F41.1
  burn-out Z73.0
  climacteric, female Z78.0
    symptomatic N95.1
  compulsive F42.8
    mixed with obsessional thoughts F42.2
  confusional (psychogenic) F44.89
    acute —*see also* Delirium
      with
        ⏵arteriosclerotic dementia *(see also*
          Dementia, vascular) F01.50
          ⏵with behavioral disturbance —*see*
            Dementia, vascular F01.51
        senility or dementia F05
        alcoholic F10.231
    epileptic F05
    reactive (from emotional stress,
      psychological trauma) F44.89
    subacute —*see* Delirium
  convulsive —*see* Convulsions
  crisis F43.0
  depressive F32.A
    neurotic F34.1
  dissociative F44.9
  emotional shock (stress) R45.7
  hypercoagulation —*see* Hypercoagulable
  locked-in G83.5
  menopausal Z78.0
    symptomatic N95.1
  neurotic F48.9
    with depersonalization F48.1
  obsessional F42.8
  oneiroid (schizophrenia-like) F23
  organic
    hallucinatory (nonalcoholic) F06.0
    paranoid (-hallucinatory) F06.2
  panic F41.0
  paranoid F22
    climacteric F22
    involutional F22
    menopausal F22
    organic F06.2
    senile F03
    simple F22
  persistent vegetative R40.3
  phobic F40.9

State *(Continued)*
  postleukotomy F07.0
  pregnant
    gestational carrier Z33.3
    incidental Z33.1
  psychogenic, twilight F44.89
  psychopathic (constitutional) F60.2
  psychotic, organic —*see also* Psychosis,
    organic
    mixed paranoid and affective F06.8
    senile or presenile F03
    transient NEC F06.8
      with
        depression F06.31
        hallucinations F06.0
  residual schizophrenic F20.5
  restlessness R45.1
  stress (emotional) R45.7
  tension (mental) F48.9
    specified NEC F48.8
  transient organic psychotic NEC F06.8
    depressive type F06.31
    hallucinatory type F06.0
  twilight
    epileptic F05
    psychogenic F44.89
  vegetative, persistent R40.3
  vital exhaustion Z73.0
  withdrawal —*see* Withdrawal, state
Status (post) —*see also* Presence (of)
  absence, epileptic —*see* Epilepsy, by type,
    with status epilepticus
  administration of tPA (rtPA) in a different
    facility within the last 24 hours prior to
    admission to the current facility Z92.82
  adrenalectomy (unilateral) (bilateral) E89.6
  anastomosis Z98.0
  anginosus I20.9
  angioplasty (peripheral) Z98.62
    with implant Z95.820
    coronary artery Z98.61
      with implant Z95.5
  aortocoronary bypass Z95.1
  arthrodesis Z98.1
  artificial opening (of) Z93.9
    gastrointestinal tract Z93.4
    specified NEC Z93.8
    urinary tract Z93.6
    vagina Z93.8
  asthmaticus —*see* Asthma, by type, with
    status asthmaticus
  awaiting organ transplant Z76.82
  bariatric surgery Z98.84
  bed confinement Z74.01
  bleb, filtering (vitreous), after glaucoma
    surgery Z98.83
  breast implant Z98.82
    removal Z98.86
  cataract extraction Z98.4-●
  cholecystectomy Z90.49
  clitorectomy N90.811
    with excision of labia minora N90.812
  colectomy (complete) (partial) Z90.49
  colonization —*see* Carrier (suspected) of
  colostomy Z93.3
  convulsivus idiopathicus —*see* Epilepsy, by
    type, with status epilepticus
  coronary artery angioplasty —*see* Status,
    angioplasty, coronary artery
  coronary artery bypass graft Z95.1
  cystectomy (urinary bladder) Z90.6
  cystostomy Z93.50
    appendico-vesicostomy Z93.52
    cutaneous Z93.51
    specified NEC Z93.59
  delinquent immunization Z28.3
  dental Z98.818
    crown Z98.811
    fillings Z98.811
    restoration Z98.811
    sealant Z98.810
    specified NEC Z98.818

Status *(Continued)*
  deployment (current) (military) Z56.82
  dialysis (hemodialysis) (peritoneal) Z99.2
  do not resuscitate (DNR) Z66
  donor —*see* Donor
  embedded fragments —*see* Retained, foreign
    body fragments (type of)
  embedded splinter —*see* Retained, foreign
    body fragments (type of)
  enterostomy Z93.4
  epileptic, epilepticus —*see also* Epilepsy, by
    type, with status epilepticus G40.901
  estrogen receptor
    negative Z17.1
    positive Z17.0
  female genital cutting —*see* Female genital
    mutilation status
  female genital mutilation —*see* Female genital
    mutilation status
  filtering (vitreous) bleb after glaucoma
    surgery Z98.83
  gastrectomy (complete) (partial) Z90.3
  gastric banding Z98.84
  gastric bypass for obesity Z98.84
  gastrostomy Z93.1
  human immunodeficiency virus (HIV)
    infection, asymptomatic Z21
  hysterectomy (complete) (total) Z90.710
    partial (with remaining cervial stump)
      Z90.711
  ileostomy Z93.2
  implant
    breast Z98.82
  infibulation N90.813
  intestinal bypass Z98.0
  jejunostomy Z93.4
  lapsed immunization schedule Z28.3
  laryngectomy Z90.02
  lymphaticus E32.8
  malignancy
    castrate resistant prostate Z19.2
    hormone resistant Z19.2
    hormone sensitive Z19.1
  marmoratus G80.3
  mastectomy (unilateral) (bilateral) Z90.1-●
  military deployment status (current)
    Z56.82
    in theater or in support of military war,
      peacekeeping and humanitarian
      operations Z56.82✹
  nephrectomy (unilateral) (bilateral) Z90.5
  nephrostomy Z93.6
  obesity surgery Z98.84
  oophorectomy
    bilateral Z90.722
    unilateral Z90.721
  organ replacement
    by artificial or mechanical device or
        prosthesis of
      artery Z95.828
      bladder Z96.0
      blood vessel Z95.828
      breast Z97.8
      eye globe Z97.0
      heart Z95.812
        valve Z95.2
      intestine Z97.8
      joint Z96.60
        hip —*see* Presence, hip joint implant
        knee —*see* Presence, knee joint
          implant
        specified site NEC Z96.698
      kidney Z97.8
      larynx Z96.3
      lens Z96.1
      limbs —*see* Presence, artificial, limb
      liver Z97.8
      lung Z97.8
      pancreas Z97.8
    by organ transplant (heterologous)
      (homologous) —*see* Transplant

▶ New ⏵ Revised ~~deleted~~ Deleted ● Use Additional Character(s)

Status (Continued)
pacemaker
brain Z96.89
cardiac Z95.0
specified NEC Z96.89
pancreatectomy Z90.410
complete Z90.410
partial Z90.411
total Z90.410
pneumonectomy (complete) (partial) Z90.2
pneumothorax, therapeutic Z98.3
postcommotio cerebri F07.81
postoperative (postprocedural) NEC
Z98.890
breast implant Z98.82
dental Z98.818
crown Z98.811
fillings Z98.811
restoration Z98.811
sealant Z98.810
specified NEC Z98.818
pneumothorax, therapeutic Z98.3
uterine scar Z98.891
postpartum (routine follow-up) Z39.2
care immediately after delivery Z39.0
postsurgical (postprocedural) NEC
Z98.890
pneumothorax, therapeutic Z98.3
pregnancy, incidental Z33.1
prosthesis coronary angioplasty Z95.5
pseudophakia Z96.1
renal dialysis (hemodialysis) (peritoneal) Z99.2
retained foreign body —see Retained, foreign
body fragments (type of)
reversed jejunal transposition (for bypass
Z98.0
salpingo-oophorectomy
bilateral Z90.722
unilateral Z90.721
sex reassignment surgery status Z87.890
shunt
arteriovenous (for dialysis) Z99.2
cerebrospinal fluid Z98.2
ventricular (communicating) (for drainage)
Z98.2
splenectomy Z90.81
thymicolymphaticus E32.8
thymicus E32.8
thymolymphaticus E32.8
thyroidectomy (hypothyroidism) E89.0
tooth (teeth) extraction —see also Absence,
teeth, acquired K08.409
tPA (rtPA) administration in a different
facility within the last 24 hours prior to
admission to current facility Z92.82
tracheostomy Z93.0
transplant —see Transplant
organ removed Z98.85
tubal ligation Z98.51
underimmunization Z28.3
ureterostomy Z93.6
urethrostomy Z93.6
vagina, artificial Z93.8
vasectomy Z98.52
wheelchair confinement Z99.3
Stealing
child problem F91.8
in company with others Z72.810
pathological (compulsive) F63.2
Steam burn —see Burn
Steatocystoma multiplex L72.2
Steatohepatitis (nonalcoholic) (NASH) K75.81
Steatoma L72.3
eyelid (cystic) —see Dermatosis, eyelid
infected —see Hordeolum
Steatorrhea (chronic) K90.9
with lacteal obstruction K90.2
idiopathic (adult) (infantile) K90.9
pancreatic K90.3
primary K90.0
tropical K90.1

Steatosis E88.89
heart —see Degeneration, myocardial
kidney N28.89
liver NEC K76.0
Steele-Richardson-Olszewski disease or
syndrome G23.1
Steinbrocker's syndrome G90.8
Steinert's disease G71.11
Stein-Leventhal syndrome E28.2
Stein's syndrome E28.2
STEMI —see also Infarct, myocardium, ST
elevation I21.3
Stenocardia I20.8
Stenocephaly Q75.8
Stenosis, stenotic (cicatricial) —see also Stricture
ampulla of Vater K83.1
anus, anal (canal) (sphincter) K62.4
and rectum K62.4
congenital Q42.3
with fistula Q42.2
aorta (ascending) (supraventricular)
(congenital) Q25.1
arteriosclerotic I70.0
calcified I70.0
supravalvular Q25.3
aortic (valve) I35.0
with insufficiency I35.2
congenital Q23.0
rheumatic I06.0
with
incompetency, insufficiency or
regurgitation I06.2
with mitral (valve) disease I08.0
with tricuspid (valve) disease
I08.3
mitral (valve) disease I08.0
with tricuspid (valve) disease I08.3
tricuspid (valve) disease I08.2
with mitral (valve) disease I08.3
specified cause NEC I35.0
syphilitic A52.03
aqueduct of Sylvius (congenital) Q03.0
with spina bifida —see Spina bifida,
by site, with hydrocephalus
acquired G91.1
artery NEC —see also Arteriosclerosis I77.1
celiac I77.4
cerebral —see Occlusion, artery, cerebral
extremities —see Arteriosclerosis,
extremities
precerebral —see Occlusion, artery,
precerebral
pulmonary (congenital) Q25.6
acquired I28.8
renal I70.1
stent
coronary T82.855
peripheral T82.856
bile duct (common) (hepatic) K83.1
congenital Q44.3
bladder-neck (acquired) N32.0
congenital Q64.31
brain G93.89
bronchus J98.09
congenital Q32.3
syphilitic A52.72
cardia (stomach) K22.2
congenital Q39.3
cardiovascular —see Disease, cardiovascular
caudal M48.08
cervix, cervical (canal) N88.2
congenital Q51.828
in pregnancy or childbirth —see
Pregnancy, complicated by, abnormal
cervix
colon —see also Obstruction, intestine
congenital Q42.9
specified NEC Q42.8
colostomy K94.03
common (bile) duct K83.1
congenital Q44.3

Stenosis, stenotic (Continued)
coronary (artery) —see Disease, heart,
ischemic, atherosclerotic
cystic duct —see Obstruction, gallbladder
due to presence of device, implant or
graft —see also Complications, by site
and type, specified NEC T85.858
arterial graft NEC T82.858
breast (implant) T85.858
catheter T85.858
dialysis (renal) T82.858
intraperitoneal T85.858
infusion NEC T82.858
spinal (epidural) (subdural)
T85.850
urinary (indwelling) T83.85
fixation, internal (orthopedic) NEC
T84.85
gastrointestinal (bile duct) (esophagus)
T85.858
genital NEC T83.85
heart NEC T82.857
joint prosthesis T84.85
ocular (corneal graft) (orbital implant)
NEC T85.858
orthopedic NEC T84.85
specified NEC T85.858
urinary NEC T83.85
vascular NEC T82.858
ventricular intracranial shunt
T85.850
duodenum K31.5
congenital Q41.0
ejaculatory duct NEC N50.89
endocervical os —see Stenosis, cervix
enterostomy K94.13
esophagus K22.2
congenital Q39.3
syphilitic A52.79
congenital A50.59 [K23]
eustachian tube —see Obstruction, eustachian
tube
external ear canal (acquired) H61.30-●
congenital Q16.1
due to
inflammation H61.32-●
trauma H61.31-●
postprocedural H95.81-●
specified cause NEC H61.39-●
gallbladder —see Obstruction, gallbladder
glottis J38.6
heart valve (see also Endocarditis) I38
aortic —see Stenosis, aortic
congenital Q24.8
mitral —see Stenosis, mitral
pulmonary —see Stenosis, pulmonary,
valve
tricuspid —see Stenosis, tricuspid Q22.4
hepatic duct K83.1
hymen N89.6
hypertrophic subaortic (idiopathic) I42.1
ileum —see also Obstruction, intestine,
specified NEC K56.699
congenital Q41.2
infundibulum cardia Q24.3
intervertebral foramina —see also Lesion,
biomechanical, specified NEC
connective tissue M99.79
abdomen M99.79
cervical region M99.71
cervicothoracic M99.71
head region M99.70
lumbar region M99.73
lumbosacral M99.73
occipitocervical M99.70
sacral region M99.74
sacrococcygeal M99.74
sacroiliac M99.74
specified NEC M99.79
thoracic region M99.72
thoracolumbar M99.72

Stenosis, stenotic *(Continued)*
  intervertebral foramina *(Continued)*
    disc M99.79
      abdomen M99.79
      cervical region M99.71
      cervicothoracic M99.71
      head region M99.70
      lower extremity M99.76
      lumbar region M99.73
      lumbosacral M99.73
      occipitocervical M99.70
      pelvic M99.75
      rib cage M99.78
      sacral region M99.74
      sacrococcygeal M99.74
      sacroiliac M99.74
      specified NEC M99.79
      thoracic region M99.72
      thoracolumbar M99.72
      upper extremity M99.77
    osseous M99.69
      abdomen M99.69
      cervical region M99.61
      cervicothoracic M99.61
      head region M99.60
      lower extremity M99.66
      lumbar region M99.63
      lumbosacral M99.63
      occipitocervical M99.60
      pelvic M99.65
      rib cage M99.68
      sacral region M99.64
      sacrococcygeal M99.64
      sacroiliac M99.64
      specified NEC M99.69
      thoracic region M99.62
      thoracolumbar M99.62
      upper extremity M99.67
    subluxation —*see* Stenosis, intervertebral
      foramina, osseous
  intestine —*see also* Obstruction, intestine
    congenital (small) Q41.9
      large Q42.9
        specified NEC Q42.8
      specified NEC Q41.8
  jejunum —*see also* Obstruction, intestine,
      specified NEC K56.699
    congenital Q41.1
  lacrimal (passage)
    canaliculi H04.54-●
    congenital Q10.5
    duct H04.55-●
    punctum H04.56-●
    sac H04.57-●
  lacrimonasal duct —*see* Stenosis, lacrimal,
      duct
    congenital Q10.5
  larynx J38.6
    congenital NEC Q31.8
      subglottic Q31.1
    syphilitic A52.73
      congenital A50.59 *[J99]*
  mitral (chronic) (inactive) (valve) I05.0
    with
      aortic valve disease I08.0
      incompetency, insufficiency or
          regurgitation I05.2
      active or acute I01.1
        with rheumatic or Sydenham's chorea
          I02.0
    congenital Q23.2
    specified cause, except rheumatic I34.2
    syphilitic A52.03
  myocardium, myocardial —*see also*
      Degeneration, myocardial
    hypertrophic subaortic (idiopathic)
      I42.1
  nares (anterior) (posterior) J34.89
    congenital Q30.0
  nasal duct —*see also* Stenosis, lacrimal, duct
    congenital Q10.5

Stenosis, stenotic *(Continued)*
  nasolacrimal duct —*see also* Stenosis, lacrimal,
      duct
    congenital Q10.5
  neural canal —*see also* Lesion, biomechanical,
      specified NEC
    connective tissue M99.49
      abdomen M99.49
      cervical region M99.41
      cervicothoracic M99.41
      head region M99.40
      lower extremity M99.46
      lumbar region M99.43
      lumbosacral M99.43
      occipitocervical M99.40
      pelvic M99.45
      rib cage M99.48
      sacral region M99.44
      sacrococcygeal M99.44
      sacroiliac M99.44
      specified NEC M99.49
      thoracic region M99.42
      thoracolumbar M99.42
      upper extremity M99.47
    intervertebral disc M99.59
      abdomen M99.59
      cervical region M99.51
      cervicothoracic M99.51
      head region M99.50
      lower extremity M99.56
      lumbar region M99.53
      lumbosacral M99.53
      occipitocervical M99.50
      pelvic M99.55
      rib cage M99.58
      sacral region M99.54
      sacrococcygeal M99.54
      sacroiliac M99.54
      specified NEC M99.59
      thoracic region M99.52
      thoracolumbar M99.52
      upper extremity M99.57
    osseous M99.39
      abdomen M99.39
      cervical region M99.31
      cervicothoracic M99.31
      head region M99.30
      lower extremity M99.36
      lumbar region M99.33
      lumbosacral M99.33
      occipitocervical M99.30
      pelvic M99.35
      rib cage M99.38
      sacral region M99.34
      sacrococcygeal M99.34
      sacroiliac M99.34
      specified NEC M99.39
      thoracic region M99.32
      thoracolumbar M99.32
      upper extremity M99.37
    subluxation M99.29
      cervical region M99.21
      cervicothoracic M99.21
      head region M99.20
      lower extremity M99.26
      lumbar region M99.23
      lumbosacral M99.23
      occipitocervical M99.20
      pelvic M99.25
      rib cage M99.28
      sacral region M99.24
      sacrococcygeal M99.24
      sacroiliac M99.24
      specified NEC M99.29
      thoracic region M99.22
      thoracolumbar M99.22
      upper extremity M99.27
  organ or site, congenital NEC —*see* Atresia,
      by site
  papilla of Vater K83.1

Stenosis, stenotic *(Continued)*
  pulmonary (artery) (congenital) Q25.6
    with ventricular septal defect,
        transposition of aorta, and
        hypertrophy of right ventricle Q21.3
    acquired I28.8
    in tetralogy of Fallot Q21.3
    infundibular Q24.3
    subvalvular Q24.3
    supravalvular Q25.6
    valve I37.0
      with insufficiency I37.2
      congenital Q22.1
      rheumatic I09.89
        with aortic, mitral or tricuspid (valve)
            disease I08.8
    vein, acquired I28.8
    vessel NEC I28.8
  pulmonic (congenital) Q22.1
    infundibular Q24.3
    subvalvular Q24.3
  pylorus (hypertrophic) (acquired) K31.1
    adult K31.1
    congenital Q40.0
    infantile Q40.0
  rectum (sphincter) —*see* Stricture, rectum
  renal artery I70.1
    congenital Q27.1
  salivary duct (any) K11.8
  sphincter of Oddi K83.1
  spinal M48.00
    cervical region M48.02
    cervicothoracic region M48.03
    lumbar region (NOS) (without neurogenic
        claudication) M48.061
      with neurogenic claudication M48.062
    lumbosacral region M48.07
    occipito-atlanto-axial region M48.01
    sacrococcygeal region M48.08
    thoracic region M48.04
    thoracolumbar region M48.05
  stent
    vascular
      end stent
        adjacent to stent —*see* Arteriosclerosis
        within the stent
          coronary T82.855
          peripheral T82.856
      in stent
        coronary vessel T82.855
        peripheral vessel T82.856
  stomach, hourglass K31.2
  subaortic (congenital) Q24.4
    hypertrophic (idiopathic) I42.1
  subglottic J38.6
    congenital Q31.1
    postprocedural J95.5
  trachea J39.8
    congenital Q32.1
    syphilitic A52.73
    tuberculous NEC A15.5
  tracheostomy J95.03
  tricuspid (valve) I07.0
    with
      aortic (valve) disease I08.2
      incompetency, insufficiency or
          regurgitation I07.2
        with aortic (valve) disease I08.2
          with mitral (valve) disease I08.3
      mitral (valve) disease I08.1
        with aortic (valve) disease I08.3
    congenital Q22.4
    nonrheumatic I36.0
      with insufficiency I36.2
  tubal N97.1
  ureter —*see* Atresia, ureter
  ureteropelvic junction, congenital
      Q62.11
  ureterovesical orifice, congenital Q62.12
  urethra (valve) —*see also* Stricture, urethra
    congenital Q64.32

▶ New   ⇒ Revised   ~~deleted~~ Deleted   ● Use Additional Character(s)

Stenosis, stenotic *(Continued)*
  urinary meatus, congenital Q64.33
  vagina N89.5
    congenital Q52.4
    in pregnancy —*see* Pregnancy, complicated
        by, abnormal vagina
      causing obstructed labor O65.5
  valve (cardiac) (heart) —*see also* Endocarditis
      I38
    congenital Q24.8
      aortic Q23.0
      mitral Q23.2
      pulmonary Q22.1
      tricuspid Q22.4
  vena cava (inferior) (superior) I87.1
    congenital Q26.0
  vesicourethral orifice Q64.31
  vulva N90.5
Stent jail T82.897
Stercolith (impaction) K56.41
  appendix K38.1
Stercoraceous, stercoral ulcer K63.3
  anus or rectum K62.6
Stereotypies NEC F98.4
Sterility —*see* Infertility
Sterilization —*see* Encounter (for), sterilization
Sternalgia —*see* Angina
Sternopagus Q89.4
Sternum bifidum Q76.7
Steroid
  effects (adverse) (adrenocortical) (iatrogenic)
    cushingoid E24.2
      correct substance properly
          administered —*see* Table of Drugs
          and Chemicals, by drug, adverse
          effect
        overdose or wrong substance given
          or taken —*see* Table of Drugs and
          Chemicals, by drug, poisoning
    diabetes —*see* category E09
      correct substance properly
          administered —*see* Table of Drugs
          and Chemicals, by drug, adverse
          effect
        overdose or wrong substance given
          or taken —*see* Table of Drugs and
          Chemicals, by drug, poisoning
    fever R50.2
    insufficiency E27.3
      correct substance properly
          administered —*see* Table of Drugs
          and Chemicals, by drug, adverse
          effect
        overdose or wrong substance given
          or taken —*see* Table of Drugs and
          Chemicals, by drug, poisoning
  responder H40.04-•
Stevens-Johnson disease or syndrome L51.1
  toxic epidermal necrolysis overlap L51.3
Stewart-Morel syndrome M85.2
Sticker's disease B08.3
Sticky eye —*see* Conjunctivitis, acute,
    mucopurulent
Stieda's disease —*see* Bursitis, tibial collateral
Stiff neck —*see* Torticollis
Stiff-man syndrome G25.82
Stiffness, joint NEC M25.60-•
  ankle M25.67-•
  ankylosis —*see* Ankylosis, joint
  contracture —*see* Contraction, joint
  elbow M25.62-•
  foot M25.67-•
  hand M25.64-•
  hip M25.65-•
  knee M25.66-•
  shoulder M25.61-•
  specified site NEC M25.69
  wrist M25.63-•
Stigmata congenital syphilis A50.59
Stillbirth P95
Still-Felty syndrome —*see* Felty's syndrome

Still's disease or syndrome (juvenile) M08.20
  adult-onset M06.1
  ankle M08.27-•
  elbow M08.22-•
  foot joint M08.27-•
  hand joint M08.24-•
  hip M08.25-•
  knee M08.26-•
  multiple site M08.29
  shoulder M08.21-•
  specified site NEC M08.2A
  vertebra M08.28
  wrist M08.23-•
Stimulation, ovary E28.1
Sting (venomous) (with allergic or anaphylactic
      shock) —*see* Table of Drugs and Chemicals,
      by animal or substance, poisoning
Stippled epiphyses Q78.8
Stitch
  abscess T81.41
  burst (in operation wound) —*see* Disruption,
      wound, operation
Stokes-Adams disease or syndrome I45.9
Stokes' disease E05.00
  with thyroid storm E05.01
Stokvis (-Talma) disease D74.8
Stoma malfunction
  colostomy K94.03
  enterostomy K94.13
  gastrostomy K94.23
  ileostomy K94.13
  tracheostomy J95.03
Stomach —*see* condition
Stomatitis (denture) (ulcerative) K12.1
  angular K13.0
    due to dietary or vitamin deficiency E53.0
  aphthous K12.0
  bovine B08.61
  candidal B37.0
  catarrhal K12.1
  diphtheritic A36.89
  due to
    dietary deficiency E53.0
    thrush B37.0
    vitamin deficiency
      B group NEC E53.9
      B2 (riboflavin) E53.0
  epidemic B08.8
  epizootic B08.8
  follicular K12.1
  gangrenous A69.0
  Geotrichum B48.3
  herpesviral, herpetic B00.2
  herpetiformis K12.0
  malignant K12.1
  membranous acute K12.1
  monilial B37.0
  mycotic B37.0
  necrotizing ulcerative A69.0
  parasitic B37.0
  septic K12.1
  spirochetal A69.1
  suppurative (acute) K12.2
  ulceromembranous A69.1
  vesicular K12.1
    with exanthem (enteroviral) B08.4
    virus disease A93.8
  Vincent's A69.1
Stomatocytosis D58.8
Stomatomycosis B37.0
Stomatorrhagia K13.79
Stone(s) —*see also* Calculus
  bladder (diverticulum) N21.0
  cystine E72.09
  heart syndrome I50.1
  kidney N20.0
  prostate N42.0
  pulpal (dental) K04.2
  renal N20.0
  salivary gland or duct (any) K11.5
  urethra (impacted) N21.1

Stone *(Continued)*
  urinary (duct) (impacted) (passage) N20.9
    bladder (diverticulum) N21.0
    lower tract N21.9
    specified NEC N21.8
  xanthine E79.8 *[N22]*
Stonecutter's lung J62.8
Stonemason's asthma, disease, lung or
    pneumoconiosis J62.8
Stoppage
  heart —*see* Arrest, cardiac
  urine —*see* Retention, urine
Storm, thyroid —*see* Thyrotoxicosis
Strabismus (congenital) (nonparalytic) H50.9
  concomitant H50.40
    convergent —*see* Strabismus, convergent
        concomitant
    divergent —*see* Strabismus, divergent
        concomitant
  convergent concomitant H50.00
    accommodative component H50.43
    alternating H50.05
      with
        A pattern H50.06
        specified nonconcomitances NEC
            H50.08
        V pattern H50.07
    monocular H50.01-•
      with
        A pattern H50.02-•
        specified nonconcomitances NEC
            H50.04-•
        V pattern H50.03-•
    intermittent H50.31-•
      alternating H50.32
  cyclotropia H50.41
  divergent concomitant H50.10
    alternating H50.15
      with
        A pattern H50.16
        specified noncomitances NEC H50.18
        V pattern H50.17
    monocular H50.11-•
      with
        A pattern H50.12-•
        specified noncomitances NEC
            H50.14-•
        V pattern H50.13-•
    intermittent H50.33-•
      alternating H50.34
  Duane's syndrome H50.81-•
  due to adhesions, scars H50.69
  heterophoria H50.50
    alternating H50.55
    cyclophoria H50.54
    esophoria H50.51
    exophoria H50.52
    vertical H50.53
  heterotropia H50.40
    intermittent H50.30
  hypertropia H50.2-•
  hypotropia —*see* Hypertropia
  latent H50.50
  mechanical H50.60
    Brown's sheath syndrome H50.61-•
    specified type NEC H50.69
  monofixation syndrome H50.42
  paralytic H49.9
    abducens nerve H49.2-•
    fourth nerve H49.1-•
    Kearns-Sayre syndrome H49.81-•
    ophthalmoplegia (external)
      progressive H49.4-•
        with pigmentary retinopathy H49.81-•
      total H49.3-•
    sixth nerve H49.2-•
    specified type NEC H49.88-•
    third nerve H49.0-•
    trochlear nerve H49.1-•
  specified type NEC H50.89
  vertical H50.2-•

Strain
  back S39.012
  cervical S16.1
  eye NEC —*see* Disturbance, vision, subjective
  heart —*see* Disease, heart
  low back S39.012
  mental NOS Z73.3
    work-related Z56.6
  muscle (tendon) —*see* Injury, muscle, by site,
    strain
  neck S16.1
  physical NOS Z73.3
    work-related Z56.6
  postural —*see also* Disorder, soft tissue, due
    to use
  psychological NEC Z73.3
  tendon —*see* Injury, muscle, by site, strain
Straining, on urination R39.16
Strand, vitreous —*see* Opacity, vitreous,
  membranes and strands
Strangulation, strangulated —*see also*
    Asphyxia, traumatic
  appendix K38.8
  bladder-neck N32.0
  bowel or colon K56.2
  food or foreign body —*see* Foreign body, by
    site
  hemorrhoids —*see* Hemorrhoids, with
    complication
  hernia —*see also* Hernia, by site, with
    obstruction
    with gangrene —*see* Hernia, by site, with
      gangrene
  intestine (large) (small) K56.2
    with hernia —*see also* Hernia, by site, with
      obstruction
      with gangrene —*see* Hernia, by site, with
        gangrene
  mesentery K56.2
  mucus —*see* Asphyxia, mucus
  omentum K56.2
  organ or site, congenital NEC —*see* Atresia,
    by site
  ovary —*see* Torsion, ovary
  penis N48.89
    foreign body T19.4
  rupture —*see* Hernia, by site, with obstruction
  stomach due to hernia —*see also* Hernia, by
    site, with obstruction
    with gangrene —*see* Hernia, by site, with
      gangrene
  vesicourethral orifice N32.0
Strangury R30.0
Straw itch B88.0
Strawberry
  gallbladder K82.4
  mark Q82.5
  tongue (red) (white) K14.3
Streak(s)
  macula, angioid H35.33
  ovarian Q50.32
Strephosymbolia F81.0
  secondary to organic lesion R48.8
Streptobacillary fever A25.1
Streptobacillosis A25.1
Streptobacillus moniliformis A25.1
Streptococcus, streptococcal —*see also* condition
  as cause of disease classified elsewhere B95.5
  group
    A, as cause of disease classified elsewhere
      B95.0
    B, as cause of disease classified elsewhere
      B95.1
    D, as cause of disease classified elsewhere
      B95.2
  pneumoniae, as cause of disease classified
    elsewhere B95.3
  specified NEC, as cause of disease classified
    elsewhere B95.4
Streptomycosis B47.1
Streptotrichosis A48.8

Stress F43.9
  family —*see* Disruption, family
  fetal P84
    complicating pregnancy O77.9
    due to drug administration O77.1
  mental NEC Z73.3
    work-related Z56.6
  physical NEC Z73.3
    work-related Z56.6
  polycythemia D75.1
  reaction —*see also* Reaction, stress F43.9
  work schedule Z56.3
Stretching, nerve —*see* Injury, nerve
Striae albicans, atrophicae or distensae
    (cutis) L90.6
Stricture —*see also* Stenosis
  ampulla of Vater K83.1
  anus (sphincter) K62.4
    congenital Q42.3
      with fistula Q42.2
    infantile Q42.3
      with fistula Q42.2
  aorta (ascending) (congenital) Q25.1
    arteriosclerotic I70.0
    calcified I70.0
    supravalvular, congenital Q25.3
  aortic (valve) —*see* Stenosis, aortic
  aqueduct of Sylvius (congenital) Q03.0
    with spina bifida —*see* Spina bifida, by site,
      with hydrocephalus
    acquired G91.1
  artery I77.1
    basilar —*see* Occlusion, artery, basilar
    carotid —*see* Occlusion, artery, carotid
    celiac I77.4
    congenital (peripheral) Q27.8
      cerebral Q28.3
      coronary Q24.5
      digestive system Q27.8
      lower limb Q27.8
      retinal Q14.1
      specified site NEC Q27.8
      umbilical Q27.0
      upper limb Q27.8
    coronary —*see* Disease, heart, ischemic,
      atherosclerotic
      congenital Q24.5
    precerebral —*see* Occlusion, artery,
      precerebral
    pulmonary (congenital) Q25.6
      acquired I28.8
    renal I70.1
    vertebral —*see* Occlusion, artery, vertebral
  auditory canal (external) (congenital)
    acquired —*see* Stenosis, external ear canal
  bile duct (common) (hepatic) K83.1
    congenital Q44.3
    postoperative K91.89
  bladder N32.89
    neck N32.0
  bowel —*see* Obstruction, intestine
  brain G93.89
  bronchus J98.09
    congenital Q32.3
    syphilitic A52.72
  cardia (stomach) K22.2
    congenital Q39.3
  cardiac —*see also* Disease, heart
    orifice (stomach) K22.2
  cecum —*see* Obstruction, intestine
  cervix, cervical (canal) N88.2
    congenital Q51.828
    in pregnancy —*see* Pregnancy, complicated
      by, abnormal cervix
      causing obstructed labor O65.5
  colon —*see also* Obstruction, intestine
    congenital Q42.9
      specified NEC Q42.8
  colostomy K94.03
  common (bile) duct K83.1
  coronary (artery) —*see* Disease, heart,
    ischemic, atherosclerotic

Stricture *(Continued)*
  cystic duct —*see* Obstruction, gallbladder
  digestive organs NEC, congenital Q45.8
  duodenum K31.5
    congenital Q41.0
  ear canal (external) (congenital) Q16.1
    acquired —*see* Stricture, auditory canal,
      acquired
  ejaculatory duct N50.89
  enterostomy K94.13
  esophagus K22.2
    congenital Q39.3
    syphilitic A52.79
      congenital A50.59 *[K23]*
  eustachian tube —*see also* Obstruction,
    eustachian tube
    congenital Q17.8
  fallopian tube N97.1
    gonococcal A54.24
    tuberculous A18.17
  gallbladder —*see* Obstruction, gallbladder
  glottis J38.6
  heart —*see also* Disease, heart
    valve (see also Endocarditis) I38
      aortic Q23.0
      mitral Q23.2
      pulmonary Q22.1
      tricuspid Q22.4
  hepatic duct K83.1
  hourglass, of stomach K31.2
  hymen N89.6
  hypopharynx J39.2
  ileum —*see also* Obstruction, intestine,
    specified NEC K56.699
    congenital Q41.2
  intestine —*see also* Obstruction, intestine
    congenital (small) Q41.9
      large Q42.9
        specified NEC Q42.8
      specified NEC Q41.8
    ischemic K55.1
  jejunum —*see also* Obstruction, intestine,
    specified NEC K56.699
    congenital Q41.1
  lacrimal passages —*see also* Stenosis, lacrimal
    congenital Q10.5
  larynx J38.6
    congenital NEC Q31.8
      subglottic Q31.1
    syphilitic A52.73
      congenital A50.59 *[J99]*
  meatus
    ear (congenital) Q16.1
      acquired —*see* Stricture, auditory canal,
        acquired
    osseous (ear) (congenital) Q16.1
      acquired —*see* Stricture, auditory canal,
        acquired
    urinarius —*see also* Stricture, urethra
      congenital Q64.33
  mitral (valve) —*see* Stenosis, mitral
  myocardium, myocardial I51.5
    hypertrophic subaortic (idiopathic) I42.1
  nares (anterior) (posterior) J34.89
    congenital Q30.0
  nasal duct —*see also* Stenosis, lacrimal, duct
    congenital Q10.5
  nasolacrimal duct —*see also* Stenosis, lacrimal,
    duct
    congenital Q10.5
  nasopharynx J39.2
    syphilitic A52.73
  nose J34.89
    congenital Q30.0
  nostril (anterior) (posterior) J34.89
    congenital Q30.0
    syphilitic A52.73
      congenital A50.59 *[J99]*
  organ or site, congenital NEC —*see* Atresia,
    by site
  os uteri —*see* Stricture, cervix

▶ New   ➡ Revised   ~~deleted~~ Deleted   ● Use Additional Character(s)

Stricture *(Continued)*
  osseous meatus (ear) (congenital) Q16.1
    acquired —*see* Stricture, auditory canal,
      acquired
  oviduct —*see* Stricture, fallopian tube
  pelviureteric junction (congenital) Q62.11
    acquired, with hydronephrosis N13.0
  penis, by foreign body T19.4
  pharynx J39.2
  prostate N42.89
  pulmonary, pulmonic
    artery (congenital) Q25.6
      acquired I28.8
      noncongenital I28.8
    infundibulum (congenital) Q24.3
    valve I37.0
      congenital Q22.1
    vein, acquired I28.8
    vessel NEC I28.8
  punctum lacrimale —*see also* Stenosis,
    lacrimal, punctum
    congenital Q10.5
  pylorus (hypertrophic) K31.1
    adult K31.1
    congenital Q40.0
    infantile Q40.0
  rectosigmoid —*see also* Obstruction, intestine,
    specified NEC K56.699
  rectum (sphincter) K62.4
    congenital Q42.1
      with fistula Q42.0
    due to
      chlamydial lymphogranuloma A55
      irradiation K91.89
      lymphogranuloma venereum A55
    gonococcal A54.6
    inflammatory (chlamydial) A55
    syphilitic A52.74
    tuberculous A18.32
  renal artery I70.1
    congenital Q27.1
  salivary duct or gland (any) K11.8
  sigmoid (flexure) —*see* Obstruction,
    intestine
  spermatic cord N50.89
  stoma (following) (of)
    colostomy K94.03
    enterostomy K94.13
    gastrostomy K94.23
    ileostomy K94.13
    tracheostomy J95.03
  stomach K31.89
    congenital Q40.2
    hourglass K31.2
  subaortic Q24.4
    hypertrophic (acquired) (idiopathic) I42.1
  subglottic J38.6
  syphilitic NEC A52.79
  trachea J39.8
    congenital Q32.1
    syphilitic A52.73
    tuberculous NEC A15.5
  tracheostomy J95.03
  tricuspid (valve) —*see* Stenosis, tricuspid
  tunica vaginalis N50.89
  ureter (postoperative) N13.5
    with
      hydronephrosis N13.1
        with infection N13.6
      pyelonephritis (chronic) N11.1
    congenital —*see* Atresia, ureter
    tuberculous A18.11
  ureteropelvic junction (congenital) Q62.11
    acquired, with hydronephrosis N13.0
  ureterovesical orifice N13.5
    with infection N13.6
  urethra (organic) (spasmodic) (*see also*
    Stricture, urethra, male N35.919
    associated with schistosomiasis B65.0 *[N37]*
    congenital Q64.39
      valvular (posterior) Q64.2

Stricture *(Continued)*
  urethra *(Continued)*
    due to
      infection —*see* Stricture, urethra,
        postinfective
      trauma —*see* Stricture, urethra,
        post-traumatic
    female N35.92
    gonococcal, gonorrheal A54.01
    infective NEC —*see* Stricture, urethra,
      postinfective
    late effect (sequelae) of injury —*see*
      Stricture, urethra, post-traumatic
    male N35.919
      anterior urethra N35.914
      bulbous urethra N35.912
      meatal N35.911
      membranous urethra N35.913
      overlapping sites N35.916
    postcatheterization —*see* Stricture, urethra,
      postprocedural
    postinfective NEC
      female N35.12
      male N35.119
        anterior urethra N35.114
        bulbous urethra N35.112
        meatal N35.111
        membranous urethra N35.113
        overlapping sites N35.116
    postobstetric N35.021
    postoperative —*see* Stricture, urethra,
      postprocedural
    postprocedural
      female N99.12
      male N99.114
        anterior bulbous urethra N99.113
        bulbous urethra N99.111
        fossa navicularis N99.115
        meatal N99.110
        membranous urethra N99.112
        overlapping sites N35.116
    post-traumatic
      female N35.028
        due to childbirth N35.021
      male N35.014
        anterior urethra N35.013
        bulbous urethra N35.011
        meatal N35.010
        membranous urethra N35.012
        overlapping sites N35.016
    sequela (late effect) of
      childbirth N35.021
      injury —*see* Stricture, urethra,
        post-traumatic
    specified cause NEC
      female N35.82
      male N35.819
        anterior urethra N35.814
        bulbous urethra N35.812
        meatal N35.811
        membranous urethra N35.813
        overlapping sites N35.816
    syphilitic A52.76
    traumatic —*see* Stricture, urethra,
      post-traumatic
    valvular (posterior), congenital Q64.2
  urinary meatus —*see* Stricture, urethra
  uterus, uterine (synechiae) N85.6
    os (external) (internal) —*see* Stricture,
      cervix
  vagina (outlet) —*see* Stenosis, vagina
  valve (cardiac) (heart) —*see also* Endocarditis
    congenital
      aortic Q23.0
      mitral Q23.2
      pulmonary Q22.1
      tricuspid Q22.4
  vas deferens N50.89
    congenital Q55.4
  vein I87.1

Stricture *(Continued)*
  vena cava (inferior) (superior) NEC I87.1
    congenital Q26.0
  vesicourethral orifice N32.0
    congenital Q64.31
  vulva (acquired) N90.5
Stridor R06.1
  congenital (larynx) P28.89
Stridulous —*see* condition
Stroke (apoplectic) (brain) (embolic) (ischemic)
    (paralytic) (thrombotic) I63.9
  cerebral, perinatal P91.82-●
  cryptogenic —*see also* infarction, cerebral I63.9
  epileptic —*see* Epilepsy
  heat T67.01
    exertional T67.02
    specified NEC T67.09
  in evolution I63.9
  intraoperative
    during cardiac surgery I97.810
    during other surgery I97.811
  ischemic, perinatal arterial P91.82-●
  lightning —*see* Lightning
  meaning
    cerebral hemorrhage — code to
      Hemorrhage, intracranial
    cerebral infarction — code to Infarction,
      cerebral
  neonatal P91.82-●
  postprocedural
    following cardiac surgery I97.820
    following other surgery I97.821
  sun T67.01
    specified NEC T67.09
  unspecified (NOS) I63.9
Stromatosis, endometrial D39.0
Strongyloidiasis, strongyloidosis B78.9
  cutaneous B78.1
  disseminated B78.7
  intestinal B78.0
Strophulus pruriginosus L28.2
Struck by lightning —*see* Lightning
Struma —*see also* Goiter
  Hashimoto E06.3
  lymphomatosa E06.3
  nodosa (simplex) E04.9
    endemic E01.2
      multinodular E01.1
    multinodular E04.2
      iodine-deficiency related E01.1
    toxic or with hyperthyroidism E05.20
      with thyroid storm E05.21
      multinodular E05.20
        with thyroid storm E05.21
      uninodular E05.10
        with thyroid storm E05.11
    toxicosa E05.20
      with thyroid storm E05.21
      multinodular E05.20
        with thyroid storm E05.21
      uninodular E05.10
        with thyroid storm E05.11
    uninodular E04.1
  ovarii D27.-●
  Riedel's E06.5
Strumipriva cachexia E03.4
Strümpell-Marie spine —*see* Spondylitis,
  ankylosing
Strümpell-Westphal pseudosclerosis E83.01
Stuart deficiency disease (factor X) D68.2
Stuart-Prower factor deficiency (factor X) D68.2
Student's elbow —*see* Bursitis, elbow, olecranon
Stump —*see* Amputation
Stunting, nutritional E45
Stupor (catatonic) R40.1
  depressive (single episode) F32.89
    recurrent episode F33.8
  dissociative F44.2
  manic F30.2
  manic-depressive F31.89
  psychogenic (anergic) F44.2
  reaction to exceptional stress (transient) F43.0

Sturge (-Weber) (-Dimitri) (-Kalischer) disease or syndrome Q85.89
Stuttering F80.81
  adult onset F98.5
  childhood onset F80.81
  following cerebrovascular disease —
    see Disorder, fluency, following
    cerebrovascular disease
  in conditions classified elsewhere R47.82
Sty, stye (external) (internal) (meibomian)
  (zeisian) —*see* Hordeolum
Subacidity, gastric K31.89
  psychogenic F45.8
Subacute —*see* condition
Subarachnoid —*see* condition
Subcortical —*see* condition
Subcostal syndrome, nerve compression —*see*
  Mononeuropathy, upper limb, specified
  site NEC
Subcutaneous, subcuticular —*see* condition
Subdural —*see* condition
Subendocardium —*see* condition
Subependymoma
  specified site —*see* Neoplasm, uncertain
    behavior, by site
  unspecified site D43.2
Suberosis J67.3
Subglossitis —*see* Glossitis
Subhemophilia D66
Subinvolution
  breast (postlactational) (postpuerperal) N64.89
    puerperal O90.89
  uterus (chronic) (nonpuerperal) N85.3
    puerperal O90.89
Sublingual —*see* condition
Sublinguitis —*see* Sialoadenitis
Subluxatable hip Q65.6
Subluxation —*see also* Dislocation
  acromioclavicular S43.11-●
  ankle S93.0-●
  atlantoaxial, recurrent M43.4
    with myelopathy M43.3
  carpometacarpal (joint) NEC S63.05-●
    thumb S63.04-●
  complex, vertebral —*see* Complex,
    subluxation
  congenital —*see also* Malposition, congenital
    hip —*see* Dislocation, hip, congenital, partial
    joint (excluding hip)
      lower limb Q68.8
      shoulder Q68.8
      upper limb Q68.8
  elbow (traumatic) S53.10-●
    anterior S53.11-●
    lateral S53.14-●
    medial S53.13-●
    posterior S53.12-●
    specified type NEC S53.19-●
  finger S63.20-●
    index S63.20-●
    interphalangeal S63.22-●
      distal S63.24-●
        index S63.24-●
        little S63.24-●
        middle S63.24-●
        ring S63.24-●
      index S63.22-●
      little S63.22-●
      middle S63.22-●
      proximal S63.23-●
        index S63.23-●
        little S63.23-●
        middle S63.23-●
        ring S63.23-●
      ring S63.22-●
    little S63.20-●
    metacarpophalangeal S63.21-●
      index S63.21-●
      little S63.21-●
      middle S63.21-●
      ring S63.21-●
    middle S63.20-●
    ring S63.20-●

Subluxation (*Continued*)
  foot S93.30-●
    specified site NEC S93.33-●
    tarsal joint S93.31-●
    tarsometatarsal joint S93.32-●
    toe —*see* Subluxation, toe
  hip S73.00-●
    anterior S73.03-●
      obturator S73.02-●
    central S73.04-●
    posterior S73.01-●
  interphalangeal (joint)
    finger S63.22-●
      distal joint S63.24-●
        index S63.24-●
        little S63.24-●
        middle S63.24-●
        ring S63.24-●
      index S63.22-●
      little S63.22-●
      middle S63.22-●
      proximal joint S63.23-●
        index S63.23-●
        little S63.23-●
        middle S63.23-●
        ring S63.23-●
      ring S63.22-●
    thumb S63.12-●
    toe S93.13-●
      great S93.13-●
      lesser S93.13-●
  joint prosthesis —*see* Complications, joint
    prosthesis, mechanical, displacement,
    by site
  knee S83.10-●
    cap —*see* Subluxation, patella
    patella —*see* Subluxation, patella
    proximal tibia
      anteriorly S83.11-●
      laterally S83.14-●
      medially S83.13-●
      posteriorly S83.12-●
    specified type NEC S83.19-●
  lens —*see* Dislocation, lens, partial
  ligament, traumatic —*see* Sprain,
    by site
  metacarpal (bone)
    proximal end S63.06-●
  metacarpophalangeal (joint)
    finger S63.21-●
      index S63.21-●
      little S63.21-●
      middle S63.21-●
      ring S63.21-●
    thumb S63.11-●
  metatarsophalangeal joint S93.14-●
    great toe S93.14-●
    lesser toe S93.14-●
  midcarpal (joint) S63.03-●
  patella S83.00-●
    lateral S83.01-●
    recurrent (nontraumatic) —*see*
      Dislocation, patella, recurrent,
      incomplete
    specified type NEC S83.09-●
  pathological —*see* Dislocation,
    pathological
  radial head S53.00-●
    anterior S53.01-●
    nursemaid's elbow S53.03-●
    posterior S53.02-●
    specified type NEC S53.09-●
  radiocarpal (joint) S63.02-●
  radioulnar (joint)
    distal S63.01-●
    proximal —*see* Subluxation, elbow
  shoulder
    congenital Q68.8
    girdle S43.30-●
      scapula S43.31-●
      specified site NEC S43.39-●

Subluxation (*Continued*)
  shoulder (*Continued*)
    traumatic S43.00-●
      anterior S43.01-●
      inferior S43.03-●
      posterior S43.02-●
      specified type NEC S43.08-●
  sternoclavicular (joint) S43.20-●
    anterior S43.21-●
    posterior S43.22-●
  symphysis (pubis) —*see also* Dislocation,
    symphysis pubis
  thumb S63.103
    interphalangeal joint —*see* Subluxation,
      interphalangeal (joint), thumb
    metacarpophalangeal joint —*see*
      Subluxation, metacarpophalangeal
      (joint), thumb
  toe(s) S93.10-●
    great S93.10-●
      interphalangeal joint S93.13-●
      metatarsophalangeal joint S93.14-●
    interphalangeal joint S93.13-●
    lesser S93.10-●
      interphalangeal joint S93.13-●
      metatarsophalangeal joint S93.14-●
    metatarsophalangeal joint S93.149
  ulnohumeral joint —*see* Subluxation, elbow
  vertebral
    recurrent NEC —*see* subcategory M43.5
    traumatic
      cervical S13.100
        atlantoaxial joint S13.120
        atlantooccipital joint S13.110
        atloidooccipital joint S13.110
        joint between
          C0 and C1 S13.110
          C1 and C2 S13.120
          C2 and C3 S13.130
          C3 and C4 S13.140
          C4 and C5 S13.150
          C5 and C6 S13.160
          C6 and C7 S13.170
          C7 and T1 S13.180
        occipitoatloid joint S13.110
      lumbar S33.100
        joint between
          L1 and L2 S33.110
          L2 and L3 S33.120
          L3 and L4 S33.130
          L4 and L5 S33.140
      thoracic S23.100
        joint between
          T1 and T2 S23.110
          T2 and T3 S23.120
          T3 and T4 S23.122
          T4 and T5 S23.130
          T5 and T6 S23.132
          T6 and T7 S23.140
          T7 and T8 S23.142
          T8 and T9 S23.150
          T9 and T10 S23.152
          T10 and T11 S23.160
          T11 and T12 S23.162
          T12 and L1 S23.170
  ulna
    distal end S63.07-●
    proximal end —*see* Subluxation, elbow
  wrist (carpal bone) S63.00-●
    carpometacarpal joint —*see* Subluxation,
      carpometacarpal (joint)
    distal radioulnar joint —*see* Subluxation,
      radioulnar (joint), distal
    metacarpal bone, proximal —*see* Subluxation,
      metacarpal (bone), proximal end
    midcarpal —*see* Subluxation, midcarpal
      (joint)
    radiocarpal joint —*see* Subluxation,
      radiocarpal (joint)
    recurrent —*see* Dislocation, recurrent, wrist
    specified site NEC S63.09-●
    ulna —*see* Subluxation, ulna, distal end

▶ New   ⇨ Revised   ~~deleted~~ Deleted   ● Use Additional Character(s)

Submaxillary —*see* condition
Submersion (fatal) (nonfatal) T75.1
Submucous —*see* condition
Subnormal, subnormality
  accommodation (old age) H52.4
  mental —*see* Disability, intellectual
  temperature (accidental) T68
Subphrenic —*see* condition
Subscapular nerve —*see* condition
Subseptus uterus Q51.28
Subsiding appendicitis K36
Substance (other psychoactive) -induced
  anxiety disorder F19.980
  bipolar and related disorder F19.94
  delirium F19.921
  depressive disorder F19.94
  major neurocognitive disorder F19.97
  mild neurocognitive disorder F19.988
  obsessive-compulsive and related disorder
    F19.988
  psychotic disorder F19.959
  sexual dysfunction F19.981
  sleep disorder F19.982
Substernal thyroid E04.9
  congenital Q89.2
Substitution disorder F44.9
Subtentorial —*see* condition
Subthyroidism (acquired) —*see also*
  Hypothyroidism
  congenital E03.1
Succenturiate placenta O43.19-●
Sucking thumb, child (excessive) F98.8
Sudamen, sudamina L74.1
Sudanese kala-azar B55.0
Sudden
  hearing loss —*see* Deafness, sudden
  heart failure —*see* Failure, heart
Sudeck's atrophy, disease, or syndrome —*see*
  Algoneurodystrophy
Suffocation —*see* Asphyxia, traumatic
Sugar
  blood
    high (transient) R73.9
    low (transient) E16.2
  in urine R81
Suicide, suicidal (attempted) T14.91
  by poisoning —*see* Table of Drugs and
    Chemicals
  history of (personal) Z91.51
    in family Z81.8
  ideation —*see* Ideation, suicidal
  risk
    meaning personal history of attempted
      suicide Z91.51
    meaning suicidal ideation —*see* Ideation,
      suicidal
  tendencies
    meaning personal history of attempted
      suicide Z91.51
    meaning suicidal ideation —*see* Ideation,
      suicidal
  trauma —*see* nature of injury by site
Suipestifer infection —*see* Infection, salmonella
Sulfhemoglobinemia, sulphemoglobinemia
  (acquired) (with methemoglobinemia) D74.8
Sumatran mite fever A75.3
Summer —*see* condition
Sunburn L55.9
  due to
    tanning bed (acute) L56.8
      chronic L57.8
    ultraviolet radiation (acute) L56.8
      chronic L57.8
  first degree L55.0
  second degree L55.1
  third degree L55.2
SUNCT (short lasting unilateral neuralgiform
    headache with conjunctival injection and
    tearing) G44.059
  intractable G44.051
  not intractable G44.059

Sundowning F05
Sunken acetabulum —*see* Derangement, joint,
    specified type NEC, hip
Sunstroke T67.01
  specified NEC T67.09
Superfecundation —*see* Pregnancy, multiple
Superfetation —*see* Pregnancy, multiple
Superinvolution (uterus) N85.8
Supernumerary (congenital)
  aortic cusps Q23.8
  auditory ossicles Q16.3
  bone Q79.8
  breast Q83.1
  carpal bones Q74.0
  cusps, heart valve NEC Q24.8
    aortic Q23.8
    mitral Q23.2
    pulmonary Q22.3
  digit(s) Q69.9
  ear (lobule) Q17.0
  fallopian tube Q50.6
  finger Q69.0
  hymen Q52.4
  kidney Q63.0
  lacrimonasal duct Q10.6
  lobule (ear) Q17.0
  mitral cusps Q23.2
  muscle Q79.8
  nipple(s) Q83.3
  organ or site not listed —*see* Accessory
  ossicles, auditory Q16.3
  ovary Q50.31
  oviduct Q50.6
  pulmonary, pulmonic cusps Q22.3
  rib Q76.6
    cervical or first (syndrome) Q76.5
  roots (of teeth) K00.2
  spleen Q89.09
  tarsal bones Q74.2
  teeth K00.1
  testis Q55.29
  thumb Q69.1
  toe Q69.2
  uterus Q51.28
  vagina Q52.1
  vertebra Q76.49
Supervision (of)
  contraceptive —*see* Prescription,
    contraceptives
  dietary (for) Z71.3
    allergy (food) Z71.3
    colitis Z71.3
    diabetes mellitus Z71.3
    food allergy or intolerance Z71.3
    gastritis Z71.3
    hypercholesterolemia Z71.3
    hypoglycemia Z71.3
    intolerance (food) Z71.3
    obesity Z71.3
    specified NEC Z71.3
  healthy infant or child Z76.2
    foundling Z76.1
  high-risk pregnancy —*see* Pregnancy,
    supervision of, high, risk
  lactation Z39.1
  pregnancy —*see* Pregnancy, supervision of
Supplemental teeth K00.1
Suppression
  binocular vision H53.34
  lactation O92.5
  menstruation N94.89
  ovarian secretion E28.39
  renal N28.9
  urine, urinary secretion R34
Suppuration, suppurative —*see also* condition
  accessory sinus (chronic) —*see* Sinusitis
  adrenal gland
  antrum (chronic) —*see* Sinusitis, maxillary
  bladder —*see* Cystitis
  brain G06.0
    sequelae G09

Suppuration, suppurative (*Continued*)
  breast N61.1
    puerperal, postpartum or gestational —*see*
      Mastitis, obstetric, purulent
  dental periosteum M27.3
  ear (middle) —*see also* Otitis, media
    external NEC —*see* Otitis, externa, infective
    internal —*see* subcategory H83.0
  ethmoidal (chronic) (sinus) —*see* Sinusitis,
    ethmoidal
  fallopian tube —*see* Salpingo-oophoritis
  frontal (chronic) (sinus) —*see* Sinusitis, frontal
  gallbladder (acute) K81.0
  gum K05.20
    generalized —*see* Periodontitis, aggressive,
      generalized
    localized —*see* Periodontitis, aggressive,
      localized
  intracranial G06.0
  joint —*see* Arthritis, pyogenic or pyemic
  labyrinthine —*see* subcategory H83.0
  lung —*see* Abscess, lung
  mammary gland N61.1
    puerperal, postpartum O91.12
      associated with lactation O91.13
  maxilla, maxillary M27.2
    sinus (chronic) —*see* Sinusitis, maxillary
  muscle —*see* Myositis, infective
  nasal sinus (chronic) —*see* Sinusitis
  pancreas, acute —*see also* Pancreatitis, acute
    K85.80
  parotid gland —*see* Sialoadenitis
  pelvis, pelvic
    female —*see* Disease, pelvis, inflammatory
    male K65.0
  pericranial —*see* Osteomyelitis
  salivary duct or gland (any) —*see*
    Sialoadenitis
  sinus (accessory) (chronic) (nasal) —*see*
    Sinusitis
  sphenoidal sinus (chronic) —*see* Sinusitis,
    sphenoidal
  thymus (gland) E32.1
  thyroid (gland) E06.0
  tonsil —*see* Tonsillitis
  uterus —*see* Endometritis
Supraeruption of tooth (teeth) M26.34
Supraglottitis J04.30
  with obstruction J04.31
Suprarenal (gland) —*see* condition
Suprascapular nerve —*see* condition
Suprasellar —*see* condition
Surfer's knots or nodules S89.8-●
Surgical
  emphysema T81.82
  procedures, complication or misadventure —
    see Complications, surgical procedures
  shock T81.10
Surveillance (of) (for) —*see also* Observation
  alcohol abuse Z71.41
  contraceptive —*see* Prescription, contraceptives
  dietary Z71.3
  drug abuse Z71.51
Susceptibility to disease, genetic Z15.89
  malignant neoplasm Z15.09
    breast Z15.01
    endometrium Z15.04
    ovary Z15.02
    prostate Z15.03
    specified NEC Z15.09
  multiple endocrine neoplasia Z15.81
Suspected condition, ruled out —*see also*
  Observation, suspected
  amniotic cavity and membrane Z03.71
  cervical shortening Z03.75
  fetal anomaly Z03.73
  fetal growth Z03.74
  maternal and fetal conditions NEC Z03.79
  newborn —*see also* Observation, newborn,
    suspected condition ruled out Z05.9
  oligohydramnios Z03.71

Syndrome *(Continued)*
androgen insensitivity E34.50
  complete E34.51
  partial E34.52
androgen resistance *(see also* Syndrome,
    androgen insensitivity) E34.50
Angelman Q93.51
anginal —*see* Angina
ankyloglossia superior Q38.1
anterior
  chest wall R07.89
  cord G83.82
  spinal artery G95.19
    compression M47.019
      cervical region M47.012
      cervicothoracic region M47.013
      lumbar region M47.016
      occipito-atlanto-axial region M47.011
      thoracic region M47.014
      thoracolumbar region M47.015
  tibial M76.81-•
antibody deficiency D80.9
  agammaglobulinemic D80.1
    hereditary D80.0
  congenital D80.0
  hypogammaglobulinemic D80.1
    hereditary D80.0
anticardiolipin (-antibody) D68.61
antidepressant discontinuation T43.205
antiphospholipid (-antibody) D68.61
aortic
  arch M31.4
  bifurcation I74.09
aortomesenteric duodenum occlusion K31.5
apical ballooning (transient left ventricular)
    I51.81
arcuate ligament I77.4
argentaffin, argintaffinoma E34.0
Arnold-Chiari —*see* Arnold-Chiari disease
Arrillaga-Ayerza I27.0
arterial tortuosity Q87.82
arteriovenous steal T82.898-•
Asherman's N85.6
aspiration, of newborn —*see* Aspiration, by
    substance, with pneumonia
  meconium P24.01
ataxia-telangiectasia G11.3
auriculotemporal G50.8
autoerythrocyte sensitization (Gardner-
    Diamond) D69.2
autoimmune lymphoproliferative [ALPS]
    D89.82
autoimmune polyglandular E31.0
autoinflammatory M04.9
  specified type NEC M04.8
autosomal —*see* Abnormal, autosomes
Avellis' G46.8
Ayerza (-Arrillaga) I27.0
Babinski-Nageotte G83.89
Bakwin-Krida Q78.5
bare lymphocyte D81.6
Barré-Guillain G61.0
Barré-Liéou M53.0
Barrett's —*see* Barrett's, esophagus
Barsony-Polgar K22.4
Barsony-Teschendorf K22.4
Barth E78.71
Bartter's E26.81
basal cell nevus Q87.89
Basedow's E05.00
  with thyroid storm E05.01
basilar artery G45.0
Batten-Steinert G71.11
battered
  baby or child —*see* Maltreatment, child,
    physical abuse
  spouse —*see* Maltreatment, adult, physical
    abuse
Beals Q87.40
Beau's I51.5
Beck's I65.8

Syndrome *(Continued)*
Benedikt's G46.3
Béquez César (-Steinbrinck-Chédiak-Higashi)
    D70.330
Bernhardt-Roth —*see* Meralgia paresthetica
Bernheim's —*see* Failure, heart, right
big spleen D73.51
bilateral polycystic ovarian E28.2
Bing-Horton's —*see* Horton's headache
Birt-Hogg-Dube syndrome Q87.89
Björck (-Thorsen) E34.0
black
  lung J60
  widow spider bite —*see* Toxicity, venom,
    spider, black widow
Blackfan-Diamond D61.01
Blau M04.8
blind loop K90.2
  congenital Q43.8
  postsurgical K91.2
blue sclera Q78.0
blue toe I75.02-•
Boder-Sedgewick G11.3
Boerhaave's K22.3
Borjeson Forssman Lehmann Q89.8
Bouillaud's I01.9
Bourneville (-Pringle) Q85.1
Bouveret (-Hoffman) I47.9
brachial plexus G54.0
bradycardia-tachycardia I49.5
brain (nonpsychotic) F09
  with psychosis, psychotic reaction F09
  acute or subacute —*see* Delirium
  congenital —*see* Disability, intellectual
  organic F09
    post-traumatic (nonpsychotic) F07.81
      psychotic F09
    personality change F07.0
    postcontusional F07.81
    post-traumatic, nonpsychotic F07.81
    psycho-organic F09
    psychotic F06.8
brain stem stroke G46.3
Brandt's (acrodermatitis enteropathica)
    E83.2
broad ligament laceration N83.8
Brock's J98.11
bronze baby P83.88
Brown-Sequard G83.81
Brugada I49.8
bubbly lung P27.0
Buchem's M85.2
Budd-Chiari I82.0
bulbar (progressive) G12.22
Bürger-Grütz E78.3
Burke's K86.89
Burnett's (milk-alkali) E83.52
burning feet E53.9
Bywaters' T79.5
Call-Fleming I67.841
carbohydrate-deficient glycoprotein (CDGS)
    E77.8
carcinogenic thrombophlebitis I82.1
carcinoid E34.0
cardiac asthma I50.1
cardiacos negros I27.0
cardiofaciocutaneous Q87.89
cardiopulmonary-obesity E66.2
cardiorenal —*see* Hypertension, cardiorenal
cardiorespiratory distress (idiopathic),
    newborn P22.0
cardiovascular renal —*see* Hypertension,
    cardiorenal
carotid
  artery (hemispheric) (internal)
    G45.1
  body G90.01
  sinus G90.01
carpal tunnel G56.0-•
Cassidy (-Scholte) E34.0
cat-cry Q93.4

Syndrome *(Continued)*
cat eye Q92.8
cauda equina G83.4
causalgia —*see* Causalgia
celiac K90.0
  artery compression I77.4
  axis I77.4
central pain G89.0
cerebellar
  hereditary G11.9
  stroke G46.4
cerebellomedullary malformation —*see* Spina
    bifida
cerebral
  artery
    anterior G46.1
    middle G46.0
    posterior G46.2
  gigantism E22.0
cervical (root) M53.1
  disc —*see* Disorder, disc, cervical, with
    neuritis
  fusion Q76.1
  posterior, sympathicus M53.0
  rib Q76.5
  sympathetic paralysis G90.2
cervicobrachial (diffuse) M53.1
cervicocranial M53.0
cervicodorsal outlet G54.2
cervicothoracic outlet G54.0
Céstan (-Raymond) I65.8
Charcot's (angina cruris) (intermittent
    claudication) I73.9
Charcot-Weiss-Baker G90.09
CHARGE Q89.8
Chédiak-Higashi (-Steinbrinck) E70.330
chest wall R07.1
Chiari's (hepatic vein thrombosis) I82.0
Chilaiditi's Q43.3
child maltreatment —*see* Maltreatment,
    child
chondrocostal junction M94.0
chondroectodermal dysplasia Q77.6
chromosome 4 short arm deletion Q93.3
chromosome 5 short arm deletion Q93.4
chronic
  infantile neurological, cutaneous and
    articular (CINCA) M04.2
  pain G89.4
    personality F68.8
Churg-Strauss M30.1
Clarke-Hadfield K86.89
Clerambault's automatism G93.89
Clouston's (hidrotic ectodermal dysplasia)
    Q82.4
clumsiness, clumsy child F82
cluster headache G44.009
  intractable G44.001
  not intractable G44.009
Coffin-Lowry Q89.8
cold injury (newborn) P80.0
combined immunity deficiency D81.9
compartment (deep) (posterior) (traumatic)
    T79.A0
  abdomen T79.A3
  lower extremity (hip, buttock, thigh, leg,
    foot, toes) T79.A2
  nontraumatic
    abdomen M79.A3
    lower extremity (hip, buttock, thigh, leg,
      foot, toes) M79.A2-•
    specified site NEC M79.A9
    upper extremity (shoulder, arm, forearm,
      wrist, hand, fingers) M79.A1-•
  postprocedural —*see* Syndrome
    compartment, nontraumatic
  specified site NEC T79.A9
  upper extremity (shoulder, arm, forearm,
    wrist, hand, fingers) T79.A1
complex regional pain —*see* Syndrome, pain,
    complex regional

S

Syndrome *(Continued)*
 compression T79.5
  anterior spinal —*see* Syndrome, anterior,
   spinal artery, compression
  cauda equina G83.4
  celiac artery I77.4
  vertebral artery M47.029
   cervical region M47.022
   occipito-atlanto-axial region M47.021
 concussion F07.81
 congenital
  affecting multiple systems NEC Q87.89
  central alveolar hypoventilation G47.35
  facial diplegia Q87.0
  muscular hypertrophy-cerebral Q87.89
  oculo-auriculovertebral Q87.0
  oculofacial diplegia (Moebius) Q87.0
  rubella (manifest) P35.0
 congestion-fibrosis (pelvic), female
  N94.89
 congestive dysmenorrhea N94.6
 Conn's E26.01
 connective tissue M35.9
  overlap NEC M35.1
 conus medullaris G95.81
 cord
  anterior G83.82
  posterior G83.83
 coronary
  acute NEC I24.9
  insufficiency or intermediate I20.0
  slow flow I20.8
 Costen's (complex) M26.69
 costochondral junction M94.0
 costoclavicular G54.0
 costovertebral E22.0
➡Cowden
 ▶PTEN related Q85.81
 ▶specified NEC Q85.82
 craniovertebral M53.0
 Creutzfeldt-Jakob —*see* Creutzfeldt-Jakob
  disease or syndrome
 cri-du-chat Q93.4
 crib death R99
 cricopharyngeal —*see* Dysphagia
 croup J05.0
 CRPS I —*see* Syndrome, pain, complex
  regional I
 crush T79.5
 cubital tunnel —*see* Lesion, nerve, ulnar
 Curschmann (-Batten) (-Steinert) G71.11
 Cushing's E24.9
  alcohol-induced E24.4
  drug-induced E24.2
  due to
   alcohol
    drugs E24.2
   ectopic ACTH E24.3
   overproduction of pituitary ACTH
    E24.0
  overdose or wrong substance given
   or taken —*see* Table of Drugs and
   Chemicals, by drug, poisoning
  pituitary-dependent E24.0
  specified type NEC E24.8
 cryopyrin-associated periodic M04.2
 cryptophthalmos Q87.0
 cystic duct stump K91.5
 cytokine release D89.839
  grade 1 D89.831
  grade 2 D89.832
  grade 3 D89.833
  grade 4 D89.834
  grade 5 D89.835
 Dana-Putnam D51.0
 Danbolt (-Cross) (acrodermatitis
  enteropathica) E83.2
 Dandy-Walker Q03.1
  with spina bifida Q07.01
 Danlos' *(see also* Syndrome, Ehlers-Danlos)
  Q79.60

Syndrome *(Continued)*
 defibrination —*see also* Fibrinolysis
  with
   antepartum hemorrhage —*see*
    Hemorrhage, antepartum, with
    coagulation defect
   intrapartum hemorrhage —*see*
    Hemorrhage, complicating,
    delivery
  newborn P60
  postpartum O72.3
 Degos' I77.8
 Déjérine-Roussy G89.0
 delayed sleep phase G47.21
 demyelinating G37.9
 dependence —*see* F10-F19 with fourth
  character .2
 depersonalization (-derealization) F48.1
 De Quervain E34.51
 de Toni-Fanconi (-Debré) E72.09
  with cystinosis E72.04
 de Vivo syndrome E74.810
 diabetes mellitus-hypertension-nephrosis —
  see Diabetes, nephrosis
 diabetes mellitus in newborn infant P70.2
 diabetes-nephrosis —*see* Diabetes, nephrosis
 diabetic amyotrophy —*see* Diabetes,
  amyotrophy
 dialysis associated steal T82.898-•
 Diamond-Blackfan D61.01
 Diamond-Gardener D69.2
 DIC (diffuse or disseminated intravascular
  coagulopathy) D65
 di George's D82.1
 Dighton's Q78.0
 disequilibrium E87.8
 Döhle body-panmyelopathic D72.0
 dorsolateral medullary G46.4
 double athetosis G80.3
 Down *(see also* Down syndrome) Q90.9
 Dravet (intractable) G40.834
  with status epilepticus G40.833
  without status epilepticus G40.834
 Dresbach's (elliptocytosis) D58.1
 DRESS (drug rash with eosinophilia and
  systemic symptoms) D72.12
 Dressler's (postmyocardial infarction) I24.1
  postcardiotomy I97.0
 drug rash with eosinophilia and systemic
  symptoms (DRESS) D72.12
 drug withdrawal, infant of dependent mother
  P96.1
 dry eye H04.12-•
 due to abnormality
  chromosomal Q99.9
   sex
    female phenotype Q97.9
    male phenotype Q98.9
   specified NEC Q99.8
 dumping (postgastrectomy) K91.1
  nonsurgical K31.89
 Dupré's (meningism) R29.1
 dysmetabolic X E88.81
 dyspraxia, developmental F82
 Eagle-Barrett Q79.4
 Eaton-Lambert —*see* Syndrome, Lambert-Eaton
 Ebstein's Q22.5
 ectopic ACTH E24.3
 eczema-thrombocytopenia D82.0
 Eddowes' Q78.0
 effort (psychogenic) F45.8
 Ehlers-Danlos Q79.60
  classical (cEDS) (classical EDS) Q79.61
  hypermobile (hEDS) (hypermobile EDS)
   Q79.62
  specified NEC Q79.69
  vascular (vascular EDS) (vEDS) Q79.63
 Eisenmenger's I27.83
 Ekman's Q78.0
 electric feet E53.8
 Ellis-van Creveld Q77.6
 empty nest Z60.0

Syndrome *(Continued)*
 endocrine-hypertensive E27.0
 entrapment —*see* Neuropathy, entrapment
 eosinophilia-myalgia M35.89
 epileptic —*see also* Epilepsy, by type
  absence G40.A09
   intractable G40.A19
    with status epilepticus G40.A11
    without status epilepticus G40.A19
   not intractable G40.A09
    with status epilepticus G40.A01
    without status epilepticus G40.A09
 Erdheim-Chester (ECD) E88.89
 Erdheim's E22.0
 erythrocyte fragmentation D59.4
 Evans D69.41
 exhaustion F48.8
 extrapyramidal G25.9
  specified NEC G25.89
 eye retraction —*see* Strabismus
 eyelid-malar-mandible Q87.0
 Faber's D50.9
 facet M47.89-•
 facet joint *(see also* Spondylosis) M47.819
 facial pain, paroxysmal G50.0
 Fallot's Q21.3
 familial cold autoinflammatory M04.2
 familial eczema-thrombocytopenia (Wiskott-
  Aldrich) D82.0
 Fanconi (-de Toni) (-Debré) E72.09
  with cystinosis E72.04
 Fanconi's (anemia) (congenital pancytopenia)
  D61.09
 fatigue
 ➡chronic G93.32
 ▶postviral G93.31
  psychogenic F48.8
 faulty bowel habit K59.39
 Feil-Klippel (brevicollis) Q76.1
 Felty's —*see* Felty's syndrome
 fertile eunuch E23.0
 fetal
  alcohol (dysmorphic) Q86.0
  hydantoin Q86.1
 Fiedler's I40.1
 first arch Q87.0
 fish odor E72.89
 Fisher's G61.0
 Fitzhugh-Curtis
  due to
   Chlamydia trachomatis A74.81
   Neisseria gonorrhorea (gonococcal
    peritonitis) A54.85
 Fitz's —*see also* Pancreatitis, acute K85.80
 Flajani (-Basedow) E05.00
  with thyroid storm E05.01
 flatback —*see* Flatback syndrome
 floppy
  baby P94.2
  iris (intraoeprative) (IFIS) H21.81
  mitral valve I34.1
 flush E34.0
 Foix-Alajouanine G95.19
 Fong's Q87.2
 food protein-induced enterocolitis (FPIES)
  K52.21
 foramen magnum G93.5
 Foster-Kennedy H47.14-•
 Foville's (peduncular) G46.3
 fragile X Q99.2
 Franceschetti Q75.4
 Frey's
  auriculotemporal G50.8
  hyperhidrosis L74.52
 Friderichsen-Waterhouse A39.1
 Froin's G95.89
 frontal lobe F07.0
 Fukuhara E88.49
 functional
  bowel K59.9
  prepubertal castrate E29.1
 Gaisböck's D75.1

Syndrome *(Continued)*
  ganglion (basal ganglia brain) G25.9
    geniculi G51.1
  Gardner-Diamond D69.2
  gastroesophageal
    junction K22.0
    laceration-hemorrhage K22.6
  gastrojejunal loop obstruction K91.89
  Gee-Herter-Heubner K90.0
  Gelineau's G47.419
    with cataplexy G47.411
  genito-anorectal A55
  Gerstmann-Sträussler-Scheinker (GSS) A81.82
  Gianotti-Crosti L44.4
  giant platelet (Bernard-Soulier) D69.1
  Gilles de la Tourette's F95.2
  Glass Q87.89
  Gleich's D72.118
  goiter-deafness E07.1
  Goldberg Q89.8
  Goldberg-Maxwell E34.51
  Good's D83.8
  Gopalan' (burning feet) E53.8
  Gorlin's Q87.89
  Gougerot-Blum L81.7
  Gouley's I31.1
  Gower's R55
  gray or grey (newborn) P93.0
    platelet D69.1
  Gubler-Millard G46.3
  Guillain-Barré (-Strohl) G61.0
  gustatory sweating G50.8
  Hadfield-Clarke K86.89
  hair tourniquet —*see* Constriction, external,
    by site
  Hamman's J98.19
  hand-foot L27.1
  hand-shoulder G90.8
  hantavirus (cardio)-pulmonary (HPS) (HCPS)
    B33.4
  happy puppet Q93.51
  Harada's H30.81-●
  Hayem-Faber D50.9
  headache NEC G44.89
    complicated NEC G44.59
  Heberden's I20.8
  Hedinger's E34.0
  Hegglin's D72.0
  HELLP (hemolysis, elevated liver enzymes
    and low platelet count) O14.2-●
    complicating
      childbirth O14.24
        puerperium O14.25
  ▶hemolytic-uremic D59.30
    ▶atypical D59.39
      ▶genetic D59.32
      ▶hereditary D59.32
      ▶infection-associated D59.31
      ▶secondary D59.39
      ▶specified NEC D59.39
    ▶due to genetic disorder D59.32
    ▶familial D59.32
    ▶hereditary D59.32
    ▶infection-associated D59.31
    ▶secondary D59.39
    ▶Shiga toxin-producing E. coli [STEC]
      related D59.31
    ▶specified NEC D59.39
    ▶typical D59.31
  hemophagocytic, infection-associated D76.2
  Henoch-Schönlein D69.0
  hepatic flexure K59.89
  hepatopulmonary K76.81
  hepatorenal K76.7
    following delivery O90.4
    postoperative or postprocedural K91.83
    postpartum, puerperal O90.4
  hepatourologic K76.7
  hereditary alpha tryptasemia D89.44
  Herter (-Gee) (nontropical sprue) K90.0
  Heubner-Herter K90.0
  Heyd's K76.7

Syndrome *(Continued)*
  Hilger's G90.09
  histamine-like (fish poisoning) —*see*
    Poisoning, fish
  histiocytic D76.3
  histiocytosis NEC D76.3
  HIV infection, acute B20
  Hoffmann-Werdnig G12.0
  Hollander-Simons E88.1
  Hoppe-Goldflam G70.00
    with exacerbation (acute) G70.01
    in crisis G70.01
  Horner's G90.2
  hungry bone E83.81
  hunterian glossitis D51.0
  Hutchinson's triad A50.53
  hyperabduction G54.0
  hyperammonemia-hyperornithinemia-
    homocitrullinemia E72.4
  hypereosinophilic (HES) D72.119
    idiopathic (IHES) D72.110
    lymphocytic variant (LHES) D72.111
    myeloid D72.118
    specified NEC D72.118
  hyperimmunoglobulin D M04.1
  hyperimmunoglobulin E (IgE) D82.4
  hyperkalemic E87.5
  hyperkinetic —*see* Hyperkinesia
  hypermobility M35.7
  hypernatremia E87.0
  hyperosmolarity E87.0
  hyperperfusion G97.82
  hypersplenic D73.1
  hypertransfusion, newborn P61.1
  hyperventilation F45.8
  hyperviscosity (of serum)
    polycythemic D75.1
    sclerothymic D58.8
  hypoglycemic (familial) (neonatal) E16.2
  hypokalemic E87.6
  hyponatremic E87.1
  hypopituitarism E23.0
  hypoplastic left-heart Q23.4
  hypopotassemia E87.6
  hyposmolality E87.1
  hypotension, maternal O26.5-●
  hypothenar hammer I73.89
  hypoventilation, obesity (OHS) E66.2
  ICF (intravascular coagulation-fibrinolysis) D65
  idiopathic
    cardiorespiratory distress, newborn P22.0
    nephrotic (infantile) N04.9
  iliotibial band M76.3-●
  immobility, immobilization (paraplegic) M62.3
  immune effector cell-associated neurotoxicity
    (ICANS) G92.00
    grade
      1 G92.01
      2 G92.02
      3 G92.03
      4 G92.04
      5 G92.05
      unspecified G92.00
  immune reconstitution D89.3
  immune reconstitution inflammatory [IRIS]
    D89.3
  immunity deficiency, combined D81.9
  immunodeficiency
    acquired —*see* Human, immunodeficiency
      virus (HIV) disease
    combined D81.9
  impending coronary I20.0
  impingement, shoulder M75.4-●
  inappropriate secretion of antidiuretic
    hormone E22.2
  infant
    gestational diabetes P70.0
    of diabetic mother P70.1
  infantilism (pituitary) E23.0
  inferior vena cava I87.1
  inspissated bile (newborn) P59.1
  institutional (childhood) F94.2
  insufficient sleep F51.12

Syndrome *(Continued)*
  intermediate coronary (artery) I20.0
  interspinous ligament —*see* Spondylopathy,
    specified NEC
  intestinal
    carcinoid E34.0
    knot K56.2
  intravascular coagulation-fibrinolysis (ICF)
    D65
  iodine-deficiency, congenital E00.9
    type
      mixed E00.2
      myxedematous E00.1
      neurological E00.0
  IRDS (idiopathic respiratory distress,
    newborn) P22.0
  irritable
    bowel K58.9
      with
        constipation K58.1
        diarrhea K58.0
      mixed K58.2
      psychogenic F45.8
      specified NEC K58.8
    heart (psychogenic) F45.8
    weakness F48.8
  ischemic
    bowel (transient) K55.9
      chronic K55.1
      due to mesenteric artery insufficiency
        K55.1
    steal T82.898
  IVC (intravascular coagulopathy) D65
  Ivemark's Q89.01
  Jaccoud's —*see* Arthropathy, postrheumatic,
    chronic
  Jackson's G83.89
  Jakob-Creutzfeldt —*see* Creutzfeldt-Jakob
    disease or syndrome
  jaw-winking Q07.8
  Jervell-Lange-Nielsen I45.81
  jet lag G47.25
  Job's D71
  Joseph-Diamond-Blackfan D61.01
  jugular foramen G52.7
  Kabuki Q89.8
  Kanner's (autism) F84.0
  Kartagener's Q89.3
  Kelly's D50.1
  Kimmelstiel-Wilson —*see* Diabetes,specified
    type, with Kimmelstiel-Wilson disease
  Klein (e)-Levine G47.13
  Klippel-Feil (brevicollis) Q76.1
  Köhler-Pellegrini-Steida —*see* Bursitis, tibial
    collateral
  König's K59.89
  Korsakoff (-Wernicke) (nonalcoholic) F04
    alcoholic F10.26
  Kostmann's D70.0
  Krabbe's congenital muscle hypoplasia Q79.8
  labyrinthine —*see* subcategory H83.2
  lacunar NEC G46.7
  Lambert-Eaton G70.80
    in
      neoplastic disease G73.1
      specified disease NEC G70.81
  Landau-Kleffner —*see* Epilepsy, specified NEC
  Larsen's Q74.8
  lateral
    cutaneous nerve of thigh G57.1-●
    medullary G46.4
  Launois' E22.0
  lazy
    leukocyte D70.8
    posture M62.3
  Lemiere I80.8
  Lennox-Gastaut G40.812
    intractable G40.814
      with status epilepticus G40.813
      without status epilepticus G40.814
    not intractable G40.812
      with status epilepticus G40.811
      without status epilepticus G40.812

Syndrome *(Continued)*
  lenticular, progressive E83.01
  Leopold-Levi's E05.90
  Lev's I44.2
  Li-Fraumeni Z15.01
  Lichtheim's D51.0
  Lightwood's N25.89
  Lignac (de Toni) (-Fanconi) (-Debré) E72.09
    with cystinosis E72.04
  Likoff's I20.8
  limbic epilepsy personality F07.0
  liver-kidney K76.7
  lobotomy F07.0
  Löffler's J82.89
  long arm 18 or 21 deletion Q93.89
  long QT I45.81
  Louis-Barré G11.3
  low
    atmospheric pressure T70.29
    back M54.50
    output (cardiac) I50.9
  lower radicular, newborn (birth injury) P14.8
  Luetscher's (dehydration) E86.0
  Lupus anticoagulant D68.62
▌ Lutembacher's Q21.19
  macrophage activation D76.1
    due to infection D76.2
  magnesium-deficiency R29.0
  Majeed M04.8
  Mal de Debarquement R42
  malabsorption K90.9
    postsurgical K91.2
  malformation, congenital, due to
    alcohol Q86.0
    exogenous cause NEC Q86.8
    hydantoin Q86.1
    warfarin Q86.2
  malignant
    carcinoid E34.0
    neuroleptic G21.0
  Mallory-Weiss K22.6
  mandibulofacial dysostosis Q75.4
  manic-depressive —*see* Disorder, bipolar
  maple-syrup-urine E71.0
  Marable's I77.4
  Marfan's Q87.40
    with
      cardiovascular manifestations Q87.418
        aortic dilation Q87.410
      ocular manifestations Q87.42
      skeletal manifestations Q87.43
  Marie's (acromegaly) E22.0
  mast cell activation —*see* Activation, mast cell
  maternal hypotension —*see* Syndrome,
      hypotension, maternal
  May (-Hegglin) D72.0
  McArdle (-Schmidt) (-Pearson) E74.04
  McQuarrie's E16.2
  meconium plug (newborn) P76.0
  median arcuate ligament I77.4
  Meekeren-Ehlers-Danlos Q79.6
  megavitamin-B6 E67.2
  Meige G24.4
  MELAS E88.41
  Mendelson's O74.0
  MERRF (myoclonic epilepsy associated with
      ragged-red fibers) E88.42
  mesenteric
    artery (superior) K55.1
    vascular insufficiency K55.1
  metabolic E88.81
  metastatic carcinoid E34.0
  micrognathia-glossoptosis Q87.0
  midbrain NEC G93.89
  middle lobe (lung) J98.19
  middle radicular G54.0
  migraine —*see also* Migraine G43.909-●
  Mikulicz' K11.8
  milk-alkali E83.52
  Millard-Gubler G46.3
  Miller-Dieker Q93.88

Syndrome *(Continued)*
  Miller-Fisher G61.0
  Minkowski-Chauffard D58.0
  Mirizzi's K83.1
  MNGIE (Mitochondrial Neurogastrointestinal
      Encephalopathy) E88.49
  Möbius, ophthalmoplegic migraine —*see*
      Migraine, ophthalmoplegic
  monofixation H50.42
  Morel-Moore M85.2
  Morel-Morgagni M85.2
  Morgagni (-Morel) (-Stewart) M85.2
  Morgagni-Adams-Stokes I45.9
  Mounier-Kuhn Q32.4
    with bronchiectasis J47.9
      with
        exacerbation (acute) J47.1
        lower respiratory infection J47.0
    acquired J98.09
      with bronchiectasis J47.9
        with
          exacerbation (acute) J47.1
          lower respiratory infection J47.0
  Muckle-Wells M04.2
  mucocutaneous lymph node (acute febrile)
      (MCLS) M30.3
  multiple endocrine neoplasia (MEN) —*see*
      Neoplasia, endocrine, multiple (MEN}
  multiple operations —*see* Disorder, factitious
  multisystem inflammatory (in adults) (in
      children) M35.81
  myasthenic G70.9
    in
      diabetes mellitus —*see* Diabetes,
          amyotrophy
      endocrine disease NEC E34.9 *[G73.3]*
      neoplastic disease —*see also* Neoplasm
          D49.9 *[G73.3]*
      thyrotoxicosis (hyperthyroidism) E05.90
          [G73.3]
        with thyroid storm E05.91 *[G73.3]*
  myelodysplastic D46.9
    with
      5q deletion D46.C
      isolated del (5q) chromosomal
          abnormality D46.C
      multilineage dysplasia D46.A
        with ringed sideroblasts D46.B
    lesions, low grade D46.20
    specified NEC D46.Z
  myeloid hypereosinophilic D72.118
  myelopathic pain G89.0
  myeloproliferative (chronic) D47.1
  myofascial pain M79.18
  Naffziger's G54.0
  nail patella Q87.2
  NARP (Neuropathy, Ataxia and Retinitis
      pigmentosa) E88.49
  neonatal abstinence P96.1
  nephritic —*see also* Nephritis
    with edema —*see* Nephrosis
    acute N00.9
    chronic N03.9
    rapidly progressive N01.9
  nephrotic (congenital) —*see also* Nephrosis
      N04.9
    with
      C3
        glomerulonephritis N04.A
        glomerulopathy N04.A
          with dense deposit disease N04.6
      dense deposit disease N04.6
    diffuse
      crescentic glomerulonephritis N04.7
      endocapillary proliferative
          glomerulonephritis N04.4
      membranous glomerulonephritis N04.2
      mesangial proliferative
          glomerulonephritis N04.3
      mesangiocapillary glomerulonephritis
          N04.5

Syndrome *(Continued)*
  nephrotic *(Continued)*
    with *(Continued)*
      focal and segmental glomerular lesions
          N04.1
      minor glomerular abnormality N04.0
      specified morphological changes NEC
          N04.8
    diabetic —*see* Diabetes, nephrosis
  neurologic neglect R41.4
  Nezelof's D81.4
  Nonne-Milroy-Meige Q82.0
  Nothnagel's vasomotor acroparesthesia I73.89
  obesity hypoventilation (OHS) E66.2
  oculomotor H51.9
  Ogilvie K59.81
  ophthalmoplegia-cerebellar ataxia —*see*
      Strabismus, paralytic, third nerve
  oral allergy T78.1
  oral-facial-digital Q87.0
  organic
    affective F06.30
    amnesic (not alcohol- or drug-induced) F04
    brain F09
    depressive F06.31
    hallucinosis F06.0
    personality F07.0
  Ormond's N13.5
  oro-facial-digital Q87.0
  os trigonum Q68.8
  Osler-Weber-Rendu I78.0
  osteoporosis-osteomalacia M83.8
  Osterreicher-Turner Q87.2
  otolith —*see* subcategory H81.8
  oto-palatal-digital Q87.0
  outlet (thoracic) G54.0
  ovary
    polycystic E28.2
    resistant E28.39
    sclerocystic E28.2
  Owren's D68.2
  Paget-Schroetter I82.890
  pain —*see also* Pain
    complex regional I G90.50
      lower limb G90.52-●
      specified site NEC G90.59
      upper limb G90.51-●
    complex regional II —*see* Causalgia
  painful
    bruising D69.2
    feet E53.8
    prostate N42.81
  paralysis agitans —*see* Parkinsonism
  paralytic G83.9
    specified NEC G83.89
  Parinaud's H51.0
  parkinsonian —*see* Parkinsonism
  Parkinson's —*see* Parkinsonism
  paroxysmal facial pain G50.0
  Parry's E05.00
    with thyroid storm E05.01
  Parsonage (-Aldren)-Turner G54.5
  patella clunk M25.86-●
  Paterson (-Brown) (-Kelly) D50.1
  pectoral girdle I77.89
  pectoralis minor I77.89
  pediatric autoimmune neuropsychiatric
      disorders associated with streptococcal
      infections (PANDAS) D89.89
  pediatric inflammatory multisystem M35.81
  Pelger-Huet D72.0
  pellagra-cerebellar ataxia-renal
      aminoaciduria E72.02
  pellagroid E52
  Pellegrini-Stieda —*see* Bursitis, tibial collateral
  pelvic congestion-fibrosis, female N94.89
  penta X Q97.1
  peptic ulcer —*see* Ulcer, peptic
  perabduction I77.89
  periodic fever M04.1
  periodic fever, aphthous stomatitis, pharyngitis,
      and adenopathy [PFAPA] M04.8

▶ New   ⇒ Revised   ~~deleted~~ Deleted   ● Use Additional Character(s)

Syndrome *(Continued)*
  periodic headache, in adults and children —
        see Headache, periodic syndromes in
        adults and children
  periurethral fibrosis N13.5
▶ Peutz-Jeghers Q85.89
  phantom limb (without pain) G54.7
        with pain G54.6
  pharyngeal pouch D82.1
  Pick's —*see* Disease, Pick's
  Pickwickian E66.2
  PIE (pulmonary infiltration with
        eosinophilia) J82.89
  pigmentary pallidal degeneration
        (progressive) G23.0
  pineal E34.8
  pituitary E22.0
  placental transfusion —*see* Pregnancy,
        complicated by, placental transfusion
        syndromes
  plantar fascia M72.2
  plateau iris (post-iridectomy)
        (postprocedural) H21.82
  Plummer-Vinson D50.1
  pluricarential of infancy E40
  plurideficiency E40
  pluriglandular (compensatory) E31.8
        autoimmune E31.0
  pneumatic hammer T75.21
  polyangiitis overlap M30.8
  polycarential of infancy E40
  polyglandular E31.8
        autoimmune E31.0
  polysplenia Q89.09
  pontine NEC G93.89
  popliteal
        artery entrapment I77.89
        web Q87.89
▶ postbacterial fatigue G93.39
  postcardiac injury
        postcardiotomy I97.0
        postmyocardial infarction I24.1
  postcardiotomy I97.0
  post chemoembolization — code to
        associated conditions
  postcholecystectomy K91.5
  postcommissurotomy I97.0
  postconcussional F07.81
  postcontusional F07.81
  post-COVID (-19) U09.9
  postencephalitic F07.89
  post endometrial ablation N99.85
  posterior
        cervical sympathetic M53.0
        cord G83.83
        fossa compression G93.5
        reversible encephalopathy (PRES) I67.83
  postgastrectomy (dumping) K91.1
  postgastric surgery K91.1
  postinfarction I24.1
▶ postinfectious fatigue G93.39
  postlaminectomy NEC M96.1
  postleukotomy F07.0
  postmastectomy lymphedema I97.2
  postmyocardial infarction I24.1
  postoperative NEC T81.9
        blind loop K90.2
  postpartum panhypopituitary (Sheehan) E23.0
  postpolio (myelitic) G14
  postthrombotic I87.009
        with
              inflammation I87.02-●
                    with ulcer I87.03-●
              specified complication NEC I87.09-●
              ulcer I87.01-●
                    with inflammation I87.03-●
        asymptomatic I87.00-●
▶ postural
  ▶ orthostatic tachycardia [POTS] G90.A
  ▶ tachycardia G90.A
  postvagotomy K91.1

Syndrome *(Continued)*
  postvalvulotomy I97.0
⇒ postviral NEC G93.31
  ⇒ fatigue G93.31
  Potain's K31.0
  potassium intoxication E87.5
  Prader-Willi Q87.11
  Prader-Willi-like Q87.19
  precerebral artery (multiple) (bilateral) G45.2
  preinfarction I20.0
  preleukemic D46.9
  premature senility E34.8
  premenstrual dysphoric F32.81
  premenstrual tension N94.3
  Prinzmetal-Massumi R07.1
  prune belly Q79.4
  pseudocarpal tunnel (sublimis) —*see*
        Syndrome, carpal tunnel
  pseudoparalytica G70.00
        with exacerbation (acute) G70.01
        in crisis G70.01
  pseudo-Turner's Q87.19
  psycho-organic (nonpsychotic severity) F07.9
        acute or subacute F05
        depressive type F06.31
        hallucinatory type F06.0
        nonpsychotic severity F07.0
        specified NEC F07.89
▶ PTEN (hamartoma) tumor Q85.81
  pulmonary
        arteriosclerosis I27.0
        dysmaturity (Wilson-Mikity) P27.0
        hypoperfusion (idiopathic) P22.0
        renal (hemorrhagic) (Goodpasture's) M31.0
  pure
        motor lacunar G46.5
        sensory lacunar G46.6
  Putnam-Dana D51.0
  pyogenic arthritis, pyoderma gangrenosum,
        and acne [PAPA] M04.8
  pyramidopallidonigral G20
  pyriformis —*see* Lesion, nerve, sciatic
  QT interval prolongation I45.81
  radicular NEC —*see* Radiculopathy
        upper limbs, newborn (birth injury) P14.3
  rapid time-zone change G47.25
  Rasmussen G04.81
  Raymond (-Céstan) I65.8
  Raynaud's I73.00
        with gangrene I73.01
  RDS (respiratory distress syndrome,
        newborn) P22.0
  reactive airways dysfunction J68.3
  Refsum's G60.1
  Reifenstein E34.52
  renal glomerulohyalinosis-diabetic —*see*
        Diabetes, nephrosis
  Rendu-Osler-Weber I78.0
  residual ovary N99.83
  resistant ovary E28.39
  respiratory
        distress
              acute J80
                    adult J80
                    child J80
                    idiopathic J84.114
              newborn (idiopathic) (type I) P22.0
                    type II P22.1
  restless legs G25.81
  retinoblastoma (familial) C69.2
  retroperitoneal fibrosis N13.5
  retroviral seroconversion (acute) Z21
  Reye's G93.7
  Richter —*see* Leukemia, chronic lymphocytic,
        B-cell type
  Ridley's I50.1
  right
        heart, hypoplastic Q22.6
        ventricular obstruction —*see* Failure, heart,
              right
  Romano-Ward (prolonged QT interval) I45.81

Syndrome *(Continued)*
  rotator cuff, shoulder —*see also* Tear, rotator
        cuff M75.10-●
  Rotes Quérol —*see* Hyperostosis, ankylosing
  Roth —*see* Meralgia paresthetica
  rubella (congenital) P35.0
  Ruvalcaba-Myhre-Smith E71.440
  Rytand-Lipsitch I44.2
  salt
        depletion E87.1
              due to heat NEC T67.8
                    causing heat exhaustion or prostration
                          T67.4
        low E87.1
  salt-losing N28.89
  SATB2-associated Q87.89
  Scaglietti-Dagnini E22.0
  scalenus anticus (anterior) G54.0
  scapulocostal —*see* Mononeuropathy, upper
        limb, specified site NEC
  scapuloperoneal G71.09
  schizophrenic, of childhood NEC F84.5
  Schnitzler D47.2
  Scholte's E34.0
  Schroeder's E27.0
  Schüller-Christian C96.5
  Schwachman's —*see* Syndrome, Shwachman's
  Schwartz (-Jampel) G71.13
  Schwartz-Bartter E22.2
  scimitar Q26.8
  sclerocystic ovary E28.2
  Seitelberger's G31.89
  septicemic adrenal hemorrhage A39.1
  seroconversion, retroviral (acute) Z21
  serous meningitis G93.2
  severe acute respiratory (SARS) J12.81
  coronavirus 2 -*see also* COVID-19 U07.1
        pneumonia J12.82
  shaken infant T74.4
  shock (traumatic) T79.4
        kidney N17.0
              following crush injury T79.5
        toxic A48.3
  shock-lung J80
  Shone's — code to specific anomalies
  short
        bowel K91.2
        rib Q77.2
  shoulder-hand —*see* Algoneurodystrophy
  Shwachman's D70.4
  sicca —*see* Syndrome, Sjögren
  sick
        cell E87.1
        sinus I49.5
  sick-euthyroid E07.81
  sideropenic D50.1
  Siemens' ectodermal dysplasia Q82.4
  Silfversköld's Q78.9
  Simons' E88.1
  sinus tarsi M25.57-●
  sinusitis-bronchiectasis-situs inversus Q89.3
  Sipple's E31.22
  sirenomelia Q87.2
  Sjögren M35.00
        with
              central nervous system involvement
                    M35.0F
              dental involvement M35.0C
              gastrointestinal involvement M35.08
              glomerular disease M35.0A
              inflammatory arthritis M35.05
              keratoconjunctivitis M35.01
              lung involvement M35.02
              myopathy M35.03
              peripheral nervous system involvement
                    M35.06
              renal tubular acidosis M35.04
              specified organ involvement, NEC
                    M35.09
              tubulo-interstitial nephropathy M35.04
              vasculitis M35.0B

Syndrome *(Continued)*
  Slocumb's E27.0
  slow flow, coronary I20.8
  Sluder's G44.89
  Smith-Magenis Q93.88
  Sneddon-Wilkinson L13.1
  Sotos' Q87.3
  South African cardiomyopathy I42.8
  spasmodic
    upward movement, eyes H51.8
    winking F95.8
  Spen's I45.9
  splenic
    agenesis Q89.01
    flexure K59.89
    neutropenia D73.81
  Spurway's Q78.0
  staphylococcal scalded skin L00
  steal
    arteriovenous T82.898-●
    ischemic T82.898-●
    subclavian G45.8
  Stein-Leventhal E28.2
  Stein's E28.2
  Stevens-Johnson syndrome L51.1
    toxic epidermal necrolysis overlap
      L51.3
  Stewart-Morel M85.2
  Stickler Q89.8
  stiff baby Q89.8
  stiff man G25.82
  Still-Felty —*see* Felty's syndrome
  Stokes (-Adams) I45.9
  stone heart I50.1
  straight back, congenital Q76.49
  ▶Sturge-Weber (-Dimitri) Q85.89
  subclavian steal G45.8
  subcoracoid-pectoralis minor G54.0
  subcostal nerve compression I77.89
  subphrenic interposition Q43.3
  superior
    cerebellar artery I63.89
    mesenteric artery K55.1
    semi-circular canal dehiscence H83.8X-●
    vena cava I87.1
  supine hypotensive (maternal) —*see*
    Syndrome, hypotension, maternal
  suprarenal cortical E27.0
  supraspinatus —*see also* Tear, rotator cuff
    M75.10-●
  Susac G93.49
  swallowed blood P78.2
  sweat retention L74.0
  Swyer Q99.1
  Symond's G93.2
  sympathetic
    cervical paralysis G90.2
    pelvic, female N94.89
  systemic inflammatory response (SIRS), of
    non-infectious origin (without organ
    dysfunction) R65.10
    with acute organ dysfunction R65.11
  tachycardia-bradycardia I49.5
  takotsubo I51.81
  TAR (thrombocytopenia with absent radius)
    Q87.2
  tarsal tunnel G57.5-●
  teething K00.7
  tegmental G93.89
  telangiectasic-pigmentation-cataract Q82.8
  temporal pyramidal apex —*see* Otitis, media,
    suppurative, acute
  temporomandibular joint-pain-dysfunction
    M26.62-●
  Terry's —*see also* Myopia, degenerative
    H44.2-●
  testicular feminization —*see also* Syndrome,
    androgen insensitivity E34.51
  thalamic pain (hyperesthetic) G89.0
  thoracic outlet (compression) G54.0
  Thorson-Björck E34.0
  thrombocytopenia with absent radius (TAR)
    Q87.2

Syndrome *(Continued)*
  ▶thrombosis with thrombocytopenia D75.84
  thyroid-adrenocortical insufficiency E31.0
  tibial
    anterior M76.81-●
    posterior M76.82-●
  Tietze's M94.0
  time-zone (rapid) G47.25
  Toni-Fanconi E72.09
    with cystinosis E72.04
  Touraine's Q79.8
  tourniquet —*see* Constriction, external, by site
  toxic shock A48.3
  transient left ventricular apical ballooning
    I51.81
  traumatic vasospastic T75.22
  Treacher Collins Q75.4
  triple X, female Q97.0
  trisomy Q92.9
    13 Q91.7
      meiotic nondisjunction Q91.4
      mitotic nondisjunction Q91.5
      mosaicism Q91.5
      translocation Q91.6
    18 Q91.3
      meiotic nondisjunction Q91.0
      mitotic nondisjunction Q91.1
      mosaicism Q91.1
      translocation Q91.2
  trisomy Q92.9
    20 (q)(p) Q92.8
    21 Q90.9
      meiotic nondisjunction Q90.0
      mitotic nondisjunction Q90.1
      mosaicism Q90.1
      translocation Q90.2
    22 Q92.8
  tropical wet feet T69.0-●
  Trousseau's I82.1
  tumor lysis (following antineoplastic
    chemotherapy) (spontaneous) NEC E88.3
  tumor necrosis factor receptor associated
    periodic (TRAPS) M04.1
  Twiddler's (due to)
    automatic implantable defibrillator T82.198
    cardiac pacemaker T82.198
  Unverricht (-Lundborg) —*see* Epilepsy,
    generalized, idiopathic
  upward gaze H51.8
  uremia, chronic —*see also* Disease, kidney,
    chronic N18.9
  urethral N34.3
  urethro-oculo-articular —*see* Reiter's disease
  urohepatic K76.7
  vago-hypoglossal G52.7
  van Buchem's M85.2
  van der Hoeve's Q78.0
  vascular NEC in cerebrovascular disease G46.8
  vasoconstriction, reversible cerebrovascular
    I67.841
  vasomotor I73.9
  vasospastic (traumatic) T75.22
  vasovagal R55
  VATER Q87.2
  velo-cardio-facial Q93.81
  vena cava (inferior) (superior) (obstruction)
    I87.1
  vertebral
    artery G45.0
      compression —*see* Syndrome, anterior,
        spinal artery, compression
      steal G45.0
  vertebro-basilar artery G45.0
  vertebrogenic (pain) (*see also* Pain,
    vertebrogenic) M54.89
  vertiginous —*see* Disorder, vestibular function
  Vinson-Plummer D50.1
  virus B34.9
  visceral larva migrans B83.0
  visual disorientation H53.8
  vitamin B6 deficiency E53.1
  vitreal corneal H59.01-●
  vitreous (touch) H59.01-●

Syndrome *(Continued)*
  Vogt-Koyanagi H20.82-●
  Volkmann's T79.6
  ▶von Hippel-Lindau Q85.83
  von Schroetter's I82.890
  ⇒von Willebrand (-Jürgen) —*see* Disease, von
    Willebrand
  ▶acquired (*see also* Disease, von Willebrand)
    D68.04
  Waldenström-Kjellberg D50.1
  Wallenberg's G46.3
  water retention E87.79
  Waterhouse (-Friderichsen) A39.1
  Weber-Gubler G46.3
  Weber-Leyden G46.3
  Weber's G46.3
  Wegener's M31.30
    with
      kidney involvement M31.31
      lung involvement M31.30
        with kidney involvement M31.31
  Weingarten's (tropical eosinophilia) J82.89
  Weiss-Baker G90.09
  Werdnig-Hoffman G12.0
  Werner's E31.21
  Werner's E34.8
  Wernicke-Korsakoff (nonalcoholic) F04
    alcoholic F10.26
  West's —*see* Epilepsy, spasms
  Westphal-Strümpell E83.01
  wet
    feet (maceration) (tropical) T69.0-●
    lung, newborn P22.1
  whiplash S13.4
  whistling face Q87.0
  Wilkie's K55.1
  Wilkinson-Sneddon L13.1
  ⇒Willebrand (-Jürgens) —*see* Disease, von
    Willebrand
  Williams Q93.82
  Wilson's (hepatolenticular degeneration)
    E83.01
  Wiskott-Aldrich D82.0
  withdrawal —*see* Withdrawal, state
    drug
      infant of dependent mother P96.1
      therapeutic use, newborn P96.2
  Woakes' (ethmoiditis) J33.1
  Wright's (hyperabduction) G54.0
  X I20.9
  XXXX Q97.1
  XXXXX Q97.1
  XXXXY Q98.1
  XXY Q98.0
  Yao M04.8
  yellow nail L60.5
  Zahorsky's B08.5
  Zellweger syndrome E71.510
  Zellweger-like syndrome E71.541
Synechia (anterior) (iris) (posterior) (pupil) —
  see also Adhesions, iris
  intra-uterine (traumatic) N85.6
Synesthesia R20.8
Syngamiasis, syngamosis B83.3
Synodontia K00.2
Synorchidism, synorchism Q55.1
Synostosis (congenital) Q78.8
  astragalo-scaphoid Q74.2
  radioulnar Q74.0
Synovial sarcoma —*see* Neoplasm, connective
  tissue, malignant
Synovioma (malignant) —*see also* Neoplasm,
  connective tissue, malignant
  benign —*see* Neoplasm, connective tissue,
    benign
Synoviosarcoma —*see* Neoplasm, connective
  tissue, malignant
Synovitis —*see also* Tenosynovitis M65.9
  crepitant
    hand M70.0-●
    wrist M70.03-●
  gonococcal A54.49
  gouty —*see* Gout

▶ New   ⇒ Revised   ~~deleted~~ Deleted   ● Use Additional Character(s)

Synovitis*(Continued)*
in (due to)
crystals M65.8-●
gonorrhea A54.49
syphilis (late) A52.78
use, overuse, pressure —*see* Disorder, soft tissue, due to use
infective NEC —*see* Tenosynovitis, infective NEC
specified NEC —*see* Tenosynovitis, specified type NEC
syphilitic A52.78
congenital (early) A50.02
toxic —*see* Synovitis, transient
transient M67.3-●
ankle M67.37-●
elbow M67.32-●
foot joint M67.37-●
hand joint M67.34-●
hip M67.35-●
knee M67.36-●
multiple site M67.39
pelvic region M67.35-●
shoulder M67.31-●
specified joint NEC M67.38
wrist M67.33-●
traumatic, current —*see* Sprain
tuberculous —*see* Tuberculosis, synovitis
villonodular (pigmented) M12.2-●
ankle M12.27-●
elbow M12.22-●
foot joint M12.27-●
hand joint M12.24-●
hip M12.25-●
knee M12.26-●
multiple site M12.29
pelvic region M12.25-●
shoulder M12.21-●
specified joint NEC M12.28
vertebrae M12.28
wrist M12.23-●
Syphilid A51.39
congenital A50.06
newborn A50.06
tubercular (late) A52.79
Syphilis, syphilitic (acquired) A53.9
abdomen (late) A52.79
acoustic nerve A52.15
adenopathy (secondary) A51.49
adrenal (gland) (with cortical hypofunction) A52.79
age under 2 years NOS —*see also* Syphilis, congenital, early
acquired A51.9
alopecia (secondary) A51.32
anemia (late) A52.79 [D63.8]
aneurysm (aorta) (ruptured) A52.01
central nervous system A52.05
congenital A50.54 [I79.0]
anus (late) A52.74
primary A51.1
secondary A51.39
aorta (arch) (abdominal) (thoracic) A52.02
aneurysm A52.01
aortic (insufficiency) (regurgitation) (stenosis)A52.03
aneurysm A52.01
arachnoid (adhesive) (cerebral) (spinal) A52.13
asymptomatic —*see* Syphilis, latent
ataxia (locomotor) A52.11
atrophoderma maculatum A51.39
auricular fibrillation A52.06
bladder (late) A52.76
bone A52.77
secondary A51.46
brain A52.17
breast (late) A52.79
bronchus (late) A52.72
bubo (primary) A51.0
bulbar palsy A52.19
bursa (late) A52.78
cardiac decompensation A52.06
cardiovascular A52.00

Syphilis, syphilitic (Continued)
central nervous system (late) (recurrent) (relapse) (tertiary) A52.3
with
ataxia A52.11
general paralysis A52.17
juvenile A50.45
paresis (general) A52.17
juvenile A50.45
tabes (dorsalis) A52.11
juvenile A50.45
taboparesis A52.17
juvenile A50.45
aneurysm A52.05
congenital A50.40
juvenile A50.40
remission in (sustained) A52.3
serology doubtful, negative, or positive A52.3
specified nature or site NEC A52.19
vascular A52.05
cerebral A52.17
meningovascular A52.13
nerves (multiple palsies) A52.15
sclerosis A52.17
thrombosis A52.05
cerebrospinal (tabetic type) A52.12
cerebrovascular A52.05
cervix (late) A52.76
chancre (multiple) A51.0
extragenital A51.2
Rollet's A51.0
Charcot's joint A52.16
chorioretinitis A51.43
congenital A50.01
late A52.71
prenatal A50.01
choroiditis —*see* Syphilitic chorioretinitis
choroidoretinitis —*see* Syphilitic chorioretinitis
ciliary body (secondary) A51.43
late A52.71
colon (late) A52.74
combined spinal sclerosis A52.11
condyloma (latum) A51.31
congenital A50.9
with
paresis (general) A50.45
tabes (dorsalis) A50.45
taboparesis A50.45
chorioretinitis, choroiditis A50.01 [H32]
early, or less than 2 years after birth NEC A50.2
with manifestations —*see* Syphilis, congenital, early, symptomatic
latent (without manifestations) A50.1
negative spinal fluid test A50.1
serology positive A50.1
symptomatic A50.09
cutaneous A50.06
mucocutaneous A50.07
oculopathy A50.01
osteochondropathy A50.02
pharyngitis A50.03
pneumonia A50.04
rhinitis A50.05
visceral A50.08
interstitial keratitis A50.31
juvenile neurosyphilis A50.45
late, or 2 years or more after birth NEC A50.7
chorioretinitis, choroiditis A50.32
interstitial keratitis A50.31
juvenile neurosyphilis A50.45
latent (without manifestations) A50.6
negative spinal fluid test A50.6
serology positive A50.6
symptomatic or with manifestations NEC A50.59
arthropathy A50.55
cardiovascular A50.54
Clutton's joints A50.51
Hutchinson's teeth A50.52
Hutchinson's triad A50.53
osteochondropathy A50.56
saddle nose A50.57

Syphilis, syphilitic (Continued)
conjugal A53.9
tabes A52.11
conjunctiva (late) A52.71
contact Z20.2
cord bladder A52.19
cornea, late A52.71
coronary (artery) (sclerosis) A52.06
coryza, congenital A50.05
cranial nerve A52.15
multiple palsies A52.15
cutaneous —*see* Syphilis, skin
dacryocystitis (late) A52.71
degeneration, spinal cord A52.12
dementia paralytica A52.17
juvenilis A50.45
destruction of bone A52.77
dilatation, aorta A52.01
due to blood transfusion A53.9
dura mater A52.13
ear A52.79
inner A52.79
nerve (eighth) A52.15
neurorecurrence A52.15
early A51.9
cardiovascular A52.00
central nervous system A52.3
latent (without manifestations) (less than 2 years after infection) A51.5
negative spinal fluid test A51.5
serological relapse after treatment A51.5
serology positive A51.5
relapse (treated, untreated) A51.9
skin A51.39
symptomatic A51.9
extragenital chancre A51.2
primary, except extragenital chancre A51.0
secondary —*see also* Syphilis, secondary A51.39
relapse (treated, untreated) A51.49
ulcer A51.39
eighth nerve (neuritis) A52.15
endemic A65
endocarditis A52.03
aortic A52.03
pulmonary A52.03
epididymis (late) A52.76
epiglottis (late) A52.73
epiphysitis (congenital) (early) A50.02
episcleritis (late) A52.71
esophagus A52.79
eustachian tube A52.73
exposure to Z20.2
eye A52.71
eyelid (late) (with gumma) A52.71
fallopian tube (late) A52.76
fracture A52.77
gallbladder (late) A52.74
gastric (polyposis) (late) A52.74
general A53.9
paralysis A52.17
juvenile A50.45
genital (primary) A51.0
glaucoma A52.71
gumma NEC A52.79
cardiovascular system A52.00
central nervous system A52.3
congenital A50.59
heart (block) (decompensation) (disease) (failure) A52.06 [I52]
valve NEC A52.03
hemianesthesia A52.19
hemianopia A52.71
hemiparesis A52.17
hemiplegia A52.17
hepatic artery A52.09
hepatis A52.74
hepatomegaly, congenital A50.08
hereditaria tarda —*see* Syphilis, congenital, late

S

Syphilis, syphilitic *(Continued)*
  hereditary —*see* Syphilis, congenital
  Hutchinson's teeth A50.52
  hyalitis A52.71
  inactive —*see* Syphilis, latent
  infantum —*see* Syphilis, congenital
  inherited —*see* Syphilis, congenital
  internal ear A52.79
  intestine (late) A52.74
  iris, iritis (secondary) A51.43
    late A52.71
  joint (late) A52.77
  keratitis (congenital) (interstitial) (late) A50.31
  kidney (late) A52.75
  lacrimal passages (late) A52.71
  larynx (late) A52.73
  late A52.9
    cardiovascular A52.00
    central nervous system A52.3
    kidney A52.75
    latent or 2 years or more after infection
        (without manifestations) A52.8
      negative spinal fluid test A52.8
      serology positive A52.8
    paresis A52.17
    specified site NEC A52.79
    symptomatic or with manifestations
        A52.79
    tabes A52.11
  latent A53.0
    with signs or symptoms - code by site and
        stage under Syphilis
    central nervous system A52.2
    date of infection unspecified A53.0
    early, or less than 2 years after infection
        A51.5
    follow-up of latent syphilis A53.0
      date of infection unspecified A53.0
      late, or 2 years or more after infection
          A52.8
    late, or 2 years or more after infection A52.8
    positive serology (only finding) A53.0
      date of infection unspecified A53.0
      early, or less than 2 years after infection
          A51.5
      late, or 2 years or more after infection
          A52.8
  lens (late) A52.71
  leukoderma A51.39
    late A52.79
  lienitis A52.79
  lip A51.39
    chancre (primary) A51.2
    late A52.79
  Lissauer's paralysis A52.17
  liver A52.74
  locomotor ataxia A52.11
  lung A52.72
  lymph gland (early) (secondary) A51.49
    late A52.79
  lymphadenitis (secondary) A51.49
  macular atrophy of skin A51.39
    striated A52.79
  mediastinum (late) A52.73
  meninges (adhesive) (brain) (spinal cord)
      A52.13
  meningitis A52.13
    acute (secondary) A51.41
    congenital A50.41
  meningoencephalitis A52.14
  meningovascular A52.13
    congenital A50.41
  mesarteritis A52.09
    brain A52.04
  middle ear A52.77
  mitral stenosis A52.03
  monoplegia A52.17
  mouth (secondary) A51.39
    late A52.79
  mucocutaneous (secondary) A51.39
    late A52.79

Syphilis, syphilitic *(Continued)*
  mucous
    membrane (secondary) A51.39
      late A52.79
    patches A51.39
      congenital A50.07
  mulberry molars A50.52
  muscle A52.78
  myocardium A52.06
  nasal sinus (late) A52.73
  neonatorum —*see* Syphilis, congenital
  nephrotic syndrome (secondary) A51.44
  nerve palsy (any cranial nerve) A52.15
    multiple A52.15
  nervous system, central A52.3
  neuritis A52.15
    acoustic A52.15
  neurorecidive of retina A52.19
  neuroretinitis A52.19
  newborn —*see* Syphilis, congenital
  nodular superficial (late) A52.79
  nonvenereal A65
  nose (late) A52.73
    saddle back deformity A50.57
  occlusive arterial disease A52.09
  oculopathy A52.71
  ophthalmic (late) A52.71
  optic nerve (atrophy) (neuritis) (papilla)
      A52.15
  orbit (late) A52.71
  organic A53.9
  osseous (late) A52.77
  osteochondritis (congenital) (early) A50.02
      [M90.80]
  osteoporosis A52.77
  ovary (late) A52.76
  oviduct (late) A52.76
  palate (late) A52.79
  pancreas (late) A52.74
  paralysis A52.17
    general A52.17
    juvenile A50.45
  paresis (general) A52.17
    juvenile A50.45
  paresthesia A52.19
  Parkinson's disease or syndrome A52.19
  paroxysmal tachycardia A52.06
  pemphigus (congenital) A50.06
  penis (chancre) A51.0
    late A52.76
  pericardium A52.06
  perichondritis, larynx (late) A52.73
  periosteum (late) A52.77
    congenital (early) A50.02 *[M90.80]*
    early (secondary) A51.46
  peripheral nerve A52.79
  petrous bone (late) A52.77
  pharynx (late) A52.73
    secondary A51.39
  pituitary (gland) A52.79
  pleura (late) A52.73
  pneumonia, white A50.04
  pontine lesion A52.17
  portal vein A52.09
  primary A51.0
    anal A51.1
    and secondary —*see* Syphilis, secondary
    central nervous system A52.3
    extragenital chancre NEC A51.2
    fingers A51.2
    genital A51.0
    lip A51.2
    specified site NEC A51.2
    tonsils A51.2
  prostate (late) A52.76
  ptosis (eyelid) A52.71
  pulmonary (late) A52.72
    artery A52.09
  pyelonephritis (late) A52.75
  recently acquired, symptomatic A51.9
  rectum (late) A52.74

Syphilis, syphilitic *(Continued)*
  respiratory tract (late) A52.73
  retina, late A52.71
  retrobulbar neuritis A52.15
  salpingitis A52.76
  sclera (late) A52.71
  sclerosis
    cerebral A52.17
    coronary A52.06
    multiple A52.11
  scotoma (central) A52.71
  scrotum (late) A52.76
  secondary (and primary) A51.49
    adenopathy A51.49
    anus A51.39
    bone A51.46
    chorioretinitis, choroiditis A51.43
    hepatitis A51.45
    liver A51.45
    lymphadenitis A51.49
    meningitis (acute) A51.41
    mouth A51.39
    mucous membranes A51.39
    periosteum, periostitis A51.46
    pharynx A51.39
    relapse (treated, untreated) A51.49
    skin A51.39
    specified form NEC A51.49
    tonsil A51.39
    ulcer A51.39
    viscera NEC A51.49
    vulva A51.39
  seminal vesicle (late) A52.76
  seronegative with signs or symptoms - code
      by site and stage under Syphilis
  seropositive
    with signs or symptoms - code by site and
        stage under Syphilis
    follow-up of latent syphilis —*see* Syphilis,
        latent
    only finding —*see* Syphilis, latent
  seventh nerve (paralysis) A52.15
  sinus, sinusitis (late) A52.73
  skeletal system A52.77
  skin (with ulceration) (early) (secondary)
      A51.39
    late or tertiary A52.79
  small intestine A52.74
  spastic spinal paralysis A52.17
  spermatic cord (late) A52.76
  spinal (cord) A52.12
  spleen A52.79
  splenomegaly A52.79
  spondylitis A52.77
  staphyloma A52.71
  stigmata (congenital) A50.59
  stomach A52.74
  synovium A52.78
  tabes dorsalis (late) A52.11
    juvenile A50.45
  tabetic type A52.11
    juvenile A50.45
  taboparesis A52.17
    juvenile A50.45
  tachycardia A52.06
  tendon (late) A52.78
  tertiary A52.9
    with symptoms NEC A52.79
    cardiovascular A52.00
    central nervous system A52.3
    multiple NEC A52.79
    specified site NEC A52.79
  testis A52.76
  thorax A52.73
  throat A52.73
  thymus (gland) (late) A52.79
  thyroid (late) A52.79
  tongue (late) A52.79
  tonsil (lingual) (late) A52.73
    primary A51.2
    secondary A51.39

▶ New   ⇒ Revised   ~~deleted~~ Deleted   • Use Additional Character(s)

Syphilis, syphilitic (Continued)
trachea (late) A52.73
tunica vaginalis (late) A52.76
ulcer (any site) (early) (secondary) A51.39
late A52.79
perforating A52.79
foot A52.11
urethra (late) A52.76
urogenital (late) A52.76
uterus (late) A52.76
uveal tract (secondary) A51.43
late A52.71
uveitis (secondary) A51.43
late A52.71
uvula (late) (perforated) A52.79
vagina A51.0
late A52.76
valvulitis NEC A52.03
vascular A52.00
brain (cerebral) A52.05

Syphilis, syphilitic (Continued)
ventriculi A52.74
vesicae urinariae (late) A52.76
viscera (abdominal) (late) A52.74
secondary A51.49
vitreous (opacities) (late) A52.71
hemorrhage A52.71
vulva A51.0
late A52.76
secondary A51.39
Syphiloma A52.79
cardiovascular system A52.00
central nervous system A52.3
circulatory system A52.00
congenital A50.59
Syphilophobia F45.29
Syringadenoma —see also Neoplasm, skin, benign
papillary —see Neoplasm, skin, benign
Syringobulbia G95.0

Syringocystadenoma —see Neoplasm, skin, benign
papillary —see Neoplasm, skin, benign
Syringoma —see also Neoplasm, skin, benign
chondroid —see Neoplasm, skin, benign
Syringomyelia G95.0
Syringomyelitis —see Encephalitis
Syringomyelocele —see Spina bifida
Syringopontia G95.0
System, systemic —see also condition
disease, combined —see Degeneration, combined
inflammatory response syndrome (SIRS) of non-infectious origin (without organ dysfunction) R65.10
with acute organ dysfunction R65.11
lupus erythematosus M32.9
inhibitor present D68.62
► Systemic exertion intolerance disease [SEID] G93.32

T

Tabacism, tabacosis, tabagism —see also
  Poisoning, tobacco
  meaning dependence (without remission)
    F17.200
    with
      disorder F17.299
        in remission F17.211
        specified disorder NEC F17.298
        withdrawal F17.203
Tabardillo A75.9
  flea-borne A75.2
  louse-borne A75.0
Tabes, tabetic A52.10
  with
    central nervous system syphilis A52.10
    Charcot's joint A52.16
    cord bladder A52.19
    crisis, viscera (any) A52.19
    paralysis, general A52.17
    paresis (general) A52.17
    perforating ulcer (foot) A52.19
  arthropathy (Charcot) A52.16
  bladder A52.19
  bone A52.11
  cerebrospinal A52.12
  congenital A50.45
  conjugal A52.10
  dorsalis A52.11
    juvenile A50.49
  juvenile A50.49
  latent A52.19
  mesenterica A18.39
  paralysis, insane, general A52.17
  spasmodic A52.17
  syphilis (cerebrospinal) A52.12
Taboparalysis A52.17
Taboparesis (remission) A52.17
  juvenile A50.45
TAC (trigeminal autonomic cephalgia) NEC
    G44.099
  intractable G44.091
  not intractable G44.099
Tache noir S60.22-●
Tachyalimentation K91.2
Tachyarrhythmia, tachyrhythmia —see
    Tachycardia
Tachycardia R00.0
  atrial (paroxysmal) I47.1
  auricular I47.1
  AV nodal re-entry (re-entrant) I47.1
  junctional (paroxysmal) I47.1
  newborn P29.11
  nodal (paroxysmal) I47.1
  non-paroxysmal AV nodal I45.89
  paroxysmal (sustained) (nonsustained) I47.9
    with sinus bradycardia I49.5
    atrial (PAT) I47.1
    atrioventricular (AV) (re-entrant) I47.1
      psychogenic F54
    junctional I47.1
      ectopic I47.1
    nodal I47.1
    psychogenic (atrial) (supraventricular)
      (ventricular) F54
    supraventricular (sustained) I47.1
      psychogenic F54
    ⮕ventricular I47.20
      psychogenic F54
      ▶specified type NEC I47.29
  psychogenic F45.8
  sick sinus I49.5
  sinoauricular NOS R00.0
    paroxysmal I47.1
  sinus [sinusal] NOS R00.0
    paroxysmal I47.1
  supraventricular I47.1
  ⮕ventricular (paroxysmal) (sustained) I47.20
    psychogenic F54
    ▶specified type NEC I47.29

Tachygastria K31.89
Tachypnea R06.82
  hysterical F45.8
  newborn (idiopathic) (transitory) P22.1
  psychogenic F45.8
  transitory, of newborn P22.1
TACO (transfusion associated circulatory
    overload) E87.71
▶TAD (transfusion-associated dyspnea) J95.87
Taenia (infection) (infestation) B68.9
  diminuta B71.0
  echinococcal infestation B67.90
  mediocanellata B68.1
  nana B71.0
  saginata B68.1
  solium (intestinal form) B68.0
    larval form —see Cysticercosis
Taeniasis (intestine) —see Taenia
Tag (hypertrophied skin) (infected) L91.8
  adenoid J35.8
  anus K64.4
  hemorrhoidal K64.4
  hymen N89.8
  perineal N90.89
  preauricular Q17.0
  sentinel K64.4
  skin L91.8
    accessory (congenital) Q82.8
    anus K64.4
    congenital Q82.8
    preauricular Q17.0
  tonsil J35.8
  urethra, urethral N36.8
  vulva N90.89
Tahyna fever B33.8
Takahara's disease E80.3
Takayasu's disease or syndrome M31.4
Talaromycosis B48.4
Talcosis (pulmonary) J62.0
Talipes (congenital) Q66.89
  acquired, planus —see Deformity, limb, flat foot
  asymmetric Q66.89
  calcaneovalgus Q66.4-●
  calcaneovarus Q66.1-●
  calcaneus Q66.89
  cavus Q66.7-●
  equinovalgus Q66.6
  equinovarus Q66.0-●
  equinus Q66.89
  percavus Q66.7-●
  planovalgus Q66.6
  planus (acquired) (any degree) —see also
      Deformity, limb, flat foot
    congenital Q66.5-●
    due to rickets (sequelae) E64.3
  valgus Q66.6
  varus Q66.3-●
Tall stature, constitutional E34.4
Talma's disease M62.89
Talon noir S90.3-●
  hand S60.22-●
  heel S90.3-●
  toe S90.1-●
Tamponade, heart I31.4
Tanapox (virus disease) B08.71
Tangier disease E78.6
Tantrum, child problem F91.8
Tapeworm (infection) (infestation) —see
    Infestation, tapeworm
Tapia's syndrome G52.7
TAR (thrombocytopenia with absent radius)
    syndrome Q87.2
Tarral-Besnier disease L44.0
Tarsal tunnel syndrome —see Syndrome, tarsal
    tunnel
Tarsalgia —see Pain, limb, lower
Tarsitis (eyelid) H01.8
  syphilitic A52.71
  tuberculous A18.4
Tartar (teeth) (dental calculus) K03.6
Tattoo (mark) L81.8
Tauri's disease E74.09

Taurodontism K00.2
Taussig-Bing syndrome Q20.1
Taybi's syndrome Q87.2
Tay-Sachs amaurotic familial idiocy or disease
    E75.02
TBI (traumatic brain injury) S06.9
Teacher's node or nodule J38.2
Tear, torn (traumatic) —see also Laceration
  with abortion —see Abortion
  annular fibrosis M51.35
  anus, anal (sphincter) S31.831
    complicating delivery
      with third degree perineal laceration —
          see also Delivery, complicated, by,
          laceration, perineum, third degree
          O70.20
        with mucosa O70.3
      without third degree perineal laceration
          O70.4
    nontraumatic (healed) (old) K62.81
  articular cartilage, old —see Derangement,
      joint, articular cartilage, by site
  bladder
    with ectopic or molar pregnancy O08.6
    following ectopic or molar pregnancy
        O08.6
    obstetrical O71.5
    traumatic —see Injury, bladder
  bowel
    with ectopic or molar pregnancy O08.6
    following ectopic or molar pregnancy
        O08.6
    obstetrical trauma O71.5
  broad ligament
    with ectopic or molar pregnancy O08.6
    following ectopic or molar pregnancy O08.6
    obstetrical trauma O71.6
  bucket handle (knee) (meniscus) —see Tear,
      meniscus
  capsule, joint —see Sprain
  cartilage —see also Sprain
    articular, old —see Derangement, joint,
        articular cartilage, by site
  cervix
    with ectopic or molar pregnancy O08.6
    following ectopic or molar pregnancy
        O08.6
    obstetrical trauma (current) O71.3
    old N88.1
    traumatic —see Injury, uterus
  dural G97.41
    nontraumatic G96.11
  internal organ —see Injury, by site
  knee cartilage
    articular (current) S83.3-●
    old —see Derangement, knee, meniscus,
        due to old tear
  ligament —see Sprain
  meniscus (knee) (current injury) S83.209
    bucket-handle S83.20-●
    lateral
      bucket-handle S83.25-●
      complex S83.27-●
      peripheral S83.26-●
      specified type NEC S83.28-●
    medial
      bucket-handle S83.21-●
      complex S83.23-●
      peripheral S83.22-●
      specified type NEC S83.24-●
    old —see Derangement, knee, meniscus,
        due to old tear
    site other than knee - code as Sprain
    specified type NEC S83.20-●
  muscle —see Strain
  pelvic
    floor, complicating delivery O70.1
    organ NEC, obstetrical trauma O71.5
      with ectopic or molar pregnancy O08.6
      following ectopic or molar pregnancy
          O08.6
  perineal, secondary O90.1

▶ New   ⮕ Revised   ~~deleted~~ Deleted   ● Use Additional Character(s)

Tear, torn *(Continued)*
  periurethral tissue, obstetrical trauma O71.82
    with ectopic or molar pregnancy O08.6
    following ectopic or molar pregnancy
      O08.6
  rectovaginal septum —*see* Laceration, vagina
  retina, retinal (without detachment)
    (horseshoe) —*see also* Break, retina,
    horseshoe
    with detachment —*see* Detachment, retina,
      with retinal, break
  rotator cuff (nontraumatic) M75.10-●
    complete M75.12-●
    incomplete M75.11-●
    traumatic S46.01-●
      capsule S43.42-●
  semilunar cartilage, knee —*see* Tear, meniscus
  supraspinatus (complete) (incomplete)
    (nontraumatic) —*see also* Tear, rotator
    cuff M75.10-●
  tendon —*see* Strain
  tentorial, at birth P10.4
  umbilical cord
    complicating delivery O69.89
  urethra
    with ectopic or molar pregnancy O08.6
    following ectopic or molar pregnancy
      O08.6
    obstetrical trauma O71.5
  uterus —*see* Injury, uterus
  vagina —*see* Laceration, vagina
  vessel, from catheter —*see* Puncture,
    accidental complicating surgery
  vulva, complicating delivery O70.0
Tear-stone —*see* Dacryolith
Teeth —*see also* condition
  grinding
    psychogenic F45.8
    sleep related G47.63
Teething (syndrome) K00.7
Telangiectasia, telangiectasis (verrucous) I78.1
  ataxic (cerebellar) (Louis-Bar) G11.3
  familial I78.0
  hemorrhagic, hereditary (congenital) (senile)
    I78.0
  hereditary, hemorrhagic (congenital) (senile)
    I78.0
  juxtafoveal H35.07-●
  macular H35.07-●
  macularis eruptiva perstans D47.01
  parafoveal H35.07-●
  retinal (idiopathic) (juxtafoveal) (macular)
    (parafoveal) H35.07-●
  spider I78.1
Telephone scatologia F65.89
Telescoped bowel or intestine K56.1
  congenital Q43.8
Temperature
  body, high (of unknown origin) R50.9
  cold, trauma from T69.9
    newborn P80.0
    specified effect NEC T69.8
Temple —*see* condition
Temporal —*see* condition
Temporomandibular joint pain-dysfunction
  syndrome M26.62-●
Temporosphenoidal —*see* condition
Tendency
  bleeding —*see* Defect, coagulation
  suicide
    meaning personal history of attempted
      suicide Z91.51
    meaning suicidal ideation —*see* Ideation,
      suicidal
  to fall R29.6
Tenderness, abdominal R10.819
  epigastric R10.816
  generalized R10.817
  left lower quadrant R10.814
  left upper quadrant R10.812
  periumbilic R10.815

Tenderness, abdominal *(Continued)*
  rebound R10.829
    epigastric R10.826
    generalized R10.827
    left lower quadrant R10.824
    left upper quadrant R10.822
    periumbilic R10.825
    right lower quadrant R10.823
    right upper quadrant R10.821
  right lower quadrant R10.813
  right upper quadrant R10.811
Tendinitis, tendonitis —*see also* Enthesopathy
  Achilles M76.6-●
  adhesive —*see* Tenosynovitis, specified type
    NEC
    shoulder —*see* Capsulitis, adhesive
  bicipital M75.2-●
  calcific M65.2-●
    ankle M65.27-●
    foot M65.27-●
    forearm M65.23-●
    hand M65.24-●
    lower leg M65.26-●
    multiple sites M65.29
    pelvic region M65.25-●
    shoulder M75.3-●
    specified site NEC M65.28
    thigh M65.25-●
    upper arm M65.22-●
  due to use, overuse, pressure —*see also*
    Disorder, soft tissue, due to use
    specified NEC —*see* Disorder, soft tissue,
      due to use, specified NEC
  gluteal M76.0-●
  patellar M76.5-●
  peroneal M76.7-●
  psoas M76.1-●
  tibial (posterior) M76.82-●
    anterior M76.81-●
  trochanteric —*see* Bursitis, hip, trochanteric
Tendon —*see* condition
Tendosynovitis —*see* Tenosynovitis
Tenesmus (rectal) R19.8
  vesical R30.1
Tennis elbow —*see* Epicondylitis, lateral
Tenonitis —*see also* Tenosynovitis
  eye (capsule) H05.04-●
Tenontosynovitis —*see* Tenosynovitis
Tenontothecitis —*see* Tenosynovitis
Tenophyte —*see* Disorder, synovium, specified
  type NEC
Tenosynovitis —*see also* Synovitis M65.9
  adhesive —*see* Tenosynovitis, specified type
    NEC
    shoulder —*see* Capsulitis, adhesive
  bicipital (calcifying) —*see* Tendinitis,
    bicipital
  gonococcal A54.49
  in (due to)
    crystals M65.8-●
    gonorrhea A54.49
    syphilis (late) A52.78
    use, overuse, pressure —*see also* Disorder,
      soft tissue, due to use
      specified NEC —*see* Disorder, soft tissue,
        due to use, specified NEC
  infective NEC M65.1-●
    ankle M65.17-●
    foot M65.17-●
    forearm M65.13-●
    hand M65.14-●
    lower leg M65.16-●
    multiple sites M65.19
    pelvic region M65.15-●
    shoulder region M65.11-●
    specified site NEC M65.18
    thigh M65.15-●
    upper arm M65.12-●
  radial styloid M65.4
  shoulder region M65.81-●
    adhesive —*see* Capsulitis, adhesive

Tenosynovitis *(Continued)*
  specified type NEC M65.88-●
    ankle M65.87-●
    foot M65.87-●
    forearm M65.83-●
    hand M65.84-●
    lower leg M65.86-●
    multiple sites M65.89
    pelvic region M65.85-●
    shoulder region M65.81-●
    specified site NEC M65.88
    thigh M65.85-●
    upper arm M65.82-●
  tuberculous —*see* Tuberculosis, tenosynovitis
Tenovaginitis —*see* Tenosynovitis
Tension
  arterial, high —*see also* Hypertension
    without diagnosis of hypertension R03.0
  headache G44.209
    intractable G44.201
    not intractable G44.209
  nervous R45.0
  pneumothorax J93.0
  premenstrual N94.3
  state (mental) F48.9
Tentorium —*see* condition
Teratencephalus Q89.8
Teratism Q89.7
Teratoblastoma (malignant) —*see* Neoplasm,
  malignant, by site
Teratocarcinoma —*see also* Neoplasm,
  malignant, by site
  liver C22.7
Teratoma (solid) —*see also* Neoplasm, uncertain
  behavior, by site
  with embryonal carcinoma, mixed —*see*
    Neoplasm, malignant, by site
  with malignant transformation —*see*
    Neoplasm, malignant, by site
  adult (cystic) —*see* Neoplasm, benign, by site
  benign —*see* Neoplasm, benign, by site
  combined with choriocarcinoma —*see*
    Neoplasm, malignant, by site
  cystic (adult) —*see* Neoplasm, benign, by site
  differentiated —*see* Neoplasm, benign, by site
  embryonal —*see also* Neoplasm, malignant,
    by site
    liver C22.7
  immature —*see* Neoplasm, malignant, by site
  liver C22.7
    adult, benign, cystic, differentiated type or
      mature D13.4
  malignant —*see also* Neoplasm, malignant,
    by site
    anaplastic —*see* Neoplasm, malignant, by
      site
    intermediate —*see* Neoplasm, malignant,
      by site
    specified site —*see* Neoplasm,
      malignant, by site
    unspecified site C62.90
    undifferentiated —*see* Neoplasm,
      malignant, by site
  mature —*see* Neoplasm, uncertain behavior,
    by site
    malignant —*see* Neoplasm, by site,
      malignant, by site
  ovary D27.-●
    embryonal, immature or malignant C56-●
  solid —*see* Neoplasm, uncertain behavior,
    by site
  testis C62.9-●
    adult, benign, cystic, differentiated type or
      mature D29.2-●
    scrotal C62.1-●
    undescended C62.0-●
Termination
  anomalous —*see also* Malposition, congenital
    right pulmonary vein Q26.3
  pregnancy, elective Z33.2
Ternidens diminutus infestation B81.8
Ternidensiasis B81.8

Terror(s) night (child) F51.4
Terrorism, victim of Z65.4
Terry's syndrome —see also Myopia,
    degenerative H44.2-●
Tertiary —see condition
Test, tests, testing (for)
    adequacy (for dialysis)
        hemodialysis Z49.31
        peritoneal Z49.32
    blood pressure Z01.30
        abnormal reading —see Blood, pressure
    blood typing Z01.83
        Rh typing Z01.83
    blood-alcohol Z02.83
        positive —see Findings, abnormal, in blood
    blood-drug Z02.83
        positive —see Findings, abnormal, in blood
    cardiac pulse generator (battery) Z45.010
    fertility Z31.41
    genetic
        disease carrier status for procreative
            management
                female Z31.430
                male Z31.440
        male partner of patient with recurrent
            pregnancy loss Z31.441
        procreative management NEC
            female Z31.438
            male Z31.448
    hearing Z01.10
        with abnormal findings NEC Z01.118
        infant or child (over 28 days old) Z00.129
            with abnormal findings Z00.121
    HIV (human immunodeficiency virus)
        nonconclusive (in infants) R75
        positive Z21
        seropositive Z21
    immunity status Z01.84
    intelligence NEC Z01.89
    laboratory (as part of a general medical
        examination) Z00.00
        with abnormal finding Z00.01
        for medicolegal reason NEC Z04.89
    male partner of patient with recurrent
        pregnancy loss Z31.441
    Mantoux (for tuberculosis) Z11.1
        abnormal result R76.11
    pregnancy, positive first pregnancy —see
        Pregnancy, normal, first
    procreative Z31.49
        fertility Z31.41
    skin, diagnostic
        allergy Z01.82
        special screening examination —see
            Screening, by name of disease
        Mantoux Z11.1
        tuberculin Z11.1
    specified NEC Z01.89
    tuberculin Z11.1
        abnormal result R76.11
    vision Z01.00
        with abnormal findings Z01.01
        following failed vision screening Z01.020
            with abnormal findings Z01.021
        infant or child (over 28 days old) Z00.129
            with abnormal findings Z00.121
    Wassermann Z11.3
        positive —see Serology for syphilis, positive
Testicle, testicular, testis —see also condition
    feminization syndrome —see also Syndrome,
        androgen insensitivity E34.51
    migrans Q55.29
Tetanus, tetanic (cephalic) (convulsions) A35
    with
        abortion A34
        ectopic or molar pregnancy O08.0
    following ectopic or molar pregnancy O08.0
    inoculation reaction (due to serum) —see
        Complications, vaccination
    neonatorum A33
    obstetrical A34
    puerperal, postpartum, childbirth A34

Tetany (due to) R29.0
    alkalosis E87.3
    associated with rickets E55.0
    convulsions R29.0
        hysterical F44.5
    functional (hysterical) F44.5
    hyperkinetic R29.0
        hysterical F44.5
    hyperpnea R06.4
        hysterical F44.5
        psychogenic F45.8
    hyperventilation —see also Hyperventilation
        R06.4
        hysterical F44.5
    neonatal (without calcium or magnesium
        deficiency) P71.3
    parathyroid (gland) E20.9
    parathyroprival E89.2
    post- (para)thyroidectomy E89.2
    postoperative E89.2
    pseudotetany R29.0
    psychogenic (conversion reaction) F44.5
Tetralogy of Fallot Q21.3
Tetraplegia (chronic) —see also Quadriplegia
    G82.50-●
Thailand hemorrhagic fever A91
Thalassanemia —see Thalassemia
Thalassemia (anemia) (disease) D56.9
    with other hemoglobinopathy D56.8
    alpha (major) (severe) (triple gene defect)
        D56.0
        minor D56.3
        silent carrier D56.3
        trait D56.3
    beta (severe) D56.1
        homozygous D56.1
        major D56.1
        minor D56.3
        trait D56.3
    delta-beta (homozygous) D56.2
        minor D56.3
        trait D56.3
    dominant D56.8
    hemoglobin
        C D56.8
        E-beta D56.5
    intermedia D56.1
    major D56.1
    minor D56.3
    mixed D56.8
    sickle-cell —see Disease, sickle-cell,
        thalassemia
    specified type NEC D56.8
    trait D56.3
    variants D56.8
Thanatophoric dwarfism or short stature Q77.1
Thaysen-Gee disease (nontropical sprue) K90.0
Thaysen's disease K90.0
Thecoma D27-●
    luteinized D27-●
    malignant C56-●
Thelarche, premature E30.8
Thelaziasis B83.8
Thelitis N61.0
    puerperal, postpartum or gestational —see
        Infection, nipple
Therapeutic —see condition
Therapy
    drug, long-term (current) (prophylactic)
        agents affecting estrogen receptors and
            estrogen levels NEC Z79.818
        anastrozole (Arimidex) Z79.811
        antibiotics Z79.2
            short-term use - omit code
        anticoagulants Z79.01
        anti-inflammatory Z79.1
        antiplatelet Z79.02
        antithrombotics Z79.02
        aromatase inhibitors Z79.811
        aspirin Z79.82
        birth control pill or patch Z79.3

Therapy (Continued)
    drug, long-term (Continued)
        bisphosphonates Z79.83
        contraceptive, oral Z79.3
        drug, specified NEC Z79.899
        estrogen receptor downregulators Z79.818
        Evista Z79.810
        exemestane (Aromasin) Z79.811
        Fareston Z79.810
        fulvestrant (Faslodex) Z79.818
        gonadotropin-releasing hormone (GnRH)
            agonist Z79.818
        goserelin acetate (Zoladex) Z79.818
        hormone replacement Z79.890
        insulin Z79.4
        letrozole (Femara) Z79.811
        leuprolide acetate (leuprorelin) (Lupron)
            Z79.818
        megestrol acetate (Megace) Z79.818
        methadone
            for pain management Z79.891
            maintenance therapy F11.20
        Nolvadex Z79.810
        opiate analgesic Z79.891
        oral contraceptive Z79.3
        raloxifene (Evista) Z79.810
        selective estrogen receptor modulators
            (SERMs) Z79.810
        short term - omit code
        steroids
            inhaled Z79.51
            systemic Z79.52
        tamoxifen (Nolvadex) Z79.810
        toremifene (Fareston) Z79.810
Thermic —see condition
Thermography (abnormal) —see also Abnormal,
    diagnostic imaging R93.89
    breast R92.8
Thermoplegia T67.01
Thesaurismosis, glycogen —see Disease,
    glycogen storage
Thiamin deficiency E51.9
    specified NEC E51.8
Thiaminic deficiency with beriberi E51.11
Thibierge-Weissenbach syndrome —see
    Sclerosis, systemic
Thickening
    bone —see Hypertrophy, bone
    breast N64.59
    endometrium R93.89
    epidermal L85.9
        specified NEC L85.8
    hymen N89.6
    larynx J38.7
    nail L60.2
        congenital Q84.5
    periosteal —see Hypertrophy, bone
    pleura J92.9
        with asbestos J92.0
    skin R23.4
    subepiglottic J38.7
    tongue K14.8
    valve, heart —see Endocarditis
Thigh —see condition
Thinning vertebra —see Spondylopathy,
    specified NEC
Thirst, excessive R63.1
    due to deprivation of water T73.1
Thomsen disease G71.12
Thoracic —see also condition
    kidney Q63.2
    outlet syndrome G54.0
Thoracogastroschisis (congenital) Q79.8
Thoracopagus Q89.4
Thorax —see condition
Thorn's syndrome N28.89
Thorson-Björck syndrome E34.0
Threadworm (infection) (infestation) B80
Threatened
    abortion O20.0
        with subsequent abortion O03.9
    job loss, anxiety concerning Z56.2

▶ New   ⟹ Revised   ~~deleted~~ Deleted   ● Use Additional Character(s)

Threatened *(Continued)*
labor (without delivery) O47.9
at or after 37 completed weeks of gestation O47.1
before 37 completed weeks of gestation O47.0-•
loss of job, anxiety concerning Z56.2
miscarriage O20.0
unemployment, anxiety concerning Z56.2
Three-day fever A93.1
Threshers' lung J67.0
Thrix annulata (congenital) Q84.1
Throat —*see* condition
Thrombasthenia (Glanzmann) (hemorrhagic) (hereditary) D69.1
Thromboangiitis I73.1
obliterans (general) I73.1
cerebral I67.89
vessels
brain I67.89
spinal cord I67.89
Thromboarteritis —*see* Arteritis
Thromboasthenia (Glanzmann) (hemorrhagic) (hereditary) D69.1
Thrombocytasthenia (Glanzmann) D69.1
Thrombocythemia (hemorrhagic) (see also Thrombocytosis) D75.839
essential D47.3
idiopathic D47.3
primary D47.3
Thrombocytopathy (dystrophic) (granulopenic) D69.1
Thrombocytopenia, thrombocytopenic D69.6
with absent radius (TAR) Q87.2
congenital D69.42
dilutional D69.59
due to
drugs D69.59
extracorporeal circulation of blood D69.59
(massive)blood transfusion D69.59
platelet alloimmunization D69.59
essential D69.3
▷heparin-associated D75.821
⮞heparin induced (HIT) D75.829
▷delayed-onset D75.828
▷immune-mediated D75.822
▷non-immune D75.821
▷persisting D75.828
▷syndrome
▷autoimmune D75.828
▷specified NEC D75.828
▷spontaneous (without heparin exposure) D75.84
▷type 1 D75.821
▷type 2 D75.822
hereditary D69.42
idiopathic D69.3
neonatal, transitory P61.0
due to
exchange transfusion P61.0
idiopathic maternal thrombocytopenia P61.0
isoimmunization P61.0
primary NEC D69.49
idiopathic D69.3
puerperal, postpartum O72.3
secondary D69.59
transient neonatal P61.0
▷vaccine-induced thrombotic D75.84
Thrombocytosis D75.839
essential D47.3
idiopathic D47.3
primary D47.3
reactive D75.838
secondary D75.838
specified NEC D75.838
Thromboembolism —*see* Embolism
Thrombopathy (Bernard-Soulier) D69.1
⮞constitutional —*see* Disease, von Willebrand
⮞Willebrand-Jurgens —*see* Disease, von Willebrand

Thrombopenia —*see* Thrombocytopenia
Thrombophilia D68.59
primary NEC D68.59
secondary NEC D68.69
specified NEC D68.69
Thrombophlebitis I80.9
antepartum O22.2-•
deep O22.3-•
superficial O22.2-•
calf muscular vein (NOS) I80.25-•
cavernous (venous) sinus G08
complicating pregnancy O22.5-•
nonpyogenic I67.6
cerebral (sinus) (vein) G08
nonpyogenic I67.6
sequelae G09
due to implanted device —*see* Complications, by site and type, specified NEC
during or resulting from a procedure NEC T81.72
femoral vein (superficial) I80.1-•
femoropopliteal vein I80.0-•
gastrocnemial vein I80.25-•
hepatic (vein) I80.8
idiopathic, recurrent I82.1
iliac vein (common) (external) (internal) I80.21-•
iliofemoral I80.1-•
intracranial venous sinus (any) G08
nonpyogenic I67.6
sequelae G09
intraspinal venous sinuses and veins G08
nonpyogenic G95.19
lateral (venous) sinus G08
nonpyogenic I67.6
leg I80.3
superficial I80.0-•
longitudinal (venous) sinus G08
nonpyogenic I67.6
lower extremity I80.299
migrans, migrating I82.1
pelvic
with ectopic or molar pregnancy O08.0
following ectopic or molar pregnancy O08.0
puerperal O87.1
peroneal vein I80.24-•
popliteal vein —*see* Phlebitis, leg, deep, popliteal
portal (vein) K75.1
postoperative T81.72
pregnancy —*see* Thrombophlebitis, antepartum
puerperal, postpartum, childbirth O87.0
deep O87.1
pelvic O87.1
septic O86.81
superficial O87.0
saphenous (greater) (lesser) I80.0-•
sinus (intracranial) G08
nonpyogenic I67.6
soleal vein I80.25-•
specified site NEC I80.8
tibial vein (anterior) (posterior) I80.23-•
Thrombosis, thrombotic (bland) (multiple) (progressive) (silent) (vessel) I82.90
anal K64.5
antepartum —*see* Thrombophlebitis, antepartum
aorta, aortic I74.10
abdominal I74.09
saddle I74.01
bifurcation I74.09
saddle I74.01
specified site NEC I74.19
terminal I74.09
thoracic I74.11
valve —*see* Endocarditis, aortic
apoplexy I63.3-•
artery, arteries (postinfectional) I74.9
auditory, internal —*see* Occlusion, artery, precerebral, specified NEC
basilar —*see* Occlusion, artery, basilar

Thrombosis, thrombotic *(Continued)*
artery, arteries *(Continued)*
carotid (common) (internal) —*see* Occlusion, artery, carotid
cerebellar (anterior inferior) (posterior inferior) (superior) —*see* Occlusion, artery, cerebellar
cerebral —*see* Occlusion, artery, cerebral
choroidal (anterior) —*see* Occlusion, artery, precerebral, specified NEC
communicating, posterior —*see* Occlusion, artery, precerebral, specified NEC
coronary —*see also* Infarct, myocardium
not resulting in infarction I24.0
hepatic I74.8
hypophyseal —*see* Occlusion, artery, precerebral, specified NEC
iliac I74.5
limb I74.4
lower I74.3
upper I74.2
meningeal, anterior or posterior —*see* Occlusion, artery, cerebral, specified NEC
mesenteric (with gangrene) —*see also* Infarct, intestine K55.069
ophthalmic —*see* Occlusion, artery, retina
pontine —*see* Occlusion, artery, precerebral, specified NEC
precerebral —*see* Occlusion, artery, precerebral
pulmonary (iatrogenic) —*see* Embolism, pulmonary
renal N28.0
retinal —*see* Occlusion, artery, retina
spinal, anterior or posterior G95.11
traumatic NEC T14.8
vertebral —*see* Occlusion, artery, vertebral
atrium, auricular —*see also* Infarct, myocardium
following acute myocardial infarction (current complication) I23.6
not resulting in infarction I51.3
old I51.3
basilar (artery) —*see* Occlusion, artery, basilar
brain (artery) (stem) —*see also* Occlusion, artery, cerebral
due to syphilis A52.05
puerperal O99.43
sinus —*see* Thrombosis, intracranial venous sinus
capillary I78.8
cardiac —*see also* Infarct, myocardium
not resulting in infarction I51.3
valve —*see* Endocarditis
old I51.3
carotid (artery) (common) (internal) —*see* Occlusion, artery, carotid
cavernous (venous) sinus —*see* Thrombosis, intracranial venous sinus
cerebellar artery (anterior inferior) (posterior inferior) (superior) I66.3
cerebral (artery) —*see* Occlusion, artery, cerebral
cerebrovenous sinus —*see also* Thrombosis, intracranial venous sinus
puerperium O87.3
chronic I82.91
coronary (artery) (vein) —*see also* Infarct, myocardium
not resulting in infarction I24.0
corpus cavernosum N48.89
cortical I66.9
deep —*see* Embolism, vein, lower extremity
due to device, implant or graft —*see also* Complications, by site and type, specified NEC T85.868
arterial graft NEC T82.868
breast (implant) T85.868
catheter NEC T85.868
dialysis (renal) T82.868
intraperitoneal T85.868
infusion NEC T82.868
spinal (epidural) (subdural) T85.860
urinary (indwelling) T83.86

Thrombosis, thrombotic *(Continued)*
  due to device, implant or graft *(Continued)*
    electronic (electrode) (pulse generator)
        (stimulator)
      bone T84.86
      cardiac T82.867
      nervous system (brain) (peripheral
          nerve) (spinal) T85.860
      urinary T83.86
    fixation, internal (orthopedic) NEC T84.86
    gastrointestinal (bile duct) (esophagus)
        T85.868
    genital NEC T83.86
    heart T82.867
    joint prosthesis T84.86
    ocular (corneal graft) (orbital implant)
        NEC T85.868
    orthopedic NEC T84.86
    specified NEC T85.868
    urinary NEC T83.86
    vascular NEC T82.868
    ventricular intracranial shunt T85.860
  during the puerperium —*see* Thrombosis,
      puerperal
  endocardial —*see also* Infarct, myocardium
    not resulting in infarction I51.3
  eye —*see* Occlusion, retina
  genital organ
    female NEC N94.89
      pregnancy —*see* Thrombophlebitis,
          antepartum
    male N50.1
  gestational —*see* Phlebopathy, gestational
  heart (chamber) —*see also* Infarct, myocardium
    not resulting in infarction I51.3
    old I51.3
  hepatic (vein) I82.0
    artery I74.8
  history (of) Z86.718
  intestine (with gangrene) —*see also* Infarct,
      intestine K55.069
  intracardiac NEC (apical) (atrial) (auricular)
      (ventricular) (old) I51.3
  intracranial (arterial) I66.9
    venous sinus (any) G08
      nonpyogenic origin I67.6
      puerperium O87.3
  intramural —*see also* Infarct, myocardium
    not resulting in infarction I51.3
    old I51.3
  intraspinal venous sinuses and veins G08
    nonpyogenic G95.19
  kidney (artery) N28.0
  lateral (venous) sinus —*see* Thrombosis,
      intracranial venous sinus
  leg —*see* Thrombosis, vein, lower extremity
    arterial I74.3
  liver (venous) I82.0
    artery I74.8
    portal vein I81
  longitudinal (venous) sinus —*see* Thrombosis,
      intracranial venous sinus
  lower limb —*see* Thrombosis, vein, lower
      extremity
  lung (iatrogenic) (postoperative) —*see*
      Embolism, pulmonary
  meninges (brain) (arterial) I66.8
  mesenteric (artery) (with gangrene) —*see also*
      Infarct, intestine K55.069
    vein (inferior) (superior) K55.0-●
  mitral I34.89
  mural —*see also* Infarct, myocardium
    due to syphilis A52.06
    not resulting in infarction I51.3
    old I51.3
  omentum (with gangrene) —*see also* Infarct,
      intestine K55.069
  ophthalmic —*see* Occlusion, retina
  pampiniform plexus (male) N50.1
  parietal —*see also* Infarct, myocardium
    not resulting in infarction I24.0

Thrombosis, thrombotic *(Continued)*
  penis, superficial vein N48.81
  perianal venous K64.5
  peripheral arteries I74.4
    upper I74.2
  personal history (of) Z86.718
  portal I81
    due to syphilis A52.09
  precerebral artery —*see* Occlusion, artery,
      precerebral
  puerperal, postpartum O87.0
    brain (artery) O99.43
      venous (sinus) O87.3
    cardiac O99.43
    cerebral (artery) O99.43
      venous (sinus) O87.3
    superficial O87.0
  pulmonary (artery) (iatrogenic)
      (postoperative) (vein) —*see* Embolism,
      pulmonary
  renal (artery) N28.0
    vein I82.3
  resulting from presence of device, implant or
      graft —*see* Complications, by site and
      type, specified NEC
  retina, retinal —*see* Occlusion, retina
  scrotum N50.1
  seminal vesicle N50.1
  sigmoid (venous) sinus —*see* Thrombosis,
      intracranial venous sinus
  sinus, intracranial (any) —*see* Thrombosis,
      intracranial venous sinus
  specified site NEC I82.890
    chronic I82.891
  spermatic cord N50.1
  spinal cord (arterial) G95.11
    due to syphilis A52.09
    pyogenic origin G06.1
  spleen, splenic D73.5
    artery I74.8
  testis N50.1
  traumatic NEC T14.8
  tricuspid I07.8
  tumor —*see* Neoplasm, by site
  tunica vaginalis N50.1
  umbilical cord (vessels), complicating
      delivery O69.5
  vas deferens N50.1
  vein (acute) I82.90
    antecubital I82.61-●
      chronic I82.71-●
    axillary I82.A1-●
      chronic I82.A2-●
    basilic I82.61-●
      chronic I82.71-●
    brachial I82.62-●
      chronic I82.72-●
    brachiocephalic (innominate) I82.290
      chronic I82.291
    cerebral, nonpyogenic I67.6
    cephalic I82.61-●
      chronic I82.71-●
    chronic I82.91
    deep (DVT) I82.40-●
      calf I82.4Z-●
        chronic I82.5Z-●
      lower leg I82.4Z-●
        chronic I82.5Z-●
      thigh I82.4Y-●
        chronic I82.5Y-●
      upper leg I82.4Y●
        chronic I82.5Y-●
    femoral I82.41-●
      chronic I82.51-●
    iliac (iliofemoral) I82.42-●
      chronic I82.52-●
    innominate I82.290
      chronic I82.291
    internal jugular I82.C1-●
      chronic I82.C2-●

Thrombosis, thrombotic *(Continued)*
  vein *(Continued)*
    lower extremity
      deep I82.40-●
        chronic I82.50-●
        specified NEC I82.49-●
          chronic NEC I82.59-●
      distal
        deep I82.4Z-●
      proximal
        deep I82.4Y-●
          chronic I82.5Y-●
      superficial I82.81-●
    perianal K64.5
    popliteal I82.43-●
      chronic I82.53-●
    radial I82.62-●
      chronic I82.72-●
    renal I82.3
    saphenous (greater) (lesser) I82.81-●
    specified NEC I82.890
      chronic NEC I82.891
    subclavian I82.B1-●
      chronic I82.B2-●
    thoracic NEC I82.290
      chronic I82.291
    tibial I82.44-●
      chronic I82.54-●
    ulnar I82.62-●
      chronic I82.72-●
    upper extremity I82.60-●
      chronic I82.70-●
      deep I82.62-●
        chronic I82.72-●
      superficial I82.61-●
        chronic I82.71-●
  vena cava
    inferior I82.220
      chronic I82.221
    superior I82.210
      chronic I82.211
  venous, perianal K64.5
  ventricle —*see also* Infarct, myocardium
    following acute myocardial infarction
        (current complication) I23.6
    not resulting in infarction I24.0
    old I51.3
Thrombus —*see* Thrombosis
Thrush —*see also* Candidiasis
  newborn P37.5
  oral B37.0
  vaginal (acute) B37.31
    chronic (recurrent) B37.32
Thumb —*see also* condition
  sucking (child problem) F98.8
Thymitis E32.8
Thymoma —*see* also Neoplasm, thymus,
    by type
  malignant C37
  metaplastic C37
  microscopic D15.0
  sclerosing C37
  type A C37
  type AB C37
  type B1 C37
  type B2 C37
  type B3 C37
Thymus, thymic (gland) —*see* condition
Thyrocele —*see* Goiter
Thyroglossal —*see also* condition
  cyst Q89.2
  duct, persistent Q89.2
Thyroid (gland) (body) —*see also* condition
  hormone resistance E07.89
  lingual Q89.2
  nodule (cystic) (nontoxic) (single) E04.1
Thyroiditis E06.9
  acute (nonsuppurative) (pyogenic)
      (suppurative) E06.0
  autoimmune E06.3

▶ New   ⇒ Revised   ~~deleted~~ Deleted   ● Use Additional Character(s)

Thyroiditis *(Continued)*
  chronic (nonspecific) (sclerosing) E06.5
    with thyrotoxicosis, transient E06.2
      fibrous E06.5
      lymphadenoid E06.3
      lymphocytic E06.3
      lymphoid E06.3
  de Quervain's E06.1
  drug-induced E06.4
  fibrous (chronic) E06.5
  giant-cell (follicular) E06.1
  granulomatous (de Quervain) (subacute) E06.1
  Hashimoto's (struma lymphomatosa) E06.3
  iatrogenic E06.4
  ligneous E06.5
  lymphocytic (chronic) E06.3
  lymphoid E06.3
  lymphomatous E06.3
  nonsuppurative E06.1
  postpartum, puerperal O90.5
  pseudotuberculous E06.1
  pyogenic E06.0
  radiation E06.4
  Riedel's E06.5
  subacute (granulomatous) E06.1
  suppurative E06.0
  tuberculous A18.81
  viral E06.1
  woody E06.5
Thyrolingual duct, persistent Q89.2
Thyromegaly E01.0
Thyrotoxic
  crisis —*see* Thyrotoxicosis
  heart disease or failure —*see also*
    Thyrotoxicosis E05.90 *[I43]*
    with thyroid storm E05.91 *[I43]*
  storm —*see* Thyrotoxicosis
Thyrotoxicosis (recurrent) E05.90
  with
    goiter (diffuse) E05.00
      with thyroid storm E05.01
      adenomatous uninodular E05.10
        with thyroid storm E05.11
      multinodular E05.20
        with thyroid storm E05.21
      nodular E05.20
        with thyroid storm E05.21
      uninodular E05.10
        with thyroid storm E05.11
    infiltrative
      dermopathy E05.00
        with thyroid storm E05.01
      ophthalmopathy E05.00
        with thyroid storm E05.01
    single thyroid nodule E05.10
      with thyroid storm E05.11
    thyroid storm E05.91
  due to
    ectopic thyroid nodule or tissue E05.30
      with thyroid storm E05.31
    ingestion of (excessive) thyroid material E05.40
      with thyroid storm E05.41
    overproduction of thyroid-stimulating hormone E05.80
      with thyroid storm E05.81
    specified cause NEC E05.80
      with thyroid storm E05.81
  factitia E05.40
    with thyroid storm E05.41
  heart —*see also* Failure, heart, high-output E05.90 *[I43]*
    with thyroid storm —*see also* Failure, heart, high-output E05.91 *[I43]*
    failure —*see also* Failure, heart, high-output E05.90 *[I43]*
  neonatal (transient) P72.1
  transient with chronic thyroiditis E06.2
Tibia vara M92.51-●
Tic (disorder) F95.9
  breathing F95.8
  child problem F95.0

Tic *(Continued)*
  compulsive F95.1
  de la Tourette F95.2
  degenerative (generalized) (localized) G25.69
    facial G25.69
  disorder
    chronic
      motor F95.1
      vocal F95.1
    combined vocal and multiple motor F95.2
    transient F95.0
  douloureux G50.0
    atypical G50.1
    postherpetic, postzoster B02.22
  drug-induced G25.61
  eyelid F95.8
  habit F95.9
    chronic F95.1
    transient of childhood F95.0
  lid, transient of childhood F95.0
  motor-verbal F95.2
  occupational F48.8
  orbicularis F95.8
    transient of childhood F95.0
  organic origin G25.69
  postchoreic G25.69
  provisional F95.0
  psychogenic, compulsive F95.1
  salaam R25.8
  spasm (motor or vocal) F95.9
    chronic F95.1
    transient of childhood F95.0
  specified NEC F95.8
Tick-borne —*see* condition
Tietze's disease or syndrome M94.0
Tight, tightness
  anus K62.89
  chest R07.89
  fascia (lata) M62.89
  foreskin (congenital) N47.1
  hymen, hymenal ring N89.6
  introitus (acquired) (congenital) N89.6
  rectal sphincter K62.89
  tendon —*see* Short, tendon
  urethral sphincter N35.919
Tilting vertebra —*see* Dorsopathy, deforming, specified NEC
Timidity, child F93.8
Tin-miner's lung J63.5
Tinea (intersecta) (tarsi) B35.9
  amiantacea L44.8
  asbestina B35.0
  barbae B35.0
  beard B35.0
  black dot B35.0
  blanca B36.2
  capitis B35.0
  corporis B35.4
  cruris B35.6
  flava B36.0
  foot B35.3
  furfuracea B36.0
  imbricata (Tokelau) B35.5
  kerion B35.0
  manuum B35.2
  microsporic —*see* Dermatophytosis
  nigra B36.1
  nodosa —*see* Piedra
  pedis B35.3
  scalp B35.0
  specified NEC B35.8
  sycosis B35.0
  tonsurans B35.0
  trichophytic —*see* Dermatophytosis
  unguium B35.1
  versicolor B36.0
Tingling sensation (skin) R20.2
Tinnitus NOS H93.1-●
  audible H93.1-●
  aurium H93.1-●
  pulsatile H93.A-●
  subjective H93.1-●

Tipped tooth (teeth) M26.33
Tipping
  pelvis M95.5
    with disproportion (fetopelvic) O33.0
      causing obstructed labor O65.0
  tooth (teeth), fully erupted M26.33
Tiredness R53.83
Tissue —*see* condition
Tobacco (nicotine)
  abuse —*see* Tobacco, use
  dependence —*see* Dependence, drug, nicotine
  harmful use Z72.0
  heart —*see* Tobacco, toxic effect
  maternal use, affecting newborn P04.2
  toxic effect —*see* Table of Drugs and Chemicals, by substance, poisoning
    chewing tobacco —*see* Table of Drugs and Chemicals, by substance, poisoning
    cigarettes —*see* Table of Drugs and Chemicals, by substance, poisoning
  use Z72.0
    complicating
      childbirth O99.334
      pregnancy O99.33-●
      puerperium O99.335
    counseling and surveillance Z71.6
    history Z87.891
  withdrawal state —*see also* Dependence, drug, nicotine F17.203
Tocopherol deficiency E56.0
Todd's
  cirrhosis K74.3
  paralysis (postepileptic) (transitory) G83.84
Toe —*see* condition
Toilet, artificial opening —*see* Attention to, artificial, opening
Tokelau (ringworm) B35.5
Tollwut —*see* Rabies
Tommaselli's disease R31.9
  correct substance properly administered —*see* Table of Drugs and Chemicals, by drug, adverse effect
  overdose or wrong substance given or taken —*see* Table of Drugs and Chemicals, by drug, poisoning
Tongue —*see also* condition
  tie Q38.1
Tonic pupil —*see* Anomaly, pupil, function, tonic pupil
Toni-Fanconi syndrome (cystinosis) E72.09
  with cystinosis E72.04
Tonsil —*see* condition
Tonsillitis (acute) (catarrhal) (croupous) (follicular) (gangrenous) (infective) (lacunar) (lingual) (malignant) (membranous) (parenchymatous) (phlegmonous) (pseudomembranous) (purulent) (septic) (subacute) (suppurative) (toxic) (ulcerative) (vesicular) (viral) J03.90
  chronic J35.01
    with adenoiditis J35.03
  diphtheritic A36.0
  hypertrophic J35.01
    with adenoiditis J35.03
  recurrent J03.91
  specified organism NEC J03.80
    recurrent J03.81
  staphylococcal J03.80
    recurrent J03.81
  streptococcal J03.00
    recurrent J03.01
  tuberculous A15.8
  Vincent's A69.1
Tooth, teeth —*see* condition
Toothache K08.89
Topagnosis R20.8
Tophi —*see* Gout, chronic
TORCH infection —*see* Infection, congenital
  without active infection P00.2
Torn —*see* Tear
Tornwaldt's cyst or disease J39.2

Torsades de pointes I47.21
Torsion
    accessory tube —see Torsion, fallopian tube
    adnexa (female) —see Torsion, fallopian tube
    aorta, acquired I77.1
    appendix epididymis N44.04
    appendix testis N44.03
    bile duct (common) (hepatic) K83.8
        congenital Q44.5
    bowel, colon or intestine K56.2
    cervix —see Malposition, uterus
    cystic duct K82.8
    dystonia —see Dystonia, torsion
    epididymis (appendix) N44.04
    fallopian tube N83.52-●
        with ovary N83.53
    gallbladder K82.8
        congenital Q44.1
    hydatid of Morgagni
        female N83.52-●
        male N44.03
    kidney (pedicle) (leading to infarction) N28.0
    Meckel's diverticulum (congenital) Q43.0
        malignant —see Table of Neoplasms, small
            intestine, malignant
    mesentery K56.2
    omentum K56.2
    organ or site, congenital NEC —see Anomaly,
        by site
    ovary (pedicle) N83.51-●
        with fallopian tube N83.53
        congenital Q50.2
    oviduct —see Torsion, fallopian tube
    penis (acquired) N48.82
        congenital Q55.63
    spasm —see Dystonia, torsion
    spermatic cord N44.02
        extravaginal N44.01
        intravaginal N44.02
    spleen D73.5
    testis, testicle N44.00
        appendix N44.03
    tibia —see Deformity, limb, specified type
        NEC, lower leg
    uterus —see Malposition, uterus
Torticollis (intermittent) (spastic) M43.6
    congenital (sternomastoid) Q68.0
    due to birth injury P15.8
    hysterical F44.4
    ocular R29.891
    psychogenic F45.8
        conversion reaction F44.4
    rheumatic M43.6
    rheumatoid M06.88
    spasmodic G24.3
    traumatic, current S13.4
Tortipelvis G24.1
Tortuous
    aortic arch Q25.46
    artery I77.1
    organ or site, congenital NEC —see Distortion
    retinal vessel, congenital Q14.1
    ureter N13.8
    urethra N36.8
    vein —see Varix
Torture, victim of Z65.4
Torula, torular (histolytica) (infection) —see
    Cryptococcosis
Torulosis —see Cryptococcosis
Torus (mandibularis) (palatinus) M27.0
    fracture —see Fracture, by site, torus
Touraine's syndrome Q79.8
Tourette's syndrome F95.2
Tourniquet syndrome —see Constriction,
    external, by site
Tower skull Q75.0
    with exophthalmos Q87.0
Toxemia R68.89
    bacterial —see Sepsis
    burn —see Burn
    eclamptic (with pre-existing hypertension) —
        see Eclampsia

Toxemia (Continued)
    erysipelatous —see Erysipelas
    fatigue R68.89
    food —see Poisoning, food
    gastrointestinal K52.1
    intestinal K52.1
    kidney —see Uremia
    malarial —see Malaria
    myocardial —see Myocarditis, toxic
    of pregnancy —see Pre-eclampsia
    pre-eclamptic —see Pre-eclampsia
    small intestine K52.1
    staphylococcal, due to food A05.0
    stasis R68.89
    uremic —see Uremia
    urinary —see Uremia
Toxemica cerebropathia psychica
        (nonalcoholic) F04
    alcoholic —see Alcohol, amnestic disorder
Toxic (poisoning) —see also condition T65.91
    effect —see Table of Drugs and Chemicals, by
        substance, poisoning
    shock syndrome A48.3
    thyroid (gland) —see Thyrotoxicosis
Toxicemia —see Toxemia
Toxicity —see Table of Drugs and Chemicals, by
        substance, poisoning
    fava bean D55.0
    food, noxious —see Poisoning, food
    from drug or nonmedicinal substance —see
        Table of Drugs and Chemicals, by drug
Toxicosis —see also Toxemia
    capillary, hemorrhagic D69.0
Toxinfection, gastrointestinal K52.1
Toxocariasis B83.0
Toxoplasma, toxoplasmosis (acquired) B58.9
    with
        hepatitis B58.1
        meningoencephalitis B58.2
        ocular involvement B58.00
        other organ involvement B58.89
        pneumonia, pneumonitis B58.3
    congenital (acute) (subacute) (chronic) P37.1
    maternal, manifest toxoplasmosis in infant
        (acute) (subacute) (chronic) P37.1
tPA (rtPA) administation in a different facility
    within the last 24 hours prior to admission
    to current facility Z92.82
Trabeculation, bladder N32.89
Trachea —see condition
Tracheitis (catarrhal) (infantile) (membranous)
        (plastic) (septal) (suppurative) (viral) J04.10
    with
        bronchitis (15 years of age and above) J40
            acute or subacute —see Bronchitis,
                acute
            chronic J42
            tuberculous NEC A15.5
            under 15 years of age J20.9
        laryngitis (acute) J04.2
            chronic J37.1
            tuberculous NEC A15.5
    acute J04.10
        with obstruction J04.11
    chronic J42
        with
            bronchitis (chronic) J42
            laryngitis (chronic) J37.1
    diphtheritic (membranous) A36.89
    due to external agent —see Inflammation,
        respiratory, upper, due to
    syphilitic A52.73
    tuberculous A15.5
Trachelitis (nonvenereal) —see Cervicitis
Tracheobronchial —see condition
Tracheobronchitis (15 years of age and
        above) —see also Bronchitis
    due to
        Bordetella bronchiseptica A37.80
            with pneumonia A37.81
        Francisella tularensis A21.8

Tracheobronchomegaly Q32.4
    with bronchiectasis J47.9
        with
            exacerbation (acute) J47.1
            lower respiratory infection J47.0
    acquired J98.09
        with bronchiectasis J47.9
            with
                exacerbation (acute) J47.1
                lower respiratory infection J47.0
Tracheobronchopneumonitis —see Pneumonia,
    broncho-●
Tracheocele (external) (internal) J39.8
    congenital Q32.1
Tracheomalacia J39.8
    congenital Q32.0
Tracheopharyngitis (acute) J06.9
    chronic J42
    due to external agent —see Inflammation,
        respiratory, upper, due to
Tracheostenosis J39.8
Tracheostomy
    complication —see Complication,
        tracheostomy
    status Z93.0
        attention to Z43.0
        malfunctioning J95.03
Trachoma, trachomatous A71.9
    active (stage) A71.1
    contraction of conjunctiva A71.1
    dubium A71.0
    healed or sequelae B94.0
    initial (stage) A71.0
    pannus A71.1
    Türck's J37.0
Traction, vitreomacular H43.82-●
Train sickness T75.3
Trait(s)
    Hb-S D57.3
    hemoglobin
        abnormal NEC D58.2
            with thalassemia D56.3
        C —see Disease, hemoglobin C
        S (Hb-S) D57.3
    Lepore D56.3
    personality, accentuated Z73.1
    sickle-cell D57.3
        with elliptocytosis or spherocytosis
            D57.3
    type A personality Z73.1
Tramp Z59.00
Trance R41.89
    hysterical F44.89
Transaminasemia R74.01
Transection
    abdomen (partial) S38.3
    aorta (incomplete) —see also Injury, aorta
        complete —see Injury, aorta, laceration,
            major
    carotid artery (incomplete) —see also Injury,
        blood vessel, carotid, laceration
        complete —see Injury, blood vessel, carotid,
            laceration, major
    celiac artery (incomplete) S35.211
        branch (incomplete) S35.291
            complete S35.292
        complete S35.212
    innominate
        artery (incomplete) —see also Injury, blood
            vessel, thoracic, innominate, artery,
            laceration
            complete —see Injury, blood vessel,
                thoracic, innominate, artery,
                laceration, major
        vein (incomplete) —see also Injury, blood
            vessel, thoracic, innominate, vein,
            laceration
            complete —see Injury, blood vessel,
                thoracic, innominate, vein,
                laceration, major

▶ New   ⇒ Revised   ~~deleted~~ Deleted   ● Use Additional Character(s)

Transection (Continued)
  jugular vein (external) (incomplete) —see
      also Injury, blood vessel, jugular vein,
      laceration
    complete —see Injury, blood vessel, jugular
        vein, laceration, major
    internal (incomplete) —see also Injury,
        blood vessel, jugular vein, internal,
        laceration
      complete —see Injury, blood vessel,
          jugular vein, internal, laceration,
          major
  mesenteric artery (incomplete) —see also
      Injury, mesenteric, artery, laceration
    complete —see Injury, mesenteric artery,
        laceration, major
  pulmonary vessel (incomplete) —see also
      Injury, blood vessel, thoracic, pulmonary,
      laceration
    complete —see Injury, blood vessel,
        thoracic, pulmonary, laceration, major
  subclavian —see Transection, innominate
  vena cava (incomplete) —see also Injury, vena
      cava
    complete —see Injury, vena cava,
        laceration, major
  vertebral artery (incomplete) —see also Injury,
      blood vessel, vertebral, laceration
    complete —see Injury, blood vessel,
        vertebral, laceration, major
Transfusion
  associated (red blood cell) hemochromatosis
      E83.111
  blood
    ABO incompatible —see Complication(s),
        transfusion, incompatibility reaction,
        ABO
    minor blood group (Duffy) (E) (K) (Kell)
        (Kidd) (Lewis) (M) (N) (P) (S) T80.89
    reaction or complication —see
        Complications, transfusion
  fetomaternal (mother) —see Pregnancy,
      complicated by, placenta, transfusion
      syndrome
  maternofetal (mother) —see Pregnancy,
      complicated by, placenta, transfusion
      syndrome
  placental (syndrome) (mother) —see
      Pregnancy, complicated by, placenta,
      transfusion syndrome
  reaction (adverse) —see Complications,
      transfusion
  related acute lung injury (TRALI) J95.84
  twin-to-twin —see Pregnancy, complicated
      by, placenta, transfusion syndrome, fetus
      to fetus
Transient (meaning homeless) —see also
    condition Z59.00
Translocation
  balanced autosomal Q95.9
    in normal individual Q95.0
  chromosomes NEC Q99.8
    balanced and insertion in normal
        individual Q95.0
  Down's syndrome Q90.2
  trisomy
    13 Q91.6
    18 Q91.2
    21 Q90.2
Translucency, iris —see Degeneration, iris
Transmission of chemical substances through
    the placenta —see Absorption, chemical,
    through placenta
Transparency, lung, unilateral J43.0
Transplant (ed) (status) Z94.9
  awaiting organ Z76.82
  bone Z94.6
    marrow Z94.81
  candidate Z76.82
  complication —see Complication, transplant
  cornea Z94.7

Transplant (Continued)
  heart Z94.1
    and lung(s) Z94.3
    valve Z95.2
      prosthetic Z95.2
      specified NEC Z95.4
      xenogenic Z95.3
  intestine Z94.82
  kidney Z94.0
  liver Z94.4
  lung(s) Z94.2
    and heart Z94.3
  organ (failure) (infection) (rejection)Z94.9
    removal status Z98.85
  pancreas Z94.83
  skin Z94.5
  social Z60.3
  specified organ or tissue NEC Z94.89
  stem cells Z94.84
  tissue Z94.9
➡ Transplants, ovarian, endometrial N80.10-●
Transposed —see Transposition
Transposition (congenital) —see also
      Malposition, congenital
  abdominal viscera Q89.3
  aorta (dextra) Q20.3
  appendix Q43.8
  colon Q43.8
  corrected Q20.5
  great vessels (complete) (partial) Q20.3
  heart Q24.0
    with complete transposition of viscera Q89.3
  intestine (large) (small) Q43.8
  reversed jejunal (for bypass) (status) Z98.0
  scrotum Q55.23
  stomach Q40.2
    with general transposition of viscera Q89.3
  tooth, teeth, fully erupted M26.30
  vessels, great (complete) (partial) Q20.3
  viscera (abdominal) (thoracic) Q89.3
Transsexualism F64.0
Transverse —see also condition
  arrest (deep), in labor O64.0
  lie (mother) O32.2
    causing obstructed labor O64.8
Transvestism, transvestitism (dual-role) F64.1
  fetishistic F65.1
Trapped placenta (with hemorrhage) O72.0
  without hemorrhage O73.0
TRAPS (tumor necrosis factor receptor
    associated periodic syndrome) M04.1
Trauma, traumatism —see also Injury
  acoustic —see subcategory H83.3
  birth —see Birth, injury
  complicating ectopic or molar pregnancy
      O08.6
  during delivery O71.9
  following ectopic or molar pregnancy O08.6
  obstetric O71.9
    specified NEC O71.89
  occlusal
    primary K08.81
    secondary K08.82
Traumatic —see also condition
  brain injury S06.9
Treacher Collins syndrome Q75.4
Treitz's hernia —see Hernia, abdomen, specified
    site NEC
Trematode infestation —see Infestation, fluke
Trematodiasis —see Infestation, fluke
Trembling paralysis —see Parkinsonism
Tremor(s) R25.1
  drug induced G25.1
  essential (benign) G25.0
  familial G25.0
  hereditary G25.0
  hysterical F44.4
  intention G25.2
  medication induced postural G25.1
  mercurial —see subcategory T56.1
  Parkinson's —see Parkinsonism

Tremor (Continued)
  psychogenic (conversion reaction) F44.4
  senilis R54
  specified type NEC G25.2
Trench
  fever A79.0
  foot —see Immersion, foot
  mouth A69.1
Treponema pallidum infection —see Syphilis
Treponematosis
  due to
    T. pallidum —see Syphilis
    T. pertenue —see Yaws
Triad
  Hutchinson's (congenital syphilis) A50.53
  Kartagener's Q89.3
  Saint's —see Hernia, diaphragm
Trichiasis (eyelid) H02.059
  with entropion —see Entropion
  left H02.056
    lower H02.055
    upper H02.054
  right H02.053
    lower H02.052
    upper H02.051
Trichinella spiralis (infection) (infestation) B75
Trichinellosis, trichiniasis, trichinelliasis,
    trichinosis B75
  with muscle disorder B75 [M63.80]
    ankle B75 [M63.87-●]
    foot B75 [M63.87-●]
    forearm B75 [M63.83-●]
    hand B75 [M63.84-●]
    lower leg B75 [M63.86-●]
    multiple sites B75 [M63.89]
    pelvic region B75 [M63.85-●]
    shoulder region B75 [M63.81-●]
    specified site NEC B75 [M63.88]
    thigh B75 [M63.85-●]
    upper arm B75 [M63.82-●]
Trichobezoar T18.9
  intestine T18.3
  stomach T18.2
Trichocephaliasis, trichocephalosis B79
Trichocephalus infestation B79
Trichoclasis L67.8
Trichoepithelioma —see also Neoplasm, skin,
    benign
  malignant —see Neoplasm, skin, malignant
Trichofolliculoma —see Neoplasm, skin, benign
Tricholemmoma —see Neoplasm, skin, benign
Trichomoniasis A59.9
  bladder A59.03
  cervix A59.09
  intestinal A07.8
  prostate A59.02
  seminal vesicles A59.09
  specified site NEC A59.8
  urethra A59.03
  urogenitalis A59.00
  vagina A59.01
  vulva A59.01
Trichomycosis
  axillaris A48.8
  nodosa, nodularis B36.8
Trichonodosis L67.8
Trichophytid, trichophyton infection —see
    Dermatophytosis
Trichophytobezoar T18.9
  intestine T18.3
  stomach T18.2
Trichophytosis —see Dermatophytosis
Trichoptilosis L67.8
Trichorrhexis (nodosa) (invaginata) L67.0
Trichosis axillaris A48.8
Trichosporosis nodosa B36.2
Trichostasis spinulosa (congenital) Q84.1
Trichostrongyliasis, trichostrongylosis (small
    intestine) B81.2
Trichostrongylus infection B81.2
Trichotillomania F63.3

Trichromat, trichromatopsia, anomalous
 (congenital) H53.55
Trichuriasis B79
Trichuris trichiura (infection) (infestation) (any
 site) B79
Tricuspid (valve) —see condition
Trifid —see also Accessory
 kidney (pelvis) Q63.8
 tongue Q38.3
Trigeminal neuralgia —see Neuralgia,
 trigeminal
Trigeminy R00.8
Trigger finger (acquired) M65.30
 congenital Q74.0
 index finger M65.32-●
 little finger M65.35-●
 middle finger M65.33-●
 ring finger M65.34-●
 thumb M65.31-●
Trigonitis (bladder) (chronic)
 (pseudomembranous) N30.30
 with hematuria N30.31
Trigonocephaly Q75.0
Trilocular heart —see Cor triloculare
Trimethylaminuria E72.52
Tripartite placenta O43.19-●
Triphalangeal thumb Q74.0
Triple —see also Accessory
 kidneys Q63.0
 uteri Q51.818
 X, female Q97.0
Triple I O41.12-●
Triplegia G83.89
 congenital G80.8
Triplet (newborn) —see also Newborn, triplet
 complicating pregnancy —see Pregnancy, triplet
Triplication —see Accessory
Triploidy Q92.7
Trismus R25.2
 neonatorum A33
 newborn A33
Trisomy (syndrome) Q92.9
 13 (partial) Q91.7
  meiotic nondisjunction Q91.4
  mitotic nondisjunction Q91.5
  mosaicism Q91.5
  translocation Q91.6
 18 (partial) Q91.3
  meiotic nondisjunction Q91.0
  mitotic nondisjunction Q91.1
  mosaicism Q91.1
  translocation Q91.2
 20 Q92.8
 21 (partial) Q90.9
  meiotic nondisjunction Q90.0
  mitotic nondisjunction Q90.1
  mosaicism Q90.1
  translocation Q90.2
 22 Q92.8
 autosomes Q92.9
 chromosome specified NEC Q92.8
  partial Q92.2
   due to unbalanced translocation Q92.5
  specified NEC Q92.8
  whole (nonsex chromosome)
   meiotic nondisjunction Q92.0
   mitotic nondisjunction Q92.1
   mosaicism Q92.1
 due to
  dicentrics —see Extra, marker chromosomes
  extra rings —see Extra, marker
   chromosomes
  isochromosomes —see Extra, marker
   chromosomes
 specified NEC Q92.8
 whole chromosome Q92.9
  meiotic nondisjunction Q92.0
  mitotic nondisjunction Q92.1
  mosaicism Q92.1
  partial Q92.9
  specified NEC Q92.8

Tritanomaly, tritanopia H53.55
Trombiculosis, trombiculiasis, trombidiosis
 B88.0
Trophedema (congenital) (hereditary) Q82.0
Trophoblastic disease —see also Mole,
 hydatidiform O01.9
Tropholymphedema Q82.0
Trophoneurosis NEC G96.89
 disseminated M34.9
Tropical —see condition
Trouble —see also Disease
 heart —see Disease, heart
 kidney —see Disease, renal
 nervous R45.0
 sinus —see Sinusitis
Trousseau's syndrome (thrombophlebitis
 migrans) I82.1
Truancy, childhood
 from school Z72.810
Truncus
 arteriosus (persistent) Q20.0
 communis Q20.0
Trunk —see condition
Trypanosomiasis
 African B56.9
  by Trypanosoma brucei
   gambiense B56.0
   rhodesiense B56.1
 American —see Chagas' disease
 Brazilian —see Chagas' disease
 by Trypanosoma
  brucei gambiense B56.0
  brucei rhodesiense B56.1
  cruzi —see Chagas' disease
 gambiensis, Gambian B56.0
 rhodesiensis, Rhodesian B56.1
 South American —see Chagas' disease
 where
  African trypanosomiasis is prevalent B56.9
  Chagas' disease is prevalent B57.2
Tryptasemia, hereditary alpha D89.44
T-shaped incisors K00.2
Tsutsugamushi (disease) (fever) A75.3
Tube, tubal, tubular —see condition
Tubercle —see also Tuberculosis
 brain, solitary A17.81
 Darwin's Q17.8
 Ghon, primary infection A15.7
Tuberculid, tuberculide (indurating,
 subcutaneous) (lichenoid) (miliary)
 (papulonecrotic) (primary) (skin) A18.4
Tuberculoma —see also Tuberculosis
 brain A17.81
 meninges (cerebral) (spinal) A17.1
 spinal cord A17.81
Tuberculosis, tubercular, tuberculous
 (calcification) (calcified) (caseous)
 (chromogenic acid-fast bacilli)
 (degeneration) (fibrocaseous) (fistula)
 (interstitial) (isolated circumscribed
 lesions) (necrosis) (parenchymatous)
 (ulcerative) A15.9
 with pneumoconiosis (any condition in
  J60-J64) J65
 abdomen (lymph gland) A18.39
 abscess (respiratory) A15.9
  bone A18.03
   hip A18.02
   knee A18.02
   sacrum A18.01
   specified site NEC A18.03
   spinal A18.01
   vertebra A18.01
  brain A17.81
  breast A18.89
  Cowper's gland A18.15
  dura (mater) (cerebral) (spinal) A17.81
  epidural (cerebral) (spinal) A17.81
  female pelvis A18.17
  frontal sinus A15.8
  genital organs NEC A18.10

Tuberculosis, tubercular, tuberculous
 (Continued)
 abscess (Continued)
  genitourinary A18.10
  gland (lymphatic) —see Tuberculosis,
   lymph gland
  hip A18.02
  intestine A18.32
  ischiorectal A18.32
  joint NEC A18.02
   hip A18.02
   knee A18.02
   specified NEC A18.02
   vertebral A18.01
  kidney A18.11
  knee A18.02
  latent Z22.7
  lumbar (spine) A18.01
  lung —see Tuberculosis, pulmonary
  meninges (cerebral) (spinal) A17.0
  muscle A18.09
  perianal (fistula) A18.32
  perinephritic A18.11
  perirectal A18.32
  rectum A18.32
  retropharyngeal A15.8
  sacrum A18.01
  scrofulous A18.2
  scrotum A18.15
  skin (primary) A18.4
  spinal cord A17.81
  spine or vertebra (column) A18.01
  subdiaphragmatic A18.31
  testis A18.15
  urinary A18.13
  uterus A18.17
 accessory sinus —see Tuberculosis, sinus
 Addison's disease A18.7
 adenitis —see Tuberculosis, lymph gland
 adenoids A15.8
 adenopathy —see Tuberculosis, lymph gland
 adherent pericardium A18.84
 adnexa (uteri) A18.17
 adrenal (capsule) (gland) A18.7
 alimentary canal A18.32
 anemia A18.89
 ankle (joint) (bone) A18.02
 anus A18.32
 apex, apical —see Tuberculosis, pulmonary
 appendicitis, appendix A18.32
 arachnoid A17.0
 artery, arteritis A18.89
  cerebral A18.89
 arthritis (chronic) (synovial) A18.02
  spine or vertebra (column) A18.01
 articular —see Tuberculosis, joint
 ascites A18.31
 asthma —see Tuberculosis, pulmonary
 axilla, axillary (gland) A18.2
 bladder A18.12
 bone A18.03
  hip A18.02
  knee A18.02
  limb NEC A18.03
  sacrum A18.01
  spine or vertebral column A18.01
 bowel (miliary) A18.32
 brain A17.81
 breast A18.89
 broad ligament A18.17
 bronchi, bronchial, bronchus A15.5
  ectasia, ectasis (bronchiectasis) —see
   Tuberculosis, pulmonary
  fistula A15.5
   primary (progressive) A15.7
  gland or node A15.4
   primary (progressive) A15.7
  lymph gland or node A15.4
   primary (progressive) A15.7
 bronchiectasis —see Tuberculosis, pulmonary
 bronchitis A15.5

▶ New   ⇒ Revised   ~~deleted~~ Deleted   ● Use Additional Character(s)

Tuberculosis, tubercular, tuberculous
(Continued)
bronchopleural A15.6
bronchopneumonia, bronchopneumonic —see Tuberculosis, pulmonary
bronchorrhagia A15.5
bronchotracheal A15.5
bronze disease A18.7
buccal cavity A18.83
bulbourethral gland A18.15
bursa A18.09
cachexia A15.9
cardiomyopathy A18.84
caries —see Tuberculosis, bone
cartilage A18.02
  intervertebral A18.01
catarrhal —see Tuberculosis, respiratory
cecum A18.32
cellulitis (primary) A18.4
cerebellum A17.81
cerebral, cerebrum A17.81
cerebrospinal A17.81
  meninges A17.0
cervical (lymph gland or node) A18.2
cervicitis, cervix (uteri) A18.16
chest —see Tuberculosis, respiratory
chorioretinitis A18.53
choroid, choroiditis A18.53
ciliary body A18.54
colitis A18.32
collier's J65
colliquativa (primary) A18.4
colon A18.32
complex, primary A15.7
congenital P37.0
conjunctiva A18.59
connective tissue (systemic) A18.89
contact Z20.1
cornea (ulcer) A18.52
Cowper's gland A18.15
coxae A18.02
coxalgia A18.02
cul-de-sac of Douglas A18.17
curvature, spine A18.01
cutis (colliquativa) (primary) A18.4
cyst, ovary A18.18
cystitis A18.12
dactylitis A18.03
diarrhea A18.32
diffuse —see Tuberculosis, miliary
digestive tract A18.32
disseminated —see Tuberculosis, miliary
duodenum A18.32
dura (mater) (cerebral) (spinal) A17.0
  abscess (cerebral) (spinal) A17.81
dysentery A18.32
ear (inner) (middle) A18.6
  bone A18.03
  external (primary) A18.4
  skin (primary) A18.4
elbow A18.02
emphysema —see Tuberculosis, pulmonary
empyema A15.6
encephalitis A17.82
endarteritis A18.89
endocarditis A18.84
  aortic A18.84
  mitral A18.84
  pulmonary A18.84
  tricuspid A18.84
endocrine glands NEC A18.82
endometrium A18.17
enteric, enterica, enteritis A18.32
enterocolitis A18.32
epididymis, epididymitis A18.15
epidural abscess (cerebral) (spinal) A17.81
epiglottis A15.5
episcleritis A18.51
erythema (induratum) (nodosum) (primary) A18.4
esophagus A18.83

Tuberculosis, tubercular, tuberculous
(Continued)
eustachian tube A18.6
exposure (to) Z20.1
exudative —see Tuberculosis, pulmonary
eye A18.50
eyelid (primary) (lupus) A18.4
fallopian tube (acute) (chronic) A18.17
fascia A18.09
fauces A15.8
female pelvic inflammatory disease A18.17
finger A18.03
first infection A15.7
gallbladder A18.83
ganglion A18.09
gastritis A18.83
gastrocolic fistula A18.32
gastroenteritis A18.32
gastrointestinal tract A18.32
general, generalized —see Tuberculosis, miliary
genital organs A18.10
genitourinary A18.10
genu A18.02
glandula suprarenalis A18.7
glandular, general A18.2
glottis A15.5
grinder's J65
gum A18.83
hand A18.03
heart A18.84
hematogenous —see Tuberculosis, miliary
hemoptysis —see Tuberculosis, pulmonary
hemorrhage NEC —see Tuberculosis, pulmonary
hemothorax A15.6
hepatitis A18.83
hilar lymph nodes A15.4
  primary (progressive) A15.7
hip (joint) (disease) (bone) A18.02
hydropneumothorax A15.6
hydrothorax A15.6
hypoadrenalism A18.7
hypopharynx A15.8
ileocecal (hyperplastic) A18.32
ileocolitis A18.32
ileum A18.32
iliac spine (superior) A18.03
immunological findings only A15.7
indurativa (primary) A18.4
infantile A15.7
infection A15.9
  without clinical manifestations A15.7
infraclavicular gland A18.2
inguinal gland A18.2
inguinalis A18.2
intestine (any part) A18.32
iridocyclitis A18.54
iris, iritis A18.54
ischiorectal A18.32
jaw A18.03
jejunum A18.32
joint A18.02
  vertebral A18.01
keratitis (interstitial) A18.52
keratoconjunctivitis A18.52
kidney A18.11
knee (joint) A18.02
kyphosis, kyphoscoliosis A18.01
laryngitis A15.5
larynx A15.5
latent Z22.7
leptomeninges, leptomeningitis (cerebral) (spinal) A17.0
lichenoides (primary) A18.4
linguae A18.83
lip A18.83
liver A18.83
lordosis A18.01
lung —see Tuberculosis, pulmonary
lupus vulgaris A18.4

Tuberculosis, tubercular, tuberculous
(Continued)
lymph gland or node (peripheral) A18.2
  abdomen A18.39
  bronchial A15.4
    primary (progressive) A15.7
  cervical A18.2
  hilar A15.4
    primary (progressive) A15.7
  intrathoracic A15.4
    primary (progressive) A15.7
  mediastinal A15.4
    primary (progressive) A15.7
  mesenteric A18.39
  retroperitoneal A18.39
  tracheobronchial A15.4
    primary (progressive) A15.7
lymphadenitis —see Tuberculosis, lymph gland
lymphangitis —see Tuberculosis, lymph gland
lymphatic (gland) (vessel) —see Tuberculosis, lymph gland
mammary gland A18.89
marasmus A15.9
mastoiditis A18.03
mediastinal lymph gland or node A15.4
  primary (progressive) A15.7
mediastinitis A15.8
  primary (progressive) A15.7
mediastinum A15.8
  primary (progressive) A15.7
medulla A17.81
melanosis, Addisonian A18.7
meninges, meningitis (basilar) (cerebral) (cerebrospinal) (spinal) A17.0
meningoencephalitis A17.82
mesentery, mesenteric (gland or node) A18.39
miliary A19.9
  acute A19.2
    multiple sites A19.1
    single specified site A19.0
  chronic A19.8
  specified NEC A19.8
millstone makers' J65
miner's J65
molder's J65
mouth A18.83
multiple A19.9
  acute A19.1
  chronic A19.8
muscle A18.09
myelitis A17.82
myocardium, myocarditis A18.84
nasal (passage) (sinus) A15.8
nasopharynx A15.8
neck gland A18.2
nephritis A18.11
nerve (mononeuropathy) A17.83
nervous system A17.9
nose (septum) A15.8
ocular A18.50
omentum A18.31
oophoritis (acute) (chronic) A18.17
optic (nerve trunk) (papilla) A18.59
orbit A18.59
orchitis A18.15
organ, specified NEC A18.89
osseous —see Tuberculosis, bone
osteitis —see Tuberculosis, bone
osteomyelitis —see Tuberculosis, bone
otitis media A18.6
ovary, ovaritis (acute) (chronic) A18.17
oviduct (acute) (chronic) A18.17
pachymeningitis A17.0
palate (soft) A18.83
pancreas A18.83
papulonecrotic (a) (primary) A18.4
parathyroid glands A18.82
paronychia (primary) A18.4
parotid gland or region A18.83

Tuberculosis, tubercular, tuberculous
(Continued)
pelvis (bony) A18.03
penis A18.15
peribronchitis A15.5
pericardium, pericarditis A18.84
perichondritis, larynx A15.5
periostitis —*see* Tuberculosis, bone
perirectal fistula A18.32
peritoneum NEC A18.31
peritonitis A18.31
pharynx, pharyngitis A15.8
phlyctenulosis (keratoconjunctivitis) A18.52
phthisis NEC —*see* Tuberculosis, pulmonary
pituitary gland A18.82
pleura, pleural, pleurisy, pleuritis (fibrinous)
     (obliterative) (purulent) (simple plastic)
     (with effusion) A15.6
     primary (progressive) A15.7
pneumonia, pneumonic —*see* Tuberculosis,
     pulmonary
pneumothorax (spontaneous) (tense
     valvular) —*see* Tuberculosis, pulmonary
polyneuropathy A17.89
polyserositis A19.9
     acute A19.1
     chronic A19.8
potter's J65
prepuce A18.15
primary (complex) A15.7
proctitis A18.32
prostate, prostatitis A18.14
pulmonalis —*see* Tuberculosis, pulmonary
pulmonary (cavitated) (fibrotic) (infiltrative)
     (nodular) A15.0
     childhood type or first infection A15.7
     primary (complex) A15.7
pyelitis A18.11
pyelonephritis A18.11
pyemia —*see* Tuberculosis, miliary
pyonephrosis A18.11
pyopneumothorax A15.6
pyothorax A15.6
rectum (fistula) (with abscess) A18.32
reinfection stage —*see* Tuberculosis,
     pulmonary
renal A18.11
renis A18.11
respiratory A15.9
     primary A15.7
     specified site NEC A15.8
retina, retinitis A18.53
retroperitoneal (lymph gland or node) A18.39
rheumatism NEC A18.09
rhinitis A15.8
sacroiliac (joint) A18.01
sacrum A18.01
salivary gland A18.83
salpingitis (acute) (chronic) A18.17
sandblaster's J65
sclera A18.51
scoliosis A18.01
scrofulous A18.2
scrotum A18.15
seminal tract or vesicle A18.15
senile A15.9
septic —*see* Tuberculosis, miliary
shoulder (joint) A18.02
     blade A18.03
sigmoid A18.32
sinus (any nasal) A15.8
     bone A18.03
     epididymis A18.15
skeletal NEC A18.03
skin (any site) (primary) A18.4
small intestine A18.32
soft palate A18.83
spermatic cord A18.15
spine, spinal (column) A18.01
     cord A17.81
     medulla A17.81
     membrane A17.0
     meninges A17.0

Tuberculosis, tubercular, tuberculous
(Continued)
spleen, splenitis A18.85
spondylitis A18.01
sternoclavicular joint A18.02
stomach A18.83
stonemason's J65
subcutaneous tissue (cellular) (primary) A18.4
subcutis (primary) A18.4
subdeltoid bursa A18.83
submaxillary (region) A18.83
supraclavicular gland A18.2
suprarenal (capsule) (gland) A18.7
swelling, joint —*see also* category M01 (*see also*
     Tuberculosis, joint) A18.02
symphysis pubis A18.02
synovitis A18.09
     articular A18.02
     spine or vertebra A18.01
systemic —*see* Tuberculosis, miliary
tarsitis A18.4
tendon (sheath) —*see* Tuberculosis,
     tenosynovitis
tenosynovitis A18.09
     spine or vertebra A18.01
testis A18.15
throat A15.8
thymus gland A18.82
thyroid gland A18.81
tongue A18.83
tonsil, tonsillitis A15.8
trachea, tracheal A15.5
     lymph gland or node A15.4
          primary (progressive) A15.7
tracheobronchial A15.5
     lymph gland or node A15.4
          primary (progressive) A15.7
tubal (acute) (chronic) A18.17
tunica vaginalis A18.15
ulcer (skin) (primary) A18.4
     bowel or intestine A18.32
     specified NEC - code under Tuberculosis,
          by site
unspecified site A15.9
ureter A18.11
urethra, urethral (gland) A18.13
urinary organ or tract A18.13
uterus A18.17
uveal tract A18.54
uvula A18.83
vagina A18.18
vas deferens A18.15
verruca, verrucosa (cutis) (primary) A18.4
vertebra (column) A18.01
vesiculitis A18.15
vulva A18.18
wrist (joint) A18.02
Tuberculum
Carabelli —*see* Note at K00.2
occlusal —*see* Note at K00.2
paramolare K00.2
Tuberosity, enitre maxillary M26.07
Tuberous sclerosis (brain) Q85.1
Tubo-ovarian —*see* condition
Tuboplasty, after previous sterilization
     Z31.0
     aftercare Z31.42
Tubotympanitis, catarrhal (chronic) —*see* Otitis,
     media, nonsuppurative, chronic, serous
Tularemia A21.9
with
     conjunctivitis A21.1
     pneumonia A21.2
abdominal A21.3
bronchopneumonic A21.2
conjunctivitis A21.1
cryptogenic A21.3
enteric A21.3
gastrointestinal A21.3
generalized A21.7
ingestion A21.3

Tularemia *(Continued)*
intestinal A21.3
oculoglandular A21.1
ophthalmic A21.1
pneumonia (any), pneumonic A21.2
pulmonary A21.2
sepsis A21.7
specified NEC A21.8
typhoidal A21.7
ulceroglandular A21.0
Tularensis conjunctivitis A21.1
Tumefaction —*see also* Swelling
liver —*see* Hypertrophy, liver
Tumor —*see also* Neoplasm, unspecified
     behavior, by site
acinar cell —*see* Neoplasm, uncertain
     behavior, by site
acinic cell —*see* Neoplasm, uncertain
     behavior, by site
adenocarcinoid —*see* Neoplasm, malignant,
     by site
adenomatoid —*see also* Neoplasm, benign,
     by site
     odontogenic —*see* Cyst, calcifying
          odontogenic
adnexal (skin) —*see* Neoplasm, skin, benign,
     by site
adrenal
     cortical (benign) D35.0-●
          malignant C74.0-●
     rest —*see* Neoplasm, benign, by site
alpha-cell
     malignant
          pancreas C25.4
          specified site NEC —*see* Neoplasm,
               malignant, by site
          unspecified site C25.4
     pancreas D13.7
     specified site NEC —*see* Neoplasm, benign,
          by site
     unspecified site D13.7
aneurysmal —*see* Aneurysm
aortic body D44.7
     malignant C75.5
Askin's —*see* Neoplasm, connective tissue,
     malignant
basal cell —*see also* Neoplasm, skin, uncertain
     behavior D48.5
Bednar —*see* Neoplasm, skin, malignant
benign (unclassified) —*see* Neoplasm, benign,
     by site
beta-cell
     malignant
          pancreas C25.4
          specified site NEC —*see* Neoplasm,
               malignant, by site
          unspecified site C25.4
     pancreas D13.7
     specified site NEC —*see* Neoplasm, benign,
          by site
     unspecified site D13.7
Brenner D27.9
     borderline malignancy D39.1-●
          malignant C56-●
     proliferating D39.1
bronchial alveolar, intravascular D38.1
Brooke's —*see* Neoplasm, skin, benign
brown fat —*see* Lipoma
Burkitt —*see* Lymphoma, Burkitt
calcifying epithelial odontogenic —*see* Cyst,
     calcifying odontogenic
carcinoid D3A.00
     benign D3A.00
          appendix D3A.020
          ascending colon D3A.022
          bronchus (lung) D3A.090
          cecum D3A.021
          colon D3A.029
          descending colon D3A.024
          duodenum D3A.010
          foregut NOS D3A.094

▶ New   ⇒ Revised   ~~deleted~~ Deleted   ● Use Additional Character(s)

Tumor *(Continued)*
  carcinoid *(Continued)*
    malignant *(Continued)*
      hindgut NOS D3A.096
      ileum D3A.012
      jejunum D3A.011
      kidney D3A.093
      large intestine D3A.029
      lung (bronchus) D3A.090
      midgut NOS D3A.095
      rectum D3A.026
      sigmoid colon D3A.025
      small intestine D3A.019
      specified NEC D3A.098
      stomach D3A.092
      thymus D3A.091
      transverse colon D3A.023
    malignant C7A.00
      appendix C7A.020
      ascending colon C7A.022
      bronchus (lung) C7A.090
      cecum C7A.021
      colon C7A.029
      descending colon C7A.024
      duodenum C7A.010
      foregut NOS C7A.094
      hindgut NOS C7A.096
      ileum C7A.012
      jejunum C7A.011
      kidney C7A.093
      large intestine C7A.029
      lung (bronchus) C7A.090
      midgut NOS C7A.095
      rectum C7A.026
      sigmoid colon C7A.025
      small intestine C7A.019
      specified NEC C7A.098
      stomach C7A.092
      thymus C7A.091
      transverse colon C7A.023
    mesentary metastasis C7B.04
    secondary C7B.00
      bone C7B.03
      distant lymph nodes C7B.01
      liver C7B.02
      peritoneum C7B.04
      specified NEC C7B.09
  carotid body D44.6
    malignant C75.4
  cells —*see also* Neoplasm, unspecified behavior, by site
    benign —*see* Neoplasm, benign, by site
    malignant —*see* Neoplasm, malignant, by site
    uncertain whether benign or malignant —*see* Neoplasm, uncertain behavior, by site
  cervix, in pregnancy or childbirth —*see* Pregnancy, complicated by, tumor, cervix
  chondromatous giant cell —*see* Neoplasm, bone, benign
  chromaffin —*see also* Neoplasm, benign, by site
    malignant —*see* Neoplasm, malignant, by site
  Cock's peculiar L72.3
  Codman's —*see* Neoplasm, bone, benign
  dentigerous, mixed —*see* Cyst, calcifying odontogenic
  dermoid —*see* Neoplasm, benign, by site
    with malignant transformation C56-●
  desmoid (extra-abdominal) —*see also* Neoplasm, connective tissue, uncertain behavior
    abdominal —*see* Neoplasm, connective tissue, uncertain behavior
  embolus —*see* Neoplasm, secondary, by site

Tumor *(Continued)*
  embryonal (mixed) —*see also* Neoplasm, uncertain behavior, by site
    liver C22.7
  endodermal sinus
    specified site —*see* Neoplasm, malignant, by site
    unspecified site
      female C56.-●
      male C62.90
  epithelial
    benign —*see* Neoplasm, benign, by site
    malignant —*see* Neoplasm, malignant, by site
  Ewing's —*see* Neoplasm, bone, malignant, by site
  fatty —*see* Lipoma
  fibroid —*see* Leiomyoma
  G cell
    malignant
      pancreas C25.4
      specified site NEC —*see* Neoplasm, malignant, by site
      unspecified site C25.4
    specified site —*see* Neoplasm, uncertain behavior, by site
    unspecified site D37.8
  germ cell —*see also* Neoplasm, malignant, by site
    mixed —*see* Neoplasm, malignant, by site
  ghost cell, odontogenic —*see* Cyst, calcifying odontogenic
  giant cell —*see also* Neoplasm, uncertain behavior, by site
    bone D48.0
      malignant —*see* Neoplasm, bone, malignant
    chondromatous —*see* Neoplasm, bone, benign
    malignant —*see* Neoplasm, malignant, by site
    soft parts —*see* Neoplasm, connective tissue, uncertain behavior
      malignant —*see* Neoplasm, connective tissue, malignant
  glomus D18.00
    intra-abdominal D18.03
    intracranial D18.02
    jugulare D44.7
      malignant C75.5
    skin D18.01
    specified site NEC D18.09
  gonadal stromal —*see* Neoplasm, uncertain behavior, by site
  granular cell —*see also* Neoplasm, connective tissue, benign
    malignant —*see* Neoplasm, connective tissue, malignant
  granulosa cell D39.1-●
    juvenile D39.1-●
    malignant C56-●
  granulosa cell-theca cell D39.1-●
    malignant C56-●
  Grawitz's C64-●
  hemorrhoidal —*see* Hemorrhoids
  hilar cell D27-●
  hilus cell D27-●
  Hurthle cell (benign) D34
    malignant C73
  hydatid —*see* Echinococcus
  hypernephroid —*see also* Neoplasm, uncertain behavior, by site
  interstitial cell —*see also* Neoplasm, uncertain behavior, by site
    benign —*see* Neoplasm, benign, by site
    malignant —*see* Neoplasm, malignant, by site
  intravascular bronchial alveolar D38.1

Tumor *(Continued)*
  islet cell —*see* Neoplasm, benign, by site
    malignant —*see* Neoplasm, malignant, by site
      pancreas C25.4
      specified site NEC —*see* Neoplasm, malignant, by site
      unspecified site C25.4
    pancreas D13.7
    specified site NEC —*see* Neoplasm, benign, by site
    unspecified site D13.7
  juxtaglomerular D41.0-●
  Klatskin's C24.0
  Krukenberg's C79.6-●
  Leydig cell —*see* Neoplasm, uncertain behavior, by site
    benign —*see* Neoplasm, benign, by site
      specified site —*see* Neoplasm, benign, by site
      unspecified site
        female D27.9
        male D29.20
    malignant —*see* Neoplasm, malignant, by site
      specified site —*see* Neoplasm, malignant, by site
      unspecified site
        female C56.9
        male C62.90
    specified site —*see* Neoplasm, uncertain behavior, by site
    unspecified site
      female D39.10
      male D40.10
  lipid cell, ovary D27-●
  lipoid cell, ovary D27-●
  malignant —*see also* Neoplasm, malignant, by site C80.1
    fusiform cell (type) C80.1
    giant cell (type) C80.1
    localized, plasma cell —*see* Plasmacytoma, solitary
    mixed NEC C80.1
    small cell (type) C80.1
    spindle cell (type) C80.1
    unclassified C80.1
  mast cell D47.09
  melanotic, neuroectodermal —*see* Neoplasm, benign, by site
  Merkel cell —*see* Carcinoma, Merkel cell
  mesenchymal
    malignant —*see* Neoplasm, connective tissue, malignant
    mixed —*see* Neoplasm, connective tissue, uncertain behavior
  mesodermal, mixed —*see also* Neoplasm, malignant, by site
    liver C22.4
  mesonephric —*see also* Neoplasm, uncertain behavior, by site
    malignant —*see* Neoplasm, malignant, by site
  metastatic
    from specified site —*see* Neoplasm, malignant, by site
    of specified site —*see* Neoplasm, malignant, by site
    to specified site —*see* Neoplasm, secondary, by site
  mixed NEC —*see also* Neoplasm, benign, by site
    malignant —*see* Neoplasm, malignant, by site
  mucinous of low malignant potential
    specified site —*see* Neoplasm, malignant, by site
    unspecified site C56.9
  mucocarcinoid
    specified site —*see* Neoplasm, malignant, by site
    unspecified site C18.1

Tumor *(Continued)*
  mucoepidermoid —*see* Neoplasm, uncertain
    behavior, by site
  Müllerian, mixed
    specified site —*see* Neoplasm, malignant,
     by site
    unspecified site C54.9
  myoepithelial —*see* Neoplasm, benign,
    by site
  neuroectodermal (peripheral) —*see*
    Neoplasm, malignant, by site
    primitive
     specified site —*see* Neoplasm,
      malignant, by site
     unspecified site C71.9
  neuroendocrine D3A.8
    malignant poorly differentiated C7A.1
    secondary NEC C7B.8
    specified NEC C7A.8
  neurogenic olfactory C30.0
  nonencapsulated sclerosing C73
  odontogenic (adenomatoid) (benign)
    (calcifying epithelial) (keratocystic)
    (squamous) —*see* Cyst, calcifying
    odontogenic
    malignant C41.1
     upper jaw (bone) C41.0
  ovarian stromal D39.1-•
  ovary, in pregnancy —*see* Pregnancy,
    complicated by
  pacinian —*see* Neoplasm, skin, benign
  Pancoast's —*see* Pancoast's syndrome
  papillary —*see also* Papilloma
    cystic D37.9
    mucinous of low malignant potential
     C56-•
     specified site —*see* Neoplasm,
      malignant, by site
     unspecified site C56.9
    serous of low malignant potential
     specified site —*see* Neoplasm,
      malignant, by site
     unspecified site C56.9
  pelvic, in pregnancy or childbirth —*see*
    Pregnancy, complicated by
  phantom F45.8
  phyllodes D48.6-•
    benign D24-•
    malignant —*see* Neoplasm, breast,
     malignant
  Pindborg —*see* Cyst, calcifying odontogenic
  placental site trophoblastic D39.2
  plasma cell (malignant) (localized) —*see*
    Plasmacytoma, solitary
  polyvesicular vitelline
    specified site —*see* Neoplasm, malignant,
     by site
    unspecified site
     female C56.9
     male C62.90
  Pott's puffy —*see* Osteomyelitis, specified
    NEC
  Rathke's pouch D44.3
  retinal anlage —*see* Neoplasm, benign, by site
  salivary gland type, mixed —*see* Neoplasm,
    salivary gland, benign
    malignant —*see* Neoplasm, salivary gland,
     malignant
  Sampson's N80.10-•
  Schmincke's —*see* Neoplasm, nasopharynx,
    malignant
  sclerosing stromal D27-•
  sebaceous —*see* Cyst, sebaceous
  secondary —*see* Neoplasm, secondary, by site
    carcinoid C7B.00
     bone C7B.03
     distant lymph nodes C7B.01
     liver C7B.02
     peritoneum C7B.04
     specified NEC C7B.09
    neuroendocrine NEC C7B.8

Tumor *(Continued)*
  serous of low malignant potential
    specified site —*see* Neoplasm, malignant,
     by site
    unspecified site C56.9
  Sertoli cell —*see* Neoplasm, benign, by site
    with lipid storage
     specified site —*see* Neoplasm, benign,
      by site
     unspecified site
      female D27.9
      male D29.20
    specified site —*see* Neoplasm, benign, by
     site
    unspecified site
     female D27.9
     male D29.20
  Sertoli-Leydig cell —*see* Neoplasm, benign,
    by site
    specified site —*see* Neoplasm, benign, by
     site
    unspecified site
     female D27.9
     male D29.20
  sex cord(-stromal) —*see* Neoplasm, uncertain
    behavior, by site
    with annular tubules D39.1-•
  skin appendage —*see* Neoplasm, skin,
    benign
  smooth muscle —*see* Neoplasm, connective
    tissue, uncertain behavior
  soft tissue
    benign —*see* Neoplasm, connective tissue,
     benign
    malignant —*see* Neoplasm, connective
     tissue, malignant
  sternomastoid (congenital) Q68.0
  stromal
    endometrial D39.0
    gastric D48.1
     benign D21.4
     malignant C16.9
     uncertain behavior D48.1
    gastrointestinal C49.A-•
     benign D21.4
     esophagus C49.A1
     large intestine C49.A4
     malignant C49.A0
      colon C49.A4
      duodenum C49.A3
      esophagus C49.A1
      ileum C49.A3
      jejunum C49.A3
      Meckel diverticulum C49.A3
      large intestine C49.A4
      omentum C49.A9
      peritoneum C49.A9
      rectum C49.A5
      small intestine C49.A3
      specified site NEC C49.A9
      stomach C49.A2
     rectum C49.A5
     small intestine C49.A3
     specified site NEC C49.A9
     stomach C49.A2
     uncertain behavior D48.1
    intestine
     benign D21.4
     malignant
      large C49.A4
      small C49.A3
     uncertain behavior D48.1
    ovarian D39.1-•
    stomach C49.A2
     benign D21.4
     malignant C49.A2
     uncertain behavior D48.1
  sweat gland —*see also* Neoplasm, skin,
    uncertain behavior
    benign —*see* Neoplasm, skin, benign
    malignant —*see* Neoplasm, skin, malignant

Tumor *(Continued)*
  syphilitic, brain A52.17
  testicular D40.10
  testicular stromal D40.1-•
  theca cell D27.-•
  theca cell-granulosa cell D39.1-•
  Triton, malignant —*see* Neoplasm, nerve,
    malignant
  trophoblastic, placental site D39.2
  turban D23.4
  uterus (body), in pregnancy or childbirth —
    see Pregnancy, complicated by, tumor,
    uterus
  vagina, in pregnancy or childbirth —*see*
    Pregnancy, complicated by
  varicose —*see* Varix
  von Recklinghausen's —*see*
    Neurofibromatosis
  vulva or perineum, in pregnancy or
    childbirth —*see* Pregnancy,
    complicated by
    causing obstructed labor O65.5
  Warthin's —*see* Neoplasm, salivary gland,
    benign
  Wilms' C64-•
  yolk sac —*see* Neoplasm, malignant, by site
    specified site —*see* Neoplasm, malignant,
     by site
    unspecified site
     female C56.9
     male C62.90
Tumor lysis syndrome (following
  antineoplastic chemotherapy)
  (spontaneous) NEC E88.3
Tumorlet —*see* Neoplasm, uncertain behavior,
  by site
Tungiasis B88.1
Tunica vasculosa lentis Q12.2
Turban tumor D23.4
Türck's trachoma J37.0
Turner-Kieser syndrome Q87.2
Turner-like syndrome Q87.19
Turner's
  hypoplasia (tooth) K00.4
  syndrome Q96.9
    specified NEC Q96.8
  tooth K00.4
Turner-Ullrich syndrome Q96.9
Tussis convulsiva —*see* Whooping cough
Twiddler's syndrome (due to)
  automatic implantable defibrillator T82.198
  cardiac pacemaker T82.198
Twilight state
  epileptic F05
  psychogenic F44.89
Twin (newborn) —*see also* Newborn, twin
  conjoined Q89.4
  pregnancy —*see* Pregnancy, twin
Twinning, teeth K00.2
Twist, twisted
  bowel, colon or intestine K56.2
  hair (congenital) Q84.1
  mesentery K56.2
  omentum K56.2
  organ or site, congenital NEC —*see* Anomaly,
    by site
  ovarian pedicle —*see* Torsion, ovary
Twitching R25.3
Tylosis (acquired) L84
  buccalis K13.29
  linguae K13.29
  palmaris et plantaris (congenital) (inherited)
    Q82.8
    acquired L85.1
Tympanism R14.0
Tympanites (abdominal) (intestinal)
  R14.0
Tympanitis —*see* Myringitis
Tympanosclerosis —*see* subcategory
  H74.0
Tympanum —*see* condition

▶ New   ⇒ Revised   ~~deleted~~ Deleted   • Use Additional Character(s)

Tympany
  abdomen R14.0
  chest R09.89
Type A behavior pattern Z73.1
Typhlitis —*see* Cecitis
Typhoenteritis —*see* Typhoid
Typhoid (abortive) (ambulant) (any site)
      (clinical) (fever) (hemorrhagic) (infection)
      (intermittent) (malignant) (rheumatic)
      (Widal negative) A01.00
  with pneumonia A01.03
  abdominal A01.09
  arthritis A01.04
  carrier (suspected) of Z22.0
  cholecystitis (current) A01.09
  endocarditis A01.02
  heart involvement A01.02
  inoculation reaction —*see* Complications,
      vaccination
  meningitis A01.01
  mesenteric lymph nodes A01.09
  myocarditis A01.02
  Orientia Tsutsugamushi (scrub typhus) A75.3
  osteomyelitis A01.05
  perichondritis, larynx A01.09
  pneumonia A01.03

Typhoid (*Continued*)
  specified NEC A01.09
  spine A01.05
  ulcer (perforating) A01.09
Typhomalaria (fever) —*see* Malaria
Typhomania A01.00
Typhoperitonitis A01.09
Typhus (fever) A75.9
  abdominal, abdominalis —*see* Typhoid
  African tick A77.1
  amarillic A95.9
  brain A75.9 [*G94*]
  cerebral A75.9 [*G94*]
  classical A75.0
  due to Rickettsia
      prowazekii A75.0
          recrudescent A75.1
      tsutsugamushi A75.3
      typhi A75.2
  endemic (flea-borne) A75.2
  epidemic (louse-borne) A75.0
  exanthematic NEC A75.0
  exanthematicus SAI A75.0
      brillii SAI A75.1
      mexicanus SAI A75.2
      typhus murinus A75.2

Typhus (*Continued*)
  flea-borne A75.2
  India tick A77.1
  Kenya (tick) A77.1
  louse-borne A75.0
  Mexican A75.2
  mite-borne A75.3
  murine A75.2
  North Asian tick-borne A77.2
  petechial A75.9
  Queensland tick A77.3
  rat A75.2
  recrudescent A75.1
  recurrens —*see* Fever, relapsing
  Sao Paulo A77.0
  scrub (China) (India) (Malaysia) (New
      Guinea) A75.3
  shop (of Malaysia) A75.2
  Siberian tick A77.2
  tick-borne A77.9
  tropical (mite-borne) A75.3
Tyrosinemia E70.21
  newborn, transitory P74.5
Tyrosinosis E70.21
Tyrosinuria E70.29

U

Uhl's anomaly or disease Q24.8
Ulcer, ulcerated, ulcerating, ulceration,
     ulcerative
  alveolar process M27.3
  amebic (intestine) A06.1
    skin A06.7
  anastomotic —*see* Ulcer, gastrojejunal
  anorectal K62.6
  antral —*see* Ulcer, stomach
  anus (sphincter) (solitary) K62.6
  aorta —*see* Aneurysm
  aphthous (oral) (recurrent) K12.0
    genital organ(s)
      female N76.6
      male N50.89
  artery I77.2
  atrophic —*see* Ulcer, skin
    decubitus —*see* Ulcer, pressure, by site
  back L98.429
    with
      bone involvement without evidence of
        necrosis L98.426
      bone necrosis L98.424
      exposed fat layer L98.422
      muscle involvement without evidence of
        necrosis L98.425
      muscle necrosis L98.423
      skin breakdown only L98.421
      specified severity NEC L98.428
  Barrett's (esophagus) K22.10
    with bleeding K22.11
  bile duct (common) (hepatic) K83.8
  bladder (solitary) (sphincter) NEC N32.89
    bilharzial B65.9 [N33]
    in schistosomiasis (bilharzial) B65.9 [N33]
    submucosal —*see* Cystitis, interstitial
    tuberculous A18.12
  bleeding K27.4
  bone —*see* Osteomyelitis, specified type NEC
  bowel —*see* Ulcer, intestine
  breast N61.1
  bronchus J98.09
  buccal (cavity) (traumatic) K12.1
  Buruli A31.1
  buttock L98.419
    with
      bone involvement without evidence of
        necrosis L98.416
      bone necrosis L98.414
      exposed fat layer L98.412
      muscle involvement without evidence of
        necrosis L98.415
      muscle necrosis L98.413
      skin breakdown only L98.411
      specified severity NEC L98.418
  cancerous —*see* Neoplasm, malignant, by site
  cardia K22.10
    with bleeding K22.11
  cardioesophageal (peptic) K22.10
    with bleeding K22.11
  cecum —*see* Ulcer, intestine
  cervix (uteri) (decubitus) (trophic) N86
    with cervicitis N72
  chancroidal A57
  chiclero B55.1
  chronic (cause unknown) —*see* Ulcer, skin
  Cochin-China B55.1
  colon —*see* Ulcer, intestine
  conjunctiva H10.89
  cornea H16.00-●
    with hypopyon H16.03-●
    central H16.01-●
    dendritic (herpes simplex) B00.52
    marginal H16.04-●
    Mooren's H16.05-●
    mycotic H16.06-●
    perforated H16.07-●
    ring H16.02-●
    tuberculous (phlyctenular) A18.52

Ulcer, ulcerated, ulcerating, ulceration,
     ulcerative (*Continued*)
  corpus cavernosum (chronic) N48.5
  crural —*see* Ulcer, lower limb
  Curling's —*see* Ulcer, peptic, acute
  Cushing's —*see* Ulcer, peptic, acute
  cystic duct K82.8
  cystitis (interstitial) —*see* Cystitis,
    interstitial
  decubitus —*see* Ulcer, pressure, by site
  dendritic, cornea (herpes simplex) B00.52
  diabetes, diabetic —*see* Diabetes, ulcer
  Dieulafoy's K25.0
  due to
    infection NEC —*see* Ulcer, skin
    radiation NEC L59.8
    trophic disturbance (any region) —*see*
      Ulcer, skin
    X-ray L58.1
  duodenum, duodenal (eroded) (peptic)
    K26.9
    with
      hemorrhage K26.4
        and perforation K26.6
      perforation K26.5
    acute K26.3
      with
        hemorrhage K26.0
          and perforation K26.2
        perforation K26.1
    chronic K26.7
      with
        hemorrhage K26.4
          and perforation K26.6
        perforation K26.5
  dysenteric A09
  elusive —*see* Cystitis, interstitial
  endocarditis (acute) (chronic) (subacute) I28.8
  epiglottis J38.7
  esophagus (peptic) K22.10
    with bleeding K22.11
    due to
      aspirin K22.10
        with bleeding K22.11
      gastrointestinal reflux disease (without
        bleeding) K21.00
        with bleeding K21.01
      ingestion of chemical or medicament
        K22.10
        with bleeding K22.11
    fungal K22.10
      with bleeding K22.11
    infective K22.10
      with bleeding K22.11
    varicose —*see* Varix, esophagus
  eyelid (region) H01.8
  fauces J39.2
  Fenwick (-Hunner) (solitary) —*see* Cystitis,
    interstitial
  fistulous —*see* Ulcer, skin
  foot (indolent) (trophic) —*see* Ulcer, lower
    limb
  frambesial, initial A66.0
  frenum (tongue) K14.0
  gallbladder or duct K82.8
  gangrenous —*see* Gangrene
  gastric —*see* Ulcer, stomach
  gastrocolic —*see* Ulcer, gastrojejunal
  gastroduodenal —*see* Ulcer, peptic
  gastroesophageal —*see* Ulcer, stomach
  gastrointestinal —*see* Ulcer, gastrojejunal
  gastrojejunal (peptic) K28.9
    with
      hemorrhage K28.4
        and perforation K28.6
      perforation K28.5
    acute K28.3
      with
        hemorrhage K28.0
          and perforation K28.2
        perforation K28.1

Ulcer, ulcerated, ulcerating, ulceration,
     ulcerative (*Continued*)
  gastrojejunal (*Continued*)
    chronic K28.7
      with
        hemorrhage K28.4
          and perforation K28.6
        perforation K28.5
  gastrojejunocolic —*see* Ulcer, gastrojejunal
  gingiva K06.8
  gingivitis K05.10
    nonplaque induced K05.11
    plaque induced K05.10
  glottis J38.7
  granuloma of pudenda A58
  gum K06.8
  gumma, due to yaws A66.4
  heel —*see* Ulcer, lower limb
  hemorrhoid —*see also* Hemorrhoids, by
    degree K64.8
  Hunner's —*see* Cystitis, interstitial
  hypopharynx J39.2
  hypopyon (chronic) (subacute) —*see* Ulcer,
    cornea, with hypopyon
  hypostaticum —*see* Ulcer, varicose
  ileum —*see* Ulcer, intestine
  intestine, intestinal K63.3
    with perforation K63.1
    amebic A06.1
    duodenal —*see* Ulcer, duodenum
    granulocytopenic (with hemorrhage) —*see*
      Neutropenia
    marginal —*see* Ulcer, gastrojejunal
    perforating K63.1
      newborn P78.0
    primary, small intestine K63.3
    rectum K62.6
    stercoraceous, stercoral K63.3
    tuberculous A18.32
    typhoid (fever) —*see* Typhoid
    varicose I86.8
  jejunum, jejunal —*see* Ulcer, gastrojejunal
  keratitis —*see* Ulcer, cornea
  knee —*see* Ulcer, lower limb
  labium (majus) (minus) N76.6
  laryngitis —*see* Laryngitis
  larynx (aphthous) (contact) J38.7
    diphtheritic A36.2
  leg —*see* Ulcer, lower limb
  lip K13.0
  Lipschütz's N76.6
  lower limb (atrophic) (chronic) (neurogenic)
    (perforating) (pyogenic) (trophic)
    (tropical) L97.909
    with
      bone involvement without evidence of
        necrosis L97.906
      bone necrosis L97.904
      exposed fat layer L97.902
      muscle involvement without evidence of
        necrosis L97.905
      muscle necrosis L97.903
      skin breakdown only L97.901
      specified severity NEC L97.908
    ankle L97.309
      with
        bone involvement without evidence of
          necrosis L97.306
        bone necrosis L97.304
        exposed fat layer L97.302
        muscle involvement without evidence
          of necrosis L97.305
        muscle necrosis L97.303
        skin breakdown only L97.301
        specified severity NEC L97.308
    left L97.329
      with
        bone involvement without evidence
          of necrosis L97.326
        bone necrosis L97.324
        exposed fat layer L97.322

▶ New   ➡ Revised   ~~deleted~~ Deleted   ● Use Additional Character(s)

Ulcer, ulcerated, ulcerating, ulceration, ulcerative *(Continued)*
  lower limb *(Continued)*
    ankle *(Continued)*
      left *(Continued)*
        with *(Continued)*
          muscle involvement without evidence of necrosis L97.325
          muscle necrosis L97.323
          skin breakdown only L97.321
          specified severity NEC L97.328
      right L97.319
        with
          bone involvement without evidence of necrosis L97.316
          bone necrosis L97.314
          exposed fat layer L97.312
          muscle involvement without evidence of necrosis L97.315
          muscle necrosis L97.313
          skin breakdown only L97.311
          specified severity NEC L97.318
    calf L97.209
      with
        bone involvement without evidence of necrosis L97.206
        bone necrosis L97.204
        exposed fat layer L97.202
        muscle involvement without evidence of necrosis L97.205
        muscle necrosis L97.203
        skin breakdown only L97.201
        specified severity NEC L97.208
      left L97.229
        with
          bone involvement without evidence of necrosis L97.226
          bone necrosis L97.224
          exposed fat layer L97.222
          muscle involvement without evidence of necrosis L97.225
          muscle necrosis L97.223
          skin breakdown only L97.221
          specified severity NEC L97.228
      right L97.219
        with
          bone involvement without evidence of necrosis L97.216
          bone necrosis L97.214
          exposed fat layer L97.212
          muscle involvement without evidence of necrosis L97.215
          muscle necrosis L97.213
          skin breakdown only L97.211
          specified severity NEC L97.218
    decubitus —*see* Ulcer, pressure, by site
    foot specified NEC L97.509
      with
        bone involvement without evidence of necrosis L97.506
        bone necrosis L97.504
        exposed fat layer L97.502
        muscle involvement without evidence of necrosis L97.505
        muscle necrosis L97.503
        skin breakdown only L97.501
        specified severity NEC L97.508
      left L97.529
        with
          bone involvement without evidence of necrosis L97.526
          bone necrosis L97.524
          exposed fat layer L97.522
          muscle involvement without evidence of necrosis L97.525
          muscle necrosis L97.523
          skin breakdown only L97.521
          specified severity NEC L97.528

Ulcer, ulcerated, ulcerating, ulceration, ulcerative *(Continued)*
  lower limb *(Continued)*
    foot specified *(Continued)*
      right L97.519
        with
          bone involvement without evidence of necrosis L97.516
          bone necrosis L97.514
          exposed fat layer L97.512
          muscle involvement without evidence of necrosis L97.515
          muscle necrosis L97.513
          skin breakdown only L97.511
          specified severity NEC L97.518
    heel L97.409
      with
        bone involvement without evidence of necrosis L97.406
        bone necrosis L97.404
        exposed fat layer L97.402
        muscle involvement without evidence of necrosis L97.405
        muscle necrosis L97.403
        skin breakdown only L97.401
        specified severity NEC L97.408
      left L97.429
        with
          bone involvement without evidence of necrosis L97.426
          bone necrosis L97.424
          exposed fat layer L97.422
          muscle involvement without evidence of necrosis L97.425
          muscle necrosis L97.423
          skin breakdown only L97.421
          specified severity NEC L97.428
      right L97.419
        with
          bone involvement without evidence of necrosis L97.416
          bone necrosis L97.414
          exposed fat layer L97.412
          muscle involvement without evidence of necrosis L97.415
          muscle necrosis L97.413
          skin breakdown only L97.411
          specified severity NEC L97.418
    left L97.929
      with
        bone involvement without evidence of necrosis L97.926
        bone necrosis L97.924
        exposed fat layer L97.922
        muscle involvement without evidence of necrosis L97.925
        muscle necrosis L97.923
        skin breakdown only L97.921
        specified severity NEC L97.928
    lower leg NOS L97.909
      with
        bone involvement without evidence of necrosis L97.906
        bone necrosis L97.904
        exposed fat layer L97.902
        muscle involvement without evidence of necrosis L97.905
        muscle necrosis L97.903
        skin breakdown only L97.901
        specified severity NEC L97.908
      left L97.929
        with
          bone involvement without evidence of necrosis L97.926
          bone necrosis L97.924
          exposed fat layer L97.922
          muscle involvement without evidence of necrosis L97.925
          muscle necrosis L97.923
          skin breakdown only L97.921
          specified severity NEC L97.928

Ulcer, ulcerated, ulcerating, ulceration, ulcerative *(Continued)*
  lower limb *(Continued)*
    lower leg NOS *(Continued)*
      right L97.919
        with
          bone involvement without evidence of necrosis L97.916
          bone necrosis L97.914
          exposed fat layer L97.912
          muscle involvement without evidence of necrosis L97.915
          muscle necrosis L97.913
          skin breakdown only L97.911
          specified severity NEC L97.918
    specified site NEC L97.809
      with
        bone involvement without evidence of necrosis L97.806
        bone necrosis L97.804
        exposed fat layer L97.802
        muscle involvement without evidence of necrosis L97.805
        muscle necrosis L97.803
        skin breakdown only L97.801
        specified severity NEC L97.808
      left L97.829
        with
          bone involvement without evidence of necrosis L97.826
          bone necrosis L97.824
          exposed fat layer L97.822
          muscle involvement without evidence of necrosis L97.825
          muscle necrosis L97.823
          skin breakdown only L97.821
          specified severity NEC L97.828
      right L97.819
        with
          bone involvement without evidence of necrosis L97.816
          bone necrosis L97.814
          exposed fat layer L97.812
          muscle involvement without evidence of necrosis L97.815
          muscle necrosis L97.813
          skin breakdown only L97.811
          specified severity NEC L97.818
    midfoot L97.409
      with
        bone involvement without evidence of necrosis L97.406
        bone necrosis L97.404
        exposed fat layer L97.402
        muscle involvement without evidence of necrosis L97.405
        muscle necrosis L97.403
        skin breakdown only L97.401
        specified severity NEC L97.408
      left L97.429
        with
          bone involvement without evidence of necrosis L97.426
          bone necrosis L97.424
          exposed fat layer L97.422
          muscle involvement without evidence of necrosis L97.425
          muscle necrosis L97.423
          skin breakdown only L97.421
          specified severity NEC L97.428
      right L97.419
        with
          bone involvement without evidence of necrosis L97.416
          bone necrosis L97.414
          exposed fat layer L97.412
          muscle involvement without evidence of necrosis L97.415
          muscle necrosis L97.413
          skin breakdown only L97.411
          specified severity NEC L97.418

Ulcer, ulcerated, ulcerating, ulceration,
   ulcerative (Continued)
  lower limb (Continued)
   right L97.919
    with
     bone involvement without evidence of
      necrosis L97.916
     bone necrosis L97.914
     exposed fat layer L97.912
     muscle involvement without evidence
      of necrosis L97.915
     muscle necrosis L97.913
     skin breakdown only L97.911
     specified severity NEC L97.918
   thigh L97.109
    with
     bone involvement without evidence of
      necrosis L97.106
     bone necrosis L97.104
     exposed fat layer L97.102
     muscle involvement without evidence
      of necrosis L97.105
     muscle necrosis L97.103
     skin breakdown only L97.101
     specified severity NEC L97.108
   left L97.129
    with
     bone involvement without evidence
      of necrosis L97.126
     bone necrosis L97.124
     exposed fat layer L97.122
     muscle involvement without
      evidence of necrosis L97.125
     muscle necrosis L97.123
     skin breakdown only L97.121
     specified severity NEC L97.128
   right L97.119
    with
     bone involvement without evidence
      of necrosis L97.116
     bone necrosis L97.114
     exposed fat layer L97.112
     muscle involvement without
      evidence of necrosis L97.115
     muscle necrosis L97.113
     skin breakdown only L97.111
     specified severity NEC L97.118
  toe L97.509
   with
    bone involvement without evidence of
     necrosis L97.506
    bone necrosis L97.504
    exposed fat layer L97.502
    muscle involvement without evidence
     of necrosis L97.505
    muscle necrosis L97.503
    skin breakdown only L97.501
    specified severity NEC L97.508
   left L97.529
    with
     bone involvement without evidence
      of necrosis L97.526
     bone necrosis L97.524
     exposed fat layer L97.522
     muscle involvement without
      evidence of necrosis L97.525
     muscle necrosis L97.523
     skin breakdown only L97.521
     specified severity NEC L97.528
   right L97.519
    with
     bone involvement without evidence
      of necrosis L97.516
     bone necrosis L97.514
     exposed fat layer L97.512
     muscle involvement without
      evidence of necrosis L97.515
     muscle necrosis L97.513
     skin breakdown only L97.511
     specified severity NEC
      L97.518

Ulcer, ulcerated, ulcerating, ulceration,
   ulcerative (Continued)
  lower limb (Continued)
   leprous A30.1
   syphilitic A52.19
   varicose —see Varix, leg, with, ulcer
  luetic —see Ulcer, syphilitic
  lung J98.4
   tuberculous —see Tuberculosis, pulmonary
  malignant —see Neoplasm, malignant, by site
  marginal NEC —see Ulcer, gastrojejunal
  meatus (urinarius) N34.2
  Meckel's diverticulum Q43.0
   malignant —see Table of Neoplasms, small
    intestine, malignant
  Meleney's (chronic undermining) —see Ulcer,
   skin
  Mooren's (cornea) —see Ulcer, cornea,
   Mooren's
  mycobacterial (skin) A31.1
  nasopharynx J39.2
  neck, uterus N86
  neurogenic NEC —see Ulcer, skin
  nose, nasal (passage) (infective) (septum) J34.0
   skin —see Ulcer, skin
   spirochetal A69.8
   varicose (bleeding) I86.8
  oral mucosa (traumatic) K12.1
  palate (soft) K12.1
  penis (chronic) N48.5
  peptic (site unspecified) K27.9
   with
    hemorrhage K27.4
     and perforation K27.6
    perforation K27.5
   acute K27.3
    with
     hemorrhage K27.0
      and perforation K27.2
     perforation K27.1
   chronic K27.7
    with
     hemorrhage K27.4
      and perforation K27.6
     perforation K27.5
   esophagus K22.10
    with bleeding K22.11
   newborn P78.82
  perforating K27.5
   skin —see Ulcer, skin
  peritonsillar J35.8
  phagedenic (tropical) —see Ulcer, skin
  pharynx J39.2
  phlebitis —see Phlebitis
  plaster —see Ulcer, pressure, by site
  popliteal space —see Ulcer, lower limb
  postpyloric —see Ulcer, duodenum
  prepuce N47.7
  prepyloric —see Ulcer, stomach
  pressure (pressure area) L89.9-●
   ankle L89.5-●
   back L89.1-●
   buttock L89.3-●
   coccyx L89.15-●
   contiguous site of back, buttock, hip
    L89.4-●
   elbow L89.0-●
   face L89.81-●
   head L89.81-●
   heel L89.6-●
   hip L89.2-●
   sacral region (tailbone) L89.15-●
   specified site NEC L89.89-●
   stage 1 (healing) (pre-ulcer skin changes
    limited to persistent focal edema)
    ankle L89.5-●
    back L89.1-●
    buttock L89.3-●
    coccyx L89.15-●
    contiguous site of back, buttock, hip
     L89.4-●

Ulcer, ulcerated, ulcerating, ulceration,
   ulcerative (Continued)
  pressure (Continued)
   stage 1 (Continued)
    elbow L89.0-●
    face L89.81-●
    head L89.81-●
    heel L89.6-●
    hip L89.2-●
    sacral region (tailbone) L89.15-●
    specified site NEC L89.89-●
   stage 2 (healing) (abrasion, blister,
    partial thickness skin loss involving
    epidermis and/or dermis)
    ankle L89.5-●
    back L89.1-●
    buttock L89.3-●
    coccyx L89.15-●
    contiguous site of back, buttock, hip
     L89.4-●
    elbow L89.0-●
    face L89.81-●
    head L89.81-●
    heel L89.6-●
    hip L89.2-●
    sacral region (tailbone) L89.15-●
    specified site NEC L89.89-●
   stage 3 (healing) (full thickness skin loss
    involving damage or necrosis of
    subcutaneous tissue)
    ankle L89.5-●
    back L89.1-●
    buttock L89.3-●
    coccyx L89.15-●
    contiguous site of back, buttock, hip
     L89.4-●
    elbow L89.0-●
    face L89.81-●
    head L89.81-●
    heel L89.6-●
    hip L89.2-●
    sacral region (tailbone) L89.15-●
    specified site NEC L89.89-●
   stage 4 (healing) (necrosis of soft tissues
    through to underlying muscle,
    tendon, or bone)
    ankle L89.5-●
    back L89.1-●
    buttock L89.3-●
    coccyx L89.15-●
    contiguous site of back, buttock, hip
     L89.4-●
    elbow L89.0-●
    face L89.81-●
    head L89.81-●
    heel L89.6-●
    hip L89.2-●
    sacral region (tailbone) L89.15-●
    specified site NEC L89.89-●
   unspecified stage
    ankle L89.5-●
    back L89.1-●
    buttock L89.3-●
    coccyx L89.15-●
    contiguous site of back, buttock, hip
     L89.4-●
    elbow L89.0-●
    face L89.81-●
    head L89.81-●
    heel L89.6-●
    hip L89.2-●
    sacral region (tailbone) L89.15-●
    specified site NEC L89.89-●
   unstageable
    ankle L89.5-●
    back L89.1-●
    buttock L89.3-●
    coccyx L89.15-●
    contiguous site of back, buttock, hip
     L89.4-●
    elbow L89.0-●

▶ New   ➡ Revised   ~~deleted~~ Deleted   ● Use Additional Character(s)

Universal mesentery Q43.3
▶ Unreliable transportation Z59.82
Unrepairable overhanging of dental
    restorative materials K08.52
▶ Unroofed coronary sinus Q21.13
▶ Unsafe transportation Z59.82
Unsatisfactory
    restoration of tooth K08.50
      specified NEC K08.59
    sample of cytologic smear
      anus R85.615
      cervix R87.615
      vagina R87.625
    surroundings Z59.1
    work Z56.5
Unsoundness of mind —see Psychosis
Unstable
    back NEC —see Instability, joint, spine
    hip (congenital) Q65.6
      acquired —see Derangement, joint,
        specified type NEC, hip
    joint —see Instability, joint
      secondary to removal of joint prosthesis
        M96.89
    lie (mother) O32.0
    lumbosacral joint (congenital) —see
      subcategory M53.2
    sacroiliac —see subcategory M53.2
    spine NEC —see Instability, joint, spine
Unsteadiness on feet R26.81
Untruthfulness, child problem F91.8
Unverricht(-Lundborg) disease or epilepsy —
    see Epilepsy, generalized, idiopathic
Unwanted
    multiple moves in the last 12 months
      Z59.81- •
    pregnancy Z64.0
Upbringing, institutional Z62.22
    away from parents NEC Z62.29
    in care of non-parental family member Z62.21
    in foster care Z62.21
    in orphanage or group home Z62.22
    in welfare custody Z62.21
Upper respiratory —see condition
Upset
    gastric K30
    gastrointestinal K30
      psychogenic F45.8
    intestinal (large) (small) K59.9
      psychogenic F45.8
    menstruation N93.9
    mental F48.9
    stomach K30
      psychogenic F45.8
Urachus —see also condition
    patent or persistent Q64.4
Urbach-Oppenheim disease (necrobiosis
    lipoidica diabeticorum) —see E08-E13 with
    .620
Urbach's lipoid proteinosis E78.89
Urbach-Wiethe disease E78.89
Urban yellow fever A95.1
Urea
    blood, high —see Uremia
    cycle metabolism disorder —see Disorder,
      urea cycle metabolism
Uremia, uremic N19
    with
      ectopic or molar pregnancy O08.4
      polyneuropathy N18.9 [G63]
    chronic NOS —see also Disease, kidney,
      chronic N18.9
      due to hypertension —see Hypertensive,
        kidney
    complicating
      ectopic or molar pregnancy O08.4
    congenital P96.0
    extrarenal R39.2
    following ectopic or molar pregnancy O08.4
    newborn P96.0
    prerenal R39.2

Ureter, ureteral —see condition
Ureteralgia N23
Ureterectasis —see Hydroureter
Ureteritis N28.89
    cystica N28.86
    due to calculus N20.1
      with calculus, kidney N20.2
        with hydronephrosis N13.2
    gonococcal (acute) (chronic) A54.21
    nonspecific N28.89
Ureterocele N28.89
    congenital (orthotopic) Q62.31
      ectopic Q62.32
Ureterolith, ureterolithiasis —see Calculus,
    ureter
Ureterostomy
    attention to Z43.6
    status Z93.6
Urethra, urethral —see condition
Urethralgia R39.89
Urethritis (anterior) (posterior) N34.2
    calculous N21.1
    candidal B37.41
    chlamydial A56.01
    diplococcal (gonococcal) A54.01
      with abscess (accessory gland)
        (periurethral) A54.1
    gonococcal A54.01
      with abscess (accessory gland)
        (periurethral) A54.1
    nongonococcal N34.1
      Reiter's —see Reiter's disease
    nonspecific N34.1
    nonvenereal N34.1
    postmenopausal N34.2
    puerperal O86.22
    Reiter's —see Reiter's disease
    specified NEC N34.2
    trichomonal or due to Trichomonas
      (vaginalis) A59.03
Urethrocele N81.0
    with
      cystocele —see Cystocele
      prolapse of uterus —see Prolapse, uterus
Urethrolithiasis (with colic or infection)
    N21.1
Urethrorectal —see condition
Urethrorrhagia N36.8
Urethrorrhea R36.9
Urethrostomy
    attention to Z43.6
    status Z93.6
Urethrotrigonitis —see Trigonitis
Urethrovaginal —see condition
Urgency
    fecal R15.2
    hypertensive —see Hypertension
    urinary N39.15
Urhidrosis, uridrosis L74.8
Uric acid in blood (increased) E79.0
Uricacidemia (asymptomatic) E79.0
Uricemia (asymptomatic) E79.0
Uricosuria R82.998
Urinary —see condition
Urination
    frequent R35.0
    painful R30.9
Urine
    blood in —see Hematuria
    discharge, excessive R35.89
    enuresis, nonorganic origin F98.0
    extravasation R39.0
    frequency R35.0
    incontinence R32
      nonorganic origin F98.0
    intermittent stream R39.198
    pus in N39.0
    retention or stasis R33.9
      organic R33.8
        drug-induced R33.0
      psychogenic F45.8

Urine (Continued)
    secretion
      deficient R34
      excessive R35.89
      frequency R35.0
    stream
      intermittent R39.198
      slowing R39.198
      splitting R39.13
      weak R39.12
Urinemia —see Uremia
Urinoma, urethra N36.8
Uroarthritis, infectious (Reiter's) —see Reiter's
    disease
Urodialysis R34
Urolithiasis —see Calculus, urinary
Uronephrosis —see Hydronephrosis
Uropathy N39.9
    obstructive N13.9
      specified NEC N13.8
    reflux N13.9
      specified NEC N13.8
    vesicoureteral reflux-associated —see Reflux,
      vesicoureteral
Urosepsis — code to condition
Urticaria L50.9
    with angioneurotic edema T78.3
      hereditary D84.1
    allergic L50.0
    cholinergic L50.5
    chronic L50.8
    cold, familial L50.2
    contact L50.6
    dermatographic L50.3
    due to
      cold or heat L50.2
      drugs L50.0
      food L50.0
      inhalants L50.0
      plants L50.6
      serum —see also Reaction, serum
        T80.69
    factitial L50.3
    familial cold M04.2
    giant T78.3
      hereditary D84.1
    gigantea T78.3
    idiopathic L50.1
    larynx T78.3
      hereditary D84.1
    neonatorum P83.88
    nonallergic L50.1
    papulosa (Hebra) L28.2
    pigmentosa D47.01
      congenital Q82.2
      of neonatal onset Q82.2
      of newborn onset Q82.2
    recurrent periodic L50.8
    serum —see also Reaction, serum T80.69
    solar L56.3
    specified type NEC L50.8
    thermal (cold) (heat) L50.2
    vibratory L50.4
    xanthelasmoidea —see Urticaria
      pigmentosa
Use (of)
▦ alcohol F10.90
    with
      intoxication F10.929
      sleep disorder F10.982
      withdrawal F10.939
        with
          perceptual disturbance
            F10.932
          delirium F10.931
          uncomplicated F10.930
      harmful —see Abuse, alcohol
   ▶ in remission F10.91
    amphetamines —see Use, stimulant NEC
    caffeine —see Use, stimulant NEC

Use *(Continued)*
cannabis F12.90
  with
    anxiety disorder F12.980
    intoxication F12.929
      with
        delirium F12.921
        perceptual disturbance F12.922
      uncomplicated F12.920
    other specified disorder F12.988
    psychosis F12.959
      delusions F12.950
      hallucinations F12.951
    unspecified disorder F12.99
    withdrawal F12.93
▶ in remission F12.91
cocaine F14.90
  with
    anxiety disorder F14.980
    intoxication F14.929
      with
        delirium F14.921
        perceptual disturbance F14.922
      uncomplicated F14.920
    other specified disorder F14.988
    psychosis F14.959
      delusions F14.950
      hallucinations F14.951
    sexual dysfunction F14.981
    sleep disorder F14.982
    unspecified disorder F14.99
    withdrawal F14.93
  harmful —*see* Abuse, drug, cocaine
▶ in remission F14.91
drug(s) NEC F19.90
  with sleep disorder F19.982
  harmful —*see* Abuse, drug, by type
hallucinogen NEC F16.90
  with
    anxiety disorder F16.980
    intoxication F16.929
      with
        delirium F16.921
      uncomplicated F16.920
    mood disorder F16.94
    other specified disorder F16.988
    perception disorder (flashbacks) F16.983
    psychosis F16.959
      delusions F16.950
      hallucinations F16.951
    unspecified disorder F16.99
  harmful —*see* Abuse, drug, hallucinogen NEC
▶ in remission F16.91
inhalants F18.90
  with
    anxiety disorder F18.980
    intoxication F18.929
      with delirium F18.921
      uncomplicated F18.920
    mood disorder F18.94
    other specified disorder F18.988
    persisting dementia F18.97
    psychosis F18.959
      delusions F18.950
      hallucinations F18.951
    unspecified disorder F18.99

Use *(Continued)*
inhalants *(Continued)*
  harmful —*see* Abuse, drug, inhalant
▶ in remission F18.91
methadone —*see* Use, opioid
nonprescribed drugs F19.90
  harmful —*see* Abuse, non-psychoactive substance
opioid F11.90
  with
    disorder F11.99
      mood F11.94
      sleep F11.982
      specified type NEC F11.988
    intoxication F11.929
      with
        delirium F11.921
        perceptual disturbance F11.922
      uncomplicated F11.920
    withdrawal F11.93
  harmful —*see* Abuse, drug, opioid
▶ in remission F11.91
patent medicines F19.90
  harmful —*see* Abuse, non-psychoactive substance
psychoactive drug NEC F19.90
  with
    anxiety disorder F19.980
    intoxication F19.929
      with
        delirium F19.921
        perceptual disturbance F19.922
      uncomplicated F19.920
    mood disorder F19.94
    other specified disorder F19.988
    persisting
      amnestic disorder F19.96
      dementia F19.97
    psychosis F19.959
      delusions F19.950
      hallucinations F19.951
    sexual dysfunction F19.981
    sleep disorder F19.982
    unspecified disorder F19.99
    withdrawal F19.939
      with
        delirium F19.931
        perceptual disturbance F19.932
      uncomplicated F19.930
  harmful —*see* Abuse, drug NEC, psychoactive NEC
▶ in remission F19.91
sedative, hypnotic, or anxiolytic F13.90
  with
    anxiety disorder F13.980
    intoxication F13.929
      with
        delirium F13.921
      uncomplicated F13.920
    other specified disorder F13.988
    persisting
      amnestic disorder F13.96
      dementia F13.97
    psychosis F13.959
      delusions F13.950
      hallucinations F13.951

Use *(Continued)*
sedative, hypnotic, or anxiolytic *(Continued)*
  with *(Continued)*
    sexual dysfunction F13.981
    sleep disorder F13.982
    unspecified disorder F13.99
  harmful —*see* Abuse, drug, sedative, hypnotic, or anxiolytic
▶ in remission F13.91
stimulant NEC F15.90
  with
    anxiety disorder F15.980
    intoxication F15.929
      with
        delirium F15.921
        perceptual disturbance F15.922
      uncomplicated F15.920
    mood disorder F15.94
    other specified disorder F15.988
    psychosis F15.959
      delusions F15.950
      hallucinations F15.951
    sexual dysfunction F15.981
    sleep disorder F15.982
    unspecified disorder F15.99
    withdrawal F15.93
  harmful —*see* Abuse, drug, stimulant NEC
▶ in remission F15.91
tobacco Z72.0
  with dependence —*see* Dependence, drug, nicotine
volatile solvents —*see also* Use, inhalant F18.90
  harmful —*see* Abuse, drug, inhalant
Usher-Senear disease or syndrome L10.4
Uta B55.1
Uteromegaly N85.2
Uterovaginal —*see* condition
Uterovesical —*see* condition
Uveal —*see* condition
Uveitis (anterior) —*see also* Iridocyclitis
  acute —*see* Iridocyclitis, acute
  chronic —*see* Iridocyclitis, chronic
  due to toxoplasmosis (acquired) B58.09
    congenital P37.1
  granulomatous —*see* Iridocyclitis, chronic
  heterochromic —*see* Cyclitis, Fuchs' heterochromic
  lens-induced —*see* Iridocyclitis, lens-induced
  posterior —*see* Chorioretinitis
  sympathetic H44.13- •
  syphilitic (secondary) A51.43
    congenital (early) A50.01
    late A52.71
  tuberculous A18.54
Uveoencephalitis —*see* Inflammation, chorioretinal
Uveokeratitis —*see* Iridocyclitis
Uveoparotitis D86.89
Uvula —*see* condition
Uvulitis (acute) (catarrhal) (chronic) (membranous) (suppurative) (ulcerative) K12.2

V

Vaccination (prophylactic)
  complication or reaction —see Complications, vaccination
  delayed Z28.9
  encounter for Z23
  not done —see Immunization, not done, because (of)
Vaccinia (generalized) (localized) T88.1
  without vaccination B08.011
  congenital P35.8
Vacuum, in sinus (accessory) (nasal) J34.89
Vagabond, vagabondage Z59.00
Vagabond's disease B85.1
Vagina, vaginal —see condition
Vaginalitis (tunica) (testis) N49.1
Vaginismus (reflex) N94.2
  functional F52.5
  nonorganic F52.5
  psychogenic F52.5
  secondary N94.2
Vaginitis (acute) (circumscribed) (diffuse) (emphysematous) (nonvenereal) (ulcerative) N76.0
  with ectopic or molar pregnancy O08.0
  amebic A06.82
  atrophic, postmenopausal N95.2
  bacterial N76.0
  blennorrhagic (gonococcal) A54.02
  candidal (acute) B37.31
  ▶chronic (recurrent) B37.32
  chlamydial A56.02
  chronic N76.1
  due to Trichomonas (vaginalis) A59.01
  following ectopic or molar pregnancy O08.0
  gonococcal A54.02
    with abscess (accessory gland) (periurethral) A54.1
  granuloma A58
  in (due to)
    candidiasis (acute) B37.31
    ▶chronic (recurrent) B37.32
    herpesviral (herpes simplex) infection A60.04
    pinworm infection B80 [N77.1]
  monilial (acute) B37.31
    ▶chronic (recurrent) B37.32
  mycotic (candidal) (acute) B37.31
    ▶chronic (recurrent) B37.32
  postmenopausal atrophic N95.2
  puerperal (postpartum) O86.13
  senile (atrophic) N95.2
  subacute or chronic N76.1
  syphilitic (early) A51.0
    late A52.76
  trichomonal A59.01
  tuberculous A18.18
Vaginosis —see Vaginitis
Vagotonia G52.2
Vagrancy Z59.00
VAIN —see Neoplasia, intraepithelial, vagina
Vallecula —see condition
Valley fever B38.0
Valsuani's disease —see Anemia, obstetric
Valve, valvular (formation) —see also condition
  cerebral ventricle (communicating) in situ Z98.2
  cervix, internal os Q51.828
  congenital NEC —see Atresia, by site
  ureter (pelvic junction) (vesical orifice) Q62.39
  urethra (congenital) (posterior) Q64.2
Valvulitis (chronic) —see Endocarditis
Valvulopathy —see Endocarditis
Van Bogaert's leukoencephalopathy (sclerosing) (subacute) A81.1
Van Bogaert-Scherer-Epstein disease or syndrome E75.5
Van Buchem's syndrome M85.2
Van Creveld-von Gierke disease E74.01

Van der Hoeve (-de Kleyn) syndrome Q78.0
Van der Woude's syndrome Q38.0
Van Neck's disease or osteochondrosis M91.0
Vanishing lung J44.9
Vapor asphyxia or suffocation T59.9
  specified agent —see Table of Drugs and Chemicals
Variance, lethal ball, prosthetic heart valve T82.09
Variants, thalassemic D56.8
Variations in hair color L67.1
Varicella B01.9
  with
    complications NEC B01.89
    encephalitis B01.11
    encephalomyelitis B01.11
    meningitis B01.0
    myelitis B01.12
    pneumonia B01.2
  congenital P35.8
Varices —see Varix
Varicocele (scrotum) (thrombosed) I86.1
  ovary I86.2
  perineum I86.3
  spermatic cord (ulcerated) I86.1
Varicose
  aneurysm (ruptured) I77.0
  dermatitis —see Varix, leg, with, inflammation
  eczema —see Varix, leg, with, inflammation
  phlebitis —see Varix, with, inflammation
  tumor —see Varix
  ulcer (lower limb, any part) —see also Varix, leg, with, ulcer
    anus —see also Hemorrhoids K64.8
    esophagus —see Varix, esophagus
    inflamed or infected —see Varix, leg, with ulcer, with inflammation
    nasal septum I86.8
    perineum I86.3
    scrotum I86.1
    specified site NEC I86.8
  vein —see Varix
  vessel —see Varix, leg
Varicosis, varicosities, varicosity —see Varix
Variola (major) (minor) B03
Varioloid B03
Varix (lower limb) I83.90
  with
    bleeding I83.899
    edema I83.899
    inflammation I83.10
      with ulcer (venous) I83.209
    pain I83.819
    rupture I83.899
    specified complication NEC I83.899
    stasis dermatitis I83.10
      with ulcer (venous) I83.209
    swelling I83.899
    ulcer I83.009
      with inflammation I83.209
  aneurysmal I77.0
  asymptomatic I83.9-●
  bladder I86.2
  broad ligament I86.2
  complicating
    childbirth (lower extremity) O87.4
      anus or rectum O87.2
      genital (vagina, vulva or perineum) O87.8
    pregnancy (lower extremity) O22.0-●
      anus or rectum O22.4-●
      genital (vagina, vulva or perineum) O22.1-●
    puerperium (lower extremity) O87.4
      anus or rectum O87.2
      genital (vagina, vulva, perineum) O87.8
  congenital (any site) Q27.8
  esophagus (idiopathic) (primary) (ulcerated) I85.00
    bleeding I85.01
    congenital Q27.8

Varix (Continued)
  esophagus (Continued)
    in (due to)
      alcoholic liver disease I85.10
        bleeding I85.11
      cirrhosis of liver I85.10
        bleeding I85.11
      portal hypertension I85.10
        bleeding I85.11
      schistosomiasis I85.10
        bleeding I85.11
      toxic liver disease I85.10
        bleeding I85.11
    secondary I85.10
      bleeding I85.11
  gastric I86.4
  inflamed or infected I83.10
    ulcerated I83.209
  labia (majora) I86.3
  leg (asymptomatic) I83.9-●
    with
      edema I83.899
      inflammation I83.10
        with ulcer —see Varix, leg, with, ulcer, with inflammation by site
      pain I83.819
      specified complication NEC I83.899
      swelling I83.899
      ulcer I83.0-●
        with inflammation I83.2-●
        ankle I83.003
          with inflammation I83.203
        calf I83.002
          with inflammation I83.202
        foot NEC I83.005
          with inflammation I83.205
        heel I83.004
          with inflammation I83.204
        lower leg NEC I83.008
          with inflammation I83.208
        midfoot I83.004
          with inflammation I83.204
        thigh I83.001
          with inflammation I83.201
  bilateral (asymptomatic) I83.93
    with
      edema I83.893
      pain I83.813
      specified complication NEC I83.893
      swelling I83.893
      ulcer I83.0-●
        with inflammation I83.209
  left (asymptomatic) I83.92
    with
      edema I83.892
      inflammation I83.12
        with ulcer —see Varix, leg, with, ulcer, with inflammation by site
      pain I83.812
      specified complication NEC I83.892
      swelling I83.892
      ulcer I83.029
        with inflammation I83.229
        ankle I83.023
          with inflammation I83.223
        calf I83.022
          with inflammation I83.222
        foot NEC I83.025
          with inflammation I83.225
        heel I83.024
          with inflammation I83.224
        lower leg NEC I83.028
          with inflammation I83.228
        midfoot I83.024
          with inflammation I83.224
        thigh I83.021
          with inflammation I83.221
  right (asymptomatic) I83.91
    with
      edema I83.891

▶ New   ⇒ Revised   ~~deleted~~ Deleted   ● Use Additional Character(s)

Varix *(Continued)*
 leg *(Continued)*
  right *(Continued)*
   with *(Continued)*
    inflammation I83.11
     with ulcer —*see* Varix, leg, with,
      ulcer, with inflammation by
      site
    pain I83.811
    specified complication NEC I83.891
    swelling I83.891
    ulcer I83.019
     with inflammation I83.219
     ankle I83.013
      with inflammation I83.213
     calf I83.012
      with inflammation I83.212
     foot NEC I83.015
      with inflammation I83.215
     heel I83.014
      with inflammation I83.214
     lower leg NEC I83.018
      with inflammation I83.218
     midfoot I83.014
      with inflammation I83.214
     thigh I83.011
      with inflammation I83.211
  nasal septum I86.8
  orbit I86.8
   congenital Q27.8
  ovary I86.2
  papillary I78.1
  pelvis I86.2
  perineum I86.3
  pharynx I86.8
  placenta O43.89-•
  renal papilla I86.8
  retina H35.09
  scrotum (ulcerated) I86.1
  sigmoid colon I86.8
  specified site NEC I86.8
  spinal (cord) (vessels) I86.8
  spleen, splenic (vein) (with phlebolith) I86.8
  stomach I86.4
  sublingual I86.0
  ulcerated I83.009
   inflamed or infected I83.209
  uterine ligament I86.2
  vagina I86.8
  vocal cord I86.8
  vulva I86.3
Vas deferens —*see* condition
Vas deferentitis N49.1
Vasa previa O69.4
 hemorrhage from, affecting newborn P50.0
Vascular —*see also* condition
 loop on optic papilla Q14.2
 spasm I73.9
 spider I78.1
Vascularization, cornea —*see*
  Neovascularization, cornea
Vasculitis I77.6
 allergic D69.0
▶ANCA (antineutrophilic cytoplasmic
  antibody) associated I77.82
▶ANCA (antineutrophilic cytoplasmic
  antibody) positive I77.82
▶antineutrophilic cytoplasmic antibody
  [ANCA] I77.82
 cryoglobulinemic D89.1
 disseminated I77.6
 hypocomplementemic M31.8
 kidney I77.89
 leukocytoclastic M31.0
 livedoid L95.0
 nodular L95.8
 retina H35.06-•
 rheumatic —*see* Fever, rheumatic
 rheumatoid —*see* Rheumatoid, vasculitis
 skin (limited to) L95.9
  specified NEC L95.8
 systemic M31.8

Vasculopathy, necrotizing M31.9
 cardiac allograft T86.290
 specified NEC M31.8
Vasitis (nodosa) N49.1
 tuberculous A18.15
Vasodilation I73.9
Vasomotor —*see* condition
Vasoplasty, after previous sterilization Z31.0
 aftercare Z31.42
Vasospasm (vasoconstriction) I73.9
 cerebral (cerebrovascular) (artery)
   I67.848
   reversible I67.841
 coronary I20.1
 nerve
  arm —*see* Mononeuropathy, upper limb
  brachial plexus G54.0
  cervical plexus G54.2
  leg —*see* Mononeuropathy, lower limb
 peripheral NOS I73.9
 retina (artery) —*see* Occlusion, artery,
   retina
Vasospastic —*see* condition
Vasovagal attack (paroxysmal) R55
 psychogenic F45.8
VATER syndrome Q87.2
Vater's ampulla —*see* condition
Vegetation, vegetative
 adenoid (nasal fossa) J35.8
 endocarditis (acute) (any valve) (subacute)
   I33.0
 heart (mycotic) (valve) I33.0
Veil
 Jackson's Q43.3
Vein, venous —*see* condition
Veldt sore —*see* Ulcer, skin
Velpeau's hernia —*see* Hernia, femoral
Venereal
 bubo A55
 disease A64
 granuloma inguinale A58
 lymphogranuloma (Durand-Nicolas-Favre)
   A55
Venofibrosis I87.8
Venom, venomous —*see* Table of Drugs and
  Chemicals, by animal or substance,
  poisoning
Venous —*see* condition
Ventilator lung, newborn P27.8
Ventral —*see* condition
Ventricle, ventricular —*see also* condition
 escape I49.3
 inversion Q20.5
Ventriculitis (cerebral) —*see also* Encephalitis
  G04.90
Ventriculostomy status Z98.2
Vernet's syndrome G52.7
Verneuil's disease (syphilitic bursitis) A52.78
Verruca (due to HPV) (filiformis) (simplex)
  (viral) (vulgaris) B07.9
 acuminata A63.0
 necrogenica (primary) (tuberculosa) A18.4
 plana B07.8
 plantaris B07.0
 seborrheica L82.1
  inflamed L82.0
 senile (seborrheic) L82.1
  inflamed L82.0
 tuberculosa (primary) A18.4
 venereal A63.0
Verrucosities —*see* Verruca
Verruga peruana, peruviana A44.1
Version
 cervix —*see* Malposition, uterus
 uterus (postinfectional) (postpartal, old) —*see*
  Malposition, uterus
Vertebra, vertebral —*see* condition
Vertical talus (congenital) Q66.80
 left foot Q66.82
 right foot Q66.81

Vertigo R42
 auditory —*see* Vertigo, aural
 aural H81.31-•
 benign paroxysmal (positional) H81.1-•
 central (origin) H81.4
 cerebral H81.4
 Dix and Hallpike (epidemic) —*see* Neuronitis,
   vestibular
 due to infrasound T75.23
 epidemic A88.1
  Dix and Hallpike —*see* Neuronitis,
    vestibular
  Pedersen's —*see* Neuronitis, vestibular
  vestibular neuronitis —*see* Neuronitis,
    vestibular
 hysterical F44.89
 infrasound T75.23
 labyrinthine —*see* subcategory H81.0
 laryngeal R05.4
 malignant positional H81.4
 Ménière's —*see* subcategory H81.40
 menopausal N95.11
 otogenic —*see* Vertigo, aural
 paroxysmal positional, benign —*see* Vertigo,
   benign paroxysmal
 Pedersen's (epidemic) —*see* Neuronitis,
   vestibular
 peripheral NEC H81.39-•
 positional
  benign paroxysmal —*see* Vertigo, benign
    paroxysmal
  malignant H81.4
Very-low-density-lipoprotein-type (VLDL)
  hyperlipoproteinemia E78.1
Vesania —*see* Psychosis
Vesical —*see* condition
Vesicle
 cutaneous R23.8
 seminal —*see* condition
 skin R23.8
Vesicocolic —*see* condition
Vesicoperineal —*see* condition
Vesicorectal —*see* condition
Vesicourethrorectal —*see* condition
Vesicovaginal —*see* condition
Vesicular —*see* condition
Vesiculitis (seminal) N49.0
 amebic A06.82
 gonorrheal (acute) (chronic) A54.23
 trichomonal A59.09
 tuberculous A18.15
Vestibulitis (ear) —*see also* subcategory
  H83.0
 nose (external) J34.89
 vulvar N94.810
Vestibulopathy, acute peripheral (recurrent) —
  see Neuronitis, vestibular
Vestige, vestigial —*see also* Persistence
 branchial Q18.0
 structures in vitreous Q14.0
Vibration
 adverse effects T75.20
  pneumatic hammer syndrome T75.21
  specified effect NEC T75.29
  vasospastic syndrome T75.22
  vertigo from infrasound T75.23
 exposure (occupational) Z57.7
 vertigo T75.23
Vibriosis A28.9
Victim (of)
 crime Z65.4
 disaster Z65.5
 terrorism Z65.4
 torture Z65.4
 war Z65.5
Vidal's disease L28.0
Villaret's syndrome G52.7
Villous —*see* condition
VIN —*see* Neoplasia, intraepithelial, vulva
Vincent's infection (angina) (gingivitis)
  A69.1
 stomatitis NEC A69.1

Vinson-Plummer syndrome D50.1
Violence, physical R45.6
Viosterol deficiency —*see* Deficiency, calciferol
Vipoma —*see* Neoplasm, malignant, by site
Viremia B34.9
Virilism (adrenal) E25.9
  congenital E25.0
Virilization (female) (suprarenal) E25.9
  congenital E25.0
  isosexual E28.2
Virulent bubo A57
Virus, viral —*see also* condition
  as cause of disease classified elsewhere B97.89
    respiratory syncytial virus (RSV) —*see* Virus,
      infection, respiratory syncytial (RSV)
  cytomegalovirus B25.9
  human immunodeficiency (HIV) —*see* Human,
    immunodeficiency virus (HIV) disease
  infection —*see* Infection, virus
  respiratory syncytial (RSV)
    as cause of disease classified elsewhere
      B97.4
    bronchiolitis J21.0
    bronchitis J20.5
    bronchopneumonia J12.1
    otitis media H65-● [B97.4]
    pneumonia J12.1
    upper respiratory infection J06.9 [B97.4]
  specified NEC B34.8
  swine influenza (viruses that normally cause
    infections in pigs) —*see also* Influenza,
    due to, identified novel influenza A virus
    J09.X2
  West Nile (fever) A92.30
    with
      complications NEC A92.39
      cranial nerve disorders A92.32
      encephalitis A92.31
      encephalomyelitis A92.31
      neurologic manifestation NEC A92.32
      optic neuritis A92.32
      polyradiculitis A92.32
Viscera, visceral —*see* condition
Visceroptosis K63.4
Visible peristalsis R19.2
Vision, visual
  binocular, suppression H53.34
  blurred, blurring H53.8
    hysterical F44.6
  defect, defective NEC H54.7
  disorientation (syndrome) H53.8
  disturbance H53.9
    hysterical F44.6
  double H53.2
  examination Z01.00
    with abnormal findings Z01.01
    following failed vision screening Z01.020
      with abnormal findings Z01.021
  field, limitation (defect) —*see* Defect, visual
    field
  hallucinations R44.1
  halos H53.19
  loss —*see* Loss, vision
    sudden —*see* Disturbance, vision,
      subjective, loss, sudden

Vision, visual *(Continued)*
  low (both eyes) —*see* Low, vision
  perception, simultaneous without fusion
    H53.33
Vitality, lack or want of R53.83
  newborn P96.89
Vitamin deficiency —*see* Deficiency, vitamin
Vitelline duct, persistent Q43.0
Vitiligo L80
  eyelid H02.739
    left H02.736
      lower H02.735
      upper H02.734
    right H02.733
      lower H02.732
      upper H02.731
  pinta A67.2
  vulva N90.89
Vitreal corneal syndrome H59.01-●
Vitreoretinopathy, proliferative —*see also*
  Retinopathy, proliferative
  with retinal detachment —*see* Detachment,
    retina, traction
Vitreous —*see also* condition
  touch syndrome —*see* Complication,
    postprocedural, following cataract
    surgery
Vocal cord —*see* condition
Vogt-Koyanagi syndrome H20.82-●
Vogt's disease or syndrome G80.3
Vogt-Spielmeyer amaurotic idiocy or disease
  E75.4
Voice
  change R49.9
    specified NEC R49.8
  loss —*see* Aphonia
Volhynian fever A79.0
Volkmann's ischemic contracture or paralysis
  (complicating trauma) T79.6
Volvulus (bowel) (colon) (intestine) K56.2
  with perforation K56.2
  congenital Q43.8
  duodenum K31.5
  fallopian tube —*see* Torsion, fallopian tube
  oviduct —*see* Torsion, fallopian tube
  stomach (due to absence of gastrocolic
    ligament) K31.89
Vomiting R11.10
  with nausea R11.2
  without nausea R11.11
  asphyxia —*see* Foreign body, by site, causing
    asphyxia, gastric contents
  bilious (cause unknown) R11.14
    following gastro-intestinal surgery K91.0
    in newborn P92.01
  blood —*see* Hematemesis
  causing asphyxia, choking, or suffocation —
    see Foreign body, by site
  cyclical, in migraine G43.A0
    with refractory migraine G43.A1
    intractable G43.A1
    not intractable G43.A0
    psychogenic F50.89
    without refractory migraine G43.A0

Vomiting *(Continued)*
  cyclical syndrome NOS (unrelated to
    migraine) R53.1
    persistent R11.15
  fecal mater R11.13
  following gastrointestinal surgery K91.0
    psychogenic F50.89
  functional K31.89
  hysterical F50.89
  nervous F50.89
  neurotic F50.89
  newborn NEC P92.09
    bilious P92.01
  periodic R11.10
    psychogenic F50.89
  projectile R11.12
  psychogenic F50.89
  uremic —*see* Uremia
Vomito negro —*see* Fever, yellow
Von Bezold's abscess —*see* Mastoiditis, acute
Von Economo-Cruchet disease A85.8
Von Eulenburg's disease G71.19
Von Gierke's disease E74.01
Von Hippel (-Lindau) disease or syndrome
  Q85.83
Von Jaksch's anemia or disease D64.89
Von Recklinghausen
  disease (neurofibromatosis) Q85.01
    bones E21.0
Von Schroetter's syndrome I82.890
Von Willebrand (-Jurgens)(-Minot) disease or
  syndrome —*see* Disease, von Willebrand
Von Zumbusch's disease L40.1
Voyeurism F65.3
Vrolik's disease Q78.0
Vulva —*see* condition
Vulvismus N94.2
Vulvitis (acute) (allergic) (atrophic)
  (hypertrophic) (intertriginous) (senile) N76.2
  with ectopic or molar pregnancy O08.0
  adhesive, congenital Q52.79
  blennorrhagic (gonococcal) A54.02
  candidal (acute) B37.31
    chronic (recurrent) B37.32
  chlamydial A56.02
  due to Haemophilus ducreyi A57
  following ectopic or molar pregnancy O08.0
  gonococcal A54.02
    with abscess (accessory gland)
      (periurethral) A54.1
  herpesviral A60.04
  leukoplakic N90.4
  monilial (acute) B37.31
  chronic (recurrent) B37.32
  puerperal (postpartum) O86.19
  subacute or chronic N76.3
  syphilitic (early) A51.0
    late A52.76
  trichomonal A59.01
  tuberculous A18.18
Vulvodynia N94.819
  specified NEC N94.818
Vulvorectal —*see* condition
Vulvovaginitis (acute) —*see* Vaginitis

▶ New   ⇒ Revised   ~~deleted~~ Deleted   ● Use Additional Character(s)

W

Waiting list, person on Z75.1
  for organ transplant Z76.82
  undergoing social agency investigation Z75.2
Waldenström
  hypergammaglobulinemia D89.0
  syndrome or macroglobulinemia C88.0
Waldenström-Kjellberg syndrome D50.1
Walking
  difficulty R26.2
    psychogenic F44.4
  sleep F51.3
    hysterical F44.89
Wall, abdominal —see condition
Wallenberg's disease or syndrome G46.3
Wallgren's disease I87.8
Wandering
  gallbladder, congenital Q44.1
  in diseases classified elsewhere Z91.83
  kidney, congenital Q63.8
  organ or site, congenital NEC —see
    Malposition, congenital, by site
  pacemaker (heart) I49.8
  spleen D73.89
War neurosis F48.8
Wart (due to HPV) (filiform) (infectious)
    (viral) B07.9
  anogenital region (venereal) A63.0
  common B07.8
  external genital organs (venereal)
    A63.0
  flat B07.8
  Hassal-Henle's (of cornea) H18.49
  Peruvian A44.1
  plantar B07.0
  prosector (tuberculous) A18.4
  seborrheic L82.1
    inflamed L82.0
  senile (seborrheic) L82.1
    inflamed L82.0
  tuberculous A18.4
  venereal A63.0
Warthin's tumor —see Neoplasm, salivary
    gland, benign
Wassilieff's disease A27.0
Wasting
  disease R64
    due to malnutrition E43
    with marasmus E41
  extreme (due to malnutrition) E43
    with marasmus E41
  muscle NEC —see Atrophy, muscle
Water
  clefts (senile cataract) —see Cataract, senile,
    incipient
  deprivation of T73.1
  intoxication E87.79
  itch B76.9
  lack of T73.1
    safe drinking Z58.6
  loading E87.70
  on
    brain —see Hydrocephalus
    chest J94.8
  poisoning E87.79
Waterbrash R12
Waterhouse(-Friderichsen) syndrome or
    disease (meningococcal) A39.1
Water-losing nephritis N25.89
Watermelon stomach K31.819
  with hemorrhage K31.811
  without hemorrhage K31.819
Watsoniasis B66.8
Wax in ear —see Impaction, cerumen
Weak, weakening, weakness (generalized)
    R53.1
  arches (acquired) —see also Deformity, limb,
    flat foot
  bladder (sphincter) R32

Weak, weakening, weakness (Continued)
  facial R29.810
    following
      cerebrovascular disease I69.992
        cerebral infarction I69.392
        intracerebral hemorrhage I69.192
        nontraumatic intracranial hemorrhage
          NEC I69.292
        specified disease NEC I69.892
        stroke I69.392
        subarachnoid hemorrhage I69.092
  foot (double) —see also Weak, arches
  heart, cardiac —see Failure, heart
  mind F70
  muscle M62.81
  myocardium —see Failure, heart
  newborn P96.89
  pelvic fundus N81.89
  pubocervical tissue N81.82
  rectovaginal tissue N81.83
  senile R54
  urinary stream R39.12
  valvular —see Endocarditis
Wear, worn (with normal or routine use)
  articular bearing surface of internal joint
    prosthesis —see Complications, joint
    prosthesis, mechanical, wear of articular
    bearing surfaces, by site
  device, implant or graft —see Complications,
    by site, mechanical complication
  tooth, teeth (approximal) (hard tissues)
    (interproximal) (occlusal) K03.0
Weather, weathered
  effects of
    cold T69.9
      specified effect NEC T69.8
    hot —see Heat
  skin L57.8
Weaver's syndrome Q87.3
Web, webbed (congenital)
  duodenal Q43.8
  esophagus Q39.4
  fingers Q70.1
  larynx (glottic) (subglottic) Q31.0
  neck (pterygium colli) Q18.3
  Paterson-Kelly D50.1
  popliteal syndrome Q87.89
  toes Q70.3
Weber-Christian disease M35.6
Weber-Cockayne syndrome (epidermolysis
    bullosa) Q81.8
Weber-Gubler syndrome G46.3
Weber-Leyden syndrome G46.3
Weber-Osler syndrome I78.0
Weber's paralysis or syndrome G46.3
Wedge-shaped or wedging vertebra —see
    Collapse, vertebra NEC
Wegener's granulomatosis or syndrome
    M31.30
  with
    kidney involvement M31.31
    lung involvement M31.30
      with kidney involvement M31.31
Wegner's disease A50.02
Weight
  1000-2499 grams at birth (low) —see Low,
    birthweight
  999 grams or less at birth (extremely low) —
    see Low, birthweight, extreme
  and length below 10th percentile for
    gestational age P05.1-●
  below but length above 10th percentile for
    gestational age P05.0-●
  gain (abnormal) (excessive) R63.5
    in pregnancy —see Pregnancy, complicated
      by, excessive weight gain
    low —see Pregnancy, complicated by,
      insufficient, weight gain
  loss (abnormal) (cause unknown) R63.4
Weightlessness (effect of) T75.82

Weil (l)-Marchesani syndrome Q87.19
Weil's disease A27.0
Weingarten's syndrome J82.89
Weir Mitchell's disease I73.81
Weiss-Baker syndrome G90.09
Wells' disease L98.3
Wen —see Cyst, sebaceous
Wenckebach's block or phenomenon I44.1
Werdnig-Hoffmann syndrome (muscular
    atrophy) G12.0
Werlhof's disease D69.3
Werner-His disease A79.0
Wermer's disease or syndrome E31.21
Werner's disease or syndrome E34.8
Wernicke-Korsakoff's syndrome or psychosis
    (alcoholic) F10.96
  with dependence F10.26
  drug-induced
    due to drug abuse —see Abuse, drug, by
      type, with amnestic disorder
    due to drug dependence —see
      Dependence, drug, by type, with
      amnestic disorder
  nonalcoholic F04
Wernicke-Posadas disease B38.9
Wernicke's
  developmental aphasia F80.2
  disease or syndrome E51.2
  encephalopathy E51.2
  polioencephalitis, superior E51.2
West African fever B50.8
Westphal-Strümpell syndrome E83.01
West's syndrome —see Epilepsy, spasms
Wet
  feet, tropical (maceration) (syndrome) —see
    Immersion, foot
  lung (syndrome), newborn P22.1
Wharton's duct —see condition
Wheal —see Urticaria
Wheezing R06.2
Whiplash injury S13.4
Whipple's disease —see also subcategory
    M14.8-● K90.81
Whipworm (disease) (infection) (infestation)
    B79
Whistling face Q87.0
White —see also condition
  kidney, small N03.9
  leg, puerperal, postpartum, childbirth O87.1
  mouth B37.0
  patches of mouth K13.29
  spot lesions, teeth
    chewing surface K02.51
    pit and fissure surface K02.51
    smooth surface K02.61
Whitehead L70.0
Whitlow —see also Cellulitis, digit
  with lymphangitis —see Lymphangitis, acute,
    digit
  herpesviral B00.89
Whitmore's disease or fever —see Melioidosis
Whooping cough A37.90
  with pneumonia A37.91
    due to Bordetella
      bronchiseptica A37.81
      parapertussis A37.11
      pertussis A37.01
      specified organism NEC A37.81
  due to
    Bordetella
      bronchiseptica A37.80
        with pneumonia A37.81
      parapertussis A37.10
        with pneumonia A37.11
      pertussis A37.00
        with pneumonia A37.01
      specified NEC A37.80
        with pneumonia A37.81
Wichman's asthma J38.5
Wide cranial sutures, newborn P96.3

Widening aorta —*see* Ectasia, aorta
  with aneurysm —*see* Aneurysm, aorta
Wilkie's disease or syndrome K55.1
Wilkinson-Sneddon disease or syndrome
  L13.1
➠Willebrand (-Jürgens) thrombopathy —*see*
  Disease, von Willebrand
Williams syndrome Q93.82
Willige-Hunt disease or syndrome G23.1
Wilms' tumor C64-●
Wilson-Mikity syndrome P27.0
Wilson's
  disease or syndrome E83.01
  hepatolenticular degeneration E83.01
  lichen ruber L43.9
Window —*see also* Imperfect, closure
  aorticopulmonary Q21.4
Winter —*see* condition
Wiskott-Aldrich syndrome D82.0
Withdrawal state —*see also* Dependence, drug
  by type, with withdrawal
  alcohol
    with perceptual disturbances F10.232
      ▶due to alcohol abuse F10.132
      ▶due to alcohol use F10.932
    ▶abuse —*see* Abuse, alcohol, with,
      withdrawal
    ▶dependence —*see* Dependence, alcohol,
      with, withdrawal
    ▶use —*see* Use, alcohol, with, withdrawal
    without perceptual disturbances F10.239
      ▶due to alcohol abuse F10.139
      ▶due to alcohol use F10.939
  caffeine F15.93
  cannabis F12.23
  newborn
    correct therapeutic substance properly
      administered P96.2
    infant of dependent mother P96.1
  therapeutic substance, neonatal P96.2
Witts' anemia D50.8
Witzelsucht F07.0
Woakes' ethmoiditis or syndrome J33.1
Wolff-Hirschorn syndrome Q93.3
Wolff-Parkinson-White syndrome I45.6
Wolhynian fever A79.0
Wolman's disease E75.5
Wood lung or pneumonitis J67.8
Woolly, wooly hair (congenital) (nevus) Q84.1
Woolsorter's disease A22.1
Word
  blindness (congenital) (developmental)
    F81.0
  deafness (congenital) (developmental)
    H93.25
Worm(s) (infection) (infestation) —*see also*
  Infestation, helminth
  guinea B72
  in intestine NEC B82.0
Worm-eaten soles A66.3
Worn out —*see* Exhaustion
  cardiac
    defibrillator (with synchronous cardiac
      pacemaker) Z45.02
    pacemaker
      battery Z45.010
      lead Z45.018
  device, implant or graft —*see* Complications,
    by site, mechanical
Worried well Z71.1
Worries R45.82
Wound check Z48.0-●
  due to injury - code to Injury, by site, using
    appropriate seventh character for
    subsequent encounter
Wound, open T14.8-●
  abdomen, abdominal
    wall S31.109
      with penetration into peritoneal cavity
        S31.609
      bite —*see* Bite, abdomen, wall

Wound, open (*Continued*)
  abdomen, abdominal (*Continued*)
    wall (*Continued*)
      epigastric region S31.102
        with penetration into peritoneal cavity
          S31.602
        bite —*see* Bite, abdomen, wall,
          epigastric region
        laceration —*see* Laceration, abdomen,
          wall, epigastric region
        puncture —*see* Puncture, abdomen,
          wall, epigastric region
      laceration —*see* Laceration, abdomen, wall
      left
        lower quadrant S31.104
          with penetration into peritoneal
            cavity S31.604
          bite —*see* Bite, abdomen, wall, left,
            lower quadrant
          laceration —*see* Laceration, abdomen,
            wall, left, lower quadrant
          puncture —*see* Puncture, abdomen,
            wall, left, lower quadrant
        upper quadrant S31.101
          with penetration into peritoneal
            cavity S31.601
          bite —*see* Bite, abdomen, wall, left,
            upper quadrant
          laceration —*see* Laceration,
            abdomen, wall, left, upper
            quadrant
          puncture —*see* Puncture, abdomen,
            wall, left, upper quadrant
      periumbilic region S31.105
        with penetration into peritoneal cavity
          S31.605
        bite —*see* Bite, abdomen, wall,
          periumbilic region
        laceration —*see* Laceration, abdomen,
          wall, periumbilic region
        puncture —*see* Puncture, abdomen,
          wall, periumbilic region
      puncture —*see* Puncture, abdomen, wall
      right
        lower quadrant S31.103
          with penetration into peritoneal
            cavity S31.603
          bite —*see* Bite, abdomen, wall, right,
            lower quadrant
          laceration —*see* Laceration,
            abdomen, wall, right, lower
            quadrant
          puncture —*see* Puncture, abdomen,
            wall, right, lower quadrant
        upper quadrant S31.100
          with penetration into peritoneal
            cavity S31.600
          bite —*see* Bite, abdomen, wall, right,
            upper quadrant
          laceration —*see* Laceration,
            abdomen, wall, right, upper
            quadrant
          puncture —*see* Puncture, abdomen,
            wall, right, upper quadrant
  alveolar (process) —*see* Wound, open, oral
    cavity
  ankle S91.00-●
    bite —*see* Bite, ankle
    laceration —*see* Laceration, ankle
    puncture —*see* Puncture, ankle
  antecubital space —*see* Wound, open, elbow
  anterior chamber, eye —*see* Wound, open,
    ocular
  anus S31.839
    bite S31.835
    laceration —*see* Laceration, anus
    puncture —*see* Puncture, anus
  arm (upper) S41.10-●
    with amputation —*see* Amputation,
      traumatic, arm
    bite —*see* Bite, arm

Wound, open (*Continued*)
  arm (*Continued*)
    forearm —*see* Wound, open, forearm
    laceration —*see* Laceration, arm
    puncture —*see* Puncture, arm
  auditory canal (external) (meatus) —*see*
    Wound, open, ear
  auricle, ear —*see* Wound, open, ear
  axilla —*see* Wound, open, arm
  back —*see also* Wound, open, thorax, back
    lower S31.000
      with penetration into retroperitoneal
        space S31.001
      bite —*see* Bite, back, lower
      laceration —*see* Laceration, back, lower
      puncture —*see* Puncture, back, lower
  bite —*see* Bite
  blood vessel —*see* Injury, blood vessel
  breast S21.00-●
    with amputation —*see* Amputation,
      traumatic, breast
    bite —*see* Bite, breast
    laceration —*see* Laceration, breast
    puncture —*see* Puncture, breast
  buttock S31.809
    bite —*see* Bite, buttock
    laceration —*see* Laceration, buttock
    left S31.829
    puncture —*see* Puncture, buttock
    right S31.819
  calf —*see* Wound, open, leg
  canaliculus lacrimalis —*see* Wound, open,
    eyelid
  canthus, eye —*see* Wound, open, eyelid
  cervical esophagus S11.20
    bite S11.25
    laceration —*see* Laceration, esophagus,
      traumatic, cervical
    puncture —*see* Puncture, cervical
      esophagus
  cheek (external) S01.40-●
    bite —*see* Bite, cheek
    internal —*see* Wound, open, oral cavity
    laceration —*see* Laceration, cheek
    puncture —*see* Puncture, cheek
  chest wall —*see* Wound, open, thorax
  chin —*see* Wound, open, head, specified site
    NEC
  choroid —*see* Wound, open, ocular
  ciliary body (eye) —*see* Wound, open,
    ocular
  clitoris S31.40
    with amputation —*see* Amputation,
      traumatic, clitoris
    bite S31.45
    laceration —*see* Laceration, vulva
    puncture —*see* Puncture, vulva
  conjunctiva —*see* Wound, open, ocular
  cornea —*see* Wound, open, ocular
  costal region —*see* Wound, open, thorax
  Descemet's membrane —*see* Wound, open,
    ocular
  digit(s)
    foot —*see* Wound, open, toe
    hand —*see* Wound, open, finger
  ear (canal) (external) S01.30-●
    with amputation —*see* Amputation,
      traumatic, ear
    bite —*see* Bite, ear
    drum S09.2-●
    laceration —*see* Laceration, ear
    puncture —*see* Puncture, ear
  elbow S51.00-●
    bite —*see* Bite, elbow
    laceration —*see* Laceration, elbow
    puncture —*see* Puncture, elbow
  epididymis —*see* Wound, open, testis
  epigastric region S31.102
    with penetration into peritoneal cavity
      S31.602
    bite —*see* Bite, abdomen, wall, epigastric
      region

▶ New   ➠ Revised   ~~deleted~~ Deleted   ● Use Additional Character(s)

Wound, open *(Continued)*
  epigastric region *(Continued)*
    laceration —*see* Laceration, abdomen, wall, epigastric region
    puncture —*see* Puncture, abdomen, wall, epigastric region
  epiglottis —*see* Wound, open, neck, specified site NEC
  esophagus (thoracic) S27.819
    cervical —*see* Wound, open, cervical esophagus
    laceration S27.813
    specified type NEC S27.818
  eye —*see* Wound, open, ocular
  eyeball —*see* Wound, open, ocular
  eyebrow —*see* Wound, open, eyelid
  eyelid S01.10-•
    bite —*see* Bite, eyelid
    laceration —*see* Laceration, eyelid
    puncture —*see* Puncture, eyelid
  face NEC —*see* Wound, open, head, specified site NEC
  finger(s) S61.209
    with
      amputation —*see* Amputation, traumatic, finger
      damage to nail S61.309
    bite —*see* Bite, finger
    index S61.208
      with
        damage to nail S61.308
      left S61.201
        with
          damage to nail S61.301
      right S61.200
        with
          damage to nail S61.300
    laceration —*see* Laceration, finger
    little S61.208
      with
        damage to nail S61.308
      left S61.207
        with damage to nail S61.307
      right S61.206
        with damage to nail S61.306
    middle S61.208
      with
        damage to nail S61.308
      left S61.203
        with damage to nail S61.303
      right S61.202
        with damage to nail S61.302
    puncture —*see* Puncture, finger
    ring S61.208
      with
        damage to nail S61.308
      left S61.205
        with damage to nail S61.305
      right S61.204
        with damage to nail S61.304
  flank —*see* Wound, open, abdomen, wall
  foot (except toe(s) alone) S91.30-•
    with amputation —*see* Amputation, traumatic, foot
    bite —*see* Bite, foot
    laceration —*see* Laceration, foot
    puncture —*see* Puncture, foot
    toe —*see* Wound, open, toe
  forearm S51.80-•
    with
      amputation —*see* Amputation, traumatic, forearm
    bite —*see* Bite, forearm
    elbow only —*see* Wound, open, elbow
    laceration —*see* Laceration, forearm
    puncture —*see* Puncture, forearm
  forehead —*see* Wound, open, head, specified site NEC
  genital organs, external
    with amputation —*see* Amputation, traumatic, genital organs

Wound, open *(Continued)*
  genital organs, external *(Continued)*
    bite —*see* Bite, genital organ
    female S31.502
      vagina S31.40
      vulva S31.40
    laceration —*see* Laceration, genital organ
    male S31.501
      penis S31.20
      scrotum S31.30
      testes S31.30
    puncture —*see* Puncture, genital organ
  globe (eye) —*see* Wound, open, ocular
  groin —*see* Wound, open, abdomen, wall
  gum —*see* Wound, open, oral cavity
  hand S61.40-•
    with
      amputation —*see* Amputation, traumatic, hand
    bite —*see* Bite, hand
    finger(s) —*see* Wound, open, finger
    laceration —*see* Laceration, hand
    puncture —*see* Puncture, hand
    thumb —*see* Wound, open, thumb
  head S01.90
    bite —*see* Bite, head
    cheek —*see* Wound, open, cheek
    ear —*see* Wound, open, ear
    eyelid —*see* Wound, open, eyelid
    laceration —*see* Laceration, head
    lip —*see* Wound, open, lip
    nose S01.20
    oral cavity —*see* Wound, open, oral cavity
    puncture —*see* Puncture, head
    scalp —*see* Wound, open, scalp
    specified site NEC S01.80
    temporomandibular area —*see* Wound, open, cheek
  heel —*see* Wound, open, foot
  hip S71.00-•
    with amputation —*see* Amputation, traumatic, hip
    bite —*see* Bite, hip
    laceration —*see* Laceration, hip
    puncture —*see* Puncture, hip
  hymen S31.40
    bite —*see* Bite, vulva
    laceration —*see* Laceration, vagina
    puncture —*see* Puncture, vagina
  hypochondrium S31.109
    bite —*see* Bite, hypochondrium
    laceration —*see* Laceration, hypochondrium
    puncture —*see* Puncture, hypochondrium
  hypogastric region S31.109
    bite —*see* Bite, hypogastric region
    laceration —*see* Laceration, hypogastric region
    puncture —*see* Puncture, hypogastric region
  iliac (region) —*see* Wound, open, inguinal region
  inguinal region S31.109
    bite —*see* Bite, abdomen, wall, lower quadrant
    laceration —*see* Laceration, inguinal region
    puncture —*see* Puncture, inguinal region
  instep —*see* Wound, open, foot
  interscapular region —*see* Wound, open, thorax, back
  intraocular —*see* Wound, open, ocular
  iris —*see* Wound, open, ocular
  jaw —*see* Wound, open, head, specified site NEC
  knee S81.00-•
    bite —*see* Bite, knee
    laceration —*see* Laceration, knee
    puncture —*see* Puncture, knee
  labium (majus) (minus) —*see* Wound, open, vulva

Wound, open *(Continued)*
  laceration —*see* Laceration, by site
  lacrimal duct —*see* Wound, open, eyelid
  larynx S11.019
    bite —*see* Bite, larynx
    laceration —*see* Laceration, larynx
    puncture —*see* Puncture, larynx
  left
    lower quadrant S31.104
      with penetration into peritoneal cavity S31.604
      bite —*see* Bite, abdomen, wall, left, lower quadrant
      laceration —*see* Laceration, abdomen, wall, left, lower quadrant
      puncture —*see* Puncture, abdomen, wall, left, lower quadrant
    upper quadrant S31.101
      with penetration into peritoneal cavity S31.601
      bite —*see* Bite, abdomen, wall, left, upper quadrant
      laceration —*see* Laceration, abdomen, wall, left, upper quadrant
      puncture —*see* Puncture, abdomen, wall, left, upper quadrant
  leg (lower) S81.80-•
    with amputation —*see* Amputation, traumatic, leg
    ankle —*see* Wound, open, ankle
    bite —*see* Bite, leg
    foot —*see* Wound, open, foot
    knee —*see* Wound, open, knee
    laceration —*see* Laceration, leg
    puncture —*see* Puncture, leg
    toe —*see* Wound, open, toe
    upper —*see* Wound, open, thigh
  lip S01.501
    bite —*see* Bite, lip
    laceration —*see* Laceration, lip
    puncture —*see* Puncture, lip
  loin S31.109
    bite —*see* Bite, abdomen, wall
    laceration —*see* Laceration, loin
    puncture —*see* Puncture, loin
  lower back —*see* Wound, open, back, lower
  lumbar region —*see* Wound, open, back, lower
  malar region —*see* Wound, open, head, specified site NEC
  mammary —*see* Wound, open, breast
  mastoid region —*see* Wound, open, head, specified site NEC
  mouth —*see* Wound, open, oral cavity
  nail
    finger —*see* Wound, open, finger, with damage to nail
    toe —*see* Wound, open, toe, with damage to nail
  nape (neck) —*see* Wound, open, neck
  nasal (septum) (sinus) —*see* Wound, open, nose
  nasopharynx —*see* Wound, open, head, specified site NEC
  neck S11.90
    bite —*see* Bite, neck
    involving
      cervical esophagus S11.20
      larynx —*see* Wound, open, larynx
      pharynx S11.20
      thyroid S11.10
      trachea (cervical) S11.029
        bite —*see* Bite, trachea
        laceration S11.021
          with foreign body S11.022
        puncture S11.023
          with foreign body S11.024
    laceration —*see* Laceration, neck
    puncture —*see* Puncture, neck
    specified site NEC S11.80
      specified type NEC S11.89

Wound, open *(Continued)*
  nose (septum) (sinus) S01.20
    with amputation —*see* Amputation,
      traumatic, nose
    bite —*see* Bite, nose
    laceration —*see* Laceration, nose
    puncture —*see* Puncture, nose
  ocular S05.90
    avulsion (traumatic enucleation) S05.7-●
    eyeball S05.6-●
      with foreign body S05.5-●
    eyelid —*see* Wound, open, eyelid
    laceration and rupture S05.3-●
      with prolapse or loss of intraocular
        tissue S05.2-●
    orbit (penetrating) (with or without foreign
      body) S05.4-●
    periocular area —*see* Wound, open, eyelid
    specified NEC S05.8X-●
  oral cavity S01.502
    bite S01.552
    laceration —*see* Laceration, oral cavity
    puncture —*see* Puncture, oral cavity
  orbit —*see* Wound, open, ocular, orbit
  palate —*see* Wound, open, oral cavity
  palm —*see* Wound, open, hand
  pelvis, pelvic —*see also* Wound, open, back,
    lower
    girdle —*see* Wound, open, hip
  penetrating —*see* Puncture, by site
  penis S31.20
    with amputation —*see* Amputation,
      traumatic, penis
    bite S31.25
    laceration —*see* Laceration, penis
    puncture —*see* Puncture, penis
  perineum
    bite —*see* Bite, perineum
    female S31.502
    laceration —*see* Laceration, perineum
    male S31.501
    puncture —*see* Puncture, perineum
  periocular area (with or without lacrimal
    passages) —*see* Wound, open, eyelid
  periumbilic region S31.105
    with penetration into peritoneal cavity
      S31.605
    bite —*see* Bite, abdomen, wall, periumbilic
      region
    laceration —*see* Laceration, abdomen, wall,
      periumbilic region
    puncture —*see* Puncture, abdomen, wall,
      periumbilic region
  phalanges
    finger —*see* Wound, open, finger
    toe —*see* Wound, open, toe
  pharynx S11.20
  pinna —*see* Wound, open, ear
  popliteal space —*see* Wound, open, knee
  prepuce —*see* Wound, open, penis
  pubic region —*see* Wound, open, back, lower
  pudendum —*see* Wound, open, genital
    organs, external
  puncture wound —*see* Puncture
  rectovaginal septum —*see* Wound, open,
    vagina
  right
    lower quadrant S31.103
      with penetration into peritoneal cavity
        S31.603
      bite —*see* Bite, abdomen, wall, right,
        lower quadrant
      laceration —*see* Laceration, abdomen,
        wall, right, lower quadrant
      puncture —*see* Puncture, abdomen, wall,
        right, lower quadrant
    upper quadrant S31.100
      with penetration into peritoneal cavity
        S31.600

Wound, open *(Continued)*
  right *(Continued)*
    upper quadrant *(Continued)*
      bite —*see* Bite, abdomen, wall, right,
        upper quadrant
      laceration —*see* Laceration, abdomen,
        wall, right, upper quadrant
      puncture —*see* Puncture, abdomen, wall,
        right, upper quadrant
  sacral region —*see* Wound, open, back, lower
  sacroiliac region —*see* Wound, open, back,
    lower
  salivary gland —*see* Wound, open, oral cavity
  scalp S01.00
    bite S01.05
    laceration —*see* Laceration, scalp
    puncture —*see* Puncture, scalp
  scalpel, newborn (birth injury) P15.8
  scapular region —*see* Wound, open, shoulder
  sclera —*see* Wound, open, ocular
  scrotum S31.30
    with amputation —*see* Amputation,
      traumatic, scrotum
    bite S31.35
    laceration —*see* Laceration, scrotum
    puncture —*see* Puncture, scrotum
  shin —*see* Wound, open, leg
  shoulder S41.00-●
    with amputation —*see* Amputation,
      traumatic, arm
    bite —*see* Bite, shoulder
    laceration —*see* Laceration, shoulder
    puncture —*see* Puncture, shoulder
  skin NOS T14.8
  spermatic cord —*see* Wound, open, testis
  sternal region —*see* Wound, open, thorax,
    front wall
  submaxillary region —*see* Wound, open,
    head, specified site NEC
  submental region —*see* Wound, open, head,
    specified site NEC
  subungual
    finger(s) —*see* Wound, open, finger
    toe(s) —*see* Wound, open, toe
  supraclavicular region —*see* Wound, open,
    neck, specified site NEC
  temple, temporal region —*see* Wound, open,
    head, specified site NEC
  temporomandibular area —*see* Wound, open,
    cheek
  testis S31.30
    with amputation —*see* Amputation,
      traumatic, testes
    bite S31.35
    laceration —*see* Laceration, testis
    puncture —*see* Puncture, testis
  thigh S71.10-●
    with amputation —*see* Amputation,
      traumatic, hip
    bite —*see* Bite, thigh
    laceration —*see* Laceration, thigh
    puncture —*see* Puncture, thigh
  thorax, thoracic (wall) S21.90
    back S21.20-●
      with penetration S21.40
    bite —*see* Bite, thorax
    breast —*see* Wound, open, breast
    front S21.10-●
      with penetration S21.30
    laceration —*see* Laceration, thorax
    puncture —*see* Puncture, thorax
  throat —*see* Wound, open, neck
  thumb S61.009
    with
      amputation —*see* Amputation,
        traumatic, thumb
      damage to nail S61.109
    bite —*see* Bite, thumb
    laceration —*see* Laceration, thumb

Wound, open *(Continued)*
  thumb *(Continued)*
    left S61.002
      with
        damage to nail S61.102
    puncture —*see* Puncture, thumb
    right S61.001
      with
        damage to nail S61.101
  thyroid (gland) —*see* Wound, open, neck,
    thyroid
  toe(s) S91.109
    with
      amputation —*see* Amputation,
        traumatic, toe
      damage to nail S91.209
    bite —*see* Bite, toe
    great S91.103
      with
        damage to nail S91.203
      left S91.102
        with
          damage to nail S91.202
      right S91.101
        with
          damage to nail S91.201
    laceration —*see* Laceration, toe
    lesser S91.106
      with
        damage to nail S91.206
      left S91.105
        with
          damage to nail S91.205
      right S91.104
        with
          damage to nail S91.204
    puncture —*see* Puncture, toe
  tongue —*see* Wound, open, oral cavity
  trachea (cervical region) —*see* Wound, open,
    neck, trachea
  tunica vaginalis —*see* Wound, open, testis
  tympanum, tympanic membrane S09.2-●
    laceration —*see* Laceration, ear, drum
    puncture —*see* Puncture, tympanum
  umbilical region —*see* Wound, open,
    abdomen, wall, periumbilic region
  uvula —*see* Wound, open, oral cavity
  vagina S31.40
    bite S31.45
    laceration —*see* Laceration, vagina
    puncture —*see* Puncture, vagina
  vitreous (humor) —*see* Wound, open, ocular
  vocal cord S11.039
    bite —*see* Bite, vocal cord
    laceration S11.031
      with foreign body S11.032
    puncture S11.033
      with foreign body S11.034
  vulva S31.40
    with amputation —*see* Amputation,
      traumatic, vulva
    bite S31.45
    laceration —*see* Laceration, vulva
    puncture —*see* Puncture, vulva
  wrist S61.50-●
    bite —*see* Bite, wrist
    laceration —*see* Laceration, wrist
    puncture —*see* Puncture, wrist
Wound, superficial —*see* Injury (*see also*
  specified injury type)
Wright's syndrome G54.0
Wrist —*see* condition
Wrong drug (by accident) (given in error) —
  see Table of Drugs and Chemicals, by
  drug, poisoning
Wry neck —*see* Torticollis
Wuchereria (bancrofti) **infestation** B74.0
Wuchereriasis B74.0
Wuchernde Struma Langhans C73

▶ New ➡ Revised ~~deleted~~ Deleted ● Use Additional Character(s)

X

Xanthelasma (eyelid) (palpebrarum) H02.60
  left H02.66
    lower H02.65
    upper H02.64
  right H02.63
    lower H02.62
    upper H02.61
Xanthelasmatosis (essential) E78.2
Xanthinuria, hereditary E79.8
Xanthoastrocytoma
  specified site —*see* Neoplasm, malignant, by site
  unspecified site C71.9
Xanthofibroma —*see* Neoplasm, connective tissue, benign
Xanthogranuloma D76.3
Xanthoma(s), xanthomatosis (primary) (familial) (hereditary) E75.5
  with
    hyperlipoproteinemia
      Type I E78.3
      Type III E78.2
      Type IV E78.1
      Type V E78.3
  bone (generalisata) C96.5
  cerebrotendinous E75.5
  cutaneotendinous E75.5

Xanthoma(s), xanthomatosis *(Continued)*
  disseminatum (skin) E78.2
  eruptive E78.2
  hypercholesterinemic E78.00
  hypercholesterolemic E78.00
  hyperlipidemic E78.5
  joint E75.5
  multiple (skin) E78.2
  tendon (sheath) E75.5
  tuberosum E78.2
  tuberous E78.2
  tubo-eruptive E78.2
  verrucous, oral mucosa K13.4
Xanthosis R23.8
Xenophobia F40.10
Xeroderma —*see also* Ichthyosis
  acquired L85.0
    eyelid H01.149
      left H01.146
        lower H01.145
        upper H01.144
      right H01.143
        lower H01.142
        upper H01.141
  pigmentosum Q82.1
  vitamin A deficiency E50.8
Xerophthalmia (vitamin A deficiency) E50.7
  unrelated to vitamin A deficiency —*see* Keratoconjunctivitis

Xerosis
  conjunctiva H11.14-●
    with Bitot's spots —*see also* Pigmentation, conjunctiva
      vitamin A deficiency E50.1
    vitamin A deficiency E50.0
  cornea H18.89-●
    with ulceration —*see* Ulcer, cornea
      vitamin A deficiency E50.3
    vitamin A deficiency E50.2
  cutis (dry skin) L85.3
  skin L85.3
Xerostomia K11.7
Xiphopagus Q89.4
XO syndrome Q96.9
X-ray (of)
  abnormal findings —*see* Abnormal, diagnostic imaging
  breast (mammogram) (routine) Z12.31
  chest
    routine (as part of a general medical examination) Z00.00
      with abnormal findings Z00.01
  routine (as part of a general medical examination) Z00.00
    with abnormal findings Z00.01
XXXXY syndrome Q98.1
XXY syndrome Q98.0

Y

Yaba pox virus disease B08.72
Yatapoxvirus B08.70
  specified NEC B08.79
Yawning R06.89
  psychogenic F45.8
Yaws A66.9
  bone lesions A66.6
  butter A66.1
  chancre A66.0
  cutaneous, less than five years after infection
      A66.2
  early (cutaneous) (macular) (maculopapular)
      (micropapular) (papular) A66.2
    frambeside A66.2
    skin lesions NEC A66.2
  eyelid A66.2
  ganglion A66.6
  gangosis, gangosa A66.5
  gumma, gummata A66.4
    bone A66.6
  gummatous
    frambeside A66.4
    osteitis A66.6
    periostitis A66.6
  hydrarthrosis —see also subcategory
      M14.8-● A66.6
  hyperkeratosis (early) (late) A66.3

Yaws (Continued)
  initial lesions A66.0
  joint lesions —see also subcategory
      M14.8-● A66.6
  juxta-articular nodules A66.7
  late nodular (ulcerated) A66.4
  latent (without clinical manifestations) (with
      positive serology) A66.8
  mother A66.0
  mucosal A66.7
  multiple papillomata A66.1
  nodular, late (ulcerated) A66.4
  osteitis A66.6
  papilloma, plantar or palmar A66.1
  periostitis (hypertrophic) A66.6
  specified NEC A66.7
  ulcers A66.4
  wet crab A66.1
Yeast infection —see also Candidiasis B37.9
Yellow
  atrophy (liver) —see Failure, hepatic
  fever —see Fever, yellow
  jack —see Fever, yellow
  jaundice —see Jaundice
  nail syndrome L60.5
Yersiniosis —see also Infection, Yersinia
  extraintestinal A28.2
  intestinal A04.6

Z

Zahorsky's syndrome (herpangina) B08.5
Zellweger's syndrome E71.510
Zenker's diverticulum (esophagus) K22.5
Ziehen-Oppenheim disease G24.1
Zieve's syndrome K70.0
Zika NOS A92.5
  congenital P35.4
Zinc
  deficiency, dietary E60
  metabolism disorder E83.2
Zollinger-Ellison syndrome E16.4
Zona —see Herpes, zoster
Zoophobia F40.218
Zoster (herpes) —see Herpes, zoster
Zygomycosis B46.9
  specified NEC B46.8
Zymotic —see condition

Y, Z

▶ New   ⟹ Revised   ~~deleted~~ Deleted   ● Use Additional Character(s)

ICD-10-CM
Table of Neoplasms

The list below gives the code numbers for neoplasms by anatomical site. For each site there are six possible code numbers according to whether the neoplasm in question is malignant, benign, in situ, of uncertain behavior, or of unspecified nature. The description of the neoplasm will often indicate which of the six columns is appropriate; e.g., malignant melanoma of skin, benign fibroadenoma of breast, carcinoma in situ of cervix uteri.

Where such descriptors are not present, the remainder of the Index should be consulted where guidance is given to the appropriate column for each morphological (histological) variety listed; e.g., Mesonephroma — *see Neoplasm, malignant;* Embryoma — *see also Neoplasm, uncertain behavior;* Disease, Bowen's — *see Neoplasm, skin, in situ.* However, the guidance in the Index can be overridden if one of the descriptors mentioned above is present; e.g., malignant adenoma of colon is coded to C18.9 and not to D12.6 as the adjective "Malignant" overrides the Index entry 'Adenoma — *see also Neoplasm, benign.*'

Codes listed with a dash -, following the code have a required additional character for laterality. The Tablular must be reviewed for the complete code.

	Malignant Primary	Malignant Secondary	Ca in situ	Benign	Uncertain Behavior	Unspecified Behavior
Neoplasm, neoplastic	C80.1	C79.9	D09.9	D36.9	D48.9	D49.9
abdomen, abdominal	C76.2	C79.8-•	D09.8	D36.7	D48.7	D49.89
cavity	C76.2	C79.8-•	D09.8	D36.7	D48.7	D49.89
organ	C76.2	C79.8-•	D09.8	D36.7	D48.7	D49.89
viscera	C76.2	C79.8-•	D09.8	D36.7	D48.7	D49.89
wall — *see also Neoplasm, abdomen, wall, skin*	C44.509	C79.2-•	D04.5	D23.5	D48.5	D49.2
connective tissue	C49.4	C79.8-•	—	D21.4	D48.1	D49.2
skin	C44.509					
basal cell carcinoma	C44.519	—	—	—	—	—
specified type NEC	C44.599	—	—	—	—	—
squamous cell carcinoma	C44.529	—	—	—	—	—
abdominopelvic	C76.8	C79.8-•	—	D36.7	D48.7	D49.89
accessory sinus — *see Neoplasm, sinus*						
acoustic nerve	C72.4-•	C79.49	—	D33.3	D43.3	D49.7
adenoid (pharynx) (tissue)	C11.1	C79.89	D00.08	D10.6	D37.05	D49.0
adipose tissue — *see also Neoplasm, connective tissue*	C49.4	C79.89	—	D21.9	D48.1	D49.2
adnexa (uterine)	C57.4	C79.89	D07.39	D28.7	D39.8	D49.59
adrenal	C74.9-•	C79.7-•	D09.3	D35.0-•	D44.1-•	D49.7
capsule	C74.9-•	C79.7-•	D09.3	D35.0-•	D44.1-•	D49.7
cortex	C74.0-•	C79.7-•	D09.3	D35.0-•	D44.1-•	D49.7
gland	C74.9-•	C79.7-•	D09.3	D35.0-•	D44.1-•	D49.7
medulla	C74.1-•	C79.7-•	D09.3	D35.0-•	D44.1-•	D49.7
ala nasi (external) — *see also Neoplasm, skin, nose*	C44.301	C79.2	D04.39	D23.39	D48.5	D49.2

	Malignant Primary	Malignant Secondary	Ca in situ	Benign	Uncertain Behavior	Unspecified Behavior
alimentary canal or tract NEC	C26.9	C78.80	D01.9	D13.9	D37.9	D49.0
alveolar	C03.9	C79.89	D00.03	D10.39	D37.09	D49.0
mucosa	C03.9	C79.89	D00.03	D10.39	D37.09	D49.0
lower	C03.1	C79.89	D00.03	D10.39	D37.09	D49.0
upper	C03.0	C79.89	D00.03	D10.39	D37.09	D49.0
ridge or process	C41.1	C79.51	—	D16.5-•	D48.0	D49.2
carcinoma	C03.9	C79.8-•	—	—	—	—
lower	C03.1	C79.8-•	—	—	—	—
upper	C03.0	C79.8-•	—	—	—	—
lower	C41.1	C79.51	—	D16.5-•	D48.0	D49.2
mucosa	C03.9	C79.89	D00.03	D10.39	D37.09	D49.0
lower	C03.1	C79.89	D00.03	D10.39	D37.09	D49.0
upper	C03.0	C79.89	D00.03	D10.39	D37.09	D49.0
upper	C41.0	C79.51	—	D16.4-•	D48.0	D49.2
sulcus	C06.1	C79.89	D00.02	D10.39	D37.09	D49.0
alveolus	C03.9	C79.89	D00.03	D10.39	D37.09	D49.0
lower	C03.1	C79.89	D00.03	D10.39	D37.09	D49.0
upper	C03.0	C79.89	D00.03	D10.39	D37.09	D49.0
ampulla of Vater	C24.1	C78.89	D01.5	D13.5	D37.6	D49.0
ankle NEC	C76.5-•	C79.89	D04.7-•	D36.7	D48.7	D49.89
anorectum, anorectal (junction)	C21.8	C78.5	D01.3	D12.9	D37.8	D49.0
antecubital fossa or space	C76.4-•	C79.89	D04.6-•	D36.7	D48.7	D49.89
antrum (Highmore) (maxillary)	C31.0	C78.39	D02.3	D14.0	D38.5	D49.1
pyloric	C16.3	C78.89	D00.2	D13.1	D37.1	D49.0
tympanicum	C30.1	C78.39	D02.3	D14.0	D38.5	D49.1
anus, anal	C21.0	C78.5	D01.3	D12.9	D37.8	D49.0
canal	C21.1	C78.5	D01.3	D12.9	D37.8	D49.0
cloacogenic zone	C21.2	C78.5	D01.3	D12.9	D37.8	D49.0
margin — *see also Neoplasm, anus, skin*	C44.500	C79.2	D04.5	D23.5	D48.5	D49.2
overlapping lesion with rectosigmoid junction or rectum	C21.8	—	—	—	—	—
skin	C44.500	C79.2	D04.5	D23.5	D48.5	D49.2
basal cell carcinoma	C44.510	—	—	—	—	—
specified type NEC	C44.590	—	—	—	—	—
squamous cell carcinoma	C44.520	—	—	—	—	—
sphincter	C21.1	C78.5	D01.3	D12.9	D37.8	D49.0
aorta (thoracic)	C49.3	C79.89	—	D21.3	D48.1	D49.2
abdominal	C49.4	C79.89	—	D21.4	D48.1	D49.2
aortic body	C75.5	C79.89	—	D35.6	D44.7	D49.7
aponeurosis	C49.9	C79.89	—	D21.9	D48.1	D49.2
palmar	C49.1-•	C79.89	—	D21.1-•	D48.1	D49.2
plantar	C49.2-•	C79.89	—	D21.2-•	D48.1	D49.2

TABLE OF NEOPLASMS

	Malignant Primary	Malignant Secondary	Ca in situ	Benign	Uncertain Behavior	Unspecified Behavior
appendix	C18.1	C78.5	D01.0	D12.1	D37.3	D49.0
arachnoid	C70.9	C79.49	—	D32.9	D42.9	D49.7
cerebral	C70.0	C79.32	—	D32.0	D42.0	D49.7
spinal	C70.1	C79.49	—	D32.1	D42.1	D49.7
areola	C50.0-●	C79.81	D05.-●	D24.-●	D48.6-●	D49.3
arm NEC	C76.4-●	C79.89	D04.6-●	D36.7	D48.7	D49.89
artery — see Neoplasm, connective tissue						
aryepiglottic fold	C13.1	C79.89	D00.08	D10.7	D37.05	D49.0
hypopharyngeal aspect	C13.1	C79.89	D00.08	D10.7	D37.05	D49.0
laryngeal aspect	C32.1	C78.39	D02.0	D14.1	D38.0	D49.1
marginal zone	C13.1	C79.89	D00.08	D10.7	D37.05	D49.0
arytenoid (cartilage)	C32.3	C78.39	D02.0	D14.1	D38.0	D49.1
fold — see Neoplasm, aryepiglottic						
associated with transplanted organ	C80.2	—	—	—	—	—
atlas	C41.2	C79.51	—	D16.6	D48.0	D49.2
atrium, cardiac	C38.0	C79.89	—	D15.1	D48.7	D49.89
auditory						
canal (external) (skin)	C44.20-●	C79.2	D04.2-●	D23.2-●	D48.5	D49.2
internal	C30.1	C78.39	D02.3	D14.0	D38.5	D49.1
nerve	C72.4-●	C79.49	—	D33.3	D43.3	D49.7
tube	C30.1	C78.39	D02.3	D14.0	D38.5	D49.1
opening	C11.2	C79.89	D00.08	D10.6	D37.05	D49.0
auricle, ear — see also Neoplasm, skin, ear	C44.20-●	C79.2	D04.2-●	D23.2-●	D48.5	D49.2
auricular canal (external) — see also Neoplasm, skin, ear	C44.20-●	C79.2	D04.2-●	D23.2-●	D48.5	D49.2
internal	C30.1	C78.39	D02.3	D14.0	D38.5	D49.2
autonomic nerve or nervous system NEC (see Neoplasm, nerve, peripheral)						
axilla, axillary	C76.1	C79.89	D09.8	D36.7	D48.7	D49.89
fold — see also Neoplasm, skin, trunk	C44.509	C79.2	D04.5	D23.5	D48.5	D49.2
back NEC	C76.8	C79.89	D04.5	D36.7	D48.7	D49.89
Bartholin's gland	C51.0	C79.82	D07.1	D28.0	D39.8	D49.59
basal ganglia	C71.0	C79.31	—	D33.0	D43.0	D49.6
basis pedunculi	C71.7	C79.31	—	D33.1	D43.1	D49.6
bile or biliary (tract)	C24.9	C78.89	D01.5	D13.5	D37.6	D49.0
canaliculi (biliferi) (intrahepatic)	C22.1	C78.7	D01.5	D13.4	D37.6	D49.0
canals, interlobular	C22.1	C78.89	D01.5	D13.4	D37.6	D49.0

	Malignant Primary	Malignant Secondary	Ca in situ	Benign	Uncertain Behavior	Unspecified Behavior
bile or biliary (Continued)						
duct or passage (common) (cystic) (extrahepatic)	C24.0	C78.89	D01.5	D13.5	D37.6	D49.0
interlobular	C22.1	C78.89	D01.5	D13.4	D37.6	D49.0
intrahepatic	C22.1	C78.7	D01.5	D13.4	D37.6	D49.0
and extrahepatic	C24.8	C78.89	D01.5	D13.5	D37.6	D49.0
bladder (urinary)	C67.9	C79.11	D09.0	D30.3	D41.4	D49.4
dome	C67.1	C79.11	D09.0	D30.3	D41.4	D49.4
neck	C67.5	C79.11	D09.0	D30.3	D41.4	D49.4
orifice	C67.9	C79.11	D09.0	D30.3	D41.4	D49.4
ureteric	C67.6	C79.11	D09.0	D30.3	D41.4	D49.4
urethral	C67.5	C79.11	D09.0	D30.3	D41.4	D49.4
overlapping lesion	C67.8	—	—	—	—	—
sphincter	C67.8	C79.11	D09.0	D30.3	D41.4	D49.4
trigone	C67.0	C79.11	D09.0	D30.3	D41.4	D49.4
urachus	C67.7	C79.11	D09.0	D30.3	D41.4	D49.4
wall	C67.9	C79.11	D09.0	D30.3	D41.4	D49.4
anterior	C67.3	C79.11	D09.0	D30.3	D41.4	D49.4
lateral	C67.2	C79.11	D09.0	D30.3	D41.4	D49.4
posterior	C67.4	C79.11	D09.0	D30.3	D41.4	D49.4
blood vessel — see Neoplasm, connective tissue						
bone (periosteum)	C41.9	C79.51	—	D16.9-●	D48.0	D49.2
acetabulum	C41.4	C79.51	—	D16.8-●	D48.0	D49.2
ankle	C40.3-●	C79.51	—	D16.3-●	—	—
arm NEC	C40.0-●	C79.51	—	D16.0-●	—	—
astragalus	C40.3-●	C79.51	—	D16.3-●	—	—
atlas	C41.2	C79.51	—	D16.6-●	D48.0	D49.2
axis	C41.2	C79.51	—	D16.6-●	D48.0	D49.2
back NEC	C41.2	C79.51	—	D16.6-●	D48.0	D49.2
calcaneus	C40.3-●	C79.51	—	D16.3-●	—	—
calvarium	C41.0	C79.51	—	D16.4-●	D48.0	D49.2
carpus (any)	C40.1-●	C79.51	—	D16.1-●	—	—
cartilage NEC	C41.9	C79.51	—	D16.9-●	D48.0	D49.2
clavicle	C41.3	C79.51	—	D16.7-●	D48.0	D49.2
clivus	C41.0	C79.51	—	D16.4-●	D48.0	D49.2
coccygeal vertebra	C41.4	C79.51	—	D16.8-●	D48.0	D49.2
coccyx	C41.4	C79.51	—	D16.8-●	D48.0	D49.2
costal cartilage	C41.3	C79.51	—	D16.7-●	D48.0	D49.2
costovertebral joint	C41.3	C79.51	—	D16.7-●	D48.0	D49.2
cranial	C41.0	C79.51	—	D16.4-●	D48.0	D49.2
cuboid	C40.3-●	C79.51	—	D16.3-●	—	—
cuneiform	C41.9	C79.51	—	D16.9-●	D48.0	D49.2
elbow	C40.0-●	C79.51	—	D16.0-●	—	—

◀ New ◀ Revised ~~deleted~~ Deleted ● Use Additional Character(s)

bone (Continued)	Malignant Primary	Malignant Secondary	Ca in situ	Benign	Uncertain Behavior	Unspecified Behavior
ethmoid (labyrinth)	C41.0	C79.51	—	D16.4-●	D48.0	D49.2
face	C41.0	C79.51	—	D16.4-●	D48.0	D49.2
femur (any part)	C40.2-●	C79.51	—	D16.2-●	—	—
fibula (any part)	C40.2-●	C79.51	—	D16.2-●	—	—
finger (any)	C40.1-●	C79.51	—	D16.1-●	—	—
foot	C40.3-●	C79.51	—	D16.3-●	—	—
forearm	C40.0-●	C79.51	—	D16.0-●	—	—
frontal	C41.0	C79.51	—	D16.4-●	D48.0	D49.2
hand	C40.1-●	C79.51	—	D16.1-●	—	—
heel	C40.3-●	C79.51	—	D16.3-●	—	—
hip	C41.4	C79.51	—	D16.8-●	D48.0	D49.2
humerus (any part)	C40.0-●	C79.51	—	D16.0-●	—	—
hyoid	C41.0	C79.51	—	D16.4-●	D48.0	D49.2
ilium	C41.4	C79.51	—	D16.8-●	D48.0	D49.2
innominate	C41.4	C79.51	—	D16.8-●	D48.0	D49.2
intervertebral cartilage or disc	C41.2	C79.51	—	D16.6-●	D48.0	D49.2
ischium	C41.4	C79.51	—	D16.8-●	D48.0	D49.2
jaw (lower)	C41.1	C79.51	—	D16.5-●	D48.0	D49.2
knee	C40.2-●	C79.51	—	D16.2-●	—	—
leg NEC	C40.2-●	C79.51	—	D16.2-●	—	—
limb NEC	C40.9-●	C79.51	—	D16.9-●	—	—
lower (long bones)	C40.2-●	C79.51	—	D16.2-●	—	—
short bones	C40.3-●	C79.51	—	D16.3-●	—	—
upper (long bones)	C40.0-●	C79.51	—	D16.0-●	—	—
short bones	C40.1-●	C79.51	—	D16.1-●	—	—
malar	C41.0	C79.51	—	D16.4-●	D48.0	D49.2
mandible	C41.1	C79.51	—	D16.5-●	D48.0	D49.2
marrow NEC (any bone)	C96.9	C79.52	—	—	D47.9	D49.89
mastoid	C41.0	C79.51	—	D16.4-●	D48.0	D49.2
maxilla, maxillary (superior)	C41.0	C79.51	—	D16.4-●	D48.0	D49.2
inferior	C41.1	C79.51	—	D16.5-●	D48.0	D49.2
metacarpus (any)	C40.1-●	C79.51	—	D16.1-●	—	—
metatarsus (any)	C40.3-●	C79.51	—	D16.3-●	—	—
overlapping sites	C40.8-●	—	—	—	—	—
navicular						
ankle	C40.3-●	C79.51	—	—	—	—
hand	C40.1-●	C79.51	—	—	—	—
nose, nasal	C41.0	C79.51	—	D16.4-●	D48.0	D49.2
occipital	C41.0	C79.51	—	D16.4-●	D48.0	D49.2
orbit	C41.0	C79.51	—	D16.4-●	D48.0	D49.2
parietal	C41.0	C79.51	—	D16.4-●	D48.0	D49.2
patella	C40.2-●	C79.51	—	—	—	—
pelvic	C41.4	C79.51	—	D16.8	D48.0	D49.2

bone (Continued)	Malignant Primary	Malignant Secondary	Ca in situ	Benign	Uncertain Behavior	Unspecified Behavior
phalanges						
foot	C40.3-●	C79.51	—	—	—	—
hand	C40.1-●	C79.51	—	—	—	—
pubic	C41.4	C79.51	—	D16.8	D48.0	D49.2
radius (any part)	C40.0-●	C79.51	—	D16.0-●	—	—
rib	C41.3	C79.51	—	D16.7	D48.0	D49.2
sacral vertebra	C41.4	C79.51	—	D16.8	D48.0	D49.2
sacrum	C41.4	C79.51	—	D16.8	D48.0	D49.2
scaphoid	—					
of ankle	C40.3-●	C79.51	—	—	—	—
of hand	C40.1-●	C79.51	—	—	—	—
scapula (any part)	C40.0-●	C79.51	—	D16.0-●	—	—
sella turcica	C41.0	C79.51	—	D16.4-●	D48.0	D49.2
shoulder	C40.0-●	C79.51	—	D16.0-●	—	—
skull	C41.0	C79.51	—	D16.4-●	D48.0	D49.2
sphenoid	C41.0	C79.51	—	D16.4-●	D48.0	D49.2
spine, spinal (column)	C41.2	C79.51	—	D16.6	D48.0	D49.2
coccyx	C41.4	C79.51	—	D16.8	D48.0	D49.2
sacrum	C41.4	C79.51	—	D16.8	D48.0	D49.2
sternum	C41.3	C79.51	—	D16.7	D48.0	D49.2
tarsus (any)	C40.3-●	C79.51	—	—	—	—
temporal	C41.0	C79.51	—	D16.4-●	D48.0	D49.2
thumb	C40.1-●	C79.51	—	—	—	—
tibia (any part)	C40.2-●	C79.51	—	—	—	—
toe (any)	C40.3-●	C79.51	—	—	—	—
trapezium	C40.1-●	C79.51	—	—	—	—
trapezoid	C40.1-●	C79.51	—	—	—	—
turbinate	C41.0	C79.51	—	D16.4-●	D48.0	D49.2
ulna (any part)	C40.0-●	C79.51	—	D16.0-●	—	—
unciform	C40.1-●	C79.51	—	—	—	—
vertebra (column)	C41.2	C79.51	—	D16.6	D48.0	D49.2
coccyx	C41.4	C79.51	—	D16.8	D48.0	D49.2
sacrum	C41.4	C79.51	—	D16.8	D48.0	D49.2
vomer	C41.0	C79.51	—	D16.4-●	D48.0	D49.2
wrist	C40.1-●	C79.51	—	—	—	—
xiphoid process	C41.3	C79.51	—	D16.7	D48.0	D49.2
zygomatic	C41.0	C79.51	—	D16.4-●	D48.0	D49.2
book-leaf (mouth)	C06.89	C79.89	D00.00	D10.39	D37.09	D49.0
bowel—see Neoplasm, intestine						
brachial plexus	C47.1-●	C79.89	—	D36.12	D48.2	D49.2
brain NEC	C71.9	C79.31	—	D33.2	D43.2	D49.6
basal ganglia	C71.0	C79.31	—	D33.0	D43.0	D49.6
cerebellopontine angle	C71.6	C79.31	—	D33.1	D43.1	D49.6

◀ New   ◀◀ Revised   ~~deleted~~ Deleted   ● Use Additional Character(s)

TABLE OF NEOPLASMS

	Malignant Primary	Malignant Secondary	Ca in situ	Benign	Uncertain Behavior	Unspecified Behavior
brain NEC *(Continued)*						
cerebellum NOS	C71.6	C79.31	—	D33.1	D43.1	D49.6
cerebrum	C71.0	C79.31	—	D33.0	D43.0	D49.6
choroid plexus	C71.7	C79.31	—	D33.1	D43.1	D49.6
corpus callosum	C71.8	C79.31	—	D33.2	D43.2	D49.6
corpus striatum	C71.0	C79.31	—	D33.0	D43.0	D49.6
cortex (cerebral)	C71.0	C79.31	—	D33.0	D43.0	D49.6
frontal lobe	C71.1	C79.31	—	D33.0	D43.0	D49.6
globus pallidus	C71.0	C79.31	—	D33.0	D43.0	D49.6
hippocampus	C71.2	C79.31	—	D33.0	D43.0	D49.6
hypothalamus	C71.0	C79.31	—	D33.0	D43.0	D49.6
internal capsule	C71.0	C79.31	—	D33.0	D43.0	D49.6
medulla oblongata	C71.7	C79.31	—	D33.1	D43.1	D49.6
meninges	C70.0	C79.32	—	D32.0	D42.0	D49.7
midbrain	C71.7	C79.31	—	D33.1	D43.1	D49.6
occipital lobe	C71.4	C79.31	—	D33.0	D43.0	D49.6
overlapping lesion	C71.8	C79.31	—	—	—	—
parietal lobe	C71.3	C79.31	—	D33.0	D43.0	D49.6
peduncle	C71.7	C79.31	—	D33.1	D43.1	D49.6
pons	C71.7	C79.31	—	D33.1	D43.1	D49.6
stem	C71.7	C79.31	—	D33.1	D43.1	D49.6
tapetum	C71.8	C79.31	—	D33.2	D43.2	D49.6
temporal lobe	C71.2	C79.31	—	D33.0	D43.0	D49.6
thalamus	C71.0	C79.31	—	D33.0	D43.0	D49.6
uncus	C71.2	C79.31	—	D33.0	D43.0	D49.6
ventricle (floor)	C71.5	C79.31	—	D33.0	D43.0	D49.6
fourth	C71.7	C79.31	—	D33.1	D43.1	D49.6
branchial (cleft) (cyst) (vestiges)	C10.4	C79.89	D00.08	D10.5	D37.05	D49.0
breast (connective tissue) (glandular tissue) (soft parts)	C50.9-●	C79.81	D05.-●	D24.-●	D48.6-●	D49.3
areola	C50.0-●	C79.81	D05.-●	D24.-●	D48.6-●	D49.3
axillary tail	C50.6-●	C79.81	D05.-●	D24.-●	D48.6-●	D49.3
central portion	C50.1-●	C79.81	D05.-●	D24.-●	D48.6-●	D49.3
inner	C50.8-●	C79.81	D05.-●	D24.-●	D48.6-●	D49.3
lower	C50.8-●	C79.81	D05.-●	D24.-●	D48.6-●	D49.3
lower-inner quadrant	C50.3-●	C79.81	D05.-●	D24.-●	D48.6-●	D49.3
lower-outer quadrant	C50.5-●	C79.81	D05.-●	D24.-●	D48.6-●	D49.3
mastectomy site (skin) — *see also Neoplasm, breast, skin*	C44.501	C79.2	—	—	—	—
specified as breast tissue	C50.8-●	C79.81	—	—	—	—
midline	C50.8-●	C79.81	D05.-●	D24.-●	D48.6-●	D49.3
nipple	C50.0-●	C79.81	D05.-●	D24.-●	D48.6-●	D49.3
outer	C50.8-●	C79.81	D05.-●	D24.-●	D48.6-●	D49.3
overlapping lesion	C50.8-●	—	—	—	—	—

	Malignant Primary	Malignant Secondary	Ca in situ	Benign	Uncertain Behavior	Unspecified Behavior
breast *(Continued)*						
skin	C44.501	C79.2	D04.5	D23.5	D48.5	D49.2
basal cell carcinoma	C44.511	—	—	—	—	—
specified type NEC	C44.591	—	—	—	—	—
squamous cell carcinoma	C44.521	—	—	—	—	—
tail (axillary)	C50.6-●	C79.81	D05.-●	D24.-●	D48.6-●	D49.3
upper	C50.8-●	C79.81	D05.-●	D24.-●	D48.6-●	D49.3
upper-inner quadrant	C50.2-●	C79.81	D05.-●	D24.-●	D48.6-●	D49.3
upper-outer quadrant	C50.4-●	C79.81	D05.-●	D24.-●	D48.6-●	D49.3
broad ligament	C57.1	C79.82	D07.39	D28.2	D39.8	D49.59
bronchiogenic, bronchogenic (lung)	C34.9-●	C78.0-●	D02.2-●	D14.3-●	D38.1	D49.1
bronchiole	C34.9-●	C78.0-●	D02.2-●	D14.3-●	D38.1	D49.1
bronchus	C34.9-●	C78.0-●	D02.2-●	D14.3-●	D38.1	D49.1
carina	C34.0-●	C78.0-●	D02.2-●	D14.3-●	D38.1	D49.1
lower lobe of lung	C34.3-●	C78.0-●	D02.2-●	D14.3-●	D38.1	D49.1
main	C34.0-●	C78.0-●	D02.2-●	D14.3-●	D38.1	D49.1
middle lobe of lung	C34.2	C78.0-●	D02.21	D14.31	D38.1	D49.1
overlapping lesion	C34.8-●	—	—	—	—	—
upper lobe of lung	C34.1-●	C78.0-●	D02.2-●	D14.3-●	D38.1	D49.1
brow	C44.309	C79.2	D04.39	D23.39	D48.5	D49.2
basal cell carcinoma	C44.319	—	—	—	—	—
specified type NEC	C44.399	—	—	—	—	—
squamous cell carcinoma	C44.329	—	—	—	—	—
buccal (cavity)	C06.9	C79.89	D00.00	D10.39	D37.09	D49.0
commissure	C06.0	C79.89	D00.02	D10.39	D37.09	D49.0
groove (lower) (upper)	C06.1	C79.89	D00.02	D10.39	D37.09	D49.0
mucosa	C06.0	C79.89	D00.02	D10.39	D37.09	D49.0
sulcus (lower) (upper)	C06.1	C79.89	D00.02	D10.39	D37.09	D49.0
bulbourethral gland	C68.0	C79.19	D09.19	D30.4	D41.3	D49.59
bursa — *see Neoplasm, connective tissue*						
buttock NEC	C76.3	C79.89	D04.5	D36.7	D48.7	D49.89
calf	C76.5-●	C79.89	D04.7-●	D36.7	D48.7	D49.89
calvarium	C41.0	C79.51	—	D16.4-●	D48.0	D49.2
calyx, renal	C65.-●	C79.0-●	D09.19	D30.1-●	D41.1-●	D49.51-●
canal						
anal	C21.1	C78.5	D01.3	D12.9	D37.8	D49.0
auditory (external) — *see also Neoplasm, skin, ear*	C44.20-●	C79.2	D04.2-●	D23.2-●	D48.5	D49.2
auricular (external) — *see also Neoplasm, skin, ear*	C44.20-●	C79.2	D04.2-●	D23.2-●	D48.5	D49.2
canaliculi, biliary (biliferi) (intrahepatic)	C22.1	C78.7	D01.5	D13.4	D37.6	D49.0

◄ New ◄ Revised ~~deleted~~ Deleted ● Use Additional Character(s)

	Malignant Primary	Malignant Secondary	Ca in situ	Benign	Uncertain Behavior	Unspecified Behavior
canthus (eye) (inner) (outer)	C44.10-•	C79.2	D04.1-•	D23.1-•	D48.5	D49.2
basal cell carcinoma	C44.11-•	—	—	—	—	—
sebaceous cell	C44.13-•	—	—	—	—	—
specified type NEC	C44.19-•	—	—	—	—	—
squamous cell carcinoma	C44.12-•	—	—	—	—	—
capillary — *see Neoplasm, connective tissue*						
caput coli	C18.0	C78.5	D01.0	D12.0	D37.4	D49.0
carcinoid — *see Tumor, carcinoid*						
cardia (gastric)	C16.0	C78.89	D00.2	D13.1	D37.1	D49.0
cardiac orifice (stomach)	C16.0	C78.89	D00.2	D13.1	D37.1	D49.0
cardio-esophageal junction	C16.0	C78.89	D00.2	D13.1	D37.1	D49.0
cardio-esophagus	C16.0	C78.89	D00.2	D13.1	D37.1	D49.0
carina (bronchus)	C34.0-•	C78.0-•	D02.2-•	D14.3-•	D38.1	D49.1
carotid (artery)	C49.0	C79.89	—	D21.0	D48.1	D49.2
body	C75.4	C79.89	—	D35.5	D44.6	D49.7
carpus (any bone)	C40.1-•	C79.51	—	D16.1-•	—	—
cartilage (articular) (joint) NEC — *see also Neoplasm, bone*	C41.9	C79.51		D16.9-•	D48.0	D49.2
arytenoid	C32.3	C78.39	D02.0	D14.1	D38.0	D49.1
auricular	C49.0	C79.89	—	D21.0	D48.1	D49.2
bronchi	C34.0-•	C78.39	—	D14.3-•	D38.1	D49.1
costal	C41.3	C79.51	—	D16.7	D48.0	D49.2
cricoid	C32.3	C78.39	D02.0	D14.1	D38.0	D49.1
cuneiform	C32.3	C78.39	D02.0	D14.1	D38.0	D49.1
ear (external)	C49.0	C79.89	—	D21.0	D48.1	D49.2
ensiform	C41.3	C79.51	—	D16.7	D48.0	D49.2
epiglottis	C32.1	C78.39	D02.0	D14.1	D38.0	D49.1
anterior surface	C10.1	C79.89	D00.08	D10.5	D37.05	D49.0
eyelid	C49.0	C79.89	—	D21.0	D48.1	D49.2
intervertebral	C41.2	C79.51	—	D16.6	D48.0	D49.2
larynx, laryngeal	C32.3	C78.39	D02.0	D14.1	D38.0	D49.1
nose, nasal	C30.0	C78.39	D02.3	D14.0	D38.5	D49.1
pinna	C49.0	C79.89	—	D21.0	D48.1	D49.2
rib	C41.3	C79.51	—	D16.7	D48.0	D49.2
semilunar (knee)	C40.2-•	C79.51	—	D16.2-•	D48.0	D49.2
thyroid	C32.3	C78.39	D02.0	D14.1	D38.0	D49.1
trachea	C33	C78.39	D02.1	D14.2	D38.1	D49.1
cauda equina	C72.1	C79.49	—	D33.4	D43.4	D49.7
cavity						
buccal	C06.9	C79.89	D00.00	D10.30	D37.09	D49.0
nasal	C30.0	C78.39	D02.3	D14.0	D38.5	D49.1
oral	C06.9	C79.89	D00.00	D10.30	D37.09	D49.0

	Malignant Primary	Malignant Secondary	Ca in situ	Benign	Uncertain Behavior	Unspecified Behavior
cavity (*Continued*)						
peritoneal	C48.2	C78.6	—	D20.1	D48.4	D49.0
tympanic	C30.1	C78.39	D02.3	D14.0	D38.5	D49.1
cecum	C18.0	C78.5	D01.0	D12.0	D37.4	D49.0
central nervous system	C72.9	C79.40	—	—	—	—
cerebellopontine (angle)	C71.6	C79.31	—	D33.1	D43.1	D49.6
cerebellum, cerebellar	C71.6	C79.31	—	D33.1	D43.1	D49.6
cerebrum, cerebra (cortex) (hemisphere) (white matter)	C71.0	C79.31	—	D33.0	D43.0	D49.6
meninges	C70.0	C79.32	—	D32.0	D42.0	D49.7
peduncle	C71.7	C79.31	—	D33.1	D43.1	D49.6
ventricle	C71.5	C79.31	—	D33.0	D43.0	D49.6
fourth	C71.7	C79.31	—	D33.1	D43.1	D49.6
cervical region	C76.0	C79.89	D09.8	D36.7	D48.7	D49.89
cervix (cervical) (uteri) (uterus)	C53.9	C79.82	D06.9	D26.0	D39.0	D49.59
canal	C53.0	C79.82	D06.0	D26.0	D39.0	D49.59
endocervix (canal) (gland)	C53.0	C79.82	D06.0	D26.0	D39.0	D49.59
exocervix	C53.1	C79.82	D06.1	D26.0	D39.0	D49.59
external os	C53.1	C79.82	D06.1	D26.0	D39.0	D49.59
internal os	C53.0	C79.82	D06.0	D26.0	D39.0	D49.59
nabothian gland	C53.0	C79.82	D06.0	D26.0	D39.0	D49.59
overlapping lesion	C53.8	—	—	—	—	—
squamocolumnar junction	C53.8	C79.82	D06.7	D26.0	D39.0	D49.59
stump	C53.8	C79.82	D06.7	D26.0	D39.0	D49.59
cheek	C76.0	C79.89	D09.8	D36.7	D48.7	D49.89
external	C44.309	C79.2	D04.39	D23.39	D48.5	D49.2
basal cell carcinoma	C44.319	—	—	—	—	—
specified type NEC	C44.399	—	—	—	—	—
squamous cell carcinoma	C44.329	—	—	—	—	—
inner aspect	C06.0	C79.89	D00.02	D10.39	D37.09	D49.0
internal	C06.0	C79.89	D00.02	D10.39	D37.09	D49.0
mucosa	C06.0	C79.89	D00.02	D10.39	D37.09	D49.0
chest (wall) NEC	C76.1	C79.89	D09.8	D36.7	D48.7	D49.89
chiasma opticum	C72.3-•	C79.49	—	D33.3	D43.3	D49.7
chin	C44.309	C79.2	D04.39	D23.39	D48.5	D49.2
basal cell carcinoma	C44.319	—	—	—	—	—
specified type NEC	C44.399	—	—	—	—	—
squamous cell carcinoma	C44.329	—	—	—	—	—
choana	C11.3	C79.89	D00.08	D10.6	D37.05	D49.0
cholangiole	C22.1	C78.89	D01.5	D13.4	D37.6	D49.0
choledochal duct	C24.0	C78.89	D01.5	D13.5	D37.6	D49.0
choroid	C69.3-•	C79.49	D09.2-•	D31.3-•	D48.7	D49.81
plexus	C71.5	C79.31	—	D33.0	D43.0	D49.6
ciliary body	C69.4-•	C79.49	D09.2-•	D31.4-•	D48.7	D49.89

TABLE OF NEOPLASMS

	Malignant Primary	Malignant Secondary	Ca in situ	Benign	Uncertain Behavior	Unspecified Behavior
clavicle	C41.3	C79.51	—	D16.7	D48.0	D49.2
clitoris	C51.2	C79.82	D07.1	D28.0	D39.8	D49.59
clivus	C41.0	C79.51	—	D16.4-●	D48.0	D49.2
cloacogenic zone	C21.2	C78.5	D01.3	D12.9	D37.8	D49.0
coccygeal						
body or glomus	C49.5	C79.89	—	D21.5	D48.1	D49.2
vertebra	C41.4	C79.51	—	D16.8	D48.0	D49.2
coccyx	C41.4	C79.51	—	D16.8	D48.0	D49.2
colon — *see also Neoplasm, intestine, large*	C18.9	C78.5	—	—	—	—
with rectum	C19	C78.5	D01.1	D12.7	D37.5	D49.0
column, spinal — *see Neoplasm, spine*						
columnella — *see also Neoplasm, skin, face*	C44.390	C79.2	D04.39	D23.39	D48.5	D49.2
commissure						
labial, lip	C00.6	C79.89	D00.01	D10.39	D37.01	D49.0
laryngeal	C32.0	C78.39	D02.0	D14.1	D38.0	D49.1
common (bile) duct	C24.0	C78.89	D01.5	D13.5	D37.6	D49.0
concha — *see also Neoplasm, skin, ear*	C44.20-●	C79.2	D04.2-●	D23.2-●	D48.5	D49.2
nose	C30.0	C78.39	D02.3	D14.0	D38.5	D49.1
conjunctiva	C69.0-●	C79.49	D09.2-●	D31.0-●	D48.7	D49.89
connective tissue NEC	C49.9	C79.89	—	D21.9	D48.1	D49.2

Note: For neoplasms of connective tissue (blood vessel, bursa, fascia, ligament, muscle, peripheral nerves, sympathetic and parasympathetic nerves and ganglia, synovia, tendon, etc.) or of morphological types that indicate connective tissue, code according to the list under "Neoplasm, connective tissue." For sites that do not appear in this list, code to neoplasm of that site; e.g., fibrosarcoma, pancreas (C25.9)

Note: Morphological types that indicate connective tissue appear in their proper place in the alphabetic index with the instruction "*see Neoplasm, connective tissue ....*"

	Malignant Primary	Malignant Secondary	Ca in situ	Benign	Uncertain Behavior	Unspecified Behavior
abdomen	C49.4	C79.89	—	D21.4	D48.1	D49.2
abdominal wall	C49.4	C79.89	—	D21.4	D48.1	D49.2
ankle	C49.2-●	C79.89	—	D21.2-●	D48.1	D49.2
antecubital fossa or space	C49.1-●	C79.89	—	D21.1-●	D48.1	D49.2
arm	C49.1-●	C79.89	—	D21.1-●	D48.1	D49.2
auricle (ear)	C49.0	C79.89	—	D21.0	D48.1	D49.2
axilla	C49.3	C79.89	—	D21.3	D48.1	D49.2
back	C49.6	C79.89	—	D21.6	D48.1	D49.2
breast — *see Neoplasm, breast*						
buttock	C49.5	C79.89	—	D21.5	D48.1	D49.2
calf	C49.2-●	C79.89	—	D21.2-●	D48.1	D49.2
cervical region	C49.0	C79.89	—	D21.0	D48.1	D49.2

	Malignant Primary	Malignant Secondary	Ca in situ	Benign	Uncertain Behavior	Unspecified Behavior
connective tissue NEC *(Continued)*						
cheek	C49.0	C79.89	—	D21.0	D48.1	D49.2
chest (wall)	C49.3	C79.89	—	D21.3	D48.1	D49.2
chin	C49.0	C79.89	—	D21.0	D48.1	D49.2
diaphragm	C49.3	C79.89	—	D21.3	D48.1	D49.2
ear (external)	C49.0	C79.89	—	D21.0	D48.1	D49.2
elbow	C49.1-●	C79.89	—	D21.1-●	D48.1	D49.2
extrarectal	C49.5	C79.89	—	D21.5	D48.1	D49.2
extremity	C49.9	C79.89	—	D21.9	D48.1	D49.2
lower	C49.2-●	C79.89	—	D21.2-●	D48.1	D49.2
upper	C49.1-●	C79.89	—	D21.1-●	D48.1	D49.2
eyelid	C49.0	C79.89	—	D21.0	D48.1	D49.2
face	C49.0	C79.89	—	D21.0	D48.1	D49.2
finger	C49.1-●	C79.89	—	D21.1-●	D48.1	D49.2
flank	C49.6	C79.89	—	D21.6	D48.1	D49.2
foot	C49.2-●	C79.89	—	D21.2-●	D48.1	D49.2
forearm	C49.1-●	C79.89	—	D21.1-●	D48.1	D49.2
forehead	C49.0	C79.89	—	D21.0	D48.1	D49.2
gastric	C49.4	C79.89	—	D21.4	D48.1	D49.2
gastrointestinal	C49.4	C79.89	—	D21.4	D48.1	D49.2
gluteal region	C49.5	C79.89	—	D21.5	D48.1	D49.2
great vessels NEC	C49.3	C79.89	—	D21.3	D48.1	D49.2
groin	C49.5	C79.89	—	D21.5	D48.1	D49.2
hand	C49.1-●	C79.89	—	D21.1-●	D48.1	D49.2
head	C49.0	C79.89	—	D21.0	D48.1	D49.2
heel	C49.2-●	C79.89	—	D21.2-●	D48.1	D49.2
hip	C49.2-●	C79.89	—	D21.2-●	D48.1	D49.2
hypochondrium	C49.4	C79.89	—	D21.4	D48.1	D49.2
iliopsoas muscle	C49.5	C79.89	—	D21.5	D48.1	D49.2
infraclavicular region	C49.3	C79.89	—	D21.3	D48.1	D49.2
inguinal (canal) (region)	C49.5	C79.89	—	D21.5	D48.1	D49.2
intestinal	C49.4	C79.89	—	D21.4	D48.1	D49.2
intrathoracic	C49.3	C79.89	—	D21.3	D48.1	D49.2
ischiorectal fossa	C49.5	C79.89	—	D21.5	D48.1	D49.2
jaw	C03.9	C79.89	D00.03	D10.39	D48.1	D49.0
knee	C49.2-●	C79.89	—	D21.2-●	D48.1	D49.2
leg	C49.2-●	C79.89	—	D21.2-●	D48.1	D49.2
limb NEC	C49.9	C79.89	—	D21.9	D48.1	D49.2
lower	C49.2-●	C79.89	—	D21.2-●	D48.1	D49.2
upper	C49.1-●	C79.89	—	D21.1-●	D48.1	D49.2
nates	C49.5	C79.89	—	D21.5	D48.1	D49.2
neck	C49.0	C79.89	—	D21.0	D48.1	D49.2
orbit	C69.6-●	C79.49	D09.2-●	D31.6-●	D48.1	D49.89
overlapping lesion	C49.8	—	—	—	—	—

◄ New   ◄ Revised   ~~deleted~~ Deleted   ● Use Additional Character(s)

	Malignant Primary	Malignant Secondary	Ca in situ	Benign	Uncertain Behavior	Unspecified Behavior
connective tissue NEC *(Continued)*						
pararectal	C49.5	C79.89	—	D21.5	D48.1	D49.2
para-urethral	C49.5	C79.89	—	D21.5	D48.1	D49.2
paravaginal	C49.5	C79.89	—	D21.5	D48.1	D49.2
pelvis (floor)	C49.5	C79.89	—	D21.5	D48.1	D49.2
pelvo-abdominal	C49.8	C79.89	—	D21.6	D48.1	D49.2
perineum	C49.5	C79.89	—	D21.5	D48.1	D49.2
perirectal (tissue)	C49.5	C79.89	—	D21.5	D48.1	D49.2
periurethral (tissue)	C49.5	C79.89	—	D21.5	D48.1	D49.2
popliteal fossa or space	C49.2-●	C79.89	—	D21.2-●	D48.1	D49.2
presacral	C49.5	C79.89	—	D21.5	D48.1	D49.2
psoas muscle	C49.4	C79.89	—	D21.4	D48.1	D49.2
pterygoid fossa	C49.0	C79.89	—	D21.0	D48.1	D49.2
rectovaginal septum or wall	C49.5	C79.89	—	D21.5	D48.1	D49.2
rectovesical	C49.5	C79.89	—	D21.5	D48.1	D49.2
retroperitoneum	C48.0	C78.6	—	D20.0	D48.3	D49.0
sacrococcygeal region	C49.5	C79.89	—	D21.5	D48.1	D49.2
scalp	C49.0	C79.89	—	D21.0	D48.1	D49.2
scapular region	C49.3	C79.89	—	D21.3	D48.1	D49.2
shoulder	C49.1-●	C79.89	—	D21.1-●	D48.1	D49.2
skin (dermis) NEC — *see also* *Neoplasm, skin, by site*	C44.90	C79.2	D04.9	D23.9	D48.5	D49.2
stomach	C49.4	C79.89	—	D21.4	D48.1	D49.2
submental	C49.0	C79.89	—	D21.0	D48.1	D49.2
supraclavicular region	C49.0	C79.89	—	D21.0	D48.1	D49.2
temple	C49.0	C79.89	—	D21.0	D48.1	D49.2
temporal region	C49.0	C79.89	—	D21.0	D48.1	D49.2
thigh	C49.2-●	C79.89	—	D21.2-●	D48.1	D49.2
thoracic (duct) (wall)	C49.3	C79.89	—	D21.3	D48.1	D49.2
thorax	C49.3	C79.89	—	D21.3	D48.1	D49.2
thumb	C49.1-●	C79.89	—	D21.1-●	D48.1	D49.2
toe	C49.2-●	C79.89	—	D21.2-●	D48.1	D49.2
trunk	C49.6	C79.89	—	D21.6	D48.1	D49.2
umbilicus	C49.4	C79.89	—	D21.4	D48.1	D49.2
vesicorectal	C49.5	C79.89	—	D21.5	D48.1	D49.2
wrist	C49.1-●	C79.89	—	D21.1-●	D48.1	D49.2
conus medullaris	C72.0	C79.49	—	D33.4	D43.4	D49.7
cord (true) (vocal)	C32.0	C78.39	D02.0	D14.1	D38.0	D49.1
false	C32.1	C78.39	D02.0	D14.1	D38.0	D49.1
spermatic	C63.1-●	C79.82	D07.69	D29.8	D40.8	D49.59
spinal (cervical) (lumbar) (thoracic)	C72.0	C79.49	—	D33.4	D43.4	D49.7
cornea (limbus)	C69.1-●	C79.49	D09.2-●	D31.1-●	D48.7	D49.89
corpus						

	Malignant Primary	Malignant Secondary	Ca in situ	Benign	Uncertain Behavior	Unspecified Behavior
corpus *(Continued)*						
albicans	C56.-●	C79.6-●	D07.39	D27.-●	D39.1-●	D49.59
callosum, brain	C71.0	C79.31	—	D33.2	D43.2	D49.6
cavernosum	C60.2	C79.82	D07.4	D29.0	D40.8	D49.59
gastric	C16.2	C78.89	D00.2	D13.1	D37.1	D49.0
overlapping sites	C54.8	—	—	—	—	—
penis	C60.2	C79.82	D07.4	D29.0	D40.8	D49.59
striatum, cerebrum	C71.0	C79.31	—	D33.0	D43.0	D49.6
uteri	C54.9	C79.82	D07.0	D26.1	D39.0	D49.59
isthmus	C54.0	C79.82	D07.0	D26.1	D39.0	D49.59
cortex						
adrenal	C74.0-●	C79.7-●	D09.3	D35.0-●	D44.1-●	D49.7
cerebral	C71.0	C79.31	—	D33.0	D43.0	D49.6
costal cartilage	C41.3	C79.51	—	D16.7	D48.0	D49.2
costovertebral joint	C41.3	C79.51	—	D16.7	D48.0	D49.2
Cowper's gland	C68.0	C79.19	D09.19	D30.4	D41.3	D49.59
cranial (fossa, any)	C71.9	C79.31	—	D33.2	D43.2	D49.6
meninges	C70.0	C79.32	—	D32.0	D42.0	D49.7
nerve	C72.50	C79.49	—	D33.3	D43.3	D49.7
specified NEC	C72.59	C79.49	—	D33.3	D43.3	D49.7
craniobuccal pouch	C75.2	C79.89	D09.3	D35.2	D44.3	D49.7
craniopharyngeal (duct) (pouch)	C75.2	C79.89	D09.3	D35.3	D44.4	D49.7
cricoid	C13.0	C79.89	D00.08	D10.7	D37.05	D49.0
cartilage	C32.3	C78.39	D02.0	D14.1	D38.0	D49.1
cricopharynx	C13.0	C79.89	D00.08	D10.7	D37.05	D49.0
crypt of Morgagni	C21.8	C78.5	D01.3	D12.9	D37.8	D49.0
crystalline lens	C69.4-●	C79.49	D09.2-●	D31.4-●	D48.7	D49.89
cul-de-sac (Douglas')	C48.1	C78.6	—	D20.1	D48.4	D49.0
cuneiform cartilage	C32.3	C78.39	D02.0	D14.1	D38.0	D49.1
cutaneous — *see Neoplasm, skin*						
cutis — *see Neoplasm, skin*						
cystic (bile) duct (common)	C24.0	C78.89	D01.5	D13.5	D37.6	D49.0
dermis — *see Neoplasm, skin*						
diaphragm	C49.3	C79.89	—	D21.3	D48.1	D49.2
digestive organs, system, tube, or tract NEC	C26.9	C78.89	D01.9	D13.9	D37.9	D49.0
disc, intervertebral	C41.2	C79.51	—	D16.6	D48.0	D49.2
disease, generalized	C80.0	—	—	—	—	—
disseminated	C80.0	—	—	—	—	—
Douglas' cul-de-sac or pouch	C48.1	C78.6	—	D20.1	D48.4	D49.0
duodenojejunal junction	C17.8	C78.4	D01.49	D13.39	D37.2	D49.0
duodenum	C17.0	C78.4	D01.49	D13.2	D37.2	D49.0

◄ New   ◄▌ Revised   ~~deleted~~ Deleted   ● Use Additional Character(s)

TABLE OF NEOPLASMS

	Malignant Primary	Malignant Secondary	Ca in situ	Benign	Uncertain Behavior	Unspecified Behavior
dura (cranial) (mater)	C70.9	C79.49	—	D32.9	D42.9	D49.7
cerebral	C70.0	C79.32	—	D32.0	D42.0	D49.7
spinal	C70.1	C79.49	—	D32.1	D42.1	D49.7
ear (external) — see also Neoplasm, skin, ear	C44.20-●	C79.2	D04.2-●	D23.2-●	D48.5	D49.2
auricle or auris — see also Neoplasm, skin, ear	C44.20-●	C79.2	D04.2-●	D23.2-●	D48.5	D49.2
canal, external — see also Neoplasm, skin, ear	C44.20-●	C79.2	D04.2-●	D23.2-●	D48.5	D49.2
cartilage	C49.0	C79.89	—	D21.0	D48.1	D49.2
external meatus — see also Neoplasm, skin, ear	C44.20-●	C79.2	D04.2-●	D23.2-●	D48.5	D49.2
inner	C30.1	C78.39	D02.3	D14.0	D38.5	D49.1
lobule — see also Neoplasm, skin, ear	C44.20-●	C79.2	D04.2-●	D23.2-●	D48.5	D49.2
middle	C30.1	C78.39	D02.3	D14.0	D38.5	D49.1
overlapping lesion with accessory sinuses	C31.8	—	—	—	—	—
skin	C44.20-●	C79.2	D04.2-●	D23.2-●	D48.5	D49.2
basal cell carcinoma	C44.21-●	—	—	—	—	—
specified type NEC	C44.29-●	—	—	—	—	—
squamous cell carcinoma	C44.22-●	—	—	—	—	—
earlobe	C44.20-●	C79.2	D04.2-●	D23.2-●	D48.5	D49.2
basal cell carcinoma	C44.21-●	—	—	—	—	—
specified type NEC	C44.29-●	—	—	—	—	—
squamous cell carcinoma	C44.22-●	—	—	—	—	—
ejaculatory duct	C63.7	C79.82	D07.69	D29.8	D40.8	D49.59
elbow NEC	C76.4-●	C79.89	D04.6-●	D36.7	D48.7	D49.89
endocardium	C38.0	C79.89	—	D15.1	D48.7	D49.89
endocervix (canal) (gland)	C53.0	C79.82	D06.0	D26.0	D39.0	D49.59
endocrine gland NEC	C75.9	C79.89	D09.3	D35.9	D44.9	D49.7
pluriglandular	C75.8	C79.89	D09.3	D35.7	D44.9	D49.7
endometrium (gland) (stroma)	C54.1	C79.82	D07.0	D26.1	D39.0	D49.59
ensiform cartilage	C41.3	C79.51	—	D16.7	D48.0	D49.2
enteric — see Neoplasm, intestine						
ependyma (brain)	C71.5	C79.31	—	D33.0	D43.0	D49.6
fourth ventricle	C71.7	C79.31	—	D33.1	D43.1	D49.6
epicardium	C38.0	C79.89	—	D15.1	D48.7	D49.89
epididymis	C63.0-●	C79.82	D07.69	D29.3-●	D40.8	D49.59
epidural	C72.9	C79.49	—	D33.9	D43.9	D49.7
epiglottis	C32.1	C78.39	D02.0	D14.1	D38.0	D49.1
anterior aspect or surface	C10.1	C79.89	D00.08	D10.5	D37.05	D49.0
cartilage	C32.3	C78.39	D02.0	D14.1	D38.0	D49.1
free border (margin)	C10.1	C79.89	D00.08	D10.5	D37.05	D49.0

	Malignant Primary	Malignant Secondary	Ca in situ	Benign	Uncertain Behavior	Unspecified Behavior
junctional region	C10.8	C79.89	D00.08	D10.5	D37.05	D49.0
posterior (laryngeal) surface	C32.1	C78.39	D02.0	D14.1	D38.0	D49.1
suprahyoid portion	C32.1	C78.39	D02.0	D14.1	D38.0	D49.1
esophagogastric junction	C16.0	C78.89	D00.2	D13.1	D37.1	D49.0
esophagus	C15.9	C78.89	D00.1	D13.0	D37.8	D49.0
abdominal	C15.5	C78.89	D00.1	D13.0	D37.8	D49.0
cervical	C15.3	C78.89	D00.1	D13.0	D37.8	D49.0
distal (third)	C15.5	C78.89	D00.1	D13.0	D37.8	D49.0
lower (third)	C15.5	C78.89	D00.1	D13.0	D37.8	D49.0
middle (third)	C15.4	C78.89	D00.1	D13.0	D37.8	D49.0
overlapping lesion	C15.8	—	—	—	—	—
proximal (third)	C15.3	C78.89	D00.1	D13.0	D37.8	D49.0
thoracic	C15.4	C78.89	D00.1	D13.0	D37.8	D49.0
upper (third)	C15.3	C78.89	D00.1	D13.0	D37.8	D49.0
ethmoid (sinus)	C31.1	C78.39	D02.3	D14.0	D38.5	D49.1
bone or labyrinth	C41.0	C79.51	—	D16.4-●	D48.0	D49.2
eustachian tube	C30.1	C78.39	D02.3	D14.0	D38.5	D49.1
exocervix	C53.1	C79.82	D06.1	D26.0	D39.0	D49.59
external						
meatus (ear) — see also Neoplasm, skin, ear	C44.20-●	C79.2	D04.2-●	D23.2-●	D48.5	D49.2
os, cervix uteri	C53.1	C79.82	D06.1	D26.0	D39.0	D49.59
extradural	C72.9	C79.49	—	D33.9	D43.9	D49.7
extrahepatic (bile) duct	C24.0	C78.89	D01.5	D13.5	D37.6	D49.0
overlapping lesion with gallbladder	C24.8	—	—	—	—	—
extraocular muscle	C69.6-●	C79.49	D09.2-●	D31.6-●	D48.7	D49.89
extrarectal	C76.3	C79.89	D09.8	D36.7	D48.7	D49.89
extremity	C76.8	C79.89	D04.8	D36.7	D48.7	D49.89
lower	C76.5-●	C79.89	D04.7-●	D36.7	D48.7	D49.89
upper	C76.4-●	C79.89	D04.6-●	D36.7	D48.7	D49.89
eye NEC	C69.9-●	C79.49	D09.2	D31.9	D48.7	D49.89
overlapping sites	C69.8	—	—	—	—	—
eyeball	C69.9-●	C79.49	D09.2-●	D31.9-●	D48.7	D49.89
eyebrow	C44.309	C79.2	D04.39	D23.39	D48.5	D49.2
basal cell carcinoma	C44.319	—	—	—	—	—
specified type NEC	C44.399	—	—	—	—	—
squamous cell carcinoma	C44.329	—	—	—	—	—
eyelid (lower) (skin) (upper)	C44.10-●	—	—	—	—	—
basal cell carcinoma	C44.11-●	—	—	—	—	—
cartilage	C49.0	C79.89	—	D21.0	D48.1	D49.2
sebaceous cell	C44.13-●	—	—	—	—	—
specified type NEC	C44.19-●	—	—	—	—	—
squamous cell carcinoma	C44.12-●	—	—	—	—	—

◀ New   ◀ Revised   ~~deleted~~ Deleted   ● Use Additional Character(s)

	Malignant Primary	Malignant Secondary	Ca in situ	Benign	Uncertain Behavior	Unspecified Behavior
face NEC	C76.0	C79.89	D04.39	D36.7	D48.7	D49.89
fallopian tube (accessory)	C57.0-●	C79.82	D07.39	D28.2	D39.8	D49.59
falx (cerebella) (cerebri)	C70.0	C79.32	—	D32.0	D42.0	D49.7
fascia — *see also Neoplasm, connective tissue*						
palmar	C49.1-●	C79.89	—	D21.1-●	D48.1	D49.2
plantar	C49.2-●	C79.89	—	D21.2-●	D48.1	D49.2
fatty tissue — *see Neoplasm, connective tissue*						
fauces, faucial NEC	C10.9	C79.89	D00.08	D10.5	D37.05	D49.0
pillars	C09.1	C79.89	D00.08	D10.5	D37.05	D49.0
tonsil	C09.9	C79.89	D00.08	D10.4	D37.05	D49.0
femur (any part)	C40.2-●	—	—	D16.2-●	—	—
fetal membrane	C58	C79.82	D07.0	D26.7	D39.2	D49.59
fibrous tissue — *see Neoplasm, connective tissue*						
fibula (any part)	C40.2-●	C79.51	—	D16.2-●	—	—
filum terminale	C72.0	C79.49	—	D33.4	D43.4	D49.7
finger NEC	C76.4-●	C79.89	D04.6-●	D36.7	D48.7	D49.89
flank NEC	C76.8	C79.89	D04.5	D36.7	D48.7	D49.89
follicle, nabothian	C53.0	C79.82	D06.0	D26.0	D39.0	D49.59
foot NEC	C76.5-●	C79.89	D04.7-●	D36.7	D48.7	D49.89
forearm NEC	C76.4-●	C79.89	D04.6-●	D36.7	D48.7	D49.89
forehead (skin)	C44.309	C79.2	D04.39	D23.39	D48.5	D49.2
basal cell carcinoma	C44.319	—	—	—	—	—
specified type NEC	C44.399	—	—	—	—	—
squamous cell carcinoma	C44.329	—	—	—	—	—
foreskin	C60.0	C79.82	D07.4	D29.0	D40.8	D49.59
fornix						
pharyngeal	C11.3	C79.89	D00.08	D10.6	D37.05	D49.0
vagina	C52	C79.82	D07.2	D28.1	D39.8	D49.59
fossa (of)						
anterior (cranial)	C71.9	C79.31	—	D33.2	D43.2	D49.6
cranial	C71.9	C79.31	—	D33.2	D43.2	D49.6
ischiorectal	C76.3	C79.89	D09.8	D36.7	D48.7	D49.89
middle (cranial)	C71.9	C79.31	—	D33.2	D43.2	D49.6
piriform	C12	C79.89	D00.08	D10.7	D37.05	D49.0
pituitary	C75.1	C79.89	D09.3	D35.2	D44.3	D49.7
posterior (cranial)	C71.9	C79.31	—	D33.2	D43.2	D49.6
pterygoid	C49.0	C79.89	—	D21.0	D48.1	D49.2
pyriform	C12	C79.89	D00.08	D10.7	D37.05	D49.0
Rosenmuller	C11.2	C79.89	D00.08	D10.6	D37.05	D49.0
tonsillar	C09.0	C79.89	D00.08	D10.5	D37.05	D49.0
fourchette	C51.9	C79.82	D07.1	D28.0	D39.8	D49.59

	Malignant Primary	Malignant Secondary	Ca in situ	Benign	Uncertain Behavior	Unspecified Behavior
frenulum						
labii — *see Neoplasm, lip, internal*						
linguae	C02.2	C79.89	D00.07	D10.1	D37.02	D49.0
frontal						
bone	C41.0	C79.51	—	D16.4-●	D48.0	D49.2
lobe, brain	C71.1	C79.31	—	D33.0	D43.0	D49.6
pole	C71.1	C79.31	—	D33.0	D43.0	D49.6
sinus	C31.2	C78.39	D02.3	D14.0	D38.5	D49.1
fundus						
stomach	C16.1	C78.89	D00.2	D13.1	D37.1	D49.0
uterus	C54.3	C79.82	D07.0	D26.1	D39.0	D49.59
gall duct (extrahepatic)	C24.0	C78.89	D01.5	D13.5	D37.6	D49.0
intrahepatic	C22.1	C78.7	D01.5	D13.4	D37.6	D49.0
gallbladder	C23	C78.89	D01.5	D13.5	D37.6	D49.0
overlapping lesion with extrahepatic bile ducts	C24.8	—	—	—	—	—
ganglia — *see also Neoplasm, nerve, peripheral*	C47.9	C79.89	—	D36.10	D48.2	D49.2
basal	C71.0	C79.31	—	D33.0	D43.0	D49.6
cranial nerve	C72.50	C79.49	—	D33.3	D43.3	D49.7
Gartner's duct	C52	C79.82	D07.2	D28.1	D39.8	D49.59
gastric — *see Neoplasm, stomach*						
gastrocolic	C26.9	C78.89	D01.9	D13.9	D37.9	D49.0
gastroesophageal junction	C16.0	C78.89	D00.2	D13.1	D37.1	D49.0
gastrointestinal (tract) NEC	C26.9	C78.89	D01.9	D13.9	D37.9	D49.0
generalized	C80.0	—	—	—	—	—
genital organ or tract						
female NEC	C57.9	C79.82	D07.30	D28.9	D39.9	D49.59
overlapping lesion	C57.8	—	—	—	—	—
specified site NEC	C57.7	C79.82	D07.39	D28.7	D39.8	D49.59
male NEC	C63.9	C79.82	D07.60	D29.9	D40.9	D49.59
overlapping lesion	C63.8	—	—	—	—	—
specified site NEC	C63.7	C79.82	D07.69	D29.8	D40.8	D49.59
genitourinary tract						
female	C57.9	C79.82	D07.30	D28.9	D39.9	D49.59
male	C63.9	C79.82	D07.60	D29.9	D40.9	D49.59
gingiva (alveolar) (marginal)	C03.9	C79.89	D00.03	D10.39	D37.09	D49.0
lower	C03.1	C79.89	D00.03	D10.39	D37.09	D49.0
mandibular	C03.1	C79.89	D00.03	D10.39	D37.09	D49.0
maxillary	C03.0	C79.89	D00.03	D10.39	D37.09	D49.0
upper	C03.0	C79.89	D00.03	D10.39	D37.09	D49.0

◀ New   ◀ Revised   ~~deleted~~ Deleted   ● Use Additional Character(s)

TABLE OF NEOPLASMS (side note, vertical)

	Malignant Primary	Malignant Secondary	Ca in situ	Benign	Uncertain Behavior	Unspecified Behavior
gland, glandular (lymphatic) (system) — see also Neoplasm, lymph gland						
endocrine NEC	C75.9	C79.89	D09.3	D35.9	D44.9	D49.7
salivary — see Neoplasm, salivary gland						
glans penis	C60.1	C79.82	D07.4	D29.0	D40.8	D49.59
globus pallidus	C71.0	C79.31	—	D33.0	D43.0	D49.6
glomus						
coccygeal	C49.5	C79.89	—	D21.5	D48.1	D49.2
jugularis	C75.5	C79.89	—	D35.6	D44.7	D49.7
glosso-epiglottic fold(s)	C10.1	C79.89	D00.08	D10.5	D37.05	D49.0
glossopalatine fold	C09.1	C79.89	D00.08	D10.5	D37.05	D49.0
glossopharyngeal sulcus	C09.0	C79.89	D00.08	D10.5	D37.05	D49.0
glottis	C32.0	C78.39	D02.0	D14.1	D38.0	D49.1
gluteal region	C76.3	C79.89	D04.5	D36.7	D48.7	D49.89
great vessels NEC	C49.3	C79.89	—	D21.3	D48.1	D49.2
groin NEC	C76.3	C79.89	D04.5	D36.7	D48.7	D49.89
gum	C03.9	C79.89	D00.03	D10.39	D37.09	D49.0
lower	C03.1	C79.89	D00.03	D10.39	D37.09	D49.0
upper	C03.0	C79.89	D00.03	D10.39	D37.09	D49.0
hand NEC	C76.4-●	C79.89	D04.6-●	D36.7	D48.7	D49.89
head NEC	C76.0	C79.89	D04.4	D36.7	D48.7	D49.89
heart	C38.0	C79.89	—	D15.1	D48.7	D49.89
heel NEC	C76.5-●	C79.89	D04.7-●	D36.7	D48.7	D49.89
helix — see also Neoplasm, skin, ear	C44.20-●	C79.2	D04.2-●	D23.2-●	D48.5	D49.2
hematopoietic, hemopoietic tissue NEC	C96.9	—	—	—	—	—
specified NEC	C96.Z	—	—	—	—	—
hemisphere, cerebral	C71.0	C79.31	—	D33.0	D43.0	D49.6
hemorrhoidal zone	C21.1	C78.5	D01.3	D12.9	D37.8	D49.0
hepatic — see also Index to disease, by histology	C22.9	C78.7	D01.5	D13.4	D37.6	D49.0
duct (bile)	C24.0	C78.89	D01.5	D13.5	D37.6	D49.0
flexure (colon)	C18.3	C78.5	D01.0	D12.3	D37.4	D49.0
primary	C22.8	C78.7	D01.5	D13.4	D37.6	D49.0
hepatobiliary	C24.9	C79.89	D01.5	D13.5	D37.6	D49.0
hepatoblastoma	C22.2	C78.7	D01.5	D13.4	D37.6	D49.0
hepatoma	C22.0	C78.7	D01.5	D13.4	D37.6	D49.0
hilus of lung	C34.0-●	C78.0-●	D02.2-●	D14.3-●	D38.1	D49.1
hip NEC	C76.5-●	C79.89	D04.7-●	D36.7	D48.7	D49.89
hippocampus, brain	C71.2	C79.31	—	D33.0	D43.0	D49.6
humerus (any part)	C40.0-●	C79.51	—	D16.0-●	—	—
hymen	C52	C79.82	D07.2	D28.1	D39.8	D49.59

	Malignant Primary	Malignant Secondary	Ca in situ	Benign	Uncertain Behavior	Unspecified Behavior
hypopharynx, hypopharyngeal NEC	C13.9	C79.89	D00.08	D10.7	D37.05	D49.0
overlapping lesion	C13.8	—	—	—	—	—
postcricoid region	C13.0	C79.89	D00.08	D10.7	D37.05	D49.0
posterior wall	C13.2	C79.89	D00.08	D10.7	D37.05	D49.0
pyriform fossa (sinus)	C12	C79.89	D00.08	D10.7	D37.05	D49.0
hypophysis	C75.1	C79.89	D09.3	D35.2	D44.3	D49.7
hypothalamus	C71.0	C79.31	—	D33.0	D43.0	D49.6
ileocecum, ileocecal (coil) (junction) (valve)	C18.0	C78.5	D01.0	D12.0	D37.4	D49.0
ileum	C17.2	C78.4	D01.49	D13.39	D37.2	D49.0
ilium	C41.4	C79.51	—	D16.8	D48.0	D49.2
immunoproliferative NEC	C88.9	—	—	—	—	—
infraclavicular (region)	C76.1	C79.89	D04.5	D36.7	D48.7	D49.89
inguinal (region)	C76.3	C79.89	D04.5	D36.7	D48.7	D49.89
insula	C71.0	C79.31	—	D33.0	D43.0	D49.6
insular tissue (pancreas)	C25.4	C78.89	D01.7	D13.7	D37.8	D49.0
brain	C71.0	C79.31	—	D33.0	D43.0	D49.6
interarytenoid fold	C13.1	C79.89	D00.08	D10.7	D37.05	D49.0
hypopharyngeal aspect	C13.1	C79.89	D00.08	D10.7	D37.05	D49.0
laryngeal aspect	C32.1	C78.39	D02.0	D14.1	D38.0	D49.1
marginal zone	C13.1	C79.89	D00.08	D10.7	D37.05	D49.0
interdental papillae	C03.9	C79.89	D00.03	D10.39	D37.09	D49.0
lower	C03.1	C79.89	D00.03	D10.39	D37.09	D49.0
upper	C03.0	C79.89	D00.03	D10.39	D37.09	D49.0
internal						
capsule	C71.0	C79.31	—	D33.0	D43.0	D49.6
os (cervix)	C53.0	C79.82	D06.0	D26.0	D39.0	D49.59
intervertebral cartilage or disc	C41.2	C79.51	—	D16.6	D48.0	D49.2
intestine, intestinal	C26.0	C78.80	D01.40	D13.9	D37.8	D49.0
large	C18.9	C78.5	D01.0	D12.6	D37.4	D49.0
appendix	C18.1	C78.5	D01.0	D12.1	D37.3	D49.0
caput coli	C18.0	C78.5	D01.0	D12.0	D37.4	D49.0
cecum	C18.0	C78.5	D01.0	D12.0	D37.4	D49.0
colon	C18.9	C78.5	D01.0	D12.6	D37.4	D49.0
and rectum	C19	C78.5	D01.1	D12.7	D37.5	D49.0
ascending	C18.2	C78.5	D01.0	D12.2	D37.4	D49.0
caput	C18.0	C78.5	D01.0	D12.0	D37.4	D49.0
descending	C18.6	C78.5	D01.0	D12.4	D37.4	D49.0
distal	C18.6	C78.5	D01.0	D12.4	D37.4	D49.0
left	C18.6	C78.5	D01.0	D12.4	D37.4	D49.0
overlapping lesion	C18.8	—	—	—	—	—
pelvic	C18.7	C78.5	D01.0	D12.5	D37.4	D49.0
right	C18.2	C78.5	D01.0	D12.2	D37.4	D49.0

◀ New   ◀ Revised   ~~deleted~~ Deleted   ● Use Additional Character(s)

	Malignant Primary	Malignant Secondary	Ca in situ	Benign	Uncertain Behavior	Unspecified Behavior
intestine, intestinal *(Continued)*						
large *(Continued)*						
colon *(Continued)*						
sigmoid (flexure)	C18.7	C78.5	D01.0	D12.5	D37.4	D49.0
transverse	C18.4	C78.5	D01.0	D12.3	D37.4	D49.0
hepatic flexure	C18.3	C78.5	D01.0	D12.3	D37.4	D49.0
ileocecum, ileocecal (coil) (valve)	C18.0	C78.5	D01.0	D12.0	D37.4	D49.0
overlapping lesion	C18.8	—	—	—	—	—
sigmoid flexure (lower) (upper)	C18.7	C78.5	D01.0	D12.5	D37.4	D49.0
splenic flexure	C18.5	C78.5	D01.0	D12.3	D37.4	D49.0
small	C17.9	C78.4	D01.40	D13.30	D37.2	D49.0
duodenum	C17.0	C78.4	D01.49	D13.2	D37.2	D49.0
ileum	C17.2	C78.4	D01.49	D13.39	D37.2	D49.0
jejunum	C17.1	C78.4	D01.49	D13.39	D37.2	D49.0
overlapping lesion	C17.8	—	—	—	—	—
tract NEC	C26.0	C78.89	D01.40	D13.9	D37.8	D49.0
intra-abdominal	C76.2	C79.89	D09.8	D36.7	D48.7	D49.89
intracranial NEC	C71.9	C79.31	—	D33.2	D43.2	D49.6
intrahepatic (bile) duct	C22.1	C78.7	D01.5	D13.4	D37.6	D49.0
intraocular	C69.9-●	C79.49	D09.2-●	D31.9-●	D48.7	D49.89
intraorbital	C69.6-●	C79.49	D09.2-●	D31.6-●	D48.7	D49.89
intrasellar	C75.1	C79.89	D09.3	D35.2	D44.3	D49.7
intrathoracic (cavity) (organs)	C76.1	C79.89	D09.8	D15.9	D48.7	D49.89
specified NEC	C76.1	C79.89	D09.8	D15.7	—	—
iris	C69.4-●	C79.49	D09.2-●	D31.4-●	D48.7	D49.89
ischiorectal (fossa)	C76.3	C79.89	D09.8	D36.7	D48.7	D49.89
ischium	C41.4	C79.51	—	D16.8	D48.0	D49.2
island of Reil	C71.0	C79.31	—	D33.0	D43.0	D49.6
islands or islets of Langerhans	C25.4	C78.89	D01.7	D13.7	D37.8	D49.0
isthmus uteri	C54.0	C79.82	D07.0	D26.1	D39.0	D49.59
jaw	C76.0	C79.89	D09.8	D36.7	D48.7	D49.89
bone	C41.1	C79.51	—	D16.5-●	D48.0	D49.2
lower	C41.1	C79.51	—	D16.5-●	—	—
upper	C41.0	C79.51	—	D16.4-●	—	—
carcinoma (any type) (lower) (upper)	C76.0	C79.89	—	—	—	—
skin — *see also Neoplasm, skin, face*	C44.309	C79.2	D04.39	D23.39	D48.5	D49.2
soft tissues	C03.9	C79.89	D00.03	D10.39	D37.09	D49.0
lower	C03.1	C79.89	D00.03	D10.39	D37.09	D49.0
upper	C03.0	C79.89	D00.03	D10.39	D37.09	D49.0
jejunum	C17.1	C78.4	D01.49	D13.39	D37.2	D49.0

	Malignant Primary	Malignant Secondary	Ca in situ	Benign	Uncertain Behavior	Unspecified Behavior
joint NEC — *see also Neoplasm, bone*	C41.9	C79.51	—	D16.9-●	D48.0	D49.2
acromioclavicular	C40.0-●	C79.51	—	D16.0-●	—	—
bursa or synovial membrane — *see Neoplasm, connective tissue*						
costovertebral	C41.3	C79.51	—	D16.7	D48.0	D49.2
sternocostal	C41.3	C79.51	—	D16.7	D48.0	D49.2
temporomandibular	C41.1	C79.51	—	D16.5-●	D48.0	D49.2
junction						
anorectal	C21.8	C78.5	D01.3	D12.9	D37.8	D49.0
cardioesophageal	C16.0	C78.89	D00.2	D13.1	D37.1	D49.0
esophagogastric	C16.0	C78.89	D00.2	D13.1	D37.1	D49.0
gastroesophageal	C16.0	C78.89	D00.2	D13.1	D37.1	D49.0
hard and soft palate	C05.9	C79.89	D00.00	D10.39	D37.09	D49.0
ileocecal	C18.0	C78.5	D01.0	D12.0	D37.4	D49.0
pelvirectal	C19	C78.5	D01.1	D12.7	D37.5	D49.0
pelviureteric	C65.-●	C79.0-●	D09.19	D30.1-●	D41.1-●	D49.59
rectosigmoid	C19	C78.5	D01.1	D12.7	D37.5	D49.0
squamocolumnar, of cervix	C53.8	C79.82	D06.7	D26.0	D39.0	D49.59
Kaposi's sarcoma — *see Kaposi's, sarcoma*						
kidney (parenchymal)	C64.-●	C79.0-●	D09.19	D30.0-●	D41.0-●	D49.51-●
calyx	C65.-●	C79.0-●	D09.19	D30.1-●	D41.1-●	D49.51-●
hilus	C65.-●	C79.0-●	D09.19	D30.1-●	D41.1-●	D49.51-●
pelvis	C65.-●	C79.0-●	D09.19	D30.1-●	D41.1-●	D49.51-●
knee NEC	C76.5-●	C79.89	D04.7-●	D36.7	D48.7	D49.89
labia (skin)	C51.9	C79.82	D07.1	D28.0	D39.8	D49.59
majora	C51.0	C79.82	D07.1	D28.0	D39.8	D49.59
minora	C51.1	C79.82	D07.1	D28.0	D39.8	D49.59
labial — *see also Neoplasm, lip*	C00.9	C79.89	D00.01	D10.0	D37.01	D49.0
sulcus (lower) (upper)	C06.1	C79.89	D00.02	D10.39	D37.09	D49.0
labium (skin)	C51.9	C79.82	D07.1	D28.0	D39.8	D49.59
majus	C51.0	C79.82	D07.1	D28.0	D39.8	D49.59
minus	C51.1	C79.82	D07.1	D28.0	D39.8	D49.59
lacrimal						
canaliculi	C69.5-●	C79.49	D09.2-●	D31.5-●	D48.7	D49.89
duct (nasal)	C69.5-●	C79.49	D09.2-●	D31.5-●	D48.7	D49.89
gland	C69.5-●	C79.49	D09.2-●	D31.5-●	D48.7	D49.89
punctum	C69.5-●	C79.49	D09.2-●	D31.5-●	D48.7	D49.89
sac	C69.5-●	C79.49	D09.2-●	D31.5-●	D48.7	D49.89
Langerhans, islands or islets	C25.4	C78.89	D01.7	D13.7	D37.8	D49.0
laryngopharynx	C13.9	C79.89	D00.08	D10.7	D37.05	D49.0

◀ New   ◀|| Revised   ~~deleted~~ Deleted   ● Use Additional Character(s)

	Malignant Primary	Malignant Secondary	Ca in situ	Benign	Uncertain Behavior	Unspecified Behavior
larynx, laryngeal NEC	C32.9	C78.39	D02.0	D14.1	D38.0	D49.1
aryepiglottic fold	C32.1	C78.39	D02.0	D14.1	D38.0	D49.1
cartilage (arytenoid) (cricoid) (cuneiform) (thyroid)	C32.3	C78.39	D02.0	D14.1	D38.0	D49.1
commissure (anterior) (posterior)	C32.0	C78.39	D02.0	D14.1	D38.0	D49.1
extrinsic NEC	C32.1	C78.39	D02.0	D14.1	D38.0	D49.1
meaning hypopharynx	C13.9	C79.89	D00.08	D10.7	D37.05	D49.0
interarytenoid fold	C32.1	C78.39	D02.0	D14.1	D38.0	D49.1
intrinsic	C32.0	C78.39	D02.0	D14.1	D38.0	D49.1
overlapping lesion	C32.8	—	—	—	—	—
ventricular band	C32.1	C78.39	D02.0	D14.1	D38.0	D49.1
leg NEC	C76.5-●	C79.89	D04.7-●	D36.7	D48.7	D49.89
lens, crystalline	C69.4-●	C79.49	D09.2-●	D31.4-●	D48.7	D49.89
lid (lower) (upper)	C44.10-●	C79.2	D04.1-●	D23.1-●	D48.5	D49.2
basal cell carcinoma	C44.11-●	—	—	—	—	—
sebaceous cell	C44.13-●	—	—	—	—	—
specified type NEC	C44.19-●	—	—	—	—	—
squamous cell carcinoma	C44.12-●	—	—	—	—	—
ligament — see also Neoplasm, connective tissue						
broad	C57.1	C79.82	D07.39	D28.2	D39.8	D49.59
Mackenrodt's	C57.7	C79.82	D07.39	D28.7	D39.8	D49.59
non-uterine — see Neoplasm, connective tissue						
round	C57.2	C79.82	—	D28.2	D39.8	D49.59
sacro-uterine	C57.3	C79.82	—	D28.2	D39.8	D49.59
uterine	C57.3	C79.82	—	D28.2	D39.8	D49.59
utero-ovarian	C57.7	C79.82	D07.39	D28.2	D39.8	D49.59
uterosacral	C57.3	C79.82		D28.2	D39.8	D49.59
limb	C76.8	C79.89	D04.8	D36.7	D48.7	D49.89
lower	C76.5-●	C79.89	D04.7-●	D36.7	D48.7	D49.89
upper	C76.4-●	C79.89	D04.6-●	D36.7	D48.7	D49.89
limbus of cornea	C69.1-●	C79.49	D09.2-●	D31.1-●	D48.7	D49.89
lingual NEC — see also Neoplasm, tongue	C02.9	C79.89	D00.07	D10.1	D37.02	D49.0
lingula, lung	C34.1-●	C78.0-●	D02.2-●	D14.3-●	D38.1	D49.1
lip	C00.9	C79.89	D00.01	D10.0	D37.01	D49.0
buccal aspect — see Neoplasm, lip, internal						
commissure	C00.6	C79.89	D00.01	D10.0	D37.01	D49.0
external	C00.2	C79.89	D00.01	D10.0	D37.01	D49.0
lower	C00.1	C79.89	D00.01	D10.0	D37.01	D49.0
upper	C00.0	C79.89	D00.01	D10.0	D37.01	D49.0
frenulum — see Neoplasm, lip, internal						

	Malignant Primary	Malignant Secondary	Ca in situ	Benign	Uncertain Behavior	Unspecified Behavior
lip (Continued)						
inner aspect — see Neoplasm, lip, internal						
internal	C00.5	C79.89	D00.01	D10.0	D37.01	D49.0
lower	C00.4	C79.89	D00.01	D10.0	D37.01	D49.0
upper	C00.3	C79.89	D00.01	D10.0	D37.01	D49.0
lipstick area	C00.2	C79.89	D00.01	D10.0	D37.01	D49.0
lower	C00.1	C79.89	D00.01	D10.0	D37.01	D49.0
upper	C00.0	C79.89	D00.01	D10.0	D37.01	D49.0
lower	C00.1	C79.89	D00.01	D10.0	D37.01	D49.0
internal	C00.4	C79.89	D00.01	D10.0	D37.01	D49.0
mucosa — see Neoplasm, lip, internal						
oral aspect — see Neoplasm, lip, internal						
overlapping lesion	C00.8	—	—	—	—	—
with oral cavity or pharynx	C14.8	—	—	—	—	—
skin (commissure) (lower) (upper)	C44.00	C79.2	D04.0	D23.0	D48.5	D49.2
basal cell carcinoma	C44.01	—	—	—	—	—
specified type NEC	C44.09	—	—	—	—	—
squamous cell carcinoma	C44.02	—	—	—	—	—
upper	C00.0	C79.89	D00.01	D10.0	D37.01	D49.0
internal	C00.3	C79.89	D00.01	D10.0	D37.01	D49.0
vermilion border	C00.2	C79.89	D00.01	D10.0	D37.01	D49.0
lower	C00.1	C79.89	D00.01	D10.0	D37.01	D49.0
upper	C00.0	C79.89	D00.01	D10.0	D37.01	D49.0
lipomatous — see Lipoma, by site						
liver — see also Index to disease, by histology	C22.9	C78.7	D01.5	D13.4	D37.6	D49.0
primary	C22.8	C78.7	D01.5	D13.4	D37.6	D49.0
lumbosacral plexus	C47.5	C79.89	—	D36.16	D48.2	D49.2
lung	C34.9-●	C78.0-●	D02.2-●	D14.3-●	D38.1	D49.1
azygos lobe	C34.1-●	C78.0-●	D02.2-●	D14.3-●	D38.1	D49.1
carina	C34.0-●	C78.0-●	D02.2-●	D14.3-●	D38.1	D49.1
hilus	C34.0-●	C78.0-●	D02.2-●	D14.3-●	D38.1	D49.1
linqula	C34.1-●	C78.0-●	D02.2-●	D14.3-●	D38.1	D49.1
lobe NEC	C34.9-●	C78.0-●	D02.2-●	D14.3-●	D38.1	D49.1
lower lobe	C34.3-●	C78.0-●	D02.2-●	D14.3-●	D38.1	D49.1
main bronchus	C34.0-●	C78.0-●	D02.2-●	D14.3-●	D38.1	D49.1
mesothelioma — see Mesothelioma						
middle lobe	C34.2	C78.0-●	D02.21	D14.31	D38.1	D49.1
overlapping lesion	C34.8-●	—	—	—	—	—
upper lobe	C34.1-●	C78.0-●	D02.2-●	D14.3-●	D38.1	D49.1

◀ New   ◀| Revised   ~~deleted~~ Deleted   ● Use Additional Character(s)

	Malignant Primary	Malignant Secondary	Ca in situ	Benign	Uncertain Behavior	Unspecified Behavior
lymph, lymphatic channel NEC	C49.9	C79.89	—	D21.9	D48.1	D49.2
gland (secondary)	—	C77.9	—	D36.0	D48.7	D49.89
abdominal	—	C77.2	—	D36.0	D48.7	D49.89
aortic	—	C77.2	—	D36.0	D48.7	D49.89
arm	—	C77.3	—	D36.0	D48.7	D49.89
auricular (anterior) (posterior)	—	C77.0	—	D36.0	D48.7	D49.89
axilla, axillary	—	C77.3	—	D36.0	D48.7	D49.89
brachial	—	C77.3	—	D36.0	D48.7	D49.89
bronchial	—	C77.1	—	D36.0	D48.7	D49.89
bronchopulmonary	—	C77.1	—	D36.0	D48.7	D49.89
celiac	—	C77.2	—	D36.0	D48.7	D49.89
cervical	—	C77.0	—	D36.0	D48.7	D49.89
cervicofacial	—	C77.0	—	D36.0	D48.7	D49.89
Cloquet	—	C77.4	—	D36.0	D48.7	D49.89
colic	—	C77.2	—	D36.0	D48.7	D49.89
common duct	—	C77.2	—	D36.0	D48.7	D49.89
cubital	—	C77.3	—	D36.0	D48.7	D49.89
diaphragmatic	—	C77.1	—	D36.0	D48.7	D49.89
epigastric, inferior	—	C77.1	—	D36.0	D48.7	D49.89
epitrochlear	—	C77.3	—	D36.0	D48.7	D49.89
esophageal	—	C77.1	—	D36.0	D48.7	D49.89
face	—	C77.0	—	D36.0	D48.7	D49.89
femoral	—	C77.4	—	D36.0	D48.7	D49.89
gastric	—	C77.2	—	D36.0	D48.7	D49.89
groin	—	C77.4	—	D36.0	D48.7	D49.89
head	—	C77.0	—	D36.0	D48.7	D49.89
hepatic	—	C77.2	—	D36.0	D48.7	D49.89
hilar (pulmonary)	—	C77.1	—	D36.0	D48.7	D49.89
splenic	—	C77.2	—	D36.0	D48.7	D49.89
hypogastric	—	C77.5	—	D36.0	D48.7	D49.89
ileocolic	—	C77.2	—	D36.0	D48.7	D49.89
iliac	—	C77.5	—	D36.0	D48.7	D49.89
infraclavicular	—	C77.3	—	D36.0	D48.7	D49.89
inguina, inguinal	—	C77.4	—	D36.0	D48.7	D49.89
innominate	—	C77.1	—	D36.0	D48.7	D49.89
intercostal	—	C77.1	—	D36.0	D48.7	D49.89
intestinal	—	C77.2	—	D36.0	D48.7	D49.89
intrabdominal	—	C77.2	—	D36.0	D48.7	D49.89
intrapelvic	—	C77.5	—	D36.0	D48.7	D49.89
intrathoracic	—	C77.1	—	D36.0	D48.7	D49.89
jugular	—	C77.0	—	D36.0	D48.7	D49.89
leg	—	C77.4	—	D36.0	D48.7	D49.89
limb						
lower	—	C77.4	—	D36.0	D48.7	D49.89
upper	—	C77.3	—	D36.0	D48.7	D49.89

	Malignant Primary	Malignant Secondary	Ca in situ	Benign	Uncertain Behavior	Unspecified Behavior
lymph, lymphatic channel NEC (Continued)						
gland (Continued)						
lower limb	—	C77.4	—	D36.0	D48.7	D49.89
lumbar	—	C77.2	—	D36.0	D48.7	D49.89
mandibular	—	C77.0	—	D36.0	D48.7	D49.89
mediastinal	—	C77.1	—	D36.0	D48.7	D49.89
mesenteric (inferior) (superior)	—	C77.2	—	D36.0	D48.7	D49.89
midcolic	—	C77.2	—	D36.0	D48.7	D49.89
multiple sites in categories C77.0 - C77.5	—	C77.8	—	D36.0	D48.7	D49.89
neck	—	C77.0	—	D36.0	D48.7	D49.89
obturator	—	C77.5	—	D36.0	D48.7	D49.89
occipital	—	C77.0	—	D36.0	D48.7	D49.89
pancreatic	—	C77.2	—	D36.0	D48.7	D49.89
para-aortic	—	C77.2	—	D36.0	D48.7	D49.89
paracervical	—	C77.5	—	D36.0	D48.7	D49.89
parametrial	—	C77.5	—	D36.0	D48.7	D49.89
parasternal	—	C77.1	—	D36.0	D48.7	D49.89
parotid	—	C77.0	—	D36.0	D48.7	D49.89
pectoral	—	C77.3	—	D36.0	D48.7	D49.89
pelvic	—	C77.5	—	D36.0	D48.7	D49.89
peri-aortic	—	C77.2	—	D36.0	D48.7	D49.89
peripancreatic	—	C77.2	—	D36.0	D48.7	D49.89
popliteal	—	C77.4	—	D36.0	D48.7	D49.89
porta hepatis	—	C77.2	—	D36.0	D48.7	D49.89
portal	—	C77.2	—	D36.0	D48.7	D49.89
preauricular	—	C77.0	—	D36.0	D48.7	D49.89
prelaryngeal	—	C77.0	—	D36.0	D48.7	D49.89
presymphysial	—	C77.5	—	D36.0	D48.7	D49.89
pretracheal	—	C77.0	—	D36.0	D48.7	D49.89
primary (any site) NEC	C96.9	—	—	—	—	D49.89
pulmonary (hiler)	—	C77.1	—	D36.0	D48.7	D49.89
pyloric	—	C77.2	—	D36.0	D48.7	D49.89
retroperitoneal	—	C77.2	—	D36.0	D48.7	D49.89
retropharyngeal	—	C77.0	—	D36.0	D48.7	D49.89
Rosenmuller's	—	C77.4	—	D36.0	D48.7	D49.89
sacral	—	C77.5	—	D36.0	D48.7	D49.89
scalene	—	C77.0	—	D36.0	D48.7	D49.89
site NEC	—	C77.9	—	D36.0	D48.7	D49.89
splenic (hilar)	—	C77.2	—	D36.0	D48.7	D49.89
subclavicular	—	C77.3	—	D36.0	D48.7	D49.89
subinguinal	—	C77.4	—	D36.0	D48.7	D49.89

◀ New   ◀ Revised   ~~deleted~~ Deleted   ● Use Additional Character(s)

	Malignant Primary	Malignant Secondary	Ca in situ	Benign	Uncertain Behavior	Unspecified Behavior
lymph, lymphatic channel NEC *(Continued)*						
gland *(Continued)*						
sublingual	—	C77.0	—	D36.0	D48.7	D49.89
submandibular	—	C77.0	—	D36.0	D48.7	D49.89
submaxillary	—	C77.0	—	D36.0	D48.7	D49.89
submental	—	C77.0	—	D36.0	D48.7	D49.89
subscapular	—	C77.3	—	D36.0	D48.7	D49.89
supraclavicular	—	C77.0	—	D36.0	D48.7	D49.89
thoracic	—	C77.1	—	D36.0	D48.7	D49.89
tibial	—	C77.4	—	D36.0	D48.7	D49.89
tracheal	—	C77.1	—	D36.0	D48.7	D49.89
tracheobronchial	—	C77.1	—	D36.0	D48.7	D49.89
upper limb	—	C77.3	—	D36.0	D48.7	D49.89
Virchow's	—	C77.0	—	D36.0	D48.7	D49.89
node — *see also Neoplasm, lymph gland*						
primary NEC	C96.9	—	—	—	—	—
vessel — *see also Neoplasm, connective tissue*	C49.9	C79.89	—	D21.9	D48.1	D49.2
Mackenrodt's ligament	C57.7	C79.82	D07.39	D28.7	D39.8	D49.59
malar	C41.0	C79.51	—	D16.4-•	D48.0	D49.2
region — *see Neoplasm, cheek*						
mammary gland — *see Neoplasm, breast*						
mandible	C41.1	C79.51	—	D16.5-•	D48.0	D49.2
alveolar						
mucosa (carcinoma)	C03.1	C79.89	D00.03	D10.39	D37.09	D49.0
ridge or process	C41.1	C79.51	—	D16.5-•	D48.0	D49.2
marrow (bone) NEC	C96.9	C79.52	—	—	D47.9	D49.89
mastectomy site (skin) — *see also Neoplasm, breast, skin*	C44.501	C79.2	—	—	—	—
specified as breast tissue	C50.8-•	C79.81				
mastoid (air cells) (antrum) (cavity)	C30.1	C78.39	D02.3	D14.0	D38.5	D49.1
bone or process	C41.0	C79.51	—	D16.4-•	D48.0	D49.2
maxilla, maxillary (superior)	C41.0	C79.51	—	D16.4-•	D48.0	D49.2
alveolar						
mucosa	C03.0	C79.89	D00.03	D10.39	D37.09	D49.0
ridge or process (carcinoma)	C41.0	C79.51	—	D16.4-•	D48.0	D49.2
antrum	C31.0	C78.39	D02.3	D14.0	D38.5	D49.1
carcinoma	C03.0	C79.51		—	—	—
inferior — *see Neoplasm, mandible*						
sinus	C31.0	C78.39	D02.3	D14.0	D38.5	D49.1

	Malignant Primary	Malignant Secondary	Ca in situ	Benign	Uncertain Behavior	Unspecified Behavior
meatus external (ear) — *see also Neoplasm, skin, ear*	C44.20-•	C79.2	D04.2-•	D23.2-•	D48.5	D49.2
Meckel diverticulum, malignant	C17.3	C78.4	D01.49	D13.39	D37.2	D49.0
mediastinum, mediastinal	C38.3	C78.1	—	D15.2	D38.3	D49.89
anterior	C38.1	C78.1	—	D15.2	D38.3	D49.89
posterior	C38.2	C78.1	—	D15.2	D38.3	D49.89
medulla						
adrenal	C74.1-•	C79.7-•	D09.3	D35.0-•	D44.1-•	D49.7
oblongata	C71.7	C79.31	—	D33.1	D43.1	D49.6
meibomian gland	C44.10-•	C79.2	D04.1-•	D23.1-•	D48.5	D49.2
basal cell carcinoma	C44.11-•	—	—	—	—	—
sebaceous cell	C44.13-•	—	—	—	—	—
specified type NEC	C44.19-•	—	—	—	—	—
squamous cell carcinoma	C44.12-•	—	—	—	—	—
melanoma — *see Melanoma*						
meninges	C70.9	C79.49	—	D32.9	D42.9	D49.7
brain	C70.0	C79.32	—	D32.0	D42.0	D49.7
cerebral	C70.0	C79.32		D32.0	D42.0	D49.7
crainial	C70.0	C79.32		D32.0	D42.0	D49.7
intracranial	C70.0	C79.32		D32.0	D42.0	D49.7
spinal (cord)	C70.1	C79.49	—	D32.1	D42.1	D49.7
meniscus, knee joint (lateral) (medial)	C40.2-•	C79.51	—	D16.2-•	D48.0	D49.2
Merkel cell — *see Carcinoma, Merkel cell*						
mesentery, mesenteric	C48.1	C78.6	—	D20.1	D48.4	D49.0
mesoappendix	C48.1	C78.6	—	D20.1	D48.4	D49.0
mesocolon	C48.1	C78.6	—	D20.1	D48.4	D49.0
mesopharynx — *see Neoplasm, oropharynx*						
mesosalpinx	C57.1	C79.82	D07.39	D28.2	D39.8	D49.59
mesothelial tissue — *see Mesothelioma*						
mesothelioma — *see Mesothelioma*						
mesovarium	C57.1	C79.82	D07.39	D28.2	D39.8	D49.59
metacarpus (any bone)	C40.1-•	C79.51	—	D16.1-•	—	—
metastatic NEC — *see also Neoplasm, by site, secondary*	—	C79.9				
metatarsus (any bone)	C40.3-•	C79.51	—	D16.3-•	—	—
midbrain	C71.7	C79.31	—	D33.1	D43.1	D49.6
milk duct — *see Neoplasm, breast*						
mons						
pubis	C51.9	C79.82	D07.1	D28.0	D39.8	D49.59
veneris	C51.9	C79.82	D07.1	D28.0	D39.8	D49.59

◀ New ◀ Revised ~~deleted~~ Deleted • Use Additional Character(s)

	Malignant Primary	Malignant Secondary	Ca in situ	Benign	Uncertain Behavior	Unspecified Behavior
motor tract	C72.9	C79.49	—	D33.9	D43.9	D49.7
brain	C71.9	C79.31	—	D33.2	D43.2	D49.6
cauda equina	C72.1	C79.49	—	D33.4	D43.4	D49.7
spinal	C72.0	C79.49	—	D33.4	D43.4	D49.7
mouth	C06.9	C79.89	D00.00	D10.30	D37.09	D49.0
book-leaf	C06.89	C79.89	—	—	—	—
floor	C04.9	C79.89	D00.06	D10.2	D37.09	D49.0
anterior portion	C04.0	C79.89	D00.06	D10.2	D37.09	D49.0
lateral portion	C04.1	C79.89	D00.06	D10.2	D37.09	D49.0
overlapping lesion	C04.8	—	—	—	—	—
overlapping NEC	C06.80	—	—	—	—	—
roof	C05.9	C79.89	D00.00	D10.39	D37.09	D49.0
specified part NEC	C06.89	C79.89	D00.00	D10.39	D37.09	D49.0
vestibule	C06.1	C79.89	D00.00	D10.39	D37.09	D49.0
mucosa						
alveolar (ridge or process)	C03.9	C79.89	D00.03	D10.39	D37.09	D49.0
lower	C03.1	C79.89	D00.03	D10.39	D37.09	D49.0
upper	C03.0	C79.89	D00.03	D10.39	D37.09	D49.0
buccal	C06.0	C79.89	D00.02	D10.39	D37.09	D49.0
cheek	C06.0	C79.89	D00.02	D10.39	D37.09	D49.0
lip — see Neoplasm, lip, internal						
nasal	C30.0	C78.39	D02.3	D14.0	D38.5	D49.1
oral	C06.0	C79.89	D00.02	D10.39	D37.09	D49.0
Mullerian duct						
female	C57.7	C79.82	D07.39	D28.7	D39.8	D49.59
male	C63.7	C79.82	D07.69	D29.8	D40.8	D49.59
muscle — see also Neoplasm, connective tissue						
extraocular	C69.6-●	C79.49	D09.2-●	D31.6-●	D48.7	D49.89
myocardium	C38.0	C79.89	—	D15.1	D48.7	D49.89
myometrium	C54.2	C79.82	D07.0	D26.1	D39.0	D49.59
myopericardium	C38.0	C79.89	—	D15.1	D48.7	D49.89
nabothian gland (follicle)	C53.0	C79.82	D06.0	D26.0	D39.0	D49.59
nail — see also Neoplasm, skin, limb	C44.90	C79.2	D04.9	D23.9	D48.5	D49.2
finger — see also Neoplasm, skin, limb, upper	C44.60-●	C79.2	D04.6-●	D23.6-●	D48.5	D49.2
toe — see also Neoplasm, skin, limb, lower	C44.70-●	C79.2	D04.7-●	D23.7-●	D48.5	D49.2
nares, naris (anterior) (posterior)	C30.0	C78.39	D02.3	D14.0	D38.5	D49.1
nasal — see Neoplasm, nose						
nasolabial groove — see also Neoplasm, skin, face	C44.309	C79.2	D04.39	D23.39	D48.5	D49.2
nasolacrimal duct	C69.5-●	C79.49	D09.2-●	D31.5-●	D48.7	D49.89

	Malignant Primary	Malignant Secondary	Ca in situ	Benign	Uncertain Behavior	Unspecified Behavior
nasopharynx, nasopharyngeal	C11.9	C79.89	D00.08	D10.6	D37.05	D49.0
floor	C11.3	C79.89	D00.08	D10.6	D37.05	D49.0
overlapping lesion	C11.8	—	—	—	—	—
roof	C11.0	C79.89	D00.08	D10.6	D37.05	D49.0
wall	C11.9	C79.89	D00.08	D10.6	D37.05	D49.0
anterior	C11.3	C79.89	D00.08	D10.6	D37.05	D49.0
lateral	C11.2	C79.89	D00.08	D10.6	D37.05	D49.0
posterior	C11.1	C79.89	D00.08	D10.6	D37.05	D49.0
superior	C11.0	C79.89	D00.08	D10.6	D37.05	D49.0
nates — see also Neoplasm, skin, trunk	C44.509	C79.2	D04.5	D23.5	D48.5	D49.2
neck NEC	C76.0	C79.89	D09.8	D36.7	D48.7	D49.89
skin	C44.40	—	—	—	—	—
basal cell carcinoma	C44.41	—	—	—	—	—
specified type NEC	C44.49	—	—	—	—	—
squamous cell carcinoma	C44.42	—	—	—	—	—
nerve (ganglion)	C47.9	C79.89	—	D36.10	D48.2	D49.2
abducens	C72.59	C79.49	—	D33.3	D43.3	D49.7
accessory (spinal)	C72.59	C79.49	—	D33.3	D43.3	D49.7
acoustic	C72.4-●	C79.49	—	D33.3	D43.3	D49.7
auditory	C72.4-●	C79.49	—	D33.3	D43.3	D49.7
autonomic NEC — see also Neoplasm, nerve, peripheral	C47.9	C79.89	—	D36.10	D48.2	D49.2
brachial	C47.1-●	C79.89	—	D36.12	D48.2	D49.2
cranial	C72.50	C79.49	—	D33.3	D43.3	D49.7
specified NEC	C72.59	C79.49	—	D33.3	D43.3	D49.7
facial	C72.59	C79.49	—	D33.3	D43.3	D49.7
femoral	C47.2-●	C79.89	—	D36.13	D48.2	D49.2
ganglion NEC — see also Neoplasm, nerve, peripheral	C47.9	C79.89	—	D36.10	D48.2	D49.2
glossopharyngeal	C72.59	C79.49	—	D33.3	D43.3	D49.7
hypoglossal	C72.59	C79.49	—	D33.3	D43.3	D49.7
intercostal	C47.3	C79.89	—	D36.14	D48.2	D49.2
lumbar	C47.6	C79.89	—	D36.17	D48.2	D49.2
median	C47.1-●	C79.89	—	D36.12	D48.2	D49.2
obturator	C47.2-●	C79.89	—	D36.13	D48.2	D49.2
oculomotor	C72.59	C79.49	—	D33.3	D43.3	D49.7
olfactory	C47.2-●	C79.49	—	D33.3	D43.3	D49.7
optic	C72.3-●	C79.49	—	D33.3	D43.3	D49.7
parasympathetic NEC	C47.9	C79.89	—	D36.10	D48.2	D49.2
peripheral NEC	C47.9	C79.89	—	D36.10	D48.2	D49.2
abdomen	C47.4	C79.89	—	D36.15	D48.2	D49.2
abdominal wall	C47.4	C79.89	—	D36.15	D48.2	D49.2

TABLE OF NEOPLASMS

	Malignant Primary	Malignant Secondary	Ca in situ	Benign	Uncertain Behavior	Unspecified Behavior
nerve *(Continued)*						
peripheral NEC *(Continued)*						
ankle	C47.2-●	C79.89	—	D36.13	D48.2	D49.2
antecubital fossa or space	C47.1-●	C79.89	—	D36.12	D48.2	D49.2
arm	C47.1-●	C79.89	—	D36.12	D48.2	D49.2
auricle (ear)	C47.0	C79.89	—	D36.11	D48.2	D49.2
axilla	C47.3	C79.89	—	D36.12	D48.2	D49.2
back	C47.6	C79.89	—	D36.17	D48.2	D49.2
buttock	C47.5	C79.89	—	D36.16	D48.2	D49.2
calf	C47.2-●	C79.89	—	D36.13	D48.2	D49.2
cervical region	C47.0	C79.89	—	D36.11	D48.2	D49.2
cheek	C47.0	C79.89	—	D36.11	D48.2	D49.2
chest (wall)	C47.3	C79.89	—	D36.14	D48.2	D49.2
chin	C47.0	C79.89	—	D36.11	D48.2	D49.2
ear (external)	C47.0	C79.89	—	D36.11	D48.2	D49.2
elbow	C47.1-●	C79.89	—	D36.12	D48.2	D49.2
extrarectal	C47.5	C79.89	—	D36.16	D48.2	D49.2
extremity	C47.9	C79.89	—	D36.10	D48.2	D49.2
lower	C47.2-●	C79.89	—	D36.13	D48.2	D49.2
upper	C47.1-●	C79.89	—	D36.12	D48.2	D49.2
eyelid	C47.0	C79.89	—	D36.11	D48.2	D49.2
face	C47.0	C79.89	—	D36.11	D48.2	D49.2
finger	C47.1-●	C79.89	—	D36.12	D48.2	D49.2
flank	C47.6	C79.89	—	D36.17	D48.2	D49.2
foot	C47.2-●	C79.89	—	D36.13	D48.2	D49.2
forearm	C47.1-●	C79.89	—	D36.12	D48.2	D49.2
forehead	C47.0	C79.89	—	D36.11	D48.2	D49.2
gluteal region	C47.5	C79.89	—	D36.16	D48.2	D49.2
groin	C47.5	C79.89	—	D36.16	D48.2	D49.2
hand	C47.1-●	C79.89	—	D36.12	D48.2	D49.2
head	C47.0	C79.89	—	D36.11	D48.2	D49.2
heel	C47.2-●	C79.89	—	D36.13	D48.2	D49.2
hip	C47.2-●	C79.89	—	D36.13	D48.2	D49.2
infraclavicular region	C47.3	C79.89	—	D36.14	D48.2	D49.2
inguinal (canal) (region)	C47.5	C79.89	—	D36.16	D48.2	D49.2
intrathoracic	C47.3	C79.89	—	D36.14	D48.2	D49.2
ischiorectal fossa	C47.5	C79.89	—	D36.16	D48.2	D49.2
knee	C47.2-●	C79.89	—	D36.13	D48.2	D49.2
leg	C47.2-●	C79.89	—	D36.13	D48.2	D49.2
limb NEC	C47.9	C79.89	—	D36.10	D48.2	D49.2
lower	C47.2-●	C79.89	—	D36.13	D48.2	D49.2
upper	C47.1-●	C79.89	—	D36.12	D48.2	D49.2
nates	C47.5	C79.89	—	D36.16	D48.2	D49.2
neck	C47.0	C79.89	—	D36.11	D48.2	D49.2

	Malignant Primary	Malignant Secondary	Ca in situ	Benign	Uncertain Behavior	Unspecified Behavior
nerve *(Continued)*						
peripheral NEC *(Continued)*						
orbit	C69.6-●	C79.49	—	D31.6-●	D48.7	D49.2
pararectal	C47.5	C79.89	—	D36.16	D48.2	D49.2
paraurethral	C47.5	C79.89	—	D36.16	D48.2	D49.2
paravaginal	C47.5	C79.89	—	D36.16	D48.2	D49.2
pelvis (floor)	C47.5	C79.89	—	D36.16	D48.2	D49.2
pelvoabdominal	C47.8	C79.89	—	D36.17	D48.2	D49.2
perineum	C47.5	C79.89	—	D36.16	D48.2	D49.2
perirectal (tissue)	C47.5	C79.89	—	D36.16	D48.2	D49.2
periurethral (tissue)	C47.5	C79.89	—	D36.16	D48.2	D49.2
popliteal fossa or space	C47.2-●	C79.89	—	D36.13	D48.2	D49.2
presacral	C47.5	C79.89	—	D36.16	D48.2	D49.2
pterygoid fossa	C47.0	C79.89	—	D36.11	D48.2	D49.2
rectovaginal septum or wall	C47.5	C79.89	—	D36.16	D48.2	D49.2
rectovesical	C47.5	C79.89	—	D36.16	D48.2	D49.2
sacrococcygeal region	C47.5	C79.89	—	D36.16	D48.2	D49.2
scalp	C47.0	C79.89	—	D36.11	D48.2	D49.2
scapular region	C47.3	C79.89	—	D36.14	D48.2	D49.2
shoulder	C47.1-●	C79.89	—	D36.12	D48.2	D49.2
submental	C47.0	C79.89	—	D36.11	D48.2	D49.2
supraclavicular region	C47.0	C79.89	—	D36.11	D48.2	D49.2
temple	C47.0	C79.89	—	D36.11	D48.2	D49.2
temporal region	C47.0	C79.89	—	D36.11	D48.2	D49.2
thigh	C47.2-●	C79.89	—	D36.13	D48.2	D49.2
thoracic (duct) (wall)	C47.3	C79.89	—	D36.14	D48.2	D49.2
thorax	C47.3	C79.89	—	D36.14	D48.2	D49.2
thumb	C47.1-●	C79.89	—	D36.12	D48.2	D49.2
toe	C47.2-●	C79.89	—	D36.13	D48.2	D49.2
trunk	C47.6	C79.89	—	D36.17	D48.2	D49.2
umbilicus	C47.4	C79.89	—	D36.15	D48.2	D49.2
vesicorectal	C47.5	C79.89	—	D36.16	D48.2	D49.2
wrist	C47.1-●	C79.89	—	D36.12	D48.2	D49.2
radial	C47.1-●	C79.89	—	D36.12	D48.2	D49.2
sacral	C47.5	C79.89	—	D36.16	D48.2	D49.2
sciatic	C47.2-●	C79.89	—	D36.13	D48.2	D49.2
spinal NEC	C47.9	C79.89	—	D36.10	D48.2	D49.2
accessory	C72.59	C79.49	—	D33.3	D43.3	D49.7
sympathetic NEC — *see also Neoplasm, nerve, peripheral*	C47.9	C79.89	—	D36.10	D48.2	D49.2
trigeminal	C72.59	C79.49	—	D33.3	D43.3	D49.7
trochlear	C72.59	C79.49	—	D33.3	D43.3	D49.7
ulnar	C47.1-●	C79.89	—	D36.12	D48.2	D49.2
vagus	C72.59	C79.49	—	D33.3	D43.3	D49.7

◀ New ◀ Revised ~~deleted~~ Deleted ● Use Additional Character(s)

	Malignant Primary	Malignant Secondary	Ca in situ	Benign	Uncertain Behavior	Unspecified Behavior
nervous system (central)	C72.9	C79.40	—	D33.9	D43.9	D49.7
autonomic — *see Neoplasm, nerve, peripheral*						
parasympathetic — *see Neoplasm, nerve, peripheral*						
specified site NEC	—	C79.49	—	D33.7	D43.8	—
sympathetic — *see Neoplasm, nerve, peripheral*						
nevus — *see Nevus*						
nipple	C50.0-●	C79.81	D05.-●	D24.-●	—	—
nose, nasal	C76.0	C79.89	D09.8	D36.7	D48.7	D49.89
ala (external) (nasi) — *see also Neoplasm, nose, skin*	C44.301	C79.2	D04.39	D23.39	D48.5	D49.2
bone	C41.0	C79.51	—	D16.4-●	D48.0	D49.2
cartilage	C30.0	C78.39	D02.3	D14.0	D38.5	D49.1
cavity	C30.0	C78.39	D02.3	D14.0	D38.5	D49.1
choana	C11.3	C79.89	D00.08	D10.6	D37.05	D49.0
external (skin) — *see also Neoplasm, nose, skin*	C44.301	C79.2	D04.39	D23.39	D48.5	D49.2
fossa	C30.0	C78.39	D02.3	D14.0	D38.5	D49.1
internal	C30.0	C78.39	D02.3	D14.0	D38.5	D49.1
mucosa	C30.0	C78.39	D02.3	D14.0	D38.5	D49.1
septum	C30.0	C78.39	D02.3	D14.0	D38.5	D49.1
posterior margin	C11.3	C79.89	D00.08	D10.6	D37.05	D49.0
sinus — *see Neoplasm, sinus*						
skin	C44.301	C79.2	D04.39	D23.39	D48.5	D49.2
basal cell carcinoma	C44.311	—	—	—	—	—
specified type NEC	C44.391	—	—	—	—	—
squamous cell carcinoma	C44.321	—	—	—	—	—
turbinate (mucosa)	C30.0	C78.39	D02.3	D14.0	D38.5	D49.1
bone	C41.0	C79.51	—	D16.4-●	D48.0	D49.2
vestibule	C30.0	C78.39	D02.3	D14.0	D38.5	D49.1
nostril	C30.0	C78.39	D02.3	D14.0	D38.5	D49.1
nucleus pulposus	C41.2	C79.51	—	D16.6	D48.0	D49.2
occipital						
bone	C41.0	C79.51	—	D16.4-●	D48.0	D49.2
lobe or pole, brain	C71.4	C79.31	—	D33.0	D43.0	D49.6
odontogenic — *see Neoplasm, jaw bone*						
olfactory nerve or bulb	C72.2-●	C79.49	—	D33.3	D43.3	D49.7
olive (brain)	C71.7	C79.31	—	D33.1	D43.1	D49.6
omentum	C48.1	C78.6		D20.1	D48.4	D49.0
operculum (brain)	C71.0	C79.31	—	D33.0	D43.0	D49.6
optic nerve, chiasm, or tract	C72.3-●	C79.49	—	D33.3	D43.3	D49.7
oral (cavity)	C06.9	C79.89	D00.00	D10.30	D37.09	D49.0
ill-defined	C14.8	C79.89	D00.00	D10.30	D37.09	D49.0
mucosa	C06.0	C79.89	D00.02	D10.39	D37.09	D49.0
orbit	C69.6-●	C79.49	D09.2-●	D31.6-●	D48.7	D49.89
autonomic nerve	C69.6-●	C79.49	—	D31.6-●	D48.7	D49.2
bone	C41.0	C79.51	—	D16.4-●	D48.0	D49.2
eye	C69.6-●	C79.49	D09.2-●	D31.6-●	D48.7	D49.89
peripheral nerves	C69.6-●	C79.49	—	D31.6-●	D48.7	D49.2
soft parts	C69.6-●	C79.49	D09.2-●	D31.6-●	D48.7	D49.89
organ of Zuckerkandl	C75.5	C79.89	—	D35.6	D44.7	D49.7
oropharynx	C10.9	C79.89	D00.08	D10.5	D37.05	D49.0
branchial cleft (vestige)	C10.4	C79.89	D00.08	D10.5	D37.05	D49.0
junctional region	C10.8	C79.89	D00.08	D10.5	D37.05	D49.0
lateral wall	C10.2	C79.89	D00.08	D10.5	D37.05	D49.0
overlapping lesion	C10.8	—	—	—	—	—
pillars or fauces	C09.1	C79.89	D00.08	D10.5	D37.05	D49.0
posterior wall	C10.3	C79.89	D00.08	D10.5	D37.05	D49.0
vallecula	C10.0	C79.89	D00.08	D10.5	D37.05	D49.0
os						
external	C53.1	C79.82	D06.1	D26.0	D39.0	D49.59
internal	C53.0	C79.82	D06.0	D26.0	D39.0	D49.59
ovary	C56.-●	C79.6-●	D07.39	D27.-●	D39.1-●	D49.59
oviduct	C57.0-●	C79.82	D07.39	D28.2	D39.8	D49.59
palate	C05.9	C79.89	D00.00	D10.39	D37.09	D49.0
hard	C05.0	C79.89	D00.05	D10.39	D37.09	D49.0
junction of hard and soft palate	C05.9	C79.89	D00.00	D10.39	D37.09	D49.0
overlapping lesions	C05.8	—	—	—	—	—
soft	C05.1	C79.89	D00.04	D10.39	D37.09	D49.0
nasopharyngeal surface	C11.3	C79.89	D00.08	D10.6	D37.05	D49.0
posterior surface	C11.3	C79.89	D00.08	D10.6	D37.05	D49.0
superior surface	C11.3	C79.89	D00.08	D10.6	D37.05	D49.0
palatoglossal arch	C09.1	C79.89	D00.00	D10.5	D37.09	D49.0
palatopharyngeal arch	C09.1	C79.89	D00.00	D10.5	D37.09	D49.0
pallium	C71.0	C79.31	—	D33.0	D43.0	D49.6
palpebra	C44.10-●	C79.2	D04.1-●	D23.1-●	D48.5	D49.2
basal cell carcinoma	C44.11-●	—	—	—	—	—
sebaceous cell	C44.13-●	—	—	—	—	—
specified type NEC	C44.19-●	—	—	—	—	—
squamous cell carcinoma	C44.12-●	—	—	—	—	—
pancreas	C25.9	C78.89	D01.7	D13.6	D37.8	D49.0
body	C25.1	C78.89	D01.7	D13.6	D37.8	D49.0
duct (of Santorini) (of Wirsung)	C25.3	C78.89	D01.7	D13.6	D37.8	D49.0
ectopic tissue	C25.7	C78.89		D13.6	D37.8	D49.0
head	C25.0	C78.89	D01.7	D13.6	D37.8	D49.0

◀ New   ◀| Revised   ~~deleted~~ Deleted   ● Use Additional Character(s)

	Malignant Primary	Malignant Secondary	Ca in situ	Benign	Uncertain Behavior	Unspecified Behavior
pancreas *(Continued)*						
islet cells	C25.4	C78.89	D01.7	D13.7	D37.8	D49.0
neck	C25.7	C78.89	D01.7	D13.6	D37.8	D49.0
overlapping lesion	C25.8	—				—
tail	C25.2	C78.89	D01.7	D13.6	D37.8	D49.0
para-aortic body	C75.5	C79.89	—	D35.6	D44.7	D49.7
paraganglion NEC	C75.5	C79.89	—	D35.6	D44.7	D49.7
parametrium	C57.3	C79.82	—	D28.2	D39.8	D49.59
paranephric	C48.0	C78.6	—	D20.0	D48.3	D49.0
pararectal	C76.3	C79.89		D36.7	D48.7	D49.89
parasagittal (region)	C76.0	C79.89	D09.8	D36.7	D48.7	D49.89
parasellar	C72.9	C79.49	—	D33.9	D43.8	D49.7
parathyroid (gland)	C75.0	C79.89	D09.3	D35.1	D44.2	D49.7
paraurethral	C76.3	C79.89	—	D36.7	D48.7	D49.89
gland	C68.1	C79.19	D09.19	D30.8	D41.8	D49.59
paravaginal	C76.3	C79.89	—	D36.7	D48.7	D49.89
parenchyma, kidney	C64.-●	C79.0-●	D09.19	D30.0-●	D41.0-●	D49.51-●
parietal						
bone	C41.0	C79.51		D16.4-●	D48.0	D49.2
lobe, brain	C71.3	C79.31	—	D33.0	D43.0	D49.6
paroophoron	C57.1	C79.82	D07.39	D28.2	D39.8	D49.59
parotid (duct) (gland)	C07	C79.89	D00.00	D11.0	D37.030	D49.0
parovarium	C57.1	C79.82	D07.39	D28.2	D39.8	D49.59
patella	C40.20	C79.51	—	—	—	—
peduncle, cerebral	C71.7	C79.31	—	D33.1	D43.1	D49.6
pelvirectal junction	C19	C78.5	D01.1	D12.7	D37.5	D49.0
pelvis, pelvic	C76.3	C79.89	D09.8	D36.7	D48.7	D49.89
bone	C41.4	C79.51		D16.8	D48.0	D49.2
floor	C76.3	C79.89	D09.8	D36.7	D48.7	D49.89
renal	C65.-●	C79.0-●	D09.19	D30.1-●	D41.1-●	D49.51-●
viscera	C76.3	C79.89	D09.8	D36.7	D48.7	D49.89
wall	C76.3	C79.89	D09.8	D36.7	D48.7	D49.89
pelvo-abdominal	C76.8	C79.89	D09.8	D36.7	D48.7	D49.89
penis	C60.9	C79.82	D07.4	D29.0	D40.8	D49.59
body	C60.2	C79.82	D07.4	D29.0	D40.8	D49.59
corpus (cavernosum)	C60.2	C79.82	D07.4	D29.0	D40.8	D49.59
glans	C60.1	C79.82	D07.4	D29.0	D40.8	D49.59
overlapping sites	C60.8	—		—	—	—
skin NEC	C60.9	C79.82	D07.4	D29.0	D40.8	D49.59
periadrenal (tissue)	C48.0	C78.6	—	D20.0	D48.3	D49.0
perianal (skin) — *see also Neoplasm, anus, skin*	C44.500	C79.2	D04.5	D23.5	D48.5	D49.2
pericardium	C38.0	C79.89	—	D15.1	D48.7	D49.89
perinephric	C48.0	C78.6	—	D20.0	D48.3	D49.0

	Malignant Primary	Malignant Secondary	Ca in situ	Benign	Uncertain Behavior	Unspecified Behavior
perineum	C76.3	C79.89	D09.8	D36.7	D48.7	D49.89
periodontal tissue NEC	C03.9	C79.89	D00.03	D10.39	D37.09	D49.0
periosteum — *see Neoplasm, bone*						
peripancreatic	C48.0	C78.6	—	D20.0	D48.3	D49.0
peripheral nerve NEC	C47.9	C79.89	—	D36.10	D48.2	D49.2
perirectal (tissue)	C76.3	C79.89	—	D36.7	D48.7	D49.89
perirenal (tissue)	C48.0	C78.6	—	D20.0	D48.3	D49.0
peritoneum, peritoneal (cavity)	C48.2	C78.6	—	D20.1	D48.4	D49.0
benign mesothelial tissue — *see Mesothelioma, benign*						
overlapping lesion	C48.8	—		—	—	—
with digestive organs	C26.9	—		—	—	—
parietal	C48.1	C78.6	—	D20.1	D48.4	D49.0
pelvic	C48.1	C78.6	—	D20.1	D48.4	D49.0
specified part NEC	C48.1	C78.6	—	D20.1	D48.4	D49.0
peritonsillar (tissue)	C76.0	C79.89	D09.8	D36.7	D48.7	D49.89
periurethral tissue	C76.3	C79.89		D36.7	D48.7	D49.89
phalanges						
foot	C40.3-●	C79.51	—	D16.3-●	—	—
hand	C40.1-●	C79.51	—	D16.1-●	—	—
pharynx, pharyngeal	C14.0	C79.89	D00.08	D10.9	D37.05	D49.0
bursa	C11.1	C79.89	D00.08	D10.6	D37.05	D49.0
fornix	C11.3	C79.89	D00.08	D10.6	D37.05	D49.0
recess	C11.2	C79.89	D00.08	D10.6	D37.05	D49.0
region	C14.0	C79.89	D00.08	D10.9	D37.05	D49.0
tonsil	C11.1	C79.89	D00.08	D10.6	D37.05	D49.0
wall (lateral) (posterior)	C14.0	C79.89	D00.08	D10.9	D37.05	D49.0
pia mater	C70.9	C79.40	—	D32.9	D42.9	D49.7
cerebral	C70.0	C79.32	—	D32.0	D42.0	D49.7
cranial	C70.0	C79.32	—	D32.0	D42.0	D49.7
spinal	C70.1	C79.49	—	D32.1	D42.1	D49.7
pillars of fauces	C09.1	C79.89	D00.08	D10.5	D37.05	D49.0
pineal (body) (gland)	C75.3	C79.89	D09.3	D35.4	D44.5	D49.7
pinna (ear) NEC — *see also Neoplasm, skin, ear*	C44.20-●	C79.2	D04.2-●	D23.2-●	D48.5	D49.2
piriform fossa or sinus	C12	C79.89	D00.08	D10.7	D37.05	D49.0
pituitary (body) (fossa) (gland) (lobe)	C75.1	C79.89	D09.3	D35.2	D44.3	D49.7
placenta	C58	C79.82	D07.0	D26.7	D39.2	D49.59
pleura, pleural (cavity)	C38.4	C78.2		D19.0	D38.2	D49.1
overlapping lesion with heart or mediastinum	C38.8	—		—	—	—
parietal	C38.4	C78.2	—	D19.0	D38.2	D49.1
visceral	C38.4	C78.2	—	D19.0	D38.2	D49.1

◄ New   ◀▌ Revised   ~~deleted~~ Deleted   ● Use Additional Character(s)

	Malignant Primary	Malignant Secondary	Ca in situ	Benign	Uncertain Behavior	Unspecified Behavior
plexus						
brachial	C47.1-●	C79.89	—	D36.12	D48.2	D49.2
cervical	C47.0	C79.89	—	D36.11	D48.2	D49.2
choroid	C71.5	C79.31	—	D33.0	D43.0	D49.6
lumbosacral	C47.5	C79.89	—	D36.16	D48.2	D49.2
sacral	C47.5	C79.89	—	D36.16	D48.2	D49.2
pluriendocrine	C75.8	C79.89	D09.3	D35.7	D44.9	D49.7
pole						
frontal	C71.1	C79.31	—	D33.0	D43.0	D49.6
occipital	C71.4	C79.31	—	D33.0	D43.0	D49.6
pons (varolii)	C71.7	C79.31	—	D33.1	D43.1	D49.6
popliteal fossa or space	C76.5-●	C79.89	D04.7-●	D36.7	D48.7	D49.89
postcricoid (region)	C13.0	C79.89	D00.08	D10.7	D37.05	D49.0
posterior fossa (cranial)	C71.9	C79.31	—	D33.2	D43.2	D49.6
postnasal space	C11.9	C79.89	D00.08	D10.6	D37.05	D49.0
prepuce	C60.0	C79.82	D07.4	D29.0	D40.8	D49.59
prepylorus	C16.4	C78.89	D00.2	D13.1	D37.1	D49.0
presacral (region)	C76.3	C79.89	—	D36.7	D48.7	D49.89
prostate (gland)	C61	C79.82	D07.5	D29.1	D40.0	D49.59
utricle	C68.0	C79.19	D09.19	D30.4	D41.3	D49.59
pterygoid fossa	C49.0	C79.89	—	D21.0	D48.1	D49.2
pubic bone	C41.4	C79.51	—	D16.8	D48.0	D49.2
pudenda, pudendum (femaie)	C51.9	C79.82	D07.1	D28.0	D39.8	D49.59
pulmonary — see also Neoplasm, lung	C34.9-●	C78.0-●	D02.2-●	D14.3-●	D38.1	D49.1
putamen	C71.0	C79.31	—	D33.0	D43.0	D49.6
pyloric						
antrum	C16.3	C78.89	D00.2	D13.1	D37.1	D49.0
canal	C16.4	C78.89	D00.2	D13.1	D37.1	D49.0
pylorus	C16.4	C78.89	D00.2	D13.1	D37.1	D49.0
pyramid (brain)	C71.7	C79.31	—	D33.1	D43.1	D49.6
pyriform fossa or sinus	C12	C79.89	D00.08	D10.7	D37.05	D49.0
radius (any part)	C40.0-●	C79.51	—	D16.0-●	—	—
Rathke's pouch	C75.1	C79.89	D09.3	D35.2	D44.3	D49.7
rectosigmoid (junction)	C19	C78.5	D01.1	D12.7	D37.5	D49.0
overlapping lesion with anus or rectum	C21.8	—	—	—	—	—
rectouterine pouch	C48.1	C78.6	—	D20.1	D48.4	D49.0
rectovaginal septum or wall	C76.3	C79.89	D09.8	D36.7	D48.7	D49.89
rectovesical septum	C76.3	C79.89	D09.8	D36.7	D48.7	D49.89
rectum (ampulla)	C20	C78.5	D01.2	D12.8	D37.5	D49.0
and colon	C19	C78.5	D01.1	D12.7	D37.5	D49.0
overlapping lesion with anus or rectosigmoid junction	C21.8	—	—	—	—	—
renal	C64.-●	C79.0-●	D09.19	D30.0-●	D41.0-●	D49.51-●
calyx	C65.-●	C79.0-●	D09.19	D30.1-●	D41.1-●	D49.51-●
hilus	C65.-●	C79.0-●	D09.19	D30.1-●	D41.1-●	D49.51-●
parenchyma	C64.-●	C79.0-●	D09.19	D30.0-●	D41.0-●	D49.51-●
pelvis	C65.-●	C79.0-●	D09.19	D30.1-●	D41.1-●	D49.51-●
respiratory						
organs or system NEC	C39.9	C78.30	D02.4	D14.4	D38.6	D49.1
tract NEC	C39.9	C78.30	D02.4	D14.4	D38.5	D49.1
upper	C39.0	C78.30	D02.4	D14.4	D38.5	D49.1
retina	C69.2-●	C79.49	D09.2-●	D31.2-●	D48.7	D49.81
retrobulbar	C69.6-●	C79.49	—	D31.6-●	D48.7	D49.89
retrocecal	C48.0	C78.6	—	D20.0	D48.3	D49.0
retromolar (area) (triangle) (trigone)	C06.2	C79.89	D00.00	D10.39	D37.09	D49.0
retro-orbital	C76.0	C79.89	D09.8	D36.7	D48.7	D49.89
retroperitoneal (space) (tissue)	C48.0	C78.6	—	D20.0	D48.3	D49.0
retroperitoneum	C48.0	C78.6	—	D20.0	D48.3	D49.0
retropharyngeal	C14.0	C79.89	D00.08	D10.9	D37.05	D49.0
retrovesical (septum)	C76.3	C79.89	D09.8	D36.7	D48.7	D49.89
rhinencephalon	C71.0	C79.31	—	D33.0	D43.0	D49.6
rib	C41.3	C79.51●	—	D16.7	D48.0	D49.2
Rosenmuller's fossa	C11.2	C79.89	D00.08	D10.6	D37.05	D49.0
round ligament	C57.2	C79.82	—	D28.2	D39.8	D49.59
sacrococcyx, sacrococcygeal	C41.4	C79.51	—	D16.8	D48.0	D49.2
region	C76.3	C79.89	D09.8	D36.7	D48.7	D49.89
sacrouterine ligament	C57.3	C79.82	—	D28.2	D39.8	D49.59
sacrum, sacral (vertebra)	C41.4	C79.51	—	D16.8	D48.0	D49.2
salivary gland or duct (major)	C08.9	C79.89	D00.00	D11.9	D37.039	D49.0
minor NEC	C06.9	C79.89	D00.00	D10.39	D37.04	D49.0
overlapping lesion	C08.9	—	—	—	—	—
parotid	C07	C79.89	D00.00	D11.0	D37.030	D49.0
pluriglandular	C08.9	C79.89	D00.00	D11.9	D37.039	D49.0
sublingual	C08.1	C79.89	D00.00	D11.7	D37.031	D49.0
submandibular	C08.0	C79.89	D00.00	D11.7	D37.032	D49.0
submaxillary	C08.0	C79.89	D00.00	D11.7	D37.032	D49.0
salpinx (uterine)	C57.0-●	C79.82	D07.39	D28.2	D39.8	D49.59
Santorini's duct	C25.3	C78.89	D01.7	D13.6	D37.8	D49.0
scalp	C44.40	C79.2	D04.4	D23.4	D48.5	D49.2
basal cell carcinoma	C44.41	—	—	—	—	—
specified type NEC	C44.49	—	—	—	—	—
squamous cell carcinoma	C44.42	—	—	—	—	—
scapula (any part)	C40.0-●	C79.51	—	D16.0-●	—	—
scapular region	C76.1	C79.89	D09.8	D36.7	D48.7	D49.89

◀ New ◀ Revised ~~deleted~~ Deleted ● Use Additional Character(s)

501

TABLE OF NEOPLASMS

	Malignant Primary	Malignant Secondary	Ca in situ	Benign	Uncertain Behavior	Unspecified Behavior
scar NEC — see also Neoplasm, skin, by site	C44.90	C79.2	D04.9	D23.9	D48.5	D49.2
sciatic nerve	C47.2-●	C79.89	—	D36.13	D48.2	D49.2
sclera	C69.4-●	C79.49	D09.2-●	D31.4-●	D48.7	D49.89
scrotum (skin)	C63.2	C79.82	D07.61	D29.4	D40.8	D49.59
sebaceous gland — see Neoplasm, skin						
sella turcica	C75.1	C79.89	D09.3	D35.2	D44.3	D49.7
bone	C41.0	C79.51	—	D16.4-●	D48.0	D49.2
semilunar cartilage (knee)	C40.2-●	C79.51	—	D16.2-●	D48.0	D49.2
seminal vesicle	C63.7	C79.82	D07.69	D29.8	D40.8	D49.59
septum						
nasal	C30.0	C78.39	D02.3	D14.0	D38.5	D49.1
posterior margin	C11.3	C79.89	D00.08	D10.6	D37.05	D49.0
rectovaginal	C76.3	C79.89	D09.8	D36.7	D48.7	D49.89
rectovesical	C76.3	C79.89	D09.8	D36.7	D48.7	D49.89
urethrovaginal	C57.9	C79.82	D07.30	D28.9	D39.9	D49.59
vesicovaginal	C57.9	C79.82	D07.30	D28.9	D39.9	D49.59
shoulder NEC	C76.4-●	C79.89	D04.6-●	D36.7	D48.7	D49.89
sigmoid flexure (lower) (upper)	C18.7	C78.5	D01.0	D12.5	D37.4	D49.0
sinus (accessory)	C31.9	C78.39	D02.3	D14.0	D38.5	D49.1
bone (any)	C41.0	C79.51	—	D16.4-●	D48.0	D49.2
ethmoidal	C31.1	C78.39	D02.3	D14.0	D38.5	D49.1
frontal	C31.2	C78.39	D02.3	D14.0	D38.5	D49.1
maxillary	C31.0	C78.39	D02.3	D14.0	D38.5	D49.1
nasal, paranasal NEC	C31.9	C78.39	D02.3	D14.0	D38.5	D49.1
overlapping lesion	C31.8	—	—	—	—	—
pyriform	C12	C79.89	D00.08	D10.7	D37.05	D49.0
sphenoid	C31.3	C78.39	D02.3	D14.0	D38.5	D49.1
skeleton, skeletal NEC	C41.9	C79.51	—	D16.9-●	D48.0	D49.2
Skene's gland	C68.1	C79.19	D09.19	D30.8	D41.8	D49.59
skin NOS	C44.90	C79.2	D04.9	D23.9	D48.5	D49.2
abdominal wall	C44.509	C79.2	D04.5	D23.5	D48.5	D49.2
basal cell carcinoma	C44.519	—	—	—	—	—
specified type NEC	C44.599	—	—	—	—	—
squamous cell carcinoma	C44.529	—	—	—	—	—
ala nasi — see also Neoplasm, nose, skin	C44.301	C79.2	D04.39	D23.39	D48.5	D49.2
ankle — see also Neoplasm, skin, limb, lower	C44.70-●	C79.2	D04.7-●	D23.7-●	D48.5	D49.2
antecubital space — see also Neoplasm, skin, limb, upper	C44.60-●	C79.2	D04.6-●	D23.6-●	D48.5	D49.2

	Malignant Primary	Malignant Secondary	Ca in situ	Benign	Uncertain Behavior	Unspecified Behavior
skin NOS (Continued)						
anus	C44.500	C79.2	D04.5	D23.5	D48.5	D49.2
basal cell carcinoma	C44.510	—	—	—	—	—
specified type NEC	C44.590	—	—	—	—	—
squamous cell carcinoma	C44.520	—	—	—	—	—
arm — see also Neoplasm, skin, limb, upper	C44.60-●	C79.2	D04.6-●	D23.6-●	D48.5	D49.2
auditory canal (external) — see also Neoplasm, skin, ear	C44.20-●	C79.2	D04.2-●	D23.2-●	D48.5	D49.2
auricle (ear) — see also Neoplasm, skin, ear	C44.20-●	C79.2	D04.2-●	D23.2-●	D48.5	D49.2
auricular canal (external) — see also Neoplasm, skin, ear	C44.20-●	C79.2	D04.2-●	D23.2-●	D48.5	D49.2
axilla, axillary fold — see also Neoplasm, skin, trunk	C44.509	C79.2	D04.5	D23.5	D48.5	D49.2
back — see also Neoplasm, skin, trunk	C44.509	C79.2	D04.5	D23.5	D48.5	D49.2
basal cell carcinoma	C44.91					
breast	C44.501	C79.2	D04.5	D23.5	D48.5	D49.2
basal cell carcinoma	C44.511	—	—	—	—	—
specified type NEC	C44.591	—	—	—	—	—
squamous cell carcinoma	C44.521	—	—	—	—	—
brow — see also Neoplasm, skin, face	C44.309	C79.2	D04.39	D23.39	D48.5	D49.2
buttock — see also Neoplasm, skin, trunk	C44.509	C79.2	D04.5	D23.5	D48.5	D49.2
calf — see also Neoplasm, skin, limb, lower	C44.70-●	C79.2	D04.7-●	D23.7-●	D48.5	D49.2
canthus (eye) (inner) (outer)	C44.10-●	C79.2	D04.1-●	D23.1-●	D48.5	D49.2
basal cell carcinoma	C44.11-●	—	—	—	—	—
sebaceous cell	C44.13-●	—	—	—	—	—
specified type NEC	C44.19-●	—	—	—	—	—
squamous cell carcinoma	C44.12-●	—	—	—	—	—
cervical region — see also Neoplasm, skin, neck	C44.40	C79.2	D04.4	D23.4	D48.5	D49.2
cheek (external) — see also Neoplasm, skin, face	C44.309	C79.2	D04.39	D23.39	D48.5	D49.2
chest (wall) — see also Neoplasm, skin, trunk	C44.509	C79.2	D04.5	D23.5	D48.5	D49.2
chin — see also Neoplasm, skin, face	C44.309	C79.2	D04.39	D23.39	D48.5	D49.2
clavicular area — see also Neoplasm, skin, trunk	C44.509	C79.2	D04.5	D23.5	D48.5	D49.2
clitoris	C51.2	C79.82	D07.1	D28.0	D39.8	D49.59

◀ New ◀ Revised ~~deleted~~ Deleted ● Use Additional Character(s)

TABLE OF NEOPLASMS

	Malignant Primary	Malignant Secondary	Ca in situ	Benign	Uncertain Behavior	Unspecified Behavior
skin NOS *(Continued)*						
columnella — *see also Neoplasm, skin, face*	C44.309	C79.2	D04.39	D23.39	D48.5	D49.2
concha — *see also Neoplasm, skin, ear*	C44.20-●	C79.2	D04.2-●	D23.2-●	D48.5	D49.2
ear (external)	C44.20-●	C79.2	D04.2-●	D23.2-●	D48.5	D49.2
basal cell carcinoma	C44.21-●	—	—	—	—	—
specified type NEC	C44.29-●	—	—	—	—	—
squamous cell carcinoma	C44.22-●	—	—	—	—	—
elbow — *see also Neoplasm, skin, limb, upper*	C44.60-●	C79.2	D04.6-●	D23.6-●	D48.5	D49.2
eyebrow — *see also Neoplasm, skin, face*	C44.309	C79.2	D04.39	D23.39	D48.5	D49.2
eyelid	C44.10-●	C79.2	D04.1-●	D23.1-●	D48.5	D49.2
basal cell carcinoma	C44.11-●	—	—	—	—	—
sebaceous cell	C44.13-●	—	—	—	—	—
specified type NEC	C44.19-●	—	—	—	—	—
squamous cell carcinoma	C44.12-●	—	—	—	—	—
face NOS	C44.300	C79.2	D04.30	D23.30	D48.5	D49.2
basal cell carcinoma	C44.310	—	—	—	—	—
specified type NEC	C44.390	—	—	—	—	—
squamous cell carcinoma	C44.320	—	—	—	—	—
female genital organs (external)	C51.9	C79.82	D07.1	D28.0	D39.8	D49.59
clitoris	C51.2	C79.82	D07.1	D28.0	D39.8	D49.59
labium NEC	C51.9	C79.82	D07.1	D28.0	D39.8	D49.59
majus	C51.0	C79.82	D07.1	D28.0	D39.8	D49.59
minus	C51.1	C79.82	D07.1	D28.0	D39.8	D49.59
pudendum	C51.9	C79.82	D07.1	D28.0	D39.8	D49.59
vulva	C51.9	C79.82	D07.1	D28.0	D39.8	D49.59
finger — *see also Neoplasm, skin, limb, upper*	C44.60-●	C79.2	D04.6-●	D23.6-●	D48.5	D49.2
flank — *see also Neoplasm, skin, trunk*	C44.509	C79.2	D04.5	D23.5	D48.5	D49.2
foot — *see also Neoplasm, skin, limb, lower*	C44.70-●	C79.2	D04.7-●	D23.7-●	D48.5	D49.2
forearm — *see also Neoplasm, skin, limb, upper*	C44.60-●	C79.2	D04.6-●	D23.6-●	D48.5	D49.2
forehead — *see also Neoplasm, skin, face*	C44.309	C79.2	D04.39	D23.39	D48.5	D49.2
glabella — *see also Neoplasm, skin, face*	C44.309	C79.2	D04.39	D23.39	D48.5	D49.2
gluteal region — *see also Neoplasm, skin, trunk*	C44.509	C79.2	D04.5	D23.5	D48.5	D49.2
groin — *see also Neoplasm, skin, trunk*	C44.509	C79.2	D04.5	D23.5	D48.5	D49.2

	Malignant Primary	Malignant Secondary	Ca in situ	Benign	Uncertain Behavior	Unspecified Behavior
skin NOS *(Continued)*						
hand — *see also Neoplasm, skin, limb, upper*	C44.60-●	C79.2	D04.6-●	D23.6-●	D48.5	D49.2
head NEC — *see also Neoplasm, skin, scalp*	C44.40	C79.2	D04.4	D23.4	D48.5	D49.2
heel — *see also Neoplasm, skin, limb, lower*	C44.70-●	C79.2	D04.7-●	D23.7-●	D48.5	D49.2
helix — *see also Neoplasm, skin, ear*	C44.20-●	C79.2	D04.2-●	D23.2-●	D48.5	D49.2
hip — *see also Neoplasm, skin, limb, lower*	C44.70-●	C79.2	D04.7-●	D23.7-●	D48.5	D49.2
infraclavicular region — *see also Neoplasm, skin, trunk*	C44.509	C79.2	D04.5	D23.5	D48.5	D49.2
inguinal region — *see also Neoplasm, skin, trunk*	C44.509	C79.2	D04.5	D23.5	D48.5	D49.2
jaw — *see also Neoplasm, skin, face*	C44.309	C79.2	D04.39	D23.39	D48.5	D49.2
Kaposi's sarcoma — *see Kaposi's, sarcoma, skin*						
knee — *see also Neoplasm, skin, limb, lower*	C44.70-●	C79.2	D04.7-●	D23.7-●	D48.5	D49.2
labia						
majora	C51.0	C79.82	D07.1	D28.0	D39.8	D49.59
minora	C51.1	C79.82	D07.1	D28.0	D39.8	D49.59
leg — *see also Neoplasm, skin, limb, lower*	C44.70-●	C79.2	D04.7-●	D23.7-●	D48.5	D49.2
lid (lower) (upper)	C44.10-●	C79.2	D04.1-●	D23.1-●	D48.5	D49.2
basal cell carcinoma	C44.11-●	—	—	—	—	—
sebaceous cell	C44.13-●	—	—	—	—	—
specified type NEC	C44.19-●	—	—	—	—	—
squamous cell carcinoma	C44.12-●	—	—	—	—	—
limb NEC	C44.90	C79.2	D04.9	D23.9	D48.5	D49.2
basal cell carcinoma	C44.91					
lower	C44.70-●	C79.2	D04.7-●	D23.7-●	D48.5	D49.2
basal cell carcinoma	C44.71-●	—	—	—	—	—
specified type NEC	C44.79-●	—	—	—	—	—
squamous cell carcinoma	C44.72-●	—	—	—	—	—
upper	C44.60-●	C79.2	D04.6-●	D23.6-●	D48.5	D49.2
basal cell carcinoma	C44.61-●	—	—	—	—	—
specified type NEC	C44.69-●	—	—	—	—	—
squamous cell carcinoma	C44.62-●	—	—	—	—	—
lip (lower) (upper)	C44.00	C79.2	D04.0	D23.0	D48.5	D49.2
basal cell carcinoma	C44.01	—	—	—	—	—
specified type NEC	C44.09	—	—	—	—	—
squamous cell carcinoma	C44.02	—	—	—	—	—

◀ New　◀ Revised　deleted Deleted　● Use Additional Character(s)

TABLE OF NEOPLASMS

TABLE OF NEOPLASMS

	Malignant Primary	Malignant Secondary	Ca in situ	Benign	Uncertain Behavior	Unspecified Behavior
skin NOS *(Continued)*						
male genital organs	C63.9	C79.82	D07.60	D29.9	D40.8	D49.59
penis	C60.9	C79.82	D07.4	D29.0	D40.8	D49.59
prepuce	C60.0	C79.82	D07.4	D29.0	D40.8	D49.59
scrotum	C63.2	C79.82	D07.61	D29.4	D40.8	D49.59
mastectomy site (skin) — *see also Neoplasm, skin, breast*	C44.501	C79.2	—			
specified as breast tissue	C50.8-●	C79.81	—			
meatus, acoustic (external) — *see also Neoplasm, skin, ear*	C44.20-●	C79.2	D04.2-●	D23.2-●	D48.5	D49.2
melanotic — *see Melanoma*						
Merkel cell — *see Carcinoma, Merkel cell*						
nates — *see also Neoplasm, skin, trunk*	C44.509	C79.2	D04.5	D23.5	D48.5	D49.2
neck	C44.40	C79.2	D04.4	D23.4	D48.5	D49.2
basal cell carcinoma	C44.41	—	—	—	—	—
specified type NEC	C44.49	—	—	—	—	—
squamous cell carcinoma	C44.42	—	—	—	—	—
nevus — *see Nevus, skin*						
nose (external) — *see also Neoplasm, nose, skin*	C44.301	C79.2	D04.39	D23.39	D48.5	D49.2
overlapping lesion	C44.80	—	—	—	—	—
basal cell carcinoma	C44.81	—	—	—	—	—
specified type NEC	C44.89	—	—	—	—	—
squamous cell carcinoma	C44.82	—	—	—	—	—
palm — *see also Neoplasm, skin, limb, upper*	C44.60-●	C79.2	D04.6-●	D23.6-●	D48.5	D49.2
palpebra	C44.10-●	C79.2	D04.1-●	D23.1-●	D48.5	D49.2
basal cell carcinoma	C44.11-●	—	—	—	—	—
sebaceous cell	C44.13-●	—	—	—	—	—
specified type NEC	C44.19-●	—	—	—	—	—
squamous cell carcinoma	C44.12-●	—	—	—	—	—
penis NEC	C60.9	C79.82	D07.4	D29.0	D40.8	D49.59
perianal — *see also Neoplasm, skin, anus*	C44.500	C79.2	D04.5	D23.5	D48.5	D49.2
perineum — *see also Neoplasm, skin, anus*	C44.500	C79.2	D04.5	D23.5	D48.5	D49.2
pinna — *see also Neoplasm, skin, ear*	C44.20-●	C79.2	D04.2-●	D23.2-●	D48.5	D49.2
plantar — *see also Neoplasm, skin, limb, lower*	C44.70-●	C79.2	D04.7-●	D23.7-●	D48.5	D49.2
popliteal fossa or space — *see also Neoplasm, skin, limb, lower*	C44.70-●	C79.2	D04.7-●	D23.7-●	D48.5	D49.2

	Malignant Primary	Malignant Secondary	Ca in situ	Benign	Uncertain Behavior	Unspecified Behavior
skin NOS *(Continued)*						
prepuce	C60.0	C79.82	D07.4	D29.0	D40.8	D49.59
pubes — *see also Neoplasm, skin, trunk*	C44.509	C79.2	D04.5	D23.5	D48.5	D49.2
sacrococcygeal region — *see also Neoplasm, skin, trunk*	C44.509	C79.2	D04.5	D23.5	D48.5	D49.2
scalp	C44.40	C79.2	D04.4	D23.4	D48.5	D49.2
basal cell carcinoma	C44.41	—	—	—	—	—
specified type NEC	C44.49	—	—	—	—	—
squamous cell carcinoma	C44.42	—	—	—	—	—
scapular region — *see also Neoplasm, skin, trunk*	C44.509	C79.2	D04.5	D23.5	D48.5	D49.2
scrotum	C63.2	C79.82	D07.61	D29.4	D40.8	D49.59
shoulder — *see also Neoplasm, skin, limb, upper*	C44.60-●	C79.2	D04.6-●	D23.6-●	D48.5	D49.2
sole (foot) — *see also Neoplasm, skin, limb, lower*	C44.70-●	C79.2	D04.7-●	D23.7-●	D48.5	D49.2
specified sites NEC	C44.80	C79.2	D04.8	D23.9	D48.5	D49.2
basal cell carcinoma	C44.81	—	—	—	—	—
specified type NEC	C44.89	—	—	—	—	—
squamous cell carcinoma	C44.82	—	—	—	—	—
specified type NEC	C44.99	—	—	—	—	—
squamous cell carcinoma	C44.92	—	—	—	—	—
submammary fold — *see also Neoplasm, skin, trunk*	C44.509	C79.2	D04.5	D23.5	D48.5	D49.2
supraclavicular region — *see also Neoplasm, skin, neck*	C44.40	C79.2	D04.4	D23.4	D48.5	D49.2
temple — *see also Neoplasm, skin, face*	C44.309	C79.2	D04.39	D23.39	D48.5	D49.2
thigh — *see also Neoplasm, skin, limb, lower*	C44.70-●	C79.2	D04.7-●	D23.7-●	D48.5	D49.2
thoracic wall — *see also Neoplasm, skin, trunk*	C44.509	C79.2	D04.5	D23.5	D48.5	D49.2
thumb — *see also Neoplasm, skin, limb, upper*	C44.60-●	C79.2	D04.6-●	D23.6-●	D48.5	D49.2
toe — *see also Neoplasm, skin, limb, lower*	C44.70-●	C79.2	D04.7-●	D23.7-●	D48.5	D49.2
tragus — *see also Neoplasm, skin, ear*	C44.20-●	C79.2	D04.2-●	D23.2-●	D48.5	D49.2
trunk	C44.509	C79.2	D04.5	D23.5	D48.5	D49.2
basal cell carcinoma	C44.519	—	—	—	—	—
specified type NEC	C44.599	—	—	—	—	—
squamous cell carcinoma	C44.529	—	—	—	—	—
umbilicus — *see also Neoplasm, skin, trunk*	C44.509	C79.2	D04.5	D23.5	D48.5	D49.2

◀ New   ◀ Revised   ~~deleted~~ Deleted   ● Use Additional Character(s)

	Malignant Primary	Malignant Secondary	Ca in situ	Benign	Uncertain Behavior	Unspecified Behavior
skin NOS *(Continued)*						
vulva	C51.9	C79.82	D07.1	D28.0	D39.8	D49.59
overlapping lesion	C51.8	—	—	—	—	—
wrist — *see also Neoplasm, skin, limb, upper*	C44.60-•	C79.2	D04.6-•	D23.6-•	D48.5	D49.2
skull	C41.0	C79.51	—	D16.4-•	D48.0	D49.2
soft parts or tissues — *see Neoplasm, connective tissue*						
specified site NEC	C76.8	C79.89	D09.8	D36.7	D48.7	D49.89
spermatic cord	C63.1-•	C79.82	D07.69	D29.8	D40.8	D49.59
sphenoid	C31.3	C78.39	D02.3	D14.0	D38.5	D49.1
bone	C41.0	C79.51	—	D16.4-•	D48.0	D49.2
sinus	C31.3	C78.39	D02.3	D14.0	D38.5	D49.1
sphincter						
anal	C21.1	C78.5	D01.3	D12.9	D37.8	D49.0
of Oddi	C24.0	C78.89	D01.5	D13.5	D37.6	D49.0
spine, spinal (column)	C41.2	C79.51	—	D16.6	D48.0	D49.2
bulb	C71.7	C79.31	—	D33.1	D43.1	D49.6
coccyx	C41.4	C79.51	—	D16.8	D48.0	D49.2
cord (cervical) (lumbar) (sacral) (thoracic)	C72.0	C79.49	—	D33.4	D43.4	D49.7
dura mater	C70.1	C79.49	—	D32.1	D42.1	D49.7
lumbosacral	C41.2	C79.51	—	D16.6	D48.0	D49.2
marrow NEC	C96.9	C79.52	—	—	D47.9	D49.89
membrane	C70.1	C79.49	—	D32.1	D42.1	D49.7
meninges	C70.1	C79.49	—	D32.1	D42.1	D49.7
nerve (root)	C47.9	C79.89	—	D36.10	D48.2	D49.2
pia mater	C70.1	C79.49	—	D32.1	D42.1	D49.7
root	C47.9	C79.89	—	D36.10	D48.2	D49.2
sacrum	C41.4	C79.51	—	D16.8	D48.0	D49.2
spleen, splenic NEC	C26.1	C78.89	D01.7	D13.9	D37.8	D49.0
flexure (colon)	C18.5	C78.5	D01.0	D12.3	D37.4	D49.0
stem, brain	C71.7	C79.31	—	D33.1	D43.1	D49.6
Stensen's duct	C07	C79.89	D00.00	D11.0	D37.030	D49.0
sternum	C41.3	C79.51	—	D16.7	D48.0	D49.2
stomach	C16.9	C78.89	D00.2	D13.1	D37.1	D49.0
antrum (pyloric)	C16.3	C78.89	D00.2	D13.1	D37.1	D49.0
body	C16.2	C78.89	D00.2	D13.1	D37.1	D49.0
cardia	C16.0	C78.89	D00.2	D13.1	D37.1	D49.0
cardiac orifice	C16.0	C78.89	D00.2	D13.1	D37.1	D49.0
corpus	C16.2	C78.89	D00.2	D13.1	D37.1	D49.0
fundus	C16.1	C78.89	D00.2	D13.1	D37.1	D49.0
greater curvature NEC	C16.6	C78.89	D00.2	D13.1	D37.1	D49.0
lesser curvature NEC	C16.5	C78.89	D00.2	D13.1	D37.1	D49.0

	Malignant Primary	Malignant Secondary	Ca in situ	Benign	Uncertain Behavior	Unspecified Behavior
stomach *(Continued)*						
overlapping lesion	C16.8	—	—	—	—	—
prepylorus	C16.4	C78.89	D00.2	D13.1	D37.1	D49.0
pylorus	C16.4	C78.89	D00.2	D13.1	D37.1	D49.0
wall NEC	C16.9	C78.89	D00.2	D13.1	D37.1	D49.0
anterior NEC	C16.8	C78.89	D00.2	D13.1	D37.1	D49.0
posterior NEC	C16.8	C78.89	D00.2	D13.1	D37.1	D49.0
stroma, endometrial	C54.1	C79.82	D07.0	D26.1	D39.0	D49.59
stump, cervical	C53.8	C79.82	D06.7	D26.0	D39.0	D49.59
subcutaneous (nodule) (tissue) NEC — *see Neoplasm, connective tissue*						
subdural	C70.9	C79.32	—	D32.9	D42.9	D49.7
subglottis, subglottic	C32.2	C78.39	D02.0	D14.1	D38.0	D49.1
sublingual	C04.9	C79.89	D00.06	D10.2	D37.09	D49.0
gland or duct	C08.1	C79.89	D00.00	D11.7	D37.031	D49.0
submandibular gland	C08.0	C79.89	D00.00	D11.7	D37.032	D49.0
submaxillary gland or duct	C08.0	C79.89	D00.00	D11.7	D37.032	D49.0
submental	C76.0	C79.89	D09.8	D36.7	D48.7	D49.89
subpleural	C34.9-•	C78.0-•	D02.2-•	D14.3-•	D38.1	D49.1
substernal	C38.1	C78.1	—	D15.2	D38.3	D49.89
sudoriferous, sudoriparous gland, site unspecified	C44.90	C79.2	D04.9	D23.9	D48.5	D49.2
specified site — *see Neoplasm, skin*						
supraclavicular region	C76.0	C79.89	D09.8	D36.7	D48.7	D49.89
supraglottis	C32.1	C78.39	D02.0	D14.1	D38.0	D49.1
suprarenal	C74.9-•	C79.7-•	D09.3	D35.0-•	D44.1-•	D49.7
capsule	C74.9-•	C79.7-•	D09.3	D35.0-•	D44.1-•	D49.7
cortex	C74.0-•	C79.7-•	D09.3	D35.0-•	D44.1-•	D49.7
gland	C74.9-•	C79.7-•	D09.3	D35.0-•	D44.1-•	D49.7
medulla	C74.1-•	C79.7-•	D09.3	D35.0-•	D44.1-•	D49.7
suprasellar (region)	C71.9	C79.31	—	D33.2	D43.2	D49.6
supratentorial (brain) NEC	C71.0	C79.31	—	D33.0	D43.0	D49.6
sweat gland (apocrine) (eccrine), site unspecified	C44.90	C79.2	D04.9	D23.9	D48.5	D49.2
specified site — *see Neoplasm, skin*						
sympathetic nerve or nervous system NEC	C47.9	C79.89	—	D36.10	D48.2	D49.2
symphysis pubis	C41.4	C79.51	—	D16.8	D48.0	D49.2
synovial membrane — *see Neoplasm, connective tissue*						
tapetum, brain	C71.8	C79.31	—	D33.2	D43.2	D49.6

◀ New ◀ Revised ~~deleted~~ Deleted • Use Additional Character(s)

	Malignant Primary	Malignant Secondary	Ca in situ	Benign	Uncertain Behavior	Unspecified Behavior
tarsus (any bone)	C40.3-●	C79.51	—	D16.3-●	—	—
temple (skin) — see also Neoplasm, skin, face	C44.309	C79.2	D04.39	D23.39	D48.5	D49.2
temporal						
bone	C41.0	C79.51	—	D16.4-●	D48.0	D49.2
lobe or pole	C71.2	C79.31	—	D33.0	D43.0	D49.6
region	C76.0	C79.89	D09.8	D36.7	D48.7	D49.89
skin — see also Neoplasm, skin, face	C44.309	C79.2	D04.39	D23.39	D48.5	D49.2
tendon (sheath) — see Neoplasm, connective tissue						
tentorium (cerebelli)	C70.0	C79.32	—	D32.0	D42.0	D49.7
testis, testes	C62.9-●	C79.82	D07.69	D29.2-●	D40.1-●	D49.59
descended	C62.1-●	C79.82	D07.69	D29.2-●	D40.1-●	D49.59
ectopic	C62.0-●	C79.82	D07.69	D29.2-●	D40.1-●	D49.59
retained	C62.0-●	C79.82	D07.69	D29.2-●	D40.1-●	D49.59
scrotal	C62.1-●	C79.82	D07.69	D29.2-●	D40.1-●	D49.59
undescended	C62.0-●	C79.82	D07.69	D29.2-●	D40.1-●	D49.59
unspecified whether descended or undescended	C62.9-●	C79.82	D07.69	D29.2-●	D40.1-●	D49.59
thalamus	C71.0	C79.31	—	D33.0	D43.0	D49.6
thigh NEC	C76.5-●	C79.89	D04.7-●	D36.7	D48.7	D49.89
thorax, thoracic (cavity) (organs NEC)	C76.1	C79.89	D09.8	D36.7	D48.7	D49.89
duct	C49.3	C79.89	—	D21.3	D48.1	D49.2
wall NEC	C76.1	C79.89	D09.8	D36.7	D48.7	D49.89
throat	C14.0	C79.89	D00.08	D10.9	D37.05	D49.0
thumb NEC	C76.4-●	C79.89	D04.6-●	D36.7	D48.7	D49.89
thymus (gland)	C37	C79.89	D09.3	D15.0	D38.4	D49.89
thyroglossal duct	C73	C79.89	D09.3	D34	D44.0	D49.7
thyroid (gland)	C73	C79.89	D09.3	D34	D44.0	D49.7
cartilage	C32.3	C78.39	D02.0	D14.1	D38.0	D49.1
tibia (any part)	C40.2-●	C79.51	—	D16.2-●	—	—
toe NEC	C76.5-●	C79.89	D04.7-●	D36.7	D48.7	D49.89
tongue	C02.9	C79.89	D00.07	D10.1	D37.02	D49.0
anterior (two-thirds) NEC	C02.3	C79.89	D00.07	D10.1	D37.02	D49.0
dorsal surface	C02.0	C79.89	D00.07	D10.1	D37.02	D49.0
ventral surface	C02.2	C79.89	D00.07	D10.1	D37.02	D49.0
base (dorsal surface)	C01	C79.89	D00.07	D10.1	D37.02	D49.0
border (lateral)	C02.1	C79.89	D00.07	D10.1	D37.02	D49.0
dorsal surface NEC	C02.0	C79.89	D00.07	D10.1	D37.02	D49.0
fixed part NEC	C01	C79.89	D00.07	D10.1	D37.02	D49.0
foreamen cecum	C02.0	C79.89	D00.07	D10.1	D37.02	D49.0
frenulum linguae	C02.2	C79.89	D00.07	D10.1	D37.02	D49.0

	Malignant Primary	Malignant Secondary	Ca in situ	Benign	Uncertain Behavior	Unspecified Behavior
tongue (Continued)						
junctional zone	C02.8	C79.89	D00.07	D10.1	D37.02	D49.0
margin (lateral)	C02.1	C79.89	D00.07	D10.1	D37.02	D49.0
midline NEC	C02.0	C79.89	D00.07	D10.1	D37.02	D49.0
mobile part NEC	C02.3	C79.89	D00.07	D10.1	D37.02	D49.0
overlapping lesion	C02.8	—	—	—	—	—
posterior (third)	C01	C79.89	D00.07	D10.1	D37.02	D49.0
root	C01	C79.89	D00.07	D10.1	D37.02	D49.0
surface (dorsal)	C02.0	C79.89	D00.07	D10.1	D37.02	D49.0
base	C01	C79.89	D00.07	D10.1	D37.02	D49.0
ventral	C02.2	C79.89	D00.07	D10.1	D37.02	D49.0
tip	C02.1	C79.89	D00.07	D10.1	D37.02	D49.0
tonsil	C02.4	C79.89	D00.07	D10.1	D37.02	D49.0
tonsil	C09.9	C79.89	D00.08	D10.4	D37.05	D49.0
fauces, faucial	C09.9	C79.89	D00.08	D10.4	D37.05	D49.0
lingual	C02.4	C79.89	D00.07	D10.1	D37.02	D49.0
overlapping sites	C09.8	—	—	—	—	—
palatine	C09.9	C79.89	D00.08	D10.4	D37.05	D49.0
pharyngeal	C11.1	C79.89	D00.08	D10.6	D37.05	D49.0
pillar (anterior) (posterior)	C09.1	C79.89	D00.08	D10.5	D37.05	D49.0
tonsillar fossa	C09.0	C79.89	D00.08	D10.5	D37.05	D49.0
tooth socket NEC	C03.9	C79.89	D00.03	D10.39	D37.09	D49.0
trachea (cartilage) (mucosa)	C33	C78.39	D02.1	D14.2	D38.1	D49.1
overlapping lesion with bronchus or lung	C34.8-●	—	—	—	—	—
tracheobronchial	C34.8-●	C78.39	D02.1	D14.2	D38.1	D49.1
overlapping lesion with lung	C34.8-●	—	—	—	—	—
tragus — see also Neoplasm, skin, ear	C44.20-●	C79.2	D04.2-●	D23.2-●	D48.5	D49.2
trunk NEC	C76.8	C79.89	D04.5	D36.7	D48.7	D49.89
tubo-ovarian	C57.8	C79.82	D07.39	D28.7	D39.8	D49.59
tunica vaginalis	C63.7	C79.82	D07.69	D29.8	D40.8	D49.59
turbinate (bone)	C41.0	C79.51	—	D16.4-●	D48.0	D49.2
nasal	C30.0	C78.39	D02.3	D14.0	D38.5	D49.1
tympanic cavity	C30.1	C78.39	D02.3	D14.0	D38.5	D49.1
ulna (any part)	C40.0-●	C79.51	—	D16.0-●	—	—
umbilicus, umbilical — see also Neoplasm, skin, trunk	C44.509	C79.2	D04.5	D23.5	D48.5	D49.2
uncus, brain	C71.2	C79.31	—	D33.0	D43.0	D49.6
unknown site or unspecified	C80.1	C79.9	D09.9	D36.9	D48.9	D49.9
urachus	C67.7	C79.11	D09.0	D30.3	D41.4	D49.4
ureter, ureteral	C66.-●	C79.19	D09.19	D30.2-●	D41.2-●	D49.59
orifice (bladder)	C67.6	C79.11	D09.0	D30.3	D41.4	D49.4
ureter-bladder (junction)	C67.6	C79.11	D09.0	D30.3	D41.4	D49.4

◀ New ◀ Revised deleted Deleted ● Use Additional Character(s)

	Malignant Primary	Malignant Secondary	Ca in situ	Benign	Uncertain Behavior	Unspecified Behavior
urethra, urethral (gland)	C68.0	C79.19	D09.19	D30.4	D41.3	D49.59
orifice, internal	C67.5	C79.11	D09.0	D30.3	D41.4	D49.4
urethrovaginal (septum)	C57.9	C79.82	D07.30	D28.9	D39.8	D49.59
urinary organ or system	C68.9	C79.10	D09.10	D30.9	D41.9	D49.59
bladder — see Neoplasm, bladder						
overlapping lesion	C68.8	—	—	—	—	—
specified sites NEC	C68.8	C79.19	D09.19	D30.8	D41.8	D49.59
utero-ovarian	C57.8	C79.82	D07.39	D28.7	D39.8	D49.59
ligament	C57.1	C79.82	D07.39	D28.2	D39.8	D49.59
uterosacral ligament	C57.3	C79.82	—	D28.2	D39.8	D49.59
uterus, uteri, uterine	C55	C79.82	D07.0	D26.9	D39.0	D49.59
adnexa NEC	C57.4	C79.82	D07.39	D28.7	D39.8	D49.59
body	C54.9	C79.82	D07.0	D26.1	D39.0	D49.59
cervix	C53.9	C79.82	D06.9	D26.0	D39.0	D49.59
cornu	C54.9	C79.82	D07.0	D26.1	D39.0	D49.59
corpus	C54.9	C79.82	D07.0	D26.1	D39.0	D49.59
endocervix (canal) (gland)	C53.0	C79.82	D06.0	D26.0	D39.0	D49.59
endometrium	C54.1	C79.82	D07.0	D26.1	D39.0	D49.59
exocervix	C53.1	C79.82	D06.1	D26.0	D39.0	D49.59
external os	C53.1	C79.82	D06.1	D26.0	D39.0	D49.59
fundus	C54.3	C79.82	D07.0	D26.1	D39.0	D49.59
internal os	C53.0	C79.82	D06.0	D26.0	D39.0	D49.59
isthmus	C54.0	C79.82	D07.0	D26.1	D39.0	D49.59
ligament	C57.3	C79.82	—	D28.2	D39.8	D49.59
broad	C57.1	C79.82	D07.39	D28.2	D39.8	D49.59
round	C57.2	C79.82	—	D28.2	D39.8	D49.59
lower segment	C54.0	C79.82	D07.0	D26.1	D39.0	D49.59
myometrium	C54.2	C79.82	D07.0	D26.1	D39.0	D49.59
overlapping sites	C54.8	—	—	—	—	—
squamocolumnar junction	C53.8	C79.82	D06.7	D26.0	D39.0	D49.59
tube	C57.0-•	C79.82	D07.39	D28.2	D39.8	D49.59
utricle, prostatic	C68.0	C79.19	D09.19	D30.4	D41.3	D49.59
uveal tract	C69.4-•	C79.49	D09.2-•	D31.4-•	D48.7	D49.89
uvula	C05.2	C79.89	D00.04	D10.39	D37.09	D49.0
vagina, vaginal (fornix) (vault) (wall)	C52	C79.82	D07.2	D28.1	D39.8	D49.59
vaginovesical	C57.9	C79.82	D07.30	D28.9	D39.9	D49.59
septum	C57.9	C79.82	D07.30	D28.9	D39.9	D49.59
vallecula (epiglottis)	C10.0	C79.89	D00.08	D10.5	D37.05	D49.0
vas deferens	C63.1-•	C79.82	D07.69	D29.8	D40.8	D49.59
vascular — see Neoplasm, connective tissue						
Vater's ampulla	C24.1	C78.89	D01.5	D13.5	D37.6	D49.0
vein, venous — see Neoplasm, connective tissue						
vena cava (abdominal) (inferior)	C49.4	C79.89	—	D21.4	D48.1	D49.2
superior	C49.3	C79.89	—	D21.3	D48.1	D49.2
ventricle (cerebral) (floor) (lateral) (third)	C71.5	C79.31	—	D33.0	D43.0	D49.6
cardiac (left) (right)	C38.0	C79.89	—	D15.1	D48.7	D49.89
fourth	C71.7	C79.31	—	D33.1	D43.1	D49.6
ventricular band of larynx	C32.1	C78.39	D02.0	D14.1	D38.0	D49.1
ventriculus — see Neoplasm, stomach						
vermillion border — see Neoplasm, lip						
vermis, cerebellum	C71.6	C79.31	—	D33.1	D43.1	D49.6
vertebra (column)	C41.2	C79.51	—	D16.6	D48.0	D49.2
coccyx	C41.4	C79.51	—	D16.8-•	D48.0	D49.2
marrow NEC	C96.9	C79.52	—	—	D47.9	D49.89
sacrum	C41.4	C79.51	—	D16.8-•	D48.0	D49.2
vesical — see Neoplasm, bladder						
vesicle, seminal	C63.7	C79.82	D07.69	D29.8	D40.8	D49.59
vesicocervical tissue	C57.9	C79.82	D07.30	D28.9	D39.9	D49.59
vesicorectal	C76.3	C79.82	D09.8	D36.7	D48.7	D49.89
vesicovaginal	C57.9	C79.82	D07.30	D28.9	D39.9	D49.59
septum	C57.9	C79.82	D07.30	D28.9	D39.9	D49.59
vessel (blood) — see Neoplasm, connective tissue						
vestibular gland, greater	C51.0	C79.82	D07.1	D28.0	D39.8	D49.59
vestibule						
mouth	C06.1	C79.89	D00.00	D10.39	D37.09	D49.0
nose	C30.0	C78.39	D02.3	D14.0	D38.5	D49.1
Virchow's gland	C77.0	C77.0	—	D36.0	D48.7	D49.89
viscera NEC	C76.8	C79.89	D09.8	D36.7	D48.7	D49.89
vocal cords (true)	C32.0	C78.39	D02.0	D14.1	D38.0	D49.1
false	C32.1	C78.39	D02.0	D14.1	D38.0	D49.1
vomer	C41.0	C79.51	—	D16.4-•	D48.0	D49.2
vulva	C51.9	C79.82	D07.1	D28.0	D39.8	D49.59
vulvovaginal gland	C51.0	C79.82	D07.1	D28.0	D39.8	D49.59
Waldeyer's ring	C14.2	C79.89	D00.08	D10.9	D37.05	D49.0
Wharton's duct	C08.0	C79.89	D00.00	D11.7	D37.032	D49.0
white matter (central) (cerebral)	C71.0	C79.31	—	D33.0	D43.0	D49.6
windpipe	C33	C78.39	D02.1	D14.2	D38.1	D49.1

◄ New   ◀ Revised   ~~deleted~~ Deleted   • Use Additional Character(s)

TABLE OF NEOPLASMS

	Malignant Primary	Malignant Secondary	Ca in situ	Benign	Uncertain Behavior	Unspecified Behavior
Wirsung's duct	C25.3	C78.89	D01.7	D13.6	D37.8	D49.0
wolffian (body) (duct)						
female	C57.7	C79.82	D07.39	D28.7	D39.8	D49.59
male	C63.7	C79.82	D07.69	D29.8	D40.8	D49.59

	Malignant Primary	Malignant Secondary	Ca in situ	Benign	Uncertain Behavior	Unspecified Behavior
womb — *see Neoplasm, uterus*						
wrist NEC	C76.4-●	C79.89	D04.6-●	D36.7	D48.7	D49.89
xiphoid process	C41.3	C79.51	—	D16.7	D48.0	D49.2
Zuckerkandl organ	C75.5	C79.89	—	D35.6	D44.7	D49.7

◀ New   ◀ Revised   ~~deleted~~ Deleted   ● Use Additional Character(s)

ICD-10-CM
Table of Drugs and Chemicals

TOD

ICD-10-CM
Table of Drugs and Chemicals

Substance	Poisoning, Accidental (Unintentional)	Poisoning, Intentional Self-Harm	Poisoning, Assault	Poisoning, Undetermined	Adverse Effect	Underdosing
#						
1-propanol	T51.3X1	T51.3X2	T51.3X3	T51.3X4	—	—
2-propanol	T51.2X1	T51.2X2	T51.2X3	T51.2X4	—	—
2,4-D (dichlorophen-oxyacetic acid)	T60.3X1	T60.3X2	T60.3X3	T60.3X4	—	—
2,4-toluene diisocyanate	T65.0X1	T65.0X2	T65.0X3	T65.0X4		
2,4,5-T (trichloro-phenoxyacetic acid)	T60.1X1	T60.1X2	T60.1X3	T60.1X4		
3,4-methylenedioxy-methamphetamine	T43.641	T43.642	T43.643	T43.644	—	—
14-hydroxydihydro-morphinone	T40.2X1	T40.2X2	T40.2X3	T40.2X4	T40.2X5	T40.2X6
A						
ABOB	T37.5X1	T37.5X2	T37.5X3	T37.5X4	T37.5X5	T37.5X6
Abrine	T62.2X1	T62.2X2	T62.2X3	T62.2X4	—	—
Abrus (seed)	T62.2X1	T62.2X2	T62.2X3	T62.2X4	—	—
Absinthe	T51.0X1	T51.0X2	T51.0X3	T51.0X4	—	—
beverage	T51.0X1	T51.0X2	T51.0X3	T51.0X4	—	—
Acaricide	T60.8X1	T60.8X2	T60.8X3	T60.8X4	—	—
Acebutolol	T44.7X1	T44.7X2	T44.7X3	T44.7X4	T44.7X5	T44.7X6
Acecarbromal	T42.6X1	T42.6X2	T42.6X3	T42.6X4	T42.6X5	T42.6X6
Aceclidine	T44.1X1	T44.1X2	T44.1X3	T44.1X4	T44.1X5	T44.1X6
Acedapsone	T37.0X1	T37.0X2	T37.0X3	T37.0X4	T37.0X5	T37.0X6
Acefylline piperazine	T48.6X1	T48.6X2	T48.6X3	T48.6X4	T48.6X5	T48.6X6
Acemorphan	T40.2X1	T40.2X2	T40.2X3	T40.2X4	T40.2X5	T40.2X6
Acenocoumarin	T45.511	T45.512	T45.513	T45.514	T45.515	T45.516
Acenocoumarol	T45.511	T45.512	T45.513	T45.514	T45.515	T45.516
Acepifylline	T48.6X1	T48.6X2	T48.6X3	T48.6X4	T48.6X5	T48.6X6
Acepromazine	T43.3X1	T43.3X2	T43.3X3	T43.3X4	T43.3X5	T43.3X6
Acesulfamethoxypyridazine	T37.0X1	T37.0X2	T37.0X3	T37.0X4	T37.0X5	T37.0X6
Acetal	T52.8X1	T52.8X2	T52.8X3	T52.8X4	—	—
Acetaldehyde (vapor)	T52.8X1	T52.8X2	T52.8X3	T52.8X4	—	—
liquid	T65.891	T65.892	T65.893	T65.894	—	—
P-Acetamidophenol	T39.1X1	T39.1X2	T39.1X3	T39.1X4	T39.1X5	T39.1X6
Acetaminophen	T39.1X1	T39.1X2	T39.1X3	T39.1X4	T39.1X5	T39.1X6
Acetaminosalol	T39.1X1	T39.1X2	T39.1X3	T39.1X4	T39.1X5	T39.1X6
Acetanilide	T39.1X1	T39.1X2	T39.1X3	T39.1X4	T39.1X5	T39.1X6
Acetarsol	T37.3X1	T37.3X2	T37.3X3	T37.3X4	T37.3X5	T37.3X6
Acetazolamide	T50.2X1	T50.2X2	T50.2X3	T50.2X4	T50.2X5	T50.2X6
Acetiamine	T45.2X1	T45.2X2	T45.2X3	T45.2X4	T45.2X5	T45.2X6
Acetic						
acid	T54.2X1	T54.2X2	T54.2X3	T54.2X4	—	—
with sodium acetate (ointment)	T49.3X1	T49.3X2	T49.3X3	T49.3X4	T49.3X5	T49.3X6

Substance	Poisoning, Accidental (Unintentional)	Poisoning, Intentional Self-Harm	Poisoning, Assault	Poisoning, Undetermined	Adverse Effect	Underdosing
Acetic (Continued)						
acid (Continued)						
ester (solvent) (vapor)	T52.8X1	T52.8X2	T52.8X3	T52.8X4	—	—
irrigating solution	T50.3X1	T50.3X2	T50.3X3	T50.3X4	T50.3X5	T50.3X6
medicinal (lotion)	T49.2X1	T49.2X2	T49.2X3	T49.2X4	T49.2X5	T49.2X6
anhydride	T65.891	T65.892	T65.893	T65.894		
ether (vapor)	T52.8X1	T52.8X2	T52.8X3	T52.8X4	—	—
Acetohexamide	T38.3X1	T38.3X2	T38.3X3	T38.3X4	T38.3X5	T38.3X6
Acetohydroxamic acid	T50.991	T50.992	T50.993	T50.994	T50.995	T50.996
Acetomenaphthone	T45.7X1	T45.7X2	T45.7X3	T45.7X4	T45.7X5	T45.7X6
Acetomorphine	T40.1X1	T40.1X2	T40.1X3	T40.1X4	—	—
Acetone (oils)	T52.4X1	T52.4X2	T52.4X3	T52.4X4	—	—
chlorinated	T52.4X1	T52.4X2	T52.4X3	T52.4X4	—	—
vapor	T52.4X1	T52.4X2	T52.4X3	T52.4X4	—	—
Acetonitrile	T52.8X1	T52.8X2	T52.8X3	T52.8X4	—	—
Acetophenazine	T43.3X1	T43.3X2	T43.3X3	T43.3X4	T43.3X5	T43.3X6
Acetophenetedin	T39.1X1	T39.1X2	T39.1X3	T39.1X4	T39.1X5	T39.1X6
Acetophenone	T52.4X1	T52.4X2	T52.4X3	T52.4X4	—	—
Acetorphine	T40.2X1	T40.2X2	T40.2X3	T40.2X4	—	—
Acetosulfone (sodium)	T37.1X1	T37.1X2	T37.1X3	T37.1X4	T37.1X5	T37.1X6
Acetrizoate (sodium)	T50.8X1	T50.8X2	T50.8X3	T50.8X4	T50.8X5	T50.8X6
Acetylcarbromal	T42.6X1	T42.6X2	T42.6X3	T42.6X4	T42.6X5	T42.6X6
Acetrizoic acid	T50.8X1	T50.8X2	T50.8X3	T50.8X4	T50.8X5	T50.8X6
Acetyl						
bromide	T53.6X1	T53.6X2	T53.6X3	T53.6X4	—	—
chloride	T53.6X1	T53.6X2	T53.6X3	T53.6X4	—	—
Acetylcholine						
chloride	T44.1X1	T44.1X2	T44.1X3	T44.1X4	T44.1X5	T44.1X6
derivative	T44.1X1	T44.1X2	T44.1X3	T44.1X4	T44.1X5	T44.1X6
Acetylcysteine	T48.4X1	T48.4X2	T48.4X3	T48.4X4	T48.4X5	T48.4X6
Acetyldigitoxin	T46.0X1	T46.0X2	T46.0X3	T46.0X4	T46.0X5	T46.0X6
Acetyldigoxin	T46.0X1	T46.0X2	T46.0X3	T46.0X4	T46.0X5	T46.0X6
Acetyldihydrocodeine	T40.2X1	T40.2X2	T40.2X3	T40.2X4	—	—
Acetyldihydrocodeinone	T40.2X1	T40.2X2	T40.2X3	T40.2X4	—	—
Acetylene (gas)	T59.891	T59.892	T59.893	T59.894	—	—
dichloride	T53.6X1	T53.6X2	T53.6X3	T53.6X4	—	—
incomplete combustion of	T58.11	T58.12	T58.13	T58.14		
industrial	T59.891	T59.892	T59.893	T59.894	—	—
tetrachloride	T53.6X1	T53.6X2	T53.6X3	T53.6X4	—	—
vapor	T53.6X1	T53.6X2	T53.6X3	T53.6X4	—	—
Acetylphenylhydrazine	T39.8X1	T39.8X2	T39.8X3	T39.8X4	T39.8X5	T39.8X6
Acetylpheneturide	T42.6X1	T42.6X2	T42.6X3	T42.6X4	T42.6X5	T42.6X6

◀ New   ◀ Revised   ~~deleted~~ Deleted

TABLE OF DRUGS AND CHEMICALS

	External Cause (T-Code)					
Substance	Poisoning, Accidental (Unintentional)	Poisoning, Intentional Self-Harm	Poisoning, Assault	Poisoning, Undetermined	Adverse Effect	Underdosing
Acetylsalicylic acid (salts)	T39.011	T39.012	T39.013	T39.014	T39.015	T39.016
enteric coated	T39.011	T39.012	T39.013	T39.014	T39.015	T39.016
Acetylsulfamethoxypyridazine	T37.0X1	T37.0X2	T37.0X3	T37.0X4	T37.0X5	T37.0X6
Achromycin	T36.4X1	T36.4X2	T36.4X3	T36.4X4	T36.4X5	T36.4X6
ophthalmic preparation	T49.5X1	T49.5X2	T49.5X3	T49.5X4	T49.5X5	T49.5X6
topical NEC	T49.0X1	T49.0X2	T49.0X3	T49.0X4	T49.0X5	T49.0X6
Aciclovir	T37.5X1	T37.5X2	T37.5X3	T37.5X4	T37.5X5	T37.5X6
Acid (corrosive) NEC	T54.2X1	T54.2X2	T54.2X3	T54.2X4	—	—
Acidifying agent NEC	T50.901	T50.902	T50.903	T50.904	T50.905	T50.906
Acipimox	T46.6X1	T46.6X2	T46.6X3	T46.6X4	T46.6X5	T46.6X6
Acitretin	T50.991	T50.992	T50.993	T50.994	T50.995	T50.996
Aclarubicin	T45.1X1	T45.1X2	T45.1X3	T45.1X4	T45.1X5	T45.1X6
Aclatonium napadisilate	T48.1X1	T48.1X2	T48.1X3	T48.1X4	T48.1X5	T48.1X6
Aconite (wild)	T46.991	T46.992	T46.993	T46.994	T46.995	T46.996
Aconitine	T46.991	T46.992	T46.993	T46.994	T46.995	T46.996
Aconitum ferox	T46.991	T46.992	T46.993	T46.994	T46.995	T46.996
Acridine	T65.6X1	T65.6X2	T65.6X3	T65.6X4	—	—
vapor	T59.891	T59.892	T59.893	T59.894	—	—
Acriflavine	T37.91	T37.92	T37.93	T37.94	T37.95	T37.96
Acriflavinium chloride	T49.0X1	T49.0X2	T49.0X3	T49.0X4	T49.0X5	T49.0X6
Acrinol	T49.0X1	T49.0X2	T49.0X3	T49.0X4	T49.0X5	T49.0X6
Acrisorcin	T49.0X1	T49.0X2	T49.0X3	T49.0X4	T49.0X5	T49.0X6
Acrivastine	T45.0X1	T45.0X2	T45.0X3	T45.0X4	T45.0X5	T45.0X6
Acrolein (gas)	T59.891	T59.892	T59.893	T59.894	—	—
liquid	T54.1X1	T54.1X2	T54.1X3	T54.1X4	—	—
Acrylamide	T65.891	T65.892	T65.893	T65.894	—	—
Acrylic resin	T49.3X1	T49.3X2	T49.3X3	T49.3X4	T49.3X5	T49.3X6
Acrylonitrile	T65.891	T65.892	T65.893	T65.894	—	—
Actaea spicata	T62.2X1	T62.2X2	T62.2X3	T62.2X4	—	—
berry	T62.1X1	T62.1X2	T62.1X3	T62.1X4	—	—
Acterol	T37.3X1	T37.3X2	T37.3X3	T37.3X4	T37.3X5	T37.3X6
ACTH	T38.811	T38.812	T38.813	T38.814	T38.815	T38.816
Actinomycin C	T45.1X1	T45.1X2	T45.1X3	T45.1X4	T45.1X5	T45.1X6
Actinomycin D	T45.1X1	T45.1X2	T45.1X3	T45.1X4	T45.1X5	T45.1X6
Activated charcoal — see also Charcoal, medicinal	T47.6X1	T47.6X2	T47.6X3	T47.6X4	T47.6X5	T47.6X6
Acyclovir	T37.5X1	T37.5X2	T37.5X3	T37.5X4	T37.5X5	T37.5X6
Adenine	T45.2X1	T45.2X2	T45.2X3	T45.2X4	T45.2X5	T45.2X6
arabinoside	T37.5X1	T37.5X2	T37.5X3	T37.5X4	T37.5X5	T37.5X6
Adenosine (phosphate)	T46.2X1	T46.2X2	T46.2X3	T46.2X4	T46.2X5	T46.2X6
ADH	T38.891	T38.892	T38.893	T38.894	T38.895	T38.896
Adhesive NEC	T65.891	T65.892	T65.893	T65.894	—	—

	External Cause (T-Code)					
Substance	Poisoning, Accidental (Unintentional)	Poisoning, Intentional Self-Harm	Poisoning, Assault	Poisoning, Undetermined	Adverse Effect	Underdosing
Adicillin	T36.0X1	T36.0X2	T36.0X3	T36.0X4	T36.0X5	T36.0X6
Adiphenine	T44.3X1	T44.3X2	T44.3X3	T44.3X4	T44.3X5	T44.3X6
Adipiodone	T50.8X1	T50.8X2	T50.8X3	T50.8X4	T50.8X5	T50.8X6
Adjunct, pharmaceutical	T50.901	T50.902	T50.903	T50.904	T50.905	T50.906
Adrenal (extract, cortex or medulla) (glucocorticoids) (hormones) (mineralo corticoids)	T38.0X1	T38.0X2	T38.0X3	T38.0X4	T38.0X5	T38.0X6
ENT agent	T49.6X1	T49.6X2	T49.6X3	T49.6X4	T49.6X5	T49.6X6
ophthalmic preparation	T49.5X1	T49.5X2	T49.5X3	T49.5X4	T49.5X5	T49.5X6
topical NEC	T49.0X1	T49.0X2	T49.0X3	T49.0X4	T49.0X5	T49.0X6
Adrenaline	T44.5X1	T44.5X2	T44.5X3	T44.5X4	T44.5X5	T44.5X6
Adrenalin — see Adrenaline						
Adrenergic NEC	T44.901	T44.902	T44.903	T44.904	T44.905	T44.906
blocking agent NEC	T44.8X1	T44.8X2	T44.8X3	T44.8X4	T44.8X5	T44.8X6
beta, heart	T44.7X1	T44.7X2	T44.7X3	T44.7X4	T44.7X5	T44.7X6
specified NEC	T44.991	T44.992	T44.993	T44.994	T44.995	T44.996
Adrenochrome						
(mono) semicarbazone	T46.991	T46.992	T46.993	T46.994	T46.995	T46.996
derivative	T46.991	T46.992	T46.993	T46.994	T46.995	T46.996
Adrenocorticotrophic hormone	T38.811	T38.812	T38.813	T38.814	T38.815	T38.816
Adrenocorticotrophin	T38.811	T38.812	T38.813	T38.814	T38.815	T38.816
Adriamycin	T45.1X1	T45.1X2	T45.1X3	T45.1X4	T45.1X5	T45.1X6
Aerosol spray NEC	T65.91	T65.92	T65.93	T65.94	—	—
Aerosporin	T36.8X1	T36.8X2	T36.8X3	T36.8X4	T36.8X5	T36.8X6
ENT agent	T49.6X1	T49.6X2	T49.6X3	T49.6X4	T49.6X5	T49.6X6
ophthalmic preparation	T49.5X1	T49.5X2	T49.5X3	T49.5X4	T49.5X5	T49.5X6
topical NEC	T49.0X1	T49.0X2	T49.0X3	T49.0X4	T49.0X5	T49.0X6
Aethusa cynapium	T62.2X1	T62.2X2	T62.2X3	T62.2X4	—	—
Afghanistan black	T40.711	T40.712	T40.713	T40.714	T40.715	T40.716
Aflatoxin	T64.01	T64.02	T64.03	T64.04	—	—
Afloqualone	T42.8X1	T42.8X2	T42.8X3	T42.8X4	T42.8X5	T42.8X6
African boxwood	T62.2X1	T62.2X2	T62.2X3	T62.2X4	—	—
Agar	T47.4X1	T47.4X2	T47.4X3	T47.4X4	T47.4X5	T47.4X6
Agonist						
predominantly						
alpha-adrenoreceptor	T44.4X1	T44.4X2	T44.4X3	T44.4X4	T44.4X5	T44.4X6
beta-adrenoreceptor	T44.5X1	T44.5X2	T44.5X3	T44.5X4	T44.5X5	T44.5X6
Agricultural agent NEC	T65.91	T65.92	T65.93	T65.94	—	—
Agrypnal	T42.3X1	T42.3X2	T42.3X3	T42.3X4	T42.3X5	T42.3X6
AHLG	T50.Z11	T50.Z12	T50.Z13	T50.Z14	T50.Z15	T50.Z16
Air contaminant(s), source/type NOS	T65.91	T65.92	T65.93	T65.94	—	—

◀ New ◀ Revised ~~deleted~~ Deleted

Substance	Poisoning, Accidental (Unintentional)	Poisoning, Intentional Self-Harm	Poisoning, Assault	Poisoning, Undetermined	Adverse Effect	Underdosing
Ajmaline	T46.2X1	T46.2X2	T46.2X3	T46.2X4	T46.2X5	T46.2X6
Akritoin	T37.8X1	T37.8X2	T37.8X3	T37.8X4	T37.8X5	T37.8X6
Akee	T62.1X1	T62.1X2	T62.1X3	T62.1X4	—	—
Akrinol	T49.0X1	T49.0X2	T49.0X3	T49.0X4	T49.0X5	T49.0X6
Alacepril	T46.4X1	T46.4X2	T46.4X3	T46.4X4	T46.4X5	T46.4X6
Alantolactone	T37.4X1	T37.4X2	T37.4X3	T37.4X4	T37.4X5	T37.4X6
Albamycin	T36.8X1	T36.8X2	T36.8X3	T36.8X4	T36.8X5	T36.8X6
Albendazole	T37.4X1	T37.4X2	T37.4X3	T37.4X4	T37.4X5	T37.4X6
Albumin						
bovine	T45.8X1	T45.8X2	T45.8X3	T45.8X4	T45.8X5	T45.8X6
human serum	T45.8X1	T45.8X2	T45.8X3	T45.8X4	T45.8X5	T45.8X6
salt-poor	T45.8X1	T45.8X2	T45.8X3	T45.8X4	T45.8X5	T45.8X6
normal human serum	T45.8X1	T45.8X2	T45.8X3	T45.8X4	T45.8X5	T45.8X6
Albuterol	T48.6X1	T48.6X2	T48.6X3	T48.6X4	T48.6X5	T48.6X6
Albutoin	T42.0X1	T42.0X2	T42.0X3	T42.0X4	T42.0X5	T42.0X6
Alclometasone	T49.0X1	T49.0X2	T49.0X3	T49.0X4	T49.0X5	T49.0X6
Alcohol	T51.91	T51.92	T51.93	T51.94	—	—
absolute	T51.0X1	T51.0X2	T51.0X3	T51.0X4		
beverage	T51.0X1	T51.0X2	T51.0X3	T51.0X4	—	—
allyl	T51.8X1	T51.8X2	T51.8X3	T51.8X4		
amyl	T51.3X1	T51.3X2	T51.3X3	T51.3X4		
antifreeze	T51.1X1	T51.1X2	T51.1X3	T51.1X4	—	—
beverage	T51.0X1	T51.0X2	T51.0X3	T51.0X4		
butyl	T51.3X1	T51.3X2	T51.3X3	T51.3X4		
dehydrated	T51.0X1	T51.0X2	T51.0X3	T51.0X4		
beverage	T51.0X1	T51.0X2	T51.0X3	T51.0X4		
denatured	T51.0X1	T51.0X2	T51.0X3	T51.0X4		
deterrent NEC	T50.6X1	T50.6X2	T50.6X3	T50.6X4	T50.6X5	T50.6X6
diagnostic (gastric function)	T50.8X1	T50.8X2	T50.8X3	T50.8X4	T50.8X5	T50.8X6
ethyl	T51.0X1	T51.0X2	T51.0X3	T51.0X4		
beverage	T51.0X1	T51.0X2	T51.0X3	T51.0X4	—	—
grain	T51.0X1	T51.0X2	T51.0X3	T51.0X4		
beverage	T51.0X1	T51.0X2	T51.0X3	T51.0X4		
industrial	T51.0X1	T51.0X2	T51.0X3	T51.0X4	—	—
isopropyl	T51.2X1	T51.2X2	T51.2X3	T51.2X4		
methyl	T51.1X1	T51.1X2	T51.1X3	T51.1X4		
preparation for consumption	T51.0X1	T51.0X2	T51.0X3	T51.0X4	—	—
propyl	T51.3X1	T51.3X2	T51.3X3	T51.3X4		
secondary	T51.2X1	T51.2X2	T51.2X3	T51.2X4		
radiator	T51.1X1	T51.1X2	T51.1X3	T51.1X4	—	—
rubbing	T51.2X1	T51.2X2	T51.2X3	T51.2X4	—	—
specified type NEC	T51.8X1	T51.8X2	T51.8X3	T51.8X4	—	—

Substance	Poisoning, Accidental (Unintentional)	Poisoning, Intentional Self-Harm	Poisoning, Assault	Poisoning, Undetermined	Adverse Effect	Underdosing
Alcohol (Continued)						
surgical	T51.0X1	T51.0X2	T51.0X3	T51.0X4	—	—
vapor (from any type of Alcohol)	T59.891	T59.892	T59.893	T59.894	—	—
wood	T51.1X1	T51.1X2	T51.1X3	T51.1X4	—	—
Alcuronium (chloride)	T48.1X1	T48.1X2	T48.1X3	T48.1X4	T48.1X5	T48.1X6
Aldactone	T50.0X1	T50.0X2	T50.0X3	T50.0X4	T50.0X5	T50.0X6
Aldesulfone sodium	T37.1X1	T37.1X2	T37.1X3	T37.1X4	T37.1X5	T37.1X6
Aldicarb	T60.0X1	T60.0X2	T60.0X3	T60.0X4	—	—
Aldomet	T46.5X1	T46.5X2	T46.5X3	T46.5X4	T46.5X5	T46.5X6
Aldosterone	T50.0X1	T50.0X2	T50.0X3	T50.0X4	T50.0X5	T50.0X6
Aldrin (dust)	T60.1X1	T60.1X2	T60.1X3	T60.1X4	—	—
Aleve — see Naproxen						
Alexitol sodium	T47.1X1	T47.1X2	T47.1X3	T47.1X4	T47.1X5	T47.1X6
Alfacalcidol	T45.2X1	T45.2X2	T45.2X3	T45.2X4	T45.2X5	T45.2X6
Alfadolone	T41.1X1	T41.1X2	T41.1X3	T41.1X4	T41.1X5	T41.1X6
Alfaxalone	T41.1X1	T41.1X2	T41.1X3	T41.1X4	T41.1X5	T41.1X6
Alfentanil	T40.411	T40.412	T40.413	T40.414	T40.415	T40.416
Alfuzosin (hydrochloride)	T44.8X1	T44.8X2	T44.8X3	T44.8X4	T44.8X5	T44.8X6
Algae (harmful) (toxin)	T65.821	T65.822	T65.823	T65.824	—	—
Algeldrate	T47.1X1	T47.1X2	T47.1X3	T47.1X4	T47.1X5	T47.1X6
Algin	T47.8X1	T47.8X2	T47.8X3	T47.8X4	T47.8X5	T47.8X6
Alglucerase	T45.3X1	T45.3X2	T45.3X3	T45.3X4	T45.3X5	T45.3X6
Alidase	T45.3X1	T45.3X2	T45.3X3	T45.3X4	T45.3X5	T45.3X6
Alimemazine	T43.3X1	T43.3X2	T43.3X3	T43.3X4	T43.3X5	T43.3X6
Aliphatic thiocyanates	T65.0X1	T65.0X2	T65.0X3	T65.0X4	—	—
Alizapride	T45.0X1	T45.0X2	T45.0X3	T45.0X4	T45.0X5	T45.0X6
Alkali (caustic)	T54.3X1	T54.3X2	T54.3X3	T54.3X4	—	—
Alkalizing agent NEC	T50.901	T50.902	T50.903	T50.904	T50.905	T50.906
Alkaline antiseptic solution (aromatic)	T49.6X1	T49.6X2	T49.6X3	T49.6X4	T49.6X5	T49.6X6
Alkalinizing agents (medicinal)	T50.901	T50.902	T50.903	T50.904	T50.905	T50.906
Alka-seltzer	T39.011	T39.012	T39.013	T39.014	T39.015	T39.016
Alkavervir	T46.5X1	T46.5X2	T46.5X3	T46.5X4	T46.5X5	T46.5X6
Alkonium (bromide)	T49.0X1	T49.0X2	T49.0X3	T49.0X4	T49.0X5	T49.0X6
Alkylating drug NEC	T45.1X1	T45.1X2	T45.1X3	T45.1X4	T45.1X5	T45.1X6
antimyeloproliferative	T45.1X1	T45.1X2	T45.1X3	T45.1X4	T45.1X5	T45.1X6
lymphatic	T45.1X1	T45.1X2	T45.1X3	T45.1X4	T45.1X5	T45.1X6
Alkylisocyanate	T65.0X1	T65.0X2	T65.0X3	T65.0X4	—	—
Allantoin	T49.411	T49.412	T49.413	T49.414	T49.415	T49.416
Allegron	T43.0X1	T43.0X2	T43.0X3	T43.0X4	T43.0X5	T43.0X6
Allethrin	T49.0X1	T49.0X2	T49.0X3	T49.0X4	T49.0X5	T49.0X6
Allobarbital	T42.3X1	T42.3X2	T42.3X3	T42.3X4	T42.3X5	T42.3X6

◀ New ◀ Revised ~~deleted~~ Deleted

TABLE OF DRUGS AND CHEMICALS

Substance	External Cause (T-Code) Poisoning, Accidental (Unintentional)	Poisoning, Intentional Self-Harm	Poisoning, Assault	Poisoning, Undetermined	Adverse Effect	Underdosing
Allopurinol	T50.4X1	T50.4X2	T50.4X3	T50.4X4	T50.4X5	T50.4X6
Allyl						
alcohol	T51.8X1	T51.8X2	T51.8X3	T51.8X4	—	—
disulfide	T46.6X1	T46.6X2	T46.6X3	T46.6X4	T46.6X5	T46.6X6
Allylestrenol	T38.5X1	T38.5X2	T38.5X3	T38.5X4	T38.5X5	T38.5X6
Allylisopropylacetylurea	T42.6X1	T42.6X2	T42.6X3	T42.6X4	T42.6X5	T42.6X6
Allylisopropylmalonylurea	T42.3X1	T42.3X2	T42.3X3	T42.3X4	T42.3X5	T42.3X6
Allylthiourea	T49.3X1	T49.3X2	T49.3X3	T49.3X4	T49.3X5	T49.3X6
Allyltribromide	T42.6X1	T42.6X2	T42.6X3	T42.6X4	T42.6X5	T42.6X6
Allypropymal	T42.3X1	T42.3X2	T42.3X3	T42.3X4	T42.3X5	T42.3X6
Almagate	T47.1X1	T47.1X2	T47.1X3	T47.1X4	T47.1X5	T47.1X6
Almasilate	T47.1X1	T47.1X2	T47.1X3	T47.1X4	T47.1X5	T47.1X6
Almitrine	T50.7X1	T50.7X2	T50.7X3	T50.7X4	T50.7X5	T50.7X6
Aloes	T47.2X1	T47.2X2	T47.2X3	T47.2X4	T47.2X5	T47.2X6
Aloglutamol	T47.1X1	T47.1X2	T47.1X3	T47.1X4	T47.1X5	T47.1X6
Aloin	T47.2X1	T47.2X2	T47.2X3	T47.2X4	T47.2X5	T47.2X6
Aloxidone	T42.2X1	T42.2X2	T42.2X3	T42.2X4	T42.2X5	T42.2X6
Alpha						
acetyldigoxin	T46.0X1	T46.0X2	T46.0X3	T46.0X4	T46.0X5	T46.0X6
adrenergic blocking drug	T44.6X1	T44.6X2	T44.6X3	T44.6X4	T44.6X5	T44.6X6
amylase	T45.3X1	T45.3X2	T45.3X3	T45.3X4	T45.3X5	T45.3X6
tocoferol (acetate)	T45.2X1	T45.2X2	T45.2X3	T45.2X4	T45.2X5	T45.2X6
tocopherol	T45.2X1	T45.2X2	T45.2X3	T45.2X4	T45.2X5	T45.2X6
Alphadolone	T41.1X1	T41.1X2	T41.1X3	T41.1X4	T41.1X5	T41.1X6
Alphaprodine	T40.491	T40.492	T40.493	T40.494	T40.495	T40.496
Alphaxalone	T41.1X1	T41.1X2	T41.1X3	T41.1X4	T41.1X5	T41.1X6
Alprazolam	T42.4X1	T42.4X2	T42.4X3	T42.4X4	T42.4X5	T42.4X6
Alprenolol	T44.7X1	T44.7X2	T44.7X3	T44.7X4	T44.7X5	T44.7X6
Alprostadil	T46.7X1	T46.7X2	T46.7X3	T46.7X4	T46.7X5	T46.7X6
Alsactide	T38.811	T38.812	T38.813	T38.814	T38.815	T38.816
Alseroxylon	T46.5X1	T46.5X2	T46.5X3	T46.5X4	T46.5X5	T46.5X6
Alteplase	T45.611	T45.612	T45.613	T45.614	T45.615	T45.616
Altizide	T50.2X1	T50.2X2	T50.2X3	T50.2X4	T50.2X5	T50.2X6
Altretamine	T45.1X1	T45.1X2	T45.1X3	T45.1X4	T45.1X5	T45.1X6
Alum (medicinal)	T49.4X1	T49.4X2	T49.4X3	T49.4X4	T49.4X5	T49.4X6
nonmedicinal (ammonium) (potassium)	T56.891	T56.892	T56.893	T56.894	—	—
Aluminium, aluminum						
acetate	T49.2X1	T49.2X2	T49.2X3	T49.2X4	T49.2X5	T49.2X6
solution	T49.0X1	T49.0X2	T49.0X3	T49.0X4	T49.0X5	T49.0X6
aspirin	T39.011	T39.012	T39.013	T39.014	T39.015	T39.016
bis (acetylsalicylate)	T39.011	T39.012	T39.013	T39.014	T39.015	T39.016

Substance	External Cause (T-Code) Poisoning, Accidental (Unintentional)	Poisoning, Intentional Self-Harm	Poisoning, Assault	Poisoning, Undetermined	Adverse Effect	Underdosing
Aluminium, aluminum (Continued)						
carbonate (gel, basic)	T47.1X1	T47.1X2	T47.1X3	T47.1X4	T47.1X5	T47.1X6
chlorhydroxide-complex	T47.1X1	T47.1X2	T47.1X3	T47.1X4	T47.1X5	T47.1X6
chloride	T49.2X1	T49.2X2	T49.2X3	T49.2X4	T49.2X5	T49.2X6
clofibrate	T46.6X1	T46.6X2	T46.6X3	T46.6X4	T46.6X5	T46.6X6
diacetate	T49.2X1	T49.2X2	T49.2X3	T49.2X4	T49.2X5	T49.2X6
glycinate	T47.1X1	T47.1X2	T47.1X3	T47.1X4	T47.1X5	T47.1X6
hydroxide (gel)	T47.1X1	T47.1X2	T47.1X3	T47.1X4	T47.1X5	T47.1X6
hydroxide-magnesium carb. gel	T47.1X1	T47.1X2	T47.1X3	T47.1X4	T47.1X5	T47.1X6
magnesium silicate	T47.1X1	T47.1X2	T47.1X3	T47.1X4	T47.1X5	T47.1X6
nicotinate	T46.7X1	T46.7X2	T46.7X3	T46.7X4	T46.7X5	T46.7X6
ointment (surgical) (topical)	T49.3X1	T49.3X2	T49.3X3	T49.3X4	T49.3X5	T49.3X6
phosphate	T47.1X1	T47.1X2	T47.1X3	T47.1X4	T47.1X5	T47.1X6
salicylate	T39.091	T39.092	T39.093	T39.094	T39.095	T39.096
silicate	T47.1X1	T47.1X2	T47.1X3	T47.1X4	T47.1X5	T47.1X6
sodium silicate	T47.1X1	T47.1X2	T47.1X3	T47.1X4	T47.1X5	T47.1X6
subacetate	T49.2X1	T49.2X2	T49.2X3	T49.2X4	T49.2X5	T49.2X6
sulfate	T49.0X1	T49.0X2	T49.0X3	T49.0X4	T49.0X5	T49.0X6
tannate	T47.6X1	T47.6X2	T47.6X3	T47.6X4	T47.6X5	T47.6X6
topical NEC	T49.3X1	T49.3X2	T49.3X3	T49.3X4	T49.3X5	T49.3X6
Alurate	T42.3X1	T42.3X2	T42.3X3	T42.3X4	T42.3X5	T42.3X6
Alverine	T44.3X1	T44.3X2	T44.3X3	T44.3X4	T44.3X5	T44.3X6
Alvodine	T40.2X1	T40.2X2	T40.2X3	T40.2X4	T40.2X5	T40.2X6
Amanita phalloides	T62.0X1	T62.0X2	T62.0X3	T62.0X4	—	—
Amanitine	T62.0X1	T62.0X2	T62.0X3	T62.0X4	—	—
Amantadine	T42.8X1	T42.8X2	T42.8X3	T42.8X4	T42.8X5	T42.8X6
Ambazone	T49.6X1	T49.6X2	T49.6X3	T49.6X4	T49.6X5	T49.6X6
Ambenonium (chloride)	T44.0X1	T44.0X2	T44.0X3	T44.0X4	T44.0X5	T44.0X6
Ambroxol	T48.4X1	T48.4X2	T48.4X3	T48.4X4	T48.4X5	T48.4X6
Ambuphylline	T48.6X1	T48.6X2	T48.6X3	T48.6X4	T48.6X5	T48.6X6
Ambutonium bromide	T44.3X1	T44.3X2	T44.3X3	T44.3X4	T44.3X5	T44.3X6
Amcinonide	T49.0X1	T49.0X2	T49.0X3	T49.0X4	T49.0X5	T49.0X6
Amdinocilline	T36.0X1	T36.0X2	T36.0X3	T36.0X4	T36.0X5	T36.0X6
Ametazole	T50.8X1	T50.8X2	T50.8X3	T50.8X4	T50.8X5	T50.8X6
Amethocaine	T41.3X1	T41.3X2	T41.3X3	T41.3X4	T41.3X5	T41.3X6
regional	T41.3X1	T41.3X2	T41.3X3	T41.3X4	T41.3X5	T41.3X6
spinal	T41.3X1	T41.3X2	T41.3X3	T41.3X4	T41.3X5	T41.3X6
Amethopterin	T45.1X1	T45.1X2	T45.1X3	T45.1X4	T45.1X5	T45.1X6
Amezinium metilsulfate	T44.991	T44.992	T44.993	T44.994	T44.995	T44.996
Amfebutamone	T43.291	T43.292	T43.293	T43.294	T43.295	T43.296
Amfepramone	T50.5X1	T50.5X2	T50.5X3	T50.5X4	T50.5X5	T50.5X6

◀ New   ◀ Revised   ~~deleted~~ Deleted

Substance	Poisoning, Accidental (Unintentional)	Poisoning, Intentional Self-Harm	Poisoning, Assault	Poisoning, Undetermined	Adverse Effect	Underdosing
Amfetamine	T43.621	T43.622	T43.623	T43.624	T43.625	T43.626
Amfetaminil	T43.621	T43.622	T43.623	T43.624	T43.625	T43.626
Amfomycin	T36.8X1	T36.8X2	T36.8X3	T36.8X4	T36.8X5	T36.8X6
Amidefrine mesilate	T48.5X1	T48.5X2	T48.5X3	T48.5X4	T48.5X5	T48.5X6
Amidone	T40.3X1	T40.3X2	T40.3X3	T40.3X4	T40.3X5	T40.3X6
Amidopyrine	T39.2X1	T39.2X2	T39.2X3	T39.2X4	T39.2X5	T39.2X6
Amidotrizoate	T50.8X1	T50.8X2	T50.8X3	T50.8X4	T50.8X5	T50.8X6
Amiflamine	T43.1X1	T43.1X2	T43.1X3	T43.1X4	T43.1X5	T43.1X6
Amikacin	T36.5X1	T36.5X2	T36.5X3	T36.5X4	T36.5X5	T36.5X6
Amikhelline	T46.3X1	T46.3X2	T46.3X3	T46.3X4	T46.3X5	T46.3X6
Amiloride	T50.2X1	T50.2X2	T50.2X3	T50.2X4	T50.2X5	T50.2X6
Aminacrine	T49.0X1	T49.0X2	T49.0X3	T49.0X4	T49.0X5	T49.0X6
Amineptine	T43.011	T43.012	T43.013	T43.014	T43.015	T43.016
Aminitrozole	T37.3X1	T37.3X2	T37.3X3	T37.3X4	T37.3X5	T37.3X6
Aminoacetic acid (derivatives)	T50.3X1	T50.3X2	T50.3X3	T50.3X4	T50.3X5	T50.3X6
Amino acids	T50.3X1	T50.3X2	T50.3X3	T50.3X4	T50.3X5	T50.3X6
Aminoacridine	T49.0X1	T49.0X2	T49.0X3	T49.0X4	T49.0X5	T49.0X6
Aminobenzoic acid (-p)	T49.3X1	T49.3X2	T49.3X3	T49.3X4	T49.3X5	T49.3X6
4-Aminobutyric acid	T43.8X1	T43.8X2	T43.8X3	T43.8X4	T43.8X5	T43.8X6
Aminocaproic acid	T45.621	T45.622	T45.623	T45.624	T45.625	T45.626
Aminofenazone	T39.2X1	T39.2X2	T39.2X3	T39.2X4	T39.2X5	T39.2X6
Aminoethylisothiourium	T45.8X1	T45.8X2	T45.8X3	T45.8X4	T45.8X5	T45.8X6
Aminoglutethimide	T45.1X1	T45.1X2	T45.1X3	T45.1X4	T45.1X5	T45.1X6
Aminohippuric acid	T50.8X1	T50.8X2	T50.8X3	T50.8X4	T50.8X5	T50.8X6
Aminomethylbenzoic acid	T45.691	T45.692	T45.693	T45.694	T45.695	T45.696
Aminometradine	T50.2X1	T50.2X2	T50.2X3	T50.2X4	T50.2X5	T50.2X6
Aminopentamide	T44.3X1	T44.3X2	T44.3X3	T44.3X4	T44.3X5	T44.3X6
Aminophenazone	T39.2X1	T39.2X2	T39.2X3	T39.2X4	T39.2X5	T39.2X6
Aminophenol	T54.0X1	T54.0X2	T54.0X3	T54.0X4	—	—
4-Aminophenol derivatives	T39.1X1	T39.1X2	T39.1X3	T39.1X4	T39.1X5	T39.1X6
Aminophenylpyridone	T43.591	T43.592	T43.593	T43.594	T43.595	T43.596
Aminophylline	T48.6X1	T48.6X2	T48.6X3	T48.6X4	T48.6X5	T48.6X6
Aminopterin sodium	T45.1X1	T45.1X2	T45.1X3	T45.1X4	T45.1X5	T45.1X6
Aminopyrine	T39.2X1	T39.2X2	T39.2X3	T39.2X4	T39.2X5	T39.2X6
8-Aminoquinoline drugs	T37.2X1	T37.2X2	T37.2X3	T37.2X4	T37.2X5	T37.2X6
Aminorex	T50.5X1	T50.5X2	T50.5X3	T50.5X4	T50.5X5	T50.5X6
Aminosalicylic acid	T37.1X1	T37.1X2	T37.1X3	T37.1X4	T37.1X5	T37.1X6
Aminosalylum	T37.1X1	T37.1X2	T37.1X3	T37.1X4	T37.1X5	T37.1X6
Amiodarone	T46.2X1	T46.2X2	T46.2X3	T46.2X4	T46.2X5	T46.2X6
Amiphenazole	T50.7X1	T50.7X2	T50.7X3	T50.7X4	T50.7X5	T50.7X6
Amiquinsin	T46.5X1	T46.5X2	T46.5X3	T46.5X4	T46.5X5	T46.5X6
Amisometradine	T50.2X1	T50.2X2	T50.2X3	T50.2X4	T50.2X5	T50.2X6

Substance	Poisoning, Accidental (Unintentional)	Poisoning, Intentional Self-Harm	Poisoning, Assault	Poisoning, Undetermined	Adverse Effect	Underdosing
Amisulpride	T43.591	T43.592	T43.593	T43.594	T43.595	T43.596
Amitriptyline	T43.021	T43.022	T43.023	T43.024	T43.025	T43.026
Amitriptylinoxide	T43.021	T43.022	T43.023	T43.024	T43.025	T43.026
Amlexanox	T48.6X1	T48.6X2	T48.6X3	T48.6X4	T48.6X5	T48.6X6
Ammonia (fumes) (gas) (vapor)	T59.891	T59.892	T59.893	T59.894	—	—
aromatic spirit	T48.991	T48.992	T48.993	T48.994	T48.995	T48.996
liquid (household)	T54.3X1	T54.3X2	T54.3X3	T54.3X4	—	—
Ammoniated mercury	T49.0X1	T49.0X2	T49.0X3	T49.0X4	T49.0X5	T49.0X6
Ammonium						
acid tartrate	T49.5X1	T49.5X2	T49.5X3	T49.5X4	T49.5X5	T49.5X6
bromide	T42.6X1	T42.6X2	T42.6X3	T42.6X4	T42.6X5	T42.6X6
carbonate	T54.3X1	T54.3X2	T54.3X3	T54.3X4	—	—
chloride	T50.991	T50.992	T50.993	T50.994	T50.995	T50.996
expectorant	T48.4X1	T48.4X2	T48.4X3	T48.4X4	T48.4X5	T48.4X6
compounds (household) NEC	T54.3X1	T54.3X2	T54.3X3	T54.3X4	—	—
fumes (any usage)	T59.891	T59.892	T59.893	T59.894	—	—
industrial	T54.3X1	T54.3X2	T54.3X3	T54.3X4	—	—
ichthyosulronate	T49.4X1	T49.4X2	T49.4X3	T49.4X4	T49.4X5	T49.4X6
mandelate	T37.91	T37.92	T37.93	T37.94	T37.95	T37.96
sulfamate	T60.3X1	T60.3X2	T60.3X3	T60.3X4	—	—
sulfonate resin	T47.8X1	T47.8X2	T47.8X3	T47.8X4	T47.8X5	T47.8X6
Amobarbital (sodium)	T42.3X1	T42.3X2	T42.3X3	T42.3X4	T42.3X5	T42.3X6
Amodiaquine	T37.2X1	T37.2X2	T37.2X3	T37.2X4	T37.2X5	T37.2X6
Amopyroquin(e)	T37.2X1	T37.2X2	T37.2X3	T37.2X4	T37.2X5	T37.2X6
Amoxapine	T43.011	T43.012	T43.013	T43.014	T43.015	T43.016
Amoxicillin	T36.0X1	T36.0X2	T36.0X3	T36.0X4	T36.0X5	T36.0X6
Amperozide	T43.591	T43.592	T43.593	T43.594	T43.595	T43.596
Amphenidone	T43.591	T43.592	T43.593	T43.594	T43.595	T43.596
Amphetamine NEC	T43.621	T43.622	T43.623	T43.624	T43.625	T43.626
Amphomycin	T36.8X1	T36.8X2	T36.8X3	T36.8X4	T36.8X5	T36.8X6
Amphotalide	T37.4X1	T37.4X2	T37.4X3	T37.4X4	T37.4X5	T37.4X6
Amphotericin B	T36.7X1	T36.7X2	T36.7X3	T36.7X4	T36.7X5	T36.7X6
topical	T49.0X1	T49.0X2	T49.0X3	T49.0X4	T49.0X5	T49.0X6
Ampicillin	T36.0X1	T36.0X2	T36.0X3	T36.0X4	T36.0X5	T36.0X6
Amprotropine	T44.3X1	T44.3X2	T44.3X3	T44.3X4	T44.3X5	T44.3X6
Amsacrine	T45.1X1	T45.1X2	T45.1X3	T45.1X4	T45.1X5	T45.1X6
Amygdaline	T62.2X1	T62.2X2	T62.2X3	T62.2X4	—	—
Amyl						
acetate	T52.8X1	T52.8X2	T52.8X3	T52.8X4	—	—
vapor	T59.891	T59.892	T59.893	T59.894	—	—
alcohol	T51.3X1	T51.3X2	T51.3X3	T51.3X4	—	—
chloride	T53.6X1	T53.6X2	T53.6X3	T53.6X4	—	—

◀ New   ◀ Revised   ~~deleted~~ Deleted

TABLE OF DRUGS AND CHEMICALS

Substance	External Cause (T-Code) Poisoning, Accidental (Unintentional)	Poisoning, Intentional Self-Harm	Poisoning, Assault	Poisoning, Undetermined	Adverse Effect	Underdosing
Amyl (Continued)						
formate	T52.8X1	T52.8X2	T52.8X3	T52.8X4	—	—
nitrite	T46.3X1	T46.3X2	T46.3X3	T46.3X4	T46.3X5	T46.3X6
propionate	T65.891	T65.892	T65.893	T65.894	—	—
Amylase	T47.5X1	T47.5X2	T47.5X3	T47.5X4	T47.5X5	T47.5X6
Amyleine, regional	T41.3X1	T41.3X2	T41.3X3	T41.3X4	T41.3X5	T41.3X6
Amylene						
dichloride	T53.6X1	T53.6X2	T53.6X3	T53.6X4	—	—
hydrate	T51.3X1	T51.3X2	T51.3X3	T51.3X4	—	—
Amylmetacresol	T49.6X1	T49.6X2	T49.6X3	T49.6X4	T49.6X5	T49.6X6
Amylobarbitone	T42.3X1	T42.3X2	T42.3X3	T42.3X4	T42.3X5	T42.3X6
Amylocaine, regional	T41.3X1	T41.3X2	T41.3X3	T41.3X4	T41.3X5	T41.3X6
infiltration (subcutaneous)	T41.3X1	T41.3X2	T41.3X3	T41.3X4	T41.3X5	T41.3X6
nerve block (peripheral) (plexus)	T41.3X1	T41.3X2	T41.3X3	T41.3X4	T41.3X5	T41.3X6
spinal	T41.3X1	T41.3X2	T41.3X3	T41.3X4	T41.3X5	T41.3X6
topical (surface)	T41.3X1	T41.3X2	T41.3X3	T41.3X4	T41.3X5	T41.3X6
Amylopectin	T47.6X1	T47.6X2	T47.6X3	T47.6X4	T47.6X5	T47.6X6
Amytal (sodium)	T42.3X1	T42.3X2	T42.3X3	T42.3X4	T42.3X5	T42.3X6
Anabolic steroid	T38.7X1	T38.7X2	T38.7X3	T38.7X4	T38.7X5	T38.7X6
Analeptic NEC	T50.7X1	T50.7X2	T50.7X3	T50.7X4	T50.7X5	T50.7X6
Analgesic	T39.91	T39.92	T39.93	T39.94	T39.95	T39.96
anti-inflammatory NEC	T39.91	T39.92	T39.93	T39.94	T39.95	T39.96
propionic acid derivative	T39.311	T39.312	T39.313	T39.314	T39.315	T39.316
antirheumatic NEC	T39.4X1	T39.4X2	T39.4X4	T39.4X4	T39.4X5	T39.4X6
aromatic NEC	T39.1X1	T39.1X2	T39.1X3	T39.1X4	T39.1X5	T39.1X6
narcotic NEC	T40.601	T40.602	T40.603	T40.604	T40.605	T40.606
combination	T40.601	T40.602	T40.603	T40.604	T40.605	T40.606
obstetric	T40.601	T40.602	T40.603	T40.604	T40.605	T40.606
non-narcotic NEC	T39.91	T39.92	T39.93	T39.94	T39.95	T39.96
combination	T39.91	T39.92	T39.93	T39.94	T39.95	T39.96
pyrazole	T39.2X1	T39.2X2	T39.2X3	T39.2X4	T39.2X5	T39.2X6
specified NEC	T39.8X1	T39.8X2	T39.8X3	T39.8X4	T39.8X5	T39.8X6
Analgin	T39.2X1	T39.2X2	T39.2X3	T39.2X4	T39.2X5	T39.2X6
Anamirta cocculus	T62.1X1	T62.1X2	T62.1X3	T62.1X4	—	—
Ancillin	T36.0X1	T36.0X2	T36.0X3	T36.0X4	T36.0X5	T36.0X6
Ancrod	T45.691	T45.692	T45.693	T45.694	T45.695	T45.696
Androgen	T38.7X1	T38.7X2	T38.7X3	T38.7X4	T38.7X5	T38.7X6
Androgen-estrogen mixture	T38.7X1	T38.7X2	T38.7X3	T38.7X4	T38.7X5	T38.7X6
Androstalone	T38.7X1	T38.7X2	T38.7X3	T38.7X4	T38.7X5	T38.7X6
Androstanolone	T38.7X1	T38.7X2	T38.7X3	T38.7X4	T38.7X5	T38.7X6
Androsterone	T38.7X1	T38.7X2	T38.7X3	T38.7X4	T38.7X5	T38.7X6

Substance	External Cause (T-Code) Poisoning, Accidental (Unintentional)	Poisoning, Intentional Self-Harm	Poisoning, Assault	Poisoning, Undetermined	Adverse Effect	Underdosing
Anemone pulsatilla	T62.2X1	T62.2X2	T62.2X3	T62.2X4	—	—
Anesthesia						
caudal	T41.3X1	T41.3X2	T41.3X3	T41.3X4	T41.3X5	T41.3X6
endotracheal	T41.0X1	T41.0X2	T41.0X3	T41.0X4	T41.0X5	T41.0X6
epidural	T41.3X1	T41.3X2	T41.3X3	T41.3X4	T41.3X5	T41.3X6
inhalation	T41.0X1	T41.0X2	T41.0X3	T41.0X4	T41.0X5	T41.0X6
local	T41.3X1	T41.3X2	T41.3X3	T41.3X4	T41.3X5	T41.3X6
mucosal	T41.3X1	T41.3X2	T41.3X3	T41.3X4	T41.3X5	T41.3X6
muscle relaxation	T48.1X1	T48.1X2	T48.1X3	T48.1X4	T48.1X5	T48.1X6
nerve blocking	T41.3X1	T41.3X2	T41.3X3	T41.3X4	T41.3X5	T41.3X6
plexus blocking	T41.3X1	T41.3X2	T41.3X3	T41.3X4	T41.3X5	T41.3X6
potentiated	T41.201	T41.202	T41.203	T41.204	T41.205	T41.206
rectal	T41.201	T41.202	T41.203	T41.204	T41.205	T41.206
general	T41.201	T41.202	T41.203	T41.204	T41.205	T41.206
local	T41.3X1	T41.3X2	T41.3X3	T41.3X4	T41.3X5	T41.3X6
regional	T41.3X1	T41.3X2	T41.3X3	T41.3X4	T41.3X5	T41.3X6
surface	T41.3X1	T41.3X2	T41.3X3	T41.3X4	T41.3X5	T41.3X6
Anesthetic NEC—see also Anesthesia	T41.41	T41.42	T41.43	T41.44	T41.45	T41.46
with muscle relaxant	T41.201	T41.202	T41.203	T41.204	T41.205	T41.206
general	T41.201	T41.202	T41.203	T41.204	T41.205	T41.206
local	T41.3X1	T41.3X2	T41.3X3	T41.3X4	T41.3X5	T41.3X6
gaseous NEC	T41.0X1	T41.0X2	T41.0X3	T41.0X4	T41.0X5	T41.0X6
general NEC	T41.201	T41.202	T41.203	T41.204	T41.205	T41.206
halogenated hydrocarbon derivatives NEC	T41.0X1	T41.0X2	T41.0X3	T41.0X4	T41.0X5	T41.0X6
infiltration NEC	T41.3X1	T41.3X2	T41.3X3	T41.3X4	T41.3X5	T41.3X6
intravenous NEC	T41.1X1	T41.1X2	T41.1X3	T41.1X4	T41.1X5	T41.1X6
local NEC	T41.3X1	T41.3X2	T41.3X3	T41.3X4	T41.3X5	T41.3X6
rectal	T41.201	T41.202	T41.203	T41.204	T41.205	T41.206
general	T41.201	T41.202	T41.203	T41.204	T41.205	T41.206
local	T41.3X1	T41.3X2	T41.3X3	T41.3X4	T41.3X5	T41.3X6
regional NEC	T41.3X1	T41.3X2	T41.3X3	T41.3X4	T41.3X5	T41.3X6
spinal NEC	T41.3X1	T41.3X2	T41.3X3	T41.3X4	T41.3X5	T41.3X6
thiobarbiturate	T41.1X1	T41.1X2	T41.1X3	T41.1X4	T41.1X5	T41.1X6
topical	T41.3X1	T41.3X2	T41.3X3	T41.3X4	T41.3X5	T41.3X6
Aneurine	T45.2X1	T45.2X2	T45.2X3	T45.2X4	T45.2X5	T45.2X6
Angio-Conray	T50.8X1	T50.8X2	T50.8X3	T50.8X4	T50.8X5	T50.8X6
Angiotensin	T44.5X1	T44.5X2	T44.5X3	T44.5X4	T44.5X5	T44.5X6
Angiotensinamide	T44.991	T44.992	T44.993	T44.994	T44.995	T44.996
Anhydrohydroxy-progesterone	T38.5X1	T38.5X2	T38.5X3	T38.5X4	T38.5X5	T38.5X6
Anhydron	T50.2X1	T50.2X2	T50.2X3	T50.2X4	T50.2X5	T50.2X6
Anileridine	T40.491	T40.492	T40.493	T40.494	T40.495	T40.496

◀ New ◀ Revised ~~deleted~~ Deleted

Substance	External Cause (T-Code) Poisoning, Accidental (Unintentional)	Poisoning, Intentional Self-Harm	Poisoning, Assault	Poisoning, Undetermined	Adverse Effect	Underdosing
Aniline (dye) (liquid)	T65.3X1	T65.3X2	T65.3X3	T65.3X4	—	—
analgesic	T39.1X1	T39.1X2	T39.1X3	T39.1X4	T39.1X5	T39.1X6
derivatives, therapeutic NEC	T39.1X1	T39.1X2	T39.1X3	T39.1X4	T39.1X5	T39.1X6
vapor	T65.3X1	T65.3X2	T65.3X3	T65.3X4	—	—
Anise oil	T47.5X1	T47.5X2	T47.5X3	T47.5X4	T47.5X5	T47.5X6
Aniscoropine	T44.3X1	T44.3X2	T44.3X3	T44.3X4	T44.3X5	T44.3X6
Anisidine	T65.3X1	T65.3X2	T65.3X3	T65.3X4	—	—
Anisindione	T45.511	T45.512	T45.513	T45.514	T45.515	T45.516
Anisotropine methyl-bromide	T44.3X1	T44.3X2	T44.3X3	T44.3X4	T44.3X5	T44.3X6
Anistreplase	T45.611	T45.612	T45.613	T45.614	T45.615	T45.616
Anorexiant (central)	T50.5X1	T50.5X2	T50.5X3	T50.5X4	T50.5X5	T50.5X6
Anorexic agents	T50.5X1	T50.5X2	T50.5X3	T50.5X4	T50.5X5	T50.5X6
Ansamycin	T36.6X1	T36.6X2	T36.6X3	T36.6X4	T36.6X5	T36.6X6
Ant (bite) (sting)	T63.421	T63.422	T63.423	T63.424	—	—
Antabuse	T50.6X1	T50.6X2	T50.6X3	T50.6X4	T50.6X5	T50.6X6
Ant poison — see Insecticide						
Antacid NEC	T47.1X1	T47.1X2	T47.1X3	T47.1X4	T47.1X5	T47.1X6
Antagonist						
Aldosterone	T50.0X1	T50.0X2	T50.0X3	T50.0X4	T50.0X5	T50.0X6
alpha-adrenoreceptor	T44.6X1	T44.6X2	T44.6X3	T44.6X4	T44.6X5	T44.6X6
anticoagulant	T45.7X1	T45.7X2	T45.7X3	T45.7X4	T45.7X5	T45.7X6
beta-adrenoreceptor	T44.7X1	T44.7X2	T44.7X3	T44.7X4	T44.7X5	T44.7X6
extrapyramidal NEC	T44.3X1	T44.3X2	T44.3X3	T44.3X4	T44.3X5	T44.3X6
folic acid	T45.1X1	T45.1X2	T45.1X3	T45.1X4	T45.1X5	T45.1X6
H2 receptor	T47.0X1	T47.0X2	T47.0X3	T47.0X4	T47.0X5	T47.0X6
heavy metal	T45.8X1	T45.8X2	T45.8X3	T45.8X4	T45.8X5	T45.8X6
narcotic analgesic	T50.7X1	T50.7X2	T50.7X3	T50.7X4	T50.7X5	T50.7X6
opiate	T50.7X1	T50.7X2	T50.7X3	T50.7X4	T50.7X5	T50.7X6
pyrimidine	T45.1X1	T45.1X2	T45.1X3	T45.1X4	T45.1X5	T45.1X6
serotonin	T46.5X1	T46.5X2	T46.5X3	T46.5X4	T46.5X5	T46.5X6
Antazolin(e)	T45.0X1	T45.0X2	T45.0X3	T45.0X4	T45.0X5	T45.0X6
Anterior pituitary hormone NEC	T38.811	T38.812	T38.813	T38.814	T38.815	T38.816
Anthelmintic NEC	T37.4X1	T37.4X2	T37.4X3	T37.4X4	T37.4X5	T37.4X6
Anthiolimine	T37.4X1	T37.4X2	T37.4X3	T37.4X4	T37.4X5	T37.4X6
Anthralin	T49.4X1	T49.4X2	T49.4X3	T49.4X4	T49.4X5	T49.4X6
Anthramycin	T45.1X1	T45.1X2	T45.1X3	T45.1X4	T45.1X5	T45.1X6
Antiadrenergic NEC	T44.8X1	T44.8X2	T44.8X3	T44.8X4	T44.8X5	T44.8X6
Antiallergic NEC	T45.0X1	T45.0X2	T45.0X3	T45.0X4	T45.0X5	T45.0X6
Anti-anemic (drug) (preparation)	T45.8X1	T45.8X2	T45.8X3	T45.8X4	T45.8X5	T45.8X6
Antiandrogen NEC	T38.6X1	T38.6X2	T38.6X3	T38.6X4	T38.6X5	T38.6X6
Antianxiety drug NEC	T43.501	T43.502	T43.503	T43.504	T43.505	T43.506
Antiaris toxicaria	T65.891	T65.892	T65.893	T65.894	—	—
Antiarteriosclerotic drug	T46.6X1	T46.6X2	T46.6X3	T46.6X4	T46.6X5	T46.6X6
Antiasthmatic drug NEC	T48.6X1	T48.6X2	T48.6X3	T48.6X4	T48.6X5	T48.6X6
Antibiotic NEC	T36.91	T36.92	T36.93	T36.94	T36.95	T36.96
aminoglycoside	T36.5X1	T36.5X2	T36.5X3	T36.5X4	T36.5X5	T36.5X6
anticancer	T45.1X1	T45.1X2	T45.1X3	T45.1X4	T45.1X5	T45.1X6
antifungal	T36.7X1	T36.7X2	T36.7X3	T36.7X4	T36.7X5	T36.7X6
antimycobacterial	T36.5X1	T36.5X2	T36.5X3	T36.5X4	T36.5X5	T36.5X6
antineoplastic	T45.1X1	T45.1X2	T45.1X3	T45.1X4	T45.1X5	T45.1X6
cephalosporin (group)	T36.1X1	T36.1X2	T36.1X3	T36.1X4	T36.1X5	T36.1X6
chloramphenicol (group)	T36.2X1	T36.2X2	T36.2X3	T36.2X4	T36.2X5	T36.2X6
ENT	T49.6X1	T49.6X2	T49.6X3	T49.6X4	T49.6X5	T49.6X6
eye	T49.5X1	T49.5X2	T49.5X3	T49.5X4	T49.5X5	T49.5X6
fungicidal (local)	T49.0X1	T49.0X2	T49.0X3	T49.0X4	T49.0X5	T49.0X6
intestinal	T36.8X1	T36.8X2	T36.8X3	T36.8X4	T36.8X5	T36.8X6
b-lactam NEC	T36.1X1	T36.1X2	T36.1X3	T36.1X4	T36.1X5	T36.1X6
local	T49.0X1	T49.0X2	T49.0X3	T49.0X4	T49.0X5	T49.0X6
macrolides	T36.3X1	T36.3X2	T36.3X3	T36.3X4	T36.3X5	T36.3X6
polypeptide	T36.8X1	T36.8X2	T36.8X3	T36.8X4	T36.8X5	T36.8X6
specified NEC	T36.8X1	T36.8X2	T36.8X3	T36.8X4	T36.8X5	T36.8X6
tetracycline (group)	T36.4X1	T36.4X2	T36.4X3	T36.4X4	T36.4X5	T36.4X6
throat	T49.6X1	T49.6X2	T49.6X3	T49.6X4	T49.6X5	T49.6X6
Anticancer agents NEC	T45.1X1	T45.1X2	T45.1X3	T45.1X4	T45.1X5	T45.1X6
Anticholesterolemic drug NEC	T46.6X1	T46.6X2	T46.6X3	T46.6X4	T46.6X5	T46.6X6
Anticholinergic NEC	T44.3X1	T44.3X2	T44.3X3	T44.3X4	T44.3X5	T44.3X6
Anticholinesterase	T44.0X1	T44.0X2	T44.0X3	T44.0X4	T44.0X5	T44.0X6
organophosphorus	T44.0X1	T44.0X2	T44.0X3	T44.0X4	T44.0X5	T44.0X6
insecticide	T60.0X1	T60.0X2	T60.0X3	T60.0X4	—	—
nerve gas	T59.891	T59.892	T59.893	T59.894	—	—
reversible	T44.0X1	T44.0X2	T44.0X3	T44.0X4	T44.0X5	T44.0X6
ophthalmological	T49.5X1	T49.5X2	T49.5X3	T49.5X4	T49.5X5	T49.5X6
Anticoagulant NEC	T45.511	T45.512	T45.513	T45.514	T45.515	T45.516
Antagonist	T45.7X1	T45.7X2	T45.7X3	T45.7X4	T45.7X5	T45.7X6
Anti-common-cold drug NEC	T48.5X1	T48.5X2	T48.5X3	T48.5X4	T48.5X5	T48.5X6
Anticonvulsant	T42.71	T42.72	T42.73	T42.74	T42.75	T42.76
barbiturate	T42.3X1	T42.3X2	T42.3X3	T42.3X4	T42.3X5	T42.3X6
combination (with barbiturate)	T42.3X1	T42.3X2	T42.3X3	T42.3X4	T42.3X5	T42.3X6
hydantoin	T42.0X1	T42.0X2	T42.0X3	T42.0X4	T42.0X5	T42.0X6
hypnotic NEC	T42.6X1	T42.6X2	T42.6X3	T42.6X4	T42.6X5	T42.6X6
oxazolidinedione	T42.2X1	T42.2X2	T42.2X3	T42.2X4	T42.2X5	T42.2X6
pyrimidinedione	T42.6X1	T42.6X2	T42.6X3	T42.6X4	T42.6X5	T42.6X6
specified NEC	T42.6X1	T42.6X2	T42.6X3	T42.6X4	T42.6X5	T42.6X6
succinimide	T42.2X1	T42.2X2	T42.2X3	T42.2X4	T42.2X5	T42.2X6

New ◀ Revised ◀ ~~deleted~~ Deleted

TABLE OF DRUGS AND CHEMICALS

Substance	External Cause (T-Code)					
	Poisoning, Accidental (Unintentional)	Poisoning, Intentional Self-Harm	Poisoning, Assault	Poisoning, Undetermined	Adverse Effect	Underdosing
Anti-D immunoglobulin (human)	T50.Z11	T50.Z12	T50.Z13	T50.Z14	T50.Z15	T50.Z16
Antidepressant NEC	T43.201	T43.202	T43.203	T43.204	T43.205	T43.206
monoamine oxidase inhibitor	T43.1X1	T43.1X2	T43.1X3	T43.1X4	T43.1X5	T43.1X6
selective serotonin norepinephrine reuptake inhibitor	T43.211	T43.212	T43.213	T43.214	T43.215	T43.216
selective serotonin reuptake inhibitor	T43.221	T43.222	T43.223	T43.224	T43.225	T43.226
specified NEC	T43.291	T43.292	T43.293	T43.294	T43.295	T43.296
tetracyclic	T43.021	T43.022	T43.023	T43.024	T43.025	T43.026
triazolopyridine	T43.221	T43.222	T43.223	T43.224	T43.225	T43.226
tricyclic	T43.011	T43.012	T43.013	T43.014	T43.015	T43.016
Antidiabetic NEC	T38.3X1	T38.3X2	T38.3X3	T38.3X4	T38.3X5	T38.3X6
biguanide	T38.3X1	T38.3X2	T38.3X3	T38.3X4	T38.3X5	T38.3X6
and sulfonyl combined	T38.3X1	T38.3X2	T38.3X3	T38.3X4	T38.3X5	T38.3X6
combined	T38.3X1	T38.3X2	T38.3X3	T38.3X4	T38.3X5	T38.3X6
sulfonylurea	T38.3X1	T38.3X2	T38.3X3	T38.3X4	T38.3X5	T38.3X6
Antidiarrheal drug NEC	T47.6X1	T47.6X2	T47.6X3	T47.6X4	T47.6X5	T47.6X6
absorbent	T47.6X1	T47.6X2	T47.6X3	T47.6X4	T47.6X5	T47.6X6
Antidiphtheria serum	T50.Z11	T50.Z12	T50.Z13	T50.Z14	T50.Z15	T50.Z16
Antidiuretic hormone	T38.891	T38.892	T38.893	T38.894	T38.895	T38.896
Antidote NEC	T50.6X1	T50.6X2	T50.6X3	T50.6X4	T50.6X5	T50.6X6
heavy metal	T45.8X1	T45.8X2	T45.8X3	T45.8X4	T45.8X5	T45.8X6
Antidysrhythmic NEC	T46.2X1	T46.2X2	T46.2X3	T46.2X4	T46.2X5	T46.2X6
Antiemetic drug	T45.0X1	T45.0X2	T45.0X3	T45.0X4	T45.0X5	T45.0X6
Antiepilepsy agent	T42.71	T42.72	T42.73	T42.74	T42.75	T42.76
combination	T42.5X1	T42.5X2	T42.5X3	T42.5X4	T42.5X5	T42.5X6
mixed	T42.5X1	T42.5X2	T42.5X3	T42.5X4	T42.5X5	T42.5X6
specified, NEC	T42.6X1	T42.6X2	T42.6X3	T42.6X4	T42.6X5	T42.6X6
Antiestrogen NEC	T38.6X1	T38.6X2	T38.6X3	T38.6X4	T38.6X5	T38.6X6
Antifertility pill	T38.4X1	T38.4X2	T38.4X3	T38.4X4	T38.4X5	T38.4X6
Antifibrinolytic drug	T45.621	T45.622	T45.623	T45.624	T45.625	T45.626
Antifilarial drug	T37.4X1	T37.4X2	T37.4X3	T37.4X4	T37.4X5	T37.4X6
Antiflatulent	T47.5X1	T47.5X2	T47.5X3	T47.5X4	T47.5X5	T47.5X6
Antifreeze	T65.91	T65.92	T65.93	T65.94	—	—
alcohol	T51.1X1	T51.1X2	T51.1X3	T51.1X4	—	—
ethylene glycol	T51.8X1	T51.8X2	T51.8X3	T51.8X4	—	—
Antifungal						
antibiotic (systemic)	T36.7X1	T36.7X2	T36.7X3	T36.7X4	T36.7X5	T36.7X6
anti-infective NEC	T37.91	T37.92	T37.93	T37.94	T37.95	T37.96
disinfectant, local	T49.0X1	T49.0X2	T49.0X3	T49.0X4	T49.0X5	T49.0X6
nonmedicinal (spray)	T60.3X1	T60.3X2	T60.3X3	T60.3X4	—	—
topical	T49.0X1	T49.0X2	T49.0X3	T49.0X4	T49.0X5	T49.0X6
Anti-gastric-secretion drug NEC	T47.1X1	T47.1X2	T47.1X3	T47.1X4	T47.1X5	T47.1X6
Antigonadotrophin NEC	T38.6X1	T38.6X2	T38.6X3	T38.6X4	T38.6X5	T38.6X6
Antihallucinogen	T43.501	T43.502	T43.503	T43.504	T43.505	T43.506
Antihelmintics	T37.4X1	T37.4X2	T37.4X3	T37.4X4	T37.4X5	T37.4X6
Antihemophilic						
factor	T45.8X1	T45.8X2	T45.8X3	T45.8X4	T45.8X5	T45.8X6
fraction	T45.8X1	T45.8X2	T45.8X3	T45.8X4	T45.8X5	T45.8X6
globulin concentrate	T45.7X1	T45.7X2	T45.7X3	T45.7X4	T45.7X5	T45.7X6
human plasma	T45.8X1	T45.8X2	T45.8X3	T45.8X4	T45.8X5	T45.8X6
plasma, dried	T45.7X1	T45.7X2	T45.7X3	T45.7X4	T45.7X5	T45.7X6
Antihemorrhoidal preparation	T49.2X1	T49.2X2	T49.2X3	T49.2X4	T49.2X5	T49.2X6
Antiheparin drug	T45.7X1	T45.7X2	T45.7X3	T45.7X4	T45.7X5	T45.7X6
Antihistamine	T45.0X1	T45.0X2	T45.0X3	T45.0X4	T45.0X5	T45.0X6
Antihookworm drug	T37.4X1	T37.4X2	T37.4X3	T37.4X4	T37.4X5	T37.4X6
Anti-human lymphocytic globulin	T50.Z11	T50.Z12	T50.Z13	T50.Z14	T50.Z15	T50.Z16
Antihyperlipidemic drug	T46.6X1	T46.6X2	T46.6X3	T46.6X4	T46.6X5	T46.6X6
Antihypertensive drug NEC	T46.5X1	T46.5X2	T46.5X3	T46.5X4	T46.5X5	T46.5X6
Anti-infective NEC	T37.91	T37.92	T37.93	T37.94	T37.95	T37.96
anthelmintic	T37.4X1	T37.4X2	T37.4X3	T37.4X4	T37.4X5	T37.4X6
antibiotics	T36.91	T36.92	T36.93	T36.94	T36.95	T36.96
specified NEC	T36.8X1	T36.8X2	T36.8X3	T36.8X4	T36.8X5	T36.8X6
antimalarial	T37.2X1	T37.2X2	T37.2X3	T37.2X4	T37.2X5	T37.2X6
antimycobacterial NEC	T37.1X1	T37.1X2	T37.1X3	T37.1X4	T37.1X5	T37.1X6
antibiotics	T36.5X1	T36.5X2	T36.5X3	T36.5X4	T36.5X5	T36.5X6
antiprotozoal NEC	T37.3X1	T37.3X2	T37.3X3	T37.3X4	T37.3X5	T37.3X6
blood	T37.2X1	T37.2X2	T37.2X3	T37.2X4	T37.2X5	T37.2X6
antiviral	T37.5X1	T37.5X2	T37.5X3	T37.5X4	T37.5X5	T37.5X6
arsenical	T37.8X1	T37.8X2	T37.8X3	T37.8X4	T37.8X5	T37.8X6
bismuth, local	T49.0X1	T49.0X2	T49.0X3	T49.0X4	T49.0X5	T49.0X6
ENT	T49.6X1	T49.6X2	T49.6X3	T49.6X4	T49.6X5	T49.6X6
eye NEC	T49.5X1	T49.5X2	T49.5X3	T49.5X4	T49.5X5	T49.5X6
heavy metals NEC	T37.8X1	T37.8X2	T37.8X3	T37.8X4	T37.8X5	T37.8X6
local NEC	T49.0X1	T49.0X2	T49.0X3	T49.0X4	T49.0X5	T49.0X6
specified NEC	T49.0X1	T49.0X2	T49.0X3	T49.0X4	T49.0X5	T49.0X6
mixed	T37.91	T37.92	T37.93	T37.94	T37.95	T37.96
ophthalmic preparation	T49.5X1	T49.5X2	T49.5X3	T49.5X4	T49.5X5	T49.5X6
topical NEC	T49.0X1	T49.0X2	T49.0X3	T49.0X4	T49.0X5	T49.0X6
Anti-inflammatory drug NEC	T49.0X1	T49.0X2	T49.0X3	T49.0X4	T49.0X5	T49.0X6
local	T49.0X1	T49.0X2	T49.0X3	T49.0X4	T49.0X5	T49.0X6
nonsteroidal NEC	T39.391	T39.392	T39.393	T39.394	T39.395	T39.396
propionic acid derivative	T39.311	T39.312	T39.313	T39.314	T39.315	T39.316
specified NEC	T39.391	T39.392	T39.393	T39.394	T39.395	T39.396

◀ New ◀ Revised ~~deleted~~ Deleted

	External Cause (T-Code)					
Substance	Poisoning, Accidental (Unintentional)	Poisoning, Intentional Self-Harm	Poisoning, Assault	Poisoning, Undetermined	Adverse Effect	Underdosing
Antikaluretic	T50.3X1	T50.3X2	T50.3X3	T50.3X4	T50.3X5	T50.3X6
Antiknock (tetraethyl lead)	T56.0X1	T56.0X2	T56.0X3	T56.0X4	—	—
Antilipemic drug NEC	T46.6X1	T46.6X2	T46.6X3	T46.6X4	T46.6X5	T46.6X6
Antimalarial	T37.2X1	T37.2X2	T37.2X3	T37.2X4	T37.2X5	T37.2X6
prophylactic NEC	T37.2X1	T37.2X2	T37.2X3	T37.2X4	T37.2X5	T37.2X6
pyrimidine derivative	T37.2X1	T37.2X2	T37.2X3	T37.2X4	T37.2X5	T37.2X6
Antimetabolite	T45.1X1	T45.1X2	T45.1X3	T45.1X4	T45.1X5	T45.1X6
Antimitotic agent	T45.1X1	T45.1X2	T45.1X3	T45.1X4	T45.1X5	T45.1X6
Antimony (compounds) (vapor) NEC	T56.891	T56.892	T56.893	T56.894	—	—
anti-infectives	T37.8X1	T37.8X2	T37.8X3	T37.8X4	T37.8X5	T37.8X6
dimercaptosuccinate	T37.3X1	T37.3X2	T37.3X3	T37.3X4	T37.3X5	T37.3X6
hydride	T56.891	T56.892	T56.893	T56.894		
pesticide (vapor)	T60.8X1	T60.8X2	T60.8X3	T60.8X4	—	—
potassium (sodium) tartrate	T37.8X1	T37.8X2	T37.8X3	T37.8X4	T37.8X5	T37.8X6
sodium dimercaptosuccinate	T37.3X1	T37.3X2	T37.3X3	T37.3X4	T37.3X5	T37.3X6
tartrated	T37.8X1	T37.8X2	T37.8X3	T37.8X4	T37.8X5	T37.8X6
Antimuscarinic NEC	T44.3X1	T44.3X2	T44.3X3	T44.3X4	T44.3X5	T44.3X6
Antimycobacterial drug NEC	T37.1X1	T37.1X2	T37.1X3	T37.1X4	T37.1X5	T37.1X6
antibiotics	T36.5X1	T36.5X2	T36.5X3	T36.5X4	T36.5X5	T36.5X6
combination	T37.1X1	T37.1X2	T37.1X3	T37.1X4	T37.1X5	T37.1X6
Antinausea drug	T45.0X1	T45.0X2	T45.0X3	T45.0X4	T45.0X5	T45.0X6
Antinematode drug	T37.4X1	T37.4X2	T37.4X3	T37.4X4	T37.4X5	T37.4X6
Antineoplastic NEC	T45.1X1	T45.1X2	T45.1X3	T45.1X4	T45.1X5	T45.1X6
alkaloidal	T45.1X1	T45.1X2	T45.1X3	T45.1X4	T45.1X5	T45.1X6
antibiotics	T45.1X1	T45.1X2	T45.1X3	T45.1X4	T45.1X5	T45.1X6
combination	T45.1X1	T45.1X2	T45.1X3	T45.1X4	T45.1X5	T45.1X6
estrogen	T38.5X1	T38.5X2	T38.5X3	T38.5X4	T38.5X5	T38.5X6
steroid	T38.7X1	T38.7X2	T38.7X3	T38.7X4	T38.7X5	T38.7X6
Antiparasitic drug (systemic)	T37.91	T37.92	T37.93	T37.94	T37.95	T37.96
local	T49.0X1	T49.0X2	T49.0X3	T49.0X4	T49.0X5	T49.0X6
specified NEC	T37.8X1	T37.8X2	T37.8X3	T37.8X4	T37.8X5	T37.8X6
Antiparkinsonism drug NEC	T42.8X1	T42.8X2	T42.8X3	T42.8X4	T42.8X5	T42.8X6
Antiperspirant NEC	T49.2X1	T49.2X2	T49.2X3	T49.2X4	T49.2X5	T49.2X6
Antiphlogistic NEC	T39.4X1	T39.4X2	T39.4X3	T39.4X4	T39.4X5	T39.4X6
Antiplatyhelmintic drug	T37.4X1	T37.4X2	T37.4X3	T37.4X4	T37.4X5	T37.4X6
Antiprotozoal drug NEC	T37.3X1	T37.3X2	T37.3X3	T37.3X4	T37.3X5	T37.3X6
blood	T37.2X1	T37.2X2	T37.2X3	T37.2X4	T37.2X5	T37.2X6
local	T49.0X1	T49.0X2	T49.0X3	T49.0X4	T49.0X5	T49.0X6
Antipruritic drug NEC	T49.1X1	T49.1X2	T49.1X3	T49.1X4	T49.1X5	T49.1X6
Antipsychotic drug	T43.501	T43.502	T43.503	T43.504	T43.505	T43.506
specified NEC	T43.591	T43.592	T43.593	T43.594	T43.595	T43.596

	External Cause (T-Code)					
Substance	Poisoning, Accidental (Unintentional)	Poisoning, Intentional Self-Harm	Poisoning, Assault	Poisoning, Undetermined	Adverse Effect	Underdosing
Antipyretic	T39.91	T39.92	T39.93	T39.94	T39.95	T39.96
specified NEC	T39.8X1	T39.8X2	T39.8X3	T39.8X4	T39.8X5	T39.8X6
Antipyrine	T39.2X1	T39.2X2	T39.2X3	T39.2X4	T39.2X5	T39.2X6
Antirabies hyperimmune serum	T50.Z11	T50.Z12	T50.Z13	T50.Z14	T50.Z15	T50.Z16
Antirheumatic NEC	T39.4X1	T39.4X2	T39.4X3	T39.4X4	T39.4X5	T39.4X6
Antirigidity drug NEC	T42.8X1	T42.8X2	T42.8X3	T42.8X4	T42.8X5	T42.8X6
Antischistosomal drug	T37.4X1	T37.4X2	T37.4X3	T37.4X4	T37.4X5	T37.4X6
Antiscorpion sera	T50.Z11	T50.Z12	T50.Z13	T50.Z14	T50.Z15	T50.Z16
Antiseborrheics	T49.4X1	T49.4X2	T49.4X3	T49.4X4	T49.4X5	T49.4X6
Antiseptics (external) (medicinal)	T49.0X1	T49.0X2	T49.0X3	T49.0X4	T49.0X5	T49.0X6
Antistine	T45.0X1	T45.0X2	T45.0X3	T45.0X4	T45.0X5	T45.0X6
Antitapeworm drug	T37.4X1	T37.4X2	T37.4X3	T37.4X4	T37.4X5	T37.4X6
Antitetanus immunoglobulin	T50.Z11	T50.Z12	T50.Z13	T50.Z14	T50.Z15	T50.Z16
Antithrombotic	T45.521	T45.522	T45.523	T45.524	T45.525	T45.526
Antithyroid drug NEC	T38.2X1	T38.2X2	T38.2X3	T38.2X4	T38.2X5	T38.2X6
Antitoxin	T50.Z11	T50.Z12	T50.Z13	T50.Z14	T50.Z15	T50.Z16
diphtheria	T50.Z11	T50.Z12	T50.Z13	T50.Z14	T50.Z15	T50.Z16
gas gangrene	T50.Z11	T50.Z12	T50.Z13	T50.Z14	T50.Z15	T50.Z16
tetanus	T50.Z11	T50.Z12	T50.Z13	T50.Z14	T50.Z15	T50.Z16
Antitoxin, any	T50.901	T50.902	T50.903	T50.904	T50.905	T50.906
Antitrichomonal drug	T37.3X1	T37.3X2	T37.3X3	T37.3X4	T37.3X5	T37.3X6
Antituberculars	T37.1X1	T37.1X2	T37.1X3	T37.1X4	T37.1X5	T37.1X6
antibiotics	T36.5X1	T36.5X2	T36.5X3	T36.5X4	T36.5X5	T36.5X6
Antitussive NEC	T48.3X1	T48.3X2	T48.3X3	T48.3X4	T48.3X5	T48.3X6
codeine mixture	T40.2X1	T40.2X2	T40.2X3	T40.2X4	T40.2X5	T40.2X6
opiate	T40.2X1	T40.2X2	T40.2X3	T40.2X4	T40.2X5	T40.2X6
Antivaricose drug	T46.8X1	T46.8X2	T46.8X3	T46.8X4	T46.8X5	T46.8X6
Antivenin, antivenom (sera)	T50.Z11	T50.Z12	T50.Z13	T50.Z14	T50.Z15	T50.Z16
crotaline	T50.Z11	T50.Z12	T50.Z13	T50.Z14	T50.Z15	T50.Z16
spider bite	T50.Z11	T50.Z12	T50.Z13	T50.Z14	T50.Z15	T50.Z16
Antivertigo drug	T45.0X1	T45.0X2	T45.0X3	T45.0X4	T45.0X5	T45.0X6
Antiviral drug NEC	T37.5X1	T37.5X2	T37.5X3	T37.5X4	T37.5X5	T37.5X6
eye	T49.5X1	T49.5X2	T49.5X3	T49.5X4	T49.5X5	T49.5X6
Antiwhipworm drug	T37.4X1	T37.4X2	T37.4X3	T37.4X4	T37.4X5	T37.4X6
Ant poisons — see Pesticides						
Antrol — see also by specific chemical substance	T60.91	T60.92	T60.93	T60.94	—	—
fungicide	T60.91	T60.92	T60.93	T60.94	—	—
ANTU (alpha naphthylthiourea)	T60.4X1	T60.4X2	T60.4X3	T60.4X4	—	—
Apalcillin	T36.0X1	T36.0X2	T36.0X3	T36.0X4	T36.0X5	T36.0X6
APC	T48.5X1	T48.5X2	T48.5X3	T48.5X4	T48.5X5	T48.5X6
Aplonidine	T44.4X1	T44.4X2	T44.4X3	T44.4X4	T44.4X5	T44.4X6
Apomorphine	T47.7X1	T47.7X2	T47.7X3	T47.7X4	T47.7X5	T47.7X6

TABLE OF DRUGS AND CHEMICALS

Substance	External Cause (T-Code)					
	Poisoning, Accidental (Unintentional)	Poisoning, Intentional Self-Harm	Poisoning, Assault	Poisoning, Undetermined	Adverse Effect	Underdosing
Appetite depressants, central	T50.5X1	T50.5X2	T50.5X3	T50.5X4	T50.5X5	T50.5X6
Apraclonidine (hydrochloride)	T44.4X1	T44.4X2	T44.4X3	T44.4X4	T44.4X5	T44.4X6
Apresoline	T46.5X1	T46.5X2	T46.5X3	T46.5X4	T46.5X5	T46.5X6
Aprindine	T46.2X1	T46.2X2	T46.2X3	T46.2X4	T46.2X5	T46.2X6
Aprobarbital	T42.3X1	T42.3X2	T42.3X3	T42.3X4	T42.3X5	T42.3X6
Apronalide	T42.6X1	T42.6X2	T42.6X3	T42.6X4	T42.6X5	T42.6X6
Aprotinin	T45.621	T45.622	T45.623	T45.624	T45.625	T45.626
Aptocaine	T41.3X1	T41.3X2	T41.3X3	T41.3X4	T41.3X5	T41.3X6
Aqua fortis	T54.2X1	T54.2X2	T54.2X3	T54.2X4	—	—
Ara-A	T37.5X1	T37.5X2	T37.5X3	T37.5X4	T37.5X5	T37.5X6
Ara-C	T45.1X1	T45.1X2	T45.1X3	T45.1X4	T45.1X5	T45.1X6
Arachis oil	T49.3X1	T49.3X2	T49.3X3	T49.3X4	T49.3X5	T49.3X6
cathartic	T47.4X1	T47.4X2	T47.4X3	T47.4X4	T47.4X5	T47.4X6
Aralen	T37.2X1	T37.2X2	T37.2X3	T37.2X4	T37.2X5	T37.2X6
Arecoline	T44.1X1	T44.1X2	T44.1X3	T44.1X4	T44.1X5	T44.1X6
Arginine	T50.991	T50.992	T50.993	T50.994	T50.995	T50.996
glutamate	T50.991	T50.992	T50.993	T50.994	T50.995	T50.996
Argyrol	T49.0X1	T49.0X2	T49.0X3	T49.0X4	T49.0X5	T49.0X6
ENT agent	T49.6X1	T49.6X2	T49.6X3	T49.6X4	T49.6X5	T49.6X6
ophthalmic preparation	T49.5X1	T49.5X2	T49.5X3	T49.5X4	T49.5X5	T49.5X6
Aristocort	T38.0X1	T38.0X2	T38.0X3	T38.0X4	T38.0X5	T38.0X6
ENT agent	T49.6X1	T49.6X2	T49.6X3	T49.6X4	T49.6X5	T49.6X6
ophthalmic preparation	T49.5X1	T49.5X2	T49.5X3	T49.5X4	T49.5X5	T49.5X6
topical NEC	T49.0X1	T49.0X2	T49.0X3	T49.0X4	T49.0X5	T49.0X6
Aromatics, corrosive	T54.1X1	T54.1X2	T54.1X3	T54.1X4	—	—
disinfectants	T54.1X1	T54.1X2	T54.1X3	T54.1X4	—	—
Arsenate of lead	T57.0X1	T57.0X2	T57.0X3	T57.0X4	—	—
herbicide	T57.0X1	T57.0X2	T57.0X3	T57.0X4	—	—
Arsenic, arsenicals (compounds) (dust) (vapor) NEC	T57.0X1	T57.0X2	T57.0X3	T57.0X4	—	—
anti-infectives	T37.8X1	T37.8X2	T37.8X3	T37.8X4	T37.8X5	T37.8X6
pesticide (dust) (fumes)	T57.0X1	T57.0X2	T57.0X3	T57.0X4	—	—
Arsine (gas)	T57.0X1	T57.0X2	T57.0X3	T57.0X4	—	—
Arsphenamine (silver)	T37.8X1	T37.8X2	T37.8X3	T37.8X4	T37.8X5	T37.8X6
Arsthinol	T37.3X1	T37.3X2	T37.3X3	T37.3X4	T37.3X5	T37.3X6
Artane	T44.3X1	T44.3X2	T44.3X3	T44.3X4	T44.3X5	T44.3X6
Arthropod (venomous) NEC	T63.481	T63.482	T63.483	T63.484	—	—
Articaine	T41.3X1	T41.3X2	T41.3X3	T41.3X4	T41.3X5	T41.3X6
Asbestos	T57.8X1	T57.8X2	T57.8X3	T57.8X4	—	—
Ascaridole	T37.4X1	T37.4X2	T37.4X3	T37.4X4	T37.4X5	T37.4X6
Ascorbic acid	T45.2X1	T45.2X2	T45.2X3	T45.2X4	T45.2X5	T45.2X6
Asiaticoside	T49.0X1	T49.0X2	T49.0X3	T49.0X4	T49.0X5	T49.0X6

Substance	External Cause (T-Code)					
	Poisoning, Accidental (Unintentional)	Poisoning, Intentional Self-Harm	Poisoning, Assault	Poisoning, Undetermined	Adverse Effect	Underdosing
Asparaginase	T45.1X1	T45.1X2	T45.1X3	T45.1X4	T45.1X5	T45.1X6
Aspidium (oleoresin)	T37.4X1	T37.4X2	T37.4X3	T37.4X4	T37.4X5	T37.4X6
Aspirin (aluminum) (soluble)	T39.011	T39.012	T39.013	T39.014	T39.015	T39.016
Aspoxicillin	T36.0X1	T36.0X2	T36.0X3	T36.0X4	T36.0X5	T36.0X6
Astemizole	T45.0X1	T45.0X2	T45.0X3	T45.0X4	T45.0X5	T45.0X6
Astringent (local)	T49.2X1	T49.2X2	T49.2X3	T49.2X4	T49.2X5	T49.2X6
specified NEC	T49.2X1	T49.2X2	T49.2X3	T49.2X4	T49.2X5	T49.2X6
Astromicin	T36.5X1	T36.5X2	T36.5X3	T36.5X4	T36.5X5	T36.5X6
Ataractic drug NEC	T43.501	T43.502	T43.503	T43.504	T43.505	T43.506
Atenolol	T44.7X1	T44.7X2	T44.7X3	T44.7X4	T44.7X5	T44.7X6
Atonia drug, intestinal	T47.4X1	T47.4X2	T47.4X3	T47.4X4	T47.4X5	T47.4X6
Atophan	T50.4X1	T50.4X2	T50.4X3	T50.4X4	T50.4X5	T50.4X6
Atracurium besilate	T48.1X1	T48.1X2	T48.1X3	T48.1X4	T48.1X5	T48.1X6
Atropine	T44.3X1	T44.3X2	T44.3X3	T44.3X4	T44.3X5	T44.3X6
derivative	T44.3X1	T44.3X2	T44.3X3	T44.3X4	T44.3X5	T44.3X6
methonitrate	T44.3X1	T44.3X2	T44.3X3	T44.3X4	T44.3X5	T44.3X6
Attapulgite	T47.6X1	T47.6X2	T47.6X3	T47.6X4	T47.6X5	T47.6X6
Attenuvax	T50.991	T50.992	T50.993	T50.994	T50.995	T50.996
Auramine	T65.891	T65.892	T65.893	T65.894	—	—
dye	T65.6X1	T65.6X2	T65.6X3	T65.6X4	—	—
fungicide	T60.3X1	T60.3X2	T60.3X3	T60.3X4	—	—
Auranofin	T39.4X1	T39.4X2	T39.4X3	T39.4X4	T39.4X5	T39.4X6
Aurantiin	T46.991	T46.992	T46.993	T46.994	T46.995	T46.996
Aureomycin	T36.4X1	T36.4X2	T36.4X3	T36.4X4	T36.4X5	T36.4X6
ophthalmic preparation	T49.5X1	T49.5X2	T49.5X3	T49.5X4	T49.5X5	T49.5X6
topical NEC	T49.0X1	T49.0X2	T49.0X3	T49.0X4	T49.0X5	T49.0X6
Aurothioglucose	T39.4X1	T39.4X2	T39.4X3	T39.4X4	T39.4X5	T39.4X6
Aurothioglycanide	T39.4X1	T39.4X2	T39.4X3	T39.4X4	T39.4X5	T39.4X6
Aurothiomalate sodium	T39.4X1	T39.4X2	T39.4X3	T39.4X4	T39.4X5	T39.4X6
Aurotioprol	T39.4X1	T39.4X2	T39.4X3	T39.4X4	T39.4X5	T39.4X6
Automobile fuel	T52.0X1	T52.0X2	T52.0X3	T52.0X4	—	—
Autonomic nervous system agent NEC	T44.901	T44.902	T44.903	T44.904	T44.905	T44.906
Avlosulfon	T37.1X1	T37.1X2	T37.1X3	T37.1X4	T37.1X5	T37.1X6
Avomine	T42.6X1	T42.6X2	T42.6X3	T42.6X4	T42.6X5	T42.6X6
Axerophthol	T45.2X1	T45.2X2	T45.2X3	T45.2X4	T45.2X5	T45.2X6
Azacitidine	T45.1X1	T45.1X2	T45.1X3	T45.1X4	T45.1X5	T45.1X6
Azacyclonol	T43.591	T43.592	T43.593	T43.594	T43.595	T43.596
Azadirachta	T60.2X1	T60.2X2	T60.2X3	T60.2X4	—	—
Azanidazole	T37.3X1	T37.3X2	T37.3X3	T37.3X4	T37.3X5	T37.3X6
Azapetine	T46.7X1	T46.7X2	T46.7X3	T46.7X4	T46.7X5	T46.7X6
Azapropazone	T39.2X1	T39.2X2	T39.2X3	T39.2X4	T39.2X5	T39.2X6

◀ New ◀ Revised ~~deleted~~ Deleted

Substance	Poisoning, Accidental (Unintentional)	Poisoning, Intentional Self-Harm	Poisoning, Assault	Poisoning, Undetermined	Adverse Effect	Underdosing
Azaribine	T45.1X1	T45.1X2	T45.1X3	T45.1X4	T45.1X5	T45.1X6
Azaserine	T45.1X1	T45.1X2	T45.1X3	T45.1X4	T45.1X5	T45.1X6
Azatadine	T45.0X1	T45.0X2	T45.0X3	T45.0X4	T45.0X5	T45.0X6
Azatepa	T45.1X1	T45.1X2	T45.1X3	T45.1X4	T45.1X5	T45.1X6
Azathioprine	T45.1X1	T45.1X2	T45.1X3	T45.1X4	T45.1X5	T45.1X6
Azelaic acid	T49.0X1	T49.0X2	T49.0X3	T49.0X4	T49.0X5	T49.0X6
Azelastine	T45.0X1	T45.0X2	T45.0X3	T45.0X4	T45.0X5	T45.0X6
Azidocillin	T36.0X1	T36.0X2	T36.0X3	T36.0X4	T36.0X5	T36.0X6
Azidothymidine	T37.5X1	T37.5X2	T37.5X3	T37.5X4	T37.5X5	T37.5X6
Azinphos (ethyl) (methyl)	T60.0X1	T60.0X2	T60.0X3	T60.0X4	—	—
Aziridine (chelating)	T54.1X1	T54.1X2	T54.1X3	T54.1X4	—	—
Azithromycin	T36.3X1	T36.3X2	T36.3X3	T36.3X4	T36.3X5	T36.3X6
Azlocillin	T36.01	T36.02	T36.03	T36.04	T36.05	T36.06
Azobenzene smoke	T65.3X1	T65.3X2	T65.3X3	T65.3X4	—	—
acaricide	T60.8X1	T60.8X2	T60.8X3	T60.8X4	—	—
Azosulfamide	T37.0X1	T37.0X2	T37.0X3	T37.0X4	T37.0X5	T37.0X6
AZT	T37.5X1	T37.5X2	T37.5X3	T37.5X4	T37.5X5	T37.5X6
Aztreonam	T36.1X1	T36.1X2	T36.1X3	T36.1X4	T36.1X5	T36.1X6
Azulfidine	T37.0X1	T37.0X2	T37.0X3	T37.0X4	T37.0X5	T37.0X6
Azuresin	T50.8X1	T50.8X2	T50.8X3	T50.8X4	T50.8X5	T50.8X6
B						
Bacampicillin	T36.0X1	T36.0X2	T36.0X3	T36.0X4	T36.0X5	T36.0X6
Bacillus						
lactobacillus	T47.8X1	T47.8X2	T47.8X3	T47.8X4	T47.8X5	T47.8X6
subtilis	T47.6X1	T47.6X2	T47.6X3	T47.6X4	T47.6X5	T47.6X6
Bacimycin	T49.0X1	T49.0X2	T49.0X3	T49.0X4	T49.0X5	T49.0X6
ophthalmic preparation	T49.5X1	T49.5X2	T49.5X3	T49.5X4	T49.5X5	T49.5X6
Bacitracin zinc	T49.0X1	T49.0X2	T49.0X3	T49.0X4	T49.0X5	T49.0X6
with neomycin	T49.0X1	T49.0X2	T49.0X3	T49.0X4	T49.0X5	T49.0X6
ENT agent	T49.6X1	T49.6X2	T49.6X3	T49.6X4	T49.6X5	T49.6X6
ophthalmic preparation	T49.5X1	T49.5X2	T49.5X3	T49.5X4	T49.5X5	T49.5X6
topical NEC	T49.0X1	T49.0X2	T49.0X3	T49.0X4	T49.0X5	T49.0X6
Baclofen	T42.8X1	T42.8X2	T42.8X3	T42.8X4	T42.8X5	T42.8X6
Baking soda	T50.991	T50.992	T50.993	T50.994	T50.995	T50.996
BAL	T45.8X1	T45.8X2	T45.8X3	T45.8X4	T45.8X5	T45.8X6
Bambuterol	T48.6X1	T48.6X2	T48.6X3	T48.6X4	T48.6X5	T48.6X6
Bamethan (sulfate)	T46.7X1	T46.7X2	T46.7X3	T46.7X4	T46.7X5	T46.7X6
Bamifylline	T48.6X1	T48.6X2	T48.6X3	T48.6X4	T48.6X5	T48.6X6
Bamipine	T45.0X1	T45.0X2	T45.0X3	T45.0X4	T45.0X5	T45.0X6
Baneberry — see Actaea spicata						
Banewort — see Belladonna						

Substance	Poisoning, Accidental (Unintentional)	Poisoning, Intentional Self-Harm	Poisoning, Assault	Poisoning, Undetermined	Adverse Effect	Underdosing
Barbenyl	T42.3X1	T42.3X2	T42.3X3	T42.3X4	T42.3X5	T42.3X6
Barbexaclone	T42.6X1	T42.6X2	T42.6X3	T42.6X4	T42.6X5	T42.6X6
Barbital	T42.3X1	T42.3X2	T42.3X3	T42.3X4	T42.3X5	T42.3X6
sodium	T42.3X1	T42.3X2	T42.3X3	T42.3X4	T42.3X5	T42.3X6
Barbitone	T42.3X1	T42.3X2	T42.3X3	T42.3X4	T42.3X5	T42.3X6
Barbiturate NEC	T42.3X1	T42.3X2	T42.3X3	T42.3X4	T42.3X5	T42.3X6
with tranquilizer	T42.3X1	T42.3X2	T42.3X3	T42.3X4	T42.3X5	T42.3X6
anesthetic (intravenous)	T41.1X1	T41.1X2	T41.1X3	T41.1X4	T41.1X5	T41.1X6
Barium (carbonate) (chloride) (sulfite)	T57.8X1	T57.8X2	T57.8X3	T57.8X4	—	—
diagnostic agent	T50.8X1	T50.8X2	T50.8X3	T50.8X4	T50.8X5	T50.8X6
pesticide	T60.4X1	T60.4X2	T60.4X3	T60.4X4	—	—
rodenticide	T60.4X1	T60.4X2	T60.4X3	T60.4X4	—	—
sulfate (medicinal)	T50.8X1	T50.8X2	T50.8X3	T50.8X4	T50.8X5	T50.8X6
Barrier cream	T49.3X1	T49.3X2	T49.3X3	T49.3X4	T49.3X5	T49.3X6
Basic fuchsin	T49.0X1	T49.0X2	T49.0X3	T49.0X4	T49.0X5	T49.0X6
Battery acid or fluid	T54.2X1	T54.2X2	T54.2X3	T54.2X4	—	—
Bay rum	T51.8X1	T51.8X2	T51.8X3	T51.8X4	—	—
BCG (vaccine)	T50.A91	T50.A92	T50.A93	T50.A94	T50.A95	T50.A96
BCNU	T45.1X1	T45.1X2	T45.1X3	T45.1X4	T45.1X5	T45.1X6
Bearsfoot	T62.2X1	T62.2X2	T62.2X3	T62.2X4	—	—
Beclamide	T42.6X1	T42.6X2	T42.6X3	T42.6X4	T42.6X5	T42.6X6
Beclomethasone	T44.5X1	T44.5X2	T44.5X3	T44.5X4	T44.5X5	T44.5X6
Bee (sting) (venom)	T63.441	T63.442	T63.443	T63.444	—	—
Befunolol	T49.5X1	T49.5X2	T49.5X3	T49.5X4	T49.5X5	T49.5X6
Bekanamycin	T36.5X1	T36.5X2	T36.5X3	T36.5X4	T36.5X5	T36.5X6
Belladonna — see also Nightshade						
alkaloids	T44.3X1	T44.3X2	T44.3X3	T44.3X4	T44.3X5	T44.3X6
extract	T44.3X1	T44.3X2	T44.3X3	T44.3X4	T44.3X5	T44.3X6
herb	T44.3X1	T44.3X2	T44.3X3	T44.3X4	T44.3X5	T44.3X6
Bemegride	T50.7X1	T50.7X2	T50.7X3	T50.7X4	T50.7X5	T50.7X6
Benactyzine	T44.3X1	T44.3X2	T44.3X3	T44.3X4	T44.3X5	T44.3X6
Benadryl	T45.0X1	T45.0X2	T45.0X3	T45.0X4	T45.0X5	T45.0X6
Benaprizine	T44.3X1	T44.3X2	T44.3X3	T44.3X4	T44.3X5	T44.3X6
Benazepril	T46.4X1	T46.4X2	T46.4X3	T46.4X4	T46.4X5	T46.4X6
Bencyclane	T46.7X1	T46.7X2	T46.7X3	T46.7X4	T46.7X5	T46.7X6
Bendazol	T46.3X1	T46.3X2	T46.3X3	T46.3X4	T46.3X5	T46.3X6
Bendrofluazide	T50.2X1	T50.2X2	T50.2X3	T50.2X4	T50.2X5	T50.2X6
Bendroflumethiazide	T50.2X1	T50.2X2	T50.2X3	T50.2X4	T50.2X5	T50.2X6
Benemid	T50.4X1	T50.4X2	T50.4X3	T50.4X4	T50.4X5	T50.4X6
Benethamine penicillin	T36.0X1	T36.0X2	T36.0X3	T36.0X4	T36.0X5	T36.0X6
Benisone	T49.0X1	T49.0X2	T49.0X3	T49.0X4	T49.0X5	T49.0X6

◀ New ◀ Revised ~~deleted~~ Deleted

TABLE OF DRUGS AND CHEMICALS

Substance	External Cause (T-Code)					
	Poisoning, Accidental (Unintentional)	Poisoning, Intentional Self-Harm	Poisoning, Assault	Poisoning, Undetermined	Adverse Effect	Underdosing
Benexate	T47.1X1	T47.1X2	T47.1X3	T47.1X4	T47.1X5	T47.1X6
Benfluorex	T46.6X1	T46.6X2	T46.6X3	T46.6X4	T46.6X5	T46.6X6
Benfotiamine	T45.2X1	T45.2X2	T45.2X3	T45.2X4	T45.2X5	T45.2X6
Benomyl	T60.0X1	T60.0X2	T60.0X3	T60.0X4	—	—
Benoquin	T49.8X1	T49.8X2	T49.8X3	T49.8X4	T49.8X5	T49.8X6
Benoxinate	T41.3X1	T41.3X2	T41.3X3	T41.3X4	T41.3X5	T41.3X6
Benperidol	T43.4X1	T43.4X2	T43.4X3	T43.4X4	T43.4X5	T43.4X6
Benproperine	T48.3X1	T48.3X2	T48.3X3	T48.3X4	T48.3X5	T48.3X6
Benserazide	T42.8X1	T42.8X2	T42.8X3	T42.8X4	T42.8X5	T42.8X6
Bentazepam	T42.4X1	T42.4X2	T42.4X3	T42.4X4	T42.4X5	T42.4X6
Bentiromide	T50.8X1	T50.8X2	T50.8X3	T50.8X4	T50.8X5	T50.8X6
Bentonite	T49.3X1	T49.3X2	T49.3X3	T49.3X4	T49.3X5	T49.3X6
Benzalbutyramide	T46.6X1	T46.6X2	T46.6X3	T46.6X4	T46.6X5	T46.6X6
Benzalkonium (chloride)	T49.0X1	T49.0X2	T49.0X3	T49.0X4	T49.0X5	T49.0X6
ophthalmic preparation	T49.5X1	T49.5X2	T49.5X3	T49.5X4	T49.5X5	T49.5X6
Benzamine	T41.3X1	T41.3X2	T41.3X3	T41.3X4	T41.3X5	T41.3X6
lactate	T49.1X1	T49.1X2	T49.1X3	T49.1X4	T49.1X5	T49.1X6
Benzamidosalicylate (calcium)	T37.1X1	T37.1X2	T37.1X3	T37.1X4	T37.1X5	T37.1X6
Benzamphetamine	T50.5X1	T50.5X2	T50.5X3	T50.5X4	T50.5X5	T50.5X6
Benzapril hydrochloride	T46.5X1	T46.5X2	T46.5X3	T46.5X4	T46.5X5	T46.5X6
Benzathine benzylpenicillin	T36.0X1	T36.0X2	T36.0X3	T36.0X4	T36.0X5	T36.0X6
Benzathine penicillin	T36.0X1	T36.0X2	T36.0X3	T36.0X4	T36.0X5	T36.0X6
Benzatropine	T42.8X1	T42.8X2	T42.8X3	T42.8X4	T42.8X5	T42.8X6
Benzbromarone	T50.4X1	T50.4X2	T50.4X3	T50.4X4	T50.4X5	T50.4X6
Benzcarbimine	T45.1X1	T45.1X2	T45.1X3	T45.1X4	T45.1X5	T45.1X6
Benzedrex	T44.991	T44.992	T44.993	T44.994	T44.995	T44.996
Benzedrine (amphetamine)	T43.621	T43.622	T43.623	T43.624	T43.625	T43.626
Benzenamine	T65.3X1	T65.3X2	T65.3X3	T65.3X4	—	—
Benzene	T52.1X1	T52.1X2	T52.1X3	T52.1X4		
homologues (acetyl) (dimethyl) (methyl) (solvent)	T52.2X1	T52.2X2	T52.2X3	T52.2X4		
Benzethonium (chloride)	T49.0X1	T49.0X2	T49.0X3	T49.0X4	T49.0X5	T49.0X6
Benzfetamine	T50.5X1	T50.5X2	T50.5X3	T50.5X4	T50.5X5	T50.5X6
Benzhexol	T44.3X1	T44.3X2	T44.3X3	T44.3X4	T44.3X5	T44.3X6
Benzhydramine (chloride)	T45.0X1	T45.0X2	T45.0X3	T45.0X4	T45.0X5	T45.0X6
Benzidine	T65.891	T65.892	T65.893	T65.894	—	—
Benzilonium bromide	T44.3X1	T44.3X2	T44.3X3	T44.3X4	T44.3X5	T44.3X6
Benzimidazole	T60.3X1	T60.3X2	T60.3X3	T60.3X4	—	—
Benzin(e) — see Ligroin						
Benziodarone	T46.3X1	T46.3X2	T46.3X3	T46.3X4	T46.3X5	T46.3X6
Benznidazole	T37.3X1	T37.3X2	T37.3X3	T37.3X4	T37.3X5	T37.3X6
Benzocaine	T41.3X1	T41.3X2	T41.3X3	T41.3X4	T41.3X5	T41.3X6

Substance	External Cause (T-Code)					
	Poisoning, Accidental (Unintentional)	Poisoning, Intentional Self-Harm	Poisoning, Assault	Poisoning, Undetermined	Adverse Effect	Underdosing
Benzoctamine	T43.0X1	T43.0X2	T43.0X3	T43.0X4	T43.0X5	T43.0X6
Benzodiapin	T42.4X1	T42.4X2	T42.4X3	T42.4X4	T42.4X5	T42.4X6
Benzodiazepine NEC	T42.4X1	T42.4X2	T42.4X3	T42.4X4	T42.4X5	T42.4X6
Benzoic acid	T49.0X1	T49.0X2	T49.0X3	T49.0X4	T49.0X5	T49.0X6
with salicylic acid	T49.0X1	T49.0X2	T49.0X3	T49.0X4	T49.0X5	T49.0X6
Benzoin (tincture)	T48.5X1	T48.5X2	T48.5X3	T48.5X4	T48.5X5	T48.5X6
Benzol (benzene)	T52.1X1	T52.1X2	T52.1X3	T52.1X4	—	—
vapor	T52.0X1	T52.0X2	T52.0X3	T52.0X4	—	—
Benzomorphan	T40.2X1	T40.2X2	T40.2X3	T40.2X4	T40.2X5	T40.2X6
Benzonatate	T48.3X1	T48.3X2	T48.3X3	T48.3X4	T48.3X5	T48.3X6
Benzophenones	T49.3X1	T49.3X2	T49.3X3	T49.3X4	T49.3X5	T49.3X6
Benzopyrone	T46.991	T46.992	T46.993	T46.994	T46.995	T46.996
Benzothiadiazides	T50.2X1	T50.2X2	T50.2X3	T50.2X4	T50.2X5	T50.2X6
Benzoxonium chloride	T49.0X1	T49.0X2	T49.0X3	T49.0X4	T49.0X5	T49.0X6
Benzoyl peroxide	T49.0X1	T49.0X2	T49.0X3	T49.0X4	T49.0X5	T49.0X6
Benzoylpas calcium	T37.1X1	T37.1X2	T37.1X3	T37.1X4	T37.1X5	T37.1X6
Benzperidin	T43.591	T43.592	T43.593	T43.594	T43.595	T43.596
Benzperidol	T43.591	T43.592	T43.593	T43.594	T43.595	T43.596
Benzphetamine	T50.5X1	T50.5X2	T50.5X3	T50.5X4	T50.5X5	T50.5X6
Benzpyrinium bromide	T44.1X1	T44.1X2	T44.1X3	T44.1X4	T44.1X5	T44.1X6
Benzquinamide	T45.0X1	T45.0X2	T45.0X3	T45.0X4	T45.0X5	T45.0X6
Benzthiazide	T50.2X1	T50.2X2	T50.2X3	T50.2X4	T50.2X5	T50.2X6
Benztropine						
anticholinergic	T44.3X1	T44.3X2	T44.3X3	T44.3X4	T44.3X5	T44.3X6
antiparkinson	T42.8X1	T42.8X2	T42.8X3	T42.8X4	T42.8X5	T42.8X6
Benzydamine	T49.0X1	T49.0X2	T49.0X3	T49.0X4	T49.0X5	T49.0X6
Benzyl						
acetate	T52.8X1	T52.8X2	T52.8X3	T52.8X4	—	—
alcohol	T49.0X1	T49.0X2	T49.0X3	T49.0X4	T49.0X5	T49.0X6
benzoate	T49.0X1	T49.0X2	T49.0X3	T49.0X4	T49.0X5	T49.0X6
Benzoic acid	T49.0X1	T49.0X2	T49.0X3	T49.0X4	T49.0X5	T49.0X6
morphine	T40.2X1	T40.2X2	T40.2X3	T40.2X4	—	—
nicotinate	T46.6X1	T46.6X2	T46.6X3	T46.6X4	T46.6X5	T46.6X6
penicillin	T36.0X1	T36.0X2	T36.0X3	T36.0X4	T36.0X5	T36.0X6
Benzylhydrochlorthia-zide	T50.2X1	T50.2X2	T50.2X3	T50.2X4	T50.2X5	T50.2X6
Benzylpenicillin	T36.0X1	T36.0X2	T36.0X3	T36.0X4	T36.0X5	T36.0X6
Benzylthiouracil	T38.2X1	T38.2X2	T38.2X3	T38.2X4	T38.2X5	T38.2X6
Bephenium hydroxy-naphthoate	T37.4X1	T37.4X2	T37.4X3	T37.4X4	T37.4X5	T37.4X6
Bepridil	T46.1X1	T46.1X2	T46.1X3	T46.1X4	T46.1X5	T46.1X6
Bergamot oil	T65.891	T65.892	T65.893	T65.894	—	—
Bergapten	T50.991	T50.992	T50.993	T50.994	T50.995	T50.996
Berries, poisonous	T62.1X1	T62.1X2	T62.1X3	T62.1X4	—	—

◀ New   ◀ Revised   ~~deleted~~ Deleted

Substance	Poisoning, Accidental (Unintentional)	Poisoning, Intentional Self-Harm	Poisoning, Assault	Poisoning, Undetermined	Adverse Effect	Underdosing
Beryllium (compounds)	T56.7X1	T56.7X2	T56.7X3	T56.7X4	—	—
b-acetyldigoxin	T46.0X1	T46.0X2	T46.0X3	T46.0X4	T46.0X5	T46.0X6
beta adrenergic blocking agent, heart	T44.7X1	T44.7X2	T44.7X3	T44.7X4	T44.7X5	T44.7X6
b-benzalbutyramide	T46.6X1	T46.6X2	T46.6X3	T46.6X4	T46.6X5	T46.6X6
Betacarotene	T45.2X1	T45.2X2	T45.2X3	T45.2X4	T45.2X5	T45.2X6
b-eucaine	T49.1X1	T49.1X2	T49.1X3	T49.1X4	T49.1X5	T49.1X6
Beta-Chlor	T42.6X1	T42.6X2	T42.6X3	T42.6X4	T42.6X5	T42.6X6
b-galactosidase	T47.5X1	T47.5X2	T47.5X3	T47.5X4	T47.5X5	T47.5X6
Betahistine	T46.7X1	T46.7X2	T46.7X3	T46.7X4	T46.7X5	T46.7X6
Betaine	T47.5X1	T47.5X2	T47.5X3	T47.5X4	T47.5X5	T47.5X6
Betamethasone	T49.0X1	T49.0X2	T49.0X3	T49.0X4	T49.0X5	T49.0X6
topical	T49.0X1	T49.0X2	T49.0X3	T49.0X4	T49.0X5	T49.0X6
Betamicin	T36.8X1	T36.8X2	T36.8X3	T36.8X4	T36.8X5	T36.8X6
Betanidine	T46.5X1	T46.5X2	T46.5X3	T46.5X4	T46.5X5	T46.5X6
b-sitosterol(s)	T46.6X1	T46.6X2	T46.6X3	T46.6X4	T46.6X5	T46.6X6
Betaxolol	T44.7X1	T44.7X2	T44.7X3	T44.7X4	T44.7X5	T44.7X6
Betazole	T50.8X1	T50.8X2	T50.8X3	T50.8X4	T50.8X5	T50.8X6
Bethanechol	T44.1X1	T44.1X2	T44.1X3	T44.1X4	T44.1X5	T44.1X6
chloride	T44.1X1	T44.1X2	T44.1X3	T44.1X4	T44.1X5	T44.1X6
Bethanidine	T46.5X1	T46.5X2	T46.5X3	T46.5X4	T46.5X5	T46.5X6
Betoxycaine	T41.3X1	T41.3X2	T41.3X3	T41.3X4	T41.3X5	T41.3X6
Betula oil	T49.3X1	T49.3X2	T49.3X3	T49.3X4	T49.3X5	T49.3X6
Bevantolol	T44.7X1	T44.7X2	T44.7X3	T44.7X4	T44.7X5	T44.7X6
Bevonium metilsulfate	T44.3X1	T44.3X2	T44.3X3	T44.3X4	T44.3X5	T44.3X6
Bezafibrate	T46.6X1	T46.6X2	T46.6X3	T46.6X4	T46.6X5	T46.6X6
Bezitramide	T40.491	T40.492	T40.493	T40.494	T40.495	T40.496
BHA	T50.991	T50.992	T50.993	T50.994	T50.995	T50.996
Bhang	T40.711	T40.712	T40.713	T40.714	T40.715	T40.716
BHC (medicinal)	T49.0X1	T49.0X2	T49.0X3	T49.0X4	T49.0X5	T49.0X6
nonmedicinal (vapor)	T53.6X1	T53.6X2	T53.6X3	T53.6X4	—	—
Bialamicol	T37.3X1	T37.3X2	T37.3X3	T37.3X4	T37.3X5	T37.3X6
Bibenzonium bromide	T48.3X1	T48.3X2	T48.3X3	T48.3X4	T48.3X5	T48.3X6
Bibrocathol	T49.5X1	T49.5X2	T49.5X3	T49.5X4	T49.5X5	T49.5X6
Bichloride of mercury — see Mercury, chloride						
Bichromates (calcium) (potassium) (sodium) (crystals)	T57.8X1	T57.8X2	T57.8X3	T57.8X4	—	—
fumes	T56.2X1	T56.2X2	T56.2X3	T56.2X4	—	—
Biclotymol	T49.6X1	T49.6X2	T49.6X3	T49.6X4	T49.6X5	T49.6X6
Bicuculline	T50.7X1	T50.7X2	T50.7X3	T50.7X4	T50.7X5	T50.7X6
Bifemelane	T43.291	T43.292	T43.293	T43.294	T43.295	T43.296
Biguanide derivatives, oral	T38.3X1	T38.3X2	T38.3X3	T38.3X4	T38.3X5	T38.3X6

Substance	Poisoning, Accidental (Unintentional)	Poisoning, Intentional Self-Harm	Poisoning, Assault	Poisoning, Undetermined	Adverse Effect	Underdosing
Biligrafin	T50.8X1	T50.8X2	T50.8X3	T50.8X4	T50.8X5	T50.8X6
Bile salts	T47.5X1	T47.5X2	T47.5X3	T47.5X4	T47.5X5	T47.5X6
Bilopaque	T50.8X1	T50.8X2	T50.8X3	T50.8X4	T50.8X5	T50.8X6
Binifibrate	T46.6X1	T46.6X2	T46.6X3	T46.6X4	T46.6X5	T46.6X6
Binitrobenzol	T65.3X1	T65.3X2	T65.3X3	T65.3X4	—	—
Bioflavonoid(s)	T46.991	T46.992	T46.993	T46.994	T46.995	T46.996
Biological substance NEC	T50.901	T50.902	T50.903	T50.904	T50.905	T50.906
Biotin	T45.2X1	T45.2X2	T45.2X3	T45.2X4	T45.2X5	T45.2X6
Biperiden	T44.3X1	T44.3X2	T44.3X3	T44.3X4	T44.3X5	T44.3X6
Bisacodyl	T47.2X1	T47.2X2	T47.2X3	T47.2X4	T47.2X5	T47.2X6
Bisbentiamine	T45.2X1	T45.2X2	T45.2X3	T45.2X4	T45.2X5	T45.2X6
Bisbutiamine	T45.2X1	T45.2X2	T45.2X3	T45.2X4	T45.2X5	T45.2X6
Bisdequalinium (salts) (diacetate)	T49.6X1	T49.6X2	T49.6X3	T49.6X4	T49.6X5	T49.6X6
Bishydroxycoumarin	T45.511	T45.512	T45.513	T45.514	T45.515	T45.516
Bismarsen	T37.8X1	T37.8X2	T37.8X3	T37.8X4	T37.8X5	T37.8X6
Bismuth salts	T47.6X1	T47.6X2	T47.6X3	T47.6X4	T47.6X5	T47.6X6
aluminate	T47.1X1	T47.1X2	T47.1X3	T47.1X4	T47.1X5	T47.1X6
anti-infectives	T37.8X1	T37.8X2	T37.8X3	T37.8X4	T37.8X5	T37.8X6
formic iodide	T49.0X1	T49.0X2	T49.0X3	T49.0X4	T49.0X5	T49.0X6
glycolylarsenate	T49.0X1	T49.0X2	T49.0X3	T49.0X4	T49.0X5	T49.0X6
nonmedicinal (compounds) NEC	T65.91	T65.92	T65.93	T65.94	—	—
subcarbonate	T47.6X1	T47.6X2	T47.6X3	T47.6X4	T47.6X5	T47.6X6
subsalicylate	T37.8X1	T37.8X2	T37.8X3	T37.8X4	T37.8X5	T37.8X6
sulfarsphenamine	T37.8X1	T37.8X2	T37.8X3	T37.8X4	T37.8X5	T37.8X6
Bisoprolol	T44.7X1	T44.7X2	T44.7X3	T44.7X4	T44.7X5	T44.7X6
Bisoxatin	T47.2X1	T47.2X2	T47.2X3	T47.2X4	T47.2X5	T47.2X6
Bisulepin (hydrochloride)	T45.0X1	T45.0X2	T45.0X3	T45.0X4	T45.0X5	T45.0X6
Bithionol	T37.8X1	T37.8X2	T37.8X3	T37.8X4	T37.8X5	T37.8X6
anthelminthic	T37.4X1	T37.4X2	T37.4X3	T37.4X4	T37.4X5	T37.4X6
Bitolterol	T48.6X1	T48.6X2	T48.6X3	T48.6X4	T48.6X5	T48.6X6
Bitoscanate	T37.4X1	T37.4X2	T37.4X3	T37.4X4	T37.4X5	T37.4X6
Bitter almond oil	T62.8X1	T62.8X2	T62.8X3	T62.8X4	—	—
Bittersweet	T62.2X1	T62.2X2	T62.2X3	T62.2X4	—	—
Black						
flag	T60.91	T60.92	T60.93	T60.94	—	—
henbane	T62.2X1	T62.2X2	T62.2X3	T62.2X4	—	—
leaf (40)	T60.91	T60.92	T60.93	T60.94	—	—
widow spider (bite)	T63.311	T63.312	T63.313	T63.314	—	—
antivenin	T50.Z11	T50.Z12	T50.Z13	T50.Z14	T50.Z15	T50.Z16
Blast furnace gas (carbon monoxide from)	T58.8X1	T58.8X2	T58.8X3	T58.8X4	—	—
Bleach	T54.91	T54.92	T54.93	T54.94	—	—

◀ New ◀ Revised ~~deleted~~ Deleted

Substance	External Cause (T-Code) Poisoning, Accidental (Unintentional)	Poisoning, Intentional Self-Harm	Poisoning, Assault	Poisoning, Undetermined	Adverse Effect	Underdosing
Bleaching agent (medicinal)	T49.4X1	T49.4X2	T49.4X3	T49.4X4	T49.4X5	T49.4X6
Bleomycin	T45.1X1	T45.1X2	T45.1X3	T45.1X4	T45.1X5	T45.1X6
Blockain	T41.3X1	T41.3X2	T41.3X3	T41.3X4	T41.3X5	T41.3X6
infiltration (subcutaneous)	T41.3X1	T41.3X2	T41.3X3	T41.3X4	T41.3X5	T41.3X6
nerve block (peripheral) (plexus)	T41.3X1	T41.3X2	T41.3X3	T41.3X4	T41.3X5	T41.3X6
topical (surface)	T41.3X1	T41.3X2	T41.3X3	T41.3X4	T41.3X5	T41.3X6
Blockers, calcium channel	T46.1X1	T46.1X2	T46.1X3	T46.1X4	T46.1X5	T46.1X6
Blood (derivatives) (natural) (plasma) (whole)	T45.8X1	T45.8X2	T45.8X3	T45.8X4	T45.8X5	T45.8X6
dried	T45.8X1	T45.8X2	T45.8X3	T45.8X4	T45.8X5	T45.8X6
drug affecting NEC	T45.91	T45.92	T45.93	T45.94	T45.95	T45.96
expander NEC	T45.8X1	T45.8X2	T45.8X3	T45.8X4	T45.8X5	T45.8X6
fraction NEC	T45.8X1	T45.8X2	T45.8X3	T45.8X4	T45.8X5	T45.8X6
substitute (macromolecular)	T45.8X1	T45.8X2	T45.8X3	T45.8X4	T45.8X5	T45.8X6
Blue velvet	T40.2X1	T40.2X2	T40.2X3	T40.2X4	—	—
Bone meal	T62.8X1	T62.8X2	T62.8X3	T62.8X4	—	—
Bonine	T45.0X1	T45.0X2	T45.0X3	T45.0X4	T45.0X5	T45.0X6
Bopindolol	T44.7X1	T44.7X2	T44.7X3	T44.7X4	T44.7X5	T44.7X6
Boracic acid	T49.0X1	T49.0X2	T49.0X3	T49.0X4	T49.0X5	T49.0X6
ENT agent	T49.6X1	T49.6X2	T49.6X3	T49.6X4	T49.6X5	T49.6X6
ophthalmic preparation	T49.5X1	T49.5X2	T49.5X3	T49.5X4	T49.5X5	T49.5X6
Borane complex	T57.8X1	T57.8X2	T57.8X3	T57.8X4	—	—
Borate(s)	T57.8X1	T57.8X2	T57.8X3	T57.8X4	—	—
buffer	T50.991	T50.992	T50.993	T50.994	T50.995	T50.996
cleanser	T54.91	T54.92	T54.93	T54.94		
sodium	T57.8X1	T57.8X2	T57.8X3	T57.8X4	—	—
Borax (cleanser)	T54.91	T54.92	T54.93	T54.94	—	—
Bordeaux mixture	T60.3X1	T60.3X2	T60.3X3	T60.3X4	—	—
Boric acid	T49.0X1	T49.0X2	T49.0X3	T49.0X4	T49.0X5	T49.0X6
ENT agent	T49.6X1	T49.6X2	T49.6X3	T49.6X4	T49.6X5	T49.6X6
ophthalmic preparation	T49.5X1	T49.5X2	T49.5X3	T49.5X4	T49.5X5	T49.5X6
Bornaprine	T44.3X1	T44.3X2	T44.3X3	T44.3X4	T44.3X5	T44.3X6
Boron	T57.8X1	T57.8X2	T57.8X3	T57.8X4	—	—
hydride NEC	T57.8X1	T57.8X2	T57.8X3	T57.8X4	—	—
fumes or gas	T57.8X1	T57.8X2	T57.8X3	T57.8X4	—	—
trifluoride	T59.891	T59.892	T59.893	T59.894	—	—
Botox	T48.291	T48.292	T48.293	T48.294	T48.295	T48.296
Botulinus anti-toxin (type A, B)	T50.Z11	T50.Z12	T50.Z13	T50.Z14	T50.Z15	T50.Z16
Brake fluid vapor	T59.891	T59.892	T59.893	T59.894	—	—
Brallobarbital	T42.3X1	T42.3X2	T42.3X3	T42.3X4	T42.3X5	T42.3X6
Bran (wheat)	T47.4X1	T47.4X2	T47.4X3	T47.4X4	T47.4X5	T47.4X6
Brass (fumes)	T56.891	T56.892	T56.893	T56.894	—	—

Substance	External Cause (T-Code) Poisoning, Accidental (Unintentional)	Poisoning, Intentional Self-Harm	Poisoning, Assault	Poisoning, Undetermined	Adverse Effect	Underdosing
Brasso	T52.0X1	T52.0X2	T52.0X3	T52.0X4	—	—
Bretylium tosilate	T46.2X1	T46.2X2	T46.2X3	T46.2X4	T46.2X5	T46.2X6
Brevital (sodium)	T41.1X1	T41.1X2	T41.1X3	T41.1X4	T41.1X5	T41.1X6
Brinase	T45.3X1	T45.3X2	T45.3X3	T45.3X4	T45.3X5	T45.3X6
British antilewisite	T45.8X1	T45.8X2	T45.8X3	T45.8X4	T45.8X5	T45.8X6
Brodifacoum	T60.4X1	T60.4X2	T60.4X3	T60.4X4	—	—
Bromal (hydrate)	T42.6X1	T42.6X2	T42.6X3	T42.6X4	T42.6X5	T42.6X6
Bromazepam	T42.4X1	T42.4X2	T42.4X3	T42.4X4	T42.4X5	T42.4X6
Bromazine	T45.0X1	T45.0X2	T45.0X3	T45.0X4	T45.0X5	T45.0X6
Brombenzylcyanide	T59.3X1	T59.3X2	T59.3X3	T59.3X4	—	—
Bromelains	T45.3X1	T45.3X2	T45.3X3	T45.3X4	T45.3X5	T45.3X6
Bromethalin	T60.4X1	T60.4X2	T60.4X3	T60.4X4	—	—
Bromhexine	T48.4X1	T48.4X2	T48.4X3	T48.4X4	T48.4X5	T48.4X6
Bromide salts	T42.6X1	T42.6X2	T42.6X3	T42.6X4	T42.6X5	T42.6X6
Bromindione	T45.511	T45.512	T45.513	T45.514	T45.515	T45.516
Bromine						
compounds (medicinal)	T42.6X1	T42.6X2	T42.6X3	T42.6X4	T42.6X5	T42.6X6
sedative	T42.6X1	T42.6X2	T42.6X3	T42.6X4	T42.6X5	T42.6X6
vapor	T59.891	T59.892	T59.893	T59.894	—	—
Bromisovalum	T42.6X1	T42.6X2	T42.6X3	T42.6X4	T42.6X5	T42.6X6
Bromisoval	T42.6X1	T42.6X2	T42.6X3	T42.6X4	T42.6X5	T42.6X6
Bromobenzylcyanide	T59.3X1	T59.3X2	T59.3X3	T59.3X4	—	—
Bromochlorosalicylani-lide	T49.0X1	T49.0X2	T49.0X3	T49.0X4	T49.0X5	T49.0X6
Bromocriptine	T42.8X1	T42.8X2	T42.8X3	T42.8X4	T42.8X5	T42.8X6
Bromodiphenhydramine	T45.0X1	T45.0X2	T45.0X3	T45.0X4	T45.0X5	T45.0X6
Bromoform	T42.6X1	T42.6X2	T42.6X3	T42.6X4	T42.6X5	T42.6X6
Bromophenol blue reagent	T50.991	T50.992	T50.993	T50.994	T50.995	T50.996
Bromopride	T47.8X1	T47.8X2	T47.8X3	T47.8X4	T47.8X5	T47.8X6
Bromosalicylchloranitide	T49.0X1	T49.0X2	T49.0X3	T49.0X4	T49.0X5	T49.0X6
Bromosalicylhydroxamic acid	T37.1X1	T37.1X2	T37.1X3	T37.1X4	T37.1X5	T37.1X6
Bromo-seltzer	T39.1X1	T39.1X2	T39.1X3	T39.1X4	T39.1X5	T39.1X6
Bromoxynil	T60.3X1	T60.3X2	T60.3X3	T60.3X4	—	—
Bromperidol	T43.4X1	T43.4X2	T43.4X3	T43.4X4	T43.4X5	T43.4X6
Brompheniramine	T45.0X1	T45.0X2	T45.0X3	T45.0X4	T45.0X5	T45.0X6
Bromsulfophthalein	T50.8X1	T50.8X2	T50.8X3	T50.8X4	T50.8X5	T50.8X6
Bromural	T42.6X1	T42.6X2	T42.6X3	T42.6X4	T42.6X5	T42.6X6
Bromvaletone	T42.6X1	T42.6X2	T42.6X3	T42.6X4	T42.6X5	T42.6X6
Bronchodilator NEC	T48.6X1	T48.6X2	T48.6X3	T48.6X4	T48.6X5	T48.6X6
Brotizolam	T42.4X1	T42.4X2	T42.4X3	T42.4X4	T42.4X5	T42.4X6
Brovincamine	T46.7X1	T46.7X2	T46.7X3	T46.7X4	T46.7X5	T46.7X6
Brown spider (bite) (venom)	T63.391	T63.392	T63.393	T63.394		

◄ New ◄ Revised ~~deleted~~ Deleted

Substance	Poisoning, Accidental (Unintentional)	Poisoning, Intentional Self-Harm	Poisoning, Assault	Poisoning, Undetermined	Adverse Effect	Underdosing
Brown recluse spider (bite) (venom)	T63.331	T63.332	T63.333	T63.334	—	—
Broxaterol	T48.6X1	T48.6X2	T48.6X3	T48.6X4	T48.6X5	T48.6X6
Broxuridine	T45.1X1	T45.1X2	T45.1X3	T45.1X4	T45.1X5	T45.1X6
Broxyquinoline	T37.8X1	T37.8X2	T37.8X3	T37.8X4	T37.8X5	T37.8X6
Bruceine	T48.291	T48.292	T48.293	T48.294	T48.295	T48.296
Brucia	T62.2X1	T62.2X2	T62.2X3	T62.2X4	—	—
Brucine	T65.1X1	T65.1X2	T65.1X3	T65.1X4	—	—
Brunswick green — see Copper						
Bruten — see Ibuprofen						
Bryonia	T47.2X1	T47.2X2	T47.2X3	T47.2X4	T47.2X5	T47.2X6
Buclizine	T45.0X1	T45.0X2	T45.0X3	T45.0X4	T45.0X5	T45.0X6
Buclosamide	T49.0X1	T49.0X2	T49.0X3	T49.0X4	T49.0X5	T49.0X6
Budesonide	T44.5X1	T44.5X2	T44.5X3	T44.5X4	T44.5X5	T44.5X6
Budralazine	T46.5X1	T46.5X2	T46.5X3	T46.5X4	T46.5X5	T46.5X6
Bufferin	T39.011	T39.012	T39.013	T39.014	T39.015	T39.016
Buflomedil	T46.7X1	T46.7X2	T46.7X3	T46.7X4	T46.7X5	T46.7X6
Buformin	T38.3X1	T38.3X2	T38.3X3	T38.3X4	T38.3X5	T38.3X6
Bufotenine	T40.991	T40.992	T40.993	T40.994	—	—
Bufrolin	T48.6X1	T48.6X2	T48.6X3	T48.6X4	T48.6X5	T48.6X6
Bufylline	T48.6X1	T48.6X2	T48.6X3	T48.6X4	T48.6X5	T48.6X6
Bulk filler	T50.5X1	T50.5X2	T50.5X3	T50.5X4	T50.5X5	T50.5X6
cathartic	T47.4X1	T47.4X2	T47.4X3	T47.4X4	T47.4X5	T47.4X6
Bumetanide	T50.1X1	T50.1X2	T50.1X3	T50.1X4	T50.1X5	T50.1X6
Bunaftine	T46.2X1	T46.2X2	T46.2X3	T46.2X4	T46.2X5	T46.2X6
Bunamiodyl	T50.8X1	T50.8X2	T50.8X3	T50.8X4	T50.8X5	T50.8X6
Bunazosin	T44.6X1	T44.6X2	T44.6X3	T44.6X4	T44.6X5	T44.6X6
Bunitrolol	T44.7X1	T44.7X2	T44.7X3	T44.7X4	T44.7X5	T44.7X6
Buphenine	T46.7X1	T46.7X2	T46.7X3	T46.7X4	T46.7X5	T46.7X6
Bupivacaine	T41.3X1	T41.3X2	T41.3X3	T41.3X4	T41.3X5	T41.3X6
infiltration (subcutaneous)	T41.3X1	T41.3X2	T41.3X3	T41.3X4	T41.3X5	T41.3X6
nerve block (peripheral) (plexus)	T41.3X1	T41.3X2	T41.3X3	T41.3X4	T41.3X5	T41.3X6
spinal	T41.3X1	T41.3X2	T41.3X3	T41.3X4	T41.3X5	T41.3X6
Bupranolol	T44.7X1	T44.7X2	T44.7X3	T44.7X4	T44.7X5	T44.7X6
Buprenorphine	T40.491	T40.492	T40.493	T40.494	T40.495	T40.496
Bupropion	T43.291	T43.292	T43.293	T43.294	T43.295	T43.296
Burimamide	T47.1X1	T47.1X2	T47.1X3	T47.1X4	T47.1X5	T47.1X6
Buserelin	T38.891	T38.892	T38.893	T38.894	T38.895	T38.896
Buspirone	T43.591	T43.592	T43.593	T43.594	T43.595	T43.596
Busulfan, busulphan	T45.1X1	T45.1X2	T45.1X3	T45.1X4	T45.1X5	T45.1X6
Butabarbital (sodium)	T42.3X1	T42.3X2	T42.3X3	T42.3X4	T42.3X5	T42.3X6
Butabarbitone	T42.3X1	T42.3X2	T42.3X3	T42.3X4	T42.3X5	T42.3X6
Butabarpal	T42.3X1	T42.3X2	T42.3X3	T42.3X4	T42.3X5	T42.3X6
Butacaine	T41.3X1	T41.3X2	T41.3X3	T41.3X4	T41.3X5	T41.3X6
Butalamine	T46.7X1	T46.7X2	T46.7X3	T46.7X4	T46.7X5	T46.7X6
Butalbital	T42.3X1	T42.3X2	T42.3X3	T42.3X4	T42.3X5	T42.3X6
Butallylonal	T42.3X1	T42.3X2	T42.3X3	T42.3X4	T42.3X5	T42.3X6
Butamben	T41.3X1	T41.3X2	T41.3X3	T41.3X4	T41.3X5	T41.3X6
Butamirate	T48.3X1	T48.3X2	T48.3X3	T48.3X4	T48.3X5	T48.3X6
Butane (distributed in mobile container)	T59.891	T59.892	T59.893	T59.894	—	—
distributed through pipes	T59.891	T59.892	T59.893	T59.894	—	—
incomplete combustion	T58.11	T58.12	T58.13	T58.14	—	—
Butanilicaine	T41.3X1	T41.3X2	T41.3X3	T41.3X4	T41.3X5	T41.3X6
Butanol	T51.3X1	T51.3X2	T51.3X3	T51.3X4	—	—
Butanone, 2-butanone	T52.4X1	T52.4X2	T52.4X3	T52.4X4	—	—
Butantrone	T49.4X1	T49.4X2	T49.4X3	T49.4X4	T49.4X5	T49.4X6
Butaperazine	T43.3X1	T43.3X2	T43.3X3	T43.3X4	T43.3X5	T43.3X6
Butazolidin	T39.2X1	T39.2X2	T39.2X3	T39.2X4	T39.2X5	T39.2X6
Butetamate	T48.6X1	T48.6X2	T48.6X3	T48.6X4	T48.6X5	T48.6X6
Butethal	T42.3X1	T42.3X2	T42.3X3	T42.3X4	T42.3X5	T42.3X6
Butethamate	T44.3X1	T44.3X2	T44.3X3	T44.3X4	T44.3X5	T44.3X6
Buthalitone (sodium)	T41.1X1	T41.1X2	T41.1X3	T41.1X4	T41.1X5	T41.1X6
Butisol (sodium)	T42.3X1	T42.3X2	T42.3X3	T42.3X4	T42.3X5	T42.3X6
Butizide	T50.2X1	T50.2X2	T50.2X3	T50.2X4	T50.2X5	T50.2X6
Butobarbital	T42.3X1	T42.3X2	T42.3X3	T42.3X4	T42.3X5	T42.3X6
sodium	T42.3X1	T42.3X2	T42.3X3	T42.3X4	T42.3X5	T42.3X6
Butobarbitone	T42.3X1	T42.3X2	T42.3X3	T42.3X4	T42.3X5	T42.3X6
Butoconazole (nitrate)	T49.0X1	T49.0X2	T49.0X3	T49.0X4	T49.0X5	T49.0X6
Butorphanol	T40.491	T40.492	T40.493	T40.494	T40.495	T40.496
Butriptyline	T43.011	T43.012	T43.013	T43.014	T43.015	T43.016
Butropium bromide	T44.3X1	T44.3X2	T44.3X3	T44.3X4	T44.3X5	T44.3X6
Buttercups	T62.2X1	T62.2X2	T62.2X3	T62.2X4	—	—
Butter of antimony — see Antimony						
Butyl						
acetate (secondary)	T52.8X1	T52.8X2	T52.8X3	T52.8X4	—	—
alcohol	T51.3X1	T51.3X2	T51.3X3	T51.3X4	—	—
aminobenzoate	T41.3X1	T41.3X2	T41.3X3	T41.3X4	T41.3X5	T41.3X6
butyrate	T52.8X1	T52.8X2	T52.8X3	T52.8X4	—	—
carbinol	T51.3X1	T51.3X2	T51.3X3	T51.3X4	—	—
carbitol	T52.3X1	T52.3X2	T52.3X3	T52.3X4	—	—
cellosolve	T52.3X1	T52.3X2	T52.3X3	T52.3X4	—	—
chloral (hydrate)	T42.6X1	T42.6X2	T42.6X3	T42.6X4	T42.6X5	T42.6X6
formate	T52.8X1	T52.8X2	T52.8X3	T52.8X4	—	—

TABLE OF DRUGS AND CHEMICALS

	External Cause (T-Code)					
Substance	Poisoning, Accidental (Unintentional)	Poisoning, Intentional Self-Harm	Poisoning, Assault	Poisoning, Undetermined	Adverse Effect	Underdosing
Butyl (Continued)						
lactate	T52.8X1	T52.8X2	T52.8X3	T52.8X4	—	—
propionate	T52.8X1	T52.8X2	T52.8X3	T52.8X4	—	—
scopolamine bromide	T44.3X1	T44.3X2	T44.3X3	T44.3X4	T44.3X5	T44.3X6
thiobarbital sodium	T41.1X1	T41.1X2	T41.1X3	T41.1X4	T41.1X5	T41.1X6
Butylated hydroxy-anisole	T50.991	T50.992	T50.993	T50.994	T50.995	T50.996
Butylchloral hydrate	T42.6X1	T42.6X2	T42.6X3	T42.6X4	T42.6X5	T42.6X6
Butyltoluene	T52.2X1	T52.2X2	T52.2X3	T52.2X4	—	—
Butyn	T41.3X1	T41.3X2	T41.3X3	T41.3X4	T41.3X5	T41.3X6
Butyrophenone (-based tranquilizers)	T43.4X1	T43.4X2	T43.4X3	T43.4X4	T43.4X5	T43.4X6

C

Substance	Poisoning, Accidental (Unintentional)	Poisoning, Intentional Self-Harm	Poisoning, Assault	Poisoning, Undetermined	Adverse Effect	Underdosing
Cabergoline	T42.8X1	T42.8X2	T42.8X3	T42.8X4	T42.8X5	T42.8X6
Cacodyl, cacodylic acid	T57.0X1	T57.0X2	T57.0X3	T57.0X4	—	—
Cactinomycin	T45.1X1	T45.1X2	T45.1X3	T45.1X4	T45.1X5	T45.1X6
Cade oil	T49.4X1	T49.4X2	T49.4X3	T49.4X4	T49.4X5	T49.4X6
Cadexomer iodine	T49.0X1	T49.0X2	T49.0X3	T49.0X4	T49.0X5	T49.0X6
Cadmium (chloride) (fumes) (oxide)	T56.3X1	T56.3X2	T56.3X3	T56.3X4	—	—
sulfide (medicinal) NEC	T49.4X1	T49.4X2	T49.4X3	T49.4X4	T49.4X5	T49.4X6
Cadralazine	T46.5X1	T46.5X2	T46.5X3	T46.5X4	T46.5X5	T46.5X6
Caffeine	T43.611	T43.612	T43.613	T43.614	T43.615	T43.616
Calabar bean	T62.2X1	T62.2X2	T62.2X3	T62.2X4	—	—
Caladium seguinum	T62.2X1	T62.2X2	T62.2X3	T62.2X4	—	—
Calamine (lotion)	T49.3X1	T49.3X2	T49.3X3	T49.3X4	T49.3X5	T49.3X6
Calcifediol	T45.2X1	T45.2X2	T45.2X3	T45.2X4	T45.2X5	T45.2X6
Calciferol	T45.2X1	T45.2X2	T45.2X3	T45.2X4	T45.2X5	T45.2X6
Calcitonin	T50.991	T50.992	T50.993	T50.994	T50.995	T50.996
Calcitriol	T45.2X1	T45.2X2	T45.2X3	T45.2X4	T45.2X5	T45.2X6
Calcium	T50.3X1	T50.3X2	T50.3X3	T50.3X4	T50.3X5	T50.3X6
actylsalicylate	T39.011	T39.012	T39.013	T39.014	T39.015	T39.016
benzamidosalicylate	T37.1X1	T37.1X2	T37.1X3	T37.1X4	T37.1X5	T37.1X6
bromide	T42.6X1	T42.6X2	T42.6X3	T42.6X4	T42.6X5	T42.6X6
bromolactobionate	T42.6X1	T42.6X2	T42.6X3	T42.6X4	T42.6X5	T42.6X6
carbaspirin	T39.011	T39.012	T39.013	T39.014	T39.015	T39.016
carbimide	T50.6X1	T50.6X2	T50.6X3	T50.6X4	T50.6X5	T50.6X6
carbonate	T47.1X1	T47.1X2	T47.1X3	T47.1X4	T47.1X5	T47.1X6
chloride	T50.991	T50.992	T50.993	T50.994	T50.995	T50.996
anhydrous	T50.991	T50.992	T50.993	T50.994	T50.995	T50.996
cyanide	T57.8X1	T57.8X2	T57.8X3	T57.8X4	—	—
dioctyl sulfosuccinate	T47.4X1	T47.4X2	T47.4X3	T47.4X4	T47.4X5	T47.4X6
disodium edathamil	T45.8X1	T45.8X2	T45.8X3	T45.8X4	T45.8X5	T45.8X6

Substance	Poisoning, Accidental (Unintentional)	Poisoning, Intentional Self-Harm	Poisoning, Assault	Poisoning, Undetermined	Adverse Effect	Underdosing
Calcium (Continued)						
disodium edetate	T45.8X1	T45.8X2	T45.8X3	T45.8X4	T45.8X5	T45.8X6
dobesilate	T46.991	T46.992	T46.993	T46.994	T46.995	T46.996
EDTA	T45.8X1	T45.8X2	T45.8X3	T45.8X4	T45.8X5	T45.8X6
ferrous citrate	T45.4X1	T45.4X2	T45.4X3	T45.4X4	T45.4X5	T45.4X6
folinate	T45.8X1	T45.8X2	T45.8X3	T45.8X4	T45.8X5	T45.8X6
glubionate	T50.3X1	T50.3X2	T50.3X3	T50.3X4	T50.3X5	T50.3X6
gluconate	T50.3X1	T50.3X2	T50.3X3	T50.3X4	T50.3X5	T50.3X6
gluconogalactogluconate	T50.3X1	T50.3X2	T50.3X3	T50.3X4	T50.3X5	T50.3X6
hydrate, hydroxide	T54.3X1	T54.3X2	T54.3X3	T54.3X4	—	—
hypochlorite	T54.3X1	T54.3X2	T54.3X3	T54.3X4	—	—
iodide	T48.4X1	T48.4X2	T48.4X3	T48.4X4	T48.4X5	T48.4X6
ipodate	T50.8X1	T50.8X2	T50.8X3	T50.8X4	T50.8X5	T50.8X6
lactate	T50.3X1	T50.3X2	T50.3X3	T50.3X4	T50.3X5	T50.3X6
leucovorin	T45.8X1	T45.8X2	T45.8X3	T45.8X4	T45.8X5	T45.8X6
mandelate	T37.91	T37.92	T37.93	T37.94	T37.95	T37.96
oxide	T54.3X1	T54.3X2	T54.3X3	T54.3X4	—	—
pantothenate	T45.2X1	T45.2X2	T45.2X3	T45.2X4	T45.2X5	T45.2X6
phosphate	T50.3X1	T50.3X2	T50.3X3	T50.3X4	T50.3X5	T50.3X6
salicylate	T39.091	T39.092	T39.093	T39.094	T39.095	T39.096
salts	T50.3X1	T50.3X2	T50.3X3	T50.3X4	T50.3X5	T50.3X6
Calculus-dissolving drug	T50.991	T50.992	T50.993	T50.994	T50.995	T50.996
Calomel	T49.0X1	T49.0X2	T49.0X3	T49.0X4	T49.0X5	T49.0X6
Caloric agent	T50.3X1	T50.3X2	T50.3X3	T50.3X4	T50.3X5	T50.3X6
Calusterone	T38.7X1	T38.7X2	T38.7X3	T38.7X4	T38.7X5	T38.7X6
Camazepam	T42.4X1	T42.4X2	T42.4X3	T42.4X4	T42.4X5	T42.4X6
Camomile	T49.0X1	T49.0X2	T49.0X3	T49.0X4	T49.0X5	T49.0X6
Camoquin	T37.2X1	T37.2X2	T37.2X3	T37.2X4	T37.2X5	T37.2X6
Camphor						
insecticide	T60.2X1	T60.2X2	T60.2X3	T60.2X4	—	—
medicinal	T49.8X1	T49.8X2	T49.8X3	T49.8X4	T49.8X5	T49.8X6
Camylofin	T44.3X1	T44.3X2	T44.3X3	T44.3X4	T44.3X5	T44.3X6
Cancer chemotherapy drug regimen	T45.1X1	T45.1X2	T45.1X3	T45.1X4	T45.1X5	T45.1X6
Candeptin	T49.0X1	T49.0X2	T49.0X3	T49.0X4	T49.0X5	T49.0X6
Candicidin	T49.0X1	T49.0X2	T49.0X3	T49.0X4	T49.0X5	T49.0X6
Cannabinoids, synthetic	T40.721	T40.722	T40.723	T40.724	T40.725	T40.726
Cannabinol	T40.711	T40.712	T40.713	T40.714	T40.715	T40.716
Cannabis (derivatives)	T40.711	T40.712	T40.713	T40.714	T40.715	T40.716
Canned heat	T51.1X1	T51.1X2	T51.1X3	T51.1X4	—	—
Canrenoic acid	T50.0X1	T50.0X2	T50.0X3	T50.0X4	T50.0X5	T50.0X6
Canrenone	T50.0X1	T50.0X2	T50.0X3	T50.0X4	T50.0X5	T50.0X6

◀ New ◀ Revised ~~deleted~~ Deleted

Substance	Poisoning, Accidental (Unintentional)	Poisoning, Intentional Self-Harm	Poisoning, Assault	Poisoning, Undetermined	Adverse Effect	Underdosing
Cantharides, cantharidin, cantharis	T49.8X1	T49.8X2	T49.8X3	T49.8X4	T49.8X5	T49.8X6
Canthaxanthin	T50.991	T50.992	T50.993	T50.994	T50.995	T50.996
Capillary-active drug NEC	T46.901	T46.902	T46.903	T46.904	T46.905	T46.906
Capreomycin	T36.8X1	T36.8X2	T36.8X3	T36.8X4	T36.8X5	T36.8X6
Capsicum	T49.4X1	T49.4X2	T49.4X3	T49.4X4	T49.4X5	T49.4X6
Captafol	T60.3X1	T60.3X2	T60.3X3	T60.3X4	—	—
Captan	T60.3X1	T60.3X2	T60.3X3	T60.3X4	—	—
Captodiame, captodiamine	T43.591	T43.592	T43.593	T43.594	T43.595	T43.596
Captopril	T46.4X1	T46.4X2	T46.4X3	T46.4X4	T46.4X5	T46.4X6
Caramiphen	T44.3X1	T44.3X2	T44.3X3	T44.3X4	T44.3X5	T44.3X6
Carazolol	T44.7X1	T44.7X2	T44.7X3	T44.7X4	T44.7X5	T44.7X6
Carbachol	T44.1X1	T44.1X2	T44.1X3	T44.1X4	T44.1X5	T44.1X6
Carbacrylamine (resin)	T50.3X1	T50.3X2	T50.3X3	T50.3X4	T50.3X5	T50.3X6
Carbamate (insecticide)	T60.0X1	T60.0X2	T60.0X3	T60.0X4	—	—
Carbamate (sedative)	T42.6X1	T42.6X2	T42.6X3	T42.6X4	T42.6X5	T42.6X6
herbicide	T60.0X1	T60.0X2	T60.0X3	T60.0X4	—	—
insecticide	T60.0X1	T60.0X2	T60.0X3	T60.0X4	—	—
Carbamazepine	T42.1X1	T42.1X2	T42.1X3	T42.1X4	T42.1X5	T42.1X6
Carbamide	T47.3X1	T47.3X2	T47.3X3	T47.3X4	T47.3X5	T47.3X6
peroxide	T49.0X1	T49.0X2	T49.0X3	T49.0X4	T49.0X5	T49.0X6
topical	T49.8X1	T49.8X2	T49.8X3	T49.8X4	T49.8X5	T49.8X6
Carbamylcholine chloride	T44.1X1	T44.1X2	T44.1X3	T44.1X4	T44.1X5	T44.1X6
Carbaril	T60.0X1	T60.0X2	T60.0X3	T60.0X4	—	—
Carbarsone	T37.3X1	T37.3X2	T37.3X3	T37.3X4	T37.3X5	T37.3X6
Carbaryl	T60.0X1	T60.0X2	T60.0X3	T60.0X4	—	—
Carbaspirin	T39.011	T39.012	T39.013	T39.014	T39.015	T39.016
Carbazochrome (salicylate) (sodium sulfonate)	T49.4X1	T49.4X2	T49.4X3	T49.4X4	T49.4X5	T49.4X6
Carbenicillin	T36.0X1	T36.0X2	T36.0X3	T36.0X4	T36.0X5	T36.0X6
Carbenoxolone	T47.1X1	T47.1X2	T47.1X3	T47.1X4	T47.1X5	T47.1X6
Carbetapentane	T48.3X1	T48.3X2	T48.3X3	T48.3X4	T48.3X5	T48.3X6
Carbethyl salicylate	T39.091	T39.092	T39.093	T39.094	T39.095	T39.096
Carbidopa (with levodopa)	T42.8X1	T42.8X2	T42.8X3	T42.8X4	T42.8X5	T42.8X6
Carbimazole	T38.2X1	T38.2X2	T38.2X3	T38.2X4	T38.2X5	T38.2X6
Carbinol	T51.1X1	T51.1X2	T51.1X3	T51.1X4	—	—
Carbinoxamine	T45.0X1	T45.0X2	T45.0X3	T45.0X4	T45.0X5	T45.0X6
Carbiphene	T39.8X1	T39.8X2	T39.8X3	T39.8X4	T39.8X5	T39.8X6
Carbitol	T52.3X1	T52.3X2	T52.3X3	T52.3X4	—	—
Carbocaine	T41.3X1	T41.3X2	T41.3X3	T41.3X4	T41.3X5	T41.3X6
infiltration (subcutaneous)	T41.3X1	T41.3X2	T41.3X3	T41.3X4	T41.3X5	T41.3X6
nerve block (peripheral) (plexus)	T41.3X1	T41.3X2	T41.3X3	T41.3X4	T41.3X5	T41.3X6
topical (surface)	T41.3X1	T41.3X2	T41.3X3	T41.3X4	T41.3X5	T41.3X6

Substance	Poisoning, Accidental (Unintentional)	Poisoning, Intentional Self-Harm	Poisoning, Assault	Poisoning, Undetermined	Adverse Effect	Underdosing
Carbo medicinalis	T47.6X1	T47.6X2	T47.6X3	T47.6X4	T47.6X5	T47.6X6
Carbomycin	T36.8X1	T36.8X2	T36.8X3	T36.8X4	T36.8X5	T36.8X6
Carbocisteine	T48.4X1	T48.4X2	T48.4X3	T48.4X4	T48.4X5	T48.4X6
Carbocromen	T46.3X1	T46.3X2	T46.3X3	T46.3X4	T46.3X5	T46.3X6
Carbol fuchsin	T49.0X1	T49.0X2	T49.0X3	T49.0X4	T49.0X5	T49.0X6
Carbolic acid — see also Phenol	T54.0X1	T54.0X2	T54.0X3	T54.0X4	—	—
Carbolonium (bromide)	T48.1X1	T48.1X2	T48.1X3	T48.1X4	T48.1X5	T48.1X6
Carbon						
bisulfide (liquid)	T65.4X1	T65.4X2	T65.4X3	T65.4X4	—	—
vapor	T65.4X1	T65.4X2	T65.4X3	T65.4X4	—	—
dioxide (gas)	T59.7X1	T59.7X2	T59.7X3	T59.7X4	—	—
medicinal	T41.5X1	T41.5X2	T41.5X3	T41.5X4	T41.5X5	T41.5X6
nonmedicinal	T59.7X1	T59.7X2	T59.7X3	T59.7X4	—	—
snow	T49.4X1	T49.4X2	T49.4X3	T49.4X4	T49.4X5	T49.4X6
disulfide (liquid)	T65.4X1	T65.4X2	T65.4X3	T65.4X4	—	—
vapor	T65.4X1	T65.4X2	T65.4X3	T65.4X4	—	—
monoxide (from incomplete combustion)	T58.91	T58.92	T58.93	T58.94	—	—
blast furnace gas	T58.8X1	T58.8X2	T58.8X3	T58.8X4	—	—
butane (distributed in mobile container)	T58.11	T58.12	T58.13	T58.14	—	—
distributed through pipes	T58.11	T58.12	T58.13	T58.14	—	—
charcoal fumes	T58.2X1	T58.2X2	T58.2X3	T58.2X4	—	—
coal	T58.2X1	T58.2X2	T58.2X3	T58.2X4	—	—
coke (in domestic stoves, fireplaces)	T58.2X1	T58.2X2	T58.2X3	T58.2X4	—	—
gas (piped)	T58.11	T58.12	T58.13	T58.14	—	—
solid (in domestic stoves, fireplaces)	T58.2X1	T58.2X2	T58.2X3	T58.2X4	—	—
exhaust gas (motor) not in transit	T58.01	T58.02	T58.03	T58.04	—	—
combustion engine, any not in watercraft	T58.01	T58.02	T58.03	T58.04	—	—
farm tractor, not in transit	T58.01	T58.02	T58.03	T58.04	—	—
gas engine	T58.01	T58.02	T58.03	T58.04	—	—
motor pump	T58.01	T58.02	T58.03	T58.04	—	—
motor vehicle, not in transit	T58.01	T58.02	T58.03	T58.04	—	—
fuel (in domestic use)	T58.2X1	T58.2X2	T58.2X3	T58.2X4	—	—
gas (piped)	T58.11	T58.12	T58.13	T58.14	—	—
in mobile container	T58.11	T58.12	T58.13	T58.14	—	—
utility	T58.11	T58.12	T58.13	T58.14	—	—
in mobile container	T58.11	T58.12	T58.13	T58.14	—	—
piped (natural)	T58.11	T58.12	T58.13	T58.14	—	—

◀ New ◀ Revised ~~deleted~~ Deleted

	External Cause (T-Code)					
Substance	Poisoning, Accidental (Unintentional)	Poisoning, Intentional Self-Harm	Poisoning, Assault	Poisoning, Undetermined	Adverse Effect	Underdosing
Carbon *(Continued)*						
monoxide *(Continued)*						
illuminating gas	T58.11	T58.12	T58.13	T58.14	—	—
industrial fuels or gases, any	T58.8X1	T58.8X2	T58.8X3	T58.8X4	—	—
kerosene (in domestic stoves, fireplaces)	T58.2X1	T58.2X2	T58.2X3	T58.2X4	—	—
kiln gas or vapor	T58.8X1	T58.8X2	T58.8X3	T58.8X4	—	—
motor exhaust gas, not in transit	T58.01	T58.02	T58.03	T58.04	—	—
piped gas (manufactured) (natural)	T58.11	T58.12	T58.13	T58.14	—	—
producer gas	T58.8X1	T58.8X2	T58.8X3	T58.8X4	—	—
propane (distributed in mobile container)	T58.11	T58.12	T58.13	T58.14	—	—
distributed through pipes	T58.11	T58.12	T58.13	T58.14	—	—
specified source NEC	T58.8X1	T58.8X2	T58.8X3	T58.8X4	—	—
stove gas	T58.11	T58.12	T58.13	T58.14	—	—
piped	T58.11	T58.12	T58.13	T58.14	—	—
utility gas	T58.11	T58.12	T58.13	T58.14	—	—
piped	T58.11	T58.12	T58.13	T58.14	—	—
water gas	T58.11	T58.12	T58.13	T58.14	—	—
wood (in domestic stoves, fireplaces)	T58.2X1	T58.2X2	T58.2X3	T58.2X4	—	—
tetrachloride (vapor) NEC	T53.0X1	T53.0X2	T53.0X3	T53.0X4	—	—
liquid (cleansing agent) NEC	T53.0X1	T53.0X2	T53.0X3	T53.0X4	—	—
solvent	T53.0X1	T53.0X2	T53.0X3	T53.0X4	—	—
Carbonic acid gas	T59.7X1	T59.7X2	T59.7X3	T59.7X4	—	—
anhydrase inhibitor NEC	T50.2X1	T50.2X2	T50.2X3	T50.2X4	T50.2X5	T50.2X6
Carbophenothion	T60.0X1	T60.0X2	T60.0X3	T60.0X4	—	—
Carboplatin	T45.1X1	T45.1X2	T45.1X3	T45.1X4	T45.1X5	T45.1X6
Carboprost	T48.0X1	T48.0X2	T48.0X3	T48.0X4	T48.0X5	T48.0X6
Carboquone	T45.1X1	T45.1X2	T45.1X3	T45.1X4	T45.1X5	T45.1X6
Carbowax	T49.3X1	T49.3X2	T49.3X3	T49.3X4	T49.3X5	T49.3X6
Carboxymethyl-cellulose	T47.4X1	T47.4X2	T47.4X3	T47.4X4	T47.4X5	T47.4X6
S-Carboxymethyl-cysteine	T48.4X1	T48.4X2	T48.4X3	T48.4X4	T48.4X5	T48.4X6
Carbrital	T42.3X1	T42.3X2	T42.3X3	T42.3X4	T42.3X5	T42.3X6
Carbromal	T42.6X1	T42.6X2	T42.6X3	T42.6X4	T42.6X5	T42.6X6
Carbutamide	T38.3X1	T38.3X2	T38.3X3	T38.3X4	T38.3X5	T38.3X6
Carbuterol	T48.6X1	T48.6X2	T48.6X3	T48.6X4	T48.6X5	T48.6X6
Cardiac						
depressants	T46.2X1	T46.2X2	T46.2X3	T46.2X4	T46.2X5	T46.2X6
rhythm regulator	T46.2X1	T46.2X2	T46.2X3	T46.2X4	T46.2X5	T46.2X6
specified NEC	T46.2X1	T46.2X2	T46.2X3	T46.2X4	T46.2X5	T46.2X6

	External Cause (T-Code)					
Substance	Poisoning, Accidental (Unintentional)	Poisoning, Intentional Self-Harm	Poisoning, Assault	Poisoning, Undetermined	Adverse Effect	Underdosing
Cardiografin	T50.8X1	T50.8X2	T50.8X3	T50.8X4	T50.8X5	T50.8X6
Cardio-green	T50.8X1	T50.8X2	T50.8X3	T50.8X4	T50.8X5	T50.8X6
Cardiotonic (glycoside) NEC	T46.0X1	T46.0X2	T46.0X3	T46.0X4	T46.0X5	T46.0X6
Cardiovascular drug NEC	T46.901	T46.902	T46.903	T46.904	T46.905	T46.906
Cardrase	T50.2X1	T50.2X2	T50.2X3	T50.2X4	T50.2X5	T50.2X6
Carfusin	T49.0X1	T49.0X2	T49.0X3	T49.0X4	T49.0X5	T49.0X6
Carfecillin	T36.0X1	T36.0X2	T36.0X3	T36.0X4	T36.0X5	T36.0X6
Carfenazine	T43.3X1	T43.3X2	T43.3X3	T43.3X4	T43.3X5	T43.3X6
Carindacillin	T36.0X1	T36.0X2	T36.0X3	T36.0X4	T36.0X5	T36.0X6
Carisoprodol	T42.8X1	T42.8X2	T42.8X3	T42.8X4	T42.8X5	T42.8X6
Carmellose	T47.4X1	T47.4X2	T47.4X3	T47.4X4	T47.4X5	T47.4X6
Carminative	T47.5X1	T47.5X2	T47.5X3	T47.5X4	T47.5X5	T47.5X6
Carmofur	T45.1X1	T45.1X2	T45.1X3	T45.1X4	T45.1X5	T45.1X6
Carmustine	T45.1X1	T45.1X2	T45.1X3	T45.1X4	T45.1X5	T45.1X6
Carotene	T45.2X1	T45.2X2	T45.2X3	T45.2X4	T45.2X5	T45.2X6
Carphenazine	T43.3X1	T43.3X2	T43.3X3	T43.3X4	T43.3X5	T43.3X6
Carpipramine	T42.4X1	T42.4X2	T42.4X3	T42.4X4	T42.4X5	T42.4X6
Carprofen	T39.311	T39.312	T39.313	T39.314	T39.315	T39.316
Carpronium chloride	T44.3X1	T44.3X2	T44.3X3	T44.3X4	T44.3X5	T44.3X6
Carrageenan	T47.8X1	T47.8X2	T47.8X3	T47.8X4	T47.8X5	T47.8X6
Carteolol	T44.7X1	T44.7X2	T44.7X3	T44.7X4	T44.7X5	T44.7X6
Carter's Little Pills	T47.2X1	T47.2X2	T47.2X3	T47.2X4	T47.2X5	T47.2X6
Cascara (sagrada)	T47.2X1	T47.2X2	T47.2X3	T47.2X4	T47.2X5	T47.2X6
Cassava	T62.2X1	T62.2X2	T62.2X3	T62.2X4	—	—
Castellani's paint	T49.0X1	T49.0X2	T49.0X3	T49.0X4	T49.0X5	T49.0X6
Castor						
bean	T62.2X1	T62.2X2	T62.2X3	T62.2X4	—	—
oil	T47.2X1	T47.2X2	T47.2X3	T47.2X4	T47.2X5	T47.2X6
Catalase	T45.3X1	T45.3X2	T45.3X3	T45.3X4	T45.3X5	T45.3X6
Caterpillar (sting)	T63.431	T63.432	T63.433	T63.434	—	—
Catha (edulis) (tea)	T43.691	T43.692	T43.693	T43.694	—	—
Cathartic NEC	T47.4X1	T47.4X2	T47.4X3	T47.4X4	T47.4X5	T47.4X6
anthacene derivative	T47.2X1	T47.2X2	T47.2X3	T47.2X4	T47.2X5	T47.2X6
bulk	T47.4X1	T47.4X2	T47.4X3	T47.4X4	T47.4X5	T47.4X6
contact	T47.2X1	T47.2X2	T47.2X3	T47.2X4	T47.2X5	T47.2X6
emollient NEC	T47.4X1	T47.4X2	T47.4X3	T47.4X4	T47.4X5	T47.4X6
irritant NEC	T47.2X1	T47.2X2	T47.2X3	T47.2X4	T47.2X5	T47.2X6
mucilage	T47.4X1	T47.4X2	T47.4X3	T47.4X4	T47.4X5	T47.4X6
saline	T47.3X1	T47.3X2	T47.3X3	T47.3X4	T47.3X5	T47.3X6
vegetable	T47.2X1	T47.2X2	T47.2X3	T47.2X4	T47.2X5	T47.2X6
Cathine	T50.5X1	T50.5X2	T50.5X3	T50.5X4	T50.5X5	T50.5X6
Cathomycin	T36.8X1	T36.8X2	T36.8X3	T36.8X4	T36.8X5	T36.8X6

◀ New ◀ Revised ~~deleted~~ Deleted

Substance	External Cause (T-Code)					
	Poisoning, Accidental (Unintentional)	Poisoning, Intentional Self-Harm	Poisoning, Assault	Poisoning, Undetermined	Adverse Effect	Underdosing
Cation exchange resin	T50.3X1	T50.3X2	T50.3X3	T50.3X4	T50.3X5	T50.3X6
Caustic(s) NEC	T54.91	T54.92	T54.93	T54.94	—	—
alkali	T54.3X1	T54.3X2	T54.3X3	T54.3X4	—	—
hydroxide	T54.3X1	T54.3X2	T54.3X3	T54.3X4	—	—
potash	T54.3X1	T54.3X2	T54.3X3	T54.3X4	—	—
soda	T54.3X1	T54.3X2	T54.3X3	T54.3X4	—	—
specified NEC	T54.91	T54.92	T54.93	T54.94	—	—
Ceepryn	T49.0X1	T49.0X2	T49.0X3	T49.0X4	T49.0X5	T49.0X6
ENT agent	T49.6X1	T49.6X2	T49.6X3	T49.6X4	T49.6X5	T49.6X6
lozenges	T49.6X1	T49.6X2	T49.6X3	T49.6X4	T49.6X5	T49.6X6
Cefacetrile	T36.1X1	T36.1X2	T36.1X3	T36.1X4	T36.1X5	T36.1X6
Cefaclor	T36.1X1	T36.1X2	T36.1X3	T36.1X4	T36.1X5	T36.1X6
Cefadroxil	T36.1X1	T36.1X2	T36.1X3	T36.1X4	T36.1X5	T36.1X6
Cefalexin	T36.1X1	T36.1X2	T36.1X3	T36.1X4	T36.1X5	T36.1X6
Cefaloglycin	T36.1X1	T36.1X2	T36.1X3	T36.1X4	T36.1X5	T36.1X6
Cefaloridine	T36.1X1	T36.1X2	T36.1X3	T36.1X4	T36.1X5	T36.1X6
Cefalosporins	T36.1X1	T36.1X2	T36.1X3	T36.1X4	T36.1X5	T36.1X6
Cefalotin	T36.1X1	T36.1X2	T36.1X3	T36.1X4	T36.1X5	T36.1X6
Cefamandole	T36.1X1	T36.1X2	T36.1X3	T36.1X4	T36.1X5	T36.1X6
Cefamycin antibiotic	T36.1X1	T36.1X2	T36.1X3	T36.1X4	T36.1X5	T36.1X6
Cefapirin	T36.1X1	T36.1X2	T36.1X3	T36.1X4	T36.1X5	T36.1X6
Cefatrizine	T36.1X1	T36.1X2	T36.1X3	T36.1X4	T36.1X5	T36.1X6
Cefazedone	T36.1X1	T36.1X2	T36.1X3	T36.1X4	T36.1X5	T36.1X6
Cefazolin	T36.1X1	T36.1X2	T36.1X3	T36.1X4	T36.1X5	T36.1X6
Cefbuperazone	T36.1X1	T36.1X2	T36.1X3	T36.1X4	T36.1X5	T36.1X6
Cefetamet	T36.1X1	T36.1X2	T36.1X3	T36.1X4	T36.1X5	T36.1X6
Cefixime	T36.1X1	T36.1X2	T36.1X3	T36.1X4	T36.1X5	T36.1X6
Cefmenoxime	T36.1X1	T36.1X2	T36.1X3	T36.1X4	T36.1X5	T36.1X6
Cefmetazole	T36.1X1	T36.1X2	T36.1X3	T36.1X4	T36.1X5	T36.1X6
Cefminox	T36.1X1	T36.1X2	T36.1X3	T36.1X4	T36.1X5	T36.1X6
Cefonicid	T36.1X1	T36.1X2	T36.1X3	T36.1X4	T36.1X5	T36.1X6
Cefoperazone	T36.1X1	T36.1X2	T36.1X3	T36.1X4	T36.1X5	T36.1X6
Ceforanide	T36.1X1	T36.1X2	T36.1X3	T36.1X4	T36.1X5	T36.1X6
Cefotaxime	T36.1X1	T36.1X2	T36.1X3	T36.1X4	T36.1X5	T36.1X6
Cefotetan	T36.1X1	T36.1X2	T36.1X3	T36.1X4	T36.1X5	T36.1X6
Cefotiam	T36.1X1	T36.1X2	T36.1X3	T36.1X4	T36.1X5	T36.1X6
Cefoxitin	T36.1X1	T36.1X2	T36.1X3	T36.1X4	T36.1X5	T36.1X6
Cefpimizole	T36.1X1	T36.1X2	T36.1X3	T36.1X4	T36.1X5	T36.1X6
Cefpiramide	T36.1X1	T36.1X2	T36.1X3	T36.1X4	T36.1X5	T36.1X6
Cefradine	T36.1X1	T36.1X2	T36.1X3	T36.1X4	T36.1X5	T36.1X6
Cefroxadine	T36.1X1	T36.1X2	T36.1X3	T36.1X4	T36.1X5	T36.1X6
Cefsulodin	T36.1X1	T36.1X2	T36.1X3	T36.1X4	T36.1X5	T36.1X6

Substance	External Cause (T-Code)					
	Poisoning, Accidental (Unintentional)	Poisoning, Intentional Self-Harm	Poisoning, Assault	Poisoning, Undetermined	Adverse Effect	Underdosing
Ceftazidime	T36.1X1	T36.1X2	T36.1X3	T36.1X4	T36.1X5	T36.1X6
Cefteram	T36.1X1	T36.1X2	T36.1X3	T36.1X4	T36.1X5	T36.1X6
Ceftezole	T36.1X1	T36.1X2	T36.1X3	T36.1X4	T36.1X5	T36.1X6
Ceftizoxime	T36.1X1	T36.1X2	T36.1X3	T36.1X4	T36.1X5	T36.1X6
Ceftriaxone	T36.1X1	T36.1X2	T36.1X3	T36.1X4	T36.1X5	T36.1X6
Cefuroxime	T36.1X1	T36.1X2	T36.1X3	T36.1X4	T36.1X5	T36.1X6
Cefuzonam	T36.1X1	T36.1X2	T36.1X3	T36.1X4	T36.1X5	T36.1X6
Celestone	T38.0X1	T38.0X2	T38.0X3	T38.0X4	T38.0X5	T38.0X6
topical	T49.0X1	T49.0X2	T49.0X3	T49.0X4	T49.0X5	T49.0X6
Celiprolol	T44.7X1	T44.7X2	T44.7X3	T44.7X4	T44.7X5	T44.7X6
Cellosolve	T52.91	T52.92	T52.93	T52.94	—	—
Cell stimulants and proliferants	T49.8X1	T49.8X2	T49.8X3	T49.8X4	T49.8X5	T49.8X6
Cellulose						
cathartic	T47.4X1	T47.4X2	T47.4X3	T47.4X4	T47.4X5	T47.4X6
hydroxyethyl	T47.4X1	T47.4X2	T47.4X3	T47.4X4	T47.4X5	T47.4X6
nitrates (topical)	T49.3X1	T49.3X2	T49.3X3	T49.3X4	T49.3X5	T49.3X6
oxidized	T49.4X1	T49.4X2	T49.4X3	T49.4X4	T49.4X5	T49.4X6
Centipede (bite)	T63.411	T63.412	T63.413	T63.414	—	—
Central nervous system						
depressants	T42.71	T42.72	T42.73	T42.74	T42.75	T42.76
anesthetic (general) NEC	T41.201	T41.202	T41.203	T41.204	T41.205	T41.206
gases NEC	T41.0X1	T41.0X2	T41.0X3	T41.0X4	T41.0X5	T41.0X6
intravenous	T41.1X1	T41.1X2	T41.1X3	T41.1X4	T41.1X5	T41.1X6
barbiturates	T42.3X1	T42.3X2	T42.3X3	T42.3X4	T42.3X5	T42.3X6
benzodiazepines	T42.4X1	T42.4X2	T42.4X3	T42.4X4	T42.4X5	T42.4X6
bromides	T42.6X1	T42.6X2	T42.6X3	T42.6X4	T42.6X5	T42.6X6
cannabis sativa	T40.711	T40.712	T40.713	T40.714	T40.715	T40.716
chloral hydrate	T42.6X1	T42.6X2	T42.6X3	T42.6X4	T42.6X5	T42.6X6
ethanol	T51.0X1	T51.0X2	T51.0X3	T51.0X4	—	—
hallucinogenics	T40.901	T40.902	T40.903	T40.904	T40.905	T40.906
hypnotics	T42.71	T42.72	T42.73	T42.74	T42.75	T42.76
specified NEC	T42.6X1	T42.6X2	T42.6X3	T42.6X4	T42.6X5	T42.6X6
muscle relaxants	T42.8X1	T42.8X2	T42.8X3	T42.8X4	T42.8X5	T42.8X6
paraldehyde	T42.6X1	T42.6X2	T42.6X3	T42.6X4	T42.6X5	T42.6X6
sedatives; sedative-hypnotics	T42.71	T42.72	T42.73	T42.74	T42.75	T42.76
mixed NEC	T42.6X1	T42.6X2	T42.6X3	T42.6X4	T42.6X5	T42.6X6
specified NEC	T42.6X1	T42.6X2	T42.6X3	T42.6X4	T42.6X5	T42.6X6
muscle-tone depressants	T42.8X1	T42.8X2	T42.8X3	T42.8X4	T42.8X5	T42.8X6
stimulants	T43.601	T43.602	T43.603	T43.604	T43.605	T43.606
amphetamines	T43.621	T43.622	T43.623	T43.624	T43.625	T43.626
analeptics	T50.7X1	T50.7X2	T50.7X3	T50.7X4	T50.7X5	T50.7X6

◄ New ◄ Revised ~~deleted~~ Deleted

TABLE OF DRUGS AND CHEMICALS

Substance	External Cause (T-Code)					
	Poisoning, Accidental (Unintentional)	Poisoning, Intentional Self-Harm	Poisoning, Assault	Poisoning, Undetermined	Adverse Effect	Underdosing
Central nervous system (Continued)						
stimulants (Continued)						
antidepressants	T43.201	T43.202	T43.203	T43.204	T43.205	T43.206
opiate antagonists	T50.7X1	T50.7X2	T50.7X3	T50.7X4	T50.7X5	T50.7X6
specified NEC	T43.691	T43.692	T43.693	T43.694	T43.695	T43.696
Cephalexin	T36.1X1	T36.1X2	T36.1X3	T36.1X4	T36.1X5	T36.1X6
Cephaloglycin	T36.1X1	T36.1X2	T36.1X3	T36.1X4	T36.1X5	T36.1X6
Cephaloridine	T36.1X1	T36.1X2	T36.1X3	T36.1X4	T36.1X5	T36.1X6
Cephalosporins	T36.1X1	T36.1X2	T36.1X3	T36.1X4	T36.1X5	T36.1X6
N (adicillin)	T36.0X1	T36.0X2	T36.0X3	T36.0X4	T36.0X5	T36.0X6
Cephalothin	T36.1X1	T36.1X2	T36.1X3	T36.1X4	T36.1X5	T36.1X6
Cephalotin	T36.1X1	T36.1X2	T36.1X3	T36.1X4	T36.1X5	T36.1X6
Cephradine	T36.1X1	T36.1X2	T36.1X3	T36.1X4	T36.1X5	T36.1X6
Cerbera (odallam)	T62.2X1	T62.2X2	T62.2X3	T62.2X4	—	—
Cerberin	T46.0X1	T46.0X2	T46.0X3	T46.0X4	T46.0X5	T46.0X6
Cerebral stimulants	T43.601	T43.602	T43.603	T43.604	T43.605	T43.606
psychotherapeutic	T43.601	T43.602	T43.603	T43.604	T43.605	T43.606
specified NEC	T43.691	T43.692	T43.693	T43.694	T43.695	T43.696
Cerium oxalate	T45.0X1	T45.0X2	T45.0X3	T45.0X4	T45.0X5	T45.0X6
Cerous oxalate	T45.0X1	T45.0X2	T45.0X3	T45.0X4	T45.0X5	T45.0X6
Ceruletide	T50.8X1	T50.8X2	T50.8X3	T50.8X4	T50.8X5	T50.8X6
Cetalkonium (chloride)	T49.0X1	T49.0X2	T49.0X3	T49.0X4	T49.0X5	T49.0X6
Cethexonium chloride	T49.0X1	T49.0X2	T49.0X3	T49.0X4	T49.0X5	T49.0X6
Cetiedil	T46.7X1	T46.7X2	T46.7X3	T46.7X4	T46.7X5	T46.7X6
Cetirizine	T45.0X1	T45.0X2	T45.0X3	T45.0X4	T45.0X5	T45.0X6
Cetomacrogol	T50.991	T50.992	T50.993	T50.994	T50.995	T50.996
Cetotiamine	T45.2X1	T45.2X2	T45.2X3	T45.2X4	T45.2X5	T45.2X6
Cetoxime	T45.0X1	T45.0X2	T45.0X3	T45.0X4	T45.0X5	T45.0X6
Cetraxate	T47.1X1	T47.1X2	T47.1X3	T47.1X4	T47.1X5	T47.1X6
Cetrimide	T49.0X1	T49.0X2	T49.0X3	T49.0X4	T49.0X5	T49.0X6
Cetrimonium (bromide)	T49.0X1	T49.0X2	T49.0X3	T49.0X4	T49.0X5	T49.0X6
Cetylpyridinium chloride	T49.0X1	T49.0X2	T49.0X3	T49.0X4	T49.0X5	T49.0X6
ENT agent	T49.6X1	T49.6X2	T49.6X3	T49.6X4	T49.6X5	T49.6X6
lozenges	T49.6X1	T49.6X2	T49.6X3	T49.6X4	T49.6X5	T49.6X6
Cevadillasee Sabadilla						
Cevitamic acid	T45.2X1	T45.2X2	T45.2X3	T45.2X4	T45.2X5	T45.2X6
Chalk, precipitated	T47.1X1	T47.1X2	T47.1X3	T47.1X4	T47.1X5	T47.1X6
Chamomile	T49.0X1	T49.0X2	T49.0X3	T49.0X4	T49.0X5	T49.0X6
Ch'an su	T46.0X1	T46.0X2	T46.0X3	T46.0X4	T46.0X5	T46.0X6
Charcoal	T47.6X1	T47.6X2	T47.6X3	T47.6X4	T47.6X5	T47.6X6
activated — see also Charcoal, medicinal	T47.6X1	T47.6X2	T47.6X3	T47.6X4	T47.6X5	T47.6X6

Substance	External Cause (T-Code)					
	Poisoning, Accidental (Unintentional)	Poisoning, Intentional Self-Harm	Poisoning, Assault	Poisoning, Undetermined	Adverse Effect	Underdosing
Charcoal (Continued)						
fumes (Carbon monoxide)	T58.2X1	T58.2X2	T58.2X3	T58.2X4	—	—
industrial	T58.8X1	T58.8X2	T58.8X3	T58.8X4	—	—
medicinal (activated)	T47.6X1	T47.6X2	T47.6X3	T47.6X4	T47.6X5	T47.6X6
antidiarrheal	T47.6X1	T47.6X2	T47.6X3	T47.6X4	T47.6X5	T47.6X6
poison control	T47.8X1	T47.8X2	T47.8X3	T47.8X4	T47.8X5	T47.8X6
specified use other than for diarrhea	T47.8X1	T47.8X2	T47.8X3	T47.8X4	T47.8X5	T47.8X6
topical	T49.8X1	T49.8X2	T49.8X3	T49.8X4	T49.8X5	T49.8X6
Chaulmosulfone	T37.1X1	T37.1X2	T37.1X3	T37.1X4	T37.1X5	T37.1X6
Chelating agent NEC	T50.6X1	T50.6X2	T50.6X3	T50.6X4	T50.6X5	T50.6X6
Chelidonium majus	T62.2X1	T62.2X2	T62.2X3	T62.2X4	—	—
Chemical substance NEC	T65.91	T65.92	T65.93	T65.94	—	—
Chenodeoxycholic acid	T47.5X1	T47.5X2	T47.5X3	T47.5X4	T47.5X5	T47.5X6
Chenodiol	T47.5X1	T47.5X2	T47.5X3	T47.5X4	T47.5X5	T47.5X6
Chenopodium	T37.4X1	T37.4X2	T37.4X3	T37.4X4	T37.4X5	T37.4X6
Cherry laurel	T62.2X1	T62.2X2	T62.2X3	T62.2X4	—	—
Chinidin(e)	T46.2X1	T46.2X2	T46.2X3	T46.2X4	T46.2X5	T46.2X6
Chiniofon	T37.8X1	T37.8X2	T37.8X3	T37.8X4	T37.8X5	T37.8X6
Chlophedianol	T48.3X1	T48.3X2	T48.3X3	T48.3X4	T48.3X5	T48.3X6
Chloral	T42.6X1	T42.6X2	T42.6X3	T42.6X4	T42.6X5	T42.6X6
derivative	T42.6X1	T42.6X2	T42.6X3	T42.6X4	T42.6X5	T42.6X6
hydrate	T42.6X1	T42.6X2	T42.6X3	T42.6X4	T42.6X5	T42.6X6
Chloralamide	T42.6X1	T42.6X2	T42.6X3	T42.6X4	T42.6X5	T42.6X6
Chloralodol	T42.6X1	T42.6X2	T42.6X3	T42.6X4	T42.6X5	T42.6X6
Chloralose	T60.4X1	T60.4X2	T60.4X3	T60.4X4	—	—
Chlorambucil	T45.1X1	T45.1X2	T45.1X3	T45.1X4	T45.1X5	T45.1X6
Chloramine	T57.8X1	T57.8X2	T57.8X3	T57.8X4	—	—
T	T49.0X1	T49.0X2	T49.0X3	T49.0X4	T49.0X5	T49.0X6
topical	T49.0X1	T49.0X2	T49.0X3	T49.0X4	T49.0X5	T49.0X6
Chloramphenicol	T36.2X1	T36.2X2	T36.2X3	T36.2X4	T36.2X5	T36.2X6
ENT agent	T49.6X1	T49.6X2	T49.6X3	T49.6X4	T49.6X5	T49.6X6
ophthalmic preparation	T49.5X1	T49.5X2	T49.5X3	T49.5X4	T49.5X5	T49.5X6
topical NEC	T49.0X1	T49.0X2	T49.0X3	T49.0X4	T49.0X5	T49.0X6
Chlorate (potassium) (sodium) NEC	T60.3X1	T60.3X2	T60.3X3	T60.3X4	—	—
herbicide	T60.3X1	T60.3X2	T60.3X3	T60.3X4	—	—
Chlorazanil	T50.2X1	T50.2X2	T50.2X3	T50.2X4	T50.2X5	T50.2X6
Chlorbenzene, chlorbenzol	T53.7X1	T53.7X2	T53.7X3	T53.7X4	—	—
Chlorbenzoxamine	T44.3X1	T44.3X2	T44.3X3	T44.3X4	T44.3X5	T44.3X6
Chlorbutol	T42.6X1	T42.6X2	T42.6X3	T42.6X4	T42.6X5	T42.6X6
Chlorcyclizine	T45.0X1	T45.0X2	T45.0X3	T45.0X4	T45.0X5	T45.0X6

◀ New ◀ Revised ~~deleted~~ Deleted

TABLE OF DRUGS AND CHEMICALS

Substance	Poisoning, Accidental (Unintentional)	Poisoning, Intentional Self-Harm	Poisoning, Assault	Poisoning, Undetermined	Adverse Effect	Underdosing
Chlordan(e) (dust)	T60.1X1	T60.1X2	T60.1X3	T60.1X4	—	—
Chlordantoin	T49.0X1	T49.0X2	T49.0X3	T49.0X4	T49.0X5	T49.0X6
Chlordiazepoxide	T42.4X1	T42.4X2	T42.4X3	T42.4X4	T42.4X5	T42.4X6
Chlordiethyl benzamide	T49.3X1	T49.3X2	T49.3X3	T49.3X4	T49.3X5	T49.3X6
Chloresium	T49.8X1	T49.8X2	T49.8X3	T49.8X4	T49.8X5	T49.8X6
Chlorethiazol	T42.6X1	T42.6X2	T42.6X3	T42.6X4	T42.6X5	T42.6X6
Chlorethyl — see Ethyl, chloride						
Chloretone	T42.6X1	T42.6X2	T42.6X3	T42.6X4	T42.6X5	T42.6X6
Chlorex	T53.6X1	T53.6X2	T53.6X3	T53.6X4	—	—
insecticide	T60.1X1	T60.1X2	T60.1X3	T60.1X4	—	—
Chlorfenvinphos	T60.0X1	T60.0X2	T60.0X3	T60.0X4	—	—
Chlorhexadol	T42.6X1	T42.6X2	T42.6X3	T42.6X4	T42.6X5	T42.6X6
Chlorhexamide	T45.1X1	T45.1X2	T45.1X3	T45.1X4	T45.1X5	T45.1X6
Chlorhexidine	T49.0X1	T49.0X2	T49.0X3	T49.0X4	T49.0X5	T49.0X6
Chlorhydroxyquinolin	T49.0X1	T49.0X2	T49.0X3	T49.0X4	T49.0X5	T49.0X6
Chloride of lime (bleach)	T54.3X1	T54.3X2	T54.3X3	T54.3X4	—	—
Chlorimipramine	T43.011	T43.012	T43.013	T43.014	T43.015	T43.016
Chlorinated						
camphene	T53.6X1	T53.6X2	T53.6X3	T53.6X4	—	—
diphenyl	T53.7X1	T53.7X2	T53.7X3	T53.7X4	—	—
hydrocarbons NEC	T53.91	T53.92	T53.93	T53.94	—	—
solvents	T53.91	T53.92	T53.93	T53.94	—	—
lime (bleach)	T54.3X1	T54.3X2	T54.3X3	T54.3X4	—	—
and boric acid solution	T49.0X1	T49.0X2	T49.0X3	T49.0X4	T49.0X5	T49.0X6
naphthalene (insecticide)	T60.1X1	T60.1X2	T60.1X3	T60.1X4	—	—
industrial (non-pesticide)	T53.7X1	T53.7X2	T53.7X3	T53.7X4	—	—
pesticide NEC	T60.8X1	T60.8X2	T60.8X3	T60.8X4	—	—
soda — see also Sodium hypochlorite						
solution	T49.0X1	T49.0X2	T49.0X3	T49.0X4	T49.0X5	T49.0X6
Chlorine (fumes) (gas)	T59.4X1	T59.4X2	T59.4X3	T59.4X4	—	—
bleach	T54.3X1	T54.3X2	T54.3X3	T54.3X4	—	—
compound gas NEC	T59.4X1	T59.4X2	T59.4X3	T59.4X4	—	—
disinfectant	T59.4X1	T59.4X2	T59.4X3	T59.4X4	—	—
releasing agents NEC	T59.4X1	T59.4X2	T59.4X3	T59.4X4	—	—
Chlorisondamine chloride	T46.991	T46.992	T46.993	T46.994	T46.995	T46.996
Chlormadinone	T38.5X1	T38.5X2	T38.5X3	T38.5X4	T38.5X5	T38.5X6
Chlormephos	T60.0X1	T60.0X2	T60.0X3	T60.0X4	—	—
Chlormerodrin	T50.2X1	T50.2X2	T50.2X3	T50.2X4	T50.2X5	T50.2X6
Chlormethiazole	T42.6X1	T42.6X2	T42.6X3	T42.6X4	T42.6X5	T42.6X6
Chlormethine	T45.1X1	T45.1X2	T45.1X3	T45.1X4	T45.1X5	T45.1X6
Chlormethylenecycline	T36.4X1	T36.4X2	T36.4X3	T36.4X4	T36.4X5	T36.4X6

Substance	Poisoning, Accidental (Unintentional)	Poisoning, Intentional Self-Harm	Poisoning, Assault	Poisoning, Undetermined	Adverse Effect	Underdosing
Chlormezanone	T42.6X1	T42.6X2	T42.6X3	T42.6X4	T42.6X5	T42.6X6
Chloroacetic acid	T60.3X1	T60.3X2	T60.3X3	T60.3X4	—	—
Chloroacetone	T59.3X1	T59.3X2	T59.3X3	T59.3X4	—	—
Chloroacetophenone	T59.3X1	T59.3X2	T59.3X3	T59.3X4	—	—
Chloroaniline	T53.7X1	T53.7X2	T53.7X3	T53.7X4	—	—
Chlorobenzene, chlorobenzol	T53.7X1	T53.7X2	T53.7X3	T53.7X4	—	—
Chlorobromomethane (fire extinguisher)	T53.6X1	T53.6X2	T53.6X3	T53.6X4	—	—
Chlorobutanol	T49.0X1	T49.0X2	T49.0X3	T49.0X4	T49.0X5	T49.0X6
Chlorocresol	T49.0X1	T49.0X2	T49.0X3	T49.0X4	T49.0X5	T49.0X6
Chlorodehydro-methyltestosterone	T38.7X1	T38.7X2	T38.7X3	T38.7X4	T38.7X5	T38.7X6
Chlorodinitrobenzene	T53.7X1	T53.7X2	T53.7X3	T53.7X4	—	—
dust or vapor	T53.7X1	T53.7X2	T53.7X3	T53.7X4	—	—
Chlorodiphenyl	T53.7X1	T53.7X2	T53.7X3	T53.7X4	—	—
Chloroethane — see Ethyl, chloride						
Chloroethylene	T53.6X1	T53.6X2	T53.6X3	T53.6X4	—	—
Chlorofluorocarbons	T53.5X1	T53.5X2	T53.5X3	T53.5X4	—	—
Chloroform (fumes) (vapor)	T53.1X1	T53.1X2	T53.1X3	T53.1X4	—	—
anesthetic	T41.0X1	T41.0X2	T41.0X3	T41.0X4	T41.0X5	T41.0X6
solvent	T53.1X1	T53.1X2	T53.1X3	T53.1X4	—	—
water, concentrated	T41.0X1	T41.0X2	T41.0X3	T41.0X4	T41.0X5	T41.0X6
Chloroguanide	T37.2X1	T37.2X2	T37.2X3	T37.2X4	T37.2X5	T37.2X6
Chloromycetin	T36.2X1	T36.2X2	T36.2X3	T36.2X4	T36.2X5	T36.2X6
ENT agent	T49.6X1	T49.6X2	T49.6X3	T49.6X4	T49.6X5	T49.6X6
ophthalmic preparation	T49.5X1	T49.5X2	T49.5X3	T49.5X4	T49.5X5	T49.5X6
otic solution	T49.6X1	T49.6X2	T49.6X3	T49.6X4	T49.6X5	T49.6X6
topical NEC	T49.0X1	T49.0X2	T49.0X3	T49.0X4	T49.0X5	T49.0X6
Chloronitrobenzene	T53.7X1	T53.7X2	T53.7X3	T53.7X4	—	—
dust or vapor	T53.7X1	T53.7X2	T53.7X3	T53.7X4	—	—
Chlorophacinone	T60.4X1	T60.4X2	T60.4X3	T60.4X4	—	—
Chlorophenol	T53.7X1	T53.7X2	T53.7X3	T53.7X4	—	—
Chlorophenothane	T60.1X1	T60.1X2	T60.1X3	T60.1X4	—	—
Chlorophyll	T50.991	T50.992	T50.993	T50.994	T50.995	T50.996
Chloropicrin (fumes)	T53.6X1	T53.6X2	T53.6X3	T53.6X4	—	—
fumigant	T60.8X1	T60.8X2	T60.8X3	T60.8X4	—	—
fungicide	T60.3X1	T60.3X2	T60.3X3	T60.3X4	—	—
pesticide	T60.8X1	T60.8X2	T60.8X3	T60.8X4	—	—
Chloroprocaine	T41.3X1	T41.3X2	T41.3X3	T41.3X4	T41.3X5	T41.3X6
infiltration (subcutaneous)	T41.3X1	T41.3X2	T41.3X3	T41.3X4	T41.3X5	T41.3X6
nerve block (peripheral) (plexus)	T41.3X1	T41.3X2	T41.3X3	T41.3X4	T41.3X5	T41.3X6
spinal	T41.3X1	T41.3X2	T41.3X3	T41.3X4	T41.3X5	T41.3X6

◀ New ◀ Revised ~~deleted~~ Deleted

TABLE OF DRUGS AND CHEMICALS

TABLE OF DRUGS AND CHEMICALS

Substance	Poisoning, Accidental (Unintentional)	Poisoning, Intentional Self-Harm	Poisoning, Assault	Poisoning, Undetermined	Adverse Effect	Underdosing
Chloroptic	T49.5X1	T49.5X2	T49.5X3	T49.5X4	T49.5X5	T49.5X6
Chloropurine	T45.1X1	T45.1X2	T45.1X3	T45.1X4	T45.1X5	T45.1X6
Chloropyramine	T45.0X1	T45.0X2	T45.0X3	T45.0X4	T45.0X5	T45.0X6
Chloropyrifos	T60.0X1	T60.0X2	T60.0X3	T60.0X4	—	—
Chloropyrilene	T45.0X1	T45.0X2	T45.0X3	T45.0X4	T45.0X5	T45.0X6
Chloroquine	T37.2X1	T37.2X2	T37.2X3	T37.2X4	T37.2X5	T37.2X6
Chlorothalonil	T60.3X1	T60.3X2	T60.3X3	T60.3X4	—	—
Chlorothen	T45.0X1	T45.0X2	T45.0X3	T45.0X4	T45.0X5	T45.0X6
Chlorothiazide	T50.2X1	T50.2X2	T50.2X3	T50.2X4	T50.2X5	T50.2X6
Chlorothymol	T49.4X1	T49.4X2	T49.4X3	T49.4X4	T49.4X5	T49.4X6
Chlorotrianisene	T38.5X1	T38.5X2	T38.5X3	T38.5X4	T38.5X5	T38.5X6
Chlorovinyldichloro-arsine, not in war	T57.0X1	T57.0X2	T57.0X3	T57.0X4	—	—
Chloroxine	T49.4X1	T49.4X2	T49.4X3	T49.4X4	T49.4X5	T49.4X6
Chloroxylenol	T49.0X1	T49.0X2	T49.0X3	T49.0X4	T49.0X5	T49.0X6
Chlorphenamine	T45.0X1	T45.0X2	T45.0X3	T45.0X4	T45.0X5	T45.0X6
Chlorphenesin	T42.8X1	T42.8X2	T42.8X3	T42.8X4	T42.8X5	T42.8X6
topical (antifungal)	T49.0X1	T49.0X2	T49.0X3	T49.0X4	T49.0X5	T49.0X6
Chlorpheniramine	T45.0X1	T45.0X2	T45.0X3	T45.0X4	T45.0X5	T45.0X6
Chlorphenoxamine	T45.0X1	T45.0X2	T45.0X3	T45.0X4	T45.0X5	T45.0X6
Chlorphentermine	T50.5X1	T50.5X2	T50.5X3	T50.5X4	T50.5X5	T50.5X6
Chlorprocaine — see Chloroprocaine						
Chlorproguanil	T37.2X1	T37.2X2	T37.2X3	T37.2X4	T37.2X5	T37.2X6
Chlorpromazine	T43.3X1	T43.3X2	T43.3X3	T43.3X4	T43.3X5	T43.3X6
Chlorpropamide	T38.3X1	T38.3X2	T38.3X3	T38.3X4	T38.3X5	T38.3X6
Chlorprothixene	T43.4X1	T43.4X2	T43.4X3	T43.4X4	T43.4X5	T43.4X6
Chlorquinaldol	T49.0X1	T49.0X2	T49.0X3	T49.0X4	T49.0X5	T49.0X6
Chlorquinol	T49.0X1	T49.0X2	T49.0X3	T49.0X4	T49.0X5	T49.0X6
Chlortalidone	T50.2X1	T50.2X2	T50.2X3	T50.2X4	T50.2X5	T50.2X6
Chlortetracycline	T36.4X1	T36.4X2	T36.4X3	T36.4X4	T36.4X5	T36.4X6
Chlorthalidone	T50.2X1	T50.2X2	T50.2X3	T50.2X4	T50.2X5	T50.2X6
Chlorthiophos	T60.0X1	T60.0X2	T60.0X3	T60.0X4	—	—
Chlorotrianisene	T38.5X1	T38.5X2	T38.5X3	T38.5X4	T38.5X5	T38.5X6
Chlor-Trimeton	T45.0X1	T45.0X2	T45.0X3	T45.0X4	T45.0X5	T45.0X6
Chlorthion	T60.0X1	T60.0X2	T60.0X3	T60.0X4	—	—
Chlorzoxazone	T42.8X1	T42.8X2	T42.8X3	T42.8X4	T42.8X5	T42.8X6
Choke damp	T59.7X1	T59.7X2	T59.7X3	T59.7X4	—	—
Cholagogues	T47.5X1	T47.5X2	T47.5X3	T47.5X4	T47.5X5	T47.5X6
Cholebrine	T50.8X1	T50.8X2	T50.8X3	T50.8X4	T50.8X5	T50.8X6
Cholecalciferol	T45.2X1	T45.2X2	T45.2X3	T45.2X4	T45.2X5	T45.2X6
Cholecystokinin	T50.8X1	T50.8X2	T50.8X3	T50.8X4	T50.8X5	T50.8X6
Cholera vaccine	T50.A91	T50.A92	T50.A93	T50.A94	T50.A95	T50.A96

Substance	Poisoning, Accidental (Unintentional)	Poisoning, Intentional Self-Harm	Poisoning, Assault	Poisoning, Undetermined	Adverse Effect	Underdosing
Choleretic	T47.5X1	T47.5X2	T47.5X3	T47.5X4	T47.5X5	T47.5X6
Cholesterol-lowering agents	T46.6X1	T46.6X2	T46.6X3	T46.6X4	T46.6X5	T46.6X6
Cholestyramine (resin)	T46.6X1	T46.6X2	T46.6X3	T46.6X4	T46.6X5	T46.6X6
Cholic acid	T47.5X1	T47.5X2	T47.5X3	T47.5X4	T47.5X5	T47.5X6
Choline	T48.6X1	T48.6X2	T48.6X3	T48.6X4	T48.6X5	T48.6X6
chloride	T50.991	T50.992	T50.993	T50.994	T50.995	T50.996
dihydrogen citrate	T50.991	T50.992	T50.993	T50.994	T50.995	T50.996
salicylate	T39.091	T39.092	T39.093	T39.094	T39.095	T39.096
theophyllinate	T48.6X1	T48.6X2	T48.6X3	T48.6X4	T48.6X5	T48.6X6
Cholinergic (drug) NEC	T44.1X1	T44.1X2	T44.1X3	T44.1X4	T44.1X5	T44.1X6
muscle tone enhancer	T44.1X1	T44.1X2	T44.1X3	T44.1X4	T44.1X5	T44.1X6
organophosphorus	T44.0X1	T44.0X2	T44.0X3	T44.0X4	T44.0X5	T44.0X6
insecticide	T60.0X1	T60.0X2	T60.0X3	T60.0X4	—	—
nerve gas	T59.891	T59.892	T59.893	T59.894		
trimethyl ammonium propanediol	T44.1X1	T44.1X2	T44.1X3	T44.1X4	T44.1X5	T44.1X6
Cholinesterase reactivator	T50.6X1	T50.6X2	T50.6X3	T50.6X4	T50.6X5	T50.6X6
Cholografin	T50.8X1	T50.8X2	T50.8X3	T50.8X4	T50.8X5	T50.8X6
Chorionic gonadotropin	T38.891	T38.892	T38.893	T38.894	T38.895	T38.896
Chromate	T56.2X1	T56.2X2	T56.2X3	T56.2X4	—	—
dust or mist	T56.2X1	T56.2X2	T56.2X3	T56.2X4	—	—
lead — see also Lead	T56.0X1	T56.0X2	T56.0X3	T56.0X4	—	—
paint	T56.0X1	T56.0X2	T56.0X3	T56.0X4		
Chromic						
acid	T56.2X1	T56.2X2	T56.2X3	T56.2X4	—	—
dust or mist	T56.2X1	T56.2X2	T56.2X3	T56.2X4	—	—
phosphate 32P	T45.1X1	T45.1X2	T45.1X3	T45.1X4	T45.1X5	T45.1X6
Chromium	T56.2X1	T56.2X2	T56.2X3	T56.2X4		
compounds — see Chromate						
sesquioxide	T50.8X1	T50.8X2	T50.8X3	T50.8X4	T50.8X5	T50.8X6
Chromomycin A3	T45.1X1	T45.1X2	T45.1X3	T45.1X4	T45.1X5	T45.1X6
Chromonar	T46.3X1	T46.3X2	T46.3X3	T46.3X4	T46.3X5	T46.3X6
Chromyl chloride	T56.2X1	T56.2X2	T56.2X3	T56.2X4	—	—
Chrysarobin	T49.4X1	T49.4X2	T49.4X3	T49.4X4	T49.4X5	T49.4X6
Chrysazin	T47.2X1	T47.2X2	T47.2X3	T47.2X4	T47.2X5	T47.2X6
Chymar	T45.3X1	T45.3X2	T45.3X3	T45.3X4	T45.3X5	T45.3X6
ophthalmic preparation	T49.5X1	T49.5X2	T49.5X3	T49.5X4	T49.5X5	T49.5X6
Chymopapain	T45.3X1	T45.3X2	T45.3X3	T45.3X4	T45.3X5	T45.3X6
Chymotrypsin	T45.3X1	T45.3X2	T45.3X3	T45.3X4	T45.3X5	T45.3X6
ophthalmic preparation	T49.5X1	T49.5X2	T49.5X3	T49.5X4	T49.5X5	T49.5X6
Cianidanol	T50.991	T50.992	T50.993	T50.994	T50.995	T50.996
Cianopramine	T43.011	T43.012	T43.013	T43.014	T43.015	T43.016
Cibenzoline	T46.2X1	T46.2X2	T46.2X3	T46.2X4	T46.2X5	T46.2X6

◀ New　◀ Revised　~~deleted~~ Deleted

	External Cause (T-Code)					
Substance	Poisoning, Accidental (Unintentional)	Poisoning, Intentional Self-Harm	Poisoning, Assault	Poisoning, Undetermined	Adverse Effect	Underdosing
Ciclacillin	T36.0X1	T36.0X2	T36.0X3	T36.0X4	T36.0X5	T36.0X6
Ciclobarbital — see Hexobarbital						
Ciclonicate	T46.7X1	T46.7X2	T46.7X3	T46.7X4	T46.7X5	T46.7X6
Ciclopirox (olamine)	T49.0X1	T49.0X2	T49.0X3	T49.0X4	T49.0X5	T49.0X6
Ciclosporin	T45.1X1	T45.1X2	T45.1X3	T45.1X4	T45.1X5	T45.1X6
Cicuta maculata or virosa	T62.2X1	T62.2X2	T62.2X3	T62.2X4	—	—
Cicutoxin	T62.2X1	T62.2X2	T62.2X3	T62.2X4	—	—
Cigarette lighter fluid	T52.0X1	T52.0X2	T52.0X3	T52.0X4	—	—
Cigarettes (tobacco)	T65.221	T65.222	T65.223	T65.224	—	—
Ciguatoxin	T61.01	T61.02	T61.03	T61.04	—	—
Cilazapril	T46.4X1	T46.4X2	T46.4X3	T46.4X4	T46.4X5	T46.4X6
Cimetidine	T47.0X1	T47.0X2	T47.0X3	T47.0X4	T47.0X5	T47.0X6
Cimetropium bromide	T44.3X1	T44.3X2	T44.3X3	T44.3X4	T44.3X5	T44.3X6
Cinchocaine	T41.3X1	T41.3X2	T41.3X3	T41.3X4	T41.3X5	T41.3X6
topical (surface)	T41.3X1	T41.3X2	T41.3X3	T41.3X4	T41.3X5	T41.3X6
Cinchona	T37.2X1	T37.2X2	T37.2X3	T37.2X4	T37.2X5	T37.2X6
Cinchonine alkaloids	T37.2X1	T37.2X2	T37.2X3	T37.2X4	T37.2X5	T37.2X6
Cinchophen	T50.4X1	T50.4X2	T50.4X3	T50.4X4	T50.4X5	T50.4X6
Cinepazide	T46.7X1	T46.7X2	T46.7X3	T46.7X4	T46.7X5	T46.7X6
Cinnamedrine	T48.5X1	T48.5X2	T48.5X3	T48.5X4	T48.5X5	T48.5X6
Cinnarizine	T45.0X1	T45.0X2	T45.0X3	T45.0X4	T45.0X5	T45.0X6
Cinoxacin	T37.8X1	T37.8X2	T37.8X3	T37.8X4	T37.8X5	T37.8X6
Ciprofibrate	T46.6X1	T46.6X2	T46.6X3	T46.6X4	T46.6X5	T46.6X6
Ciprofloxacin	T36.8X1	T36.8X2	T36.8X3	T36.8X4	T36.8X5	T36.8X6
Cisapride	T47.8X1	T47.8X2	T47.8X3	T47.8X4	T47.8X5	T47.8X6
Cisplatin	T45.1X1	T45.1X2	T45.1X3	T45.1X4	T45.1X5	T45.1X6
Citalopram	T43.221	T43.222	T43.223	T43.224	T43.225	T43.226
Citanest	T41.3X1	T41.3X2	T41.3X3	T41.3X4	T41.3X5	T41.3X6
infiltration (subcutaneous)	T41.3X1	T41.3X2	T41.3X3	T41.3X4	T41.3X5	T41.3X6
nerve block (peripheral) (plexus)	T41.3X1	T41.3X2	T41.3X3	T41.3X4	T41.3X5	T41.3X6
Citric acid	T47.5X1	T47.5X2	T47.5X3	T47.5X4	T47.5X5	T47.5X6
Citrovorum (factor)	T45.8X1	T45.8X2	T45.8X3	T45.8X4	T45.8X5	T45.8X6
Claviceps purpurea	T62.2X1	T62.2X2	T62.2X3	T62.2X4	—	—
Clavulanic acid	T36.1X1	T36.1X2	T36.1X3	T36.1X4	T36.1X5	T36.1X6
Cleaner, cleansing agent, type not specified	T65.891	T65.892	T65.893	T65.894	—	—
of paint or varnish	T52.91	T52.92	T52.93	T52.94	—	—
specified type NEC	T65.891	T65.892	T65.893	T65.894	—	—
Clebopride	T47.8X1	T47.8X2	T47.8X3	T47.8X4	T47.8X5	T47.8X6
Clefamide	T37.3X1	T37.3X2	T37.3X3	T37.3X4	T37.3X5	T37.3X6
Clemastine	T45.0X1	T45.0X2	T45.0X3	T45.0X4	T45.0X5	T45.0X6
Clematis vitalba	T62.2X1	T62.2X2	T62.2X3	T62.2X4	—	—

	External Cause (T-Code)					
Substance	Poisoning, Accidental (Unintentional)	Poisoning, Intentional Self-Harm	Poisoning, Assault	Poisoning, Undetermined	Adverse Effect	Underdosing
Clemizole	T45.0X1	T45.0X2	T45.0X3	T45.0X4	T45.0X5	T45.0X6
penicillin	T36.0X1	T36.0X2	T36.0X3	T36.0X4	T36.0X5	T36.0X6
Clenbuterol	T48.6X1	T48.6X2	T48.6X3	T48.6X4	T48.6X5	T48.6X6
Clidinium bromide	T44.3X1	T44.3X2	T44.3X3	T44.3X4	T44.3X5	T44.3X6
Clindamycin	T36.8X1	T36.8X2	T36.8X3	T36.8X4	T36.8X5	T36.8X6
Clinofibrate	T46.6X1	T46.6X2	T46.6X3	T46.6X4	T46.6X5	T46.6X6
Clioquinol	T37.8X1	T37.8X2	T37.8X3	T37.8X4	T37.8X5	T37.8X6
Cliradon	T40.2X1	T40.2X2	T40.2X3	T40.2X4	—	—
Clobazam	T42.4X1	T42.4X2	T42.4X3	T42.4X4	T42.4X5	T42.4X6
Clobenzorex	T50.5X1	T50.5X2	T50.5X3	T50.5X4	T50.5X5	T50.5X6
Clobetasol	T49.0X1	T49.0X2	T49.0X3	T49.0X4	T49.0X5	T49.0X6
Clobetasone	T49.0X1	T49.0X2	T49.0X3	T49.0X4	T49.0X5	T49.0X6
Clobutinol	T48.3X1	T48.3X2	T48.3X3	T48.3X4	T48.3X5	T48.3X6
Clocapramine	T43.0X1	T43.0X2	T43.0X3	T43.0X4	T43.0X5	T43.0X6
Clocortolone	T38.0X1	T38.0X2	T38.0X3	T38.0X4	T38.0X5	T38.0X6
Clodantoin	T49.0X1	T49.0X2	T49.0X3	T49.0X4	T49.0X5	T49.0X6
Clodronic acid	T50.991	T50.992	T50.993	T50.994	T50.995	T50.996
Clofazimine	T37.1X1	T37.1X2	T37.1X3	T37.1X4	T37.1X5	T37.1X6
Clofedanol	T48.3X1	T48.3X2	T48.3X3	T48.3X4	T48.3X5	T48.3X6
Clofenamide	T50.2X1	T50.2X2	T50.2X3	T50.2X4	T50.2X5	T50.2X6
Clofenotane	T49.0X1	T49.0X2	T49.0X3	T49.0X4	T49.0X5	T49.0X6
Clofezone	T39.2X1	T39.2X2	T39.2X3	T39.2X4	T39.2X5	T39.2X6
Clofibrate	T46.6X1	T46.6X2	T46.6X3	T46.6X4	T46.6X5	T46.6X6
Clofibride	T46.6X1	T46.6X2	T46.6X3	T46.6X4	T46.6X5	T46.6X6
Cloforex	T50.5X1	T50.5X2	T50.5X3	T50.5X4	T50.5X5	T50.5X6
Clomacran	T43.0X1	T43.0X2	T43.0X3	T43.0X4	T43.0X5	T43.0X6
Clomethiazole	T42.6X1	T42.6X2	T42.6X3	T42.6X4	T42.6X5	T42.6X6
Clometocillin	T36.0X1	T36.0X2	T36.0X3	T36.0X4	T36.0X5	T36.0X6
Clomifene	T38.5X1	T38.5X2	T38.5X3	T38.5X4	T38.5X5	T38.5X6
Clomiphene	T38.5X1	T38.5X2	T38.5X3	T38.5X4	T38.5X5	T38.5X6
Clomipramine	T43.011	T43.012	T43.013	T43.014	T43.015	T43.016
Clomocycline	T36.4X1	T36.4X2	T36.4X3	T36.4X4	T36.4X5	T36.4X6
Clonazepam	T42.4X1	T42.4X2	T42.4X3	T42.4X4	T42.4X5	T42.4X6
Clonidine	T46.5X1	T46.5X2	T46.5X3	T46.5X4	T46.5X5	T46.5X6
Clonixin	T39.8X1	T39.8X2	T39.8X3	T39.8X4	T39.8X5	T39.8X6
Clopamide	T50.2X1	T50.2X2	T50.2X3	T50.2X4	T50.2X5	T50.2X6
Clopenthixol	T43.4X1	T43.4X2	T43.4X3	T43.4X4	T43.4X5	T43.4X6
Cloperastine	T48.3X1	T48.3X2	T48.3X3	T48.3X4	T48.3X5	T48.3X6
Clophedianol	T48.3X1	T48.3X2	T48.3X3	T48.3X4	T48.3X5	T48.3X6
Cloponone	T36.2X1	T36.2X2	T36.2X3	T36.2X4	T36.2X5	T36.2X6
Cloprednol	T38.0X1	T38.0X2	T38.0X3	T38.0X4	T38.0X5	T38.0X6
Cloral betaine	T42.6X1	T42.6X2	T42.6X3	T42.6X4	T42.6X5	T42.6X6

TABLE OF DRUGS AND CHEMICALS

	External Cause (T-Code)					
Substance	Poisoning, Accidental (Unintentional)	Poisoning, Intentional Self-Harm	Poisoning, Assault	Poisoning, Undetermined	Adverse Effect	Underdosing
Cloramfenicol	T36.2X1	T36.2X2	T36.2X3	T36.2X4	T36.2X5	T36.2X6
Clorazepate (dipotassium)	T42.4X1	T42.4X2	T42.4X3	T42.4X4	T42.4X5	T42.4X6
Clorexolone	T50.2X1	T50.2X2	T50.2X3	T50.2X4	T50.2X5	T50.2X6
Clorox (bleach)	T54.91	T54.92	T54.93	T54.94	—	—
Clorfenamine	T45.0X1	T45.0X2	T45.0X3	T45.0X4	T45.0X5	T45.0X6
Clorgiline	T43.1X1	T43.1X2	T43.1X3	T43.1X4	T43.1X5	T43.1X6
Clorotepine	T44.3X1	T44.3X2	T44.3X3	T44.3X4	T44.3X5	T44.3X6
Clorprenaline	T48.6X1	T48.6X2	T48.6X3	T48.6X4	T48.6X5	T48.6X6
Clortermine	T50.5X1	T50.5X2	T50.5X3	T50.5X4	T50.5X5	T50.5X6
Clotiapine	T43.591	T43.592	T43.593	T43.594	T43.595	T43.596
Clotiazepam	T42.4X1	T42.4X2	T42.4X3	T42.4X4	T42.4X5	T42.4X6
Clotibric acid	T46.6X1	T46.6X2	T46.6X3	T46.6X4	T46.6X5	T46.6X6
Clotrimazole	T49.0X1	T49.0X2	T49.0X3	T49.0X4	T49.0X5	T49.0X6
Cloxacillin	T36.0X1	T36.0X2	T36.0X3	T36.0X4	T36.0X5	T36.0X6
Cloxazolam	T42.4X1	T42.4X2	T42.4X3	T42.4X4	T42.4X5	T42.4X6
Cloxiquine	T49.0X1	T49.0X2	T49.0X3	T49.0X4	T49.0X5	T49.0X6
Clozapine	T42.4X1	T42.4X2	T42.4X3	T42.4X4	T42.4X5	T42.4X6
Coagulant NEC	T45.7X1	T45.7X2	T45.7X3	T45.7X4	T45.7X5	T45.7X6
Coal (carbon monoxide from) — see also Carbon, monoxide, coal	T58.2X1	T58.2X2	T58.2X3	T58.2X4	—	—
oil — see Kerosene						
tar	T49.1X1	T49.1X2	T49.1X3	T49.1X4	T49.1X5	T49.1X6
fumes	T59.891	T59.892	T59.893	T59.894	—	—
medicinal (ointment)	T49.4X1	T49.4X2	T49.4X3	T49.4X4	T49.4X5	T49.4X6
analgesics NEC	T39.2X1	T39.2X2	T39.2X3	T39.2X4	T39.2X5	T39.2X6
naphtha (solvent)	T52.0X1	T52.0X2	T52.0X3	T52.0X4		
Cobalamine	T45.2X1	T45.2X2	T45.2X3	T45.2X4	T45.2X5	T45.2X6
Cobalt (nonmedicinal) (fumes) (industrial)	T56.891	T56.892	T56.893	T56.894		
medicinal (trace) (chloride)	T45.8X1	T45.8X2	T45.8X3	T45.8X4	T45.8X5	T45.8X6
Cobra (venom)	T63.041	T63.042	T63.043	T63.044		
Coca (leaf)	T40.5X1	T40.5X2	T40.5X3	T40.5X4	T40.5X5	T40.5X6
Cocaine	T40.5X1	T40.5X2	T40.5X3	T40.5X4	T40.5X5	T40.5X6
topical anesthetic	T41.3X1	T41.3X2	T41.3X3	T41.3X4	T41.3X5	T41.3X6
Cocarboxylase	T45.3X1	T45.3X2	T45.3X3	T45.3X4	T45.3X5	T45.3X6
Coccidioidin	T50.8X1	T50.8X2	T50.8X3	T50.8X4	T50.8X5	T50.8X6
Cocculus indicus	T62.1X1	T62.1X2	T62.1X3	T62.1X4		
Cochineal	T65.6X1	T65.6X2	T65.6X3	T65.6X4		
medicinal products	T50.991	T50.992	T50.993	T50.994	T50.995	T50.996
Codeine	T40.2X1	T40.2X2	T40.2X3	T40.2X4	T40.2X5	T40.2X6
Cod-liver oil	T45.2X1	T45.2X2	T45.2X3	T45.2X4	T45.2X5	T45.2X6

	External Cause (T-Code)					
Substance	Poisoning, Accidental (Unintentional)	Poisoning, Intentional Self-Harm	Poisoning, Assault	Poisoning, Undetermined	Adverse Effect	Underdosing
Coenzyme A	T50.991	T50.992	T50.993	T50.994	T50.995	T50.996
Coffee	T62.8X1	T62.8X2	T62.8X3	T62.8X4	—	—
Cogalactoisomerase	T50.991	T50.992	T50.993	T50.994	T50.995	T50.996
Cogentin	T44.3X1	T44.3X2	T44.3X3	T44.3X4	T44.3X5	T44.3X6
Coke fumes or gas (carbon monoxide)	T58.2X1	T58.2X2	T58.2X3	T58.2X4	—	—
industrial use	T58.8X1	T58.8X2	T58.8X3	T58.8X4		
Colace	T47.4X1	T47.4X2	T47.4X3	T47.4X4	T47.4X5	T47.4X6
Colaspase	T45.1X1	T45.1X2	T45.1X3	T45.1X4	T45.1X5	T45.1X6
Colchicine	T50.4X1	T50.4X2	T50.4X3	T50.4X4	T50.4X5	T50.4X6
Colchicum	T62.2X1	T62.2X2	T62.2X3	T62.2X4	—	—
Cold cream	T49.3X1	T49.3X2	T49.3X3	T49.3X4	T49.3X5	T49.3X6
Colecalciferol	T45.2X1	T45.2X2	T45.2X3	T45.2X4	T45.2X5	T45.2X6
Colestipol	T46.6X1	T46.6X2	T46.6X3	T46.6X4	T46.6X5	T46.6X6
Colestyramine	T46.6X1	T46.6X2	T46.6X3	T46.6X4	T46.6X5	T46.6X6
Colimycin	T36.8X1	T36.8X2	T36.8X3	T36.8X4	T36.8X5	T36.8X6
Colistimethate	T36.8X1	T36.8X2	T36.8X3	T36.8X4	T36.8X5	T36.8X6
Colistin	T36.8X1	T36.8X2	T36.8X3	T36.8X4	T36.8X5	T36.8X6
sulfate (eye preparation)	T49.5X1	T49.5X2	T49.5X3	T49.5X4	T49.5X5	T49.5X6
Collagen	T50.991	T50.992	T50.993	T50.994	T50.995	T50.996
Collagenase	T49.4X1	T49.4X2	T49.4X3	T49.4X4	T49.4X5	T49.4X6
Collodion	T49.3X1	T49.3X2	T49.3X3	T49.3X4	T49.3X5	T49.3X6
Colocynth	T47.2X1	T47.2X2	T47.2X3	T47.2X4	T47.2X5	T47.2X6
Colophony adhesive	T49.3X1	T49.3X2	T49.3X3	T49.3X4	T49.3X5	T49.3X6
Colorant — see also Dye	T50.991	T50.992	T50.993	T50.994	T50.995	T50.996
Coloring matter — see Dye(s)						
Combustion gas (after combustion) — see Carbon, monoxide						
prior to combustion	T59.891	T59.892	T59.893	T59.894	—	—
Compazine	T43.3X1	T43.3X2	T43.3X3	T43.3X4	T43.3X5	T43.3X6
Compound						
42 (warfarin)	T60.4X1	T60.4X2	T60.4X3	T60.4X4	—	—
269 (endrin)	T60.1X1	T60.1X2	T60.1X3	T60.1X4	—	—
497 (dieldrin)	T60.1X1	T60.1X2	T60.1X3	T60.1X4	—	—
1080 (sodium fluoroacetate)	T60.4X1	T60.4X2	T60.4X3	T60.4X4	—	—
3422 (parathion)	T60.0X1	T60.0X2	T60.0X3	T60.0X4	—	—
3911 (phorate)	T60.0X1	T60.0X2	T60.0X3	T60.0X4	—	—
3956 (toxaphene)	T60.1X1	T60.1X2	T60.1X3	T60.1X4	—	—
4049 (malathion)	T60.0X1	T60.0X2	T60.0X3	T60.0X4	—	—
4069 (malathion)	T60.0X1	T60.0X2	T60.0X3	T60.0X4	—	—
4124 (dicapthon)	T60.0X1	T60.0X2	T60.0X3	T60.0X4	—	—

◀ New ◀ Revised ~~deleted~~ Deleted

Substance	Poisoning, Accidental (Unintentional)	Poisoning, Intentional Self-Harm	Poisoning, Assault	Poisoning, Undetermined	Adverse Effect	Underdosing
Compound *(Continued)*						
E (cortisone)	T38.0X1	T38.0X2	T38.0X3	T38.0X4	T38.0X5	T38.0X6
F (hydrocortisone)	T38.0X1	T38.0X2	T38.0X3	T38.0X4	T38.0X5	T38.0X6
Congener, anabolic	T38.7X1	T38.7X2	T38.7X3	T38.7X4	T38.7X5	T38.7X6
Congo red	T50.8X1	T50.8X2	T50.8X3	T50.8X4	T50.8X5	T50.8X6
Coniine, conine	T62.2X1	T62.2X2	T62.2X3	T62.2X4	—	—
Conium (maculatum)	T62.2X1	T62.2X2	T62.2X3	T62.2X4	—	—
Conjugated estrogenic substances	T38.5X1	T38.5X2	T38.5X3	T38.5X4	T38.5X5	T38.5X6
Contac	T48.5X1	T48.5X2	T48.5X3	T48.5X4	T48.5X5	T48.5X6
Contact lens solution	T49.5X1	T49.5X2	T49.5X3	T49.5X4	T49.5X5	T49.5X6
Contraceptive (oral)	T38.4X1	T38.4X2	T38.4X3	T38.4X4	T38.4X5	T38.4X6
vaginal	T49.8X1	T49.8X2	T49.8X3	T49.8X4	T49.8X5	T49.8X6
Contrast medium, radiography	T50.8X1	T50.8X2	T50.8X3	T50.8X4	T50.8X5	T50.8X6
Convallaria glycosides	T46.0X1	T46.0X2	T46.0X3	T46.0X4	T46.0X5	T46.0X6
Convallaria majalis	T62.2X1	T62.2X2	T62.2X3	T62.2X4	—	—
berry	T62.1X1	T62.1X2	T62.1X3	T62.1X4	—	—
Copper (dust) (fumes) (nonmedicinal) NEC	T56.4X1	T56.4X2	T56.4X3	T56.4X4	—	—
arsenate, arsenite	T57.0X1	T57.0X2	T57.0X3	T57.0X4	—	—
insecticide	T60.2X1	T60.2X2	T60.2X3	T60.2X4	—	—
emetic	T47.7X1	T47.7X2	T47.7X3	T47.7X4	T47.7X5	T47.7X6
fungicide	T60.3X1	T60.3X2	T60.3X3	T60.3X4	—	—
gluconate	T49.0X1	T49.0X2	T49.0X3	T49.0X4	T49.0X5	T49.0X6
insecticide	T60.2X1	T60.2X2	T60.2X3	T60.2X4	—	—
medicinal (trace)	T45.8X1	T45.8X2	T45.8X3	T45.8X4	T45.8X5	T45.8X6
oleate	T49.0X1	T49.0X2	T49.0X3	T49.0X4	T49.0X5	T49.0X6
sulfate	T56.4X1	T56.4X2	T56.4X3	T56.4X4	—	—
cupric	T56.4X1	T56.4X2	T56.4X3	T56.4X4	—	—
fungicide	T60.3X1	T60.3X2	T60.3X3	T60.3X4	—	—
medicinal						
ear	T49.6X1	T49.6X2	T49.6X3	T49.6X4	T49.6X5	T49.6X6
emetic	T47.7X1	T47.7X2	T47.7X3	T47.7X4	T47.7X5	T47.7X6
eye	T49.5X1	T49.5X2	T49.5X3	T49.5X4	T49.5X5	T49.5X6
cuprous	T56.4X1	T56.4X2	T56.4X3	T56.4X4	—	—
fungicide	T60.3X1	T60.3X2	T60.3X3	T60.3X4	—	—
medicinal						
ear	T49.6X1	T49.6X2	T49.6X3	T49.6X4	T49.6X5	T49.6X6
emetic	T47.7X1	T47.7X2	T47.7X3	T47.7X4	T47.7X5	T47.7X6
eye	T49.5X1	T49.5X2	T49.5X3	T49.5X4	T49.5X5	T49.5X6
Copperhead snake (bite) (venom)	T63.061	T63.062	T63.063	T63.064	—	—
Coral (sting)	T63.691	T63.692	T63.693	T63.694	—	—
snake (bite) (venom)	T63.021	T63.022	T63.023	T63.024	—	—

Substance	Poisoning, Accidental (Unintentional)	Poisoning, Intentional Self-Harm	Poisoning, Assault	Poisoning, Undetermined	Adverse Effect	Underdosing
Corbadrine	T49.6X1	T49.6X2	T49.6X3	T49.6X4	T49.6X5	T49.6X6
Cordran	T49.0X1	T49.0X2	T49.0X3	T49.0X4	T49.0X5	T49.0X6
Cordite	T65.891	T65.892	T65.893	T65.894	—	—
vapor	T59.891	T59.892	T59.893	T59.894	—	—
Corn cures	T49.4X1	T49.4X2	T49.4X3	T49.4X4	T49.4X5	T49.4X6
Cornhusker's lotion	T49.3X1	T49.3X2	T49.3X3	T49.3X4	T49.3X5	T49.3X6
Corn starch	T49.3X1	T49.3X2	T49.3X3	T49.3X4	T49.3X5	T49.3X6
Coronary vasodilator NEC	T46.3X1	T46.3X2	T46.3X3	T46.3X4	T46.3X5	T46.3X6
Corrosive NEC	T54.91	T54.92	T54.93	T54.94	—	—
acid NEC	T54.2X1	T54.2X2	T54.2X3	T54.2X4	—	—
aromatics	T54.1X1	T54.1X2	T54.1X3	T54.1X4	—	—
disinfectant	T54.1X1	T54.1X2	T54.1X3	T54.1X4	—	—
fumes NEC	T54.91	T54.92	T54.93	T54.94	—	—
specified NEC	T54.91	T54.92	T54.93	T54.94	—	—
sublimate	T56.1X1	T56.1X2	T56.1X3	T56.1X4	—	—
Cortate	T38.0X1	T38.0X2	T38.0X3	T38.0X4	T38.0X5	T38.0X6
Cort-Dome	T38.0X1	T38.0X2	T38.0X3	T38.0X4	T38.0X5	T38.0X6
ENT agent	T49.6X1	T49.6X2	T49.6X3	T49.6X4	T49.6X5	T49.6X6
ophthalmic preparation	T49.5X1	T49.5X2	T49.5X3	T49.5X4	T49.5X5	T49.5X6
topical NEC	T49.0X1	T49.0X2	T49.0X3	T49.0X4	T49.0X5	T49.0X6
Cortef	T38.0X1	T38.0X2	T38.0X3	T38.0X4	T38.0X5	T38.0X6
ENT agent	T49.6X1	T49.6X2	T49.6X3	T49.6X4	T49.6X5	T49.6X6
ophthalmic preparation	T49.5X1	T49.5X2	T49.5X3	T49.5X4	T49.5X5	T49.5X6
topical NEC	T49.0X1	T49.0X2	T49.0X3	T49.0X4	T49.0X5	T49.0X6
Corticosteroid	T38.0X1	T38.0X2	T38.0X3	T38.0X4	T38.0X5	T38.0X6
ENT agent	T49.6X1	T49.6X2	T49.6X3	T49.6X4	T49.6X5	T49.6X6
mineral	T50.0X1	T50.0X2	T50.0X3	T50.0X4	T50.0X5	T50.0X6
ophthalmic	T49.5X1	T49.5X2	T49.5X3	T49.5X4	T49.5X5	T49.5X6
topical NEC	T49.0X1	T49.0X2	T49.0X3	T49.0X4	T49.0X5	T49.0X6
Corticotropin	T38.811	T38.812	T38.813	T38.814	T38.815	T38.816
Cortisol	T49.0X1	T49.0X2	T49.0X3	T49.0X4	T49.0X5	T49.0X6
ENT agent	T49.6X1	T49.6X2	T49.6X3	T49.6X4	T49.6X5	T49.6X6
ophthalmic preparation	T49.5X1	T49.5X2	T49.5X3	T49.5X4	T49.5X5	T49.5X6
topical NEC	T49.0X1	T49.0X2	T49.0X3	T49.0X4	T49.0X5	T49.0X6
Cortisone (acetate)	T38.0X1	T38.0X2	T38.0X3	T38.0X4	T38.0X5	T38.0X6
ENT agent	T49.6X1	T49.6X2	T49.6X3	T49.6X4	T49.6X5	T49.6X6
ophthalmic preparation	T49.5X1	T49.5X2	T49.5X3	T49.5X4	T49.5X5	T49.5X6
topical NEC	T49.0X1	T49.0X2	T49.0X3	T49.0X4	T49.0X5	T49.0X6
Cortivazol	T38.0X1	T38.0X2	T38.0X3	T38.0X4	T38.0X5	T38.0X6
Cortogen	T38.0X1	T38.0X2	T38.0X3	T38.0X4	T38.0X5	T38.0X6
ENT agent	T49.6X1	T49.6X2	T49.6X3	T49.6X4	T49.6X5	T49.6X6
ophthalmic preparation	T49.5X1	T49.5X2	T49.5X3	T49.5X4	T49.5X5	T49.5X6

◀ New   ◀ Revised   ~~deleted~~ Deleted

TABLE OF DRUGS AND CHEMICALS

Substance	Poisoning, Accidental (Unintentional)	Poisoning, Intentional Self-Harm	Poisoning, Assault	Poisoning, Undetermined	Adverse Effect	Underdosing
	External Cause (T-Code)					
Cortone	T38.0X1	T38.0X2	T38.0X3	T38.0X4	T38.0X5	T38.0X6
ENT agent	T49.6X1	T49.6X2	T49.6X3	T49.6X4	T49.6X5	T49.6X6
ophthalmic preparation	T49.5X1	T49.5X2	T49.5X3	T49.5X4	T49.5X5	T49.5X6
Cortril	T38.0X1	T38.0X2	T38.0X3	T38.0X4	T38.0X5	T38.0X6
ENT agent	T49.6X1	T49.6X2	T49.6X3	T49.6X4	T49.6X5	T49.6X6
ophthalmic preparation	T49.5X1	T49.5X2	T49.5X3	T49.5X4	T49.5X5	T49.5X6
topical NEC	T49.0X1	T49.0X2	T49.0X3	T49.0X4	T49.0X5	T49.0X6
Corynebacterium parvum	T45.1X1	T45.1X2	T45.1X3	T45.1X4	T45.1X5	T45.1X6
Cosmetic preparation	T49.8X1	T49.8X2	T49.8X3	T49.8X4	T49.8X5	T49.8X6
Cosmetics	T49.8X1	T49.8X2	T49.8X3	T49.8X4	T49.8X5	T49.8X6
Cosyntropin	T38.811	T38.812	T38.813	T38.814	T38.815	T38.816
Cotarnine	T45.7X1	T45.7X2	T45.7X3	T45.7X4	T45.7X5	T45.7X6
Co-trimoxazole	T36.8X1	T36.8X2	T36.8X3	T36.8X4	T36.8X5	T36.8X6
Cottonseed oil	T49.3X1	T49.3X2	T49.3X3	T49.3X4	T49.3X5	T49.3X6
Cough mixture (syrup)	T48.4X1	T48.4X2	T48.4X3	T48.4X4	T48.4X5	T48.4X6
containing opiates	T40.2X1	T40.2X2	T40.2X3	T40.2X4	T40.2X5	T40.2X6
expectorants	T48.4X1	T48.4X2	T48.4X3	T48.4X4	T48.4X5	T48.4X6
Coumadin	T45.511	T45.512	T45.513	T45.514	T45.515	T45.516
rodenticide	T60.4X1	T60.4X2	T60.4X3	T60.4X4	—	—
Coumaphos	T60.0X1	T60.0X2	T60.0X3	T60.0X4	—	—
Coumarin	T45.511	T45.512	T45.513	T45.514	T45.515	T45.516
Coumetarol	T45.511	T45.512	T45.513	T45.514	T45.515	T45.516
Cowbane	T62.2X1	T62.2X2	T62.2X3	T62.2X4	—	—
Cozyme	T45.2X1	T45.2X2	T45.2X3	T45.2X4	T45.2X5	T45.2X6
Crack	T40.5X1	T40.5X2	T40.5X3	T40.5X4		
Crataegus extract	T46.0X1	T46.0X2	T46.0X3	T46.0X4	T46.0X5	T46.0X6
Creolin	T54.1X1	T54.1X2	T54.1X3	T54.1X4		
disinfectant	T54.1X1	T54.1X2	T54.1X3	T54.1X4	—	—
Creosol (compound)	T49.0X1	T49.0X2	T49.0X3	T49.0X4	T49.0X5	T49.0X6
Creosote (coal tar) (beechwood)	T49.0X1	T49.0X2	T49.0X3	T49.0X4	T49.0X5	T49.0X6
medicinal (expectorant)	T48.4X1	T48.4X2	T48.4X3	T48.4X4	T48.4X5	T48.4X6
syrup	T48.4X1	T48.4X2	T48.4X3	T48.4X4	T48.4X5	T48.4X6
Cresol(s)	T49.0X1	T49.0X2	T49.0X3	T49.0X4	T49.0X5	T49.0X6
and soap solution	T49.0X1	T49.0X2	T49.0X3	T49.0X4	T49.0X5	T49.0X6
Cresyl acetate	T49.0X1	T49.0X2	T49.0X3	T49.0X4	T49.0X5	T49.0X6
Cresylic acid	T49.0X1	T49.0X2	T49.0X3	T49.0X4	T49.0X5	T49.0X6
Crimidine	T60.4X1	T60.4X2	T60.4X3	T60.4X4	—	—
Croconazole	T37.8X1	T37.8X2	T37.8X3	T37.8X4	T37.8X5	T37.8X6
Cromoglicic acid	T48.6X1	T48.6X2	T48.6X3	T48.6X4	T48.6X5	T48.6X6
Cromolyn	T48.6X1	T48.6X2	T48.6X3	T48.6X4	T48.6X5	T48.6X6
Cromonar	T46.3X1	T46.3X2	T46.3X3	T46.3X4	T46.3X5	T46.3X6

Substance	Poisoning, Accidental (Unintentional)	Poisoning, Intentional Self-Harm	Poisoning, Assault	Poisoning, Undetermined	Adverse Effect	Underdosing
	External Cause (T-Code)					
Cropropamide	T39.8X1	T39.8X2	T39.8X3	T39.8X4	T39.8X5	T39.8X6
with crotethamide	T50.7X1	T50.7X2	T50.7X3	T50.7X4	T50.7X5	T50.7X6
Crotamiton	T49.0X1	T49.0X2	T49.0X3	T49.0X4	T49.0X5	T49.0X6
Crotethamide	T39.8X1	T39.8X2	T39.8X3	T39.8X4	T39.8X5	T39.8X6
with cropropamide	T50.7X1	T50.7X2	T50.7X3	T50.7X4	T50.7X5	T50.7X6
Croton (oil)	T47.2X1	T47.2X2	T47.2X3	T47.2X4	T47.2X5	T47.2X6
chloral	T42.6X1	T42.6X2	T42.6X3	T42.6X4	T42.6X5	T42.6X6
Crude oil	T52.0X1	T52.0X2	T52.0X3	T52.0X4	—	—
Cryogenine	T39.8X1	T39.8X2	T39.8X3	T39.8X4	T39.8X5	T39.8X6
Cryolite (vapor)	T60.1X1	T60.1X2	T60.1X3	T60.1X4	—	—
insecticide	T60.1X1	T60.1X2	T60.1X3	T60.1X4	—	—
Cryptenamine (tannates)	T46.5X1	T46.5X2	T46.5X3	T46.5X4	T46.5X5	T46.5X6
Crystal violet	T49.0X1	T49.0X2	T49.0X3	T49.0X4	T49.0X5	T49.0X6
Cuckoopint	T62.2X1	T62.2X2	T62.2X3	T62.2X4	—	—
Cumetharol	T45.511	T45.512	T45.513	T45.514	T45.515	T45.516
Cupric						
acetate	T60.3X1	T60.3X2	T60.3X3	T60.3X4	—	—
acetoarsenite	T57.0X1	T57.0X2	T57.0X3	T57.0X4	—	—
arsenate	T57.0X1	T57.0X2	T57.0X3	T57.0X4	—	—
gluconate	T49.0X1	T49.0X2	T49.0X3	T49.0X4	T49.0X5	T49.0X6
oleate	T49.0X1	T49.0X2	T49.0X3	T49.0X4	T49.0X5	T49.0X6
sulfate	T56.4X1	T56.4X2	T56.4X3	T56.4X4	—	—
Cuprous sulfate — see also Copper, sulfate	T56.4X1	T56.4X2	T56.4X3	T56.4X4	—	—
Curare, curarine	T48.1X1	T48.1X2	T48.1X3	T48.1X4	T48.1X5	T48.1X6
Cyamemazine	T43.3X1	T43.3X2	T43.3X3	T43.3X4	T43.3X5	T43.3X6
Cyamopsis tetragono-loba	T46.6X1	T46.6X2	T46.6X3	T46.6X4	T46.6X5	T46.6X6
Cyanacetyl hydrazide	T37.1X1	T37.1X2	T37.1X3	T37.1X4	T37.1X5	T37.1X6
Cyanic acid (gas)	T59.891	T59.892	T59.893	T59.894	—	—
Cyanide(s) (compounds) (potassium) (sodium) NEC	T65.0X1	T65.0X2	T65.0X3	T65.0X4	—	—
dust or gas (inhalation) NEC	T57.3X1	T57.3X2	T57.3X3	T57.3X4	—	—
fumigant	T65.0X1	T65.0X2	T65.0X3	T65.0X4	—	—
hydrogen	T57.3X1	T57.3X2	T57.3X3	T57.3X4	—	—
mercuric — see Mercury						
pesticide (dust) (fumes)	T65.0X1	T65.0X2	T65.0X3	T65.0X4	—	—
Cyanoacrylate adhesive	T49.3X1	T49.3X2	T49.3X3	T49.3X4	T49.3X5	T49.3X6
Cyanocobalamin	T45.8X1	T45.8X2	T45.8X3	T45.8X4	T45.8X5	T45.8X6
Cyanogen (chloride) (gas) NEC	T59.891	T59.892	T59.893	T59.894	—	—
Cyclacillin	T36.0X1	T36.0X2	T36.0X3	T36.0X4	T36.0X5	T36.0X6
Cyclaine	T41.3X1	T41.3X2	T41.3X3	T41.3X4	T41.3X5	T41.3X6
Cyclamate	T50.991	T50.992	T50.993	T50.994	T50.995	T50.996

◀ New   ◀ Revised   ~~deleted~~ Deleted

	External Cause (T-Code)					
Substance	Poisoning, Accidental (Unintentional)	Poisoning, Intentional Self-Harm	Poisoning, Assault	Poisoning, Undetermined	Adverse Effect	Underdosing
Cyclamen europaeum	T62.2X1	T62.2X2	T62.2X3	T62.2X4	—	—
Cyclandelate	T46.7X1	T46.7X2	T46.7X3	T46.7X4	T46.7X5	T46.7X6
Cyclazocine	T50.7X1	T50.7X2	T50.7X3	T50.7X4	T50.7X5	T50.7X6
Cyclizine	T45.0X1	T45.0X2	T45.0X3	T45.0X4	T45.0X5	T45.0X6
Cyclobarbital	T42.3X1	T42.3X2	T42.3X3	T42.3X4	T42.3X5	T42.3X6
Cyclobarbitone	T42.3X1	T42.3X2	T42.3X3	T42.3X4	T42.3X5	T42.3X6
Cyclobenzaprine	T48.1X1	T48.1X2	T48.1X3	T48.1X4	T48.1X5	T48.1X6
Cyclodrine	T44.3X1	T44.3X2	T44.3X3	T44.3X4	T44.3X5	T44.3X6
Cycloguanil embonate	T37.2X1	T37.2X2	T37.2X3	T37.2X4	T37.2X5	T37.2X6
Cycloheptadiene	T43.291	T43.292	T43.293	T43.294	T43.295	T43.296
Cyclohexane	T52.8X1	T52.8X2	T52.8X3	T52.8X4	—	—
Cyclohexanol	T51.8X1	T51.8X2	T51.8X3	T51.8X4	—	—
Cyclohexanone	T52.4X1	T52.4X2	T52.4X3	T52.4X4	—	—
Cycloheximide	T60.3X1	T60.3X2	T60.3X3	T60.3X4	—	—
Cyclohexyl acetate	T52.8X1	T52.8X2	T52.8X3	T52.8X4	—	—
Cycloleucin	T45.1X1	T45.1X2	T45.1X3	T45.1X4	T45.1X5	T45.1X6
Cyclomethycaine	T41.3X1	T41.3X2	T41.3X3	T41.3X4	T41.3X5	T41.3X6
Cyclopentamine	T44.4X1	T44.4X2	T44.4X3	T44.4X4	T44.4X5	T44.4X6
Cyclopenthiazide	T50.2X1	T50.2X2	T50.2X3	T50.2X4	T50.2X5	T50.2X6
Cyclopentolate	T44.3X1	T44.3X2	T44.3X3	T44.3X4	T44.3X5	T44.3X6
Cyclophosphamide	T45.1X1	T45.1X2	T45.1X3	T45.1X4	T45.1X5	T45.1X6
Cycloplegic drug	T49.5X1	T49.5X2	T49.5X3	T49.5X4	T49.5X5	T49.5X6
Cyclopropane	T41.291	T41.292	T41.293	T41.294	T41.295	T41.296
Cyclopyrabital	T39.8X1	T39.8X2	T39.8X3	T39.8X4	T39.8X5	T39.8X6
Cycloserine	T37.1X1	T37.1X2	T37.1X3	T37.1X4	T37.1X5	T37.1X6
Cyclosporin	T45.1X1	T45.1X2	T45.1X3	T45.1X4	T45.1X5	T45.1X6
Cyclothiazide	T50.2X1	T50.2X2	T50.2X3	T50.2X4	T50.2X5	T50.2X6
Cycrimine	T44.3X1	T44.3X2	T44.3X3	T44.3X4	T44.3X5	T44.3X6
Cyhalothrin	T60.1X1	T60.1X2	T60.1X3	T60.1X4	—	—
Cymarin	T46.0X1	T46.0X2	T46.0X3	T46.0X4	T46.0X5	T46.0X6
Cypermethrin	T60.1X1	T60.1X2	T60.1X3	T60.1X4	—	—
Cyphenothrin	T60.2X1	T60.2X2	T60.2X3	T60.2X4	—	—
Cyproheptadine	T45.0X1	T45.0X2	T45.0X3	T45.0X4	T45.0X5	T45.0X6
Cyprolidol	T43.291	T43.292	T43.293	T43.294	T43.295	T43.296
Cyproterone	T38.6X1	T38.6X2	T38.6X3	T38.6X4	T38.6X5	T38.6X6
Cysteamine	T50.6X1	T50.6X2	T50.6X3	T50.6X4	T50.6X5	T50.6X6
Cytarabine	T45.1X1	T45.1X2	T45.1X3	T45.1X4	T45.1X5	T45.1X6
Cytisus						
laburnum	T62.2X1	T62.2X2	T62.2X3	T62.2X4	—	—
scoparius	T62.2X1	T62.2X2	T62.2X3	T62.2X4	—	—
Cytochrome C	T47.5X1	T47.5X2	T47.5X3	T47.5X4	T47.5X5	T47.5X6
Cytomel	T38.1X1	T38.1X2	T38.1X3	T38.1X4	T38.1X5	T38.1X6

	External Cause (T-Code)					
Substance	Poisoning, Accidental (Unintentional)	Poisoning, Intentional Self-Harm	Poisoning, Assault	Poisoning, Undetermined	Adverse Effect	Underdosing
Cytosine arabinoside	T45.1X1	T45.1X2	T45.1X3	T45.1X4	T45.1X5	T45.1X6
Cytoxan	T45.1X1	T45.1X2	T45.1X3	T45.1X4	T45.1X5	T45.1X6
Cytozyme	T45.7X1	T45.7X2	T45.7X3	T45.7X4	T45.7X5	T45.7X6
2,4-D	T60.3X1	T60.3X2	T60.3X3	T60.3X4	—	—
D						
Dacarbazine	T45.1X1	T45.1X2	T45.1X3	T45.1X4	T45.1X5	T45.1X6
Dactinomycin	T45.1X1	T45.1X2	T45.1X3	T45.1X4	T45.1X5	T45.1X6
DADPS	T37.1X1	T37.1X2	T37.1X3	T37.1X4	T37.1X5	T37.1X6
Dakin's solution	T49.0X1	T49.0X2	T49.0X3	T49.0X4	T49.0X5	T49.0X6
Dalapon (sodium)	T60.3X1	T60.3X2	T60.3X3	T60.3X4	—	—
Dalmane	T42.4X1	T42.4X2	T42.4X3	T42.4X4	T42.4X5	T42.4X6
Danazol	T38.6X1	T38.6X2	T38.6X3	T38.6X4	T38.6X5	T38.6X6
Danilone	T45.511	T45.512	T45.513	T45.514	T45.515	T45.516
Danthron	T47.2X1	T47.2X2	T47.2X3	T47.2X4	T47.2X5	T47.2X6
Dantrolene	T42.8X1	T42.8X2	T42.8X3	T42.8X4	T42.8X5	T42.8X6
Dantron	T47.2X1	T47.2X2	T47.2X3	T47.2X4	T47.2X5	T47.2X6
Daphne (gnidium) (mezereum)	T62.2X1	T62.2X2	T62.2X3	T62.2X4	—	—
berry	T62.1X1	T62.1X2	T62.1X3	T62.1X4		
Dapsone	T37.1X1	T37.1X2	T37.1X3	T37.1X4	T37.1X5	T37.1X6
Daraprim	T37.2X1	T37.2X2	T37.2X3	T37.2X4	T37.2X5	T37.2X6
Darnel	T62.2X1	T62.2X2	T62.2X3	T62.2X4	—	—
Darvon	T39.8X1	T39.8X2	T39.8X3	T39.8X4	T39.8X5	T39.8X6
Daunomycin	T45.1X1	T45.1X2	T45.1X3	T45.1X4	T45.1X5	T45.1X6
Daunorubicin	T45.1X1	T45.1X2	T45.1X3	T45.1X4	T45.1X5	T45.1X6
DBI	T38.3X1	T38.3X2	T38.3X3	T38.3X4	T38.3X5	T38.3X6
D-Con	T60.91	T60.92	T60.93	T60.94	—	—
insecticide	T60.2X1	T60.2X2	T60.2X3	T60.2X4	—	—
rodenticide	T60.4X1	T60.4X2	T60.4X3	T60.4X4	—	—
DDAVP	T38.891	T38.892	T38.893	T38.894	T38.895	T38.896
DDE (bis(chlorophenyl)-dichloroethylene)	T60.2X1	T60.2X2	T60.2X3	T60.2X4	—	—
DDS	T37.1X1	T37.1X2	T37.1X3	T37.1X4	T37.1X5	T37.1X6
DDT (dust)	T60.1X1	T60.1X2	T60.1X3	T60.1X4	—	—
Deadly nightshade—*see also* Belladonna	T62.2X1	T62.2X2	T62.2X3	T62.2X4	—	—
berry	T62.1X1	T62.1X2	T62.1X3	T62.1X4		
Deamino-D-arginine vasopressin	T38.891	T38.892	T38.893	T38.894	T38.895	T38.896
Deanol (aceglumate)	T50.991	T50.992	T50.993	T50.994	T50.995	T50.996
Debrisoquine	T46.5X1	T46.5X2	T46.5X3	T46.5X4	T46.5X5	T46.5X6
Decaborane	T57.8X1	T57.8X2	T57.8X3	T57.8X4	—	—
fumes	T59.891	T59.892	T59.893	T59.894	—	—

◀ New   ◀ Revised   ~~deleted~~ Deleted

TABLE OF DRUGS AND CHEMICALS

Substance	External Cause (T-Code)					
	Poisoning, Accidental (Unintentional)	Poisoning, Intentional Self-Harm	Poisoning, Assault	Poisoning, Undetermined	Adverse Effect	Underdosing
Decadron	T38.0X1	T38.0X2	T38.0X3	T38.0X4	T38.0X5	T38.0X6
ENT agent	T49.6X1	T49.6X2	T49.6X3	T49.6X4	T49.6X5	T49.6X6
ophthalmic preparation	T49.5X1	T49.5X2	T49.5X3	T49.5X4	T49.5X5	T49.5X6
topical NEC	T49.0X1	T49.0X2	T49.0X3	T49.0X4	T49.0X5	T49.0X6
Decahydronaphthalene	T52.8X1	T52.8X2	T52.8X3	T52.8X4	—	—
Decalin	T52.8X1	T52.8X2	T52.8X3	T52.8X4	—	—
Decamethonium (bromide)	T48.1X1	T48.1X2	T48.1X3	T48.1X4	T48.1X5	T48.1X6
Decholin	T47.5X1	T47.5X2	T47.5X3	T47.5X4	T47.5X5	T47.5X6
Declomycin	T36.4X1	T36.4X2	T36.4X3	T36.4X4	T36.4X5	T36.4X6
Decongestant, nasal (mucosa)	T48.5X1	T48.5X2	T48.5X3	T48.5X4	T48.5X5	T48.5X6
combination	T48.5X1	T48.5X2	T48.5X3	T48.5X4	T48.5X5	T48.5X6
Deet	T60.8X1	T60.8X2	T60.8X3	T60.8X4	—	—
Deferoxamine	T45.8X1	T45.8X2	T45.8X3	T45.8X4	T45.8X5	T45.8X6
Deflazacort	T38.0X1	T38.0X2	T38.0X3	T38.0X4	T38.0X5	T38.0X6
Deglycyrrhizinized extract of licorice	T48.4X1	T48.4X2	T48.4X3	T48.4X4	T48.4X5	T48.4X6
Dehydrocholic acid	T47.5X1	T47.5X2	T47.5X3	T47.5X4	T47.5X5	T47.5X6
Dehydroemetine	T37.3X1	T37.3X2	T37.3X3	T37.3X4	T37.3X5	T37.3X6
Dekalin	T52.8X1	T52.8X2	T52.8X3	T52.8X4	—	—
Delalutin	T38.5X1	T38.5X2	T38.5X3	T38.5X4	T38.5X5	T38.5X6
Delphinium	T62.2X1	T62.2X2	T62.2X3	T62.2X4	—	—
Deltasone	T38.0X1	T38.0X2	T38.0X3	T38.0X4	T38.0X5	T38.0X6
Deltra	T38.0X1	T38.0X2	T38.0X3	T38.0X4	T38.0X5	T38.0X6
Delvinal	T42.3X1	T42.3X2	T42.3X3	T42.3X4	T42.3X5	T42.3X6
Delorazepam	T42.4X1	T42.4X2	T42.4X3	T42.4X4	T42.4X5	T42.4X6
Deltamethrin	T60.1X1	T60.1X2	T60.1X3	T60.1X4	—	—
Demecarium (bromide)	T49.5X1	T49.5X2	T49.5X3	T49.5X4	T49.5X5	T49.5X6
Demeclocycline	T36.4X1	T36.4X2	T36.4X3	T36.4X4	T36.4X5	T36.4X6
Demecolcine	T45.1X1	T45.1X2	T45.1X3	T45.1X4	T45.1X5	T45.1X6
Demegestone	T38.5X1	T38.5X2	T38.5X3	T38.5X4	T38.5X5	T38.5X6
Demelanizing agents	T49.8X1	T49.8X2	T49.8X3	T49.8X4	T49.8X5	T49.8X6
Demephion -O and -S	T60.0X1	T60.0X2	T60.0X3	T60.0X4	—	—
Demerol	T40.2X1	T40.2X2	T40.2X3	T40.2X4	T40.2X5	T40.2X6
Demethylchlortetracycline	T36.4X1	T36.4X2	T36.4X3	T36.4X4	T36.4X5	T36.4X6
Demethyltetracycline	T36.4X1	T36.4X2	T36.4X3	T36.4X4	T36.4X5	T36.4X6
Demeton -O and -S	T60.0X1	T60.0X2	T60.0X3	T60.0X4	—	—
Demulcent (external)	T49.3X1	T49.3X2	T49.3X3	T49.3X4	T49.3X5	T49.3X6
specified NEC	T49.3X1	T49.3X2	T49.3X3	T49.3X4	T49.3X5	T49.3X6
Demulen	T38.4X1	T38.4X2	T38.4X3	T38.4X4	T38.4X5	T38.4X6
Denatured alcohol	T51.0X1	T51.0X2	T51.0X3	T51.0X4	—	—
Dendrid	T49.5X1	T49.5X2	T49.5X3	T49.5X4	T49.5X5	T49.5X6
Dental drug, topical application NEC	T49.7X1	T49.7X2	T49.7X3	T49.7X4	T49.7X5	T49.7X6

Substance	External Cause (T-Code)					
	Poisoning, Accidental (Unintentional)	Poisoning, Intentional Self-Harm	Poisoning, Assault	Poisoning, Undetermined	Adverse Effect	Underdosing
Dentifrice	T49.7X1	T49.7X2	T49.7X3	T49.7X4	T49.7X5	T49.7X6
Deodorant spray (feminine hygiene)	T49.8X1	T49.8X2	T49.8X3	T49.8X4	T49.8X5	T49.8X6
Deoxycortone	T50.0X1	T50.0X2	T50.0X3	T50.0X4	T50.0X5	T50.0X6
2-Deoxy-5-fluorouridine	T45.1X1	T45.1X2	T45.1X3	T45.1X4	T45.1X5	T45.1X6
5-Deoxy-5-fluorouridine	T45.1X1	T45.1X2	T45.1X3	T45.1X4	T45.1X5	T45.1X6
Deoxyribonuclease (pancreatic)	T45.3X1	T45.3X2	T45.3X3	T45.3X4	T45.3X5	T45.3X6
Depilatory	T49.4X1	T49.4X2	T49.4X3	T49.4X4	T49.4X5	T49.4X6
Deprenalin	T42.8X1	T42.8X2	T42.8X3	T42.8X4	T42.8X5	T42.8X6
Deprenyl	T42.8X1	T42.8X2	T42.8X3	T42.8X4	T42.8X5	T42.8X6
Depressant, appetite	T50.5X1	T50.5X2	T50.5X3	T50.5X4	T50.5X5	T50.5X6
Depressant						
appetite, central	T50.5X1	T50.5X2	T50.5X3	T50.5X4	T50.5X5	T50.5X6
cardiac	T46.2X1	T46.2X2	T46.2X3	T46.2X4	T46.2X5	T46.2X6
central nervous system (anesthetic) — see also Central nervous system, depressants	T42.71	T42.72	T42.73	T42.74	T42.75	T42.76
general anesthetic	T41.201	T41.202	T41.203	T41.204	T41.205	T41.206
muscle tone	T42.8X1	T42.8X2	T42.8X3	T42.8X4	T42.8X5	T42.8X6
muscle tone, central	T42.8X1	T42.8X2	T42.8X3	T42.8X4	T42.8X5	T42.8X6
psychotherapeutic	T43.501	T43.502	T43.503	T43.504	T43.505	T43.506
Deptropine	T45.0X1	T45.0X2	T45.0X3	T45.0X4	T45.0X5	T45.0X6
Dequalinium (chloride)	T49.0X1	T49.0X2	T49.0X3	T49.0X4	T49.0X5	T49.0X6
Derris root	T60.2X1	T60.2X2	T60.2X3	T60.2X4	—	—
Deserpidine	T43.011	T43.012	T43.013	T43.014	T43.015	T43.016
Desferrioxamine	T45.8X1	T45.8X2	T45.8X3	T45.8X4	T45.8X5	T45.8X6
Desipramine	T43.0X1	T43.0X2	T43.0X3	T43.0X4	T43.0X5	T43.0X6
Deslanoside	T46.0X1	T46.0X2	T46.0X3	T46.0X4	T46.0X5	T46.0X6
Desloughing agent	T49.4X1	T49.4X2	T49.4X3	T49.4X4	T49.4X5	T49.4X6
Desmethylimipramine	T43.011	T43.012	T43.013	T43.014	T43.015	T43.016
Desmopressin	T38.891	T38.892	T38.893	T38.894	T38.895	T38.896
Desocodeine	T40.2X1	T40.2X2	T40.2X3	T40.2X4	T40.2X5	T40.2X6
Desogestrel	T38.5X1	T38.5X2	T38.5X3	T38.5X4	T38.5X5	T38.5X6
Desomorphine	T40.2X1	T40.2X2	T40.2X3	T40.2X4	—	—
Desonide	T49.0X1	T49.0X2	T49.0X3	T49.0X4	T49.0X5	T49.0X6
Desoximetasone	T49.0X1	T49.0X2	T49.0X3	T49.0X4	T49.0X5	T49.0X6
Desoxycorticosteroid	T50.0X1	T50.0X2	T50.0X3	T50.0X4	T50.0X5	T50.0X6
Desoxycortone	T50.0X1	T50.0X2	T50.0X3	T50.0X4	T50.0X5	T50.0X6
Desoxyephedrine	T43.651	T43.652	T43.652	T43.654	T43.655	T43.656
Detaxtran	T46.6X1	T46.6X2	T46.6X3	T46.6X4	T46.6X5	T46.6X6
Detergent	T49.2X1	T49.2X2	T49.2X3	T49.2X4	T49.2X5	T49.2X6
external medication	T49.2X1	T49.2X2	T49.2X3	T49.2X4	T49.2X5	T49.2X6
local	T49.2X1	T49.2X2	T49.2X3	T49.2X4	T49.2X5	T49.2X6

◀ New ◀ Revised ~~deleted~~ Deleted

	External Cause (T-Code)					
Substance	Poisoning, Accidental (Unintentional)	Poisoning, Intentional Self-Harm	Poisoning, Assault	Poisoning, Undetermined	Adverse Effect	Underdosing
Detergent *(Continued)*						
medicinal	T49.2X1	T49.2X2	T49.2X3	T49.2X4	T49.2X5	T49.2X6
nonmedicinal	T55.1X1	T55.1X2	T55.1X3	T55.1X4	—	—
specified NEC	T55.1X1	T55.1X2	T55.1X3	T55.1X4	T55.1X5	T55.1X6
Deterrent, alcohol	T50.6X1	T50.6X2	T50.6X3	T50.6X4	T50.6X5	T50.6X6
Detoxifying agent	T50.6X1	T50.6X2	T50.6X3	T50.6X4	T50.6X5	T50.6X6
Detrothyronine	T38.1X1	T38.1X2	T38.1X3	T38.1X4	T38.1X5	T38.1X6
Dettol (external medication)	T49.0X1	T49.0X2	T49.0X3	T49.0X4	T49.0X5	T49.0X6
Dexamethasone	T38.0X1	T38.0X2	T38.0X3	T38.0X4	T38.0X5	T38.0X6
ENT agent	T49.6X1	T49.6X2	T49.6X3	T49.6X4	T49.6X5	T49.6X6
ophthalmic preparation	T49.5X1	T49.5X2	T49.5X3	T49.5X4	T49.5X5	T49.5X6
topical NEC	T49.0X1	T49.0X2	T49.0X3	T49.0X4	T49.0X5	T49.0X6
Dexamfetamine	T43.621	T43.622	T43.623	T43.624	T43.625	T43.626
Dexamphetamine	T43.621	T43.622	T43.623	T43.624	T43.625	T43.626
Dexbrompheniramine	T45.0X1	T45.0X2	T45.0X3	T45.0X4	T45.0X5	T45.0X6
Dexchlorpheniramine	T45.0X1	T45.0X2	T45.0X3	T45.0X4	T45.0X5	T45.0X6
Dexedrine	T43.621	T43.622	T43.623	T43.624	T43.625	T43.626
Dexetimide	T44.3X1	T44.3X2	T44.3X3	T44.3X4	T44.3X5	T44.3X6
Dexfenfluramine	T50.5X1	T50.5X2	T50.5X3	T50.5X4	T50.5X5	T50.5X6
Dexpanthenol	T45.2X1	T45.2X2	T45.2X3	T45.2X4	T45.2X5	T45.2X6
Dextran (40) (70) (150)	T45.8X1	T45.8X2	T45.8X3	T45.8X4	T45.8X5	T45.8X6
Dextriferron	T45.4X1	T45.4X2	T45.4X3	T45.4X4	T45.4X5	T45.4X6
Dextroamphetamine	T43.621	T43.622	T43.623	T43.624	T43.625	T43.626
Dextro calcium pantothenate	T45.2X1	T45.2X2	T45.2X3	T45.2X4	T45.2X5	T45.2X6
Dextromethorphan	T48.3X1	T48.3X2	T48.3X3	T48.3X4	T48.3X5	T48.3X6
Dextromoramide	T40.491	T40.492	T40.493	T40.494	—	—
topical	T49.8X1	T49.8X2	T49.8X3	T49.8X4	T49.8X5	T49.8X6
Dextro pantothenyl alcohol	T45.2X1	T45.2X2	T45.2X3	T45.2X4	T45.2X5	T45.2X6
Dextropropoxyphene	T40.491	T40.492	T40.493	T40.494	T40.495	T40.496
Dextrorphan	T40.2X1	T40.2X2	T40.2X3	T40.2X4	T40.2X5	T40.2X6
Dextrose	T50.3X1	T50.3X2	T50.3X3	T50.3X4	T50.3X5	T50.3X6
concentrated solution, intravenous	T46.8X1	T46.8X2	T46.8X3	T46.8X4	T46.8X5	T46.8X6
Dextrothyroxin	T38.1X1	T38.1X2	T38.1X3	T38.1X4	T38.1X5	T38.1X6
Dextrothyroxine sodium	T38.1X1	T38.1X2	T38.1X3	T38.1X4	T38.1X5	T38.1X6
DFP	T44.0X1	T44.0X2	T44.0X3	T44.0X4	T44.0X5	T44.0X6
DHE	T37.3X1	T37.3X2	T37.3X3	T37.3X4	T37.3X5	T37.3X6
45	T46.5X1	T46.5X2	T46.5X3	T46.5X4	T46.5X5	T46.5X6
Diabinese	T38.3X1	T38.3X2	T38.3X3	T38.3X4	T38.3X5	T38.3X6
Diacetone alcohol	T52.4X1	T52.4X2	T52.4X3	T52.4X4	—	—
Diacetyl monoxime	T50.991	T50.992	T50.993	T50.994	—	—
Diacetylmorphine	T40.1X1	T40.1X2	T40.1X3	T40.1X4	—	—

	External Cause (T-Code)					
Substance	Poisoning, Accidental (Unintentional)	Poisoning, Intentional Self-Harm	Poisoning, Assault	Poisoning, Undetermined	Adverse Effect	Underdosing
Diachylon plaster	T49.4X1	T49.4X2	T49.4X3	T49.4X4	T49.4X5	T49.4X6
Diaethylstilboestrolum	T38.5X1	T38.5X2	T38.5X3	T38.5X4	T38.5X5	T38.5X6
Diagnostic agent NEC	T50.8X1	T50.8X2	T50.8X3	T50.8X4	T50.8X5	T50.8X6
Dial (soap)	T49.2X1	T49.2X2	T49.2X3	T49.2X4	T49.2X5	T49.2X6
sedative	T42.3X1	T42.3X2	T42.3X3	T42.3X4	T42.3X5	T42.3X6
Dialkyl carbonate	T52.91	T52.92	T52.93	T52.94	—	—
Diallylbarbituric acid	T42.3X1	T42.3X2	T42.3X3	T42.3X4	T42.3X5	T42.3X6
Diallymal	T42.3X1	T42.3X2	T42.3X3	T42.3X4	T42.3X5	T42.3X6
Dialysis solution (intraperitoneal)	T50.3X1	T50.3X2	T50.3X3	T50.3X4	T50.3X5	T50.3X6
Diaminodiphenylsulfone	T37.1X1	T37.1X2	T37.1X3	T37.1X4	T37.1X5	T37.1X6
Diamorphine	T40.1X1	T40.1X2	T40.1X3	T40.1X4	—	—
Diamox	T50.2X1	T50.2X2	T50.2X3	T50.2X4	T50.2X5	T50.2X6
Diamthazole	T49.0X1	T49.0X2	T49.0X3	T49.0X4	T49.0X5	T49.0X6
Dianthone	T47.2X1	T47.2X2	T47.2X3	T47.2X4	T47.2X5	T47.2X6
Diaphenylsulfone	T37.0X1	T37.0X2	T37.0X3	T37.0X4	T37.0X5	T37.0X6
Diasone (sodium)	T37.1X1	T37.1X2	T37.1X3	T37.1X4	T37.1X5	T37.1X6
Diastase	T47.5X1	T47.5X2	T47.5X3	T47.5X4	T47.5X5	T47.5X6
Diatrizoate	T50.8X1	T50.8X2	T50.8X3	T50.8X4	T50.8X5	T50.8X6
Diazepam	T42.4X1	T42.4X2	T42.4X3	T42.4X4	T42.4X5	T42.4X6
Diazinon	T60.0X1	T60.0X2	T60.0X3	T60.0X4	—	—
Diazomethane (gas)	T59.891	T59.892	T59.893	T59.894	—	—
Diazoxide	T46.5X1	T46.5X2	T46.5X3	T46.5X4	T46.5X5	T46.5X6
Dibekacin	T36.5X1	T36.5X2	T36.5X3	T36.5X4	T36.5X5	T36.5X6
Dibenamine	T44.6X1	T44.6X2	T44.6X3	T44.6X4	T44.6X5	T44.6X6
Dibenzepin	T43.011	T43.012	T43.013	T43.014	T43.015	T43.016
Dibenzheptropine	T45.0X1	T45.0X2	T45.0X3	T45.0X4	T45.0X5	T45.0X6
Dibenzyline	T44.6X1	T44.6X2	T44.6X3	T44.6X4	T44.6X5	T44.6X6
Diborane (gas)	T59.891	T59.892	T59.893	T59.894	—	—
Dibromochloropropane	T60.8X1	T60.8X2	T60.8X3	T60.8X4	—	—
Dibromodulcitol	T45.1X1	T45.1X2	T45.1X3	T45.1X4	T45.1X5	T45.1X6
Dibromoethane	T53.6X1	T53.6X2	T53.6X3	T53.6X4	—	—
Dibromomannitol	T45.1X1	T45.1X2	T45.1X3	T45.1X4	T45.1X5	T45.1X6
Dibromopropamidine isethionate	T49.0X1	T49.0X2	T49.0X3	T49.0X4	T49.0X5	T49.0X6
Dibrompropamidine	T49.0X1	T49.0X2	T49.0X3	T49.0X4	T49.0X5	T49.0X6
Dibucaine	T41.3X1	T41.3X2	T41.3X3	T41.3X4	T41.3X5	T41.3X6
topical (surface)	T41.3X1	T41.3X2	T41.3X3	T41.3X4	T41.3X5	T41.3X6
Dibunate sodium	T48.3X1	T48.3X2	T48.3X3	T48.3X4	T48.3X5	T48.3X6
Dibutoline sulfate	T44.3X1	T44.3X2	T44.3X3	T44.3X4	T44.3X5	T44.3X6
Dicamba	T60.3X1	T60.3X2	T60.3X3	T60.3X4	—	—
Dicapthon	T60.0X1	T60.0X2	T60.0X3	T60.0X4	—	—
Dichlobenil	T60.3X1	T60.3X2	T60.3X3	T60.3X4	—	—
Dichlone	T60.3X1	T60.3X2	T60.3X3	T60.3X4	—	—

TABLE OF DRUGS AND CHEMICALS

	External Cause (T-Code)					
Substance	Poisoning, Accidental (Unintentional)	Poisoning, Intentional Self-Harm	Poisoning, Assault	Poisoning, Undetermined	Adverse Effect	Underdosing
Dichloralphenozone	T42.6X1	T42.6X2	T42.6X3	T42.6X4	T42.6X5	T42.6X6
Dichlorbenzidine	T65.3X1	T65.3X2	T65.3X3	T65.3X4	—	—
Dichlorhydrin	T52.8X1	T52.8X2	T52.8X3	T52.8X4	—	—
Dichlorhydroxyquinoline	T37.8X1	T37.8X2	T37.8X3	T37.8X4	T37.8X5	T37.8X6
Dichlorobenzene	T53.7X1	T53.7X2	T53.7X3	T53.7X4	—	—
Dichlorobenzyl alcohol	T49.6X1	T49.6X2	T49.6X3	T49.6X4	T49.6X5	T49.6X6
Dichlorodifluoromethane	T53.5X1	T53.5X2	T53.5X3	T53.5X4	—	—
Dichloroethane	T52.8X1	T52.8X2	T52.8X3	T52.8X4	—	—
Sym-Dichloroethyl ether	T53.6X1	T53.6X2	T53.6X3	T53.6X4	—	—
Dichloroethyl sulfide, not in war	T59.891	T59.892	T59.893	T59.894	—	—
Dichloroethylene	T53.6X1	T53.6X2	T53.6X3	T53.6X4	—	—
Dichloroformoxine, not in war	T59.891	T59.892	T59.893	T59.894	—	—
Dichlorohydrin, alpha-dichlorohydrin	T52.8X1	T52.8X2	T52.8X3	T52.8X4	—	—
Dichloromethane (solvent)	T53.4X1	T53.4X2	T53.4X3	T53.4X4	—	—
vapor	T53.4X1	T53.4X2	T53.4X3	T53.4X4	—	—
Dichloronaphthoquinone	T60.3X1	T60.3X2	T60.3X3	T60.3X4	—	—
Dichlorophen	T37.4X1	T37.4X2	T37.4X3	T37.4X4	T37.4X5	T37.4X6
2,4-Dichlorophenoxy-acetic acid	T60.3X1	T60.3X2	T60.3X3	T60.3X4	—	—
Dichloropropene	T60.3X1	T60.3X2	T60.3X3	T60.3X4	—	—
Dichloropropionic acid	T60.3X1	T60.3X2	T60.3X3	T60.3X4	—	—
Dichlorphenamide	T50.2X1	T50.2X2	T50.2X3	T50.2X4	T50.2X5	T50.2X6
Dichlorvos	T60.0X1	T60.0X2	T60.0X3	T60.0X4	—	—
Diclofenac	T39.391	T39.392	T39.393	T39.394	T39.395	T39.396
Diclofenamide	T50.2X1	T50.2X2	T50.2X3	T50.2X4	T50.2X5	T50.2X6
Diclofensine	T43.291	T43.292	T43.293	T43.294	T43.295	T43.296
Diclonixine	T39.8X1	T39.8X2	T39.8X3	T39.8X4	T39.8X5	T39.8X6
Dicloxacillin	T36.0X1	T36.0X2	T36.0X3	T36.0X4	T36.0X5	T36.0X6
Dicophane	T49.0X1	T49.0X2	T49.0X3	T49.0X4	T49.0X5	T49.0X6
Dicoumarol, dicoumarin, dicumarol	T45.511	T45.512	T45.513	T45.514	T45.515	T45.516
Dicrotophos	T60.0X1	T60.0X2	T60.0X3	T60.0X4	—	—
Dicyanogen (gas)	T65.0X1	T65.0X2	T65.0X3	T65.0X4	—	—
Dicyclomine	T44.3X1	T44.3X2	T44.3X3	T44.3X4	T44.3X5	T44.3X6
Dicycloverine	T44.3X1	T44.3X2	T44.3X3	T44.3X4	T44.3X5	T44.3X6
Dideoxycytidine	T37.5X1	T37.5X2	T37.5X3	T37.5X4	T37.5X5	T37.5X6
Dideoxyinosine	T37.5X1	T37.5X2	T37.5X3	T37.5X4	T37.5X5	T37.5X6
Dieldrin (vapor)	T60.1X1	T60.1X2	T60.1X3	T60.1X4	—	—
Diemal	T42.3X1	T42.3X2	T42.3X3	T42.3X4	T42.3X5	T42.3X6
Dienestrol	T38.5X1	T38.5X2	T38.5X3	T38.5X4	T38.5X5	T38.5X6
Dienoestrol	T38.5X1	T38.5X2	T38.5X3	T38.5X4	T38.5X5	T38.5X6
Dietetic drug NEC	T50.901	T50.902	T50.903	T50.904	T50.905	T50.906
Diethazine	T42.8X1	T42.8X2	T42.8X3	T42.8X4	T42.8X5	T42.8X6

	External Cause (T-Code)					
Substance	Poisoning, Accidental (Unintentional)	Poisoning, Intentional Self-Harm	Poisoning, Assault	Poisoning, Undetermined	Adverse Effect	Underdosing
Diethyl						
barbituric acid	T42.3X1	T42.3X2	T42.3X3	T42.3X4	T42.3X5	T42.3X6
carbamazine	T37.4X1	T37.4X2	T37.4X3	T37.4X4	T37.4X5	T37.4X6
carbinol	T51.3X1	T51.3X2	T51.3X3	T51.3X4	—	—
carbonate	T52.8X1	T52.8X2	T52.8X3	T52.8X4	—	—
ether (vapor) — see also Ether	T41.0X1	T41.0X2	T41.0X3	T41.0X4	T41.0X5	T41.0X6
oxide	T52.8X1	T52.8X2	T52.8X3	T52.8X4	—	—
propion	T50.5X1	T50.5X2	T50.5X3	T50.5X4	T50.5X5	T50.5X6
stilbestrol	T38.5X1	T38.5X2	T38.5X3	T38.5X4	T38.5X5	T38.5X6
toluamide (nonmedicinal)	T60.8X1	T60.8X2	T60.8X3	T60.8X4	—	—
medicinal	T49.3X1	T49.3X2	T49.3X3	T49.3X4	T49.3X5	T49.3X6
Diethylcarbamazine	T37.4X1	T37.4X2	T37.4X3	T37.4X4	T37.4X5	T37.4X6
Diethylene						
dioxide	T52.8X1	T52.8X2	T52.8X3	T52.8X4	—	—
glycol (monoacetate) (monobutyl ether) (monoethyl ether)	T52.3X1	T52.3X2	T52.3X3	T52.3X4	—	—
Diethylhexylphthalate	T65.891	T65.892	T65.893	T65.894	—	—
Diethylpropion	T50.5X1	T50.5X2	T50.5X3	T50.5X4	T50.5X5	T50.5X6
Diethylstilbestrol	T38.5X1	T38.5X2	T38.5X3	T38.5X4	T38.5X5	T38.5X6
Diethylstilboestrol	T38.5X1	T38.5X2	T38.5X3	T38.5X4	T38.5X5	T38.5X6
Diethylsulfone-diethylmethane	T42.6X1	T42.6X2	T42.6X3	T42.6X4	T42.6X5	T42.6X6
Diethyltoluamide	T49.0X1	T49.0X2	T49.0X3	T49.0X4	T49.0X5	T49.0X6
Diethyltryptamine (DET)	T40.991	T40.992	T40.993	T40.994	—	—
Difebarbamate	T42.3X1	T42.3X2	T42.3X3	T42.3X4	T42.3X5	T42.3X6
Difencloxazine	T40.2X1	T40.2X2	T40.2X3	T40.2X4	T40.2X5	T40.2X6
Difenidol	T45.0X1	T45.0X2	T45.0X3	T45.0X4	T45.0X5	T45.0X6
Difenoxin	T47.6X1	T47.6X2	T47.6X3	T47.6X4	T47.6X5	T47.6X6
Difetarsone	T37.3X1	T37.3X2	T37.3X3	T37.3X4	T37.3X5	T37.3X6
Diffusin	T45.3X1	T45.3X2	T45.3X3	T45.3X4	T45.3X5	T45.3X6
Diflorasone	T49.0X1	T49.0X2	T49.0X3	T49.0X4	T49.0X5	T49.0X6
Diflubenzuron	T60.1X1	T60.1X2	T60.1X3	T60.1X4	—	—
Diflos	T44.0X1	T44.0X2	T44.0X3	T44.0X4	T44.0X5	T44.0X6
Diflucortolone	T49.0X1	T49.0X2	T49.0X3	T49.0X4	T49.0X5	T49.0X6
Diflunisal	T39.091	T39.092	T39.093	T39.094	T39.095	T39.096
Difluoromethyldopa	T42.8X1	T42.8X2	T42.8X3	T42.8X4	T42.8X5	T42.8X6
Difluorophate	T44.0X1	T44.0X2	T44.0X3	T44.0X4	T44.0X5	T44.0X6
Digestant NEC	T47.5X1	T47.5X2	T47.5X3	T47.5X4	T47.5X5	T47.5X6
Digitalin(e)	T46.0X1	T46.0X2	T46.0X3	T46.0X4	T46.0X5	T46.0X6
Digitalis (leaf) (glycoside)	T46.0X1	T46.0X2	T46.0X3	T46.0X4	T46.0X5	T46.0X6
lanata	T46.0X1	T46.0X2	T46.0X3	T46.0X4	T46.0X5	T46.0X6
purpurea	T46.0X1	T46.0X2	T46.0X3	T46.0X4	T46.0X5	T46.0X6
Digitoxin	T46.0X1	T46.0X2	T46.0X3	T46.0X4	T46.0X5	T46.0X6

◀ New ◀ Revised ~~deleted~~ Deleted

Substance	External Cause (T-Code)					
	Poisoning, Accidental (Unintentional)	Poisoning, Intentional Self-Harm	Poisoning, Assault	Poisoning, Undetermined	Adverse Effect	Underdosing
Digitoxose	T46.0X1	T46.0X2	T46.0X3	T46.0X4	T46.0X5	T46.0X6
Digoxin	T46.0X1	T46.0X2	T46.0X3	T46.0X4	T46.0X5	T46.0X6
Digoxine	T46.0X1	T46.0X2	T46.0X3	T46.0X4	T46.0X5	T46.0X6
Dihydralazine	T46.5X1	T46.5X2	T46.5X3	T46.5X4	T46.5X5	T46.5X6
Dihydrazine	T46.5X1	T46.5X2	T46.5X3	T46.5X4	T46.5X5	T46.5X6
Dihydrocodeinone	T40.2X1	T40.2X2	T40.2X3	T40.2X4	T40.2X5	T40.2X6
Dihydroergocornine	T46.7X1	T46.7X2	T46.7X3	T46.7X4	T46.7X5	T46.7X6
Dihydroergocristine (mesilate)	T46.7X1	T46.7X2	T46.7X3	T46.7X4	T46.7X5	T46.7X6
Dihydroergokryptine	T46.7X1	T46.7X2	T46.7X3	T46.7X4	T46.7X5	T46.7X6
Dihydroergotamine	T46.5X1	T46.5X2	T46.5X3	T46.5X4	T46.5X5	T46.5X6
Dihydroergotoxine	T46.7X1	T46.7X2	T46.7X3	T46.7X4	T46.7X5	T46.7X6
mesilate	T46.7X1	T46.7X2	T46.7X3	T46.7X4	T46.7X5	T46.7X6
Dihydrohydroxycodein-one	T40.2X1	T40.2X2	T40.2X3	T40.2X4	T40.2X5	T40.2X6
Dihydrohydroxymorphinone	T40.2X1	T40.2X2	T40.2X3	T40.2X4	T40.2X5	T40.2X6
Dihydroisocodeine	T40.2X1	T40.2X2	T40.2X3	T40.2X4	T40.2X5	T40.2X6
Dihydromorphine	T40.2X1	T40.2X2	T40.2X3	T40.2X4	—	—
Dihydromorphinone	T40.2X1	T40.2X2	T40.2X3	T40.2X4	T40.2X5	T40.2X6
Dihydrostreptomycin	T36.5X1	T36.5X2	T36.5X3	T36.5X4	T36.5X5	T36.5X6
Dihydrotachysterol	T45.2X1	T45.2X2	T45.2X3	T45.2X4	T45.2X5	T45.2X6
Dihydroxyaluminum aminoacetate	T47.1X1	T47.1X2	T47.1X3	T47.1X4	T47.1X5	T47.1X6
Dihydroxyaluminum sodium carbonate	T47.1X1	T47.1X2	T47.1X3	T47.1X4	T47.1X5	T47.1X6
Dihydroxyanthraquinone	T47.2X1	T47.2X2	T47.2X3	T47.2X4	T47.2X5	T47.2X6
Dihydroxycodeinone	T40.2X1	T40.2X2	T40.2X3	T40.2X4	T40.2X5	T40.2X6
Dihydroxypropyl theophylline	T50.2X1	T50.2X2	T50.2X3	T50.2X4	T50.2X5	T50.2X6
Diiodohydroxyquin	T37.8X1	T37.8X2	T37.8X3	T37.8X4	T37.8X5	T37.8X6
topical	T49.0X1	T49.0X2	T49.0X3	T49.0X4	T49.0X5	T49.0X6
Diiodohydroxyquinoline	T37.8X1	T37.8X2	T37.8X3	T37.8X4	T37.8X5	T37.8X6
Diiodotyrosine	T38.2X1	T38.2X2	T38.2X3	T38.2X4	T38.2X5	T38.2X6
Diisopromine	T44.3X1	T44.3X2	T44.3X3	T44.3X4	T44.3X5	T44.3X6
Diisopropylamine	T46.3X1	T46.3X2	T46.3X3	T46.3X4	T46.3X5	T46.3X6
Diisopropylfluorophosphonate	T44.0X1	T44.0X2	T44.0X3	T44.0X4	T44.0X5	T44.0X6
Dilantin	T42.0X1	T42.0X2	T42.0X3	T42.0X4	T42.0X5	T42.0X6
Dilaudid	T40.2X1	T40.2X2	T40.2X3	T40.2X4	T40.2X5	T40.2X6
Dilazep	T46.3X1	T46.3X2	T46.3X3	T46.3X4	T46.3X5	T46.3X6
Dill	T47.5X1	T47.5X2	T47.5X3	T47.5X4	T47.5X5	T47.5X6
Diloxanide	T37.3X1	T37.3X2	T37.3X3	T37.3X4	T37.3X5	T37.3X6
Diltiazem	T46.1X1	T46.1X2	T46.1X3	T46.1X4	T46.1X5	T46.1X6
Dimazole	T49.0X1	T49.0X2	T49.0X3	T49.0X4	T49.0X5	T49.0X6
Dimefline	T50.7X1	T50.7X2	T50.7X3	T50.7X4	T50.7X5	T50.7X6
Dimefox	T60.0X1	T60.0X2	T60.0X3	T60.0X4	—	—

Substance	External Cause (T-Code)					
	Poisoning, Accidental (Unintentional)	Poisoning, Intentional Self-Harm	Poisoning, Assault	Poisoning, Undetermined	Adverse Effect	Underdosing
Dimemorfan	T48.3X1	T48.3X2	T48.3X3	T48.3X4	T48.3X5	T48.3X6
Dimenhydrinate	T45.0X1	T45.0X2	T45.0X3	T45.0X4	T45.0X5	T45.0X6
Dimercaprol (British anti-lewisite)	T45.8X1	T45.8X2	T45.8X3	T45.8X4	T45.8X5	T45.8X6
Dimercaptopropanol	T45.8X1	T45.8X2	T45.8X3	T45.8X4	T45.8X5	T45.8X6
Dimestrol	T38.5X1	T38.5X2	T38.5X3	T38.5X4	T38.5X5	T38.5X6
Dimetane	T45.0X1	T45.0X2	T45.0X3	T45.0X4	T45.0X5	T45.0X6
Dimethicone	T47.1X1	T47.1X2	T47.1X3	T47.1X4	T47.1X5	T47.1X6
Dimethindene	T45.0X1	T45.0X2	T45.0X3	T45.0X4	T45.0X5	T45.0X6
Dimethisoquin	T49.1X1	T49.1X2	T49.1X3	T49.1X4	T49.1X5	T49.1X6
Dimethisterone	T38.5X1	T38.5X2	T38.5X3	T38.5X4	T38.5X5	T38.5X6
Dimethoate	T60.0X1	T60.0X2	T60.0X3	T60.0X4	—	—
Dimethocaine	T41.3X1	T41.3X2	T41.3X3	T41.3X4	T41.3X5	T41.3X6
Dimethoxanate	T48.3X1	T48.3X2	T48.3X3	T48.3X4	T48.3X5	T48.3X6
Dimethyl						
arsine, arsinic acid	T57.0X1	T57.0X2	T57.0X3	T57.0X4	—	—
carbinol	T51.2X1	T51.2X2	T51.2X3	T51.2X4	—	—
carbonate	T52.8X1	T52.8X2	T52.8X3	T52.8X4	—	—
diguanide	T38.3X1	T38.3X2	T38.3X3	T38.3X4	T38.3X5	T38.3X6
ketone	T52.4X1	T52.4X2	T52.4X3	T52.4X4	—	—
vapor	T52.4X1	T52.4X2	T52.4X3	T52.4X4	—	—
meperidine	T40.2X1	T40.2X2	T40.2X3	T40.2X4	T40.2X5	T40.2X6
parathion	T60.0X1	T60.0X2	T60.0X3	T60.0X4	—	—
phthlate	T49.3X1	T49.3X2	T49.3X3	T49.3X4	T49.3X5	T49.3X6
polysiloxane	T47.8X1	T47.8X2	T47.8X3	T47.8X4	T47.8X5	T47.8X6
sulfate (fumes)	T59.891	T59.892	T59.893	T59.894	—	—
liquid	T65.891	T65.892	T65.893	T65.894	—	—
sulfoxide (nonmedicinal)	T52.8X1	T52.8X2	T52.8X3	T52.8X4	—	—
medicinal	T49.4X1	T49.4X2	T49.4X3	T49.4X4	T49.4X5	T49.4X6
tryptamine	T40.991	T40.992	T40.993	T40.994	—	—
tubocurarine	T48.1X1	T48.1X2	T48.1X3	T48.1X4	T48.1X5	T48.1X6
Dimethylamine sulfate	T49.4X1	T49.4X2	T49.4X3	T49.4X4	T49.4X5	T49.4X6
Dimethylformamide	T52.8X1	T52.8X2	T52.8X3	T52.8X4	—	—
Dimethyltubocurarinium chloride	T48.1X1	T48.1X2	T48.1X3	T48.1X4	T48.1X5	T48.1X6
Dimeticone	T47.1X1	T47.1X2	T47.1X3	T47.1X4	T47.1X5	T47.1X6
Dimetilan	T60.0X1	T60.0X2	T60.0X3	T60.0X4	—	—
Dimetindene	T45.0X1	T45.0X2	T45.0X3	T45.0X4	T45.0X5	T45.0X6
Dimetotiazine	T43.3X1	T43.3X2	T43.3X3	T43.3X4	T43.3X5	T43.3X6
Dimorpholamine	T50.7X1	T50.7X2	T50.7X3	T50.7X4	T50.7X5	T50.7X6
Dimoxyline	T46.3X1	T46.3X2	T46.3X3	T46.3X4	T46.3X5	T46.3X6
Dinitrobenzene	T65.3X1	T65.3X2	T65.3X3	T65.3X4	—	—
vapor	T59.891	T59.892	T59.893	T59.894	—	—

◀ New ◀ Revised ~~deleted~~ Deleted

Substance	External Cause (T-Code) Poisoning, Accidental (Unintentional)	Poisoning, Intentional Self-Harm	Poisoning, Assault	Poisoning, Undetermined	Adverse Effect	Underdosing
Dinitrobenzol	T65.3X1	T65.3X2	T65.3X3	T65.3X4	—	—
vapor	T59.891	T59.892	T59.893	T59.894	—	—
Dinitrobutylphenol	T65.3X1	T65.3X2	T65.3X3	T65.3X4	—	—
Dinitro (-ortho-)cresol (pesticide) (spray)	T65.3X1	T65.3X2	T65.3X3	T65.3X4	—	—
Dinitrocyclohexylphenol	T65.3X1	T65.3X2	T65.3X3	T65.3X4	—	—
Dinitrophenol	T65.3X1	T65.3X2	T65.3X3	T65.3X4	—	—
Dinoprost	T48.0X1	T48.0X2	T48.0X3	T48.0X4	T48.0X5	T48.0X6
Dinoprostone	T48.0X1	T48.0X2	T48.0X3	T48.0X4	T48.0X5	T48.0X6
Dinoseb	T60.3X1	T60.3X2	T60.3X3	T60.3X4		
Dioctyl sulfosuccinate (calcium) (sodium)	T47.4X1	T47.4X2	T47.4X3	T47.4X4	T47.4X5	T47.4X6
Diodone	T50.8X1	T50.8X2	T50.8X3	T50.8X4	T50.8X5	T50.8X6
Diodoquin	T37.8X1	T37.8X2	T37.8X3	T37.8X4	T37.8X5	T37.8X6
Dionin	T40.2X1	T40.2X2	T40.2X3	T40.2X4	T40.2X5	T40.2X6
Diosmin	T46.991	T46.992	T46.993	T46.994	T46.995	T46.996
Dioxane	T52.8X1	T52.8X2	T52.8X3	T52.8X4	—	—
Dioxathion	T60.0X1	T60.0X2	T60.0X3	T60.0X4	—	—
Dioxin	T53.7X1	T53.7X2	T53.7X3	T53.7X4	—	—
Dioxopromethazine	T43.3X1	T43.3X2	T43.3X3	T43.3X4	T43.3X5	T43.3X6
Dioxyline	T46.3X1	T46.3X2	T46.3X3	T46.3X4	T46.3X5	T46.3X6
Dipentene	T52.8X1	T52.8X2	T52.8X3	T52.8X4	—	—
Diperodon	T41.3X1	T41.3X2	T41.3X3	T41.3X4	T41.3X5	T41.3X6
Diphacinone	T60.4X1	T60.4X2	T60.4X3	T60.4X4		
Diphemanil	T44.3X1	T44.3X2	T44.3X3	T44.3X4	T44.3X5	T44.3X6
metilsulfate	T44.3X1	T44.3X2	T44.3X3	T44.3X4	T44.3X5	T44.3X6
Diphenadione	T45.511	T45.512	T45.513	T45.514	T45.515	T45.516
rodenticide	T60.4X1	T60.4X2	T60.4X3	T60.4X4	—	—
Diphenhydramine	T45.0X1	T45.0X2	T45.0X3	T45.0X4	T45.0X5	T45.0X6
Diphenidol	T45.0X1	T45.0X2	T45.0X3	T45.0X4	T45.0X5	T45.0X6
Diphenoxylate	T47.6X1	T47.6X2	T47.6X3	T47.6X4	T47.6X5	T47.6X6
Diphenylamine	T65.3X1	T65.3X2	T65.3X3	T65.3X4	—	—
Diphenylbutazone	T39.2X1	T39.2X2	T39.2X3	T39.2X4	T39.2X5	T39.2X6
Diphenylchloroarsine, not in war	T57.0X1	T57.0X2	T57.0X3	T57.0X4	—	—
Diphenylhydantoin	T42.0X1	T42.0X2	T42.0X3	T42.0X4	T42.0X5	T42.0X6
Diphenylmethane dye	T52.1X1	T52.1X2	T52.1X3	T52.1X4	—	—
Diphenylpyraline	T45.0X1	T45.0X2	T45.0X3	T45.0X4	T45.0X5	T45.0X6
Diphtheria						
antitoxin	T50.Z11	T50.Z12	T50.Z13	T50.Z14	T50.Z15	T50.Z16
toxoid	T50.A91	T50.A92	T50.A93	T50.A94	T50.A95	T50.A96
with tetanus toxoid	T50.A21	T50.A22	T50.A23	T50.A24	T50.A25	T50.A26
with pertussis component	T50.A11	T50.A12	T50.A13	T50.A14	T50.A15	T50.A16

Substance	External Cause (T-Code) Poisoning, Accidental (Unintentional)	Poisoning, Intentional Self-Harm	Poisoning, Assault	Poisoning, Undetermined	Adverse Effect	Underdosing
Diphtheria *(Continued)*						
vaccine (combination)	T50.A91	T50.A92	T50.A93	T50.A94	T50.A95	T50.A96
combination						
including pertussis	T50.A11	T50.A12	T50.A13	T50.A14	T50.A15	T50.A16
without pertussis	T50.A21	T50.A22	T50.A23	T50.A24	T50.A25	T50.A26
Diphylline	T50.2X1	T50.2X2	T50.2X3	T50.2X4	T50.2X5	T50.2X6
Dipipanone	T40.491	T40.492	T40.493	T40.494	—	—
Dipivefrine	T49.5X1	T49.5X2	T49.5X3	T49.5X4	T49.5X5	T49.5X6
Diplovax	T50.B91	T50.B92	T50.B93	T50.B94	T50.B95	T50.B96
Diprophylline	T50.2X1	T50.2X2	T50.2X3	T50.2X4	T50.2X5	T50.2X6
Dipropyline	T48.291	T48.292	T48.293	T48.294	T48.295	T48.296
Dipyridamole	T46.3X1	T46.3X2	T46.3X3	T46.3X4	T46.3X5	T46.3X6
Dipyrone	T39.2X1	T39.2X2	T39.2X3	T39.2X4	T39.2X5	T39.2X6
Diquat (dibromide)	T60.3X1	T60.3X2	T60.3X3	T60.3X4	—	—
Disinfectant	T65.891	T65.892	T65.893	T65.894	—	—
alkaline	T54.3X1	T54.3X2	T54.3X3	T54.3X4	—	—
aromatic	T54.1X1	T54.1X2	T54.1X3	T54.1X4	—	—
intestinal	T37.8X1	T37.8X2	T37.8X3	T37.8X4	T37.8X5	T37.8X6
Disipal	T42.8X1	T42.8X2	T42.8X3	T42.8X4	T42.8X5	T42.8X6
Disodium edetate	T50.6X1	T50.6X2	T50.6X3	T50.6X4	T50.6X5	T50.6X6
Disoprofol	T41.291	T41.292	T41.293	T41.294	T41.295	T41.296
Disopyramide	T46.2X1	T46.2X2	T46.2X3	T46.2X4	T46.2X5	T46.2X6
Distigmine (bromide)	T44.0X1	T44.0X2	T44.0X3	T44.0X4	T44.0X5	T44.0X6
Disulfamide	T50.2X1	T50.2X2	T50.2X3	T50.2X4	T50.2X5	T50.2X6
Disulfanilamide	T37.0X1	T37.0X2	T37.0X3	T37.0X4	T37.0X5	T37.0X6
Disulfiram	T50.6X1	T50.6X2	T50.6X3	T50.6X4	T50.6X5	T50.6X6
Disulfoton	T60.0X1	T60.0X2	T60.0X3	T60.0X4	—	—
Dithiazanine iodide	T37.4X1	T37.4X2	T37.4X3	T37.4X4	T37.4X5	T37.4X6
Dithiocarbamate	T60.0X1	T60.0X2	T60.0X3	T60.0X4	—	—
Dithranol	T49.4X1	T49.4X2	T49.4X3	T49.4X4	T49.4X5	T49.4X6
Diucardin	T50.2X1	T50.2X2	T50.2X3	T50.2X4	T50.2X5	T50.2X6
Diupres	T50.2X1	T50.2X2	T50.2X3	T50.2X4	T50.2X5	T50.2X6
Diuretic NEC	T50.2X1	T50.2X2	T50.2X3	T50.2X4	T50.2X5	T50.2X6
benzothiadiazine	T50.2X1	T50.2X2	T50.2X3	T50.2X4	T50.2X5	T50.2X6
carbonic acid anhydrase inhibitors	T50.2X1	T50.2X2	T50.2X3	T50.2X4	T50.2X5	T50.2X6
furfuryl NEC	T50.2X1	T50.2X2	T50.2X3	T50.2X4	T50.2X5	T50.2X6
loop (high-ceiling)	T50.1X1	T50.1X2	T50.1X3	T50.1X4	T50.1X5	T50.1X6
mercurial NEC	T50.2X1	T50.2X2	T50.2X3	T50.2X4	T50.2X5	T50.2X6
osmotic	T50.2X1	T50.2X2	T50.2X3	T50.2X4	T50.2X5	T50.2X6
purine NEC	T50.2X1	T50.2X2	T50.2X3	T50.2X4	T50.2X5	T50.2X6
saluretic NEC	T50.2X1	T50.2X2	T50.2X3	T50.2X4	T50.2X5	T50.2X6

◄ New ◄ Revised ~~deleted~~ Deleted

Substance	Poisoning, Accidental (Unintentional)	Poisoning, Intentional Self-Harm	Poisoning, Assault	Poisoning, Undetermined	Adverse Effect	Underdosing
Diuretic NEC *(Continued)*						
sulfonamide	T50.2X1	T50.2X2	T50.2X3	T50.2X4	T50.2X5	T50.2X6
thiazide NEC	T50.2X1	T50.2X2	T50.2X3	T50.2X4	T50.2X5	T50.2X6
xanthine	T50.2X1	T50.2X2	T50.2X3	T50.2X4	T50.2X5	T50.2X6
Diurgin	T50.2X1	T50.2X2	T50.2X3	T50.2X4	T50.2X5	T50.2X6
Diuril	T50.2X1	T50.2X2	T50.2X3	T50.2X4	T50.2X5	T50.2X6
Diuron	T60.3X1	T60.3X2	T60.3X3	T60.3X4	—	—
Divalproex	T42.6X1	T42.6X2	T42.6X3	T42.6X4	T42.6X5	T42.6X6
Divinyl ether	T41.0X1	T41.0X2	T41.0X3	T41.0X4	T41.0X5	T41.0X6
Dixanthogen	T49.0X1	T49.0X2	T49.0X3	T49.0X4	T49.0X5	T49.0X6
Dixyrazine	T43.3X1	T43.3X2	T43.3X3	T43.3X4	T43.3X5	T43.3X6
D-lysergic acid diethylamide	T40.8X1	T40.8X2	T40.8X3	T40.8X4	—	—
DMCT	T36.4X1	T36.4X2	T36.4X3	T36.4X4	T36.4X5	T36.4X6
DMSO — *see Dimethyl, sulfoxide*						
DNBP	T60.3X1	T60.3X2	T60.3X3	T60.3X4	—	—
DNOC	T65.3X1	T65.3X2	T65.3X3	T65.3X4	—	—
DOCA	T38.0X1	T38.0X2	T38.0X3	T38.0X4	T38.0X5	T38.0X6
Dobutamine	T44.5X1	T44.5X2	T44.5X3	T44.5X4	T44.5X5	T44.5X6
Docusate sodium	T47.4X1	T47.4X2	T47.4X3	T47.4X4	T47.4X5	T47.4X6
Dodicin	T49.0X1	T49.0X2	T49.0X3	T49.0X4	T49.0X5	T49.0X6
Dofamium chloride	T49.0X1	T49.0X2	T49.0X3	T49.0X4	T49.0X5	T49.0X6
Dolophine	T40.3X1	T40.3X2	T40.3X3	T40.3X4	T40.3X5	T40.3X6
Doloxene	T39.8X1	T39.8X2	T39.8X3	T39.8X4	T39.8X5	T39.8X6
Domestic gas (after combustion) — *see Gas, utility*						
prior to combustion	T59.891	T59.892	T59.893	T59.894	—	—
Domiodol	T48.4X1	T48.4X2	T48.4X3	T48.4X4	T48.4X5	T48.4X6
Domiphen (bromide)	T49.0X1	T49.0X2	T49.0X3	T49.0X4	T49.0X5	T49.0X6
Domperidone	T45.0X1	T45.0X2	T45.0X3	T45.0X4	T45.0X5	T45.0X6
Dopa	T42.8X1	T42.8X2	T42.8X3	T42.8X4	T42.8X5	T42.8X6
Dopamine	T44.991	T44.992	T44.993	T44.994	T44.995	T44.996
Doriden	T42.6X1	T42.6X2	T42.6X3	T42.6X4	T42.6X5	T42.6X6
Dormiral	T42.3X1	T42.3X2	T42.3X3	T42.3X4	T42.3X5	T42.3X6
Dormison	T42.6X1	T42.6X2	T42.6X3	T42.6X4	T42.6X5	T42.6X6
Dornase	T48.4X1	T48.4X2	T48.4X3	T48.4X4	T48.4X5	T48.4X6
Dorsacaine	T41.3X1	T41.3X2	T41.3X3	T41.3X4	T41.3X5	T41.3X6
Dosulepin	T43.011	T43.012	T43.013	T43.014	T43.015	T43.016
Dothiepin	T43.011	T43.012	T43.013	T43.014	T43.015	T43.016
Doxantrazole	T48.6X1	T48.6X2	T48.6X3	T48.6X4	T48.6X5	T48.6X6
Doxapram	T50.7X1	T50.7X2	T50.7X3	T50.7X4	T50.7X5	T50.7X6
Doxazosin	T44.6X1	T44.6X2	T44.6X3	T44.6X4	T44.6X5	T44.6X6
Doxepin	T43.011	T43.012	T43.013	T43.014	T43.015	T43.016

Substance	Poisoning, Accidental (Unintentional)	Poisoning, Intentional Self-Harm	Poisoning, Assault	Poisoning, Undetermined	Adverse Effect	Underdosing
Doxifluridine	T45.1X1	T45.1X2	T45.1X3	T45.1X4	T45.1X5	T45.1X6
Doxorubicin	T45.1X1	T45.1X2	T45.1X3	T45.1X4	T45.1X5	T45.1X6
Doxycycline	T36.4X1	T36.4X2	T36.4X3	T36.4X4	T36.4X5	T36.4X6
Doxylamine	T45.0X1	T45.0X2	T45.0X3	T45.0X4	T45.0X5	T45.0X6
Dramamine	T45.0X1	T45.0X2	T45.0X3	T45.0X4	T45.0X5	T45.0X6
Drano (drain cleaner)	T54.3X1	T54.3X2	T54.3X3	T54.3X4	—	—
Dressing, live pulp	T49.7X1	T49.7X2	T49.7X3	T49.7X4	T49.7X5	T49.7X6
Drocode	T40.2X1	T40.2X2	T40.2X3	T40.2X4	T40.2X5	T40.2X6
Dromoran	T40.2X1	T40.2X2	T40.2X3	T40.2X4	T40.2X5	T40.2X6
Dromostanolone	T38.7X1	T38.7X2	T38.7X3	T38.7X4	T38.7X5	T38.7X6
Dronabinol	T40.711	T40.712	T40.713	T40.714	T40.715	T40.716
Droperidol	T43.591	T43.592	T43.593	T43.594	T43.595	T43.596
Dropropizine	T48.3X1	T48.3X2	T48.3X3	T48.3X4	T48.3X5	T48.3X6
Drostanolone	T38.7X1	T38.7X2	T38.7X3	T38.7X4	T38.7X5	T38.7X6
Drotaverine	T44.3X1	T44.3X2	T44.3X3	T44.3X4	T44.3X5	T44.3X6
Drotrecogin alfa	T45.511	T45.512	T45.513	T45.514	T45.515	T45.516
Drug NEC	T50.901	T50.902	T50.903	T50.904	T50.905	T50.906
specified NEC	T50.991	T50.992	T50.993	T50.994	T50.995	T50.996
DTIC	T45.1X1	T45.1X2	T45.1X3	T45.1X4	T45.1X5	T45.1X6
Duboisine	T44.3X1	T44.3X2	T44.3X3	T44.3X4	T44.3X5	T44.3X6
Dulcolax	T47.2X1	T47.2X2	T47.2X3	T47.2X4	T47.2X5	T47.2X6
Duponol (C) (EP)	T49.2X1	T49.2X2	T49.2X3	T49.2X4	T49.2X5	T49.2X6
Durabolin	T38.7X1	T38.7X2	T38.7X3	T38.7X4	T38.7X5	T38.7X6
Dyclone	T41.3X1	T41.3X2	T41.3X3	T41.3X4	T41.3X5	T41.3X6
Dyclonine	T41.3X1	T41.3X2	T41.3X3	T41.3X4	T41.3X5	T41.3X6
Dydrogesterone	T38.5X1	T38.5X2	T38.5X3	T38.5X4	T38.5X5	T38.5X6
Dye NEC	T65.6X1	T65.6X2	T65.6X3	T65.6X4	—	—
antiseptic	T49.0X1	T49.0X2	T49.0X3	T49.0X4	T49.0X5	T49.0X6
diagnostic agents	T50.8X1	T50.8X2	T50.8X3	T50.8X4	T50.8X5	T50.8X6
pharmaceutical NEC	T50.901	T50.902	T50.903	T50.904	T50.905	T50.906
Dyflos	T44.0X1	T44.0X2	T44.0X3	T44.0X4	T44.0X5	T44.0X6
Dymelor	T38.3X1	T38.3X2	T38.3X3	T38.3X4	T38.3X5	T38.3X6
Dynamite	T65.3X1	T65.3X2	T65.3X3	T65.3X4	—	—
fumes	T59.891	T59.892	T59.893	T59.894	—	—
Dyphylline	T44.3X1	T44.3X2	T44.3X3	T44.3X4	T44.3X5	T44.3X6
E						
Ear drug NEC	T49.6X1	T49.6X2	T49.6X3	T49.6X4	T49.6X5	T49.6X6
Ear preparations	T49.6X1	T49.6X2	T49.6X3	T49.6X4	T49.6X5	T49.6X6
Econazole	T49.0X1	T49.0X2	T49.0X3	T49.0X4	T49.0X5	T49.0X6
Ecothiopate iodide	T49.5X1	T49.5X2	T49.5X3	T49.5X4	T49.5X5	T49.5X6
Echothiophate, echothiopate, ecothiopate	T49.5X1	T49.5X2	T49.5X3	T49.5X4	T49.5X5	T49.5X6

Substance	Poisoning, Accidental (Unintentional)	Poisoning, Intentional Self-Harm	Poisoning, Assault	Poisoning, Undetermined	Adverse Effect	Underdosing
Ecstasy	T43.641	T43.642	T43.643	T43.644	—	—
Ectylurea	T42.6X1	T42.6X2	T42.6X3	T42.6X4	T42.6X5	T42.6X6
Edathamil disodium	T45.8X1	T45.8X2	T45.8X3	T45.8X4	T45.8X5	T45.8X6
Edecrin	T50.1X1	T50.1X2	T50.1X3	T50.1X4	T50.1X5	T50.1X6
Edetate, disodium (calcium)	T45.8X1	T45.8X2	T45.8X3	T45.8X4	T45.8X5	T45.8X6
Edoxudine	T49.5X1	T49.5X2	T49.5X3	T49.5X4	T49.5X5	T49.5X6
Edrophonium	T44.0X1	T44.0X2	T44.0X3	T44.0X4	T44.0X5	T44.0X6
chloride	T44.0X1	T44.0X2	T44.0X3	T44.0X4	T44.0X5	T44.0X6
EDTA	T50.6X1	T50.6X2	T50.6X3	T50.6X4	T50.6X5	T50.6X6
Eflornithine	T37.2X1	T37.2X2	T37.2X3	T37.2X4	T37.2X5	T37.2X6
Efloxate	T46.3X1	T46.3X2	T46.3X3	T46.3X4	T46.3X5	T46.3X6
Elase	T49.8X1	T49.8X2	T49.8X3	T49.8X4	T49.8X5	T49.8X6
Elastase	T47.5X1	T47.5X2	T47.5X3	T47.5X4	T47.5X5	T47.5X6
Elaterium	T47.2X1	T47.2X2	T47.2X3	T47.2X4	T47.2X5	T47.2X6
Elcatonin	T50.991	T50.992	T50.993	T50.994	T50.995	T50.996
Elder	T62.2X1	T62.2X2	T62.2X3	T62.2X4	—	—
berry (unripe)	T62.1X1	T62.1X2	T62.1X3	T62.1X4	—	—
Electrolyte balance drug	T50.3X1	T50.3X2	T50.3X3	T50.3X4	T50.3X5	T50.3X6
Electrolytes NEC	T50.3X1	T50.3X2	T50.3X3	T50.3X4	T50.3X5	T50.3X6
Electrolytic agent NEC	T50.3X1	T50.3X2	T50.3X3	T50.3X4	T50.3X5	T50.3X6
Elemental diet	T50.901	T50.902	T50.903	T50.904	T50.905	T50.906
Elliptinium acetate	T45.1X1	T45.1X2	T45.1X3	T45.1X4	T45.1X5	T45.1X6
Embramine	T45.0X1	T45.0X2	T45.0X3	T45.0X4	T45.0X5	T45.0X6
Emepronium (salts)	T44.3X1	T44.3X2	T44.3X3	T44.3X4	T44.3X5	T44.3X6
bromide	T44.3X1	T44.3X2	T44.3X3	T44.3X4	T44.3X5	T44.3X6
Emetic NEC	T47.7X1	T47.7X2	T47.7X3	T47.7X4	T47.7X5	T47.7X6
Emetine	T37.3X1	T37.3X2	T37.3X3	T37.3X4	T37.3X5	T37.3X6
Emollient NEC	T49.3X1	T49.3X2	T49.3X3	T49.3X4	T49.3X5	T49.3X6
Emorfazone	T39.8X1	T39.8X2	T39.8X3	T39.8X4	T39.8X5	T39.8X6
Emylcamate	T43.591	T43.592	T43.593	T43.594	T43.595	T43.596
Enalapril	T46.4X1	T46.4X2	T46.4X3	T46.4X4	T46.4X5	T46.4X6
Enalaprilat	T46.4X1	T46.4X2	T46.4X3	T46.4X4	T46.4X5	T46.4X6
Encainide	T46.2X1	T46.2X2	T46.2X3	T46.2X4	T46.2X5	T46.2X6
Endocaine	T41.3X1	T41.3X2	T41.3X3	T41.3X4	T41.3X5	T41.3X6
Endosulfan	T60.2X1	T60.2X2	T60.2X3	T60.2X4	—	—
Endothall	T60.3X1	T60.3X2	T60.3X3	T60.3X4	—	—
Endralazine	T46.5X1	T46.5X2	T46.5X3	T46.5X4	T46.5X5	T46.5X6
Endrin	T60.1X1	T60.1X2	T60.1X3	T60.1X4	—	—
Enflurane	T41.0X1	T41.0X2	T41.0X3	T41.0X4	T41.0X5	T41.0X6
Enhexymal	T42.3X1	T42.3X2	T42.3X3	T42.3X4	T42.3X5	T42.3X6
Enocitabine	T45.1X1	T45.1X2	T45.1X3	T45.1X4	T45.1X5	T45.1X6
Enovid	T38.4X1	T38.4X2	T38.4X3	T38.4X4	T38.4X5	T38.4X6

Substance	Poisoning, Accidental (Unintentional)	Poisoning, Intentional Self-Harm	Poisoning, Assault	Poisoning, Undetermined	Adverse Effect	Underdosing
Enoxacin	T36.8X1	T36.8X2	T36.8X3	T36.8X4	T36.8X5	T36.8X6
Enoxaparin (sodium)	T45.511	T45.512	T45.513	T45.514	T45.515	T45.516
Enpiprazole	T43.591	T43.592	T43.593	T43.594	T43.595	T43.596
Enprofylline	T48.6X1	T48.6X2	T48.6X3	T48.6X4	T48.6X5	T48.6X6
Enprostil	T47.1X1	T47.1X2	T47.1X3	T47.1X4	T47.1X5	T47.1X6
ENT preparations (anti-infectives)	T49.6X1	T49.6X2	T49.6X3	T49.6X4	T49.6X5	T49.6X6
Enviomycin	T36.8X1	T36.8X2	T36.8X3	T36.8X4	T36.8X5	T36.8X6
Enzodase	T45.3X1	T45.3X2	T45.3X3	T45.3X4	T45.3X5	T45.3X6
Enzyme NEC	T45.3X1	T45.3X2	T45.3X3	T45.3X4	T45.3X5	T45.3X6
depolymerizing	T49.8X1	T49.8X2	T49.8X3	T49.8X4	T49.8X5	T49.8X6
fibrolytic	T45.3X1	T45.3X2	T45.3X3	T45.3X4	T45.3X5	T45.3X6
gastric	T47.5X1	T47.5X2	T47.5X3	T47.5X4	T47.5X5	T47.5X6
intestinal	T47.5X1	T47.5X2	T47.5X3	T47.5X4	T47.5X5	T47.5X6
local action	T49.4X1	T49.4X2	T49.4X3	T49.4X4	T49.4X5	T49.4X6
proteolytic	T49.4X1	T49.4X2	T49.4X3	T49.4X4	T49.4X5	T49.4X6
thrombolytic	T45.3X1	T45.3X2	T45.3X3	T45.3X4	T45.3X5	T45.3X6
EPAB	T41.3X1	T41.3X2	T41.3X3	T41.3X4	T41.3X5	T41.3X6
Epanutin	T42.0X1	T42.0X2	T42.0X3	T42.0X4	T42.0X5	T42.0X6
Ephedra	T44.991	T44.992	T44.993	T44.994	T44.995	T44.996
Ephedrine	T44.991	T44.992	T44.993	T44.994	T44.995	T44.996
Epichlorhydrin, epichlorohydrin	T52.8X1	T52.8X2	T52.8X3	T52.8X4	—	—
Epicillin	T36.0X1	T36.0X2	T36.0X3	T36.0X4	T36.0X5	T36.0X6
Epiestriol	T38.5X1	T38.5X2	T38.5X3	T38.5X4	T38.5X5	T38.5X6
Epilim — see Sodium, valproate						
Epimestrol	T38.5X1	T38.5X2	T38.5X3	T38.5X4	T38.5X5	T38.5X6
Epinephrine	T44.5X1	T44.5X2	T44.5X3	T44.5X4	T44.5X5	T44.5X6
Epirubicin	T45.1X1	T45.1X2	T45.1X3	T45.1X4	T45.1X5	T45.1X6
Epitiostanol	T38.7X1	T38.7X2	T38.7X3	T38.7X4	T38.7X5	T38.7X6
Epitizide	T50.2X1	T50.2X2	T50.2X3	T50.2X4	T50.2X5	T50.2X6
EPN	T60.0X1	T60.0X2	T60.0X3	T60.0X4	—	—
EPO	T45.8X1	T45.8X2	T45.8X3	T45.8X4	T45.8X5	T45.8X6
Epoetin alpha	T45.8X1	T45.8X2	T45.8X3	T45.8X4	T45.8X5	T45.8X6
Epomediol	T50.991	T50.992	T50.993	T50.994	T50.995	T50.996
Epoprostenol	T45.521	T45.522	T45.523	T45.524	T45.525	T45.526
Epoxy resin	T65.891	T65.892	T65.893	T65.894	—	—
Eprazinone	T48.4X1	T48.4X2	T48.4X3	T48.4X4	T48.4X5	T48.4X6
Epsilon amino-caproic acid	T45.621	T45.622	T45.623	T45.624	T45.625	T45.626
Epsom salt	T47.3X1	T47.3X2	T47.3X3	T47.3X4	T47.3X5	T47.3X6
Eptazocine	T40.491	T40.492	T40.493	T40.494	T40.495	T40.496
Equanil	T43.591	T43.592	T43.593	T43.594	T43.595	T43.596
Equisetum	T62.2X1	T62.2X2	T62.2X3	T62.2X4	—	—
diuretic	T50.2X1	T50.2X2	T50.2X3	T50.2X4	T50.2X5	T50.2X6

◀ New ◀ Revised ~~deleted~~ Deleted

	External Cause (T-Code)					
Substance	Poisoning, Accidental (Unintentional)	Poisoning, Intentional Self-Harm	Poisoning, Assault	Poisoning, Undetermined	Adverse Effect	Underdosing
Ergobasine	T48.0X1	T48.0X2	T48.0X3	T48.0X4	T48.0X5	T48.0X6
Ergocalciferol	T45.2X1	T45.2X2	T45.2X3	T45.2X4	T45.2X5	T45.2X6
Ergoloid mesylates	T46.7X1	T46.7X2	T46.7X3	T46.7X4	T46.7X5	T46.7X6
Ergometrine	T48.0X1	T48.0X2	T48.0X3	T48.0X4	T48.0X5	T48.0X6
Ergonovine	T48.0X1	T48.0X2	T48.0X3	T48.0X4	T48.0X5	T48.0X6
Ergot NEC	T64.81	T64.82	T64.83	T64.84	—	—
derivative	T48.0X1	T48.0X2	T48.0X3	T48.0X4	T48.0X5	T48.0X6
medicinal (alkaloids)	T48.0X1	T48.0X2	T48.0X3	T48.0X4	T48.0X5	T48.0X6
prepared	T48.0X1	T48.0X2	T48.0X3	T48.0X4	T48.0X5	T48.0X6
Ergotamine	T46.5X1	T46.5X2	T46.5X3	T46.5X4	T46.5X5	T46.5X6
Ergotocine	T48.0X1	T48.0X2	T48.0X3	T48.0X4	T48.0X5	T48.0X6
Ergotrate	T48.0X1	T48.0X2	T48.0X3	T48.0X4	T48.0X5	T48.0X6
Eritrityl tetranitrate	T46.3X1	T46.3X2	T46.3X3	T46.3X4	T46.3X5	T46.3X6
Erythrityl tetranitrate	T46.3X1	T46.3X2	T46.3X3	T46.3X4	T46.3X5	T46.3X6
Erythrol tetranitrate	T46.3X1	T46.3X2	T46.3X3	T46.3X4	T46.3X5	T46.3X6
Erythromycin (salts)	T36.3X1	T36.3X2	T36.3X3	T36.3X4	T36.3X5	T36.3X6
ophthalmic preparation	T49.5X1	T49.5X2	T49.5X3	T49.5X4	T49.5X5	T49.5X6
topical NEC	T49.0X1	T49.0X2	T49.0X3	T49.0X4	T49.0X5	T49.0X6
Erythropoietin	T45.8X1	T45.8X2	T45.8X3	T45.8X4	T45.8X5	T45.8X6
human	T45.8X1	T45.8X2	T45.8X3	T45.8X4	T45.8X5	T45.8X6
Escin	T46.991	T46.992	T46.993	T46.994	T46.995	T46.996
Esculin	T45.2X1	T45.2X2	T45.2X3	T45.2X4	T45.2X5	T45.2X6
Esculoside	T45.2X1	T45.2X2	T45.2X3	T45.2X4	T45.2X5	T45.2X6
ESDT (ether-soluble tar distillate)	T49.1X1	T49.1X2	T49.1X3	T49.1X4	T49.1X5	T49.1X6
Eserine	T49.5X1	T49.5X2	T49.5X3	T49.5X4	T49.5X5	T49.5X6
Esflurbiprofen	T39.311	T39.312	T39.313	T39.314	T39.315	T39.316
Eskabarb	T42.3X1	T42.3X2	T42.3X3	T42.3X4	T42.3X5	T42.3X6
Eskalith	T43.8X1	T43.8X2	T43.8X3	T43.8X4	T43.8X5	T43.8X6
Esmolol	T44.7X1	T44.7X2	T44.7X3	T44.7X4	T44.7X5	T44.7X6
Estanozolol	T38.7X1	T38.7X2	T38.7X3	T38.7X4	T38.7X5	T38.7X6
Estazolam	T42.4X1	T42.4X2	T42.4X3	T42.4X4	T42.4X5	T42.4X6
Estradiol	T38.5X1	T38.5X2	T38.5X3	T38.5X4	T38.5X5	T38.5X6
with testosterone	T38.7X1	T38.7X2	T38.7X3	T38.7X4	T38.7X5	T38.7X6
benzoate	T38.5X1	T38.5X2	T38.5X3	T38.5X4	T38.5X5	T38.5X6
Estramustine	T45.1X1	T45.1X2	T45.1X3	T45.1X4	T45.1X5	T45.1X6
Estriol	T38.5X1	T38.5X2	T38.5X3	T38.5X4	T38.5X5	T38.5X6
Estrogen	T38.5X1	T38.5X2	T38.5X3	T38.5X4	T38.5X5	T38.5X6
with progesterone	T38.5X1	T38.5X2	T38.5X3	T38.5X4	T38.5X5	T38.5X6
conjugated	T38.5X1	T38.5X2	T38.5X3	T38.5X4	T38.5X5	T38.5X6
Estrone	T38.5X1	T38.5X2	T38.5X3	T38.5X4	T38.5X5	T38.5X6
Estropipate	T38.5X1	T38.5X2	T38.5X3	T38.5X4	T38.5X5	T38.5X6

	External Cause (T-Code)					
Substance	Poisoning, Accidental (Unintentional)	Poisoning, Intentional Self-Harm	Poisoning, Assault	Poisoning, Undetermined	Adverse Effect	Underdosing
Etacrynate sodium	T50.1X1	T50.1X2	T50.1X3	T50.1X4	T50.1X5	T50.1X6
Etacrynic acid	T50.1X1	T50.1X2	T50.1X3	T50.1X4	T50.1X5	T50.1X6
Etafedrine	T48.6X1	T48.6X2	T48.6X3	T48.6X4	T48.6X5	T48.6X6
Etafenone	T46.3X1	T46.3X2	T46.3X3	T46.3X4	T46.3X5	T46.3X6
Etambutol	T37.1X1	T37.1X2	T37.1X3	T37.1X4	T37.1X5	T37.1X6
Etamiphyllin	T48.6X1	T48.6X2	T48.6X3	T48.6X4	T48.6X5	T48.6X6
Etamivan	T50.7X1	T50.7X2	T50.7X3	T50.7X4	T50.7X5	T50.7X6
Etamsylate	T45.7X1	T45.7X2	T45.7X3	T45.7X4	T45.7X5	T45.7X6
Etebenecid	T50.4X1	T50.4X2	T50.4X3	T50.4X4	T50.4X5	T50.4X6
Ethacridine	T49.0X1	T49.0X2	T49.0X3	T49.0X4	T49.0X5	T49.0X6
Ethacrynic acid	T50.1X1	T50.1X2	T50.1X3	T50.1X4	T50.1X5	T50.1X6
Ethadione	T42.2X1	T42.2X2	T42.2X3	T42.2X4	T42.2X5	T42.2X6
Ethambutol	T37.1X1	T37.1X2	T37.1X3	T37.1X4	T37.1X5	T37.1X6
Ethamide	T50.2X1	T50.2X2	T50.2X3	T50.2X4	T50.2X5	T50.2X6
Ethamivan	T50.7X1	T50.7X2	T50.7X3	T50.7X4	T50.7X5	T50.7X6
Ethamsylate	T45.7X1	T45.7X2	T45.7X3	T45.7X4	T45.7X5	T45.7X6
Ethanol	T51.0X1	T51.0X2	T51.0X3	T51.0X4	—	—
beverage	T51.0X1	T51.0X2	T51.0X3	T51.0X4	—	—
Ethanolamine oleate	T46.8X1	T46.8X2	T46.8X3	T46.8X4	T46.8X5	T46.8X6
Ethaverine	T44.3X1	T44.3X2	T44.3X3	T44.3X4	T44.3X5	T44.3X6
Ethchlorvynol	T42.6X1	T42.6X2	T42.6X3	T42.6X4	T42.6X5	T42.6X6
Ethebenecid	T50.4X1	T50.4X2	T50.4X3	T50.4X4	T50.4X5	T50.4X6
Ether (vapor)	T41.0X1	T41.0X2	T41.0X3	T41.0X4	T41.0X5	T41.0X6
anesthetic	T41.0X1	T41.0X2	T41.0X3	T41.0X4	T41.0X5	T41.0X6
divinyl	T41.0X1	T41.0X2	T41.0X3	T41.0X4	T41.0X5	T41.0X6
ethyl (medicinal)	T41.0X1	T41.0X2	T41.0X3	T41.0X4	T41.0X5	T41.0X6
nonmedicinal	T52.8X1	T52.8X2	T52.8X3	T52.8X4	—	—
petroleum — *see* Ligroin						
solvent	T52.8X1	T52.8X2	T52.8X3	T52.8X4	—	—
Ethiazide	T50.2X1	T50.2X2	T50.2X3	T50.2X4	T50.2X5	T50.2X6
Ethidium chloride (vapor)	T59.891	T59.892	T59.893	T59.894	—	—
Ethinamate	T42.6X1	T42.6X2	T42.6X3	T42.6X4	T42.6X5	T42.6X6
Ethinylestradiol, ethinyloestradiol	T38.5X1	T38.5X2	T38.5X3	T38.5X4	T38.5X5	T38.5X6
with						
levonorgestrel	T38.4X1	T38.4X2	T38.4X3	T38.4X4	T38.4X5	T38.4X6
norethisterone	T38.4X1	T38.4X2	T38.4X3	T38.4X4	T38.4X5	T38.4X6
Ethiodized oil (131 I)	T50.8X1	T50.8X2	T50.8X3	T50.8X4	T50.8X5	T50.8X6
Ethion	T60.0X1	T60.0X2	T60.0X3	T60.0X4	—	—
Ethionamide	T37.1X1	T37.1X2	T37.1X3	T37.1X4	T37.1X5	T37.1X6
Ethioniamide	T37.1X1	T37.1X2	T37.1X3	T37.1X4	T37.1X5	T37.1X6
Ethisterone	T38.5X1	T38.5X2	T38.5X3	T38.5X4	T38.5X5	T38.5X6
Ethobral	T42.3X1	T42.3X2	T42.3X3	T42.3X4	T42.3X5	T42.3X6

◀ New   ◀ Revised   ~~deleted~~ Deleted

	External Cause (T-Code)					
Substance	Poisoning, Accidental (Unintentional)	Poisoning, Intentional Self-Harm	Poisoning, Assault	Poisoning, Undetermined	Adverse Effect	Underdosing
Ethocaine (infiltration) (topical)	T41.3X1	T41.3X2	T41.3X3	T41.3X4	T41.3X5	T41.3X6
nerve block (peripheral) (plexus)	T41.3X1	T41.3X2	T41.3X3	T41.3X4	T41.3X5	T41.3X6
spinal	T41.3X1	T41.3X2	T41.3X3	T41.3X4	T41.3X5	T41.3X6
Ethoheptazine	T40.491	T40.492	T40.493	T40.494	T40.495	T40.496
Ethopropazine	T44.3X1	T44.3X2	T44.3X3	T44.3X4	T44.3X5	T44.3X6
Ethosuximide	T42.2X1	T42.2X2	T42.2X3	T42.2X4	T42.2X5	T42.2X6
Ethotoin	T42.0X1	T42.0X2	T42.0X3	T42.0X4	T42.0X5	T42.0X6
Ethoxazene	T37.91	T37.92	T37.93	T37.94	T37.95	T37.96
Ethoxazorutoside	T46.991	T46.992	T46.993	T46.994	T46.995	T46.996
2-Ethoxyethanol	T52.3X1	T52.3X2	T52.3X3	T52.3X4	—	—
Ethoxzolamide	T50.2X1	T50.2X2	T50.2X3	T50.2X4	T50.2X5	T50.2X6
Ethyl						
acetate	T52.8X1	T52.8X2	T52.8X3	T52.8X4	—	—
alcohol	T51.0X1	T51.0X2	T51.0X3	T51.0X4	—	—
beverage	T51.0X1	T51.0X2	T51.0X3	T51.0X4	—	—
aldehyde (vapor)	T59.891	T59.892	T59.893	T59.894	—	—
liquid	T52.8X1	T52.8X2	T52.8X3	T52.8X4	—	—
aminobenzoate	T41.3X1	T41.3X2	T41.3X3	T41.3X4	T41.3X5	T41.3X6
aminophenothiazine	T43.3X1	T43.3X2	T43.3X3	T43.3X4	T43.3X5	T43.3X6
benzoate	T52.8X1	T52.8X2	T52.8X3	T52.8X4	—	—
biscoumacetate	T45.511	T45.512	T45.513	T45.514	T45.515	T45.516
bromide (anesthetic)	T41.0X1	T41.0X2	T41.0X3	T41.0X4	T41.0X5	T41.0X6
carbamate	T45.1X1	T45.1X2	T45.1X3	T45.1X4	T45.1X5	T45.1X6
carbinol	T51.3X1	T51.3X2	T51.3X3	T51.3X4	—	—
carbonate	T52.8X1	T52.8X2	T52.8X3	T52.8X4	—	—
chaulmoograte	T37.1X1	T37.1X2	T37.1X3	T37.1X4	T37.1X5	T37.1X6
chloride (anesthetic)	T41.0X1	T41.0X2	T41.0X3	T41.0X4	T41.0X5	T41.0X6
anesthetic (local)	T41.3X1	T41.3X2	T41.3X3	T41.3X4	T41.3X5	T41.3X6
inhaled	T41.0X1	T41.0X2	T41.0X3	T41.0X4	T41.0X5	T41.0X6
local	T49.4X1	T49.4X2	T49.4X3	T49.4X4	T49.4X5	T49.4X6
solvent	T53.6X1	T53.6X2	T53.6X3	T53.6X4	—	—
dibunate	T48.3X1	T48.3X2	T48.3X3	T48.3X4	T48.3X5	T48.3X6
dichloroarsine (vapor)	T57.0X1	T57.0X2	T57.0X3	T57.0X4		
estranol	T38.7X1	T38.7X2	T38.7X3	T38.7X4	T38.7X5	T38.7X6
ether — see also Ether	T52.8X1	T52.8X2	T52.8X3	T52.8X4	—	—
formate NEC (solvent)	T52.0X1	T52.0X2	T52.0X3	T52.0X4	—	—
fumarate	T49.4X1	T49.4X2	T49.4X3	T49.4X4	T49.4X5	T49.4X6
hydroxyisobutyrate NEC (solvent)	T52.8X1	T52.8X2	T52.8X3	T52.8X4	—	—
iodoacetate	T59.3X1	T59.3X2	T59.3X3	T59.3X4		
lactate NEC (solvent)	T52.8X1	T52.8X2	T52.8X3	T52.8X4		
loflazepate	T42.4X1	T42.4X2	T42.4X3	T42.4X4	T42.4X5	T42.4X6

	External Cause (T-Code)					
Substance	Poisoning, Accidental (Unintentional)	Poisoning, Intentional Self-Harm	Poisoning, Assault	Poisoning, Undetermined	Adverse Effect	Underdosing
Ethyl (Continued)						
mercuric chloride	T56.1X1	T56.1X2	T56.1X3	T56.1X4	—	—
methylcarbinol	T51.8X1	T51.8X2	T51.8X3	T51.8X4	—	—
morphine	T40.2X1	T40.2X2	T40.2X3	T40.2X4	T40.2X5	T40.2X6
noradrenaline	T48.6X1	T48.6X2	T48.6X3	T48.6X4	T48.6X5	T48.6X6
oxybutyrate NEC (solvent)	T52.8X1	T52.8X2	T52.8X3	T52.8X4		
Ethylene (gas)	T59.891	T59.892	T59.893	T59.894	—	—
anesthetic (general)	T41.0X1	T41.0X2	T41.0X3	T41.0X4	T41.0X5	T41.0X6
chlorohydrin	T52.8X1	T52.8X2	T52.8X3	T52.8X4		
vapor	T53.6X1	T53.6X2	T53.6X3	T53.6X4	—	—
dichloride	T52.8X1	T52.8X2	T52.8X3	T52.8X4		
vapor	T53.6X1	T53.6X2	T53.6X3	T53.6X4		
dinitrate	T52.3X1	T52.3X2	T52.3X3	T52.3X4	—	—
glycol(s)	T52.8X1	T52.8X2	T52.8X3	T52.8X4		
dinitrate	T52.3X1	T52.3X2	T52.3X3	T52.3X4		
monobutyl ether	T52.3X1	T52.3X2	T52.3X3	T52.3X4	—	—
imine	T54.1X1	T54.1X2	T54.1X3	T54.1X4		
oxide (fumigant) (nonmedicinal)	T59.891	T59.892	T59.893	T59.894		
medicinal	T49.0X1	T49.0X2	T49.0X3	T49.0X4	T49.0X5	T49.0X6
Ethylenediamine theophylline	T48.6X1	T48.6X2	T48.6X3	T48.6X4	T48.6X5	T48.6X6
Ethylenediaminetetra-acetic acid	T50.6X1	T50.6X2	T50.6X3	T50.6X4	T50.6X5	T50.6X6
Ethylenedinitrilotetra-acetate	T50.6X1	T50.6X2	T50.6X3	T50.6X4	T50.6X5	T50.6X6
Ethylestrenol	T38.7X1	T38.7X2	T38.7X3	T38.7X4	T38.7X5	T38.7X6
Ethylhydroxycellulose	T47.4X1	T47.4X2	T47.4X3	T47.4X4	T47.4X5	T47.4X6
Ethylidene						
chloride NEC	T53.6X1	T53.6X2	T53.6X3	T53.6X4	—	—
diacetate	T60.3X1	T60.3X2	T60.3X3	T60.3X4	—	—
dicoumarin	T45.511	T45.512	T45.513	T45.514	T45.515	T45.516
dicoumarol	T45.511	T45.512	T45.513	T45.514	T45.515	T45.516
diethyl ether	T52.0X1	T52.0X2	T52.0X3	T52.0X4	—	—
Ethylmorphine	T40.2X1	T40.2X2	T40.2X3	T40.2X4	T40.2X5	T40.2X6
Ethylnorepinephrine	T48.6X1	T48.6X2	T48.6X3	T48.6X4	T48.6X5	T48.6X6
Ethylparachlorophen- oxyisobutyrate	T46.6X1	T46.6X2	T46.6X3	T46.6X4	T46.6X5	T46.6X6
Ethynodiol	T38.4X1	T38.4X2	T38.4X3	T38.4X4	T38.4X5	T38.4X6
with mestranol diacetate	T38.4X1	T38.4X2	T38.4X3	T38.4X4	T38.4X5	T38.4X6
Etidocaine	T41.3X1	T41.3X2	T41.3X3	T41.3X4	T41.3X5	T41.3X6
infiltration (subcutaneous)	T41.3X1	T41.3X2	T41.3X3	T41.3X4	T41.3X5	T41.3X6
nerve (peripheral) (plexus)	T41.3X1	T41.3X2	T41.3X3	T41.3X4	T41.3X5	T41.3X6
Etidronate	T50.991	T50.992	T50.993	T50.994	T50.995	T50.996
Etidronic acid (disodium salt)	T50.991	T50.992	T50.993	T50.994	T50.995	T50.996
Etifoxine	T42.6X1	T42.6X2	T42.6X3	T42.6X4	T42.6X5	T42.6X6

Substance	Poisoning, Accidental (Unintentional)	Poisoning, Intentional Self-Harm	Poisoning, Assault	Poisoning, Undetermined	Adverse Effect	Underdosing
	External Cause (T-Code)					
Etilefrine	T44.4X1	T44.4X2	T44.4X3	T44.4X4	T44.4X5	T44.4X6
Etilfen	T42.3X1	T42.3X2	T42.3X3	T42.3X4	T42.3X5	T42.3X6
Etinodiol	T38.4X1	T38.4X2	T38.4X3	T38.4X4	T38.4X5	T38.4X6
Etiroxate	T46.6X1	T46.6X2	T46.6X3	T46.6X4	T46.6X5	T46.6X6
Etizolam	T42.4X1	T42.4X2	T42.4X3	T42.4X4	T42.4X5	T42.4X6
Etodolac	T39.391	T39.392	T39.393	T39.394	T39.395	T39.396
Etofamide	T37.3X1	T37.3X2	T37.3X3	T37.3X4	T37.3X5	T37.3X6
Etofibrate	T46.6X1	T46.6X2	T46.6X3	T46.6X4	T46.6X5	T46.6X6
Etofylline	T46.7X1	T46.7X2	T46.7X3	T46.7X4	T46.7X5	T46.7X6
clofibrate	T46.6X1	T46.6X2	T46.6X3	T46.6X4	T46.6X5	T46.6X6
Etoglucid	T45.1X1	T45.1X2	T45.1X3	T45.1X4	T45.1X5	T45.1X6
Etomidate	T41.1X1	T41.1X2	T41.1X3	T41.1X4	T41.1X5	T41.1X6
Etomide	T39.8X1	T39.8X2	T39.8X3	T39.8X4	T39.8X5	T39.8X6
Etomidoline	T44.3X1	T44.3X2	T44.3X3	T44.3X4	T44.3X5	T44.3X6
Etoposide	T45.1X1	T45.1X2	T45.1X3	T45.1X4	T45.1X5	T45.1X6
Etorphine	T40.2X1	T40.2X2	T40.2X3	T40.2X4	T40.2X5	T40.2X6
Etoval	T42.3X1	T42.3X2	T42.3X3	T42.3X4	T42.3X5	T42.3X6
Etozolin	T50.1X1	T50.1X2	T50.1X3	T50.1X4	T50.1X5	T50.1X6
Etretinate	T50.991	T50.992	T50.993	T50.994	T50.995	T50.996
Etryptamine	T43.691	T43.692	T43.693	T43.694	T43.695	T43.696
Etybenzatropine	T44.3X1	T44.3X2	T44.3X3	T44.3X4	T44.3X5	T44.3X6
Etynodiol	T38.4X1	T38.4X2	T38.4X3	T38.4X4	T38.4X5	T38.4X6
Eucaine	T41.3X1	T41.3X2	T41.3X3	T41.3X4	T41.3X5	T41.3X6
Eucalyptus oil	T49.7X1	T49.7X2	T49.7X3	T49.7X4	T49.7X5	T49.7X6
Eucatropine	T49.5X1	T49.5X2	T49.5X3	T49.5X4	T49.5X5	T49.5X6
Eucodal	T40.2X1	T40.2X2	T40.2X3	T40.2X4	T40.2X5	T40.2X6
Euneryl	T42.3X1	T42.3X2	T42.3X3	T42.3X4	T42.3X5	T42.3X6
Euphthalmine	T44.3X1	T44.3X2	T44.3X3	T44.3X4	T44.3X5	T44.3X6
Eurax	T49.0X1	T49.0X2	T49.0X3	T49.0X4	T49.0X5	T49.0X6
Euresol	T49.4X1	T49.4X2	T49.4X3	T49.4X4	T49.4X5	T49.4X6
Euthroid	T38.1X1	T38.1X2	T38.1X3	T38.1X4	T38.1X5	T38.1X6
Evans blue	T50.8X1	T50.8X2	T50.8X3	T50.8X4	T50.8X5	T50.8X6
Evipal	T42.3X1	T42.3X2	T42.3X3	T42.3X4	T42.3X5	T42.3X6
sodium	T41.1X1	T41.1X2	T41.1X3	T41.1X4	T41.1X5	T41.1X6
Evipan	T42.3X1	T42.3X2	T42.3X3	T42.3X4	T42.3X5	T42.3X6
sodium	T41.1X1	T41.1X2	T41.1X3	T41.1X4	T41.1X5	T41.1X6
Exalamide	T49.0X1	T49.0X2	T49.0X3	T49.0X4	T49.0X5	T49.0X6
Exalgin	T39.1X1	T39.1X2	T39.1X3	T39.1X4	T39.1X5	T39.1X6
Excipients, pharmaceutical	T50.901	T50.902	T50.903	T50.904	T50.905	T50.906
Exhaust gas (engine) (motor vehicle)	T58.01	T58.02	T58.03	T58.04	—	—
Ex-Lax (phenolphthalein)	T47.2X1	T47.2X2	T47.2X3	T47.2X4	T47.2X5	T47.2X6
Expectorant NEC	T48.4X1	T48.4X2	T48.4X3	T48.4X4	T48.4X5	T48.4X6

Substance	Poisoning, Accidental (Unintentional)	Poisoning, Intentional Self-Harm	Poisoning, Assault	Poisoning, Undetermined	Adverse Effect	Underdosing
	External Cause (T-Code)					
Extended insulin zinc suspension	T38.3X1	T38.3X2	T38.3X3	T38.3X4	T38.3X5	T38.3X6
External medications (skin) (mucous membrane)	T49.91	T49.92	T49.93	T49.94	T49.95	T49.96
dental agent	T49.7X1	T49.7X2	T49.7X3	T49.7X4	T49.7X5	T49.7X6
ENT agent	T49.6X1	T49.6X2	T49.6X3	T49.6X4	T49.6X5	T49.6X6
ophthalmic preparation	T49.5X1	T49.5X2	T49.5X3	T49.5X4	T49.5X5	T49.5X6
specified NEC	T49.8X1	T49.8X2	T49.8X3	T49.8X4	T49.8X5	T49.8X6
Extrapyramidal antagonist NEC	T44.3X1	T44.3X2	T44.3X3	T44.3X4	T44.3X5	T44.3X6
Eye agents (anti-infective)	T49.5X1	T49.5X2	T49.5X3	T49.5X4	T49.5X5	T49.5X6
Eye drug NEC	T49.5X1	T49.5X2	T49.5X3	T49.5X4	T49.5X5	T49.5X6
F						
FAC (fluorouracil + doxorubicin + cyclophosphamide)	T45.1X1	T45.1X2	T45.1X3	T45.1X4	T45.1X5	T45.1X6
Factor						
I (fibrinogen)	T45.8X1	T45.8X2	T45.8X3	T45.8X4	T45.8X5	T45.8X6
III (thromboplastin)	T45.8X1	T45.8X2	T45.8X3	T45.8X4	T45.8X5	T45.8X6
VIII (antihemophilic Factor) (Concentrate)	T45.8X1	T45.8X2	T45.8X3	T45.8X4	T45.8X5	T45.8X6
IX complex	T45.7X1	T45.7X2	T45.7X3	T45.7X4	T45.7X5	T45.7X6
human	T45.8X1	T45.8X2	T45.8X3	T45.8X4	T45.8X5	T45.8X6
Famotidine	T47.0X1	T47.0X2	T47.0X3	T47.0X4	T47.0X5	T47.0X6
Fat suspension, intravenous	T50.991	T50.992	T50.993	T50.994	T50.995	T50.996
Fazadinium bromide	T48.1X1	T48.1X2	T48.1X3	T48.1X4	T48.1X5	T48.1X6
Febarbamate	T42.3X1	T42.3X2	T42.3X3	T42.3X4	T42.3X5	T42.3X6
Fecal softener	T47.4X1	T47.4X2	T47.4X3	T47.4X4	T47.4X5	T47.4X6
Fedrilate	T48.3X1	T48.3X2	T48.3X3	T48.3X4	T48.3X5	T48.3X6
Felodipine	T46.1X1	T46.1X2	T46.1X3	T46.1X4	T46.1X5	T46.1X6
Felypressin	T38.891	T38.892	T38.893	T38.894	T38.895	T38.896
Femoxetine	T43.221	T43.222	T43.223	T43.224	T43.225	T43.226
Fenalcomine	T46.3X1	T46.3X2	T46.3X3	T46.3X4	T46.3X5	T46.3X6
Fenamisal	T37.1X1	T37.1X2	T37.1X3	T37.1X4	T37.1X5	T37.1X6
Fenazone	T39.2X1	T39.2X2	T39.2X3	T39.2X4	T39.2X5	T39.2X6
Fenbendazole	T37.4X1	T37.4X2	T37.4X3	T37.4X4	T37.4X5	T37.4X6
Fenbutrazate	T50.5X1	T50.5X2	T50.5X3	T50.5X4	T50.5X5	T50.5X6
Fencamfamine	T43.691	T43.692	T43.693	T43.694	T43.695	T43.696
Fendiline	T46.1X1	T46.1X2	T46.1X3	T46.1X4	T46.1X5	T46.1X6
Fenetylline	T43.691	T43.692	T43.693	T43.694	T43.695	T43.696
Fenflumizole	T39.391	T39.392	T39.393	T39.394	T39.395	T39.396
Fenfluramine	T50.5X1	T50.5X2	T50.5X3	T50.5X4	T50.5X5	T50.5X6
Fenobarbital	T42.3X1	T42.3X2	T42.3X3	T42.3X4	T42.3X5	T42.3X6
Fenofibrate	T46.6X1	T46.6X2	T46.6X3	T46.6X4	T46.6X5	T46.6X6
Fenoprofen	T39.311	T39.312	T39.313	T39.314	T39.315	T39.316
Fenoterol	T48.6X1	T48.6X2	T48.6X3	T48.6X4	T48.6X5	T48.6X6

◀ New   ◀ Revised   ~~deleted~~ Deleted

Substance	External Cause (T-Code)					
	Poisoning, Accidental (Unintentional)	Poisoning, Intentional Self-Harm	Poisoning, Assault	Poisoning, Undetermined	Adverse Effect	Underdosing
Fenoverine	T44.3X1	T44.3X2	T44.3X3	T44.3X4	T44.3X5	T44.3X6
Fenoxazoline	T48.5X1	T48.5X2	T48.5X3	T48.5X4	T48.5X5	T48.5X6
Fenproporex	T50.5X1	T50.5X2	T50.5X3	T50.5X4	T50.5X5	T50.5X6
Fenquizone	T50.2X1	T50.2X2	T50.2X3	T50.2X4	T50.2X5	T50.2X6
Fentanyl (analogs)	T40.411	T40.412	T40.413	T40.414	T40.415	T40.416
Fentazin	T43.3X1	T43.3X2	T43.3X3	T43.3X4	T43.3X5	T43.3X6
Fenthion	T60.0X1	T60.0X2	T60.0X3	T60.0X4	—	—
Fenticlor	T49.0X1	T49.0X2	T49.0X3	T49.0X4	T49.0X5	T49.0X6
Fenylbutazone	T39.2X1	T39.2X2	T39.2X3	T39.2X4	T39.2X5	T39.2X6
Feprazone	T39.2X1	T39.2X2	T39.2X3	T39.2X4	T39.2X5	T39.2X6
Fer de lance (bite) (venom)	T63.061	T63.062	T63.063	T63.064	—	—
Ferric — see also Iron						
chloride	T45.4X1	T45.4X2	T45.4X3	T45.4X4	T45.4X5	T45.4X6
citrate	T45.4X1	T45.4X2	T45.4X3	T45.4X4	T45.4X5	T45.4X6
hydroxide						
colloidal	T45.4X1	T45.4X2	T45.4X3	T45.4X4	T45.4X5	T45.4X6
polymaltose	T45.4X1	T45.4X2	T45.4X3	T45.4X4	T45.4X5	T45.4X6
pyrophosphate	T45.4X1	T45.4X2	T45.4X3	T45.4X4	T45.4X5	T45.4X6
Ferritin	T45.4X1	T45.4X2	T45.4X3	T45.4X4	T45.4X5	T45.4X6
Ferrocholinate	T45.4X1	T45.4X2	T45.4X3	T45.4X4	T45.4X5	T45.4X6
Ferrodextrane	T45.4X1	T45.4X2	T45.4X3	T45.4X4	T45.4X5	T45.4X6
Ferropolimaler	T45.4X1	T45.4X2	T45.4X3	T45.4X4	T45.4X5	T45.4X6
Ferrous — see also Iron						
phosphate	T45.4X1	T45.4X2	T45.4X3	T45.4X4	T45.4X5	T45.4X6
salt	T45.4X1	T45.4X2	T45.4X3	T45.4X4	T45.4X5	T45.4X6
with folic acid	T45.4X1	T45.4X2	T45.4X3	T45.4X4	T45.4X5	T45.4X6
Ferrous fumarate, gluconate, lactate, salt NEC, sulfate (medicinal)	T45.4X1	T45.4X2	T45.4X3	T45.4X4	T45.4X5	T45.4X6
Ferrovanadium (fumes)	T59.891	T59.892	T59.893	T59.894	—	—
Ferrum — see Iron						
Fertilizers NEC	T65.891	T65.892	T65.893	T65.894	—	—
with herbicide mixture	T60.3X1	T60.3X2	T60.3X3	T60.3X4	—	—
Fetoxilate	T47.6X1	T47.6X2	T47.6X3	T47.6X4	T47.6X5	T47.6X6
Fiber, dietary	T47.4X1	T47.4X2	T47.4X3	T47.4X4	T47.4X5	T47.4X6
Fibrinogen (human)	T45.8X1	T45.8X2	T45.8X3	T45.8X4	T45.8X5	T45.8X6
Fibrinolysin (human)	T45.691	T45.692	T45.693	T45.694	T45.695	T45.696
Fibrinolysis						
affecting drug	T45.601	T45.602	T45.603	T45.604	T45.605	T45.606
inhibitor NEC	T45.621	T45.622	T45.623	T45.624	T45.625	T45.626
Fibrinolytic drug	T45.611	T45.612	T45.613	T45.614	T45.615	T45.616
Filix mas	T37.4X1	T37.4X2	T37.4X3	T37.4X4	T37.4X5	T37.4X6
Filtering cream	T49.3X1	T49.3X2	T49.3X3	T49.3X4	T49.3X5	T49.3X6

Substance	External Cause (T-Code)					
	Poisoning, Accidental (Unintentional)	Poisoning, Intentional Self-Harm	Poisoning, Assault	Poisoning, Undetermined	Adverse Effect	Underdosing
Fiorinal	T39.011	T39.012	T39.013	T39.014	T39.015	T39.016
Firedamp	T59.891	T59.892	T59.893	T59.894	—	—
Fish, noxious, nonbacterial	T61.91	T61.92	T61.93	T61.94	—	—
ciguatera	T61.01	T61.02	T61.03	T61.04	—	—
scombroid	T61.11	T61.12	T61.13	T61.14	—	—
shell	T61.781	T61.782	T61.783	T61.784	—	—
specified NEC	T61.771	T61.772	T61.773	T61.774	—	—
Flagyl	T37.3X1	T37.3X2	T37.3X3	T37.3X4	T37.3X5	T37.3X6
Flavine adenine dinucleotide	T45.2X1	T45.2X2	T45.2X3	T45.2X4	T45.2X5	T45.2X6
Flavodic acid	T46.991	T46.992	T46.993	T46.994	T46.995	T46.996
Flavoxate	T44.3X1	T44.3X2	T44.3X3	T44.3X4	T44.3X5	T44.3X6
Flaxedil	T48.1X1	T48.1X2	T48.1X3	T48.1X4	T48.1X5	T48.1X6
Flaxseed (medicinal)	T49.3X1	T49.3X2	T49.3X3	T49.3X4	T49.3X5	T49.3X6
Flecainide	T46.2X1	T46.2X2	T46.2X3	T46.2X4	T46.2X5	T46.2X6
Fleroxacin	T36.8X1	T36.8X2	T36.8X3	T36.8X4	T36.8X5	T36.8X6
Floctafenine	T39.8X1	T39.8X2	T39.8X3	T39.8X4	T39.8X5	T39.8X6
Flomax	T44.6X1	T44.6X2	T44.6X3	T44.6X4	T44.6X5	T44.6X6
Flomoxef	T36.1X1	T36.1X2	T36.1X3	T36.1X4	T36.1X5	T36.1X6
Flopropione	T44.3X1	T44.3X2	T44.3X3	T44.3X4	T44.3X5	T44.3X6
Florantyrone	T47.5X1	T47.5X2	T47.5X3	T47.5X4	T47.5X5	T47.5X6
Floraquin	T37.8X1	T37.8X2	T37.8X3	T37.8X4	T37.8X5	T37.8X6
Florinef	T38.0X1	T38.0X2	T38.0X3	T38.0X4	T38.0X5	T38.0X6
ENT agent	T49.6X1	T49.6X2	T49.6X3	T49.6X4	T49.6X5	T49.6X6
ophthalmic preparation	T49.5X1	T49.5X2	T49.5X3	T49.5X4	T49.5X5	T49.5X6
topical NEC	T49.0X1	T49.0X2	T49.0X3	T49.0X4	T49.0X5	T49.0X6
Flowers of sulfur	T49.4X1	T49.4X2	T49.4X3	T49.4X4	T49.4X5	T49.4X6
Floxuridine	T45.1X1	T45.1X2	T45.1X3	T45.1X4	T45.1X5	T45.1X6
Fluanisone	T43.4X1	T43.4X2	T43.4X3	T43.4X4	T43.4X5	T43.4X6
Flubendazole	T37.4X1	T37.4X2	T37.4X3	T37.4X4	T37.4X5	T37.4X6
Fluclorolone acetonide	T49.0X1	T49.0X2	T49.0X3	T49.0X4	T49.0X5	T49.0X6
Flucloxacillin	T36.0X1	T36.0X2	T36.0X3	T36.0X4	T36.0X5	T36.0X6
Fluconazole	T37.8X1	T37.8X2	T37.8X3	T37.8X4	T37.8X5	T37.8X6
Flucytosine	T37.8X1	T37.8X2	T37.8X3	T37.8X4	T37.8X5	T37.8X6
Fludeoxyglucose (18F)	T50.8X1	T50.8X2	T50.8X3	T50.8X4	T50.8X5	T50.8X6
Fludiazepam	T42.4X1	T42.4X2	T42.4X3	T42.4X4	T42.4X5	T42.4X6
Fludrocortisone	T50.0X1	T50.0X2	T50.0X3	T50.0X4	T50.0X5	T50.0X6
ENT agent	T49.6X1	T49.6X2	T49.6X3	T49.6X4	T49.6X5	T49.6X6
ophthalmic preparation	T49.5X1	T49.5X2	T49.5X3	T49.5X4	T49.5X5	T49.5X6
topical NEC	T49.0X1	T49.0X2	T49.0X3	T49.0X4	T49.0X5	T49.0X6
Fludroxycortide	T49.0X1	T49.0X2	T49.0X3	T49.0X4	T49.0X5	T49.0X6
Flufenamic acid	T39.391	T39.392	T39.393	T39.394	T39.395	T39.396
Fluindione	T45.511	T45.512	T45.513	T45.514	T45.515	T45.516

◄ New   ◄ Revised   ~~deleted~~ Deleted

Substance	Poisoning, Accidental (Unintentional)	Poisoning, Intentional Self-Harm	Poisoning, Assault	Poisoning, Undetermined	Adverse Effect	Underdosing
Flumequine	T37.8X1	T37.8X2	T37.8X3	T37.8X4	T37.8X5	T37.8X6
Flumethasone	T49.0X1	T49.0X2	T49.0X3	T49.0X4	T49.0X5	T49.0X6
Flumethiazide	T50.2X1	T50.2X2	T50.2X3	T50.2X4	T50.2X5	T50.2X6
Flumidin	T37.5X1	T37.5X2	T37.5X3	T37.5X4	T37.5X5	T37.5X6
Flunarizine	T46.7X1	T46.7X2	T46.7X3	T46.7X4	T46.7X5	T46.7X6
Flunidazole	T37.8X1	T37.8X2	T37.8X3	T37.8X4	T37.8X5	T37.8X6
Flunisolide	T48.6X1	T48.6X2	T48.6X3	T48.6X4	T48.6X5	T48.6X6
Flunitrazepam	T42.4X1	T42.4X2	T42.4X3	T42.4X4	T42.4X5	T42.4X6
Fluocinolone (acetonide)	T49.0X1	T49.0X2	T49.0X3	T49.0X4	T49.0X5	T49.0X6
Fluocinonide	T49.0X1	T49.0X2	T49.0X3	T49.0X4	T49.0X5	T49.0X6
Fluocortin (butyl)	T49.0X1	T49.0X2	T49.0X3	T49.0X4	T49.0X5	T49.0X6
Fluocortolone	T49.0X1	T49.0X2	T49.0X3	T49.0X4	T49.0X5	T49.0X6
Fluohydrocortisone	T38.0X1	T38.0X2	T38.0X3	T38.0X4	T38.0X5	T38.0X6
ENT agent	T49.6X1	T49.6X2	T49.6X3	T49.6X4	T49.6X5	T49.6X6
ophthalmic preparation	T49.5X1	T49.5X2	T49.5X3	T49.5X4	T49.5X5	T49.5X6
topical NEC	T49.0X1	T49.0X2	T49.0X3	T49.0X4	T49.0X5	T49.0X6
Fluonid	T49.0X1	T49.0X2	T49.0X3	T49.0X4	T49.0X5	T49.0X6
Fluopromazine	T43.3X1	T43.3X2	T43.3X3	T43.3X4	T43.3X5	T43.3X6
Fluoroacetate	T60.8X1	T60.8X2	T60.8X3	T60.8X4	—	—
Fluorescein	T50.8X1	T50.8X2	T50.8X3	T50.8X4	T50.8X5	T50.8X6
Fluorhydrocortisone	T50.0X1	T50.0X2	T50.0X3	T50.0X4	T50.0X5	T50.0X6
Fluoride (nonmedicinal) (pesticide) (sodium) NEC	T60.8X1	T60.8X2	T60.8X3	T60.8X4	—	—
hydrogen — *see Hydrofluoric acid*						
medicinal NEC	T50.991	T50.992	T50.993	T50.994	T50.995	T50.996
dental use	T49.7X1	T49.7X2	T49.7X3	T49.7X4	T49.7X5	T49.7X6
not pesticide NEC	T54.91	T54.92	T54.93	T54.94	—	—
stannous	T49.7X1	T49.7X2	T49.7X3	T49.7X4	T49.7X5	T49.7X6
Fluorinated corticosteroids	T38.0X1	T38.0X2	T38.0X3	T38.0X4	T38.0X5	T38.0X6
Fluorine (gas)	T59.5X1	T59.5X2	T59.5X3	T59.5X4	—	—
salt — *see Fluoride(s)*						
Fluoristan	T49.7X1	T49.7X2	T49.7X3	T49.7X4	T49.7X5	T49.7X6
Fluormetholone	T49.0X1	T49.0X2	T49.0X3	T49.0X4	T49.0X5	T49.0X6
Fluoroacetate	T60.8X1	T60.8X2	T60.8X3	T60.8X4	—	—
Fluorocarbon monomer	T53.6X1	T53.6X2	T53.6X3	T53.6X4	—	—
Fluorocytosine	T37.8X1	T37.8X2	T37.8X3	T37.8X4	T37.8X5	T37.8X6
Fluorodeoxyuridine	T45.1X1	T45.1X2	T45.1X3	T45.1X4	T45.1X5	T45.1X6
Fluorometholone	T49.0X1	T49.0X2	T49.0X3	T49.0X4	T49.0X5	T49.0X6
ophthalmic preparation	T49.5X1	T49.5X2	T49.5X3	T49.5X4	T49.5X5	T49.5X6
Fluorophosphate insecticide	T60.0X1	T60.0X2	T60.0X3	T60.0X4	—	—
Fluorosol	T46.3X1	T46.3X2	T46.3X3	T46.3X4	T46.3X5	T46.3X6
Fluorouracil	T45.1X1	T45.1X2	T45.1X3	T45.1X4	T45.1X5	T45.1X6

Substance	Poisoning, Accidental (Unintentional)	Poisoning, Intentional Self-Harm	Poisoning, Assault	Poisoning, Undetermined	Adverse Effect	Underdosing
Fluorphenylalanine	T49.5X1	T49.5X2	T49.5X3	T49.5X4	T49.5X5	T49.5X6
Fluothane	T41.0X1	T41.0X2	T41.0X3	T41.0X4	T41.0X5	T41.0X6
Fluoxetine	T43.221	T43.222	T43.223	T43.224	T43.225	T43.226
Fluoxymesterone	T38.7X1	T38.7X2	T38.7X3	T38.7X4	T38.7X5	T38.7X6
Flupenthixol	T43.4X1	T43.4X2	T43.4X3	T43.4X4	T43.4X5	T43.4X6
Flupentixol	T43.4X1	T43.4X2	T43.4X3	T43.4X4	T43.4X5	T43.4X6
Fluphenazine	T43.3X1	T43.3X2	T43.3X3	T43.3X4	T43.3X5	T43.3X6
Fluprednidene	T49.0X1	T49.0X2	T49.0X3	T49.0X4	T49.0X5	T49.0X6
Fluprednisolone	T38.0X1	T38.0X2	T38.0X3	T38.0X4	T38.0X5	T38.0X6
Fluradoline	T39.8X1	T39.8X2	T39.8X3	T39.8X4	T39.8X5	T39.8X6
Flurandrenolide	T49.0X1	T49.0X2	T49.0X3	T49.0X4	T49.0X5	T49.0X6
Flurandrenolone	T49.0X1	T49.0X2	T49.0X3	T49.0X4	T49.0X5	T49.0X6
Flurazepam	T42.4X1	T42.4X2	T42.4X3	T42.4X4	T42.4X5	T42.4X6
Flurbiprofen	T39.311	T39.312	T39.313	T39.314	T39.315	T39.316
Flurobate	T49.0X1	T49.0X2	T49.0X3	T49.0X4	T49.0X5	T49.0X6
Flurotyl	T43.291	T43.292	T43.293	T43.294	T43.295	T43.296
Fluroxene	T41.0X1	T41.0X2	T41.0X3	T41.0X4	T41.0X5	T41.0X6
Fluspirilene	T43.591	T43.592	T43.593	T43.594	T43.595	T43.596
Flutamide	T38.6X1	T38.6X2	T38.6X3	T38.6X4	T38.6X5	T38.6X6
Flutazolam	T42.4X1	T42.4X2	T42.4X3	T42.4X4	T42.4X5	T42.4X6
Fluticasone propionate	T38.0X1	T38.0X2	T38.0X3	T38.0X4	T38.0X5	T38.0X6
Flutoprazepam	T42.4X1	T42.4X2	T42.4X3	T42.4X4	T42.4X5	T42.4X6
Flutropium bromide	T48.6X1	T48.6X2	T48.6X3	T48.6X4	T48.6X5	T48.6X6
Fluvoxamine	T43.221	T43.222	T43.223	T43.224	T43.225	T43.226
Folacin	T45.8X1	T45.8X2	T45.8X3	T45.8X4	T45.8X5	T45.8X6
Folic acid	T45.8X1	T45.8X2	T45.8X3	T45.8X4	T45.8X5	T45.8X6
with ferrous salt	T45.2X1	T45.2X2	T45.2X3	T45.2X4	T45.2X5	T45.2X6
antagonist	T45.1X1	T45.1X2	T45.1X3	T45.1X4	T45.1X5	T45.1X6
Folinic acid	T45.8X1	T45.8X2	T45.8X3	T45.8X4	T45.8X5	T45.8X6
Folium stramoniae	T48.6X1	T48.6X2	T48.6X3	T48.6X4	T48.6X5	T48.6X6
Follicle-stimulating hormone, human	T38.811	T38.812	T38.813	T38.814	T38.815	T38.816
Folpet	T60.3X1	T60.3X2	T60.3X3	T60.3X4	—	—
Fominoben	T48.3X1	T48.3X2	T48.3X3	T48.3X4	T48.3X5	T48.3X6
Food, foodstuffs, noxious, nonbacterial, NEC	T62.91	T62.92	T62.93	T62.94		
berries	T62.1X1	T62.1X2	T62.1X3	T62.1X4	—	—
fish — *see also Fish*	T61.91	T61.92	T61.93	T61.94	—	—
mushrooms	T62.0X1	T62.0X2	T62.0X3	T62.0X4	—	—
plants	T62.2X1	T62.2X2	T62.2X3	T62.2X4	—	—
seafood	T61.91	T61.92	T61.93	T61.94	—	—
specified NEC	T61.8X1	T61.8X2	T61.8X3	T61.8X4	—	—
seeds	T62.2X1	T62.2X2	T62.2X3	T62.2X4	—	—

◀ New   ◀ Revised   ~~deleted~~ Deleted

Substance	Poisoning, Accidental (Unintentional)	Poisoning, Intentional Self-Harm	Poisoning, Assault	Poisoning, Undetermined	Adverse Effect	Underdosing
External Cause (T-Code)						
Food, foodstuffs, noxious, nonbacterial, NEC *(Continued)*						
shellfish	T61.781	T61.782	T61.783	T61.784	—	—
specified NEC	T62.8X1	T62.8X2	T62.8X3	T62.8X4	—	—
Fool's parsley	T62.2X1	T62.2X2	T62.2X3	T62.2X4	—	—
Formaldehyde (solution), gas or vapor	T59.2X1	T59.2X2	T59.2X3	T59.2X4	—	—
fungicide	T60.3X1	T60.3X2	T60.3X3	T60.3X4	—	—
Formalin	T59.2X1	T59.2X2	T59.2X3	T59.2X4	—	—
fungicide	T60.3X1	T60.3X2	T60.3X3	T60.3X4	—	—
vapor	T59.2X1	T59.2X2	T59.2X3	T59.2X4	—	—
Formic acid	T54.2X1	T54.2X2	T54.2X3	T54.2X4	—	—
vapor	T59.891	T59.892	T59.893	T59.894	—	—
Foscarnet sodium	T37.5X1	T37.5X2	T37.5X3	T37.5X4	T37.5X5	T37.5X6
Fosfestrol	T38.5X1	T38.5X2	T38.5X3	T38.5X4	T38.5X5	T38.5X6
Fosfomycin	T36.8X1	T36.8X2	T36.8X3	T36.8X4	T36.8X5	T36.8X6
Fosfonet sodium	T37.5X1	T37.5X2	T37.5X3	T37.5X4	T37.5X5	T37.5X6
Fosinopril	T46.4X1	T46.4X2	T46.4X3	T46.4X4	T46.4X5	T46.4X6
sodium	T46.4X1	T46.4X2	T46.4X3	T46.4X4	T46.4X5	T46.4X6
Fowler's solution	T57.0X1	T57.0X2	T57.0X3	T57.0X4	—	—
Foxglove	T62.2X1	T62.2X2	T62.2X3	T62.2X4	—	—
Framycetin	T36.5X1	T36.5X2	T36.5X3	T36.5X4	T36.5X5	T36.5X6
Frangula	T47.2X1	T47.2X2	T47.2X3	T47.2X4	T47.2X5	T47.2X6
extract	T47.2X1	T47.2X2	T47.2X3	T47.2X4	T47.2X5	T47.2X6
Frei antigen	T50.8X1	T50.8X2	T50.8X3	T50.8X4	T50.8X5	T50.8X6
Freon	T53.5X1	T53.5X2	T53.5X3	T53.5X4	—	—
Fructose	T50.3X1	T50.3X2	T50.3X3	T50.3X4	T50.3X5	T50.3X6
Frusemide	T50.1X1	T50.1X2	T50.1X3	T50.1X4	T50.1X5	T50.1X6
FSH	T38.811	T38.812	T38.813	T38.814	T38.815	T38.816
Ftorafur	T45.1X1	T45.1X2	T45.1X3	T45.1X4	T45.1X5	T45.1X6
Fuel						
automobile	T52.0X1	T52.0X2	T52.0X3	T52.0X4	—	—
exhaust gas, not in transit	T58.01	T58.02	T58.03	T58.04	—	—
vapor NEC	T52.0X1	T52.0X2	T52.0X3	T52.0X4	—	—
gas (domestic use) — *see also Carbon, monoxide, fuel, utility*	T59.891	T59.892	T59.893	T59.894	—	—
utility	T59.891	T59.892	T59.893	T59.894	—	—
in mobile container	T59.891	T59.892	T59.893	T59.894	—	—
incomplete combustion of — *see Carbon, monoxide, fuel, utility*						
piped (natural)	T59.891	T59.892	T59.893	T59.894	—	—
industrial, incomplete combustion	T58.8X1	T58.8X2	T58.8X3	T58.8X4	—	—

Substance	Poisoning, Accidental (Unintentional)	Poisoning, Intentional Self-Harm	Poisoning, Assault	Poisoning, Undetermined	Adverse Effect	Underdosing
External Cause (T-Code)						
Fugillin	T36.8X1	T36.8X2	T36.8X3	T36.8X4	T36.8X5	T36.8X6
Fulminate of mercury	T56.1X1	T56.1X2	T56.1X3	T56.1X4	—	—
Fulvicin	T36.7X1	T36.7X2	T36.7X3	T36.7X4	T36.7X5	T36.7X6
Fumadil	T36.8X1	T36.8X2	T36.8X3	T36.8X4	T36.8X5	T36.8X6
Fumagillin	T36.8X1	T36.8X2	T36.8X3	T36.8X4	T36.8X5	T36.8X6
Fumaric acid	T49.4X1	T49.4X2	T49.4X3	T49.4X4	T49.4X5	T49.4X6
Fumes (from)	T59.91	T59.92	T59.93	T59.94	—	—
carbon monoxide — *see Carbon, monoxide*						
charcoal (domestic use) — *see Charcoal, fumes*						
chloroform — *see Chloroform*						
coke (in domestic stoves, fireplaces) — *see Coke, fumes*						
corrosive NEC	T54.91	T54.92	T54.93	T54.94	—	—
ether — *see Ether*						
freons	T53.5X1	T53.5X2	T53.5X3	T53.5X4	—	—
hydrocarbons	T59.891	T59.892	T59.893	T59.894	—	—
petroleum (liquefied)	T59.891	T59.892	T59.893	T59.894	—	—
distributed through pipes (pure or mixed with air)	T59.891	T59.892	T59.893	T59.894	—	—
lead — *see Lead*						
metal — *see Metals, or the specified metal*						
nitrogen dioxide	T59.0X1	T59.0X2	T59.0X3	T59.0X4	—	—
pesticides — *see Pesticide*						
petroleum (liquefied)	T59.891	T59.892	T59.893	T59.894	—	—
distributed through pipes (pure or mixed with air)	T59.891	T59.892	T59.893	T59.894	—	—
polyester	T59.891	T59.892	T59.893	T59.894	—	—
specified source NEC — *see also substance specified*	T59.891	T59.892	T59.893	T59.894	—	—
sulfur dioxide	T59.1X1	T59.1X2	T59.1X3	T59.1X4	—	—
Fumigant NEC	T60.91	T60.92	T60.93	T60.94	—	—
Fungi, noxious, used as food	T62.0X1	T62.0X2	T62.0X3	T62.0X4	—	—
Fungicide NEC (nonmedicinal)	T60.3X1	T60.3X2	T60.3X3	T60.3X4	—	—
Fungizone	T36.7X1	T36.7X2	T36.7X3	T36.7X4	T36.7X5	T36.7X6
topical	T49.0X1	T49.0X2	T49.0X3	T49.0X4	T49.0X5	T49.0X6
Furacin	T49.0X1	T49.0X2	T49.0X3	T49.0X4	T49.0X5	T49.0X6
Furadantin	T37.91	T37.92	T37.93	T37.94	T37.95	T37.96
Furazolidone	T37.8X1	T37.8X2	T37.8X3	T37.8X4	T37.8X5	T37.8X6
Furazolium chloride	T49.0X1	T49.0X2	T49.0X3	T49.0X4	T49.0X5	T49.0X6
Furfural	T52.8X1	T52.8X2	T52.8X3	T52.8X4	—	—

◄ New ◄ Revised ~~deleted~~ Deleted

Substance	Poisoning, Accidental (Unintentional)	Poisoning, Intentional Self-Harm	Poisoning, Assault	Poisoning, Undetermined	Adverse Effect	Underdosing
Furnace (coal burning) (domestic), gas from industrial	T58.2X1	T58.2X2	T58.2X3	T58.2X4	—	—
industrial	T58.8X1	T58.8X2	T58.8X3	T58.8X4	—	—
Furniture polish	T65.891	T65.892	T65.893	T65.894	—	—
Furosemide	T50.1X1	T50.1X2	T50.1X3	T50.1X4	T50.1X5	T50.1X6
Furoxone	T37.91	T37.92	T37.93	T37.94	T37.95	T37.96
Fursultiamine	T45.2X1	T45.2X2	T45.2X3	T45.2X4	T45.2X5	T45.2X6
Fusafungine	T36.8X1	T36.8X2	T36.8X3	T36.8X4	T36.8X5	T36.8X6
Fusel oil (any) (amyl) (butyl) (propyl), vapor	T51.3X1	T51.3X2	T51.3X3	T51.3X4	—	—
Fusidate (ethanolamine) (sodium)	T36.8X1	T36.8X2	T36.8X3	T36.8X4	T36.8X5	T36.8X6
Fusidic acid	T36.8X1	T36.8X2	T36.8X3	T36.8X4	T36.8X5	T36.8X6
Fytic acid, nonasodium	T50.6X1	T50.6X2	T50.6X3	T50.6X4	T50.6X5	T50.6X6
G						
GABA	T43.8X1	T43.8X2	T43.8X3	T43.8X4	T43.8X5	T43.8X6
Gadopentetic acid	T50.8X1	T50.8X2	T50.8X3	T50.8X4	T50.8X5	T50.8X6
Galactose	T50.3X1	T50.3X2	T50.3X3	T50.3X4	T50.3X5	T50.3X6
b-Galactosidase	T47.5X1	T47.5X2	T47.5X3	T47.5X4	T47.5X5	T47.5X6
Galantamine	T44.0X1	T44.0X2	T44.0X3	T44.0X4	T44.0X5	T44.0X6
Gallamine (triethiodide)	T48.1X1	T48.1X2	T48.1X3	T48.1X4	T48.1X5	T48.1X6
Gallium citrate	T50.991	T50.992	T50.993	T50.994	T50.995	T50.996
Gallopamil	T46.1X1	T46.1X2	T46.1X3	T46.1X4	T46.1X5	T46.1X6
Gamboge	T47.2X1	T47.2X2	T47.2X3	T47.2X4	T47.2X5	T47.2X6
Gamimune	T50.Z11	T50.Z12	T50.Z13	T50.Z14	T50.Z15	T50.Z16
Gamma-aminobutyric acid	T43.8X1	T43.8X2	T43.8X3	T43.8X4	T43.8X5	T43.8X6
Gamma-benzene hexachloride (medicinal)	T49.0X1	T49.0X2	T49.0X3	T49.0X4	T49.0X5	T49.0X6
nonmedicinal, vapor	T53.6X1	T53.6X2	T53.6X3	T53.6X4	—	—
Gamma-BHC (medicinal) — see also Gamma-benzene hexachloride	T49.0X1	T49.0X2	T49.0X3	T49.0X4	T49.0X5	T49.0X6
Gamma globulin	T50.Z11	T50.Z12	T50.Z13	T50.Z14	T50.Z15	T50.Z16
Gamulin	T50.Z11	T50.Z12	T50.Z13	T50.Z14	T50.Z15	T50.Z16
Ganciclovir (sodium)	T37.5X1	T37.5X2	T37.5X3	T37.5X4	T37.5X5	T37.5X6
Ganglionic blocking drug NEC	T44.2X1	T44.2X2	T44.2X3	T44.2X4	T44.2X5	T44.2X6
specified NEC	T44.2X1	T44.2X2	T44.2X3	T44.2X4	T44.2X5	T44.2X6
Ganja	T40.711	T40.712	T40.713	T40.714	T40.715	T40.716
Garamycin	T36.5X1	T36.5X2	T36.5X3	T36.5X4	T36.5X5	T36.5X6
ophthalmic preparation	T49.5X1	T49.5X2	T49.5X3	T49.5X4	T49.5X5	T49.5X6
topical NEC	T49.0X1	T49.0X2	T49.0X3	T49.0X4	T49.0X5	T49.0X6
Gardenal	T42.3X1	T42.3X2	T42.3X3	T42.3X4	T42.3X5	T42.3X6
Gardepanyl	T42.3X1	T42.3X2	T42.3X3	T42.3X4	T42.3X5	T42.3X6

Substance	Poisoning, Accidental (Unintentional)	Poisoning, Intentional Self-Harm	Poisoning, Assault	Poisoning, Undetermined	Adverse Effect	Underdosing
Gas NEC	T59.91	T59.92	T59.93	T59.94	—	—
acetylene	T59.891	T59.892	T59.893	T59.894	—	—
incomplete combustion of	T58.11	T58.12	T58.13	T58.14	—	—
air contaminants, source or type not specified	T59.91	T59.92	T59.93	T59.94	—	—
anesthetic	T41.0X1	T41.0X2	T41.0X3	T41.0X4	T41.0X5	T41.0X6
blast furnace	T58.8X1	T58.8X2	T58.8X3	T58.8X4	—	—
butane — see Butane						
carbon monoxide — see Carbon, monoxide						
chlorine	T59.4X1	T59.4X2	T59.4X3	T59.4X4	—	—
coal	T58.2X1	T58.2X2	T58.2X3	T58.2X4	—	—
cyanide	T57.3X1	T57.3X2	T57.3X3	T57.3X4	—	—
dicyanogen	T65.0X1	T65.0X2	T65.0X3	T65.0X4	—	—
domestic — see Domestic gas	T57.91	T57.92	T57.93	T57.94	—	—
exhaust	T57.91	T57.92	T57.93	T57.94	—	—
from utility (for cooking, heating, or lighting) (after combustion) — see Carbon, monoxide, fuel, utility						
prior to combustion	T59.891	T59.892	T59.893	T59.894	—	—
from wood or coal-burning stove or fireplace	T57.91	T57.92	T57.93	T57.94	—	—
fuel (domestic use) (after combustion) — see also Carbon, monoxide, fuel	T57.91	T57.92	T57.93	T57.94	—	—
industrial use	T58.8X1	T58.8X2	T58.8X3	T58.8X4	—	—
prior to combustion	T59.891	T59.892	T59.893	T59.894	—	—
utility	T59.891	T59.892	T59.893	T59.894	—	—
in mobile container	T59.891	T59.892	T59.893	T59.894	—	—
incomplete combustion of — see Carbon, monoxide, fuel, utility						
piped (natural)	T59.891	T59.892	T59.893	T59.894	—	—
garage	T58.01	T58.02	T58.03	T58.04	—	—
hydrocarbon NEC	T59.891	T59.892	T59.893	T59.894	—	—
incomplete combustion of — see Carbon, monoxide, fuel, utility						
liquefied — see Butane						
piped	T59.891	T59.892	T59.893	T59.894	—	—
hydrocyanic acid	T65.0X1	T65.0X2	T65.0X3	T65.0X4	—	—

TABLE OF DRUGS AND CHEMICALS

Substance	External Cause (T-Code)					
	Poisoning, Accidental (Unintentional)	Poisoning, Intentional Self-Harm	Poisoning, Assault	Poisoning, Undetermined	Adverse Effect	Underdosing
Gas NEC (Continued)						
illuminating (after combustion)	T58.11	T58.12	T58.13	T58.14	—	—
prior to combustion	T59.891	T59.892	T59.893	T59.894		
incomplete combustion, any — see Carbon, monoxide						
kiln	T58.8X1	T58.8X2	T58.8X3	T58.8X4	—	—
lacrimogenic	T59.3X1	T59.3X2	T59.3X3	T59.3X4	—	—
liquefied petroleum — see Butane						
marsh	T59.891	T59.892	T59.893	T59.894		
motor exhaust, not in transit	T58.01	T58.02	T58.03	T58.04	—	—
mustard, not in war	T59.891	T59.892	T59.893	T59.894		
natural	T59.891	T59.892	T59.893	T59.894		
nerve, not in war	T59.91	T59.92	T59.93	T59.94		
oil	T52.0X1	T52.0X2	T52.0X3	T52.0X4		
petroleum (liquefied) (distributed in mobile containers)	T59.891	T59.892	T59.893	T59.894		
piped (pure or mixed with air)	T59.891	T59.892	T59.893	T59.894		
piped (manufactured) (natural) NEC	T59.891	T59.892	T59.893	T59.894		
producer	T58.8X1	T58.8X2	T58.8X3	T58.8X4	—	—
propane — see Propane						
refrigerant (chlorofluoro-carbon)	T53.5X1	T53.5X2	T53.5X3	T53.5X4		
not chlorofluoro-carbon	T59.891	T59.892	T59.893	T59.894	—	—
sewer	T59.91	T59.92	T59.93	T59.94		
specified source NEC	T59.91	T59.92	T59.93	T59.94		
stove (after combustion)	T58.11	T58.12	T58.13	T58.14	—	—
tear	T59.3X1	T59.3X2	T59.3X3	T59.3X4		
therapeutic	T41.5X1	T41.5X2	T41.5X3	T41.5X4	T41.5X5	T41.5X6
utility (for cooking, heating, or lighting) (piped) NEC	T59.891	T59.892	T59.893	T59.894	—	—
in mobile container	T59.891	T59.892	T59.893	T59.894	—	—
incomplete combustion of — see Carbon, monoxide, fuel, utility						
piped (natural)	T59.891	T59.892	T59.893	T59.894	—	—
water	T58.11	T58.12	T58.13	T58.14	—	—
incomplete combustion of — see Carbon, monoxide, fuel, utility						

Substance	External Cause (T-Code)					
	Poisoning, Accidental (Unintentional)	Poisoning, Intentional Self-Harm	Poisoning, Assault	Poisoning, Undetermined	Adverse Effect	Underdosing
Gaseous substance — see Gas						
Gasoline	T52.0X1	T52.0X2	T52.0X3	T52.0X4	—	—
vapor	T52.0X1	T52.0X2	T52.0X3	T52.0X4	—	—
Gastric enzymes	T47.5X1	T47.5X2	T47.5X3	T47.5X4	T47.5X5	T47.5X6
Gastrografin	T50.8X1	T50.8X2	T50.8X3	T50.8X4	T50.8X5	T50.8X6
Gastrointestinal drug	T47.91	T47.92	T47.93	T47.94	T47.95	T47.96
biological	T47.8X1	T47.8X2	T47.8X3	T47.8X4	T47.8X5	T47.8X6
specified NEC	T47.8X1	T47.8X2	T47.8X3	T47.8X4	T47.8X5	T47.8X6
Gaultheria procumbens	T62.2X1	T62.2X2	T62.2X3	T62.2X4	—	—
Gelatin (intravenous)	T45.8X1	T45.8X2	T45.8X3	T45.8X4	T45.8X5	T45.8X6
absorbable (sponge)	T45.7X1	T45.7X2	T45.7X3	T45.7X4	T45.7X5	T45.7X6
Gefarnate	T44.3X1	T44.3X2	T44.3X3	T44.3X4	T44.3X5	T44.3X6
Gelfilm	T49.8X1	T49.8X2	T49.8X3	T49.8X4	T49.8X5	T49.8X6
Gelfoam	T45.7X1	T45.7X2	T45.7X3	T45.7X4	T45.7X5	T45.7X6
Gelsemine	T50.991	T50.992	T50.993	T50.994	T50.995	T50.996
Gelsemium (sempervirens)	T62.2X1	T62.2X2	T62.2X3	T62.2X4	—	—
Gemeprost	T48.0X1	T48.0X2	T48.0X3	T48.0X4	T48.0X5	T48.0X6
Gemfibrozil	T46.6X1	T46.6X2	T46.6X3	T46.6X4	T46.6X5	T46.6X6
Gemonil	T42.3X1	T42.3X2	T42.3X3	T42.3X4	T42.3X5	T42.3X6
Gentamicin	T36.5X1	T36.5X2	T36.5X3	T36.5X4	T36.5X5	T36.5X6
ophthalmic preparation	T49.5X1	T49.5X2	T49.5X3	T49.5X4	T49.5X5	T49.5X6
topical NEC	T49.0X1	T49.0X2	T49.0X3	T49.0X4	T49.0X5	T49.0X6
Gentian	T47.5X1	T47.5X2	T47.5X3	T47.5X4	T47.5X5	T47.5X6
violet	T49.0X1	T49.0X2	T49.0X3	T49.0X4	T49.0X5	T49.0X6
Gepefrine	T44.4X1	T44.4X2	T44.4X3	T44.4X4	T44.4X5	T44.4X6
Gestonorone caproate	T38.5X1	T38.5X2	T38.5X3	T38.5X4	T38.5X5	T38.5X6
Gexane	T49.0X1	T49.0X2	T49.0X3	T49.0X4	T49.0X5	T49.0X6
Gila monster (venom)	T63.111	T63.112	T63.113	T63.114	—	—
Ginger	T47.5X1	T47.5X2	T47.5X3	T47.5X4	T47.5X5	T47.5X6
Jamaica — see Jamaica, ginger						
Gitalin	T46.0X1	T46.0X2	T46.0X3	T46.0X4	T46.0X5	T46.0X6
amorphous	T46.0X1	T46.0X2	T46.0X3	T46.0X4	T46.0X5	T46.0X6
Gitaloxin	T46.0X1	T46.0X2	T46.0X3	T46.0X4	T46.0X5	T46.0X6
Gitoxin	T46.0X1	T46.0X2	T46.0X3	T46.0X4	T46.0X5	T46.0X6
Glafenine	T39.8X1	T39.8X2	T39.8X3	T39.8X4	T39.8X5	T39.8X6
Glandular extract (medicinal) NEC	T50.Z91	T50.Z92	T50.Z93	T50.Z94	T50.Z95	T50.Z96
Glaucarubin	T37.3X1	T37.3X2	T37.3X3	T37.3X4	T37.3X5	T37.3X6
Glibenclamide	T38.3X1	T38.3X2	T38.3X3	T38.3X4	T38.3X5	T38.3X6
Glibornuride	T38.3X1	T38.3X2	T38.3X3	T38.3X4	T38.3X5	T38.3X6
Gliclazide	T38.3X1	T38.3X2	T38.3X3	T38.3X4	T38.3X5	T38.3X6
Glimidine	T38.3X1	T38.3X2	T38.3X3	T38.3X4	T38.3X5	T38.3X6

◀ New ◀ Revised ~~deleted~~ Deleted

Substance	Poisoning, Accidental (Unintentional)	Poisoning, Intentional Self-Harm	Poisoning, Assault	Poisoning, Undetermined	Adverse Effect	Underdosing
Glipizide	T38.3X1	T38.3X2	T38.3X3	T38.3X4	T38.3X5	T38.3X6
Gliquidone	T38.3X1	T38.3X2	T38.3X3	T38.3X4	T38.3X5	T38.3X6
Glisolamide	T38.3X1	T38.3X2	T38.3X3	T38.3X4	T38.3X5	T38.3X6
Glisoxepide	T38.3X1	T38.3X2	T38.3X3	T38.3X4	T38.3X5	T38.3X6
Globin zinc insulin	T38.3X1	T38.3X2	T38.3X3	T38.3X4	T38.3X5	T38.3X6
Globulin						
antilymphocytic	T50.Z11	T50.Z12	T50.Z13	T50.Z14	T50.Z15	T50.Z16
antirhesus	T50.Z11	T50.Z12	T50.Z13	T50.Z14	T50.Z15	T50.Z16
antivenin	T50.Z11	T50.Z12	T50.Z13	T50.Z14	T50.Z15	T50.Z16
antiviral	T50.Z11	T50.Z12	T50.Z13	T50.Z14	T50.Z15	T50.Z16
Glucagon	T38.3X1	T38.3X2	T38.3X3	T38.3X4	T38.3X5	T38.3X6
Glucocorticoids	T38.0X1	T38.0X2	T38.0X3	T38.0X4	T38.0X5	T38.0X6
Glucocorticosteroid	T38.0X1	T38.0X2	T38.0X3	T38.0X4	T38.0X5	T38.0X6
Gluconic acid	T50.991	T50.992	T50.993	T50.994	T50.995	T50.996
Glucosamine sulfate	T39.4X1	T39.4X2	T39.4X3	T39.4X4	T39.4X5	T39.4X6
Glucose	T50.3X1	T50.3X2	T50.3X3	T50.3X4	T50.3X5	T50.3X6
with sodium chloride	T50.3X1	T50.3X2	T50.3X3	T50.3X4	T50.3X5	T50.3X6
Glucosulfone sodium	T37.1X1	T37.1X2	T37.1X3	T37.1X4	T37.1X5	T37.1X6
Glucurolactone	T47.8X1	T47.8X2	T47.8X3	T47.8X4	T47.8X5	T47.8X6
Glue NEC	T52.8X1	T52.8X2	T52.8X3	T52.8X4	—	—
Glutamic acid	T47.5X1	T47.5X2	T47.5X3	T47.5X4	T47.5X5	T47.5X6
Glutaral (medicinal)	T49.0X1	T49.0X2	T49.0X3	T49.0X4	T49.0X5	T49.0X6
nonmedicinal	T65.891	T65.892	T65.893	T65.894	—	—
Glutaraldehyde (nonmedicinal)	T65.891	T65.892	T65.893	T65.894	—	—
medicinal	T49.0X1	T49.0X2	T49.0X3	T49.0X4	T49.0X5	T49.0X6
Glutathione	T50.6X1	T50.6X2	T50.6X3	T50.6X4	T50.6X5	T50.6X6
Glutethimide	T42.6X1	T42.6X2	T42.6X3	T42.6X4	T42.6X5	T42.6X6
Glyburide	T38.3X1	T38.3X2	T38.3X3	T38.3X4	T38.3X5	T38.3X6
Glycerin	T47.4X1	T47.4X2	T47.4X3	T47.4X4	T47.4X5	T47.4X6
Glycerol	T47.4X1	T47.4X2	T47.4X3	T47.4X4	T47.4X5	T47.4X6
borax	T49.6X1	T49.6X2	T49.6X3	T49.6X4	T49.6X5	T49.6X6
intravenous	T50.3X1	T50.3X2	T50.3X3	T50.3X4	T50.3X5	T50.3X6
iodinated	T48.4X1	T48.4X2	T48.4X3	T48.4X4	T48.4X5	T48.4X6
Glycerophosphate	T50.991	T50.992	T50.993	T50.994	T50.995	T50.996
Glyceryl						
gualacolate	T48.4X1	T48.4X2	T48.4X3	T48.4X4	T48.4X5	T48.4X6
nitrate	T46.3X1	T46.3X2	T46.3X3	T46.3X4	T46.3X5	T46.3X6
triacetate (topical)	T49.0X1	T49.0X2	T49.0X3	T49.0X4	T49.0X5	T49.0X6
trinitrate	T46.3X1	T46.3X2	T46.3X3	T46.3X4	T46.3X5	T46.3X6
Glycine	T50.3X1	T50.3X2	T50.3X3	T50.3X4	T50.3X5	T50.3X6
Glyclopyramide	T38.3X1	T38.3X2	T38.3X3	T38.3X4	T38.3X5	T38.3X6
Glycobiarsol	T37.3X1	T37.3X2	T37.3X3	T37.3X4	T37.3X5	T37.3X6

Substance	Poisoning, Accidental (Unintentional)	Poisoning, Intentional Self-Harm	Poisoning, Assault	Poisoning, Undetermined	Adverse Effect	Underdosing
Glycols (ether)	T52.3X1	T52.3X2	T52.3X3	T52.3X4	—	—
Glyconiazide	T37.1X1	T37.1X2	T37.1X3	T37.1X4	T37.1X5	T37.1X6
Glycopyrrolate	T44.3X1	T44.3X2	T44.3X3	T44.3X4	T44.3X5	T44.3X6
Glycopyrronium	T44.3X1	T44.3X2	T44.3X3	T44.3X4	T44.3X5	T44.3X6
bromide	T44.3X1	T44.3X2	T44.3X3	T44.3X4	T44.3X5	T44.3X6
Glycoside, cardiac (stimulant)	T46.0X1	T46.0X2	T46.0X3	T46.0X4	T46.0X5	T46.0X6
Glycyclamide	T38.3X1	T38.3X2	T38.3X3	T38.3X4	T38.3X5	T38.3X6
Glycyrrhiza extract	T48.4X1	T48.4X2	T48.4X3	T48.4X4	T48.4X5	T48.4X6
Glycyrrhizic acid	T48.4X1	T48.4X2	T48.4X3	T48.4X4	T48.4X5	T48.4X6
Glycyrrhizinate potassium	T48.4X1	T48.4X2	T48.4X3	T48.4X4	T48.4X5	T48.4X6
Glymidine sodium	T38.3X1	T38.3X2	T38.3X3	T38.3X4	T38.3X5	T38.3X6
Glyphosate	T60.3X1	T60.3X2	T60.3X3	T60.3X4	—	—
Glyphylline	T48.6X1	T48.6X2	T48.6X3	T48.6X4	T48.6X5	T48.6X6
Gold						
colloidal (I98Au)	T45.1X1	T45.1X2	T45.1X3	T45.1X4	T45.1X5	T45.1X6
salts	T39.4X1	T39.4X2	T39.4X3	T39.4X4	T39.4X5	T39.4X6
Golden sulfide of antimony	T56.891	T56.892	T56.893	T56.894	—	—
Goldylocks	T62.2X1	T62.2X2	T62.2X3	T62.2X4	—	—
Gonadal tissue extract	T38.901	T38.902	T38.903	T38.904	T38.905	T38.906
female	T38.5X1	T38.5X2	T38.5X3	T38.5X4	T38.5X5	T38.5X6
male	T38.7X1	T38.7X2	T38.7X3	T38.7X4	T38.7X5	T38.7X6
Gonadorelin	T38.891	T38.892	T38.893	T38.894	T38.895	T38.896
Gonadotropin	T38.891	T38.892	T38.893	T38.894	T38.895	T38.896
chorionic	T38.891	T38.892	T38.893	T38.894	T38.895	T38.896
pituitary	T38.811	T38.812	T38.813	T38.814	T38.815	T38.816
Goserelin	T45.1X1	T45.1X2	T45.1X3	T45.1X4	T45.1X5	T45.1X6
Grain alcohol	T51.0X1	T51.0X2	T51.0X3	T51.0X4	—	—
Gramicidin	T49.0X1	T49.0X2	T49.0X3	T49.0X4	T49.0X5	T49.0X6
Granisetron	T45.0X1	T45.0X2	T45.0X3	T45.0X4	T45.0X5	T45.0X6
Gratiola officinalis	T62.2X1	T62.2X2	T62.2X3	T62.2X4	—	—
Grease	T65.891	T65.892	T65.893	T65.894	—	—
Green hellebore	T62.2X1	T62.2X2	T62.2X3	T62.2X4	—	—
Green soap	T49.2X1	T49.2X2	T49.2X3	T49.2X4	T49.2X5	T49.2X6
Grifulvin	T36.7X1	T36.7X2	T36.7X3	T36.7X4	T36.7X5	T36.7X6
Griseofulvin	T36.7X1	T36.7X2	T36.7X3	T36.7X4	T36.7X5	T36.7X6
Growth hormone	T38.811	T38.812	T38.813	T38.814	T38.815	T38.816
Guaiacol derivatives	T48.4X1	T48.4X2	T48.4X3	T48.4X4	T48.4X5	T48.4X6
Guaiac reagent	T50.991	T50.992	T50.993	T50.994	T50.995	T50.996
Guaifenesin	T48.4X1	T48.4X2	T48.4X3	T48.4X4	T48.4X5	T48.4X6
Guaimesal	T48.4X1	T48.4X2	T48.4X3	T48.4X4	T48.4X5	T48.4X6
Guaiphenesin	T48.4X1	T48.4X2	T48.4X3	T48.4X4	T48.4X5	T48.4X6
Guamecycline	T36.4X1	T36.4X2	T36.4X3	T36.4X4	T36.4X5	T36.4X6

◀ New   ◀ Revised   ~~deleted~~ Deleted

TABLE OF DRUGS AND CHEMICALS

Substance	External Cause (T-Code) Poisoning, Accidental (Unintentional)	Poisoning, Intentional Self-Harm	Poisoning, Assault	Poisoning, Undetermined	Adverse Effect	Underdosing
Guanabenz	T46.5X1	T46.5X2	T46.5X3	T46.5X4	T46.5X5	T46.5X6
Guanacline	T46.5X1	T46.5X2	T46.5X3	T46.5X4	T46.5X5	T46.5X6
Guanadrel	T46.5X1	T46.5X2	T46.5X3	T46.5X4	T46.5X5	T46.5X6
Guanatol	T37.2X1	T37.2X2	T37.2X3	T37.2X4	T37.2X5	T37.2X6
Guanethidine	T46.5X1	T46.5X2	T46.5X3	T46.5X4	T46.5X5	T46.5X6
Guanfacine	T46.5X1	T46.5X2	T46.5X3	T46.5X4	T46.5X5	T46.5X6
Guano	T65.891	T65.892	T65.893	T65.894	—	—
Guanochlor	T46.5X1	T46.5X2	T46.5X3	T46.5X4	T46.5X5	T46.5X6
Guanoclor	T46.5X1	T46.5X2	T46.5X3	T46.5X4	T46.5X5	T46.5X6
Guanoctine	T46.5X1	T46.5X2	T46.5X3	T46.5X4	T46.5X5	T46.5X6
Guanoxabenz	T46.5X1	T46.5X2	T46.5X3	T46.5X4	T46.5X5	T46.5X6
Guanoxan	T46.5X1	T46.5X2	T46.5X3	T46.5X4	T46.5X5	T46.5X6
Guar gum (medicinal)	T46.6X1	T46.6X2	T46.6X3	T46.6X4	T46.6X5	T46.6X6
H						
Hachimycin	T36.7X1	T36.7X2	T36.7X3	T36.7X4	T36.7X5	T36.7X6
Hair						
dye	T49.4X1	T49.4X2	T49.4X3	T49.4X4	T49.4X5	T49.4X6
preparation NEC	T49.4X1	T49.4X2	T49.4X3	T49.4X4	T49.4X5	T49.4X6
Halazepam	T42.4X1	T42.4X2	T42.4X3	T42.4X4	T42.4X5	T42.4X6
Halcinolone	T49.0X1	T49.0X2	T49.0X3	T49.0X4	T49.0X5	T49.0X6
Halcinonide	T49.0X1	T49.0X2	T49.0X3	T49.0X4	T49.0X5	T49.0X6
Halethazole	T49.0X1	T49.0X2	T49.0X3	T49.0X4	T49.0X5	T49.0X6
Hallucinogen NOS	T40.901	T40.902	T40.903	T40.904	T40.905	T40.906
specified NEC	T40.991	T40.992	T40.993	T40.994	T40.995	T40.996
Halofantrine	T37.2X1	T37.2X2	T37.2X3	T37.2X4	T37.2X5	T37.2X6
Halofenate	T46.6X1	T46.6X2	T46.6X3	T46.6X4	T46.6X5	T46.6X6
Halometasone	T49.0X1	T49.0X2	T49.0X3	T49.0X4	T49.0X5	T49.0X6
Haloperidol	T43.4X1	T43.4X2	T43.4X3	T43.4X4	T43.4X5	T43.4X6
Haloprogin	T49.0X1	T49.0X2	T49.0X3	T49.0X4	T49.0X5	T49.0X6
Halotex	T49.0X1	T49.0X2	T49.0X3	T49.0X4	T49.0X5	T49.0X6
Halothane	T41.0X1	T41.0X2	T41.0X3	T41.0X4	T41.0X5	T41.0X6
Haloxazolam	T42.4X1	T42.4X2	T42.4X3	T42.4X4	T42.4X5	T42.4X6
Halquinols	T49.0X1	T49.0X2	T49.0X3	T49.0X4	T49.0X5	T49.0X6
Hamamelis	T49.2X1	T49.2X2	T49.2X3	T49.2X4	T49.2X5	T49.2X6
Haptendextran	T45.8X1	T45.8X2	T45.8X3	T45.8X4	T45.8X5	T45.8X6
Harmonyl	T46.5X1	T46.5X2	T46.5X3	T46.5X4	T46.5X5	T46.5X6
Hartmann's solution	T50.3X1	T50.3X2	T50.3X3	T50.3X4	T50.3X5	T50.3X6
Hashish	T40.711	T40.712	T40.713	T40.714	T40.715	T40.716
Hawaiian Woodrose seeds	T40.991	T40.992	T40.993	T40.994	—	—
HCB	T60.3X1	T60.3X2	T60.3X3	T60.3X4	—	—
HCH	T53.6X1	T53.6X2	T53.6X3	T53.6X4	—	—
medicinal	T49.0X1	T49.0X2	T49.0X3	T49.0X4	T49.0X5	T49.0X6

Substance	External Cause (T-Code) Poisoning, Accidental (Unintentional)	Poisoning, Intentional Self-Harm	Poisoning, Assault	Poisoning, Undetermined	Adverse Effect	Underdosing
HCN	T57.3X1	T57.3X2	T57.3X3	T57.3X4	—	—
Headache cures, drugs, powders NEC	T50.901	T50.902	T50.903	T50.904	T50.905	T50.906
Heavenly Blue (morning glory)	T40.991	T40.992	T40.993	T40.994		
Heavy metal antidote	T45.8X1	T45.8X2	T45.8X3	T45.8X4	T45.8X5	T45.8X6
Hedaquinium	T49.0X1	T49.0X2	T49.0X3	T49.0X4	T49.0X5	T49.0X6
Hedge hyssop	T62.2X1	T62.2X2	T62.2X3	T62.2X4	—	—
Heet	T49.8X1	T49.8X2	T49.8X3	T49.8X4	T49.8X5	T49.8X6
Helium	T48.991	T48.992	T48.993	T48.994	T48.995	T48.996
Helenin	T37.4X1	T37.4X2	T37.4X3	T37.4X4	T37.4X5	T37.4X6
Hellebore (black) (green) (white)	T62.2X1	T62.2X2	T62.2X3	T62.2X4	—	—
Helium (nonmedicinal) NEC	T59.891	T59.892	T59.893	T59.894	—	—
medicinal	T48.991	T48.992	T48.993	T48.994	T48.995	T48.996
Hematin	T45.8X1	T45.8X2	T45.8X3	T45.8X4	T45.8X5	T45.8X6
Hematinic preparation	T45.8X1	T45.8X2	T45.8X3	T45.8X4	T45.8X5	T45.8X6
Hemlock	T62.2X1	T62.2X2	T62.2X3	T62.2X4	—	—
Hemostatic	T45.621	T45.622	T45.623	T45.624	T45.625	T45.626
drug, systemic	T45.621	T45.622	T45.623	T45.624	T45.625	T45.626
Hemostyptic	T49.4X1	T49.4X2	T49.4X3	T49.4X4	T49.4X5	T49.4X6
Henbane	T62.2X1	T62.2X2	T62.2X3	T62.2X4	—	—
Heparin (sodium)	T45.511	T45.512	T45.513	T45.514	T45.515	T45.516
action reverser	T45.7X1	T45.7X2	T45.7X3	T45.7X4	T45.7X5	T45.7X6
Heparin-fraction	T45.511	T45.512	T45.513	T45.514	T45.515	T45.516
Heparinoid (systemic)	T45.511	T45.512	T45.513	T45.514	T45.515	T45.516
Hepatic secretion stimulant	T47.8X1	T47.8X2	T47.8X3	T47.8X4	T47.8X5	T47.8X6
Hepatitis B						
immune globulin	T50.Z11	T50.Z12	T50.Z13	T50.Z14	T50.Z15	T50.Z16
vaccine	T50.B91	T50.B92	T50.B93	T50.B94	T50.B95	T50.B96
Hepronicate	T46.7X1	T46.7X2	T46.7X3	T46.7X4	T46.7X5	T46.7X6
Heptabarb	T42.3X1	T42.3X2	T42.3X3	T42.3X4	T42.3X5	T42.3X6
Heptabarbitone	T42.3X1	T42.3X2	T42.3X3	T42.3X4	T42.3X5	T42.3X6
Heptabarbital	T42.3X1	T42.3X2	T42.3X3	T42.3X4	T42.3X5	T42.3X6
Heptachlor	T60.1X1	T60.1X2	T60.1X3	T60.1X4	—	—
Heptalgin	T40.2X1	T40.2X2	T40.2X3	T40.2X4	T40.2X5	T40.2X6
Heptaminol	T46.3X1	T46.3X2	T46.3X3	T46.3X4	T46.3X5	T46.3X6
Herbicide NEC	T60.3X1	T60.3X2	T60.3X3	T60.3X4	—	—
Heroin	T40.1X1	T40.1X2	T40.1X3	T40.1X4	—	—
Herplex	T49.5X1	T49.5X2	T49.5X3	T49.5X4	T49.5X5	T49.5X6
HES	T45.8X1	T45.8X2	T45.8X3	T45.8X4	T45.8X5	T45.8X6
Hesperidin	T46.991	T46.992	T46.993	T46.994	T46.995	T46.996
Hetacillin	T36.0X1	T36.0X2	T36.0X3	T36.0X4	T36.0X5	T36.0X6

◀ New   ◀ Revised   ~~deleted~~ Deleted

Substance	External Cause (T-Code)					
	Poisoning, Accidental (Unintentional)	Poisoning, Intentional Self-Harm	Poisoning, Assault	Poisoning, Undetermined	Adverse Effect	Underdosing
Hetastarch	T45.8X1	T45.8X2	T45.8X3	T45.8X4	T45.8X5	T45.8X6
HETP	T60.0X1	T60.0X2	T60.0X3	T60.0X4	—	—
Hexachlorobenzene (vapor)	T60.3X1	T60.3X2	T60.3X3	T60.3X4	—	—
Hexachlorocyclohexane	T53.6X1	T53.6X2	T53.6X3	T53.6X4	—	—
Hexachlorophene	T49.0X1	T49.0X2	T49.0X3	T49.0X4	T49.0X5	T49.0X6
Hexadiline	T46.3X1	T46.3X2	T46.3X3	T46.3X4	T46.3X5	T46.3X6
Hexadimethrine (bromide)	T45.7X1	T45.7X2	T45.7X3	T45.7X4	T45.7X5	T45.7X6
Hexadylamine	T46.3X1	T46.3X2	T46.3X3	T46.3X4	T46.3X5	T46.3X6
Hexaethyl tetraphosphate	T60.0X1	T60.0X2	T60.0X3	T60.0X4	—	—
Hexafluorenium bromide	T48.1X1	T48.1X2	T48.1X3	T48.1X4	T48.1X5	T48.1X6
Hexafluorodiethyl ether	T43.291	T43.292	T43.293	T43.294	T43.295	T43.296
Hexafluronium (bromide)	T48.1X1	T48.1X2	T48.1X3	T48.1X4	T48.1X5	T48.1X6
Hexahydrobenzol	T52.8X1	T52.8X2	T52.8X3	T52.8X4	—	—
Hexahydrocresol(s)	T51.8X1	T51.8X2	T51.8X3	T51.8X4	—	—
arsenide	T57.0X1	T57.0X2	T57.0X3	T57.0X4	—	—
arseniurated	T57.0X1	T57.0X2	T57.0X3	T57.0X4	—	—
cyanide	T57.3X1	T57.3X2	T57.3X3	T57.3X4	—	—
gas	T59.891	T59.892	T59.893	T59.894	—	—
Fluoride (liquid)	T57.8X1	T57.8X2	T57.8X3	T57.8X4	—	—
vapor	T59.891	T59.892	T59.893	T59.894	—	—
phophorated	T60.0X1	T60.0X2	T60.0X3	T60.0X4	—	—
sulfate	T57.8X1	T57.8X2	T57.8X3	T57.8X4	—	—
sulfide (gas)	T59.6X1	T59.6X2	T59.6X3	T59.6X4	—	—
arseniurated	T57.0X1	T57.0X2	T57.0X3	T57.0X4	—	—
sulfurated	T57.8X1	T57.8X2	T57.8X3	T57.8X4	—	—
Hexahydrophenol	T51.8X1	T51.8X2	T51.8X3	T51.8X4	—	—
Hexa-germ	T49.2X1	T49.2X2	T49.2X3	T49.2X4	T49.2X5	T49.2X6
Hexalen	T51.8X1	T51.8X2	T51.8X3	T51.8X4	—	—
Hexamethonium bromide	T44.2X1	T44.2X2	T44.2X3	T44.2X4	T44.2X5	T44.2X6
Hexamethylene	T52.8X1	T52.8X2	T52.8X3	T52.8X4	—	—
Hexamethylmelamine	T45.1X1	T45.1X2	T45.1X3	T45.1X4	T45.1X5	T45.1X6
Hexamidine	T49.0X1	T49.0X2	T49.0X3	T49.0X4	T49.0X5	T49.0X6
Hexamine (mandelate)	T37.8X1	T37.8X2	T37.8X3	T37.8X4	T37.8X5	T37.8X6
Hexanone, 2-hexanone	T52.4X1	T52.4X2	T52.4X3	T52.4X4	—	—
Hexanuorenium	T48.1X1	T48.1X2	T48.1X3	T48.1X4	T48.1X5	T48.1X6
Hexapropymate	T42.6X1	T42.6X2	T42.6X3	T42.6X4	T42.6X5	T42.6X6
Hexasonium iodide	T44.3X1	T44.3X2	T44.3X3	T44.3X4	T44.3X5	T44.3X6
Hexcarbacholine bromide	T48.1X1	T48.1X2	T48.1X3	T48.1X4	T48.1X5	T48.1X6
Hexemal	T42.3X1	T42.3X2	T42.3X3	T42.3X4	T42.3X5	T42.3X6
Hexestrol	T38.5X1	T38.5X2	T38.5X3	T38.5X4	T38.5X5	T38.5X6
Hexethal (sodium)	T42.3X1	T42.3X2	T42.3X3	T42.3X4	T42.3X5	T42.3X6
Hexetidine	T37.8X1	T37.8X2	T37.8X3	T37.8X4	T37.8X5	T37.8X6

Substance	External Cause (T-Code)					
	Poisoning, Accidental (Unintentional)	Poisoning, Intentional Self-Harm	Poisoning, Assault	Poisoning, Undetermined	Adverse Effect	Underdosing
Hexobarbital	T42.3X1	T42.3X2	T42.3X3	T42.3X4	T42.3X5	T42.3X6
rectal	T41.291	T41.292	T41.293	T41.294	T41.295	T41.296
sodium	T41.1X1	T41.1X2	T41.1X4	T41.1X4	T41.1X5	T41.1X6
Hexobendine	T46.3X1	T46.3X2	T46.3X3	T46.3X4	T46.3X5	T46.3X6
Hexocyclium	T44.3X1	T44.3X2	T44.3X3	T44.3X4	T44.3X5	T44.3X6
metilsulfate	T44.3X1	T44.3X2	T44.3X3	T44.3X4	T44.3X5	T44.3X6
Hexoestrol	T38.5X1	T38.5X2	T38.5X3	T38.5X4	T38.5X5	T38.5X6
Hexone	T52.4X1	T52.4X2	T52.4X3	T52.4X4	—	—
Hexoprenaline	T48.6X1	T48.6X2	T48.6X3	T48.6X4	T48.6X5	T48.6X6
Hexylcaine	T41.3X1	T41.3X2	T41.3X3	T41.3X4	T41.3X5	T41.3X6
Hexylresorcinol	T52.2X1	T52.2X2	T52.2X3	T52.2X4	—	—
HGH (human growth hormone)	T38.811	T38.812	T38.813	T38.814	T38.815	T38.816
Hinkle's pills	T47.2X1	T47.2X2	T47.2X3	T47.2X4	T47.2X5	T47.2X6
Histalog	T50.8X1	T50.8X2	T50.8X3	T50.8X4	T50.8X5	T50.8X6
Histamine (phosphate)	T50.8X1	T50.8X2	T50.8X3	T50.8X4	T50.8X5	T50.8X6
Histoplasmin	T50.8X1	T50.8X2	T50.8X3	T50.8X4	T50.8X5	T50.8X6
Holly berries	T62.2X1	T62.2X2	T62.2X3	T62.2X4	—	—
Homatropine	T44.3X1	T44.3X2	T44.3X3	T44.3X4	T44.3X5	T44.3X6
methylbromide	T44.3X1	T44.3X2	T44.3X3	T44.3X4	T44.3X5	T44.3X6
Homochlorcyclizine	T45.0X1	T45.0X2	T45.0X3	T45.0X4	T45.0X5	T45.0X6
Homosalate	T49.3X1	T49.3X2	T49.3X3	T49.3X4	T49.3X5	T49.3X6
Homo-tet	T50.Z11	T50.Z12	T50.Z13	T50.Z14	T50.Z15	T50.Z16
Hormone	T38.801	T38.802	T38.803	T38.804	T38.805	T38.806
adrenal cortical steroids	T38.0X1	T38.0X2	T38.0X3	T38.0X4	T38.0X5	T38.0X6
androgenic	T38.7X1	T38.7X2	T38.7X3	T38.7X4	T38.7X5	T38.7X6
anterior pituitary NEC	T38.811	T38.812	T38.813	T38.814	T38.815	T38.816
antidiabetic agents	T38.3X1	T38.3X2	T38.3X3	T38.3X4	T38.3X5	T38.3X6
antidiuretic	T38.891	T38.892	T38.893	T38.894	T38.895	T38.896
cancer therapy	T45.1X1	T45.1X2	T45.1X3	T45.1X4	T45.1X5	T45.1X6
follicle stimulating	T38.811	T38.812	T38.813	T38.814	T38.815	T38.816
gonadotropic	T38.891	T38.892	T38.893	T38.894	T38.895	T38.896
pituitary	T38.811	T38.812	T38.813	T38.814	T38.815	T38.816
growth	T38.811	T38.812	T38.813	T38.814	T38.815	T38.816
luteinizing	T38.811	T38.812	T38.813	T38.814	T38.815	T38.816
ovarian	T38.5X1	T38.5X2	T38.5X3	T38.5X4	T38.5X5	T38.5X6
oxytocic	T48.0X1	T48.0X2	T48.0X3	T48.0X4	T48.0X5	T48.0X6
parathyroid (derivatives)	T50.991	T50.992	T50.993	T50.994	T50.995	T50.996
pituitary (posterior) NEC	T38.891	T38.892	T38.893	T38.894	T38.895	T38.896
anterior	T38.811	T38.812	T38.813	T38.814	T38.815	T38.816
specified, NEC	T38.891	T38.892	T38.893	T38.894	T38.895	T38.896
thyroid	T38.1X1	T38.1X2	T38.1X3	T38.1X4	T38.1X5	T38.1X6
Hornet (sting)	T63.451	T63.452	T63.453	T63.454	—	—

◀ New ◀ Revised ~~deleted~~ Deleted

TABLE OF DRUGS AND CHEMICALS

	External Cause (T-Code)					
Substance	Poisoning, Accidental (Unintentional)	Poisoning, Intentional Self-Harm	Poisoning, Assault	Poisoning, Undetermined	Adverse Effect	Underdosing
Horse anti-human lymphocytic serum	T50.Z11	T50.Z12	T50.Z13	T50.Z14	T50.Z15	T50.Z16
Horticulture agent NEC	T65.91	T65.92	T65.93	T65.94	—	—
with pesticide	T60.91	T60.92	T60.93	T60.94	—	—
Human						
albumin	T45.8X1	T45.8X2	T45.8X3	T45.8X4	T45.8X5	T45.8X6
growth hormone (HGH)	T38.811	T38.812	T38.813	T38.814	T38.815	T38.816
immune serum	T50.Z11	T50.Z12	T50.Z13	T50.Z14	T50.Z15	T50.Z16
Hyaluronidase	T45.3X1	T45.3X2	T45.3X3	T45.3X4	T45.3X5	T45.3X6
Hyazyme	T45.3X1	T45.3X2	T45.3X3	T45.3X4	T45.3X5	T45.3X6
Hycodan	T40.2X1	T40.2X2	T40.2X3	T40.2X4	T40.2X5	T40.2X6
Hydantoin derivative NEC	T42.0X1	T42.0X2	T42.0X3	T42.0X4	T42.0X5	T42.0X6
Hydeltra	T38.0X1	T38.0X2	T38.0X3	T38.0X4	T38.0X5	T38.0X6
Hydergine	T44.6X1	T44.6X2	T44.6X3	T44.6X4	T44.6X5	T44.6X6
Hydrabamine penicillin	T36.0X1	T36.0X2	T36.0X3	T36.0X4	T36.0X5	T36.0X6
Hydralazine	T46.5X1	T46.5X2	T46.5X3	T46.5X4	T46.5X5	T46.5X6
Hydrargaphen	T49.0X1	T49.0X2	T49.0X3	T49.0X4	T49.0X5	T49.0X6
Hydrargyri amino-chloridum	T49.0X1	T49.0X2	T49.0X3	T49.0X4	T49.0X5	T49.0X6
Hydrastine	T48.291	T48.292	T48.293	T48.294	T48.295	T48.296
Hydrazine	T54.1X1	T54.1X2	T54.1X3	T54.1X4	—	—
monoamine oxidase inhibitors	T43.1X1	T43.1X2	T43.1X3	T43.1X4	T43.1X5	T43.1X6
Hydrazoic acid, azides	T54.2X1	T54.2X2	T54.2X3	T54.2X4	—	—
Hydriodic acid	T48.4X1	T48.4X2	T48.4X3	T48.4X4	T48.4X5	T48.4X6
Hydrocarbon gas	T59.891	T59.892	T59.893	T59.894	—	—
incomplete combustion of — see Carbon, monoxide, fuel, utility						
liquefied (mobile container)	T59.891	T59.892	T59.893	T59.894	—	—
piped (natural)	T59.891	T59.892	T59.893	T59.894	—	—
Hydrochloric acid (liquid)	T54.2X1	T54.2X2	T54.2X3	T54.2X4	—	—
medicinal (digestant)	T47.5X1	T47.5X2	T47.5X3	T47.5X4	T47.5X5	T47.5X6
vapor	T59.891	T59.892	T59.893	T59.894	—	—
Hydrochlorothiazide	T50.2X1	T50.2X2	T50.2X3	T50.2X4	T50.2X5	T50.2X6
Hydrocodone	T40.2X1	T40.2X2	T40.2X3	T40.2X4	T40.2X5	T40.2X6
Hydrocortisone (derivatives)	T38.0X1	T38.0X2	T38.0X3	T38.0X4	T38.0X5	T38.0X6
aceponate	T49.0X1	T49.0X2	T49.0X3	T49.0X4	T49.0X5	T49.0X6
ENT agent	T49.6X1	T49.6X2	T49.6X3	T49.6X4	T49.6X5	T49.6X6
ophthalmic preparation	T49.5X1	T49.5X2	T49.5X3	T49.5X4	T49.5X5	T49.5X6
topical NEC	T49.0X1	T49.0X2	T49.0X3	T49.0X4	T49.0X5	T49.0X6
Hydrocortone	T38.0X1	T38.0X2	T38.0X3	T38.0X4	T38.0X5	T38.0X6
ENT agent	T49.6X1	T49.6X2	T49.6X3	T49.6X4	T49.6X5	T49.6X6
ophthalmic preparation	T49.5X1	T49.5X2	T49.5X3	T49.5X4	T49.5X5	T49.5X6
topical NEC	T49.0X1	T49.0X2	T49.0X3	T49.0X4	T49.0X5	T49.0X6

	External Cause (T-Code)					
Substance	Poisoning, Accidental (Unintentional)	Poisoning, Intentional Self-Harm	Poisoning, Assault	Poisoning, Undetermined	Adverse Effect	Underdosing
Hydrocyanic acid (liquid)	T57.3X1	T57.3X2	T57.3X3	T57.3X4	—	—
gas	T65.0X1	T65.0X2	T65.0X3	T65.0X4	—	—
Hydroflumethiazide	T50.2X1	T50.2X2	T50.2X3	T50.2X4	T50.2X5	T50.2X6
Hydrofluoric acid (liquid)	T54.2X1	T54.2X2	T54.2X3	T54.2X4	—	—
vapor	T59.891	T59.892	T59.893	T59.894	—	—
Hydrogen	T59.891	T59.892	T59.893	T59.894	—	—
arsenide	T57.0X1	T57.0X2	T57.0X3	T57.0X4	—	—
arseniureted	T57.0X1	T57.0X2	T57.0X3	T57.0X4	—	—
chloride	T57.8X1	T57.8X2	T57.8X3	T57.8X4	—	—
cyanide (salts)	T57.3X1	T57.3X2	T57.3X3	T57.3X4	—	—
gas	T57.3X1	T57.3X2	T57.3X3	T57.3X4	—	—
Fluoride	T59.5X1	T59.5X2	T59.5X3	T59.5X4	—	—
vapor	T59.5X1	T59.5X2	T59.5X3	T59.5X4	—	—
peroxide	T49.0X1	T49.0X2	T49.0X3	T49.0X4	T49.0X5	T49.0X6
phosphureted	T57.1X1	T57.1X2	T57.1X3	T57.1X4	—	—
sulfide	T59.6X1	T59.6X2	T59.6X3	T59.6X4	—	—
arseniureted	T57.0X1	T57.0X2	T57.0X3	T57.0X4	—	—
sulfureted	T59.6X1	T59.6X2	T59.6X3	T59.6X4	—	—
Hydromethylpyridine	T46.7X1	T46.7X2	T46.7X3	T46.7X4	T46.7X5	T46.7X6
Hydromorphinol	T40.2X1	T40.2X2	T40.2X3	T40.2X4	—	—
Hydromorphinone	T40.2X1	T40.2X2	T40.2X3	T40.2X4	T40.2X5	T40.2X6
Hydromorphone	T40.2X1	T40.2X2	T40.2X3	T40.2X4	T40.2X5	T40.2X6
Hydromox	T50.2X1	T50.2X2	T50.2X3	T50.2X4	T50.2X5	T50.2X6
Hydrophilic lotion	T49.3X1	T49.3X2	T49.3X3	T49.3X4	T49.3X5	T49.3X6
Hydroquinidine	T46.2X1	T46.2X2	T46.2X3	T46.2X4	T46.2X5	T46.2X6
Hydroquinone	T52.2X1	T52.2X2	T52.2X3	T52.2X4	—	—
vapor	T59.891	T59.892	T59.893	T59.894	—	—
Hydrosulfuric acid (gas)	T59.6X1	T59.6X2	T59.6X3	T59.6X4	—	—
Hydrotalcite	T47.1X1	T47.1X2	T47.1X3	T47.1X4	T47.1X5	T47.1X6
Hydrous wool fat	T49.3X1	T49.3X2	T49.3X3	T49.3X4	T49.3X5	T49.3X6
Hydroxide, caustic	T54.3X1	T54.3X2	T54.3X3	T54.3X4	—	—
Hydroxocobalamin	T45.8X1	T45.8X2	T45.8X3	T45.8X4	T45.8X5	T45.8X6
Hydroxyamphetamine	T49.5X1	T49.5X2	T49.5X3	T49.5X4	T49.5X5	T49.5X6
Hydroxycarbamide	T45.1X1	T45.1X2	T45.1X3	T45.1X4	T45.1X5	T45.1X6
Hydroxychloroquine	T37.8X1	T37.8X2	T37.8X3	T37.8X4	T37.8X5	T37.8X6
Hydroxydihydrocodeinone	T40.2X1	T40.2X2	T40.2X3	T40.2X4	T40.2X5	T40.2X6
Hydroxyestrone	T38.5X1	T38.5X2	T38.5X3	T38.5X4	T38.5X5	T38.5X6
Hydroxyethyl starch	T45.8X1	T45.8X2	T45.8X3	T45.8X4	T45.8X5	T45.8X6
Hydroxymethylpentanone	T52.4X1	T52.4X2	T52.4X3	T52.4X4	—	—
Hydroxyphenamate	T43.591	T43.592	T43.593	T43.594	T43.595	T43.596
Hydroxyphenylbutazone	T39.2X1	T39.2X2	T39.2X3	T39.2X4	T39.2X5	T39.2X6

◀ New ◀ Revised ~~deleted~~ Deleted

Substance	Poisoning, Accidental (Unintentional)	Poisoning, Intentional Self-Harm	Poisoning, Assault	Poisoning, Undetermined	Adverse Effect	Underdosing
Hydroxyprogesterone	T38.5X1	T38.5X2	T38.5X3	T38.5X4	T38.5X5	T38.5X6
caproate	T38.5X1	T38.5X2	T38.5X3	T38.5X4	T38.5X5	T38.5X6
Hydroxyquinoline (derivatives) NEC	T37.8X1	T37.8X2	T37.8X3	T37.8X4	T37.8X5	T37.8X6
Hydroxystilbamidine	T37.3X1	T37.3X2	T37.3X3	T37.3X4	T37.3X5	T37.3X6
Hydroxytoluene (nonmedicinal)	T54.0X1	T54.0X2	T54.0X3	T54.0X4	—	—
medicinal	T49.0X1	T49.0X2	T49.0X3	T49.0X4	T49.0X5	T49.0X6
Hydroxyurea	T45.1X1	T45.1X2	T45.1X3	T45.1X4	T45.1X5	T45.1X6
Hydroxyzine	T43.591	T43.592	T43.593	T43.594	T43.595	T43.596
Hyoscine	T44.3X1	T44.3X2	T44.3X3	T44.3X4	T44.3X5	T44.3X6
Hyoscyamine	T44.3X1	T44.3X2	T44.3X3	T44.3X4	T44.3X5	T44.3X6
Hyoscyamus	T44.3X1	T44.3X2	T44.3X3	T44.3X4	T44.3X5	T44.3X6
dry extract	T44.3X1	T44.3X2	T44.3X3	T44.3X4	T44.3X5	T44.3X6
Hypaque	T50.8X1	T50.8X2	T50.8X3	T50.8X4	T50.8X5	T50.8X6
Hypertussis	T50.Z11	T50.Z12	T50.Z13	T50.Z14	T50.Z15	T50.Z16
Hypnotic	T42.71	T42.72	T42.73	T42.74	T42.75	T42.76
anticonvulsant	T42.71	T42.72	T42.73	T42.74	T42.75	T42.76
specified NEC	T42.6X1	T42.6X2	T42.6X3	T42.6X4	T42.6X5	T42.6X6
Hypochlorite	T49.0X1	T49.0X2	T49.0X3	T49.0X4	T49.0X5	T49.0X6
Hypophysis, posterior	T38.891	T38.892	T38.893	T38.894	T38.895	T38.896
Hypotensive NEC	T46.5X1	T46.5X2	T46.5X3	T46.5X4	T46.5X5	T46.5X6
Hypromellose	T49.5X1	T49.5X2	T49.5X3	T49.5X4	T49.5X5	T49.5X6

I

Substance	Poisoning, Accidental (Unintentional)	Poisoning, Intentional Self-Harm	Poisoning, Assault	Poisoning, Undetermined	Adverse Effect	Underdosing
Ibacitabine	T37.5X1	T37.5X2	T37.5X3	T37.5X4	T37.5X5	T37.5X6
Ibopamine	T44.991	T44.992	T44.993	T44.994	T44.995	T44.996
Ibufenac	T39.311	T39.312	T39.313	T39.314	T39.315	T39.316
Ibuprofen	T39.311	T39.312	T39.313	T39.314	T39.315	T39.316
Ibuproxam	T39.311	T39.312	T39.313	T39.314	T39.315	T39.316
Ibuterol	T48.6X1	T48.6X2	T48.6X3	T48.6X4	T48.6X5	T48.6X6
Ichthammol	T49.0X1	T49.0X2	T49.0X3	T49.0X4	T49.0X5	T49.0X6
Ichthyol	T49.4X1	T49.4X2	T49.4X3	T49.4X4	T49.4X5	T49.4X6
Idarubicin	T45.1X1	T45.1X2	T45.1X3	T45.1X4	T45.1X5	T45.1X6
Idrocilamide	T42.8X1	T42.8X2	T42.8X3	T42.8X4	T42.8X5	T42.8X6
Ifenprodil	T46.7X1	T46.7X2	T46.7X3	T46.7X4	T46.7X5	T46.7X6
Ifosfamide	T45.1X1	T45.1X2	T45.1X3	T45.1X4	T45.1X5	T45.1X6
Iletin	T38.3X1	T38.3X2	T38.3X3	T38.3X4	T38.3X5	T38.3X6
Ilex	T62.2X1	T62.2X2	T62.2X3	T62.2X4	—	—
Illuminating gas (after combustion)	T58.11	T58.12	T58.13	T58.14	—	—
prior to combustion	T59.891	T59.892	T59.893	T59.894	—	—
Ilopan	T45.2X1	T45.2X2	T45.2X3	T45.2X4	T45.2X5	T45.2X6
Iloprost	T46.7X1	T46.7X2	T46.7X3	T46.7X4	T46.7X5	T46.7X6

Substance	Poisoning, Accidental (Unintentional)	Poisoning, Intentional Self-Harm	Poisoning, Assault	Poisoning, Undetermined	Adverse Effect	Underdosing
Ilotycin	T36.3X1	T36.3X2	T36.3X3	T36.3X4	T36.3X5	T36.3X6
ophthalmic preparation	T49.5X1	T49.5X2	T49.5X3	T49.5X4	T49.5X5	T49.5X6
topical NEC	T49.0X1	T49.0X2	T49.0X3	T49.0X4	T49.0X5	T49.0X6
Imidazole-4-carboxamide	T45.1X1	T45.1X2	T45.1X3	T45.1X4	T45.1X5	T45.1X6
Imipenem	T36.0X1	T36.0X2	T36.0X3	T36.0X4	T36.0X5	T36.0X6
Imipramine	T43.011	T43.012	T43.013	T43.014	T43.015	T43.016
Iminostilbene	T42.1X1	T42.1X2	T42.1X3	T42.1X4	T42.1X5	T42.1X6
Immu-G	T50.Z11	T50.Z12	T50.Z13	T50.Z14	T50.Z15	T50.Z16
Immuglobin	T50.Z11	T50.Z12	T50.Z13	T50.Z14	T50.Z15	T50.Z16
Immune						
globulin	T50.Z11	T50.Z12	T50.Z13	T50.Z14	T50.Z15	T50.Z16
serum globulin	T50.Z11	T50.Z12	T50.Z13	T50.Z14	T50.Z15	T50.Z16
Immunoglobin human (intravenous) (normal)	T50.Z11	T50.Z12	T50.Z13	T50.Z14	T50.Z15	T50.Z16
unmodified	T50.Z11	T50.Z12	T50.Z13	T50.Z14	T50.Z15	T50.Z16
Immunosuppressive drug	T45.1X1	T45.1X2	T45.1X3	T45.1X4	T45.1X5	T45.1X6
Immu-tetanus	T50.Z11	T50.Z12	T50.Z13	T50.Z14	T50.Z15	T50.Z16
Indalpine	T43.221	T43.222	T43.223	T43.224	T43.225	T43.226
Indanazoline	T48.5X1	T48.5X2	T48.5X3	T48.5X4	T48.5X5	T48.5X6
Indandione (derivatives)	T45.511	T45.512	T45.513	T45.514	T45.515	T45.516
Indapamide	T46.5X1	T46.5X2	T46.5X3	T46.5X4	T46.5X5	T46.5X6
Indendione (derivatives)	T45.511	T45.512	T45.513	T45.514	T45.515	T45.516
Indenolol	T44.7X1	T44.7X2	T44.7X3	T44.7X4	T44.7X5	T44.7X6
Inderal	T44.7X1	T44.7X2	T44.7X3	T44.7X4	T44.7X5	T44.7X6
Indian						
hemp	T40.711	T40.712	T40.713	T40.714	T40.715	T40.716
tobacco	T62.2X1	T62.2X2	T62.2X3	T62.2X4	—	—
Indigo carmine	T50.8X1	T50.8X2	T50.8X3	T50.8X4	T50.8X5	T50.8X6
Indobufen	T45.521	T45.522	T45.523	T45.524	T45.525	T45.526
Indocin	T39.2X1	T39.2X2	T39.2X3	T39.2X4	T39.2X5	T39.2X6
Indocyanine green	T50.8X1	T50.8X2	T50.8X3	T50.8X4	T50.8X5	T50.8X6
Indometacin	T39.391	T39.392	T39.393	T39.394	T39.395	T39.396
Indomethacin	T39.391	T39.392	T39.393	T39.394	T39.395	T39.396
farnesil	T39.4X1	T39.4X2	T39.4X3	T39.4X4	T39.4X5	T39.4X6
Indoramin	T44.6X1	T44.6X2	T44.6X3	T44.6X4	T44.6X5	T44.6X6
Industrial						
alcohol	T51.0X1	T51.0X2	T51.0X3	T51.0X4	—	—
fumes	T59.891	T59.892	T59.893	T59.894	—	—
solvents (fumes) (vapors)	T52.91	T52.92	T52.93	T52.94	—	—
Influenza vaccine	T50.B91	T50.B92	T50.B93	T50.B94	T50.B95	T50.B96
Ingested substance NEC	T65.91	T65.92	T65.93	T65.94		
INH	T37.1X1	T37.1X2	T37.1X3	T37.1X4	T37.1X5	T37.1X6

TABLE OF DRUGS AND CHEMICALS

Substance	Poisoning, Accidental (Unintentional)	Poisoning, Intentional Self-Harm	Poisoning, Assault	Poisoning, Undetermined	Adverse Effect	Underdosing
Inhalation, gas (noxious)—*see Gas*						
Inhibitor						
angiotensin-converting enzyme	T46.4X1	T46.4X2	T46.4X3	T46.4X4	T46.4X5	T46.4X6
carbonic anhydrase	T50.2X1	T50.2X2	T50.2X3	T50.2X4	T50.2X5	T50.2X6
fibrinolysis	T45.621	T45.622	T45.623	T45.624	T45.625	T45.626
monoamine oxidase NEC	T43.1X1	T43.1X2	T43.1X3	T43.1X4	T43.1X5	T43.1X6
hydrazine	T43.1X1	T43.1X2	T43.1X3	T43.1X4	T43.1X5	T43.1X6
postsynaptic	T43.8X1	T43.8X2	T43.8X3	T43.8X4	T43.8X5	T43.8X6
prothrombin synthesis	T45.511	T45.512	T45.513	T45.514	T45.515	T45.516
Ink	T65.891	T65.892	T65.893	T65.894	—	—
Inorganic substance NEC	T57.91	T57.92	T57.93	T57.94	—	—
Inosine pranobex	T37.5X1	T37.5X2	T37.5X3	T37.5X4	T37.5X5	T37.5X6
Inositol	T50.991	T50.992	T50.993	T50.994	T50.995	T50.996
nicotinate	T46.7X1	T46.7X2	T46.7X3	T46.7X4	T46.7X5	T46.7X6
Inproquone	T45.1X1	T45.1X2	T45.1X3	T45.1X4	T45.1X5	T45.1X6
Insect (sting), venomous	T63.481	T63.482	T63.483	T63.484	—	—
ant	T63.421	T63.422	T63.423	T63.424	—	—
bee	T63.441	T63.442	T63.443	T63.444	—	—
caterpillar	T63.431	T63.432	T63.433	T63.434	—	—
hornet	T63.451	T63.452	T63.453	T63.454	—	—
wasp	T63.461	T63.462	T63.463	T63.464	—	—
Insecticide NEC	T60.91	T60.92	T60.93	T60.94	—	—
carbamate	T60.0X1	T60.0X2	T60.0X3	T60.0X4	—	—
chlorinated	T60.1X1	T60.1X2	T60.1X3	T60.1X4	—	—
mixed	T60.91	T60.92	T60.93	T60.94	—	—
organochlorine	T60.1X1	T60.1X2	T60.1X3	T60.1X4	—	—
organophosphorus	T60.0X1	T60.0X2	T60.0X3	T60.0X4	—	—
Insular tissue extract	T38.3X1	T38.3X2	T38.3X3	T38.3X4	T38.3X5	T38.3X6
Insulin (amorphous) (globin) (isophane) (Lente) (NPH) (Semilente) (Ultralente)	T38.3X1	T38.3X2	T38.3X3	T38.3X4	T38.3X5	T38.3X6
defalan	T38.3X1	T38.3X2	T38.3X3	T38.3X4	T38.3X5	T38.3X6
human	T38.3X1	T38.3X2	T38.3X3	T38.3X4	T38.3X5	T38.3X6
injection, soluble	T38.3X1	T38.3X2	T38.3X3	T38.3X4	T38.3X5	T38.3X6
biphasic	T38.3X1	T38.3X2	T38.3X3	T38.3X4	T38.3X5	T38.3X6
intermediate acting	T38.3X1	T38.3X2	T38.3X3	T38.3X4	T38.3X5	T38.3X6
protamine zinc	T38.3X1	T38.3X2	T38.3X3	T38.3X4	T38.3X5	T38.3X6
slow acting	T38.3X1	T38.3X2	T38.3X3	T38.3X4	T38.3X5	T38.3X6
zinc						
protamine injection	T38.3X1	T38.3X2	T38.3X3	T38.3X4	T38.3X5	T38.3X6
suspension (amorphous) (crystalline)	T38.3X1	T38.3X2	T38.3X3	T38.3X4	T38.3X5	T38.3X6

Substance	Poisoning, Accidental (Unintentional)	Poisoning, Intentional Self-Harm	Poisoning, Assault	Poisoning, Undetermined	Adverse Effect	Underdosing
Interferon (alpha) (beta) (gamma)	T37.5X1	T37.5X2	T37.5X3	T37.5X4	T37.5X5	T37.5X6
Intestinal motility control drug	T47.6X1	T47.6X2	T47.6X3	T47.6X4	T47.6X5	T47.6X6
biological	T47.8X1	T47.8X2	T47.8X3	T47.8X4	T47.8X5	T47.8X6
Intranarcon	T41.1X1	T41.1X2	T41.1X3	T41.1X4	T41.1X5	T41.1X6
Intravenous						
amino acids	T50.991	T50.992	T50.993	T50.994	T50.995	T50.996
fat suspension	T50.991	T50.992	T50.993	T50.994	T50.995	T50.996
Inulin	T50.8X1	T50.8X2	T50.8X3	T50.8X4	T50.8X5	T50.8X6
Invert sugar	T50.3X1	T50.3X2	T50.3X3	T50.3X4	T50.3X5	T50.3X6
Inza—*see Naproxen*						
Iobenzamic acid	T50.8X1	T50.8X2	T50.8X3	T50.8X4	T50.8X5	T50.8X6
Iocarmic acid	T50.8X1	T50.8X2	T50.8X3	T50.8X4	T50.8X5	T50.8X6
Iocetamic acid	T50.8X1	T50.8X2	T50.8X3	T50.8X4	T50.8X5	T50.8X6
Iodamide	T50.8X1	T50.8X2	T50.8X3	T50.8X4	T50.8X5	T50.8X6
Iodide NEC—*see also Iodine*	T49.0X1	T49.0X2	T49.0X3	T49.0X4	T49.0X5	T49.0X6
mercury (ointment)	T49.0X1	T49.0X2	T49.0X3	T49.0X4	T49.0X5	T49.0X6
methylate	T49.0X1	T49.0X2	T49.0X3	T49.0X4	T49.0X5	T49.0X6
potassium (expectorant) NEC	T48.4X1	T48.4X2	T48.4X3	T48.4X4	T48.4X5	T48.4X6
Iodinated						
contrast medium	T50.8X1	T50.8X2	T50.8X3	T50.8X4	T50.8X5	T50.8X6
glycerol	T48.4X1	T48.4X2	T48.4X3	T48.4X4	T48.4X5	T48.4X6
human serum albumin (131I)	T50.8X1	T50.8X2	T50.8X3	T50.8X4	T50.8X5	T50.8X6
Iodine (antiseptic, external) (tincture) NEC	T49.0X1	T49.0X2	T49.0X3	T49.0X4	T49.0X5	T49.0X6
125—*see also Radiation sickness, and Exposure to radioactive isotopes*						
therapeutic	T50.991	T50.992	T50.993	T50.994	T50.995	T50.996
131—*see also Radiation sickness, and Exposure to radioactive isotopes*						
therapeutic	T38.2X1	T38.2X2	T38.2X3	T38.2X4	T38.2X5	T38.2X6
diagnostic	T50.8X1	T50.8X2	T50.8X3	T50.8X4	T50.8X5	T50.8X6
for thyroid conditions (antithyroid)	T38.2X1	T38.2X2	T38.2X3	T38.2X4	T38.2X5	T38.2X6
solution	T49.0X1	T49.0X2	T49.0X3	T49.0X4	T49.0X5	T49.0X6
vapor	T59.891	T59.892	T59.893	T59.894	—	—
Iodipamide	T50.8X1	T50.8X2	T50.8X3	T50.8X4	T50.8X5	T50.8X6
Iodized (poppy seed) oil	T50.8X1	T50.8X2	T50.8X3	T50.8X4	T50.8X5	T50.8X6
Iodobismitol	T37.8X1	T37.8X2	T37.8X3	T37.8X4	T37.8X5	T37.8X6
Iodochlorhydroxyquin	T37.8X1	T37.8X2	T37.8X3	T37.8X4	T37.8X5	T37.8X6
topical	T49.0X1	T49.0X2	T49.0X3	T49.0X4	T49.0X5	T49.0X6
Iodochlorhydroxyquino-line	T37.8X1	T37.8X2	T37.8X3	T37.8X4	T37.8X5	T37.8X6
Iodocholesterol (131I)	T50.8X1	T50.8X2	T50.8X3	T50.8X4	T50.8X5	T50.8X6

◀ New   ◀ Revised   ~~deleted~~ Deleted

Substance	External Cause (T-Code) Poisoning, Accidental (Unintentional)	Poisoning, Intentional Self-Harm	Poisoning, Assault	Poisoning, Undetermined	Adverse Effect	Underdosing
Iodoform	T49.0X1	T49.0X2	T49.0X3	T49.0X4	T49.0X5	T49.0X6
Iodohippuric acid	T50.8X1	T50.8X2	T50.8X3	T50.8X4	T50.8X5	T50.8X6
Iodopanoic acid	T50.8X1	T50.8X2	T50.8X3	T50.8X4	T50.8X5	T50.8X6
Iodophthalein (sodium)	T50.8X1	T50.8X2	T50.8X3	T50.8X4	T50.8X5	T50.8X6
Iodopyracet	T50.8X1	T50.8X2	T50.8X3	T50.8X4	T50.8X5	T50.8X6
Iodoquinol	T37.8X1	T37.8X2	T37.8X3	T37.8X4	T37.8X5	T37.8X6
Iodoxamic acid	T50.8X1	T50.8X2	T50.8X3	T50.8X4	T50.8X5	T50.8X6
Iofendylate	T50.8X1	T50.8X2	T50.8X3	T50.8X4	T50.8X5	T50.8X6
Ioglycamic acid	T50.8X1	T50.8X2	T50.8X3	T50.8X4	T50.8X5	T50.8X6
Iohexol	T50.8X1	T50.8X2	T50.8X3	T50.8X4	T50.8X5	T50.8X6
Ion exchange resin						
anion	T47.8X1	T47.8X2	T47.8X3	T47.8X4	T47.8X5	T47.8X6
cation	T50.3X1	T50.3X2	T50.3X3	T50.3X4	T50.3X5	T50.3X6
cholestyramine	T46.6X1	T46.6X2	T46.6X3	T46.6X4	T46.6X5	T46.6X6
intestinal	T47.8X1	T47.8X2	T47.8X3	T47.8X4	T47.8X5	T47.8X6
Iopamidol	T50.8X1	T50.8X2	T50.8X3	T50.8X4	T50.8X5	T50.8X6
Iopanoic acid	T50.8X1	T50.8X2	T50.8X3	T50.8X4	T50.8X5	T50.8X6
Iophenoic acid	T50.8X1	T50.8X2	T50.8X3	T50.8X4	T50.8X5	T50.8X6
Iopodate, sodium	T50.8X1	T50.8X2	T50.8X3	T50.8X4	T50.8X5	T50.8X6
Iopodic acid	T50.8X1	T50.8X2	T50.8X3	T50.8X4	T50.8X5	T50.8X6
Iopromide	T50.8X1	T50.8X2	T50.8X3	T50.8X4	T50.8X5	T50.8X6
Iopydol	T50.8X1	T50.8X2	T50.8X3	T50.8X4	T50.8X5	T50.8X6
Iotalamic acid	T50.8X1	T50.8X2	T50.8X3	T50.8X4	T50.8X5	T50.8X6
Iothalamate	T50.8X1	T50.8X2	T50.8X3	T50.8X4	T50.8X5	T50.8X6
Iothiouracil	T38.2X1	T38.2X2	T38.2X3	T38.2X4	T38.2X5	T38.2X6
Iotrol	T50.8X1	T50.8X2	T50.8X3	T50.8X4	T50.8X5	T50.8X6
Iotrolan	T50.8X1	T50.8X2	T50.8X3	T50.8X4	T50.8X5	T50.8X6
Iotroxate	T50.8X1	T50.8X2	T50.8X3	T50.8X4	T50.8X5	T50.8X6
Iotroxic acid	T50.8X1	T50.8X2	T50.8X3	T50.8X4	T50.8X5	T50.8X6
Ioversol	T50.8X1	T50.8X2	T50.8X3	T50.8X4	T50.8X5	T50.8X6
Ioxaglate	T50.8X1	T50.8X2	T50.8X3	T50.8X4	T50.8X5	T50.8X6
Ioxaglic acid	T50.8X1	T50.8X2	T50.8X3	T50.8X4	T50.8X5	T50.8X6
Ioxitalamic acid	T50.8X1	T50.8X2	T50.8X3	T50.8X4	T50.8X5	T50.8X6
Ipecac	T47.7X1	T47.7X2	T47.7X3	T47.7X4	T47.7X5	T47.7X6
Ipecacuanha	T48.4X1	T48.4X2	T48.4X3	T48.4X4	T48.4X5	T48.4X6
Ipodate, calcium	T50.8X1	T50.8X2	T50.8X3	T50.8X4	T50.8X5	T50.8X6
Ipral	T42.3X1	T42.3X2	T42.3X3	T42.3X4	T42.3X5	T42.3X6
Ipratropium (bromide)	T48.6X1	T48.6X2	T48.6X3	T48.6X4	T48.6X5	T48.6X6
Ipriflavone	T46.3X1	T46.3X2	T46.3X3	T46.3X4	T46.3X5	T46.3X6
Iprindole	T43.011	T43.012	T43.013	T43.014	T43.015	T43.016
Iproclozide	T43.1X1	T43.1X2	T43.1X3	T43.1X4	T43.1X5	T43.1X6
Iprofenin	T50.8X1	T50.8X2	T50.8X3	T50.8X4	T50.8X5	T50.8X6

Substance	External Cause (T-Code) Poisoning, Accidental (Unintentional)	Poisoning, Intentional Self-Harm	Poisoning, Assault	Poisoning, Undetermined	Adverse Effect	Underdosing
Iproheptine	T49.2X1	T49.2X2	T49.2X3	T49.2X4	T49.2X5	T49.2X6
Iproniazid	T43.1X1	T43.1X2	T43.1X3	T43.1X4	T43.1X5	T43.1X6
Iproplatin	T45.1X1	T45.1X2	T45.1X3	T45.1X4	T45.1X5	T45.1X6
Iproveratril	T46.1X1	T46.1X2	T46.1X3	T46.1X4	T46.1X5	T46.1X6
Iron (compounds) (medicinal) NEC	T45.4X1	T45.4X2	T45.4X3	T45.4X4	T45.4X5	T45.4X6
ammonium	T45.4X1	T45.4X2	T45.4X3	T45.4X4	T45.4X5	T45.4X6
dextran injection	T45.4X1	T45.4X2	T45.4X3	T45.4X4	T45.4X5	T45.4X6
nonmedicinal	T56.891	T56.892	T56.893	T56.894	—	—
salts	T45.4X1	T45.4X2	T45.4X3	T45.4X4	T45.4X5	T45.4X6
sorbitex	T45.4X1	T45.4X2	T45.4X3	T45.4X4	T45.4X5	T45.4X6
sorbitol citric acid complex	T45.4X1	T45.4X2	T45.4X3	T45.4X4	T45.4X5	T45.4X6
Irrigating fluid (vaginal)	T49.8X1	T49.8X2	T49.8X3	T49.8X4	T49.8X5	T49.8X6
eye	T49.5X1	T49.5X2	T49.5X3	T49.5X4	T49.5X5	T49.5X6
Isepamicin	T36.5X1	T36.5X2	T36.5X3	T36.5X4	T36.5X5	T36.5X6
Isoaminile (citrate)	T48.3X1	T48.3X2	T48.3X3	T48.3X4	T48.3X5	T48.3X6
Isoamyl nitrite	T46.3X1	T46.3X2	T46.3X3	T46.3X4	T46.3X5	T46.3X6
Isobenzan	T60.1X1	T60.1X2	T60.1X3	T60.1X4	—	—
Isobutyl acetate	T52.8X1	T52.8X2	T52.8X3	T52.8X4	—	—
Isocarboxazid	T43.1X1	T43.1X2	T43.1X3	T43.1X4	T43.1X5	T43.1X6
Isoconazole	T49.0X1	T49.0X2	T49.0X3	T49.0X4	T49.0X5	T49.0X6
Isocyanate	T65.0X1	T65.0X2	T65.0X3	T65.0X4	—	—
Isoephedrine	T44.991	T44.992	T44.993	T44.994	T44.995	T44.996
Isoetarine	T48.6X1	T48.6X2	T48.6X3	T48.6X4	T48.6X5	T48.6X6
Isoethadione	T42.2X1	T42.2X2	T42.2X3	T42.2X4	T42.2X5	T42.2X6
Isoetharine	T44.5X1	T44.5X2	T44.5X3	T44.5X4	T44.5X5	T44.5X6
Isoflurane	T41.0X1	T41.0X2	T41.0X3	T41.0X4	T41.0X5	T41.0X6
Isoflurophate	T44.0X1	T44.0X2	T44.0X3	T44.0X4	T44.0X5	T44.0X6
Isomaltose, ferric complex	T45.4X1	T45.4X2	T45.4X3	T45.4X4	T45.4X5	T45.4X6
Isometheptene	T44.3X1	T44.3X2	T44.3X3	T44.3X4	T44.3X5	T44.3X6
Isoniazid	T37.1X1	T37.1X2	T37.1X3	T37.1X4	T37.1X5	T37.1X6
with						
rifampicin	T36.6X1	T36.6X2	T36.6X3	T36.6X4	T36.6X5	T36.6X6
thioacetazone	T37.1X1	T37.1X2	T37.1X3	T37.1X4	T37.1X5	T37.1X6
Isonicotinic acid hydrazide	T37.1X1	T37.1X2	T37.1X3	T37.1X4	T37.1X5	T37.1X6
Isonipecaine	T40.491	T40.492	T40.493	T40.494	T40.495	T40.496
Isopentaquine	T37.2X1	T37.2X2	T37.2X3	T37.2X4	T37.2X5	T37.2X6
Isophane insulin	T38.3X1	T38.3X2	T38.3X3	T38.3X4	T38.3X5	T38.3X6
Isophorone	T65.891	T65.892	T65.893	T65.894	—	—
Isophosphamide	T45.1X1	T45.1X2	T45.1X3	T45.1X4	T45.1X5	T45.1X6
Isopregnenone	T38.5X1	T38.5X2	T38.5X3	T38.5X4	T38.5X5	T38.5X6
Isoprenaline	T48.6X1	T48.6X2	T48.6X3	T48.6X4	T48.6X5	T48.6X6
Isopromethazine	T43.3X1	T43.3X2	T43.3X3	T43.3X4	T43.3X5	T43.3X6

◀ New   ◀ Revised   ~~deleted~~ Deleted

Substance	Poisoning, Accidental (Unintentional)	Poisoning, Intentional Self-Harm	Poisoning, Assault	Poisoning, Undetermined	Adverse Effect	Underdosing
Isopropamide	T44.3X1	T44.3X2	T44.3X3	T44.3X4	T44.3X5	T44.3X6
iodide	T44.3X1	T44.3X2	T44.3X3	T44.3X4	T44.3X5	T44.3X6
Isopropanol	T51.2X1	T51.2X2	T51.2X3	T51.2X4	—	—
Isopropyl						
acetate	T52.8X1	T52.8X2	T52.8X3	T52.8X4	—	—
alcohol	T51.2X1	T51.2X2	T51.2X3	T51.2X4	—	—
medicinal	T49.4X1	T49.4X2	T49.4X3	T49.4X4	T49.4X5	T49.4X6
ether	T52.8X1	T52.8X2	T52.8X3	T52.8X4	—	—
Isopropylaminophena-zone	T39.2X1	T39.2X2	T39.2X3	T39.2X4	T39.2X5	T39.2X6
Isoproterenol	T48.6X1	T48.6X2	T48.6X3	T48.6X4	T48.6X5	T48.6X6
Isosorbide dinitrate	T46.3X1	T46.3X2	T46.3X3	T46.3X4	T46.3X5	T46.3X6
Isothipendyl	T45.0X1	T45.0X2	T45.0X3	T45.0X4	T45.0X5	T45.0X6
Isotretinoin	T50.991	T50.992	T50.993	T50.994	T50.995	T50.996
Isoxazolyl penicillin	T36.0X1	T36.0X2	T36.0X3	T36.0X4	T36.0X5	T36.0X6
Isoxicam	T39.391	T39.392	T39.393	T39.394	T39.395	T39.396
Isoxsuprine	T46.7X1	T46.7X2	T46.7X3	T46.7X4	T46.7X5	T46.7X6
Ispagula	T47.4X1	T47.4X2	T47.4X3	T47.4X4	T47.4X5	T47.4X6
husk	T47.4X1	T47.4X2	T47.4X3	T47.4X4	T47.4X5	T47.4X6
Isradipine	T46.1X1	T46.1X2	T46.1X3	T46.1X4	T46.1X5	T46.1X6
I-thyroxine sodium	T38.1X1	T38.1X2	T38.1X3	T38.1X4	T38.1X5	T38.1X6
Itraconazole	T37.8X1	T37.8X2	T37.8X3	T37.8X4	T37.8X5	T37.8X6
Itramin tosilate	T46.3X1	T46.3X2	T46.3X3	T46.3X4	T46.3X5	T46.3X6
Ivermectin	T37.4X1	T37.4X2	T37.4X3	T37.4X4	T37.4X5	T37.4X6
Izoniazid	T37.1X1	T37.1X2	T37.1X3	T37.1X4	T37.1X5	T37.1X6
with thioacetazone	T37.1X1	T37.1X2	T37.1X3	T37.1X4	T37.1X5	T37.1X6
J						
Jalap	T47.2X1	T47.2X2	T47.2X3	T47.2X4	T47.2X5	T47.2X6
Jamaica						
dogwood (bark)	T39.8X1	T39.8X2	T39.8X3	T39.8X4	T39.8X5	T39.8X6
ginger	T65.891	T65.892	T65.893	T65.894	—	—
root	T62.2X1	T62.2X2	T62.2X3	T62.2X4	—	—
Jatropha	T62.2X1	T62.2X2	T62.2X3	T62.2X4	—	—
curcas	T62.2X1	T62.2X2	T62.2X3	T62.2X4	—	—
Jectofer	T45.4X1	T45.4X2	T45.4X3	T45.4X4	T45.4X5	T45.4X6
Jellyfish (sting)	T63.621	T63.622	T63.623	T63.624	—	—
Jequirity (bean)	T62.2X1	T62.2X2	T62.2X3	T62.2X4	—	—
Jimson weed (stramonium)	T62.2X1	T62.2X2	T62.2X3	T62.2X4	—	—
seeds	T62.2X1	T62.2X2	T62.2X3	T62.2X4	—	—
Josamycin	T36.3X1	T36.3X2	T36.3X3	T36.3X4	T36.3X5	T36.3X6
Juniper tar	T49.1X1	T49.1X2	T49.1X3	T49.1X4	T49.1X5	T49.1X6

Substance	Poisoning, Accidental (Unintentional)	Poisoning, Intentional Self-Harm	Poisoning, Assault	Poisoning, Undetermined	Adverse Effect	Underdosing
K						
Kallidinogenase	T46.7X1	T46.7X2	T46.7X3	T46.7X4	T46.7X5	T46.7X6
Kallikrein	T46.7X1	T46.7X2	T46.7X3	T46.7X4	T46.7X5	T46.7X6
Kanamycin	T36.5X1	T36.5X2	T36.5X3	T36.5X4	T36.5X5	T36.5X6
Kantrex	T36.5X1	T36.5X2	T36.5X3	T36.5X4	T36.5X5	T36.5X6
Kaolin	T47.6X1	T47.6X2	T47.6X3	T47.6X4	T47.6X5	T47.6X6
light	T47.6X1	T47.6X2	T47.6X3	T47.6X4	T47.6X5	T47.6X6
Karaya (gum)	T47.4X1	T47.4X2	T47.4X3	T47.4X4	T47.4X5	T47.4X6
Kebuzone	T39.2X1	T39.2X2	T39.2X3	T39.2X4	T39.2X5	T39.2X6
Kelevan	T60.1X1	T60.1X2	T60.1X3	T60.1X4	—	—
Kemithal	T41.1X1	T41.1X2	T41.1X3	T41.1X4	T41.1X5	T41.1X6
Kenacort	T38.0X1	T38.0X2	T38.0X3	T38.0X4	T38.0X5	T38.0X6
Keratolytic drug NEC	T49.4X1	T49.4X2	T49.4X3	T49.4X4	T49.4X5	T49.4X6
anthracene	T49.4X1	T49.4X2	T49.4X3	T49.4X4	T49.4X5	T49.4X6
Keratoplastic NEC	T49.4X1	T49.4X2	T49.4X3	T49.4X4	T49.4X5	T49.4X6
Kerosene, kerosine (fuel) (solvent) NEC	T52.0X1	T52.0X2	T52.0X3	T52.0X4	—	—
insecticide	T52.0X1	T52.0X2	T52.0X3	T52.0X4	—	—
vapor	T52.0X1	T52.0X2	T52.0X3	T52.0X4	—	—
Ketamine	T41.291	T41.292	T41.293	T41.294	T41.295	T41.296
Ketazolam	T42.4X1	T42.4X2	T42.4X3	T42.4X4	T42.4X5	T42.4X6
Ketazon	T39.2X1	T39.2X2	T39.2X3	T39.2X4	T39.2X5	T39.2X6
Ketobemidone	T40.491	T40.492	T40.493	T40.494	—	—
Ketoconazole	T49.0X1	T49.0X2	T49.0X3	T49.0X4	T49.0X5	T49.0X6
Ketols	T52.4X1	T52.4X2	T52.4X3	T52.4X4	—	—
Ketone oils	T52.4X1	T52.4X2	T52.4X3	T52.4X4	—	—
Ketoprofen	T39.311	T39.312	T39.313	T39.314	T39.315	T39.316
Ketorolac	T39.8X1	T39.8X2	T39.8X3	T39.8X4	T39.8X5	T39.8X6
Ketotifen	T45.0X1	T45.0X2	T45.0X3	T45.0X4	T45.0X5	T45.0X6
Khat	T43.691	T43.692	T43.693	T43.694		
Khellin	T46.3X1	T46.3X2	T46.3X3	T46.3X4	T46.3X5	T46.3X6
Khelloside	T46.3X1	T46.3X2	T46.3X3	T46.3X4	T46.3X5	T46.3X6
Kiln gas or vapor (carbon monoxide)	T58.8X1	T58.8X2	T58.8X3	T58.8X4	—	—
Kitasamycin	T36.3X1	T36.3X2	T36.3X3	T36.3X4	T36.3X5	T36.3X6
Konsyl	T47.4X1	T47.4X2	T47.4X3	T47.4X4	T47.4X5	T47.4X6
Kosam seed	T62.2X1	T62.2X2	T62.2X3	T62.2X4	—	—
Krait (venom)	T63.091	T63.092	T63.093	T63.094	—	—
Kwell (insecticide)	T60.1X1	T60.1X2	T60.1X3	T60.1X4	—	—
anti-infective (topical)	T49.0X1	T49.0X2	T49.0X3	T49.0X4	T49.0X5	T49.0X6

◀ New ◀ Revised ~~deleted~~ Deleted

Substance	Poisoning, Accidental (Unintentional)	Poisoning, Intentional Self-Harm	Poisoning, Assault	Poisoning, Undetermined	Adverse Effect	Underdosing
L						
Labetalol	T44.8X1	T44.8X2	T44.8X3	T44.8X4	T44.8X5	T44.8X6
Laburnum (seeds)	T62.2X1	T62.2X2	T62.2X3	T62.2X4	—	—
leaves	T62.2X1	T62.2X2	T62.2X3	T62.2X4	—	—
Lachesine	T49.5X1	T49.5X2	T49.5X3	T49.5X4	T49.5X5	T49.5X6
Lacidipine	T46.5X1	T46.5X2	T46.5X3	T46.5X4	T46.5X5	T46.5X6
Lacquer	T65.6X1	T65.6X2	T65.6X3	T65.6X4	—	—
Lacrimogenic gas	T59.3X1	T59.3X2	T59.3X3	T59.3X4		
Lactated potassic saline	T50.3X1	T50.3X2	T50.3X3	T50.3X4	T50.3X5	T50.3X6
Lactic acid	T49.8X1	T49.8X2	T49.8X3	T49.8X4	T49.8X5	T49.8X6
Lactobacillus						
acidophilus	T47.6X1	T47.6X2	T47.6X3	T47.6X4	T47.6X5	T47.6X6
compound	T47.6X1	T47.6X2	T47.6X3	T47.6X4	T47.6X5	T47.6X6
bifidus, lyophilized	T47.6X1	T47.6X2	T47.6X3	T47.6X4	T47.6X5	T47.6X6
bulgaricus	T47.6X1	T47.6X2	T47.6X3	T47.6X4	T47.6X5	T47.6X6
sporogenes	T47.6X1	T47.6X2	T47.6X3	T47.6X4	T47.6X5	T47.6X6
Lactoflavin	T45.2X1	T45.2X2	T45.2X3	T45.2X4	T45.2X5	T45.2X6
Lactose (as excipient)	T50.901	T50.902	T50.903	T50.904	T50.905	T50.906
Lactuca (virosa) (extract)	T42.6X1	T42.6X2	T42.6X3	T42.6X4	T42.6X5	T42.6X6
Lactucarium	T42.6X1	T42.6X2	T42.6X3	T42.6X4	T42.6X5	T42.6X6
Lactulose	T47.3X1	T47.3X2	T47.3X3	T47.3X4	T47.3X5	T47.3X6
Laevo — see Levo-						
Lanatosides	T46.0X1	T46.0X2	T46.0X3	T46.0X4	T46.0X5	T46.0X6
Lanolin	T49.3X1	T49.3X2	T49.3X3	T49.3X4	T49.3X5	T49.3X6
Largactil	T43.3X1	T43.3X2	T43.3X3	T43.3X4	T43.3X5	T43.3X6
Larkspur	T62.2X1	T62.2X2	T62.2X3	T62.2X4	—	—
Laroxyl	T43.011	T43.012	T43.013	T43.014	T43.015	T43.016
Lassar's paste	T49.4X1	T49.4X2	T49.4X3	T49.4X4	T49.4X5	T49.4X6
Lasix	T50.1X1	T50.1X2	T50.1X3	T50.1X4	T50.1X5	T50.1X6
Latamoxef	T36.1X1	T36.1X2	T36.1X3	T36.1X4	T36.1X5	T36.1X6
Latex	T65.811	T65.812	T65.813	T65.814	—	—
Lathyrus (seed)	T62.2X1	T62.2X2	T62.2X3	T62.2X4	—	—
Laudanum	T40.0X1	T40.0X2	T40.0X3	T40.0X4	T40.0X5	T40.0X6
Laudexium	T48.1X1	T48.1X2	T48.1X3	T48.1X4	T48.1X5	T48.1X6
Laughing gas	T41.0X1	T41.0X2	T41.0X3	T41.0X4	T41.0X5	T41.0X6
Laurel, black or cherry	T62.2X1	T62.2X2	T62.2X3	T62.2X4	—	—
Laurolinium	T49.0X1	T49.0X2	T49.0X3	T49.0X4	T49.0X5	T49.0X6
Lauryl sulfoacetate	T49.2X1	T49.2X2	T49.2X3	T49.2X4	T49.2X5	T49.2X6

Substance	Poisoning, Accidental (Unintentional)	Poisoning, Intentional Self-Harm	Poisoning, Assault	Poisoning, Undetermined	Adverse Effect	Underdosing
Laxative NEC	T47.4X1	T47.4X2	T47.4X3	T47.4X4	T47.4X5	T47.4X6
osmotic	T47.3X1	T47.3X2	T47.3X3	T47.3X4	T47.3X5	T47.3X6
saline	T47.3X1	T47.3X2	T47.3X3	T47.3X4	T47.3X5	T47.3X6
stimulant	T47.2X1	T47.2X2	T47.2X3	T47.2X4	T47.2X5	T47.2X6
L-dopa	T42.8X1	T42.8X2	T42.8X3	T42.8X4	T42.8X5	T42.8X6
Lead (dust) (fumes) (vapor) NEC	T56.0X1	T56.0X2	T56.0X3	T56.0X4	—	—
acetate	T49.2X1	T49.2X2	T49.2X3	T49.2X4	T49.2X5	T49.2X6
alkyl (fuel additive)	T56.0X1	T56.0X2	T56.0X3	T56.0X4	—	—
anti-infectives	T37.8X1	T37.8X2	T37.8X3	T37.8X4	T37.8X5	T37.8X6
antiknock compound (tetraethyl)	T56.0X1	T56.0X2	T56.0X3	T56.0X4	—	—
arsenate, arsenite (dust) (herbicide) (insecticide) (vapor)	T57.0X1	T57.0X2	T57.0X3	T57.0X4	—	—
carbonate	T56.0X1	T56.0X2	T56.0X3	T56.0X4	—	—
paint	T56.0X1	T56.0X2	T56.0X3	T56.0X4	—	—
chromate	T56.0X1	T56.0X2	T56.0X3	T56.0X4	—	—
paint	T56.0X1	T56.0X2	T56.0X3	T56.0X4	—	—
dioxide	T56.0X1	T56.0X2	T56.0X3	T56.0X4	—	—
inorganic	T56.0X1	T56.0X2	T56.0X3	T56.0X4	—	—
iodide	T56.0X1	T56.0X2	T56.0X3	T56.0X4	—	—
pigment (paint)	T56.0X1	T56.0X2	T56.0X3	T56.0X4	—	—
monoxide (dust)	T56.0X1	T56.0X2	T56.0X3	T56.0X4	—	—
paint	T56.0X1	T56.0X2	T56.0X3	T56.0X4	—	—
organic	T56.0X1	T56.0X2	T56.0X3	T56.0X4	—	—
oxide	T56.0X1	T56.0X2	T56.0X3	T56.0X4	—	—
paint	T56.0X1	T56.0X2	T56.0X3	T56.0X4	—	—
paint	T56.0X1	T56.0X2	T56.0X3	T56.0X4	—	—
salts	T56.0X1	T56.0X2	T56.0X3	T56.0X4	—	—
specified compound NEC	T56.0X1	T56.0X2	T56.0X3	T56.0X4	—	—
tetra-ethyl	T56.0X1	T56.0X2	T56.0X3	T56.0X4	—	—
Lebanese red	T40.711	T40.712	T40.713	T40.714	T40.715	T40.716
Lefetamine	T39.8X1	T39.8X2	T39.8X3	T39.8X4	T39.8X5	T39.8X6
Lenperone	T43.4X1	T43.4X2	T43.4X3	T43.4X4	T43.4X5	T43.4X6
Lente lietin (insulin)	T38.3X1	T38.3X2	T38.3X3	T38.3X4	T38.3X5	T38.3X6
Leptazol	T50.7X1	T50.7X2	T50.7X3	T50.7X4	T50.7X5	T50.7X6
Leptophos	T60.0X1	T60.0X2	T60.0X3	T60.0X4	—	—
Leritine	T40.2X1	T40.2X2	T40.2X3	T40.2X4	T40.2X5	T40.2X6
Letosteine	T48.4X1	T48.4X2	T48.4X3	T48.4X4	T48.4X5	T48.4X6
Letter	T38.1X1	T38.1X2	T38.1X3	T38.1X4	T38.1X5	T38.1X6
Lettuce opium	T42.6X1	T42.6X2	T42.6X3	T42.6X4	T42.6X5	T42.6X6
Leucinocaine	T41.3X1	T41.3X2	T41.3X3	T41.3X4	T41.3X5	T41.3X6

◀ New   ◀ Revised   ~~deleted~~ Deleted

TABLE OF DRUGS AND CHEMICALS

TABLE OF DRUGS AND CHEMICALS

Substance	External Cause (T-Code)					
	Poisoning, Accidental (Unintentional)	Poisoning, Intentional Self-Harm	Poisoning, Assault	Poisoning, Undetermined	Adverse Effect	Underdosing
Leucocianidol	T46.991	T46.992	T46.993	T46.994	T46.995	T46.996
Leucovorin (factor)	T45.8X1	T45.8X2	T45.8X3	T45.8X4	T45.8X5	T45.8X6
Leukeran	T45.1X1	T45.1X2	T45.1X3	T45.1X4	T45.1X5	T45.1X6
Leuprolide	T38.891	T38.892	T38.893	T38.894	T38.895	T38.896
Levalbuterol	T48.6X1	T48.6X2	T48.6X3	T48.6X4	T48.6X5	T48.6X6
Levallorphan	T50.7X1	T50.7X2	T50.7X3	T50.7X4	T50.7X5	T50.7X6
Levamisole	T37.4X1	T37.4X2	T37.4X3	T37.4X4	T37.4X5	T37.4X6
Levanil	T42.6X1	T42.6X2	T42.6X3	T42.6X4	T42.6X5	T42.6X6
Levarterenol	T44.4X1	T44.4X2	T44.4X3	T44.4X4	T44.4X5	T44.4X6
Levdropropizine	T48.3X1	T48.3X2	T48.3X3	T48.3X4	T48.3X5	T48.3X6
Levobunolol	T49.5X1	T49.5X2	T49.5X3	T49.5X4	T49.5X5	T49.5X6
Levocabastine (hydrochloride)	T45.0X1	T45.0X2	T45.0X3	T45.0X4	T45.0X5	T45.0X6
Levocarnitine	T50.991	T50.992	T50.993	T50.994	T50.995	T50.996
Levodopa	T42.8X1	T42.8X2	T42.8X3	T42.8X4	T42.8X5	T42.8X6
with carbidopa	T42.8X1	T42.8X2	T42.8X3	T42.8X4	T42.8X5	T42.8X6
Levo-dromoran	T40.2X1	T40.2X2	T40.2X3	T40.2X4	T40.2X5	T40.2X6
Levoglutamide	T50.991	T50.992	T50.993	T50.994	T50.995	T50.996
Levoid	T38.1X1	T38.1X2	T38.1X3	T38.1X4	T38.1X5	T38.1X6
Levo-iso-methadone	T40.3X1	T40.3X2	T40.3X3	T40.3X4	T40.3X5	T40.3X6
Levomepromazine	T43.3X1	T43.3X2	T43.3X3	T43.3X4	T43.3X5	T43.3X6
Levonordefrin	T49.6X1	T49.6X2	T49.6X3	T49.6X4	T49.6X5	T49.6X6
Levonorgestrel	T38.4X1	T38.4X2	T38.4X3	T38.4X4	T38.4X5	T38.4X6
with ethinylestradiol	T38.5X1	T38.5X2	T38.5X3	T38.5X4	T38.5X5	T38.5X6
Levopromazine	T43.3X1	T43.3X2	T43.3X3	T43.3X4	T43.3X5	T43.3X6
Levoprome	T42.6X1	T42.6X2	T42.6X3	T42.6X4	T42.6X5	T42.6X6
Levopropoxyphene	T40.491	T40.492	T40.493	T40.494	T40.495	T40.496
Levopropylhexedrine	T50.5X1	T50.5X2	T50.5X3	T50.5X4	T50.5X5	T50.5X6
Levoproxyphylline	T48.6X1	T48.6X2	T48.6X3	T48.6X4	T48.6X5	T48.6X6
Levorphanol	T40.491	T40.492	T40.493	T40.494	T40.495	T40.496
Levothyroxine	T38.1X1	T38.1X2	T38.1X3	T38.1X4	T38.1X5	T38.1X6
sodium	T38.1X1	T38.1X2	T38.1X3	T38.1X4	T38.1X5	T38.1X6
Levsin	T44.3X1	T44.3X2	T44.3X3	T44.3X4	T44.3X5	T44.3X6
Levulose	T50.3X1	T50.3X2	T50.3X3	T50.3X4	T50.3X5	T50.3X6
Lewisite (gas), not in war	T57.0X1	T57.0X2	T57.0X3	T57.0X4	—	—
Librium	T42.4X1	T42.4X2	T42.4X3	T42.4X4	T42.4X5	T42.4X6
Lidex	T49.0X1	T49.0X2	T49.0X3	T49.0X4	T49.0X5	T49.0X6
Lidocaine	T41.3X1	T41.3X2	T41.3X3	T41.3X4	T41.3X5	T41.3X6
regional	T41.3X1	T41.3X2	T41.3X3	T41.3X4	T41.3X5	T41.3X6
spinal	T41.3X1	T41.3X2	T41.3X3	T41.3X4	T41.3X5	T41.3X6
Lidofenin	T50.8X1	T50.8X2	T50.8X3	T50.8X4	T50.8X5	T50.8X6
Lidoflazine	T46.1X1	T46.1X2	T46.1X3	T46.1X4	T46.1X5	T46.1X6
Lighter fluid	T52.0X1	T52.0X2	T52.0X3	T52.0X4	—	—

Substance	External Cause (T-Code)					
	Poisoning, Accidental (Unintentional)	Poisoning, Intentional Self-Harm	Poisoning, Assault	Poisoning, Undetermined	Adverse Effect	Underdosing
Lignin hemicellulose	T47.6X1	T47.6X2	T47.6X3	T47.6X4	T47.6X5	T47.6X6
Lignocaine	T41.3X1	T41.3X2	T41.3X3	T41.3X4	T41.3X5	T41.3X6
regional	T41.3X1	T41.3X2	T41.3X3	T41.3X4	T41.3X5	T41.3X6
spinal	T41.3X1	T41.3X2	T41.3X3	T41.3X4	T41.3X5	T41.3X6
Ligroin(e) (solvent)	T52.0X1	T52.0X2	T52.0X3	T52.0X4	—	—
vapor	T59.891	T59.892	T59.893	T59.894	—	—
Ligustrum vulgare	T62.2X1	T62.2X2	T62.2X3	T62.2X4	—	—
Lily of the valley	T62.2X1	T62.2X2	T62.2X3	T62.2X4	—	—
Lime (chloride)	T54.3X1	T54.3X2	T54.3X3	T54.3X4	—	—
Limonene	T52.8X1	T52.8X2	T52.8X3	T52.8X4	—	—
Lincomycin	T36.8X1	T36.8X2	T36.8X3	T36.8X4	T36.8X5	T36.8X6
Lindane (insecticide) (nonmedicinal) (vapor)	T53.6X1	T53.6X2	T53.6X3	T53.6X4	—	—
medicinal	T49.0X1	T49.0X2	T49.0X3	T49.0X4	T49.0X5	T49.0X6
Liniments NEC	T49.91	T49.92	T49.93	T49.94	T49.95	T49.96
Linoleic acid	T46.6X1	T46.6X2	T46.6X3	T46.6X4	T46.6X5	T46.6X6
Linolenic acid	T46.6X1	T46.6X2	T46.6X3	T46.6X4	T46.6X5	T46.6X6
Linseed	T47.4X1	T47.4X2	T47.4X3	T47.4X4	T47.4X5	T47.4X6
Liothyronine	T38.1X1	T38.1X2	T38.1X3	T38.1X4	T38.1X5	T38.1X6
Liotrix	T38.1X1	T38.1X2	T38.1X3	T38.1X4	T38.1X5	T38.1X6
Lipancreatin	T47.5X1	T47.5X2	T47.5X3	T47.5X4	T47.5X5	T47.5X6
Lipo-alprostadil	T46.7X1	T46.7X2	T46.7X3	T46.7X4	T46.7X5	T46.7X6
Lipo-Lutin	T38.5X1	T38.5X2	T38.5X3	T38.5X4	T38.5X5	T38.5X6
Lipotropic drug NEC	T50.901	T50.902	T50.903	T50.904	T50.905	T50.906
Liquefied petroleum gases	T59.891	T59.892	T59.893	T59.894	—	—
piped (pure or mixed with air)	T59.891	T59.892	T59.893	T59.894	—	—
Liquid						
paraffin	T47.4X1	T47.4X2	T47.4X3	T47.4X4	T47.4X5	T47.4X6
petrolatum	T47.4X1	T47.4X2	T47.4X3	T47.4X4	T47.4X5	T47.4X6
topical	T49.3X1	T49.3X2	T49.3X3	T49.3X4	T49.3X5	T49.3X6
specified NEC	T65.891	T65.892	T65.893	T65.894	—	—
substance	T65.91	T65.92	T65.93	T65.94	—	—
Liquor creosolis compositus	T65.891	T65.892	T65.893	T65.894	—	—
Liquorice	T48.4X1	T48.4X2	T48.4X3	T48.4X4	T48.4X5	T48.4X6
extract	T47.8X1	T47.8X2	T47.8X3	T47.8X4	T47.8X5	T47.8X6
Lirugen	T50.991	T50.992	T50.993	T50.994	T50.995	T50.996
Lisinopril	T46.4X1	T46.4X2	T46.4X3	T46.4X4	T46.4X5	T46.4X6
Lisuride	T42.8X1	T42.8X2	T42.8X3	T42.8X4	T42.8X5	T42.8X6
Lithane	T43.8X1	T43.8X2	T43.8X3	T43.8X4	T43.8X5	T43.8X6
Lithium	T56.891	T56.892	T56.893	T56.894		
gluconate	T43.591	T43.592	T43.593	T43.594	T43.595	T43.596
salts (carbonate)	T43.591	T43.592	T43.593	T43.594	T43.595	T43.596

◀ New ◀ Revised ~~deleted~~ Deleted

Substance	External Cause (T-Code)					
	Poisoning, Accidental (Unintentional)	Poisoning, Intentional Self-Harm	Poisoning, Assault	Poisoning, Undetermined	Adverse Effect	Underdosing
Lithonate	T43.8X1	T43.8X2	T43.8X3	T43.8X4	T43.8X5	T43.8X6
Liver						
extract	T45.8X1	T45.8X2	T45.8X3	T45.8X4	T45.8X5	T45.8X6
for parenteral use	T45.8X1	T45.8X2	T45.8X3	T45.8X4	T45.8X5	T45.8X6
fraction 1	T45.8X1	T45.8X2	T45.8X3	T45.8X4	T45.8X5	T45.8X6
hydrolysate	T45.8X1	T45.8X2	T45.8X3	T45.8X4	T45.8X5	T45.8X6
Lizard (bite) (venom)	T63.121	T63.122	T63.123	T63.124	—	—
LMD	T45.8X1	T45.8X2	T45.8X3	T45.8X4	T45.8X5	T45.8X6
Lobelia	T62.2X1	T62.2X2	T62.2X3	T62.2X4	—	
Lobeline	T50.7X1	T50.7X2	T50.7X3	T50.7X4	T50.7X5	T50.7X6
Local action drug NEC	T49.8X1	T49.8X2	T49.8X3	T49.8X4	T49.8X5	T49.8X6
Locorten	T49.0X1	T49.0X2	T49.0X3	T49.0X4	T49.0X5	T49.0X6
Lofepramine	T43.011	T43.012	T43.013	T43.014	T43.015	T43.016
Lolium temulentum	T62.2X1	T62.2X2	T62.2X3	T62.2X4	—	
Lomotil	T47.6X1	T47.6X2	T47.6X3	T47.6X4	T47.6X5	T47.6X6
Lomustine	T45.1X1	T45.1X2	T45.1X4	T45.1X4	T45.1X5	T45.1X6
Lonidamine	T45.1X1	T45.1X2	T45.1X3	T45.1X4	T45.1X5	T45.1X6
Loperamide	T47.6X1	T47.6X2	T47.6X3	T47.6X4	T47.6X5	T47.6X6
Loprazolam	T42.4X1	T42.4X2	T42.4X3	T42.4X4	T42.4X5	T42.4X6
Lorajmine	T46.2X1	T46.2X2	T46.2X3	T46.2X4	T46.2X5	T46.2X6
Loratidine	T45.0X1	T45.0X2	T45.0X3	T45.0X4	T45.0X5	T45.0X6
Lorazepam	T42.4X1	T42.4X2	T42.4X3	T42.4X4	T42.4X5	T42.4X6
Lorcainide	T46.2X1	T46.2X2	T46.2X3	T46.2X4	T46.2X5	T46.2X6
Lormetazepam	T42.4X1	T42.4X2	T42.4X3	T42.4X4	T42.4X5	T42.4X6
Lotions NEC	T49.91	T49.92	T49.93	T49.94	T49.95	T49.96
Lotusate	T42.3X1	T42.3X2	T42.3X3	T42.3X4	T42.3X5	T42.3X6
Lovastatin	T46.6X1	T46.6X2	T46.6X3	T46.6X4	T46.6X5	T46.6X6
Loxapine	T43.591	T43.592	T43.593	T43.594	T43.595	T43.596
Lowila	T49.2X1	T49.2X2	T49.2X3	T49.2X4	T49.2X5	T49.2X6
Lozenges (throat)	T49.6X1	T49.6X2	T49.6X3	T49.6X4	T49.6X5	T49.6X6
LSD	T40.8X1	T40.8X2	T40.8X3	T40.8X4	—	—
L-Tryptophan — see Amino acid						
Lubricant, eye	T49.5X1	T49.5X2	T49.5X3	T49.5X4	T49.5X5	T49.5X6
Lubricating oil NEC	T52.0X1	T52.0X2	T52.0X3	T52.0X4	—	—
Lucanthone	T37.4X1	T37.4X2	T37.4X3	T37.4X4	T37.4X5	T37.4X6
Luminal	T42.3X1	T42.3X2	T42.3X3	T42.3X4	T42.3X5	T42.3X6
Lung irritant (gas) NEC	T59.91	T59.92	T59.93	T59.94	—	—
Luteinizing hormone	T38.811	T38.812	T38.813	T38.814	T38.815	T38.816
Lutocylol	T38.5X1	T38.5X2	T38.5X3	T38.5X4	T38.5X5	T38.5X6
Lutromone	T38.5X1	T38.5X2	T38.5X3	T38.5X4	T38.5X5	T38.5X6
Lututrin	T48.291	T48.292	T48.293	T48.294	T48.295	T48.296
Lye (Concentrated)	T54.3X1	T54.3X2	T54.3X3	T54.3X4	—	—

Substance	External Cause (T-Code)					
	Poisoning, Accidental (Unintentional)	Poisoning, Intentional Self-Harm	Poisoning, Assault	Poisoning, Undetermined	Adverse Effect	Underdosing
Lygranum (skin test)	T50.8X1	T50.8X2	T50.8X3	T50.8X4	T50.8X5	T50.8X6
Lymecycline	T36.4X1	T36.4X2	T36.4X3	T36.4X4	T36.4X5	T36.4X6
Lymphogranuloma venereum antigen	T50.8X1	T50.8X2	T50.8X3	T50.8X4	T50.8X5	T50.8X6
Lynestrenol	T38.4X1	T38.4X2	T38.4X3	T38.4X4	T38.4X5	T38.4X6
Lypressin	T38.891	T38.892	T38.893	T38.894	T38.895	T38.896
Lyovac Sodium Edecrin	T50.1X1	T50.1X2	T50.1X3	T50.1X4	T50.1X5	T50.1X6
Lysergic acid diethylamide	T40.8X1	T40.8X2	T40.8X3	T40.8X4	—	—
Lysergide	T40.8X1	T40.8X2	T40.8X3	T40.8X4	—	—
Lysine vasopressin	T38.891	T38.892	T38.893	T38.894	T38.895	T38.896
Lysol	T54.1X1	T54.1X2	T54.1X3	T54.1X4	—	—
Lysozyme	T49.0X1	T49.0X2	T49.0X3	T49.0X4	T49.0X5	T49.0X6
Lytta (vitatta)	T49.8X1	T49.8X2	T49.8X3	T49.8X4	T49.8X5	T49.8X6
M						
Mace	T59.3X1	T59.3X2	T59.3X3	T59.3X4	—	—
Macrogol	T50.991	T50.992	T50.993	T50.994	T50.995	T50.996
Macrolide						
anabolic drug	T38.7X1	T38.7X2	T38.7X3	T38.7X4	T38.7X5	T38.7X6
antibiotic	T36.3X1	T36.3X2	T36.3X3	T36.3X4	T36.3X5	T36.3X6
Mafenide	T49.0X1	T49.0X2	T49.0X3	T49.0X4	T49.0X5	T49.0X6
Magaldrate	T47.1X1	T47.1X2	T47.1X3	T47.1X4	T47.1X5	T47.1X6
Magic mushroom	T40.991	T40.992	T40.993	T40.994	—	—
Magnamycin	T36.8X1	T36.8X2	T36.8X3	T36.8X4	T36.8X5	T36.8X6
Magnesia magma	T47.1X1	T47.1X2	T47.1X3	T47.1X4	T47.1X5	T47.1X6
Magnesium NEC	T56.891	T56.892	T56.893	T56.894		
carbonate	T47.1X1	T47.1X2	T47.1X3	T47.1X4	T47.1X5	T47.1X6
citrate	T47.4X1	T47.4X2	T47.4X3	T47.4X4	T47.4X5	T47.4X6
hydroxide	T47.1X1	T47.1X2	T47.1X3	T47.1X4	T47.1X5	T47.1X6
oxide	T47.1X1	T47.1X2	T47.1X3	T47.1X4	T47.1X5	T47.1X6
peroxide	T49.0X1	T49.0X2	T49.0X3	T49.0X4	T49.0X5	T49.0X6
salicylate	T39.091	T39.092	T39.093	T39.094	T39.095	T39.096
silicofluoride	T50.3X1	T50.3X2	T50.3X3	T50.3X4	T50.3X5	T50.3X6
sulfate	T47.4X1	T47.4X2	T47.4X3	T47.4X4	T47.4X5	T47.4X6
thiosulfate	T45.0X1	T45.0X2	T45.0X3	T45.0X4	T45.0X5	T45.0X6
trisilicate	T47.1X1	T47.1X2	T47.1X3	T47.1X4	T47.1X5	T47.1X6
Malathion (medicinal)	T49.0X1	T49.0X2	T49.0X3	T49.0X4	T49.0X5	T49.0X6
insecticide	T60.0X1	T60.0X2	T60.0X3	T60.0X4	—	—
Male fern extract	T37.4X1	T37.4X2	T37.4X3	T37.4X4	T37.4X5	T37.4X6
M-AMSA	T45.1X1	T45.1X2	T45.1X3	T45.1X4	T45.1X5	T45.1X6
Mandelic acid	T37.8X1	T37.8X2	T37.8X3	T37.8X4	T37.8X5	T37.8X6
Manganese (dioxide) (salts)	T57.2X1	T57.2X2	T57.2X3	T57.2X4	—	—
medicinal	T50.991	T50.992	T50.993	T50.994	T50.995	T50.996

◀ New   ◀ Revised   ~~deleted~~ Deleted

Substance	Poisoning, Accidental (Unintentional)	Poisoning, Intentional Self-Harm	Poisoning, Assault	Poisoning, Undetermined	Adverse Effect	Underdosing
Mannitol	T47.3X1	T47.3X2	T47.3X3	T47.3X4	T47.3X5	T47.3X6
hexanitrate	T46.3X1	T46.3X2	T46.3X3	T46.3X4	T46.3X5	T46.3X6
Mannomustine	T45.1X1	T45.1X2	T45.1X3	T45.1X4	T45.1X5	T45.1X6
MAO inhibitors	T43.1X1	T43.1X2	T43.1X3	T43.1X4	T43.1X5	T43.1X6
Mapharsen	T37.8X1	T37.8X2	T37.8X3	T37.8X4	T37.8X5	T37.8X6
Maphenide	T49.0X1	T49.0X2	T49.0X3	T49.0X4	T49.0X5	T49.0X6
Maprotiline	T43.021	T43.022	T43.023	T43.024	T43.025	T43.026
Marcaine	T41.3X1	T41.3X2	T41.3X3	T41.3X4	T41.3X5	T41.3X6
infiltration (subcutaneous)	T41.3X1	T41.3X2	T41.3X3	T41.3X4	T41.3X5	T41.3X6
nerve block (peripheral) (plexus)	T41.3X1	T41.3X2	T41.3X3	T41.3X4	T41.3X5	T41.3X6
Marezine	T45.0X1	T45.0X2	T45.0X3	T45.0X4	T45.0X5	T45.0X6
Marihuana	T40.711	T40.712	T40.713	T40.714	T40.715	T40.716
Marijuana	T40.711	T40.712	T40.713	T40.714	T40.715	T40.716
Marine (sting)	T63.691	T63.692	T63.693	T63.694	—	—
animals (sting)	T63.691	T63.692	T63.693	T63.694	—	—
plants (sting)	T63.711	T63.712	T63.713	T63.714	—	—
Marplan	T43.1X1	T43.1X2	T43.1X3	T43.1X4	T43.1X5	T43.1X6
Marsh gas	T59.891	T59.892	T59.893	T59.894		
Marsilid	T43.1X1	T43.1X2	T43.1X3	T43.1X4	T43.1X5	T43.1X6
Matulane	T45.1X1	T45.1X2	T45.1X3	T45.1X4	T45.1X5	T45.1X6
Mazindol	T50.5X1	T50.5X2	T50.5X3	T50.5X4	T50.5X5	T50.5X6
MCPA	T60.3X1	T60.3X2	T60.3X3	T60.3X4	—	—
MDMA	T43.641	T43.642	T43.643	T43.644	—	—
Meadow saffron	T62.2X1	T62.2X2	T62.2X3	T62.2X4	—	—
Measles virus vaccine (attenuated)	T50.B91	T50.B92	T50.B93	T50.B94	T50.B95	T50.B96
Meat, noxious	T62.8X1	T62.8X2	T62.8X3	T62.8X4	—	—
Meballymal	T42.3X1	T42.3X2	T42.3X3	T42.3X4	T42.3X5	T42.3X6
Mebanazine	T43.1X1	T43.1X2	T43.1X3	T43.1X4	T43.1X5	T43.1X6
Mebaral	T42.3X1	T42.3X2	T42.3X3	T42.3X4	T42.3X5	T42.3X6
Mebendazole	T37.4X1	T37.4X2	T37.4X3	T37.4X4	T37.4X5	T37.4X6
Mebeverine	T44.3X1	T44.3X2	T44.3X3	T44.3X4	T44.3X5	T44.3X6
Mebhydrolin	T45.0X1	T45.0X2	T45.0X3	T45.0X4	T45.0X5	T45.0X6
Mebumal	T42.3X1	T42.3X2	T42.3X3	T42.3X4	T42.3X5	T42.3X6
Mebutamate	T43.591	T43.592	T43.593	T43.594	T43.595	T43.596
Mecamylamine	T44.2X1	T44.2X2	T44.2X3	T44.2X4	T44.2X5	T44.2X6
Mechlorethamine	T45.1X1	T45.1X2	T45.1X3	T45.1X4	T45.1X5	T45.1X6
Mecillinam	T36.0X1	T36.0X2	T36.0X3	T36.0X4	T36.0X5	T36.0X6
Meclizine (hydrochloride)	T45.0X1	T45.0X2	T45.0X3	T45.0X4	T45.0X5	T45.0X6
Meclocycline	T36.4X1	T36.4X2	T36.4X3	T36.4X4	T36.4X5	T36.4X6
Meclofenamate	T39.391	T39.392	T39.393	T39.394	T39.395	T39.396
Meclofenamic acid	T39.391	T39.392	T39.393	T39.394	T39.395	T39.396

Substance	Poisoning, Accidental (Unintentional)	Poisoning, Intentional Self-Harm	Poisoning, Assault	Poisoning, Undetermined	Adverse Effect	Underdosing
Meclofenoxate	T43.691	T43.692	T43.693	T43.694	T43.695	T43.696
Meclozine	T45.0X1	T45.0X2	T45.0X3	T45.0X4	T45.0X5	T45.0X6
Mecobalamin	T45.8X1	T45.8X2	T45.8X3	T45.8X4	T45.8X5	T45.8X6
Mecoprop	T60.3X1	T60.3X2	T60.3X3	T60.3X4	—	—
Mecrilate	T49.3X1	T49.3X2	T49.3X3	T49.3X4	T49.3X5	T49.3X6
Mecysteine	T48.4X1	T48.4X2	T48.4X3	T48.4X4	T48.4X5	T48.4X6
Medazepam	T42.4X1	T42.4X2	T42.4X3	T42.4X4	T42.4X5	T42.4X6
Medicament NEC	T50.901	T50.902	T50.903	T50.904	T50.905	T50.906
Medinal	T42.3X1	T42.3X2	T42.3X3	T42.3X4	T42.3X5	T42.3X6
Medomin	T42.3X1	T42.3X2	T42.3X3	T42.3X4	T42.3X5	T42.3X6
Medrogestone	T38.5X1	T38.5X2	T38.5X3	T38.5X4	T38.5X5	T38.5X6
Medroxalol	T44.8X1	T44.8X2	T44.8X3	T44.8X4	T44.8X5	T44.8X6
Medroxyprogesterone acetate (depot)	T38.5X1	T38.5X2	T38.5X3	T38.5X4	T38.5X5	T38.5X6
Medrysone	T49.0X1	T49.0X2	T49.0X3	T49.0X4	T49.0X5	T49.0X6
Mefenamic acid	T39.391	T39.392	T39.393	T39.394	T39.395	T39.396
Mefenorex	T50.5X1	T50.5X2	T50.5X3	T50.5X4	T50.5X5	T50.5X6
Mefloquine	T37.2X1	T37.2X2	T37.2X3	T37.2X4	T37.2X5	T37.2X6
Mefruside	T50.2X1	T50.2X2	T50.2X3	T50.2X4	T50.2X5	T50.2X6
Megahallucinogen	T40.901	T40.902	T40.903	T40.904	T40.905	T40.906
Megestrol	T38.5X1	T38.5X2	T38.5X3	T38.5X4	T38.5X5	T38.5X6
Meglumine						
antimoniate	T37.8X1	T37.8X2	T37.8X3	T37.8X4	T37.8X5	T37.8X6
diatrizoate	T50.8X1	T50.8X2	T50.8X3	T50.8X4	T50.8X5	T50.8X6
iodipamide	T50.8X1	T50.8X2	T50.8X3	T50.8X4	T50.8X5	T50.8X6
iotroxate	T50.8X1	T50.8X2	T50.8X3	T50.8X4	T50.8X5	T50.8X6
MEK (methyl ethyl ketone)	T52.4X1	T52.4X2	T52.4X3	T52.4X4	—	—
Meladrazine	T44.3X1	T44.3X2	T44.3X3	T44.3X4	T44.3X5	T44.3X6
Meladinin	T49.3X1	T49.3X2	T49.3X3	T49.3X4	T49.3X5	T49.3X6
Melaleuca alternifolia oil	T49.0X1	T49.0X2	T49.0X3	T49.0X4	T49.0X5	T49.0X6
Melanizing agents	T49.3X1	T49.3X2	T49.3X3	T49.3X4	T49.3X5	T49.3X6
Melanocyte-stimulating hormone	T38.891	T38.892	T38.893	T38.894	T38.895	T38.896
Melarsonyl potassium	T37.3X1	T37.3X2	T37.3X3	T37.3X4	T37.3X5	T37.3X6
Melarsoprol	T37.3X1	T37.3X2	T37.3X3	T37.3X4	T37.3X5	T37.3X6
Melia azedarach	T62.2X1	T62.2X2	T62.2X3	T62.2X4	—	—
Melitracen	T43.011	T43.012	T43.013	T43.014	T43.015	T43.016
Mellaril	T43.3X1	T43.3X2	T43.3X3	T43.3X4	T43.3X5	T43.3X6
Meloxine	T49.3X1	T49.3X2	T49.3X3	T49.3X4	T49.3X5	T49.3X6
Melperone	T43.4X1	T43.4X2	T43.4X3	T43.4X4	T43.4X5	T43.4X6
Melphalan	T45.1X1	T45.1X2	T45.1X3	T45.1X4	T45.1X5	T45.1X6
Memantine	T43.8X1	T43.8X2	T43.8X3	T43.8X4	T43.8X5	T43.8X6

◀ New ◀ Revised ~~deleted~~ Deleted

Substance	External Cause (T-Code)					
	Poisoning, Accidental (Unintentional)	Poisoning, Intentional Self-Harm	Poisoning, Assault	Poisoning, Undetermined	Adverse Effect	Underdosing
Menadiol	T45.7X1	T45.7X2	T45.7X3	T45.7X4	T45.7X5	T45.7X6
sodium sulfate	T45.7X1	T45.7X2	T45.7X3	T45.7X4	T45.7X5	T45.7X6
Menadione	T45.7X1	T45.7X2	T45.7X3	T45.7X4	T45.7X5	T45.7X6
sodium bisulfite	T45.7X1	T45.7X2	T45.7X3	T45.7X4	T45.7X5	T45.7X6
Menaphthone	T45.7X1	T45.7X2	T45.7X3	T45.7X4	T45.7X5	T45.7X6
Menaquinone	T45.7X1	T45.7X2	T45.7X3	T45.7X4	T45.7X5	T45.7X6
Menatetrenone	T45.7X1	T45.7X2	T45.7X3	T45.7X4	T45.7X5	T45.7X6
Meningococcal vaccine	T50.A91	T50.A92	T50.A93	T50.A94	T50.A95	T50.A96
Menningovax (-AC) (-C)	T50.A91	T50.A92	T50.A93	T50.A94	T50.A95	T50.A96
Menotropins	T38.811	T38.812	T38.813	T38.814	T38.815	T38.816
Menthol	T48.5X1	T48.5X2	T48.5X3	T48.5X4	T48.5X5	T48.5X6
Mepacrine	T37.2X1	T37.2X2	T37.2X3	T37.2X4	T37.2X5	T37.2X6
Meparfynol	T42.6X1	T42.6X2	T42.6X3	T42.6X4	T42.6X5	T42.6X6
Mepartricin	T36.7X1	T36.7X2	T36.7X3	T36.7X4	T36.7X5	T36.7X6
Mepazine	T43.3X1	T43.3X2	T43.3X3	T43.3X4	T43.3X5	T43.3X6
Mepenzolate	T44.3X1	T44.3X2	T44.3X3	T44.3X4	T44.3X5	T44.3X6
bromide	T44.3X1	T44.3X2	T44.3X3	T44.3X4	T44.3X5	T44.3X6
Meperidine	T40.491	T40.492	T40.493	T40.494	T40.495	T40.496
Mephebarbital	T42.3X1	T42.3X2	T42.3X3	T42.3X4	T42.3X5	T42.3X6
Mephenamin(e)	T42.8X1	T42.8X2	T42.8X3	T42.8X4	T42.8X5	T42.8X6
Mephenesin	T42.8X1	T42.8X2	T42.8X3	T42.8X4	T42.8X5	T42.8X6
Mephenhydramine	T45.0X1	T45.0X2	T45.0X3	T45.0X4	T45.0X5	T45.0X6
Mephenoxalone	T42.8X1	T42.8X2	T42.8X3	T42.8X4	T42.8X5	T42.8X6
Mephentermine	T44.991	T44.992	T44.993	T44.994	T44.995	T44.996
Mephenytoin	T42.0X1	T42.0X2	T42.0X3	T42.0X4	T42.0X5	T42.0X6
with phenobarbital	T42.3X1	T42.3X2	T42.3X3	T42.3X4	T42.3X5	T42.3X6
Mephobarbital	T42.3X1	T42.3X2	T42.3X3	T42.3X4	T42.3X5	T42.3X6
Mephosfolan	T60.0X1	T60.0X2	T60.0X3	T60.0X4	—	—
Mepindolol	T44.7X1	T44.7X2	T44.7X3	T44.7X4	T44.7X5	T44.7X6
Mepiperphenidol	T44.3X1	T44.3X2	T44.3X3	T44.3X4	T44.3X5	T44.3X6
Mepitiostane	T38.7X1	T38.7X2	T38.7X3	T38.7X4	T38.7X5	T38.7X6
Mepivacaine	T41.3X1	T41.3X2	T41.3X3	T41.3X4	T41.3X5	T41.3X6
epidural	T41.3X1	T41.3X2	T41.3X3	T41.3X4	T41.3X5	T41.3X6
Meprednisone	T38.0X1	T38.0X2	T38.0X3	T38.0X4	T38.0X5	T38.0X6
Meprobam	T43.591	T43.592	T43.593	T43.594	T43.595	T43.596
Meprobamate	T43.591	T43.592	T43.593	T43.594	T43.595	T43.596
Meproscillarin	T46.0X1	T46.0X2	T46.0X3	T46.0X4	T46.0X5	T46.0X6
Meprylcaine	T41.3X1	T41.3X2	T41.3X3	T41.3X4	T41.3X5	T41.3X6
Meptazinol	T39.8X1	T39.8X2	T39.8X3	T39.8X4	T39.8X5	T39.8X6
Mepyramine	T45.0X1	T45.0X2	T45.0X3	T45.0X4	T45.0X5	T45.0X6
Mequitazine	T43.3X1	T43.3X2	T43.3X3	T43.3X4	T43.3X5	T43.3X6
Meralluride	T50.2X1	T50.2X2	T50.2X3	T50.2X4	T50.2X5	T50.2X6

Substance	External Cause (T-Code)					
	Poisoning, Accidental (Unintentional)	Poisoning, Intentional Self-Harm	Poisoning, Assault	Poisoning, Undetermined	Adverse Effect	Underdosing
Merbaphen	T50.2X1	T50.2X2	T50.2X3	T50.2X4	T50.2X5	T50.2X6
Merbromin	T49.0X1	T49.0X2	T49.0X3	T49.0X4	T49.0X5	T49.0X6
Mercaptobenzothiazole salts	T49.0X1	T49.0X2	T49.0X3	T49.0X4	T49.0X5	T49.0X6
Mercaptomerin	T50.2X1	T50.2X2	T50.2X3	T50.2X4	T50.2X5	T50.2X6
Mercaptopurine	T45.1X1	T45.1X2	T45.1X3	T45.1X4	T45.1X5	T45.1X6
Mercumatilin	T50.2X1	T50.2X2	T50.2X3	T50.2X4	T50.2X5	T50.2X6
Mercuramide	T50.2X1	T50.2X2	T50.2X3	T50.2X4	T50.2X5	T50.2X6
Mercurochrome	T49.0X1	T49.0X2	T49.0X3	T49.0X4	T49.0X5	T49.0X6
Mercurophylline	T50.2X1	T50.2X2	T50.2X3	T50.2X4	T50.2X5	T50.2X6
Mercury, mercurial, mercuric, mercurous (compounds) (cyanide) (fumes) (nonmedicinal) (vapor) NEC	T56.1X1	T56.1X2	T56.1X3	T56.1X4	—	—
ammoniated	T49.0X1	T49.0X2	T49.0X3	T49.0X4	T49.0X5	T49.0X6
anti-infective						
local	T49.0X1	T49.0X2	T49.0X3	T49.0X4	T49.0X5	T49.0X6
systemic	T37.8X1	T37.8X2	T37.8X3	T37.8X4	T37.8X5	T37.8X6
topical	T49.0X1	T49.0X2	T49.0X3	T49.0X4	T49.0X5	T49.0X6
chloride (ammoniated)	T49.0X1	T49.0X2	T49.0X3	T49.0X4	T49.0X5	T49.0X6
fungicide	T56.1X1	T56.1X2	T56.1X3	T56.1X4	—	—
diuretic NEC	T50.2X1	T50.2X2	T50.2X3	T50.2X4	T50.2X5	T50.2X6
fungicide	T56.1X1	T56.1X2	T56.1X3	T56.1X4	—	—
organic (fungicide)	T56.1X1	T56.1X2	T56.1X3	T56.1X4	—	—
oxide, yellow	T49.0X1	T49.0X2	T49.0X3	T49.0X4	T49.0X5	T49.0X6
Mersalyl	T50.2X1	T50.2X2	T50.2X3	T50.2X4	T50.2X5	T50.2X6
Merthiolate	T49.0X1	T49.0X2	T49.0X3	T49.0X4	T49.0X5	T49.0X6
ophthalmic preparation	T49.5X1	T49.5X2	T49.5X3	T49.5X4	T49.5X5	T49.5X6
Meruvax	T50.B91	T50.B92	T50.B93	T50.B94	T50.B95	T50.B96
Mesalazine	T47.8X1	T47.8X2	T47.8X3	T47.8X4	T47.8X5	T47.8X6
Mescal buttons	T40.991	T40.992	T40.993	T40.994	—	—
Mescaline	T40.991	T40.992	T40.993	T40.994	—	—
Mesna	T48.4X1	T48.4X2	T48.4X3	T48.4X4	T48.4X5	T48.4X6
Mesoglycan	T46.6X1	T46.6X2	T46.6X3	T46.6X4	T46.6X5	T46.6X6
Mesoridazine	T43.3X1	T43.3X2	T43.3X3	T43.3X4	T43.3X5	T43.3X6
Mestanolone	T38.7X1	T38.7X2	T38.7X3	T38.7X4	T38.7X5	T38.7X6
Mesterolone	T38.7X1	T38.7X2	T38.7X3	T38.7X4	T38.7X5	T38.7X6
Mestranol	T38.5X1	T38.5X2	T38.5X3	T38.5X4	T38.5X5	T38.5X6
Mesulergine	T42.8X1	T42.8X2	T42.8X3	T42.8X4	T42.8X5	T42.8X6
Mesulfen	T49.0X1	T49.0X2	T49.0X3	T49.0X4	T49.0X5	T49.0X6
Mesuximide	T42.2X1	T42.2X2	T42.2X3	T42.2X4	T42.2X5	T42.2X6
Metabutethamine	T41.3X1	T41.3X2	T41.3X3	T41.3X4	T41.3X5	T41.3X6
Metactesylacetate	T49.0X1	T49.0X2	T49.0X3	T49.0X4	T49.0X5	T49.0X6

◀ New   ◀|| Revised   ~~deleted~~ Deleted

	External Cause (T-Code)					
Substance	Poisoning, Accidental (Unintentional)	Poisoning, Intentional Self-Harm	Poisoning, Assault	Poisoning, Undetermined	Adverse Effect	Underdosing
Metacycline	T36.4X1	T36.4X2	T36.4X3	T36.4X4	T36.4X5	T36.4X6
Metaldehyde (snail killer) NEC	T60.8X1	T60.8X2	T60.8X3	T60.8X4	—	—
Metals (heavy) (nonmedicinal)	T56.91	T56.92	T56.93	T56.94	—	—
dust, fumes, or vapor NEC	T56.91	T56.92	T56.93	T56.94	—	—
light NEC	T56.91	T56.92	T56.93	T56.94	—	—
dust, fumes, or vapor NEC	T56.91	T56.92	T56.93	T56.94	—	—
specified NEC	T56.891	T56.892	T56.893	T56.894	—	—
thallium	T56.811	T56.812	T56.813	T56.814	—	—
Metamfetamine	T43.651	T43.652	T43.652	T43.654	T43.655	T43.656
Metamizole sodium	T39.2X1	T39.2X2	T39.2X3	T39.2X4	T39.2X5	T39.2X6
Metampicillin	T36.0X1	T36.0X2	T36.0X3	T36.0X4	T36.0X5	T36.0X6
Metamucil	T47.4X1	T47.4X2	T47.4X3	T47.4X4	T47.4X5	T47.4X6
Metaphen	T49.0X1	T49.0X2	T49.0X3	T49.0X4	T49.0X5	T49.0X6
Metandienone	T38.7X1	T38.7X2	T38.7X3	T38.7X4	T38.7X5	T38.7X6
Metandrostenolone	T38.7X1	T38.7X2	T38.7X3	T38.7X4	T38.7X5	T38.7X6
Metaphos	T60.0X1	T60.0X2	T60.0X3	T60.0X4	—	—
Metapramine	T43.011	T43.012	T43.013	T43.014	T43.015	T43.016
Metaproterenol	T48.291	T48.292	T48.293	T48.294	T48.295	T48.296
Metaraminol	T44.4X1	T44.4X2	T44.4X3	T44.4X4	T44.4X5	T44.4X6
Metaxalone	T42.8X1	T42.8X2	T42.8X3	T42.8X4	T42.8X5	T42.8X6
Metenolone	T38.7X1	T38.7X2	T38.7X3	T38.7X4	T38.7X5	T38.7X6
Metergoline	T42.8X1	T42.8X2	T42.8X3	T42.8X4	T42.8X5	T42.8X6
Metescufylline	T46.991	T46.992	T46.993	T46.994	T46.995	T46.996
Metetoin	T42.0X1	T42.0X2	T42.0X3	T42.0X4	T42.0X5	T42.0X6
Metformin	T38.3X1	T38.3X2	T38.3X3	T38.3X4	T38.3X5	T38.3X6
Methacholine	T44.1X1	T44.1X2	T44.1X3	T44.1X4	T44.1X5	T44.1X6
Methacycline	T36.4X1	T36.4X2	T36.4X3	T36.4X4	T36.4X5	T36.4X6
Methadone	T40.3X1	T40.3X2	T40.3X3	T40.3X4	T40.3X5	T40.3X6
Methallenestril	T38.5X1	T38.5X2	T38.5X3	T38.5X4	T38.5X5	T38.5X6
Methallenoestril	T38.5X1	T38.5X2	T38.5X3	T38.5X4	T38.5X5	T38.5X6
Methamphetamine	T43.651	T43.652	T43.652	T43.654	T43.655	T43.656
Methampyrone	T39.2X1	T39.2X2	T39.2X3	T39.2X4	T39.2X5	T39.2X6
Methandienone	T38.7X1	T38.7X2	T38.7X3	T38.7X4	T38.7X5	T38.7X6
Methandriol	T38.7X1	T38.7X2	T38.7X3	T38.7X4	T38.7X5	T38.7X6
Methandrostenolone	T38.7X1	T38.7X2	T38.7X3	T38.7X4	T38.7X5	T38.7X6
Methane	T59.891	T59.892	T59.893	T59.894	—	—
Methanethiol	T59.891	T59.892	T59.893	T59.894	—	—
Methaniazide	T37.1X1	T37.1X2	T37.1X3	T37.1X4	T37.1X5	T37.1X6
Methanol (vapor)	T51.1X1	T51.1X2	T51.1X3	T51.1X4	—	—
Methantheline	T44.3X1	T44.3X2	T44.3X3	T44.3X4	T44.3X5	T44.3X6
Methanthelinium bromide	T44.3X1	T44.3X2	T44.3X3	T44.3X4	T44.3X5	T44.3X6
Methaphenilene	T45.0X1	T45.0X2	T45.0X3	T45.0X4	T45.0X5	T45.0X6

	External Cause (T-Code)					
Substance	Poisoning, Accidental (Unintentional)	Poisoning, Intentional Self-Harm	Poisoning, Assault	Poisoning, Undetermined	Adverse Effect	Underdosing
Methapyrilene	T45.0X1	T45.0X2	T45.0X3	T45.0X4	T45.0X5	T45.0X6
Methaqualone (compound)	T42.6X1	T42.6X2	T42.6X3	T42.6X4	T42.6X5	T42.6X6
Metharbital	T42.3X1	T42.3X2	T42.3X3	T42.3X4	T42.3X5	T42.3X6
Methazolamide	T50.2X1	T50.2X2	T50.2X3	T50.2X4	T50.2X5	T50.2X6
Methdilazine	T43.3X1	T43.3X2	T43.3X3	T43.3X4	T43.3X5	T43.3X6
Methedrine	T43.651	T43.652	T43.652	T43.654	T43.655	T43.656 ◄
Methenamine (mandelate)	T37.8X1	T37.8X2	T37.8X3	T37.8X4	T37.8X5	T37.8X6
Methenolone	T38.7X1	T38.7X2	T38.7X3	T38.7X4	T38.7X5	T38.7X6
Methergine	T48.0X1	T48.0X2	T48.0X3	T48.0X4	T48.0X5	T48.0X6
Methetoin	T42.0X1	T42.0X2	T42.0X3	T42.0X4	T42.0X5	T42.0X6
Methiacil	T38.2X1	T38.2X2	T38.2X3	T38.2X4	T38.2X5	T38.2X6
Methicillin	T36.0X1	T36.0X2	T36.0X3	T36.0X4	T36.0X5	T36.0X6
Methimazole	T38.2X1	T38.2X2	T38.2X3	T38.2X4	T38.2X5	T38.2X6
Methiodal sodium	T50.8X1	T50.8X2	T50.8X3	T50.8X4	T50.8X5	T50.8X6
Methionine	T50.991	T50.992	T50.993	T50.994	T50.995	T50.996
Methisazone	T37.5X1	T37.5X2	T37.5X3	T37.5X4	T37.5X5	T37.5X6
Methisoprinol	T37.5X1	T37.5X2	T37.5X3	T37.5X4	T37.5X5	T37.5X6
Methitural	T42.3X1	T42.3X2	T42.3X3	T42.3X4	T42.3X5	T42.3X6
Methixene	T44.3X1	T44.3X2	T44.3X3	T44.3X4	T44.3X5	T44.3X6
Methobarbital, methobarbitone	T42.3X1	T42.3X2	T42.3X3	T42.3X4	T42.3X5	T42.3X6
Methocarbamol	T42.8X1	T42.8X2	T42.8X3	T42.8X4	T42.8X5	T42.8X6
skeletal muscle relaxant	T48.1X1	T48.1X2	T48.1X3	T48.1X4	T48.1X5	T48.1X6
Methohexital	T41.1X1	T41.1X2	T41.1X3	T41.1X4	T41.1X5	T41.1X6
Methohexitone	T41.1X1	T41.1X2	T41.1X3	T41.1X4	T41.1X5	T41.1X6
Methoin	T42.0X1	T42.0X2	T42.0X3	T42.0X4	T42.0X5	T42.0X6
Methopholine	T39.8X1	T39.8X2	T39.8X3	T39.8X4	T39.8X5	T39.8X6
Methopromazine	T43.3X1	T43.3X2	T43.3X3	T43.3X4	T43.3X5	T43.3X6
Methorate	T48.3X1	T48.3X2	T48.3X3	T48.3X4	T48.3X5	T48.3X6
Methoserpidine	T46.5X1	T46.5X2	T46.5X3	T46.5X4	T46.5X5	T46.5X6
Methotrexate	T45.1X1	T45.1X2	T45.1X3	T45.1X4	T45.1X5	T45.1X6
Methotrimeprazine	T43.3X1	T43.3X2	T43.3X3	T43.3X4	T43.3X5	T43.3X6
Methoxa-Dome	T49.3X1	T49.3X2	T49.3X3	T49.3X4	T49.3X5	T49.3X6
Methoxamine	T44.4X1	T44.4X2	T44.4X3	T44.4X4	T44.4X5	T44.4X6
Methoxsalen	T50.991	T50.992	T50.993	T50.994	T50.995	T50.996
Methoxyaniline	T65.3X1	T65.3X2	T65.3X3	T65.3X4	—	—
Methoxybenzyl penicillin	T36.0X1	T36.0X2	T36.0X3	T36.0X4	T36.0X5	T36.0X6
Methoxychlor	T53.7X1	T53.7X2	T53.7X3	T53.7X4	—	—
Methoxy-DDT	T53.7X1	T53.7X2	T53.7X3	T53.7X4	—	—
2-Methoxyethanol	T52.3X1	T52.3X2	T52.3X3	T52.3X4	—	—
Methoxyflurane	T41.0X1	T41.0X2	T41.0X3	T41.0X4	T41.0X5	T41.0X6
Methoxyphenamine	T48.6X1	T48.6X2	T48.6X3	T48.6X4	T48.6X5	T48.6X6
Methoxypromazine	T43.3X1	T43.3X2	T43.3X3	T43.3X4	T43.3X5	T43.3X6

◄ New ◄◄ Revised ~~deleted~~ Deleted

	External Cause (T-Code)					
Substance	Poisoning, Accidental (Unintentional)	Poisoning, Intentional Self-Harm	Poisoning, Assault	Poisoning, Undetermined	Adverse Effect	Underdosing
5-Methoxypsoralen (5-MOP)	T50.991	T50.992	T50.993	T50.994	T50.995	T50.996
8-Methoxypsoralen (8-MOP)	T50.991	T50.992	T50.993	T50.994	T50.995	T50.996
Methscopolamine bromide	T44.3X1	T44.3X2	T44.3X3	T44.3X4	T44.3X5	T44.3X6
Methsuximide	T42.2X1	T42.2X2	T42.2X3	T42.2X4	T42.2X5	T42.2X6
Methyclothiazide	T50.2X1	T50.2X2	T50.2X3	T50.2X4	T50.2X5	T50.2X6
Methyl						
acetate	T52.4X1	T52.4X2	T52.4X3	T52.4X4	—	—
acetone	T52.4X1	T52.4X2	T52.4X3	T52.4X4	—	—
acrylate	T65.891	T65.892	T65.893	T65.894	—	—
alcohol	T51.1X1	T51.1X2	T51.1X3	T51.1X4	—	—
aminophenol	T65.3X1	T65.3X2	T65.3X3	T65.3X4	—	—
amphetamine	T43.651	T43.652	T43.652	T43.654	T43.655	T43.656
androstanolone	T38.7X1	T38.7X2	T38.7X3	T38.7X4	T38.7X5	T38.7X6
atropine	T44.3X1	T44.3X2	T44.3X3	T44.3X4	T44.3X5	T44.3X6
benzene	T52.2X1	T52.2X2	T52.2X3	T52.2X4	—	—
benzoate	T52.8X1	T52.8X2	T52.8X3	T52.8X4	—	—
benzol	T52.2X1	T52.2X2	T52.2X3	T52.2X4	—	—
bromide (gas)	T59.891	T59.892	T59.893	T59.894	—	—
fumigant	T60.8X1	T60.8X2	T60.8X3	T60.8X4	—	—
butanol	T51.3X1	T51.3X2	T51.3X3	T51.3X4	—	—
carbinol	T51.1X1	T51.1X2	T51.1X3	T51.1X4	—	—
carbonate	T52.8X1	T52.8X2	T52.8X3	T52.8X4	—	—
CCNU	T45.1X1	T45.1X2	T45.1X3	T45.1X4	T45.1X5	T45.1X6
cellosolve	T52.91	T52.92	T52.93	T52.94	—	—
cellulose	T47.4X1	T47.4X2	T47.4X3	T47.4X4	T47.4X5	T47.4X6
chloride (gas)	T59.891	T59.892	T59.893	T59.894	—	—
chloroformate	T59.3X1	T59.3X2	T59.3X3	T59.3X4	—	—
cyclohexane	T52.8X1	T52.8X2	T52.8X3	T52.8X4	—	—
cyclohexanol	T51.8X1	T51.8X2	T51.8X3	T51.8X4	—	—
cyclohexanone	T52.8X1	T52.8X2	T52.8X3	T52.8X4	—	—
cyclohexyl acetate	T52.8X1	T52.8X2	T52.8X3	T52.8X4	—	—
demeton	T60.0X1	T60.0X2	T60.0X3	T60.0X4	—	—
dihydromorphinone	T40.2X1	T40.2X2	T40.2X3	T40.2X4	T40.2X5	T40.2X6
ergometrine	T48.0X1	T48.0X2	T48.0X3	T48.0X4	T48.0X5	T48.0X6
ergonovine	T48.0X1	T48.0X2	T48.0X3	T48.0X4	T48.0X5	T48.0X6
ethyl ketone	T52.4X1	T52.4X2	T52.4X3	T52.4X4	—	—
glucamine antimonate	T37.8X1	T37.8X2	T37.8X3	T37.8X4	T37.8X5	T37.8X6
hydrazine	T65.891	T65.892	T65.893	T65.894	—	—
iodide	T65.891	T65.892	T65.893	T65.894	—	—
isobutyl ketone	T52.4X1	T52.4X2	T52.4X3	T52.4X4	—	—
isothiocyanate	T60.3X1	T60.3X2	T60.3X3	T60.3X4	—	—
mercaptan	T59.891	T59.892	T59.893	T59.894	—	—

	External Cause (T-Code)					
Substance	Poisoning, Accidental (Unintentional)	Poisoning, Intentional Self-Harm	Poisoning, Assault	Poisoning, Undetermined	Adverse Effect	Underdosing
Methyl (Continued)						
morphine NEC	T40.2X1	T40.2X2	T40.2X3	T40.2X4	T40.2X5	T40.2X6
nicotinate	T49.4X1	T49.4X2	T49.4X3	T49.4X4	T49.4X5	T49.4X6
paraben	T49.0X1	T49.0X2	T49.0X3	T49.0X4	T49.0X5	T49.0X6
parafynol	T42.6X1	T42.6X2	T42.6X3	T42.6X4	T42.6X5	T42.6X6
parathion	T60.0X1	T60.0X2	T60.0X3	T60.0X4	—	—
peridol	T43.4X1	T43.4X2	T43.4X3	T43.4X4	T43.4X5	T43.4X6
phenidate	T43.631	T43.632	T43.633	T43.634	T43.635	T43.636
prednisolone	T38.0X1	T38.0X2	T38.0X3	T38.0X4	T38.0X5	T38.0X6
ENT agent	T49.6X1	T49.6X2	T49.6X3	T49.6X4	T49.6X5	T49.6X6
ophthalmic preparation	T49.5X1	T49.5X2	T49.5X3	T49.5X4	T49.5X5	T49.5X6
topical NEC	T49.0X1	T49.0X2	T49.0X3	T49.0X4	T49.0X5	T49.0X6
propylcarbinol	T51.3X1	T51.3X2	T51.3X3	T51.3X4	—	—
rosaniline NEC	T49.0X1	T49.0X2	T49.0X3	T49.0X4	T49.0X5	T49.0X6
salicylate	T49.2X1	T49.2X2	T49.2X3	T49.2X4	T49.2X5	T49.2X6
sulfate (fumes)	T59.891	T59.892	T59.893	T59.894	—	—
liquid	T52.8X1	T52.8X2	T52.8X3	T52.8X4	—	—
sulfonal	T42.6X1	T42.6X2	T42.6X3	T42.6X4	T42.6X5	T42.6X6
testosterone	T38.7X1	T38.7X2	T38.7X3	T38.7X4	T38.7X5	T38.7X6
thiouracil	T38.2X1	T38.2X2	T38.2X3	T38.2X4	T38.2X5	T38.2X6
Methylamphetamine	T43.651	T43.652	T43.652	T43.654	T43.655	T43.656
Methylated spirit	T51.1X1	T51.1X2	T51.1X3	T51.1X4	—	—
Methylatropine nitrate	T44.3X1	T44.3X2	T44.3X3	T44.3X4	T44.3X5	T44.3X6
Methylbenactyzium bromide	T44.3X1	T44.3X2	T44.3X3	T44.3X4	T44.3X5	T44.3X6
Methylbenzethonium chloride	T49.0X1	T49.0X2	T49.0X3	T49.0X4	T49.0X5	T49.0X6
Methylcellulose	T47.4X1	T47.4X2	T47.4X3	T47.4X4	T47.4X5	T47.4X6
laxative	T47.4X1	T47.4X2	T47.4X3	T47.4X4	T47.4X5	T47.4X6
Methylchlorophenoxy-acetic acid	T60.3X1	T60.3X2	T60.3X3	T60.3X4	—	—
Methyldopa	T46.5X1	T46.5X2	T46.5X3	T46.5X4	T46.5X5	T46.5X6
Methyldopate	T46.5X1	T46.5X2	T46.5X3	T46.5X4	T46.5X5	T46.5X6
Methylene						
blue	T50.6X1	T50.6X2	T50.6X3	T50.6X4	T50.6X5	T50.6X6
chloride or dichloride (solvent) NEC	T53.4X1	T53.4X2	T53.4X3	T53.4X4	—	—
Methylenedioxyamphet-amine	T43.621	T43.622	T43.623	T43.624	T43.625	T43.626
Methylenedioxymethamphetamine	T43.641	T43.642	T43.643	T43.644	—	—
Methylergometrine	T48.0X1	T48.0X2	T48.0X3	T48.0X4	T48.0X5	T48.0X6
Methylergonovine	T48.0X1	T48.0X2	T48.0X3	T48.0X4	T48.0X5	T48.0X6
Methylestrenolone	T38.5X1	T38.5X2	T38.5X3	T38.5X4	T38.5X5	T38.5X6
Methylethyl cellulose	T50.991	T50.992	T50.993	T50.994	T50.995	T50.996
Methylhexabital	T42.3X1	T42.3X2	T42.3X3	T42.3X4	T42.3X5	T42.3X6
Methylmorphine	T40.2X1	T40.2X2	T40.2X3	T40.2X4	T40.2X5	T40.2X6

◀ New   ◀╫ Revised   deleted Deleted

	External Cause (T-Code)					
Substance	Poisoning, Accidental (Unintentional)	Poisoning, Intentional Self-Harm	Poisoning, Assault	Poisoning, Undetermined	Adverse Effect	Underdosing
Methylparaben (ophthalmic)	T49.5X1	T49.5X2	T49.5X3	T49.5X4	T49.5X5	T49.5X6
Methylparafynol	T42.6X1	T42.6X2	T42.6X3	T42.6X4	T42.6X5	T42.6X6
Methylpentynol, methylpenthynol	T42.6X1	T42.6X2	T42.6X3	T42.6X4	T42.6X5	T42.6X6
Methylphenidate	T43.631	T43.632	T43.633	T43.634	T43.635	T43.636
Methylphenobarbital	T42.3X1	T42.3X2	T42.3X3	T42.3X4	T42.3X5	T42.3X6
Methylpolysiloxane	T47.1X1	T47.1X2	T47.1X3	T47.1X4	T47.1X5	T47.1X6
Methylprednisolone — see Methyl, prednisolone						
Methylrosaniline	T49.0X1	T49.0X2	T49.0X3	T49.0X4	T49.0X5	T49.0X6
Methylrosanilinium chloride	T49.0X1	T49.0X2	T49.0X3	T49.0X4	T49.0X5	T49.0X6
Methyltestosterone	T38.7X1	T38.7X2	T38.7X3	T38.7X4	T38.7X5	T38.7X6
Methylthionine chloride	T50.6X1	T50.6X2	T50.6X3	T50.6X4	T50.6X5	T50.6X6
Methylthioninium chloride	T50.6X1	T50.6X2	T50.6X3	T50.6X4	T50.6X5	T50.6X6
Methylthiouracil	T38.2X1	T38.2X2	T38.2X3	T38.2X4	T38.2X5	T38.2X6
Methyprylon	T42.6X1	T42.6X2	T42.6X3	T42.6X4	T42.6X5	T42.6X6
Methysergide	T46.5X1	T46.5X2	T46.5X3	T46.5X4	T46.5X5	T46.5X6
Metiamide	T47.1X1	T47.1X2	T47.1X3	T47.1X4	T47.1X5	T47.1X6
Meticillin	T36.0X1	T36.0X2	T36.0X3	T36.0X4	T36.0X5	T36.0X6
Meticrane	T50.2X1	T50.2X2	T50.2X3	T50.2X4	T50.2X5	T50.2X6
Metildigoxin	T46.0X1	T46.0X2	T46.0X3	T46.0X4	T46.0X5	T46.0X6
Metipranolol	T49.5X1	T49.5X2	T49.5X3	T49.5X4	T49.5X5	T49.5X6
Metirosine	T46.5X1	T46.5X2	T46.5X3	T46.5X4	T46.5X5	T46.5X6
Metisazone	T37.5X1	T37.5X2	T37.5X3	T37.5X4	T37.5X5	T37.5X6
Metixene	T44.3X1	T44.3X2	T44.3X3	T44.3X4	T44.3X5	T44.3X6
Metizoline	T48.5X1	T48.5X2	T48.5X3	T48.5X4	T48.5X5	T48.5X6
Metoclopramide	T45.0X1	T45.0X2	T45.0X3	T45.0X4	T45.0X5	T45.0X6
Metofenazate	T43.3X1	T43.3X2	T43.3X3	T43.3X4	T43.3X5	T43.3X6
Metofoline	T39.8X1	T39.8X2	T39.8X3	T39.8X4	T39.8X5	T39.8X6
Metolazone	T50.2X1	T50.2X2	T50.2X3	T50.2X4	T50.2X5	T50.2X6
Metopon	T40.2X1	T40.2X2	T40.2X3	T40.2X4	T40.2X5	T40.2X6
Metoprine	T45.1X1	T45.1X2	T45.1X3	T45.1X4	T45.1X5	T45.1X6
Metoprolol	T44.7X1	T44.7X2	T44.7X3	T44.7X4	T44.7X5	T44.7X6
Metrifonate	T60.0X1	T60.0X2	T60.0X3	T60.0X4	—	—
Metrizamide	T50.8X1	T50.8X2	T50.8X3	T50.8X4	T50.8X5	T50.8X6
Metrizoic acid	T50.8X1	T50.8X2	T50.8X3	T50.8X4	T50.8X5	T50.8X6
Metronidazole	T37.8X1	T37.8X2	T37.8X3	T37.8X4	T37.8X5	T37.8X6
Metycaine	T41.3X1	T41.3X2	T41.3X3	T41.3X4	T41.3X5	T41.3X6
infiltration (subcutaneous)	T41.3X1	T41.3X2	T41.3X3	T41.3X4	T41.3X5	T41.3X6
nerve block (peripheral) (plexus)	T41.3X1	T41.3X2	T41.3X3	T41.3X4	T41.3X5	T41.3X6
topical (surface)	T41.3X1	T41.3X2	T41.3X3	T41.3X4	T41.3X5	T41.3X6
Metyrapone	T50.8X1	T50.8X2	T50.8X3	T50.8X4	T50.8X5	T50.8X6
Mevinphos	T60.0X1	T60.0X2	T60.0X3	T60.0X4	—	—

	External Cause (T-Code)					
Substance	Poisoning, Accidental (Unintentional)	Poisoning, Intentional Self-Harm	Poisoning, Assault	Poisoning, Undetermined	Adverse Effect	Underdosing
Mexazolam	T42.4X1	T42.4X2	T42.4X3	T42.4X4	T42.4X5	T42.4X6
Mexenone	T49.3X1	T49.3X2	T49.3X3	T49.3X4	T49.3X5	T49.3X6
Mexiletine	T46.2X1	T46.2X2	T46.2X3	T46.2X4	T46.2X5	T46.2X6
Mezereon	T62.2X1	T62.2X2	T62.2X3	T62.2X4	—	—
berries	T62.1X1	T62.1X2	T62.1X3	T62.1X4	—	—
Mezlocillin	T36.0X1	T36.0X2	T36.0X3	T36.0X4	T36.0X5	T36.0X6
Mianserin	T43.021	T43.022	T43.023	T43.024	T43.025	T43.026
Micatin	T49.0X1	T49.0X2	T49.0X3	T49.0X4	T49.0X5	T49.0X6
Miconazole	T49.0X1	T49.0X2	T49.0X3	T49.0X4	T49.0X5	T49.0X6
Micronomicin	T36.5X1	T36.5X2	T36.5X3	T36.5X4	T36.5X5	T36.5X6
Midazolam	T42.4X1	T42.4X2	T42.4X3	T42.4X4	T42.4X5	T42.4X6
Midecamycin	T36.3X1	T36.3X2	T36.3X3	T36.3X4	T36.3X5	T36.3X6
Mifepristone	T38.6X1	T38.6X2	T38.6X3	T38.6X4	T38.6X5	T38.6X6
Milk of magnesia	T47.1X1	T47.1X2	T47.1X3	T47.1X4	T47.1X5	T47.1X6
Millipede (tropical) (venomous)	T63.411	T63.412	T63.413	T63.414	—	—
Miltown	T43.591	T43.592	T43.593	T43.594	T43.595	T43.596
Milverine	T44.3X1	T44.3X2	T44.3X3	T44.3X4	T44.3X5	T44.3X6
Minaprine	T43.291	T43.292	T43.293	T43.294	T43.295	T43.296
Minaxolone	T41.291	T41.292	T41.293	T41.294	T41.295	T41.296
Mineral						
acids	T54.2X1	T54.2X2	T54.2X3	T54.2X4	—	—
oil (laxative) (medicinal)	T47.4X1	T47.4X2	T47.4X3	T47.4X4	T47.4X5	T47.4X6
emulsion	T47.2X1	T47.2X2	T47.2X3	T47.2X4	T47.2X5	T47.2X6
nonmedicinal	T52.0X1	T52.0X2	T52.0X3	T52.0X4	—	—
topical	T49.3X1	T49.3X2	T49.3X3	T49.3X4	T49.3X5	T49.3X6
salt NEC	T50.3X1	T50.3X2	T50.3X3	T50.3X4	T50.3X5	T50.3X6
spirits	T52.0X1	T52.0X2	T52.0X3	T52.0X4	—	—
Mineralocorticosteroid	T50.0X1	T50.0X2	T50.0X3	T50.0X4	T50.0X5	T50.0X6
Minocycline	T36.4X1	T36.4X2	T36.4X3	T36.4X4	T36.4X5	T36.4X6
Minoxidil	T46.7X1	T46.7X2	T46.7X3	T46.7X4	T46.7X5	T46.7X6
Miokamycin	T36.3X1	T36.3X2	T36.3X3	T36.3X4	T36.3X5	T36.3X6
Miotic drug	T49.5X1	T49.5X2	T49.5X3	T49.5X4	T49.5X5	T49.5X6
Mipafox	T60.0X1	T60.0X2	T60.0X3	T60.0X4	—	—
Mirex	T60.1X1	T60.1X2	T60.1X3	T60.1X4	—	—
Mirtazapine	T43.021	T43.022	T43.023	T43.024	T43.025	T43.026
Misonidazole	T37.3X1	T37.3X2	T37.3X3	T37.3X4	T37.3X5	T37.3X6
Misoprostol	T47.1X1	T47.1X2	T47.1X3	T47.1X4	T47.1X5	T47.1X6
Mithramycin	T45.1X1	T45.1X2	T45.1X3	T45.1X4	T45.1X5	T45.1X6
Mitobronitol	T45.1X1	T45.1X2	T45.1X3	T45.1X4	T45.1X5	T45.1X6
Mitoguazone	T45.1X1	T45.1X2	T45.1X3	T45.1X4	T45.1X5	T45.1X6
Mitolactol	T45.1X1	T45.1X2	T45.1X3	T45.1X4	T45.1X5	T45.1X6
Mitomycin	T45.1X1	T45.1X2	T45.1X3	T45.1X4	T45.1X5	T45.1X6

◀ New   ◀ Revised   deleted Deleted

Substance	Poisoning, Accidental (Unintentional)	Poisoning, Intentional Self-Harm	Poisoning, Assault	Poisoning, Undetermined	Adverse Effect	Underdosing
Mitopodozide	T45.1X1	T45.1X2	T45.1X3	T45.1X4	T45.1X5	T45.1X6
Mitotane	T45.1X1	T45.1X2	T45.1X3	T45.1X4	T45.1X5	T45.1X6
Mitoxantrone	T45.1X1	T45.1X2	T45.1X3	T45.1X4	T45.1X5	T45.1X6
Mivacurium chloride	T48.1X1	T48.1X2	T48.1X3	T48.1X4	T48.1X5	T48.1X6
Miyari bacteria	T47.6X1	T47.6X2	T47.6X3	T47.6X4	T47.6X5	T47.6X6
Moclobemide	T43.1X1	T43.1X2	T43.1X3	T43.1X4	T43.1X5	T43.1X6
Moderil	T46.5X1	T46.5X2	T46.5X3	T46.5X4	T46.5X5	T46.5X6
Mofebutazone	T39.2X1	T39.2X2	T39.2X3	T39.2X4	T39.2X5	T39.2X6
Mogadon — see Nitrazepam						
Molindone	T43.591	T43.592	T43.593	T43.594	T43.595	T43.596
Molsidomine	T46.3X1	T46.3X2	T46.3X3	T46.3X4	T46.3X5	T46.3X6
Mometasone	T49.0X1	T49.0X2	T49.0X3	T49.0X4	T49.0X5	T49.0X6
Monistat	T49.0X1	T49.0X2	T49.0X3	T49.0X4	T49.0X5	T49.0X6
Monkshood	T62.2X1	T62.2X2	T62.2X3	T62.2X4	—	—
Monoamine oxidase inhibitor NEC	T43.1X1	T43.1X2	T43.1X3	T43.1X4	T43.1X5	T43.1X6
hydrazine	T43.1X1	T43.1X2	T43.1X3	T43.1X4	T43.1X5	T43.1X6
Monobenzone	T49.4X1	T49.4X2	T49.4X3	T49.4X4	T49.4X5	T49.4X6
Monochloroacetic acid	T60.3X1	T60.3X2	T60.3X3	T60.3X4	—	—
Monochlorobenzene	T53.7X1	T53.7X2	T53.7X3	T53.7X4	—	—
Monoethanolamine	T46.8X1	T46.8X2	T46.8X3	T46.8X4	T46.8X5	T46.8X6
oleate	T46.8X1	T46.8X2	T46.8X3	T46.8X4	T46.8X5	T46.8X6
Monooctanoin	T50.991	T50.992	T50.993	T50.994	T50.995	T50.996
Monophenylbutazone	T39.2X1	T39.2X2	T39.2X3	T39.2X4	T39.2X5	T39.2X6
Monosodium glutamate	T65.891	T65.892	T65.893	T65.894	—	—
Monosulfiram	T49.0X1	T49.0X2	T49.0X3	T49.0X4	T49.0X5	T49.0X6
Monoxide, carbon — see Carbon, monoxide	T57.91	T57.92	T57.93	T57.94	—	—
Monoxidine hydrochloride	T46.1X1	T46.1X2	T46.1X3	T46.1X4	T46.1X5	T46.1X6
Monuron	T60.3X1	T60.3X2	T60.3X3	T60.3X4	—	—
Moperone	T43.4X1	T43.4X2	T43.4X3	T43.4X4	T43.4X5	T43.4X6
Mopidamol	T45.1X1	T45.1X2	T45.1X3	T45.1X4	T45.1X5	T45.1X6
MOPP (mechlorethamine + vincristine + prednisone + procarbazine)	T45.1X1	T45.1X2	T45.1X3	T45.1X4	T45.1X5	T45.1X6
Morfin	T40.2X1	T40.2X2	T40.2X3	T40.2X4	T40.2X5	T40.2X6
Morinamide	T37.1X1	T37.1X2	T37.1X3	T37.1X4	T37.1X5	T37.1X6
Morning glory seeds	T40.991	T40.992	T40.993	T40.994	—	—
Moroxydine	T37.5X1	T37.5X2	T37.5X3	T37.5X4	T37.5X5	T37.5X6
Morphazinamide	T37.1X1	T37.1X2	T37.1X3	T37.1X4	T37.1X5	T37.1X6
Morphine	T40.2X1	T40.2X2	T40.2X3	T40.2X4	T40.2X5	T40.2X6
antagonist	T50.7X1	T50.7X2	T50.7X3	T50.7X4	T50.7X5	T50.7X6
Morpholinylethylmorphine	T40.2X1	T40.2X2	T40.2X3	T40.2X4	—	—
Morsuximide	T42.2X1	T42.2X2	T42.2X3	T42.2X4	T42.2X5	T42.2X6

Substance	Poisoning, Accidental (Unintentional)	Poisoning, Intentional Self-Harm	Poisoning, Assault	Poisoning, Undetermined	Adverse Effect	Underdosing
Mosapramine	T43.591	T43.592	T43.593	T43.594	T43.595	T43.596
Moth balls — see also Pesticide	T60.2X1	T60.2X2	T60.2X3	T60.2X4	—	—
naphthalene	T60.2X1	T60.2X2	T60.2X3	T60.2X4	—	—
paradichlorobenzene	T60.1X1	T60.1X2	T60.1X3	T60.1X4	—	—
Motor exhaust gas	T58.01	T58.02	T58.03	T58.04		
Mouthwash (antiseptic) (zinc chloride)	T49.6X1	T49.6X2	T49.6X3	T49.6X4	T49.6X5	T49.6X6
Moxastine	T45.0X1	T45.0X2	T45.0X3	T45.0X4	T45.0X5	T45.0X6
Moxaverine	T44.3X1	T44.3X2	T44.3X3	T44.3X4	T44.3X5	T44.3X6
Moxifensine	T43.291	T43.292	T43.293	T43.294	T43.295	T43.296
Moxisylyte	T46.7X1	T46.7X2	T46.7X3	T46.7X4	T46.7X5	T46.7X6
Mucilage, plant	T47.4X1	T47.4X2	T47.4X3	T47.4X4	T47.4X5	T47.4X6
Mucolytic drug	T48.4X1	T48.4X2	T48.4X3	T48.4X4	T48.4X5	T48.4X6
Mucomyst	T48.4X1	T48.4X2	T48.4X3	T48.4X4	T48.4X5	T48.4X6
Mucous membrane agents (external)	T49.91	T49.92	T49.93	T49.94	T49.95	T49.96
specified NEC	T49.8X1	T49.8X2	T49.8X3	T49.8X4	T49.8X5	T49.8X6
Multiple unspecified drugs, medicaments and biological substances	T50.911	T50.912	T50.913	T50.914	T50.915	T50.916
Mumps						
immune globulin (human)	T50.Z11	T50.Z12	T50.Z13	T50.Z14	T50.Z15	T50.Z16
skin test antigen	T50.8X1	T50.8X2	T50.8X3	T50.8X4	T50.8X5	T50.8X6
vaccine	T50.B91	T50.B92	T50.B93	T50.B94	T50.B95	T50.B96
Mumpsvax	T50.B91	T50.B92	T50.B93	T50.B94	T50.B95	T50.B96
Mupirocin	T49.0X1	T49.0X2	T49.0X3	T49.0X4	T49.0X5	T49.0X6
Muriatic acid — see Hydrochloric acid						
Muromonab-CD3	T45.1X1	T45.1X2	T45.1X3	T45.1X4	T45.1X5	T45.1X6
Muscle relaxant — see Relaxant, muscle						
Muscle-action drug NEC	T48.201	T48.202	T48.203	T48.204	T48.205	T48.206
Muscle affecting agents NEC	T48.201	T48.202	T48.203	T48.204	T48.205	T48.206
oxytocic	T48.0X1	T48.0X2	T48.0X3	T48.0X4	T48.0X5	T48.0X6
relaxants	T48.201	T48.202	T48.203	T48.204	T48.205	T48.206
central nervous system	T42.8X1	T42.8X2	T42.8X3	T42.8X4	T42.8X5	T42.8X6
skeletal	T48.1X1	T48.1X2	T48.1X3	T48.1X4	T48.1X5	T48.1X6
smooth	T44.3X1	T44.3X2	T44.3X3	T44.3X4	T44.3X5	T44.3X6
Muscle-tone depressant, central NEC	T42.8X1	T42.8X2	T42.8X3	T42.8X4	T42.8X5	T42.8X6
specified NEC	T42.8X1	T42.8X2	T42.8X3	T42.8X4	T42.8X5	T42.8X6
Mushroom, noxious	T62.0X1	T62.0X2	T62.0X3	T62.0X4	—	—
Mussel, noxious	T61.781	T61.782	T61.783	T61.784	—	—

◀ New ◀ Revised deleted Deleted

TABLE OF DRUGS AND CHEMICALS

Substance	External Cause (T-Code) Poisoning, Accidental (Unintentional)	Poisoning, Intentional Self-Harm	Poisoning, Assault	Poisoning, Undetermined	Adverse Effect	Underdosing
Mustard (emetic)	T47.7X1	T47.7X2	T47.7X3	T47.7X4	T47.7X5	T47.7X6
black	T47.7X1	T47.7X2	T47.7X3	T47.7X4	T47.7X5	T47.7X6
gas, not in war	T59.91	T59.92	T59.93	T59.94	—	—
nitrogen	T45.1X1	T45.1X2	T45.1X3	T45.1X4	T45.1X5	T45.1X6
Mustine	T45.1X1	T45.1X2	T45.1X3	T45.1X4	T45.1X5	T45.1X6
M-vac	T45.1X1	T45.1X2	T45.1X3	T45.1X4	T45.1X5	T45.1X6
Mycifradin	T36.5X1	T36.5X2	T36.5X3	T36.5X4	T36.5X5	T36.5X6
topical	T49.0X1	T49.0X2	T49.0X3	T49.0X4	T49.0X5	T49.0X6
Mycitracin	T36.8X1	T36.8X2	T36.8X3	T36.8X4	T36.8X5	T36.8X6
ophthalmic preparation	T49.5X1	T49.5X2	T49.5X3	T49.5X4	T49.5X5	T49.5X6
Mycostatin	T36.7X1	T36.7X2	T36.7X3	T36.7X4	T36.7X5	T36.7X6
topical	T49.0X1	T49.0X2	T49.0X3	T49.0X4	T49.0X5	T49.0X6
Mycotoxins	T64.81	T64.82	T64.83	T64.84	—	—
aflatoxin	T64.01	T64.02	T64.03	T64.04	—	—
specified NEC	T64.81	T64.82	T64.83	T64.84	—	—
Mydriacyl	T44.3X1	T44.3X2	T44.3X3	T44.3X4	T44.3X5	T44.3X6
Mydriatic drug	T49.5X1	T49.5X2	T49.5X3	T49.5X4	T49.5X5	T49.5X6
Myelobromal	T45.1X1	T45.1X2	T45.1X3	T45.1X4	T45.1X5	T45.1X6
Myleran	T45.1X1	T45.1X2	T45.1X3	T45.1X4	T45.1X5	T45.1X6
Myochrysin(e)	T39.2X1	T39.2X2	T39.2X3	T39.2X4	T39.2X5	T39.2X6
Myoneural blocking agents	T48.1X1	T48.1X2	T48.1X3	T48.1X4	T48.1X5	T48.1X6
Myralact	T49.0X1	T49.0X2	T49.0X3	T49.0X4	T49.0X5	T49.0X6
Myristica fragrans	T62.2X1	T62.2X2	T62.2X3	T62.2X4	—	—
Myristicin	T65.891	T65.892	T65.893	T65.894	—	—
Mysoline	T42.3X1	T42.3X2	T42.3X3	T42.3X4	T42.3X5	T42.3X6
N						
Nabilone	T40.711	T40.712	T40.713	T40.714	T40.715	T40.716
Nabumetone	T39.391	T39.392	T39.393	T39.394	T39.395	T39.396
Nadolol	T44.7X1	T44.7X2	T44.7X3	T44.7X4	T44.7X5	T44.7X6
Nafcillin	T36.0X1	T36.0X2	T36.0X3	T36.0X4	T36.0X5	T36.0X6
Nafoxidine	T38.6X1	T38.6X2	T38.6X3	T38.6X4	T38.6X5	T38.6X6
Naftazone	T46.991	T46.992	T46.993	T46.994	T46.995	T46.996
Naftidrofuryl (oxalate)	T46.7X1	T46.7X2	T46.7X3	T46.7X4	T46.7X5	T46.7X6
Naftifine	T49.0X1	T49.0X2	T49.0X3	T49.0X4	T49.0X5	T49.0X6
Nail polish remover	T52.91	T52.92	T52.93	T52.94	—	—
Nalbuphine	T40.491	T40.492	T40.493	T40.494	T40.495	T40.496
Naled	T60.0X1	T60.0X2	T60.0X3	T60.0X4	—	—
Nalidixic acid	T37.8X1	T37.8X2	T37.8X3	T37.8X4	T37.8X5	T37.8X6
Nalorphine	T50.7X1	T50.7X2	T50.7X3	T50.7X4	T50.7X5	T50.7X6
Naloxone	T50.7X1	T50.7X2	T50.7X3	T50.7X4	T50.7X5	T50.7X6
Naltrexone	T50.7X1	T50.7X2	T50.7X3	T50.7X4	T50.7X5	T50.7X6
Namenda	T43.8X1	T43.8X2	T43.8X3	T43.8X4	T43.8X5	T43.8X6

Substance	External Cause (T-Code) Poisoning, Accidental (Unintentional)	Poisoning, Intentional Self-Harm	Poisoning, Assault	Poisoning, Undetermined	Adverse Effect	Underdosing
Nandrolone	T38.7X1	T38.7X2	T38.7X3	T38.7X4	T38.7X5	T38.7X6
Naphazoline	T48.5X1	T48.5X2	T48.5X3	T48.5X4	T48.5X5	T48.5X6
Naphtha (painters') (petroleum)	T52.0X1	T52.0X2	T52.0X3	T52.0X4	—	—
solvent	T52.0X1	T52.0X2	T52.0X3	T52.0X4	—	—
vapor	T52.0X1	T52.0X2	T52.0X3	T52.0X4	—	—
Naphthalene (non-chlorinated)	T60.2X1	T60.2X2	T60.2X3	T60.2X4	—	—
chlorinated	T60.1X1	T60.1X2	T60.1X3	T60.1X4	—	—
vapor	T60.1X1	T60.1X2	T60.1X3	T60.1X4	—	—
insecticide or moth repellent	T60.2X1	T60.2X2	T60.2X3	T60.2X4	—	—
chlorinated	T60.1X1	T60.1X2	T60.1X3	T60.1X4	—	—
vapor	T60.2X1	T60.2X2	T60.2X3	T60.2X4	—	—
chlorinated	T60.1X1	T60.1X2	T60.1X3	T60.1X4	—	—
Naphthol	T65.891	T65.892	T65.893	T65.894	—	—
Naphthylamine	T65.891	T65.892	T65.893	T65.894	—	—
Naphthylthiourea (ANTU)	T60.4X1	T60.4X2	T60.4X3	T60.4X4	—	—
Naprosyn— see Naproxen						
Naproxen	T39.311	T39.312	T39.313	T39.314	T39.315	T39.316
Narcotic (drug)	T40.601	T40.602	T40.603	T40.604	T40.605	T40.606
analgesic NEC	T40.601	T40.602	T40.603	T40.604	T40.605	T40.606
antagonist	T50.7X1	T50.7X2	T50.7X3	T50.7X4	T50.7X5	T50.7X6
specified NEC	T40.691	T40.692	T40.693	T40.694	T40.695	T40.696
synthetic	T40.491	T40.492	T40.493	T40.494	T40.495	T40.496
Narcotine	T48.3X1	T48.3X2	T48.3X3	T48.3X4	T48.3X5	T48.3X6
Nardil	T43.1X1	T43.1X2	T43.1X3	T43.1X4	T43.1X5	T43.1X6
Nasal drug NEC	T49.6X1	T49.6X2	T49.6X3	T49.6X4	T49.6X5	T49.6X6
Natamycin	T49.0X1	T49.0X2	T49.0X3	T49.0X4	T49.0X5	T49.0X6
Natrium cyanide— see Cyanide(s)						
Natural gas	T59.891	T59.892	T59.893	T59.894	—	—
incomplete combustion	T57.91	T57.92	T57.93	T57.94	—	—
Natural						
blood (product)	T45.8X1	T45.8X2	T45.8X3	T45.8X4	T45.8X5	T45.8X6
gas (piped)	T59.891	T59.892	T59.893	T59.894	—	—
incomplete combustion	T58.11	T58.12	T58.13	T58.14	—	—
Nealbarbital	T42.3X1	T42.3X2	T42.3X3	T42.3X4	T42.3X5	T42.3X6
Nectadon	T48.3X1	T48.3X2	T48.3X3	T48.3X4	T48.3X5	T48.3X6
Nedocromil	T48.6X1	T48.6X2	T48.6X3	T48.6X4	T48.6X5	T48.6X6
Nefopam	T39.8X1	T39.8X2	T39.8X3	T39.8X4	T39.8X5	T39.8X6
Nematocyst (sting)	T63.691	T63.692	T63.693	T63.694	—	—
Nembutal	T42.3X1	T42.3X2	T42.3X3	T42.3X4	T42.3X5	T42.3X6
Nemonapride	T43.591	T43.592	T43.593	T43.594	T43.595	T43.596
Neoarsphenamine	T37.8X1	T37.8X2	T37.8X3	T37.8X4	T37.8X5	T37.8X6

◀ New ◀ Revised deleted Deleted

Substance	Poisoning, Accidental (Unintentional)	Poisoning, Intentional Self-Harm	Poisoning, Assault	Poisoning, Undetermined	Adverse Effect	Underdosing
Neocinchophen	T50.4X1	T50.4X2	T50.4X3	T50.4X4	T50.4X5	T50.4X6
Neomycin (derivatives)	T36.5X1	T36.5X2	T36.5X3	T36.5X4	T36.5X5	T36.5X6
with						
bacitracin	T49.0X1	T49.0X2	T49.0X3	T49.0X4	T49.0X5	T49.0X6
neostigmine	T44.0X1	T44.0X2	T44.0X3	T44.0X4	T44.0X5	T44.0X6
ENT agent	T49.6X1	T49.6X2	T49.6X3	T49.6X4	T49.6X5	T49.6X6
ophthalmic preparation	T49.5X1	T49.5X2	T49.5X3	T49.5X4	T49.5X5	T49.5X6
topical NEC	T49.0X1	T49.0X2	T49.0X3	T49.0X4	T49.0X5	T49.0X6
Neonal	T42.3X1	T42.3X2	T42.3X3	T42.3X4	T42.3X5	T42.3X6
Neoprontosil	T37.0X1	T37.0X2	T37.0X3	T37.0X4	T37.0X5	T37.0X6
Neosalvarsan	T37.8X1	T37.8X2	T37.8X3	T37.8X4	T37.8X5	T37.8X6
Neosilversalvarsan	T37.8X1	T37.8X2	T37.8X3	T37.8X4	T37.8X5	T37.8X6
Neosporin	T36.8X1	T36.8X2	T36.8X3	T36.8X4	T36.8X5	T36.8X6
ENT agent	T49.6X1	T49.6X2	T49.6X3	T49.6X4	T49.6X5	T49.6X6
opthalmic preparation	T49.5X1	T49.5X2	T49.5X3	T49.5X4	T49.5X5	T49.5X6
topical NEC	T49.0X1	T49.0X2	T49.0X3	T49.0X4	T49.0X5	T49.0X6
Neostigmine bromide	T44.0X1	T44.0X2	T44.0X3	T44.0X4	T44.0X5	T44.0X6
Neraval	T42.3X1	T42.3X2	T42.3X3	T42.3X4	T42.3X5	T42.3X6
Neravan	T42.3X1	T42.3X2	T42.3X3	T42.3X4	T42.3X5	T42.3X6
Nerium oleander	T62.2X1	T62.2X2	T62.2X3	T62.2X4	—	—
Nerve gas, not in war	T59.91	T59.92	T59.93	T59.94	—	—
Nesacaine	T41.3X1	T41.3X2	T41.3X3	T41.3X4	T41.3X5	T41.3X6
infiltration (subcutaneous)	T41.3X1	T41.3X2	T41.3X3	T41.3X4	T41.3X5	T41.3X6
nerve block (peripheral) (plexus)	T41.3X1	T41.3X2	T41.3X3	T41.3X4	T41.3X5	T41.3X6
Netilmicin	T36.5X1	T36.5X2	T36.5X3	T36.5X4	T36.5X5	T36.5X6
Neurobarb	T42.3X1	T42.3X2	T42.3X3	T42.3X4	T42.3X5	T42.3X6
Neuroleptic drug NEC	T43.501	T43.502	T43.503	T43.504	T43.505	T43.506
Neuromuscular blocking drug	T48.1X1	T48.1X2	T48.1X3	T48.1X4	T48.1X5	T48.1X6
Neutral insulin injection	T38.3X1	T38.3X2	T38.3X3	T38.3X4	T38.3X5	T38.3X6
Neutral spirits	T51.0X1	T51.0X2	T51.0X3	T51.0X4	—	—
beverage	T51.0X1	T51.0X2	T51.0X3	T51.0X4	—	—
Niacin	T46.7X1	T46.7X2	T46.7X3	T46.7X4	T46.7X5	T46.7X6
Niacinamide	T45.2X1	T45.2X2	T45.2X3	T45.2X4	T45.2X5	T45.2X6
Nialamide	T43.1X1	T43.1X2	T43.1X3	T43.1X4	T43.1X5	T43.1X6
Niaprazine	T42.6X1	T42.6X2	T42.6X3	T42.6X4	T42.6X5	T42.6X6
Nicametate	T46.7X1	T46.7X2	T46.7X3	T46.7X4	T46.7X5	T46.7X6
Nicardipine	T46.1X1	T46.1X2	T46.1X3	T46.1X4	T46.1X5	T46.1X6
Nicergoline	T46.7X1	T46.7X2	T46.7X3	T46.7X4	T46.7X5	T46.7X6
Nickel (carbonyl) (tetra-carbonyl) (fumes) (vapor)	T56.891	T56.892	T56.893	T56.894	—	—

Substance	Poisoning, Accidental (Unintentional)	Poisoning, Intentional Self-Harm	Poisoning, Assault	Poisoning, Undetermined	Adverse Effect	Underdosing
Nickelocene	T56.891	T56.892	T56.893	T56.894	—	—
Niclosamide	T37.4X1	T37.4X2	T37.4X3	T37.4X4	T37.4X5	T37.4X6
Nicofuranose	T46.7X1	T46.7X2	T46.7X3	T46.7X4	T46.7X5	T46.7X6
Nicomorphine	T40.2X1	T40.2X2	T40.2X3	T40.2X4	—	—
Nicorandil	T46.3X1	T46.3X2	T46.3X3	T46.3X4	T46.3X5	T46.3X6
Nicotiana (plant)	T62.2X1	T62.2X2	T62.2X3	T62.2X4	—	—
Nicotinamide	T45.2X1	T45.2X2	T45.2X3	T45.2X4	T45.2X5	T45.2X6
Nicotine (insecticide) (spray) (sulfate) NEC	T60.2X1	T60.2X2	T60.2X3	T60.2X4	—	—
from tobacco	T65.291	T65.292	T65.293	T65.294	—	—
cigarettes	T65.221	T65.222	T65.223	T65.224	—	—
not insecticide	T65.291	T65.292	T65.293	T65.294	—	—
Nicotinic acid	T46.7X1	T46.7X2	T46.7X3	T46.7X4	T46.7X5	T46.7X6
Nicotinyl alcohol	T46.7X1	T46.7X2	T46.7X3	T46.7X4	T46.7X5	T46.7X6
Nicoumalone	T45.511	T45.512	T45.513	T45.514	T45.515	T45.516
Nifedipine	T46.1X1	T46.1X2	T46.1X3	T46.1X4	T46.1X5	T46.1X6
Nifenazone	T39.2X1	T39.2X2	T39.2X3	T39.2X4	T39.2X5	T39.2X6
Nifuraldezone	T37.91	T37.92	T37.93	T37.94	T37.95	T37.96
Nifuratel	T37.8X1	T37.8X2	T37.8X3	T37.8X4	T37.8X5	T37.8X6
Nifurtimox	T37.3X1	T37.3X2	T37.3X3	T37.3X4	T37.3X5	T37.3X6
Nifurtoinol	T37.8X1	T37.8X2	T37.8X3	T37.8X4	T37.8X5	T37.8X6
Nightshade, deadly (solanum) — see also Belladonna	T62.2X1	T62.2X2	T62.2X3	T62.2X4	—	—
berry	T62.1X1	T62.1X2	T62.1X3	T62.1X4	—	—
Nikethamide	T50.7X1	T50.7X2	T50.7X3	T50.7X4	T50.7X5	T50.7X6
Nilstat	T36.7X1	T36.7X2	T36.7X3	T36.7X4	T36.7X5	T36.7X6
topical	T49.0X1	T49.0X2	T49.0X3	T49.0X4	T49.0X5	T49.0X6
Nilutamide	T38.6X1	T38.6X2	T38.6X3	T38.6X4	T38.6X5	T38.6X6
Nimesulide	T39.391	T39.392	T39.393	T39.394	T39.395	T39.396
Nimetazepam	T42.4X1	T42.4X2	T42.4X3	T42.4X4	T42.4X5	T42.4X6
Nimodipine	T46.1X1	T46.1X2	T46.1X3	T46.1X4	T46.1X5	T46.1X6
Nimorazole	T37.3X1	T37.3X2	T37.3X3	T37.3X4	T37.3X5	T37.3X6
Nimustine	T45.1X1	T45.1X2	T45.1X3	T45.1X4	T45.1X5	T45.1X6
Niridazole	T37.4X1	T37.4X2	T37.4X3	T37.4X4	T37.4X5	T37.4X6
Nisentil	T40.2X1	T40.2X2	T40.2X3	T40.2X4	T40.2X5	T40.2X6
Nisoldipine	T46.1X1	T46.1X2	T46.1X3	T46.1X4	T46.1X5	T46.1X6
Nitramine	T65.3X1	T65.3X2	T65.3X3	T65.3X4	—	—
Nitrate, organic	T46.3X1	T46.3X2	T46.3X3	T46.3X4	T46.3X5	T46.3X6
Nitrazepam	T42.4X1	T42.4X2	T42.4X3	T42.4X4	T42.4X5	T42.4X6
Nitrefazole	T50.6X1	T50.6X2	T50.6X3	T50.6X4	T50.6X5	T50.6X6
Nitrendipine	T46.1X1	T46.1X2	T46.1X3	T46.1X4	T46.1X5	T46.1X6

TABLE OF DRUGS AND CHEMICALS

	External Cause (T-Code)					
Substance	Poisoning, Accidental (Unintentional)	Poisoning, Intentional Self-Harm	Poisoning, Assault	Poisoning, Undetermined	Adverse Effect	Underdosing
Nitric						
acid (liquid)	T54.2X1	T54.2X2	T54.2X3	T54.2X4	—	—
vapor	T59.891	T59.892	T59.893	T59.894	—	—
oxide (gas)	T59.0X1	T59.0X2	T59.0X3	T59.0X4	—	—
Nitrimidazine	T37.3X1	T37.3X2	T37.3X3	T37.3X4	T37.3X5	T37.3X6
Nitrite, amyl (medicinal) (vapor)	T46.3X1	T46.3X2	T46.3X3	T46.3X4	T46.3X5	T46.3X6
Nitroaniline	T65.3X1	T65.3X2	T65.3X3	T65.3X4	—	—
vapor	T59.891	T59.892	T59.893	T59.894	—	—
Nitrobenzene, nitrobenzol	T65.3X1	T65.3X2	T65.3X3	T65.3X4	—	—
vapor	T65.3X1	T65.3X2	T65.3X3	T65.3X4	—	—
Nitrocellulose	T65.891	T65.892	T65.893	T65.894	—	—
lacquer	T65.891	T65.892	T65.893	T65.894	—	—
Nitrodiphenyl	T65.3X1	T65.3X2	T65.3X3	T65.3X4	—	—
Nitrofural	T49.0X1	T49.0X2	T49.0X3	T49.0X4	T49.0X5	T49.0X6
Nitrofurantoin	T37.8X1	T37.8X2	T37.8X3	T37.8X4	T37.8X5	T37.8X6
Nitrofurazone	T49.0X1	T49.0X2	T49.0X3	T49.0X4	T49.0X5	T49.0X6
Nitrogen	T59.0X1	T59.0X2	T59.0X3	T59.0X4	—	—
mustard	T45.1X1	T45.1X2	T45.1X3	T45.1X4	T45.1X5	T45.1X6
Nitroglycerin, nitro-glycerol (medicinal)	T46.3X1	T46.3X2	T46.3X3	T46.3X4	T46.3X5	T46.3X6
nonmedicinal	T65.5X1	T65.5X2	T65.5X3	T65.5X4	—	—
fumes	T65.5X1	T65.5X2	T65.5X3	T65.5X4	—	—
Nitroglycol	T52.3X1	T52.3X2	T52.3X3	T52.3X4	—	—
Nitrohydrochloric acid	T54.2X1	T54.2X2	T54.2X3	T54.2X4	—	—
Nitromersol	T49.0X1	T49.0X2	T49.0X3	T49.0X4	T49.0X5	T49.0X6
Nitronaphthalene	T65.891	T65.892	T65.893	T65.894	—	—
Nitrophenol	T54.0X1	T54.0X2	T54.0X3	T54.0X4	—	—
Nitropropane	T52.8X1	T52.8X2	T52.8X3	T52.8X4	—	—
Nitroprusside	T46.5X1	T46.5X2	T46.5X3	T46.5X4	T46.5X5	T46.5X6
Nitrosodimethylamine	T65.3X1	T65.3X2	T65.3X3	T65.3X4	—	—
Nitrothiazol	T37.4X1	T37.4X2	T37.4X3	T37.4X4	T37.4X5	T37.4X6
Nitrotoluene, nitrotoluol	T65.3X1	T65.3X2	T65.3X3	T65.3X4	—	—
vapor	T65.3X1	T65.3X2	T65.3X3	T65.3X4	—	—
Nitrous						
acid (liquid)	T54.2X1	T54.2X2	T54.2X3	T54.2X4	—	—
fumes	T59.891	T59.892	T59.893	T59.894	—	—
ether spirit	T46.3X1	T46.3X2	T46.3X3	T46.3X4	T46.3X5	T46.3X6
oxide	T41.0X1	T41.0X2	T41.0X3	T41.0X4	T41.0X5	T41.0X6
Nitroxoline	T37.8X1	T37.8X2	T37.8X3	T37.8X4	T37.8X5	T37.8X6
Nitrozone	T49.0X1	T49.0X2	T49.0X3	T49.0X4	T49.0X5	T49.0X6
Nizatidine	T47.0X1	T47.0X2	T47.0X3	T47.0X4	T47.0X5	T47.0X6

	External Cause (T-Code)					
Substance	Poisoning, Accidental (Unintentional)	Poisoning, Intentional Self-Harm	Poisoning, Assault	Poisoning, Undetermined	Adverse Effect	Underdosing
Nizofenone	T43.8X1	T43.8X2	T43.8X3	T43.8X4	T43.8X5	T43.8X6
Noctec	T42.6X1	T42.6X2	T42.6X3	T42.6X4	T42.6X5	T42.6X6
Noludar	T42.6X1	T42.6X2	T42.6X3	T42.6X4	T42.6X5	T42.6X6
Noptil	T42.3X1	T42.3X2	T42.3X3	T42.3X4	T42.3X5	T42.3X6
Nomegestrol	T38.5X1	T38.5X2	T38.5X3	T38.5X4	T38.5X5	T38.5X6
Nomifensine	T43.291	T43.292	T43.293	T43.294	T43.295	T43.296
Nonoxinol	T49.8X1	T49.8X2	T49.8X3	T49.8X4	T49.8X5	T49.8X6
Nonylphenoxy (polyethoxy-ethanol)	T49.8X1	T49.8X2	T49.8X3	T49.8X4	T49.8X5	T49.8X6
Noptil	T42.3X1	T42.3X2	T42.3X3	T42.3X4	T42.3X5	T42.3X6
Noradrenaline	T44.4X1	T44.4X2	T44.4X3	T44.4X4	T44.4X5	T44.4X6
Noramidopyrine	T39.2X1	T39.2X2	T39.2X3	T39.2X4	T39.2X5	T39.2X6
methanesulfonate sodium	T39.2X1	T39.2X2	T39.2X3	T39.2X4	T39.2X5	T39.2X6
Norbormide	T60.4X1	T60.4X2	T60.4X3	T60.4X4	—	—
Nordazepam	T42.4X1	T42.4X2	T42.4X3	T42.4X4	T42.4X5	T42.4X6
Norepinephrine	T44.4X1	T44.4X2	T44.4X3	T44.4X4	T44.4X5	T44.4X6
Norethandrolone	T38.7X1	T38.7X2	T38.7X3	T38.7X4	T38.7X5	T38.7X6
Norethindrone	T38.4X1	T38.4X2	T38.4X3	T38.4X4	T38.4X5	T38.4X6
Norethisterone (acetate) (enantate)	T38.4X1	T38.4X2	T38.4X3	T38.4X4	T38.4X5	T38.4X6
with ethinylestradiol	T38.5X1	T38.5X2	T38.5X3	T38.5X4	T38.5X5	T38.5X6
Noretynodrel	T38.5X1	T38.5X2	T38.5X3	T38.5X4	T38.5X5	T38.5X6
Norfenefrine	T44.4X1	T44.4X2	T44.4X3	T44.4X4	T44.4X5	T44.4X6
Norfloxacin	T36.8X1	T36.8X2	T36.8X3	T36.8X4	T36.8X5	T36.8X6
Norgestrel	T38.4X1	T38.4X2	T38.4X3	T38.4X4	T38.4X5	T38.4X6
Norgestrienone	T38.4X1	T38.4X2	T38.4X3	T38.4X4	T38.4X5	T38.4X6
Norlestrin	T38.4X1	T38.4X2	T38.4X3	T38.4X4	T38.4X5	T38.4X6
Norlutin	T38.4X1	T38.4X2	T38.4X3	T38.4X4	T38.4X5	T38.4X6
Normal serum albumin (human), salt-poor	T45.8X1	T45.8X2	T45.8X3	T45.8X4	T45.8X5	T45.8X6
Normethandrone	T38.5X1	T38.5X2	T38.5X3	T38.5X4	T38.5X5	T38.5X6
Normison — *see Benzodiazepines*						
Normorphine	T40.2X1	T40.2X2	T40.2X3	T40.2X4	—	—
Norpseudoephedrine	T50.5X1	T50.5X2	T50.5X3	T50.5X4	T50.5X5	T50.5X6
Nortestosterone (furanpropionate)	T38.7X1	T38.7X2	T38.7X3	T38.7X4	T38.7X5	T38.7X6
Nortriptyline	T43.011	T43.012	T43.013	T43.014	T43.015	T43.016
Noscapine	T48.3X1	T48.3X2	T48.3X3	T48.3X4	T48.3X5	T48.3X6
Nose preparations	T49.6X1	T49.6X2	T49.6X3	T49.6X4	T49.6X5	T49.6X6
Novobiocin	T36.5X1	T36.5X2	T36.5X3	T36.5X4	T36.5X5	T36.5X6
Novocain (infiltration) (topical)	T41.3X1	T41.3X2	T41.3X3	T41.3X4	T41.3X5	T41.3X6
nerve block (peripheral) (plexus)	T41.3X1	T41.3X2	T41.3X3	T41.3X4	T41.3X5	T41.3X6
spinal	T41.3X1	T41.3X2	T41.3X3	T41.3X4	T41.3X5	T41.3X6

◀ New   ◀ Revised   ~~deleted~~ Deleted

Substance	External Cause (T-Code) Poisoning, Accidental (Unintentional)	Poisoning, Intentional Self-Harm	Poisoning, Assault	Poisoning, Undetermined	Adverse Effect	Underdosing
Noxious foodstuff	T62.91	T62.92	T62.93	T62.94	—	—
specified NEC	T62.8X1	T62.8X2	T62.8X3	T62.8X4	—	—
Noxiptiline	T43.011	T43.012	T43.013	T43.014	T43.015	T43.016
Noxytiolin	T49.0X1	T49.0X2	T49.0X3	T49.0X4	T49.0X5	T49.0X6
NPH Iletin (insulin)	T38.3X1	T38.3X2	T38.3X3	T38.3X4	T38.3X5	T38.3X6
Numorphan	T40.2X1	T40.2X2	T40.2X3	T40.2X4	T40.2X5	T40.2X6
Nunol	T42.3X1	T42.3X2	T42.3X3	T42.3X4	T42.3X5	T42.3X6
Nupercaine (spinal anesthetic)	T41.3X1	T41.3X2	T41.3X3	T41.3X4	T41.3X5	T41.3X6
topical (surface)	T41.3X1	T41.3X2	T41.3X3	T41.3X4	T41.3X5	T41.3X6
Nutmeg oil (liniment)	T49.3X1	T49.3X2	T49.3X3	T49.3X4	T49.3X5	T49.3X6
Nutritional supplement	T50.901	T50.902	T50.903	T50.904	T50.905	T50.906
Nux vomica	T65.1X1	T65.1X2	T65.1X3	T65.1X4	—	—
Nydrazid	T37.1X1	T37.1X2	T37.1X3	T37.1X4	T37.1X5	T37.1X6
Nylidrin	T46.7X1	T46.7X2	T46.7X3	T46.7X4	T46.7X5	T46.7X6
Nystatin	T36.7X1	T36.7X2	T36.7X3	T36.7X4	T36.7X5	T36.7X6
topical	T49.0X1	T49.0X2	T49.0X3	T49.0X4	T49.0X5	T49.0X6
Nytol	T45.0X1	T45.0X2	T45.0X3	T45.0X4	T45.0X5	T45.0X6
O						
Obidoxime chloride	T50.6X1	T50.6X2	T50.6X3	T50.6X4	T50.6X5	T50.6X6
Octafonium (chloride)	T49.3X1	T49.3X2	T49.3X3	T49.3X4	T49.3X5	T49.3X6
Octamethyl pyrophos-phoramide	T60.0X1	T60.0X2	T60.0X3	T60.0X4	—	—
Octanoin	T50.991	T50.992	T50.993	T50.994	T50.995	T50.996
Octatropine methyl-bromide	T44.3X1	T44.3X2	T44.3X3	T44.3X4	T44.3X5	T44.3X6
Octotiamine	T45.2X1	T45.2X2	T45.2X3	T45.2X4	T45.2X5	T45.2X6
Octoxinol (9)	T49.8X1	T49.8X2	T49.8X3	T49.8X4	T49.8X5	T49.8X6
Octreotide	T38.991	T38.992	T38.993	T38.994	T38.995	T38.996
Octyl nitrite	T46.3X1	T46.3X2	T46.3X3	T46.3X4	T46.3X5	T46.3X6
Oestradiol	T38.5X1	T38.5X2	T38.5X3	T38.5X4	T38.5X5	T38.5X6
Oestriol	T38.5X1	T38.5X2	T38.5X3	T38.5X4	T38.5X5	T38.5X6
Oestrogen	T38.5X1	T38.5X2	T38.5X3	T38.5X4	T38.5X5	T38.5X6
Oestrone	T38.5X1	T38.5X2	T38.5X3	T38.5X4	T38.5X5	T38.5X6
Ofloxacin	T36.8X1	T36.8X2	T36.8X3	T36.8X4	T36.8X5	T36.8X6
Oil (of)	T65.891	T65.892	T65.893	T65.894	—	—
bitter almond	T62.8X1	T62.8X2	T62.8X3	T62.8X4	—	—
cloves	T49.7X1	T49.7X2	T49.7X3	T49.7X4	T49.7X5	T49.7X6
colors	T65.6X1	T65.6X2	T65.6X3	T65.6X4	—	—
fumes	T59.891	T59.892	T59.893	T59.894	—	—
lubricating	T52.0X1	T52.0X2	T52.0X3	T52.0X4	—	—
Niobe	T52.8X1	T52.8X2	T52.8X3	T52.8X4	—	—

Substance	External Cause (T-Code) Poisoning, Accidental (Unintentional)	Poisoning, Intentional Self-Harm	Poisoning, Assault	Poisoning, Undetermined	Adverse Effect	Underdosing
Oil (of) *(Continued)*						
vitriol (liquid)	T54.2X1	T54.2X2	T54.2X3	T54.2X4	—	—
fumes	T54.2X1	T54.2X2	T54.2X3	T54.2X4	—	—
wintergreen (bitter) NEC	T49.3X1	T49.3X2	T49.3X3	T49.3X4	T49.3X5	T49.3X6
Oily preparation (for skin)	T49.3X1	T49.3X2	T49.3X3	T49.3X4	T49.3X5	T49.3X6
Ointment NEC	T49.3X1	T49.3X2	T49.3X3	T49.3X4	T49.3X5	T49.3X6
Olanzapine	T43.591	T43.592	T43.593	T43.594	T43.595	T43.596
Oleander	T62.2X1	T62.2X2	T62.2X3	T62.2X4	—	—
Oleandomycin	T36.3X1	T36.3X2	T36.3X3	T36.3X4	T36.3X5	T36.3X6
Oleandrin	T46.0X1	T46.0X2	T46.0X3	T46.0X4	T46.0X5	T46.0X6
Oleic acid	T46.6X1	T46.6X2	T46.6X3	T46.6X4	T46.6X5	T46.6X6
Oleovitamin A	T45.2X1	T45.2X2	T45.2X3	T45.2X4	T45.2X5	T45.2X6
Oleum ricini	T47.2X1	T47.2X2	T47.2X3	T47.2X4	T47.2X5	T47.2X6
Olive oil (medicinal) NEC	T47.4X1	T47.4X2	T47.4X3	T47.4X4	T47.4X5	T47.4X6
Olivomycin	T45.1X1	T45.1X2	T45.1X3	T45.1X4	T45.1X5	T45.1X6
Olsalazine	T47.8X1	T47.8X2	T47.8X3	T47.8X4	T47.8X5	T47.8X6
Omeprazole	T47.1X1	T47.1X2	T47.1X3	T47.1X4	T47.1X5	T47.1X6
OMPA	T60.0X1	T60.0X2	T60.0X3	T60.0X4	—	—
Ondansetron	T45.0X1	T45.0X2	T45.0X3	T45.0X4	T45.0X5	T45.0X6
Oncovin	T45.1X1	T45.1X2	T45.1X3	T45.1X4	T45.1X5	T45.1X6
Ophthaine	T41.3X1	T41.3X2	T41.3X3	T41.3X4	T41.3X5	T41.3X6
Ophthetic	T41.3X1	T41.3X2	T41.3X3	T41.3X4	T41.3X5	T41.3X6
Opiate NEC	T40.601	T40.602	T40.603	T40.604	T40.605	T40.606
antagonists	T50.7X1	T50.7X2	T50.7X3	T50.7X4	T50.7X5	T50.7X6
Opioid NEC	T40.2X1	T40.2X2	T40.2X3	T40.2X4	T40.2X5	T40.2X6
Opipramol	T43.011	T43.012	T43.013	T43.014	T43.015	T43.016
Opium alkaloids (total)	T40.0X1	T40.0X2	T40.0X3	T40.0X4	T40.0X5	T40.0X6
standardized powdered	T40.0X1	T40.0X2	T40.0X3	T40.0X4	T40.0X5	T40.0X6
tincture (camphorated)	T40.0X1	T40.0X2	T40.0X3	T40.0X4	T40.0X5	T40.0X6
Oracon	T38.4X1	T38.4X2	T38.4X3	T38.4X4	T38.4X5	T38.4X6
Oragrafin	T50.8X1	T50.8X2	T50.8X3	T50.8X4	T50.8X5	T50.8X6
Oral contraceptives	T38.4X1	T38.4X2	T38.4X3	T38.4X4	T38.4X5	T38.4X6
Oral rehydration salts	T50.3X1	T50.3X2	T50.3X3	T50.3X4	T50.3X5	T50.3X6
Orazamide	T50.991	T50.992	T50.993	T50.994	T50.995	T50.996
Orciprenaline	T48.291	T48.292	T48.293	T48.294	T48.295	T48.296
Organidin	T48.4X1	T48.4X2	T48.4X3	T48.4X4	T48.4X5	T48.4X6
Organonitrate NEC	T46.3X1	T46.3X2	T46.3X3	T46.3X4	T46.3X5	T46.3X6
Organophosphates	T60.0X1	T60.0X2	T60.0X3	T60.0X4	—	—
Orimune	T50.B91	T50.B92	T50.B93	T50.B94	T50.B95	T50.B96
Orinase	T38.3X1	T38.3X2	T38.3X3	T38.3X4	T38.3X5	T38.3X6
Ormeloxifene	T38.6X1	T38.6X2	T38.6X3	T38.6X4	T38.6X5	T38.6X6

TABLE OF DRUGS AND CHEMICALS

Substance	External Cause (T-Code)					
	Poisoning, Accidental (Unintentional)	Poisoning, Intentional Self-Harm	Poisoning, Assault	Poisoning, Undetermined	Adverse Effect	Underdosing
Ornidazole	T37.3X1	T37.3X2	T37.3X3	T37.3X4	T37.3X5	T37.3X6
Ornithine aspartate	T50.991	T50.992	T50.993	T50.994	T50.995	T50.996
Ornoprostil	T47.1X1	T47.1X2	T47.1X3	T47.1X4	T47.1X5	T47.1X6
Orphenadrine (hydrochloride)	T42.8X1	T42.8X2	T42.8X3	T42.8X4	T42.8X5	T42.8X6
Ortal (sodium)	T42.3X1	T42.3X2	T42.3X3	T42.3X4	T42.3X5	T42.3X6
Orthoboric acid	T49.0X1	T49.0X2	T49.0X3	T49.0X4	T49.0X5	T49.0X6
ENT agent	T49.6X1	T49.6X2	T49.6X3	T49.6X4	T49.6X5	T49.6X6
ophthalmic preparation	T49.5X1	T49.5X2	T49.5X3	T49.5X4	T49.5X5	T49.5X6
Orthocaine	T41.3X1	T41.3X2	T41.3X3	T41.3X4	T41.3X5	T41.3X6
Orthodichlorobenzene	T53.7X1	T53.7X2	T53.7X3	T53.7X4	—	—
Ortho-Novum	T38.4X1	T38.4X2	T38.4X3	T38.4X4	T38.4X5	T38.4X6
Orthotolidine (reagent)	T54.2X1	T54.2X2	T54.2X3	T54.2X4	—	—
Osmic acid (liquid)	T54.2X1	T54.2X2	T54.2X3	T54.2X4	—	—
fumes	T54.2X1	T54.2X2	T54.2X3	T54.2X4	—	—
Osmotic diuretics	T50.2X1	T50.2X2	T50.2X3	T50.2X4	T50.2X5	T50.2X6
Otilonium bromide	T44.3X1	T44.3X2	T44.3X3	T44.3X4	T44.3X5	T44.3X6
Otorhinolaryngological drug NEC	T49.6X1	T49.6X2	T49.6X3	T49.6X4	T49.6X5	T49.6X6
Ouabain(e)	T46.0X1	T46.0X2	T46.0X3	T46.0X4	T46.0X5	T46.0X6
Ovarian						
hormone	T38.5X1	T38.5X2	T38.5X3	T38.5X4	T38.5X5	T38.5X6
stimulant	T38.5X1	T38.5X2	T38.5X3	T38.5X4	T38.5X5	T38.5X6
Ovral	T38.4X1	T38.4X2	T38.4X3	T38.4X4	T38.4X5	T38.4X6
Ovulen	T38.4X1	T38.4X2	T38.4X3	T38.4X4	T38.4X5	T38.4X6
Oxacillin	T36.0X1	T36.0X2	T36.0X3	T36.0X4	T36.0X5	T36.0X6
Oxalic acid	T54.2X1	T54.2X2	T54.2X3	T54.2X4	—	—
ammonium salt	T50.991	T50.992	T50.993	T50.994	T50.995	T50.996
Oxamniquine	T37.4X1	T37.4X2	T37.4X3	T37.4X4	T37.4X5	T37.4X6
Oxanamide	T43.591	T43.592	T43.593	T43.594	T43.595	T43.596
Oxandrolone	T38.7X1	T38.7X2	T38.7X3	T38.7X4	T38.7X5	T38.7X6
Oxantel	T37.4X1	T37.4X2	T37.4X3	T37.4X4	T37.4X5	T37.4X6
Oxapium iodide	T44.3X1	T44.3X2	T44.3X3	T44.3X4	T44.3X5	T44.3X6
Oxaprotiline	T43.021	T43.022	T43.023	T43.024	T43.025	T43.026
Oxaprozin	T39.311	T39.312	T39.313	T39.314	T39.315	T39.316
Oxatomide	T45.0X1	T45.0X2	T45.0X3	T45.0X4	T45.0X5	T45.0X6
Oxazepam	T42.4X1	T42.4X2	T42.4X3	T42.4X4	T42.4X5	T42.4X6
Oxazimedrine	T50.5X1	T50.5X2	T50.5X3	T50.5X4	T50.5X5	T50.5X6
Oxazolam	T42.4X1	T42.4X2	T42.4X3	T42.4X4	T42.4X5	T42.4X6
Oxazolidine derivatives	T42.2X1	T42.2X2	T42.2X3	T42.2X4	T42.2X5	T42.2X6
Oxazolidinedione (derivative)	T42.2X1	T42.2X2	T42.2X3	T42.2X4	T42.2X5	T42.2X6
Ox bile extract	T47.5X1	T47.5X2	T47.5X3	T47.5X4	T47.5X5	T47.5X6
Oxcarbazepine	T42.1X1	T42.1X2	T42.1X3	T42.1X4	T42.1X5	T42.1X6
Oxedrine	T44.4X1	T44.4X2	T44.4X3	T44.4X4	T44.4X5	T44.4X6

Substance	External Cause (T-Code)					
	Poisoning, Accidental (Unintentional)	Poisoning, Intentional Self-Harm	Poisoning, Assault	Poisoning, Undetermined	Adverse Effect	Underdosing
Oxeladin (citrate)	T48.3X1	T48.3X2	T48.3X3	T48.3X4	T48.3X5	T48.3X6
Oxendolone	T38.5X1	T38.5X2	T38.5X3	T38.5X4	T38.5X5	T38.5X6
Oxetacaine	T41.3X1	T41.3X2	T41.3X3	T41.3X4	T41.3X5	T41.3X6
Oxethazine	T41.3X1	T41.3X2	T41.3X3	T41.3X4	T41.3X5	T41.3X6
Oxetorone	T39.8X1	T39.8X2	T39.8X3	T39.8X4	T39.8X5	T39.8X6
Oxiconazole	T49.0X1	T49.0X2	T49.0X3	T49.0X4	T49.0X5	T49.0X6
Oxidizing agent NEC	T54.91	T54.92	T54.93	T54.94	—	—
Oxipurinol	T50.4X1	T50.4X2	T50.4X3	T50.4X4	T50.4X5	T50.4X6
Oxitriptan	T43.291	T43.292	T43.293	T43.294	T43.295	T43.296
Oxitropium bromide	T48.6X1	T48.6X2	T48.6X3	T48.6X4	T48.6X5	T48.6X6
Oxodipine	T46.1X1	T46.1X2	T46.1X3	T46.1X4	T46.1X5	T46.1X6
Oxolamine	T48.3X1	T48.3X2	T48.3X3	T48.3X4	T48.3X5	T48.3X6
Oxolinic acid	T37.8X1	T37.8X2	T37.8X3	T37.8X4	T37.8X5	T37.8X6
Oxomemazine	T43.3X1	T43.3X2	T43.3X3	T43.3X4	T43.3X5	T43.3X6
Oxophenarsine	T37.3X1	T37.3X2	T37.3X3	T37.3X4	T37.3X5	T37.3X6
Oxprenolol	T44.7X1	T44.7X2	T44.7X3	T44.7X4	T44.7X5	T44.7X6
Oxsoralen	T49.3X1	T49.3X2	T49.3X3	T49.3X4	T49.3X5	T49.3X6
Oxtriphylline	T48.6X1	T48.6X2	T48.6X3	T48.6X4	T48.6X5	T48.6X6
Oxybate sodium	T41.291	T41.292	T41.293	T41.294	T41.295	T41.296
Oxybuprocaine	T41.3X1	T41.3X2	T41.3X3	T41.3X4	T41.3X5	T41.3X6
Oxybutynin	T44.3X1	T44.3X2	T44.3X3	T44.3X4	T44.3X5	T44.3X6
Oxychlorosene	T49.0X1	T49.0X2	T49.0X3	T49.0X4	T49.0X5	T49.0X6
Oxycodone	T40.2X1	T40.2X2	T40.2X3	T40.2X4	T40.2X5	T40.2X6
Oxyfedrine	T46.3X1	T46.3X2	T46.3X3	T46.3X4	T46.3X5	T46.3X6
Oxygen	T41.5X1	T41.5X2	T41.5X3	T41.5X4	T41.5X5	T41.5X6
Oxylone	T49.0X1	T49.0X2	T49.0X3	T49.0X4	T49.0X5	T49.0X6
ophthalmic preparation	T49.5X1	T49.5X2	T49.5X3	T49.5X4	T49.5X5	T49.5X6
Oxymesterone	T38.7X1	T38.7X2	T38.7X3	T38.7X4	T38.7X5	T38.7X6
Oxymetazoline	T48.5X1	T48.5X2	T48.5X3	T48.5X4	T48.5X5	T48.5X6
Oxymetholone	T38.7X1	T38.7X2	T38.7X3	T38.7X4	T38.7X5	T38.7X6
Oxymorphone	T40.2X1	T40.2X2	T40.2X3	T40.2X4	T40.2X5	T40.2X6
Oxypertine	T43.591	T43.592	T43.593	T43.594	T43.595	T43.596
Oxyphenbutazone	T39.2X1	T39.2X2	T39.2X3	T39.2X4	T39.2X5	T39.2X6
Oxyphencyclimine	T44.3X1	T44.3X2	T44.3X3	T44.3X4	T44.3X5	T44.3X6
Oxyphenisatine	T47.2X1	T47.2X2	T47.2X3	T47.2X4	T47.2X5	T47.2X6
Oxyphenonium bromide	T44.3X1	T44.3X2	T44.3X3	T44.3X4	T44.3X5	T44.3X6
Oxypolygelatin	T45.8X1	T45.8X2	T45.8X3	T45.8X4	T45.8X5	T45.8X6
Oxyquinoline (derivatives)	T37.8X1	T37.8X2	T37.8X3	T37.8X4	T37.8X5	T37.8X6
Oxytetracycline	T36.4X1	T36.4X2	T36.4X3	T36.4X4	T36.4X5	T36.4X6
Oxytocic drug NEC	T48.0X1	T48.0X2	T48.0X3	T48.0X4	T48.0X5	T48.0X6
Oxytocin (synthetic)	T48.0X1	T48.0X2	T48.0X3	T48.0X4	T48.0X5	T48.0X6
Ozone	T59.891	T59.892	T59.893	T59.894	—	—

◀ New   ◀ Revised   ~~deleted~~ Deleted

Substance	Poisoning, Accidental (Unintentional)	Poisoning, Intentional Self-Harm	Poisoning, Assault	Poisoning, Undetermined	Adverse Effect	Underdosing
P						
PABA	T49.3X1	T49.3X2	T49.3X3	T49.3X4	T49.3X5	T49.3X6
Packed red cells	T45.8X1	T45.8X2	T45.8X3	T45.8X4	T45.8X5	T45.8X6
Padimate	T49.3X1	T49.3X2	T49.3X3	T49.3X4	T49.3X5	T49.3X6
Paint NEC	T65.6X1	T65.6X2	T65.6X3	T65.6X4	—	—
cleaner	T52.91	T52.92	T52.93	T52.94	—	—
fumes NEC	T59.891	T59.892	T59.893	T59.894	—	—
lead (fumes)	T56.0X1	T56.0X2	T56.0X3	T56.0X4	—	—
solvent NEC	T52.8X1	T52.8X2	T52.8X3	T52.8X4	—	—
stripper	T52.8X1	T52.8X2	T52.8X3	T52.8X4	—	—
Palfium	T40.2X1	T40.2X2	T40.2X3	T40.2X4	—	—
Palm kernel oil	T50.991	T50.992	T50.993	T50.994	T50.995	T50.996
Paludrine	T37.2X1	T37.2X2	T37.2X3	T37.2X4	T37.2X5	T37.2X6
PAM (pralidoxime)	T50.6X1	T50.6X2	T50.6X3	T50.6X4	T50.6X5	T50.6X6
Pamaquine (naphthoute)	T37.2X1	T37.2X2	T37.2X3	T37.2X4	T37.2X5	T37.2X6
Panadol	T39.1X1	T39.1X2	T39.1X3	T39.1X4	T39.1X5	T39.1X6
Pancreatic						
digestive secretion stimulant	T47.8X1	T47.8X2	T47.8X3	T47.8X4	T47.8X5	T47.8X6
dornase	T45.3X1	T45.3X2	T45.3X3	T45.3X4	T45.3X5	T45.3X6
Pancreatin	T47.5X1	T47.5X2	T47.5X3	T47.5X4	T47.5X5	T47.5X6
Pancrelipase	T47.5X1	T47.5X2	T47.5X3	T47.5X4	T47.5X5	T47.5X6
Pancuronium (bromide)	T48.1X1	T48.1X2	T48.1X3	T48.1X4	T48.1X5	T48.1X6
Pangamic acid	T45.2X1	T45.2X2	T45.2X3	T45.2X4	T45.2X5	T45.2X6
Panthenol	T45.2X1	T45.2X2	T45.2X3	T45.2X4	T45.2X5	T45.2X6
topical	T49.8X1	T49.8X2	T49.8X3	T49.8X4	T49.8X5	T49.8X6
Pantopon	T40.0X1	T40.0X2	T40.0X3	T40.0X4	T40.0X5	T40.0X6
Pantothenic acid	T45.2X1	T45.2X2	T45.2X3	T45.2X4	T45.2X5	T45.2X6
Panwarfin	T45.511	T45.512	T45.513	T45.514	T45.515	T45.516
Papain	T47.5X1	T47.5X2	T47.5X3	T47.5X4	T47.5X5	T47.5X6
digestant	T47.5X1	T47.5X2	T47.5X3	T47.5X4	T47.5X5	T47.5X6
Papaveretum	T40.0X1	T40.0X2	T40.0X3	T40.0X4	T40.0X5	T40.0X6
Papaverine	T44.3X1	T44.3X2	T44.3X3	T44.3X4	T44.3X5	T44.3X6
Para-acetamidophenol	T39.1X1	T39.1X2	T39.1X3	T39.1X4	T39.1X5	T39.1X6
Para-aminobenzoic acid	T49.3X1	T49.3X2	T49.3X3	T49.3X4	T49.3X5	T49.3X6
Para-aminophenol derivatives	T39.1X1	T39.1X2	T39.1X3	T39.1X4	T39.1X5	T39.1X6
Para-aminosalicylic acid	T37.1X1	T37.1X2	T37.1X3	T37.1X4	T37.1X5	T37.1X6
Paracetaldehyde	T42.6X1	T42.6X2	T42.6X3	T42.6X4	T42.6X5	T42.6X6
Paracetamol	T39.1X1	T39.1X2	T39.1X3	T39.1X4	T39.1X5	T39.1X6
Parachlorophenol (camphorated)	T49.0X1	T49.0X2	T49.0X3	T49.0X4	T49.0X5	T49.0X6
Paracodin	T40.2X1	T40.2X2	T40.2X3	T40.2X4	T40.2X5	T40.2X6
Paradione	T42.2X1	T42.2X2	T42.2X3	T42.2X4	T42.2X5	T42.2X6

Substance	Poisoning, Accidental (Unintentional)	Poisoning, Intentional Self-Harm	Poisoning, Assault	Poisoning, Undetermined	Adverse Effect	Underdosing
Paraffin(s) (wax)	T52.0X1	T52.0X2	T52.0X3	T52.0X4	—	—
liquid (medicinal)	T47.4X1	T47.4X2	T47.4X3	T47.4X4	T47.4X5	T47.4X6
nonmedicinal	T52.0X1	T52.0X2	T52.0X3	T52.0X4	—	—
Paraformaldehyde	T60.3X1	T60.3X2	T60.3X3	T60.3X4	—	—
Paraldehyde	T42.6X1	T42.6X2	T42.6X3	T42.6X4	T42.6X5	T42.6X6
Paramethadione	T42.2X1	T42.2X2	T42.2X3	T42.2X4	T42.2X5	T42.2X6
Paramethasone	T38.0X1	T38.0X2	T38.0X3	T38.0X4	T38.0X5	T38.0X6
acetate	T49.0X1	T49.0X2	T49.0X3	T49.0X4	T49.0X5	T49.0X6
Paraoxon	T60.0X1	T60.0X2	T60.0X3	T60.0X4	—	—
Paraquat	T60.3X1	T60.3X2	T60.3X3	T60.3X4	—	—
Parasympatholytic NEC	T44.3X1	T44.3X2	T44.3X3	T44.3X4	T44.3X5	T44.3X6
Parasympathomimetic drug NEC	T44.1X1	T44.1X2	T44.1X3	T44.1X4	T44.1X5	T44.1X6
Parathion	T60.0X1	T60.0X2	T60.0X3	T60.0X4	—	—
Parathormone	T50.991	T50.992	T50.993	T50.994	T50.995	T50.996
Parathyroid extract	T50.991	T50.992	T50.993	T50.994	T50.995	T50.996
Paratyphoid vaccine	T50.A91	T50.A92	T50.A93	T50.A94	T50.A95	T50.A96
Paredrine	T44.4X1	T44.4X2	T44.4X3	T44.4X4	T44.4X5	T44.4X6
Paregoric	T40.0X1	T40.0X2	T40.0X3	T40.0X4	T40.0X5	T40.0X6
Pargyline	T46.5X1	T46.5X2	T46.5X3	T46.5X4	T46.5X5	T46.5X6
Paris green	T57.0X1	T57.0X2	T57.0X3	T57.0X4	—	—
insecticide	T57.0X1	T57.0X2	T57.0X3	T57.0X4	—	—
Parnate	T43.1X1	T43.1X2	T43.1X3	T43.1X4	T43.1X5	T43.1X6
Paromomycin	T36.5X1	T36.5X2	T36.5X3	T36.5X4	T36.5X5	T36.5X6
Paroxypropione	T45.1X1	T45.1X2	T45.1X3	T45.1X4	T45.1X5	T45.1X6
Parzone	T40.2X1	T40.2X2	T40.2X3	T40.2X4	T40.2X5	T40.2X6
PAS	T37.1X1	T37.1X2	T37.1X3	T37.1X4	T37.1X5	T37.1X6
Pasiniazid	T37.1X1	T37.1X2	T37.1X3	T37.1X4	T37.1X5	T37.1X6
PBB (polybrominated biphenyls)	T65.891	T65.892	T65.893	T65.894	—	—
PCB	T65.891	T65.892	T65.893	T65.894	—	—
PCP						
meaning pentachlorophenol	T60.1X1	T60.1X2	T60.1X3	T60.1X4	—	—
fungicide	T60.3X1	T60.3X2	T60.3X3	T60.3X4	—	—
herbicide	T60.3X1	T60.3X2	T60.3X3	T60.3X4	—	—
insecticide	T60.1X1	T60.1X2	T60.1X3	T60.1X4	—	—
meaning phencyclidine	T40.991	T40.992	T40.993	T40.994		
Peach kernel oil (emulsion)	T47.4X1	T47.4X2	T47.4X3	T47.4X4	T47.4X5	T47.4X6
Peanut oil (emulsion) NEC	T47.4X1	T47.4X2	T47.4X3	T47.4X4	T47.4X5	T47.4X6
topical	T49.3X1	T49.3X2	T49.3X3	T49.3X4	T49.3X5	T49.3X6
Pearly Gates (morning glory seeds)	T40.991	T40.992	T40.993	T40.994	—	—
Pecazine	T43.3X1	T43.3X2	T43.3X3	T43.3X4	T43.3X5	T43.3X6
Pectin	T47.6X1	T47.6X2	T47.6X3	T47.6X4	T47.6X5	T47.6X6

◀ New ◀ Revised ~~deleted~~ Deleted

TABLE OF DRUGS AND CHEMICALS

TABLE OF DRUGS AND CHEMICALS

	External Cause (T-Code)					
Substance	Poisoning, Accidental (Unintentional)	Poisoning, Intentional Self-Harm	Poisoning, Assault	Poisoning, Undetermined	Adverse Effect	Underdosing
Pefloxacin	T37.8X1	T37.8X2	T37.8X3	T37.8X4	T37.8X5	T37.8X6
Pegademase, bovine	T50.Z91	T50.Z92	T50.Z93	T50.Z94	T50.Z95	T50.Z96
Pelletierine tannate	T37.4X1	T37.4X2	T37.4X3	T37.4X4	T37.4X5	T37.4X6
Pemirolast (potassium)	T48.6X1	T48.6X2	T48.6X3	T48.6X4	T48.6X5	T48.6X6
Pemoline	T50.7X1	T50.7X2	T50.7X3	T50.7X4	T50.7X5	T50.7X6
Pempidine	T44.2X1	T44.2X2	T44.2X3	T44.2X4	T44.2X5	T44.2X6
Penamecillin	T36.0X1	T36.0X2	T36.0X3	T36.0X4	T36.0X5	T36.0X6
Penbutolol	T44.7X1	T44.7X2	T44.7X3	T44.7X4	T44.7X5	T44.7X6
Penethamate	T36.0X1	T36.0X2	T36.0X3	T36.0X4	T36.0X5	T36.0X6
Penfluridol	T43.591	T43.592	T43.593	T43.594	T43.595	T43.596
Penflutizide	T50.2X1	T50.2X2	T50.2X3	T50.2X4	T50.2X5	T50.2X6
Pengitoxin	T46.0X1	T46.0X2	T46.0X3	T46.0X4	T46.0X5	T46.0X6
Penicillamine	T50.6X1	T50.6X2	T50.6X3	T50.6X4	T50.6X5	T50.6X6
Penicillin (any)	T36.0X1	T36.0X2	T36.0X3	T36.0X4	T36.0X5	T36.0X6
Penicillinase	T45.3X1	T45.3X2	T45.3X3	T45.3X4	T45.3X5	T45.3X6
Penicilloyl polylysine	T50.8X1	T50.8X2	T50.8X3	T50.8X4	T50.8X5	T50.8X6
Penimepicycline	T36.4X1	T36.4X2	T36.4X3	T36.4X4	T36.4X5	T36.4X6
Pentachloroethane	T53.6X1	T53.6X2	T53.6X3	T53.6X4	—	—
Pentachloronaphthalene	T53.7X1	T53.7X2	T53.7X3	T53.7X4	—	—
Pentachlorophenol (pesticide)	T60.1X1	T60.1X2	T60.1X3	T60.1X4	—	—
fungicide	T60.3X1	T60.3X2	T60.3X3	T60.3X4	—	—
herbicide	T60.3X1	T60.3X2	T60.3X3	T60.3X4	—	—
insecticide	T60.1X1	T60.1X2	T60.1X3	T60.1X4	—	—
Pentaerythritol tetranitrate	T46.3X1	T46.3X2	T46.3X3	T46.3X4	T46.3X5	T46.3X6
Pentaerythritol	T46.3X1	T46.3X2	T46.3X3	T46.3X4	T46.3X5	T46.3X6
chloral	T42.6X1	T42.6X2	T42.6X3	T42.6X4	T42.6X5	T42.6X6
tetranitrate NEC	T46.3X1	T46.3X2	T46.3X3	T46.3X4	T46.3X5	T46.3X6
Pentagastrin	T50.8X1	T50.8X2	T50.8X3	T50.8X4	T50.8X5	T50.8X6
Pentalin	T53.6X1	T53.6X2	T53.6X3	T53.6X4	—	—
Pentamethonium bromide	T44.2X1	T44.2X2	T44.2X3	T44.2X4	T44.2X5	T44.2X6
Pentamidine	T37.3X1	T37.3X2	T37.3X3	T37.3X4	T37.3X5	T37.3X6
Pentanol	T51.3X1	T51.3X2	T51.3X3	T51.3X4	—	—
Pentapyrrolinium (bitartrate)	T44.2X1	T44.2X2	T44.2X3	T44.2X4	T44.2X5	T44.2X6
Pentaquine	T37.2X1	T37.2X2	T37.2X3	T37.2X4	T37.2X5	T37.2X6
Pentazocine	T40.491	T40.492	T40.493	T40.494	T40.495	T40.496
Pentetrazole	T50.7X1	T50.7X2	T50.7X3	T50.7X4	T50.7X5	T50.7X6
Penthienate bromide	T44.3X1	T44.3X2	T44.3X3	T44.3X4	T44.3X5	T44.3X6
Pentifylline	T46.7X1	T46.7X2	T46.7X3	T46.7X4	T46.7X5	T46.7X6
Pentobarbital	T42.3X1	T42.3X2	T42.3X3	T42.3X4	T42.3X5	T42.3X6
sodium	T42.3X1	T42.3X2	T42.3X3	T42.3X4	T42.3X5	T42.3X6
Pentobarbitone	T42.3X1	T42.3X2	T42.3X3	T42.3X4	T42.3X5	T42.3X6
Pentolonium tartrate	T44.2X1	T44.2X2	T44.2X3	T44.2X4	T44.2X5	T44.2X6

	External Cause (T-Code)					
Substance	Poisoning, Accidental (Unintentional)	Poisoning, Intentional Self-Harm	Poisoning, Assault	Poisoning, Undetermined	Adverse Effect	Underdosing
Pentosan polysulfate (sodium)	T39.8X1	T39.8X2	T39.8X3	T39.8X4	T39.8X5	T39.8X6
Pentostatin	T45.1X1	T45.1X2	T45.1X3	T45.1X4	T45.1X5	T45.1X6
Pentothal	T41.1X1	T41.1X2	T41.1X3	T41.1X4	T41.1X5	T41.1X6
Pentoxifylline	T46.7X1	T46.7X2	T46.7X3	T46.7X4	T46.7X5	T46.7X6
Pentoxyverine	T48.3X1	T48.3X2	T48.3X3	T48.3X4	T48.3X5	T48.3X6
Pentrinat	T46.3X1	T46.3X2	T46.3X3	T46.3X4	T46.3X5	T46.3X6
Pentylenetetrazole	T50.7X1	T50.7X2	T50.7X3	T50.7X4	T50.7X5	T50.7X6
Pentylsalicylamide	T37.1X1	T37.1X2	T37.1X3	T37.1X4	T37.1X5	T37.1X6
Pentymal	T42.3X1	T42.3X2	T42.3X3	T42.3X4	T42.3X5	T42.3X6
Peplomycin	T45.1X1	T45.1X2	T45.1X3	T45.1X4	T45.1X5	T45.1X6
Peppermint (oil)	T47.5X1	T47.5X2	T47.5X3	T47.5X4	T47.5X5	T47.5X6
Pepsin	T47.5X1	T47.5X2	T47.5X3	T47.5X4	T47.5X5	T47.5X6
digestant	T47.5X1	T47.5X2	T47.5X3	T47.5X4	T47.5X5	T47.5X6
Pepstatin	T47.1X1	T47.1X2	T47.1X3	T47.1X4	T47.1X5	T47.1X6
Peptavlon	T50.8X1	T50.8X2	T50.8X3	T50.8X4	T50.8X5	T50.8X6
Perazine	T43.3X1	T43.3X2	T43.3X3	T43.3X4	T43.3X5	T43.3X6
Percaine (spinal)	T41.3X1	T41.3X2	T41.3X3	T41.3X4	T41.3X5	T41.3X6
topical (surface)	T41.3X1	T41.3X2	T41.3X3	T41.3X4	T41.3X5	T41.3X6
Perchloroethylene	T53.3X1	T53.3X2	T53.3X3	T53.3X4	—	—
medicinal	T37.4X1	T37.4X2	T37.4X3	T37.4X4	T37.4X5	T37.4X6
vapor	T53.3X1	T53.3X2	T53.3X3	T53.3X4	—	—
Percodan	T40.2X1	T40.2X2	T40.2X3	T40.2X4	T40.2X5	T40.2X6
Percogesic — see also Acetaminophen	T45.0X1	T45.0X2	T45.0X3	T45.0X4	T45.0X5	T45.0X6
Percorten	T38.0X1	T38.0X2	T38.0X3	T38.0X4	T38.0X5	T38.0X6
Pergolide	T42.8X1	T42.8X2	T42.8X3	T42.8X4	T42.8X5	T42.8X6
Pergonal	T38.811	T38.812	T38.813	T38.814	T38.815	T38.816
Perhexilene	T46.3X1	T46.3X2	T46.3X3	T46.3X4	T46.3X5	T46.3X6
Perhexiline (maleate)	T46.3X1	T46.3X2	T46.3X3	T46.3X4	T46.3X5	T46.3X6
Periactin	T45.0X1	T45.0X2	T45.0X3	T45.0X4	T45.0X5	T45.0X6
Periciazine	T43.3X1	T43.3X2	T43.3X3	T43.3X4	T43.3X5	T43.3X6
Periclor	T42.6X1	T42.6X2	T42.6X3	T42.6X4	T42.6X5	T42.6X6
Perindopril	T46.4X1	T46.4X2	T46.4X3	T46.4X4	T46.4X5	T46.4X6
Perisoxal	T39.8X1	T39.8X2	T39.8X3	T39.8X4	T39.8X5	T39.8X6
Peritrate	T46.3X1	T46.3X2	T46.3X3	T46.3X4	T46.3X5	T46.3X6
Peritoneal dialysis solution	T50.3X1	T50.3X2	T50.3X3	T50.3X4	T50.3X5	T50.3X6
Perlapine	T42.4X1	T42.4X2	T42.4X3	T42.4X4	T42.4X5	T42.4X6
Permanganate	T65.891	T65.892	T65.893	T65.894	—	—
Permethrin	T60.1X1	T60.1X2	T60.1X3	T60.1X4	—	—
Pernocton	T42.3X1	T42.3X2	T42.3X3	T42.3X4	T42.3X5	T42.3X6
Pernoston	T42.3X1	T42.3X2	T42.3X3	T42.3X4	T42.3X5	T42.3X6
Peronine	T40.2X1	T40.2X2	T40.2X3	T40.2X4	—	—
Perphenazine	T43.3X1	T43.3X2	T43.3X3	T43.3X4	T43.3X5	T43.3X6

◄ New   ◄ Revised   ~~deleted~~ Deleted

	External Cause (T-Code)					
Substance	Poisoning, Accidental (Unintentional)	Poisoning, Intentional Self-Harm	Poisoning, Assault	Poisoning, Undetermined	Adverse Effect	Underdosing
Pertofrane	T43.011	T43.012	T43.013	T43.014	T43.015	T43.016
Pertussis						
immune serum (human)	T50.Z11	T50.Z12	T50.Z13	T50.Z14	T50.Z15	T50.Z16
vaccine (with diphtheria toxoid) (with tetanus toxoid)	T50.A11	T50.A12	T50.A13	T50.A14	T50.A15	T50.A16
Peruvian balsam	T49.0X1	T49.0X2	T49.0X3	T49.0X4	T49.0X5	T49.0X6
Peruvoside	T46.0X1	T46.0X2	T46.0X3	T46.0X4	T46.0X5	T46.0X6
Pesticide (dust) (fumes) (vapor) NEC	T60.91	T60.92	T60.93	T60.94	—	—
arsenic	T57.0X1	T57.0X2	T57.0X3	T57.0X4	—	—
chlorinated	T60.1X1	T60.1X2	T60.1X3	T60.1X4	—	—
cyanide	T65.0X1	T65.0X2	T65.0X3	T65.0X4	—	—
kerosene	T52.0X1	T52.0X2	T52.0X3	T52.0X4	—	—
mixture (of compounds)	T60.91	T60.92	T60.93	T60.94	—	—
naphthalene	T60.2X1	T60.2X2	T60.2X3	T60.2X4	—	—
organochlorine (compounds)	T60.1X1	T60.1X2	T60.1X3	T60.1X4	—	—
petroleum (distillate) (products) NEC	T60.8X1	T60.8X2	T60.8X3	T60.8X4	—	—
specified ingredient NEC	T60.8X1	T60.8X2	T60.8X3	T60.8X4	—	—
strychnine	T65.1X1	T65.1X2	T65.1X3	T65.1X4	—	—
thallium	T60.4X1	T60.4X2	T60.4X3	T60.4X4	—	—
Pethidine	T40.491	T40.492	T40.493	T40.494	T40.495	T40.496
Petrichloral	T42.6X1	T42.6X2	T42.6X3	T42.6X4	T42.6X5	T42.6X6
Petrol	T52.0X1	T52.0X2	T52.0X3	T52.0X4	—	—
vapor	T52.0X1	T52.0X2	T52.0X3	T52.0X4	—	—
Petrolatum	T49.3X1	T49.3X2	T49.3X3	T49.3X4	T49.3X5	T49.3X6
hydrophilic	T49.3X1	T49.3X2	T49.3X3	T49.3X4	T49.3X5	T49.3X6
liquid	T47.4X1	T47.4X2	T47.4X3	T47.4X4	T47.4X5	T47.4X6
topical	T49.3X1	T49.3X2	T49.3X3	T49.3X4	T49.3X5	T49.3X6
nonmedicinal	T52.0X1	T52.0X2	T52.0X3	T52.0X4	—	—
red veterinary	T49.3X1	T49.3X2	T49.3X3	T49.3X4	T49.3X5	T49.3X6
white	T49.3X1	T49.3X2	T49.3X3	T49.3X4	T49.3X5	T49.3X6
Petroleum (products) NEC	T52.0X1	T52.0X2	T52.0X3	T52.0X4	—	—
benzine(s) — see Ligroin						
ether — see Ligroin						
jelly — see Petrolatum						
naphtha — see Ligroin						
pesticide	T60.8X1	T60.8X2	T60.8X3	T60.8X4	—	—
solids	T52.0X1	T52.0X2	T52.0X3	T52.0X4	—	—
solvents	T52.0X1	T52.0X2	T52.0X3	T52.0X4	—	—
vapor	T52.0X1	T52.0X2	T52.0X3	T52.0X4	—	—
Peyote	T40.991	T40.992	T40.993	T40.994	—	—
Phanodorm, phanodorn	T42.3X1	T42.3X2	T42.3X3	T42.3X4	T42.3X5	T42.3X6

	External Cause (T-Code)					
Substance	Poisoning, Accidental (Unintentional)	Poisoning, Intentional Self-Harm	Poisoning, Assault	Poisoning, Undetermined	Adverse Effect	Underdosing
Phanquinone	T37.3X1	T37.3X2	T37.3X3	T37.3X4	T37.3X5	T37.3X6
Phanquone	T37.3X1	T37.3X2	T37.3X3	T37.3X4	T37.3X5	T37.3X6
Pharmaceutical						
adjunct NEC	T50.901	T50.902	T50.903	T50.904	T50.905	T50.906
excipient NEC	T50.901	T50.902	T50.903	T50.904	T50.905	T50.906
sweetener	T50.901	T50.902	T50.903	T50.904	T50.905	T50.906
viscous agent	T50.901	T50.902	T50.903	T50.904	T50.905	T50.906
Phemitone	T42.3X1	T42.3X2	T42.3X3	T42.3X4	T42.3X5	T42.3X6
Phenacaine	T41.3X1	T41.3X2	T41.3X3	T41.3X4	T41.3X5	T41.3X6
Phenacemide	T42.6X1	T42.6X2	T42.6X3	T42.6X4	T42.6X5	T42.6X6
Phenacetin	T39.1X1	T39.1X2	T39.1X3	T39.1X4	T39.1X5	T39.1X6
Phenadoxone	T40.2X1	T40.2X2	T40.2X3	T40.2X4	—	—
Phenaglycodol	T43.591	T43.592	T43.593	T43.594	T43.595	T43.596
Phenantoin	T42.0X1	T42.0X2	T42.0X3	T42.0X4	T42.0X5	T42.0X6
Phenaphthazine reagent	T50.991	T50.992	T50.993	T50.994	T50.995	T50.996
Phenazocine	T40.491	T40.492	T40.493	T40.494	T40.495	T40.496
Phenazone	T39.2X1	T39.2X2	T39.2X3	T39.2X4	T39.2X5	T39.2X6
Phenazopyridine	T39.8X1	T39.8X2	T39.8X3	T39.8X4	T39.8X5	T39.8X6
Phenbenicillin	T36.0X1	T36.0X2	T36.0X3	T36.0X4	T36.0X5	T36.0X6
Phenbutrazate	T50.5X1	T50.5X2	T50.5X3	T50.5X4	T50.5X5	T50.5X6
Phencyclidine	T40.991	T40.992	T40.993	T40.994	T40.995	T40.996
Phendimetrazine	T50.5X1	T50.5X2	T50.5X3	T50.5X4	T50.5X5	T50.5X6
Phenelzine	T43.1X1	T43.1X2	T43.1X3	T43.1X4	T43.1X5	T43.1X6
Phenemal	T42.3X1	T42.3X2	T42.3X3	T42.3X4	T42.3X5	T42.3X6
Phenergan	T42.6X1	T42.6X2	T42.6X3	T42.6X4	T42.6X5	T42.6X6
Pheneticillin	T36.0X1	T36.0X2	T36.0X3	T36.0X4	T36.0X5	T36.0X6
Pheneturide	T42.6X1	T42.6X2	T42.6X3	T42.6X4	T42.6X5	T42.6X6
Phenformin	T38.3X1	T38.3X2	T38.3X3	T38.3X4	T38.3X5	T38.3X6
Phenglutarimide	T44.3X1	T44.3X2	T44.3X3	T44.3X4	T44.3X5	T44.3X6
Phenicarbazide	T39.8X1	T39.8X2	T39.8X3	T39.8X4	T39.8X5	T39.8X6
Phenindamine	T45.0X1	T45.0X2	T45.0X3	T45.0X4	T45.0X5	T45.0X6
Phenindione	T45.511	T45.512	T45.513	T45.514	T45.515	T45.516
Pheniprazine	T43.1X1	T43.1X2	T43.1X3	T43.1X4	T43.1X5	T43.1X6
Pheniramine	T45.0X1	T45.0X2	T45.0X3	T45.0X4	T45.0X5	T45.0X6
Phenisatin	T47.2X1	T47.2X2	T47.2X3	T47.2X4	T47.2X5	T47.2X6
Phenmetrazine	T50.5X1	T50.5X2	T50.5X3	T50.5X4	T50.5X5	T50.5X6
Phenobal	T42.3X1	T42.3X2	T42.3X3	T42.3X4	T42.3X5	T42.3X6
Phenobarbital	T42.3X1	T42.3X2	T42.3X3	T42.3X4	T42.3X5	T42.3X6
with						
mephenytoin	T42.3X1	T42.3X2	T42.3X3	T42.3X4	T42.3X5	T42.3X6
phenytoin	T42.3X1	T42.3X2	T42.3X3	T42.3X4	T42.3X5	T42.3X6
sodium	T42.3X1	T42.3X2	T42.3X3	T42.3X4	T42.3X5	T42.3X6

TABLE OF DRUGS AND CHEMICALS

Substance	External Cause (T-Code)					
	Poisoning, Accidental (Unintentional)	Poisoning, Intentional Self-Harm	Poisoning, Assault	Poisoning, Undetermined	Adverse Effect	Underdosing
Phenobarbitone	T42.3X1	T42.3X2	T42.3X3	T42.3X4	T42.3X5	T42.3X6
Phenobutiodil	T50.8X1	T50.8X2	T50.8X3	T50.8X4	T50.8X5	T50.8X6
Phenoctide	T49.0X1	T49.0X2	T49.0X3	T49.0X4	T49.0X5	T49.0X6
Phenol	T49.0X1	T49.0X2	T49.0X3	T49.0X4	T49.0X5	T49.0X6
disinfectant	T54.0X1	T54.0X2	T54.0X3	T54.0X4	—	—
in oil injection	T46.8X1	T46.8X2	T46.8X3	T46.8X4	T46.8X5	T46.8X6
medicinal	T49.1X1	T49.1X2	T49.1X3	T49.1X4	T49.1X5	T49.1X6
nonmedicinal NEC	T54.0X1	T54.0X2	T54.0X3	T54.0X4	—	—
pesticide	T60.8X1	T60.8X2	T60.8X3	T60.8X4	—	—
red	T50.8X1	T50.8X2	T50.8X3	T50.8X4	T50.8X5	T50.8X6
Phenolic preparation	T49.1X1	T49.1X2	T49.1X3	T49.1X4	T49.1X5	T49.1X6
Phenolphthalein	T47.2X1	T47.2X2	T47.2X3	T47.2X4	T47.2X5	T47.2X6
Phenolsulfonphthalein	T50.8X1	T50.8X2	T50.8X3	T50.8X4	T50.8X5	T50.8X6
Phenomorphan	T40.2X1	T40.2X2	T40.2X3	T40.2X4	—	—
Phenonyl	T42.3X1	T42.3X2	T42.3X3	T42.3X4	T42.3X5	T42.3X6
Phenoperidine	T40.491	T40.492	T40.493	T40.494	—	—
Phenopyrazone	T46.991	T46.992	T46.993	T46.994	T46.995	T46.996
Phenoquin	T50.4X1	T50.4X2	T50.4X3	T50.4X4	T50.4X5	T50.4X6
Phenothiazine (psychotropic) NEC	T43.3X1	T43.3X2	T43.3X3	T43.3X4	T43.3X5	T43.3X6
insecticide	T60.2X1	T60.2X2	T60.2X3	T60.2X4	—	—
Phenothrin	T49.0X1	T49.0X2	T49.0X3	T49.0X4	T49.0X5	T49.0X6
Phenoxybenzamine	T46.7X1	T46.7X2	T46.7X3	T46.7X4	T46.7X5	T46.7X6
Phenoxyethanol	T49.0X1	T49.0X2	T49.0X3	T49.0X4	T49.0X5	T49.0X6
Phenoxymethyl penicillin	T36.0X1	T36.0X2	T36.0X3	T36.0X4	T36.0X5	T36.0X6
Phenprobamate	T42.8X1	T42.8X2	T42.8X3	T42.8X4	T42.8X5	T42.8X6
Phenprocoumon	T45.511	T45.512	T45.513	T45.514	T45.515	T45.516
Phensuximide	T42.2X1	T42.2X2	T42.2X3	T42.2X4	T42.2X5	T42.2X6
Phentermine	T50.5X1	T50.5X2	T50.5X3	T50.5X4	T50.5X5	T50.5X6
Phenthicillin	T36.0X1	T36.0X2	T36.0X3	T36.0X4	T36.0X5	T36.0X6
Phentolamine	T46.7X1	T46.7X2	T46.7X3	T46.7X4	T46.7X5	T46.7X6
Phenyl						
butazone	T39.2X1	T39.2X2	T39.2X3	T39.2X4	T39.2X5	T39.2X6
enediamine	T65.3X1	T65.3X2	T65.3X3	T65.3X4	—	—
hydrazine	T65.3X1	T65.3X2	T65.3X3	T65.3X4	—	—
antineoplastic	T45.1X1	T45.1X2	T45.1X3	T45.1X4	T45.1X5	T45.1X6
mercuric compounds — see Mercury						
salicylate	T49.3X1	T49.3X2	T49.3X3	T49.3X4	T49.3X5	T49.3X6
Phenylalanine mustard	T45.1X1	T45.1X2	T45.1X3	T45.1X4	T45.1X5	T45.1X6
Phenylbutazone	T39.2X1	T39.2X2	T39.2X3	T39.2X4	T39.2X5	T39.2X6
Phenylenediamine	T65.3X1	T65.3X2	T65.3X3	T65.3X4	—	—
Phenylephrine	T44.4X1	T44.4X2	T44.4X3	T44.4X4	T44.4X5	T44.4X6

Substance	External Cause (T-Code)					
	Poisoning, Accidental (Unintentional)	Poisoning, Intentional Self-Harm	Poisoning, Assault	Poisoning, Undetermined	Adverse Effect	Underdosing
Phenylethylbiguanide	T38.3X1	T38.3X2	T38.3X3	T38.3X4	T38.3X5	T38.3X6
Phenylmercuric						
acetate	T49.0X1	T49.0X2	T49.0X3	T49.0X4	T49.0X5	T49.0X6
borate	T49.0X1	T49.0X2	T49.0X3	T49.0X4	T49.0X5	T49.0X6
nitrate	T49.0X1	T49.0X2	T49.0X3	T49.0X4	T49.0X5	T49.0X6
Phenylmethylbarbitone	T42.3X1	T42.3X2	T42.3X3	T42.3X4	T42.3X5	T42.3X6
Phenylpropanol	T47.5X1	T47.5X2	T47.5X3	T47.5X4	T47.5X5	T47.5X6
Phenylpropanolamine	T44.991	T44.992	T44.993	T44.994	T44.995	T44.996
Phenylsulfthion	T60.0X1	T60.0X2	T60.0X3	T60.0X4	—	—
Phenyltoloxamine	T45.0X1	T45.0X2	T45.0X3	T45.0X4	T45.0X5	T45.0X6
Phenyramidol, phenyramidon	T39.8X1	T39.8X2	T39.8X3	T39.8X4	T39.8X5	T39.8X6
Phenytoin	T42.0X1	T42.0X2	T42.0X3	T42.0X4	T42.0X5	T42.0X6
with Phenobarbital	T42.3X1	T42.3X2	T42.3X3	T42.3X4	T42.3X5	T42.3X6
pHisoHex	T49.2X1	T49.2X2	T49.2X3	T49.2X4	T49.2X5	T49.2X6
Pholcodine	T48.3X1	T48.3X2	T48.3X3	T48.3X4	T48.3X5	T48.3X6
Pholedrine	T46.991	T46.992	T46.993	T46.994	T46.995	T46.996
Phorate	T60.0X1	T60.0X2	T60.0X3	T60.0X4	—	—
Phosdrin	T60.0X1	T60.0X2	T60.0X3	T60.0X4	—	—
Phosfolan	T60.0X1	T60.0X2	T60.0X3	T60.0X4	—	—
Phosgene (gas)	T59.891	T59.892	T59.893	T59.894		
Phosphamidon	T60.0X1	T60.0X2	T60.0X3	T60.0X4	—	—
Phosphate	T65.891	T65.892	T65.893	T65.894		
laxative	T47.4X1	T47.4X2	T47.4X3	T47.4X4	T47.4X5	T47.4X6
organic	T60.0X1	T60.0X2	T60.0X3	T60.0X4	—	—
solvent	T52.91	T52.92	T52.93	T52.94	—	—
tricresyl	T65.891	T65.892	T65.893	T65.894		
Phosphine	T57.1X1	T57.1X2	T57.1X3	T57.1X4		
fumigant	T57.1X1	T57.1X2	T57.1X3	T57.1X4		
Phospholine	T49.5X1	T49.5X2	T49.5X3	T49.5X4	T49.5X5	T49.5X6
Phosphoric acid	T54.2X1	T54.2X2	T54.2X3	T54.2X4		
Phosphorus (compound) NEC	T57.1X1	T57.1X2	T57.1X3	T57.1X4		
pesticide	T60.0X1	T60.0X2	T60.0X3	T60.0X4	—	—
Phthalates	T65.891	T65.892	T65.893	T65.894		
Phthalic anhydride	T65.891	T65.892	T65.893	T65.894		
Phthalimidoglutarimide	T42.6X1	T42.6X2	T42.6X3	T42.6X4	T42.6X5	T42.6X6
Phthalylsulfathiazole	T37.0X1	T37.0X2	T37.0X3	T37.0X4	T37.0X5	T37.0X6
Phylloquinone	T45.7X1	T45.7X2	T45.7X3	T45.7X4	T45.7X5	T45.7X6
Physeptone	T40.3X1	T40.3X2	T40.3X3	T40.3X4	T40.3X5	T40.3X6
Physostigma venenosum	T62.2X1	T62.2X2	T62.2X3	T62.2X4	—	—
Physostigmine	T49.5X1	T49.5X2	T49.5X3	T49.5X4	T49.5X5	T49.5X6
Phytolacca decandra	T62.2X1	T62.2X2	T62.2X3	T62.2X4	—	—
berries	T62.1X1	T62.1X2	T62.1X3	T62.1X4	—	—

◀ New   ◀ Revised   ~~deleted~~ Deleted

Substance	Poisoning, Accidental (Unintentional)	Poisoning, Intentional Self-Harm	Poisoning, Assault	Poisoning, Undetermined	Adverse Effect	Underdosing
Phytomenadione	T45.7X1	T45.7X2	T45.7X3	T45.7X4	T45.7X5	T45.7X6
Phytonadione	T45.7X1	T45.7X2	T45.7X3	T45.7X4	T45.7X5	T45.7X6
Picoperine	T48.3X1	T48.3X2	T48.3X3	T48.3X4	T48.3X5	T48.3X6
Picosulfate (sodium)	T47.2X1	T47.2X2	T47.2X3	T47.2X4	T47.2X5	T47.2X6
Picric (acid)	T54.2X1	T54.2X2	T54.2X3	T54.2X4	—	—
Picrotoxin	T50.7X1	T50.7X2	T50.7X3	T50.7X4	T50.7X5	T50.7X6
Piketoprofen	T49.0X1	T49.0X2	T49.0X3	T49.0X4	T49.0X5	T49.0X6
Pilocarpine	T44.1X1	T44.1X2	T44.1X3	T44.1X4	T44.1X5	T44.1X6
Pilocarpus (jaborandi) extract	T44.1X1	T44.1X2	T44.1X3	T44.1X4	T44.1X5	T44.1X6
Pilsicainide (hydrochloride)	T46.2X1	T46.2X2	T46.2X3	T46.2X4	T46.2X5	T46.2X6
Pimaricin	T36.7X1	T36.7X2	T36.7X3	T36.7X4	T36.7X5	T36.7X6
Pimeclone	T50.7X1	T50.7X2	T50.7X3	T50.7X4	T50.7X5	T50.7X6
Pimelic ketone	T52.8X1	T52.8X2	T52.8X3	T52.8X4	—	—
Pimethixene	T45.0X1	T45.0X2	T45.0X3	T45.0X4	T45.0X5	T45.0X6
Piminodine	T40.2X1	T40.2X2	T40.2X3	T40.2X4	T40.2X5	T40.2X6
Pimozide	T43.591	T43.592	T43.593	T43.594	T43.595	T43.596
Pinacidil	T46.5X1	T46.5X2	T46.5X3	T46.5X4	T46.5X5	T46.5X6
Pinaverium bromide	T44.3X1	T44.3X2	T44.3X3	T44.3X4	T44.3X5	T44.3X6
Pinazepam	T42.4X1	T42.4X2	T42.4X3	T42.4X4	T42.4X5	T42.4X6
Pindolol	T44.7X1	T44.7X2	T44.7X3	T44.7X4	T44.7X5	T44.7X6
Pindone	T60.4X1	T60.4X2	T60.4X3	T60.4X4	—	—
Pine oil (disinfectant)	T65.891	T65.892	T65.893	T65.894	—	—
Pinkroot	T37.4X1	T37.4X2	T37.4X3	T37.4X4	T37.4X5	T37.4X6
Pipadone	T40.2X1	T40.2X2	T40.2X3	T40.2X4	—	—
Pipamazine	T45.0X1	T45.0X2	T45.0X3	T45.0X4	T45.0X5	T45.0X6
Pipamperone	T43.4X1	T43.4X2	T43.4X3	T43.4X4	T43.4X5	T43.4X6
Pipazetate	T48.3X1	T48.3X2	T48.3X3	T48.3X4	T48.3X5	T48.3X6
Pipemidic acid	T37.8X1	T37.8X2	T37.8X3	T37.8X4	T37.8X5	T37.8X6
Pipenzolate bromide	T44.3X1	T44.3X2	T44.3X3	T44.3X4	T44.3X5	T44.3X6
Piperacetazine	T43.3X1	T43.3X2	T43.3X3	T43.3X4	T43.3X5	T43.3X6
Piperacillin	T36.0X1	T36.0X2	T36.0X3	T36.0X4	T36.0X5	T36.0X6
Piperazine	T37.4X1	T37.4X2	T37.4X3	T37.4X4	T37.4X5	T37.4X6
estrone sulfate	T38.5X1	T38.5X2	T38.5X3	T38.5X4	T38.5X5	T38.5X6
Piper cubeba	T62.2X1	T62.2X2	T62.2X3	T62.2X4	—	—
Piperidione	T48.3X1	T48.3X2	T48.3X3	T48.3X4	—	—
Piperidolate	T44.3X1	T44.3X2	T44.3X3	T44.3X4	T44.3X5	T44.3X6
Piperocaine	T41.3X1	T41.3X2	T41.3X3	T41.3X4	T41.3X5	T41.3X6
infiltration (subcutaneous)	T41.3X1	T41.3X2	T41.3X3	T41.3X4	T41.3X5	T41.3X6
nerve block (peripheral) (plexus)	T41.3X1	T41.3X2	T41.3X3	T41.3X4	T41.3X5	T41.3X6
topical (surface)	T41.3X1	T41.3X2	T41.3X3	T41.3X4	T41.3X5	T41.3X6
Piperonyl butoxide	T60.8X1	T60.8X2	T60.8X3	T60.8X4	—	—
Pipethanate	T44.3X1	T44.3X2	T44.3X3	T44.3X4	T44.3X5	T44.3X6

Substance	Poisoning, Accidental (Unintentional)	Poisoning, Intentional Self-Harm	Poisoning, Assault	Poisoning, Undetermined	Adverse Effect	Underdosing
Pipobroman	T45.1X1	T45.1X2	T45.1X3	T45.1X4	T45.1X5	T45.1X6
Pipofezine	T43.0X1	T43.0X2	T43.0X3	T43.0X4	T43.0X5	T43.0X6
Pipotiazine	T43.3X1	T43.3X2	T43.3X3	T43.3X4	T43.3X5	T43.3X6
Pipoxizine	T45.0X1	T45.0X2	T45.0X3	T45.0X4	T45.0X5	T45.0X6
Pipradrol	T43.691	T43.692	T43.693	T43.694	T43.695	T43.696
Piprinhydrinate	T45.0X1	T45.0X2	T45.0X3	T45.0X4	T45.0X5	T45.0X6
Pirarubicin	T45.1X1	T45.1X2	T45.1X3	T45.1X4	T45.1X5	T45.1X6
Pirazinamide	T37.1X1	T37.1X2	T37.1X3	T37.1X4	T37.1X5	T37.1X6
Pirbuterol	T48.6X1	T48.6X2	T48.6X3	T48.6X4	T48.6X5	T48.6X6
Pirenzepine	T47.1X1	T47.1X2	T47.1X3	T47.1X4	T47.1X5	T47.1X6
Piretanide	T50.1X1	T50.1X2	T50.1X3	T50.1X4	T50.1X5	T50.1X6
Piribedil	T42.8X1	T42.8X2	T42.8X3	T42.8X4	T42.8X5	T42.8X6
Piridoxilate	T46.3X1	T46.3X2	T46.3X3	T46.3X4	T46.3X5	T46.3X6
Piritramide	T40.491	T40.492	T40.493	T40.494	—	—
Pirlindole	T43.0X1	T43.0X2	T43.0X3	T43.0X4	T43.0X5	T43.0X6
Piromidic acid	T37.8X1	T37.8X2	T37.8X3	T37.8X4	T37.8X5	T37.8X6
Piroxicam	T39.391	T39.392	T39.393	T39.394	T39.395	T39.396
beta-cyclodextrin complex	T39.8X1	T39.8X2	T39.8X3	T39.8X4	T39.8X5	T39.8X6
Pirozadil	T46.6X1	T46.6X2	T46.6X3	T46.6X4	T46.6X5	T46.6X6
Piscidia (bark) (erythrina)	T39.8X1	T39.8X2	T39.8X3	T39.8X4	T39.8X5	T39.8X6
Pitch	T65.891	T65.892	T65.893	T65.894	—	—
Pitkin's solution	T41.3X1	T41.3X2	T41.3X3	T41.3X4	T41.3X5	T41.3X6
Pitocin	T48.0X1	T48.0X2	T48.0X3	T48.0X4	T48.0X5	T48.0X6
Pitressin (tannate)	T38.891	T38.892	T38.893	T38.894	T38.895	T38.896
Pituitary extracts (posterior)	T38.891	T38.892	T38.893	T38.894	T38.895	T38.896
anterior	T38.811	T38.812	T38.813	T38.814	T38.815	T38.816
Pituitrin	T38.891	T38.892	T38.893	T38.894	T38.895	T38.896
Pivampicillin	T36.0X1	T36.0X2	T36.0X3	T36.0X4	T36.0X5	T36.0X6
Pivmecillinam	T36.0X1	T36.0X2	T36.0X3	T36.0X4	T36.0X5	T36.0X6
Placental hormone	T38.891	T38.892	T38.893	T38.894	T38.895	T38.896
Placidyl	T42.6X1	T42.6X2	T42.6X3	T42.6X4	T42.6X5	T42.6X6
Plague vaccine	T50.A91	T50.A92	T50.A93	T50.A94	T50.A95	T50.A96
Plant						
food or fertilizer NEC	T65.891	T65.892	T65.893	T65.894	—	—
containing herbicide	T60.3X1	T60.3X2	T60.3X3	T60.3X4	—	—
noxious, used as food	T62.2X1	T62.2X2	T62.2X3	T62.2X4	—	—
berries	T62.1X1	T62.1X2	T62.1X3	T62.1X4	—	—
seeds	T62.2X1	T62.2X2	T62.2X3	T62.2X4	—	—
specified type NEC	T62.2X1	T62.2X2	T62.2X3	T62.2X4	—	—
Plasma	T45.8X1	T45.8X2	T45.8X3	T45.8X4	T45.8X5	T45.8X6
expander NEC	T45.8X1	T45.8X2	T45.8X3	T45.8X4	T45.8X5	T45.8X6
protein fraction (human)	T45.8X1	T45.8X2	T45.8X3	T45.8X4	T45.8X5	T45.8X6

◀ New ◀ Revised ~~deleted~~ Deleted

Substance	Poisoning, Accidental (Unintentional)	Poisoning, Intentional Self-Harm	Poisoning, Assault	Poisoning, Undetermined	Adverse Effect	Underdosing
Plasmanate	T45.8X1	T45.8X2	T45.8X3	T45.8X4	T45.8X5	T45.8X6
Plasminogen (tissue) activator	T45.611	T45.612	T45.613	T45.614	T45.615	T45.616
Plaster dressing	T49.3X1	T49.3X2	T49.3X3	T49.3X4	T49.3X5	T49.3X6
Plastic dressing	T49.3X1	T49.3X2	T49.3X3	T49.3X4	T49.3X5	T49.3X6
Plegicil	T43.3X1	T43.3X2	T43.3X3	T43.3X4	T43.3X5	T43.3X6
Plicamycin	T45.1X1	T45.1X2	T45.1X3	T45.1X4	T45.1X5	T45.1X6
Podophyllotoxin	T49.8X1	T49.8X2	T49.8X3	T49.8X4	T49.8X5	T49.8X6
Podophyllum (resin)	T49.4X1	T49.4X2	T49.4X3	T49.4X4	T49.4X5	T49.4X6
Poison NEC	T65.91	T65.92	T65.93	T65.94	—	—
Poisonous berries	T62.1X1	T62.1X2	T62.1X3	T62.1X4	—	—
Pokeweed (any part)	T62.2X1	T62.2X2	T62.2X3	T62.2X4	—	—
Poldine metilsulfate	T44.3X1	T44.3X2	T44.3X3	T44.3X4	T44.3X5	T44.3X6
Polidexide (sulfate)	T46.6X1	T46.6X2	T46.6X3	T46.6X4	T46.6X5	T46.6X6
Polidocanol	T46.8X1	T46.8X2	T46.8X3	T46.8X4	T46.8X5	T46.8X6
Poliomyelitis vaccine	T50.B91	T50.B92	T50.B93	T50.B94	T50.B95	T50.B96
Polish (car) (floor) (furniture) (metal) (porcelain) (silver)	T65.891	T65.892	T65.893	T65.894	—	—
abrasive	T65.891	T65.892	T65.893	T65.894	—	—
porcelain	T65.891	T65.892	T65.893	T65.894	—	—
Poloxalkol	T47.4X1	T47.4X2	T47.4X3	T47.4X4	T47.4X5	T47.4X6
Poloxamer	T47.4X1	T47.4X2	T47.4X3	T47.4X4	T47.4X5	T47.4X6
Polyaminostyrene resins	T50.3X1	T50.3X2	T50.3X3	T50.3X4	T50.3X5	T50.3X6
Polycarbophil	T47.4X1	T47.4X2	T47.4X3	T47.4X4	T47.4X5	T47.4X6
Polychlorinated biphenyl	T65.891	T65.892	T65.893	T65.894	—	—
Polycycline	T36.4X1	T36.4X2	T36.4X3	T36.4X4	T36.4X5	T36.4X6
Polyester fumes	T59.891	T59.892	T59.893	T59.894	—	—
Polyester resin hardener	T52.91	T52.92	T52.93	T52.94	—	—
fumes	T59.891	T59.892	T59.893	T59.894	—	—
Polyestradiol phosphate	T38.5X1	T38.5X2	T38.5X3	T38.5X4	T38.5X5	T38.5X6
Polyethanolamine alkyl sulfate	T49.2X1	T49.2X2	T49.2X3	T49.2X4	T49.2X5	T49.2X6
Polyethylene adhesive	T49.3X1	T49.3X2	T49.3X3	T49.3X4	T49.3X5	T49.3X6
Polyferose	T45.4X1	T45.4X2	T45.4X3	T45.4X4	T45.4X5	T45.4X6
Polygeline	T45.8X1	T45.8X2	T45.8X3	T45.8X4	T45.8X5	T45.8X6
Polymyxin	T36.8X1	T36.8X2	T36.8X3	T36.8X4	T36.8X5	T36.8X6
B	T36.8X1	T36.8X2	T36.8X3	T36.8X4	T36.8X5	T36.8X6
ENT agent	T49.6X1	T49.6X2	T49.6X3	T49.6X4	T49.6X5	T49.6X6
ophthalmic preparation	T49.5X1	T49.5X2	T49.5X3	T49.5X4	T49.5X5	T49.5X6
topical NEC	T49.0X1	T49.0X2	T49.0X3	T49.0X4	T49.0X5	T49.0X6
E sulfate (eye preparation)	T49.5X1	T49.5X2	T49.5X3	T49.5X4	T49.5X5	T49.5X6
Polynoxylin	T49.0X1	T49.0X2	T49.0X3	T49.0X4	T49.0X5	T49.0X6
Polyoestradiol phosphate	T38.5X1	T38.5X2	T38.5X3	T38.5X4	T38.5X5	T38.5X6
Polyoxymethyleneurea	T49.0X1	T49.0X2	T49.0X3	T49.0X4	T49.0X5	T49.0X6

Substance	Poisoning, Accidental (Unintentional)	Poisoning, Intentional Self-Harm	Poisoning, Assault	Poisoning, Undetermined	Adverse Effect	Underdosing
Polysilane	T47.8X1	T47.8X2	T47.8X3	T47.8X4	T47.8X5	T47.8X6
Polytetrafluoroethylene (inhaled)	T59.891	T59.892	T59.893	T59.894	—	—
Polythiazide	T50.2X1	T50.2X2	T50.2X3	T50.2X4	T50.2X5	T50.2X6
Polyvidone	T45.8X1	T45.8X2	T45.8X3	T45.8X4	T45.8X5	T45.8X6
Polyvinylpyrrolidone	T45.8X1	T45.8X2	T45.8X3	T45.8X4	T45.8X5	T45.8X6
Pontocaine (hydrochloride) (infiltration) (topical)	T41.3X1	T41.3X2	T41.3X3	T41.3X4	T41.3X5	T41.3X6
nerve block (peripheral) (plexus)	T41.3X1	T41.3X2	T41.3X3	T41.3X4	T41.3X5	T41.3X6
spinal	T41.3X1	T41.3X2	T41.3X3	T41.3X4	T41.3X5	T41.3X6
Porfiromycin	T45.1X1	T45.1X2	T45.1X3	T45.1X4	T45.1X5	T45.1X6
Posterior pituitary hormone NEC	T38.891	T38.892	T38.893	T38.894	T38.895	T38.896
Pot	T40.711	T40.712	T40.713	T40.714	T40.715	T40.716
Potash (caustic)	T54.3X1	T54.3X2	T54.3X3	T54.3X4	—	—
Potassic saline injection (lactated)	T50.3X1	T50.3X2	T50.3X3	T50.3X4	T50.3X5	T50.3X6
Potassium (salts) NEC	T50.3X1	T50.3X2	T50.3X3	T50.3X4	T50.3X5	T50.3X6
aminobenzoate	T45.8X1	T45.8X2	T45.8X3	T45.8X4	T45.8X5	T45.8X6
aminosalicylate	T37.1X1	T37.1X2	T37.1X3	T37.1X4	T37.1X5	T37.1X6
antimony 'tartrate'	T37.8X1	T37.8X2	T37.8X3	T37.8X4	T37.8X5	T37.8X6
arsenite (solution)	T57.0X1	T57.0X2	T57.0X3	T57.0X4	—	—
bichromate	T56.2X1	T56.2X2	T56.2X3	T56.2X4	—	—
bisulfate	T47.3X1	T47.3X2	T47.3X3	T47.3X4	T47.3X5	T47.3X6
bromide	T42.6X1	T42.6X2	T42.6X3	T42.6X4	T42.6X5	T42.6X6
canrenoate	T50.0X1	T50.0X2	T50.0X3	T50.0X4	T50.0X5	T50.0X6
carbonate	T54.3X1	T54.3X2	T54.3X3	T54.3X4	—	—
chlorate NEC	T65.891	T65.892	T65.893	T65.894	—	—
chloride	T50.3X1	T50.3X2	T50.3X3	T50.3X4	T50.3X5	T50.3X6
citrate	T50.991	T50.992	T50.993	T50.994	T50.995	T50.996
cyanide	T65.0X1	T65.0X2	T65.0X3	T65.0X4	—	—
ferric hexacyanoferrate (medicinal)	T50.6X1	T50.6X2	T50.6X3	T50.6X4	T50.6X5	T50.6X6
nonmedicinal	T65.891	T65.892	T65.893	T65.894	—	—
Fluoride	T57.8X1	T57.8X2	T57.8X3	T57.8X4	—	—
glucaldrate	T47.1X1	T47.1X2	T47.1X3	T47.1X4	T47.1X5	T47.1X6
hydroxide	T54.3X1	T54.3X2	T54.3X3	T54.3X4	—	—
iodate	T49.0X1	T49.0X2	T49.0X3	T49.0X4	T49.0X5	T49.0X6
iodide	T48.4X1	T48.4X2	T48.4X3	T48.4X4	T48.4X5	T48.4X6
nitrate	T57.8X1	T57.8X2	T57.8X3	T57.8X4	—	—
oxalate	T65.891	T65.892	T65.893	T65.894	—	—
perchlorate (nonmedicinal) NEC	T65.891	T65.892	T65.893	T65.894	—	—
antithyroid	T38.2X1	T38.2X2	T38.2X3	T38.2X4	T38.2X5	T38.2X6
medicinal	T38.2X1	T38.2X2	T38.2X3	T38.2X4	T38.2X5	T38.2X6

◀ New ◀ Revised ~~deleted~~ Deleted

Substance	Poisoning, Accidental (Unintentional)	Poisoning, Intentional Self-Harm	Poisoning, Assault	Poisoning, Undetermined	Adverse Effect	Underdosing
Permanganate (nonmedicinal)	T65.891	T65.892	T65.893	T65.894	—	—
medicinal	T49.0X1	T49.0X2	T49.0X3	T49.0X4	T49.0X5	T49.0X6
sulfate	T47.2X1	T47.2X2	T47.2X3	T47.2X4	T47.2X5	T47.2X6
Potassium-removing resin	T50.3X1	T50.3X2	T50.3X3	T50.3X4	T50.3X5	T50.3X6
Potassium-retaining drug	T50.3X1	T50.3X2	T50.3X3	T50.3X4	T50.3X5	T50.3X6
Povidone	T45.8X1	T45.8X2	T45.8X3	T45.8X4	T45.8X5	T45.8X6
iodine	T49.0X1	T49.0X2	T49.0X3	T49.0X4	T49.0X5	T49.0X6
Practolol	T44.7X1	T44.7X2	T44.7X3	T44.7X4	T44.7X5	T44.7X6
Prajmalium bitartrate	T46.2X1	T46.2X2	T46.2X3	T46.2X4	T46.2X5	T46.2X6
Pralidoxime (iodide)	T50.6X1	T50.6X2	T50.6X3	T50.6X4	T50.6X5	T50.6X6
chloride	T50.6X1	T50.6X2	T50.6X3	T50.6X4	T50.6X5	T50.6X6
Pramiverine	T44.3X1	T44.3X2	T44.3X3	T44.3X4	T44.3X5	T44.3X6
Pramocaine	T49.1X1	T49.1X2	T49.1X3	T49.1X4	T49.1X5	T49.1X6
Pramoxine	T49.1X1	T49.1X2	T49.1X3	T49.1X4	T49.1X5	T49.1X6
Prasterone	T38.7X1	T38.7X2	T38.7X3	T38.7X4	T38.7X5	T38.7X6
Pravastatin	T46.6X1	T46.6X2	T46.6X3	T46.6X4	T46.6X5	T46.6X6
Prazepam	T42.4X1	T42.4X2	T42.4X3	T42.4X4	T42.4X5	T42.4X6
Praziquantel	T37.4X1	T37.4X2	T37.4X3	T37.4X4	T37.4X5	T37.4X6
Prazitone	T43.291	T43.292	T43.293	T43.294	T43.295	T43.296
Prazosin	T44.6X1	T44.6X2	T44.6X3	T44.6X4	T44.6X5	T44.6X6
Prednicarbate	T49.0X1	T49.0X2	T49.0X3	T49.0X4	T49.0X5	T49.0X6
Prednimustine	T45.1X1	T45.1X2	T45.1X3	T45.1X4	T45.1X5	T45.1X6
Prednisolone	T38.0X1	T38.0X2	T38.0X3	T38.0X4	T38.0X5	T38.0X6
ENT agent	T49.6X1	T49.6X2	T49.6X3	T49.6X4	T49.6X5	T49.6X6
ophthalmic preparation	T49.5X1	T49.5X2	T49.5X3	T49.5X4	T49.5X5	T49.5X6
steaglate	T49.0X1	T49.0X2	T49.0X3	T49.0X4	T49.0X5	T49.0X6
topical NEC	T49.0X1	T49.0X2	T49.0X3	T49.0X4	T49.0X5	T49.0X6
Prednisone	T38.0X1	T38.0X2	T38.0X3	T38.0X4	T38.0X5	T38.0X6
Prednylidene	T38.0X1	T38.0X2	T38.0X3	T38.0X4	T38.0X5	T38.0X6
Pregnandiol	T38.5X1	T38.5X2	T38.5X3	T38.5X4	T38.5X5	T38.5X6
Pregneninolone	T38.5X1	T38.5X2	T38.5X3	T38.5X4	T38.5X5	T38.5X6
Preludin	T43.691	T43.692	T43.693	T43.694	T43.695	T43.696
Premarin	T38.5X1	T38.5X2	T38.5X3	T38.5X4	T38.5X5	T38.5X6
Premedication anesthetic	T41.201	T41.202	T41.203	T41.204	T41.205	T41.206
Prenalterol	T44.5X1	T44.5X2	T44.5X3	T44.5X4	T44.5X5	T44.5X6
Prenoxdiazine	T48.3X1	T48.3X2	T48.3X3	T48.3X4	T48.3X5	T48.3X6
Prenylamine	T46.3X1	T46.3X2	T46.3X3	T46.3X4	T46.3X5	T46.3X6
Preparation, local	T49.4X1	T49.4X2	T49.4X3	T49.4X4	T49.4X5	T49.4X6
Preparation H	T49.8X1	T49.8X2	T49.8X3	T49.8X4	T49.8X5	T49.8X6
Preservative (nonmedicinal)	T65.891	T65.892	T65.893	T65.894	—	—
medicinal	T50.901	T50.902	T50.903	T50.904	T50.905	T50.906
wood	T60.91	T60.92	T60.93	T60.94	—	—

Substance	Poisoning, Accidental (Unintentional)	Poisoning, Intentional Self-Harm	Poisoning, Assault	Poisoning, Undetermined	Adverse Effect	Underdosing
Prethcamide	T50.7X1	T50.7X2	T50.7X3	T50.7X4	T50.7X5	T50.7X6
Pride of China	T62.2X1	T62.2X2	T62.2X3	T62.2X4	—	—
Pridinol	T44.3X1	T44.3X2	T44.3X3	T44.3X4	T44.3X5	T44.3X6
Prifinium bromide	T44.3X1	T44.3X2	T44.3X3	T44.3X4	T44.3X5	T44.3X6
Prilocaine	T41.3X1	T41.3X2	T41.3X3	T41.3X4	T41.3X5	T41.3X6
infiltration (subcutaneous)	T41.3X1	T41.3X2	T41.3X3	T41.3X4	T41.3X5	T41.3X6
nerve block (peripheral) (plexus)	T41.3X1	T41.3X2	T41.3X3	T41.3X4	T41.3X5	T41.3X6
regional	T41.3X1	T41.3X2	T41.3X3	T41.3X4	T41.3X5	T41.3X6
Primaquine	T37.2X1	T37.2X2	T37.2X3	T37.2X4	T37.2X5	T37.2X6
Primidone	T42.6X1	T42.6X2	T42.6X3	T42.6X4	T42.6X5	T42.6X6
Primula (veris)	T62.2X1	T62.2X2	T62.2X3	T62.2X4	—	—
Prinadol	T40.2X1	T40.2X2	T40.2X3	T40.2X4	T40.2X5	T40.2X6
Priscol, Priscoline	T44.6X1	T44.6X2	T44.6X3	T44.6X4	T44.6X5	T44.6X6
Pristinamycin	T36.3X1	T36.3X2	T36.3X3	T36.3X4	T36.3X5	T36.3X6
Privet	T62.2X1	T62.2X2	T62.2X3	T62.2X4	—	—
berries	T62.1X1	T62.1X2	T62.1X3	T62.1X4	—	—
Privine	T44.4X1	T44.4X2	T44.4X3	T44.4X4	T44.4X5	T44.4X6
Pro-Banthine	T44.3X1	T44.3X2	T44.3X3	T44.3X4	T44.3X5	T44.3X6
Probarbital	T42.3X1	T42.3X2	T42.3X3	T42.3X4	T42.3X5	T42.3X6
Probenecid	T50.4X1	T50.4X2	T50.4X3	T50.4X4	T50.4X5	T50.4X6
Probucol	T46.6X1	T46.6X2	T46.6X3	T46.6X4	T46.6X5	T46.6X6
Procainamide	T46.2X1	T46.2X2	T46.2X3	T46.2X4	T46.2X5	T46.2X6
Procaine	T41.3X1	T41.3X2	T41.3X3	T41.3X4	T41.3X5	T41.3X6
benzylpenicillin	T36.0X1	T36.0X2	T36.0X3	T36.0X4	T36.0X5	T36.0X6
nerve block (periphreal) (plexus)	T41.3X1	T41.3X2	T41.3X3	T41.3X4	T41.3X5	T41.3X6
penicillin G	T36.0X1	T36.0X2	T36.0X3	T36.0X4	T36.0X5	T36.0X6
regional	T41.3X1	T41.3X2	T41.3X3	T41.3X4	T41.3X5	T41.3X6
spinal	T41.3X1	T41.3X2	T41.3X3	T41.3X4	T41.3X5	T41.3X6
Procalmidol	T43.591	T43.592	T43.593	T43.594	T43.595	T43.596
Procarbazine	T45.1X1	T45.1X2	T45.1X3	T45.1X4	T45.1X5	T45.1X6
Procaterol	T44.5X1	T44.5X2	T44.5X3	T44.5X4	T44.5X5	T44.5X6
Prochlorperazine	T43.3X1	T43.3X2	T43.3X3	T43.3X4	T43.3X5	T43.3X6
Procyclidine	T44.3X1	T44.3X2	T44.3X3	T44.3X4	T44.3X5	T44.3X6
Producer gas	T58.8X1	T58.8X2	T58.8X3	T58.8X4	—	—
Profadol	T40.491	T40.492	T40.493	T40.494	T40.495	T40.496
Profenamine	T44.3X1	T44.3X2	T44.3X3	T44.3X4	T44.3X5	T44.3X6
Profenil	T44.3X1	T44.3X2	T44.3X3	T44.3X4	T44.3X5	T44.3X6
Proflavine	T49.0X1	T49.0X2	T49.0X3	T49.0X4	T49.0X5	T49.0X6
Progabide	T42.6X1	T42.6X2	T42.6X3	T42.6X4	T42.6X5	T42.6X6
Progestin	T38.5X1	T38.5X2	T38.5X3	T38.5X4	T38.5X5	T38.5X6
oral contraceptive	T38.4X1	T38.4X2	T38.4X3	T38.4X4	T38.4X5	T38.4X6

TABLE OF DRUGS AND CHEMICALS

Substance	Poisoning, Accidental (Unintentional)	Poisoning, Intentional Self-Harm	Poisoning, Assault	Poisoning, Undetermined	Adverse Effect	Underdosing
Progesterone	T38.5X1	T38.5X2	T38.5X3	T38.5X4	T38.5X5	T38.5X6
Progestogen NEC	T38.5X1	T38.5X2	T38.5X3	T38.5X4	T38.5X5	T38.5X6
Progestone	T38.5X1	T38.5X2	T38.5X3	T38.5X4	T38.5X5	T38.5X6
Proglumide	T47.1X1	T47.1X2	T47.1X3	T47.1X4	T47.1X5	T47.1X6
Proguanil	T37.2X1	T37.2X2	T37.2X3	T37.2X4	T37.2X5	T37.2X6
Prolactin	T38.811	T38.812	T38.813	T38.814	T38.815	T38.816
Prolintane	T43.691	T43.692	T43.693	T43.694	T43.695	T43.696
Proloid	T38.1X1	T38.1X2	T38.1X3	T38.1X4	T38.1X5	T38.1X6
Proluton	T38.5X1	T38.5X2	T38.5X3	T38.5X4	T38.5X5	T38.5X6
Promacetin	T37.1X1	T37.1X2	T37.1X3	T37.1X4	T37.1X5	T37.1X6
Promazine	T43.3X1	T43.3X2	T43.3X3	T43.3X4	T43.3X5	T43.3X6
Promedol	T40.2X1	T40.2X2	T40.2X3	T40.2X4	—	—
Promegestone	T38.5X1	T38.5X2	T38.5X3	T38.5X4	T38.5X5	T38.5X6
Promethazine (teoclate)	T43.3X1	T43.3X2	T43.3X3	T43.3X4	T43.3X5	T43.3X6
Promin	T37.1X1	T37.1X2	T37.1X3	T37.1X4	T37.1X5	T37.1X6
Pronase	T45.3X1	T45.3X2	T45.3X3	T45.3X4	T45.3X5	T45.3X6
Pronestyl (hydrochloride)	T46.2X1	T46.2X2	T46.2X3	T46.2X4	T46.2X5	T46.2X6
Pronetalol	T44.7X1	T44.7X2	T44.7X3	T44.7X4	T44.7X5	T44.7X6
Prontosil	T37.0X1	T37.0X2	T37.0X3	T37.0X4	T37.0X5	T37.0X6
Propachlor	T60.3X1	T60.3X2	T60.3X3	T60.3X4	—	—
Propafenone	T46.2X1	T46.2X2	T46.2X3	T46.2X4	T46.2X5	T46.2X6
Propallylonal	T42.3X1	T42.3X2	T42.3X3	T42.3X4	T42.3X5	T42.3X6
Propamidine	T49.0X1	T49.0X2	T49.0X3	T49.0X4	T49.0X5	T49.0X6
Propane (distributed in mobile container)	T59.891	T59.892	T59.893	T59.894	—	—
distributed through pipes	T59.891	T59.892	T59.893	T59.894	—	—
incomplete combustion	T57.11	T57.12	T57.13	T57.14	—	—
Propanidid	T41.291	T41.292	T41.293	T41.294	T41.295	T41.296
Propanil	T60.3X1	T60.3X2	T60.3X3	T60.3X4	—	—
1-Propanol	T51.3X1	T51.3X2	T51.3X3	T51.3X4	—	—
2-Propanol	T51.2X1	T51.2X2	T51.2X3	T51.2X4	—	—
Propantheline	T44.3X1	T44.3X2	T44.3X3	T44.3X4	T44.3X5	T44.3X6
bromide	T44.3X1	T44.3X2	T44.3X3	T44.3X4	T44.3X5	T44.3X6
Proparacaine	T41.3X1	T41.3X2	T41.3X3	T41.3X4	T41.3X5	T41.3X6
Propatylnitrate	T46.3X1	T46.3X2	T46.3X3	T46.3X4	T46.3X5	T46.3X6
Propicillin	T36.0X1	T36.0X2	T36.0X3	T36.0X4	T36.0X5	T36.0X6
Propiolactone	T49.0X1	T49.0X2	T49.0X3	T49.0X4	T49.0X5	T49.0X6
Propiomazine	T45.0X1	T45.0X2	T45.0X3	T45.0X4	T45.0X5	T45.0X6
Propionaldehyde (medicinal)	T42.6X1	T42.6X2	T42.6X3	T42.6X4	T42.6X5	T42.6X6
Propionate (calcium) (sodium)	T49.0X1	T49.0X2	T49.0X3	T49.0X4	T49.0X5	T49.0X6
Propion gel	T49.0X1	T49.0X2	T49.0X3	T49.0X4	T49.0X5	T49.0X6

Substance	Poisoning, Accidental (Unintentional)	Poisoning, Intentional Self-Harm	Poisoning, Assault	Poisoning, Undetermined	Adverse Effect	Underdosing
Propitocaine	T41.3X1	T41.3X2	T41.3X3	T41.3X4	T41.3X5	T41.3X6
infiltration (subcutaneous)	T41.3X1	T41.3X2	T41.3X3	T41.3X4	T41.3X5	T41.3X6
nerve block (peripheral) (plexus)	T41.3X1	T41.3X2	T41.3X3	T41.3X4	T41.3X5	T41.3X6
Propofol	T41.291	T41.292	T41.293	T41.294	T41.295	T41.296
Propoxur	T60.0X1	T60.0X2	T60.0X3	T60.0X4	—	—
Propoxycaine	T41.3X1	T41.3X2	T41.3X3	T41.3X4	T41.3X5	T41.3X6
infiltration (subcutaneous)	T41.3X1	T41.3X2	T41.3X3	T41.3X4	T41.3X5	T41.3X6
nerve block (peripheral) (plexus)	T41.3X1	T41.3X2	T41.3X3	T41.3X4	T41.3X5	T41.3X6
topical (surface)	T41.3X1	T41.3X2	T41.3X3	T41.3X4	T41.3X5	T41.3X6
Propoxyphene	T40.491	T40.492	T40.493	T40.494	T40.495	T40.496
Propranolol	T44.7X1	T44.7X2	T44.7X3	T44.7X4	T44.7X5	T44.7X6
Propyl						
alcohol	T51.3X1	T51.3X2	T51.3X3	T51.3X4	—	—
carbinol	T51.3X1	T51.3X2	T51.3X3	T51.3X4	—	—
hexadrine	T44.4X1	T44.4X2	T44.4X3	T44.4X4	T44.4X5	T44.4X6
iodone	T50.8X1	T50.8X2	T50.8X3	T50.8X4	T50.8X5	T50.8X6
thiouracil	T38.2X1	T38.2X2	T38.2X3	T38.2X4	T38.2X5	T38.2X6
Propylaminophenothiazine	T43.3X1	T43.3X2	T43.3X3	T43.3X4	T43.3X5	T43.3X6
Propylene	T59.891	T59.892	T59.893	T59.894	—	—
Propylhexedrine	T48.5X1	T48.5X2	T48.5X3	T48.5X4	T48.5X5	T48.5X6
Propyliodone	T50.8X1	T50.8X2	T50.8X3	T50.8X4	T50.8X5	T50.8X6
Propylthiouracil	T38.2X1	T38.2X2	T38.2X3	T38.2X4	T38.2X5	T38.2X6
Propylparaben (ophthalmic)	T49.5X1	T49.5X2	T49.5X3	T49.5X4	T49.5X5	T49.5X6
Propyphenazone	T39.2X1	T39.2X2	T39.2X3	T39.2X4	T39.2X5	T39.2X6
Proquazone	T39.391	T39.392	T39.393	T39.394	T39.395	T39.396
Proscillaridin	T46.0X1	T46.0X2	T46.0X3	T46.0X4	T46.0X5	T46.0X6
Prostacyclin	T45.521	T45.522	T45.523	T45.524	T45.525	T45.526
Prostaglandin (I2)	T45.521	T45.522	T45.523	T45.524	T45.525	T45.526
E1	T46.7X1	T46.7X2	T46.7X3	T46.7X4	T46.7X5	T46.7X6
E2	T48.0X1	T48.0X2	T48.0X3	T48.0X4	T48.0X5	T48.0X6
F2 alpha	T48.0X1	T48.0X2	T48.0X3	T48.0X4	T48.0X5	T48.0X6
Prostigmin	T44.0X1	T44.0X2	T44.0X3	T44.0X4	T44.0X5	T44.0X6
Prosultiamine	T45.2X1	T45.2X2	T45.2X3	T45.2X4	T45.2X5	T45.2X6
Protamine sulfate	T45.7X1	T45.7X2	T45.7X3	T45.7X4	T45.7X5	T45.7X6
zinc insulin	T38.3X1	T38.3X2	T38.3X3	T38.3X4	T38.3X5	T38.3X6
Protease	T47.5X1	T47.5X2	T47.5X3	T47.5X4	T47.5X5	T47.5X6
Protectant, skin NEC	T49.3X1	T49.3X2	T49.3X3	T49.3X4	T49.3X5	T49.3X6
Protein hydrolysate	T50.991	T50.992	T50.993	T50.994	T50.995	T50.996
Prothiaden — see Dothiepin hydrochloride						
Prothionamide	T37.1X1	T37.1X2	T37.1X3	T37.1X4	T37.1X5	T37.1X6

◄ New ◄ Revised deleted Deleted

	External Cause (T-Code)					
Substance	Poisoning, Accidental (Unintentional)	Poisoning, Intentional Self-Harm	Poisoning, Assault	Poisoning, Undetermined	Adverse Effect	Underdosing
Prothipendyl	T43.591	T43.592	T43.593	T43.594	T43.595	T43.596
Prothoate	T60.0X1	T60.0X2	T60.0X3	T60.0X4	—	—
Prothrombin						
activator	T45.7X1	T45.7X2	T45.7X3	T45.7X4	T45.7X5	T45.7X6
synthesis inhibitor	T45.511	T45.512	T45.513	T45.514	T45.515	T45.516
Protionamide	T37.1X1	T37.1X2	T37.1X3	T37.1X4	T37.1X5	T37.1X6
Protirelin	T38.891	T38.892	T38.893	T38.894	T38.895	T38.896
Protokylol	T48.6X1	T48.6X2	T48.6X4	T48.6X4	T48.6X5	T48.6X6
Protopam	T50.6X1	T50.6X2	T50.6X3	T50.6X4	T50.6X5	T50.6X6
Protoveratrine(s) (A) (B)	T46.5X1	T46.5X2	T46.5X3	T46.5X4	T46.5X5	T46.5X6
Protriptyline	T43.011	T43.012	T43.013	T43.014	T43.015	T43.016
Provera	T38.5X1	T38.5X2	T38.5X3	T38.5X4	T38.5X5	T38.5X6
Provitamin A	T45.2X1	T45.2X2	T45.2X3	T45.2X4	T45.2X5	T45.2X6
Proxibarbal	T42.3X1	T42.3X2	T42.3X3	T42.3X4	T42.3X5	T42.3X6
Proxymetacaine	T41.3X1	T41.3X2	T41.3X3	T41.3X4	T41.3X5	T41.3X6
Proxyphylline	T48.6X1	T48.6X2	T48.6X4	T48.6X4	T48.6X5	T48.6X6
Prozac — see Fluoxetine hydrochloride						
Prunus						
laurocerasus	T62.2X1	T62.2X2	T62.2X3	T62.2X4	—	—
virginiana	T62.2X1	T62.2X2	T62.2X3	T62.2X4	—	—
Prussian blue						
commercial	T65.891	T65.892	T65.893	T65.894		
therapeutic	T50.6X1	T50.6X2	T50.6X3	T50.6X4	T50.6X5	T50.6X6
Prussic acid	T65.0X1	T65.0X2	T65.0X3	T65.0X4		
vapor	T57.3X1	T57.3X2	T57.3X3	T57.3X4	—	—
Pseudoephedrine	T44.991	T44.992	T44.993	T44.994	T44.995	T44.996
Psilocin	T40.991	T40.992	T40.993	T40.994		
Psilocybin	T40.991	T40.992	T40.993	T40.994	—	—
Psilocybine	T40.991	T40.992	T40.993	T40.994	—	—
Psoralene (nonmedicinal)	T65.891	T65.892	T65.893	T65.894		
Psoralens (medicinal)	T50.991	T50.992	T50.993	T50.994	T50.995	T50.996
PSP (phenolsulfonphthalein)	T50.8X1	T50.8X2	T50.8X3	T50.8X4	T50.8X5	T50.8X6
Psychodysleptic drug NOS	T40.901	T40.902	T40.903	T40.904	T40.905	T40.906
specified NEC	T40.991	T40.992	T40.993	T40.994	T40.995	T40.996
Psychostimulant	T43.601	T43.602	T43.603	T43.604	T43.605	T43.606
amphetamine	T43.621	T43.622	T43.623	T43.624	T43.625	T43.626
caffeine	T43.611	T43.612	T43.613	T43.614	T43.615	T43.616
methylphenidate	T43.631	T43.632	T43.633	T43.634	T43.635	T43.636
specified NEC	T43.691	T43.692	T43.693	T43.694	T43.695	T43.696
Psychotherapeutic drug NEC	T43.91	T43.92	T43.93	T43.94	T43.95	T43.96
antidepressants — see also Antidepressant	T43.201	T43.202	T43.203	T43.204	T43.205	T43.206

	External Cause (T-Code)					
Substance	Poisoning, Accidental (Unintentional)	Poisoning, Intentional Self-Harm	Poisoning, Assault	Poisoning, Undetermined	Adverse Effect	Underdosing
Psychotherapeutic drug NEC (Continued)						
specified NEC	T43.8X1	T43.8X2	T43.8X3	T43.8X4	T43.8X5	T43.8X6
tranquilizers NEC	T43.501	T43.502	T43.503	T43.504	T43.505	T43.506
Psychotomimetic agents	T40.901	T40.902	T40.903	T40.904	T40.905	T40.906
Psychotropic drug NEC	T43.91	T43.92	T43.93	T43.94	T43.95	T43.96
specified NEC	T43.8X1	T43.8X2	T43.8X3	T43.8X4	T43.8X5	T43.8X6
Psyllium hydrophilic mucilloid	T47.4X1	T47.4X2	T47.4X3	T47.4X4	T47.4X5	T47.4X6
Pteroylglutamic acid	T45.8X1	T45.8X2	T45.8X3	T45.8X4	T45.8X5	T45.8X6
Pteroyltriglutamate	T45.1X1	T45.1X2	T45.1X3	T45.1X4	T45.1X5	T45.1X6
PTFE — see Polytetrafluoroethylene						
Pulp						
devitalizing paste	T49.7X1	T49.7X2	T49.7X3	T49.7X4	T49.7X5	T49.7X6
dressing	T49.7X1	T49.7X2	T49.7X3	T49.7X4	T49.7X5	T49.7X6
Pulsatilla	T62.2X1	T62.2X2	T62.2X3	T62.2X4	—	—
Pumpkin seed extract	T37.4X1	T37.4X2	T37.4X3	T37.4X4	T37.4X5	T37.4X6
Purex (bleach)	T54.91	T54.92	T54.93	T54.94		—
Purgative NEC — see also Cathartic	T47.4X1	T47.4X2	T47.4X3	T47.4X4	T47.4X5	T47.4X6
Purine analogue (antineoplastic)	T45.1X1	T45.1X2	T45.1X3	T45.1X4	T45.1X5	T45.1X6
Purine diuretics	T50.2X1	T50.2X2	T50.2X3	T50.2X4	T50.2X5	T50.2X6
Purinethol	T45.1X1	T45.1X2	T45.1X3	T45.1X4	T45.1X5	T45.1X6
PVP	T45.8X1	T45.8X2	T45.8X3	T45.8X4	T45.8X5	T45.8X6
Pyrabital	T39.8X1	T39.8X2	T39.8X3	T39.8X4	T39.8X5	T39.8X6
Pyramidon	T39.2X1	T39.2X2	T39.2X3	T39.2X4	T39.2X5	T39.2X6
Pyrantel	T37.4X1	T37.4X2	T37.4X3	T37.4X4	T37.4X5	T37.4X6
Pyrathiazine	T45.0X1	T45.0X2	T45.0X3	T45.0X4	T45.0X5	T45.0X6
Pyrazinamide	T37.1X1	T37.1X2	T37.1X3	T37.1X4	T37.1X5	T37.1X6
Pyrazinoic acid (amide)	T37.1X1	T37.1X2	T37.1X3	T37.1X4	T37.1X5	T37.1X6
Pyrazole (derivatives)	T39.2X1	T39.2X2	T39.2X3	T39.2X4	T39.2X5	T39.2X6
Pyrazolone analgesic NEC	T39.2X1	T39.2X2	T39.2X3	T39.2X4	T39.2X5	T39.2X6
Pyrethrin, pyrethrum (nonmedicinal)	T60.2X1	T60.2X2	T60.2X3	T60.2X4	—	—
Pyrethrum extract	T49.0X1	T49.0X2	T49.0X3	T49.0X4	T49.0X5	T49.0X6
Pyribenzamine	T45.0X1	T45.0X2	T45.0X3	T45.0X4	T45.0X5	T45.0X6
Pyridine	T52.8X1	T52.8X2	T52.8X3	T52.8X4	—	—
aldoxime methiodide	T50.6X1	T50.6X2	T50.6X3	T50.6X4	T50.6X5	T50.6X6
aldoxime methyl chloride	T50.6X1	T50.6X2	T50.6X3	T50.6X4	T50.6X5	T50.6X6
vapor	T59.891	T59.892	T59.893	T59.894	—	—
Pyridium	T39.8X1	T39.8X2	T39.8X3	T39.8X4	T39.8X5	T39.8X6
Pyridostigmine bromide	T44.0X1	T44.0X2	T44.0X3	T44.0X4	T44.0X5	T44.0X6
Pyridoxal phosphate	T45.2X1	T45.2X2	T45.2X3	T45.2X4	T45.2X5	T45.2X6

TABLE OF DRUGS AND CHEMICALS

TABLE OF DRUGS AND CHEMICALS

Substance	Poisoning, Accidental (Unintentional)	Poisoning, Intentional Self-Harm	Poisoning, Assault	Poisoning, Undetermined	Adverse Effect	Underdosing
Pyridoxine	T45.2X1	T45.2X2	T45.2X3	T45.2X4	T45.2X5	T45.2X6
Pyrilamine	T45.0X1	T45.0X2	T45.0X3	T45.0X4	T45.0X5	T45.0X6
Pyrimethamine	T37.2X1	T37.2X2	T37.2X3	T37.2X4	T37.2X5	T37.2X6
with sulfadoxine	T37.2X1	T37.2X2	T37.2X3	T37.2X4	T37.2X5	T37.2X6
Pyrimidine antagonist	T45.1X1	T45.1X2	T45.1X3	T45.1X4	T45.1X5	T45.1X6
Pyriminil	T60.4X1	T60.4X2	T60.4X3	T60.4X4	—	—
Pyrithione zinc	T49.4X1	T49.4X2	T49.4X3	T49.4X4	T49.4X5	T49.4X6
Pyrithyldione	T42.6X1	T42.6X2	T42.6X3	T42.6X4	T42.6X5	T42.6X6
Pyrogallic acid	T49.0X1	T49.0X2	T49.0X3	T49.0X4	T49.0X5	T49.0X6
Pyrogallol	T49.0X1	T49.0X2	T49.0X3	T49.0X4	T49.0X5	T49.0X6
Pyroxylin	T49.3X1	T49.3X2	T49.3X3	T49.3X4	T49.3X5	T49.3X6
Pyrrobutamine	T45.0X1	T45.0X2	T45.0X3	T45.0X4	T45.0X5	T45.0X6
Pyrrolizidine alkaloids	T62.8X1	T62.8X2	T62.8X3	T62.8X4	—	—
Pyrvinium chloride	T37.4X1	T37.4X2	T37.4X3	T37.4X4	T37.4X5	T37.4X6
PZI	T38.3X1	T38.3X2	T38.3X3	T38.3X4	T38.3X5	T38.3X6
Q						
Quaalude	T42.6X1	T42.6X2	T42.6X3	T42.6X4	T42.6X5	T42.6X6
Quarternary ammonium						
anti-infective	T49.0X1	T49.0X2	T49.0X3	T49.0X4	T49.0X5	T49.0X6
ganglion blocking	T44.2X1	T44.2X2	T44.2X3	T44.2X4	T44.2X5	T44.2X6
parasympatholytic	T44.3X1	T44.3X2	T44.3X3	T44.3X4	T44.3X5	T44.3X6
Quazepam	T42.4X1	T42.4X2	T42.4X3	T42.4X4	T42.4X5	T42.4X6
Quicklime	T54.3X1	T54.3X2	T54.3X3	T54.3X4	—	—
Quillaja extract	T48.4X1	T48.4X2	T48.4X3	T48.4X4	T48.4X5	T48.4X6
Quinacrine	T37.2X1	T37.2X2	T37.2X3	T37.2X4	T37.2X5	T37.2X6
Quinaglute	T46.2X1	T46.2X2	T46.2X3	T46.2X4	T46.2X5	T46.2X6
Quinalbarbital	T42.3X1	T42.3X2	T42.3X3	T42.3X4	T42.3X5	T42.3X6
Quinalbarbitone sodium	T42.3X1	T42.3X2	T42.3X3	T42.3X4	T42.3X5	T42.3X6
Quinalphos	T60.0X1	T60.0X2	T60.0X3	T60.0X4	—	—
Quinapril	T46.4X1	T46.4X2	T46.4X3	T46.4X4	T46.4X5	T46.4X6
Quinestradiol	T38.5X1	T38.5X2	T38.5X3	T38.5X4	T38.5X5	T38.5X6
Quinestradol	T38.5X1	T38.5X2	T38.5X3	T38.5X4	T38.5X5	T38.5X6
Quinestrol	T38.5X1	T38.5X2	T38.5X3	T38.5X4	T38.5X5	T38.5X6
Quinethazone	T50.2X1	T50.2X2	T50.2X3	T50.2X4	T50.2X5	T50.2X6
Quingestanol	T38.4X1	T38.4X2	T38.4X3	T38.4X4	T38.4X5	T38.4X6
Quinidine	T46.2X1	T46.2X2	T46.2X3	T46.2X4	T46.2X5	T46.2X6
Quinine	T37.2X1	T37.2X2	T37.2X3	T37.2X4	T37.2X5	T37.2X6
Quiniobine	T37.8X1	T37.8X2	T37.8X3	T37.8X4	T37.8X5	T37.8X6
Quinisocaine	T49.1X1	T49.1X2	T49.1X3	T49.1X4	T49.1X5	T49.1X6
Quinocide	T37.2X1	T37.2X2	T37.2X3	T37.2X4	T37.2X5	T37.2X6
Quinoline (derivatives) NEC	T37.8X1	T37.8X2	T37.8X3	T37.8X4	T37.8X5	T37.8X6

Substance	Poisoning, Accidental (Unintentional)	Poisoning, Intentional Self-Harm	Poisoning, Assault	Poisoning, Undetermined	Adverse Effect	Underdosing
Quinupramine	T43.011	T43.012	T43.013	T43.014	T43.015	T43.016
Quotane	T41.3X1	T41.3X2	T41.3X3	T41.3X4	T41.3X5	T41.3X6
R						
Rabies						
immune globulin (human)	T50.Z11	T50.Z12	T50.Z13	T50.Z14	T50.Z15	T50.Z16
vaccine	T50.B91	T50.B92	T50.B93	T50.B94	T50.B95	T50.B96
Racemoramide	T40.2X1	T40.2X2	T40.2X3	T40.2X4	—	—
Racemorphan	T40.2X1	T40.2X2	T40.2X3	T40.2X4	T40.2X5	T40.2X6
Racepinefrin	T44.5X1	T44.5X2	T44.5X3	T44.5X4	T44.5X5	T44.5X6
Raclopride	T43.591	T43.592	T43.593	T43.594	T43.595	T43.596
Radiator alcohol	T51.1X1	T51.1X2	T51.1X3	T51.1X4	—	—
Radioactive drug NEC	T50.8X1	T50.8X2	T50.8X3	T50.8X4	T50.8X5	T50.8X6
Radio-opaque (drugs) (materials)	T50.8X1	T50.8X2	T50.8X3	T50.8X4	T50.8X5	T50.8X6
Ramifenazone	T39.2X1	T39.2X2	T39.2X3	T39.2X4	T39.2X5	T39.2X6
Ramipril	T46.4X1	T46.4X2	T46.4X3	T46.4X4	T46.4X5	T46.4X6
Ranitidine	T47.0X1	T47.0X2	T47.0X3	T47.0X4	T47.0X5	T47.0X6
Ranunculus	T62.2X1	T62.2X2	T62.2X3	T62.2X4	—	—
Rat poison NEC	T60.4X1	T60.4X2	T60.4X3	T60.4X4	—	—
Rattlesnake (venom)	T63.011	T63.012	T63.013	T63.014	—	—
Raubasine	T46.7X1	T46.7X2	T46.7X3	T46.7X4	T46.7X5	T46.7X6
Raudixin	T46.5X1	T46.5X2	T46.5X3	T46.5X4	T46.5X5	T46.5X6
Rautensin	T46.5X1	T46.5X2	T46.5X3	T46.5X4	T46.5X5	T46.5X6
Rautina	T46.5X1	T46.5X2	T46.5X3	T46.5X4	T46.5X5	T46.5X6
Rautotal	T46.5X1	T46.5X2	T46.5X3	T46.5X4	T46.5X5	T46.5X6
Rauwiloid	T46.5X1	T46.5X2	T46.5X3	T46.5X4	T46.5X5	T46.5X6
Rauwoldin	T46.5X1	T46.5X2	T46.5X3	T46.5X4	T46.5X5	T46.5X6
Rauwolfia (alkaloids)	T46.5X1	T46.5X2	T46.5X3	T46.5X4	T46.5X5	T46.5X6
Razoxane	T45.1X1	T45.1X2	T45.1X3	T45.1X4	T45.1X5	T45.1X6
Realgar	T57.0X1	T57.0X2	T57.0X3	T57.0X4	—	—
Recombinant (R) — *see specific protein*						
Red blood cells, packed	T45.8X1	T45.8X2	T45.8X3	T45.8X4	T45.8X5	T45.8X6
Red squill (scilliroside)	T60.4X1	T60.4X2	T60.4X3	T60.4X4	—	—
Reducing agent, industrial NEC	T65.891	T65.892	T65.893	T65.894		
Refrigerant gas (chlorofluoro-carbon)	T53.5X1	T53.5X2	T53.5X3	T53.5X4		
not chlorofluoro-carbon	T59.891	T59.892	T59.893	T59.894	—	—
Regroton	T50.2X1	T50.2X2	T50.2X3	T50.2X4	T50.2X5	T50.2X6
Rehydration salts (oral)	T50.3X1	T50.3X2	T50.3X3	T50.3X4	T50.3X5	T50.3X6
Rela	T42.8X1	T42.8X2	T42.8X3	T42.8X4	T42.8X5	T42.8X6

◀ New ◀ Revised ~~deleted~~ Deleted

	External Cause (T-Code)					
Substance	Poisoning, Accidental (Unintentional)	Poisoning, Intentional Self-Harm	Poisoning, Assault	Poisoning, Undetermined	Adverse Effect	Underdosing
Relaxant, muscle						
anesthetic	T48.1X1	T48.1X2	T48.1X3	T48.1X4	T48.1X5	T48.1X6
central nervous system	T42.8X1	T42.8X2	T42.8X3	T42.8X4	T42.8X5	T42.8X6
skeletal NEC	T48.1X1	T48.1X2	T48.1X3	T48.1X4	T48.1X5	T48.1X6
smooth NEC	T44.3X1	T44.3X2	T44.3X3	T44.3X4	T44.3X5	T44.3X6
Remoxipride	T43.591	T43.592	T43.593	T43.594	T43.595	T43.596
Renese	T50.2X1	T50.2X2	T50.2X3	T50.2X4	T50.2X5	T50.2X6
Renografin	T50.8X1	T50.8X2	T50.8X3	T50.8X4	T50.8X5	T50.8X6
Replacement solution	T50.3X1	T50.3X2	T50.3X3	T50.3X4	T50.3X5	T50.3X6
Reproterol	T48.6X1	T48.6X2	T48.6X3	T48.6X4	T48.6X5	T48.6X6
Rescinnamine	T46.5X1	T46.5X2	T46.5X3	T46.5X4	T46.5X5	T46.5X6
Reserpin(e)	T46.5X1	T46.5X2	T46.5X3	T46.5X4	T46.5X5	T46.5X6
Resorcin, resorcinol (nonmedicinal)	T65.891	T65.892	T65.893	T65.894	—	—
medicinal	T49.4X1	T49.4X2	T49.4X3	T49.4X4	T49.4X5	T49.4X6
Respaire	T48.4X1	T48.4X2	T48.4X3	T48.4X4	T48.4X5	T48.4X6
Respiratory drug NEC	T48.901	T48.902	T48.903	T48.904	T48.905	T48.906
antiasthmatic NEC	T48.6X1	T48.6X2	T48.6X3	T48.6X4	T48.6X5	T48.6X6
anti-common-cold NEC	T48.5X1	T48.5X2	T48.5X3	T48.5X4	T48.5X5	T48.5X6
expectorant NEC	T48.4X1	T48.4X2	T48.4X3	T48.4X4	T48.4X5	T48.4X6
stimulant	T48.901	T48.902	T48.903	T48.904	T48.905	T48.906
Retinoic acid	T49.0X1	T49.0X2	T49.0X3	T49.0X4	T49.0X5	T49.0X6
Retinol	T45.2X1	T45.2X2	T45.2X3	T45.2X4	T45.2X5	T45.2X6
Rh (D) immune globulin (human)	T50.Z11	T50.Z12	T50.Z13	T50.Z14	T50.Z15	T50.Z16
Rhodine	T39.011	T39.012	T39.013	T39.014	T39.015	T39.016
RhoGAM	T50.Z11	T50.Z12	T50.Z13	T50.Z14	T50.Z15	T50.Z16
Rhubarb						
dry extract	T47.2X1	T47.2X2	T47.2X3	T47.2X4	T47.2X5	T47.2X6
tincture, compound	T47.2X1	T47.2X2	T47.2X3	T47.2X4	T47.2X5	T47.2X6
Ribavirin	T37.5X1	T37.5X2	T37.5X3	T37.5X4	T37.5X5	T37.5X6
Riboflavin	T45.2X1	T45.2X2	T45.2X3	T45.2X4	T45.2X5	T45.2X6
Ribostamycin	T36.5X1	T36.5X2	T36.5X3	T36.5X4	T36.5X5	T36.5X6
Ricin	T62.2X1	T62.2X2	T62.2X3	T62.2X4	—	—
Ricinus communis	T62.2X1	T62.2X2	T62.2X3	T62.2X4	—	—
Rickettsial vaccine NEC	T50.A91	T50.A92	T50.A93	T50.A94	T50.A95	T50.A96
Rifabutin	T36.6X1	T36.6X2	T36.6X3	T36.6X4	T36.6X5	T36.6X6
Rifamide	T36.6X1	T36.6X2	T36.6X3	T36.6X4	T36.6X5	T36.6X6
Rifampicin	T36.6X1	T36.6X2	T36.6X3	T36.6X4	T36.6X5	T36.6X6
with isoniazid	T37.1X1	T37.1X2	T37.1X3	T37.1X4	T37.1X5	T37.1X6
Rifampin	T36.6X1	T36.6X2	T36.6X3	T36.6X4	T36.6X5	T36.6X6
Rifamycin	T36.6X1	T36.6X2	T36.6X3	T36.6X4	T36.6X5	T36.6X6
Rifaximin	T36.6X1	T36.6X2	T36.6X3	T36.6X4	T36.6X5	T36.6X6

	External Cause (T-Code)					
Substance	Poisoning, Accidental (Unintentional)	Poisoning, Intentional Self-Harm	Poisoning, Assault	Poisoning, Undetermined	Adverse Effect	Underdosing
Rimantadine	T37.5X1	T37.5X2	T37.5X3	T37.5X4	T37.5X5	T37.5X6
Rimazolium metilsulfate	T39.8X1	T39.8X2	T39.8X3	T39.8X4	T39.8X5	T39.8X6
Rimifon	T37.1X1	T37.1X2	T37.1X3	T37.1X4	T37.1X5	T37.1X6
Rimiterol	T48.6X1	T48.6X2	T48.6X3	T48.6X4	T48.6X5	T48.6X6
Ringer (lactate) solution	T50.3X1	T50.3X2	T50.3X3	T50.3X4	T50.3X5	T50.3X6
Ristocetin	T36.8X1	T36.8X2	T36.8X3	T36.8X4	T36.8X5	T36.8X6
Ritalin	T43.631	T43.632	T43.633	T43.634	T43.635	T43.636
Ritodrine	T44.5X1	T44.5X2	T44.5X3	T44.5X4	T44.5X5	T44.5X6
Roach killer — see Insecticide						
Rociverine	T44.3X1	T44.3X2	T44.3X3	T44.3X4	T44.3X5	T44.3X6
Rocky Mountain spotted fever vaccine	T50.A91	T50.A92	T50.A93	T50.A94	T50.A95	T50.A96
Rodenticide NEC	T60.4X1	T60.4X2	T60.4X3	T60.4X4	—	—
Rohypnol	T42.4X1	T42.4X2	T42.4X3	T42.4X4	T42.4X5	T42.4X6
Rokitamycin	T36.3X1	T36.3X2	T36.3X3	T36.3X4	T36.3X5	T36.3X6
Rolaids	T47.1X1	T47.1X2	T47.1X3	T47.1X4	T47.1X5	T47.1X6
Rolitetracycline	T36.4X1	T36.4X2	T36.4X3	T36.4X4	T36.4X5	T36.4X6
Romilar	T48.3X1	T48.3X2	T48.3X3	T48.3X4	T48.3X5	T48.3X6
Ronifibrate	T46.6X1	T46.6X2	T46.6X3	T46.6X4	T46.6X5	T46.6X6
Rosaprostol	T47.1X1	T47.1X2	T47.1X3	T47.1X4	T47.1X5	T47.1X6
Rose bengal sodium (131I)	T50.8X1	T50.8X2	T50.8X3	T50.8X4	T50.8X5	T50.8X6
Rose water ointment	T49.3X1	T49.3X2	T49.3X3	T49.3X4	T49.3X5	T49.3X6
Rosoxacin	T37.8X1	T37.8X2	T37.8X3	T37.8X4	T37.8X5	T37.8X6
Rotenone	T60.2X1	T60.2X2	T60.2X3	T60.2X4	—	—
Rotoxamine	T45.0X1	T45.0X2	T45.0X3	T45.0X4	T45.0X5	T45.0X6
Rough-on-rats	T60.4X1	T60.4X2	T60.4X3	T60.4X4	—	—
Roxatidine	T47.0X1	T47.0X2	T47.0X3	T47.0X4	T47.0X5	T47.0X6
Roxithromycin	T36.3X1	T36.3X2	T36.3X3	T36.3X4	T36.3X5	T36.3X6
Rt-PA	T45.611	T45.612	T45.613	T45.614	T45.615	T45.616
Rubbing alcohol	T51.2X1	T51.2X2	T51.2X3	T51.2X4	—	—
Rubefacient	T49.4X1	T49.4X2	T49.4X3	T49.4X4	T49.4X5	T49.4X6
Rubella vaccine	T50.B91	T50.B92	T50.B93	T50.B94	T50.B95	T50.B96
Rubelogen	T50.B91	T50.B92	T50.B93	T50.B94	T50.B95	T50.B96
Rubeovax	T50.991	T50.992	T50.993	T50.994	T50.995	T50.996
Rubidium chloride Rb82	T50.8X1	T50.8X2	T50.8X3	T50.8X4	T50.8X5	T50.8X6
Rubidomycin	T45.1X1	T45.1X2	T45.1X3	T45.1X4	T45.1X5	T45.1X6
Rue	T62.2X1	T62.2X2	T62.2X3	T62.2X4	—	—
Rufocromomycin	T45.1X1	T45.1X2	T45.1X3	T45.1X4	T45.1X5	T45.1X6
Russel's viper venin	T45.7X1	T45.7X2	T45.7X3	T45.7X4	T45.7X5	T45.7X6
Ruta (graveolens)	T62.2X1	T62.2X2	T62.2X3	T62.2X4	—	—
Rutinum	T46.991	T46.992	T46.993	T46.994	T46.995	T46.996
Rutoside	T46.991	T46.992	T46.993	T46.994	T46.995	T46.996

TABLE OF DRUGS AND CHEMICALS

Substance	External Cause (T-Code)					
	Poisoning, Accidental (Unintentional)	Poisoning, Intentional Self-Harm	Poisoning, Assault	Poisoning, Undetermined	Adverse Effect	Underdosing
S						
Sabadilla (plant)	T62.2X1	T62.2X2	T62.2X3	T62.2X4	—	—
pesticide	T60.2X1	T60.2X2	T60.2X3	T60.2X4	—	—
Saccharated iron oxide	T45.8X1	T45.8X2	T45.8X3	T45.8X4	T45.8X5	T45.8X6
Saccharin	T50.901	T50.902	T50.903	T50.904	T50.905	T50.906
Saccharomyces boulardii	T47.6X1	T47.6X2	T47.6X3	T47.6X4	T47.6X5	T47.6X6
Safflower oil	T46.6X1	T46.6X2	T46.6X3	T46.6X4	T46.6X5	T46.6X6
Safrazine	T43.1X1	T43.1X2	T43.1X3	T43.1X4	T43.1X5	T43.1X6
Salazosulfapyridine	T37.0X1	T37.0X2	T37.0X3	T37.0X4	T37.0X5	T37.0X6
Salbutamol	T48.6X1	T48.6X2	T48.6X3	T48.6X4	T48.6X5	T48.6X6
Salicylamide	T39.091	T39.092	T39.093	T39.094	T39.095	T39.096
Salicylate NEC	T39.091	T39.092	T39.093	T39.094	T39.095	T39.096
methyl	T49.3X1	T49.3X2	T49.3X3	T49.3X4	T49.3X5	T49.3X6
theobromine calcium	T50.2X1	T50.2X2	T50.2X3	T50.2X4	T50.2X5	T50.2X6
Salicylazosulfapyridine	T37.0X1	T37.0X2	T37.0X3	T37.0X4	T37.0X5	T37.0X6
Salicylhydroxamic acid	T49.0X1	T49.0X2	T49.0X3	T49.0X4	T49.0X5	T49.0X6
Salicylic acid	T49.4X1	T49.4X2	T49.4X3	T49.4X4	T49.4X5	T49.4X6
with benzoic acid	T49.4X1	T49.4X2	T49.4X3	T49.4X4	T49.4X5	T49.4X6
congeners	T39.091	T39.092	T39.093	T39.094	T39.095	T39.096
derivative	T39.091	T39.092	T39.093	T39.094	T39.095	T39.096
salts	T39.091	T39.092	T39.093	T39.094	T39.095	T39.096
Salinazid	T37.1X1	T37.1X2	T37.1X3	T37.1X4	T37.1X5	T37.1X6
Salmeterol	T48.6X1	T48.6X2	T48.6X3	T48.6X4	T48.6X5	T48.6X6
Salol	T49.3X1	T49.3X2	T49.3X3	T49.3X4	T49.3X5	T49.3X6
Salsalate	T39.091	T39.092	T39.093	T39.094	T39.095	T39.096
Salt substitute	T50.901	T50.902	T50.903	T50.904	T50.905	T50.906
Salt-replacing drug	T50.901	T50.902	T50.903	T50.904	T50.905	T50.906
Salt-retaining mineralocorticoid	T50.0X1	T50.0X2	T50.0X3	T50.0X4	T50.0X5	T50.0X6
Saluretic NEC	T50.2X1	T50.2X2	T50.2X3	T50.2X4	T50.2X5	T50.2X6
Saluron	T50.2X1	T50.2X2	T50.2X3	T50.2X4	T50.2X5	T50.2X6
Salvarsan 606 (neosilver) (silver)	T37.8X1	T37.8X2	T37.8X3	T37.8X4	T37.8X5	T37.8X6
Sambucus canadensis	T62.2X1	T62.2X2	T62.2X3	T62.2X4	—	—
berry	T62.1X1	T62.1X2	T62.1X3	T62.1X4	—	—
Sandril	T46.5X1	T46.5X2	T46.5X3	T46.5X4	T46.5X5	T46.5X6
Sanguinaria canadensis	T62.2X1	T62.2X2	T62.2X3	T62.2X4	—	—
Saniflush (cleaner)	T54.2X1	T54.2X2	T54.2X3	T54.2X4	—	—
Santonin	T37.4X1	T37.4X2	T37.4X3	T37.4X4	T37.4X5	T37.4X6
Santyl	T49.8X1	T49.8X2	T49.8X3	T49.8X4	T49.8X5	T49.8X6
Saralasin	T46.5X1	T46.5X2	T46.5X3	T46.5X4	T46.5X5	T46.5X6
Sarcolysin	T45.1X1	T45.1X2	T45.1X3	T45.1X4	T45.1X5	T45.1X6
Sarkomycin	T45.1X1	T45.1X2	T45.1X3	T45.1X4	T45.1X5	T45.1X6
Saroten	T43.011	T43.012	T43.013	T43.014	T43.015	T43.016

Substance	External Cause (T-Code)					
	Poisoning, Accidental (Unintentional)	Poisoning, Intentional Self-Harm	Poisoning, Assault	Poisoning, Undetermined	Adverse Effect	Underdosing
Saturnine — see Lead						
Savin (oil)	T49.4X1	T49.4X2	T49.4X3	T49.4X4	T49.4X5	T49.4X6
Scammony	T47.2X1	T47.2X2	T47.2X3	T47.2X4	T47.2X5	T47.2X6
Scarlet red	T49.8X1	T49.8X2	T49.8X3	T49.8X4	T49.8X5	T49.8X6
Scheele's green	T57.0X1	T57.0X2	T57.0X3	T57.0X4	—	—
insecticide	T57.0X1	T57.0X2	T57.0X3	T57.0X4	—	—
Schizontozide (blood) (tissue)	T37.2X1	T37.2X2	T37.2X3	T37.2X4	T37.2X5	T37.2X6
Schradan	T60.0X1	T60.0X2	T60.0X3	T60.0X4	—	—
Schweinfurth green	T57.0X1	T57.0X2	T57.0X3	T57.0X4	—	—
insecticide	T57.0X1	T57.0X2	T57.0X3	T57.0X4	—	—
Scilla, rat poison	T60.4X1	T60.4X2	T60.4X3	T60.4X4	—	—
Scillaren	T60.4X1	T60.4X2	T60.4X3	T60.4X4	—	—
Sclerosing agent	T46.8X1	T46.8X2	T46.8X3	T46.8X4	T46.8X5	T46.8X6
Scombrotoxin	T61.11	T61.12	T61.13	T61.14		
Scopolamine	T44.3X1	T44.3X2	T44.3X3	T44.3X4	T44.3X5	T44.3X6
Scopolia extract	T44.3X1	T44.3X2	T44.3X3	T44.3X4	T44.3X5	T44.3X6
Scouring powder	T65.891	T65.892	T65.893	T65.894	—	—
Sea						
anemone (sting)	T63.631	T63.632	T63.633	T63.634	—	—
cucumber (sting)	T63.691	T63.692	T63.693	T63.694	—	—
snake (bite) (venom)	T63.091	T63.092	T63.093	T63.094	—	—
urchin spine (puncture)	T63.691	T63.692	T63.693	T63.694	—	—
Seafood	T61.91	T61.92	T61.93	T61.94		
specified NEC	T61.8X1	T61.8X2	T61.8X3	T61.8X4		
Secbutabarbital	T42.3X1	T42.3X2	T42.3X3	T42.3X4	T42.3X5	T42.3X6
Secbutabarbitone	T42.3X1	T42.3X2	T42.3X3	T42.3X4	T42.3X5	T42.3X6
Secnidazole	T37.3X1	T37.3X2	T37.3X3	T37.3X4	T37.3X5	T37.3X6
Secobarbital	T42.3X1	T42.3X2	T42.3X3	T42.3X4	T42.3X5	T42.3X6
Seconal	T42.3X1	T42.3X2	T42.3X3	T42.3X4	T42.3X5	T42.3X6
Secretin	T50.8X1	T50.8X2	T50.8X3	T50.8X4	T50.8X5	T50.8X6
Sedative NEC	T42.71	T42.72	T42.73	T42.74	T42.75	T42.76
mixed NEC	T42.6X1	T42.6X2	T42.6X3	T42.6X4	T42.6X5	T42.6X6
Sedormid	T42.6X1	T42.6X2	T42.6X3	T42.6X4	T42.6X5	T42.6X6
Seed disinfectant or dressing	T60.8X1	T60.8X2	T60.8X3	T60.8X4	—	—
Seeds (poisonous)	T62.2X1	T62.2X2	T62.2X3	T62.2X4	—	—
Selegiline	T42.8X1	T42.8X2	T42.8X3	T42.8X4	T42.8X5	T42.8X6
Selenium NEC	T56.891	T56.892	T56.893	T56.894	—	—
disulfide or sulfide	T49.4X1	T49.4X2	T49.4X3	T49.4X4	T49.4X5	T49.4X6
fumes	T59.891	T59.892	T59.893	T59.894	—	—
sulfide	T49.4X1	T49.4X2	T49.4X3	T49.4X4	T49.4X5	T49.4X6
Selenomethionine (75Se)	T50.8X1	T50.8X2	T50.8X3	T50.8X4	T50.8X5	T50.8X6
Selsun	T49.4X1	T49.4X2	T49.4X3	T49.4X4	T49.4X5	T49.4X6

◀ New ◀ Revised ~~deleted~~ Deleted

Substance	Poisoning, Accidental (Unintentional)	Poisoning, Intentional Self-Harm	Poisoning, Assault	Poisoning, Undetermined	Adverse Effect	Underdosing
		External Cause (T-Code)				
Semustine	T45.1X1	T45.1X2	T45.1X3	T45.1X4	T45.1X5	T45.1X6
Senega syrup	T48.4X1	T48.4X2	T48.4X3	T48.4X4	T48.4X5	T48.4X6
Senna	T47.2X1	T47.2X2	T47.2X3	T47.2X4	T47.2X5	T47.2X6
Sennoside A+B	T47.2X1	T47.2X2	T47.2X3	T47.2X4	T47.2X5	T47.2X6
Septisol	T49.2X1	T49.2X2	T49.2X3	T49.2X4	T49.2X5	T49.2X6
Seractide	T38.811	T38.812	T38.813	T38.814	T38.815	T38.816
Serax	T42.4X1	T42.4X2	T42.4X3	T42.4X4	T42.4X5	T42.4X6
Serenesil	T42.6X1	T42.6X2	T42.6X3	T42.6X4	T42.6X5	T42.6X6
Serenium (hydrochloride)	T37.91	T37.92	T37.93	T37.94	T37.95	T37.96
Serepax — see Oxazepam						
Sermorelin	T38.891	T38.892	T38.893	T38.894	T38.895	T38.896
Sernyl	T41.1X1	T41.1X2	T41.1X3	T41.1X4	T41.1X5	T41.1X6
Serotonin	T50.991	T50.992	T50.993	T50.994	T50.995	T50.996
Serpasil	T46.5X1	T46.5X2	T46.5X3	T46.5X4	T46.5X5	T46.5X6
Serrapeptase	T45.3X1	T45.3X2	T45.3X3	T45.3X4	T45.3X5	T45.3X6
Serum						
antibotulinus	T50.Z11	T50.Z12	T50.Z13	T50.Z14	T50.Z15	T50.Z16
anticytotoxic	T50.Z11	T50.Z12	T50.Z13	T50.Z14	T50.Z15	T50.Z16
antidiphtheria	T50.Z11	T50.Z12	T50.Z13	T50.Z14	T50.Z15	T50.Z16
antimeningococcus	T50.Z11	T50.Z12	T50.Z13	T50.Z14	T50.Z15	T50.Z16
anti-Rh	T50.Z11	T50.Z12	T50.Z13	T50.Z14	T50.Z15	T50.Z16
anti-snake-bite	T50.Z11	T50.Z12	T50.Z13	T50.Z14	T50.Z15	T50.Z16
antitetanic	T50.Z11	T50.Z12	T50.Z13	T50.Z14	T50.Z15	T50.Z16
antitoxic	T50.Z11	T50.Z12	T50.Z13	T50.Z14	T50.Z15	T50.Z16
complement (inhibitor)	T45.8X1	T45.8X2	T45.8X3	T45.8X4	T45.8X5	T45.8X6
convalescent	T50.Z11	T50.Z12	T50.Z13	T50.Z14	T50.Z15	T50.Z16
hemolytic complement	T45.8X1	T45.8X2	T45.8X3	T45.8X4	T45.8X5	T45.8X6
immune (human)	T50.Z11	T50.Z12	T50.Z13	T50.Z14	T50.Z15	T50.Z16
protective NEC	T50.Z11	T50.Z12	T50.Z13	T50.Z14	T50.Z15	T50.Z16
Setastine	T45.0X1	T45.0X2	T45.0X3	T45.0X4	T45.0X5	T45.0X6
Setoperone	T43.591	T43.592	T43.593	T43.594	T43.595	T43.596
Sewer gas	T59.91	T59.92	T59.93	T59.94	—	—
Shampoo	T55.0X1	T55.0X2	T55.0X3	T55.0X4	—	—
Shellfish, noxious, nonbacterial	T61.781	T61.782	T61.783	T61.784	—	—
Sildenafil	T46.7X1	T46.7X2	T46.7X3	T46.7X4	T46.7X5	T46.7X6
Silibinin	T50.991	T50.992	T50.993	T50.994	T50.995	T50.996
Silicone NEC	T65.891	T65.892	T65.893	T65.894	—	—
medicinal	T49.3X1	T49.3X2	T49.3X3	T49.3X4	T49.3X5	T49.3X6
Silvadene	T49.0X1	T49.0X2	T49.0X3	T49.0X4	T49.0X5	T49.0X6
Silver	T49.0X1	T49.0X2	T49.0X3	T49.0X4	T49.0X5	T49.0X6
anti-infectives	T49.0X1	T49.0X2	T49.0X3	T49.0X4	T49.0X5	T49.0X6
arsphenamine	T37.8X1	T37.8X2	T37.8X3	T37.8X4	T37.8X5	T37.8X6

Substance	Poisoning, Accidental (Unintentional)	Poisoning, Intentional Self-Harm	Poisoning, Assault	Poisoning, Undetermined	Adverse Effect	Underdosing
		External Cause (T-Code)				
Silver (Continued)						
colloidal	T49.0X1	T49.0X2	T49.0X3	T49.0X4	T49.0X5	T49.0X6
nitrate	T49.0X1	T49.0X2	T49.0X3	T49.0X4	T49.0X5	T49.0X6
ophthalmic preparation	T49.5X1	T49.5X2	T49.5X3	T49.5X4	T49.5X5	T49.5X6
toughened (keratolytic)	T49.4X1	T49.4X2	T49.4X3	T49.4X4	T49.4X5	T49.4X6
nonmedicinal (dust)	T56.891	T56.892	T56.893	T56.894	—	—
protein	T49.5X1	T49.5X2	T49.5X3	T49.5X4	T49.5X5	T49.5X6
salvarsan	T37.8X1	T37.8X2	T37.8X3	T37.8X4	T37.8X5	T37.8X6
sulfadiazine	T49.4X1	T49.4X2	T49.4X3	T49.4X4	T49.4X5	T49.4X6
Silymarin	T50.991	T50.992	T50.993	T50.994	T50.995	T50.996
Simaldrate	T47.1X1	T47.1X2	T47.1X3	T47.1X4	T47.1X5	T47.1X6
Simazine	T60.3X1	T60.3X2	T60.3X3	T60.3X4	—	—
Simethicone	T47.1X1	T47.1X2	T47.1X3	T47.1X4	T47.1X5	T47.1X6
Simfibrate	T46.6X1	T46.6X2	T46.6X3	T46.6X4	T46.6X5	T46.6X6
Simvastatin	T46.6X1	T46.6X2	T46.6X3	T46.6X4	T46.6X5	T46.6X6
Sincalide	T50.8X1	T50.8X2	T50.8X3	T50.8X4	T50.8X5	T50.8X6
Sinequan	T43.011	T43.012	T43.013	T43.014	T43.015	T43.016
Singoserp	T46.5X1	T46.5X2	T46.5X3	T46.5X4	T46.5X5	T46.5X6
Sintrom	T45.511	T45.512	T45.513	T45.514	T45.515	T45.516
Sisomicin	T36.5X1	T36.5X2	T36.5X3	T36.5X4	T36.5X5	T36.5X6
Sitosterols	T46.6X1	T46.6X2	T46.6X3	T46.6X4	T46.6X5	T46.6X6
Skeletal muscle relaxants	T48.1X1	T48.1X2	T48.1X3	T48.1X4	T48.1X5	T48.1X6
Skin						
agents (external)	T49.91	T49.92	T49.93	T49.94	T49.95	T49.96
specified NEC	T49.8X1	T49.8X2	T49.8X3	T49.8X4	T49.8X5	T49.8X6
test antigen	T50.8X1	T50.8X2	T50.8X3	T50.8X4	T50.8X5	T50.8X6
Sleep-eze	T45.0X1	T45.0X2	T45.0X3	T45.0X4	T45.0X5	T45.0X6
Sleeping draught, pill	T42.71	T42.72	T42.73	T42.74	T42.75	T42.76
Smallpox vaccine	T50.B11	T50.B12	T50.B13	T50.B14	T50.B15	T50.B16
Smelter fumes NEC	T56.91	T56.92	T56.93	T56.94	—	—
Smog	T59.1X1	T59.1X2	T59.1X3	T59.1X4	—	—
Smoke NEC	T59.811	T59.812	T59.813	T59.814	—	—
Smooth muscle relaxant	T44.3X1	T44.3X2	T44.3X3	T44.3X4	T44.3X5	T44.3X6
Snail killer NEC	T60.8X1	T60.8X2	T60.8X3	T60.8X4	—	—
Snake venom or bite	T63.001	T63.002	T63.003	T63.004	—	—
hemocoagulase	T45.7X1	T45.7X2	T45.7X3	T45.7X4	T45.7X5	T45.7X6
Snuff	T65.211	T65.212	T65.213	T65.214	—	—
Soap (powder) (product)	T55.0X1	T55.0X2	T55.0X3	T55.0X4	—	—
enema	T47.4X1	T47.4X2	T47.4X3	T47.4X4	T47.4X5	T47.4X6
medicinal, soft	T49.2X1	T49.2X2	T49.2X3	T49.2X4	T49.2X5	T49.2X6
superfatted	T49.2X1	T49.2X2	T49.2X3	T49.2X4	T49.2X5	T49.2X6
Sobrerol	T48.4X1	T48.4X2	T48.4X3	T48.4X4	T48.4X5	T48.4X6

◀ New ◀ Revised ~~deleted~~ Deleted

TABLE OF DRUGS AND CHEMICALS

Substance	Poisoning, Accidental (Unintentional)	Poisoning, Intentional Self-Harm	Poisoning, Assault	Poisoning, Undetermined	Adverse Effect	Underdosing
Soda (caustic)	T54.3X1	T54.3X2	T54.3X3	T54.3X4	—	—
bicarb	T47.1X1	T47.1X2	T47.1X3	T47.1X4	T47.1X5	T47.1X6
chlorinated — *see Sodium, hypochlorite*						
Sodium						
acetosulfone	T37.1X1	T37.1X2	T37.1X3	T37.1X4	T37.1X5	T37.1X6
acetrizoate	T50.8X1	T50.8X2	T50.8X3	T50.8X4	T50.8X5	T50.8X6
acid phosphate	T50.3X1	T50.3X2	T50.3X3	T50.3X4	T50.3X5	T50.3X6
alginate	T47.8X1	T47.8X2	T47.8X3	T47.8X4	T47.8X5	T47.8X6
amidotrizoate	T50.8X1	T50.8X2	T50.8X3	T50.8X4	T50.8X5	T50.8X6
aminopterin	T45.1X1	T45.1X2	T45.1X3	T45.1X4	T45.1X5	T45.1X6
amylosulfate	T47.8X1	T47.8X2	T47.8X3	T47.8X4	T47.8X5	T47.8X6
amytal	T42.3X1	T42.3X2	T42.3X3	T42.3X4	T42.3X5	T42.3X6
antimony gluconate	T37.3X1	T37.3X2	T37.3X3	T37.3X4	T37.3X5	T37.3X6
arsenate	T57.0X1	T57.0X2	T57.0X3	T57.0X4	—	—
aurothiomalate	T39.4X1	T39.4X2	T39.4X3	T39.4X4	T39.4X5	T39.4X6
aurothiosulfate	T39.4X1	T39.4X2	T39.4X3	T39.4X4	T39.4X5	T39.4X6
barbiturate	T42.3X1	T42.3X2	T42.3X3	T42.3X4	T42.3X5	T42.3X6
basic phosphate	T47.4X1	T47.4X2	T47.4X3	T47.4X4	T47.4X5	T47.4X6
bicarbonate	T47.1X1	T47.1X2	T47.1X3	T47.1X4	T47.1X5	T47.1X6
bichromate	T57.8X1	T57.8X2	T57.8X3	T57.8X4	—	—
biphosphate	T50.3X1	T50.3X2	T50.3X3	T50.3X4	T50.3X5	T50.3X6
bisulfate	T65.891	T65.892	T65.893	T65.894	—	—
borate						
cleanser	T57.8X1	T57.8X2	T57.8X3	T57.8X4	—	—
eye	T49.5X1	T49.5X2	T49.5X3	T49.5X4	T49.5X5	T49.5X6
therapeutic	T49.8X1	T49.8X2	T49.8X3	T49.8X4	T49.8X5	T49.8X6
bromide	T42.6X1	T42.6X2	T42.6X3	T42.6X4	T42.6X5	T42.6X6
cacodylate (nonmedicinal) NEC	T50.8X1	T50.8X2	T50.8X3	T50.8X4	T50.8X5	T50.8X6
anti-infective	T37.8X1	T37.8X2	T37.8X3	T37.8X4	T37.8X5	T37.8X6
herbicide	T60.3X1	T60.3X2	T60.3X3	T60.3X4	—	—
calcium edetate	T45.8X1	T45.8X2	T45.8X3	T45.8X4	T45.8X5	T45.8X6
carbonate NEC	T54.3X1	T54.3X2	T54.3X3	T54.3X4	—	—
chlorate NEC	T65.891	T65.892	T65.893	T65.894	—	—
herbicide	T54.91	T54.92	T54.93	T54.94	—	—
chloride	T50.3X1	T50.3X2	T50.3X3	T50.3X4	T50.3X5	T50.3X6
with glucose	T50.3X1	T50.3X2	T50.3X3	T50.3X4	T50.3X5	T50.3X6
chromate	T65.891	T65.892	T65.893	T65.894	—	—
citrate	T50.991	T50.992	T50.993	T50.994	T50.995	T50.996
cromoglicate	T48.6X1	T48.6X2	T48.6X3	T48.6X4	T48.6X5	T48.6X6
cyanide	T65.0X1	T65.0X2	T65.0X3	T65.0X4	—	—
cyclamate	T50.3X1	T50.3X2	T50.3X3	T50.3X4	T50.3X5	T50.3X6

Substance	Poisoning, Accidental (Unintentional)	Poisoning, Intentional Self-Harm	Poisoning, Assault	Poisoning, Undetermined	Adverse Effect	Underdosing
Sodium *(Continued)*						
dehydrocholate	T45.8X1	T45.8X2	T45.8X3	T45.8X4	T45.8X5	T45.8X6
diatrizoate	T50.8X1	T50.8X2	T50.8X3	T50.8X4	T50.8X5	T50.8X6
dibunate	T48.4X1	T48.4X2	T48.4X3	T48.4X4	T48.4X5	T48.4X6
dioctyl sulfosuccinate	T47.4X1	T47.4X2	T47.4X3	T47.4X4	T47.4X5	T47.4X6
dipantoyl ferrate	T45.8X1	T45.8X2	T45.8X3	T45.8X4	T45.8X5	T45.8X6
edetate	T45.8X1	T45.8X2	T45.8X3	T45.8X4	T45.8X5	T45.8X6
ethacrynate	T50.1X1	T50.1X2	T50.1X3	T50.1X4	T50.1X5	T50.1X6
feredetate	T45.8X1	T45.8X2	T45.8X3	T45.8X4	T45.8X5	T45.8X6
Fluoride — *see Fluoride*						
fluoroacetate (dust) (pesticide)	T60.4X1	T60.4X2	T60.4X3	T60.4X4	—	—
free salt	T50.3X1	T50.3X2	T50.3X3	T50.3X4	T50.3X5	T50.3X6
fusidate	T36.8X1	T36.8X2	T36.8X3	T36.8X4	T36.8X5	T36.8X6
glucaldrate	T47.1X1	T47.1X2	T47.1X3	T47.1X4	T47.1X5	T47.1X6
glucosulfone	T37.1X1	T37.1X2	T37.1X3	T37.1X4	T37.1X5	T37.1X6
glutamate	T45.8X1	T45.8X2	T45.8X3	T45.8X4	T45.8X5	T45.8X6
hydrogen carbonate	T50.3X1	T50.3X2	T50.3X3	T50.3X4	T50.3X5	T50.3X6
hydroxide	T54.3X1	T54.3X2	T54.3X3	T54.3X4	—	—
hypochlorite (bleach) NEC	T54.3X1	T54.3X2	T54.3X3	T54.3X4	—	—
disinfectant	T54.3X1	T54.3X2	T54.3X3	T54.3X4	—	—
medicinal (anti-infective) (external)	T49.0X1	T49.0X2	T49.0X3	T49.0X4	T49.0X5	T49.0X6
vapor	T54.3X1	T54.3X2	T54.3X3	T54.3X4	—	—
hyposulfite	T49.0X1	T49.0X2	T49.0X3	T49.0X4	T49.0X5	T49.0X6
indigotin disulfonate	T50.8X1	T50.8X2	T50.8X3	T50.8X4	T50.8X5	T50.8X6
iodide	T50.991	T50.992	T50.993	T50.994	T50.995	T50.996
I-131	T50.8X1	T50.8X2	T50.8X3	T50.8X4	T50.8X5	T50.8X6
therapeutic	T38.2X1	T38.2X2	T38.2X3	T38.2X4	T38.2X5	T38.2X6
iodohippurate (131I)	T50.8X1	T50.8X2	T50.8X3	T50.8X4	T50.8X5	T50.8X6
iopodate	T50.8X1	T50.8X2	T50.8X3	T50.8X4	T50.8X5	T50.8X6
iothalamate	T50.8X1	T50.8X2	T50.8X3	T50.8X4	T50.8X5	T50.8X6
iron edetate	T45.4X1	T45.4X2	T45.4X3	T45.4X4	T45.4X5	T45.4X6
lactate (compound solution)	T45.8X1	T45.8X2	T45.8X3	T45.8X4	T45.8X5	T45.8X6
lauryl (sulfate)	T49.2X1	T49.2X2	T49.2X3	T49.2X4	T49.2X5	T49.2X6
(L)-triiodothyronine	T38.1X1	T38.1X2	T38.1X3	T38.1X4	T38.1X5	T38.1X6
magnesium citrate	T50.991	T50.992	T50.993	T50.994	T50.995	T50.996
mersalate	T50.2X1	T50.2X2	T50.2X3	T50.2X4	T50.2X5	T50.2X6
metasilicate	T65.891	T65.892	T65.893	T65.894	—	—
metrizoate	T50.8X1	T50.8X2	T50.8X3	T50.8X4	T50.8X5	T50.8X6
monofluoroacetate (pesticide)	T60.1X1	T60.1X2	T60.1X3	T60.1X4	—	—
morrhuate	T46.8X1	T46.8X2	T46.8X3	T46.8X4	T46.8X5	T46.8X6
nafcillin	T36.0X1	T36.0X2	T36.0X3	T36.0X4	T36.0X5	T36.0X6

◀ New ◀ Revised ~~deleted~~ Deleted

Substance	External Cause (T-Code)					
	Poisoning, Accidental (Unintentional)	Poisoning, Intentional Self-Harm	Poisoning, Assault	Poisoning, Undetermined	Adverse Effect	Underdosing
Sodium *(Continued)*						
nitrate (oxidizing agent)	T65.891	T65.892	T65.893	T65.894	—	—
nitrite	T50.6X1	T50.6X2	T50.6X3	T50.6X4	T50.6X5	T50.6X6
nitroferricyanide	T46.5X1	T46.5X2	T46.5X3	T46.5X4	T46.5X5	T46.5X6
nitroprusside	T46.5X1	T46.5X2	T46.5X3	T46.5X4	T46.5X5	T46.5X6
oxalate	T65.891	T65.892	T65.893	T65.894	—	—
oxide/peroxide	T65.891	T65.892	T65.893	T65.894	—	—
oxybate	T41.291	T41.292	T41.293	T41.294	T41.295	T41.296
para-aminohippurate	T50.8X1	T50.8X2	T50.8X3	T50.8X4	T50.8X5	T50.8X6
perborate (nonmedicinal) NEC	T65.891	T65.892	T65.893	T65.894	—	—
medicinal	T49.0X1	T49.0X2	T49.0X3	T49.0X4	T49.0X5	T49.0X6
soap	T55.0X1	T55.0X2	T55.0X3	T55.0X4	—	—
percarbonate — *see Sodium, perborate*						
pertechnetate Tc99m	T50.8X1	T50.8X2	T50.8X3	T50.8X4	T50.8X5	T50.8X6
phosphate						
cellulose	T45.8X1	T45.8X2	T45.8X3	T45.8X4	T45.8X5	T45.8X6
dibasic	T47.2X1	T47.2X2	T47.2X3	T47.2X4	T47.2X5	T47.2X6
monobasic	T47.2X1	T47.2X2	T47.2X3	T47.2X4	T47.2X5	T47.2X6
phytate	T50.6X1	T50.6X2	T50.6X3	T50.6X4	T50.6X5	T50.6X6
picosulfate	T47.2X1	T47.2X2	T47.2X3	T47.2X4	T47.2X5	T47.2X6
polyhydroxyaluminium monocarbonate	T47.1X1	T47.1X2	T47.1X3	T47.1X4	T47.1X5	T47.1X6
polystyrene sulfonate	T50.3X1	T50.3X2	T50.3X3	T50.3X4	T50.3X5	T50.3X6
propionate	T49.0X1	T49.0X2	T49.0X3	T49.0X4	T49.0X5	T49.0X6
propyl hydroxybenzoate	T50.991	T50.992	T50.993	T50.994	T50.995	T50.996
psylliate	T46.8X1	T46.8X2	T46.8X3	T46.8X4	T46.8X5	T46.8X6
removing resins	T50.3X1	T50.3X2	T50.3X3	T50.3X4	T50.3X5	T50.3X6
salicylate	T39.091	T39.092	T39.093	T39.094	T39.095	T39.096
salt NEC	T50.3X1	T50.3X2	T50.3X3	T50.3X4	T50.3X5	T50.3X6
selenate	T60.2X1	T60.2X2	T60.2X3	T60.2X4	—	—
stibogluconate	T37.3X1	T37.3X2	T37.3X3	T37.3X4	T37.3X5	T37.3X6
sulfate	T47.4X1	T47.4X2	T47.4X3	T47.4X4	T47.4X5	T47.4X6
sulfoxone	T37.1X1	T37.1X2	T37.1X3	T37.1X4	T37.1X5	T37.1X6
tetradecyl sulfate	T46.8X1	T46.8X2	T46.8X3	T46.8X4	T46.8X5	T46.8X6
thiopental	T41.1X1	T41.1X2	T41.1X3	T41.1X4	T41.1X5	T41.1X6
thiosalicylate	T39.091	T39.092	T39.093	T39.094	T39.095	T39.096
thiosulfate	T50.6X1	T50.6X2	T50.6X3	T50.6X4	T50.6X5	T50.6X6
tolbutamide	T38.3X1	T38.3X2	T38.3X3	T38.3X4	T38.3X5	T38.3X6
l-triiodothyronine	T38.1X1	T38.1X2	T38.1X3	T38.1X4	T38.1X5	T38.1X6
tyropanoate	T50.8X1	T50.8X2	T50.8X3	T50.8X4	T50.8X5	T50.8X6
valproate	T42.6X1	T42.6X2	T42.6X3	T42.6X4	T42.6X5	T42.6X6
versenate	T50.6X1	T50.6X2	T50.6X3	T50.6X4	T50.6X5	T50.6X6

Substance	External Cause (T-Code)					
	Poisoning, Accidental (Unintentional)	Poisoning, Intentional Self-Harm	Poisoning, Assault	Poisoning, Undetermined	Adverse Effect	Underdosing
Sodium-free salt	T50.901	T50.902	T50.903	T50.904	T50.905	T50.906
Sodium-removing resin	T50.3X1	T50.3X2	T50.3X3	T50.3X4	T50.3X5	T50.3X6
Soft soap	T55.0X1	T55.0X2	T55.0X3	T55.0X4	—	—
Solanine	T62.2X1	T62.2X2	T62.2X3	T62.2X4	—	—
berries	T62.1X1	T62.1X2	T62.1X3	T62.1X4	—	—
Solanum dulcamara	T62.2X1	T62.2X2	T62.2X3	T62.2X4	—	—
berries	T62.1X1	T62.1X2	T62.1X3	T62.1X4	—	—
Solapsone	T37.1X1	T37.1X2	T37.1X3	T37.1X4	T37.1X5	T37.1X6
Solar lotion	T49.3X1	T49.3X2	T49.3X3	T49.3X4	T49.3X5	T49.3X6
Solasulfone	T37.1X1	T37.1X2	T37.1X3	T37.1X4	T37.1X5	T37.1X6
Soldering fluid	T65.891	T65.892	T65.893	T65.894	—	—
Solid substance	T65.91	T65.92	T65.93	T65.94		
specified NEC	T65.891	T65.892	T65.893	T65.894	—	—
Solvent, industrial NEC	T52.91	T52.92	T52.93	T52.94		
naphtha	T52.0X1	T52.0X2	T52.0X3	T52.0X4		—
petroleum	T52.0X1	T52.0X2	T52.0X3	T52.0X4		—
specified NEC	T52.8X1	T52.8X2	T52.8X3	T52.8X4		—
Soma	T42.8X1	T42.8X2	T42.8X3	T42.8X4	T42.8X5	T42.8X6
Somatorelin	T38.891	T38.892	T38.893	T38.894	T38.895	T38.896
Somatostatin	T38.991	T38.992	T38.993	T38.994	T38.995	T38.996
Somatotropin	T38.811	T38.812	T38.813	T38.814	T38.815	T38.816
Somatrem	T38.811	T38.812	T38.813	T38.814	T38.815	T38.816
Somatropin	T38.811	T38.812	T38.813	T38.814	T38.815	T38.816
Sominex	T45.0X1	T45.0X2	T45.0X3	T45.0X4	T45.0X5	T45.0X6
Somnos	T42.6X1	T42.6X2	T42.6X3	T42.6X4	T42.6X5	T42.6X6
Somonal	T42.3X1	T42.3X2	T42.3X3	T42.3X4	T42.3X5	T42.3X6
Soneryl	T42.3X1	T42.3X2	T42.3X3	T42.3X4	T42.3X5	T42.3X6
Soothing syrup	T50.901	T50.902	T50.903	T50.904	T50.905	T50.906
Sopor	T42.6X1	T42.6X2	T42.6X3	T42.6X4	T42.6X5	T42.6X6
Soporific	T42.71	T42.72	T42.73	T42.74	T42.75	T42.76
Soporific drug	T42.71	T42.72	T42.73	T42.74	T42.75	T42.76
specified type NEC	T42.6X1	T42.6X2	T42.6X3	T42.6X4	T42.6X5	T42.6X6
Sorbide nitrate	T46.3X1	T46.3X2	T46.3X3	T46.3X4	T46.3X5	T46.3X6
Sorbitol	T47.4X1	T47.4X2	T47.4X3	T47.4X4	T47.4X5	T47.4X6
Sotalol	T44.7X1	T44.7X2	T44.7X3	T44.7X4	T44.7X5	T44.7X6
Sotradecol	T46.8X1	T46.8X2	T46.8X3	T46.8X4	T46.8X5	T46.8X6
Soysterol	T46.6X1	T46.6X2	T46.6X3	T46.6X4	T46.6X5	T46.6X6
Spacoline	T44.3X1	T44.3X2	T44.3X3	T44.3X4	T44.3X5	T44.3X6
Spanish fly	T49.8X1	T49.8X2	T49.8X3	T49.8X4	T49.8X5	T49.8X6
Sparine	T43.3X1	T43.3X2	T43.3X3	T43.3X4	T43.3X5	T43.3X6
Sparteine	T48.0X1	T48.0X2	T48.0X3	T48.0X4	T48.0X5	T48.0X6

◀ New　◀ Revised　~~deleted~~ Deleted

Substance	External Cause (T-Code) Poisoning, Accidental (Unintentional)	Poisoning, Intentional Self-Harm	Poisoning, Assault	Poisoning, Undetermined	Adverse Effect	Underdosing
Spasmolytic						
anticholinergics	T44.3X1	T44.3X2	T44.3X3	T44.3X4	T44.3X5	T44.3X6
autonomic	T44.3X1	T44.3X2	T44.3X3	T44.3X4	T44.3X5	T44.3X6
bronchial NEC	T48.6X1	T48.6X2	T48.6X3	T48.6X4	T48.6X5	T48.6X6
quaternary ammonium	T44.3X1	T44.3X2	T44.3X3	T44.3X4	T44.3X5	T44.3X6
skeletal muscle NEC	T48.1X1	T48.1X2	T48.1X3	T48.1X4	T48.1X5	T48.1X6
Spectinomycin	T36.5X1	T36.5X2	T36.5X3	T36.5X4	T36.5X5	T36.5X6
Speed	T43.651	T43.652	T43.652	T43.654	T43.655	T43.656
Spermicide	T49.8X1	T49.8X2	T49.8X3	T49.8X4	T49.8X5	T49.8X6
Spider (bite) (venom)	T63.391	T63.392	T63.393	T63.394	—	—
antivenin	T50.Z11	T50.Z12	T50.Z13	T50.Z14	T50.Z15	T50.Z16
Spigelia (root)	T37.4X1	T37.4X2	T37.4X3	T37.4X4	T37.4X5	T37.4X6
Spindle inactivator	T50.4X1	T50.4X2	T50.4X3	T50.4X4	T50.4X5	T50.4X6
Spiperone	T43.4X1	T43.4X2	T43.4X3	T43.4X4	T43.4X5	T43.4X6
Spiramycin	T36.3X1	T36.3X2	T36.3X3	T36.3X4	T36.3X5	T36.3X6
Spirapril	T46.4X1	T46.4X2	T46.4X3	T46.4X4	T46.4X5	T46.4X6
Spirilene	T43.591	T43.592	T43.593	T43.594	T43.595	T43.596
Spirit(s) (neutral) NEC	T51.0X1	T51.0X2	T51.0X3	T51.0X4		
beverage	T51.0X1	T51.0X2	T51.0X3	T51.0X4	—	—
industrial	T51.0X1	T51.0X2	T51.0X3	T51.0X4		
mineral	T52.0X1	T52.0X2	T52.0X3	T52.0X4		
of salt — see Hydrochloric acid						
surgical	T51.0X1	T51.0X2	T51.0X3	T51.0X4		
Spironolactone	T50.0X1	T50.0X2	T50.0X3	T50.0X4	T50.0X5	T50.0X6
Spiroperidol	T43.4X1	T43.4X2	T43.4X3	T43.4X4	T43.4X5	T43.4X6
Sponge, absorbable (gelatin)	T45.7X1	T45.7X2	T45.7X3	T45.7X4	T45.7X5	T45.7X6
Sporostacin	T49.0X1	T49.0X2	T49.0X3	T49.0X4	T49.0X5	T49.0X6
Spray (aerosol)	T65.91	T65.92	T65.93	T65.94	—	—
cosmetic	T65.891	T65.892	T65.893	T65.894	—	—
medicinal NEC	T50.901	T50.902	T50.903	T50.904	T50.905	T50.906
pesticides — see Pesticide						
specified content — see specific substance						
Spurge flax	T62.2X1	T62.2X2	T62.2X3	T62.2X4	—	—
Spurges	T62.2X1	T62.2X2	T62.2X3	T62.2X4	—	—
Sputum viscosity-lowering drug	T48.4X1	T48.4X2	T48.4X3	T48.4X4	T48.4X5	T48.4X6
Squill	T46.0X1	T46.0X2	T46.0X3	T46.0X4	T46.0X5	T46.0X6
rat poison	T60.4X1	T60.4X2	T60.4X3	T60.4X4	—	—
Squirting cucumber (cathartic)	T47.2X1	T47.2X2	T47.2X3	T47.2X4	T47.2X5	T47.2X6
Stains	T65.6X1	T65.6X2	T65.6X3	T65.6X4	—	—
Stannous fluoride	T49.7X1	T49.7X2	T49.7X3	T49.7X4	T49.7X5	T49.7X6
Stanolone	T38.7X1	T38.7X2	T38.7X3	T38.7X4	T38.7X5	T38.7X6

Substance	External Cause (T-Code) Poisoning, Accidental (Unintentional)	Poisoning, Intentional Self-Harm	Poisoning, Assault	Poisoning, Undetermined	Adverse Effect	Underdosing
Stanozolol	T38.7X1	T38.7X2	T38.7X3	T38.7X4	T38.7X5	T38.7X6
Staphisagria or stavesacre (pediculicide)	T49.0X1	T49.0X2	T49.0X3	T49.0X4	T49.0X5	T49.0X6
Starch	T50.901	T50.902	T50.903	T50.904	T50.905	T50.906
Stelazine	T43.3X1	T43.3X2	T43.3X3	T43.3X4	T43.3X5	T43.3X6
Stemetil	T43.3X1	T43.3X2	T43.3X3	T43.3X4	T43.3X5	T43.3X6
Stepronin	T48.4X1	T48.4X2	T48.4X3	T48.4X4	T48.4X5	T48.4X6
Sterculia	T47.4X1	T47.4X2	T47.4X3	T47.4X4	T47.4X5	T47.4X6
Sternutator gas	T59.891	T59.892	T59.893	T59.894	—	—
Steroid	T38.0X1	T38.0X2	T38.0X3	T38.0X4	T38.0X5	T38.0X6
anabolic	T38.7X1	T38.7X2	T38.7X3	T38.7X4	T38.7X5	T38.7X6
androgenic	T38.7X1	T38.7X2	T38.7X3	T38.7X4	T38.7X5	T38.7X6
antineoplastic, hormone	T38.7X1	T38.7X2	T38.7X3	T38.7X4	T38.7X5	T38.7X6
estrogen	T38.5X1	T38.5X2	T38.5X3	T38.5X4	T38.5X5	T38.5X6
ENT agent	T49.6X1	T49.6X2	T49.6X3	T49.6X4	T49.6X5	T49.6X6
ophthalmic preparation	T49.5X1	T49.5X2	T49.5X3	T49.5X4	T49.5X5	T49.5X6
topical NEC	T49.0X1	T49.0X2	T49.0X3	T49.0X4	T49.0X5	T49.0X6
Stibine	T56.891	T56.892	T56.893	T56.894	—	—
Stibogluconate	T37.3X1	T37.3X2	T37.3X3	T37.3X4	T37.3X5	T37.3X6
Stibophen	T37.4X1	T37.4X2	T37.4X3	T37.4X4	T37.4X5	T37.4X6
Stilbamidine (isetionate)	T37.3X1	T37.3X2	T37.3X3	T37.3X4	T37.3X5	T37.3X6
Stilbestrol	T38.5X1	T38.5X2	T38.5X3	T38.5X4	T38.5X5	T38.5X6
Stilboestrol	T38.5X1	T38.5X2	T38.5X3	T38.5X4	T38.5X5	T38.5X6
Stimulant						
central nervous system — see also Psychostimulant	T43.601	T43.602	T43.603	T43.604	T43.605	T43.606
analeptics	T50.7X1	T50.7X2	T50.7X3	T50.7X4	T50.7X5	T50.7X6
opiate antagonist	T50.7X1	T50.7X2	T50.7X3	T50.7X4	T50.7X5	T50.7X6
psychotherapeutic NEC — see also Psychotherapeutic drug	T43.601	T43.602	T43.603	T43.604	T43.605	T43.606
specified NEC	T43.691	T43.692	T43.693	T43.694	T43.695	T43.696
respiratory	T48.901	T48.902	T48.903	T48.904	T48.905	T48.906
Stone-dissolving drug	T50.901	T50.902	T50.903	T50.904	T50.905	T50.906
Storage battery (cells) (acid)	T54.2X1	T54.2X2	T54.2X3	T54.2X4	—	—
Stovaine	T41.3X1	T41.3X2	T41.3X3	T41.3X4	T41.3X5	T41.3X6
infiltration (subcutaneous)	T41.3X1	T41.3X2	T41.3X3	T41.3X4	T41.3X5	T41.3X6
nerve block (peripheral) (plexus)	T41.3X1	T41.3X2	T41.3X3	T41.3X4	T41.3X5	T41.3X6
spinal	T41.3X1	T41.3X2	T41.3X3	T41.3X4	T41.3X5	T41.3X6
topical (surface)	T41.3X1	T41.3X2	T41.3X3	T41.3X4	T41.3X5	T41.3X6
Stovarsal	T37.8X1	T37.8X2	T37.8X3	T37.8X4	T37.8X5	T37.8X6
Stove gas — see Gas, stove	T57.91	T57.92	T57.93	T57.94		

◀ New ◀| Revised ~~deleted~~ Deleted

	External Cause (T-Code)					
Substance	Poisoning, Accidental (Unintentional)	Poisoning, Intentional Self-Harm	Poisoning, Assault	Poisoning, Undetermined	Adverse Effect	Underdosing
Stoxil	T49.5X1	T49.5X2	T49.5X3	T49.5X4	T49.5X5	T49.5X6
Stramonium	T48.6X1	T48.6X2	T48.6X3	T48.6X4	T48.6X5	T48.6X6
natural state	T62.2X1	T62.2X2	T62.2X3	T62.2X4	—	—
Streptodornase	T45.3X1	T45.3X2	T45.3X3	T45.3X4	T45.3X5	T45.3X6
Streptoduocin	T36.5X1	T36.5X2	T36.5X3	T36.5X4	T36.5X5	T36.5X6
Streptokinase	T45.611	T45.612	T45.613	T45.614	T45.615	T45.616
Streptomycin (derivative)	T36.5X1	T36.5X2	T36.5X3	T36.5X4	T36.5X5	T36.5X6
Streptonivicin	T36.5X1	T36.5X2	T36.5X3	T36.5X4	T36.5X5	T36.5X6
Streptovarycin	T36.5X1	T36.5X2	T36.5X3	T36.5X4	T36.5X5	T36.5X6
Streptozocin	T45.1X1	T45.1X2	T45.1X3	T45.1X4	T45.1X5	T45.1X6
Streptozotocin	T45.1X1	T45.1X2	T45.1X3	T45.1X4	T45.1X5	T45.1X6
Stripper (paint) (solvent)	T52.8X1	T52.8X2	T52.8X3	T52.8X4	—	—
Strobane	T60.1X1	T60.1X2	T60.1X3	T60.1X4	—	—
Strofantina	T46.0X1	T46.0X2	T46.0X3	T46.0X4	T46.0X5	T46.0X6
Strophanthin (g) (k)	T46.0X1	T46.0X2	T46.0X3	T46.0X4	T46.0X5	T46.0X6
Strophanthus	T46.0X1	T46.0X2	T46.0X3	T46.0X4	T46.0X5	T46.0X6
Strophantin	T46.0X1	T46.0X2	T46.0X3	T46.0X4	T46.0X5	T46.0X6
Strophantin-g	T46.0X1	T46.0X2	T46.0X3	T46.0X4	T46.0X5	T46.0X6
Strychnine (nonmedicinal) (pesticide) (salts)	T65.1X1	T65.1X2	T65.1X3	T65.1X4	—	—
medicinal	T48.291	T48.292	T48.293	T48.294	T48.295	T48.296
Strychnos (ignatii) — *see* Strychnine						
Styramate	T42.8X1	T42.8X2	T42.8X3	T42.8X4	T42.8X5	T42.8X6
Styrene	T65.891	T65.892	T65.893	T65.894	—	—
Succinimide, antiepileptic or anticonvulsant	T42.2X1	T42.2X2	T42.2X3	T42.2X4	T42.2X5	T42.2X6
mercuric — *see* Mercury						
Succinylcholine	T48.1X1	T48.1X2	T48.1X3	T48.1X4	T48.1X5	T48.1X6
Succinylsulfathiazole	T37.0X1	T37.0X2	T37.0X3	T37.0X4	T37.0X5	T37.0X6
Sucralfate	T47.1X1	T47.1X2	T47.1X3	T47.1X4	T47.1X5	T47.1X6
Sucrose	T50.3X1	T50.3X2	T50.3X3	T50.3X4	T50.3X5	T50.3X6
Sufentanil	T40.411	T40.412	T40.413	T40.414	T40.415	T40.416
Sulbactam	T36.0X1	T36.0X2	T36.0X3	T36.0X4	T36.0X5	T36.0X6
Sulbenicillin	T36.0X1	T36.0X2	T36.0X3	T36.0X4	T36.0X5	T36.0X6
Sulbentine	T49.0X1	T49.0X2	T49.0X3	T49.0X4	T49.0X5	T49.0X6
Sulfacetamide	T49.0X1	T49.0X2	T49.0X3	T49.0X4	T49.0X5	T49.0X6
ophthalmic preparation	T49.5X1	T49.5X2	T49.5X3	T49.5X4	T49.5X5	T49.5X6
Sulfachlorpyridazine	T37.0X1	T37.0X2	T37.0X3	T37.0X4	T37.0X5	T37.0X6
Sulfacitine	T37.0X1	T37.0X2	T37.0X3	T37.0X4	T37.0X5	T37.0X6
Sulfadiasulfone sodium	T37.0X1	T37.0X2	T37.0X3	T37.0X4	T37.0X5	T37.0X6
Sulfadiazine	T37.0X1	T37.0X2	T37.0X3	T37.0X4	T37.0X5	T37.0X6
silver (topical)	T49.0X1	T49.0X2	T49.0X3	T49.0X4	T49.0X5	T49.0X6

	External Cause (T-Code)					
Substance	Poisoning, Accidental (Unintentional)	Poisoning, Intentional Self-Harm	Poisoning, Assault	Poisoning, Undetermined	Adverse Effect	Underdosing
Sulfadimethoxine	T37.0X1	T37.0X2	T37.0X3	T37.0X4	T37.0X5	T37.0X6
Sulfadimidine	T37.0X1	T37.0X2	T37.0X3	T37.0X4	T37.0X5	T37.0X6
Sulfadoxine	T37.0X1	T37.0X2	T37.0X3	T37.0X4	T37.0X5	T37.0X6
with pyrimethamine	T37.2X1	T37.2X2	T37.2X3	T37.2X4	T37.2X5	T37.2X6
Sulfaethidole	T37.0X1	T37.0X2	T37.0X3	T37.0X4	T37.0X5	T37.0X6
Sulfafurazole	T37.0X1	T37.0X2	T37.0X3	T37.0X4	T37.0X5	T37.0X6
Sulfaguanidine	T37.0X1	T37.0X2	T37.0X3	T37.0X4	T37.0X5	T37.0X6
Sulfalene	T37.0X1	T37.0X2	T37.0X3	T37.0X4	T37.0X5	T37.0X6
Sulfaloxate	T37.0X1	T37.0X2	T37.0X3	T37.0X4	T37.0X5	T37.0X6
Sulfaloxic acid	T37.0X1	T37.0X2	T37.0X3	T37.0X4	T37.0X5	T37.0X6
Sulfamazone	T39.2X1	T39.2X2	T39.2X3	T39.2X4	T39.2X5	T39.2X6
Sulfamerazine	T37.0X1	T37.0X2	T37.0X3	T37.0X4	T37.0X5	T37.0X6
Sulfameter	T37.0X1	T37.0X2	T37.0X3	T37.0X4	T37.0X5	T37.0X6
Sulfamethazine	T37.0X1	T37.0X2	T37.0X3	T37.0X4	T37.0X5	T37.0X6
Sulfamethizole	T37.0X1	T37.0X2	T37.0X3	T37.0X4	T37.0X5	T37.0X6
Sulfamethoxazole	T37.0X1	T37.0X2	T37.0X3	T37.0X4	T37.0X5	T37.0X6
with trimethoprim	T36.8X1	T36.8X2	T36.8X3	T36.8X4	T36.8X5	T36.8X6
Sulfamethoxydiazine	T37.0X1	T37.0X2	T37.0X3	T37.0X4	T37.0X5	T37.0X6
Sulfamethoxypyridazine	T37.0X1	T37.0X2	T37.0X3	T37.0X4	T37.0X5	T37.0X6
Sulfamethylthiazole	T37.0X1	T37.0X2	T37.0X3	T37.0X4	T37.0X5	T37.0X6
Sulfametoxydiazine	T37.0X1	T37.0X2	T37.0X3	T37.0X4	T37.0X5	T37.0X6
Sulfamidopyrine	T39.2X1	T39.2X2	T39.2X3	T39.2X4	T39.2X5	T39.2X6
Sulfamonomethoxine	T37.0X1	T37.0X2	T37.0X3	T37.0X4	T37.0X5	T37.0X6
Sulfamoxole	T37.0X1	T37.0X2	T37.0X3	T37.0X4	T37.0X5	T37.0X6
Sulfamylon	T49.0X1	T49.0X2	T49.0X3	T49.0X4	T49.0X5	T49.0X6
Sulfan blue (diagnostic dye)	T50.8X1	T50.8X2	T50.8X3	T50.8X4	T50.8X5	T50.8X6
Sulfanilamide	T37.0X1	T37.0X2	T37.0X3	T37.0X4	T37.0X5	T37.0X6
Sulfanilylguanidine	T37.0X1	T37.0X2	T37.0X3	T37.0X4	T37.0X5	T37.0X6
Sulfaperin	T37.0X1	T37.0X2	T37.0X3	T37.0X4	T37.0X5	T37.0X6
Sulfaphenazole	T37.0X1	T37.0X2	T37.0X3	T37.0X4	T37.0X5	T37.0X6
Sulfaphenylthiazole	T37.0X1	T37.0X2	T37.0X3	T37.0X4	T37.0X5	T37.0X6
Sulfaproxyline	T37.0X1	T37.0X2	T37.0X3	T37.0X4	T37.0X5	T37.0X6
Sulfapyridine	T37.0X1	T37.0X2	T37.0X3	T37.0X4	T37.0X5	T37.0X6
Sulfapyrimidine	T37.0X1	T37.0X2	T37.0X3	T37.0X4	T37.0X5	T37.0X6
Sulfarsphenamine	T37.8X1	T37.8X2	T37.8X3	T37.8X4	T37.8X5	T37.8X6
Sulfasalazine	T37.0X1	T37.0X2	T37.0X3	T37.0X4	T37.0X5	T37.0X6
Sulfasuxidine	T37.0X1	T37.0X2	T37.0X3	T37.0X4	T37.0X5	T37.0X6
Sulfasymazine	T37.0X1	T37.0X2	T37.0X3	T37.0X4	T37.0X5	T37.0X6
Sulfated amylopectin	T47.8X1	T47.8X2	T47.8X3	T47.8X4	T47.8X5	T47.8X6
Sulfathiazole	T37.0X1	T37.0X2	T37.0X3	T37.0X4	T37.0X5	T37.0X6
Sulfatostearate	T49.2X1	T49.2X2	T49.2X3	T49.2X4	T49.2X5	T49.2X6
Sulfinpyrazone	T50.4X1	T50.4X2	T50.4X3	T50.4X4	T50.4X5	T50.4X6

TABLE OF DRUGS AND CHEMICALS

TABLE OF DRUGS AND CHEMICALS

Substance	External Cause (T-Code)					
	Poisoning, Accidental (Unintentional)	Poisoning, Intentional Self-Harm	Poisoning, Assault	Poisoning, Undetermined	Adverse Effect	Underdosing
Sulfiram	T49.0X1	T49.0X2	T49.0X3	T49.0X4	T49.0X5	T49.0X6
Sulfisomidine	T37.0X1	T37.0X2	T37.0X3	T37.0X4	T37.0X5	T37.0X6
Sulfisoxazole	T37.0X1	T37.0X2	T37.0X3	T37.0X4	T37.0X5	T37.0X6
ophthalmic preparation	T49.5X1	T49.5X2	T49.5X3	T49.5X4	T49.5X5	T49.5X6
Sulfobromophthalein (sodium)	T50.8X1	T50.8X2	T50.8X3	T50.8X4	T50.8X5	T50.8X6
Sulfobromphthalein	T50.8X1	T50.8X2	T50.8X3	T50.8X4	T50.8X5	T50.8X6
Sulfogaiacol	T48.4X1	T48.4X2	T48.4X3	T48.4X4	T48.4X5	T48.4X6
Sulfomyxin	T36.8X1	T36.8X2	T36.8X3	T36.8X4	T36.8X5	T36.8X6
Sulfonal	T42.6X1	T42.6X2	T42.6X3	T42.6X4	T42.6X5	T42.6X6
Sulfonamide NEC	T37.0X1	T37.0X2	T37.0X3	T37.0X4	T37.0X5	T37.0X6
eye	T49.5X1	T49.5X2	T49.5X3	T49.5X4	T49.5X5	T49.5X6
Sulfonazide	T37.1X1	T37.1X2	T37.1X3	T37.1X4	T37.1X5	T37.1X6
Sulfones	T37.1X1	T37.1X2	T37.1X3	T37.1X4	T37.1X5	T37.1X6
Sulfonethylmethane	T42.6X1	T42.6X2	T42.6X3	T42.6X4	T42.6X5	T42.6X6
Sulfonmethane	T42.6X1	T42.6X2	T42.6X3	T42.6X4	T42.6X5	T42.6X6
Sulfonphthal, sulfonphthol	T50.8X1	T50.8X2	T50.8X3	T50.8X4	T50.8X5	T50.8X6
Sulfonylurea derivatives, oral	T38.3X1	T38.3X2	T38.3X3	T38.3X4	T38.3X5	T38.3X6
Sulforidazine	T43.3X1	T43.3X2	T43.3X3	T43.3X4	T43.3X5	T43.3X6
Sulfoxone	T37.1X1	T37.1X2	T37.1X3	T37.1X4	T37.1X5	T37.1X6
Sulfur, sulfurated, sulfuric, sulfurous, sulfuryl (compounds NEC) (medicinal)	T49.4X1	T49.4X2	T49.4X3	T49.4X4	T49.4X5	T49.4X6
acid	T54.2X1	T54.2X2	T54.2X3	T54.2X4	—	—
dioxide (gas)	T59.1X1	T59.1X2	T59.1X3	T59.1X4	—	—
ether — see Ether(s)						
hydrogen	T59.6X1	T59.6X2	T59.6X3	T59.6X4	—	—
medicinal (keratolytic) (ointment) NEC	T49.4X1	T49.4X2	T49.4X3	T49.4X4	T49.4X5	T49.4X6
ointment	T49.0X1	T49.0X2	T49.0X3	T49.0X4	T49.0X5	T49.0X6
pesticide (vapor)	T60.91	T60.92	T60.93	T60.94	—	—
vapor NEC	T59.891	T59.892	T59.893	T59.894	—	—
Sulfuric acid	T54.2X1	T54.2X2	T54.2X3	T54.2X4		
Sulglicotide	T47.1X1	T47.1X2	T47.1X3	T47.1X4	T47.1X5	T47.1X6
Sulindac	T39.391	T39.392	T39.393	T39.394	T39.395	T39.396
Sulisatin	T47.2X1	T47.2X2	T47.2X3	T47.2X4	T47.2X5	T47.2X6
Sulisobenzone	T49.3X1	T49.3X2	T49.3X3	T49.3X4	T49.3X5	T49.3X6
Sulkowitch's reagent	T50.8X1	T50.8X2	T50.8X3	T50.8X4	T50.8X5	T50.8X6
Sulmetozine	T44.3X1	T44.3X2	T44.3X3	T44.3X4	T44.3X5	T44.3X6
Suloctidil	T46.7X1	T46.7X2	T46.7X3	T46.7X4	T46.7X5	T46.7X6
Sulph — see also Sulf-						
Sulphadiazine	T37.0X1	T37.0X2	T37.0X3	T37.0X4	T37.0X5	T37.0X6
Sulphadimethoxine	T37.0X1	T37.0X2	T37.0X3	T37.0X4	T37.0X5	T37.0X6

Substance	External Cause (T-Code)					
	Poisoning, Accidental (Unintentional)	Poisoning, Intentional Self-Harm	Poisoning, Assault	Poisoning, Undetermined	Adverse Effect	Underdosing
Sulphadimidine	T37.0X1	T37.0X2	T37.0X3	T37.0X4	T37.0X5	T37.0X6
Sulphadione	T37.1X1	T37.1X2	T37.1X3	T37.1X4	T37.1X5	T37.1X6
Sulphafurazole	T37.0X1	T37.0X2	T37.0X3	T37.0X4	T37.0X5	T37.0X6
Sulphamethizole	T37.0X1	T37.0X2	T37.0X3	T37.0X4	T37.0X5	T37.0X6
Sulphamethoxazole	T37.0X1	T37.0X2	T37.0X3	T37.0X4	T37.0X5	T37.0X6
Sulphan blue	T50.8X1	T50.8X2	T50.8X3	T50.8X4	T50.8X5	T50.8X6
Sulphaphenazole	T37.0X1	T37.0X2	T37.0X3	T37.0X4	T37.0X5	T37.0X6
Sulphapyridine	T37.0X1	T37.0X2	T37.0X3	T37.0X4	T37.0X5	T37.0X6
Sulphasalazine	T37.0X1	T37.0X2	T37.0X3	T37.0X4	T37.0X5	T37.0X6
Sulphinpyrazone	T50.4X1	T50.4X2	T50.4X3	T50.4X4	T50.4X5	T50.4X6
Sulpiride	T43.591	T43.592	T43.593	T43.594	T43.595	T43.596
Sulprostone	T48.0X1	T48.0X2	T48.0X3	T48.0X4	T48.0X5	T48.0X6
Sulpyrine	T39.2X1	T39.2X2	T39.2X3	T39.2X4	T39.2X5	T39.2X6
Sultamicillin	T36.0X1	T36.0X2	T36.0X3	T36.0X4	T36.0X5	T36.0X6
Sulthiame	T42.6X1	T42.6X2	T42.6X3	T42.6X4	T42.6X5	T42.6X6
Sultiame	T42.6X1	T42.6X2	T42.6X3	T42.6X4	T42.6X5	T42.6X6
Sultopride	T43.591	T43.592	T43.593	T43.594	T43.595	T43.596
Sumatriptan	T39.8X1	T39.8X2	T39.8X3	T39.8X4	T39.8X5	T39.8X6
Sunflower seed oil	T46.6X1	T46.6X2	T46.6X3	T46.6X4	T46.6X5	T46.6X6
Superinone	T48.4X1	T48.4X2	T48.4X3	T48.4X4	T48.4X5	T48.4X6
Suprofen	T39.311	T39.312	T39.313	T39.314	T39.315	T39.316
Suramin (sodium)	T37.4X1	T37.4X2	T37.4X3	T37.4X4	T37.4X5	T37.4X6
Surfacaine	T41.3X1	T41.3X2	T41.3X3	T41.3X4	T41.3X5	T41.3X6
Surital	T41.1X1	T41.1X2	T41.1X3	T41.1X4	T41.1X5	T41.1X6
Sutilains	T45.3X1	T45.3X2	T45.3X3	T45.3X4	T45.3X5	T45.3X6
Suxamethonium (chloride)	T48.1X1	T48.1X2	T48.1X3	T48.1X4	T48.1X5	T48.1X6
Suxethonium (chloride)	T48.1X1	T48.1X2	T48.1X3	T48.1X4	T48.1X5	T48.1X6
Suxibuzone	T39.2X1	T39.2X2	T39.2X3	T39.2X4	T39.2X5	T39.2X6
Sweet oil (birch)	T49.3X1	T49.3X2	T49.3X3	T49.3X4	T49.3X5	T49.3X6
Sweet niter spirit	T46.3X1	T46.3X2	T46.3X3	T46.3X4	T46.3X5	T46.3X6
Sweetener	T50.901	T50.902	T50.903	T50.904	T50.905	T50.906
Sym-dichloroethyl ether	T53.6X1	T53.6X2	T53.6X3	T53.6X4	—	—
Sympatholytic NEC	T44.8X1	T44.8X2	T44.8X3	T44.8X4	T44.8X5	T44.8X6
haloalkylamine	T44.8X1	T44.8X2	T44.8X3	T44.8X4	T44.8X5	T44.8X6
Sympathomimetic NEC	T44.901	T44.902	T44.903	T44.904	T44.905	T44.906
anti-common-cold	T48.5X1	T48.5X2	T48.5X3	T48.5X4	T48.5X5	T48.5X6
bronchodilator	T48.6X1	T48.6X2	T48.6X3	T48.6X4	T48.6X5	T48.6X6
specified NEC	T44.991	T44.992	T44.993	T44.994	T44.995	T44.996
Synagis	T50.B91	T50.B92	T50.B93	T50.B94	T50.B95	T50.B96
Synalar	T49.0X1	T49.0X2	T49.0X3	T49.0X4	T49.0X5	T49.0X6
Synthetic cannabinoids	T40.721	T40.722	T40.723	T40.724	T40.725	T40.726
Synthroid	T38.1X1	T38.1X2	T38.1X3	T38.1X4	T38.1X5	T38.1X6

◀ New ◀ Revised ~~deleted~~ Deleted

	External Cause (T-Code)					
Substance	Poisoning, Accidental (Unintentional)	Poisoning, Intentional Self-Harm	Poisoning, Assault	Poisoning, Undetermined	Adverse Effect	Underdosing
Syntocinon	T48.0X1	T48.0X2	T48.0X3	T48.0X4	T48.0X5	T48.0X6
Syrosingopine	T46.5X1	T46.5X2	T46.5X3	T46.5X4	T46.5X5	T46.5X6
Systemic drug	T45.91	T45.92	T45.93	T45.94	T45.95	T45.96
specified NEC	T45.8X1	T45.8X2	T45.8X3	T45.8X4	T45.8X5	T45.8X6
2,4,5-T	T60.3X1	T60.3X2	T60.3X3	T60.3X4	—	—
T						
Tablets — see also specified substance	T50.901	T50.902	T50.903	T50.904	T50.905	T50.906
Tace	T38.5X1	T38.5X2	T38.5X3	T38.5X4	T38.5X5	T38.5X6
Tacrine	T44.0X1	T44.0X2	T44.0X3	T44.0X4	T44.0X5	T44.0X6
Tadalafil	T46.7X1	T46.7X2	T46.7X3	T46.7X4	T46.7X5	T46.7X6
Talampicillin	T36.0X1	T36.0X2	T36.0X3	T36.0X4	T36.0X5	T36.0X6
Talbutal	T42.3X1	T42.3X2	T42.3X3	T42.3X4	T42.3X5	T42.3X6
Talc powder	T49.3X1	T49.3X2	T49.3X3	T49.3X4	T49.3X5	T49.3X6
Talcum	T49.3X1	T49.3X2	T49.3X3	T49.3X4	T49.3X5	T49.3X6
Taleranol	T38.6X1	T38.6X2	T38.6X3	T38.6X4	T38.6X5	T38.6X6
Tamoxifen	T38.6X1	T38.6X2	T38.6X3	T38.6X4	T38.6X5	T38.6X6
Tamsulosin	T44.6X1	T44.6X2	T44.6X3	T44.6X4	T44.6X5	T44.6X6
Tandearil, tanderil	T39.2X1	T39.2X2	T39.2X3	T39.2X4	T39.2X5	T39.2X6
Tannic acid	T49.2X1	T49.2X2	T49.2X3	T49.2X4	T49.2X5	T49.2X6
medicinal (astringent)	T49.2X1	T49.2X2	T49.2X3	T49.2X4	T49.2X5	T49.2X6
Tannin — see Tannic acid						
Tansy	T62.2X1	T62.2X2	T62.2X3	T62.2X4	—	—
TAO	T36.3X1	T36.3X2	T36.3X3	T36.3X4	T36.3X5	T36.3X6
Tapazole	T38.2X1	T38.2X2	T38.2X3	T38.2X4	T38.2X5	T38.2X6
Tar NEC	T52.0X1	T52.0X2	T52.0X3	T52.0X4	—	—
camphor	T60.1X1	T60.1X2	T60.1X3	T60.1X4	—	—
distillate	T49.1X1	T49.1X2	T49.1X3	T49.1X4	T49.1X5	T49.1X6
fumes	T59.891	T59.892	T59.893	T59.894	—	—
medicinal	T49.1X1	T49.1X2	T49.1X3	T49.1X4	T49.1X5	T49.1X6
ointment	T49.1X1	T49.1X2	T49.1X3	T49.1X4	T49.1X5	T49.1X6
Taractan	T43.591	T43.592	T43.593	T43.594	T43.595	T43.596
Tarantula (venomous)	T63.321	T63.322	T63.323	T63.324	—	—
Tartar emetic	T37.8X1	T37.8X2	T37.8X3	T37.8X4	T37.8X5	T37.8X6
Tartaric acid	T65.891	T65.892	T65.893	T65.894	—	—
Tartrated antimony (anti-infective)	T37.8X1	T37.8X2	T37.8X3	T37.8X4	T37.8X5	T37.8X6
Tartrate, laxative	T47.4X1	T47.4X2	T47.4X3	T47.4X4	T47.4X5	T47.4X6
Tauromustine	T45.1X1	T45.1X2	T45.1X3	T45.1X4	T45.1X5	T45.1X6
TCA — see Trichloroacetic acid						
TCDD	T53.7X1	T53.7X2	T53.7X3	T53.7X4	—	—
TDI (vapor)	T65.0X1	T65.0X2	T65.0X3	T65.0X4	—	—

	External Cause (T-Code)					
Substance	Poisoning, Accidental (Unintentional)	Poisoning, Intentional Self-Harm	Poisoning, Assault	Poisoning, Undetermined	Adverse Effect	Underdosing
Tear						
gas	T59.3X1	T59.3X2	T59.3X3	T59.3X4	—	—
solution	T49.5X1	T49.5X2	T49.5X3	T49.5X4	T49.5X5	T49.5X6
Teclothiazide	T50.2X1	T50.2X2	T50.2X3	T50.2X4	T50.2X5	T50.2X6
Teclozan	T37.3X1	T37.3X2	T37.3X3	T37.3X4	T37.3X5	T37.3X6
Tegafur	T45.1X1	T45.1X2	T45.1X3	T45.1X4	T45.1X5	T45.1X6
Tegretol	T42.1X1	T42.1X2	T42.1X3	T42.1X4	T42.1X5	T42.1X6
Teicoplanin	T36.8X1	T36.8X2	T36.8X3	T36.8X4	T36.8X5	T36.8X6
Telepaque	T50.8X1	T50.8X2	T50.8X3	T50.8X4	T50.8X5	T50.8X6
Tellurium	T56.891	T56.892	T56.893	T56.894	—	—
fumes	T56.891	T56.892	T56.893	T56.894	—	—
TEM	T45.1X1	T45.1X2	T45.1X3	T45.1X4	T45.1X5	T45.1X6
Temazepam	T42.4X1	T42.4X2	T42.4X3	T42.4X4	T42.4X5	T42.4X6
Temocillin	T36.0X1	T36.0X2	T36.0X3	T36.0X4	T36.0X5	T36.0X6
Tenamfetamine	T43.621	T43.622	T43.623	T43.624	T43.625	T43.626
Teniposide	T45.1X1	T45.1X2	T45.1X3	T45.1X4	T45.1X5	T45.1X6
Tenitramine	T46.3X1	T46.3X2	T46.3X3	T46.3X4	T46.3X5	T46.3X6
Tenoglicin	T48.4X1	T48.4X2	T48.4X3	T48.4X4	T48.4X5	T48.4X6
Tenonitrozole	T37.3X1	T37.3X2	T37.3X3	T37.3X4	T37.3X5	T37.3X6
Tenoxicam	T39.391	T39.392	T39.393	T39.394	T39.395	T39.396
TEPA	T45.1X1	T45.1X2	T45.1X3	T45.1X4	T45.1X5	T45.1X6
TEPP	T60.0X1	T60.0X2	T60.0X3	T60.0X4	—	—
Teprotide	T46.5X1	T46.5X2	T46.5X3	T46.5X4	T46.5X5	T46.5X6
Terazosin	T44.6X1	T44.6X2	T44.6X3	T44.6X4	T44.6X5	T44.6X6
Terbufos	T60.0X1	T60.0X2	T60.0X3	T60.0X4	—	—
Terbutaline	T48.6X1	T48.6X2	T48.6X3	T48.6X4	T48.6X5	T48.6X6
Terconazole	T49.0X1	T49.0X2	T49.0X3	T49.0X4	T49.0X5	T49.0X6
Terfenadine	T45.0X1	T45.0X2	T45.0X3	T45.0X4	T45.0X5	T45.0X6
Teriparatide (acetate)	T50.991	T50.992	T50.993	T50.994	T50.995	T50.996
Terizidone	T37.1X1	T37.1X2	T37.1X3	T37.1X4	T37.1X5	T37.1X6
Terlipressin	T38.891	T38.892	T38.893	T38.894	T38.895	T38.896
Terodiline	T46.3X1	T46.3X2	T46.3X3	T46.3X4	T46.3X5	T46.3X6
Teroxalene	T37.4X1	T37.4X2	T37.4X3	T37.4X4	T37.4X5	T37.4X6
Terpin(cis) hydrate	T48.4X1	T48.4X2	T48.4X3	T48.4X4	T48.4X5	T48.4X6
Terramycin	T36.4X1	T36.4X2	T36.4X3	T36.4X4	T36.4X5	T36.4X6
Tertatolol	T44.7X1	T44.7X2	T44.7X3	T44.7X4	T44.7X5	T44.7X6
Tessalon	T48.3X1	T48.3X2	T48.3X3	T48.3X4	T48.3X5	T48.3X6
Testolactone	T38.7X1	T38.7X2	T38.7X3	T38.7X4	T38.7X5	T38.7X6
Testosterone	T38.7X1	T38.7X2	T38.7X3	T38.7X4	T38.7X5	T38.7X6
Tetanus toxoid or vaccine	T50.A91	T50.A92	T50.A93	T50.A94	T50.A95	T50.A96
antitoxin	T50.Z11	T50.Z12	T50.Z13	T50.Z14	T50.Z15	T50.Z16
immune globulin (human)	T50.Z11	T50.Z12	T50.Z13	T50.Z14	T50.Z15	T50.Z16

◀ New   ◀ Revised   ~~deleted~~ Deleted

TABLE OF DRUGS AND CHEMICALS

TABLE OF DRUGS AND CHEMICALS

Substance	External Cause (T-Code)					
	Poisoning, Accidental (Unintentional)	Poisoning, Intentional Self-Harm	Poisoning, Assault	Poisoning, Undetermined	Adverse Effect	Underdosing
Tetanus toxoid or vaccine (Continued)						
toxoid	T50.A91	T50.A92	T50.A93	T50.A94	T50.A95	T50.A96
with diphtheria toxoid	T50.A21	T50.A22	T50.A23	T50.A24	T50.A25	T50.A26
with pertussis	T50.A11	T50.A12	T50.A13	T50.A14	T50.A15	T50.A16
Tetrabenazine	T43.591	T43.592	T43.593	T43.594	T43.595	T43.596
Tetracaine	T41.3X1	T41.3X2	T41.3X3	T41.3X4	T41.3X5	T41.3X6
nerve block (peripheral) (plexus)	T41.3X1	T41.3X2	T41.3X3	T41.3X4	T41.3X5	T41.3X6
regional	T41.3X1	T41.3X2	T41.3X3	T41.3X4	T41.3X5	T41.3X6
spinal	T41.3X1	T41.3X2	T41.3X3	T41.3X4	T41.3X5	T41.3X6
Tetrachlorethylene — see Tetrachloroethylene						
Tetrachlormethiazide	T50.2X1	T50.2X2	T50.2X3	T50.2X4	T50.2X5	T50.2X6
2,3,7,8-Tetrachlorodibenzo-p-dioxin	T53.7X1	T53.7X2	T53.7X3	T53.7X4	—	—
Tetrachloroethane	T53.6X1	T53.6X2	T53.6X3	T53.6X4	—	—
vapor	T53.6X1	T53.6X2	T53.6X3	T53.6X4	—	—
paint or varnish	T53.6X1	T53.6X2	T53.6X3	T53.6X4	—	—
Tetrachloroethylene (liquid)	T53.3X1	T53.3X2	T53.3X3	T53.3X4	—	—
medicinal	T37.4X1	T37.4X2	T37.4X3	T37.4X4	T37.4X5	T37.4X6
vapor	T53.3X1	T53.3X2	T53.3X3	T53.3X4	—	—
Tetrachloromethane — see Carbon tetrachloride						
Tetracosactide	T38.811	T38.812	T38.813	T38.814	T38.815	T38.816
Tetracosactrin	T38.811	T38.812	T38.813	T38.814	T38.815	T38.816
Tetracycline	T36.4X1	T36.4X2	T36.4X3	T36.4X4	T36.4X5	T36.4X6
ophthalmic preparation	T49.5X1	T49.5X2	T49.5X3	T49.5X4	T49.5X5	T49.5X6
topical NEC	T49.0X1	T49.0X2	T49.0X3	T49.0X4	T49.0X5	T49.0X6
Tetradifon	T60.8X1	T60.8X2	T60.8X3	T60.8X4	—	—
Tetradotoxin	T61.771	T61.772	T61.773	T61.774		
Tetraethyl						
lead	T56.0X1	T56.0X2	T56.0X3	T56.0X4	—	—
pyrophosphate	T60.0X1	T60.0X2	T60.0X3	T60.0X4	—	—
Tetraethylammonium chloride	T44.2X1	T44.2X2	T44.2X3	T44.2X4	T44.2X5	T44.2X6
Tetraethylthiuram disulfide	T50.6X1	T50.6X2	T50.6X3	T50.6X4	T50.6X5	T50.6X6
Tetrahydroaminoacridine	T44.0X1	T44.0X2	T44.0X3	T44.0X4	T44.0X5	T44.0X6
Tetrahydrocannabinol	T40.711	T40.712	T40.713	T40.714	T40.715	T40.716
Tetrahydrofuran	T52.8X1	T52.8X2	T52.8X3	T52.8X4	—	—
Tetrahydronaphthalene	T52.8X1	T52.8X2	T52.8X3	T52.8X4	—	—
Tetrahydrozoline	T49.5X1	T49.5X2	T49.5X3	T49.5X4	T49.5X5	T49.5X6
Tetralin	T52.8X1	T52.8X2	T52.8X3	T52.8X4	—	—
Tetramethrin	T60.2X1	T60.2X2	T60.2X3	T60.2X4	—	—

Substance	External Cause (T-Code)					
	Poisoning, Accidental (Unintentional)	Poisoning, Intentional Self-Harm	Poisoning, Assault	Poisoning, Undetermined	Adverse Effect	Underdosing
Tetramethylthiuram (disulfide) NEC	T60.3X1	T60.3X2	T60.3X3	T60.3X4	—	—
medicinal	T49.0X1	T49.0X2	T49.0X3	T49.0X4	T49.0X5	T49.0X6
Tetramisole	T37.4X1	T37.4X2	T37.4X3	T37.4X4	T37.4X5	T37.4X6
Tetranicotinoyl fructose	T46.7X1	T46.7X2	T46.7X3	T46.7X4	T46.7X5	T46.7X6
Tetronal	T42.6X1	T42.6X2	T42.6X3	T42.6X4	T42.6X5	T42.6X6
Tetrazepam	T42.4X1	T42.4X2	T42.4X3	T42.4X4	T42.4X5	T42.4X6
Tetryl	T65.3X1	T65.3X2	T65.3X3	T65.3X4	—	—
Tetrylammonium chloride	T44.2X1	T44.2X2	T44.2X3	T44.2X4	T44.2X5	T44.2X6
Tetryzoline	T49.5X1	T49.5X2	T49.5X3	T49.5X4	T49.5X5	T49.5X6
Thalidomide	T45.1X1	T45.1X2	T45.1X3	T45.1X4	T45.1X5	T45.1X6
Thallium (compounds) (dust) NEC	T56.811	T56.812	T56.813	T56.814	—	—
pesticide	T60.4X1	T60.4X2	T60.4X3	T60.4X4	—	—
THC	T40.711	T40.712	T40.713	T40.714	T40.715	T40.716
Thebacon	T48.3X1	T48.3X2	T48.3X3	T48.3X4	T48.3X5	T48.3X6
Thebaine	T40.2X1	T40.2X2	T40.2X3	T40.2X4	T40.2X5	T40.2X6
Thenoic acid	T49.6X1	T49.6X2	T49.6X3	T49.6X4	T49.6X5	T49.6X6
Thenyldiamine	T45.0X1	T45.0X2	T45.0X3	T45.0X4	T45.0X5	T45.0X6
Theobromine (calcium salicylate)	T48.6X1	T48.6X2	T48.6X3	T48.6X4	T48.6X5	T48.6X6
sodium salicylate	T48.6X1	T48.6X2	T48.6X3	T48.6X4	T48.6X5	T48.6X6
Theophyllamine	T48.6X1	T48.6X2	T48.6X3	T48.6X4	T48.6X5	T48.6X6
Theophylline	T48.6X1	T48.6X2	T48.6X3	T48.6X4	T48.6X5	T48.6X6
aminobenzoic acid	T48.6X1	T48.6X2	T48.6X3	T48.6X4	T48.6X5	T48.6X6
ethylenediamine	T48.6X1	T48.6X2	T48.6X3	T48.6X4	T48.6X5	T48.6X6
piperazine p-amino-benzoate	T48.6X1	T48.6X2	T48.6X3	T48.6X4	T48.6X5	T48.6X6
Thiabendazole	T37.4X1	T37.4X2	T37.4X3	T37.4X4	T37.4X5	T37.4X6
Thialbarbital	T41.1X1	T41.1X2	T41.1X3	T41.1X4	T41.1X5	T41.1X6
Thiamazole	T38.2X1	T38.2X2	T38.2X3	T38.2X4	T38.2X5	T38.2X6
Thiambutosine	T37.1X1	T37.1X2	T37.1X3	T37.1X4	T37.1X5	T37.1X6
Thiamine	T45.2X1	T45.2X2	T45.2X3	T45.2X4	T45.2X5	T45.2X6
Thiamphenicol	T36.2X1	T36.2X2	T36.2X3	T36.2X4	T36.2X5	T36.2X6
Thiamylal	T41.1X1	T41.1X2	T41.1X3	T41.1X4	T41.1X5	T41.1X6
sodium	T41.1X1	T41.1X2	T41.1X3	T41.1X4	T41.1X5	T41.1X6
Thiazesim	T43.291	T43.292	T43.293	T43.294	T43.295	T43.296
Thiazides (diuretics)	T50.2X1	T50.2X2	T50.2X3	T50.2X4	T50.2X5	T50.2X6
Thiazinamium metilsulfate	T43.3X1	T43.3X2	T43.3X3	T43.3X4	T43.3X5	T43.3X6
Thiethylperazine	T43.3X1	T43.3X2	T43.3X3	T43.3X4	T43.3X5	T43.3X6
Thimerosal	T49.0X1	T49.0X2	T49.0X3	T49.0X4	T49.0X5	T49.0X6
ophthalmic preparation	T49.5X1	T49.5X2	T49.5X3	T49.5X4	T49.5X5	T49.5X6
Thioacetazone	T37.1X1	T37.1X2	T37.1X3	T37.1X4	T37.1X5	T37.1X6
with isoniazid	T37.1X1	T37.1X2	T37.1X3	T37.1X4	T37.1X5	T37.1X6
Thiobarbital sodium	T41.1X1	T41.1X2	T41.1X3	T41.1X4	T41.1X5	T41.1X6

◀ New ◀ Revised ~~deleted~~ Deleted

Substance	Poisoning, Accidental (Unintentional)	Poisoning, Intentional Self-Harm	Poisoning, Assault	Poisoning, Undetermined	Adverse Effect	Underdosing
Thiobarbiturate anesthetic	T41.1X1	T41.1X2	T41.1X3	T41.1X4	T41.1X5	T41.1X6
Thiobismol	T37.8X1	T37.8X2	T37.8X3	T37.8X4	T37.8X5	T37.8X6
Thiobutabarbital sodium	T41.1X1	T41.1X2	T41.1X3	T41.1X4	T41.1X5	T41.1X6
Thiocarbamate (insecticide)	T60.0X1	T60.0X2	T60.0X3	T60.0X4	—	—
Thiocarbamide	T38.2X1	T38.2X2	T38.2X3	T38.2X4	T38.2X5	T38.2X6
Thiocarbarsone	T37.8X1	T37.8X2	T37.8X3	T37.8X4	T37.8X5	T37.8X6
Thiocarlide	T37.1X1	T37.1X2	T37.1X3	T37.1X4	T37.1X5	T37.1X6
Thioctamide	T50.991	T50.992	T50.993	T50.994	T50.995	T50.996
Thioctic acid	T50.991	T50.992	T50.993	T50.994	T50.995	T50.996
Thiofos	T60.0X1	T60.0X2	T60.0X3	T60.0X4	—	—
Thioglycolate	T49.4X1	T49.4X2	T49.4X3	T49.4X4	T49.4X5	T49.4X6
Thioglycolic acid	T65.891	T65.892	T65.893	T65.894	—	—
Thioguanine	T45.1X1	T45.1X2	T45.1X3	T45.1X4	T45.1X5	T45.1X6
Thiomercaptomerin	T50.2X1	T50.2X2	T50.2X3	T50.2X4	T50.2X5	T50.2X6
Thiomerin	T50.2X1	T50.2X2	T50.2X3	T50.2X4	T50.2X5	T50.2X6
Thiomersal	T49.0X1	T49.0X2	T49.0X3	T49.0X4	T49.0X5	T49.0X6
Thionazin	T60.0X1	T60.0X2	T60.0X3	T60.0X4	—	—
Thiopental (sodium)	T41.1X1	T41.1X2	T41.1X3	T41.1X4	T41.1X5	T41.1X6
Thiopentone (sodium)	T41.1X1	T41.1X2	T41.1X3	T41.1X4	T41.1X5	T41.1X6
Thiopropazate	T43.3X1	T43.3X2	T43.3X3	T43.3X4	T43.3X5	T43.3X6
Thioproperazine	T43.3X1	T43.3X2	T43.3X3	T43.3X4	T43.3X5	T43.3X6
Thioridazine	T43.3X1	T43.3X2	T43.3X3	T43.3X4	T43.3X5	T43.3X6
Thiosinamine	T49.3X1	T49.3X2	T49.3X3	T49.3X4	T49.3X5	T49.3X6
Thiotepa	T45.1X1	T45.1X2	T45.1X3	T45.1X4	T45.1X5	T45.1X6
Thiothixene	T43.4X1	T43.4X2	T43.4X3	T43.4X4	T43.4X5	T43.4X6
Thiouracil (benzyl) (methyl) (propyl)	T38.2X1	T38.2X2	T38.2X3	T38.2X4	T38.2X5	T38.2X6
Thiourea	T38.2X1	T38.2X2	T38.2X3	T38.2X4	T38.2X5	T38.2X6
Thiphenamil	T44.3X1	T44.3X2	T44.3X3	T44.3X4	T44.3X5	T44.3X6
Thiram	T60.3X1	T60.3X2	T60.3X3	T60.3X4	—	—
medicinal	T49.2X1	T49.2X2	T49.2X3	T49.2X4	T49.2X5	T49.2X6
Thonzylamine (systemic)	T45.0X1	T45.0X2	T45.0X3	T45.0X4	T45.0X5	T45.0X6
mucosal decongestant	T48.5X1	T48.5X2	T48.5X3	T48.5X4	T48.5X5	T48.5X6
Thorazine	T43.3X1	T43.3X2	T43.3X3	T43.3X4	T43.3X5	T43.3X6
Thorium dioxide suspension	T50.8X1	T50.8X2	T50.8X3	T50.8X4	T50.8X5	T50.8X6
Thornapple	T62.2X1	T62.2X2	T62.2X3	T62.2X4	—	—
Throat drug NEC	T49.6X1	T49.6X2	T49.6X3	T49.6X4	T49.6X5	T49.6X6
Thrombin	T45.7X1	T45.7X2	T45.7X3	T45.7X4	T45.7X5	T45.7X6
Thrombolysin	T45.611	T45.612	T45.613	T45.614	T45.615	T45.616
Thromboplastin	T45.7X1	T45.7X2	T45.7X3	T45.7X4	T45.7X5	T45.7X6
Thurfyl nicotinate	T46.7X1	T46.7X2	T46.7X3	T46.7X4	T46.7X5	T46.7X6
Thymol	T49.0X1	T49.0X2	T49.0X3	T49.0X4	T49.0X5	T49.0X6

Substance	Poisoning, Accidental (Unintentional)	Poisoning, Intentional Self-Harm	Poisoning, Assault	Poisoning, Undetermined	Adverse Effect	Underdosing
Thymopentin	T37.5X1	T37.5X2	T37.5X3	T37.5X4	T37.5X5	T37.5X6
Thymoxamine	T46.7X1	T46.7X2	T46.7X3	T46.7X4	T46.7X5	T46.7X6
Thymus extract	T38.891	T38.892	T38.893	T38.894	T38.895	T38.896
Thyreotrophic hormone	T38.811	T38.812	T38.813	T38.814	T38.815	T38.816
Thyroglobulin	T38.1X1	T38.1X2	T38.1X3	T38.1X4	T38.1X5	T38.1X6
Thyroid (hormone)	T38.1X1	T38.1X2	T38.1X3	T38.1X4	T38.1X5	T38.1X6
Thyrolar	T38.1X1	T38.1X2	T38.1X3	T38.1X4	T38.1X5	T38.1X6
Thyrotrophin	T38.811	T38.812	T38.813	T38.814	T38.815	T38.816
Thyrotropic hormone	T38.811	T38.812	T38.813	T38.814	T38.815	T38.816
Thyroxine	T38.1X1	T38.1X2	T38.1X3	T38.1X4	T38.1X5	T38.1X6
Tiabendazole	T37.4X1	T37.4X2	T37.4X3	T37.4X4	T37.4X5	T37.4X6
Tiamizide	T50.2X1	T50.2X2	T50.2X3	T50.2X4	T50.2X5	T50.2X6
Tianeptine	T43.291	T43.292	T43.293	T43.294	T43.295	T43.296
Tiapamil	T46.1X1	T46.1X2	T46.1X3	T46.1X4	T46.1X5	T46.1X6
Tiapride	T43.591	T43.592	T43.593	T43.594	T43.595	T43.596
Tiaprofenic acid	T39.311	T39.312	T39.313	T39.314	T39.315	T39.316
Tiaramide	T39.8X1	T39.8X2	T39.8X3	T39.8X4	T39.8X5	T39.8X6
Ticarcillin	T36.0X1	T36.0X2	T36.0X3	T36.0X4	T36.0X5	T36.0X6
Ticlatone	T49.0X1	T49.0X2	T49.0X3	T49.0X4	T49.0X5	T49.0X6
Ticlopidine	T45.521	T45.522	T45.523	T45.524	T45.525	T45.526
Ticrynafen	T50.1X1	T50.1X2	T50.1X3	T50.1X4	T50.1X5	T50.1X6
Tidiacic	T50.991	T50.992	T50.993	T50.994	T50.995	T50.996
Tiemonium	T44.3X1	T44.3X2	T44.3X3	T44.3X4	T44.3X5	T44.3X6
iodide	T44.3X1	T44.3X2	T44.3X3	T44.3X4	T44.3X5	T44.3X6
Tienilic acid	T50.1X1	T50.1X2	T50.1X3	T50.1X4	T50.1X5	T50.1X6
Tifenamil	T44.3X1	T44.3X2	T44.3X3	T44.3X4	T44.3X5	T44.3X6
Tigan	T45.0X1	T45.0X2	T45.0X3	T45.0X4	T45.0X5	T45.0X6
Tigloidine	T44.3X1	T44.3X2	T44.3X3	T44.3X4	T44.3X5	T44.3X6
Tilactase	T47.5X1	T47.5X2	T47.5X3	T47.5X4	T47.5X5	T47.5X6
Tiletamine	T41.291	T41.292	T41.293	T41.294	T41.295	T41.296
Tilidine	T40.441	T40.442	T40.443	T40.444	—	—
Timepidium bromide	T44.3X1	T44.3X2	T44.3X3	T44.3X4	T44.3X5	T44.3X6
Timiperone	T43.4X1	T43.4X2	T43.4X3	T43.4X4	T43.4X5	T43.4X6
Timolol	T44.7X1	T44.7X2	T44.7X3	T44.7X4	T44.7X5	T44.7X6
Tin (chloride) (dust) (oxide) NEC	T56.6X1	T56.6X2	T56.6X3	T56.6X4	—	—
anti-infectives	T37.8X1	T37.8X2	T37.8X3	T37.8X4	T37.8X5	T37.8X6
Tincture, iodine—see Iodine						
Tindal	T43.3X1	T43.3X2	T43.3X3	T43.3X4	T43.3X5	T43.3X6
Tinidazole	T37.3X1	T37.3X2	T37.3X3	T37.3X4	T37.3X5	T37.3X6
Tinoridine	T39.8X1	T39.8X2	T39.8X3	T39.8X4	T39.8X5	T39.8X6
Tiocarlide	T37.1X1	T37.1X2	T37.1X3	T37.1X4	T37.1X5	T37.1X6
Tioclomarol	T45.511	T45.512	T45.513	T45.514	T45.515	T45.516

◀ New　◀ Revised　deleted Deleted

TABLE OF DRUGS AND CHEMICALS

Substance	External Cause (T-Code)					
	Poisoning, Accidental (Unintentional)	Poisoning, Intentional Self-Harm	Poisoning, Assault	Poisoning, Undetermined	Adverse Effect	Underdosing
Tioconazole	T49.0X1	T49.0X2	T49.0X3	T49.0X4	T49.0X5	T49.0X6
Tioguanine	T45.1X1	T45.1X2	T45.1X3	T45.1X4	T45.1X5	T45.1X6
Tiopronin	T50.991	T50.992	T50.993	T50.994	T50.995	T50.996
Tiotixene	T43.4X1	T43.4X2	T43.4X3	T43.4X4	T43.4X5	T43.4X6
Tioxolone	T49.4X1	T49.4X2	T49.4X3	T49.4X4	T49.4X5	T49.4X6
Tipepidine	T48.3X1	T48.3X2	T48.3X3	T48.3X4	T48.3X5	T48.3X6
Tiquizium bromide	T44.3X1	T44.3X2	T44.3X3	T44.3X4	T44.3X5	T44.3X6
Tiratricol	T38.1X1	T38.1X2	T38.1X3	T38.1X4	T38.1X5	T38.1X6
Tisopurine	T50.4X1	T50.4X2	T50.4X3	T50.4X4	T50.4X5	T50.4X6
Titanium (compounds) (vapor)	T56.891	T56.892	T56.893	T56.894	—	—
dioxide	T49.3X1	T49.3X2	T49.3X3	T49.3X4	T49.3X5	T49.3X6
ointment	T49.3X1	T49.3X2	T49.3X3	T49.3X4	T49.3X5	T49.3X6
oxide	T49.3X1	T49.3X2	T49.3X3	T49.3X4	T49.3X5	T49.3X6
tetrachloride	T56.891	T56.892	T56.893	T56.894	—	—
Titanocene	T56.891	T56.892	T56.893	T56.894	—	—
Titroid	T38.1X1	T38.1X2	T38.1X3	T38.1X4	T38.1X5	T38.1X6
Tizanidine	T42.8X1	T42.8X2	T42.8X3	T42.8X4	T42.8X5	T42.8X6
TMTD	T60.3X1	T60.3X2	T60.3X3	T60.3X4		
TNT (fumes)	T65.3X1	T65.3X2	T65.3X3	T65.3X4	—	—
Toadstool	T62.0X1	T62.0X2	T62.0X3	T62.0X4		
Tobacco NEC	T65.291	T65.292	T65.293	T65.294	—	—
cigarettes	T65.221	T65.222	T65.223	T65.224	—	—
Indian	T62.2X1	T62.2X2	T62.2X3	T62.2X4		
smoke, second-hand	T65.221	T65.222	T65.223	T65.224	—	—
Tobramycin	T36.5X1	T36.5X2	T36.5X3	T36.5X4	T36.5X5	T36.5X6
Tocainide	T46.2X1	T46.2X2	T46.2X3	T46.2X4	T46.2X5	T46.2X6
Tocoferol	T45.2X1	T45.2X2	T45.2X3	T45.2X4	T45.2X5	T45.2X6
Tocopherol	T45.2X1	T45.2X2	T45.2X3	T45.2X4	T45.2X5	T45.2X6
acetate	T45.2X1	T45.2X2	T45.2X3	T45.2X4	T45.2X5	T45.2X6
Tocosamine	T48.0X1	T48.0X2	T48.0X3	T48.0X4	T48.0X5	T48.0X6
Todralazine	T46.5X1	T46.5X2	T46.5X3	T46.5X4	T46.5X5	T46.5X6
Tofisopam	T42.4X1	T42.4X2	T42.4X3	T42.4X4	T42.4X5	T42.4X6
Tofranil	T43.011	T43.012	T43.013	T43.014	T43.015	T43.016
Toilet deodorizer	T65.891	T65.892	T65.893	T65.894	—	—
Tolamolol	T44.7X1	T44.7X2	T44.7X3	T44.7X4	T44.7X5	T44.7X6
Tolazamide	T38.3X1	T38.3X2	T38.3X3	T38.3X4	T38.3X5	T38.3X6
Tolazoline	T46.7X1	T46.7X2	T46.7X3	T46.7X4	T46.7X5	T46.7X6
Tolbutamide (sodium)	T38.3X1	T38.3X2	T38.3X3	T38.3X4	T38.3X5	T38.3X6
Tolciclate	T49.0X1	T49.0X2	T49.0X3	T49.0X4	T49.0X5	T49.0X6
Tolmetin	T39.391	T39.392	T39.393	T39.394	T39.395	T39.396
Tolnaftate	T49.0X1	T49.0X2	T49.0X3	T49.0X4	T49.0X5	T49.0X6
Tolonidine	T46.5X1	T46.5X2	T46.5X3	T46.5X4	T46.5X5	T46.5X6

Substance	External Cause (T-Code)					
	Poisoning, Accidental (Unintentional)	Poisoning, Intentional Self-Harm	Poisoning, Assault	Poisoning, Undetermined	Adverse Effect	Underdosing
Toloxatone	T42.6X1	T42.6X2	T42.6X3	T42.6X4	T42.6X5	T42.6X6
Tolperisone	T44.3X1	T44.3X2	T44.3X3	T44.3X4	T44.3X5	T44.3X6
Tolserol	T42.8X1	T42.8X2	T42.8X3	T42.8X4	T42.8X5	T42.8X6
Toluene (liquid)	T52.2X1	T52.2X2	T52.2X3	T52.2X4	—	—
diisocyanate	T65.0X1	T65.0X2	T65.0X3	T65.0X4	—	—
Toluidine	T65.891	T65.892	T65.893	T65.894	—	—
vapor	T59.891	T59.892	T59.893	T59.894	—	—
Toluol (liquid)	T52.2X1	T52.2X2	T52.2X3	T52.2X4	—	—
vapor	T52.2X1	T52.2X2	T52.2X3	T52.2X4	—	—
Toluylenediamine	T65.3X1	T65.3X2	T65.3X3	T65.3X4	—	—
Tolylene-2,4-diisocyanate	T65.0X1	T65.0X2	T65.0X3	T65.0X4	—	—
Tonic NEC	T50.901	T50.902	T50.903	T50.904	T50.905	T50.906
Topical action drug NEC	T49.91	T49.92	T49.93	T49.94	T49.95	T49.96
ear, nose or throat	T49.6X1	T49.6X2	T49.6X3	T49.6X4	T49.6X5	T49.6X6
eye	T49.5X1	T49.5X2	T49.5X3	T49.5X4	T49.5X5	T49.5X6
skin	T49.91	T49.92	T49.93	T49.94	T49.95	T49.96
specified NEC	T49.8X1	T49.8X2	T49.8X3	T49.8X4	T49.8X5	T49.8X6
Toquizine	T44.3X1	T44.3X2	T44.3X3	T44.3X4	T44.3X5	T44.3X6
Toremifene	T38.6X1	T38.6X2	T38.6X3	T38.6X4	T38.6X5	T38.6X6
Tosylchloramide sodium	T49.8X1	T49.8X2	T49.8X3	T49.8X4	T49.8X5	T49.8X6
Toxaphene (dust) (spray)	T60.1X1	T60.1X2	T60.1X3	T60.1X4	—	—
Toxin, diphtheria (Schick Test)	T50.8X1	T50.8X2	T50.8X3	T50.8X4	T50.8X5	T50.8X6
Toxoid						
combined	T50.A21	T50.A22	T50.A23	T50.A24	T50.A25	T50.A26
diphtheria	T50.A91	T50.A92	T50.A93	T50.A94	T50.A95	T50.A96
tetanus	T50.A91	T50.A92	T50.A93	T50.A94	T50.A95	T50.A96
Trace element NEC	T45.8X1	T45.8X2	T45.8X3	T45.8X4	T45.8X5	T45.8X6
Tractor fuel NEC	T52.0X1	T52.0X2	T52.0X3	T52.0X4	—	—
Tragacanth	T50.991	T50.992	T50.993	T50.994	T50.995	T50.996
Tramadol	T40.421	T40.422	T40.423	T40.424	T40.425	T40.426
Tramazoline	T48.5X1	T48.5X2	T48.5X3	T48.5X4	T48.5X5	T48.5X6
Tranexamic acid	T45.621	T45.622	T45.623	T45.624	T45.625	T45.626
Tranilast	T45.0X1	T45.0X2	T45.0X3	T45.0X4	T45.0X5	T45.0X6
Tranquilizer NEC	T43.501	T43.502	T43.503	T43.504	T43.505	T43.506
with hypnotic or sedative	T42.6X1	T42.6X2	T42.6X3	T42.6X4	T42.6X5	T42.6X6
benzodiazepine NEC	T42.4X1	T42.4X2	T42.4X3	T42.4X4	T42.4X5	T42.4X6
butyrophenone NEC	T43.4X1	T43.4X2	T43.4X3	T43.4X4	T43.4X5	T43.4X6
carbamate	T43.591	T43.592	T43.593	T43.594	T43.595	T43.596
dimethylamine	T43.3X1	T43.3X2	T43.3X3	T43.3X4	T43.3X5	T43.3X6
ethylamine	T43.3X1	T43.3X2	T43.3X3	T43.3X4	T43.3X5	T43.3X6
hydroxyzine	T43.591	T43.592	T43.593	T43.594	T43.595	T43.596
major NEC	T43.501	T43.502	T43.503	T43.504	T43.505	T43.506

◀ New ◀ Revised ~~deleted~~ Deleted

Substance	Poisoning, Accidental (Unintentional)	Poisoning, Intentional Self-Harm	Poisoning, Assault	Poisoning, Undetermined	Adverse Effect	Underdosing
Tranquilizer NEC *(Continued)*						
penothiazine NEC	T43.3X1	T43.3X2	T43.3X3	T43.3X4	T43.3X5	T43.3X6
phenothiazine-based	T43.3X1	T43.3X2	T43.3X3	T43.3X4	T43.3X5	T43.3X6
piperazine NEC	T43.3X1	T43.3X2	T43.3X3	T43.3X4	T43.3X5	T43.3X6
piperidine	T43.3X1	T43.3X2	T43.3X3	T43.3X4	T43.3X5	T43.3X6
propylamine	T43.3X1	T43.3X2	T43.3X3	T43.3X4	T43.3X5	T43.3X6
specified NEC	T43.591	T43.592	T43.593	T43.594	T43.595	T43.596
thioxanthene NEC	T43.591	T43.592	T43.593	T43.594	T43.595	T43.596
Tranxene	T42.4X1	T42.4X2	T42.4X3	T42.4X4	T42.4X5	T42.4X6
Tranylcypromine	T43.1X1	T43.1X2	T43.1X3	T43.1X4	T43.1X5	T43.1X6
Trapidil	T46.3X1	T46.3X2	T46.3X3	T46.3X4	T46.3X5	T46.3X6
Trasentine	T44.3X1	T44.3X2	T44.3X3	T44.3X4	T44.3X5	T44.3X6
Travert	T50.3X1	T50.3X2	T50.3X3	T50.3X4	T50.3X5	T50.3X6
Trazodone	T43.211	T43.212	T43.213	T43.214	T43.215	T43.216
Trecator	T37.1X1	T37.1X2	T37.1X3	T37.1X4	T37.1X5	T37.1X6
Treosulfan	T45.1X1	T45.1X2	T45.1X3	T45.1X4	T45.1X5	T45.1X6
Tretamine	T45.1X1	T45.1X2	T45.1X3	T45.1X4	T45.1X5	T45.1X6
Tretinoin	T49.0X1	T49.0X2	T49.0X3	T49.0X4	T49.0X5	T49.0X6
Tretoquinol	T48.6X1	T48.6X2	T48.6X3	T48.6X4	T48.6X5	T48.6X6
Triacetin	T49.0X1	T49.0X2	T49.0X3	T49.0X4	T49.0X5	T49.0X6
Triacetoxyanthracene	T49.4X1	T49.4X2	T49.4X3	T49.4X4	T49.4X5	T49.4X6
Triacetyloleandomycin	T36.3X1	T36.3X2	T36.3X3	T36.3X4	T36.3X5	T36.3X6
Triamcinolone	T38.0X1	T38.0X2	T38.0X3	T38.0X4	T38.0X5	T38.0X6
ENT agent	T49.6X1	T49.6X2	T49.6X3	T49.6X4	T49.6X5	T49.6X6
hexacetonide	T49.0X1	T49.0X2	T49.0X3	T49.0X4	T49.0X5	T49.0X6
ophthalmic preparation	T49.5X1	T49.5X2	T49.5X3	T49.5X4	T49.5X5	T49.5X6
topical NEC	T49.0X1	T49.0X2	T49.0X3	T49.0X4	T49.0X5	T49.0X6
Triampyzine	T44.3X1	T44.3X2	T44.3X3	T44.3X4	T44.3X5	T44.3X6
Triamterene	T50.2X1	T50.2X2	T50.2X3	T50.2X4	T50.2X5	T50.2X6
Triazine (herbicide)	T60.3X1	T60.3X2	T60.3X3	T60.3X4	—	—
Triaziquone	T45.1X1	T45.1X2	T45.1X3	T45.1X4	T45.1X5	T45.1X6
Triazolam	T42.4X1	T42.4X2	T42.4X3	T42.4X4	T42.4X5	T42.4X6
Triazole (herbicide)	T60.3X1	T60.3X2	T60.3X3	T60.3X4	—	—
Tribenoside	T46.991	T46.992	T46.993	T46.994	T46.995	T46.996
Tribromacetaldehyde	T42.6X1	T42.6X2	T42.6X3	T42.6X4	T42.6X5	T42.6X6
Tribromoethanol, rectal	T41.291	T41.292	T41.293	T41.294	T41.295	T41.296
Tribromomethane	T42.6X1	T42.6X2	T42.6X3	T42.6X4	T42.6X5	T42.6X6
Trichlorethane	T53.2X1	T53.2X2	T53.2X3	T53.2X4	—	—
Trichlorethylene	T53.2X1	T53.2X2	T53.2X3	T53.2X4	—	—
Trichlorfon	T60.0X1	T60.0X2	T60.0X3	T60.0X4	—	—
Trichlormethiazide	T50.2X1	T50.2X2	T50.2X3	T50.2X4	T50.2X5	T50.2X6
Trichlormethine	T45.1X1	T45.1X2	T45.1X3	T45.1X4	T45.1X5	T45.1X6

Substance	Poisoning, Accidental (Unintentional)	Poisoning, Intentional Self-Harm	Poisoning, Assault	Poisoning, Undetermined	Adverse Effect	Underdosing
Trichloroacetic acid, Trichloracetic acid	T54.2X1	T54.2X2	T54.2X3	T54.2X4	—	—
medicinal	T49.4X1	T49.4X2	T49.4X3	T49.4X4	T49.4X5	T49.4X6
Trichloroethane	T53.2X1	T53.2X2	T53.2X3	T53.2X4	—	—
Trichloroethanol	T42.6X1	T42.6X2	T42.6X3	T42.6X4	T42.6X5	T42.6X6
Trichloroethylene (liquid) (vapor)	T53.2X1	T53.2X2	T53.2X3	T53.2X4	—	—
anesthetic (gas)	T41.0X1	T41.0X2	T41.0X3	T41.0X4	T41.0X5	T41.0X6
vapor NEC	T53.2X1	T53.2X2	T53.2X3	T53.2X4		
Trichloroethyl phosphate	T42.6X1	T42.6X2	T42.6X3	T42.6X4	T42.6X5	T42.6X6
Trichlorofluoromethane NEC	T53.5X1	T53.5X2	T53.5X3	T53.5X4	—	—
Trichloronate	T60.0X1	T60.0X2	T60.0X3	T60.0X4		
2,4,5-Trichlorophen-oxyacetic acid	T60.3X1	T60.3X2	T60.3X3	T60.3X4		
Trichloropropane	T53.6X1	T53.6X2	T53.6X3	T53.6X4		
Trichlorotriethylamine	T45.1X1	T45.1X2	T45.1X3	T45.1X4	T45.1X5	T45.1X6
Trichomonacides NEC	T37.3X1	T37.3X2	T37.3X3	T37.3X4	T37.3X5	T37.3X6
Trichomycin	T36.7X1	T36.7X2	T36.7X3	T36.7X4	T36.7X5	T36.7X6
Triclobisonium chloride	T49.0X1	T49.0X2	T49.0X3	T49.0X4	T49.0X5	T49.0X6
Triclocarban	T49.0X1	T49.0X2	T49.0X3	T49.0X4	T49.0X5	T49.0X6
Triclofos	T42.6X1	T42.6X2	T42.6X3	T42.6X4	T42.6X5	T42.6X6
Triclosan	T49.0X1	T49.0X2	T49.0X3	T49.0X4	T49.0X5	T49.0X6
Tricresyl phosphate	T65.891	T65.892	T65.893	T65.894	—	—
solvent	T52.91	T52.92	T52.93	T52.94		
Tricyclamol chloride	T44.3X1	T44.3X2	T44.3X3	T44.3X4	T44.3X5	T44.3X6
Tridesilon	T49.0X1	T49.0X2	T49.0X3	T49.0X4	T49.0X5	T49.0X6
Tridihexethyl iodide	T44.3X1	T44.3X2	T44.3X3	T44.3X4	T44.3X5	T44.3X6
Tridione	T42.2X1	T42.2X2	T42.2X3	T42.2X4	T42.2X5	T42.2X6
Trientine	T45.8X1	T45.8X2	T45.8X3	T45.8X4	T45.8X5	T45.8X6
Triethanolamine NEC	T54.3X1	T54.3X2	T54.3X3	T54.3X4	—	—
detergent	T54.3X1	T54.3X2	T54.3X3	T54.3X4		
trinitrate (biphosphate)	T46.3X1	T46.3X2	T46.3X3	T46.3X4	T46.3X5	T46.3X6
Triethanomelamine	T45.1X1	T45.1X2	T45.1X3	T45.1X4	T45.1X5	T45.1X6
Triethylenemelamine	T45.1X1	T45.1X2	T45.1X3	T45.1X4	T45.1X5	T45.1X6
Triethylenephosphoramide	T45.1X1	T45.1X2	T45.1X3	T45.1X4	T45.1X5	T45.1X6
Triethylenethiophosphoramide	T45.1X1	T45.1X2	T45.1X3	T45.1X4	T45.1X5	T45.1X6
Trifluoperazine	T43.3X1	T43.3X2	T43.3X3	T43.3X4	T43.3X5	T43.3X6
Trifluoroethyl vinyl ether	T41.0X1	T41.0X2	T41.0X3	T41.0X4	T41.0X5	T41.0X6
Trifluperidol	T43.4X1	T43.4X2	T43.4X3	T43.4X4	T43.4X5	T43.4X6
Triflupromazine	T43.3X1	T43.3X2	T43.3X3	T43.3X4	T43.3X5	T43.3X6
Trifluridine	T37.5X1	T37.5X2	T37.5X3	T37.5X4	T37.5X5	T37.5X6
Triflusal	T45.521	T45.522	T45.523	T45.524	T45.525	T45.526
Trihexyphenidyl	T44.3X1	T44.3X2	T44.3X3	T44.3X4	T44.3X5	T44.3X6
Triiodothyronine	T38.1X1	T38.1X2	T38.1X3	T38.1X4	T38.1X5	T38.1X6

Substance	Poisoning, Accidental (Unintentional)	Poisoning, Intentional Self-Harm	Poisoning, Assault	Poisoning, Undetermined	Adverse Effect	Underdosing
Trilene	T41.0X1	T41.0X2	T41.0X3	T41.0X4	T41.0X5	T41.0X6
Trilostane	T38.991	T38.992	T38.993	T38.994	T38.995	T38.996
Trimebutine	T44.3X1	T44.3X2	T44.3X3	T44.3X4	T44.3X5	T44.3X6
Trimecaine	T41.3X1	T41.3X2	T41.3X3	T41.3X4	T41.3X5	T41.3X6
Trimeprazine (tartrate)	T44.3X1	T44.3X2	T44.3X3	T44.3X4	T44.3X5	T44.3X6
Trimetaphan camsilate	T44.2X1	T44.2X2	T44.2X3	T44.2X4	T44.2X5	T44.2X6
Trimetazidine	T46.7X1	T46.7X2	T46.7X3	T46.7X4	T46.7X5	T46.7X6
Trimethadione	T42.2X1	T42.2X2	T42.2X3	T42.2X4	T42.2X5	T42.2X6
Trimethaphan	T44.2X1	T44.2X2	T44.2X3	T44.2X4	T44.2X5	T44.2X6
Trimethidinium	T44.2X1	T44.2X2	T44.2X3	T44.2X4	T44.2X5	T44.2X6
Trimethobenzamide	T45.0X1	T45.0X2	T45.0X3	T45.0X4	T45.0X5	T45.0X6
Trimethoprim	T37.8X1	T37.8X2	T37.8X3	T37.8X4	T37.8X5	T37.8X6
with sulfamethoxazole	T36.8X1	T36.8X2	T36.8X3	T36.8X4	T36.8X5	T36.8X6
Trimethylcarbinol	T51.3X1	T51.3X2	T51.3X3	T51.3X4	—	—
Trimethylpsoralen	T49.3X1	T49.3X2	T49.3X3	T49.3X4	T49.3X5	T49.3X6
Trimeton	T45.0X1	T45.0X2	T45.0X3	T45.0X4	T45.0X5	T45.0X6
Trimetrexate	T45.1X1	T45.1X2	T45.1X3	T45.1X4	T45.1X5	T45.1X6
Trimipramine	T43.011	T43.012	T43.013	T43.014	T43.015	T43.016
Trimustine	T45.1X1	T45.1X2	T45.1X3	T45.1X4	T45.1X5	T45.1X6
Trinitrine	T46.3X1	T46.3X2	T46.3X3	T46.3X4	T46.3X5	T46.3X6
Trinitrobenzol	T65.3X1	T65.3X2	T65.3X3	T65.3X4	—	—
Trinitrophenol	T65.3X1	T65.3X2	T65.3X3	T65.3X4	—	—
Trinitrotoluene (fumes)	T65.3X1	T65.3X2	T65.3X3	T65.3X4	—	—
Trional	T42.6X1	T42.6X2	T42.6X3	T42.6X4	T42.6X5	T42.6X6
Triorthocresyl phosphate	T65.891	T65.892	T65.893	T65.894	—	—
Trioxide of arsenic	T57.0X1	T57.0X2	T57.0X3	T57.0X4	—	—
Trioxysalen	T49.4X1	T49.4X2	T49.4X3	T49.4X4	T49.4X5	T49.4X6
Tripamide	T50.2X1	T50.2X2	T50.2X3	T50.2X4	T50.2X5	T50.2X6
Triparanol	T46.6X1	T46.6X2	T46.6X3	T46.6X4	T46.6X5	T46.6X6
Tripelennamine	T45.0X1	T45.0X2	T45.0X3	T45.0X4	T45.0X5	T45.0X6
Triperiden	T44.3X1	T44.3X2	T44.3X3	T44.3X4	T44.3X5	T44.3X6
Triperidol	T43.4X1	T43.4X2	T43.4X3	T43.4X4	T43.4X5	T43.4X6
Triphenylphosphate	T65.891	T65.892	T65.893	T65.894	—	—
Triple						
bromides	T42.6X1	T42.6X2	T42.6X3	T42.6X4	T42.6X5	T42.6X6
carbonate	T47.1X1	T47.1X2	T47.1X3	T47.1X4	T47.1X5	T47.1X6
vaccine						
DPT	T50.A11	T50.A12	T50.A13	T50.A14	T50.A15	T50.A16
including pertussis	T50.A11	T50.A12	T50.A13	T50.A14	T50.A15	T50.A16
MMR	T50.B91	T50.B92	—	—	—	—
Triprolidine	T45.0X1	T45.0X2	T45.0X3	T45.0X4	T45.0X5	T45.0X6
Trisodium hydrogen edetate	T50.6X1	T50.6X2	T50.6X3	T50.6X4	T50.6X5	T50.6X6
Trisoralen	T49.3X1	T49.3X2	T49.3X3	T49.3X4	T49.3X5	T49.3X6
Trisulfapyrimidines	T37.0X1	T37.0X2	T37.0X3	T37.0X4	T37.0X5	T37.0X6
Trithiozine	T44.3X1	T44.3X2	T44.3X3	T44.3X4	T44.3X5	T44.3X6
Tritiozine	T44.3X1	T44.3X2	T44.3X3	T44.3X4	T44.3X5	T44.3X6
Tritoqualine	T45.0X1	T45.0X2	T45.0X3	T45.0X4	T45.0X5	T45.0X6
Trofosfamide	T45.1X1	T45.1X2	T45.1X3	T45.1X4	T45.1X5	T45.1X6
Troleandomycin	T36.3X1	T36.3X2	T36.3X3	T36.3X4	T36.3X5	T36.3X6
Trolnitrate (phosphate)	T46.3X1	T46.3X2	T46.3X3	T46.3X4	T46.3X5	T46.3X6
Tromantadine	T37.5X1	T37.5X2	T37.5X3	T37.5X4	T37.5X5	T37.5X6
Trometamol	T50.2X1	T50.2X2	T50.2X3	T50.2X4	T50.2X5	T50.2X6
Tromethamine	T50.2X1	T50.2X2	T50.2X3	T50.2X4	T50.2X5	T50.2X6
Tronothane	T41.3X1	T41.3X2	T41.3X3	T41.3X4	T41.3X5	T41.3X6
Tropacine	T44.3X1	T44.3X2	T44.3X3	T44.3X4	T44.3X5	T44.3X6
Tropatepine	T44.3X1	T44.3X2	T44.3X3	T44.3X4	T44.3X5	T44.3X6
Tropicamide	T44.3X1	T44.3X2	T44.3X3	T44.3X4	T44.3X5	T44.3X6
Trospium chloride	T44.3X1	T44.3X2	T44.3X3	T44.3X4	T44.3X5	T44.3X6
Troxerutin	T46.991	T46.992	T46.993	T46.994	T46.995	T46.996
Troxidone	T42.2X1	T42.2X2	T42.2X3	T42.2X4	T42.2X5	T42.2X6
Tryparsamide	T37.3X1	T37.3X2	T37.3X3	T37.3X4	T37.3X5	T37.3X6
Trypsin	T45.3X1	T45.3X2	T45.3X3	T45.3X4	T45.3X5	T45.3X6
Tryptizol	T43.011	T43.012	T43.013	T43.014	T43.015	T43.016
TSH	T38.811	T38.812	T38.813	T38.814	T38.815	T38.816
Tuaminoheptane	T48.5X1	T48.5X2	T48.5X3	T48.5X4	T48.5X5	T48.5X6
Tuberculin, purified protein derivative (PPD)	T50.8X1	T50.8X2	T50.8X3	T50.8X4	T50.8X5	T50.8X6
Tubocurare	T48.1X1	T48.1X2	T48.1X3	T48.1X4	T48.1X5	T48.1X6
Tubocurarine (chloride)	T48.1X1	T48.1X2	T48.1X3	T48.1X4	T48.1X5	T48.1X6
Tulobuterol	T48.6X1	T48.6X2	T48.6X3	T48.6X4	T48.6X5	T48.6X6
Turpentine (spirits of)	T52.8X1	T52.8X2	T52.8X3	T52.8X4	—	—
vapor	T52.8X1	T52.8X2	T52.8X3	T52.8X4	—	—
Tybamate	T43.591	T43.592	T43.593	T43.594	T43.595	T43.596
Tyloxapol	T48.4X1	T48.4X2	T48.4X3	T48.4X4	T48.4X5	T48.4X6
Tymazoline	T48.5X1	T48.5X2	T48.5X3	T48.5X4	T48.5X5	T48.5X6
Typhoid-paratyphoid vaccine	T50.A91	T50.A92	T50.A93	T50.A94	T50.A95	T50.A96
Typhus vaccine	T50.A91	T50.A92	T50.A93	T50.A94	T50.A95	T50.A96
Tyropanoate	T50.8X1	T50.8X2	T50.8X3	T50.8X4	T50.8X5	T50.8X6
Tyrothricin	T49.6X1	T49.6X2	T49.6X3	T49.6X4	T49.6X5	T49.6X6
ENT agent	T49.6X1	T49.6X2	T49.6X3	T49.6X4	T49.6X5	T49.6X6
ophthalmic preparation	T49.5X1	T49.5X2	T49.5X3	T49.5X4	T49.5X5	T49.5X6

U

Substance	Poisoning, Accidental (Unintentional)	Poisoning, Intentional Self-Harm	Poisoning, Assault	Poisoning, Undetermined	Adverse Effect	Underdosing
Ufenamate	T39.391	T39.392	T39.393	T39.394	T39.395	T39.396
Ultraviolet light protectant	T49.3X1	T49.3X2	T49.3X3	T49.3X4	T49.3X5	T49.3X6

◀ New ◀ Revised ~~deleted~~ Deleted

Substance	Poisoning, Accidental (Unintentional)	Poisoning, Intentional Self-Harm	Poisoning, Assault	Poisoning, Undetermined	Adverse Effect	Underdosing
Undecenoic acid	T49.0X1	T49.0X2	T49.0X3	T49.0X4	T49.0X5	T49.0X6
Undecoylium	T49.0X1	T49.0X2	T49.0X3	T49.0X4	T49.0X5	T49.0X6
Undecylenic acid (derivatives)	T49.0X1	T49.0X2	T49.0X3	T49.0X4	T49.0X5	T49.0X6
Unna's boot	T49.3X1	T49.3X2	T49.3X3	T49.3X4	T49.3X5	T49.3X6
Unsaturated fatty acid	T46.6X1	T46.6X2	T46.6X3	T46.6X4	T46.6X5	T46.6X6
Uracil mustard	T45.1X1	T45.1X2	T45.1X3	T45.1X4	T45.1X5	T45.1X6
Uramustine	T45.1X1	T45.1X2	T45.1X3	T45.1X4	T45.1X5	T45.1X6
Urapidil	T46.5X1	T46.5X2	T46.5X3	T46.5X4	T46.5X5	T46.5X6
Urari	T48.1X1	T48.1X2	T48.1X3	T48.1X4	T48.1X5	T48.1X6
Urate oxidase	T50.4X1	T50.4X2	T50.4X3	T50.4X4	T50.4X5	T50.4X6
Urea	T47.3X1	T47.3X2	T47.3X3	T47.3X4	T47.3X5	T47.3X6
peroxide	T49.0X1	T49.0X2	T49.0X3	T49.0X4	T49.0X5	T49.0X6
stibamine	T37.4X1	T37.4X2	T37.4X3	T37.4X4	T37.4X5	T37.4X6
topical	T49.8X1	T49.8X2	T49.8X3	T49.8X4	T49.8X5	T49.8X6
Urethane	T45.1X1	T45.1X2	T45.1X3	T45.1X4	T45.1X5	T45.1X6
Urginea (maritima) (scilla) — see Squill						
Uric acid metabolism drug NEC	T50.4X1	T50.4X2	T50.4X3	T50.4X4	T50.4X5	T50.4X6
Uricosuric agent	T50.4X1	T50.4X2	T50.4X3	T50.4X4	T50.4X5	T50.4X6
Urinary anti-infective	T37.8X1	T37.8X2	T37.8X3	T37.8X4	T37.8X5	T37.8X6
Urofollitropin	T38.811	T38.812	T38.813	T38.814	T38.815	T38.816
Urokinase	T45.611	T45.612	T45.613	T45.614	T45.615	T45.616
Urokon	T50.8X1	T50.8X2	T50.8X3	T50.8X4	T50.8X5	T50.8X6
Ursodeoxycholic acid	T50.991	T50.992	T50.993	T50.994	T50.995	T50.996
Ursodiol	T50.991	T50.992	T50.993	T50.994	T50.995	T50.996
Urtica	T62.2X1	T62.2X2	T62.2X3	T62.2X4	—	—
Utility gas — see Gas, utility						

V

Substance	Poisoning, Accidental (Unintentional)	Poisoning, Intentional Self-Harm	Poisoning, Assault	Poisoning, Undetermined	Adverse Effect	Underdosing
Vaccine NEC	T50.Z91	T50.Z92	T50.Z93	T50.Z94	T50.Z95	T50.Z96
antineoplastic	T50.Z91	T50.Z92	T50.Z93	T50.Z94	T50.Z95	T50.Z96
bacterial NEC	T50.A91	T50.A92	T50.A93	T50.A94	T50.A95	T50.A96
with						
other bacterial component	T50.A91	T50.A92	T50.A93	T50.A94	T50.A95	T50.A96
pertussis component	T50.A91	T50.A92	T50.A93	T50.A94	T50.A95	T50.A96
viral-rickettsial component	T50.A91	T50.A92	T50.A93	T50.A94	T50.A95	T50.A96
mixed NEC	T50.A91	T50.A92	T50.A93	T50.A94	T50.A95	T50.A96
BCG	T50.A91	T50.A92	T50.A93	T50.A94	T50.A95	T50.A96
cholera	T50.A91	T50.A92	T50.A93	T50.A94	T50.A95	T50.A96
diphtheria	T50.A91	T50.A92	T50.A93	T50.A94	T50.A95	T50.A96
with tetanus	T50.A21	T50.A22	T50.A23	T50.A24	T50.A25	T50.A26
and pertussis	T50.A11	T50.A12	T50.A13	T50.A14	T50.A15	T50.A16

Substance	Poisoning, Accidental (Unintentional)	Poisoning, Intentional Self-Harm	Poisoning, Assault	Poisoning, Undetermined	Adverse Effect	Underdosing
Vaccine NEC (Continued)						
influenza	T50.B91	T50.B92	T50.B93	T50.B94	T50.B95	T50.B96
measles	T50.B91	T50.B92	T50.B93	T50.B94	T50.B95	T50.B96
with mumps and rubella	T50.B91	T50.B92	T50.B93	T50.B94	T50.B95	T50.B96
meningococcal	T50.A91	T50.A92	T50.A93	T50.A94	T50.A95	T50.A96
mumps	T50.B91	T50.B92	T50.B93	T50.B94	T50.B95	T50.B96
paratyphoid	T50.A91	T50.A92	T50.A93	T50.A94	T50.A95	T50.A96
pertussis	T50.A11	T50.A12	T50.A13	T50.A14	T50.A15	T50.A16
with diphtheria	T50.A11	T50.A12	T50.A13	T50.A14	T50.A15	T50.A16
and tetanus	T50.A11	T50.A12	T50.A13	T50.A14	T50.A15	T50.A16
plague	T50.A91	T50.A92	T50.A93	T50.A94	T50.A95	T50.A96
poliomyelitis	T50.B91	T50.B92	T50.B93	T50.B94	T50.B95	T50.B96
poliovirus	T50.B91	T50.B92	T50.B93	T50.B94	T50.B95	T50.B96
rabies	T50.B91	T50.B92	T50.B93	T50.B94	T50.B95	T50.B96
respiratory syncytial virus	T50.B91	T50.B92	T50.B93	T50.B94	T50.B95	T50.B96
rickettsial NEC	T50.A91	T50.A92	T50.A93	T50.A94	T50.A95	T50.A96
with						
bacterial component	T50.A21	T50.A22	T50.A23	T50.A24	T50.A25	T50.A26
Rocky Mountain spotted fever	T50.A91	T50.A92	T50.A93	T50.A94	T50.A95	T50.A96
rubella	T50.B91	T50.B92	T50.B93	T50.B94	T50.B95	T50.B96
sabin oral	T50.B91	T50.B92	T50.B93	T50.B94	T50.B95	T50.B96
smallpox	T50.B11	T50.B12	T50.B13	T50.B14	T50.B15	T50.B16
TAB	T50.A91	T50.A92	T50.A93	T50.A94	T50.A95	T50.A96
tetanus	T50.A91	T50.A92	T50.A93	T50.A94	T50.A95	T50.A96
typhoid	T50.A91	T50.A92	T50.A93	T50.A94	T50.A95	T50.A96
typhus	T50.A91	T50.A92	T50.A93	T50.A94	T50.A95	T50.A96
viral NEC	T50.B91	T50.B92	T50.B93	T50.B94	T50.B95	T50.B96
yellow fever	T50.B91	T50.B92	T50.B93	T50.B94	T50.B95	T50.B96
Vaccinia immune globulin	T50.Z11	T50.Z12	T50.Z13	T50.Z14	T50.Z15	T50.Z16
Vaginal contraceptives	T49.8X1	T49.8X2	T49.8X3	T49.8X4	T49.8X5	T49.8X6
Valerian						
root	T42.6X1	T42.6X2	T42.6X3	T42.6X4	T42.6X5	T42.6X6
tincture	T42.6X1	T42.6X2	T42.6X3	T42.6X4	T42.6X5	T42.6X6
Valethamate bromide	T44.3X1	T44.3X2	T44.3X3	T44.3X4	T44.3X5	T44.3X6
Valisone	T49.0X1	T49.0X2	T49.0X3	T49.0X4	T49.0X5	T49.0X6
Valium	T42.4X1	T42.4X2	T42.4X3	T42.4X4	T42.4X5	T42.4X6
Valmid	T42.6X1	T42.6X2	T42.6X3	T42.6X4	T42.6X5	T42.6X6
Valnoctamide	T42.6X1	T42.6X2	T42.6X3	T42.6X4	T42.6X5	T42.6X6
Valproate (sodium)	T42.6X1	T42.6X2	T42.6X3	T42.6X4	T42.6X5	T42.6X6
Valproic acid	T42.6X1	T42.6X2	T42.6X3	T42.6X4	T42.6X5	T42.6X6
Valpromide	T42.6X1	T42.6X2	T42.6X3	T42.6X4	T42.6X5	T42.6X6
Vanadium	T56.891	T56.892	T56.893	T56.894	—	—

◀ New ◀ Revised ~~deleted~~ Deleted

TABLE OF DRUGS AND CHEMICALS

Substance	External Cause (T-Code)					
	Poisoning, Accidental (Unintentional)	Poisoning, Intentional Self-Harm	Poisoning, Assault	Poisoning, Undetermined	Adverse Effect	Underdosing
Vancomycin	T36.8X1	T36.8X2	T36.8X3	T36.8X4	T36.8X5	T36.8X6
Vapor — see also Gas	T59.91	T59.92	T59.93	T59.94	—	—
kiln (carbon monoxide)	T58.8X1	T58.8X2	T58.8X3	T58.8X4	—	—
lead — see Lead						
specified source NEC	T59.891	T59.892	T59.893	T59.894	—	—
Vardenafil	T46.7X1	T46.7X2	T46.7X3	T46.7X4	T46.7X5	T46.7X6
Varicose reduction drug	T46.8X1	T46.8X2	T46.8X3	T46.8X4	T46.8X5	T46.8X6
Varnish	T65.4X1	T65.4X2	T65.4X3	T65.4X4	—	—
cleaner	T52.91	T52.92	T52.93	T52.94	—	—
Vaseline	T49.3X1	T49.3X2	T49.3X3	T49.3X4	T49.3X5	T49.3X6
Vasodilan	T46.7X1	T46.7X2	T46.7X3	T46.7X4	T46.7X5	T46.7X6
Vasodilator						
coronary NEC	T46.3X1	T46.3X2	T46.3X3	T46.3X4	T46.3X5	T46.3X6
peripheral NEC	T46.7X1	T46.7X2	T46.7X3	T46.7X4	T46.7X5	T46.7X6
Vasopressin	T38.891	T38.892	T38.893	T38.894	T38.895	T38.896
Vasopressor drugs	T38.891	T38.892	T38.893	T38.894	T38.895	T38.896
Vecuronium bromide	T48.1X1	T48.1X2	T48.1X3	T48.1X4	T48.1X5	T48.1X6
Vegetable extract, astringent	T49.2X1	T49.2X2	T49.2X3	T49.2X4	T49.2X5	T49.2X6
Venlafaxine	T43.211	T43.212	T43.213	T43.214	T43.215	T43.216
Venom, venomous (bite) (sting)	T63.91	T63.92	T63.93	T63.94	—	—
amphibian NEC	T63.831	T63.832	T63.833	T63.834	—	—
animal NEC	T63.891	T63.892	T63.893	T63.894	—	—
ant	T63.421	T63.422	T63.423	T63.424	—	—
arthropod NEC	T63.481	T63.482	T63.483	T63.484	—	—
bee	T63.441	T63.442	T63.443	T63.444	—	—
centipede	T63.411	T63.412	T63.413	T63.414	—	—
fish	T63.591	T63.592	T63.593	T63.594	—	—
frog	T63.811	T63.812	T63.813	T63.814	—	—
hornet	T63.451	T63.452	T63.453	T63.454	—	—
insect NEC	T63.481	T63.482	T63.483	T63.484	—	—
lizard	T63.121	T63.122	T63.123	T63.124	—	—
marine						
animals	T63.691	T63.692	T63.693	T63.694	—	—
bluebottle	T63.611	T63.612	T63.613	T63.614	—	—
jellyfish NEC	T63.621	T63.622	T63.623	T63.624	—	—
Portuguese Man-o-war	T63.611	T63.612	T63.613	T63.614	—	—
sea anemone	T63.631	T63.632	T63.633	T63.634	—	—
specified NEC	T63.691	T63.692	T63.693	T63.694	—	—
fish	T63.591	T63.592	T63.593	T63.594	—	—
plants	T63.711	T63.712	T63.713	T63.714	—	—
sting ray	T63.511	T63.512	T63.513	T63.514	—	—

Substance	External Cause (T-Code)					
	Poisoning, Accidental (Unintentional)	Poisoning, Intentional Self-Harm	Poisoning, Assault	Poisoning, Undetermined	Adverse Effect	Underdosing
Venom, venomous (Continued)						
millipede (tropical)	T63.411	T63.412	T63.413	T63.414	—	—
plant NEC	T63.791	T63.792	T63.793	T63.794	—	—
marine	T63.711	T63.712	T63.713	T63.714	—	—
reptile	T63.191	T63.192	T63.193	T63.194	—	—
gila monster	T63.111	T63.112	T63.113	T63.114	—	—
lizard NEC	T63.121	T63.122	T63.123	T63.124	—	—
scorpion	T63.2X1	T63.2X2	T63.2X3	T63.2X4	—	—
snake	T63.001	T63.002	T63.003	T63.004	—	—
African NEC	T63.081	T63.082	T63.083	T63.084	—	—
American (North) (South) NEC	T63.061	T63.062	T63.063	T63.064	—	—
Asian	T63.081	T63.082	T63.083	T63.084	—	—
Australian	T63.071	T63.072	T63.073	T63.074	—	—
cobra	T63.041	T63.042	T63.043	T63.044	—	—
coral snake	T63.021	T63.022	T63.023	T63.024	—	—
rattlesnake	T63.011	T63.012	T63.013	T63.014	—	—
specified NEC	T63.091	T63.092	T63.093	T63.094	—	—
taipan	T63.031	T63.032	T63.033	T63.034	—	—
specified NEC	T63.891	T63.892	T63.893	T63.894	—	—
spider	T63.301	T63.302	T63.303	T63.304	—	—
black widow	T63.311	T63.312	T63.313	T63.314	—	—
brown recluse	T63.331	T63.332	T63.333	T63.334	—	—
specified NEC	T63.391	T63.392	T63.393	T63.394	—	—
tarantula	T63.321	T63.322	T63.323	T63.324	—	—
sting ray	T63.511	T63.512	T63.513	T63.514	—	—
toad	T63.821	T63.822	T63.823	T63.824	—	—
wasp	T63.461	T63.462	T63.463	T63.464	—	—
Venous sclerosing drug NEC	T46.8X1	T46.8X2	T46.8X3	T46.8X4	T46.8X5	T46.8X6
Ventolin — see Albuterol						
Verapamil	T46.1X1	T46.1X2	T46.1X3	T46.1X4	T46.1X5	T46.1X6
Veramon	T42.3X1	T42.3X2	T42.3X3	T42.3X4	T42.3X5	T42.3X6
Veratrine	T46.5X1	T46.5X2	T46.5X3	T46.5X4	T46.5X5	T46.5X6
Veratrum						
album	T62.2X1	T62.2X2	T62.2X3	T62.2X4	—	—
alkaloids	T46.5X1	T46.5X2	T46.5X3	T46.5X4	T46.5X5	T46.5X6
viride	T62.2X1	T62.2X2	T62.2X3	T62.2X4	—	—
Verdigris	T60.3X1	T60.3X2	T60.3X3	T60.3X4	—	—
Veronal	T42.3X1	T42.3X2	T42.3X3	T42.3X4	T42.3X5	T42.3X6
Veroxil	T37.4X1	T37.4X2	T37.4X3	T37.4X4	T37.4X5	T37.4X6
Versenate	T50.6X1	T50.6X2	T50.6X3	T50.6X4	T50.6X5	T50.6X6

◀ New ◀◀ Revised ~~deleted~~ Deleted

Substance	Poisoning, Accidental (Unintentional)	Poisoning, Intentional Self-Harm	Poisoning, Assault	Poisoning, Undetermined	Adverse Effect	Underdosing
Versidyne	T39.8X1	T39.8X2	T39.8X3	T39.8X4	T39.8X5	T39.8X6
Vetrabutine	T48.0X1	T48.0X2	T48.0X3	T48.0X4	T48.0X5	T48.0X6
Vidarabine	T37.5X1	T37.5X2	T37.5X3	T37.5X4	T37.5X5	T37.5X6
Vienna						
green	T57.0X1	T57.0X2	T57.0X3	T57.0X4	—	—
insecticide	T60.2X1	T60.2X2	T60.2X3	T60.2X4	—	—
red	T57.0X1	T57.0X2	T57.0X3	T57.0X4	—	—
pharmaceutical dye	T50.991	T50.992	T50.993	T50.994	T50.995	T50.996
Vigabatrin	T42.6X1	T42.6X2	T42.6X3	T42.6X4	T42.6X5	T42.6X6
Viloxazine	T43.291	T43.292	T43.293	T43.294	T43.295	T43.296
Viminol	T39.8X1	T39.8X2	T39.8X3	T39.8X4	T39.8X5	T39.8X6
Vinbarbital, vinbarbitone	T42.3X1	T42.3X2	T42.3X3	T42.3X4	T42.3X5	T42.3X6
Vinblastine	T45.1X1	T45.1X2	T45.1X3	T45.1X4	T45.1X5	T45.1X6
Vinburnine	T46.7X1	T46.7X2	T46.7X3	T46.7X4	T46.7X5	T46.7X6
Vincamine	T45.1X1	T45.1X2	T45.1X3	T45.1X4	T45.1X5	T45.1X6
Vincristine	T45.1X1	T45.1X2	T45.1X3	T45.1X4	T45.1X5	T45.1X6
Vindesine	T45.1X1	T45.1X2	T45.1X3	T45.1X4	T45.1X5	T45.1X6
Vinesthene, vinethene	T41.0X1	T41.0X2	T41.0X3	T41.0X4	T41.0X5	T41.0X6
Vinorelbine tartrate	T45.1X1	T45.1X2	T45.1X3	T45.1X4	T45.1X5	T45.1X6
Vinpocetine	T46.7X1	T46.7X2	T46.7X3	T46.7X4	T46.7X5	T46.7X6
Vinyl						
acetate	T65.891	T65.892	T65.893	T65.894	—	—
bital	T42.3X1	T42.3X2	T42.3X3	T42.3X4	T42.3X5	T42.3X6
bromide	T65.891	T65.892	T65.893	T65.894	—	—
chloride	T59.891	T59.892	T59.893	T59.894	—	—
ether	T41.0X1	T41.0X2	T41.0X3	T41.0X4	T41.0X5	T41.0X6
Vinylbital	T42.3X1	T42.3X2	T42.3X3	T42.3X4	T42.3X5	T42.3X6
Vinylidene chloride	T65.891	T65.892	T65.893	T65.894	—	—
Vioform	T37.8X1	T37.8X2	T37.8X3	T37.8X4	T37.8X5	T37.8X6
topical	T49.0X1	T49.0X2	T49.0X3	T49.0X4	T49.0X5	T49.0X6
Viomycin	T36.8X1	T36.8X2	T36.8X3	T36.8X4	T36.8X5	T36.8X6
Viosterol	T45.2X1	T45.2X2	T45.2X3	T45.2X4	T45.2X5	T45.2X6
Viper (venom)	T63.091	T63.092	T63.093	T63.094	—	—
Viprynium	T37.4X1	T37.4X2	T37.4X3	T37.4X4	T37.4X5	T37.4X6
Viquidil	T46.7X1	T46.7X2	T46.7X3	T46.7X4	T46.7X5	T46.7X6
Viral vaccine NEC	T50.B91	T50.B92	T50.B93	T50.B94	T50.B95	T50.B96
Virginiamycin	T36.8X1	T36.8X2	T36.8X3	T36.8X4	T36.8X5	T36.8X6
Virugon	T37.5X1	T37.5X2	T37.5X3	T37.5X4	T37.5X5	T37.5X6
Viscous agent	T50.901	T50.902	T50.903	T50.904	T50.905	T50.906
Visine	T49.5X1	T49.5X2	T49.5X3	T49.5X4	T49.5X5	T49.5X6
Visnadine	T46.3X1	T46.3X2	T46.3X3	T46.3X4	T46.3X5	T46.3X6

Substance	Poisoning, Accidental (Unintentional)	Poisoning, Intentional Self-Harm	Poisoning, Assault	Poisoning, Undetermined	Adverse Effect	Underdosing
Vitamin NEC	T45.2X1	T45.2X2	T45.2X3	T45.2X4	T45.2X5	T45.2X6
A	T45.2X1	T45.2X2	T45.2X3	T45.2X4	T45.2X5	T45.2X6
B NEC	T45.2X1	T45.2X2	T45.2X3	T45.2X4	T45.2X5	T45.2X6
nicotinic acid	T46.7X1	T46.7X2	T46.7X3	T46.7X4	T46.7X5	T46.7X6
B1	T45.2X1	T45.2X2	T45.2X3	T45.2X4	T45.2X5	T45.2X6
B2	T45.2X1	T45.2X2	T45.2X3	T45.2X4	T45.2X5	T45.2X6
B6	T45.2X1	T45.2X2	T45.2X3	T45.2X4	T45.2X5	T45.2X6
B12	T45.2X1	T45.2X2	T45.2X3	T45.2X4	T45.2X5	T45.2X6
B15	T45.2X1	T45.2X2	T45.2X3	T45.2X4	T45.2X5	T45.2X6
C	T45.2X1	T45.2X2	T45.2X3	T45.2X4	T45.2X5	T45.2X6
D	T45.2X1	T45.2X2	T45.2X3	T45.2X4	T45.2X5	T45.2X6
D2	T45.2X1	T45.2X2	T45.2X3	T45.2X4	T45.2X5	T45.2X6
D3	T45.2X1	T45.2X2	T45.2X3	T45.2X4	T45.2X5	T45.2X6
E	T45.2X1	T45.2X2	T45.2X3	T45.2X4	T45.2X5	T45.2X6
E acetate	T45.2X1	T45.2X2	T45.2X3	T45.2X4	T45.2X5	T45.2X6
hematopoietic	T45.8X1	T45.8X2	T45.8X3	T45.8X4	T45.8X5	T45.8X6
K NEC	T45.7X1	T45.7X2	T45.7X3	T45.7X4	T45.7X5	T45.7X6
K1	T45.7X1	T45.7X2	T45.7X3	T45.7X4	T45.7X5	T45.7X6
K2	T45.7X1	T45.7X2	T45.7X3	T45.7X4	T45.7X5	T45.7X6
PP	T45.2X1	T45.2X2	T45.2X3	T45.2X4	T45.2X5	T45.2X6
ulceroprotectant	T47.1X1	T47.1X2	T47.1X3	T47.1X4	T47.1X5	T47.1X6
Vleminckx's solution	T49.4X1	T49.4X2	T49.4X3	T49.4X4	T49.4X5	T49.4X6
Voltaren — *see Diclofenac sodium*						
W						
Warfarin	T45.511	T45.512	T45.513	T45.514	T45.515	T45.516
rodenticide	T60.4X1	T60.4X2	T60.4X3	T60.4X4	—	—
sodium	T45.511	T45.512	T45.513	T45.514	T45.515	T45.516
Wasp (sting)	T63.461	T63.462	T63.463	T63.464	—	—
Water						
balance drug	T50.3X1	T50.3X2	T50.3X3	T50.3X4	T50.3X5	T50.3X6
distilled	T50.3X1	T50.3X2	T50.3X3	T50.3X4	T50.3X5	T50.3X6
gas — *see Gas, water*						
incomplete combustion of — *see Carbon, monoxide, fuel, utility*						
hemlock	T62.2X1	T62.2X2	T62.2X3	T62.2X4	—	—
moccasin (venom)	T63.061	T63.062	T63.063	T63.064	—	—
purified	T50.3X1	T50.3X2	T50.3X3	T50.3X4	T50.3X5	T50.3X6
Wax (paraffin) (petroleum)	T52.0X1	T52.0X2	T52.0X3	T52.0X4	—	—
automobile	T65.891	T65.892	T65.893	T65.894	—	—
floor	T52.0X1	T52.0X2	T52.0X3	T52.0X4	—	—

◀ New　◀ Revised　~~deleted~~ Deleted

TABLE OF DRUGS AND CHEMICALS

Substance	External Cause (T-Code)					
	Poisoning, Accidental (Unintentional)	Poisoning, Intentional Self-Harm	Poisoning, Assault	Poisoning, Undetermined	Adverse Effect	Underdosing
Weed killers NEC	T60.3X1	T60.3X2	T60.3X3	T60.3X4	—	—
Welldorm	T42.6X1	T42.6X2	T42.6X3	T42.6X4	T42.6X5	T42.6X6
White						
arsenic	T57.0X1	T57.0X2	T57.0X3	T57.0X4	—	—
hellebore	T62.2X1	T62.2X2	T62.2X3	T62.2X4	—	—
lotion (keratolytic)	T49.4X1	T49.4X2	T49.4X3	T49.4X4	T49.4X5	T49.4X6
spirit	T52.0X1	T52.0X2	T52.0X3	T52.0X4	—	—
Whitewash	T65.891	T65.892	T65.893	T65.894	—	—
Whole blood (human)	T45.8X1	T45.8X2	T45.8X3	T45.8X4	T45.8X5	T45.8X6
Wild						
black cherry	T62.2X1	T62.2X2	T62.2X3	T62.2X4	—	—
poisonous plants NEC	T62.2X1	T62.2X2	T62.2X3	T62.2X4	—	—
Window cleaning fluid	T65.891	T65.892	T65.893	T65.894	—	—
Wintergreen (oil)	T49.3X1	T49.3X2	T49.3X3	T49.3X4	T49.3X5	T49.3X6
Wisterine	T62.2X1	T62.2X2	T62.2X3	T62.2X4	—	—
Witch hazel	T49.2X1	T49.2X2	T49.2X3	T49.2X4	T49.2X5	T49.2X6
Wood alcohol or spirit	T51.1X1	T51.1X2	T51.1X3	T51.1X4	—	—
Wool fat (hydrous)	T49.3X1	T49.3X2	T49.3X3	T49.3X4	T49.3X5	T49.3X6
Woorali	T48.1X1	T48.1X2	T48.1X3	T48.1X4	T48.1X5	T48.1X6
Wormseed, American	T37.4X1	T37.4X2	T37.4X3	T37.4X4	T37.4X5	T37.4X6
X						
Xamoterol	T44.5X1	T44.5X2	T44.5X3	T44.5X4	T44.5X5	T44.5X6
Xanthine diuretics	T50.2X1	T50.2X2	T50.2X3	T50.2X4	T50.2X5	T50.2X6
Xanthinol nicotinate	T46.7X1	T46.7X2	T46.7X3	T46.7X4	T46.7X5	T46.7X6
Xanthotoxin	T49.3X1	T49.3X2	T49.3X3	T49.3X4	T49.3X5	T49.3X6
Xantinol nicotinate	T46.7X1	T46.7X2	T46.7X3	T46.7X4	T46.7X5	T46.7X6
Xantocillin	T36.0X1	T36.0X2	T36.0X3	T36.0X4	T36.0X5	T36.0X6
Xenon (127Xe) (133Xe)	T50.8X1	T50.8X2	T50.8X3	T50.8X4	T50.8X5	T50.8X6
Xenysalate	T49.4X1	T49.4X2	T49.4X3	T49.4X4	T49.4X5	T49.4X6
Xibornol	T37.8X1	T37.8X2	T37.8X3	T37.8X4	T37.8X5	T37.8X6
Xigris	T45.511	T45.512	T45.513	T45.514	T45.515	T45.516
Xipamide	T50.2X1	T50.2X2	T50.2X3	T50.2X4	T50.2X5	T50.2X6
Xylene (vapor)	T52.2X1	T52.2X2	T52.2X3	T52.2X4	—	—
Xylocaine (infiltration) (topical)	T41.3X1	T41.3X2	T41.3X3	T41.3X4	T41.3X5	T41.3X6
nerve block (peripheral) (plexus)	T41.3X1	T41.3X2	T41.3X3	T41.3X4	T41.3X5	T41.3X6
spinal	T41.3X1	T41.3X2	T41.3X3	T41.3X4	T41.3X5	T41.3X6
Xylol (vapor)	T52.2X1	T52.2X2	T52.2X3	T52.2X4	—	—
Xylometazoline	T48.5X1	T48.5X2	T48.5X3	T48.5X4	T48.5X5	T48.5X6

Substance	External Cause (T-Code)					
	Poisoning, Accidental (Unintentional)	Poisoning, Intentional Self-Harm	Poisoning, Assault	Poisoning, Undetermined	Adverse Effect	Underdosing
Y						
Yeast	T45.2X1	T45.2X2	T45.2X3	T45.2X4	T45.2X5	T45.2X6
dried	T45.2X1	T45.2X2	T45.2X3	T45.2X4	T45.2X5	T45.2X6
Yellow						
fever vaccine	T50.B91	T50.B92	T50.B93	T50.B94	T50.B95	T50.B96
jasmine	T62.2X1	T62.2X2	T62.2X3	T62.2X4	—	—
phenolphthalein	T47.2X1	T47.2X2	T47.2X3	T47.2X4	T47.2X5	T47.2X6
Yew	T62.2X1	T62.2X2	T62.2X3	T62.2X4	—	—
Yohimbic acid	T40.991	T40.992	T40.993	T40.994	T40.995	T40.996
Z						
Zactane	T39.8X1	T39.8X2	T39.8X3	T39.8X4	T39.8X5	T39.8X6
Zalcitabine	T37.5X1	T37.5X2	T37.5X3	T37.5X4	T37.5X5	T37.5X6
Zaroxolyn	T50.2X1	T50.2X2	T50.2X3	T50.2X4	T50.2X5	T50.2X6
Zephiran (topical)	T49.0X1	T49.0X2	T49.0X3	T49.0X4	T49.0X5	T49.0X6
ophthalmic preparation	T49.5X1	T49.5X2	T49.5X3	T49.5X4	T49.5X5	T49.5X6
Zeranol	T38.7X1	T38.7X2	T38.7X3	T38.7X4	T38.7X5	T38.7X6
Zerone	T51.1X1	T51.1X2	T51.1X3	T51.1X4	—	—
Zidovudine	T37.5X1	T37.5X2	T37.5X3	T37.5X4	T37.5X5	T37.5X6
Zimeldine	T43.221	T43.222	T43.223	T43.224	T43.225	T43.226
Zinc (compounds) (fumes) (vapor) NEC	T56.5X1	T56.5X2	T56.5X3	T56.5X4	—	—
anti-infectives	T49.0X1	T49.0X2	T49.0X3	T49.0X4	T49.0X5	T49.0X6
antivaricose	T46.8X1	T46.8X2	T46.8X3	T46.8X4	T46.8X5	T46.8X6
bacitracin	T49.0X1	T49.0X2	T49.0X3	T49.0X4	T49.0X5	T49.0X6
chloride (mouthwash)	T49.6X1	T49.6X2	T49.6X3	T49.6X4	T49.6X5	T49.6X6
chromate	T56.5X1	T56.5X2	T56.5X3	T56.5X4	—	—
gelatin	T49.3X1	T49.3X2	T49.3X3	T49.3X4	T49.3X5	T49.3X6
oxide	T49.3X1	T49.3X2	T49.3X3	T49.3X4	T49.3X5	T49.3X6
plaster	T49.3X1	T49.3X2	T49.3X3	T49.3X4	T49.3X5	T49.3X6
peroxide	T49.0X1	T49.0X2	T49.0X3	T49.0X4	T49.0X5	T49.0X6
pesticides	T56.5X1	T56.5X2	T56.5X3	T56.5X4	—	—
phosphide	T60.4X1	T60.4X2	T60.4X3	T60.4X4	—	—
pyrithionate	T49.4X1	T49.4X2	T49.4X3	T49.4X4	T49.4X5	T49.4X6
stearate	T49.3X1	T49.3X2	T49.3X3	T49.3X4	T49.3X5	T49.3X6
sulfate	T49.5X1	T49.5X2	T49.5X3	T49.5X4	T49.5X5	T49.5X6
ENT agent	T49.6X1	T49.6X2	T49.6X3	T49.6X4	T49.6X5	T49.6X6
ophthalmic solution	T49.5X1	T49.5X2	T49.5X3	T49.5X4	T49.5X5	T49.5X6
topical NEC	T49.0X1	T49.0X2	T49.0X3	T49.0X4	T49.0X5	T49.0X6
undecylenate	T49.0X1	T49.0X2	T49.0X3	T49.0X4	T49.0X5	T49.0X6

◀ New   ◀ Revised   ~~deleted~~ Deleted

Substance	External Cause (T-Code)					
	Poisoning, Accidental (Unintentional)	Poisoning, Intentional Self-Harm	Poisoning, Assault	Poisoning, Undetermined	Adverse Effect	Underdosing
Zineb	T60.0X1	T60.0X2	T60.0X3	T60.0X4	—	—
Zinostatin	T45.1X1	T45.1X2	T45.1X3	T45.1X4	T45.1X5	T45.1X6
Zipeprol	T48.3X1	T48.3X2	T48.3X3	T48.3X4	T48.3X5	T48.3X6
Zofenopril	T46.4X1	T46.4X2	T46.4X3	T46.4X4	T46.4X5	T46.4X6
Zolpidem	T42.6X1	T42.6X2	T42.6X3	T42.6X4	T42.6X5	T42.6X6
Zomepirac	T39.391	T39.392	T39.393	T39.394	T39.395	T39.396
Zopiclone	T42.6X1	T42.6X2	T42.6X3	T42.6X4	T42.6X5	T42.6X6

Substance	External Cause (T-Code)					
	Poisoning, Accidental (Unintentional)	Poisoning, Intentional Self-Harm	Poisoning, Assault	Poisoning, Undetermined	Adverse Effect	Underdosing
Zorubicin	T45.1X1	T45.1X2	T45.1X3	T45.1X4	T45.1X5	T45.1X6
Zotepine	T43.591	T43.592	T43.593	T43.594	T43.595	T43.596
Zovant	T45.511	T45.512	T45.513	T45.514	T45.515	T45.516
Zoxazolamine	T42.8X1	T42.8X2	T42.8X3	T42.8X4	T42.8X5	T42.8X6
Zuclopenthixol	T43.4X1	T43.4X2	T43.4X3	T43.4X4	T43.4X5	T43.4X6
Zygadenus (venenosus)	T62.2X1	T62.2X2	T62.2X3	T62.2X4	—	—
Zyprexa	T43.591	T43.592	T43.593	T43.594	T43.595	T43.596

TABLE OF DRUGS AND CHEMICALS

ECI

External Cause
of Injuries Index

ICD-10-CM EXTERNAL CAUSE OF INJURIES INDEX

A

Abandonment (causing exposure to weather conditions) (with intent to injure or kill) NEC X58

Abuse (adult) (child) (mental) (physical) (sexual) X58

Accident (to) X58
- aircraft (in transit) (powered) —*see also* Accident, transport, aircraft
  - due to, caused by cataclysm —*see* Forces of nature, by type
- animal-drawn vehicle —*see* Accident, transport, animal-drawn vehicle occupant
- animal-rider —*see* Accident, transport, animal-rider
- automobile —*see* Accident, transport, car occupant
- bare foot water skiier V94.4
- boat, boating —*see also* Accident, watercraft
  - striking swimmer
    - powered V94.11
    - unpowered V94.12
- bus —*see* Accident, transport, bus occupant
- cable car, not on rails V98.0
  - on rails —*see* Accident, transport, streetcar occupant
- car —*see* Accident, transport, car occupant
- caused by, due to
  - animal NEC W64
  - chain hoist W24.0
  - cold (excessive) —*see* Exposure, cold
  - corrosive liquid, substance —*see* Table of Drugs and Chemicals
  - cutting or piercing instrument —*see* Contact, with, by type of instrument
  - drive belt W24.0
  - electric
    - current —*see* Exposure, electric current
    - motor —*see also* Contact, with, by type of machine W31.3
      - current (of) W86.8
  - environmental factor NEC X58
  - explosive material —*see* Explosion
  - fire, flames —*see* Exposure, fire
  - firearm missile —*see* Discharge, firearm by type
  - heat (excessive) —*see* Heat
  - hot —*see* Contact, with, hot
  - ignition —*see* Ignition
  - lifting device W24.0
  - lightning —*see* subcategory T75.0
    - causing fire —*see* Exposure, fire
  - machine, machinery —*see* Contact, with, by type of machine
  - natural factor NEC X58
  - pulley (block) W24.0
  - radiation —*see* Radiation
  - steam X13.1
    - inhalation X13.0
    - pipe X16
  - thunderbolt —*see* subcategory T75.0
    - causing fire —*see* Exposure, fire
  - transmission device W24.1
- coach —*see* Accident, transport, bus occupant
- coal car —*see* Accident, transport, industrial vehicle occupant
- diving —*see also* Fall, into, water
  - with
    - drowning or submersion —*see* Drowning
- forklift —*see* Accident, transport, industrial vehicle occupant
- heavy transport vehicle NOS —*see* Accident, transport, truck occupant
- ice yacht V98.2

Accident (Continued)
- in
  - medical, surgical procedure
    - as, or due to misadventure —*see* Misadventure
    - causing an abnormal reaction or later complication without mention of misadventure —*see also* Complication of or following, by type of procedure Y84.9
- land yacht V98.1
- late effect of —*see* W00-X58 with 7th character S
- logging car —*see* Accident, transport, industrial vehicle occupant
- machine, machinery —*see also* Contact, with, by type of machine
  - on board watercraft V93.69
    - explosion —*see* Explosion, in, watercraft
    - fire —*see* Burn, on board watercraft
    - powered craft V93.63
      - ferry boat V93.61
      - fishing boat V93.62
      - jet ski V93.63
      - liner V93.61
      - merchant ship V93.60
      - passenger ship V93.61
      - sailboat V93.64
- mine tram —*see* Accident, transport, industrial vehicle occupant
- mobility scooter (motorized) —*see* Accident, transport, pedestrian, conveyance, specified type NEC
- motor scooter —*see* Accident, transport, motorcyclist
- motor vehicle NOS (traffic) —*see also* Accident, transport V89.2
  - nontraffic V89.0
  - three-wheeled NOS —*see* Accident, transport, three-wheeled motor vehicle occupant
- motorcycle NOS —*see* Accident, transport, motorcyclist
- nonmotor vehicle NOS (nontraffic) —*see also* Accident, transport V89.1
  - traffic NOS V89.3
- nontraffic (victim's mode of transport NOS) V88.9
  - collision (between) V88.7
    - bus and truck V88.5
    - car and:
      - bus V88.3
      - pickup V88.2
      - three-wheeled motor vehicle V88.0
      - train V88.6
      - truck V88.4
      - two-wheeled motor vehicle V88.0
      - van V88.2
    - specified vehicle NEC and:
      - three-wheeled motor vehicle V88.1
      - two-wheeled motor vehicle V88.1
  - known mode of transport —*see* Accident, transport, by type of vehicle
  - noncollision V88.8
- on board watercraft V93.89
  - powered craft V93.83
    - ferry boat V93.81
    - fishing boat V93.82
    - jet ski V93.83
    - liner V93.81
    - merchant ship V93.80
    - passenger ship V93.81
  - unpowered craft V93.88
    - canoe V93.85
    - inflatable V93.86
      - in tow
        - recreational V94.31
        - specified NEC V94.32
    - kayak V93.85

Accident (Continued)
- on board watercraft (Continued)
  - unpowered craft (Continued)
    - sailboat V93.84
    - surf-board V93.88
    - water skis V93.87
    - windsurfer V93.88
- parachutist V97.29
  - entangled in object V97.21
  - injured on landing V97.22
- pedal cycle —*see* Accident, transport, pedal cyclist
- pedestrian (on foot)
  - with
    - another pedestrian W51
      - with fall W03
        - due to ice or snow W00.0
      - on pedestrian conveyance NEC V00.09
    - rider of
      - hoverboard V00.038
      - Segway V00.038
      - standing
        - electric scooter V00.031
        - micro-mobility pedestrian conveyance NEC V00.038
    - roller skater (in-line) V00.01
    - skate boarder V00.02
    - transport vehicle —*see* Accident, transport
  - on pedestrian conveyance —*see* Accident, transport, pedestrian, conveyance
- pick-up truck or van —*see* Accident, transport, pickup truck occupant
- quarry truck —*see* Accident, transport, industrial vehicle occupant
- railway vehicle (any) (in motion) —*see* Accident, transport, railway vehicle occupant
  - due to cataclysm —*see* Forces of nature, by type
- scooter (non-motorized) —*see* Accident, transport, pedestrian, conveyance, scooter
- sequelae of —*see* W00-X58 with 7th character S
- skateboard —*see* Accident, transport, pedestrian, conveyance, skateboard
- ski (ing) —*see* Accident, transport, pedestrian, conveyance
  - lift V98.3
- specified cause NEC X58
- streetcar —*see* Accident, transport, streetcar occupant
- traffic (victim's mode of transport NOS) V87.9
  - collision (between) V87.7
    - bus and truck V87.5
    - car and:
      - bus V87.3
      - pickup V87.2
      - three-wheeled motor vehicle V87.0
      - train V87.6
      - truck V87.4
      - two-wheeled motor vehicle V87.0
      - van V87.2
    - specified vehicle NEC V86.39
      - and
        - three-wheeled motor vehicle V87.1
        - two-wheeled motor vehicle V87.1
      - driver V86.09
      - person on outside V86.29
      - passenger V86.19
      - while boarding or alighting V86.49
  - known mode of transport —*see* Accident, transport, by type of vehicle
  - noncollision V87.8

606

▶ New   ⇒ Revised   ~~deleted~~ Deleted   • Use Additional Character(s)

Accident (Continued)
  transport (involving injury to) V99
    18 wheeler —see Accident, transport, truck occupant
    agricultural vehicle occupant (nontraffic) V84.9
      driver V84.5
      hanger-on V84.7
      passenger V84.6
      traffic V84.3
        driver V84.0
        hanger-on V84.2
        passenger V84.1
      while boarding or alighting V84.4
    aircraft NEC V97.89
      military NEC V97.818
        with civilian aircraft V97.810
        civilian injured by V97.811
      occupant injured (in)
        nonpowered craft accident V96.9
          balloon V96.00
            collision V96.03
            crash V96.01
            explosion V96.05
            fire V96.04
            forced landing V96.02
            specified type NEC V96.09
          glider V96.20
            collision V96.23
            crash V96.21
            explosion V96.25
            fire V96.24
            forced landing V96.22
            specified type NEC V96.29
          hang glider V96.10
            collision V96.13
            crash V96.11
            explosion V96.15
            fire V96.14
            forced landing V96.12
            specified type NEC V96.19
          specified craft NEC V96.8
        powered craft accident V95.9
          fixed wing NEC
            commercial V95.30
              collision V95.33
              crash V95.31
              explosion V95.35
              fire V95.34
              forced landing V95.32
              specified type NEC V95.39
            private V95.20
              collision V95.23
              crash V95.21
              explosion V95.25
              fire V95.24
              forced landing V95.22
              specified type NEC V95.29
          glider V95.10
            collision V95.13
            crash V95.11
            explosion V95.15
            fire V95.14
            forced landing V95.12
            specified type NEC V95.19
          helicopter V95.00
            collision V95.03
            crash V95.01
            explosion V95.05
            fire V95.04
            forced landing V95.02
            specified type NEC V95.09
          spacecraft V95.40
            collision V95.43
            crash V95.41
            explosion V95.45
            fire V95.44
            forced landing V95.42
            specified type NEC V95.49
          specified craft NEC V95.8

Accident (Continued)
  transport (Continued)
    aircraft NEC (Continued)
      occupant injured (Continued)
        powered craft accident (Continued)
          ultralight V95.10
            collision V95.13
            crash V95.11
            explosion V95.15
            fire V95.14
            forced landing V95.12
            specified type NEC V95.19
        specified accident NEC V97.0
        while boarding or alighting V97.1
      person (injured by)
        falling from, in or on aircraft V97.0
        machinery on aircraft V97.89
        on ground with aircraft involvement V97.39
        rotating propeller V97.32
        struck by object falling from aircraft V97.31
        sucked into aircraft jet V97.33
        while boarding or alighting aircraft V97.1
    airport (battery-powered) passenger vehicle —see Accident, transport, industrial vehicle occupant
    all-terrain vehicle occupant (nontraffic) V86.95
      driver V86.55
      dune buggy —see Accident, transport, dune buggy occupant
      hanger-on V86.75
      passenger V86.65
      snowmobile —see Accident, transport, snowmobile occupant
      specified type NEC V86.99
        driver V86.59
        passenger V86.69
        person on outside V86.79
      traffic V86.35
        driver V86.05
        hanger-on V86.25
        passenger V86.15
      while boarding or alighting V86.45
    ambulance occupant (traffic) V86.31
      driver V86.01
      hanger-on V86.21
      nontraffic V86.91
        driver V86.51
        hanger-on V86.71
        passenger V86.61
      passenger V86.11
      while boarding or alighting V86.41
    animal-drawn vehicle occupant (in) V80.929
      collision (with)
        animal V80.12
          being ridden V80.711
        animal-drawn vehicle V80.721
        bus V80.42
        car V80.42
        fixed or stationary object V80.82
        military vehicle V80.920
        nonmotor vehicle V80.791
        pedal cycle V80.22
        pedestrian V80.12
        pickup V80.42
        railway train or vehicle V80.62
        specified motor vehicle NEC V80.52
        streetcar V80.731
        truck V80.42
        two-or three-wheeled motor vehicle V80.32
        van V80.42
      noncollision V80.02
      specified circumstance NEC V80. 928
    animal-rider V80.919
      collision (with)
        animal V80.11
          being ridden V80.710

Accident (Continued)
  transport (Continued)
    animal-rider (Continued)
      collision (Continued)
        animal-drawn vehicle V80.720
        bus V80.41
        car V80.41
        fixed or stationary object V80.81
        military vehicle V80.910
        nonmotor vehicle V80.790
        pedal cycle V80.21
        pedestrian V80.11
        pickup V80.41
        railway train or vehicle V80.61
        specified motor vehicle NEC V80.51
        streetcar V80.730
        truck V80.41
        two- or three-wheeled motor vehicle V80.31
        van V80.41
      noncollision V80.018
        specified as horse rider V80.010
        specified circumstance NEC V80.918
    armored car —see Accident, transport, truck occupant
    battery-powered truck (baggage) (mail) — see Accident, transport, industrial vehicle occupant
    bus occupant V79.9
      collision (with)
        animal (traffic) V70.9
          being ridden (traffic) V76.9
            nontraffic V76.3
            while boarding or alighting V76.4
          nontraffic V70.3
          while boarding or alighting V70.4
        animal-drawn vehicle (traffic) V76.9
          nontraffic V76.3
          while boarding or alighting V76.4
        bus (traffic) V74.9
          nontraffic V74.3
          while boarding or alighting V74.4
        car (traffic) V73.9
          nontraffic V73.3
          while boarding or alighting V73.4
        motor vehicle NOS (traffic) V79.60
          nontraffic V79.20
          specified type NEC (traffic) V79.69
            nontraffic V79.29
        pedal cycle (traffic) V71.9
          nontraffic V71.3
          while boarding or alighting V71.4
        pickup truck (traffic) V73.9
          nontraffic V73.3
          while boarding or alighting V73.4
        railway vehicle (traffic) V75.9
          nontraffic V75.3
          while boarding or alighting V75.4
        specified vehicle NEC (traffic) V76.9
          nontraffic V76.3
          while boarding or alighting V76.4
        stationary object (traffic) V77.9
          nontraffic V77.3
          while boarding or alighting V77.4
        streetcar (traffic) V76.9
          nontraffic V76.3
          while boarding or alighting V76.4
        three wheeled motor vehicle (traffic) V72.9
          nontraffic V72.3
          while boarding or alighting V72.4
        truck (traffic) V74.9
          nontraffic V74.3
          while boarding or alighting V74.4
        two wheeled motor vehicle (traffic) V72.9
          nontraffic V72.3
          while boarding or alighting V72.4
        van (traffic) V73.9
          nontraffic V73.3
          while boarding or alighting V73.4

Accident *(Continued)*
  transport *(Continued)*
    bus occupant *(Continued)*
      driver
        collision (with)
          animal (traffic) V70.5
            being ridden (traffic) V76.5
              nontraffic V76.0
            nontraffic V70.0
          animal-drawn vehicle (traffic) V76.5
            nontraffic V76.0
          bus (traffic) V74.5
            nontraffic V74.0
          car (traffic) V73.5
            nontraffic V73.0
          motor vehicle NOS (traffic) V79.40
            nontraffic V79.00
            specified type NEC (traffic) V79.49
              nontraffic V79.09
          pedal cycle (traffic) V71.5
            nontraffic V71.0
          pickup truck (traffic) V73.5
            nontraffic V73.0
          railway vehicle (traffic) V75.5
            nontraffic V75.0
          specified vehicle NEC (traffic) V76.5
            nontraffic V76.0
          stationary object (traffic) V77.5
            nontraffic V77.0
          streetcar (traffic) V76.5
            nontraffic V76.0
          three wheeled motor vehicle (traffic) V72.5
            nontraffic V72.0
          truck (traffic) V74.5
            nontraffic V74.0
          two wheeled motor vehicle (traffic) V72.5
            nontraffic V72.0
          van (traffic) V73.5
            nontraffic V73.0
        noncollision accident (traffic) V78.5
          nontraffic V78.0
      hanger-on
        collision (with)
          animal (traffic) V70.7
            being ridden (traffic) V76.7
              nontraffic V76.2
            nontraffic V70.2
          animal-drawn vehicle (traffic) V76.7
            nontraffic V76.2
          bus (traffic) V74.7
            nontraffic V74.2
          car (traffic) V73.7
            nontraffic V73.2
          pedal cycle (traffic) V71.7
            nontraffic V71.2
          pickup truck (traffic) V73.7
            nontraffic V73.2
          railway vehicle (traffic) V75.7
            nontraffic V75.2
          specified vehicle NEC (traffic) V76.7
            nontraffic V76.2
          stationary object (traffic) V77.7
            nontraffic V77.2
          streetcar (traffic) V76.7
            nontraffic V76.2
          three wheeled motor vehicle (traffic) V72.7
            nontraffic V72.2
          truck (traffic) V74.7
            nontraffic V74.2
          two wheeled motor vehicle (traffic) V72.7
            nontraffic V72.2
          van (traffic) V73.7
            nontraffic V73.2
        noncollision accident (traffic) V78.7
          nontraffic V78.2

Accident *(Continued)*
  transport *(Continued)*
    bus occupant *(Continued)*
      noncollision accident (traffic) V78.9
        nontraffic V78.3
        while boarding or alighting V78.4
      nontraffic V79.3
      passenger
        collision (with)
          animal (traffic) V70.6
            being ridden (traffic) V76.6
              nontraffic V76.1
            nontraffic V70.1
          animal-drawn vehicle (traffic) V76.6
            nontraffic V76.1
          bus (traffic) V74.6
            nontraffic V74.1
          car (traffic) V73.6
            nontraffic V73.1
          motor vehicle NOS (traffic) V79.50
            nontraffic V79.10
            specified type NEC (traffic) V79.59
              nontraffic V79.19
          pedal cycle (traffic) V71.6
            nontraffic V71.1
          pickup truck (traffic) V73.6
            nontraffic V73.1
          railway vehicle (traffic) V75.6
            nontraffic V75.1
          specified vehicle NEC (traffic) V76.6
            nontraffic V76.1
          stationary object (traffic) V77.6
            nontraffic V77.1
          streetcar (traffic) V76.6
            nontraffic V76.1
          three wheeled motor vehicle (traffic) V72.6
            nontraffic V72.1
          truck (traffic) V74.6
            nontraffic V74.1
          two wheeled motor vehicle (traffic) V72.6
            nontraffic V72.1
          van (traffic) V73.6
            nontraffic V73.1
        noncollision accident (traffic) V78.6
          nontraffic V78.1
      specified type NEC V79.88
      military vehicle V79.81
    cable car, not on rails V98.0
      on rails —*see* Accident, transport, streetcar occupant
    car occupant V49.9
      ambulance occupant —*see* Accident, transport, ambulance occupant
      collision (with)
        animal (traffic) V40.9
          being ridden (traffic) V46.9
            nontraffic V46.3
            while boarding or alighting V46.4
          nontraffic V40.3
          while boarding or alighting V40.4
        animal-drawn vehicle (traffic) V46.9
          nontraffic V46.3
          while boarding or alighting V46.4
        bus (traffic) V44.9
          nontraffic V44.3
          while boarding or alighting V44.4
        car (traffic) V43.92
          nontraffic V43.32
          while boarding or alighting V43.42
        motor vehicle NOS (traffic) V49.60
          nontraffic V49.20
          specified type NEC (traffic) V49.69
           nontraffic V49.29
        pedal cycle (traffic) V41.9
          nontraffic V41.3
          while boarding or alighting V41.4

Accident *(Continued)*
  transport *(Continued)*
    car occupant *(Continued)*
      collision *(Continued)*
        pickup truck (traffic) V43.93
          nontraffic V43.33
          while boarding or alighting V43.43
        railway vehicle (traffic) V45.9
          nontraffic V45.3
          while boarding or alighting V45.4
        specified vehicle NEC (traffic) V46.9
          nontraffic V46.3
          while boarding or alighting V46.4
        sport utility vehicle (traffic) V43.91
          nontraffic V43.31
          while boarding or alighting V43.41
        stationary object (traffic) V47.9
          nontraffic V47.3
          while boarding or alighting V47.4
        streetcar (traffic) V46.9
          nontraffic V46.3
          while boarding or alighting V46.4
        three wheeled motor vehicle (traffic) V42.9
          nontraffic V42.3
          while boarding or alighting V42.4
        truck (traffic) V44.9
          nontraffic V44.3
          while boarding or alighting V44.4
        two wheeled motor vehicle (traffic) V42.9
          nontraffic V42.3
          while boarding or alighting V42.4
        van (traffic) V43.94
          nontraffic V43.34
          while boarding or alighting V43.44
    driver
      collision (with)
        animal (traffic) V40.5
          being ridden (traffic) V46.5
            nontraffic V46.0
          nontraffic V40.0
        animal-drawn vehicle (traffic) V46.5
          nontraffic V46.0
        bus (traffic) V44.5
          nontraffic V44.0
        car (traffic) V43.52
          nontraffic V43.02
        motor vehicle NOS (traffic) V49.40
          nontraffic V49.00
          specified type NEC (traffic) V49.49
           nontraffic V49.09
        pedal cycle (traffic) V41.5
          nontraffic V41.0
        pickup truck (traffic) V43.53
          nontraffic V43.03
        railway vehicle (traffic) V45.5
          nontraffic V45.0
        specified vehicle NEC (traffic) V46.5
          nontraffic V46.0
        sport utility vehicle (traffic) V43.51
          nontraffic V43.01
        stationary object (traffic) V47.5
          nontraffic V47.0
        streetcar (traffic) V46.5
          nontraffic V46.0
        three wheeled motor vehicle (traffic) V42.5
          nontraffic V42.0
        truck (traffic) V44.5
          nontraffic V44.0
        two wheeled motor vehicle (traffic) V42.5
          nontraffic V42.0
        van (traffic) V43.54
          nontraffic V43.04
      noncollision accident (traffic) V48.5
        nontraffic V48.0

▶ New   ▦ Revised   ~~deleted~~ Deleted   ● Use Additional Character(s)

Accident *(Continued)*
  transport *(Continued)*
    car occupant *(Continued)*
      hanger-on
        collision (with)
          animal (traffic) V40.7
            being ridden (traffic) V46.7
              nontraffic V46.2
            nontraffic V40.2
          animal-drawn vehicle (traffic) V46.7
            nontraffic V46.2
          bus (traffic) V44.7
            nontraffic V44.2
          car (traffic) V43.72
            nontraffic V43.22
          pedal cycle (traffic) V41.7
            nontraffic V41.2
          pickup truck (traffic) V43.73
            nontraffic V43.23
          railway vehicle (traffic) V45.7
            nontraffic V45.2
          specified vehicle NEC (traffic) V46.7
            nontraffic V46.2
          sport utility vehicle (traffic) V43.71
            nontraffic V43.21
          stationary object (traffic) V47.7
            nontraffic V47.2
          streetcar (traffic) V46.7
            nontraffic V46.2
          three wheeled motor vehicle (traffic) V42.7
            nontraffic V42.2
          truck (traffic) V44.7
            nontraffic V44.2
          two wheeled motor vehicle (traffic) V42.7
            nontraffic V42.2
          van (traffic) V43.74
            nontraffic V43.24
        noncollision accident (traffic) V48.7
         nontraffic V48.2
      noncollision accident (traffic) V48.9
        nontraffic V48.3
        while boarding or alighting V48.4
      nontraffic V49.3
      passenger
        collision (with)
          animal (traffic) V40.6
            being ridden (traffic) V46.6
              nontraffic V46.1
            nontraffic V40.1
          animal-drawn vehicle (traffic) V46.6
            nontraffic V46.1
          bus (traffic) V44.6
            nontraffic V44.1
          car (traffic) V43.62
            nontraffic V43.12
          motor vehicle NOS (traffic) V49.50
            nontraffic V49.10
            specified type NEC (traffic) V49.59
              nontraffic V49.19
          pedal cycle (traffic) V41.6
            nontraffic V41.1
          pickup truck (traffic) V43.63
            nontraffic V43.13
          railway vehicle (traffic) V45.6
            nontraffic V45.1
          specified vehicle NEC (traffic) V46.6
            nontraffic V46.1
          sport utility vehicle (traffic) V43.61
            nontraffic V43.11
          stationary object (traffic) V47.6
            nontraffic V47.1
          streetcar (traffic) V46.6
            nontraffic V46.1
          three wheeled motor vehicle (traffic) V42.6
            nontraffic V42.1
          truck (traffic) V44.6
            nontraffic V44.1

Accident *(Continued)*
  transport *(Continued)*
    car occupant *(Continued)*
      passenger *(Continued)*
        collision *(Continued)*
          two wheeled motor vehicle (traffic) V42.6
            nontraffic V42.1
          van (traffic) V43.64
            nontraffic V43.14
        noncollision accident (traffic) V48.6
         nontraffic V48.1
        specified type NEC V49.88
         military vehicle V49.81
    coal car —*see* Accident, transport, industrial vehicle occupant
    construction vehicle occupant (nontraffic) V85.9
      driver V85.5
      hanger-on V85.7
      passenger V85.6
      traffic V85.3
        driver V85.0
        hanger-on V85.2
        passenger V85.1
      while boarding or alighting V85.4
    dirt bike rider (nontraffic) V86.96
      driver V86.56
      hanger-on V86.76
      passenger V86.66
      traffic V86.36
        driver V86.06
        hanger-on V86.26
        passenger V86.16
      while boarding or alighting V86.46
    due to cataclysm —*see* Forces of nature, by type
    dune buggy occupant (nontraffic) V86.93
      driver V86.53
      hanger-on V86.73
      passenger V86.63
      traffic V86.33
        driver V86.03
        hanger-on V86.23
        passenger V86.13
      while boarding or alighting V86.43
    ▶e-bicycle —*see* Accident, transport, electric (assisted) bicylist
    ▶e-bike —*see* Accident, transport, electric (assisted) bicylist
    ▶electric (assisted) bicyclist V29.91
      ▶collision (with)
        ▶animal (traffic) V20.91
          ▶being ridden (traffic) V26.91
            ▶nontraffic V26.21
            ▶while boarding or alighting V26.31
          ▶nontraffic V20.21
          ▶while boarding or alighting V20.31
        ▶animal-drawn vehicle (traffic) V26.91
          ▶nontraffic V26.21
          ▶while boarding or alighting V26.31
        ▶bus (traffic) V24.91
          ▶nontraffic V24.21
          ▶while boarding or alighting V24.31
        ▶car (traffic) V23.91
          ▶nontraffic V23.21
          ▶while boarding or alighting V23.31
        ▶motor vehicle NOS (traffic) V29.601
          ▶nontraffic V29.201
          ▶specified type NEC (traffic) V29.691
          ▶nontraffic V29.291
        ▶pedal cycle (traffic) V21.91
          ▶nontraffic V21.21
          ▶while boarding or alighting V21.31
        ▶pedestrian V20.91
          ▶nontraffic V20.01
          ▶while boarding or alighting V20.31
        ▶pickup truck (traffic) V23.91
          ▶nontraffic V23.21
          ▶while boarding or alighting V23.31

Accident *(Continued)*
  transport *(Continued)*
    e-bike *(Continued)*
      electric (assisted) bicyclist *(Continued)*
        collision *(Continued)*
          ▶railway vehicle (traffic) V25.91
            ▶nontraffic V25.21
            ▶while boarding or alighting V25.31
          ▶specified vehicle NEC (traffic) V26.91
            ▶nontraffic V26.21
            ▶while boarding or alighting V26.31
          ▶stationary object (traffic) V27.91
            ▶nontraffic V27.21
            ▶while boarding or alighting V27.31
          ▶streetcar (traffic) V26.91
            ▶nontraffic V26.21
            ▶while boarding or alighting V26.31
          ▶three wheeled motor vehicle (traffic) V22.91
            ▶nontraffic V22.21
            ▶while boarding or alighting V22.31
          ▶truck (traffic) V24.91
            ▶nontraffic V24.21
            ▶while boarding or alighting V24.31
          ▶two wheeled motor vehicle (traffic) V22.91
            ▶nontraffic V22.21
            ▶while boarding or alighting V22.31
          ▶van (traffic) V23.91
            ▶nontraffic V23.21
            ▶while boarding or alighting V23.31
      ▶driver
        ▶collision (with)
          ▶animal (traffic) V20.41
            ▶being ridden (traffic) V26.41
              ▶nontraffic V26.01
            ▶nontraffic V20.01
          ▶animal-drawn vehicle (traffic) V26.41
            ▶nontraffic V26.01
          ▶bus (traffic) V24.41
            ▶nontraffic V24.01
          ▶car (traffic) V23.41
            ▶nontraffic V23.01
          ▶motor vehicle NOS (traffic) V29.401
            ▶nontraffic V29.001
            ▶specified type NEC (traffic) V29.491
              ▶nontraffic V29.091
          ▶pedal cycle (traffic) V21.41
            ▶nontraffic V21.01
          ▶pedestrian
            ▶nontraffic V20.01
            ▶traffic V20.41
          ▶pickup truck (traffic) V23.41
            ▶nontraffic V23.01
          ▶railway vehicle (traffic) V25.41
            ▶nontraffic V25.01
          ▶specified vehicle NEC (traffic) V26.41
            ▶nontraffic V26.01
          ▶stationary object (traffic) V27.41
            ▶nontraffic V27.01
          ▶streetcar (traffic) V26.41
            ▶nontraffic V26.01
          ▶three wheeled motor vehicle (traffic) V22.41
            ▶nontraffic V22.01
          ▶truck (traffic) V24.41
            ▶nontraffic V24.01
          ▶two wheeled motor vehicle (traffic) V22.41
            ▶nontraffic V22.01
          ▶van (traffic) V23.41
            ▶nontraffic V23.01
        ▶noncollision accident (traffic) V28.41
          ▶nontraffic V28.01
      ▶noncollision accident (traffic) V28.91
        ▶nontraffic V28.21
        ▶while boarding or alighting V28.31
      ▶nontraffic V29.31

▶ New   ⇒ Revised   ~~deleted~~ Deleted   ● Use Additional Character(s)

Accident (*Continued*)
transport (*Continued*)
e-bike (*Continued*)
▶passenger
▶collision (with)
▶animal (traffic) V20.51
▶being ridden (traffic) V26.51
▶nontraffic V26.11
▶nontraffic V20.11
▶animal-drawn vehicle (traffic) V26.51
▶nontraffic V26.11
▶bus (traffic) V24.51
▶nontraffic V24.11
▶car (traffic) V23.51
▶nontraffic V23.11
▶motor vehicle NOS (traffic) V29.501
▶nontraffic V29.101
▶specified type NEC (traffic) V29.591
▶nontraffic V29.191
▶pedal cycle (traffic) V21.51
▶nontraffic V21.11
▶pedestrian
▶nontraffic V20.11
▶traffic V20.51
▶pickup truck (traffic) V23.51
▶nontraffic V23.11
▶railway vehicle (traffic) V25.51
▶nontraffic 25.11
▶specified vehicle NEC (traffic) V26.51
▶nontraffic V26.11
▶stationary object (traffic) V27.51
▶nontraffic V27.11
▶streetcar (traffic) V26.51
▶nontraffic V26.11
▶three wheeled motor vehicle (traffic) V22.51
▶nontraffic V22.11
▶truck (traffic) V24.51
▶nontraffic V24.11
▶two wheeled motor vehicle (traffic) V22.51
▶nontraffic V22.11
▶van (traffic) V23.51
▶nontraffic V23.11
▶noncollision accident (traffic) V28.51
▶nontraffic V28.11
▶specified type NEC V29.881
▶military vehicle V29.811
forklift —*see* Accident, transport, industrial vehicle occupant
go cart —*see* Accident, transport, all-terrain vehicle occupant
golf cart —*see* Accident, transport, all-terrain vehicle occupant
heavy transport vehicle occupant — *see* Accident, transport, truck occupant
hoverboard V00.848
ice yacht V98.2
industrial vehicle occupant (nontraffic) V83.9
driver V83.5
hanger-on V83.7
passenger V83.6
traffic V83.3
driver V83.0
hanger-on V83.2
passenger V83.1
while boarding or alighting V83.4
interurban electric car —*see* Accident, transport, streetcar
land yacht V98.1
logging car —*see* Accident, transport, industrial vehicle occupant
military vehicle occupant (traffic) V86.34
driver V86.04
hanger-on V86.24
nontraffic V86.94
driver V86.54
hanger-on V86.74
passenger V86.64

Accident (*Continued*)
transport (*Continued*)
military vehicle occupant (traffic) (*Continued*)
passenger V86.14
while boarding or alighting V86.44
mine tram —*see* Accident, transport, industrial vehicle occupant
motor vehicle NEC occupant (traffic) V89.2
motorcoach —*see* Accident, transport, bus occupant
motor/cross bike rider —*see also* Accident, transport, dirt bike rider V86.96
▦motorcyclist V29.99
collision (with)
▦animal (traffic) V20.99
▦being ridden (traffic) V26.99
▦nontraffic V26.29
▦while boarding or alighting V26.39
▦nontraffic V20.29
▦while boarding or alighting V20.39
▦animal-drawn vehicle (traffic) V26.99
▦nontraffic V26.29
▦while boarding or alighting V26.39
▦bus (traffic) V24.99
▦nontraffic V24.29
▦while boarding or alighting V24.39
▦car (traffic) V23.99
▦nontraffic V23.29
▦while boarding or alighting V23.39
▦motor vehicle NOS (traffic) V29.608
▦nontraffic V29.208
▦specified type NEC (traffic) V29.698
▦nontraffic V29.298
▦pedal cycle (traffic) V21.99
▦nontraffic V21.29
▦while boarding or alighting V21.39
▦pickup truck (traffic) V23.99
▦nontraffic V23.29
▦while boarding or alighting V23.39
▦railway vehicle (traffic) V25.99
▦nontraffic V25.29
▦while boarding or alighting V25.39
▦specified vehicle NEC (traffic) V26.99
▦nontraffic V26.29
▦while boarding or alighting V26.39
▦stationary object (traffic) V27.99
▦nontraffic V27.29
▦while boarding or alighting V27.39
▦streetcar (traffic) V26.99
▦nontraffic V26.29
▦while boarding or alighting V26.39
▦three wheeled motor vehicle (traffic) V22.99
▦nontraffic V22.29
▦while boarding or alighting V22.39
▦truck (traffic) V24.99
▦nontraffic V24.29
▦while boarding or alighting V24.39
▦two wheeled motor vehicle (traffic) V22.99
▦nontraffic V22.29
▦while boarding or alighting V22.39
▦van (traffic) V23.99
▦nontraffic V23.29
▦while boarding or alighting V23.39
driver
collision (with)
▦animal (traffic) V20.49
▦being ridden (traffic) V26.49
▦nontraffic V26.09
▦nontraffic V20.09
▦animal-drawn vehicle (traffic) V26.49
▦nontraffic V26.09
▦bus (traffic) V24.49
▦nontraffic V24.09
▦car (traffic) V23.49
▦nontraffic V23.09
▦motor vehicle NOS (traffic) V29.408
▦nontraffic V29.008
▦specified type NEC (traffic) V29.498
▦nontraffic V29.098

Accident (*Continued*)
transport (*Continued*)
motorcyclist (*Continued*)
driver (*Continued*)
collision (with) (*Continued*)
▦pedal cycle (traffic) V21.49
▦nontraffic V21.09
▶pedestrian
▶nontraffic V20.09
▶traffic V20.49
▦pickup truck (traffic) V23.49
▦nontraffic V23.09
▦railway vehicle (traffic) V25.49
▦nontraffic V25.09
▦specified vehicle NEC (traffic) V26.49
▦nontraffic V26.09
▦stationary object (traffic) V27.49
▦nontraffic V27.09
▦streetcar (traffic) V26.49
▦nontraffic V26.09
▦three wheeled motor vehicle (traffic) V22.49
▦nontraffic V22.09
▦truck (traffic) V24.49
▦nontraffic V24.09
▦two wheeled motor vehicle (traffic) V22.49
▦nontraffic V22.09
▦van (traffic) V23.49
▦nontraffic V23.09
▦noncollision accident (traffic) V28.49
▦nontraffic V28.09
▦noncollision accident (traffic) V28.99
▦nontraffic V28.29
▦while boarding or alighting V28.39
▦nontraffic V29.39
passenger
collision (with)
▦animal (traffic) V20.59
▦being ridden (traffic) V26.59
▦nontraffic V26.19
▦nontraffic V20.19
▦animal-drawn vehicle (traffic) V26.59
▦nontraffic V26.19
▦bus (traffic) V24.59
▦nontraffic V24.19
▦car (traffic) V23.59
▦nontraffic V23.19
▦motor vehicle NOS (traffic) V29.508
▦nontraffic V29.108
▦specified type NEC (traffic) V29.598
▦nontraffic V29.198
▦pedal cycle (traffic) V21.59
▦nontraffic V21.19
▶pedestrian
▶nontraffic V20.19
▶traffic V20.59
▦pickup truck (traffic) V23.59
▦nontraffic V23.19
▦railway vehicle (traffic) V25.59
▦nontraffic V25.19
▦specified vehicle NEC (traffic) V26.59
▦nontraffic V26.19
▦stationary object (traffic) V27.59
▦nontraffic V27.19
▦streetcar (traffic) V26.59
▦nontraffic V26.19
▦three wheeled motor vehicle (traffic) V22.59
▦nontraffic V22.19
▦truck (traffic) V24.59
▦nontraffic V24.19
▦two wheeled motor vehicle (traffic) V22.59
▦nontraffic V22.19
▦van (traffic) V23.59
▦nontraffic V23.19
▦noncollision accident (traffic) V28.59
▦nontraffic V28.19
▦specified type NEC V29.888
▦military vehicle V29.818

▶ New   ⇒ Revised   ~~deleted~~ Deleted   ● Use Additional Character(s)

Accident (Continued)
  transport (Continued)
    occupant (of)
      aircraft (powered) V95.9
        fixed wing
          commercial —see Accident,
            transport, aircraft, occupant,
            powered, fixed wing,
            commercial
          private —see Accident, transport,
            aircraft, occupant, powered,
            fixed wing, private
        nonpowered V96.9
        specified NEC V95.8
      airport battery-powered vehicle —see
        Accident, transport, industrial
        vehicle occupant
      all-terrain vehicle (ATV) —see Accident,
        transport, all-terrain vehicle
        occupant
      animal-drawn vehicle —see Accident,
        transport, animal-drawn vehicle
        occupant
      automobile —see Accident, transport, car
        occupant
      balloon V96.00
      battery-powered vehicle —see Accident,
        transport, industrial vehicle
        occupant
      bicycle —see Accident, transport, pedal
        cyclist
        motorized —see Accident, transport,
          motorcycle rider
      boat NEC —see Accident, watercraft
      bulldozer —see Accident, transport,
        construction vehicle occupant
      bus —see Accident, transport, bus
        occupant
      cable car (on rails) —see also Accident,
        transport, streetcar occupant
        not on rails V98.0
      car —see also Accident, transport, car
        occupant
        cable (on rails) —see also Accident,
          transport, streetcar occupant
          not on rails V98.0
      coach —see Accident, transport, bus
        occupant
      coal-car —see Accident, transport,
        industrial vehicle occupant
      digger —see Accident, transport,
        construction vehicle occupant
      dump truck —see Accident, transport,
        construction vehicle occupant
      earth-leveler —see Accident, transport,
        construction vehicle occupant
      farm machinery (self-propelled) —see
        Accident, transport, agricultural
        vehicle occupant
      forklift —see Accident, transport,
        industrial vehicle occupant
      glider (unpowered) V96.20
        hang V96.10
        powered (microlight) (ultralight) —see
          Accident, transport, aircraft,
          occupant, powered, glider
      glider (unpowered) NEC V96.20
      hang-glider V96.10
      harvester —see Accident, transport,
        agricultural vehicle occupant
      heavy (transport) vehicle —see Accident,
        transport, truck occupant
      helicopter —see Accident, transport,
        aircraft, occupant, helicopter
      ice-yacht V98.2
      kite (carrying person) V96.8
      land-yacht V98.1
      logging car —see Accident, transport,
        industrial vehicle occupant
      mechanical shovel —see Accident,
        transport, construction vehicle
        occupant

Accident (Continued)
  transport (Continued)
    occupant (Continued)
      microlight —see Accident, transport,
        aircraft, occupant, powered, glider
      minibus —see Accident, transport,
        pickup truck occupant
      minivan —see Accident, transport,
        pickup truck occupant
      moped —see Accident, transport,
        motorcycle
      motor scooter —see Accident, transport,
        motorcycle
      motorcycle (with sidecar) —see Accident,
        transport, motorcycle
      off-road motor-vehicle —see also
        Accident, transport, all-terrain
        vehicle occupant V86.99
      pedal cycle —see also Accident,
        transport, pedal cyclist
      pick-up (truck) —see Accident, transport,
        pickup truck occupant
      railway (train) (vehicle) (subterranean)
        (elevated) —see Accident, transport,
        railway vehicle occupant
      rickshaw —see Accident, transport,
        pedal cycle
        pedal driven —see Accident, transport,
          pedal cyclist
      road-roller —see Accident, transport,
        construction vehicle occupant
      ship NOS V94.9
      ski-lift (chair) (gondola) V98.3
      snowmobile —see Accident, transport,
        snowmobile occupant
      spacecraft, spaceship —see Accident,
        transport, aircraft, occupant,
        spacecraft
      sport utility vehicle —see Accident,
        transport, pickup truck occupant
      streetcar (interurban) (operating on
        public street or highway) —see
        Accident, transport, streetcar
        occupant
      SUV —see Accident, transport, pickup
        truck occupant
      téléférique V98.0
      three-wheeled vehicle (motorized) —see
        also Accident, transport, three-
        wheeled motor vehicle occupant
        nonmotorized —see Accident,
          transport, pedal cycle
      tractor (farm) (and trailer) —see
        Accident, transport, agricultural
        vehicle occupant
      train —see Accident, transport, railway
        vehicle occupant
      tram —see Accident, transport, streetcar
        occupant
        in mine or quarry —see Accident,
          transport, industrial vehicle
          occupant
      tricycle —see Accident, transport, pedal
        cycle
        motorized —see Accident, transport,
          three-wheeled motor vehicle
      trolley —see Accident, transport,
        streetcar occupant
        in mine or quarry —see Accident,
          transport, industrial vehicle
          occupant
      tub, in mine or quarry —see Accident,
        transport, industrial vehicle
        occupant
      ultralight —see Accident, transport,
        aircraft, occupant, powered, glider
      van —see Accident, transport, van
        occupant
      vehicle NEC V89.9
        heavy transport —see Accident,
          transport, truck occupant

Accident (Continued)
  transport (Continued)
    occupant (Continued)
      vehicle NEC (Continued)
        motor (traffic) NEC V89.2
        nontraffic NEC V89.0
      watercraft NOS V94.9
        causing drowning —see Drowning,
          resulting from accident to boat
      off-road motor-vehicle —see also Accident,
        transport, all-terrain vehicle occupant
        V86.99
    parachutist V97.29
      after accident to aircraft —see Accident,
        transport, aircraft
      entangled in object V97.21
      injured on landing V97.22
    pedal cyclist V19.9
      collision (with)
        animal (traffic) V10.9
          being ridden (traffic) V16.9
            nontraffic V16.2
            while boarding or alighting V16.3
          nontraffic V10.2
          while boarding or alighting V10.3
        animal-drawn vehicle (traffic) V16.9
          nontraffic V16.2
          while boarding or alighting V16.3
        bus (traffic) V14.9
          nontraffic V14.2
          while boarding or alighting V14.3
        car (traffic) V13.9
          nontraffic V13.2
          while boarding or alighting V13.3
        motor vehicle NOS (traffic) V19.60
          nontraffic V19.20
          specified type NEC (traffic) V19.69
            nontraffic V19.29
        pedal cycle (traffic) V11.9
          nontraffic V11.2
          while boarding or alighting V11.3
        pickup truck (traffic) V13.9
          nontraffic V13.2
          while boarding or alighting V13.3
        railway vehicle (traffic) V15.9
          nontraffic V15.2
          while boarding or alighting V15.3
        specified vehicle NEC (traffic) V16.9
          nontraffic V16.2
          while boarding or alighting V16.3
        stationary object (traffic) V17.9
          nontraffic V17.2
          while boarding or alighting V17.3
        streetcar (traffic) V16.9
          nontraffic V16.2
          while boarding or alighting V16.3
        three wheeled motor vehicle (traffic)
          V12.9
          nontraffic V12.2
          while boarding or alighting V12.3
        truck (traffic) V14.9
          nontraffic V14.2
          while boarding or alighting V14.3
        two wheeled motor vehicle (traffic)
          V12.9
          nontraffic V12.2
          while boarding or alighting V12.3
        van (traffic) V13.9
          nontraffic V13.2
          while boarding or alighting V13.3
      driver
        collision (with)
          animal (traffic) V10.4
            being ridden (traffic) V16.4
              nontraffic V16.0
            nontraffic V10.0
          animal-drawn vehicle (traffic) V16.4
            nontraffic V16.0
          bus (traffic) V14.4
            nontraffic V14.0
          car (traffic) V13.4
            nontraffic V13.0

Accident *(Continued)*
  transport *(Continued)*
    pedal cyclist *(Continued)*
      driver *(Continued)*
        collision *(Continued)*
          motor vehicle NOS (traffic) V19.40
            nontraffic V19.00
            specified type NEC (traffic) V19.49
              nontraffic V19.09
          pedal cycle (traffic) V11.4
            nontraffic V11.0
          pickup truck (traffic) V13.4
            nontraffic V13.0
          railway vehicle (traffic) V15.4
            nontraffic V15.0
          specified vehicle NEC (traffic) V16.4
            nontraffic V16.0
          stationary object (traffic) V17.4
            nontraffic V17.0
          streetcar (traffic) V16.4
            nontraffic V16.0
          three wheeled motor vehicle
              (traffic) V12.4
            nontraffic V12.0
          truck (traffic) V14.4
            nontraffic V14.0
          two wheeled motor vehicle (traffic)
              V12.4
            nontraffic V12.0
          van (traffic) V13.4
            nontraffic V13.0
        noncollision accident (traffic) V18.4
          nontraffic V18.0
      noncollision accident (traffic) V18.9
        nontraffic V18.2
        while boarding or alighting V18.3
      nontraffic V19.3
      passenger
        collision (with)
          animal (traffic) V10.5
            being ridden (traffic) V16.5
              nontraffic V16.1
            nontraffic V10.1
          animal-drawn vehicle (traffic) V16.5
            nontraffic V16.1
          bus (traffic) V14.5
            nontraffic V14.1
          car (traffic) V13.5
            nontraffic V13.1
          motor vehicle NOS (traffic) V19.50
            nontraffic V19.10
            specified type NEC (traffic)
              V19.59
              nontraffic V19.19
          pedal cycle (traffic) V11.5
            nontraffic V11.1
          pickup truck (traffic) V13.5
            nontraffic V13.1
          railway vehicle (traffic) V15.5
            nontraffic V15.1
          specified vehicle NEC (traffic) V16.5
            nontraffic V16.1
          stationary object (traffic) V17.5
            nontraffic V17.1
          streetcar (traffic) V16.5
            nontraffic V16.1
          three wheeled motor vehicle
              (traffic) V12.5
            nontraffic V12.1
          truck (traffic) V14.5
            nontraffic V14.1
          two wheeled motor vehicle (traffic)
              V12.5
            nontraffic V12.1
          van (traffic) V13.5
            nontraffic V13.1
        noncollision accident (traffic) V18.5
          nontraffic V18.1
      specified type NEC V19.88
        military vehicle V19.81
    pedestrian

  transport *(Continued)*
    pedestrian *(Continued)*
      conveyance (occupant) V09.9
        baby stroller V00.828
          collision (with) V09.9
            animal being ridden or animal
                drawn vehicle V06.99
              nontraffic V06.09
              traffic V06.19
            bus or heavy transport V04.99
              nontraffic V04.09
              traffic V04.19
            car V03.99
              nontraffic V03.09
              traffic V03.19
            pedal cycle V01.99
              nontraffic V01.09
              traffic V01.19
            pick-up truck or van V03.99
              nontraffic V03.09
              traffic V03.19
            railway (train) (vehicle)
                V05.99
              nontraffic V05.09
              traffic V05.19
            stationary object V00.822
            streetcar V06.99
              nontraffic V06.09
              traffic V06.19
            two- or three-wheeled motor
                vehicle V02.99
              nontraffic V02.09
              traffic V02.19
            vehicle V09.9
              animal-drawn V06.99
                nontraffic V06.09
                traffic V06.19
              motor
                nontraffic V09.00
                traffic V09.20
          fall V00.821
          nontraffic V09.1
            involving motor vehicle NEC
                V09.00
          traffic V09.3
            involving motor vehicle NEC
                V09.20
        flat-bottomed NEC V00.388
          collision (with) V09.9
            animal being ridden or animal
                drawn vehicle V06.99
              nontraffic V06.09
              traffic V06.19
            bus or heavy transport V04.99
              nontraffic V04.09
              traffic V04.19
            car V03.99
              nontraffic V03.09
              traffic V03.19
            pedal cycle V01.99
              nontraffic V01.09
              traffic V01.19
            pick-up truck or van V03.99
              nontraffic V03.09
              traffic V03.19
            railway (train) (vehicle) V05.99
              nontraffic V05.09
              traffic V05.19
            stationary object V00.382
            streetcar V06.99
              nontraffic V06.09
              traffic V06.19
            two-or three-wheeled motor
                vehicle V02.99
              nontraffic V02.09
              traffic V02.19
            vehicle V09.9
              animal-drawn V06.99
                nontraffic V06.09
                traffic V06.19

  transport *(Continued)*
    pedestrian *(Continued)*
      conveyance *(Continued)*
        flat-bottomed NEC *(Continued)*
          collision *(Continued)*
            vehicle *(Continued)*
              motor
                nontraffic V09.00
                traffic V09.20
          fall V00.381
          nontraffic V09.1
            involving motor vehicle NEC
                V09.00
          snow
            board —*see* Accident, transport,
                pedestrian, conveyance,
                snow board
            ski —*see* Accident, transport,
                pedestrian, conveyance, skis
                (snow)
          traffic V09.3
            involving motor vehicle NEC
                V09.20
        gliding type NEC V00.288
          collision (with) V09.9
            animal being ridden or animal
                drawn vehicle V06.99
              nontraffic V06.09
              traffic V06.19
            bus or heavy transport
                V04.99
              nontraffic V04.09
              traffic V04.19
            car V03.99
              nontraffic V03.09
              traffic V03.19
            pedal cycle V01.99
              nontraffic V01.09
              traffic V01.19
            pick-up truck or van V03.99
              nontraffic V03.09
              traffic V03.19
            railway (train) (vehicle) V05.99
              nontraffic V05.09
              traffic V05.19
            stationary object V00.282
            streetcar V06.99
              nontraffic V06.09
              traffic V06.19
            two- or three-wheeled motor
                vehicle V02.99
              nontraffic V02.09
              traffic V02.19
            vehicle V09.9
              animal-drawn V06.99
                nontraffic V06.09
                traffic V06.19
              motor
                nontraffic V09.00
                traffic V09.20
          fall V00.281
          heelies —*see* Accident, transport,
              pedestrian, conveyance,
              heelies
        hoverboard
          collision with
            animal being ridden or animal
                drawn vehicle V06.938
              nontraffic V06.038
              traffic V06.138
            bus or heavy transport
                V04.938
              nontraffic V04.038
              traffic V04.138
            car V03.938
              nontraffic V03.038
              traffic V03.138
            pedal cycle V01.938
              nontraffic V01.038
              traffic V01.138

▶ New   ⇒ Revised   ~~deleted~~ Deleted   ● Use Additional Character(s)

Accident *(Continued)*
  transport *(Continued)*
    pedestrian *(Continued)*
      conveyance *(Continued)*
        gliding type NEC *(Continued)*
          hoverboard *(Continued)*
            collision with *(Continued)*
              pick-up or van V03.938
                nontraffic V03.038
                traffic V03.138
              railway (train) (vehicle) V05.938
                nontraffic V05.038
                traffic V05.138
              streetcar V06.938
                nontraffic V06.038
                traffic V06.138
              three-wheeled motor vehicle
                V02.938
                nontraffic V02.038
                traffic V02.138
              two-wheeled motor vehicle
                V02.938
                nontraffic V02.038
                traffic V02.138
              vehicle, nonmotor, specified
                NEC V06.938
                nontraffic V06.038
                traffic V06.138
            fall V00.848
          ice skate —*see* Accident, transport,
            pedestrian, conveyance, ice
            skate
          nontraffic V09.1
            involving motor vehicle NEC
              V09.00
          Segway
            collision with
              animal being ridden or animal
                drawn vehicle V06.938
                nontraffic V06.038
                traffic V06.138
              bus or heavy transport V04.938
                nontraffic V04.038
                traffic V04.138
              car V03.938
                nontraffic V03.038
                traffic V03.138
              pedal cycle V01.938
                nontraffic V01.038
                traffic V01.138
              pick-up or van V03.038
                nontraffic V01.038
                traffic V03.138
              railway (train) (vehicle) V05.938
                nontraffic V05.038
                traffic V05.138
              streetcar V06.938
                nontraffic V06.038
                traffic V06.138
              three-wheeled motor vehicle
                V02.938
                nontraffic V02.038
                traffic V02.138
              two-wheeled motor vehicle
                V02.938
                nontraffic V02.038
                traffic V02.138
              vehicle, nonmotor, specified
                NEC V06.938
                nontraffic V06.038
                traffic V06.138
            fall V00.848
          sled —*see* Accident, transport,
            pedestrian, conveyance, sled
        standing
          electric scooter
            collision with
              animal being ridden or
                animal drawn vehicle
                V06.931
                nontraffic V06.031
                traffic V06.131

Accident *(Continued)*
  transport *(Continued)*
    pedestrian *(Continued)*
      conveyance *(Continued)*
        gliding type NEC *(Continued)*
          standing *(Continued)*
            electric scooter *(Continued)*
              collision with *(Continued)*
                bus or heavy transport
                  V04.931
                  nontraffic V04.031
                  traffic V04.131
                car V03.931
                  nontraffic V03.031
                  traffic V03.131
                pedal cycle V01.931
                  nontraffic V01.031
                  traffic V01.131
                pick-up or van V03.931
                  nontraffic V03.031
                  traffic V03.131
                railway (train) (vehicle)
                  V05.931
                  nontraffic V05.031
                  traffic V05.131
                streetcar V06.931
                  nontraffic V06.031
                  traffic V06.131
                three-wheeled motor vehicle
                  V02.931
                  nontraffic V02.031
                  traffic V02.131
                two-wheeled motor vehicle
                  V02.931
                  nontraffic V02.031
                  traffic V02.131
                vehicle, nonmotor, specified
                  NEC V06.931
                  nontraffic V06.031
                  traffic V06.131
              fall V00.841
          micro-mobility pedestrian
            conveyance
          collision with
            animal being ridden or
              animal drawn vehicle
              V06.938
              nontraffic V06.038
              traffic V06.138
            bus or heavy transport
              V04.938
              nontraffic V04.038
              traffic V04.138
            car V03.938
              nontraffic V03.038
              traffic V03.138
            pedal cycle V01.938
              nontraffic V01.038
              traffic V01.138
            pick-up or van V03.938
              nontraffic V03.038
              traffic V03.138
            railway (train) (vehicle)
              V05.938
              nontraffic V05.038
              traffic V05.138
            stationary object V00.842
            streetcar V06.938
              nontraffic V06.038
              traffic V06.138
            three-wheeled motor vehicle
              V02.938
              nontraffic V02.038
              traffic V02.138
            two-wheeled motor vehicle
              V02.938
              nontraffic V02.038
              traffic V02.138
            vehicle, nonmotor, specified
              NEC V06.938
              nontraffic V06.038
              traffic V06.138
          fall V00.848

Accident *(Continued)*
  transport *(Continued)*
    pedestrian *(Continued)*
      conveyance *(Continued)*
        gliding type NEC *(Continued)*
          traffic V09.3
            involving motor vehicle NEC
              V09.20
          wheelies —*see* Accident,
            transport, pedestrian,
            conveyance, heelies
        heelies V00.158
          colliding with stationary object
            V00.152
          fall V00.151
        ice skates V00.218
          collision (with) V09.9
            animal being ridden or animal
              drawn vehicle V06.99
              nontraffic V06.09
              traffic V06.19
            bus or heavy transport V04.99
              nontraffic V04.09
              traffic V04.19
            car V03.99
              nontraffic V03.09
              traffic V03.19
            pedal cycle V01.99
              nontraffic V01.09
              traffic V01.19
            pick-up truck or van V03.99
              nontraffic V03.09
              traffic V03.19
            railway (train) (vehicle)
              V05.99
              nontraffic V05.09
              traffic V05.19
            stationary object V00.212
            streetcar V06.99
              nontraffic V06.09
              traffic V06.19
            two- or three-wheeled motor
              vehicle V02.99
              nontraffic V02.09
              traffic V02.19
            vehicle V09.9
              animal-drawn V06.99
                nontraffic V06.09
                traffic V06.19
              motor
                nontraffic V09.00
                traffic V09.20
          fall V00.211
          nontraffic V09.1
            involving motor vehicle NEC
              V09.00
          traffic V09.3
            involving motor vehicle NEC
              V09.20
        motorized mobility scooter
          V00.838
          collision with stationary object
            V00.832
          fall from V00.831
          nontraffic V09.1
            involving motor vehicle
              V09.00
              military V09.01
              specified type NEC V09.09
        roller skates (non in-line) V00.128
          collision (with) V09.9
            animal being ridden or animal
              drawn vehicle V06.91
              nontraffic V06.01
              traffic V06.11
            bus or heavy transport V04.91
              nontraffic V04.01
              traffic V04.11
            car V03.91
              nontraffic V03.01
              traffic V03.11

Accident *(Continued)*
  transport *(Continued)*
    pedestrian *(Continued)*
      conveyance *(Continued)*
        roller skates *(Continued)*
          collision *(Continued)*
            pedal cycle V01.91
              nontraffic V01.01
              traffic V01.11
            pick-up truck or van V03.91
              nontraffic V03.01
              traffic V03.11
            railway (train) (vehicle) V05.91
              nontraffic V05.01
              traffic V05.11
            stationary object V00.122
            streetcar V06.91
              nontraffic V06.01
              traffic V06.11
            two- or three-wheeled motor vehicle V02.91
              nontraffic V02.01
              traffic V02.11
            vehicle V09.9
              animal-drawn V06.91
                nontraffic V06.01
                traffic V06.11
              motor
                nontraffic V09.00
                traffic V09.20
        fall V00.121
        in-line V00.118
          collision —*see also* Accident, transport, pedestrian, conveyance occupant, roller skates, collision
            with stationary object V00.112
          fall V00.111
          nontraffic V09.1
            involving motor vehicle NEC V09.00
          traffic V09.3
            involving motor vehicle NEC V09.20
         rolling shoes V00.158
          colliding with stationary object V00.152
          fall V00.151
         rolling type NEC V00.188
          collision (with) V09.9
            animal being ridden or animal drawn vehicle V06.99
              nontraffic V06.09
              traffic V06.19
            bus or heavy transport V04.99
              nontraffic V04.09
              traffic V04.19
            car V03.99
              nontraffic V03.09
              traffic V03.19
            pedal cycle V01.99
              nontraffic V01.09
              traffic V01.19
            pick-up truck or van V03.99
              nontraffic V03.09
              traffic V03.19
            railway (train) (vehicle) V05.99
              nontraffic V05.09
              traffic V05.19
            stationary object V00.182
            streetcar V06.99
              nontraffic V06.09
              traffic V06.19
            two- or three-wheeled motor vehicle V02.99
              nontraffic V02.09
              traffic V02.19

Accident *(Continued)*
  transport *(Continued)*
    pedestrian *(Continued)*
      conveyance *(Continued)*
        rolling type NEC *(Continued)*
          collision *(Continued)*
            vehicle V09.9
              animal-drawn V06.99
                nontraffic V06.09
                traffic V06.19
              motor
                nontraffic V09.00
                traffic V09.20
          fall V00.181
          in-line roller skate —*see* Accident, transport, pedestrian, conveyance, roller skate, in-line
          nontraffic V09.1
            involving motor vehicle NEC V09.00
          roller skate —*see* Accident, transport, pedestrian, conveyance, roller skate
          scooter (non-motorized) — *see* Accident, transport, pedestrian, conveyance, scooter
          skateboard —*see* Accident, transport, pedestrian, conveyance, skateboard
          traffic V09.3
            involving motor vehicle NEC V09.20
         scooter (non-motorized) V00.148
          collision (with) V09.9
            animal being ridden or animal drawn vehicle V06.99
              nontraffic V06.09
              traffic V06.19
            bus or heavy transport V04.99
              nontraffic V04.09
              traffic V04.19
            car V03.99
              nontraffic V03.09
              traffic V03.19
            pedal cycle V01.99
              nontraffic V01.09
              traffic V01.19
            pick-up truck or van V03.99
              nontraffic V03.09
              traffic V03.19
            railway (train) (vehicle) V05.99
              nontraffic V05.09
              traffic V05.19
            stationary object V00.142
            streetcar V06.99
              nontraffic V06.09
              traffic V06.19
            two- or three-wheeled motor vehicle V02.99
              nontraffic V02.09
              traffic V02.19
            vehicle V09.9
              animal-drawn V06.99
                nontraffic V06.09
                traffic V06.19
              motor
                nontraffic V09.00
                traffic V09.20
          fall V00.141
          nontraffic V09.1
            involving motor vehicle NEC V09.00
          traffic V09.3
            involving motor vehicle NEC V09.20

Accident *(Continued)*
  transport *(Continued)*
    pedestrian *(Continued)*
      conveyance *(Continued)*
        ▶ skateboard V00.138
          collision (with) V09.9
            animal being ridden or animal drawn vehicle V06.92
              nontraffic V06.02
              traffic V06.12
            bus or heavy transport V04.92
              nontraffic V04.02
              traffic V04.12
            car V03.92
              nontraffic V03.02
              traffic V03.12
            pedal cycle V01.92
              nontraffic V01.02
              traffic V01.12
            pick-up truck or van V03.92
              nontraffic V03.02
              traffic V03.12
            railway (train) (vehicle) V05.92
              nontraffic V05.02
              traffic V05.12
            stationary object V00.132
            streetcar V06.92
              nontraffic V06.02
              traffic V06.12
            two- or three-wheeled motor vehicle V02.92
              nontraffic V02.02
              traffic V02.12
            vehicle V09.9
              animal-drawn V06.92
                nontraffic V06.02
                traffic V06.12
              motor
                nontraffic V09.00
                traffic V09.20
          fall V00.131
          nontraffic V09.1
            involving motor vehicle NEC V09.00
          traffic V09.3
            involving motor vehicle NEC V09.20
         skis (snow) V00.328
          collision (with) V09.9
            animal being ridden or animal drawn vehicle V06.99
              nontraffic V06.09
              traffic V06.19
            bus or heavy transport V04.99
              nontraffic V04.09
              traffic V04.19
            car V03.99
              nontraffic V03.09
              traffic V03.19
            pedal cycle V01.99
              nontraffic V01.09
              traffic V01.19
            pick-up truck or van V03.99
              nontraffic V03.09
              traffic V03.19
            railway (train) (vehicle) V05.99
              nontraffic V05.09
              traffic V05.19
            stationary object V00.322
            streetcar V06.99
              nontraffic V06.09
              traffic V06.19
            two- or three-wheeled motor vehicle V02.99
              nontraffic V02.09
              traffic V02.19
            vehicle V09.9
              animal-drawn V06.99
                nontraffic V06.09
                traffic V06.19

▶ New   ⇒ Revised   ~~deleted~~ Deleted   ● Use Additional Character(s)

Accident *(Continued)*
 transport *(Continued)*
  pedestrian *(Continued)*
   conveyance *(Continued)*
    sled *(Continued)*
     collision *(Continued)*
      vehicle *(Continued)*
       motor
        nontraffic V09.00
        traffic V09.20
      fall V00.321
      nontraffic V09.1
       involving motor vehicle NEC
        V09.00
      traffic V09.3
       involving motor vehicle NEC
        V09.20
    sled V00.228
     collision (with) V09.9
      animal being ridden or animal
       drawn vehicle V06.99
       nontraffic V06.09
       traffic V06.19
      bus or heavy transport V04.99
       nontraffic V04.09
       traffic V04.19
      car V03.99
       nontraffic V03.09
       traffic V03.19
      pedal cycle V01.99
       nontraffic V01.09
       traffic V01.19
      pick-up truck or van V03.99
       nontraffic V03.09
       traffic V03.19
      railway (train) (vehicle) V05.99
       nontraffic V05.09
       traffic V05.19
      stationary object V00.222
      streetcar V06.99
       nontraffic V06.09
       traffic V06.19
      two- or three-wheeled motor
       vehicle V02.99
       nontraffic V02.09
       traffic V02.19
      vehicle V09.9
       animal-drawn V06.99
        nontraffic V06.09
        traffic V06.19
       motor
        nontraffic V09.00
        traffic V09.20
     fall V00.221
     nontraffic V09.1
      involving motor vehicle NEC
       V09.00
     traffic V09.3
      involving motor vehicle NEC
       V09.20
    snow board V00.318
     collision (with) V09.9
      animal being ridden or animal
       drawn vehicle V06.99
       nontraffic V06.09
       traffic V06.19
      bus or heavy transport V04.99
       nontraffic V04.09
       traffic V04.19
      car V03.99
       nontraffic V03.09
       traffic V03.19
      pedal cycle V01.99
       nontraffic V01.09
       traffic V01.19
      pick-up truck or van V03.99
       nontraffic V03.09
       traffic V03.19
      railway (train) (vehicle) V05.99
       nontraffic V05.09
       traffic V05.19

Accident *(Continued)*
 transport *(Continued)*
  pedestrian *(Continued)*
   conveyance *(Continued)*
    snow board *(Continued)*
     collision *(Continued)*
      stationary object V00.312
      streetcar V06.99
       nontraffic V06.09
       traffic V06.19
      two- or three-wheeled motor
       vehicle V02.99
       nontraffic V02.09
       traffic V02.19
      vehicle V09.9
       animal-drawn V06.99
        nontraffic V06.09
        traffic V06.19
       motor
        nontraffic V09.00
        traffic V09.20
     fall V00.311
     nontraffic V09.1
      involving motor vehicle NEC
       V09.00
     traffic V09.3
      involving motor vehicle NEC
       V09.20
    specified type NEC V00.898
     collision (with) V09.9
      animal being ridden or animal
       drawn vehicle V06.99
       nontraffic V06.09
       traffic V06.19
      bus or heavy transport V04.99
       nontraffic V04.09
       traffic V04.19
      car V03.99
       nontraffic V03.09
       traffic V03.19
      pedal cycle V01.99
       nontraffic V01.09
       traffic V01.19
      pick-up truck or van V03.99
       nontraffic V03.09
       traffic V03.19
      railway (train) (vehicle) V05.99
       nontraffic V05.09
       traffic V05.19
      stationary object V00.892
      streetcar V06.99
       nontraffic V06.09
       traffic V06.19
      two- or three-wheeled motor
       vehicle V02.99
       nontraffic V02.09
       traffic V02.19
      vehicle V09.9
       animal-drawn V06.99
        nontraffic V06.09
        traffic V06.19
       motor
        nontraffic V09.00
        traffic V09.20
     fall V00.891
     nontraffic V09.1
      involving motor vehicle NEC
       V09.00
     traffic V09.3
      involving motor vehicle NEC
       V09.20
    traffic V09.3
     involving motor vehicle V09.20
      military V09.21
      specified type NEC V09.29
    wheelchair (powered) V00.818
     collision (with) V09.9
      animal being ridden or animal
       drawn vehicle V06.99
       nontraffic V06.09
       traffic V06.19

Accident *(Continued)*
 transport *(Continued)*
  pedestrian *(Continued)*
   conveyance *(Continued)*
    wheelchair *(Continued)*
     collision *(Continued)*
      bus or heavy transport V04.99
       nontraffic V04.09
       traffic V04.19
      car V03.99
       nontraffic V03.09
       traffic V03.19
      pedal cycle V01.99
       nontraffic V01.09
       traffic V01.19
      pick-up truck or van V03.99
       nontraffic V03.09
       traffic V03.19
      railway (train) (vehicle) V05.99
       nontraffic V05.09
       traffic V05.19
      stationary object V00.812
      streetcar V06.99
       nontraffic V06.09
       traffic V06.19
      two- or three-wheeled motor
       vehicle V02.99
       nontraffic V02.09
       traffic V02.19
      vehicle V09.9
       animal-drawn V06.99
        nontraffic V06.09
        traffic V06.19
       motor
        nontraffic V09.00
        traffic V09.20
     fall V00.811
     nontraffic V09.1
      involving motor vehicle NEC
       V09.00
     traffic V09.3
      involving motor vehicle NEC
       V09.20
    wheeled shoe V00.158
     colliding with stationary object
      V00.152
     fall V00.151
   on foot —*see also* Accident, pedestrian
    collision (with)
     animal being ridden or animal
      drawn vehicle V06.90
      nontraffic V06.00
      traffic V06.10
     bus or heavy transport V04.90
      nontraffic V04.00
      traffic V04.10
     car V03.90
      nontraffic V03.00
      traffic V03.10
     pedal cycle V01.90
      nontraffic V01.00
      traffic V01.10
     pick-up truck or van V03.90
      nontraffic V03.00
      traffic V03.10
     railway (train) (vehicle) V05.90
      nontraffic V05.00
      traffic V05.10
     streetcar V06.90
      nontraffic V06.00
      traffic V06.10
     two- or three-wheeled motor
      vehicle V02.90
      nontraffic V02.00
      traffic V02.10
     vehicle V09.9
      animal-drawn V06.90
       nontraffic V06.00
       traffic V06.10
      motor
       nontraffic V09.00
       traffic V09.20

Accident (*Continued*)
transport (*Continued*)
  pedestrian (*Continued*)
    on foot (*Continued*)
      nontraffic V09.1
        involving motor vehicle V09.00
          military V09.01
          specified type NEC V09.09
        traffic V09.3
          involving motor vehicle V09.20
            military V09.21
            specified type NEC V09.29
    person NEC (unknown way or
      transportation) V99
    collision (between)
      bus (with)
        heavy transport vehicle (traffic)
          V87.5
          nontraffic V88.5
      car (with)
        nontraffic V88.5
        bus (traffic) V87.3
          nontraffic V88.3
        heavy transport vehicle (traffic)
          V87.4
          nontraffic V88.4
        pick-up truck or van (traffic)
          V87.2
          nontraffic V88.2
        train or railway vehicle (traffic)
          V87.6
          nontraffic V88.6
        two- or three-wheeled motor
          vehicle (traffic) V87.0
          nontraffic V88.0
      motor vehicle (traffic) NEC V87.7
        nontraffic V88.7
      two- or three-wheeled vehicle (with)
        (traffic)
        motor vehicle NEC V87.1
          nontraffic V88.1
      nonmotor vehicle (collision)
        (noncollision) (traffic) V87.9
        nontraffic V88.9
    pickup truck occupant V59.9
      collision (with)
        animal (traffic) V50.9
          being ridden (traffic) V56.9
            nontraffic V56.3
            while boarding or alighting
              V56.4
          nontraffic V50.3
          while boarding or alighting V50.4
        animal-drawn vehicle (traffic) V56.9
          nontraffic V56.3
          while boarding or alighting V56.4
        bus (traffic) V54.9
          nontraffic V54.3
          while boarding or alighting V54.4
        car (traffic) V53.9
          nontraffic V53.3
          while boarding or alighting V53.4
        motor vehicle NOS (traffic) V59.60
          nontraffic V59.20
          specified type NEC (traffic) V59.69
            nontraffic V59.29
        pedal cycle (traffic) V51.9
          nontraffic V51.3
          while boarding or alighting V51.4
        pickup truck (traffic) V53.9
          nontraffic V53.3
          while boarding or alighting V53.4
        railway vehicle (traffic) V55.9
          nontraffic V55.3
          while boarding or alighting V55.4
        specified vehicle NEC (traffic) V56.9
          nontraffic V56.3
          while boarding or alighting V56.4
        stationary object (traffic) V57.9
          nontraffic V57.3
          while boarding or alighting V57.4

Accident (*Continued*)
transport (*Continued*)
  pickup truck occupant (*Continued*)
    collision (with) (*Continued*)
      streetcar (traffic) V56.9
        nontraffic V56.3
        while boarding or alighting V56.4
      three wheeled motor vehicle (traffic)
        V52.9
        nontraffic V52.3
        while boarding or alighting V52.4
      truck (traffic) V54.9
        nontraffic V54.3
        while boarding or alighting V54.4
      two wheeled motor vehicle (traffic)
        V52.9
        nontraffic V52.3
        while boarding or alighting V52.4
      van (traffic) V53.9
        nontraffic V53.3
        while boarding or alighting V53.4
    driver
      collision (with)
        animal (traffic) V50.5
          being ridden (traffic) V56.5
            nontraffic V56.0
          nontraffic V50.0
        animal-drawn vehicle (traffic)
          V56.5
          nontraffic V56.0
        bus (traffic) V54.5
          nontraffic V54.0
        car (traffic) V53.5
          nontraffic V53.0
        motor vehicle NOS (traffic) V59.40
          nontraffic V59.00
          specified type NEC (traffic)
            V59.49
            nontraffic V59.09
        pedal cycle (traffic) V51.5
          · nontraffic V51.0
        pickup truck (traffic) V53.5
          nontraffic V53.0
        railway vehicle (traffic) V55.5
          nontraffic V55.0
        specified vehicle NEC (traffic) V56.5
          nontraffic V56.0
        stationary object (traffic) V57.5
          nontraffic V57.0
        streetcar (traffic) V56.5
          nontraffic V56.0
        three wheeled motor vehicle
          (traffic) V52.5
          nontraffic V52.0
        truck (traffic) V54.5
          nontraffic V54.0
        two wheeled motor vehicle (traffic)
          V52.5
          nontraffic V52.0
        van (traffic) V53.5
          nontraffic V53.0
      noncollision accident (traffic) V58.5
        nontraffic V58.0
    hanger-on
      collision (with)
        animal (traffic) V50.7
          being ridden (traffic) V56.7
            nontraffic V56.2
          nontraffic V50.2
        animal-drawn vehicle (traffic) V56.7
          nontraffic V56.2
        bus (traffic) V54.7
          nontraffic V54.2
        car (traffic) V53.7
          nontraffic V53.2
        pedal cycle (traffic) V51.7
          nontraffic V51.2
        pickup truck (traffic) V53.7
          nontraffic V53.2
        railway vehicle (traffic) V55.7
          nontraffic V55.2

Accident (*Continued*)
transport (*Continued*)
  pickup truck occupant (*Continued*)
    hanger-on (*Continued*)
      collision (*Continued*)
        specified vehicle NEC (traffic) V56.7
          nontraffic V56.2
        stationary object (traffic) V57.7
          nontraffic V57.2
        streetcar (traffic) V56.7
          nontraffic V56.2
        three wheeled motor vehicle
          (traffic) V52.7
          nontraffic V52.2
        truck (traffic) V54.7
          nontraffic V54.2
        two wheeled motor vehicle (traffic)
          V52.7
          nontraffic V52.2
        van (traffic) V53.7
          nontraffic V53.2
      noncollision accident (traffic) V58.7
        nontraffic V58.2
    noncollision accident (traffic) V58.9
      nontraffic V58.3
      while boarding or alighting V58.4
    nontraffic V59.3
    passenger
      collision (with)
        animal (traffic) V50.6
          being ridden (traffic) V56.6
            nontraffic V56.1
          nontraffic V50.1
        animal-drawn vehicle (traffic) V56.6
          nontraffic V56.1
        bus (traffic) V54.6
          nontraffic V54.1
        car (traffic) V53.6
          nontraffic V53.1
        motor vehicle NOS (traffic) V59.50
          nontraffic V59.10
          specified type NEC (traffic) V59.59
            nontraffic V59.19
        pedal cycle (traffic) V51.6
          nontraffic V51.1
        pickup truck (traffic) V53.6
          nontraffic V53.1
        railway vehicle (traffic) V55.6
          nontraffic V55.1
        specified vehicle NEC (traffic) V56.6
          nontraffic V56.1
        stationary object (traffic) V57.6
          nontraffic V57.1
        streetcar (traffic) V56.6
          nontraffic V56.1
        three wheeled motor vehicle
          (traffic) V52.6
          nontraffic V52.1
        truck (traffic) V54.6
          nontraffic V54.1
        two wheeled motor vehicle (traffic)
          V52.6
          nontraffic V52.1
        van (traffic) V53.6
          nontraffic V53.1
      noncollision accident (traffic) V58.6
        nontraffic V58.1
    specified type NEC V59.88
      military vehicle V59.81
    quarry truck —*see* Accident, transport,
      industrial vehicle occupant
    race car —*see* Accident, transport, motor
      vehicle NEC occupant
    railway vehicle occupant V81.9
      collision (with) V81.3
        motor vehicle (non-military) (traffic)
          V81.1
          military V81.83
          nontraffic V81.0
        rolling stock V81.2
        specified object NEC V81.3

▶ New   ⇒ Revised   ~~deleted~~ Deleted   ● Use Additional Character(s)

Accident *(Continued)*
  transport *(Continued)*
    railway vehicle occupant *(Continued)*
      during derailment V81.7
        with antecedent collision —*see*
          Accident, transport, railway
          vehicle occupant, collision
      explosion V81.81
      fall (in railway vehicle) V81.5
        during derailment V81.7
          with antecedent collision —*see*
            Accident, transport, railway
            vehicle occupant, collision
        from railway vehicle V81.6
          during derailment V81.7
            with antecedent collision —*see*
              Accident, transport,
              railway vehicle occupant,
              collision
        while boarding or alighting V81.4
      fire V81.81
      object falling onto train V81.82
      specified type NEC V81.89
      while boarding or alighting V81.4
    Segway V00.848
    ski lift V98.3
    snowmobile occupant (nontraffic) V86.92
      driver V86.52
      hanger-on V86.72
      passenger V86.62
      traffic V86.32
        driver V86.02
        hanger-on V86.22
        passenger V86.12
      while boarding or alighting V86.42
    specified NEC V98.8
    sport utility vehicle occupant —*see also*
      Accident, transport, pickup truck
      occupant
    streetcar occupant V82.9
      collision (with) V82.3
        motor vehicle (traffic) V82.1
          nontraffic V82.0
        rolling stock V82.2
      during derailment V82.7
        with antecedent collision —*see*
          Accident, transport, streetcar
          occupant, collision
      fall (in streetcar) V82.5
        during derailment V82.7
          with antecedent collision —*see*
            Accident, transport, streetcar
            occupant, collision
        from streetcar V82.6
          during derailment V82.7
            with antecedent collision —*see*
              Accident, transport, streetcar
              occupant, collision
          while boarding or alighting
          V82.4
        while boarding or alighting V82.4
      specified type NEC V82.8
      while boarding or alighting V82.4
    three-wheeled motor vehicle occupant
      V39.9
      collision (with)
        animal (traffic) V30.9
          being ridden (traffic) V36.9
            nontraffic V36.3
            while boarding or alighting V36.4
          nontraffic V30.3
          while boarding or alighting V30.4
        animal-drawn vehicle (traffic) V36.9
          nontraffic V36.3
          while boarding or alighting V36.4
        bus (traffic) V34.9
          nontraffic V34.3
          while boarding or alighting V34.4
        car (traffic) V33.9
          nontraffic V33.3
          while boarding or alighting V33.4

Accident *(Continued)*
  transport *(Continued)*
    three-wheeled motor vehicle occupant
      (Continued)
      collision *(Continued)*
        motor vehicle NOS (traffic) V39.60
          nontraffic V39.20
          specified type NEC (traffic)
            V39.69
            nontraffic V39.29
        pedal cycle (traffic) V31.9
          nontraffic V31.3
          while boarding or alighting
            V31.4
        pickup truck (traffic) V33.9
          nontraffic V33.3
          while boarding or alighting
            V33.4
        railway vehicle (traffic) V35.9
          nontraffic V35.3
          while boarding or alighting
            V35.4
        specified vehicle NEC (traffic) V36.9
          nontraffic V36.3
          while boarding or alighting V36.4
        stationary object (traffic) V37.9
          nontraffic V37.3
          while boarding or alighting V37.4
        streetcar (traffic) V36.9
          nontraffic V36.3
          while boarding or alighting V36.4
        three wheeled motor vehicle (traffic)
          V32.9
          nontraffic V32.3
          while boarding or alighting V32.4
        truck (traffic) V34.9
          nontraffic V34.3
          while boarding or alighting V34.4
        two wheeled motor vehicle (traffic)
          V32.9
          nontraffic V32.3
          while boarding or alighting V32.4
        van (traffic) V33.9
          nontraffic V33.3
          while boarding or alighting V33.4
      driver
        collision (with)
          animal (traffic) V30.5
            being ridden (traffic) V36.5
              nontraffic V36.0
            nontraffic V30.0
          animal-drawn vehicle (traffic) V36.5
            nontraffic V36.0
          bus (traffic) V34.5
            nontraffic V34.0
          car (traffic) V33.5
            nontraffic V33.0
          motor vehicle NOS (traffic)
            V39.40
            nontraffic V39.00
            specified type NEC (traffic)
              V39.49
              nontraffic V39.09
          pedal cycle (traffic) V31.5
            nontraffic V31.0
          pickup truck (traffic) V33.5
            nontraffic V33.0
          railway vehicle (traffic) V35.5
            nontraffic V35.0
          specified vehicle NEC (traffic)
            V36.5
            nontraffic V36.0
          stationary object (traffic) V37.5
            nontraffic V37.0
          streetcar (traffic) V36.5
            nontraffic V36.0
          three wheeled motor vehicle
            (traffic) V32.5
            nontraffic V32.0
          truck (traffic) V34.5
            nontraffic V34.0

Accident *(Continued)*
  transport *(Continued)*
    three-wheeled motor vehicle occupant
      (Continued)
      driver *(Continued)*
        collision *(Continued)*
          two wheeled motor vehicle (traffic)
            V32.5
            nontraffic V32.0
          van (traffic) V33.5
            nontraffic V33.0
        noncollision accident (traffic) V38.5
          nontraffic V38.0
      hanger-on
        collision (with)
          animal (traffic) V30.7
            being ridden (traffic) V36.7
              nontraffic V36.2
            nontraffic V30.2
          animal-drawn vehicle (traffic) V36.7
            nontraffic V36.2
          bus (traffic) V34.7
            nontraffic V34.2
          car (traffic) V33.7
            nontraffic V33.2
          pedal cycle (traffic) V31.7
            nontraffic V31.2
          pickup truck (traffic) V33.7
            nontraffic V33.2
          railway vehicle (traffic) V35.7
            nontraffic V35.2
          specified vehicle NEC (traffic) V36.7
            nontraffic V36.2
          stationary object (traffic) V37.7
            nontraffic V37.2
          streetcar (traffic) V36.7
            nontraffic V36.2
          three wheeled motor vehicle
            (traffic) V32.7
            nontraffic V32.2
          truck (traffic) V34.7
            nontraffic V34.2
          two wheeled motor vehicle (traffic)
            V32.7
            nontraffic V32.2
          van (traffic) V33.7
            nontraffic V33.2
        noncollision accident (traffic) V38.7
          nontraffic V38.2
      noncollision accident (traffic) V38.9
        nontraffic V38.3
      while boarding or alighting V38.4
      nontraffic V39.3
      passenger
        collision (with)
          animal (traffic) V30.6
            being ridden (traffic) V36.6
              nontraffic V36.1
            nontraffic V30.1
          animal-drawn vehicle (traffic) V36.6
            nontraffic V36.1
          bus (traffic) V34.6
            nontraffic V34.1
          car (traffic) V33.6
            nontraffic V33.1
          motor vehicle NOS (traffic) V39.50
            nontraffic V39.10
            specified type NEC (traffic)
              V39.59
              nontraffic V39.19
          pedal cycle (traffic) V31.6
            nontraffic V31.1
          pickup truck (traffic) V33.6
            nontraffic V33.1
          railway vehicle (traffic) V35.6
            nontraffic V35.1
          specified vehicle NEC (traffic)
            V36.6
            nontraffic V36.1
          stationary object (traffic) V37.6
            nontraffic V37.1

Accident *(Continued)*
  transport *(Continued)*
    three-wheeled motor vehicle occupant
        (Continued)
      passenger *(Continued)*
        collision *(Continued)*
          streetcar (traffic) V36.6
            nontraffic V36.1
          three wheeled motor vehicle
              (traffic) V32.6
            nontraffic V32.1
          truck (traffic) V34.6
            nontraffic V34.1
          two wheeled motor vehicle (traffic)
              V32.6
            nontraffic V32.1
          van (traffic) V33.6
            nontraffic V33.1
          noncollision accident (traffic)
              V38.6
            nontraffic V38.1
        specified type NEC V39.89
        military vehicle V39.81
    tractor (farm) (and trailer) —*see* Accident,
        transport, agricultural vehicle
        occupant
    tram —*see* Accident, transport, streetcar
    in mine or quarry —*see* Accident,
        transport, industrial vehicle
        occupant
    trolley —*see* Accident, transport, streetcar
    in mine or quarry —*see* Accident,
        transport, industrial vehicle
        occupant
    truck (heavy) occupant V69.9
      collision (with)
        animal (traffic) V60.9
          being ridden (traffic) V66.9
            nontraffic V66.3
            while boarding or alighting
                V66.4
          nontraffic V60.3
          while boarding or alighting V60.4
        animal-drawn vehicle (traffic) V66.9
          nontraffic V66.3
          while boarding or alighting V66.4
        bus (traffic) V64.9
          nontraffic V64.3
          while boarding or alighting V64.4
        car (traffic) V63.9
          nontraffic V63.3
          while boarding or alighting V63.4
        motor vehicle NOS (traffic) V69.60
          nontraffic V69.20
          specified type NEC (traffic) V69.69
            nontraffic V69.29
        pedal cycle (traffic) V61.9
          nontraffic V61.3
          while boarding or alighting V61.4
        pickup truck (traffic) V63.9
          nontraffic V63.3
          while boarding or alighting V63.4
        railway vehicle (traffic) V65.9
          nontraffic V65.3
          while boarding or alighting V65.4
        specified vehicle NEC (traffic) V66.9
          nontraffic V66.3
          while boarding or alighting V66.4
        stationary object (traffic) V67.9
          nontraffic V67.3
          while boarding or alighting V67.4
        streetcar (traffic) V66.9
          nontraffic V66.3
          while boarding or alighting V66.4
        three wheeled motor vehicle (traffic)
            V62.9
          nontraffic V62.3
          while boarding or alighting V62.4
        truck (traffic) V64.9
          nontraffic V64.3
          while boarding or alighting V64.4

Accident *(Continued)*
  transport *(Continued)*
    truck occupant *(Continued)*
      collision *(Continued)*
        two wheeled motor vehicle (traffic)
            V62.9
          nontraffic V62.3
          while boarding or alighting V62.4
        van (traffic) V63.9
          nontraffic V63.3
          while boarding or alighting V63.4
      driver
        collision (with)
          animal (traffic) V60.5
            being ridden (traffic) V66.5
              nontraffic V66.0
            nontraffic V60.0
          animal-drawn vehicle (traffic) V66.5
            nontraffic V66.0
          bus (traffic) V64.5
            nontraffic V64.0
          car (traffic) V63.5
            nontraffic V63.0
          motor vehicle NOS (traffic) V69.40
            nontraffic V69.00
            specified type NEC (traffic)
                V69.49
              nontraffic V69.09
          pedal cycle (traffic) V61.5
            nontraffic V61.0
          pickup truck (traffic) V63.5
            nontraffic V63.0
          railway vehicle (traffic) V65.5
            nontraffic V65.0
          specified vehicle NEC (traffic) V66.5
            nontraffic V66.0
          stationary object (traffic) V67.5
            nontraffic V67.0
          streetcar (traffic) V66.5
            nontraffic V66.0
          three wheeled motor vehicle
              (traffic) V62.5
            nontraffic V62.0
          truck (traffic) V64.5
            nontraffic V64.0
          two wheeled motor vehicle (traffic)
              V62.5
            nontraffic V62.0
          van (traffic) V63.5
            nontraffic V63.0
        noncollision accident (traffic) V68.5
          nontraffic V68.0
      dump —*see* Accident, transport,
          construction vehicle occupant
      hanger-on
        collision (with)
          animal (traffic) V60.7
            being ridden (traffic) V66.7
              nontraffic V66.2
            nontraffic V60.2
          animal-drawn vehicle (traffic) V66.7
            nontraffic V66.2
          bus (traffic) V64.7
            nontraffic V64.2
          car (traffic) V63.7
            nontraffic V63.2
          pedal cycle (traffic) V61.7
            nontraffic V61.2
          pickup truck (traffic) V63.7
            nontraffic V63.2
          railway vehicle (traffic) V65.7
            nontraffic V65.2
          specified vehicle NEC (traffic) V66.7
            nontraffic V66.2
          stationary object (traffic) V67.7
            nontraffic V67.2
          streetcar (traffic) V66.7
            nontraffic V66.2
          three wheeled motor vehicle
              (traffic) V62.7
            nontraffic V62.2

Accident *(Continued)*
  transport *(Continued)*
    truck occupant *(Continued)*
      hanger-on *(Continued)*
        collision *(Continued)*
          truck (traffic) V64.7
            nontraffic V64.2
          two wheeled motor vehicle (traffic)
              V62.7
            nontraffic V62.2
          van (traffic) V63.7
            nontraffic V63.2
          noncollision accident (traffic) V68.7
            nontraffic V68.2
        noncollision accident (traffic) V68.9
          nontraffic V68.3
          while boarding or alighting V68.4
      nontraffic V69.3
      passenger
        collision (with)
          animal (traffic) V60.6
            being ridden (traffic) V66.6
              nontraffic V66.1
            nontraffic V60.1
          animal-drawn vehicle (traffic) V66.6
            nontraffic V66.1
          bus (traffic) V64.6
            nontraffic V64.1
          car (traffic) V63.6
            nontraffic V63.1
          motor vehicle NOS (traffic) V69.50
            nontraffic V69.10
            specified type NEC (traffic)
                V69.59
              nontraffic V69.19
          pedal cycle (traffic) V61.6
            nontraffic V61.1
          pickup truck (traffic) V63.6
            nontraffic V63.1
          railway vehicle (traffic) V65.6
            nontraffic V65.1
          specified vehicle NEC (traffic) V66.6
            nontraffic V66.1
          stationary object (traffic) V67.6
            nontraffic V67.1
          streetcar (traffic) V66.6
            nontraffic V66.1
          three wheeled motor vehicle
              (traffic) V62.6
            nontraffic V62.1
          truck (traffic) V64.6
            nontraffic V64.1
          two wheeled motor vehicle (traffic)
              V62.6
            nontraffic V62.1
          van (traffic) V63.6
            nontraffic V63.1
        noncollision accident (traffic) V68.6
          nontraffic V68.1
      pickup —*see* Accident, transport, pickup
          truck occupant
      specified type NEC V69.88
      military vehicle V69.81
    van occupant V59.9
      collision (with)
        animal (traffic) V50.9
          being ridden (traffic) V56.9
            nontraffic V56.3
            while boarding or alighting
                V56.4
          nontraffic V50.3
          while boarding or alighting V50.4
        animal-drawn vehicle (traffic) V56.9
          nontraffic V56.3
          while boarding or alighting V56.4
        bus (traffic) V54.9
          nontraffic V54.3
          while boarding or alighting V54.4
        car (traffic) V53.9
          nontraffic V53.3
          while boarding or alighting V53.4

▶ New   ⇒ Revised   ~~deleted~~ Deleted   ● Use Additional Character(s)

Accident *(Continued)*
  transport *(Continued)*
    van occupant *(Continued)*
      collision *(Continued)*
        motor vehicle NOS (traffic) V59.60
          nontraffic V59.20
          specified type NEC (traffic) V59.69
            nontraffic V59.29
        pedal cycle (traffic) V51.9
          nontraffic V51.3
          while boarding or alighting V51.4
        pickup truck (traffic) V53.9
          nontraffic V53.3
          while boarding or alighting V53.4
        railway vehicle (traffic) V55.9
          nontraffic V55.3
          while boarding or alighting V55.4
        specified vehicle NEC (traffic) V56.9
          nontraffic V56.3
          while boarding or alighting V56.4
        stationary object (traffic) V57.9
          nontraffic V57.3
          while boarding or alighting V57.4
        streetcar (traffic) V56.9
          nontraffic V56.3
          while boarding or alighting V56.4
        three wheeled motor vehicle (traffic) V52.9
          nontraffic V52.3
          while boarding or alighting V52.4
        truck (traffic) V54.9
          nontraffic V54.3
          while boarding or alighting V54.4
        two wheeled motor vehicle (traffic) V52.9
          nontraffic V52.3
          while boarding or alighting V52.4
        van (traffic) V53.9
          nontraffic V53.3
          while boarding or alighting V53.4
      driver
        collision (with)
          animal (traffic) V50.5
            being ridden (traffic) V56.5
              nontraffic V56.0
            nontraffic V50.0
          animal-drawn vehicle (traffic) V56.5
            nontraffic V56.0
          bus (traffic) V54.5
            nontraffic V54.0
          car (traffic) V53.5
            nontraffic V53.0
          motor vehicle NOS (traffic) V59.40
            nontraffic V59.00
            specified type NEC (traffic) V59.49
              nontraffic V59.09
          pedal cycle (traffic) V51.5
            nontraffic V51.0
          pickup truck (traffic) V53.5
            nontraffic V53.0
          railway vehicle (traffic) V55.5
            nontraffic V55.0
          specified vehicle NEC (traffic) V56.5
            nontraffic V56.0
          stationary object (traffic) V57.5
            nontraffic V57.0
          streetcar (traffic) V56.5
            nontraffic V56.0
          three wheeled motor vehicle (traffic) V52.5
            nontraffic V52.0
          truck (traffic) V54.5
            nontraffic V54.0
          two wheeled motor vehicle (traffic) V52.5
            nontraffic V52.0
          van (traffic) V53.5
            nontraffic V53.0
        noncollision accident (traffic) V58.5
          nontraffic V58.0

Accident *(Continued)*
  transport *(Continued)*
    van occupant *(Continued)*
      hanger-on
        collision (with)
          animal (traffic) V50.7
            being ridden (traffic) V56.7
              nontraffic V56.2
            nontraffic V50.2
          animal-drawn vehicle (traffic) V56.7
            nontraffic V56.2
          bus (traffic) V54.7
            nontraffic V54.2
          car (traffic) V53.7
            nontraffic V53.2
          pedal cycle (traffic) V51.7
            nontraffic V51.2
          pickup truck (traffic) V53.7
            nontraffic V53.2
          railway vehicle (traffic) V55.7
            nontraffic V55.2
          specified vehicle NEC (traffic) V56.7
            nontraffic V56.2
          stationary object (traffic) V57.7
            nontraffic V57.2
          streetcar (traffic) V56.7
            nontraffic V56.2
          three wheeled motor vehicle (traffic) V52.7
            nontraffic V52.2
          truck (traffic) V54.7
            nontraffic V54.2
          two wheeled motor vehicle (traffic) V52.7
            nontraffic V52.2
          van (traffic) V53.7
            nontraffic V53.2
        noncollision accident (traffic) V58.7
          nontraffic V58.2
      noncollision accident (traffic) V58.9
        nontraffic V58.3
        while boarding or alighting V58.4
      nontraffic V59.3
      passenger
        collision (with)
          animal (traffic) V50.6
            being ridden (traffic) V56.6
              nontraffic V56.1
            nontraffic V50.1
          animal-drawn vehicle (traffic) V56.6
            nontraffic V56.1
          bus (traffic) V54.6
            nontraffic V54.1
          car (traffic) V53.6
            nontraffic V53.1
          motor vehicle NOS (traffic) V59.50
            nontraffic V59.10
            specified type NEC (traffic) V59.59
              nontraffic V59.19
          pedal cycle (traffic) V51.6
            nontraffic V51.1
          pickup truck (traffic) V53.6
            nontraffic V53.1
          railway vehicle (traffic) V55.6
            nontraffic V55.1
          specified vehicle NEC (traffic) V56.6
            nontraffic V56.1
          stationary object (traffic) V57.6
            nontraffic V57.1
          streetcar (traffic) V56.6
            nontraffic V56.1
          three wheeled motor vehicle (traffic) V52.6
            nontraffic V52.1
          truck (traffic) V54.6
            nontraffic V54.1
          two wheeled motor vehicle (traffic) V52.6
          van (traffic) V53.6
            nontraffic V53.1

Accident *(Continued)*
  transport *(Continued)*
    van occupant *(Continued)*
      passenger *(Continued)*
        noncollision accident (traffic) V58.6
          nontraffic V58.1
      specified type NEC V59.88
        military vehicle V59.81
    watercraft occupant —*see* Accident, watercraft
    vehicle NEC V89.9
      animal-drawn NEC —*see* Accident, transport, animal-drawn vehicle occupant
      special
        agricultural —*see* Accident, transport, agricultural vehicle occupant
        construction —*see* Accident, transport, construction vehicle occupant
        industrial —*see* Accident, transport, industrial vehicle occupant
      three-wheeled NEC (motorized) —*see* Accident, transport, three-wheeled motor vehicle occupant
  watercraft V94.9
    causing
      drowning —*see* Drowning, due to, accident to, watercraft
      injury NEC V91.89
        crushed between craft and object V91.19
          powered craft V91.13
            ferry boat V91.11
            fishing boat V91.12
            jet ski V91.13
            liner V91.11
            merchant ship V91.10
            passenger ship V91.11
          unpowered craft V91.18
            canoe V91.15
            inflatable V91.16
            kayak V91.15
            sailboat V91.14
            surf-board V91.18
            windsurfer V91.18
        fall on board V91.29
          powered craft V91.23
            ferry boat V91.21
            fishing boat V91.22
            jet ski V91.23
            liner V91.21
            merchant ship V91.20
            passenger ship V91.21
          unpowered craft
            canoe V91.25
            inflatable V91.26
            kayak V91.25
            sailboat V91.24
        fire on board causing burn V91.09
          powered craft V91.03
            ferry boat V91.01
            fishing boat V91.02
            jet ski V91.03
            liner V91.01
            merchant ship V91.00
            passenger ship V91.01
          unpowered craft V91.08
            canoe V91.05
            inflatable V91.06
            kayak V91.05
            sailboat V91.04
            surf-board V91.08
            water skis V91.07
            windsurfer V91.08
        hit by falling object V91.39
          powered craft V91.33
            ferry boat V91.31
            fishing boat V91.32
            jet skis V91.33
            liner V91.31
            merchant ship V91.30
            passenger ship V91.31

Accident *(Continued)*
  watercraft *(Continued)*
    causing *(Continued)*
      injury NEC *(Continued)*
        hit by falling object *(Continued)*
          unpowered craft V91.38
            canoe V91.35
            inflatable V91.36
            kayak V91.35
            sailboat V91.34
            surf-board V91.38
            water skis V91.37
            windsurfer V91.38
        specified type NEC V91.89
          powered craft V91.83
            ferry boat V91.81
            fishing boat V91.82
            jet ski V91.83
            liner V91.81
            merchant ship V91.80
            passenger ship V91.81
          unpowered craft V91.88
            canoe V91.85
            inflatable V91.86
            kayak V91.85
            sailboat V91.84
            surf-board V91.88
            water skis V91.87
            windsurfer V91.88
      due to, caused by cataclysm —*see* Forces of nature, by type
      military NEC V94.818
        with civilian watercraft V94.810
          civilian in water injured by V94.811
      nonpowered, struck by
        nonpowered vessel V94.22
        powered vessel V94.21
      specified type NEC V94.89
      striking swimmer
        powered V94.11
        unpowered V94.12
Acid throwing (assault) Y08.89
Activity (involving) (of victim at time of event) Y93.9
  aerobic and step exercise (class) Y93.A3
  alpine skiing Y93.23
  animal care NEC Y93.K9
  arts and handcrafts NEC Y93.D9
  athletics NEC Y93.79
  athletics played as a team or group NEC Y93.69
  athletics played individually NEC Y93.59
  baking Y93.G3
  ballet Y93.41
  barbells Y93.B3
  BASE (Building, Antenna, Span, Earth) jumping Y93.33
  baseball Y93.64
  basketball Y93.67
  bathing (personal) Y93.E1
  beach volleyball Y93.68
  bike riding Y93.55
  blackout game Y93.85
  boogie boarding Y93.18
  bowling Y93.54
  boxing Y93.71
  brass instrument playing Y93.J4
  building construction Y93.H3
  bungee jumping Y93.34
  calisthenics Y93.A2
  canoeing (in calm and turbulent water) Y93.16
  capture the flag Y93.6A
  cardiorespiratory exercise NEC Y93.A9
  caregiving (providing) NEC Y93.F9
    bathing Y93.F1
    lifting Y93.F2
  cellular
    communication device Y93.C2
    telephone Y93.C2
  challenge course Y93.A5
  cheerleading Y93.45

Activity *(Continued)*
  choking game Y93.85
  circuit training Y93.A4
  cleaning
    floor Y93.E5
  climbing NEC Y93.39
    mountain Y93.31
    rock Y93.31
    wall Y93.31
  clothing care and maintenance NEC Y93.E9
  combatives Y93.75
  computer
    keyboarding Y93.C1
    technology NEC Y93.C9
  confidence course Y93.A5
  construction (building) Y93.H3
  cooking and baking Y93.G3
  cool down exercises Y93.A2
  cricket Y93.69
  crocheting Y93.D1
  cross country skiing Y93.24
  dancing (all types) Y93.41
  digging
    dirt Y93.H1
  dirt digging Y93.H1
  dishwashing Y93.G1
  diving (platform) (springboard) Y93.12
    underwater Y93.15
  dodge ball Y93.6A
  downhill skiing Y93.23
  drum playing Y93.J2
  dumbbells Y93.B3
  electronic
    devices NEC Y93.C9
      hand held interactive Y93.C2
    game playing (using) (with)
      interactive device Y93.C2
      keyboard or other stationary device Y93.C1
  elliptical machine Y93.A1
  exercise(s)
    machines ((primarily) for)
      cardiorespiratory conditioning Y93.A1
      muscle strengthening Y93.B1
    muscle strengthening (non-machine) NEC Y93.B9
  external motion NEC Y93.I9
    rollercoaster Y93.I1
  fainting game Y93.85
  field hockey Y93.65
  figure skating (pairs) (singles) Y93.21
  flag football Y93.62
  floor mopping and cleaning Y93.E5
  food preparation and clean up Y93.G1
  football (American) NOS Y93.61
    flag Y93.62
    tackle Y93.61
    touch Y93.62
  four square Y93.6A
  free weights Y93.B3
  frisbee (ultimate) Y93.74
  furniture
    building Y93.D3
    finishing Y93.D3
    repair Y93.D3
  game playing (electronic)
    using interactive device Y93.C2
    using keyboard or other stationary device Y93.C1
  gardening Y93.H2
  golf Y93.53
  grass drills Y93.A6
  grilling and smoking food Y93.G2
  grooming and shearing an animal Y93.K3
  guerilla drills Y93.A6
  gymnastics (rhythmic) Y93.43
  hand held interactive electronic device Y93.C2
  handball Y93.73
  handcrafts NEC Y93.D9
  hang gliding Y93.35
  hiking (on level or elevated terrain) Y93.01

Activity *(Continued)*
  hockey (ice) Y93.22
    field Y93.65
  horseback riding Y93.52
  household (interior) maintenance NEC Y93.E9
  ice NEC Y93.29
    dancing Y93.21
    hockey Y93.22
    skating Y93.21
  inline roller skating Y93.51
  ironing Y93.E4
  judo Y93.75
  jumping (off) NEC Y93.39
    BASE (Building, Antenna, Span, Earth) Y93.33
    bungee Y93.34
    jacks Y93.A2
    rope Y93.56
  jumping jacks Y93.A2
  jumping rope Y93.56
  karate Y93.75
  kayaking (in calm and turbulent water) Y93.16
  keyboarding (computer) Y93.C1
  kickball Y93.6A
  knitting Y93.D1
  lacrosse Y93.65
  land maintenance NEC Y93.H9
  landscaping Y93.H2
  laundry Y93.E2
  machines (exercise)
    primarily for cardiorespiratory conditioning Y93.A1
    primarily for muscle strengthening Y93.B1
  maintenance
    exterior building NEC Y93.H9
    household (interior) NEC Y93.E9
    land Y93.H9
    property Y93.H9
  marching (on level or elevated terrain) Y93.01
  martial arts Y93.75
  microwave oven Y93.G3
  milking an animal Y93.K2
  mopping (floor) Y93.E5
  mountain climbing Y93.31
  muscle strengthening
    exercises (non-machine) NEC Y93.B9
    machines Y93.B1
  musical keyboard (electronic) playing Y93.J1
  nordic skiing Y93.24
  obstacle course Y93.A5
  oven (microwave) Y93.G3
  packing up and unpacking in moving to a new residence Y93.E6
  parasailing Y93.19
  pass out game Y93.85
  percussion instrument playing NEC Y93.J2
  personal
    bathing and showering Y93.E1
    hygiene NEC Y93.E8
    showering Y93.E1
  physical games generally associated with school recess, summer camp and children Y93.6A
  physical training NEC Y93.A9
  piano playing Y93.J1
  pilates Y93.B4
  platform diving Y93.12
  playing musical instrument
    brass instrument Y93.J4
    drum Y93.J2
    musical keyboard (electronic) Y93.J1
    percussion instrument NEC Y93.J2
    piano Y93.J1
    string instrument Y93.J3
    winds instrument Y93.J4
  property maintenance
    exterior NEC Y93.H9
    interior NEC Y93.E9
  pruning (garden and lawn) Y93.H2

▶ New ⇒ Revised ~~deleted~~ Deleted ● Use Additional Character(s)

Activity *(Continued)*
- pull-ups Y93.B2
- push-ups Y93.B2
- racquetball Y93.73
- rafting (in calm and turbulent water) Y93.16
- raking (leaves) Y93.H1
- rappelling Y93.32
- refereeing a sports activity Y93.81
- residential relocation Y93.E6
- rhythmic gymnastics Y93.43
- rhythmic movement NEC Y93.49
- riding
    - horseback Y93.52
    - rollercoaster Y93.I1
- rock climbing Y93.31
- roller skating (inline) Y93.51
- rollercoaster riding Y93.I1
- rough housing and horseplay Y93.83
- rowing (in calm and turbulent water) Y93.16
- rugby Y93.63
- SCUBA diving Y93.15
- sewing Y93.D2
- shoveling Y93.H1
    - dirt Y93.H1
    - snow Y93.H1
- showering (personal) Y93.E1
- sit-ups Y93.B2
- skateboarding Y93.51
- skating (ice) Y93.21
    - roller Y93.51
- skiing (alpine) (downhill) Y93.23
    - cross country Y93.24
    - nordic Y93.24
    - water Y93.17
- sledding (snow) Y93.23
- sleeping (sleep) Y93.84
- smoking and grilling food Y93.G2
- snorkeling Y93.15
- snow NEC Y93.29
    - boarding Y93.23
    - shoveling Y93.H1
    - sledding Y93.23
    - tubing Y93.23
- soccer Y93.66
- softball Y93.64
- specified NEC Y93.89
- spectator at an event Y93.82
- sports NEC Y93.79
    - sports played as a team or group NEC Y93.69
    - sports played individually NEC Y93.59
- springboard diving Y93.12
- squash Y93.73
- stationary bike Y93.A1
- step (stepping) exercise (class) Y93.A3
- stepper machine Y93.A1
- stove Y93.G3
- string instrument playing Y93.J3
- surfing Y93.18
    - wind Y93.18
- swimming Y93.11
- tackle football Y93.61
- tap dancing Y93.41
- tennis Y93.73
- tobogganing Y93.23
- touch football Y93.62
- track and field events (non-running) Y93.57
    - running Y93.02
- trampoline Y93.44
- treadmill Y93.A1
- trimming shrubs Y93.H2
- tubing (in calm and turbulent water) Y93.16
    - snow Y93.23
- ultimate frisbee Y93.74
- underwater diving Y93.15
- unpacking in moving to a new residence Y93.E6
- use of stove, oven and microwave oven Y93.G3

Activity *(Continued)*
- vacuuming Y93.E3
- volleyball (beach) (court) Y93.68
- wake boarding Y93.17
- walking (on level or elevated terrain) Y93.01
    - an animal Y93.K1
- walking an animal Y93.K1
- wall climbing Y93.31
- warm up and cool down exercises Y93.A2
- water NEC Y93.19
    - aerobics Y93.14
    - craft NEC Y93.19
    - exercise Y93.14
    - polo Y93.13
    - skiing Y93.17
    - sliding Y93.18
    - survival training and testing Y93.19
- weeding (garden and lawn) Y93.H2
- wind instrument playing Y93.J4
- windsurfing Y93.18
- wrestling Y93.72
- yoga Y93.42

Adverse effect of drugs —*see* Table of Drugs and Chemicals

Aerosinusitis —*see* Air, pressure

After-effect, late —*see* Sequelae

Air
- blast in war operations —*see* War operations, air blast
- pressure
    - change, rapid
        - during
            - ascent W94.29
                - while (in) (surfacing from)
                    - aircraft W94.23
                    - deep water diving W94.21
                    - underground W94.22
            - descent W94.39
                - in
                    - aircraft W94.31
                    - water W94.32
        - high, prolonged W94.0
        - low, prolonged W94.12
            - due to residence or long visit at high altitude W94.11

Alpine sickness W94.11

Altitude sickness W94.11

Anaphylactic shock, anaphylaxis —*see* Table of Drugs and Chemicals

Andes disease W94.11

Arachnidism, arachnoidism X58

Arson (with intent to injure or kill) X97

Asphyxia, asphyxiation
- by
    - food (bone) (seed) —*see* categories T17 and T18
    - gas —*see also* Table of Drugs and Chemicals
        - legal
            - execution —*see* Legal, intervention, gas
            - intervention —*see* Legal, intervention, gas
- from
    - fire —*see also* Exposure, fire
        - in war operations —*see* War operations, fire
    - ignition —*see* Ignition
    - vomitus T17.81
- in war operations —*see* War operations, restriction of airway

Aspiration
- food (any type) (into respiratory tract) (with asphyxia, obstruction respiratory tract, suffocation) —*see* categories T17 and T18
- foreign body —*see* Foreign body, aspiration
- vomitus (with asphyxia, obstruction respiratory tract, suffocation) T17.81

Assassination (attempt) —*see* Assault

Assault (homicidal) (by) (in) Y09
- arson X97
- bite (of human being) Y04.1
- bodily force Y04.8
    - bite Y04.1
    - bumping into Y04.2
    - sexual —*see* subcategories T74.0, T76.0
    - unarmed fight Y04.0
- bomb X96.9
    - antipersonnel X96.0
    - fertilizer X96.3
    - gasoline X96.1
    - letter X96.2
    - petrol X96.1
    - pipe X96.3
    - specified NEC X96.8
- brawl (hand) (fists) (foot) (unarmed) Y04.0
- burning, burns (by fire) NEC X97
    - acid Y08.89
    - caustic, corrosive substance Y08.89
    - chemical from swallowing caustic, corrosive substance —*see* Table of Drugs and Chemicals
    - cigarette(s) X97
    - hot object X98.9
        - fluid NEC X98.2
        - household appliance X98.3
        - specified NEC X98.8
        - steam X98.0
        - tap water X98.1
        - vapors X98.0
    - scalding —*see* Assault, burning
    - steam X98.0
    - vitriol Y08.89
- caustic, corrosive substance (gas) Y08.89
- crashing of
    - aircraft Y08.81
    - motor vehicle Y03.8
        - pushed in front of Y02.0
        - run over Y03.0
        - specified NEC Y03.8
- cutting or piercing instrument X99.9
    - dagger X99.2
    - glass X99.0
    - knife X99.1
    - specified NEC X99.8
    - sword X99.2
- dagger X99.2
- drowning (in) X92.9
    - bathtub Y92.0
    - natural water X92.3
    - specified NEC X92.8
    - swimming pool X92.1
        - following fall X92.2
- dynamite X96.8
- explosive(s) (material) X96.9
- fight (hand) (fists) (foot) (unarmed) Y04.0
    - with weapon —*see* Assault, by type of weapon
- fire X97
- firearm X95.9
    - airgun X95.01
    - handgun X93
    - hunting rifle X94.1
    - larger X94.9
        - specified NEC X94.8
    - machine gun X94.2
    - shotgun X94.0
    - specified NEC X95.8
- from high place Y01
- gunshot (wound) NEC —*see* Assault, firearm, by type
- incendiary device X97
- injury Y09
    - to child due to criminal abortion attempt NEC Y08.89
- knife X99.1

Assault *(Continued)*
    late effect of —*see* X92-Y08 with 7th
        character S
    placing before moving object NEC Y02.8
        motor vehicle Y02.0
    poisoning —*see* categories T36-T65 with 7th
        character S
    puncture, any part of body —*see* Assault,
        cutting or piercing instrument
    pushing
        before moving object NEC Y02.8
            motor vehicle Y02.0
            subway train Y02.1
            train Y02.1
    rape T74.2-●
    scalding —*see* Assault, burning
    sequelae of —*see* X92-Y08 with 7th character S
    sexual (by bodily force) T74.2-●
    shooting —*see* Assault, firearm
    specified means NEC Y08.89

Assault *(Continued)*
    stab, any part of body —*see* Assault, cutting
        or piercing instrument
    steam X98.0
    striking against
        other person Y04.2
        sports equipment Y08.09
            baseball bat Y08.02
            hockey stick Y08.01
    struck by
        sports equipment Y08.09
            baseball bat Y08.02
            hockey stick Y08.01
    submersion —*see* Assault, drowning
    violence Y09
    weapon Y09
        blunt Y00
        cutting or piercing —*see* Assault, cutting or
            piercing instrument
        firearm —*see* Assault, firearm

Assault *(Continued)*
    wound Y09
        cutting —*see* Assault, cutting or piercing
            instrument
        gunshot —*see* Assault, firearm
        knife X99.1
        piercing —*see* Assault, cutting or piercing
            instrument
        puncture —*see* Assault, cutting or piercing
            instrument
        stab —*see* Assault, cutting or piercing
            instrument
Attack by mammals NEC W55.89
Avalanche —*see* Landslide
Aviator's disease —*see* Air, pressure

▶ New   ⇒ Revised   ~~deleted~~ Deleted   ● Use Additional Character(s)

B

Barotitis, barodontalgia, barosinusitis, barotrauma (otitic) (sinus) —see Air, pressure
Battered (baby) (child) (person) (syndrome) X58
Bayonet wound W26.1
  in
    legal intervention —see Legal, intervention, sharp object, bayonet
    war operations —see War operations, combat
  stated as undetermined whether accidental or intentional Y28.8
  suicide (attempt) X78.2
Bean in nose —see categories T17 and T18
Bed set on fire NEC —see Exposure, fire, uncontrolled, building, bed
Beheading (by guillotine)
  homicide X99.9
  legal execution —see Legal, intervention
Bending, injury in (prolonged) (static) X50.1
Bends —see Air, pressure, change
Bite, bitten by
  alligator W58.01
  arthropod (nonvenomous) NEC W57
  bull W55.21
  cat W55.01
  cow W55.21
  crocodile W58.11
  dog W54.0
  goat W55.31
  hoof stock NEC W55.31
  horse W55.11
  human being (accidentally) W50.3
    with intent to injure or kill Y04.1
    as, or caused by, a crowd or human stampede (with fall) W52
    assault Y04.1
    homicide (attempt) Y04.1
    in
      fight Y04.1
  insect (nonvenomous) W57
  lizard (nonvenomous) W59.01
  mammal NEC W55.81
    marine W56.31
  marine animal (nonvenomous) W56.81
  millipede W57
  moray eel W56.51
  mouse W53.01
  person(s) (accidentally) W50.3
    with intent to injure or kill Y04.1
    as, or caused by, a crowd or human stampede (with fall) W52
    assault Y04.1
    homicide (attempt) Y04.1
    in
      fight Y04.1
  pig W55.41
  raccoon W55.51
  rat W53.11
  reptile W59.81
    lizard W59.01
    snake W59.11
    turtle W59.21
    terrestrial W59.81
  rodent W53.81
    mouse W53.01
    rat W53.11
    specified NEC W53.81
    squirrel W53.21
  shark W56.41
  sheep W55.31
  snake (nonvenomous) W59.11
  spider (nonvenomous) W57
  squirrel W53.21
Blast (air) in war operations —see War operations, blast
Blizzard X37.2

Blood alcohol level Y90.9
  20-39mg/100ml Y90.1
  40-59mg/100ml Y90.2
  60-79mg/100ml Y90.3
  80-99mg/100ml Y90.4
  100-119mg/100ml Y90.5
  120-199mg/100ml Y90.6
  200-239mg/100ml Y90.7
  less than 20mg/100ml Y90.0
  presence in blood, level not specified Y90.9
Blow X58
  by law-enforcing agent, police (on duty) —see Legal, intervention, manhandling
    blunt object —see Legal, intervention, blunt object
Blowing up —see Explosion
Brawl (hand) (fists) (foot) Y04.0
Breakage (accidental) (part of)
  ladder (causing fall) W11
  scaffolding (causing fall) W12
Broken
  glass, contact with —see Contact, with, glass
  power line (causing electric shock) W85
Bumping against, into (accidentally)
  object NEC W22.8
    with fall —see Fall, due to, bumping against, object
    caused by crowd or human stampede (with fall) W52
    sports equipment W21.9
  person(s) W51
    with fall W03
      due to ice or snow W00.0
    assault Y04.2
    caused by, a crowd or human stampede (with fall) W52
    homicide (attempt) Y04.2
  sports equipment W21.9
Burn, burned, burning (accidental) (by) (from) (on)
  acid NEC —see Table of Drugs and Chemicals
  bed linen —see Exposure, fire, uncontrolled, in building, bed
  blowtorch X08.8
    with ignition of clothing NEC X06.2
      nightwear X05
  bonfire, campfire (controlled) —see also Exposure, fire, controlled, not in building
    uncontrolled —see Exposure, fire, uncontrolled, not in building
  candle X08.8
    with ignition of clothing NEC X06.2
      nightwear X05
  caustic liquid, substance (external) (internal) NEC —see Table of Drugs and Chemicals
  chemical (external) (internal) —see also Table of Drugs and Chemicals
    in war operations —see War operations, fire
  cigar(s) or cigarette(s) X08.8
    with ignition of clothing NEC X06.2
      nightwear X05
  clothes, clothing NEC (from controlled fire) X06.2
    with conflagration —see Exposure, fire, uncontrolled, building
    not in building or structure —see Exposure, fire, uncontrolled, not in building
  cooker (hot) X15.8
    stated as undetermined whether accidental or intentional Y27.3
    suicide (attempt) X77.3
  electric blanket X16
  engine (hot) X17
  fire, flames —see Exposure, fire
  flare, Very pistol —see Discharge, firearm NEC

Burn, burned, burning (Continued)
  heat
    from appliance (electrical) (household) X15.8
      cooker X15.8
      hotplate X15.2
      kettle X15.8
      light bulb X15.8
      saucepan X15.3
      skillet X15.3
      stated as undetermined whether accidental or intentional Y27.3
      stove X15.0
      suicide (attempt) X77.3
      toaster X15.1
    in local application or packing during medical or surgical procedure Y63.5
  heating
    appliance, radiator or pipe X16
  homicide (attempt) —see Assault, burning
  hot
    air X14.1
    cooker X15.8
    drink X10.0
    engine X17
    fat X10.2
    fluid NEC X12
    food X10.1
    gases X14.1
    heating appliance X16
    household appliance NEC X15.8
    kettle X15.8
    liquid NEC X12
    machinery X17
    metal (molten) (liquid) NEC X18
    object (not producing fire or flames) NEC X19
    oil (cooking) X10.2
    pipe(s) X16
    radiator X16
    saucepan (glass) (metal) X15.3
    stove (kitchen) X15.0
    substance NEC X19
      caustic or corrosive NEC —see Table of Drugs and Chemicals
    toaster X15.1
    tool X17
    vapor X13.1
    water (tap) —see Contact, with, hot, tap water
  hotplate X15.2
    suicide (attempt) X77.3
  ignition —see Ignition
  in war operations —see War operations, fire
  inflicted by other person X97
    by hot objects, hot vapor, and steam —see Assault, burning, hot object
  internal, from swallowed caustic, corrosive liquid, substance —see Table of Drugs and Chemicals
  iron (hot) X15.8
    stated as undetermined whether accidental or intentional Y27.3
    suicide (attempt) X77.3
  kettle (hot) X15.8
    stated as undetermined whether accidental or intentional Y27.3
    suicide (attempt) X77.3
  lamp (flame) X08.8
    with ignition of clothing NEC X06.2
      nightwear X05
  lighter (cigar) (cigarette) X08.8
    with ignition of clothing NEC X06.2
      nightwear X05
  lightning —see subcategory T75.0
    causing fire —see Exposure, fire
  liquid (boiling) (hot) NEC X12
    stated as undetermined whether accidental or intentional Y27.2
    suicide (attempt) X77.2

Burn, burned, burning (Continued)
local application of externally applied
  substance in medical or surgical care
  Y63.5
machinery (hot) X17
matches X08.8
  with ignition of clothing NEC X06.2
    nightwear X05
mattress —see Exposure, fire, uncontrolled,
  building, bed
medicament, externally applied Y63.5
metal (hot) (liquid) (molten) NEC X18
nightwear (nightclothes, nightdress, gown,
  pajamas, robe) X05
object (hot) NEC X19
on board watercraft
  due to
    accident to watercraft V91.09
      powered craft V91.03
        ferry boat V91.01
        fishing boat V91.02
        jet ski V91.03
        liner V91.01
        merchant ship V91.00
        passenger ship V91.01
      unpowered craft V91.08
        canoe V91.05
        inflatable V91.06
        kayak V91.05
        sailboat V91.04
        surf-board V91.08
        water skis V91.07
        windsurfer V91.08
    fire on board V93.09
      ferry boat V93.01
      fishing boat V93.02
      jet ski V93.03
      liner V93.01
      merchant ship V93.00
      passenger ship V93.01
      powered craft NEC V93.03
      sailboat V93.04

Burn, burned, burning (Continued)
on board watercraft (Continued)
  due to (Continued)
    specified heat source NEC on board
      V93.19
      ferry boat V93.11
      fishing boat V93.12
      jet ski V93.13
      liner V93.11
      merchant ship V93.10
      passenger ship V93.11
      powered craft NEC V93.13
      sailboat V93.14
pipe (hot) X16
  smoking X08.8
    with ignition of clothing NEC X06.2
      nightwear X05
powder —see Powder burn
radiator (hot) X16
saucepan (hot) (glass) (metal) X15.3
  stated as undetermined whether
    accidental or intentional
    Y27.3
  suicide (attempt) X77.3
self-inflicted X76
  stated as undetermined whether
    accidental or intentional
    Y26
stated as undetermined whether
  accidental or intentional Y27.0
steam X13.1
  pipe X16
    stated as undetermined whether
      accidental or intentional
      Y27.8
  stated as undetermined whether
    accidental or intentional Y27.0
  suicide (attempt) X77.0
stove (hot) (kitchen) X15.0
  stated as undetermined whether
    accidental or intentional Y27.3
  suicide (attempt) X77.3

Burn, burned, burning (Continued)
substance (hot) NEC X19
  boiling X12
    stated as undetermined whether
      accidental or intentional Y27.2
    suicide (attempt) X77.2
  molten (metal) X18
suicide (attempt) NEC X76
  hot
    household appliance X77.3
    object X77.9
stated as undetermined whether accidental or
  intentional Y27.0
therapeutic misadventure
  heat in local application or packing during
    medical or surgical procedure Y63.5
  overdose of radiation Y63.2
toaster (hot) X15.1
  stated as undetermined whether accidental
    or intentional Y27.3
  suicide (attempt) X77.3
tool (hot) X17
torch, welding X08.8
  with ignition of clothing NEC X06.2
    nightwear X05
trash fire (controlled) —see Exposure, fire,
  controlled, not in building
  uncontrolled —see Exposure, fire,
    uncontrolled, not in building
vapor (hot) X13.1
  stated as undetermined whether accidental
    or intentional Y27.0
  suicide (attempt) X77.0
Very pistol —see Discharge, firearm NEC
Butted by animal W55.82
bull W55.22
cow W55.22
goat W55.32
horse W55.12
pig W55.42
sheep W55.32

C

Caisson disease —*see* Air, pressure, change
Campfire (exposure to) (controlled) —*see also*
    Exposure, fire, controlled, not in building
uncontrolled —*see* Exposure, fire,
    uncontrolled, not in building
Capital punishment (any means) —*see* Legal,
    intervention
Car sickness T75.3
Casualty (not due to war) NEC X58
    war —*see* War operations
Cat
    bite W55.01
    scratch W55.03
Cataclysm, cataclysmic (any injury) NEC —*see*
    Forces of nature
Catching fire —*see* Exposure, fire
Caught
    between
        folding object W23.0
      ▶objects (moving) W23.0
        ▶and
          ▶machinery —*see* Contact, with, by
            type of machine
          ▶stationary W23.2
        stationary W23.1
        ▶and moving W23.2
        sliding door and door frame W23.0
    by, in
        machinery (moving parts of) —*see* Contact,
          with, by type of machine
        washing-machine wringer W23.0
    under packing crate (due to losing grip) W23.1
Cave-in caused by cataclysmic earth surface
    movement or eruption —*see* Landslide
Change(s) in air pressure —*see* Air, pressure,
    change
Choked, choking (on) (any object except food
    or vomitus)
    food (bone) (seed) —*see* categories T17 and
        T18
    vomitus T17.81-•
Civil insurrection —*see* War operations
Cloudburst (any injury) X37.8
Cold, exposure to (accidental) (excessive)
    (extreme) (natural) (place) NEC —*see*
    Exposure, cold
Collapse
    building W20.1
        burning (uncontrolled fire) X00.2
    dam or man-made structure (causing earth
        movement) X36.0
    machinery —*see* Contact, with, by type of
        machine
    structure W20.1
        burning (uncontrolled fire) X00.2
Collision (accidental) NEC —*see also* Accident,
    transport V89.9
    pedestrian W51
        with fall W03
          due to ice or snow W00.0
          involving pedestrian conveyance —*see*
            Accident, transport, pedestrian,
            conveyance
        and
          crowd or human stampede (with fall)
            W52
          object W22.8
            with fall —*see* Fall, due to, bumping
              against, object
    person(s) —*see* Collision, pedestrian
    transport vehicle NEC V89.9
        and
          avalanche, fallen or not moving —*see*
            Accident, transport
            falling or moving —*see* Landslide
          landslide, fallen or not moving —*see*
            Accident, transport
            falling or moving —*see* Landslide

Collision NEC *(Continued)*
    transport vehicle NEC *(Continued)*
        due to cataclysm —*see* Forces of nature,
          by type
        intentional, purposeful suicide (attempt) —
          see Suicide, collision
Combustion, spontaneous —*see* Ignition
Complication (delayed) of or following
    (medical or surgical procedure) Y84.9
    with misadventure —*see* Misadventure
    amputation of limb(s) Y83.5
    anastomosis (arteriovenous) (blood vessel)
        (gastrojejunal) (tendon) (natural or
        artificial material) Y83.2
    aspiration (of fluid) Y84.4
        tissue Y84.8
    biopsy Y84.8
    blood
        sampling Y84.7
        transfusion
          procedure Y84.8
    bypass Y83.2
    catheterization (urinary) Y84.6
        cardiac Y84.0
    colostomy Y83.3
    cystostomy Y83.3
    dialysis (kidney) Y84.1
    drug —*see* Table of Drugs and Chemicals
    due to misadventure —*see* Misadventure
    duodenostomy Y83.3
    electroshock therapy Y84.3
    external stoma, creation of Y83.3
    formation of external stoma Y83.3
    gastrostomy Y83.3
    graft Y83.2
    hypothermia (medically-induced) Y84.8
    implant, implantation (of)
        artificial
          internal device (cardiac pacemaker)
            (electrodes in brain) (heart valve
            prosthesis) (orthopedic) Y83.1
          material or tissue (for anastomosis or
            bypass) Y83.2
            with creation of external stoma Y83.3
        natural tissues (for anastomosis or bypass)
          Y83.2
          with creation of external stoma Y83.3
    infusion
        procedure Y84.8
    injection —*see* Table of Drugs and
        Chemicals
        procedure Y84.8
    insertion of gastric or duodenal sound Y84.5
    insulin-shock therapy Y84.3
    paracentesis (abdominal) (thoracic)
        (aspirative) Y84.4
    procedures other than surgical operation —
        see Complication of or following, by type
        of procedure
    radiological procedure or therapy Y84.2
    removal of organ (partial) (total) NEC Y83.6
    sampling
        blood Y84.7
        fluid NEC Y84.4
        tissue Y84.8
    shock therapy Y84.3
    surgical operation NEC —*see also*
        Complication of or following, by type of
        operation Y83.9
        reconstructive NEC Y83.4
          with
            anastomosis, bypass or graft Y83.2
            formation of external stoma Y83.3
        specified NEC Y83.8
    transfusion —*see also* Table of Drugs and
        Chemicals
        procedure Y84.8
    transplant, transplantation (heart) (kidney)
        (liver) (whole organ, any) Y83.0
        partial organ Y83.4
    ureterostomy Y83.3

Complication of or following *(Continued)*
    vaccination —*see also* Table of Drugs and
        Chemicals
        procedure Y84.8
Compression
    divers' squeeze —*see* Air, pressure, change
    trachea by
        food (lodged in esophagus) —*see* categories
          T17 and T18
        vomitus (lodged in esophagus) T17.81-•
Conflagration —*see* Exposure, fire, uncontrolled
Constriction (external)
    hair W49.01
    jewelry W49.04
    ring W49.04
    rubber band W49.03
    specified item NEC W49.09
    string W49.02
    thread W49.02
Contact (accidental)
    with
        abrasive wheel (metalworking) W31.1
        alligator W58.09
          bite W58.01
          crushing W58.03
          strike W58.02
        amphibian W62.9
          frog W62.0
          toad W62.1
        animal (nonvenomous) NEC W64
          marine W56.89
            bite W56.81
            dolphin —*see* Contact, with, dolphin
            fish NEC —*see* Contact, with, fish
            mammal —*see* Contact, with,
             mammal, marine
            orca —*see* Contact, with, orca
            sea lion —*see* Contact, with, sea lion
            shark —*see* Contact, with, shark
            strike W56.82
        animate mechanical force NEC W64
        arrow W21.89
          not thrown, projected or falling W45.8
        arthropods (nonvenomous) W57
        axe W27.0
        band-saw (industrial) W31.2
        bayonet —*see* Bayonet wound
        bee(s) X58
        bench-saw (industrial) W31.2
        bird W61.99
          bite W61.91
          chicken —*see* Contact, with, chicken
          duck —*see* Contact, with, duck
          goose —*see* Contact, with, goose
          macaw —*see* Contact, with, macaw
          parrot —*see* Contact, with, parrot
          psittacine —*see* Contact, with, psittacine
          strike W61.92
          turkey —*see* Contact, with, turkey
        blender W29.0
        boiling water X12
          stated as undetermined whether
            accidental or intentional Y27.2
          suicide (attempt) X77.2
        bore, earth-drilling or mining (land)
          (seabed) W31.0
        buffalo —*see* Contact, with, hoof stock NEC
        bull W55.29
          bite W55.21
          gored W55.22
          strike W55.22
        bumper cars W31.81
        camel —*see* Contact, with, hoof stock NEC
        can
          lid W26.8
          opener W27.4
            powered W29.0
        cat W55.09
          bite W55.01
          scratch W55.03
        caterpillar (venomous) X58

Contact *(Continued)*
  with *(Continued)*
    centipede (venomous) X58
    chain
      hoist W24.0
        agricultural operations W30.89
      saw W29.3
    chicken W61.39
      peck W61.33
      strike W61.32
    chisel W27.0
    circular saw W31.2
    cobra X58
    combine (harvester) W30.0
    conveyer belt W24.1
    cooker (hot) X15.8
      stated as undetermined whether
        accidental or intentional Y27.3
      suicide (attempt) X77.3
    coral X58
    cotton gin W31.82
    cow W55.29
      bite W55.21
      strike W55.22
    crane W24.0
      agricultural operations W30.89
    crocodile W58.19
      bite W58.11
      crushing W58.13
      strike W58.12
    dagger W26.1
      stated as undetermined whether
        accidental or intentional Y28.2
      suicide (attempt) X78.2
    dairy equipment W31.82
    dart W21.89
      not thrown, projected or falling W45.8
    deer —*see* Contact, with, hoof stock
      NEC
    derrick W24.0
      agricultural operations W30.89
        hay W30.2
    dog W54.8
      bite W54.0
      strike W54.1
    dolphin W56.09
      bite W56.01
      strike W56.02
    donkey —*see* Contact, with, hoof stock
      NEC
    drill (powered) W29.8
      earth (land) (seabed) W31.0
      nonpowered W27.8
    drive belt W24.0
      agricultural operations W30.89
    dry ice —*see* Exposure, cold, man-made
    dryer (clothes) (powered) (spin) W29.2
    duck W61.69
      bite W61.61
      strike W61.62
    earth(-)
      drilling machine (industrial) W31.0
      scraping machine in stationary use
        W31.83
    edge of stiff paper W26.2
    electric
      beater W29.0
      blanket X16
      fan W29.2
        commercial W31.82
      knife W29.1
      mixer W29.0
    elevator (building) W24.0
      agricultural operations W30.89
        grain W30.3
    engine(s), hot NEC X17
    excavating machine W31.0
    farm machine W30.9
    feces —*see* Contact, with, by type of
      animal
    fer de lance X58

Contact *(Continued)*
  with *(Continued)*
    fish W56.59
      bite W56.51
      shark —*see* Contact, with, shark
      strike W56.52
    flying horses W31.81
    forging (metalworking) machine W31.1
    fork W27.4
    forklift (truck) W24.0
      agricultural operations W30.89
    frog W62.0
    garden
      cultivator (powered) W29.3
        riding W30.89
      fork W27.1
    gas turbine W31.3
    Gila monster X58
    giraffe —*see* Contact, with, hoof stock NEC
    glass (sharp) (broken) W25
      with subsequent fall W18.02
      assault X99.0
      due to fall —*see* Fall, by type
      stated as undetermined whether
        accidental or intentional Y28. 0
      suicide (attempt) X78.0
    goat W55.39
      bite W55.31
      strike W55.32
    goose W61.59
      bite W61.51
      strike W61.52
    hand
      saw W27.0
      tool (not powered) NEC W27.8
        powered W29.8
    harvester W30.0
    hay-derrick W30.2
    heat NEC X19
      from appliance (electrical)
        (household) —*see* Contact, with,
        hot, household appliance
      heating appliance X16
    heating
      appliance (hot) X16
      pad (electric) X16
    hedge-trimmer (powered) W29.3
    hoe W27.1
    hoist (chain) (shaft) NEC W24.0
      agricultural W30.89
    hoof stock NEC W55.39
      bite W55.31
      strike W55.32
    hornet(s) X58
    horse W55.19
      bite W55.11
      strike W55.12
    hot
      air X14.1
        inhalation X14.0
      cooker X15.8
    ▶ cooking
      ▶ pan X15.3
      ▶ pot X15.3
      drinks X10.0
      engine X17
      fats X10.2
      fluids NEC X12
        assault X98.2
        suicide (attempt) X77.2
        undetermined whether accidental or
          intentional Y27.2
      food X10.1
      gases X14.1
        inhalation X14.0
      heating appliance X16
      household appliance X15.8
        assault X98.3
        cooker X15.8
        hotplate X15.2
        kettle X15.8
        light bulb X15.8

Contact *(Continued)*
  with *(Continued)*
    hot *(Continued)*
      household appliance *(Continued)*
        object NEC X19
          assault X98.8
          stated as undetermined whether
            accidental or intentional Y27.9
          suicide (attempt) X77.8
        saucepan X15.3
        skillet X15.3
        stated as undetermined whether
          accidental or intentional Y27.3
        stove X15.0
        suicide (attempt) X77.3
        toaster X15.1
      kettle X15.8
      light bulb X15.8
      liquid NEC —*see also* Burn X12
        drinks X10.0
        stated as undetermined whether
          accidental or intentional Y27.2
        suicide (attempt) X77.2
        tap water X11.8
          stated as undetermined whether
            accidental or intentional Y27.1
          suicide (attempt) X77.1
      machinery X17
      metal (molten) (liquid) NEC X18
      object (not producing fire or flames)
        NEC X19
      oil (cooking) X10.2
      pipe X16
      plate X15.2
      radiator X16
      saucepan (glass) (metal) X15.3
      skillet X15.3
      stove (kitchen) X15.0
      substance NEC X19
      tap-water X11.8
        assault X98.1
        heated on stove X12
          stated as undetermined whether
            accidental or intentional Y27.2
          suicide (attempt) X77.2
        in bathtub X11.0
        running X11.1
        stated as undetermined whether
          accidental or intentional Y27.1
        suicide (attempt) X77.1
      toaster X15.1
      tool X17
      vapors X13.1
        inhalation X13.0
      water (tap) X11.8
        boiling X12
          stated as undetermined whether
            accidental or intentional Y27.2
          suicide (attempt) X77.2
        heated on stove X12
          stated as undetermined whether
            accidental or intentional Y27.2
          suicide (attempt) X77.2
        in bathtub X11.0
        running X11.1
        stated as undetermined whether
          accidental or intentional Y27.1
        suicide (attempt) X77.1
    hotplate X15.2
    ice-pick W27.4
    insect (nonvenomous) NEC W57
    kettle (hot) X15.8
    knife W26.0
      assault X99.1
      electric W29.1
      stated as undetermined whether
        accidental or intentional Y28.1
      suicide (attempt) X78.1
    lathe (metalworking) W31.1
      turnings W45.8
      woodworking W31.2

Contact (Continued)
  with (Continued)
    lawnmower (powered) (ridden) W28
      causing electrocution W86.8
        suicide (attempt) X83.1
      unpowered W27.1
    lift, lifting (devices) W24.0
      agricultural operations W30.89
      shaft W24.0
    liquefied gas —see Exposure, cold,
        man-made
    liquid air, hydrogen, nitrogen —see
        Exposure, cold, man-made
    lizard (nonvenomous) W59.09
      bite W59.01
      strike W59.02
    llama —see Contact, with, hoof stock NEC
    macaw W61.19
      bite W61.11
      strike W61.12
    machine, machinery W31.9
      abrasive wheel W31.1
      agricultural including animal-powered
          W30.9
        combine harvester W30.0
        grain storage elevator W30.3
        hay derrick W30.2
        power take-off device W30.1
        reaper W30.0
        specified NEC W30.89
        thresher W30.0
        transport vehicle, stationary W30.81
      band saw W31.2
      bench saw W31.2
      circular saw W31.2
      commercial NEC W31.82
      drilling, metal (industrial) W31.1
      earth-drilling W31.0
      earthmoving or scraping W31.89
      excavating W31.89
      forging machine W31.1
      gas turbine W31.3
      hot X17
      internal combustion engine W31.3
      land drill W31.0
      lathe W31.1
      lifting (devices) W24.0
      metal drill W31.1
      metalworking (industrial) W31.1
      milling, metal W31.1
      mining W31.0
      molding W31.2
      overhead plane W31.2
      power press, metal W31.1
      prime mover W31.3
      printing W31.89
      radial saw W31.2
      recreational W31.81
      roller-coaster W31.81
      rolling mill, metal W31.1
      sander W31.2
      seabed drill W31.0
      shaft
        hoist W31.0
        lift W31.0
      specified NEC W31.89
      spinning W31.89
      steam engine W31.3
      transmission W24.1
      undercutter W31.0
      water driven turbine W31.3
      weaving W31.89
      woodworking or forming (industrial)
          W31.2
    mammal (feces) (urine) W55.89
      bull —see Contact, with, bull
      cat —see Contact, with, cat
      cow —see Contact, with, cow
      goat —see Contact, with, goat
      hoof stock —see Contact, with, hoof
          stock

Contact (Continued)
  with (Continued)
    mammal (Continued)
      horse —see Contact, with, horse
      marine W56.39
        dolphin —see Contact, with, dolphin
        orca —see Contact, with, orca
        sea lion —see Contact, with, sea lion
        specified NEC W56.39
          bite W56.31
          strike W56.32
      pig —see Contact, with, pig
      raccoon —see Contact, with, raccoon
      rodent —see Contact, with, rodent
      sheep —see Contact, with, sheep
      specified NEC W55.89
        bite W55.81
        strike W55.82
    marine
      animal W56.89
        bite W56.81
        dolphin —see Contact, with, dolphin
        fish NEC —see Contact, with, fish
        mammal —see Contact, with,
            mammal, marine
        orca —see Contact, with, orca
        sea lion —see Contact, with, sea lion
        shark —see Contact, with, shark
        strike W56.82
    meat
      grinder (domestic) W29.0
        industrial W31.82
        nonpowered W27.4
      slicer (domestic) W29.0
        industrial W31.82
    merry go round W31.81
    metal, (hot) (liquid) (molten) NEC X18
    millipede W57
    nail W45.0
      gun W29.4
    needle (sewing) W27.3
      hypodermic W46.0
        contaminated W46.1
    object (blunt) NEC
      hot NEC X19
      legal intervention —see Legal,
          intervention, blunt object
      sharp NEC W45.8
        inflicted by other person NEC W45.8
          stated as
            intentional homicide (attempt) —
                see Assault, cutting or
                piercing instrument
        legal intervention —see Legal,
            intervention, sharp object
        self-inflicted X78.9
    orca W56.29
      bite W56.21
      strike W56.22
    overhead plane W31.2
    paper (as sharp object) W26.2
    paper-cutter W27.5
    parrot W61.09
      bite W61.01
      strike W61.02
    pig W55.49
      bite W55.41
      strike W55.42
    pipe, hot X16
    pitchfork W27.1
    plane (metal) (wood) W27.0
      overhead W31.2
    plant thorns, spines, sharp leaves or other
        mechanisms W60
    powered
      garden cultivator W29.3
      household appliance, implement, or
          machine W29.8
      saw (industrial) W31.2
        hand W29.8
    printing machine W31.89

Contact (Continued)
  with (Continued)
    psittacine bird W61.29
      bite W61.21
      macaw —see Contact, with, macaw
      parrot —see Contact, with, parrot
      strike W61.22
    pulley (block) (transmission) W24.0
      agricultural operations W30.89
    raccoon W55.59
      bite W55.51
      strike W55.52
    radial-saw (industrial) W31.2
    radiator (hot) X16
    rake W27.1
    rattlesnake X58
    reaper W30.0
    reptile W59.89
      lizard —see Contact, with, lizard
      snake —see Contact, with, snake
      specified NEC W59.89
        bite W59.81
        crushing W59.83
        strike W59.82
      turtle —see Contact, with, turtle
    rivet gun (powered) W29.4
    road scraper —see Accident, transport,
        construction vehicle
    rodent (feces) (urine) W53.89
      bite W53.81
      mouse W53.09
        bite W53.01
      rat W53.19
        bite W53.11
      specified NEC W53.89
        bite W53.81
      squirrel W53.29
        bite W53.21
    roller coaster W31.81
    rope NEC W24.0
      agricultural operations W30.89
    saliva —see Contact, with, by type of
        animal
    sander W29.8
      industrial W31.2
    saucepan (hot) (glass) (metal) X15.3
    saw W27.0
      band (industrial) W31.2
      bench (industrial) W31.2
      chain W29.3
      hand W27.0
    sawing machine, metal W31.1
    scissors W27.2
    scorpion X58
    screwdriver W27.0
      powered W29.8
    sea
      anemone, cucumber or urchin (spine)
          X58
      lion W56.19
        bite W56.11
        strike W56.12
    serpent —see Contact, with, snake, by type
    sewing-machine (electric) (powered) W29.2
      not powered W27.8
    shaft (hoist) (lift) (transmission) NEC W24.0
      agricultural W30.89
    shark W56.49
      bite W56.41
      strike W56.42
    sharp object(s) W26.9
      specified NEC W26.8
    shears (hand) W27.2
      powered (industrial) W31.1
        domestic W29.2
    sheep W55.39
      bite W55.31
      strike W55.32
    shovel W27.8
      steam —see Accident, transport,
          construction vehicle

Contact *(Continued)*
　with *(Continued)*
　　snake (nonvenomous) W59.19
　　　bite W59.11
　　　crushing W59.13
　　　strike W59.12
　　spade W27.1
　　spider (venomous) X58
　　spin-drier W29.2
　　spinning machine W31.89
　　splinter W45.8
　　sports equipment W21.9
　　staple gun (powered) W29.8
　　steam X13.1
　　　engine W31.3
　　　inhalation X13.0
　　　pipe X16
　　　shovel W31.89
　　stove (hot) (kitchen) X15.0
　　substance, hot NEC X19
　　　molten (metal) X18
　　sword W26.1
　　　assault X99.2
　　　stated as undetermined whether
　　　　accidental or intentional
　　　　Y28.2
　　　suicide (attempt) X78.2
　　tarantula X58
　　thresher W30.0
　　tin can lid W26.8
　　toad W62.1
　　toaster (hot) X15.1
　　tool W27.8
　　　hand (not powered) W27.8
　　　　auger W27.0
　　　　axe W27.0
　　　　can opener W27.4
　　　　chisel W27.0
　　　　fork W27.4
　　　　garden W27.1
　　　　handsaw W27.0
　　　　hoe W27.1
　　　　ice-pick W27.4
　　　　kitchen utensil W27.4
　　　　manual
　　　　　lawn mower W27.1
　　　　　sewing machine W27.8
　　　　meat grinder W27.4
　　　　needle (sewing) W27.3
　　　　　hypodermic W46.0
　　　　　　contaminated W46.1
　　　　paper cutter W27.5
　　　　pitchfork W27.1
　　　　rake W27.1
　　　　scissors W27.2
　　　　screwdriver W27.0
　　　　specified NEC W27.8
　　　　workbench W27.0
　　　hot X17
　　　powered W29.8
　　　　blender W29.0
　　　　　commercial W31.82
　　　　can opener W29.0
　　　　　commercial W31.82
　　　　chainsaw W29.3
　　　　clothes dryer W29.2
　　　　　commercial W31.82
　　　　dishwasher W29.2
　　　　　commercial W31.82
　　　　edger W29.3
　　　　electric fan W29.2
　　　　　commercial W31.82
　　　　electric knife W29.1
　　　　food processor W29.0
　　　　　commercial W31.82
　　　　garbage disposal W29.0
　　　　　commercial W31.82

Contact *(Continued)*
　with *(Continued)*
　　tool *(Continued)*
　　　powered *(Continued)*
　　　　garden tool W29.3
　　　　hedge trimmer W29.3
　　　　ice maker W29.0
　　　　　commercial W31.82
　　　　kitchen appliance W29.0
　　　　　commercial W31.82
　　　　lawn mower W28
　　　　meat grinder W29.0
　　　　　commercial W31.82
　　　　mixer W29.0
　　　　　commercial W31.82
　　　　rototiller W29.3
　　　　sewing machine W29.2
　　　　　commercial W31.82
　　　　washing machine W29.2
　　　　　commercial W31.82
　　transmission device (belt, cable, chain,
　　　gear, pinion, shaft) W24.1
　　　agricultural operations W30.89
　　turbine (gas) (water-driven) W31.3
　　turkey W61.49
　　　peck W61.43
　　　strike W61.42
　　turtle (nonvenomous) W59.29
　　　bite W59.21
　　　strike W59.22
　　　terrestrial W59.89
　　　　bite W59.81
　　　　crushing W59.83
　　　　strike W59.82
　　under-cutter W31.0
　　urine —*see* Contact, with, by type of animal
　　vehicle
　　　agricultural use (transport) —*see*
　　　　Accident, transport, agricultural
　　　　vehicle
　　　　not on public highway W30.81
　　　industrial use (transport) —*see*
　　　　Accident, transport, industrial
　　　　vehicle
　　　　not on public highway W31.83
　　　off-road use (transport) —*see* Accident,
　　　　transport, all-terrain or off-road
　　　　vehicle
　　　　not on public highway W31.83
　　　special construction use (transport) —*see*
　　　　Accident, transport, construction
　　　　vehicle
　　　　not on public highway W31.83
　　venomous
　　　animal X58
　　　arthropods X58
　　　lizard X58
　　　marine animal NEC X58
　　　marine plant NEC X58
　　　millipedes (tropical) X58
　　　plant(s) X58
　　　snake X58
　　　spider X58
　　viper X58
　　washing-machine (powered) W29.2
　　wasp X58
　　weaving-machine W31.89
　　winch W24.0
　　　agricultural operations W30.89
　　wire NEC W24.0
　　　agricultural operations W30.89
　　wood slivers W45.8
　　yellow jacket X58
　　zebra —*see* Contact, with, hoof stock NEC
　pressure X50.9
　stress X50.9
Coup de soleil X32

Crash
　aircraft (in transit) (powered) V95.9
　　balloon V96.01
　　fixed wing NEC (private) V95.21
　　　commercial V95.31
　　glider V96.21
　　　hang V96.11
　　　powered V95.11
　　helicopter V95.01
　　in war operations —*see* War operations,
　　　destruction of aircraft
　　microlight V95.11
　　nonpowered V96.9
　　　specified NEC V96.8
　　powered NEC V95.8
　　stated as
　　　homicide (attempt) Y08.81
　　　suicide (attempt) X83.0
　　ultralight V95.11
　spacecraft V95.41
　transport vehicle NEC —*see also* Accident,
　　transport V89.9
　　homicide (attempt) Y03.8
　　motor NEC (traffic) V89.2
　　　homicide (attempt) Y03.8
　　　suicide (attempt) —*see* Suicide, collision
Cruelty (mental) (physical) (sexual) X58
Crushed (accidentally) X58
　between objects (moving) (stationary and
　　moving) W23.0
　　stationary W23.1
　by
　　alligator W58.03
　　avalanche NEC —*see* Landslide
　　cave-in W20.0
　　　caused by cataclysmic earth surface
　　　　movement —*see* Landslide
　　crocodile W58.13
　　crowd or human stampede W52
　　falling
　　　aircraft V97.39
　　　　in war operations —*see* War
　　　　　operations, destruction of aircraft
　　　earth, material W20.0
　　　　caused by cataclysmic earth surface
　　　　　movement —*see* Landslide
　　　object NEC W20.8
　　landslide NEC —*see* Landslide
　　lizard (nonvenomous) W59.09
　　machinery —*see* Contact, with, by type of
　　　machine
　　reptile NEC W59.89
　　snake (nonvenomous) W59.13
　in
　　machinery —*see* Contact, with, by type of
　　　machine
Cut, cutting (any part of body) (accidental) —
　see also Contact, with, by object or machine
　during medical or surgical treatment as
　　misadventure —*see* Index to Diseases
　　and Injuries, Complications
　homicide (attempt) —*see* Assault, cutting or
　　piercing instrument
　inflicted by other person —*see* Assault,
　　cutting or piercing instrument
　legal
　　execution —*see* Legal, intervention
　　intervention —*see* Legal, intervention,
　　　sharp object
　machine NEC —*see also* Contact, with, by
　　type of machine W31.9
　self-inflicted —*see* Suicide, cutting or piercing
　　instrument
　suicide (attempt) —*see* Suicide, cutting or
　　piercing instrument
Cyclone (any injury) X37.1

D

Decapitation (accidental circumstances)
NEC X58
homicide X99.9
legal execution —see Legal, intervention
Dehydration from lack of water X58
Deprivation X58
Derailment (accidental)
railway (rolling stock) (train) (vehicle)
(without antecedent collision) V81.7
with antecedent collision —see Accident,
transport, railway vehicle occupant
streetcar (without antecedent collision) V82.7
with antecedent collision —see Accident,
transport, streetcar occupant
Descent
parachute (voluntary) (without accident to
aircraft) V97.29
due to accident to aircraft —see Accident,
transport, aircraft
Desertion X58
Destitution X58
Disability, late effect or sequela of injury —see
Sequelae
Discharge (accidental)
airgun W34.010
assault X95.01
homicide (attempt) X95.01
stated as undetermined whether accidental
or intentional Y24.0
suicide (attempt) X74.01
BB gun —see Discharge, airgun
firearm (accidental) W34.00
assault X95.9
handgun (pistol) (revolver) W32.0
assault X93
homicide (attempt) X93
legal intervention —see Legal,
intervention, firearm, handgun
stated as undetermined whether
accidental or intentional Y22
suicide (attempt) X72
homicide (attempt) X95.9
hunting rifle W33.02
assault X94.1
homicide (attempt) X94.1
legal intervention
injuring
bystander Y35.032
law enforcement personnel Y35.031
suspect Y35.033
unspecified person Y35.039
stated as undetermined whether
accidental or intentional Y23.1
suicide (attempt) X73.1
larger W33.00
assault X94.9
homicide (attempt) X94.9
hunting rifle —see Discharge, firearm,
hunting rifle
legal intervention —see Legal,
intervention, firearm by type of
firearm
machine gun —see Discharge, firearm,
machine gun
shotgun —see Discharge, firearm,
shotgun
specified NEC W33.09
assault X94.8
homicide (attempt) X94.8
legal intervention
injuring
bystander Y35.092
law enforcement personnel
Y35.091
suspect Y35.093
unspecified person Y35.099
stated as undetermined whether
accidental or intentional Y23.8
suicide (attempt) X73.8

Discharge (Continued)
firearm (Continued)
larger (Continued)
stated as undetermined whether
accidental or intentional Y23.9
suicide (attempt) X73.9
legal intervention
injuring
bystander Y35.002
law enforcement personnel Y35.001
suspect Y35.03
unspecified person Y35.009
using rubber bullet
injuring
bystander Y35.042
law enforcement personnel Y35.041
suspect Y35.043
unspecified person Y35.049
machine gun W33.03
assault X94.2
homicide (attempt) X94.2
legal intervention —see Legal,
intervention, firearm, machine gun
stated as undetermined whether
accidental or intentional Y23.3
suicide (attempt) X73.2
pellet gun —see Discharge, airgun
shotgun W33.01
assault X94.0
homicide (attempt) X94.0
legal intervention —see Legal,
intervention, firearm, specified NEC
stated as undetermined whether
accidental or intentional Y23.0
suicide (attempt) X73.0
specified NEC W34.09
assault X95.8
homicide (attempt) X95.8
legal intervention —see Legal,
intervention, firearm, specified NEC
stated as undetermined whether
accidental or intentional Y24.8
suicide (attempt) X74.9
stated as undetermined whether accidental
or intentional Y24.9
suicide (attempt) X74.9
Very pistol W34.09
assault X95.8
homicide (attempt) X95.8
stated as undetermined whether
accidental or intentional Y24.8
suicide (attempt) X74.8
firework(s) W39
stated as undetermined whether accidental
or intentional Y25
gas-operated gun NEC W34.018
airgun —see Discharge, airgun
assault X95.09
homicide (attempt) X95.09
paintball gun —see Discharge, paintball gun
stated as undetermined whether accidental
or intentional Y24.8
suicide (attempt) X74.09
gun NEC —see also Discharge, firearm NEC
air —see Discharge, airgun
BB —see Discharge, airgun
for single hand use —see Discharge,
firearm, handgun
hand —see Discharge, firearm, handgun
machine —see Discharge, firearm, machine
gun
other specified —see Discharge, firearm
NEC
paintball —see Discharge, paintball gun
pellet —see Discharge, airgun
handgun —see Discharge, firearm, handgun
machine gun —see Discharge, firearm,
machine gun
paintball gun W34.011
assault X95.02
homicide (attempt) X95.02

Discharge (Continued)
paintball gun (Continued)
stated as undetermined whether accidental
or intentional Y24.8
suicide (attempt) X74.02
pistol —see Discharge, firearm, handgun
flare —see Discharge, firearm, Very pistol
pellet —see Discharge, airgun
Very —see Discharge, firearm, Very pistol
revolver —see Discharge, firearm, handgun
rifle (hunting) —see Discharge, firearm,
hunting rifle
shotgun —see Discharge, firearm, shotgun
spring-operated gun NEC W34.018
assault X95.09
homicide (attempt) X95.09
stated as undetermined whether accidental
or intentional Y24.8
suicide (attempt) X74.09
Disease
Andes W94.11
aviator's —see Air, pressure
range W94.11
Diver's disease, palsy, paralysis, squeeze —see
Air, pressure
Diving (into water) —see Accident, diving
Dog bite W54.0
Dragged by transport vehicle NEC —see also
Accident, transport V09.9
Drinking poison (accidental) —see Table of
Drugs and Chemicals
Dropped (accidentally) while being carried or
supported by other person W04
Drowning (accidental) W74
assault X92.9
due to
accident (to)
machinery —see Contact, with, by type
of machine
watercraft V90.89
burning V90.29
powered V90.23
fishing boat V90.22
jet ski V90.23
merchant ship V90.20
passenger ship V90.21
unpowered V90.28
canoe V90.25
inflatable V90.26
kayak V90.25
sailboat V90.24
water skis V90.27
crushed V90.39
powered V90.33
fishing boat V90.32
jet ski V90.33
merchant ship V90.30
passenger ship V90.31
unpowered V90.38
canoe V90.35
inflatable V90.36
kayak V90.35
sailboat V90.34
water skis V90.37
overturning V90.09
powered V90.03
fishing boat V90.02
jet ski V90.03
merchant ship V90.00
passenger ship V90.01
unpowered V90.08
canoe V90.05
inflatable V90.06
kayak V90.05
sailboat V90.04
sinking V90.19
powered V90.13
fishing boat V90.12
jet ski V90.13
merchant ship V90.10
passenger ship V90.11

Drowning (Continued)
  due to (Continued)
    accident (Continued)
      watercraft (Continued)
        sinking (Continued)
          unpowered V90.18
            canoe V90.15
            inflatable V90.16
            kayak V90.15
            sailboat V90.14
            specified type NEC V90.89
          powered V90.83
            fishing boat V90.82
            jet ski V90.83
            merchant ship V90.80
            passenger ship V90.81
          unpowered V90.88
            canoe V90.85
            inflatable V90.86
            kayak V90.85
            sailboat V90.84
            water skis V90.87
    avalanche —see Landslide
    cataclysmic
      earth surface movement NEC —see
        Forces of nature, earth movement
      storm —see Forces of nature, cataclysmic
        storm
    cloudburst X37.8
    cyclone X37.1
    fall overboard (from) V92.09
      powered craft V92.03
        ferry boat V92.01
        fishing boat V92.02
        jet ski V92.03
        liner V92.01
        merchant ship V92.00
        passenger ship V92.01
      resulting from
        accident to watercraft —see Drowning,
          due to, accident to, watercraft
        being washed overboard (from)
          V92.29
          powered craft V92.23
            ferry boat V92.21
            fishing boat V92.22
            jet ski V92.23
            liner V92.21
            merchant ship V92.20
            passenger ship V92.21
          unpowered craft V92.28
            canoe V92.25
            inflatable V92.26
            kayak V92.25
            sailboat V92.24
            surf-board V92.28
            water skis V92.27
            windsurfer V92.28
        motion of watercraft V92.19
          powered craft V92.13
            ferry boat V92.11
            fishing boat V92.12
            jet ski V92.13
            liner V92.11
            merchant ship V92.10
            passenger ship V92.11
          unpowered craft
            canoe V92.15
            inflatable V92.16
            kayak V92.15
            sailboat V92.14
      unpowered craft V92.08
        canoe V92.05
        inflatable V92.06
        kayak V92.05

Drowning (Continued)
  due to (Continued)
    fall overboard (Continued)
      unpowered craft (Continued)
        sailboat V92.04
        surf-board V92.08
        water skis V92.07
        windsurfer V92.08
    hurricane X37.0
    jumping into water from watercraft
      (involved in accident) —see also
      Drowning, due to, accident to,
      watercraft
      without accident to or on watercraft
        W16.711
    tidal wave NEC —see Forces of nature,
      tidal wave
    torrential rain X37.8
  following
    fall
      into
        bathtub W16.211
        bucket W16.221
        fountain —see Drowning, following,
          fall, into, water, specified NEC
        quarry —see Drowning, following,
          fall, into, water, specified NEC
        reservoir —see Drowning, following,
          fall, into, water, specified NEC
        swimming-pool W16.011
          stated as undetermined whether
            accidental or intentional
            Y21.3
          striking
            bottom W16.021
            wall W16.031
          suicide (attempt) X71.2
        water NOS W16.41
          natural (lake) (open sea) (river)
            (stream) (pond) W16.111
            striking
              bottom W16.121
              side W16.131
          specified NEC W16.311
            striking
              bottom W16.321
              wall W16.331
    overboard NEC —see Drowning, due to,
      fall overboard
    jump or dive
      from boat W16.711
        striking bottom W16.721
      into
        fountain —see Drowning, following,
          jump or dive, into, water,
          specified NEC
        quarry —see Drowning, following,
          jump or dive, into, water,
          specified NEC
        reservoir —see Drowning, following,
          jump or dive, into, water,
          specified NEC
        swimming-pool W16.511
          striking
            bottom W16.521
            wall W16.531
          suicide (attempt) X71.2
        water NOS W16.91
          natural (lake) (open sea) (river)
            (stream) (pond) W16.611
          specified NEC W16.811
            striking
             bottom W16.821
             wall W16.831
          striking bottom W16.621

Drowning (Continued)
  homicide (attempt) X92.9
  in
    bathtub (accidental) W65
      assault X92.0
      following fall W16.211
        stated as undetermined whether
          accidental or intentional
          Y21.1
      stated as undetermined whether
        accidental or intentional Y21.0
      suicide (attempt) X71.0
    lake —see Drowning, in, natural water
    natural water (lake) (open sea) (river)
      (stream) (pond) W69
      assault X92.3
      following
        dive or jump W16.611
          striking bottom W16.621
         fall W16.111
          striking
            bottom W16.121
            side W16.131
      stated as undetermined whether
        accidental or intentional Y21.4
      suicide (attempt) X71.3
    quarry —see Drowning, in, specified place
      NEC
    quenching tank —see Drowning, in,
      specified place NEC
    reservoir —see Drowning, in, specified
      place NEC
    river —see Drowning, in, natural water
    sea —see Drowning, in, natural water
    specified place NEC W73
      assault X92.8
      following
        dive or jump W16.811
          striking
            bottom W16.821
            wall W16.831
         fall W16.311
          striking
            bottom W16.321
            wall W16.331
      stated as undetermined whether
        accidental or intentional Y21.8
      suicide (attempt) X71.8
    stream —see Drowning, in, natural water
    swimming-pool W67
      assault X92.1
        following fall X92.2
      following
        dive or jump W16.511
          striking
            bottom W16.521
            wall W16.531
         fall W16.011
          striking
            bottom W16.021
            wall W16.031
      stated as undetermined whether
        accidental or intentional Y21.2
        following fall Y21.3
      suicide (attempt) X71.1
        following fall X71.2
    war operations —see War operations,
      restriction of airway
  resulting from accident to watercraft —see
    Drowning, due to, accident, watercraft
  self-inflicted X71.9
  stated as undetermined whether accidental or
    intentional Y21.9
  suicide (attempt) X71.9

▶ New   ➡ Revised   ~~deleted~~ Deleted   ● Use Additional Character(s)

E

Earth (surface) movement NEC —*see* Forces of nature, earth movement
Earth falling (on) W20.0
  caused by cataclysmic earth surface movement or eruption —*see* Landslide
Earthquake (any injury) X34
Effect(s) (adverse) of
  air pressure (any) —*see* Air, pressure
  cold, excessive (exposure to) —*see* Exposure, cold
  heat (excessive) —*see* Heat
  hot place (weather) —*see* Heat
  insolation X30
  late —*see* Sequelae
  motion —*see* Motion
  nuclear explosion or weapon in war operations —*see* War operations, nuclear weapon
  radiation —*see* Radiation
  travel —*see* Travel
Electric shock (accidental) (by) (in) —*see* Exposure, electric current
Electrocution (accidental) —*see* Exposure, electric current
Endotracheal tube wrongly placed during anesthetic procedure Y65.3
Entanglement
  in
    bed linen, causing suffocation —*see* category T71
    wheel of pedal cycle V19.88
Entry of foreign body or material —*see* Foreign body
Environmental pollution related condition —*see* Z57
Execution, legal (any method) —*see* Legal, intervention
Exhaustion
  cold —*see* Exposure, cold
  due to excessive exertion —*see also* Overexertion X50.9
  heat —*see* Heat
Explosion (accidental) (of) (with secondary fire) W40.9
  acetylene W40.1
  aerosol can W36.1
  air tank (compressed) (in machinery) W36.2
  aircraft (in transit) (powered) NEC V95.9
    balloon V96.05
    fixed wing NEC (private) V95.25
      commercial V95.35
    glider V96.25
      hang V96.15
      powered V95.15
    helicopter V95.05
    in war operations —*see* War operations, destruction of aircraft
    microlight V95.15
    nonpowered V96.9
      specified NEC V96.8
    powered NEC V95.8
    stated as
      homicide (attempt) Y03.8
      suicide (attempt) X83.0
    ultralight V95.15
  anesthetic gas in operating room W40.1
  antipersonnel bomb W40.8
    assault X96.0
    homicide (attempt) X96.0
    suicide (attempt) X75
  assault X96.9
  bicycle tire W37.0
  blasting (cap) (materials) W40.0
  boiler (machinery), not on transport vehicle W35
    on watercraft —*see* Explosion, in, watercraft
  butane W40.1
  caused by other person X96.9
  coal gas W40.1

Explosion *(Continued)*
  detonator W40.0
  dump (munitions) W40.8
  dynamite W40.0
    in
      assault X96.8
      homicide (attempt) X96.8
      legal intervention
        injuring
          bystander Y35.112
          law enforcement personnel Y35.111
          suspect Y35.113
          unspecified person Y35.119
      suicide (attempt) X75
  explosive (material) W40.9
    gas W40.1
    in blasting operation W40.0
    specified NEC W40.8
      in
        assault X96.8
        homicide (attempt) X96.8
        legal intervention
          injuring
            bystander Y35.192
            law enforcement personnel Y35.191
            suspect Y35.193
            unspecified person Y35.199
        suicide (attempt) X75
  factory (munitions) W40.8
  fertilizer bomb W40.8
    assault X96.3
    homicide (attempt) X96.3
    suicide (attempt) X75
  fire-damp W40.1
  firearm (parts) NEC W34.19
    airgun W34.110
    BB gun W34.110
    gas, air or spring-operated gun NEC W34.118
    handgun W32.1
    hunting rifle W33.12
    larger firearm W33.10
      specified NEC W33.19
    machine gun W33.13
    paintball gun W34.111
    pellet gun W34.110
    shotgun W33.11
    Very pistol [flare] W34.19
  fireworks W39
  gas (coal) (explosive) W40.1
    cylinder W36.9
      aerosol can W36.1
      air tank W36.2
      pressurized W36.3
      specified NEC W36.8
  gasoline (fumes) (tank) not in moving motor vehicle W40.1
    bomb W40.8
      assault X96.1
      homicide (attempt) X96.1
      suicide (attempt) X75
    in motor vehicle —*see* Accident, transport, by type of vehicle
  grain store W40.8
  grenade W40.8
    in
      assault X96.8
      homicide (attempt) X96.8
      legal intervention
        injuring
          bystander Y35.192
          law enforcement personnel Y35.191
          suspect Y35.193
          unspecified person Y35.199
      suicide (attempt) X75
  handgun (parts) —*see* Explosion, firearm, handgun (parts)
  homicide (attempt) X96.9
    antipersonnel bomb —*see* Explosion, antipersonnel bomb
    fertilizer bomb —*see* Explosion, fertilizer bomb

Explosion *(Continued)*
  homicide *(Continued)*
    gasoline bomb —*see* Explosion, gasoline bomb
    letter bomb —*see* Explosion, letter bomb
    pipe bomb —*see* Explosion, pipe bomb
    specified NEC X96.8
  hose, pressurized W37.8
  hot water heater, tank (in machinery) W35
    on watercraft —*see* Explosion, in, watercraft
  in, on
    dump W40.8
    factory W40.8
    mine (of explosive gases) NEC W40.1
    watercraft V93.59
      powered craft V93.53
        ferry boat V93.51
        fishing boat V93.52
        jet ski V93.53
        liner V93.51
        merchant ship V93.50
        passenger ship V93.51
        sailboat V93.54
  letter bomb W40.8
    assault X96.2
    homicide (attempt) X96.2
    suicide (attempt) X75
  machinery —*see also* Contact, with, by type of machine
    on board watercraft —*see* Explosion, in, watercraft
    pressure vessel —*see* Explosion, by type of vessel
  methane W40.1
  mine W40.1
  missile NEC W40.8
  mortar bomb W40.8
    in
      assault X96.8
      homicide (attempt) X96.8
      legal intervention
        injuring
          bystander Y35.192
          law enforcement personnel Y35.191
          suspect Y35.193
          unspecified person Y35.199
      suicide (attempt) X75
  munitions (dump) (factory) W40.8
  pipe, pressurized W37.8
    bomb W40.8
      assault X96.4
      homicide (attempt) X96.4
      suicide (attempt) X75
  pressure, pressurized
    cooker W38
    gas tank (in machinery) W36.3
    hose W37.8
    pipe W37.8
    specified device NEC W38
    tire W37.8
      bicycle W37.0
    vessel (in machinery) W38
  propane W40.1
  self-inflicted X75
  shell (artillery) NEC W40.8
    during war operations —*see* War operations, explosion
    in
      legal intervention
        injuring
          bystander Y35.122
          law enforcement personnel Y35.121
          suspect Y35.123
          unspecified person Y35.129
    war —*see* War operations, explosion
  spacecraft V95.45
  stated as undetermined whether accidental or intentional Y25
  steam or water lines (in machinery) W37.8
  stove W40.9
  suicide (attempt) X75

Explosion (Continued)
 tire, pressurized W37.8
  bicycle W37.0
 undetermined whether accidental or
   intentional Y25
 vehicle tire NEC W37.8
  bicycle W37.0
 war operations —see War operations,
   explosion

Exposure (to) X58
 air pressure change —see Air, pressure
 cold (accidental) (excessive) (extreme)
   (natural) (place) X31
  assault Y08.89
  due to
   man-made conditions W93.8
    dry ice (contact) W93.01
     inhalation W93.02
    liquid air (contact) (hydrogen)
      (nitrogen) W93.11
     inhalation W93.12
    refrigeration unit (deep freeze)
      W93.2
   suicide (attempt) X83.2
   weather (conditions) X31
  homicide (attempt) Y08.89
  self-inflicted X83.2
 due to abandonment or neglect X58
 electric current W86.8
  appliance (faulty) W86.8
   domestic W86.0
  caused by other person Y08.89
  conductor (faulty) W86.1
  control apparatus (faulty) W86.1
  electric power generating plant,
    distribution station W86.1
  electroshock gun —see Exposure, electric
    current, taser
  high-voltage cable W85
  homicide (attempt) Y08.89
  legal execution —see Legal, intervention,
    specified means NEC
  lightning —see subcategory T75.0
  live rail W86.8
  misadventure in medical or surgical
    procedure in electroshock therapy
    Y63.4
  motor (electric) (faulty) W86.8
   domestic W86.0
  self-inflicted X83.1
  specified NEC W86.8
   domestic W86.0
  stun gun —see Exposure, electric current,
    taser
  suicide (attempt) X83.1
  taser W86.8
   assault Y08.89
   legal intervention —see category Y35
   self-harm (intentional) X83.8
   undetermined intent Y33
  third rail W86.8
  transformer (faulty) W86.1
  transmission lines W85
 environmental tobacco smoke X58
 excessive
  cold —see Exposure, cold
  heat (natural) NEC X30
   man-made W92
 factor(s) NOS X58
  environmental NEC X58
   man-made NEC W99
  natural NEC —see Forces of nature
  specified NEC X58
 fire, flames (accidental) X08.8
  assault X97
  campfire —see Exposure, fire, controlled,
    not in building
  controlled (in)
   with ignition (of) clothing —see also
     Ignition, clothes X06.2
    nightwear X05

Exposure (Continued)
 fire, flames (Continued)
  controlled (Continued)
   bonfire —see Exposure, fire, controlled,
     not in building
   brazier (in building or structure) —see
     also Exposure, fire, controlled,
     building
    not in building or structure —see
      Exposure, fire, controlled, not in
      building
   building or structure X02.0
    with
     fall from building X02.3
     from building X02.5
     injury due to building collapse
       X02.2
     smoke inhalation X02.1
    hit by object from building X02.4
    specified mode of injury NEC X02.8
   fireplace, furnace or stove —see
     Exposure, fire, controlled, building
   not in building or structure X03.0
    with
     fall X03.3
     smoke inhalation X03.1
    hit by object X03.4
    specified mode of injury NEC X03.8
   trash —see Exposure, fire, controlled, not
     in building
  fireplace —see Exposure, fire, controlled,
    building
  fittings or furniture (in building or
    structure) (uncontrolled) —see
    Exposure, fire, uncontrolled, building
  forest (uncontrolled) —see Exposure, fire,
    uncontrolled, not in building
  grass (uncontrolled) —see Exposure, fire,
    uncontrolled, not in building
  hay (uncontrolled) —see Exposure, fire,
    uncontrolled, not in building
  homicide (attempt) X97
  ignition of highly flammable material X04
  in, of, on, starting in
   machinery —see Contact, with, by type
     of machine
   motor vehicle (in motion) —see also
     Accident, transport, occupant by
     type of vehicle V87.8
    with collision —see Collision
   railway rolling stock, train, vehicle
     V81.81
    with collision —see Accident,
      transport, railway vehicle
      occupant
   street car (in motion) V82.8
    with collision —see Accident,
      transport, streetcar occupant
   transport vehicle NEC —see also
     Accident, transport
    with collision —see Collision
   war operations —see also War operations,
     fire
    from nuclear explosion —see War
      operations, nuclear weapons
   watercraft (in transit) (not in transit)
     V91.09
    localized —see Burn, on board
      watercraft, due to, fire on board
    powered craft V91.03
     ferry boat V91.01
     fishing boat V91.02
     jet skis V91.03
     liner V91.01
     merchant ship V91.00
     passenger ship V91.01
    unpowered craft V91.08
     canoe V91.05
     inflatable V91.06
     kayak V91.05
     sailboat V91.04

Exposure (Continued)
 fire, flames (Continued)
  in, of, on, starting in (Continued)
   watercraft (Continued)
    unpowered craft (Continued)
     surf-board V91.08
     waterskis V91.07
     windsurfer V91.08
  lumber (uncontrolled) —see Exposure, fire,
    uncontrolled, not in building
  mine (uncontrolled) —see Exposure, fire,
    uncontrolled, not in building
  prairie (uncontrolled) —see Exposure, fire,
    uncontrolled, not in building
  resulting from
   explosion —see Explosion
   lightning X08.8
  self-inflicted X76
  specified NEC X08.8
  started by other person X97
  stated as undetermined whether accidental
    or intentional Y26
  stove —see Exposure, fire, controlled,
    building
  suicide (attempt) X76
  tunnel (uncontrolled) —see Exposure, fire,
    uncontrolled, not in building
  uncontrolled
   in building or structure X00.0
    with
     fall from building X00.3
     injury due to building collapse
       X00.2
     jump from building X00.5
     smoke inhalation X00.1
    bed X08.00
     due to
      cigarette X08.01
      specified material NEC X08.09
    furniture NEC X08.20
     due to
      cigarette X08.21
      specified material NEC X08.29
    hit by object from building X00.4
    sofa X08.10
     due to
      cigarette X08.11
      specified material NEC
        X08.19
    specified mode of injury NEC
      X00.8
   not in building or structure (any)
     X01.0
    with
     fall X01.3
     smoke inhalation X01.1
    hit by object X01.4
    specified mode of injury NEC
      X01.8
  undetermined whether accidental or
    intentional Y26
 forces of nature NEC —see Forces of nature
 G-forces (abnormal) W49.9
 gravitational forces (abnormal) W49.9
 heat (natural) NEC —see Heat
 high-pressure jet (hydraulic) (pneumatic)
   W49.9
 hydraulic jet W49.9
 inanimate mechanical force W49.9
 jet, high-pressure (hydraulic) (pneumatic)
   W49.9
 lightning —see subcategory T75.0
  causing fire —see Exposure, fire
 mechanical forces NEC W49.9
  animate NEC W64
  inanimate NEC W49.9
 noise W42.9
  supersonic W42.0
 noxious substance —see Table of Drugs and
   Chemicals
 pneumatic jet W49.9

▶ New   ➡ Revised   ~~deleted~~ Deleted   ● Use Additional Character(s)

Exposure *(Continued)*
    prolonged in deep-freeze unit or refrigerator W93.2
    radiation —*see* Radiation
    smoke —*see also* Exposure, fire
        tobacco, second hand Z77.22
    specified factors NEC X58
    sunlight X32
        man-made (sun lamp) W89.8
            tanning bed W89.1
    supersonic waves W42.0
    transmission line(s), electric W85
    vibration W49.9

Exposure *(Continued)*
    waves
        infrasound W49.9
        sound W42.9
        supersonic W42.0
    weather NEC —*see* Forces of nature
External cause status Y99.9
    child assisting in compensated work for family Y99.8
    civilian activity done for financial or other compensation Y99.0
    civilian activity done for income or pay Y99.0

External cause status *(Continued)*
    family member assisting in compensated work for other family member Y99.8
    hobby not done for income Y99.8
    leisure activity Y99.8
    military activity Y99.1
    off-duty activity of military personnel Y99.8
    recreation or sport not for income or while a student Y99.8
    specified NEC Y99.8
    student activity Y99.8
    volunteer activity Y99.2

F

Factors, supplemental
  alcohol
    blood level
      less than 20mg/100ml Y90.0
      presence in blood, level not specified
        Y90.9
      20-39mg/100ml Y90.1
      40-59mg/100ml Y90.2
      60-79mg/100ml Y90.3
      80-99mg/100ml Y90.4
      100-119mg/100ml Y90.5
      120-199mg/100ml Y90.6
      200-239mg/100ml Y90.7
      240mg/100ml or more Y90.8
      presence in blood, but level not specified
        Y90.9
  environmental-pollution-related condition —
    see Z57
  nosocomial condition Y95
  work-related condition Y99.0

Failure
  in suture or ligature during surgical
    procedure Y65.2
  mechanical, of instrument or apparatus
    (any) (during any medical or surgical
    procedure) Y65.8
  sterile precautions (during medical and
    surgical care) —see Misadventure,
    failure, sterile precautions, by type of
    procedure
  to
    introduce tube or instrument Y65.4
      endotracheal tube during anesthesia Y65.3
    make curve (transport vehicle) NEC —see
      Accident, transport
    remove tube or instrument Y65.4

Fall, falling (accidental) W19
  building W20.1
    burning (uncontrolled fire) X00.3
  down
    embankment W17.81
    escalator W10.0
    hill W17.81
    ladder W11
    ramp W10.2
    stairs, steps W10.9
  due to
    bumping against
      object W18.00
        sharp glass W18.02
        specified NEC W18.09
        sports equipment W18.01
      person W03
        due to ice or snow W00.0
        on pedestrian conveyance —see
          Accident, transport, pedestrian,
          conveyance
    collision with another person W03
      due to ice or snow W00.0
      involving pedestrian conveyance —see
        Accident, transport, pedestrian,
        conveyance
    grocery cart tipping over W17.82
    ice or snow W00.9
      from one level to another W00.2
        on stairs or steps W00.1
      involving pedestrian conveyance —see
        Accident, transport, pedestrian,
        conveyance
      on same level W00.0
    slipping (on moving sidewalk) W01.0
      with subsequent striking against object
        W01.10
        furniture W01.190
        sharp object W01.119
          glass W01.110
          power tool or machine W01.111
          specified NEC W01.118
        specified NEC W01.198

Fall, falling (Continued)
  due to (Continued)
    striking against
      object W18.00
        sharp glass W18.02
        specified NEC W18.09
        sports equipment W18.01
      person W03
        due to ice or snow W00.0
        on pedestrian conveyance —see
          Accident, transport, pedestrian,
          conveyance
  earth (with asphyxia or suffocation (by
    pressure)) —see Earth, falling
  from, off, out of
    aircraft NEC (with accident to aircraft
      NEC) V97.0
      while boarding or alighting V97.1
    balcony W13.0
    bed W06
    boat, ship, watercraft NEC (with drowning
      or submersion) —see Drowning, due
      to, fall overboard
      with hitting bottom or object V94.0
    bridge W13.1
    building W13.9
      burning (uncontrolled fire) X00.3
    cavity W17.2
    chair W07
    cherry picker W17.89
    cliff W15
    dock W17.4
    embankment W17.81
    escalator W10.0
    flagpole W13.8
    furniture NEC W08
    grocery cart W17.82
    haystack W17.89
    high place NEC W17.89
      stated as undetermined whether
        accidental or intentional Y30
    hole W17.2
    incline W10.2
    ladder W11
    lifting device W17.89
    machine, machinery —see also Contact,
      with, by type of machine
      not in operation W17.89
    manhole W17.1
    mobile elevated work platform [MEWP]
      W17.89
    motorized mobility scooter W05.2
    one level to another NEC W17.89
      intentional, purposeful, suicide
        (attempt) X80
      stated as undetermined whether
        accidental or intentional Y30
    pit W17.2
    playground equipment W09.8
      jungle gym W09.2
      slide W09.0
      swing W09.1
    quarry W17.89
    railing W13.9
    ramp W10.2
    roof W13.2
    scaffolding W12
    scooter (nonmotorized) W05.1
      motorized mobility W05.2
    sky lift W17.89
    stairs, steps W10.9
      curb W10.1
      due to ice or snow W00.1
      escalator W10.0
      incline W10.2
      ramp W10.2
      sidewalk curb W10.1
      specified NEC W10.8
    Standing
      electric scooter V00.841
      micro-mobility pedestrian conveyance
        V00.848

Fall, falling (Continued)
  from, off, out of (Continued)
    stepladder W11
    ▶ stool W08
    storm drain W17.1
    streetcar NEC V82.6
      with antecedent collision —see
        Accident, transport, streetcar
        occupant
      while boarding or alighting V82.4
    structure NEC W13.8
      burning (uncontrolled fire) X00.3
    table W08
    toilet W18.11
      with subsequent striking against object
        W18.12
    train NEC V81.6
      during derailment (without antecedent
        collision) V81.7
        with antecedent collision —see
          Accident, transport, railway
          vehicle occupant
      while boarding or alighting V81.4
    transport vehicle after collision —see
      Accident, transport, by type of
      vehicle, collision
    tree W14
    vehicle (in motion) NEC —see also
      Accident, transport V89.9
      motor NEC —see also Accident,
        transport, occupant, by type of
        vehicle V87.8
      stationary W17.89
        while boarding or alighting —see
          Accident, transport, by type of
          vehicle, while boarding or
          alighting
    viaduct W13.8
    wall W13.8
    watercraft —see also Drowning, due to, fall
      overboard
      with hitting bottom or object V94.0
    well W17.0
    wheelchair, non-moving W05.0
      powered —see Accident, transport,
        pedestrian, conveyance occupant,
        specified type NEC
    window W13.4
  in, on
    aircraft NEC V97.0
      with accident to aircraft V97.0
      while boarding or alighting V97.1
    bathtub (empty) W18.2
      filled W16.212
        causing drowning W16.211
    escalator W10.0
    incline W10.2
    ladder W11
    machine, machinery —see Contact, with,
      by type of machine
    object, edged, pointed or sharp (with
      cut) —see Fall, by type
    playground equipment W09.8
      jungle gym W09.2
      slide W09.0
      swing W09.1
    ramp W10.2
    scaffolding W12
    shower W18.2
      causing drowning W16.211
    staircase, stairs, steps W10.9
      curb W10.1
      due to ice or snow W00.1
      escalator W10.0
      incline W10.2
      specified NEC W10.8
    streetcar (without antecedent collision)
      V82.5
      with antecedent collision —see Accident,
        transport, streetcar occupant
      while boarding or alighting V82.4

▶ New   ⇒ Revised   ~~deleted~~ Deleted   ● Use Additional Character(s)

Fall, falling (Continued)
in, on (Continued)
 train (without antecedent collision) V81.5
  with antecedent collision —see Accident,
   transport, railway vehicle occupant
  during derailment (without antecedent
   collision) V81.7
   with antecedent collision —see
    Accident, transport, railway
    vehicle occupant
  while boarding or alighting V81.4
 transport vehicle after collision —see
  Accident, transport, by type of
  vehicle, collision
 watercraft V93.39
  due to
   accident to craft V91.29
    powered craft V91.23
     ferry boat V91.21
     fishing boat V91.22
     jet ski V91.23
     liner V91.21
     merchant ship V91.20
     passenger ship V91.21
    unpowered craft
     canoe V91.25
     inflatable V91.26
     kayak V91.25
     sailboat V91.24
   powered craft V93.33
    ferry boat V93.31
    fishing boat V93.32
    jet ski V93.33
    liner V93.31
    merchant ship V93.30
    passenger ship V93.31
   unpowered craft V93.38
    canoe V93.35
    inflatable V93.36
    kayak V93.35
    sailboat V93.34
    surf-board V93.38
    windsurfer V93.38
into
 cavity W17.2
 dock W17.4
 fire —see Exposure, fire, by type
 haystack W17.89
 hole W17.2
 manhole W17.1
 moving part of machinery —see Contact,
  with, by type of machine
 ocean —see Fall, into, water
 opening in surface NEC W17.89
 pit W17.2
 pond —see Fall, into, water
 quarry W17.89
 river —see Fall, into, water
 shaft W17.89
 storm drain W17.1
 stream —see Fall, into, water
 swimming pool —see also Fall, into, water,
  in, swimming pool
  empty W17.3
 tank W17.89
 water W16.42
  causing drowning W16.41
  from watercraft —see Drowning, due to,
   fall overboard
  hitting diving board W21.4
  in
   bathtub W16.212
    causing drowning W16.211
   bucket W16.222
    causing drowning W16.221
   natural body of water W16.112
    causing drowning W16.111
    striking
     bottom W16.122
      causing drowning
       W16.121

Fall, falling (Continued)
into (Continued)
 water (Continued)
  in (Continued)
   natural body of water (Continued)
    striking (Continued)
     side W16.132
      causing drowning W16.131
   specified water NEC W16.312
    causing drowning W16.311
    striking
     bottom W16.322
      causing drowning W16.321
     wall W16.332
      causing drowning W16.331
   swimming pool W16.012
    causing drowning W16.011
    striking
     bottom W16.022
      causing drowning W16.021
     wall W16.032
      causing drowning W16.031
   utility bucket W16.222
    causing drowning W16.221
 well W17.0
involving
 bed W06
 chair W07
 furniture NEC W08
 glass —see Fall, by type
 playground equipment W09.8
  jungle gym W09.2
  slide W09.0
  swing W09.1
 roller blades —see Accident, transport,
  pedestrian, conveyance
 skateboard(s) —see Accident, transport,
  pedestrian, conveyance
 skates (ice) (in line) (roller) —see
  Accident, transport, pedestrian,
  conveyance
 skis —see Accident, transport, pedestrian,
  conveyance
 table W08
 wheelchair, non-moving W05.0
  powered —see Accident, transport,
   pedestrian, conveyance, specified
   type NEC
object —see Struck by, object, falling
off
 toilet W18.11
  with subsequent striking against object
   W18.12
on same level W18.30
 due to
  specified NEC W18.39
  stepping on an object W18.31
out of
 bed W06
 building NEC W13.8
 chair W07
 furniture NEC W08
 wheelchair, non-moving W05.0
  powered —see Accident, transport,
   pedestrian, conveyance, specified
   type NEC
 window W13.4
over
 animal W01.0
 cliff W15
 embankment W17.81
 small object W01.0
rock W20.8
same level W18.30
 from
  being crushed, pushed, or stepped on
   by a crowd or human stampede
   W52
  collision, pushing, shoving, by or with
   other person W03
  slipping, stumbling, tripping W01.0

Fall, falling (Continued)
same level (Continued)
 involving ice or snow W00.0
  involving skates (ice) (roller),
   skateboard, skis —see Accident,
   transport, pedestrian, conveyance
snowslide (avalanche) —see Landslide
stone W20.8
structure W20.1
 burning (uncontrolled fire) X00.3
through
 bridge W13.1
 floor W13.3
 roof W13.2
 wall W13.8
 window W13.4
timber W20.8
tree (caused by lightning) W20.8
while being carried or supported by other
 person(s) W04
Fallen on by
 animal (not being ridden) NEC W55.89
Felo-de-se —see Suicide
Fight (hand) (fists) (foot) —see Assault, fight
Fire (accidental) —see Exposure, fire
Firearm discharge —see Discharge, firearm
Fireball effects from nuclear explosion in war
 operations —see War operations, nuclear
 weapons
Fireworks (explosion) W39
Flash burns from explosion —see Explosion
Flood (any injury) (caused by) X38
 collapse of man-made structure causing earth
  movement X36.0
 tidal wave —see Forces of nature, tidal wave
Food (any type) in
 air passages (with asphyxia, obstruction, or
  suffocation) —see categories T17 and T18
 alimentary tract causing asphyxia (due to
  compression of trachea) —see categories
  T17 and T18
Forces of nature X39.8
 avalanche X36.1
  causing transport accident —see Accident,
   transport, by type of vehicle
 blizzard X37.2
 cataclysmic storm X37.9
  with flood X38
  blizzard X37.2
  cloudburst X37.8
  cyclone X37.1
  dust storm X37.3
  hurricane X37.0
  specified storm NEC X37.8
  storm surge X37.0
  tornado X37.1
  twister X37.1
  typhoon X37.0
 cloudburst X37.8
 cold (natural) X31
 cyclone X37.1
 dam collapse causing earth movement X36.0
 dust storm X37.3
 earth movement X36.1
  caused by dam or structure collapse X36.0
  earthquake X34
 earthquake X34
 flood (caused by) X38
  dam collapse X36.0
  tidal wave —see Forces of nature, tidal
   wave
 heat (natural) X30
 hurricane X37.0
 landslide X36.1
  causing transport accident —see Accident,
   transport, by type of vehicle
 lightning —see subcategory T75.0
  causing fire —see Exposure, fire
 mudslide X36.1
  causing transport accident —see Accident,
   transport, by type of vehicle

Forces of nature *(Continued)*
  radiation (natural) X39.08
    radon X39.01
  radon X39.01
  specified force NEC X39.8
  storm surge X37.0
  structure collapse causing
    earth movement
    X36.0
  sunlight X32
  tidal wave X37.41
    due to
      earthquake X37.41
      landslide X37.43
      storm X37.42
      volcanic eruption X37.41
  tornado X37.1

Forces of nature *(Continued)*
  tsunami X37.41
  twister X37.1
  typhoon X37.0
  volcanic eruption X35
Foreign body
  aspiration —*see* Index to Diseases and
    Injuries, Foreign body, respitory
    tract
  embedded in skin W45
  entering through skin W45.8
    can lid W26.2
    nail W45.0
    paper W26.2
    specified NEC 45.8
    splinter W45.8

Forest fire (exposure to) —*see* Exposure, fire,
  uncontrolled, not in building
Found injured X58
  from exposure (to) —*see* Exposure
  on
    highway, road(way), street V89.9
    railway right of way V81.9
Fracture (circumstances unknown or
  unspecified) X58
  due to specified cause NEC X58
Freezing —*see* Exposure, cold
Frostbite X31
  due to man-made conditions —*see* Exposure,
    cold, man-made
Frozen —*see* Exposure, cold

G

Gored by bull W55.22
Gunshot wound W34.00

H

Hailstones, injured by X39.8
Hanged herself or himself —*see* Hanging,
  self-inflicted
Hanging (accidental) —*see also* category T71
  legal execution —*see* Legal, intervention,
    specified means NEC
Heat (effects of) (excessive) X30
  due to
    man-made conditions W92
      on board watercraft V93.29
        fishing boat V93.22
        merchant ship V93.20
        passenger ship V93.21
        sailboat V93.24
        specified powered craft NEC V93.23
    weather (conditions) X30

Heat *(Continued)*
  from
    electric heating apparatus causing
      burning X16
    nuclear explosion in war operations —
      see War operations, nuclear
      weapons
  inappropriate in local application or
    packing in medical or surgical
    procedure Y63.5
Hemorrhage
  delayed following medical or surgical
    treatment without mention of
    misadventure —*see* Index to Diseases
    and Injuries, Complication(s)
  during medical or surgical treatment as
    misadventure —*see* Index to Diseases
    and Injuries, Complication(s)

High
  altitude (effects) —*see* Air, pressure, low
  level of radioactivity, effects —*see* Radiation
  pressure (effects) —*see* Air, pressure, high
  temperature, effects —*see* Heat
Hit, hitting (accidental) by —*see* Struck by
Hitting against —*see* Striking against
Homicide (attempt) (justifiable) —*see* Assault
Hot
  place, effects —*see also* Heat
  weather, effects X30
House fire (uncontrolled) —*see* Exposure, fire,
  uncontrolled, building
Humidity, causing problem X39.8
Hunger X58
Hurricane (any injury) X37.0
Hypobarism, hypobaropathy —*see* Air,
  pressure, low

▶ New   ⇒ Revised   ~~deleted~~ Deleted   ● Use Additional Character(s)

F, G, & H

I

Ictus
  caloris —*see also* Heat
  solaris X30
Ignition (accidental) —*see also* Exposure, fire
    X08.8
  anesthetic gas in operating room W40.1
  apparel X06.2
    from highly flammable material X04
    nightwear X05
  bed linen (sheets) (spreads) (pillows)
    (mattress) —*see* Exposure, fire,
    uncontrolled, building, bed
  benzine X04
  clothes, clothing NEC (from controlled fire)
    X06.2
    from
      highly flammable material X04
  ether X04
    in operating room W40.1
  explosive material —*see* Explosion
  gasoline X04
  jewelry (plastic) (any) X06.0
  kerosene X04
  material
    explosive —*see* Explosion
    highly flammable with secondary
      explosion X04
  nightwear X05
  paraffin X04
  petrol X04
Immersion (accidental) —*see also* Drowning
  hand or foot due to cold (excessive) X31
Implantation of quills of porcupine W55.89
Inanition (from) (hunger) X58
  thirst X58.8
Inappropriate operation performed
  correct operation on wrong side or body part
    (wrong side) (wrong site) Y65.53
  operation intended for another patient done
    on wrong patient Y65.52
  wrong operation performed on correct
    patient Y65.51
Inattention after, at birth (homicidal intent)
    (infanticidal intent) X58
Incident, adverse
  device
    anesthesiology Y70.8
      accessory Y70.2
      diagnostic Y70.0
      miscellaneous Y70.8
      monitoring Y70.0
      prosthetic Y70.2
      rehabilitative Y70.1
      surgical Y70.3
      therapeutic Y70.1
    cardiovascular Y71.8
      accessory Y71.2
      diagnostic Y71.0
      miscellaneous Y71.8
      monitoring Y71.0
      prosthetic Y71.2
      rehabilitative Y71.1
      surgical Y71.3
      therapeutic Y71.1
    gastroenterology Y73.8
      accessory Y73.2
      diagnostic Y73.0
      miscellaneous Y73.8
      monitoring Y73.0
      prosthetic Y73.2
      rehabilitative Y73.1
      surgical Y73.3
      therapeutic Y73.1
    general
      hospital Y74.8
        accessory Y74.2
        diagnostic Y74.0
        miscellaneous Y74.8
        monitoring Y74.0

Incident, adverse (Continued)
  device (Continued)
    general (Continued)
      hospital (Continued)
        prosthetic Y74.2
        rehabilitative Y74.1
        surgical Y74.3
        therapeutic Y74.1
      surgical Y81.8
        accessory Y81.2
        diagnostic Y81.0
        miscellaneous Y81.8
        monitoring Y81.0
        prosthetic Y81.2
        rehabilitative Y81.1
        surgical Y81.3
        therapeutic Y81.1
    gynecological Y76.8
      accessory Y76.2
      diagnostic Y76.0
      miscellaneous Y76.8
      monitoring Y76.0
      prosthetic Y76.2
      rehabilitative Y76.1
      surgical Y76.3
      therapeutic Y76.1
    medical Y82.9
      specified type NEC Y82.8
    neurological Y75.8
      accessory Y75.2
      diagnostic Y75.0
      miscellaneous Y75.8
      monitoring Y75.0
      prosthetic Y75.2
      rehabilitative Y75.1
      surgical Y75.3
      therapeutic Y75.1
    obstetrical Y76.8
      accessory Y76.2
      diagnostic Y76.0
      miscellaneous Y76.8
      monitoring Y76.0
      prosthetic Y76.2
      rehabilitative Y76.1
      surgical Y76.3
      therapeutic Y76.1
    ophthalmic Y77.8
      accessory Y77.2
      contact lens (rigid gas permeable)
        (soft) (hydrophilic)) Y77.11
      diagnostic Y77.0
      miscellaneous Y77.8
      monitoring Y77.0
      prosthetic Y77.2
      rehabilitative Y77.19
      surgical Y77.3
      therapeutic Y77.19
    orthopedic Y79.8
      accessory Y79.2
      diagnostic Y79.0
      miscellaneous Y79.8
      monitoring Y79.0
      prosthetic Y79.2
      rehabilitative Y79.1
      surgical Y79.3
      therapeutic Y79.1
    otorhinolaryngological Y72.8
      accessory Y72.2
      diagnostic Y72.0
      miscellaneous Y72.8
      monitoring Y72.0
      prosthetic Y72.2
      rehabilitative Y72.1
      surgical Y72.3
      therapeutic Y72.1
    personal use Y74.8
      accessory Y74.2
      diagnostic Y74.0
      miscellaneous Y74.8
      monitoring Y74.0
      prosthetic Y74.2

Incident, adverse (Continued)
  device (Continued)
    personal use (Continued)
      rehabilitative Y74.1
      surgical Y74.3
      therapeutic Y74.1
    physical medicine Y80.8
      accessory Y80.2
      diagnostic Y80.0
      miscellaneous Y80.8
      monitoring Y80.0
      prosthetic Y80.2
      rehabilitative Y80.1
      surgical Y80.3
      therapeutic Y80.1
    plastic surgical Y81.8
      accessory Y81.2
      diagnostic Y81.0
      miscellaneous Y81.8
      monitoring Y81.0
      prosthetic Y81.2
      rehabilitative Y81.1
      surgical Y81.3
      therapeutic Y81.1
    radiological Y78.8
      accessory Y78.2
      diagnostic Y78.0
      miscellaneous Y78.8
      monitoring Y78.0
      prosthetic Y78.2
      rehabilitative Y78.1
      surgical Y78.3
      therapeutic Y78.1
    urology Y73.8
      accessory Y73.2
      diagnostic Y73.0
      miscellaneous Y73.8
      monitoring Y73.0
      prosthetic Y73.2
      rehabilitative Y73.1
      surgical Y73.3
      therapeutic Y73.1
Incineration (accidental) —*see* Exposure, fire
Infanticide —*see* Assault
Infrasound waves (causing injury) W49.9
Ingestion
  foreign body (causing injury) (with
    obstruction) —*see* Foreign body,
    alimentary canal
  poisonous
    plant(s) X58
    substance NEC —*see* Table of Drugs and
      Chemicals
Inhalation
  excessively cold substance, man-made —*see*
    Exposure, cold, man-made
  food (any type) (into respiratory tract) (with
    asphyxia, obstruction respiratory tract,
    suffocation) —*see* categories T17 and T18
  foreign body —*see* Foreign body, aspiration
  gastric contents (with asphyxia, obstruction
    respiratory passage, suffocation) T17.81-●
  hot air or gases X14.0
  liquid air, hydrogen, nitrogen W93.12
    suicide (attempt) X83.2
  steam X13.0
    assault X98.0
    stated as undetermined whether accidental
      or intentional Y27.0
    suicide (attempt) X77.0
  toxic gas —*see* Table of Drugs and
    Chemicals
  vomitus (with asphyxia, obstruction
    respiratory passage, suffocation) T17.81-●
Injury, injured (accidental(ly)) NOS X58
  by, caused by, from
    assault —*see* Assault
    law-enforcing agent, police, in course
      of legal intervention —*see* Legal
      intervention
    suicide (attempt) X83.8

Injury, injured NOS *(Continued)*
 due to, in
  civil insurrection —*see* War
   operations
  fight —*see also* Assault, fight
   Y04.0
  war operations —*see* War
   operations
 homicide —*see also* Assault Y09
 inflicted (by)
  in course of arrest (attempted), suppression
   of disturbance, maintenance of order,
   by law-enforcing agents —*see* Legal
   intervention

Injury, injured NOS *(Continued)*
 inflicted *(Continued)*
  other person
   stated as
    accidental X58
    intentional, homicide (attempt) —*see*
     Assault
    undetermined whether accidental or
     intentional Y33
  purposely (inflicted) by other person(s) —*see*
   Assault
  self-inflicted X83.8
   stated as accidental X58
  specified cause NEC X58

Injury, injured NOS *(Continued)*
 undetermined whether accidental or
  intentional Y33
Insolation, effects X30
Insufficient nourishment X58
Interruption of respiration (by)
 food (lodged in esophagus) —*see* categories
  T17 and T18
 vomitus (lodged in esophagus) T17.81-●
Intervention, legal —*see* Legal intervention
Intoxication
 drug —*see* Table of Drugs and Chemicals
 poison —*see* Table of Drugs and
  Chemicals

J

Jammed (accidentally)
 between objects (moving) (stationary and
  moving) W23.0
 stationary W23.1
Jumped, jumping
 before moving object NEC X81.8
  motor vehicle X81.0
  subway train X81.1
  train X81.1
  undetermined whether accidental or
   intentional Y31
 from
  boat (into water) voluntarily,
   without accident (to or on boat)
   W16.712
   with
    accident to or on boat —*see* Accident,
     watercraft
    drowning or submersion W16.711
     suicide (attempt) X71.3

Jumped, jumping *(Continued)*
 from *(Continued)*
  boat voluntarily, without accident
   (Continued)
   striking bottom W16.722
    causing drowning W16.721
  building —*see also* Jumped, from,
   high place W13.9
   burning (uncontrolled fire)
    X00.5
  high place NEC W17.89
   suicide (attempt) X80
   undetermined whether accidental or
    intentional Y30
  structure —*see also* Jumped, from, high
   place W13.9
   burning (uncontrolled fire)
    X00.5
 into water W16.92
  causing drowning W16.91
  from, off watercraft —*see* Jumped, from,
   boat

Jumped, jumping *(Continued)*
 into water *(Continued)*
  in
   natural body W16.612
    causing drowning W16.611
    striking bottom W16.622
     causing drowning W16.621
   specified place NEC W16.812
    causing drowning W16.811
    striking
     bottom W16.822
      causing drowning W16.821
     wall W16.832
      causing drowning W16.831
   swimming pool W16.512
    causing drowning W16.511
    striking
     bottom W16.522
      causing drowning W16.521
     wall W16.532
      causing drowning W16.531
  suicide (attempt) X71.3

K

Kicked by
 animal NEC W55.82
 person(s) (accidentally) W50.1
  with intent to injure or kill Y04.0
  as, or caused by, a crowd or human
   stampede (with fall) W52
  assault Y04.0
  homicide (attempt) Y04.0
  in
   fight Y04.0
   legal intervention
    injuring
     bystander Y35.812
     law enforcement personnel
      Y35.811
     suspect Y35.813
     unspecified person Y35.819

Kicking
 against
  object W22.8
   sports equipment W21.9
   stationary W22.09
    sports equipment W21.89
  person —*see* Striking against, person
  sports equipment W21.9
 carpet stretcher with knee X50.3
Killed, killing (accidentally) NOS —*see also*
 Injury X58
 in
  action —*see* War operations
  brawl, fight (hand) (fists) (foot) Y04.0
   by weapon —*see also* Assault
    cutting, piercing —*see* Assault, cutting
     or piercing instrument
    firearm —*see* Discharge, firearm, by
     type, homicide

Killed, killing NOS *(Continued)*
 self
  stated as
   accident NOS X58
   suicide —*see* Suicide
   undetermined whether accidental or
    intentional Y33
Kneeling (prolonged) (static) X50.1
Knocked down (accidentally) (by) NOS X58
 animal (not being ridden) NEC —*see also*
  Struck by, by type of animal
 crowd or human stampede W52
 person W51
  in brawl, fight Y04.0
 transport vehicle NEC —*see also* Accident,
  transport V09.9

▶ New   ⇒ Revised   ~~deleted~~ Deleted   ● Use Additional Character(s)

L

Laceration NEC —*see* Injury
Lack of
  care (helpless person) (infant) (newborn) X58
  food except as result of abandonment or
    neglect X58
    due to abandonment or neglect X58
  water except as result of transport accident
    X58
    due to transport accident —*see* Accident,
      transport, by type
  helpless person, infant, newborn X58
Landslide (falling on transport vehicle) X36.1
  caused by collapse of man-made structure
    X36.0
Late effect —*see* Sequelae
Legal
  execution (any method) —*see* Legal,
    intervention
  intervention (by)
    baton —*see* Legal, intervention, blunt
      object, baton
    bayonet —*see* Legal, intervention, sharp
      object, bayonet
    blow —*see* Legal, intervention,
      manhandling
    blunt object
      baton
        injuring
          bystander Y35.312
          law enforcement personnel Y35.311
          suspect Y35.313
          unspecified person Y35.319
      injuring
        bystander Y35.302
        law enforcement personnel Y35.301
        suspect Y35.303
        unspecified person Y35.309
      specified NEC
        injuring
          bystander Y35.392
          law enforcement personnel Y35.391
          suspect Y35.393
          unspecified person Y35.399
      stave
        injuring
          bystander Y35.392
          law enforcement personnel Y35.391
          suspect Y35.393
          unspecified person Y35.399
    bomb —*see* Legal, intervention, explosive
    conducted energy device
      injuring
        bystander Y35.832
        law enforcement personnel Y35.831
        suspect Y35.833
        unspecified person Y35.839
    cutting or piercing instrument —*see* Legal,
      intervention, sharp object
    dynamite —*see* Legal, intervention,
      explosive, dynamite
    electroshock device (taser)
      injuring
        bystander Y35.832
        law enforcement personnel Y35.831
        suspect Y35.833
        unspecified person Y35.839
    explosive(s)
      dynamite
        injuring
          bystander Y35.112
          law enforcement personnel Y35.111
          suspect Y35.113
          unspecified person Y35.119
      grenade
        injuring
          bystander Y35.192
          law enforcement personnel Y35.191
          suspect Y35.193
          unspecified person Y35.199

Legal *(Continued)*
  intervention *(Continued)*
    explosive *(Continued)*
      injuring
        bystander Y35.102
        law enforcement personnel Y35.101
        suspect Y35.103
        unspecified person Y35.109
      mortar bomb
        injuring
          bystander Y35.192
          law enforcement personnel Y35.191
          suspect Y35.193
          unspecified person Y35.199
      shell
        injuring
          bystander Y35.122
          law enforcement personnel Y35.121
          suspect Y35.123
          unspecified person Y35.129
      specified NEC
        injuring
          bystander Y35.192
          law enforcement personnel Y35.191
          suspect Y35.193
          unspecified person Y35.199
    firearm(s) (discharge)
      handgun
        injuring
          bystander Y35.022
          law enforcement personnel Y35.021
          suspect Y35.023
          unspecified person Y35.029
      injuring
        bystander Y35.002
        law enforcement personnel Y35.001
        suspect Y35.003
        unspecified person Y35.009
      machine gun
        injuring
          bystander Y35.012
          law enforcement personnel Y35.011
          suspect Y35.013
          unspecified person Y35.019
      rifle pellet
        injuring
          bystander Y35.032
          law enforcement personnel Y35.031
          suspect Y35.033
          unspecified person Y35.039
      rubber bullet
        injuring
          bystander Y35.042
          law enforcement personnel Y35.041
          suspect Y35.043
          unspecified person Y35.049
      shotgun —*see* Legal, intervention,
        firearm, specified NEC
      specified NEC
        injuring
          bystander Y35.092
          law enforcement personnel Y35.091
          suspect Y35.093
          unspecified person Y35.099
    gas (asphyxiation) (poisoning)
      injuring
        bystander Y35.202
        law enforcement personnel Y35.201
        suspect Y35.203
        unspecified person Y35.209
      specified NEC
        injuring
          bystander Y35.292
          law enforcement personnel Y35.291
          suspect Y35.293
          unspecified person Y35.299
      tear gas
        injuring
          bystander Y35.212
          law enforcement personnel Y35.211
          suspect Y35.213
          unspecified person Y35.219

Legal *(Continued)*
  intervention *(Continued)*
    grenade —*see* Legal, intervention,
      explosive, grenade
    injuring
      bystander Y35.92
      law enforcement personnel Y35.91
      suspect Y35.93
      unspecified person Y35.99
    late effect (of) —*see* with 7th character S
      Y35
    manhandling
      injuring
        bystander Y35.812
        law enforcement personnel Y35.811
        suspect Y35.813
        unspecified person Y35.819
    sequelae (of) —*see* with 7th character S Y35
    sharp objects
      bayonet
        injuring
          bystander Y35.412
          law enforcement personnel
            Y35.411
          suspect Y35.413
          unspecified person Y35.419
      injuring
        bystander Y35.402
        law enforcement personnel Y35.401
        suspect Y35.403
        unspecified person Y35.409
      specified NEC
        injuring
          bystander Y35.492
          law enforcement personnel Y35.491
          suspect Y35.493
          unspecified person Y35.499
    specified means NEC
      injuring
        bystander Y35.892
        law enforcement personnel Y35.891
        suspect Y35.893
        unspecified person Y35.899
    stabbing —*see* Legal, intervention, sharp
      object
    stave —*see* Legal, intervention, blunt
      object, stave
    stun gun
      injuring
        bystander Y35.832
        law enforcement personnel Y35.831
        suspect Y35.833
        unspecified person Y35.839
    taser
      injuring
        bystander Y35.832
        law enforcement personnel Y35.831
        suspect Y35.833
        unspecified person Y35.839
    tear gas —*see* Legal, intervention, gas, tear
      gas
    truncheon —*see* Legal, intervention, blunt
      object, stave
Lifting —*see also* Overexertion
  heavy objects X50.0
  weights X50.0
Lightning (shock) (stroke) (struck by) —*see*
  subcategory T75.0
  causing fire —*see* Exposure, fire
Loss of control (transport vehicle) NEC —*see*
  Accident, transport
Lost at sea NOS —*see* Drowning, due to, fall
  overboard
Low
  pressure (effects) —*see* Air, pressure, low
  temperature (effects) —*see* Exposure, cold
Lying before train, vehicle or other moving
  object X81.8
  subway train X81.1
  train X81.1
  undetermined whether accidental or
    intentional Y31
Lynching —*see* Assault

M

▶ New   ⇒ Revised   ~~deleted~~ Deleted   • Use Additional Character(s)

Misadventure(s) to patient(s) during surgical or medical care *(Continued)*
  failure *(Continued)*
    sterile precautions *(Continued)*
      puncture (lumbar) Y62.6
      removal of catheter or packing Y62.8
      specified procedure NEC Y62.8
      surgical operation Y62.0
      transfusion Y62.1
      vaccination Y62.3
    suture or ligature during surgical procedure Y65.2
    to introduce or to remove tube or instrument —*see* Failure, to
  hemorrhage —*see* Index to Diseases and Injuries, Complication(s)
  inadvertent exposure of patient to radiation Y63.3
  inappropriate
    operation performed —*see* Inappropriate operation performed
    temperature (too hot or too cold) in local application or packing Y63.5

Misadventure(s) to patient(s) during surgical or medical care *(Continued)*
  infusion —*see also* Misadventure, by type, infusion Y69
    excessive amount of fluid Y63.0
    incorrect dilution of fluid Y63.1
    wrong fluid Y65.1
  mismatched blood in transfusion Y65.0
  nonadministration of necessary drug or biological substance Y63.6
  overdose —*see* Table of Drugs and Chemicals
    radiation (in therapy) Y63.2
  perforation —*see* Index to Diseases and Injuries, Complication(s)
  performance of inappropriate operation —*see* Inappropriate operation performed
  puncture —*see* Index to Diseases and Injuries, Complication(s)
  specified type NEC Y65.8
    failure
      suture or ligature during surgical operation Y65.2
      to introduce or to remove tube or instrument —*see* Failure, to
    infusion of wrong fluid Y65.1

Misadventure(s) to patient(s) during surgical or medical care *(Continued)*
  specified type NEC *(Continued)*
    performance of inappropriate operation —*see* Inappropriate operation performed
    transfusion of mismatched blood Y65.0
    wrong
      fluid in infusion Y65.1
      placement of endotracheal tube during anesthetic procedure Y65.3
  transfusion —*see* Misadventure, by type, transfusion
    excessive amount of blood Y63.0
    mismatched blood Y65.0
  wrong
    drug given in error —*see* Table of Drugs and Chemicals
    fluid in infusion Y65.1
    placement of endotracheal tube during anesthetic procedure Y65.3
Mismatched blood in transfusion Y65.0
Motion sickness T75.3
Mountain sickness W94.11
Mudslide (of cataclysmic nature) —*see* Landslide
Murder (attempt) —*see* Assault

N

Nail
  contact with W45.0
    gun W29.4
  embedded in skin W45.0
Neglect (criminal) (homicidal intent) X58

Noise (causing injury) (pollution) W42.9
  supersonic W42.0
Nonadministration (of)
  drug or biological substance (necessary) Y63.6
  surgical and medical care Y66
Nosocomial condition Y95

O

Object
  falling
    from, in, on, hitting
      machinery —*see* Contact, with, by type of machine
  set in motion by
    accidental explosion or rupture of pressure vessel W38
    firearm —*see* Discharge, firearm, by type
    machine (ry) —*see* Contact, with, by type of machine
Overdose (drug) —*see* Table of Drugs and Chemicals
  radiation Y63.2

Overexertion X50.9
  from
    prolonged static or awkward postures X50.1
    repetitive movements X50.3
    specified strenuous movements or postures NEC X50.9
    strenuous movement or load X50.0
Overexposure (accidental) (to)
  cold —*see also* Exposure, cold X31
    due to man-made conditions —*see* Exposure, cold, man-made
  heat —*see also* Heat X30
  radiation —*see* Radiation
  radioactivity W88.0
  sun (sunburn) X32

Overexposure *(Continued)*
  weather NEC —*see* Forces of nature
  wind NEC —*see* Forces of nature
Overheated —*see* Heat
Overturning (accidental)
  machinery —*see* Contact, with, by type of machine
  transport vehicle NEC —*see also* Accident, transport V89.9
  watercraft (causing drowning, submersion) —*see also* Drowning, due to, accident to, watercraft, overturning
    causing injury except drowning or submersion —*see* Accident, watercraft, causing, injury NEC

M, N, & O

P

Parachute descent (voluntary) (without accident to aircraft) V97.29
  due to accident to aircraft —see Accident, transport, aircraft
Pecked by bird W61.99
Perforation during medical or surgical treatment as misadventure —see Index to Diseases and Injuries, Complication(s)
Perpetrator, perpetration, of assault, maltreatment and neglect (by) Y07.9
  boyfriend Y07.03
  brother Y07.410
    stepbrother Y07.435
  coach Y07.53
  cousin
    female Y07.491
    male Y07.490
  daycare provider Y07.519
    at-home
      adult care Y07.512
      childcare Y07.510
    care center
      adult care Y07.513
      childcare Y07.511
  family member NEC Y07.499
  father Y07.11
    adoptive Y07.13
    foster Y07.420
    stepfather Y07.430
  foster father Y07.420
  foster mother Y07.421
  girl friend Y07.04
  healthcare provider Y07.529
    mental health Y07.521
    specified NEC Y07.528
  husband Y07.01
  instructor Y07.53
  mother Y07.12
    adoptive Y07.14
    foster Y07.421
    stepmother Y07.433
  nonfamily member Y07.50
    specified NEC Y07.59
  nurse Y07.528
  occupational therapist Y07.528
  partner of parent
    female Y07.434
    male Y07.432
  physical therapist Y07.528
  sister Y07.411
  speech therapist Y07.528
  stepbrother Y07.435
  stepfather Y07.430
  stepmother Y07.433
  stepsister Y07.436
  teacher Y07.53
  wife Y07.02
Piercing —see Contact, with, by type of object or machine
Pinched
  between objects (moving) (stationary and moving) W23.0
    stationary W23.1
Pinned under machine (ry) —see Contact, with, by type of machine
Place of occurrence Y92.9
  abandoned house Y92.89
  airplane Y92.813
  airport Y92.520
  ambulatory health services establishment NEC Y92.538
  ambulatory surgery center Y92.530
  amusement park Y92.831
  apartment (co-op) —see Place of occurrence, residence, apartment
  assembly hall Y92.29
  bank Y92.510
  barn Y92.71
  baseball field Y92.320

Place of occurrence (Continued)
  basketball court Y92.310
  beach Y92.832
  boarding house —see Place of occurrence, residence, boarding house
  boat Y92.814
  bowling alley Y92.39
  bridge Y92.89
  building under construction Y92.61
  bus Y92.811
    station Y92.521
  cafe Y92.511
  campsite Y92.833
  campus —see Place of occurrence, school
  canal Y92.89
  car Y92.810
  casino Y92.59
  children's home —see Place of occurrence, residence, institutional, orphanage
  church Y92.22
  cinema Y92.26
  clubhouse Y92.29
  coal pit Y92.64
  college (community) Y92.214
  condominium —see Place of occurrence, residence, apartment
  construction area —see Place of occurrence, industrial and construction area
  convalescent home —see Place of occurrence, residence, institutional, nursing home
  court-house Y92.240
  cricket ground Y92.328
  cultural building Y92.258
    art gallery Y92.250
    museum Y92.251
    music hall Y92.252
    opera house Y92.253
    specified NEC Y92.258
    theater Y92.254
  dancehall Y92.252
  day nursery Y92.210
  dentist office Y92.531
  derelict house Y92.89
  desert Y92.820
  dock NOS Y92.89
  dockyard Y92.62
  doctor's office Y92.531
  dormitory —see Place of occurrence, residence, institutional, school dormitory
  dry dock Y92.62
  factory (building) (premises) Y92.63
  farm (land under cultivation) (outbuildings) Y92.79
    barn Y92.71
    chicken coop Y92.72
    field Y92.73
    hen house Y92.72
    house —see Place of occurrence, residence, house
    orchard Y92.74
    specified NEC Y92.79
  football field Y92.321
  forest Y92.821
  freeway Y92.411
  gallery Y92.250
  garage (commercial) Y92.59
    boarding house Y92.044
    military base Y92.135
    mobile home Y92.025
    nursing home Y92.124
    orphanage Y92.114
    private house Y92.015
    reform school Y92.155
  gas station Y92.524
  gasworks Y92.69
  golf course Y92.39
  gravel pit Y92.64
  grocery Y92.512
  gymnasium Y92.39
  handball court Y92.318
  harbor Y92.89
  harness racing course Y92.39

Place of occurrence (Continued)
  healthcare provider office Y92.531
  highway Y92.411
    interstate Y92.411
  interstate Y92.411
  hill Y92.828
  hockey rink Y92.330
  home —see Place of occurrence, residence
  hospice —see Place of occurrence, residence, institutional, nursing home
  hospital Y92.239
    cafeteria Y92.233
    corridor Y92.232
    operating room Y92.234
    patient
      bathroom Y92.231
      room Y92.230
    specified NEC Y92.238
  hotel Y92.59
  house —see also Place of occurrence, residence
    abandoned Y92.89
    under construction Y92.61
  industrial and construction area (yard) Y92.69
    building under construction Y92.61
    dock Y92.62
    dry dock Y92.62
    factory Y92.63
    gasworks Y92.69
    mine Y92.64
    oil rig Y92.65
    pit Y92.64
    power station Y92.69
    shipyard Y92.62
    specified NEC Y92.69
    tunnel under construction Y92.69
    workshop Y92.69
  kindergarten Y92.211
  lacrosse field Y92.328
  lake Y92.838
  wilderness Y92.828
  library Y92.241
  mall Y92.59
  market Y92.512
  marsh Y92.828
  military
    base —see Place of occurrence, residence, institutional, military base
    training ground Y92.84
  mine Y92.64
  mosque Y92.22
  motel Y92.59
  motorway (interstate) Y92.411
  mountain Y92.828
  movie-house Y92.26
  museum Y92.251
  music-hall Y92.252
  not applicable Y92.9
  nuclear power station Y92.69
  nursing home —see Place of occurrence, residence, institutional, nursing home
  office building Y92.59
  offshore installation Y92.65
  oil rig Y92.65
  old people's home —see Place of occurrence, residence, institutional, specified NEC
  opera-house Y92.253
  orphanage —see Place of occurrence, residence, institutional, orphanage
  outpatient surgery center Y92.530
  park (public) Y92.830
    amusement Y92.831
  parking garage Y92.89
    lot Y92.481
  pavement Y92.480
  physician office Y92.531
  polo field Y92.328
  pond Y92.828
  post office Y92.242
  power station Y92.69
  prairie Y92.828
  prison —see Place of occurrence, residence, institutional, prison

▶ New   ⇒ Revised   deleted Deleted   • Use Additional Character(s)

Place of occurrence *(Continued)*
  public
    administration building Y92.248
      city hall Y92.243
      courthouse Y92.240
      library Y92.241
      post office Y92.242
      specified NEC Y92.248
    building NEC Y92.29
    hall Y92.29
    place NOS Y92.89
  race course Y92.39
  radio station Y92.59
  railway line (bridge) Y92.85
  ranch (outbuildings) —*see* Place of occurrence, farm
  recreation area Y92.838
    amusement park Y92.831
    beach Y92.832
    campsite Y92.833
    park (public) Y92.830
    seashore Y92.832
    specified NEC Y92.838
  reform school —*see* Place of occurrence, residence, institutional, reform school
  religious institution Y92.22
  residence (non-institutional) (private) Y92.009
    apartment Y92.039
      bathroom Y92.031
      bedroom Y92.032
      kitchen Y92.030
      specified NEC Y92.038
    bathroom Y92.002
    bedroom Y92.003
    boarding house Y92.049
      bathroom Y92.041
      bedroom Y92.042
      driveway Y92.043
      garage Y92.044
      garden Y92.046
      kitchen Y92.040
      specified NEC Y92.048
      swimming pool Y92.045
      yard Y92.046
    dining room Y92.001
    garden Y92.007
    home Y92.009
    house, single family Y92.019
      bathroom Y92.012
      bedroom Y92.013
      dining room Y92.011
      driveway Y92.014
      garage Y92.015
      garden Y92.017
      kitchen Y92.010
      specified NEC Y92.018
      swimming pool Y92.016
      yard Y92.017
    institutional Y92.10
      children's home —*see* Place of occurrence, residence, institutional, orphanage
      hospice —*see* Place of occurrence, residence, institutional, nursing home
      military base Y92.139
        barracks Y92.133
        garage Y92.135
        garden Y92.137
        kitchen Y92.130
        mess hall Y92.131
        specified NEC Y92.138
        swimming pool Y92.136
        yard Y92.137
      nursing home Y92.129
        bathroom Y92.121
        bedroom Y92.122
        driveway Y92.123
        garage Y92.124
        garden Y92.126
        kitchen Y92.120

Place of occurrence *(Continued)*
  residence *(Continued)*
    institutional *(Continued)*
      nursing home *(Continued)*
        specified NEC Y92.128
        swimming pool Y92.125
        yard Y92.126
      orphanage Y92.119
        bathroom Y92.111
        bedroom Y92.112
        driveway Y92.113
        garage Y92.114
        garden Y92.116
        kitchen Y92.110
        specified NEC Y92.118
        swimming pool Y92.115
        yard Y92.116
      prison Y92.149
        bathroom Y92.142
        cell Y92.143
        courtyard Y92.147
        dining room Y92.141
        kitchen Y92.140
        specified NEC Y92.148
        swimming pool Y92.146
      reform school Y92.159
        bathroom Y92.152
        bedroom Y92.153
        dining room Y92.151
        driveway Y92.154
        garage Y92.155
        garden Y92.157
        kitchen Y92.150
        specified NEC Y92.158
        swimming pool Y92.156
        yard Y92.157
      school dormitory Y92.169
        bathroom Y92.162
        bedroom Y92.163
        dining room Y92.161
        kitchen Y92.160
        specified NEC Y92.168
      specified NEC Y92.199
        bathroom Y92.192
        bedroom Y92.193
        dining room Y92.191
        driveway Y92.194
        garage Y92.195
        garden Y92.197
        kitchen Y92.190
        specified NEC Y92.198
        swimming pool Y92.196
        yard Y92.197
    kitchen Y92.000
    mobile home Y92.029
      bathroom Y92.022
      bedroom Y92.023
      dining room Y92.021
      driveway Y92.024
      garage Y92.025
      garden Y92.027
      kitchen Y92.020
      specified NEC Y92.028
      swimming pool Y92.026
      yard Y92.027
    specified place in residence NEC Y92.008
    specified residence type NEC Y92.099
      bathroom Y92.091
      bedroom Y92.092
      driveway Y92.093
      garage Y92.094
      garden Y92.096
      kitchen Y92.090
      specified NEC Y92.098
      swimming pool Y92.095
      yard Y92.096
  restaurant Y92.511
  riding school Y92.39
  river Y92.828
  road Y92.410
  rodeo ring Y92.39

Place of occurrence *(Continued)*
  rugby field Y92.328
  same day surgery center Y92.530
  sand pit Y92.64
  school (private) (public) (state) Y92.219
    college Y92.214
    daycare center Y92.210
    elementary school Y92.211
    high school Y92.213
    kindergarten Y92.211
    middle school Y92.212
    specified NEC Y92.218
    trace school Y92.215
    university Y92.214
    vocational school Y92.215
  sea (shore) Y92.832
  senior citizen center Y92.29
  service area
    airport Y92.520
    bus station Y92.521
    gas station Y92.524
    highway rest stop Y92.523
    railway station Y92.522
  shipyard Y92.62
  shop(commercial) Y92.513
  sidewalk Y92.480
  silo Y92.79
  skating rink (roller) Y92.331
    ice Y92.330
  slaughter house Y92.86
  soccer field Y92.322
  specified place NEC Y92.89
  sports area Y92.39
    athletic
      court Y92.318
        basketball Y92.310
        specified NEC Y92.318
        squash Y92.311
        tennis Y92.312
      field Y92.328
        baseball Y92.320
        cricket ground Y92.328
        football Y92.321
        hockey Y92.328
        soccer Y92.322
        specified NEC Y92.328
    golf course Y92.39
    gymnasium Y92.39
    riding school Y92.39
    skating rink (roller) Y92.331
      ice Y92.330
    stadium Y92.39
    swimming pool Y92.34
  squash court Y92.311
  stadium Y92.39
  steeplechasing course Y92.39
  store Y92.512
  stream Y92.828
  street and highway Y92.410
    bike path Y92.482
    freeway Y92.411
    highway ramp Y92.415
    interstate highway Y92.411
    local residential or business street Y92.414
    motorway Y92.411
    parking lot Y92.481
    parkway Y92.412
    sidewalk Y92.480
    specified NEC Y92.488
    state road Y92.413
  subway car Y92.816
  supermarket Y92.512
  swamp Y92.828
  swimming pool (public) Y92.34
    private (at) Y92.095
      boarding house Y92.045
      military base Y92.136
      mobile home Y92.026
      nursing home Y92.125
      orphanage Y92.115

▶ New   ⇒ Revised   ~~deleted~~ Deleted   • Use Additional Character(s)

Place of occurrence *(Continued)*
  swimming pool *(Continued)*
    private *(Continued)*
      prison Y92.146
      reform school Y92.156
      single family residence
        Y92.016
  synagogue Y92.22
  television station Y92.59
  tennis court Y92.312
  theater Y92.254
  trade area Y92.59
    bank Y92.510
    cafe Y92.511
    casino Y92.59
    garage Y92.59
    hotel Y92.59
    market Y92.512
    office building Y92.59
    radio station Y92.59
    restaurant Y92.511
    shop Y92.513
    shopping mall Y92.59
    store Y92.512
    supermarket Y92.512
    television station Y92.59
    warehouse Y92.59
  trailer park, residential —*see* Place of
    occurrence, residence, mobile
    home
  trailer site NOS Y92.89
  train Y92.815
    station Y92.522
  truck Y92.812
  tunnel under construction Y92. 69
  university Y92.214
  urgent (health) care center Y92.532
  vehicle (transport) Y92.818
    airplane Y92.813
    boat Y92.814
    bus Y92.811
    car Y92.810
    specified NEC Y92.818
    subway car Y92.816
    train Y92.815
    truck Y92.812
  warehouse Y92.59
  water reservoir Y92.89
  wilderness area Y92.828
    desert Y92.820
    forest Y92.821
    marsh Y92.828
    mountain Y92.828
    prairie Y92.828
    specified NEC Y92.828
    swamp Y92.828
  workshop Y92.69
  yard, private Y92.096
    boarding house Y92.046
    mobile home Y92.027
    single family house Y92.017

Place of occurrence *(Continued)*
  youth center Y92.29
  zoo (zoological garden) Y92.834
Plumbism —*see* Table of Drugs and Chemicals,
  lead
Poisoning (accidental) (by) —*see also* Table of
  Drugs and Chemicals
  by plant, thorns, spines, sharp leaves or other
    mechanisms NEC X58
  carbon monoxide
    generated by
      motor vehicle —*see* Accident, transport
      watercraft (in transit) (not in transit)
        V93.89
        ferry boat V93.81
        fishing boat V93.82
        jet skis V93.83
        liner V93.81
        merchant ship V93.80
        passenger ship V93.81
        powered craft NEC V93.83
  caused by injection of poisons into skin by
    plant thorns, spines, sharp leaves X58
    marine or sea plants (venomous) X58
  exhaust gas
    generated by
      motor vehicle —*see* Accident, transport
      watercraft (in transit) (not in transit)
        V93.89
        ferry boat V93.81
        fishing boat V93.82
        jet skis V93.83
        liner V93.81
        merchant ship V93.80
        passenger ship V93.81
        powered craft NEC V93.83
  fumes or smoke due to
    explosion —*see also* Explosion W40.9
    fire —*see* Exposure, fire
    ignition —*see* Ignition
  gas
    in legal intervention —*see* Legal,
      intervention, gas
    legal execution —*see* Legal, intervention,
      gas
  in war operations —*see* War operations
  legal
  execution —*see* Legal, intervention, gas
    intervention
      by gas —*see* Legal, intervention, gas
      other specified means —*see* Legal,
        intervention, specified means
        NEC
Powder burn (by) (from)
  airgun W34.110
  BB gun W34.110
  firearm NEC W34.19
  gas, air or spring-operated gun NEC
    W34.118
  handgun W32.1
  hunting rifle W33.12

Powder burn *(Continued)*
  larger firearm W33.10
    specified NEC W33.19
  machine gun W33.13
  paintball gun W34.111
  pellet gun W34.110
  shotgun W33.11
  Very pistol [flare] W34.19
Premature cessation (of) surgical and medical
  care Y66
Privation (food) (water) X58
Procedure (operation)
  correct, on wrong side or body part (wrong
    side) (wrong site) Y65.53
  intended for another patient done on wrong
    patient Y65.52
  performed on patient not scheduled for
    surgery Y65.52
  performed on wrong patient Y65.52
  wrong, performed on correct patient Y65.51
Prolonged
  sitting in transport vehicle —*see* Travel, by
    type of vehicle
  stay in
    high altitude as cause of anoxia,
      barodontalgia, barotitis or hypoxia
      W94.11
    weightless environment X52
Pulling, excessive —*see also* Overexertion
  X50.9
Puncture, puncturing —*see also* Contact, with,
  by type of object or machine
  by
    plant thorns, spines, sharp leaves or other
      mechanisms NEC W60
  during medical or surgical treatment as
    misadventure —*see* Index to Diseases
    and Injuries, Complication(s)
Pushed, pushing (accidental) (injury in)
  by other person(s) (accidental) W51
    with fall W03
      due to ice or snow W00.0
    as, or caused by, a crowd or human
      stampede (with fall) W52
    before moving object NEC Y02.8
      motor vehicle Y02.0
      subway train Y02.1
      train Y02.1
    from
      high place NEC
        in accidental circumstances W17.89
        stated as
          intentional, homicide (attempt) Y01
          undetermined whether accidental
            or intentional Y30
      transport vehicle NEC —*see also*
        Accident, transport V89.9
        stated as
          intentional, homicide (attempt)
            Y08.89
    overexertion X50.9

▶ New   ⟹ Revised   ~~deleted~~ Deleted   ● Use Additional Character(s)

R

Radiation (exposure to)
arc lamps W89.0
atomic power plant (malfunction) NEC
W88.1
complication of or abnormal reaction to
medical radiotherapy Y84.2
electromagnetic, ionizing W88.0
gamma rays W88.1
in
war operations (from or following
nuclear explosion) —*see also* War
operations
inadvertent exposure of patient (receiving
test or therapy) Y63.3
infrared (heaters and lamps) W90.1
excessive heat from W92
ionized, ionizing (particles, artificially
accelerated)
radioisotopes W88.1
specified NEC W88.8
x-rays W88.0
isotopes, radioactive —*see* Radiation,
radioactive isotopes
laser(s) W90.2
in war operations —*see* War operations
misadventure in medical care Y63.2
light sources (man-made visible and
ultraviolet) W89.9
natural X32
specified NEC W89.8
tanning bed W89.1
welding light W89.0
man-made visible light W89.9
specified NEC W89.8
tanning bed W89.1
welding light W89.0
microwave W90.8
misadventure in medical or surgical
procedure Y63.2

Radiation *(Continued)*
natural NEC X39.08
radon X39.01
overdose (in medical or surgical procedure)
Y63.2
radar W90.0
radioactive isotopes (any) W88.1
atomic power plant malfunction W88.1
misadventure in medical or surgical
treatment Y63.2
radiofrequency W90.0
radium NEC W88.1
sun X32
ultraviolet (light) (man-made) W89.9
natural X32
specified NEC W89.8
tanning bed W89.1
welding light W89.0
welding arc, torch, or light W89.0
excessive heat from W92
x-rays (hard) (soft) W88.0
Range disease W94.11
Rape (attempted) T74.2-●
Rat bite W53.11
Reaching (prolonged) (static) X50.1
Reaction, abnormal to medical procedure —*see
also* Complication of or following, by type
of procedure Y84.9
with misadventure —*see* Misadventure
biologicals —*see* Table of Drugs and
Chemicals
drugs —*see* Table of Drugs and Chemicals
vaccine —*see* Table of Drugs and
Chemicals
Recoil
airgun W34.110
BB gun W34.110
firearm NEC W34.19
gas, air or spring-operated gun NEC W34.118

Recoil *(Continued)*
handgun W32.1
hunting rifle W33.12
larger firearm W33.10
specified NEC W33.19
machine gun W33.13
paintball gun W34.111
pellet W34.110
shotgun W33.11
Very pistol [flare] W34.19
Reduction in
atmospheric pressure —*see* Air, pressure,
change
Rock falling on or hitting (accidentally)
(person) W20.8
in cave-in W20.0
Run over (accidentally) (by)
animal (not being ridden) NEC W55.89
machinery —*see* Contact, with, by specified
type of machine
transport vehicle NEC —*see also* Accident,
transport V09.9
intentional homicide (attempt) Y03.0
motor NEC V09.20
intentional homicide (attempt) Y03.0
Running
before moving object X81.8
motor vehicle X81.0
Running off, away
animal (being ridden) —*see also* Accident,
transport V80.918
not being ridden W55.89
animal-drawn vehicle NEC —*see also*
Accident, transport V80.928
highway, road(way), street
transport vehicle NEC —*see also* Accident,
transport V89.9
Rupture pressurized devices —*see* Explosion,
by type of device

S

Saturnism —see Table of Drugs and Chemicals, lead
Scald, scalding (accidental) (by) (from) (in) X19
  air (hot) X14.1
  gases (hot) X14.1
  homicide (attempt) —see Assault, burning, hot object
  inflicted by other person
    stated as intentional, homicide (attempt) — see Assault, burning, hot object
  liquid (boiling) (hot) NEC X12
    stated as undetermined whether accidental or intentional Y27.2
    suicide (attempt) X77.2
  local application of externally applied substance in medical or surgical care Y63.5
  metal (molten) (liquid) (hot) NEC X18
  self-inflicted X77.9
  stated as undetermined whether accidental or intentional Y27.8
  steam X13.1
    assault X98.0
    stated as undetermined whether accidental or intentional Y27.0
    suicide (attempt) X77.0
  suicide (attempt) X77.9
  vapor (hot) X13.1
    assault X98.0
    stated as undetermined whether accidental or intentional Y27.0
    suicide (attempt) X77.0
Scratched by
  cat W55.03
  person(s) (accidentally) W50.4
    with intent to injure or kill Y04.0
    as, or caused by, a crowd or human stampede (with fall) W52
    assault Y04.0
    homicide (attempt) Y04.0
    in
      fight Y04.0
      legal intervention
        injuring
          bystander Y35.892
          law enforcement personnel Y35.891
          suspect Y35.893
          unspecified person Y35.899
Seasickness T75.3
Self-harm NEC —see also External cause by type, undetermined whether accidental or intentional
  intentional —see Suicide
  poisoning NEC —see Table of drugs and biologicals, accident
Self-inflicted (injury) NEC —see also External cause by type, undetermined whether accidental or intentional
  intentional —see Suicide
  poisoning NEC —see Table of drugs and biologicals, accident
Sequelae (of)
  accident NEC —see W00-X58 with 7th character S
  assault (homicidal) (any means) —see X92-Y08 with 7th character S
  homicide, attempt (any means) —see X92-Y08 with 7th character S
  injury undetermined whether accidentally or purposely inflicted —see Y21-Y33 with 7th character S
  intentional self-harm (classifiable to X71-X83) —see X71-X83 with 7th character S
  legal intervention (see with 7th character S Y35)
  motor vehicle accident —see V00-V99 with 7th character S
  suicide, attempt (any means) —see X71-X83 with 7th character S

Sequelae (Continued)
  transport accident —see V00-V99 with 7th character S
  war operations —see War operations
Shock
  electric —see Exposure, electric current
  from electric appliance (any) (faulty) W86.8
    domestic W86.0
  suicide (attempt) X83.1
Shooting, shot (accidental) (ly)) —see also Discharge, firearm, by type
  herself or himself —see Discharge, firearm by type, self-inflicted
  homicide (attempt) —see Discharge, firearm by type, homicide
  in war operations —see War operations
  inflicted by other person —see Discharge, firearm by type, homicide
    accidental —see Discharge, firearm, by type of firearm
  legal
    execution —see Legal, intervention, firearm
    intervention —see Legal, intervention, firearm
  self-inflicted —see Discharge, firearm by type, suicide
    accidental —see Discharge, firearm, by type of firearm
  suicide (attempt) —see Discharge, firearm by type, suicide
Shoving (accidentally) by other person —see Pushed, by other person
Sickness
  alpine W94.11
  motion —see Motion
  mountain W94.11
Sinking (accidental)
  watercraft (causing drowning, submersion) —see also Drowning, due to, accident to, watercraft, sinking
    causing injury except drowning or submersion —see Accident, watercraft, causing, injury NEC
Siriasis X32
Sitting (prolonged) (static) X50.1
Slashed wrists —see Cut, self-inflicted
Slipping (accidental) (on same level) (with fall) W01.0
  without fall W18.40
    due to
      specified NEC W18.49
      stepping from one level to another W18.43
      stepping into hole or opening W18.42
      stepping on object W18.41
  on
    ice W00.0
      with skates —see Accident, transport, pedestrian, conveyance
    mud W01.0
    oil W01.0
    snow W00.0
      with skis —see Accident, transport, pedestrian, conveyance
    surface (slippery) (wet) NEC W01.0
Sliver, wood, contact with W45.8
Smoldering (due to fire) —see Exposure, fire
Sodomy (attempt) by force T74.2-•
Sound waves (causing injury) W42.9
  supersonic W42.0
Splinter, contact with W45.8
Stab, stabbing —see Cut
Standing (prolonged) (static) X50.1
Starvation X58
Status of external cause Y99.9
  child assisting in compensated work for family Y99.8
  civilian activity done for financial or other compensation Y99.0
  civilian activity done for income or pay Y99.0

Status of external cause (Continued)
  family member assisting in compensated work for other family member Y99.8
  hobby not done for income Y99.8
  leisure activity Y99.8
  military activity Y99.1
  off-duty activity of military personnel Y99.8
  recreation or sport not for income or while a student Y99.8
  specified NEC Y99.8
  student activity Y99.8
  volunteer activity Y99.2
Stepped on
  by
    animal (not being ridden) NEC W55.89
    crowd or human stampede W52
    person W50.0
Stepping on
  object W22.8
    with fall W18.31
      sports equipment W21.9
    stationary W22.09
      sports equipment W21.89
  person W51
    by crowd or human stampede W52
  sports equipment W21.9
Sting
  arthropod, nonvenomous W57
  insect, nonvenomous W57
Storm (cataclysmic) —see Forces of nature, cataclysmic storm
Straining, excessive —see also Overexertion X50.9
Strangling —see Strangulation
Strangulation (accidental) —see category T71
Strenuous movements —see also Overexertion X50.9
Striking against
  airbag (automobile) W22.10
    driver side W22.11
    front passenger side W22.12
    specified NEC W22.19
  bottom when
    diving or jumping into water (in) W16.822
      causing drowning W16.821
      from boat W16.722
        causing drowning W16.721
      natural body W16.622
        causing drowning W16.821
      swimming pool W16.522
        causing drowning W16.521
    falling into water (in) W16.322
      causing drowning W16.321
      fountain —see Striking against, bottom when, falling into water, specified NEC
      natural body W16.122
        causing drowning W16.121
      reservoir —see Striking against, bottom when, falling into water, specified NEC
      specified NEC W16.322
        causing drowning W16.321
      swimming pool W16.022
        causing drowning W16.021
  diving board (swimming-pool) W21.4
  object W22.8
    with
      drowning or submersion —see Drowning
      fall —see Fall, due to, bumping against, object
    caused by crowd or human stampede (with fall) W52
    furniture W22.03
    lamppost W22.02
    sports equipment W21.9
    stationary W22.09
      sports equipment W21.89
    wall W22.01

▶ New   ⟹ Revised   ~~deleted~~ Deleted   ● Use Additional Character(s)

Striking against (Continued)
person(s) W51
with fall W03
due to ice or snow W00.0
as, or caused by, a crowd or human
stampede (with fall) W52
assault Y04.2
homicide (attempt) Y04.2
sports equipment W21.9
wall (when) W22.01
diving or jumping into water (in) W16.832
causing drowning W16.831
swimming pool W16.532
causing drowning W16.531
falling into water (in) W16.332
causing drowning W16.331
fountain —see Striking against, wall
when, falling into water, specified
NEC
natural body W16.132
causing drowning W16.131
reservoir —see Striking against, wall
when, falling into water, specified
NEC
specified NEC W16.332
causing drowning W16.331
swimming pool W16.032
causing drowning W16.031
swimming pool (when) W22.042
causing drowning W22.041
diving or jumping into water W16.532
causing drowning W16.531
falling into water W16.032
causing drowning W16.031
Struck (accidentally) by
airbag (automobile) W22.10
driver side W22.11
front passenger side W22.12
specified NEC W22.19
alligator W58.02
animal (not being ridden) NEC W55.89
avalanche —see Landslide
ball (hit) (thrown) W21.00
assault Y08.09
baseball W21.03
basketball W21.05
football W21.01
golf ball W21.04
football W21.01
soccer W21.02
softball W21.07
specified NEC W21.09
volleyball W21.06
bat or racquet
baseball bat W21.11
assault Y08.02
golf club W21.13
assault Y08.09
specified NEC W21.19
assault Y08.09
tennis racquet W21.12
assault Y08.09
bullet —see also Discharge, firearm by type
in war operations —see War operations
crocodile W58.12
dog W54.1
flare, Very pistol —see Discharge, firearm
NEC
hailstones X39.8
hockey (ice)
field
puck W21.221
stick W21.211
puck W21.220
stick W21.210
assault Y08.01
landslide —see Landslide
law-enforcement agent (on duty) —see Legal,
intervention, manhandling
with blunt object —see Legal, intervention,
blunt object

Struck by (Continued)
lightning —see subcategory T75.0
causing fire —see Exposure, fire
machine —see Contact, with, by type of
machine
mammal NEC W55.89
marine W56.32
marine animal W56.82
missile
firearm —see Discharge, firearm by type
in war operations —see War operations,
missile
object W22.8
blunt W22.8
assault Y00
suicide (attempt) X79
undetermined whether accidental or
intentional Y29
falling W20.8
from, in, on
building W20.1
burning (uncontrolled fire) X00.4
cataclysmic
earth surface movement NEC —see
Landslide
storm —see Forces of nature,
cataclysmic storm
cave-in W20.0
earthquake X34
machine (in operation) —see Contact,
with, by type of machine
structure W20.1
burning X00.4
transport vehicle (in motion) —see
Accident, transport, by type of
vehicle
watercraft V93.49
due to
accident to craft V91.39
powered craft V91.33
ferry boat V91.31
fishing boat V91.32
jet ski V91.33
liner V91.31
merchant ship V91.30
passenger ship V91.31
unpowered craft V91.38
canoe V91.35
inflatable V91.36
kayak V91.35
sailboat V91.34
surf-board V91.38
windsurfer V91.38
powered craft V93.43
ferry boat V93.41
fishing boat V93.42
jet ski V93.43
liner V93.41
merchant ship V93.40
passenger ship V93.41
unpowered craft V93.48
sailboat V93.44
surf-board V93.48
windsurfer V93.48
moving NEC W20.8
projected W20.8
assault Y00
in sports W21.9
assault Y08.09
ball W21.00
baseball W21.03
basketball W21.05
football W21.01
golf ball W21.04
soccer W21.02
softball W21.07
specified NEC W21.09
volleyball W21.06
bat or racquet
baseball bat W21.11
assault Y08.02

Struck by (Continued)
object (Continued)
projected (Continued)
in sports (Continued)
bat or racquet (Continued)
golf club W21.13
assault Y08.09-●
specified NEC W21.19
assault Y08.09
tennis racquet W21.12
assault Y08.09
hockey (ice)
field
puck W21.221
stick W21.211
puck W21.220
stick W21.210
assault Y08.01
specified NEC W21.89
set in motion by explosion —see Explosion
thrown W20.8
assault Y00
in sports W21.9
assault Y08.09
ball W21.00
baseball W21.03
basketball W21.05
football W21.01
golf ball W21.04
soccer W21.02
soft ball W21.07
specified NEC W21.09
volleyball W21.06
bat or racquet
baseball bat W21.11
assault Y08.02
golf club W21.13
assault Y08.09
specified NEC W21.19
assault Y08.09
tennis racquet W21.12
assault Y08.09
hockey (ice)
field
puck W21.221
stick W21.211
puck W21.220
stick W21.210
assault Y08.01
specified NEC W21.89
other person(s) W50.0
with
blunt object W22.8
intentional, homicide (attempt) Y00
sports equipment W21.9
undetermined whether accidental or
intentional Y29
fall W03
due to ice or snow W00.0
as, or caused by, a crowd or human
stampede (with fall) W52
assault Y04.2
homicide (attempt) Y04.2
in legal intervention
injuring
bystander Y35.812
law enforcement personnel Y35.811
suspect Y35.813
unspecified person Y35.819
sports equipment W21.9
police (on duty) —see Legal, intervention,
manhandling
with blunt object —see Legal, intervention,
blunt object
sports equipment W21.9
assault Y08.09
ball W21.00
baseball W21.03
basketball W21.05
football W21.01
golf ball W21.04
soccer W21.02

Struck by *(Continued)*
  sports equipment *(Continued)*
    ball *(Continued)*
      soft ball W21.07
      specified NEC W21.09
      volleyball W21.06
    bat or racquet
      baseball bat W21.11
        assault Y08.02
      golf club W21.13
        assault Y08.09
      specified NEC W21.19
      tennis racquet W21.12
        assault Y08.09
    cleats (shoe) W21.31
    foot wear NEC W21.39
    football helmet W21.81
    hockey (ice)
      field
        puck W21.221
        stick W21.211
      puck W21.220
      stick W21.210
        assault Y08.01
    skate blades W21.32
    specified NEC W21.89
      assault Y08.09
  thunderbolt —*see* subcategory
    T75.0
  causing fire —*see* Exposure, fire
  transport vehicle NEC —*see also* Accident,
    transport V09.9
    intentional, homicide (attempt) Y03.0
    motor NEC —*see also* Accident, transport
      V09.20
      homicide Y03.0
  vehicle (transport) NEC —*see* Accident,
    transport, by type of vehicle
    stationary (falling from jack,
      hydraulic lift, ramp)
      W20.8
Stumbling
  without fall W18.40
    due to
      specified NEC W18.49
      stepping from one level to another
        W18.43
      stepping into hole or opening W18.42
      stepping on object W18.41
  over
    animal NEC W01.0
      with fall W18.09
    carpet, rug or (small) object W22.8
      with fall W18.09
    person W51
      with fall W03
        due to ice or snow W00.0

Submersion (accidental) —*see* Drowning
Suffocation (accidental) (by external means)
  (by pressure) (mechanical) —*see also*
    category T71
  due to, by
    avalanche —*see* Landslide
    explosion —*see* Explosion
    fire —*see* Exposure, fire
    food, any type (aspiration) (ingestion)
      (inhalation) —*see* categories T17 and
      T18
    ignition —*see* Ignition
    landslide —*see* Landslide
    machine (ry) —*see* Contact, with, by type
      of machine
    vomitus (aspiration) (inhalation)
      T17.81-●
  in
    burning building X00.8
Suicide, suicidal (attempted) (by) X83.8
  blunt object X79
  burning, burns X76
    hot object X77.9
      fluid NEC X77.2
      household appliance X77.3
      specified NEC X77.8
      steam X77.0
      tap water X77.1
      vapors X77.0
  caustic substance —*see* Table of Drugs and
    Chemicals
  cold, extreme X83.2
  collision of motor vehicle with
    motor vehicle X82.0
    specified NEC X82.8
    train X82.1
    tree X82.2
  crashing of aircraft X83.0
  cut (any part of body) X78.9
  cutting or piercing instrument X78.9
    dagger X78.2
    glass X78.0
    knife X78.1
    specified NEC X78.8
    sword X78.2
  drowning (in) X71.9
    bathtub X71.0
    natural water X71.3
    specified NEC X71.8
    swimming pool X71.1
      following fall X71.2
  electrocution X83.1
  explosive(s) (material) X75
  fire, flames X76
  firearm X74.9
    airgun X74.01
    handgun X72

Suicide, suicidal *(Continued)*
  firearm *(Continued)*
    hunting rifle X73.1
    larger X73.9
      specified NEC X73.8
    machine gun X73.2
    shotgun X73.0
    specified NEC X74.8
  hanging X83.8
  hot object —*see* Suicide, burning, hot object
  jumping
    before moving object X81.8
      motor vehicle X81.0
      subway train X81.1
      train X81.1
    from high place X80
  late effect of attempt —*see* X71-X83 with 7th
    character S
  lying before moving object, train, vehicle X81.8
  poisoning —*see* Table of Drugs and
    Chemicals
  puncture (any part of body) —*see* Suicide,
    cutting or piercing instrument
  scald —*see* Suicide, burning, hot object
  sequelae of attempt —*see* X71-X83 with 7th
    character S
  sharp object (any) —*see* Suicide, cutting or
    piercing instrument
  shooting —*see* Suicide, firearm
  specified means NEC X83.8
  stab (any part of body) —*see* Suicide, cutting
    or piercing instrument
  steam, hot vapors X77.0
  strangulation X83.8
  submersion —*see* Suicide, drowning
  suffocation X83.8
  wound NEC X83.8
Sunstroke X32
Supersonic waves (causing injury) W42.0
Surgical procedure, complication of (delayed
  or as an abnormal reaction without
  mention of misadventure) —*see also*
  Complication of or following, by type of
  procedure
  due to or as a result of misadventure —*see*
    Misadventure
Swallowed, swallowing
  foreign body —*see* Foreign body, alimentary
    canal
  poison —*see* Table of Drugs and Chemicals
  substance
    caustic or corrosive —*see* Table of Drugs
      and Chemicals
    poisonous —*see* Table of Drugs and
      Chemicals

T

Tackle in sport W03
Terrorism (involving) Y38.80
  biological weapons Y38.6X-●
  chemical weapons Y38.7X-●
  conflagration Y38.3X-●
  drowning and submersion Y38.89-●
  explosion Y38.2X-●
    destruction of aircraft Y38.1X-●
    marine weapons Y38.0X-●
  fire Y38.3X-●
  firearms Y38.4X-●
  hot substances Y38.3X-●
  lasers Y38.89-●
  nuclear weapons Y38.5X-●
  piercing or stabbing instruments
    Y38.89-●
  secondary effects Y38.9X-●
  specified method NEC Y38.89-●
  suicide bomber Y38.81-●
Thirst X58
Threat to breathing
  aspiration —*see* Aspiration
  due to cave-in, falling earth or substance
    NEC —*see* category T71
Thrown (accidentally)
  against part (any) of or object in transport
    vehicle (in motion) NEC —*see also*
    Accident, transport

Thrown (Continued)
  from
    high place, homicide (attempt) Y01
    machinery —*see* Contact, with, by type of
      machine
    transport vehicle NEC —*see also* Accident,
      transport V89.9
  off —*see* Thrown, from
Thunderbolt —*see* subcategory T75.0
  causing fire —*see* Exposure, fire
Tidal wave (any injury) NEC —*see* Forces of
  nature, tidal wave
Took
  overdose (drug) —*see* Table of Drugs and
    Chemicals
  poison —*see* Table of Drugs and Chemicals
Tornado (any injury) X37.1
Torrential rain (any injury) X37.8
Torture X58
Trampled by animal NEC W55.89
Trapped (accidentally)
  between objects (moving) (stationary and
    moving) —*see* Caught
  by part (any) of
  ▶electric (assisted) bicycle V29.881
  ⇒motorcycle V29.888
    pedal cycle V19.88
    transport vehicle NEC —*see also* Accident,
      transport V89.9
Travel (effects) (sickness) T75.3

Tree falling on or hitting (accidentally)
  (person) W20.8
Tripping
  without fall W18.40
    due to
      specified NEC W18.49
      stepping from one level to another
        W18.43
      stepping into hole or opening
        W18.42
      stepping on object W18.41
  over
    animal W01.0
      with fall W01.0
    carpet, rug or (small) object W22.8
      with fall W18.09
    person W51
      with fall W03
        due to ice or snow W00.0
Twisted by person(s) (accidentally) W50.2
  with intent to injure or kill Y04.0
  as, or caused by, a crowd or human stampede
    (with fall) W52
  assault Y04.0
  homicide (attempt) Y04.0
  in
    fight Y04.0
    legal intervention —*see* Legal, intervention,
      manhandling
Twisting (prolonged) (static) X50.1

U

Underdosing of necessary drugs, medicaments
  or biological substances Y63.6
Undetermined intent (contact)
  (exposure)
  automobile collision Y32
  blunt object Y29
  drowning (submersion) (in) Y21.9
    bathtub Y21.0
      after fall Y21.1
    natural water (lake) (ocean) (pond) (river)
      (stream) Y21.4
    specified place NEC Y21.8
    swimming pool Y21.2
      after fall Y21.3
  explosive material Y25
  fall, jump or push from high place Y30
  falling, lying or running before moving object
    Y31
  fire Y26

Undetermined intent (Continued)
  firearm discharge Y24.9
    airgun (BB) (pellet) Y24.0
    handgun (pistol) (revolver)
      Y22
    hunting rifle Y23.1
    larger Y23.9
      hunting rifle Y23.1
      machine gun Y23.3
      military Y23.2
      shotgun Y23.0
      specified type NEC Y23.8
    machine gun Y23.3
    military Y23.2
    shotgun Y23.0
    specified type NEC Y24.8
    Very pistol Y24.8
  hot object Y27.9
    fluid NEC Y27.2
    household appliance Y27.3
    specified object NEC Y27.8

Undetermined intent (Continued)
  hot object (Continued)
    steam Y27.0
    tap water Y27.1
    vapor Y27.0
  jump, fall or push from high place Y30
  lying, falling or running before moving object
    Y31
  motor vehicle crash Y32
  push, fall or jump from high place Y30
  running, falling or lying before moving object
    Y31
  sharp object Y28.9
    dagger Y28.2
    glass Y28.0
    knife Y28.1
    specified object NEC Y28.8
    sword Y28.2
  smoke Y26
  specified event NEC Y33
Use of hand as hammer X50.3

V

Vibration (causing injury) W49.9
Victim (of)
  avalanche —*see* Landslide
  earth movements NEC —*see* Forces of nature,
    earth movement
  earthquake X34

Victim (Continued)
  flood —*see* Flood
  landslide —*see* Landslide
  lightning —*see* subcategory T75.0
    causing fire —*see* Exposure, fire
  storm (cataclysmic) NEC —*see* Forces of
    nature, cataclysmic storm
  volcanic eruption X35

Volcanic eruption (any injury) X35
Vomitus, gastric contents in air passages (with
  asphyxia, obstruction or
  suffocation) T17.81-●

T, U, & V

W

Walked into stationary object (any) W22.09
  furniture W22.03
  lamppost W22.02
  wall W22.01
War operations (injuries to military personnel
    and civilians during war, civil insurrection
    and peacekeeping missions) (by) (from)
    (involving) Y36.90-●
  after cessation of hostilities Y36.89-●
    explosion (of)
      bomb placed during war operations
        Y36.82-●
      mine placed during war operations
        Y36.81-●
    specified NEC Y36.88-●
  air blast Y36.20-●
  aircraft
    destruction —see War operations,
      destruction of aircraft
  airway restriction —see War operations,
    restriction of airways
  asphyxiation —see War operations, restriction
    of airways
  biological weapons Y36.6X-●
  blast Y36.20-●
  blast fragments Y36.20-●
  blast wave Y36.20-●
  blast wind Y36.20-●
  bomb Y36.20-●
    dirty Y36.50-●
    gasoline Y36.31-●
    incendiary Y36.31-●
    petrol Y36.31-●
  bullet Y36.43-●
    incendiary Y36.32-●
    rubber Y36.41-●
  chemical weapons Y36.7X-●
  combat
    hand to hand (unarmed) combat Y36.44-●
    using blunt or piercing object Y36.45-●
  conflagration —see War operations, fire
  conventional warfare NEC Y36.49-●
  depth-charge Y36.01-●
  destruction of aircraft Y36.10-●
    due to
      air to air missile Y36.11-●
      collision with other aircraft Y36.12-●
      detonation (accidental) of onboard
        munitions and explosives Y36.14-●
      enemy fire or explosives Y36.11-●
      explosive placed on aircraft Y36.11-●
      onboard fire Y36.13-●
      rocket propelled grenade [RPG] Y36.11-●
      small arms fire Y36.11-●
      surface to air missile Y36.11-●
      specified NEC Y36.19-●
  detonation (accidental) of
    onboard marine weapons Y36.05-●
    own munitions or munitions launch device
      Y36.24-●

War operations (Continued)
  dirty bomb Y36.50-●
  explosion (of) Y36.20-●
    aerial bomb Y36.21-●
    after cessation of hostilities
      bomb placed during war operations
        Y36.82-●
      mine placed during war operations
        Y36.81-●
    bomb NOS —see also War operations,
      bomb(s) Y36.20-●
    fragments Y36.20-●
    grenade Y36.29-●
    guided missile Y36.22-●
    improvised explosive device [IED]
      (person-borne) (roadside)
      (vehicle-borne) Y36.23-●
    land mine Y36.29-●
    marine mine (at sea) (in harbor)
      Y36.02-●
    marine weapon Y36.00-●
      specified NEC Y36.09-●
    own munitions or munitions launch
      device (accidental) Y36.24-●
    sea-based artillery shell Y36.03-●
    specified NEC Y36.29-●
    torpedo Y36.04-●
  fire Y36.30-●
    specified NEC Y36.39-●
  firearms
    discharge Y36.43-●
    pellets Y36.42-●
  flamethrower Y36.33-●
  fragments (from) (of)
    improvised explosive device [IED]
      (person-borne) (roadside)
      (vehicle-borne) Y36.26-●
    munitions Y36.25-●
    specified NEC Y36.29-●
    weapons Y36.27-●
  friendly fire Y36.92
  hand to hand (unarmed) combat
    Y36.44-●
  hot substances —see War operations,
    fire
  incendiary bullet Y36.32-●
  nuclear weapon (effects of) Y36.50-●
    acute radiation exposure Y36.54-●
    blast pressure Y36.51-●
    direct blast Y36.51-●
    direct heat Y36.53-●
    fallout exposure Y36.54-●
    fireball Y36.53-●
    indirect blast (struck or crushed by blast
      debris) (being thrown by blast)
      Y36.52-●
    ionizing radiation (immediate exposure)
      Y36.54-●
    nuclear radiation Y36.54-●
    radiation
      ionizing (immediate exposure)
        Y36.54-●

War operations (Continued)
  nuclear weapon (Continued)
    radiation (Continued)
      nuclear Y36.54-●
      thermal Y36.53-●
    secondary effects Y36.54-●
    specified NEC Y36.59-●
    thermal radiation Y36.53-●
  restriction of air (airway)
    intentional Y36.46-●
    unintentional Y36.47-●
  rubber bullets Y36.41-●
  shrapnel NOS Y36.29-●
  suffocation —see War operations, restriction
    of airways
  unconventional warfare NEC Y36.7X-●
  underwater blast NOS Y36.00-●
  warfare
    conventional NEC Y36.49-●
    unconventional NEC Y36.7X-●
  weapon of mass destruction [WMD] Y36.91
  weapons
    biological weapons Y36.6X-●
    chemical Y36.7X-●
    nuclear (effects of) Y36.50-●
      acute radiation exposure Y36.54-●
      blast pressure Y36.51-●
      direct blast Y36.51-●
      direct heat Y36.53-●
      fallout exposure Y36.54-●
      fireball Y36.53-●
      radiation
        ionizing (immediate exposure)
          Y36.54-●
        nuclear Y36.54-●
        thermal Y36.53-●
      secondary effects Y36.54-●
      specified NEC Y36.59-●
    of mass destruction [WMD] Y36.91-●
Washed
  away by flood —see Flood
  off road by storm (transport vehicle) —see
    Forces of nature, cataclysmic storm
Weather exposure NEC —see Forces of nature
Weightlessness (causing injury) (effects of) (in
    spacecraft, real or simulated) X52
Work related condition Y99.0
Wound (accidental) NEC —see also Injury X58
  battle —see also War operations Y36.90
  gunshot —see Discharge, firearm by type
Wreck transport vehicle NEC —see also
    Accident, transport V89.9
Wrong
  device implanted into correct surgical site
    Y65.51
  fluid in infusion Y65.1
  patient, procedure performed on Y65.52
  procedure (operation) on correct patient
    Y65.51

▶ New   ⇛ Revised   ~~deleted~~ Deleted   ● Use Additional Character(s)

PART III

ICD-10-CM Tabular List of Diseases and Injuries

CHAPTER 1

CERTAIN INFECTIOUS AND PARASITIC DISEASES (A00-B99)

OGCR Chapter-Specific Coding Guidelines

1. Chapter 1: Certain Infectious and Parasitic Diseases (A00-B99)

   a. Human Immunodeficiency Virus (HIV) Infections

      1) Code only confirmed cases

   Code only confirmed cases of HIV infection/illness. This is an exception to the hospital inpatient guideline Section II, H.

   In this context, "confirmation" does not require documentation of positive serology or culture for HIV; the provider's diagnostic statement that the patient is HIV positive, or has an HIV-related illness is sufficient.

      2) Selection and sequencing of HIV codes

         (a) Patient admitted for HIV-related condition

   If a patient is admitted for an HIV-related condition, the principal diagnosis should be B20, Human immunodeficiency virus [HIV] disease followed by additional diagnosis codes for all reported HIV-related conditions.

         (b) Patient with HIV disease admitted for unrelated condition

   If a patient with HIV disease is admitted for an unrelated condition (such as a traumatic injury), the code for the unrelated condition (e.g., the nature of injury code) should be the principal diagnosis. Other diagnoses would be B20 followed by additional diagnosis codes for all reported HIV-related conditions.

         (c) Whether the patient is newly diagnosed

   Whether the patient is newly diagnosed or has had previous admissions/encounters for HIV conditions is irrelevant to the sequencing decision.

         (d) Asymptomatic human immunodeficiency virus

   Z21, Asymptomatic human immunodeficiency virus [HIV] infection status, is to be applied when the patient without any documentation of symptoms is listed as being "HIV positive," "known HIV," "HIV test positive," or similar terminology. Do not use this code if the term "AIDS" is used or if the patient is treated for any HIV-related illness or is described as having any condition(s) resulting from his/her HIV positive status; use B20 in these cases.

         (e) Patients with inconclusive HIV serology

   Patients with inconclusive HIV serology, but no definitive diagnosis or manifestations of the illness, may be assigned code R75, Inconclusive laboratory evidence of human immunodeficiency virus [HIV].

         (f) Previously diagnosed HIV-related illness

   Patients with any known prior diagnosis of an HIV-related illness should be coded to B20. Once a patient has developed an HIV-related illness, the patient should always be assigned code B20 on every subsequent admission/encounter. Patients previously diagnosed with any HIV illness (B20) should never be assigned to R75 or Z21, Asymptomatic human immunodeficiency virus [HIV] infection status.

         (g) HIV Infection in Pregnancy, Childbirth and the Puerperium

   During pregnancy, childbirth or the puerperium, a patient admitted (or presenting for a health care encounter) because of an HIV-related illness should receive a principal diagnosis code of O98.7-, Human immunodeficiency [HIV] disease complicating pregnancy, childbirth and the puerperium, followed by B20 and the code(s) for the HIV-related illness(es). Codes from Chapter 15 always take sequencing priority.

   Patients with asymptomatic HIV infection status admitted (or presenting for a health care encounter) during pregnancy, childbirth, or the puerperium should receive codes of O98.7- and Z21.

         (h) Encounters for testing for HIV

   If a patient is being seen to determine his/her HIV status, use code Z11.4, Encounter for screening for human immunodeficiency virus [HIV]. Use additional codes for any associated high-risk behavior.

   If a patient with signs or symptoms is being seen for HIV testing, code the signs and symptoms. An additional counseling code Z71.7, Human immunodeficiency virus [HIV] counseling, may be used if counseling is provided during the encounter for the test.

   When a patient returns to be informed of his/her HIV test results and the test result is negative, use code Z71.7, Human immunodeficiency virus [HIV] counseling.

If the results are positive, see previous guidelines and assign codes as appropriate.

   b. Infectious agents as the cause of diseases classified to other chapters

   Certain infections are classified in chapters other than Chapter 1 and no organism is identified as part of the infection code. In these instances, it is necessary to use an additional code from Chapter 1 to identify the organism. A code from category B95, Streptococcus, Staphylococcus, and Enterococcus as the cause of diseases classified to other chapters, B96, Other bacterial agents as the cause of diseases classified to other chapters, or B97, Viral agents as the cause of diseases classified to other chapters, is to be used as an additional code to identify the organism. An instructional note will be found at the infection code advising that an additional organism code is required.

   c. Infections resistant to antibiotics

   Many bacterial infections are resistant to current antibiotics. It is necessary to identify all infections documented as antibiotic resistant. Assign a code from category Z16, Resistance to antimicrobial drugs, following the infection code only if the infection code does not identify drug resistance.

   d. Sepsis, Severe Sepsis, and Septic Shock

      1) Coding of Sepsis and Severe Sepsis

         (a) Sepsis

   For a diagnosis of sepsis, assign the appropriate code for the underlying systemic infection. If the type of infection or causal organism is not further specified, assign code A41.9, Sepsis, unspecified organism.

   A code from subcategory R65.2, Severe sepsis, should not be assigned unless severe sepsis or an associated acute organ dysfunction is documented.

            (i) Negative or inconclusive blood cultures and sepsis

   Negative or inconclusive blood cultures do not preclude a diagnosis of sepsis in patients with clinical evidence of the condition, however, the provider should be queried.

            (ii) Urosepsis

   The term urosepsis is a nonspecific term. It is not to be considered synonymous with sepsis. It has no default code in the Alphabetic Index. Should a provider use this term, he/she must be queried for clarification.

            (iii) Sepsis with organ dysfunction

   If a patient has sepsis and associated acute organ dysfunction or multiple organ dysfunction (MOD), follow the instructions for coding severe sepsis.

            (iv) Acute organ dysfunction that is not clearly associated with the sepsis

   If a patient has sepsis and an acute organ dysfunction, but the medical record documentation indicates that the acute organ dysfunction is related to a medical condition other than the sepsis, do not assign a code from subcategory R65.2, Severe sepsis. An acute organ dysfunction must be associated with the sepsis in order to assign the severe sepsis code. If the documentation is not clear as to whether an acute organ dysfunction is related to the sepsis or another medical condition, query the provider.

         (b) Severe sepsis

   The coding of severe sepsis requires a minimum of 2 codes: first a code for the underlying systemic infection, followed by a code from subcategory R65.2, Severe sepsis. If the causal organism is not documented, assign code A41.9, Sepsis, unspecified organism, for the infection. Additional code(s) for the associated acute organ dysfunction are also required.

   Due to the complex nature of severe sepsis, some cases may require querying the provider prior to assignment of the codes.

      2) Septic shock

         (a) Septic shock generally refers to circulatory failure associated with severe sepsis, and therefore, it represents a type of acute organ dysfunction.

   For all cases of septic shock, the code for the systemic infection should be sequenced first, followed by code R65.21, Severe sepsis with septic shock or code T81.12, Postprocedural septic shock.

Any additional codes for the other acute organ dysfunctions should also be assigned. As noted in the sequencing instructions in the Tabular List, the code for septic shock cannot be assigned as a principal diagnosis.

3) Sequencing of severe sepsis

If severe sepsis is present on admission, and meets the definition of principal diagnosis, the underlying systemic infection should be assigned as principal diagnosis followed by the appropriate code from subcategory R65.2 as required by the sequencing rules in the Tabular List. A code from subcategory R65.2 can never be assigned as a principal diagnosis.

When severe sepsis develops during an encounter (it was not present on admission) the underlying systemic infection and the appropriate code from subcategory R65.2 should be assigned as secondary diagnoses.

Severe sepsis may be present on admission but the diagnosis may not be confirmed until sometime after admission. If the documentation is not clear whether severe sepsis was present on admission, the provider should be queried.

4) Sepsis and severe sepsis with a localized infection

If the reason for admission is both sepsis or severe sepsis and a localized infection, such as pneumonia or cellulitis, a code(s) for the underlying systemic infection should be assigned first and the code for the localized infection should be assigned as a secondary diagnosis. If the patient has severe sepsis, a code from subcategory R65.2 should also be assigned as a secondary diagnosis. If the patient is admitted with a localized infection, such as pneumonia, and sepsis/severe sepsis doesn't develop until after admission, the localized infection should be assigned first, followed by the appropriate sepsis/severe sepsis codes.

5) Sepsis due to a postprocedural infection

(a) Documentation of causal relationship

As with all postprocedural complications, code assignment is based on the provider's documentation of the relationship between the infection and the procedure.

(b) Sepsis due to a postprocedural infection

For infections following a procedure, a code from T81.40, to T81.43. Infection following a procedure, or O86.00 to O86.03, Infection of obstetric surgical wound, that identifies the site of the infection should be coded first, if known. Assign an additional code for sepsis following a procedure (T81.44) or sepsis following an obstetrical procedure (O86.04). Use an additional code to identify the infectious agent. If the patient has severe sepsis the appropriate code from subcategory R65.2 should also be assigned with the additional code(s) for any acute organ dysfunction.

For infections following infusion, transfusion, therapeutic injection, or immunization, a code from subcategory T80.2, Infections following infusion, transfusion, and therapeutic injection, or code T88.0-, Infection following immunization, should be coded first, followed by the code for the specific infection. If the patient has severe sepsis, the appropriate code from subcategory R65.2 should also be assigned, with the additional codes(s) for any acute organ dysfunction.

(c) Postprocedural infection and postprocedural septic shock

If a postprocedural infection has resulted in postprocedural septic shock, assign the codes indicated above for sepsis due to a postprocedural infection, followed by code T81.12-, Postprocedural septic shock. Do not assign code R65.21, Severe sepsis with septic shock. Additional code(s) should be assigned for any acute organ dysfunction.

6) Sepsis and severe sepsis associated with a noninfectious process (condition)

In some cases a noninfectious process (condition), such as trauma, may lead to an infection which can result in sepsis or severe sepsis. If sepsis or severe sepsis is documented as associated with a noninfectious condition, such as a burn or serious injury, and this condition meets the definition for principal diagnosis, the code for the noninfectious condition should be sequenced first, followed by the code for the resulting infection. If severe sepsis is present, a code from subcategory R65.2 should also be assigned with any associated organ dysfunction(s) codes. It is not necessary to assign a code from subcategory R65.1, Systemic inflammatory response syndrome (SIRS) of noninfectious origin, for these cases.

If the infection meets the definition of principal diagnosis it should be sequenced before the noninfectious condition. When both the associated noninfectious condition and the infection meet the definition of principal diagnosis either may be assigned as principal diagnosis.

Only one code from category R65, Symptoms and signs specifically associated with systemic inflammation and infection, should be assigned. Therefore, when a noninfectious condition leads to an infection resulting in severe sepsis, assign the appropriate code from subcategory R65.2, Severe sepsis. Do not additionally assign a code from subcategory R65.1, Systemic inflammatory response syndrome (SIRS) of noninfectious origin.
See Section I.C.18. SIRS due to non-infectious process

7) Sepsis and septic shock complicating abortion, pregnancy, childbirth, and the puerperium

See Section I.C.15. Sepsis and septic shock complicating abortion, pregnancy, childbirth and the puerperium

8) Newborn sepsis

See Section I.C.16. f. Bacterial sepsis of Newborn

e. Methicillin Resistant Staphylococcus aureus (MRSA) Conditions

1) Selection and sequencing of MRSA codes

(a) Combination codes for MRSA infection

When a patient is diagnosed with an infection that is due to methicillin resistant *Staphylococcus aureus* (MRSA), and that infection has a combination code that includes the causal organism (e.g., sepsis, pneumonia) assign the appropriate combination code for the condition (e.g., code A41.02, Sepsis due to Methicillin resistant Staphylococcus aureus or code J15.212, Pneumonia due to Methicillin resistant Staphylococcus aureus). Do not assign code B95.62, Methicillin resistant Staphylococcus aureus infection as the cause of diseases classified elsewhere, as an additional code because the combination code includes the type of infection and the MRSA organism. Do not assign a code from subcategory Z16.11, Resistance to penicillins, as an additional diagnosis.
See Section C.1. for instructions on coding and sequencing of sepsis and severe sepsis.

(b) Other codes for MRSA infection

When there is documentation of a current infection (e.g., wound infection, stitch abscess, urinary tract infection) due to MRSA, and that infection does not have a combination code that includes the causal organism, assign the appropriate code to identify the condition along with code B95.62, Methicillin resistant Staphylococcus aureus infection as the cause of diseases classified elsewhere for the MRSA infection. Do not assign a code from subcategory Z16.11, Resistance to penicillins.

(c) Methicillin susceptible Staphylococcus aureus (MSSA) and MRSA colonization

The condition or state of being colonized or carrying MSSA or MRSA is called colonization or carriage, while an individual person is described as being colonized or being a carrier. Colonization means that MSSA or MSRA is present on or in the body without necessarily causing illness. A positive MRSA colonization test might be documented by the provider as "MRSA screen positive" or "MRSA nasal swab positive".

Assign code Z22.322, Carrier or suspected carrier of Methicillin resistant Staphylococcus aureus, for patients documented as having MRSA colonization. Assign code Z22.321, Carrier or suspected carrier of Methicillin susceptible Staphylococcus aureus, for patient documented as having MSSA colonization. Colonization is not necessarily indicative of a disease process or as the cause of a specific condition the patient may have unless documented as such by the provider.

(d) MRSA colonization and infection

If a patient is documented as having both MRSA colonization and infection during a hospital admission, code Z22.322, Carrier or suspected carrier of Methicillin resistant Staphylococcus aureus, and a code for the MRSA infection may both be assigned.

f. Zika virus infections

1) Code only confirmed cases

Code only a confirmed diagnosis of Zika virus (A92.5, Zika virus disease) as documented by the provider. This is an exception to the hospital inpatient guideline Section II, H.

In this context, "confirmation" does not require documentation of the type of test performed; the physician's diagnostic statement that the condition is confirmed is sufficient. This code should be assigned regardless of the stated mode of transmission.

If the provider documents "suspected", "possible" or "probable" Zika, do not assign code A92.5. Assign a code(s) explaining the reason for encounter (such as fever, rash, or joint pain) or Z20.821, Contact with and (suspected) exposure to Zika virus.

CHAPTER 1

CERTAIN INFECTIOUS AND PARASITIC DISEASES (A00-B99)

Includes   diseases generally recognized as communicable or transmissible

Use additional code to identify resistance to antimicrobial drugs (Z16.-)

Excludes1   certain localized infections - see body system-related chapters

Excludes2   carrier or suspected carrier of infectious disease (Z22.-)

infectious and parasitic diseases complicating pregnancy, childbirth and the puerperium (O98.-)

infectious and parasitic diseases specific to the perinatal period (P35-P39)

influenza and other acute respiratory infections (J00-J22)

This chapter contains the following blocks:

A00-A09	Intestinal infectious diseases
A15-A19	Tuberculosis
A20-A28	Certain zoonotic bacterial diseases
A30-A49	Other bacterial diseases
A50-A64	Infections with a predominantly sexual mode of transmission
A65-A69	Other spirochetal diseases
A70-A74	Other diseases caused by chlamydiae
A75-A79	Rickettsioses
A80-A89	Viral and prion infections of the central nervous system
A90-A99	Arthropod-borne viral fevers and viral hemorrhagic fevers
B00-B09	Viral infections characterized by skin and mucous membrane lesions
B10	Other human herpesviruses
B15-B19	Viral hepatitis
B20	Human immunodeficiency virus [HIV] disease
B25-B34	Other viral diseases
B35-B49	Mycoses
B50-B64	Protozoal diseases
B65-B83	Helminthiases
B85-B89	Pediculosis, acariasis and other infestations
B90-B94	Sequelae of infectious and parasitic diseases
B95-B97	Bacterial and viral infectious agents
B99	Other infectious diseases

INTESTINAL INFECTIOUS DISEASES (A00-A09)

● **A00**   **Cholera**
A serious, often deadly, infectious disease of the small intestine

   A00.0   **Cholera due to Vibrio cholerae 01, biovar cholerae**
       Classical cholera

   A00.1   **Cholera due to Vibrio cholerae 01, biovar eltor**
       Cholera eltor

   A00.9   **Cholera, unspecified**

● **A01**   **Typhoid and paratyphoid fevers**
Caused by Salmonella typhi and Salmonella paratyphi A, B, and C bacteria

   ● **A01.0**   **Typhoid fever**
       Infection due to Salmonella typhi

     A01.00   **Typhoid fever, unspecified**

     A01.01   **Typhoid meningitis**

     A01.02   **Typhoid fever with heart involvement**
         Typhoid endocarditis
         Typhoid myocarditis

     A01.03   **Typhoid pneumonia** 🐾

     A01.04   **Typhoid arthritis** 🐾

     A01.05   **Typhoid osteomyelitis** 🐾

     A01.09   **Typhoid fever with other complications**

   A01.1   **Paratyphoid fever A**

   A01.2   **Paratyphoid fever B**

   A01.3   **Paratyphoid fever C**

   A01.4   **Paratyphoid fever, unspecified**
       Infection due to Salmonella paratyphi NOS

● **A02**   **Other salmonella infections**

     Includes   infection or foodborne intoxication due to any Salmonella species other than S. typhi and S. paratyphi

   A02.0   **Salmonella enteritis**
       Salmonellosis

   A02.1   **Salmonella sepsis** 🐾

   ● **A02.2**   **Localized salmonella infections**

     A02.20   **Localized salmonella infection, unspecified**
         Specified in the documentation as localized, but unspecified as to type

     A02.21   **Salmonella meningitis**
         Specified as localized in the meninges

     A02.22   **Salmonella pneumonia** 🐾
         Specified as localized in the lungs

     A02.23   **Salmonella arthritis** 🐾
         Specified as localized in the joints

     A02.24   **Salmonella osteomyelitis** 🐾
         Specified as localized in bone

     A02.25   **Salmonella pyelonephritis**
         Salmonella tubulo-interstitial nephropathy

     A02.29   **Salmonella with other localized infection**
         Specified as localized (because it is still under localized heading) but does not assign into any of the above codes

   A02.8   **Other specified salmonella infections**
       Any specified salmonella infection which does NOT assign into any of the above codes (not specified as localized)

   A02.9   **Salmonella infection, unspecified**
       Unspecified in the documentation as to specific type of salmonella

● **A03**   **Shigellosis**
An infectious disease caused by bacteria (Shigella)

   A03.0   **Shigellosis due to Shigella dysenteriae**
       Group A shigellosis [Shiga-Kruse dysentery]

   A03.1   **Shigellosis due to Shigella flexneri**
       Group B shigellosis

   A03.2   **Shigellosis due to Shigella boydii**
       Group C shigellosis

   A03.3   **Shigellosis due to Shigella sonnei**
       Group D shigellosis

   A03.8   **Other shigellosis**

   A03.9   **Shigellosis, unspecified**
       Bacillary dysentery NOS

Item 1-1   **Salmonella** is a bacterium that lives in the intestines of fowl and mammals and can spread to humans through improper food preparation and cooking. Salmonellosis is an infection with the bacterium. Symptoms include diarrhea, fever, and abdominal cramps 12 to 72 hours after infection. The illness usually lasts 4 to 7 days, and most persons recover without treatment. The diarrhea may be so severe that the patient needs to be hospitalized. Patients with immunocompromised systems in chronic, ill health are more likely to have the infection invade their bloodstream with life-threatening results. For example, patients with sickle cell disease are more prone to salmonella osteomyelitis than others.

▶ New   ⇒ Revised   ~~deleted~~ Deleted   Excludes 1   Excludes 2   Includes   Use additional   Code first   Code also   Key words

OGCR Official Guidelines   X Assign placeholder X   ● Use Additional Character(s)   ▶ Manifestation Code   🐾 Hierarchical Condition Category   **Coding Clinic**

CHAPTER 1 (A00-B99)

Figure 1-1 Electron micrograph of escherichia coli (E. coli) expressing P fimbriae. (Getty Image)

Item 1-2 *Escherichia coli [E. coli]* is a Gram-negative bacterium found in the intestinal tracts of humans and animals and is usually nonpathogenic. Pathogenic strains can cause diarrhea or pyogenic (pus-producing) infections. Can be a threat to food safety.

● **A04   Other bacterial intestinal infections**
    Excludes1   bacterial foodborne intoxications, NEC (A05.-)
                 tuberculous enteritis (A18.32)

  A04.0   Enteropathogenic Escherichia coli infection
      Pertaining to or producing intestinal disease

  A04.1   Enterotoxigenic Escherichia coli infection
      Producing or containing intestinal toxin

  A04.2   Enteroinvasive Escherichia coli infection
      Capable of penetrating and spreading through intestinal mucosal epithelium

  A04.3   Enterohemorrhagic Escherichia coli infection
      Causing bloody diarrhea, resulting from microorganisms

  A04.4   Other intestinal Escherichia coli infections
      Escherichia coli enteritis NOS

  A04.5   Campylobacter enteritis
      Spiral shaped bacterium

  A04.6   Enteritis due to Yersinia enterocolitica
      Excludes1   extraintestinal yersiniosis (A28.2)
      Transmitted by infected food/water and person-to-person contact, affecting intestinal tract

● **A04.7   Enterocolitis due to Clostridium difficile**
      Foodborne intoxication by Clostridium difficile
      Pseudomembraneous colitis
      Marked by fibrinous deposit (false membrane) with enmeshed necrotic cells

    A04.71   Enterocolitis due to Clostridium difficile, recurrent
        Coding Clinic: 2020, Q1, P18

    A04.72   Enterocolitis due to Clostridium difficile, not specified as recurrent

  A04.8   Other specified bacterial intestinal infections

  A04.9   Bacterial intestinal infection, unspecified
      Bacterial enteritis NOS

● **A05   Other bacterial foodborne intoxications, not elsewhere classified**
    Excludes1   Clostridium difficile foodborne intoxication and infection (A04.7-)
                Escherichia coli infection (A04.0-A04.4)
                listeriosis (A32.-)
                salmonella foodborne intoxication and infection (A02.-)
                toxic effect of noxious foodstuffs (T61-T62)

  A05.0   Foodborne staphylococcal intoxication

  A05.1   Botulism food poisoning
      Botulism NOS
      Classical foodborne intoxication due to Clostridium botulinum
      Excludes1   infant botulism (A48.51)
                wound botulism (A48.52)

  A05.2   Foodborne Clostridium perfringens [Clostridium welchii] intoxication
      Type A causes gas gangrene and necrotizing colitis; major cause of food poisoning in humans
      Enteritis necroticans
      Pig-bel

  A05.3   Foodborne Vibrio parahaemolyticus intoxication
      Organism that survives only in high salt environment (halophilic), major cause of gastroenteritis due to consumption of raw or improperly cooked fish/seafood

  A05.4   Foodborne Bacillus cereus intoxication
      Spore-forming species commonly found in soil, causes food poisoning from formation of intestinal toxins in contaminated foods

  A05.5   Foodborne Vibrio vulnificus intoxication
      Species that survives in high salt environment (halophilic) with infection by eating raw seafood causes septicemia and cellulitis

  A05.8   Other specified bacterial foodborne intoxications

  A05.9   Bacterial foodborne intoxication, unspecified

● **A06   Amebiasis**
    An intestinal illness caused by the microscopic parasite Entamoeba histolytica
    Includes   infection due to Entamoeba histolytica
    Excludes1   other protozoal intestinal diseases (A07.-)
    Excludes2   acanthamebiasis (B60.1-)
              Naegleriasis (B60.2)

  A06.0   Acute amebic dysentery
      Acute amebiasis
      Intestinal amebiasis NOS

  A06.1   Chronic intestinal amebiasis

  A06.2   Amebic nondysenteric colitis
      Pertaining to single cell microorganism

  A06.3   Ameboma of intestine
      Tumorlike mass produced by localized inflammation often in intestine
      Ameboma NOS

  A06.4   Amebic liver abscess
      Hepatic amebiasis

  A06.5   Amebic lung abscess 🔗
      Amebic abscess of lung (and liver)

  A06.6   Amebic brain abscess
      Amebic abscess of brain (and liver) (and lung)

  A06.7   Cutaneous amebiasis

● **A06.8   Amebic infection of other sites**

    A06.81   Amebic cystitis

    A06.82   Other amebic genitourinary infections
        Amebic balanitis
        Amebic vesiculitis
        Amebic vulvovaginitis

    A06.89   Other amebic infections
        Amebic appendicitis
        Amebic splenic abscess

  A06.9   Amebiasis, unspecified

⬤ **A07**   **Other protozoal intestinal diseases**

     A07.0   **Balantidiasis**
          Balantidial dysentery
          Infection by protozoa that may cause diarrhea and dysentery,
          with ulceration of colonic mucous membranes

     A07.1   **Giardiasis [lambliasis]**
          Common infection in small intestine spread by contaminated
          food, water, or direct person-to-person contact

     A07.2   **Cryptosporidiosis** 🦠
          Human infection with protozoa usually seen as self-limited
          diarrhea in those who work with cattle

     A07.3   **Isosporiasis**
          Human intestinal disease caused by protozoa
          Infection due to Isospora belli and Isospora hominis
          Intestinal coccidiosis
          Isosporosis

     A07.4   **Cyclosporiasis**
          Infection by protozoa with most common species infecting
          humans being C cayetanensis

     A07.8   **Other specified protozoal intestinal diseases**
          Intestinal microsporidiosis
          Intestinal trichomoniasis
          Sarcocystosis
          Sarcosporidiosis

     A07.9   **Protozoal intestinal disease, unspecified**
          Flagellate diarrhea
          Protozoal colitis
          Protozoal diarrhea
          Protozoal dysentery

⬤ **A08**   **Viral and other specified intestinal infections**

     Excludes1   influenza with involvement of gastrointestinal
              tract (J09.X3, J10.2, J11.2)

     A08.0   **Rotaviral enteritis**

⬤   **A08.1**   **Acute gastroenteropathy due to Norwalk agent and**
          other small round viruses

          A08.11   **Acute gastroenteropathy due to Norwalk agent**
                 Acute gastroenteropathy due to Norovirus
                 Acute gastroenteropathy due to Norwalk-like
                   agent

          A08.19   **Acute gastroenteropathy due to other small**
               round viruses
                 Acute gastroenteropathy due to small round
                   virus [SRV] NOS

     A08.2   **Adenoviral enteritis**

⬤   **A08.3**   **Other viral enteritis**

          A08.31   **Calicivirus enteritis**

          A08.32   **Astrovirus enteritis**

          A08.39   **Other viral enteritis**
                 Coxsackie virus enteritis
                 Echovirus enteritis
                 Enterovirus enteritis NEC
                 Torovirus enteritis

     A08.4   **Viral intestinal infection, unspecified**
          Viral enteritis NOS
          Viral gastroenteritis NOS
          Viral gastroenteropathy NOS
          Coding Clinic: 2016, Q3, P12

     A08.8   **Other specified intestinal infections**

A09   **Infectious gastroenteritis and colitis, unspecified**
       Infectious colitis NOS
       Infectious enteritis NOS
       Infectious gastroenteritis NOS

     Excludes1   colitis NOS (K52.9)
              diarrhea NOS (R19.7)
              enteritis NOS (K52.9)
              gastroenteritis NOS (K52.9)
              noninfective gastroenteritis and colitis,
                 unspecified (K52.9)

Figure 1-2   Far advanced bilateral pulmonary tuberculosis before and after 8 months of treatment with streptomycin, PAS, and isoniazid. (Getty Image)

Item 1–3   **Tuberculosis** is a common and deadly infectious disease caused by the *Mycobacterium tuberculosis* organism. The first tuberculosis infection is called the **primary infection** and most commonly attacks the lungs but can affect the central nervous system, lymphatic system, circulatory system, genitourinary system, bones, joints, and even the skin. A **Ghon** lesion is the **initial lesion.** A **secondary lesion** occurs when the tubercle bacilli are carried to other areas.

Item 1–4   Although it primarily affects the lungs, the bacteria *Mycobacterium tuberculosis* can travel from the pulmonary circulation to virtually any organ in the body, much as a cancer metastasizes to a secondary site. If the immune system becomes compromised by age or disease, what would otherwise be a self-limiting primary tuberculosis in the lungs will develop in other organs. These are known as extrapulmonary sites.

TUBERCULOSIS (A15-A19)

     Includes   infections due to Mycobacterium tuberculosis
               and Mycobacterium bovis

     Excludes1   congenital tuberculosis (P37.0)
              nonspecific reaction to test for tuberculosis
                 without active tuberculosis (R76.1-)
              pneumoconiosis associated with tuberculosis, any
                 type in A15 (J65)
              positive PPD (R76.11)
              positive tuberculin skin test without active
                 tuberculosis (R76.11)
              sequelae of tuberculosis (B90.-)
              silicotuberculosis (J65)

⬤ **A15**   **Respiratory tuberculosis**

     A15.0   **Tuberculosis of lung**
          Tuberculous bronchiectasis
          Chronic dilatation of bronchi
          Tuberculous fibrosis of lung
          Tuberculous pneumonia
          Tuberculous pneumothorax

     A15.4   **Tuberculosis of intrathoracic lymph nodes**
          Tuberculosis of hilar lymph nodes
          Tuberculosis of mediastinal lymph nodes
          Tuberculosis of tracheobronchial lymph nodes

          Excludes1   tuberculosis specified as primary (A15.7)

     A15.5   **Tuberculosis of larynx, trachea and bronchus**
          Tuberculosis of bronchus
          Tuberculosis of glottis
          Tuberculosis of larynx
          Tuberculosis of trachea

     A15.6   **Tuberculous pleurisy**
          Tuberculosis of pleura
          Tuberculous empyema

          Excludes1   primary respiratory tuberculosis (A15.7)

     A15.7   **Primary respiratory tuberculosis**

     A15.8   **Other respiratory tuberculosis**
          Mediastinal tuberculosis
          Nasopharyngeal tuberculosis
          Tuberculosis of nose
          Tuberculosis of sinus [any nasal]

     A15.9   **Respiratory tuberculosis unspecified**

▶ New   ➡ Revised   ~~deleted~~ Deleted   Excludes 1   Excludes 2   Includes   Use additional   Code first   Code also   Key words

OGCR Official Guidelines   X Assign placeholder X   ⬤ Use Additional Character(s)   ▶ Manifestation Code   🦠 Hierarchical Condition Category   **Coding Clinic**

● **A17 Tuberculosis of nervous system**
    A17.0 Tuberculous meningitis
        Tuberculosis of meninges (cerebral) (spinal)
        Tuberculous leptomeningitis
        Excludes1 tuberculous meningoencephalitis
                        (A17.82)

    A17.1 Meningeal tuberculoma
        Tuberculoma of meninges (cerebral) (spinal)
        Excludes2 tuberculoma of brain and spinal cord
                        (A17.81)

● **A17.8 Other tuberculosis of nervous system**
    A17.81 Tuberculoma of brain and spinal cord
        Tuberculous abscess of brain and spinal cord

    A17.82 Tuberculous meningoencephalitis
        Inflammation of brain and meninges; AKA
            cerebromeningitis and encephalomeningitis
        Tuberculous myelitis

    A17.83 Tuberculous neuritis
        Tuberculous mononeuropathy

    A17.89 Other tuberculosis of nervous system
        Tuberculous polyneuropathy

    A17.9 Tuberculosis of nervous system, unspecified

● **A18 Tuberculosis of other organs**
● **A18.0 Tuberculosis of bones and joints**
    A18.01 Tuberculosis of spine
        Pott's disease or curvature of spine
        Tuberculous arthritis
        Tuberculous osteomyelitis of spine
        Tuberculous spondylitis

    A18.02 Tuberculous arthritis of other joints
        Tuberculosis of hip (joint)
        Tuberculosis of knee (joint)

    A18.03 Tuberculosis of other bones
        Tuberculous mastoiditis
        Tuberculous osteomyelitis

    A18.09 Other musculoskeletal tuberculosis
        Tuberculous myositis
        Tuberculous synovitis
        Tuberculous tenosynovitis

● **A18.1 Tuberculosis of genitourinary system**
    A18.10 Tuberculosis of genitourinary system, unspecified

    A18.11 Tuberculosis of kidney and ureter
    A18.12 Tuberculosis of bladder
    A18.13 Tuberculosis of other urinary organs
        Tuberculous urethritis

    A18.14 Tuberculosis of prostate ♂   **A**
    A18.15 Tuberculosis of other male genital organs ♂
    A18.16 Tuberculosis of cervix ♀
    A18.17 Tuberculous female pelvic inflammatory disease ♀
        Tuberculous endometritis
        Tuberculous oophoritis and salpingitis
          Oophoritis = inflammation of ovary
          Salpingitis = inflammation of fallopian tube

    A18.18 Tuberculosis of other female genital organs ♀
        Tuberculous ulceration of vulva

    A18.2 Tuberculous peripheral lymphadenopathy
        Tuberculous adenitis
        Excludes2 tuberculosis of bronchial and mediastinal
                lymph nodes (A15.4)
                tuberculosis of mesenteric and
                  retroperitoneal lymph nodes
                  (A18.39)
                tuberculous tracheobronchial adenopathy
                  (A15.4)

● **A18.3 Tuberculosis of intestines, peritoneum and mesenteric glands**
    A18.31 Tuberculous peritonitis
        Tuberculous ascites

    A18.32 Tuberculous enteritis
        Tuberculosis of anus and rectum
        Tuberculosis of intestine (large) (small)

    A18.39 Retroperitoneal tuberculosis
        Tuberculosis of mesenteric glands
        Tuberculosis of retroperitoneal (lymph glands)

    A18.4 Tuberculosis of skin and subcutaneous tissue
        Erythema induratum, tuberculous
        Lupus excedens
        Lupus vulgaris NOS
        Lupus vulgaris of eyelid
          Cutaneous tuberculosis characterized by reddish brown
            plaque on skin surrounded by papules and nodules
        Scrofuloderma
          Type of cutaneous tuberculosis, with direct extension of
            tuberculosis into skin from underlying structures;
            AKA tuberculosis colliquativa
        Tuberculosis of external ear
        Excludes2 lupus erythematosus (L93.-)
                      systemic lupus erythematosus (M32.-)

● **A18.5 Tuberculosis of eye**
        Excludes2 lupus vulgaris of eyelid (A18.4)

    A18.50 Tuberculosis of eye, unspecified
    A18.51 Tuberculous episcleritis
        Inflammation of episclera and adjacent tissues

    A18.52 Tuberculous keratitis
        Tuberculous interstitial keratitis
        Tuberculous keratoconjunctivitis (interstitial)
          (phlyctenular)
        Inflammation of cornea and conjunctiva

    A18.53 Tuberculous chorioretinitis
        Inflammation of choroid and retina;
          retinochoroiditis

    A18.54 Tuberculous iridocyclitis
        Inflammation of iris and ciliary body

    A18.59 Other tuberculosis of eye
        Tuberculous conjunctivitis

    A18.6 Tuberculosis of (inner) (middle) ear
        Tuberculous otitis media
        Excludes2 tuberculosis of external ear (A18.4)
                      tuberculous mastoiditis (A18.03)

    A18.7 Tuberculosis of adrenal glands
        Tuberculous Addison's disease

● **A18.8 Tuberculosis of other specified organs**
    A18.81 Tuberculosis of thyroid gland
    A18.82 Tuberculosis of other endocrine glands
        Tuberculosis of pituitary gland
        Tuberculosis of thymus gland

    A18.83 Tuberculosis of digestive tract organs, not elsewhere classified
        Excludes1 tuberculosis of intestine (A18.32)

    A18.84 Tuberculosis of heart
        Tuberculous cardiomyopathy
        Tuberculous endocarditis
        Tuberculous myocarditis
        Tuberculous pericarditis

    A18.85 Tuberculosis of spleen
    A18.89 Tuberculosis of other sites
        Tuberculosis of muscle
        Tuberculous cerebral arteritis

CHAPTER 1 (A00-B99)

Item 1-5 Miliary tuberculosis can be a life-threatening condition. If a tuberculous lesion enters a blood vessel, immense dissemination of tuberculous organisms can occur if the immune system is weak. High-risk populations— children under 4 years of age, the elderly, or the immunocompromised— are particularly prone to this type of infection. The lesions will have a millet seedlike appearance on chest x-ray. Bronchial washings and biopsy may aid in diagnosis.

● **A19   Miliary tuberculosis**

   Includes   disseminated tuberculosis
                  generalized tuberculosis
                  tuberculous polyserositis

   A19.0   **Acute miliary tuberculosis of a single specified site**

   A19.1   **Acute miliary tuberculosis of multiple sites**

   A19.2   **Acute miliary tuberculosis, unspecified**

   A19.8   **Other miliary tuberculosis**

   A19.9   **Miliary tuberculosis, unspecified**

CERTAIN ZOONOTIC BACTERIAL DISEASES (A20-A28)

● **A20   Plague**

   Infectious disease caused by a Yersinia pestis bacterium, transmitted by a rodent flea bite or handling of infected animal

   Includes   infection due to Yersinia pestis

   A20.0   **Bubonic plague**

   A20.1   **Cellulocutaneous plague**
           Skin and subcutaneous tissue plague

   A20.2   **Pneumonic plague** 🝔

   A20.3   **Plague meningitis**

   A20.7   **Septicemic plague** 🝔

   A20.8   **Other forms of plague**
           Abortive plague
           Asymptomatic plague
           Pestis minor
             Systemic bacterial disease

   A20.9   **Plague, unspecified**

● **A21   Tularemia**

   Caused by Francisella tularensis bacterium found in rodents, rabbits, and hares and transmitted to humans by contact with infected animal tissues or by ticks, biting flies, or mosquitoes

   Includes   deer-fly fever
                  infection due to Francisella tularensis
                  rabbit fever

   Coding Clinic: 2016, Q4, P25

   A21.0   **Ulceroglandular tularemia**
           Most common form of tularemia in humans is painful, swollen, erythematous papule at point of inoculation that ruptures to form shallow ulcer

   A21.1   **Oculoglandular tularemia**
           Primary site of entry is conjunctival sac, results in granulomatous corneal lesions
           Ophthalmic tularemia

   A21.2   **Pulmonary tularemia** 🝔

   A21.3   **Gastrointestinal tularemia**
           Abdominal tularemia

   A21.7   **Generalized tularemia**

   A21.8   **Other forms of tularemia**

   A21.9   **Tularemia, unspecified**

● **A22   Anthrax**
   An acute infectious disease caused by the spore-forming Bacillus anthracis; occurs in humans exposed to infected animals or tissue from infected animals

   Includes   infection due to Bacillus anthracis

   A22.0   **Cutaneous anthrax**
           Malignant carbuncle
           Malignant pustule

   A22.1   **Pulmonary anthrax** 🝔
           Inhalation anthrax
           Ragpicker's disease
           Woolsorter's disease

   A22.2   **Gastrointestinal anthrax**

   A22.7   **Anthrax sepsis** 🝔
           Infectious bacterial disease

   A22.8   **Other forms of anthrax**
           Anthrax meningitis

   A22.9   **Anthrax, unspecified**

● **A23   Brucellosis**

   Includes   Malta fever
                  Mediterranean fever
                  undulant fever

   A23.0   **Brucellosis due to Brucella melitensis**
           Resulting in flu-like symptoms that may lead to chronic symptoms that include recurrent fevers, joint pain, and fatigue

   A23.1   **Brucellosis due to Brucella abortus**
           Most common cause of brucellosis in humans; AKA Bang bacillus

   A23.2   **Brucellosis due to Brucella suis**
           Species found primarily in pigs, rabbits, and reindeer

   A23.3   **Brucellosis due to Brucella canis**
           Species that causes respiratory tract infection in humans

   A23.8   **Other brucellosis**

   A23.9   **Brucellosis, unspecified**

● **A24   Glanders and melioidosis**
   Infection, usually of rodents, which spreads to other animals and humans, caused by Burkholderia pseudomallei through break in skin contaminated with infested soil or water

   A24.0   **Glanders**
           Infection due to Pseudomonas mallei
           Malleus

   A24.1   **Acute and fulminating melioidosis**
           Melioidosis pneumonia
           Melioidosis sepsis

   A24.2   **Subacute and chronic melioidosis**

   A24.3   **Other melioidosis**

   A24.9   **Melioidosis, unspecified**
           Infection due to Pseudomonas pseudomallei NOS
           Whitmore's disease

Item 1-6 Brucellosis: An infectious disease caused by the bacterium Brucella. Humans are infected by contact with contaminated animals or animal products. In humans brucellosis symptoms that are similar to the flu include fever, sweats, headaches, back pains, and physical weakness. Severe infections of the central nervous system or lining of the heart may occur. Brucellosis can also cause chronic symptoms that include recurrent fevers, joint pain, and fatigue.

▶ New   ⇒ Revised   ~~deleted~~ Deleted   Excludes 1   Excludes 2   Includes   Use additional   Code first   Code also   Key words

OGCR Official Guidelines   X Assign placeholder X   ● Use Additional Character(s)   ▶ Manifestation Code   🝔 Hierarchical Condition Category   Coding Clinic

● **A25   Rat-bite fevers**
RBF, infectious disease caused by Streptobacillus moniliformis or Spirillum minus.

     A25.0   Spirillosis
         Any disease condition caused by spirilla
         Sodoku

     A25.1   Streptobacillosis
         Acute, febrile human illness caused by bacteria transmitted by rats in most cases, passed from rodent to human via rodent's urine or mucous secretions; AKA rat fever
         Epidemic arthritic erythema
         Haverhill fever
         Streptobacillary rat-bite fever

     A25.9   Rat-bite fever, unspecified

● **A26   Erysipeloid**
Infection with Erysipelothrix rhusiopathiae, *occurring often as occupational disease resulting from handling infected fish, shellfish, meat, or poultry*

     A26.0   Cutaneous erysipeloid
         Erythema migrans

     A26.7   Erysipelothrix sepsis 🦠

     A26.8   Other forms of erysipeloid

     A26.9   Erysipeloid, unspecified

● **A27   Leptospirosis**
Occurs most commonly in the tropics

     A27.0   Leptospirosis icterohemorrhagica
         Leptospiral or spirochetal jaundice (hemorrhagic)
         Weil's disease

     ● **A27.8   Other forms of leptospirosis**
         A27.81   Aseptic meningitis in leptospirosis
         A27.89   Other forms of leptospirosis

     A27.9   Leptospirosis, unspecified

● **A28   Other zoonotic bacterial diseases, not elsewhere classified**

     A28.0   Pasteurellosis
         Infection of humans or other animals by species of Pasteurella

     A28.1   Cat-scratch disease
         Cat-scratch fever

     A28.2   Extraintestinal yersiniosis
         Infection from Yersinia enterocolitica; *AKA enteric yersiniosis, intestinal yersiniosis, Yersinia enteritis*
         Excludes1   enteritis due to Yersinia enterocolitica (A04.6)
                     plague (A20.-)

     A28.8   Other specified zoonotic bacterial diseases, not elsewhere classified

     A28.9   Zoonotic bacterial disease, unspecified

OTHER BACTERIAL DISEASES (A30-A49)

● **A30   Leprosy [Hansen's disease]**
Chronic infectious disease attacking the skin, peripheral nerves, and mucous membranes

     Includes   infection due to Mycobacterium leprae
     Excludes1   sequelae of leprosy (B92)

     A30.0   Indeterminate leprosy
         I leprosy

     A30.1   Tuberculoid leprosy
         TT leprosy

     A30.2   Borderline tuberculoid leprosy
         BT leprosy

     A30.3   Borderline leprosy
         BB leprosy

     A30.4   Borderline lepromatous leprosy
         BL leprosy

     A30.5   Lepromatous leprosy
         LL leprosy

     A30.8   Other forms of leprosy

     A30.9   Leprosy, unspecified

● **A31   Infection due to other mycobacteria**

     Excludes2   leprosy (A30.-)
                   tuberculosis (A15-A19)

     A31.0   Pulmonary mycobacterial infection 🦠
         Infection due to Mycobacterium avium
         Infection due to Mycobacterium intracellulare [Battey bacillus]
         Infection due to Mycobacterium kansasii

     A31.1   Cutaneous mycobacterial infection
         Buruli ulcer
         Infection due to Mycobacterium marinum
         Infection due to Mycobacterium ulcerans

     A31.2   Disseminated mycobacterium avium-intracellulare complex (DMAC) 🦠
         MAC sepsis

     A31.8   Other mycobacterial infections

     A31.9   Mycobacterial infection, unspecified
         Atypical mycobacterial infection NOS
         Mycobacteriosis NOS

● **A32   Listeriosis**
Infection caused by Listeria monocytogenes

     Includes   listerial foodborne infection
     Excludes1   neonatal (disseminated) listeriosis (P37.2)

     A32.0   Cutaneous listeriosis

     ● **A32.1   Listerial meningitis and meningoencephalitis**
         A32.11   Listerial meningitis
         A32.12   Listerial meningoencephalitis

     A32.7   Listerial sepsis 🦠

     ● **A32.8   Other forms of listeriosis**
         A32.81   Oculoglandular listeriosis
            Primary infection site is conjunctival sac, which if untreated may result in perforation of cornea and optic atrophy
         A32.82   Listerial endocarditis
            Exudative and proliferative inflammatory condition of endocardium caused by listeria bacteria
         A32.89   Other forms of listeriosis
            Listerial cerebral arteritis

     A32.9   Listeriosis, unspecified

     A33   Tetanus neonatorum   N
         Neonate = newborn

     A34   Obstetrical tetanus ♀   M

     A35   Other tetanus
         Tetanus NOS
     Excludes1   tetanus neonatorum (A33)
                   obstetrical tetanus (A34)

● **A36   Diphtheria**

     A36.0   Pharyngeal diphtheria
         Diphtheritic membranous angina
         Tonsillar diphtheria

     A36.1   Nasopharyngeal diphtheria

     A36.2   Laryngeal diphtheria
         Diphtheritic laryngotracheitis

     A36.3   Cutaneous diphtheria
         Excludes2   erythrasma (L08.1)

Item 1-7 Diphtheria: A highly contagious bacterial disease that results in the formation of an adherent membrane in the throat that may lead to suffocation. In its most poisonous form, it attacks the heart and lungs. It is spread by direct physical contact or breathing the aerosolized secretions of infected individuals. The exact location is specified in the codes.

CHAPTER 1 (A00-B99)

● **A36.8   Other diphtheria**

     A36.81   Diphtheritic cardiomyopathy 🐾
            Diphtheritic myocarditis

     A36.82   Diphtheritic radiculomyelitis

     A36.83   Diphtheritic polyneuritis

     A36.84   Diphtheritic tubulo-interstitial nephropathy

     A36.85   Diphtheritic cystitis

     A36.86   Diphtheritic conjunctivitis

     A36.89   Other diphtheritic complications
            Diphtheritic peritonitis

A36.9   Diphtheria, unspecified

● **A37   Whooping cough**
     Pertussis is a highly contagious disease caused by the bacterium Bordetella pertussis and results in a whooping sounding cough.

  ● **A37.0   Whooping cough due to Bordetella pertussis**

     A37.00   Whooping cough due to Bordetella pertussis without pneumonia
            Paroxysmal cough due to Bordetella pertussis without pneumonia

     A37.01   Whooping cough due to Bordetella pertussis with pneumonia
            Paroxysmal cough due to Bordetella pertussis without pneumonia

  ● **A37.1   Whooping cough due to Bordetella parapertussis**

     A37.10   Whooping cough due to Bordetella parapertussis without pneumonia

     A37.11   Whooping cough due to Bordetella parapertussis with pneumonia

  ● **A37.8   Whooping cough due to other Bordetella species**

     A37.80   Whooping cough due to other Bordetella species without pneumonia

     A37.81   Whooping cough due to other Bordetella species with pneumonia

  ● **A37.9   Whooping cough, unspecified species**

     A37.90   Whooping cough, unspecified species without pneumonia

     A37.91   Whooping cough, unspecified species with pneumonia

● **A38   Scarlet fever**
     Most commonly caused by the bacteria Streptococcus pneumoniae and Neisseria meningitides

     Includes   scarlatina
     Excludes2   streptococcal sore throat (J02.0)

A38.0   Scarlet fever with otitis media

A38.1   Scarlet fever with myocarditis

A38.8   Scarlet fever with other complications

A38.9   Scarlet fever, uncomplicated
     Scarlet fever, NOS

● **A39   Meningococcal infection**
     Most commonly caused by the bacteria Streptococcus pneumoniae and Neisseria meningitides

A39.0   Meningococcal meningitis

A39.1   Waterhouse-Friderichsen syndrome 🐾
     Fulminating complication of meningococcemia
     Meningococcal hemorrhagic adrenalitis
     Meningococcic adrenal syndrome

A39.2   Acute meningococcemia 🐾

A39.3   Chronic meningococcemia 🐾

A39.4   Meningococcemia, unspecified 🐾

  ● **A39.5   Meningococcal heart disease**

     A39.50   Meningococcal carditis, unspecified

     A39.51   Meningococcal endocarditis

     A39.52   Meningococcal myocarditis

     A39.53   Meningococcal pericarditis

● **A39.8   Other meningococcal infections**

     A39.81   Meningococcal encephalitis

     A39.82   Meningococcal retrobulbar neuritis
            Optic neuritis in portion of optic nerve posterior to eyeball; AKA postocular optic neuritis

     A39.83   Meningococcal arthritis 🐾

     A39.84   Postmeningococcal arthritis 🐾

     A39.89   Other meningococcal infections
            Meningococcal conjunctivitis

A39.9   Meningococcal infection, unspecified
     Meningococcal disease NOS

● **A40   Streptococcal sepsis**
     Code first
       postprocedural streptococcal sepsis (T81.44)
       streptococcal sepsis during labor (O75.3)
       streptococcal sepsis following abortion or ectopic or molar pregnancy (O03-O07, O08.0)
       streptococcal sepsis following immunization (T88.0)
       streptococcal sepsis following infusion, transfusion or therapeutic injection (T80.2-)

     Excludes1   neonatal (P36.0-P36.1)
                 puerperal sepsis (O85)
                 sepsis due to Streptococcus, group D (A41.81)

A40.0   Sepsis due to streptococcus, group A 🐾

A40.1   Sepsis due to streptococcus, group B 🐾
     Coding Clinic: 2019, Q1, P14

A40.3   Sepsis due to Streptococcus pneumoniae 🐾
     Pneumococcal sepsis

A40.8   Other streptococcal sepsis 🐾

A40.9   Streptococcal sepsis, unspecified 🐾

● **A41   Other sepsis**
     Code first
       postprocedural sepsis (T81.44)
       sepsis during labor (O75.3)
       sepsis following abortion, ectopic or molar pregnancy (O03-O07, O08.0)
       sepsis following immunization (T88.0)
       sepsis following infusion, transfusion or therapeutic injection (T80.2-)

     Excludes1   bacteremia NOS (R78.81)
                 neonatal (P36.-)
                 puerperal sepsis (O85)
                 streptococcal sepsis (A40.-)

     Excludes2   sepsis (due to) (in) actinomycotic (A42.7)
                 sepsis (due to) (in) anthrax (A22.7)
                 sepsis (due to) (in) candidal (B37.7)
                 sepsis (due to) (in) Erysipelothrix (A26.7)
                 sepsis (due to) (in) extraintestinal yersiniosis (A28.2)
                 sepsis (due to) (in) gonococcal (A54.86)
                 sepsis (due to) (in) herpesviral (B00.7)
                 sepsis (due to) (in) listerial (A32.7)
                 sepsis (due to) (in) melioidosis (A24.1)
                 sepsis (due to) (in) meningococcal (A39.2-A39.4)
                 sepsis (due to) (in) plague (A20.7)
                 sepsis (due to) (in) tularemia (A21.7)
                 toxic shock syndrome (A48.3)
     Coding Clinic: 2022, Q1, P35; 2016, Q1, P39

● **A41.0   Sepsis due to Staphylococcus aureus**

     A41.01   Sepsis due to Methicillin susceptible Staphylococcus aureus 🐾
            MSSA sepsis
            Staphylococcus aureus sepsis NOS

     A41.02   Sepsis due to Methicillin resistant Staphylococcus aureus 🐾

▶ New   ⇒ Revised   ~~deleted~~ Deleted   Excludes 1   Excludes 2   Includes   Use additional   Code first   Code also   Key words

OGCR Official Guidelines   X Assign placeholder X   ● Use Additional Character(s)   ▶ Manifestation Code   🐾 Hierarchical Condition Category   **Coding Clinic**

Item 1–8 Gas gangrene is a necrotizing subcutaneous infection that will cause tissue death. Patients with poor circulation (e.g., diabetes, peripheral nephropathy) will have low oxygen content in their tissues (hypoxia), which allows the Clostridium bacteria to flourish. Gas gangrene often occurs at the site of a surgical wound or trauma. Onset is sudden and dramatic. Treatment can include debridement, amputation, and/or hyperbaric oxygen treatments.

A41.1   **Sepsis due to other specified staphylococcus** 🦠
     Coagulase negative staphylococcus sepsis

A41.2   **Sepsis due to unspecified staphylococcus** 🦠

A41.3   **Sepsis due to Hemophilus influenzae** 🦠

A41.4   **Sepsis due to anaerobes** 🦠
     Excludes1   gas gangrene (A48.0)

● A41.5   **Sepsis due to other Gram-negative organisms**

   A41.50   **Gram-negative sepsis, unspecified** 🦠
       Gram-negative sepsis NOS

   A41.51   **Sepsis due to Escherichia coli [E. coli]** 🦠
       Coding Clinic: 2018, Q1, P16

   A41.52   **Sepsis due to Pseudomonas** 🦠
       Pseudomonas aeroginosa

   A41.53   **Sepsis due to Serratia** 🦠

   A41.59   **Other Gram-negative sepsis** 🦠
       Coding Clinic: 2019, Q1, P13

● A41.8   **Other specified sepsis**

   A41.81   **Sepsis due to Enterococcus** 🦠

   A41.89   **Other specified sepsis** 🦠
       Coding Clinic: 2021, Q1, P33; 2016, Q3, P8-14

A41.9   **Sepsis, unspecified organism** 🦠
     Septicemia NOS
     Coding Clinic: 2022, Q2, P5; Q1, P30; 2018, Q4, P18

● A42   **Actinomycosis**
     Excludes1   actinomycetoma (B47.1)

A42.0   **Pulmonary actinomycosis** 🦠

A42.1   **Abdominal actinomycosis**

A42.2   **Cervicofacial actinomycosis**

A42.7   **Actinomycotic sepsis** 🦠

● A42.8   **Other forms of actinomycosis**

   A42.81   **Actinomycotic meningitis**

   A42.82   **Actinomycotic encephalitis**

   A42.89   **Other forms of actinomycosis**

A42.9   **Actinomycosis, unspecified**

● A43   **Nocardiosis**

A43.0   **Pulmonary nocardiosis** 🦠

A43.1   **Cutaneous nocardiosis**

A43.8   **Other forms of nocardiosis**

A43.9   **Nocardiosis, unspecified**

● A44   **Bartonellosis**

A44.0   **Systemic bartonellosis**
     Oroya fever

A44.1   **Cutaneous and mucocutaneous bartonellosis**
     Verruga peruana

A44.8   **Other forms of bartonellosis**

A44.9   **Bartonellosis, unspecified**

A46   **Erysipelas**
     Excludes1   postpartum or puerperal erysipelas (O86.89)

● A48   **Other bacterial diseases, not elsewhere classified**
     Excludes1   actinomycetoma (B47.1)

A48.0   **Gas gangrene** 🦠
     Clostridial cellulitis
     Clostridial myonecrosis
     Coding Clinic: 2017, Q4, P102

A48.1   **Legionnaires' disease** 🦠

A48.2   **Nonpneumonic Legionnaires' disease [Pontiac fever]**

A48.3   **Toxic shock syndrome** 🦠
     Use additional code to identify the organism (B95, B96)
     Excludes1   endotoxic shock NOS (R57.8)
                sepsis NOS (A41.9)
     Coding Clinic: 2022, Q1, P35

A48.4   **Brazilian purpuric fever**
     Systemic Hemophilus aegyptius infection

● A48.5   **Other specified botulism**
     Non-foodborne intoxication due to toxins of Clostridium botulinum [C. botulinum]
     Excludes1   food poisoning due to toxins of Clostridium botulinum (A05.1)

   A48.51   **Infant botulism**   P

   A48.52   **Wound botulism**
       Non-foodborne botulism NOS
       Use additional code for associated wound

A48.8   **Other specified bacterial diseases**

● A49   **Bacterial infection of unspecified site**
     Excludes1   bacterial agents as the cause of diseases classified elsewhere (B95-B96)
       chlamydial infection NOS (A74.9)
       meningococcal infection NOS (A39.9)
       rickettsial infection NOS (A79.9)
       spirochetal infection NOS (A69.9)

● A49.0   **Staphylococcal infection, unspecified site**

   A49.01   **Methicillin susceptible Staphylococcus aureus infection, unspecified site**
       Methicillin susceptible Staphylococcus aureus (MSSA) infection
       Staphylococcus aureus infection NOS

   A49.02   **Methicillin resistant Staphylococcus aureus infection, unspecified site**
       Methicillin resistant Staphylococcus aureus (MRSA) infection

A49.1   **Streptococcal infection, unspecified site**

A49.2   **Hemophilus influenzae infection, unspecified site**
     Any of seven bacterium of genus Haemophilus

A49.3   **Mycoplasma infection, unspecified site**
     Bacterium of class Mollicutes, unusual group of bacteria distinguished by absence of cell wall

A49.8   **Other bacterial infections of unspecified site**

A49.9   **Bacterial infection, unspecified**
     Excludes1   bacteremia NOS (R78.81)

INFECTIONS WITH A PREDOMINANTLY SEXUAL MODE OF TRANSMISSION (A50-A64)

     Excludes1   human immunodeficiency virus [HIV] disease (B20)
       nonspecific and nongonococcal urethritis (N34.1)
       Reiter's disease (M02.3-)

● A50   **Congenital syphilis**

● A50.0   **Early congenital syphilis, symptomatic**
     Any congenital syphilitic condition specified as early or manifest less than two years after birth

   A50.01   **Early congenital syphilitic oculopathy**

   A50.02   **Early congenital syphilitic osteochondropathy**

   A50.03   **Early congenital syphilitic pharyngitis**
       Early congenital syphilitic laryngitis

   A50.04   **Early congenital syphilitic pneumonia**

   A50.05   **Early congenital syphilitic rhinitis**

   A50.06   **Early cutaneous congenital syphilis**

   A50.07   **Early mucocutaneous congenital syphilis**

   A50.08   **Early visceral congenital syphilis**

   A50.09   **Other early congenital syphilis, symptomatic**

Figure 1-3 Chancre of primary syphilis. (From James WD, Berger TG, Elston DM: Andrews' Diseases of the Skin: Clinical Dermatology, Philadelphia, Saunders Elsevier, 2006)

Item 1–9 Syphilis, also known as lues, is the most serious of the venereal diseases caused by *Treponema pallidum.* The **primary** stage is characterized by an ulceration known as **chancre,** which usually appears on the genitals but can also develop on the anus, lips, tonsils, breasts, or fingers. Syphilis is easy to cure in its early stages. A single intramuscular injection of penicillin will usually cure a person who has had syphilis for less than a year.

The **secondary** stage is characterized by a rash that can affect any area of the body. **Latent** syphilis is divided into **early,** which is diagnosed within two years of infection, and **late,** which is diagnosed two years or more after infection. Additional doses of penicillin or another antibiotic are needed to treat someone who has had syphilis for longer than a year. For those allergic to penicillin, there are other antibiotic treatments. **Congenital** syphilis is also labeled **early** or **late** based on the time of diagnosis.

A50.1 **Early congenital syphilis, latent**
Congenital syphilis without clinical manifestations, with positive serological reaction and negative spinal fluid test, less than two years after birth

A50.2 **Early congenital syphilis, unspecified**
Congenital syphilis NOS less than two years after birth

● A50.3 **Late congenital syphilitic oculopathy**
Excludes1   Hutchinson's triad (A50.53)

A50.30 **Late congenital syphilitic oculopathy, unspecified**

A50.31 **Late congenital syphilitic interstitial keratitis**

A50.32 **Late congenital syphilitic chorioretinitis**

A50.39 **Other late congenital syphilitic oculopathy**

● A50.4 **Late congenital neurosyphilis [juvenile neurosyphilis]**
Use additional code to identify any associated mental disorder
Excludes1   Hutchinson's triad (A50.53)

A50.40 **Late congenital neurosyphilis, unspecified**
Juvenile neurosyphilis NOS

A50.41 **Late congenital syphilitic meningitis**

A50.42 **Late congenital syphilitic encephalitis**

A50.43 **Late congenital syphilitic polyneuropathy**

A50.44 **Late congenital syphilitic optic nerve atrophy**

A50.45 **Juvenile general paresis**
Dementia paralytica juvenilis
Juvenile tabetoparetic neurosyphilis

A50.49 **Other late congenital neurosyphilis**
Juvenile tabes dorsalis

● A50.5 **Other late congenital syphilis, symptomatic**
Any congenital syphilitic condition specified as late or manifest two years or more after birth

A50.51 **Clutton's joints**

A50.52 **Hutchinson's teeth**

A50.53 **Hutchinson's triad**

A50.54 **Late congenital cardiovascular syphilis**

A50.55 **Late congenital syphilitic arthropathy** 🔖

A50.56 **Late congenital syphilitic osteochondropathy**

A50.57 **Syphilitic saddle nose**

A50.59 **Other late congenital syphilis, symptomatic**

A50.6 **Late congenital syphilis, latent**
Congenital syphilis without clinical manifestations, with positive serological reaction and negative spinal fluid test, two years or more after birth.

A50.7 **Late congenital syphilis, unspecified**
Congenital syphilis NOS two years or more after birth.

A50.9 **Congenital syphilis, unspecified**

● A51 **Early syphilis**
A51.0 **Primary genital syphilis**
Syphilitic chancre NOS

A51.1 **Primary anal syphilis**

A51.2 **Primary syphilis of other sites**

● A51.3 **Secondary syphilis of skin and mucous membranes**

A51.31 **Condyloma latum**

A51.32 **Syphilitic alopecia**

A51.39 **Other secondary syphilis of skin**
Syphilitic leukoderma
Syphilitic mucous patch
Excludes1   late syphilitic leukoderma (A52.79)

● A51.4 **Other secondary syphilis**

A51.41 **Secondary syphilitic meningitis**

A51.42 **Secondary syphilitic female pelvic disease** ♀

A51.43 **Secondary syphilitic oculopathy**
Secondary syphilitic chorioretinitis
Secondary syphilitic iridocyclitis, iritis
Secondary syphilitic uveitis

A51.44 **Secondary syphilitic nephritis**

A51.45 **Secondary syphilitic hepatitis**

A51.46 **Secondary syphilitic osteopathy**

A51.49 **Other secondary syphilitic conditions**
Secondary syphilitic lymphadenopathy
Secondary syphilitic myositis

A51.5 **Early syphilis, latent**
Syphilis (acquired) without clinical manifestations, with positive serological reaction and negative spinal fluid test, less than two years after infection.

A51.9 **Early syphilis, unspecified**

● A52 **Late syphilis**
● A52.0 **Cardiovascular and cerebrovascular syphilis**

A52.00 **Cardiovascular syphilis, unspecified**

A52.01 **Syphilitic aneurysm of aorta**

A52.02 **Syphilitic aortitis**

A52.03 **Syphilitic endocarditis**
Syphilitic aortic valve incompetence or stenosis
Syphilitic mitral valve stenosis
Syphilitic pulmonary valve regurgitation

A52.04 **Syphilitic cerebral arteritis**

A52.05 **Other cerebrovascular syphilis**
Syphilitic cerebral aneurysm (ruptured) (non-ruptured)
Syphilitic cerebral thrombosis

A52.06 **Other syphilitic heart involvement**
Syphilitic coronary artery disease
Syphilitic myocarditis
Syphilitic pericarditis

A52.09 **Other cardiovascular syphilis**

● A52.1 **Symptomatic neurosyphilis**

A52.10 **Symptomatic neurosyphilis, unspecified**

A52.11 **Tabes dorsalis**
Cognitive decline with progressive degeneration of posterior columns, roots, and ganglia of spinal cord, occur 15-20 years after initial infection of syphilis; AKA Duchenne disease
Locomotor ataxia (progressive)
Tabetic neurosyphilis

A52.12 **Other cerebrospinal syphilis**

A52.13 **Late syphilitic meningitis**

A52.14 **Late syphilitic encephalitis**

A52.15 **Late syphilitic neuropathy**
Late syphilitic acoustic neuritis
Late syphilitic optic (nerve) atrophy
Late syphilitic polyneuropathy
Late syphilitic retrobulbar neuritis

▶ New   ⇒ Revised   ~~deleted~~ Deleted   Excludes 1   Excludes 2   Includes   Use additional   Code first   Code also   Key words

OGCR Official Guidelines   X Assign placeholder X   ● Use Additional Character(s)   ▌ Manifestation Code   🔖 Hierarchical Condition Category   **Coding Clinic**

A52.16   Charcôt's arthropathy (tabetic)
Progressive musculoskeletal condition characterized by joint dislocation, fractures, and deformities, results in progressive destruction of bone and soft tissue of weight-bearing joints

A52.17   General paresis
Chronic meningoencephalitis results in loss of cortical function, or progressive dementia and generalized paralysis, occurring 10-20 years after initial infection of syphilis; AKA Bayle disease, dementia paralytica, paralytic dementiaparetic neurosyphilis, syphilitic meningoencephalitis
Dementia paralytica

A52.19   Other symptomatic neurosyphilis
Syphilitic parkinsonism

A52.2   Asymptomatic neurosyphilis

A52.3   Neurosyphilis, unspecified
Gumma (syphilitic)
Destructive lesions of syphilis
Syphilis (late)
Syphiloma
Coding Clinic: 2021, Q2, P6

● **A52.7   Other symptomatic late syphilis**

A52.71   Late syphilitic oculopathy
Late syphilitic chorioretinitis
Late syphilitic episcleritis

A52.72   Syphilis of lung and bronchus

A52.73   Symptomatic late syphilis of other respiratory organs

A52.74   Syphilis of liver and other viscera
Late syphilitic peritonitis

A52.75   Syphilis of kidney and ureter
Syphilitic glomerular disease

A52.76   Other genitourinary symptomatic late syphilis ♀
Late syphilitic female pelvic inflammatory disease

A52.77   Syphilis of bone and joint

A52.78   Syphilis of other musculoskeletal tissue
Late syphilitic bursitis
Syphilis [stage unspecified] of bursa
Syphilis [stage unspecified] of muscle
Syphilis [stage unspecified] of synovium
Syphilis [stage unspecified] of tendon

A52.79   Other symptomatic late syphilis
Late syphilitic leukoderma
Syphilis of adrenal gland
Syphilis of pituitary gland
Syphilis of thyroid gland
Syphilitic splenomegaly
> **Excludes1**   syphilitic leukoderma (secondary) (A51.39)

A52.8   Late syphilis, latent
Syphilis (acquired) without clinical manifestations, with positive serological reaction and negative spinal fluid test, two years or more after infection

A52.9   Late syphilis, unspecified

● **A53   Other and unspecified syphilis**

A53.0   Latent syphilis, unspecified as early or late
Latent syphilis NOS
Positive serological reaction for syphilis

A53.9   Syphilis, unspecified
Infection due to Treponema pallidum NOS
Syphilis (acquired) NOS
> **Excludes1**   syphilis NOS under two years of age (A50.2)

● **A54   Gonococcal infection**

● **A54.0   Gonococcal infection of lower genitourinary tract without periurethral or accessory gland abscess**
> **Excludes1**   gonococcal infection with genitourinary gland abscess (A54.1)
> gonococcal infection with periurethral abscess (A54.1)

A54.00   Gonococcal infection of lower genitourinary tract, unspecified

A54.01   Gonococcal cystitis and urethritis, unspecified

A54.02   Gonococcal vulvovaginitis, unspecified ♀

A54.03   Gonococcal cervicitis, unspecified ♀

A54.09   Other gonococcal infection of lower genitourinary tract

Item 1-10 An STD (sexually transmitted disease) caused by **Neisseria gonorrhoeae** that flourishes in the warm, moist areas of the reproductive tract. Untreated gonorrhea spreads to other parts of the body, causing inflammation of the testes or prostate or pelvic inflammatory disease (PID).

A54.1   Gonococcal infection of lower genitourinary tract with periurethral and accessory gland abscess
Gonococcal Bartholin's gland abscess

● **A54.2   Gonococcal pelviperitonitis and other gonococcal genitourinary infection**

A54.21   Gonococcal infection of kidney and ureter

A54.22   Gonococcal prostatitis ♂

A54.23   Gonococcal infection of other male genital organs ♂
Gonococcal epididymitis
Gonococcal orchitis

A54.24   Gonococcal female pelvic inflammatory disease ♀
Gonococcal pelviperitonitis
> **Excludes1**   gonococcal peritonitis (A54.85)

A54.29   Other gonococcal genitourinary infections

● **A54.3   Gonococcal infection of eye**

A54.30   Gonococcal infection of eye, unspecified

A54.31   Gonococcal conjunctivitis
Form of bacterial conjunctivitis contracted by newborns during delivery; AKA neonatal conjunctivitis
Ophthalmia neonatorum due to gonococcus

A54.32   Gonococcal iridocyclitis
Inflammation of iris and of ciliary body due to gonococcal infection

A54.33   Gonococcal keratitis
Inflammation of cornea due to gonococcal infection; AKA keratoconjunctivitis, keratopathy

A54.39   Other gonococcal eye infection
Gonococcal endophthalmia

● **A54.4   Gonococcal infection of musculoskeletal system**

A54.40   Gonococcal infection of musculoskeletal system, unspecified 🦠

A54.41   Gonococcal spondylopathy 🦠
Disorder of vertebrae due to gonococcal infection; AKA rachiopathy

A54.42   Gonococcal arthritis 🦠
> **Excludes2**   gonococcal infection of spine (A54.41)

A54.43   Gonococcal osteomyelitis 🦠
> **Excludes2**   gonococcal infection of spine (A54.41)

A54.49   Gonococcal infection of other musculoskeletal tissue 🦠
Gonococcal bursitis
Gonococcal myositis
Gonococcal synovitis
Gonococcal tenosynovitis

CHAPTER 1 (A00–B99)

CHAPTER 1 (A00–B99)

A54.5   Gonococcal **pharyngitis**

A54.6   Gonococcal infection of **anus and rectum**

● A54.8   **Other gonococcal infections**

    A54.81   Gonococcal **meningitis**

    A54.82   Gonococcal **brain abscess**

    A54.83   Gonococcal **heart infection**
        Gonococcal endocarditis
        Gonococcal myocarditis
        Gonococcal pericarditis

    A54.84   Gonococcal **pneumonia** 🦠

    A54.85   Gonococcal **peritonitis** 🦠
        Excludes1   gonococcal pelviperitonitis
               (A54.24)

    A54.86   Gonococcal **sepsis** 🦠

    A54.89   **Other** gonococcal infections
        Gonococcal keratoderma
        Gonococcal lymphadenitis

A54.9   Gonococcal infection, **unspecified**

A55   **Chlamydial lymphogranuloma (venereum)**
    Climatic or tropical bubo
    Durand-Nicolas-Favre disease
    Esthiomene
    Lymphogranuloma inguinale

● A56   **Other sexually transmitted chlamydial diseases**
    Includes   sexually transmitted diseases due to Chlamydia
            trachomatis

    Excludes1   neonatal chlamydial conjunctivitis (P39.1)
            neonatal chlamydial pneumonia (P23.1)

    Excludes2   chlamydial lymphogranuloma (A55)
            conditions classified to A74.-

  ● A56.0   **Chlamydial infection of lower genitourinary tract**

    A56.00   **Chlamydial infection of lower genitourinary
        tract, unspecified**

    A56.01   **Chlamydial cystitis and urethritis**

    A56.02   **Chlamydial vulvovaginitis** ♀

    A56.09   **Other** chlamydial infection of lower
        genitourinary tract
        Chlamydial cervicitis

  ● A56.1   **Chlamydial infection of pelviperitoneum and other
        genitourinary organs**

    A56.11   **Chlamydial female pelvic inflammatory
        disease** ♀

    A56.19   **Other** chlamydial genitourinary infection
        Chlamydial epididymitis
        Chlamydial orchitis

  A56.2   **Chlamydial infection of genitourinary tract, unspecified**

  A56.3   **Chlamydial infection of anus and rectum**

  A56.4   **Chlamydial infection of pharynx**

  A56.8   **Sexually transmitted chlamydial infection of other sites**

A57   **Chancroid**
    Ulcus molle
    *Sexually transmitted infection caused by bacteria, Haemophilus
      ducreyi*

A58   **Granuloma inguinale**
    Chronic, progressive, ulcerative granulomatous disease
    Donovanosis

● A59   **Trichomoniasis**
    Excludes2   intestinal trichomoniasis (A07.8)
    A common STD caused by a parasite, Trichomonas vaginalis

  ● A59.0   **Urogenital trichomoniasis**

    A59.00   **Urogenital trichomoniasis, unspecified**
        Fluor (vaginalis) due to Trichomonas
        Leukorrhea (vaginalis) due to Trichomonas

    A59.01   **Trichomonal vulvovaginitis** ♀

    A59.02   **Trichomonal prostatitis** ♂

    A59.03   **Trichomonal cystitis and urethritis**

    A59.09   **Other urogenital trichomoniasis**
        *Common sexually transmitted disease (STD)
          caused by single-celled protozoan parasite;
          AKA trich*
        Trichomonas cervicitis

  A59.8   **Trichomoniasis of other sites**

  A59.9   **Trichomoniasis, unspecified**

● A60   **Anogenital herpesviral [herpes simplex] infections**

  ● A60.0   **Herpesviral infection of genitalia and urogenital tract**

    A60.00   **Herpesviral infection of urogenital system,
        unspecified**

    A60.01   **Herpesviral infection of penis** ♂

    A60.02   **Herpesviral infection of other male genital
        organs** ♂

    A60.03   **Herpesviral cervicitis** ♀

    A60.04   **Herpesviral vulvovaginitis** ♀
        Herpesviral [herpes simplex] ulceration
        Herpesviral [herpes simplex] vaginitis
        Herpesviral [herpes simplex] vulvitis

    A60.09   **Herpesviral infection of other urogenital tract**
        Coding Clinic: 2020, Q1, P20

  A60.1   **Herpesviral infection of perianal skin and rectum**

  A60.9   **Anogenital herpesviral infection, unspecified**

● A63   **Other predominantly sexually transmitted diseases, not
    elsewhere classified**

    Excludes2   molluscum contagiosum (B08.1)
            papilloma of cervix (D26.0)

  A63.0   **Anogenital (venereal) warts**
    Anogenital warts due to (human) papillomavirus
      [HPV]
    Condyloma acuminatum

  A63.8   **Other specified predominantly sexually transmitted
    diseases**

A64   **Unspecified sexually transmitted disease**

OTHER SPIROCHETAL DISEASES (A65-A69)

    Excludes2   leptospirosis (A27.-)
            syphilis (A50-A53)

A65   **Nonvenereal syphilis**
    Bejel
    Endemic syphilis
    Njovera

● A66   **Yaws**
    *Endemic, infectious, tropical disease caused by spirochete, spread by
      direct contact; AKA frambesia, framboesia, frambesia tropica*

    Includes   bouba
            frambesia (tropica)
            pian

  A66.0   **Initial lesions of yaws**
    Chancre of yaws
    Frambesia, initial or primary
    Initial frambesial ulcer
    Mother yaw

  A66.1   **Multiple papillomata and wet crab yaws**
    Frambesioma
    Pianoma
    Plantar or palmar papilloma of yaws

  A66.2   **Other early skin lesions of yaws**
    Cutaneous yaws, less than five years after infection
    Early yaws (cutaneous)(macular)(maculopapular)
      (micropapular)(papular)
    Frambeside of early yaws

▶ New   ⇒ Revised   ~~deleted~~ Deleted   Excludes 1   Excludes 2   Includes   Use additional   Code first   Code also   Key words

OGCR Official Guidelines   X Assign placeholder X   ● Use Additional Character(s)   ❱ Manifestation Code   🦠 Hierarchical Condition Category   **Coding Clinic**

A66.3 Hyperkeratosis of yaws
Hypertrophy of stratum corneum of skin in which there are small, hard, verrucous scales
Ghoul hand
Hyperkeratosis, palmar or plantar (early) (late) due to yaws
Worm-eaten soles

A66.4 Gummata and ulcers of yaws
Small, rubbery granuloma with necrotic center and inflamed characteristic of advanced stage of syphilis; AKA syphiloma
Gummatous frambeside
Nodular late yaws (ulcerated)

A66.5 Gangosa
Manifestation of yaws that develops in the soft palate and spreads eroding bone, cartilage, and soft tissue
Rhinopharyngitis mutilans

A66.6 Bone and joint lesions of yaws 🔾
Yaws ganglion
Yaws goundou
Yaws gumma, bone
Yaws gummatous osteitis or periostitis
Yaws hydrarthrosis
Yaws osteitis
Yaws periostitis (hypertrophic)

A66.7 Other manifestations of yaws
Juxta-articular nodules of yaws
Mucosal yaws

A66.8 Latent yaws
Yaws without clinical manifestations, with positive serology

A66.9 Yaws, unspecified

● **A67 Pinta [carate]**
Group of nonvenereal diseases caused by Treponema species

A67.0 Primary lesions of pinta
Chancre (primary) of pinta
Papule (primary) of pinta

A67.1 Intermediate lesions of pinta
Erythematous plaques of pinta
Hyperchromic lesions of pinta
Hyperkeratosis of pinta
Pintids

A67.2 Late lesions of pinta
Achromic skin lesions of pinta
Cicatricial skin lesions of pinta
Dyschromic skin lesions of pinta

A67.3 Mixed lesions of pinta
Achromic with hyperchromic skin lesions of pinta [carate]

A67.9 Pinta, unspecified

● **A68 Relapsing fevers**
Includes   recurrent fever
Excludes2   Lyme disease (A69.2-)

A68.0 Louse-borne relapsing fever
Relapsing fever due to Borrelia recurrentis

A68.1 Tick-borne relapsing fever
Relapsing fever due to any Borrelia species other than Borrelia recurrentis

A68.9 Relapsing fever, unspecified

Item 1-11 Cancrum oris, also known as **noma** or **gangrenous stomatitis,** begins as an ulcer of the gingiva and results in a progressive gangrenous process.

● **A69 Other spirochetal infections**

A69.0 Necrotizing ulcerative stomatitis
Cancrum oris
Fusospirochetal gangrene
Noma
Stomatitis gangrenosa

A69.1 Other Vincent's infections
Fusospirochetal pharyngitis
Necrotizing ulcerative (acute) gingivitis
Necrotizing ulcerative (acute) gingivostomatitis
Spirochetal stomatitis
Trench mouth
Vincent's angina
Vincent's gingivitis

● **A69.2 Lyme disease**
Erythema chronicum migrans due to Borrelia burgdorferi

A69.20 Lyme disease, unspecified
Coding Clinic: 2021, Q4, P5

A69.21 Meningitis due to Lyme disease

A69.22 Other neurologic disorders in Lyme disease
Cranial neuritis
Meningoencephalitis
Polyneuropathy

A69.23 Arthritis due to Lyme disease 🔾

A69.29 Other conditions associated with Lyme disease
Myopericarditis due to Lyme disease
Coding Clinic: 2016, Q3, P12

A69.8 Other specified spirochetal infections

A69.9 Spirochetal infection, unspecified

OTHER DISEASES CAUSED BY CHLAMYDIAE (A70-A74)

Excludes1   sexually transmitted chlamydial diseases (A55-A56)

A70 Chlamydia psittaci infections
Ornithosis
Parrot fever
Psittacosis

● **A71 Trachoma**
Excludes1   sequelae of trachoma (B94.0)

A71.0 Initial stage of trachoma
Trachoma dubium

A71.1 Active stage of trachoma
Granular conjunctivitis (trachomatous)
Trachomatous follicular conjunctivitis
Trachomatous pannus

A71.9 Trachoma, unspecified

● **A74 Other diseases caused by chlamydiae**
Excludes1   neonatal chlamydial conjunctivitis (P39.1)
neonatal chlamydial pneumonia (P23.1)
Reiter's disease (M02.3-)
sexually transmitted chlamydial diseases (A55-A56)

Excludes2   chlamydial pneumonia (J16.0)

A74.0 Chlamydial conjunctivitis
Paratrachoma

● **A74.8 Other chlamydial diseases**

A74.81 Chlamydial peritonitis

A74.89 Other chlamydial diseases

A74.9 Chlamydial infection, unspecified
Chlamydiosis NOS

CHAPTER 1 (A00-B99)

CHAPTER 1 (A00-B99)

Item 1–12 **Rickettsioses** are diseases spread from ticks, lice, fleas, or mites to humans.

Typhus is spread to humans chiefly by the fleas of rats.

Endemic identifies a disease as being present in low numbers of humans at all times, whereas **epidemic** identifies a disease as being present in high numbers of humans at a specific time. Morbidity (death) is higher in epidemic diseases.

Brill's disease, also known as **Brill-Zinsser disease,** is spread from human to human by body lice and also from the lice of flying squirrels. **Scrub typhus** is spread in the same ways as Brill's disease.

Malaria is spread to humans by mosquitoes.

RICKETTSIOSES (A75-A79)

● **A75** **Typhus fever**
> **Excludes1**   rickettsiosis due to Ehrlichia sennetsu (A79.81)

    A75.0 **Epidemic louse-borne typhus fever due to Rickettsia prowazekii**
       Organisms transmitted between humans via louse
       Classical typhus (fever)
       Epidemic (louse-borne) typhus

    A75.1 **Recrudescent typhus [Brill's disease]**
       Brill-Zinsser disease

    A75.2 **Typhus fever due to Rickettsia typhi**
       Murine (flea-borne) typhus

    A75.3 **Typhus fever due to Rickettsia tsutsugamushi**
       Scrub (mite-borne) typhus
       Tsutsugamushi fever
       Typhus fever due to Orientia Tsutsugamushi (scrub typhus)

    A75.9 **Typhus fever, unspecified**
       Typhus (fever) NOS

● **A77** **Spotted fever [tick-borne rickettsioses]**
    A77.0 **Spotted fever due to Rickettsia rickettsii**
       Rocky Mountain spotted fever
       Sao Paulo fever

    A77.1 **Spotted fever due to Rickettsia conorii**
       African tick typhus
       Boutonneuse fever
       India tick typhus
       Kenya tick typhus
       Marseilles fever
       Mediterranean tick fever

    A77.2 **Spotted fever due to Rickettsia siberica**
       North Asian tick fever
       Siberian tick typhus

    A77.3 **Spotted fever due to Rickettsia australis**
       Queensland tick typhus

●   **A77.4** **Ehrlichiosis**
       Type of tick-borne fever caused by bacteria infection
> **Excludes1**   anaplasmosis [A. phagocytophilum] (A79.82)
>   rickettsiosis due to Ehrlichia sennetsu (A79.81)
>   **Coding Clinic: 2021, Q4, P5**

       A77.40 **Ehrlichiosis, unspecified**
          Coding Clinic: 2021, Q4, P5

       A77.41 **Ehrlichiosis chafeensis [E. chafeensis]**

       A77.49 **Other ehrlichiosis**
          Ehrlichiosis due to E. ewingii
          Ehrlichiosis due to E. muris euclairensis

    A77.8 **Other spotted fevers**
       Rickettsia 364D/R. philipii (Pacific Coast tick fever)
       Spotted fever due to Rickettsia africae (African tick bite fever)
       Spotted fever due to Rickettsia parkeri]

    A77.9 **Spotted fever, unspecified**
       Tick-borne typhus NOS

   A78 **Q fever**
       Infection due to Coxiella burnetii
       Nine Mile fever
       Quadrilateral fever

● **A79** **Other rickettsioses**
    A79.0 **Trench fever**
       Quintan fever
       Wolhynian fever

    A79.1 **Rickettsialpox due to Rickettsia akari**
       Kew Garden fever
       Vesicular rickettsiosis

● **A79.8** **Other specified rickettsioses**
       A79.81 **Rickettsiosis due to Ehrlichia sennetsu**
          Rickettsiosis due to Neorickettsia sennetsu

       A79.82 Anaplasmosis [A. phagocytophilum]
          Transfusion transmitted A. phagocytophilum
          Coding Clinic: 2021, Q4, P5

       A79.89 **Other specified rickettsioses**

    A79.9 **Rickettsiosis, unspecified**
       Rickettsial infection NOS

VIRAL AND PRION INFECTIONS OF THE CENTRAL NERVOUS SYSTEM (A80-A89)

> **Excludes1**   postpolio syndrome (G14)
>   sequelae of poliomyelitis (B91)
>   sequelae of viral encephalitis (B94.1)

● **A80** **Acute poliomyelitis**
> **Excludes1**   acute flaccid myelitis (G04.82)

    A80.0 **Acute paralytic poliomyelitis, vaccine-associated**

    A80.1 **Acute paralytic poliomyelitis, wild virus, imported**

    A80.2 **Acute paralytic poliomyelitis, wild virus, indigenous**

● **A80.3** **Acute paralytic poliomyelitis, other and unspecified**
       A80.30 **Acute paralytic poliomyelitis, unspecified**

       A80.39 **Other acute paralytic poliomyelitis**

    A80.4 **Acute nonparalytic poliomyelitis**

    A80.9 **Acute poliomyelitis, unspecified**

● **A81** **Atypical virus infections of central nervous system**
> **Includes**   diseases of the central nervous system caused by prions

⇒ Use additional , if applicable, code to identify:
    dementia with anxiety (F02.84, F02.A4, F02.B4, F02.C4)
    dementia without behavioral disturbance (F02.80)
▶ dementia with behavioral disturbance (F02.81-, F02.A1-, F02.B1-, F02.C1-)
▶ dementia with mood disturbance (F02.83, F02.A3, F02.B3, F02.C3)
▶ dementia with psychotic disturbance (F02.82, F02.A2, F02.B2, F02.C2)
▶ dementia without behavioral disturbance (F02.80, F02.A0, F02.B0, F02.C0)
▶ mild neurocognitive disorder due to known physiological condition (F06.7-)

● **A81.0** **Creutzfeldt-Jakob disease**
       A81.00 **Creutzfeldt-Jakob disease, unspecified**
          Jakob-Creutzfeldt disease, unspecified

       A81.01 **Variant Creutzfeldt-Jakob disease**
          vCJD

       A81.09 **Other Creutzfeldt-Jakob disease**
          CJD
          Familial Creutzfeldt-Jakob disease
          Iatrogenic Creutzfeldt-Jakob disease
          Sporadic Creutzfeldt-Jakob disease
          Subacute spongiform encephalopathy (with dementia)

    A81.1 **Subacute sclerosing panencephalitis**
       Type of viral encephalitis that causes parenchymatous lesions in gray and white matter of brain
       Dawson's inclusion body encephalitis
       Van Bogaert's sclerosing leukoencephalopathy

Item 1-13 **Acute Poliomyelitis:** Also called infantile paralysis and is caused by the poliovirus, which enters the body orally and infects the intestinal wall and then enters the blood stream and central nervous system, causing muscle weakness and paralysis. This disease has been nearly eradicated with the polio vaccine.

▶ New   ⇒ Revised   ~~deleted~~ Deleted   Excludes 1   Excludes 2   Includes   Use additional   Code first   Code also   Key words

OGCR Official Guidelines   **X** Assign placeholder X   ● Use Additional Character(s)   ▶ Manifestation Code   🐷 Hierarchical Condition Category   **Coding Clinic**

A81.2 **Progressive multifocal leukoencephalopathy**
Group of diseases affecting white matter of brain
Multifocal leukoencephalopathy NOS

● A81.8 **Other atypical virus infections of central nervous system**

A81.81 **Kuru**

A81.82 **Gerstmann-Sträussler-Scheinker syndrome**
GSS syndrome

A81.83 **Fatal familial insomnia**
FFI

A81.89 **Other atypical virus infections of central
nervous system**

A81.9 **Atypical virus infection of central nervous system,
unspecified**
Prion diseases of the central nervous system NOS

● **A82 Rabies**
*Viral disease affecting the central nervous system and transmitted
from infected mammals to man*

A82.0 **Sylvatic rabies**

A82.1 **Urban rabies**

A82.9 **Rabies, unspecified**

● **A83 Mosquito-borne viral encephalitis**
*Inflammation of the brain caused most commonly by Herpes Simplex
virus*

Includes mosquito-borne viral meningoencephalitis

Excludes2 Venezuelan equine encephalitis (A92.2)
West Nile fever (A92.3-)
West Nile virus (A92.3-)

A83.0 **Japanese encephalitis**

A83.1 **Western equine encephalitis**

A83.2 **Eastern equine encephalitis**

A83.3 **St. Louis encephalitis**

A83.4 **Australian encephalitis**
Kunjin virus disease

A83.5 **California encephalitis**
California meningoencephalitis
La Crosse encephalitis

A83.6 **Rocio virus disease**
Mosquito-borne virus

A83.8 **Other mosquito-borne viral encephalitis**

A83.9 **Mosquito-borne viral encephalitis, unspecified**

● **A84 Tick-borne viral encephalitis**

Includes tick-borne viral meningoencephalitis

A84.0 **Far Eastern tick-borne encephalitis [Russian
spring-summer encephalitis]**

A84.1 **Central European tick-borne encephalitis**

A84.8 **Other tick-borne viral encephalitis**

A84.81 **Powassan virus disease**

A84.89 **Other tick-borne viral encephalitis**
Louping ill

*Code first, if applicable, transfusion related
infection (T80.22-)*

A84.9 **Tick-borne viral encephalitis, unspecified**

● **A85 Other viral encephalitis, not elsewhere classified**

Includes specified viral encephalomyelitis NEC
specified viral meningoencephalitis NEC

Excludes1 ~~benign myalgic encephalomyelitis (G93.3)~~
encephalitis due to cytomegalovirus (B25.8)
encephalitis due to herpesvirus NEC (B10.0-)
encephalitis due to herpesvirus [herpes simplex]
(B00.4)
encephalitis due to measles virus (B05.0)
encephalitis due to mumps virus (B26.2)
encephalitis due to poliomyelitis virus (A80.-)
encephalitis due to zoster (B02.0)
lymphocytic choriomeningitis (A87.2)
▶ myalgic encephalomyelitis (G93.32)

A85.0 **Enteroviral encephalitis**
Enteroviral encephalomyelitis

A85.1 **Adenoviral encephalitis**
Adenoviral meningoencephalitis

A85.2 **Arthropod-borne viral encephalitis, unspecified**

Excludes1 West nile virus with encephalitis (A92.31)

A85.8 **Other specified viral encephalitis**
Encephalitis lethargica
Von Economo-Cruchet disease

● **A86 Unspecified viral encephalitis**
Viral encephalomyelitis NOS
Viral meningoencephalitis NOS

● **A87 Viral meningitis**

Excludes1 meningitis due to herpesvirus [herpes simplex]
(B00.3)
meningitis due to measles virus (B05.1)
meningitis due to mumps virus (B26.1)
meningitis due to poliomyelitis virus (A80.-)
meningitis due to zoster (B02.1)

A87.0 **Enteroviral meningitis**
*Group of common viruses responsible for the majority of viral
meningitis*
Coxsackievirus meningitis
Echovirus meningitis

A87.1 **Adenoviral meningitis**

A87.2 **Lymphocytic choriomeningitis**
Lymphocytic meningoencephalitis

A87.8 **Other viral meningitis**

A87.9 **Viral meningitis, unspecified**

● **A88 Other viral infections of central nervous system, not elsewhere
classified**

Excludes1 viral encephalitis NOS (A86)
viral meningitis NOS (A87.9)

A88.0 **Enteroviral exanthematous fever [Boston exanthem]**
Infectious skin eruption

A88.1 **Epidemic vertigo**

A88.8 **Other specified viral infections of central nervous
system**

A89 **Unspecified viral infection of central nervous system**

OGCR Section I. C.1.f.

Certain Infectious and Parasitic Diseases (A00-B99)

Zika virus infections

Code only confirmed cases

Code only a confirmed diagnosis of Zika virus (A92.5, Zika virus
disease) as documented by the provider. This is an exception to the
hospital inpatient guideline Section II, H.

In this context, "confirmation" does not require documentation of
the type of test performed; the physician's diagnostic statement that
the condition is confirmed is sufficient. This code should be assigned
regardless of the stated mode of transmission.

If the provider documents "suspected", "possible" or "probable" Zika,
do not assign code A92.5. Assign a code(s) explaining the reason for
encounter (such as fever, rash, or joint pain) or Z20.828, Contact with
and (suspected) exposure to other viral communicable diseases.

CHAPTER 1 (A00-B99)

Item 1-14 Encephalitis is an inflammation of the brain most often caused
by a virus but may also be caused by a bacteria and most commonly transmitted
by a mosquito. **Myelitis** is an inflammation of the spinal cord that may disrupt
CNS function. Untreated myelitis may rapidly lead to permanent damage to the
spinal cord. **Encephalomyelitis** is a general term for an inflammation of the
brain and spinal cord.

ARTHROPOD-BORNE VIRAL FEVERS AND VIRAL HEMORRHAGIC FEVERS (A90-A99)

A90   Dengue fever [classical dengue]
Acute, self-limited disease, characterized by fever, prostration, severe muscle pains, headache, rash, lymphadenopathy, and leukopenia, caused by dengue virus; AKA breakbone, dandy

> **Excludes1**   dengue hemorrhagic fever (A91)

Coding Clinic: 2016, Q3, P13

A91   Dengue hemorrhagic fever
Serious follow-up to regular dengue, with symptoms of hemorrhage

●**A92   Other mosquito-borne viral fevers**

> **Excludes1**   Ross River disease (B33.1)

A92.0   Chikungunya virus disease
Transmitted by mosquitoes
Chikungunya (hemorrhagic) fever

A92.1   O'nyong-nyong fever
Acute, nonfatal febrile disease transmitted by mosquitoes, which clinically resembles dengue and chikungunya

A92.2   Venezuelan equine fever
Venezuelan equine encephalitis
Venezuelan equine encephalomyelitis virus disease

●**A92.3   West Nile virus infection**
West Nile fever

    A92.30   West Nile virus infection, unspecified
West Nile fever NOS
West Nile fever without complications
West Nile virus NOS

    A92.31   West Nile virus infection with encephalitis
West Nile encephalitis
West Nile encephalomyelitis
Coding Clinic: 2016, Q3, P13

    A92.32   West Nile virus infection with other neurologic manifestation
Use additional code to specify the neurologic manifestation

    A92.39   West Nile virus infection with other complications
Use additional code to specify the other conditions

A92.4   Rift Valley fever

A92.5   Zika virus disease
Zika virus fever
Zika virus infection
Zika NOS

> **Excludes1**   congenital Zika virus disease (P35.4)

Coding Clinic: 2016, Q4, P4-7, 121

A92.8   Other specified mosquito-borne viral fevers

A92.9   Mosquito-borne viral fever, unspecified

●**A93   Other arthropod-borne viral fevers, not elsewhere classified**

A93.0   Oropouche virus disease
Tropical viral infection
Oropouche fever

A93.1   Sandfly fever
Pappataci fever
Phlebotomus fever

A93.2   Colorado tick fever

A93.8   Other specified arthropod-borne viral fevers
Piry virus disease
Vesicular stomatitis virus disease [Indiana fever]

A94   Unspecified arthropod-borne viral fever
Arboviral fever NOS
Arbovirus infection NOS

●**A95   Yellow fever**
Acute infectious disease transmitted by mosquitoes

A95.0   Sylvatic yellow fever
Jungle yellow fever

A95.1   Urban yellow fever

A95.9   Yellow fever, unspecified

●**A96   Arenaviral hemorrhagic fever**
Virus that causes various hemorrhagic fevers

A96.0   Junin hemorrhagic fever

Argentinian hemorrhagic fever

A96.1   Machupo hemorrhagic fever
Transmitted by contact with infected rodents
Bolivian hemorrhagic fever

A96.2   Lassa fever
Acute type of hemorrhagic fever caused by contact with disease carrying mouse or person

A96.8   Other arenaviral hemorrhagic fevers

A96.9   Arenaviral hemorrhagic fever, unspecified

●**A98   Other viral hemorrhagic fevers, not elsewhere classified**

> **Excludes1**   chikungunya hemorrhagic fever (A92.0)
> dengue hemorrhagic fever (A91)

A98.0   Crimean-Congo hemorrhagic fever
Virus transmitted by ticks and contact with blood, secretions, or fluids from infected humans or animals
Central Asian hemorrhagic fever

A98.1   Omsk hemorrhagic fever
Transmitted to humans by bites of infected ticks or contact with infected muskrats

A98.2   Kyasanur Forest disease
Transmitted via infected monkeys, voles, ticks

A98.3   Marburg virus disease
Rare, acute, often fatal type of hemorrhagic fever

A98.4   Ebola virus disease

A98.5   Hemorrhagic fever with renal syndrome
Epidemic hemorrhagic fever
Korean hemorrhagic fever
Russian hemorrhagic fever
Hantaan virus disease
Hantavirus disease with renal manifestations
Nephropathia epidemica
Songo fever

> **Excludes1**   hantavirus (cardio)-pulmonary syndrome (B33.4)

A98.8   Other specified viral hemorrhagic fevers

A99   Unspecified viral hemorrhagic fever

VIRAL INFECTIONS CHARACTERIZED BY SKIN AND MUCOUS MEMBRANE LESIONS (B00-B09)

●**B00   Herpesviral [herpes simplex] infections**

> **Excludes1**   congenital herpesviral infections (P35.2)
> **Excludes2**   anogenital herpesviral infection (A60.-)
> gammaherpesviral mononucleosis (B27.0-)
> herpangina (B08.5)

B00.0   Eczema herpeticum
Cutaneous eruption caused by herpes simplex virus (HSV) type 1, HSV-2, coxsackievirus A16, or vaccinia virus
Kaposi's varicelliform eruption

B00.1   Herpesviral vesicular dermatitis
Vesicle formation; characteristics include formation of blisters and scabs on feet and legs
Herpes simplex facialis
Herpes simplex labialis
Herpes simplex otitis externa
Vesicular dermatitis of ear
Vesicular dermatitis of lip

Figure 1-4   Primary herpes simplex in and around the mouth. The infection is usually acquired from siblings or parents and is readily transmitted to other direct contacts. (Getty Image)

Item 1-15   Herpes is a viral disease for which there is no cure. There are two types of the herpes simplex virus: **Type I** causes **cold sores** or **fever blisters,** and **Type II** causes **genital herpes.** The virus can be spread from a sore on the lips to the genitals or from the genitals to the lips.

▶ New   ⇒ Revised   ~~deleted~~ Deleted   Excludes 1   Excludes 2   Includes   Use additional   Code first   Code also   Key words

OGCR Official Guidelines   X Assign placeholder X   ● Use Additional Character(s)   ▶ Manifestation Code   🐾 Hierarchical Condition Category   **Coding Clinic**

B00.2 **Herpesviral gingivostomatitis and pharyngotonsillitis**
Inflammation involving both gingivae and oral mucosa
Herpesviral pharyngitis
Inflammation of pharynx and tonsils; AKA tonsillopharyngitis

B00.3 **Herpesviral meningitis**

B00.4 **Herpesviral encephalitis**
Herpesviral meningoencephalitis
Simian B disease

> **Excludes1** herpesviral encephalitis due to herpesvirus 6 and 7 (B10.01, B10.09)
> non-simplex herpesviral encephalitis (B10.0-)

● **B00.5** **Herpesviral ocular disease**

  B00.50 **Herpesviral ocular disease, unspecified**

  B00.51 **Herpesviral iridocyclitis**
      Herpesviral iritis
      Herpesviral uveitis, anterior

  B00.52 **Herpesviral keratitis**
      Herpesviral keratoconjunctivitis

  B00.53 **Herpesviral conjunctivitis**

  B00.59 **Other herpesviral disease of eye**
      Herpesviral dermatitis of eyelid

B00.7 **Disseminated herpesviral disease** 🔒
Herpesviral sepsis

● **B00.8** **Other forms of herpesviral infections**

  B00.81 **Herpesviral hepatitis**

  B00.82 **Herpes simplex myelitis** 🔒

  B00.89 **Other herpesviral infection**
      Herpesviral whitlow

B00.9 **Herpesviral infection, unspecified**
Herpes simplex infection NOS

● **B01** **Varicella [chickenpox]**
Very contagious disease caused by the varicella zoster virus that results in an itchy outbreak of skin blisters (varicella). The same virus causes shingles (zoster).

  B01.0 **Varicella meningitis**

● **B01.1** **Varicella encephalitis, myelitis and encephalomyelitis**
Postchickenpox encephalitis, myelitis and encephalomyelitis

  B01.11 **Varicella encephalitis and encephalomyelitis**
      Postchickenpox encephalitis and encephalomyelitis

  B01.12 **Varicella myelitis** 🔒
      Postchickenpox myelitis

  B01.2 **Varicella pneumonia**

● **B01.8** **Varicella with other complications**

  B01.81 **Varicella keratitis**

  B01.89 **Other varicella complications**

  B01.9 **Varicella without complication**
Varicella NOS

● **B02** **Zoster [herpes zoster]**

> **Includes** shingles
> zona

  B02.0 **Zoster encephalitis**
Zoster meningoencephalitis

  B02.1 **Zoster meningitis**

● **B02.2** **Zoster with other nervous system involvement**
Coding Clinic: 2019, Q1, P18

  B02.21 **Postherpetic geniculate ganglionitis**

  B02.22 **Postherpetic trigeminal neuralgia**

  B02.23 **Postherpetic polyneuropathy**

Item 1-16 Zoster: Also known as ***shingles*** and is caused by the same virus as chickenpox. After exposure, the virus lies dormant in nerve tissue and is activated by factors including aging, stress, suppression of the immune system, and certain medication. It begins as a unilateral rash that leads to blisters and sores on the skin. It may involve the nerve pathways of the eye, forehead, nose, and eyelids and may be very painful with long-term systemic effects.

Figure 1-5 Photograph of eyelids with marginal blepharitis. (From Hoyt CS, Taylor D: Pediatric Ophthalmology and Strabismus, London, Elsevier Saunders, 2005)

Item 1–17 Blepharitis is a common condition in which the eyelid is swollen and yellow scaling and conjunctivitis develop. Usually the hair on the scalp and brow is involved.

  B02.24 **Postherpetic myelitis** 🔒
      Herpes zoster myelitis

  B02.29 **Other postherpetic nervous system involvement**
      Postherpetic radiculopathy

● **B02.3** **Zoster ocular disease**

  B02.30 **Zoster ocular disease, unspecified**

  B02.31 **Zoster conjunctivitis**

  B02.32 **Zoster iridocyclitis**

  B02.33 **Zoster keratitis**
      Herpes zoster keratoconjunctivitis

  B02.34 **Zoster scleritis**

  B02.39 **Other herpes zoster eye disease**
      Zoster blepharitis

B02.7 **Disseminated zoster**

B02.8 **Zoster with other complications**
Herpes zoster otitis externa

B02.9 **Zoster without complications**
Zoster NOS

B03 **Smallpox**
Note: In 1980 the 33rd World Health Assembly declared that smallpox had been eradicated. The classification is maintained for surveillance purposes.

B04 **Monkeypox**
Disease occurring in captive monkeys and other mammals that may be transmitted to humans, clinically similar to smallpox

● **B05** **Measles**

> **Includes** morbilli
> **Excludes1** subacute sclerosing panencephalitis (A81.1)

  B05.0 **Measles complicated by encephalitis**
      Postmeasles encephalitis

  B05.1 **Measles complicated by meningitis**
      Postmeasles meningitis

  B05.2 **Measles complicated by pneumonia**
      Postmeasles pneumonia

  B05.3 **Measles complicated by otitis media**
      Postmeasles otitis media

  B05.4 **Measles with intestinal complications**

● **B05.8** **Measles with other complications**

  B05.81 **Measles keratitis and keratoconjunctivitis**

  B05.89 **Other measles complications**

  B05.9 **Measles without complication**
      Measles NOS

● **B06** **Rubella [German measles]**

> **Excludes1** congenital rubella (P35.0)

● **B06.0** **Rubella with neurological complications**

  B06.00 **Rubella with neurological complication, unspecified**

  B06.01 **Rubella encephalitis**
      Rubella meningoencephalitis

  B06.02 **Rubella meningitis**

  B06.09 **Other neurological complications of rubella**

● **B06.8** **Rubella with other complications**

  B06.81 **Rubella pneumonia**

  B06.82 **Rubella arthritis** 🔒

  B06.89 **Other rubella complications**

  B06.9 **Rubella without complication**
      Rubella NOS

CHAPTER 1 (A00-B99)

CHAPTER 1 (A00-B99)

● **B07**   **Viral warts**

    Includes   verruca simplex
                       verruca vulgaris
                       viral warts due to human papillomavirus

    Excludes2   anogenital (venereal) warts (A63.0)
                       papilloma of bladder (D41.4)
                       papilloma of cervix (D26.0)
                       papilloma of larynx (D14.1)

    B07.0   **Plantar wart**
            Verruca plantaris

    B07.8   **Other viral warts**
            Common wart
            Flat wart
            Verruca plana

    B07.9   **Viral wart, unspecified**

● **B08**   **Other viral infections characterized by skin and mucous membrane lesions, not elsewhere classified**

    Excludes1   vesicular stomatitis virus disease (A93.8)

● **B08.0**   **Other orthopoxvirus infections**

       Excludes2   monkeypox (B04)

    ● **B08.01**   **Cowpox and vaccinia not from vaccine**

        B08.010   **Cowpox**

        B08.011   **Vaccinia not from vaccine**

            Excludes1   vaccinia (from vaccination) (generalized) (T88.1)

    B08.02   **Orf virus disease**
            Contagious pustular dermatitis
            Ecthyma contagiosum

    B08.03   **Pseudocowpox [milker's node]**

    B08.04   **Paravaccinia, unspecified**

    B08.09   **Other orthopoxvirus infections**
            Orthopoxvirus infection NOS

    B08.1   **Molluscum contagiosum**
        Various skin diseases characterized by soft, rounded, cutaneous lesions

● **B08.2**   **Exanthema subitum [sixth disease] Roseola infantum**
        Acute, short-lived high fever in infants and young children followed by a rash mainly on the trunk, caused by human herpesvirus 6

    B08.20   **Exanthema subitum [sixth disease], unspecified Roseola infantum, unspecified**   P

    B08.21   **Exanthema subitum [sixth disease] due to human herpesvirus 6 Roseola infantum due to human herpesvirus 6**   P
        Virus results in sudden rash; infection results in lifelong persistence

    B08.22   **Exanthema subitum [sixth disease] due to human herpesvirus 7 Roseola infantum due to human herpesvirus 7**   P

    B08.3   **Erythema infectiosum [fifth disease]**
        Moderately contagious, epidemic disease in children caused by B19 virus; onset of rash that begins as redness of cheeks, later there is rash on trunk and limbs; when this fades, there may be central clearing that leaves lacelike pattern

    B08.4   **Enteroviral vesicular stomatitis with exanthem**
        Hand, foot and mouth disease
        Check your documentation—this code is HAND, foot, and mouth disease. Code B08.8 is foot and mouth disease.

    B08.5   **Enteroviral vesicular pharyngitis**
        Herpangina

● **B08.6**   **Parapoxvirus infections**

    B08.60   **Parapoxvirus infection, unspecified**

    B08.61   **Bovine stomatitis**

    B08.62   **Sealpox**

    B08.69   **Other parapoxvirus infections**

● **B08.7**   **Yatapoxvirus infections**

    B08.70   **Yatapoxvirus infection, unspecified**

    B08.71   **Tanapox virus disease**

    B08.72   **Yaba pox virus disease**
        Yaba monkey tumor disease

    B08.79   **Other yatapoxvirus infections**

  B08.8   **Other specified viral infections characterized by skin and mucous membrane lesions**
      Enteroviral lymphonodular pharyngitis
      Foot-and-mouth disease
        Check your documentation. Code B08.4 is for HAND, foot, and mouth disease.
      Poxvirus NEC

B09   **Unspecified viral infection characterized by skin and mucous membrane lesions**
    Viral enanthema NOS
    Viral exanthema NOS

OTHER HUMAN HERPESVIRUSES (B10)

● **B10**   **Other human herpesviruses**

    Excludes2   cytomegalovirus (B25.9)
                 Epstein-Barr virus (B27.0-)
                 herpes NOS (B00.9)
                 herpes simplex (B00.-)
                 herpes zoster (B02.-)
                 human herpesvirus NOS (B00.-)
                 human herpesvirus 1 and 2 (B00.-)
                 human herpesvirus 3 (B01.-, B02.-)
                 human herpesvirus 4 (B27.0-)
                 human herpesvirus 5 (B25.-)
                 varicella (B01.-)
                 zoster (B02.-)

● **B10.0**   **Other human herpesvirus encephalitis**

     Excludes2   herpes encephalitis NOS (B00.4)
               herpes simplex encephalitis (B00.4)
               human herpesvirus encephalitis (B00.4)
               simian B herpes virus encephalitis (B00.4)

    B10.01   **Human herpesvirus 6 encephalitis**
        Sudden rash or roseola

    B10.09   **Other human herpesvirus encephalitis**
        Human herpesvirus 7 encephalitis
        Virus closely related to human herpesvirus 6, but not known to cause any disease
        Causative agent of exanthema subitum that results in sudden rash

● **B10.8**   **Other human herpesvirus infection**

    B10.81   **Human herpesvirus 6 infection**

    B10.82   **Human herpesvirus 7 infection**
        Closely related to human herpesvirus 6, but not known cause any disease

    B10.89   **Other human herpesvirus infection**
        Human herpesvirus 8 infection
        May be the cause of Kaposi sarcoma, a malignant tumor
        Kaposi's sarcoma-associated herpesvirus infection

Figure 1-6 Hepatitis B viral infection. **A.** Liver parenchyma showing hepatocytes with diffuse granular cytoplasm, so-called ground glass hepatocytes (H&E). **B.** Immunoperoxidase stains from the same case, showing cytoplasmic inclusions of viral particles. (From Kumar: Robbins and Cotran: Pathologic Basis of Disease, ed 8, Saunders, An Imprint of Elsevier, 2009)

▶ New   ⇒ Revised   ~~deleted~~ Deleted   Excludes 1   Excludes 2   Includes   Use additional   Code first   Code also   Key words

OGCR Official Guidelines   X Assign placeholder X   ● Use Additional Character(s)   ▶ Manifestation Code   🐾 Hierarchical Condition Category   **Coding Clinic**

Item 1–18 Hepatitis A (HAV) was formerly called epidemic, infectious, short-incubation, or acute catarrhal jaundice hepatitis. The primary transmission mode is the oral–fecal route. **Hepatitis B (HBV)** was formerly called long-incubation period, serum, or homologous serum hepatitis. Transmission modes are through blood from infected persons and from body fluids of infected mother to neonate. **Hepatitis C (HCV),** caused by the hepatitis C virus, is primarily transfusion associated. **Hepatitis D (HDV),** also called delta hepatitis, is caused by the hepatitis D virus in patients formerly or currently infected with hepatitis B. **Hepatitis E (HEV)** is also called enterically transmitted non-A, non-B hepatitis. The primary transmission mode is the oral–fecal route, usually through contaminated water.

Figure 1-7 Kaposi's sarcoma. There are large confluent hyperpigmented patch-stage lesions with lymphedema. (From Kanski, JJ: Clinical Diagnosis in Ophthalmology, London, Elsevier Mosby, 2006)

Item 1–19 AIDS (acquired immune deficiency syndrome) is caused by **HIV** (human immunodeficiency virus). HIV affects certain white blood cells (T-4 lymphocytes) and destroys the ability of the cells to fight infections, making patients susceptible to a host of infectious diseases (e.g., ***Pneumocystis carinii pneumonia [PCP], Kaposi's sarcoma,*** and ***lymphoma).*** ***AIDS-related complex (ARC)*** is an early stage of AIDS in which tests for HIV are positive but the symptoms are mild.

OGCR Section I. C.1.a.

Certain Infectious and Parasitic Diseases (A00-B99)

a. Human Immunodeficiency Virus (HIV) Infections

1) Code only confirmed cases

Code only confirmed cases of HIV infection illness. This is an exception to the hospital inpatient guideline Section II, H.

In this context, "confirmation" does not require documentation of positive serology or culture for HIV; the provider's diagnostic statement that the patient is HIV positive or has an HIV-related illness is sufficient.

VIRAL HEPATITIS (B15-B19)

Excludes1	sequelae of viral hepatitis (B94.2)
Excludes2	cytomegaloviral hepatitis (B25.1)
	herpesviral [herpes simplex] hepatitis (B00.81)

● **B15   Acute hepatitis A**

   B15.0   Hepatitis A with hepatic coma

   B15.9   Hepatitis A without hepatic coma
       Hepatitis A (acute) (viral) NOS

● **B16   Acute hepatitis B**

   B16.0   Acute hepatitis B with delta-agent with hepatic coma

   B16.1   Acute hepatitis B with delta-agent without hepatic coma

   B16.2   Acute hepatitis B without delta-agent with hepatic coma

   B16.9   Acute hepatitis B without delta-agent and without hepatic coma
       Hepatitis B (acute) (viral) NOS
       Coding Clinic: 2016, Q3, P13

● **B17   Other acute viral hepatitis**

   B17.0   Acute delta-(super) infection of hepatitis B carrier

 ● **B17.1   Acute hepatitis C**

     B17.10   Acute hepatitis C without hepatic coma
        Acute hepatitis C NOS

     B17.11   Acute hepatitis C with hepatic coma

   B17.2   Acute hepatitis E

   B17.8   Other specified acute viral hepatitis
       Hepatitis non-A non-B (acute) (viral) NEC

   B17.9   Acute viral hepatitis, unspecified
       Acute hepatitis NOS
       Acute infectious hepatitis NOS

● **B18   Chronic viral hepatitis**

   Includes   Carrier of viral hepatitis

   B18.0   Chronic viral hepatitis B with delta-agent 🔹

   B18.1   Chronic viral hepatitis B without delta-agent 🔹
       Carrier of viral hepatitis B
       Chronic (viral) hepatitis B

   B18.2   Chronic viral hepatitis C 🔹
       Carrier of viral hepatitis C
       Coding Clinic: 2018, Q1, P4; 2017, Q1, P41

   B18.8   Other chronic viral hepatitis 🔹
       Carrier of other viral hepatitis

   B18.9   Chronic viral hepatitis, unspecified 🔹
       Carrier of unspecified viral hepatitis

● **B19   Unspecified viral hepatitis**

   B19.0   Unspecified viral hepatitis with hepatic coma

 ● **B19.1   Unspecified viral hepatitis B**

     B19.10   Unspecified viral hepatitis B without hepatic coma
        Unspecified viral hepatitis B NOS

     B19.11   Unspecified viral hepatitis B with hepatic coma

 ● **B19.2   Unspecified viral hepatitis C**

     B19.20   Unspecified viral hepatitis C without hepatic coma
        Viral hepatitis C NOS

     B19.21   Unspecified viral hepatitis C with hepatic coma

   B19.9   Unspecified viral hepatitis without hepatic coma
       Viral hepatitis NOS

HUMAN IMMUNODEFICIENCY VIRUS [HIV] DISEASE (B20)

  B20   **Human immunodeficiency virus [HIV] disease** 🔹

     Includes   acquired immune deficiency syndrome [AIDS]
           AIDS-related complex [ARC]
           HIV infection, symptomatic

     Code first Human immunodeficiency virus [HIV] disease
        complicating pregnancy, childbirth and the puerperium, if
        applicable (O98.7-)

     Use additional code(s) to identify all manifestations of HIV
     infection

     Excludes1   asymptomatic human immunodeficiency virus
           [HIV] infection status (Z21)
           exposure to HIV virus (Z20.6)
           inconclusive serologic evidence of HIV (R75)
     Coding Clinic: 2022, Q1, P36; 2021, Q2, P6; 2019, Q1, P9-11

OTHER VIRAL DISEASES (B25-B34)

● **B25   Cytomegaloviral disease**
   AKA: HCMV or Human Herpesvirus 5 (HHV-5)

   Excludes1   congenital cytomegalovirus infection (P35.1)
         cytomegaloviral mononucleosis (B27.1-)

   B25.0   Cytomegaloviral pneumonitis 🔹

   B25.1   Cytomegaloviral hepatitis 🔹

   B25.2   Cytomegaloviral pancreatitis 🔹

   B25.8   Other cytomegaloviral diseases 🔹
       Cytomegaloviral encephalitis

   B25.9   Cytomegaloviral disease, unspecified 🔹

● **B26   Mumps**

   Includes   epidemic parotitis
          infectious parotitis
     Acute, contagious, viral disease

   B26.0   Mumps orchitis ♂

   B26.1   Mumps meningitis

   B26.2   Mumps encephalitis

   B26.3   Mumps pancreatitis

● B26.8   **Mumps with other complications**

     B26.81   **Mumps hepatitis**

     B26.82   **Mumps myocarditis**

     B26.83   **Mumps nephritis**

     B26.84   **Mumps polyneuropathy**

     B26.85   **Mumps arthritis** 🐾

     B26.89   **Other mumps complications**

● B26.9   **Mumps without complication**
     Mumps NOS
     Mumps parotitis NOS

● B27   **Infectious mononucleosis**

     Includes   glandular fever
                 monocytic angina
                 Pfeiffer's disease

● B27.0   **Gammaherpesviral mononucleosis**
     AKA: Pfeiffer's disease, infective mononucleosis
     Mononucleosis due to Epstein-Barr virus

     B27.00   **Gammaherpesviral mononucleosis without complication**
             Infective mononucleosis

     B27.01   **Gammaherpesviral mononucleosis with polyneuropathy**

     B27.02   **Gammaherpesviral mononucleosis with meningitis**

     B27.09   **Gammaherpesviral mononucleosis with other complications**
             Hepatomegaly in gammaherpesviral mononucleosis

● B27.1   **Cytomegaloviral mononucleosis**
     Infectious disease resembling infectious mononucleosis

     B27.10   **Cytomegaloviral mononucleosis without complications**

     B27.11   **Cytomegaloviral mononucleosis with polyneuropathy**

     B27.12   **Cytomegaloviral mononucleosis with meningitis**

     B27.19   **Cytomegaloviral mononucleosis with other complication**
             Hepatomegaly in cytomegaloviral mononucleosis

● B27.8   **Other infectious mononucleosis**

     B27.80   **Other infectious mononucleosis without complication**

     B27.81   **Other infectious mononucleosis with polyneuropathy**

     B27.82   **Other infectious mononucleosis with meningitis**

     B27.89   **Other infectious mononucleosis with other complication**
             Hepatomegaly in other infectious mononucleosis

● B27.9   **Infectious mononucleosis, unspecified**

     B27.90   **Infectious mononucleosis, unspecified without complication**

     B27.91   **Infectious mononucleosis, unspecified with polyneuropathy**

     B27.92   **Infectious mononucleosis, unspecified with meningitis**

     B27.99   **Infectious mononucleosis, unspecified with other complication**
             Hepatomegaly in unspecified infectious mononucleosis

● B30   **Viral conjunctivitis**

     Excludes 1   herpesviral [herpes simplex] ocular disease (B00.5)
                    ocular zoster (B02.3)

     B30.0   **Keratoconjunctivitis due to adenovirus**
            Epidemic keratoconjunctivitis
            Shipyard eye

     B30.1   **Conjunctivitis due to adenovirus**
            Acute adenoviral follicular conjunctivitis
            Swimming-pool conjunctivitis

     B30.2   **Viral pharyngoconjunctivitis**

     B30.3   **Acute epidemic hemorrhagic conjunctivitis (enteroviral)**
            Conjunctivitis due to coxsackievirus 24
            Conjunctivitis due to enterovirus 70
            Hemorrhagic conjunctivitis (acute)(epidemic)

     B30.8   **Other viral conjunctivitis**
            Newcastle conjunctivitis

     B30.9   **Viral conjunctivitis, unspecified**

● B33   **Other viral diseases, not elsewhere classified**

     B33.0   **Epidemic myalgia**
            Acute infectious disease, caused by group A coxsackie viruses or other enteroviruses with symptoms that include sudden pain in chest or upper abdomen with fever
            Bornholm disease

     B33.1   **Ross River disease**
            Epidemic polyarthritis and exanthema
            Ross River fever

● B33.2   **Viral carditis**
     Coxsackie (virus) carditis

     B33.20   **Viral carditis, unspecified**

     B33.21   **Viral endocarditis**

     B33.22   **Viral myocarditis**

     B33.23   **Viral pericarditis**

     B33.24   **Viral cardiomyopathy** 🐾

     B33.3   **Retrovirus infections, not elsewhere classified**
            Retrovirus infection NOS

     B33.4   **Hantavirus (cardio)-pulmonary syndrome [HPS] [HCPS]**
            Hantavirus disease with pulmonary manifestations
            Sin nombre virus disease

            Use additional code to identify any associated acute kidney failure (N17.9)

         Excludes 1   hantavirus disease with renal manifestations (A98.5)
                     hemorrhagic fever with renal manifestations (A98.5)

     B33.8   **Other specified viral diseases**

         Excludes 1   anogenital human papillomavirus infection (A63.0)
                     viral warts due to human papillomavirus infection (B07)

● B34   **Viral infection of unspecified site**

     Excludes 1   anogenital human papillomavirus infection (A63.0)
                  cytomegaloviral disease NOS (B25.9)
                  herpesvirus [herpes simplex] infection NOS (B00.9)
                  retrovirus infection NOS (B33.3)
                  viral agents as the cause of diseases classified elsewhere (B97.-)
                  viral warts due to human papillomavirus infection (B07)

     B34.0   **Adenovirus infection, unspecified**

     B34.1   **Enterovirus infection, unspecified**
            Intestinal tract infection
            Coxsackievirus infection NOS
            Echovirus infection NOS

     B34.2   **Coronavirus infection, unspecified**

         Excludes 1   COVID-19 (U07.1)
                     pneumonia due to SARS-associated coronavirus (J12.81)

▶ New   ⟹ Revised   ~~deleted~~ Deleted   Excludes 1   Excludes 2   Includes   Use additional   Code first   Code also   Key words

OGCR Official Guidelines   X Assign placeholder X   ● Use Additional Character(s)   ▶ Manifestation Code   🐾 Hierarchical Condition Category   **Coding Clinic**

B34.3   **Parvovirus infection, unspecified**
B34.4   **Papovavirus infection, unspecified**
B34.8   **Other viral infections of unspecified site**
B34.9   **Viral infection, unspecified**
      Viremia NOS
      Coding Clinic: 2016, Q3, P10

MYCOSES (B35-B49)

> **Excludes2**   hypersensitivity pneumonitis due to organic dust
>   (J67.-)
>   mycosis fungoides (C84.0-)

● **B35**   **Dermatophytosis**
    AKA tinea or ringworm

> **Includes**   favus
>   infections due to species of Epidermophyton,
>   Micro-sporum and Trichophyton
>   tinea, any type except those in B36.-

B35.0   **Tinea barbae and tinea capitis**
    Beard ringworm
    Kerion
    Scalp ringworm
    Sycosis, mycotic

B35.1   **Tinea unguium**
    White patches or pits on surface or edges of nails, followed by
      infection under nail plate
    Dermatophytic onychia
    Dermatophytosis of nail
    Onychomycosis
    Ringworm of nails

B35.2   **Tinea manuum**
    Tinea of hands
    Dermatophytosis of hand
    Hand ringworm

B35.3   **Tinea pedis**
    Tinea affecting feet
    Athlete's foot
    Dermatophytosis of foot
    Foot ringworm

B35.4   **Tinea corporis**
    Infecting skin areas other than hands
    Ringworm of the body

B35.5   **Tinea imbricata**
    Chronic tropical tinea corporis; AKA Oriental ringworm,
      tinea inguinalis, tinea cruris
    Tokelau

B35.6   **Tinea cruris**
    In groin or perineal area, spreading to adjacent regions; AKA
      jock itch, eczema marginatum, ringworm of groin, or
      tinea inguinalis
    Dhobi itch
    Groin ringworm
    Jock itch

B35.8   **Other dermatophytoses**
    Disseminated dermatophytosis
    Granulomatous dermatophytosis

B35.9   **Dermatophytosis, unspecified**
    Ringworm NOS

● **B36**   **Other superficial mycoses**
    B36.0   **Pityriasis versicolor**
      Common, chronic, symptomless disorder that includes
        macular patches of various sizes and shapes; AKA liver
        spots
      Tinea flava
      Tinea versicolor

    B36.1   **Tinea nigra**
      Minor fungal infection, with dark lesions, usually on skin of
        hands
      Keratomycosis nigricans palmaris
      Microsporosis nigra
      Pityriasis nigra

Figure 1-8   Oral candidiasis (thrush). (From James WD, Berger T, Elston D: Andrews' Diseases of the Skin: Clinical Dermatology, 11e, Saunders, 2011)

Item 1-20 Candidiasis, also called oidiomycosis or moniliasis, is a fungal infection. It most often appears on moist cutaneous areas of the body but can also be responsible for a variety of systemic infections such as endocarditis, meningitis, arthritis, and myositis. Antifungal medications cure most yeast infections.

B36.2   **White piedra**
    White to light brown nodules on hair of beard, axilla, or
      groin; AKA trichosporosis
    Tinea blanca

B36.3   **Black piedra**
    Characterized by small black or brown nodules on shafts of
      scalp hair

B36.8   **Other specified superficial mycoses**
B36.9   **Superficial mycosis, unspecified**

● **B37**   **Candidiasis**
> **Includes**   candidosis
>   moniliasis

> **Excludes1**   neonatal candidiasis (P37.5)

B37.0   **Candidal stomatitis**
    Oral thrush

B37.1   **Pulmonary candidiasis** 🦠
    Candidal bronchitis
    Candidal pneumonia

B37.2   **Candidiasis of skin and nail**
    Candidal onychia
    Candidal paronychia

> **Excludes2**   diaper dermatitis (L22)

B37.3   **Candidiasis of vulva and vagina** ♀
    Candidal vulvovaginitis
    Monilial vulvovaginitis
    Vaginal thrush

  ▶ B37.31   **Acute candidiasis of vulva and vagina**
      ▶Candidiasis of vulva and vagina NOS

  ▶ B37.32   **Chronic candidiasis of vulva and vagina**
      ▶Recurrent candidiasis of vulva and vagina

● B37.4   **Candidiasis of other urogenital sites**
    B37.41   **Candidal cystitis and urethritis**
    B37.42   **Candidal balanitis** ♂
      Male condition only
    B37.49   **Other urogenital candidiasis**
      Candidal pyelonephritis

B37.5   **Candidal meningitis**
B37.6   **Candidal endocarditis**
B37.7   **Candidal sepsis** 🦠
    Disseminated candidiasis systemic candidiasis

● B37.8   **Candidiasis of other sites**
    B37.81   **Candidal esophagitis** 🦠
    B37.82   **Candidal enteritis**
      Candidal proctitis
    B37.83   **Candidal cheilitis**
      Inflammation affecting lip
    B37.84   **Candidal otitis externa**
      Inflammation of external auditory canal
    B37.89   **Other sites of candidiasis**
      Infection manifested by invasive candidiasis
      Candidal osteomyelitis

B37.9   **Candidiasis, unspecified**
    Thrush NOS

Item 1-21 Bird and bat droppings that fall into the soil give rise to a fungus that can spread airborne spores. When inhaled into the lungs, these spores divide and multiply into lesions. Histoplasmosis capsulatum takes three forms: primary (lodged in the lungs only), chronic (resembles TB), and disseminated (infection has moved to other organs). This is an opportunistic infection in immunosuppressed patients.

● **B38**   **Coccidioidomycosis**
Fungal disease; AKA coccidioidosis, coccidioidal granuloma, Posadas, or Posadas-Wernicke disease

    B38.0   **Acute pulmonary coccidioidomycosis** 🐾

    B38.1   **Chronic pulmonary coccidioidomycosis** 🐾

    B38.2   **Pulmonary coccidioidomycosis, unspecified** 🐾

    B38.3   **Cutaneous coccidioidomycosis**

    B38.4   **Coccidioidomycosis meningitis**

    B38.7   **Disseminated coccidioidomycosis**
          Generalized coccidioidomycosis

 ● **B38.8**   **Other forms of coccidioidomycosis**

      B38.81   **Prostatic coccidioidomycosis** ♂

      B38.89   **Other forms of coccidioidomycosis**

    B38.9   **Coccidioidomycosis, unspecified**

● **B39**   **Histoplasmosis**
Infection resulting from inhalation or ingestion of spores; AKA Darling disease

    Code first associated AIDS (B20)

    Use additional code for any associated manifestations, such as:
       endocarditis (I39)
       meningitis (G02)
       pericarditis (I32)
       retinitis (H32)

    B39.0   **Acute pulmonary histoplasmosis capsulati** 🐾

    B39.1   **Chronic pulmonary histoplasmosis capsulati** 🐾

    B39.2   **Pulmonary histoplasmosis capsulati, unspecified** 🐾

    B39.3   **Disseminated histoplasmosis capsulati**
          Generalized histoplasmosis capsulati

    B39.4   **Histoplasmosis capsulati, unspecified**
          American histoplasmosis

    B39.5   **Histoplasmosis duboisii**
          African histoplasmosis

    B39.9   **Histoplasmosis, unspecified**

● **B40**   **Blastomycosis**
Rare and potentially fatal infection caused by inhaling fungus found in moist soil in temperate climates.

    Excludes1   Brazilian blastomycosis (B41.-)
               keloidal blastomycosis (B48.0)

    B40.0   **Acute pulmonary blastomycosis** 🐾

    B40.1   **Chronic pulmonary blastomycosis** 🐾

    B40.2   **Pulmonary blastomycosis, unspecified** 🐾

    B40.3   **Cutaneous blastomycosis**

    B40.7   **Disseminated blastomycosis**
          Generalized blastomycosis

 ● **B40.8**   **Other forms of blastomycosis**

      B40.81   **Blastomycotic meningoencephalitis**
            Meningomyelitis due to blastomycosis

      B40.89   **Other forms of blastomycosis**

    B40.9   **Blastomycosis, unspecified**

● **B41**   **Paracoccidioidomycosis**
Fungal infection usually chronic that begins in lungs, spreads to mucocutaneous areas which may extend to skin, tonsils, gastrointestinal lymphatics, liver, and spleen; AKA Almeida or Lutz-Splendore-Almeida disease, Brazilian or South American blastomycosis, or paracoccidioidal granuloma

    Includes   Brazilian blastomycosis
              Lutz' disease

    B41.0   **Pulmonary paracoccidioidomycosis** 🐾

    B41.7   **Disseminated paracoccidioidomycosis**
          Generalized paracoccidioidomycosis

    B41.8   **Other forms of paracoccidioidomycosis**

    B41.9   **Paracoccidioidomycosis, unspecified**

● **B42**   **Sporotrichosis**
Chronic fungal infection with nodular lesions

    B42.0   **Pulmonary sporotrichosis**

    B42.1   **Lymphocutaneous sporotrichosis**

    B42.7   **Disseminated sporotrichosis**
          Generalized sporotrichosis

 ● **B42.8**   **Other forms of sporotrichosis**

      B42.81   **Cerebral sporotrichosis**
            Meningitis due to sporotrichosis

      B42.82   **Sporotrichosis arthritis** 🐾

      B42.89   **Other forms of sporotrichosis**

    B42.9   **Sporotrichosis, unspecified**

● **B43**   **Chromomycosis and pheomycotic abscess**
Chronic fungal infection of skin, initiated at site of puncture affecting lower limb or foot (mossy foot)

    B43.0   **Cutaneous chromomycosis**
          Dermatitis verrucosa

    B43.1   **Pheomycotic brain abscess**
          Cerebral chromomycosis

    B43.2   **Subcutaneous pheomycotic abscess and cyst**

    B43.8   **Other forms of chromomycosis**

    B43.9   **Chromomycosis, unspecified**

● **B44**   **Aspergillosis**
Infection marked by inflammatory lesions in skin, ear, orbit, nasal sinuses, lungs, and occasionally bones and meninges

    Includes   aspergilloma

    B44.0   **Invasive pulmonary aspergillosis** 🐾

    B44.1   **Other pulmonary aspergillosis** 🐾

    B44.2   **Tonsillar aspergillosis** 🐾

    B44.7   **Disseminated aspergillosis** 🐾
          Generalized aspergillosis

 ● **B44.8**   **Other forms of aspergillosis**

      B44.81   **Allergic bronchopulmonary aspergillosis** 🐾

      B44.89   **Other forms of aspergillosis** 🐾

    B44.9   **Aspergillosis, unspecified** 🐾

● **B45**   **Cryptococcosis**
Infection in the immunocompromised and fatal if left untreated; AKA torulosis, Buschke, or Busse-Buschke disease

    B45.0   **Pulmonary cryptococcosis** 🐾

    B45.1   **Cerebral cryptococcosis** 🐾
          Cryptococcal meningitis
          Cryptococcosis meningocerebralis

    B45.2   **Cutaneous cryptococcosis** 🐾

    B45.3   **Osseous cryptococcosis** 🐾

    B45.7   **Disseminated cryptococcosis** 🐾
          Generalized cryptococcosis

    B45.8   **Other forms of cryptococcosis** 🐾

    B45.9   **Cryptococcosis, unspecified** 🐾

● **B46**   **Zygomycosis**
Fungal infections including subcutaneous lesions and infection of sinuses, brain, or lungs

    B46.0   **Pulmonary mucormycosis** 🐾
          Fungal infection affecting lung

    B46.1   **Rhinocerebral mucormycosis** 🐾

    B46.2   **Gastrointestinal mucormycosis** 🐾

    B46.3   **Cutaneous mucormycosis** 🐾
          Subcutaneous mucormycosis

    B46.4   **Disseminated mucormycosis** 🐾
          Generalized mucormycosis

    B46.5   **Mucormycosis, unspecified** 🐾

    B46.8   **Other zygomycoses** 🐾
          Entomophthoromycosis

    B46.9   **Zygomycosis, unspecified** 🐾
          Phycomycosis NOS

CHAPTER 1 (A00-B99)

▶ New   ⇒ Revised   ~~deleted~~ Deleted   Excludes 1   Excludes 2   Includes   Use additional   Code first   Code also   Key words

OGCR Official Guidelines   X Assign placeholder X   ● Use Additional Character(s)   ▶ Manifestation Code   🐾 Hierarchical Condition Category   **Coding Clinic**

● **B47   Mycetoma**
Slow progressive, destructive fungal infection of cutaneous and subcutaneous tissues, fascia, and bone, primarily seen in foot (Madura foot) or leg

   B47.0   Eumycetoma
   Madura foot, mycotic Maduromycosis

   B47.1   Actinomycetoma

   B47.9   Mycetoma, unspecified
   Madura foot NOS

● **B48   Other mycoses, not elsewhere classified**

   B48.0   Lobomycosis
   Infection with symptoms of red, smooth, hard cutaneous nodules resembling keloids
   Keloidal blastomycosis
   Lobo's disease

   B48.1   Rhinosporidiosis
   Chronic, localized granulomatous fungal infection, affecting mucocutaneous tissues, usually of nose characterized by polyps, papillomas, and wartlike lesions

   B48.2   Allescheriasis
   Fungal infection
   Infection due to Pseudallescheria boydii
   Excludes1   eumycetoma (B47.0)

   B48.3   Geotrichosis
   Fungal infection usually of bronchi, lungs, mouth, or intestinal tract
   Geotrichum stomatitis

   B48.4   Penicillosis ⊛
   Fungal infection
   Talaromycosis

   B48.8   Other specified mycoses ⊛
   Adiaspiromycosis
   Infection of tissue and organs by Alternaria
   Infection of tissue and organs by Drechslera
   Infection of tissue and organs by Fusarium
   Infection of tissue and organs by saprophytic fungi NEC

● **B49   Unspecified mycosis**
   Fungemia NOS

PROTOZOAL DISEASES (B50-B64)

   Excludes1   amebiasis (A06.-)
   other protozoal intestinal diseases (A07.-)

● **B50   Plasmodium falciparum malaria**
   Severe form of malaria that can be fatal
   Includes   mixed infections of Plasmodium falciparum with any other Plasmodium species

   B50.0   Plasmodium falciparum malaria with cerebral complications
   Cerebral malaria NOS

   B50.8   Other severe and complicated Plasmodium falciparum malaria
   Severe or complicated Plasmodium falciparum malaria NOS

   B50.9   Plasmodium falciparum malaria, unspecified

● **B51   Plasmodium vivax malaria**
   Includes   mixed infections of Plasmodium vivax with other Plasmodium species, except Plasmodium falciparum
   Excludes1   plasmodium vivax with Plasmodium falciparum (B50.-)

   B51.0   Plasmodium vivax malaria with rupture of spleen

   B51.8   Plasmodium vivax malaria with other complications

   B51.9   Plasmodium vivax malaria without complication
   Plasmodium vivax malaria NOS

● **B52   Plasmodium malariae malaria**
   Causes fever that recurs at approximately three-day intervals (quartan fever), longer than two-day (tertian) intervals of other malarial parasites
   Includes   mixed infections of Plasmodium malariae with other Plasmodium species, except Plasmodium falciparum and Plasmodium vivax
   Excludes1   plasmodium falciparum (B50.-)
   plasmodium vivax (B51.-)

   B52.0   Plasmodium malariae malaria with nephropathy

   B52.8   Plasmodium malariae malaria with other complications

   B52.9   Plasmodium malariae malaria without complication
   Plasmodium malariae malaria NOS

● **B53   Other specified malaria**

   B53.0   Plasmodium ovale malaria
   Least diagnosed type of malaria spread by female mosquitoes of rare species
   Excludes1   plasmodium ovale with Plasmodium falciparum (B50.-)
   plasmodium ovale with Plasmodium malariae (B52.-)
   plasmodium ovale with Plasmodium vivax (B51.-)

   B53.1   Malaria due to simian plasmodia
   Malaria-like disease (parasite infection)
   Excludes1   malaria due to simian plasmodia with Plasmodium falciparum (B50.-)
   malaria due to simian plasmodia with Plasmodium malariae (B52.-)
   malaria due to simian plasmodia with Plasmodium ovale (B53.0)
   malaria due to simian plasmodia with Plasmodium vivax (B51.-)

   B53.8   Other malaria, not elsewhere classified

   B54   Unspecified malaria

● **B55   Leishmaniasis**
   Protozoal infection

   B55.0   Visceral leishmaniasis
   Kala-azar
   Post-kala-azar dermal leishmaniasis

   B55.1   Cutaneous leishmaniasis

   B55.2   Mucocutaneous leishmaniasis

   B55.9   Leishmaniasis, unspecified

● **B56   African trypanosomiasis**
   Human African trypanosomiasis (HAT) is transmitted by fly bites

   B56.0   Gambiense trypanosomiasis
   Infection due to Trypanosoma brucei gambiense
   West African sleeping sickness

   B56.1   Rhodesiense trypanosomiasis
   East African sleeping sickness
   Infection due to Trypanosoma brucei rhodesiense

   B56.9   African trypanosomiasis, unspecified
   Sleeping sickness NOS

● **B57   Chagas' disease**
   Tropical parasitic disease
   Includes   American trypanosomiasis
   infection due to Trypanosoma cruzi

   B57.0   Acute Chagas' disease with heart involvement
   Acute Chagas' disease with myocarditis

   B57.1   Acute Chagas' disease without heart involvement
   Acute Chagas' disease NOS

   B57.2   Chagas' disease (chronic) with heart involvement
   American trypanosomiasis NOS
   Chagas' disease (chronic) NOS
   Chagas' disease (chronic) with myocarditis
   Trypanosomiasis NOS

CHAPTER 1 (A00-B99)

CHAPTER 1 (A00-B99)

● **B57.3 Chagas' disease (chronic) with digestive system involvement**
  - B57.30 Chagas' disease with digestive system involvement, **unspecified**
  - B57.31 **Megaesophagus** in Chagas' disease
  - B57.32 **Megacolon** in Chagas' disease
  - B57.39 Other digestive system involvement in Chagas' disease

● **B57.4 Chagas' disease (chronic) with nervous system involvement**
  - B57.40 Chagas' disease with nervous system involvement, **unspecified**
  - B57.41 **Meningitis** in Chagas' disease
  - B57.42 **Meningoencephalitis** in Chagas' disease
  - B57.49 Other nervous system involvement in Chagas' disease

B57.5 Chagas' disease (chronic) **with other organ involvement**

● **B58 Toxoplasmosis**
  Infection by protozoon transmitted in cysts in feces of cats
  Includes infection due to Toxoplasma gondii
  Excludes1 congenital toxoplasmosis (P37.1)

  ● **B58.0 Toxoplasma oculopathy**
  - B58.00 Toxoplasma oculopathy, **unspecified**
  - B58.01 Toxoplasma **chorioretinitis**
  - B58.09 Other toxoplasma oculopathy
    Toxoplasma uveitis

  B58.1 Toxoplasma **hepatitis**
  B58.2 Toxoplasma **meningoencephalitis** 🦠
  B58.3 **Pulmonary toxoplasmosis** 🦠

  ● **B58.8 Toxoplasmosis with other organ involvement**
  - B58.81 **Toxoplasma myocarditis**
  - B58.82 **Toxoplasma myositis**
  - B58.83 **Toxoplasma tubulo-interstitial nephropathy**
    Toxoplasma pyelonephritis
  - B58.89 Toxoplasmosis with **other organ involvement**

  B58.9 Toxoplasmosis, **unspecified**

B59 **Pneumocystosis** 🦠
  Caused by fungus
  Pneumonia due to Pneumocystis carinii
  Pneumonia due to Pneumocystis jiroveci

● **B60 Other protozoal diseases, not elsewhere classified**
  Excludes1 cryptosporidiosis (A07.2)
  intestinal microsporidiosis (A07.8)
  isosporiasis (A07.3)

  B60.0 **Babesiosis**
    Tickborne disease caused by microscopic organisms
  - B60.00 **Babesiosis, unspecified**
    Babesiosis due to unspecified Babesia species
    Piroplasmosis, unspecified
  - B60.01 **Babesiosis due to Babesia microti**
    Infection due to B. microti
  - B60.02 **Babesiosis due to Babesia duncani**
    Infection due to B. duncani and B. duncani-type species
  - B60.03 **Babesiosis due to Babesia divergens**
    Babesiosis due to Babesia MO-1
    Infection due to B. divergens and B. divergens-like strains
  - B60.09 **Other babesiosis**
    Babesiosis due to Babesia KO-1
    Babesiosis due to Babesia venatorum
    Infection due to other Babesia species
    Infection due to other protozoa of the order Piroplasmida
    Other piroplasmosis

Item 1-22 Toxoplasmosis is caused by the protozoa **Toxoplasma gondii,** of which the house cat can be a host. Human infection occurs when contact is made with materials containing the pathogen, such as feces, contaminated soil, or ingestion of infected lamb, goat, or pork. Of the infected, very few have symptoms because a healthy person's immune system keeps the parasite from causing illness. When the immune system is compromised, symptoms may occur. Clinical symptoms include flu-like symptoms, but the disease progresses to include the eyes and the brain in babies.

● **B60.1 Acanthamebiasis**
  - B60.10 **Acanthamebiasis, unspecified**
  - B60.11 **Meningoencephalitis** due to Acanthamoeba (culbertsoni)
  - B60.12 **Conjunctivitis** due to Acanthamoeba
  - B60.13 **Keratoconjunctivitis** due to Acanthamoeba
  - B60.19 **Other acanthamebic disease**

  B60.2 **Naegleriasis**
    Infection with microscopic organisms
    Primary amebic meningoencephalitis

  B60.8 **Other specified protozoal diseases**
    Microsporidiosis

B64 **Unspecified protozoal disease**

HELMINTHIASES (B65-B83)

Diseases or infestations caused by parasitic worms

● **B65 Schistosomiasis [bilharziasis]**
  Infection with flukes (flat parasitic worms)
  Includes snail fever

  B65.0 **Schistosomiasis due to Schistosoma haematobium [urinary schistosomiasis]**
  B65.1 **Schistosomiasis due to Schistosoma mansoni [intestinal schistosomiasis]**
  B65.2 **Schistosomiasis due to Schistosoma japonicum**
    Asiatic schistosomiasis
  B65.3 **Cercarial dermatitis**
    Swimmer's itch
  B65.8 **Other schistosomiasis**
    Infection due to Schistosoma intercalatum
    Infection due to Schistosoma mattheei
    Infection due to Schistosoma mekongi
  B65.9 **Schistosomiasis, unspecified**

● **B66 Other fluke infections**
  Trematode (parasitic worms)
  B66.0 **Opisthorchiasis**
    Infection due to cat liver fluke
    Infection due to Opisthorchis (felineus)(viverrini)
  B66.1 **Clonorchiasis**
    Chinese liver fluke disease
    Infection due to Clonorchis sinensis
    Oriental liver fluke disease
  B66.2 **Dicroceliasis**
    Liver fluke
    Infection due to Dicrocoelium dendriticum
    Lancet fluke infection
  B66.3 **Fascioliasis**
    Infection due to Fasciola gigantica
    Infection due to Fasciola hepatica
    Infection due to Fasciola indica
    Sheep liver fluke disease
  B66.4 **Paragonimiasis** 🦠
    Infection due to Paragonimus species
    Lung fluke disease
    Pulmonary distomiasis
  B66.5 **Fasciolopsiasis**
    Largest intestinal fluke in humans
    Infection due to Fasciolopsis buski
    Intestinal distomiasis

▶ New   ⇒ Revised   ~~deleted~~ Deleted   Excludes 1   Excludes 2   Includes   Use additional   Code first   Code also   Key words

OGCR Official Guidelines   X Assign placeholder X   ● Use Additional Character(s)   ▶ Manifestation Code   🦠 Hierarchical Condition Category   **Coding Clinic**

Item 1-23 Echinococcosis: Also known as hydatid disease; is caused by Echinococcus granulosus, E. multilocularis, and E. vogeli tapeworms; and is contracted from infected food. Found in southern South America, the Mediterranean, the Middle East, central Asia, and Africa and uncommon in the United States but has been reported in California, New Mexico, Arizona and Utah. The disease is treated with medication over a long course, as it is resistive.

B66.8   **Other specified fluke infections**
     Echinostomiasis
     Heterophyiasis
     Metagonimiasis
     Nanophyetiasis
     Watsoniasis

B66.9   **Fluke infection, unspecified**

● **B67**   **Echinococcosis**
     Larval forms of tapeworms usually of liver or lungs
     Includes   hydatidosis

B67.0   **Echinococcus granulosus infection of liver**

B67.1   **Echinococcus granulosus infection of lung** 🔊

B67.2   **Echinococcus granulosus infection of bone**

● **B67.3**   **Echinococcus granulosus infection, other and multiple sites**

     B67.31   **Echinococcus granulosus infection, thyroid gland**

     B67.32   **Echinococcus granulosus infection, multiple sites**

     B67.39   **Echinococcus granulosus infection, other sites**

B67.4   **Echinococcus granulosus infection, unspecified**
     Dog tapeworm (infection)

B67.5   **Echinococcus multilocularis infection of liver**

● **B67.6**   **Echinococcus multilocularis infection, other and multiple sites**

     B67.61   **Echinococcus multilocularis infection, multiple sites**

     B67.69   **Echinococcus multilocularis infection, other sites**

B67.7   **Echinococcus multilocularis infection, unspecified**

B67.8   **Echinococcosis, unspecified, of liver**

● **B67.9**   **Echinococcosis, other and unspecified**

     B67.90   **Echinococcosis, unspecified**
        Echinococcosis NOS

     B67.99   **Other echinococcosis**

● **B68**   **Taeniasis**
     Intestinal tapeworm (cestode) infection from raw or undercooked meat of infected animal
     Excludes1   cysticercosis (B69.-)

B68.0   **Taenia solium taeniasis**
     Pork tapeworm (infection)

B68.1   **Taenia saginata taeniasis**
     Beef tapeworm (infection)
     Infection due to adult tapeworm Taenia saginata

B68.9   **Taeniasis, unspecified**

● **B69**   **Cysticercosis**
     Systemic illness caused by the larvae of pork tapeworm
     Includes   cysticerciasis infection due to larval form of Taenia solium

B69.0   **Cysticercosis of central nervous system**

B69.1   **Cysticercosis of eye**

● **B69.8**   **Cysticercosis of other sites**

     B69.81   **Myositis in cysticercosis**

     B69.89   **Cysticercosis of other sites**

B69.9   **Cysticercosis, unspecified**

● **B70**   **Diphyllobothriasis and sparganosis**
     Infection with tapeworms seen most often from inadequately cooked fish

B70.0   **Diphyllobothriasis**
     Diphyllobothrium (adult) (latum) (pacificum) infection
     Fish tapeworm (infection)
     Excludes2   larval diphyllobothriasis (B70.1)

B70.1   **Sparganosis**
     Infection with migrating tapeworm larvae, which invade subcutaneous tissues, causing inflammation and fibrosis that resembles cellulitis
     Infection due to Sparganum (mansoni) (proliferum)
     Infection due to Spirometra larva
     Larval diphyllobothriasis
     Spirometrosis

● **B71**   **Other cestode infections**

B71.0   **Hymenolepiasis**
     Intestinal infestation with tapeworms
     Dwarf tapeworm infection
     Rat tapeworm (infection)

B71.1   **Dipylidiasis**
     Infection with tapeworm common to dogs and cats and seen in children having close contact with infected pets

B71.8   **Other specified cestode infections**
     Infection by the larval stage of a tapeworm, usually through fruit or vegetables
     Coenurosis

B71.9   **Cestode infection, unspecified**
     Tapeworm (infection) NOS

● **B72**   **Dracunculiasis**
     Infection with roundworms
     Includes   guinea worm infection
        infection due to Dracunculus medinensis

● **B73**   **Onchocerciasis**
     Infection with parasitic worm
     Includes   onchocerca volvulus infection
        onchocercosis
        river blindness

● **B73.0**   **Onchocerciasis with eye disease**

     B73.00   **Onchocerciasis with eye involvement, unspecified**

     B73.01   **Onchocerciasis with endophthalmitis**

     B73.02   **Onchocerciasis with glaucoma**

     B73.09   **Onchocerciasis with other eye involvement**
        Infestation of eyelid due to onchocerciasis

B73.1   **Onchocerciasis without eye disease**

● **B74**   **Filariasis**
     Infestation with slender threadlike worms
     Excludes2   onchocerciasis (B73)
        tropical (pulmonary) eosinophilia NOS (J82.89)

B74.0   **Filariasis due to Wuchereria bancrofti**
     Bancroftian elephantiasis
     Bancroftian filariasis

B74.1   **Filariasis due to Brugia malayi**

B74.2   **Filariasis due to Brugia timori**

B74.3   **Loiasis**
     Infection with round worms growing in subcutaneous connective tissue
     Calabar swelling
     Eyeworm disease of Africa
     Loa loa infection

B74.4   **Mansonelliasis**
     Infection with filarial parasite
     Infection due to Mansonella ozzardi
     Infection due to Mansonella perstans
     Infection due to Mansonella streptocerca

B74.8   **Other filariases**
     Dirofilariasis

B74.9   **Filariasis, unspecified**

CHAPTER 1 (A00-B99)

B75   **Trichinellosis**
Infestation with parasitic roundworms ingested in undercooked contaminated meat
> **Includes**   infection due to Trichinella species trichiniasis

● B76   **Hookworm diseases**
Occurs in hot, humid parts of world where larvae are soil borne, enter digestive tract through skin of feet/legs or in contaminated food/ water; AKA ground itch
> **Includes**   uncinariasis

    B76.0   **Ancylostomiasis**
         Infection due to Ancylostoma species

    B76.1   **Necatoriasis**
         Infection due to Necator americanus

    B76.8   **Other hookworm diseases**

    B76.9   **Hookworm disease, unspecified**
         Cutaneous larva migrans NOS

● B77   **Ascariasis**
Infection by roundworm in small intestine
> **Includes**   ascaridiasis
>   roundworm infection

    B77.0   **Ascariasis with intestinal complications**

● B77.8   **Ascariasis with other complications**

         B77.81   **Ascariasis pneumonia**

         B77.89   **Ascariasis with other complications**

    B77.9   **Ascariasis, unspecified**

● B78   **Strongyloidiasis**
Infection with adult female roundworms
> **Excludes1**   trichostrongyliasis (B81.2)

    B78.0   **Intestinal strongyloidiasis**

    B78.1   **Cutaneous strongyloidiasis**

    B78.7   **Disseminated strongyloidiasis**

    B78.9   **Strongyloidiasis, unspecified**

B79   **Trichuriasis**
Intestinal infection with roundworms
> **Includes**   trichocephaliasis
>   whipworm (disease)(infection)

B80   **Enterobiasis**
Intestinal infection with pinworms
> **Includes**   oxyuriasis
>   pinworm infection
>   threadworm infection

● B81   **Other intestinal helminthiases, not elsewhere classified**
Diseases or infestations caused by parasitic worms
> **Excludes1**   angiostrongyliasis due to:
>   Angiostrongylus cantonensis (B83.2)
>   Parastrongylus cantonensis (B83.2)

    B81.0   **Anisakiasis**
Roundworm infection via contaminated undercooked infected fish or marine mammals
         Infection due to Anisakis larva

    B81.1   **Intestinal capillariasis**
Infestation with of parasites (nematodes)
         Capillariasis NOS
         Infection due to Capillaria philippinensis
> **Excludes2**   hepatic capillariasis (B83.8)

    B81.2   **Trichostrongyliasis**

    B81.3   **Intestinal angiostrongyliasis**
         Angiostrongyliasis due to:
           Angiostrongylus costaricensis (B83.2)
           Parastrongylus costaricensis (B83.2)

    B81.4   **Mixed intestinal helminthiases**
         Infection due to intestinal helminths classified to more than one of the categories B65.0-B81.3 and B81.8
         Mixed helminthiasis NOS

    B81.8   **Other specified intestinal helminthiases**
         Infection due to Oesophagostomum species [esophagostomiasis]
         Infection due to Ternidens diminutus [ternidensiasis]

● B82   **Unspecified intestinal parasitism**

    B82.0   **Intestinal helminthiasis, unspecified**
Infected with worms

    B82.9   **Intestinal parasitism, unspecified**

● B83   **Other helminthiases**
Caused by parasitic worms
> **Excludes1**   capillariasis NOS (B81.1)
> **Excludes2**   intestinal capillariasis (B81.1)

    B83.0   **Visceral larva migrans**
Prolonged migration of nematode larvae
         Toxocariasis

    B83.1   **Gnathostomiasis**
Infection with nematode occurring from ingested undercooked fish contaminated with larvae; larvae migrate to subcutaneous tissue or deeper tissues, results are abscesses
         Wandering swelling

    B83.2   **Angiostrongyliasis due to Parastrongylus cantonensis**
Nematode infection caused by eating contaminated raw snails, slugs, or paratenic hosts such as prawns or crabs; larval worms migrate to central nervous system resulting in eosinophilic meningitis
         Eosinophilic meningoencephalitis due to Parastrongylus cantonensis
> **Excludes2**   intestinal angiostrongyliasis (B81.3)

    B83.3   **Syngamiasis**
Infestation with gapeworm from turkey, pheasant, guinea fowl, goose, and wild birds
         Syngamosis

    B83.4   **Internal hirudiniasis**
Infestation by leeches
> **Excludes2**   external hirudiniasis (B88.3)

    B83.8   **Other specified helminthiases**
Parasitic worm infestation
         Acanthocephaliasis
         Gongylonemiasis
         Hepatic capillariasis
         Metastrongyliasis
         Thelaziasis

    B83.9   **Helminthiasis, unspecified**
         Worms NOS
> **Excludes1**   intestinal helminthiasis NOS (B82.0)

PEDICULOSIS, ACARIASIS AND OTHER INFESTATIONS (B85-B89)

● B85   **Pediculosis and phthiriasis**
Infestation of lice

    B85.0   **Pediculosis due to Pediculus humanus capitis**
         Head-louse infestation

    B85.1   **Pediculosis due to Pediculus humanus corporis**
         Body-louse infestation

    B85.2   **Pediculosis, unspecified**

    B85.3   **Phthiriasis**
Crab or pubic lice
         Infestation by crab-louse
         Infestation by Phthirus pubis

    B85.4   **Mixed pediculosis and phthiriasis**
         Infestation classifiable to more than one of the categories B85.0-B85.3

B86   **Scabies**
Contagious dermatitis caused by mites
Sarcoptic itch

▶ New   ⇛ Revised   ~~deleted~~ Deleted   Excludes 1   Excludes 2   Includes   Use additional   Code first   Code also   Key words

OGCR Official Guidelines   X Assign placeholder X   ● Use Additional Character(s)   ▶ Manifestation Code   🍬 Hierarchical Condition Category   **Coding Clinic**

● **B87   Myiasis**
Infestation by fly maggots
> **Includes**   infestation by larva of flies

    B87.0   Cutaneous myiasis
        Creeping myiasis

    B87.1   Wound myiasis
        Traumatic myiasis

    B87.2   Ocular myiasis

    B87.3   Nasopharyngeal myiasis
        Laryngeal myiasis

    B87.4   Aural myiasis

●   **B87.8   Myiasis of other sites**
      B87.81   Genitourinary myiasis
      B87.82   Intestinal myiasis
      B87.89   Myiasis of other sites

    B87.9   Myiasis, unspecified

● **B88   Other infestations**

    B88.0   Other acariasis
        Acarine dermatitis
        Dermatitis due to Demodex species
        Dermatitis due to Dermanyssus gallinae
        Dermatitis due to Liponyssoides sanguineus
        Trombiculosis
> **Excludes2**   scabies (B86)

    B88.1   Tungiasis [sandflea infestation]
        Inflammatory skin disease caused by infestation of fleas

    B88.2   Other arthropod infestations
        Scarabiasis

    B88.3   External hirudiniasis
        Leech infestation NOS
> **Excludes2**   internal hirudiniasis (B83.4)

    B88.8   Other specified infestations
        Infection of topical fresh water fish parasite
        Ichthyoparasitism due to Vandellia cirrhosa
        Linguatulosis
        Porocephaliasis

    B88.9   Infestation, unspecified
        Infestation (skin) NOS
        Infestation by mites NOS
        Skin parasites NOS

  B89   Unspecified parasitic disease

SEQUELAE OF INFECTIOUS AND PARASITIC DISEASES (B90-B94)

Note: Categories B90-B94 are to be used to indicate conditions in categories A00-B89 as the cause of sequelae, which are themselves classified elsewhere. The 'sequelae' include conditions specified as such; they also include residuals of diseases classifiable to the above categories if there is evidence that the disease itself is no longer present. Codes from these categories are not to be used for chronic infections. Code chronic current infections to active infectious disease as appropriate.

Code first condition resulting from (sequela) the infectious or parasitic disease

● **B90   Sequelae of tuberculosis**
Condition resulting from tuberculosis

    B90.0   Sequelae of central nervous system tuberculosis

    B90.1   Sequelae of genitourinary tuberculosis

    B90.2   Sequelae of tuberculosis of bones and joints

    B90.8   Sequelae of tuberculosis of other organs
> **Excludes2**   sequelae of respiratory tuberculosis (B90.9)

    B90.9   Sequelae of respiratory and unspecified tuberculosis
        Sequelae of tuberculosis NOS

  B91   Sequelae of poliomyelitis
> **Excludes1**   postpolio syndrome (G14)

  B92   Sequelae of leprosy

● **B94   Sequelae of other and unspecified infectious and parasitic diseases**

    B94.0   Sequelae of trachoma

    B94.1   Sequelae of viral encephalitis

    B94.2   Sequelae of viral hepatitis

    B94.8   Sequelae of other specified infectious and parasitic diseases
        Coding Clinic: 2021, Q4, P102-106; 2021, Q1, P34,37,41,44,46,48

    B94.9   Sequelae of unspecified infectious and parasitic disease
> **Excludes2**   post COVID-19 condition (U09.9)
        Coding Clinic: 2017, Q4, P109

OGCR Section I.C.1.b.

> Certain infectious and parasitic diseases
> Infectious agents as the cause of diseases classified to other chapters
> Certain infections are classified in chapters other than Chapter 1 and no organism is identified as part of the infection code. In these instances, it is necessary to use an additional code from Chapter 1 to identify the organism. A code from category B95, Streptococcus, Staphylococcus, and Enterococcus as the cause of diseases classified to other chapters, B96, Other bacterial agents as the cause of diseases classified to other chapters, or B97, Viral agents as the cause of diseases classified to other chapters, is to be used as an additional code to identify the organism. An instructional note will be found at the infection code advising that an additional organism code is required.

BACTERIAL AND VIRAL INFECTIOUS AGENTS (B95-B97)

Note: These categories are provided for use as supplementary or additional codes to identify the infectious agent(s) in diseases classified elsewhere.
Code the disease first, then the bacterium. Do not report codes from B95-B97 for sepsis.

● **B95   Streptococcus, Staphylococcus, and Enterococcus as the cause of diseases classified elsewhere**

    B95.0   Streptococcus, group A, as the cause of diseases classified elsewhere

    B95.1   Streptococcus, group B, as the cause of diseases classified elsewhere
        Coding Clinic: 2020, Q1, P10; 2019, Q2, P9-10; 2018, Q4, P23

    B95.2   Enterococcus as the cause of diseases classified elsewhere

    B95.3   Streptococcus pneumoniae as the cause of diseases classified elsewhere

    B95.4   Other streptococcus as the cause of diseases classified elsewhere

    B95.5   Unspecified streptococcus as the cause of diseases classified elsewhere

●   **B95.6   Staphylococcus aureus as the cause of diseases classified elsewhere**
      B95.61   Methicillin susceptible Staphylococcus aureus infection as the cause of diseases classified elsewhere
          Methicillin susceptible Staphylococcus aureus (MSSA) infection as the cause of diseases classified elsewhere
          Staphylococcus aureus infection NOS as the cause of diseases classified elsewhere

      B95.62   Methicillin resistant Staphylococcus aureus infection as the cause of diseases classified elsewhere
          Methicillin resistant staphylococcus aureus (MRSA) infection as the cause of diseases classified elsewhere
          Coding Clinic: 2016, Q1, P13

    B95.7   Other staphylococcus as the cause of diseases classified elsewhere

    B95.8   Unspecified staphylococcus as the cause of diseases classified elsewhere

CHAPTER 1 (A00-B99)

● **B96** **Other bacterial agents as the cause of diseases classified elsewhere**

B96.0 Mycoplasma pneumoniae [M. pneumoniae] as the cause of diseases classified elsewhere
Pleuro-pneumonia-like-organism [PPLO]

B96.1 Klebsiella pneumoniae [K. pneumoniae] as the cause of diseases classified elsewhere

● **B96.2** Escherichia coli [E. coli] as the cause of diseases classified elsewhere

B96.20 Unspecified Escherichia coli [E. coli] as the cause of diseases classified elsewhere
Escherichia coli [E. coli] NOS
Coding Clinic: 2022, Q1, P31; 2018, Q4, P34; 2018, Q1, P16

B96.21 Shiga toxin-producing Escherichia coli [E. coli] [STEC] O157 as the cause of diseases classified elsewhere
E. coli O157:H- (nonmotile) with confirmation of Shiga toxin
E. coli O157 with confirmation of Shiga toxin when H antigen is unknown, or is not H7
O157:H7 Escherichia coli [E.coli] with or without confirmation of Shiga toxin-production
Shiga toxin-producing Escherichia coli [E.coli] O157:H7 with or without confirmation of Shiga toxin-production
STEC O157:H7 with or without confirmation of Shiga toxin-production

B96.22 Other specified Shiga toxin-producing Escherichia coli [E. coli] [STEC] as the cause of diseases classified elsewhere
Non-O157 Shiga toxin-producing Escherichia coli [E.coli]
Non-O157 Shiga toxin-producing Escherichia coli [E.coli] with known O group

B96.23 Unspecified Shiga toxin-producing Escherichia coli [E. coli] [STEC] as the cause of diseases classified elsewhere
Shiga toxin-producing Escherichia coli [E. coli] with unspecified O group
STEC NOS

B96.29 Other Escherichia coli [E. coli] as the cause of diseases classified elsewhere
Non-Shiga toxin-producing E. coli

B96.3 Hemophilus influenzae [H. influenzae] as the cause of diseases classified elsewhere

B96.4 Proteus (mirabilis) (morganii) as the cause of diseases classified elsewhere

B96.5 Pseudomonas (aeruginosa) (mallei) (pseudomallei) as the cause of diseases classified elsewhere
Coding Clinic: 2015, Q1, P18

B96.6 Bacteroides fragilis [B. fragilis] as the cause of diseases classified elsewhere

B96.7 Clostridium perfringens [C. perfringens] as the cause of diseases classified elsewhere

● **B96.8** Other specified bacterial agents as the cause of diseases classified elsewhere

B96.81 Helicobacter pylori [H. pylori] as the cause of diseases classified elsewhere

B96.82 Vibrio vulnificus as the cause of diseases classified elsewhere

B96.89 Other specified bacterial agents as the cause of diseases classified elsewhere

● **B97** **Viral agents as the cause of diseases classified elsewhere**

B97.0 Adenovirus as the cause of diseases classified elsewhere

● **B97.1** Enterovirus as the cause of diseases classified elsewhere

B97.10 Unspecified enterovirus as the cause of diseases classified elsewhere

B97.11 Coxsackievirus as the cause of diseases classified elsewhere

B97.12 Echovirus as the cause of diseases classified elsewhere

B97.19 Other enterovirus as the cause of diseases classified elsewhere

Item 1–24 **Retrovirus** develops by copying its RNA, genetic materials, into the DNA, which then produces new virus particles. It is from the Retroviridae virus family. **Human T-cell lymphotropic virus, Type I (HTLV-I)**, is also called human T-cell leukemia virus, Type I, and is a retrovirus thought to cause T-cell leukemia/lymphoma. **Human T-cell lymphotropic virus, Type II (HTLV-II)**, is also called human T-cell leukemia virus, Type II, and is a retrovirus associated with hematologic disorders.

HIV-2 is one of the serotypes of HIV and is usually confined to West Africa, whereas **HIV-1** is found worldwide.

● **B97.2** Coronavirus as the cause of diseases classified elsewhere

B97.21 SARS-associated coronavirus as the cause of diseases classified elsewhere
Excludes1 pneumonia due to SARS-associated coronavirus (J12.81)

B97.29 Other coronavirus as the cause of diseases classified elsewhere

● **B97.3** Retrovirus as the cause of diseases classified elsewhere
Excludes1 human immunodeficiency virus [HIV] disease (B20)

B97.30 Unspecified retrovirus as the cause of diseases classified elsewhere

B97.31 Lentivirus as the cause of diseases classified elsewhere

B97.32 Oncovirus as the cause of diseases classified elsewhere

B97.33 Human T-cell lymphotrophic virus, type I [HTLV-I] as the cause of diseases classified elsewhere

B97.34 Human T-cell lymphotrophic virus, type II [HTLV-II] as the cause of diseases classified elsewhere

B97.35 Human immunodeficiency virus, type 2 [HIV 2] as the cause of diseases classified elsewhere 🔴

B97.39 Other retrovirus as the cause of diseases classified elsewhere

B97.4 Respiratory syncytial virus as the cause of diseases classified elsewhere
RSV as the cause of diseases classified elsewhere
Code first related disorders, such as:
otitis media (H65.-)
upper respiratory infection (J06.9)
Excludes1 acute bronchiolitis due to respiratory syncytial virus (RSV) (J21.0)
acute bronchitis due to respiratory syncytial virus (RSV) (J20.5)
respiratory syncytial virus (RSV) pneumonia (J12.1)

B97.5 Reovirus as the cause of diseases classified elsewhere

B97.6 Parvovirus as the cause of diseases classified elsewhere

B97.7 Papillomavirus as the cause of diseases classified elsewhere

● **B97.8** Other viral agents as the cause of diseases classified elsewhere

B97.81 Human metapneumovirus as the cause of diseases classified elsewhere

B97.89 Other viral agents as the cause of diseases classified elsewhere
Coding Clinic: 2016, Q3, P8-10, 14

OTHER INFECTIOUS DISEASES (B99)

● **B99** **Other and unspecified infectious diseases**

B99.8 Other infectious disease

B99.9 Unspecified infectious disease

▶ New ⇒ Revised ~~deleted~~ Deleted Excludes 1 Excludes 2 Includes Use additional Code first Code also Key words
OGCR Official Guidelines X Assign placeholder X ● Use Additional Character(s) ▸ Manifestation Code 🔴 Hierarchical Condition Category Coding Clinic

CHAPTER 2

NEOPLASMS (C00-D49)

OGCR Chapter-Specific Coding Guidelines

2. **Chapter 2: Neoplasms (C00-D49)**
General guidelines
Chapter 2 of the ICD-10-CM contains the codes for most benign and all malignant neoplasms. Certain benign neoplasms, such as prostatic adenomas, may be found in the specific body system chapters. To properly code a neoplasm it is necessary to determine from the record if the neoplasm is benign, in-situ, malignant, or of uncertain histologic behavior. If malignant, any secondary (metastatic) sites should also be determined.

Primary malignant neoplasms overlapping site boundaries
A primary malignant neoplasm that overlaps two or more contiguous (next to each other) sites should be classified to the subcategory/code .8 ('overlapping lesion'), unless the combination is specifically indexed elsewhere. For multiple neoplasms of the same site that are not contiguous such as tumors in different quadrants of the same breast, codes for each site should be assigned.

Malignant neoplasm of ectopic tissue
Malignant neoplasms of ectopic tissue are to be coded to the site of origin mentioned, e.g., ectopic pancreatic malignant neoplasms involving the stomach are coded to malignant neoplasm of pancreas, unspecified (C25.9).

The neoplasm table in the Alphabetic Index should be referenced first. However, if the histological term is documented, that term should be referenced first, rather than going immediately to the Neoplasm Table, in order to determine which column in the Neoplasm Table is appropriate. For example, if the documentation indicates "adenoma," refer to the term in the Alphabetic Index to review the entries under this term and the instructional note to "see also neoplasm, by site, benign." The table provides the proper code based on the type of neoplasm and the site. It is important to select the proper column in the table that corresponds to the type of neoplasm. The Tabular List should then be referenced to verify that the correct code has been selected from the table and that a more specific site code does not exist.

See Section I.C.21. Factors influencing health status and contact with health services, Status, for information regarding Z15.0, codes for genetic susceptibility to cancer.

a. **Treatment directed at the malignancy**
If the treatment is directed at the malignancy, designate the malignancy as the principal diagnosis.

The only exception to this guideline is if a patient admission/encounter is solely for the administration of chemotherapy, immunotherapy or external beam radiation therapy, assign the appropriate Z51.— code as the first-listed or principal diagnosis, and the diagnosis or problem for which the service is being performed as a secondary diagnosis.

b. **Treatment of secondary site**
When a patient is admitted because of a primary neoplasm with metastasis and treatment is directed toward the secondary site only, the secondary neoplasm is designated as the principal diagnosis even though the primary malignancy is still present.

c. **Coding and sequencing of complications**
Coding and sequencing of complications associated with the malignancies or with the therapy thereof are subject to the following guidelines:

1) **Anemia associated with malignancy**
When admission/encounter is for management of an anemia associated with the malignancy, and the treatment is only for anemia, the appropriate code for the malignancy is sequenced as the principal or first-listed diagnosis followed by the appropriate code for the anemia (such as code D63.0, Anemia in neoplastic disease).

2) **Anemia associated with chemotherapy, immunotherapy and radiation therapy**
When the admission/encounter is for management of an anemia associated with an adverse effect of the administration of chemotherapy or immunotherapy and the only treatment is for the anemia, the anemia code is sequenced first followed by

the appropriate codes for the neoplasm and the adverse effect (T45.1X5, Adverse effect of antineoplastic and immunosuppressive drugs).

When the admission/encounter is for management of an anemia associated with an adverse effect of radiotherapy, the anemia code should be sequenced first, followed by the appropriate neoplasm code and code Y84.2, Radiological procedure and radiotherapy as the cause of abnormal reaction of the patient, or of later complication, without mention of misadventure at the time of the procedure.

3) **Management of dehydration due to the malignancy**
When the admission/encounter is for management of dehydration due to the malignancy and only the dehydration is being treated (intravenous rehydration), the dehydration is sequenced first, followed by the code(s) for the malignancy.

4) **Treatment of a complication resulting from a surgical procedure**
When the admission/encounter is for treatment of a complication resulting from a surgical procedure, designate the complication as the principal or first-listed diagnosis if treatment is directed at resolving the complication.

d. **Primary malignancy previously excised**
When a primary malignancy has been previously excised or eradicated from its site and there is no further treatment directed to that site and there is no evidence of any existing primary malignancy at that site, a code from category Z85, Personal history of malignant neoplasm, should be used to indicate the former site of the malignancy. Any mention of extension, invasion, or metastasis to another site is coded as a secondary malignant neoplasm to that site. The secondary site may be the principal or first-listed with the Z85 code used as a secondary code.

e. **Admissions/Encounters involving chemotherapy, immunotherapy and radiation therapy**

1) **Episode of care involves surgical removal of neoplasm**
When an episode of care involves the surgical removal of a neoplasm, primary or secondary site, followed by adjunct chemotherapy or radiation treatment during the same episode of care, the code for the neoplasm should be assigned as principal or first-listed diagnosis.

2) **Patient admission/encounter solely for administration of chemotherapy, immunotherapy and radiation therapy**
If a patient admission/encounter is solely for the administration of chemotherapy, immunotherapy or external beam radiation therapy assign code Z51.0, Encounter for antineoplastic radiation therapy, or Z51.11, Encounter for antineoplastic chemotherapy, or Z51.12, Encounter for antineoplastic immunotherapy as the first-listed or principal diagnosis. If a patient receives more than one of these therapies during the same admission more than one of these codes may be assigned, in any sequence.

The malignancy for which the therapy is being administered should be assigned as a secondary diagnosis.

If a patient admission/encounter is for the insertion or implantation of radioactive elements (e.g., brachytherapy) the appropriate code for the malignancy is sequenced as the principal or first-listed diagnosis. Code Z51.0 should not be assigned.

3) **Patient admitted for radiation therapy, chemotherapy or immunotherapy and develops complications**
When a patient is admitted for the purpose of external beam radiotherapy, immunotherapy or chemotherapy and develops complications such as uncontrolled nausea and vomiting or dehydration, the principal or first-listed diagnosis is Z51.0, Encounter for antineoplastic radiation therapy, or Z51.11, Encounter for antineoplastic chemotherapy, or Z51.12, Encounter for antineoplastic immunotherapy followed by any codes for the complications.

When a patient is admitted for the purpose of insertion or implantation of radioactive elements (e.g., brachytherapy) and develops complications such as uncontrolled nausea and vomiting or dehydration, the principal or first-listed diagnosis is the appropriate code for the malignancy followed by any codes for the complications.

f. **Admission/encounter to determine extent of malignancy**
When the reason for admission/encounter is to determine the extent of the malignancy, or for a procedure such as paracentesis

or thoracentesis, the primary malignancy or appropriate metastatic site is designated as the principal or first-listed diagnosis, even though chemotherapy or radiotherapy is administered.

g. Symptoms, signs, and abnormal findings listed in Chapter 18 associated with neoplasms

Symptoms, signs, and ill-defined conditions listed in Chapter 18 characteristic of, or associated with, an existing primary or secondary site malignancy cannot be used to replace the malignancy as principal or first-listed diagnosis, regardless of the number of admissions or encounters for treatment and care of the neoplasm.

See Section I.C.21. Factors influencing health status and contact with health services, Encounter for prophylactic organ removal.

h. Admission/encounter for pain control/management

See Section I.C.6. for information on coding admission/encounter for pain control/management.

i. Malignancy in two or more noncontiguous sites

A patient may have more than one malignant tumor in the same organ. These tumors may represent different primaries or metastatic disease, depending on the site. Should the documentation be unclear, the provider should be queried as to the status of each tumor so that the correct codes can be assigned.

j. Disseminated malignant neoplasm, unspecified

Code C80.0, Disseminated malignant neoplasm, unspecified, is for use only in those cases where the patient has advanced metastatic disease and no known primary or secondary sites are specified. It should not be used in place of assigning codes for the primary site and all known secondary sites.

k. Malignant neoplasm without specification of site

Code C80.1, Malignant (primary) neoplasm, unspecified, equates to Cancer, unspecified. This code should only be used when no determination can be made as to the primary site of a malignancy. This code should rarely be used in the inpatient setting.

l. Sequencing of neoplasm codes

1) Encounter for treatment of primary malignancy

If the reason for the encounter is for treatment of a primary malignancy, assign the malignancy as the principal/first-listed diagnosis. The primary site is to be sequenced first, followed by any metastatic sites.

2) Encounter for treatment of secondary malignancy

When an encounter is for a primary malignancy with metastasis and treatment is directed toward the metastatic (secondary) site(s) only, the metastatic site(s) is designated as the principal/first-listed diagnosis. The primary malignancy is coded as an additional code.

3) Malignant neoplasm in a pregnant patient

When a pregnant woman has a malignant neoplasm, a code from subcategory O9A.1-, Malignant neoplasm complicating pregnancy, childbirth, and the puerperium, should be sequenced first, followed by the appropriate code from Chapter 2 to indicate the type of neoplasm.

4) Encounter for complication associated with a neoplasm

When an encounter is for management of a complication associated with a neoplasm, such as dehydration, and the treatment is only for the complication, the complication is coded first, followed by the appropriate code(s) for the neoplasm.

The exception to this guideline is anemia. When the admission/encounter is for management of an anemia associated with the malignancy, and the treatment is only for anemia, the appropriate code for the malignancy is sequenced as the principal or first-listed diagnosis followed by code D63.0, Anemia in neoplastic disease.

5) Complication from surgical procedure for treatment of a neoplasm

When an encounter is for treatment of a complication resulting from a surgical procedure performed for the treatment of the neoplasm, designate the complication as the principal/first-listed diagnosis. See guideline regarding the coding of a current malignancy versus personal history to determine if the code for the neoplasm should also be assigned.

6) Pathologic fracture due to a neoplasm

When an encounter is for a pathological fracture due to a neoplasm, and the focus of treatment is the fracture, a code from subcategory M84.5, Pathological fracture in neoplastic disease, should be sequenced first, followed by the code for the neoplasm.

If the focus of treatment is the neoplasm with an associated pathological fracture, the neoplasm code should be sequenced first, followed by a code from M84.5 for the pathological fracture.

m. Current malignancy versus personal history of malignancy

When a primary malignancy has been excised but further treatment, such as an additional surgery for the malignancy, radiation therapy or chemotherapy is directed to that site, the primary malignancy code should be used until treatment is completed.

When a primary malignancy has been previously excised or eradicated from its site, there is no further treatment (of the malignancy) directed to that site, and there is no evidence of any existing primary malignancy at that site, a code from category Z85, Personal history of malignant neoplasm, should be used to indicate the former site of the malignancy.

Subcategories Z85.0–Z85.7 should only be assigned for the former site of a primary malignancy, not the site of a secondary malignancy. Codes from subcategory Z85.8-, may be assigned for the former site(s) of either a primary or secondary malignancy included in this subcategory.

See Section I.C.21. Factors influencing health status and contact with health services, History (of)

n. Leukemia, Multiple Myeloma, and Malignant Plasma Cell Neoplasms in remission versus personal history

The categories for leukemia, and category C90, Multiple myeloma and malignant plasma cell neoplasms, have codes indicating whether or not the leukemia has achieved remission. There are also codes Z85.6, Personal history of leukemia, and Z85.79, Personal history of other malignant neoplasms of lymphoid, hematopoietic and related tissues. If the documentation is unclear, as to whether the leukemia has achieved remission, the provider should be queried.

See Section I.C.21. Factors influencing health status and contact with health services, History (of)

o. Aftercare following surgery for neoplasm

See Section I.C.21. Factors influencing health status and contact with health services, Aftercare

p. Follow-up care for completed treatment of a malignancy

See Section I.C.21. Factors influencing health status and contact with health services, Follow-up

q. Prophylactic organ removal for prevention of malignancy

See Section I.C. 21, Factors influencing health status and contact with health services, Prophylactic organ removal

r. Malignant neoplasm associated with transplanted organ

A malignant neoplasm of a transplanted organ should be coded as a transplant complication. Assign first the appropriate code from category T86.-, Complications of transplanted organs and tissue, followed by code C80.2, Malignant neoplasm associated with transplanted organ. Use an additional code for the specific malignancy.

Item 2–1 Neoplasm: Neo = new, plasm = growth, development, formation. This new growth (mass, tumor) can be malignant or benign, which is confirmed by the pathology report. Do not assign a code to a neoplasm until you review the pathology report. Certain CPT codes will specify benign or malignant lesion, so be certain the diagnosis code supports the procedure code.

CHAPTER 2

NEOPLASMS (C00-D49)

This chapter contains the following blocks:

C00-C14	Malignant neoplasms of lip, oral cavity and pharynx
C15-C26	Malignant neoplasms of digestive organs
C30-C39	Malignant neoplasms of respiratory and intrathoracic organs
C40-C41	Malignant neoplasms of bone and articular cartilage
C43-C44	Melanoma and other malignant neoplasms of skin
C45-C49	Malignant neoplasms of mesothelial and soft tissue
C50	Malignant neoplasms of breast
C51-C58	Malignant neoplasms of female genital organs
C60-C63	Malignant neoplasms of male genital organs
C64-C68	Malignant neoplasms of urinary tract
C69-C72	Malignant neoplasms of eye, brain and other parts of central nervous system
C73-C75	Malignant neoplasms of thyroid and other endocrine glands
C7A	Malignant neuroendocrine tumors
C7B	Secondary neuroendocrine tumors
C76-C80	Malignant neoplasms of ill-defined, other secondary and unspecified sites
C81-C96	Malignant neoplasms of lymphoid, hematopoietic and related tissue
D00-D09	In situ neoplasms
D10-D36	Benign neoplasms, except benign neuroendocrine tumors
D3A	Benign neuroendocrine tumors
D37-D48	Neoplasms of uncertain behavior, polycythemia vera and myelodysplastic syndromes
D49	Neoplasms of unspecified behavior

Notes: Functional activity

All neoplasms are classified in this chapter, whether they are functionally active or not. An additional code from Chapter 4 may be used, to identify functional activity associated with any neoplasm.

Morphology [Histology]

Chapter 2 classifies neoplasms primarily by site (topography), with broad groupings for behavior, malignant, in situ, benign, etc. The Table of Neoplasms should be used to identify the correct topography code. In a few cases, such as for malignant melanoma and certain neuroendocrine tumors, the morphology (histologic type) is included in the category and codes.

Primary malignant neoplasms overlapping site boundaries

A primary malignant neoplasm that overlaps two or more contiguous (next to each other) sites should be classified to the subcategory/code .8 ("overlapping lesion"), unless the combination is specifically indexed elsewhere. For multiple neoplasms of the same site that are not contiguous, such as tumors in different quadrants of the same breast, codes for each site should be assigned.

Malignant neoplasm of ectopic tissue

Malignant neoplasms of ectopic tissue are to be coded to the site mentioned, e.g., ectopic pancreatic malignant neoplasms are coded to pancreas, unspecified (C25.9).

MALIGNANT NEOPLASMS (C00-C96)

MALIGNANT NEOPLASMS, STATED OR PRESUMED TO BE PRIMARY (OF SPECIFIED SITES), AND CERTAIN SPECIFIED HISTOLOGIES, EXCEPT NEUROENDOCRINE, AND OF LYMPHOID, HEMATOPOIETIC AND RELATED TISSUE (C00-C75)

MALIGNANT NEOPLASMS OF LIP, ORAL CAVITY AND PHARYNX (C00-C14)

● **C00 Malignant neoplasm of lip**

Use additional code to identify:
alcohol abuse and dependence (F10.-)
history of tobacco dependence (Z87.891)
tobacco dependence (F17.-)
tobacco use (Z72.0)

Excludes1 malignant melanoma of lip (C43.0)
Merkel cell carcinoma of lip (C4A.0)
other and unspecified malignant neoplasm of skin of lip (C44.0-)

C00.0 Malignant neoplasm of external upper lip
Malignant neoplasm of lipstick area of upper lip
Malignant neoplasm of upper lip NOS
Malignant neoplasm of vermilion border of upper lip

C00.1 Malignant neoplasm of external lower lip
Malignant neoplasm of lower lip NOS
Malignant neoplasm of lipstick area of lower lip
Malignant neoplasm of vermilion border of lower lip

C00.2 Malignant neoplasm of external lip, unspecified
Malignant neoplasm of vermilion border of lip NOS

C00.3 Malignant neoplasm of upper lip, inner aspect
Malignant neoplasm of buccal aspect of upper lip
Malignant neoplasm of frenulum of upper lip
Malignant neoplasm of mucosa of upper lip
Malignant neoplasm of oral aspect of upper lip

C00.4 Malignant neoplasm of lower lip, inner aspect
Malignant neoplasm of buccal aspect of lower lip
Malignant neoplasm of frenulum of lower lip
Malignant neoplasm of mucosa of lower lip
Malignant neoplasm of oral aspect of lower lip

C00.5 Malignant neoplasm of lip, unspecified, inner aspect
Malignant neoplasm of buccal aspect of lip, unspecified
Malignant neoplasm of frenulum of lip, unspecified
Malignant neoplasm of mucosa of lip, unspecified
Malignant neoplasm of oral aspect of lip, unspecified

C00.6 Malignant neoplasm of commissure of lip, unspecified
Commissure: Site of union of corresponding parts

C00.8 Malignant neoplasm of overlapping sites of lip

C00.9 Malignant neoplasm of lip, unspecified

CHAPTER 2 (C00-D49)

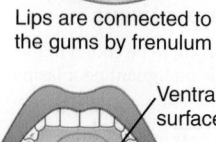

Hard palate
Soft palate
Vestibule
Uvula
Tonsil
Dorsal surface (anterior two-thirds of tongue)

Transitional or vermilion surfaces

A Lips are connected to the gums by frenulum

B

Ventral surface

Lingual frenum

C

Figure 2-1 Anatomical structures of the mouth and lips. **A.** Transitional or vermilion borders. Lips are connected to the gums by frenulum. **B.** Dorsal surface. **C.** Ventral surface.

C01 Malignant neoplasm of base of tongue 🦠
  Malignant neoplasm of dorsal surface of base of tongue
  Malignant neoplasm of fixed part of tongue NOS
  Malignant neoplasm of posterior third of tongue
  Use additional code to identify:
    alcohol abuse and dependence (F10.-)
    history of tobacco dependence (Z87.891)
    tobacco dependence (F17.-)
    tobacco use (Z72.0)

● C02 Malignant neoplasm of other and unspecified parts of tongue
  Use additional code to identify:
    alcohol abuse and dependence (F10.-)
    history of tobacco dependence (Z87.891)
    tobacco dependence (F17.-)
    tobacco use (Z72.0)

  C02.0 Malignant neoplasm of dorsal surface of tongue 🦠
    Malignant neoplasm of anterior two-thirds of tongue, dorsal surface
    Excludes2 malignant neoplasm of dorsal surface of base of tongue (C01)

  C02.1 Malignant neoplasm of border of tongue 🦠
    Malignant neoplasm of tip of tongue

  C02.2 Malignant neoplasm of ventral surface of tongue 🦠
    Malignant neoplasm of anterior two-thirds of tongue, ventral surface
    Malignant neoplasm of frenulum linguae

  C02.3 Malignant neoplasm of anterior two-thirds of tongue, part unspecified 🦠
    Malignant neoplasm of middle third of tongue NOS
    Malignant neoplasm of mobile part of tongue NOS

  C02.4 Malignant neoplasm of lingual tonsil 🦠
    Lingual tonsil: Aggregation of lymph follicles at root of tongue
    Excludes2 malignant neoplasm of tonsil NOS (C09.9)

  C02.8 Malignant neoplasm of overlapping sites of tongue 🦠
    Malignant neoplasm of two or more contiguous sites of tongue

  C02.9 Malignant neoplasm of tongue, unspecified 🦠

● C03 Malignant neoplasm of gum
  Includes malignant neoplasm of alveolar (ridge) mucosa
    malignant neoplasm of gingiva
  Use additional code to identify:
    alcohol abuse and dependence (F10.-)
    history of tobacco dependence (Z87.891)
    tobacco dependence (F17.-)
    tobacco use (Z72.0)
  Excludes2 malignant odontogenic neoplasms (C41.0-C41.1)

  C03.0 Malignant neoplasm of upper gum 🦠
  C03.1 Malignant neoplasm of lower gum 🦠
  C03.9 Malignant neoplasm of gum, unspecified 🦠

● C04 Malignant neoplasm of floor of mouth
  Use additional code to identify:
    alcohol abuse and dependence (F10.-)
    history of tobacco dependence (Z87.891)
    tobacco dependence (F17.-)
    tobacco use (Z72.0)

  C04.0 Malignant neoplasm of anterior floor of mouth 🦠
    Malignant neoplasm of anterior to the premolar-canine junction
  C04.1 Malignant neoplasm of lateral floor of mouth 🦠
  C04.8 Malignant neoplasm of overlapping sites of floor of mouth 🦠
  C04.9 Malignant neoplasm of floor of mouth, unspecified 🦠

● C05 Malignant neoplasm of palate
  Use additional code to identify:
    alcohol abuse and dependence (F10.-)
    history of tobacco dependence (Z87.891)
    tobacco dependence (F17.-)
    tobacco use (Z72.0)
  Excludes1 Kaposi's sarcoma of palate (C46.2)

  C05.0 Malignant neoplasm of hard palate 🦠
  C05.1 Malignant neoplasm of soft palate 🦠
    Excludes2 malignant neoplasm of nasopharyngeal surface of soft palate (C11.3)
  C05.2 Malignant neoplasm of uvula 🦠
  C05.8 Malignant neoplasm of overlapping sites of palate 🦠
  C05.9 Malignant neoplasm of palate, unspecified 🦠
    Malignant neoplasm of roof of mouth

● C06 Malignant neoplasm of other and unspecified parts of mouth
  Use additional code to identify:
    alcohol abuse and dependence (F10.-)
    history of tobacco dependence (Z87.891)
    tobacco dependence (F17.-)
    tobacco use (Z72.0)

  C06.0 Malignant neoplasm of cheek mucosa 🦠
    Malignant neoplasm of buccal mucosa NOS
    Malignant neoplasm of internal cheek
  C06.1 Malignant neoplasm of vestibule of mouth 🦠
    Malignant neoplasm of buccal sulcus (upper) (lower)
    Malignant neoplasm of labial sulcus (upper) (lower)
  C06.2 Malignant neoplasm of retromolar area 🦠
  ● C06.8 Malignant neoplasm of overlapping sites of other and unspecified parts of mouth
    C06.80 Malignant neoplasm of overlapping sites of unspecified parts of mouth 🦠
    C06.89 Malignant neoplasm of overlapping sites of other parts of mouth 🦠
      'book leaf' neoplasm [ventral surface of tongue and floor of mouth]
  C06.9 Malignant neoplasm of mouth, unspecified 🦠
    Malignant neoplasm of minor salivary gland, unspecified site
    Malignant neoplasm of oral cavity NOS

▶ New   ⇒ Revised   ~~deleted~~ Deleted   Excludes 1   Excludes 2   Includes   Use additional   Code first   Code also   Key words
OGCR Official Guidelines   X Assign placeholder X   ● Use Additional Character(s)   ▶ Manifestation Code   🦠 Hierarchical Condition Category   **Coding Clinic**

Figure 2-2   Major salivary glands.

Parotid gland
Sublingual gland
Submandibular gland

C07   Malignant neoplasm of parotid gland 🔍
Use additional code to identify:
alcohol abuse and dependence (F10.-)
exposure to environmental tobacco smoke (Z77.22)
exposure to tobacco smoke in the perinatal period (P96.81)
history of tobacco dependence (Z87.891)
occupational exposure to environmental tobacco smoke (Z57.31)
tobacco dependence (F17.-)
tobacco use (Z72.0)

● **C08   Malignant neoplasm of other and unspecified major salivary glands**
   Includes   malignant neoplasm of salivary ducts
Use additional code to identify:
alcohol abuse and dependence (F10.-)
exposure to environmental tobacco smoke (Z77.22)
exposure to tobacco smoke in the perinatal period (P96.81)
history of tobacco dependence (Z87.891)
occupational exposure to environmental tobacco smoke (Z57.31)
tobacco dependence (F17.-)
tobacco use (Z72.0)
   Excludes1   malignant neoplasms of specified minor salivary glands which are classified according to their anatomical location
   Excludes2   malignant neoplasms of minor salivary glands NOS (C06.9)
               malignant neoplasm of parotid gland (C07)
C08.0   Malignant neoplasm of submandibular gland 🔍
     Malignant neoplasm of submaxillary gland
C08.1   Malignant neoplasm of sublingual gland 🔍
C08.9   Malignant neoplasm of major salivary gland, unspecified 🔍
     Malignant neoplasm of salivary gland (major) NOS

★**(See Plate 28 of the Anatomy Illustrations.)**

● **C09   Malignant neoplasm of tonsil**
Use additional code to identify:
alcohol abuse and dependence (F10.-)
exposure to environmental tobacco smoke (Z77.22)
exposure to tobacco smoke in the perinatal period (P96.81)
history of tobacco dependence (Z87.891)
occupational exposure to environmental tobacco smoke (Z57.31)
tobacco dependence (F17.-)
tobacco use (Z72.0)
   Excludes2   malignant neoplasm of lingual tonsil (C02.4)
               malignant neoplasm of pharyngeal tonsil (C11.1)
C09.0   Malignant neoplasm of tonsillar fossa 🔍
     Surface of palatine (two masses of lymphatic tissue on sides of throat) tonsils
C09.1   Malignant neoplasm of tonsillar pillar (anterior) (posterior) 🔍
     Extension from palatine (two masses of lymphatic tissue on sides of throat) tonsils
C09.8   Malignant neoplasm of overlapping sites of tonsil 🔍
C09.9   Malignant neoplasm of tonsil, unspecified 🔍
     Malignant neoplasm of tonsil NOS
     Malignant neoplasm of faucial tonsils
     Malignant neoplasm of palatine tonsils

● **C10   Malignant neoplasm of oropharynx**
     Area of throat at back of mouth
Use additional code to identify:
alcohol abuse and dependence (F10.-)
exposure to environmental tobacco smoke (Z77.22)
exposure to tobacco smoke in the perinatal period (P96.81)
history of tobacco dependence (Z87.891)
occupational exposure to environmental tobacco smoke (Z57.31)
tobacco dependence (F17.-)
tobacco use (Z72.0)
   Excludes2   malignant neoplasm of tonsil (C09.-)
C10.0   Malignant neoplasm of vallecula 🔍
     Vallecula, depression or furrow
C10.1   Malignant neoplasm of anterior surface of epiglottis 🔍
     Malignant neoplasm of epiglottis, free border [margin]
     Malignant neoplasm of glossoepiglottic fold(s)
   Excludes2   malignant neoplasm of epiglottis (suprahyoid portion) NOS (C32.1)
C10.2   Malignant neoplasm of lateral wall of oropharynx 🔍
C10.3   Malignant neoplasm of posterior wall of oropharynx 🔍
C10.4   Malignant neoplasm of branchial cleft 🔍
     Congenital slitlike openings formed between branchial arches pharyngeal groove
     Malignant neoplasm of branchial cyst [site of neoplasm]
C10.8   Malignant neoplasm of overlapping sites of oropharynx 🔍
     Malignant neoplasm of junctional region of oropharynx
C10.9   Malignant neoplasm of oropharynx, unspecified 🔍

● **C11   Malignant neoplasm of nasopharynx**
Use additional code to identify:
exposure to environmental tobacco smoke (Z77.22)
exposure to tobacco smoke in the perinatal period (P96.81)
history of tobacco dependence (Z87.891)
occupational exposure to environmental tobacco smoke (Z57.31)
tobacco dependence (F17.-)
tobacco use (Z72.0)
C11.0   Malignant neoplasm of superior wall of nasopharynx 🔍
     Part of pharynx that lies above soft palate
     Malignant neoplasm of roof of nasopharynx
C11.1   Malignant neoplasm of posterior wall of nasopharynx 🔍
     Malignant neoplasm of adenoid
     Malignant neoplasm of pharyngeal tonsil
C11.2   Malignant neoplasm of lateral wall of nasopharynx 🔍
     Malignant neoplasm of fossa of Rosenmüller
     Malignant neoplasm of opening of auditory tube
     Malignant neoplasm of pharyngeal recess
C11.3   Malignant neoplasm of anterior wall of nasopharynx 🔍
     Malignant neoplasm of floor of nasopharynx
     Malignant neoplasm of nasopharyngeal (anterior) (posterior) surface of soft palate
     Malignant neoplasm of posterior margin of nasal choana
     Malignant neoplasm of posterior margin of nasal septum
C11.8   Malignant neoplasm of overlapping sites of nasopharynx 🔍
C11.9   Malignant neoplasm of nasopharynx, unspecified 🔍
     Malignant neoplasm of nasopharyngeal wall NOS

C12   Malignant neoplasm of pyriform sinus 🔍
     Malignant neoplasm of pyriform fossa
Use additional code to identify:
exposure to environmental tobacco smoke (Z77.22)
exposure to tobacco smoke in the perinatal period (P96.81)
history of tobacco dependence (Z87.891)
occupational exposure to environmental tobacco smoke (Z57.31)
tobacco dependence (F17.-)
tobacco use (Z72.0)

● **C13**   **Malignant neoplasm of hypopharynx**

Use additional code to identify:
exposure to environmental tobacco smoke (Z77.22)
exposure to tobacco smoke in the perinatal period (P96.81)
history of tobacco dependence (Z87.891)
occupational exposure to environmental tobacco smoke (Z57.31)
tobacco dependence (F17.-)
tobacco use (Z72.0)

Excludes2   malignant neoplasm of pyriform sinus (C12)

C13.0   **Malignant neoplasm of postcricoid region** 🐾
Behind the cricoid cartilage of neck

C13.1   **Malignant neoplasm of aryepiglottic fold, hypopharyngeal aspect** 🐾
Arytenoepiglottic fold, triangular opening between side of epiglottis and apex of arytenoid cartilage
Malignant neoplasm of aryepiglottic fold, marginal zone
Malignant neoplasm of aryepiglottic fold NOS
Malignant neoplasm of interarytenoid fold, marginal zone
Malignant neoplasm of interarytenoid fold NOS

Excludes2   malignant neoplasm of aryepiglottic fold or interarytenoid fold, laryngeal aspect (C32.1)

C13.2   **Malignant neoplasm of posterior wall of hypopharynx** 🐾

C13.8   **Malignant neoplasm of overlapping sites of hypopharynx** 🐾

C13.9   **Malignant neoplasm of hypopharynx, unspecified** 🐾
Malignant neoplasm of hypopharyngeal wall NOS

● **C14**   **Malignant neoplasm of other and ill-defined sites in the lip, oral cavity and pharynx**

Use additional code to identify:
alcohol abuse and dependence (F10.-)
exposure to environmental tobacco smoke (Z77.22)
exposure to tobacco smoke in the perinatal period (P96.81)
history of tobacco dependence (Z87.891)
occupational exposure to environmental tobacco smoke (Z57.31)
tobacco dependence (F17.-)
tobacco use (Z72.0)

Excludes1   malignant neoplasm of oral cavity NOS (C06.9)

C14.0   **Malignant neoplasm of pharynx, unspecified** 🐾

C14.2   **Malignant neoplasm of Waldeyer's ring** 🐾

C14.8   **Malignant neoplasm of overlapping sites of lip, oral cavity and pharynx** 🐾
Primary malignant neoplasm of two or more contiguous sites of lip, oral cavity and pharynx

Excludes1   'book leaf' neoplasm [ventral surface of tongue and floor of mouth] (C06.89)

MALIGNANT NEOPLASM OF DIGESTIVE ORGANS (C15-C26)

Excludes1   Kaposi's sarcoma of gastrointestinal sites (C46.4)

Excludes2   gastrointestinal stromal tumors (C49.A-)

● **C15**   **Malignant neoplasms of esophagus**

Use additional code to identify:
alcohol abuse and dependence (F10.-)

C15.3   **Malignant neoplasm of upper third of esophagus** 🐾

C15.4   **Malignant neoplasm of middle third of esophagus** 🐾

C15.5   **Malignant neoplasm of lower third of esophagus** 🐾

Excludes1   malignant neoplasm of cardio-esophageal junction (C16.0)

C15.8   **Malignant neoplasm of overlapping sites of esophagus** 🐾

C15.9   **Malignant neoplasm of esophagus, unspecified** 🐾

● **C16**   **Malignant neoplasm of stomach**

Use additional code to identify:
alcohol abuse and dependence (F10.-)

Excludes2   malignant carcinoid tumor of the stomach (C7A.092)

C16.0   **Malignant neoplasm of cardia** 🐾
Malignant neoplasm of cardiac orifice
Malignant neoplasm of cardio-esophageal junction
Malignant neoplasm of esophagus and stomach
Malignant neoplasm of gastro-esophageal junction

C16.1   **Malignant neoplasm of fundus of stomach** 🐾

C16.2   **Malignant neoplasm of body of stomach** 🐾

C16.3   **Malignant neoplasm of pyloric antrum** 🐾
Malignant neoplasm of gastric antrum

C16.4   **Malignant neoplasm of pylorus** 🐾
Malignant neoplasm of prepylorus
Malignant neoplasm of pyloric canal

C16.5   **Malignant neoplasm of lesser curvature of stomach, unspecified** 🐾
Malignant neoplasm of lesser curvature of stomach, not classifiable to C16.1-C16.4

C16.6   **Malignant neoplasm of greater curvature of stomach, unspecified** 🐾
Malignant neoplasm of greater curvature of stomach, not classifiable to C16.0-C16.4

C16.8   **Malignant neoplasm of overlapping sites of stomach** 🐾

C16.9   **Malignant neoplasm of stomach, unspecified** 🐾
Gastric cancer NOS

CERVICAL ESOPHAGUS
Left subclavian artery
First rib
Arch of aorta
Diaphragm
THORACIC ESOPHAGUS
ABDOMINAL ESOPHAGUS
Stomach

Figure 2-3   The esophagus is the muscular tube that connects the pharynx and the stomach. The 10 inch (25 cm) long esophagus is divided into three parts: **cervical, thoracic,** and **abdominal.**

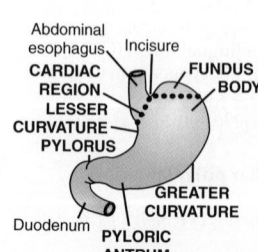

Abdominal esophagus   Incisure
CARDIAC REGION   **FUNDUS**   **BODY**
LESSER CURVATURE
PYLORUS
GREATER CURVATURE
Duodenum   **PYLORIC ANTRUM**

Figure 2-4   Parts of the stomach.

Item 2-2   The esophagus opens into the stomach through the **cardiac orifice,** also called the **cardioesophageal junction.** The **cardia** is adjacent to the cardiac orifice. The stomach widens into the **greater** and **lesser curvatures.** The **pyloric antrum** precedes the **pylorus,** which opens to the duodenum.

▶ New   ⇒ Revised   ~~deleted~~ Deleted   Excludes 1   Excludes 2   Includes   Use additional   Code first   Code also   Key words
OGCR Official Guidelines   X Assign placeholder X   ● Use Additional Character(s)   ▶ Manifestation Code   🐾 Hierarchical Condition Category   **Coding Clinic**

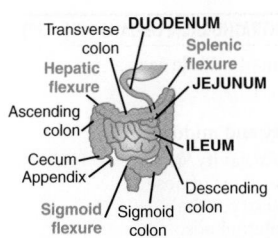

Figure 2-5 Small intestine and colon.

● **C17** Malignant neoplasm of small intestine
  > **Excludes1** malignant carcinoid tumor of the small intestine (C7A.01)

  C17.0 **Malignant neoplasm of duodenum** 🔍
  > *First or proximal portion of small intestine, extending from pylorus to jejunum*

  C17.1 **Malignant neoplasm of jejunum** 🔍
  > *Second section of small intestine, extending from duodenum to ileum*

  C17.2 **Malignant neoplasm of ileum** 🔍
  > *Distal and longest portion of small intestine, extending from jejunum to cecum*
  > > **Excludes1** malignant neoplasm of ileocecal valve (C18.0)

  C17.3 **Meckel's diverticulum, malignant** 🔍
  > *Appendage of ileum*
  > > **Excludes1** Meckel's diverticulum, congenital (Q43.0)

  C17.8 **Malignant neoplasm of overlapping sites of small intestine** 🔍

  C17.9 **Malignant neoplasm of small intestine, unspecified** 🔍

● **C18** Malignant neoplasm of colon
  > **Excludes1** malignant carcinoid tumors of the colon (C7A.02)

  C18.0 **Malignant neoplasm of cecum** 🔍
  > *First section of large intestine*
  > Malignant neoplasm of ileocecal valve

  C18.1 **Malignant neoplasm of appendix** 🔍
  > *Blind ended tube connected to the cecum; AKA vermiform appendix*

  C18.2 **Malignant neoplasm of ascending colon** 🔍
  > *Ascending colon is between cecum and right colic flexure*

  C18.3 **Malignant neoplasm of hepatic flexure** 🔍
  > *A flexure is a bending in a structure or organ. Note the three flexures illustrated in Figure 2–5.*

  C18.4 **Malignant neoplasm of transverse colon** 🔍
  > *Portion of colon that runs transversely across upper part of abdomen, between right and left colic flexures*

  C18.5 **Malignant neoplasm of splenic flexure** 🔍
  > *Bend at junction of transverse and descending colon*

  C18.6 **Malignant neoplasm of descending colon** 🔍
  > *Portion between left colic flexure and sigmoid colon at pelvic brim; AKA iliac colon*

  C18.7 **Malignant neoplasm of sigmoid colon** 🔍
  > *S-shaped part of colon extending from pelvic brim to third segment of sacrum*
  > Malignant neoplasm of sigmoid (flexure)
  > > **Excludes1** malignant neoplasm of rectosigmoid junction (C19)

  C18.8 **Malignant neoplasm of overlapping sites of colon** 🔍

  C18.9 **Malignant neoplasm of colon, unspecified** 🔍
  > Malignant neoplasm of large intestine NOS

● **C19** Malignant neoplasm of rectosigmoid junction 🔍
  > Malignant neoplasm of colon with rectum
  > Malignant neoplasm of rectosigmoid (colon)
  > > **Excludes1** malignant carcinoid tumors of the colon (C7A.02-)

● **C20** Malignant neoplasm of rectum 🔍
  > Malignant neoplasm of rectal ampulla
  > > **Excludes1** malignant carcinoid tumor of the rectum (C7A.026)

● **C21** Malignant neoplasm of anus and anal canal
  > **Excludes2** malignant carcinoid tumors of the colon (C7A.02-)
  > malignant melanoma of anal margin (C43.51)
  > malignant melanoma of anal skin (C43.51)
  > malignant melanoma of perianal skin (C43.51)
  > other and unspecified malignant neoplasm of anal margin (C44.500, C44.510, C44.520, C44.590)
  > other and unspecified malignant neoplasm of anal skin (C44.500, C44.510, C44.520, C44.590)
  > other and unspecified malignant neoplasm of perianal skin (C44.500, C44.510, C44.520, C44.590)

  C21.0 **Malignant neoplasm of anus, unspecified** 🔍

  C21.1 **Malignant neoplasm of anal canal** 🔍
  > *Terminal part of large intestine*
  > Malignant neoplasm of anal sphincter

  C21.2 **Malignant neoplasm of cloacogenic zone** 🔍

  C21.8 **Malignant neoplasm of overlapping sites of rectum, anus and anal canal** 🔍
  > Malignant neoplasm of anorectal junction
  > Malignant neoplasm of anorectum
  > Primary malignant neoplasm of two or more contiguous sites of rectum, anus and anal canal

● **C22** Malignant neoplasm of liver and intrahepatic bile ducts
  > *Intrahepatic: Within liver*
  > Use additional code to identify:
  > alcohol abuse and dependence (F10.-)
  > hepatitis B (B16.-, B18.0-B18.1) hepatitis C (B17.1-, B18.2)
  > > **Excludes1** malignant neoplasm of biliary tract NOS (C24.9)
  > > secondary malignant neoplasm of liver and intrahepatic bile duct (C78.7)

  C22.0 **Liver cell carcinoma** 🔍
  > Hepatocellular carcinoma
  > Hepatoma

  C22.1 **Intrahepatic bile duct carcinoma** 🔍
  > Cholangiocarcinoma
  > *Adenocarcinoma (cancer that originates in glandular tissue) arising from epithelium of intrahepatic bile ducts*
  > > **Excludes1** malignant neoplasm of hepatic duct (C24.0)

  C22.2 **Hepatoblastoma** 🔍
  > *Malignant intrahepatic tumor*

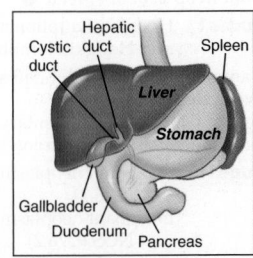

Figure 2-6 Diagram of liver, gallbladder, hepatic duct, pancreas, and spleen. (From Thibodeau and Patton: Anatomy and Physiology, ed 7, Mosby, 2010)

CHAPTER 2 (C00-D49)

C22.3   **Angiosarcoma of liver** 🧬
     Kupffer cell sarcoma

C22.4   **Other sarcomas of liver** 🧬

C22.7   **Other specified carcinomas of liver** 🧬

C22.8   **Malignant neoplasm of liver, primary, unspecified as to type** 🧬

C22.9   **Malignant neoplasm of liver, not specified as primary or secondary** 🧬

C23   **Malignant neoplasm of gallbladder** 🧬

● **C24**   **Malignant neoplasm of other and unspecified parts of biliary tract**
     Excludes1   malignant neoplasm of intrahepatic bile duct (C22.1)

C24.0   **Malignant neoplasm of extrahepatic bile duct** 🧬
     Extrahepatic = outside the liver
     Malignant neoplasm of biliary duct or passage NOS
     Malignant neoplasm of common bile duct
     Malignant neoplasm of cystic duct
     Malignant neoplasm of hepatic duct

C24.1   **Malignant neoplasm of ampulla of Vater** 🧬
     Union of pancreatic duct and common bile duct

C24.8   **Malignant neoplasm of overlapping sites of biliary tract** 🧬
     Malignant neoplasm involving both intrahepatic and extrahepatic bile ducts
     Primary malignant neoplasm of two or more contiguous sites of biliary tract

C24.9   **Malignant neoplasm of biliary tract, unspecified** 🧬

● **C25**   **Malignant neoplasm of pancreas**
     Check documentation for specific site.
     Code also if applicable exocrine pancreatic insufficiency (K86.81)
     Use additional code to identify:
     alcohol abuse and dependence (F10.-)

C25.0   **Malignant neoplasm of head of pancreas** 🧬

C25.1   **Malignant neoplasm of body of pancreas** 🧬
     Coding Clinic: 2018, Q4, P40

C25.2   **Malignant neoplasm of tail of pancreas** 🧬

C25.3   **Malignant neoplasm of pancreatic duct** 🧬

C25.4   **Malignant neoplasm of endocrine pancreas** 🧬
     Malignant neoplasm of islets of Langerhans
     That part of the pancreas that acts as endocrine gland and consists of islets of Langerhans
     Use additional code to identify any functional activity.

C25.7   **Malignant neoplasm of other parts of pancreas** 🧬
     Malignant neoplasm of neck of pancreas

C25.8   **Malignant neoplasm of overlapping sites of pancreas** 🧬

C25.9   **Malignant neoplasm of pancreas, unspecified** 🧬

● **C26**   **Malignant neoplasm of other and ill-defined digestive organs**
     Excludes1   malignant neoplasm of peritoneum and retroperitoneum (C48.-)

C26.0   **Malignant neoplasm of intestinal tract, part unspecified** 🧬
     Malignant neoplasm of intestine NOS

C26.1   **Malignant neoplasm of spleen** 🧬
     Excludes1   Hodgkin lymphoma (C81.-)
               non-Hodgkin lymphoma (C82-C85)

C26.9   **Malignant neoplasm of ill-defined sites within the digestive system** 🧬
     Malignant neoplasm of alimentary canal or tract NOS
     Malignant neoplasm of gastrointestinal tract NOS
     Excludes1   malignant neoplasm of abdominal NOS (C76.2)
               malignant neoplasm of intra-abdominal NOS (C76.2)

MALIGNANT NEOPLASMS OF RESPIRATORY AND INTRATHORACIC ORGANS (C30-C39)

     Includes   malignant neoplasm of middle ear
     Excludes1   mesothelioma (C45.-)

● **C30**   **Malignant neoplasm of nasal cavity and middle ear**

C30.0   **Malignant neoplasm of nasal cavity** 🧬
     Malignant neoplasm of cartilage of nose
     Malignant neoplasm of nasal concha
     Malignant neoplasm of internal nose
     Malignant neoplasm of septum of nose
     Malignant neoplasm of vestibule of nose
     Anterior part of nasal cavity
     Excludes1   malignant neoplasm of nasal bone (C41.0)
               malignant neoplasm of nose NOS (C76.0)
               malignant neoplasm of olfactory bulb (C72.2-)
               malignant neoplasm of posterior margin of nasal septum and choana (C11.3)
               malignant melanoma of skin of nose (C43.31)
               malignant neoplasm of turbinates (C41.0)
               other and unspecified malignant neoplasm of skin of nose (C44.301, C44.311, C44.321, C44.391)

C30.1   **Malignant neoplasm of middle ear** 🧬
     Malignant neoplasm of antrum tympanicum
     Boney cavity or chamber
     Malignant neoplasm of auditory tube
     Malignant neoplasm of eustachian tube
     Malignant neoplasm of inner ear
     Malignant neoplasm of mastoid air cells
     Malignant neoplasm of tympanic cavity
     Excludes1   malignant neoplasm of auricular canal (external) (C43.2-, C44.2-)
               malignant neoplasm of bone of ear (meatus) (C41.0)
               malignant neoplasm of cartilage of ear (C49.0)
               malignant melanoma of skin of (external) ear (C43.2-)
               other and unspecified malignant neoplasm of skin of (external) ear (C44.2-)

● **C31**   **Malignant neoplasm of accessory sinuses**
     Paired sinuses in bones of face

C31.0   **Malignant neoplasm of maxillary sinus** 🧬
     Malignant neoplasm of antrum (Highmore) (maxillary)

C31.1   **Malignant neoplasm of ethmoidal sinus** 🧬

C31.2   **Malignant neoplasm of frontal sinus** 🧬

C31.3   **Malignant neoplasm of sphenoid sinus** 🧬

C31.8   **Malignant neoplasm of overlapping sites of accessory sinuses** 🧬

C31.9   **Malignant neoplasm of accessory sinus, unspecified** 🧬

Item 2–3   **Islets** of Langerhans (endocrine producing cells comprising 1% to 2% of the pancreatic mass) make and secrete hormones that regulate the body's production of insulin, glucagon, and stomach acid. Breakdown of the insulin-producing cells can cause diabetes mellitus. Islet cell tumors can be benign or malignant and include glucagonomas, insulinomas, gastrinomas, and neuroendocrine tumor. The neoplasm table must be consulted for the correct neoplasm code.

Figure 2-7   Paranasal sinuses. (From Buck CJ: Step-by-Step Medical Coding, ed 2016, St. Louis, Elsevier, 2016)

▶ New   ➡ Revised   ~~deleted~~ Deleted   Excludes 1   Excludes 2   Includes   Use additional   Code first   Code also   Key words
OGCR Official Guidelines   X Assign placeholder X   ● Use Additional Character(s)   ▶ Manifestation Code   🧬 Hierarchical Condition Category   **Coding Clinic**

● **C32**   **Malignant neoplasm of** larynx

     Use additional code to identify:
        alcohol abuse and dependence (F10.-)
        exposure to environmental tobacco smoke (Z77.22)
        exposure to tobacco smoke in the perinatal period (P96.81)
        history of tobacco dependence (Z87.891)
        occupational exposure to environmental tobacco smoke
          (Z57.31)
        tobacco dependence (F17.-)
        tobacco use (Z72.0)

    C32.0   **Malignant neoplasm of** glottis 🔎

        Vocal apparatus of larynx, consisting of true vocal cords
          (plicae vocales) and opening between them (rima
          glottidis)
        Malignant neoplasm of intrinsic larynx
        Malignant neoplasm of laryngeal commissure (anterior)
          (posterior)
        Malignant neoplasm of vocal cord (true) NOS
          True vocal cords ("lower vocal folds") produce vocalization
           when air from the lungs passes between them. Check
           your documentation. Code C32.1 is for malignant
           *neoplasm of the **false** vocal cords.*

    C32.1   **Malignant neoplasm of** supraglottis 🔎

        Area of pharynx above glottis
        Malignant neoplasm of aryepiglottic fold or
          interarytenoid fold, laryngeal aspect
        Malignant neoplasm of epiglottis (suprahyoid portion)
          NOS
        Malignant neoplasm of extrinsic larynx
        Malignant neoplasm of false vocal cord
          ***False** vocal cords ("upper vocal folds") are not involved in*
           vocalization. Check your documentation. Code C32.0 is
           for true vocal cords.
        Malignant neoplasm of posterior (laryngeal) surface of
          epiglottis
        Malignant neoplasm of ventricular bands

        Excludes2   malignant neoplasm of anterior surface of
                 epiglottis (C10.1)
               malignant neoplasm of aryepiglottic
                 fold or interarytenoid fold,
                 hypopharyngeal aspect (C13.1)
               malignant neoplasm of aryepiglottic fold
                 or interarytenoid fold, marginal zone
                 (C13.1)
               malignant neoplasm of aryepiglottic fold
                 or interarytenoid fold NOS (C13.1)

    C32.2   **Malignant neoplasm of** subglottis 🔎

        Lowest part of larynx from just below vocal cords down to top
          of trachea

    C32.3   **Malignant neoplasm of laryngeal** cartilage 🔎

        Cartilages of larynx, including cricoid, thyroid, and
          epiglottic, and two each of arytenoid, corniculate, and
          cuneiform

    C32.8   **Malignant neoplasm of** overlapping sites **of larynx** 🔎

    C32.9   **Malignant neoplasm of larynx,** unspecified 🔎

● **C33**   **Malignant neoplasm of** trachea 🔎

     Use additional code to identify:
        exposure to environmental tobacco smoke (Z77.22)
        exposure to tobacco smoke in the perinatal period (P96.81)
        history of tobacco dependence (Z87.891)
        occupational exposure to environmental tobacco smoke
          (Z57.31)
        tobacco dependence (F17.-)
        tobacco use (Z72.0)

● **C34**   **Malignant neoplasm of** bronchus and lung

     Use additional code to identify:
        exposure to environmental tobacco smoke (Z77.22)
        exposure to tobacco smoke in the perinatal period (P96.81)
        history of tobacco dependence (Z87.891)
        occupational exposure to environmental tobacco smoke
          (Z57.31)
        tobacco dependence (F17.-)
        tobacco use (Z72.0)

     Excludes1   Kaposi's sarcoma of lung (C46.5-)
               malignant carcinoid tumor of the bronchus and
                 lung (C7A.090)

● **C34.0**   **Malignant neoplasm of** main bronchus

        Malignant neoplasm of carina
          Ridgelike structure
        Malignant neoplasm of hilus (of lung)
          Anatomic depression or pit

     C34.00   **Malignant neoplasm of** unspecified **main**
              bronchus 🔎

     C34.01   **Malignant neoplasm of** right **main bronchus** 🔎

     C34.02   **Malignant neoplasm of** left **main bronchus** 🔎

● **C34.1**   **Malignant neoplasm of** upper lobe, **bronchus or lung**

     C34.10   **Malignant neoplasm of** unspecified **bronchus**
              or lung 🔎

     C34.11   **Malignant neoplasm of upper lobe,** right
              bronchus or lung 🔎

     C34.12   **Malignant neoplasm of upper lobe,** left
              bronchus or lung 🔎

    C34.2   **Malignant neoplasm of** middle lobe, **bronchus or**
         lung 🔎

● **C34.3**   **Malignant neoplasm of** lower lobe, **bronchus or lung**

     C34.30   **Malignant neoplasm of lower lobe,** unspecified
              bronchus or lung 🔎

     C34.31   **Malignant neoplasm of lower lobe,** right
              bronchus or lung 🔎

     C34.32   **Malignant neoplasm of lower lobe,** left
              bronchus or lung 🔎

● **C34.8**   **Malignant neoplasm of** overlapping sites **of bronchus**
       and lung

     C34.80   **Malignant neoplasm of overlapping sites**
              of unspecified **bronchus and lung** 🔎

     C34.81   **Malignant neoplasm of overlapping sites of**
              right **bronchus and lung** 🔎

     C34.82   **Malignant neoplasm of overlapping sites of** left
              bronchus and lung 🔎

● **C34.9**   **Malignant neoplasm of** unspecified part **of bronchus or**
       lung

     C34.90   **Malignant neoplasm of unspecified part of**
              unspecified **bronchus or lung** 🔎
              Lung cancer NOS

     C34.91   **Malignant neoplasm of unspecified part of**
              right **bronchus or lung** 🔎

     C34.92   **Malignant neoplasm of unspecified part of** left
              bronchus or lung 🔎

C37   **Malignant neoplasm of thymus** 🔎

     Excludes1   malignant carcinoid tumor of the thymus
               (C7A.091)

CHAPTER 2 (C00–D49)

● **C38 Malignant neoplasm of heart, mediastinum and pleura**
> **Excludes1**   mesothelioma (C45.-)

  C38.0 Malignant neoplasm of heart 🐾
     Malignant neoplasm of pericardium
> **Excludes1**   malignant neoplasm of great vessels (C49.3)

  C38.1 Malignant neoplasm of anterior mediastinum 🐾
  C38.2 Malignant neoplasm of posterior mediastinum 🐾
  C38.3 Malignant neoplasm of mediastinum, part unspecified 🐾
  C38.4 Malignant neoplasm of pleura 🐾
  C38.8 Malignant neoplasm of overlapping sites of heart, mediastinum and pleura 🐾
> *Pleura are comprised of serous membrane that lines the thoracic cavity (parietal) and covers the lungs (visceral).*

● **C39 Malignant neoplasm of other and ill-defined sites in the respiratory system and intrathoracic organs**
Intrathoracic: within thorax/chest

Use additional code to identify:
  exposure to environmental tobacco smoke (Z77.22)
  exposure to tobacco smoke in the perinatal period (P96.81)
  history of tobacco dependence (Z87.891)
  occupational exposure to environmental tobacco smoke (Z57.31)
  tobacco dependence (F17.-)
  tobacco use (Z72.0)
> **Excludes1**   intrathoracic malignant neoplasm NOS (C76.1)
>   thoracic malignant neoplasm NOS (C76.1)

  C39.0 Malignant neoplasm of upper respiratory tract, part unspecified 🐾
  C39.9 Malignant neoplasm of lower respiratory tract, part unspecified 🐾
     Malignant neoplasm of respiratory tract NOS

MALIGNANT NEOPLASMS OF BONE AND ARTICULAR CARTILAGE (C40-C41)

> **Includes**   malignant neoplasm of cartilage (articular) (joint)
>   malignant neoplasm of periosteum
> **Excludes1**   malignant neoplasm of bone marrow NOS (C96.9)
>   malignant neoplasm of synovia (C49.-)

● **C40 Malignant neoplasm of bone and articular cartilage of limbs**
Use additional code to identify major osseous defect, if applicable (M89.7-)

  ● **C40.0 Malignant neoplasm of scapula and long bones of upper limb**
    C40.00 Malignant neoplasm of scapula and long bones of unspecified upper limb 🐾
    C40.01 Malignant neoplasm of scapula and long bones of right upper limb 🐾
    C40.02 Malignant neoplasm of scapula and long bones of left upper limb 🐾

  ● **C40.1 Malignant neoplasm of short bones of upper limb**
    C40.10 Malignant neoplasm of short bones of unspecified upper limb 🐾
    C40.11 Malignant neoplasm of short bones of right upper limb 🐾
    C40.12 Malignant neoplasm of short bones of left upper limb 🐾

  ● **C40.2 Malignant neoplasm of long bones of lower limb**
    C40.20 Malignant neoplasm of long bones of unspecified lower limb 🐾
    C40.21 Malignant neoplasm of long bones of right lower limb 🐾
    C40.22 Malignant neoplasm of long bones of left lower limb 🐾

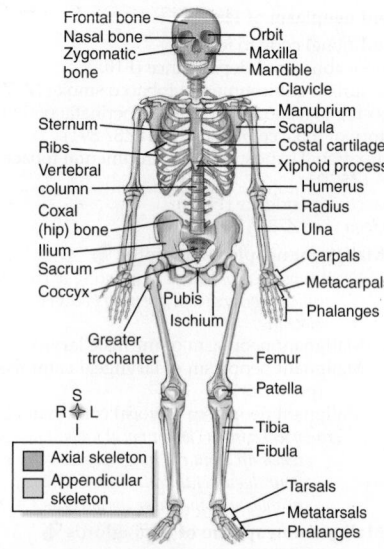

Figure 2-8   Diagram of skeleton of trunk and limbs with bones labeled. (From Thibodeau and Patton: Anatomy and Physiology, ed 7, Mosby, 2010)

  ● **C40.3 Malignant neoplasm of short bones of lower limb**
    C40.30 Malignant neoplasm of short bones of unspecified lower limb 🐾
    C40.31 Malignant neoplasm of short bones of right lower limb 🐾
    C40.32 Malignant neoplasm of short bones of left lower limb 🐾

  ● **C40.8 Malignant neoplasm of overlapping sites of bone and articular cartilage of limb**
    C40.80 Malignant neoplasm of overlapping sites of bone and articular cartilage of unspecified limb 🐾
    C40.81 Malignant neoplasm of overlapping sites of bone and articular cartilage of right limb 🐾
    C40.82 Malignant neoplasm of overlapping sites of bone and articular cartilage of left limb 🐾

  ● **C40.9 Malignant neoplasm of unspecified bones and articular cartilage of limb**
    C40.90 Malignant neoplasm of unspecified bones and articular cartilage of unspecified limb 🐾
    C40.91 Malignant neoplasm of unspecified bones and articular cartilage of right limb 🐾
    C40.92 Malignant neoplasm of unspecified bones and articular cartilage of left limb 🐾

● **C41 Malignant neoplasm of bone and articular cartilage of other and unspecified sites**
> **Excludes1**   malignant neoplasm of bones of limbs (C40.-)
>   malignant neoplasm of cartilage of ear (C49.0)
>   malignant neoplasm of cartilage of eyelid (C49.0)
>   malignant neoplasm of cartilage of larynx (C32.3)
>   malignant neoplasm of cartilage of limbs (C40.-)
>   malignant neoplasm of cartilage of nose (C30.0)

  C41.0 Malignant neoplasm of bones of skull and face 🐾
    Malignant neoplasm of maxilla (superior)
    Malignant neoplasm of orbital bone
> **Excludes2**   carcinoma, any type except intraosseous or odontogenic of:
>   maxillary sinus (C31.0)
>   upper jaw (C03.0)
>   malignant neoplasm of jaw bone (lower) (C41.1)

▶ New   ⇒ Revised   ~~deleted~~ Deleted   Excludes 1   Excludes 2   Includes   Use additional   Code first   Code also   Key words
OGCR Official Guidelines   **X** Assign placeholder X   ● Use Additional Character(s)   ) Manifestation Code   🐾 Hierarchical Condition Category   **Coding Clinic**

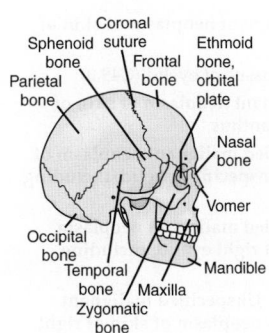

Figure 2-9   Bones of the skull.

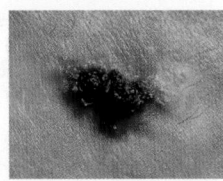

Figure 2-10   Malignant melanoma of skin. (Getty Image)

Item 2–4   Malignant melanoma is a serious form of skin cancer that affects the melanocytes (pigment-forming cells) and is caused by ultraviolet (UV) rays from the sun that damage skin. It is most commonly seen in the 40- to 60-year-olds with fair skin, blue or green eyes, and red or blond hair who sunburn easily.

Melanoma can spread very rapidly and is the most deadly form of skin cancer. It is less common than other types of skin cancer. The rate of melanoma is increasing and currently is the leading cause of death from skin disease.

C41.1   Malignant neoplasm of mandible 🔧
Malignant neoplasm of inferior maxilla
Malignant neoplasm of lower jaw bone

     Excludes2   carcinoma, any type except intraosseous or odontogenic of:
jaw NOS (C03.9)
lower (C03.1)
malignant neoplasm of upper jaw bone (C41.0)

C41.2   Malignant neoplasm of vertebral column 🔧

     Excludes1   malignant neoplasm of sacrum and coccyx (C41.4)

C41.3   Malignant neoplasm of ribs, sternum and clavicle 🔧

C41.4   Malignant neoplasm of pelvic bones, sacrum and coccyx 🔧

C41.9   Malignant neoplasm of bone and articular cartilage, unspecified 🔧

MELANOMA AND OTHER MALIGNANT NEOPLASMS OF SKIN (C43-C44)

● **C43   Malignant melanoma of skin**

     Excludes1   melanoma in situ (D03.-)

     Excludes2   malignant melanoma of skin of genital organs (C51-C52, C60.-, C63.-)
Merkel cell carcinoma (C4A.-)
sites other than skin-code to malignant neoplasm of the site

C43.0   Malignant melanoma of lip 🔧

     Excludes1   malignant neoplasm of vermilion border of lip (C00.0-C00.2)

● **C43.1   Malignant melanoma of eyelid, including canthus**
Canthus: Either corner of eye where upper and lower eyelids meet

     C43.10   Malignant melanoma of unspecified eyelid, including canthus 🔧

     ● **C43.11   Malignant melanoma of right eyelid, including canthus** 🔧

         C43.111   Malignant melanoma of right upper eyelid, including canthus 🔧

         C43.112   Malignant melanoma of right lower eyelid, including canthus 🔧

     ● **C43.12   Malignant melanoma of left eyelid, including canthus** 🔧

         C43.121   Malignant melanoma of left upper eyelid, including canthus 🔧

         C43.122   Malignant melanoma of left lower eyelid, including canthus 🔧

● **C43.2   Malignant melanoma of ear and external auricular canal**

     C43.20   Malignant melanoma of unspecified ear and external auricular canal 🔧

     C43.21   Malignant melanoma of right ear and external auricular canal 🔧

     C43.22   Malignant melanoma of left ear and external auricular canal 🔧

● **C43.3   Malignant melanoma of other and unspecified parts of face**

     C43.30   Malignant melanoma of unspecified part of face 🔧

     C43.31   Malignant melanoma of nose 🔧

     C43.39   Malignant melanoma of other parts of face 🔧

C43.4   Malignant melanoma of scalp and neck 🔧

● **C43.5   Malignant melanoma of trunk**

     Excludes2   malignant neoplasm of anus NOS (C21.0)
malignant neoplasm of scrotum (C63.2)

     C43.51   Malignant melanoma of anal skin 🔧
Malignant melanoma of anal margin
Malignant melanoma of perianal skin

     C43.52   Malignant melanoma of skin of breast 🔧

     C43.59   Malignant melanoma of other part of trunk 🔧

● **C43.6   Malignant melanoma of upper limb, including shoulder**

     C43.60   Malignant melanoma of upper limb, including shoulder, unspecified side 🔧

     C43.61   Malignant melanoma of right upper limb, including shoulder 🔧

     C43.62   Malignant melanoma of left upper limb, including shoulder 🔧

● **C43.7   Malignant melanoma of lower limb, including hip**

     C43.70   Malignant melanoma of unspecified lower limb, including hip 🔧

     C43.71   Malignant melanoma of right lower limb, including hip 🔧

     C43.72   Malignant melanoma of left lower limb, including hip 🔧

C43.8   Malignant melanoma of overlapping sites of skin 🔧

C43.9   Malignant melanoma of skin, unspecified 🔧
Malignant melanoma of unspecified site of skin
Melanoma (malignant) NOS

● **C4A   Merkel cell carcinoma**

C4A.0   Merkel cell carcinoma of lip 🔧

     Excludes1   malignant neoplasm of vermilion border of lip (C00.0-C00.2)

● **C4A.1   Merkel cell carcinoma of eyelid, including canthus**

     C4A.10   Merkel cell carcinoma of unspecified eyelid, including canthus 🔧

     ● **C4A.11   Merkel cell carcinoma of right eyelid, including canthus** 🔧

         C4A.111   Merkel cell carcinoma of right upper eyelid, including canthus 🔧

         C4A.112   Merkel cell carcinoma of right lower eyelid, including canthus 🔧

     ● **C4A.12   Merkel cell carcinoma of left eyelid, including canthus** 🔧

         C4A.121   Merkel cell carcinoma of left upper eyelid, including canthus 🔧

         C4A.122   Merkel cell carcinoma of left lower eyelid, including canthus 🔧

CHAPTER 2 (C00-D49)

● C4A.2 Merkel cell carcinoma of ear and external auricular canal
    C4A.20 Merkel cell carcinoma of unspecified ear and external auricular canal 🦠
    C4A.21 Merkel cell carcinoma of right ear and external auricular canal 🦠
    C4A.22 Merkel cell carcinoma of left ear and external auricular canal 🦠
● C4A.3 Merkel cell carcinoma of other and unspecified parts of face
    C4A.30 Merkel cell carcinoma of unspecified part of face 🦠
    C4A.31 Merkel cell carcinoma of nose 🦠
    C4A.39 Merkel cell carcinoma of other parts of face 🦠
● C4A.4 Merkel cell carcinoma of scalp and neck 🦠
● C4A.5 Merkel cell carcinoma of trunk
    Excludes2 malignant neoplasm of anus NOS (C21.0)
                  malignant neoplasm of scrotum (C63.2)
    C4A.51 Merkel cell carcinoma of anal skin 🦠
          Merkel cell carcinoma of anal margin
          Merkel cell carcinoma of perianal skin
    C4A.52 Merkel cell carcinoma of skin of breast 🦠
    C4A.59 Merkel cell carcinoma of other part of trunk 🦠
● C4A.6 Merkel cell carcinoma of upper limb, including shoulder
    C4A.60 Merkel cell carcinoma of unspecified upper limb, including shoulder 🦠
    C4A.61 Merkel cell carcinoma of right upper limb, including shoulder 🦠
    C4A.62 Merkel cell carcinoma of left upper limb, including shoulder 🦠
● C4A.7 Merkel cell carcinoma of lower limb, including hip
    C4A.70 Merkel cell carcinoma of unspecified lower limb, including hip 🦠
    C4A.71 Merkel cell carcinoma of right lower limb, including hip 🦠
    C4A.72 Merkel cell carcinoma of left lower limb, including hip 🦠
    C4A.8 Merkel cell carcinoma of overlapping sites 🦠
    C4A.9 Merkel cell carcinoma, unspecified 🦠
          Merkel cell carcinoma of unspecified site
          Merkel cell carcinoma NOS

● **C44** Other and unspecified malignant neoplasm of skin
    Includes malignant neoplasm of sebaceous glands
              malignant neoplasm of sweat glands
    Excludes1 Kaposi's sarcoma of skin (C46.0)
             malignant melanoma of skin (C43.-)
             malignant neoplasm of skin of genital organs (C51-C52, C60.-, C63.2)
             Merkel cell carcinoma (C4A.-)
● C44.0 Other and unspecified malignant neoplasm of skin of lip
    Excludes1 malignant neoplasm of lip (C00.-)
    C44.00 Unspecified malignant neoplasm of skin of lip
    C44.01 Basal cell carcinoma of skin of lip
    C44.02 Squamous cell carcinoma of skin of lip
    C44.09 Other specified malignant neoplasm of skin of lip

● C44.1 Other and unspecified malignant neoplasm of skin of eyelid, including canthus
    Excludes1 connective tissue of eyelid (C49.0)
● C44.10 Unspecified malignant neoplasm of skin of eyelid, including canthus
    C44.101 Unspecified malignant neoplasm of skin of unspecified eyelid, including canthus
    C44.102 Unspecified malignant neoplasm of skin of right eyelid, including canthus
          C44.1021 Unspecified malignant neoplasm of skin of right upper eyelid, including canthus
          C44.1022 Unspecified malignant neoplasm of skin of right lower eyelid, including canthus
    C44.109 Unspecified malignant neoplasm of skin of left eyelid, including canthus
          C44.1091 Unspecified malignant neoplasm of skin of left upper eyelid, including canthus
          C44.1092 Unspecified malignant neoplasm of skin of left lower eyelid, including canthus
● C44.11 Basal cell carcinoma of skin of eyelid, including canthus
    C44.111 Basal cell carcinoma of skin of unspecified eyelid, including canthus
    C44.112 Basal cell carcinoma of skin of right eyelid, including canthus
          C44.1121 Basal cell carcinoma of skin of right upper eyelid, including canthus
          C44.1122 Basal cell carcinoma of skin of right lower eyelid, including canthus
    C44.119 Basal cell carcinoma of skin of left eyelid, including canthus
          C44.1191 Basal cell carcinoma of skin of left upper eyelid, including canthus
          C44.1192 Basal cell carcinoma of skin of left lower eyelid, including canthus
● C44.12 Squamous cell carcinoma of skin of eyelid, including canthus
    C44.121 Squamous cell carcinoma of skin of unspecified eyelid, including canthus
    C44.122 Squamous cell carcinoma of skin of right eyelid, including canthus
          C44.1221 Squamous cell carcinoma of skin of right upper eyelid, including canthus
          C44.1222 Squamous cell carcinoma of skin of right lower eyelid, including canthus
    C44.129 Squamous cell carcinoma of skin of left eyelid, including canthus
          C44.1291 Squamous cell carcinoma of skin of left upper eyelid, including canthus
          C44.1292 Squamous cell carcinoma of skin of left lower eyelid, including canthus

▶ New   ⇒ Revised   ~~deleted~~ Deleted   Excludes 1   Excludes 2   Includes   Use additional   Code first   Code also   Key words
OGCR Official Guidelines   X Assign placeholder X   ● Use Additional Character(s)   ▶ Manifestation Code   🦠 Hierarchical Condition Category   **Coding Clinic**

● C44.13   Sebaceous cell carcinoma of skin of eyelid, including canthus

    C44.131   Sebaceous cell carcinoma of skin of unspecified eyelid, including canthus

    ● C44.132   Sebaceous cell carcinoma of skin of right eyelid, including canthus

        C44.1321   Sebaceous cell carcinoma of skin of right upper eyelid, including canthus

        C44.1322   Sebaceous cell carcinoma of skin of right lower eyelid, including canthus

    ● C44.139   Sebaceous cell carcinoma of skin of left eyelid, including canthus

        C44.1391   Sebaceous cell carcinoma of skin of left upper eyelid, including canthus

        C44.1392   Sebaceous cell carcinoma of skin of left lower eyelid, including canthus

● C44.19   Other specified malignant neoplasm of skin of eyelid, including canthus

    C44.191   Other specified malignant neoplasm of skin of unspecified eyelid, including canthus

    ● C44.192   Other specified malignant neoplasm of skin of right eyelid, including canthus

        C44.1921   Other specified malignant neoplasm of skin of right upper eyelid, including canthus

        C44.1922   Other specified malignant neoplasm of skin of right lower eyelid, including canthus

    ● C44.199   Other specified malignant neoplasm of skin of left eyelid, including canthus

        C44.1991   Other specified malignant neoplasm of skin of left upper eyelid, including canthus

        C44.1992   Other specified malignant neoplasm of skin of left lower eyelid, including canthus

● C44.2   Other and unspecified malignant neoplasm of skin of ear and external auricular canal

    Excludes1   connective tissue of ear (C49.0)

● C44.20   Unspecified malignant neoplasm of skin of ear and external auricular canal

    C44.201   Unspecified malignant neoplasm of skin of unspecified ear and external auricular canal

    C44.202   Unspecified malignant neoplasm of skin of right ear and external auricular canal

    C44.209   Unspecified malignant neoplasm of skin of left ear and external auricular canal

● C44.21   Basal cell carcinoma of skin of ear and external auricular canal

    C44.211   Basal cell carcinoma of skin of unspecified ear and external auricular canal

    C44.212   Basal cell carcinoma of skin of right ear and external auricular canal

    C44.219   Basal cell carcinoma of skin of left ear and external auricular canal

● C44.22   Squamous cell carcinoma of skin of ear and external auricular canal

    C44.221   Squamous cell carcinoma of skin of unspecified ear and external auricular canal

    C44.222   Squamous cell carcinoma of skin of right ear and external auricular canal

    C44.229   Squamous cell carcinoma of skin of left ear and external auricular canal

● C44.29   Other specified malignant neoplasm of skin of ear and external auricular canal

    C44.291   Other specified malignant neoplasm of skin of unspecified ear and external auricular canal

    C44.292   Other specified malignant neoplasm of skin of right ear and external auricular canal

    C44.299   Other specified malignant neoplasm of skin of left ear and external auricular canal

● C44.3   Other and unspecified malignant neoplasm of skin of other and unspecified parts of face

● C44.30   Unspecified malignant neoplasm of skin of other and unspecified parts of face

    C44.300   Unspecified malignant neoplasm of skin of unspecified part of face

    C44.301   Unspecified malignant neoplasm of skin of nose

    C44.309   Unspecified malignant neoplasm of skin of other parts of face

● C44.31   Basal cell carcinoma of skin of other and unspecified parts of face

    C44.310   Basal cell carcinoma of skin of unspecified parts of face

    C44.311   Basal cell carcinoma of skin of nose

    C44.319   Basal cell carcinoma of skin of other parts of face

        Coding Clinic: 2017, Q1, P4

● C44.32   Squamous cell carcinoma of skin of other and unspecified parts of face

    C44.320   Squamous cell carcinoma of skin of unspecified parts of face

    C44.321   Squamous cell carcinoma of skin of nose

    C44.329   Squamous cell carcinoma of skin of other parts of face

● C44.39   Other specified malignant neoplasm of skin of other and unspecified parts of face

    C44.390   Other specified malignant neoplasm of skin of unspecified parts of face

    C44.391   Other specified malignant neoplasm of skin of nose

    C44.399   Other specified malignant neoplasm of skin of other parts of face

● C44.4   Other and unspecified malignant neoplasm of skin of scalp and neck

    C44.40   Unspecified malignant neoplasm of skin of scalp and neck

    C44.41   Basal cell carcinoma of skin of scalp and neck

    C44.42   Squamous cell carcinoma of skin of scalp and neck

    C44.49   Other specified malignant neoplasm of skin of scalp and neck

● **C44.5　Other and unspecified malignant neoplasm of skin of trunk**

   Excludes1　anus NOS (C21.0)
              scrotum (C63.2)

● C44.50　**Unspecified malignant neoplasm of skin of trunk**

  C44.500　**Unspecified malignant neoplasm of anal skin**
      Unspecified malignant neoplasm of anal margin
      Unspecified malignant neoplasm of perianal skin

  C44.501　**Unspecified malignant neoplasm of skin of breast**

  C44.509　**Unspecified malignant neoplasm of skin of other part of trunk**

● C44.51　**Basal cell carcinoma of skin of trunk**

  C44.510　**Basal cell carcinoma of anal skin**
      Basal cell carcinoma of anal margin
      Basal cell carcinoma of perianal skin

  C44.511　**Basal cell carcinoma of skin of breast**

  C44.519　**Basal cell carcinoma of skin of other part of trunk**

● C44.52　**Squamous cell carcinoma of skin of trunk**

  C44.520　**Squamous cell carcinoma of anal skin**
      Squamous cell carcinoma of anal margin
      Squamous cell carcinoma of perianal skin

  C44.521　**Squamous cell carcinoma of skin of breast**

  C44.529　**Squamous cell carcinoma of skin of other part of trunk**

● C44.59　**Other specified malignant neoplasm of skin of trunk**

  C44.590　**Other specified malignant neoplasm of anal skin**
      Other specified malignant neoplasm of anal margin
      Other specified malignant neoplasm of perianal skin

  C44.591　**Other specified malignant neoplasm of skin of breast**

  C44.599　**Other specified malignant neoplasm of skin of other part of trunk**

● **C44.6　Other and unspecified malignant neoplasm of skin of upper limb, including shoulder**

● C44.60　**Unspecified malignant neoplasm of skin of upper limb, including shoulder**

  C44.601　**Unspecified malignant neoplasm of skin of unspecified upper limb, including shoulder**

  C44.602　**Unspecified malignant neoplasm of skin of right upper limb, including shoulder**

  C44.609　**Unspecified malignant neoplasm of skin of left upper limb, including shoulder**

● C44.61　**Basal cell carcinoma of skin of upper limb, including shoulder**

  C44.611　**Basal cell carcinoma of skin of unspecified upper limb, including shoulder**

  C44.612　**Basal cell carcinoma of skin of right upper limb, including shoulder**

  C44.619　**Basal cell carcinoma of skin of left upper limb, including shoulder**

● C44.62　**Squamous cell carcinoma of skin of upper limb, including shoulder**

  C44.621　**Squamous cell carcinoma of skin of unspecified upper limb, including shoulder**

  C44.622　**Squamous cell carcinoma of skin of right upper limb, including shoulder**

  C44.629　**Squamous cell carcinoma of skin of left upper limb, including shoulder**

● C44.69　**Other specified malignant neoplasm of skin of upper limb, including shoulder**

  C44.691　**Other specified malignant neoplasm of skin of unspecified upper limb, including shoulder**

  C44.692　**Other specified malignant neoplasm of skin of right upper limb, including shoulder**

  C44.699　**Other specified malignant neoplasm of skin of left upper limb, including shoulder**

● **C44.7　Other and unspecified malignant neoplasm of skin of lower limb, including hip**

● C44.70　**Unspecified malignant neoplasm of skin of lower limb, including hip**

  C44.701　**Unspecified malignant neoplasm of skin of unspecified lower limb, including hip**

  C44.702　**Unspecified malignant neoplasm of skin of right lower limb, including hip**

  C44.709　**Unspecified malignant neoplasm of skin of left lower limb, including hip**

● C44.71　**Basal cell carcinoma of skin of lower limb, including hip**

  C44.711　**Basal cell carcinoma of skin of unspecified lower limb, including hip**

  C44.712　**Basal cell carcinoma of skin of right lower limb, including hip**

  C44.719　**Basal cell carcinoma of skin of left lower limb, including hip**

● C44.72　**Squamous cell carcinoma of skin of lower limb, including hip**

  C44.721　**Squamous cell carcinoma of skin of unspecified lower limb, including hip**

  C44.722　**Squamous cell carcinoma of skin of right lower limb, including hip**

  C44.729　**Squamous cell carcinoma of skin of left lower limb, including hip**

● C44.79　**Other specified malignant neoplasm of skin of lower limb, including hip**

  C44.791　**Other specified malignant neoplasm of skin of unspecified lower limb, including hip**

  C44.792　**Other specified malignant neoplasm of skin of right lower limb, including hip**

  C44.799　**Other specified malignant neoplasm of skin of left lower limb, including hip**

● **C44.8　Other and unspecified malignant neoplasm of overlapping sites of skin**

  C44.80　**Unspecified malignant neoplasm of overlapping sites of skin**

  C44.81　**Basal cell carcinoma of overlapping sites of skin**

  C44.82　**Squamous cell carcinoma of overlapping sites of skin**

  C44.89　**Other specified malignant neoplasm of overlapping sites of skin**

● **C44.9** **Other and unspecified malignant neoplasm of skin, unspecified**

    C44.90 **Unspecified malignant neoplasm of skin, unspecified**

        Malignant neoplasm of unspecified site of skin

    C44.91 **Basal cell carcinoma of skin, unspecified**

    C44.92 **Squamous cell carcinoma of skin, unspecified**

    C44.99 **Other specified malignant neoplasm of skin, unspecified**

MALIGNANT NEOPLASMS OF MESOTHELIAL AND SOFT TISSUE (C45-C49)

● **C45** **Mesothelioma**

    Malignant cells develop in protective lining that covers internal organs (mesothelium) caused by exposure to asbestos

    C45.0 **Mesothelioma of pleura** 🔍

        Excludes1   other malignant neoplasm of pleura (C38.4)

        Coding Clinic: 2017, Q2, P11

    C45.1 **Mesothelioma of peritoneum** 🔍

        Mesothelioma of cul-de-sac

        Mesothelioma of mesentery

        Mesothelioma of mesocolon

        Mesothelioma of omentum

        Mesothelioma of peritoneum (parietal) (pelvic)

        Excludes1   other malignant neoplasm of soft tissue of peritoneum (C48.-)

    C45.2 **Mesothelioma of pericardium** 🔍

        Excludes1   other malignant neoplasm of pericardium (C38.0)

    C45.7 **Mesothelioma of other sites** 🔍

    C45.9 **Mesothelioma, unspecified** 🔍

● **C46** **Kaposi's sarcoma**

    Code first any human immunodeficiency virus [HIV] disease (B20)

    C46.0 **Kaposi's sarcoma of skin** 🔍

    C46.1 **Kaposi's sarcoma of soft tissue** 🔍

        Kaposi's sarcoma of blood vessel

        Kaposi's sarcoma of connective tissue

        Kaposi's sarcoma of fascia

        Kaposi's sarcoma of ligament

        Kaposi's sarcoma of lymphatic(s) NEC

        Kaposi's sarcoma of muscle

        Excludes2   Kaposi's sarcoma of lymph glands and nodes (C46.3)

    C46.2 **Kaposi's sarcoma of palate** 🔍

    C46.3 **Kaposi's sarcoma of lymph nodes** 🔍

    C46.4 **Kaposi's sarcoma of gastrointestinal sites** 🔍

●   **C46.5** **Kaposi's sarcoma of lung**

    C46.50 **Kaposi's sarcoma of unspecified lung** 🔍

    C46.51 **Kaposi's sarcoma of right lung** 🔍

    C46.52 **Kaposi's sarcoma of left lung** 🔍

    C46.7 **Kaposi's sarcoma of other sites** 🔍

    C46.9 **Kaposi's sarcoma, unspecified** 🔍

        Kaposi's sarcoma of unspecified site

Figure 2-11 Kaposi's sarcoma. There are large confluent hyperpigmented patch-stage lesions with lymphedema. (From Goldman L, Ausiello D, Arend W, Armitage J, Clemmons D, Drazen J, Griggs R, et al: Cecil Medicine: Expert Consult, 23e, Saunders, 2007)

● **C47** **Malignant neoplasm of peripheral nerves and autonomic nervous system**

    Includes   malignant neoplasm of sympathetic and parasympathetic nerves and ganglia

    Excludes1   Kaposi's sarcoma of soft tissue (C46.1)

    C47.0 **Malignant neoplasm of peripheral nerves of head, face and neck** 🔍

        Excludes1   malignant neoplasm of peripheral nerves of orbit (C69.6-)

●   **C47.1** **Malignant neoplasm of peripheral nerves of upper limb, including shoulder**

    C47.10 **Malignant neoplasm of peripheral nerves of unspecified upper limb, including shoulder** 🔍

    C47.11 **Malignant neoplasm of peripheral nerves of right upper limb, including shoulder** 🔍

    C47.12 **Malignant neoplasm of peripheral nerves of left upper limb, including shoulder** 🔍

●   **C47.2** **Malignant neoplasm of peripheral nerves of lower limb, including hip**

    C47.20 **Malignant neoplasm of peripheral nerves of unspecified lower limb, including hip** 🔍

    C47.21 **Malignant neoplasm of peripheral nerves of right lower limb, including hip** 🔍

    C47.22 **Malignant neoplasm of peripheral nerves of left lower limb, including hip** 🔍

    C47.3 **Malignant neoplasm of peripheral nerves of thorax** 🔍

    C47.4 **Malignant neoplasm of peripheral nerves of abdomen** 🔍

    C47.5 **Malignant neoplasm of peripheral nerves of pelvis** 🔍

    C47.6 **Malignant neoplasm of peripheral nerves of trunk, unspecified** 🔍

        Malignant neoplasm of peripheral nerves of unspecified part of trunk

    C47.8 **Malignant neoplasm of overlapping sites of peripheral nerves and autonomic nervous system** 🔍

    C47.9 **Malignant neoplasm of peripheral nerves and autonomic nervous system, unspecified** 🔍

        Malignant neoplasm of unspecified site of peripheral nerves and autonomic nervous system

● **C48** **Malignant neoplasm of retroperitoneum and peritoneum**

    Excludes1   Kaposi's sarcoma of connective tissue (C46.1) mesothelioma (C45.-)

    C48.0 **Malignant neoplasm of retroperitoneum** 🔍

        Behind/outside of peritoneum

    C48.1 **Malignant neoplasm of specified parts of peritoneum** 🔍

        Serous membrane lining abdominopelvic walls and covering viscera

        Malignant neoplasm of cul-de-sac

        Malignant neoplasm of mesentery

        Malignant neoplasm of mesocolon

        Malignant neoplasm of omentum

        Malignant neoplasm of parietal peritoneum

        Malignant neoplasm of pelvic peritoneum

    C48.2 **Malignant neoplasm of peritoneum, unspecified** 🔍

    C48.8 **Malignant neoplasm of overlapping sites of retroperitoneum and peritoneum** 🔍

CHAPTER 2 (C00-D49)

Item 2-5 Kaposi's sarcoma is a cancer that causes patches of abnormal tissue to grow under the skin; in the lining of the mouth, nose, and throat; or in other organs, often beginning and spreading to other organs. Patients who have had organ transplants or patients with AIDS are at high risk for this malignancy.

● **C49**   **Malignant neoplasm of other connective and soft tissue**

     Includes   malignant neoplasm of blood vessel
                      malignant neoplasm of bursa
                      malignant neoplasm of cartilage
                      malignant neoplasm of fascia
                      malignant neoplasm of fat
                      malignant neoplasm of ligament, except uterine
                      malignant neoplasm of lymphatic vessel
                      malignant neoplasm of muscle
                      malignant neoplasm of synovia
                      malignant neoplasm of tendon (sheath)

     Excludes1   malignant neoplasm of cartilage (of):
                      articular (C40-C41)
                      larynx (C32.3)
                      nose (C30.0)
                      malignant neoplasm of connective tissue of breast (C50.-)

     Excludes2   Kaposi's sarcoma of soft tissue (C46.1)
                      malignant neoplasm of heart (C38.0)
                      malignant neoplasm of peripheral nerves and autonomic nervous system (C47.-)
                      malignant neoplasm of peritoneum (C48.2)
                      malignant neoplasm of retroperitoneum (C48.0)
                      malignant neoplasm of uterine ligament (C57.3)
                      mesothelioma (C45.-)

C49.0   **Malignant neoplasm of connective and soft tissue of head, face and neck** 🅱
      Malignant neoplasm of connective tissue of ear
      Malignant neoplasm of connective tissue of eyelid

     Excludes1   connective tissue of orbit (C69.6-)

● **C49.1**   **Malignant neoplasm of connective and soft tissue of upper limb, including shoulder**

     C49.10   **Malignant neoplasm of connective and soft tissue of unspecified upper limb, including shoulder** 🅱

     C49.11   **Malignant neoplasm of connective and soft tissue of right upper limb, including shoulder** 🅱

     C49.12   **Malignant neoplasm of connective and soft tissue of left upper limb, including shoulder** 🅱

● **C49.2**   **Malignant neoplasm of connective and soft tissue of lower limb, including hip**

     C49.20   **Malignant neoplasm of connective and soft tissue of unspecified lower limb, including hip** 🅱

     C49.21   **Malignant neoplasm of connective and soft tissue of right lower limb, including hip** 🅱

     C49.22   **Malignant neoplasm of connective and soft tissue of left lower limb, including hip** 🅱

C49.3   **Malignant neoplasm of connective and soft tissue of thorax** 🅱
      Malignant neoplasm of axilla
      Malignant neoplasm of diaphragm
      Malignant neoplasm of great vessels

     Excludes1   malignant neoplasm of breast (C50.-)
                      malignant neoplasm of heart (C38.0)
                      malignant neoplasm of mediastinum (C38.1-C38.3)
                      malignant neoplasm of thymus (C37)

     Coding Clinic: 2015, Q3, P19

C49.4   **Malignant neoplasm of connective and soft tissue of abdomen** 🅱
      Malignant neoplasm of abdominal wall
      Malignant neoplasm of hypochondrium
     Coding Clinic: 2019, Q4, P44

C49.5   **Malignant neoplasm of connective and soft tissue of pelvis** 🅱
      Malignant neoplasm of buttock
      Malignant neoplasm of groin
      Malignant neoplasm of perineum

C49.6   **Malignant neoplasm of connective and soft tissue of trunk, unspecified** 🅱
      Malignant neoplasm of back NOS

C49.8   **Malignant neoplasm of overlapping sites of connective and soft tissue** 🅱
      Primary malignant neoplasm of two or more contiguous sites of connective and soft tissue

C49.9   **Malignant neoplasm of connective and soft tissue, unspecified** 🅱

● **C49.A**   **Gastrointestinal stromal tumor**
     Coding Clinic: 2016, Q4, P8

     C49.A0   **Gastrointestinal stromal tumor, unspecified site** 🅱

     C49.A1   **Gastrointestinal stromal tumor of esophagus** 🅱

     C49.A2   **Gastrointestinal stromal tumor of stomach** 🅱

     C49.A3   **Gastrointestinal stromal tumor of small intestine** 🅱

     C49.A4   **Gastrointestinal stromal tumor of large intestine** 🅱

     C49.A5   **Gastrointestinal stromal tumor of rectum** 🅱

     C49.A9   **Gastrointestinal stromal tumor of other sites** 🅱

MALIGNANT NEOPLASMS OF BREAST (C50)

● **C50**   **Malignant neoplasm of breast**

     Includes   connective tissue of breast
                      Paget's disease of breast
                      Paget's disease of nipple
                      Intraductal carcinoma of breast characterized by eczema-like inflammatory skin changes

     Use additional code to identify estrogen receptor status (Z17.0, Z17.1)

     Excludes1   skin of breast (C44.501, C44.511, C44.521, C44.591)

● **C50.0**   **Malignant neoplasm of nipple and areola**

     ● **C50.01**   **Malignant neoplasm of nipple and areola, female**

         C50.011   **Malignant neoplasm of nipple and areola, right female breast** ♀ 🅱

         C50.012   **Malignant neoplasm of nipple and areola, left female breast** ♀ 🅱

         C50.019   **Malignant neoplasm of nipple and areola, unspecified female breast** ♀ 🅱

     ● **C50.02**   **Malignant neoplasm of nipple and areola, male**

         C50.021   **Malignant neoplasm of nipple and areola, right male breast** ♂ 🅱

         C50.022   **Malignant neoplasm of nipple and areola, left male breast** ♂ 🅱

         C50.029   **Malignant neoplasm of nipple and areola, unspecified male breast** ♂ 🅱

● **C50.1**   **Malignant neoplasm of central portion of breast**

     ● **C50.11**   **Malignant neoplasm of central portion of breast, female**

         C50.111   **Malignant neoplasm of central portion of right female breast** ♀ 🅱

         C50.112   **Malignant neoplasm of central portion of left female breast** ♀ 🅱

         C50.119   **Malignant neoplasm of central portion of unspecified female breast** ♀ 🅱

     ● **C50.12**   **Malignant neoplasm of central portion of breast, male**

         C50.121   **Malignant neoplasm of central portion of right male breast** ♂ 🅱

         C50.122   **Malignant neoplasm of central portion of left male breast** ♂ 🅱

         C50.129   **Malignant neoplasm of central portion of unspecified male breast** ♂ 🅱

Figure 2-12 Female breast quadrants and axillary tail.

● **C50.2** Malignant neoplasm of upper-inner quadrant of breast
   ● **C50.21** Malignant neoplasm of upper-inner quadrant of breast, female
     C50.211 Malignant neoplasm of upper-inner quadrant of right female breast ♀ 🐾
     C50.212 Malignant neoplasm of upper-inner quadrant of left female breast ♀ 🐾
     C50.219 Malignant neoplasm of upper-inner quadrant of unspecified female breast ♀ 🐾
   ● **C50.22** Malignant neoplasm of upper-inner quadrant of breast, male
     C50.221 Malignant neoplasm of upper-inner quadrant of right male breast ♂ 🐾
     C50.222 Malignant neoplasm of upper-inner quadrant of left male breast ♂ 🐾
     C50.229 Malignant neoplasm of upper-inner quadrant of unspecified male breast ♂ 🐾

● **C50.3** Malignant neoplasm of lower-inner quadrant of breast
   ● **C50.31** Malignant neoplasm of lower-inner quadrant of breast, female
     C50.311 Malignant neoplasm of lower-inner quadrant of right female breast ♀ 🐾
     C50.312 Malignant neoplasm of lower-inner quadrant of left female breast ♀ 🐾
     C50.319 Malignant neoplasm of lower-inner quadrant of unspecified female breast ♀ 🐾
   ● **C50.32** Malignant neoplasm of lower-inner quadrant of breast, male
     C50.321 Malignant neoplasm of lower-inner quadrant of right male breast ♂ 🐾
     C50.322 Malignant neoplasm of lower-inner quadrant of left male breast ♂ 🐾
     C50.329 Malignant neoplasm of lower-inner quadrant of unspecified male breast ♂ 🐾

● **C50.4** Malignant neoplasm of upper-outer quadrant of breast
   ● **C50.41** Malignant neoplasm of upper-outer quadrant of breast, female
     C50.411 Malignant neoplasm of upper-outer quadrant of right female breast ♀ 🐾
     C50.412 Malignant neoplasm of upper-outer quadrant of left female breast ♀ 🐾
     C50.419 Malignant neoplasm of upper-outer quadrant of unspecified female breast ♀ 🐾
   ● **C50.42** Malignant neoplasm of upper-outer quadrant of breast, male
     C50.421 Malignant neoplasm of upper-outer quadrant of right male breast ♂ 🐾
     C50.422 Malignant neoplasm of upper-outer quadrant of left male breast ♂ 🐾
     C50.429 Malignant neoplasm of upper-outer quadrant of unspecified male breast ♂ 🐾

● **C50.5** Malignant neoplasm of lower-outer quadrant of breast
   ● **C50.51** Malignant neoplasm of lower-outer quadrant of breast, female
     C50.511 Malignant neoplasm of lower-outer quadrant of right female breast ♀ 🐾
     C50.512 Malignant neoplasm of lower-outer quadrant of left female breast ♀ 🐾
     C50.519 Malignant neoplasm of lower-outer quadrant of unspecified female breast ♀ 🐾
   ● **C50.52** Malignant neoplasm of lower-outer quadrant of breast, male
     C50.521 Malignant neoplasm of lower-outer quadrant of right male breast ♂ 🐾
     C50.522 Malignant neoplasm of lower-outer quadrant of left male breast ♂ 🐾
     C50.529 Malignant neoplasm of lower-outer quadrant of unspecified male breast ♂ 🐾

● **C50.6** Malignant neoplasm of axillary tail of breast
   ● **C50.61** Malignant neoplasm of axillary tail of breast, female
     C50.611 Malignant neoplasm of axillary tail of right female breast ♀ 🐾
     C50.612 Malignant neoplasm of axillary tail of left female breast ♀ 🐾
     C50.619 Malignant neoplasm of axillary tail of unspecified female breast ♀ 🐾
   ● **C50.62** Malignant neoplasm of axillary tail of breast, male
     C50.621 Malignant neoplasm of axillary tail of right male breast ♂ 🐾
     C50.622 Malignant neoplasm of axillary tail of left male breast ♂ 🐾
     C50.629 Malignant neoplasm of axillary tail of unspecified male breast ♂ 🐾

● **C50.8** Malignant neoplasm of overlapping sites of breast
   ● **C50.81** Malignant neoplasm of overlapping sites of breast, female
     C50.811 Malignant neoplasm of overlapping sites of right female breast ♀ 🐾
     C50.812 Malignant neoplasm of overlapping sites of left female breast ♀ 🐾
     C50.819 Malignant neoplasm of overlapping sites of unspecified female breast ♀ 🐾
   ● **C50.82** Malignant neoplasm of overlapping sites of breast, male
     C50.821 Malignant neoplasm of overlapping sites of right male breast ♂ 🐾
     C50.822 Malignant neoplasm of overlapping sites of left male breast ♂ 🐾
     C50.829 Malignant neoplasm of overlapping sites of unspecified male breast ♂ 🐾

● **C50.9** Malignant neoplasm of breast of unspecified site
   ● **C50.91** Malignant neoplasm of breast of unspecified site, female
     C50.911 Malignant neoplasm of unspecified site of right female breast ♀ 🐾
     C50.912 Malignant neoplasm of unspecified site of left female breast ♀ 🐾
     C50.919 Malignant neoplasm of unspecified site of unspecified female breast ♀ 🐾
   ● **C50.92** Malignant neoplasm of breast of unspecified site, male
     C50.921 Malignant neoplasm of unspecified site of right male breast ♂ 🐾
     C50.922 Malignant neoplasm of unspecified site of left male breast ♂ 🐾
     C50.929 Malignant neoplasm of unspecified site of unspecified male breast ♂ 🐾

MALIGNANT NEOPLASMS OF FEMALE GENITAL ORGANS (C51-C58)

Includes   malignant neoplasm of skin of female genital organs

● **C51   Malignant neoplasm of vulva**

     Excludes1   carcinoma in situ of vulva (D07.1)

     C51.0   Malignant neoplasm of labium majus ♀ 🐾
          Outer folds of skin external female genitalia
          Malignant neoplasm of Bartholin's [greater vestibular] gland

     C51.1   Malignant neoplasm of labium minus ♀ 🐾
          Two inner folds surrounding vulva in female genitalia

     C51.2   Malignant neoplasm of clitoris ♀ 🐾

     C51.8   Malignant neoplasm of overlapping sites of vulva ♀ 🐾

     C51.9   Malignant neoplasm of vulva, unspecified ♀ 🐾
          Malignant neoplasm of external female genitalia NOS
          Malignant neoplasm of pudendum

C52   Malignant neoplasm of vagina ♀ 🐾

     Excludes1   carcinoma in situ of vagina (D07.2)

● **C53   Malignant neoplasm of cervix uteri**

     Excludes1   carcinoma in situ of cervix uteri (D06.-)

     C53.0   Malignant neoplasm of endocervix ♀ 🐾
          Inside the cervix

     C53.1   Malignant neoplasm of exocervix ♀ 🐾
          Outside the cervix

     C53.8   Malignant neoplasm of overlapping sites of cervix uteri ♀ 🐾

     C53.9   Malignant neoplasm of cervix uteri, unspecified ♀ 🐾
          Coding Clinic: 2017, Q4, P103

● **C54   Malignant neoplasm of corpus uteri**

     C54.0   Malignant neoplasm of isthmus uteri ♀ 🐾
          Constricted part of uterus between cervix and body
          Malignant neoplasm of lower uterine segment

     C54.1   Malignant neoplasm of endometrium ♀ 🐾
          Lining of uterus

     C54.2   Malignant neoplasm of myometrium ♀ 🐾
          Middle layer of uterine wall consisting of smooth muscle supporting stromal and vascular tissue

     C54.3   Malignant neoplasm of fundus uteri ♀ 🐾
          Top rounded portion of uterus

     C54.8   Malignant neoplasm of overlapping sites of corpus uteri ♀ 🐾
          Main body of uterus

     C54.9   Malignant neoplasm of corpus uteri, unspecified ♀ 🐾

C55   Malignant neoplasm of uterus, part unspecified ♀ 🐾

● **C56   Malignant neoplasm of ovary**

     Use additional code to identify any functional activity

     C56.1   Malignant neoplasm of right ovary ♀ 🐾

     C56.2   Malignant neoplasm of left ovary ♀ 🐾

     C56.3   Malignant neoplasm of bilateral ovaries ♀

     C56.9   Malignant neoplasm of unspecified ovary ♀ 🐾

Figure 2-13   Cervix uteri.

● **C57   Malignant neoplasm of other and unspecified female genital organs**

     ● **C57.0   Malignant neoplasm of fallopian tube**
          Malignant neoplasm of oviduct
          Malignant neoplasm of uterine tube

         C57.00   Malignant neoplasm of unspecified fallopian tube ♀ 🐾

         C57.01   Malignant neoplasm of right fallopian tube ♀ 🐾

         C57.02   Malignant neoplasm of left fallopian tube ♀ 🐾

     ● **C57.1   Malignant neoplasm of broad ligament**

         C57.10   Malignant neoplasm of unspecified broad ligament ♀ 🐾

         C57.11   Malignant neoplasm of right broad ligament ♀ 🐾

         C57.12   Malignant neoplasm of left broad ligament ♀ 🐾

     ● **C57.2   Malignant neoplasm of round ligament**

         C57.20   Malignant neoplasm of unspecified round ligament ♀ 🐾

         C57.21   Malignant neoplasm of right round ligament ♀ 🐾

         C57.22   Malignant neoplasm of left round ligament ♀ 🐾

     C57.3   Malignant neoplasm of parametrium ♀ 🐾
          Malignant neoplasm of uterine ligament NOS

     C57.4   Malignant neoplasm of uterine adnexa, unspecified ♀ 🐾

     C57.7   Malignant neoplasm of other specified female genital organs ♀ 🐾
          Malignant neoplasm of wolffian body or duct

     C57.8   Malignant neoplasm of overlapping sites of female genital organs ♀ 🐾
          Primary malignant neoplasm of two or more contiguous sites of the female genital organs whose point of origin cannot be determined
          Primary tubo-ovarian malignant neoplasm whose point of origin cannot be determined
          Primary utero-ovarian malignant neoplasm whose point of origin cannot be determined

     C57.9   Malignant neoplasm of female genital organ, unspecified ♀ 🐾
          Malignant neoplasm of female genitourinary tract NOS

C58   Malignant neoplasm of placenta ♀ 🐾   M

     Includes   choriocarcinoma NOS
             chorionepithelioma NOS

     Excludes1   chorioadenoma (destruens) (D39.2)
             hydatidiform mole NOS (O01.9)
             invasive hydatidiform mole (D39.2)
             male choriocarcinoma NOS (C62.9-)
             malignant hydatidiform mole (D39.2)

MALIGNANT NEOPLASMS OF MALE GENITAL ORGANS (C60-C63)

Includes   malignant neoplasm of skin of male genital organs

● **C60   Malignant neoplasm of penis**

     C60.0   Malignant neoplasm of prepuce ♂ 🐾
          Malignant neoplasm of foreskin

     C60.1   Malignant neoplasm of glans penis ♂ 🐾

     C60.2   Malignant neoplasm of body of penis ♂ 🐾
          Malignant neoplasm of corpus cavernosum

     C60.8   Malignant neoplasm of overlapping sites of penis ♂ 🐾

     C60.9   Malignant neoplasm of penis, unspecified ♂ 🐾
          Malignant neoplasm of skin of penis NOS

C61   Malignant neoplasm of prostate ♂ 🐾

     ⇨ Use additional , if applicable, code to identify:
         hormone sensitivity status (Z19.1-Z19.2)
         rising PSA following treatment for malignant neoplasm of prostate (R97.21)

     Excludes1   malignant neoplasm of seminal vesicle (C63.7)

CHAPTER 2 (C00-D49)

▶ New   ⇨ Revised   ~~deleted~~ Deleted   Excludes 1   Excludes 2   Includes   Use additional   Code first   Code also   Key words
OGCR Official Guidelines   X Assign placeholder X   ● Use Additional Character(s)   ) Manifestation Code   🐾 Hierarchical Condition Category   **Coding Clinic**

Figure 2-14 Penis and other male genital organs.

C62 **Malignant neoplasm of testis**
  Use additional code to identify any functional activity.
  C62.0 **Malignant neoplasm of undescended testis**
    Malignant neoplasm of ectopic testis
    Malignant neoplasm of retained testis
    C62.00 **Malignant neoplasm of unspecified undescended testis** ♂ 🐾
    C62.01 **Malignant neoplasm of undescended right testis** ♂ 🐾
    C62.02 **Malignant neoplasm of undescended left testis** ♂ 🐾
  C62.1 **Malignant neoplasm of descended testis**
    Malignant neoplasm of scrotal testis
    C62.10 **Malignant neoplasm of unspecified descended testis, unspecified side** ♂ 🐾
    C62.11 **Malignant neoplasm of descended right testis** ♂ 🐾
    C62.12 **Malignant neoplasm of descended left testis** ♂ 🐾
  C62.9 **Malignant neoplasm of testis, unspecified whether descended or undescended**
    C62.90 **Malignant neoplasm of unspecified testis, unspecified whether descended or undescended** ♂ 🐾
      Malignant neoplasm of testis NOS
    C62.91 **Malignant neoplasm of right testis, unspecified whether descended or undescended** ♂ 🐾
    C62.92 **Malignant neoplasm of left testis, unspecified whether descended or undescended** ♂ 🐾

C63 **Malignant neoplasm of other and unspecified male genital organs**
  C63.0 **Malignant neoplasm of epididymis**
    C63.00 **Malignant neoplasm of unspecified epididymis** ♂ 🐾
    C63.01 **Malignant neoplasm of right epididymis** ♂ 🐾
    C63.02 **Malignant neoplasm of left epididymis** ♂ 🐾
  C63.1 **Malignant neoplasm of spermatic cord**
    C63.10 **Malignant neoplasm of unspecified spermatic cord** ♂ 🐾
    C63.11 **Malignant neoplasm of right spermatic cord** ♂ 🐾
    C63.12 **Malignant neoplasm of left spermatic cord** ♂ 🐾
  C63.2 **Malignant neoplasm of scrotum** ♂ 🐾
    Malignant neoplasm of skin of scrotum
  C63.7 **Malignant neoplasm of other specified male genital organs** ♂ 🐾
    Malignant neoplasm of seminal vesicle
    Malignant neoplasm of tunica vaginalis
  C63.8 **Malignant neoplasm of overlapping sites of male genital organs** ♂ 🐾
    Primary malignant neoplasm of two or more contiguous sites of male genital organs whose point of origin cannot be determined
  C63.9 **Malignant neoplasm of male genital organ, unspecified** ♂ 🐾
    Malignant neoplasm of male genitourinary tract NOS

MALIGNANT NEOPLASMS OF URINARY TRACT (C64-C68)

C64 **Malignant neoplasm of kidney, except renal pelvis**
  Excludes1 malignant carcinoid tumor of the kidney (C7A.093)
    malignant neoplasm of renal calyces (C65.-)
    malignant neoplasm of renal pelvis (C65.-)
  C64.1 **Malignant neoplasm of right kidney, except renal pelvis** 🐾
  C64.2 **Malignant neoplasm of left kidney, except renal pelvis** 🐾
  C64.9 **Malignant neoplasm of unspecified kidney, except renal pelvis** 🐾

C65 **Malignant neoplasm of renal pelvis**
  Includes malignant neoplasm of pelviureteric junction
    malignant neoplasm of renal calyces
  C65.1 **Malignant neoplasm of right renal pelvis** 🐾
  C65.2 **Malignant neoplasm of left renal pelvis** 🐾
  C65.9 **Malignant neoplasm of unspecified renal pelvis** 🐾

C66 **Malignant neoplasm of ureter**
  Excludes1 malignant neoplasm of ureteric orifice of bladder (C67.6)
  C66.1 **Malignant neoplasm of right ureter** 🐾
  C66.2 **Malignant neoplasm of left ureter** 🐾
  C66.9 **Malignant neoplasm of unspecified ureter** 🐾

C67 **Malignant neoplasm of bladder**
  C67.0 **Malignant neoplasm of trigone of bladder** 🐾
    Triangular area formed by three openings in the floor of urinary bladder
  C67.1 **Malignant neoplasm of dome of bladder** 🐾
    Vaulted roof
  C67.2 **Malignant neoplasm of lateral wall of bladder** 🐾
    Side walls
  C67.3 **Malignant neoplasm of anterior wall of bladder** 🐾
    Front wall
  C67.4 **Malignant neoplasm of posterior wall of bladder** 🐾
    Back wall
  C67.5 **Malignant neoplasm of bladder neck** 🐾
    Joining of bladder and urethra
    Malignant neoplasm of internal urethral orifice
  C67.6 **Malignant neoplasm of ureteric orifice** 🐾
    Opening from bladder to ureters
  C67.7 **Malignant neoplasm of urachus** 🐾
    Embryonic canal that connects the urinary bladder with the structure that forms the umbilical cord (allantois)
  C67.8 **Malignant neoplasm of overlapping sites of bladder** 🐾
  C67.9 **Malignant neoplasm of bladder, unspecified** 🐾
    Coding Clinic: 2017, Q1, P6; 2016, Q1, P19

C68 **Malignant neoplasm of other and unspecified urinary organs**
  Excludes1 malignant neoplasm of female genitourinary tract NOS (C57.9)
    malignant neoplasm of male genitourinary tract NOS (C63.9)
  C68.0 **Malignant neoplasm of urethra** 🐾
    Excludes1 malignant neoplasm of urethral orifice of bladder (C67.5)
  C68.1 **Malignant neoplasm of paraurethral glands** 🐾
    Group of glands of female urethra drained by paraurethral ducts; AKA Skene glands, female prostate
  C68.8 **Malignant neoplasm of overlapping sites of urinary organs** 🐾
    Primary malignant neoplasm of two or more contiguous sites of urinary organs whose point of origin cannot be determined
  C68.9 **Malignant neoplasm of urinary organ, unspecified** 🐾
    Malignant neoplasm of urinary system NOS

CHAPTER 2 (C00-D49)

MALIGNANT NEOPLASMS OF EYE, BRAIN AND OTHER PARTS OF CENTRAL NERVOUS SYSTEM (C69-C72)

● C69   Malignant neoplasm of eye and adnexa
  Excludes1   malignant neoplasm of connective tissue of eyelid (C49.0)
  malignant neoplasm of eyelid (skin) (C43.1-, C44.1-)
  malignant neoplasm of optic nerve (C72.3-)

● C69.0   Malignant neoplasm of conjunctiva
  C69.00   Malignant neoplasm of unspecified conjunctiva
  C69.01   Malignant neoplasm of right conjunctiva
  C69.02   Malignant neoplasm of left conjunctiva

● C69.1   Malignant neoplasm of cornea
  C69.10   Malignant neoplasm of unspecified cornea
  C69.11   Malignant neoplasm of right cornea
  C69.12   Malignant neoplasm of left cornea

● C69.2   Malignant neoplasm of retina
  Excludes1   dark area on retina (D49.81)
  neoplasm of unspecified behavior of retina and choroid (D49.81)
  retinal freckle (D49.81)
  C69.20   Malignant neoplasm of unspecified retina
  C69.21   Malignant neoplasm of right retina
  C69.22   Malignant neoplasm of left retina

● C69.3   Malignant neoplasm of choroid
  C69.30   Malignant neoplasm of unspecified choroid
  C69.31   Malignant neoplasm of right choroid
  C69.32   Malignant neoplasm of left choroid

● C69.4   Malignant neoplasm of ciliary body
  C69.40   Malignant neoplasm of unspecified ciliary body
  C69.41   Malignant neoplasm of right ciliary body
  C69.42   Malignant neoplasm of left ciliary body

● C69.5   Malignant neoplasm of lacrimal gland and duct
  Malignant neoplasm of lacrimal sac
  Malignant neoplasm of nasolacrimal duct
  C69.50   Malignant neoplasm of unspecified lacrimal gland and duct
  C69.51   Malignant neoplasm of right lacrimal gland and duct
  C69.52   Malignant neoplasm of left lacrimal gland and duct

● C69.6   Malignant neoplasm of orbit
  Malignant neoplasm of connective tissue of orbit
  Malignant neoplasm of extraocular muscle
  Malignant neoplasm of peripheral nerves of orbit
  Malignant neoplasm of retrobulbar tissue
  Malignant neoplasm of retro-ocular tissue
  Excludes1   malignant neoplasm of orbital bone (C41.0)
  C69.60   Malignant neoplasm of unspecified orbit
  C69.61   Malignant neoplasm of right orbit
  C69.62   Malignant neoplasm of left orbit

● C69.8   Malignant neoplasm of overlapping sites of eye and adnexa
  C69.80   Malignant neoplasm of overlapping sites of unspecified eye and adnexa
  C69.81   Malignant neoplasm of overlapping sites of right eye and adnexa
  C69.82   Malignant neoplasm of overlapping sites of left eye and adnexa

● C69.9   Malignant neoplasm of unspecified site of eye
  Malignant neoplasm of eyeball
  C69.90   Malignant neoplasm of unspecified site of unspecified eye
  C69.91   Malignant neoplasm of unspecified site of right eye
  C69.92   Malignant neoplasm of unspecified site of left eye

Figure 2-15   The brain.

● C70   Malignant neoplasm of meninges
  C70.0   Malignant neoplasm of cerebral meninges
  C70.1   Malignant neoplasm of spinal meninges
  C70.9   Malignant neoplasm of meninges, unspecified

● C71   Malignant neoplasm of brain
  Excludes1   malignant neoplasm of cranial nerves (C72.2-C72.5)
  retrobulbar malignant neoplasm (C69.6-)
  C71.0   Malignant neoplasm of cerebrum, except lobes and ventricles
  Malignant neoplasm of supratentorial NOS
  C71.1   Malignant neoplasm of frontal lobe
  C71.2   Malignant neoplasm of temporal lobe
  C71.3   Malignant neoplasm of parietal lobe
  C71.4   Malignant neoplasm of occipital lobe
  C71.5   Malignant neoplasm of cerebral ventricle
  Excludes1   malignant neoplasm of fourth cerebral ventricle (C71.7)
  C71.6   Malignant neoplasm of cerebellum
  C71.7   Malignant neoplasm of brain stem
  Malignant neoplasm of fourth cerebral ventricle
  Infratentorial malignant neoplasm NOS
  C71.8   Malignant neoplasm of overlapping sites of brain
  C71.9   Malignant neoplasm of brain, unspecified

● C72   Malignant neoplasm of spinal cord, cranial nerves and other parts of central nervous system
  Excludes1   malignant neoplasm of meninges (C70.-)
  malignant neoplasm of peripheral nerves and autonomic nervous system (C47.-)
  C72.0   Malignant neoplasm of spinal cord
  C72.1   Malignant neoplasm of cauda equina
  Lower end of spinal column
● C72.2   Malignant neoplasm of olfactory nerve
  Malignant neoplasm of olfactory bulb
  C72.20   Malignant neoplasm of unspecified olfactory nerve
  C72.21   Malignant neoplasm of right olfactory nerve
  C72.22   Malignant neoplasm of left olfactory nerve
● C72.3   Malignant neoplasm of optic nerve
  C72.30   Malignant neoplasm of unspecified optic nerve
  C72.31   Malignant neoplasm of right optic nerve
  C72.32   Malignant neoplasm of left optic nerve
● C72.4   Malignant neoplasm of acoustic nerve
  C72.40   Malignant neoplasm of unspecified acoustic nerve
  C72.41   Malignant neoplasm of right acoustic nerve
  C72.42   Malignant neoplasm of left acoustic nerve

● **C72.5** Malignant neoplasm of other and unspecified cranial nerves

    C72.50 Malignant neoplasm of unspecified cranial nerve
       Malignant neoplasm of cranial nerve NOS

    C72.59 Malignant neoplasm of other cranial nerves

C72.9 Malignant neoplasm of central nervous system, unspecified
    Malignant neoplasm of unspecified site of central nervous system
    Malignant neoplasm of nervous system NOS

MALIGNANT NEOPLASMS OF THYROID AND OTHER ENDOCRINE GLANDS (C73-C75)

C73 Malignant neoplasm of thyroid gland
    Use additional code to identify any functional activity

● **C74** Malignant neoplasm of adrenal gland

● **C74.0** Malignant neoplasm of cortex of adrenal gland

    C74.00 Malignant neoplasm of cortex of unspecified adrenal gland

    C74.01 Malignant neoplasm of cortex of right adrenal gland

    C74.02 Malignant neoplasm of cortex of left adrenal gland

● **C74.1** Malignant neoplasm of medulla of adrenal gland
    Pair of glands situated on top of or above each kidney ("suprarenal")

    C74.10 Malignant neoplasm of medulla of unspecified adrenal gland

    C74.11 Malignant neoplasm of medulla of right adrenal gland

    C74.12 Malignant neoplasm of medulla of left adrenal gland

● **C74.9** Malignant neoplasm of unspecified part of adrenal gland

    C74.90 Malignant neoplasm of unspecified part of unspecified adrenal gland

    C74.91 Malignant neoplasm of unspecified part of right adrenal gland

    C74.92 Malignant neoplasm of unspecified part of left adrenal gland

● **C75** Malignant neoplasm of other endocrine glands and related structures

    Excludes1   malignant carcinoid tumors (C7A.0-)
       malignant neoplasm of adrenal gland (C74.-)
       malignant neoplasm of endocrine pancreas (C25.4)
       malignant neoplasm of islets of Langerhans (C25.4)
       malignant neoplasm of ovary (C56.-)
       malignant neoplasm of testis (C62.-)
       malignant neoplasm of thymus (C37)
       malignant neoplasm of thyroid gland (C73)
       malignant neuroendocrine tumors (C7A.-)

C75.0 Malignant neoplasm of parathyroid gland

C75.1 Malignant neoplasm of pituitary gland

C75.2 Malignant neoplasm of craniopharyngeal duct

C75.3 Malignant neoplasm of pineal gland

C75.4 Malignant neoplasm of carotid body

C75.5 Malignant neoplasm of aortic body and other paraganglia

C75.8 Malignant neoplasm with pluriglandular involvement, unspecified

C75.9 Malignant neoplasm of endocrine gland, unspecified

MALIGNANT NEOPLASMS OF ILL-DEFINED, OTHER SECONDARY AND UNSPECIFIED SITES (C76-C80)

● **C76** Malignant neoplasm of other and ill-defined sites

    Excludes1   malignant neoplasm of female genitourinary tract NOS (C57.9)
       malignant neoplasm of male genitourinary tract NOS (C63.9)
       malignant neoplasm of lymphoid, hematopoietic and related tissue (C81-C96)
       malignant neoplasm of skin (C44.-)
       malignant neoplasm of unspecified site NOS (C80.1)

C76.0 Malignant neoplasm of head, face and neck
    Malignant neoplasm of cheek NOS
    Malignant neoplasm of nose NOS

C76.1 Malignant neoplasm of thorax
    Intrathoracic malignant neoplasm NOS
    Malignant neoplasm of axilla NOS
    Thoracic malignant neoplasm NOS

C76.2 Malignant neoplasm of abdomen

C76.3 Malignant neoplasm of pelvis
    Malignant neoplasm of groin NOS
    Malignant neoplasm of sites overlapping systems within the pelvis
    Rectovaginal (septum) malignant neoplasm
       Between rectum and vagina
    Rectovesical (septum) malignant neoplasm
       Between rectum and urinary bladder; AKA vesicorectal

● **C76.4** Malignant neoplasm of upper limb

    C76.40 Malignant neoplasm of unspecified upper limb

    C76.41 Malignant neoplasm of right upper limb

    C76.42 Malignant neoplasm of left upper limb

● **C76.5** Malignant neoplasm of lower limb

    C76.50 Malignant neoplasm of unspecified lower limb

    C76.51 Malignant neoplasm of right lower limb

    C76.52 Malignant neoplasm of left lower limb

C76.8 Malignant neoplasm of other specified ill-defined sites
    Malignant neoplasm of overlapping ill-defined sites

● **C77** Secondary and unspecified malignant neoplasm of lymph nodes

    Excludes1   malignant neoplasm of lymph nodes, specified as primary (C81-C86, C88, C96.-)
       mesentery metastasis of carcinoid tumor (C7B.04)
       secondary carcinoid tumors of distant lymph nodes (C7B.01)

C77.0 Secondary and unspecified malignant neoplasm of lymph nodes of head, face and neck
    Secondary and unspecified malignant neoplasm of supraclavicular lymph nodes

C77.1 Secondary and unspecified malignant neoplasm of intrathoracic lymph nodes

C77.2 Secondary and unspecified malignant neoplasm of intra-abdominal lymph nodes

C77.3 Secondary and unspecified malignant neoplasm of axilla and upper limb lymph nodes
    Secondary and unspecified malignant neoplasm of pectoral lymph nodes

C77.4 Secondary and unspecified malignant neoplasm of inguinal and lower limb lymph nodes

C77.5 Secondary and unspecified malignant neoplasm of intrapelvic lymph nodes

C77.8 Secondary and unspecified malignant neoplasm of lymph nodes of multiple regions

C77.9 Secondary and unspecified malignant neoplasm of lymph node, unspecified

Item 2–6 The adrenal glands are a pair of glands situated on top of or above each kidney ("suprarenal") and chiefly responsible for regulating the stress response through the synthesis of corticosteroids and catecholamines, including cortisol and adrenaline.

● C78　**Secondary malignant neoplasm of respiratory and digestive organs**

　　　Excludes1　secondary carcinoid tumors of liver (C7B.02)
　　　　　　　　secondary carcinoid tumors of peritoneum (C7B.04)

　　　Excludes2　lymph node metastases (C77.0)

● C78.0　**Secondary malignant neoplasm of lung**

　　　C78.00　Secondary malignant neoplasm of unspecified lung

　　　C78.01　Secondary malignant neoplasm of right lung 🐾

　　　C78.02　Secondary malignant neoplasm of left lung 🐾

　　C78.1　**Secondary malignant neoplasm of mediastinum** 🐾
　　　　Thoracic cavity between pleural cavities

　　C78.2　**Secondary malignant neoplasm of pleura** 🐾
　　　　Serous membrane covering lungs and lining thoracic cavity

● C78.3　**Secondary malignant neoplasm of other and unspecified respiratory organs**

　　　C78.30　Secondary malignant neoplasm of unspecified respiratory organ 🐾

　　　C78.39　Secondary malignant neoplasm of other respiratory organs 🐾

　　C78.4　**Secondary malignant neoplasm of small intestine** 🐾

　　C78.5　**Secondary malignant neoplasm of large intestine and rectum** 🐾

　　C78.6　**Secondary malignant neoplasm of retroperitoneum and peritoneum** 🐾
　　　　Coding Clinic: 2017, Q2, P12

　　C78.7　**Secondary malignant neoplasm of liver and intrahepatic bile duct** 🐾

● C78.8　**Secondary malignant neoplasm of other and unspecified digestive organs**

　　　C78.80　Secondary malignant neoplasm of unspecified digestive organ 🐾

　　　C78.89　Secondary malignant neoplasm of other digestive organs 🐾
　　　　　Code also exocrine pancreatic insufficiency (K86.81)

● C79　**Secondary malignant neoplasm of other and unspecified sites**

　　　Excludes1　secondary carcinoid tumors (C7B.-)
　　　　　　　　secondary neuroendocrine tumors (C7B.-)

● C79.0　**Secondary malignant neoplasm of kidney and renal pelvis**

　　　C79.00　Secondary malignant neoplasm of unspecified kidney and renal pelvis 🐾

　　　C79.01　Secondary malignant neoplasm of right kidney and renal pelvis 🐾

　　　C79.02　Secondary malignant neoplasm of left kidney and renal pelvis 🐾

● C79.1　**Secondary malignant neoplasm of bladder and other and unspecified urinary organs**

　　　C79.10　Secondary malignant neoplasm of unspecified urinary organs 🐾

　　　C79.11　Secondary malignant neoplasm of bladder 🐾
　　　　　Excludes2　lymph node metastases (C77.0)

　　　C79.19　Secondary malignant neoplasm of other urinary organs 🐾

　　C79.2　**Secondary malignant neoplasm of skin** 🐾
　　　　Excludes1　secondary Merkel cell carcinoma (C7B.1)

● C79.3　**Secondary malignant neoplasm of brain and cerebral meninges**

　　　C79.31　Secondary malignant neoplasm of brain 🐾

　　　C79.32　Secondary malignant neoplasm of cerebral meninges 🐾
　　　　　Coding Clinic: 2020, Q1, P13

● C79.4　**Secondary malignant neoplasm of other and unspecified parts of nervous system**

　　　C79.40　Secondary malignant neoplasm of unspecified part of nervous system 🐾

　　　C79.49　Secondary malignant neoplasm of other parts of nervous system 🐾

● C79.5　**Secondary malignant neoplasm of bone and bone marrow**

　　　Excludes1　secondary carcinoid tumors of bone (C7B.03)

　　　C79.51　Secondary malignant neoplasm of bone 🐾

　　　C79.52　Secondary malignant neoplasm of bone marrow 🐾

● C79.6　**Secondary malignant neoplasm of ovary**

　　　C79.60　Secondary malignant neoplasm of unspecified ovary ♀ 🐾

　　　C79.61　Secondary malignant neoplasm of right ovary ♀ 🐾

　　　C79.62　Secondary malignant neoplasm of left ovary ♀ 🐾

　　　C79.63　Secondary malignant neoplasm of bilateral ovaries ♀

● C79.7　**Secondary malignant neoplasm of adrenal gland**

　　　C79.70　Secondary malignant neoplasm of unspecified adrenal gland 🐾

　　　C79.71　Secondary malignant neoplasm of right adrenal gland 🐾

　　　C79.72　Secondary malignant neoplasm of left adrenal gland 🐾

● C79.8　**Secondary malignant neoplasm of other specified sites**

　　　C79.81　Secondary malignant neoplasm of breast 🐾

　　　C79.82　Secondary malignant neoplasm of genital organs 🐾

　　　C79.89　Secondary malignant neoplasm of other specified sites 🐾
　　　　　Coding Clinic: 2017, Q2, P11

　　C79.9　**Secondary malignant neoplasm of unspecified site** 🐾
　　　　Metastatic cancer NOS
　　　　Metastatic disease NOS

　　　　Excludes1　carcinomatosis NOS (C80.0)
　　　　　　　　generalized cancer NOS (C80.0)
　　　　　　　　malignant (primary) neoplasm of unspecified site (C80.1)

MALIGNANT NEUROENDOCRINE TUMORS (C7A)

● C7A　**Malignant neuroendocrine tumors**

　　Code also any associated multiple endocrine neoplasia [MEN] syndromes (E31.2-)

　　Use additional code to identify any associated endocrine syndrome, such as:
　　carcinoid syndrome (E34.0)

　　　Excludes2　malignant pancreatic islet cell tumors (C25.4)
　　　　　　　　Merkel cell carcinoma (C4A.-)

● C7A.0　**Malignant carcinoid tumors**

　　　C7A.00　Malignant carcinoid tumor of unspecified site 🐾

● 　C7A.01　**Malignant carcinoid tumors of the small intestine**

　　　　　C7A.010　Malignant carcinoid tumor of the duodenum 🐾

　　　　　C7A.011　Malignant carcinoid tumor of the jejunum 🐾

　　　　　C7A.012　Malignant carcinoid tumor of the ileum 🐾

　　　　　C7A.019　Malignant carcinoid tumor of the small intestine, unspecified portion 🐾

- **C7A.02　Malignant carcinoid tumors of the appendix, large intestine, and rectum**
  - C7A.020　Malignant carcinoid tumor of the appendix 🔗
  - C7A.021　Malignant carcinoid tumor of the cecum 🔗
  - C7A.022　Malignant carcinoid tumor of the ascending colon 🔗
  - C7A.023　Malignant carcinoid tumor of the transverse colon 🔗
  - C7A.024　Malignant carcinoid tumor of the descending colon 🔗
  - C7A.025　Malignant carcinoid tumor of the sigmoid colon 🔗
  - C7A.026　Malignant carcinoid tumor of the rectum 🔗
  - C7A.029　Malignant carcinoid tumor of the large intestine, unspecified portion 🔗
    Malignant carcinoid tumor of the colon NOS
- **C7A.09　Malignant carcinoid tumors of other sites**
  - C7A.090　Malignant carcinoid tumor of the bronchus and lung 🔗
  - C7A.091　Malignant carcinoid tumor of the thymus 🔗
  - C7A.092　Malignant carcinoid tumor of the stomach 🔗
  - C7A.093　Malignant carcinoid tumor of the kidney 🔗
  - C7A.094　Malignant carcinoid tumor of the foregut, unspecified 🔗
  - C7A.095　Malignant carcinoid tumor of the midgut, unspecified 🔗
  - C7A.096　Malignant carcinoid tumor of the hindgut, unspecified 🔗
  - C7A.098　Malignant carcinoid tumors of other sites 🔗

C7A.1　**Malignant poorly differentiated neuroendocrine tumors** 🔗
　Malignant poorly differentiated neuroendocrine tumor NOS
　Malignant poorly differentiated neuroendocrine carcinoma, any site
　High grade neuroendocrine carcinoma, any site

C7A.8　**Other malignant neuroendocrine tumors** 🔗
　Secondary neuroendocrine tumors (C7B)
　Coding Clinic: 2019, Q3, P7

SECONDARY NEUROENDOCRINE TUMORS (C7B)

- **C7B　Secondary neuroendocrine tumors**
  Use additional code to identify any functional activity
  - **C7B.0　Secondary carcinoid tumors**
    - C7B.00　Secondary carcinoid tumors, unspecified site 🔗
    - C7B.01　Secondary carcinoid tumors of distant lymph nodes 🔗
    - C7B.02　Secondary carcinoid tumors of liver 🔗
    - C7B.03　Secondary carcinoid tumors of bone 🔗
    - C7B.04　Secondary carcinoid tumors of peritoneum 🔗
      Mesentary metastasis of carcinoid tumor
    - C7B.09　Secondary carcinoid tumors of other sites 🔗

C7B.1　**Secondary Merkel cell carcinoma** 🔗
　Merkel cell carcinoma nodal presentation
　Merkel cell carcinoma visceral metastatic presentation

C7B.8　**Other secondary neuroendocrine tumors** 🔗
　Coding Clinic: 2019, Q3, P7

OGCR Section I.C.2.j and k

Disseminated malignant neoplasm, unspecified

j. Code C80.0, Disseminated malignant neoplasm, unspecified, is for use only in those cases where the patient has advanced metastatic disease and no known primary or secondary sites are specified. It should not be used in place of assigning codes for the primary site and all known secondary sites.

Malignant neoplasm without specification of site

k. Code C80.1, Malignant (primary) neoplasm, unspecified, equates to Cancer, unspecified. This code should only be used when no determination can be made as to the primary site of a malignancy. This code should rarely be used in the inpatient setting.

- **C80　Malignant neoplasm without specification of site**
  - **Excludes1**　malignant carcinoid tumor of unspecified site (C7A.00)
    malignant neoplasm of specified multiple sites-code to each site
  - C80.0　**Disseminated malignant neoplasm, unspecified** 🔗
    Carcinomatosis NOS
    Generalized cancer, unspecified site (primary) (secondary)
    Generalized malignancy, unspecified site (primary) (secondary)
  - C80.1　**Malignant (primary) neoplasm, unspecified** 🔗
    Cancer NOS
    Cancer unspecified site (primary)
    Carcinoma unspecified site (primary)
    Malignancy unspecified site (primary)
    - **Excludes1**　secondary malignant neoplasm of unspecified site (C79.9)
  - C80.2　**Malignant neoplasm associated with transplanted organ** 🔗
    Code first complication of transplanted organ (T86.-)
    Use additional code to identify the specific malignancy

★ **(See Plate 1 of the Anatomy Illustrations.)**

MALIGNANT NEOPLASMS OF LYMPHOID, HEMATOPOIETIC AND RELATED TISSUE (C81-C96)

- **Excludes2**　Kaposi's sarcoma of lymph nodes (C46.3)
  secondary and unspecified neoplasm of lymph nodes (C77.-)
  secondary neoplasm of bone marrow (C79.52)
  secondary neoplasm of spleen (C78.89)
- **C81　Hodgkin lymphoma**
  Form of malignant lymphoma with four types, nodular sclerosis, mixed cellularity, lymphocyte depleted, and lymphocyte predominant
  - **Excludes1**　personal history of Hodgkin lymphoma (Z85.71)
- **C81.0　Nodular lymphocyte predominant Hodgkin lymphoma**
  Least aggressive, least common, typically no symptoms
  Lymphocytic-histiocytic predominance Hodgkin's disease
  - C81.00　Nodular lymphocyte predominant Hodgkin lymphoma, unspecified site 🔗
  - C81.01　Nodular lymphocyte predominant Hodgkin lymphoma, lymph nodes of head, face, and neck 🔗
  - C81.02　Nodular lymphocyte predominant Hodgkin lymphoma, intrathoracic lymph nodes 🔗
  - C81.03　Nodular lymphocyte predominant Hodgkin lymphoma, intra-abdominal lymph nodes 🔗
  - C81.04　Nodular lymphocyte predominant Hodgkin lymphoma, lymph nodes of axilla and upper limb 🔗
  - C81.05　Nodular lymphocyte predominant Hodgkin lymphoma, lymph nodes of inguinal region and lower limb 🔗
  - C81.06　Nodular lymphocyte predominant Hodgkin lymphoma, intrapelvic lymph nodes 🔗
  - C81.07　Nodular lymphocyte predominant Hodgkin lymphoma, spleen 🔗

C81.08 Nodular lymphocyte predominant Hodgkin lymphoma, lymph nodes of multiple sites 🐾

C81.09 Nodular lymphocyte predominant Hodgkin lymphoma, extranodal and solid organ sites 🐾

● C81.1 Nodular sclerosis Hodgkin lymphoma
Nodular sclerosis classical Hodgkin lymphoma
Moderately aggressive; most common in young adults

C81.10 Nodular sclerosis Hodgkin lymphoma, unspecified site 🐾

C81.11 Nodular sclerosis Hodgkin lymphoma, lymph nodes of head, face, and neck 🐾

C81.12 Nodular sclerosis Hodgkin lymphoma, intrathoracic lymph nodes 🐾

C81.13 Nodular sclerosis Hodgkin lymphoma, intra-abdominal lymph nodes 🐾

C81.14 Nodular sclerosis Hodgkin lymphoma, lymph nodes of axilla and upper limb 🐾

C81.15 Nodular sclerosis Hodgkin lymphoma, lymph nodes of inguinal region and lower limb 🐾

C81.16 Nodular sclerosis Hodgkin lymphoma, intrapelvic lymph nodes 🐾

C81.17 Nodular sclerosis Hodgkin lymphoma, spleen 🐾

C81.18 Nodular sclerosis Hodgkin lymphoma, lymph nodes of multiple sites 🐾

C81.19 Nodular sclerosis Hodgkin lymphoma, extranodal and solid organ sites 🐾

● C81.2 Mixed cellularity Hodgkin lymphoma
Mixed cellularity classical Hodgkin lymphoma
A type of Hodgkin's that is moderately aggressive with mixed cell types

C81.20 Mixed cellularity Hodgkin lymphoma, unspecified site 🐾

C81.21 Mixed cellularity Hodgkin lymphoma, lymph nodes of head, face, and neck 🐾

C81.22 Mixed cellularity Hodgkin lymphoma, intrathoracic lymph nodes 🐾

C81.23 Mixed cellularity Hodgkin lymphoma, intra-abdominal lymph nodes 🐾

C81.24 Mixed cellularity Hodgkin lymphoma, lymph nodes of axilla and upper limb 🐾

C81.25 Mixed cellularity Hodgkin lymphoma, lymph nodes of inguinal region and lower limb 🐾

C81.26 Mixed cellularity Hodgkin lymphoma, intrapelvic lymph nodes 🐾

C81.27 Mixed cellularity Hodgkin lymphoma, spleen 🐾

C81.28 Mixed cellularity Hodgkin lymphoma, lymph nodes of multiple sites 🐾

C81.29 Mixed cellularity Hodgkin lymphoma, extranodal and solid organ sites 🐾

● C81.3 Lymphocyte depleted Hodgkin lymphoma
Lymphocyte depleted classical Hodgkin lymphoma
Most aggressive type with poor prognosis

C81.30 Lymphocyte depleted Hodgkin lymphoma, unspecified site 🐾

C81.31 Lymphocyte depleted Hodgkin lymphoma, lymph nodes of head, face, and neck 🐾

C81.32 Lymphocyte depleted Hodgkin lymphoma, intrathoracic lymph nodes 🐾

C81.33 Lymphocyte depleted Hodgkin lymphoma, intra-abdominal lymph nodes 🐾

C81.34 Lymphocyte depleted Hodgkin lymphoma, lymph nodes of axilla and upper limb 🐾

C81.35 Lymphocyte depleted Hodgkin lymphoma, lymph nodes of inguinal region and lower limb 🐾

C81.36 Lymphocyte depleted Hodgkin lymphoma, intrapelvic lymph nodes 🐾

C81.37 Lymphocyte depleted Hodgkin lymphoma, spleen 🐾

C81.38 Lymphocyte depleted Hodgkin lymphoma, lymph nodes of multiple sites 🐾

C81.39 Lymphocyte depleted Hodgkin lymphoma, extranodal and solid organ sites 🐾

● C81.4 Lymphocyte-rich Hodgkin lymphoma
Lymphocyte-rich classical Hodgkin lymphoma

Excludes1 nodular lymphocyte predominant Hodgkin lymphoma (C81.0-)

C81.40 Lymphocyte-rich Hodgkin lymphoma, unspecified site 🐾

C81.41 Lymphocyte-rich Hodgkin lymphoma, lymph nodes of head, face, and neck 🐾

C81.42 Lymphocyte-rich Hodgkin lymphoma, intrathoracic lymph nodes 🐾

C81.43 Lymphocyte-rich Hodgkin lymphoma, intra-abdominal lymph nodes 🐾

C81.44 Lymphocyte-rich Hodgkin lymphoma, lymph nodes of axilla and upper limb 🐾

C81.45 Lymphocyte-rich Hodgkin lymphoma, lymph nodes of inguinal region and lower limb 🐾

C81.46 Lymphocyte-rich Hodgkin lymphoma, intrapelvic lymph nodes 🐾

C81.47 Lymphocyte-rich Hodgkin lymphoma, spleen 🐾

C81.48 Lymphocyte-rich Hodgkin lymphoma, lymph nodes of multiple sites 🐾

C81.49 Lymphocyte-rich Hodgkin lymphoma, extranodal and solid organ sites 🐾

● C81.7 Other Hodgkin lymphoma
Classical Hodgkin lymphoma NOS
Other classical Hodgkin lymphoma

C81.70 Other Hodgkin lymphoma, unspecified site 🐾

C81.71 Other Hodgkin lymphoma, lymph nodes of head, face, and neck 🐾

C81.72 Other Hodgkin lymphoma, intrathoracic lymph nodes 🐾

C81.73 Other Hodgkin lymphoma, intra-abdominal lymph nodes 🐾

C81.74 Other Hodgkin lymphoma, lymph nodes of axilla and upper limb 🐾

C81.75 Other Hodgkin lymphoma, lymph nodes of inguinal region and lower limb 🐾

C81.76 Other Hodgkin lymphoma, intrapelvic lymph nodes 🐾

C81.77 Other Hodgkin lymphoma, spleen 🐾

C81.78 Other Hodgkin lymphoma, lymph nodes of multiple sites 🐾

C81.79 Other Hodgkin lymphoma, extranodal and solid organ sites 🐾

● C81.9 Hodgkin lymphoma, unspecified

C81.90 Hodgkin lymphoma, unspecified, unspecified site 🐾

C81.91 Hodgkin lymphoma, unspecified, lymph nodes of head, face, and neck 🐾

C81.92 Hodgkin lymphoma, unspecified, intrathoracic lymph nodes 🐾

C81.93 Hodgkin lymphoma, unspecified, intra-abdominal lymph nodes 🐾

C81.94 Hodgkin lymphoma, unspecified, lymph nodes of axilla and upper limb 🐾

C81.95 Hodgkin lymphoma, unspecified, lymph nodes of inguinal region and lower limb 🐾

C81.96 Hodgkin lymphoma, unspecified, intrapelvic lymph nodes 🐾

C81.97 Hodgkin lymphoma, unspecified, spleen 🐾

C81.98 Hodgkin lymphoma, unspecified, lymph nodes of multiple sites 🐾

C81.99 Hodgkin lymphoma, unspecified, extranodal and solid organ sites 🐾

▶ New ⇒ Revised ~~deleted~~ Deleted Excludes 1 Excludes 2 Includes Use additional Code first Code also Key words
OGCR Official Guidelines X Assign placeholder X ● Use Additional Character(s) ▶ Manifestation Code 🐾 Hierarchical Condition Category **Coding Clinic**

● **C82**   **Follicular lymphoma**
     Group of malignant lymphomas

     Includes   follicular lymphoma with or without diffuse areas

     Excludes1   mature T/NK-cell lymphomas (C84.-)
                 personal history of non-Hodgkin lymphoma (Z85.72)

● **C82.0**   **Follicular lymphoma grade I**
     C82.00   Follicular lymphoma grade I, unspecified site 🔖
     C82.01   Follicular lymphoma grade I, lymph nodes of head, face, and neck 🔖
     C82.02   Follicular lymphoma grade I, intrathoracic lymph nodes 🔖
     C82.03   Follicular lymphoma grade I, intra-abdominal lymph nodes 🔖
     C82.04   Follicular lymphoma grade I, lymph nodes of axilla and upper limb 🔖
     C82.05   Follicular lymphoma grade I, lymph nodes of inguinal region and lower limb 🔖
     C82.06   Follicular lymphoma grade I, intrapelvic lymph nodes 🔖
     C82.07   Follicular lymphoma grade I, spleen 🔖
     C82.08   Follicular lymphoma grade I, lymph nodes of multiple sites 🔖
     C82.09   Follicular lymphoma grade I, extranodal and solid organ sites 🔖

● **C82.1**   **Follicular lymphoma grade II**
     C82.10   Follicular lymphoma grade II, unspecified site 🔖
     C82.11   Follicular lymphoma grade II, lymph nodes of head, face, and neck 🔖
     C82.12   Follicular lymphoma grade II, intrathoracic lymph nodes 🔖
     C82.13   Follicular lymphoma grade II, intra-abdominal lymph nodes 🔖
     C82.14   Follicular lymphoma grade II, lymph nodes of axilla and upper limb 🔖
     C82.15   Follicular lymphoma grade II, lymph nodes of inguinal region and lower limb 🔖
     C82.16   Follicular lymphoma grade II, intrapelvic lymph nodes 🔖
     C82.17   Follicular lymphoma grade II, spleen 🔖
     C82.18   Follicular lymphoma grade II, lymph nodes of multiple sites 🔖
     C82.19   Follicular lymphoma grade II, extranodal and solid organ sites 🔖

● **C82.2**   **Follicular lymphoma grade III, unspecified**
     C82.20   Follicular lymphoma grade III, unspecified, unspecified site 🔖
     C82.21   Follicular lymphoma grade III, unspecified, lymph nodes of head, face, and neck 🔖
     C82.22   Follicular lymphoma grade III, unspecified, intrathoracic lymph nodes 🔖
     C82.23   Follicular lymphoma grade III, unspecified, intra-abdominal lymph nodes 🔖
     C82.24   Follicular lymphoma grade III, unspecified, lymph nodes of axilla and upper limb 🔖
     C82.25   Follicular lymphoma grade III, unspecified, lymph nodes of inguinal region and lower limb 🔖
     C82.26   Follicular lymphoma grade III, unspecified, intrapelvic lymph nodes 🔖
     C82.27   Follicular lymphoma grade III, unspecified, spleen 🔖
     C82.28   Follicular lymphoma grade III, unspecified, lymph nodes of multiple sites 🔖
     C82.29   Follicular lymphoma grade III, unspecified, extranodal and solid organ sites 🔖

● **C82.3**   **Follicular lymphoma grade IIIa**
     C82.30   Follicular lymphoma grade IIIa, unspecified site 🔖
     C82.31   Follicular lymphoma grade IIIa, lymph nodes of head, face, and neck 🔖
     C82.32   Follicular lymphoma grade IIIa, intrathoracic lymph nodes 🔖
     C82.33   Follicular lymphoma grade IIIa, intra-abdominal lymph nodes 🔖
     C82.34   Follicular lymphoma grade IIIa, lymph nodes of axilla and upper limb 🔖
     C82.35   Follicular lymphoma grade IIIa, lymph nodes of inguinal region and lower limb 🔖
     C82.36   Follicular lymphoma grade IIIa, intrapelvic lymph nodes 🔖
     C82.37   Follicular lymphoma grade IIIa, spleen 🔖
     C82.38   Follicular lymphoma grade IIIa, lymph nodes of multiple sites 🔖
     C82.39   Follicular lymphoma grade IIIa, extranodal and solid organ sites 🔖

● **C82.4**   **Follicular lymphoma grade IIIb**
     C82.40   Follicular lymphoma grade IIIb, unspecified site 🔖
     C82.41   Follicular lymphoma grade IIIb, lymph nodes of head, face, and neck 🔖
     C82.42   Follicular lymphoma grade IIIb, intrathoracic lymph nodes 🔖
     C82.43   Follicular lymphoma grade IIIb, intra-abdominal lymph nodes 🔖
     C82.44   Follicular lymphoma grade IIIb, lymph nodes of axilla and upper limb 🔖
     C82.45   Follicular lymphoma grade IIIb, lymph nodes of inguinal region and lower limb 🔖
     C82.46   Follicular lymphoma grade IIIb, intrapelvic lymph nodes 🔖
     C82.47   Follicular lymphoma grade IIIb, spleen 🔖
     C82.48   Follicular lymphoma grade IIIb, lymph nodes of multiple sites 🔖
     C82.49   Follicular lymphoma grade IIIb, extranodal and solid organ sites 🔖

● **C82.5**   **Diffuse follicle center lymphoma**
     C82.50   Diffuse follicle center lymphoma, unspecified site 🔖
     C82.51   Diffuse follicle center lymphoma, lymph nodes of head, face, and neck 🔖
     C82.52   Diffuse follicle center lymphoma, intrathoracic lymph nodes 🔖
     C82.53   Diffuse follicle center lymphoma, intra-abdominal lymph nodes 🔖
     C82.54   Diffuse follicle center lymphoma, lymph nodes of axilla and upper limb 🔖
     C82.55   Diffuse follicle center lymphoma, lymph nodes of inguinal region and lower limb 🔖
     C82.56   Diffuse follicle center lymphoma, intrapelvic lymph nodes 🔖
     C82.57   Diffuse follicle center lymphoma, spleen 🔖
     C82.58   Diffuse follicle center lymphoma, lymph nodes of multiple sites 🔖
     C82.59   Diffuse follicle center lymphoma, extranodal and solid organ sites 🔖

● **C82.6**   **Cutaneous follicle center lymphoma**
     C82.60   Cutaneous follicle center lymphoma, unspecified site 🔖
     C82.61   Cutaneous follicle center lymphoma, lymph nodes of head, face, and neck 🔖
     C82.62   Cutaneous follicle center lymphoma, intrathoracic lymph nodes 🔖
     C82.63   Cutaneous follicle center lymphoma, intra-abdominal lymph nodes 🔖

CHAPTER 2 (C00-D49)

CHAPTER 2 (C00-D49)

C82.64   Cutaneous follicle center lymphoma, lymph nodes of axilla and upper limb 🦠

C82.65   Cutaneous follicle center lymphoma, lymph nodes of inguinal region and lower limb 🦠

C82.66   Cutaneous follicle center lymphoma, intrapelvic lymph nodes 🦠

C82.67   Cutaneous follicle center lymphoma, spleen 🦠

C82.68   Cutaneous follicle center lymphoma, lymph nodes of multiple sites 🦠

C82.69   Cutaneous follicle center lymphoma, extranodal and solid organ sites 🦠

● C82.8   Other types of follicular lymphoma

C82.80   Other types of follicular lymphoma, unspecified site 🦠

C82.81   Other types of follicular lymphoma, lymph nodes of head, face, and neck 🦠

C82.82   Other types of follicular lymphoma, intrathoracic lymph nodes 🦠

C82.83   Other types of follicular lymphoma, intra-abdominal lymph nodes 🦠

C82.84   Other types of follicular lymphoma, lymph nodes of axilla and upper limb 🦠

C82.85   Other types of follicular lymphoma, lymph nodes of inguinal region and lower limb 🦠

C82.86   Other types of follicular lymphoma, intrapelvic lymph nodes 🦠

C82.87   Other types of follicular lymphoma, spleen 🦠

C82.88   Other types of follicular lymphoma, lymph nodes of multiple sites 🦠

C82.89   Other types of follicular lymphoma, extranodal and solid organ sites 🦠

● C82.9   Follicular lymphoma, unspecified

C82.90   Follicular lymphoma, unspecified, unspecified site 🦠

C82.91   Follicular lymphoma, unspecified, lymph nodes of head, face, and neck 🦠

C82.92   Follicular lymphoma, unspecified, intrathoracic lymph nodes 🦠

C82.93   Follicular lymphoma, unspecified, intra-abdominal lymph nodes 🦠

C82.94   Follicular lymphoma, unspecified, lymph nodes of axilla and upper limb 🦠

C82.95   Follicular lymphoma, unspecified, lymph nodes of inguinal region and lower limb 🦠

C82.96   Follicular lymphoma, unspecified, intrapelvic lymph nodes 🦠

C82.97   Follicular lymphoma, unspecified, spleen 🦠

C82.98   Follicular lymphoma, unspecified, lymph nodes of multiple sites 🦠

C82.99   Follicular lymphoma, unspecified, extranodal and solid organ sites 🦠

● C83   Non-follicular lymphoma

   Excludes1   personal history of non-Hodgkin lymphoma (Z85.72)

● C83.0   Small cell B-cell lymphoma

   Lymphoplasmacytic lymphoma
   Nodal marginal zone lymphoma
   Non-leukemic variant of B-CLL
   Splenic marginal zone lymphoma

   Excludes1   chronic lymphocytic leukemia (C91.1)
                   mature T/NK-cell lymphomas (C84.-)
                   Waldenström macroglobulinemia (C88.0)

C83.00   Small cell B-cell lymphoma, unspecified site 🦠

C83.01   Small cell B-cell lymphoma, lymph nodes of head, face, and neck 🦠

C83.02   Small cell B-cell lymphoma, intrathoracic lymph nodes 🦠

C83.03   Small cell B-cell lymphoma, intra-abdominal lymph nodes 🦠

C83.04   Small cell B-cell lymphoma, lymph nodes of axilla and upper limb 🦠

C83.05   Small cell B-cell lymphoma, lymph nodes of inguinal region and lower limb 🦠

C83.06   Small cell B-cell lymphoma, intrapelvic lymph nodes 🦠

C83.07   Small cell B-cell lymphoma, spleen 🦠

C83.08   Small cell B-cell lymphoma, lymph nodes of multiple sites 🦠

C83.09   Small cell B-cell lymphoma, extranodal and solid organ sites 🦠

● C83.1   Mantle cell lymphoma

   Centrocytic lymphoma
   Malignant lymphomatous polyposis

C83.10   Mantle cell lymphoma, unspecified site 🦠

C83.11   Mantle cell lymphoma, lymph nodes of head, face, and neck 🦠

C83.12   Mantle cell lymphoma, intrathoracic lymph nodes 🦠

C83.13   Mantle cell lymphoma, intra-abdominal lymph nodes 🦠

C83.14   Mantle cell lymphoma, lymph nodes of axilla and upper limb 🦠

C83.15   Mantle cell lymphoma, lymph nodes of inguinal region and lower limb 🦠

C83.16   Mantle cell lymphoma, intrapelvic lymph nodes 🦠

C83.17   Mantle cell lymphoma, spleen 🦠

C83.18   Mantle cell lymphoma, lymph nodes of multiple sites 🦠

C83.19   Mantle cell lymphoma, extranodal and solid organ sites 🦠

● C83.3   Diffuse large B-cell lymphoma

   Anaplastic diffuse large B-cell lymphoma
   CD30-positive diffuse large B-cell lymphoma
   Centroblastic diffuse large B-cell lymphoma
   Diffuse large B-cell lymphoma, subtype not specified
   Immunoblastic diffuse large B-cell lymphoma
   Plasmablastic diffuse large B-cell lymphoma
   Diffuse large B-cell lymphoma, subtype not specified
   T-cell rich diffuse large B-cell lymphoma

   Excludes1   mediastinal (thymic) large B-cell lymphoma (C85.2-)
                   mature T/NK-cell lymphomas (C84.-)

C83.30   Diffuse large B-cell lymphoma, unspecified site 🦠

C83.31   Diffuse large B-cell lymphoma, lymph nodes of head, face, and neck 🦠

C83.32   Diffuse large B-cell lymphoma, intrathoracic lymph nodes 🦠

C83.33   Diffuse large B-cell lymphoma, intra-abdominal lymph nodes 🦠

C83.34   Diffuse large B-cell lymphoma, lymph nodes of axilla and upper limb 🦠

C83.35   Diffuse large B-cell lymphoma, lymph nodes of inguinal region and lower limb 🦠

C83.36   Diffuse large B-cell lymphoma, intrapelvic lymph nodes 🦠

C83.37   Diffuse large B-cell lymphoma, spleen 🦠

C83.38   Diffuse large B-cell lymphoma, lymph nodes of multiple sites 🦠

C83.39   Diffuse large B-cell lymphoma, extranodal and solid organ sites 🦠

● **C83.5**   **Lymphoblastic (diffuse) lymphoma**
     Highly malignant type of non-Hodgkin lymphoma with
        diffuse infiltration
     B-precursor lymphoma
     Lymphoblastic B-cell lymphoma
     Lymphoblastic lymphoma NOS
     Lymphoblastic T-cell lymphoma
     T-precursor lymphoma

     C83.50   Lymphoblastic (diffuse) lymphoma, unspecified site 🔍

     C83.51   Lymphoblastic (diffuse) lymphoma, lymph nodes of head, face, and neck 🔍

     C83.52   Lymphoblastic (diffuse) lymphoma, intrathoracic lymph nodes 🔍

     C83.53   Lymphoblastic (diffuse) lymphoma, intra-abdominal lymph nodes 🔍

     C83.54   Lymphoblastic (diffuse) lymphoma, lymph nodes of axilla and upper limb 🔍

     C83.55   Lymphoblastic (diffuse) lymphoma, lymph nodes of inguinal region and lower limb 🔍

     C83.56   Lymphoblastic (diffuse) lymphoma, intrapelvic lymph nodes 🔍

     C83.57   Lymphoblastic (diffuse) lymphoma, spleen 🔍

     C83.58   Lymphoblastic (diffuse) lymphoma, lymph nodes of multiple sites 🔍

     C83.59   Lymphoblastic (diffuse) lymphoma, extranodal and solid organ sites 🔍

● **C83.7**   **Burkitt lymphoma**
     Form of small cell lymphoma
     Atypical Burkitt lymphoma
     Burkitt-like lymphoma

     Excludes1   mature B-cell leukemia Burkitt type (C91.A-)

     C83.70   Burkitt lymphoma, unspecified site 🔍
     C83.71   Burkitt lymphoma, lymph nodes of head, face, and neck 🔍
     C83.72   Burkitt lymphoma, intrathoracic lymph nodes 🔍
     C83.73   Burkitt lymphoma, intra-abdominal lymph nodes 🔍
     C83.74   Burkitt lymphoma, lymph nodes of axilla and upper limb 🔍
     C83.75   Burkitt lymphoma, lymph nodes of inguinal region and lower limb 🔍
     C83.76   Burkitt lymphoma, intrapelvic lymph nodes 🔍
     C83.77   Burkitt lymphoma, spleen 🔍
     C83.78   Burkitt lymphoma, lymph nodes of multiple sites 🔍
     C83.79   Burkitt lymphoma, extranodal and solid organ sites 🔍

● **C83.8**   **Other non-follicular lymphoma**
     Intravascular large B-cell lymphoma
     Lymphoid granulomatosis
     Primary effusion B-cell lymphoma

     Excludes1   mediastinal (thymic) large B-cell lymphoma (C85.2-)
               T-cell rich B-cell lymphoma (C83.3-)

     C83.80   Other non-follicular lymphoma, unspecified site 🔍
     C83.81   Other non-follicular lymphoma, lymph nodes of head, face, and neck 🔍
     C83.82   Other non-follicular lymphoma, intrathoracic lymph nodes 🔍
     C83.83   Other non-follicular lymphoma, intra-abdominal lymph nodes 🔍
     C83.84   Other non-follicular lymphoma, lymph nodes of axilla and upper limb 🔍
     C83.85   Other non-follicular lymphoma, lymph nodes of inguinal region and lower limb 🔍
     C83.86   Other non-follicular lymphoma, intrapelvic lymph nodes 🔍

     C83.87   Other non-follicular lymphoma, spleen 🔍
     C83.88   Other non-follicular lymphoma, lymph nodes of multiple sites 🔍
     C83.89   Other non-follicular lymphoma, extranodal and solid organ sites 🔍

● **C83.9**   **Non-follicular (diffuse) lymphoma, unspecified**
     C83.90   Non-follicular (diffuse) lymphoma, unspecified, unspecified site 🔍
     C83.91   Non-follicular (diffuse) lymphoma, unspecified, lymph nodes of head, face, and neck 🔍
     C83.92   Non-follicular (diffuse) lymphoma, unspecified, intrathoracic lymph nodes 🔍
     C83.93   Non-follicular (diffuse) lymphoma, unspecified, intra-abdominal lymph nodes 🔍
     C83.94   Non-follicular (diffuse) lymphoma, unspecified, lymph nodes of axilla and upper limb 🔍
     C83.95   Non-follicular (diffuse) lymphoma, unspecified, lymph nodes of inguinal region and lower limb 🔍
     C83.96   Non-follicular (diffuse) lymphoma, unspecified, intrapelvic lymph nodes 🔍
     C83.97   Non-follicular (diffuse) lymphoma, unspecified, spleen 🔍
     C83.98   Non-follicular (diffuse) lymphoma, unspecified, lymph nodes of multiple sites 🔍
     C83.99   Non-follicular (diffuse) lymphoma, unspecified, extranodal and solid organ sites 🔍

● **C84**   **Mature T/NK-cell lymphomas**
     Excludes1   personal history of non-Hodgkin lymphoma (Z85.72)

● **C84.0**   **Mycosis fungoides**
     Chronic or rapidly progressive form of cutaneous T-cell lymphoma; AKA granuloma fungoides

     ➡ **Excludes1**   peripheral T-cell lymphoma, not elsewhere classified (C84.4-)

     C84.00   Mycosis fungoides, unspecified site 🔍
     C84.01   Mycosis fungoides, lymph nodes of head, face, and neck 🔍
     C84.02   Mycosis fungoides, intrathoracic lymph nodes 🔍
     C84.03   Mycosis fungoides, intra-abdominal lymph nodes 🔍
     C84.04   Mycosis fungoides, lymph nodes of axilla and upper limb 🔍
     C84.05   Mycosis fungoides, lymph nodes of inguinal region and lower limb 🔍
     C84.06   Mycosis fungoides, intrapelvic lymph nodes 🔍
     C84.07   Mycosis fungoides, spleen 🔍
     C84.08   Mycosis fungoides, lymph nodes of multiple sites 🔍
     C84.09   Mycosis fungoides, extranodal and solid organ sites 🔍

● **C84.1**   **Sézary disease**
     Type of cutaneous lymphoma affecting T-cells
     C84.10   Sézary disease, unspecified site 🔍
     C84.11   Sézary disease, lymph nodes of head, face, and neck 🔍
     C84.12   Sézary disease, intrathoracic lymph nodes 🔍
     C84.13   Sézary disease, intra-abdominal lymph nodes 🔍
     C84.14   Sézary disease, lymph nodes of axilla and upper limb 🔍
     C84.15   Sézary disease, lymph nodes of inguinal region and lower limb 🔍
     C84.16   Sézary disease, intrapelvic lymph nodes 🔍
     C84.17   Sézary disease, spleen 🔍
     C84.18   Sézary disease, lymph nodes of multiple sites 🔍
     C84.19   Sézary disease, extranodal and solid organ sites 🔍

CHAPTER 2 (C00-D49)

▶●C84.4   Peripheral T-cell lymphoma, not elsewhere classified
Diverse group of blood carcinomas originating from T-cells, requiring aggressive chemotherapy
Lennert's lymphoma
Lymphoepithelioid lymphoma
Mature T-cell lymphoma, not elsewhere classified

➡ C84.40   Peripheral T-cell lymphoma, not elsewhere classified, unspecified site 🦠

➡ C84.41   Peripheral T-cell lymphoma, not elsewhere classified, lymph nodes of head, face, and neck 🦠

➡ C84.42   Peripheral T-cell lymphoma, not elsewhere classified, intrathoracic lymph nodes 🦠

➡ C84.43   Peripheral T-cell lymphoma, not elsewhere classified, intra-abdominal lymph nodes 🦠

➡ C84.44   Peripheral T-cell lymphoma, not elsewhere classified, lymph nodes of axilla and upper limb 🦠

➡ C84.45   Peripheral T-cell lymphoma, not elsewhere classified, lymph nodes of inguinal region and lower limb 🦠

➡ C84.46   Peripheral T-cell lymphoma, not elsewhere classified, intrapelvic lymph nodes 🦠

➡ C84.47   Peripheral T-cell lymphoma, not elsewhere classified, spleen 🦠

➡ C84.48   Peripheral T-cell lymphoma, not elsewhere classified, lymph nodes of multiple sites 🦠

➡ C84.49   Peripheral T-cell lymphoma, not elsewhere classified, extranodal and solid organ sites 🦠

●C84.6   Anaplastic large cell lymphoma, ALK-positive
Anaplastic large cell lymphoma, CD30-positive

C84.60   Anaplastic large cell lymphoma, ALK-positive, unspecified site 🦠

C84.61   Anaplastic large cell lymphoma, ALK-positive, lymph nodes of head, face, and neck 🦠

C84.62   Anaplastic large cell lymphoma, ALK-positive, intrathoracic lymph nodes 🦠

C84.63   Anaplastic large cell lymphoma, ALK-positive, intra-abdominal lymph nodes 🦠

C84.64   Anaplastic large cell lymphoma, ALK-positive, lymph nodes of axilla and upper limb 🦠

C84.65   Anaplastic large cell lymphoma, ALK-positive, lymph nodes of inguinal region and lower limb 🦠

C84.66   Anaplastic large cell lymphoma, ALK-positive, intrapelvic lymph nodes 🦠

C84.67   Anaplastic large cell lymphoma, ALK-positive, spleen 🦠

C84.68   Anaplastic large cell lymphoma, ALK-positive, lymph nodes of multiple sites 🦠

C84.69   Anaplastic large cell lymphoma, ALK-positive, extranodal and solid organ sites 🦠

●C84.7   Anaplastic large cell lymphoma, ALK-negative

Excludes1   primary cutaneous CD30-positive T-cell proliferations (C86.6-)

C84.70   Anaplastic large cell lymphoma, ALK-negative, unspecified site 🦠

C84.71   Anaplastic large cell lymphoma, ALK-negative, lymph nodes of head, face, and neck 🦠

C84.72   Anaplastic large cell lymphoma, ALK-negative, intrathoracic lymph nodes 🦠

C84.73   Anaplastic large cell lymphoma, ALK-negative, intra-abdominal lymph nodes 🦠

C84.74   Anaplastic large cell lymphoma, ALK-negative, lymph nodes of axilla and upper limb 🦠

C84.75   Anaplastic large cell lymphoma, ALK-negative, lymph nodes of inguinal region and lower limb 🦠

C84.76   Anaplastic large cell lymphoma, ALK-negative, intrapelvic lymph nodes 🦠

Item 2-7   Lymphosarcoma, also known as malignant lymphoma, is a cancer of the lymph system exhibiting abnormal cells encompassing an entire lymph node creating a diffuse pattern without any definite organization. Diffuse pattern lymphoma has a more unfavorable survival outlook than those with a follicular or nodular pattern. Reticulosarcoma is the most common aggressive form of non-Hodgkin lymphoma.

C84.77   Anaplastic large cell lymphoma, ALK-negative, spleen 🦠

C84.78   Anaplastic large cell lymphoma, ALK-negative, lymph nodes of multiple sites 🦠

C84.79   Anaplastic large cell lymphoma, ALK-negative, extranodal and solid organ sites 🦠

C84.7A   Anaplastic large cell lymphoma, ALK-negative, breast
Breast implant associated anaplastic large cell lymphoma (BIA-ALCL)

Use additional code to identify:
breast implant status (Z98.82)
personal history of breast implant removal (Z98.86)

●C84.9   Mature T/NK-cell lymphomas, unspecified
NK/T cell lymphoma NOS

Excludes1   mature T-cell lymphoma, not elsewhere classified (C84.4-)

C84.90   Mature T/NK-cell lymphomas, unspecified, unspecified site 🦠

C84.91   Mature T/NK-cell lymphomas, unspecified, lymph nodes of head, face, and neck 🦠

C84.92   Mature T/NK-cell lymphomas, unspecified, intrathoracic lymph nodes 🦠

C84.93   Mature T/NK-cell lymphomas, unspecified, intra-abdominal lymph nodes 🦠

C84.94   Mature T/NK-cell lymphomas, unspecified, lymph nodes of axilla and upper limb 🦠

C84.95   Mature T/NK-cell lymphomas, unspecified, lymph nodes of inguinal region and lower limb 🦠

C84.96   Mature T/NK-cell lymphomas, unspecified, intrapelvic lymph nodes 🦠

C84.97   Mature T/NK-cell lymphomas, unspecified, spleen 🦠

C84.98   Mature T/NK-cell lymphomas, unspecified, lymph nodes of multiple sites 🦠

C84.99   Mature T/NK-cell lymphomas, unspecified, extranodal and solid organ sites 🦠

●C84.A   Cutaneous T-cell lymphoma, unspecified

C84.A0   Cutaneous T-cell lymphoma, unspecified, unspecified site 🦠

C84.A1   Cutaneous T-cell lymphoma, unspecified lymph nodes of head, face, and neck 🦠

C84.A2   Cutaneous T-cell lymphoma, unspecified, intrathoracic lymph nodes 🦠

C84.A3   Cutaneous T-cell lymphoma, unspecified, intra-abdominal lymph nodes 🦠

C84.A4   Cutaneous T-cell lymphoma, unspecified, lymph nodes of axilla and upper limb 🦠

C84.A5   Cutaneous T-cell lymphoma, unspecified, lymph nodes of inguinal region and lower limb 🦠

C84.A6   Cutaneous T-cell lymphoma, unspecified, intrapelvic lymph nodes 🦠

C84.A7   Cutaneous T-cell lymphoma, unspecified, spleen 🦠
Coding Clinic: 2021, Q2, P7

C84.A8   Cutaneous T-cell lymphoma, unspecified, lymph nodes of multiple sites 🦠
Coding Clinic: 2021, Q2, P7

C84.A9   Cutaneous T-cell lymphoma, unspecified, extranodal and solid organ sites 🦠

▶ New   ➡ Revised   ~~deleted~~ Deleted   Excludes 1   Excludes 2   Includes   Use additional   Code first   Code also   Key words

OGCR Official Guidelines   X Assign placeholder X   ● Use Additional Character(s)   ▶ Manifestation Code   🦠 Hierarchical Condition Category   **Coding Clinic**

● **C84.Z   Other mature T/NK-cell lymphomas**

Note: If T-cell lineage or involvement is mentioned in conjunction with a specific lymphoma, code to the more specific description.

Excludes1   angioimmunoblastic T-cell lymphoma (C86.5)
blastic NK-cell lymphoma (C86.4)
enteropathy-type T-cell lymphoma (C86.2)
extranodal NK-cell lymphoma, nasal type (C86.0)
hepatosplenic T-cell lymphoma (C86.1)
primary cutaneous CD30-positive T-cell proliferations (C86.6)
subcutaneous panniculitis-like T-cell lymphoma (C86.3)
T-cell leukemia (C91.1-)

C84.Z0   Other mature T/NK-cell lymphomas, **unspecified site** 🦠

C84.Z1   Other mature T/NK-cell lymphomas, lymph nodes of **head, face, and neck** 🦠

C84.Z2   Other mature T/NK-cell lymphomas, **intrathoracic lymph nodes** 🦠

C84.Z3   Other mature T/NK-cell lymphomas, **intra-abdominal** lymph nodes 🦠

C84.Z4   Other mature T/NK-cell lymphomas, lymph nodes of **axilla and upper limb** 🦠

C84.Z5   Other mature T/NK-cell lymphomas, lymph nodes of **inguinal region and lower limb** 🦠

C84.Z6   Other mature T/NK-cell lymphomas, **intrapelvic** lymph nodes 🦠

C84.Z7   Other mature T/NK-cell lymphomas, **spleen** 🦠

C84.Z8   Other mature T/NK-cell lymphomas, lymph nodes of **multiple sites** 🦠

C84.Z9   Other mature T/NK-cell lymphomas, **extranodal and solid organ sites** 🦠

● **C85   Other specified and unspecified types of non-Hodgkin lymphoma**

Excludes1   other specified types of T/NK-cell lymphoma (C86.-)
personal history of non-Hodgkin lymphoma (Z85.72)

● **C85.1   Unspecified B-cell lymphoma**

Note: If B-cell lineage or involvement is mentioned in conjunction with a specific lymphoma, code to the more specific description.

C85.10   Unspecified B-cell lymphoma, **unspecified site** 🦠

C85.11   Unspecified B-cell lymphoma, lymph nodes of **head, face, and neck** 🦠

C85.12   Unspecified B-cell lymphoma, **intrathoracic lymph nodes** 🦠

C85.13   Unspecified B-cell lymphoma, **intra-abdominal lymph nodes** 🦠

C85.14   Unspecified B-cell lymphoma, lymph nodes of **axilla and upper limb** 🦠

C85.15   Unspecified B-cell lymphoma, lymph nodes of **inguinal region and lower limb** 🦠

C85.16   Unspecified B-cell lymphoma, **intrapelvic lymph nodes** 🦠

C85.17   Unspecified B-cell lymphoma, **spleen** 🦠

C85.18   Unspecified B-cell lymphoma, lymph nodes of **multiple sites** 🦠

C85.19   Unspecified B-cell lymphoma, **extranodal and solid organ sites** 🦠

● **C85.2   Mediastinal (thymic) large B-cell lymphoma**

C85.20   Mediastinal (thymic) large B-cell lymphoma, **unspecified site** 🦠

C85.21   Mediastinal (thymic) large B-cell lymphoma, **lymph nodes of head, face, and neck** 🦠

C85.22   Mediastinal (thymic) large B-cell lymphoma, **intrathoracic lymph nodes** 🦠

C85.23   Mediastinal (thymic) large B-cell lymphoma, **intra-abdominal lymph nodes** 🦠

C85.24   Mediastinal (thymic) large B-cell lymphoma, lymph nodes of **axilla and upper limb** 🦠

C85.25   Mediastinal (thymic) large B-cell lymphoma, lymph nodes of **inguinal region and lower limb** 🦠

C85.26   Mediastinal (thymic) large B-cell lymphoma, **intrapelvic lymph nodes** 🦠

C85.27   Mediastinal (thymic) large B-cell lymphoma, **spleen** 🦠

C85.28   Mediastinal (thymic) large B-cell lymphoma, lymph nodes of **multiple sites** 🦠

C85.29   Mediastinal (thymic) large B-cell lymphoma, **extranodal and solid organ sites** 🦠

● **C85.8   Other specified types of non-Hodgkin lymphoma**

C85.80   Other specified types of non-Hodgkin lymphoma, **unspecified site** 🦠

C85.81   Other specified types of non-Hodgkin lymphoma, lymph nodes of **head, face, and neck** 🦠

C85.82   Other specified types of non-Hodgkin lymphoma, **intrathoracic lymph nodes** 🦠

C85.83   Other specified types of non-Hodgkin lymphoma, **intra-abdominal lymph nodes** 🦠

C85.84   Other specified types of non-Hodgkin lymphoma, lymph nodes of **axilla and upper limb** 🦠

C85.85   Other specified types of non-Hodgkin lymphoma, lymph nodes of **inguinal region and lower limb** 🦠

C85.86   Other specified types of non-Hodgkin lymphoma, **intrapelvic lymph nodes** 🦠

C85.87   Other specified types of non-Hodgkin lymphoma, **spleen** 🦠

C85.88   Other specified types of non-Hodgkin lymphoma, lymph nodes of **multiple sites** 🦠

C85.89   Other specified types of non-Hodgkin lymphoma, **extranodal and solid organ sites** 🦠

● **C85.9   Non-Hodgkin lymphoma, unspecified**

Lymphoma NOS
Malignant lymphoma NOS
Non-Hodgkin lymphoma NOS

C85.90   Non-Hodgkin lymphoma, unspecified, **unspecified site** 🦠

C85.91   Non-Hodgkin lymphoma, unspecified, lymph nodes of **head, face, and neck** 🦠

C85.92   Non-Hodgkin lymphoma, unspecified, **intrathoracic lymph nodes** 🦠

C85.93   Non-Hodgkin lymphoma, unspecified, **intra-abdominal lymph nodes** 🦠

C85.94   Non-Hodgkin lymphoma, unspecified, lymph nodes of **axilla and upper limb** 🦠

C85.95   Non-Hodgkin lymphoma, unspecified, lymph nodes of **inguinal region and lower limb** 🦠

C85.96   Non-Hodgkin lymphoma, unspecified, **intrapelvic lymph nodes** 🦠

C85.97   Non-Hodgkin lymphoma, unspecified, **spleen** 🦠

C85.98   Non-Hodgkin lymphoma, unspecified, lymph nodes of **multiple sites** 🦠

C85.99   Non-Hodgkin lymphoma, unspecified, **extranodal and solid organ sites** 🦠

CHAPTER 2 (C00-D49)

● **C86** **Other specified types of T/NK-cell lymphoma**

    Excludes1   anaplastic large cell lymphoma, ALK negative (C84.7-)
                   anaplastic large cell lymphoma, ALK positive (C84.6-)
                   mature T/NK-cell lymphomas (C84.-)
                   other specified types of non-Hodgkin lymphoma (C85.8-)

    C86.0   **Extranodal NK/T-cell lymphoma, nasal type** 🔖

    C86.1   **Hepatosplenic T-cell lymphoma** 🔖
            Alpha-beta and gamma delta types

    C86.2   **Enteropathy-type (intestinal) T-cell lymphoma** 🔖
            Enteropathy associated T-cell lymphoma

    C86.3   **Subcutaneous panniculitis-like T-cell lymphoma** 🔖

    C86.4   **Blastic NK-cell lymphoma** 🔖
            Blastic plasmacytoid dendritic cell neoplasm (BPDCN)

    C86.5   **Angioimmunoblastic T-cell lymphoma** 🔖
            Angioimmunoblastic lymphadenopathy with dysproteinemia (AILD)

    C86.6   **Primary cutaneous CD30-positive T-cell proliferations** 🔖
            Lymphomatoid papulosis
            Primary cutaneous anaplastic large cell lymphoma
            Primary cutaneous CD30-positive large T-cell lymphoma

● **C88** **Malignant immunoproliferative diseases and certain other B-cell lymphomas**
    Diseases involving immune system

    Excludes1   B-cell lymphoma, unspecified (C85.1-)
                   personal history of other malignant neoplasms of lymphoid, hematopoietic and related tissues (Z85.79)

    C88.0   **Waldenström's macroglobulinemia** 🔖
            Lymphoplasmacytic lymphoma with IgM-production
            Macroglobulinemia (idiopathic) (primary)
            Excludes1   small cell B-cell lymphoma (C83.0)

    C88.2   **Heavy chain disease** 🔖
            Franklin disease
            Gamma heavy chain disease
            Mu heavy chain disease

    C88.3   **Immunoproliferative small intestinal disease** 🔖
            Alpha heavy chain disease
            Mediterranean lymphoma

    C88.4   **Extranodal marginal zone B-cell lymphoma of mucosa-associated lymphoid tissue [MALT-lymphoma]** 🔖
            Lymphoma of skin-associated lymphoid tissue [SALT-lymphoma]
            Lymphoma of bronchial-associated lymphoid tissue [BALT-lymphoma]
            Excludes1   high malignant (diffuse large B-cell) lymphoma (C83.3-)

    C88.8   **Other malignant immunoproliferative diseases** 🔖

    C88.9   **Malignant immunoproliferative disease, unspecified** 🔖
            Immunoproliferative disease NOS

● **C90** **Multiple myeloma and malignant plasma cell neoplasms**

    Excludes1   personal history of other malignant neoplasms of lymphoid, hematopoietic and related tissues (Z85.79)

  ● **C90.0**   **Multiple myeloma**
            Kahler's disease
            Medullary plasmacytoma
            Myelomatosis
            Plasma cell myeloma
            Excludes1   solitary myeloma (C90.3-)
                        solitary plasmacytoma (C90.3-)

      C90.00   **Multiple myeloma not having achieved remission** 🔖
              Multiple myeloma with failed remission
              Multiple myeloma NOS

    C90.01   **Multiple myeloma in remission** 🔖
    C90.02   **Multiple myeloma in relapse** 🔖

● **C90.1** **Plasma cell leukemia**
    Rare type of acute leukemia
    Plasmacytic leukemia
    Coding Clinic: 2019, Q2, P30

    C90.10   **Plasma cell leukemia not having achieved remission**
            Plasma cell leukemia with failed remission
            Plasma cell leukemia NOS
            Coding Clinic: 2019, Q2, P30

    C90.11   **Plasma cell leukemia in remission** 🔖
    C90.12   **Plasma cell leukemia in relapse** 🔖

● **C90.2** **Extramedullary plasmacytoma**
    Malignant monoclonal plasma cell tumor growing in soft tissue; AKA plasma cell dyscrasias

    C90.20   **Extramedullary plasmacytoma not having achieved remission**
            Extramedullary plasmacytoma with failed remission
            Extramedullary plasmacytoma NOS

    C90.21   **Extramedullary plasmacytoma in remission** 🔖
    C90.22   **Extramedullary plasmacytoma in relapse** 🔖

● **C90.3** **Solitary plasmacytoma**
    Localized malignant plasma cell tumor NOS
    Plasmacytoma NOS
    Solitary myeloma

    C90.30   **Solitary plasmacytoma not having achieved remission** 🔖
            Solitary plasmacytoma with failed remission
            Solitary plasmacytoma NOS

    C90.31   **Solitary plasmacytoma in remission** 🔖
    C90.32   **Solitary plasmacytoma in relapse** 🔖

● **C91** **Lymphoid leukemia**
    Type of leukemia affecting circulating cells of lymphoid origin
    Excludes1   personal history of leukemia (Z85.6)

● **C91.0** **Acute lymphoblastic leukemia [ALL]**
    Note: Codes in subcategory C91.0 should only be used for T-cell and B-cell precursor leukemia

    C91.00   **Acute lymphoblastic leukemia not having achieved remission** 🔖
            Acute lymphoblastic leukemia with failed remission
            Acute lymphoblastic leukemia NOS
            Coding Clinic: 2022, Q1, P16

    C91.01   **Acute lymphoblastic leukemia, in remission** 🔖
    C91.02   **Acute lymphoblastic leukemia, in relapse** 🔖

● **C91.1** **Chronic lymphocytic leukemia of B-cell type**
    Lymphoplasmacytic leukemia
    Richter syndrome
    Excludes1   lymphoplasmacytic lymphoma (C83.0-)

    C91.10   **Chronic lymphocytic leukemia of B-cell type not having achieved remission** 🔖
            Chronic lymphocytic leukemia of B-cell type with failed remission
            Chronic lymphocytic leukemia of B-cell type NOS

    C91.11   **Chronic lymphocytic leukemia of B-cell type in remission** 🔖

    C91.12   **Chronic lymphocytic leukemia of B-cell type in relapse** 🔖

Item 2–8 **Multiple myeloma** is a cancer of a plasma cell (a type of white blood cell) and is an incurable but treatable disease. Immunoproliferative neoplasm is a term for diseases (mostly cancers) in which the immune system cells proliferate.

Item 2–9 Leukemia is a cancer (acute or chronic) of the blood-forming tissues of the bone marrow. Blood cells all start out as stem cells. They mature and become red cells, white cells, or platelets. There are three main types of leukocytes (white cells that fight infection): monocytes, lymphocytes, and granulocytes. **Acute monocytic leukemia** (AML) affects monocytes. **Acute lymphoid leukemia** (ALL) affects lymphocytes, and **acute myeloid leukemia** (AML) affects cells that typically develop into white blood cells (not lymphocytes), though it may develop in other blood cells.

▶ New   ⟾ Revised   ~~deleted~~ Deleted   Excludes 1   Excludes 2   Includes   Use additional   Code first   Code also   Key words

OGCR Official Guidelines   X Assign placeholder X   ● Use Additional Character(s)   ▶ Manifestation Code   🔖 Hierarchical Condition Category   **Coding Clinic**

● **C91.3**   **Prolymphocytic leukemia of B-cell type**
Chronic leukemia with symptoms of large number of circulating lymphocytes

    C91.30   **Prolymphocytic leukemia of B-cell type not having achieved remission** 🐾
Prolymphocytic leukemia of B-cell type with failed remission
Prolymphocytic leukemia of B-cell type NOS

    C91.31   **Prolymphocytic leukemia of B-cell type, in remission** 🐾

    C91.32   **Prolymphocytic leukemia of B-cell type, in relapse** 🐾

● **C91.4**   **Hairy cell leukemia**
Chronic leukemia with splenomegaly and excessive number of abnormal large mononuclear cells covered by hairlike villi
Leukemic reticuloendotheliosis

    C91.40   **Hairy cell leukemia not having achieved remission** 🐾
Hairy cell leukemia with failed remission
Hairy cell leukemia NOS

    C91.41   **Hairy cell leukemia, in remission** 🐾

    C91.42   **Hairy cell leukemia, in relapse** 🐾

● **C91.5**   **Adult T-cell lymphoma/leukemia (HTLV-1-associated)**
Acute variant of adult T-cell lymphoma/leukemia (HTLV-1-associated)
Chronic variant of adult T-cell lymphoma/leukemia (HTLV-1-associated)
Lymphomatoid variant of adult T-cell lymphoma/leukemia (HTLV-1-associated)
Smouldering variant of adult T-cell lymphoma/leukemia (HTLV-1-associated)

    C91.50   **Adult T-cell lymphoma/leukemia (HTLV-1-associated) not having achieved remission** 🐾   **A**
Adult T-cell lymphoma/leukemia (HTLV-1-associated) with failed remission
Adult T-cell lymphoma/leukemia (HTLV-1-associated) NOS

    C91.51   **Adult T-cell lymphoma/leukemia (HTLV-1-associated), in remission** 🐾   **A**

    C91.52   **Adult T-cell lymphoma/leukemia (HTLV-1-associated), in relapse** 🐾   **A**

● **C91.6**   **Prolymphocytic leukemia of T-cell type**

    C91.60   **Prolymphocytic leukemia of T-cell type not having achieved remission** 🐾
Prolymphocytic leukemia of T-cell type with failed remission
Prolymphocytic leukemia of T-cell type NOS

    C91.61   **Prolymphocytic leukemia of T-cell type, in remission** 🐾

    C91.62   **Prolymphocytic leukemia of T-cell type, in relapse** 🐾

● **C91.A**   **Mature B-cell leukemia Burkitt-type**

    Excludes1   Burkitt lymphoma (C83.7-)

    C91.A0   **Mature B-cell leukemia Burkitt-type not having achieved remission** 🐾
Mature B-cell leukemia Burkitt-type with failed remission
Mature B-cell leukemia Burkitt-type NOS

    C91.A1   **Mature B-cell leukemia Burkitt-type, in remission** 🐾

    C91.A2   **Mature B-cell leukemia Burkitt-type, in relapse** 🐾

● **C91.Z**   **Other lymphoid leukemia**
T-cell large granular lymphocytic leukemia (associated with rheumatoid arthritis)

    C91.Z0   **Other lymphoid leukemia not having achieved remission** 🐾
Other lymphoid leukemia with failed remission
Other lymphoid leukemia NOS
Coding Clinic: 2019, Q2, P25

    C91.Z1   **Other lymphoid leukemia, in remission** 🐾

    C91.Z2   **Other lymphoid leukemia, in relapse** 🐾

● **C91.9**   **Lymphoid leukemia, unspecified**

    C91.90   **Lymphoid leukemia, unspecified not having achieved remission** 🐾
Lymphoid leukemia with failed remission
Lymphoid leukemia NOS

    C91.91   **Lymphoid leukemia, unspecified, in remission** 🐾

    C91.92   **Lymphoid leukemia, unspecified, in relapse** 🐾

● **C92**   **Myeloid leukemia**

    Includes   granulocytic leukemia
myelogenous leukemia

    Excludes1   personal history of leukemia (Z85.6)

    Coding Clinic: 2019, Q1, P16

● **C92.0**   **Acute myeloblastic leukemia**
Acute myeloblastic leukemia, minimal differentiation
Acute myeloblastic leukemia (with maturation)
Acute myeloblastic leukemia 1/ETO
Acute myeloblastic leukemia M0
Acute myeloblastic leukemia M1
Acute myeloblastic leukemia M2
Acute myeloblastic leukemia with t(8;21)
Acute myeloblastic leukemia (without a FAB classification) NOS
Refractory anemia with excess blasts in transformation [RAEB T]

    Excludes1   acute exacerbation of chronic myeloid leukemia (C92.10)
refractory anemia with excess of blasts not in transformation (D46.2-)

    Coding Clinic: 2018, Q4, P87

    C92.00   **Acute myeloblastic leukemia, not having achieved remission** 🐾
Acute myeloblastic leukemia with failed remission
Acute myeloblastic leukemia NOS

    C92.01   **Acute myeloblastic leukemia, in remission** 🐾
Coding Clinic: 2021, Q3, P4

    C92.02   **Acute myeloblastic leukemia, in relapse** 🐾

● **C92.1**   **Chronic myeloid leukemia, BCR/ABL-positive**
Chronic myelogenous leukemia, Philadelphia chromosome (Ph1) positive
Chronic myelogenous leukemia, t(9;22) (q34;q11)
Chronic myelogenous leukemia with crisis of blast cells

    Excludes1   atypical chronic myeloid leukemia BCR/ABL-negative (C92.2-)
chronic myelomonocytic leukemia (C93.1-)
chronic myeloproliferative disease (D47.1)

    C92.10   **Chronic myeloid leukemia, BCR/ABL-positive, not having achieved remission** 🐾
Chronic myeloid leukemia, BCR/ABL-positive with failed remission
Chronic myeloid leukemia, BCR/ABL-positive NOS
Coding Clinic: 2017, Q1, P7

    C92.11   **Chronic myeloid leukemia, BCR/ABL-positive, in remission** 🐾

    C92.12   **Chronic myeloid leukemia, BCR/ABL-positive, in relapse** 🐾

● **C92.2**   **Atypical chronic myeloid leukemia, BCR/ABL-negative**

    C92.20   **Atypical chronic myeloid leukemia, BCR/ABL-negative, not having achieved remission** 🐾
Atypical chronic myeloid leukemia, BCR/ABL-negative with failed remission
Atypical chronic myeloid leukemia, BCR/ABL-negative NOS

    C92.21   **Atypical chronic myeloid leukemia, BCR/ABL-negative, in remission** 🐾

    C92.22   **Atypical chronic myeloid leukemia, BCR/ABL-negative, in relapse** 🐾

CHAPTER 2 (C00-D49)

CHAPTER 2 (C00-D49)

● **C92.3**   Myeloid sarcoma
    A malignant tumor of immature myeloid cells
    Chloroma
    Granulocytic sarcoma

   C92.30   Myeloid sarcoma, not having achieved remission 🔖
     Myeloid sarcoma with failed remission
     Myeloid sarcoma NOS

   C92.31   Myeloid sarcoma, in remission 🔖

   C92.32   Myeloid sarcoma, in relapse 🔖

● **C92.4**   Acute promyelocytic leukemia
    AML M3
    AML Me with t(15;17) and variants

   C92.40   Acute promyelocytic leukemia, not having achieved remission 🔖
     Acute promyelocytic leukemia with failed remission
     Acute promyelocytic leukemia NOS

   C92.41   Acute promyelocytic leukemia, in remission 🔖

   C92.42   Acute promyelocytic leukemia, in relapse 🔖

● **C92.5**   Acute myelomonocytic leukemia
    AML M4
    AML M4 Eo with inv(16) or t(16;16)

   C92.50   Acute myelomonocytic leukemia, not having achieved remission 🔖
     Acute myelomonocytic leukemia with failed remission
     Acute myelomonocytic leukemia NOS

   C92.51   Acute myelomonocytic leukemia, in remission 🔖

   C92.52   Acute myelomonocytic leukemia, in relapse 🔖

● **C92.6**   Acute myeloid leukemia with 11q23-abnormality
    Acute myeloid leukemia with variation of MLL-gene

   C92.60   Acute myeloid leukemia with 11q23-abnormality not having achieved remission 🔖
     Acute myeloid leukemia with 11q23-abnormality with failed remission
     Acute myeloid leukemia with 11q23-abnormality NOS

   C92.61   Acute myeloid leukemia with 11q23-abnormality in remission 🔖

   C92.62   Acute myeloid leukemia with 11q23-abnormality in relapse 🔖

● **C92.A**   Acute myeloid leukemia with multilineage dysplasia
    Acute myeloid leukemia with dysplasia of remaining hematopoesis and/or myelodysplastic disease in its history

   C92.A0   Acute myeloid leukemia with multilineage dysplasia, not having achieved remission 🔖
     Acute myeloid leukemia with multilineage dysplasia with failed remission
     Acute myeloid leukemia with multilineage dysplasia NOS

   C92.A1   Acute myeloid leukemia with multilineage dysplasia, in remission 🔖

   C92.A2   Acute myeloid leukemia with multilineage dysplasia, in relapse 🔖

● **C92.Z**   Other myeloid leukemia

   C92.Z0   Other myeloid leukemia not having achieved remission 🔖
     Myeloid leukemia NEC with failed remission
     Myeloid leukemia NEC

   C92.Z1   Other myeloid leukemia, in remission 🔖

   C92.Z2   Other myeloid leukemia, in relapse 🔖

● **C92.9**   Myeloid leukemia, unspecified

   C92.90   Myeloid leukemia, unspecified, not having achieved remission 🔖
     Myeloid leukemia, unspecified with failed remission
     Myeloid leukemia, unspecified NOS

   C92.91   Myeloid leukemia, unspecified in remission 🔖

   C92.92   Myeloid leukemia, unspecified in relapse 🔖

● **C93**   Monocytic leukemia
   Includes   monocytoid leukemia
   Excludes1   personal history of leukemia (Z85.6)

● **C93.0**   Acute monoblastic/monocytic leukemia
    AML M5
    AML M5a
    AML M5b

   C93.00   Acute monoblastic/monocytic leukemia, not having achieved remission 🔖
     Acute monoblastic/monocytic leukemia with failed remission
     Acute monoblastic/monocytic leukemia NOS

   C93.01   Acute monoblastic/monocytic leukemia, in remission 🔖

   C93.02   Acute monoblastic/monocytic leukemia, in relapse 🔖

● **C93.1**   Chronic myelomonocytic leukemia
    Chronic monocytic leukemia
    CMML-1
    CMML-2
    CMML with eosinophilia
    Code also, if applicable, eosinophilia (D72.18)

   C93.10   Chronic myelomonocytic leukemia not having achieved remission 🔖
     Chronic myelomonocytic leukemia with failed remission
     Chronic myelomonocytic leukemia NOS

   C93.11   Chronic myelomonocytic leukemia, in remission 🔖

   C93.12   Chronic myelomonocytic leukemia, in relapse 🔖

● **C93.3**   Juvenile myelomonocytic leukemia

   C93.30   Juvenile myelomonocytic leukemia, not having achieved remission 🔖   P
     Juvenile myelomonocytic leukemia with failed remission
     Juvenile myelomonocytic leukemia NOS

   C93.31   Juvenile myelomonocytic leukemia, in remission 🔖   P

   C93.32   Juvenile myelomonocytic leukemia, in relapse 🔖   P

● **C93.Z**   Other monocytic leukemia

   C93.Z0   Other monocytic leukemia, not having achieved remission 🔖
     Other monocytic leukemia NOS

   C93.Z1   Other monocytic leukemia, in remission 🔖

   C93.Z2   Other monocytic leukemia, in relapse 🔖

● **C93.9**   Monocytic leukemia, unspecified

   C93.90   Monocytic leukemia, unspecified, not having achieved remission 🔖
     Monocytic leukemia, unspecified with failed remission
     Monocytic leukemia, unspecified NOS

   C93.91   Monocytic leukemia, unspecified in remission 🔖

   C93.92   Monocytic leukemia, unspecified in relapse 🔖

● **C94**   Other leukemias of specified cell type
   Excludes1   leukemic reticuloendotheliosis (C91.4-)
     myelodysplastic syndromes (D46.-)
     personal history of leukemia (Z85.6)
     plasma cell leukemia (C90.1-)

● **C94.0**   Acute erythroid leukemia
    Acute myeloid leukemia M6(a)(b)
    Erythroleukemia

   C94.00   Acute erythroid leukemia, not having achieved remission 🔖
     Acute erythroid leukemia with failed remission
     Acute erythroid leukemia NOS

   C94.01   Acute erythroid leukemia, in remission 🔖

   C94.02   Acute erythroid leukemia, in relapse 🔖

● **C94.2 Acute megakaryoblastic leukemia**
　　Acute myeloid leukemia M7
　　Acute megakaryocytic leukemia

　　C94.20 Acute megakaryoblastic leukemia not having achieved remission 🔖
　　　　Acute megakaryoblastic leukemia with failed remission
　　　　Acute megakaryoblastic leukemia NOS

　　C94.21 Acute megakaryoblastic leukemia, in remission 🔖

　　C94.22 Acute megakaryoblastic leukemia, in relapse 🔖

● **C94.3 Mast cell leukemia**

　　C94.30 Mast cell leukemia not having achieved remission 🔖
　　　　Mast cell leukemia with failed remission
　　　　Mast cell leukemia NOS

　　C94.31 Mast cell leukemia, in remission 🔖

　　C94.32 Mast cell leukemia, in relapse 🔖

● **C94.4 Acute panmyelosis with myelofibrosis**
　　Acute myelofibrosis

　　Excludes1 myelofibrosis NOS (D75.81)
　　　　secondary myelofibrosis NOS (D75.81)

　　C94.40 Acute panmyelosis with myelofibrosis not having achieved remission 🔖
　　　　Acute myelofibrosis NOS
　　　　Acute panmyelosis with myelofibrosis with failed remission
　　　　Acute panmyelosis NOS

　　C94.41 Acute panmyelosis with myelofibrosis, in remission 🔖

　　C94.42 Acute panmyelosis with myelofibrosis, in relapse 🔖

⫸ **C94.6 Myelodysplastic disease, not elsewhere classified** 🔖
　　~~Myeloproliferative disease, not classified~~
　　▶Myelodysplastic/myeloproliferative neoplasm, unclassifiable
　　▶Myeloproliferative disease, not elsewhere classified

● **C94.8 Other specified leukemias**
　　Aggressive NK-cell leukemia
　　Acute basophilic leukemia

　　C94.80 Other specified leukemias not having achieved remission 🔖
　　　　Other specified leukemia with failed remission
　　　　Other specified leukemias NOS

　　C94.81 Other specified leukemias, in remission 🔖

　　C94.82 Other specified leukemias, in relapse 🔖

● **C95 Leukemia of unspecified cell type**

　　Excludes1 personal history of leukemia (Z85.6)

● **C95.0 Acute leukemia of unspecified cell type**
　　Acute bilineal leukemia
　　Acute mixed lineage leukemia
　　Biphenotypic acute leukemia
　　Stem cell leukemia of unclear lineage

　　Excludes1 acute exacerbation of unspecified chronic leukemia (C95.10)

　　C95.00 Acute leukemia of unspecified cell type not having achieved remission 🔖
　　　　Acute leukemia of unspecified cell type with failed remission
　　　　Acute leukemia NOS

　　C95.01 Acute leukemia of unspecified cell type, in remission 🔖

　　C95.02 Acute leukemia of unspecified cell type, in relapse 🔖

● **C95.1 Chronic leukemia of unspecified cell type**

　　C95.10 Chronic leukemia of unspecified cell type not having achieved remission 🔖
　　　　Chronic leukemia of unspecified cell type with failed remission
　　　　Chronic leukemia NOS

　　C95.11 Chronic leukemia of unspecified cell type, in remission 🔖

　　C95.12 Chronic leukemia of unspecified cell type, in relapse 🔖

● **C95.9 Leukemia, unspecified**

　　C95.90 Leukemia, unspecified not having achieved remission 🔖
　　　　Leukemia, unspecified with failed remission
　　　　Leukemia NOS

　　C95.91 Leukemia, unspecified, in remission 🔖

　　C95.92 Leukemia, unspecified, in relapse 🔖

● **C96 Other and unspecified malignant neoplasms of lymphoid, hematopoietic and related tissue**

　　Excludes1 personal history of other malignant neoplasms of lymphoid, hematopoietic and related tissues (Z85.79)

● **C96.0 Multifocal and multisystemic (disseminated) Langerhans-cell histiocytosis** 🔖
　　Histiocytosis X, multisystemic
　　Letterer-Siwe disease

　　Excludes1 adult pulmonary Langerhans cell histiocytosis (J84.82)
　　　　multifocal and unisystemic Langerhans-cell histiocytosis (C96.5)
　　　　unifocal Langerhans-cell histiocytosis (C96.6)

● **C96.2 Malignant mast cell neoplasm**

　　Excludes1 indolent mastocytosis (D47.02)
　　　　mast cell leukemia (C94.30)
　　　　mastocytosis (congenital) (cutaneous) (Q82.2)

　　C96.20 Malignant mast cell neoplasm, unspecified 🔖

　　C96.21 Aggressive systemic mastocytosis 🔖

　　C96.22 Mast cell sarcoma 🔖

　　C96.29 Other malignant mast cell neoplasm 🔖

● **C96.4 Sarcoma of dendritic cells (accessory cells)** 🔖
　　Follicular dendritic cell sarcoma
　　Interdigitating dendritic cell sarcoma
　　Langerhans cell sarcoma

● **C96.5 Multifocal and unisystemic Langerhans-cell histiocytosis** 🔖
　　Hand-Schüller-Christian disease
　　Histiocytosis X, multifocal

　　Excludes1 multifocal and multisystemic (disseminated) Langerhans-cell histiocytosis (C96.0)
　　　　unifocal Langerhans-cell histiocytosis (C96.6)

● **C96.6 Unifocal Langerhans-cell histiocytosis** 🔖
　　Eosinophilic granuloma
　　Histiocytosis X, unifocal
　　Histiocytosis X NOS
　　Langerhans-cell histiocytosis NOS

　　Excludes1 multifocal and multisysemic (disseminated) Langerhans-cell histiocytosis (C96.0)
　　　　multifocal and unisystemic Langerhans-cell histiocytosis (C96.5)

● **C96.A Histiocytic sarcoma** 🔖
　　Malignant histiocytosis

● **C96.Z Other specified malignant neoplasms of lymphoid, hematopoietic and related tissue** 🔖

● **C96.9 Malignant neoplasm of lymphoid, hematopoietic and related tissue, unspecified** 🔖

CHAPTER 2 (C00–D49)

IN SITU NEOPLASMS (D00-D09)

In situ is carcinoma involving cells in localized tissues that has not spread to nearby tissues

Includes	Bowen's disease
	erythroplasia
	grade III intraepithelial neoplasia
	Queyrat's erythroplasia

● **D00 Carcinoma in situ of oral cavity, esophagus and stomach**

Excludes1   melanoma in situ (D03.-)

● **D00.0 Carcinoma in situ of lip, oral cavity and pharynx**

Use additional code to identify:
exposure to environmental tobacco smoke (Z77.22)
exposure to tobacco smoke in the perinatal period (P96.81)
history of tobacco dependence (Z87.891)
occupational exposure to environmental tobacco smoke (Z57.31)
tobacco dependence (F17.-)
tobacco use (Z72.0)

Excludes1   carcinoma in situ of aryepiglottic fold or interarytenoid fold, laryngeal aspect (D02.0)
carcinoma in situ of epiglottis NOS (D02.0)
carcinoma in situ of epiglottis suprahyoid portion (D02.0)
carcinoma in situ of skin of lip (D03.0, D04.0)

D00.00 Carcinoma in situ of oral cavity, unspecified site

D00.01 Carcinoma in situ of labial mucosa and vermilion border

D00.02 Carcinoma in situ of buccal mucosa

D00.03 Carcinoma in situ of gingiva and edentulous alveolar ridge

D00.04 Carcinoma in situ of soft palate

D00.05 Carcinoma in situ of hard palate

D00.06 Carcinoma in situ of floor of mouth

D00.07 Carcinoma in situ of tongue

D00.08 Carcinoma in situ of pharynx
Carcinoma in situ of aryepiglottic fold NOS
Carcinoma in situ of hypopharyngeal aspect of aryepiglottic fold
Carcinoma in situ of marginal zone of aryepiglottic fold

D00.1 Carcinoma in situ of esophagus

D00.2 Carcinoma in situ of stomach

● **D01 Carcinoma in situ of other and unspecified digestive organs**

Excludes1   melanoma in situ (D03.-)

D01.0 Carcinoma in situ of colon

Excludes1   carcinoma in situ of rectosigmoid junction (D01.1)

D01.1 Carcinoma in situ of rectosigmoid junction

D01.2 Carcinoma in situ of rectum

D01.3 Carcinoma in situ of anus and anal canal
Anal intraepithelial neoplasia III [AIN III]
Severe dysplasia of anus

Excludes1   anal intraepithelial neoplasia I and II [AIN I and AIN II] (K62.82)
carcinoma in situ of anal margin (D04.5)
carcinoma in situ of anal skin (D04.5)
carcinoma in situ of perianal skin (D04.5)

● **D01.4 Carcinoma in situ of other and unspecified parts of intestine**

Excludes1   carcinoma in situ of ampulla of Vater (D01.5)

D01.40 Carcinoma in situ of unspecified part of intestine

D01.49 Carcinoma in situ of other parts of intestine

D01.5 Carcinoma in situ of liver, gallbladder and bile ducts
Carcinoma in situ of ampulla of Vater

D01.7 Carcinoma in situ of other specified digestive organs
Carcinoma in situ of pancreas

D01.9 Carcinoma in situ of digestive organ, unspecified

● **D02 Carcinoma in situ of middle ear and respiratory system**

Use additional code to identify:
exposure to environmental tobacco smoke (Z77.22)
exposure to tobacco smoke in the perinatal period (P96.81)
history of tobacco dependence (Z87.891)
occupational exposure to environmental tobacco smoke (Z57.31)
tobacco dependence (F17.-)
tobacco use (Z72.0)

Excludes1   melanoma in situ (D03.-)

D02.0 Carcinoma in situ of larynx
Carcinoma in situ of aryepiglottic fold or interarytenoid fold, laryngeal aspect
Carcinoma in situ of epiglottis (suprahyoid portion)

Excludes1   carcinoma in situ of aryepiglottic fold or interarytenoid fold NOS (D00.08)
carcinoma in situ of hypopharyngeal aspect (D00.08)
carcinoma in situ of marginal zone (D00.08)

D02.1 Carcinoma in situ of trachea

● **D02.2 Carcinoma in situ of bronchus and lung**

D02.20 Carcinoma in situ of unspecified bronchus and lung

D02.21 Carcinoma in situ of right bronchus and lung

D02.22 Carcinoma in situ of left bronchus and lung

D02.3 Carcinoma in situ of other parts of respiratory system
Carcinoma in situ of accessory sinuses
Carcinoma in situ of middle ear
Carcinoma in situ of nasal cavities

Excludes1   carcinoma in situ of ear (external) (skin) (D04.2-)
carcinoma in situ of nose NOS (D09.8)
carcinoma in situ of skin of nose (D04.3)

D02.4 Carcinoma in situ of respiratory system, unspecified

● **D03 Melanoma in situ**

D03.0 Melanoma in situ of lip 🐾

● **D03.1 Melanoma in situ of eyelid, including canthus**

D03.10 Melanoma in situ of unspecified eyelid, including canthus 🐾

● **D03.11 Melanoma in situ of right eyelid, including canthus** 🐾

D03.111 Melanoma in situ of right upper eyelid, including canthus 🐾

D03.112 Melanoma in situ of right lower eyelid, including canthus 🐾

● **D03.12 Melanoma in situ of left eyelid, including canthus** 🐾

D03.121 Melanoma in situ of left upper eyelid, including canthus 🐾

D03.122 Melanoma in situ of left lower eyelid, including canthus 🐾

● **D03.2 Melanoma in situ of ear and external auricular canal**

D03.20 Melanoma in situ of unspecified ear and external auricular canal 🐾

D03.21 Melanoma in situ of right ear and external auricular canal 🐾

D03.22 Melanoma in situ of left ear and external auricular canal 🐾

● **D03.3 Melanoma in situ of other and unspecified parts of face**

D03.30 Melanoma in situ of unspecified part of face 🐾

D03.39 Melanoma in situ of other parts of face 🐾

D03.4 Melanoma in situ of scalp and neck 🐾

- **D03.5 Melanoma in situ of trunk**
  - **D03.51 Melanoma in situ of anal skin** 🔖
    - Melanoma in situ of anal margin
    - Melanoma in situ of perianal skin
  - **D03.52 Melanoma in situ of breast (skin) (soft tissue)** 🔖
  - **D03.59 Melanoma in situ of other part of trunk** 🔖
- **D03.6 Melanoma in situ of upper limb, including shoulder**
  - **D03.60 Melanoma in situ of unspecified upper limb, including shoulder** 🔖
  - **D03.61 Melanoma in situ of right upper limb, including shoulder** 🔖
  - **D03.62 Melanoma in situ of left upper limb, including shoulder** 🔖
- **D03.7 Melanoma in situ of lower limb, including hip**
  - **D03.70 Melanoma in situ of unspecified lower limb, including hip** 🔖
  - **D03.71 Melanoma in situ of right lower limb, including hip** 🔖
  - **D03.72 Melanoma in situ of left lower limb, including hip** 🔖
- **D03.8 Melanoma in situ of other sites** 🔖
  - Melanoma in situ of scrotum
  - **Excludes1** carcinoma in situ of scrotum (D07.61)
- **D03.9 Melanoma in situ, unspecified** 🔖

- **D04 Carcinoma in situ of skin**
  - **Excludes1** erythroplasia of Queyrat (penis) NOS (D07.4)
    melanoma in situ (D03.-)
  - **D04.0 Carcinoma in situ of skin of lip**
  - **Excludes2** carcinoma in situ of vermilion border of lip (D00.01)
  - **D04.1 Carcinoma in situ of skin of eyelid, including canthus**
    - **D04.10 Carcinoma in situ of skin of unspecified eyelid, including canthus**
    - **D04.11 Carcinoma in situ of skin of right eyelid, including canthus**
      - **D04.111 Carcinoma in situ of skin of right upper eyelid, including canthus**
      - **D04.112 Carcinoma in situ of skin of right lower eyelid, including canthus**
    - **D04.12 Carcinoma in situ of skin of left eyelid, including canthus**
      - **D04.121 Carcinoma in situ of skin of left upper eyelid, including canthus**
      - **D04.122 Carcinoma in situ of skin of left lower eyelid, including canthus**
  - **D04.2 Carcinoma in situ of skin of ear and external auricular canal**
    - **D04.20 Carcinoma in situ of skin of unspecified ear and external auricular canal**
    - **D04.21 Carcinoma in situ of skin of right ear and external auricular canal**
    - **D04.22 Carcinoma in situ of skin of left ear and external auricular canal**
  - **D04.3 Carcinoma in situ of skin of other and unspecified parts of face**
    - **D04.30 Carcinoma in situ of skin of unspecified part of face**
    - **D04.39 Carcinoma in situ of skin of other parts of face**
  - **D04.4 Carcinoma in situ of skin of scalp and neck**
  - **D04.5 Carcinoma in situ of skin of trunk**
    - Carcinoma in situ of anal margin
    - Carcinoma in situ of anal skin
    - Carcinoma in situ of perianal skin
    - Carcinoma in situ of skin of breast
    - **Excludes1** carcinoma in situ of anus NOS (D01.3)
      carcinoma in situ of scrotum (D07.61)
      carcinoma in situ of skin of genital organs (D07.-)

- **D04.6 Carcinoma in situ of skin of upper limb, including shoulder**
  - **D04.60 Carcinoma in situ of skin of unspecified upper limb, including shoulder**
  - **D04.61 Carcinoma in situ of skin of right upper limb, including shoulder**
  - **D04.62 Carcinoma in situ of skin of left upper limb, including shoulder**
- **D04.7 Carcinoma in situ of skin of lower limb, including hip**
  - **D04.70 Carcinoma in situ of skin of unspecified lower limb, including hip**
  - **D04.71 Carcinoma in situ of skin of right lower limb, including hip**
  - **D04.72 Carcinoma in situ of skin of left lower limb, including hip**
  - **D04.8 Carcinoma in situ of skin of other sites**
  - **D04.9 Carcinoma in situ of skin, unspecified**

- **D05 Carcinoma in situ of breast**
  - **Excludes1** carcinoma in situ of skin of breast (D04.5)
    melanoma in situ of breast (skin) (D03.5)
    Paget's disease of breast or nipple (C50.-)
  - **D05.0 Lobular carcinoma in situ of breast**
    - **D05.00 Lobular carcinoma in situ of unspecified breast**
    - **D05.01 Lobular carcinoma in situ of right breast**
    - **D05.02 Lobular carcinoma in situ of left breast**
  - **D05.1 Intraductal carcinoma in situ of breast**
    - **D05.10 Intraductal carcinoma in situ of unspecified breast**
    - **D05.11 Intraductal carcinoma in situ of right breast**
    - **D05.12 Intraductal carcinoma in situ of left breast**
  - **D05.8 Other specified type of carcinoma in situ of breast**
    - **D05.80 Other specified type of carcinoma in situ of unspecified breast**
    - **D05.81 Other specified type of carcinoma in situ of right breast**
    - **D05.82 Other specified type of carcinoma in situ of left breast**
  - **D05.9 Unspecified type of carcinoma in situ of breast**
    - **D05.90 Unspecified type of carcinoma in situ of unspecified breast**
    - **D05.91 Unspecified type of carcinoma in situ of right breast**
    - **D05.92 Unspecified type of carcinoma in situ of left breast**

- **D06 Carcinoma in situ of cervix uteri**
  - **Includes** cervical adenocarcinoma in situ
    cervical intraepithelial glandular neoplasia
    cervical intraepithelial neoplasia III [CIN III]
    severe dysplasia of cervix uteri
  - **Excludes1** cervical intraepithelial neoplasia II [CIN II] (N87.1)
    cytologic evidence of malignancy of cervix without histologic confirmation (R87.614)
    high grade squamous intraepithelial lesion (HGSIL) of cervix (R87.613)
    melanoma in situ of cervix (D03.5)
    moderate cervical dysplasia (N87.1)
  - **D06.0 Carcinoma in situ of endocervix** ♀
  - **D06.1 Carcinoma in situ of exocervix** ♀
  - **D06.7 Carcinoma in situ of other parts of cervix** ♀
  - **D06.9 Carcinoma in situ of cervix, unspecified** ♀

CHAPTER 2 (C00-D49)

● **D07 Carcinoma in situ of other and unspecified genital organs**
> **Excludes1**   melanoma in situ of trunk (D03.5)

D07.0 Carcinoma in situ of endometrium ♀

D07.1 Carcinoma in situ of vulva ♀
Severe dysplasia of vulva
Vulvar intraepithelial neoplasia III [VIN III]
> **Excludes1**   moderate dysplasia of vulva (N90.1)
> vulvar intraepithelial neoplasia II [VIN II] (N90.1)

D07.2 Carcinoma in situ of vagina ♀
Severe dysplasia of vagina
Vaginal intraepithelial neoplasia III [VIN III]
> **Excludes1**   moderate dysplasia of vagina (N89.1)
> vaginal intraepithelial neoplasia II [VIN II] (N89.1)

● **D07.3 Carcinoma in situ of other and unspecified female genital organs**

     D07.30 Carcinoma in situ of unspecified female genital organs ♀

     D07.39 Carcinoma in situ of other female genital organs ♀

D07.4 Carcinoma in situ of penis ♂
Erythroplasia of Queyrat NOS

D07.5 Carcinoma in situ of prostate ♂
Prostatic intraepithelial neoplasia III (PIN III)
Severe dysplasia of prostate
> **Excludes1**   dysplasia (mild) (moderate) of prostate (N42.3-)
> prostatic intraepithelial neoplasia II [PIN II] (N42.3-)

● **D07.6 Carcinoma in situ of other and unspecified male genital organs**

     D07.60 Carcinoma in situ of unspecified male genital organs ♂

     D07.61 Carcinoma in situ of scrotum ♂

     D07.69 Carcinoma in situ of other male genital organs ♂

● **D09 Carcinoma in situ of other and unspecified sites**
> **Excludes1**   melanoma in situ (D03.-)

D09.0 Carcinoma in situ of bladder

● **D09.1 Carcinoma in situ of other and unspecified urinary organs**

     D09.10 Carcinoma in situ of unspecified urinary organ

     D09.19 Carcinoma in situ of other urinary organs

● **D09.2 Carcinoma in situ of eye**
> **Excludes1**   carcinoma in situ of skin of eyelid (D04.1-)

     D09.20 Carcinoma in situ of unspecified eye

     D09.21 Carcinoma in situ of right eye

     D09.22 Carcinoma in situ of left eye

D09.3 Carcinoma in situ of thyroid and other endocrine glands
> **Excludes1**   carcinoma in situ of endocrine pancreas (D01.7)
> carcinoma in situ of ovary (D07.39)
> carcinoma in situ of testis (D07.69)

D09.8 Carcinoma in situ of other specified sites

D09.9 Carcinoma in situ, unspecified

Figure 2-16 The esophagus is the muscular tube that connects the pharynx and the stomach. The 10 inch (25 cm) long esophagus is divided into three parts: **cervical, thoracic,** and **abdominal.**

BENIGN NEOPLASMS, EXCEPT BENIGN NEUROENDOCRINE TUMORS (D10-D36)

● **D10 Benign neoplasm of mouth and pharynx**

D10.0 Benign neoplasm of lip
Benign neoplasm of lip (frenulum) (inner aspect) (mucosa) (vermilion border)
> **Excludes1**   benign neoplasm of skin of lip (D22.0, D23.0)

D10.1 Benign neoplasm of tongue
Benign neoplasm of lingual tonsil

D10.2 Benign neoplasm of floor of mouth

● **D10.3 Benign neoplasm of other and unspecified parts of mouth**

     D10.30 Benign neoplasm of unspecified part of mouth

     D10.39 Benign neoplasm of other parts of mouth
Benign neoplasm of minor salivary gland NOS
> **Excludes1**   benign odontogenic neoplasms (D16.4-D16.5)
> benign neoplasm of mucosa of lip (D10.0)
> benign neoplasm of nasopharyngeal surface of soft palate (D10.6)

D10.4 Benign neoplasm of tonsil
Benign neoplasm of tonsil (faucial) (palatine)
> **Excludes1**   benign neoplasm of lingual tonsil (D10.1)
> benign neoplasm of pharyngeal tonsil (D10.6)
> benign neoplasm of tonsillar fossa (D10.5)
> benign neoplasm of tonsillar pillars (D10.5)

D10.5 Benign neoplasm of other parts of oropharynx
Division of pharynx lying between soft palate and upper edge of epiglottis
Benign neoplasm of epiglottis, anterior aspect
Benign neoplasm of tonsillar fossa
Benign neoplasm of tonsillar pillars
Benign neoplasm of vallecula
> **Excludes1**   benign neoplasm of epiglottis NOS (D14.1)
> benign neoplasm of epiglottis, suprahyoid portion (D14.1)

D10.6 Benign neoplasm of nasopharynx
Segment of pharynx that lies above soft palate
Benign neoplasm of pharyngeal tonsil
Benign neoplasm of posterior margin of septum and choanae

D10.7 **Benign neoplasm of hypopharynx**
Segment of pharynx that lies below upper edge of epiglottis and opens into larynx and esophagus

D10.9 **Benign neoplasm of pharynx, unspecified**

● **D11** **Benign neoplasm of major salivary glands**

     Excludes1   benign neoplasms of specified minor salivary glands which are classified according to their anatomical location
           benign neoplasms of minor salivary glands NOS (D10.39)

D11.0 **Benign neoplasm of parotid gland**

D11.7 **Benign neoplasm of other major salivary glands**
Benign neoplasm of sublingual salivary gland
Benign neoplasm of submandibular salivary gland

D11.9 **Benign neoplasm of major salivary gland, unspecified**

● **D12** **Benign neoplasm of colon, rectum, anus and anal canal**

     Excludes1   benign carcinoid tumors of the large intestine, and rectum (D3A.02-)
           polyp of colon NOS (K63.5)

Coding Clinic: 2017, Q1, P15; 2015, Q2, P14

D12.0 **Benign neoplasm of cecum**
Benign neoplasm of ileocecal valve

D12.1 **Benign neoplasm of appendix**

     Excludes1   benign carcinoid tumor of the appendix (D3A.020)

D12.2 **Benign neoplasm of ascending colon**
Coding Clinic: 2018, Q2, P14; 2017, Q1, P15

D12.3 **Benign neoplasm of transverse colon**
Benign neoplasm of hepatic flexure
Benign neoplasm of splenic flexure
Flexure is a bending in a structure or organ. Note the three flexures illustrated in Figure 2–17. Hepatic = liver, sigmoid = colon, splenic = spleen.
Coding Clinic: 2017, Q1, P16

D12.4 **Benign neoplasm of descending colon**
Coding Clinic: 2015, Q2, P14

D12.5 **Benign neoplasm of sigmoid colon**

D12.6 **Benign neoplasm of colon, unspecified**
Adenomatosis of colon
Benign neoplasm of large intestine NOS
Polyposis (hereditary) of colon

     Excludes1   inflammatory polyp of colon (K51.4-)
Coding Clinic: 2017, Q1, P8-9

D12.7 **Benign neoplasm of rectosigmoid junction**
Angle where sigmoid colon becomes rectum

D12.8 **Benign neoplasm of rectum**

     Excludes1   benign carcinoid tumor of the rectum (D3A.026)
Coding Clinic: 2018, Q1, P7

D12.9 **Benign neoplasm of anus and anal canal**
Benign neoplasm of anus NOS

     Excludes1   benign neoplasm of anal margin (D22.5, D23.5)
           benign neoplasm of anal skin (D22.5, D23.5)
           benign neoplasm of perianal skin (D22.5, D23.5)

● **D13** **Benign neoplasm of other and ill-defined parts of digestive system**

     Excludes1   benign stromal tumors of digestive system (D21.4)

D13.0 **Benign neoplasm of esophagus**

D13.1 **Benign neoplasm of stomach**

     Excludes1   benign carcinoid tumor of the stomach (D3A.092)

D13.2 **Benign neoplasm of duodenum**

     Excludes1   benign carcinoid tumor of the duodenum (D3A.010)

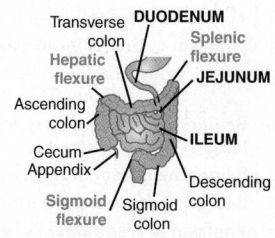

Figure 2-17   Small intestine and colon.

● **D13.3** **Benign neoplasm of other and unspecified parts of small intestine**

     Excludes1   benign carcinoid tumors of the small intestine (D3A.01-)
           benign neoplasm of ileocecal valve (D12.0)

D13.30 **Benign neoplasm of unspecified part of small intestine**

D13.39 **Benign neoplasm of other parts of small intestine**

D13.4 **Benign neoplasm of liver**
Benign neoplasm of intrahepatic bile ducts

D13.5 **Benign neoplasm of extrahepatic bile ducts**
Extensions of common hepatic bile duct (tube that collects bile from liver)

D13.6 **Benign neoplasm of pancreas**

     Excludes1   benign neoplasm of endocrine pancreas (D13.7)

D13.7 **Benign neoplasm of endocrine pancreas**
Pancreatic islets: Cells scattered throughout pancreas
Islet cell tumor
Benign neoplasm of islets of Langerhans

     Use additional code to identify any functional activity.

D13.9 **Benign neoplasm of ill-defined sites within the digestive system**
Benign neoplasm of digestive system NOS
Benign neoplasm of intestine NOS
Benign neoplasm of spleen

● **D14** **Benign neoplasm of middle ear and respiratory system**

D14.0 **Benign neoplasm of middle ear, nasal cavity and accessory sinuses**
Benign neoplasm of cartilage of nose

     Excludes1   benign neoplasm of auricular canal (external) (D22.2-, D23.2-)
           benign neoplasm of bone of ear (D16.4)
           benign neoplasm of bone of nose (D16.4)
           benign neoplasm of cartilage of ear (D21.0)
           benign neoplasm of ear (external) (skin) (D22.2-, D23.2-)
           benign neoplasm of nose NOS (D36.7)
           benign neoplasm of skin of nose (D22.39, D23.39)
           benign neoplasm of olfactory bulb (D33.3)
           benign neoplasm of posterior margin of septum and choanae (D10.6)
           polyp of accessory sinus (J33.8)
           polyp of ear (middle) (H74.4)
           polyp of nasal (cavity) (J33.-)

D14.1 **Benign neoplasm of larynx**
Adenomatous polyp of larynx
Benign neoplasm of epiglottis (suprahyoid portion)
Horseshoe-shaped bone in anterior midline of neck between chin and thyroid cartilage

     Excludes1   benign neoplasm of epiglottis, anterior aspect (D10.5)
           polyp (nonadenomatous) of vocal cord or larynx (J38.1)

CHAPTER 2 (C00-D49)

D14.2   Benign neoplasm of trachea

● D14.3   Benign neoplasm of bronchus and lung

Excludes1   benign carcinoid tumor of the bronchus
              and lung (D3A.090)

   D14.30   Benign neoplasm of unspecified bronchus and
             lung

   D14.31   Benign neoplasm of right bronchus and lung

   D14.32   Benign neoplasm of left bronchus and lung

D14.4   Benign neoplasm of respiratory system, unspecified

● D15   Benign neoplasm of other and unspecified intrathoracic organs

Excludes1   benign neoplasm of mesothelial tissue (D19.-)

D15.0   Benign neoplasm of thymus

Excludes1   benign carcinoid tumor of the thymus
              (D3A.091)

D15.1   Benign neoplasm of heart

Excludes1   benign neoplasm of great vessels (D21.3)

D15.2   Benign neoplasm of mediastinum

D15.7   Benign neoplasm of other specified intrathoracic organs

D15.9   Benign neoplasm of intrathoracic organ, unspecified

● D16   Benign neoplasm of bone and articular cartilage

Excludes1   benign neoplasm of connective tissue of ear
              (D21.0)
              benign neoplasm of connective tissue of eyelid
              (D21.0)
              benign neoplasm of connective tissue of larynx
              (D14.1)
              benign neoplasm of connective tissue of nose
              (D14.0)
              benign neoplasm of synovia (D21.-)

● D16.0   Benign neoplasm of scapula and long bones of upper
          limb

   D16.00   Benign neoplasm of scapula and long bones
             of unspecified upper limb

   D16.01   Benign neoplasm of scapula and long bones of
             right upper limb

   D16.02   Benign neoplasm of scapula and long bones of
             left upper limb

● D16.1   Benign neoplasm of short bones of upper limb

   D16.10   Benign neoplasm of short bones of unspecified
             upper limb

   D16.11   Benign neoplasm of short bones of right upper
             limb

   D16.12   Benign neoplasm of short bones of left upper
             limb

● D16.2   Benign neoplasm of long bones of lower limb

   D16.20   Benign neoplasm of long bones of unspecified
             lower limb

   D16.21   Benign neoplasm of long bones of right lower
             limb

   D16.22   Benign neoplasm of long bones of left lower
             limb

● D16.3   Benign neoplasm of short bones of lower limb

   D16.30   Benign neoplasm of short bones of unspecified
             lower limb

   D16.31   Benign neoplasm of short bones of right lower
             limb

   D16.32   Benign neoplasm of short bones of left lower
             limb

D16.4   Benign neoplasm of bones of skull and face
         Benign neoplasm of maxilla (superior)
         Benign neoplasm of orbital bone
         *Cavity or socket of skull in which eye and its appendages
         are located*
         Keratocyst of maxilla
         Keratocystic odontogenic tumor of maxilla

Excludes2   benign neoplasm of lower jaw bone
              (D16.5)

D16.5   Benign neoplasm of lower jaw bone
         Keratocyst of mandible
         Keratocystic odontogenic tumor of mandible

D16.6   Benign neoplasm of vertebral column

Excludes1   benign neoplasm of sacrum and coccyx
              (D16.8)

D16.7   Benign neoplasm of ribs, sternum and clavicle

D16.8   Benign neoplasm of pelvic bones, sacrum and coccyx

D16.9   Benign neoplasm of bone and articular
         cartilage, unspecified

● D17   Benign lipomatous neoplasm
         *Slow-growing benign tumors (rubbery masses) of mature fat cells
         enclosed in a thin fibrous capsule*

D17.0   Benign lipomatous neoplasm of skin and subcutaneous
         tissue of head, face and neck

D17.1   Benign lipomatous neoplasm of skin and subcutaneous
         tissue of trunk

● D17.2   Benign lipomatous neoplasm of skin and subcutaneous
          tissue of limb

   D17.20   Benign lipomatous neoplasm of skin and
             subcutaneous tissue of unspecified limb

   D17.21   Benign lipomatous neoplasm of skin and
             subcutaneous tissue of right arm

   D17.22   Benign lipomatous neoplasm of skin and
             subcutaneous tissue of left arm

   D17.23   Benign lipomatous neoplasm of skin and
             subcutaneous tissue of right leg

   D17.24   Benign lipomatous neoplasm of skin and
             subcutaneous tissue of left leg

● D17.3   Benign lipomatous neoplasm of skin and subcutaneous
          tissue of other and unspecified sites

   D17.30   Benign lipomatous neoplasm of skin and
             subcutaneous tissue of unspecified sites

   D17.39   Benign lipomatous neoplasm of skin and
             subcutaneous tissue of other sites

D17.4   Benign lipomatous neoplasm of intrathoracic organs

D17.5   Benign lipomatous neoplasm of intra-abdominal organs

Excludes1   benign lipomatous neoplasm of
              peritoneum and retroperitoneum
              (D17.79)

D17.6   Benign lipomatous neoplasm of spermatic cord ♂

● D17.7   Benign lipomatous neoplasm of other sites

   D17.71   Benign lipomatous neoplasm of kidney

   D17.72   Benign lipomatous neoplasm of other
             genitourinary organ

   D17.79   Benign lipomatous neoplasm of other sites
             Benign lipomatous neoplasm of peritoneum
             Benign lipomatous neoplasm of
             retroperitoneum

D17.9   Benign lipomatous neoplasm, unspecified
         Lipoma NOS

● D18   Hemangioma and lymphangioma, any site

Excludes1   benign neoplasm of glomus jugulare (D35.6)
              blue or pigmented nevus (D22.-)
              nevus NOS (D22.-)
              vascular nevus (Q82.5)

● D18.0   Hemangioma
          Common type of vascular malformation
          Angioma NOS
          Cavernous nevus

   D18.00   Hemangioma unspecified site

   D18.01   Hemangioma of skin and subcutaneous tissue

   D18.02   Hemangioma of intracranial structures 🅗

   D18.03   Hemangioma of intra-abdominal structures

   D18.09   Hemangioma of other sites

D18.1   Lymphangioma, any site
         Coding Clinic: 2018, Q2, P13

▶ New   ⇒ Revised   ~~deleted~~ Deleted   Excludes 1   Excludes 2   Includes   Use additional   Code first   Code also   Key words

OGCR Official Guidelines   X Assign placeholder X   ● Use Additional Character(s)   ▶ Manifestation Code   🅗 Hierarchical Condition Category   **Coding Clinic**

Figure 2-18   Hemangioma of skin and subcutaneous tissue. (Getty Image)

Item 2-10   **Hemangiomas** are abnormally dense collections of dilated capillaries that occur on the skin or in internal organs. Hemangiomas are both deep and superficial and undergo a rapid growth phase when the size increases rapidly, followed by a rest phase, in which the tumor changes very little, followed by an involutional phase in which the tumor begins to and can disappear altogether. **Lymphangiomas** or cystic hygroma are benign collections of overgrown lymph vessels and, although rare, may occur anywhere but most commonly on the head and neck of children and infants. Visceral organs, lungs, and gastrointestinal tract may also be involved.

● **D19**   **Benign neoplasm of mesothelial tissue**
     Mesothelial tissue is the membrane lining several body cavities
     D19.0   Benign neoplasm of mesothelial tissue of pleura
     D19.1   Benign neoplasm of mesothelial tissue of peritoneum
     D19.7   Benign neoplasm of mesothelial tissue of other sites
     D19.9   Benign neoplasm of mesothelial tissue, unspecified
         Benign mesothelioma NOS

● **D20**   **Benign neoplasm of soft tissue of retroperitoneum and peritoneum**
     Excludes 1   benign lipomatous neoplasm of peritoneum and retroperitoneum (D17.79)
                 benign neoplasm of mesothelial tissue (D19.-)
     D20.0   Benign neoplasm of soft tissue of retroperitoneum
     D20.1   Benign neoplasm of soft tissue of peritoneum

● **D21**   **Other benign neoplasms of connective and other soft tissue**
     Includes   benign neoplasm of blood vessel
           benign neoplasm of bursa
           benign neoplasm of cartilage
           benign neoplasm of fascia
           benign neoplasm of fat
           benign neoplasm of ligament, except uterine
           benign neoplasm of lymphatic channel
           benign neoplasm of muscle
           benign neoplasm of synovia
           benign neoplasm of tendon (sheath)
           benign stromal tumors
     Excludes 1   benign neoplasm of articular cartilage (D16.-)
               benign neoplasm of cartilage of larynx (D14.1)
               benign neoplasm of cartilage of nose (D14.0)
               benign neoplasm of connective tissue of breast (D24.-)
               benign neoplasm of peripheral nerves and autonomic nervous system (D36.1-)
               benign neoplasm of peritoneum (D20.1)
               benign neoplasm of retroperitoneum (D20.0)
               benign neoplasm of uterine ligament, any (D28.2)
               benign neoplasm of vascular tissue (D18.-)
               hemangioma (D18.0-)
               lipomatous neoplasm (D17.-)
               lymphangioma (D18.1)
               uterine leiomyoma (D25.-)
     D21.0   Benign neoplasm of connective and other soft tissue of head, face and neck
         Benign neoplasm of connective tissue of ear
         Benign neoplasm of connective tissue of eyelid
         Excludes 1   benign neoplasm of connective tissue of orbit (D31.6-)

● **D21.1**   **Benign neoplasm of connective and other soft tissue of upper limb, including shoulder**
     D21.10   Benign neoplasm of connective and other soft tissue of unspecified upper limb, including shoulder
     D21.11   Benign neoplasm of connective and other soft tissue of right upper limb, including shoulder
     D21.12   Benign neoplasm of connective and other soft tissue of left upper limb, including shoulder

● **D21.2**   **Benign neoplasm of connective and other soft tissue of lower limb, including hip**
     D21.20   Benign neoplasm of connective and other soft tissue of unspecified lower limb, including hip
     D21.21   Benign neoplasm of connective and other soft tissue of right lower limb, including hip
     D21.22   Benign neoplasm of connective and other soft tissue of left lower limb, including hip

     D21.3   Benign neoplasm of connective and other soft tissue of thorax
         Benign neoplasm of axilla
         Benign neoplasm of diaphragm
         Benign neoplasm of great vessels
         Excludes 1   benign neoplasm of heart (D15.1)
                 benign neoplasm of mediastinum (D15.2)
                 benign neoplasm of thymus (D15.0)

     D21.4   Benign neoplasm of connective and other soft tissue of abdomen
         Benign stromal tumors of abdomen

     D21.5   Benign neoplasm of connective and other soft tissue of pelvis
         Excludes 1   benign neoplasm of any uterine ligament (D28.2)
                 uterine leiomyoma (D25.-)

     D21.6   Benign neoplasm of connective and other soft tissue of trunk, unspecified
         Benign neoplasm of connective and other soft tissue of back NOS

     D21.9   Benign neoplasm of connective and other soft tissue, unspecified

● **D22**   **Melanocytic nevi**
     Includes   atypical nevus
           blue hairy pigmented nevus
           nevus NOS
     D22.0   Melanocytic nevi of lip
         Skin lesions composed of nests of nevus cells with macules/papules

● **D22.1**   **Melanocytic nevi of eyelid, including canthus**
     D22.10   Melanocytic nevi of unspecified eyelid, including canthus
     ● **D22.11**   Melanocytic nevi of right eyelid, including canthus
         D22.111   Melanocytic nevi of right upper eyelid, including canthus
         D22.112   Melanocytic nevi of right lower eyelid, including canthus
     ● **D22.12**   Melanocytic nevi of left eyelid, including canthus
         D22.121   Melanocytic nevi of left upper eyelid, including canthus
         D22.122   Melanocytic nevi of left lower eyelid, including canthus

● **D22.2**   **Melanocytic nevi of ear and external auricular canal**
     D22.20   Melanocytic nevi of unspecified ear and external auricular canal
     D22.21   Melanocytic nevi of right ear and external auricular canal
     D22.22   Melanocytic nevi of left ear and external auricular canal

CHAPTER 2 (C00-D49)

CHAPTER 2 (C00-D49)

● **D22.3** Melanocytic nevi of other and unspecified parts of face
     D22.30 Melanocytic nevi of unspecified part of face
     D22.39 Melanocytic nevi of other parts of face
   D22.4 Melanocytic nevi of scalp and neck
   D22.5 Melanocytic nevi of trunk
     Melanocytic nevi of anal margin
     Melanocytic nevi of anal skin
     Melanocytic nevi of perianal skin
     Melanocytic nevi of skin of breast
● **D22.6** Melanocytic nevi of upper limb, including shoulder
     D22.60 Melanocytic nevi of unspecified upper limb, including shoulder
     D22.61 Melanocytic nevi of right upper limb, including shoulder
     D22.62 Melanocytic nevi of left upper limb, including shoulder
● **D22.7** Melanocytic nevi of lower limb, including hip
     D22.70 Melanocytic nevi of unspecified lower limb, including hip
     D22.71 Melanocytic nevi of right lower limb, including hip
     D22.72 Melanocytic nevi of left lower limb, including hip
   D22.9 Melanocytic nevi, unspecified

● **D23** **Other benign neoplasms of skin**
     Includes   benign neoplasm of hair follicles
                benign neoplasm of sebaceous glands
                benign neoplasm of sweat glands
     Excludes1   benign lipomatous neoplasms of skin (D17.0-D17.3)
     Excludes2   melanocytic nevi (D22.-)
   D23.0 Other benign neoplasm of skin of lip
     Excludes1   benign neoplasm of vermilion border of lip (D10.0)
● **D23.1** Other benign neoplasm of skin of eyelid, including canthus
     D23.10 Other benign neoplasm of skin unspecified of eyelid, including canthus
   ● **D23.11** Other benign neoplasm of skin of right eyelid, including canthus
       D23.111 Other benign neoplasm of skin of right upper eyelid, including canthus
       D23.112 Other benign neoplasm of skin of right lower eyelid, including canthus
   ● **D23.12** Other benign neoplasm of skin of left eyelid, including canthus
       D23.121 Other benign neoplasm of skin of left upper eyelid, including canthus
       D23.122 Other benign neoplasm of skin of left lower eyelid, including canthus
● **D23.2** Other benign neoplasm of skin of ear and external auricular canal
     D23.20 Other benign neoplasm of skin of unspecified ear and external auricular canal
     D23.21 Other benign neoplasm of skin of right ear and external auricular canal
     D23.22 Other benign neoplasm of skin of left ear and external auricular canal
● **D23.3** Other benign neoplasm of skin of other and unspecified parts of face
     D23.30 Other benign neoplasm of skin of unspecified part of face
     D23.39 Other benign neoplasm of skin of other parts of face
   D23.4 Other benign neoplasm of skin of scalp and neck

   D23.5 Other benign neoplasm of skin of trunk
     Other benign neoplasm of anal margin
     Other benign neoplasm of anal skin
     Other benign neoplasm of perianal skin
     Other benign neoplasm of skin of breast
     Excludes1   benign neoplasm of anus NOS (D12.9)
● **D23.6** Other benign neoplasm of skin of upper limb, including shoulder
     D23.60 Other benign neoplasm of skin of unspecified upper limb, including shoulder
     D23.61 Other benign neoplasm of skin of right upper limb, including shoulder
     D23.62 Other benign neoplasm of skin of left upper limb, including shoulder
● **D23.7** Other benign neoplasm of skin of lower limb, including hip
     D23.70 Other benign neoplasm of skin of unspecified lower limb, including hip
     D23.71 Other benign neoplasm of skin of right lower limb, including hip
     D23.72 Other benign neoplasm of skin of left lower limb, including hip
   D23.9 Other benign neoplasm of skin, unspecified

● **D24** **Benign neoplasm of breast**
     Includes   benign neoplasm of connective tissue of breast
                benign neoplasm of soft parts of breast
                fibroadenoma of breast
     Excludes2   adenofibrosis of breast (N60.2)
                benign cyst of breast (N60.-)
                benign mammary dysplasia (N60.-)
                benign neoplasm of skin of breast (D22.5, D23.5)
                fibrocystic disease of breast (N60.-)
   D24.1 Benign neoplasm of right breast
     Coding Clinic: 2017, Q1, P5
   D24.2 Benign neoplasm of left breast
   D24.9 Benign neoplasm of unspecified breast

● **D25** **Leiomyoma of uterus**
     Benign tumors or nodules of the uterine wall
     Includes   uterine fibroid
                uterine fibromyoma
                uterine myoma
   D25.0 Submucous leiomyoma of uterus ♀
   D25.1 Intramural leiomyoma of uterus ♀
     Interstitial leiomyoma of uterus
   D25.2 Subserosal leiomyoma of uterus ♀
     Subperitoneal leiomyoma of uterus
   D25.9 Leiomyoma of uterus, unspecified ♀

● **D26** **Other benign neoplasms of uterus**
   D26.0 Other benign neoplasm of cervix uteri ♀
   D26.1 Other benign neoplasm of corpus uteri ♀
   D26.7 Other benign neoplasm of other parts of uterus ♀
   D26.9 Other benign neoplasm of uterus, unspecified ♀

● **D27** **Benign neoplasm of ovary**
     Use additional code to identify any functional activity.
     Excludes2   corpus albicans cyst (N83.2-)
                corpus luteum cyst (N83.1-)
                ⇒endometrial cyst (N80.1-)
                follicular (atretic) cyst (N83.0-)
                graafian follicle cyst (N83.0-)
                ovarian cyst NEC (N83.2-)
                ovarian retention cyst (N83.2-)
   D27.0 Benign neoplasm of right ovary ♀
   D27.1 Benign neoplasm of left ovary ♀
   D27.9 Benign neoplasm of unspecified ovary ♀
     Ovarian teratoma

▶ New   ⇒ Revised   ~~deleted~~ Deleted   Excludes 1   Excludes 2   Includes   Use additional   Code first   Code also   Key words
OGCR Official Guidelines   X Assign placeholder X   ● Use Additional Character(s)   ▷ Manifestation Code   🔖 Hierarchical Condition Category   **Coding Clinic**

Item 2-11 Teratoma: terat = monster, oma = mass, tumor. Alternate terms: dermoid cyst of the ovary, ovarian teratoma. Teratomas are neoplasms and arise from germ cells (ovaries in female and testes in male) and can be benign or malignant. Teratomas have been known to contain hair, nails, and teeth, giving them a bizarre ("monster") appearance.

● **D28   Benign neoplasm of other and unspecified female genital organs**

> **Includes**   adenomatous polyp
> benign neoplasm of skin of female genital organs
> benign teratoma

> **Excludes1**   epoophoron cyst (Q50.5)
> fimbrial cyst (Q50.4)
> Gartner's duct cyst (Q52.4)
> parovarian cyst (Q50.5)

D28.0   Benign neoplasm of vulva ♀

D28.1   Benign neoplasm of vagina ♀

D28.2   Benign neoplasm of uterine tubes and ligaments ♀
> Benign neoplasm of fallopian tube
> Benign neoplasm of uterine ligament (broad) (round)

D28.7   Benign neoplasm of other specified female genital organs ♀

D28.9   Benign neoplasm of female genital organ, unspecified ♀

● **D29   Benign neoplasm of male genital organs**

> **Includes**   benign neoplasm of skin of male genital organs

D29.0   Benign neoplasm of penis ♂

D29.1   Benign neoplasm of prostate ♂
> **Excludes1**   enlarged prostate (N40.-)

● **D29.2**   Benign neoplasm of testis
> Use additional code to identify any functional activity.

D29.20   Benign neoplasm of unspecified testis ♂

D29.21   Benign neoplasm of right testis ♂

D29.22   Benign neoplasm of left testis ♂

● **D29.3**   Benign neoplasm of epididymis

D29.30   Benign neoplasm of unspecified epididymis ♂

D29.31   Benign neoplasm of right epididymis ♂

D29.32   Benign neoplasm of left epididymis ♂

D29.4   Benign neoplasm of scrotum ♂
> Benign neoplasm of skin of scrotum

D29.8   Benign neoplasm of other specified male genital organs ♂
> Benign neoplasm of seminal vesicle
> Benign neoplasm of spermatic cord
> Benign neoplasm of tunica vaginalis

D29.9   Benign neoplasm of male genital organ, unspecified ♂

● **D30   Benign neoplasm of urinary organs**

● **D30.0**   Benign neoplasm of kidney
> **Excludes1**   benign carcinoid tumor of the kidney (D3A.093)
> benign neoplasm of renal calyces (D30.1-)
> benign neoplasm of renal pelvis (D30.1-)

D30.00   Benign neoplasm of unspecified kidney

D30.01   Benign neoplasm of right kidney

D30.02   Benign neoplasm of left kidney

● **D30.1**   Benign neoplasm of renal pelvis

D30.10   Benign neoplasm of unspecified renal pelvis

D30.11   Benign neoplasm of right renal pelvis

D30.12   Benign neoplasm of left renal pelvis

● **D30.2**   Benign neoplasm of ureter
> **Excludes1**   benign neoplasm of ureteric orifice of bladder (D30.3)

D30.20   Benign neoplasm of unspecified ureter

D30.21   Benign neoplasm of right ureter

D30.22   Benign neoplasm of left ureter

D30.3   Benign neoplasm of bladder
> Benign neoplasm of ureteric orifice of bladder
> Benign neoplasm of urethral orifice of bladder

D30.4   Benign neoplasm of urethra
> **Excludes1**   benign neoplasm of urethral orifice of bladder (D30.3)

D30.8   Benign neoplasm of other specified urinary organs
> Benign neoplasm of paraurethral glands

D30.9   Benign neoplasm of urinary organ, unspecified
> Benign neoplasm of urinary system NOS

● **D31   Benign neoplasm of eye and adnexa**
> **Excludes1**   benign neoplasm of connective tissue of eyelid (D21.0)
> benign neoplasm of optic nerve (D33.3)
> benign neoplasm of skin of eyelid (D22.1-, D23.1-)

● **D31.0**   Benign neoplasm of conjunctiva

D31.00   Benign neoplasm of unspecified conjunctiva

D31.01   Benign neoplasm of right conjunctiva

D31.02   Benign neoplasm of left conjunctiva

● **D31.1**   Benign neoplasm of cornea

D31.10   Benign neoplasm of unspecified cornea

D31.11   Benign neoplasm of right cornea

D31.12   Benign neoplasm of left cornea

● **D31.2**   Benign neoplasm of retina
> **Excludes1**   dark area on retina (D49.81)
> hemangioma of retina (D49.81)
> neoplasm of unspecified behavior of retina and choroid (D49.81)
> retinal freckle (D49.81)

D31.20   Benign neoplasm of unspecified retina

D31.21   Benign neoplasm of right retina

D31.22   Benign neoplasm of left retina

● **D31.3**   Benign neoplasm of choroid

D31.30   Benign neoplasm of unspecified choroid

D31.31   Benign neoplasm of right choroid

D31.32   Benign neoplasm of left choroid

● **D31.4**   Benign neoplasm of ciliary body

D31.40   Benign neoplasm of unspecified ciliary body

D31.41   Benign neoplasm of right ciliary body

D31.42   Benign neoplasm of left ciliary body

● **D31.5**   Benign neoplasm of lacrimal gland and duct
> Benign neoplasm of lacrimal sac
> Benign neoplasm of nasolacrimal duct

D31.50   Benign neoplasm of unspecified lacrimal gland and duct

D31.51   Benign neoplasm of right lacrimal gland and duct

D31.52   Benign neoplasm of left lacrimal gland and duct

● **D31.6**   Benign neoplasm of unspecified site of orbit
> Benign neoplasm of connective tissue of orbit
> Benign neoplasm of extraocular muscle
> Benign neoplasm of peripheral nerves of orbit
> Benign neoplasm of retrobulbar tissue
> Benign neoplasm of retro-ocular tissue

> **Excludes1**   benign neoplasm of orbital bone (D16.4)

D31.60   Benign neoplasm of unspecified site of unspecified orbit

D31.61   Benign neoplasm of unspecified site of right orbit

D31.62   Benign neoplasm of unspecified site of left orbit

● **D31.9**   Benign neoplasm of unspecified part of eye
> Benign neoplasm of eyeball

D31.90   Benign neoplasm of unspecified part of unspecified eye

D31.91   Benign neoplasm of unspecified part of right eye

D31.92   Benign neoplasm of unspecified part of left eye

CHAPTER 2 (C00-D49)

● **D32** **Benign neoplasm of** meninges
    D32.0 Benign neoplasm of cerebral meninges 🐾
    D32.1 Benign neoplasm of spinal meninges 🐾
    D32.9 Benign neoplasm of meninges, unspecified 🐾
         Meningioma NOS

● **D33** **Benign neoplasm of** brain and other parts of central nervous system
    Excludes1   angioma (D18.0-)
         benign neoplasm of meninges (D32.-)
         benign neoplasm of peripheral nerves and autonomic nervous system (D36.1-)
         hemangioma (D18.0-)
         neurofibromatosis (Q85.0-)
         retro-ocular benign neoplasm (D31.6-)
    D33.0 Benign neoplasm of brain, supratentorial 🐾
         Benign neoplasm of cerebral ventricle
         Benign neoplasm of cerebrum
         Benign neoplasm of frontal lobe
         Benign neoplasm of occipital lobe
         Benign neoplasm of parietal lobe
         Benign neoplasm of temporal lobe
        Excludes1   benign neoplasm of fourth ventricle (D33.1)
    D33.1 Benign neoplasm of brain, infratentorial 🐾
         Benign neoplasm of brain stem
         Benign neoplasm of cerebellum
         Benign neoplasm of fourth ventricle
    D33.2 Benign neoplasm of brain, unspecified 🐾
    D33.3 Benign neoplasm of cranial nerves 🐾
         Benign neoplasm of olfactory bulb
    D33.4 Benign neoplasm of spinal cord 🐾
    D33.7 Benign neoplasm of other specified parts of central nervous system 🐾
    D33.9 Benign neoplasm of central nervous system, unspecified 🐾
         Benign neoplasm of nervous system (central) NOS

D34 **Benign neoplasm of** thyroid gland
     Use additional code to identify any functional activity.

● **D35** **Benign neoplasm of** other and unspecified endocrine glands
     Use additional code to identify any functional activity.
    Excludes1   benign neoplasm of endocrine pancreas (D13.7)
         benign neoplasm of ovary (D27.-)
         benign neoplasm of testis (D29.2.-)
         benign neoplasm of thymus (D15.0)
    ● **D35.0** Benign neoplasm of adrenal gland
        D35.00 Benign neoplasm of unspecified adrenal gland
        D35.01 Benign neoplasm of right adrenal gland
        D35.02 Benign neoplasm of left adrenal gland
    D35.1 Benign neoplasm of parathyroid gland
    D35.2 Benign neoplasm of pituitary gland 🐾
    D35.3 Benign neoplasm of craniopharyngeal duct 🐾
    D35.4 Benign neoplasm of pineal gland 🐾
    D35.5 Benign neoplasm of carotid body
    D35.6 Benign neoplasm of aortic body and other paraganglia
         Benign tumor of glomus jugulare
    D35.7 Benign neoplasm of other specified endocrine glands
    D35.9 Benign neoplasm of endocrine gland, unspecified
         Benign neoplasm of unspecified endocrine gland

● **D36** **Benign neoplasm of** other and unspecified sites
    D36.0 Benign neoplasm of lymph nodes
        Excludes1   lymphangioma (D18.1)
    ● **D36.1** Benign neoplasm of peripheral nerves and autonomic nervous system
        Excludes1   benign neoplasm of peripheral nerves of orbit (D31.6-)
             neurofibromatosis (Q85.0-)
        D36.10 Benign neoplasm of peripheral nerves and autonomic nervous system, unspecified
        D36.11 Benign neoplasm of peripheral nerves and autonomic nervous system of face, head, and neck
        D36.12 Benign neoplasm of peripheral nerves and autonomic nervous system, upper limb, including shoulder
        D36.13 Benign neoplasm of peripheral nerves and autonomic nervous system of lower limb, including hip
        D36.14 Benign neoplasm of peripheral nerves and autonomic nervous system of thorax
        D36.15 Benign neoplasm of peripheral nerves and autonomic nervous system of abdomen
        D36.16 Benign neoplasm of peripheral nerves and autonomic nervous system of pelvis
        D36.17 Benign neoplasm of peripheral nerves and autonomic nervous system of trunk, unspecified
    D36.7 Benign neoplasm of other specified sites
         Benign neoplasm of nose NOS
         Benign neoplasm of back NOS
    D36.9 Benign neoplasm, unspecified site

BENIGN NEUROENDOCRINE TUMORS (D3A)

● **D3A** **Benign neuroendocrine tumors**
     Code also any associated multiple endocrine neoplasia [MEN] syndromes (E31.2-)
     Use additional code to identify any associated endocrine syndrome, such as:
     carcinoid syndrome (E34.0)
    Excludes2   benign pancreatic islet cell tumors (D13.7)
    ● **D3A.0** Benign carcinoid tumors
        D3A.00 Benign carcinoid tumor of unspecified site
             Carcinoid tumor NOS
        ● **D3A.01** Benign carcinoid tumors of the small intestine
            D3A.010 Benign carcinoid tumor of the duodenum
            D3A.011 Benign carcinoid tumor of the jejunum
            D3A.012 Benign carcinoid tumor of the ileum
            D3A.019 Benign carcinoid tumor of the small intestine, unspecified portion
        ● **D3A.02** Benign carcinoid tumors of the appendix, large intestine, and rectum
            D3A.020 Benign carcinoid tumor of the appendix
            D3A.021 Benign carcinoid tumor of the cecum
            D3A.022 Benign carcinoid tumor of the ascending colon
            D3A.023 Benign carcinoid tumor of the transverse colon
            D3A.024 Benign carcinoid tumor of the descending colon
            D3A.025 Benign carcinoid tumor of the sigmoid colon
            D3A.026 Benign carcinoid tumor of the rectum
            D3A.029 Benign carcinoid tumor of the large intestine, unspecified portion
                 Benign carcinoid tumor of the colon NOS

▶ New   ⇒ Revised   ~~deleted~~ Deleted   Excludes 1   Excludes 2   Includes   Use additional   Code first   Code also   Key words
OGCR Official Guidelines   X Assign placeholder X   ● Use Additional Character(s)   ▶ Manifestation Code   🐾 Hierarchical Condition Category   **Coding Clinic**

● **D3A.09** **Benign carcinoid tumors of other sites**

    D3A.090 **Benign carcinoid tumor of the bronchus and lung**

    D3A.091 **Benign carcinoid tumor of the thymus**

    D3A.092 **Benign carcinoid tumor of the stomach**

    D3A.093 **Benign carcinoid tumor of the kidney**

    D3A.094 **Benign carcinoid tumor of the foregut, unspecified**

    D3A.095 **Benign carcinoid tumor of the midgut, unspecified**

    D3A.096 **Benign carcinoid tumor of the hindgut, unspecified**

    D3A.098 **Benign carcinoid tumors of other sites**

 D3A.8 **Other benign neuroendocrine tumors**
    Neuroendocrine tumor NOS

NEOPLASMS OF UNCERTAIN BEHAVIOR, POLYCYTHEMIA VERA AND MYELODYSPLASTIC SYNDROMES (D37-D48)

Note: Categories D37-D44, and D48 classify by site neoplasms of uncertain behavior, i.e., histologic confirmation whether the neoplasm is malignant or benign cannot be made.

Excludes1	neoplasms of unspecified behavior (D49.-)

● **D37** **Neoplasm of uncertain behavior of oral cavity and digestive organs**

Excludes1	stromal tumors of uncertain behavior of digestive system (D48.1)

 ● **D37.0** **Neoplasm of uncertain behavior of lip, oral cavity and pharynx**

Excludes1	neoplasm of uncertain behavior of aryepiglottic fold or interarytenoid fold, laryngeal aspect (D38.0)
	neoplasm of uncertain behavior of epiglottis NOS (D38.0)
	neoplasm of uncertain behavior of skin of lip (D48.5)
	neoplasm of uncertain behavior of suprahyoid portion of epiglottis (D38.0)

    D37.01 **Neoplasm of uncertain behavior of lip**
       Neoplasm of uncertain behavior of vermilion border of lip

    D37.02 **Neoplasm of uncertain behavior of tongue**

    ● **D37.03** **Neoplasm of uncertain behavior of the major salivary glands**

       D37.030 **Neoplasm of uncertain behavior of the parotid salivary glands**

       D37.031 **Neoplasm of uncertain behavior of the sublingual salivary glands**

       D37.032 **Neoplasm of uncertain behavior of the submandibular salivary glands**

       D37.039 **Neoplasm of uncertain behavior of the major salivary glands, unspecified**

    D37.04 **Neoplasm of uncertain behavior of the minor salivary glands**
       Neoplasm of uncertain behavior of submucosal salivary glands of lip
       Neoplasm of uncertain behavior of submucosal salivary glands of cheek
       Neoplasm of uncertain behavior of submucosal salivary glands of hard palate
       Neoplasm of uncertain behavior of submucosal salivary glands of soft palate

    D37.05 **Neoplasm of uncertain behavior of pharynx**
       Neoplasm of uncertain behavior of aryepiglottic fold of pharynx NOS
       Neoplasm of uncertain behavior of hypopharyngeal aspect of aryepiglottic fold of pharynx
       Neoplasm of uncertain behavior of marginal zone of aryepiglottic fold of pharynx

    D37.09 **Neoplasm of uncertain behavior of other specified sites of the oral cavity**

 D37.1 **Neoplasm of uncertain behavior of stomach**

 D37.2 **Neoplasm of uncertain behavior of small intestine**

 D37.3 **Neoplasm of uncertain behavior of appendix**

 D37.4 **Neoplasm of uncertain behavior of colon**

 D37.5 **Neoplasm of uncertain behavior of rectum**
    Neoplasm of uncertain behavior of rectosigmoid junction
    Rectosigmoid junction: Angle where sigmoid colon becomes rectum

 D37.6 **Neoplasm of uncertain behavior of liver, gallbladder and bile ducts**
    Neoplasm of uncertain behavior of ampulla of Vater
    Ampulla of Vater: Enlarged segment of ducts from liver and pancreas at entry point to small intestine

 D37.8 **Neoplasm of uncertain behavior of other specified digestive organs**
    Neoplasm of uncertain behavior of anal canal
    Neoplasm of uncertain behavior of anal sphincter
    Neoplasm of uncertain behavior of anus NOS
    Neoplasm of uncertain behavior of esophagus
    Neoplasm of uncertain behavior of intestine NOS
    Neoplasm of uncertain behavior of pancreas

Excludes1	neoplasm of uncertain behavior of anal margin (D48.5)
	neoplasm of uncertain behavior of anal skin (D48.5)
	neoplasm of uncertain behavior of perianal skin (D48.5)

 D37.9 **Neoplasm of uncertain behavior of digestive organ, unspecified**

Figure 2-19 Major salivary glands.

Parotid gland
Sublingual gland
Submandibular gland

CHAPTER 2 (C00-D49)

● **D38   Neoplasm of uncertain behavior of middle ear and respiratory and intrathoracic organs**

> **Excludes1**   neoplasm of uncertain behavior of heart (D48.7)

D38.0   Neoplasm of uncertain behavior of larynx
> Neoplasm of uncertain behavior of aryepiglottic fold or interarytenoid fold, laryngeal aspect
> Neoplasm of uncertain behavior of epiglottis (suprahyoid portion)
>
> > **Excludes1**   neoplasm of uncertain behavior of aryepiglottic fold or interarytenoid fold NOS (D37.05)
> > neoplasm of uncertain behavior of hypopharyngeal aspect of aryepiglottic fold (D37.05)
> > neoplasm of uncertain behavior of marginal zone of aryepiglottic fold (D37.05)

D38.1   Neoplasm of uncertain behavior of trachea, bronchus and lung

D38.2   Neoplasm of uncertain behavior of pleura

D38.3   Neoplasm of uncertain behavior of mediastinum

D38.4   Neoplasm of uncertain behavior of thymus

D38.5   Neoplasm of uncertain behavior of other respiratory organs
> Neoplasm of uncertain behavior of accessory sinuses
> Neoplasm of uncertain behavior of cartilage of nose
> Neoplasm of uncertain behavior of middle ear
> Neoplasm of uncertain behavior of nasal cavities
>
> > **Excludes1**   neoplasm of uncertain behavior of ear (external) (skin) (D48.5)
> > neoplasm of uncertain behavior of nose NOS (D48.7)
> > neoplasm of uncertain behavior of skin of nose (D48.5)

D38.6   Neoplasm of uncertain behavior of respiratory organ, unspecified

● **D39   Neoplasm of uncertain behavior of female genital organs**

D39.0   Neoplasm of uncertain behavior of uterus ♀

● **D39.1   Neoplasm of uncertain behavior of ovary**
> Use additional code to identify any functional activity.
>
> **D39.10   Neoplasm of uncertain behavior of unspecified ovary ♀**
>
> **D39.11   Neoplasm of uncertain behavior of right ovary ♀**
>
> **D39.12   Neoplasm of uncertain behavior of left ovary ♀**

D39.2   Neoplasm of uncertain behavior of placenta ♀M
> Chorioadenoma destruens
> Invasive hydatidiform mole
> Malignant hydatidiform mole
>
> > **Excludes1**   hydatidiform mole NOS (O01.9)

D39.8   Neoplasm of uncertain behavior of other specified female genital organs ♀
> Neoplasm of uncertain behavior of skin of female genital organs

D39.9   Neoplasm of uncertain behavior of female genital organ, unspecified ♀

● **D40   Neoplasm of uncertain behavior of male genital organs**

D40.0   Neoplasm of uncertain behavior of prostate ♂

● **D40.1   Neoplasm of uncertain behavior of testis**
> **D40.10   Neoplasm of uncertain behavior of unspecified testis ♂**
>
> **D40.11   Neoplasm of uncertain behavior of right testis ♂**
>
> **D40.12   Neoplasm of uncertain behavior of left testis ♂**

D40.8   Neoplasm of uncertain behavior of other specified male genital organs ♂
> Neoplasm of uncertain behavior of skin of male genital organs

D40.9   Neoplasm of uncertain behavior of male genital organ, unspecified ♂

● **D41   Neoplasm of uncertain behavior of urinary organs**

● **D41.0   Neoplasm of uncertain behavior of kidney**
> > **Excludes1**   neoplasm of uncertain behavior of renal pelvis (D41.1-)
>
> **D41.00   Neoplasm of uncertain behavior of unspecified kidney**
>
> **D41.01   Neoplasm of uncertain behavior of right kidney**
>
> **D41.02   Neoplasm of uncertain behavior of left kidney**

● **D41.1   Neoplasm of uncertain behavior of renal pelvis**
> **D41.10   Neoplasm of uncertain behavior of unspecified renal pelvis**
>
> **D41.11   Neoplasm of uncertain behavior of right renal pelvis**
>
> **D41.12   Neoplasm of uncertain behavior of left renal pelvis**

● **D41.2   Neoplasm of uncertain behavior of ureter**
> **D41.20   Neoplasm of uncertain behavior of unspecified ureter**
>
> **D41.21   Neoplasm of uncertain behavior of right ureter**
>
> **D41.22   Neoplasm of uncertain behavior of left ureter**

D41.3   Neoplasm of uncertain behavior of urethra

D41.4   Neoplasm of uncertain behavior of bladder

D41.8   Neoplasm of uncertain behavior of other specified urinary organs

D41.9   Neoplasm of uncertain behavior of unspecified urinary organ

● **D42   Neoplasm of uncertain behavior of meninges**

D42.0   Neoplasm of uncertain behavior of cerebral meninges 🅗

D42.1   Neoplasm of uncertain behavior of spinal meninges 🅗

D42.9   Neoplasm of uncertain behavior of meninges, unspecified 🅗

● **D43   Neoplasm of uncertain behavior of brain and central nervous system**

> **Excludes1**   neoplasm of uncertain behavior of peripheral nerves and autonomic nervous system (D48.2)

D43.0   Neoplasm of uncertain behavior of brain, supratentorial 🅗
> *Superior to tentorium of cerebellum*
> Neoplasm of uncertain behavior of cerebral ventricle
> Neoplasm of uncertain behavior of cerebrum
> Neoplasm of uncertain behavior of frontal lobe
> Neoplasm of uncertain behavior of occipital lobe
> Neoplasm of uncertain behavior of parietal lobe
> Neoplasm of uncertain behavior of temporal lobe
>
> > **Excludes1**   neoplasm of uncertain behavior of fourth ventricle (D43.1)

D43.1   Neoplasm of uncertain behavior of brain, infratentorial 🅗
> *Beneath the tentorium of cerebellum*
> Neoplasm of uncertain behavior of brain stem
> Neoplasm of uncertain behavior of cerebellum
> Neoplasm of uncertain behavior of fourth ventricle

D43.2   Neoplasm of uncertain behavior of brain, unspecified 🅗

D43.3   Neoplasm of uncertain behavior of cranial nerves 🅗

D43.4   Neoplasm of uncertain behavior of spinal cord 🅗

D43.8   Neoplasm of uncertain behavior of other specified parts of central nervous system 🅗

D43.9   Neoplasm of uncertain behavior of central nervous system, unspecified 🅗
> Neoplasm of uncertain behavior of nervous system (central) NOS

▶ New   ⇒ Revised   ~~deleted~~ Deleted   Excludes 1   Excludes 2   Includes   Use additional   Code first   Code also   Key words
OGCR Official Guidelines   X Assign placeholder X   ● Use Additional Character(s)   ▶ Manifestation Code   🅗 Hierarchical Condition Category   Coding Clinic

● **D44   Neoplasm of uncertain behavior of endocrine glands**

Excludes1   multiple endocrine adenomatosis (E31.2-)
multiple endocrine neoplasia (E31.2-)
neoplasm of uncertain behavior of endocrine pancreas (D37.8)
neoplasm of uncertain behavior of ovary (D39.1-)
neoplasm of uncertain behavior of testis (D40.1-)
neoplasm of uncertain behavior of thymus (D38.4)

D44.0   Neoplasm of uncertain behavior of thyroid gland

● **D44.1   Neoplasm of uncertain behavior of adrenal gland**
Use additional code to identify any functional activity.

D44.10   Neoplasm of uncertain behavior of unspecified adrenal gland

D44.11   Neoplasm of uncertain behavior of right adrenal gland

D44.12   Neoplasm of uncertain behavior of left adrenal gland

D44.2   Neoplasm of uncertain behavior of parathyroid gland

D44.3   Neoplasm of uncertain behavior of pituitary gland 🔵
Use additional code to identify any functional activity.

D44.4   Neoplasm of uncertain behavior of craniopharyngeal duct 🔵

D44.5   Neoplasm of uncertain behavior of pineal gland 🔵

D44.6   Neoplasm of uncertain behavior of carotid body 🔵

D44.7   Neoplasm of uncertain behavior of aortic body and other paraganglia 🔵
Coding Clinic: 2016, Q4, P26

D44.9   Neoplasm of uncertain behavior of unspecified endocrine gland

● **D45   Polycythemia vera** 🔵

Excludes1   familial polycythemia (D75.0)
secondary polycythemia (D75.1)

Primary polycythemia. Secondary polycythemia is D75.1. Check your documentation. Polycythemia is caused by too many red blood cells, which increase the thickness of blood (viscosity). This can cause engorgement of the spleen (splenomegaly) with extra RBCs and potential clot formation.

● **D46   Myelodysplastic syndromes**
Use additional code for adverse effect, if applicable, to identify drug (T36-T50 with fifth or sixth character 5)

Excludes2   drug-induced aplastic anemia (D61.1)

D46.0   Refractory anemia without ring sideroblasts, so stated 🔵
Refractory anemia without sideroblasts, without excess of blasts

D46.1   Refractory anemia with ring sideroblasts RARS 🔵

● **D46.2   Refractory anemia with excess of blasts [RAEB]**
Form of myelodysplasia with increased immature white blood cells (blasts) in bone marrow

D46.20   Refractory anemia with excess of blasts, unspecified RAEB NOS 🔵

D46.21   Refractory anemia with excess of blasts 1 RAEB 1 🔵
Bone marrow disease which results in insufficient RBCs (anemia) in which level of blasts is less than 10%

D46.22   Refractory anemia with excess of blasts 2 RAEB 2 🔵
Bone marrow disease manifested by insufficient numbers of RBCs (anemia) with level of blasts 10-20%

D46.A   Refractory cytopenia with multilineage dysplasia 🔵

D46.B   Refractory cytopenia with multilineage dysplasia and ring sideroblasts 🔵
RCMD RS

D46.C   Myelodysplastic syndrome with isolated del(5q) chromosomal abnormality 🔵
Myelodysplastic syndrome with 5q deletion
5q minus syndrome NOS

D46.4   Refractory anemia, unspecified 🔵

D46.Z   Other myelodysplastic syndromes 🔵

Excludes1   chronic myelomonocytic leukemia (C93.1-)

D46.9   Myelodysplastic syndrome, unspecified 🔵
Myelodysplasia NOS

● **D47   Other neoplasms of uncertain behavior of lymphoid, hematopoietic and related tissue**

● **D47.0   Mast cell neoplasms of uncertain behavior**

Excludes1   congenital cutaneous mastocytosis (Q82.2)
histiocytic neoplasms of uncertain behavior (D47.Z9)
malignant mast cell neoplasm (C96.2-)

D47.01   Cutaneous mastocytosis
Diffuse cutaneous mastocytosis
Maculopapular cutaneous mastocytosis
Solitary mastocytoma
Telangiectasia macularis eruptiva perstans
Urticaria pigmentosa

Excludes1   congenitᵃl (diffuse) (maculopapular) cutaneous mastocytosis (Q82.2)
congenital urticaria pigmentosa (Q82.2)
extracutaneous mastocytoma (D47.09)

D47.02   Systemic mastocytosis
Indolent systemic mastocytosis
Isolated bone marrow mastocytosis
Smoldering systemic mastocytosis
Systemic mastocytosis, with an associated hematological non-mast cell lineage disease (SM-AHNMD)

Code also if applicable, any associated hematological non-mast cell lineage disease, such as:
acute myeloid leukemia (C92.6-, C92.A-)
chronic myelomonocytic leukemia (C93.1-)
essential thrombocytosis (D47.3)
hypereosinophilic syndrome (D72.1)
myelodysplastic syndrome (D46.9)
myeloproliferative syndrome (D47.1)
non-Hodgkin lymphoma (C82-C85)
plasma cell myeloma (C90.0-)
polycythemia vera (D45)

Excludes1   aggressive systemic mastocytosis (C96.21)
mast cell leukemia (C94.3-)

D47.09   Other mast cell neoplasms of uncertain behavior
Extracutaneous mastocytoma
Mast cell tumor NOS
Mastocytoma NOS
Mastocytosis NOS

D47.1   Chronic myeloproliferative disease 🔵
Chronic neutrophilic leukemia
Myeloproliferative disease, unspecified

Excludes1   atypical chronic myeloid leukemia BCR/ABL-negative (C92.2-)
chronic myeloid leukemia BCR/ABL-positive (C92.1-)
myelofibrosis NOS (D75.81)
myelophthisic anemia (D61.82)
myelophthisis (D61.82)
secondary myelofibrosis NOS (D75.81)

D47.2   Monoclonal gammopathy
Monoclonal gammopathy of undetermined significance [MGUS]
Coding Clinic: 2021, Q3, P5

CHAPTER 2 (C00-D49)

D47.3 **Essential (hemorrhagic) thrombocythemia** 🔲
Essential thrombocytosis
Idiopathic hemorrhagic thrombocythemia
Primary thrombocytosis
   Excludes2   reactive thrombocytosis (D75.838)
                 secondary thrombocytosis (D75.838)
                 thrombocythemia NOS (D75.839)
                 thrombocytosis NOS (D75.839)

D47.4 **Osteomyelofibrosis** 🔲
Chronic idiopathic myelofibrosis
Myelofibrosis (idiopathic) (with myeloid metaplasia)
Myelosclerosis (megakaryocytic) with myeloid metaplasia
Secondary myelofibrosis in myeloproliferative disease
   Excludes1   acute myelofibrosis (C94.4-)

● D47.Z **Other specified neoplasms of uncertain behavior of lymphoid, hematopoietic and related tissue**
  D47.Z1 **Post-transplant lymphoproliferative disorder (PTLD)** 🔲
    Code first complications of transplanted organs and tissue (T86.-)
  D47.Z2 **Castleman disease** 🔲
    Code also if applicable, human herpesvirus 8 infection (B10.89)
      Excludes2   Kaposi's sarcoma (C46.-)
    Coding Clinic: 2016, Q4, P8
  D47.Z9 **Other specified neoplasms of uncertain behavior of lymphoid, hematopoietic and related tissue** 🔲
    Histiocytic tumors of uncertain behavior

D47.9 **Neoplasm of uncertain behavior of lymphoid, hematopoietic and related tissue, unspecified** 🔲
Lymphoproliferative disease NOS

● D48 **Neoplasm of uncertain behavior of other and unspecified sites**
  Excludes1   neurofibromatosis (nonmalignant) (Q85.0-)

D48.0 **Neoplasm of uncertain behavior of bone and articular cartilage**
  Excludes1   neoplasm of uncertain behavior of cartilage of ear (D48.1)
       neoplasm of uncertain behavior of cartilage of larynx (D38.0)
       neoplasm of uncertain behavior of cartilage of nose (D38.5)
       neoplasm of uncertain behavior of connective tissue of eyelid (D48.1)
       neoplasm of uncertain behavior of synovia (D48.1)

D48.1 **Neoplasm of uncertain behavior of connective and other soft tissue**
Neoplasm of uncertain behavior of connective tissue of ear
Neoplasm of uncertain behavior of connective tissue of eyelid
Stromal tumors of uncertain behavior of digestive system
  Excludes1   neoplasm of uncertain behavior of articular cartilage (D48.0)
       neoplasm of uncertain behavior of cartilage of larynx (D38.0)
       neoplasm of uncertain behavior of cartilage of nose (D38.5)
       neoplasm of uncertain behavior of connective tissue of breast (D48.6-)

D48.2 **Neoplasm of uncertain behavior of peripheral nerves and autonomic nervous system**
  Excludes1   neoplasm of uncertain behavior of peripheral nerves of orbit (D48.7)

D48.3 **Neoplasm of uncertain behavior of retroperitoneum**

D48.4 **Neoplasm of uncertain behavior of peritoneum**

D48.5 **Neoplasm of uncertain behavior of skin**
Neoplasm of uncertain behavior of anal margin
Neoplasm of uncertain behavior of anal skin
Neoplasm of uncertain behavior of perianal skin
Neoplasm of uncertain behavior of skin of breast
  Excludes1   neoplasm of uncertain behavior of anus NOS (D37.8)
       neoplasm of uncertain behavior of skin of genital organs (D39.8, D40.8)
       neoplasm of uncertain behavior of vermilion border of lip (D37.0)

● D48.6 **Neoplasm of uncertain behavior of breast**
Neoplasm of uncertain behavior of connective tissue of breast
Cystosarcoma phyllodes
  Excludes1   neoplasm of uncertain behavior of skin of breast (D48.5)
  D48.60 **Neoplasm of uncertain behavior of unspecified breast**
  D48.61 **Neoplasm of uncertain behavior of right breast**
  D48.62 **Neoplasm of uncertain behavior of left breast**

D48.7 **Neoplasm of uncertain behavior of other specified sites**
Neoplasm of uncertain behavior of eye
Neoplasm of uncertain behavior of heart
Neoplasm of uncertain behavior of peripheral nerves of orbit
  Excludes1   neoplasm of uncertain behavior of connective tissue (D48.1)
       neoplasm of uncertain behavior of skin of eyelid (D48.5)

D48.9 **Neoplasm of uncertain behavior, unspecified**

● D49 **Neoplasms of unspecified behavior**
Note: Category D49 classifies by site neoplasms of unspecified morphology and behavior. The term "mass," unless otherwise stated, is not to be regarded as a neoplastic growth.
  Includes   'growth' NOS
       neoplasm NOS
       new growth NOS
       tumor NOS
  Excludes1   neoplasms of uncertain behavior (D37-D44, D48)

D49.0 **Neoplasm of unspecified behavior of digestive system**
  Excludes1   neoplasm of unspecified behavior of margin of anus (D49.2)
       neoplasm of unspecified behavior of perianal skin (D49.2)
       neoplasm of unspecified behavior of skin of anus (D49.2)

D49.1 **Neoplasm of unspecified behavior of respiratory system**

D49.2 **Neoplasm of unspecified behavior of bone, soft tissue, and skin**
  Excludes1   neoplasm of unspecified behavior of anal canal (D49.0)
       neoplasm of unspecified behavior of anus NOS (D49.0)
       neoplasm of unspecified behavior of bone marrow (D49.89)
       neoplasm of unspecified behavior of cartilage of larynx (D49.1)
       neoplasm of unspecified behavior of cartilage of nose (D49.1)
       neoplasm of unspecified behavior of connective tissue of breast (D49.3)
       neoplasm of unspecified behavior of skin of genital organs (D49.59)
       neoplasm of unspecified behavior of vermilion border of lip (D49.0)

▶ New   ⇒ Revised   deleted Deleted   Excludes 1   Excludes 2   Includes   Use additional   Code first   Code also   Key words
OGCR Official Guidelines   X Assign placeholder X   ● Use Additional Character(s)   ▶ Manifestation Code   🔲 Hierarchical Condition Category   Coding Clinic

D49.3   **Neoplasm of unspecified behavior of breast**

     Excludes1   neoplasm of unspecified behavior of skin of breast (D49.2)

D49.4   **Neoplasm of unspecified behavior of bladder**

● **D49.5**   **Neoplasm of unspecified behavior of other genitourinary organs**

   ● **D49.51**   **Neoplasm of unspecified behavior of kidney**

       D49.511   **Neoplasm of unspecified behavior of right kidney**
          Coding Clinic: 2016, Q4, P9

       D49.512   **Neoplasm of unspecified behavior of left kidney**
          Coding Clinic: 2016, Q4, P9

       D49.519   **Neoplasm of unspecified behavior of unspecified kidney**
          Coding Clinic: 2016, Q4, P9

   D49.59   **Neoplasm of unspecified behavior of other genitourinary organ**
      Coding Clinic: 2016, Q4, P9

D49.6   **Neoplasm of unspecified behavior of brain** 🔗

     Excludes1   neoplasm of unspecified behavior of cerebral meninges (D49.7)
           neoplasm of unspecified behavior of cranial nerves (D49.7)

D49.7   **Neoplasm of unspecified behavior of endocrine glands and other parts of nervous system**

     Excludes1   neoplasm of unspecified behavior of peripheral, sympathetic, and parasympathetic nerves and ganglia (D49.2)

● **D49.8**   **Neoplasm of unspecified behavior of other specified sites**

     Excludes1   neoplasm of unspecified behavior of eyelid (skin) (D49.2)
           neoplasm of unspecified behavior of eyelid cartilage (D49.2)
           neoplasm of unspecified behavior of great vessels (D49.2)
           neoplasm of unspecified behavior of optic nerve (D49.7)

   D49.81   **Neoplasm of unspecified behavior of retina and choroid**
      Dark area on retina
      Retinal freckle

   D49.89   **Neoplasm of unspecified behavior of other specified sites**

D49.9   **Neoplasm of unspecified behavior of unspecified site**

CHAPTER 3

DISEASES OF THE BLOOD AND BLOOD-FORMING ORGANS AND CERTAIN DISORDERS INVOLVING THE IMMUNE MECHANISM (D50-D89)

Excludes2   autoimmune disease (systemic) NOS (M35.9)
certain conditions originating in the perinatal period (P00-P96)
complications of pregnancy, childbirth and the puerperium (O00-O9A)
congenital malformations, deformations and chromosomal abnormalities (Q00-Q99)
endocrine, nutritional and metabolic diseases (E00-E88)
human immunodeficiency virus [HIV] disease (B20)
injury, poisoning and certain other consequences of external causes (S00-T88)
neoplasms (C00-D49)
symptoms, signs and abnormal clinical and laboratory findings, not elsewhere classified (R00-R94)

This chapter contains the following blocks:

D50-D53	Nutritional anemias
D55-D59	Hemolytic anemias
D60-D64	Aplastic and other anemias and other bone marrow failure syndromes
D65-D69	Coagulation defects, purpura and other hemorrhagic conditions
D70-D77	Other disorders of blood and blood-forming organs
D78	Intraoperative and postprocedural complications of the spleen
D80-D89	Certain disorders involving the immune mechanism

NUTRITIONAL ANEMIAS (D50-D53)

● **D50**   **Iron deficiency anemia**
A disease characterized by a decrease in the number of red cells (hemoglobin) in the blood.

Includes   asiderotic anemia
hypochromic anemia

D50.0   **Iron deficiency anemia secondary to blood loss (chronic)**
Posthemorrhagic anemia (chronic)

Excludes1   acute posthemorrhagic anemia (D62)
congenital anemia from fetal blood loss (P61.3)

Coding Clinic: 2019, Q3, P17

D50.1   **Sideropenic dysphagia**
Weblike growth of membranes in throat that makes swallowing difficult
Kelly-Paterson syndrome
Plummer-Vinson syndrome

D50.8   **Other iron deficiency anemias**
Iron deficiency anemia due to inadequate dietary iron intake

D50.9   **Iron deficiency anemia, unspecified**

● **D51**   **Vitamin B12 deficiency anemia**

Excludes1   vitamin B12 deficiency (E53.8)

D51.0   **Vitamin B12 deficiency anemia due to intrinsic factor deficiency**
Addison anemia
Biermer anemia
Pernicious (congenital) anemia
Congenital intrinsic factor deficiency

D51.1   **Vitamin B12 deficiency anemia due to selective vitamin B12 malabsorption with proteinuria**
Imerslund (Gräsbeck) syndrome
Megaloblastic hereditary anemia

D51.2   **Transcobalamin II deficiency**

D51.3   **Other dietary vitamin B12 deficiency anemia**
Vegan anemia

D51.8   **Other vitamin B12 deficiency anemias**

D51.9   **Vitamin B12 deficiency anemia, unspecified**

● **D52**   **Folate deficiency anemia**

Excludes1   folate deficiency without anemia (E53.8)

D52.0   **Dietary folate deficiency anemia**
Nutritional megaloblastic anemia

D52.1   **Drug-induced folate deficiency anemia**
Use additional code for adverse effect, if applicable, to identify drug (T36-T50 with fifth or sixth character 5)

D52.8   **Other folate deficiency anemias**

D52.9   **Folate deficiency anemia, unspecified**
Folic acid deficiency anemia NOS

● **D53**   **Other nutritional anemias**

Includes   megaloblastic anemia unresponsive to vitamin B12 or folate therapy

D53.0   **Protein deficiency anemia**
Amino-acid deficiency anemia
Orotaciduric anemia

Excludes1   Lesch-Nyhan syndrome (E79.1)

D53.1   **Other megaloblastic anemias, not elsewhere classified**
Megaloblastic anemia NOS

Excludes1   Di Guglielmo's disease (C94.0)

D53.2   **Scorbutic anemia**
Anemia resulting from deficiency of ascorbic acid (vitamin C)

Excludes1   scurvy (E54)

D53.8   **Other specified nutritional anemias**
Anemia associated with deficiency of copper
Anemia associated with deficiency of molybdenum
Anemia associated with deficiency of zinc

Excludes1   nutritional deficiencies without anemia, such as:
copper deficiency NOS (E61.0)
molybdenum deficiency NOS (E61.5)
zinc deficiency NOS (E60)

D53.9   **Nutritional anemia, unspecified**
Simple chronic anemia

Excludes1   anemia NOS (D64.9)

Coding Clinic: 2018, Q4, P88

HEMOLYTIC ANEMIAS (D55-D59)

● **D55**   **Anemia due to enzyme disorders**

Excludes1   drug-induced enzyme deficiency anemia (D59.2)

D55.0   **Anemia due to glucose-6-phosphate dehydrogenase [G6PD] deficiency** 🍩
Favism
G6PD deficiency anemia

Excludes1   glucose-6-phosphate dehydrogenase (G6PD) deficiency without anemia (D75.A)

D55.1   **Anemia due to other disorders of glutathione metabolism** 🍩
Anemia (due to) enzyme deficiencies, except G6PD, related to the hexose monophosphate [HMP] shunt pathway
Anemia (due to) hemolytic nonspherocytic (hereditary), type I

● **D55.2**   **Anemia due to disorders of glycolytic enzymes** 🍩

D55.21 Anemia due to pyruvate kinase deficiency
PK deficiency anemia
Pyruvate kinase deficiency anemia

D55.29 Anemia due to other disorders of glycolytic enzymes
Hexokinase deficiency anemia
Triose-phosphate isomerase deficiency anemia

> **Excludes1**   disorders of glycolysis not associated with anemia (E74.81-)

D55.3   Anemia due to disorders of nucleotide metabolism 🦠

D55.8   Other anemias due to enzyme disorders 🦠

D55.9   Anemia due to enzyme disorder, unspecified 🦠

● **D56   Thalassemia**
Hereditary disorders characterized by low production of hemoglobin or excessive destruction of red blood cells

> **Excludes1**   sickle-cell thalassemia (D57.4-)

D56.0   Alpha thalassemia 🦠
Alpha thalassemia major
Hemoglobin H Constant Spring
Hemoglobin H disease
Hydrops fetalis due to alpha thalassemia
Severe alpha thalassemia
Triple gene defect alpha thalassemia

Use additional code, if applicable, for hydrops fetalis due to alpha thalassemia (P56.99)

> **Excludes1**   alpha thalassemia trait or minor (D56.3)
> asymptomatic alpha thalassemia (D56.3)
> hydrops fetalis due to isoimmunization (P56.0)
> hydrops fetalis not due to immune hemolysis (P83.2)

D56.1   Beta thalassemia 🦠
Beta thalassemia major
Cooley's anemia
Homozygous beta thalassemia
Severe beta thalassemia
Thalassemia intermedia
Thalassemia major

> **Excludes1**   beta thalassemia minor (D56.3)
> beta thalassemia trait (D56.3)
> delta-beta thalassemia (D56.2)
> hemoglobin E-beta thalassemia (D56.5)
> sickle-cell beta thalassemia (D57.4-)

D56.2   Delta-beta thalassemia
Homozygous delta-beta thalassemia

> **Excludes1**   delta-beta thalassemia minor (D56.3)
> delta-beta thalassemia trait (D56.3)

D56.3   Thalassemia minor
Genetic disorders that have in common defective production of hemoglobin
Alpha thalassemia minor
Alpha thalassemia silent carrier
Alpha thalassemia trait
Beta thalassemia minor
Beta thalassemia trait
Delta-beta thalassemia minor
Delta-beta thalassemia trait
Thalassemia trait NOS

> **Excludes1**   alpha thalassemia (D56.0)
> beta thalassemia (D56.1)
> delta-beta thalassemia (D56.2)
> hemoglobin E-beta thalassemia (D56.5)
> sickle-cell trait (D57.3)

D56.4   Hereditary persistence of fetal hemoglobin [HPFH] 🦠
Persistent production of hemoglobin

D56.5   Hemoglobin E-beta thalassemia 🦠

> **Excludes1**   beta thalassemia (D56.1)
> beta thalassemia minor (D56.3)
> beta thalassemia trait (D56.3)
> delta-beta thalassemia (D56.2)
> delta-beta thalassemia trait (D56.3)
> hemoglobin E disease (D58.2)
> other hemoglobinopathies (D58.2)
> sickle-cell beta thalassemia (D57.4-)

D56.8   Other thalassemias 🦠
Dominant thalassemia
Hemoglobin C thalassemia
Mixed thalassemia
Thalassemia with other hemoglobinopathy

> **Excludes1**   hemoglobin C disease (D58.2)
> hemoglobin E disease (D58.2)
> other hemoglobinopathies (D58.2)
> sickle cell anemia (D57.-)
> sickle-cell thalassemia (D57.4)

D56.9   Thalassemia, unspecified
Mediterranean anemia (with other hemoglobinopathy)

● **D57   Sickle-cell disorders**
Inherited disease in which red blood cells, normally disc-shaped, become crescent shaped

Use additional code for any associated fever (R50.81)

> **Excludes1**   other hemoglobinopathies (D58.-)

Coding Clinic: 2022, Q2, P29

● **D57.0   Hb-SS disease with crisis**
Sickle-cell disease with crisis
Hb-SS disease with vasoocclusive pain

D57.00   Hb-SS disease with crisis, unspecified 🦠
Hb-SS disease with (painful) crisis NOS
Hb-SS disease with vasoocclusive pain NOS

D57.01   Hb-SS disease with acute chest syndrome 🦠

D57.02   Hb-SS disease with splenic sequestration 🦠

D57.03   Hb-SS disease with cerebral vascular involvement
Code also, if applicable, cerebral infarction (I63.-)

D57.09   Hb-SS disease with crisis with other specified complication
Use additional code to identify complications, such as:
cholelithiasis (K80.-)
priapism (N48.32)

D57.1   Sickle-cell disease without crisis Hb-SS disease without crisis 🦠
Sickle-cell anemia NOS
Sickle-cell disease NOS
Sickle-cell disorder NOS

● **D57.2   Sickle-cell/Hb-C disease**
Hb-SC disease
Hb-S/Hb-C disease

D57.20   Sickle-cell/Hb-C disease without crisis 🦠

● **D57.21   Sickle-cell/Hb-C disease with crisis**

D57.211   Sickle-cell/Hb-C disease with acute chest syndrome 🦠

D57.212   Sickle-cell/Hb-C disease with splenic sequestration 🦠

D57.213   Sickle-cell/Hb-C disease with cerebral vascular involvement
Code also, if applicable, cerebral infarction (I63.-)

D57.218   Sickle-cell/Hb-C disease with crisis with other specified complication
Use additional code to identify complications, such as:
cholelithiasis (K80.-)
priapism (N48.32)

D57.219   Sickle-cell/Hb-C disease with crisis, unspecified 🦠
Sickle-cell/Hb-C disease with crisis NOS
Sickle-cell/Hb-C disease with vasoocclusive pain NOS

D57.3   Sickle-cell trait 🦠
Hb-S trait
Heterozygous hemoglobin S

CHAPTER 3 (D50–D89)

● **D57.4**   **Sickle-cell thalassemia**
Sickle-cell beta thalassemia
Thalassemia Hb-S disease

     D57.40   **Sickle-cell thalassemia without crisis** 🔗
            Microdrepanocytosis
            Sickle-cell thalassemia NOS

     ● **D57.41**   **Sickle-cell thalassemia, unspecified, with crisis**
            Sickle-cell "crisis" is precipitated when abnormally crescent-shaped red blood cells form clots and interrupt blood flow to major organs, causing severe pain and organ damage.
            Sickle-cell thalassemia with (painful) crisis NOS
            Sickle-cell thalassemia with vasoocclusive pain NOS

         D57.411   **Sickle-cell thalassemia, unspecified, with acute chest syndrome** 🔗

         D57.412   **Sickle-cell thalassemia with, unspecified, splenic sequestration** 🔗

         D57.413   **Sickle-cell thalassemia, unspecified, with cerebral vascular involvement**
                Code also, if applicable cerebral infarction (I63.-)

         D57.418   **Sickle-cell thalassemia, unspecified, with crisis with other specified complication**
                Use additional code to identify complications, such as:
                     cholelithiasis (K80.-)
                     priapism (N48.32)

         D57.419   **Sickle-cell thalassemia with, unspecified, crisis** 🔗
                Sickle-cell thalassemia with (painful) crisis NOS
                Sickle-cell thalassemia with vasoocclusive pain NOS

     D57.42   **Sickle-cell thalassemia beta zero without crisis**
            HbS-beta zero without crisis
            Sickle-cell beta zero without crisis

     ● **D57.43**   **Sickle-cell thalassemia beta zero with crisis**
            HbS-beta zero with crisis
            Sickle-cell beta zero with crisis

         D57.431   **Sickle-cell thalassemia beta zero with acute chest syndrome**
                HbS-beta zero with acute chest syndrome
                Sickle-cell beta zero with acute chest syndrome

         D57.432   **Sickle-cell thalassemia beta zero with splenic sequestration**
                HbS-beta zero with splenic sequestration
                Sickle-cell beta zero with splenic sequestration

         D57.433   **Sickle-cell thalassemia beta zero with cerebral vascular involvement**
                HbS-beta zero with cerebral vascular involvement
                Sickle-cell beta zero with cerebral vascular involvement
                Code also, if applicable cerebral infarction (I63.-)

D57.438   **Sickle-cell thalassemia beta zero with crisis with other specified complication**
            HbS-beta zero with other specified complication
            Sickle-cell beta zero with other specified complication
            Use additional code to identify complications, such as:
                cholelithiasis (K80.-)
                priapism (N48.32)

D57.439   **Sickle-cell thalassemia beta zero with crisis, unspecified**
            HbS-beta zero with other specified complication
            Sickle-cell beta zero with crisis unspecified
            Sickle-cell thalassemia beta zero with (painful) crisis NOS
            Sickle-cell thalassemia beta zero with vasoocclusive pain NOS

     D57.44   **Sickle-cell thalassemia beta plus without crisis**
            HbS-beta plus without crisis
            Sickle-cell beta plus without crisis

     ● **D57.45**   **Sickle-cell thalassemia beta plus with crisis**
            HbS-beta plus with crisis
            Sickle-cell beta plus with crisis

         D57.451   **Sickle-cell thalassemia beta plus with acute chest syndrome**
                HbS-beta plus with acute chest syndrome
                Sickle-cell beta plus with acute chest syndrome

         D57.452   **Sickle-cell thalassemia beta plus with splenic sequestration**
                HbS-beta plus with splenic sequestration
                Sickle-cell beta plus with splenic sequestration

         D57.453   **Sickle-cell thalassemia beta plus with cerebral vascular involvement**
                HbS-beta plus with cerebral vascular involvement
                Sickle-cell beta plus with cerebral vascular involvement
                Code also, if applicable cerebral infarction (I63.-)

         D57.458   **Sickle-cell thalassemia beta plus with crisis with other specified complication**
                HbS-beta plus with crisis with other specified complication
                Sickle-cell beta plus with crisis with other specified complication
                Use additional code to identify complications, such as:
                     cholelithiasis (K80.-)
                     priapism (N48.32)

         D57.459   **Sickle-cell thalassemia beta plus with crisis, unspecified**
                HbS-beta plus with crisis with unspecified complication
                Sickle-cell beta plus with crisis with unspecified complication
                Sickle-cell thalassemia beta plus with (painful) crisis NOS
                Sickle-cell thalassemia beta plus with vasoocclusive pain NOS

▶ New   ⟹ Revised   ~~deleted~~ Deleted   Excludes 1   Excludes 2   Includes   Use additional   Code first   Code also   Key words
OGCR Official Guidelines   X Assign placeholder X   ● Use Additional Character(s)   ▶ Manifestation Code   🔗 Hierarchical Condition Category   **Coding Clinic**

● **D57.8**   **Other sickle-cell disorders**
     Hb-SD disease
     Hb-SE disease

     D57.80   **Other sickle-cell disorders without crisis** 🔖

●   **D57.81**   **Other sickle-cell disorders with crisis**

        D57.811   **Other sickle-cell disorders with acute chest syndrome** 🔖

        D57.812   **Other sickle-cell disorders with splenic sequestration** 🔖

        D57.813   **Other sickle-cell disorders with cerebral vascular involvement**

           Code also, if applicable: cerebral infarction (I63.-)

        D57.818   **Other sickle-cell disorders with crisis with other specified complication**

           Use additional code to identify complications, such as:
             cholelithiasis (K80.-)
             priapism (N48.32)

        D57.819   **Other sickle-cell disorders with crisis, unspecified** 🔖

           Other sickle-cell disorders with crisis NOS
           Other sickle-cell disorders with vasooclusive pain NOS

● **D58**   **Other hereditary hemolytic anemias**
     Genetic condition in which bone marrow is unable to compensate for premature destruction of red blood cells

     Excludes1   hemolytic anemia of the newborn (P55.-)

   D58.0   **Hereditary spherocytosis** 🔖
     Presence of spherocytes (spherically shaped red blood cells)
     Acholuric (familial) jaundice
     Congenital (spherocytic) hemolytic icterus
     Minkowski-Chauffard syndrome

   D58.1   **Hereditary elliptocytosis** 🔖
     Presence of large numbers of elliptocytes in blood
     Elliptocytosis (congenital)
     Ovalocytosis (congenital) (hereditary)

   D58.2   **Other hemoglobinopathies** 🔖
     Abnormal hemoglobin NOS
     Congenital Heinz body anemia
     Hb-C disease
     Hb-D disease
     Hb-E disease
     Hemoglobinopathy NOS
     Unstable hemoglobin hemolytic disease

     Excludes1   familial polycythemia (D75.0)
               Hb-M disease (D74.0)
               hemoglobin E-beta thalassemia (D56.5)
               hereditary persistence of fetal hemoglobin [HPFH] (D56.4)
               high-altitude polycythemia (D75.1)
               methemoglobinemia (D74.-)
               other hemoglobinopathies with thalassemia (D56.8)

   D58.8   **Other specified hereditary hemolytic anemias** 🔖
     Stomatocytosis

   D58.9   **Hereditary hemolytic anemia, unspecified** 🔖

● **D59**   **Acquired hemolytic anemia**

   D59.0   **Drug-induced autoimmune hemolytic anemia** 🔖
     Use additional code for adverse effect, if applicable, to identify drug (T36-T50 with fifth or sixth character 5)

   D59.1   **Other autoimmune hemolytic anemias** 🔖

     Excludes2   Evans syndrome (D69.41)
               hemolytic disease of newborn (P55.-)
               paroxysmal cold hemoglobinuria (D59.6)

     D59.10   **Autoimmune hemolytic anemia, unspecified**

     D59.11   **Warm autoimmune hemolytic anemia**
        Warm type (primary) (secondary) (symptomatic) autoimmune hemolytic anemia
        Warm type autoimmune hemolytic disease

     D59.12   **Cold autoimmune hemolytic anemia**
        Chronic cold hemagglutinin disease
        Cold agglutinin disease
        Cold agglutinin hemoglobinuria
        Cold type (primary) (secondary) (symptomatic) autoimmune hemolytic anemia
        Cold type autoimmune hemolytic disease

     D59.13   **Mixed type autoimmune hemolytic anemia**
        Mixed type autoimmune hemolytic disease
        Mixed type, cold and warm, (primary) (secondary) (symptomatic) autoimmune hemolyticanemia

     D59.19   **Other autoimmune hemolytic anemia**

   D59.2   **Drug-induced nonautoimmune hemolytic anemia** 🔖
     Drug-induced enzyme deficiency anemia
     Use additional code for adverse effect, if applicable, to identify drug (T36-T50 with fifth or sixth character 5)

   D59.3   **Hemolytic-uremic syndrome** 🔖
     ~~Use additional code to identify associated:~~
       ~~E. coli infection (B96.2-)~~
       ~~Pneumococcal pneumonia (J13)~~
       ~~Shigella dysenteriae (A03.9)~~
     ▶ Code also, if applicable, any associated:
       ▶ acute kidney failure (N17.-)
       ▶ chronic kidney disease (N18.-)

     ▶ **D59.30**   **Hemolytic-uremic syndrome, unspecified**
        ▶ Hemolytic-uremic syndrome NOS

     ▶ **D59.31**   **Infection-associated hemolytic-uremic syndrome**
        ▶ Shiga toxin-producing E. coli [STEC] related hemolytic uremic syndrome
        ▶ Typical hemolytic uremic syndrome
        ▶ Use Additional code to identify associated infection, such as:
          ▶ E. coli infection (B96.2-)
          ▶ Human immunodeficiency virus [HIV] disease (B20)
          ▶ Pneumococcal meningitis (G00.1)
          ▶ Pneumococcal pneumonia (J13)
          ▶ Sepsis due to Streptococcus pneumoniae (A40.3)
          ▶ Shigella dysenteriae (A03.9)
          ▶ Streptococcus pneumoniae as the cause of diseases classified elsewhere (B95.3)

     ▶ **D59.32**   **Hereditary hemolytic-uremic syndrome**
        ▶ Atypical hemolytic uremic syndrome with an identified genetic cause

        ▶ Code also, if applicable:
          ▶ defects in the complement system (D84.1)
          ▶ methylmalonic acidemia (E71.120)

     ▶ **D59.39**   **Other hemolytic-uremic syndrome**
        ▶ Atypical (nongenetic) hemolytic uremic syndrome
        ▶ Secondary hemolytic-uremic syndrome
        ▶ *Code first, if applicable, any associated:*
          ▶ COVID-19 (U07.1)
          ▶ complications of kidney transplant (T86.1-)
          ▶ complications of heart transplant (T86.2-)
          ▶ complications of liver transplant (T86.4-)
        ▶ Code also, if applicable, any associated condition, such as:
          ▶ hypertensive emergency (I16.1)
          ▶ malignant neoplasm (C00-C96)
          ▶ systemic lupus erythematosus (M32.-)
        ▶ Use Additional code, if applicable, for adverse effect to identify drug (T36-T50 with fifth or sixth character 5)

CHAPTER 3 (D50-D89)

CHAPTER 3 (D50-D89)

D59.4   **Other nonautoimmune hemolytic anemias** 🩸
     Mechanical hemolytic anemia
     Microangiopathic hemolytic anemia
     Toxic hemolytic anemia

D59.5   **Paroxysmal nocturnal hemoglobinuria [Marchiafava-Micheli]**
     Excludes 1   hemoglobinuria NOS (R82.3)

D59.6   **Hemoglobinuria due to hemolysis from other external causes** 🩸
     Hemoglobinuria from exertion
     March hemoglobinuria
     Paroxysmal cold hemoglobinuria
     Use additional code (Chapter 20) to identify external cause
     Excludes 1   hemoglobinuria NOS (R82.3)

D59.8   **Other acquired hemolytic anemias** 🩸

D59.9   **Acquired hemolytic anemia, unspecified** 🩸
     Idiopathic hemolytic anemia, chronic

APLASTIC AND OTHER ANEMIAS AND OTHER BONE MARROW FAILURE SYNDROMES (D60-D64)

● **D60**   **Acquired pure red cell aplasia [erythroblastopenia]**
     Deficiency of erythroblasts
     Includes   red cell aplasia (acquired) (adult) (with thymoma)
     Excludes 1   congenital red cell aplasia (D61.01)

D60.0   **Chronic acquired pure red cell aplasia** 🩸
     Lack of development of blood cell

D60.1   **Transient acquired pure red cell aplasia** 🩸

D60.8   **Other acquired pure red cell aplasias** 🩸

D60.9   **Acquired pure red cell aplasia, unspecified** 🩸

● **D61**   **Other aplastic anemias and other bone marrow failure syndromes**
     Excludes 2   neutropenia (D70.-)

● D61.0   **Constitutional aplastic anemia**
     Condition where bone marrow is unable to produce blood cells

     D61.01   **Constitutional (pure) red blood cell aplasia** 🩸
         Blackfan-Diamond syndrome
         Congenital (pure) red cell aplasia
         Familial hypoplastic anemia
         Primary (pure) red cell aplasia
         Red cell (pure) aplasia of infants
         Excludes 1   acquired red cell aplasia (D60.9)

     D61.09   **Other constitutional aplastic anemia** 🩸
         Fanconi's anemia
         Pancytopenia with malformations

D61.1   **Drug-induced aplastic anemia** 🩸
     Use additional code for adverse effect, if applicable, to identify drug (T36-T50 with fifth or sixth character 5)

D61.2   **Aplastic anemia due to other external agents** 🩸
     Code first, if applicable, toxic effects of substances chiefly nonmedicinal as to source (T51-T65)

D61.3   **Idiopathic aplastic anemia** 🩸

● D61.8   **Other specified aplastic anemias and other bone marrow failure syndromes**

     ● D61.81   **Pancytopenia**
         Marked deficiency of all the blood elements: Red blood cells (erythrocytes), white blood cells (leukocytes), and platelets (thrombocytes). Check laboratory results.

         Excludes 1   pancytopenia (due to) (with) aplastic anemia (D61.9)
                    pancytopenia (due to) (with) bone marrow infiltration (D61.82)
                    pancytopenia (due to) (with) congenital (pure) red cell aplasia (D61.01)
                    pancytopenia (due to) (with) hairy cell leukemia (C91.4-)
                    pancytopenia (due to) (with) human immunodeficiency virus disease (B20.-)
                    pancytopenia (due to) (with) leukoerythroblastic anemia (D61.82)
                    pancytopenia (due to) (with) myeloproliferative disease (D47.1)

         Excludes 2   pancytopenia (due to) (with) myelodysplastic syndromes (D46.-)

     D61.810   **Antineoplastic chemotherapy induced pancytopenia** 🩸
         Excludes 2   aplastic anemia due to antineoplastic chemotherapy (D61.1)

     D61.811   **Other drug-induced pancytopenia** 🩸
         Excludes 2   aplastic anemia due to drugs (D61.1)

     D61.818   **Other pancytopenia** 🩸
         Coding Clinic: 2019, Q1, P16

     D61.82   **Myelophthisis** 🩸
         Leukoerythroblastic anemia
         Myelophthisic anemia
         Panmyelophthisis
         Code also the underlying disorder, such as: malignant neoplasm of breast (C50.-) tuberculosis (A15.-)
         Excludes 1   idiopathic myelofibrosis (D47.1)
                    myelofibrosis NOS (D75.81)
                    myelofibrosis with myeloid metaplasia (D47.4)
                    primary myelofibrosis (D47.1)
                    secondary myelofibrosis (D75.81)

     D61.89   **Other specified aplastic anemias and other bone marrow failure syndromes** 🩸

D61.9   **Aplastic anemia, unspecified** 🩸
     Hypoplastic anemia NOS
     Medullary hypoplasia

D62   **Acute posthemorrhagic anemia**
     Excludes 1   anemia due to chronic blood loss (D50.0)
                    blood loss anemia NOS (D50.0)
                    congenital anemia from fetal blood loss (P61.3)
     Coding Clinic: 2019, Q3, P13,17

▶ New   ⇒ Revised   ~~deleted~~ Deleted   Excludes 1   Excludes 2   Includes   Use additional   Code first   Code also   Key words
OGCR Official Guidelines   **X** Assign placeholder X   ● Use Additional Character(s)   ▶ Manifestation Code   🩸 Hierarchical Condition Category   **Coding Clinic**

● **D63   Anemia in chronic diseases classified elsewhere**

▶ **D63.0**   *Anemia in neoplastic disease*

     Code first neoplasm (C00-D49)

     Excludes1   aplastic anemia due to antineoplastic chemotherapy (D61.1)

     Excludes2   anemia due to antineoplastic chemotherapy (D64.81)

     OGCR   Section I.C.2.e.2.

> 2) Anemia associated with chemotherapy, immunotherapy and radiation therapy
>
> When the admission/encounter is for management of an anemia associated with an adverse effect of the administration of chemotherapy or immunotherapy and the only treatment is for the anemia, the anemia code is sequenced first followed by the appropriate codes for the neoplasm and the adverse effect (T45.1X5, Adverse effect of antineoplastic and immunosuppressive drugs).

▶ **D63.1**   *Anemia in chronic kidney disease*

     Erythropoietin resistant anemia (EPO resistant anemia)

     Code first underlying chronic kidney disease (CKD) (N18.-)

▶ **D63.8**   *Anemia in other chronic diseases classified elsewhere*

     Code first underlying disease, such as:
       diphyllobothriasis (B70.0)
       hookworm disease (B76.0-B76.9)
       hypothyroidism (E00.0-E03.9)
       malaria (B50.0-B54)
       symptomatic late syphilis (A52.79)
       tuberculosis (A18.89)

● **D64   Other anemias**

     Excludes1   refractory anemia (D46.-)
          refractory anemia with excess blasts in transformation [RAEB T] (C92.0-)

D64.0   **Hereditary sideroblastic anemia** 🔖
     Abnormal production RBCs (erythrocytes)
     Sex-linked hypochromic sideroblastic anemia

▶ **D64.1**   **Secondary sideroblastic anemia due to disease** 🔖
     Code first underlying disease

D64.2   **Secondary sideroblastic anemia due to drugs and toxins** 🔖
     Code first poisoning due to drug or toxin, if applicable (T36-T65 with fifth or sixth character 1-4 or 6)
     Use additional code for adverse effect, if applicable, to identify drug (T36-T50 with fifth or sixth character 5)

D64.3   **Other sideroblastic anemias** 🔖
     Sideroblastic anemia NOS
     Pyridoxine-responsive sideroblastic anemia NEC

D64.4   **Congenital dyserythropoietic anemia**
     Any of several rare hereditary anemias, mostly types of macrocytic anemia
     Dyshematopoietic anemia (congenital)

     Excludes1   Blackfan-Diamond syndrome (D61.01)
          Di Guglielmo's disease (C94.0)

● **D64.8**   **Other specified anemias**

     D64.81   **Anemia due to antineoplastic chemotherapy**
          Antineoplastic chemotherapy induced anemia
          aplastic anemia due to antineoplastic chemotherapy (D61.1)

          Excludes2   anemia in neoplastic disease (D63.0)
          Coding Clinic: 2021, Q3, P4

     D64.89   **Other specified anemias**
          Infantile pseudoleukemia

D64.9   **Anemia, unspecified**
     Coding Clinic: 2018, Q4, P88; 2017, Q1, P7

COAGULATION DEFECTS, PURPURA AND OTHER HEMORRHAGIC CONDITIONS (D65-D69)

D65   Disseminated intravascular coagulation [defibrination syndrome] 🔖
     Blood clots form and consume all coagulation proteins and platelets and disrupt normal coagulation, resulting in abnormal bleeding
     Afibrinogenemia, acquired
     Consumption coagulopathy
     Diffuse or disseminated intravascular coagulation [DIC]
     Fibrinolytic hemorrhage, acquired
     Fibrinolytic purpura
     Purpura fulminans

     Excludes1   disseminated intravascular coagulation (complicating):
          abortion or ectopic or molar pregnancy (O00-O07, O08.1)
          in newborn (P60)
          pregnancy, childbirth and the puerperium (O45.0, O46.0, O67.0, O72.3)

     Coding Clinic: 2021, Q1, P39; 2019, Q2, P25

D66   Hereditary factor VIII deficiency 🔖
     Inherited coagulation disorder carried by females but most often affecting males
     Classical hemophilia
     Deficiency factor VIII (with functional defect)
     Hemophilia NOS
     Hemophilia A

     Excludes1   factor VIII deficiency with vascular defect (D68.0-)

D67   Hereditary factor IX deficiency 🔖
     Christmas disease
     Factor IX deficiency (with functional defect)
     Hemophilia B
     Plasma thromboplastin component [PTC] deficiency

● **D68   Other coagulation defects**

     Excludes1   abnormal coagulation profile NOS (R79.1)
          ~~coagulation defects complicating abortion or ectopic or molar pregnancy (O00-O07, O08.1)~~
          ~~coagulation defects complicating pregnancy, childbirth and the puerperium (O45.0, O46.0, O67.0, O72.3)~~

     Excludes2   coagulation defects complicating abortion or ectopic or molar pregnancy (O00-O07, O08.1)
          coagulation defects complicating pregnancy, childbirth and the puerperium (O45.0, O46.0, O67.0, O72.3)

     Coding Clinic: 2016, Q1, P14

▶ **D68.0   Von Willebrand disease** 🔖
     Congenital bleeding disorder
     ~~Angiohemophilia~~
     ~~Factor VIII deficiency with vascular defect~~
     ~~Vascular hemophilia~~

     Excludes1   capillary fragility (hereditary) (D69.8)
          factor VIII deficiency NOS (D66)
          factor VIII deficiency with functional defect (D66)

     ▶ **D68.00**   **Von Willebrand disease, unspecified**

     ▶ **D68.01**   **Von Willebrand disease, type 1**
          ▶ Partial quantitative deficiency of von Willebrand factor
          ▶ Type 1C von Willebrand disease

     ▶ ● **D68.02**   **Von Willebrand disease, type 2**
          ▶ Qualitative defects of von Willebrand factor

          ▶ **D68.020**   **Von Willebrand disease, type 2A**
               ▶ Qualitative defects of von Willebrand factor with decreased platelet adhesion and selective deficiency of high-molecular-weight multimers

CHAPTER 3 (D50-D89)

▶**D68.021   Von Willebrand disease, type 2B**
　▶Qualitative defects of von Willebrand factor with high-molecular-weight von Willebrand factor loss
　▶Qualitative defects of von Willebrand factor with hyper-adhesive forms
　▶Qualitative defects of von Willebrand factor with increased affinity for platelet glycoprotein lb

▶**D68.022   Von Willebrand disease, type 2M**
　▶Qualitative defects of von Willebrand factor with defective platelet adhesion with anormal size distribution of von Willebrand factor multimers

▶**D68.023   Von Willebrand disease, type 2N**
　▶Qualitative defects of von Willebrand factor with defective von Willebrand factor to factor VIII binding
　▶Qualitative defects of von Willebrand factor with markedly decreased affinity for factor VIII

▶**D68.029   Von Willebrand disease, type 2, unspecified**
　▶Qualitative defect in von Willebrand factor function, with no further subtyping

▶**D68.03   Von Willebrand disease, type 3**
　▶(Near) complete absence of von Willebrand factor
　▶Total quantitative deficiency of von Willebrand factor

▶**D68.04   Acquired von Willebrand disease**
　▶Acquired von Willebrand syndrome

▶**D68.09   Other von Willebrand disease**
　▶Platelet-type von Willebrand disease
　▶Pseudo-von Willebrand disease
　▶ Code also, if applicable, qualitative platelet defects (D69.1)

D68.1   Hereditary factor XI deficiency 🔲
　Deficiency of blood coagulation resulting in systemic blood-clotting defect
　Hemophilia C
　Plasma thromboplastin antecedent [PTA] deficiency
　Rosenthal's disease

D68.2   Hereditary deficiency of other clotting factors 🔲
　Blood clotting disorders caused by hereditary deficiencies of one or more clotting factors
　AC globulin deficiency
　Congenital afibrinogenemia
　Deficiency of factor I [fibrinogen]
　Deficiency of factor II [prothrombin]
　Deficiency of factor V [labile]
　Deficiency of factor VII [stable]
　Deficiency of factor X [Stuart-Prower]
　Deficiency of factor XII [Hageman]
　Deficiency of factor XIII [fibrin stabilizing]
　Dysfibrinogenemia (congenital)
　Hypoproconvertinemia
　Owren's disease
　Proaccelerin deficiency

●**D68.3   Hemorrhagic disorder due to circulating anticoagulants**
　Blood clotting disorders caused by anticoagulants (warfarin and heparin)

●**D68.31   Hemorrhagic disorder due to intrinsic circulating anticoagulants, antibodies, or inhibitors**

　D68.311   Acquired hemophilia 🔲
　　Autoimmune hemophilia
　　Autoimmune inhibitors to clotting factors
　　Secondary hemophilia

　D68.312   Antiphospholipid antibody with hemorrhagic disorder 🔲
　　Lupus anticoagulant (LAC) with hemorrhagic disorder
　　Systemic lupus erythematosus [SLE] inhibitor with hemorrhagic disorder

　　Excludes1   antiphospholipid antibody, finding without diagnosis (R76.0)
　　　antiphospholipid antibody syndrome (D68.61)
　　　antiphospholipid antibody with hypercoagulable state (D68.61)
　　　lupus anticoagulant (LAC) finding without diagnosis (R76.0)
　　　lupus anticoagulant (LAC) with hypercoagulable state (D68.62)
　　　systemic lupus erythematosus [SLE] inhibitor finding without diagnosis (R76.0)
　　　systemic lupus erythematosus [SLE] inhibitor with hypercoagulable state (D68.62)

　D68.318   Other hemorrhagic disorder due to intrinsic circulating anticoagulants, antibodies, or inhibitors 🔲
　　Antithromboplastinemia
　　Antithromboplastinogenemia
　　Hemorrhagic disorder due to intrinsic increase in antithrombin
　　Hemorrhagic disorder due to intrinsic increase in anti-VIIIa
　　Hemorrhagic disorder due to intrinsic increase in anti-IXa
　　Hemorrhagic disorder due to intrinsic increase in anti-XIa

D68.32   **Hemorrhagic disorder due to extrinsic circulating anticoagulants** 🔍
Drug-induced hemorrhagic disorder
Hemorrhagic disorder due to increase in anti-IIa
Hemorrhagic disorder due to increase in anti-Xa
Hyperheparinemia
Use additional code for adverse effect, if applicable, to identify drug (T45.515, T45.525)
Coding Clinic: 2021, Q1, P5; 2016, Q1, P14-15

D68.4   **Acquired coagulation factor deficiency** 🔍
Deficiency of coagulation factor due to liver disease
Deficiency of coagulation factor due to vitamin K deficiency
Excludes1   vitamin K deficiency of newborn (P53)

● **D68.5**   **Primary thrombophilia**
AKA idiopathic thrombocytopenia, may be acquired or congenital and is a common cause of coagulation disorders.
Primary hypercoagulable states
Excludes1   antiphospholipid syndrome (D68.61)
lupus anticoagulant (D68.62)
secondary activated protein C resistance (D68.69)
secondary antiphospholipid antibody syndrome (D68.69)
secondary lupus anticoagulant with hypercoagulable state (D68.69)
secondary systemic lupus erythematosus [SLE] inhibitor with hypercoagulable state (D68.69)
systemic lupus erythematosus [SLE] inhibitor finding without diagnosis (R76.0)
systemic lupus erythematosus [SLE] inhibitor with hemorrhagic disorder (D68.312)
thrombotic thrombocytopenic purpura (M31.19)

     D68.51   **Activated protein C resistance** 🔍
Factor V Leiden mutation

     D68.52   **Prothrombin gene mutation** 🔍

     D68.59   **Other primary thrombophilia** 🔍
Antithrombin III deficiency
Hypercoagulable state NOS
Primary hypercoagulable state NEC
Primary thrombophilia NEC
Protein C deficiency
Protein S deficiency
Thrombophilia NOS
Coding Clinic: 2021, Q2, P8-9

● **D68.6**   **Other thrombophilia**
Other hypercoagulable states
Excludes1   diffuse or disseminated intravascular coagulation [DIC] (D65)
heparin induced thrombocytopenia (HIT) (D75.82-)
hyperhomocysteinemia (E72.11)

     D68.61   **Antiphospholipid syndrome** 🔍
Anticardiolipin syndrome
Antiphospholipid antibody syndrome
Excludes1   anti-phospholipid antibody, finding without diagnosis (R76.0)
anti-phospholipid antibody with hemorrhagic disorder (D68.312)
lupus anticoagulant syndrome (D68.62)

     D68.62   **Lupus anticoagulant syndrome** 🔍
Lupus anticoagulant
Presence of systemic lupus erythematosus [SLE] inhibitor
Excludes1   anticardiolipin syndrome (D68.61)
antiphospholipid syndrome (D68.61)
lupus anticoagulant (LAC) finding without diagnosis (R76.0)
lupus anticoagulant (LAC) with hemorrhagic disorder (D68.312)

     D68.69   **Other thrombophilia** 🔍
Hypercoagulable states NEC
Secondary hypercoagulable state NOS
Coding Clinic: 2021, Q2, P8

D68.8   **Other specified coagulation defects** 🔍
Excludes1   hemorrhagic disease of newborn (P53)
Coding Clinic: 2021, Q1, P39-40

D68.9   **Coagulation defect, unspecified** 🔍

● **D69**   **Purpura and other hemorrhagic conditions**
Group of conditions characterized by small hemorrhages in skin, mucous membranes, or serosal surfaces
Excludes1   benign hypergammaglobulinemic purpura (D89.0)
cryoglobulinemic purpura (D89.1)
essential (hemorrhagic) thrombocythemia (D47.3)
hemorrhagic thrombocythemia (D47.3)
purpura fulminans (D65)
thrombotic thrombocytopenic purpura (M31.19)
Waldenström hypergammaglobulinemic purpura (D89.0)

D69.0   **Allergic purpura** 🔍
Allergic vasculitis
Nonthrombocytopenic hemorrhagic purpura
Nonthrombocytopenic idiopathic purpura
Purpura anaphylactoid
Purpura Henoch(-Schönlein)
Purpura rheumatica
Vascular purpura
Excludes1   thrombocytopenic hemorrhagic purpura (D69.3)

D69.1   **Qualitative platelet defects** 🔍
Bernard-Soulier [giant platelet] syndrome
Glanzmann's disease
Grey platelet syndrome
Thromboasthenia (hemorrhagic) (hereditary)
Thrombocytopathy
Excludes1   ~~von Willebrand's disease (D68.0)~~
► hemolytic-uremic syndrome (D59.3-)
► **Excludes2**   von Willebrand disease (D68.0-)

D69.2   **Other nonthrombocytopenic purpura** 🔍
Purpura NOS
Purpura simplex
Senile purpura

D69.3   **Immune thrombocytopenic purpura** 🔍
Hemorrhagic (thrombocytopenic) purpura
Idiopathic thrombocytopenic purpura
Tidal platelet dysgenesis

● **D69.4**   **Other primary thrombocytopenia**
Excludes1   transient neonatal thrombocytopenia (P61.0)
Wiskott-Aldrich syndrome (D82.0)

     D69.41   **Evans syndrome** 🔍
Acquired hemolytic anemia and thrombocytopenia

CHAPTER 3 (D50-D89)

D69.42 Congenital and hereditary thrombocytopenia purpura 🐾
Congenital thrombocytopenia
Hereditary thrombocytopenia
Code first congenital or hereditary disorder, such as:
thrombocytopenia with absent radius (TAR syndrome) (Q87.2)

D69.49 Other primary thrombocytopenia 🐾
Megakaryocytic hypoplasia
Primary thrombocytopenia NOS

D69.5 Secondary thrombocytopenia
Acquired reduction of number of platelets required for blood clotting

Excludes1 heparin induced thrombocytopenia (HIT) (D75.82-)
transient thrombocytopenia of newborn (P61.0)

D69.51 Posttransfusion purpura
Posttransfusion purpura from whole blood (fresh) or blood products PTP

D69.59 Other secondary thrombocytopenia

D69.6 Thrombocytopenia, unspecified 🐾

D69.8 Other specified hemorrhagic conditions 🐾
Capillary fragility (hereditary)
Vascular pseudohemophilia

D69.9 Hemorrhagic condition, unspecified 🐾

OTHER DISORDERS OF BLOOD AND BLOOD-FORMING ORGANS (D70-D77)

D70 Neutropenia
Decrease in number of neutrophils (type of white blood cell)

Includes agranulocytosis
decreased absolute neurophile count (ANC)
Use additional code for any associated:
fever (R50.81)
mucositis (J34.81, K12.3-, K92.81, N76.81)

Excludes1 neutropenic splenomegaly (D73.81)
transient neonatal neutropenia (P61.5)

D70.0 Congenital agranulocytosis 🐾
Reduced numbers of neutrophils (type of white blood cell)
Congenital neutropenia
Infantile genetic agranulocytosis
Kostmann's disease

D70.1 Agranulocytosis secondary to cancer chemotherapy 🐾
Decreased numbers of granulocytes (type of white blood cell)
Code also *underlying neoplasm*
Use additional code for adverse effect, if applicable, to identify drug (T45.1X5)

D70.2 Other drug-induced agranulocytosis 🐾
Use additional code for adverse effect, if applicable, to identify drug (T36-T50 with fifth or sixth character 5)

D70.3 Neutropenia due to infection 🐾

D70.4 Cyclic neutropenia 🐾
Chronic neutropenia (low number of type of white blood cell)
Cyclic hematopoiesis
Periodic neutropenia

D70.8 Other neutropenia 🐾

D70.9 Neutropenia, unspecified 🐾
Coding Clinic: 2019, Q2, P25

D71 Functional disorders of polymorphonuclear neutrophils 🐾
Polymorphonuclear: varying shapes of nucleus; AKA PMNs
Cell membrane receptor complex [CR3] defect
Chronic (childhood) granulomatous disease
Congenital dysphagocytosis
Progressive septic granulomatosis

D72 Other disorders of white blood cells
Excludes1 basophilia (D72.824)
immunity disorders (D80-D89)
neutropenia (D70)
preleukemia (syndrome) (D46.9)

D72.0 Genetic anomalies of leukocytes 🐾
Alder (granulation) (granulocyte) anomaly
Alder syndrome
Hereditary leukocytic hypersegmentation
Hereditary leukocytic hyposegmentation
Hereditary leukomelanopathy
May-Hegglin (granulation) (granulocyte) anomaly
May-Hegglin syndrome
Pelger-Huët (granulation) (granulocyte) anomaly
Pelger-Huët syndrome
Excludes1 Chédiak (-Steinbrinck)-Higashi syndrome (E70.330)

D72.1 Eosinophilia
Formation and accumulation of high number of white cells in blood/tissue
Excludes2 Löffler's syndrome (J82.89)
pulmonary eosinophilia (J82.-)

D72.10 Eosinophilia, unspecified

D72.11 Hypereosinophilic syndrome [HES]

D72.110 Idiopathic hypereosinophilic syndrome [IHES]

D72.111 Lymphocytic Variant Hypereosinophilic Syndrome [LHES]
Lymphocyte variant hypereosinophilia
Code also, if applicable, any associated lymphocytic neoplastic disorder

D72.118 Other hypereosinophilic syndrome
Episodic angioedema with eosinophilia
Gleich's syndrome

D72.119 Hypereosinophilic syndrome [HES], unspecified

D72.12 Drug rash with eosinophilia and systemic symptoms syndrome
DRESS syndrome
Use additional code for adverse effect, if applicable, to identify drug (T36-T50 with fifth or sixth character 5)

D72.18 Eosinophilia in diseases classified elsewhere
Code first underlying disease, such as:
chronic myelomonocytic leukemia (C93.1-)

D72.19 Other eosinophilia
Familial eosinophilia
Hereditary eosinophilia

D72.8 Other specified disorders of white blood cells
Excludes1 leukemia (C91-C95)

D72.81 Decreased white blood cell count
Excludes1 neutropenia (D70.-)

D72.810 Lymphocytopenia
Decreased lymphocytes
Reduction in number of lympho cytes in blood

D72.818 Other decreased white blood cell count
Basophilic leukopenia
Eosinophilic leukopenia
Monocytopenia
Other decreased leukocytes
Plasmacytopenia

D72.819 Decreased white blood cell count, unspecified
Decreased leukocytes, unspecified
Leukocytopenia, unspecified
Leukopenia
Excludes1 malignant leukopenia (D70.9)

● **D72.82 Elevated white blood cell count**
> **Excludes1**   eosinophilia (D72.1)

D72.820 Lymphocytosis (symptomatic)
> Elevated lymphocytes
> *Excess of normal lymphocytes*

D72.821 Monocytosis (symptomatic)
> **Excludes1**   infectious
> mononucleosis
> (B27.-)

D72.822 Plasmacytosis
> *Presence of excess plasma cells*

D72.823 Leukemoid reaction
> Basophilic leukemoid reaction
> Leukemoid reaction NOS
> Lymphocytic leukemoid reaction
> Monocytic leukemoid reaction
> Myelocytic leukemoid reaction
> Neutrophilic leukemoid reaction

D72.824 Basophilia
> *Increase of basophils in blood*

D72.825 Bandemia
> Bandemia without diagnosis of
> specific infection
> *Excess number of band cells (immature
> white blood cells) released by bone
> marrow*
>> **Excludes1**   confirmed infection
>> -code to infection
>> leukemia (C91.-,
>> C92.-, C93.-,
>> C94.-, C95.-)

D72.828 Other elevated white blood cell count

**D72.829 Elevated white blood cell
count, unspecified**
> Elevated leukocytes, unspecified
> Leukocytosis, unspecified

D72.89 Other specified disorders of white blood cells
> Abnormality of white blood cells NEC

D72.9 Disorder of white blood cells, unspecified
> Abnormal leukocyte differential NOS

● **D73 Diseases of spleen**

D73.0 Hyposplenism
> *Diminished functioning of spleen*
> Atrophy of spleen
>> **Excludes1**   asplenia (congenital) (Q89.01)
>> postsurgical absence of spleen (Z90.81)

D73.1 Hypersplenism
> *Accelerated function of spleen*
>> **Excludes1**   neutropenic splenomegaly (D73.81)
>> primary splenic neutropenia (D73.81)
>> splenitis, splenomegaly in late syphilis
>> (A52.79)
>> splenitis, splenomegaly in tuberculosis
>> (A18.85)
>> splenomegaly NOS (R16.1)
>> splenomegaly congenital (Q89.0)

D73.2 Chronic congestive splenomegaly
> *Enlargement of spleen*

D73.3 Abscess of spleen

D73.4 Cyst of spleen

D73.5 Infarction of spleen
> Splenic rupture, nontraumatic
> Torsion of spleen
>> **Excludes1**   rupture of spleen due to Plasmodium
>> vivax malaria (B51.0)
>> traumatic rupture of spleen (S36.03-)

● **D73.8 Other diseases of spleen**

D73.81 Neutropenic splenomegaly
> Werner-Schultz disease
> *Enlarged spleen responding to inadequate number
> of neutrophils*

D73.89 Other diseases of spleen
> Fibrosis of spleen NOS
> Perisplenitis
> Splenitis NOS

D73.9 Disease of spleen, unspecified

● **D74 Methemoglobinemia**
> *Excessive methemoglobin (form of hemoglobin)*

D74.0 Congenital methemoglobinemia
> Congenital NADH-methemoglobin reductase
> deficiency
> Hemoglobin-M [Hb-M] disease
> Methemoglobinemia, hereditary

D74.8 Other methemoglobinemias
> Acquired methemoglobinemia (with
> sulfhemoglobinemia)
> Toxic methemoglobinemia

D74.9 Methemoglobinemia, unspecified

● **D75 Other and unspecified diseases of blood and blood-forming
organs**
> **Excludes2**   acute lymphadenitis (L04.-)
> chronic lymphadenitis (I88.1)
> enlarged lymph nodes (R59.-)
> hypergammaglobulinemia NOS (D89.2)
> lymphadenitis NOS (I88.9)
> mesenteric lymphadenitis (acute) (chronic) (I88.0)

**D75.A Glucose-6-phosphate dehydrogenase (G6PD) deficiency
without anemia**
> **Excludes1**   glucose-6-phosphate dehydrogenase
> (G6PD) deficiency with anemia
> (D55.0)

D75.0 Familial erythrocytosis
> *Genetic mutation of gene that results in increased circulating
> RBCs*
> Benign polycythemia
> Familial polycythemia
>> **Excludes1**   hereditary ovalocytosis (D58.1)

D75.1 Secondary polycythemia
> *Increase in total red cell mass*
> Acquired polycythemia
> Emotional polycythemia
> Erythrocytosis NOS
> Hypoxemic polycythemia
> Nephrogenous polycythemia
> Polycythemia due to erythropoietin
> Polycythemia due to fall in plasma volume
> Polycythemia due to high altitude
> Polycythemia due to stress
> Polycythemia NOS
> Relative polycythemia
>> **Excludes1**   polycythemia neonatorum (P61.1)
>> polycythemia vera (D45)

CHAPTER 3 (D50-D89)

CHAPTER 3 (D50-D89)

● **D75.8** **Other specified diseases of blood and blood-forming organs**

▷ *D75.81* *Myelofibrosis* 🐾
  Replacing bone marrow by fibrous tissue
  Myelofibrosis NOS
  Secondary myelofibrosis NOS

  Code first the underlying disorder, such as:
  malignant neoplasm of breast (C50.-)

  Use additional code, if applicable, for associated therapy-related myelodysplastic syndrome (D46.-)

  Use additional code for adverse effect, if applicable, to identify drug (T45.1X5)

  Excludes1 acute myelofibrosis (C94.4-)
  idiopathic myelofibrosis (D47.1)
  leukoerythroblastic anemia (D61.82)
  myelofibrosis with myeloid metaplasia (D47.4)
  myelophthisic anemia (D61.82)
  myelophthisis (D61.82)
  primary myelofibrosis (D47.1)

D75.82 **Heparin induced thrombocytopenia (HIT)** 🐾

▶ Use Additional code, if applicable, for adverse effect of heparin (T45.515-)

▷ **D75.821** **Non-immune heparin-induced thrombocytopenia**
  ▶Non-immune HIT
  ▶Type 1 heparin-induced thrombocytopenia

▷ **D75.822** **Immune-mediated heparin-induced thrombocytopenia**
  ▶Immune-mediated HIT
  ▶Type 2 heparin-induced thrombocytopenia

▷ **D75.828** **Other heparin-induced thrombocytopenia syndrome**
  ▶Autoimmune heparin-induced thrombocytopenia syndrome
  ▶Delayed-onset heparin-induced thrombocytopenia
  ▶Persisting heparin-induced thrombocytopenia

▷ **D75.829** **Heparin-induced thrombocytopenia, unspecified**

● **D75.83** **Thrombocytosis**
  Excludes2 essential thrombocythemia (D47.3)

  D75.838 **Other thrombocytosis**
  Reactive thrombocytosis
  Secondary thrombocytosis
  Code also, underlying condition, if known and applicable

  D75.839 **Thrombocytosis, unspecified**
  Thrombocythemia NOS
  Thrombocytosis NOS

▷ **D75.84** **Other platelet-activating anti-PF4 disorders**
  ▶Spontaneous heparin-induced thrombocytopenia syndrome (without heparin exposure)
  ▶Thrombosis with thrombocytopenia syndrome
  ▶Vaccine-induced thrombotic thrombocytopenia
  ▶ Use Additional code, if applicable, for adverse effect of other viral vaccine (T50.B95-)

D75.89 **Other specified diseases of blood and blood-forming organs**

D75.9 **Disease of blood and blood-forming organs, unspecified**

● **D76** **Other specified diseases with participation of lymphoreticular and reticulohistiocytic tissue**
  Excludes1 (Abt-) Letterer-Siwe disease (C96.0)
  eosinophilic granuloma (C96.6)
  Hand-Schüller-Christian disease (C96.5)
  histiocytic medullary reticulosis (C96.9)
  histiocytic sarcoma (C96.A)
  histiocytosis X, multifocal (C96.5)
  histiocytosis X, unifocal (C96.6)
  Langerhans-cell histiocytosis, multifocal (C96.5)
  Langerhans-cell histiocytosis NOS (C96.6)
  Langerhans-cell histiocytosis, unifocal (C96.6)
  leukemic reticuloendotheliosis (C91.4-)
  lipomelanotic reticulosis (I89.8)
  malignant histiocytosis (C96.A)
  malignant reticulosis (C86.0)
  nonlipid reticuloendotheliosis (C96.0)

D76.1 **Hemophagocytic lymphohistiocytosis** 🐾
  Familial hemophagocytic reticulosis
  Histiocytoses of mononuclear phagocytes

D76.2 **Hemophagocytic syndrome, infection-associated** 🐾
  Use additional code to identify infectious agent or disease.

D76.3 **Other histiocytosis syndromes** 🐾
  Reticulohistiocytoma (giant-cell)
  Sinus histiocytosis with massive lymphadenopathy
  Xanthogranuloma

▷ **D77** *Other disorders of blood and blood-forming organs in diseases classified elsewhere*
  Code first underlying disease, such as:
  amyloidosis (E85.-)
  congenital early syphilis (A50.0)
  echinococcosis (B67.0-B67.9)
  malaria (B50.0-B54)
  schistosomiasis [bilharziasis] (B65.0-B65.9)
  vitamin C deficiency (E54)
  Excludes1 rupture of spleen due to Plasmodium vivax malaria (B51.0)
  splenitis, splenomegaly in late syphilis (A52.79)
  splenitis, splenomegaly in tuberculosis (A18.85)

INTRAOPERATIVE AND POSTPROCEDURAL COMPLICATIONS OF THE SPLEEN (D78)

● **D78** **Intraoperative and postprocedural complications of the spleen**
  Coding Clinic: 2016, Q4, P9

  ● **D78.0** **Intraoperative hemorrhage and hematoma of the spleen complicating a procedure**
  Excludes1 intraoperative hemorrhage and hematoma of the spleen due to accidental puncture or laceration during a procedure (D78.1-)

  D78.01 **Intraoperative hemorrhage and hematoma of the spleen complicating a procedure on the spleen**

  D78.02 **Intraoperative hemorrhage and hematoma of the spleen complicating other procedure**

  ● **D78.1** **Accidental puncture and laceration of the spleen during a procedure**
  D78.11 **Accidental puncture and laceration of the spleen during a procedure on the spleen**
  D78.12 **Accidental puncture and laceration of the spleen during other procedure**
  Coding Clinic: 2022, Q1, P22-23

  ● **D78.2** **Postprocedural hemorrhage of the spleen following a procedure**
  D78.21 **Postprocedural hemorrhage of the spleen following a procedure on the spleen**
  D78.22 **Postprocedural hemorrhage of the spleen following other procedure**

▶ New ⟹ Revised ~~deleted~~ Deleted Excludes 1 Excludes 2 Includes Use additional Code first Code also Key words
OGCR Official Guidelines X Assign placeholder X ● Use Additional Character(s) ▷ Manifestation Code 🐾 Hierarchical Condition Category Coding Clinic

● **D78.3** Postprocedural hematoma and seroma of the spleen following a procedure

    D78.31 Postprocedural hematoma of the spleen following a procedure on the spleen

    D78.32 Postprocedural hematoma of the spleen following other procedure

    D78.33 Postprocedural seroma of the spleen following a procedure on the spleen

    D78.34 Postprocedural seroma of the spleen following other procedure

● **D78.8** Other intraoperative and postprocedural complications of the spleen

    Use additional code, if applicable, to further specify disorder

    D78.81 Other intraoperative complications of the spleen

    D78.89 Other postprocedural complications of the spleen

CERTAIN DISORDERS INVOLVING THE IMMUNE MECHANISM (D80–D89)

Includes	defects in the complement system immunodeficiency disorders, except human immunodeficiency virus [HIV] disease sarcoidosis
Excludes1	autoimmune disease (systemic) NOS (M35.9) functional disorders of polymorphonuclear neutrophils (D71) human immunodeficiency virus [HIV] disease (B20)

● **D80** Immunodeficiency with predominantly antibody defects

    D80.0 Hereditary hypogammaglobulinemia 🐾
        Autosomal recessive agammaglobulinemia (Swiss type)
        X-linked agammaglobulinemia [Bruton] (with growth hormone deficiency)

    D80.1 Nonfamilial hypogammaglobulinemia 🐾
        Abnormally low levels of all classes of immunoglobulins
        Agammaglobulinemia with immunoglobulin-bearing B-lymphocytes
        Common variable agammaglobulinemia [CVAgamma]
        Hypogammaglobulinemia NOS

    D80.2 Selective deficiency of immunoglobulin A [IgA] 🐾

    D80.3 Selective deficiency of immunoglobulin G [IgG] subclasses 🐾

    D80.4 Selective deficiency of immunoglobulin M [IgM] 🐾

    D80.5 Immunodeficiency with increased immunoglobulin M [IgM] 🐾

    D80.6 Antibody deficiency with near-normal immunoglobulins or with hyperimmunoglobulinemia 🐾
        Abnormally high levels of immunoglobulins in serum

    D80.7 Transient hypogammaglobulinemia of infancy 🐾

    D80.8 Other immunodeficiencies with predominantly antibody defects 🐾
        Kappa light chain deficiency

    D80.9 Immunodeficiency with predominantly antibody defects, unspecified 🐾

● **D81** Combined immunodeficiencies

Excludes1	autosomal recessive agammaglobulinemia (Swiss type) (D80.0)

    D81.0 Severe combined immunodeficiency [SCID] with reticular dysgenesis 🐾

    D81.1 Severe combined immunodeficiency [SCID] with low T- and B-cell numbers 🐾

    D81.2 Severe combined immunodeficiency [SCID] with low or normal B-cell numbers 🐾

●   **D81.3** Adenosine deaminase [ADA] deficiency 🐾

    D81.30 Adenosine deaminase deficiency, unspecified
        ADA deficiency NOS

    D81.31 Severe combined immunodeficiency due to adenosine deaminase deficiency
        ADA deficiency with SCID
        Adenosine deaminase [ADA] deficiency with severe combined immunodeficiency

    D81.32 Adenosine deaminase 2 deficiency
        ADA2 deficiency
        Adenosine deaminase deficiency type 2
        Code also, if applicable, any associated manifestations, such as:
          polyarteritis nodosa (M30.0)
          stroke (I63.-)

    D81.39 Other adenosine deaminase deficiency
        Adenosine deaminase [ADA] deficiency type 1, NOS
        Adenosine deaminase [ADA] deficiency type 1, without SCID
        Adenosine deaminase [ADA] deficiency type 1, without severe combined immunodeficiency
        Partial ADA deficiency (type 1)
        Partial adenosine deaminase deficiency (type 1)

  D81.4 Nezelof's syndrome 🐾

  D81.5 Purine nucleoside phosphorylase [PNP] deficiency 🐾

  D81.6 Major histocompatibility complex class I deficiency 🐾
    Bare lymphocyte syndrome

  D81.7 Major histocompatibility complex class II deficiency 🐾

● **D81.8** Other combined immunodeficiencies

●   **D81.81** Biotin-dependent carboxylase deficiency
        Multiple carboxylase deficiency

Excludes1	biotin-dependent carboxylase deficiency due to dietary deficiency of biotin (E53.8)

    D81.810 Biotinidase deficiency

    D81.818 Other biotin-dependent carboxylase deficiency
        Holocarboxylase synthetase deficiency
        Other multiple carboxylase deficiency

    D81.819 Biotin-dependent carboxylase deficiency, unspecified
        Multiple carboxylase deficiency, unspecified

▶**D81.82** Activated Phosphoinositide 3-kinase Delta Syndrome [APDS]
    ▶p110d-activating mutation causing senescent T cells, lymphadenopathy, and immunodeficiency [PASLI] disease
    ▶*Code also, if applicable, any associated manifestations, such as:*
      ▶bronchiectasis (J47.-)
      ▶herpes virus infections (B00.-)
      ▶other acute respiratory tract infections (J00-J06; J20-J22)
      ▶other infections (A00-B99)
      ▶pneumonia (J12-J18)

    D81.89 Other combined immunodeficiencies 🐾

  D81.9 Combined immunodeficiency, unspecified 🐾
    Severe combined immunodeficiency disorder [SCID] NOS

● **D82** Immunodeficiency associated with other major defects

Excludes1	ataxia telangiectasia [Louis-Bar] (G11.3)

  D82.0 Wiskott-Aldrich syndrome 🐾
    X-linked immunodeficiency
    Immunodeficiency with thrombocytopenia and eczema

  D82.1 Di George's syndrome 🐾
    Congenital disorder with defective development of third and fourth pharyngeal pouches
    Pharyngeal pouch syndrome
    Thymic alymphoplasia
    Thymic aplasia or hypoplasia with immunodeficiency
    Coding Clinic: 2019, Q3, P14

  D82.2 Immunodeficiency with short-limbed stature 🐾

  D82.3 Immunodeficiency following hereditary defective response to Epstein-Barr virus 🐾
    X-linked lymphoproliferative disease

CHAPTER 3 (D50–D89)

D82.4   Hyperimmunoglobulin E [IgE] syndrome 🐾
> *Suspected genetic defect that produces high levels of antibody immunoglobulin (IgE) that causes skin and lung infections and eczema*

D82.8   Immunodeficiency associated with other specified major defects 🐾

D82.9   Immunodeficiency associated with major defect, unspecified 🐾

● **D83   Common variable immunodeficiency**

D83.0   Common variable immunodeficiency with predominant abnormalities of B-cell numbers and function 🐾

D83.1   Common variable immunodeficiency with predominant immunoregulatory T-cell disorders 🐾

D83.2   Common variable immunodeficiency with autoantibodies to B- or T-cells 🐾

D83.8   Other common variable immunodeficiencies 🐾

D83.9   Common variable immunodeficiency, unspecified 🐾

● **D84   Other immunodeficiencies**

D84.0   Lymphocyte function antigen-1 [LFA-1] defect 🐾

● **D84.1   Defects in the complement system** 🐾
> C1 esterase inhibitor [C1-INH] deficiency

D84.8   Other specified immunodeficiencies 🐾

▷ *D84.81   Immunodeficiency due to conditions classified elsewhere*

> Code first underlying condition, such as:
> chromosomal abnormalities (Q90-Q99)
> diabetes mellitus (E08-E13)
> malignant neoplasms (C00-C96)

> **Excludes1**   certain disorders involving the immune mechanism (D80-D83, D84.0, D84.1, D84.9)
> human immunodeficiency virus [HIV] disease (B20)

● **D84.82   Immunodeficiency due to drugs and external causes**

D84.821   Immunodeficiency due to drugs
> Immunodeficiency due to (current or past) medication

> Use additional code for adverse effect if applicable, to identify adverse effect of drug (T36-T50 with fifth or six character 5)

> Use additional code, if applicable, for associated long term (current) drug therapy drug or medication such as:
> long term (current) drug therapy systemic steroids (Z79.52)
> other long term (current) drug therapy (Z79.899)

D84.822   Immunodeficiency due to external causes
> Code also, if applicable, radiological procedure and radiotherapy (Y84.2)

> Use additional code for external cause such as:
> exposure to ionizing radiation (W88)

D84.89   Other immunodeficiencies

D84.9   Immunodeficiency, unspecified 🐾
> Immunocompromised NOS
> Immunodeficient NOS
> Immunosuppressed NOS]

Item 3-1 Sarcoidosis: A symptom of an inflammation producing tiny lumps of cells (granulomas) in various organs, most commonly the lungs and lymph nodes, that affect organ function. Cause is unknown occurring primarily in 20- to 40-year-olds, African-American, especially women, and those of Asian, German, Irish, Scandinavian, and Puerto Rican heritage.

● **D86   Sarcoidosis**

D86.0   Sarcoidosis of lung 🐾

D86.1   Sarcoidosis of lymph nodes

D86.2   Sarcoidosis of lung with sarcoidosis of lymph nodes 🐾

D86.3   Sarcoidosis of skin

● **D86.8   Sarcoidosis of other sites**

D86.81   Sarcoid meningitis

D86.82   Multiple cranial nerve palsies in sarcoidosis 🐾

D86.83   Sarcoid iridocyclitis
> *Rare large tumor with irregular surface of iris*

D86.84   Sarcoid pyelonephritis
> *Systemic disease of unknown etiology characterized by chronic granulomatous inflammation with tissue destruction of pelvis kidney*
> Tubulo-interstitial nephropathy in sarcoidosis

D86.85   Sarcoid myocarditis

D86.86   Sarcoid arthropathy
> Polyarthritis in sarcoidosis

D86.87   Sarcoid myositis
> *Granumloma of muscle*

D86.89   Sarcoidosis of other sites
> Hepatic granuloma
> Uveoparotid fever [Heerfordt]

D86.9   Sarcoidosis, unspecified

● **D89   Other disorders involving the immune mechanism, not elsewhere classified**

> **Excludes1**   hyperglobulinemia NOS (R77.1)
> monoclonal gammopathy (of undetermined significance) (D47.2)

> **Excludes2**   transplant failure and rejection (T86.-)

D89.0   Polyclonal hypergammaglobulinemia
> Benign hypergammaglobulinemic purpura
> Polyclonal gammopathy NOS

D89.1   Cryoglobulinemia 🐾
> *Cryoglobulin (proteins) in blood that precipitate temperatures below 98.6° F; usually symptomatic of underlying disease*
> Cryoglobulinemic purpura
> Cryoglobulinemic vasculitis
> Essential cryoglobulinemia
> Idiopathic cryoglobulinemia
> Mixed cryoglobulinemia
> Primary cryoglobulinemia
> Secondary cryoglobulinemia

D89.2   Hypergammaglobulinemia, unspecified

D89.3   Immune reconstitution syndrome 🐾
> Immune reconstitution inflammatory syndrome [IRIS]

> Use additional code for adverse effect, if applicable, to identify drug (T36-T50 with fifth or sixth character 5)

▶ New   ➡ Revised   ~~deleted~~ Deleted   Excludes 1   Excludes 2   Includes   Use additional   Code first   Code also   Key words

OGCR Official Guidelines   X Assign placeholder X   ● Use Additional Character(s)   ▷ Manifestation Code   🐾 Hierarchical Condition Category   **Coding Clinic**

● D89.4　Mast cell activation syndrome and related disorders
　　　Excludes1　aggressive systemic mastocytosis (C96.21)
　　　　　　　　congenital cutaneous mastocytosis (Q82.2)
　　　　　　　　(non-congenital) cutaneous mastocytosis
　　　　　　　　　　(D47.01)
　　　　　　　　(indolent) systemic mastocytosis (D47.02)
　　　　　　　　malignant mast cell neoplasm (C96.2-)
　　　　　　　　malignant mastocytoma (C96.29)
　　　　　　　　mast cell leukemia (C94.3-)
　　　　　　　　mast cell sarcoma (C96.22)
　　　　　　　　mastocytoma NOS (D47.09)
　　　　　　　　other mast cell neoplasms of uncertain
　　　　　　　　　　behavior (D47.09)
　　　　　　　　systemic mastocytosis associated with
　　　　　　　　　　a clonal hematologic non-mast
　　　　　　　　　　cell lineage disease (SM-AHNMD)
　　　　　　　　　　(D47.02)
　　　Coding Clinic: 2016, Q4, P11

　　D89.40　Mast cell activation, unspecified 🔍
　　　　　Mast cell activation disorder, unspecified
　　　　　Mast cell activation syndrome, NOS

　　D89.41　Monoclonal mast cell activation syndrome 🔍
　　　　　Coding Clinic: 2016, Q4, P11

　　D89.42　Idiopathic mast cell activation syndrome 🔍
　　　　　Coding Clinic: 2016, Q4, P11

　　D89.44　Hereditary alpha tryptasemia
　　　　　Use additional code, if applicable, for:
　　　　　　allergy status, other than to drugs and
　　　　　　　biological substances (Z91.0-)
　　　　　　personal history of anaphylaxis (Z87.892)

　　D89.43　Secondary mast cell activation 🔍
　　　　　Secondary mast cell activation syndrome
　　　　　Code also underlying etiology, if known
　　　　　Coding Clinic: 2016, Q4, P11

　　D89.49　Other mast cell activation disorder 🔍
　　　　　Other mast cell activation syndrome
　　　　　Coding Clinic: 2016, Q4, P11

● D89.8　Other specified disorders involving the immune
　　　mechanism, not elsewhere classified

● D89.81　Graft-versus-host disease
　　　　　Code first underlying cause, such as:
　　　　　　complications of transplanted organs and
　　　　　　　tissue (T86.-)
　　　　　　complications of blood transfusion (T80.89)
　　　　　Use additional code to identify associated
　　　　　　manifestations, such as:
　　　　　　desquamative dermatitis (L30.8)
　　　　　　diarrhea (R19.7)
　　　　　　elevated bilirubin (R17)
　　　　　　hair loss (L65.9)

　　D89.810　Acute graft-versus-host disease 🔍
　　D89.811　Chronic graft-versus-host disease 🔍

　　D89.812　Acute on chronic graft-versus-host
　　　　　disease 🔍
　　D89.813　Graft-versus-host disease,
　　　　　unspecified 🔍

　D89.82　Autoimmune lymphoproliferative syndrome
　　　[ALPS] 🔍

● D89.83　Cytokine release syndrome
　　　　　Code first underlying cause, such as:
　　　　　　complications following infusion,
　　　　　　　transfusion and therapeutic injection
　　　　　　　(T80.89-)
　　　　　　complications of transplanted organs and
　　　　　　　tissue (T86.-)
　　　　　Use additional code to identify associated
　　　　　　manifestations

　　D89.831　Cytokine release syndrome, grade 1
　　D89.832　Cytokine release syndrome, grade 2
　　D89.833　Cytokine release syndrome,
　　　　　grade 3
　　D89.834　Cytokine release syndrome,
　　　　　grade 4
　　D89.835　Cytokine release syndrome,
　　　　　grade 5
　　D89.839　Cytokine release syndrome, grade
　　　　　unspecified

　D89.89　Other specified disorders involving the
　　　immune mechanism, not elsewhere classified 🔍
　　　　　Excludes1　human immunodeficiency virus
　　　　　　　　　　disease (B20)
　　　　　Coding Clinic: 2017, Q4, P109

D89.9　Disorder involving the immune
　　mechanism, unspecified 🔍
　　　Immune disease NOS
　　　Coding Clinic: 2015, Q3, P22

CHAPTER 3 (D50-D89)

CHAPTER 4

ENDOCRINE, NUTRITIONAL AND METABOLIC DISEASES (E00-E89)

OGCR Chapter-Specific Coding Guidelines

4. **Chapter 4: Endocrine, Nutritional, and Metabolic Diseases (E00-E89)**

a. **Diabetes mellitus**
The diabetes mellitus codes are combination codes that include the type of diabetes mellitus, the body system affected, and the complications affecting that body system. As many codes within a particular category as are necessary to describe all of the complications of the disease may be used. They should be sequenced based on the reason for a particular encounter. Assign as many codes from categories E08 – E13 as needed to identify all of the associated conditions that the patient has.

1) **Type of diabetes**
The age of a patient is not the sole determining factor, though most type 1 diabetics develop the condition before reaching puberty. For this reason type 1 diabetes mellitus is also referred to as juvenile diabetes.

2) **Type of diabetes mellitus not documented**
If the type of diabetes mellitus is not documented in the medical record the default is E11.-, Type 2 diabetes mellitus.

3) **Diabetes mellitus and the use of insulin oral hypoglycemics**
If the documentation in a medical record does not indicate the type of diabetes but does indicate that the patient uses insulin, code E11, Type 2 diabetes mellitus, should be assigned. An additional code should be assigned from category Z79 to identify the long-term (current) use of insulin or oral hypoglycemic drugs. If the patient is treated with both oral medications and insulin, only the code for long-term (current) use of insulin should be assigned. Code Z79.4 should not be assigned if insulin is given temporarily to bring a type 2 patient's blood sugar under control during an encounter.

4) **Diabetes mellitus in pregnancy and gestational diabetes**
See Section I.C.15. Diabetes mellitus in pregnancy.
See Section I.C.15. Gestational (pregnancy induced) diabetes

5) **Complications due to insulin pump malfunction**

(a) **Underdose of insulin due to insulin pump failure**
An underdose of insulin due to an insulin pump failure should be assigned to a code from subcategory T85.6, Mechanical complication of other specified internal and external prosthetic devices, implants and grafts, that specifies the type of pump malfunction, as the principal or first-listed code, followed by code T38.3X6-, Underdosing of insulin and oral hypoglycemic [antidiabetic] drugs. Additional codes for the type of diabetes mellitus and any associated complications due to the underdosing should also be assigned.

(b) **Overdose of insulin due to insulin pump failure**
The principal or first-listed code for an encounter due to an insulin pump malfunction resulting in an overdose of insulin, should also be T85.6-, Mechanical complication of other specified internal and external prosthetic devices, implants and grafts, followed by code T38.3X1-, Poisoning by insulin and oral hypoglycemic [antidiabetic] drugs, accidental (unintentional).

6) **Secondary diabetes mellitus**
Codes under categories E08, Diabetes mellitus due to underlying condition, E09, Drug or chemical induced diabetes mellitus and E13, Other specified diabetes mellitus, identify complications/ manifestations associated with secondary diabetes mellitus. Secondary diabetes is always caused by another condition or event (e.g., cystic fibrosis, malignant neoplasm of pancreas, pancreatectomy, adverse effect of drug, or poisoning).

(a) **Secondary diabetes mellitus and the use of insulin** or hypoglycemic drugs
For patients with secondary diabetes mellitus who routinely use insulin or oral hypoglycemic drugs, an additional code from category Z79 should be assigned to identify the long-term (current) use of insulin or oral hypoglycemic drugs. If the patient is treated with both oral medications and insulin, only the code for long-term (current) use of insulin should be assigned. Code Z79.4 should not be assigned if insulin is given temporarily to bring a type 2 patient's blood sugar under control during an encounter.

(b) **Assigning and sequencing secondary diabetes codes and its causes**
The sequencing of the secondary diabetes codes in relationship to codes for the cause of the diabetes is based on the Tabular List instructions for categories E08, E09 and E13.

(i) **Secondary diabetes mellitus due to pancreatectomy** For postpancreatectomy diabetes mellitus (lack of insulin due to the surgical removal of all or part of the pancreas), assign code E89.1, Postprocedural hypoinsulinemia. Assign a code from category E13 and a code from subcategory Z90.41-, Acquired absence of pancreas, as additional codes.

(ii) **Secondary diabetes due to drugs** Secondary diabetes may be caused by an adverse effect of correctly administered medications, poisoning or sequela of poisoning.
See Section I.C.19.e for coding of adverse effects and poisoning, and Section I.C.20 for external cause code reporting.

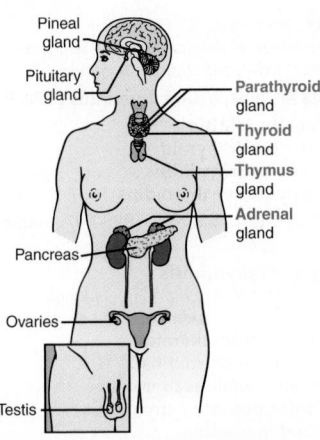

Figure 4-1 The endocrine system. (From Buck CJ: Step-by-Step Medical Coding, ed 2016, St. Louis, Elsevier, 2016)

CHAPTER 4

ENDOCRINE, NUTRITIONAL AND METABOLIC DISEASES (E00-E89)

All neoplasms, whether functionally active or not, are classified in Chapter 2. Appropriate codes in this chapter (i.e., E05.8, E07.0, E16-E31, E34.-) may be used as additional codes to indicate either functional activity by neoplasms and ectopic endocrine tissue or hyperfunction and hypofunction of endocrine glands associated with neoplasms and other conditions classified elsewhere.

Excludes1   transitory endocrine and metabolic disorders specific to newborn (P70-P74)

This chapter contains the following blocks:

E00-E07	Disorders of thyroid gland
E08-E13	Diabetes mellitus
E15-E16	Other disorders of glucose regulation and pancreatic internal secretion
E20-E35	Disorders of other endocrine glands
E36	Intraoperative complications of endocrine system
E40-E46	Malnutrition
E50-E64	Other nutritional deficiencies
E65-E68	Overweight, obesity and other hyperalimentation
E70-E88	Metabolic disorders
E89	Postprocedural endocrine and metabolic complications and disorders, not elsewhere classified

DISORDERS OF THYROID GLAND (E00-E07)

● **E00   Congenital iodine-deficiency syndrome**

Use additional code (F70-F79) to identify associated intellectual disabilities.

Excludes1   subclinical iodine-deficiency hypothyroidism (E02)

E00.0   Congenital iodine-deficiency syndrome, neurological type
Endemic cretinism, neurological type

E00.1   Congenital iodine-deficiency syndrome, myxedematous type
Dry, waxy type of swelling (nonpitting edema) with abnormal deposits of mucin in skin (mucinosis) and other tissues
Endemic hypothyroid cretinism
Endemic cretinism, myxedematous type

E00.2   Congenital iodine-deficiency syndrome, mixed type
Endemic cretinism, mixed type

E00.9   Congenital iodine-deficiency syndrome, unspecified
Congenital iodine-deficiency hypothyroidism NOS
Endemic cretinism NOS

Figure 4-2   Goiter is an enlargement of the thyroid gland.

Item 4–1   Simple goiter indicates no nodules are present. The most common type of goiter is a **diffuse colloidal**, also called a **nontoxic** or **endemic** goiter.

● **E01   Iodine-deficiency related thyroid disorders and allied conditions**

Excludes1   congenital iodine-deficiency syndrome (E00.-) subclinical iodine-deficiency hypothyroidism (E02)

E01.0   Iodine-deficiency related diffuse (endemic) goiter
Thyroid gland is enlarged

E01.1   Iodine-deficiency related multinodular (endemic) goiter
Iodine-deficiency related nodular goiter

E01.2   Iodine-deficiency related (endemic) goiter, unspecified
Endemic goiter NOS

E01.8   Other iodine-deficiency related thyroid disorders and allied conditions
Acquired iodine-deficiency hypothyroidism NOS

E02   Subclinical iodine-deficiency hypothyroidism
Coding Clinic: 2021, Q1, P8-9

● **E03   Other hypothyroidism**

Excludes1   iodine-deficiency related hypothyroidism (E00-E02) postprocedural hypothyroidism (E89.0)

E03.0   Congenital hypothyroidism with diffuse goiter
Congenital parenchymatous goiter (nontoxic)
Congenital goiter (nontoxic) NOS

     Excludes1   transitory congenital goiter with normal function (P72.0)

E03.1   Congenital hypothyroidism without goiter
Aplasia of thyroid (with myxedema)
Congenital atrophy of thyroid
Congenital hypothyroidism NOS

E03.2   Hypothyroidism due to medicaments and other exogenous substances
Code first poisoning due to drug or toxin, if applicable (T36-T65 with fifth or sixth character 1-4 or 6)

Use additional code for adverse effect, if applicable, to identify drug (T36-T50 with fifth or sixth character 5)

E03.3   Postinfectious hypothyroidism

E03.4   Atrophy of thyroid (acquired)

     Excludes1   congenital atrophy of thyroid (E03.1)

E03.5   Myxedema coma ●
Often fatal complication of long-term hypothyroidism

E03.8   Other specified hypothyroidism

E03.9   Hypothyroidism, unspecified
Myxedema NOS
Coding Clinic: 2021, Q1, P9

● **E04   Other nontoxic goiter**

Excludes1   congenital goiter (NOS) (diffuse) (parenchymatous) (E03.0)
iodine-deficiency related goiter (E00-E02)

E04.0   Nontoxic diffuse goiter
Thyroid gland is enlarged
Diffuse (colloid) nontoxic goiter
Simple nontoxic goiter

E04.1   Nontoxic single thyroid nodule
Colloid nodule (cystic) (thyroid)
Nontoxic uninodular goiter
Thyroid (cystic) nodule NOS

Item 4–2   Hypothyroidism is a condition in which there are insufficient levels of thyroxine. **Cretinism** is congenital hypothyroidism, which can result in mental and physical retardation.

CHAPTER 4 (E00-E89)

E04.2   **Nontoxic multinodular goiter**
         Enlarged thyroid gland with multiple nodules
         Cystic goiter NOS
         Multinodular (cystic) goiter NOS

E04.8   **Other specified nontoxic goiter**

E04.9   **Nontoxic goiter, unspecified**
         Goiter NOS
         Nodular goiter (nontoxic) NOS

● E05   **Thyrotoxicosis [hyperthyroidism]**
         Enlarged thyroid gland with multiple nodules

         Excludes1   chronic thyroiditis with transient thyrotoxicosis
                         (E06.2)
                         neonatal thyrotoxicosis (P72.1)

● E05.0   **Thyrotoxicosis with diffuse goiter**
           Exophthalmic or toxic goiter NOS
           Graves' disease
           Toxic diffuse goiter

           E05.00   **Thyrotoxicosis with diffuse goiter without
                     thyrotoxic crisis or storm**

           E05.01   **Thyrotoxicosis with diffuse goiter with
                     thyrotoxic crisis or storm**

● E05.1   **Thyrotoxicosis with toxic single thyroid nodule**
           Thyrotoxicosis with toxic uninodular goiter

           E05.10   **Thyrotoxicosis with toxic single thyroid nodule
                     without thyrotoxic crisis or storm**

           E05.11   **Thyrotoxicosis with toxic single thyroid nodule
                     with thyrotoxic crisis or storm**

● E05.2   **Thyrotoxicosis with toxic multinodular goiter**
           Toxic nodular goiter NOS

           E05.20   **Thyrotoxicosis with toxic multinodular goiter
                     without thyrotoxic crisis or storm**

           E05.21   **Thyrotoxicosis with toxic multinodular goiter
                     with thyrotoxic crisis or storm**

● E05.3   **Thyrotoxicosis from ectopic thyroid tissue**

           E05.30   **Thyrotoxicosis from ectopic thyroid tissue
                     without thyrotoxic crisis or storm**

           E05.31   **Thyrotoxicosis from ectopic thyroid tissue with
                     thyrotoxic crisis or storm**

● E05.4   **Thyrotoxicosis factitia**

           E05.40   **Thyrotoxicosis factitia without thyrotoxic crisis
                     or storm**

           E05.41   **Thyrotoxicosis factitia with thyrotoxic crisis or
                     storm**

● E05.8   **Other thyrotoxicosis**
           Overproduction of thyroid-stimulating hormone

           E05.80   **Other thyrotoxicosis without thyrotoxic crisis or
                     storm**

           E05.81   **Other thyrotoxicosis with thyrotoxic crisis or
                     storm**

● E05.9   **Thyrotoxicosis, unspecified**
           Hyperthyroidism NOS

           E05.90   **Thyrotoxicosis, unspecified without thyrotoxic
                     crisis or storm**

           E05.91   **Thyrotoxicosis, unspecified with thyrotoxic
                     crisis or storm**

● E06   **Thyroiditis**
         *An inflammation of the thyroid gland which results in an inability to
         convert iodine into thyroid hormone*

         Excludes1   postpartum thyroiditis (O90.5)

E06.0   **Acute thyroiditis**
         Abscess of thyroid
         Pyogenic thyroiditis
         Suppurative thyroiditis

         Use additional code (B95-B97) to identify infectious
         agent.

E06.1   **Subacute thyroiditis**
         *Inflammation of thyroid gland following viral upper
         respiratory infection*
         de Quervain thyroiditis
         Giant-cell thyroiditis
         Granulomatous thyroiditis
         Nonsuppurative thyroiditis
         Viral thyroiditis

         Excludes1   autoimmune thyroiditis (E06.3)

E06.2   **Chronic thyroiditis with transient thyrotoxicosis**
         *Chronic inflammation of thyroid gland with intermittent
         overproduction of thyroid hormone*

         Excludes1   autoimmune thyroiditis (E06.3)

E06.3   **Autoimmune thyroiditis**
         Hashimoto's thyroiditis
         Hashitoxicosis (transient)
         Lymphadenoid goiter
         Lymphocytic thyroiditis
         Struma lymphomatosa

E06.4   **Drug-induced thyroiditis**
         Use additional code for adverse effect, if applicable,
         to identify drug (T36-T50 with fifth or sixth
         character 5)

E06.5   **Other chronic thyroiditis**
         Chronic fibrous thyroiditis
         Chronic thyroiditis NOS
         Ligneous thyroiditis
         Riedel thyroiditis

E06.9   **Thyroiditis, unspecified**

● E07   **Other disorders of thyroid**

E07.0   **Hypersecretion of calcitonin**
         C-cell hyperplasia of thyroid
         Hypersecretion of thyrocalcitonin

E07.1   **Dyshormogenetic goiter**
         *Group of several types of goiter resulting from enzyme defects
         in hormone synthesis*
         Familial dyshormogenetic goiter
         Pendred's syndrome

         Excludes1   transitory congenital goiter with normal
                         function (P72.0)

● E07.8   **Other specified disorders of thyroid**

           E07.81   **Sick-euthyroid syndrome**
                     Euthyroid sick-syndrome

           E07.89   **Other specified disorders of thyroid**
                     Abnormality of thyroid-binding globulin
                     Hemorrhage of thyroid
                     Infarction of thyroid

E07.9   **Disorder of thyroid, unspecified**

OGCR   Section I.C.4.a.

Diabetes mellitus

The diabetes mellitus codes are combination codes that
include the type of diabetes mellitus, body system affected,
and the complications affecting that body system. As many
codes within a particular category as are necessary to describe
all of the complications of the disease may be used. They
should be sequenced based on the reason for a particular visit.
Assign as many codes from categories E08–E13 as needed to
identify all of the associated conditions that the patient has.

Figure 4-3 Graves' disease. In Graves'
disease, exophthalmos often looks more
pronounced than it actually is because of the
extreme lid retraction that may occur. This
patient, for instance, had minimal proptosis
of the left eye but marked lid retraction. (From
Lissauer T, Clayden G, and Craft A: Illustrated
Textbook of Paediatrics, Edinburgh, Mosby,
2015)

Item 4–3 Thyrotoxicosis is a condition caused by excessive amounts
of the thyroid hormone thyroxine production or hyperthyroidism. **Graves'
disease is associated with hyperthyroidism** (known as **Basedow's
disease** in Europe).

▶ New   ⇒ Revised   ~~deleted~~ Deleted   Excludes 1   Excludes 2   Includes   Use additional   Code first   Code also   Key words

OGCR Official Guidelines   X Assign placeholder X   ● Use Additional Character(s)   ▶ Manifestation Code   🐄 Hierarchical Condition Category   **Coding Clinic**

DIABETES MELLITUS (E08-E13)

A metabolic disease that results in persistent hyperglycemia
Coding Clinic: 2016, Q4, P142

● **E08**   **Diabetes mellitus due to underlying condition**

Code first the underlying condition, such as:
congenital rubella (P35.0)
Cushing's syndrome (E24.-)
cystic fibrosis (E84.-)
malignant neoplasm (C00-C96)
malnutrition (E40-E46)
pancreatitis and other diseases of the pancreas (K85-K86.-)

Use additional code to identify control using:
insulin (Z79.4)
oral antidiabetic drugs (Z79.84)
oral hypoglycemic drugs (Z79.84)

Excludes1	drug or chemical induced diabetes mellitus (E09.-)
	gestational diabetes (O24.4-)
	neonatal diabetes mellitus (P70.2)
	postpancreatectomy diabetes mellitus (E13.-)
	postprocedural diabetes mellitus (E13.-)
	secondary diabetes mellitus NEC (E13.-)
	type 1 diabetes mellitus (E10.-)
	type 2 diabetes mellitus (E11.-)

● **E08.0**   **Diabetes mellitus due to underlying condition with hyperosmolarity**

▹ *E08.00*   *Diabetes mellitus due to underlying condition with hyperosmolarity without nonketotic hyperglycemic-hyperosmolar coma (NKHHC)* 🔍

▹ *E08.01*   *Diabetes mellitus due to underlying condition with hyperosmolarity with coma* 🔍

● **E08.1**   **Diabetes mellitus due to underlying condition with ketoacidosis**

▹ *E08.10*   *Diabetes mellitus due to underlying condition with ketoacidosis without coma* 🔍

▹ *E08.11*   *Diabetes mellitus due to underlying condition with ketoacidosis with coma* 🔍

● **E08.2**   **Diabetes mellitus due to underlying condition with kidney complications**

▹ *E08.21*   *Diabetes mellitus due to underlying condition with diabetic nephropathy* 🔍
Diabetes mellitus due to underlying condition with intercapillary glomerulosclerosis
Diabetes mellitus due to underlying condition with intracapillary glomerulonephrosis
Diabetes mellitus due to underlying condition with Kimmelstiel-Wilson disease

▹ *E08.22*   *Diabetes mellitus due to underlying condition with diabetic chronic kidney disease* 🔍
Use additional code to identify stage of chronic kidney disease (N18.1-N18.6)

▹ *E08.29*   *Diabetes mellitus due to underlying condition with other diabetic kidney complication* 🔍
Renal tubular degeneration in diabetes mellitus due to underlying condition

● **E08.3**   **Diabetes mellitus due to underlying condition with ophthalmic complications**
Changes in blood vessels of retina in which blood vessels swell and leak fluid into retinal surface.
Coding Clinic: 2016, Q4, P11

  ● **E08.31**   **Diabetes mellitus due to underlying condition with unspecified diabetic retinopathy**

    ▹ *E08.311*   *Diabetes mellitus due to underlying condition with unspecified diabetic retinopathy with macular edema* 🔍

    ▹ *E08.319*   *Diabetes mellitus due to underlying condition with unspecified diabetic retinopathy without macular edema* 🔍

  ● **E08.32**   **Diabetes mellitus due to underlying condition with mild nonproliferative diabetic retinopathy**
Diabetes mellitus due to underlying condition with nonproliferative diabetic retinopathy NOS
One of the following 7th characters is to be assigned to codes in subcategory E08.32 to designate laterality of the disease:

1	right eye
2	left eye
3	bilateral
9	unspecified eye

    ● *E08.321*   *Diabetes mellitus due to underlying condition with mild nonproliferative diabetic retinopathy with macular edema* 🔍

    ● *E08.329*   *Diabetes mellitus due to underlying condition with mild nonproliferative diabetic retinopathy without macular edema* 🔍

  ● **E08.33**   **Diabetes mellitus due to underlying condition with moderate nonproliferative diabetic retinopathy**
One of the following 7th characters is to be assigned to codes in subcategory E08.33 to designate laterality of the disease:

1	right eye
2	left eye
3	bilateral
9	unspecified eye

    ● *E08.331*   *Diabetes mellitus due to underlying condition with moderate nonproliferative diabetic retinopathy with macular edema* 🔍

    ● *E08.339*   *Diabetes mellitus due to underlying condition with moderate nonproliferative diabetic retinopathy without macular edema* 🔍

  ● **E08.34**   **Diabetes mellitus due to underlying condition with severe nonproliferative diabetic retinopathy**
One of the following 7th characters is to be assigned to codes in subcategory E08.34 to designate laterality of the disease:

1	right eye
2	left eye
3	bilateral
9	unspecified eye

    ● *E08.341*   *Diabetes mellitus due to underlying condition with severe nonproliferative diabetic retinopathy with macular edema* 🔍

    ● *E08.349*   *Diabetes mellitus due to underlying condition with severe nonproliferative diabetic retinopathy without macular edema* 🔍

  ● **E08.35**   **Diabetes mellitus due to underlying condition with proliferative diabetic retinopathy**
One of the following 7th characters is to be assigned to codes in subcategory E08.35 to designate laterality of the disease:

1	right eye
2	left eye
3	bilateral
9	unspecified eye

CHAPTER 4 (E00-E89)

CHAPTER 4 (E00-E89)

E08.351   *Diabetes mellitus due to underlying condition with proliferative diabetic retinopathy with macular edema* 🐾

E08.352   *Diabetes mellitus due to underlying condition with proliferative diabetic retinopathy with traction retinal detachment involving the macula* 🐾

E08.353   *Diabetes mellitus due to underlying condition with proliferative diabetic retinopathy with traction retinal detachment not involving the macula* 🐾

E08.354   *Diabetes mellitus due to underlying condition with proliferative diabetic retinopathy with combined traction retinal detachment and rhegmatogenous retinal detachment* 🐾

E08.355   *Diabetes mellitus due to underlying condition with stable proliferative diabetic retinopathy* 🐾

E08.359   *Diabetes mellitus due to underlying condition with proliferative diabetic retinopathy without macular edema* 🐾

E08.36   *Diabetes mellitus due to underlying condition with diabetic cataract* 🐾

X ● E08.37   *Diabetes mellitus due to underlying condition with diabetic macular edema, resolved following treatment* 🐾

One of the following 7th characters is to be assigned to code E08.37 to designate laterality of the disease:

1	right eye
2	left eye
3	bilateral
9	unspecified eye

E08.39   *Diabetes mellitus due to underlying condition with other diabetic ophthalmic complication* 🐾

Use additional code to identify manifestation, such as:
diabetic glaucoma (H40-H42)

● E08.4   **Diabetes mellitus due to underlying condition with neurological complications**

E08.40   *Diabetes mellitus due to underlying condition with diabetic neuropathy, unspecified* 🐾

E08.41   *Diabetes mellitus due to underlying condition with diabetic mononeuropathy* 🐾

E08.42   *Diabetes mellitus due to underlying condition with diabetic polyneuropathy* 🐾
Diabetes mellitus due to underlying condition with diabetic neuralgia

E08.43   *Diabetes mellitus due to underlying condition with diabetic autonomic (poly)neuropathy* 🐾
Diabetes mellitus due to underlying condition with diabetic gastroparesis

E08.44   *Diabetes mellitus due to underlying condition with diabetic amyotrophy* 🐾

E08.49   *Diabetes mellitus due to underlying condition with other diabetic neurological complication* 🐾

● E08.5   **Diabetes mellitus due to underlying condition with circulatory complications**

E08.51   *Diabetes mellitus due to underlying condition with diabetic peripheral angiopathy without gangrene* 🐾

E08.52   *Diabetes mellitus due to underlying condition with diabetic peripheral angiopathy with gangrene* 🐾
Diabetes mellitus due to underlying condition with diabetic gangrene

E08.59   *Diabetes mellitus due to underlying condition with other circulatory complications* 🐾

● E08.6   **Diabetes mellitus due to underlying condition with other specified complications**

● E08.61   **Diabetes mellitus due to underlying condition with diabetic arthropathy**

E08.610   *Diabetes mellitus due to underlying condition with diabetic neuropathic arthropathy* 🐾
Diabetes mellitus due to underlying condition with Charcôt's joints

E08.618   *Diabetes mellitus due to underlying condition with other diabetic arthropathy* 🐾

● E08.62   **Diabetes mellitus due to underlying condition with skin complications**

E08.620   *Diabetes mellitus due to underlying condition with diabetic dermatitis* 🐾
Diabetes mellitus due to underlying condition with diabetic necrobiosis lipoidica

E08.621   *Diabetes mellitus due to underlying condition with foot ulcer* 🐾
Use additional code to identify site of ulcer (L97.4-, L97.5-)

E08.622   *Diabetes mellitus due to underlying condition with other skin ulcer* 🐾
Use additional code to identify site of ulcer (L97.1-L97.9, L98.41-L98.49)

E08.628   *Diabetes mellitus due to underlying condition with other skin complications* 🐾

● E08.63   **Diabetes mellitus due to underlying condition with oral complications**

E08.630   *Diabetes mellitus due to underlying condition with periodontal disease* 🐾

E08.638   *Diabetes mellitus due to underlying condition with other oral complications* 🐾

● E08.64   **Diabetes mellitus due to underlying condition with hypoglycemia**

E08.641   *Diabetes mellitus due to underlying condition with hypoglycemia with coma* 🐾

E08.649   *Diabetes mellitus due to underlying condition with hypoglycemia without coma* 🐾

E08.65   *Diabetes mellitus due to underlying condition with hyperglycemia* 🐾

E08.69   *Diabetes mellitus due to underlying condition with other specified complication* 🐾
Use additional code to identify complication

E08.8   *Diabetes mellitus due to underlying condition with unspecified complications* 🐾

E08.9   *Diabetes mellitus due to underlying condition without complications* 🐾

● E09   **Drug or chemical induced diabetes mellitus**

Code first poisoning due to drug or toxin, if applicable (T36-T65 with fifth or sixth character 1-4 or 6)

Use additional code for adverse effect, if applicable, to identify drug (T36-T50 with fifth or sixth character 5)

Use additional code to identify control using:
insulin (Z79.4)
oral antidiabetic drugs (Z79.84)
oral hypoglycemic drugs (Z79.84)

Excludes1   diabetes mellitus due to underlying condition (E08.-)
gestational diabetes (O24.4-)
neonatal diabetes mellitus (P70.2)
postpancreatectomy diabetes mellitus (E13.-)
postprocedural diabetes mellitus (E13.-)
secondary diabetes mellitus NEC (E13.-)
type 1 diabetes mellitus (E10.-)
type 2 diabetes mellitus (E11.-)

▶ New   ⇒ Revised   ~~deleted~~ Deleted   Excludes 1   Excludes 2   Includes   Use additional   Code first   Code also   Key words

OGCR Official Guidelines   X Assign placeholder X   ● Use Additional Character(s)   ▶ Manifestation Code   🐾 Hierarchical Condition Category   **Coding Clinic**

● **E09.0** **Drug or chemical induced diabetes mellitus with hyperosmolarity**

    E09.00 **Drug or chemical induced diabetes mellitus with hyperosmolarity without nonketotic hyperglycemic-hyperosmolar coma (NKHHC)** 🔎

    E09.01 **Drug or chemical induced diabetes mellitus with hyperosmolarity with coma** 🔎

● **E09.1** **Drug or chemical induced diabetes mellitus with ketoacidosis**

    E09.10 **Drug or chemical induced diabetes mellitus with ketoacidosis without coma** 🔎

    E09.11 **Drug or chemical induced diabetes mellitus with ketoacidosis with coma** 🔎

● **E09.2** **Drug or chemical induced diabetes mellitus with kidney complications**

    E09.21 **Drug or chemical induced diabetes mellitus with diabetic nephropathy** 🔎

        Drug or chemical induced diabetes mellitus with intercapillary glomerulosclerosis

        Drug or chemical induced diabetes mellitus with intracapillary glomerulonephrosis

        Drug or chemical induced diabetes mellitus with Kimmelstiel-Wilson disease

    E09.22 **Drug or chemical induced diabetes mellitus with diabetic chronic kidney disease** 🔎

        Use additional code to identify stage of chronic kidney disease (N18.1-N18.6)

    E09.29 **Drug or chemical induced diabetes mellitus with other diabetic kidney complication** 🔎

        Drug or chemical induced diabetes mellitus with renal tubular degeneration

● **E09.3** **Drug or chemical induced diabetes mellitus with ophthalmic complications**
    Coding Clinic: 2016, Q4, P11

  ● **E09.31** **Drug or chemical induced diabetes mellitus with unspecified diabetic retinopathy**

    E09.311 **Drug or chemical induced diabetes mellitus with unspecified diabetic retinopathy with macular edema** 🔎

    E09.319 **Drug or chemical induced diabetes mellitus with unspecified diabetic retinopathy without macular edema** 🔎

  ● **E09.32** **Drug or chemical induced diabetes mellitus with mild nonproliferative diabetic retinopathy**

    Drug or chemical induced diabetes mellitus with nonproliferative diabetic retinopathy NOS

    One of the following 7th characters is to be assigned to codes in subcategory E09.32 to designate laterality of the disease:

1	right eye
2	left eye
3	bilateral
9	unspecified eye

    ● **E09.321** **Drug or chemical induced diabetes mellitus with mild nonproliferative diabetic retinopathy with macular edema** 🔎

    ● **E09.329** **Drug or chemical induced diabetes mellitus with mild nonproliferative diabetic retinopathy without macular edema** 🔎

● **E09.33** **Drug or chemical induced diabetes mellitus with moderate nonproliferative diabetic retinopathy**

    One of the following 7th characters is to be assigned to codes in subcategory E09.33 to designate laterality of the disease:

1	right eye
2	left eye
3	bilateral
9	unspecified eye

  ● **E09.331** **Drug or chemical induced diabetes mellitus with moderate nonproliferative diabetic retinopathy with macular edema** 🔎

  ● **E09.339** **Drug or chemical induced diabetes mellitus with moderate nonproliferative diabetic retinopathy without macular edema** 🔎

● **E09.34** **Drug or chemical induced diabetes mellitus with severe nonproliferative diabetic retinopathy**

    One of the following 7th characters is to be assigned to codes in subcategory E09.34 to designate laterality of the disease:

1	right eye
2	left eye
3	bilateral
9	unspecified eye

  ● **E09.341** **Drug or chemical induced diabetes mellitus with severe nonproliferative diabetic retinopathy with macular edema** 🔎

  ● **E09.349** **Drug or chemical induced diabetes mellitus with severe nonproliferative diabetic retinopathy without macular edema** 🔎

● **E09.35** **Drug or chemical induced diabetes mellitus with proliferative diabetic retinopathy**

    One of the following 7th characters is to be assigned to codes in subcategory E09.35 to designate laterality of the disease:

1	right eye
2	left eye
3	bilateral
9	unspecified eye

  ● **E09.351** **Drug or chemical induced diabetes mellitus with proliferative diabetic retinopathy with macular edema** 🔎

  ● **E09.352** **Drug or chemical induced diabetes mellitus with proliferative diabetic retinopathy with traction retinal detachment involving the macula** 🔎

  ● **E09.353** **Drug or chemical induced diabetes mellitus with proliferative diabetic retinopathy with traction retinal detachment not involving the macula** 🔎

  ● **E09.354** **Drug or chemical induced diabetes mellitus with proliferative diabetic retinopathy with combined traction retinal detachment and rhegmatogenous retinal detachment** 🔎

  ● **E09.355** **Drug or chemical induced diabetes mellitus with stable proliferative diabetic retinopathy** 🔎

  ● **E09.359** **Drug or chemical induced diabetes mellitus with proliferative diabetic retinopathy without macular edema** 🔎

CHAPTER 4 (E00-E89)

E09.36　Drug or chemical induced diabetes mellitus with diabetic cataract 🐾

X ● E09.37　Drug or chemical induced diabetes mellitus with diabetic macular edema, resolved following treatment 🐾

One of the following 7th characters is to be assigned to code E09.37 to designate laterality of the disease:

1	right eye
2	left eye
3	bilateral
9	unspecified eye

E09.39　Drug or chemical induced diabetes mellitus with other diabetic ophthalmic complication 🐾

Use additional code to identify manifestation, such as:
diabetic glaucoma (H40-H42)

● E09.4　Drug or chemical induced diabetes mellitus with neurological complications

E09.40　Drug or chemical induced diabetes mellitus with neurological complications with diabetic neuropathy, unspecified 🐾

E09.41　Drug or chemical induced diabetes mellitus with neurological complications with diabetic mononeuropathy 🐾

E09.42　Drug or chemical induced diabetes mellitus with neurological complications with diabetic polyneuropathy 🐾
Drug or chemical induced diabetes mellitus with diabetic neuralgia

E09.43　Drug or chemical induced diabetes mellitus with neurological complications with diabetic autonomic (poly)neuropathy 🐾
Drug or chemical induced diabetes mellitus with diabetic gastroparesis

E09.44　Drug or chemical induced diabetes mellitus with neurological complications with diabetic amyotrophy 🐾

E09.49　Drug or chemical induced diabetes mellitus with neurological complications with other diabetic neurological complication 🐾

● E09.5　Drug or chemical induced diabetes mellitus with circulatory complications

E09.51　Drug or chemical induced diabetes mellitus with diabetic peripheral angiopathy without gangrene 🐾

E09.52　Drug or chemical induced diabetes mellitus with diabetic peripheral angiopathy with gangrene 🐾
Drug or chemical induced diabetes mellitus with diabetic gangrene

E09.59　Drug or chemical induced diabetes mellitus with other circulatory complications 🐾

● E09.6　Drug or chemical induced diabetes mellitus with other specified complications

● E09.61　Drug or chemical induced diabetes mellitus with diabetic arthropathy

E09.610　Drug or chemical induced diabetes mellitus with diabetic neuropathic arthropathy 🐾
Drug or chemical induced diabetes mellitus with Charcôt's joints
Progressive degeneration of weight-bearing joint

E09.618　Drug or chemical induced diabetes mellitus with other diabetic arthropathy 🐾

● E09.62　Drug or chemical induced diabetes mellitus with skin complications

E09.620　Drug or chemical induced diabetes mellitus with diabetic dermatitis 🐾
Drug or chemical induced diabetes mellitus with diabetic necrobiosis lipoidica
Necrotizing skin condition

E09.621　Drug or chemical induced diabetes mellitus with foot ulcer 🐾
Use additional code to identify site of ulcer (L97.4-, L97.5-)

E09.622　Drug or chemical induced diabetes mellitus with other skin ulcer 🐾
Use additional code to identify site of ulcer (L97.1-L97.9, L98.41-L98.49)

E09.628　Drug or chemical induced diabetes mellitus with other skin complications 🐾

● E09.63　Drug or chemical induced diabetes mellitus with oral complications

E09.630　Drug or chemical induced diabetes mellitus with periodontal disease 🐾

E09.638　Drug or chemical induced diabetes mellitus with other oral complications 🐾

● E09.64　Drug or chemical induced diabetes mellitus with hypoglycemia

E09.641　Drug or chemical induced diabetes mellitus with hypoglycemia with coma 🐾

E09.649　Drug or chemical induced diabetes mellitus with hypoglycemia without coma 🐾

E09.65　Drug or chemical induced diabetes mellitus with hyperglycemia 🐾

E09.69　Drug or chemical induced diabetes mellitus with other specified complication 🐾
Use additional code to identify complication

E09.8　Drug or chemical induced diabetes mellitus with unspecified complications 🐾

E09.9　Drug or chemical induced diabetes mellitus without complications 🐾

● E10　Type 1 diabetes mellitus

Includes　brittle diabetes (mellitus)
diabetes (mellitus) due to autoimmune process
diabetes (mellitus) due to immune mediated pancreatic islet beta-cell destruction
idiopathic diabetes (mellitus)
juvenile onset diabetes (mellitus)
ketosis-prone diabetes (mellitus)

Excludes1　diabetes mellitus due to underlying condition (E08.-)
drug or chemical induced diabetes mellitus (E09.-)
gestational diabetes (O24.4-)
hyperglycemia NOS (R73.9)
neonatal diabetes mellitus (P70.2)
postpancreatectomy diabetes mellitus (E13.-)
postprocedural diabetes mellitus (E13.-)
secondary diabetes mellitus NEC (E13.-)
type 2 diabetes mellitus (E11.-)

● E10.1　Type 1 diabetes mellitus with ketoacidosis
Acidosis accompanied by accumulation of ketone bodies (ketosis) in body tissues and fluids

E10.10　Type 1 diabetes mellitus with ketoacidosis without coma 🐾
Coding Clinic: 2013, Q3, P20

E10.11　Type 1 diabetes mellitus with ketoacidosis with coma 🐾

▶ New　⇒ Revised　deleted Deleted　Excludes 1　Excludes 2　Includes　Use additional　Code first　Code also　Key words
OGCR Official Guidelines　X Assign placeholder X　● Use Additional Character(s)　▷ Manifestation Code　🐾 Hierarchical Condition Category　**Coding Clinic**

● **E10.2**   **Type 1 diabetes mellitus with kidney complications**

     E10.21   **Type 1 diabetes mellitus with diabetic nephropathy** 🔍

         Type 1 diabetes mellitus with intercapillary glomerulosclerosis

         Type 1 diabetes mellitus with intracapillary glomerulonephrosis

         Type 1 diabetes mellitus with Kimmelstiel-Wilson disease

     E10.22   **Type 1 diabetes mellitus with diabetic chronic kidney disease** 🔍

         Use additional code to identify stage of chronic kidney disease (N18.1-N18.6)

     E10.29   **Type 1 diabetes mellitus with other diabetic kidney complication** 🔍

         Type 1 diabetes mellitus with renal tubular degeneration

         Coding Clinic: 2016, Q1, P13

● **E10.3**   **Type 1 diabetes mellitus with ophthalmic complications**

         Coding Clinic: 2016, Q4, P11

 ● **E10.31**   **Type 1 diabetes mellitus with unspecified diabetic retinopathy**

     E10.311   **Type 1 diabetes mellitus with unspecified diabetic retinopathy with macular edema** 🔍

     E10.319   **Type 1 diabetes mellitus with unspecified diabetic retinopathy without macular edema** 🔍

 ● **E10.32**   **Type 1 diabetes mellitus with mild nonproliferative diabetic retinopathy**

         Type 1 diabetes mellitus with nonproliferative diabetic retinopathy NOS

         One of the following 7th characters is to be assigned to codes in subcategory E10.32 to designate laterality of the disease:

1	right eye
2	left eye
3	bilateral
9	unspecified eye

     ● **E10.321**   **Type 1 diabetes mellitus with mild nonproliferative diabetic retinopathy with macular edema** 🔍

     ● **E10.329**   **Type 1 diabetes mellitus with mild nonproliferative diabetic retinopathy without macular edema** 🔍

 ● **E10.33**   **Type 1 diabetes mellitus with moderate nonproliferative diabetic retinopathy**

         One of the following 7th characters is to be assigned to codes in subcategory E10.33 to designate laterality of the disease:

1	right eye
2	left eye
3	bilateral
9	unspecified eye

     ● **E10.331**   **Type 1 diabetes mellitus with moderate nonproliferative diabetic retinopathy with macular edema** 🔍

     ● **E10.339**   **Type 1 diabetes mellitus with moderate nonproliferative diabetic retinopathy without macular edema** 🔍

 ● **E10.34**   **Type 1 diabetes mellitus with severe nonproliferative diabetic retinopathy**

         One of the following 7th characters is to be assigned to codes in subcategory E10.34 to designate laterality of the disease:

1	right eye
2	left eye
3	bilateral
9	unspecified eye

     ● **E10.341**   **Type 1 diabetes mellitus with severe nonproliferative diabetic retinopathy with macular edema** 🔍

     ● **E10.349**   **Type 1 diabetes mellitus with severe nonproliferative diabetic retinopathy without macular edema** 🔍

 ● **E10.35**   **Type 1 diabetes mellitus with proliferative diabetic retinopathy**

         One of the following 7th characters is to be assigned to codes in subcategory E10.35 to designate laterality of the disease:

1	right eye
2	left eye
3	bilateral
9	unspecified eye

     ● **E10.351**   **Type 1 diabetes mellitus with proliferative diabetic retinopathy with macular edema** 🔍

     ● **E10.352**   **Type 1 diabetes mellitus with proliferative diabetic retinopathy with traction retinal detachment involving the macula** 🔍

     ● **E10.353**   **Type 1 diabetes mellitus with proliferative diabetic retinopathy with traction retinal detachment not involving the macula** 🔍

     ● **E10.354**   **Type 1 diabetes mellitus with proliferative diabetic retinopathy with combined traction retinal detachment and rhegmatogenous retinal detachment** 🔍

     ● **E10.355**   **Type 1 diabetes mellitus with stable proliferative diabetic retinopathy** 🔍

     ● **E10.359**   **Type 1 diabetes mellitus with proliferative diabetic retinopathy without macular edema** 🔍

     E10.36   **Type 1 diabetes mellitus with diabetic cataract** 🔍

X ● **E10.37**   **Type 1 diabetes mellitus with diabetic macular edema, resolved following treatment** 🔍

         One of the following 7th characters is to be assigned to code E10.37 to designate laterality of the disease:

1	right eye
2	left eye
3	bilateral
9	unspecified eye

     E10.39   **Type 1 diabetes mellitus with other diabetic ophthalmic complication** 🔍

         Use additional code to identify manifestation, such as:

         diabetic glaucoma (H40-H42)

● **E10.4**   **Type 1 diabetes mellitus with neurological complications**

     E10.40   **Type 1 diabetes mellitus with diabetic neuropathy, unspecified** 🔍

     E10.41   **Type 1 diabetes mellitus with diabetic mononeuropathy** 🔍

     E10.42   **Type 1 diabetes mellitus with diabetic polyneuropathy** 🔍

         Type 1 diabetes mellitus with diabetic neuralgia

     E10.43   **Type 1 diabetes mellitus with diabetic autonomic (poly)neuropathy** 🔍

         Type 1 diabetes mellitus with diabetic gastroparesis

     E10.44   **Type 1 diabetes mellitus with diabetic amyotrophy** 🔍

     E10.49   **Type 1 diabetes mellitus with other diabetic neurological complication** 🔍

N Newborn Age: 0   **P** Pediatric Age: 0–17   **M** Maternity DX: 9–64   **A** Adult Age: 15–124   ♀ Females Only   ♂ Males Only

749

CHAPTER 4 (E00-E89)

● **E10.5 Type 1 diabetes mellitus with circulatory complications**
  E10.51 Type 1 diabetes mellitus with diabetic peripheral angiopathy without gangrene 🖥
  E10.52 Type 1 diabetes mellitus with diabetic peripheral angiopathy with gangrene 🖥
    Type 1 diabetes mellitus with diabetic gangrene
  E10.59 Type 1 diabetes mellitus with other circulatory complications 🖥

● **E10.6 Type 1 diabetes mellitus with other specified complications**
  ● E10.61 Type 1 diabetes mellitus with diabetic arthropathy
    E10.610 Type 1 diabetes mellitus with diabetic neuropathic arthropathy 🖥
      Type 1 diabetes mellitus with Charcôt's joints
    E10.618 Type 1 diabetes mellitus with other diabetic arthropathy 🖥
  ● E10.62 Type 1 diabetes mellitus with skin complications
    E10.620 Type 1 diabetes mellitus with diabetic dermatitis 🖥
      Type 1 diabetes mellitus with diabetic necrobiosis lipoidica
    E10.621 Type 1 diabetes mellitus with foot ulcer 🖥
      Use additional code to identify site of ulcer (L97.4-, L97.5-)
    E10.622 Type 1 diabetes mellitus with other skin ulcer 🖥
      Use additional code to identify site of ulcer (L97.1-L97.9, L98.41-L98.49)
    E10.628 Type 1 diabetes mellitus with other skin complications 🖥
  ● E10.63 Type 1 diabetes mellitus with oral complications
    E10.630 Type 1 diabetes mellitus with periodontal disease 🖥
    E10.638 Type 1 diabetes mellitus with other oral complications 🖥
  ● E10.64 Type 1 diabetes mellitus with hypoglycemia
    E10.641 Type 1 diabetes mellitus with hypoglycemia with coma 🖥
    E10.649 Type 1 diabetes mellitus with hypoglycemia without coma 🖥
      Coding Clinic: 2016, Q1, P13
  E10.65 Type 1 diabetes mellitus with hyperglycemia 🖥
    Coding Clinic: 2022, Q1, P29; 2013, Q3, P20
  E10.69 Type 1 diabetes mellitus with other specified complication 🖥
    Use additional code to identify complication
    Coding Clinic: 2022, Q1, P29

E10.8 Type 1 diabetes mellitus with unspecified complications 🖥
E10.9 Type 1 diabetes mellitus without complications 🖥

● **E11 Type 2 diabetes mellitus**
  Includes diabetes (mellitus) due to insulin secretory defect
    diabetes NOS
    insulin resistant diabetes (mellitus)
  Use additional code to identify control using:
    insulin (Z79.4)
    oral antidiabetic drugs (Z79.84)
    oral hypoglycemic drugs (Z79.84)
  Excludes1 diabetes mellitus due to underlying condition (E08.-)
    drug or chemical induced diabetes mellitus (E09.-)
    gestational diabetes (O24.4-)
    neonatal diabetes mellitus (P70.2)
    postpancreatectomy diabetes mellitus (E13.-)
    postprocedural diabetes mellitus (E13.-)
    secondary diabetes mellitus NEC (E13.-)
    type 1 diabetes mellitus (E10.-)
  Coding Clinic: 2020, Q1, P12; 2016, Q4, P121, Q2, P10

● **E11.0 Type 2 diabetes mellitus with hyperosmolarity**
  E11.00 Type 2 diabetes mellitus with hyperosmolarity without nonketotic hyperglycemic-hyperosmolar coma (NKHHC) 🖥
    Coding Clinic: 2022, Q1, P28
  E11.01 Type 2 diabetes mellitus with hyperosmolarity with coma 🖥

● **E11.1 Type 2 diabetes mellitus with ketoacidosis**
  E11.10 Type 2 diabetes mellitus with ketoacidosis without coma 🖥
    Coding Clinic: 2017, Q4, P6
  E11.11 Type 2 diabetes mellitus with ketoacidosis with coma 🖥

● **E11.2 Type 2 diabetes mellitus with kidney complications**
  E11.21 Type 2 diabetes mellitus with diabetic nephropathy 🖥
    Type 2 diabetes mellitus with intercapillary glomerulosclerosis
    Type 2 diabetes mellitus with intracapillary glomerulonephrosis
    Type 2 diabetes mellitus with Kimmelstiel-Wilson disease
    Coding Clinic: 2019, Q3, P3
  E11.22 Type 2 diabetes mellitus with diabetic chronic kidney disease 🖥
    Use additional code to identify stage of chronic kidney disease (N18.1-N18.6)
    Coding Clinic: 2019, Q3, P3; 2018, Q4, P88; 2016, Q2, P36, Q1, P13
  E11.29 Type 2 diabetes mellitus with other diabetic kidney complication 🖥
    Type 2 diabetes mellitus with renal tubular degeneration

● **E11.3 Type 2 diabetes mellitus with ophthalmic complications**
  Coding Clinic: 2016, Q4, P11
  ● E11.31 Type 2 diabetes mellitus with unspecified diabetic retinopathy
    E11.311 Type 2 diabetes mellitus with unspecified diabetic retinopathy with macular edema 🖥
    E11.319 Type 2 diabetes mellitus with unspecified diabetic retinopathy without macular edema 🖥
      Coding Clinic: 2013, Q3, P20
  ● E11.32 Type 2 diabetes mellitus with mild nonproliferative diabetic retinopathy
    Type 2 diabetes mellitus with nonproliferative diabetic retinopathy NOS
    One of the following 7th characters is to be assigned to codes in subcategory E11.32 to designate laterality of the disease:

1	right eye
2	left eye
3	bilateral
9	unspecified eye

  ● E11.321 Type 2 diabetes mellitus with mild nonproliferative diabetic retinopathy with macular edema 🖥
  ● E11.329 Type 2 diabetes mellitus with mild nonproliferative diabetic retinopathy without macular edema 🖥
● E11.33 Type 2 diabetes mellitus with moderate nonproliferative diabetic retinopathy
  One of the following 7th characters is to be assigned to codes in subcategory E11.33 to designate laterality of the disease:

1	right eye
2	left eye
3	bilateral
9	unspecified eye

● E11.331   Type 2 diabetes mellitus with moderate nonproliferative diabetic retinopathy with macular edema 🔎

● E11.339   Type 2 diabetes mellitus with moderate nonproliferative diabetic retinopathy without macular edema 🔎

● E11.34   Type 2 diabetes mellitus with severe nonproliferative diabetic retinopathy

One of the following 7th characters is to be assigned to codes in subcategory E11.34 to designate laterality of the disease:

1	right eye
2	left eye
3	bilateral
9	unspecified eye

● E11.341   Type 2 diabetes mellitus with severe nonproliferative diabetic retinopathy with macular edema 🔎

● E11.349   Type 2 diabetes mellitus with severe nonproliferative diabetic retinopathy without macular edema 🔎

● E11.35   Type 2 diabetes mellitus with proliferative diabetic retinopathy

One of the following 7th characters is to be assigned to codes in subcategory E11.35 to designate laterality of the disease:

1	right eye
2	left eye
3	bilateral
9	unspecified eye

● E11.351   Type 2 diabetes mellitus with proliferative diabetic retinopathy with macular edema 🔎

● E11.352   Type 2 diabetes mellitus with proliferative diabetic retinopathy with traction retinal detachment involving the macula 🔎

● E11.353   Type 2 diabetes mellitus with proliferative diabetic retinopathy with traction retinal detachment not involving the macula 🔎

● E11.354   Type 2 diabetes mellitus with proliferative diabetic retinopathy with combined traction retinal detachment and rhegmatogenous retinal detachment 🔎

● E11.355   Type 2 diabetes mellitus with stable proliferative diabetic retinopathy 🔎

● E11.359   Type 2 diabetes mellitus with proliferative diabetic retinopathy without macular edema 🔎

E11.36   Type 2 diabetes mellitus with diabetic cataract 🔎
Coding Clinic: 2019, Q2, P30-31; 2016, Q2, P36

X ● E11.37   Type 2 diabetes mellitus with diabetic macular edema, resolved following treatment 🔎

One of the following 7th characters is to be assigned to code E11.37 to designate laterality of the disease:

1	right eye
2	left eye
3	bilateral
9	unspecified eye

E11.39   Type 2 diabetes mellitus with other diabetic ophthalmic complication 🔎
Use additional code to identify manifestation, such as:
diabetic glaucoma (H40-H42)

● E11.4   Type 2 diabetes mellitus with neurological complications

E11.40   Type 2 diabetes mellitus with diabetic neuropathy, unspecified 🔎

E11.41   Type 2 diabetes mellitus with diabetic mononeuropathy 🔎

E11.42   Type 2 diabetes mellitus with diabetic polyneuropathy 🔎
Type 2 diabetes mellitus with diabetic neuralgia
Coding Clinic: 2020, Q1, P12; 2016, Q1, P13

E11.43   Type 2 diabetes mellitus with diabetic autonomic (poly)neuropathy 🔎
Type 2 diabetes mellitus with diabetic gastroparesis
Coding Clinic: 2016, Q2, P36

E11.44   Type 2 diabetes mellitus with diabetic amyotrophy 🔎
Coding Clinic: 2016, Q2, P36

E11.49   Type 2 diabetes mellitus with other diabetic neurological complication 🔎

● E11.5   Type 2 diabetes mellitus with circulatory complications

E11.51   Type 2 diabetes mellitus with diabetic peripheral angiopathy without gangrene 🔎

E11.52   Type 2 diabetes mellitus with diabetic peripheral angiopathy with gangrene 🔎
Type 2 diabetes mellitus with diabetic gangrene
Coding Clinic: 2017, Q4, P102

E11.59   Type 2 diabetes mellitus with other circulatory complications 🔎

● E11.6   Type 2 diabetes mellitus with other specified complications

● E11.61   Type 2 diabetes mellitus with diabetic arthropathy

E11.610   Type 2 diabetes mellitus with diabetic neuropathic arthropathy 🔎
Type 2 diabetes mellitus with Charcôt's joints
Coding Clinic: 2016, Q2, P36

E11.618   Type 2 diabetes mellitus with other diabetic arthropathy 🔎
Coding Clinic: 2018, Q2, P7; 2016, Q2, P36

● E11.62   Type 2 diabetes mellitus with skin complications

E11.620   Type 2 diabetes mellitus with diabetic dermatitis 🔎
Type 2 diabetes mellitus with diabetic necrobiosis lipoidica

E11.621   Type 2 diabetes mellitus with foot ulcer 🔎
Use additional code to identify site of ulcer (L97.4-, L97.5-)
Coding Clinic: 2020, Q1, P12; 2016, Q1, P12

E11.622   Type 2 diabetes mellitus with other skin ulcer 🔎
Use additional code to identify site of ulcer (L97.1-L97.9, L98.41-L98.49)
Coding Clinic: 2021, Q1, P8; 2017, Q4, P17

E11.628   Type 2 diabetes mellitus with other skin complications 🔎

● E11.63   Type 2 diabetes mellitus with oral complications

E11.630   Type 2 diabetes mellitus with periodontal disease 🔎

E11.638   Type 2 diabetes mellitus with other oral complications 🔎

● E11.64   Type 2 diabetes mellitus with hypoglycemia

E11.641   Type 2 diabetes mellitus with hypoglycemia with coma 🔎

E11.649   Type 2 diabetes mellitus with hypoglycemia without coma 🔎
Coding Clinic: 2016, Q3, P42; 2015, Q3, P21

CHAPTER 4 (E00-E89)

E11.65   Type 2 diabetes mellitus with hyperglycemia 🏷
     Coding Clinic: 2022, Q1, P28; 2013, Q3, P20

E11.69   Type 2 diabetes mellitus with other specified complication 🏷
     Use additional code to identify complication
     Coding Clinic: 2020, Q1, P12; 2016, Q4, P142

E11.8   Type 2 diabetes mellitus with unspecified complications 🏷

E11.9   Type 2 diabetes mellitus without complications 🏷
     Coding Clinic: 2016, Q4, P142, Q2, P36

● **E13**   **Other specified diabetes mellitus**

     Includes   diabetes mellitus due to genetic defects of beta-cell function
         diabetes mellitus due to genetic defects in insulin action
         postpancreatectomy diabetes mellitus
         postprocedural diabetes mellitus
         secondary diabetes mellitus NEC

     Use additional code to identify control using:
       insulin (Z79.4)
       oral antidiabetic drugs (Z79.84)
       oral hypoglycemic drugs (Z79.84)

     Excludes1   diabetes (mellitus) due to autoimmune process (E10.-)
         diabetes (mellitus) due to immune mediated pancreatic islet beta-cell destruction (E10.-)
         diabetes mellitus due to underlying condition (E08.-)
         drug or chemical induced diabetes mellitus (E09.-)
         gestational diabetes (O24.4-)
         neonatal diabetes mellitus (P70.2)
         type 1 diabetes mellitus (E10.-)

● **E13.0**   Other specified diabetes mellitus with hyperosmolarity

     E13.00   Other specified diabetes mellitus with hyperosmolarity without nonketotic hyperglycemic-hyperosmolar coma (NKHHC) 🏷
         Excludes2   type 2 diabetes mellitus (E11.-)

     E13.01   Other specified diabetes mellitus with hyperosmolarity with coma 🏷

● **E13.1**   Other specified diabetes mellitus with ketoacidosis

     E13.10   Other specified diabetes mellitus with ketoacidosis without coma 🏷
         Coding Clinic: 2016, Q2, P10; 2013, Q1, P26

     E13.11   Other specified diabetes mellitus with ketoacidosis with coma 🏷

● **E13.2**   Other specified diabetes mellitus with kidney complications

     E13.21   Other specified diabetes mellitus with diabetic nephropathy 🏷
         Other specified diabetes mellitus with intercapillary glomerulosclerosis
         Other specified diabetes mellitus with intracapillary glomerulonephrosis
         Other specified diabetes mellitus with Kimmelstiel-Wilson disease

     E13.22   Other specified diabetes mellitus with diabetic chronic kidney disease 🏷
         Use additional code to identify stage of chronic kidney disease (N18.1-N18.6)

     E13.29   Other specified diabetes mellitus with other diabetic kidney complication 🏷
         Other specified diabetes mellitus with renal tubular degeneration

● **E13.3**   Other specified diabetes mellitus with ophthalmic complications
     Coding Clinic: 2016, Q4, P11

     ● **E13.31**   Other specified diabetes mellitus with unspecified diabetic retinopathy

         E13.311   Other specified diabetes mellitus with unspecified diabetic retinopathy with macular edema 🏷

E13.319   Other specified diabetes mellitus with unspecified diabetic retinopathy without macular edema 🏷

● **E13.32**   Other specified diabetes mellitus with mild nonproliferative diabetic retinopathy
     Other specified diabetes mellitus with nonproliferative diabetic retinopathy NOS
     One of the following 7th characters is to be assigned to codes in subcategory E13.32 to designate laterality of the disease:

1	right eye
2	left eye
3	bilateral
9	unspecified eye

     ● **E13.321**   Other specified diabetes mellitus with mild nonproliferative diabetic retinopathy with macular edema 🏷

     ● **E13.329**   Other specified diabetes mellitus with mild nonproliferative diabetic retinopathy without macular edema 🏷

● **E13.33**   Other specified diabetes mellitus with moderate nonproliferative diabetic retinopathy
     One of the following 7th characters is to be assigned to codes in subcategory E13.33 to designate laterality of the disease:

1	right eye
2	left eye
3	bilateral
9	unspecified eye

     ● **E13.331**   Other specified diabetes mellitus with moderate nonproliferative diabetic retinopathy with macular edema 🏷

     ● **E13.339**   Other specified diabetes mellitus with moderate nonproliferative diabetic retinopathy without macular edema 🏷

● **E13.34**   Other specified diabetes mellitus with severe nonproliferative diabetic retinopathy
     One of the following 7th characters is to be assigned to codes in subcategory E13.34 to designate laterality of the disease:

1	right eye
2	left eye
3	bilateral
9	unspecified eye

     ● **E13.341**   Other specified diabetes mellitus with severe nonproliferative diabetic retinopathy with macular edema 🏷

     ● **E13.349**   Other specified diabetes mellitus with severe nonproliferative diabetic retinopathy without macular edema 🏷

● **E13.35**   Other specified diabetes mellitus with proliferative diabetic retinopathy
     One of the following 7th characters is to be assigned to codes in subcategory E13.35 to designate laterality of the disease:

1	right eye
2	left eye
3	bilateral
9	unspecified eye

     ● **E13.351**   Other specified diabetes mellitus with proliferative diabetic retinopathy with macular edema 🏷

     ● **E13.352**   Other specified diabetes mellitus with proliferative diabetic retinopathy with traction retinal detachment involving the macula 🏷

▶ New   ⇒ Revised   ~~deleted~~ Deleted   Excludes 1   Excludes 2   Includes   Use additional   Code first   Code also   Key words
OGCR Official Guidelines   X Assign placeholder X   ● Use Additional Character(s)   ▶ Manifestation Code   🏷 Hierarchical Condition Category   Coding Clinic

● E13.353 Other specified diabetes mellitus with proliferative diabetic retinopathy with traction retinal detachment not involving the macula 🔍

● E13.354 Other specified diabetes mellitus with proliferative diabetic retinopathy with combined traction retinal detachment and rhegmatogenous retinal detachment 🔍

● E13.355 Other specified diabetes mellitus with stable proliferative diabetic retinopathy 🔍

● E13.359 Other specified diabetes mellitus with proliferative diabetic retinopathy without macular edema 🔍

E13.36 Other specified diabetes mellitus with diabetic cataract 🔍

X ● E13.37 Other specified diabetes mellitus with diabetic macular edema, resolved following treatment 🔍

One of the following 7th characters is to be assigned to code E13.37 to designate laterality of the disease:

1	right eye
2	left eye
3	bilateral
9	unspecified eye

E13.39 Other specified diabetes mellitus with other diabetic ophthalmic complication 🔍

Use additional code to identify manifestation, such as:
diabetic glaucoma (H40-H42)

● E13.4 Other specified diabetes mellitus with neurological complications

E13.40 Other specified diabetes mellitus with diabetic neuropathy, unspecified 🔍

E13.41 Other specified diabetes mellitus with diabetic mononeuropathy 🔍

E13.42 Other specified diabetes mellitus with diabetic polyneuropathy 🔍
Other specified diabetes mellitus with diabetic neuralgia

E13.43 Other specified diabetes mellitus with diabetic autonomic (poly)neuropathy 🔍
Other specified diabetes mellitus with diabetic gastroparesis

E13.44 Other specified diabetes mellitus with diabetic amyotrophy 🔍

E13.49 Other specified diabetes mellitus with other diabetic neurological complication 🔍

● E13.5 Other specified diabetes mellitus with circulatory complications

E13.51 Other specified diabetes mellitus with diabetic peripheral angiopathy without gangrene 🔍

E13.52 Other specified diabetes mellitus with diabetic peripheral angiopathy with gangrene 🔍
Other specified diabetes mellitus with diabetic gangrene

E13.59 Other specified diabetes mellitus with other circulatory complications 🔍

● E13.6 Other specified diabetes mellitus with other specified complications

● E13.61 Other specified diabetes mellitus with diabetic arthropathy

E13.610 Other specified diabetes mellitus with diabetic neuropathic arthropathy 🔍
Other specified diabetes mellitus with Charcôt's joints

E13.618 Other specified diabetes mellitus with other diabetic arthropathy 🔍

● E13.62 Other specified diabetes mellitus with skin complications

E13.620 Other specified diabetes mellitus with diabetic dermatitis 🔍
Other specified diabetes mellitus with diabetic necrobiosis lipoidica

E13.621 Other specified diabetes mellitus with foot ulcer 🔍
Use additional code to identify site of ulcer (L97.4-, L97.5-)

E13.622 Other specified diabetes mellitus with other skin ulcer 🔍
Use additional code to identify site of ulcer (L97.1-L97.9, L98.41-L98.49)

E13.628 Other specified diabetes mellitus with other skin complications 🔍

● E13.63 Other specified diabetes mellitus with oral complications

E13.630 Other specified diabetes mellitus with periodontal disease 🔍

E13.638 Other specified diabetes mellitus with other oral complications 🔍

● E13.64 Other specified diabetes mellitus with hypoglycemia

E13.641 Other specified diabetes mellitus with hypoglycemia with coma 🔍

E13.649 Other specified diabetes mellitus with hypoglycemia without coma 🔍

E13.65 Other specified diabetes mellitus with hyperglycemia 🔍

E13.69 Other specified diabetes mellitus with other specified complication 🔍
Use additional code to identify complication

E13.8 Other specified diabetes mellitus with unspecified complications 🔍

E13.9 Other specified diabetes mellitus without complications 🔍

OTHER DISORDERS OF GLUCOSE REGULATION AND PANCREATIC INTERNAL SECRETION (E15-E16)

E15 Nondiabetic hypoglycemic coma 🔍
Includes drug-induced insulin coma in nondiabetic hyperinsulinism with hypoglycemic coma
hypoglycemic coma NOS

● E16 Other disorders of pancreatic internal secretion

E16.0 Drug-induced hypoglycemia without coma
Excludes1 diabetes with hypoglycemia without coma (E09.649)

Use additional code for adverse effect, if applicable, to identify drug (T36-T50 with fifth or sixth character 5)

E16.1 Other hypoglycemia
Functional hyperinsulinism
Functional nonhyperinsulinemic hypoglycemia
Hyperinsulinism NOS
Hyperplasia of pancreatic islet beta cells NOS
Excludes1 diabetes with hypoglycemia (E08.649, E10.649, E11.649, E13.649)
hypoglycemia in infant of diabetic mother (P70.1)
neonatal hypoglycemia (P70.4)

E16.2 Hypoglycemia, unspecified
Excludes1 diabetes with hypoglycemia (E08.649, E10.649, E11.649, E13.649)
Coding Clinic: 2016, Q3, P42

E16.3 Increased secretion of glucagon
Hyperplasia of pancreatic endocrine cells with glucagon excess

CHAPTER 4 (E00-E89)

Item 4–4 Hyperparathyroidism is an overactive parathyroid gland that secretes excessive parathormone, causing increased levels of circulating calcium. This results in a loss of calcium in the bone (osteoporosis).

Hypoparathyroidism is an underactive parathyroid gland that results in decreased levels of circulating calcium. The primary manifestation is **tetany**, a continuous muscle spasm.

Figure 4-4 Tetany caused by hypoparathyroidism.

E16.4   **Increased secretion of gastrin**
     Hypergastrinemia
     Hyperplasia of pancreatic endocrine cells with gastrin excess
     Zollinger-Ellison syndrome

E16.8   **Other specified disorders of pancreatic internal secretion**
     Increased secretion from endocrine pancreas of growth hormone-releasing hormone
     Increased secretion from endocrine pancreas of pancreatic polypeptide
     Increased secretion from endocrine pancreas of somatostatin
     Increased secretion from endocrine pancreas of vasoactive-intestinal polypeptide

E16.9   **Disorder of pancreatic internal secretion, unspecified**
     Islet-cell hyperplasia NOS
     Pancreatic endocrine cell hyperplasia NOS

DISORDERS OF OTHER ENDOCRINE GLANDS (E20-E35)

Excludes1   galactorrhea (N64.3)
              gynecomastia (N62)

● E20   **Hypoparathyroidism**
     Greatly reduced function of parathyroid glands; AKA parathyroid insufficiency
     Excludes1   Di George's syndrome (D82.1)
                  postprocedural hypoparathyroidism (E89.2)
                  tetany NOS (R29.0)
                  transitory neonatal hypoparathyroidism (P71.4)

E20.0   **Idiopathic hypoparathyroidism** 🔖
     Rare condition, unknown cause; short dwarf-like with round face

E20.1   **Pseudohypoparathyroidism**
     Hereditary condition resembling hypoparathyroidism, but caused by inability to respond to parathyroid hormone

E20.8   **Other hypoparathyroidism** 🔖

E20.9   **Hypoparathyroidism, unspecified** 🔖
     Parathyroid tetany

● E21   **Hyperparathyroidism and other disorders of parathyroid gland**
     Excludes1   adult osteomalacia (M83.-)
                  ectopic hyperparathyroidism (E34.2)
                  hungry bone syndrome (E83.81)
                  infantile and juvenile osteomalacia (E55.0)
     Excludes2   familial hypocalciuric hypercalcemia (E83.52)

E21.0   **Primary hyperparathyroidism** 🔖
     Hyperplasia of parathyroid
     Osteitis fibrosa cystica generalisata [von Recklinghausen's disease of bone]

E21.1   **Secondary hyperparathyroidism, not elsewhere classified** 🔖
     Excludes1   secondary hyperparathyroidism of renal origin (N25.81)

Item 4–5 Hyperadrenalism is overactivity of the adrenal cortex, which secretes corticosteroid hormones. Excessive glucocorticoid hormone results in hyperglycemia (**Cushing's syndrome**), and excessive aldosterone results in **Conn's syndrome. Adrenogenital syndrome** is the result of excessive secretion of androgens, male hormones, which stimulates premature sexual development. **Hypoadrenalism, Addison's disease,** is a condition in which the adrenal glands atrophy.

E21.2   **Other hyperparathyroidism** 🔖
     Tertiary hyperparathyroidism
     Excludes1   familial hypocalciuric hypercalcemia (E83.52)

E21.3   **Hyperparathyroidism, unspecified** 🔖
E21.4   **Other specified disorders of parathyroid gland** 🔖
E21.5   **Disorder of parathyroid gland, unspecified** 🔖

● E22   **Hyperfunction of pituitary gland**
     Excludes1   Cushing's syndrome (E24.-)
                  Nelson's syndrome (E24.1)
                  overproduction of ACTH not associated with Cushing's disease (E27.0)
                  overproduction of pituitary ACTH (E24.0)
                  overproduction of thyroid-stimulating hormone (E05.8-)

E22.0   **Acromegaly and pituitary gigantism** 🔖
     Chronic disease caused by hypersecretion of growth hormone
     Overproduction of growth hormone
     Excludes1   constitutional gigantism (E34.4)
                  constitutional tall stature (E34.4)
                  increased secretion from endocrine pancreas of growth hormone-releasing hormone (E16.8)

E22.1   **Hyperprolactinemia** 🔖
     Increased levels of prolactin
     Use additional code for adverse effect, if applicable, to identify drug (T36-T50 with fifth or sixth character 5)

E22.2   **Syndrome of inappropriate secretion of antidiuretic hormone** 🔖

E22.8   **Other hyperfunction of pituitary gland** 🔖
     Central precocious puberty

E22.9   **Hyperfunction of pituitary gland, unspecified** 🔖

● E23   **Hypofunction and other disorders of the pituitary gland**
     Includes   the listed conditions whether the disorder is in the pituitary or the hypothalamus
     Excludes1   postprocedural hypopituitarism (E89.3)

E23.0   **Hypopituitarism** 🔖
     Fertile eunuch syndrome
     Hypogonadotropic hypogonadism
     Idiopathic growth hormone deficiency
     Isolated deficiency of gonadotropin
     Isolated deficiency of growth hormone
     Isolated deficiency of pituitary hormone
     Kallmann's syndrome
     Lorain-Levi short stature
     Necrosis of pituitary gland (postpartum)
     Panhypopituitarism
     Pituitary cachexia
     Pituitary insufficiency NOS
     Pituitary short stature
     Sheehan's syndrome
     Simmonds' disease

E23.1   **Drug-induced hypopituitarism** 🔖
     Use additional code for adverse effect, if applicable, to identify drug (T36-T50 with fifth or sixth character 5)

E23.2   **Diabetes insipidus** 🔖
     Excludes1   nephrogenic diabetes insipidus (N25.1)

E23.3   **Hypothalamic dysfunction, not elsewhere classified** 🔖
     Excludes1   Prader-Willi syndrome (Q87.11)
                  Russell-Silver syndrome (Q87.19)

E23.6   **Other disorders of pituitary gland** 🔖
     Abscess of pituitary
     Adiposogenital dystrophy

E23.7   **Disorder of pituitary gland, unspecified** 🔖

CHAPTER 4 (E00-E89)

▶ New   ⇒ Revised   ~~deleted~~ Deleted   Excludes 1   Excludes 2   Includes   Use additional   Code first   Code also   Key words
OGCR Official Guidelines   X Assign placeholder X   ● Use Additional Character(s)   ▶ Manifestation Code   🔖 Hierarchical Condition Category   **Coding Clinic**

Figure 4-5 Centripetal and generalized obesity and dorsal kyphosis in a woman with Cushing's disease. (From Salvo SG: Mosby's Pathology for Massage Therapists, St. Louis, MO: Mosby/Elsevier, 2009)

● **E24   Cushing's syndrome**

> **Excludes1**   congenital adrenal hyperplasia (E25.0)

   E24.0   Pituitary-dependent Cushing's disease 🔖
   Overproduction of pituitary ACTH
   Pituitary-dependent hypercorticalism

   E24.1   Nelson's syndrome 🔖

   E24.2   Drug-induced Cushing's syndrome 🔖
   > Use additional code for adverse effect, if applicable, to identify drug (T36-T50 with fifth or sixth character 5)

   E24.3   Ectopic ACTH syndrome 🔖

   E24.4   Alcohol-induced pseudo-Cushing's syndrome 🔖

   E24.8   Other Cushing's syndrome 🔖

   E24.9   Cushing's syndrome, unspecified 🔖

● **E25   Adrenogenital disorders**

   Disorder of production of steroid hormone in adrenal gland

   > **Includes**   adrenogenital syndromes, virilizing or feminizing, whether acquired or due to adrenal hyperplasia consequent on inborn enzyme defects in hormone synthesis
   > female adrenal pseudohermaphroditism
   > female heterosexual precocious pseudopuberty
   > male isosexual precocious pseudopuberty
   > male macrogenitosomia praecox
   > male sexual precocity with adrenal hyperplasia
   > male virilization (female)

   > **Excludes1**   indeterminate sex and pseudohermaphroditism (Q56)
   > chromosomal abnormalities (Q90-Q99)

   E25.0   Congenital adrenogenital disorders associated with enzyme deficiency 🔖
   Congenital adrenal hyperplasia
   21-Hydroxylase deficiency
   Salt-losing congenital adrenal hyperplasia

   E25.8   Other adrenogenital disorders 🔖
   Idiopathic adrenogenital disorder
   > Use additional code for adverse effect, if applicable, to identify drug (T36-T50 with fifth or sixth character 5)

   E25.9   Adrenogenital disorder, unspecified 🔖
   Adrenogenital syndrome NOS

● **E26   Hyperaldosteronism**

   Abnormality of electrolyte metabolism caused by excessive secretion of aldosterone

● **E26.0   Primary hyperaldosteronism**

   E26.01   Conn's syndrome 🔖
   Code also adrenal adenoma (D35.0-)

   E26.02   Glucocorticoid-remediable aldosteronism 🔖
   Familial aldosteronism type I

   E26.09   Other primary hyperaldosteronism 🔖
   Primary aldosteronism due to adrenal hyperplasia (bilateral)

   E26.1   Secondary hyperaldosteronism 🔖

● **E26.8   Other hyperaldosteronism**

   E26.81   Bartter's syndrome 🔖

   E26.89   Other hyperaldosteronism 🔖

   E26.9   Hyperaldosteronism, unspecified 🔖
   Aldosteronism NOS
   Hyperaldosteronism NOS

● **E27   Other disorders of adrenal gland**

   E27.0   Other adrenocortical overactivity 🔖
   Overproduction of ACTH, not associated with Cushing's disease
   Premature adrenarche
   > **Excludes1**   Cushing's syndrome (E24.-)

   E27.1   Primary adrenocortical insufficiency 🔖
   Addison's disease
   Autoimmune adrenalitis
   > **Excludes1**   Addison only phenotype adrenoleukodystrophy (E71.528)
   > amyloidosis (E85.-)
   > tuberculous Addison's disease (A18.7)
   > Waterhouse-Friderichsen syndrome (A39.1)

   E27.2   Addisonian crisis 🔖
   Acute onset of adrenocortical insufficiency
   Adrenal crisis
   Adrenocortical crisis

   E27.3   Drug-induced adrenocortical insufficiency 🔖
   > Use additional code for adverse effect, if applicable, to identify drug (T36-T50 with fifth or sixth character 5)

● **E27.4   Other and unspecified adrenocortical insufficiency**
   > **Excludes1**   adrenoleukodystrophy [Addison-Schilder] (E71.528)
   > Waterhouse-Friderichsen syndrome (A39.1)

   E27.40   Unspecified adrenocortical insufficiency 🔖
   Adrenocortical insufficiency NOS
   Hypoaldosteronism

   E27.49   Other adrenocortical insufficiency 🔖
   Adrenal hemorrhage
   Adrenal infarction

   E27.5   Adrenomedullary hyperfunction 🔖
   Adrenomedullary hyperplasia
   Catecholamine hypersecretion

   E27.8   Other specified disorders of adrenal gland 🔖
   Abnormality of cortisol-binding globulin

   E27.9   Disorder of adrenal gland, unspecified 🔖

● **E28   Ovarian dysfunction**

   > **Excludes1**   isolated gonadotropin deficiency (E23.0)
   > postprocedural ovarian failure (E89.4-)

   E28.0   Estrogen excess ♀
   > Use additional code for adverse effect, if applicable, to identify drug (T36-T50 with fifth or sixth character 5)

   E28.1   Androgen excess ♀
   Hypersecretion of ovarian androgens
   > Use additional code for adverse effect, if applicable, to identify drug (T36-T50 with fifth or sixth character 5)

   E28.2   Polycystic ovarian syndrome ♀
   Sclerocystic ovary syndrome
   Stein-Leventhal syndrome

● **E28.3   Primary ovarian failure**
   > **Excludes1**   pure gonadal dysgenesis (Q99.1)
   > Turner's syndrome (Q96.-)

● **E28.31   Premature menopause**

   E28.310   Symptomatic premature menopause ♀   A
   Symptoms such as flushing, sleeplessness, headache, lack of concentration, associated with premature menopause

   E28.319   Asymptomatic premature menopause ♀   A
   Premature menopause NOS

   E28.39   Other primary ovarian failure ♀
   Decreased estrogen
   Resistant ovary syndrome

CHAPTER 4 (E00-E89)

CHAPTER 4 (E00-E89)

E28.8   **Other ovarian dysfunction** ♀
Ovarian hyperfunction NOS

> **Excludes1**   postprocedural ovarian failure (E89.4-)

E28.9   **Ovarian dysfunction, unspecified** ♀

● E29   **Testicular dysfunction**

> **Excludes1**   androgen insensitivity syndrome (E34.5-)
> azoospermia or oligospermia NOS (N46.0-N46.1)
> isolated gonadotropin deficiency (E23.0)
> Klinefelter's syndrome (Q98.0-Q98.1, Q98.4)

E29.0   **Testicular hyperfunction** ♂
Hypersecretion of testicular hormones

E29.1   **Testicular hypofunction** ♂
Defective biosynthesis of testicular androgen NOS
5-delta-Reductase deficiency (with male pseudohermaphroditism)
Testicular hypogonadism NOS

> Use additional code for adverse effect, if applicable, to identify drug (T36-T50 with fifth or sixth character 5)

> **Excludes1**   postprocedural testicular hypofunction (E89.5)

E29.8   **Other testicular dysfunction** ♂
E29.9   **Testicular dysfunction, unspecified** ♂

● E30   **Disorders of puberty, not elsewhere classified**

E30.0   **Delayed puberty**
Constitutional delay of puberty
Delayed sexual development

E30.1   **Precocious puberty**   P
Sexual maturation at earlier age than normal, or before age 8 in girls and 9 in boys, usually hormonal; AKA sexual precocity or pubertas praecox
Precocious menstruation

> **Excludes1**   Albright (-McCune) (-Sternberg) syndrome (Q78.1)
> central precocious puberty (E22.8)
> congenital adrenal hyperplasia (E25.0)
> female heterosexual precocious pseudopuberty (E25.-)
> male isosexual precocious pseudopuberty (E25.-)

E30.8   **Other disorders of puberty**   P
Premature thelarche

E30.9   **Disorder of puberty, unspecified**

● E31   **Polyglandular dysfunction**

> **Excludes1**   ataxia telangiectasia [Louis-Bar] (G11.3)
> dystrophia myotonica [Steinert] (G71.11)
> pseudohypoparathyroidism (E20.1)

E31.0   **Autoimmune polyglandular failure** 🐾
Schmidt's syndrome

E31.1   **Polyglandular hyperfunction** 🐾

> **Excludes1**   multiple endocrine adenomatosis (E31.2-)
> multiple endocrine neoplasia (E31.2-)

● E31.2   **Multiple endocrine neoplasia [MEN] syndromes**
Adenomatous hyperplasia and malignant tumors in endocrine glands
Multiple endocrine adenomatosis

> Code also any associated malignancies and other conditions associated with the syndromes

E31.20   **Multiple endocrine neoplasia [MEN] syndrome, unspecified** 🐾
Multiple endocrine adenomatosis NOS
Multiple endocrine neoplasia [MEN] syndrome NOS

E31.21   **Multiple endocrine neoplasia [MEN] type I** 🐾
Wermer's syndrome

E31.22   **Multiple endocrine neoplasia [MEN] type IIA** 🐾
Sipple's syndrome

E31.23   **Multiple endocrine neoplasia [MEN] type IIB** 🐾

E31.8   **Other polyglandular dysfunction** 🐾
E31.9   **Polyglandular dysfunction, unspecified** 🐾

● E32   **Diseases of thymus**

> **Excludes1**   aplasia or hypoplasia of thymus with immunodeficiency (D82.1)
> myasthenia gravis (G70.0)

E32.0   **Persistent hyperplasia of thymus** 🐾
Hypertrophy of thymus

E32.1   **Abscess of thymus** 🐾

E32.8   **Other diseases of thymus** 🐾

> **Excludes1**   aplasia or hypoplasia with immunodeficiency (D82.1)
> thymoma (D15.0)

E32.9   **Disease of thymus, unspecified** 🐾

● E34   **Other endocrine disorders**

> **Excludes1**   pseudohypoparathyroidism (E20.1)

E34.0   **Carcinoid syndrome** 🐾

> **Note:** May be used as an additional code to identify functional activity associated with a carcinoid tumor.

E34.1   **Other hypersecretion of intestinal hormones**

E34.2   **Ectopic hormone secretion, not elsewhere classified**

> **Excludes1**   ectopic ACTH syndrome (E24.3)

E34.3   **Short stature due to endocrine disorder**
~~Constitutional short stature~~
~~Laron-type short stature~~

> **Excludes1**   achondroplastic short stature (Q77.4)
> hypochondroplastic short stature (Q77.4)
> nutritional short stature (E45)
> pituitary short stature (E23.0)
> progeria (E34.8)
> renal short stature (N25.0)
> Russell-Silver syndrome (Q87.19)
> short-limbed stature with immunodeficiency (D82.2)
> ▶ short stature due to endocrine disorder (E34.3-)
> short stature in specific dysmorphic syndromes - code to syndrome - see Alphabetical Index
> short stature NOS (R62.52)

▶ E34.30   **Short stature due to endocrine disorder, unspecified**

▶ E34.31   **Constitutional short stature**
▶ Constitutional delay of growth, puberty, or maturation

▶ ● E34.32   **Genetic causes of short stature**

▶ E34.321   **Primary insulin-like growth factor-1 (IGF-1) deficiency**
▶ Acid-labile subunit gene (IGFALS) defect
▶ Growth hormone gene 1 (GH1) defect with growth hormone neutralizing antibodies
▶ Growth hormone insensitivity syndrome (GHIS)
▶ Insulin-like growth factor 1 gene (IGF1) defect
▶ Laron type short stature
▶ Severe primary insulin-like growth factor-1 deficiency (SPIGFD)
▶ Signal transducer and activator of transcription 5B gene (STAT5b) defect

▶ E34.322   **Insulin-like growth factor-1 (IGF-1) resistance**
▶ Genetic syndrome with resistance to insulin-like growth factor-1
▶ Insulin-like growth factor-1 receptor (IGF-1R) defect
▶ Post-insulin-like growth factor-1 receptor signaling defect

▶ New   ⇒ Revised   ~~deleted~~ Deleted   Excludes 1   Excludes 2   Includes   Use additional   Code first   Code also   Key words

OGCR Official Guidelines   X Assign placeholder X   ● Use Additional Character(s)   ▶ Manifestation Code   🐾 Hierarchical Condition Category   **Coding Clinic**

▶E34.328   **Other genetic causes of short stature**
   ▶Short stature due to ACAN gene variant
   ▶Short stature due to aggrecan deficiency
   ▶Short stature due to NPR-2 gene variant

▶E34.329   **Unspecified genetic causes of short stature**

▶● E34.39   **Other short stature due to endocrine disorder**

E34.4   **Constitutional tall stature** 🐾
   Constitutional gigantism

● E34.5   **Androgen insensitivity syndrome**

   E34.50   **Androgen insensitivity syndrome, unspecified**
     Androgen insensitivity NOS

   E34.51   **Complete androgen insensitivity syndrome**
     Complete androgen insensitivity
     de Quervain syndrome
     Goldberg-Maxwell syndrome

   E34.52   **Partial androgen insensitivity syndrome**
     Partial androgen insensitivity
     Reifenstein syndrome

E34.8   **Other specified endocrine disorders**
   Pineal gland dysfunction
   Progeria
   Excludes2   pseudohypoparathyroidism (E20.1)

E34.9   **Endocrine disorder, unspecified**
   Endocrine disturbance NOS
   Hormone disturbance NOS

▷ E35   *Disorders of endocrine glands in diseases classified elsewhere*
   Code first underlying disease, such as:
     late congenital syphilis of thymus gland [Dubois disease] (A50.5)
   Use additional code, if applicable, to identify:
     sequelae of tuberculosis of other organs (B90.8)
   Excludes1   Echinococcus granulosus infection of thyroid gland (B67.3)
     meningococcal hemorrhagic adrenalitis (A39.1)
     syphilis of endocrine gland (A52.79)
     tuberculosis of adrenal gland, except calcification (A18.7)
     tuberculosis of endocrine gland NEC (A18.82)
     tuberculosis of thyroid gland (A18.81)
     Waterhouse-Friderichsen syndrome (A39.1)

INTRAOPERATIVE COMPLICATIONS OF ENDOCRINE SYSTEM (E36)

● E36   **Intraoperative complications of endocrine system**
   Excludes2   postprocedural endocrine and metabolic complications and disorders, not elsewhere classified (E89.-)

● E36.0   **Intraoperative hemorrhage and hematoma of an endocrine system organ or structure complicating a procedure**
   Excludes1   intraoperative hemorrhage and hematoma of an endocrine system organ or structure due to accidental puncture or laceration during a procedure (E36.1-)

   E36.01   **Intraoperative hemorrhage and hematoma of an endocrine system organ or structure complicating an endocrine system procedure**
     Coding Clinic: 2020, Q1, P19

   E36.02   **Intraoperative hemorrhage and hematoma of an endocrine system organ or structure complicating other procedure**

● E36.1   **Accidental puncture and laceration of an endocrine system organ or structure during a procedure**

   E36.11   **Accidental puncture and laceration of an endocrine system organ or structure during an endocrine system procedure**

   E36.12   **Accidental puncture and laceration of an endocrine system organ or structure during other procedure**

E36.8   **Other intraoperative complications of endocrine system**
   Use additional code, if applicable, to further specify disorder

MALNUTRITION (E40-E46)

   Excludes1   intestinal malabsorption (K90.-)
     sequelae of protein-calorie malnutrition (E64.0)
   Excludes2   nutritional anemias (D50-D53)
     starvation (T73.0)

E40   **Kwashiorkor** 🐾
   Malnutrition produced by severe protein deficiency
   Severe malnutrition with nutritional edema with dyspigmentation of skin and hair
   Excludes1   marasmic kwashiorkor (E42)
   Coding Clinic: 22017, Q3, P25

E41   **Nutritional marasmus** 🐾
   Severe malnutrition with marasmus
   Excludes1   marasmic kwashiorkor (E42)
   Coding Clinic: 2017, Q3, P24-25

E42   **Marasmic kwashiorkor** 🐾
   Severe protein malnutrition
   Intermediate form severe protein-calorie malnutrition
   Severe protein-calorie malnutrition with signs of both kwashiorkor and marasmus
   Coding Clinic: 2017, Q3, P25

E43   **Unspecified severe protein-calorie malnutrition** 🐾
   Starvation edema
   Coding Clinic: 2022, Q1, P13; 2020, Q1, P5-6; 2017, Q4, P108-109; 2017, Q3, P25

● E44   **Protein-calorie malnutrition of moderate and mild degree**

   E44.0   **Moderate protein-calorie malnutrition** 🐾
   E44.1   **Mild protein-calorie malnutrition** 🐾

E45   **Retarded development following protein-calorie malnutrition** 🐾
   Nutritional short stature
   Nutritional stunting
   Physical retardation due to malnutrition

E46   **Unspecified protein-calorie malnutrition** 🐾
   Malnutrition NOS
   Protein-calorie imbalance NOS
   Excludes1   nutritional deficiency NOS (E63.9)
   Coding Clinic: 2017, Q3, P25

OTHER NUTRITIONAL DEFICIENCIES (E50-E64)

   Excludes2   nutritional anemias (D50-D53)

● E50   **Vitamin A deficiency**
   Excludes1   sequelae of vitamin A deficiency (E64.1)
   E50.0   **Vitamin A deficiency with conjunctival xerosis**
   E50.1   **Vitamin A deficiency with Bitot's spot and conjunctival xerosis**
     Bitot's spot in the young child
   E50.2   **Vitamin A deficiency with corneal xerosis**
   E50.3   **Vitamin A deficiency with corneal ulceration and xerosis**

Item 4-6   **Bitot's spots** are the result of a buildup of keratin debris found on the superficial surface the conjunctiva; oval, triangular, or irregular in shape; and a sign of vitamin A deficiency and associated with night blindness. The disease may progress to **keratomalacia**, which can result in eventual prolapse of the iris and loss of the lens.

Figure 4-6   Bitot's spot on the conjunctiva.

CHAPTER 4 (E00-E89)

Figure 4-7 The sharply demarcated, characteristic scaling dermatitis of pellagra. (From James WD, Berger TG, Elston DM: Andrews' Diseases of the Skin: Clinical Dermatology, Philadelphia, Saunders Elsevier, 2006)

Item 4–7 Pellagra is associated with a deficiency of niacin and its precursor, **tryptophan.** Characteristics of the condition include diarrhea, dermatitis on exposed skin surfaces, dementia, and death. It is prevalent in developing countries where nutrition is inadequate. **Beriberi** is associated with thiamine deficiency.

E50.4 Vitamin A deficiency with keratomalacia
Eye disorder that results in dry cornea caused by vitamin A deficiency

E50.5 Vitamin A deficiency with night blindness

E50.6 Vitamin A deficiency with xerophthalmic scars of cornea
Abnormal dryness and thickening of conjunctiva and cornea due to vitamin A deficiency

E50.7 Other ocular manifestations of vitamin A deficiency
Xerophthalmia NOS

E50.8 Other manifestations of vitamin A deficiency
Follicular keratosis
Xeroderma

E50.9 Vitamin A deficiency, unspecified
Hypovitaminosis A NOS

● **E51 Thiamine deficiency**
Excludes1 sequelae of thiamine deficiency (E64.8)

  ● **E51.1 Beriberi**

   E51.11 Dry beriberi
   Thiamine deficiency with nervous system manifestation most often caused by excessive alcohol consumption
   Beriberi NOS
   Beriberi with polyneuropathy

   E51.12 Wet beriberi
   Thiamine deficiency with cardiovascular manifestation most often caused by excessive alcohol consumption
   Beriberi with cardiovascular manifestations
   Cardiovascular beriberi
   Shoshin disease

  E51.2 Wernicke's encephalopathy
  Acute disease of brain due to thiamine deficiency most often associated with excessive alcohol consumption

  E51.8 Other manifestations of thiamine deficiency

  E51.9 Thiamine deficiency, unspecified

E52 Niacin deficiency [pellagra]
Niacin (-tryptophan) deficiency
Nicotinamide deficiency
Pellagra (alcoholic)
Excludes1 sequelae of niacin deficiency (E64.8)

● **E53 Deficiency of other B group vitamins**
Excludes1 sequelae of vitamin B deficiency (E64.8)

  E53.0 Riboflavin deficiency
  Ariboflavinosis
  Vitamin B2 deficiency

  E53.1 Pyridoxine deficiency
  Vitamin B6 deficiency
  Excludes1 pyridoxine-responsive sideroblastic anemia (D64.3)

  E53.8 Deficiency of other specified B group vitamins
  Biotin deficiency
  Cyanocobalamin deficiency
  Folate deficiency
  Folic acid deficiency
  Pantothenic acid deficiency
  Vitamin B12 deficiency
  Excludes1 folate deficiency anemia (D52.-)
  vitamin B12 deficiency anemia (D51.-)

  E53.9 Vitamin B deficiency, unspecified

E54 Ascorbic acid deficiency
Deficiency of vitamin C
Scurvy
Excludes1 scorbutic anemia (D53.2)
sequelae of vitamin C deficiency (E64.2)

● **E55 Vitamin D deficiency**
Excludes1 adult osteomalacia (M83.-)
osteoporosis (M80.-)
sequelae of rickets (E64.3)

  E55.0 Rickets, active
  Infantile osteomalacia
  Juvenile osteomalacia
  Softening of bone
  Excludes1 celiac rickets (K90.0)
  Crohn's rickets (K50.-)
  hereditary vitamin D-dependent rickets (E83.32)
  inactive rickets (E64.3)
  renal rickets (N25.0)
  sequelae of rickets (E64.3)
  vitamin D-resistant rickets (E83.31)

  E55.9 Vitamin D deficiency, unspecified
  Avitaminosis D

● **E56 Other vitamin deficiencies**
Excludes1 sequelae of other vitamin deficiencies (E64.8)

  E56.0 Deficiency of vitamin E
  E56.1 Deficiency of vitamin K
  Excludes1 deficiency of coagulation factor due to vitamin K deficiency (D68.4)
  vitamin K deficiency of newborn (P53)

  E56.8 Deficiency of other vitamins
  E56.9 Vitamin deficiency, unspecified

E58 Dietary calcium deficiency
Excludes1 disorders of calcium metabolism (E83.5-)
sequelae of calcium deficiency (E64.8)

E59 Dietary selenium deficiency
Keshan disease
Excludes1 sequelae of selenium deficiency (E64.8)

E60 Dietary zinc deficiency

● **E61 Deficiency of other nutrient elements**
Use additional code for adverse effect, if applicable, to identify drug (T36-T50 with fifth or sixth character 5)
Excludes1 disorders of mineral metabolism (E83.-)
iodine deficiency related thyroid disorders (E00-E02)
sequelae of malnutrition and other nutritional deficiencies (E64.-)

  E61.0 Copper deficiency
  E61.1 Iron deficiency
  Excludes1 iron deficiency anemia (D50.-)
  E61.2 Magnesium deficiency
  E61.3 Manganese deficiency
  E61.4 Chromium deficiency
  E61.5 Molybdenum deficiency
  E61.6 Vanadium deficiency
  E61.7 Deficiency of multiple nutrient elements
  E61.8 Deficiency of other specified nutrient elements
  E61.9 Deficiency of nutrient element, unspecified

- **E63   Other nutritional deficiencies**

   Excludes2   dehydration (E86.0)
   failure to thrive, adult (R62.7)
   failure to thrive, child (R62.51)
   feeding problems in newborn (P92.-)
   sequelae of malnutrition and other nutritional
       deficiencies (E64.-)

   E63.0   Essential fatty acid [EFA] deficiency
   E63.1   Imbalance of constituents of food intake
   E63.8   Other specified nutritional deficiencies
   E63.9   Nutritional deficiency, unspecified

- **E64   Sequelae of malnutrition and other nutritional deficiencies**
   Pathological condition resulting from disease, injury, or other trauma

   Note: This category is to be used to indicate conditions in
   categories E43, E44, E46, E50-E63 as the cause of sequelae,
   which are themselves classified elsewhere. The "sequelae"
   include conditions specified as such; they also include the
   late effects of diseases classifiable to the above categories if
   the disease itself is no longer present

   *Code first condition resulting from (sequela) of malnutrition and
   other nutritional deficiencies*

   E64.0   Sequelae of protein-calorie malnutrition 🔖

      Excludes2   retarded development following protein-
          calorie malnutrition (E45)

   E64.1   Sequelae of vitamin A deficiency
   E64.2   Sequelae of vitamin C deficiency
   E64.3   Sequelae of rickets
   E64.8   Sequelae of other nutritional deficiencies
   E64.9   Sequelae of unspecified nutritional deficiency

OVERWEIGHT, OBESITY AND OTHER HYPERALIMENTATION (E65-E68)

- **E65   Localized adiposity**
   Fat pad

- **E66   Overweight and obesity**

   *Code first obesity complicating pregnancy, childbirth and the
   puerperium, if applicable (O99.21-)*

   Use additional code to identify body mass index (BMI), if
   known (Z68.-)

   Excludes1   adiposogenital dystrophy (E23.6)
   lipomatosis NOS (E88.2)
   lipomatosis dolorosa [Dercum] (E88.2)
   Prader-Willi syndrome (Q87.11)

   Coding Clinic: 2018, Q4, P80

- **E66.0   Obesity due to excess calories**

   **E66.01   Morbid (severe) obesity due to excess
       calories 🔖**

      Excludes1   morbid (severe) obesity with
          alveolar hypoventilation
          (E66.2)
      Coding Clinic: 2022, Q2, P9; 2018, Q4, P79

   E66.09   Other obesity due to excess calories

   E66.1   Drug-induced obesity

   Use additional code for adverse effect, if applicable,
   to identify drug (T36-T50 with fifth or sixth
   character 5)

   **E66.2   Morbid (severe) obesity with alveolar
       hypoventilation 🔖**

   *Uncommon condition of unknown cause leading to
   inadequate ventilation in lungs, even though lungs and
   airways are normal*

   Obesity hypoventilation syndrome (OHS)
   Pickwickian syndrome

   E66.3   Overweight
   E66.8   Other obesity
   E66.9   Obesity, unspecified
   Obesity NOS
   Coding Clinic: 2021, Q2, P10-11

- **E67   Other hyperalimentation**
   Ingestion of more than optimal amount of nutrients

   Excludes1   hyperalimentation NOS (R63.2)
   sequelae of hyperalimentation (E68)

   E67.0   Hypervitaminosis A
   E67.1   Hypercarotenemia
   E67.2   Megavitamin-B6 syndrome
   E67.3   Hypervitaminosis D
   E67.8   Other specified hyperalimentation

- **E68   Sequelae of hyperalimentation**
   Code first condition resulting from (sequela) of hyperalimentation

METABOLIC DISORDERS (E70-E88)

   Excludes1   androgen insensitivity syndrome (E34.5-)
   congenital adrenal hyperplasia (E25.0)
   hemolytic anemias attributable to enzyme
       disorders (D55.-)
   Marfan's syndrome (Q87.4)
   5-alpha-reductase deficiency (E29.1)

   Excludes2   Ehlers-Danlos syndromes (Q79.6-)

- **E70   Disorders of aromatic amino-acid metabolism**

   E70.0   Classical phenylketonuria 🔖
   *Inherited disorder that increases to harmful levels amino acid
   phenylalanine*

   E70.1   Other hyperphenylalaninemias 🔖

- **E70.2   Disorders of tyrosine metabolism**

   Excludes1   transitory tyrosinemia of newborn (P74.5)

   E70.20   Disorder of tyrosine metabolism, unspecified 🔖
   *Tyrosine: Nonessential amino acid occurring in
   most proteins*

   E70.21   Tyrosinemia 🔖
   Congenital amino acid metabolism
   Hypertyrosinemia

   E70.29   Other disorders of tyrosine metabolism 🔖
   Alkaptonuria
   Ochronosis

- **E70.3   Albinism**
   *Congenital condition of reduced or absent pigment in eyes,
   skin, and hair*

   E70.30   Albinism, unspecified 🔖

- **E70.31   Ocular albinism**

   E70.310   X-linked ocular albinism 🔖
   **E70.311   Autosomal recessive ocular
       albinism 🔖**
   E70.318   Other ocular albinism 🔖
   E70.319   Ocular albinism, unspecified 🔖

- **E70.32   Oculocutaneous albinism**
   Partial or total lack of melanin pigment in eyes

   Excludes1   Chediak-Higashi syndrome
       (E70.330)
   Hermansky-Pudlak syndrome
       (E70.331)

   **E70.320   Tyrosinase negative oculocutaneous
       albinism 🔖**
   Albinism I
   Oculocutaneous albinism ty-neg

   **E70.321   Tyrosinase positive oculocutaneous
       albinism 🔖**
   Albinism II
   Oculocutaneous albinism ty-pos

   E70.328   Other oculocutaneous albinism 🔖
   Cross syndrome

   **E70.329   Oculocutaneous
       albinism, unspecified 🔖**

N Newborn Age: 0   **P** Pediatric Age: 0–17   **M** Maternity DX: 9–64   **A** Adult Age: 15–124   ♀ Females Only   ♂ Males Only

759

● E70.33   Albinism with hematologic abnormality
     E70.330   Chediak-Higashi syndrome 🅒
     E70.331   Hermansky-Pudlak syndrome 🅒
     E70.338   Other albinism with hematologic abnormality 🅒
     E70.339   Albinism with hematologic abnormality, unspecified 🅒
   E70.39   Other specified albinism 🅒
       Piebaldism
● E70.4   Disorders of histidine metabolism
   E70.40   Disorders of histidine metabolism, unspecified 🅒
   E70.41   Histidinemia 🅒
   E70.49   Other disorders of histidine metabolism 🅒
● E70.5   Disorders of tryptophan metabolism 🅒
● E70.8   Other disorders of aromatic amino-acid metabolism 🅒
   E70.81   Aromatic L-amino acid decarboxylase deficiency
       AADC deficiency
   E70.89   Other disorders of aromatic amino-acid metabolism
   E70.9   Disorder of aromatic amino-acid metabolism, unspecified 🅒

● E71   Disorders of branched-chain amino-acid metabolism and fatty-acid metabolism
   E71.0   Maple-syrup-urine disease 🅒
       Due to defect in amino acid catabolism, causing severe ketoacidosis with smell of maple syrup in urine and on body
● E71.1   Other disorders of branched-chain amino-acid metabolism
   ● E71.11   Branched-chain organic acidurias
     E71.110   Isovaleric acidemia 🅒
     E71.111   3-methylglutaconic aciduria 🅒
     E71.118   Other branched-chain organic acidurias
   ● E71.12   Disorders of propionate metabolism
     E71.120   Methylmalonic acidemia 🅒
     E71.121   Propionic acidemia 🅒
     E71.128   Other disorders of propionate metabolism 🅒
   E71.19   Other disorders of branched-chain amino-acid metabolism 🅒
       Hyperleucine-isoleucinemia
       Hypervalinemia
   E71.2   Disorder of branched-chain amino-acid metabolism, unspecified 🅒
● E71.3   Disorders of fatty-acid metabolism
   Excludes1   peroxisomal disorders (E71.5)
       Refsum's disease (G60.1)
       Schilder's disease (G37.0)
   Excludes2   carnitine deficiency due to inborn error of metabolism (E71.42)
   E71.30   Disorder of fatty-acid metabolism, unspecified
   ● E71.31   Disorders of fatty-acid oxidation
     E71.310   Long chain/very long chain acyl CoA dehydrogenase deficiency 🅒
       LCAD
       VLCAD
     E71.311   Medium chain acyl CoA dehydrogenase deficiency 🅒
       MCAD

     E71.312   Short chain acyl CoA dehydrogenase deficiency 🅒
       SCAD
     E71.313   Glutaric aciduria type II 🅒
       Glutaric aciduria type II A
       Glutaric aciduria type II B
       Glutaric aciduria type II C
       Excludes1   glutaric aciduria (type 1) NOS (E72.3)
     E71.314   Muscle carnitine palmitoyltransferase deficiency 🅒
     E71.318   Other disorders of fatty-acid oxidation 🅒
   E71.32   Disorders of ketone metabolism 🅒
   E71.39   Other disorders of fatty-acid metabolism 🅒
● E71.4   Disorders of carnitine metabolism
   Excludes1   muscle carnitine palmitoyltransferase deficiency (E71.314)
   E71.40   Disorder of carnitine metabolism, unspecified 🅒
   E71.41   Primary carnitine deficiency 🅒
   E71.42   Carnitine deficiency due to inborn errors of metabolism 🅒
       Code also associated inborn error or metabolism
   E71.43   Iatrogenic carnitine deficiency 🅒
       Iatrogenic: Outcomes from activity of physicians
       Carnitine deficiency due to hemodialysis
       Carnitine deficiency due to Valproic acid therapy
   ● E71.44   Other secondary carnitine deficiency
     E71.440   Ruvalcaba-Myhre-Smith syndrome 🅒
     E71.448   Other secondary carnitine deficiency 🅒
● E71.5   Peroxisomal disorders
   Class of conditions which lead to disorders of lipid metabolism
   Excludes1   Schilder's disease (G37.0)
   E71.50   Peroxisomal disorder, unspecified 🅒
   ● E71.51   Disorders of peroxisome biogenesis
       Group 1 peroxisomal disorders
     Excludes1   Refsum's disease (G60.1)
     E71.510   Zellweger syndrome 🅒
     E71.511   Neonatal adrenoleukodystrophy 🅒
       Excludes1   X-linked adrenoleuko-dystrophy (E71.42-)
     E71.518   Other disorders of peroxisome biogenesis 🅒
   ● E71.52   X-linked adrenoleukodystrophy
     E71.520   Childhood cerebral X-linked adrenoleukodystrophy 🅒
     E71.521   Adolescent X-linked adrenoleukodystrophy 🅒
     E71.522   Adrenomyeloneuropathy 🅒
     E71.528   Other X-linked adrenoleukodystrophy 🅒
       Addison only phenotype adrenoleukodystrophy
       Addison-Schilder adrenoleukodystrophy
     E71.529   X-linked adrenoleukodystrophy, unspecified type 🅒

E71.53   **Other group 2 peroxisomal disorders** 🔎

● E71.54   **Other peroxisomal disorders**

    E71.540   **Rhizomelic chondrodysplasia punctata** 🔎
      Rare, severe, inherited disorder with limb shortening, bone and cartilage abnormalities, abnormal facial appearance, severe mental retardation, psychomotor retardation, and cataracts

      Excludes 1   chondrodysplasia punctata NOS (Q77.3)

    E71.541   **Zellweger-like syndrome** 🔎

    E71.542   **Other group 3 peroxisomal disorders** 🔎

    E71.548   **Other peroxisomal disorders** 🔎

● **E72**   **Other disorders of amino-acid metabolism**

    Excludes 1   disorders of:
      aromatic amino-acid metabolism (E70.-)
      branched-chain amino-acid metabolism (E71.0-E71.2)
      fatty-acid metabolism (E71.3)
      purine and pyrimidine metabolism (E79.-)
      gout (M1A.-, M10.-)

● **E72.0**   **Disorders of amino-acid transport**

    Excludes 1   disorders of tryptophan metabolism (E70.5)

    E72.00   **Disorders of amino-acid transport, unspecified** 🔎

    E72.01   **Cystinuria** 🔎
      Hereditary aminoaciduria due to impairment of renal transport with predominant symptom of urinary cystine calculi

    E72.02   **Hartnup's disease** 🔎
      Inborn error of metabolism

    E72.03   **Lowe's syndrome** 🔎
      X-linked disorder with rickets, hydrophthalmia, congenital glaucoma, cataracts, mental retardation, and renal tubule dysfunction

      Use additional code for associated glaucoma (H42)

    E72.04   **Cystinosis** 🔎
      Genetic disease with excessive deposits of amino acid cystine in cells
      Fanconi (-de Toni) (-Debré) syndrome with cystinosis

      Excludes 1   Fanconi (-de Toni) (-Debré) syndrome without cystinosis (E72.09)

    E72.09   **Other disorders of amino-acid transport** 🔎
      Fanconi (-de Toni) (-Debré) syndrome, unspecified

● **E72.1**   **Disorders of sulfur-bearing amino-acid metabolism**

    Excludes 1   cystinosis (E72.04)
      cystinuria (E72.01)
      transcobalamin II deficiency (D51.2)

    E72.10   **Disorders of sulfur-bearing amino-acid metabolism, unspecified** 🔎

    E72.11   **Homocystinuria** 🔎
      Cystathionine synthase deficiency

    E72.12   **Methylenetetrahydrofolate reductase deficiency** 🔎

    E72.19   **Other disorders of sulfur-bearing amino-acid metabolism** 🔎
      Cystathioninuria
      Methioninemia
      Sulfite oxidase deficiency

● E72.2   **Disorders of urea cycle metabolism**

    Excludes 1   disorders of ornithine metabolism (E72.4)

    E72.20   **Disorder of urea cycle metabolism, unspecified** 🔎
      Hyperammonemia
      Elevated levels of ammonia

      Excludes 1   hyperammonemia-hyperornithinemia-homocitrullinemia syndrome E72.4
       transient hyperammonemia of newborn (P74.6)

    E72.21   **Argininemia** 🔎
      Disorder in which deficiency of enzyme arginase causes build-up of arginine and ammonia in blood

    E72.22   **Arginosuccinic aciduria** 🔎
      Gene disorder of urea cycle resulting accumulation of ammonia

    E72.23   **Citrullinemia** 🔎
      Urea cycle disorder that causes ammonia and other toxic substances to accumulate in blood

    E72.29   **Other disorders of urea cycle metabolism** 🔎

E72.3   **Disorders of lysine and hydroxylysine metabolism** 🔎
    Glutaric aciduria NOS
    Glutaric aciduria (type I)
    Hydroxylysinemia
    Hyperlysinemia

    Excludes 1   glutaric aciduria type II (E71.313)
      Refsum's disease (G60.1)
      Zellweger syndrome (E71.510)

E72.4   **Disorders of ornithine metabolism** 🔎
    Hyperammonemia-Hyperornithinemia-Homocitrullinemia syndrome
    Ornithinemia (types I, II)
    Ornithine transcarbamylase deficiency

    Excludes 1   hereditary choroidal dystrophy (H31.2-)

● E72.5   **Disorders of glycine metabolism**

    E72.50   **Disorder of glycine metabolism, unspecified** 🔎

    E72.51   **Non-ketotic hyperglycinemia** 🔎

    E72.52   **Trimethylaminuria** 🔎

    E72.53   **Primary hyperoxaluria** 🔎
      Oxalosis
      Oxaluria

    E72.59   **Other disorders of glycine metabolism** 🔎
      D-glycericacidemia
      Hyperhydroxyprolinemia
      Hyperprolinemia (types I, II)
      Sarcosinemia

● E72.8   **Other specified disorders of amino-acid metabolism** 🔎

    E72.81   **Disorders of gamma aminobutyric acid metabolism** 🔎
      4-hydroxybutyric aciduria
      Disorders of GABA metabolism
      GABA metabolic defect
      GABA transaminase deficiency
      GABA-T deficiency
      Gamma-hydroxybutyric aciduria
      SSADHD
      Succinic semialdehyde dehydrogenase deficiency

    E72.89   **Other specified disorders of amino-acid metabolism** 🔎
      Disorders of beta-amino-acid metabolism
      Disorders of gamma-glutamyl cycle

E72.9   **Disorder of amino-acid metabolism, unspecified** 🔎

● **E73** **Lactose intolerance**
Intolerance for lactose, due to inherited deficiency of lactase activity in intestinal mucosa

     E73.0   **Congenital lactase deficiency**

     E73.1   **Secondary lactase deficiency**

     E73.8   **Other lactose intolerance**

     E73.9   **Lactose intolerance, unspecified**

● **E74** **Other disorders of carbohydrate metabolism**
     Excludes1   diabetes mellitus (E08-E13)
                  hypoglycemia NOS (E16.2)
                  increased secretion of glucagon (E16.3)
                  mucopolysaccharidosis (E76.0-E76.3)

  ● **E74.0** **Glycogen storage disease**

     E74.00   **Glycogen storage disease, unspecified** 🐾

     E74.01   **von Gierke's disease** 🐾
                 Type I glycogen storage disease

     E74.02   **Pompe disease** 🐾
                 Cardiac glycogenosis
                 Type II glycogen storage disease

     E74.03   **Cori disease** 🐾
                 Forbes' disease
                 Type III glycogen storage disease

     E74.04   **McArdle disease** 🐾
                 Type V glycogen storage disease

     E74.09   **Other glycogen storage disease** 🐾
                 Andersen disease
                 Hers disease
                 Tauri disease
                 Glycogen storage disease, types 0, IV, VI-XI
                 Liver phosphorylase deficiency
                 Muscle phosphofructokinase deficiency

  ● **E74.1** **Disorders of fructose metabolism**
       Excludes1   muscle phosphofructokinase deficiency (E74.09)

     E74.10   **Disorder of fructose metabolism, unspecified**

     E74.11   **Essential fructosuria**
                 Fructokinase deficiency

     E74.12   **Hereditary fructose intolerance**
                 Fructosemia

     E74.19   **Other disorders of fructose metabolism**
                 Fructose-1, 6-diphosphatase deficiency

  ● **E74.2** **Disorders of galactose metabolism**

     E74.20   **Disorders of galactose metabolism, unspecified** 🐾

     E74.21   **Galactosemia** 🐾
                 Genetic disorders resulting from defective simple sugar (galactose) metabolism

     E74.29   **Other disorders of galactose metabolism** 🐾
                 Galactokinase deficiency

  ● **E74.3** **Other disorders of intestinal carbohydrate absorption**
       Excludes2   lactose intolerance (E73.-)

     E74.31   **Sucrase-isomaltase deficiency**
                 Deficiency in metabolism in intestinal mucosa results in malabsorption of sucrose and starch

     E74.39   **Other disorders of intestinal carbohydrate absorption**
                 Disorder of intestinal carbohydrate absorption NOS
                 Glucose-galactose malabsorption
                 Sucrase deficiency

     E74.4   **Disorders of pyruvate metabolism and gluconeogenesis** 🐾
                 Deficiency of phosphoenolpyruvate carboxykinase
                 Deficiency of pyruvate carboxylase
                 Deficiency of pyruvate dehydrogenase
       Excludes1   disorders of pyruvate metabolism and gluconeogenesis with anemia (D55.-)
                 Leigh's syndrome (G31.82)

     E74.8   **Other specified disorders of carbohydrate metabolism** 🐾

      ● **E74.81** **Disorders of glucose transport, not elsewhere classified**

          E74.810   **Glucose transporter protein type 1 deficiency**
                    De Vivo syndrome
                    Glucose transport defect, blood-brain barrier
                    GLUT1 deficiency
                    GLUT1 deficiency syndrome 1, infantile onset
                    GLUT1 deficiency syndrome 2, childhood onset

          E74.818   **Other disorders of glucose transport**
                    (Familial) renal glycosuria

          E74.819   **Disorders of glucose transport, unspecified**

       E74.89   **Other specified disorders of carbohydrate metabolism**
                 Essential pentosuria

     E74.9   **Disorder of carbohydrate metabolism, unspecified** 🐾

● **E75** **Disorders of sphingolipid metabolism and other lipid storage disorders**
     Excludes1   mucolipidosis, types I-III (E77.0-E77.1)
                  Refsum's disease (G60.1)

  ● **E75.0** **GM2 gangliosidosis**
       Rare metabolic disorder that causes destruction of nerve cells of brain and spinal cord

     E75.00   **GM2 gangliosidosis, unspecified**

     E75.01   **Sandhoff disease**

     E75.02   **Tay-Sachs disease**

     E75.09   **Other GM2 gangliosidosis**
                 Adult GM2 gangliosidosis
                 Juvenile GM2 gangliosidosis

  ● **E75.1** **Other and unspecified gangliosidosis**

     E75.10   **Unspecified gangliosidosis**
                 Gangliosidosis NOS

     E75.11   **Mucolipidosis IV**
                 Disorder with symptoms of psychomotor retardation and severe visual impairment

     E75.19   **Other gangliosidosis**
                 GM1 gangliosidosis
                 GM3 gangliosidosis

  ● **E75.2** **Other sphingolipidosis**
       Lysosomal (a particle in a cytoplasm cell that contains digestive enzymes) storage diseases with symptoms of abnormal storage of amino acids
       Excludes1   adrenoleukodystrophy [Addison-Schilder] (E71.528)

     E75.21   **Fabry (-Anderson) disease** 🐾

     E75.22   **Gaucher disease** 🐾

     E75.23   **Krabbe disease**

  ● **E75.24** **Niemann-Pick disease**
                 Acid sphingomyelinase deficiency (ASMD)

       E75.240   **Niemann-Pick disease type A** 🐾
                    Acid sphingomyelinase deficiency type A (ASMD type A)
                    Infantile neurovisceral acid sphingomyelinase deficiency

       E75.241   **Niemann-Pick disease type B** 🐾
                    Acid sphingomyelinase deficiency type B (ASMD type B)
                    Chronic visceral acid sphingomyelinase deficiency

Item 4-8 Leukodystrophy is characterized by degeneration and/or failure of the myelin formation of the central nervous system and sometimes of the peripheral nervous system. The disease is inherited and progressive.

CHAPTER 4 (E00-E89)

▶ New   ⇒ Revised   ~~deleted~~ Deleted   Excludes 1   Excludes 2   Includes   Use additional   Code first   Code also   Key words

OGCR Official Guidelines   X Assign placeholder X   ● Use Additional Character(s)   ▸ Manifestation Code   🐾 Hierarchical Condition Category   **Coding Clinic**

         E75.242   **Niemann-Pick disease type C** 🔒

         E75.243   **Niemann-Pick disease type D** 🔒

         E75.244   **Niemann-Pick disease type A/B**
                   Acid sphingomyelinase deficiency
                       type A/B (ASMD type A/B)
                   Chronic neurovisceral acid
                       sphingomyelinase deficiency

         E75.248   **Other Niemann-Pick disease** 🔒

         E75.249   **Niemann-Pick disease, unspecified** 🔒
                   Acid sphingomyelinase deficiency
                       (ASMD) NOS

     E75.25   **Metachromatic leukodystrophy**

     E75.26   **Sulfatase deficiency**
               Multiple sulfatase deficiency (MSD)

     E75.29   **Other sphingolipidosis**
               Farber's syndrome
               Sulfatide lipidosis

   E75.3   **Sphingolipidosis, unspecified** 🔒

   E75.4   **Neuronal ceroid lipofuscinosis**
            Batten disease
            Bielschowsky-Jansky disease
            Kufs disease
            Spielmeyer-Vogt disease

   E75.5   **Other lipid storage disorders**
            Cerebrotendinous cholesterosis [van Bogaert-Scherer-
               Epstein]
            Wolman's disease

   E75.6   **Lipid storage disorder, unspecified**

● **E76**   **Disorders of glycosaminoglycan metabolism**

●   **E76.0**   **Mucopolysaccharidosis, type I**
           Inborn metabolic disorder of enzymes that break down
              carbohydrates

     E76.01   **Hurler's syndrome** 🔒

     E76.02   **Hurler-Scheie syndrome** 🔒

     E76.03   **Scheie's syndrome** 🔒

   E76.1   **Mucopolysaccharidosis, type II** 🔒
           Inborn metabolic disorder of enzymes that break down
              carbohydrates occurs in 2-4 year old males
           Hunter's syndrome

●   **E76.2**   **Other mucopolysaccharidoses**

   ●   **E76.21**   **Morquio mucopolysaccharidoses**

         E76.210   **Morquio A mucopolysaccharidoses** 🔒
                   Classic Morquio syndrome
                   Morquio syndrome A
                   Mucopolysaccharidosis, type IVA

         E76.211   **Morquio B mucopolysaccharidoses** 🔒
                   Morquio-like
                       mucopolysaccharidoses
                   Morquio-like syndrome
                   Morquio syndrome B
                   Mucopolysaccharidosis, type IVB

         E76.219   **Morquio mucopolysaccharidoses, unspecified** 🔒
                   Morquio syndrome
                   Mucopolysaccharidosis, type IV

     E76.22   **Sanfilippo mucopolysaccharidoses** 🔒
               Mucopolysaccharidosis, type III (A) (B) (C) (D)
               Sanfilippo A syndrome
               Sanfilippo B syndrome
               Sanfilippo C syndrome
               Sanfilippo D syndrome

     E76.29   **Other mucopolysaccharidoses** 🔒
               beta-Glucuronidase deficiency
               Maroteaux-Lamy (mild) (severe) syndrome
               Mucopolysaccharidosis, types VI, VII

   E76.3   **Mucopolysaccharidosis, unspecified** 🔒

   E76.8   **Other disorders of glucosaminoglycan metabolism** 🔒

   E76.9   **Glucosaminoglycan metabolism disorder, unspecified** 🔒

● **E77**   **Disorders of glycoprotein metabolism**

   E77.0   **Defects in post-translational modification of lysosomal enzymes** 🔒
           Mucolipidosis II [I-cell disease]
           Mucolipidosis III [pseudo-Hurler polydystrophy]

   E77.1   **Defects in glycoprotein degradation** 🔒
           Aspartylglucosaminuria
           Fucosidosis
           Mannosidosis
           Sialidosis [mucolipidosis I]

   E77.8   **Other disorders of glycoprotein metabolism** 🔒

   E77.9   **Disorder of glycoprotein metabolism, unspecified** 🔒

● **E78**   **Disorders of lipoprotein metabolism and other lipidemias**
       Excludes1   sphingolipidosis (E75.0-E75.3)

●   **E78.0**   **Pure hypercholesterolemia**
       Coding Clinic: 2016, Q4, P13

     E78.00   **Pure hypercholesterolemia, unspecified**
               Fredrickson's hyperlipoproteinemia, type IIa
               Hyperbetalipoproteinemia
               Low-density-lipoprotein-type [LDL]
                   hyperlipoproteinemia
               (Pure) hypercholesterolemia NOS
               Coding Clinic: 2022, Q2, P6; 2016, Q4, P13

     E78.01   **Familial hypercholesterolemia**
               Coding Clinic: 2016, Q4, P13

   E78.1   **Pure hyperglyceridemia**
           Elevated fasting triglycerides
           Endogenous hyperglyceridemia
           Fredrickson's hyperlipoproteinemia, type IV
           Hyperlipidemia, group B
           Hyperprebetalipoproteinemia
           Very-low-density-lipoprotein-type [VLDL]
              hyperlipoproteinemia

   E78.2   **Mixed hyperlipidemia**
           Broad- or floating-betalipoproteinemia
           Combined hyperlipidemia NOS
           Elevated cholesterol with elevated triglycerides NEC
           Fredrickson's hyperlipoproteinemia, type IIb or III
           Hyperbetalipoproteinemia with prebetalipoproteinemia
           Hypercholesteremia with endogenous hyperglyceridemia
           Hyperlipidemia, group C
           Tubo-eruptive xanthoma
           Xanthoma tuberosum

       Excludes1   cerebrotendinous cholesterosis [van
                   Bogaert-Scherer-Epstein] (E75.5)
                   familial combined hyperlipidemia (E78.49)
       Coding Clinic: 2022, Q2, P6-7

   E78.3   **Hyperchylomicronemia**
           Chylomicron retention disease
           Fredrickson's hyperlipoproteinemia, type I or V
           Hyperlipidemia, group D
           Mixed hyperglyceridemia

●   **E78.4**   **Other hyperlipidemia**

     E78.41   **Elevated Lipoprotein(a)**
               Elevated Lp(a)

     E78.49   **Other hyperlipidemia**
               Familial combined hyperlipidemia

   E78.5   **Hyperlipidemia, unspecified**
       Coding Clinic: 2022, Q2, P6

   E78.6   **Lipoprotein deficiency**
           Abetalipoproteinemia
           Depressed HDL cholesterol
           High-density lipoprotein deficiency
           Hypoalphalipoproteinemia
           Hypobetalipoproteinemia (familial)
           Lecithin cholesterol acyltransferase deficiency
           Tangier disease

CHAPTER 4 (E00-E89)

CHAPTER 4 (E00-E89)

● **E78.7** Disorders of **bile acid** and **cholesterol metabolism**

    Excludes1   Niemann-Pick disease type C (E75.242)

    E78.70 Disorder of bile acid and cholesterol metabolism, **unspecified**

    E78.71 **Barth syndrome**

    E78.72 **Smith-Lemli-Opitz syndrome**

    E78.79 **Other disorders of bile acid and cholesterol metabolism**

● **E78.8** Other disorders of lipoprotein metabolism

    E78.81 **Lipoid dermatoarthritis**

    E78.89 **Other lipoprotein metabolism disorders**

    E78.9 Disorder of lipoprotein metabolism, **unspecified**

● **E79** Disorders of **purine and pyrimidine metabolism**

    Purines, along with pyrimidines, signal RNA and DNA production

    Excludes1   Ataxia-telangiectasia (Q87.19)
           Bloom's syndrome (Q82.8)
           Cockayne's syndrome (Q87.19)
           calculus of kidney (N20.0)
           combined immunodeficiency disorders (D81.-)
           Fanconi's anemia (D61.09)
           gout (M1A.-, M10.-)
           orotaciduric anemia (D53.0)
           progeria (E34.8)
           Werner's syndrome (E34.8)
           xeroderma pigmentosum (Q82.1)

    E79.0 **Hyperuricemia without signs of inflammatory arthritis and tophaceous disease**
           Asymptomatic hyperuricemia

    E79.1 **Lesch-Nyhan syndrome** 🦠
           HGPRT deficiency

    E79.2 **Myoadenylate deaminase deficiency** 🦠

    E79.8 **Other disorders of purine and pyrimidine metabolism** 🦠
           Hereditary xanthinuria

    E79.9 Disorder of purine and pyrimidine metabolism, **unspecified** 🦠

● **E80** Disorders of **porphyrin and bilirubin metabolism**

    Group of chemical compounds in RBCs that combine with iron to form heme

    Includes   defects of catalase and peroxidase

    E80.0 **Hereditary erythropoietic porphyria** 🦠
           Congenital erythropoietic porphyria
           Erythropoietic protoporphyria

    E80.1 **Porphyria cutanea tarda** 🦠

●   **E80.2** **Other and unspecified porphyria**

        E80.20 **Unspecified porphyria** 🦠
                Porphyria NOS

        E80.21 **Acute intermittent (hepatic) porphyria** 🦠

        E80.29 **Other porphyria** 🦠
                Hereditary coproporphyria

    E80.3 **Defects of catalase and peroxidase** 🦠
           Acatalasia [Takahara]

    E80.4 **Gilbert syndrome**

    E80.5 **Crigler-Najjar syndrome**

    E80.6 **Other disorders of bilirubin metabolism**
           Dubin-Johnson syndrome
           Rotor's syndrome

    E80.7 Disorder of bilirubin metabolism, **unspecified**

● **E83** Disorders of **mineral metabolism**

    Excludes1   dietary mineral deficiency (E58-E61)
           parathyroid disorders (E20-E21)
           vitamin D deficiency (E55.-)

●   **E83.0** Disorders of **copper metabolism**

        E83.00 **Disorder of copper metabolism, unspecified**

        E83.01 **Wilson's disease**
                Code also associated Kayser Fleischer ring (H18.04-)

        E83.09 **Other disorders of copper metabolism**
                Menkes' (kinky hair) (steely hair) disease

● **E83.1** Disorders of **iron metabolism**

    Excludes1   iron deficiency anemia (D50.-)
           sideroblastic anemia (D64.0-D64.3)

    E83.10 **Disorder of iron metabolism, unspecified**

●   **E83.11** **Hemochromatosis**

        Excludes1   GALD (P78.84)
                Gestational alloimmune liver disease (P78.84)
                Neonatal hemochromatosis (P78.84)

        E83.110 **Hereditary hemochromatosis** 🦠
                Bronzed diabetes
                Pigmentary cirrhosis (of liver)
                Primary (hereditary) hemochromatosis

        E83.111 **Hemochromatosis due to repeated red blood cell transfusions**
                Iron overload due to repeated red blood cell transfusions
                Transfusion (red blood cell) associated hemochromatosis

        E83.118 **Other hemochromatosis**

        E83.119 **Hemochromatosis, unspecified**

    E83.19 **Other disorders of iron metabolism**
           Use additional code, if applicable, for idiopathic pulmonary hemosiderosis (J84.03)

    E83.2 Disorders of **zinc metabolism**
        Acrodermatitis enteropathica

● **E83.3** Disorders of **phosphorus metabolism** and **phosphatases**

    Excludes1   adult osteomalacia (M83.-)
           osteoporosis (M80.-)

    E83.30 **Disorder of phosphorus metabolism, unspecified**

    E83.31 **Familial hypophosphatemia**
           Vitamin D-resistant osteomalacia
           Vitamin D-resistant rickets

        Excludes1   vitamin D-deficiency rickets (E55.0)

    E83.32 **Hereditary vitamin D-dependent rickets (type 1) (type 2)**
           25-hydroxyvitamin D 1-alpha-hydroxylase deficiency
           Pseudovitamin D deficiency
           Vitamin D receptor defect

    E83.39 **Other disorders of phosphorus metabolism**
           Acid phosphatase deficiency
           Hypophosphatasia

● **E83.4** Disorders of **magnesium metabolism**

    E83.40 **Disorders of magnesium metabolism, unspecified**

    E83.41 **Hypermagnesemia**
           Coding Clinic: 2016, Q4, P55

    E83.42 **Hypomagnesemia**

    E83.49 **Other disorders of magnesium metabolism**

● **E83.5** Disorders of **calcium metabolism**

    Excludes1   chondrocalcinosis (M11.1-M11.2)
           hungry bone syndrome (E83.81)
           hyperparathyroidism (E21.0-E21.3)

    E83.50 **Unspecified disorder of calcium metabolism**

    E83.51 **Hypocalcemia**

    E83.52 **Hypercalcemia**
           Familial hypocalciuric hypercalcemia

    E83.59 **Other disorders of calcium metabolism**
           Idiopathic hypercalciuria

● **E83.8** Other disorders of **mineral metabolism**

    E83.81 **Hungry bone syndrome**

    E83.89 **Other disorders of mineral metabolism**

    E83.9 Disorder of mineral metabolism, **unspecified**

▶ New   ➡ Revised   ~~deleted~~ Deleted   Excludes 1   Excludes 2   Includes   Use additional   Code first   Code also   Key words

OGCR Official Guidelines   **X** Assign placeholder X   ● Use Additional Character(s)   ▶ Manifestation Code   🦠 Hierarchical Condition Category   **Coding Clinic**

● **E84**   **Cystic fibrosis**

      Includes   mucoviscidosis

      Code also exocrine pancreatic insufficiency (K86.81)

   E84.0   **Cystic fibrosis with pulmonary manifestations** 🔗

        Use additional code to identify any infectious organism present, such as:
          Pseudomonas (B96.5)
          Coding Clinic: 2021, Q1, P24

●   **E84.1**   **Cystic fibrosis with intestinal manifestations**

      E84.11   **Meconium ileus in cystic fibrosis** 🔗   **N**

         Excludes1   meconium ileus not due to cystic fibrosis (P76.0)

      E84.19   **Cystic fibrosis with other intestinal manifestations** 🔗
         Distal intestinal obstruction syndrome

   E84.8   **Cystic fibrosis with other manifestations** 🔗

   E84.9   **Cystic fibrosis, unspecified** 🔗

● **E85**   **Amyloidosis**

      A disorder resulting from the abnormal deposition of a particular protein (amyloid) into tissues of the body

      Excludes2   Alzheimer's disease (G30.0-)

   E85.0   **Non-neuropathic heredofamilial amyloidosis** 🔗
        Hereditary amyloid nephropathy

        Code also associated disorders, such as:
         autoinflammatory syndromes (M04.-)

        Excludes2   Transthyretin-related (ATTR) familial amyloid cardiomyopathy (E85.4)

   E85.1   **Neuropathic heredofamilial amyloidosis** 🔗
        Amyloid polyneuropathy (Portuguese)
        Transthyretin-related (ATTR) familial amyloid polyneuropathy
        Coding Clinic: 2012, Q4, P100

   E85.2   **Heredofamilial amyloidosis, unspecified** 🔗

   E85.3   **Secondary systemic amyloidosis** 🔗
        Hemodialysis-associated amyloidosis

   E85.4   **Organ-limited amyloidosis** 🔗
        Localized amyloidosis
        Transthyretin-related (ATTR) familial amyloid cardiomyopathy

●   **E85.8**   **Other amyloidosis**

      E85.81   **Light chain (AL) amyloidosis** 🔗

      E85.82   **Wild-type transthyretin-related (ATTR) amyloidosis** 🔗
         Senile systemic amyloidosis (SSA)

      E85.89   **Other amyloidosis** 🔗

   E85.9   **Amyloidosis, unspecified** 🔗

● **E86**   **Volume depletion**

      Excludes1   dehydration of newborn (P74.1)
          postprocedural hypovolemic shock (T81.19)
          traumatic hypovolemic shock (T79.4)

      Excludes2   hypovolemic shock NOS (R57.1)

      Use additional code(s) for any associated disorders of electrolyte and acid-base balance (E87.-)
      Coding Clinic: 2019, Q2, P7

   E86.0   **Dehydration**
        Excessive loss of body water
        Coding Clinic: 2019, Q2, P7-8

   E86.1   **Hypovolemia**
        Diminished volume of circulating blood
        Depletion of volume of plasma

   E86.9   **Volume depletion, unspecified**
        Coding Clinic: 2019, Q2, P7-8

● **E87**   **Other disorders of fluid, electrolyte and acid-base balance**

      Excludes1   diabetes insipidus (E23.2)
          electrolyte imbalance associated with hyperemesis gravidarum (O21.1)
          electrolyte imbalance following ectopic or molar pregnancy (O08.5)
          familial periodic paralysis (G72.3)

   E87.0   **Hyperosmolality and hypernatremia**
        Sodium [Na] excess
        Sodium [Na] overload
        Coding Clinic: 2022, Q1, P29; 2018, Q2, P6

   E87.1   **Hypo-osmolality and hyponatremia**
        Sodium [Na] deficiency

        Excludes1   syndrome of inappropriate secretion of antidiuretic hormone (E22.2)

        Coding Clinic: 2018, Q2, P6

●   **E87.2**   **Acidosis**

        ~~Acidosis NOS~~
        ~~Lactic acidosis~~
        ~~Metabolic acidosis~~
        ~~Respiratory acidosis~~

        Excludes1   diabetic acidosis - see categories E08-E10, E11, E13 with ketoacidosis

▶ **E87.20**   **Acidosis, unspecified**
      ▶ Lactic acidosis NOS
      ▶ Metabolic acidosis NOS

      ▶ Code also, if applicable, respiratory failure with hypercapnia (J96. with 5th character 2)

▶ **E87.21**   **Acute metabolic acidosis**
      ▶ Acute lactic acidosis

▶ **E87.22**   **Chronic metabolic acidosis**
      ▶ Chronic lactic acidosis

      ▶ *Code first* underlying etiology, if applicable

▶ **E87.29**   **Other acidosis**
      ▶ Respiratory acidosis NOS

      ▶ **Excludes2**   acute respiratory acidosis (J96.02)
        ▶ chronic respiratory acidosis (J96.12)

   E87.3   **Alkalosis**
        Alkalosis NOS
        Metabolic alkalosis
        Respiratory alkalosis

   E87.4   **Mixed disorder of acid-base balance**

   E87.5   **Hyperkalemia**
        Potassium [K] excess
        Potassium [K] overload

   E87.6   **Hypokalemia**
        Potassium [K] deficiency

●   **E87.7**   **Fluid overload**

        Excludes1   edema NOS (R60.9)
          fluid retention (R60.9)

      E87.70   **Fluid overload, unspecified**

      E87.71   **Transfusion associated circulatory overload**
         Fluid overload due to transfusion (blood) (blood components) TACO

      E87.79   **Other fluid overload**

   E87.8   **Other disorders of electrolyte and fluid balance, not elsewhere classified**
        Electrolyte imbalance NOS
        Hyperchloremia
        Hypochloremia

Item 4–9 Circulating fluid volume is regulated by the amount of water and sodium ingested, excreted by the kidneys into the urine, and lost through the gastrointestinal tract, lungs, and skin. To maintain blood volume within a normal range, the kidneys regulate the amount of water and sodium lost into the urine. Too much (**fluid overload**) or too little fluid volume (**volume depletion**) will affect blood pressure. Severe cases of vomiting, diarrhea, bleeding, and burns (fluid loss through exposed burn surface area) can contribute to fluid loss. Internal body environment must maintain a precise balance (homeostasis) between too much fluid and too little fluid. This complex balancing mechanism is critical to good health.

CHAPTER 4 (E00-E89)

E88   Other and unspecified metabolic disorders
　　　Use additional codes for associated conditions
　　　　Excludes1　histiocytosis X (chronic) (C96.6)
　●　**E88.0   Disorders of plasma-protein metabolism, not elsewhere classified**
　　　　Excludes1　monoclonal gammopathy (of undetermined significance) (D47.2)
　　　　　　　　polyclonal hypergammaglobulinemia (D89.0)
　　　　　　　　Waldenström macroglobulinemia (C88.0)
　　　　Excludes2　disorder of lipoprotein metabolism (E78.-)

　　　　E88.01   Alpha-1-antitrypsin deficiency AAT deficiency 🐾
　　　　E88.02   Plasminogen deficiency
　　　　　　Dysplasminogenemia
　　　　　　Hypoplasminogenemia
　　　　　　Type 1 plasminogen deficiency
　　　　　　Type 2 plasminogen deficiency
　　　　　　Code also, if applicable, ligneous conjunctivitis (H10.51)
　　　　　　Use additional code for associated findings, such as:
　　　　　　　hydrocephalus (G91.4)
　　　　　　　otitis media (H67.-)
　　　　　　　respiratory disorder related to plasminogen deficiency (J99)
　　　　E88.09   Other disorders of plasma-protein metabolism, not elsewhere classified
　　　　　　Bisalbuminemia

　　E88.1   Lipodystrophy, not elsewhere classified
　　　　Defective fat metabolism resulting in absence of subcutaneous fat
　　　　Lipodystrophy NOS
　　　　Excludes1　Whipple's disease (K90.81)

　　E88.2   Lipomatosis, not elsewhere classified
　　　　Abnormal tumorlike accumulations of fat in tissue
　　　　Lipomatosis NOS
　　　　Lipomatosis (Check) dolorosa [Dercum]

　　E88.3   Tumor lysis syndrome
　　　　Tumor lysis syndrome (spontaneous)
　　　　Tumor lysis syndrome following antineoplastic drug chemotherapy
　　　　Use additional code for adverse effect, if applicable, to identify drug (T45.1X5)
　　　　Coding Clinic: 2019, Q2, P25

　●　**E88.4   Mitochondrial metabolism disorders**
　　　　Congenital disorder of metabolism
　　　　Excludes1　disorders of pyruvate metabolism (E74.4)
　　　　　　　　Kearns-Sayre syndrome (H49.81)
　　　　　　　　Leber's disease (H47.22)
　　　　　　　　Leigh's encephalopathy (G31.82)
　　　　　　　　Mitochondrial myopathy, NEC (G71.3)
　　　　　　　　Reye's syndrome (G93.7)
　　　　E88.40   Mitochondrial metabolism disorder, unspecified 🐾
　　　　E88.41   MELAS syndrome 🐾
　　　　　　Mitochondrial myopathy, encephalopathy, lactic acidosis and stroke-like episodes
　　　　E88.42   MERRF syndrome 🐾
　　　　　　Myoclonic epilepsy associated with ragged-red fibers
　　　　　　Code also progressive myoclonic epilepsy (G40.3-)
　　　　E88.49   Other mitochondrial metabolism disorders 🐾
　●　**E88.8   Other specified metabolic disorders**
　　　　E88.81   Metabolic syndrome
　　　　　　Dysmetabolic syndrome X
　　　　　　Use additional codes for associated manifestations, such as:
　　　　　　　obesity (E66.-)
　　　　E88.89   Other specified metabolic disorders 🐾
　　　　　　Launois-Bensaude adenolipomatosis
　　　　　　Excludes1　adult pulmonary Langerhans cell histiocytosis (J84.82)

　　E88.9   Metabolic disorder, unspecified

POSTPROCEDURAL ENDOCRINE AND METABOLIC COMPLICATIONS AND DISORDERS, NOT ELSEWHERE CLASSIFIED (E89)

　●　**E89   Postprocedural endocrine and metabolic complications and disorders, not elsewhere classified**
　　　　Excludes2　intraoperative complications of endocrine system organ or structure (E36.0-, E36.1-, E36.8)

　　E89.0   Postprocedural hypothyroidism
　　　　Postirradiation hypothyroidism
　　　　Postsurgical hypothyroidism

　　E89.1   Postprocedural hypoinsulinemia
　　　　Postpancreatectomy hyperglycemia
　　　　Postsurgical hypoinsulinemia
　　　　Use additional code, if applicable, to identify:
　　　　　acquired absence of pancreas (Z90.41-)
　　　　　diabetes mellitus (postpancreatectomy) (postprocedural) (E13.-)
　　　　　insulin use (Z79.4)
　　　　Excludes1　transient postprocedural hyperglycemia (R73.9)
　　　　　　　　transient postprocedural hypoglycemia (E16.2)

　　E89.2   Postprocedural hypoparathyroidism 🐾
　　　　Parathyroprival tetany

　　E89.3   Postprocedural hypopituitarism 🐾
　　　　Postirradiation hypopituitarism

　●　**E89.4   Postprocedural ovarian failure**
　　　　E89.40   Asymptomatic postprocedural ovarian failure ♀
　　　　　　Postprocedural ovarian failure NOS
　　　　E89.41   Symptomatic postprocedural ovarian failure ♀
　　　　　　Symptoms such as flushing, sleeplessness, headache, lack of concentration, associated with postprocedural menopause

　　E89.5   Postprocedural testicular hypofunction ♂

　　E89.6   Postprocedural adrenocortical (-medullary) hypofunction 🐾

　●　**E89.8   Other postprocedural endocrine and metabolic complications and disorders**
　　　　Coding Clinic: 2016, Q4, P9
　　　　●　**E89.81   Postprocedural hemorrhage of an endocrine system organ or structure following a procedure**
　　　　　　E89.810   Postprocedural hemorrhage of an endocrine system organ or structure following an endocrine system procedure
　　　　　　E89.811   Postprocedural hemorrhage of an endocrine system organ or structure following other procedure
　　　　●　**E89.82   Postprocedural hematoma and seroma of an endocrine system organ or structure**
　　　　　　E89.820   Postprocedural hematoma of an endocrine system organ or structure following an endocrine system procedure
　　　　　　E89.821   Postprocedural hematoma of an endocrine system organ or structure following other procedure
　　　　　　E89.822   Postprocedural seroma of an endocrine system organ or structure following an endocrine system procedure
　　　　　　E89.823   Postprocedural seroma of an endocrine system organ or structure following other procedure
　　　　E89.89   Other postprocedural endocrine and metabolic complications and disorders
　　　　　　Use additional code, if applicable, to further specify disorder

▶ New　⇒ Revised　~~deleted~~ Deleted　Excludes 1　Excludes 2　Includes　Use additional　Code first　Code also　Key words
OGCR Official Guidelines　X Assign placeholder X　● Use Additional Character(s)　▷ Manifestation Code　🐾 Hierarchical Condition Category　Coding Clinic

CHAPTER 5

MENTAL, BEHAVIORAL AND NEURODEVELOPMENTAL DISORDERS (F01-F99)

OGCR Chapter-Specific Coding Guidelines

5. Chapter 5: Mental, Behavioral and Neurodevelopmental disorders (F01 – F99)

a. Pain disorders related to psychological factors

Assign code F45.41, for pain that is exclusively related to psychological disorders. As indicated by the Excludes 1 note under category G89, a code from category G89 should not be assigned with code F45.41

Code F45.42, Pain disorders with related psychological factors, should be used with a code from category G89, Pain, not elsewhere classified, if there is documentation of a psychological component for a patient with acute or chronic pain.

See Section I.C.6. Pain

b. Mental and behavioral disorders due to psychoactive substance use

1) In Remission

Selection of codes for "in remission" for categories F10-F19, Mental and behavioral disorders due to psychoactive substance use (categories F10-F19 with -11, -.21) requires the provider's clinical judgment. The appropriate codes for "in remission" are assigned only on the basis of provider documentation (as defined in the Official Guidelines for Coding and Reporting), unless otherwise instructed by the classification.

Mild substance use disorders in early or sustained remission are classified to the appropriate codes for substance abuse in remission, and moderate or severe substance use disorders in early or sustained remission are classified to the appropriate codes for substance dependence in remission.

2) Psychoactive Substance Use, Abuse and Dependence

When the provider documentation refers to use, abuse and dependence of the same substance (e.g., alcohol, opioid, cannabis, etc.), only one code should be assigned to identify the pattern of use based on the following hierarchy:

- If both use and abuse are documented, assign only the code for abuse
- If both abuse and dependence are documented, assign only the code for dependence
- If use, abuse and dependence are all documented, assign only the code for dependence
- If both use and dependence are documented, assign only the code for dependence

3) Psychoactive Substance Use, Unspecified

As with all other unspecified diagnoses, the codes for unspecified psychoactive substance use disorders (F10.9-, F11.9-, F12.9-, F13.9-, F14.9-, F15.9-, F16.9-, F19.9-) should only be assigned based on provider documentation and when they meet the definition of a reportable diagnosis (see Section III, Reporting Additional Diagnoses). These codes are to be used only when the psychoactive substance use is associated with a physical, mental or behavioral disorder, and such a relationship is documented by the provider.

c. Factitious Disorder

Factitious disorder imposed on self or Munchausen's syndrome is a disorder in which a person falsely reports or causes his or her own physical or psychological signs or symptoms. For patients with documented factitious disorder on self or Munchausen's syndrome, assign the appropriate code from subcategory F68.1-, Factitious disorder imposed on self.

Munchausen's syndrome by proxy (MSBP) is a disorder in which a caregiver (perpetrator) falsely reports or causes an illness or injury in another person (victim) under his or her care, such as a child, an elderly adult, or a person who has a disability. The condition is also referred to as "factitious disorder imposed on another" or "factitious disorder by proxy." The perpetrator, not the victim, receives this diagnosis. Assign code F68.A, Factitious disorder imposed on another, to the perpetrator's record. For the victim of a patient suffering from MSBP, assign the appropriate code from categories T74, Adult and child abuse, neglect and other maltreatment, confirmed, or T76, Adult and child abuse, neglect and other maltreatment, suspected.

See Section I.C.19.f. Adult and child abuse, neglect and other maltreatment

CHAPTER 5

MENTAL, BEHAVIORAL AND NEURODEVELOPMENTAL DISORDERS (F01-F99)

Includes disorders of psychological development
Excludes2 symptoms, signs and abnormal clinical laboratory findings, not elsewhere classified (R00-R99)

This chapter contains the following blocks:

F01-F09	Mental disorders due to known physiological conditions
F10-F19	Mental and behavioral disorders due to psychoactive substance use
F20-F29	Schizophrenia, schizotypal, delusional, and other non-mood psychotic disorders
F30-F39	Mood [affective] disorders
F40-F48	Anxiety, dissociative, stress-related, somatoform and other nonpsychotic mental disorders
F50-F59	Behavioral syndromes associated with physiological disturbances and physical factors
F60-F69	Disorders of adult personality and behavior
F70-F79	Intellectual disabilities
F80-F89	Pervasive and specific developmental disorders
F90-F98	Behavioral and emotional disorders with onset usually occurring in childhood and adolescence
F99	Unspecified mental disorder

MENTAL DISORDERS DUE TO KNOWN PHYSIOLOGICAL CONDITIONS (F01-F09)

This block comprises a range of mental disorders grouped together on the basis of their having in common a demonstrable etiology in cerebral disease, brain injury, or other insult leading to cerebral dysfunction. The dysfunction may be primary, as in diseases, injuries, and insults that affect the brain directly and selectively; or secondary, as in systemic diseases and disorders that attack the brain only as one of the multiple organs or systems of the body that are involved.

● **F01**   **Vascular dementia**

Vascular dementia as a result of infarction of the brain due to vascular disease, including hypertensive cerebrovascular disease.

Includes   arteriosclerotic dementia

▶major neurocognitive disorder due to vascular disease
▶multi-infarct dementia

Code first the underlying physiological condition or sequelae of cerebrovascular disease.

➡ ● **F01.5**   **Vascular dementia, unspecified severity**

➡ **F01.50**   **Vascular dementia, unspecified severity, without behavioral disturbance, psychotic disturbance, mood disturbance, and anxiety**   A

➡Major neurocognitive disorder due to vascular disease NOS
▶Vascular dementia NOS
Coding Clinic: 2021, Q2, P4

➡ ● **F01.51**   **Vascular dementia, unspecified severity, with behavioral disturbance**   A

~~Major neurocognitive disorder due to vascular disease, with behavioral disturbance~~
~~Major neurocognitive disorder with aggressive behavior~~
~~Major neurocognitive disorder with combative behavior~~
~~Major neurocognitive disorder with violent behavior~~
~~Vascular dementia with aggressive behavior~~
~~Vascular dementia with combative behavior~~
~~Vascular dementia with violent behavior~~
~~Use additional code, if applicable, to identify wandering in vascular dementia (Z91.83)~~

CHAPTER 5 (F01-F99)

▶ **F01.511** **Vascular dementia, unspecified severity, with agitation**
  ▶ Major neurocognitive disorder due to vascular disease, unspecified severity, with aberrant motor behavior such as restlessness, rocking, pacing, or exit-seeking
  ▶ Major neurocognitive disorder due to vascular disease, unspecified severity, with verbal or physical behaviors such as profanity, shouting, threatening, anger, aggression, combativeness, or violence
  ▶ Vascular dementia, unspecified severity, with aberrant motor behavior such as restlessness, rocking, pacing, or exit-seeking
  ▶ Vascular dementia, unspecified severity, with verbal or physical behaviors such as profanity, shouting, threatening, anger, aggression, combativeness, or violence

▶ **F01.518** **Vascular dementia, unspecified severity, with other behavioral disturbance**
  ▶ Major neurocognitive disorder due to vascular disease, unspecified severity, with behavioral disturbances such as sleep disturbance, social disinhibition, or sexual disinhibition
  ▶ Vascular dementia, unspecified severity, with behavioral disturbances such as sleep disturbance, social disinhibition, or sexual disinhibition
  ▶ Use Additional code, if applicable, to identify wandering in vascular dementia (Z91.83)

▶ **F01.52** **Vascular dementia, unspecified severity, with psychotic disturbance**
  ▶ Major neurocognitive disorder due to vascular disease, unspecified severity, with psychotic disturbance such as hallucinations, paranoia, suspiciousness, or delusional state
  ▶ Vascular dementia, unspecified severity, with psychotic disturbance such as hallucinations, paranoia, suspiciousness, or delusional state

▶ **F01.53** **Vascular dementia, unspecified severity, with mood disturbance**
  ▶ Major neurocognitive disorder due to vascular disease, unspecified severity, with mood disturbance such as depression, apathy, or anhedonia
  ▶ Vascular dementia, unspecified severity, with mood disturbance such as depression, apathy, or anhedonia

▶ **F01.54** **Vascular dementia, unspecified severity, with anxiety**
  ▶ Major neurocognitive disorder due to vascular disease, unspecified severity, with anxiety

▶ ● **F01.A** **Vascular dementia, mild**
  ▶ **Excludes1**   mild neurocognitive disorder due to known physiological condition with or without behavioral disturbance (F06.7-)

▶ **F01.A0** **Vascular dementia, mild, without behavioral disturbance, psychotic disturbance, mood disturbance, and anxiety**
  ▶ Major neurocognitive disorder due to vascular disease, mild, NOS
  ▶ Vascular dementia, mild, NOS

▶ ● **F01.A1** **Vascular dementia, mild, with behavioral disturbance**
  ▶ **F01.A11** **Vascular dementia, mild, with agitation**
    ▶ Major neurocognitive disorder due to vascular disease, mild, with aberrant motor behavior such as restlessness, rocking, pacing, or exit-seeking
    ▶ Major neurocognitive disorder due to vascular disease, mild, with verbal or physical behaviors such as profanity, shouting, threatening, anger, aggression, combativeness, or violence
    ▶ Vascular dementia, mild, with aberrant motor behavior such as restlessness, rocking, pacing, or exit-seeking
    ▶ Vascular dementia, mild, with verbal or physical behaviors such as profanity, shouting, threatening, anger, aggression, combativeness, or violence
  ▶ **F01.A18** **Vascular dementia, mild, with other behavioral disturbance**
    ▶ Major neurocognitive disorder due to vascular disease, mild, with behavioral disturbances such as sleep disturbance, social disinhibition, or sexual disinhibition
    ▶ Vascular dementia, mild, with behavioral disturbances such as sleep disturbance, social disinhibition, or sexual disinhibition
  ▶ Use Additional code, if applicable, to identify wandering in vascular dementia (Z91.83)

▶ **F01.A2** **Vascular dementia, mild, with psychotic disturbance**
  ▶ Major neurocognitive disorder due to vascular disease, mild, with psychotic disturbance such as hallucinations, paranoia, suspiciousness, or delusional state
  ▶ Vascular dementia, mild, with psychotic disturbance such as hallucinations, paranoia, suspiciousness, or delusional state

▶ **F01.A3** **Vascular dementia, mild, with mood disturbance**
  ▶ Major neurocognitive disorder due to vascular disease, mild, with mood disturbance such as depression, apathy, or anhedonia
  ▶ Vascular dementia, mild, with mood disturbance such as depression, apathy, or anhedonia

▶ **F01.A4** **Vascular dementia, mild, with anxiety**
  ▶ Major neurocognitive disorder due to vascular disease, mild, with anxiety

▶ ● **F01.B** **Vascular dementia, moderate**
  ▶ **F01.B0** **Vascular dementia, moderate, without behavioral disturbance, psychotic disturbance, mood disturbance, and anxiety**
    ▶ Major neurocognitive disorder due to vascular disease, moderate, NOS
    ▶ Vascular dementia, moderate, NOS

▶ New   ⇒ Revised   ~~deleted~~ Deleted   Excludes 1   Excludes 2   Includes   Use additional   Code first   Code also   Key words

OGCR Official Guidelines   X Assign placeholder X   ● Use Additional Character(s)   ▌ Manifestation Code   🔾 Hierarchical Condition Category   **Coding Clinic**

▶ ● **F01.B1** **Vascular dementia, moderate, with behavioral disturbance**
    ▶ **F01.B11** **Vascular dementia, moderate, with agitation**
        ▶ Major neurocognitive disorder due to vascular disease, moderate, with aberrant motor behavior such as restlessness, rocking, pacing, or exit-seeking
        ▶ Major neurocognitive disorder due to vascular disease, moderate, with verbal or physical behaviors such as profanity, shouting, threatening, anger, aggression, combativeness, or violence
        ▶ Vascular dementia, moderate, with aberrant motor behavior such as restlessness, rocking, pacing, or exit-seeking
        ▶ Vascular dementia, moderate, with verbal or physical behaviors such as profanity, shouting, threatening, anger, aggression, combativeness, or violence
    ▶ **F01.B18** **Vascular dementia, moderate, with other behavioral disturbance**
        ▶ Major neurocognitive disorder due to vascular disease, moderate, with behavioral disturbances such as sleep disturbance, social disinhibition, or sexual disinhibition
        ▶ Vascular dementia, moderate, with behavioral disturbances such as sleep disturbance, social disinhibition, or sexual disinhibition
    ▶ Use Additional code, if applicable, to identify wandering in vascular dementia (Z91.83)

▶ **F01.B2** **Vascular dementia, moderate, with psychotic disturbance**
    ▶ Major neurocognitive disorder due to vascular disease, moderate, with psychotic disturbance such as hallucinations, paranoia, suspiciousness, or delusional state
    ▶ Vascular dementia, moderate, with psychotic disturbance such as hallucinations, paranoia, suspiciousness, or delusional state

▶ **F01.B3** **Vascular dementia, moderate, with mood disturbance**
    ▶ Major neurocognitive disorder due to vascular disease, moderate, with mood disturbance such as depression, apathy, or anhedonia
    ▶ Vascular dementia, moderate, with mood disturbance such as depression, apathy, or anhedonia

▶ **F01.B4** **Vascular dementia, moderate, with anxiety**
    ▶ Major neurocognitive disorder due to vascular disease, moderate, with anxiety

▶ ● **F01.C** **Vascular dementia, severe**
    ▶ **F01.C0** **Vascular dementia, severe, without behavioral disturbance, psychotic disturbance, mood disturbance, and anxiety**
        ▶ Major neurocognitive disorder due to vascular disease, severe, NOS
        ▶ Vascular dementia, severe, NOS

▶ ● **F01.C1** **Vascular dementia, severe, with behavioral disturbance**
    ▶ **F01.C11** **Vascular dementia, severe, with agitation**
        ▶ Major neurocognitive disorder due to vascular disease, severe, with aberrant motor behavior such as restlessness, rocking, pacing, or exit-seeking
        ▶ Major neurocognitive disorder due to vascular disease, severe, with verbal or physical behaviors such as profanity, shouting, threatening, anger, aggression, combativeness, or violence
        ▶ Vascular dementia, severe, with aberrant motor behavior such as restlessness, rocking, pacing, or exit-seeking
        ▶ Vascular dementia, severe, with verbal or physical behaviors such as profanity, shouting, threatening, anger, aggression, combativeness, or violence
    ▶ **F01.C18** **Vascular dementia, severe, with other behavioral disturbance**
        ▶ Major neurocognitive disorder due to vascular disease, severe, with behavioral disturbances such as sleep disturbance, social disinhibition, or sexual disinhibition
        ▶ Vascular dementia, severe, with behavioral disturbances such as sleep disturbance, social disinhibition, or sexual disinhibition
    ▶ Use Additional code, if applicable, to identify wandering in vascular dementia (Z91.83)

▶ **F01.C2** **Vascular dementia, severe, with psychotic disturbance**
    ▶ Major neurocognitive disorder due to vascular disease, severe, with psychotic disturbance such as hallucinations, paranoia, suspiciousness, or delusional state
    ▶ Vascular dementia, severe, with psychotic disturbance such as hallucinations, paranoia, suspiciousness, or delusional state

▶ **F01.C3** **Vascular dementia, severe, with mood disturbance**
    ▶ Major neurocognitive disorder due to vascular disease, severe, with mood disturbance such as depression, apathy, or anhedonia
    ▶ Vascular dementia, severe, with mood disturbance such as depression, apathy, or anhedonia

▶ **F01.C4** **Vascular dementia, severe, with anxiety**
    ▶ Major neurocognitive disorder due to vascular disease, severe, with anxiety

CHAPTER 5 (F01-F99)

● **F02   Dementia in other diseases classified elsewhere**

Code first the underlying physiological condition, such as:
   Alzheimer's (G30.-)
   cerebral lipidosis (E75.4)
   Creutzfeldt-Jakob disease (A81.0-)
   dementia with Lewy bodies (G31.83)
   dementia with Parkinsonism (G31.83)
   epilepsy and recurrent seizures (G40.-)
   frontotemporal dementia (G31.09)
   hepatolenticular degeneration (E83.0)
   human immunodeficiency virus [HIV] disease (B20)
   Huntington's disease (G10)
   hypercalcemia (E83.52)
   hypothyroidism, acquired (E00-E03.-)
   intoxications (T36-T65)
   Jakob-Creutzfeldt disease (A81.0-)
   multiple sclerosis (G35)
   neurosyphilis (A52.17)
   niacin deficiency [pellagra] (E52)
   Parkinson's disease (G20)
   Pick's disease (G31.01)
   polyarteritis nodosa (M30.0)
   prion disease (A81.9)
   systemic lupus erythematosus (M32.-)
   traumatic brain injury (S06.-)
   trypanosomiasis (B56.-, B57.-)
   vitamin B deficiency (E53.8)

Includes   Major neurocognitive disorder in other diseases classified elsewhere

▶ **Excludes1**   mild neurocognitive disorder due to known physiological condition with or without behavioral disturbance (F06.7-)

Excludes2   dementia in alcohol and psychoactive substance disorders (F10-F19, with .17, .27, .97)
➡ vascular dementia (F01.5-, F01.A-, F01.B-, F01.C-)
Coding Clinic: 2016, Q4, P141

➡● **F02.8   Dementia in other diseases classified elsewhere, unspecified severity**

➡▷ *F02.80   Dementia in other diseases classified elsewhere, unspecified severity, without behavioral disturbance, psychotic disturbance, mood disturbance, and anxiety*
   Dementia in other diseases classified elsewhere NOS
➡ Major neurocognitive disorder in other diseases classified elsewhere NOS
   Coding Clinic: 2017, Q1, P43; 2016, Q2, P6

●▷ *F02.81   Dementia in other diseases classified elsewhere, unspecified severity, with behavioral disturbance*
   ~~Dementia in other diseases classified elsewhere with aggressive behavior~~
   ~~Dementia in other diseases classified elsewhere with combative behavior~~
   ~~Dementia in other diseases classified elsewhere with violent behavior~~
   ~~Major neurocognitive disorder in other diseases classified elsewhere with aggressive behavior~~
   ~~Major neurocognitive disorder in other diseases classified elsewhere with combative behavior~~
   ~~Major neurocognitive disorder in other diseases classified elsewhere with violent behavior~~
   ~~Use additional code, if applicable, to identify wandering in dementia in conditions classified elsewhere (Z91.83)~~
   Coding Clinic: 2017, Q2, P8, Q1, P43

▷ **F02.811   Dementia in other diseases classified elsewhere, unspecified severity, with agitation**
   ▶Dementia in other diseases classified elsewhere, unspecified severity, with aberrant motor behavior such as restlessness, rocking, pacing, or exit-seeking
   ▶Dementia in other diseases classified elsewhere, unspecified severity, with verbal or physical behaviors such as profanity, shouting, threatening, anger, aggression, combativeness, or violence
   ▶Major neurocognitive disorder in other diseases classified elsewhere, unspecified severity, with aberrant motor behavior such as restlessness, rocking, pacing, or exit-seeking
   ▶Major neurocognitive disorder in other diseases classified elsewhere, unspecified severity, with verbal or physical behaviors such as profanity, shouting, threatening, anger, aggression, combativeness, or violence

▷ **F02.818   Dementia in other diseases classified elsewhere, unspecified severity, with other behavioral disturbance**
   ▶Dementia in other diseases classified elsewhere with sleep disturbance, social disinhibition, or sexual disinhibition
   ▶Major neurocognitive disorder in other diseases classified elsewhere with sleep disturbance, social disinhibition, or sexual disinhibition

▷ Use Additional code, if applicable, to identify wandering in dementia in conditions classified elsewhere (Z91.83)

▶ **F02.82   Dementia in other diseases classified elsewhere, unspecified severity, with psychotic disturbance**
   ▶Dementia in other diseases classified elsewhere, unspecified severity, with psychotic disturbance such as hallucinations, paranoia, suspiciousness, or delusional state
   ▶Major neurocognitive disorder in other diseases classified elsewhere, unspecified, with psychotic disturbance such as hallucinations, paranoia, suspiciousness, or delusional state

▶ **F02.83   Dementia in other diseases classified elsewhere, unspecified severity, with mood disturbance**
   ▶Dementia in other diseases classified elsewhere, unspecified severity, with mood disturbance such as depression, apathy, or anhedonia
   ▶Major neurocognitive disorder in other diseases classified elsewhere unspecified severity, with mood disturbance such as with depression, apathy, or anhedonia

▶ **F02.84   Dementia in other diseases classified elsewhere, unspecified severity, with anxiety**
   ▶Major neurocognitive disorder in other diseases classified elsewhere unspecified severity, with anxiety

▶● **F02.A   Dementia in other diseases classified elsewhere, mild**
   ▶ **Excludes1**   mild neurocognitive disorder due to known physiological condition with or without behavioral disturbance (F06.7-)

▶ New   ➡ Revised   ~~deleted~~ Deleted   Excludes 1   Excludes 2   Includes   Use additional   Code first   Code also   Key words
OGCR Official Guidelines   X Assign placeholder X   ● Use Additional Character(s)   ▷ Manifestation Code   🐾 Hierarchical Condition Category   **Coding Clinic**

▶ **F02.A0 Dementia in other diseases classified elsewhere, mild, without behavioral disturbance, psychotic disturbance, mood disturbance, and anxiety**
　▶ Dementia in other diseases classified elsewhere, mild, NOS
　▶ Major neurocognitive disorder in other diseases classified elsewhere, mild, NOS

▶● **F02.A1 Dementia in other diseases classified elsewhere, mild, with behavioral disturbance**
　▶ **F02.A11 Dementia in other diseases classified elsewhere, mild, with agitation**
　　▶ Dementia in other diseases classified elsewhere, mild, with aberrant motor behavior such as restlessness, rocking, pacing, or exit-seeking
　　▶ Dementia in other diseases classified elsewhere, mild, with verbal or physical behaviors such as profanity, shouting, threatening, anger, aggression, combativeness, or violence
　　▶ Major neurocognitive disorder in other diseases classified elsewhere, mild, with aberrant motor behavior such as restlessness, rocking, pacing, or exit-seeking
　　▶ Major neurocognitive disorder in other diseases classified elsewhere, mild, with verbal or physical behaviors such as profanity, shouting, threatening, anger, aggression, combativeness, or violence
　▶ **F02.A18 Dementia in other diseases classified elsewhere, mild, with other behavioral disturbance**
　　▶ Dementia in other diseases classified elsewhere, mild, with behavioral disturbances such as sleep disturbance, social disinhibition, or sexual disinhibition
　　▶ Major neurocognitive disorder in other diseases classified elsewhere, mild, with behavioral disturbances such as sleep disturbance, social disinhibition, or sexual disinhibition
　▶ Use Additional code, if applicable, to identify wandering in dementia in conditions classified elsewhere (Z91.83)

▶ **F02.A2 Dementia in other diseases classified elsewhere, mild, with psychotic disturbance**
　▶ Dementia in other diseases classified elsewhere, mild, with psychotic disturbance such as hallucinations, paranoia, suspiciousness, or delusional state
　▶ Major neurocognitive disorder in other diseases classified elsewhere, mild, with psychotic disturbance such as hallucinations, paranoia, suspiciousness, or delusional state

▶ **F02.A3 Dementia in other diseases classified elsewhere, mild, with mood disturbance**
　▶ Dementia in other diseases classified elsewhere, mild, with mood disturbance such as depression, apathy, or anhedonia
　▶ Major neurocognitive disorder in other diseases classified elsewhere, mild, with mood disturbance such as depression, apathy, or anhedonia

▶ **F02.A4 Dementia in other diseases classified elsewhere, mild, with anxiety**
　▶ Major neurocognitive disorder in other diseases classified elsewhere, mild, with anxiety

▶● **F02.B Dementia in other diseases classified elsewhere, moderate**
　▶ **F02.B0 Dementia in other diseases classified elsewhere, moderate, without behavioral disturbance, psychotic disturbance, mood disturbance, and anxiety**
　　▶ Dementia in other diseases classified elsewhere, moderate, NOS
　　▶ Major neurocognitive disorder in other diseases classified elsewhere, moderate, NOS

▶● **F02.B1 Dementia in other diseases classified elsewhere, moderate, with behavioral disturbance**
　▶ **F02.B11 Dementia in other diseases classified elsewhere, moderate, with agitation**
　　▶ Dementia in other diseases classified elsewhere, moderate, with aberrant motor behavior such as restlessness, rocking, pacing, or exit-seeking
　　▶ Dementia in other diseases classified elsewhere, moderate, with verbal or physical behaviors such as profanity, shouting, threatening, anger, aggression, combativeness, or violence
　　▶ Major neurocognitive disorder in other diseases classified elsewhere, moderate, with aberrant motor behavior such as restlessness, rocking, pacing, or exit- seeking
　　▶ Major neurocognitive disorder in other diseases classified elsewhere, moderate, with verbal or physical behaviors such as profanity, shouting, threatening, anger, aggression, combativeness, or violence
　▶ **F02.B18 Dementia in other diseases classified elsewhere, moderate, with other behavioral disturbance**
　　▶ Dementia in other diseases classified elsewhere, moderate, with behavioral disturbances such as sleep disturbance, social disinhibition, or sexual disinhibition
　　▶ Major neurocognitive disorder in other diseases classified elsewhere, moderate, with behavioral disturbance such as sleep disturbance, social disinhibition, or sexual disinhibition
　▶ Use Additional code, if applicable, to identify wandering in dementia in conditions classified elsewhere (Z91.83)

　▶ **F02.B2 Dementia in other diseases classified elsewhere, moderate, with psychotic disturbance**
　　▶ Dementia in other diseases classified elsewhere, moderate, with psychotic disturbance such as hallucinations, paranoia, suspiciousness, or delusional state
　　▶ Major neurocognitive disorder in other diseases classified elsewhere, moderate, with psychotic disturbance such as hallucinations, paranoia, suspiciousness, or delusional state

▶F02.B3 **Dementia in other diseases classified elsewhere, moderate, with mood disturbance**
  ▶Dementia in other diseases classified elsewhere, moderate, with mood disturbance such as depression, apathy, or anhedonia
  ▶Major neurocognitive disorder in other diseases classified elsewhere, moderate, with mood disturbance such as depression, apathy, or anhedonia

▶F02.B4 **Dementia in other diseases classified elsewhere, moderate, with anxiety**
  ▶Major neurocognitive disorder in other diseases classified elsewhere, moderate, with anxiety

▶●F02.C **Dementia in other diseases classified elsewhere, severe**

▶F02.C0 **Dementia in other diseases classified elsewhere, severe, without behavioral disturbance, psychotic disturbance, mood disturbance, and anxiety**
  ▶Dementia in other diseases classified elsewhere, severe, NOS
  ▶Major neurocognitive disorder in other diseases classified elsewhere, severe, NOS

▶●F02.C1 **Dementia in other diseases classified elsewhere, severe, with behavioral disturbance**

▶F02.C11 **Dementia in other diseases classified elsewhere, severe, with agitation**
  ▶Dementia in other diseases classified elsewhere, severe, with aberrant motor behavior such as restlessness, rocking, pacing, or exit-seeking
  ▶Dementia in other diseases classified elsewhere, severe, with verbal or physical behaviors such as profanity, shouting, threatening, anger, aggression, combativeness, or violence
  ▶Major neurocognitive disorder in other diseases classified elsewhere, severe, with aberrant motor behavior such as restlessness, rocking, pacing, or exit-seeking
  ▶Major neurocognitive disorder in other diseases classified elsewhere, severe, with verbal or physical behaviors such as profanity, shouting, threatening, anger, aggression, combativeness, or violence

▶F02.C18 **Dementia in other diseases classified elsewhere, severe, with other behavioral disturbance**
  ▶Dementia in other diseases classified elsewhere, severe, with behavioral disturbances such as sleep disturbance, social disinhibition, or sexual disinhibition
  ▶Major neurocognitive disorder in other diseases classified elsewhere, severe, with behavioral disturbances such as sleep disturbance, social disinhibition, or sexual disinhibition

▶ Use Additional code, if applicable, to identify wandering in dementia in conditions classified elsewhere (Z91.83)

▶F02.C2 **Dementia in other diseases classified elsewhere, severe, with psychotic disturbance**
  ▶Dementia in other diseases classified elsewhere, severe, with psychotic disturbance such as hallucinations, paranoia, suspiciousness, or delusional state
  ▶Major neurocognitive disorder in other diseases classified elsewhere, severe, with psychotic disturbance such as hallucinations, paranoia, suspiciousness, or delusional state

F02.C3 **Dementia in other diseases classified elsewhere, severe, with mood disturbance**
  ▶Dementia in other diseases classified elsewhere, severe, with mood disturbance such as depression, apathy, or anhedonia
  ▶Major neurocognitive disorder in other diseases classified elsewhere, severe, with mood disturbance such as depression, apathy, or anhedonia

▶F02.C4 **Dementia in other diseases classified elsewhere, severe, with anxiety**
  ▶Major neurocognitive disorder in other diseases classified elsewhere, severe, with anxiety

●F03 **Unspecified dementia**
  ▶Major neurocognitive disorder NOS
  Presenile dementia NOS
  Presenile psychosis NOS
  Primary degenerative dementia NOS
  Senile dementia NOS
  Senile dementia depressed or paranoid type
  Senile psychosis NOS
  Excludes1 senility NOS (R41.81)
  Excludes2 mild memory disturbance due to known physiological condition (F06.8)
  senile dementia with delirium or acute confusional state (F05)

⇒●F03.9 **Unspecified dementia, unspecified severity**

⇒F03.90 **Unspecified dementia, unspecified severity, without behavioral disturbance, psychotic disturbance, mood disturbance, and anxiety** A
  Dementia NOS
  Coding Clinic: 2021, Q2, P4; 2012, Q4, P92

⇒●F03.91 **Unspecified dementia with, unspecified severity, behavioral disturbance** A
  ~~Unspecified dementia with aggressive behavior~~
  ~~Unspecified dementia with combative behavior~~
  ~~Unspecified dementia with violent behavior~~
  ~~Use additional code, if applicable, to identify wandering in unspecified dementia (Z91.83)~~

  ▶F03.911 **Unspecified dementia, unspecified severity, with agitation**
    ▶Unspecified dementia, unspecified severity, with aberrant motor behavior such as restlessness, rocking, pacing, or exit-seeking
    ▶Unspecified dementia, unspecified severity, with verbal or physical behaviors such as profanity, shouting, threatening, anger, aggression, combativeness, or violence

Item 5-1 Psychosis was a term formerly applied to any mental disorder but is now restricted to disturbances of a great magnitude in which there is a personality disintegration and loss of contact with reality.

CHAPTER 5 (F01–F99)

772

▶ New   ⇒ Revised   ~~deleted~~ Deleted   Excludes 1   Excludes 2   Includes   Use additional   Code first   Code also   Key words
OGCR Official Guidelines   X Assign placeholder X   ● Use Additional Character(s)   ▶ Manifestation Code   🏷 Hierarchical Condition Category   Coding Clinic

▶F03.918   **Unspecified dementia, unspecified severity, with other behavioral disturbance**
▶ Unspecified dementia, unspecified severity, with behavioral disturbances such as sleep disturbance, social disinhibition, or sexual disinhibition
▶ Use Additional code, if applicable, to identify wandering in unspecified dementia (Z91.83)

▶F03.92   **Unspecified dementia, unspecified severity, with psychotic disturbance**
▶ Unspecified dementia, unspecified severity, with psychotic disturbance such as hallucinations, paranoia, suspiciousness, or delusional state

▶F03.93   **Unspecified dementia, unspecified severity, with mood disturbance**
▶ Unspecified dementia, unspecified severity, with mood disturbance such as depression, apathy, or anhedonia

▶F03.94   **Unspecified dementia, unspecified severity, with anxiety**

▶ ● **F03.A**   **Unspecified dementia, mild**

▶ **Excludes1**   mild neurocognitive disorder due to known physiological condition with or without behavioral disturbance (F06.7-)

▶F03.A0   **Unspecified dementia, mild, without behavioral disturbance, psychotic disturbance, mood disturbance, and anxiety**
▶ Dementia, mild, NOS

▶ ● **F03.A1**   **Unspecified dementia, mild, with behavioral disturbance**

▶F03.A11   **Unspecified dementia, mild, with agitation**
▶ Unspecified dementia, mild, with aberrant motor behavior such as restlessness, rocking, pacing, or exit-seeking
▶ Unspecified dementia, mild, with verbal or physical behaviors such as profanity, shouting, threatening, anger, aggression, combativeness, or violence

▶F03.A18   **Unspecified dementia, mild, with other behavioral disturbance**
▶ Unspecified dementia, mild, with behavioral disturbances such as sleep disturbance, social disinhibition, or sexual disinhibition

▶ Use Additional code, if applicable, to identify wandering in unspecified dementia (Z91.83)

▶F03.A2   **Unspecified dementia, mild, with psychotic disturbance**
▶ Unspecified dementia, mild, with psychotic disturbance such as hallucinations, paranoia, suspiciousness, or delusional state

▶F03.A3   **Unspecified dementia, mild, with mood disturbance**
▶ Unspecified dementia, mild, with mood disturbance such as depression, apathy, or anhedonia

▶F03.A4   **Unspecified dementia, mild, with anxiety**

▶ ● **F03.B**   **Unspecified dementia, moderate**

▶F03.B0   **Unspecified dementia, moderate, without behavioral disturbance, psychotic disturbance, mood disturbance, and anxiety**
▶ Dementia, moderate, NOS

▶ ● **F03.B1**   **Unspecified dementia, moderate, with behavioral disturbance**

▶F03.B11   **Unspecified dementia, moderate, with agitation**
▶ Unspecified dementia, moderate, with aberrant motor behavior such as restlessness, rocking, pacing, or exit-seeking
▶ Unspecified dementia, moderate, with verbal or physical behaviors such as profanity, shouting, threatening, anger, aggression, combativeness, or violence

▶F03.B18   **Unspecified dementia, moderate, with other behavioral disturbance**
▶ Unspecified dementia, moderate, with behavioral disturbances such as sleep disturbance, social disinhibition, or sexual disinhibition

▶ Use Additional code, if applicable, to identify wandering in unspecified dementia (Z91.83)

▶F03.B2   **Unspecified dementia, moderate, with psychotic disturbance**
▶ Unspecified dementia, moderate, with psychotic disturbance such as hallucinations, paranoia, suspiciousness, or delusional state

▶F03.B3   **Unspecified dementia, moderate, with mood disturbance**
▶ Unspecified dementia, moderate, with mood disturbance such as depression, apathy, or anhedonia

▶F03.B4   **Unspecified dementia, moderate, with anxiety**

▶ ● **F03.C**   **Unspecified dementia, severe**

▶F03.C0   **Unspecified dementia, severe, without behavioral disturbance, psychotic disturbance, mood disturbance, and anxiety**
▶ Dementia, severe, NOS

▶ ● **F03.C1**   **Unspecified dementia, severe, with behavioral disturbance**

▶F03.C11   **Unspecified dementia, severe, with agitation**
▶ Unspecified dementia, severe, with aberrant motor behavior such as restlessness, rocking, pacing, or exit-seeking
▶ Unspecified dementia, severe, with verbal or physical behaviors such as profanity, shouting, threatening, anger, aggression, combativeness, or violence

▶F03.C18   **Unspecified dementia, severe, with other behavioral disturbance**
▶ Unspecified dementia, severe, with behavioral disturbances such as sleep disturbance, social disinhibition, or sexual disinhibition

▶ Use Additional code, if applicable, to identify wandering in unspecified dementia (Z91.83)

▶F03.C2   **Unspecified dementia, severe, with psychotic disturbance**
▶ Unspecified dementia, severe, with psychotic disturbance such as hallucinations, paranoia, suspiciousness, or delusional state

▶F03.C3   **Unspecified dementia, severe, with mood disturbance**
▶ Unspecified dementia, severe, with mood disturbance such as depression, apathy, or anhedonia

▶F03.C4   **Unspecified dementia, severe, with anxiety**

CHAPTER 5 (F01-F99)

F04   **Amnestic disorder due to known physiological condition**
Korsakov's psychosis or syndrome, nonalcoholic
Code first the underlying physiological condition
   Excludes1   amnesia NOS (R41.3)
anterograde amnesia (R41.1)
dissociative amnesia (F44.0)
retrograde amnesia (R41.2)
   Excludes2   alcohol-induced or unspecified Korsakov's syndrome (F10.26, F10.96)
Korsakov's syndrome induced by other psychoactive substances (F13.26, F13.96, F19.16, F19.26, F19.96)

F05   **Delirium due to known physiological condition**
Acute or subacute brain syndrome
Acute or subacute confusional state (nonalcoholic)
Acute or subacute infective psychosis
Acute or subacute organic reaction
Acute or subacute psycho-organic syndrome
Delirium of mixed etiology
Delirium superimposed on dementia
Sundowning
Code first the underlying physiological condition
   Excludes1   delirium NOS (R41.0)
   Excludes2   delirium tremens alcohol-induced or unspecified (F10.231, F10.921)
Coding Clinic: 2019, Q2, P34

● **F06**   **Other mental disorders due to known physiological condition**
   Includes   mental disorders due to endocrine disorder
mental disorders due to exogenous hormone
mental disorders due to exogenous toxic substance
mental disorders due to primary cerebral disease
mental disorders due to somatic illness
mental disorders due to systemic disease affecting the brain
Code first the underlying physiological condition
   Excludes1   unspecified dementia (F03)
   Excludes2   delirium due to known physiological condition (F05)
dementia as classified in F01-F02
other mental disorders associated with alcohol and other psychoactive substances (F10-F19)

F06.0   **Psychotic disorder with hallucinations due to known physiological condition**
Organic hallucinatory state (nonalcoholic)
   Excludes2   hallucinations and perceptual disturbance induced by alcohol and other psychoactive substances (F10-F19 with .151, .251, .951)
schizophrenia (F20.-)

F06.1   **Catatonic disorder due to known physiological condition**
Catatonia associated with another mental disorder
Catatonia NOS
   Excludes1   catatonic stupor (R40.1)
stupor NOS (R40.1)
   Excludes2   catatonic schizophrenia (F20.2)
dissociative stupor (F44.2)

F06.2   **Psychotic disorder with delusions due to known physiological condition**
Paranoid and paranoid-hallucinatory organic states
Schizophrenia-like psychosis in epilepsy
   Excludes2   alcohol and drug-induced psychotic disorder (F10-F19 with .150, .250, .950)
brief psychotic disorder (F23)
delusional disorder (F22)
schizophrenia (F20.-)

● **F06.3**   **Mood disorder due to known physiological condition**
   Excludes2   mood disorders due to alcohol and other psychoactive substances (F10-F19 with .14, .24, .94)
mood disorders, not due to known physiological condition or unspecified (F30-F39)
F06.30   Mood disorder due to known physiological condition, **unspecified**
F06.31   Mood disorder due to known physiological condition **with depressive features**
Depressive disorder due to known physiological condition, with depressive features
F06.32   Mood disorder due to known physiological condition **with major depressive-like episode**
Depressive disorder due to known physiological condition, with major depressive-like episode
F06.33   Mood disorder due to known physiological condition **with manic features**
Bipolar and related disorder due to a known physiological condition, with manic features
Bipolar and related disorder due to known physiological condition, with manic- or hypomanic-like episodes
F06.34   Mood disorder due to known physiological condition **with mixed features**
Bipolar and related disorder due to known physiological condition, with mixed features
Depressive disorder due to known physiological condition, with mixed features

F06.4   **Anxiety disorder due to known physiological condition**
   Excludes2   anxiety disorders due to alcohol and other psychoactive substances (F10-F19 with .180, .280, .980)
anxiety disorders, not due to known physiological condition or unspecified (F40.-, F41.-)

▶ ● **F06.7**   **Mild neurocognitive disorder due to known physiological condition**
▶ Mild neurocognitive impairment due to a known physiological condition
▶ *Code first the underlying physiological condition, such as:*
▶ Alzheimer's disease (G30.-)
▶ frontotemporal neurocognitive disorder (G31.09)
▶ human immunodeficiency virus [HIV] disease (B20)
▶ Huntington's disease (G10)
▶ Neurocognitive disorder with Lewy bodies (G31.83)
▶ Parkinson's disease (G20)
▶ systemic lupus erythematosus (M32.-)
▶ traumatic brain injury (S06.-)
▶ vitamin B deficiency (E53-)
▶   **Excludes1**   age related cognitive decline (R41.81)
altered mental status (R41.82)
cerebral degeneration (G31.9)
change in mental status (R41.82)
cognitive deficits following (sequelae of) cerebral hemorrhage or infarction (I69.01- I69.11-, I69.21-I69.31-, I69.81-I69.91-)
dementia (F01.-, F02.-, F03)
mild cognitive impairment due to unknown or unspecified etiology (G31.84)
neurologic neglect syndrome (R41.4)
personality change, nonpsychotic (F68.8)
▶ **F06.70**   Mild neurocognitive disorder due to known physiological condition without behavioral disturbance
▶ Mild neurocognitive disorder due to known physiological condition, NOS
▶ **F06.71**   Mild neurocognitive disorder due to known physiological condition with behavioral disturbance

▶ New   ⇒ Revised   ~~deleted~~ Deleted   Excludes 1   Excludes 2   Includes   Use additional   Code first   Code also   Key words
OGCR Official Guidelines   X Assign placeholder X   ● Use Additional Character(s)   ▶ Manifestation Code   🝆 Hierarchical Condition Category   **Coding Clinic**

F06.8   **Other specified mental disorders due to known physiological condition**
Epileptic psychosis NOS
Obsessive-compulsive and related disorder due to a known physiological condition
Organic dissociative disorder
Organic emotionally labile [asthenic] disorder

● **F07**   **Personality and behavioral disorders due to known physiological condition**
Code first the underlying physiological condition

F07.0   **Personality change due to known physiological condition**
Frontal lobe syndrome
Limbic epilepsy personality syndrome
Lobotomy syndrome
Organic personality disorder
Organic pseudopsychopathic personality
Organic pseudoretarded personality
Postleucotomy syndrome
~~Code first underlying physiological condition~~

> **Excludes1**   mild cognitive impairment (G31.84)
> postconcussional syndrome (F07.81)
> postencephalitic syndrome (F07.89)
> signs and symptoms involving emotional state (R45.-)

> **Excludes2**   specific personality disorder (F60.-)

● **F07.8**   **Other personality and behavioral disorders due to known physiological condition**

F07.81   **Postconcussional syndrome**
Postcontusional syndrome (encephalopathy)
Post-traumatic brain syndrome, nonpsychotic
Use additional code to identify associated post-traumatic headache, if applicable (G44.3-)

> **Excludes1**   current concussion (brain) (S06.0-)
> postencephalitic syndrome (F07.89)

F07.89   **Other personality and behavioral disorders due to known physiological condition**
Postencephalitic syndrome
Damage to temporal brain lobes with memory loss and abnormal behavior
Right hemispheric organic affective disorder

F07.9   **Unspecified personality and behavioral disorder due to known physiological condition**
Organic psychosyndrome
Due to exposure to organic solvents

F09   **Unspecified mental disorder due to known physiological condition**
Mental disorder NOS due to known physiological condition
Organic brain syndrome NOS
Organic mental disorder NOS
Organic psychosis NOS
Symptomatic psychosis NOS
Code first the underlying physiological condition

▶ **Excludes1**   mild neurocognitive disorder due to known physiological condition (F06.7-)
psychosis NOS (F29)

MENTAL AND BEHAVIORAL DISORDERS DUE TO PSYCHOACTIVE SUBSTANCE USE (F10-F19)

● **F10**   **Alcohol related disorders**
Use additional code for blood alcohol level, if applicable (Y90.-)
Coding Clinic: 2019, Q3, P8

● **F10.1**   **Alcohol abuse**

> **Excludes1**   alcohol dependence (F10.2-)
> alcohol use, unspecified (F10.9-)

F10.10   **Alcohol abuse, uncomplicated**
Alcohol use disorder, mild

F10.11   **Alcohol abuse, in remission**
Alcohol use disorder, mild, in early remission
Alcohol use disorder, mild, in sustained remission
Coding Clinic: 2022, Q1, P25

● **F10.12**   **Alcohol abuse with intoxication**

F10.120   **Alcohol abuse with intoxication, uncomplicated** 🔗

F10.121   **Alcohol abuse with intoxication, delirium** 🔗

F10.129   **Alcohol abuse with intoxication, unspecified** 🔗

● **F10.13**   **Alcohol abuse, with withdrawal**

F10.130   **Alcohol abuse with withdrawal, uncomplicated**

F10.131   **Alcohol abuse with withdrawal delirium**

F10.132   **Alcohol abuse with withdrawal with perceptual disturbance**

F10.139   **Alcohol abuse with withdrawal, unspecified**

● **F10.14**   **Alcohol abuse with alcohol-induced mood disorder** 🔗
Alcohol use disorder, mild, with alcohol-induced bipolar or related disorder
Alcohol use disorder, mild, with alcohol-induced depressive disorder

● **F10.15**   **Alcohol abuse with alcohol-induced psychotic disorder**

F10.150   **Alcohol abuse with alcohol-induced psychotic disorder with delusions** 🔗

F10.151   **Alcohol abuse with alcohol-induced psychotic disorder with hallucinations** 🔗

F10.159   **Alcohol abuse with alcohol-induced psychotic disorder, unspecified** 🔗

● **F10.18**   **Alcohol abuse with other alcohol-induced disorders**
Coding Clinic: 2022, Q1, P33

F10.180   **Alcohol abuse with alcohol-induced anxiety disorder** 🔗
Coding Clinic: 2022, Q1, P33

F10.181   **Alcohol abuse with alcohol-induced sexual dysfunction** 🔗

F10.182   **Alcohol abuse with alcohol-induced sleep disorder** 🔗

F10.188   **Alcohol abuse with other alcohol-induced disorder** 🔗
Coding Clinic: 2022, Q1, P25

F10.19   **Alcohol abuse with unspecified alcohol-induced disorder** 🔗

● **F10.2**   **Alcohol dependence**

> **Excludes1**   alcohol abuse (F10.1-)
> alcohol use, unspecified (F10.9-)

> **Excludes2**   toxic effect of alcohol (T51.0-)

Coding Clinic: 2019, Q3, P8

F10.20   **Alcohol dependence, uncomplicated** 🔗
Alcohol use disorder, moderate
Alcohol use disorder, severe
Coding Clinic: 2020, Q1, P9

F10.21   **Alcohol dependence, in remission** 🔗
Alcohol use disorder, moderate, in early remission
Alcohol use disorder, moderate, in sustained remission
Alcohol use disorder, severe, in early remission
Alcohol use disorder, severe, in sustained remission

● **F10.22**   **Alcohol dependence with intoxication**
Acute drunkenness (in alcoholism)

> **Excludes2**   alcohol dependence with withdrawal (F10.23-)

F10.220   **Alcohol dependence with intoxication, uncomplicated** 🔗

CHAPTER 5 (F01-F99)

F10.221   Alcohol dependence with intoxication delirium

F10.229   Alcohol dependence with intoxication, unspecified

● F10.23   Alcohol dependence with withdrawal

Excludes2   alcohol dependence with intoxication (F10.22-)

F10.230   Alcohol dependence with withdrawal, uncomplicated

F10.231   Alcohol dependence with withdrawal delirium

F10.232   Alcohol dependence with withdrawal with perceptual disturbance

F10.239   Alcohol dependence with withdrawal, unspecified

Coding Clinic: 2015, Q2, P15

F10.24   Alcohol dependence with alcohol-induced mood disorder

Alcohol use disorder, moderate, with alcohol-induced bipolar or related disorder

Alcohol use disorder, moderate, with alcohol-induced depressive disorder

Alcohol use disorder, severe, with alcohol-induced bipolar or related disorder

Alcohol use disorder, severe, with alcohol-induced depressive disorder

● F10.25   Alcohol dependence with alcohol-induced psychotic disorder

F10.250   Alcohol dependence with alcohol-induced psychotic disorder with delusions

F10.251   Alcohol dependence with alcohol-induced psychotic disorder with hallucinations

F10.259   Alcohol dependence with alcohol-induced psychotic disorder, unspecified

F10.26   Alcohol dependence with alcohol-induced persisting amnestic disorder

Alcohol use disorder, moderate, with alcohol-induced major neurocognitive disorder, amnestic-confabulatory type

Alcohol use disorder, severe, with alcohol-induced major neurocognitive disorder, amnestic-confabulatory type

F10.27   Alcohol dependence with alcohol-induced persisting dementia

Alcohol use disorder, moderate, with alcohol-induced major neurocognitive disorder, nonamnestic-confabulatory type

Alcohol use disorder, severe, with alcohol-induced major neurocognitive disorder, nonamnestic-confabulatory type

● F10.28   Alcohol dependence with other alcohol-induced disorders

F10.280   Alcohol dependence with alcohol-induced anxiety disorder

F10.281   Alcohol dependence with alcohol-induced sexual dysfunction

F10.282   Alcohol dependence with alcohol-induced sleep disorder

F10.288   Alcohol dependence with other alcohol-induced disorder

Alcohol use disorder, moderate, with alcohol-induced mild neurocognitive disorder

Alcohol use disorder, severe, with alcohol-induced mild neurocognitive disorder

Coding Clinic: 2020, Q1, P9

F10.29   Alcohol dependence with unspecified alcohol-induced disorder

● F10.9   Alcohol use, unspecified

Excludes1   alcohol abuse (F10.1-)
alcohol dependence (F10.2-)

▶ F10.90   Alcohol use, unspecified, uncomplicated

▶ F10.91   Alcohol use, unspecified, in remission

● F10.92   Alcohol use, unspecified with intoxication

F10.920   Alcohol use, unspecified with intoxication, uncomplicated

F10.921   Alcohol use, unspecified with intoxication delirium

F10.929   Alcohol use, unspecified with intoxication, unspecified

● F10.93   Alcohol use, unspecified with withdrawal

F10.930   Alcohol use, unspecified with withdrawal, uncomplicated

F10.931   Alcohol use, unspecified with withdrawal delirium

F10.932   Alcohol use, unspecified with withdrawal with perceptual disturbance

F10.939   Alcohol use, unspecified with withdrawal, unspecified

F10.94   Alcohol use, unspecified with alcohol-induced mood disorder

Alcohol-induced bipolar or related disorder, without use disorder

Alcohol-induced depressive disorder, without use disorder

● F10.95   Alcohol use, unspecified with alcohol-induced psychotic disorder

F10.950   Alcohol use, unspecified with alcohol-induced psychotic disorder with delusions

F10.951   Alcohol use, unspecified with alcohol-induced psychotic disorder with hallucinations

F10.959   Alcohol use, unspecified with alcohol-induced psychotic disorder, unspecified

Alcohol-induced psychotic disorder without use disorder

F10.96   Alcohol use, unspecified with alcohol-induced persisting amnestic disorder

Alcohol-induced major neurocognitive disorder, amnestic-confabulatory type, without use disorder

F10.97   Alcohol use, unspecified with alcohol-induced persisting dementia

Alcohol-induced major neurocognitive disorder, nonamnestic-confabulatory type, without use disorder

● F10.98   Alcohol use, unspecified with other alcohol-induced disorders

F10.980   Alcohol use, unspecified with alcohol-induced anxiety disorder

Alcohol-induced anxiety disorder, without use disorder

F10.981   Alcohol use, unspecified with alcohol-induced sexual dysfunction

Alcohol-induced sexual dysfunction, without use disorder

F10.982   Alcohol use, unspecified with alcohol-induced sleep disorder

Alcohol-induced sleep disorder, without use disorder

F10.988   Alcohol use, unspecified with other alcohol-induced disorder

Alcohol-induced mild neurocognitive disorder, without use disorder

Coding Clinic: 2019, Q3, P8

F10.99   Alcohol use, unspecified with unspecified alcohol-induced disorder

▶ New   ⮕ Revised   ~~deleted~~ Deleted | Excludes 1 | | Excludes 2 | | Includes | | Use additional | | Code first | | Code also | | Key words |

OGCR Official Guidelines   X Assign placeholder X   ● Use Additional Character(s)   ▶ Manifestation Code   Hierarchical Condition Category | Coding Clinic |

● **F11**   **Opioid related disorders**
  ● **F11.1**   **Opioid abuse**
       Excludes1   opioid dependence (F11.2-)
                  opioid use, unspecified (F11.9-)

    F11.10   **Opioid abuse, uncomplicated**
           Opioid use disorder, mild

    F11.11   **Opioid abuse, in remission**
           Opioid use disorder, mild, in early remission
           Opioid use disorder, mild, in sustained remission

  ● **F11.12**   **Opioid abuse with intoxication**
        F11.120   **Opioid abuse with intoxication, uncomplicated** 🔎

        F11.121   **Opioid abuse with intoxication delirium** 🔎

        F11.122   **Opioid abuse with intoxication with perceptual disturbance** 🔎

        F11.129   **Opioid abuse with intoxication, unspecified** 🔎

    F11.13   **Opioid abuse with withdrawal**

    F11.14   **Opioid abuse with opioid-induced mood disorder** 🔎
           Opioid use disorder, mild, with opioid-induced depressive disorder

  ● **F11.15**   **Opioid abuse with opioid-induced psychotic disorder**
        F11.150   **Opioid abuse with opioid-induced psychotic disorder with delusions** 🔎

        F11.151   **Opioid abuse with opioid-induced psychotic disorder with hallucinations** 🔎

        F11.159   **Opioid abuse with opioid-induced psychotic disorder, unspecified** 🔎

  ● **F11.18**   **Opioid abuse with other opioid-induced disorder**
        F11.181   **Opioid abuse with opioid-induced sexual dysfunction** 🔎

        F11.182   **Opioid abuse with opioid-induced sleep disorder** 🔎

        F11.188   **Opioid abuse with other opioid-induced disorder** 🔎

    F11.19   **Opioid abuse with unspecified opioid-induced disorder** 🔎

  ● **F11.2**   **Opioid dependence**
       Excludes1   opioid abuse (F11.1-)
                  opioid use, unspecified (F11.9-)
       Excludes2   opioid poisoning (T40.0—T40.2-)

    F11.20   **Opioid dependence, uncomplicated** 🔎
           Opioid use disorder, moderate
           Opioid use disorder, severe

    F11.21   **Opioid dependence, in remission** 🔎
           Opioid use disorder, moderate, in early remission
           Opioid use disorder, moderate, in sustained remission
           Opioid use disorder, severe, in early remission
           Opioid use disorder, severe, in sustained remission

  ● **F11.22**   **Opioid dependence with intoxication**
       Excludes1   opioid dependence with withdrawal (F11.23)

        F11.220   **Opioid dependence with intoxication, uncomplicated** 🔎

        F11.221   **Opioid dependence with intoxication delirium** 🔎

        F11.222   **Opioid dependence with intoxication with perceptual disturbance** 🔎

        F11.229   **Opioid dependence with intoxication, unspecified** 🔎

    F11.23   **Opioid dependence with withdrawal** 🔎
       Excludes1   opioid dependence with intoxication (F11.22-)

    F11.24   **Opioid dependence with opioid-induced mood disorder** 🔎
           Opioid use disorder, moderate, with opioid-induced depressive disorder

  ● **F11.25**   **Opioid dependence with opioid-induced psychotic disorder**
        F11.250   **Opioid dependence with opioid-induced psychotic disorder with delusions** 🔎

        F11.251   **Opioid dependence with opioid-induced psychotic disorder with hallucinations** 🔎

        F11.259   **Opioid dependence with opioid-induced psychotic disorder, unspecified** 🔎

  ● **F11.28**   **Opioid dependence with other opioid-induced disorder**
        F11.281   **Opioid dependence with opioid-induced sexual dysfunction** 🔎

        F11.282   **Opioid dependence with opioid-induced sleep disorder** 🔎

        F11.288   **Opioid dependence with other opioid-induced disorder** 🔎

    F11.29   **Opioid dependence with unspecified opioid-induced disorder** 🔎

  ● **F11.9**   **Opioid use, unspecified**
       Excludes1   opioid abuse (F11.1-)
                  opioid dependence (F11.2-)

    F11.90   **Opioid use, unspecified, uncomplicated**

  ▶**F11.91**   **Opioid use, unspecified, in remission**

  ● **F11.92**   **Opioid use, unspecified with intoxication**
       Excludes1   opioid use, unspecified with withdrawal (F11.93)

        F11.920   **Opioid use, unspecified with intoxication, uncomplicated** 🔎

        F11.921   **Opioid use, unspecified with intoxication delirium** 🔎
             Opioid-induced delirium

        F11.922   **Opioid use, unspecified with intoxication with perceptual disturbance** 🔎

        F11.929   **Opioid use, unspecified with intoxication, unspecified** 🔎

    F11.93   **Opioid use, unspecified with withdrawal** 🔎
       Excludes1   opioid use, unspecified with intoxication (F11.92-)

    F11.94   **Opioid use, unspecified with opioid-induced mood disorder** 🔎
           Opioid-induced depressive disorder, without use disorder

  ● **F11.95**   **Opioid use, unspecified with opioid-induced psychotic disorder**
        F11.950   **Opioid use, unspecified with opioid-induced psychotic disorder with delusions** 🔎

        F11.951   **Opioid use, unspecified with opioid-induced psychotic disorder with hallucinations** 🔎

        F11.959   **Opioid use, unspecified with opioid-induced psychotic disorder, unspecified** 🔎

  ● **F11.98**   **Opioid use, unspecified with other specified opioid-induced disorder**
        F11.981   **Opioid use, unspecified with opioid-induced sexual dysfunction** 🔎
             Opioid-induced sexual dysfunction, without use disorder

CHAPTER 5 (F01-F99)

F11.982   Opioid use, unspecified with
           opioid-induced sleep disorder 🐾
               Opioid-induced sleep disorder,
               without use disorder

F11.988   Opioid use, unspecified with other
           opioid-induced disorder 🐾
               Opioid-induced anxiety disorder,
               without use disorder

F11.99   Opioid use, unspecified with unspecified
           opioid-induced disorder 🐾

● F12   Cannabis related disorders
            Includes   marijuana
            Coding Clinic: 2020, Q1, P8

● F12.1   Cannabis abuse
            Excludes1   cannabis dependence (F12.2-)
                             cannabis use, unspecified (F12.9-)

    F12.10   Cannabis abuse, uncomplicated
                  Cannabis use disorder, mild

    F12.11   Cannabis abuse, in remission
                  Cannabis use disorder, mild, in early remission
                  Cannabis use disorder, mild, in sustained
                  remission

  ● F12.12   Cannabis abuse with intoxication
        F12.120   Cannabis abuse with intoxication,
                   uncomplicated 🐾
        F12.121   Cannabis abuse with intoxication
                   delirium 🐾
        F12.122   Cannabis abuse with intoxication
                   with perceptual disturbance 🐾
        F12.129   Cannabis abuse with
                   intoxication, unspecified 🐾

    F12.13   Cannabis abuse with withdrawal

  ● F12.15   Cannabis abuse with psychotic disorder
        F12.150   Cannabis abuse with psychotic
                   disorder with delusions 🐾
        F12.151   Cannabis abuse with psychotic
                   disorder with hallucinations 🐾
        F12.159   Cannabis abuse with psychotic
                   disorder, unspecified 🐾

  ● F12.18   Cannabis abuse with other cannabis-induced
             disorder
        F12.180   Cannabis abuse with cannabis-
                   induced anxiety disorder 🐾
        F12.188   Cannabis abuse with other cannabis-
                   induced disorder 🐾
                       Cannabis use disorder, mild,
                           with cannabis-induced sleep
                           disorder

    F12.19   Cannabis abuse with unspecified cannabis-
              induced disorder 🐾

● F12.2   Cannabis dependence
            Excludes1   cannabis abuse (F12.1-)
                             cannabis use, unspecified (F12.9-)
            Excludes2   cannabis poisoning (T40.7-)

    F12.20   Cannabis dependence, uncomplicated 🐾
                  Cannabis use disorder, moderate
                  Cannabis use disorder, severe

    F12.21   Cannabis dependence, in remission 🐾
                  Cannabis use disorder, moderate, in early
                  remission
                  Cannabis use disorder, moderate, in sustained
                  remission
                  Cannabis use disorder, severe, in early
                  remission
                  Cannabis use disorder, severe, in sustained
                  remission

  ● F12.22   Cannabis dependence with intoxication
        F12.220   Cannabis dependence with
                   intoxication, uncomplicated 🐾
        F12.221   Cannabis dependence with
                   intoxication delirium 🐾

        F12.222   Cannabis dependence with
                   intoxication with perceptual
                   disturbance 🐾
        F12.229   Cannabis dependence with
                   intoxication, unspecified 🐾

    F12.23   Cannabis dependence with withdrawal 🐾

  ● F12.25   Cannabis dependence with psychotic disorder
        F12.250   Cannabis dependence with psychotic
                   disorder with delusions 🐾
        F12.251   Cannabis dependence with psychotic
                   disorder with hallucinations 🐾
        F12.259   Cannabis dependence with psychotic
                   disorder, unspecified 🐾

  ● F12.28   Cannabis dependence with other cannabis-
             induced disorder
        F12.280   Cannabis dependence with cannabis-
                   induced anxiety disorder 🐾
        F12.288   Cannabis dependence with other
                   cannabis-induced disorder 🐾
                       Cannabis use disorder, moderate,
                           with cannabis-induced sleep
                           disorder
                       Cannabis use disorder, severe,
                           with cannabis-induced sleep
                           disorder

    F12.29   Cannabis dependence with unspecified
              cannabis-induced disorder 🐾

● F12.9   Cannabis use, unspecified
            Excludes1   cannabis abuse (F12.1-)
                             cannabis dependence (F12.2-)

    F12.90   Cannabis use, unspecified, uncomplicated

  ▶ F12.91   Cannabis use, unspecified, in remission

  ● F12.92   Cannabis use, unspecified with intoxication
        F12.920   Cannabis use, unspecified with
                   intoxication, uncomplicated 🐾
        F12.921   Cannabis use, unspecified with
                   intoxication delirium 🐾
        F12.922   Cannabis use, unspecified with
                   intoxication with perceptual
                   disturbance 🐾
        F12.929   Cannabis use, unspecified with
                   intoxication, unspecified 🐾

    F12.93   Cannabis use, unspecified with withdrawal 🐾

  ● F12.95   Cannabis use, unspecified with psychotic
             disorder
        F12.950   Cannabis use, unspecified with
                   psychotic disorder with delusions 🐾
        F12.951   Cannabis use, unspecified with
                   psychotic disorder with
                   hallucinations 🐾
        F12.959   Cannabis use, unspecified with
                   psychotic disorder, unspecified 🐾
                       Cannabis-induced psychotic
                           disorder, without use disorder

  ● F12.98   Cannabis use, unspecified with other cannabis-
             induced disorder
        F12.980   Cannabis use, unspecified with
                   anxiety disorder 🐾
                       Cannabis-induced anxiety disorder,
                           without use disorder
        F12.988   Cannabis use, unspecified with other
                   cannabis-induced disorder 🐾
                       Cannabis-induced sleep disorder,
                           without use disorder

    F12.99   Cannabis use, unspecified with unspecified
              cannabis-induced disorder 🐾

● **F13   Sedative, hypnotic, or anxiolytic related disorders**
   ● **F13.1   Sedative, hypnotic or anxiolytic-related abuse**
       Excludes1   sedative, hypnotic or anxiolytic-related
           dependence (F13.2-)
           sedative, hypnotic, or anxiolytic use,
           unspecified (F13.9-)

       F13.10   Sedative, hypnotic or anxiolytic abuse, uncomplicated
           Sedative, hypnotic, or anxiolytic use disorder, mild

       F13.11   Sedative, hypnotic or anxiolytic abuse, in remission
           Sedative, hypnotic or anxiolytic use disorder, mild, in early remission
           Sedative, hypnotic or anxiolytic use disorder, mild, in sustained remission

      ● **F13.12   Sedative, hypnotic or anxiolytic abuse with intoxication**
         F13.120   Sedative, hypnotic or anxiolytic abuse with intoxication, uncomplicated 🔍
         F13.121   Sedative, hypnotic or anxiolytic abuse with intoxication delirium 🔍
         F13.129   Sedative, hypnotic or anxiolytic abuse with intoxication, unspecified 🔍

      ● **F13.13   Sedative, hypnotic or anxiolytic abuse with withdrawal**
         F13.130   Sedative, hypnotic or anxiolytic abuse with withdrawal, uncomplicated
         F13.131   Sedative, hypnotic or anxiolytic abuse with withdrawal delirium
         F13.132   Sedative, hypnotic or anxiolytic abuse with withdrawal with perceptual disturbance
         F13.139   Sedative, hypnotic or anxiolytic abuse with withdrawal, unspecified

       F13.14   Sedative, hypnotic or anxiolytic abuse with sedative, hypnotic or anxiolytic-induced mood disorder 🔍
           Sedative, hypnotic, or anxiolytic use disorder, mild, with sedative, hypnotic, or anxiolytic-induced bipolar or related disorder
           Sedative, hypnotic, or anxiolytic use disorder, mild, with sedative, hypnotic, or anxiolytic-induced depressive disorder

      ● **F13.15   Sedative, hypnotic or anxiolytic abuse with sedative, hypnotic or anxiolytic-induced psychotic disorder**
         F13.150   Sedative, hypnotic or anxiolytic abuse with sedative, hypnotic or anxiolytic-induced psychotic disorder with delusions 🔍
         F13.151   Sedative, hypnotic or anxiolytic abuse with sedative, hypnotic or anxiolytic-induced psychotic disorder with hallucinations 🔍
         F13.159   Sedative, hypnotic or anxiolytic abuse with sedative, hypnotic or anxiolytic-induced psychotic disorder, unspecified 🔍

      ● **F13.18   Sedative, hypnotic or anxiolytic abuse with other sedative, hypnotic or anxiolytic-induced disorders**
         F13.180   Sedative, hypnotic or anxiolytic abuse with sedative, hypnotic or anxiolytic-induced anxiety disorder 🔍
         F13.181   Sedative, hypnotic or anxiolytic abuse with sedative, hypnotic or anxiolytic-induced sexual dysfunction 🔍

         F13.182   Sedative, hypnotic or anxiolytic abuse with sedative, hypnotic or anxiolytic-induced sleep disorder 🔍
         F13.188   Sedative, hypnotic or anxiolytic abuse with other sedative, hypnotic or anxiolytic-induced disorder 🔍

       F13.19   Sedative, hypnotic or anxiolytic abuse with unspecified sedative, hypnotic or anxiolytic-induced disorder 🔍

   ● **F13.2   Sedative, hypnotic or anxiolytic-related dependence**
       Excludes1   sedative, hypnotic or anxiolytic-related
           abuse (F13.1-)
           sedative, hypnotic, or anxiolytic use,
           unspecified (F13.9-)
       Excludes2   sedative, hypnotic, or anxiolytic
           poisoning (T42.-)

       F13.20   Sedative, hypnotic or anxiolytic dependence, uncomplicated 🔍

       F13.21   Sedative, hypnotic or anxiolytic dependence, in remission 🔍
           Sedative, hypnotic or anxiolytic use disorder, moderate, in early remission
           Sedative, hypnotic or anxiolytic use disorder, moderate, in sustained remission
           Sedative, hypnotic or anxiolytic use disorder, severe, in early remission
           Sedative, hypnotic or anxiolytic use disorder, severe, in sustained remission

      ● **F13.22   Sedative, hypnotic or anxiolytic dependence with intoxication**
         Excludes1   sedative, hypnotic or anxiolytic
             dependence with
             withdrawal (F13.23-)
         F13.220   Sedative, hypnotic or anxiolytic dependence with intoxication, uncomplicated 🔍
         F13.221   Sedative, hypnotic or anxiolytic dependence with intoxication delirium 🔍
         F13.229   Sedative, hypnotic or anxiolytic dependence with intoxication, unspecified 🔍

      ● **F13.23   Sedative, hypnotic or anxiolytic dependence with withdrawal**
           Sedative, hypnotic, or anxiolytic use disorder, moderate
           Sedative, hypnotic, or anxiolytic use disorder, severe
         Excludes1   sedative, hypnotic or anxiolytic
             dependence with
             intoxication (F13.22-)
         F13.230   Sedative, hypnotic or anxiolytic dependence with withdrawal, uncomplicated 🔍
         F13.231   Sedative, hypnotic or anxiolytic dependence with withdrawal delirium 🔍
         F13.232   Sedative, hypnotic or anxiolytic dependence with withdrawal with perceptual disturbance 🔍
           Sedative, hypnotic, or anxiolytic withdrawal with perceptual disturbances
         F13.239   Sedative, hypnotic or anxiolytic dependence with withdrawal, unspecified 🔍
           Sedative, hypnotic, or anxiolytic withdrawal without perceptual disturbances

CHAPTER 5 (F01-F99)

F13.24   **Sedative, hypnotic or anxiolytic dependence with sedative, hypnotic or anxiolytic-induced mood disorder** 🐾
     Sedative, hypnotic, or anxiolytic use disorder, moderate, with sedative, hypnotic, or anxiolytic-induced bipolar or related disorder
     Sedative, hypnotic, or anxiolytic use disorder, moderate, with sedative, hypnotic, or anxiolytic-induced depressive disorder
     Sedative, hypnotic, or anxiolytic use disorder, severe, with sedative, hypnotic, or anxiolytic-induced bipolar or related disorder
     Sedative, hypnotic, or anxiolytic use disorder, severe, with sedative, hypnotic, or anxiolytic-induced depressive disorder

● **F13.25**   **Sedative, hypnotic or anxiolytic dependence with sedative, hypnotic or anxiolytic-induced psychotic disorder**
    F13.250   Sedative, hypnotic or anxiolytic dependence with sedative, hypnotic or anxiolytic-induced psychotic disorder with **delusions** 🐾
    F13.251   Sedative, hypnotic or anxiolytic dependence with sedative, hypnotic or anxiolytic-induced psychotic disorder with **hallucinations** 🐾
    F13.259   Sedative, hypnotic or anxiolytic dependence with sedative, hypnotic or anxiolytic-induced psychotic disorder, **unspecified** 🐾

F13.26   **Sedative, hypnotic or anxiolytic dependence with sedative, hypnotic or anxiolytic-induced persisting amnestic disorder** 🐾

F13.27   **Sedative, hypnotic or anxiolytic dependence with sedative, hypnotic or anxiolytic-induced persisting dementia** 🐾
     Sedative, hypnotic, or anxiolytic use disorder, moderate, with sedative, hypnotic, or anxiolytic-induced major neurocognitive disorder
     Sedative, hypnotic, or anxiolytic use disorder, severe, with sedative, hypnotic, or anxiolytic-induced major neurocognitive disorder

● **F13.28**   **Sedative, hypnotic or anxiolytic dependence with other sedative, hypnotic or anxiolytic-induced disorders**
    F13.280   Sedative, hypnotic or anxiolytic dependence with sedative, hypnotic or anxiolytic-induced **anxiety disorder** 🐾
    F13.281   Sedative, hypnotic or anxiolytic dependence with sedative, hypnotic or anxiolytic-induced **sexual dysfunction** 🐾
    F13.282   Sedative, hypnotic or anxiolytic dependence with sedative, hypnotic or anxiolytic-induced **sleep disorder** 🐾
    F13.288   Sedative, hypnotic or anxiolytic dependence with **other** sedative, hypnotic or anxiolytic-induced disorder 🐾
       Sedative, hypnotic, or anxiolytic use disorder, moderate, with sedative, hypnotic, or anxiolytic-induced mild neurocognitive disorder
       Sedative, hypnotic, or anxiolytic use disorder, severe, with sedative, hypnotic, or anxiolytic-induced mild neurocognitive disorder

F13.29   **Sedative, hypnotic or anxiolytic dependence with unspecified sedative, hypnotic or anxiolytic-induced disorder** 🐾

● **F13.9**   **Sedative, hypnotic or anxiolytic-related use, unspecified**
    Excludes1   sedative, hypnotic or anxiolytic-related abuse (F13.1-)
                sedative, hypnotic or anxiolytic-related dependence (F13.2-)

F13.90   **Sedative, hypnotic, or anxiolytic use, unspecified, uncomplicated**

▶ **F13.91**   **Sedative, hypnotic or anxiolytic use, unspecified, in remission**

● **F13.92**   **Sedative, hypnotic or anxiolytic use, unspecified with intoxication**
    Excludes1   sedative, hypnotic or anxiolytic use, unspecified with withdrawal (F13.93-)
    F13.920   Sedative, hypnotic or anxiolytic use, unspecified with intoxication, **uncomplicated** 🐾
    F13.921   Sedative, hypnotic or anxiolytic use, unspecified with intoxication **delirium** 🐾
       Sedative, hypnotic, or anxiolytic-induced delirium
    F13.929   Sedative, hypnotic or anxiolytic use, unspecified with intoxication, **unspecified** 🐾

● **F13.93**   **Sedative, hypnotic or anxiolytic use, unspecified with withdrawal**
    Excludes1   sedative, hypnotic or anxiolytic use, unspecified with intoxication (F13.92-)
    F13.930   Sedative, hypnotic or anxiolytic use, unspecified with withdrawal, **uncomplicated** 🐾
    F13.931   Sedative, hypnotic or anxiolytic use, unspecified with withdrawal **delirium** 🐾
    F13.932   **Sedative, hypnotic or anxiolytic use, unspecified with withdrawal with perceptual disturbances** 🐾
    F13.939   Sedative, hypnotic or anxiolytic use, unspecified with withdrawal, **unspecified** 🐾

F13.94   **Sedative, hypnotic or anxiolytic use, unspecified with sedative, hypnotic or anxiolytic-induced mood disorder** 🐾
     Sedative, hypnotic, or anxiolytic-induced bipolar or related disorder, without use disorder
     Sedative, hypnotic, or anxiolytic-induced depressive disorder, without use disorder

● **F13.95**   **Sedative, hypnotic or anxiolytic use, unspecified with sedative, hypnotic or anxiolytic-induced psychotic disorder**
    F13.950   Sedative, hypnotic or anxiolytic use, unspecified with sedative, hypnotic or anxiolytic-induced psychotic disorder with **delusions** 🐾
    F13.951   Sedative, hypnotic or anxiolytic use, unspecified with sedative, hypnotic or anxiolytic-induced psychotic disorder with **hallucinations** 🐾
    F13.959   Sedative, hypnotic or anxiolytic use, unspecified with sedative, hypnotic or anxiolytic-induced psychotic disorder, **unspecified** 🐾
       Sedative, hypnotic, or anxiolytic-induced psychotic disorder, without use disorder

F13.96   **Sedative, hypnotic or anxiolytic use, unspecified with sedative, hypnotic or anxiolytic-induced persisting amnestic disorder** 🐾

▶ New   ⏪ Revised   ~~deleted~~ Deleted   Excludes 1   Excludes 2   Includes   Use additional   Code first   Code also   Key words

OGCR Official Guidelines   X Assign placeholder X   ● Use Additional Character(s)   ▶ Manifestation Code   🐾 Hierarchical Condition Category   **Coding Clinic**

F13.97   **Sedative, hypnotic or anxiolytic use, unspecified with sedative, hypnotic or anxiolytic-induced persisting dementia** 🔍
     Sedative, hypnotic, or anxiolytic-induced major neurocognitive disorder, without use disorder

● F13.98   **Sedative, hypnotic or anxiolytic use, unspecified with other sedative, hypnotic or anxiolytic-induced disorders**

     F13.980   **Sedative, hypnotic or anxiolytic use, unspecified with sedative, hypnotic or anxiolytic-induced anxiety disorder** 🔍
        Sedative, hypnotic, or anxiolytic-induced anxiety disorder, without use disorder

     F13.981   **Sedative, hypnotic or anxiolytic use, unspecified with sedative, hypnotic or anxiolytic-induced sexual dysfunction** 🔍
        Sedative, hypnotic, or anxiolytic-induced sexual dysfunction disorder, without use disorder

     F13.982   **Sedative, hypnotic or anxiolytic use, unspecified with sedative, hypnotic or anxiolytic-induced sleep disorder** 🔍
        Sedative, hypnotic, or anxiolytic-induced sleep disorder, without use disorder

     F13.988   **Sedative, hypnotic or anxiolytic use, unspecified with other sedative, hypnotic or anxiolytic-induced disorder** 🔍
        Sedative, hypnotic, or anxiolytic-induced mild neurocognitive disorder

F13.99   **Sedative, hypnotic or anxiolytic use, unspecified with unspecified sedative, hypnotic or anxiolytic-induced disorder** 🔍

● F14   **Cocaine related disorders**
    Excludes2   other stimulant-related disorders (F15.-)

● F14.1   **Cocaine abuse**
    Excludes1   cocaine dependence (F14.2-)
               cocaine use, unspecified (F14.9-)

F14.10   **Cocaine abuse, uncomplicated**
     Cocaine use disorder, mild

F14.11   **Cocaine abuse, in remission**
     Cocaine use disorder, mild, in early remission
     Cocaine use disorder, mild, in sustained remission

● F14.12   **Cocaine abuse with intoxication**

     F14.120   **Cocaine abuse with intoxication, uncomplicated** 🔍

     F14.121   **Cocaine abuse with intoxication with delirium** 🔍

     F14.122   **Cocaine abuse with intoxication with perceptual disturbance** 🔍

     F14.129   **Cocaine abuse with intoxication, unspecified** 🔍

F14.13   **Cocaine abuse, unspecified with withdrawal**

F14.14   **Cocaine abuse with cocaine-induced mood disorder** 🔍
     Cocaine use disorder, mild, with cocaine-induced bipolar or related disorder
     Cocaine use disorder, mild, with cocaine-induced depressive disorder

● F14.15   **Cocaine abuse with cocaine-induced psychotic disorder**

     F14.150   **Cocaine abuse with cocaine-induced psychotic disorder with delusions** 🔍

     F14.151   **Cocaine abuse with cocaine-induced psychotic disorder with hallucinations** 🔍

     F14.159   **Cocaine abuse with cocaine-induced psychotic disorder, unspecified** 🔍

● F14.18   **Cocaine abuse with other cocaine-induced disorder**

     F14.180   **Cocaine abuse with cocaine-induced anxiety disorder** 🔍

     F14.181   **Cocaine abuse with cocaine-induced sexual dysfunction** 🔍

     F14.182   **Cocaine abuse with cocaine-induced sleep disorder** 🔍

     F14.188   **Cocaine abuse with other cocaine-induced disorder** 🔍
        Cocaine use disorder, mild, with cocaine-induced obsessive-compulsive or related disorder

F14.19   **Cocaine abuse with unspecified cocaine-induced disorder** 🔍

● F14.2   **Cocaine dependence**
    Excludes1   cocaine abuse (F14.1-)
               cocaine use, unspecified (F14.9-)
    Excludes2   cocaine poisoning (T40.5-)

F14.20   **Cocaine dependence, uncomplicated** 🔍
     Cocaine use disorder, moderate
     Cocaine use disorder, severe

F14.21   **Cocaine dependence, in remission** 🔍
     Cocaine use disorder, moderate, in early remission
     Cocaine use disorder, moderate, in sustained remission
     Cocaine use disorder, severe, in early remission
     Cocaine use disorder, severe, in sustained remission
     Coding Clinic: 2017, Q2, P27

● F14.22   **Cocaine dependence with intoxication**
    Excludes1   cocaine dependence with withdrawal (F14.23)

     F14.220   **Cocaine dependence with intoxication, uncomplicated** 🔍

     F14.221   **Cocaine dependence with intoxication delirium** 🔍

     F14.222   **Cocaine dependence with intoxication with perceptual disturbance** 🔍

     F14.229   **Cocaine dependence with intoxication, unspecified** 🔍

F14.23   **Cocaine dependence with withdrawal** 🔍
    Excludes1   cocaine dependence with intoxication (F14.22-)

F14.24   **Cocaine dependence with cocaine-induced mood disorder** 🔍
     Cocaine use disorder, moderate, with cocaine-induced bipolar or related disorder
     Cocaine use disorder, moderate, with cocaine-induced depressive disorder
     Cocaine use disorder, severe, with cocaine-induced bipolar or related disorder
     Cocaine use disorder, severe, with cocaine-induced depressive disorder

● F14.25   **Cocaine dependence with cocaine-induced psychotic disorder**

     F14.250   **Cocaine dependence with cocaine-induced psychotic disorder with delusions** 🔍

     F14.251   **Cocaine dependence with cocaine-induced psychotic disorder with hallucinations** 🔍

     F14.259   **Cocaine dependence with cocaine-induced psychotic disorder, unspecified** 🔍

● **F14.28 Cocaine dependence with other cocaine-induced disorder**

    F14.280 Cocaine dependence with cocaine-induced anxiety disorder 🐾

    F14.281 Cocaine dependence with cocaine-induced sexual dysfunction 🐾

    F14.282 Cocaine dependence with cocaine-induced sleep disorder 🐾

    F14.288 Cocaine dependence with other cocaine-induced disorder 🐾
        Cocaine use disorder, moderate, with cocaine-induced obsessive-compulsive or related disorder
        Cocaine use disorder, severe, with cocaine-induced obsessive-compulsive or related disorder

F14.29 Cocaine dependence with unspecified cocaine-induced disorder 🐾

● **F14.9 Cocaine use, unspecified**

    Excludes1 cocaine abuse (F14.1-)
               cocaine dependence (F14.2-)

    F14.90 Cocaine use, unspecified, uncomplicated
        Coding Clinic: 2018, Q2, P11

▶ **F14.91 Cocaine use, unspecified, in remission**

● **F14.92 Cocaine use, unspecified with intoxication**

    F14.920 Cocaine use, unspecified with intoxication, uncomplicated 🐾

    F14.921 Cocaine use, unspecified with intoxication delirium 🐾

    F14.922 Cocaine use, unspecified with intoxication with perceptual disturbance 🐾

    F14.929 Cocaine use, unspecified with intoxication, unspecified 🐾

F14.93 Cocaine use, unspecified with withdrawal

F14.94 Cocaine use, unspecified with cocaine-induced mood disorder 🐾
    Cocaine-induced bipolar or related disorder, without use disorder
    Cocaine-induced depressive disorder, without use disorder

● **F14.95 Cocaine use, unspecified with cocaine-induced psychotic disorder**

    F14.950 Cocaine use, unspecified with cocaine-induced psychotic disorder with delusions 🐾

    F14.951 Cocaine use, unspecified with cocaine-induced psychotic disorder with hallucinations 🐾

    F14.959 Cocaine use, unspecified with cocaine-induced psychotic disorder, unspecified 🐾
        Cocaine-induced psychotic disorder, without use disorder

● **F14.98 Cocaine use, unspecified with other specified cocaine-induced disorder**

    F14.980 Cocaine use, unspecified with cocaine-induced anxiety disorder 🐾
        Cocaine-induced anxiety disorder, without use disorder

    F14.981 Cocaine use, unspecified with cocaine-induced sexual dysfunction 🐾
        Cocaine-induced sexual dysfunction, without use disorder

    F14.982 Cocaine use, unspecified with cocaine-induced sleep disorder 🐾
        Cocaine-induced sleep disorder, without use disorder

    F14.988 Cocaine use, unspecified with other cocaine-induced disorder 🐾
        Cocaine-induced obsessive-compulsive or related disorder

F14.99 Cocaine use, unspecified with unspecified cocaine-induced disorder 🐾

● **F15 Other stimulant related disorders**

    Includes amphetamine-related disorders
            caffeine

    Excludes2 cocaine-related disorders (F14.-)

● **F15.1 Other stimulant abuse**

    Excludes1 other stimulant dependence (F15.2-)
              other stimulant use, unspecified (F15.9-)

    F15.10 Other stimulant abuse, uncomplicated
        Amphetamine type substance use disorder, mild
        Other or unspecified stimulant use disorder, mild

    F15.11 Other stimulant abuse, in remission
        Amphetamine type substance use disorder, mild, in early remission
        Amphetamine type substance use disorder, mild, in sustained remission
        Other or unspecified stimulant use disorder, mild, in early remission
        Other or unspecified stimulant use disorder, mild, in sustained remission
        Coding Clinic: 2021, Q3, P8

● **F15.12 Other stimulant abuse with intoxication**

    F15.120 Other stimulant abuse with intoxication, uncomplicated 🐾

    F15.121 Other stimulant abuse with intoxication delirium 🐾

    F15.122 Other stimulant abuse with intoxication with perceptual disturbance 🐾
        Amphetamine or other stimulant use disorder, mild, with amphetamine or other stimulant intoxication, with perceptual disturbances

    F15.129 Other stimulant abuse with intoxication, unspecified 🐾
        Amphetamine or other stimulant use disorder, mild, with amphetamine or other stimulant intoxication, without perceptual disturbances

F15.13 Other stimulant abuse with withdrawal

F15.14 Other stimulant abuse with stimulant-induced mood disorder 🐾
    Amphetamine or other stimulant use disorder, mild, with amphetamine or other stimulant-induced bipolar or related disorder
    Amphetamine or other stimulant use disorder, mild, with amphetamine or other stimulant-induced depressive disorder

● **F15.15 Other stimulant abuse with stimulant-induced psychotic disorder**

    F15.150 Other stimulant abuse with stimulant-induced psychotic disorder with delusions 🐾

    F15.151 Other stimulant abuse with stimulant-induced psychotic disorder with hallucinations 🐾

    F15.159 Other stimulant abuse with stimulant-induced psychotic disorder, unspecified 🐾

● **F15.18**   **Other stimulant abuse with other stimulant-induced disorder**

     F15.180   Other stimulant abuse with stimulant-induced anxiety disorder 🐾

     F15.181   Other stimulant abuse with stimulant-induced sexual dysfunction 🐾

     F15.182   Other stimulant abuse with stimulant-induced sleep disorder 🐾

     F15.188   Other stimulant abuse with other stimulant-induced disorder 🐾

        Amphetamine or other stimulant use disorder, mild, with amphetamine or other stimulant-induced obsessive-compulsive or related disorder

     F15.19   **Other stimulant abuse with unspecified stimulant-induced disorder** 🐾

● **F15.2**   **Other stimulant dependence**

     Excludes1   other stimulant abuse (F15.1-)
                other stimulant use, unspecified (F15.9-)

     F15.20   **Other stimulant dependence, uncomplicated** 🐾

        Amphetamine type substance use disorder, moderate

        Amphetamine type substance use disorder, severe

        Other or unspecified stimulant use disorder, moderate

        Other or unspecified stimulant use disorder, severe

     F15.21   **Other stimulant dependence, in remission** 🐾

        Amphetamine type substance use disorder, moderate, in early remission

        Amphetamine type substance use disorder, moderate, in sustained remission

        Amphetamine type substance use disorder, severe, in early remission

        Amphetamine type substance use disorder, severe, in sustained remission

        Other or unspecified stimulant use disorder, moderate, in early remission

        Other or unspecified stimulant use disorder, moderate, in sustained remission

        Other or unspecified stimulant use disorder, severe, in early remission

        Other or unspecified stimulant use disorder, severe, in sustained remission

● **F15.22**   **Other stimulant dependence with intoxication**

     Excludes1   other stimulant dependence with withdrawal (F15.23)

     F15.220   Other stimulant dependence with intoxication, uncomplicated 🐾

     F15.221   Other stimulant dependence with intoxication delirium 🐾

     F15.222   Other stimulant dependence with intoxication with perceptual disturbance 🐾

        Amphetamine or other stimulant use disorder, moderate, with amphetamine or other stimulant intoxication, with perceptual disturbances

        Amphetamine or other stimulant use disorder, severe, with amphetamine or other stimulant intoxication, with perceptual disturbances

     F15.229   Other stimulant dependence with intoxication, unspecified 🐾

        Amphetamine or other stimulant use disorder, moderate, with amphetamine or other stimulant intoxication, without perceptual disturbances

        Amphetamine or other stimulant use disorder, severe, with amphetamine or other stimulant intoxication, without perceptual disturbances

     F15.23   **Other stimulant dependence with withdrawal** 🐾

        Amphetamine or other stimulant withdrawal

        Excludes1   other stimulant dependence with intoxication (F15.22-)

     F15.24   **Other stimulant dependence with stimulant-induced mood disorder** 🐾

        Amphetamine or other stimulant use disorder, moderate, with amphetamine or other stimulant-induced bipolar or related disorder

        Amphetamine or other stimulant use disorder, moderate, with amphetamine or other stimulant-induced depressive disorder

        Amphetamine or other stimulant use disorder, severe, with amphetamine or other stimulant-induced bipolar or related disorder

        Amphetamine or other stimulant use disorder, severe, with amphetamine or other stimulant-induced depressive disorder

● **F15.25**   **Other stimulant dependence with stimulant-induced psychotic disorder**

     F15.250   Other stimulant dependence with stimulant-induced psychotic disorder with delusions 🐾

     F15.251   Other stimulant dependence with stimulant-induced psychotic disorder with hallucinations 🐾

     F15.259   Other stimulant dependence with stimulant-induced psychotic disorder, unspecified 🐾

● **F15.28**   **Other stimulant dependence with other stimulant-induced disorder**

     F15.280   Other stimulant dependence with stimulant-induced anxiety disorder 🐾

     F15.281   Other stimulant dependence with stimulant-induced sexual dysfunction 🐾

     F15.282   Other stimulant dependence with stimulant-induced sleep disorder 🐾

     F15.288   Other stimulant dependence with other stimulant-induced disorder 🐾

        Amphetamine or other stimulant use disorder, moderate, with amphetamine or other stimulant-induced obsessive-compulsive or related disorder

        Amphetamine or other stimulant use disorder, severe, with amphetamine or other stimulant-induced obsessive-compulsive or related disorder

     F15.29   **Other stimulant dependence with unspecified stimulant-induced disorder** 🐾

● **F15.9 Other stimulant use, unspecified**
  Excludes1 other stimulant abuse (F15.1-)
            other stimulant dependence (F15.2-)

  F15.90 Other stimulant use, unspecified, uncomplicated

▶ **F15.91 Other stimulant use, unspecified, in remission**

● **F15.92 Other stimulant use, unspecified with intoxication**
  Excludes1 other stimulant use, unspecified with withdrawal (F15.93)

  F15.920 Other stimulant use, unspecified with intoxication, uncomplicated 🐾

  F15.921 Other stimulant use, unspecified with intoxication delirium 🐾
    Amphetamine or other stimulant-induced delirium

  F15.922 Other stimulant use, unspecified with intoxication with perceptual disturbance 🐾

  F15.929 Other stimulant use, unspecified with intoxication, unspecified 🐾
    Caffeine intoxication

  F15.93 Other stimulant use, unspecified with withdrawal 🐾
    Caffeine withdrawal
    Excludes1 other stimulant use, unspecified with intoxication (F15.92-)

  F15.94 Other stimulant use, unspecified with stimulant-induced mood disorder 🐾
    Amphetamine or other stimulant-induced bipolar or related disorder, without use disorder
    Amphetamine or other stimulant-induced depressive disorder, without use disorder

● **F15.95 Other stimulant use, unspecified with stimulant-induced psychotic disorder**

  F15.950 Other stimulant use, unspecified with stimulant-induced psychotic disorder with delusions 🐾

  F15.951 Other stimulant use, unspecified with stimulant-induced psychotic disorder with hallucinations 🐾

  F15.959 Other stimulant use, unspecified with stimulant-induced psychotic disorder, unspecified 🐾
    Amphetamine or other stimulant-induced psychotic disorder, without use disorder

● **F15.98 Other stimulant use, unspecified with other stimulant-induced disorder**

  F15.980 Other stimulant use, unspecified with stimulant-induced anxiety disorder 🐾
    Amphetamine or other stimulant-induced anxiety disorder, without use disorder
    Caffeine-induced anxiety disorder, without use disorder

  F15.981 Other stimulant use, unspecified with stimulant-induced sexual dysfunction 🐾
    Amphetamine or other stimulant-induced sexual dysfunction, without use disorder

  F15.982 Other stimulant use, unspecified with stimulant-induced sleep disorder 🐾
    Amphetamine or other stimulant-induced sleep disorder, without use disorder
    Caffeine-induced sleep disorder, without use disorder

  F15.988 Other stimulant use, unspecified with other stimulant-induced disorder 🐾
    Amphetamine or other stimulant-induced obsessive-compulsive or related disorder, without use disorder

  F15.99 Other stimulant use, unspecified with unspecified stimulant-induced disorder 🐾

● **F16 Hallucinogen related disorders**
  Includes ecstasy
            PCP
            phencyclidine

● **F16.1 Hallucinogen abuse**
  Excludes1 hallucinogen dependence (F16.2-)
            hallucinogen use, unspecified (F16.9-)

  F16.10 Hallucinogen abuse, uncomplicated
    Other hallucinogen use disorder, mild
    Phencyclidine use disorder, mild
    Coding Clinic: 2018, Q4, P31

  F16.11 Hallucinogen abuse, in remission
    Other hallucinogen use disorder, mild, in early remission
    Other hallucinogen use disorder, mild, in sustained remission
    Phencyclidine use disorder, mild, in early remission
    Phencyclidine use disorder, mild, in sustained remission

● **F16.12 Hallucinogen abuse with intoxication**

  F16.120 Hallucinogen abuse with intoxication, uncomplicated 🐾

  F16.121 Hallucinogen abuse with intoxication with delirium 🐾

  F16.122 Hallucinogen abuse with intoxication with perceptual disturbance 🐾

  F16.129 Hallucinogen abuse with intoxication, unspecified 🐾

  F16.14 Hallucinogen abuse with hallucinogen-induced mood disorder 🐾
    Other hallucinogen use disorder, mild, with other hallucinogen-induced bipolar or related disorder
    Other hallucinogen use disorder, mild, with other hallucinogen-induced depressive disorder
    Phencyclidine use disorder, mild, with phencyclidine-induced bipolar or related disorder
    Phencyclidine use disorder, mild, with phencyclidine-induced depressive disorder

● **F16.15 Hallucinogen abuse with hallucinogen-induced psychotic disorder**

  F16.150 Hallucinogen abuse with hallucinogen-induced psychotic disorder with delusions 🐾

  F16.151 Hallucinogen abuse with hallucinogen-induced psychotic disorder with hallucinations 🐾

  F16.159 Hallucinogen abuse with hallucinogen-induced psychotic disorder, unspecified 🐾

● F16.18   **Hallucinogen abuse with other hallucinogen-induced disorder**
    F16.180   **Hallucinogen abuse with hallucinogen-induced anxiety disorder** 🔖
    F16.183   **Hallucinogen abuse with hallucinogen persisting perception disorder (flashbacks)** 🔖
    F16.188   **Hallucinogen abuse with other hallucinogen-induced disorder** 🔖
  F16.19   **Hallucinogen abuse with unspecified hallucinogen-induced disorder** 🔖
● F16.2   **Hallucinogen dependence**
    Excludes1   hallucinogen abuse (F16.1-)
                 hallucinogen use, unspecified (F16.9-)
  F16.20   **Hallucinogen dependence, uncomplicated** 🔖
    Other hallucinogen use disorder, moderate
    Other hallucinogen use disorder, severe
    Phencyclidine use disorder, moderate
    Phencyclidine use disorder, severe
  F16.21   **Hallucinogen dependence, in remission** 🔖
    Other hallucinogen use disorder, moderate, in early remission
    Other hallucinogen use disorder, moderate, in sustained remission
    Other hallucinogen use disorder, severe, in early remission
    Other hallucinogen use disorder, severe, in sustained remission
    Phencyclidine use disorder, moderate, in early remission
    Phencyclidine use disorder, moderate, in sustained remission
    Phencyclidine use disorder, severe, in early remission
    Phencyclidine use disorder, severe, in sustained remission
● F16.22   **Hallucinogen dependence with intoxication**
    F16.220   **Hallucinogen dependence with intoxication, uncomplicated** 🔖
    F16.221   **Hallucinogen dependence with intoxication with delirium** 🔖
    F16.229   **Hallucinogen dependence with intoxication, unspecified** 🔖
  F16.24   **Hallucinogen dependence with hallucinogen-induced mood disorder** 🔖
    Other hallucinogen use disorder, moderate, with other hallucinogen-induced bipolar or related disorder
    Other hallucinogen use disorder, moderate, with other hallucinogen-induced depressive disorder
    Other hallucinogen use disorder, severe, with other hallucinogen-induced bipolar or related disorder
    Other hallucinogen use disorder, severe, with other hallucinogen-induced depressive disorder
    Phencyclidine use disorder, moderate, with phencyclidine-induced bipolar or related disorder
    Phencyclidine use disorder, moderate, with phencyclidine-induced depressive disorder
    Phencyclidine use disorder, severe, with phencyclidine-induced bipolar or related disorder
    Phencyclidine use disorder, severe, with phencyclidine-induced depressive disorder

● F16.25   **Hallucinogen dependence with hallucinogen-induced psychotic disorder**
    F16.250   **Hallucinogen dependence with hallucinogen-induced psychotic disorder with delusions** 🔖
    F16.251   **Hallucinogen dependence with hallucinogen-induced psychotic disorder with hallucinations** 🔖
    F16.259   **Hallucinogen dependence with hallucinogen-induced psychotic disorder, unspecified** 🔖
● F16.28   **Hallucinogen dependence with other hallucinogen-induced disorder**
    F16.280   **Hallucinogen dependence with hallucinogen-induced anxiety disorder** 🔖
    F16.283   **Hallucinogen dependence with hallucinogen persisting perception disorder (flashbacks)** 🔖
    F16.288   **Hallucinogen dependence with other hallucinogen-induced disorder** 🔖
  F16.29   **Hallucinogen dependence with unspecified hallucinogen-induced disorder** 🔖
● F16.9   **Hallucinogen use, unspecified**
    Excludes1   hallucinogen abuse (F16.1-)
                 hallucinogen dependence (F16.2-)
  F16.90   **Hallucinogen use, unspecified, uncomplicated**
▶ F16.91   **Hallucinogen use, unspecified, in remission**
● F16.92   **Hallucinogen use, unspecified with intoxication**
    F16.920   **Hallucinogen use, unspecified with intoxication, uncomplicated** 🔖
    F16.921   **Hallucinogen use, unspecified with intoxication with delirium** 🔖
        Other hallucinogen intoxication delirium
    F16.929   **Hallucinogen use, unspecified with intoxication, unspecified** 🔖
  F16.94   **Hallucinogen use, unspecified with hallucinogen-induced mood disorder** 🔖
    Other hallucinogen-induced bipolar or related disorder, without use disorder
    Other hallucinogen-induced depressive disorder, without use disorder
    Phencyclidine-induced bipolar or related disorder, without use disorder
    Phencyclidine-induced depressive disorder, without use disorder
● F16.95   **Hallucinogen use, unspecified with hallucinogen-induced psychotic disorder**
    F16.950   **Hallucinogen use, unspecified with hallucinogen-induced psychotic disorder with delusions** 🔖
    F16.951   **Hallucinogen use, unspecified with hallucinogen-induced psychotic disorder with hallucinations** 🔖
    F16.959   **Hallucinogen use, unspecified with hallucinogen-induced psychotic disorder, unspecified** 🔖
        Other hallucinogen-induced psychotic disorder, without use disorder
        Phencyclidine-induced psychotic disorder, without use disorder
● F16.98   **Hallucinogen use, unspecified with other specified hallucinogen-induced disorder**
    F16.980   **Hallucinogen use, unspecified with hallucinogen-induced anxiety disorder** 🔖
        Other hallucinogen-induced anxiety disorder, without use disorder
        Phencyclidine-induced anxiety disorder, without use disorder

CHAPTER 5 (F01-F99)

CHAPTER 5 (F01-F99)

F16.983   **Hallucinogen use, unspecified with hallucinogen persisting perception disorder (flashbacks)** 🗝

F16.988   **Hallucinogen use, unspecified with other hallucinogen-induced disorder** 🗝

F16.99   **Hallucinogen use, unspecified with unspecified hallucinogen-induced disorder** 🗝

● **F17**   **Nicotine dependence**

     Excludes1   history of tobacco dependence (Z87.891)
                  tobacco use NOS (Z72.0)

     Excludes2   tobacco use (smoking) during pregnancy, childbirth and the puerperium (O99.33-)
                  toxic effect of nicotine (T65.2-)

   ● **F17.2**   **Nicotine dependence**

     ● **F17.20**   **Nicotine dependence, unspecified**

        F17.200   **Nicotine dependence, unspecified, uncomplicated**
                Tobacco use disorder, mild
                Tobacco use disorder, moderate
                Tobacco use disorder, severe
                Coding Clinic: 2016, Q1, P37

        F17.201   **Nicotine dependence, unspecified, in remission**
                Tobacco use disorder, mild, in early remission
                Tobacco use disorder, mild, in sustained remission
                Tobacco use disorder, moderate, in early remission
                Tobacco use disorder, moderate, in sustained remission
                Tobacco use disorder, severe, in early remission
                Tobacco use disorder, severe, in sustained remission

        F17.203   **Nicotine dependence unspecified, with withdrawal**
                Tobacco withdrawal

        F17.208   **Nicotine dependence, unspecified, with other nicotine-induced disorders**

        F17.209   **Nicotine dependence, unspecified, with unspecified nicotine-induced disorders**

     ● **F17.21**   **Nicotine dependence, cigarettes**

        F17.210   **Nicotine dependence, cigarettes, uncomplicated**
                Coding Clinic: 2017, Q2, P28-29

        F17.211   **Nicotine dependence, cigarettes, in remission**
                Tobacco use disorder, cigarettes, mild, in early remission
                Tobacco use disorder, cigarettes, mild, in sustained remission
                Tobacco use disorder, cigarettes, moderate, in early remission
                Tobacco use disorder, cigarettes, moderate, in sustained remission
                Tobacco use disorder, cigarettes, severe, in early remission
                Tobacco use disorder, cigarettes, severe, in sustained remission

        F17.213   **Nicotine dependence, cigarettes, with withdrawal**

        F17.218   **Nicotine dependence, cigarettes, with other nicotine-induced disorders**

        F17.219   **Nicotine dependence, cigarettes, with unspecified nicotine-induced disorders**

     ● **F17.22**   **Nicotine dependence, chewing tobacco**

        F17.220   **Nicotine dependence, chewing tobacco, uncomplicated**

        F17.221   **Nicotine dependence, chewing tobacco, in remission**
                Tobacco use disorder, chewing tobacco, mild, in early remission
                Tobacco use disorder, chewing tobacco, mild, in sustained remission
                Tobacco use disorder, chewing tobacco, moderate, in early remission
                Tobacco use disorder, chewing tobacco, moderate, in sustained remission
                Tobacco use disorder, chewing tobacco, severe, in early remission
                Tobacco use disorder, chewing tobacco, severe, in sustained remission

        F17.223   **Nicotine dependence, chewing tobacco, with withdrawal**

        F17.228   **Nicotine dependence, chewing tobacco, with other nicotine-induced disorders**

        F17.229   **Nicotine dependence, chewing tobacco, with unspecified nicotine-induced disorders**

     ● **F17.29**   **Nicotine dependence, other tobacco product**

        F17.290   **Nicotine dependence, other tobacco product, uncomplicated**
                Coding Clinic: 2017, Q2, P28-29

        F17.291   **Nicotine dependence, other tobacco product, in remission**
                Tobacco use disorder, other tobacco product, mild, in early remission
                Tobacco use disorder, other tobacco product, mild, in sustained remission
                Tobacco use disorder, other tobacco product, moderate, in early remission
                Tobacco use disorder, other tobacco product, moderate, in sustained remission
                Tobacco use disorder, other tobacco product, severe, in early remission
                Tobacco use disorder, other tobacco product, severe, in sustained remission

        F17.293   **Nicotine dependence, other tobacco product, with withdrawal**

        F17.298   **Nicotine dependence, other tobacco product, with other nicotine-induced disorders**

        F17.299   **Nicotine dependence, other tobacco product, with unspecified nicotine-induced disorders**

● **F18**   **Inhalant related disorders**

     Includes   volatile solvents

   ● **F18.1**   **Inhalant abuse**

     Excludes1   inhalant dependence (F18.2-)
                  inhalant use, unspecified (F18.9-)

        F18.10   **Inhalant abuse, uncomplicated**
                Inhalant use disorder, mild

        F18.11   **Inhalant abuse, in remission**
                Inhalant use disorder, mild, in early remission
                Inhalant use disorder, mild, in sustained remission

▶ New   ⇒ Revised   ~~deleted~~ Deleted   Excludes 1   Excludes 2   Includes   Use additional   Code first   Code also   Key words

OGCR Official Guidelines   X Assign placeholder X   ● Use Additional Character(s)   ▶ Manifestation Code   🗝 Hierarchical Condition Category   Coding Clinic

● **F18.12   Inhalant abuse with intoxication**
   F18.120   Inhalant abuse with intoxication, uncomplicated
   F18.121   Inhalant abuse with intoxication delirium
   F18.129   Inhalant abuse with intoxication, unspecified
  F18.14   Inhalant abuse with inhalant-induced mood disorder
    Inhalant use disorder, mild, with inhalant-induced depressive disorder
● **F18.15   Inhalant abuse with inhalant-induced psychotic disorder**
   F18.150   Inhalant abuse with inhalant-induced psychotic disorder with delusions
   F18.151   Inhalant abuse with inhalant-induced psychotic disorder with hallucinations
   F18.159   Inhalant abuse with inhalant-induced psychotic disorder, unspecified
  F18.17   Inhalant abuse with inhalant-induced dementia
    Inhalant use disorder, mild, with inhalant-induced major neurocognitive disorder
● **F18.18   Inhalant abuse with other inhalant-induced disorders**
   F18.180   Inhalant abuse with inhalant-induced anxiety disorder
   F18.188   Inhalant abuse with other inhalant-induced disorder
    Inhalant use disorder, mild, with inhalant-induced mild neurocognitive disorder
  F18.19   Inhalant abuse with unspecified inhalant-induced disorder
● **F18.2   Inhalant dependence**
   Excludes1   inhalant abuse (F18.1-)
     inhalant use, unspecified (F18.9-)
  F18.20   Inhalant dependence, uncomplicated
    Inhalant use disorder, moderate
    Inhalant use disorder, severe
  F18.21   Inhalant dependence, in remission
    Inhalant use disorder, moderate, in early remission
    Inhalant use disorder, moderate, in sustained remission
    Inhalant use disorder, severe, in early remission
    Inhalant use disorder, severe, in sustained remission
● **F18.22   Inhalant dependence with intoxication**
   F18.220   Inhalant dependence with intoxication, uncomplicated
   F18.221   Inhalant dependence with intoxication delirium
   F18.229   Inhalant dependence with intoxication, unspecified
  F18.24   Inhalant dependence with inhalant-induced mood disorder
    Inhalant use disorder, moderate, with inhalant-induced depressive disorder
    Inhalant use disorder, severe, with inhalant-induced depressive disorder
● **F18.25   Inhalant dependence with inhalant-induced psychotic disorder**
   F18.250   Inhalant dependence with inhalant-induced psychotic disorder with delusions

   F18.251   Inhalant dependence with inhalant-induced psychotic disorder with hallucinations
   F18.259   Inhalant dependence with inhalant-induced psychotic disorder, unspecified
  F18.27   Inhalant dependence with inhalant-induced dementia
    Inhalant use disorder, moderate, with inhalant-induced major neurocognitive disorder
    Inhalant use disorder, severe, with inhalant-induced major neurocognitive disorder
● **F18.28   Inhalant dependence with other inhalant-induced disorders**
   F18.280   Inhalant dependence with inhalant-induced anxiety disorder
   F18.288   Inhalant dependence with other inhalant-induced disorder
    Inhalant use disorder, moderate, with inhalant-induced mild neurocognitive disorder
    Inhalant use disorder, severe, with inhalant-induced mild neurocognitive disorder
  F18.29   Inhalant dependence with unspecified inhalant-induced disorder
● **F18.9   Inhalant use, unspecified**
   Excludes1   inhalant abuse (F18.1-)
     inhalant dependence (F18.2-)
  F18.90   Inhalant use, unspecified, uncomplicated
▶ **F18.91   Inhalant use, unspecified, in remission**
● **F18.92   Inhalant use, unspecified with intoxication**
   F18.920   Inhalant use, unspecified with intoxication, uncomplicated
   F18.921   Inhalant use, unspecified with intoxication with delirium
   F18.929   Inhalant use, unspecified with intoxication, unspecified
  F18.94   Inhalant use, unspecified with inhalant-induced mood disorder
    Inhalant-induced depressive disorder
● **F18.95   Inhalant use, unspecified with inhalant-induced psychotic disorder**
   F18.950   Inhalant use, unspecified with inhalant-induced psychotic disorder with delusions
   F18.951   Inhalant use, unspecified with inhalant-induced psychotic disorder with hallucinations
   F18.959   Inhalant use, unspecified with inhalant-induced psychotic disorder, unspecified
  F18.97   Inhalant use, unspecified with inhalant-induced persisting dementia
    Inhalant-induced major neurocognitive disorder
● **F18.98   Inhalant use, unspecified with other inhalant-induced disorders**
   F18.980   Inhalant use, unspecified with inhalant-induced anxiety disorder
   F18.988   Inhalant use, unspecified with other inhalant-induced disorder
    Inhalant-induced mild neurocognitive disorder
  F18.99   Inhalant use, unspecified with unspecified inhalant-induced disorder

● **F19**   **Other psychoactive substance related disorders**

    Includes   polysubstance drug use (indiscriminate drug use)

● **F19.1**   **Other psychoactive substance abuse**

    Excludes1   other psychoactive substance dependence (F19.2-)

                    other psychoactive substance use, unspecified (F19.9-)

  F19.10   **Other psychoactive substance abuse, uncomplicated**

      Other (or unknown) substance use disorder, mild

  F19.11   **Other psychoactive substance abuse, in remission**

      Other (or unknown) substance use disorder, mild, in early remission

      Other (or unknown) substance use disorder, mild, in sustained remission

● **F19.12**   **Other psychoactive substance abuse with intoxication**

    F19.120   **Other psychoactive substance abuse with intoxication, uncomplicated** 🖭

    F19.121   **Other psychoactive substance abuse with intoxication delirium** 🖭

    F19.122   **Other psychoactive substance abuse with intoxication with perceptual disturbances** 🖭

    F19.129   **Other psychoactive substance abuse with intoxication, unspecified** 🖭

● **F19.13**   **Other psychoactive substance abuse with withdrawal**

    F19.130   **Other psychoactive substance abuse with withdrawal, uncomplicated**

    F19.131   **Other psychoactive substance abuse with withdrawal delirium**

    F19.132   **Other psychoactive substance abuse with withdrawal with perceptual disturbance**

    F19.139   **Other psychoactive substance abuse with withdrawal, unspecified**

  F19.14   **Other psychoactive substance abuse with psychoactive substance-induced mood disorder** 🖭

      Other (or unknown) substance use disorder, mild, with other (or unknown) substance-induced bipolar or related disorder

      Other (or unknown) substance use disorder, mild, with other (or unknown) substance-induced depressive disorder

● **F19.15**   **Other psychoactive substance abuse with psychoactive substance-induced psychotic disorder**

    F19.150   **Other psychoactive substance abuse with psychoactive substance-induced psychotic disorder with delusions** 🖭

    F19.151   **Other psychoactive substance abuse with psychoactive substance-induced psychotic disorder with hallucinations** 🖭

    F19.159   **Other psychoactive substance abuse with psychoactive substance-induced psychotic disorder, unspecified** 🖭

  F19.16   **Other psychoactive substance abuse with psychoactive substance-induced persisting amnestic disorder** 🖭

  F19.17   **Other psychoactive substance abuse with psychoactive substance-induced persisting dementia** 🖭

      Other (or unknown) substance use disorder, mild, with other (or unknown) substance-induced major neurocognitive disorder

● **F19.18**   **Other psychoactive substance abuse with other psychoactive substance-induced disorders**

  F19.180   **Other psychoactive substance abuse with psychoactive substance-induced anxiety disorder** 🖭

  F19.181   **Other psychoactive substance abuse with psychoactive substance-induced sexual dysfunction** 🖭

  F19.182   **Other psychoactive substance abuse with psychoactive substance-induced sleep disorder** 🖭

  F19.188   **Other psychoactive substance abuse with other psychoactive substance-induced disorder** 🖭

      Other (or unknown) substance use disorder, mild, with other (or unknown) substance-induced mild neurocognitive disorder

      Other (or unknown) substance use disorder, mild, with other (or unknown) substance-induced obsessive-compulsive or related disorder

  F19.19   **Other psychoactive substance abuse with unspecified psychoactive substance-induced disorder** 🖭

● **F19.2**   **Other psychoactive substance dependence**

    Excludes1   other psychoactive substance abuse (F19.1-)

                    other psychoactive substance use, unspecified (F19.9-)

  F19.20   **Other psychoactive substance dependence, uncomplicated** 🖭

      Other (or unknown) substance use disorder, moderate

      Other (or unknown) substance use disorder, severe

  F19.21   **Other psychoactive substance dependence, in remission** 🖭

      Other (or unknown) substance use disorder, moderate, in early remission

      Other (or unknown) substance use disorder, moderate, in sustained remission

      Other (or unknown) substance use disorder, severe, in early remission

      Other (or unknown) substance use disorder, severe, in sustained remission

● **F19.22**   **Other psychoactive substance dependence with intoxication**

    Excludes1   other psychoactive substance dependence with withdrawal (F19.23-)

  F19.220   **Other psychoactive substance dependence with intoxication, uncomplicated** 🖭

  F19.221   **Other psychoactive substance dependence with intoxication delirium** 🖭

  F19.222   **Other psychoactive substance dependence with intoxication with perceptual disturbance** 🖭

  F19.229   **Other psychoactive substance dependence with intoxication, unspecified** 🖭

● F19.23 Other psychoactive substance dependence with withdrawal

  Excludes1   other psychoactive substance dependence with intoxication (F19.22-)

  F19.230 Other psychoactive substance dependence with withdrawal, uncomplicated 🦠

  F19.231 Other psychoactive substance dependence with withdrawal delirium 🦠

  F19.232 Other psychoactive substance dependence with withdrawal with perceptual disturbance 🦠

  F19.239 Other psychoactive substance dependence with withdrawal, unspecified 🦠

F19.24 Other psychoactive substance dependence with psychoactive substance-induced mood disorder 🦠

  Other (or unknown) substance use disorder, moderate, with other (or unknown) substance-induced bipolar or related disorder

  Other (or unknown) substance use disorder, moderate, with other (or unknown) substance-induced depressive disorder

  Other (or unknown) substance use disorder, severe, with other (or unknown) substance-induced bipolar or related disorder

  Other (or unknown) substance use disorder, severe, with other (or unknown) substance-induced depressive disorder

● F19.25 Other psychoactive substance dependence with psychoactive substance-induced psychotic disorder

  F19.250 Other psychoactive substance dependence with psychoactive substance-induced psychotic disorder with delusions 🦠

  F19.251 Other psychoactive substance dependence with psychoactive substance-induced psychotic disorder with hallucinations 🦠

  F19.259 Other psychoactive substance dependence with psychoactive substance-induced psychotic disorder, unspecified 🦠

F19.26 Other psychoactive substance dependence with psychoactive substance-induced persisting amnestic disorder 🦠

F19.27 Other psychoactive substance dependence with psychoactive substance-induced persisting dementia 🦠

  Other (or unknown) substance use disorder, moderate, with other (or unknown) substance-induced major neurocognitive disorder

  Other (or unknown) substance use disorder, severe, with other (or unknown) substance-induced major neurocognitive disorder

● F19.28 Other psychoactive substance dependence with other psychoactive substance-induced disorders

  F19.280 Other psychoactive substance dependence with psychoactive substance-induced anxiety disorder 🦠

  F19.281 Other psychoactive substance dependence with psychoactive substance-induced sexual dysfunction 🦠

  F19.282 Other psychoactive substance dependence with psychoactive substance-induced sleep disorder 🦠

F19.288 Other psychoactive substance dependence with other psychoactive substance-induced disorder 🦠

  Other (or unknown) substance use disorder, moderate, with other (or unknown) substance-induced mild neurocognitive disorder

  Other (or unknown) substance use disorder, severe, with other (or unknown) substance-induced mild neurocognitive disorder

  Other (or unknown) substance use disorder, moderate, with other (or unknown) substance-induced obsessive-compulsive or related disorder

  Other (or unknown) substance use disorder, severe, with other (or unknown) substance-induced obsessive-compulsive or related disorder

F19.29 Other psychoactive substance dependence with unspecified psychoactive substance-induced disorder 🦠

● F19.9 Other psychoactive substance use, unspecified

  Excludes1   other psychoactive substance abuse (F19.1-)
              other psychoactive substance dependence (F19.2-)

  F19.90 Other psychoactive substance use, unspecified, uncomplicated

▶ F19.91 Other psychoactive substance use, unspecified, in remission

● F19.92 Other psychoactive substance use, unspecified with intoxication

  Excludes1   other psychoactive substance use, unspecified with withdrawal (F19.93)

  F19.920 Other psychoactive substance use, unspecified with intoxication, uncomplicated 🦠

  F19.921 Other psychoactive substance use, unspecified with intoxication with delirium 🦠

    Other (or unknown) substance-induced delirium

  F19.922 Other psychoactive substance use, unspecified with intoxication with perceptual disturbance 🦠

  F19.929 Other psychoactive substance use, unspecified with intoxication, unspecified 🦠

● F19.93 Other psychoactive substance use, unspecified with withdrawal

  Excludes1   other psychoactive substance use, unspecified with intoxication (F19.92-)

  F19.930 Other psychoactive substance use, unspecified with withdrawal, uncomplicated 🦠

  F19.931 Other psychoactive substance use, unspecified with withdrawal delirium 🦠

  F19.932 Other psychoactive substance use, unspecified with withdrawal with perceptual disturbance 🦠

  F19.939 Other psychoactive substance use, unspecified with withdrawal, unspecified 🦠

CHAPTER 5 (F01-F99)

F19.94 **Other psychoactive substance use, unspecified with psychoactive substance-induced mood disorder** 🜀
    Other (or unknown) substance-induced bipolar or related disorder, without use disorder
    Other (or unknown) substance-induced depressive disorder, without use disorder

● **F19.95** **Other psychoactive substance use, unspecified with psychoactive substance-induced psychotic disorder**

    F19.950 **Other psychoactive substance use, unspecified with psychoactive substance-induced psychotic disorder with delusions** 🜀

    F19.951 **Other psychoactive substance use, unspecified with psychoactive substance-induced psychotic disorder with hallucinations** 🜀

    F19.959 **Other psychoactive substance use, unspecified with psychoactive substance-induced psychotic disorder, unspecified** 🜀
        Other or unknown substance-induced psychotic disorder, without use disorder

F19.96 **Other psychoactive substance use, unspecified with psychoactive substance-induced persisting amnestic disorder** 🜀

F19.97 **Other psychoactive substance use, unspecified with psychoactive substance-induced persisting dementia** 🜀
    Other (or unknown) substance-induced major neurocognitive disorder, without use disorder

● **F19.98** **Other psychoactive substance use, unspecified with other psychoactive substance-induced disorders**

    F19.980 **Other psychoactive substance use, unspecified with psychoactive substance-induced anxiety disorder** 🜀
        Other (or unknown) substance-induced anxiety disorder, without use disorder

    F19.981 **Other psychoactive substance use, unspecified with psychoactive substance-induced sexual dysfunction** 🜀
        Other (or unknown) substance-induced sexual dysfunction, without use disorder

    F19.982 **Other psychoactive substance use, unspecified with psychoactive substance-induced sleep disorder** 🜀
        Other (or unknown) substance-induced sleep disorder, without use disorder

    F19.988 **Other psychoactive substance use, unspecified with other psychoactive substance-induced disorder** 🜀
        Other (or unknown) substance-induced mild neurocognitive disorder, without use disorder
        Other (or unknown) substance-induced obsessive-compulsive or related disorder, without use disorder

F19.99 **Other psychoactive substance use, unspecified with unspecified psychoactive substance-induced disorder** 🜀

SCHIZOPHRENIA, SCHIZOTYPAL, DELUSIONAL, AND OTHER NON-MOOD PSYCHOTIC DISORDERS (F20-F29)

● **F20** **Schizophrenia**
Personality disorders characterized by multiple mental and behavioral irregularities (may exhibit disorganized thinking, delusions, and auditory hallucinations)

    Excludes1 brief psychotic disorder (F23)
        cyclic schizophrenia (F25.0)
        mood [affective] disorders with psychotic symptoms (F30.2, F31.2, F31.5, F31.64, F32.3, F33.3)
        schizoaffective disorder (F25.-)
        schizophrenic reaction NOS (F23)

    Excludes2 schizophrenic reaction in:
        alcoholism (F10.15-, F10.25-, F10.95-)
        brain disease (F06.2)
        epilepsy (F06.2)
        psychoactive drug use (F11-F19 with .15, .25, .95)
        schizotypal disorder (F21)
    Coding Clinic: 2019, Q2, P32

F20.0 **Paranoid schizophrenia** 🜀
    Paraphrenic schizophrenia
    Excludes1 involutional paranoid state (F22)
        paranoia (F22)

F20.1 **Disorganized schizophrenia** 🜀
    Hebephrenic schizophrenia
    Hebephrenia

F20.2 **Catatonic schizophrenia** 🜀
    Schizophrenic catalepsy
    Schizophrenic catatonia
    Schizophrenic flexibilitas cerea
    Excludes1 catatonic stupor (R40.1)

F20.3 **Undifferentiated schizophrenia** 🜀
    Atypical schizophrenia
    Excludes1 acute schizophrenia-like psychotic disorder (F23)
    Excludes2 post-schizophrenic depression (F32.89)

F20.5 **Residual schizophrenia** 🜀
    Restzustand (schizophrenic)
    Schizophrenic residual state

● **F20.8** **Other schizophrenia**

    F20.81 **Schizophreniform disorder** 🜀
        Schizophreniform psychosis NOS

    F20.89 **Other schizophrenia** 🜀
        Cenesthopathic schizophrenia
        Simple schizophrenia

F20.9 **Schizophrenia, unspecified** 🜀
    Coding Clinic: 2019, Q2, P32

F21 **Schizotypal disorder**
Personality disorder characterized by need for social isolation, odd behavior and thinking, and often unconventional beliefs
    Borderline schizophrenia
    Latent schizophrenia
    Latent schizophrenic reaction
    Prepsychotic schizophrenia
    Prodromal schizophrenia
    Pseudoneurotic schizophrenia
    Pseudopsychopathic schizophrenia
    Schizotypal personality disorder
    Excludes2 Asperger's syndrome (F84.5)
        schizoid personality disorder (F60.1)

▶ New   ⇒ Revised   ~~deleted~~ Deleted   Excludes 1   Excludes 2   Includes   Use additional   Code first   Code also   Key words
OGCR Official Guidelines   X Assign placeholder X   ● Use Additional Character(s)   ▷ Manifestation Code   🜀 Hierarchical Condition Category   Coding Clinic

F22   **Delusional disorders** 🔍
    Delusional dysmorphophobia
    Involutional paranoid state
    Paranoia
    Paranoia querulans
    Paranoid psychosis
    Paranoid state
    Paraphrenia (late)
    Sensitiver Beziehungswahn

> **Excludes1**   mood [affective] disorders with psychotic symptoms (F30.2, F31.2, F31.5, F31.64, F32.3, F33.3)
>   paranoid schizophrenia (F20.0)
> **Excludes2**   paranoid personality disorder (F60.0)
>   paranoid psychosis, psychogenic (F23)
>   paranoid reaction (F23)

F23   **Brief psychotic disorder**
    Paranoid reaction
    Psychogenic paranoid psychosis

> **Excludes2**   mood [affective] disorders with psychotic symptoms (F30.2, F31.2, F31.5, F31.64, F32.3, F33.3)

    Coding Clinic: 2019, Q2, P32

F24   **Shared psychotic disorder** 🔍
    Folie à deux
    Induced paranoid disorder
    Induced psychotic disorder

● **F25**   **Schizoaffective disorders**
    Mental disorder exhibiting major depressive episode, manic episode, or mixed episode occurs with symptoms of schizophrenia, and mood disorder

> **Excludes1**   mood [affective] disorders with psychotic symptoms (F30.2, F31.2, F31.5, F31.64, F32.3, F33.3)
>   schizophrenia (F20.-)

    F25.0   **Schizoaffective disorder, bipolar type** 🔍
        Cyclic schizophrenia
        Schizoaffective disorder, manic type
        Schizoaffective disorder, mixed type
        Schizoaffective psychosis, bipolar type

    F25.1   **Schizoaffective disorder, depressive type** 🔍
        Schizoaffective psychosis, depressive type

    F25.8   **Other schizoaffective disorders** 🔍

    F25.9   **Schizoaffective disorder, unspecified** 🔍
        Schizoaffective psychosis NOS

F28   **Other psychotic disorder not due to a substance or known physiological condition**
    Chronic hallucinatory psychosis
    Other specified schizophrenia spectrum and other psychotic disorder

F29   **Unspecified psychosis not due to a substance or known physiological condition**
    Psychosis NOS
    Unspecified schizophrenia spectrum and other psychotic disorder

> **Excludes1**   mental disorder NOS (F99)
>   unspecified mental disorder due to known physiological condition (F09)

MOOD [AFFECTIVE] DISORDERS (F30-F39)

● **F30**   **Manic episode**
    Elevated, expansive, or irritable mood

> **Includes**   bipolar disorder, single manic episode
>   mixed affective episode
> **Excludes1**   bipolar disorder (F31.-)
>   major depressive disorder, single episode (F32.-)
>   major depressive disorder, recurrent (F33.-)

    ● **F30.1**   **Manic episode without psychotic symptoms**
        F30.10   Manic episode without psychotic symptoms, unspecified 🔍
        F30.11   Manic episode without psychotic symptoms, mild 🔍

        F30.12   Manic episode without psychotic symptoms, moderate 🔍
        F30.13   Manic episode, severe, without psychotic symptoms 🔍

    F30.2   **Manic episode, severe with psychotic symptoms** 🔍
        Manic stupor
        Mania with mood-congruent psychotic symptoms
        Mania with mood-incongruent psychotic symptoms

    F30.3   **Manic episode in partial remission** 🔍

    F30.4   **Manic episode in full remission** 🔍

    F30.8   **Other manic episodes** 🔍
        Abnormality of mood resembling mania but less intense
        Hypomania

    F30.9   **Manic episode, unspecified** 🔍
        Mania NOS

● **F31**   **Bipolar disorder**
    Mood disorders with history of manic, mixed, or hypomanic episodes

> **Includes**   bipolar I disorder
>   bipolar type I disorder
>   manic-depressive illness
>   manic-depressive psychosis
>   manic-depressive reaction
> ▶   seasonal bipolar disorder
> **Excludes1**   bipolar disorder, single manic episode (F30.-)
>   major depressive disorder, single episode (F32.-)
>   major depressive disorder, recurrent (F33.-)
> **Excludes2**   cyclothymia (F34.0)

    Coding Clinic: 2020, Q1, P23

    F31.0   **Bipolar disorder, current episode hypomanic** 🔍

    ● **F31.1**   **Bipolar disorder, current episode manic without psychotic features**
        F31.10   Bipolar disorder, current episode manic without psychotic features, unspecified 🔍
        F31.11   Bipolar disorder, current episode manic without psychotic features, mild 🔍
        F31.12   Bipolar disorder, current episode manic without psychotic features, moderate 🔍
        F31.13   Bipolar disorder, current episode manic without psychotic features, severe 🔍

    F31.2   **Bipolar disorder, current episode manic severe with psychotic features** 🔍
        Bipolar disorder, current episode manic with mood-congruent psychotic symptoms
        Bipolar disorder, current episode manic with mood-incongruent psychotic symptoms
        Bipolar I disorder, current or most recent episode manic with psychotic features

    ● **F31.3**   **Bipolar disorder, current episode depressed, mild or moderate severity**
        F31.30   Bipolar disorder, current episode depressed, mild or moderate severity, unspecified 🔍
        F31.31   Bipolar disorder, current episode depressed, mild 🔍
        F31.32   Bipolar disorder, current episode depressed, moderate 🔍

    F31.4   **Bipolar disorder, current episode depressed, severe, without psychotic features** 🔍

    F31.5   **Bipolar disorder, current episode depressed, severe, with psychotic features** 🔍
        Bipolar disorder, current episode depressed with mood-incongruent psychotic symptoms
        Bipolar disorder, current episode depressed with mood-congruent psychotic symptoms
        Bipolar I disorder, current or most recent episode depressed, with psychotic features

    ● **F31.6**   **Bipolar disorder, current episode mixed**
        F31.60   Bipolar disorder, current episode mixed, unspecified 🔍
        F31.61   Bipolar disorder, current episode mixed, mild 🔍

F31.62   Bipolar disorder, current episode mixed, moderate 🐾

F31.63   Bipolar disorder, current episode mixed, severe, without psychotic features 🐾

F31.64   Bipolar disorder, current episode mixed, severe, with psychotic features 🐾
　　　　　Bipolar disorder, current episode mixed with mood-congruent psychotic symptoms
　　　　　Bipolar disorder, current episode mixed with mood-incongruent psychotic symptoms

● F31.7   Bipolar disorder, currently in remission

F31.70   Bipolar disorder, currently in remission, most recent episode unspecified 🐾

F31.71   Bipolar disorder, in partial remission, most recent episode hypomanic 🐾

F31.72   Bipolar disorder, in full remission, most recent episode hypomanic 🐾

F31.73   Bipolar disorder, in partial remission, most recent episode manic 🐾

F31.74   Bipolar disorder, in full remission, most recent episode manic 🐾

F31.75   Bipolar disorder, in partial remission, most recent episode depressed 🐾

F31.76   Bipolar disorder, in full remission, most recent episode depressed 🐾

F31.77   Bipolar disorder, in partial remission, most recent episode mixed 🐾

F31.78   Bipolar disorder, in full remission, most recent episode mixed 🐾

● F31.8   Other bipolar disorders

F31.81   Bipolar II disorder 🐾
　　　　　Bipolar disorder, type 2

F31.89   Other bipolar disorder 🐾
　　　　　Recurrent manic episodes NOS

F31.9   Bipolar disorder, unspecified 🐾
　　　　Manic depression
　　　　Coding Clinic: 2020, Q1, P23

● F32   Depressive episode

Includes   single episode of agitated depression
　　　　　single episode of depressive reaction
　　　　　single episode of major depression
　　　　　single episode of psychogenic depression
　　　　　single episode of reactive depression
　　　　　single episode of vital depression

Excludes1   bipolar disorder (F31.-)
　　　　　　manic episode (F30.-)
　　　　　　recurrent depressive disorder (F33.-)

Excludes2   adjustment disorder (F43.2)

F32.0   Major depressive disorder, single episode, mild 🐾

F32.1   Major depressive disorder, single episode, moderate 🐾

F32.2   Major depressive disorder, single episode, severe without psychotic features 🐾

F32.3   Major depressive disorder, single episode, severe with psychotic features 🐾
　　　　Single episode of major depression with mood-congruent psychotic symptoms
　　　　Single episode of major depression with mood-incongruent psychotic symptoms
　　　　Single episode of major depression with psychotic symptoms
　　　　Single episode of psychogenic depressive psychosis
　　　　Single episode of psychotic depression
　　　　Single episode of reactive depressive psychosis

F32.4   Major depressive disorder, single episode, in partial remission 🐾

F32.5   Major depressive disorder, single episode, in full remission 🐾

● F32.8   Other depressive episodes

F32.81   Premenstrual dysphoric disorder ♀

Excludes1   premenstrual tension syndrome (N94.3)
Coding Clinic: 2016, Q4, P14

Figure 5-1 PET scan of depressed individual's brain before and after recovery. (From Fortinash KM: Psychiatric Mental Health Nursing, ed 4, St. Louis, Mosby, 2008)

F32.89   Other specified depressive episodes
　　　　Atypical depression
　　　　Post-schizophrenic depression
　　　　Single episode of 'masked' depression NOS
　　　　Coding Clinic: 2016, Q4, P14

F32.9   Major depressive disorder, single episode, unspecified
　　　　Major depression NOS
　　　　Coding Clinic: 2021, Q1, P10

F32.A   Depression, unspecified
　　　　Depression NOS
　　　　Depressive disorder NOS
　　　　Coding Clinic: 2021, Q4, P10

● F33   Major depressive disorder, recurrent

Includes   recurrent episodes of depressive reaction
　　　　　recurrent episodes of endogenous depression
　　　　　recurrent episodes of major depression
　　　　　recurrent episodes of psychogenic depression
　　　　　recurrent episodes of reactive depression
　　　　▶recurrent episodes of seasonal affective disorder
　　　　　recurrent episodes of seasonal depressive disorder
　　　　　recurrent episodes of vital depression

Excludes1   bipolar disorder (F31.-)
　　　　　　manic episode (F30.-)
Coding Clinic: 2020, Q1, P23

F33.0   Major depressive disorder, recurrent, mild 🐾

F33.1   Major depressive disorder, recurrent, moderate 🐾

F33.2   Major depressive disorder, recurrent severe without psychotic features 🐾

F33.3   Major depressive disorder, recurrent, severe with psychotic symptoms 🐾
　　　　Endogenous depression with psychotic symptoms
　　　　Major depressive disorder, recurrent, with psychotic features
　　　　Recurrent severe episodes of major depression with mood-congruent psychotic symptoms
　　　　Recurrent severe episodes of major depression with mood-incongruent psychotic symptoms
　　　　Recurrent severe episodes of major depression with psychotic symptoms
　　　　Recurrent severe episodes of psychogenic depressive psychosis
　　　　Recurrent severe episodes of psychotic depression
　　　　Recurrent severe episodes of reactive depressive psychosis

● F33.4   Major depressive disorder, recurrent, in remission

F33.40   Major depressive disorder, recurrent, in remission, unspecified 🐾

F33.41   Major depressive disorder, recurrent, in partial remission 🐾

F33.42   Major depressive disorder, recurrent, in full remission 🐾

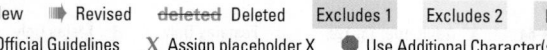

▶ New   ⇒ Revised   ~~deleted~~ Deleted   Excludes 1   Excludes 2   Includes   Use additional   Code first   Code also   Key words
OGCR Official Guidelines   X Assign placeholder X   ● Use Additional Character(s)   ▶ Manifestation Code   🐾 Hierarchical Condition Category   Coding Clinic

F33.8   **Other recurrent depressive disorders** 🗷
     Recurrent brief depressive episodes

F33.9   **Major depressive disorder, recurrent, unspecified** 🗷
     Monopolar depression NOS

● **F34**   **Persistent mood [affective] disorders**

F34.0   **Cyclothymic disorder**
     Affective personality disorder
     Cycloid personality
     Cyclothymia
     Cyclothymic personality

F34.1   **Dysthymic disorder**
     Depressive neurosis
     Depressive personality disorder
     Dysthymia
     Neurotic depression
     Persistent anxiety depression
     Persistent depressive disorder

     Excludes2   anxiety depression (mild or not persistent) (F41.8)

● **F34.8**   **Other persistent mood [affective] disorders**

F34.81   **Disruptive mood dysregulation disorder** 🗷
     Coding Clinic: 2016, Q4, P14

F34.89   **Other specified persistent mood disorders** 🗷
     Coding Clinic: 2016, Q4, P14

F34.9   **Persistent mood [affective] disorder, unspecified** 🗷

F39   **Unspecified mood [affective] disorder** 🗷
     Affective psychosis NOS

ANXIETY, DISSOCIATIVE, STRESS-RELATED, SOMATOFORM AND OTHER NONPSYCHOTIC MENTAL DISORDERS (F40-F48)

● **F40**   **Phobic anxiety disorders**
Irrational fear with avoidance of the feared subject, activity, or situation even though the individual knows that the reaction is excessive

● **F40.0**   **Agoraphobia**
Intense, irrational fear of open spaces

F40.00   **Agoraphobia, unspecified**

F40.01   **Agoraphobia with panic disorder**
     Panic disorder with agoraphobia

     Excludes1   panic disorder without agoraphobia (F41.0)

F40.02   **Agoraphobia without panic disorder**

● **F40.1**   **Social phobias**
     Anthropophobia
     Social anxiety disorder
     Social anxiety disorder of childhood
     Social neurosis

F40.10   **Social phobia, unspecified**

F40.11   **Social phobia, generalized**

● **F40.2**   **Specific (isolated) phobias**

     Excludes2   dysmorphophobia (nondelusional) (F45.22)
                nosophobia (F45.22)

● **F40.21**   **Animal type phobia**

F40.210   **Arachnophobia**
     Fear of spiders

F40.218   **Other animal type phobia**

● **F40.22**   **Natural environment type phobia**

F40.220   **Fear of thunderstorms**

F40.228   **Other natural environment type phobia**

● **F40.23**   **Blood, injection, injury type phobia**

F40.230   **Fear of blood**

F40.231   **Fear of injections and transfusions**

F40.232   **Fear of other medical care**

F40.233   **Fear of injury**

● **F40.24**   **Situational type phobia**

F40.240   **Claustrophobia**
     Fear of closed spaces

F40.241   **Acrophobia**
     Fear of heights

F40.242   **Fear of bridges**

F40.243   **Fear of flying**

F40.248   **Other situational type phobia**

● **F40.29**   **Other specified phobia**

F40.290   **Androphobia**
     Fear of men

F40.291   **Gynephobia**
     Fear of women

F40.298   **Other specified phobia**

F40.8   **Other phobic anxiety disorders**
     Phobic anxiety disorder of childhood

F40.9   **Phobic anxiety disorder, unspecified**
     Phobia NOS
     Phobic state NOS

● **F41**   **Other anxiety disorders**

     Excludes2   anxiety in:
                acute stress reaction (F43.0)
                transient adjustment reaction (F43.2)
                neurasthenia (F48.8)
                psychophysiologic disorders (F45.-)
                separation anxiety (F93.0)

F41.0   **Panic disorder [episodic paroxysmal anxiety]**
     Panic attack
     Panic state

     Excludes1   panic disorder with agoraphobia (F40.01)

F41.1   **Generalized anxiety disorder**
     Anxiety neurosis
     Anxiety reaction
     Anxiety state
     Overanxious disorder

     Excludes2   neurasthenia (F48.8)

F41.3   **Other mixed anxiety disorders**

F41.8   **Other specified anxiety disorders**
     Anxiety depression (mild or not persistent)
     Anxiety hysteria
     Mixed anxiety and depressive disorder
     Coding Clinic: 2021, Q1, P11

F41.9   **Anxiety disorder, unspecified**
     Anxiety NOS
     Coding Clinic: 2021, Q1, P11

● **F42**   **Obsessive-compulsive disorder**
Anxiety disorder with recurrent obsessions or compulsions

     Excludes2   obsessive-compulsive personality (disorder) (F60.5)
                obsessive-compulsive symptoms occurring in depression (F32-F33)
                obsessive-compulsive symptoms occurring in schizophrenia (F20.-)

F42.2   **Mixed obsessional thoughts and acts**
     Coding Clinic: 2016, Q4, P15

F42.3   **Hoarding disorder**
     Coding Clinic: 2016, Q4, P14-15

F42.4   **Excoriation (skin-picking) disorder**

     Excludes1   factitial dermatitis (L98.1)
                other specified behavioral and emotional disorders with onset usually occurring in early childhood and adolescence (F98.8)
     Coding Clinic: 2016, Q4, P14-15

F42.8   **Other obsessive-compulsive disorder**
     Anancastic neurosis
     Obsessive-compulsive neurosis
     Coding Clinic: 2016, Q4, P15

F42.9   **Obsessive-compulsive disorder, unspecified**
     Coding Clinic: 2016, Q4, P15

CHAPTER 5 (F01-F99)

● **F43　Reaction to severe stress and adjustment disorders**

F43.0　Acute stress reaction
Acute crisis reaction
Acute reaction to stress
Combat and operational stress reaction
Combat fatigue
Crisis state
Psychic shock

● **F43.1　Post-traumatic stress disorder (PTSD)**
Traumatic neurosis

F43.10　Post-traumatic stress disorder, unspecified

F43.11　Post-traumatic stress disorder, acute

F43.12　Post-traumatic stress disorder, chronic

● **F43.2　Adjustment disorders**
Culture shock
Grief reaction
Hospitalism in children

> **Excludes2**　separation anxiety disorder of childhood (F93.0)

F43.20　Adjustment disorder, unspecified

F43.21　Adjustment disorder with depressed mood

F43.22　Adjustment disorder with anxiety

F43.23　Adjustment disorder with mixed anxiety and depressed mood

F43.24　Adjustment disorder with disturbance of conduct

F43.25　Adjustment disorder with mixed disturbance of emotions and conduct

F43.29　Adjustment disorder with other symptoms

● **F43.8　Other reactions to severe stress**
Other specified trauma and stressor-related disorder

▶ **F43.81　Prolonged grief disorder**
▶ Complicated grief
▶ Complicated grief disorder
▶ Persistent complex bereavement disorder

▶ **F43.89　Other reactions to severe stress**

F43.9　Reaction to severe stress, unspecified
Trauma and stressor-related disorder, NOS

● **F44　Dissociative and conversion disorders**

> **Includes**　conversion hysteria
> conversion reaction
> hysteria
> hysterical psychosis

> **Excludes2**　malingering [conscious simulation] (Z76.5)

F44.0　Dissociative amnesia
Sudden loss of memory for personal information

> **Excludes1**　amnesia NOS (R41.3)
> anterograde amnesia (R41.1)
> dissociative amnesia with dissociative fugue (F44.1)
> retrograde amnesia (R41.2)

> **Excludes2**　alcohol or other psychoactive substance-induced amnestic disorder (F10, F13, F19 with .26, .96)
> amnestic disorder due to known physiological condition (F04)
> postictal amnesia in epilepsy (G40.-)

F44.1　Dissociative fugue
Characterized by episode of sudden, unexpected travel with amnesia for past and partial to total confusion about identity or assumption of new identity
Dissociative amnesia with dissociative fugue

> **Excludes2**　postictal fugue in epilepsy (G40.-)

F44.2　Dissociative stupor
Profound diminution or absence of voluntary movement and responsiveness to external stimuli

> **Excludes1**　catatonic stupor (R40.1)
> stupor NOS (R40.1)

> **Excludes2**　catatonic disorder due to known physiological condition (F06.1)
> depressive stupor (F32, F33)
> manic stupor (F30, F31)

F44.4　Conversion disorder with motor symptom or deficit
Conversion disorder with abnormal movement
Conversion disorder with speech symptoms
Conversion disorder with swallowing symptoms
Conversion disorder with weakness/paralysis
Dissociative motor disorders
Psychogenic aphonia
Psychogenic dysphonia

F44.5　Conversion disorder with seizures or convulsions
Conversion disorder with attacks or seizures
Dissociative convulsions
Coding Clinic: 2019, Q1, P19

F44.6　Conversion disorder with sensory symptom or deficit
Conversion disorder with anesthesia or sensory loss
Conversion disorder with special sensory symptoms
Dissociative anesthesia and sensory loss
Psychogenic deafness

F44.7　Conversion disorder with mixed symptom presentation

● **F44.8　Other dissociative and conversion disorders**

F44.81　Dissociative identity disorder
Multiple personality disorder

F44.89　Other dissociative and conversion disorders
Ganser's syndrome
Psychogenic confusion
Psychogenic twilight state
Trance and possession disorders

F44.9　Dissociative and conversion disorder, unspecified
Dissociative disorder NOS

OGCR Section I.C.5.a.

Pain disorders related to psychological factors

Assign code F45.41, for pain that is exclusively related to psychological disorders. As indicated by the Excludes 1 note under category G89, a code from category G89 should not be assigned with code F45.41 Code F45.42, Pain disorders with related psychological factors, should be used with a code from category G89, Pain, not elsewhere classified, if there is documentation of a psychological component for a patient with acute or chronic pain.

See Section I.C.6. Pain

● **F45　Somatoform disorders**
Mental disorders characterized by symptoms suggesting general medical condition

> **Excludes2**　dissociative and conversion disorders (F44.-)
> factitious disorders (F68.1-, F68.A)
> hair-plucking (F63.3)
> lalling (F80.0)
> lisping (F80.0)
> malingering [conscious simulation] (Z76.5)
> nail-biting (F98.8)
> psychological or behavioral factors associated with disorders or diseases classified elsewhere (F54)
> sexual dysfunction, not due to a substance or known physiological condition (F52.-)
> thumb-sucking (F98.8)
> tic disorders (in childhood and adolescence) (F95.-)
> Tourette's syndrome (F95.2)
> trichotillomania (F63.3)

F45.0　Somatization disorder
Briquet's disorder
Multiple psychosomatic disorder

F45.1　Undifferentiated somatoform disorder
Somatic symptom disorder
Undifferentiated psychosomatic disorder

▶ New　⇒ Revised　~~deleted~~ Deleted　Excludes 1　Excludes 2　Includes　Use additional　Code first　Code also　Key words

OGCR Official Guidelines　X Assign placeholder X　● Use Additional Character(s)　▷ Manifestation Code　⚛ Hierarchical Condition Category　**Coding Clinic**

● **F45.2**   **Hypochondriacal disorders**
Persistent, unrealistic preoccupation with possibility of having serious disease

     Excludes2   delusional dysmorphophobia (F22)
             fixed delusions about bodily functions or shape (F22)

     F45.20   **Hypochondriacal disorder, unspecified**

     F45.21   **Hypochondriasis**
             Hypochondriacal neurosis
             Illness anxiety disorder

     F45.22   **Body dysmorphic disorder**
             Dysmorphophobia (nondelusional)
             Nosophobia

     F45.29   **Other hypochondriacal disorders**

● **F45.4**   **Pain disorders related to psychological factors**
     Excludes1   pain NOS (R52)

     F45.41   **Pain disorder exclusively related to psychological factors**
             Somatoform pain disorder (persistent)

     F45.42   **Pain disorder with related psychological factors**
             Code also associated acute or chronic pain (G89.-)

  F45.8   **Other somatoform disorders**
     Psychogenic dysmenorrhea
     Psychogenic dysphagia, including 'globus hystericus'
     Psychogenic pruritus
     Psychogenic torticollis
     Somatoform autonomic dysfunction
     Teeth grinding
     Excludes1   sleep related teeth grinding (G47.63)
     Coding Clinic: 2016, Q4, P118

  F45.9   **Somatoform disorder, unspecified**
     Psychosomatic disorder NOS

● **F48**   **Other nonpsychotic mental disorders**

  F48.1   **Depersonalization-derealization syndrome**

  F48.2   **Pseudobulbar affect**
     Involuntary emotional expression disorder
     Code first underlying cause, if known, such as:
         amyotrophic lateral sclerosis (G12.21)
         multiple sclerosis (G35)
         sequelae of cerebrovascular disease (I69.-)
         sequelae of traumatic intracranial injury (S06.-)

  F48.8   **Other specified nonpsychotic mental disorders**
     Dhat syndrome
     Neurasthenia
     Occupational neurosis, including writer's cramp
     Psychasthenia
     Psychasthenic neurosis
     Psychogenic syncope

  F48.9   **Nonpsychotic mental disorder, unspecified**
     Neurosis NOS

BEHAVIORAL SYNDROMES ASSOCIATED WITH PHYSIOLOGICAL DISTURBANCES AND PHYSICAL FACTORS (F50-F59)

● **F50**   **Eating disorders**
     Excludes1   anorexia NOS (R63.0)
             feeding problems of newborn (P92.-)
             polyphagia (R63.2)
     Excludes2   feeding difficulties (R63.3)
             feeding disorder in infancy or childhood (F98.2-)

● **F50.0**   **Anorexia nervosa**
     Excludes1   loss of appetite (R63.0)
             psychogenic loss of appetite (F50.89)

     F50.00   **Anorexia nervosa, unspecified**

     F50.01   **Anorexia nervosa, restricting type**

     F50.02   **Anorexia nervosa, binge eating/purging type**
         Excludes1   bulimia nervosa (F50.2)
         Coding Clinic: 2022, Q1, P13

● **F50.2**   **Bulimia nervosa**
     Bulimia NOS
     Hyperorexia nervosa
     Excludes1   anorexia nervosa, binge eating/purging type (F50.02)

● **F50.8**   **Other eating disorders**
     Excludes2   pica of infancy and childhood (F98.3)

     F50.81   **Binge eating disorder**
         Coding Clinic: 2016, Q4, P15

     F50.82   **Avoidant/restrictive food intake disorder**

     F50.89   **Other specified eating disorder**
         Pica in adults
         Psychogenic loss of appetite
         Coding Clinic: 2016, Q4, P16

  F50.9   **Eating disorder, unspecified**
     Atypical anorexia nervosa
     Atypical bulimia nervosa
     Feeding or eating disorder, unspecified
     Other specified feeding disorder

● **F51**   **Sleep disorders not due to a substance or known physiological condition**
     Excludes2   organic sleep disorders (G47.-)

● **F51.0**   **Insomnia not due to a substance or known physiological condition**
     Excludes2   alcohol related insomnia (F10.182, F10.282, F10.982)
             drug-related insomnia (F11.182, F11.282, F11.982, F13.182, F13.282, F13.982, F14.182, F14.282, F14.982, F15.182, F15.282, F15.982, F19.182, F19.282, F19.982)
             insomnia NOS (G47.0-)
             insomnia due to known physiological condition (G47.0-)
             organic insomnia (G47.0-)
             sleep deprivation (Z72.820)

     F51.01   **Primary insomnia**
         Idiopathic insomnia

     F51.02   **Adjustment insomnia**

     F51.03   **Paradoxical insomnia**

     F51.04   **Psychophysiologic insomnia**

     F51.05   **Insomnia due to other mental disorder**
         Code also associated mental disorder

     F51.09   **Other insomnia not due to a substance or known physiological condition**

● **F51.1**   **Hypersomnia not due to a substance or known physiological condition**
     Hypersomnia: Excessive sleeping/sleepiness
     Excludes2   alcohol related hypersomnia (F10.182, F10.282, F10.982)
             drug-related hypersomnia (F11.182, F11.282, F11.982, F13.182, F13.282, F13.982, F14.182, F14.282, F14.982, F15.182, F15.282, F15.982, F19.182, F19.282, F19.982)
             hypersomnia NOS (G47.10)
             hypersomnia due to known physiological condition (G47.10)
             idiopathic hypersomnia (G47.11, G47.12)
             narcolepsy (G47.4-)

     F51.11   **Primary hypersomnia**

     F51.12   **Insufficient sleep syndrome**
         Excludes1   sleep deprivation (Z72.820)

     F51.13   **Hypersomnia due to other mental disorder**
         Code also associated mental disorder

     F51.19   **Other hypersomnia not due to a substance or known physiological condition**

CHAPTER 5 (F01-F99)

F51.3   **Sleepwalking [somnambulism]**
Non-rapid eye movement sleep arousal disorders, sleepwalking type

F51.4   **Sleep terrors [night terrors]**
Non-rapid eye movement sleep arousal disorders, sleep terror type

F51.5   **Nightmare disorder**
Dream anxiety disorder

F51.8   **Other sleep disorders not due to a substance or known physiological condition**

F51.9   **Sleep disorder not due to a substance or known physiological condition, unspecified**
Emotional sleep disorder NOS

● **F52**   **Sexual dysfunction not due to a substance or known physiological condition**
     Excludes2   Dhat syndrome (F48.8)

F52.0   **Hypoactive sexual desire disorder**
Total loss of feeling of sexual pleasure
Lack or loss of sexual desire
Male hypoactive sexual desire disorder
Sexual anhedonia
     Excludes1   decreased libido (R68.82)

F52.1   **Sexual aversion disorder**
Sexual aversion and lack of sexual enjoyment

● **F52.2**   **Sexual arousal disorders**
Failure of genital response

     F52.21   **Male erectile disorder** ♂
Erectile disorder
Psychogenic impotence
         Excludes1   impotence of organic origin (N52.-)
                        impotence NOS (N52.-)

     F52.22   **Female sexual arousal disorder** ♀
Female sexual interest/arousal disorder

● **F52.3**   **Orgasmic disorder**
Inhibited orgasm
Psychogenic anorgasmy

     F52.31   **Female orgasmic disorder** ♀

     F52.32   **Male orgasmic disorder** ♂
Delayed ejaculation

F52.4   **Premature ejaculation** ♂

F52.5   **Vaginismus not due to a substance or known physiological condition** ♀
Psychogenic vaginismus
     Excludes2   vaginismus (due to a known physiological condition) (N94.2)

F52.6   **Dyspareunia not due to a substance or known physiological condition**
Dyspareunia: Difficult or painful sexual intercourse
Genito-pelvic pain penetration disorder
Psychogenic dyspareunia
     Excludes2   dyspareunia (due to a known physiological condition) (N94.1-)

F52.8   **Other sexual dysfunction not due to a substance or known physiological condition**
Excessive sexual drive
Nymphomania
Satyriasis

F52.9   **Unspecified sexual dysfunction not due to a substance or known physiological condition**
Sexual dysfunction NOS

● **F53**   **Mental and behavioral disorders associated with the puerperium, not elsewhere classified**
Acute mental illness with sudden onset following childbirth with symptoms of affective psychosis, disorientation, and confusion are prevalent
     Excludes1   mood disorders with psychotic features (F30.2, F31.2, F31.5, F31.64, F32.3, F33.3)
                       postpartum dysphoria (O90.6)
                       psychosis in schizophrenia, schizotypal, delusional, and other psychotic disorders (F20-F29)

F53.0   **Postpartum depression** ♀   M
Postnatal depression, NOS
Postpartum depression, NOS
Coding Clinic: 2018, Q4, P8

F53.1   **Puerperal psychosis** ♀   M
Postpartum psychosis
Puerperal psychosis, NOS
Coding Clinic: 2018, Q4, P9

▷ **F54**   *Psychological and behavioral factors associated with disorders or diseases classified elsewhere*
Psychological factors affecting physical conditions
     Code first the associated physical disorder, such as:
         asthma (J45.-)
         dermatitis (L23-L25)
         gastric ulcer (K25.-)
         mucous colitis (K58.-)
         ulcerative colitis (K51.-)
         urticaria (L50.-)
     Excludes2   tension-type headache (G44.2)

● **F55**   **Abuse of non-psychoactive substances**
     Excludes2   abuse of psychoactive substances (F10-F19)

F55.0   **Abuse of antacids**

F55.1   **Abuse of herbal or folk remedies**

F55.2   **Abuse of laxatives**

F55.3   **Abuse of steroids or hormones**

F55.4   **Abuse of vitamins**

F55.8   **Abuse of other non-psychoactive substances**

F59   **Unspecified behavioral syndromes associated with physiological disturbances and physical factors**
Psychogenic physiological dysfunction NOS

DISORDERS OF ADULT PERSONALITY AND BEHAVIOR (F60-F69)

● **F60**   **Specific personality disorders**
Long-term patterns of thoughts and behaviors causing serious problems with relationships and work

F60.0   **Paranoid personality disorder**
Hostile, devious, and combative response to disappointments
Expansive paranoid personality (disorder)
Fanatic personality (disorder)
Querulant personality (disorder)
Paranoid personality (disorder)
Sensitive paranoid personality (disorder)
     Excludes2   paranoia (F22)
                   paranoia querulans (F22)
                   paranoid psychosis (F22)
                   paranoid schizophrenia (F20.0)
                   paranoid state (F22)

F60.1   **Schizoid personality disorder**
Detachment from social relationships with minimal emotional experiences and expressions
     Excludes2   Asperger's syndrome (F84.5)
                   delusional disorder (F22)
                   schizoid disorder of childhood (F84.5)
                   schizophrenia (F20.-)
                   schizotypal disorder (F21)

▶ New   ⇒ Revised   ~~deleted~~ Deleted   Excludes 1   Excludes 2   Includes   Use additional   Code first   Code also   Key words
OGCR Official Guidelines   X Assign placeholder X   ● Use Additional Character(s)   ▷ Manifestation Code   🅗 Hierarchical Condition Category   **Coding Clinic**

F60.2   Antisocial personality disorder
Continuous and chronic antisocial behavior
Amoral personality (disorder)
Asocial personality (disorder)
Dissocial personality disorder
Psychopathic personality (disorder)
Sociopathic personality (disorder)
> **Excludes1**   conduct disorders (F91.-)
> **Excludes2**   borderline personality disorder (F60.3)

F60.3   Borderline personality disorder
*Instability of mood, self-image or sense of self, and
   interpersonal relationships*
Aggressive personality (disorder)
Emotionally unstable personality disorder
Explosive personality (disorder)
> **Excludes2**   antisocial personality disorder (F60.2)

F60.4   Histrionic personality disorder
*Personality disorder with excessive emotional and attention-
   seeking behavior*
Hysterical personality (disorder)
Psychoinfantile personality (disorder)

F60.5   Obsessive-compulsive personality disorder
Anankastic personality (disorder)
Compulsive personality (disorder)
Obsessional personality (disorder)
> **Excludes2**   obsessive-compulsive disorder (F42.-)

F60.6   Avoidant personality disorder
Anxious personality disorder

F60.7   Dependent personality disorder
Asthenic personality (disorder)
Inadequate personality (disorder)
Passive personality (disorder)

● **F60.8   Other specific personality disorders**
F60.81   Narcissistic personality disorder
*Vanity, conceit, egotism or indifference to plight
   of others*

F60.89   Other specific personality disorders
Eccentric personality disorder
'Haltlose' type personality disorder
Immature personality disorder
Passive-aggressive personality disorder
Psychoneurotic personality disorder
Self-defeating personality disorder

F60.9   Personality disorder, unspecified
Character disorder NOS
Character neurosis NOS
Pathological personality NOS

● **F63   Impulse disorders**
> **Excludes2**   habitual excessive use of alcohol or psychoactive
>   substances (F10-F19)
>   impulse disorders involving sexual behavior (F65.-)

F63.0   Pathological gambling
Compulsive gambling
Gambling disorder
> **Excludes1**   gambling and betting NOS (Z72.6)
> **Excludes2**   excessive gambling by manic patients
>   (F30, F31)
>   gambling in antisocial personality
>   disorder (F60.2)

F63.1   Pyromania
Pathological fire-setting
> **Excludes2**   fire-setting (by) (in):
>   adult with antisocial personality
>   disorder (F60.2)
>   alcohol or psychoactive substance
>   intoxication (F10-F19)
>   conduct disorders (F91.-)
>   mental disorders due to known
>   physiological condition (F01-F09)
>   schizophrenia (F20.-)

F63.2   Kleptomania
Pathological stealing
> **Excludes1**   shoplifting as the reason for observation
>   for suspected mental disorder
>   (Z03.8)
> **Excludes2**   depressive disorder with stealing
>   (F31-F33)
>   stealing due to underlying mental
>   condition-code to mental condition
>   stealing in mental disorders due to known
>   physiological condition (F01-F09)

F63.3   Trichotillomania
Hair plucking
> **Excludes2**   other stereotyped movement disorder
>   (F98.4)

● **F63.8   Other impulse disorders**
F63.81   Intermittent explosive disorder
F63.89   Other impulse disorders

F63.9   Impulse disorder, unspecified
Impulse control disorder NOS

● **F64   Gender identity disorders**
F64.0   Transsexualism
Gender identity disorder in adolescence and adulthood
Gender dysphoria in adolescents and adults
Coding Clinic: 2016, Q4, P16

F64.1   Dual role transvestism
Use additional code to identify sex reassignment status
   (Z87.890)
> **Excludes1**   gender identity disorder in childhood
>   (F64.2)
> **Excludes2**   fetishistic transvestism (F65.1)
Coding Clinic: 2016, Q4, P16

F64.2   Gender identity disorder of childhood   P
Gender dysphoria in children
> **Excludes1**   gender identity disorder in adolescence
>   and adulthood (F64.0)
> **Excludes2**   sexual maturation disorder (F66)

F64.8   Other gender identity disorders
Other specified gender dysphoria

F64.9   Gender identity disorder, unspecified
Gender dysphoria, unspecified
Gender-role disorder NOS

● **F65   Paraphilias**
F65.0   Fetishism
*Intense sexual urges and arousing fantasies using inanimate
   objects*
Fetishistic disorder

F65.1   Transvestic fetishism
*Intense sexual urges, arousal, or orgasm associated with
   fantasized/actual cross-dressing*
Fetishistic transvestism
Transvestic disorder

F65.2   Exhibitionism
Exhibitionistic disorder

F65.3   Voyeurism
*Sexual urges or arousal involving real or fantasized
   observation of unsuspecting people who are naked,
   disrobing, or engaging in sexual activity*
Voyeuristic disorder

F65.4   Pedophilia
Pedophilic disorder

● **F65.5   Sadomasochism**
F65.50   Sadomasochism, unspecified
F65.51   Sexual masochism
Sexual masochism disorder
F65.52   Sexual sadism
Sexual sadism disorder

CHAPTER 5 (F01-F99)

● **F65.8**   **Other paraphilias**

     F65.81   **Frotteurism**
Sexual arousal or orgasm is achieved by rubbing up against another person (or fantasies of), in crowded place with unsuspecting victim
Frotteuristic disorder

     F65.89   **Other paraphilias**
Necrophilia
Other specified paraphilic disorder

   F65.9   **Paraphilia, unspecified**
Paraphilic disorder, unspecified
Sexual deviation NOS

F66   **Other sexual disorders**
Sexual maturation disorder
Sexual relationship disorder

● **F68**   **Other disorders of adult personality and behavior**

   ● **F68.1**   **Factitious disorder imposed on self**
Compensation neurosis
Elaboration of physical symptoms for psychological reasons
Hospital hopper syndrome
Münchhausen's syndrome
Peregrinating patient

> **Excludes2**   factitial dermatitis (L98.1)
> person feigning illness (with obvious motivation) (Z76.5)

     F68.10   **Factitious disorder imposed on self, unspecified**

     F68.11   **Factitious disorder imposed on self with predominantly psychological signs and symptoms**

     F68.12   **Factitious disorder imposed on self with predominantly physical signs and symptoms**

     F68.13   **Factitious disorder imposed on self with combined psychological and physical signs and symptoms**

   F68.8   **Other specified disorders of adult personality and behavior**

   F68.A   **Factitious disorder imposed on another**
Factitious disorder by proxy
Münchausen's by proxy

F69   **Unspecified disorder of adult personality and behavior**   A

INTELLECTUAL DISABILITIES (F70-F79)

Code first any associated physical or developmental disorders

> **Excludes1**   borderline intellectual functioning, IQ above 70 to 84 (R41.83)

F70   **Mild intellectual disabilities**
IQ level 50-55 to approximately 70
Mild mental subnormality

F71   **Moderate intellectual disabilities**
IQ level 35-40 to 50-55
Moderate mental subnormality

F72   **Severe intellectual disabilities**
IQ 20-25 to 35-40
Severe mental subnormality

F73   **Profound intellectual disabilities**
IQ level below 20-25
Profound mental subnormality

● **F78**   **Other intellectual disabilities**

   ● **F78.A**   **Other genetic related intellectual disabilities**

     F78.A1   **SYNGAP1-related intellectual disability**
Code also, if applicable, any associated:
autism spectrum disorder (F84.0)
autistic disorder (F84.0)
encephalopathy (G93.4-)
epilepsy and recurrent seizures (G40.-)
other pervasive developmental disorders (F84.8)
pervasive developmental disorder, NOS (F84.9)

     F78.A9   **Other genetic related intellectual disability**
Code also, if applicable, any associated disorders

F79   **Unspecified intellectual disabilities**
Mental deficiency NOS
Mental subnormality NOS

PERVASIVE AND SPECIFIC DEVELOPMENTAL DISORDERS (F80-F89)

● **F80**   **Specific developmental disorders of speech and language**

   F80.0   **Phonological disorder**
Communication disorder of unknown cause, characterized by failure to use age-appropriate sounds
Dyslalia
Functional speech articulation disorder
Lalling
Lisping
Phonological developmental disorder
Speech articulation developmental disorder
Speech-sound disorder

> **Excludes1**   speech articulation impairment due to aphasia NOS (R47.01)
> speech articulation impairment due to apraxia (R48.2)

> **Excludes2**   speech articulation impairment due to hearing loss (F80.4)
> speech articulation impairment due to intellectual disabilities (F70-F79)
> speech articulation impairment with expressive language developmental disorder (F80.1)
> speech articulation impairment with mixed receptive expressive language developmental disorder (F80.2)

   F80.1   **Expressive language disorder**
Developmental dysphasia or aphasia, expressive type

> **Excludes1**   mixed receptive-expressive language disorder (F80.2)
> dysphasia and aphasia NOS (R47.-)

> **Excludes2**   acquired aphasia with epilepsy [Landau-Kleffner] (G40.80-)
> intellectual disabilities (F70-F79)
> pervasive developmental disorders (F84.-)
> selective mutism (F94.0)

   F80.2   **Mixed receptive-expressive language disorder**
Developmental dysphasia or aphasia, receptive type
Developmental Wernicke's aphasia

> **Excludes1**   central auditory processing disorder (H93.25)
> dysphasia or aphasia NOS (R47.-)
> expressive language disorder (F80.1)
> expressive type dysphasia or aphasia (F80.1)
> word deafness (H93.25)

> **Excludes2**   acquired aphasia with epilepsy [Landau-Kleffner] (G40.80-)
> intellectual disabilities (F70-F79)
> pervasive developmental disorders (F84.-)
> selective mutism (F94.0)

   F80.4   **Speech and language development delay due to hearing loss**
Code also type of hearing loss (H90.-, H91.-)

   ● **F80.8**   **Other developmental disorders of speech or language**

     F80.81   **Childhood onset fluency disorder**
Cluttering NOS
Stuttering NOS

> **Excludes1**   adult onset fluency disorder (F98.5)
> fluency disorder in conditions classified elsewhere (R47.82)
> fluency disorder (stuttering) following cerebrovascular disease (I69. with final characters -23)

F80.82   Social pragmatic communication disorder
> **Excludes1**   Asperger's syndrome (F84.5)
>   autistic disorder (F84.0)
> Coding Clinic: 2016, Q4, P16

F80.89   Other developmental disorders of speech and language
> Coding Clinic: 2017, Q1, P27

F80.9   Developmental disorder of speech and language, unspecified
> Communication disorder NOS
> Language disorder NOS

F81   Specific developmental disorders of scholastic skills

F81.0   Specific reading disorder
> 'Backward reading'
> Developmental dyslexia
> Specific learning disorder, with impairment in reading
> Specific reading retardation
> **Excludes1**   alexia NOS (R48.0)
>   dyslexia NOS (R48.0)

F81.2   Mathematics disorder
> Developmental acalculia
> Developmental arithmetical disorder
> Developmental Gerstmann's syndrome
> Specific learning disorder, with impairment in mathematics
> **Excludes1**   acalculia NOS (R48.8)
> **Excludes2**   arithmetical difficulties associated with a reading disorder (F81.0)
>   arithmetical difficulties associated with a spelling disorder (F81.81)
>   arithmetical difficulties due to inadequate teaching (Z55.8)

F81.8   Other developmental disorders of scholastic skills

F81.81   Disorder of written expression
> Specific learning disorder, with impairment in written expression
> Specific spelling disorder

F81.89   Other developmental disorders of scholastic skills

F81.9   Developmental disorder of scholastic skills, unspecified
> Knowledge acquisition disability NOS
> Learning disability NOS
> Learning disorder NOS

F82   Specific developmental disorder of motor function
> Clumsy child syndrome
> Developmental coordination disorder
> Developmental dyspraxia
> **Excludes1**   abnormalities of gait and mobility (R26.-)
>   lack of coordination (R27.-)
> **Excludes2**   lack of coordination secondary to intellectual disabilities (F70-F79)

F84   Pervasive developmental disorders
> Code also any associated medical condition and intellectual disabilities

F84.0   Autistic disorder
> Autism spectrum disorder
> Infantile autism
> Infantile psychosis
> Kanner's syndrome
> **Excludes1**   Asperger's syndrome (F84.5)
> Coding Clinic: 2017, Q1, P27

F84.2   Rett's syndrome
> *Neurodevelopmental disorder*
> **Excludes1**   Asperger's syndrome (F84.5)
>   Autistic disorder (F84.0)
>   other childhood disintegrative disorder (F84.3)

F84.3   Other childhood disintegrative disorder   P
> Dementia infantilis
> *At least two years of normal development followed by significant loss of language abilities, social skills, bowel/bladder control, motor skills*
> Disintegrative psychosis
> Heller's syndrome
> *At least two years of normal development followed by significant loss of language abilities, social skills, bowel/bladder control, motor skills*
> Symbiotic psychosis
> *Abnormal relationship to mothering figure, characterized by intense separation anxiety, severe regression, giving up of useful speech, and autism*
> Use additional code to identify any associated neurological condition.
> **Excludes1**   Asperger's syndrome (F84.5)
>   Autistic disorder (F84.0)
>   Rett's syndrome (F84.2)

F84.5   Asperger's syndrome
> *Developmental disorder*
> Asperger's disorder
> Autistic psychopathy
> Schizoid disorder of childhood

F84.8   Other pervasive developmental disorders
> Overactive disorder associated with intellectual disabilities and stereotyped movements

F84.9   Pervasive developmental disorder, unspecified
> Atypical autism

F88   Other disorders of psychological development
> Developmental agnosia
> Global developmental delay
> Other specified neurodevelopmental disorder

F89   Unspecified disorder of psychological development
> Developmental disorder NOS
> Neurodevelopmental disorder NOS

BEHAVIORAL AND EMOTIONAL DISORDERS WITH ONSET USUALLY OCCURRING IN CHILDHOOD AND ADOLESCENCE (F90-F98)

Note: Codes within categories F90-F98 may be used regardless of the age of a patient. These disorders generally have onset within the childhood or adolescent years, but may continue throughout life or not be diagnosed until adulthood.

F90   Attention-deficit hyperactivity disorders
> *Attention deficit disorder with hyperactivity=ADHD*
> **Includes**   attention deficit disorder with hyperactivity
>   attention deficit syndrome with hyperactivity
> **Excludes2**   anxiety disorders (F40.-, F41.-)
>   mood [affective] disorders (F30-F39)
>   pervasive developmental disorders (F84.-)
>   schizophrenia (F20.-)

F90.0   Attention-deficit hyperactivity disorder, predominantly inattentive type
> Attention-deficit/hyperactivity disorder, predominantly inattentive presentation

F90.1   Attention-deficit hyperactivity disorder, predominantly hyperactive type
> Attention-deficit/hyperactivity disorder, predominantly hyperactive impulsive presentation

F90.2   Attention-deficit hyperactivity disorder, combined type
> Attention-deficit/hyperactivity disorder, combined presentation

F90.8   Attention-deficit hyperactivity disorder, other type

F90.9   Attention-deficit hyperactivity disorder, unspecified type
> Attention-deficit hyperactivity disorder of childhood or adolescence NOS
> Attention-deficit hyperactivity disorder NOS

F91   Conduct disorders
Childhood/adolescence disruptive behavior disorder

> **Excludes1**   antisocial behavior (Z72.81-)
> antisocial personality disorder (F60.2)
>
> **Excludes2**   conduct problems associated with attention-deficit hyperactivity disorder (F90.-)
> mood [affective] disorders (F30-F39)
> pervasive developmental disorders (F84.-)
> schizophrenia (F20.-)

F91.0   Conduct disorder confined to family context

F91.1   Conduct disorder, childhood-onset type
Unsocialized conduct disorder
Conduct disorder, solitary aggressive type
Unsocialized aggressive disorder

F91.2   Conduct disorder, adolescent-onset type
Socialized conduct disorder
Conduct disorder, group type

F91.3   Oppositional defiant disorder

F91.8   Other conduct disorders
Other specified conduct disorder
Other specified disruptive disorder

F91.9   Conduct disorder, unspecified
Behavioral disorder NOS
Conduct disorder NOS
Disruptive behavior disorder NOS
Disruptive disorder NOS

F93   Emotional disorders with onset specific to childhood

F93.0   Separation anxiety disorder of childhood

> **Excludes2**   mood [affective] disorders (F30-F39)
> nonpsychotic mental disorders (F40-F48)
> phobic anxiety disorder of childhood (F40.8)
> social phobia (F40.1)

F93.8   Other childhood emotional disorders
Identity disorder

> **Excludes2**   gender identity disorder of childhood (F64.2)

F93.9   Childhood emotional disorder, unspecified

F94   Disorders of social functioning with onset specific to childhood and adolescence

F94.0   Selective mutism
Elective mutism

> **Excludes2**   pervasive developmental disorders (F84.-)
> schizophrenia (F20.-)
> specific developmental disorders of speech and language (F80.-)
> transient mutism as part of separation anxiety in young children (F93.0)

F94.1   Reactive attachment disorder of childhood
Use additional code to identify any associated failure to thrive or growth retardation

> **Excludes1**   disinhibited attachment disorder of childhood (F94.2)
> normal variation in pattern of selective attachment
>
> **Excludes2**   Asperger's syndrome (F84.5)
> maltreatment syndromes (T74.-)
> sexual or physical abuse in childhood, resulting in psychosocial problems (Z62.81-)

Item 5-2 Enuresis: Bed wetting by children at night. Causes can be either psychological or medical (diabetes, urinary tract infections, or abnormalities). **Encopresis:** Overflow incontinence of bowels sometimes resulting from chronic constipation or fecal impaction. Check the documentation for additional diagnoses.

F94.2   Disinhibited attachment disorder of childhood
Affectionless psychopathy
Institutional syndrome

> **Excludes1**   reactive attachment disorder of childhood (F94.1)
>
> **Excludes2**   Asperger's syndrome (F84.5)
> attention-deficit hyperactivity disorders (F90.-)
> hospitalism in children (F43.2-)

F94.8   Other childhood disorders of social functioning

F94.9   Childhood disorder of social functioning, unspecified

F95   Tic disorder
Involuntary twitch

F95.0   Transient tic disorder
Provisional tic disorder

F95.1   Chronic motor or vocal tic disorder

F95.2   Tourette's disorder
Combined vocal and multiple motor tic disorder [de la Tourette]
Tourette's syndrome

F95.8   Other tic disorders

F95.9   Tic disorder, unspecified
Tic NOS

F98   Other behavioral and emotional disorders with onset usually occurring in childhood and adolescence

> **Excludes2**   breath-holding spells (R06.89)
> gender identity disorder of childhood (F64.2)
> Kleine-Levin syndrome (G47.13)
> obsessive-compulsive disorder (F42.3-)
> sleep disorders not due to a substance or known physiological condition (F51.-)

F98.0   Enuresis not due to a substance or known physiological condition
Enuresis: Urinary incontinence
Enuresis (primary) (secondary) of nonorganic origin
Functional enuresis
Psychogenic enuresis
Urinary incontinence of nonorganic origin

> **Excludes1**   enuresis NOS (R32)

F98.1   Encopresis not due to a substance or known physiological condition
Encopresis: Fecal incontinence
Functional encopresis
Incontinence of feces of nonorganic origin
Psychogenic encopresis

Use additional code to identify the cause of any coexisting constipation.

> **Excludes1**   encopresis NOS (R15.-)

F98.2   Other feeding disorders of infancy and childhood

> **Excludes2**   anorexia nervosa and other eating disorders (F50.-)
> feeding difficulties (R63.3)
> feeding problems of newborn (P92.-)
> pica of infancy or childhood (F98.3)

F98.21   Rumination disorder of infancy

F98.29   Other feeding disorders of infancy and early childhood

F98.3   Pica of infancy and childhood
Craving and eating substances such as paint, clay, or dirt to replace a nutritional deficit in the body.

▶ New   ⇒ Revised   ~~deleted~~ Deleted   Excludes 1   Excludes 2   Includes   Use additional   Code first   Code also   Key words

OGCR Official Guidelines   X Assign placeholder X   ● Use Additional Character(s)   ▶ Manifestation Code   🔖 Hierarchical Condition Category   Coding Clinic

F98.4   **Stereotyped movement disorders**
Stereotype/habit disorder

> **Excludes1**   abnormal involuntary movements (R25.-)

> **Excludes2**   compulsions in obsessive-compulsive disorder (F42.-)
> hair plucking (F63.3)
> movement disorders of organic origin (G20-G25)
> nail-biting (F98.8)
> nose-picking (F98.8)
> stereotypies that are part of a broader psychiatric condition (F01-F95)
> thumb-sucking (F98.8)
> tic disorders (F95.-)
> trichotillomania (F63.3)

F98.5   **Adult onset fluency disorder**

> **Excludes1**   childhood onset fluency disorder (F80.81)
> dysphasia (R47.02)
> fluency disorder in conditions classified elsewhere (R47.82)
> fluency disorder (stuttering) following cerebrovascular disease (I69. with final characters -23)
> tic disorders (F95.-)

F98.8   **Other specified behavioral and emotional disorders with onset usually occurring in childhood and adolescence**
Excessive masturbation
Nail-biting
Nose-picking
Thumb-sucking

F98.9   **Unspecified behavioral and emotional disorders with onset usually occurring in childhood and adolescence**

UNSPECIFIED MENTAL DISORDER (F99)

F99   **Mental disorder, not otherwise specified**
Mental illness NOS

> **Excludes1**   unspecified mental disorder due to known physiological condition (F09)

CHAPTER 6

DISEASES OF THE NERVOUS SYSTEM (G00-G99)

OGCR Chapter-Specific Coding Guidelines

6. **Chapter 6: Diseases of the Nervous System (G00-G99)**

   a. **Dominant/nondominant side**

   Codes from category G81, Hemiplegia and hemiparesis, and subcategories, G83.1, Monoplegia of lower limb, G83.2, Monoplegia of upper limb, and G83.3, Monoplegia, unspecified, identify whether the dominant or nondominant side is affected. Should the affected side be documented, but not specified as dominant or nondominant, and the classification system does not indicate a default, code selection is as follows:
   - For ambidextrous patients, the default should be dominant.
   - If the left side is affected, the default is nondominant.
   - If the right side is affected, the default is dominant.

   b. **Pain - Category G89**

   1) **General coding information**

   Codes in category G89, Pain, not elsewhere classified, may be used in conjunction with codes from other categories and chapters to provide more detail about acute or chronic pain and neoplasm-related pain, unless otherwise indicated below.

   If the pain is not specified as acute or chronic, post-thoracotomy, postprocedural, or neoplasm-related, do not assign codes from category G89.

   A code from category G89 should not be assigned if the underlying (definitive) diagnosis is known, unless the reason for the encounter is pain control/management and not management of the underlying condition.

   When an admission or encounter is for a procedure aimed at treating the underlying condition (e.g., spinal fusion, kyphoplasty), a code for the underlying condition (e.g., vertebral fracture, spinal stenosis) should be assigned as the principal diagnosis. No code from category G89 should be assigned.

   (a) **Category G89 Codes as Principal or First-Listed Diagnosis**

   Category G89 codes are acceptable as principal diagnosis or the first-listed code:
   - When pain control or pain management is the reason for the admission/encounter (e.g., a patient with displaced intervertebral disc, nerve impingement and severe back pain presents for injection of steroid into the spinal canal). The underlying cause of the pain should be reported as an additional diagnosis, if known.
   - When a patient is admitted for the insertion of a neurostimulator for pain control, assign the appropriate pain code as the principal or first-listed diagnosis. When an admission or encounter is for a procedure aimed at treating the underlying condition and a neurostimulator is inserted for pain control during the same admission/encounter, a code for the underlying condition should be assigned as the principal diagnosis and the appropriate pain code should be assigned as a secondary diagnosis.

   (b) **Use of Category G89 Codes in Conjunction with Site Specific Pain Codes**

   (i) **Assigning Category G89 and Site-Specific Pain Codes**

   Codes from category G89 may be used in conjunction with codes that identify the site of pain (including codes from Chapter 18) if the category G89 code provides additional information. For example, if the code describes the site of the pain, but does not fully describe whether the pain is acute or chronic, then both codes should be assigned.

   (ii) **Sequencing of Category G89 Codes with Site-Specific Pain Codes**

The sequencing of category G89 codes with site-specific pain codes (including Chapter 18 codes), is dependent on the circumstances of the encounter/admission as follows:
   - If the encounter is for pain control or pain management, assign the code from category G89 followed by the code identifying the specific site of pain (e.g., encounter for pain management for acute neck pain from trauma is assigned code G89.11, Acute pain due to trauma, followed by code M54.2, Cervicalgia, to identify the site of pain).
   - If the encounter is for any other reason except pain control or pain management, and a related definitive diagnosis has not been established (confirmed) by the provider, assign the code for the specific site of pain first, followed by the appropriate code from category G89.

   2) **Pain due to devices, implants and grafts**

   See Section I.C.19. Pain due to medical devices

   3) **Postoperative Pain**

   The provider's documentation should be used to guide the coding of postoperative pain, as well as *Section III. Reporting Additional Diagnoses* and *Section IV. Diagnostic Coding and Reporting in the Outpatient Setting.*

   The default for post-thoracotomy and other postoperative pain not specified as acute or chronic is the code for the acute form.

   Routine or expected postoperative pain immediately after surgery should not be coded.

   (a) **Postoperative pain not associated with specific postoperative complication**

   Postoperative pain not associated with a specific postoperative complication is assigned to the appropriate postoperative pain code in category G89.

   (b) **Postoperative pain associated with specific postoperative complication**

   Postoperative pain associated with a specific postoperative complication (such as painful wire sutures) is assigned to the appropriate code(s) found in Chapter 19, Injury, poisoning, and certain other consequences of external causes. If appropriate, use additional code(s) from category G89 to identify acute or chronic pain (G89.18 or G89.28).

   4) **Chronic pain**

   Chronic pain is classified to subcategory G89.2. There is no time frame defining when pain becomes chronic pain. The provider's documentation should be used to guide use of these codes.

   5) **Neoplasm Related Pain**

   Code G89.3 is assigned to pain documented as being related, associated or due to cancer, primary or secondary malignancy, or tumor. This code is assigned regardless of whether the pain is acute or chronic.

   This code may be assigned as the principal or first-listed code when the stated reason for the admission/encounter is documented as pain control/pain management. The underlying neoplasm should be reported as an additional diagnosis.

   When the reason for the admission/encounter is management of the neoplasm and the pain associated with the neoplasm is also documented, code G89.3 may be assigned as an additional diagnosis. It is not necessary to assign an additional code for the site of the pain.

   See Section I.C.2 for instructions on the sequencing of neoplasms for all other stated reasons for the admission/encounter (except for pain control/pain management).

   6) **Chronic pain syndrome**

   Central pain syndrome (G89.0) and chronic pain syndrome (G89.4) are different than the term "chronic pain," and therefore codes should only be used when the provider has specifically documented this condition.

   See Section I.C.5. Pain disorders related to psychological factors

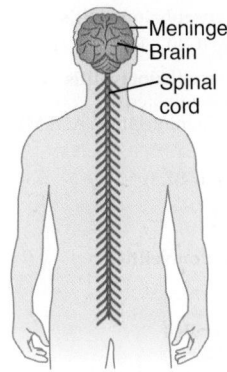

-Meninges
-Brain
-Spinal cord

Figure 6-1 The brain and spinal cord make up the central nervous system.

Item 6-1 The two major classifications of the nervous system are the peripheral nervous system and the central nervous system (CNS). The central nervous system is composed of the brain and the spinal cord. The peripheral nervous system is composed of the parasympathetic and sympathetic systems. **Encephalitis** is the swelling of the brain. **Meningitis** is swelling of the covering of the brain, the meninges. Types and causes of brain infections are:

Type	Cause
purulent	bacterial
aseptic/abacterial	viral
chronic meningitis	mycobacterial and fungal

CHAPTER 6

DISEASES OF THE NERVOUS SYSTEM (G00-G99)

Excludes2   certain conditions originating in the perinatal period (P04-P96)
certain infectious and parasitic diseases (A00-B99)
complications of pregnancy, childbirth and the puerperium (O00-O9A)
congenital malformations, deformations, and chromosomal abnormalities (Q00-Q99)
endocrine, nutritional and metabolic diseases (E00-E88)
injury, poisoning and certain other consequences of external causes (S00-T88)
neoplasms (C00-D49)
symptoms, signs and abnormal clinical and laboratory findings, not elsewhere classified (R00-R94)

This chapter contains the following blocks:

G00-G09	Inflammatory diseases of the central nervous system
G10-G14	Systemic atrophies primarily affecting the central nervous system
G20-G26	Extrapyramidal and movement disorders
G30-G32	Other degenerative diseases of the nervous system
G35-G37	Demyelinating diseases of the central nervous system
G40-G47	Episodic and paroxysmal disorders
G50-G59	Nerve, nerve root and plexus disorders
G60-G65	Polyneuropathies and other disorders of the peripheral nervous system
G70-G73	Diseases of myoneural junction and muscle
G80-G83	Cerebral palsy and other paralytic syndromes
G89-G99	Other disorders of the nervous system

INFLAMMATORY DISEASES OF THE CENTRAL NERVOUS SYSTEM (G00-G09)

● **G00**   **Bacterial meningitis, not elsewhere classified**
An infection of the cerebrospinal fluid surrounding the spinal cord and brain.

    Includes   bacterial arachnoiditis
bacterial leptomeningitis
bacterial meningitis
bacterial pachymeningitis

    Excludes1   bacterial meningoencephalitis (G04.2)
bacterial meningomyelitis (G04.2)

G00.0   **Hemophilus meningitis**
Meningitis due to Hemophilus influenzae

G00.1   **Pneumococcal meningitis**
Meningitis due to Streptococcal pneumoniae

G00.2   **Streptococcal meningitis**
Use additional code to further identify organism (B95.0-B95.5)

G00.3   **Staphylococcal meningitis**
Use additional code to further identify organism (B95.61-B95.8)

G00.8   **Other bacterial meningitis**
Meningitis due to Escherichia coli
Meningitis due to Friedländer bacillus
Meningitis due to Klebsiella
Use additional code to further identify organism (B96.-)

G00.9   **Bacterial meningitis, unspecified**
Meningitis due to gram-negative bacteria, unspecified
Purulent meningitis NOS
Pyogenic meningitis NOS
Suppurative meningitis NOS

▷ **G01**   *Meningitis in bacterial diseases classified elsewhere*
Code first underlying disease

    Excludes1   meningitis (in):
gonococcal (A54.81)
leptospirosis (A27.81)
listeriosis (A32.11)
Lyme disease (A69.21)
meningococcal (A39.0)
neurosyphilis (A52.13)
tuberculosis (A17.0)
meningoencephalitis and meningomyelitis in bacterial diseases classified elsewhere (G05)

▷ **G02**   *Meningitis in other infectious and parasitic diseases classified elsewhere*
Code first underlying disease, such as:
African trypanosomiasis (B56.-)
poliovirus infection (A80.-)

    Excludes1   candidal meningitis (B37.5)
coccidioidomycosis meningitis (B38.4)
cryptococcal meningitis (B45.1)
herpesviral [herpes simplex] meningitis (B00.3)
infectious mononucleosis complicated by meningitis (B27.- with fourth character 2)
measles complicated by meningitis (B05.1)
meningoencephalitis and meningomyelitis in other infectious and parasitic diseases classified elsewhere (G05)
mumps meningitis (B26.1)
rubella meningitis (B06.02)
varicella [chickenpox] meningitis (B01.0)
zoster meningitis (B02.1)

● **G03** **Meningitis due to other and unspecified causes**

Includes   arachnoiditis NOS
leptomeningitis NOS
meningitis NOS
pachymeningitis NOS

Excludes1   meningoencephalitis (G04.-)
meningomyelitis (G04.-)

G03.0 **Nonpyogenic meningitis**
Aseptic meningitis
Nonbacterial meningitis

G03.1 **Chronic meningitis**

G03.2 **Benign recurrent meningitis [Mollaret]**

G03.8 **Meningitis due to other specified causes**

G03.9 **Meningitis, unspecified**
Arachnoiditis (spinal) NOS

● **G04** **Encephalitis, myelitis and encephalomyelitis**

Includes   acute ascending myelitis
meningoencephalitis
meningomyelitis

Excludes1   encephalopathy NOS (G93.40)
other noninfectious acute disseminated
encephalomyelitis (noninfectious ADEM)
(G04.81)

Excludes2   acute transverse myelitis (G37.3-)
alcoholic encephalopathy (G31.2)
benign myalgic encephalomyelitis (G93.3)
multiple sclerosis (G35)
▶ myalgic encephalomyelitis (G93.32)
subacute necrotizing myelitis (G37.4)
toxic encephalitis (G92.8)
toxic encephalopathy (G92.8)

● **G04.0** **Acute disseminated encephalitis and encephalomyelitis (ADEM)**

Excludes1   acute necrotizing hemorrhagic
encephalopathy (G04.3-)

G04.00 **Acute disseminated encephalitis and encephalomyelitis, unspecified**

▶ **G04.01** *Postinfectious acute disseminated encephalitis and encephalomyelitis (postinfectious ADEM)*

Excludes1   post chickenpox encephalitis
(B01.1)
post measles encephalitis (B05.0)
post measles myelitis (B05.1)

G04.02 **Postimmunization acute disseminated encephalitis, myelitis and encephalomyelitis**
Encephalitis, post immunization
Encephalomyelitis, post immunization

Use additional code to identify the vaccine
(T50.A-, T50.B-, T50.Z-)

G04.1 **Tropical spastic paraplegia** 🝕

G04.2 **Bacterial meningoencephalitis and meningomyelitis, not elsewhere classified**

● **G04.3** **Acute necrotizing hemorrhagic encephalopathy**
Sudden and severe CNS disease with pathology of hemorrhages and necrosis of white matter

Excludes1   acute disseminated encephalitis and
encephalomyelitis (G04.0-)

G04.30 **Acute necrotizing hemorrhagic encephalopathy, unspecified**

G04.31 **Postinfectious acute necrotizing hemorrhagic encephalopathy**

G04.32 **Postimmunization acute necrotizing hemorrhagic encephalopathy**
Use additional code to identify vaccine
(T50.A-, T50.B-, T50.Z-)

G04.39 **Other acute necrotizing hemorrhagic encephalopathy**
Code also underlying etiology, if applicable

● **G04.8** **Other encephalitis, myelitis and encephalomyelitis**
Code also any associated seizure (G40.-, R56.9)

G04.81 **Other encephalitis and encephalomyelitis**
Noninfectious acute disseminated
encephalomyelitis (noninfectious ADEM)

G04.82 **Acute flaccid myelitis**
Excludes1   transverse myelitis (G37.3)

G04.89 **Other myelitis** 🝕
Coding Clinic: 2020, Q1, P14

● **G04.9** **Encephalitis, myelitis and encephalomyelitis, unspecified**

G04.90 **Encephalitis and encephalomyelitis, unspecified**
Ventriculitis (cerebral) NOS

G04.91 **Myelitis, unspecified** 🝕

● **G05** **Encephalitis, myelitis and encephalomyelitis in diseases classified elsewhere**
Code first underlying disease, such as:
congenital toxoplasmosis encephalitis, myelitis and
encephalomyelitis (P37.1)
cytomegaloviral encephalitis, myelitis and encephalomyelitis
(B25.8)
encephalitis, myelitis and encephalomyelitis (in) systemic
lupus erythematosus (M32.19)
eosinophilic meningoencephalitis (B83.2)
human immunodeficiency virus [HIV] disease (B20)
poliovirus (A80.-)
suppurative otitis media (H66.01-H66.4)
trichinellosis (B75)

Excludes1   adenoviral encephalitis, myelitis and
encephalomyelitis (A85.1)
encephalitis, myelitis and encephalomyelitis (in)
measles (B05.0)
enteroviral encephalitis, myelitis and
encephalomyelitis (A85.0)
herpesviral [herpes simplex] encephalitis,
myelitis and encephalomyelitis (B00.4)
listerial encephalitis, myelitis and
encephalomyelitis (A32.12)
meningococcal encephalitis, myelitis and
encephalomyelitis (A39.81)
mumps encephalitis, myelitis and
encephalomyelitis (B26.2)
postchickenpox encephalitis, myelitis and
encephalomyelitis (B01.1-)
rubella encephalitis, myelitis and
encephalomyelitis (B06.01)
toxoplasmosis encephalitis, myelitis and
encephalomyelitis (B58.2)
zoster encephalitis, myelitis and
encephalomyelitis (B02.0)

▶ **G05.3** *Encephalitis and encephalomyelitis in diseases classified elsewhere*
Meningoencephalitis in diseases classified elsewhere

▶ **G05.4** *Myelitis in diseases classified elsewhere* 🝕
Meningomyelitis in diseases classified elsewhere

● **G06** **Intracranial and intraspinal abscess and granuloma**
An accumulation of pus in either the brain or spinal cord
Use additional code (B95-B97) to identify infectious agent.

G06.0 **Intracranial abscess and granuloma**
Brain [any part] abscess (embolic)
Cerebellar abscess (embolic)
Cerebral abscess (embolic)
Intracranial epidural abscess or granuloma
Intracranial extradural abscess or granuloma
Intracranial subdural abscess or granuloma
Otogenic abscess (embolic)

Excludes1   tuberculous intracranial abscess and
granuloma (A17.81)

G06.1 Intraspinal abscess and granuloma
Abscess (embolic) of spinal cord [any part]
Intraspinal epidural abscess or granuloma
Intraspinal extradural abscess or granuloma
Intraspinal subdural abscess or granuloma
Excludes1   tuberculous intraspinal abscess and
granuloma (A17.81)

G06.2 Extradural and subdural abscess, unspecified

**G07 Intracranial and intraspinal abscess and granuloma in diseases
classified elsewhere**
Code first underlying disease, such as:
schistosomiasis granuloma of brain (B65.-)
Excludes1   abscess of brain:
amebic (A06.6)
chromomycotic (B43.1)
gonococcal (A54.82)
tuberculous (A17.81)
tuberculoma of meninges (A17.1)

G08 Intracranial and intraspinal phlebitis and thrombophlebitis
Septic embolism of intracranial or intraspinal venous sinuses
and veins
Septic endophlebitis of intracranial or intraspinal venous
sinuses and veins
Septic phlebitis of intracranial or intraspinal venous sinuses
and veins
Septic thrombophlebitis of intracranial or intraspinal venous
sinuses and veins
Septic thrombosis of intracranial or intraspinal venous sinuses
and veins
Excludes1   intracranial phlebitis and thrombophlebitis
complicating:
abortion, ectopic or molar pregnancy
(O00-O07, O08.7)
pregnancy, childbirth and the puerperium
(O22.5, O87.3)
nonpyogenic intracranial phlebitis and
thrombophlebitis (I67.6)
Excludes2   intracranial phlebitis and thrombophlebitis
complicating nonpyogenic intraspinal
phlebitis and thrombophlebitis (G95.1)

G09 Sequelae of inflammatory diseases of central nervous system
Note: Category G09 is to be used to indicate conditions
whose primary classification is to G00-G08 as the cause of
sequelae, themselves classifiable elsewhere. The 'sequelae'
include conditions specified as residuals.
*Code first condition resulting from (sequela) of inflammatory diseases
of central nervous system*

**SYSTEMIC ATROPHIES PRIMARILY AFFECTING
THE CENTRAL NERVOUS SYSTEM (G10-G14)**

G10 Huntington's disease 🔎
*Genetic disease with degeneration of cells of the nervous system,
including brain*
Huntington's chorea
Huntington's dementia
~~Code also dementia in other diseases classified elsewhere
without behavioral disturbance (F02.80)~~
▶ Use Additional code, if applicable, to identify:
▶ dementia with anxiety (F02.84, F02.A4, F02.B4, F02.C4)
▶ dementia with behavioral disturbance (F02.81-, F02.A1-, F02.
B1-, F02.C1-)
▶ dementia with mood disturbance (F02.83, F02.A3, F02.B3,
F02.C3)
▶ dementia with psychotic disturbance (F02.82, F02.A2, F02.B2,
F02.C2)
▶ dementia without behavioral disturbance (F02.80, F02.A0,
F02.B0, F02.C0)
▶ mild neurocognitive disorder due to known physiological
condition (F06.7-)

Item 6-2 Huntington's chorea is an inherited degenerative disorder of
the central nervous system and is characterized by ceaseless, jerky movements
and progressive cognitive and behavioral deterioration.

G11 Hereditary ataxia
Genetic neurological disorder affecting coordination
Excludes2   cerebral palsy (G80.-)
hereditary and idiopathic neuropathy (G60.-)
metabolic disorders (E70-E88)

G11.0 Congenital nonprogressive ataxia 🔎

G11.1 Early-onset cerebellar ataxia 🔎
G11.10 Early-onset cerebellar ataxia, unspecified
G11.11 Friedreich ataxia
Autosomal recessive Friedreich ataxia
Friedreich ataxia with retained reflexes
G11.19 Other early-onset cerebellar ataxia
Early-onset cerebellar ataxia with essential
tremor
Early-onset cerebellar ataxia with myoclonus
[Hunt's ataxia]
Early-onset cerebellar ataxia with retained
tendon reflexes
X-linked recessive spinocerebellar ataxia

G11.2 Late-onset cerebellar ataxia 🔎   A

G11.3 Cerebellar ataxia with defective DNA repair 🔎
Ataxia telangiectasia [Louis-Bar]
Excludes2   Cockayne's syndrome (Q87.19)
other disorders of purine and pyrimidine
metabolism (E79.-)
xeroderma pigmentosum (Q82.1)

G11.4 Hereditary spastic paraplegia 🔎
G11.8 Other hereditary ataxias 🔎
G11.9 Hereditary ataxia, unspecified 🔎
Hereditary cerebellar ataxia NOS
Hereditary cerebellar degeneration
Hereditary cerebellar disease
Hereditary cerebellar syndrome

G12 Spinal muscular atrophy and related syndromes
**G12.0 Infantile spinal muscular atrophy, type I
[Werdnig-Hoffman]** 🔎

G12.1 Other inherited spinal muscular atrophy 🔎
Adult form spinal muscular atrophy
Childhood form, type II spinal muscular atrophy
Distal spinal muscular atrophy
Juvenile form, type III spinal muscular atrophy
[Kugelberg-Welander]
Progressive bulbar palsy of childhood [Fazio-Londe]
Scapuloperoneal form spinal muscular atrophy

G12.2 Motor neuron disease
*Progressive disease of motor neurons that carry impluses to
muscles to move*
G12.20 Motor neuron disease, unspecified 🔎
G12.21 Amyotrophic lateral sclerosis 🔎   A
Lou Gehrig's disease (ALS)
G12.22 Progressive bulbar palsy 🔎
G12.23 Primary lateral sclerosis 🔎
G12.24 Familial motor neuron disease 🔎
G12.25 Progressive spinal muscle atrophy 🔎
G12.29 Other motor neuron disease 🔎
**G12.8 Other spinal muscular atrophies and related
syndromes** 🔎
G12.9 Spinal muscular atrophy, unspecified 🔎

**G13 Systemic atrophies primarily affecting central nervous system
in diseases classified elsewhere**
G13.0 Paraneoplastic neuromyopathy and neuropathy 🔎
Carcinomatous neuromyopathy
Sensorial paraneoplastic neuropathy [Denny Brown]
Code first underlying neoplasm (C00-D49)
**G13.1 Other systemic atrophy primarily affecting central
nervous system in neoplastic disease** 🔎
Paraneoplastic limbic encephalopathy
Code first underlying neoplasm (C00-D49)

▶ G13.2 **Systemic atrophy primarily affecting the central nervous system in myxedema**
    Code first underlying disease, such as:
      hypothyroidism (E03.-)
      myxedematous congenital iodine deficiency (E00.1)

▶ G13.8 **Systemic atrophy primarily affecting central nervous system in other diseases classified elsewhere**
    Code first underlying disease

G14 **Postpolio syndrome**
  Includes   Postpolio myelitic syndrome
  Excludes1   sequelae of poliomyelitis (B91)

EXTRAPYRAMIDAL AND MOVEMENT DISORDERS (G20-G26)

G20 **Parkinson's disease** 🐾
   Progressive disease of the nervous system that affects muscle coordination
   Hemiparkinsonism
   Idiopathic Parkinsonism or Parkinson's disease
   Paralysis agitans
   Parkinsonism or Parkinson's disease NOS
   Primary Parkinsonism or Parkinson's disease
  ⟹ Use additional code, if applicable, to identify:
    ⟹ dementia with anxiety (F02.84, F02.A4, F02.B4, F02.C4)
    ~~dementia without behavioral disturbance (F02.80)~~
    ▶ dementia with behavioral disturbance (F02.81-, F02.A1-, F02.B1-, F02.C1-)
    ▶ dementia with mood disturbance (F02.83, F02.A3, F02.B3, F02.C3)
    ▶ dementia with psychotic disturbance (F02.82, F02.A2, F02.B2, F02.C2)
    ▶ dementia without behavioral disturbance (F02.80, F02.A0, F02.B0, F02.C0)
    ▶ mild neurocognitive disorder due to known physiological condition (F06.7-)
    ~~Excludes1   dementia with Parkinsonism (G31.83)~~
   Coding Clinic: 2017, Q2, P7-8; 2016, Q2, P7

● G21 **Secondary parkinsonism**
   Symptoms of Parkinson's caused by medicines, illness, or other nervous system disorder
  Excludes1   dementia with Parkinsonism (G31.83)
             Huntington's disease (G10)
             Shy-Drager syndrome (G90.3)
             syphilitic Parkinsonism (A52.19)

  G21.0 **Malignant neuroleptic syndrome**
     Use additional code for adverse effect, if applicable, to identify drug (T43.3X5, T43.4X5, T43.505, T43.595)
    Excludes1   neuroleptic induced parkinsonism (G21.11)

● G21.1 **Other drug-induced secondary parkinsonism**
   G21.11 **Neuroleptic induced parkinsonism** 🐾
     Use additional code for adverse effect, if applicable, to identify drug (T43.3X5, T43.4X5, T43.505, T43.595)
     Excludes1   malignant neuroleptic syndrome (G21.0)
   G21.19 **Other drug induced secondary parkinsonism** 🐾
     Other medication-induced parkinsonism
     Use additional code for adverse effect, if applicable, to identify drug (T36-T50 with fifth or sixth character 5)

  G21.2 **Secondary parkinsonism due to other external agents** 🐾
    Code first (T51-T65) to identify external agent

  G21.3 **Postencephalitic parkinsonism** 🐾

G21.4 **Vascular parkinsonism** 🐾
G21.8 **Other secondary parkinsonism** 🐾
G21.9 **Secondary parkinsonism, unspecified** 🐾

● G23 **Other degenerative diseases of basal ganglia**
  Excludes2   multi-system degeneration of the autonomic nervous system (G90.3)

  G23.0 **Hallervorden-Spatz disease** 🐾
     Pigmentary pallidal degeneration

  G23.1 **Progressive supranuclear ophthalmoplegia [Steele-Richardson-Olszewski]** 🐾
     Progressive supranuclear palsy

  G23.2 **Striatonigral degeneration** 🐾

  G23.8 **Other specified degenerative diseases of basal ganglia** 🐾
     Calcification of basal ganglia

  G23.9 **Degenerative disease of basal ganglia, unspecified** 🐾

● G24 **Dystonia**
   Involuntary movements
  Includes   dyskinesia
  Excludes2   athetoid cerebral palsy (G80.3)

● G24.0 **Drug induced dystonia**
     Use additional code for adverse effect, if applicable, to identify drug (T36-T50 with fifth or sixth character 5)
   G24.01 **Drug induced subacute dyskinesia**
     Drug induced blepharospasm
     Drug induced orofacial dyskinesia
     Neuroleptic induced tardive dyskinesia
     Tardive dyskinesia
   G24.02 **Drug induced acute dystonia**
     Acute dystonic reaction to drugs
     Neuroleptic induced acute dystonia
   G24.09 **Other drug induced dystonia**

  G24.1 **Genetic torsion dystonia**
     Dystonia deformans progressiva
     Dystonia musculorum deformans
     Familial torsion dystonia
     Idiopathic familial dystonia
     Idiopathic (torsion) dystonia NOS
     (Schwalbe-) Ziehen-Oppenheim disease

  G24.2 **Idiopathic nonfamilial dystonia**

  G24.3 **Spasmodic torticollis**
    Head tilts toward one side and chin is elevated and turned toward opposite side (wry neck)
    Excludes1   congenital torticollis (Q68.0)
             hysterical torticollis (F44.4)
             ocular torticollis (R29.891)
             psychogenic torticollis (F45.8)
             torticollis NOS (M43.6)
             traumatic recurrent torticollis (S13.4)

  G24.4 **Idiopathic orofacial dystonia**
     Orofacial dyskinesia
    Excludes1   drug induced orofacial dyskinesia (G24.01)

  G24.5 **Blepharospasm**
    Tonic spasm of orbicularis oculi muscle, producing closure of eyelids
    Excludes1   drug induced blepharospasm (G24.01)

  G24.8 **Other dystonia**
     Acquired torsion dystonia NOS

  G24.9 **Dystonia, unspecified**
     Dyskinesia NOS

▶ New ⟹ Revised ~~deleted~~ Deleted Excludes 1 Excludes 2 Includes Use additional Code first Code also Key words
OGCR Official Guidelines X Assign placeholder X ● Use Additional Character(s) ▶ Manifestation Code 🐾 Hierarchical Condition Category **Coding Clinic**

● **G25**   **Other extrapyramidal and movement disorders**
Extrapyramidal: Other than pyramidal tracts

    Excludes2   sleep related movement disorders (G47.6-)

   G25.0   **Essential tremor**
      Familial tremor
      Excludes1   tremor NOS (R25.1)

   G25.1   **Drug-induced tremor**
      Use additional code for adverse effect, if applicable, to identify drug (T36-T50 with fifth or sixth character 5)

   G25.2   **Other specified forms of tremor**
      Intention tremor

   G25.3   **Myoclonus**
      Shocklike contractions muscle(s)
      Drug-induced myoclonus
      Palatal myoclonus
      Use additional code for adverse effect, if applicable, to identify drug (T36-T50 with fifth or sixth character 5)
      Excludes1   facial myokymia (G51.4)
                  myoclonic epilepsy (G40.-)

   G25.4   **Drug-induced chorea**
      Use additional code for adverse effect, if applicable, to identify drug (T36-T50 with fifth or sixth character 5)

   G25.5   **Other chorea**
      Continual, involuntary, jerky, movements
      Chorea NOS
      Excludes1   chorea NOS with heart involvement (I02.0)
                  Huntington's chorea (G10)
                  rheumatic chorea (I02.-)
                  Sydenham's chorea (I02.-)

● **G25.6**   **Drug induced tics and other tics of organic origin**

    G25.61   **Drug induced tics**
        Use additional code for adverse effect, if applicable, to identify drug (T36-T50 with fifth or sixth character 5)

    G25.69   **Other tics of organic origin**
        Excludes1   habit spasm (F95.9)
                    tic NOS (F95.9)
                    Tourette's syndrome (F95.2)

● **G25.7**   **Other and unspecified drug induced movement disorders**
      Use additional code for adverse effect, if applicable, to identify drug (T36-T50 with fifth or sixth character 5)

    G25.70   **Drug induced movement disorder, unspecified**

    G25.71   **Drug induced akathisia**
        Drug induced acathisia
        Neuroleptic induced acute akathisia
        Tardive akathisia

    G25.79   **Other drug induced movement disorders**

● **G25.8**   **Other specified extrapyramidal and movement disorders**

    G25.81   **Restless legs syndrome**

    G25.82   **Stiff-man syndrome**

    G25.83   **Benign shuddering attacks**

    G25.89   **Other specified extrapyramidal and movement disorders**

   G25.9   **Extrapyramidal and movement disorder, unspecified**

▷ **G26**   *Extrapyramidal and movement disorders in diseases classified elsewhere*
      Code first underlying disease

OTHER DEGENERATIVE DISEASES OF THE NERVOUS SYSTEM (G30-G32)

● **G30**   **Alzheimer's disease**
Progressive central neurodegenerative disorder

    Includes   Alzheimer's dementia senile and presenile forms

➡ Use additional code, if applicable, to identify:
    delirium, if applicable (F05)
➡   dementia with anxiety (F02.84, F02.A4, F02.B4, F02.C4)
   ~~dementia without behavioral disturbance (F02.80)~~
▶ dementia with behavioral disturbance (F02.81-, F02.A1-, F02.B1-, F02.C1-)
▶ dementia with mood disturbance (F02.83, F02.A3, F02.B3, F02.C3)
▶ dementia with psychotic disturbance (F02.82, F02.A2, F02.B2, F02.C2)
▶ dementia without behavioral disturbance (F02.80, F02.A0, F02.B0, F02.C0)
▶ mild neurocognitive disorder due to known physiological condition (F06.7-)

    Excludes1   senile degeneration of brain NEC (G31.1)
                  senile dementia NOS (F03)
                  senility NOS (R41.81)

   G30.0   **Alzheimer's disease with early onset**

   G30.1   **Alzheimer's disease with late onset**   A

   G30.8   **Other Alzheimer's disease**

   G30.9   **Alzheimer's disease, unspecified**
      Coding Clinic: 2017, Q1, P43; 2016, Q2, P6; 2012, Q4, P95

● **G31**   **Other degenerative diseases of nervous system, not elsewhere classified**

    Use additional
    ~~For codes G31.0-G31.83, G31.85-G31.9, use additional code to identify:~~
    ~~dementia with behavioral disturbance (F02.81)~~
    ~~dementia without behavioral disturbance (F02.80)~~
▶ dementia with behavioral disturbance (F02.81-, F02.A1-, F02.B1-, F02.C1-)
▶ dementia with mood disturbance (F02.83, F02.A3, F02.B3, F02.C3)
▶ dementia with psychotic disturbance (F02.82, F02.A2, F02.B2, F02.C2)
▶ dementia without behavioral disturbance (F02.80, F02.A0, F02.B0, F02.C0)
▶ mild neurocognitive disorder due to known physiological condition (F06.7-)

    Excludes2   Reye's syndrome (G93.7)

● **G31.0**   **Frontotemporal dementia**

    G31.01   **Pick's disease**
        Primary progressive aphasia
        Progressive isolated aphasia

  ➡ **G31.09**   **Other frontotemporal neurocognitive disorder**
        Frontal dementia
      ▶ Use Additional code, if applicable, to identify mild neurocognitive disorders due to known physiological condition (F06.7-)

   G31.1   **Senile degeneration of brain, not elsewhere classified**
      Excludes1   Alzheimer's disease (G30.-)
                  senility NOS (R41.81)

   G31.2   **Degeneration of nervous system due to alcohol**
      Alcoholic cerebellar ataxia
      Alcoholic cerebellar degeneration
      Alcoholic cerebral degeneration
      Alcoholic encephalopathy
      Dysfunction of the autonomic nervous system due to alcohol
      Code also associated alcoholism (F10.-)

● **G31.8**   **Other specified degenerative diseases of nervous system**

    G31.81   **Alpers' disease**
        Rare neuronal degeneration of cerebral cortex disease of young children
        Grey-matter degeneration
        Coding Clinic: 2017, Q2, P7

    G31.82   **Leigh's disease**
        Rare neurometabolic disorder that affects central nervous system
        Subacute necrotizing encephalopathy

CHAPTER 6 (G00-G99)

➡️ ⬭**G31.83** **Neurocognitive disorder with Lewy bodies**
Closely allied to Parkinson's Disease
~~Dementia with Parkinsonism~~
Lewy body dementia
Lewy body disease
▶ Use Additional code, if applicable, to identify mild neurocognitive disorders due to known physiological condition (F06.7-)
Coding Clinic: 2017, Q2, P7; 2016, Q4, P141

➡️**G31.84** **Mild cognitive impairment of uncertain or unknown etiology**
~~Mild neurocognitive disorder~~
▶ Mild cognitive disorder NOS
▶ Mild neurocognitive disorder of uncertain or unknown etiology
▶ Use Additional code to identify presence of:
▶ alcohol abuse and dependence (F10.-)
▶ exposure to environmental tobacco smoke (Z77.22)
▶ history of tobacco dependence (Z87.891)
▶ hypertension (I10-I16)
▶ occupational exposure to environmental tobacco smoke (Z57.31)
▶ tobacco dependence (F17.-)
▶ tobacco use (Z72.0)

Excludes1   age related cognitive decline (R41.81)
altered mental status (R41.82)
cerebral degeneration (G31.9)
▶ cerebrovascular diseases (I60-I69)
change in mental status (R41.82)
cognitive deficits following (sequelae of) cerebral hemorrhage or infarction (I69.01-, I69.11-, I69.21-, I69.31-, I69.81-, I69.91-)
cognitive impairment due to intracranial or head injury (S06.-)
dementia (F01.-, F02.-, F03)
~~mild memory disturbance (F06.8)~~
▶ mild neurocognitive disorder due to a known physiological condition (F06.7-)
neurologic neglect syndrome (R41.4)
personality change, nonpsychotic (F68.8)
Coding Clinic: 2021, Q3, P3

G31.85 **Corticobasal degeneration**

G31.89 **Other specified degenerative diseases of nervous system**

G31.9 **Degenerative disease of nervous system, unspecified**
Coding Clinic: 2021, Q3, P3

⬤ **G32** **Other degenerative disorders of nervous system in diseases classified elsewhere**

▷ *G32.0* *Subacute combined degeneration of spinal cord in diseases classified elsewhere* 🐾
Dana-Putnam syndrome
Sclerosis of spinal cord (combined) (dorsolateral) (posterolateral)
Code first underlying disease, such as:
anemia (D51.9)
dietary (D51.3)
pernicious (D51.0)
vitamin B12 deficiency (E53.8)
Excludes1   syphilitic combined degeneration of spinal cord (A52.11)

⬤ **G32.8** **Other specified degenerative disorders of nervous system in diseases classified elsewhere**
Code first underlying disease, such as:
amyloidosis cerebral degeneration (E85.-)
cerebral degeneration (due to) hypothyroidism (E00.0-E03.9)
cerebral degeneration (due to) neoplasm (C00-D49)
cerebral degeneration (due to) vitamin B deficiency, except thiamine (E52-E53.-)
Excludes1   superior hemorrhagic polioencephalitis [Wernicke's encephalopathy] (E51.2)

▷ *G32.81* *Cerebellar ataxia in diseases classified elsewhere* 🐾
Code first underlying disease, such as:
celiac disease (with gluten ataxia) (K90.0)
cerebellar ataxia (in) neoplastic disease (paraneoplastic cerebellar degeneration) (C00-D49)
non-celiac gluten ataxia (M35.9)
Excludes1   systemic atrophy primarily affecting the central nervous system in alcoholic cerebellar ataxia (G31.2)
systemic atrophy primarily affecting the central nervous system in myxedema (G13.2)

▷ *G32.89* *Other specified degenerative disorders of nervous system in diseases classified elsewhere*
Degenerative encephalopathy in diseases classified elsewhere

DEMYELINATING DISEASES OF THE CENTRAL NERVOUS SYSTEM (G35-G37)

G35 **Multiple sclerosis** 🐾
Destruction of central nervous system; four types: relapsing remitting, secondary progressive, primary progressive, and progressive relapsing
Disseminated multiple sclerosis
Generalized multiple sclerosis
Multiple sclerosis NOS
Multiple sclerosis of brain stem
Multiple sclerosis of cord
Coding Clinic: 2021, Q1, P7

⬤ **G36** **Other acute disseminated demyelination**
Excludes1   postinfectious encephalitis and encephalomyelitis NOS (G04.01)

G36.0 **Neuromyelitis optica [Devic]** 🐾
Inflammatory disorder in which immune system attacks optic nerves and spinal cord producing inflammation of optic nerve (optic neuritis) and spinal cord (myelitis)
Demyelination in optic neuritis
Excludes1   optic neuritis NOS (H46)

G36.1 **Acute and subacute hemorrhagic leukoencephalitis [Hurst]** 🐾

G36.8 **Other specified acute disseminated demyelination** 🐾

G36.9 **Acute disseminated demyelination, unspecified** 🐾

⬤ **G37** **Other demyelinating diseases of central nervous system**
Destruction of central nervous system

G37.0 **Diffuse sclerosis of central nervous system** 🐾
Periaxial encephalitis
Schilder's disease
Excludes1   X linked adrenoleukodystrophy (E71.52-)

G37.1 **Central demyelination of corpus callosum** 🐾

Item 6–3   **Multiple sclerosis** (MS) is a nervous system disease affecting the brain and spinal cord by damaging the myelin sheath surrounding and protecting nerve cells. The damage slows down/blocks messages between the brain and body. Symptoms are visual disturbances, muscle weakness, coordination and balance issues, numbness, prickling, thinking and memory problems. The cause is unknown, though it is thought that it may be an autoimmune disease. It affects women more than men, between 20 and 40 years of age. MS can be mild, but it may cause the loss of ability to write, walk, and speak. There is no cure, but medication may slow or control symptoms.

| ▶ New | ⇒ Revised | ~~deleted~~ Deleted | Excludes 1 | Excludes 2 | Includes | Use additional | Code first | Code also | Key words |

808   OGCR Official Guidelines   X Assign placeholder X   ⬤ Use Additional Character(s)   ▷ Manifestation Code   🐾 Hierarchical Condition Category   Coding Clinic

G37.2   **Central pontine myelinolysis** 🔖
     Coding Clinic: 2022, Q2, P11

G37.3   **Acute transverse myelitis in demyelinating disease of central nervous system** 🔖
     Acute transverse myelitis NOS
     Acute transverse myelopathy

     Excludes1   acute flaccid myelitis (G04.82)
                  multiple sclerosis (G35)
                  neuromyelitis optica [Devic] (G36.0)

G37.4   **Subacute necrotizing myelitis of central nervous system** 🔖

G37.5   **Concentric sclerosis [Baló] of central nervous system** 🔖

G37.8   **Other specified demyelinating diseases of central nervous system** 🔖

G37.9   **Demyelinating disease of central nervous system, unspecified** 🔖

EPISODIC AND PAROXYSMAL DISORDERS (G40-G47)

● **G40**   **Epilepsy and recurrent seizures**
     Note: The following terms are to be considered equivalent to intractable: pharmacoresistant (pharmacologically resistant), treatment resistant, refractory (medically) and poorly controlled

     Excludes1   conversion disorder with seizures (F44.5)
                  convulsions NOS (R56.9)
                  post traumatic seizures (R56.1)
                  seizure (convulsive) NOS (R56.9)
                  seizure of newborn (P90)

     Excludes2   hippocampal sclerosis (G93.81)
                  mesial temporal sclerosis (G93.81)
                  temporal sclerosis (G93.81)
                  Todd's paralysis (G83.84)

● **G40.0**   **Localization-related (focal) (partial) idiopathic epilepsy and epileptic syndromes with seizures of localized onset**
     Benign childhood epilepsy with centrotemporal EEG spikes
     Childhood epilepsy with occipital EEG paroxysms

     Excludes1   adult onset localization-related epilepsy (G40.1-, G40.2-)

   ● **G40.00**   **Localization-related (focal) (partial) idiopathic epilepsy and epileptic syndromes with seizures of localized onset, not intractable**
       Localization-related (focal) (partial) idiopathic epilepsy and epileptic syndromes with seizures of localized onset without intractability

       G40.001   Localization-related (focal) (partial) idiopathic epilepsy and epileptic syndromes with seizures of localized onset, not intractable, with status epilepticus 🔖

       G40.009   Localization-related (focal) (partial) idiopathic epilepsy and epileptic syndromes with seizures of localized onset, not intractable, without status epilepticus 🔖
           Localization-related (focal) (partial) idiopathic epilepsy and epileptic syndromes with seizures of localized onset NOS

   ● **G40.01**   **Localization-related (focal) (partial) idiopathic epilepsy and epileptic syndromes with seizures of localized onset, intractable**

       G40.011   Localization-related (focal) (partial) idiopathic epilepsy and epileptic syndromes with seizures of localized onset, intractable, with status epilepticus 🔖

       G40.019   Localization-related (focal) (partial) idiopathic epilepsy and epileptic syndromes with seizures of localized onset, intractable, without status epilepticus 🔖

● **G40.1**   **Localization-related (focal) (partial) symptomatic epilepsy and epileptic syndromes with simple partial seizures**
     Attacks without alteration of consciousness
     Epilepsia partialis continua [Kozhevnikof]
     Simple partial seizures developing into secondarily generalized seizures

   ● **G40.10**   **Localization-related (focal) (partial) symptomatic epilepsy and epileptic syndromes with simple partial seizures, not intractable**
       Localization-related (focal) (partial) symptomatic epilepsy and epileptic syndromes with simple partial seizures without intractability

       G40.101   Localization-related (focal) (partial) symptomatic epilepsy and epileptic syndromes with simple partial seizures, not intractable, with status epilepticus

       G40.109   Localization-related (focal) (partial) symptomatic epilepsy and epileptic syndromes with simple partial seizures, not intractable, without status epilepticus 🔖
           Localization-related (focal) (partial) symptomatic epilepsy and epileptic syndromes with simple partial seizures NOS

   ● **G40.11**   **Localization-related (focal) (partial) symptomatic epilepsy and epileptic syndromes with simple partial seizures, intractable**

       G40.111   Localization-related (focal) (partial) symptomatic epilepsy and epileptic syndromes with simple partial seizures, intractable, with status epilepticus 🔖

       G40.119   Localization-related (focal) (partial) symptomatic epilepsy and epileptic syndromes with simple partial seizures, intractable, without status epilepticus 🔖

● **G40.2**   **Localization-related (focal) (partial) symptomatic epilepsy and epileptic syndromes with complex partial seizures**
     Attacks with alteration of consciousness, often with automatisms
     Complex partial seizures developing into secondarily generalized seizures

   ● **G40.20**   **Localization-related (focal) (partial) symptomatic epilepsy and epileptic syndromes with complex partial seizures, not intractable**
       Localization-related (focal) (partial) symptomatic epilepsy and epileptic syndromes with complex partial seizures without intractability

       G40.201   Localization-related (focal) (partial) symptomatic epilepsy and epileptic syndromes with complex partial seizures, not intractable, with status epilepticus 🔖

       G40.209   Localization-related (focal) (partial) symptomatic epilepsy and epileptic syndromes with complex partial seizures, not intractable, without status epilepticus 🔖
           Localization-related (focal) (partial) symptomatic epilepsy and epileptic syndromes with complex partial seizures NOS

G40.21 **Localization-related (focal) (partial) symptomatic epilepsy and epileptic syndromes with complex partial seizures, intractable**

    G40.211 **Localization-related (focal) (partial) symptomatic epilepsy and epileptic syndromes with complex partial seizures, intractable, with status epilepticus** 🐾

    G40.219 **Localization-related (focal) (partial) symptomatic epilepsy and epileptic syndromes with complex partial seizures, intractable, without status epilepticus** 🐾

● G40.3 **Generalized idiopathic epilepsy and epileptic syndromes**

    Code also MERRF syndrome, if applicable (E88.42)

  ● G40.30 **Generalized idiopathic epilepsy and epileptic syndromes, not intractable**

    Generalized idiopathic epilepsy and epileptic syndromes without intractability

    G40.301 **Generalized idiopathic epilepsy and epileptic syndromes, not intractable, with status epilepticus** 🐾

    G40.309 **Generalized idiopathic epilepsy and epileptic syndromes, not intractable, without status epilepticus** 🐾

      Generalized idiopathic epilepsy and epileptic syndromes NOS

  ● G40.31 **Generalized idiopathic epilepsy and epileptic syndromes, intractable**

    G40.311 **Generalized idiopathic epilepsy and epileptic syndromes, intractable, with status epilepticus** 🐾

    G40.319 **Generalized idiopathic epilepsy and epileptic syndromes, intractable, without status epilepticus** 🐾

● G40.4 **Other generalized epilepsy and epileptic syndromes**

    Epilepsy with grand mal seizures on awakening
    Epilepsy with myoclonic absences
    Epilepsy with myoclonic-astatic seizures
    Grand mal seizure NOS
    Nonspecific atonic epileptic seizures
    Nonspecific clonic epileptic seizures
    Nonspecific myoclonic epileptic seizures
    Nonspecific tonic epileptic seizures
    Nonspecific tonic-clonic epileptic seizures
    Symptomatic early myoclonic encephalopathy

  ● G40.40 **Other generalized epilepsy and epileptic syndromes, not intractable**

    Other generalized epilepsy and epileptic syndromes without intractability
    Other generalized epilepsy and epileptic syndromes NOS

    G40.401 **Other generalized epilepsy and epileptic syndromes, not intractable, with status epilepticus** 🐾

    G40.409 **Other generalized epilepsy and epileptic syndromes, not intractable, without status epilepticus** 🐾

  ● G40.41 **Other generalized epilepsy and epileptic syndromes, intractable**

    G40.411 **Other generalized epilepsy and epileptic syndromes, intractable, with status epilepticus** 🐾

    G40.419 **Other generalized epilepsy and epileptic syndromes, intractable, without status epilepticus** 🐾

   G40.42 **Cyclin-Dependent Kinase-Like 5 Deficiency Disorder**
    CDKL5

    Use additional code, if known, to identify associated manifestations, such as:
      cortical blindness (H47.61-)
      global developmental delay (F88)

● G40.5 **Epileptic seizures related to external causes**

    Epileptic seizures related to alcohol
    Epileptic seizures related to drugs
    Epileptic seizures related to hormonal changes
    Epileptic seizures related to sleep deprivation
    Epileptic seizures related to stress

    Code also, if applicable, associated epilepsy and recurrent seizures (G40.-)

    Use additional code for adverse effect, if applicable, to identify drug (T36-T50 with fifth or sixth character 5)

  ● G40.50 **Epileptic seizures related to external causes, not intractable**

    G40.501 **Epileptic seizures related to external causes, not intractable, with status epilepticus** 🐾

    G40.509 **Epileptic seizures related to external causes, not intractable, without status epilepticus** 🐾
      Epileptic seizures related to external causes, NOS

● G40.8 **Other epilepsy and recurrent seizures**

    Epilepsies and epileptic syndromes undetermined as to whether they are focal or generalized
    Landau-Kleffner syndrome

  ● G40.80 **Other epilepsy**

    G40.801 **Other epilepsy, not intractable, with status epilepticus** 🐾
      Other epilepsy without intractability with status epilepticus

    G40.802 **Other epilepsy, not intractable, without status epilepticus** 🐾
      Other epilepsy NOS
      Other epilepsy without intractability without status epilepticus

    G40.803 **Other epilepsy, intractable, with status epilepticus** 🐾

    G40.804 **Other epilepsy, intractable, without status epilepticus** 🐾

  ● G40.81 **Lennox-Gastaut syndrome**

    G40.811 **Lennox-Gastaut syndrome, not intractable, with status epilepticus** 🐾

    G40.812 **Lennox-Gastaut syndrome, not intractable, without status epilepticus** 🐾

    G40.813 **Lennox-Gastaut syndrome, intractable, with status epilepticus** 🐾

    G40.814 **Lennox-Gastaut syndrome, intractable, without status epilepticus** 🐾

  ● G40.82 **Epileptic spasms**
    Infantile spasms
    Salaam attacks
    West's syndrome

    G40.821 **Epileptic spasms, not intractable, with status epilepticus** 🐾

    G40.822 **Epileptic spasms, not intractable, without status epilepticus** 🐾

    G40.823 **Epileptic spasms, intractable, with status epilepticus** 🐾

    G40.824 **Epileptic spasms, intractable, without status epilepticus** 🐾

  ● G40.83 **Dravet syndrome**
    Polymorphic epilepsy in infancy (PMEI)
    Severe myoclonic epilepsy in infancy (SMEI)

    G40.833 **Dravet syndrome, intractable, with status epilepticus**

    G40.834 **Dravet syndrome, intractable, without status epilepticus**
      Dravet syndrome NOS

   G40.89 **Other seizures** 🐾

    Excludes1   post traumatic seizures (R56.1)
               recurrent seizures NOS (G40.909)
               seizure NOS (R56.9)

▶ New   ⇒ Revised   ~~deleted~~ Deleted   Excludes 1   Excludes 2   Includes   Use additional   Code first   Code also   Key words

OGCR Official Guidelines   X Assign placeholder X   ● Use Additional Character(s)   ▶ Manifestation Code   🐾 Hierarchical Condition Category   **Coding Clinic**

● **G40.9   Epilepsy, unspecified**
  ● **G40.90   Epilepsy, unspecified, not intractable**
      Epilepsy, unspecified, without intractability
    G40.901   Epilepsy, unspecified, not intractable, with status epilepticus 🔖
    G40.909   Epilepsy, unspecified, not intractable, without status epilepticus 🔖
      Epilepsy NOS
      Epileptic convulsions NOS
      Epileptic fits NOS
      Epileptic seizures NOS
      Recurrent seizures NOS
      Seizure disorder NOS
      Coding Clinic: 2021, Q2, P3
  ● **G40.91   Epilepsy, unspecified, intractable**
      Intractable seizure disorder NOS
    G40.911   Epilepsy, unspecified, intractable, with status epilepticus 🔖
    G40.919   Epilepsy, unspecified, intractable, without status epilepticus 🔖
● **G40.A   Absence epileptic syndrome**
      Childhood absence epilepsy [pyknolepsy]
      Juvenile absence epilepsy
      Absence epileptic syndrome, NOS
  ● **G40.A0   Absence epileptic syndrome, not intractable**
    G40.A01   Absence epileptic syndrome, not intractable, with status epilepticus 🔖
    G40.A09   Absence epileptic syndrome, not intractable, without status epilepticus 🔖
  ● **G40.A1   Absence epileptic syndrome, intractable**
    G40.A11   Absence epileptic syndrome, intractable, with status epilepticus 🔖
    G40.A19   Absence epileptic syndrome, intractable, without status epilepticus 🔖
● **G40.B   Juvenile myoclonic epilepsy [impulsive petit mal]**
  ● **G40.B0   Juvenile myoclonic epilepsy, not intractable**
    G40.B01   Juvenile myoclonic epilepsy, not intractable, with status epilepticus 🔖
    G40.B09   Juvenile myoclonic epilepsy, not intractable, without status epilepticus 🔖
  ● **G40.B1   Juvenile myoclonic epilepsy, intractable**
    G40.B11   Juvenile myoclonic epilepsy, intractable, with status epilepticus 🔖
    G40.B19   Juvenile myoclonic epilepsy, intractable, without status epilepticus 🔖

● **G43   Migraine**
  Note: The following terms are to be considered equivalent to intractable: pharmacoresistant (pharmacologically resistant), treatment resistant, refractory (medically) and poorly controlled
  Use additional code for adverse effect, if applicable, to identify drug (T36-T50 with fifth or sixth character 5)
  Excludes1   headache NOS (R51.9)
          lower half migraine (G44.00)
  Excludes2   headache syndromes (G44.-)
  ● **G43.0   Migraine without aura**
      Neurological disorder, generally recurring headaches without early symptom (aura)
      Common migraine
    Excludes1   chronic migraine without aura (G43.7-)
    ● **G43.00   Migraine without aura, not intractable**
      Neurological disorder, generally recurring headaches without early symptom (aura); resistant to cure, relief, or control
      Migraine without aura without mention of refractory migraine
      G43.001   Migraine without aura, not intractable, with status migrainosus

Item 6–4   Migraine headache is described as an intense pulsing or throbbing pain in one area of the head. It can be accompanied by extreme sensitivity to light (photophobic) and sound and is three times more common in women than in men. Symptoms include nausea and vomiting. Research indicates migraine headaches are caused by inherited abnormalities in genes that control the activities of certain cell populations in the brain.

      G43.009   Migraine without aura, not intractable, without status migrainosus
        Migraine without aura NOS
    ● **G43.01   Migraine without aura, intractable**
      Intractable migraine: Not easily cured or managed; relentless pain from a migraine
      Migraine without aura with refractory migraine
      G43.011   Migraine without aura, intractable, with status migrainosus
      G43.019   Migraine without aura, intractable, without status migrainosus
  ● **G43.1   Migraine with aura**
      Basilar migraine
      Classical migraine
      Migraine equivalents
      Migraine preceded or accompanied by transient focal neurological phenomena
      Migraine triggered seizures
      Migraine with acute-onset aura
      Migraine with aura without headache (migraine equivalents)
      Migraine with prolonged aura
      Migraine with typical aura
      Retinal migraine
      Code also any associated seizure (G40.-, R56.9)
    Excludes1   persistent migraine aura (G43.5-, G43.6-)
    ● **G43.10   Migraine with aura, not intractable**
      Migraine with aura without mention of refractory migraine
      G43.101   Migraine with aura, not intractable, with status migrainosus
      G43.109   Migraine with aura, not intractable, without status migrainosus
        Migraine with aura NOS
    ● **G43.11   Migraine with aura, intractable**
      Migraine with aura with refractory migraine
      G43.111   Migraine with aura, intractable, with status migrainosus
      G43.119   Migraine with aura, intractable, without status migrainosus
  ● **G43.4   Hemiplegic migraine**
      Inherited migraine disorder causing temporary paralysis of one side of body followed by severe headache and nausea
      Familial migraine
      Sporadic migraine
    ● **G43.40   Hemiplegic migraine, not intractable**
      Hemiplegic migraine without refractory migraine
      G43.401   Hemiplegic migraine, not intractable, with status migrainosus
      G43.409   Hemiplegic migraine, not intractable, without status migrainosus
        Hemiplegic migraine NOS
    ● **G43.41   Hemiplegic migraine, intractable**
      Hemiplegic migraine with refractory migraine
      G43.411   Hemiplegic migraine, intractable, with status migrainosus
      G43.419   Hemiplegic migraine, intractable, without status migrainosus
  ● **G43.5   Persistent migraine aura without cerebral infarction**
    ● **G43.50   Persistent migraine aura without cerebral infarction, not intractable**
      Persistent migraine aura without cerebral infarction, without refractory migraine

CHAPTER 6 (G00-G99)

G43.501   Persistent migraine aura without cerebral infarction, not intractable, with status migrainosus

G43.509   Persistent migraine aura without cerebral infarction, not intractable, without status migrainosus
    Persistent migraine aura NOS

● **G43.51**   Persistent migraine aura without cerebral infarction, intractable
    Persistent migraine aura without cerebral infarction, with refractory migraine

G43.511   Persistent migraine aura without cerebral infarction, intractable, with status migrainosus

G43.519   Persistent migraine aura without cerebral infarction, intractable, without status migrainosus

● **G43.6**   Persistent migraine aura with cerebral infarction
    Visual, motor, or psychic disturbances, paresthesias, and related neurologic abnormalities accompanying migraine
    Code also the type of cerebral infarction (I63.-)

● **G43.60**   Persistent migraine aura with cerebral infarction, not intractable
    Persistent migraine aura with cerebral infarction, without refractory migraine

G43.601   Persistent migraine aura with cerebral infarction, not intractable, with status migrainosus

G43.609   Persistent migraine aura with cerebral infarction, not intractable, without status migrainosus

● **G43.61**   Persistent migraine aura with cerebral infarction, intractable
    Persistent migraine aura with cerebral infarction, with refractory migraine

G43.611   Persistent migraine aura with cerebral infarction, intractable, with status migrainosus

G43.619   Persistent migraine aura with cerebral infarction, intractable, without status migrainosus

● **G43.7**   Chronic migraine without aura
    Transformed migraine
    Excludes1   migraine without aura (G43.0-)

● **G43.70**   Chronic migraine without aura, not intractable
    Chronic migraine without aura, without refractory migraine

G43.701   Chronic migraine without aura, not intractable, with status migrainosus

G43.709   Chronic migraine without aura, not intractable, without status migrainosus
    Chronic migraine without aura NOS

● **G43.71**   Chronic migraine without aura, intractable
    Chronic migraine without aura, with refractory migraine

G43.711   Chronic migraine without aura, intractable, with status migrainosus

G43.719   Chronic migraine without aura, intractable, without status migrainosus

● **G43.A**   Cyclical vomiting
    Excludes1   cyclical vomiting syndrome unrelated to migraine (R11.15)

G43.A0   Cyclical vomiting, in migraine, not intractable
    Cyclical vomiting, without refractory migraine

G43.A1   Cyclical vomiting, in migraine, intractable
    Cyclical vomiting, with refractory migraine

● **G43.B**   Ophthalmoplegic migraine

G43.B0   Ophthalmoplegic migraine, not intractable
    Ophthalmoplegic migraine, without refractory migraine

G43.B1   Ophthalmoplegic migraine, intractable
    Ophthalmoplegic migraine, with refractory migraine

● **G43.C**   Periodic headache syndromes in child or adult

G43.C0   Periodic headache syndromes in child or adult, not intractable
    Periodic headache syndromes in child or adult, without refractory migraine

G43.C1   Periodic headache syndromes in child or adult, intractable
    Periodic headache syndromes in child or adult, with refractory migraine

● **G43.D**   Abdominal migraine

G43.D0   Abdominal migraine, not intractable
    Abdominal migraine, without refractory migraine

G43.D1   Abdominal migraine, intractable
    Abdominal migraine, with refractory migraine

● **G43.8**   Other migraine

● **G43.80**   Other migraine, not intractable
    Other migraine, without refractory migraine

G43.801   Other migraine, not intractable, with status migrainosus

G43.809   Other migraine, not intractable, without status migrainosus

● **G43.81**   Other migraine, intractable
    Other migraine, with refractory migraine

G43.811   Other migraine, intractable, with status migrainosus

G43.819   Other migraine, intractable, without status migrainosus

● **G43.82**   Menstrual migraine, not intractable
    Menstrual headache, not intractable
    Menstrual migraine, without refractory migraine
    Menstrually related migraine, not intractable
    Pre-menstrual headache, not intractable
    Pre-menstrual migraine, not intractable
    Pure menstrual migraine, not intractable
    Code also associated premenstrual tension syndrome (N94.3)

G43.821   Menstrual migraine, not intractable, with status migrainosus ♀

G43.829   Menstrual migraine, not intractable, without status migrainosus ♀
    Menstrual migraine NOS

● **G43.83**   Menstrual migraine, intractable
    Menstrual headache, intractable
    Menstrual migraine, with refractory migraine
    Menstrually related migraine, intractable
    Pre-menstrual headache, intractable
    Pre-menstrual migraine, intractable
    Pure menstrual migraine, intractable
    Code also associated premenstrual tension syndrome (N94.3)

G43.831   Menstrual migraine, intractable, with status migrainosus ♀

G43.839   Menstrual migraine, intractable, without status migrainosus ♀

● **G43.9**   Migraine, unspecified

● **G43.90**   Migraine, unspecified, not intractable
    Migraine, unspecified, without refractory migraine

G43.901   Migraine, unspecified, not intractable, with status migrainosus
    Status migrainosus NOS

G43.909   Migraine, unspecified, not intractable, without status migrainosus
    Migraine NOS

▶ New   ⇒ Revised   ~~deleted~~ Deleted   Excludes 1   Excludes 2   Includes   Use additional   Code first   Code also   Key words

OGCR Official Guidelines   X Assign placeholder X   ● Use Additional Character(s)   ▷ Manifestation Code   ✿ Hierarchical Condition Category   **Coding Clinic**

● **G43.91**   **Migraine, unspecified, intractable**
     Migraine, unspecified, with refractory
       migraine
     G43.911   **Migraine, unspecified, intractable,
         with status migrainosus**
     G43.919   **Migraine, unspecified, intractable,
         without status migrainosus**

● **G44**   **Other headache syndromes**
     Excludes1   headache NOS (R51.9)
     Excludes2   atypical facial pain (G50.1)
         headache due to lumbar puncture (G97.1)
         migraines (G43.-)
         trigeminal neuralgia (G50.0)

● **G44.0**   **Cluster headaches and other trigeminal autonomic
     cephalgias (TAC)**
     ● **G44.00**   **Cluster headache syndrome, unspecified**
         Ciliary neuralgia
         Cluster headache NOS
         Histamine cephalgia
         Lower half migraine
         Migrainous neuralgia
         G44.001   **Cluster headache
           syndrome, unspecified, intractable**
         G44.009   **Cluster headache
           syndrome, unspecified, not intractable**
           Cluster headache syndrome NOS
     ● **G44.01**   **Episodic cluster headache**
         G44.011   **Episodic cluster headache, intractable**
         G44.019   **Episodic cluster headache, not
           intractable**
           Episodic cluster headache NOS
     ● **G44.02**   **Chronic cluster headache**
         G44.021   **Chronic cluster headache, intractable**
         G44.029   **Chronic cluster headache, not
           intractable**
           Chronic cluster headache NOS
     ● **G44.03**   **Episodic paroxysmal hemicrania**
         Paroxysmal hemicrania NOS
         G44.031   **Episodic paroxysmal hemicrania,
           intractable**
         G44.039   **Episodic paroxysmal hemicrania, not
           intractable**
           Episodic paroxysmal hemicrania NOS
     ● **G44.04**   **Chronic paroxysmal hemicrania**
         Unilateral headache
         G44.041   **Chronic paroxysmal hemicrania,
           intractable**
         G44.049   **Chronic paroxysmal hemicrania, not
           intractable**
           Chronic paroxysmal hemicrania NOS
     ● **G44.05**   **Short lasting unilateral neuralgiform headache
         with conjunctival injection and tearing
         (SUNCT)**
         G44.051   **Short lasting unilateral neuralgiform
           headache with conjunctival injection
           and tearing (SUNCT), intractable**
         G44.059   **Short lasting unilateral neuralgiform
           headache with conjunctival injection
           and tearing (SUNCT), not intractable**
           Short lasting unilateral neuralgiform
            headache with conjunctival
            injection and tearing (SUNCT)
            NOS
     ● **G44.09**   **Other trigeminal autonomic cephalgias (TAC)**
         Cluster headaches
         G44.091   **Other trigeminal autonomic
           cephalgias (TAC), intractable**
         G44.099   **Other trigeminal autonomic
           cephalgias (TAC), not intractable**

● **G44.1**   **Vascular headache, not elsewhere classified**
     Excludes2   cluster headache (G44.0)
         complicated headache syndromes (G44.5-)
         drug-induced headache (G44.4-)
         migraine (G43.-)
         other specified headache syndromes
           (G44.8-)
         post-traumatic headache (G44.3-)
         tension-type headache (G44.2-)

● **G44.2**   **Tension-type headache**
     ● **G44.20**   **Tension-type headache, unspecified**
         G44.201   **Tension-type headache, unspecified,
           intractable**
         G44.209   **Tension-type headache, unspecified,
           not intractable**
           Tension headache NOS
     ● **G44.21**   **Episodic tension-type headache**
         G44.211   **Episodic tension-type headache,
           intractable**
         G44.219   **Episodic tension-type headache, not
           intractable**
           Episodic tension-type headache NOS
     ● **G44.22**   **Chronic tension-type headache**
         G44.221   **Chronic tension-type headache,
           intractable**
         G44.229   **Chronic tension-type headache, not
           intractable**
           Chronic tension-type headache NOS

● **G44.3**   **Post-traumatic headache**
     ● **G44.30**   **Post-traumatic headache, unspecified**
         G44.301   **Post-traumatic headache, unspecified,
           intractable**
         G44.309   **Post-traumatic headache, unspecified,
           not intractable**
           Post-traumatic headache NOS
     ● **G44.31**   **Acute post-traumatic headache**
         G44.311   **Acute post-traumatic headache,
           intractable**
         G44.319   **Acute post-traumatic headache, not
           intractable**
           Acute post-traumatic headache NOS
     ● **G44.32**   **Chronic post-traumatic headache**
         G44.321   **Chronic post-traumatic headache,
           intractable**
         G44.329   **Chronic post-traumatic headache, not
           intractable**
           Chronic post-traumatic headache NOS

● **G44.4**   **Drug-induced headache, not elsewhere classified**
     Medication overuse headache
     Use additional code for adverse effect, if applicable,
       to identify drug (T36-T50 with fifth or sixth
       character 5)
     G44.40   **Drug-induced headache, not elsewhere
         classified, not intractable**
     G44.41   **Drug-induced headache, not elsewhere
         classified, intractable**

● **G44.5**   **Complicated headache syndromes**
     G44.51   **Hemicrania continua**
         Persistent unilateral headache
     G44.52   **New daily persistent headache (NDPH)**
     G44.53   **Primary thunderclap headache**
     G44.59   **Other complicated headache syndrome**

● **G44.8**   **Other specified headache syndromes**
     Excludes2   headache with orthostatic or positional
           component, not elsewhere classified
           (R51.0)
     G44.81   **Hypnic headache**
         Benign primary headaches
     G44.82   **Headache associated with sexual activity**
         Orgasmic headache
         Preorgasmic headache

(right margin) **CHAPTER 6 (G00-G99)**

CHAPTER 6 (G00-G99)

G44.83   **Primary cough headache**

G44.84   **Primary exertional headache**

G44.85   **Primary stabbing headache**

G44.86   **Cervicogenic headache**
Code also associated cervical spinal condition, if known
Coding Clinic: 2021, Q4, P12

G44.89   **Other headache syndrome**

● G45   **Transient cerebral ischemic attacks and related syndromes**
Excludes1 neonatal cerebral ischemia (P91.0)
transient retinal artery occlusion (H34.0-)
Coding Clinic: 2018, Q2, P9

G45.0   **Vertebro-basilar artery syndrome**

G45.1   **Carotid artery syndrome (hemispheric)**

G45.2   **Multiple and bilateral precerebral artery syndromes**

G45.3   **Amaurosis fugax**
Transient visual loss in one eye

G45.4   **Transient global amnesia**
Episode of short-term memory loss, nonrecurrent, lasting few hours
Excludes1 amnesia NOS (R41.3)

G45.8   **Other transient cerebral ischemic attacks and related syndromes**

G45.9   **Transient cerebral ischemic attack, unspecified**
Spasm of cerebral artery
TIA
Transient cerebral ischemia NOS

● G46   **Vascular syndromes of brain in cerebrovascular diseases**
Code first underlying cerebrovascular disease (I60-I69)

G46.0   **Middle cerebral artery syndrome**

G46.1   **Anterior cerebral artery syndrome**

G46.2   **Posterior cerebral artery syndrome**

G46.3   **Brain stem stroke syndrome**
Benedikt syndrome
Claude syndrome
Foville syndrome
Millard-Gubler syndrome
Wallenberg syndrome
Weber syndrome

G46.4   **Cerebellar stroke syndrome**

G46.5   **Pure motor lacunar syndrome**
Occlusion of single deep penetrating artery

G46.6   **Pure sensory lacunar syndrome**

G46.7   **Other lacunar syndromes**

G46.8   **Other vascular syndromes of brain in cerebrovascular diseases**

● G47   **Sleep disorders**
Excludes2 nightmares (F51.5)
nonorganic sleep disorders (F51.-)
sleep terrors (F51.4)
sleepwalking (F51.3)

● G47.0   **Insomnia**
Excludes2 alcohol related insomnia (F10.182, F10.282, F10.982)
drug-related insomnia (F11.182, F11.282, F11.982, F13.182, F13.282, F13.982, F14.182, F14.282, F14.982, F15.182, F15.282, F15.982, F19.182, F19.282, F19.982)
idiopathic insomnia (F51.01)
insomnia due to a mental disorder (F51.05)
insomnia not due to a substance or known physiological condition (F51.0-)
nonorganic insomnia (F51.0-)
primary insomnia (F51.01)
sleep apnea (G47.3-)

G47.00   **Insomnia, unspecified**
Insomnia NOS

G47.01   **Insomnia due to medical condition**
Code also associated medical condition

G47.09   **Other insomnia**

● G47.1   **Hypersomnia**
Excludes2 alcohol-related hypersomnia (F10.182, F10.282, F10.982)
drug-related hypersomnia (F11.182, F11.282, F11.982, F13.182, F13.282, F13.982, F14.182, F14.282, F14.982, F15.182, F15.282, F15.982, F19.182, F19.282, F19.982)
hypersomnia due to a mental disorder (F51.13)
hypersomnia not due to a substance or known physiological condition (F51.1-)
primary hypersomnia (F51.11)
sleep apnea (G47.3-)

G47.10   **Hypersomnia, unspecified**
Hypersomnia NOS

G47.11   **Idiopathic hypersomnia with long sleep time**
Idiopathic hypersomnia NOS

G47.12   **Idiopathic hypersomnia without long sleep time**

G47.13   **Recurrent hypersomnia**
Kleine-Levin syndrome
Menstrual related hypersomnia

G47.14   **Hypersomnia due to medical condition**
Code also associated medical condition

G47.19   **Other hypersomnia**

● G47.2   **Circadian rhythm sleep disorders**
Disorders of the sleep wake schedule
Inversion of nyctohemeral rhythm
Inversion of sleep rhythm

G47.20   **Circadian rhythm sleep disorder, unspecified type**
Sleep wake schedule disorder NOS

G47.21   **Circadian rhythm sleep disorder, delayed sleep phase type**
Delayed sleep phase syndrome

G47.22   **Circadian rhythm sleep disorder, advanced sleep phase type**

G47.23   **Circadian rhythm sleep disorder, irregular sleep wake type**
Irregular sleep-wake pattern

G47.24   **Circadian rhythm sleep disorder, free running type**
Circadian rhythm sleep disorder, non-24-hour sleep-wake type

G47.25   **Circadian rhythm sleep disorder, jet lag type**

G47.26   **Circadian rhythm sleep disorder, shift work type**

❱ G47.27   *Circadian rhythm sleep disorder in conditions classified elsewhere*
Code first underlying condition

G47.29   **Other circadian rhythm sleep disorder**

● G47.3   **Sleep apnea**
Characterized by episodes in which breathing stops during sleep
Code also any associated underlying condition
Excludes1 apnea NOS (R06.81)
Cheyne-Stokes breathing (R06.3)
pickwickian syndrome (E66.2)
➥ sleep apnea of newborn (P28.3-)

G47.30   **Sleep apnea, unspecified**
Sleep apnea NOS

G47.31   **Primary central sleep apnea**
Idiopathic central sleep apnea

G47.32   **High altitude periodic breathing**

G47.33   **Obstructive sleep apnea (adult) (pediatric)**
Obstructive sleep apnea hypopnea
➥ **Excludes1** obstructive sleep apnea of newborn (P28.3-)

G47.34   **Idiopathic sleep related nonobstructive alveolar hypoventilation**
Sleep related hypoxia

▶ New   ➥ Revised   ~~deleted~~ Deleted   Excludes 1   Excludes 2   Includes   Use additional   Code first   Code also   Key words
OGCR Official Guidelines   X Assign placeholder X   ● Use Additional Character(s)   ❱ Manifestation Code   🔗 Hierarchical Condition Category   Coding Clinic

G47.35   **Congenital central alveolar hypoventilation syndrome**

▷ *G47.36*   *Sleep related hypoventilation in conditions classified elsewhere*
    Sleep related hypoxemia in conditions classified elsewhere
    Code first underlying condition

▷ *G47.37*   **Central** *sleep apnea in conditions classified elsewhere*
    Code first underlying condition

G47.39   **Other sleep apnea**

● **G47.4**   **Narcolepsy and cataplexy**
    *Cataplexy is a disorder evidenced by seizures including minor slacking of the facial muscles to complete collapse and often affects people who have **narcolepsy**, a disorder in which there is great difficulty remaining awake during the daytime.*

   ● **G47.41**   **Narcolepsy**
     G47.411   **Narcolepsy with cataplexy**
     G47.419   **Narcolepsy without cataplexy**
      Narcolepsy NOS

   ● **G47.42**   **Narcolepsy in conditions classified elsewhere**
     Code first underlying condition
     ▷ *G47.421*   *Narcolepsy in conditions classified elsewhere with cataplexy*
     ▷ *G47.429*   *Narcolepsy in conditions classified elsewhere without cataplexy*

● **G47.5**   **Parasomnia**
   Excludes1   alcohol induced parasomnia (F10.182, F10.282, F10.982)
     drug induced parasomnia (F11.182, F11.282, F11.982, F13.182, F13.282, F13.982, F14.182, F14.282, F14.982, F15.182, F15.282, F15.982, F19.182, F19.282, F19.982)
     parasomnia not due to a substance or known physiological condition (F51.8)

   G47.50   **Parasomnia, unspecified**
     Parasomnia NOS
   G47.51   **Confusional arousals**
   G47.52   **REM sleep behavior disorder**
   G47.53   **Recurrent isolated sleep paralysis**
   ▷ *G47.54*   *Parasomnia in conditions classified elsewhere*
     Code first underlying condition
   G47.59   **Other parasomnia**

● **G47.6**   **Sleep related movement disorders**
   Excludes2   restless legs syndrome (G25.81)
   G47.61   **Periodic limb movement disorder**
   G47.62   **Sleep related leg cramps**
   G47.63   **Sleep related bruxism**
     Excludes1   psychogenic bruxism (F45.8)
     Coding Clinic: 2016, Q4, P118
   G47.69   **Other sleep related movement disorders**

G47.8   **Other sleep disorders**
   Other specified sleep-wake disorder

G47.9   **Sleep disorder, unspecified**
   Sleep disorder NOS
   Unspecified sleep-wake disorder

★ **(See Plate 6 of the Anatomy Illustrations.)**

NERVE, NERVE ROOT AND PLEXUS DISORDERS (G50-G59)

   Excludes1   current traumatic nerve, nerve root and plexus disorders - see Injury, nerve by body region
     neuralgia NOS (M79.2)
     neuritis NOS (M79.2)
     peripheral neuritis in pregnancy (O26.82-)
     radiculitis NOS (M54.1-)

Item 6-5   **Trigeminal neuralgia,** tic douloureux, is a pain syndrome diagnosed from the patient's history alone. The condition is characterized by pain and a brief facial spasm or tic. Pain is unilateral and follows the sensory distribution of cranial nerve V, typically radiating to the maxillary (V2) or mandibular (V3) area.

Item 6-6   The most common facial nerve disorder is **Bell's Palsy,** which occurs suddenly and results in facial drooping unilaterally. This disorder is the result of a reaction to a virus that causes the facial nerve in the ear to swell, resulting in pressure in the bony canal.

● **G50**   **Disorders of trigeminal nerve**
   Includes   disorders of 5th cranial nerve
   G50.0   **Trigeminal neuralgia**
     Syndrome of paroxysmal facial pain
     Tic douloureux
   G50.1   **Atypical facial pain**
   G50.8   **Other disorders of trigeminal nerve**
   G50.9   **Disorder of trigeminal nerve, unspecified**

● **G51**   **Facial nerve disorders**
   Includes   disorders of 7th cranial nerve
   G51.0   **Bell's palsy**
     Facial palsy
   G51.1   **Geniculate ganglionitis**
     Rare disorder with symptoms of severe pain deep in ear, spreading to ear canal, outer ear, mastoid or eye regions
     Excludes1   postherpetic geniculate ganglionitis (B02.21)
   G51.2   **Melkersson's syndrome**
     Melkersson-Rosenthal syndrome
   ● **G51.3**   **Clonic hemifacial spasm**
     G51.31   **Clonic hemifacial spasm, right**
     G51.32   **Clonic hemifacial spasm, left**
     Coding Clinic: 2018, Q4, P10
     G51.33   **Clonic hemifacial spasm, bilateral**
     G51.39   **Clonic hemifacial spasm, unspecified**
   G51.4   **Facial myokymia**
     Involuntary facial muscle movement
   G51.8   **Other disorders of facial nerve**
   G51.9   **Disorder of facial nerve, unspecified**

● **G52**   **Disorders of other cranial nerves**
   Excludes2   disorders of acoustic [8th] nerve (H93.3)
     disorders of optic [2nd] nerve (H46, H47.0)
     paralytic strabismus due to nerve palsy (H49.0-H49.2)
   G52.0   **Disorders of olfactory nerve**
     Disorders of 1st cranial nerve
   G52.1   **Disorders of glossopharyngeal nerve**
     Disorder of 9th cranial nerve
     Glossopharyngeal neuralgia
   G52.2   **Disorders of vagus nerve**
     Disorders of pneumogastric [10th] nerve
   G52.3   **Disorders of hypoglossal nerve**
     Disorders of 12th cranial nerve
   G52.7   **Disorders of multiple cranial nerves**
     Polyneuritis cranialis
   G52.8   **Disorders of other specified cranial nerves**
   G52.9   **Cranial nerve disorder, unspecified**

▷ *G53*   *Cranial nerve disorders in diseases classified elsewhere*
   Code first underlying disease, such as:
     neoplasm (C00-D49)
   Excludes1   multiple cranial nerve palsy in sarcoidosis (D86.82)
     multiple cranial nerve palsy in syphilis (A52.15)
     postherpetic geniculate ganglionitis (B02.21)
     postherpetic trigeminal neuralgia (B02.22)

G54   Nerve root and plexus disorders

Radiculopathy (nerve root disorder) caused by pressure on nerve root, most common cause is herniation of intervertebral disk. Plexus disorders (plexopathies) are due to compression or injury.

Excludes1   current traumatic nerve root and plexus disorders - see nerve injury by body region
intervertebral disc disorders (M50-M51)
neuralgia or neuritis NOS (M79.2)
neuritis or radiculitis brachial NOS (M54.13)
neuritis or radiculitis lumbar NOS (M54.16)
neuritis or radiculitis lumbosacral NOS (M54.17)
neuritis or radiculitis thoracic NOS (M54.14)
radiculitis NOS (M54.10)
radiculopathy NOS (M54.10)
spondylosis (M47.-)

G54.0   Brachial plexus disorders
Thoracic outlet syndrome

G54.1   Lumbosacral plexus disorders

G54.2   Cervical root disorders, not elsewhere classified

G54.3   Thoracic root disorders, not elsewhere classified

G54.4   Lumbosacral root disorders, not elsewhere classified

G54.5   Neuralgic amyotrophy
Parsonage-Aldren-Turner syndrome
Shoulder-girdle neuritis

     Excludes1   neuralgic amyotrophy in diabetes mellitus (E08-E13 with .44)

G54.6   Phantom limb syndrome with pain
Sensations (cramping, itching) in a limb that no longer exists

G54.7   Phantom limb syndrome without pain
Phantom limb syndrome NOS

G54.8   Other nerve root and plexus disorders

G54.9   Nerve root and plexus disorder, unspecified

G55   *Nerve root and plexus compressions in diseases classified elsewhere*

Code first underlying disease, such as:
neoplasm (C00-D49)

Excludes1   nerve root compression (due to) (in) ankylosing spondylitis (M45.-)
nerve root compression (due to) (in)dorsopathies (M53.-, M54.-)
nerve root compression (due to) (in)intervertebral disc disorders (M50.1-, M51.1-)
nerve root compression (due to) (in) spondylopathies (M46.-, M48.-)
nerve root compression (due to) (in) spondylosis (M47.0-, M47.2.-)

★ **(See Plates 472 and 473 on pages 56 and 57.)**

G56   Mononeuropathies of upper limb

Excludes1   current traumatic nerve disorder - see nerve injury by body region

G56.0   Carpal tunnel syndrome

   G56.00   Carpal tunnel syndrome, unspecified upper limb

   G56.01   Carpal tunnel syndrome, right upper limb

   G56.02   Carpal tunnel syndrome, left upper limb

   G56.03   Carpal tunnel syndrome, bilateral upper limbs
Coding Clinic: 2016, Q4, P17

G56.1   Other lesions of median nerve

   G56.10   Other lesions of median nerve, unspecified side

   G56.11   Other lesions of median nerve, right upper limb

   G56.12   Other lesions of median nerve, left upper limb

   G56.13   Other lesions of median nerve, bilateral upper limbs
Coding Clinic: 2016, Q4, P17

G56.2   Lesion of ulnar nerve
Tardy ulnar nerve palsy

   G56.20   Lesion of ulnar nerve, unspecified upper limb

   G56.21   Lesion of ulnar nerve, right upper limb

   G56.22   Lesion of ulnar nerve, left upper limb

   G56.23   Lesion of ulnar nerve, bilateral upper limbs
Coding Clinic: 2016, Q4, P17

G56.3   Lesion of radial nerve

   G56.30   Lesion of radial nerve, unspecified upper limb

   G56.31   Lesion of radial nerve, right upper limb

   G56.32   Lesion of radial nerve, left upper limb

   G56.33   Lesion of radial nerve, bilateral upper limbs
Coding Clinic: 2016, Q4, P17

G56.4   Causalgia of upper limb
Intense burning pain and sensitivity to slight touch
Complex regional pain syndrome II of upper limb

     Excludes1   complex regional pain syndrome I of lower limb (G90.52-)
complex regional pain syndrome I of upper limb (G90.51-)
complex regional pain syndrome II of lower limb (G57.7-)
reflex sympathetic dystrophy of lower limb (G90.52-)
reflex sympathetic dystrophy (G90.51-)

   G56.40   Causalgia of unspecified upper limb

   G56.41   Causalgia of right upper limb

   G56.42   Causalgia of left upper limb

   G56.43   Causalgia of bilateral upper limbs
Coding Clinic: 2016, Q4, P17

G56.8   Other specified mononeuropathies of upper limb
Disease of a single nerve
Interdigital neuroma of upper limb

   G56.80   Other specified mononeuropathies of unspecified upper limb

   G56.81   Other specified mononeuropathies of right upper limb

   G56.82   Other specified mononeuropathies of left upper limb

   G56.83   Other specified mononeuropathies of bilateral upper limbs
Coding Clinic: 2016, Q4, P17

G56.9   Unspecified mononeuropathy of upper limb
Disease of a single nerve

   G56.90   Unspecified mononeuropathy of unspecified upper limb

   G56.91   Unspecified mononeuropathy of right upper limb

   G56.92   Unspecified mononeuropathy of left upper limb

   G56.93   Unspecified mononeuropathy of bilateral upper limbs
Coding Clinic: 2016, Q4, P17

G57   Mononeuropathies of lower limb

Excludes1   current traumatic nerve disorder - see nerve injury by body region

★ **(See Plates 544 and 545 on pages 58 and 59.)**

G57.0   Lesion of sciatic nerve

     Excludes1   sciatica NOS (M54.3-)

     Excludes2   sciatica attributed to intervertebral disc disorder (M51.1.-)

   G57.00   Lesion of sciatic nerve, unspecified lower limb

   G57.01   Lesion of sciatic nerve, right lower limb

   G57.02   Lesion of sciatic nerve, left lower limb

   G57.03   Lesion of sciatic nerve, bilateral lower limbs
Coding Clinic: 2016, Q4, P1

G57.1   Meralgia paresthetica
Numbness or pain in outer thigh caused by injury to nerve
Lateral cutaneous nerve of thigh syndrome

   G57.10   Meralgia paresthetica, unspecified lower limb

   G57.11   Meralgia paresthetica, right lower limb

   G57.12   Meralgia paresthetica, left lower limb

   G57.13   Meralgia paresthetica, bilateral lower limbs
Coding Clinic: 2016, Q4, P1

▶ New   ⇒ Revised   deleted Deleted   Excludes 1   Excludes 2   Includes   Use additional   Code first   Code also   Key words
OGCR Official Guidelines   X Assign placeholder X   ● Use Additional Character(s)   ▶ Manifestation Code   Hierarchical Condition Category   Coding Clinic

CHAPTER 6 (G00-G99)

● **G57.2** **Lesion of** femoral nerve
　　G57.20 Lesion of femoral nerve, unspecified lower limb
　　G57.21 Lesion of femoral nerve, right lower limb
　　G57.22 Lesion of femoral nerve, left lower limb
　　G57.23 Lesion of femoral nerve, bilateral lower limbs
　　　　Coding Clinic: 2016, Q4, P1

● **G57.3** **Lesion of** lateral popliteal nerve
　　Peroneal nerve palsy
　　G57.30 Lesion of lateral popliteal nerve, unspecified lower limb
　　G57.31 Lesion of lateral popliteal nerve, right lower limb
　　G57.32 Lesion of lateral popliteal nerve, left lower limb
　　G57.33 Lesion of lateral popliteal nerve, bilateral lower limbs
　　　　Coding Clinic: 2016, Q4, P1

● **G57.4** **Lesion of** medial popliteal nerve
　　G57.40 Lesion of medial popliteal nerve, unspecified lower limb
　　G57.41 Lesion of medial popliteal nerve, right lower limb
　　G57.42 Lesion of medial popliteal nerve, left lower limb
　　G57.43 Lesion of medial popliteal nerve, bilateral lower limbs
　　　　Coding Clinic: 2016, Q4, P1

● **G57.5** **Tarsal tunnel** syndrome
　　G57.50 Tarsal tunnel syndrome, unspecified lower limb
　　G57.51 Tarsal tunnel syndrome, right lower limb
　　G57.52 Tarsal tunnel syndrome, left lower limb
　　G57.53 Tarsal tunnel syndrome, bilateral lower limbs
　　　　Coding Clinic: 2016, Q4, P1

● **G57.6** **Lesion of** plantar nerve
　　Morton's metatarsalgia
　　G57.60 Lesion of plantar nerve, unspecified lower limb
　　G57.61 Lesion of plantar nerve, right lower limb
　　G57.62 Lesion of plantar nerve, left lower limb
　　G57.63 Lesion of plantar nerve, bilateral lower limbs
　　　　Coding Clinic: 2016, Q4, P1

● **G57.7** **Causalgia of lower limb**
　　Complex regional pain syndrome II of lower limb
　　Excludes1 complex regional pain syndrome I of lower limb (G90.52-)
　　　　complex regional pain syndrome I of upper limb (G90.51-)
　　　　complex regional pain syndrome II of upper limb (G56.4-)
　　　　reflex sympathetic dystrophy of lower limb (G90.52-)
　　　　reflex sympathetic dystrophy of upper limb (G90.51-)
　　G57.70 Causalgia of unspecified lower limb
　　G57.71 Causalgia of right lower limb
　　G57.72 Causalgia of left lower limb
　　G57.73 Causalgia of bilateral lower limbs
　　　　Coding Clinic: 2016, Q4, P1

● **G57.8** **Other specified mononeuropathies of lower limb**
　　Interdigital neuroma of lower limb
　　G57.80 Other specified mononeuropathies of unspecified lower limb
　　G57.81 Other specified mononeuropathies of right lower limb
　　G57.82 Other specified mononeuropathies of left lower limb
　　G57.83 Other specified mononeuropathies of bilateral lower limbs
　　　　Coding Clinic: 2016, Q4, P17

● **G57.9** **Unspecified mononeuropathy of lower limb**
　　G57.90 Unspecified mononeuropathy of unspecified lower limb
　　G57.91 Unspecified mononeuropathy of right lower limb

　　G57.92 Unspecified mononeuropathy of left lower limb
　　G57.93 Unspecified mononeuropathy of bilateral lower limbs
　　　　Coding Clinic: 2016, Q4, P17

● **G58** **Other mononeuropathies**
　　G58.0 Intercostal neuropathy
　　G58.7 Mononeuritis multiplex
　　G58.8 Other specified mononeuropathies
　　G58.9 Mononeuropathy, unspecified

▶ **G59** *Mononeuropathy in diseases classified elsewhere*
　　Code first underlying disease
　　Excludes1 diabetic mononeuropathy (E08-E13 with .41)
　　　　syphilitic nerve paralysis (A52.19)
　　　　syphilitic neuritis (A52.15)
　　　　tuberculous mononeuropathy (A17.83)

POLYNEUROPATHIES AND OTHER DISORDERS OF THE PERIPHERAL NERVOUS SYSTEM (G60-G65)

　　Excludes1 neuralgia NOS (M79.2)
　　　　neuritis NOS (M79.2)
　　　　peripheral neuritis in pregnancy (O26.82-)
　　　　radiculitis NOS (M54.10)

● **G60** **Hereditary and idiopathic neuropathy**
　　G60.0 Hereditary motor and sensory neuropathy
　　　　Charcot-Marie-Tooth disease
　　　　Déjerine-Sottas disease
　　　　Hereditary motor and sensory neuropathy, types I-IV
　　　　Hypertrophic neuropathy of infancy
　　　　Peroneal muscular atrophy (axonal type) (hypertrophic type)
　　　　Roussy-Lévy syndrome
　　G60.1 Refsum's disease
　　　　Genetic disorder affecting fatty acid metabolism
　　　　Infantile Refsum disease
　　G60.2 Neuropathy in association with hereditary ataxia
　　G60.3 Idiopathic progressive neuropathy
　　G60.8 Other hereditary and idiopathic neuropathies
　　　　Dominantly inherited sensory neuropathy
　　　　Morvan's disease
　　　　Nelaton's syndrome
　　　　Recessively inherited sensory neuropathy
　　G60.9 Hereditary and idiopathic neuropathy, unspecified

● **G61** **Inflammatory polyneuropathy**
　　G61.0 Guillain-Barré syndrome 🔎
　　　　Autoimmune disease affecting peripheral nervous system
　　　　Acute (post-)infective polyneuritis
　　　　Miller Fisher Syndrome
　　G61.1 Serum neuropathy 🔎
　　　　Use additional code for adverse effect, if applicable, to identify serum (T50.-)
　　● **G61.8** Other inflammatory polyneuropathies
　　　　G61.81 Chronic inflammatory demyelinating polyneuritis 🔎
　　　　G61.82 Multifocal motor neuropathy 🔎
　　　　　　MMN
　　　　G61.89 Other inflammatory polyneuropathies 🔎
　　G61.9 Inflammatory polyneuropathy, unspecified 🔎

● **G62** **Other and unspecified polyneuropathies**
　　G62.0 Drug-induced polyneuropathy 🔎
　　　　Use additional code for adverse effect, if applicable, to identify drug (T36-T50 with fifth or sixth character 5)
　　G62.1 Alcoholic polyneuropathy 🔎
　　　　Malfunction of many peripheral nerves throughout the body
　　　　Coding Clinic: 2019, Q3, P8
　　G62.2 Polyneuropathy due to other toxic agents 🔎
　　　　Code first (T51-T65) to identify toxic agent

SYMPATHETIC | PARASYMPATHETIC

Pupils dilated — Pupils constricted
Salivation inhibited — Salivation stimulated
Increased respiration — Decreased respiration
Bronchial passages dilated — Bronchial passages constricted
Increased heart rate — Decreased heart rate
Increased secretion by sweat glands
Hair follicles raised; goose bumps — Secretion of adrenal hormones
Digestion inhibited — Digestion stimulated
Bladder muscles relaxed (filling) — Bladder muscles contracted (emptying)

Figure 6-2 Actions of parasympathetic and sympathetic nerves. (From Chabner: The Language of Medicine, ed 9, St. Louis, Saunders, 2011)

Item 6–7 The **peripheral nervous system** consists of 31 pairs of spinal nerves, 12 pairs of cranial nerves, and the autonomic nerves, which are divided into the parasympathetic and sympathetic nerves. The cranial nerves are: olfactory (I), optic (II), oculomotor (III), trochlear (IV), trigeminal (V), abducens (VI), facial (VII), vestibulocochlear (VIII), glossopharyngeal (IX), vagus (X), accessory (XI), and hypoglossal (XII).

● **G62.8** **Other specified polyneuropathies**
　　G62.81 **Critical illness polyneuropathy** 🅗
　　　　Acute motor neuropathy
　　G62.82 **Radiation-induced polyneuropathy** 🅗
　　　　Use additional external cause code (W88-W90, X39.0-) to identify cause
　　　　Coding Clinic: 2016, Q4, P18
　　G62.89 **Other specified polyneuropathies**
　　　　Coding Clinic: 2016, Q2, P11

G62.9 **Polyneuropathy, unspecified**
　　Neuropathy NOS

▹ **G63** *Polyneuropathy in diseases classified elsewhere* 🅗
　　Code first underlying disease, such as:
　　amyloidosis (E85.-)
　　endocrine disease, except diabetes (E00-E07, E15-E16, E20-E34)
　　metabolic diseases (E70-E88)
　　neoplasm (C00-D49)
　　nutritional deficiency (E40-E64)
　　Excludes1 polyneuropathy (in):
　　　　diabetes mellitus (E08-E13 with .42)
　　　　diphtheria (A36.83)
　　　　infectious mononucleosis complicated by polyneuropathy (B27.0-B27.9 with fifth character 1)
　　　　Lyme disease (A69.22)
　　　　mumps (B26.84)
　　　　postherpetic (B02.23)
　　　　rheumatoid arthritis (M05.5-)
　　　　scleroderma (M34.83)
　　　　systemic lupus erythematosus (M32.19)

Coding Clinic: 2021, Q1, P7; 2012, Q4, P100

● **G64** **Other disorders of peripheral nervous system**
　　Disorder of peripheral nervous system NOS

● **G65** **Sequelae of inflammatory and toxic polyneuropathies**
　　Code first condition resulting from (sequela) of inflammatory and toxic polyneuropathies
　　G65.0 **Sequelae of Guillain-Barré syndrome** 🅗
　　G65.1 **Sequelae of other inflammatory polyneuropathy** 🅗
　　G65.2 **Sequelae of toxic polyneuropathy** 🅗

DISEASES OF MYONEURAL JUNCTION AND MUSCLE (G70-G73)

● **G70** **Myasthenia gravis and other myoneural disorders**
　　Excludes1 botulism (A05.1, A48.51-A48.52)
　　　　transient neonatal myasthenia gravis (P94.0)
　　● **G70.0** **Myasthenia gravis**
　　　　Acquired and results in fatigable muscle weakness exacerbated by activity and improved with rest
　　　　G70.00 **Myasthenia gravis without (acute) exacerbation** 🅗
　　　　　　Myasthenia gravis NOS
　　　　G70.01 **Myasthenia gravis with (acute) exacerbation** 🅗
　　　　　　Myasthenia gravis in crisis
　　G70.1 **Toxic myoneural disorders** 🅗
　　　　Dysfunction at junction of muscle and motor nerve (myoneural junction)
　　　　Code first (T51-T65) to identify toxic agent
　　G70.2 **Congenital and developmental myasthenia** 🅗
　　● **G70.8** **Other specified myoneural disorders**
　　　　G70.80 **Lambert-Eaton syndrome, unspecified** 🅗
　　　　　　Lambert-Eaton syndrome NOS
　　　▹ **G70.81** *Lambert-Eaton syndrome in disease classified elsewhere* 🅗
　　　　　　Code first underlying disease
　　　　　　Excludes1 Lambert-Eaton syndrome in neoplastic disease (G73.1)
　　　　G70.89 **Other specified myoneural disorders** 🅗
　　G70.9 **Myoneural disorder, unspecified** 🅗

● **G71** **Primary disorders of muscles**
　　Excludes2 arthrogryposis multiplex congenita (Q74.3)
　　　　metabolic disorders (E70-E88)
　　　　myositis (M60.-)
　　● **G71.0** **Muscular dystrophy** 🅗
　　　　G71.00 **Muscular dystrophy, unspecified** 🅗
　　　　G71.01 **Duchenne or Becker muscular dystrophy** 🅗
　　　　　　Autosomal recessive, childhood type, muscular dystrophy resembling Duchenne or Becker muscular dystrophy
　　　　　　Benign [Becker] muscular dystrophy
　　　　　　Severe [Duchenne] muscular dystrophy
　　　　G71.02 **Facioscapulohumeral muscular dystrophy** 🅗
　　　　　　Scapulohumeral muscular dystrophy
　　　　　　Coding Clinic: 2018, Q4, P12
　　▶● **G71.03** **Limb girdle muscular dystrophies**
　　　　　▶**G71.031** **Autosomal dominant limb girdle muscular dystrophy**
　　　　　　▶LGMD D4 calpain-3-related
　　　　　　▶LGMD D5 collagen 6-related
　　　　　　▶Limb girdle muscular dystrophy type 1

Item 6–8 Muscular dystrophies (MD) are a group of rare inherited muscle diseases. Voluntary muscles become progressively weaker. In the late stages of MD, fat and connective tissue replace muscle fibers. In some types of muscular dystrophy, heart muscles, other involuntary muscles, and other organs are affected. **Myopathies** is a general term for neuromuscular diseases in which the muscle fibers dysfunction for any one of many reasons, resulting in muscular weakness.

▶ New　➡ Revised　deleted Deleted　Excludes 1　Excludes 2　Includes　Use additional　Code first　Code also　Key words
OGCR Official Guidelines　X Assign placeholder X　● Use Additional Character(s)　▹ Manifestation Code　🅗 Hierarchical Condition Category　Coding Clinic

CHAPTER 6 (G00-G99)

▶G71.Ø32   **Autosomal recessive limb girdle muscular dystrophy due to calpain-3 dysfunction**
　　　▶Limb girdle muscular dystrophy type 2A
　　　▶LGMD R1 calpain-3-related
　　　▶Primary calpainopathy

▶G71.Ø33   **Limb girdle muscular dystrophy due to dysferlin dysfunction**
　　　▶Dysferlinopathy
　　　▶LGMD R2 dysferlin-related
　　　▶Limb girdle muscular dystrophy type 2B
　　　▶Miyoshi Myopathy type 1

▶●G71.Ø34   **Limb girdle muscular dystrophy due to sarcoglycan dysfunction**

　　▶G71.Ø34Ø   **Limb girdle muscular dystrophy due to sarcoglycan dysfunction, unspecified**
　　　　▶Sarcoglycanopathy, NOS

　　▶G71.Ø341   **Limb girdle muscular dystrophy due to alpha sarcoglycan dysfunction**
　　　　▶Alpha sarcoglycanopathy
　　　　▶Limb-girdle muscular dystrophy due to alpha-sarcoglycan deficiency
　　　　▶Limb girdle muscular dystrophy type 2D

　　▶G71.Ø342   **Limb girdle muscular dystrophy due to beta sarcoglycan dysfunction**
　　　　▶Beta sarcoglycanopathy
　　　　▶Limb girdle muscular dystrophy due to beta-sarcoglycan deficiency
　　　　▶Limb girdle muscular dystrophy type 2E

　　▶G71.Ø349   **Limb girdle muscular dystrophy due to other sarcoglycan dysfunction**
　　　　▶Delta sarcoglycanopathy
　　　　▶Delta-sarcoglycan-related LGMD R6
　　　　▶Gamma sarcoglycanopathy
　　　　▶Gamma-sarcoglycan-related LGMD R5
　　　　▶Limb girdle muscular dystrophy type 2C
　　　　▶Limb girdle muscular dystrophy type 2F

▶G71.Ø35   **Limb girdle muscular dystrophy due to anoctamin-5 dysfunction**
　　　▶Anoctamin-5-related LGMD R12
　　　▶Anoctaminopathy
　　　▶Autosomal recessive limb girdle muscular dystrophy type 2L
　　　▶Miyoshi myopathy type 3

▶G71.Ø38   **Other limb girdle muscular dystrophy**
　　　▶LGMD R9 FKRP-related
　　　▶LGMD R22 collagen 6-related
　　　▶Limb girdle muscular dystrophy due to fukutin related protein dysfunction
　　　▶Limb girdle muscular dystrophy type 2I
　　　▶Other autosomal recessive limb girdle muscular dystrophy

▶G71.Ø39   **Limb girdle muscular dystrophy, unspecified**

G71.Ø9   **Other specified muscular dystrophies** 🔗
　　　Benign scapuloperoneal muscular dystrophy with early contractures [Emery-Dreifuss]
　　　Congenital muscular dystrophy NOS
　　　Congenital muscular dystrophy with specific morphological abnormalities of the muscle fiber
　　　Distal muscular dystrophy
　　　~~Limb-girdle muscular dystrophy~~
　　　Ocular muscular dystrophy
　　　Oculopharyngeal muscular dystrophy
　　　Scapuloperoneal muscular dystrophy

●G71.1   **Myotonic disorders**
　　　Inherited disorder that affects muscles tone

　　G71.11   **Myotonic muscular dystrophy** 🔗
　　　　Dystrophia myotonica [Steinert]
　　　　Myotonia atrophica
　　　　Myotonic dystrophy
　　　　Proximal myotonic myopathy (PROMM)
　　　　Steinert disease

　　G71.12   **Myotonia congenita**
　　　　Acetazolamide responsive myotonia congenita
　　　　Dominant myotonia congenita [Thomsen disease]
　　　　Myotonia levior
　　　　Recessive myotonia congenita [Becker disease]

　　G71.13   **Myotonic chondrodystrophy**
　　　　Chondrodystrophic myotonia
　　　　Congenital myotonic chondrodystrophy
　　　　Schwartz-Jampel disease

　　G71.14   **Drug induced myotonia**
　　　　Use additional code for adverse effect, if applicable, to identify drug (T36-T50 with fifth or sixth character 5)

　　G71.19   **Other specified myotonic disorders**
　　　　Myotonia fluctuans
　　　　Myotonia permanens
　　　　Neuromyotonia [Isaacs]
　　　　Paramyotonia congenita (of von Eulenburg)
　　　　Pseudomyotonia
　　　　Symptomatic myotonia

G71.2   **Congenital myopathies** 🔗

　　Excludes2   arthrogryposis multiplex congenita (Q74.3)

　　G71.2Ø   **Congenital myopathy, unspecified**
　　G71.21   **Nemaline myopathy**
　●G71.22   **Centronuclear myopathy**

　　　G71.22Ø   **X-linked myotubular myopathy**
　　　　　Myotubular (centronuclear) myopathy

　　　G71.228   **Other centronuclear myopathy**
　　　　　Autosomal centronuclear myopathy
　　　　　Autosomal dominant centronuclear myopathy
　　　　　Autosomal recessive centronuclear myopathy
　　　　　Centronuclear myopathy, NOS

　　G71.29   **Other congenital myopathy**
　　　　Central core disease
　　　　Minicore disease
　　　　Multicore disease
　　　　Multiminicore disease

G71.3   **Mitochondrial myopathy, not elsewhere classified**
　　　Myopathies associated with increased number of enlarged, often abnormal, mitochondria in muscle fibers

　　Excludes1   Kearns-Sayre syndrome (H49.81)
　　　　Leber's disease (H47.21)
　　　　Leigh's encephalopathy (G31.82)
　　　　mitochondrial metabolism disorders (E88.4.-)
　　　　Reye's syndrome (G93.7)

G71.8   **Other primary disorders of muscles**

G71.9   **Primary disorder of muscle, unspecified**
　　　Hereditary myopathy NOS

● **G72 Other and unspecified myopathies**

> **Excludes1** arthrogryposis multiplex congenita (Q74.3)
> dermatopolymyositis (M33.-)
> ischemic infarction of muscle (M62.2-)
> myositis (M60.-)
> polymyositis (M33.2-)

G72.0 Drug-induced myopathy

> Use additional code for adverse effect, if applicable, to identify drug (T36-T50 with fifth or sixth character 5)

G72.1 Alcoholic myopathy

> Use additional code to identify alcoholism (F10.-)

G72.2 Myopathy due to other toxic agents

> Code first (T51-T65) to identify toxic agent

G72.3 Periodic paralysis

> Familial periodic paralysis
> Hyperkalemic periodic paralysis (familial)
> Hypokalemic periodic paralysis (familial)
> Myotonic periodic paralysis (familial)
> Normokalemic paralysis (familial)
> Potassium sensitive periodic paralysis
>
> > **Excludes1** paramyotonia congenita (of von Eulenburg) (G71.19)

● **G72.4 Inflammatory and immune myopathies, not elsewhere classified**

> **G72.41 Inclusion body myositis [IBM]**
>
> **G72.49 Other inflammatory and immune myopathies, not elsewhere classified**
> > Inflammatory myopathy NOS

● **G72.8 Other specified myopathies**

> **G72.81 Critical illness myopathy**
> > Acute necrotizing myopathy
> > Acute quadriplegic myopathy
> > Intensive care (ICU) myopathy
> > Myopathy of critical illness
>
> **G72.89 Other specified myopathies**

G72.9 Myopathy, unspecified

● **G73 Disorders of myoneural junction and muscle in diseases classified elsewhere**

▶ *G73.1 Lambert-Eaton syndrome in neoplastic disease* 🐾

> *Rare autoimmune disorder affecting calcium channels of nerve-muscle (neuromuscular) junction*
>
> *Code first underlying neoplasm (C00-D49)*
> > **Excludes1** Lambert-Eaton syndrome not associated with neoplasm (G70.80-G70.81)

▶ *G73.3 Myasthenic syndromes in other diseases classified elsewhere* 🐾

> *Code first underlying disease, such as:*
> > neoplasm (C00-D49)
> > thyrotoxicosis (E05.-)

▶ *G73.7 Myopathy in diseases classified elsewhere*

> *Code first underlying disease, such as:*
> > hyperparathyroidism (E21.0, E21.3)
> > hypoparathyroidism (E20.-)
> > glycogen storage disease (E74.0)
> > lipid storage disorders (E75.-)
> > > **Excludes1** myopathy in:
> > > rheumatoid arthritis (M05.32)
> > > sarcoidosis (D86.87)
> > > scleroderma (M34.82)
> > > Sjögren syndrome (M35.03)
> > > systemic lupus erythematosus (M32.19)

CEREBRAL PALSY AND OTHER PARALYTIC SYNDROMES (G80-G83)

● **G80 Cerebral palsy**

> **Excludes1** hereditary spastic paraplegia (G11.4)

G80.0 Spastic quadriplegic cerebral palsy 🐾
> Congenital spastic paralysis (cerebral)

G80.1 Spastic diplegic cerebral palsy 🐾
> Spastic cerebral palsy NOS

G80.2 Spastic hemiplegic cerebral palsy 🐾

G80.3 Athetoid cerebral palsy 🐾
> *Result of damage to cerebellum or basal ganglia responsible for processing neuromuscular signals*
> Double athetosis (syndrome)
> Dyskinetic cerebral palsy
> Dystonic cerebral palsy
> Vogt disease

G80.4 Ataxic cerebral palsy 🐾
> *Poor muscle tone and coordination*

G80.8 Other cerebral palsy 🐾
> Mixed cerebral palsy syndromes

G80.9 Cerebral palsy, unspecified 🐾
> Cerebral palsy NOS

OGCR Section I.C.6.a.

> Dominant/nondominant side
>
> Codes from category G81, Hemiplegia and hemiparesis, and subcategories, G83.1, Monoplegia of lower limb, G83.2, Monoplegia of upper limb, and G83.3, Monoplegia, unspecified, identify whether the dominant and nondominant side is affected. Should the affected side be documented, but not specified as dominant or nondominant, and the classification system does not indicate a default, code selection is as follows:
>
> • For ambidextrous patients, the default should be dominant.
> • If the left side is affected, the default is nondominant.
> • If the right side is affected, the default is dominant.

● **G81 Hemiplegia and hemiparesis**

> **Note:** This category is to be used only when hemiplegia (complete)(incomplete) is reported without further specification, or is stated to be old or longstanding but of unspecified cause. The category is also for use in multiple coding to identify these types of hemiplegia resulting from any cause.
>
> > **Excludes1** congenital cerebral palsy (G80.-)
> > hemiplegia and hemiparesis due to sequela of cerebrovascular disease (I69.05-, I69.15-, I69.25-, I69.35-, I69.85-, I69.95-)
>
> Coding Clinic: 2012, Q4, P106

● **G81.0 Flaccid hemiplegia**

> *Paralysis of half of body with loss of tone of muscles of paralyzed part and absence of tendon reflexes*
>
> **G81.00 Flaccid hemiplegia affecting unspecified side** 🐾
> **G81.01 Flaccid hemiplegia affecting right dominant side** 🐾
> **G81.02 Flaccid hemiplegia affecting left dominant side** 🐾
> **G81.03 Flaccid hemiplegia affecting right nondominant side** 🐾
> **G81.04 Flaccid hemiplegia affecting left nondominant side** 🐾

● **G81.1 Spastic hemiplegia**

> *Paralysis of half of body with spasticity of muscles of paralyzed part and increased tendon reflexes*
>
> **G81.10 Spastic hemiplegia affecting unspecified side** 🐾
> **G81.11 Spastic hemiplegia affecting right dominant side** 🐾
> **G81.12 Spastic hemiplegia affecting left dominant side** 🐾

CHAPTER 6 (G00-G99)

Item 6–9 Hemiplegia is complete paralysis of one side of the body—arm, leg, and trunk. **Hemiparesis** is a generalized weakness or incomplete paralysis of one side of the body. If most activities (eating, writing) are performed with the right hand, the right is the dominant side, and the left is the nondominant side. **Quadriplegia,** also called tetraplegia, is the complete paralysis of all four limbs. **Quadriparesis** is the incomplete paralysis of all four limbs. Nerve damage in C1–C4 is associated with lower limb paralysis, and C5–C7 damage is associated with upper limb paralysis. **Diplegia** is the paralysis of the upper limbs. **Monoplegia** is the complete paralysis of one limb.

> **G81.13**   Spastic hemiplegia affecting right nondominant side 🦠
>
> **G81.14**   Spastic hemiplegia affecting left nondominant side 🦠

● **G81.9**   Hemiplegia, unspecified
> **G81.90**   Hemiplegia, unspecified affecting unspecified side 🦠
>
> **G81.91**   Hemiplegia, unspecified affecting right dominant side 🦠
>
> **G81.92**   Hemiplegia, unspecified affecting left dominant side 🦠
>
> **G81.93**   Hemiplegia, unspecified affecting right nondominant side 🦠
>
> **G81.94**   Hemiplegia, unspecified affecting left nondominant side 🦠
> > Coding Clinic: 2015, Q1, P26

● **G82**   **Paraplegia (paraparesis) and quadriplegia (quadriparesis)**
> **Note:** This category is to be used only when the listed conditions are reported without further specification, or are stated to be old or longstanding but of unspecified cause. The category is also for use in multiple coding to identify these conditions resulting from any cause.
>
> **Excludes1**   congenital cerebral palsy (G80.-)
> functional quadriplegia (R53.2)
> hysterical paralysis (F44.4)

● **G82.2**   **Paraplegia**
> Paralysis of both lower limbs NOS
> Paraparesis (lower) NOS
> Paraplegia (lower) NOS
>
> **G82.20**   Paraplegia, unspecified 🦠
> > Coding Clinic: 2017, Q3, P3
>
> **G82.21**   Paraplegia, complete 🦠
> **G82.22**   Paraplegia, incomplete 🦠

● **G82.5**   **Quadriplegia**
> *Paralysis of all limbs; AKA tetraplegia*
>
> **G82.50**   Quadriplegia, unspecified 🦠
> **G82.51**   Quadriplegia, C1-C4 complete 🦠
> **G82.52**   Quadriplegia, C1-C4 incomplete 🦠
> **G82.53**   Quadriplegia, C5-C7 complete 🦠
> **G82.54**   Quadriplegia, C5-C7 incomplete 🦠

● **G83**   **Other paralytic syndromes**
> **Note:** This category is to be used only when the listed conditions are reported without further specification, or are stated to be old or longstanding but of unspecified cause. The category is also for use in multiple coding to identify these conditions resulting from any cause.
>
> **Includes**   paralysis (complete) (incomplete), except as in G80-G82

G83.0   **Diplegia of upper limbs** 🦠
> *Paralysis affecting limbs on both sides; AKA bilateral paralysis*
> Diplegia (upper)
> Paralysis of both upper limbs

● **G83.1**   **Monoplegia of lower limb**
> *Paralysis of limb on one side*
> Paralysis of lower limb
>
> **Excludes1**   monoplegia of lower limbs due to sequela of cerebrovascular disease (I69.04-, I69.14-, I69.24-, I69.34-, I69.84-, I69.94-)
> > Coding Clinic: 2012, Q4, P106
>
> **G83.10**   Monoplegia of lower limb affecting unspecified side 🦠
>
> **G83.11**   Monoplegia of lower limb affecting right dominant side 🦠
>
> **G83.12**   Monoplegia of lower limb affecting left dominant side 🦠
>
> **G83.13**   Monoplegia of lower limb affecting right nondominant side 🦠
>
> **G83.14**   Monoplegia of lower limb affecting left nondominant side 🦠

● **G83.2**   **Monoplegia of upper limb**
> Paralysis of upper limb
>
> **Excludes1**   monoplegia of upper limbs due to sequela of cerebrovascular disease (I69.03-, I69.13-, I69.23-, I69.33-, I69.83-, I69.93-)
> > Coding Clinic: 2012, Q4, P106
>
> **G83.20**   Monoplegia of upper limb affecting unspecified side 🦠
>
> **G83.21**   Monoplegia of upper limb affecting right dominant side 🦠
>
> **G83.22**   Monoplegia of upper limb affecting left dominant side 🦠
>
> **G83.23**   Monoplegia of upper limb affecting right nondominant side 🦠
>
> **G83.24**   Monoplegia of upper limb affecting left nondominant side 🦠

● **G83.3**   **Monoplegia, unspecified**
> > Coding Clinic: 2012, Q4, P106
>
> **G83.30**   Monoplegia, unspecified affecting unspecified side 🦠
>
> **G83.31**   Monoplegia, unspecified affecting right dominant side 🦠
>
> **G83.32**   Monoplegia, unspecified affecting left dominant side 🦠
>
> **G83.33**   Monoplegia, unspecified affecting right nondominant side 🦠
>
> **G83.34**   Monoplegia, unspecified affecting left nondominant side 🦠

G83.4   **Cauda equina syndrome** 🦠
> *Aching pain due to compression of spinal nerve roots*
> Neurogenic bladder due to cauda equina syndrome
>
> **Excludes1**   cord bladder NOS (G95.89)
> neurogenic bladder NOS (N31.9)

G83.5   **Locked-in state** 🦠
> > Coding Clinic: 2022, Q2, P11

● **G83.8**   **Other specified paralytic syndromes**
> **Excludes1**   paralytic syndromes due to current spinal cord injury-code to spinal cord injury (S14, S24, S34)
>
> **G83.81**   **Brown-Séquard syndrome** 🦠
> **G83.82**   **Anterior cord syndrome** 🦠
> **G83.83**   **Posterior cord syndrome** 🦠
> **G83.84**   **Todd's paralysis (postepileptic)** 🦠
> **G83.89**   **Other specified paralytic syndromes** 🦠

G83.9   **Paralytic syndrome, unspecified** 🦠

CHAPTER 6 (G00-G99)

CHAPTER 6 (G00-G99)

OTHER DISORDERS OF THE NERVOUS SYSTEM (G89-G99)

● **G89   Pain, not elsewhere classified**

Code also related psychological factors associated with pain (F45.42)

Excludes1   generalized pain NOS (R52)
pain disorders exclusively related to psychological factors (F45.41)
pain NOS (R52)

Excludes2   atypical face pain (G50.1)
headache syndromes (G44.-)
localized pain, unspecified type - code to pain by site, such as:
abdomen pain (R10.-)
back pain (M54.9)
breast pain (N64.4)
chest pain (R07.1-R07.9)
ear pain (H92.0-)
eye pain (H57.1)
headache (R51.9)
joint pain (M25.5-)
limb pain (M79.6-)
lumbar region pain (M54.5-)
painful urination (R30.9)
pelvic and perineal pain (R10.2)
shoulder pain (M25.51-)
spine pain (M54.-)
throat pain (R07.0)
tongue pain (K14.6)
tooth pain (K08.8)
renal colic (N23)
migraines (G43.-)
myalgia (M79.1-)
pain from prosthetic devices, implants, and grafts (T82.84, T83.84, T84.84, T85.84-)
phantom limb syndrome with pain (G54.6)
vulvar vestibulitis (N94.810)
vulvodynia (N94.81-)

G89.0   Central pain syndrome
Neurological condition causing intractable pain resulting from damage to CNS
Déjérine-Roussy syndrome
Myelopathic pain syndrome
Thalamic pain syndrome (hyperesthetic)

● **G89.1   Acute pain, not elsewhere classified**

G89.11   Acute pain due to trauma

G89.12   Acute post-thoracotomy pain
Post-thoracotomy pain NOS

G89.18   Other acute postprocedural pain
Postoperative pain NOS
Postprocedural pain NOS

● **G89.2   Chronic pain, not elsewhere classified**

Excludes1   causalgia, lower limb (G57.7-)
causalgia, upper limb (G56.4-)
central pain syndrome (G89.0)
chronic pain syndrome (G89.4)
complex regional pain syndrome II, lower limb (G57.7-)
complex regional pain syndrome II, upper limb (G56.4-)
neoplasm related chronic pain (G89.3)
reflex sympathetic dystrophy (G90.5-)

G89.21   Chronic pain due to trauma

G89.22   Chronic post-thoracotomy pain

G89.28   Other chronic postprocedural pain
Other chronic postoperative pain

G89.29   Other chronic pain

G89.3   Neoplasm related pain (acute) (chronic)
Cancer associated pain
Pain due to malignancy (primary) (secondary)
Tumor associated pain

G89.4   Chronic pain syndrome
Chronic pain associated with significant psychosocial dysfunction

● **G90   Disorders of autonomic nervous system**

Excludes1   dysfunction of the autonomic nervous system due to alcohol (G31.2)

● **G90.0   Idiopathic peripheral autonomic neuropathy**

G90.01   Carotid sinus syncope
Carotid sinus syndrome

G90.09   Other idiopathic peripheral autonomic neuropathy
Idiopathic peripheral autonomic neuropathy NOS

G90.1   Familial dysautonomia [Riley-Day] 🐾
Inherited disorder that affects nerve function

G90.2   Horner's syndrome
Due to damage of the sympathetic nervous system
Bernard(-Horner) syndrome
Cervical sympathetic dystrophy or paralysis

G90.3   Multi-system degeneration of the autonomic nervous system 🐾
Neurogenic orthostatic hypotension [Shy-Drager]
Excludes1   orthostatic hypotension NOS (I95.1)

G90.4   Autonomic dysreflexia
Syndrome resulting from lesions of spinal cord
Use additional code to identify the cause, such as:
fecal impaction (K56.41)
pressure ulcer (pressure area) (L89.-)
urinary tract infection (N39.0)

● **G90.5   Complex regional pain syndrome I (CRPS I)**
Reflex sympathetic dystrophy
Excludes1   causalgia of lower limb (G57.7-)
causalgia of upper limb (G56.4-)
complex regional pain syndrome II of lower limb (G57.7-)
complex regional pain syndrome II of upper limb (G56.4-)

G90.50   Complex regional pain syndrome I, unspecified

● **G90.51   Complex regional pain syndrome I of upper limb**

G90.511   Complex regional pain syndrome I of right upper limb

G90.512   Complex regional pain syndrome I of left upper limb

G90.513   Complex regional pain syndrome I of upper limb, bilateral

G90.519   Complex regional pain syndrome I of unspecified upper limb

● **G90.52   Complex regional pain syndrome I of lower limb**

G90.521   Complex regional pain syndrome I of right lower limb

G90.522   Complex regional pain syndrome I of left lower limb

G90.523   Complex regional pain syndrome I of lower limb, bilateral

G90.529   Complex regional pain syndrome I of unspecified lower limb

G90.59   Complex regional pain syndrome I of other specified site

G90.8   Other disorders of autonomic nervous system

G90.9   Disorder of the autonomic nervous system, unspecified

▶ **G90.A   Postural orthostatic tachycardia syndrome [POTS]**
▶Chronic orthostatic intolerance
▶Postural tachycardia syndrome

▶ New   ➡ Revised   ~~deleted~~ Deleted   Excludes 1   Excludes 2   Includes   Use additional   Code first   Code also   Key words

OGCR Official Guidelines   X Assign placeholder X   ● Use Additional Character(s)   ▌ Manifestation Code   🐾 Hierarchical Condition Category   Coding Clinic

● **G91   Hydrocephalus**
    Dilatation of cerebral ventricles, accompanied by accumulation of cerebrospinal fluid

    | **Includes** | acquired hydrocephalus |
    | **Excludes1** | Arnold-Chiari syndrome with hydrocephalus (Q07.-) |
    | | congenital hydrocephalus (Q03.-) |
    | | spina bifida with hydrocephalus (Q05.-) |

  G91.0   Communicating hydrocephalus
      Secondary normal pressure hydrocephalus

  G91.1   Obstructive hydrocephalus

  G91.2   (Idiopathic) normal pressure hydrocephalus
      Normal pressure hydrocephalus NOS

  G91.3   Post-traumatic hydrocephalus, unspecified

▸ **G91.4   *Hydrocephalus in diseases classified elsewhere***
      Code first underlying condition, such as:
        congenital syphilis (A50.4-)
        neoplasm (C00-D49)
        plasminogen deficiency (E88.02)

      | **Excludes1** | hydrocephalus due to congenital toxoplasmosis (P37.1) |

  G91.8   Other hydrocephalus

  G91.9   Hydrocephalus, unspecified

● **G92   Toxic encephalopathy**

  ● **G92.0   Immune effector cell-associated neurotoxicity syndrome**
      Code first underlying cause such as:
        complications of immune effector cellular therapy (T80.82)

      Code also associated signs and symptoms, such as seizures and cerebral edema

      Code also, if applicable:
        cerebral edema (G93.6)
        unspecified convulsions (R56.9)

    G92.00   Immune effector cell-associated neurotoxicity syndrome, grade unspecified
        ICANS, grade unspecified

    G92.01   Immune effector cell-associated neurotoxicity syndrome, grade 1
        ICANS, grade 1

    G92.02   Immune effector cell-associated neurotoxicity syndrome, grade 2
        ICANS, grade 2

    G92.03   Immune effector cell-associated neurotoxicity syndrome, grade 3
        ICANS, grade 3

    G92.04   Immune effector cell-associated neurotoxicity syndrome, grade 4
        ICANS, grade 4

    G92.05   Immune effector cell-associated neurotoxicity syndrome, grade 5
        ICANS, grade 5

  G92.8   Other toxic encephalopathy
      Toxic encephalitis
      Toxic metabolic encephalopathy

      Code first poisoning due to drug or toxin, if applicable, (T36-T65 with fifth or sixth character 1-4 or 6)

      Use Additional code for adverse effect, if applicable, to identify drug (T36-T50 with fifth or sixth character 5)
      Coding Clinic: 2022, Q1, P53

  G92.9   Unspecified toxic encephalopathy
      Code first poisoning due to drug or toxin, if applicable, (T36-T65 with fifth or sixth character 1-4 or 6)

      Use Additional code for adverse effect, if applicable, to identify drug (T36-T50 with fifth or sixth character 5)

    Disorder or disease of brain caused by chemicals
    Coding Clinic: 2021, Q1, P13; 2017, Q1, P39-40

● **G93   Other disorders of brain**

  G93.0   Cerebral cysts
      Arachnoid cyst
      Porencephalic cyst, acquired

      | **Excludes1** | acquired periventricular cysts of newborn (P91.1) |
      | | congenital cerebral cysts (Q04.6) |

  G93.1   Anoxic brain damage, not elsewhere classified 🔖
      Permanent brain damage by lack of oxygen perfusion through brain tissues.

      | **Excludes1** | cerebral anoxia due to anesthesia during labor and delivery (O74.3) |
      | | cerebral anoxia due to anesthesia during the puerperium (O89.2) |
      | | neonatal anoxia (P84) |

  G93.2   Benign intracranial hypertension
      Pseudotumor

      | **Excludes1** | hypertensive encephalopathy (I67.4) |
      | | obstructive hydrocephalus (G91.1) |

➡ ● **G93.3   Postviral and related fatigue syndromes**
      ~~Benign myalgic encephalomyelitis~~

      | **Excludes1** | chronic fatigue syndrome NOS (R53.82) |

    ▸ Use Additional code, if applicable, for post COVID-19 condition, unspecified (U09.9)

    ▸ | **Excludes1** | neurasthenia (F48.8) |

  ▸ **G93.31   Postviral fatigue syndrome**

  ▸ **G93.32   Myalgic encephalomyelitis/chronic fatigue syndrome**
      ▸ Chronic fatigue syndrome
      ▸ ME/CFS
      ▸ Myalgic encephalomyelitis

  ▸ **G93.39   Other post infection and related fatigue syndromes**

  ● **G93.4   Other and unspecified encephalopathy**
      | **Excludes1** | alcoholic encephalopathy (G31.2) |
      | | encephalopathy in diseases classified elsewhere (G94) |
      | | hypertensive encephalopathy (I67.4) |

      | **Excludes2** | toxic (metabolic) encephalopathy (G92.8) |
      Coding Clinic: 2017, Q2, P9

    G93.40   Encephalopathy, unspecified

    G93.41   Metabolic encephalopathy
        Septic encephalopathy
        Coding Clinic: 2017, Q2, P8; 2016, Q3, P42; 2015, Q3, P21

    G93.49   Other encephalopathy
        Encephalopathy NEC
        Coding Clinic: 2021, Q2, P3; 2018, Q4, P16; 2018, Q2, P22; 2017, Q2, P9

  G93.5   Compression of brain 🔖
      Arnold-Chiari type 1 compression of brain
      Compression of brain (stem)
      Herniation of brain (stem)

      | **Excludes1** | traumatic compression of brain (S06.A-) |

  G93.6   Cerebral edema 🔖
      | **Excludes1** | cerebral edema due to birth injury (P11.0) |
      | | traumatic cerebral edema (S06.1-) |

  G93.7   Reye's syndrome   P
    Life-threatening neurological condition, usually follows viral illness

    Code first (poisoning due to salicylates, if applicable (T39.0-, with sixth character 1-4)

    Use additional code for adverse effect due to salicylates, if applicable (T39.0-, with sixth character 5)

CHAPTER 6 (G00-G99)

● **G93.8   Other specified disorders of brain**
    G93.81   Temporal sclerosis
       Hippocampal sclerosis
       Mesial temporal sclerosis
    G93.82   Brain death
    G93.89   Other specified disorders of brain
       Postradiation encephalopathy
       Coding Clinic: 2019, Q3, P9; 2016, Q4, P7

    G93.9   Disorder of brain, unspecified

▷ *G94   Other disorders of brain in diseases classified elsewhere*
      Code first underlying disease
      Excludes1   encephalopathy in congenital syphilis (A50.49)
                encephalopathy in influenza (J09.X9, J10.81, J11.81)
                encephalopathy in syphilis (A52.19)
                hydrocephalus in diseases classified elsewhere (G91.4)
      Coding Clinic: 2018, Q2, P22; 2017, Q2, P8

● **G95   Other and unspecified diseases of spinal cord**
      Excludes2   myelitis (G04.-)
    G95.0   Syringomyelia and syringobulbia 🅗
   ● **G95.1   Vascular myelopathies**
       Excludes2   intraspinal phlebitis and thrombophlebitis, except non-pyogenic (G08)
    G95.11   Acute infarction of spinal cord (embolic) (nonembolic) 🅗
       Anoxia of spinal cord
       Arterial thrombosis of spinal cord
    G95.19   Other vascular myelopathies 🅗
       Edema of spinal cord
       Hematomyelia
       Nonpyogenic intraspinal phlebitis and thrombophlebitis
       Subacute necrotic myelopathy
   ● **G95.2   Other and unspecified cord compression**
    G95.20   Unspecified cord compression 🅗
    G95.29   Other cord compression 🅗
   ● **G95.8   Other specified diseases of spinal cord**
       Excludes1   neurogenic bladder NOS (N31.9)
                neurogenic bladder due to cauda equina syndrome (G83.4)
                neuromuscular dysfunction of bladder without spinal cord lesion (N31.-)
    G95.81   Conus medullaris syndrome 🅗
       Damage to gray matter and/or nerve roots in lower end of spinal cord
    G95.89   Other specified diseases of spinal cord 🅗
       Cord bladder NOS
       Drug-induced myelopathy
       Radiation-induced myelopathy
       Excludes1   myelopathy NOS (G95.9)
    G95.9   Disease of spinal cord, unspecified 🅗
       Myelopathy NOS

● **G96   Other disorders of central nervous system**
   ● **G96.0   Cerebrospinal fluid leak**
      Code also if applicable:
       intracranial hypotension (G96.81-)
      Excludes1   cerebrospinal fluid leak from spinal puncture (G97.0)
      Coding Clinic: 2018, Q2, P13
    G96.00   Cerebrospinal fluid leak, unspecified
       Code also if applicable:
       ▶ head injury (S00-S09)

    G96.01   Cranial cerebrospinal fluid leak, spontaneous
       Otorrhea due to spontaneous cerebrospinal fluid CSF leak
       Rhinorrhea due to spontaneous cerebrospinal fluid CSF leak
       Spontaneous cerebrospinal fluid leak from skull base
    G96.02   Spinal cerebrospinal fluid leak, spontaneous
       Spontaneous cerebrospinal fluid leak from spine
    G96.08   Other cranial cerebrospinal fluid leak
       Postoperative cranial cerebrospinal fluid leak
       Traumatic cranial cerebrospinal fluid leak
      Code also if applicable:
       head injury (S00.- to S09.-)
    G96.09   Other spinal cerebrospinal fluid leak
       Other spinal CSF leak
       Postoperative spinal cerebrospinal fluid leak
       Traumatic spinal cerebrospinal fluid leak
      Code also if applicable:
       head injury (S00.- to S09.-)
   ● **G96.1   Disorders of meninges, not elsewhere classified**
    G96.11   Dural tear
       Code also intracranial hypotension, if applicable (G96.81-)
       Excludes1   accidental puncture or laceration of dura during a procedure (G97.41)
    G96.12   Meningeal adhesions (cerebral) (spinal)
   ● **G96.19   Other disorders of meninges, not elsewhere classified**
    G96.191   Perineural cyst
       Cervical nerve root cyst
       Lumbar nerve root cyst
       Sacral nerve root cyst
       Tarlov cyst
       Thoracic nerve root cyst
    G96.198   Other disorders of meninges, not elsewhere classified
   ● **G96.8   Other specified disorders of central nervous system**
   ● **G96.81   Intracranial hypotension**
      Code also any associated diagnoses, such as:
       Brachial amyotrophy (G54.5)
       Cerebrospinal fluid leak from spine (G96.02)
       Cranial nerve disorders in diseases classified elsewhere (G53)
       Nerve root and compressions in diseases classified elsewhere (G55)
       Nonpyogenic thrombosis of intracranial venous system (I67.6)
       Nontraumatic intracerebral hemorrhage (I61.-)
       Nontraumatic subdural hemorrhage (I62.0-)
       Other and unspecified cord compression (G95.2-)
       Other secondary parkinsonism (G21.8)
       Reversible cerebrovascular vasoconstriction syndrome (I67.841)
       Spinal cord herniation (G95.89)
       Stroke (I63.-)
       Syringomyelia (G95.0)
    G96.810   Intracranial hypotension, unspecified
    G96.811   Intracranial hypotension, spontaneous
    G96.819   Other intracranial hypotension
    G96.89   Other specified disorders of central nervous system
    G96.9   Disorder of central nervous system, unspecified

▶ New   ⇒ Revised   ~~deleted~~ Deleted   Excludes 1   Excludes 2   Includes   Use additional   Code first   Code also   Key words
OGCR Official Guidelines   X Assign placeholder X   ● Use Additional Character(s)   ▷ Manifestation Code   🅗 Hierarchical Condition Category   **Coding Clinic**

G97 **Intraoperative and postprocedural complications and disorders of nervous system, not elsewhere classified**

    Excludes2   intraoperative and postprocedural cerebrovascular infarction (I97.81-, I97.82-)

    Coding Clinic: 2016, Q4, P9

    G97.0 **Cerebrospinal fluid leak from spinal puncture**

         Code also any associated diagnoses or complications, such as:

            intracranial hypotension following a procedure (G97.83-G97.84)

    G97.1 **Other reaction to spinal and lumbar puncture**

         Headache due to lumbar puncture

         Other reaction to spinal dural puncture

         Code also, if applicable, any associated headache with orthostatic component (R51.0)

    G97.2 **Intracranial hypotension following ventricular shunting**

         Code also any associated diagnoses or complications

    ● **G97.3** **Intraoperative hemorrhage and hematoma of a nervous system organ or structure complicating a procedure**

        Excludes1   intraoperative hemorrhage and hematoma of a nervous system organ or structure due to accidental puncture and laceration during a procedure (G97.4-)

         G97.31 **Intraoperative hemorrhage and hematoma of a nervous system organ or structure complicating a nervous system procedure**

         G97.32 **Intraoperative hemorrhage and hematoma of a nervous system organ or structure complicating other procedure**

    ● **G97.4** **Accidental puncture and laceration of a nervous system organ or structure during a procedure**

         G97.41 **Accidental puncture or laceration of dura during a procedure**

            Incidental (inadvertent) durotomy

            Code also any associated diagnoses or complications

         G97.48 **Accidental puncture and laceration of other nervous system organ or structure during a nervous system procedure**

         G97.49 **Accidental puncture and laceration of other nervous system organ or structure during other procedure**

    ● **G97.5** **Postprocedural hemorrhage of a nervous system organ or structure following a procedure**

         G97.51 **Postprocedural hemorrhage of a nervous system organ or structure following a nervous system procedure**

         G97.52 **Postprocedural hemorrhage of a nervous system organ or structure following other procedure**

    ● **G97.6** **Postprocedural hematoma and seroma of a nervous system organ or structure following a procedure**

         G97.61 **Postprocedural hematoma of a nervous system organ or structure following a nervous system procedure**

         G97.62 **Postprocedural hematoma of a nervous system organ or structure following other procedure**

         G97.63 **Postprocedural seroma of a nervous system organ or structure following a nervous system procedure**

         G97.64 **Postprocedural seroma of a nervous system organ or structure following other procedure**

● **G97.8** **Other intraoperative and postprocedural complications and disorders of nervous system**

     Use additional code to further specify disorder

    G97.81 **Other intraoperative complications of nervous system**

    G97.82 **Other postprocedural complications and disorders of nervous system**

        Coding Clinic: 2022, Q1, P35

    G97.83 **Intracranial hypotension following lumbar cerebrospinal fluid shunting**

         Code also any associated diagnoses or complications

    G97.84 **Intracranial hypotension following other procedure**

         Code also, if applicable:

            accidental puncture or laceration of dura during a procedure (G97.41)

            cerebrospinal fluid leak from spinal puncture (G97.0)

● **G98** **Other disorders of nervous system not elsewhere classified**

    Includes   nervous system disorder NOS

    G98.0 **Neurogenic arthritis, not elsewhere classified**

         Nonsyphilitic neurogenic arthropathy NEC

         Nonsyphilitic neurogenic spondylopathy NEC

        Excludes1   spondylopathy (in):

            syringomyelia and syringobulbia (G95.0)

            tabes dorsalis (A52.11)

    G98.8 **Other disorders of nervous system**

         Nervous system disorder NOS

● **G99** **Other disorders of nervous system in diseases classified elsewhere**

    ▌ *G99.0* *Autonomic neuropathy in diseases classified elsewhere*

         Code first underlying disease, such as:

            amyloidosis (E85.-)

            gout (M1A.-, M10.-)

            hyperthyroidism (E05.-)

        Excludes1   diabetic autonomic neuropathy (E08-E13 with .43)

    ▌ *G99.2* *Myelopathy in diseases classified elsewhere* 🔗

         Code first underlying disease, such as:

            neoplasm (C00-D49)

        Excludes1   myelopathy in:

            intervertebral disease (M50.0-, M51.0-)

            spondylosis (M47.0-, M47.1-)

    ▌ *G99.8* *Other specified disorders of nervous system in diseases classified elsewhere*

         Code first underlying disorder, such as:

            amyloidosis (E85.-)

            avitaminosis (E56.9)

        Excludes1   nervous system involvement in:

            cysticercosis (B69.0)

            rubella (B06.0-)

            syphilis (A52.1-)

CHAPTER 6 (G00-G99)

CHAPTER 7

DISEASES OF THE EYE AND ADNEXA (H00-H59)

OGCR Chapter-Specific Coding Guidelines

7. **Chapter 7: Diseases of the Eye and Adnexa (H00-H59)**

a. **Glaucoma**

1) **Assigning Glaucoma Codes**

Assign as many codes from category H40, Glaucoma, as needed to identify the type of glaucoma, the affected eye, and the glaucoma stage.

2) **Bilateral glaucoma with same type and stage**

When a patient has bilateral glaucoma and both eyes are documented as being the same type and stage, and there is a code for bilateral glaucoma, report only the code for the type of glaucoma, bilateral, with the seventh character for the stage.

When a patient has bilateral glaucoma and both eyes are documented as being the same type and stage, and the classification does not provide a code for bilateral glaucoma (i.e., subcategories H40.10, H40.11, and H40.20) report only one code for the type of glaucoma with the appropriate seventh character for the stage.

3) **Bilateral glaucoma stage with different types or stages**

When a patient has bilateral glaucoma and each eye is documented as having a different type or stage, and the classification distinguishes laterality, assign the appropriate code for each eye rather than the code for bilateral glaucoma.

When a patient has bilateral glaucoma and each eye is documented as having a different type, and the classification does not distinguish laterality (i.e., subcategories H40.10, H40.11 and H40.20), assign one code for each type of glaucoma with the appropriate seventh character for the stage.

When a patient has bilateral glaucoma and each eye is documented as having the same type, but different stage, and the classification does not distinguish laterality (i.e., subcategories H40.10, H40.11, and H40.20), assign a code for the type of glaucoma for each eye with the seventh character for the specific glaucoma stage documented for each eye.

4) **Patient admitted with glaucoma and stage evolves during the admission**

If a patient is admitted with glaucoma and the stage progresses during the admission, assign the code for highest stage documented.

5) **Indeterminate stage glaucoma**

Assignment of the seventh character "4" for "indeterminate stage" should be based on the clinical documentation. The seventh character "4" is used for glaucomas whose stage cannot be clinically determined. This seventh character should not be confused with the seventh character "0", unspecified, which should be assigned when there is no documentation regarding the stage of the glaucoma.

b. **Blindness**

If "blindness" or "low vision" of both eyes is documented but the visual impairment category is not documented, assign code H54.3, Unqualified visual loss, both eyes. If "blindness" or "low vision" in one eye is documented but the visual impairment category is not documented, assign a code from H54.6-, Unqualified visual loss, one eye. If "blindness" or "visual loss" is documented without any information about whether one or both eyes are affected, assign code H54.7, Unspecified visual loss.

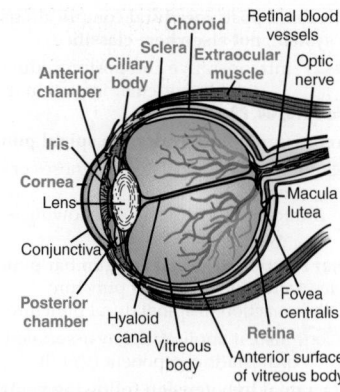

Figure 7-1 Eye and ocular adnexa. (From Buck CJ: Step-by-Step Medical Coding, ed 2016, St. Louis, Elsevier, 2016)

★ **(See Plate 15 of the Anatomy Illustrations.)**

CHAPTER 7

DISEASES OF THE EYE AND ADNEXA (H00-H59)

Note: Use an external cause code following the code for the eye condition, if applicable, to identify the cause of the eye condition

Excludes2 certain conditions originating in the perinatal period (P04-P96)

certain infectious and parasitic diseases (A00-B99)

complications of pregnancy, childbirth and the puerperium (O00-O9A)

congenital malformations, deformations, and chromosomal abnormalities (Q00-Q99)

diabetes mellitus related eye conditions (E09.3-, E10.3-, E11.3-, E13.3-)

endocrine, nutritional and metabolic diseases (E00-E88)

injury (trauma) of eye and orbit (S05.-)

injury, poisoning and certain other consequences of external causes (S00-T88)

neoplasms (C00-D49)

symptoms, signs and abnormal clinical and laboratory findings, not elsewhere classified (R00-R94)

syphilis related eye disorders (A50.01, A50.3-, A51.43, A52.71)

This chapter contains the following blocks:

H00-H05	Disorders of eyelid, lacrimal system and orbit
H10-H11	Disorders of conjunctiva
H15-H22	Disorders of sclera, cornea, iris and ciliary body
H25-H28	Disorders of lens
H30-H36	Disorders of choroid and retina
H40-H42	Glaucoma
H43-H44	Disorders of vitreous body and globe
H46-H47	Disorders of optic nerve and visual pathways
H49-H52	Disorders of ocular muscles, binocular movement, accommodation and refraction
H53-H54	Visual disturbances and blindness
H55-H57	Other disorders of eye and adnexa
H59	Intraoperative and postprocedural complications and disorders of eye and adnexa, not elsewhere classified

▶ New ⟹ Revised deleted Deleted Excludes 1 Excludes 2 Includes Use additional Code first Code also Key words

OGCR Official Guidelines X Assign placeholder X ● Use Additional Character(s) ▶ Manifestation Code 🐾 Hierarchical Condition Category Coding Clinic

DISORDERS OF EYELID, LACRIMAL SYSTEM AND ORBIT (H00-H05)

> **Excludes2**   open wound of eyelid (S01.1-)
> superficial injury of eyelid (S00.1-, S00.2-)

● **H00**   **Hordeolum and chalazion**
Hordeolum: inflammatory staphylococcal infection of sebaceous glands of eyelids; AKA stye. Chalazion: eyelid mass

● **H00.0**   **Hordeolum (externum) (internum) of eyelid**
Bacterial infection (staphylococcus) of the sebaceous gland of the eyelid (stye)

  ● **H00.01**   **Hordeolum externum**
     Hordeolum NOS
     Stye

     H00.011   Hordeolum externum right upper eyelid
     H00.012   Hordeolum externum right lower eyelid
     H00.013   Hordeolum externum right eye, unspecified eyelid
     H00.014   Hordeolum externum left upper eyelid
     H00.015   Hordeolum externum left lower eyelid
     H00.016   Hordeolum externum left eye, unspecified eyelid
     H00.019   Hordeolum externum unspecified eye, unspecified eyelid

  ● **H00.02**   **Hordeolum internum**
     Infection of meibomian gland

     H00.021   Hordeolum internum right upper eyelid
     H00.022   Hordeolum internum right lower eyelid
     H00.023   Hordeolum internum right eye, unspecified eyelid
     H00.024   Hordeolum internum left upper eyelid
     H00.025   Hordeolum internum left lower eyelid
     H00.026   Hordeolum internum left eye, unspecified eyelid
     H00.029   Hordeolum internum unspecified eye, unspecified eyelid

  ● **H00.03**   **Abscess of eyelid**
     Furuncle of eyelid

     H00.031   Abscess of right upper eyelid
     H00.032   Abscess of right lower eyelid
     H00.033   Abscess of eyelid right eye, unspecified eyelid
     H00.034   Abscess of left upper eyelid
     H00.035   Abscess of left lower eyelid
     H00.036   Abscess of eyelid left eye, unspecified eyelid
     H00.039   Abscess of eyelid unspecified eye, unspecified eyelid

● **H00.1**   **Chalazion**
Often caused by accumulation of meibomian gland secretions resulting from a blockage of duct.
     Meibomian (gland) cyst

> **Excludes2**   infected meibomian gland (H00.02-)

     H00.11   Chalazion right upper eyelid
     H00.12   Chalazion right lower eyelid
     H00.13   Chalazion right eye, unspecified eyelid
     H00.14   Chalazion left upper eyelid
     H00.15   Chalazion left lower eyelid
     H00.16   Chalazion left eye, unspecified eyelid
     H00.19   Chalazion unspecified eye, unspecified eyelid

● **H01**   **Other inflammation of eyelid**

● **H01.0**   **Blepharitis**
Inflammation of eyelids

> **Excludes1**   blepharoconjunctivitis (H10.5-)

  ● **H01.00**   **Unspecified blepharitis**

     H01.001   Unspecified blepharitis right upper eyelid
     H01.002   Unspecified blepharitis right lower eyelid
     H01.003   Unspecified blepharitis right eye, unspecified eyelid
     H01.004   Unspecified blepharitis left upper eyelid
     H01.005   Unspecified blepharitis left lower eyelid
     H01.006   Unspecified blepharitis left eye, unspecified eyelid
     H01.009   Unspecified blepharitis unspecified eye, unspecified eyelid
     H01.00A   Unspecified blepharitis right eye, upper and lower eyelids
     H01.00B   Unspecified blepharitis left eye, upper and lower eyelids

  ● **H01.01**   **Ulcerative blepharitis**

     H01.011   Ulcerative blepharitis right upper eyelid
     H01.012   Ulcerative blepharitis right lower eyelid
     H01.013   Ulcerative blepharitis right eye, unspecified eyelid
     H01.014   Ulcerative blepharitis left upper eyelid
     H01.015   Ulcerative blepharitis left lower eyelid
     H01.016   Ulcerative blepharitis left eye, unspecified eyelid
     H01.019   Ulcerative blepharitis unspecified eye, unspecified eyelid
     H01.01A   Ulcerative blepharitis right eye, upper and lower eyelids
     H01.01B   Ulcerative blepharitis left eye, upper and lower eyelids

  ● **H01.02**   **Squamous blepharitis**

     H01.021   Squamous blepharitis right upper eyelid
     H01.022   Squamous blepharitis right lower eyelid
     H01.023   Squamous blepharitis right eye, unspecified eyelid
     H01.024   Squamous blepharitis left upper eyelid
     H01.025   Squamous blepharitis left lower eyelid
     H01.026   Squamous blepharitis left eye, unspecified eyelid
     H01.029   Squamous blepharitis unspecified eye, unspecified eyelid
     H01.02A   Squamous blepharitis right eye, upper and lower eyelids
     H01.02B   Squamous blepharitis left eye, upper and lower eyelids

● **H01.1**   **Noninfectious dermatoses of eyelid**

  ● **H01.11**   **Allergic dermatitis of eyelid**
     Contact dermatitis of eyelid

     H01.111   Allergic dermatitis of right upper eyelid
     H01.112   Allergic dermatitis of right lower eyelid
     H01.113   Allergic dermatitis of right eye, unspecified eyelid

H01.114   Allergic dermatitis of left upper eyelid

H01.115   Allergic dermatitis of left lower eyelid

H01.116   Allergic dermatitis of left eye, unspecified eyelid

H01.119   Allergic dermatitis of unspecified eye, unspecified eyelid

● H01.12   Discoid lupus erythematosus of eyelid

H01.121   Discoid lupus erythematosus of right upper eyelid

H01.122   Discoid lupus erythematosus of right lower eyelid

H01.123   Discoid lupus erythematosus of right eye, unspecified eyelid

H01.124   Discoid lupus erythematosus of left upper eyelid

H01.125   Discoid lupus erythematosus of left lower eyelid

H01.126   Discoid lupus erythematosus of left eye, unspecified eyelid

H01.129   Discoid lupus erythematosus of unspecified eye, unspecified eyelid

● H01.13   Eczematous dermatitis of eyelid

H01.131   Eczematous dermatitis of right upper eyelid

H01.132   Eczematous dermatitis of right lower eyelid

H01.133   Eczematous dermatitis of right eye, unspecified eyelid

H01.134   Eczematous dermatitis of left upper eyelid

H01.135   Eczematous dermatitis of left lower eyelid

H01.136   Eczematous dermatitis of left eye, unspecified eyelid

H01.139   Eczematous dermatitis of unspecified eye, unspecified eyelid

● H01.14   Xeroderma of eyelid
          Abnormally dry

H01.141   Xeroderma of right upper eyelid

H01.142   Xeroderma of right lower eyelid

H01.143   Xeroderma of right eye, unspecified eyelid

H01.144   Xeroderma of left upper eyelid

H01.145   Xeroderma of left lower eyelid

H01.146   Xeroderma of left eye, unspecified eyelid

H01.149   Xeroderma of unspecified eye, unspecified eyelid

H01.8   Other specified inflammations of eyelid

H01.9   Unspecified inflammation of eyelid
       Inflammation of eyelid NOS

● H02   Other disorders of eyelid
       Turning inward (inversion) of eyelid margin and ingrowing eyelashes
       Excludes1   congenital malformations of eyelid (Q10.0-Q10.3)

● H02.0   Entropion and trichiasis of eyelid

● H02.00   Unspecified entropion of eyelid

H02.001   Unspecified entropion of right upper eyelid

H02.002   Unspecified entropion of right lower eyelid

H02.003   Unspecified entropion of right eye, unspecified eyelid

H02.004   Unspecified entropion of left upper eyelid

H02.005   Unspecified entropion of left lower eyelid

Figure 7-2 Right lower eyelid entropion. Note the inward rotation of the tarsal plate about the horizontal axis and the resultant contact between the mucocutaneous junction and ocular surface. (From Glynn M, Drake WM, Hutchison R: Hutchison's Clinical Methods: An Integrated Approach to Clinical Practice, Edinburgh, Saunders/Elsevier, 2012)

H02.006   Unspecified entropion of left eye, unspecified eyelid

H02.009   Unspecified entropion of unspecified eye, unspecified eyelid

● H02.01   Cicatricial entropion of eyelid
          Scar

H02.011   Cicatricial entropion of right upper eyelid

H02.012   Cicatricial entropion of right lower eyelid

H02.013   Cicatricial entropion of right eye, unspecified eyelid

H02.014   Cicatricial entropion of left upper eyelid

H02.015   Cicatricial entropion of left lower eyelid

H02.016   Cicatricial entropion of left eye, unspecified eyelid

H02.019   Cicatricial entropion of unspecified eye, unspecified eyelid

● H02.02   Mechanical entropion of eyelid
          Turning inward (inversion) of eyelid margin due to lack of support

H02.021   Mechanical entropion of right upper eyelid

H02.022   Mechanical entropion of right lower eyelid

H02.023   Mechanical entropion of right eye, unspecified eyelid

H02.024   Mechanical entropion of left upper eyelid

H02.025   Mechanical entropion of left lower eyelid

H02.026   Mechanical entropion of left eye, unspecified eyelid

H02.029   Mechanical entropion of unspecified eye, unspecified eyelid

● H02.03   Senile entropion of eyelid
          Turning inward (inversion) of eyelid margin due to aging

H02.031   Senile entropion of right upper eyelid   A

H02.032   Senile entropion of right lower eyelid   A

H02.033   Senile entropion of right eye, unspecified eyelid   A

H02.034   Senile entropion of left upper eyelid A

H02.035   Senile entropion of left lower eyelid A

H02.036   Senile entropion of left eye, unspecified eyelid   A

H02.039   Senile entropion of unspecified eye, unspecified eyelid   A

● H02.04   Spastic entropion of eyelid
          Turning inward (inversion) of eyelid margin caused by spasm of muscle

H02.041   Spastic entropion of right upper eyelid

H02.042   Spastic entropion of right lower eyelid

H02.043   Spastic entropion of right eye, unspecified eyelid

▶ New   ▐▶ Revised   ~~deleted~~ Deleted   Excludes 1   Excludes 2   Includes   Use additional   Code first   Code also   Key words

OGCR Official Guidelines   X Assign placeholder X   ● Use Additional Character(s)   ▶ Manifestation Code   🔖 Hierarchical Condition Category   Coding Clinic

H02.044 Spastic entropion of left upper eyelid

H02.045 Spastic entropion of left lower eyelid

H02.046 Spastic entropion of left eye, unspecified eyelid

H02.049 Spastic entropion of unspecified eye, unspecified eyelid

● **H02.05** Trichiasis without entropion
Ingrowing hairs of eyelashes

H02.051 Trichiasis without entropion right upper eyelid

H02.052 Trichiasis without entropion right lower eyelid

H02.053 Trichiasis without entropion right eye, unspecified eyelid

H02.054 Trichiasis without entropion left upper eyelid

H02.055 Trichiasis without entropion left lower eyelid

H02.056 Trichiasis without entropion left eye, unspecified eyelid

H02.059 Trichiasis without entropion unspecified eye, unspecified eyelid

● **H02.1** Ectropion of eyelid
Eversion (pulling away) of eyelid

● **H02.10** Unspecified ectropion of eyelid

H02.101 Unspecified ectropion of right upper eyelid

H02.102 Unspecified ectropion of right lower eyelid

H02.103 Unspecified ectropion of right eye, unspecified eyelid

H02.104 Unspecified ectropion of left upper eyelid

H02.105 Unspecified ectropion of left lower eyelid

H02.106 Unspecified ectropion of left eye, unspecified eyelid

H02.109 Unspecified ectropion of unspecified eye, unspecified eyelid

● **H02.11** Cicatricial ectropion of eyelid
Pulling of eyelid down and away from eye due to scar or tightening

H02.111 Cicatricial ectropion of right upper eyelid

H02.112 Cicatricial ectropion of right lower eyelid

H02.113 Cicatricial ectropion of right eye, unspecified eyelid

H02.114 Cicatricial ectropion of left upper eyelid

H02.115 Cicatricial ectropion of left lower eyelid

H02.116 Cicatricial ectropion of left eye, unspecified eyelid

H02.119 Cicatricial ectropion of unspecified eye, unspecified eyelid

● **H02.12** Mechanical ectropion of eyelid
Eversion (pulling away) of eyelid due to lack of support

H02.121 Mechanical ectropion of right upper eyelid

H02.122 Mechanical ectropion of right lower eyelid

H02.123 Mechanical ectropion of right eye, unspecified eyelid

H02.124 Mechanical ectropion of left upper eyelid

H02.125 Mechanical ectropion of left lower eyelid

H02.126 Mechanical ectropion of left eye, unspecified eyelid

H02.129 Mechanical ectropion of unspecified eye, unspecified eyelid

● **H02.13** Senile ectropion of eyelid
Eversion (pulling away) of eyelid due to age

H02.131 Senile ectropion of right upper eyelid   A

H02.132 Senile ectropion of right lower eyelid   A

H02.133 Senile ectropion of right eye, unspecified eyelid   A

H02.134 Senile ectropion of left upper eyelid A

H02.135 Senile ectropion of left lower eyelid A

H02.136 Senile ectropion of left eye, unspecified eyelid   A

H02.139 Senile ectropion of unspecified eye, unspecified eyelid   A

● **H02.14** Spastic ectropion of eyelid
Eversion (pulling away) of eyelid due to tonic muscle spasm

H02.141 Spastic ectropion of right upper eyelid

H02.142 Spastic ectropion of right lower eyelid

H02.143 Spastic ectropion of right eye, unspecified eyelid

H02.144 Spastic ectropion of left upper eyelid

H02.145 Spastic ectropion of left lower eyelid

H02.146 Spastic ectropion of left eye, unspecified eyelid

H02.149 Spastic ectropion of unspecified eye, unspecified eyelid

● **H02.15** Paralytic ectropion of eyelid

H02.151 Paralytic ectropion of right upper eyelid

H02.152 Paralytic ectropion of right lower eyelid

H02.153 Paralytic ectropion of right eye, unspecified eyelid

H02.154 Paralytic ectropion of left upper eyelid

H02.155 Paralytic ectropion of left lower eyelid

H02.156 Paralytic ectropion of left eye, unspecified eyelid

H02.159 Paralytic ectropion of unspecified eye, unspecified eyelid

● **H02.2** Lagophthalmos
Condition in which eye cannot completely close

● **H02.20** Unspecified lagophthalmos

H02.201 Unspecified lagophthalmos right upper eyelid

H02.202 Unspecified lagophthalmos right lower eyelid

H02.203 Unspecified lagophthalmos right eye, unspecified eyelid

H02.204 Unspecified lagophthalmos left upper eyelid

H02.205 Unspecified lagophthalmos left lower eyelid

H02.206 Unspecified lagophthalmos left eye, unspecified eyelid

H02.209 Unspecified lagophthalmos unspecified eye, unspecified eyelid

H02.20A Unspecified lagophthalmos right eye, upper and lower eyelids

H02.20B Unspecified lagophthalmos left eye, upper and lower eyelids

H02.20C Unspecified lagophthalmos, bilateral, upper and lower eyelids

● H02.21   **Cicatricial lagophthalmos**
              Upper or lower eyelid does not close due to scar or
              tightening
        H02.211   Cicatricial lagophthalmos right upper
                  eyelid
        H02.212   Cicatricial lagophthalmos right lower
                  eyelid
        H02.213   Cicatricial lagophthalmos right eye,
                  unspecified eyelid
        H02.214   Cicatricial lagophthalmos left upper
                  eyelid
        H02.215   Cicatricial lagophthalmos left lower
                  eyelid
        H02.216   Cicatricial lagophthalmos left eye,
                  unspecified eyelid
        H02.219   Cicatricial lagophthalmos unspecified
                  eye, unspecified eyelid
        H02.21A   Cicatricial lagophthalmos right eye,
                  upper and lower eyelids
        H02.21B   Cicatricial lagophthalmos left eye,
                  upper and lower eyelids
        H02.21C   Cicatricial lagophthalmos, bilateral,
                  upper and lower eyelids

● H02.22   **Mechanical lagophthalmos**
              Inability to close lids due to structural disorder
        H02.221   Mechanical lagophthalmos right
                  upper eyelid
        H02.222   Mechanical lagophthalmos right
                  lower eyelid
        H02.223   Mechanical lagophthalmos right eye,
                  unspecified eyelid
        H02.224   Mechanical lagophthalmos left upper
                  eyelid
        H02.225   Mechanical lagophthalmos left lower
                  eyelid
        H02.226   Mechanical lagophthalmos left eye,
                  unspecified eyelid
        H02.229   Mechanical lagophthalmos
                  unspecified eye, unspecified eyelid
        H02.22A   Mechanical lagophthalmos right eye,
                  upper and lower eyelids
        H02.22B   Mechanical lagophthalmos left eye,
                  upper and lower eyelids
        H02.22C   Mechanical lagophthalmos, bilateral,
                  upper and lower eyelids

● H02.23   **Paralytic lagophthalmos**
              Eyelids do not close due to paralysis
        H02.231   Paralytic lagophthalmos right upper
                  eyelid
        H02.232   Paralytic lagophthalmos right lower
                  eyelid
        H02.233   Paralytic lagophthalmos right eye,
                  unspecified eyelid
        H02.234   Paralytic lagophthalmos left upper
                  eyelid
        H02.235   Paralytic lagophthalmos left lower
                  eyelid
        H02.236   Paralytic lagophthalmos left eye,
                  unspecified eyelid
        H02.239   Paralytic lagophthalmos unspecified
                  eye, unspecified eyelid
        H02.23A   Paralytic lagophthalmos right eye,
                  upper and lower eyelids
        H02.23B   Paralytic lagophthalmos left eye,
                  upper and lower eyelids
        H02.23C   Paralytic lagophthalmos, bilateral,
                  upper and lower eyelids

Figure 7-3   Ptosis of eyelid. (From Kanski JJ:
Clinical Diagnosis in Ophthalmology, London,
Elsevier Mosby, 2006)

Item 7-1   Ptosis of eyelid is drooping of the upper eyelid over the pupil when
the eyes are fully opened resulting from nerve or muscle damage, which may
require surgical correction.

★ **(See Plate 17 of the Anatomy Illustrations.)**

● H02.3   **Blepharochalasis**
              Relaxation of skin of eyelid, due to atrophy of intercellular
              tissue
              Pseudoptosis
        H02.30   Blepharochalasis unspecified eye, unspecified
                 eyelid
        H02.31   Blepharochalasis right upper eyelid
        H02.32   Blepharochalasis right lower eyelid
        H02.33   Blepharochalasis right eye, unspecified eyelid
        H02.34   Blepharochalasis left upper eyelid
        H02.35   Blepharochalasis left lower eyelid
        H02.36   Blepharochalasis left eye, unspecified eyelid

● H02.4   **Ptosis of eyelid**
              Falling forward, drooping, sagging of eyelid
    ● H02.40   **Unspecified ptosis of eyelid**
            H02.401   Unspecified ptosis of right eyelid
            H02.402   Unspecified ptosis of left eyelid
            H02.403   Unspecified ptosis of bilateral eyelids
            H02.409   Unspecified ptosis of unspecified
                      eyelid
    ● H02.41   **Mechanical ptosis of eyelid**
            H02.411   Mechanical ptosis of right eyelid
            H02.412   Mechanical ptosis of left eyelid
            H02.413   Mechanical ptosis of bilateral eyelids
            H02.419   Mechanical ptosis of unspecified
                      eyelid
    ● H02.42   **Myogenic ptosis of eyelid**
            H02.421   Myogenic ptosis of right eyelid
            H02.422   Myogenic ptosis of left eyelid
            H02.423   Myogenic ptosis of bilateral eyelids
            H02.429   Myogenic ptosis of unspecified eyelid
    ● H02.43   **Paralytic ptosis of eyelid**
              Neurogenic ptosis of eyelid
            H02.431   Paralytic ptosis of right eyelid
            H02.432   Paralytic ptosis of left eyelid
            H02.433   Paralytic ptosis of bilateral eyelids
            H02.439   Paralytic ptosis unspecified eyelid

● H02.5   **Other disorders affecting eyelid function**
        Excludes2   blepharospasm (G24.5)
                    organic tic (G25.69)
                    psychogenic tic (F95.-)
    ● H02.51   **Abnormal innervation syndrome**
            H02.511   Abnormal innervation syndrome
                      right upper eyelid
            H02.512   Abnormal innervation syndrome
                      right lower eyelid
            H02.513   Abnormal innervation syndrome
                      right eye, unspecified eyelid
            H02.514   Abnormal innervation syndrome left
                      upper eyelid
            H02.515   Abnormal innervation syndrome left
                      lower eyelid
            H02.516   Abnormal innervation syndrome left
                      eye, unspecified eyelid
            H02.519   Abnormal innervation syndrome
                      unspecified eye, unspecified eyelid

▶ New   ⇒ Revised   ~~deleted~~ Deleted   Excludes 1   Excludes 2   Includes   Use additional   Code first   Code also   Key words

830   OGCR Official Guidelines   X Assign placeholder X   ● Use Additional Character(s)   ▷ Manifestation Code   🝙 Hierarchical Condition Category   Coding Clinic

CHAPTER 7 (H00-H59)

● **H02.52 Blepharophimosis**
Drooping of eyelid with reduced lid size
Ankyloblepharon

H02.521 Blepharophimosis right upper eyelid

H02.522 Blepharophimosis right lower eyelid

H02.523 Blepharophimosis right eye, unspecified eyelid

H02.524 Blepharophimosis left upper eyelid

H02.525 Blepharophimosis left lower eyelid

H02.526 Blepharophimosis left eye, unspecified eyelid

H02.529 Blepharophimosis unspecified eye, unspecified lid

● **H02.53 Eyelid retraction**
Eyelid lag

H02.531 Eyelid retraction right upper eyelid

H02.532 Eyelid retraction right lower eyelid

H02.533 Eyelid retraction right eye, unspecified eyelid

H02.534 Eyelid retraction left upper eyelid

H02.535 Eyelid retraction left lower eyelid

H02.536 Eyelid retraction left eye, unspecified eyelid

H02.539 Eyelid retraction unspecified eye, unspecified lid

H02.59 **Other disorders affecting eyelid function**
Deficient blink reflex
Sensory disorders

● **H02.6 Xanthelasma of eyelid**
Yellow-to-orange patches or pimples clustered together on eyelid

H02.60 Xanthelasma of unspecified eye, unspecified eyelid

H02.61 Xanthelasma of right upper eyelid

H02.62 Xanthelasma of right lower eyelid

H02.63 Xanthelasma of right eye, unspecified eyelid

H02.64 Xanthelasma of left upper eyelid

H02.65 Xanthelasma of left lower eyelid

H02.66 Xanthelasma of left eye, unspecified eyelid

● **H02.7 Other and unspecified degenerative disorders of eyelid and periocular area**

H02.70 **Unspecified degenerative disorders of eyelid and periocular area**

● **H02.71 Chloasma of eyelid and periocular area**
Dyspigmentation of eyelid
Hyperpigmentation of eyelid

H02.711 Chloasma of right upper eyelid and periocular area

H02.712 Chloasma of right lower eyelid and periocular area

H02.713 Chloasma of right eye, unspecified eyelid and periocular area

H02.714 Chloasma of left upper eyelid and periocular area

H02.715 Chloasma of left lower eyelid and periocular area

H02.716 Chloasma of left eye, unspecified eyelid and periocular area

H02.719 Chloasma of unspecified eye, unspecified eyelid and periocular area

● **H02.72 Madarosis of eyelid and periocular area**
Loss of eyelashes and/or eyebrows
Hypotrichosis of eyelid

H02.721 Madarosis of right upper eyelid and periocular area

H02.722 Madarosis of right lower eyelid and periocular area

H02.723 Madarosis of right eye, unspecified eyelid and periocular area

H02.724 Madarosis of left upper eyelid and periocular area

H02.725 Madarosis of left lower eyelid and periocular area

H02.726 Madarosis of left eye, unspecified eyelid and periocular area

H02.729 Madarosis of unspecified eye, unspecified eyelid and periocular area

● **H02.73 Vitiligo of eyelid and periocular area**
Skin pigmentation disease characterized by white patches
Hypopigmentation of eyelid

H02.731 Vitiligo of right upper eyelid and periocular area

H02.732 Vitiligo of right lower eyelid and periocular area

H02.733 Vitiligo of right eye, unspecified eyelid and periocular area

H02.734 Vitiligo of left upper eyelid and periocular area

H02.735 Vitiligo of left lower eyelid and periocular area

H02.736 Vitiligo of left eye, unspecified eyelid and periocular area

H02.739 Vitiligo of unspecified eye, unspecified eyelid and periocular area

H02.79 **Other degenerative disorders of eyelid and periocular area**

● **H02.8 Other specified disorders of eyelid**

● **H02.81 Retained foreign body in eyelid**
Use additional code to identify the type of retained foreign body (Z18.-)

   Excludes1 laceration of eyelid with foreign body (S01.12-)
retained intraocular foreign body (H44.6-, H44.7-)
superficial foreign body of eyelid and periocular area (S00.25-)

H02.811 Retained foreign body in right upper eyelid

H02.812 Retained foreign body in right lower eyelid

H02.813 Retained foreign body in right eye, unspecified eyelid

H02.814 Retained foreign body in left upper eyelid

H02.815 Retained foreign body in left lower eyelid

H02.816 Retained foreign body in left eye, unspecified eyelid

H02.819 Retained foreign body in unspecified eye, unspecified eyelid

● **H02.82 Cysts of eyelid**
Sebaceous cyst of eyelid

H02.821 Cysts of right upper eyelid

H02.822 Cysts of right lower eyelid

H02.823 Cysts of right eye, unspecified eyelid

H02.824 Cysts of left upper eyelid

H02.825 Cysts of left lower eyelid

H02.826 Cysts of left eye, unspecified eyelid

H02.829 Cysts of unspecified eye, unspecified eyelid

● **H02.83 Dermatochalasis of eyelid**
Skin is inelastic and hangs loosely in folds

H02.831 Dermatochalasis of right upper eyelid

H02.832 Dermatochalasis of right lower eyelid

H02.833 Dermatochalasis of right eye, unspecified eyelid

H02.834 Dermatochalasis of left upper eyelid

H02.835   Dermatochalasis of left lower eyelid

H02.836   Dermatochalasis of left eye, unspecified eyelid

H02.839   Dermatochalasis of unspecified eye, unspecified eyelid

● H02.84   Edema of eyelid
      Hyperemia of eyelid

H02.841   Edema of right upper eyelid

H02.842   Edema of right lower eyelid

H02.843   Edema of right eye, unspecified eyelid

H02.844   Edema of left upper eyelid

H02.845   Edema of left lower eyelid

H02.846   Edema of left eye, unspecified eyelid

H02.849   Edema of unspecified eye, unspecified eyelid

● H02.85   Elephantiasis of eyelid
      Massive secondary lymphedema with hypertrophy of skin and subcutaneous tissues (pachyderma)

H02.851   Elephantiasis of right upper eyelid

H02.852   Elephantiasis of right lower eyelid

H02.853   Elephantiasis of right eye, unspecified eyelid

H02.854   Elephantiasis of left upper eyelid

H02.855   Elephantiasis of left lower eyelid

H02.856   Elephantiasis of left eye, unspecified eyelid

H02.859   Elephantiasis of unspecified eye, unspecified eyelid

● H02.86   Hypertrichosis of eyelid
      Excessive growth of hair

H02.861   Hypertrichosis of right upper eyelid

H02.862   Hypertrichosis of right lower eyelid

H02.863   Hypertrichosis of right eye, unspecified eyelid

H02.864   Hypertrichosis of left upper eyelid

H02.865   Hypertrichosis of left lower eyelid

H02.866   Hypertrichosis of left eye, unspecified eyelid

H02.869   Hypertrichosis of unspecified eye, unspecified eyelid

● H02.87   Vascular anomalies of eyelid

H02.871   Vascular anomalies of right upper eyelid

H02.872   Vascular anomalies of right lower eyelid

H02.873   Vascular anomalies of right eye, unspecified eyelid

H02.874   Vascular anomalies of left upper eyelid

H02.875   Vascular anomalies of left lower eyelid

H02.876   Vascular anomalies of left eye, unspecified eyelid

H02.879   Vascular anomalies of unspecified eye, unspecified eyelid

● H02.88   Meibomian gland dysfunction of eyelid

H02.881   Meibomian gland dysfunction right upper eyelid

H02.882   Meibomian gland dysfunction right lower eyelid

H02.883   Meibomian gland dysfunction of right eye, unspecified eyelid

H02.884   Meibomian gland dysfunction left upper eyelid

H02.885   Meibomian gland dysfunction left lower eyelid

H02.886   Meibomian gland dysfunction of left eye, unspecified eyelid

H02.889   Meibomian gland dysfunction of unspecified eye, unspecified eyelid

H02.88A   Meibomian gland dysfunction right eye, upper and lower eyelids

H02.88B   Meibomian gland dysfunction left eye, upper and lower eyelids

H02.89   Other specified disorders of eyelid
      Hemorrhage of eyelid

H02.9   Unspecified disorder of eyelid
      Disorder of eyelid NOS

● H04   Disorders of lacrimal system

   Excludes1   congenital malformations of lacrimal system (Q10.4-Q10.6)

● H04.0   Dacryoadenitis
      Inflammation of lacrimal gland

● H04.00   Unspecified dacryoadenitis

H04.001   Unspecified dacryoadenitis, right lacrimal gland

H04.002   Unspecified dacryoadenitis, left lacrimal gland

H04.003   Unspecified dacryoadenitis, bilateral lacrimal glands

H04.009   Unspecified dacryoadenitis, unspecified lacrimal gland

● H04.01   Acute dacryoadenitis

H04.011   Acute dacryoadenitis, right lacrimal gland

H04.012   Acute dacryoadenitis, left lacrimal gland

H04.013   Acute dacryoadenitis, bilateral lacrimal glands

H04.019   Acute dacryoadenitis, unspecified lacrimal gland

★ **(See Plate 19 of the Anatomy Illustrations.)**

● H04.02   Chronic dacryoadenitis

H04.021   Chronic dacryoadenitis, right lacrimal gland

H04.022   Chronic dacryoadenitis, left lacrimal gland

H04.023   Chronic dacryoadenitis, bilateral lacrimal gland

H04.029   Chronic dacryoadenitis, unspecified lacrimal gland

● H04.03   Chronic enlargement of lacrimal gland

H04.031   Chronic enlargement of right lacrimal gland

H04.032   Chronic enlargement of left lacrimal gland

H04.033   Chronic enlargement of bilateral lacrimal glands

H04.039   Chronic enlargement of unspecified lacrimal gland

● H04.1   Other disorders of lacrimal gland

● H04.11   Dacryops
      Watery eye or distention of lacrimal duct due to fluid

H04.111   Dacryops of right lacrimal gland

H04.112   Dacryops of left lacrimal gland

H04.113   Dacryops of bilateral lacrimal glands

H04.119   Dacryops of unspecified lacrimal gland

Figure 7-4   Lacrimal apparatus. (From Buck CJ: Step-by-Step Medical Coding, 2016, St. Louis, Elsevier, 2016)

▶ New   ⇒ Revised   ~~deleted~~ Deleted   Excludes 1   Excludes 2   Includes   Use additional   Code first   Code also   Key words

OGCR Official Guidelines   X Assign placeholder X   ● Use Additional Character(s)   ▶ Manifestation Code   🏷 Hierarchical Condition Category   **Coding Clinic**

● **H04.12 Dry eye syndrome**
Tear film insufficiency, NOS

- H04.121 Dry eye syndrome of right lacrimal gland
- H04.122 Dry eye syndrome of left lacrimal gland
- H04.123 Dry eye syndrome of bilateral lacrimal glands
- H04.129 Dry eye syndrome of unspecified lacrimal gland

● **H04.13 Lacrimal cyst**
Lacrimal cystic degeneration

- H04.131 Lacrimal cyst right lacrimal gland
- H04.132 Lacrimal cyst left lacrimal gland
- H04.133 Lacrimal cyst bilateral lacrimal glands
- H04.139 Lacrimal cyst unspecified lacrimal gland

● **H04.14 Primary lacrimal gland atrophy**

- H04.141 Primary lacrimal gland atrophy, right lacrimal gland
- H04.142 Primary lacrimal gland atrophy, left lacrimal gland
- H04.143 Primary lacrimal gland atrophy, bilateral lacrimal glands
- H04.149 Primary lacrimal gland atrophy, unspecified lacrimal gland

● **H04.15 Secondary lacrimal gland atrophy**

- H04.151 Secondary lacrimal gland atrophy, right lacrimal gland
- H04.152 Secondary lacrimal gland atrophy, left lacrimal gland
- H04.153 Secondary lacrimal gland atrophy, bilateral lacrimal glands
- H04.159 Secondary lacrimal gland atrophy, unspecified lacrimal gland

● **H04.16 Lacrimal gland dislocation**

- H04.161 Lacrimal gland dislocation, right lacrimal gland
- H04.162 Lacrimal gland dislocation, left lacrimal gland
- H04.163 Lacrimal gland dislocation, bilateral lacrimal glands
- H04.169 Lacrimal gland dislocation, unspecified lacrimal gland

- H04.19 Other specified disorders of lacrimal gland

● **H04.2 Epiphora**
Overflow of tears due to stricture of lacrimal passages; AKA lacrimation

● **H04.20 Unspecified epiphora**

- H04.201 Unspecified epiphora, right side
- H04.202 Unspecified epiphora, left side
- H04.203 Unspecified epiphora, bilateral
- H04.209 Unspecified epiphora, unspecified side

● **H04.21 Epiphora due to excess lacrimation**

- H04.211 Epiphora due to excess lacrimation, right lacrimal gland
- H04.212 Epiphora due to excess lacrimation, left lacrimal gland
- H04.213 Epiphora due to excess lacrimation, bilateral lacrimal glands
- H04.219 Epiphora due to excess lacrimation, unspecified lacrimal gland

● **H04.22 Epiphora due to insufficient drainage**

- H04.221 Epiphora due to insufficient drainage, right side
- H04.222 Epiphora due to insufficient drainage, left side
- H04.223 Epiphora due to insufficient drainage, bilateral
- H04.229 Epiphora due to insufficient drainage, unspecified side

● **H04.3 Acute and unspecified inflammation of lacrimal passages**

Excludes1 neonatal dacryocystitis (P39.1)

● **H04.30 Unspecified dacryocystitis**

- H04.301 Unspecified dacryocystitis of right lacrimal passage
- H04.302 Unspecified dacryocystitis of left lacrimal passage
- H04.303 Unspecified dacryocystitis of bilateral lacrimal passages
- H04.309 Unspecified dacryocystitis of unspecified lacrimal passage

● **H04.31 Phlegmonous dacryocystitis**
Cellulitis of lacrimal sac

- H04.311 Phlegmonous dacryocystitis of right lacrimal passage
- H04.312 Phlegmonous dacryocystitis of left lacrimal passage
- H04.313 Phlegmonous dacryocystitis of bilateral lacrimal passages
- H04.319 Phlegmonous dacryocystitis of unspecified lacrimal passage

● **H04.32 Acute dacryocystitis**
Acute dacryopericystitis

- H04.321 Acute dacryocystitis of right lacrimal passage
- H04.322 Acute dacryocystitis of left lacrimal passage
- H04.323 Acute dacryocystitis of bilateral lacrimal passages
- H04.329 Acute dacryocystitis of unspecified lacrimal passage

● **H04.33 Acute lacrimal canaliculitis**

- H04.331 Acute lacrimal canaliculitis of right lacrimal passage
- H04.332 Acute lacrimal canaliculitis of left lacrimal passage
- H04.333 Acute lacrimal canaliculitis of bilateral lacrimal passages
- H04.339 Acute lacrimal canaliculitis of unspecified lacrimal passage

● **H04.4 Chronic inflammation of lacrimal passages**

● **H04.41 Chronic dacryocystitis**
Inflammation of lacrimal sac

- H04.411 Chronic dacryocystitis of right lacrimal passage
- H04.412 Chronic dacryocystitis of left lacrimal passage
- H04.413 Chronic dacryocystitis of bilateral lacrimal passages
- H04.419 Chronic dacryocystitis of unspecified lacrimal passage

● **H04.42 Chronic lacrimal canaliculitis**
Inflammation of lacrimal ducts

- H04.421 Chronic lacrimal canaliculitis of right lacrimal passage
- H04.422 Chronic lacrimal canaliculitis of left lacrimal passage
- H04.423 Chronic lacrimal canaliculitis of bilateral lacrimal passages
- H04.429 Chronic lacrimal canaliculitis of unspecified lacrimal passage

● **H04.43 Chronic lacrimal mucocele**
Accumulation of mucous secretion

- H04.431 Chronic lacrimal mucocele of right lacrimal passage
- H04.432 Chronic lacrimal mucocele of left lacrimal passage
- H04.433 Chronic lacrimal mucocele of bilateral lacrimal passages
- H04.439 Chronic lacrimal mucocele of unspecified lacrimal passage

CHAPTER 7 (H00-H59)

CHAPTER 7 (H00-H59)

● **H04.5 Stenosis and insufficiency of lacrimal passages**
  ● **H04.51 Dacryolith**
    Concretion in lacrimal sac/duct; AKA lacrimal calculus
    H04.511 Dacryolith of right lacrimal passage
    H04.512 Dacryolith of left lacrimal passage
    H04.513 Dacryolith of bilateral lacrimal passages
    H04.519 Dacryolith of unspecified lacrimal passage
  ● **H04.52 Eversion of lacrimal punctum**
    Turning out of lacrimal drainage opening
    H04.521 Eversion of right lacrimal punctum
    H04.522 Eversion of left lacrimal punctum
    H04.523 Eversion of bilateral lacrimal punctum
    H04.529 Eversion of unspecified lacrimal punctum
  ● **H04.53 Neonatal obstruction of nasolacrimal duct**
    Excludes1 congenital stenosis and stricture of lacrimal duct (Q10.5)
    H04.531 Neonatal obstruction of right nasolacrimal duct   N
    H04.532 Neonatal obstruction of left nasolacrimal duct   N
    H04.533 Neonatal obstruction of bilateral nasolacrimal duct   N
    H04.539 Neonatal obstruction of unspecified nasolacrimal duct   N
  ● **H04.54 Stenosis of lacrimal canaliculi**
    H04.541 Stenosis of right lacrimal canaliculi
    H04.542 Stenosis of left lacrimal canaliculi
    H04.543 Stenosis of bilateral lacrimal canaliculi
    H04.549 Stenosis of unspecified lacrimal canaliculi
  ● **H04.55 Acquired stenosis of nasolacrimal duct**
    H04.551 Acquired stenosis of right nasolacrimal duct
    H04.552 Acquired stenosis of left nasolacrimal duct
    H04.553 Acquired stenosis of bilateral nasolacrimal duct
    H04.559 Acquired stenosis of unspecified nasolacrimal duct
  ● **H04.56 Stenosis of lacrimal punctum**
    H04.561 Stenosis of right lacrimal punctum
    H04.562 Stenosis of left lacrimal punctum
    H04.563 Stenosis of bilateral lacrimal punctum
    H04.569 Stenosis of unspecified lacrimal punctum
  ● **H04.57 Stenosis of lacrimal sac**
    H04.571 Stenosis of right lacrimal sac
    H04.572 Stenosis of left lacrimal sac
    H04.573 Stenosis of bilateral lacrimal sac
    H04.579 Stenosis of unspecified lacrimal sac
● **H04.6 Other changes of lacrimal passages**
  ● **H04.61 Lacrimal fistula**
    H04.611 Lacrimal fistula right lacrimal passage
    H04.612 Lacrimal fistula left lacrimal passage
    H04.613 Lacrimal fistula bilateral lacrimal passages
    H04.619 Lacrimal fistula unspecified lacrimal passage
  H04.69 Other changes of lacrimal passages

● **H04.8 Other disorders of lacrimal system**
  ● **H04.81 Granuloma of lacrimal passages**
    Inflammatory response due to infectious or noninfectious agents
    H04.811 Granuloma of right lacrimal passage
    H04.812 Granuloma of left lacrimal passage
    H04.813 Granuloma of bilateral lacrimal passages
    H04.819 Granuloma of unspecified lacrimal passage
  H04.89 Other disorders of lacrimal system
  H04.9 Disorder of lacrimal system, unspecified
● **H05 Disorders of orbit**
    Excludes1 congenital malformation of orbit (Q10.7)
  ● **H05.0 Acute inflammation of orbit**
    H05.00 Unspecified acute inflammation of orbit
    ● **H05.01 Cellulitis of orbit**
      Infection of soft tissue of orbit
      Abscess of orbit
      H05.011 Cellulitis of right orbit
      H05.012 Cellulitis of left orbit
      H05.013 Cellulitis of bilateral orbits
      H05.019 Cellulitis of unspecified orbit
    ● **H05.02 Osteomyelitis of orbit**
      Infection of boney orbit of eye
      H05.021 Osteomyelitis of right orbit
      H05.022 Osteomyelitis of left orbit
      H05.023 Osteomyelitis of bilateral orbits
      H05.029 Osteomyelitis of unspecified orbit
    ● **H05.03 Periostitis of orbit**
      Inflammation of periosteum (membrane covering bone surface)
      H05.031 Periostitis of right orbit
      H05.032 Periostitis of left orbit
      H05.033 Periostitis of bilateral orbits
      H05.039 Periostitis of unspecified orbit
    ● **H05.04 Tenonitis of orbit**
      Inflammation of tenon capsule (space enclosing fascia of Tenon between eyeball and fat of orbit)
      H05.041 Tenonitis of right orbit
      H05.042 Tenonitis of left orbit
      H05.043 Tenonitis of bilateral orbits
      H05.049 Tenonitis of unspecified orbit
  ● **H05.1 Chronic inflammatory disorders of orbit**
    H05.10 Unspecified chronic inflammatory disorders of orbit
    ● **H05.11 Granuloma of orbit**
      Pseudotumor (inflammatory) of orbit
      H05.111 Granuloma of right orbit
      H05.112 Granuloma of left orbit
      H05.113 Granuloma of bilateral orbits
      H05.119 Granuloma of unspecified orbit
    ● **H05.12 Orbital myositis**
      Inflammation of extraocular muscles of orbit
      H05.121 Orbital myositis, right orbit
      H05.122 Orbital myositis, left orbit
      H05.123 Orbital myositis, bilateral
      H05.129 Orbital myositis, unspecified orbit
  ● **H05.2 Exophthalmic conditions**
      Bulging eyes
    H05.20 Unspecified exophthalmos
    ● **H05.21 Displacement (lateral) of globe**
      H05.211 Displacement (lateral) of globe, right eye
      H05.212 Displacement (lateral) of globe, left eye

▶ New   ⇒ Revised   ~~deleted~~ Deleted   Excludes 1   Excludes 2   Includes   Use additional   Code first   Code also   Key words

834   OGCR Official Guidelines   X Assign placeholder X   ● Use Additional Character(s)   ▌ Manifestation Code   🜲 Hierarchical Condition Category   Coding Clinic

Figure 7-5 Exophthalmos. (From Black JM, Hokanson JH: Medical-Surgical Nursing: Clinical Management for Positive Outcomes, St. Louis, Saunders Elsevier, 2009)

H05.213 Displacement (lateral) of globe, bilateral

H05.219 Displacement (lateral) of globe, unspecified eye

● H05.22 Edema of orbit
Orbital congestion

H05.221 Edema of right orbit

H05.222 Edema of left orbit

H05.223 Edema of bilateral orbit

H05.229 Edema of unspecified orbit

● H05.23 Hemorrhage of orbit

H05.231 Hemorrhage of right orbit

H05.232 Hemorrhage of left orbit

H05.233 Hemorrhage of bilateral orbit

H05.239 Hemorrhage of unspecified orbit

● H05.24 Constant exophthalmos
Constant bulging eyes, often symptom of Graves disease

H05.241 Constant exophthalmos, right eye

H05.242 Constant exophthalmos, left eye

H05.243 Constant exophthalmos, bilateral

H05.249 Constant exophthalmos, unspecified eye

● H05.25 Intermittent exophthalmos
Intermittent bulging eye occurring with bending forward or sharp turning of head

H05.251 Intermittent exophthalmos, right eye

H05.252 Intermittent exophthalmos, left eye

H05.253 Intermittent exophthalmos, bilateral

H05.259 Intermittent exophthalmos, unspecified eye

● H05.26 Pulsating exophthalmos
Bulging eyes with pulsation and bruit, often due to aneurysm pushing eye forward

H05.261 Pulsating exophthalmos, right eye

H05.262 Pulsating exophthalmos, left eye

H05.263 Pulsating exophthalmos, bilateral

H05.269 Pulsating exophthalmos, unspecified eye

● H05.3 Deformity of orbit

Excludes1 congenital deformity of orbit (Q10.7)
hypertelorism (Q75.2)

H05.30 Unspecified deformity of orbit

● H05.31 Atrophy of orbit

H05.311 Atrophy of right orbit

H05.312 Atrophy of left orbit

H05.313 Atrophy of bilateral orbit

H05.319 Atrophy of unspecified orbit

● H05.32 Deformity of orbit due to bone disease
Code also associated bone disease

H05.321 Deformity of right orbit due to bone disease

H05.322 Deformity of left orbit due to bone disease

H05.323 Deformity of bilateral orbits due to bone disease

H05.329 Deformity of unspecified orbit due to bone disease

● H05.33 Deformity of orbit due to trauma or surgery

H05.331 Deformity of right orbit due to trauma or surgery

H05.332 Deformity of left orbit due to trauma or surgery

H05.333 Deformity of bilateral orbits due to trauma or surgery

H05.339 Deformity of unspecified orbit due to trauma or surgery

● H05.34 Enlargement of orbit

H05.341 Enlargement of right orbit

H05.342 Enlargement of left orbit

H05.343 Enlargement of bilateral orbits

H05.349 Enlargement of unspecified orbit

● H05.35 Exostosis of orbit

H05.351 Exostosis of right orbit

H05.352 Exostosis of left orbit

H05.353 Exostosis of bilateral orbits

H05.359 Exostosis of unspecified orbit

● H05.4 Enophthalmos
Recessed eyeball into orbit

● H05.40 Unspecified enophthalmos

H05.401 Unspecified enophthalmos, right eye

H05.402 Unspecified enophthalmos, left eye

H05.403 Unspecified enophthalmos, bilateral

H05.409 Unspecified enophthalmos, unspecified eye

● H05.41 Enophthalmos due to atrophy of orbital tissue

H05.411 Enophthalmos due to atrophy of orbital tissue, right eye

H05.412 Enophthalmos due to atrophy of orbital tissue, left eye

H05.413 Enophthalmos due to atrophy of orbital tissue, bilateral

H05.419 Enophthalmos due to atrophy of orbital tissue, unspecified eye

● H05.42 Enophthalmos due to trauma or surgery

H05.421 Enophthalmos due to trauma or surgery, right eye

H05.422 Enophthalmos due to trauma or surgery, left eye

H05.423 Enophthalmos due to trauma or surgery, bilateral

H05.429 Enophthalmos due to trauma or surgery, unspecified eye

● H05.5 Retained (old) foreign body following penetrating wound of orbit
Retrobulbar foreign body

Use additional code to identify the type of retained foreign body (Z18.-)

Excludes1 current penetrating wound of orbit (S05.4-)

Excludes2 retained foreign body of eyelid (H02.81-)
retained intraocular foreign body (H44.6-, H44.7-)

H05.50 Retained (old) foreign body following penetrating wound of unspecified orbit

H05.51 Retained (old) foreign body following penetrating wound of right orbit

H05.52   Retained (old) foreign body following penetrating wound of left orbit

H05.53   Retained (old) foreign body following penetrating wound of bilateral orbits

- H05.8   Other disorders of orbit
  - H05.81   Cyst of orbit
    Encephalocele of orbit
    - H05.811   Cyst of right orbit
    - H05.812   Cyst of left orbit
    - H05.813   Cyst of bilateral orbits
    - H05.819   Cyst of unspecified orbit
  - H05.82   Myopathy of extraocular muscles
    Weakness of muscles of eye
    - H05.821   Myopathy of extraocular muscles, right orbit
    - H05.822   Myopathy of extraocular muscles, left orbit
    - H05.823   Myopathy of extraocular muscles, bilateral
    - H05.829   Myopathy of extraocular muscles, unspecified orbit
  - H05.89   Other disorders of orbit
- H05.9   Unspecified disorder of orbit

DISORDERS OF CONJUNCTIVA (H10-H11)

★ **(See Plate 18 of the Anatomy Illustrations.)**

- H10   Conjunctivitis
  Inflammation of membrane of the inside of the eyelid or on surface of eye (conjunctiva)
  Excludes1   keratoconjunctivitis (H16.2-)
  - H10.0   Mucopurulent conjunctivitis
    - H10.01   Acute follicular conjunctivitis
      - H10.011   Acute follicular conjunctivitis, right eye
      - H10.012   Acute follicular conjunctivitis, left eye
      - H10.013   Acute follicular conjunctivitis, bilateral
      - H10.019   Acute follicular conjunctivitis, unspecified eye
    - H10.02   Other mucopurulent conjunctivitis
      - H10.021   Other mucopurulent conjunctivitis, right eye
      - H10.022   Other mucopurulent conjunctivitis, left eye
      - H10.023   Other mucopurulent conjunctivitis, bilateral
      - H10.029   Other mucopurulent conjunctivitis, unspecified eye
  - H10.1   Acute atopic conjunctivitis
    Acute papillary conjunctivitis
    - H10.10   Acute atopic conjunctivitis, unspecified eye
    - H10.11   Acute atopic conjunctivitis, right eye
    - H10.12   Acute atopic conjunctivitis, left eye
    - H10.13   Acute atopic conjunctivitis, bilateral
  - H10.2   Other acute conjunctivitis
    - H10.21   Acute toxic conjunctivitis
      Acute chemical conjunctivitis
      Code first (T51-T65) to identify chemical and intent
      Excludes1   burn and corrosion of eye and adnexa (T26.-)
      - H10.211   Acute toxic conjunctivitis, right eye
      - H10.212   Acute toxic conjunctivitis, left eye
      - H10.213   Acute toxic conjunctivitis, bilateral
      - H10.219   Acute toxic conjunctivitis, unspecified eye

- H10.22   Pseudomembranous conjunctivitis
  - H10.221   Pseudomembranous conjunctivitis, right eye
  - H10.222   Pseudomembranous conjunctivitis, left eye
  - H10.223   Pseudomembranous conjunctivitis, bilateral
  - H10.229   Pseudomembranous conjunctivitis, unspecified eye
- H10.23   Serous conjunctivitis, except viral
  Excludes1   viral conjunctivitis (B30.-)
  - H10.231   Serous conjunctivitis, except viral, right eye
  - H10.232   Serous conjunctivitis, except viral, left eye
  - H10.233   Serous conjunctivitis, except viral, bilateral
  - H10.239   Serous conjunctivitis, except viral, unspecified eye
- H10.3   Unspecified acute conjunctivitis
  Excludes1   ophthalmia neonatorum NOS (P39.1)
  - H10.30   Unspecified acute conjunctivitis, unspecified eye
  - H10.31   Unspecified acute conjunctivitis, right eye
  - H10.32   Unspecified acute conjunctivitis, left eye
  - H10.33   Unspecified acute conjunctivitis, bilateral
- H10.4   Chronic conjunctivitis
  - H10.40   Unspecified chronic conjunctivitis
    - H10.401   Unspecified chronic conjunctivitis, right eye
    - H10.402   Unspecified chronic conjunctivitis, left eye
    - H10.403   Unspecified chronic conjunctivitis, bilateral
    - H10.409   Unspecified chronic conjunctivitis, unspecified eye
  - H10.41   Chronic giant papillary conjunctivitis
    Inflammation of membrane of the inside of the eyelid or on surface of eye often associated with contact lens wear
    - H10.411   Chronic giant papillary conjunctivitis, right eye
    - H10.412   Chronic giant papillary conjunctivitis, left eye
    - H10.413   Chronic giant papillary conjunctivitis, bilateral
    - H10.419   Chronic giant papillary conjunctivitis, unspecified eye
  - H10.42   Simple chronic conjunctivitis
    - H10.421   Simple chronic conjunctivitis, right eye
    - H10.422   Simple chronic conjunctivitis, left eye
    - H10.423   Simple chronic conjunctivitis, bilateral
    - H10.429   Simple chronic conjunctivitis, unspecified eye
  - H10.43   Chronic follicular conjunctivitis
    Inflammation of membrane of the inside of the eyelid or on surface of eye due to topical medications or infection
    - H10.431   Chronic follicular conjunctivitis, right eye
    - H10.432   Chronic follicular conjunctivitis, left eye
    - H10.433   Chronic follicular conjunctivitis, bilateral
    - H10.439   Chronic follicular conjunctivitis, unspecified eye

H10.44   **Vernal conjunctivitis**
Affecting children, especially boys in which there are flattened papules with thick, gelatinous exudate on conjunctivae on inside of upper lid

Excludes1   vernal keratoconjunctivitis with limbar and corneal involvement (H16.26-)

H10.45   **Other chronic allergic conjunctivitis**

H10.5   **Blepharoconjunctivitis**
Inflammation of eyelids and conjunctiva

H10.50   **Unspecified blepharoconjunctivitis**

H10.501   Unspecified blepharoconjunctivitis, right eye

H10.502   Unspecified blepharoconjunctivitis, left eye

H10.503   Unspecified blepharoconjunctivitis, bilateral

H10.509   Unspecified blepharoconjunctivitis, unspecified eye

H10.51   **Ligneous conjunctivitis**
Code also underlying condition if known, such as:
plasminogen deficiency (E88.02)

H10.511   Ligneous conjunctivitis, right eye

H10.512   Ligneous conjunctivitis, left eye

H10.513   Ligneous conjunctivitis, bilateral

H10.519   Ligneous conjunctivitis, unspecified eye

H10.52   **Angular blepharoconjunctivitis**

H10.521   Angular blepharoconjunctivitis, right eye

H10.522   Angular blepharoconjunctivitis, left eye

H10.523   Angular blepharoconjunctivitis, bilateral

H10.529   Angular blepharoconjunctivitis, unspecified eye

H10.53   **Contact blepharoconjunctivitis**

H10.531   Contact blepharoconjunctivitis, right eye

H10.532   Contact blepharoconjunctivitis, left eye

H10.533   Contact blepharoconjunctivitis, bilateral

H10.539   Contact blepharoconjunctivitis, unspecified eye

H10.8   **Other conjunctivitis**

H10.81   **Pingueculitis**
Inflammation of a yellow, raised thickening on the white of the eye associated with chronic dry eyes

Excludes1   pinguecula (H11.15-)

H10.811   Pingueculitis, right eye

H10.812   Pingueculitis, left eye

H10.813   Pingueculitis, bilateral

H10.819   Pingueculitis, unspecified eye

H10.82   **Rosacea conjunctivitis**
Code first underlying rosacea dermatitis (L71.-)

H10.821   Rosacea conjunctivitis, right eye

H10.822   Rosacea conjunctivitis, left eye

H10.823   Rosacea conjunctivitis, bilateral
Coding Clinic: 2018, Q4, P15

H10.829   Rosacea conjunctivitis, unspecified eye

H10.89   **Other conjunctivitis**

H10.9   **Unspecified conjunctivitis**

Figure 7-6   Double pterygium. Note both nasal and temporal pterygia in a 57-year-old farmer. (From Brightbill FS, McDonnell PJ: Corneal Surgery: Theory, Technique and Tissue, S.l., Mosby Elsevier, 2009)

Item 7–2   Pterygium is Greek for batlike. The condition is characterized by a membrane that extends from the limbus to the center of the cornea and resembles a wing.

H11   **Other disorders of conjunctiva**

Excludes1   keratoconjunctivitis (H16.2-)

H11.0   **Pterygium of eye**

Excludes1   pseudopterygium (H11.81-)

H11.00   **Unspecified pterygium of eye**

H11.001   Unspecified pterygium of right eye

H11.002   Unspecified pterygium of left eye

H11.003   Unspecified pterygium of eye, bilateral

H11.009   Unspecified pterygium of unspecified eye

H11.01   **Amyloid pterygium**

H11.011   Amyloid pterygium of right eye

H11.012   Amyloid pterygium of left eye

H11.013   Amyloid pterygium of eye, bilateral

H11.019   Amyloid pterygium of unspecified eye

H11.02   **Central pterygium of eye**

H11.021   Central pterygium of right eye

H11.022   Central pterygium of left eye

H11.023   Central pterygium of eye, bilateral

H11.029   Central pterygium of unspecified eye

H11.03   **Double pterygium of eye**

H11.031   Double pterygium of right eye

H11.032   Double pterygium of left eye

H11.033   Double pterygium of eye, bilateral

H11.039   Double pterygium of unspecified eye

H11.04   **Peripheral pterygium of eye, stationary**

H11.041   Peripheral pterygium, stationary, right eye

H11.042   Peripheral pterygium, stationary, left eye

H11.043   Peripheral pterygium, stationary, bilateral

H11.049   Peripheral pterygium, stationary, unspecified eye

H11.05   **Peripheral pterygium of eye, progressive**

H11.051   Peripheral pterygium, progressive, right eye

H11.052   Peripheral pterygium, progressive, left eye

H11.053   Peripheral pterygium, progressive, bilateral

H11.059   Peripheral pterygium, progressive, unspecified eye

H11.06   **Recurrent pterygium of eye**

H11.061   Recurrent pterygium of right eye

H11.062   Recurrent pterygium of left eye

H11.063   Recurrent pterygium of eye, bilateral

H11.069   Recurrent pterygium of unspecified eye

H11.1   **Conjunctival degenerations and deposits**

Excludes2   pseudopterygium (H11.81)

H11.10   **Unspecified conjunctival degenerations**

H11.11   **Conjunctival deposits**

H11.111   Conjunctival deposits, right eye

H11.112   Conjunctival deposits, left eye

H11.113   Conjunctival deposits, bilateral

H11.119   Conjunctival deposits, unspecified eye

● H11.12   Conjunctival concretions
White to yellow nodules within or beneath conjunctiva
    H11.121   Conjunctival concretions, right eye
    H11.122   Conjunctival concretions, left eye
    H11.123   Conjunctival concretions, bilateral
    H11.129   Conjunctival concretions, unspecified eye

● H11.13   Conjunctival pigmentations
Conjunctival argyrosis [argyria]
    H11.131   Conjunctival pigmentations, right eye
    H11.132   Conjunctival pigmentations, left eye
    H11.133   Conjunctival pigmentations, bilateral
    H11.139   Conjunctival pigmentations, unspecified eye

● H11.14   Conjunctival xerosis, unspecified
    Excludes1   xerosis of conjunctiva due to vitamin A deficiency (E50.0, E50.1)
    H11.141   Conjunctival xerosis, unspecified, right eye
    H11.142   Conjunctival xerosis, unspecified, left eye
    H11.143   Conjunctival xerosis, unspecified, bilateral
    H11.149   Conjunctival xerosis, unspecified, unspecified eye

● H11.15   Pinguecula
Yellowish spot near sclerocorneal junction, usually on nasal side; associated with aging
    Excludes1   pingueculitis (H10.81-)
    H11.151   Pinguecula, right eye
    H11.152   Pinguecula, left eye
    H11.153   Pinguecula, bilateral
    H11.159   Pinguecula, unspecified eye

● H11.2   Conjunctival scars
● H11.21   Conjunctival adhesions and strands (localized)
    H11.211   Conjunctival adhesions and strands (localized), right eye
    H11.212   Conjunctival adhesions and strands (localized), left eye
    H11.213   Conjunctival adhesions and strands (localized), bilateral
    H11.219   Conjunctival adhesions and strands (localized), unspecified eye

● H11.22   Conjunctival granuloma
    H11.221   Conjunctival granuloma, right eye
    H11.222   Conjunctival granuloma, left eye
    H11.223   Conjunctival granuloma, bilateral
    H11.229   Conjunctival granuloma, unspecified

● H11.23   Symblepharon
Adhesion between tarsal conjunctiva and bulbar conjunctiva
    H11.231   Symblepharon, right eye
    H11.232   Symblepharon, left eye
    H11.233   Symblepharon, bilateral
    H11.239   Symblepharon, unspecified eye

● H11.24   Scarring of conjunctiva
    H11.241   Scarring of conjunctiva, right eye
    H11.242   Scarring of conjunctiva, left eye
    H11.243   Scarring of conjunctiva, bilateral
    H11.249   Scarring of conjunctiva, unspecified eye

● H11.3   Conjunctival hemorrhage
Subconjunctival hemorrhage
    H11.30   Conjunctival hemorrhage, unspecified eye
    H11.31   Conjunctival hemorrhage, right eye

    H11.32   Conjunctival hemorrhage, left eye
    H11.33   Conjunctival hemorrhage, bilateral

● H11.4   Other conjunctival vascular disorders and cysts
● H11.41   Vascular abnormalities of conjunctiva
Conjunctival aneurysm
    H11.411   Vascular abnormalities of conjunctiva, right eye
    H11.412   Vascular abnormalities of conjunctiva, left eye
    H11.413   Vascular abnormalities of conjunctiva, bilateral
    H11.419   Vascular abnormalities of conjunctiva, unspecified eye

● H11.42   Conjunctival edema
    H11.421   Conjunctival edema, right eye
    H11.422   Conjunctival edema, left eye
    H11.423   Conjunctival edema, bilateral
    H11.429   Conjunctival edema, unspecified eye

● H11.43   Conjunctival hyperemia
    H11.431   Conjunctival hyperemia, right eye
    H11.432   Conjunctival hyperemia, left eye
    H11.433   Conjunctival hyperemia, bilateral
    H11.439   Conjunctival hyperemia, unspecified eye

● H11.44   Conjunctival cysts
    H11.441   Conjunctival cysts, right eye
    H11.442   Conjunctival cysts, left eye
    H11.443   Conjunctival cysts, bilateral
    H11.449   Conjunctival cysts, unspecified eye

● H11.8   Other specified disorders of conjunctiva
● H11.81   Pseudopterygium of conjunctiva
Conjunctival scar attached to cornea
    H11.811   Pseudopterygium of conjunctiva, right eye
    H11.812   Pseudopterygium of conjunctiva, left eye
    H11.813   Pseudopterygium of conjunctiva, bilateral
    H11.819   Pseudopterygium of conjunctiva, unspecified eye

● H11.82   Conjunctivochalasis
Conjunctiva bulges over eyelid margin or covers lower punctum
    H11.821   Conjunctivochalasis, right eye
    H11.822   Conjunctivochalasis, left eye
    H11.823   Conjunctivochalasis, bilateral
    H11.829   Conjunctivochalasis, unspecified eye

    H11.89   Other specified disorders of conjunctiva
H11.9   Unspecified disorder of conjunctiva

DISORDERS OF SCLERA, CORNEA, IRIS AND CILIARY BODY (H15-H22)

● H15   Disorders of sclera
● H15.0   Scleritis
Inflammation of the white (sclera and episclera) of the eye.
● H15.00   Unspecified scleritis
    H15.001   Unspecified scleritis, right eye
    H15.002   Unspecified scleritis, left eye
    H15.003   Unspecified scleritis, bilateral
    H15.009   Unspecified scleritis, unspecified eye

● H15.01   Anterior scleritis
    H15.011   Anterior scleritis, right eye
    H15.012   Anterior scleritis, left eye
    H15.013   Anterior scleritis, bilateral
    H15.019   Anterior scleritis, unspecified eye

▶ New   ⟹ Revised   ~~deleted~~ Deleted   Excludes 1   Excludes 2   Includes   Use additional   Code first   Code also   Key words
OGCR Official Guidelines   X Assign placeholder X   ● Use Additional Character(s)   ⟩ Manifestation Code   🅗 Hierarchical Condition Category   Coding Clinic

● **H15.02** Brawny scleritis
   *Swelling around the cornea that is gelantinous in
   appearance*
   H15.021   Brawny scleritis, **right eye**
   H15.022   Brawny scleritis, **left eye**
   H15.023   Brawny scleritis, **bilateral**
   H15.029   Brawny scleritis, **unspecified** eye
● **H15.03** Posterior scleritis
   Sclerotenonitis
   H15.031   Posterior scleritis, **right eye**
   H15.032   Posterior scleritis, **left eye**
   H15.033   Posterior scleritis, **bilateral**
   H15.039   Posterior scleritis, **unspecified** eye
● **H15.04** Scleritis with corneal involvement
   H15.041   Scleritis with corneal involvement,
             right eye
   H15.042   Scleritis with corneal involvement,
             left eye
   H15.043   Scleritis with corneal involvement,
             bilateral
   H15.049   Scleritis with corneal involvement,
             unspecified eye
● **H15.05** Scleromalacia perforans
   *Necrotic without inflammation; usually associated
   with rheumatoid arthritis*
   H15.051   Scleromalacia perforans, **right eye**
   H15.052   Scleromalacia perforans, **left eye**
   H15.053   Scleromalacia perforans, **bilateral**
   H15.059   Scleromalacia perforans, **unspecified**
             eye
● **H15.09** Other scleritis
   Scleral abscess
   H15.091   Other scleritis, **right eye**
   H15.092   Other scleritis, **left eye**
   H15.093   Other scleritis, **bilateral**
   H15.099   Other scleritis, **unspecified** eye
● **H15.1** Episcleritis
   Inflammation of the white (sclera and episclera) of the eye.
   ● **H15.10** Unspecified episcleritis
      H15.101   Unspecified episcleritis, **right eye**
      H15.102   Unspecified episcleritis, **left eye**
      H15.103   Unspecified episcleritis, **bilateral**
      H15.109   Unspecified episcleritis, **unspecified**
                eye
   ● **H15.11** Episcleritis periodica fugax
      *Transient, recurrent inflammation of portion of
      episclera (connective tissue on the surface of
      the sclera)*
      H15.111   Episcleritis periodica fugax, **right eye**
      H15.112   Episcleritis periodica fugax, **left eye**
      H15.113   Episcleritis periodica fugax, **bilateral**
      H15.119   Episcleritis periodica fugax,
                unspecified eye
   ● **H15.12** Nodular episcleritis
      *Characterized by tender, localized, moveable nodule
      within inflamed area*
      H15.121   Nodular episcleritis, **right eye**
      H15.122   Nodular episcleritis, **left eye**
      H15.123   Nodular episcleritis, **bilateral**
      H15.129   Nodular episcleritis, **unspecified** eye
● **H15.8** Other disorders of sclera
   Excludes2   blue sclera (Q13.5)
                   degenerative myopia (H44.2-)
   ● **H15.81** Equatorial staphyloma
      H15.811   Equatorial staphyloma, **right eye**
      H15.812   Equatorial staphyloma, **left eye**
      H15.813   Equatorial staphyloma, **bilateral**
      H15.819   Equatorial staphyloma, **unspecified eye**

● **H15.82** Localized anterior staphyloma
      H15.821   Localized anterior staphyloma, **right
                eye**
      H15.822   Localized anterior staphyloma, **left eye**
      H15.823   Localized anterior staphyloma,
                bilateral
      H15.829   Localized anterior staphyloma,
                unspecified eye
● **H15.83** Staphyloma posticum
      H15.831   Staphyloma posticum, **right eye**
      H15.832   Staphyloma posticum, **left eye**
      H15.833   Staphyloma posticum, **bilateral**
      H15.839   Staphyloma posticum, **unspecified** eye
● **H15.84** Scleral ectasia
      H15.841   Scleral ectasia, **right eye**
      H15.842   Scleral ectasia, **left eye**
      H15.843   Scleral ectasia, **bilateral**
      H15.849   Scleral ectasia, **unspecified** eye
● **H15.85** Ring staphyloma
      H15.851   Ring staphyloma, **right eye**
      H15.852   Ring staphyloma, **left eye**
      H15.853   Ring staphyloma, **bilateral**
      H15.859   Ring staphyloma, **unspecified** eye
   H15.89   Other disorders of sclera
H15.9   Unspecified disorder of sclera
● **H16** Keratitis
   ● **H16.0** Corneal ulcer
      ● **H16.00** Unspecified corneal ulcer
         H16.001   Unspecified corneal ulcer, **right eye**
         H16.002   Unspecified corneal ulcer, **left eye**
         H16.003   Unspecified corneal ulcer, **bilateral**
         H16.009   Unspecified corneal ulcer, **unspecified**
                   eye
      ● **H16.01** Central corneal ulcer
         H16.011   Central corneal ulcer, **right eye**
         H16.012   Central corneal ulcer, **left eye**
         H16.013   Central corneal ulcer, **bilateral**
         H16.019   Central corneal ulcer, **unspecified eye**
      ● **H16.02** Ring corneal ulcer
         H16.021   Ring corneal ulcer, **right eye**
         H16.022   Ring corneal ulcer, **left eye**
         H16.023   Ring corneal ulcer, **bilateral**
         H16.029   Ring corneal ulcer, **unspecified eye**
      ● **H16.03** Corneal ulcer with hypopyon
         H16.031   Corneal ulcer with hypopyon, **right
                   eye**
         H16.032   Corneal ulcer with hypopyon, **left eye**

Marginal | Ring | Central | Rosacea | Mooren's
(catarrhal) ulcer | ulcer | corneal ulcer | ulcer | (rodent) ulcer

Figure 7-7 Corneal ulcers: marginal, ring, central corneal, rosacea, and
Mooren's.

Item 7–3 An infected ulcer is usually called a **serpiginous** or **hypopyon**
ulcer, which is a pus sac in the anterior chamber of the eye. **Marginal** ulcers
are usually asymptomatic, not primary, and are often superficial and simple.
More severe marginal ulcers spread to form a ring ulcer. **Ring** ulcers can
extend around the entire corneal periphery. **Central corneal** ulcers develop
when there is an abrasion to the epithelium and an infection develops in the
eroded area. The **pyocyaneal** ulcer is the most serious corneal infection,
which, if left untreated, can lead to loss of the eye.

CHAPTER 7 (HØØ-H59)

- H16.Ø33   Corneal ulcer with hypopyon, bilateral
- H16.Ø39   Corneal ulcer with hypopyon, unspecified eye
- ● H16.Ø4   Marginal corneal ulcer
  - H16.Ø41   Marginal corneal ulcer, right eye
  - H16.Ø42   Marginal corneal ulcer, left eye
  - H16.Ø43   Marginal corneal ulcer, bilateral
  - H16.Ø49   Marginal corneal ulcer, unspecified eye
- ● H16.Ø5   Mooren's corneal ulcer
  - H16.Ø51   Mooren's corneal ulcer, right eye
  - H16.Ø52   Mooren's corneal ulcer, left eye
  - H16.Ø53   Mooren's corneal ulcer, bilateral
  - H16.Ø59   Mooren's corneal ulcer, unspecified eye
- ● H16.Ø6   Mycotic corneal ulcer
  - H16.Ø61   Mycotic corneal ulcer, right eye
  - H16.Ø62   Mycotic corneal ulcer, left eye
  - H16.Ø63   Mycotic corneal ulcer, bilateral
  - H16.Ø69   Mycotic corneal ulcer, unspecified eye
- ● H16.Ø7   Perforated corneal ulcer
  - H16.Ø71   Perforated corneal ulcer, right eye
  - H16.Ø72   Perforated corneal ulcer, left eye
  - H16.Ø73   Perforated corneal ulcer, bilateral
  - H16.Ø79   Perforated corneal ulcer, unspecified eye
- ● H16.1   Other and unspecified superficial keratitis without conjunctivitis
  - ● H16.1Ø   Unspecified superficial keratitis
    - H16.1Ø1   Unspecified superficial keratitis, right eye
    - H16.1Ø2   Unspecified superficial keratitis, left eye
    - H16.1Ø3   Unspecified superficial keratitis, bilateral
    - H16.1Ø9   Unspecified superficial keratitis, unspecified eye
  - ● H16.11   Macular keratitis
    - Areolar keratitis
    - Nummular keratitis
    - Stellate keratitis
    - Striate keratitis
    - H16.111   Macular keratitis, right eye
    - H16.112   Macular keratitis, left eye
    - H16.113   Macular keratitis, bilateral
    - H16.119   Macular keratitis, unspecified eye
  - ● H16.12   Filamentary keratitis
    - H16.121   Filamentary keratitis, right eye
    - H16.122   Filamentary keratitis, left eye
    - H16.123   Filamentary keratitis, bilateral
    - H16.129   Filamentary keratitis, unspecified eye
  - ● H16.13   Photokeratitis
    - Snow blindness
    - Welders' keratitis
    - H16.131   Photokeratitis, right eye
    - H16.132   Photokeratitis, left eye
    - H16.133   Photokeratitis, bilateral
    - H16.139   Photokeratitis, unspecified eye
  - ● H16.14   Punctate keratitis
    - H16.141   Punctate keratitis, right eye
    - H16.142   Punctate keratitis, left eye
    - H16.143   Punctate keratitis, bilateral
    - H16.149   Punctate keratitis, unspecified eye

- ● H16.2   Keratoconjunctivitis
  - ● H16.2Ø   Unspecified keratoconjunctivitis
    - Superficial keratitis with conjunctivitis NOS
    - H16.2Ø1   Unspecified keratoconjunctivitis, right eye
    - H16.2Ø2   Unspecified keratoconjunctivitis, left eye
    - H16.2Ø3   Unspecified keratoconjunctivitis, bilateral
    - H16.2Ø9   Unspecified keratoconjunctivitis, unspecified eye
  - ● H16.21   Exposure keratoconjunctivitis
    - H16.211   Exposure keratoconjunctivitis, right eye
    - H16.212   Exposure keratoconjunctivitis, left eye
    - H16.213   Exposure keratoconjunctivitis, bilateral
    - H16.219   Exposure keratoconjunctivitis, unspecified eye
  - ● H16.22   Keratoconjunctivitis sicca, not specified as Sjögren's
    - **Excludes1**   Sjogren's syndrome (M35.Ø1)
    - H16.221   Keratoconjunctivitis sicca, not specified as Sjögren's, right eye
    - H16.222   Keratoconjunctivitis sicca, not specified as Sjögren's, left eye
    - H16.223   Keratoconjunctivitis sicca, not specified as Sjögren's, bilateral
    - H16.229   Keratoconjunctivitis sicca, not specified as Sjögren's, unspecified eye
  - ● H16.23   Neurotrophic keratoconjunctivitis
    - H16.231   Neurotrophic keratoconjunctivitis, right eye
    - H16.232   Neurotrophic keratoconjunctivitis, left eye
    - H16.233   Neurotrophic keratoconjunctivitis, bilateral
    - H16.239   Neurotrophic keratoconjunctivitis, unspecified eye
  - ● H16.24   Ophthalmia nodosa
    - H16.241   Ophthalmia nodosa, right eye
    - H16.242   Ophthalmia nodosa, left eye
    - H16.243   Ophthalmia nodosa, bilateral
    - H16.249   Ophthalmia nodosa, unspecified eye
  - ● H16.25   Phlyctenular keratoconjunctivitis
    - H16.251   Phlyctenular keratoconjunctivitis, right eye
    - H16.252   Phlyctenular keratoconjunctivitis, left eye
    - H16.253   Phlyctenular keratoconjunctivitis, bilateral
    - H16.259   Phlyctenular keratoconjunctivitis, unspecified eye
  - ● H16.26   Vernal keratoconjunctivitis, with limbar and corneal involvement
    - **Excludes1**   vernal conjunctivitis without limbar and corneal involvement (H1Ø.44)
    - H16.261   Vernal keratoconjunctivitis, with limbar and corneal involvement, right eye
    - H16.262   Vernal keratoconjunctivitis, with limbar and corneal involvement, left eye

---

▶ New   ▣ Revised   ~~deleted~~ Deleted   Excludes 1   Excludes 2   Includes   Use additional   Code first   Code also   Key words

OGCR Official Guidelines   X Assign placeholder X   ● Use Additional Character(s)   ▌ Manifestation Code   🦘 Hierarchical Condition Category   Coding Clinic

H16.263   Vernal keratoconjunctivitis, with limbar and corneal involvement, bilateral

H16.269   Vernal keratoconjunctivitis, with limbar and corneal involvement, unspecified eye

● H16.29   Other keratoconjunctivitis

     H16.291   Other keratoconjunctivitis, right eye

     H16.292   Other keratoconjunctivitis, left eye

     H16.293   Other keratoconjunctivitis, bilateral

     H16.299   Other keratoconjunctivitis, unspecified eye

● H16.3   Interstitial and deep keratitis

   ● H16.30   Unspecified interstitial keratitis

     H16.301   Unspecified interstitial keratitis, right eye

     H16.302   Unspecified interstitial keratitis, left eye

     H16.303   Unspecified interstitial keratitis, bilateral

     H16.309   Unspecified interstitial keratitis, unspecified eye

   ● H16.31   Corneal abscess

     H16.311   Corneal abscess, right eye

     H16.312   Corneal abscess, left eye

     H16.313   Corneal abscess, bilateral

     H16.319   Corneal abscess, unspecified eye

   ● H16.32   Diffuse interstitial keratitis

      Cogan's syndrome

     H16.321   Diffuse interstitial keratitis, right eye

     H16.322   Diffuse interstitial keratitis, left eye

     H16.323   Diffuse interstitial keratitis, bilateral

     H16.329   Diffuse interstitial keratitis, unspecified eye

   ● H16.33   Sclerosing keratitis

     H16.331   Sclerosing keratitis, right eye

     H16.332   Sclerosing keratitis, left eye

     H16.333   Sclerosing keratitis, bilateral

     H16.339   Sclerosing keratitis, unspecified eye

   ● H16.39   Other interstitial and deep keratitis

     H16.391   Other interstitial and deep keratitis, right eye

     H16.392   Other interstitial and deep keratitis, left eye

     H16.393   Other interstitial and deep keratitis, bilateral

     H16.399   Other interstitial and deep keratitis, unspecified eye

● H16.4   Corneal neovascularization

   ● H16.40   Unspecified corneal neovascularization

     H16.401   Unspecified corneal neovascularization, right eye

     H16.402   Unspecified corneal neovascularization, left eye

     H16.403   Unspecified corneal neovascularization, bilateral

     H16.409   Unspecified corneal neovascularization, unspecified eye

   ● H16.41   Ghost vessels (corneal)

     H16.411   Ghost vessels (corneal), right eye

     H16.412   Ghost vessels (corneal), left eye

     H16.413   Ghost vessels (corneal), bilateral

     H16.419   Ghost vessels (corneal), unspecified eye

   ● H16.42   Pannus (corneal)

     H16.421   Pannus (corneal), right eye

     H16.422   Pannus (corneal), left eye

H16.423   Pannus (corneal), bilateral

H16.429   Pannus (corneal), unspecified eye

● H16.43   Localized vascularization of cornea

     H16.431   Localized vascularization of cornea, right eye

     H16.432   Localized vascularization of cornea, left eye

     H16.433   Localized vascularization of cornea, bilateral

     H16.439   Localized vascularization of cornea, unspecified eye

● H16.44   Deep vascularization of cornea

     H16.441   Deep vascularization of cornea, right eye

     H16.442   Deep vascularization of cornea, left eye

     H16.443   Deep vascularization of cornea, bilateral

     H16.449   Deep vascularization of cornea, unspecified eye

H16.8   Other keratitis

H16.9   Unspecified keratitis

● H17   Corneal scars and opacities

   ● H17.0   Adherent leukoma

     H17.00   Adherent leukoma, unspecified eye

     H17.01   Adherent leukoma, right eye

     H17.02   Adherent leukoma, left eye

     H17.03   Adherent leukoma, bilateral

   ● H17.1   Central corneal opacity

     H17.10   Central corneal opacity, unspecified eye

     H17.11   Central corneal opacity, right eye

     H17.12   Central corneal opacity, left eye

     H17.13   Central corneal opacity, bilateral

   ● H17.8   Other corneal scars and opacities

     ● H17.81   Minor opacity of cornea

       Corneal nebula

      H17.811   Minor opacity of cornea, right eye

      H17.812   Minor opacity of cornea, left eye

      H17.813   Minor opacity of cornea, bilateral

      H17.819   Minor opacity of cornea, unspecified eye

     ● H17.82   Peripheral opacity of cornea

      H17.821   Peripheral opacity of cornea, right eye

      H17.822   Peripheral opacity of cornea, left eye

      H17.823   Peripheral opacity of cornea, bilateral

      H17.829   Peripheral opacity of cornea, unspecified eye

     H17.89   Other corneal scars and opacities

   H17.9   Unspecified corneal scar and opacity

● H18   Other disorders of cornea

   ● H18.0   Corneal pigmentations and deposits

     ● H18.00   Unspecified corneal deposit

      H18.001   Unspecified corneal deposit, right eye

      H18.002   Unspecified corneal deposit, left eye

      H18.003   Unspecified corneal deposit, bilateral

      H18.009   Unspecified corneal deposit, unspecified eye

     ● H18.01   Anterior corneal pigmentations

       Staehli's line

      H18.011   Anterior corneal pigmentations, right eye

      H18.012   Anterior corneal pigmentations, left eye

      H18.013   Anterior corneal pigmentations, bilateral

      H18.019   Anterior corneal pigmentations, unspecified eye

CHAPTER 7 (H00–H59)

● H18.02   **Argentous corneal deposits**
     H18.021   **Argentous corneal deposits, right eye**
     H18.022   **Argentous corneal deposits, left eye**
     H18.023   **Argentous corneal deposits, bilateral**
     H18.029   **Argentous corneal deposits, unspecified eye**

● H18.03   **Corneal deposits in metabolic disorders**
     Code also associated metabolic disorder
     H18.031   **Corneal deposits in metabolic disorders, right eye**
     H18.032   **Corneal deposits in metabolic disorders, left eye**
     H18.033   **Corneal deposits in metabolic disorders, bilateral**
     H18.039   **Corneal deposits in metabolic disorders, unspecified eye**

● H18.04   **Kayser-Fleischer ring**
     Code also associated Wilson's disease (E83.01)
     H18.041   **Kayser-Fleischer ring, right eye**
     H18.042   **Kayser-Fleischer ring, left eye**
     H18.043   **Kayser-Fleischer ring, bilateral**
     H18.049   **Kayser-Fleischer ring, unspecified eye**

● H18.05   **Posterior corneal pigmentations**
     Krukenberg's spindle
     H18.051   **Posterior corneal pigmentations, right eye**
     H18.052   **Posterior corneal pigmentations, left eye**
     H18.053   **Posterior corneal pigmentations, bilateral**
     H18.059   **Posterior corneal pigmentations, unspecified eye**

● H18.06   **Stromal corneal pigmentations**
     Hematocornea
     H18.061   **Stromal corneal pigmentations, right eye**
     H18.062   **Stromal corneal pigmentations, left eye**
     H18.063   **Stromal corneal pigmentations, bilateral**
     H18.069   **Stromal corneal pigmentations, unspecified eye**

● H18.1   **Bullous keratopathy**
     H18.10   **Bullous keratopathy, unspecified eye**
     H18.11   **Bullous keratopathy, right eye**
     H18.12   **Bullous keratopathy, left eye**
     H18.13   **Bullous keratopathy, bilateral**

● H18.2   **Other and unspecified corneal edema**
     H18.20   **Unspecified corneal edema**
     ● H18.21   **Corneal edema secondary to contact lens**
         Excludes2   other corneal disorders due to contact lens (H18.82-)
         H18.211   **Corneal edema secondary to contact lens, right eye**
         H18.212   **Corneal edema secondary to contact lens, left eye**
         H18.213   **Corneal edema secondary to contact lens, bilateral**
         H18.219   **Corneal edema secondary to contact lens, unspecified eye**
     ● H18.22   **Idiopathic corneal edema**
         H18.221   **Idiopathic corneal edema, right eye**
         H18.222   **Idiopathic corneal edema, left eye**
         H18.223   **Idiopathic corneal edema, bilateral**
         H18.229   **Idiopathic corneal edema, unspecified eye**

● H18.23   **Secondary corneal edema**
     H18.231   **Secondary corneal edema, right eye**
     H18.232   **Secondary corneal edema, left eye**
     H18.233   **Secondary corneal edema, bilateral**
     H18.239   **Secondary corneal edema, unspecified eye**

● H18.3   **Changes of corneal membranes**
     H18.30   **Unspecified corneal membrane change**
     ● H18.31   **Folds and rupture in Bowman's membrane**
         H18.311   **Folds and rupture in Bowman's membrane, right eye**
         H18.312   **Folds and rupture in Bowman's membrane, left eye**
         H18.313   **Folds and rupture in Bowman's membrane, bilateral**
         H18.319   **Folds and rupture in Bowman's membrane, unspecified eye**
     ● H18.32   **Folds in Descemet's membrane**
         H18.321   **Folds in Descemet's membrane, right eye**
         H18.322   **Folds in Descemet's membrane, left eye**
         H18.323   **Folds in Descemet's membrane, bilateral**
         H18.329   **Folds in Descemet's membrane, unspecified eye**
     ● H18.33   **Rupture in Descemet's membrane**
         H18.331   **Rupture in Descemet's membrane, right eye**
         H18.332   **Rupture in Descemet's membrane, left eye**
         H18.333   **Rupture in Descemet's membrane, bilateral**
         H18.339   **Rupture in Descemet's membrane, unspecified eye**

● H18.4   **Corneal degeneration**
     Excludes1   Mooren's ulcer (H16.0-)
                 recurrent erosion of cornea (H18.83-)
     H18.40   **Unspecified corneal degeneration**
     ● H18.41   **Arcus senilis**
         Senile corneal changes
         H18.411   **Arcus senilis, right eye**
         H18.412   **Arcus senilis, left eye**
         H18.413   **Arcus senilis, bilateral**
         H18.419   **Arcus senilis, unspecified eye**
     ● H18.42   **Band keratopathy**
         H18.421   **Band keratopathy, right eye**
         H18.422   **Band keratopathy, left eye**
         H18.423   **Band keratopathy, bilateral**
         H18.429   **Band keratopathy, unspecified eye**
     H18.43   **Other calcerous corneal degeneration**
     ● H18.44   **Keratomalacia**
         Excludes1   keratomalacia due to vitamin A deficiency (E50.4)
         H18.441   **Keratomalacia, right eye**
         H18.442   **Keratomalacia, left eye**
         H18.443   **Keratomalacia, bilateral**
         H18.449   **Keratomalacia, unspecified eye**
     ● H18.45   **Nodular corneal degeneration**
         H18.451   **Nodular corneal degeneration, right eye**
         H18.452   **Nodular corneal degeneration, left eye**
         H18.453   **Nodular corneal degeneration, bilateral**
         H18.459   **Nodular corneal degeneration, unspecified eye**

▶ New   ⇒ Revised   ~~deleted~~ Deleted   Excludes 1   Excludes 2   Includes   Use additional   Code first   Code also   Key words

OGCR Official Guidelines   X Assign placeholder X   ● Use Additional Character(s)   ▶ Manifestation Code   ❤ Hierarchical Condition Category   Coding Clinic

- **H18.46 Peripheral** corneal degeneration
  - H18.461 Peripheral corneal degeneration, **right** eye
  - H18.462 Peripheral corneal degeneration, **left** eye
  - H18.463 Peripheral corneal degeneration, **bilateral**
  - H18.469 Peripheral corneal degeneration, **unspecified eye**
  - H18.49 Other corneal degeneration
- **H18.5 Hereditary** corneal dystrophies
  - **H18.50 Unspecified** hereditary corneal dystrophies
    - H18.501 Unspecified hereditary corneal dystrophies, right eye
    - H18.502 Unspecified hereditary corneal dystrophies, left eye
    - H18.503 Unspecified hereditary corneal dystrophies, bilateral
    - H18.509 Unspecified hereditary corneal dystrophies, unspecified eye
  - **H18.51 Endothelial** corneal dystrophy
    Fuchs' dystrophy
    - H18.511 Endothelial corneal dystrophy, right eye
    - H18.512 Endothelial corneal dystrophy, left eye
    - H18.513 Endothelial corneal dystrophy, bilateral
    - H18.519 Endothelial corneal dystrophy, unspecified eye
  - **H18.52 Epithelial** (juvenile) corneal dystrophy
    - H18.521 Epithelial (juvenile) corneal dystrophy, right eye
    - H18.522 Epithelial (juvenile) corneal dystrophy, left eye
    - H18.523 Epithelial (juvenile) corneal dystrophy, bilateral
    - H18.529 Epithelial (juvenile) corneal dystrophy, unspecified eye
  - **H18.53 Granular** corneal dystrophy
    - H18.531 Granular corneal dystrophy, right eye
    - H18.532 Granular corneal dystrophy, left eye
    - H18.533 Granular corneal dystrophy, bilateral
    - H18.539 Granular corneal dystrophy, unspecified eye
  - **H18.54 Lattice** corneal dystrophy
    - H18.541 Lattice corneal dystrophy, right eye
    - H18.542 Lattice corneal dystrophy, left eye
    - H18.543 Lattice corneal dystrophy, bilateral
    - H18.549 Lattice corneal dystrophy, unspecified eye
  - **H18.55 Macular** corneal dystrophy
    - H18.551 Macular corneal dystrophy, right eye
    - H18.552 Macular corneal dystrophy, left eye
    - H18.553 Macular corneal dystrophy, bilateral
    - H18.559 Macular corneal dystrophy, unspecified eye
  - **H18.59 Other** hereditary corneal dystrophies
    - H18.591 Other hereditary corneal dystrophies, right eye
    - H18.592 Other hereditary corneal dystrophies, left eye
    - H18.593 Other hereditary corneal dystrophies, bilateral
    - H18.599 Other hereditary corneal dystrophies, unspecified eye

Figure 7-8 *Lateral view of the displacement of the cone apex in keratoconus. (From Yanoff: Ophthalmology, ed 3, Mosby, Inc., 2008)*

Item 7–4 Keratoconus results in corneal degeneration that begins in childhood, gradually changes the cornea from a round to cone shape, decreasing visual acuity. Treatment includes contact lenses. In severe cases the need for corneal transplant may be the treatment of choice; however, newer technologies may use high-frequency radio energy to shrink the edges of the cornea, pulling the central area back to a more normal shape. It can help delay or avoid the need for a corneal transplantation.

- **H18.6 Keratoconus**
  - **H18.60 Keratoconus, unspecified**
    - H18.601 Keratoconus, unspecified, **right eye**
    - H18.602 Keratoconus, unspecified, **left eye**
    - H18.603 Keratoconus, unspecified, **bilateral**
    - H18.609 Keratoconus, unspecified, **unspecified eye**
  - **H18.61 Keratoconus, stable**
    - H18.611 Keratoconus, stable, **right eye**
    - H18.612 Keratoconus, stable, **left eye**
    - H18.613 Keratoconus, stable, **bilateral**
    - H18.619 Keratoconus, stable, **unspecified eye**
  - **H18.62 Keratoconus, unstable**
    Acute hydrops
    - H18.621 Keratoconus, unstable, **right eye**
    - H18.622 Keratoconus, unstable, **left eye**
    - H18.623 Keratoconus, unstable, **bilateral**
    - H18.629 Keratoconus, unstable, **unspecified eye**
- **H18.7 Other and unspecified corneal deformities**
  - **Excludes1**   congenital malformations of cornea (Q13.3-Q13.4)
  - H18.70 **Unspecified corneal deformity**
  - **H18.71 Corneal ectasia**
    - H18.711 Corneal ectasia, **right eye**
    - H18.712 Corneal ectasia, **left eye**
    - H18.713 Corneal ectasia, **bilateral**
    - H18.719 Corneal ectasia, **unspecified eye**
  - **H18.72 Corneal staphyloma**
    - H18.721 Corneal staphyloma, **right eye**
    - H18.722 Corneal staphyloma, **left eye**
    - H18.723 Corneal staphyloma, **bilateral**
    - H18.729 Corneal staphyloma, **unspecified eye**
  - **H18.73 Descemetocele**
    - H18.731 Descemetocele, **right eye**
    - H18.732 Descemetocele, **left eye**
    - H18.733 Descemetocele, **bilateral**
    - H18.739 Descemetocele, **unspecified eye**
  - **H18.79 Other corneal deformities**
    - H18.791 Other corneal deformities, **right eye**
    - H18.792 Other corneal deformities, **left eye**
    - H18.793 Other corneal deformities, **bilateral**
    - H18.799 Other corneal deformities, **unspecified eye**
- **H18.8 Other specified disorders of cornea**
  - **H18.81 Anesthesia and hypoesthesia of cornea**
    - H18.811 Anesthesia and hypoesthesia of cornea, **right eye**
    - H18.812 Anesthesia and hypoesthesia of cornea, **left eye**
    - H18.813 Anesthesia and hypoesthesia of cornea, **bilateral**
    - H18.819 Anesthesia and hypoesthesia of cornea, **unspecified eye**

CHAPTER 7 (H00-H59)

● **H18.82 Corneal disorder due to contact lens**

    Excludes2 corneal edema due to contact lens (H18.21-)

    H18.821 Corneal disorder due to contact lens, right eye

    H18.822 Corneal disorder due to contact lens, left eye

    H18.823 Corneal disorder due to contact lens, bilateral

    H18.829 Corneal disorder due to contact lens, unspecified eye

● **H18.83 Recurrent erosion of cornea**

    H18.831 Recurrent erosion of cornea, right eye

    H18.832 Recurrent erosion of cornea, left eye

    H18.833 Recurrent erosion of cornea, bilateral

    H18.839 Recurrent erosion of cornea, unspecified eye

● **H18.89 Other specified disorders of cornea**

    H18.891 Other specified disorders of cornea, right eye

    H18.892 Other specified disorders of cornea, left eye

    H18.893 Other specified disorders of cornea, bilateral

    H18.899 Other specified disorders of cornea, unspecified eye

H18.9 Unspecified disorder of cornea

● **H20 Iridocyclitis**

● **H20.0 Acute and subacute iridocyclitis**

    Acute anterior uveitis
    Acute cyclitis
    Acute iritis
    Subacute anterior uveitis
    Subacute cyclitis
    Subacute iritis

    Excludes1 iridocyclitis, iritis, uveitis (due to) (in) diabetes mellitus (E08-E13 with .39)
    iridocyclitis, iritis, uveitis (due to) (in) diphtheria (A36.89)
    iridocyclitis, iritis, uveitis (due to) (in) gonococcal (A54.32)
    iridocyclitis, iritis, uveitis (due to) (in) herpes (simplex) (B00.51)
    iridocyclitis, iritis, uveitis (due to) (in) herpes zoster (B02.32)
    iridocyclitis, iritis, uveitis (due to) (in) late congenital syphilis (A50.39)
    iridocyclitis, iritis, uveitis (due to) (in) late syphilis (A52.71)
    iridocyclitis, iritis, uveitis (due to) (in) sarcoidosis (D86.83)
    iridocyclitis, iritis, uveitis (due to) (in) syphilis (A51.43)
    iridocyclitis, iritis, uveitis (due to) (in) toxoplasmosis (B58.09)
    iridocyclitis, iritis, uveitis (due to) (in) tuberculosis (A18.54)

    H20.00 Unspecified acute and subacute iridocyclitis

●   H20.01 Primary iridocyclitis

    H20.011 Primary iridocyclitis, right eye

    H20.012 Primary iridocyclitis, left eye

    H20.013 Primary iridocyclitis, bilateral

    H20.019 Primary iridocyclitis, unspecified eye

●   H20.02 Recurrent acute iridocyclitis

    H20.021 Recurrent acute iridocyclitis, right eye

    H20.022 Recurrent acute iridocyclitis, left eye

    H20.023 Recurrent acute iridocyclitis, bilateral

    H20.029 Recurrent acute iridocyclitis, unspecified eye

● **H20.03 Secondary infectious iridocyclitis**

    H20.031 Secondary infectious iridocyclitis, right eye

    H20.032 Secondary infectious iridocyclitis, left eye

    H20.033 Secondary infectious iridocyclitis, bilateral

    H20.039 Secondary infectious iridocyclitis, unspecified eye

● **H20.04 Secondary noninfectious iridocyclitis**

    H20.041 Secondary noninfectious iridocyclitis, right eye

    H20.042 Secondary noninfectious iridocyclitis, left eye

    H20.043 Secondary noninfectious iridocyclitis, bilateral

    H20.049 Secondary noninfectious iridocyclitis, unspecified eye

● **H20.05 Hypopyon**

    H20.051 Hypopyon, right eye

    H20.052 Hypopyon, left eye

    H20.053 Hypopyon, bilateral

    H20.059 Hypopyon, unspecified eye

● **H20.1 Chronic iridocyclitis**

    Use additional code for any associated cataract (H26.21-)

    Excludes2 posterior cyclitis (H30.2-)

    H20.10 Chronic iridocyclitis, unspecified eye

    H20.11 Chronic iridocyclitis, right eye

    H20.12 Chronic iridocyclitis, left eye

    H20.13 Chronic iridocyclitis, bilateral

● **H20.2 Lens-induced iridocyclitis**

    H20.20 Lens-induced iridocyclitis, unspecified eye

    H20.21 Lens-induced iridocyclitis, right eye

    H20.22 Lens-induced iridocyclitis, left eye

    H20.23 Lens-induced iridocyclitis, bilateral

● **H20.8 Other iridocyclitis**

    Excludes2 glaucomatocyclitis crises (H40.4-)
    posterior cyclitis (H30.2-)
    sympathetic uveitis (H44.13-)

●   H20.81 Fuchs' heterochromic cyclitis

    H20.811 Fuchs' heterochromic cyclitis, right eye

    H20.812 Fuchs' heterochromic cyclitis, left eye

    H20.813 Fuchs' heterochromic cyclitis, bilateral

    H20.819 Fuchs' heterochromic cyclitis, unspecified eye

●   H20.82 Vogt-Koyanagi syndrome

    H20.821 Vogt-Koyanagi syndrome, right eye

    H20.822 Vogt-Koyanagi syndrome, left eye

    H20.823 Vogt-Koyanagi syndrome, bilateral

    H20.829 Vogt-Koyanagi syndrome, unspecified eye

H20.9 Unspecified iridocyclitis

    Uveitis NOS

● **H21 Other disorders of iris and ciliary body**

    Excludes2 sympathetic uveitis (H44.1-)

● **H21.0 Hyphema**

    Excludes1 traumatic hyphema (S05.1-)

    H21.00 Hyphema, unspecified eye

    H21.01 Hyphema, right eye

    H21.02 Hyphema, left eye

    H21.03 Hyphema, bilateral

▶ New   ⇒ Revised   deleted Deleted   Excludes 1   Excludes 2   Includes   Use additional   Code first   Code also   Key words

OGCR Official Guidelines   X Assign placeholder X   ● Use Additional Character(s)   ▶ Manifestation Code   Ⓒ Hierarchical Condition Category   Coding Clinic

● **H21.1**   **Other vascular disorders of iris and ciliary body**
Neovascularization of iris or ciliary body
Rubeosis iridis
Rubeosis of iris

  ● **H21.1X**   **Other vascular disorders of iris and ciliary body**

      H21.1X1   **Other vascular disorders of iris and ciliary body, right eye**

      H21.1X2   **Other vascular disorders of iris and ciliary body, left eye**

      H21.1X3   **Other vascular disorders of iris and ciliary body, bilateral**

      H21.1X9   **Other vascular disorders of iris and ciliary body, unspecified eye**

● **H21.2**   **Degeneration of iris and ciliary body**

  ● **H21.21**   **Degeneration of chamber angle**

      H21.211   **Degeneration of chamber angle, right eye**

      H21.212   **Degeneration of chamber angle, left eye**

      H21.213   **Degeneration of chamber angle, bilateral**

      H21.219   **Degeneration of chamber angle, unspecified eye**

  ● **H21.22**   **Degeneration of ciliary body**

      H21.221   **Degeneration of ciliary body, right eye**

      H21.222   **Degeneration of ciliary body, left eye**

      H21.223   **Degeneration of ciliary body, bilateral**

      H21.229   **Degeneration of ciliary body, unspecified eye**

  ● **H21.23**   **Degeneration of iris (pigmentary)**
      Translucency of iris

      H21.231   **Degeneration of iris (pigmentary), right eye**

      H21.232   **Degeneration of iris (pigmentary), left eye**

      H21.233   **Degeneration of iris (pigmentary), bilateral**

      H21.239   **Degeneration of iris (pigmentary), unspecified eye**

  ● **H21.24**   **Degeneration of pupillary margin**

      H21.241   **Degeneration of pupillary margin, right eye**

      H21.242   **Degeneration of pupillary margin, left eye**

      H21.243   **Degeneration of pupillary margin, bilateral**

      H21.249   **Degeneration of pupillary margin, unspecified eye**

  ● **H21.25**   **Iridoschisis**

      H21.251   **Iridoschisis, right eye**

      H21.252   **Iridoschisis, left eye**

      H21.253   **Iridoschisis, bilateral**

      H21.259   **Iridoschisis, unspecified eye**

  ● **H21.26**   **Iris atrophy (essential) (progressive)**

      H21.261   **Iris atrophy (essential) (progressive), right eye**

      H21.262   **Iris atrophy (essential) (progressive), left eye**

      H21.263   **Iris atrophy (essential) (progressive), bilateral**

      H21.269   **Iris atrophy (essential) (progressive), unspecified eye**

  ● **H21.27**   **Miotic pupillary cyst**

      H21.271   **Miotic pupillary cyst, right eye**

      H21.272   **Miotic pupillary cyst, left eye**

      H21.273   **Miotic pupillary cyst, bilateral**

      H21.279   **Miotic pupillary cyst, unspecified eye**

    H21.29   **Other iris atrophy**

● **H21.3**   **Cyst of iris, ciliary body and anterior chamber**
      Excludes2   miotic pupillary cyst (H21.27-)

  ● **H21.30**   **Idiopathic cysts of iris, ciliary body or anterior chamber**
      Cyst of iris, ciliary body or anterior chamber NOS

      H21.301   **Idiopathic cysts of iris, ciliary body or anterior chamber, right eye**

      H21.302   **Idiopathic cysts of iris, ciliary body or anterior chamber, left eye**

      H21.303   **Idiopathic cysts of iris, ciliary body or anterior chamber, bilateral**

      H21.309   **Idiopathic cysts of iris, ciliary body or anterior chamber, unspecified eye**

  ● **H21.31**   **Exudative cysts of iris or anterior chamber**

      H21.311   **Exudative cysts of iris or anterior chamber, right eye**

      H21.312   **Exudative cysts of iris or anterior chamber, left eye**

      H21.313   **Exudative cysts of iris or anterior chamber, bilateral**

      H21.319   **Exudative cysts of iris or anterior chamber, unspecified eye**

  ● **H21.32**   **Implantation cysts of iris, ciliary body or anterior chamber**

      H21.321   **Implantation cysts of iris, ciliary body or anterior chamber, right eye**

      H21.322   **Implantation cysts of iris, ciliary body or anterior chamber, left eye**

      H21.323   **Implantation cysts of iris, ciliary body or anterior chamber, bilateral**

      H21.329   **Implantation cysts of iris, ciliary body or anterior chamber, unspecified eye**

  ● **H21.33**   **Parasitic cyst of iris, ciliary body or anterior chamber**

      H21.331   **Parasitic cyst of iris, ciliary body or anterior chamber, right eye**

      H21.332   **Parasitic cyst of iris, ciliary body or anterior chamber, left eye**

      H21.333   **Parasitic cyst of iris, ciliary body or anterior chamber, bilateral**

      H21.339   **Parasitic cyst of iris, ciliary body or anterior chamber, unspecified eye**

  ● **H21.34**   **Primary cyst of pars plana**

      H21.341   **Primary cyst of pars plana, right eye**

      H21.342   **Primary cyst of pars plana, left eye**

      H21.343   **Primary cyst of pars plana, bilateral**

      H21.349   **Primary cyst of pars plana, unspecified eye**

  ● **H21.35**   **Exudative cyst of pars plana**

      H21.351   **Exudative cyst of pars plana, right eye**

      H21.352   **Exudative cyst of pars plana, left eye**

      H21.353   **Exudative cyst of pars plana, bilateral**

      H21.359   **Exudative cyst of pars plana, unspecified eye**

● **H21.4**   **Pupillary membranes**
      Iris bombé
      Pupillary occlusion
      Pupillary seclusion
      Excludes1   congenital pupillary membranes (Q13.8)

    H21.40   **Pupillary membranes, unspecified eye**

    H21.41   **Pupillary membranes, right eye**

    H21.42   **Pupillary membranes, left eye**

    H21.43   **Pupillary membranes, bilateral**

CHAPTER 7 (H00-H59)

CHAPTER 7 (H00-H59)

● **H21.5 Other and unspecified adhesions and disruptions of iris and ciliary body**

    Excludes1 corectopia (Q13.2)

● **H21.50 Unspecified adhesions of iris**
    Synechia (iris) NOS

    H21.501 Unspecified adhesions of iris, right eye

    H21.502 Unspecified adhesions of iris, left eye

    H21.503 Unspecified adhesions of iris, bilateral

    H21.509 Unspecified adhesions of iris and ciliary body, unspecified eye

● **H21.51 Anterior synechiae (iris)**

    H21.511 Anterior synechiae (iris), right eye

    H21.512 Anterior synechiae (iris), left eye

    H21.513 Anterior synechiae (iris), bilateral

    H21.519 Anterior synechiae (iris), unspecified eye

● **H21.52 Goniosynechiae**

    H21.521 Goniosynechiae, right eye

    H21.522 Goniosynechiae, left eye

    H21.523 Goniosynechiae, bilateral

    H21.529 Goniosynechiae, unspecified eye

● **H21.53 Iridodialysis**

    H21.531 Iridodialysis, right eye

    H21.532 Iridodialysis, left eye

    H21.533 Iridodialysis, bilateral

    H21.539 Iridodialysis, unspecified eye

● **H21.54 Posterior synechiae (iris)**

    H21.541 Posterior synechiae (iris), right eye

    H21.542 Posterior synechiae (iris), left eye

    H21.543 Posterior synechiae (iris), bilateral

    H21.549 Posterior synechiae (iris), unspecified eye

● **H21.55 Recession of chamber angle**

    H21.551 Recession of chamber angle, right eye

    H21.552 Recession of chamber angle, left eye

    H21.553 Recession of chamber angle, bilateral

    H21.559 Recession of chamber angle, unspecified eye

● **H21.56 Pupillary abnormalities**
    Deformed pupil
    Ectopic pupil
    Rupture of sphincter, pupil

    Excludes1 congenital deformity of pupil (Q13.2-)

    H21.561 Pupillary abnormality, right eye

    H21.562 Pupillary abnormality, left eye

    H21.563 Pupillary abnormality, bilateral

    H21.569 Pupillary abnormality, unspecified eye

● **H21.8 Other specified disorders of iris and ciliary body**

    H21.81 Floppy iris syndrome
    Intraoperative floppy iris syndrome (IFIS)

    Use additional code for adverse effect, if applicable, to identify drug (T36-T50 with fifth or sixth character 5)

    H21.82 Plateau iris syndrome (post-iridectomy) (postprocedural)

    H21.89 Other specified disorders of iris and ciliary body

H21.9 Unspecified disorder of iris and ciliary body

▷ **H22 Disorders of iris and ciliary body in diseases classified elsewhere**

    Code first underlying disease, such as:
    gout (M1A.-, M10.-)
    leprosy (A30.-)
    parasitic disease (B89)

DISORDERS OF LENS (H25-H28)

● **H25 Age-related cataract**
    Senile cataract

    Excludes2 capsular glaucoma with pseudoexfoliation of lens (H40.1-)

● **H25.0 Age-related incipient cataract**

● **H25.01 Cortical age-related cataract**

    H25.011 Cortical age-related cataract, right eye   A

    H25.012 Cortical age-related cataract, left eye   A

    H25.013 Cortical age-related cataract, bilateral   A

    H25.019 Cortical age-related cataract, unspecified eye   A

● **H25.03 Anterior subcapsular polar age-related cataract**

    H25.031 Anterior subcapsular polar age-related cataract, right eye   A

    H25.032 Anterior subcapsular polar age-related cataract, left eye   A

    H25.033 Anterior subcapsular polar age-related cataract, bilateral   A

    H25.039 Anterior subcapsular polar age-related cataract, unspecified eye   A

● **H25.04 Posterior subcapsular polar age-related cataract**

    H25.041 Posterior subcapsular polar age-related cataract, right eye   A

    H25.042 Posterior subcapsular polar age-related cataract, left eye   A

    H25.043 Posterior subcapsular polar age-related cataract, bilateral   A

    H25.049 Posterior subcapsular polar age-related cataract, unspecified eye   A

● **H25.09 Other age-related incipient cataract**
    Coronary age-related cataract
    Punctate age-related cataract
    Water clefts

    H25.091 Other age-related incipient cataract, right eye   A

    H25.092 Other age-related incipient cataract, left eye   A

    H25.093 Other age-related incipient cataract, bilateral   A

    H25.099 Other age-related incipient cataract, unspecified eye   A

Figure 7-9 Age-related cataract. Nuclear sclerosis and cortical lens opacities are present. (From Ignatavicius DD, Workman ML: Medical-Surgical Nursing: Patient-Centered Collaborative Care, St. Louis, MO, Saunders/Elsevier, 2010)

Item 7-5 Senile cataracts are linked to the aging process. The most common area for the formation of a cataract is the cortical area of the lens. **Polar cataracts** can be either anterior or posterior. **Anterior polar cataracts** are more common and are small, white, capsular cataracts located on the anterior portion of the lens. **Total cataracts,** also called **complete** or **mature,** cause an opacity of all fibers of the lens. **Hypermature** describes a mature cataract with a swollen, milky cortex that covers the entire lens. **Immature,** also called **incipient,** cataracts have a clear cortex and are only slightly opaque. Treatment for all cataracts is the removal of the lens.

▶ New   ➡ Revised   ~~deleted~~ Deleted   Excludes 1   Excludes 2   Includes   Use additional   Code first   Code also   Key words

OGCR Official Guidelines   X Assign placeholder X   ● Use Additional Character(s)   ▷ Manifestation Code   🔖 Hierarchical Condition Category   Coding Clinic

● **H25.1   Age-related nuclear cataract**
      Cataracta brunescens
      Nuclear sclerosis cataract
     H25.10   Age-related nuclear cataract, unspecified eye   A
     H25.11   Age-related nuclear cataract, right eye   A
           Coding Clinic: 2019, Q2, P30
     H25.12   Age-related nuclear cataract, left eye   A
           Coding Clinic: 2016, Q1, P33
     H25.13   Age-related nuclear cataract, bilateral   A
           Coding Clinic: 2016, Q1, P32

● **H25.2   Age-related cataract, morgagnian type**
      Age-related hypermature cataract
     H25.20   Age-related cataract, morgagnian type, unspecified eye   A
     H25.21   Age-related cataract, morgagnian type, right eye   A
     H25.22   Age-related cataract, morgagnian type, left eye   A
     H25.23   Age-related cataract, morgagnian type, bilateral   A

● **H25.8   Other age-related cataract**
    ● **H25.81   Combined forms of age-related cataract**
         H25.811   Combined forms of age-related cataract, right eye   A
         H25.812   Combined forms of age-related cataract, left eye   A
         H25.813   Combined forms of age-related cataract, bilateral   A
                Coding Clinic: 2019, Q2, P30
         H25.819   Combined forms of age-related cataract, unspecified eye   A
     H25.89   Other age-related cataract   A

     H25.9   Unspecified age-related cataract   A

● **H26   Other cataract**
     Excludes1   congenital cataract (Q12.0)
   ● **H26.0   Infantile and juvenile cataract**
    ● **H26.00   Unspecified infantile and juvenile cataract**
         H26.001   Unspecified infantile and juvenile cataract, right eye   P
         H26.002   Unspecified infantile and juvenile cataract, left eye   P
         H26.003   Unspecified infantile and juvenile cataract, bilateral   P
         H26.009   Unspecified infantile and juvenile cataract, unspecified eye   P
    ● **H26.01   Infantile and juvenile cortical, lamellar, or zonular cataract**
         H26.011   Infantile and juvenile cortical, lamellar, or zonular cataract, right eye   P
         H26.012   Infantile and juvenile cortical, lamellar, or zonular cataract, left eye   P
         H26.013   Infantile and juvenile cortical, lamellar, or zonular cataract, bilateral   P
         H26.019   Infantile and juvenile cortical, lamellar, or zonular cataract, unspecified eye   P
    ● **H26.03   Infantile and juvenile nuclear cataract**
         H26.031   Infantile and juvenile nuclear cataract, right eye   P
         H26.032   Infantile and juvenile nuclear cataract, left eye   P
         H26.033   Infantile and juvenile nuclear cataract, bilateral   P
         H26.039   Infantile and juvenile nuclear cataract, unspecified eye   P

    ● **H26.04   Anterior subcapsular polar infantile and juvenile cataract**
         H26.041   Anterior subcapsular polar infantile and juvenile cataract, right eye   P
         H26.042   Anterior subcapsular polar infantile and juvenile cataract, left eye   P
         H26.043   Anterior subcapsular polar infantile and juvenile cataract, bilateral   P
         H26.049   Anterior subcapsular polar infantile and juvenile cataract, unspecified eye   P
    ● **H26.05   Posterior subcapsular polar infantile and juvenile cataract**
         H26.051   Posterior subcapsular polar infantile and juvenile cataract, right eye   P
         H26.052   Posterior subcapsular polar infantile and juvenile cataract, left eye   P
         H26.053   Posterior subcapsular polar infantile and juvenile cataract, bilateral   P
         H26.059   Posterior subcapsular polar infantile and juvenile cataract, unspecified eye   P
    ● **H26.06   Combined forms of infantile and juvenile cataract**
         H26.061   Combined forms of infantile and juvenile cataract, right eye   P
         H26.062   Combined forms of infantile and juvenile cataract, left eye   P
         H26.063   Combined forms of infantile and juvenile cataract bilateral   P
         H26.069   Combined forms of infantile and juvenile cataract, unspecified eye   P
     H26.09   Other infantile and juvenile cataract   P

   ● **H26.1   Traumatic cataract**
      Use additional code (Chapter 20) to identify external cause
    ● **H26.10   Unspecified traumatic cataract**
         H26.101   Unspecified traumatic cataract, right eye
         H26.102   Unspecified traumatic cataract, left eye
         H26.103   Unspecified traumatic cataract, bilateral
         H26.109   Unspecified traumatic cataract, unspecified eye
    ● **H26.11   Localized traumatic opacities**
         H26.111   Localized traumatic opacities, right eye
         H26.112   Localized traumatic opacities, left eye
         H26.113   Localized traumatic opacities, bilateral
         H26.119   Localized traumatic opacities, unspecified eye
    ● **H26.12   Partially resolved traumatic cataract**
         H26.121   Partially resolved traumatic cataract, right eye
         H26.122   Partially resolved traumatic cataract, left eye
         H26.123   Partially resolved traumatic cataract, bilateral
         H26.129   Partially resolved traumatic cataract, unspecified eye
    ● **H26.13   Total traumatic cataract**
         H26.131   Total traumatic cataract, right eye
         H26.132   Total traumatic cataract, left eye
         H26.133   Total traumatic cataract, bilateral
         H26.139   Total traumatic cataract, unspecified eye

CHAPTER 7 (H00–H59)

● **H26.2**   **Complicated cataract**

    H26.20   **Unspecified complicated cataract**
         Cataracta complicata NOS

    ● **H26.21**   **Cataract with neovascularization**
         Code also associated condition, such as:
           chronic iridocyclitis (H20.1-)

       H26.211   **Cataract with neovascularization, right eye**

       H26.212   **Cataract with neovascularization, left eye**

       H26.213   **Cataract with neovascularization, bilateral**

       H26.219   **Cataract with neovascularization, unspecified eye**

    ● **H26.22**   **Cataract secondary to ocular disorders (degenerative) (inflammatory)**
         Code also associated ocular disorder

       H26.221   **Cataract secondary to ocular disorders (degenerative) (inflammatory), right eye**

       H26.222   **Cataract secondary to ocular disorders (degenerative) (inflammatory), left eye**

       H26.223   **Cataract secondary to ocular disorders (degenerative) (inflammatory), bilateral**

       H26.229   **Cataract secondary to ocular disorders (degenerative) (inflammatory), unspecified eye**

    ● **H26.23**   **Glaucomatous flecks (subcapsular)**
         Code first underlying glaucoma (H40-H42)

       H26.231   **Glaucomatous flecks (subcapsular), right eye**

       H26.232   **Glaucomatous flecks (subcapsular), left eye**

       H26.233   **Glaucomatous flecks (subcapsular), bilateral**

       H26.239   **Glaucomatous flecks (subcapsular), unspecified eye**

● **H26.3**   **Drug-induced cataract**
      Toxic cataract
      Use additional code for adverse effect, if applicable, to identify drug (T36-T50 with fifth or sixth character 5)

    H26.30   **Drug-induced cataract, unspecified eye**

    H26.31   **Drug-induced cataract, right eye**

    H26.32   **Drug-induced cataract, left eye**

    H26.33   **Drug-induced cataract, bilateral**

● **H26.4**   **Secondary cataract**
      Coding Clinic: 2018, Q2, P14

    H26.40   **Unspecified secondary cataract**

    ● **H26.41**   **Soemmering's ring**

       H26.411   **Soemmering's ring, right eye**

       H26.412   **Soemmering's ring, left eye**

       H26.413   **Soemmering's ring, bilateral**

       H26.419   **Soemmering's ring, unspecified eye**

    ● **H26.49**   **Other secondary cataract**

       H26.491   **Other secondary cataract, right eye**

       H26.492   **Other secondary cataract, left eye**
         Coding Clinic: 2018, Q2, P13

       H26.493   **Other secondary cataract, bilateral**

       H26.499   **Other secondary cataract, unspecified eye**

H26.8   **Other specified cataract**

H26.9   **Unspecified cataract**

● **H27**   **Other disorders of lens**

    Excludes1   congenital lens malformations (Q12.-)
         mechanical complications of intraocular lens implant (T85.2)
         pseudophakia (Z96.1)

    ● **H27.0**   **Aphakia**
       Acquired absence of lens
       Acquired aphakia
       Aphakia due to trauma

       Excludes1   cataract extraction status (Z98.4-)
          congenital absence of lens (Q12.3)
          congenital aphakia (Q12.3)

       H27.00   **Aphakia, unspecified eye**

       H27.01   **Aphakia, right eye**

       H27.02   **Aphakia, left eye**

       H27.03   **Aphakia, bilateral**

    ● **H27.1**   **Dislocation of lens**

       H27.10   **Unspecified dislocation of lens**

       ● **H27.11**   **Subluxation of lens**

          H27.111   **Subluxation of lens, right eye**

          H27.112   **Subluxation of lens, left eye**

          H27.113   **Subluxation of lens, bilateral**

          H27.119   **Subluxation of lens, unspecified eye**

       ● **H27.12**   **Anterior dislocation of lens**

          H27.121   **Anterior dislocation of lens, right eye**

          H27.122   **Anterior dislocation of lens, left eye**

          H27.123   **Anterior dislocation of lens, bilateral**

          H27.129   **Anterior dislocation of lens, unspecified eye**

       ● **H27.13**   **Posterior dislocation of lens**

          H27.131   **Posterior dislocation of lens, right eye**

          H27.132   **Posterior dislocation of lens, left eye**

          H27.133   **Posterior dislocation of lens, bilateral**

          H27.139   **Posterior dislocation of lens, unspecified eye**

    H27.8   **Other specified disorders of lens**

    H27.9   **Unspecified disorder of lens**

▷ *H28*   *Cataract in diseases classified elsewhere*
      Code first underlying disease, such as:
        hypoparathyroidism (E20.-)
        myotonia (G71.1-)
        myxedema (E03.-)
        protein-calorie malnutrition (E40-E46)

    Excludes1   cataract in diabetes mellitus (E08.36, E09.36, E10.36, E11.36, E13.36)

DISORDERS OF CHOROID AND RETINA (H30-H36)

★ **(See Plate 16 of the Anatomy Illustrations.)**

● **H30**   **Chorioretinal inflammation**

    ● **H30.0**   **Focal chorioretinal inflammation**
       Focal chorioretinitis
       Focal choroiditis
       Focal retinitis
       Focal retinochoroiditis

       ● **H30.00**   **Unspecified focal chorioretinal inflammation**
          Focal chorioretinitis NOS
          Focal choroiditis NOS
          Focal retinitis NOS
          Focal retinochoroiditis NOS

          H30.001   **Unspecified focal chorioretinal inflammation, right eye**

          H30.002   **Unspecified focal chorioretinal inflammation, left eye**

          H30.003   **Unspecified focal chorioretinal inflammation, bilateral**

          H30.009   **Unspecified focal chorioretinal inflammation, unspecified eye**

● H30.01   Focal chorioretinal inflammation, juxtapapillary

    H30.011   Focal chorioretinal inflammation, juxtapapillary, right eye

    H30.012   Focal chorioretinal inflammation, juxtapapillary, left eye

    H30.013   Focal chorioretinal inflammation, juxtapapillary, bilateral

    H30.019   Focal chorioretinal inflammation, juxtapapillary, unspecified eye

● H30.02   Focal chorioretinal inflammation of posterior pole

    H30.021   Focal chorioretinal inflammation of posterior pole, right eye

    H30.022   Focal chorioretinal inflammation of posterior pole, left eye

    H30.023   Focal chorioretinal inflammation of posterior pole, bilateral

    H30.029   Focal chorioretinal inflammation of posterior pole, unspecified eye

● H30.03   Focal chorioretinal inflammation, peripheral

    H30.031   Focal chorioretinal inflammation, peripheral, right eye

    H30.032   Focal chorioretinal inflammation, peripheral, left eye

    H30.033   Focal chorioretinal inflammation, peripheral, bilateral

    H30.039   Focal chorioretinal inflammation, peripheral, unspecified eye

● H30.04   Focal chorioretinal inflammation, macular or paramacular

    H30.041   Focal chorioretinal inflammation, macular or paramacular, right eye

    H30.042   Focal chorioretinal inflammation, macular or paramacular, left eye

    H30.043   Focal chorioretinal inflammation, macular or paramacular, bilateral

    H30.049   Focal chorioretinal inflammation, macular or paramacular, unspecified eye

● H30.1   Disseminated chorioretinal inflammation

    Disseminated chorioretinitis
    Disseminated choroiditis
    Disseminated retinitis
    Disseminated retinochoroiditis

    Excludes2   exudative retinopathy (H35.02-)

● H30.10   Unspecified disseminated chorioretinal inflammation

    Disseminated chorioretinitis NOS
    Disseminated choroiditis NOS
    Disseminated retinitis NOS
    Disseminated retinochoroiditis NOS

    H30.101   Unspecified disseminated chorioretinal inflammation, right eye

    H30.102   Unspecified disseminated chorioretinal inflammation, left eye

    H30.103   Unspecified disseminated chorioretinal inflammation, bilateral

    H30.109   Unspecified disseminated chorioretinal inflammation, unspecified eye

● H30.11   Disseminated chorioretinal inflammation of posterior pole

    H30.111   Disseminated chorioretinal inflammation of posterior pole, right eye

    H30.112   Disseminated chorioretinal inflammation of posterior pole, left eye

    H30.113   Disseminated chorioretinal inflammation of posterior pole, bilateral

    H30.119   Disseminated chorioretinal inflammation of posterior pole, unspecified eye

● H30.12   Disseminated chorioretinal inflammation, peripheral

    H30.121   Disseminated chorioretinal inflammation, peripheral right eye

    H30.122   Disseminated chorioretinal inflammation, peripheral, left eye

    H30.123   Disseminated chorioretinal inflammation, peripheral, bilateral

    H30.129   Disseminated chorioretinal inflammation, peripheral, unspecified eye

● H30.13   Disseminated chorioretinal inflammation, generalized

    H30.131   Disseminated chorioretinal inflammation, generalized, right eye

    H30.132   Disseminated chorioretinal inflammation, generalized, left eye

    H30.133   Disseminated chorioretinal inflammation, generalized, bilateral

    H30.139   Disseminated chorioretinal inflammation, generalized, unspecified eye

● H30.14   Acute posterior multifocal placoid pigment epitheliopathy

    H30.141   Acute posterior multifocal placoid pigment epitheliopathy, right eye

    H30.142   Acute posterior multifocal placoid pigment epitheliopathy, left eye

    H30.143   Acute posterior multifocal placoid pigment epitheliopathy, bilateral

    H30.149   Acute posterior multifocal placoid pigment epitheliopathy, unspecified eye

● H30.2   Posterior cyclitis

    Pars planitis

    H30.20   Posterior cyclitis, unspecified eye

    H30.21   Posterior cyclitis, right eye

    H30.22   Posterior cyclitis, left eye

    H30.23   Posterior cyclitis, bilateral

● H30.8   Other chorioretinal inflammations

● H30.81   Harada's disease

    H30.811   Harada's disease, right eye

    H30.812   Harada's disease, left eye

    H30.813   Harada's disease, bilateral

    H30.819   Harada's disease, unspecified eye

● H30.89   Other chorioretinal inflammations

    H30.891   Other chorioretinal inflammations, right eye

    H30.892   Other chorioretinal inflammations, left eye

    H30.893   Other chorioretinal inflammations, bilateral

    H30.899   Other chorioretinal inflammations, unspecified eye

● H30.9   Unspecified chorioretinal inflammation

    Chorioretinitis NOS
    Choroiditis NOS
    Neuroretinitis NOS
    Retinitis NOS
    Retinochoroiditis NOS

    H30.90   Unspecified chorioretinal inflammation, unspecified eye

    H30.91   Unspecified chorioretinal inflammation, right eye

CHAPTER 7 (H00-H59)

CHAPTER 7 (H00-H59)

H30.92   Unspecified chorioretinal inflammation, left eye

H30.93   Unspecified chorioretinal inflammation, bilateral

● H31   Other disorders of choroid

   ● H31.0   Chorioretinal scars

     Excludes2   postsurgical chorioretinal scars (H59.81-)

     ● H31.00   Unspecified chorioretinal scars

       H31.001   Unspecified chorioretinal scars, right eye

       H31.002   Unspecified chorioretinal scars, left eye

       H31.003   Unspecified chorioretinal scars, bilateral

       H31.009   Unspecified chorioretinal scars, unspecified eye

     ● H31.01   Macula scars of posterior pole (postinflammatory) (post-traumatic)

       Excludes1   postprocedural choriorentinal scar (H59.81-)

       H31.011   Macula scars of posterior pole (postinflammatory) (post-traumatic), right eye

       H31.012   Macula scars of posterior pole (postinflammatory) (post-traumatic), left eye

       H31.013   Macula scars of posterior pole (postinflammatory) (post-traumatic), bilateral

       H31.019   Macula scars of posterior pole (postinflammatory) (post-traumatic), unspecified eye

     ● H31.02   Solar retinopathy

       H31.021   Solar retinopathy, right eye

       H31.022   Solar retinopathy, left eye

       H31.023   Solar retinopathy, bilateral

       H31.029   Solar retinopathy, unspecified eye

     ● H31.09   Other chorioretinal scars

       H31.091   Other chorioretinal scars, right eye

       H31.092   Other chorioretinal scars, left eye

       H31.093   Other chorioretinal scars, bilateral

       H31.099   Other chorioretinal scars, unspecified eye

   ● H31.1   Choroidal degeneration

     Excludes2   angioid streaks of macula (H35.33)

     ● H31.10   Unspecified choroidal degeneration
       Choroidal sclerosis NOS

       H31.101   Choroidal degeneration, unspecified, right eye

       H31.102   Choroidal degeneration, unspecified, left eye

       H31.103   Choroidal degeneration, unspecified, bilateral

       H31.109   Choroidal degeneration, unspecified, unspecified eye

     ● H31.11   Age-related choroidal atrophy

       H31.111   Age-related choroidal atrophy, right eye   A

       H31.112   Age-related choroidal atrophy, left eye   A

       H31.113   Age-related choroidal atrophy, bilateral   A

       H31.119   Age-related choroidal atrophy, unspecified eye   A

     ● H31.12   Diffuse secondary atrophy of choroid

       H31.121   Diffuse secondary atrophy of choroid, right eye

       H31.122   Diffuse secondary atrophy of choroid, left eye

       H31.123   Diffuse secondary atrophy of choroid, bilateral

       H31.129   Diffuse secondary atrophy of choroid, unspecified eye

   ● H31.2   Hereditary choroidal dystrophy

     Excludes2   hyperornithinemia (E72.4)
                    ornithinemia (E72.4)

     H31.20   Hereditary choroidal dystrophy, unspecified

     H31.21   Choroideremia

     H31.22   Choroidal dystrophy (central areolar) (generalized) (peripapillary)

     H31.23   Gyrate atrophy, choroid

     H31.29   Other hereditary choroidal dystrophy

   ● H31.3   Choroidal hemorrhage and rupture

     ● H31.30   Unspecified choroidal hemorrhage

       H31.301   Unspecified choroidal hemorrhage, right eye

       H31.302   Unspecified choroidal hemorrhage, left eye

       H31.303   Unspecified choroidal hemorrhage, bilateral

       H31.309   Unspecified choroidal hemorrhage, unspecified eye

     ● H31.31   Expulsive choroidal hemorrhage

       H31.311   Expulsive choroidal hemorrhage, right eye

       H31.312   Expulsive choroidal hemorrhage, left eye

       H31.313   Expulsive choroidal hemorrhage, bilateral

       H31.319   Expulsive choroidal hemorrhage, unspecified eye

     ● H31.32   Choroidal rupture

       H31.321   Choroidal rupture, right eye

       H31.322   Choroidal rupture, left eye

       H31.323   Choroidal rupture, bilateral

       H31.329   Choroidal rupture, unspecified eye

   ● H31.4   Choroidal detachment

     ● H31.40   Unspecified choroidal detachment

       H31.401   Unspecified choroidal detachment, right eye

       H31.402   Unspecified choroidal detachment, left eye

       H31.403   Unspecified choroidal detachment, bilateral

       H31.409   Unspecified choroidal detachment, unspecified eye

     ● H31.41   Hemorrhagic choroidal detachment

       H31.411   Hemorrhagic choroidal detachment, right eye

       H31.412   Hemorrhagic choroidal detachment, left eye

       H31.413   Hemorrhagic choroidal detachment, bilateral

       H31.419   Hemorrhagic choroidal detachment, unspecified eye

     ● H31.42   Serous choroidal detachment

       H31.421   Serous choroidal detachment, right eye

       H31.422   Serous choroidal detachment, left eye

       H31.423   Serous choroidal detachment, bilateral

       H31.429   Serous choroidal detachment, unspecified eye

   H31.8   Other specified disorders of choroid

   H31.9   Unspecified disorder of choroid

▶ New   ⇒ Revised   ~~deleted~~ Deleted   Excludes 1   Excludes 2   Includes   Use additional   Code first   Code also   Key words

OGCR Official Guidelines   X Assign placeholder X   ● Use Additional Character(s)   ▌ Manifestation Code   🐛 Hierarchical Condition Category   **Coding Clinic**

▶ *H32*   *Chorioretinal disorders in diseases classified elsewhere*
     Code first underlying disease, such as:
       congenital toxoplasmosis (P37.1)
       histoplasmosis (B39.-)
       leprosy (A30.-)
     Excludes1   chorioretinitis (in):
                toxoplasmosis (acquired) (B58.01)
                tuberculosis (A18.53)

● **H33**   **Retinal detachments and breaks**
     Excludes1   detachment of retinal pigment epithelium
                (H35.72-, H35.73-)

   ● **H33.0**   **Retinal detachment with retinal break**
         Rhegmatogenous retinal detachment
       Excludes1   serous retinal detachment (without retinal
                break) (H33.2-)

     ● **H33.00**   **Unspecified retinal detachment with retinal break**
         H33.001   Unspecified retinal detachment with retinal break, **right eye**
         H33.002   Unspecified retinal detachment with retinal break, **left eye**
         H33.003   Unspecified retinal detachment with retinal break, **bilateral**
         H33.009   Unspecified retinal detachment with retinal break, **unspecified eye**

     ● **H33.01**   Retinal detachment with **single break**
         H33.011   Retinal detachment with single break, **right eye**
         H33.012   Retinal detachment with single break, **left eye**

NON-RHEGMATOGENOUS RETINAL DETACHMENT

Vitreous
Retina
Protein-rich fluid in sub-retinal space
Retinal pigment epithelium

VITREOUS DETACHMENT

Vitreous
Posterior hyaloid
Internal limiting membrane

RHEGMATOGENOUS RETINAL DETACHMENT

Blood
Vitreous
Posterior hyaloid
Retina
Retinal tear
Liquified vitreous
Retinal pigment epithelium

Figure 7-10   Retinal detachment. (From Kumar: Robbins and Cotran: Pathologic Basis of Disease, ed 7, Saunders, 2005)

Item 7-6   Retinal detachments and defects are conditions of the eye in which the retina separates from the underlying tissue. Initial detachment may be localized, requiring rapid treatment (medical emergency) to avoid the entire retina from detaching, which leads to vision loss and blindness.

         H33.013   Retinal detachment with single break, **bilateral**
         H33.019   Retinal detachment with single break, **unspecified eye**

     ● **H33.02**   Retinal detachment with **multiple breaks**
         H33.021   Retinal detachment with multiple breaks, **right eye**
         H33.022   Retinal detachment with multiple breaks, **left eye**
         H33.023   Retinal detachment with multiple breaks, **bilateral**
         H33.029   Retinal detachment with multiple breaks, **unspecified eye**

     ● **H33.03**   Retinal detachment with **giant retinal tear**
         H33.031   Retinal detachment with giant retinal tear, **right eye**
         H33.032   Retinal detachment with giant retinal tear, **left eye**
         H33.033   Retinal detachment with giant retinal tear, **bilateral**
         H33.039   Retinal detachment with giant retinal tear, **unspecified eye**

     ● **H33.04**   Retinal detachment with **retinal dialysis**
         H33.041   Retinal detachment with retinal dialysis, **right eye**
         H33.042   Retinal detachment with retinal dialysis, **left eye**
         H33.043   Retinal detachment with retinal dialysis, **bilateral**
         H33.049   Retinal detachment with retinal dialysis, **unspecified** eye

     ● **H33.05**   **Total retinal detachment**
         H33.051   Total retinal detachment, **right eye**
         H33.052   Total retinal detachment, **left eye**
         H33.053   Total retinal detachment, **bilateral**
         H33.059   Total retinal detachment, **unspecified eye**

   ● **H33.1**   **Retinoschisis and retinal cysts**
       Excludes1   congenital retinoschisis (Q14.1)
                microcystoid degeneration of retina (H35.42-)

     ● **H33.10**   **Unspecified retinoschisis**
         H33.101   Unspecified retinoschisis, **right eye**
         H33.102   Unspecified retinoschisis, **left eye**
         H33.103   Unspecified retinoschisis, **bilateral**
         H33.109   Unspecified retinoschisis, **unspecified** eye

     ● **H33.11**   Cyst of **ora serrata**
         H33.111   Cyst of ora serrata, **right eye**
         H33.112   Cyst of ora serrata, **left eye**
         H33.113   Cyst of ora serrata, **bilateral**
         H33.119   Cyst of ora serrata, **unspecified eye**

     ● **H33.12**   **Parasitic cyst of retina**
         H33.121   Parasitic cyst of retina, **right eye**
         H33.122   Parasitic cyst of retina, **left eye**
         H33.123   Parasitic cyst of retina, **bilateral**
         H33.129   Parasitic cyst of retina, **unspecified** eye

     ● **H33.19**   **Other retinoschisis and retinal cysts**
         Pseudocyst of retina
         H33.191   Other retinoschisis and retinal cysts, **right eye**
         H33.192   Other retinoschisis and retinal cysts, **left eye**
         H33.193   Other retinoschisis and retinal cysts, **bilateral**
         H33.199   Other retinoschisis and retinal cysts, **unspecified eye**

● **H33.2 Serous retinal detachment**
Retinal detachment NOS
Retinal detachment without retinal break
> **Excludes1** central serous chorioretinopathy
> (H35.71-)
     H33.20 Serous retinal detachment, unspecified eye
     H33.21 Serous retinal detachment, right eye
     H33.22 Serous retinal detachment, left eye
     H33.23 Serous retinal detachment, bilateral
● **H33.3 Retinal breaks without detachment**
> **Excludes1** chorioretinal scars after surgery for
> detachment (H59.81-)
> peripheral retinal degeneration without
> break (H35.4-)
  ● **H33.30 Unspecified retinal break**
     H33.301 Unspecified retinal break, right eye
     H33.302 Unspecified retinal break, left eye
     H33.303 Unspecified retinal break, bilateral
     H33.309 Unspecified retinal break, unspecified eye
  ● **H33.31 Horseshoe tear of retina without detachment**
     Operculum of retina without detachment
     H33.311 Horseshoe tear of retina without detachment, right eye
     H33.312 Horseshoe tear of retina without detachment, left eye
     H33.313 Horseshoe tear of retina without detachment, bilateral
     H33.319 Horseshoe tear of retina without detachment, unspecified eye
  ● **H33.32 Round hole of retina without detachment**
     H33.321 Round hole, right eye
     H33.322 Round hole, left eye
     H33.323 Round hole, bilateral
     H33.329 Round hole, unspecified eye
  ● **H33.33 Multiple defects of retina without detachment**
     H33.331 Multiple defects of retina without detachment, right eye
     H33.332 Multiple defects of retina without detachment, left eye
     H33.333 Multiple defects of retina without detachment, bilateral
     H33.339 Multiple defects of retina without detachment, unspecified eye
● **H33.4 Traction detachment of retina**
Proliferative vitreo-retinopathy with retinal detachment
     H33.40 Traction detachment of retina, unspecified eye
     H33.41 Traction detachment of retina, right eye
     H33.42 Traction detachment of retina, left eye
     H33.43 Traction detachment of retina, bilateral
   H33.8 Other retinal detachments

● **H34 Retinal vascular occlusions**
Blockage in vessel of the retina
> **Excludes1** amaurosis fugax (G45.3)
● **H34.0 Transient retinal artery occlusion**
     H34.00 Transient retinal artery occlusion, unspecified eye
     H34.01 Transient retinal artery occlusion, right eye
     H34.02 Transient retinal artery occlusion, left eye
     H34.03 Transient retinal artery occlusion, bilateral
● **H34.1 Central retinal artery occlusion**
     H34.10 Central retinal artery occlusion, unspecified eye
     H34.11 Central retinal artery occlusion, right eye
     H34.12 Central retinal artery occlusion, left eye
     H34.13 Central retinal artery occlusion, bilateral

● **H34.2 Other retinal artery occlusions**
  ● **H34.21 Partial retinal artery occlusion**
     Hollenhorst's plaque
     Retinal microembolism
     H34.211 Partial retinal artery occlusion, right eye
     H34.212 Partial retinal artery occlusion, left eye
     H34.213 Partial retinal artery occlusion, bilateral
     H34.219 Partial retinal artery occlusion, unspecified eye
  ● **H34.23 Retinal artery branch occlusion**
     H34.231 Retinal artery branch occlusion, right eye
     H34.232 Retinal artery branch occlusion, left eye
     H34.233 Retinal artery branch occlusion, bilateral
     H34.239 Retinal artery branch occlusion, unspecified eye
● **H34.8 Other retinal vascular occlusions**
     Coding Clinic: 2016, Q4, P19
  ● **H34.81 Central retinal vein occlusion**
> One of the following 7th characters is to
> be assigned to codes in subcategory
> H34.81 to designate the severity of the
> occlusion:

> 0   with macular edema
> 1   with retinal neovascularization
> 2   stable
>   Old central retinal vein occlusion

     ● H34.811 Central retinal vein occlusion, right eye
     ● H34.812 Central retinal vein occlusion, left eye
     ● H34.813 Central retinal vein occlusion, bilateral
     ● H34.819 Central retinal vein occlusion, unspecified eye
  ● **H34.82 Venous engorgement**
     Incipient retinal vein occlusion
     Partial retinal vein occlusion
     H34.821 Venous engorgement, right eye
     H34.822 Venous engorgement, left eye
     H34.823 Venous engorgement, bilateral
     H34.829 Venous engorgement, unspecified eye
  ● **H34.83 Tributary (branch) retinal vein occlusion**
> One of the following 7th characters is to
> be assigned to codes in subcategory
> H34.83 to designate the severity of the
> occlusion:

> 0   with macular edema
> 1   with retinal neovascularization
> 2   stable
>   Old tributary (branch) retinal vein
>   occlusion

     ● H34.831 Tributary (branch) retinal vein occlusion, right eye
     ● H34.832 Tributary (branch) retinal vein occlusion, left eye
     ● H34.833 Tributary (branch) retinal vein occlusion, bilateral
     ● H34.839 Tributary (branch) retinal vein occlusion, unspecified eye
   H34.9 Unspecified retinal vascular occlusion

▶ New   ⇒ Revised   ~~deleted~~ Deleted   Excludes 1   Excludes 2   Includes   Use additional   Code first   Code also   Key words
OGCR Official Guidelines   X Assign placeholder X   ● Use Additional Character(s)   ▌ Manifestation Code   Hierarchical Condition Category   **Coding Clinic**

● **H35   Other retinal disorders**

    Excludes2   diabetic retinal disorders (E08.311-E08.359,
                        E09.311-E09.359, E10.311-E10.359,
                        E11.311-E11.359, E13.311-E13.359)

   ● **H35.0   Background retinopathy and retinal vascular changes**

       Code also any associated hypertension (I10)

       OGCR Section I. C.9.a.5.

       Hypertensive Retinopathy
       Subcategory H35.0, Background retinopathy and
       retinal vascular changes, should be used with a
       code from category I10–I15, Hypertensive disease to
       include the systemic hypertension. The sequencing is
       based on the reason for the encounter.

      H35.00   Unspecified background retinopathy

    ● **H35.01   Changes in retinal vascular appearance**
           Retinal vascular sheathing

          H35.011   Changes in retinal vascular
                   appearance, right eye

          H35.012   Changes in retinal vascular
                   appearance, left eye

          H35.013   Changes in retinal vascular
                   appearance, bilateral

          H35.019   Changes in retinal vascular
                   appearance, unspecified eye

    ● **H35.02   Exudative retinopathy**
           Coats retinopathy

          H35.021   Exudative retinopathy, right eye
          H35.022   Exudative retinopathy, left eye
          H35.023   Exudative retinopathy, bilateral
          H35.029   Exudative retinopathy, unspecified eye

    ● **H35.03   Hypertensive retinopathy**

          H35.031   Hypertensive retinopathy, right eye
          H35.032   Hypertensive retinopathy, left eye
          H35.033   Hypertensive retinopathy, bilateral
          H35.039   Hypertensive retinopathy, unspecified
                   eye

    ● **H35.04   Retinal micro-aneurysms, unspecified**

          H35.041   Retinal micro-aneurysms,
                   unspecified, right eye

          H35.042   Retinal micro-aneurysms,
                   unspecified, left eye

          H35.043   Retinal micro-aneurysms,
                   unspecified, bilateral

          H35.049   Retinal micro-aneurysms,
                   unspecified, unspecified eye

    ● **H35.05   Retinal neovascularization, unspecified**

          H35.051   Retinal neovascularization,
                   unspecified, right eye

          H35.052   Retinal neovascularization,
                   unspecified, left eye

          H35.053   Retinal neovascularization,
                   unspecified, bilateral

          H35.059   Retinal neovascularization,
                   unspecified, unspecified eye

    ● **H35.06   Retinal vasculitis**
          Eales disease
          Retinal perivasculitis

          H35.061   Retinal vasculitis, right eye
          H35.062   Retinal vasculitis, left eye
          H35.063   Retinal vasculitis, bilateral
          H35.069   Retinal vasculitis, unspecified eye

    ● **H35.07   Retinal telangiectasis**

          H35.071   Retinal telangiectasis, right eye
          H35.072   Retinal telangiectasis, left eye
          H35.073   Retinal telangiectasis, bilateral
          H35.079   Retinal telangiectasis, unspecified eye

      H35.09   Other intraretinal microvascular abnormalities
           Retinal varices

   ● **H35.1   Retinopathy of prematurity**

    ● **H35.10   Retinopathy of prematurity, unspecified**
           Retinopathy of prematurity NOS

          H35.101   Retinopathy of prematurity,
                   unspecified, right eye

          H35.102   Retinopathy of prematurity,
                   unspecified, left eye

          H35.103   Retinopathy of prematurity,
                   unspecified, bilateral

          H35.109   Retinopathy of prematurity,
                   unspecified, unspecified eye

    ● **H35.11   Retinopathy of prematurity, stage 0**

          H35.111   Retinopathy of prematurity, stage 0,
                   right eye

          H35.112   Retinopathy of prematurity, stage 0,
                   left eye

          H35.113   Retinopathy of prematurity, stage 0,
                   bilateral

          H35.119   Retinopathy of prematurity, stage 0,
                   unspecified eye

    ● **H35.12   Retinopathy of prematurity, stage 1**

          H35.121   Retinopathy of prematurity, stage 1,
                   right eye

          H35.122   Retinopathy of prematurity, stage 1,
                   left eye

          H35.123   Retinopathy of prematurity, stage 1,
                   bilateral

          H35.129   Retinopathy of prematurity, stage 1,
                   unspecified eye

    ● **H35.13   Retinopathy of prematurity, stage 2**

          H35.131   Retinopathy of prematurity, stage 2,
                   right eye

          H35.132   Retinopathy of prematurity, stage 2,
                   left eye

          H35.133   Retinopathy of prematurity, stage 2,
                   bilateral

          H35.139   Retinopathy of prematurity, stage 2,
                   unspecified eye

    ● **H35.14   Retinopathy of prematurity, stage 3**

          H35.141   Retinopathy of prematurity, stage 3,
                   right eye

          H35.142   Retinopathy of prematurity, stage 3,
                   left eye

          H35.143   Retinopathy of prematurity, stage 3,
                   bilateral

          H35.149   Retinopathy of prematurity, stage 3,
                   unspecified eye

    ● **H35.15   Retinopathy of prematurity, stage 4**

          H35.151   Retinopathy of prematurity, stage 4,
                   right eye

          H35.152   Retinopathy of prematurity, stage 4,
                   left eye

          H35.153   Retinopathy of prematurity, stage 4,
                   bilateral

          H35.159   Retinopathy of prematurity, stage 4,
                   unspecified eye

    ● **H35.16   Retinopathy of prematurity, stage 5**

          H35.161   Retinopathy of prematurity, stage 5,
                   right eye

          H35.162   Retinopathy of prematurity, stage 5,
                   left eye

          H35.163   Retinopathy of prematurity, stage 5,
                   bilateral

          H35.169   Retinopathy of prematurity, stage 5,
                   unspecified eye

    ● **H35.17   Retrolental fibroplasia**

          H35.171   Retrolental fibroplasia, right eye
          H35.172   Retrolental fibroplasia, left eye
          H35.173   Retrolental fibroplasia, bilateral
          H35.179   Retrolental fibroplasia, unspecified
                   eye

● **H35.2   Other non-diabetic proliferative retinopathy**
         Proliferative vitreo-retinopathy

       Excludes1   proliferative vitreo-retinopathy with retinal detachment (H33.4-)

    H35.20   Other non-diabetic proliferative retinopathy, unspecified eye

    H35.21   Other non-diabetic proliferative retinopathy, right eye

    H35.22   Other non-diabetic proliferative retinopathy, left eye

    H35.23   Other non-diabetic proliferative retinopathy, bilateral

● **H35.3   Degeneration of macula and posterior pole**

    H35.30   Unspecified macular degeneration   A
             Age-related macular degeneration

  ● **H35.31   Nonexudative age-related macular degeneration**
             Atrophic age-related macular degeneration
             Dry age-related macular degeneration

             One of the following 7th characters is to be assigned to codes in subcategory H35.31 to designate the stage of the disease:

0	stage unspecified
1	early dry stage
2	intermediate dry stage
3	advanced atrophic without subfoveal involvement
	advanced dry stage
4	advanced atrophic with subfoveal involvement

     ● **H35.311   Nonexudative age-related macular degeneration, right eye**   A
                Coding Clinic: 2016, Q4, P20-21

     ● **H35.312   Nonexudative age-related macular degeneration, left eye**   A
                Coding Clinic: 2016, Q4, P20-21

     ● **H35.313   Nonexudative age-related macular degeneration, bilateral**   A
                Coding Clinic: 2016, Q4, P20

     ● **H35.319   Nonexudative age-related macular degeneration, unspecified eye**   A
                Coding Clinic: 2016, Q4, P20

  ● **H35.32   Exudative age-related macular degeneration**
             Wet age-related macular degeneration

             One of the following 7th characters is to be assigned to codes in subcategory H35.32 to designate the stage of the disease:

0	stage unspecified
1	with active choroidal neovascularization
2	with inactive choroidal neovascularization
	with involuted or regressed neovascularization
3	with inactive scar

           Coding Clinic: 2016, Q4, P20

     ● **H35.321   Exudative age-related macular degeneration, right eye** 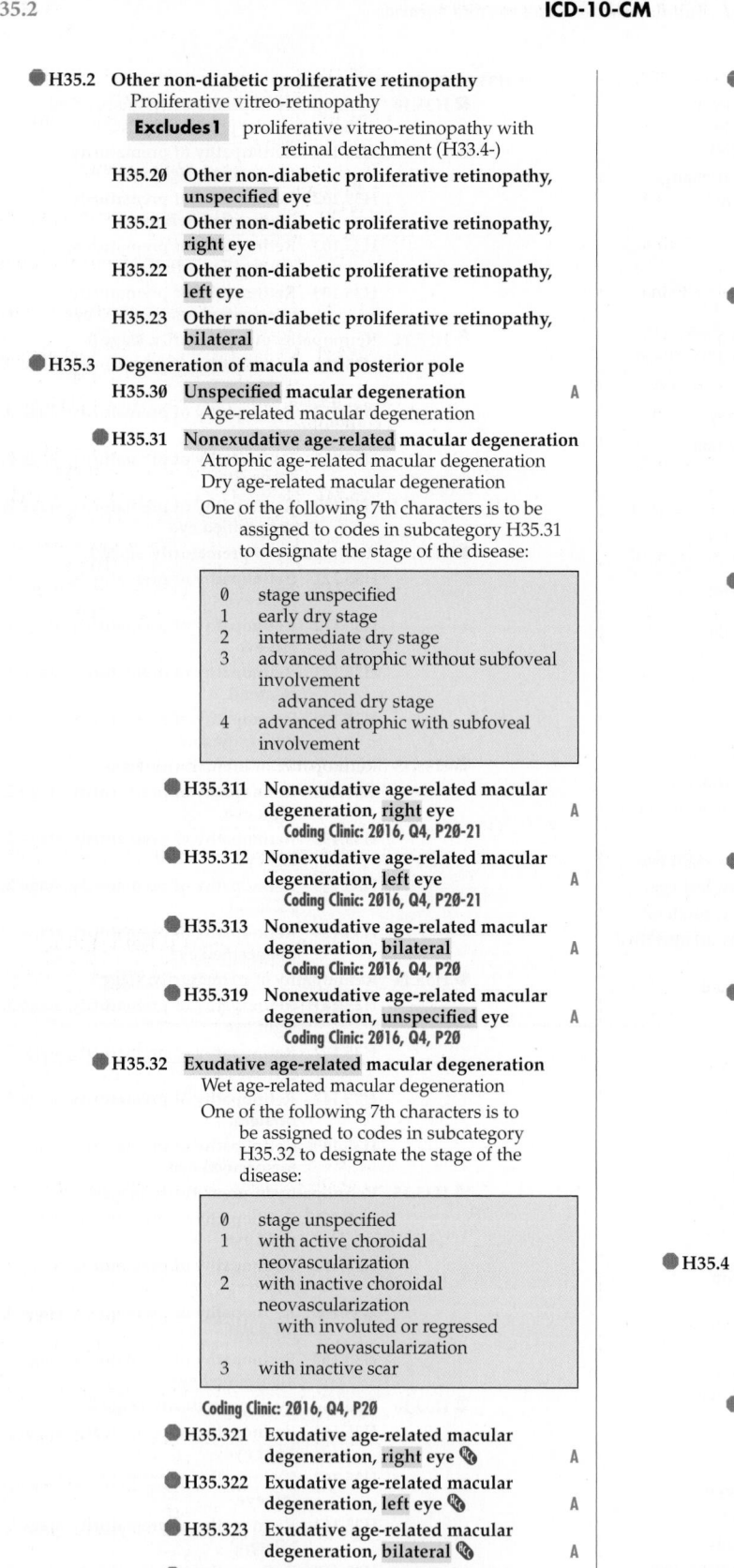   A

     ● **H35.322   Exudative age-related macular degeneration, left eye**   A

     ● **H35.323   Exudative age-related macular degeneration, bilateral**   A

     ● **H35.329   Exudative age-related macular degeneration, unspecified eye**   A

    H35.33   Angioid streaks of macula

● **H35.34   Macular cyst, hole, or pseudohole**

    H35.341   Macular cyst, hole, or pseudohole, right eye

    H35.342   Macular cyst, hole, or pseudohole, left eye

    H35.343   Macular cyst, hole, or pseudohole, bilateral

    H35.349   Macular cyst, hole, or pseudohole, unspecified eye

● **H35.35   Cystoid macular degeneration**

       Excludes1   cystoid macular edema following cataract surgery (H59.03-)

    H35.351   Cystoid macular degeneration, right eye

    H35.352   Cystoid macular degeneration, left eye

    H35.353   Cystoid macular degeneration, bilateral

    H35.359   Cystoid macular degeneration, unspecified eye

● **H35.36   Drusen (degenerative) of macula**

    H35.361   Drusen (degenerative) of macula, right eye
                Coding Clinic: 2016, Q4, P21

    H35.362   Drusen (degenerative) of macula, left eye
                Coding Clinic: 2016, Q4, P21

    H35.363   Drusen (degenerative) of macula, bilateral
                Coding Clinic: 2017, Q1, P51

    H35.369   Drusen (degenerative) of macula, unspecified eye

● **H35.37   Puckering of macula**

    H35.371   Puckering of macula, right eye

    H35.372   Puckering of macula, left eye

    H35.373   Puckering of macula, bilateral

    H35.379   Puckering of macula, unspecified eye

● **H35.38   Toxic maculopathy**

       Code first poisoning due to drug or toxin, if applicable (T36-T65 with fifth or sixth character 1-4 or 6)

       Use additional code for adverse effect, if applicable, to identify drug (T36-T50 with fifth or sixth character 5)

    H35.381   Toxic maculopathy, right eye

    H35.382   Toxic maculopathy, left eye

    H35.383   Toxic maculopathy, bilateral

    H35.389   Toxic maculopathy, unspecified eye

● **H35.4   Peripheral retinal degeneration**

       Excludes1   hereditary retinal degeneration (dystrophy) (H35.5-)
               peripheral retinal degeneration with retinal break (H33.3-)

    H35.40   Unspecified peripheral retinal degeneration

  ● **H35.41   Lattice degeneration of retina**
             Palisade degeneration of retina

    H35.411   Lattice degeneration of retina, right eye

    H35.412   Lattice degeneration of retina, left eye

    H35.413   Lattice degeneration of retina, bilateral

    H35.419   Lattice degeneration of retina, unspecified eye

  ● **H35.42   Microcystoid degeneration of retina**

    H35.421   Microcystoid degeneration of retina, right eye

    H35.422   Microcystoid degeneration of retina, left eye

Item 7-7 Macular degeneration is typically age-related, chronic, and is evidenced by deterioration of the macula (the part of the retina that provides for central field vision), resulting in blurred vision or a blind spot in the center of visual field while not affecting peripheral vision.

▶ New   ⇒ Revised   ~~deleted~~ Deleted   Excludes 1   Excludes 2   Includes   Use additional   Code first   Code also   Key words

OGCR Official Guidelines   X Assign placeholder X   ● Use Additional Character(s)   ▌ Manifestation Code   🐾 Hierarchical Condition Category   **Coding Clinic**

H35.423　Microcystoid degeneration of retina, bilateral

H35.429　Microcystoid degeneration of retina, unspecified eye

●H35.43　Paving stone degeneration of retina

H35.431　Paving stone degeneration of retina, right eye

H35.432　Paving stone degeneration of retina, left eye

H35.433　Paving stone degeneration of retina, bilateral

H35.439　Paving stone degeneration of retina, unspecified eye

●H35.44　Age-related reticular degeneration of retina

H35.441　Age-related reticular degeneration of retina, right eye　　　　A

H35.442　Age-related reticular degeneration of retina, left eye　　　　A

H35.443　Age-related reticular degeneration of retina, bilateral　　　　A

H35.449　Age-related reticular degeneration of retina, unspecified eye　　　　A

●H35.45　Secondary pigmentary degeneration

H35.451　Secondary pigmentary degeneration, right eye

H35.452　Secondary pigmentary degeneration, left eye

H35.453　Secondary pigmentary degeneration, bilateral

H35.459　Secondary pigmentary degeneration, unspecified eye

●H35.46　Secondary vitreoretinal degeneration

H35.461　Secondary vitreoretinal degeneration, right eye

H35.462　Secondary vitreoretinal degeneration, left eye

H35.463　Secondary vitreoretinal degeneration, bilateral

H35.469　Secondary vitreoretinal degeneration, unspecified eye

●H35.5　Hereditary retinal dystrophy

Excludes1　dystrophies primarily involving Bruch's membrane (H31.1-)

H35.50　Unspecified hereditary retinal dystrophy

H35.51　Vitreoretinal dystrophy

H35.52　Pigmentary retinal dystrophy
Albipunctate retinal dystrophy
Retinitis pigmentosa
Tapetoretinal dystrophy

H35.53　Other dystrophies primarily involving the sensory retina
Stargardt's disease

H35.54　Dystrophies primarily involving the retinal pigment epithelium
Vitelliform retinal dystrophy

●H35.6　Retinal hemorrhage

H35.60　Retinal hemorrhage, unspecified eye

H35.61　Retinal hemorrhage, right eye

H35.62　Retinal hemorrhage, left eye

H35.63　Retinal hemorrhage, bilateral

●H35.7　Separation of retinal layers

Excludes1　retinal detachment (serous) (H33.2-)
rhegmatogenous retinal detachment (H33.0-)

H35.70　Unspecified separation of retinal layers

●H35.71　Central serous chorioretinopathy

H35.711　Central serous chorioretinopathy, right eye

H35.712　Central serous chorioretinopathy, left eye

H35.713　Central serous chorioretinopathy, bilateral

H35.719　Central serous chorioretinopathy, unspecified eye

●H35.72　Serous detachment of retinal pigment epithelium

H35.721　Serous detachment of retinal pigment epithelium, right eye

H35.722　Serous detachment of retinal pigment epithelium, left eye

H35.723　Serous detachment of retinal pigment epithelium, bilateral

H35.729　Serous detachment of retinal pigment epithelium, unspecified eye

●H35.73　Hemorrhagic detachment of retinal pigment epithelium

H35.731　Hemorrhagic detachment of retinal pigment epithelium, right eye

H35.732　Hemorrhagic detachment of retinal pigment epithelium, left eye

H35.733　Hemorrhagic detachment of retinal pigment epithelium, bilateral

H35.739　Hemorrhagic detachment of retinal pigment epithelium, unspecified eye

●H35.8　Other specified retinal disorders

Excludes2　retinal hemorrhage (H35.6-)

H35.81　Retinal edema
Retinal cotton wool spots

H35.82　Retinal ischemia

H35.89　Other specified retinal disorders

H35.9　Unspecified retinal disorder

▷H36　*Retinal disorders in diseases classified elsewhere*
Code first underlying disease, such as:
lipid storage disorders (E75.-)
sickle-cell disorders (D57.-)

Excludes1　arteriosclerotic retinopathy (H35.0-)
diabetic retinopathy (E08.3-, E09.3-, E10.3-, E11.3-, E13.3-)

GLAUCOMA (H40-H42)

●H40　Glaucoma
Intraocular pressure (IOP) that is too high results from too much aqueous humor and because of excess production or inadequate drainage, optic nerve damage and vision loss may occur.

Excludes1　absolute glaucoma (H44.51-)
congenital glaucoma (Q15.0)
traumatic glaucoma due to birth injury (P15.3)

●H40.0　Glaucoma suspect

●H40.00　Preglaucoma, unspecified

H40.001　Preglaucoma, unspecified, right eye

H40.002　Preglaucoma, unspecified, left eye

H40.003　Preglaucoma, unspecified, bilateral

H40.009　Preglaucoma, unspecified, unspecified eye

●H40.01　Open angle with borderline findings, low risk
Open angle, low risk

H40.011　Open angle with borderline findings, low risk, right eye

H40.012　Open angle with borderline findings, low risk, left eye

H40.013　Open angle with borderline findings, low risk, bilateral

H40.019　Open angle with borderline findings, low risk, unspecified eye

CHAPTER 7 (H00-H59)

- **H40.02** Open angle with borderline findings, **high risk**
  - Open angle, high risk
  - H40.021 Open angle with borderline findings, high risk, **right eye**
  - H40.022 Open angle with borderline findings, high risk, **left eye**
  - H40.023 Open angle with borderline findings, high risk, **bilateral**
  - H40.029 Open angle with borderline findings, high risk, **unspecified** eye
- **H40.03** Anatomical narrow angle
  - Primary angle closure suspect
  - H40.031 Anatomical narrow angle, **right eye**
  - H40.032 Anatomical narrow angle, **left eye**
  - H40.033 Anatomical narrow angle, **bilateral**
  - H40.039 Anatomical narrow angle, **unspecified** eye
- **H40.04** Steroid responder
  - H40.041 Steroid responder, **right eye**
  - H40.042 Steroid responder, **left eye**
  - H40.043 Steroid responder, **bilateral**
  - H40.049 Steroid responder, **unspecified** eye
- **H40.05** Ocular **hypertension**
  - H40.051 Ocular hypertension, **right eye**
  - H40.052 Ocular hypertension, **left eye**
  - H40.053 Ocular hypertension, **bilateral**
  - H40.059 Ocular hypertension, **unspecified** eye
- **H40.06** Primary angle closure **without glaucoma damage**
  - H40.061 Primary angle closure without glaucoma damage, **right eye**
  - H40.062 Primary angle closure without glaucoma damage, **left eye**
  - H40.063 Primary angle closure without glaucoma damage, **bilateral**
  - H40.069 Primary angle closure without glaucoma damage, **unspecified** eye
- **H40.1** Open-angle glaucoma
  - X **H40.10** Unspecified open-angle glaucoma
    - One of the following 7th characters is to be assigned to code H40.10 to designate the stage of glaucoma
0	stage unspecified
1	mild stage
2	moderate stage
3	severe stage
4	indeterminate stage
  - **H40.11** Primary open-angle glaucoma
    - Chronic simple glaucoma
    - One of the following 7th characters is to be assigned to each code in subcategory H40.11 to designate the stage of glaucoma
0	stage unspecified
1	mild stage
2	moderate stage
3	severe stage
4	indeterminate stage
    - **Coding Clinic: 2016, Q4, P22**
    - H40.111 Primary open-angle glaucoma, right eye
      - **Coding Clinic: 2019, Q2, P31**
    - H40.112 Primary open-angle glaucoma, left eye
    - H40.113 Primary open-angle glaucoma, bilateral
    - H40.119 Primary open-angle glaucoma, unspecified eye

- **H40.12** Low-tension glaucoma
  - One of the following 7th characters is to be assigned to each code in subcategory H40.12 to designate the stage of glaucoma
0	stage unspecified
1	mild stage
2	moderate stage
3	severe stage
4	indeterminate stage
  - H40.121 Low-tension glaucoma, **right eye**
  - H40.122 Low-tension glaucoma, **left eye**
  - H40.123 Low-tension glaucoma, **bilateral**
  - H40.129 Low-tension glaucoma, **unspecified** eye
- **H40.13** Pigmentary glaucoma
  - One of the following 7th characters is to be assigned to each code in subcategory H40.13 to designate the stage of glaucoma
0	stage unspecified
1	mild stage
2	moderate stage
3	severe stage
4	indeterminate stage
  - H40.131 Pigmentary glaucoma, **right eye**
  - H40.132 Pigmentary glaucoma, **left eye**
  - H40.133 Pigmentary glaucoma, **bilateral**
  - H40.139 Pigmentary glaucoma, **unspecified** eye
- **H40.14** Capsular glaucoma **with pseudoexfoliation of lens**
  - One of the following 7th characters is to be assigned to each code in subcategory H40.14 to designate the stage of glaucoma
0	stage unspecified
1	mild stage
2	moderate stage
3	severe stage
4	indeterminate stage
  - H40.141 Capsular glaucoma with pseudoexfoliation of lens, **right eye**
  - H40.142 Capsular glaucoma with pseudoexfoliation of lens, **left eye**
  - H40.143 Capsular glaucoma with pseudoexfoliation of lens, **bilateral**
  - H40.149 Capsular glaucoma with pseudoexfoliation of lens, **unspecified** eye
- **H40.15** Residual stage of open-angle glaucoma
  - H40.151 Residual stage of open-angle glaucoma, **right eye**
  - H40.152 Residual stage of open-angle glaucoma, **left eye**
  - H40.153 Residual stage of open-angle glaucoma, **bilateral**
  - H40.159 Residual stage of open-angle glaucoma, **unspecified** eye
- **H40.2** Primary angle-closure glaucoma
  - **Excludes1** aqueous misdirection (H40.83-)
    - malignant glaucoma (H40.83-)
  - X **H40.20** Unspecified primary angle-closure glaucoma
    - One of the following 7th characters is to be assigned to code H40.20 to designate the stage of glaucoma
0	stage unspecified
1	mild stage
2	moderate stage
3	severe stage
4	indeterminate stage

▶ New ⇒ Revised ~~deleted~~ Deleted Excludes 1 Excludes 2 Includes Use additional Code first Code also Key words
OGCR Official Guidelines X Assign placeholder X ● Use Additional Character(s) ▷ Manifestation Code Hierarchical Condition Category **Coding Clinic**

● **H40.21** **Acute angle-closure glaucoma**
      Acute angle-closure glaucoma attack
      Acute angle-closure glaucoma crisis

    H40.211 **Acute angle-closure glaucoma, right eye**

    H40.212 **Acute angle-closure glaucoma, left eye**

    H40.213 **Acute angle-closure glaucoma, bilateral**

    H40.219 **Acute angle-closure glaucoma, unspecified eye**

● **H40.22** **Chronic angle-closure glaucoma**
      Chronic primary angle closure glaucoma

      One of the following 7th characters is to be assigned to each code in subcategory H40.22 to designate the stage of glaucoma

0	stage unspecified
1	mild stage
2	moderate stage
3	severe stage
4	indeterminate stage

  ● **H40.221** **Chronic angle-closure glaucoma, right eye**

  ● **H40.222** **Chronic angle-closure glaucoma, left eye**

  ● **H40.223** **Chronic angle-closure glaucoma, bilateral**

  ● **H40.229** **Chronic angle-closure glaucoma, unspecified eye**

● **H40.23** **Intermittent angle-closure glaucoma**

    H40.231 **Intermittent angle-closure glaucoma, right eye**

    H40.232 **Intermittent angle-closure glaucoma, left eye**

    H40.233 **Intermittent angle-closure glaucoma, bilateral**

    H40.239 **Intermittent angle-closure glaucoma, unspecified eye**

● **H40.24** **Residual stage of angle-closure glaucoma**

    H40.241 **Residual stage of angle-closure glaucoma, right eye**

    H40.242 **Residual stage of angle-closure glaucoma, left eye**

    H40.243 **Residual stage of angle-closure glaucoma, bilateral**

    H40.249 **Residual stage of angle-closure glaucoma, unspecified eye**

● **H40.3** **Glaucoma secondary to eye trauma**
      Code also underlying condition

      One of the following 7th characters is to be assigned to each code in subcategory H40.3 to designate the stage of glaucoma

0	stage unspecified
1	mild stage
2	moderate stage
3	severe stage
4	indeterminate stage

  X ● **H40.30** **Glaucoma secondary to eye trauma, unspecified eye**

  X ● **H40.31** **Glaucoma secondary to eye trauma, right eye**

  X ● **H40.32** **Glaucoma secondary to eye trauma, left eye**

  X ● **H40.33** **Glaucoma secondary to eye trauma, bilateral**

● **H40.4** **Glaucoma secondary to eye inflammation**
      Code also underlying condition

      One of the following 7th characters is to be assigned to each code in subcategory H40.4 to designate the stage of glaucoma

0	stage unspecified
1	mild stage
2	moderate stage
3	severe stage
4	indeterminate stage

  X ● **H40.40** **Glaucoma secondary to eye inflammation, unspecified eye**

  X ● **H40.41** **Glaucoma secondary to eye inflammation, right eye**

  X ● **H40.42** **Glaucoma secondary to eye inflammation, left eye**

  X ● **H40.43** **Glaucoma secondary to eye inflammation, bilateral**

● **H40.5** **Glaucoma secondary to other eye disorders**
      Code also underlying eye disorder

      One of the following 7th characters is to be assigned to each code in subcategory H40.5 to designate the stage of glaucoma

0	stage unspecified
1	mild stage
2	moderate stage
3	severe stage
4	indeterminate stage

  X ● **H40.50** **Glaucoma secondary to other eye disorders, unspecified eye**

  X ● **H40.51** **Glaucoma secondary to other eye disorders, right eye**

  X ● **H40.52** **Glaucoma secondary to other eye disorders, left eye**

  X ● **H40.53** **Glaucoma secondary to other eye disorders, bilateral**

● **H40.6** **Glaucoma secondary to drugs**
      Use additional code for adverse effect, if applicable, to identify drug (T36-T50 with fifth or sixth character 5)

      One of the following 7th characters is to be assigned to each code in subcategory H40.6 to designate the stage of glaucoma

0	stage unspecified
1	mild stage
2	moderate stage
3	severe stage
4	indeterminate stage

  X ● **H40.60** **Glaucoma secondary to drugs, unspecified eye**

  X ● **H40.61** **Glaucoma secondary to drugs, right eye**

  X ● **H40.62** **Glaucoma secondary to drugs, left eye**

  X ● **H40.63** **Glaucoma secondary to drugs, bilateral**

● **H40.8** **Other glaucoma**

  ● **H40.81** **Glaucoma with increased episcleral venous pressure**

    H40.811 **Glaucoma with increased episcleral venous pressure, right eye**

    H40.812 **Glaucoma with increased episcleral venous pressure, left eye**

    H40.813 **Glaucoma with increased episcleral venous pressure, bilateral**

    H40.819 **Glaucoma with increased episcleral venous pressure, unspecified eye**

CHAPTER 7 (H00-H59)

● H40.82   Hypersecretion glaucoma
    H40.821   Hypersecretion glaucoma, right eye
    H40.822   Hypersecretion glaucoma, left eye
    H40.823   Hypersecretion glaucoma, bilateral
    H40.829   Hypersecretion glaucoma, unspecified eye

● H40.83   Aqueous misdirection
    Malignant glaucoma
    H40.831   Aqueous misdirection, right eye
    H40.832   Aqueous misdirection, left eye
    H40.833   Aqueous misdirection, bilateral
    H40.839   Aqueous misdirection, unspecified eye

   H40.89   Other specified glaucoma

  H40.9   Unspecified glaucoma

� *H42*   *Glaucoma in diseases classified elsewhere*
    Code first underlying condition, such as:
      amyloidosis (E85.-)
      aniridia (Q13.1)
      glaucoma (in) diabetes mellitus (E08.39, E09.39, E10.39, E11.39, E13.39)
      Lowe's syndrome (E72.03)
      Reiger's anomaly (Q13.81)
      specified metabolic disorder (E70-E88)
    Excludes1   glaucoma (in) onchocerciasis (B73.02)
        glaucoma (in) syphilis (A52.71)
        glaucoma (in) tuberculous (A18.59)

DISORDERS OF VITREOUS BODY AND GLOBE (H43-H44)

● H43   **Disorders of vitreous body**
 ● H43.0   Vitreous prolapse
    Excludes1   vitreous syndrome following cataract surgery (H59.0-)
        traumatic vitreous prolapse (S05.2-)
    H43.00   Vitreous prolapse, unspecified eye
    H43.01   Vitreous prolapse, right eye
    H43.02   Vitreous prolapse, left eye
    H43.03   Vitreous prolapse, bilateral

 ● H43.1   Vitreous hemorrhage
    H43.10   Vitreous hemorrhage, unspecified eye 🐾
    H43.11   Vitreous hemorrhage, right eye 🐾
    H43.12   Vitreous hemorrhage, left eye 🐾
    H43.13   Vitreous hemorrhage, bilateral 🐾

 ● H43.2   Crystalline deposits in vitreous body
    H43.20   Crystalline deposits in vitreous body, unspecified eye
    H43.21   Crystalline deposits in vitreous body, right eye
    H43.22   Crystalline deposits in vitreous body, left eye
    H43.23   Crystalline deposits in vitreous body, bilateral

 ● H43.3   Other vitreous opacities
  ● H43.31   Vitreous membranes and strands
    H43.311   Vitreous membranes and strands, right eye
    H43.312   Vitreous membranes and strands, left eye
    H43.313   Vitreous membranes and strands, bilateral
    H43.319   Vitreous membranes and strands, unspecified eye

  ● H43.39   Other vitreous opacities
    Vitreous floaters
    Small clumps of cells that float in the vitreous of the eye, appearing as black specks or dots in the field of vision and common in the aging eye.
    H43.391   Other vitreous opacities, right eye
    H43.392   Other vitreous opacities, left eye

    H43.393   Other vitreous opacities, bilateral
    H43.399   Other vitreous opacities, unspecified eye

 ● H43.8   Other disorders of vitreous body
    Excludes1   proliferative vitreo-retinopathy with retinal detachment (H33.4)
    Excludes2   vitreous abscess (H44.02-)
  ● H43.81   Vitreous degeneration
    Vitreous detachment
    H43.811   Vitreous degeneration, right eye
    H43.812   Vitreous degeneration, left eye
    H43.813   Vitreous degeneration, bilateral
    H43.819   Vitreous degeneration, unspecified eye

  ● H43.82   Vitreomacular adhesion
    Vitreomacular traction
    H43.821   Vitreomacular adhesion, right eye   A
    H43.822   Vitreomacular adhesion, left eye   A
    H43.823   Vitreomacular adhesion, bilateral   A
    H43.829   Vitreomacular adhesion, unspecified eye   A

  H43.89   Other disorders of vitreous body
  H43.9   Unspecified disorder of vitreous body

● H44   **Disorders of globe**
  Includes   disorders affecting multiple structures of eye
 ● H44.0   Purulent endophthalmitis
    Use additional code to identify organism
    Excludes1   bleb associated endophthalmitis (H59.4-)
  ● H44.00   Unspecified purulent endophthalmitis
    H44.001   Unspecified purulent endophthalmitis, right eye
    H44.002   Unspecified purulent endophthalmitis, left eye
    H44.003   Unspecified purulent endophthalmitis, bilateral
    H44.009   Unspecified purulent endophthalmitis, unspecified eye

  ● H44.01   Panophthalmitis (acute)
    H44.011   Panophthalmitis (acute), right eye
    H44.012   Panophthalmitis (acute), left eye
    H44.013   Panophthalmitis (acute), bilateral
    H44.019   Panophthalmitis (acute), unspecified eye

  ● H44.02   Vitreous abscess (chronic)
    H44.021   Vitreous abscess (chronic), right eye
    H44.022   Vitreous abscess (chronic), left eye
    H44.023   Vitreous abscess (chronic), bilateral
    H44.029   Vitreous abscess (chronic), unspecified eye

 ● H44.1   Other endophthalmitis
    Excludes1   bleb associated endophthalmitis (H59.4-)
    Excludes2   ophthalmia nodosa (H16.2-)
  ● H44.11   Panuveitis
    H44.111   Panuveitis, right eye
    H44.112   Panuveitis, left eye
    H44.113   Panuveitis, bilateral
    H44.119   Panuveitis, unspecified eye

  ● H44.12   Parasitic endophthalmitis, unspecified
    H44.121   Parasitic endophthalmitis, unspecified, right eye
    H44.122   Parasitic endophthalmitis, unspecified, left eye
    H44.123   Parasitic endophthalmitis, unspecified, bilateral
    H44.129   Parasitic endophthalmitis, unspecified, unspecified eye

CHAPTER 7 (H00-H59)

- **H44.13**   Sympathetic uveitis
  - H44.131   Sympathetic uveitis, right eye
  - H44.132   Sympathetic uveitis, left eye
  - H44.133   Sympathetic uveitis, bilateral
  - H44.139   Sympathetic uveitis, unspecified eye
  - H44.19   Other endophthalmitis
- **H44.2**   Degenerative myopia
  - Malignant myopia
  - H44.20   Degenerative myopia, unspecified eye
  - H44.21   Degenerative myopia, right eye
  - H44.22   Degenerative myopia, left eye
  - H44.23   Degenerative myopia, bilateral
- **H44.2A**   Degenerative myopia with choroidal neovascularization
  - Use Additional code for any associated choroid disorders (H31.-)
  - H44.2A1   Degenerative myopia with choroidal neovascularization, right eye
  - H44.2A2   Degenerative myopia with choroidal neovascularization, left eye
  - H44.2A3   Degenerative myopia with choroidal neovascularization, bilateral eye
  - H44.2A9   Degenerative myopia with choroidal neovascularization, unspecified eye
- **H44.2B**   Degenerative myopia with macular hole
  - H44.2B1   Degenerative myopia with macular hole, right eye
  - H44.2B2   Degenerative myopia with macular hole, left eye
  - H44.2B3   Degenerative myopia with macular hole, bilateral eye
  - H44.2B9   Degenerative myopia with macular hole, unspecified eye
- **H44.2C**   Degenerative myopia with retinal detachment
  - Use Additional code to identify the retinal detachment (H33.-)
  - H44.2C1   Degenerative myopia with retinal detachment, right eye
  - H44.2C2   Degenerative myopia with retinal detachment, left eye
  - H44.2C3   Degenerative myopia with retinal detachment, bilateral eye
  - H44.2C9   Degenerative myopia with retinal detachment, unspecified eye
- **H44.2D**   Degenerative myopia with foveoschisis
  - H44.2D1   Degenerative myopia with foveoschisis, right eye
  - H44.2D2   Degenerative myopia with foveoschisis, left eye
  - H44.2D3   Degenerative myopia with foveoschisis, bilateral eye
  - H44.2D9   Degenerative myopia with foveoschisis, unspecified eye
- **H44.2E**   Degenerative myopia with other maculopathy
  - H44.2E1   Degenerative myopia with other maculopathy, right eye
  - H44.2E2   Degenerative myopia with other maculopathy, left eye
  - H44.2E3   Degenerative myopia with other maculopathy, bilateral eye
  - H44.2E9   Degenerative myopia with other maculopathy, unspecified eye
- **H44.3**   Other and unspecified degenerative disorders of globe
  - H44.30   Unspecified degenerative disorder of globe
- **H44.31**   Chalcosis
  - H44.311   Chalcosis, right eye
  - H44.312   Chalcosis, left eye
  - H44.313   Chalcosis, bilateral
  - H44.319   Chalcosis, unspecified eye

- **H44.32**   Siderosis of eye
  - H44.321   Siderosis of eye, right eye
  - H44.322   Siderosis of eye, left eye
  - H44.323   Siderosis of eye, bilateral
  - H44.329   Siderosis of eye, unspecified eye
- **H44.39**   Other degenerative disorders of globe
  - H44.391   Other degenerative disorders of globe, right eye
  - H44.392   Other degenerative disorders of globe, left eye
  - H44.393   Other degenerative disorders of globe, bilateral
  - H44.399   Other degenerative disorders of globe, unspecified eye
- **H44.4**   Hypotony of eye
  - H44.40   Unspecified hypotony of eye
- **H44.41**   Flat anterior chamber hypotony of eye
  - H44.411   Flat anterior chamber hypotony of right eye
  - H44.412   Flat anterior chamber hypotony of left eye
  - H44.413   Flat anterior chamber hypotony of eye, bilateral
  - H44.419   Flat anterior chamber hypotony of unspecified eye
- **H44.42**   Hypotony of eye due to ocular fistula
  - H44.421   Hypotony of right eye due to ocular fistula
  - H44.422   Hypotony of left eye due to ocular fistula
  - H44.423   Hypotony of eye due to ocular fistula, bilateral
  - H44.429   Hypotony of unspecified eye due to ocular fistula
- **H44.43**   Hypotony of eye due to other ocular disorders
  - H44.431   Hypotony of eye due to other ocular disorders, right eye
  - H44.432   Hypotony of eye due to other ocular disorders, left eye
  - H44.433   Hypotony of eye due to other ocular disorders, bilateral
  - H44.439   Hypotony of eye due to other ocular disorders, unspecified eye
- **H44.44**   Primary hypotony of eye
  - H44.441   Primary hypotony of right eye
  - H44.442   Primary hypotony of left eye
  - H44.443   Primary hypotony of eye, bilateral
  - H44.449   Primary hypotony of unspecified eye
- **H44.5**   Degenerated conditions of globe
  - H44.50   Unspecified degenerated conditions of globe
- **H44.51**   Absolute glaucoma
  - H44.511   Absolute glaucoma, right eye
  - H44.512   Absolute glaucoma, left eye
  - H44.513   Absolute glaucoma, bilateral
  - H44.519   Absolute glaucoma, unspecified eye
- **H44.52**   Atrophy of globe
  - Phthisis bulbi
  - H44.521   Atrophy of globe, right eye
  - H44.522   Atrophy of globe, left eye
  - H44.523   Atrophy of globe, bilateral
  - H44.529   Atrophy of globe, unspecified eye
- **H44.53**   Leucocoria
  - H44.531   Leucocoria, right eye
  - H44.532   Leucocoria, left eye
  - H44.533   Leucocoria, bilateral
  - H44.539   Leucocoria, unspecified eye

CHAPTER 7 (H00-H59)

● H44.6   Retained (old) intraocular foreign body, magnetic

Use additional code to identify magnetic foreign body (Z18.11)

Excludes1   current intraocular foreign body (S05.-)

Excludes2   retained foreign body in eyelid (H02.81-)
retained (old) foreign body following penetrating wound of orbit (H05.5-)
retained (old) intraocular foreign body, nonmagnetic (H44.7-)

● H44.60   Unspecified retained (old) intraocular foreign body, magnetic

H44.601   Unspecified retained (old) intraocular foreign body, magnetic, right eye

H44.602   Unspecified retained (old) intraocular foreign body, magnetic, left eye

H44.603   Unspecified retained (old) intraocular foreign body, magnetic, bilateral

H44.609   Unspecified retained (old) intraocular foreign body, magnetic, unspecified eye

● H44.61   Retained (old) magnetic foreign body in anterior chamber

H44.611   Retained (old) magnetic foreign body in anterior chamber, right eye

H44.612   Retained (old) magnetic foreign body in anterior chamber, left eye

H44.613   Retained (old) magnetic foreign body in anterior chamber, bilateral

H44.619   Retained (old) magnetic foreign body in anterior chamber, unspecified eye

● H44.62   Retained (old) magnetic foreign body in iris or ciliary body

H44.621   Retained (old) magnetic foreign body in iris or ciliary body, right eye

H44.622   Retained (old) magnetic foreign body in iris or ciliary body, left eye

H44.623   Retained (old) magnetic foreign body in iris or ciliary body, bilateral

H44.629   Retained (old) magnetic foreign body in iris or ciliary body, unspecified eye

● H44.63   Retained (old) magnetic foreign body in lens

H44.631   Retained (old) magnetic foreign body in lens, right eye

H44.632   Retained (old) magnetic foreign body in lens, left eye

H44.633   Retained (old) magnetic foreign body in lens, bilateral

H44.639   Retained (old) magnetic foreign body in lens, unspecified eye

● H44.64   Retained (old) magnetic foreign body in posterior wall of globe

H44.641   Retained (old) magnetic foreign body in posterior wall of globe, right eye

H44.642   Retained (old) magnetic foreign body in posterior wall of globe, left eye

H44.643   Retained (old) magnetic foreign body in posterior wall of globe, bilateral

H44.649   Retained (old) magnetic foreign body in posterior wall of globe, unspecified eye

● H44.65   Retained (old) magnetic foreign body in vitreous body

H44.651   Retained (old) magnetic foreign body in vitreous body, right eye

H44.652   Retained (old) magnetic foreign body in vitreous body, left eye

H44.653   Retained (old) magnetic foreign body in vitreous body, bilateral

H44.659   Retained (old) magnetic foreign body in vitreous body, unspecified eye

● H44.69   Retained (old) intraocular foreign body, magnetic, in other or multiple sites

H44.691   Retained (old) intraocular foreign body, magnetic, in other or multiple sites, right eye

H44.692   Retained (old) intraocular foreign body, magnetic, in other or multiple sites, left eye

H44.693   Retained (old) intraocular foreign body, magnetic, in other or multiple sites, bilateral

H44.699   Retained (old) intraocular foreign body, magnetic, in other or multiple sites, unspecified eye

● H44.7   Retained (old) intraocular foreign body, nonmagnetic

Use additional code to identify nonmagnetic foreign body (Z18.01-Z18.10, Z18.12, Z18.2-Z18.9)

Excludes1   current intraocular foreign body (S05.-)

Excludes2   retained foreign body in eyelid (H02.81-)
retained (old) foreign body following penetrating wound of orbit (H05.5-)
retained (old) intraocular foreign body, magnetic (H44.6-)

● H44.70   Unspecified retained (old) intraocular foreign body, nonmagnetic

H44.701   Unspecified retained (old) intraocular foreign body, nonmagnetic, right eye

H44.702   Unspecified retained (old) intraocular foreign body, nonmagnetic, left eye

H44.703   Unspecified retained (old) intraocular foreign body, nonmagnetic, bilateral

H44.709   Unspecified retained (old) intraocular foreign body, nonmagnetic, unspecified eye

Retained (old) intraocular foreign body NOS

● H44.71   Retained (nonmagnetic) (old) foreign body in anterior chamber

H44.711   Retained (nonmagnetic) (old) foreign body in anterior chamber, right eye

H44.712   Retained (nonmagnetic) (old) foreign body in anterior chamber, left eye

H44.713   Retained (nonmagnetic) (old) foreign body in anterior chamber, bilateral

H44.719   Retained (nonmagnetic) (old) foreign body in anterior chamber, unspecified eye

● H44.72   Retained (nonmagnetic) (old) foreign body in iris or ciliary body

H44.721   Retained (nonmagnetic) (old) foreign body in iris or ciliary body, right eye

H44.722   Retained (nonmagnetic) (old) foreign body in iris or ciliary body, left eye

H44.723   Retained (nonmagnetic) (old) foreign body in iris or ciliary body, bilateral

H44.729   Retained (nonmagnetic) (old) foreign body in iris or ciliary body, unspecified eye

● H44.73   Retained (nonmagnetic) (old) foreign body in lens

H44.731   Retained (nonmagnetic) (old) foreign body in lens, right eye

H44.732   Retained (nonmagnetic) (old) foreign body in lens, left eye

H44.733   Retained (nonmagnetic) (old) foreign body in lens, bilateral

H44.739   Retained (nonmagnetic) (old) foreign body in lens, unspecified eye

▶ New   ⟹ Revised   ~~deleted~~ Deleted   Excludes 1   Excludes 2   Includes   Use additional   Code first   Code also   Key words

OGCR Official Guidelines   X Assign placeholder X   ● Use Additional Character(s)   ▶ Manifestation Code   🄗 Hierarchical Condition Category   Coding Clinic

● H44.74 Retained (nonmagnetic) (old) foreign body in posterior wall of globe

  H44.741 Retained (nonmagnetic) (old) foreign body in posterior wall of globe, right eye

  H44.742 Retained (nonmagnetic) (old) foreign body in posterior wall of globe, left eye

  H44.743 Retained (nonmagnetic) (old) foreign body in posterior wall of globe, bilateral

  H44.749 Retained (nonmagnetic) (old) foreign body in posterior wall of globe, unspecified eye

● H44.75 Retained (nonmagnetic) (old) foreign body in vitreous body

  H44.751 Retained (nonmagnetic) (old) foreign body in vitreous body, right eye

  H44.752 Retained (nonmagnetic) (old) foreign body in vitreous body, left eye

  H44.753 Retained (nonmagnetic) (old) foreign body in vitreous body, bilateral

  H44.759 Retained (nonmagnetic) (old) foreign body in vitreous body, unspecified eye

● H44.79 Retained (old) intraocular foreign body, nonmagnetic, in other or multiple sites

  H44.791 Retained (old) intraocular foreign body, nonmagnetic, in other or multiple sites, right eye

  H44.792 Retained (old) intraocular foreign body, nonmagnetic, in other or multiple sites, left eye

  H44.793 Retained (old) intraocular foreign body, nonmagnetic, in other or multiple sites, bilateral

  H44.799 Retained (old) intraocular foreign body, nonmagnetic, in other or multiple sites, unspecified eye

● H44.8 Other disorders of globe

  ● H44.81 Hemophthalmos

    H44.811 Hemophthalmos, right eye

    H44.812 Hemophthalmos, left eye

    H44.813 Hemophthalmos, bilateral

    H44.819 Hemophthalmos, unspecified eye

  ● H44.82 Luxation of globe

    H44.821 Luxation of globe, right eye

    H44.822 Luxation of globe, left eye

    H44.823 Luxation of globe, bilateral

    H44.829 Luxation of globe, unspecified eye

  H44.89 Other disorders of globe

  H44.9 Unspecified disorder of globe

★ (See Plate 7 of the Anatomy Illustrations.)

DISORDERS OF OPTIC NERVE AND VISUAL PATHWAYS (H46-H47)

● H46 Optic neuritis

  Excludes2 ischemic optic neuropathy (H47.01-)
  neuromyelitis optica [Devic] (G36.0)

● H46.0 Optic papillitis

  H46.00 Optic papillitis, unspecified eye

  H46.01 Optic papillitis, right eye

  H46.02 Optic papillitis, left eye

  H46.03 Optic papillitis, bilateral

● H46.1 Retrobulbar neuritis

  Retrobulbar neuritis NOS

  Excludes1 syphilitic retrobulbar neuritis (A52.15)

  H46.10 Retrobulbar neuritis, unspecified eye

  H46.11 Retrobulbar neuritis, right eye

  H46.12 Retrobulbar neuritis, left eye

  H46.13 Retrobulbar neuritis, bilateral

H46.2 Nutritional optic neuropathy

H46.3 Toxic optic neuropathy

  Code first (T51-T65) to identify cause

H46.8 Other optic neuritis

H46.9 Unspecified optic neuritis

● H47 Other disorders of optic [2nd] nerve and visual pathways

● H47.0 Disorders of optic nerve, not elsewhere classified

  ● H47.01 Ischemic optic neuropathy

    H47.011 Ischemic optic neuropathy, right eye

    H47.012 Ischemic optic neuropathy, left eye

    H47.013 Ischemic optic neuropathy, bilateral

    H47.019 Ischemic optic neuropathy, unspecified eye

  ● H47.02 Hemorrhage in optic nerve sheath

    H47.021 Hemorrhage in optic nerve sheath, right eye

    H47.022 Hemorrhage in optic nerve sheath, left eye

    H47.023 Hemorrhage in optic nerve sheath, bilateral

    H47.029 Hemorrhage in optic nerve sheath, unspecified eye

  ● H47.03 Optic nerve hypoplasia

    H47.031 Optic nerve hypoplasia, right eye

    H47.032 Optic nerve hypoplasia, left eye

    H47.033 Optic nerve hypoplasia, bilateral

    H47.039 Optic nerve hypoplasia, unspecified eye

  ● H47.09 Other disorders of optic nerve, not elsewhere classified

    Compression of optic nerve

    H47.091 Other disorders of optic nerve, not elsewhere classified, right eye

    H47.092 Other disorders of optic nerve, not elsewhere classified, left eye

    H47.093 Other disorders of optic nerve, not elsewhere classified, bilateral

    H47.099 Other disorders of optic nerve, not elsewhere classified, unspecified eye

● H47.1 Papilledema

  H47.10 Unspecified papilledema

  H47.11 Papilledema associated with increased intracranial pressure

Figure 7-11 Stages of papilledema according to the Frisén grading scale. **A,** Very eary papilledema (Frisén stage 1). **B,** Early papilledema (Frisén stage 2). **C,** Moderate papilledema (Frisén stage 3). **D,** Marked papilledema (Frisén stage 4). **E,** Severe papilledema. (From Youmans JR, Winn HR: Youmans Neurological Surgery, Philadelphia, PA, Elsevier/Saunders, 2011)

Item 7-8 Papilledema is swelling of the optic disc caused by increased intracranial pressure. It is most often bilateral and occurs quickly (hours) or over weeks of time. It is a common symptom of a brain tumor. The term should not be used to describe optic disc swelling with underlying infectious, infiltrative, or inflammatory etiologies.

CHAPTER 7 (H00-H59)

H47.12   Papilledema associated with decreased ocular pressure

H47.13   Papilledema associated with retinal disorder

● H47.14   Foster-Kennedy syndrome

     H47.141   Foster-Kennedy syndrome, right eye

     H47.142   Foster-Kennedy syndrome, left eye

     H47.143   Foster-Kennedy syndrome, bilateral

     H47.149   Foster-Kennedy syndrome, unspecified eye

● H47.2   Optic atrophy

   H47.20   Unspecified optic atrophy

● H47.21   Primary optic atrophy

     H47.211   Primary optic atrophy, right eye

     H47.212   Primary optic atrophy, left eye

     H47.213   Primary optic atrophy, bilateral

     H47.219   Primary optic atrophy, unspecified eye

   H47.22   Hereditary optic atrophy
        Leber's optic atrophy

● H47.23   Glaucomatous optic atrophy

     H47.231   Glaucomatous optic atrophy, right eye

     H47.232   Glaucomatous optic atrophy, left eye

     H47.233   Glaucomatous optic atrophy, bilateral

     H47.239   Glaucomatous optic atrophy, unspecified eye

● H47.29   Other optic atrophy
        Temporal pallor of optic disc

     H47.291   Other optic atrophy, right eye

     H47.292   Other optic atrophy, left eye

     H47.293   Other optic atrophy, bilateral

     H47.299   Other optic atrophy, unspecified eye

● H47.3   Other disorders of optic disc

● H47.31   Coloboma of optic disc

     H47.311   Coloboma of optic disc, right eye

     H47.312   Coloboma of optic disc, left eye

     H47.313   Coloboma of optic disc, bilateral

     H47.319   Coloboma of optic disc, unspecified eye

● H47.32   Drusen of optic disc

     H47.321   Drusen of optic disc, right eye

     H47.322   Drusen of optic disc, left eye

     H47.323   Drusen of optic disc, bilateral

     H47.329   Drusen of optic disc, unspecified eye

● H47.33   Pseudopapilledema of optic disc

     H47.331   Pseudopapilledema of optic disc, right eye

     H47.332   Pseudopapilledema of optic disc, left eye

     H47.333   Pseudopapilledema of optic disc, bilateral

     H47.339   Pseudopapilledema of optic disc, unspecified eye

● H47.39   Other disorders of optic disc

     H47.391   Other disorders of optic disc, right eye

     H47.392   Other disorders of optic disc, left eye

     H47.393   Other disorders of optic disc, bilateral

     H47.399   Other disorders of optic disc, unspecified eye

● H47.4   Disorders of optic chiasm
     Code also underlying condition

   H47.41   Disorders of optic chiasm in (due to) inflammatory disorders

   H47.42   Disorders of optic chiasm in (due to) neoplasm

H47.43   Disorders of optic chiasm in (due to) vascular disorders

H47.49   Disorders of optic chiasm in (due to) other disorders

● H47.5   Disorders of other visual pathways
     Disorders of optic tracts, geniculate nuclei and optic radiations
     Code also underlying condition

● H47.51   Disorders of visual pathways in (due to) inflammatory disorders

     H47.511   Disorders of visual pathways in (due to) inflammatory disorders, right side

     H47.512   Disorders of visual pathways in (due to) inflammatory disorders, left side

     H47.519   Disorders of visual pathways in (due to) inflammatory disorders, unspecified side

● H47.52   Disorders of visual pathways in (due to) neoplasm

     H47.521   Disorders of visual pathways in (due to) neoplasm, right side

     H47.522   Disorders of visual pathways in (due to) neoplasm, left side

     H47.529   Disorders of visual pathways in (due to) neoplasm, unspecified side

● H47.53   Disorders of visual pathways in (due to) vascular disorders

     H47.531   Disorders of visual pathways in (due to) vascular disorders, right side

     H47.532   Disorders of visual pathways in (due to) vascular disorders, left side

     H47.539   Disorders of visual pathways in (due to) vascular disorders, unspecified side

● H47.6   Disorders of visual cortex
     Code also underlying condition
     Excludes1   injury to visual cortex S04.04-

● H47.61   Cortical blindness

     H47.611   Cortical blindness, right side of brain

     H47.612   Cortical blindness, left side of brain

     H47.619   Cortical blindness, unspecified side of brain

● H47.62   Disorders of visual cortex in (due to) inflammatory disorders

     H47.621   Disorders of visual cortex in (due to) inflammatory disorders, right side of brain

     H47.622   Disorders of visual cortex in (due to) inflammatory disorders, left side of brain

     H47.629   Disorders of visual cortex in (due to) inflammatory disorders, unspecified side of brain

● H47.63   Disorders of visual cortex in (due to) neoplasm

     H47.631   Disorders of visual cortex in (due to) neoplasm, right side of brain

     H47.632   Disorders of visual cortex in (due to) neoplasm, left side of brain

     H47.639   Disorders of visual cortex in (due to) neoplasm, unspecified side of brain

● H47.64   Disorders of visual cortex in (due to) vascular disorders

     H47.641   Disorders of visual cortex in (due to) vascular disorders, right side of brain

     H47.642   Disorders of visual cortex in (due to) vascular disorders, left side of brain

     H47.649   Disorders of visual cortex in (due to) vascular disorders, unspecified side of brain

H47.9   Unspecified disorder of visual pathways

▶ New   ⇒ Revised   ~~deleted~~ Deleted   Excludes 1   Excludes 2   Includes   Use additional   Code first   Code also   Key words

OGCR Official Guidelines   X Assign placeholder X   ● Use Additional Character(s)   ▶ Manifestation Code   🔖 Hierarchical Condition Category   **Coding Clinic**

Figure 7-12   A. Image of strabismus. **B.** Exotropia. (**A** from Yanoff: *Ophthalmology,* ed 3, Mosby, Inc., 2008. **B** from Zitelli BJ, Davis HW, *Pediatric Physical Diagnosis: Atlas of Pediatric Physical Diagnosis,* Philadelphia, Elsevier Saunders, 2012)

Item 7–9 Strabismus or esotropia (crossed eyes) is a condition of the extraocular eye muscles, resulting in an inability of the eyes to focus and also affects depth perception.

DISORDERS OF OCULAR MUSCLES, BINOCULAR MOVEMENT, ACCOMMODATION AND REFRACTION (H49-H52)

> **Excludes2**   nystagmus and other irregular eye movements (H55)

● H49   **Paralytic strabismus**
> **Excludes2**   internal ophthalmoplegia (H52.51-)
> internuclear ophthalmoplegia (H51.2-)
> progressive supranuclear ophthalmoplegia (G23.1)

● H49.0   Third [oculomotor] nerve palsy
    H49.00   Third [oculomotor] nerve palsy, unspecified eye
    H49.01   Third [oculomotor] nerve palsy, right eye
    H49.02   Third [oculomotor] nerve palsy, left eye
    H49.03   Third [oculomotor] nerve palsy, bilateral

● H49.1   Fourth [trochlear] nerve palsy
    H49.10   Fourth [trochlear] nerve palsy, unspecified eye
    H49.11   Fourth [trochlear] nerve palsy, right eye
    H49.12   Fourth [trochlear] nerve palsy, left eye
    H49.13   Fourth [trochlear] nerve palsy, bilateral

● H49.2   Sixth [abducent] nerve palsy
    H49.20   Sixth [abducent] nerve palsy, unspecified eye
    H49.21   Sixth [abducent] nerve palsy, right eye
    H49.22   Sixth [abducent] nerve palsy, left eye
    H49.23   Sixth [abducent] nerve palsy, bilateral

● H49.3   Total (external) ophthalmoplegia
    H49.30   Total (external) ophthalmoplegia, unspecified eye
    H49.31   Total (external) ophthalmoplegia, right eye
    H49.32   Total (external) ophthalmoplegia, left eye
    H49.33   Total (external) ophthalmoplegia, bilateral

● H49.4   Progressive external ophthalmoplegia
> **Excludes1**   Kearns-Sayre syndrome (H49.81-)

    H49.40   Progressive external ophthalmoplegia, unspecified eye
    H49.41   Progressive external ophthalmoplegia, right eye
    H49.42   Progressive external ophthalmoplegia, left eye
    H49.43   Progressive external ophthalmoplegia, bilateral

● H49.8   Other paralytic strabismus
  ● H49.81   Kearns-Sayre syndrome
      Progressive external ophthalmoplegia with pigmentary retinopathy
      Use additional code for other manifestation, such as:
       heart block (I45.9)
      H49.811   Kearns-Sayre syndrome, right eye
      H49.812   Kearns-Sayre syndrome, left eye

      H49.813   Kearns-Sayre syndrome, bilateral
      H49.819   Kearns-Sayre syndrome, unspecified eye
  ● H49.88   Other paralytic strabismus
      External ophthalmoplegia NOS
      H49.881   Other paralytic strabismus, right eye
      H49.882   Other paralytic strabismus, left eye
      H49.883   Other paralytic strabismus, bilateral
      H49.889   Other paralytic strabismus, unspecified eye
   H49.9   Unspecified paralytic strabismus

● H50   Other strabismus
  ● H50.0   Esotropia
      Convergent concomitant strabismus
> **Excludes1**   intermittent esotropia (H50.31-, H50.32)

    H50.00   Unspecified esotropia
  ● H50.01   Monocular esotropia
      H50.011   Monocular esotropia, right eye
      H50.012   Monocular esotropia, left eye
  ● H50.02   Monocular esotropia with A pattern
      H50.021   Monocular esotropia with A pattern, right eye
      H50.022   Monocular esotropia with A pattern, left eye
  ● H50.03   Monocular esotropia with V pattern
      H50.031   Monocular esotropia with V pattern, right eye
      H50.032   Monocular esotropia with V pattern, left eye
  ● H50.04   Monocular esotropia with other noncomitancies
      H50.041   Monocular esotropia with other noncomitancies, right eye
      H50.042   Monocular esotropia with other noncomitancies, left eye
    H50.05   Alternating esotropia
    H50.06   Alternating esotropia with A pattern
    H50.07   Alternating esotropia with V pattern
    H50.08   Alternating esotropia with other noncomitancies

  ● H50.1   Exotropia
> *Misalignment in which one eye deviates outward (away from nose) while the other fixates normally*
      Divergent concomitant strabismus
> **Excludes1**   intermittent exotropia (H50.33-, H50.34)

    H50.10   Unspecified exotropia
  ● H50.11   Monocular exotropia
      H50.111   Monocular exotropia, right eye
      H50.112   Monocular exotropia, left eye
  ● H50.12   Monocular exotropia with A pattern
      H50.121   Monocular exotropia with A pattern, right eye
      H50.122   Monocular exotropia with A pattern, left eye
  ● H50.13   Monocular exotropia with V pattern
      H50.131   Monocular exotropia with V pattern, right eye
      H50.132   Monocular exotropia with V pattern, left eye
  ● H50.14   Monocular exotropia with other noncomitancies
      H50.141   Monocular exotropia with other noncomitancies, right eye
      H50.142   Monocular exotropia with other noncomitancies, left eye
    H50.15   Alternating exotropia
    H50.16   Alternating exotropia with A pattern
    H50.17   Alternating exotropia with V pattern
    H50.18   Alternating exotropia with other noncomitancies

CHAPTER 7 (H00-H59)

- **H50.2 Vertical strabismus**
  Hypertropia
  - H50.21 Vertical strabismus, right eye
  - H50.22 Vertical strabismus, left eye
- **H50.3 Intermittent heterotropia**
  Displacement of an organ or part of an organ from its normal position
  - H50.30 Unspecified intermittent heterotropia
  - **H50.31 Intermittent monocular esotropia**
    - H50.311 Intermittent monocular esotropia, right eye
    - H50.312 Intermittent monocular esotropia, left eye
  - H50.32 Intermittent alternating esotropia
  - **H50.33 Intermittent monocular exotropia**
    - H50.331 Intermittent monocular exotropia, right eye
    - H50.332 Intermittent monocular exotropia, left eye
  - H50.34 Intermittent alternating exotropia
- **H50.4 Other and unspecified heterotropia**
  - H50.40 Unspecified heterotropia
  - **H50.41 Cyclotropia**
    - H50.411 Cyclotropia, right eye
    - H50.412 Cyclotropia, left eye
  - H50.42 Monofixation syndrome
  - H50.43 Accommodative component in esotropia
- **H50.5 Heterophoria**
  One or both eyes wander away from the position where both eyes are looking together in the same direction
  - H50.50 Unspecified heterophoria
  - H50.51 Esophoria
    Eye deviates inward (toward the nose)
  - H50.52 Exophoria
    Eye deviates outward (toward the ear)
  - H50.53 Vertical heterophoria
  - H50.54 Cyclophoria
  - H50.55 Alternating heterophoria
- **H50.6 Mechanical strabismus**
  - H50.60 Mechanical strabismus, unspecified
  - **H50.61 Brown's sheath syndrome**
    - H50.611 Brown's sheath syndrome, right eye
    - H50.612 Brown's sheath syndrome, left eye
  - H50.69 Other mechanical strabismus
    Strabismus due to adhesions
    Traumatic limitation of duction of eye muscle
- **H50.8 Other specified strabismus**
  - **H50.81 Duane's syndrome**
    - H50.811 Duane's syndrome, right eye
    - H50.812 Duane's syndrome, left eye
  - H50.89 Other specified strabismus
  - H50.9 Unspecified strabismus
- **H51 Other disorders of binocular movement**
  - H51.0 Palsy (spasm) of conjugate gaze
  - **H51.1 Convergence insufficiency and excess**
    - H51.11 Convergence insufficiency
    - H51.12 Convergence excess
  - **H51.2 Internuclear ophthalmoplegia**
    - H51.20 Internuclear ophthalmoplegia, unspecified eye
    - H51.21 Internuclear ophthalmoplegia, right eye
    - H51.22 Internuclear ophthalmoplegia, left eye
    - H51.23 Internuclear ophthalmoplegia, bilateral
  - H51.8 Other specified disorders of binocular movement
  - H51.9 Unspecified disorder of binocular movement

Item 7-10 Disorders of refraction: **Hypermetropia,** or farsightedness, means focus at a distance is adequate but not on close objects. **Myopia** is near-sightedness or short-sightedness and means the focus on nearby objects is clear but distant objects appear blurred. **Astigmatism** is warping of the curvature of the cornea so light rays entering do not meet a single focal point, resulting in a distorted image. **Anisometropia** is unequal refractive power in which one eye may be myopic (near-sighted) and the other hyperopic (far-sighted). **Presbyopia** is the loss of focus on near objects, which occurs with age because the lens loses elasticity.

- **H52 Disorders of refraction and accommodation**
  - **H52.0 Hypermetropia**
    - H52.00 Hypermetropia, unspecified eye
    - H52.01 Hypermetropia, right eye
    - H52.02 Hypermetropia, left eye
    - H52.03 Hypermetropia, bilateral
  - **H52.1 Myopia**
    - **Excludes1** degenerative myopia (H44.2-)
    - H52.10 Myopia, unspecified eye
    - H52.11 Myopia, right eye
    - H52.12 Myopia, left eye
    - H52.13 Myopia, bilateral
  - **H52.2 Astigmatism**
    - **H52.20 Unspecified astigmatism**
      - H52.201 Unspecified astigmatism, right eye
      - H52.202 Unspecified astigmatism, left eye
      - H52.203 Unspecified astigmatism, bilateral
      - H52.209 Unspecified astigmatism, unspecified eye
    - **H52.21 Irregular astigmatism**
      - H52.211 Irregular astigmatism, right eye
      - H52.212 Irregular astigmatism, left eye
      - H52.213 Irregular astigmatism, bilateral
      - H52.219 Irregular astigmatism, unspecified eye
    - **H52.22 Regular astigmatism**
      - H52.221 Regular astigmatism, right eye
      - H52.222 Regular astigmatism, left eye
      - H52.223 Regular astigmatism, bilateral
      - H52.229 Regular astigmatism, unspecified eye
  - **H52.3 Anisometropia and aniseikonia**
    - H52.31 Anisometropia
    - H52.32 Aniseikonia
  - H52.4 Presbyopia
  - **H52.5 Disorders of accommodation**
    - **H52.51 Internal ophthalmoplegia (complete) (total)**
      - H52.511 Internal ophthalmoplegia (complete) (total), right eye
      - H52.512 Internal ophthalmoplegia (complete) (total), left eye
      - H52.513 Internal ophthalmoplegia (complete) (total), bilateral
      - H52.519 Internal ophthalmoplegia (complete) (total), unspecified eye
    - **H52.52 Paresis of accommodation**
      - H52.521 Paresis of accommodation, right eye
      - H52.522 Paresis of accommodation, left eye
      - H52.523 Paresis of accommodation, bilateral
      - H52.529 Paresis of accommodation, unspecified eye
    - **H52.53 Spasm of accommodation**
      - H52.531 Spasm of accommodation, right eye
      - H52.532 Spasm of accommodation, left eye
      - H52.533 Spasm of accommodation, bilateral
      - H52.539 Spasm of accommodation, unspecified eye
  - H52.6 Other disorders of refraction
  - H52.7 Unspecified disorder of refraction

▶ New   ⟾ Revised   ~~deleted~~ Deleted   Excludes 1   Excludes 2   Includes   Use additional   Code first   Code also   Key words

OGCR Official Guidelines   X Assign placeholder X   ● Use Additional Character(s)   ▌ Manifestation Code   🗘 Hierarchical Condition Category   **Coding Clinic**

VISUAL DISTURBANCES AND BLINDNESS (H53-H54)

- **H53 Visual disturbances**
  - **H53.0 Amblyopia ex anopsia**
    - **Excludes1**   amblyopia due to vitamin A deficiency (E50.5)
    - **H53.00 Unspecified amblyopia**
      - H53.001   Unspecified amblyopia, right eye
      - H53.002   Unspecified amblyopia, left eye
      - H53.003   Unspecified amblyopia, bilateral
      - H53.009   Unspecified amblyopia, unspecified eye
    - **H53.01 Deprivation amblyopia**
      - H53.011   Deprivation amblyopia, right eye
      - H53.012   Deprivation amblyopia, left eye
      - H53.013   Deprivation amblyopia, bilateral
      - H53.019   Deprivation amblyopia, unspecified eye
    - **H53.02 Refractive amblyopia**
      - H53.021   Refractive amblyopia, right eye
      - H53.022   Refractive amblyopia, left eye
      - H53.023   Refractive amblyopia, bilateral
      - H53.029   Refractive amblyopia, unspecified eye
    - **H53.03 Strabismic amblyopia**
      - **Excludes1**   strabismus (H50.-)
      - H53.031   Strabismic amblyopia, right eye
      - H53.032   Strabismic amblyopia, left eye
      - H53.033   Strabismic amblyopia, bilateral
      - H53.039   Strabismic amblyopia, unspecified eye
    - **H53.04 Amblyopia suspect**
      - Coding Clinic: 2016, Q4, P22
      - H53.041   Amblyopia suspect, right eye
      - H53.042   Amblyopia suspect, left eye
      - H53.043   Amblyopia suspect, bilateral
      - H53.049   Amblyopia suspect, unspecified eye
  - **H53.1 Subjective visual disturbances**
    - **Excludes1**   subjective visual disturbances due to vitamin A deficiency (E50.5)
      - visual hallucinations (R44.1)
    - **H53.10 Unspecified subjective visual disturbances**
    - **H53.11 Day blindness**
      - Hemeralopia
    - **H53.12 Transient visual loss**
      - Scintillating scotoma
      - **Excludes1**   amaurosis fugax (G45.3-)
        - transient retinal artery occlusion (H34.0-)
      - Coding Clinic: 2022, Q1, P30
      - H53.121   Transient visual loss, right eye
      - H53.122   Transient visual loss, left eye
      - H53.123   Transient visual loss, bilateral
      - H53.129   Transient visual loss, unspecified eye
    - **H53.13 Sudden visual loss**
      - H53.131   Sudden visual loss, right eye
      - H53.132   Sudden visual loss, left eye
      - H53.133   Sudden visual loss, bilateral
      - H53.139   Sudden visual loss, unspecified eye
    - **H53.14 Visual discomfort**
      - Asthenopia
      - Photophobia
      - H53.141   Visual discomfort, right eye
      - H53.142   Visual discomfort, left eye
      - H53.143   Visual discomfort, bilateral
      - H53.149   Visual discomfort, unspecified
    - **H53.15 Visual distortions of shape and size**
      - Metamorphopsia
    - **H53.16 Psychophysical visual disturbances**
    - **H53.19 Other subjective visual disturbances**
      - Visual halos
      - Coding Clinic: 2022, Q1, P30
  - **H53.2 Diplopia**
    - Double vision
  - **H53.3 Other and unspecified disorders of binocular vision**
    - **H53.30 Unspecified disorder of binocular vision**
    - **H53.31 Abnormal retinal correspondence**
    - **H53.32 Fusion with defective stereopsis**
    - **H53.33 Simultaneous visual perception without fusion**
    - **H53.34 Suppression of binocular vision**
  - **H53.4 Visual field defects**
    - **H53.40 Unspecified visual field defects**
    - **H53.41 Scotoma involving central area**
      - Central scotoma
      - H53.411   Scotoma involving central area, right eye
      - H53.412   Scotoma involving central area, left eye
      - H53.413   Scotoma involving central area, bilateral
      - H53.419   Scotoma involving central area, unspecified eye
    - **H53.42 Scotoma of blind spot area**
      - Enlarged blind spot
      - H53.421   Scotoma of blind spot area, right eye
      - H53.422   Scotoma of blind spot area, left eye
      - H53.423   Scotoma of blind spot area, bilateral
      - H53.429   Scotoma of blind spot area, unspecified eye
    - **H53.43 Sector or arcuate defects**
      - Arcuate scotoma
      - Bjerrum scotoma
      - H53.431   Sector or arcuate defects, right eye
      - H53.432   Sector or arcuate defects, left eye
      - H53.433   Sector or arcuate defects, bilateral
      - H53.439   Sector or arcuate defects, unspecified eye
    - **H53.45 Other localized visual field defect**
      - Peripheral visual field defect
      - Ring scotoma NOS
      - Scotoma NOS
      - H53.451   Other localized visual field defect, right eye
      - H53.452   Other localized visual field defect, left eye
      - H53.453   Other localized visual field defect, bilateral
      - H53.459   Other localized visual field defect, unspecified eye
    - **H53.46 Homonymous bilateral field defects**
      - Homonymous hemianopia
      - Homonymous hemianopsia
      - Quadrant anopia
      - Quadrant anopsia
      - H53.461   Homonymous bilateral field defects, right side
      - H53.462   Homonymous bilateral field defects, left side
      - H53.469   Homonymous bilateral field defects, unspecified side
        - Homonymous bilateral field defects NOS
    - **H53.47 Heteronymous bilateral field defects**
      - Heteronymous hemianop(s)ia

CHAPTER 7 (H00–H59)

● H53.48   Generalized contraction of visual field

     H53.481   Generalized contraction of visual field, right eye

     H53.482   Generalized contraction of visual field, left eye

     H53.483   Generalized contraction of visual field, bilateral

     H53.489   Generalized contraction of visual field, unspecified eye

● H53.5   Color vision deficiencies
     Color blindness

     Excludes2   day blindness (H53.11)

     H53.50   Unspecified color vision deficiencies
         Color blindness NOS

     H53.51   Achromatopsia

     H53.52   Acquired color vision deficiency

     H53.53   Deuteranomaly
         Deuteranopia

     H53.54   Protanomaly
         Protanopia

     H53.55   Tritanomaly
         Tritanopia

     H53.59   Other color vision deficiencies

● H53.6   Night blindness

     Excludes1   night blindness due to vitamin A deficiency (E50.5)

     H53.60   Unspecified night blindness

     H53.61   Abnormal dark adaptation curve

     H53.62   Acquired night blindness

     H53.63   Congenital night blindness

     H53.69   Other night blindness

● H53.7   Vision sensitivity deficiencies

     H53.71   Glare sensitivity

     H53.72   Impaired contrast sensitivity

   H53.8   Other visual disturbances

   H53.9   Unspecified visual disturbance

● H54   Blindness and low vision

     Note: For definition of visual impairment categories see table below.

     Code first any associated underlying cause of the blindness

     Excludes1   amaurosis fugax (G45.3)

● H54.0   Blindness, both eyes
     Visual impairment categories 3, 4, 5 in both eyes.

   ● H54.0X   Blindness, both eyes, different category levels

     H54.0X3   Blindness right eye, category 3

         H54.0X33   Blindness right eye category 3, blindness left eye category 3

         H54.0X34   Blindness right eye category 3, blindness left eye category 4

         H54.0X35   Blindness right eye category 3, blindness left eye category 5

   ● H54.0X4   Blindness right eye, category 4

         H54.0X43   Blindness right eye category 4, blindness left eye category 3

         H54.0X44   Blindness right eye category 4, blindness left eye category 4

         H54.0X45   Blindness right eye category 4, blindness left eye category 5

   ● H54.0X5   Blindness right eye, category 5

         H54.0X53   Blindness right eye category 5, blindness left eye category 3

         H54.0X54   Blindness right eye category 5, blindness left eye category 4

         H54.0X55   Blindness right eye category 5, blindness left eye category 5

● H54.1   Blindness, one eye, low vision other eye
     Visual impairment categories 3, 4, 5 in one eye, with categories 1 or 2 in the other eye.

     H54.10   Blindness, one eye, low vision other eye, unspecified eyes

   ● H54.11   Blindness, right eye, low vision left eye

   ● H54.113   Blindness right eye category 3, low vision left eye

         H54.1131   Blindness right eye category 3, low vision left eye category 1

         H54.1132   Blindness right eye category 3, low vision left eye category 2

   ● H54.114   Blindness right eye category 4, low vision left eye

         H54.1141   Blindness right eye category 4, low vision left eye category 1

         H54.1142   Blindness right eye category 4, low vision left eye category 2

   ● H54.115   Blindness right eye category 5, low vision left eye

         H54.1151   Blindness right eye category 5, low vision left eye category 1

         H54.1152   Blindness right eye category 5, low vision left eye category 2

   ● H54.12   Blindness, left eye, low vision right eye

   ● H54.121   Low vision right eye category 1, blindness left eye

         H54.1213   Low vision right eye category 1, blindness left eye category 3

         H54.1214   Low vision right eye category 1, blindness left eye category 4

         H54.1215   Low vision right eye category 1, blindness left eye category 5

   ● H54.122   Low vision right eye category 2, blindness left eye

         H54.1223   Low vision right eye category 2, blindness left eye category 3

         H54.1224   Low vision right eye category 2, blindness left eye category 4

         H54.1225   Low vision right eye category 2, blindness left eye category 5

● **H54.2**   **Low vision, both eyes**
Visual impairment categories 1 or 2 in both eyes.

    ● **H54.2X**   **Low vision, both eyes, different category levels**

       ● **H54.2X1**   **Low vision, right eye, category 1**

          H54.2X11   **Low vision right eye category 1, low vision left eye category 1**

          H54.2X12   **Low vision right eye category 1, low vision left eye category 2**

       ● **H54.2X2**   **Low vision, right eye, category 2**

          H54.2X21   **Low vision right eye category 2, low vision left eye category 1**

          H54.2X22   **Low vision right eye category 2, low vision left eye category 2**

● **H54.3**   **Unqualified visual loss, both eyes**
Visual impairment category 9 in both eyes.

● **H54.4**   **Blindness, one eye**
Visual impairment categories 3, 4, 5 in one eye [normal vision in other eye]

    H54.40   **Blindness, one eye, unspecified eye**

    ● **H54.41**   **Blindness, right eye, normal vision left eye**

       ● **H54.413**   **Blindness, right eye, category 3**

          H54.413A   **Blindness right eye category 3, normal vision left eye**

       ● **H54.414**   **Blindness, right eye, category 4**

          H54.414A   **Blindness right eye category 4, normal vision left eye**

       ● **H54.415**   **Blindness, right eye, category 5**

          H54.415A   **Blindness right eye category 5, normal vision left eye**

    ● **H54.42**   **Blindness, left eye, normal vision right eye**

       ● **H54.42A**   **Blindness, left eye, category 3-5**

          H54.42A3   **Blindness left eye category 3, normal vision right eye**

          H54.42A4   **Blindness left eye category 4, normal vision right eye**

          H54.42A5   **Blindness left eye category 5, normal vision right eye**

● **H54.5**   **Low vision, one eye**
Visual impairment categories 1 or 2 in one eye [normal vision in other eye].

    H54.50   **Low vision, one eye, unspecified eye**

    ● **H54.51**   **Low vision, right eye, normal vision left eye**

       ● **H54.511**   **Low vision, right eye, category 1-2**

          H54.511A   **Low vision right eye category 1, normal vision left eye**

          H54.512A   **Low vision right eye category 2, normal vision left eye**

    ● **H54.52**   **Low vision, left eye, normal vision right eye**

       ● **H54.52A**   **Low vision, left eye, category 1-2**

          H54.52A1   **Low vision left eye category 1, normal vision right eye**

          H54.52A2   **Low vision left eye category 2, normal vision right eye**

● **H54.6**   **Unqualified visual loss, one eye**
Visual impairment category 9 in one eye [normal vision in other eye].

    H54.60   **Unqualified visual loss, one eye, unspecified**

    H54.61   **Unqualified visual loss, right eye, normal vision left eye**

    H54.62   **Unqualified visual loss, left eye, normal vision right eye**

OGCR Section I.C.7.b.

> **Blindness**
>
> If "blindness" or "low vision" of both eyes is documented but the visual impairment category is not documented, assign code H54.3, Unqualified visual loss, both eyes. If "blindness" or "low vision" in one eye is documented but the visual impairment category is not documented, assign a code from H54.6-, Unqualified visual loss, one eye. If "blindness" or "visual loss" is documented without any information about whether one or both eyes are affected, assign code H54.7, Unspecified visual loss.

    H54.7   **Unspecified visual loss**
Visual impairment category 9 NOS

    H54.8   **Legal blindness, as defined in USA**
Blindness NOS according to USA definition

       Excludes1   legal blindness with specification of impairment level (H54.0-H54.7)

       Note: The table below gives a classification of severity of visual impairment recommended by a WHO Study Group on the Prevention of Blindness, Geneva, 6-10 November 1972.

       The term "low vision" in category H54 comprises categories 1 and 2 of the table, the term "blindness" categories 3, 4, and 5, and the term "unqualified visual loss" category 9.

       If the extent of the visual field is taken into account, patients with a field no greater than 10 but greater than 5 around central fixation should be placed in category 3 and patients with a field no greater than 5 around central fixation should be placed in category 4, even if the central acuity is not impaired.

(Document 508 compliance requires all cells in the following table to be filled.)

Category of visual impairment	Visual acuity with best possible correction	
	Maximum less than:	**Minimum equal to or better than:**
—	6/18	6/60
3/10 (0.3)	1/10 (0.1)	—
20/70	20/200	—
—	6/60	3/60
1/10 (0.1)	1/20 (0.05)	—
20/200	20/400	—
—	3/60	1/60 (finger counting at one meter)
1/20 (0.05)	1/50 (0.02)	—
20/400	5/300 (20/1200)	—
—	1/60 (finger counting at one meter)	Light perception
1/50 (0.02)	—	—
5/300	—	—
—	No light perception	
—	Undetermined or unspecified	

CHAPTER 7 (H00-H59)

CHAPTER 7 (H00-H59)

OTHER DISORDERS OF EYE AND ADNEXA (H55-H57)

● H55 **Nystagmus and other irregular eye movements**
- ● H55.0 **Nystagmus**
  - *Rapid, involuntary movements of the eyes in the horizontal or vertical direction*
  - H55.00 **Unspecified** nystagmus
  - H55.01 **Congenital** nystagmus
  - H55.02 **Latent** nystagmus
  - H55.03 **Visual deprivation** nystagmus
  - H55.04 **Dissociated** nystagmus
  - H55.09 **Other forms** of nystagmus
- H55.8 **Other irregular eye movements**
  - H55.81 Deficient **saccadic** eye movements
  - H55.82 Deficient **smooth pursuit** eye movements
  - H55.89 **Other** irregular eye movements

● H57 **Other disorders of eye and adnexa**
- ● H57.0 **Anomalies of pupillary function**
  - H57.00 **Unspecified** anomaly of pupillary function
  - H57.01 **Argyll Robertson pupil, atypical**
    - **Excludes1** syphilitic Argyll Robertson pupil (A52.19)
  - H57.02 **Anisocoria**
  - H57.03 **Miosis**
  - H57.04 **Mydriasis**
  - ● H57.05 **Tonic pupil**
    - H57.051 Tonic pupil, **right eye**
    - H57.052 Tonic pupil, **left eye**
    - H57.053 Tonic pupil, **bilateral**
    - H57.059 Tonic pupil, **unspecified eye**
  - H57.09 **Other** anomalies of pupillary function
- ● H57.1 **Ocular pain**
  - H57.10 Ocular pain, **unspecified eye**
  - H57.11 Ocular pain, **right eye**
  - H57.12 Ocular pain, **left eye**
  - H57.13 Ocular pain, **bilateral**
- ● H57.8 **Other specified disorders of eye and adnexa**
  - ● H57.81 **Brow ptosis**
    - H57.811 Brow ptosis, right
    - H57.812 Brow ptosis, left
    - H57.813 Brow ptosis, bilateral
    - H57.819 Brow ptosis, unspecified
  - H57.89 **Other** specified disorders of eye and adnexa
- H57.9 **Unspecified** disorder of eye and adnexa

INTRAOPERATIVE AND POSTPROCEDURAL COMPLICATIONS AND DISORDERS OF EYE AND ADNEXA, NOT ELSEWHERE CLASSIFIED (H59)

● H59 **Intraoperative and postprocedural complications and disorders of eye and adnexa, not elsewhere classified**
- **Excludes1** mechanical complication of intraocular lens (T85.2)
  - mechanical complication of other ocular prosthetic devices, implants and grafts (T85.3)
  - pseudophakia (Z96.1)
  - secondary cataracts (H26.4-)
- ● H59.0 **Disorders of the eye following** cataract surgery
  - ● H59.01 **Keratopathy (bullous aphakic) following** cataract surgery
    - Vitreal corneal syndrome
    - Vitreous (touch) syndrome
    - H59.011 Keratopathy (bullous aphakic) following cataract surgery, **right eye**
    - H59.012 Keratopathy (bullous aphakic) following cataract surgery, **left eye**
    - H59.013 Keratopathy (bullous aphakic) following cataract surgery, **bilateral**
    - H59.019 Keratopathy (bullous aphakic) following cataract surgery, **unspecified eye**

- ● H59.02 **Cataract (lens) fragments in eye following** cataract surgery
  - H59.021 Cataract (lens) fragments in eye following cataract surgery, **right eye**
  - H59.022 Cataract (lens) fragments in eye following cataract surgery, **left eye**
  - H59.023 Cataract (lens) fragments in eye following cataract surgery, **bilateral**
  - H59.029 Cataract (lens) fragments in eye following cataract surgery, **unspecified eye**
- ● H59.03 **Cystoid macular edema following** cataract surgery
  - H59.031 Cystoid macular edema following cataract surgery, **right eye**
  - H59.032 Cystoid macular edema following cataract surgery, **left eye**
  - H59.033 Cystoid macular edema following cataract surgery, **bilateral**
  - H59.039 Cystoid macular edema following cataract surgery, **unspecified eye**
- ● H59.09 **Other disorders of the eye following** cataract surgery
  - H59.091 Other disorders of the **right eye** following cataract surgery
  - H59.092 Other disorders of the **left eye** following cataract surgery
  - H59.093 Other disorders of the eye following cataract surgery, **bilateral**
  - H59.099 Other disorders of **unspecified eye** following cataract surgery
- ● H59.1 **Intraoperative hemorrhage and hematoma of eye and adnexa complicating a procedure**
  - **Excludes1** intraoperative hemorrhage and hematoma of eye and adnexa due to accidental puncture or laceration during a procedure (H59.2-)
  - ● H59.11 **Intraoperative hemorrhage and hematoma of eye and adnexa complicating an ophthalmic procedure**
    - H59.111 Intraoperative hemorrhage and hematoma of **right eye** and adnexa complicating an ophthalmic procedure
    - H59.112 Intraoperative hemorrhage and hematoma of **left eye** and adnexa complicating an ophthalmic procedure
    - H59.113 Intraoperative hemorrhage and hematoma of eye and adnexa complicating an ophthalmic procedure, **bilateral**
    - H59.119 Intraoperative hemorrhage and hematoma of **unspecified** eye and adnexa complicating an ophthalmic procedure
  - ● H59.12 **Intraoperative hemorrhage and hematoma of eye and adnexa complicating other procedure**
    - H59.121 Intraoperative hemorrhage and hematoma of **right eye** and adnexa complicating other procedure
    - H59.122 Intraoperative hemorrhage and hematoma of **left eye** and adnexa complicating other procedure
    - H59.123 Intraoperative hemorrhage and hematoma of eye and adnexa complicating other procedure, **bilateral**
    - H59.129 Intraoperative hemorrhage and hematoma of **unspecified** eye and adnexa complicating other procedure

▶ New   ⬛▶ Revised   ~~deleted~~ Deleted   Excludes 1   Excludes 2   Includes   Use additional   Code first   Code also   Key words

OGCR Official Guidelines   X Assign placeholder X   ● Use Additional Character(s)   ▶ Manifestation Code   🝊 Hierarchical Condition Category   **Coding Clinic**

● H59.2   **Accidental puncture and laceration** of eye and adnexa during a procedure

  ● H59.21   Accidental puncture and laceration of eye and adnexa during an **ophthalmic procedure**

     H59.211   Accidental puncture and laceration of **right** eye and adnexa during an ophthalmic procedure

     H59.212   Accidental puncture and laceration of **left** eye and adnexa during an ophthalmic procedure

     H59.213   Accidental puncture and laceration of eye and adnexa during an ophthalmic procedure, **bilateral**

     H59.219   Accidental puncture and laceration of **unspecified** eye and adnexa during an ophthalmic procedure

  ● H59.22   Accidental puncture and laceration of eye and adnexa during **other procedure**

     H59.221   Accidental puncture and laceration of **right** eye and adnexa during other procedure

     H59.222   Accidental puncture and laceration of **left** eye and adnexa during other procedure

     H59.223   Accidental puncture and laceration of eye and adnexa during other procedure, **bilateral**

     H59.229   Accidental puncture and laceration of **unspecified** eye and adnexa during other procedure

● H59.3   **Postprocedural hemorrhage, hematoma, and seroma** of eye and adnexa following other procedure

     Coding Clinic: 2016, Q4, P10

  ● H59.31   Postprocedural **hemorrhage** of eye and adnexa following an **ophthalmic procedure**

     H59.311   Postprocedural hemorrhage of **right** eye and adnexa following an ophthalmic procedure

     H59.312   Postprocedural hemorrhage of **left** eye and adnexa following an ophthalmic procedure

     H59.313   Postprocedural hemorrhage of eye and adnexa following an ophthalmic procedure, **bilateral**

     H59.319   Postprocedural hemorrhage of **unspecified** eye and adnexa following an ophthalmic procedure

  ● H59.32   Postprocedural **hemorrhage** of eye and adnexa following **other procedure**

     H59.321   Postprocedural hemorrhage of **right** eye and adnexa following other procedure

     H59.322   Postprocedural hemorrhage of **left** eye and adnexa following other procedure

     H59.323   Postprocedural hemorrhage of eye and adnexa following other procedure, **bilateral**

     H59.329   Postprocedural hemorrhage of **unspecified** eye and adnexa following other procedure

  ● H59.33   Postprocedural **hematoma** of eye and adnexa following an **ophthalmic procedure**

     H59.331   Postprocedural hematoma of **right** eye and adnexa following an ophthalmic procedure

     H59.332   Postprocedural hematoma of **left** eye and adnexa following an ophthalmic procedure

     H59.333   Postprocedural hematoma of eye and adnexa following an ophthalmic procedure, **bilateral**

     H59.339   Postprocedural hematoma of **unspecified** eye and adnexa following an ophthalmic procedure

  ● H59.34   Postprocedural **hematoma** of eye and adnexa following **other procedure**

     H59.341   Postprocedural hematoma of **right** eye and adnexa following other procedure

     H59.342   Postprocedural hematoma of **left** eye and adnexa following other procedure

     H59.343   Postprocedural hematoma of eye and adnexa following other procedure, **bilateral**

     H59.349   Postprocedural hematoma of **unspecified** eye and adnexa following other procedure

  ● H59.35   Postprocedural **seroma** of eye and adnexa following an **ophthalmic procedure**

     H59.351   Postprocedural seroma of **right** eye and adnexa following an ophthalmic procedure

     H59.352   Postprocedural seroma of **left** eye and adnexa following an ophthalmic procedure

     H59.353   Postprocedural seroma of eye and adnexa following an ophthalmic procedure, **bilateral**

     H59.359   Postprocedural seroma of **unspecified** eye and adnexa following an ophthalmic procedure

  ● H59.36   Postprocedural **seroma** of eye and adnexa following **other procedure**

     H59.361   Postprocedural seroma of **right** eye and adnexa following other procedure

     H59.362   Postprocedural seroma of **left** eye and adnexa following other procedure

     H59.363   Postprocedural seroma of eye and adnexa following other procedure, **bilateral**

     H59.369   Postprocedural seroma of **unspecified** eye and adnexa following other procedure

● H59.4   **Inflammation (infection)** of **postprocedural bleb**

     Postprocedural blebitis

     Excludes1   filtering (vitreous) bleb after glaucoma surgery status (Z98.83)

   H59.40   Inflammation (infection) of postprocedural bleb, **unspecified**

   H59.41   Inflammation (infection) of postprocedural bleb, **stage 1**

   H59.42   Inflammation (infection) of postprocedural bleb, **stage 2**

   H59.43   Inflammation (infection) of postprocedural bleb, **stage 3**

     Bleb endophthalmitis

● H59.8   **Other intraoperative** and **postprocedural** complications and disorders of eye and adnexa, not elsewhere classified

  ● H59.81   Chorioretinal scars after surgery for detachment

     H59.811   Chorioretinal scars after surgery for detachment, **right eye**

     H59.812   Chorioretinal scars after surgery for detachment, left eye

     H59.813   Chorioretinal scars after surgery for detachment, **bilateral**

     H59.819   Chorioretinal scars after surgery for detachment, **unspecified** eye

   H59.88   **Other intraoperative** complications of eye and adnexa, not elsewhere classified

   H59.89   **Other postprocedural** complications and disorders of eye and adnexa, not elsewhere classified

CHAPTER 7 (H00–H59)

CHAPTER 8

DISEASES OF THE EAR AND MASTOID PROCESS (H60-H95)

OGCR Chapter-Specific Coding Guidelines

> 8. Chapter 8: Diseases of the Ear and Mastoid Process (H60-H95)
> Reserved for future guideline expansion

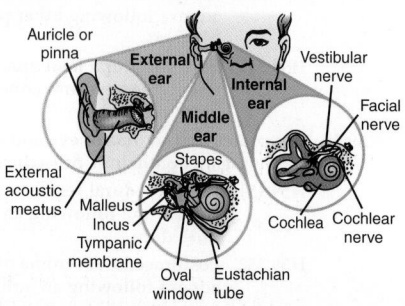

Figure 8-1 Auditory system. (From Buck CJ: Step-by-Step Medical Coding, ed 2016, St. Louis, Elsevier, 2016)

★ **(See Plate 20 of the Anatomy Illustrations.)**

CHAPTER 8

DISEASES OF THE EAR AND MASTOID PROCESS (H60-H95)

Note: Use an external cause code following the code for the ear condition, if applicable, to identify the cause of the ear condition

Excludes2   certain conditions originating in the perinatal period (P04-P96)
certain infectious and parasitic diseases (A00-B99)
complications of pregnancy, childbirth and the puerperium (O00-O9A)
congenital malformations, deformations and chromosomal abnormalities (Q00-Q99)
endocrine, nutritional and metabolic diseases (E00-E88)
injury, poisoning and certain other consequences of external causes (S00-T88)
neoplasms (C00-D49)
symptoms, signs and abnormal clinical and laboratory findings, not elsewhere classified (R00-R94)

This chapter contains the following blocks:

H60-H62	Diseases of external ear
H65-H75	Diseases of middle ear and mastoid
H80-H83	Diseases of inner ear
H90-H94	Other disorders of ear
H95	Intraoperative and postprocedural complications and disorders of ear and mastoid process, not elsewhere classified

DISEASES OF EXTERNAL EAR (H60-H62)

● **H60**   Otitis externa

   ● **H60.0**   **Abscess** of external ear
      Boil of external ear
      Carbuncle of auricle or external auditory canal
      Furuncle of external ear

     H60.00   Abscess of external ear, **unspecified ear**
     H60.01   Abscess of **right** external ear
     H60.02   Abscess of **left** external ear
     H60.03   Abscess of external ear, **bilateral**

● **H60.1**   Cellulitis of external ear
      Cellulitis of auricle
      Cellulitis of external auditory canal

     H60.10   Cellulitis of external ear, **unspecified ear**
     H60.11   Cellulitis of **right** external ear
     H60.12   Cellulitis of **left** external ear
     H60.13   Cellulitis of external ear, **bilateral**

● **H60.2**   **Malignant** otitis externa
     H60.20   Malignant otitis externa, **unspecified ear**
     H60.21   Malignant otitis externa, **right ear**
     H60.22   Malignant otitis externa, **left ear**
     H60.23   Malignant otitis externa, **bilateral**

● **H60.3**   Other infective otitis externa

   ● **H60.31**   **Diffuse** otitis externa
      H60.311   Diffuse otitis externa, **right ear**
      H60.312   Diffuse otitis externa, **left ear**
      H60.313   Diffuse otitis externa, **bilateral**
      H60.319   Diffuse otitis externa, **unspecified ear**

   ● **H60.32**   **Hemorrhagic** otitis externa
      H60.321   Hemorrhagic otitis externa, **right ear**
      H60.322   Hemorrhagic otitis externa, **left ear**
      H60.323   Hemorrhagic otitis externa, **bilateral**
      H60.329   Hemorrhagic otitis externa, **unspecified** ear

   ● **H60.33**   **Swimmer's ear**
      H60.331   Swimmer's ear, **right ear**
      H60.332   Swimmer's ear, **left ear**
      H60.333   Swimmer's ear, **bilateral**
      H60.339   Swimmer's ear, **unspecified ear**

   ● **H60.39**   Other infective otitis externa
      H60.391   Other infective otitis externa, **right ear**
      H60.392   Other infective otitis externa, **left ear**
      H60.393   Other infective otitis externa, **bilateral**
      H60.399   Other infective otitis externa, **unspecified** ear

● **H60.4**   Cholesteatoma of external ear
      Keratosis obturans of external ear (canal)

     Excludes2   cholesteatoma of middle ear (H71.-)
              recurrent cholesteatoma of postmastoidectomy cavity (H95.0-)

     H60.40   Cholesteatoma of external ear, **unspecified ear**
     H60.41   Cholesteatoma of **right** external ear
     H60.42   Cholesteatoma of **left** external ear
     H60.43   Cholesteatoma of external ear, **bilateral**

● **H60.5**   **Acute noninfective** otitis externa

   ● **H60.50**   **Unspecified** acute noninfective otitis externa
      Acute otitis externa NOS
      H60.501   Unspecified acute noninfective otitis externa, **right ear**
      H60.502   Unspecified acute noninfective otitis externa, **left ear**
      H60.503   Unspecified acute noninfective otitis externa, **bilateral**
      H60.509   Unspecified acute noninfective otitis externa, **unspecified ear**

   ● **H60.51**   Acute **actinic** otitis externa
      H60.511   Acute actinic otitis externa, **right ear**
      H60.512   Acute actinic otitis externa, **left ear**
      H60.513   Acute actinic otitis externa, **bilateral**
      H60.519   Acute actinic otitis externa, **unspecified** ear

   ● **H60.52**   Acute **chemical** otitis externa
      H60.521   Acute chemical otitis externa, **right** ear
      H60.522   Acute chemical otitis externa, **left** ear

▶ New   ➡ Revised   ~~deleted~~ Deleted   Excludes 1   Excludes 2   Includes   Use additional   Code first   Code also   Key words

OGCR Official Guidelines   X Assign placeholder X   ● Use Additional Character(s)   ▶ Manifestation Code   🏥 Hierarchical Condition Category   **Coding Clinic**

H60.523   Acute chemical otitis externa, bilateral

H60.529   Acute chemical otitis externa, unspecified ear

● H60.53   Acute contact otitis externa

H60.531   Acute contact otitis externa, right ear

H60.532   Acute contact otitis externa, left ear

H60.533   Acute contact otitis externa, bilateral

H60.539   Acute contact otitis externa, unspecified ear

● H60.54   Acute eczematoid otitis externa

H60.541   Acute eczematoid otitis externa, right ear

H60.542   Acute eczematoid otitis externa, left ear

H60.543   Acute eczematoid otitis externa, bilateral

H60.549   Acute eczematoid otitis externa, unspecified ear

● H60.55   Acute reactive otitis externa

H60.551   Acute reactive otitis externa, right ear

H60.552   Acute reactive otitis externa, left ear

H60.553   Acute reactive otitis externa, bilateral

H60.559   Acute reactive otitis externa, unspecified ear

● H60.59   Other noninfective acute otitis externa

H60.591   Other noninfective acute otitis externa, right ear

H60.592   Other noninfective acute otitis externa, left ear

H60.593   Other noninfective acute otitis externa, bilateral

H60.599   Other noninfective acute otitis externa, unspecified ear

● H60.6   Unspecified chronic otitis externa

H60.60   Unspecified chronic otitis externa, unspecified ear

H60.61   Unspecified chronic otitis externa, right ear

H60.62   Unspecified chronic otitis externa, left ear

H60.63   Unspecified chronic otitis externa, bilateral

● H60.8   Other otitis externa

● H60.8X   Other otitis externa

H60.8X1   Other otitis externa, right ear

H60.8X2   Other otitis externa, left ear

H60.8X3   Other otitis externa, bilateral

H60.8X9   Other otitis externa, unspecified ear

● H60.9   Unspecified otitis externa

H60.90   Unspecified otitis externa, unspecified ear

H60.91   Unspecified otitis externa, right ear

H60.92   Unspecified otitis externa, left ear

H60.93   Unspecified otitis externa, bilateral

● H61   Other disorders of external ear

● H61.0   Chondritis and perichondritis of external ear
   Chondrodermatitis nodularis chronica helicis
   Perichondritis of auricle
   Perichondritis of pinna

● H61.00   Unspecified perichondritis of external ear

H61.001   Unspecified perichondritis of right external ear

H61.002   Unspecified perichondritis of left external ear

H61.003   Unspecified perichondritis of external ear, bilateral

H61.009   Unspecified perichondritis of external ear, unspecified ear

● H61.01   Acute perichondritis of external ear

H61.011   Acute perichondritis of right external ear

H61.012   Acute perichondritis of left external ear

H61.013   Acute perichondritis of external ear, bilateral

H61.019   Acute perichondritis of external ear, unspecified ear

● H61.02   Chronic perichondritis of external ear

H61.021   Chronic perichondritis of right external ear

H61.022   Chronic perichondritis of left external ear

H61.023   Chronic perichondritis of external ear, bilateral

H61.029   Chronic perichondritis of external ear, unspecified ear

● H61.03   Chondritis of external ear
   Chondritis of auricle
   Chondritis of pinna

H61.031   Chondritis of right external ear

H61.032   Chondritis of left external ear
   Coding Clinic: 2015, Q1, P18

H61.033   Chondritis of external ear, bilateral

H61.039   Chondritis of external ear, unspecified ear

● H61.1   Noninfective disorders of pinna

Excludes2   cauliflower ear (M95.1-)
   gouty tophi of ear (M1A.-)

● H61.10   Unspecified noninfective disorders of pinna
   Disorder of pinna NOS

H61.101   Unspecified noninfective disorders of pinna, right ear

H61.102   Unspecified noninfective disorders of pinna, left ear

H61.103   Unspecified noninfective disorders of pinna, bilateral

H61.109   Unspecified noninfective disorders of pinna, unspecified ear

● H61.11   Acquired deformity of pinna
   Acquired deformity of auricle

Excludes2   cauliflower ear (M95.1-)

H61.111   Acquired deformity of pinna, right ear

H61.112   Acquired deformity of pinna, left ear

H61.113   Acquired deformity of pinna, bilateral

H61.119   Acquired deformity of pinna, unspecified ear

● H61.12   Hematoma of pinna
   Hematoma of auricle

H61.121   Hematoma of pinna, right ear

H61.122   Hematoma of pinna, left ear

H61.123   Hematoma of pinna, bilateral

H61.129   Hematoma of pinna, unspecified ear

● H61.19   Other noninfective disorders of pinna

H61.191   Noninfective disorders of pinna, right ear

H61.192   Noninfective disorders of pinna, left ear

H61.193   Noninfective disorders of pinna, bilateral

H61.199   Noninfective disorders of pinna, unspecified ear

● H61.2   Impacted cerumen
   Wax in ear

H61.20   Impacted cerumen, unspecified ear

H61.21   Impacted cerumen, right ear

H61.22   Impacted cerumen, left ear

H61.23   Impacted cerumen, bilateral

CHAPTER 8 (H60-H95)

● **H61.3** Acquired stenosis of external ear canal
Collapse of external ear canal
Excludes1 postprocedural stenosis of external ear
canal (H95.81-)

● **H61.30** Acquired stenosis of external ear canal,
unspecified
   H61.301 Acquired stenosis of right external ear
   canal, unspecified
   H61.302 Acquired stenosis of left external ear
   canal, unspecified
   H61.303 Acquired stenosis of external ear
   canal, unspecified, bilateral
   H61.309 Acquired stenosis of external ear
   canal, unspecified, unspecified ear

● **H61.31** Acquired stenosis of external ear canal
secondary to trauma
   H61.311 Acquired stenosis of right external ear
   canal secondary to trauma
   H61.312 Acquired stenosis of left external ear
   canal secondary to trauma
   H61.313 Acquired stenosis of external ear
   canal secondary to trauma, bilateral
   H61.319 Acquired stenosis of external
   ear canal secondary to trauma,
   unspecified ear

● **H61.32** Acquired stenosis of external ear canal
secondary to inflammation and infection
   H61.321 Acquired stenosis of right external ear
   canal secondary to inflammation and
   infection
   H61.322 Acquired stenosis of left external
   ear canal secondary to inflammation and
   infection
   H61.323 Acquired stenosis of external ear
   canal secondary to inflammation and
   infection, bilateral
   H61.329 Acquired stenosis of external ear
   canal secondary to inflammation and
   infection, unspecified ear

● **H61.39** Other acquired stenosis of external ear canal
   H61.391 Other acquired stenosis of right
   external ear canal
   H61.392 Other acquired stenosis of left
   external ear canal
   H61.393 Other acquired stenosis of external
   ear canal, bilateral
   H61.399 Other acquired stenosis of external
   ear canal, unspecified ear

● **H61.8** Other specified disorders of external ear
● **H61.81** Exostosis of external canal
   H61.811 Exostosis of right external canal
   H61.812 Exostosis of left external canal
   H61.813 Exostosis of external canal, bilateral
   H61.819 Exostosis of external canal,
   unspecified ear

● **H61.89** Other specified disorders of external ear
   H61.891 Other specified disorders of right
   external ear
   H61.892 Other specified disorders of left
   external ear
   H61.893 Other specified disorders of external
   ear, bilateral
   H61.899 Other specified disorders of external
   ear, unspecified ear

● **H61.9** Disorder of external ear, unspecified
   H61.90 Disorder of external ear, unspecified,
   unspecified ear
   H61.91 Disorder of right external ear, unspecified
   H61.92 Disorder of left external ear, unspecified
   H61.93 Disorder of external ear, unspecified, bilateral

● **H62** Disorders of external ear in diseases classified elsewhere
● **H62.4** Otitis externa in other diseases classified elsewhere
Code first underlying disease, such as:
   erysipelas (A46)
   impetigo (L01.0)
   Excludes1 otitis externa (in):
   candidiasis (B37.84)
   herpes viral [herpes simplex] (B00.1)
   herpes zoster (B02.8)

▎ *H62.40* *Otitis externa in other diseases classified
elsewhere, unspecified ear*
▎ *H62.41* *Otitis externa in other diseases classified
elsewhere, right ear*
▎ *H62.42* *Otitis externa in other diseases classified
elsewhere, left ear*
▎ *H62.43* *Otitis externa in other diseases classified
elsewhere, bilateral*

● **H62.8** Other disorders of external ear in diseases classified
elsewhere
Code first underlying disease, such as:
   gout (M1A.-, M10.-)
● **H62.8X** Other disorders of external ear in diseases
classified elsewhere
   ▎ *H62.8X1* *Other disorders of right external ear in
   diseases classified elsewhere*
   ▎ *H62.8X2* *Other disorders of left external ear in
   diseases classified elsewhere*
   ▎ *H62.8X3* *Other disorders of external ear in
   diseases classified elsewhere, bilateral*
   ▎ *H62.8X9* *Other disorders of external ear
   in diseases classified elsewhere,
   unspecified ear*

DISEASES OF MIDDLE EAR AND MASTOID (H65-H75)

★**(See Plate 21 of the Anatomy Illustrations.)**

● **H65** Nonsuppurative otitis media
*Bacterial or viral infection or inflammation of the middle ear; may result
in fluid accumulation with pain and temporary hearing loss.*
   Includes nonsuppurative otitis media with myringitis
   Use additional code for any associated perforated tympanic
   membrane (H72.-)
   Use additional code to identify:
   exposure to environmental tobacco smoke (Z77.22)
   exposure to tobacco smoke in the perinatal period (P96.81)
   history of tobacco dependence (Z87.891)
   infectious agent (B95-B97)
   occupational exposure to environmental tobacco smoke
   (Z57.31)
   tobacco dependence (F17.-)
   tobacco use (Z72.0)

● **H65.0** Acute serous otitis media
Acute and subacute secretory otitis
   H65.00 Acute serous otitis media, unspecified ear
   H65.01 Acute serous otitis media, right ear
   H65.02 Acute serous otitis media, left ear
   H65.03 Acute serous otitis media, bilateral
   H65.04 Acute serous otitis media, recurrent, right ear
   H65.05 Acute serous otitis media, recurrent, left ear
   H65.06 Acute serous otitis media, recurrent, bilateral
   H65.07 Acute serous otitis media, recurrent,
   unspecified ear

● **H65.1** Other acute nonsuppurative otitis media
   Excludes1 otitic barotrauma (T70.0)
   otitis media (acute) NOS (H66.9)
● **H65.11** Acute and subacute allergic otitis media
(mucoid) (sanguinous) (serous)
   H65.111 Acute and subacute allergic otitis
   media (mucoid) (sanguinous)
   (serous), right ear
   H65.112 Acute and subacute allergic otitis
   media (mucoid) (sanguinous)
   (serous), left ear

▶ New   ⇒ Revised   ~~deleted~~ Deleted   Excludes 1   Excludes 2   Includes   Use additional   Code first   Code also   Key words

872   OGCR Official Guidelines   X Assign placeholder X   ● Use Additional Character(s)   ▎ Manifestation Code   🗐 Hierarchical Condition Category   **Coding Clinic**

H65.113 Acute and subacute allergic otitis media (mucoid) (sanguinous) (serous), bilateral

H65.114 Acute and subacute allergic otitis media (mucoid) (sanguinous) (serous), recurrent, right ear

H65.115 Acute and subacute allergic otitis media (mucoid) (sanguinous) (serous), recurrent, left ear

H65.116 Acute and subacute allergic otitis media (mucoid) (sanguinous) (serous), recurrent, bilateral

H65.117 Acute and subacute allergic otitis media (mucoid) (sanguinous) (serous), recurrent, unspecified ear

H65.119 Acute and subacute allergic otitis media (mucoid) (sanguinous) (serous), unspecified ear

● H65.19 Other acute nonsuppurative otitis media
Acute and subacute mucoid otitis media
Acute and subacute nonsuppurative otitis media NOS
Acute and subacute sanguinous otitis media
Acute and subacute seromucinous otitis media

H65.191 Other acute nonsuppurative otitis media, right ear
H65.192 Other acute nonsuppurative otitis media, left ear
H65.193 Other acute nonsuppurative otitis media, bilateral
H65.194 Other acute nonsuppurative otitis media, recurrent, right ear
H65.195 Other acute nonsuppurative otitis media, recurrent, left ear
H65.196 Other acute nonsuppurative otitis media, recurrent, bilateral
H65.197 Other acute nonsuppurative otitis media recurrent, unspecified ear
H65.199 Other acute nonsuppurative otitis media, unspecified ear

● H65.2 Chronic serous otitis media
Chronic tubotympanal catarrh
H65.20 Chronic serous otitis media, unspecified ear
H65.21 Chronic serous otitis media, right ear
H65.22 Chronic serous otitis media, left ear
H65.23 Chronic serous otitis media, bilateral

● H65.3 Chronic mucoid otitis media
Chronic mucinous otitis media
Chronic secretory otitis media
Chronic transudative otitis media
Glue ear
Excludes1 adhesive middle ear disease (H74.1)
H65.30 Chronic mucoid otitis media, unspecified ear
H65.31 Chronic mucoid otitis media, right ear
H65.32 Chronic mucoid otitis media, left ear
H65.33 Chronic mucoid otitis media, bilateral

● H65.4 Other chronic nonsuppurative otitis media
● H65.41 Chronic allergic otitis media
H65.411 Chronic allergic otitis media, right ear
H65.412 Chronic allergic otitis media, left ear
H65.413 Chronic allergic otitis media, bilateral
H65.419 Chronic allergic otitis media, unspecified ear

● H65.49 Other chronic nonsuppurative otitis media
Chronic exudative otitis media
Chronic nonsuppurative otitis media NOS
Chronic otitis media with effusion (nonpurulent)
Chronic seromucinous otitis media
H65.491 Other chronic nonsuppurative otitis media, right ear
H65.492 Other chronic nonsuppurative otitis media, left ear

H65.493 Other chronic nonsuppurative otitis media, bilateral
H65.499 Other chronic nonsuppurative otitis media, unspecified ear

● H65.9 Unspecified nonsuppurative otitis media
Allergic otitis media NOS
Catarrhal otitis media NOS
Exudative otitis media NOS
Mucoid otitis media NOS
Otitis media with effusion (nonpurulent) NOS
Secretory otitis media NOS
Seromucinous otitis media NOS
Serous otitis media NOS
Transudative otitis media NOS

H65.90 Unspecified nonsuppurative otitis media, unspecified ear
H65.91 Unspecified nonsuppurative otitis media, right ear
H65.92 Unspecified nonsuppurative otitis media, left ear
H65.93 Unspecified nonsuppurative otitis media, bilateral

● H66 Suppurative and unspecified otitis media
Suppurative: Discharging pus
Includes suppurative and unspecified otitis media with myringitis
Use additional code to identify:
exposure to environmental tobacco smoke (Z77.22)
exposure to tobacco smoke in the perinatal period (P96.81)
history of tobacco dependence (Z87.891)
occupational exposure to environmental tobacco smoke (Z57.31)
tobacco dependence (F17.-)
tobacco use (Z72.0)

● H66.0 Acute suppurative otitis media
● H66.00 Acute suppurative otitis media without spontaneous rupture of ear drum
H66.001 Acute suppurative otitis media without spontaneous rupture of ear drum, right ear
Coding Clinic: 2016, Q1, P34
H66.002 Acute suppurative otitis media without spontaneous rupture of ear drum, left ear
H66.003 Acute suppurative otitis media without spontaneous rupture of ear drum, bilateral
H66.004 Acute suppurative otitis media without spontaneous rupture of ear drum, recurrent, right ear
H66.005 Acute suppurative otitis media without spontaneous rupture of ear drum, recurrent, left ear
H66.006 Acute suppurative otitis media without spontaneous rupture of ear drum, recurrent, bilateral
H66.007 Acute suppurative otitis media without spontaneous rupture of ear drum, recurrent, unspecified ear
H66.009 Acute suppurative otitis media without spontaneous rupture of ear drum, unspecified ear

● H66.01 Acute suppurative otitis media with spontaneous rupture of ear drum
H66.011 Acute suppurative otitis media with spontaneous rupture of ear drum, right ear
H66.012 Acute suppurative otitis media with spontaneous rupture of ear drum, left ear
H66.013 Acute suppurative otitis media with spontaneous rupture of ear drum, bilateral
H66.014 Acute suppurative otitis media with spontaneous rupture of ear drum, recurrent, right ear

CHAPTER 8 (H60-H95)

H66.015   Acute suppurative otitis media with spontaneous rupture of ear drum, recurrent, left ear

H66.016   Acute suppurative otitis media with spontaneous rupture of ear drum, recurrent, bilateral

H66.017   Acute suppurative otitis media with spontaneous rupture of ear drum, recurrent, unspecified ear

H66.019   Acute suppurative otitis media with spontaneous rupture of ear drum, unspecified ear

● **H66.1   Chronic tubotympanic suppurative otitis media**
Benign chronic suppurative otitis media
Chronic tubotympanic disease
Use additional code for any associated perforated tympanic membrane (H72.-)

H66.10   Chronic tubotympanic suppurative otitis media, unspecified

H66.11   Chronic tubotympanic suppurative otitis media, right ear

H66.12   Chronic tubotympanic suppurative otitis media, left ear

H66.13   Chronic tubotympanic suppurative otitis media, bilateral

● **H66.2   Chronic atticoantral suppurative otitis media**
Chronic atticoantral disease
Use additional code for any associated perforated tympanic membrane (H72.-)

H66.20   Chronic atticoantral suppurative otitis media, unspecified ear

H66.21   Chronic atticoantral suppurative otitis media, right ear

H66.22   Chronic atticoantral suppurative otitis media, left ear

H66.23   Chronic atticoantral suppurative otitis media, bilateral

● **H66.3   Other chronic suppurative otitis media**
Chronic suppurative otitis media NOS
Use additional code for any associated perforated tympanic membrane (H72.-)

    Excludes1   tuberculous otitis media (A18.6)

● **H66.3X   Other chronic suppurative otitis media**

H66.3X1   Other chronic suppurative otitis media, right ear

H66.3X2   Other chronic suppurative otitis media, left ear

H66.3X3   Other chronic suppurative otitis media, bilateral

H66.3X9   Other chronic suppurative otitis media, unspecified ear

● **H66.4   Suppurative otitis media, unspecified**
Purulent otitis media NOS
Use additional code for any associated perforated tympanic membrane (H72.-)

H66.40   Suppurative otitis media, unspecified, unspecified ear

H66.41   Suppurative otitis media, unspecified, right ear

H66.42   Suppurative otitis media, unspecified, left ear

H66.43   Suppurative otitis media, unspecified, bilateral

● **H66.9   Otitis media, unspecified**
Otitis media NOS
Acute otitis media NOS
Chronic otitis media NOS
Use additional code for any associated perforated tympanic membrane (H72.-)

H66.90   Otitis media, unspecified, unspecified ear

H66.91   Otitis media, unspecified, right ear

H66.92   Otitis media, unspecified, left ear

H66.93   Otitis media, unspecified, bilateral

● **H67   Otitis media in diseases classified elsewhere**
Code first underlying disease, such as:
plasminogen deficiency (E88.02)
viral disease NEC (B00-B34)
Use additional code for any associated perforated tympanic membrane (H72.-)

    Excludes1   otitis media in:
influenza (J09.X9, J10.83, J11.83)
measles (B05.3)
scarlet fever (A38.0)
tuberculosis (A18.6)

▶ H67.1   *Otitis media in diseases classified elsewhere, right ear*

▶ H67.2   *Otitis media in diseases classified elsewhere, left ear*

▶ H67.3   *Otitis media in diseases classified elsewhere, bilateral*

▶ H67.9   *Otitis media in diseases classified elsewhere, unspecified ear*

● **H68   Eustachian salpingitis and obstruction**

● **H68.0   Eustachian salpingitis**

● **H68.00   Unspecified Eustachian salpingitis**

H68.001   Unspecified Eustachian salpingitis, right ear

H68.002   Unspecified Eustachian salpingitis, left ear

H68.003   Unspecified Eustachian salpingitis, bilateral

H68.009   Unspecified Eustachian salpingitis, unspecified ear

● **H68.01   Acute Eustachian salpingitis**

H68.011   Acute Eustachian salpingitis, right ear

H68.012   Acute Eustachian salpingitis, left ear

H68.013   Acute Eustachian salpingitis, bilateral

H68.019   Acute Eustachian salpingitis, unspecified ear

● **H68.02   Chronic Eustachian salpingitis**

H68.021   Chronic Eustachian salpingitis, right ear

H68.022   Chronic Eustachian salpingitis, left ear

H68.023   Chronic Eustachian salpingitis, bilateral

H68.029   Chronic Eustachian salpingitis, unspecified ear

● **H68.1   Obstruction of Eustachian tube**
Stenosis of Eustachian tube
Stricture of Eustachian tube

● **H68.10   Unspecified obstruction of Eustachian tube**

H68.101   Unspecified obstruction of Eustachian tube, right ear

H68.102   Unspecified obstruction of Eustachian tube, left ear

H68.103   Unspecified obstruction of Eustachian tube, bilateral

H68.109   Unspecified obstruction of Eustachian tube, unspecified ear

● **H68.11   Osseous obstruction of Eustachian tube**

H68.111   Osseous obstruction of Eustachian tube, right ear

H68.112   Osseous obstruction of Eustachian tube, left ear

H68.113   Osseous obstruction of Eustachian tube, bilateral

H68.119   Osseous obstruction of Eustachian tube, unspecified ear

● **H68.12   Intrinsic cartilagenous obstruction of Eustachian tube**

H68.121   Intrinsic cartilagenous obstruction of Eustachian tube, right ear

H68.122   Intrinsic cartilagenous obstruction of Eustachian tube, left ear

H68.123   Intrinsic cartilagenous obstruction of Eustachian tube, bilateral

H68.129   Intrinsic cartilagenous obstruction of Eustachian tube, unspecified ear

● H68.13   Extrinsic cartilagenous obstruction of Eustachian tube
    Compression of Eustachian tube

H68.131   Extrinsic cartilagenous obstruction of Eustachian tube, right ear

H68.132   Extrinsic cartilagenous obstruction of Eustachian tube, left ear

H68.133   Extrinsic cartilagenous obstruction of Eustachian tube, bilateral

H68.139   Extrinsic cartilagenous obstruction of Eustachian tube, unspecified ear

● H69   Other and unspecified disorders of Eustachian tube

   ● H69.0   Patulous Eustachian tube

H69.00   Patulous Eustachian tube, unspecified ear

H69.01   Patulous Eustachian tube, right ear

H69.02   Patulous Eustachian tube, left ear

H69.03   Patulous Eustachian tube, bilateral

   ● H69.8   Other specified disorders of Eustachian tube

H69.80   Other specified disorders of Eustachian tube, unspecified ear

H69.81   Other specified disorders of Eustachian tube, right ear

H69.82   Other specified disorders of Eustachian tube, left ear

H69.83   Other specified disorders of Eustachian tube, bilateral

   ● H69.9   Unspecified Eustachian tube disorder

H69.90   Unspecified Eustachian tube disorder, unspecified ear

H69.91   Unspecified Eustachian tube disorder, right ear

H69.92   Unspecified Eustachian tube disorder, left ear

H69.93   Unspecified Eustachian tube disorder, bilateral

● H70   Mastoiditis and related conditions

   ● H70.0   Acute mastoiditis
     Abscess of mastoid
     Empyema of mastoid

    ● H70.00   Acute mastoiditis without complications

H70.001   Acute mastoiditis without complications, right ear

H70.002   Acute mastoiditis without complications, left ear

H70.003   Acute mastoiditis without complications, bilateral

H70.009   Acute mastoiditis without complications, unspecified ear

    ● H70.01   Subperiosteal abscess of mastoid

H70.011   Subperiosteal abscess of mastoid, right ear

H70.012   Subperiosteal abscess of mastoid, left ear

H70.013   Subperiosteal abscess of mastoid, bilateral

H70.019   Subperiosteal abscess of mastoid, unspecified ear

    ● H70.09   Acute mastoiditis with other complications

H70.091   Acute mastoiditis with other complications, right ear

H70.092   Acute mastoiditis with other complications, left ear

H70.093   Acute mastoiditis with other complications, bilateral

H70.099   Acute mastoiditis with other complications, unspecified ear

Item 8-1   Mastoiditis is an infection of the portion of the temporal bone of the skull that is behind the ear (mastoid process) caused by an untreated otitis media, leading to an infection of the surrounding structures which may include the brain.

   ● H70.1   Chronic mastoiditis
     Caries of mastoid
     Fistula of mastoid

     Excludes1   tuberculous mastoiditis (A18.03)

H70.10   Chronic mastoiditis, unspecified ear

H70.11   Chronic mastoiditis, right ear

H70.12   Chronic mastoiditis, left ear

H70.13   Chronic mastoiditis, bilateral

   ● H70.2   Petrositis
     Inflammation of petrous bone

    ● H70.20   Unspecified petrositis

H70.201   Unspecified petrositis, right ear

H70.202   Unspecified petrositis, left ear

H70.203   Unspecified petrositis, bilateral

H70.209   Unspecified petrositis, unspecified ear

    ● H70.21   Acute petrositis

H70.211   Acute petrositis, right ear

H70.212   Acute petrositis, left ear

H70.213   Acute petrositis, bilateral

H70.219   Acute petrositis, unspecified ear

    ● H70.22   Chronic petrositis

H70.221   Chronic petrositis, right ear

H70.222   Chronic petrositis, left ear

H70.223   Chronic petrositis, bilateral

H70.229   Chronic petrositis, unspecified ear

   ● H70.8   Other mastoiditis and related conditions

     Excludes1   preauricular sinus and cyst (Q18.1)
       sinus, fistula, and cyst of branchial cleft (Q18.0)

    ● H70.81   Postauricular fistula

H70.811   Postauricular fistula, right ear

H70.812   Postauricular fistula, left ear

H70.813   Postauricular fistula, bilateral

H70.819   Postauricular fistula, unspecified ear

    ● H70.89   Other mastoiditis and related conditions

H70.891   Other mastoiditis and related conditions, right ear

H70.892   Other mastoiditis and related conditions, left ear

H70.893   Other mastoiditis and related conditions, bilateral

H70.899   Other mastoiditis and related conditions, unspecified ear

   ● H70.9   Unspecified mastoiditis

H70.90   Unspecified mastoiditis, unspecified ear

H70.91   Unspecified mastoiditis, right ear

H70.92   Unspecified mastoiditis, left ear

H70.93   Unspecified mastoiditis, bilateral

● H71   Cholesteatoma of middle ear

     Excludes2   cholesteatoma of external ear (H60.4-)
       recurrent cholesteatoma of postmastoidectomy cavity (H95.0-)

   ● H71.0   Cholesteatoma of attic

H71.00   Cholesteatoma of attic, unspecified ear

H71.01   Cholesteatoma of attic, right ear

H71.02   Cholesteatoma of attic, left ear
     Coding Clinic: 2021, Q3, P9

H71.03   Cholesteatoma of attic, bilateral

   ● H71.1   Cholesteatoma of tympanum

H71.10   Cholesteatoma of tympanum, unspecified ear

H71.11   Cholesteatoma of tympanum, right ear

H71.12   Cholesteatoma of tympanum, left ear

H71.13   Cholesteatoma of tympanum, bilateral

● **H71.2**   Cholesteatoma of mastoid
    H71.20   Cholesteatoma of mastoid, unspecified ear
    H71.21   Cholesteatoma of mastoid, right ear
    H71.22   Cholesteatoma of mastoid, left ear
       Coding Clinic: 2021, Q3, P9
    H71.23   Cholesteatoma of mastoid, bilateral
● **H71.3**   Diffuse cholesteatosis
       Coding Clinic: 2021, Q3, P9
    H71.30   Diffuse cholesteatosis, unspecified ear
    H71.31   Diffuse cholesteatosis, right ear
    H71.32   Diffuse cholesteatosis, left ear
    H71.33   Diffuse cholesteatosis, bilateral
● **H71.9**   Unspecified cholesteatoma
    H71.90   Unspecified cholesteatoma, unspecified ear
    H71.91   Unspecified cholesteatoma, right ear
    H71.92   Unspecified cholesteatoma, left ear
    H71.93   Unspecified cholesteatoma, bilateral

★ **(See Plate 22 of the Anatomy Illustrations.)**

● **H72**   Perforation of tympanic membrane
    Hole or rupture in ear drum
    Includes   persistent post-traumatic perforation of ear drum
                postinflammatory perforation of ear drum
    Code first any associated otitis media (H65.-, H66.1-, H66.2-, H66.3-, H66.4-, H66.9-, H67.-)
    Excludes1   acute suppurative otitis media with rupture of the tympanic membrane (H66.01-)
                traumatic rupture of ear drum (S09.2-)
● **H72.0**   Central perforation of tympanic membrane
    H72.00   Central perforation of tympanic membrane, unspecified ear
    H72.01   Central perforation of tympanic membrane, right ear
    H72.02   Central perforation of tympanic membrane, left ear
    H72.03   Central perforation of tympanic membrane, bilateral
● **H72.1**   Attic perforation of tympanic membrane
    Perforation of pars flaccida
    H72.10   Attic perforation of tympanic membrane, unspecified ear
    H72.11   Attic perforation of tympanic membrane, right ear
    H72.12   Attic perforation of tympanic membrane, left ear
    H72.13   Attic perforation of tympanic membrane, bilateral
● **H72.2**   Other marginal perforations of tympanic membrane
   ● **H72.2X**   Other marginal perforations of tympanic membrane
      H72.2X1   Other marginal perforations of tympanic membrane, right ear
      H72.2X2   Other marginal perforations of tympanic membrane, left ear
      H72.2X3   Other marginal perforations of tympanic membrane, bilateral
      H72.2X9   Other marginal perforations of tympanic membrane, unspecified ear
● **H72.8**   Other perforations of tympanic membrane
   ● **H72.81**   Multiple perforations of tympanic membrane
      H72.811   Multiple perforations of tympanic membrane, right ear
      H72.812   Multiple perforations of tympanic membrane, left ear
      H72.813   Multiple perforations of tympanic membrane, bilateral
      H72.819   Multiple perforations of tympanic membrane, unspecified ear

   ● **H72.82**   Total perforations of tympanic membrane
      H72.821   Total perforations of tympanic membrane, right ear
      H72.822   Total perforations of tympanic membrane, left ear
      H72.823   Total perforations of tympanic membrane, bilateral
      H72.829   Total perforations of tympanic membrane, unspecified ear
● **H72.9**   Unspecified perforation of tympanic membrane
    H72.90   Unspecified perforation of tympanic membrane, unspecified ear
    H72.91   Unspecified perforation of tympanic membrane, right ear
    H72.92   Unspecified perforation of tympanic membrane, left ear
    H72.93   Unspecified perforation of tympanic membrane, bilateral
● **H73**   Other disorders of tympanic membrane
   ● **H73.0**   Acute myringitis
     Excludes1   acute myringitis with otitis media (H65, H66)
    ● **H73.00**   Unspecified acute myringitis
      Acute tympanitis NOS
      H73.001   Acute myringitis, right ear
      H73.002   Acute myringitis, left ear
      H73.003   Acute myringitis, bilateral
      H73.009   Acute myringitis, unspecified ear
    ● **H73.01**   Bullous myringitis
      H73.011   Bullous myringitis, right ear
      H73.012   Bullous myringitis, left ear
      H73.013   Bullous myringitis, bilateral
      H73.019   Bullous myringitis, unspecified ear
    ● **H73.09**   Other acute myringitis
      H73.091   Other acute myringitis, right ear
      H73.092   Other acute myringitis, left ear
      H73.093   Other acute myringitis, bilateral
      H73.099   Other acute myringitis, unspecified ear
   ● **H73.1**   Chronic myringitis
    Chronic tympanitis
    Excludes1   chronic myringitis with otitis media (H65, H66)
    H73.10   Chronic myringitis, unspecified ear
    H73.11   Chronic myringitis, right ear
    H73.12   Chronic myringitis, left ear
    H73.13   Chronic myringitis, bilateral
   ● **H73.2**   Unspecified myringitis
    H73.20   Unspecified myringitis, unspecified ear
    H73.21   Unspecified myringitis, right ear
    H73.22   Unspecified myringitis, left ear
    H73.23   Unspecified myringitis, bilateral
   ● **H73.8**   Other specified disorders of tympanic membrane
    ● **H73.81**   Atrophic flaccid tympanic membrane
      H73.811   Atrophic flaccid tympanic membrane, right ear
      H73.812   Atrophic flaccid tympanic membrane, left ear
      H73.813   Atrophic flaccid tympanic membrane, bilateral
      H73.819   Atrophic flaccid tympanic membrane, unspecified ear
    ● **H73.82**   Atrophic nonflaccid tympanic membrane
      H73.821   Atrophic nonflaccid tympanic membrane, right ear
      H73.822   Atrophic nonflaccid tympanic membrane, left ear

▶ New   ⇒ Revised   ~~deleted~~ Deleted   Excludes 1   Excludes 2   Includes   Use additional   Code first   Code also   Key words
OGCR Official Guidelines   X Assign placeholder X   ● Use Additional Character(s)   ▌ Manifestation Code   🐾 Hierarchical Condition Category   **Coding Clinic**

H73.823 Atrophic nonflaccid tympanic membrane, bilateral

H73.829 Atrophic nonflaccid tympanic membrane, unspecified ear

● H73.89 Other specified disorders of tympanic membrane

H73.891 Other specified disorders of tympanic membrane, right ear

H73.892 Other specified disorders of tympanic membrane, left ear

H73.893 Other specified disorders of tympanic membrane, bilateral

H73.899 Other specified disorders of tympanic membrane, unspecified ear

● H73.9 Unspecified disorder of tympanic membrane

H73.90 Unspecified disorder of tympanic membrane, unspecified ear

H73.91 Unspecified disorder of tympanic membrane, right ear

H73.92 Unspecified disorder of tympanic membrane, left ear

H73.93 Unspecified disorder of tympanic membrane, bilateral

● H74 Other disorders of middle ear mastoid

    Excludes2 mastoiditis (H70.-)

● H74.0 Tympanosclerosis

H74.01 Tympanosclerosis, right ear

H74.02 Tympanosclerosis, left ear

H74.03 Tympanosclerosis, bilateral

H74.09 Tympanosclerosis, unspecified ear

● H74.1 Adhesive middle ear disease

    Adhesive otitis

    Excludes1 glue ear (H65.3-)

H74.11 Adhesive right middle ear disease

H74.12 Adhesive left middle ear disease

H74.13 Adhesive middle ear disease, bilateral

H74.19 Adhesive middle ear disease, unspecified ear

● H74.2 Discontinuity and dislocation of ear ossicles

H74.20 Discontinuity and dislocation of ear ossicles, unspecified ear

H74.21 Discontinuity and dislocation of right ear ossicles

H74.22 Discontinuity and dislocation of left ear ossicles

H74.23 Discontinuity and dislocation of ear ossicles, bilateral

● H74.3 Other acquired abnormalities of ear ossicles

● H74.31 Ankylosis of ear ossicles

H74.311 Ankylosis of ear ossicles, right ear

H74.312 Ankylosis of ear ossicles, left ear

H74.313 Ankylosis of ear ossicles, bilateral

H74.319 Ankylosis of ear ossicles, unspecified ear

● H74.32 Partial loss of ear ossicles

H74.321 Partial loss of ear ossicles, right ear

H74.322 Partial loss of ear ossicles, left ear

H74.323 Partial loss of ear ossicles, bilateral

H74.329 Partial loss of ear ossicles, unspecified ear

● H74.39 Other acquired abnormalities of ear ossicles

H74.391 Other acquired abnormalities of right ear ossicles

H74.392 Other acquired abnormalities of left ear ossicles

H74.393 Other acquired abnormalities of ear ossicles, bilateral

H74.399 Other acquired abnormalities of ear ossicles, unspecified ear

● H74.4 Polyp of middle ear

H74.40 Polyp of middle ear, unspecified ear

H74.41 Polyp of right middle ear

H74.42 Polyp of left middle ear

H74.43 Polyp of middle ear, bilateral

● H74.8 Other specified disorders of middle ear and mastoid

● H74.8X Other specified disorders of middle ear and mastoid

H74.8X1 Other specified disorders of right middle ear and mastoid

H74.8X2 Other specified disorders of left middle ear and mastoid

H74.8X3 Other specified disorders of middle ear and mastoid, bilateral

H74.8X9 Other specified disorders of middle ear and mastoid, unspecified ear

● H74.9 Unspecified disorder of middle ear and mastoid

H74.90 Unspecified disorder of middle ear and mastoid, unspecified ear

H74.91 Unspecified disorder of right middle ear and mastoid

H74.92 Unspecified disorder of left middle ear and mastoid

H74.93 Unspecified disorder of middle ear and mastoid, bilateral

● H75 Other disorders of middle ear and mastoid in diseases classified elsewhere

    Code first underlying disease

● H75.0 Mastoiditis in infectious and parasitic diseases classified elsewhere

    Excludes1 mastoiditis (in):
        syphilis (A52.77)
        tuberculosis (A18.03)

H75.00 *Mastoiditis in infectious and parasitic diseases classified elsewhere, unspecified ear*

H75.01 *Mastoiditis in infectious and parasitic diseases classified elsewhere, right ear*

H75.02 *Mastoiditis in infectious and parasitic diseases classified elsewhere, left ear*

H75.03 *Mastoiditis in infectious and parasitic diseases classified elsewhere, bilateral*

● H75.8 Other specified disorders of middle ear and mastoid in diseases classified elsewhere

H75.80 *Other specified disorders of middle ear and mastoid in diseases classified elsewhere, unspecified ear*

H75.81 *Other specified disorders of right middle ear and mastoid in diseases classified elsewhere*

H75.82 *Other specified disorders of left middle ear and mastoid in diseases classified elsewhere*

H75.83 *Other specified disorders of middle ear and mastoid in diseases classified elsewhere, bilateral*

DISEASES OF INNER EAR (H80-H83)

★**(See Plate 23 of the Anatomy Illustrations.)**

● H80 Otosclerosis

    Inherited middle ear spongelike bone growth causing hearing loss

    Includes Otospongiosis

● H80.0 Otosclerosis involving oval window, nonobliterative

H80.00 Otosclerosis involving oval window, nonobliterative, unspecified ear

H80.01 Otosclerosis involving oval window, nonobliterative, right ear

H80.02 Otosclerosis involving oval window, nonobliterative, left ear

H80.03 Otosclerosis involving oval window, nonobliterative, bilateral

● **H80.1**   Otosclerosis involving oval window, obliterative

    H80.10   Otosclerosis involving oval window, obliterative, unspecified ear

    H80.11   Otosclerosis involving oval window, obliterative, right ear

    H80.12   Otosclerosis involving oval window, obliterative, left ear

    H80.13   Otosclerosis involving oval window, obliterative, bilateral

● **H80.2**   Cochlear otosclerosis

    Otosclerosis involving otic capsule
    Otosclerosis involving round window

    H80.20   Cochlear otosclerosis, unspecified ear

    H80.21   Cochlear otosclerosis, right ear

    H80.22   Cochlear otosclerosis, left ear

    H80.23   Cochlear otosclerosis, bilateral

● **H80.8**   Other otosclerosis

    H80.80   Other otosclerosis, unspecified ear

    H80.81   Other otosclerosis, right ear

    H80.82   Other otosclerosis, left ear

    H80.83   Other otosclerosis, bilateral

● **H80.9**   Unspecified otosclerosis

    H80.90   Unspecified otosclerosis, unspecified ear

    H80.91   Unspecified otosclerosis, right ear

    H80.92   Unspecified otosclerosis, left ear

    H80.93   Unspecified otosclerosis, bilateral

● **H81**   Disorders of vestibular function

    Excludes1   epidemic vertigo (A88.1)
               vertigo NOS (R42)

● **H81.0**   Ménière's disease

    Vestibular disorder that produces recurring symptoms including severe and intermittent hearing loss including the feeling of ear pressure or pain

    Labyrinthine hydrops
    Ménière's syndrome or vertigo

    H81.01   Ménière's disease, right ear

    H81.02   Ménière's disease, left ear

    H81.03   Ménière's disease, bilateral

    H81.09   Ménière's disease, unspecified ear

● **H81.1**   Benign paroxysmal vertigo

    H81.10   Benign paroxysmal vertigo, unspecified ear

    H81.11   Benign paroxysmal vertigo, right ear

    H81.12   Benign paroxysmal vertigo, left ear

    H81.13   Benign paroxysmal vertigo, bilateral

● **H81.2**   Vestibular neuronitis

    H81.20   Vestibular neuronitis, unspecified ear

    H81.21   Vestibular neuronitis, right ear

    H81.22   Vestibular neuronitis, left ear

    H81.23   Vestibular neuronitis, bilateral

● **H81.3**   Other peripheral vertigo

    ● **H81.31**   Aural vertigo

       H81.311   Aural vertigo, right ear

       H81.312   Aural vertigo, left ear

       H81.313   Aural vertigo, bilateral

       H81.319   Aural vertigo, unspecified ear

    ● **H81.39**   Other peripheral vertigo

       Lermoyez' syndrome
       Otogenic vertigo
       Peripheral vertigo NOS

       H81.391   Other peripheral vertigo, right ear

       H81.392   Other peripheral vertigo, left ear

       H81.393   Other peripheral vertigo, bilateral

       H81.399   Other peripheral vertigo, unspecified ear

    H81.4   Vertigo of central origin

       Central positional nystagmus

● **H81.8**   Other disorders of vestibular function

    ● **H81.8X**   Other disorders of vestibular function

       H81.8X1   Other disorders of vestibular function, right ear

       H81.8X2   Other disorders of vestibular function, left ear

       H81.8X3   Other disorders of vestibular function, bilateral

       H81.8X9   Other disorders of vestibular function, unspecified ear

       Coding Clinic: 2022, Q2, P12

● **H81.9**   Unspecified disorder of vestibular function

    Vertiginous syndrome NOS

    H81.90   Unspecified disorder of vestibular function, unspecified ear

    H81.91   Unspecified disorder of vestibular function, right ear

    H81.92   Unspecified disorder of vestibular function, left ear

    H81.93   Unspecified disorder of vestibular function, bilateral

● **H82**   Vertiginous syndromes in diseases classified elsewhere

    Code first underlying disease

    Excludes1   epidemic vertigo (A88.1)

▷ *H82.1*   *Vertiginous syndromes in diseases classified elsewhere, right ear*

▷ *H82.2*   *Vertiginous syndromes in diseases classified elsewhere, left ear*

▷ *H82.3*   *Vertiginous syndromes in diseases classified elsewhere, bilateral*

▷ *H82.9*   *Vertiginous syndromes in diseases classified elsewhere, unspecified ear*

● **H83**   Other diseases of inner ear

    ● **H83.0**   Labyrinthitis

       Balance disorder that follows URI or head injury

       H83.01   Labyrinthitis, right ear

       H83.02   Labyrinthitis, left ear

       H83.03   Labyrinthitis, bilateral

       H83.09   Labyrinthitis, unspecified ear

    ● **H83.1**   Labyrinthine fistula

       H83.11   Labyrinthine fistula, right ear

       H83.12   Labyrinthine fistula, left ear

       H83.13   Labyrinthine fistula, bilateral

       H83.19   Labyrinthine fistula, unspecified ear

    ● **H83.2**   Labyrinthine dysfunction

       Labyrinthine hypersensitivity
       Labyrinthine hypofunction
       Labyrinthine loss of function

      ● **H83.2X**   Labyrinthine dysfunction

         H83.2X1   Labyrinthine dysfunction, right ear

         H83.2X2   Labyrinthine dysfunction, left ear

         H83.2X3   Labyrinthine dysfunction, bilateral

         H83.2X9   Labyrinthine dysfunction, unspecified ear

    ● **H83.3**   Noise effects on inner ear

       Acoustic trauma of inner ear
       Noise-induced hearing loss of inner ear

      ● **H83.3X**   Noise effects on inner ear

         H83.3X1   Noise effects on right inner ear

         H83.3X2   Noise effects on left inner ear

         H83.3X3   Noise effects on inner ear, bilateral

         H83.3X9   Noise effects on inner ear, unspecified ear

    ● **H83.8**   Other specified diseases of inner ear

      ● **H83.8X**   Other specified diseases of inner ear

         H83.8X1   Other specified diseases of right inner ear

         H83.8X2   Other specified diseases of left inner ear

▶ New   ⇒ Revised   ~~deleted~~ Deleted   Excludes 1   Excludes 2   Includes   Use additional   Code first   Code also   Key words

OGCR Official Guidelines   X Assign placeholder X   ● Use Additional Character(s)   ▷ Manifestation Code   🔗 Hierarchical Condition Category   Coding Clinic

H83.8X3   Other specified diseases of inner ear, bilateral

H83.8X9   Other specified diseases of inner ear, unspecified ear

● H83.9   Unspecified disease of inner ear

H83.90   Unspecified disease of inner ear, unspecified ear

H83.91   Unspecified disease of right inner ear

H83.92   Unspecified disease of left inner ear

H83.93   Unspecified disease of inner ear, bilateral

OTHER DISORDERS OF EAR (H90–H94)

● H90   Conductive and sensorineural hearing loss

> **Excludes1**   deaf nonspeaking NEC (H91.3)
> deafness NOS (H91.9-)
> hearing loss NOS (H91.9-)
> noise-induced hearing loss (H83.3-)
> ototoxic hearing loss (H91.0-)
> sudden (idiopathic) hearing loss (H91.2-)

H90.0   Conductive hearing loss, bilateral

● H90.1   Conductive hearing loss, unilateral with unrestricted hearing on the contralateral side

H90.11   Conductive hearing loss, unilateral, right ear, with unrestricted hearing on the contralateral side

H90.12   Conductive hearing loss, unilateral, left ear, with unrestricted hearing on the contralateral side

H90.2   Conductive hearing loss, unspecified
Conductive deafness NOS

H90.3   Sensorineural hearing loss, bilateral

● H90.4   Sensorineural hearing loss, unilateral with unrestricted hearing on the contralateral side

H90.41   Sensorineural hearing loss, unilateral, right ear, with unrestricted hearing on the contralateral side

H90.42   Sensorineural hearing loss, unilateral, left ear, with unrestricted hearing on the contralateral side

H90.5   Unspecified sensorineural hearing loss
Central hearing loss NOS
Congenital deafness NOS
Neural hearing loss NOS
Perceptive hearing loss NOS
Sensorineural deafness NOS
Sensory hearing loss NOS

> **Excludes1**   abnormal auditory perception (H93.2-)
> psychogenic deafness (F44.6)

H90.6   Mixed conductive and sensorineural hearing loss, bilateral
Coding Clinic: 2015, Q2, P7

● H90.7   Mixed conductive and sensorineural hearing loss, unilateral with unrestricted hearing on the contralateral side

H90.71   Mixed conductive and sensorineural hearing loss, unilateral, right ear, with unrestricted hearing on the contralateral side

H90.72   Mixed conductive and sensorineural hearing loss, unilateral, left ear, with unrestricted hearing on the contralateral side

H90.8   Mixed conductive and sensorineural hearing loss, unspecified

● H90.A   Conductive and sensorineural hearing loss with restricted hearing on the contralateral side
Coding Clinic: 2016, Q4, P23-24

● H90.A1   Conductive hearing loss, unilateral, with restricted hearing on the contralateral side

H90.A11   Conductive hearing loss, unilateral, right ear with restricted hearing on the contralateral side

H90.A12   Conductive hearing loss, unilateral, left ear with restricted hearing on the contralateral side
Coding Clinic: 2016, Q4, P25

● H90.A2   Sensorineural hearing loss, unilateral, with restricted hearing on the contralateral side

H90.A21   Sensorineural hearing loss, unilateral, right ear, with restricted hearing on the contralateral side

H90.A22   Sensorineural hearing loss, unilateral, left ear, with restricted hearing on the contralateral side

● H90.A3   Mixed conductive and sensorineural hearing loss, unilateral with restricted hearing on the contralateral side

H90.A31   Mixed conductive and sensorineural hearing loss, unilateral, right ear with restricted hearing on the contralateral side

H90.A32   Mixed conductive and sensorineural hearing loss, unilateral, left ear with restricted hearing on the contralateral side

● H91   Other and unspecified hearing loss

> **Excludes1**   abnormal auditory perception (H93.2-)
> hearing loss as classified in H90.-
> impacted cerumen (H61.2-)
> noise-induced hearing loss (H83.3-)
> psychogenic deafness (F44.6)
> transient ischemic deafness (H93.01-)

● H91.0   Ototoxic hearing loss

> *Code first poisoning due to drug or toxin, if applicable (T36-T65 with fifth or sixth character 1-4 or 6)*
>
> Use additional code for adverse effect, if applicable, to identify drug (T36-T50 with fifth or sixth character 5)

H91.01   Ototoxic hearing loss, right ear

H91.02   Ototoxic hearing loss, left ear

H91.03   Ototoxic hearing loss, bilateral

H91.09   Ototoxic hearing loss, unspecified ear

● H91.1   Presbycusis
Presbyacusia

H91.10   Presbycusis, unspecified ear

H91.11   Presbycusis, right ear

H91.12   Presbycusis, left ear

H91.13   Presbycusis, bilateral

● H91.2   Sudden idiopathic hearing loss
Sudden hearing loss NOS

H91.20   Sudden idiopathic hearing loss, unspecified ear

H91.21   Sudden idiopathic hearing loss, right ear

H91.22   Sudden idiopathic hearing loss, left ear

H91.23   Sudden idiopathic hearing loss, bilateral

H91.3   Deaf nonspeaking, not elsewhere classified

● H91.8   Other specified hearing loss

● H91.8X   Other specified hearing loss

H91.8X1   Other specified hearing loss, right ear

H91.8X2   Other specified hearing loss, left ear

H91.8X3   Other specified hearing loss, bilateral

H91.8X9   Other specified hearing loss, unspecified ear

● H91.9   Unspecified hearing loss
Deafness NOS
High frequency deafness
Low frequency deafness

H91.90   Unspecified hearing loss, unspecified ear

H91.91   Unspecified hearing loss, right ear

H91.92   Unspecified hearing loss, left ear

H91.93   Unspecified hearing loss, bilateral

CHAPTER 8 (H60–H95)

● **H92**   **Otalgia and effusion of ear**
   ● **H92.0**   Otalgia
      H92.01   Otalgia, right ear
      H92.02   Otalgia, left ear
      H92.03   Otalgia, bilateral
      H92.09   Otalgia, unspecified ear
   ● **H92.1**   Otorrhea
      Excludes1   leakage of cerebrospinal fluid through ear (G96.0)
      H92.10   Otorrhea, unspecified ear
      H92.11   Otorrhea, right ear
      H92.12   Otorrhea, left ear
      H92.13   Otorrhea, bilateral
   ● **H92.2**   Otorrhagia
      Excludes1   traumatic otorrhagia - code to injury
      H92.20   Otorrhagia, unspecified ear
      H92.21   Otorrhagia, right ear
      H92.22   Otorrhagia, left ear
      H92.23   Otorrhagia, bilateral

● **H93**   **Other disorders of ear, not elsewhere classified**
   ● **H93.0**   Degenerative and vascular disorders of ear
      Excludes1   presbycusis (H91.1)
     ● **H93.01**   Transient ischemic deafness
       H93.011   Transient ischemic deafness, right ear
       H93.012   Transient ischemic deafness, left ear
       H93.013   Transient ischemic deafness, bilateral
       H93.019   Transient ischemic deafness, unspecified ear
     ● **H93.09**   Unspecified degenerative and vascular disorders of ear
       H93.091   Unspecified degenerative and vascular disorders of right ear
       H93.092   Unspecified degenerative and vascular disorders of left ear
       H93.093   Unspecified degenerative and vascular disorders of ear, bilateral
       H93.099   Unspecified degenerative and vascular disorders of unspecified ear
   ● **H93.1**   Tinnitus
      Perception of sound (ringing, buzzing, humming, whistling tunes, or singing)
      H93.11   Tinnitus, right ear
      H93.12   Tinnitus, left ear
      H93.13   Tinnitus, bilateral
      H93.19   Tinnitus, unspecified ear
   ● **H93.A**   Pulsatile tinnitus
      Coding Clinic: 2016, Q4, P25
      H93.A1   Pulsatile tinnitus, right ear
       Coding Clinic: 2016, Q4, P26
      H93.A2   Pulsatile tinnitus, left ear
      H93.A3   Pulsatile tinnitus, bilateral
      H93.A9   Pulsatile tinnitus, unspecified ear
   ● **H93.2**   Other abnormal auditory perceptions
      Excludes2   auditory hallucinations (R44.0)
     ● **H93.21**   Auditory recruitment
       H93.211   Auditory recruitment, right ear
       H93.212   Auditory recruitment, left ear
       H93.213   Auditory recruitment, bilateral
       H93.219   Auditory recruitment, unspecified ear
     ● **H93.22**   Diplacusis
       H93.221   Diplacusis, right ear
       H93.222   Diplacusis, left ear
       H93.223   Diplacusis, bilateral
       H93.229   Diplacusis, unspecified ear

     ● **H93.23**   Hyperacusis
       H93.231   Hyperacusis, right ear
       H93.232   Hyperacusis, left ear
       H93.233   Hyperacusis, bilateral
       H93.239   Hyperacusis, unspecified ear
     ● **H93.24**   Temporary auditory threshold shift
       H93.241   Temporary auditory threshold shift, right ear
       H93.242   Temporary auditory threshold shift, left ear
       H93.243   Temporary auditory threshold shift, bilateral
       H93.249   Temporary auditory threshold shift, unspecified ear
     H93.25   Central auditory processing disorder
      Congenital auditory imperception
      Word deafness
      Excludes1   mixed receptive-expressive language disorder (F80.2)
     ● **H93.29**   Other abnormal auditory perceptions
       H93.291   Other abnormal auditory perceptions, right ear
       H93.292   Other abnormal auditory perceptions, left ear
       H93.293   Other abnormal auditory perceptions, bilateral
       H93.299   Other abnormal auditory perceptions, unspecified ear
   ● **H93.3**   Disorders of acoustic nerve
      Disorder of 8th cranial nerve
      Excludes1   acoustic neuroma (D33.3)
         syphilitic acoustic neuritis (A52.15)
     ● **H93.3X**   Disorders of acoustic nerve
       H93.3X1   Disorders of right acoustic nerve
       H93.3X2   Disorders of left acoustic nerve
       H93.3X3   Disorders of bilateral acoustic nerves
       H93.3X9   Disorders of unspecified acoustic nerve
   ● **H93.8**   Other specified disorders of ear
     ● **H93.8X**   Other specified disorders of ear
       H93.8X1   Other specified disorders of right ear
       H93.8X2   Other specified disorders of left ear
       H93.8X3   Other specified disorders of ear, bilateral
       H93.8X9   Other specified disorders of ear, unspecified ear
   ● **H93.9**   Unspecified disorder of ear
      H93.90   Unspecified disorder of ear, unspecified ear
      H93.91   Unspecified disorder of right ear
      H93.92   Unspecified disorder of left ear
      H93.93   Unspecified disorder of ear, bilateral

● **H94**   **Other disorders of ear in diseases classified elsewhere**
   ● **H94.0**   Acoustic neuritis in infectious and parasitic diseases classified elsewhere
      Code first underlying disease, such as:
      parasitic disease (B65-B89)
      Excludes1   acoustic neuritis (in):
         herpes zoster (B02.29)
         syphilis (A52.15)
      ▷ *H94.00*   *Acoustic neuritis in infectious and parasitic diseases classified elsewhere, unspecified ear*
      ▷ *H94.01*   *Acoustic neuritis in infectious and parasitic diseases classified elsewhere, right ear*
      ▷ *H94.02*   *Acoustic neuritis in infectious and parasitic diseases classified elsewhere, left ear*
      ▷ *H94.03*   *Acoustic neuritis in infectious and parasitic diseases classified elsewhere, bilateral*

▶ New   ⇛ Revised   ~~deleted~~ Deleted   Excludes 1   Excludes 2   Includes   Use additional   Code first   Code also   Key words
OGCR Official Guidelines   X Assign placeholder X   ● Use Additional Character(s)   ▷ Manifestation Code   🍎 Hierarchical Condition Category   **Coding Clinic**

- H94.8   Other specified disorders of ear in diseases classified elsewhere

    Code first underlying disease, such as:
    congenital syphilis (A50.0)

    Excludes1   aural myiasis (B87.4)
    syphilitic labyrinthitis (A52.79)

    - H94.80   *Other specified disorders of ear in diseases classified elsewhere, unspecified ear*
    - H94.81   *Other specified disorders of right ear in diseases classified elsewhere*
    - H94.82   *Other specified disorders of left ear in diseases classified elsewhere*
    - H94.83   *Other specified disorders of ear in diseases classified elsewhere, bilateral*

INTRAOPERATIVE AND POSTPROCEDURAL COMPLICATIONS AND DISORDERS OF EAR AND MASTOID PROCESS, NOT ELSEWHERE CLASSIFIED (H95)

- H95   Intraoperative and postprocedural complications and disorders of ear and mastoid process, not elsewhere classified

    Coding Clinic: 2016, Q4, P10

    - H95.0   Recurrent cholesteatoma of postmastoidectomy cavity
        - H95.00   Recurrent cholesteatoma of postmastoidectomy cavity, unspecified ear
        - H95.01   Recurrent cholesteatoma of postmastoidectomy cavity, right ear
        - H95.02   Recurrent cholesteatoma of postmastoidectomy cavity, left ear
        - H95.03   Recurrent cholesteatoma of postmastoidectomy cavity, bilateral ears
    - H95.1   Other disorders of ear and mastoid process following mastoidectomy
        - H95.11   Chronic inflammation of postmastoidectomy cavity
            - H95.111   Chronic inflammation of postmastoidectomy cavity, right ear
            - H95.112   Chronic inflammation of postmastoidectomy cavity, left ear
            - H95.113   Chronic inflammation of postmastoidectomy cavity, bilateral ears
            - H95.119   Chronic inflammation of postmastoidectomy cavity, unspecified ear
        - H95.12   Granulation of postmastoidectomy cavity
            - H95.121   Granulation of postmastoidectomy cavity, right ear
            - H95.122   Granulation of postmastoidectomy cavity, left ear
            - H95.123   Granulation of postmastoidectomy cavity, bilateral ears
            - H95.129   Granulation of postmastoidectomy cavity, unspecified ear
        - H95.13   Mucosal cyst of postmastoidectomy cavity
            - H95.131   Mucosal cyst of postmastoidectomy cavity, right ear
            - H95.132   Mucosal cyst of postmastoidectomy cavity, left ear
            - H95.133   Mucosal cyst of postmastoidectomy cavity, bilateral ears
            - H95.139   Mucosal cyst of postmastoidectomy cavity, unspecified ear
        - H95.19   Other disorders following mastoidectomy
            - H95.191   Other disorders following mastoidectomy, right ear
            - H95.192   Other disorders following mastoidectomy, left ear

- H95.193   Other disorders following mastoidectomy, bilateral ears
- H95.199   Other disorders following mastoidectomy, unspecified ear

- H95.2   Intraoperative hemorrhage and hematoma of ear and mastoid process complicating a procedure

    Excludes1   intraoperative hemorrhage and hematoma of ear and mastoid process due to accidental puncture or laceration during a procedure (H95.3-)

    - H95.21   Intraoperative hemorrhage and hematoma of ear and mastoid process complicating a procedure on the ear and mastoid process
    - H95.22   Intraoperative hemorrhage and hematoma of ear and mastoid process complicating other procedure
- H95.3   Accidental puncture and laceration of ear and mastoid process during a procedure
    - H95.31   Accidental puncture and laceration of the ear and mastoid process during a procedure on the ear and mastoid process
    - H95.32   Accidental puncture and laceration of the ear and mastoid process during other procedure
- H95.4   Postprocedural hemorrhage of ear and mastoid process following a procedure
    - H95.41   Postprocedural hemorrhage of ear and mastoid process following a procedure on the ear and mastoid process
    - H95.42   Postprocedural hemorrhage of ear and mastoid process following other procedure
- H95.5   Postprocedural hematoma and seroma of ear and mastoid process following a procedure
    - H95.51   Postprocedural hematoma of ear and mastoid process following a procedure on the ear and mastoid process
    - H95.52   Postprocedural hematoma of ear and mastoid process following other procedure
    - H95.53   Postprocedural seroma of ear and mastoid process following a procedure on the ear and mastoid process
    - H95.54   Postprocedural seroma of ear and mastoid process following other procedure
- H95.8   Other intraoperative and postprocedural complications and disorders of the ear and mastoid process, not elsewhere classified

    Excludes2   postprocedural complications and disorders following mastoidectomy (H95.0-, H95.1-)

    - H95.81   Postprocedural stenosis of external ear canal
        - H95.811   Postprocedural stenosis of right external ear canal
        - H95.812   Postprocedural stenosis of left external ear canal
        - H95.813   Postprocedural stenosis of external ear canal, bilateral
        - H95.819   Postprocedural stenosis of unspecified external ear canal
    - H95.88   Other intraoperative complications and disorders of the ear and mastoid process, not elsewhere classified

        Use additional code, if applicable, to further specify disorder
    - H95.89   Other postprocedural complications and disorders of the ear and mastoid process, not elsewhere classified

        Use additional code, if applicable, to further specify disorder

CHAPTER 9

DISEASES OF THE CIRCULATORY SYSTEM
(I00–I99)

OGCR Chapter-Specific Coding Guidelines

9. Chapter 9: Diseases of the Circulatory System (I00–I99)

a. Hypertension

The classification presumes a causal relationship between hypertension and heart involvement and between hypertension and kidney involvement, as the two conditions are linked by the term "with" in the Alphabetic Index. These conditions should be coded as related even in the absence of provider documentation explicitly linking them, unless the documentation clearly states the conditions are unrelated.

For hypertension and conditions not specifically linked by relational terms such as "with," "associated with" or "due to" in the classification, provider documentation must link the conditions in order to code them as related.

1) Hypertension with Heart Disease

Hypertension with heart conditions classified to I50.- or I51.4-I51.7, I51.89, I51.9, are assigned to, a code from category I11, Hypertensive heart disease. Use additional code(s) from category I50, Heart failure, to identify the type(s) of heart failure in those patients with heart failure.

The same heart conditions (I50.-, I51.4-I51.7, I51.89, I51.9) with hypertension, are coded separately if the provider has documented they are unrelated to the hypertension. Sequence according to the circumstances of the admission/encounter.

2) Hypertensive Chronic Kidney Disease

Assign codes from category I12, Hypertensive chronic kidney disease, when both hypertension and a condition classifiable to category N18, Chronic kidney disease (CKD), are present. CKD should not be coded as hypertensive if the provider indicates the CKD is not related to the hypertension.

The appropriate code from category N18 should be used as a secondary code with a code from category I12 to identify the stage of chronic kidney disease.

See Section I.C.14. Chronic kidney disease.

If a patient has hypertensive chronic kidney disease and acute renal failure, an additional code for the acute renal failure is required.

3) Hypertensive Heart and Chronic Kidney Disease

Assign codes from combination category I13, Hypertensive heart and chronic kidney disease, when there is hypertension with both heart and kidney involvement. If heart failure is present, assign an additional code from category I50 to identify the type of heart failure.

The appropriate code from category N18, Chronic kidney disease, should be used as a secondary code with a code from category I13 to identify the stage of chronic kidney disease.

See Section I.C.14. Chronic kidney disease.

The codes in category I13, Hypertensive heart and chronic kidney disease, are combination codes that include hypertension, heart disease and chronic kidney disease. The Includes note at I13 specifies that the conditions included at I11 and I12 are included together in I13. If a patient has hypertension, heart disease and chronic kidney disease then a code from I13 should be used, not individual codes for hypertension, heart disease and chronic kidney disease, or codes from I11 or I12.

For patients with both acute renal failure and chronic kidney disease an additional code for acute renal failure is required.

4) Hypertensive Cerebrovascular Disease

For hypertensive cerebrovascular disease, first assign the appropriate code from categories I60-I69, followed by the appropriate hypertension code.

5) Hypertensive Retinopathy

Subcategory H35.0, Background retinopathy and retinal vascular changes, should be used with a code from category I10 – I15, Hypertensive disease to include the systemic hypertension. The sequencing is based on the reason for the encounter.

6) Hypertension, Secondary

Secondary hypertension is due to an underlying condition. Two codes are required: one to identify the underlying etiology and one from category I15 to identify the hypertension. Sequencing of codes is determined by the reason for admission/encounter.

7) Hypertension, Transient

Assign code R03.0, Elevated blood pressure reading without diagnosis of hypertension, unless patient has an established diagnosis of hypertension. Assign code O13.-, Gestational [pregnancy-induced] hypertension without significant proteinuria, or O14.-, Pre-eclampsia, for transient hypertension of pregnancy.

8) Hypertension, Controlled

This diagnostic statement usually refers to an existing state of hypertension under control by therapy. Assign the appropriate code from categories I10-I15, Hypertensive diseases.

9) Hypertension, Uncontrolled

Uncontrolled hypertension may refer to untreated hypertension or hypertension not responding to current therapeutic regimen. In either case, assign the appropriate code from categories I10-I15, Hypertensive diseases.

10) Hypertensive Crisis

Assign a code from category I16, Hypertensive crisis, for documented hypertensive urgency, hypertensive emergency or unspecified hypertensive crisis. Code also any identified hypertensive disease (I10-I15). The sequencing is based on the reason for the encounter.

11) Pulmonary Hypertension

Pulmonary hypertension is classified to category I27, Other pulmonary heart diseases. For secondary pulmonary hypertension (I27.1, I27.2-), code also any associated conditions or adverse effects of drugs or toxins. The sequencing is based on the reason for the encounter, except for adverse effects of drugs.

See Section I.C.19.e Adverse Effects, Poisoning, Underdosing and Toxic Effects.

b. Atherosclerotic Coronary Artery Disease and Angina

ICD-10-CM has combination codes for atherosclerotic heart disease with angina pectoris. The subcategories for these codes are I25.11, Atherosclerotic heart disease of native coronary artery with angina pectoris and I25.7, Atherosclerosis of coronary artery bypass graft(s) and coronary artery of transplanted heart with angina pectoris.

When using one of these combination codes it is not necessary to use an additional code for angina pectoris. A causal relationship can be assumed in a patient with both atherosclerosis and angina pectoris, unless the documentation indicates the angina is due to something other than the atherosclerosis.

If a patient with coronary artery disease is admitted due to an acute myocardial infarction (AMI), the AMI should be sequenced before the coronary artery disease.

See Section I.C.9. Acute myocardial infarction (AMI).

c. Intraoperative and Postprocedural Cerebrovascular Accident

Medical record documentation should clearly specify the cause-and-effect relationship between the medical intervention and the cerebrovascular accident in order to assign a code for intraoperative or postprocedural cerebrovascular accident.

Proper code assignment depends on whether it was an infarction or hemorrhage and whether it occurred intraoperatively or postoperatively. If it was a cerebral hemorrhage, code assignment depends on the type of procedure performed.

d. Sequelae of Cerebrovascular Disease

1) Category I69, Sequelae of Cerebrovascular disease

Category I69 is used to indicate conditions classifiable to categories I60-I67 as the causes of sequela (neurologic deficits), themselves classified elsewhere. These "late effects" include neurologic deficits that persist after initial onset of conditions classifiable to categories I60-I67. The neurologic deficits caused by cerebrovascular disease may be present from the onset or may arise at any time after the onset of the condition classifiable to categories I60-I67.

Codes from category I69, Sequelae of cerebrovascular disease, that specify hemiplegia, hemiparesis and monoplegia identify whether the dominant or nondominant side is affected. Should the affected side be documented, but not specified as dominant or nondominant, and the classification system does not indicate a default, code selection is as follows:

- For ambidextrous patients, the default should be dominant.
- If the left side is affected, the default is nondominant.
- If the right side is affected, the default is dominant.

2) Codes from category I69 with codes from I60-I67

Codes from category I69 may be assigned on a health care record with codes from I60-I67, if the patient has a current cerebrovascular disease and deficits from an old cerebrovascular disease.

3) **Codes from category I69 and Personal history of transient ischemic attack (TIA) and cerebral infarction (Z86.73)**

Codes from category I69 should not be assigned if the patient does not have neurologic deficits.

See Section I.C.21. 4. History (of) for use of personal history codes.

e. Acute myocardial infarction (AMI)

1) Type 1 ST elevation myocardial infarction (STEMI) and non-ST elevation myocardial infarction (NSTEMI)

The ICD-10-CM codes for acute type 1 myocardial infarction (AMI) identify the site, such as anterolateral wall or true posterior wall. Subcategories I21.0-I21.2 and code I21.3 are used for type 1 ST elevation myocardial infarction (STEMI). Code I21.4, non-ST elevation (NSTEMI) myocardial infarction, is used for type 1 non-ST elevation myocardial infarction (NSTEMI) and nontransmural MIs.

If a type 1 NSTEMI evolves to STEMI, assign the STEMI code. If a type 1 STEMI converts to NSTEMI due to thrombolytic therapy, it is still coded as STEMI.

For encounters occurring while the myocardial infarction is equal to, or less than, four weeks old, including transfers to another acute setting or a postacute setting, and the myocardial infarction meets the definition for "other diagnoses" (see Section III, Reporting Additional Diagnoses), codes from category I21 may continue to be reported. For encounters after the 4-week time frame and the patient is still receiving care related to the myocardial infarction, the appropriate aftercare code should be assigned, rather than a code from category I21. For old or healed myocardial infarctions not requiring further care, code I25.2, Old myocardial infarction, may be assigned.

2) Acute myocardial infarction, unspecified

Code I21.9, Acute myocardial infarction, unspecified, is the default for unspecified acute myocardial infarction or unspecified type. If only type 1 STEMI or transmural MI without the site is documented, assign code I21.3, ST elevation (STEMI) myocardial infarction of unspecified site.

3) AMI documented as nontransmural or subendocardial but site provided

If an AMI is documented as nontransmural or subendocardial, but the site is provided, it is still coded as a subendocardial AMI.

See Section I.C.21.3 for information on coding status post administration of tPA in a different facility within the last 24 hours.

4) Subsequent acute myocardial infarction

A code from category I22, Subsequent ST elevation (STEMI) and non-ST elevation (NSTEMI) myocardial infarction, is to be used when a patient who has suffered a type 1 or unspecified AMI has a new AMI within the 4-week time frame of the initial AMI. A code from category I22 must be used in conjunction with a code from category I21. The sequencing of the I22 and I21 codes depends on the circumstances of the encounter.

Do not assign code I22 for subsequent myocardial infarctions other than type 1 or unspecified. For subsequent type 2 AMI assign only code I21.A1. For subsequent type 4 or type 5 AMI, assign only code I21.A9.

If a subsequent myocardial infarction of one type occurs within 4 weeks of a myocardial infarction of a different type, assign the appropriate codes from category I21 to identify each type. Do not assign a code from I22. Codes from category I22 should only be assigned if both the initial and subsequent myocardial infarctions are type 1 or unspecified.

5) Other Types of Myocardial Infarction

The ICD-10-CM provides codes for different types of myocardial infarction. Type 1 myocardial infarctions are assigned to codes I21.0-I21.4 and I21.9.

Type 2 myocardial infarction, and myocardial infarction due to demand ischemia or secondary to ischemic balance, is assigned to code I21.A1, Myocardial infarction type 2 with a code for the underlying cause. Do not assign code I24.8, Other forms of acute ischemic heart disease for the demand ischemia. Sequencing of type 2 AMI or the underlying cause is dependent on the circumstances of admission. When a type 2 AMI code is described as NSTEMI or STEMI, only assign code I21.A1. Codes I21.01-I21.4 should only be assigned for type 1 AMIs.

Acute myocardial infarctions type 3, 4a, 4b, 4c, and 5 are assigned to code I21.A9, Other myocardial infarction type.

The "Code also" and "Code first" notes should be followed related to complications, and for coding of postprocedural myocardial infarctions during or following cardiac surgery.

Figure 9-1 Cardiovascular valves.

Item 9–1 Rheumatic fever is the inflammation of the valve(s) of the heart, usually the mitral or aortic, which leads to valve damage. Rheumatic heart inflammations are usually **pericarditis** (sac surrounding heart), **endocarditis** (heart cavity), or **myocarditis** (heart muscle).

CHAPTER 9

DISEASES OF THE CIRCULATORY SYSTEM (I00-I99)

Excludes2	certain conditions originating in the perinatal period (P04-P96)
	certain infectious and parasitic diseases (A00-B99)
	complications of pregnancy, childbirth and the puerperium (O00-O9A)
	congenital malformations, deformations, and chromosomal abnormalities (Q00-Q99)
	endocrine, nutritional and metabolic diseases (E00-E88)
	injury, poisoning and certain other consequences of external causes (S00-T88)
	neoplasms (C00-D49)
	symptoms, signs and abnormal clinical and laboratory findings, not elsewhere classified (R00-R94)
	systemic connective tissue disorders (M30-M36)
	transient cerebral ischemic attacks and related syndromes (G45.-)

This chapter contains the following blocks:

I00-I02	Acute rheumatic fever
I05-I09	Chronic rheumatic heart diseases
I10-I16	Hypertensive diseases
I20-I25	Ischemic heart diseases
I26-I28	Pulmonary heart disease and diseases of pulmonary circulation
I30-I5A	Other forms of heart disease
I60-I69	Cerebrovascular diseases
I70-I79	Diseases of arteries, arterioles and capillaries
I80-I89	Diseases of veins, lymphatic vessels and lymph nodes, not elsewhere classified
I95-I99	Other and unspecified disorders of the circulatory system

ACUTE RHEUMATIC FEVER (I00-I02)

I00   **Rheumatic fever without heart involvement**

     Includes   arthritis, rheumatic, acute or subacute

     Excludes1   rheumatic fever with heart involvement (I01.0-I01.9)

●**I01**   **Rheumatic fever with heart involvement**

     Excludes1   chronic diseases of rheumatic origin (I05-I09) unless rheumatic fever is also present or there is evidence of reactivation or activity of the rheumatic process.

   I01.0   **Acute rheumatic pericarditis**

       Any condition in I00 with pericarditis

       Rheumatic pericarditis (acute)

       Excludes1   acute pericarditis not specified as rheumatic (I30.-)

   I01.1   **Acute rheumatic endocarditis**

       Any condition in I00 with endocarditis or valvulitis

       Acute rheumatic valvulitis

Item 9–2 Rheumatic chorea, also called Sydenham's, juvenile, minor, simple, or St. Vitus' dance, is a major symptom of rheumatic fever and is characterized by ceaseless, involuntary, jerky, purposeless movements.

I01.2   **Acute rheumatic myocarditis**
Any condition in I00 with myocarditis

I01.8   **Other acute rheumatic heart disease**
Any condition in I00 with other or multiple types of heart involvement
Acute rheumatic pancarditis

I01.9   **Acute rheumatic heart disease, unspecified**
Any condition in I00 with unspecified type of heart involvement
Rheumatic carditis, acute
Rheumatic heart disease, active or acute

● **I02**   **Rheumatic chorea**
     Includes   Sydenham's chorea
     Excludes1   chorea NOS (G25.5)
                  Huntington's chorea (G10)

I02.0   **Rheumatic chorea with heart involvement**
Chorea NOS with heart involvement
Rheumatic chorea with heart involvement of any type classifiable under I01.-

I02.9   **Rheumatic chorea without heart involvement**
Rheumatic chorea NOS

CHRONIC RHEUMATIC HEART DISEASES (I05-I09)

● **I05**   **Rheumatic mitral valve diseases**
     Includes   conditions classifiable to both I05.0 and I05.2-I05.9, whether specified as rheumatic or not
     Excludes1   mitral valve disease specified as nonrheumatic (I34.-)
                  mitral valve disease with aortic and/or tricuspid valve involvement (I08.-)

I05.0   **Rheumatic mitral stenosis**
Mitral (valve) obstruction (rheumatic)

I05.1   **Rheumatic mitral insufficiency**
Rheumatic mitral incompetence
Rheumatic mitral regurgitation
     Excludes1   mitral insufficiency not specified as rheumatic (I34.0)

I05.2   **Rheumatic mitral stenosis with insufficiency**
Rheumatic mitral stenosis with incompetence or regurgitation

I05.8   **Other rheumatic mitral valve diseases**
Rheumatic mitral (valve) failure

I05.9   **Rheumatic mitral valve disease, unspecified**
Rheumatic mitral (valve) disorder (chronic) NOS

● **I06**   **Rheumatic aortic valve diseases**
     Excludes1   aortic valve disease not specified as rheumatic (I35.-)
                  aortic valve disease with mitral and/or tricuspid valve involvement (I08.-)

I06.0   **Rheumatic aortic stenosis**
Rheumatic aortic (valve) obstruction

I06.1   **Rheumatic aortic insufficiency**
Rheumatic aortic incompetence
Rheumatic aortic regurgitation

I06.2   **Rheumatic aortic stenosis with insufficiency**
Rheumatic aortic stenosis with incompetence or regurgitation

★ **(See Plate 33 of the Anatomy Illustrations.)**

Item 9–3 Mitral stenosis is the narrowing of the mitral valve separating the left atrium from the left ventricle. **Mitral insufficiency** is the improper closure of the mitral valve, which may lead to enlargement (hypertrophy) of the left atrium.

Item 9–4 Aortic stenosis is the narrowing of the aortic valve located between the left ventricle and the aorta. **Aortic insufficiency** is the improper closure of the aortic valve, which may lead to enlargement (hypertrophy) of the left ventricle.

I06.8   **Other rheumatic aortic valve diseases**

I06.9   **Rheumatic aortic valve disease, unspecified**
Rheumatic aortic (valve) disease NOS

● **I07**   **Rheumatic tricuspid valve diseases**
     Includes   rheumatic tricuspid valve diseases specified as rheumatic or unspecified
     Excludes1   tricuspid valve disease specified as nonrheumatic (I36.-)
                  tricuspid valve disease with aortic and/or mitral valve involvement (I08.-)

I07.0   **Rheumatic tricuspid stenosis**
Tricuspid (valve) stenosis (rheumatic)

I07.1   **Rheumatic tricuspid insufficiency**
Tricuspid (valve) insufficiency (rheumatic)

I07.2   **Rheumatic tricuspid stenosis and insufficiency**

I07.8   **Other rheumatic tricuspid valve diseases**

I07.9   **Rheumatic tricuspid valve disease, unspecified**
Rheumatic tricuspid valve disorder NOS

● **I08**   **Multiple valve diseases**
     Includes   multiple valve diseases specified as rheumatic or unspecified
     Excludes1   endocarditis, valve unspecified (I38)
                  multiple valve disease specified a nonrheumatic (I34.-, I35.-, I36.-, I37.-, I38.-, Q22.-, Q23.-, Q24.8-)
                  rheumatic valve disease NOS (I09.1)
     Coding Clinic: 2019, Q2, P5

I08.0   **Rheumatic disorders of both mitral and aortic valves**
Involvement of both mitral and aortic valves specified as rheumatic or unspecified
     Coding Clinic: 2019, Q2, P5

I08.1   **Rheumatic disorders of both mitral and tricuspid valves**

I08.2   **Rheumatic disorders of both aortic and tricuspid valves**

I08.3   **Combined rheumatic disorders of mitral, aortic and tricuspid valves**

I08.8   **Other rheumatic multiple valve diseases**

I08.9   **Rheumatic multiple valve disease, unspecified**

● **I09**   **Other rheumatic heart diseases**

I09.0   **Rheumatic myocarditis**
     Excludes1   myocarditis not specified as rheumatic (I51.4)

I09.1   **Rheumatic diseases of endocardium, valve unspecified**
Rheumatic endocarditis (chronic)
Rheumatic valvulitis (chronic)
     Excludes1   endocarditis, valve unspecified (I38)

I09.2   **Chronic rheumatic pericarditis**
Adherent pericardium, rheumatic
Chronic rheumatic mediastinopericarditis
Chronic rheumatic myopericarditis
     Excludes1   chronic pericarditis not specified as rheumatic (I31.-)

● **I09.8**   **Other specified rheumatic heart diseases**

I09.81   **Rheumatic heart failure** 🅗
Use additional code to identify type of heart failure (I50.-)

I09.89   **Other specified rheumatic heart diseases**
Rheumatic disease of pulmonary valve

I09.9   **Rheumatic heart disease, unspecified**
Rheumatic carditis
     Excludes1   rheumatoid carditis (M05.31)

▶ New   ⮕ Revised   ~~deleted~~ Deleted   Excludes 1   Excludes 2   Includes   Use additional   Code first   Code also   Key words

OGCR Official Guidelines   X Assign placeholder X   ● Use Additional Character(s)   ▶ Manifestation Code   🅗 Hierarchical Condition Category   **Coding Clinic**

Item 9–5 Hypertension is caused by high arterial blood pressure in the arteries. **Essential, primary,** or **idiopathic** hypertension occurs without identifiable organic cause. **Secondary** hypertension is that which has an organic cause. **Malignant** hypertension is severely elevated blood pressure. **Benign** hypertension is mildly elevated blood pressure.

HYPERTENSIVE DISEASES (I10-I16)

Use additional code to identify:
exposure to environmental tobacco smoke (Z77.22)
history of tobacco dependence (Z87.891)
occupational exposure to environmental tobacco smoke (Z57.31)
tobacco dependence (F17.-)
tobacco use (Z72.0)

Excludes1   neonatal hypertension (P29.2)
primary pulmonary hypertension (I27.0)

Excludes2   hypertensive disease complicating pregnancy, childbirth and the puerperium (O10-O11, O13-O16)

I10   Essential (primary) hypertension

Includes   high blood pressure
hypertension (arterial) (benign) (essential) (malignant) (primary) (systemic)

Excludes1   hypertensive disease complicating pregnancy, childbirth and the puerperium (O10-O11, O13-O16)

Excludes2   essential (primary) hypertension involving vessels of brain (I60-I69)
essential (primary) hypertension involving vessels of eye (H35.0-)

●**I11   Hypertensive heart disease**

Includes   any condition in I50.- or I51.4-I51.7, I51.89, I51.9 due to hypertension

I11.0   Hypertensive heart disease with heart failure 🔎
Hypertensive heart failure
Use additional code to identify type of heart failure (I50.-)
Coding Clinic: 2017, Q1, P47

I11.9   Hypertensive heart disease without heart failure
Hypertensive heart disease NOS

OGCR Section I.C.9.a.2.

Hypertensive Chronic Kidney Disease

Assign codes from category I12, Hypertensive chronic kidney disease, when both hypertension and a condition classifiable to category N18, Chronic kidney disease (CKD), are present. CKD should not be coded as hypertensive if the physician has specifically documented a different cause.

The appropriate code from category N18 should be used as a secondary code with a code from category I12 to identify the stage of chronic kidney disease.

See Section I.C.14. Chronic kidney disease.

If a patient has hypertensive chronic kidney disease and acute renal failure, an additional code for the acute renal failure is required.

●**I12   Hypertensive chronic kidney disease**

Includes   any condition in N18 and N26 - due to hypertension
arteriosclerosis of kidney
arteriosclerotic nephritis (chronic) (interstitial)
hypertensive nephropathy
nephrosclerosis

Excludes1   hypertension due to kidney disease (I15.0, I15.1)
renovascular hypertension (I15.0)
secondary hypertension (I15.-)

Excludes2   acute kidney failure (N17.-)

Coding Clinic: 2018, Q4, P89; 2016, Q4, P123

I12.0   Hypertensive chronic kidney disease with stage 5 chronic kidney disease or end stage renal disease 🔎
Use additional code to identify the stage of chronic kidney disease (N18.5, N18.6)
Coding Clinic: 2016, Q3, P23

I12.9   Hypertensive chronic kidney disease with stage 1 through stage 4 chronic kidney disease, or unspecified chronic kidney disease
Hypertensive chronic kidney disease NOS
Hypertensive renal disease NOS
Use additional code to identify the stage of chronic kidney disease (N18.1-N18.4, N18.9)
Coding Clinic: 2018, Q4, P88

OGCR Section I.c.9.a.3.

Hypertensive Heart and Chronic Kidney Disease

Assign codes from combination category I13, Hypertensive heart and chronic kidney disease, when **there is hypertension with both heart and kidney involvement.** If heart failure is present, assign an additional code from category I50 to identify the type of heart failure.

The appropriate code from category N18, Chronic kidney disease, should be used as a secondary code with a code from category I13 to identify the stage of chronic kidney disease.
See Section I.C.14. Chronic kidney disease.

The codes in category I13, Hypertensive heart and chronic kidney disease, are combination codes that include hypertension, heart disease and chronic kidney disease. The Includes note at I13 specifies that the conditions included at I11 and I12 are included together in I13. If a patient has hypertension, heart disease and chronic kidney disease then a code from I13 should be used, not individual codes for hypertension, heart disease and chronic kidney disease, or codes from I11 or I12.

For patients with both acute renal failure and chronic kidney disease an additional code for acute renal failure is required.

●**I13   Hypertensive heart and chronic kidney disease**

Includes   any condition in I11.- with any condition in I12.-
cardiorenal disease
cardiovascular renal disease

Coding Clinic: 2016, Q4, P123

I13.0   Hypertensive heart and chronic kidney disease with heart failure and stage 1 through stage 4 chronic kidney disease, or unspecified chronic kidney disease 🔎
Use additional code to identify type of heart failure (I50.-)
Use additional code to identify stage of chronic kidney disease (N18.1-N18.4, N18.9)

●**I13.1   Hypertensive heart and chronic kidney disease without heart failure**

I13.10   Hypertensive heart and chronic kidney disease without heart failure, with stage 1 through stage 4 chronic kidney disease, or unspecified chronic kidney disease
Hypertensive heart disease and hypertensive chronic kidney disease NOS
Use additional code to identify the stage of chronic kidney disease (N18.1-N18.4, N18.9)

I13.11   Hypertensive heart and chronic kidney disease without heart failure, with stage 5 chronic kidney disease, or end stage renal disease 🔎
Use additional code to identify the stage of chronic kidney disease (N18.5, N18.6)

I13.2   Hypertensive heart and chronic kidney disease with heart failure and with stage 5 chronic kidney disease, or end stage renal disease 🔎
Use additional code to identify type of heart failure (I50.-)
Use additional code to identify the stage of chronic kidney disease (N18.5, N18.6)

CHAPTER 9 (I00-I99)

Hypertension, Secondary
Secondary hypertension is due to an underlying condition. Two codes are required: one to identify the underlying etiology and one from category I15 to identify the hypertension. Sequencing of codes is determined by the reason for admission/encounter.

● **I15   Secondary hypertension**
Code also underlying condition
Excludes1   postprocedural hypertension (I97.3)
Excludes2   secondary hypertension involving vessels of brain (I60-I69)
secondary hypertension involving vessels of eye (H35.0-)

I15.0   **Renovascular hypertension**
I15.1   **Hypertension secondary to other renal disorders**
Coding Clinic: 2016, Q3, P23
I15.2   **Hypertension secondary to endocrine disorders**
I15.8   **Other secondary hypertension**
I15.9   **Secondary hypertension, unspecified**

● **I16   Hypertensive crisis**
Code also any identified hypertensive disease (I10-I15)
Coding Clinic: 2016, Q4, P26-27, 123
I16.0   **Hypertensive urgency**
I16.1   **Hypertensive emergency**
I16.9   **Hypertensive crisis, unspecified**

ISCHEMIC HEART DISEASES (I20-I25)
Code also the presence of hypertension (I10-I16)

● **I20   Angina pectoris**
Chest pain/discomfort due to lack of oxygen to the heart muscle. Principal symptom of myocardial infarction.
Use additional code to identify:
exposure to environmental tobacco smoke (Z77.22)
history of tobacco dependence (Z87.891)
occupational exposure to environmental tobacco smoke (Z57.31)
tobacco dependence (F17.-)
tobacco use (Z72.0)
Excludes1   angina pectoris with atherosclerotic heart disease of native coronary arteries (I25.1-)
atherosclerosis of coronary artery bypass graft(s) and coronary artery of transplanted heart with angina pectoris (I25.7-)
postinfarction angina (I23.7)

I20.0   **Unstable angina** 🏥
Accelerated angina
Crescendo angina
De novo effort angina
Intermediate coronary syndrome
Preinfarction syndrome
Worsening effort angina
I20.1   **Angina pectoris with documented spasm** 🏥
Angiospastic angina
Prinzmetal angina
Spasm-induced angina
Variant angina
▶I20.2   **Refractory angina pectoris**
I20.8   **Other forms of angina pectoris** 🏥
Angina equivalent
Angina of effort
Coronary slow flow syndrome
Stable angina
Stenocardia
Use additional code(s) for symptoms associated with angina equivalent
I20.9   **Angina pectoris, unspecified** 🏥
Angina NOS
Anginal syndrome
Cardiac angina
Ischemic chest pain

● **I21   Acute myocardial infarction**
Includes   cardiac infarction
coronary (artery) embolism
coronary (artery) occlusion
coronary (artery) rupture
coronary (artery) thrombosis
infarction of heart, myocardium, or ventricle
myocardial infarction specified as acute or with a stated duration of 4 weeks (28 days) or less from onset
Use additional code, if applicable, to identify:
exposure to environmental tobacco smoke (Z77.22)
history of tobacco dependence (Z87.891)
occupational exposure to environmental tobacco smoke (Z57.31)
status post administration of tPA (rtPA) in a different facility within the last 24 hours prior to admission to current facility (Z92.82)
tobacco dependence (F17.-)
tobacco use (Z72.0)
Excludes2   old myocardial infarction (I25.2)
postmyocardial infarction syndrome (I24.1)
subsequent type 1 myocardial infarction (I22.-)
Coding Clinic: 2016, Q4, P140; 2013, Q1, P25-26; 2012, Q4, P103

● **I21.0   ST elevation (STEMI) myocardial infarction of anterior wall**
Type 1 ST elevation myocardial infarction of anterior wall
Coding Clinic: 2013, Q1, P26
I21.01   **ST elevation (STEMI) myocardial infarction involving left main coronary artery** 🏥
I21.02   **ST elevation (STEMI) myocardial infarction involving left anterior descending coronary artery** 🏥
ST elevation (STEMI) myocardial infarction involving diagonal coronary artery
Coding Clinic: 2013, Q1, P26
I21.09   **ST elevation (STEMI) myocardial infarction involving other coronary artery of anterior wall** 🏥
Acute transmural myocardial infarction of anterior wall
Anteroapical transmural (Q wave) infarction (acute)
Anterolateral transmural (Q wave) infarction (acute)
Anteroseptal transmural (Q wave) infarction (acute)
Transmural (Q wave) infarction (acute) (of) anterior (wall) NOS
Coding Clinic: 2012, Q4, P102, 104

● **I21.1   ST elevation (STEMI) myocardial infarction of inferior wall**
Type 1 ST elevation myocardial infarction of inferior wall
Coding Clinic: 2013, Q1, P26
I21.11   **ST elevation (STEMI) myocardial infarction involving right coronary artery** 🏥
Inferoposterior transmural (Q wave) infarction (acute)
I21.19   **ST elevation (STEMI) myocardial infarction involving other coronary artery of inferior wall** 🏥
Acute transmural myocardial infarction of inferior wall
Inferolateral transmural (Q wave) infarction (acute)
Transmural (Q wave) infarction (acute) (of) diaphragmatic wall
Transmural (Q wave) infarction (acute) (of) inferior (wall) NOS
Excludes2   ST elevation (STEMI) myocardial infarction involving left circumflex coronary artery (I21.21)
Coding Clinic: 2012, Q4, P97

● **I21.2**   **ST elevation (STEMI) myocardial infarction of other sites**
Type 1 ST elevation myocardial infarction of other sites
Coding Clinic: 2013, Q1, P26

     I21.21   **ST elevation (STEMI) myocardial infarction involving left circumflex coronary artery** 🔧
ST elevation (STEMI) myocardial infarction involving oblique marginal coronary artery

     I21.29   **ST elevation (STEMI) myocardial infarction involving other sites** 🔧
Acute transmural myocardial infarction of other sites
Apical-lateral transmural (Q wave) infarction (acute)
Basal-lateral transmural (Q wave) infarction (acute)
High lateral transmural (Q wave) infarction (acute)
Lateral (wall) NOS transmural (Q wave) infarction (acute)
Posterior (true) transmural (Q wave) infarction (acute)
Posterobasal transmural (Q wave) infarction (acute)
Posterolateral transmural (Q wave) infarction (acute)
Posteroseptal transmural (Q wave) infarction (acute)
Septal transmural (Q wave) infarction (acute) NOS

OGCR Section I.c.9.e.2.

Acute myocardial infarction, unspecified

Code I21.9, Acute myocardial infarction, unspecified, is the default for unspecified acute myocardial infarction or unspecified type. If only type 1 STEMI or transmural MI without the site is documented, assign I21.3, ST elevation (STEMI) myocardial infarction of unspecified site.

     I21.3   **ST elevation (STEMI) myocardial infarction of unspecified site** 🔧
Acute transmural myocardial infarction of unspecified site
Transmural (Q wave) myocardial infarction NOS
Type 1 ST elevation myocardial infarction of unspecified site
Coding Clinic: 2013, Q1, P26

     I21.4   **Non-ST elevation (NSTEMI) myocardial infarction** 🔧
Acute subendocardial myocardial infarction
Non-Q wave myocardial infarction NOS
Nontransmural myocardial infarction NOS
Type 1 non-ST elevation myocardial infarction
Coding Clinic: 2021, Q3, P7; 2017, Q1, P44; 2015, Q2, P16; 2013, Q1, P26

     I21.9   **Acute myocardial infarction, unspecified** 🔧
Myocardial infarction (acute) NOS

● **I21.A**   **Other type of myocardial infarction**

     I21.A1   **Myocardial infarction type 2** 🔧
Myocardial infarction due to demand ischemia
Myocardial infarction secondary to ischemic imbalance

Code first the underlying cause, such as:
anemia (D50.0-D64.9)
chronic obstructive pulmonary disease (J44.-)
paroxysmal tachycardia (I47.0-I47.9)
shock (R57.0-R57.9)
Coding Clinic: 2017, Q4, P13-14

     I21.A9   **Other myocardial infarction type** 🔧
Myocardial infarction associated with revascularization procedure
Myocardial infarction type 3
Myocardial infarction type 4a
Myocardial infarction type 4b
Myocardial infarction type 4c
Myocardial infarction type 5

Code first, if applicable, postprocedural myocardial infarction following cardiac surgery (I97.190), or postprocedural myocardial infarction during cardiac surgery (I97.790)

Code also complication, if known and applicable, such as:
(acute) stent occlusion (T82.897-)
(acute) stent stenosis (T82.857-)
(acute) stent thrombosis (T82.865-)
cardiac arrest due to underlying cardiac condition (I46.2)
complication of percutaneous coronary intervention (PCI) (I97.89)
occlusion of coronary artery bypass graft (T82.218-)
Coding Clinic: 2021, Q3, P6-7; 2019, Q2, P32-33

● **I22**   **Subsequent ST elevation (STEMI) and non-ST elevation (NSTEMI) myocardial infarction**

     Includes   acute myocardial infarction occurring within four weeks (28 days) of a previous acute myocardial infarction, regardless of site
cardiac infarction
coronary (artery) embolism
coronary (artery) occlusion
coronary (artery) rupture
coronary (artery) thrombosis
infarction of heart, myocardium, or ventricle
recurrent myocardial infarction
reinfarction of myocardium
rupture of heart, myocardium, or ventricle
subsequent type 1 myocardial infarction

     Excludes1   subsequent myocardial infarction, type 2 (I21.A1)
subsequent myocardial infarction of other type (type 3) (type 4) (type 5) (I21.A9)

Use additional code, if applicable, to identify:
exposure to environmental tobacco smoke (Z77.22)
history of tobacco dependence (Z87.891)
occupational exposure to environmental tobacco smoke (Z57.31)
status post administration of tPA (rtPA) in a different facility within the last 24 hours prior to admission to current facility (Z92.82)
tobacco dependence (F17.-)
tobacco use (Z72.0)
Coding Clinic: 2017, Q4, P14; 2013, Q1, P25; 2012, Q4, P103

     I22.0   **Subsequent ST elevation (STEMI) myocardial infarction of anterior wall** 🔧
Subsequent acute transmural myocardial infarction of anterior wall
Subsequent transmural (Q wave) infarction (acute)(of) anterior (wall) NOS
Subsequent anteroapical transmural (Q wave) infarction (acute)
Subsequent anterolateral transmural (Q wave) infarction (acute)
Subsequent anteroseptal transmural (Q wave) infarction (acute)

CHAPTER 9 (I00-I99)

I22.1   Subsequent ST elevation (STEMI) myocardial infarction of inferior wall 🦠
Subsequent acute transmural myocardial infarction of inferior wall
Subsequent transmural (Q wave) infarction (acute)(of) diaphragmatic wall
Subsequent transmural (Q wave) infarction (acute)(of) inferior (wall) NOS
Subsequent inferolateral transmural (Q wave) infarction (acute)
Subsequent inferoposterior transmural (Q wave) infarction (acute)
Coding Clinic: 2012, Q4, P97, 102, 104

I22.2   Subsequent non-ST elevation (NSTEMI) myocardial infarction 🦠
Subsequent acute subendocardial myocardial infarction
Subsequent non-Q wave myocardial infarction NOS
Subsequent nontransmural myocardial infarction NOS

I22.8   Subsequent ST elevation (STEMI) myocardial infarction of other sites 🦠
Subsequent acute transmural myocardial infarction of other sites
Subsequent apical-lateral transmural (Q wave) myocardial infarction (acute)
Subsequent basal-lateral transmural (Q wave) myocardial infarction (acute)
Subsequent high lateral transmural (Q wave) myocardial infarction (acute)
Subsequent transmural (Q wave) myocardial infarction (acute)(of) lateral (wall) NOS
Subsequent posterior (true) transmural (Q wave) myocardial infarction (acute)
Subsequent posterobasal transmural (Q wave) myocardial infarction (acute)
Subsequent posterolateral transmural (Q wave) myocardial infarction (acute)
Subsequent posteroseptal transmural (Q wave) myocardial infarction (acute)
Subsequent septal NOS transmural (Q wave) myocardial infarction (acute)

I22.9   Subsequent ST elevation (STEMI) myocardial infarction of unspecified site 🦠
Subsequent acute myocardial infarction of unspecified site
Subsequent myocardial infarction (acute) NOS

● **I23   Certain current complications following ST elevation (STEMI) and non-ST elevation (NSTEMI) myocardial infarction (within the 28 day period)**
Coding Clinic: 2017, Q2, P11

I23.0   Hemopericardium as current complication following acute myocardial infarction 🦠   A
Excludes1   hemopericardium not specified as current complication following acute myocardial infarction (I31.2)

I23.1   Atrial septal defect as current complication following acute myocardial infarction 🦠   A
Excludes1   acquired atrial septal defect not specified as current complication following acute myocardial infarction (I51.0)

I23.2   Ventricular septal defect as current complication following acute myocardial infarction 🦠   A
Excludes1   acquired ventricular septal defect not specified as current complication following acute myocardial infarction (I51.0)

I23.3   Rupture of cardiac wall without hemopericardium as current complication following acute myocardial infarction 🦠   A
Coding Clinic: 2017, Q2, P11

I23.4   Rupture of chordae tendineae as current complication following acute myocardial infarction 🦠
Excludes1   rupture of chordae tendineae not specified as current complication following acute myocardial infarction (I51.1)

I23.5   Rupture of papillary muscle as current complication following acute myocardial infarction 🦠
Excludes1   rupture of papillary muscle not specified as current complication following acute myocardial infarction (I51.2)

I23.6   Thrombosis of atrium, auricular appendage, and ventricle as current complications following acute myocardial infarction 🦠   A
Excludes1   thrombosis of atrium, auricular appendage, and ventricle not specified as current complication following acute myocardial infarction (I51.3)

I23.7   Postinfarction angina 🦠   A
Coding Clinic: 2015, Q2, P16-17

I23.8   Other current complications following acute myocardial infarction 🦠   A

● **I24   Other acute ischemic heart diseases**
Excludes1   angina pectoris (I20.-)
transient myocardial ischemia in newborn (P29.4)
Excludes2   non-ischemic myocardial injury (I5A)

I24.0   Acute coronary thrombosis not resulting in myocardial infarction 🦠
Acute coronary (artery) (vein) embolism not resulting in myocardial infarction
Acute coronary (artery) (vein) occlusion not resulting in myocardial infarction
Acute coronary (artery) (vein) thromboembolism not resulting in myocardial infarction
Excludes1   atherosclerotic heart disease (I25.1-)
Coding Clinic: 2013, Q1, P24

I24.1   Dressler's syndrome
Postmyocardial infarction syndrome
Excludes1   postinfarction angina (I23.7)

I24.8   Other forms of acute ischemic heart disease 🦠
Excludes1   myocardial infarction due to demand ischemia (I21.A1)
Coding Clinic: 2017, Q4, P13

I24.9   Acute ischemic heart disease, unspecified 🦠
Excludes1   ischemic heart disease (chronic) NOS (I25.9)

● **I25   Chronic ischemic heart disease**
Excludes2   non-ischemic myocardial injury (I5A)

Use additional code to identify:
chronic total occlusion of coronary artery (I25.82)
exposure to environmental tobacco smoke (Z77.22)
history of tobacco dependence (Z87.891)
occupational exposure to environmental tobacco smoke (Z57.31)
tobacco dependence (F17.-)
tobacco use (Z72.0)

★ **(See Plates 218 and 219 on pages 74 and 75.)**

● **I25.1   Atherosclerotic heart disease of native coronary artery**
Disease in which fatty deposits form on the walls of arteries
Atherosclerotic cardiovascular disease
Coronary (artery) atheroma
Coronary (artery) atherosclerosis
Coronary (artery) disease
Coronary (artery) sclerosis
Use additional code, if applicable, to identify:
coronary atherosclerosis due to calcified coronary lesion (I25.84)
coronary atherosclerosis due to lipid rich plaque (I25.83)
Excludes2   atheroembolism (I75.-)
atherosclerosis of coronary artery bypass graft(s) and transplanted heart (I25.7-)

I25.10   Atherosclerotic heart disease of native coronary artery without angina pectoris   A
Atherosclerotic heart disease NOS
Coding Clinic: 2021, Q3, P6-7; 2015, Q2, P17; 2012, Q4, P92

▶ New   ⏩ Revised   ~~deleted~~ Deleted   Excludes 1   Excludes 2   Includes   Use additional   Code first   Code also   Key words

OGCR Official Guidelines   X Assign placeholder X   ● Use Additional Character(s)   ▶ Manifestation Code   🦠 Hierarchical Condition Category   Coding Clinic

Item 9–6 Classification is based on the location of the atherosclerosis. **"Of native coronary artery"** indicates the atherosclerosis is within an original heart artery. **"Of autologous vein bypass graft"** indicates that the atherosclerosis is within a vein graft that was taken from within the patient. **"Of nonautologous biological bypass graft"** indicates the atherosclerosis is within a vessel grafted from other than the patient. **"Of artery bypass graft"** indicates the atherosclerosis is within an artery that was grafted from within the patient.

Figure 9-2 Atherosclerotic plaque.

Atherosclerotic plaque (atheromas)

OGCR See Section I.9.b.

Atherosclerotic Coronary Artery Disease and Angina

ICD-10-CM has combination codes for atherosclerotic heart disease with angina pectoris. The subcategories for these codes are I25.11, Atherosclerotic heart disease of native coronary artery with angina pectoris and I25.7, Atherosclerosis of coronary artery bypass graft(s) and coronary artery of transplanted heart with angina pectoris.

When using one of these combination codes it is not necessary to use an additional code for angina pectoris. A causal relationship can be assumed in a patient with both atherosclerosis and angina pectoris, unless the documentation indicates the angina is due to something other than the atherosclerosis.

If a patient with coronary artery disease is admitted due to an acute myocardial infarction (AMI), the AMI should be sequenced before the coronary artery disease.

See Section I.C.9. Acute myocardial infarction (AMI).

● **I25.11**   **Atherosclerotic heart disease of native coronary artery with angina pectoris**

    I25.110   **Atherosclerotic heart disease of native coronary artery with unstable angina pectoris** 🔍   A

        Excludes1   unstable angina without atherosclerotic heart disease (I20.0)

    I25.111   **Atherosclerotic heart disease of native coronary artery with angina pectoris with documented spasm** 🔍   A

        Excludes1   angina pectoris with documented spasm without atherosclerotic heart disease (I20.1)

    ▶ **I25.112**   **Atherosclerosic heart disease of native coronary artery with refractory angina pectoris**

    I25.118   **Atherosclerotic heart disease of native coronary artery with other forms of angina pectoris** 🔍   A

        Excludes1   other forms of angina pectoris without atherosclerotic heart disease (I20.8)

        Coding Clinic: 2015, Q2, P16-17

    I25.119   **Atherosclerotic heart disease of native coronary artery with unspecified angina pectoris** 🔍   A

        Atherosclerotic heart disease with angina NOS

        Atherosclerotic heart disease with ischemic chest pain

        Excludes1   unspecified angina pectoris without atherosclerotic heart disease (I20.9)

I25.2   **Old myocardial infarction**

    Healed myocardial infarction

    Past myocardial infarction diagnosed by ECG or other investigation, but currently presenting no symptoms

I25.3   **Aneurysm of heart**

    Mural aneurysm

    Ventricular aneurysm

● **I25.4**   **Coronary artery aneurysm and dissection**

    I25.41   **Coronary artery aneurysm**

        Coronary arteriovenous fistula, acquired

        Excludes1   congenital coronary (artery) aneurysm (Q24.5)

    I25.42   **Coronary artery dissection**

I25.5   **Ischemic cardiomyopathy**

    Excludes2   coronary atherosclerosis (I25.1-, I25.7-)

I25.6   **Silent myocardial ischemia**

● **I25.7**   **Atherosclerosis of coronary artery bypass graft(s) and coronary artery of transplanted heart with angina pectoris**

    Use additional code, if applicable, to identify:

       coronary atherosclerosis due to calcified coronary lesion (I25.84)

       coronary atherosclerosis due to lipid rich plaque (I25.83)

    Excludes1   atherosclerosis of bypass graft(s) of transplanted heart without angina pectoris (I25.812)

           atherosclerosis of coronary artery bypass graft(s) without angina pectoris (I25.810)

           atherosclerosis of native coronary artery of transplanted heart without angina pectoris (I25.811)

● **I25.70**   **Atherosclerosis of coronary artery bypass graft(s), unspecified, with angina pectoris**

    I25.700   **Atherosclerosis of coronary artery bypass graft(s), unspecified, with unstable angina pectoris** 🔍   A

        Excludes1   unstable angina pectoris without atherosclerosis of coronary artery bypass graft (I20.0)

    I25.701   **Atherosclerosis of coronary artery bypass graft(s), unspecified, with angina pectoris with documented spasm** 🔍   A

        Excludes1   angina pectoris with documented spasm without atherosclerosis of coronary artery bypass graft (I20.1)

    ▶ **I25.702**   **Atherosclerosis of coronary artery bypass graft(s), unspecified, with refractory angina pectoris**

CHAPTER 9 (I00-I99)

I25.708　Atherosclerosis of coronary artery bypass graft(s), unspecified, with other forms of angina pectoris 🔖　A

Excludes1　other forms of angina pectoris without atherosclerosis of coronary artery bypass graft (I20.8)

I25.709　Atherosclerosis of coronary artery bypass graft(s), unspecified, with unspecified angina pectoris 🔖　A

Excludes1　unspecified angina pectoris without atherosclerosis of coronary artery bypass graft (I20.9)

● I25.71　Atherosclerosis of autologous vein coronary artery bypass graft(s) with angina pectoris

I25.710　Atherosclerosis of autologous vein coronary artery bypass graft(s) with unstable angina pectoris 🔖　A

Excludes1　unstable angina without atherosclerosis of autologous vein coronary artery bypass graft(s) (I20.0)

Excludes2　embolism or thrombus of coronary artery bypass graft(s) (T82.8-)

I25.711　Atherosclerosis of autologous vein coronary artery bypass graft(s) with angina pectoris with documented spasm 🔖　A

Excludes1　angina pectoris with documented spasm without atherosclerosis of autologous vein coronary artery bypass graft(s) (I20.1)

▶I25.712　Atherosclerosis of autologous vein coronary artery bypass graft(s) with refractory angina pectoris

I25.718　Atherosclerosis of autologous vein coronary artery bypass graft(s) with other forms of angina pectoris 🔖　A

Excludes1　other forms of angina pectoris without atherosclerosis of autologous vein coronary artery bypass graft(s) (I20.8)

I25.719　Atherosclerosis of autologous vein coronary artery bypass graft(s) with unspecified angina pectoris 🔖　A

Excludes1　unspecified angina pectoris without atherosclerosis of autologous vein coronary artery bypass graft(s) (I20.9)

● I25.72　Atherosclerosis of autologous artery coronary artery bypass graft(s) with angina pectoris
Atherosclerosis of internal mammary artery graft with angina pectoris

I25.720　Atherosclerosis of autologous artery coronary artery bypass graft(s) with unstable angina pectoris 🔖　A

Excludes1　unstable angina without atherosclerosis of autologous artery coronary artery bypass graft(s) (I20.0)

I25.721　Atherosclerosis of autologous artery coronary artery bypass graft(s) with angina pectoris with documented spasm 🔖　A

Excludes1　angina pectoris with documented spasm without atherosclerosis of autologous artery coronary artery bypass graft(s) (I20.1)

▶I25.722　Atherosclerosis of autologous artery coronary artery bypass graft(s) with refractory angina pectoris

I25.728　Atherosclerosis of autologous artery coronary artery bypass graft(s) with other forms of angina pectoris 🔖　A

Excludes1　other forms of angina pectoris without atherosclerosis of autologous artery coronary artery bypass graft(s) (I20.8)

I25.729　Atherosclerosis of autologous artery coronary artery bypass graft(s) with unspecified angina pectoris 🔖　A

Excludes1　unspecified angina pectoris without atherosclerosis of autologous artery coronary artery bypass graft(s) (I20.9)

● I25.73　Atherosclerosis of nonautologous biological coronary artery bypass graft(s) with angina pectoris

I25.730　Atherosclerosis of nonautologous biological coronary artery bypass graft(s) with unstable angina pectoris 🔖　A

Excludes1　unstable angina without atherosclerosis of nonautologous biological coronary artery bypass graft(s) (I20.0)

CHAPTER 9 (I00-I99)

▶ New　⇒ Revised　deleted Deleted　Excludes 1　Excludes 2　Includes　Use additional　Code first　Code also　Key words
OGCR Official Guidelines　X Assign placeholder X　● Use Additional Character(s)　▶ Manifestation Code　🔖 Hierarchical Condition Category　Coding Clinic

I25.731　Atherosclerosis of nonautologous biological coronary artery bypass graft(s) with angina pectoris with documented spasm 🔊　　A

    Excludes1　angina pectoris with documented spasm without atherosclerosis of nonautologous biological coronary artery bypass graft(s) (I20.1)

▶I25.732　Atherosclerosis of nonautologous biological coronary artery bypass graft(s)with refractory angina pectoris

I25.738　Atherosclerosis of nonautologous biological coronary artery bypass graft(s) with other forms of angina pectoris 🔊　　A

    Excludes1　other forms of angina pectoris without atherosclerosis of nonautologous biological coronary artery bypass graft(s) (I20.8)

I25.739　Atherosclerosis of nonautologous biological coronary artery bypass graft(s) with unspecified angina pectoris 🔊　　A

    Excludes1　unspecified angina pectoris without atherosclerosis of nonautologous biological coronary artery bypass graft(s) (I20.9)

● I25.75　Atherosclerosis of native coronary artery of transplanted heart with angina pectoris

    Excludes1　atherosclerosis of native coronary artery of transplanted heart without angina pectoris (I25.811)

I25.750　Atherosclerosis of native coronary artery of transplanted heart with unstable angina 🔊

I25.751　Atherosclerosis of native coronary artery of transplanted heart with angina pectoris with documented spasm 🔊

▶I25.752　Atherosclerosis of native coronary artery of transplanted heart with refractory angina pectoris

I25.758　Atherosclerosis of native coronary artery of transplanted heart with other forms of angina pectoris 🔊

I25.759　Atherosclerosis of native coronary artery of transplanted heart with unspecified angina pectoris 🔊

● I25.76　Atherosclerosis of bypass graft of coronary artery of transplanted heart with angina pectoris

    Excludes1　atherosclerosis of bypass graft of coronary artery of transplanted heart without angina pectoris (I25.812)

I25.760　Atherosclerosis of bypass graft of coronary artery of transplanted heart with unstable angina 🔊　　A

I25.761　Atherosclerosis of bypass graft of coronary artery of transplanted heart with angina pectoris with documented spasm 🔊　　A

▶I25.762　Atherosclerosis of bypass graft of coronary artery of transplanted heart with refractory angina pectoris

I25.768　Atherosclerosis of bypass graft of coronary artery of transplanted heart with other forms of angina pectoris 🔊　　A

I25.769　Atherosclerosis of bypass graft of coronary artery of transplanted heart with unspecified angina pectoris 🔊　　A

● I25.79　Atherosclerosis of other coronary artery bypass graft(s) with angina pectoris　　A

I25.790　Atherosclerosis of other coronary artery bypass graft(s) with unstable angina pectoris 🔊

    Excludes1　unstable angina without atherosclerosis of other coronary artery bypass graft(s) (I20.0)

I25.791　Atherosclerosis of other coronary artery bypass graft(s) with angina pectoris with documented spasm 🔊　　A

    Excludes1　angina pectoris with documented spasm without atherosclerosis of other coronary artery bypass graft(s) (I20.1)

▶I25.792　Atherosclerosis of other coronary artery bypass graft(s) with refractory angina pectoris

I25.798　Atherosclerosis of other coronary artery bypass graft(s) with other forms of angina pectoris 🔊　　A

    Excludes1　other forms of angina pectoris without atherosclerosis of other coronary artery bypass graft(s) (I20.8)

I25.799　Atherosclerosis of other coronary artery bypass graft(s) with unspecified angina pectoris 🔊　　A

    Excludes1　unspecified angina pectoris without atherosclerosis of other coronary artery bypass graft(s) (I20.9)

CHAPTER 9 (IØØ-I99)

● **I25.8**   **Other forms of chronic ischemic heart disease**

  ● **I25.81**   **Atherosclerosis of other coronary vessels without angina pectoris**

     Use additional code, if applicable, to identify:
coronary atherosclerosis due to calcified coronary lesion (I25.84)
coronary atherosclerosis due to lipid rich plaque (I25.83)

     Excludes2   atherosclerotic heart disease of native coronary artery without angina pectoris (I25.10)

     I25.810   **Atherosclerosis of coronary artery bypass graft(s) without angina pectoris**   A

       Atherosclerosis of coronary artery bypass graft NOS

       Excludes1   atherosclerosis of coronary bypass graft(s) with angina pectoris (I25.70- -I25.73-, I25.79-)

       Coding Clinic: 2016, Q4, P86

     I25.811   **Atherosclerosis of native coronary artery of transplanted heart without angina pectoris**

       Atherosclerosis of native coronary artery of transplanted heart NOS

       Excludes1   atherosclerosis of native coronary artery of transplanted heart with angina pectoris (I25.75-)

     I25.812   **Atherosclerosis of bypass graft of coronary artery of transplanted heart without angina pectoris**   A

       Atherosclerosis of bypass graft of transplanted heart NOS

       Excludes1   atherosclerosis of bypass graft of transplanted heart with angina pectoris (I25.76)

  ● **I25.82**   **Chronic total occlusion of coronary artery**

     Complete occlusion of coronary artery
Total occlusion of coronary artery

     Code first coronary atherosclerosis (I25.1-, I25.7-, I25.81-)

     Excludes1   acute coronary occlusion with myocardial infarction (I21.0-I21.9, I22.-)
acute coronary occlusion without myocardial infarction (I24.0)

  ● **I25.83**   **Coronary atherosclerosis due to lipid rich plaque**   A

     Code first coronary atherosclerosis (I25.1-, I25.7-, I25.81-)

  ● **I25.84**   **Coronary atherosclerosis due to calcified coronary lesion**

     Coronary atherosclerosis due to severely calcified coronary lesion

     Code first coronary atherosclerosis (I25.1-, I25.7-, I25.81-)

  ● **I25.89**   **Other forms of chronic ischemic heart disease**

● **I25.9**   **Chronic ischemic heart disease, unspecified**

     Ischemic heart disease (chronic) NOS

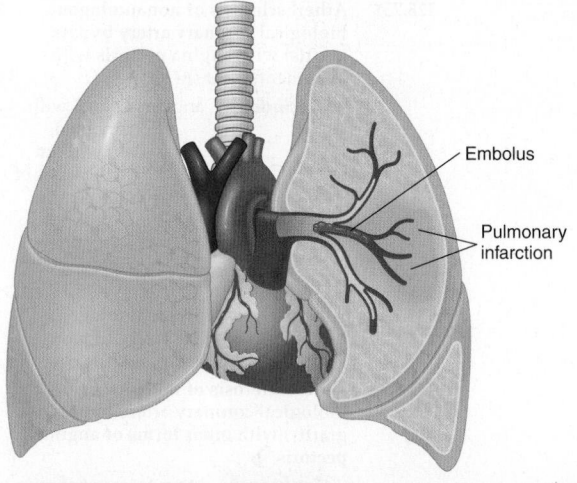

Figure 9-3   Pulmonary embolism. (From Chabner: The Language of Medicine, ed 8, St. Louis, Saunders, 2007)

Item 9–7   Pulmonary heart disease or **cor pulmonale** is right ventricle hypertrophy or RVH as a result of a respiratory disorder increasing back flow pressure to the right ventricle. Left untreated, cor pulmonale leads to right-heart failure and death.

PULMONARY HEART DISEASE AND DISEASES OF PULMONARY CIRCULATION (I26-I28)

● **I26**   **Pulmonary embolism**

   Includes   pulmonary (acute)(artery)(vein) infarction
pulmonary (acute)(artery)(vein) thromboembolism
pulmonary (acute)(artery)(vein) thrombosis

   Excludes2   chronic pulmonary embolism (I27.82)
personal history of pulmonary embolism (Z86.711)
pulmonary embolism due to trauma (T79.0, T79.1)
pulmonary embolism due to complications of surgical and medical care (T80.0, T81.7-, T82.8-)
pulmonary embolism complicating abortion, ectopic or molar pregnancy (O00-O07, O08.2)
pulmonary embolism complicating pregnancy, childbirth and the puerperium (O88.-)
septic (non-pulmonary) arterial embolism (I76)

   Coding Clinic: 2021, Q2, P10

● **I26.0**   **Pulmonary embolism with acute cor pulmonale**

   I26.01   **Septic pulmonary embolism with acute cor pulmonale** 🏵

     Code first underlying infection

   I26.02   **Saddle embolus of pulmonary artery with acute cor pulmonale** 🏵

   I26.09   **Other pulmonary embolism with acute cor pulmonale** 🏵

     Acute cor pulmonale NOS

● **I26.9**   **Pulmonary embolism without acute cor pulmonale**

   I26.90   **Septic pulmonary embolism without acute cor pulmonale** 🏵

     Code first underlying infection

   I26.92   **Saddle embolus of pulmonary artery without acute cor pulmonale** 🏵

   I26.93   **Single subsegmental pulmonary embolism without acute cor pulmonale** 🏵

     Subsegmental pulmonary embolism NOS

   I26.94   **Multiple subsegmental pulmonary emboli without acute cor pulmonale** 🏵

     Coding Clinic: 2022, Q2, P13; 2021, Q2, P10

   I26.99   **Other pulmonary embolism without acute cor pulmonale** 🏵

     Acute pulmonary embolism NOS
Pulmonary embolism NOS

     Coding Clinic: 2022, Q2, P13; 2019, Q2, P22-23

▶ New   ⇒ Revised   ~~deleted~~ Deleted   Excludes 1   Excludes 2   Includes   Use additional   Code first   Code also   Key words

OGCR Official Guidelines   X Assign placeholder X   ● Use Additional Character(s)   ▶ Manifestation Code   🏵 Hierarchical Condition Category   Coding Clinic

● **I27   Other pulmonary heart diseases**

I27.0   Primary pulmonary hypertension 🔗
   Heritable pulmonary arterial hypertension
   Idiopathic pulmonary arterial hypertension
   Primary group 1 pulmonary hypertension
   Primary pulmonary arterial hypertension
   Excludes1   persistent pulmonary hypertension of
       newborn (P29.30)
       pulmonary hypertension NOS (I27.20)
       secondary pulmonary arterial
        hypertension (I27.21)
       secondary pulmonary hypertension
        (I27.29)

I27.1   Kyphoscoliotic heart disease 🔗

● **I27.2   Other secondary pulmonary hypertension**
   Code also associated underlying condition
   Excludes1   Eisenmenger's syndrome (I27.83)
   Coding Clinic: 2016, Q2, P8

I27.20   Pulmonary hypertension, unspecified 🔗
   Pulmonary hypertension NOS

I27.21   Secondary pulmonary arterial hypertension 🔗
   (Associated) (drug-induced) (toxin-induced)
     pulmonary arterial hypertension NOS
   (Associated) (drug-induced) (toxin-induced)
     (secondary) group 1 pulmonary
     hypertension
   Code also associated conditions if applicable, or
     adverse effects of drugs or toxins, such as:
     adverse effect of appetite depressants
      (T50.5X5)
     congenital heart disease (Q20-Q28)
     human immunodeficiency virus [HIV]
      disease (B20)
     polymyositis (M33.2-)
     portal hypertension (K76.6)
     rheumatoid arthritis (M05.-)
     schistosomiasis (B65.-)
     Sjögren syndrome (M35.0-)
     systemic sclerosis (M34.-)

I27.22   Pulmonary hypertension due to left heart disease 🔗
   Group 2 pulmonary hypertension
   Code also associated left heart disease, if
     known, such as:
     multiple valve disease (I08.-)
     rheumatic mitral valve diseases (I05.-)
     rheumatic aortic valve diseases (I06.-)

I27.23   Pulmonary hypertension due to lung diseases and hypoxia 🔗
   Group 3 pulmonary hypertension
   Code also associated lung disease, if known,
     such as:
     bronchiectasis (J47.-)
     cystic fibrosis with pulmonary
      manifestations (E84.0)
     interstitial lung disease (J84.-)
     pleural effusion (J90)
     sleep apnea (G47.3-)

I27.24   Chronic thromboembolic pulmonary hypertension 🔗
   Group 4 pulmonary hypertension
   Code also associated pulmonary embolism, if
     applicable (I26.-, I27.82)

I27.29   Other secondary pulmonary hypertension 🔗
   Group 5 pulmonary hypertension
   Pulmonary hypertension with unclear
     multifactorial mechanisms
   Pulmonary hypertension due to hematologic
     disorders
   Pulmonary hypertension due to metabolic
     disorders
   Pulmonary hypertension due to other systemic
     disorders
   Code also other associated disorders, if known,
     such as:
     chronic myeloid leukemia (C92.10-C92.22)
     essential thrombocythemia (D47.3)
     Gaucher disease (E75.22)
     hypertensive chronic kidney disease
      with end stage renal disease (I12.0,
      I13.11,I13.2)
     hyperthyroidism (E05.-)
     hypothyroidism (E00-E03)
     polycythemia vera (D45)
     sarcoidosis (D86.-)

● **I27.8   Other specified pulmonary heart diseases**

I27.81   Cor pulmonale (chronic) 🔗
   Cor pulmonale NOS
   Excludes1   acute cor pulmonale (I26.0-)

I27.82   Chronic pulmonary embolism 🔗
   Use additional code, if applicable, for
     associated long-term (current) use of
     anticoagulants (Z79.01)
   Excludes1   personal history of pulmonary
     embolism (Z86.711)
   Coding Clinic: 2021, Q2, P10

I27.83   Eisenmenger's syndrome 🔗
   Eisenmenger's complex
   (Irreversible) Eisenmenger's disease
   Pulmonary hypertension with right to left
     shunt related to congenital heart disease
   Code also underlying heart defect, if known,
     such as:
     atrial septal defect (Q21.1-)
     Eisenmenger's defect (Q21.8)
     patent ductus arteriosus (Q25.0)
     ventricular septal defect (Q21.0)

I27.89   Other specified pulmonary heart diseases 🔗

I27.9   Pulmonary heart disease, unspecified 🔗
   Chronic cardiopulmonary disease

● **I28   Other diseases of pulmonary vessels**

I28.0   Arteriovenous fistula of pulmonary vessels 🔗
   Excludes1   congenital arteriovenous fistula (Q25.72)

I28.1   Aneurysm of pulmonary artery 🔗
   Excludes1   congenital aneurysm (Q25.79)
     congenital arteriovenous aneurysm
      (Q25.72)

I28.8   Other diseases of pulmonary vessels 🔗
   Pulmonary arteritis
   Pulmonary endarteritis
   Rupture of pulmonary vessels
   Stenosis of pulmonary vessels
   Stricture of pulmonary vessels

I28.9   Disease of pulmonary vessels, unspecified 🔗

CHAPTER 9 (I00-I99)

OTHER FORMS OF HEART DISEASE (I30-I5A)

● **I30   Acute pericarditis**
Inflammation of pericardium (sac surrounding the heart) caused by an infection

Includes acute mediastinopericarditis
acute myopericarditis
acute pericardial effusion
acute pleuropericarditis
acute pneumopericarditis

Excludes1 Dressler's syndrome (I24.1)
rheumatic pericarditis (acute) (I01.0)
viral pericarditis due to Coxsakie virus (B33.23)

I30.0   Acute nonspecific idiopathic pericarditis

I30.1   Infective pericarditis
Pneumococcal pericarditis
Pneumopyopericardium
Purulent pericarditis
Pyopericarditis
Pyopericardium
Pyopneumopericardium
Staphylococcal pericarditis
Streptococcal pericarditis
Suppurative pericarditis
Viral pericarditis
Use additional code (B95-B97) to identify infectious agent

I30.8   Other forms of acute pericarditis

I30.9   Acute pericarditis, unspecified

● **I31   Other diseases of pericardium**
Excludes1 diseases of pericardium specified as rheumatic (I09.2)
postcardiotomy syndrome (I97.0)
traumatic injury to pericardium (S26.-)

I31.0   Chronic adhesive pericarditis
Accretio cordis
Adherent pericardium
Adhesive mediastinopericarditis

I31.1   Chronic constrictive pericarditis
Concretio cordis
Pericardial calcification

I31.2   Hemopericardium, not elsewhere classified
Excludes1 hemopericardium as current complication following acute myocardial infarction (I23.0)

● **I31.3   Pericardial effusion (noninflammatory)**
~~Chylopericardium~~
Excludes1 acute pericardial effusion (I30.9)
Coding Clinic: 2019, Q1, P16

▶**I31.31   Malignant pericardial effusion in diseases classified elsewhere**
▶ *Code first underlying neoplasm (C00-D49)*

▶**I31.39   Other pericardial effusion (noninflammatory)**
▶Chylopericardium

I31.4   Cardiac tamponade
Code first underlying cause

I31.8   Other specified diseases of pericardium
Epicardial plaques
Focal pericardial adhesions

I31.9   Disease of pericardium, unspecified
Pericarditis (chronic) NOS

▷ **I32   Pericarditis in diseases classified elsewhere**
Code first underlying disease
Excludes1 pericarditis (in):
coxsackie (virus) (B33.23)
gonococcal (A54.83)
meningococcal (A39.53)
rheumatoid (arthritis) (M05.31)
syphilitic (A52.06)
systemic lupus erythematosus (M32.12)
tuberculosis (A18.84)

● **I33   Acute and subacute endocarditis**
Inflammation/infection of lining of heart, affecting heart valves including replacement valves and is usually caused by a bacterial infection
Excludes1 acute rheumatic endocarditis (I01.1)
endocarditis NOS (I38)

I33.0   Acute and subacute infective endocarditis
Bacterial endocarditis (acute) (subacute)
Infective endocarditis (acute) (subacute) NOS
Endocarditis lenta (acute) (subacute)
Malignant endocarditis (acute) (subacute)
Purulent endocarditis (acute) (subacute)
Septic endocarditis (acute) (subacute)
Ulcerative endocarditis (acute) (subacute)
Vegetative endocarditis (acute) (subacute)
Use additional code (B95-B97) to identify infectious agent

I33.9   Acute and subacute endocarditis, unspecified
Acute endocarditis NOS
Acute myoendocarditis NOS
Acute periendocarditis NOS
Subacute endocarditis NOS
Subacute myoendocarditis NOS
Subacute periendocarditis NOS

● **I34   Nonrheumatic mitral valve disorders**
▶Code also, if applicable:
▶nonrheumatic mitral (valve) annulus calcification (I34.81)
Excludes1 mitral valve disease (I05.9)
mitral valve failure (I05.8)
mitral valve stenosis (I05.0)
mitral valve disorder of unspecified cause with diseases of aortic and/or tricuspid valve(s) (I08.-)
mitral valve disorder of unspecified cause with mitral stenosis or obstruction (I05.0)
mitral valve disorder specified as congenital (Q23.2, Q23.9)
mitral valve disorder specified as rheumatic (I05.-)

I34.0   Nonrheumatic mitral (valve) insufficiency
Nonrheumatic mitral (valve) incompetence NOS
Nonrheumatic mitral (valve) regurgitation NOS

I34.1   Nonrheumatic mitral (valve) prolapse
Floppy nonrheumatic mitral valve syndrome
Excludes1 Marfan's syndrome (Q87.4-)

I34.2   Nonrheumatic mitral (valve) stenosis
▶Code also, if applicable:
▶nonrheumatic mitral (valve) annulus calcification (I34.81)

● **I34.8   Other nonrheumatic mitral valve disorders**
▶**I34.81   Nonrheumatic mitral (valve) annulus calcification**
▶Nonrheumatic mitral (valve) annular calcification
▶Mitral (valve) annulus calcification NOS
▶ Code also, if applicable:
▶nonrheumatic mitral (valve) insufficiency (I34.0)
▶nonrheumatic mitral (valve) stenosis (I34.2)
▶**I34.89   Other nonrheumatic mitral valve disorders**

I34.9   Nonrheumatic mitral valve disorder, unspecified

● **I35   Nonrheumatic aortic valve disorders**
Excludes1 aortic valve disorder of unspecified cause but with diseases of mitral and/or tricuspid valve(s) (I08.-)
aortic valve disorder specified as congenital (Q23.0, Q23.1)
aortic valve disorder specified as rheumatic (I06.-)
hypertrophic subaortic stenosis (I42.1)

I35.0   Nonrheumatic aortic (valve) stenosis

I35.1   Nonrheumatic aortic (valve) insufficiency
Nonrheumatic aortic (valve) incompetence NOS
Nonrheumatic aortic (valve) regurgitation NOS

I35.2   **Nonrheumatic aortic (valve) stenosis with insufficiency**

I35.8   **Other nonrheumatic aortic valve disorders**

I35.9   **Nonrheumatic aortic valve disorder, unspecified**

● **I36**   **Nonrheumatic tricuspid valve disorders**

Excludes1	tricuspid valve disorders of unspecified cause (I07.-)
	tricuspid valve disorders specified as congenital (Q22.4, Q22.8, Q22.9)
	tricuspid valve disorders specified as rheumatic (I07.-)
	tricuspid valve disorders with aortic and/or mitral valve involvement (I08.-)

I36.0   **Nonrheumatic tricuspid (valve) stenosis**

I36.1   **Nonrheumatic tricuspid (valve) insufficiency**
Nonrheumatic tricuspid (valve) incompetence
Nonrheumatic tricuspid (valve) regurgitation

I36.2   **Nonrheumatic tricuspid (valve) stenosis with insufficiency**

I36.8   **Other nonrheumatic tricuspid valve disorders**

I36.9   **Nonrheumatic tricuspid valve disorder, unspecified**

● **I37**   **Nonrheumatic pulmonary valve disorders**

Excludes1	pulmonary valve disorder specified as congenital (Q22.1, Q22.2, Q22.3)
	pulmonary valve disorder specified as rheumatic (I09.89)

I37.0   **Nonrheumatic pulmonary valve stenosis**

I37.1   **Nonrheumatic pulmonary valve insufficiency**
Nonrheumatic pulmonary valve incompetence
Nonrheumatic pulmonary valve regurgitation

I37.2   **Nonrheumatic pulmonary valve stenosis with insufficiency**

I37.8   **Other nonrheumatic pulmonary valve disorders**

I37.9   **Nonrheumatic pulmonary valve disorder, unspecified**

I38   **Endocarditis, valve unspecified**

Includes	endocarditis (chronic) NOS
	valvular incompetence NOS
	valvular insufficiency NOS
	valvular regurgitation NOS
	valvular stenosis NOS
	valvulitis (chronic) NOS

Excludes1	congenital insufficiency of cardiac valve NOS (Q24.8)
	congenital stenosis of cardiac valve NOS (Q24.8)
	endocardial fibroelastosis (I42.4)
	endocarditis specified as rheumatic (I09.1)

▶ *I39*   *Endocarditis and heart valve disorders in diseases classified elsewhere*

Code first underlying disease, such as:
Q fever (A78)

Excludes1	endocardial involvement in:
	candidiasis (B37.6)
	gonococcal infection (A54.83)
	Libman-Sacks disease (M32.11)
	listerosis (A32.82)
	meningococcal infection (A39.51)
	rheumatoid arthritis (M05.31)
	syphilis (A52.03)
	tuberculosis (A18.84)
	typhoid fever (A01.02)

● **I40**   **Acute myocarditis**

Inflammation of heart muscle due to infection (viral/bacterial)

Includes	subacute myocarditis
Excludes1	acute rheumatic myocarditis (I01.2)

I40.0   **Infective myocarditis**
Septic myocarditis
Use additional code (B95-B97) to identify infectious agent

I40.1   **Isolated myocarditis**
Fiedler's myocarditis
Giant cell myocarditis
Idiopathic myocarditis

I40.8   **Other acute myocarditis**

I40.9   **Acute myocarditis, unspecified**

▶ *I41*   *Myocarditis in diseases classified elsewhere*

Code first underlying disease, such as:
typhus (A75.0-A75.9)

Excludes1	myocarditis (in):
	Chagas' disease (chronic) (B57.2)
	acute (B57.0)
	coxsackie (virus) infection (B33.22)
	diphtheritic (A36.81)
	gonococcal (A54.83)
	influenzal (J09.X9, J10.82, J11.82)
	meningococcal (A39.52)
	mumps (B26.82)
	rheumatoid arthritis (M05.31)
	sarcoid (D86.85)
	syphilis (A52.06)
	toxoplasmosis (B58.81)
	tuberculous (A18.84)

● **I42**   **Cardiomyopathy**

Disease of the heart muscle resulting in an abnormally enlarged, weakened, thickened, and/or stiffened muscles

Includes	myocardiopathy

Code first pre-existing cardiomyopathy complicating pregnancy and puerperium (O99.4)

Excludes2	ischemic cardiomyopathy (I25.5)
	peripartum cardiomyopathy (O90.3)
	ventricular hypertrophy (I51.7)

I42.0   **Dilated cardiomyopathy** 🐾
Congestive cardiomyopathy

I42.1   **Obstructive hypertrophic cardiomyopathy** 🐾
Hypertrophic subaortic stenosis (idiopathic)

I42.2   **Other hypertrophic cardiomyopathy** 🐾
Nonobstructive hypertrophic cardiomyopathy

I42.3   **Endomyocardial (eosinophilic) disease** 🐾
Endomyocardial (tropical) fibrosis
Löffler's endocarditis

I42.4   **Endocardial fibroelastosis** 🐾
Congenital cardiomyopathy
Elastomyofibrosis

I42.5   **Other restrictive cardiomyopathy** 🐾
Constrictive cardiomyopathy NOS

I42.6   **Alcoholic cardiomyopathy** 🐾
Code also presence of alcoholism (F10.-)

I42.7   **Cardiomyopathy due to drug and external agent** 🐾
Code first poisoning due to drug or toxin, if applicable (T36-T65 with fifth or sixth character 1-4 or 6)
Use additional code for adverse effect, if applicable, to identify drug (T36-T50 with fifth or sixth character 5)
Coding Clinic: 2021, Q3, P8

I42.8   **Other cardiomyopathies** 🐾

I42.9   **Cardiomyopathy, unspecified** 🐾
Cardiomyopathy (primary) (secondary) NOS

▶ *I43*   *Cardiomyopathy in diseases classified elsewhere* 🐾

Code first underlying disease, such as:
amyloidosis (E85.-)
glycogen storage disease (E74.0)
gout (M10.0-)
thyrotoxicosis (E05.0-E05.9-)

Excludes1	cardiomyopathy (in):
	coxsackie (virus) (B33.24)
	diphtheria (A36.81)
	sarcoidosis (D86.85)
	tuberculosis (A18.84)

CHAPTER 9 (I00-I99)

CHAPTER 9 (I00-I99)

● **I44** **Atrioventricular and left bundle-branch block**
Conduction problem resulting in arrhythmias/dysrhythmias due to a lack of electrical impulses being transmitted normally through the heart

    I44.0 **Atrioventricular block, first degree**

    I44.1 **Atrioventricular block, second degree**
        Atrioventricular block, type I and II
        Möbitz block, type I and II
        Second degree block, type I and II
        Wenckebach's block

    I44.2 **Atrioventricular block, complete** 🏷
        Complete heart block NOS
        Third degree block
        Coding Clinic: 2019, Q2, P4

  ● **I44.3** **Other and unspecified atrioventricular block**
        Atrioventricular block NOS

        I44.30 **Unspecified atrioventricular block**

        I44.39 **Other atrioventricular block**

    I44.4 **Left anterior fascicular block**

    I44.5 **Left posterior fascicular block**

  ● **I44.6** **Other and unspecified fascicular block**

        I44.60 **Unspecified fascicular block**
            Left bundle-branch hemiblock NOS

        I44.69 **Other fascicular block**

    I44.7 **Left bundle-branch block, unspecified**

● **I45** **Other conduction disorders**

    I45.0 **Right fascicular block**

  ● **I45.1** **Other and unspecified right bundle-branch block**

        I45.10 **Unspecified right bundle-branch block**
            Right bundle-branch block NOS

        I45.19 **Other right bundle-branch block**

    I45.2 **Bifascicular block**

    I45.3 **Trifascicular block**

    I45.4 **Nonspecific intraventricular block**
        Bundle-branch block NOS

    I45.5 **Other specified heart block**
        Sinoatrial block
        Sinoauricular block

        Excludes1 heart block NOS (I45.9)

    I45.6 **Pre-excitation syndrome**
        Accelerated atrioventricular conduction
        Accessory atrioventricular conduction
        Anomalous atrioventricular excitation
        Lown-Ganong-Levine syndrome
        Pre-excitation atrioventricular conduction
        Wolff-Parkinson-White syndrome

  ● **I45.8** **Other specified conduction disorders**

        I45.81 **Long QT syndrome**

        I45.89 **Other specified conduction disorders**
            Atrioventricular [AV] dissociation
            Interference dissociation
            Isorhythmic dissociation
            Nonparoxysmal AV nodal tachycardia
            Coding Clinic: 2013, Q2, P32

    I45.9 **Conduction disorder, unspecified**
        Heart block NOS
        Stokes-Adams syndrome

● **I46** **Cardiac arrest**
    Excludes2 cardiogenic shock (R57.0)

    I46.2 **Cardiac arrest due to underlying cardiac condition** 🏷
        Code first underlying cardiac condition

    I46.8 **Cardiac arrest due to other underlying condition** 🏷
        Code first underlying condition

    I46.9 **Cardiac arrest, cause unspecified** 🏷

● **I47** **Paroxysmal tachycardia**
Code first tachycardia complicating:
    abortion or ectopic or molar pregnancy (O00-O07, O08.8)
    obstetric surgery and procedures (O75.4)

    Excludes1 tachycardia NOS (R00.0)
            sinoauricular tachycardia NOS (R00.0)
            sinus [sinusal] tachycardia NOS (R00.0)

    I47.0 **Re-entry ventricular arrhythmia** 🏷

    I47.1 **Supraventricular tachycardia** 🏷
        Atrial (paroxysmal) tachycardia
        Atrioventricular [AV] (paroxysmal) tachycardia
        Atrioventricular re-entrant (nodal) tachycardia
        [AVNRT] [AVRT]
        Junctional (paroxysmal) tachycardia
        Nodal (paroxysmal) tachycardia

  ● **I47.2** **Ventricular tachycardia** 🏷

    ▶**I47.20** **Ventricular tachycardia, unspecified**

    ▶**I47.21** **Torsades de pointes**
        ▶ Code also, if applicable, long QT syndrome (I45.81)
        ▶ Use Additional code for adverse effect, if applicable, to identify drug (T36-T50 with fifth or sixth character 5)

    ▶**I47.29** **Other ventricular tachycardia**
        Coding Clinic: 2021, Q3, P12; 2013, Q3, P23

    I47.9 **Paroxysmal tachycardia, unspecified** 🏷
        Bouveret (-Hoffman) syndrome

● **I48** **Atrial fibrillation and flutter**
Most common abnormal heart rhythm (arrhythmia) presenting as irregular, rapid beating (tachycardia) of the heart's upper chamber.

    I48.0 **Paroxysmal atrial fibrillation** 🏷

  ● **I48.1** **Persistent atrial fibrillation** 🏷
        Rapid contractions of the upper heart chamber

        Excludes1 Permanent atrial fibrillation (I48.21)
        Coding Clinic: 2019, Q2, P3-4

        I48.11 **Longstanding persistent atrial fibrillation**

        I48.19 **Other persistent atrial fibrillation**
            Chronic persistent atrial fibrillation
            Persistent atrial fibrillation, NOS

  ● **I48.2** **Chronic atrial fibrillation** 🏷
        Coding Clinic: 2019, Q2, P3

        I48.20 **Chronic atrial fibrillation, unspecified**
            Excludes1 Chronic persistent atrial fibrillation (I48.19)

        I48.21 **Permanent atrial fibrillation**

    I48.3 **Typical atrial flutter** 🏷
        Type I atrial flutter

    I48.4 **Atypical atrial flutter** 🏷
        Type II atrial flutter

  ● **I48.9** **Unspecified atrial fibrillation and atrial flutter**

        I48.91 **Unspecified atrial fibrillation** 🏷

        I48.92 **Unspecified atrial flutter** 🏷

● **I49** **Other cardiac arrhythmias**
Code first cardiac arrhythmia complicating:
    abortion or ectopic or molar pregnancy (O00-O07, O08.8)
    obstetric surgery and procedures (O75.4)

    Excludes1 neonatal dysrhythmia (P29.1-)
            sinoatrial bradycardia (R00.1)
            sinus bradycardia (R00.1)
            vagal bradycardia (R00.1)

    Excludes2 bradycardia NOS (R00.1)

  ● **I49.0** **Ventricular fibrillation and flutter**

        I49.01 **Ventricular fibrillation** 🏷

        I49.02 **Ventricular flutter** 🏷

    I49.1 **Atrial premature depolarization**
        Atrial premature beats

▶ New   ➠ Revised   ~~deleted~~ Deleted   Excludes 1   Excludes 2   Includes   Use additional   Code first   Code also   Key words
OGCR Official Guidelines   X Assign placeholder X   ● Use Additional Character(s)   ▶ Manifestation Code   🏷 Hierarchical Condition Category   **Coding Clinic**

I49.2 Junctional premature depolarization 🔊

I49.3 Ventricular premature depolarization

● I49.4 Other and unspecified premature depolarization

    I49.40 **Unspecified premature depolarization**
        Premature beats NOS

    I49.49 **Other premature depolarization**
        Ectopic beats
        Extrasystoles
        Extrasystolic arrhythmias
        Premature contractions

I49.5 **Sick sinus syndrome** 🔊
    Tachycardia-bradycardia syndrome
    Coding Clinic: 2019, Q1, P33

I49.8 **Other specified cardiac arrhythmias**
    Brugada syndrome
    Coronary sinus rhythm disorder
    Ectopic rhythm disorder
    Nodal rhythm disorder

I49.9 **Cardiac arrhythmia, unspecified**
    Arrhythmia (cardiac) NOS

● **I50 Heart failure**

    Code first heart failure complicating abortion or ectopic or molar
        pregnancy (O00-O07, O08.8)
    heart failure due to hypertension (I11.0)
    heart failure due to hypertension with chronic kidney disease
        (I13.-)
    heart failure following surgery (I97.13-)
    obstetric surgery and procedures (O75.4)
    rheumatic heart failure (I09.81)

    Excludes2   cardiac arrest (I46.-)
                 neonatal cardiac failure (P20.0)

    Coding Clinic: 2017, Q1, P47; 2016, Q4, P122-123, Q1, P38; 2015, Q2, P15

I50.1 **Left ventricular failure, unspecified** 🔊
    Cardiac asthma
    Edema of lung with heart disease NOS
    Edema of lung with heart failure
    Left heart failure
    Pulmonary edema with heart disease NOS
    Pulmonary edema with heart failure

    Excludes1   edema of lung without heart disease or
                 heart failure (J81.-)
                 pulmonary edema without heart disease
                 or failure (J81.-)

● I50.2 **Systolic (congestive) heart failure**
    Heart failure with reduced ejection fraction [HFrEF]
    Systolic left ventricular heart failure

    Code also end stage heart failure, if applicable (I50.84)

    Excludes1   combined systolic (congestive) and
                 diastolic (congestive) heart failure
                 (I50.4-)

    I50.20 **Unspecified systolic (congestive) heart**
        failure 🔊

    I50.21 **Acute systolic (congestive) heart failure** 🔊
        Presenting a short and relatively severe episode

    I50.22 **Chronic systolic (congestive) heart failure** 🔊
        Long-lasting, presenting over time

    I50.23 **Acute on chronic systolic (congestive) heart**
        failure 🔊
        Combination code. What was a chronic condition
            now has an acute exacerbation (to make more
            severe).
        Coding Clinic: 2013, Q2, P33

● I50.3 **Diastolic (congestive) heart failure**
    Diastolic left ventricular heart failure
    Heart failure with normal ejection fraction
    Heart failure with preserved ejection fraction [HFpEF]

    Code also end stage heart failure, if applicable (I50.84)

    Excludes1   combined systolic (congestive) and diastolic
                 (congestive) heart failure (I50.4-)

    I50.30 **Unspecified diastolic (congestive) heart**
        failure 🔊

    I50.31 **Acute diastolic (congestive) heart failure** 🔊
        Coding Clinic: 2017, Q1, P46

    I50.32 **Chronic diastolic (congestive) heart failure** 🔊

    I50.33 **Acute on chronic diastolic (congestive) heart**
        failure 🔊

● I50.4 **Combined systolic (congestive) and diastolic**
    (congestive) heart failure
    Combined systolic and diastolic left ventricular heart
        failure
    Heart failure with reduced ejection fraction and
        diastolic dysfunction

    Code also end stage heart failure, if applicable (I50.84)

    I50.40 **Unspecified combined systolic (congestive) and**
        diastolic (congestive) heart failure 🔊

    I50.41 **Acute combined systolic (congestive) and**
        diastolic (congestive) heart failure 🔊

    I50.42 **Chronic combined systolic (congestive) and**
        diastolic (congestive) heart failure 🔊

    I50.43 **Acute on chronic combined systolic**
        (congestive) and diastolic (congestive) heart
        failure 🔊

● I50.8 **Other heart failure**

    ● I50.81 **Right heart failure**
        Right ventricular failure

        I50.810 **Right heart failure, unspecified** 🔊
            Right heart failure without mention
                of left heart failure
            Right ventricular failure NOS

        I50.811 **Acute right heart failure** 🔊
            Acute isolated right heart failure
            Acute (isolated) right ventricular
                 failure

        I50.812 **Chronic right heart failure** 🔊
            Chronic isolated right heart failure
            Chronic (isolated) right ventricular
                 failure

        I50.813 **Acute on chronic right heart failure** 🔊
            Acute on chronic isolated right heart
                 failure
            Acute on chronic (isolated) right
                 ventricular failure
            Acute decompensation of chronic
                 (isolated) right ventricular
                 failure
            Acute exacerbation of chronic
                 (isolated) right ventricular
                 failure

        I50.814 **Right heart failure due to left heart**
            failure
            Right ventricular failure secondary
                 to left ventricular failure

            Code also the type of left ventricular
                 failure, if known (I50.2-I50.43)

            Excludes1   Right heart failure
                     with but not
                     due to left heart
                     failure (I50.82)

    I50.82 **Biventricular heart failure** 🔊
        Code also the type of left ventricular failure as
            systolic, diastolic, or combined, if known
            (I50.2-I50.43)

Item 9-8 Congestive heart failure (CHF) is a condition in which the left ventricle of the heart cannot pump enough blood to the body. The blood flow from the heart slows or returns to the heart from the venous system (back flow) resulting in congestion (fluid accumulation) particularly in the abdomen. Most commonly, fluid collects in the lungs and results in shortness of breath, especially when in a reclining position.

I50.83   High output heart failure 🔖

I50.84   End stage heart failure 🔖
> Stage D heart failure
>> Code also the type of heart failure as systolic, diastolic, or combined, if known (I50.2-I50.43)

I50.89   Other heart failure 🔖

I50.9   Heart failure, unspecified 🔖
> Cardiac, heart or myocardial failure NOS
> Congestive heart disease
> Congestive heart failure NOS
>> **Excludes2**   fluid overload unrelated to congestive heart failure (E87.70)
>
> Coding Clinic: 2017, Q1, P45-46; 2015, Q2, P15; 2012, Q4, P92

● **I51**   Complications and ill-defined descriptions of heart disease
> **Excludes1**   any condition in I51.4-I51.9 due to hypertension (I11.-)
>> any condition in I51.4-I51.9 due to hypertension and chronic kidney disease (I13.-)
>> heart disease specified as rheumatic (I00-I09)

I51.0   Cardiac septal defect, acquired   A
> Acquired septal atrial defect (old)
> Acquired septal auricular defect (old)
> Acquired septal ventricular defect (old)
>> **Excludes1**   cardiac septal defect as current complication following acute myocardial infarction (I23.1, I23.2)

I51.1   Rupture of chordae tendineae, not elsewhere classified 🔖
>> **Excludes1**   rupture of chordae tendineae as current complication following acute myocardial infarction (I23.4)

I51.2   Rupture of papillary muscle, not elsewhere classified 🔖
>> **Excludes1**   rupture of papillary muscle as current complication following acute myocardial infarction (I23.5)

I51.3   Intracardiac thrombosis, not elsewhere classified
> Apical thrombosis (old)
> Atrial thrombosis (old)
> Auricular thrombosis (old)
> Mural thrombosis (old)
> Ventricular thrombosis (old)
>> **Excludes1**   intracardiac thrombosis as current complication following acute myocardial infarction (I23.6)
>
> Coding Clinic: 2013, Q1, P24

I51.4   Myocarditis, unspecified 🔖
> Chronic (interstitial) myocarditis
> Myocardial fibrosis
> Myocarditis NOS
>> **Excludes1**   acute or subacute myocarditis (I40.-)
>
> Coding Clinic: 2016, Q4, P122

I51.5   Myocardial degeneration 🔖
> Fatty degeneration of heart or myocardium
> Myocardial disease
> Senile degeneration of heart or myocardium
> Coding Clinic: 2016, Q4, P122

I51.7   Cardiomegaly
> Cardiac dilatation
> Cardiac hypertrophy
> Ventricular dilatation
> Coding Clinic: 2016, Q4, P122

● **I51.8**   Other ill-defined heart diseases
> Coding Clinic: 2016, Q4, P122

I51.81   Takotsubo syndrome
> Reversible left ventricular dysfunction following sudden emotional stress
> Stress induced cardiomyopathy
> Takotsubo cardiomyopathy
> Transient left ventricular apical ballooning syndrome

I51.89   Other ill-defined heart diseases
> Carditis (acute)(chronic)
> Pancarditis (acute)(chronic)
> Coding Clinic: 2019, Q2, P6

I51.9   Heart disease, unspecified
> Coding Clinic: 2016, Q4, P122

▶ **I52**   *Other heart disorders in diseases classified elsewhere*
> *Code first underlying disease, such as:*
> congenital syphilis (A50.5)
> mucopolysaccharidosis (E76.3)
> schistosomiasis (B65.0-B65.9)
>> **Excludes1**   heart disease (in):
>>> gonococcal infection (A54.83)
>>> meningococcal infection (A39.50)
>>> rheumatoid arthritis (M05.31)
>>> syphilis (A52.06)

CEREBROVASCULAR DISEASES (I60-I69)

Use additional code to identify presence of:
> alcohol abuse and dependence (F10.-)
> exposure to environmental tobacco smoke (Z77.22)
> history of tobacco dependence (Z87.891)
> hypertension (I10-I16)
> occupational exposure to environmental tobacco smoke (Z57.31)
> tobacco dependence (F17.-)
> tobacco use (Z72.0)
>> **Excludes1**   traumatic intracranial hemorrhage (S06.-)
>
> Coding Clinic: 2015, Q4, P40

I5A   Non-ischemic myocardial injury (non-traumatic)
> Acute (non-ischemic) myocardial injury
> Chronic (non-ischemic) myocardial injury
> Unspecified (non-ischemic) myocardial injury
> *Code first the underlying cause, if known and applicable, such as:*
>> acute kidney failure (N17.-)
>> acute myocarditis (I40.-)
>> cardiomyopathy (I42.-)
>> chronic kidney disease (CKD) (N18.-)
>> heart failure (I50.-)
>> hypertensive urgency (I16.0)
>> nonrheumatic aortic valve disorders (I35.-)
>> paroxysmal tachycardia (I47.-)
>> pulmonary embolism (I26.-)
>> pulmonary hypertension (I27.0, I27.2-)
>> sepsis (A41.-)
>> takotsubo syndrome (I51.81)
>
>> **Excludes1**   acute myocardial infarction (I21.-)
>>> injury of heart (S26.-)
>
>> **Excludes2**   other acute ischemic heart diseases (I24.-)
>
> Coding Clinic: 2021, Q4, P15

● **I60**   Nontraumatic subarachnoid hemorrhage
> **Excludes1**   syphilitic ruptured cerebral aneurysm (A52.05)
>
> **Excludes2**   sequelae of subarachnoid hemorrhage (I69.0-)

● **I60.0**   Nontraumatic subarachnoid hemorrhage from carotid siphon and bifurcation

I60.00   Nontraumatic subarachnoid hemorrhage from unspecified carotid siphon and bifurcation 🔖

I60.01   Nontraumatic subarachnoid hemorrhage from right carotid siphon and bifurcation 🔖

I60.02   Nontraumatic subarachnoid hemorrhage from left carotid siphon and bifurcation 🔖

● **I60.1**   Nontraumatic subarachnoid hemorrhage from middle cerebral artery

I60.10   Nontraumatic subarachnoid hemorrhage from unspecified middle cerebral artery 🔖

I60.11   Nontraumatic subarachnoid hemorrhage from right middle cerebral artery 🔖

I60.12   Nontraumatic subarachnoid hemorrhage from left middle cerebral artery 🔖

I60.2   Nontraumatic subarachnoid hemorrhage from anterior communicating artery 🔖

▶ New   ⇒ Revised   ~~deleted~~ Deleted   Excludes 1   Excludes 2   Includes   Use additional   Code first   Code also   Key words

OGCR Official Guidelines   X Assign placeholder X   ● Use Additional Character(s)   ▶ Manifestation Code   🔖 Hierarchical Condition Category   Coding Clinic

● I60.3   Nontraumatic subarachnoid hemorrhage from posterior communicating artery

　　　I60.30   Nontraumatic subarachnoid hemorrhage from unspecified posterior communicating artery

　　　I60.31   Nontraumatic subarachnoid hemorrhage from right posterior communicating artery

　　　I60.32   Nontraumatic subarachnoid hemorrhage from left posterior communicating artery

I60.4   Nontraumatic subarachnoid hemorrhage from basilar artery

● I60.5   Nontraumatic subarachnoid hemorrhage from vertebral artery

　　　I60.50   Nontraumatic subarachnoid hemorrhage from unspecified vertebral artery

　　　I60.51   Nontraumatic subarachnoid hemorrhage from right vertebral artery

　　　I60.52   Nontraumatic subarachnoid hemorrhage from left vertebral artery

I60.6   Nontraumatic subarachnoid hemorrhage from other intracranial arteries

I60.7   Nontraumatic subarachnoid hemorrhage from unspecified intracranial artery
　　　Ruptured (congenital) berry aneurysm
　　　Ruptured (congenital) cerebral aneurysm
　　　Subarachnoid hemorrhage (nontraumatic) from cerebral artery NOS
　　　Subarachnoid hemorrhage (nontraumatic) from communicating artery NOS

　　　Excludes1   berry aneurysm, nonruptured (I67.1)

I60.8   Other nontraumatic subarachnoid hemorrhage
　　　Meningeal hemorrhage
　　　Rupture of cerebral arteriovenous malformation

I60.9   Nontraumatic subarachnoid hemorrhage, unspecified

● I61   Nontraumatic intracerebral hemorrhage

　　Excludes2   sequelae of intracerebral hemorrhage (I69.1-)

　　Coding Clinic: 2017, Q2, P10

I61.0   Nontraumatic intracerebral hemorrhage in hemisphere, subcortical
　　　Deep intracerebral hemorrhage (nontraumatic)
　　　Coding Clinic: 2016, Q4, P27

I61.1   Nontraumatic intracerebral hemorrhage in hemisphere, cortical
　　　Cerebral lobe hemorrhage (nontraumatic)
　　　Superficial intracerebral hemorrhage (nontraumatic)
　　　Coding Clinic: 2016, Q4, P28

I61.2   Nontraumatic intracerebral hemorrhage in hemisphere, unspecified

I61.3   Nontraumatic intracerebral hemorrhage in brain stem

I61.4   Nontraumatic intracerebral hemorrhage in cerebellum

I61.5   Nontraumatic intracerebral hemorrhage, intraventricular

I61.6   Nontraumatic intracerebral hemorrhage, multiple localized

I61.8   Other nontraumatic intracerebral hemorrhage

I61.9   Nontraumatic intracerebral hemorrhage, unspecified

● I62   Other and unspecified nontraumatic intracranial hemorrhage

　　Excludes2   sequelae of intracranial hemorrhage (I69.2)

● I62.0   Nontraumatic subdural hemorrhage

　　　I62.00   Nontraumatic subdural hemorrhage, unspecified

　　　I62.01   Nontraumatic acute subdural hemorrhage

　　　I62.02   Nontraumatic subacute subdural hemorrhage

　　　I62.03   Nontraumatic chronic subdural hemorrhage

I62.1   Nontraumatic extradural hemorrhage
　　　Nontraumatic epidural hemorrhage

I62.9   Nontraumatic intracranial hemorrhage, unspecified

★ **(See Plate 31 of the Anatomy Illustrations.)**

● I63   Cerebral infarction

　　Excludes1   neonatal cerebral infarction (P91.82-)

　　Includes   occlusion and stenosis of cerebral and precerebral arteries, resulting in cerebral infarction

　　Use additional code, if applicable, to identify status post administration of tPA (rtPA) in a different facility within the last 24 hours prior to admission to current facility (Z92.82)

　　Use additional code, if known, to indicate National Institutes of Health Stroke Scale (NIHSS) score (R29.7-)

　　Excludes2   sequelae of cerebral infarction (I69.3-)

　　Coding Clinic: 2016, Q4, P28, 61, 127

● I63.0   Cerebral infarction due to thrombosis of precerebral arteries

　　　I63.00   Cerebral infarction due to thrombosis of unspecified precerebral artery

　　● I63.01   Cerebral infarction due to thrombosis of vertebral artery

　　　　I63.011   Cerebral infarction due to thrombosis of right vertebral artery

　　　　I63.012   Cerebral infarction due to thrombosis of left vertebral artery

　　　　I63.013   Cerebral infarction due to thrombosis of bilateral vertebral arteries

　　　　I63.019   Cerebral infarction due to thrombosis of unspecified vertebral artery

　　　I63.02   Cerebral infarction due to thrombosis of basilar artery

　　● I63.03   Cerebral infarction due to thrombosis of carotid artery

　　　　I63.031   Cerebral infarction due to thrombosis of right carotid artery

　　　　I63.032   Cerebral infarction due to thrombosis of left carotid artery

　　　　I63.033   Cerebral infarction due to thrombosis of bilateral carotid arteries

　　　　I63.039   Cerebral infarction due to thrombosis of unspecified carotid artery

　　　I63.09   Cerebral infarction due to thrombosis of other precerebral artery

Figure 9-4 Events causing a stroke. (From Shiland: Mastering Healthcare Terminology, ed 1, St. Louis, Mosby, 2003)

CHAPTER 9 (I00-I99)

● I63.1   Cerebral infarction due to embolism of precerebral arteries

    I63.10   Cerebral infarction due to embolism of unspecified precerebral artery 🦠

    ● I63.11   Cerebral infarction due to embolism of vertebral artery

        I63.111   Cerebral infarction due to embolism of right vertebral artery 🦠

        I63.112   Cerebral infarction due to embolism of left vertebral artery 🦠

        I63.113   Cerebral infarction due to embolism of bilateral vertebral arteries 🦠

        I63.119   Cerebral infarction due to embolism of unspecified vertebral artery 🦠

    I63.12   Cerebral infarction due to embolism of basilar artery 🦠

    ● I63.13   Cerebral infarction due to embolism of carotid artery

        I63.131   Cerebral infarction due to embolism of right carotid artery 🦠

        I63.132   Cerebral infarction due to embolism of left carotid artery 🦠

        I63.133   Cerebral infarction due to embolism of bilateral carotid arteries 🦠

        I63.139   Cerebral infarction due to embolism of unspecified carotid artery 🦠

    I63.19   Cerebral infarction due to embolism of other precerebral artery 🦠

● I63.2   Cerebral infarction due to unspecified occlusion or stenosis of precerebral arteries

    I63.20   Cerebral infarction due to unspecified occlusion or stenosis of unspecified precerebral arteries 🦠

    ● I63.21   Cerebral infarction due to unspecified occlusion or stenosis of vertebral arteries

        I63.211   Cerebral infarction due to unspecified occlusion or stenosis of right vertebral artery 🦠

        I63.212   Cerebral infarction due to unspecified occlusion or stenosis of left vertebral artery 🦠

        I63.213   Cerebral infarction due to unspecified occlusion or stenosis of bilateral vertebral arteries 🦠

        I63.219   Cerebral infarction due to unspecified occlusion or stenosis of unspecified vertebral artery 🦠

    I63.22   Cerebral infarction due to unspecified occlusion or stenosis of basilar artery 🦠

    ● I63.23   Cerebral infarction due to unspecified occlusion or stenosis of carotid arteries

        I63.231   Cerebral infarction due to unspecified occlusion or stenosis of right carotid arteries 🦠

        I63.232   Cerebral infarction due to unspecified occlusion or stenosis of left carotid arteries 🦠

        I63.233   Cerebral infarction due to unspecified occlusion or stenosis of bilateral carotid arteries 🦠

        I63.239   Cerebral infarction due to unspecified occlusion or stenosis of unspecified carotid artery 🦠

    I63.29   Cerebral infarction due to unspecified occlusion or stenosis of other precerebral arteries 🦠

● I63.3   Cerebral infarction due to thrombosis of cerebral arteries

    I63.30   Cerebral infarction due to thrombosis of unspecified cerebral artery 🦠

    ● I63.31   Cerebral infarction due to thrombosis of middle cerebral artery

        I63.311   Cerebral infarction due to thrombosis of right middle cerebral artery 🦠

        I63.312   Cerebral infarction due to thrombosis of left middle cerebral artery 🦠

        I63.313   Cerebral infarction due to thrombosis of bilateral middle cerebral arteries 🦠

        I63.319   Cerebral infarction due to thrombosis of unspecified middle cerebral artery 🦠

    ● I63.32   Cerebral infarction due to thrombosis of anterior cerebral artery

        I63.321   Cerebral infarction due to thrombosis of right anterior cerebral artery 🦠

        I63.322   Cerebral infarction due to thrombosis of left anterior cerebral artery 🦠

        I63.323   Cerebral infarction due to thrombosis of bilateral anterior cerebral arteries 🦠

        I63.329   Cerebral infarction due to thrombosis of unspecified anterior cerebral artery 🦠

    ● I63.33   Cerebral infarction due to thrombosis of posterior cerebral artery

        I63.331   Cerebral infarction due to thrombosis of right posterior cerebral artery 🦠

        I63.332   Cerebral infarction due to thrombosis of left posterior cerebral artery 🦠

        I63.333   Cerebral infarction due to thrombosis of bilateral posterior cerebral arteries 🦠

        I63.339   Cerebral infarction due to thrombosis of unspecified posterior cerebral artery 🦠

    ● I63.34   Cerebral infarction due to thrombosis of cerebellar artery

        I63.341   Cerebral infarction due to thrombosis of right cerebellar artery 🦠

        I63.342   Cerebral infarction due to thrombosis of left cerebellar artery 🦠

        I63.343   Cerebral infarction due to thrombosis of bilateral cerebellar arteries 🦠

        I63.349   Cerebral infarction due to thrombosis of unspecified cerebellar artery 🦠

    I63.39   Cerebral infarction due to thrombosis of other cerebral artery 🦠

● I63.4   Cerebral infarction due to embolism of cerebral arteries

    I63.40   Cerebral infarction due to embolism of unspecified cerebral artery 🦠

    ● I63.41   Cerebral infarction due to embolism of middle cerebral artery

        I63.411   Cerebral infarction due to embolism of right middle cerebral artery 🦠

        I63.412   Cerebral infarction due to embolism of left middle cerebral artery 🦠

        I63.413   Cerebral infarction due to embolism of bilateral middle cerebral arteries 🦠

        I63.419   Cerebral infarction due to embolism of unspecified middle cerebral artery 🦠

    ● I63.42   Cerebral infarction due to embolism of anterior cerebral artery

        I63.421   Cerebral infarction due to embolism of right anterior cerebral artery 🦠

        I63.422   Cerebral infarction due to embolism of left anterior cerebral artery 🦠

        I63.423   Cerebral infarction due to embolism of bilateral anterior cerebral arteries 🦠

        I63.429   Cerebral infarction due to embolism of unspecified anterior cerebral artery 🦠

▶ New   ⇒ Revised   ~~deleted~~ Deleted   Excludes 1   Excludes 2   Includes   Use additional   Code first   Code also   Key words

OGCR Official Guidelines   X Assign placeholder X   ● Use Additional Character(s)   ▶ Manifestation Code   🦠 Hierarchical Condition Category   Coding Clinic

● I63.43   Cerebral infarction due to embolism of posterior cerebral artery
    I63.431   Cerebral infarction due to embolism of right posterior cerebral artery 🔎
    I63.432   Cerebral infarction due to embolism of left posterior cerebral artery 🔎
    I63.433   Cerebral infarction due to embolism of bilateral posterior cerebral arteries 🔎
    I63.439   Cerebral infarction due to embolism of unspecified posterior cerebral artery 🔎

● I63.44   Cerebral infarction due to embolism of cerebellar artery
    I63.441   Cerebral infarction due to embolism of right cerebellar artery 🔎
    I63.442   Cerebral infarction due to embolism of left cerebellar artery 🔎
    I63.443   Cerebral infarction due to embolism of bilateral cerebellar arteries 🔎
    I63.449   Cerebral infarction due to embolism of unspecified cerebellar artery 🔎

    I63.49   Cerebral infarction due to embolism of other cerebral artery 🔎

● I63.5   Cerebral infarction due to unspecified occlusion or stenosis of cerebral arteries
    I63.50   Cerebral infarction due to unspecified occlusion or stenosis of unspecified cerebral artery 🔎

● I63.51   Cerebral infarction due to unspecified occlusion or stenosis of middle cerebral artery
    I63.511   Cerebral infarction due to unspecified occlusion or stenosis of right middle cerebral artery 🔎
    I63.512   Cerebral infarction due to unspecified occlusion or stenosis of left middle cerebral artery 🔎
    I63.513   Cerebral infarction due to unspecified occlusion or stenosis of bilateral middle cerebral arteries 🔎
    I63.519   Cerebral infarction due to unspecified occlusion or stenosis of unspecified middle cerebral artery 🔎

● I63.52   Cerebral infarction due to unspecified occlusion or stenosis of anterior cerebral artery
    I63.521   Cerebral infarction due to unspecified occlusion or stenosis of right anterior cerebral artery 🔎
    I63.522   Cerebral infarction due to unspecified occlusion or stenosis of left anterior cerebral artery 🔎
    I63.523   Cerebral infarction due to unspecified occlusion or stenosis of bilateral anterior cerebral arteries 🔎
    I63.529   Cerebral infarction due to unspecified occlusion or stenosis of unspecified anterior cerebral artery 🔎

● I63.53   Cerebral infarction due to unspecified occlusion or stenosis of posterior cerebral artery
    I63.531   Cerebral infarction due to unspecified occlusion or stenosis of right posterior cerebral artery 🔎
    I63.532   Cerebral infarction due to unspecified occlusion or stenosis of left posterior cerebral artery 🔎
        Coding Clinic: 2017, Q2, P10

    I63.533   Cerebral infarction due to unspecified occlusion or stenosis of bilateral posterior cerebral arteries 🔎
    I63.539   Cerebral infarction due to unspecified occlusion or stenosis of unspecified posterior cerebral artery 🔎

● I63.54   Cerebral infarction due to unspecified occlusion or stenosis of cerebellar artery
    I63.541   Cerebral infarction due to unspecified occlusion or stenosis of right cerebellar artery 🔎
    I63.542   Cerebral infarction due to unspecified occlusion or stenosis of left cerebellar artery 🔎
    I63.543   Cerebral infarction due to unspecified occlusion or stenosis of bilateral cerebellar arteries 🔎
    I63.549   Cerebral infarction due to unspecified occlusion or stenosis of unspecified cerebellar artery 🔎

    I63.59   Cerebral infarction due to unspecified occlusion or stenosis of other cerebral artery 🔎

I63.6   Cerebral infarction due to cerebral venous thrombosis, nonpyogenic 🔎

● I63.8   Other cerebral infarction 🔎
    I63.81   Other cerebral infarction due to occlusion or stenosis of small artery 🔎
        Lacunar infarction
        Coding Clinic: 2018, Q4, P16
    I63.89   Other cerebral infarction 🔎
        Coding Clinic: 2022, Q1, P25; 2017, Q2, P9

I63.9   Cerebral infarction, unspecified 🔎
    Stroke NOS
    Excludes2   transient cerebral ischemic attacks and related syndromes (G45.-)
    Coding Clinic: 2016, Q4, P62; 2015, Q1, P26

● I65   Occlusion and stenosis of precerebral arteries, not resulting in cerebral infarction
    Includes   embolism of precerebral artery
        narrowing of precerebral artery
        obstruction (complete) (partial) of precerebral artery
        thrombosis of precerebral artery
    Excludes1   insufficiency, NOS, of precerebral artery (G45.-)
        insufficiency of precerebral arteries causing cerebral infarction (I63.0-I63.2)

● I65.0   Occlusion and stenosis of vertebral artery
    I65.01   Occlusion and stenosis of right vertebral artery
    I65.02   Occlusion and stenosis of left vertebral artery
    I65.03   Occlusion and stenosis of bilateral vertebral arteries
    I65.09   Occlusion and stenosis of unspecified vertebral artery

I65.1   Occlusion and stenosis of basilar artery

● I65.2   Occlusion and stenosis of carotid artery
    I65.21   Occlusion and stenosis of right carotid artery
    I65.22   Occlusion and stenosis of left carotid artery
    I65.23   Occlusion and stenosis of bilateral carotid arteries
        Coding Clinic: 2021, Q1, P4
    I65.29   Occlusion and stenosis of unspecified carotid artery

I65.8   Occlusion and stenosis of other precerebral arteries

I65.9   Occlusion and stenosis of unspecified precerebral artery
    Occlusion and stenosis of precerebral artery NOS

● **I66   Occlusion and stenosis of cerebral arteries, not resulting in cerebral infarction**

     Includes   embolism of cerebral artery
                       narrowing of cerebral artery
                       obstruction (complete) (partial) of cerebral artery
                       thrombosis of cerebral artery

     Excludes1   occlusion and stenosis of cerebral artery causing cerebral infarction (I63.3-I63.5)

● **I66.0   Occlusion and stenosis of middle cerebral artery**

     I66.01   Occlusion and stenosis of right middle cerebral artery

     I66.02   Occlusion and stenosis of left middle cerebral artery

     I66.03   Occlusion and stenosis of bilateral middle cerebral arteries

     I66.09   Occlusion and stenosis of unspecified middle cerebral artery

● **I66.1   Occlusion and stenosis of anterior cerebral artery**

     I66.11   Occlusion and stenosis of right anterior cerebral artery

     I66.12   Occlusion and stenosis of left anterior cerebral artery

     I66.13   Occlusion and stenosis of bilateral anterior cerebral arteries

     I66.19   Occlusion and stenosis of unspecified anterior cerebral artery

● **I66.2   Occlusion and stenosis of posterior cerebral artery**

     I66.21   Occlusion and stenosis of right posterior cerebral artery

     I66.22   Occlusion and stenosis of left posterior cerebral artery

     I66.23   Occlusion and stenosis of bilateral posterior cerebral arteries

     I66.29   Occlusion and stenosis of unspecified posterior cerebral artery

   I66.3   Occlusion and stenosis of cerebellar arteries

   I66.8   Occlusion and stenosis of other cerebral arteries
           Occlusion and stenosis of perforating arteries

   I66.9   Occlusion and stenosis of unspecified cerebral artery

● **I67   Other cerebrovascular diseases**

     Excludes2   sequelae of the listed conditions (I69.8)

   I67.0   Dissection of cerebral arteries, nonruptured 🖻

       Excludes1   ruptured cerebral arteries (I60.7)

       Coding Clinic: 2021, Q3, P5

   I67.1   Cerebral aneurysm, nonruptured
           Cerebral aneurysm NOS
           Cerebral arteriovenous fistula, acquired
           Internal carotid artery aneurysm, intracranial portion
           Internal carotid artery aneurysm, NOS

       Excludes1   congenital cerebral aneurysm, nonruptured (Q28.-)
                       ruptured cerebral aneurysm (I60.7)

   I67.2   Cerebral atherosclerosis   A
           Atheroma of cerebral and precerebral arteries

   I67.3   Progressive vascular leukoencephalopathy
           Binswanger's disease

   I67.4   Hypertensive encephalopathy

       Excludes2   insufficiency, NOS, of precerebral arteries (G45.2)

   I67.5   Moyamoya disease

   I67.6   Nonpyogenic thrombosis of intracranial venous system
           Nonpyogenic thrombosis of cerebral vein
           Nonpyogenic thrombosis of intracranial venous sinus

       Excludes1   nonpyogenic thrombosis of intracranial venous system causing infarction (I63.6)

   I67.7   Cerebral arteritis, not elsewhere classified
           Granulomatous angiitis of the nervous system

       Excludes1   allergic granulomatous angiitis (M30.1)

● **I67.8   Other specified cerebrovascular diseases**

     I67.81   Acute cerebrovascular insufficiency
           Acute cerebrovascular insufficiency unspecified as to location or reversibility

     I67.82   Cerebral ischemia
           Chronic cerebral ischemia

     I67.83   Posterior reversible encephalopathy syndrome
           PRES

●   **I67.84**   Cerebral vasospasm and vasoconstriction

         I67.841   Reversible cerebrovascular vasoconstriction syndrome
              Call-Fleming syndrome

              Code first underlying condition, if applicable, such as eclampsia (O15.00-O15.9)

         I67.848   Other cerebrovascular vasospasm and vasoconstriction

●   **I67.85**   Hereditary cerebrovascular diseases

         I67.850   Cerebral autosomal dominant arteriopathy with subcortical infarcts and leukoencephalopathy
              CADASIL

              Code also any associated diagnoses, such as:
                 epilepsy (G40.-), stroke (I63.-)
                 vascular dementia (F01.-)

         I67.858   Other hereditary cerebrovascular disease

     I67.89   Other cerebrovascular disease

   I67.9   Cerebrovascular disease, unspecified

● **I68   Cerebrovascular disorders in diseases classified elsewhere**

▷   **I68.0   *Cerebral amyloid angiopathy***
         Code first underlying amyloidosis (E85.-)

▷   **I68.2   *Cerebral arteritis in other diseases classified elsewhere***
         Code first underlying disease

       Excludes1   cerebral arteritis (in):
                     listerosis (A32.89)
                     systemic lupus erythematosus (M32.19)
                     syphilis (A52.04)
                     tuberculosis (A18.89)

▷   **I68.8   *Other cerebrovascular disorders in diseases classified elsewhere***

         Code first underlying disease

       Excludes1   syphilitic cerebral aneurysm (A52.05)

OGCR   Section I.c.9.d.

Sequelae of Cerebrovascular Disease

1) Category I69, Sequelae of Cerebrovascular disease

Category I69 is used to indicate conditions classifiable to categories I60-I67 as the causes of sequela (neurologic deficits), themselves classified elsewhere. These "late effects" include neurologic deficits that persist after initial onset of conditions classifiable to categories I60-I67. The neurologic deficits caused by cerebrovascular disease may be present from the onset of may arise at any time after the onset of the condition classifiable to categories I60-I67.

Codes from category I69, Sequelae of cerebrovascular disease, that specify hemiplegia, hemiparesis and monoplegia identify whether the dominant or nondominant side is affected. Should the affected side be documented, but not specified as dominant or nondominant, and the classification system does not indicate a default, code selection is as follows:

For ambidextrous patients, the default should be dominant.

If the left side is affected, the default is nondominant.

If the right side is affected, the default is dominant.

2) Codes from category I69 with codes from I60-I67

Codes from category I69 may be assigned on a health care record with codes from I60-I67, if the patient has a current cerebrovascular disease and deficits from an old cerebrovascular disease.

▶ New   ➾ Revised   ~~deleted~~ Deleted   Excludes 1   Excludes 2   Includes   Use additional   Code first   Code also   Key words

OGCR Official Guidelines   X Assign placeholder X   ● Use Additional Character(s)   ▷ Manifestation Code   🖻 Hierarchical Condition Category   **Coding Clinic**

● **I69   Sequelae of cerebrovascular disease**

　　Note: Category I69 is to be used to indicate conditions in I60-I67 as the cause of sequelae. The 'sequelae' include conditions specified as such or as residuals which may occur at any time after the onset of the causal condition.

　　Excludes1　personal history of cerebral infarction without residual deficit (Z86.73)
　　　　　personal history of prolonged reversible ischemic neurologic deficit (PRIND) (Z86.73)
　　　　　personal history of reversible ischemic neurologcial deficit (RIND) (Z86.73)
　　　　　sequelae of traumatic intracranial injury (S06.-)

　　Coding Clinic: 2016, Q4, P28; 2015, Q4, P40; 2012, Q4, P107

● **I69.0   Sequelae of nontraumatic subarachnoid hemorrhage**

　　I69.00　Unspecified sequelae of nontraumatic subarachnoid hemorrhage

●　I69.01　Cognitive deficits following nontraumatic subarachnoid hemorrhage

　　　　I69.010　**Attention and concentration** deficit following nontraumatic subarachnoid hemorrhage

　　　　I69.011　**Memory** deficit following nontraumatic subarachnoid hemorrhage

　　　　I69.012　**Visuospatial** deficit and spatial neglect following nontraumatic subarachnoid hemorrhage

　　　　I69.013　**Psychomotor** deficit following nontraumatic subarachnoid hemorrhage

　　　　I69.014　**Frontal lobe and executive function** deficit following nontraumatic subarachnoid hemorrhage

　　　　I69.015　**Cognitive social or emotional** deficit following nontraumatic subarachnoid hemorrhage

　　　　I69.018　**Other symptoms and signs** involving cognitive functions following nontraumatic subarachnoid hemorrhage

　　　　I69.019　**Unspecified** symptoms and signs involving cognitive functions following nontraumatic subarachnoid hemorrhage

●　I69.02　**Speech and language deficits** following nontraumatic subarachnoid hemorrhage

　　　　I69.020　**Aphasia** following nontraumatic subarachnoid hemorrhage

　　　　I69.021　**Dysphasia** following nontraumatic subarachnoid hemorrhage

　　　　I69.022　**Dysarthria** following nontraumatic subarachnoid hemorrhage

　　　　I69.023　**Fluency disorder** following nontraumatic subarachnoid hemorrhage
　　　　　　Stuttering following nontraumatic subarachnoid hemorrhage

　　　　I69.028　**Other speech and language deficits** following nontraumatic subarachnoid hemorrhage

●　I69.03　**Monoplegia of upper limb** following nontraumatic subarachnoid hemorrhage

　　　　I69.031　**Monoplegia of upper limb** following nontraumatic subarachnoid hemorrhage affecting **right dominant side** 🔍

　　　　I69.032　**Monoplegia of upper limb** following nontraumatic subarachnoid hemorrhage affecting **left dominant side** 🔍

　　　　I69.033　**Monoplegia of upper limb** following nontraumatic subarachnoid hemorrhage affecting **right non-dominant side** 🔍

　　　　I69.034　**Monoplegia of upper limb** following nontraumatic subarachnoid hemorrhage affecting **left non-dominant side** 🔍

　　　　I69.039　**Monoplegia of upper limb** following nontraumatic subarachnoid hemorrhage affecting **unspecified side** 🔍

●　I69.04　**Monoplegia of lower limb** following nontraumatic subarachnoid hemorrhage

　　　　I69.041　**Monoplegia of lower limb** following nontraumatic subarachnoid hemorrhage affecting **right dominant side** 🔍

　　　　I69.042　**Monoplegia of lower limb** following nontraumatic subarachnoid hemorrhage affecting **left dominant side** 🔍

　　　　I69.043　**Monoplegia of lower limb** following nontraumatic subarachnoid hemorrhage affecting **right non-dominant side** 🔍

　　　　I69.044　**Monoplegia of lower limb** following nontraumatic subarachnoid hemorrhage affecting **left non-dominant side** 🔍

　　　　I69.049　**Monoplegia of lower limb** following nontraumatic subarachnoid hemorrhage affecting **unspecified side** 🔍

●　I69.05　**Hemiplegia and hemiparesis** following nontraumatic subarachnoid hemorrhage

　　　　I69.051　**Hemiplegia and hemiparesis** following nontraumatic subarachnoid hemorrhage affecting **right dominant side** 🔍

　　　　I69.052　**Hemiplegia and hemiparesis** following nontraumatic subarachnoid hemorrhage affecting **left dominant side** 🔍

　　　　I69.053　**Hemiplegia and hemiparesis** following nontraumatic subarachnoid hemorrhage affecting **right non-dominant side** 🔍

　　　　I69.054　**Hemiplegia and hemiparesis** following nontraumatic subarachnoid hemorrhage affecting **left non-dominant side** 🔍

　　　　I69.059　**Hemiplegia and hemiparesis** following nontraumatic subarachnoid hemorrhage affecting **unspecified side** 🔍

●　I69.06　**Other paralytic syndrome** following nontraumatic subarachnoid hemorrhage

　　　　Use additional code to identify type of paralytic syndrome, such as:
　　　　locked-in state (G83.5)
　　　　quadriplegia (G82.5-)

　　　　Excludes1　hemiplegia/hemiparesis following nontraumatic subarachnoid hemorrhage (I69.05-)
　　　　　　monoplegia of lower limb following nontraumatic subarachnoid hemorrhage (I69.04-)
　　　　　　monoplegia of upper limb following nontraumatic subarachnoid hemorrhage (I69.03-)

　　　　I69.061　**Other paralytic syndrome** following nontraumatic subarachnoid hemorrhage affecting **right dominant side** 🔍

N Newborn Age: 0　　**P** Pediatric Age: 0–17　　**M** Maternity DX: 9–64　　**A** Adult Age: 15–124　　♀ Females Only　　♂ Males Only

903

CHAPTER 9 (I00-I99)

I69.062   Other paralytic syndrome following nontraumatic subarachnoid hemorrhage affecting left dominant side 🦠

I69.063   Other paralytic syndrome following nontraumatic subarachnoid hemorrhage affecting right non-dominant side 🦠

I69.064   Other paralytic syndrome following nontraumatic subarachnoid hemorrhage affecting left non-dominant side 🦠

I69.065   Other paralytic syndrome following nontraumatic subarachnoid hemorrhage, bilateral 🦠

I69.069   Other paralytic syndrome following nontraumatic subarachnoid hemorrhage affecting unspecified side 🦠

● I69.09   Other sequelae of nontraumatic subarachnoid hemorrhage

I69.090   Apraxia following nontraumatic subarachnoid hemorrhage

I69.091   Dysphagia following nontraumatic subarachnoid hemorrhage

⇨ Use additional code to identify the type of dysphagia, if known (R13.11-R13.19)

I69.092   Facial weakness following nontraumatic subarachnoid hemorrhage

Facial droop following nontraumatic subarachnoid hemorrhage

I69.093   Ataxia following nontraumatic subarachnoid hemorrhage

I69.098   Other sequelae following nontraumatic subarachnoid hemorrhage

Alterations of sensation following nontraumatic subarachnoid hemorrhage

Disturbance of vision following nontraumatic subarachnoid hemorrhage

Use additional code to identify the sequelae

● I69.1 Sequelae of nontraumatic intracerebral hemorrhage

I69.10   Unspecified sequelae of nontraumatic intracerebral hemorrhage

● I69.11   Cognitive deficits following nontraumatic intracerebral hemorrhage

I69.110   Attention and concentration deficit following nontraumatic intracerebral hemorrhage

I69.111   Memory deficit following nontraumatic intracerebral hemorrhage

I69.112   Visuospatial deficit and spatial neglect following nontraumatic intracerebral hemorrhage

I69.113   Psychomotor deficit following nontraumatic intracerebral hemorrhage

I69.114   Frontal lobe and executive function deficit following nontraumatic intracerebral hemorrhage

I69.115   Cognitive social or emotional deficit following nontraumatic intracerebral hemorrhage

I69.118   Other symptoms and signs involving cognitive functions following nontraumatic intracerebral hemorrhage

I69.119   Unspecified symptoms and signs involving cognitive functions following nontraumatic intracerebral hemorrhage

● I69.12   Speech and language deficits following nontraumatic intracerebral hemorrhage

I69.120   Aphasia following nontraumatic intracerebral hemorrhage

I69.121   Dysphasia following nontraumatic intracerebral hemorrhage

I69.122   Dysarthria following nontraumatic intracerebral hemorrhage

I69.123   Fluency disorder following nontraumatic intracerebral hemorrhage

Stuttering following nontraumatic intracerebral hemorrhage

I69.128   Other speech and language deficits following nontraumatic intracerebral hemorrhage

● I69.13   Monoplegia of upper limb following nontraumatic intracerebral hemorrhage

I69.131   Monoplegia of upper limb following nontraumatic intracerebral hemorrhage affecting right dominant side 🦠

I69.132   Monoplegia of upper limb following nontraumatic intracerebral hemorrhage affecting left dominant side 🦠

I69.133   Monoplegia of upper limb following nontraumatic intracerebral hemorrhage affecting right non-dominant side 🦠

I69.134   Monoplegia of upper limb following nontraumatic intracerebral hemorrhage affecting left non-dominant side 🦠

I69.139   Monoplegia of upper limb following nontraumatic intracerebral hemorrhage affecting unspecified side 🦠

● I69.14   Monoplegia of lower limb following nontraumatic intracerebral hemorrhage

I69.141   Monoplegia of lower limb following nontraumatic intracerebral hemorrhage affecting right dominant side 🦠

I69.142   Monoplegia of lower limb following nontraumatic intracerebral hemorrhage affecting left dominant side 🦠

I69.143   Monoplegia of lower limb following nontraumatic intracerebral hemorrhage affecting right non-dominant side 🦠

I69.144   Monoplegia of lower limb following nontraumatic intracerebral hemorrhage affecting left non-dominant side 🦠

I69.149   Monoplegia of lower limb following nontraumatic intracerebral hemorrhage affecting unspecified side 🦠

● I69.15   Hemiplegia and hemiparesis following nontraumatic intracerebral hemorrhage

I69.151   Hemiplegia and hemiparesis following nontraumatic intracerebral hemorrhage affecting right dominant side 🦠

I69.152   Hemiplegia and hemiparesis following nontraumatic intracerebral hemorrhage affecting left dominant side 🦠

I69.153   Hemiplegia and hemiparesis following nontraumatic intracerebral hemorrhage affecting right non-dominant side 🦠

▶ New   ⇨ Revised   ~~deleted~~ Deleted   Excludes 1   Excludes 2   Includes   Use additional   Code first   Code also   Key words
OGCR Official Guidelines   X Assign placeholder X   ● Use Additional Character(s)   ▶ Manifestation Code   🦠 Hierarchical Condition Category   Coding Clinic

I69.154   **Hemiplegia and hemiparesis following nontraumatic intracerebral hemorrhage affecting left non-dominant side** 🗝

I69.159   **Hemiplegia and hemiparesis following nontraumatic intracerebral hemorrhage affecting unspecified side** 🗝

● I69.16   **Other paralytic syndrome following nontraumatic intracerebral hemorrhage**

Use additional code to identify type of paralytic syndrome, such as:
locked-in state (G83.5)
quadriplegia (G82.5-)

> **Excludes1**   hemiplegia/hemiparesis following nontraumatic intracerebral hemorrhage (I69.15-)
> monoplegia of lower limb following nontraumatic intracerebral hemorrhage (I69.14-)
> monoplegia of upper limb following nontraumatic intracerebral hemorrhage (I69.13-)

I69.161   **Other paralytic syndrome following nontraumatic intracerebral hemorrhage affecting right dominant side** 🗝

I69.162   **Other paralytic syndrome following nontraumatic intracerebral hemorrhage affecting left dominant side** 🗝

I69.163   **Other paralytic syndrome following nontraumatic intracerebral hemorrhage affecting right non-dominant side** 🗝

I69.164   **Other paralytic syndrome following nontraumatic intracerebral hemorrhage affecting left non-dominant side** 🗝

I69.165   **Other paralytic syndrome following nontraumatic intracerebral hemorrhage, bilateral** 🗝

I69.169   **Other paralytic syndrome following nontraumatic intracerebral hemorrhage affecting unspecified side** 🗝

● I69.19   **Other sequelae of nontraumatic intracerebral hemorrhage**

I69.190   **Apraxia following nontraumatic intracerebral hemorrhage**

I69.191   **Dysphagia following nontraumatic intracerebral hemorrhage**

➡ Use additional code to identify the type of dysphagia, if known (R13.11-R13.19)

I69.192   **Facial weakness following nontraumatic intracerebral hemorrhage**
Facial droop following nontraumatic intracerebral hemorrhage

I69.193   **Ataxia following nontraumatic intracerebral hemorrhage**

I69.198   **Other sequelae of nontraumatic intracerebral hemorrhage**
Alteration of sensations following nontraumatic intracerebral hemorrhage
Disturbance of vision following nontraumatic intracerebral hemorrhage

Use additional code to identify the sequelae

● I69.2   **Sequelae of other nontraumatic intracranial hemorrhage**

I69.20   **Unspecified sequelae of other nontraumatic intracranial hemorrhage**

● I69.21   **Cognitive deficits following other nontraumatic intracranial hemorrhage**

I69.210   **Attention and concentration deficit following other nontraumatic intracranial hemorrhage**

I69.211   **Memory deficit following other nontraumatic intracranial hemorrhage**

I69.212   **Visuospatial deficit and spatial neglect following other nontraumatic intracranial hemorrhage**

I69.213   **Psychomotor deficit following other nontraumatic intracranial hemorrhage**

I69.214   **Frontal lobe and executive function deficit following other nontraumatic intracranial hemorrhage**

I69.215   **Cognitive social or emotional deficit following other nontraumatic intracranial hemorrhage**

I69.218   **Other symptoms and signs involving cognitive functions following other nontraumatic intracranial hemorrhage**

I69.219   **Unspecified symptoms and signs involving cognitive functions following other nontraumatic intracranial hemorrhage**

● I69.22   **Speech and language deficits following other nontraumatic intracranial hemorrhage**

I69.220   **Aphasia following other nontraumatic intracranial hemorrhage**

I69.221   **Dysphasia following other nontraumatic intracranial hemorrhage**

I69.222   **Dysarthria following other nontraumatic intracranial hemorrhage**

I69.223   **Fluency disorder following other nontraumatic intracranial hemorrhage**
Stuttering following other nontraumatic intracranial hemorrhage

I69.228   **Other speech and language deficits following other nontraumatic intracranial hemorrhage**

● I69.23   **Monoplegia of upper limb following other nontraumatic intracranial hemorrhage**

I69.231   **Monoplegia of upper limb following other nontraumatic intracranial hemorrhage affecting right dominant side** 🗝

I69.232   **Monoplegia of upper limb following other nontraumatic intracranial hemorrhage affecting left dominant side** 🗝

I69.233   **Monoplegia of upper limb following other nontraumatic intracranial hemorrhage affecting right non-dominant side** 🗝

I69.234   **Monoplegia of upper limb following other nontraumatic intracranial hemorrhage affecting left non-dominant side** 🗝

I69.239   **Monoplegia of upper limb following other nontraumatic intracranial hemorrhage affecting unspecified side** 🗝

● I69.24   **Monoplegia of lower limb following other nontraumatic intracranial hemorrhage**

I69.241   **Monoplegia of lower limb following other nontraumatic intracranial hemorrhage affecting right dominant side** 🗝

I69.242   **Monoplegia of lower limb following other nontraumatic intracranial hemorrhage affecting left dominant side** 🐾

I69.243   **Monoplegia of lower limb following other nontraumatic intracranial hemorrhage affecting right non-dominant side** 🐾

I69.244   **Monoplegia of lower limb following other nontraumatic intracranial hemorrhage affecting left non-dominant side** 🐾

I69.249   **Monoplegia of lower limb following other nontraumatic intracranial hemorrhage affecting unspecified side** 🐾

● I69.25   **Hemiplegia and hemiparesis following other nontraumatic intracranial hemorrhage**

I69.251   **Hemiplegia and hemiparesis following other nontraumatic intracranial hemorrhage affecting right dominant side** 🐾

I69.252   **Hemiplegia and hemiparesis following other nontraumatic intracranial hemorrhage affecting left dominant side** 🐾

I69.253   **Hemiplegia and hemiparesis following other nontraumatic intracranial hemorrhage affecting right non-dominant side** 🐾

I69.254   **Hemiplegia and hemiparesis following other nontraumatic intracranial hemorrhage affecting left non-dominant side** 🐾

I69.259   **Hemiplegia and hemiparesis following other nontraumatic intracranial hemorrhage affecting unspecified side** 🐾

● I69.26   **Other paralytic syndrome following other nontraumatic intracranial hemorrhage**

Use additional code to identify type of paralytic syndrome, such as:
locked-in state (G83.5)
quadriplegia (G82.5-)

Excludes1   hemiplegia/hemiparesis following other nontraumatic intracranial hemorrhage (I69.25-)
monoplegia of lower limb following other nontraumatic intracranial hemorrhage (I69.24-)
monoplegia of upper limb following other nontraumatic intracranial hemorrhage (I69.23-)

I69.261   **Other paralytic syndrome following other nontraumatic intracranial hemorrhage affecting right dominant side** 🐾

I69.262   **Other paralytic syndrome following other nontraumatic intracranial hemorrhage affecting left dominant side** 🐾

I69.263   **Other paralytic syndrome following other nontraumatic intracranial hemorrhage affecting right non-dominant side** 🐾

I69.264   **Other paralytic syndrome following other nontraumatic intracranial hemorrhage affecting left non-dominant side** 🐾

I69.265   **Other paralytic syndrome following other nontraumatic intracranial hemorrhage, bilateral** 🐾

I69.269   **Other paralytic syndrome following other nontraumatic intracranial hemorrhage affecting unspecified side** 🐾

● I69.29   **Other sequelae of other nontraumatic intracranial hemorrhage**

I69.290   **Apraxia following other nontraumatic intracranial hemorrhage**

I69.291   **Dysphagia following other nontraumatic intracranial hemorrhage**
➡ Use additional code to identify the type of dysphagia, if known (R13.11-R13.19)

I69.292   **Facial weakness following other nontraumatic intracranial hemorrhage**
Facial droop following other nontraumatic intracranial hemorrhage

I69.293   **Ataxia following other nontraumatic intracranial hemorrhage**

I69.298   **Other sequelae of other nontraumatic intracranial hemorrhage**
Alteration of sensation following other nontraumatic intracranial hemorrhage
Disturbance of vision following other nontraumatic intracranial hemorrhage
Use additional code to identify the sequelae

● I69.3   **Sequelae of cerebral infarction**
Sequelae of stroke NOS
Coding Clinic: 2012, Q4, P92, 95

I69.30   **Unspecified sequelae of cerebral infarction**

● I69.31   **Cognitive deficits following cerebral infarction**

I69.310   **Attention and concentration deficit following cerebral infarction**

I69.311   **Memory deficit following cerebral infarction**

I69.312   **Visuospatial deficit and spatial neglect following cerebral infarction**

I69.313   **Psychomotor deficit following cerebral infarction**

I69.314   **Frontal lobe and executive function deficit following cerebral infarction**

I69.315   **Cognitive social or emotional deficit following cerebral infarction**

I69.318   **Other symptoms and signs involving cognitive functions following cerebral infarction**

I69.319   **Unspecified symptoms and signs involving cognitive functions following cerebral infarction**

● I69.32   **Speech and language deficits following cerebral infarction**

I69.320   **Aphasia following cerebral infarction**

I69.321   **Dysphasia following cerebral infarction**
Coding Clinic: 2012, Q4, P91

I69.322   **Dysarthria following cerebral infarction**
Excludes2   transient ischemic attack (TIA) (G45.9)

I69.323   **Fluency disorder following cerebral infarction**
Stuttering following cerebral infarction

I69.328   **Other speech and language deficits following cerebral infarction**

● **I69.33**   **Monoplegia of upper limb following cerebral infarction**
Coding Clinic: 2017, Q1, P47

I69.331   **Monoplegia of upper limb following cerebral infarction affecting right dominant side** 🔧

I69.332   **Monoplegia of upper limb following cerebral infarction affecting left dominant side** 🔧

I69.333   **Monoplegia of upper limb following cerebral infarction affecting right non-dominant side** 🔧

I69.334   **Monoplegia of upper limb following cerebral infarction affecting left non-dominant side** 🔧

I69.339   **Monoplegia of upper limb following cerebral infarction affecting unspecified side** 🔧

● **I69.34**   **Monoplegia of lower limb following cerebral infarction**
Coding Clinic: 2017, Q1, P47

I69.341   **Monoplegia of lower limb following cerebral infarction affecting right dominant side** 🔧

I69.342   **Monoplegia of lower limb following cerebral infarction affecting left dominant side** 🔧

I69.343   **Monoplegia of lower limb following cerebral infarction affecting right non-dominant side** 🔧

I69.344   **Monoplegia of lower limb following cerebral infarction affecting left non-dominant side** 🔧

I69.349   **Monoplegia of lower limb following cerebral infarction affecting unspecified side** 🔧

● **I69.35**   **Hemiplegia and hemiparesis following cerebral infarction**

I69.351   **Hemiplegia and hemiparesis following cerebral infarction affecting right dominant side** 🔧

> **Excludes2**   transient ischemic attack (TIA) (G45.9)
> *Coding Clinic: 2015, Q1, P25*

I69.352   **Hemiplegia and hemiparesis following cerebral infarction affecting left dominant side** 🔧

I69.353   **Hemiplegia and hemiparesis following cerebral infarction affecting right non-dominant side** 🔧

I69.354   **Hemiplegia and hemiparesis following cerebral infarction affecting left non-dominant side** 🔧
Coding Clinic: 2012, Q4, P91

I69.359   **Hemiplegia and hemiparesis following cerebral infarction affecting unspecified side** 🔧

● **I69.36**   **Other paralytic syndrome following cerebral infarction**

Use additional code to identify type of paralytic syndrome, such as:
locked-in state (G83.5)
quadriplegia (G82.5-)

> **Excludes1**   hemiplegia/hemiparesis following cerebral infarction (I69.35-)
> monoplegia of lower limb following cerebral infarction (I69.34-)
> monoplegia of upper limb following cerebral infarction (I69.33-)

I69.361   **Other paralytic syndrome following cerebral infarction affecting right dominant side** 🔧

I69.362   **Other paralytic syndrome following cerebral infarction affecting left dominant side** 🔧

I69.363   **Other paralytic syndrome following cerebral infarction affecting right non-dominant side** 🔧

I69.364   **Other paralytic syndrome following cerebral infarction affecting left non-dominant side** 🔧

I69.365   **Other paralytic syndrome following cerebral infarction, bilateral** 🔧

I69.369   **Other paralytic syndrome following cerebral infarction affecting unspecified side** 🔧

● **I69.39**   **Other sequelae of cerebral infarction**

I69.390   **Apraxia following cerebral infarction**

I69.391   **Dysphagia following cerebral infarction**

> ➠ Use additional code to identify the type of dysphagia, if known (R13.11-R13.19)

I69.392   **Facial weakness following cerebral infarction**
Facial droop following cerebral infarction

I69.393   **Ataxia following cerebral infarction**

I69.398   **Other sequelae of cerebral infarction**
Alteration of sensation following cerebral infarction
Disturbance of vision following cerebral infarction
Use additional code to identify the sequelae

● **I69.8**   **Sequelae of other cerebrovascular diseases**

> **Excludes1**   sequelae of traumatic intracranial injury (S06.-)

I69.80   **Unspecified sequelae of other cerebrovascular disease**

● **I69.81**   **Cognitive deficits following other cerebrovascular disease**

I69.810   **Attention and concentration deficit following other cerebrovascular disease**

I69.811   **Memory deficit following other cerebrovascular disease**

I69.812   **Visuospatial deficit and spatial neglect following other cerebrovascular disease**

I69.813   **Psychomotor deficit following other cerebrovascular disease**

I69.814   **Frontal lobe and executive function deficit following other cerebrovascular disease**

CHAPTER 9 (I00-I99)

I69.815 Cognitive social or emotional deficit following other cerebrovascular disease

I69.818 Other symptoms and signs involving cognitive functions following other cerebrovascular disease

I69.819 Unspecified symptoms and signs involving cognitive functions following other cerebrovascular disease

● **I69.82** Speech and language deficits following other cerebrovascular disease

I69.820 Aphasia following other cerebrovascular disease

I69.821 Dysphasia following other cerebrovascular disease

I69.822 Dysarthria following other cerebrovascular disease

I69.823 Fluency disorder following other cerebrovascular disease
Stuttering following other cerebrovascular disease

I69.828 Other speech and language deficits following other cerebrovascular disease
Coding Clinic: 2019, Q3, P9

● **I69.83** Monoplegia of upper limb following other cerebrovascular disease

I69.831 Monoplegia of upper limb following other cerebrovascular disease affecting right dominant side 🦥

I69.832 Monoplegia of upper limb following other cerebrovascular disease affecting left dominant side 🦥

I69.833 Monoplegia of upper limb following other cerebrovascular disease affecting right non-dominant side 🦥

I69.834 Monoplegia of upper limb following other cerebrovascular disease affecting left non-dominant side 🦥

I69.839 Monoplegia of upper limb following other cerebrovascular disease affecting unspecified side 🦥

● **I69.84** Monoplegia of lower limb following other cerebrovascular disease

I69.841 Monoplegia of lower limb following other cerebrovascular disease affecting right dominant side 🦥

I69.842 Monoplegia of lower limb following other cerebrovascular disease affecting left dominant side 🦥

I69.843 Monoplegia of lower limb following other cerebrovascular disease affecting right non-dominant side 🦥

I69.844 Monoplegia of lower limb following other cerebrovascular disease affecting left non-dominant side 🦥

I69.849 Monoplegia of lower limb following other cerebrovascular disease affecting unspecified side 🦥

● **I69.85** Hemiplegia and hemiparesis following other cerebrovascular disease

I69.851 Hemiplegia and hemiparesis following other cerebrovascular disease affecting right dominant side 🦥

I69.852 Hemiplegia and hemiparesis following other cerebrovascular disease affecting left dominant side 🦥

I69.853 Hemiplegia and hemiparesis following other cerebrovascular disease affecting right non-dominant side 🦥

I69.854 Hemiplegia and hemiparesis following other cerebrovascular disease affecting left non-dominant side 🦥

I69.859 Hemiplegia and hemiparesis following other cerebrovascular disease affecting unspecified side 🦥

● **I69.86** Other paralytic syndrome following other cerebrovascular disease
Use additional code to identify type of paralytic syndrome, such as:
locked-in state (G83.5)
quadriplegia (G82.5-)

Excludes 1   hemiplegia/hemiparesis following other cerebrovascular disease (I69.85-)
monoplegia of lower limb following other cerebrovascular disease (I69.84-)
monoplegia of upper limb following other cerebrovascular disease (I69.83-)

I69.861 Other paralytic syndrome following other cerebrovascular disease affecting right dominant side 🦥

I69.862 Other paralytic syndrome following other cerebrovascular disease affecting left dominant side 🦥

I69.863 Other paralytic syndrome following other cerebrovascular disease affecting right non-dominant side 🦥

I69.864 Other paralytic syndrome following other cerebrovascular disease affecting left non-dominant side 🦥

I69.865 Other paralytic syndrome following other cerebrovascular disease, bilateral 🦥

I69.869 Other paralytic syndrome following other cerebrovascular disease affecting unspecified side 🦥

● **I69.89** Other sequelae of other cerebrovascular disease

I69.890 Apraxia following other cerebrovascular disease

I69.891 Dysphagia following other cerebrovascular disease
⮕ Use additional code to identify the type of dysphagia, if known (R13.11-R13.19)

I69.892 Facial weakness following other cerebrovascular disease
Facial droop following other cerebrovascular disease

I69.893 Ataxia following other cerebrovascular disease

I69.898 Other sequelae of other cerebrovascular disease
Alteration of sensation following other cerebrovascular disease
Disturbance of vision following other cerebrovascular disease
Use additional code to identify the sequelae

● **I69.9   Sequelae of unspecified cerebrovascular diseases**

    Excludes1   sequelae of stroke (I69.3)
                     sequelae of traumatic intracranial injury
                        (S06.-)

    I69.90   **Unspecified sequelae of unspecified cerebrovascular disease**

● **I69.91**   **Cognitive deficits following unspecified cerebrovascular disease**

      I69.910   **Attention and concentration deficit following unspecified cerebrovascular disease**

      I69.911   **Memory deficit following unspecified cerebrovascular disease**

      I69.912   **Visuospatial deficit and spatial neglect following unspecified cerebrovascular disease**

      I69.913   **Psychomotor deficit following unspecified cerebrovascular disease**

      I69.914   **Frontal lobe and executive function deficit following unspecified cerebrovascular disease**

      I69.915   **Cognitive social or emotional deficit following unspecified cerebrovascular disease**

      I69.918   **Other symptoms and signs involving cognitive functions following unspecified cerebrovascular disease**

      I69.919   **Unspecified symptoms and signs involving cognitive functions following unspecified cerebrovascular disease**

● **I69.92**   **Speech and language deficits following unspecified cerebrovascular disease**

      I69.920   **Aphasia following unspecified cerebrovascular disease**

      I69.921   **Dysphasia following unspecified cerebrovascular disease**

      I69.922   **Dysarthria following unspecified cerebrovascular disease**

      I69.923   **Fluency disorder following unspecified cerebrovascular disease**
               Stuttering following unspecified cerebrovascular disease

      I69.928   **Other speech and language deficits following unspecified cerebrovascular disease**

● **I69.93**   **Monoplegia of upper limb following unspecified cerebrovascular disease**

      I69.931   **Monoplegia of upper limb following unspecified cerebrovascular disease affecting right dominant side** 🖑

      I69.932   **Monoplegia of upper limb following unspecified cerebrovascular disease affecting left dominant side** 🖑

      I69.933   **Monoplegia of upper limb following unspecified cerebrovascular disease affecting right non-dominant side** 🖑

      I69.934   **Monoplegia of upper limb following unspecified cerebrovascular disease affecting left non-dominant side** 🖑

      I69.939   **Monoplegia of upper limb following unspecified cerebrovascular disease affecting unspecified side** 🖑

● **I69.94**   **Monoplegia of lower limb following unspecified cerebrovascular disease**

      I69.941   **Monoplegia of lower limb following unspecified cerebrovascular disease affecting right dominant side** 🖑

      I69.942   **Monoplegia of lower limb following unspecified cerebrovascular disease affecting left dominant side** 🖑

      I69.943   **Monoplegia of lower limb following unspecified cerebrovascular disease affecting right non-dominant side** 🖑

      I69.944   **Monoplegia of lower limb following unspecified cerebrovascular disease affecting left non-dominant side** 🖑

      I69.949   **Monoplegia of lower limb following unspecified cerebrovascular disease affecting unspecified side** 🖑

● **I69.95**   **Hemiplegia and hemiparesis following unspecified cerebrovascular disease**

      I69.951   **Hemiplegia and hemiparesis following unspecified cerebrovascular disease affecting right dominant side** 🖑

      I69.952   **Hemiplegia and hemiparesis following unspecified cerebrovascular disease affecting left dominant side** 🖑

      I69.953   **Hemiplegia and hemiparesis following unspecified cerebrovascular disease affecting right non-dominant side** 🖑

      I69.954   **Hemiplegia and hemiparesis following unspecified cerebrovascular disease affecting left non-dominant side** 🖑

      I69.959   **Hemiplegia and hemiparesis following unspecified cerebrovascular disease affecting unspecified side** 🖑

● **I69.96**   **Other paralytic syndrome following unspecified cerebrovascular disease**

     Use additional code to identify type of paralytic syndrome, such as:
       locked-in state (G83.5)
       quadriplegia (G82.5-)

     Excludes1   hemiplegia/hemiparesis following unspecified cerebrovascular disease (I69.95-)
               monoplegia of lower limb following unspecified cerebrovascular disease (I69.94-)
               monoplegia of upper limb following unspecified cerebrovascular disease (I69.93-)

      I69.961   **Other paralytic syndrome following unspecified cerebrovascular disease affecting right dominant side** 🖑

      I69.962   **Other paralytic syndrome following unspecified cerebrovascular disease affecting left dominant side** 🖑

      I69.963   **Other paralytic syndrome following unspecified cerebrovascular disease affecting right non-dominant side** 🖑

      I69.964   **Other paralytic syndrome following unspecified cerebrovascular disease affecting left non-dominant side** 🖑

      I69.965   **Other paralytic syndrome following unspecified cerebrovascular disease, bilateral** 🖑

      I69.969   **Other paralytic syndrome following unspecified cerebrovascular disease affecting unspecified side** 🖑

● **I69.99**   **Other sequelae of unspecified cerebrovascular disease**

      I69.990   **Apraxia following unspecified cerebrovascular disease**

      I69.991   **Dysphagia following unspecified cerebrovascular disease**

       ➡ Use additional code to identify the type of dysphagia, if known (R13.11-R13.19)

I69.992   **Facial weakness following unspecified cerebrovascular disease**
     Facial droop following unspecified cerebrovascular disease

I69.993   **Ataxia following unspecified cerebrovascular disease**

I69.998   **Other sequelae following unspecified cerebrovascular disease**
     Alteration in sensation following unspecified cerebrovascular disease
     Disturbance of vision following unspecified cerebrovascular disease
     Use additional code to identify the sequelae

DISEASES OF ARTERIES, ARTERIOLES AND CAPILLARIES (I70-I79)

● **I70**   **Atherosclerosis**

> **Includes**   arteriolosclerosis
> arterial degeneration
> arteriosclerosis
> arteriosclerotic vascular disease
> arteriovascular degeneration
> atheroma
> endarteritis deformans or obliterans
> senile arteritis
> senile endarteritis
> vascular degeneration

Use additional code to identify:
   exposure to environmental tobacco smoke (Z77.22)
   history of tobacco dependence (Z87.891)
   occupational exposure to environmental tobacco smoke (Z57.31)
   tobacco dependence (F17.-)
   tobacco use (Z72.0)

> **Excludes2**   arteriosclerotic cardiovascular disease (I25.1-)
> arteriosclerotic heart disease (I25.1-)
> atheroembolism (I75.-)
> cerebral atherosclerosis (I67.2)
> coronary atherosclerosis (I25.1-)
> mesenteric atherosclerosis (K55.1)
> precerebral atherosclerosis (I67.2)
> primary pulmonary atherosclerosis (I27.0)

I70.0   **Atherosclerosis of aorta** 🖾   A

I70.1   **Atherosclerosis of renal artery** 🖾   A
     Goldblatt's kidney

> **Excludes2**   atherosclerosis of renal arterioles (I12.-)

★ **(See Plates 500, 501, and 502 on pages 60 – 62.)**

● **I70.2**   **Atherosclerosis of native arteries of the extremities**
     Mönckeberg's (medial) sclerosis

Use additional code, if applicable, to identify chronic total occlusion of artery of extremity (I70.92)

> **Excludes2**   atherosclerosis of bypass graft of extremities (I70.30-I70.79)

● **I70.20**   **Unspecified atherosclerosis of native arteries of extremities**

I70.201   **Unspecified atherosclerosis of native arteries of extremities, right leg** 🖾   A

I70.202   **Unspecified atherosclerosis of native arteries of extremities, left leg** 🖾   A

I70.203   **Unspecified atherosclerosis of native arteries of extremities, bilateral legs** 🖾   A

I70.208   **Unspecified atherosclerosis of native arteries of extremities, other extremity** 🖾   A

I70.209   **Unspecified atherosclerosis of native arteries of extremities, unspecified extremity** 🖾   A

● **I70.21**   **Atherosclerosis of native arteries of extremities with intermittent claudication**

I70.211   **Atherosclerosis of native arteries of extremities with intermittent claudication, right leg** 🖾   A

I70.212   **Atherosclerosis of native arteries of extremities with intermittent claudication, left leg** 🖾   A

I70.213   **Atherosclerosis of native arteries of extremities with intermittent claudication, bilateral legs** 🖾   A

I70.218   **Atherosclerosis of native arteries of extremities with intermittent claudication, other extremity** 🖾   A

I70.219   **Atherosclerosis of native arteries of extremities with intermittent claudication, unspecified extremity** 🖾   A

● **I70.22**   **Atherosclerosis of native arteries of extremities with rest pain**

> **Includes**   any condition classifiable to I70.21-
> chronic limb-threatening ischemia NOS of native arteries of extremities
> chronic limb-threatening ischemia of native arteries of extremities with rest pain
> critical limb ischemia NOS of native arteries of extremities
> critical limb ischemia of native arteries of extremities with rest pain

I70.221   **Atherosclerosis of native arteries of extremities with rest pain, right leg** 🖾   A

I70.222   **Atherosclerosis of native arteries of extremities with rest pain, left leg** 🖾 A

I70.223   **Atherosclerosis of native arteries of extremities with rest pain, bilateral legs** 🖾   A

I70.228   **Atherosclerosis of native arteries of extremities with rest pain, other extremity** 🖾   A

I70.229   **Atherosclerosis of native arteries of extremities with rest pain, unspecified extremity** 🖾   A

● **I70.23**   **Atherosclerosis of native arteries of right leg with ulceration**

> **Includes**   any condition classifiable to I70.211 and I70.221
> chronic limb-threatening ischemia of native arteries of right leg with ulceration
> critical limb ischemia of native arteries of right leg with ulceration

Use additional code to identify severity of ulcer (L97.-)

I70.231   **Atherosclerosis of native arteries of right leg with ulceration of thigh** 🖾   A

I70.232   **Atherosclerosis of native arteries of right leg with ulceration of calf** 🖾   A

I70.233   **Atherosclerosis of native arteries of right leg with ulceration of ankle** 🖾   A

I70.234   **Atherosclerosis of native arteries of right leg with ulceration of heel and midfoot** 🖾
     Atherosclerosis of native arteries of right leg with ulceration of plantar surface of midfoot

---

▶ New   ⏵▶ Revised   ~~deleted~~ Deleted   Excludes 1   Excludes 2   Includes   Use additional   Code first   Code also   Key words

OGCR Official Guidelines   X Assign placeholder X   ● Use Additional Character(s)   ▸ Manifestation Code   🖾 Hierarchical Condition Category   **Coding Clinic**

I70.235   **Atherosclerosis of native arteries of right leg with ulceration of** other part of foot 🦠   A

Atherosclerosis of native arteries of right leg extremities with ulceration of toe

I70.238   **Atherosclerosis of native arteries of right leg with ulceration of** other part of lower leg 🦠   A

I70.239   **Atherosclerosis of native arteries of right leg with ulceration of** unspecified site 🦠   A

● **I70.24**   **Atherosclerosis of native arteries of** left leg with ulceration

     Includes   any condition classifiable to I70.212 and I70.222

chronic limb-threatening ischemia of native arteries of left leg with ulceration

critical limb ischemia of native arteries of left leg with ulceration

Use additional code to identify severity of ulcer (L97.-)

I70.241   **Atherosclerosis of native arteries of left leg with ulceration of** thigh 🦠   A

I70.242   **Atherosclerosis of native arteries of left leg with ulceration of** calf 🦠   A

I70.243   **Atherosclerosis of native arteries of left leg with ulceration of** ankle 🦠   A

I70.244   **Atherosclerosis of native arteries of left leg with ulceration of** heel and midfoot 🦠   A

Atherosclerosis of native arteries of left leg with ulceration of plantar surface of midfoot

I70.245   **Atherosclerosis of native arteries of left leg with ulceration of** other part of foot 🦠   A

Atherosclerosis of native arteries of left leg extremities with ulceration of toe

I70.248   **Atherosclerosis of native arteries of left leg with ulceration of** other part of lower leg 🦠   A

I70.249   **Atherosclerosis of native arteries of left leg with ulceration of** unspecified site 🦠   A

I70.25   **Atherosclerosis of native arteries of** other extremities with ulceration 🦠   A

     Includes   any condition classifiable to I70.218 and I70.228

Use additional code to identify the severity of the ulcer (L98.49-)

● **I70.26**   **Atherosclerosis of native arteries of extremities with gangrene**

     Includes   any condition classifiable to I70.21-, I70.22-, I70.23-, I70.24-, and I70.25-

chronic limb-threatening ischemia of native arteries of extremities with gangrene

critical limb ischemia of native arteries of extremities with gangrene

Use additional code to identify the severity of any ulcer (L97.-, L98.49-), if applicable

I70.261   **Atherosclerosis of native arteries of extremities with gangrene,** right leg   A

I70.262   **Atherosclerosis of native arteries of extremities with gangrene,** left leg 🦠A

I70.263   **Atherosclerosis of native arteries of extremities with gangrene,** bilateral legs 🦠   A

I70.268   **Atherosclerosis of native arteries of extremities with gangrene,** other extremity 🦠   A

I70.269   **Atherosclerosis of native arteries of extremities with gangrene,** unspecified extremity 🦠   A

● **I70.29**   **Other atherosclerosis of native arteries of extremities**

I70.291   **Other atherosclerosis of native arteries of extremities,** right leg 🦠   A

I70.292   **Other atherosclerosis of native arteries of extremities,** left leg 🦠   A

I70.293   **Other atherosclerosis of native arteries of extremities,** bilateral legs 🦠   A

I70.298   **Other atherosclerosis of native arteries of extremities,** other extremity 🦠   A

I70.299   **Other atherosclerosis of native arteries of extremities,** unspecified extremity 🦠   A

● **I70.3**   **Atherosclerosis of** unspecified type of bypass graft(s) of the extremities

Use additional code, if applicable, to identify chronic total occlusion of artery of extremity (I70.92)

     Excludes1   embolism or thrombus of bypass graft(s) of extremities (T82.8-)

● **I70.30**   **Unspecified atherosclerosis of** unspecified type of bypass graft(s) of the extremities

I70.301   **Unspecified atherosclerosis of unspecified type of bypass graft(s) of the extremities,** right leg 🦠   A

I70.302   **Unspecified atherosclerosis of unspecified type of bypass graft(s) of the extremities,** left leg 🦠   A

I70.303   **Unspecified atherosclerosis of unspecified type of bypass graft(s) of the extremities,** bilateral legs 🦠   A

I70.308   **Unspecified atherosclerosis of unspecified type of bypass graft(s) of the extremities,** other extremity 🦠   A

I70.309   **Unspecified atherosclerosis of unspecified type of bypass graft(s) of the extremities,** unspecified extremity 🦠   A

● **I70.31**   **Atherosclerosis of** unspecified type of bypass graft(s) of the extremities with intermittent claudication

I70.311   **Atherosclerosis of unspecified type of bypass graft(s) of the extremities with intermittent claudication,** right leg 🦠   A

I70.312   **Atherosclerosis of unspecified type of bypass graft(s) of the extremities with intermittent claudication,** left leg 🦠 A

I70.313   **Atherosclerosis of unspecified type of bypass graft(s) of the extremities with intermittent claudication,** bilateral legs 🦠   A

I70.318   **Atherosclerosis of unspecified type of bypass graft(s) of the extremities with intermittent claudication,** other extremity 🦠   A

I70.319   **Atherosclerosis of unspecified type of bypass graft(s) of the extremities with intermittent claudication,** unspecified extremity 🦠   A

● **I70.32** **Atherosclerosis of unspecified type of bypass graft(s) of the extremities with rest pain**

Includes any condition classifiable to I70.31-
chronic limb-threatening ischemia NOS of unspecified type of bypass graft(s) of the extremities
chronic limb-threatening ischemia of unspecified type of bypass graft(s) of the extremities with rest pain, right leg
critical limb ischemia NOS of unspecified type of bypass graft(s) of the extremities
critical limb ischemia of unspecified type of bypass graft(s) of the extremities with rest pain

I70.321 Atherosclerosis of unspecified type of bypass graft(s) of the extremities with rest pain, right leg 🐾   A

I70.322 Atherosclerosis of unspecified type of bypass graft(s) of the extremities with rest pain, left leg 🐾   A

I70.323 Atherosclerosis of unspecified type of bypass graft(s) of the extremities with rest pain, bilateral legs 🐾   A

I70.328 Atherosclerosis of unspecified type of bypass graft(s) of the extremities with rest pain, other extremity 🐾   A

I70.329 Atherosclerosis of unspecified type of bypass graft(s) of the extremities with rest pain, unspecified extremity 🐾   A

● **I70.33** **Atherosclerosis of unspecified type of bypass graft(s) of the right leg with ulceration**

Includes any condition classifiable to I70.311 and I70.321
chronic limb-threatening ischemia of unspecified type of bypass graft(s) of the right leg with ulceration
critical limb ischemia of unspecified type of bypass graft(s) of the right leg with ulceration

Use additional code to identify severity of ulcer (L97.-)

I70.331 Atherosclerosis of unspecified type of bypass graft(s) of the right leg with ulceration of thigh 🐾   A

I70.332 Atherosclerosis of unspecified type of bypass graft(s) of the right leg with ulceration of calf 🐾   A

I70.333 Atherosclerosis of unspecified type of bypass graft(s) of the right leg with ulceration of ankle 🐾   A

I70.334 Atherosclerosis of unspecified type of bypass graft(s) of the right leg with ulceration of heel and midfoot 🐾   A
Atherosclerosis of unspecified type of bypass graft(s) of right leg with ulceration of plantar surface of midfoot

I70.335 Atherosclerosis of unspecified type of bypass graft(s) of the right leg with ulceration of other part of foot 🐾   A
Atherosclerosis of unspecified type of bypass graft(s) of the right leg with ulceration of toe

I70.338 Atherosclerosis of unspecified type of bypass graft(s) of the right leg with ulceration of other part of lower leg 🐾   A

I70.339 Atherosclerosis of unspecified type of bypass graft(s) of the right leg with ulceration of unspecified site 🐾   A

● **I70.34** **Atherosclerosis of unspecified type of bypass graft(s) of the left leg with ulceration**

Includes any condition classifiable to I70.312 and I70.322
chronic limb-threatening ischemia of unspecified type of bypass graft(s) of the left leg with ulceration
critical limb ischemia of unspecified type of bypass graft(s) of the left leg with ulceration

Use additional code to identify severity of ulcer (L97.-)

I70.341 Atherosclerosis of unspecified type of bypass graft(s) of the left leg with ulceration of thigh 🐾   A

I70.342 Atherosclerosis of unspecified type of bypass graft(s) of the left leg with ulceration of calf 🐾   A

I70.343 Atherosclerosis of unspecified type of bypass graft(s) of the left leg with ulceration of ankle 🐾   A

I70.344 Atherosclerosis of unspecified type of bypass graft(s) of the left leg with ulceration of heel and midfoot 🐾   A
Atherosclerosis of unspecified type of bypass graft(s) of left leg with ulceration of plantar surface of midfoot

I70.345 Atherosclerosis of unspecified type of bypass graft(s) of the left leg with ulceration of other part of foot 🐾   A
Atherosclerosis of unspecified type of bypass graft(s) of the left leg with ulceration of toe

I70.348 Atherosclerosis of unspecified type of bypass graft(s) of the left leg with ulceration of other part of lower leg 🐾   A

I70.349 Atherosclerosis of unspecified type of bypass graft(s) of the left leg with ulceration of unspecified site 🐾   A

I70.35 Atherosclerosis of unspecified type of bypass graft(s) of other extremity with ulceration 🐾   A

Includes any condition classifiable to I70.318 and I70.328

Use additional code to identify severity of ulcer (L98.49-)

● **I70.36** **Atherosclerosis of unspecified type of bypass graft(s) of the extremities with gangrene**

Includes any condition classifiable to I70.31-, I70.32-, I70.33-, I70.34-, I70.35
chronic limb-threatening ischemia of unspecified type of bypass graft(s) of the extremities with gangrene
critical limb ischemia of unspecified type of bypass graft(s) of the extremities with gangrene

Use additional code to identify the severity of any ulcer (L97.-, L98.49-), if applicable

I70.361 Atherosclerosis of unspecified type of bypass graft(s) of the extremities with gangrene, right leg 🐾   A

I70.362   Atherosclerosis of unspecified type of bypass graft(s) of the extremities with gangrene, left leg 🦠   A

I70.363   Atherosclerosis of unspecified type of bypass graft(s) of the extremities with gangrene, bilateral legs 🦠   A

I70.368   Atherosclerosis of unspecified type of bypass graft(s) of the extremities with gangrene, other extremity 🦠   A

I70.369   Atherosclerosis of unspecified type of bypass graft(s) of the extremities with gangrene, unspecified extremity 🦠   A

● I70.39   Other atherosclerosis of unspecified type of bypass graft(s) of the extremities

I70.391   Other atherosclerosis of unspecified type of bypass graft(s) of the extremities, right leg 🦠   A

I70.392   Other atherosclerosis of unspecified type of bypass graft(s) of the extremities, left leg 🦠   A

I70.393   Other atherosclerosis of unspecified type of bypass graft(s) of the extremities, bilateral legs 🦠   A

I70.398   Other atherosclerosis of unspecified type of bypass graft(s) of the extremities, other extremity 🦠   A

I70.399   Other atherosclerosis of unspecified type of bypass graft(s) of the extremities, unspecified extremity 🦠 A

● I70.4   Atherosclerosis of autologous vein bypass graft(s) of the extremities

Use additional code, if applicable, to identify chronic total occlusion of artery of extremity (I70.92)

● I70.40   Unspecified atherosclerosis of autologous vein bypass graft(s) of the extremities

I70.401   Unspecified atherosclerosis of autologous vein bypass graft(s) of the extremities, right leg 🦠   A

I70.402   Unspecified atherosclerosis of autologous vein bypass graft(s) of the extremities, left leg 🦠   A

I70.403   Unspecified atherosclerosis of autologous vein bypass graft(s) of the extremities, bilateral legs 🦠   A

I70.408   Unspecified atherosclerosis of autologous vein bypass graft(s) of the extremities, other extremity 🦠   A

I70.409   Unspecified atherosclerosis of autologous vein bypass graft(s) of the extremities, unspecified extremity 🦠 A

● I70.41   Atherosclerosis of autologous vein bypass graft(s) of the extremities with intermittent claudication

I70.411   Atherosclerosis of autologous vein bypass graft(s) of the extremities ith intermittent claudication, right leg 🦠   A

I70.412   Atherosclerosis of autologous vein bypass graft(s) of the extremities with intermittent claudication, left leg 🦠   A

I70.413   Atherosclerosis of autologous vein bypass graft(s) of the extremities with intermittent claudication, bilateral legs 🦠   A

I70.418   Atherosclerosis of autologous vein bypass graft(s) of the extremities with intermittent claudication, other extremity 🦠   A

I70.419   Atherosclerosis of autologous vein bypass graft(s) of the extremities with intermittent claudication, unspecified extremity 🦠   A

● I70.42   Atherosclerosis of autologous vein bypass graft(s) of the extremities with rest pain

Includes   any condition classifiable to I70.41-
chronic limb-threatening ischemia NOS of autologous vein bypass graft(s) of the extremities
chronic limb-threatening ischemia of autologous vein bypass graft(s) of the extremities with rest pain
critical limb ischemia NOS of autologous vein bypass graft(s) of the extremities
critical limb ischemia of autologous vein bypass graft(s) of the extremities with rest pain

I70.421   Atherosclerosis of autologous vein bypass graft(s) of the extremities with rest pain, right leg 🦠   A

I70.422   Atherosclerosis of autologous vein bypass graft(s) of the extremities with rest pain, left leg 🦠   A

I70.423   Atherosclerosis of autologous vein bypass graft(s) of the extremities with rest pain, bilateral legs 🦠   A

I70.428   Atherosclerosis of autologous vein bypass graft(s) of the extremities with rest pain, other extremity 🦠   A

I70.429   Atherosclerosis of autologous vein bypass graft(s) of the extremities with rest pain, unspecified extremity 🦠   A

● I70.43   Atherosclerosis of autologous vein bypass graft(s) of the right leg with ulceration

Includes   any condition classifiable to I70.411 and I70.421
chronic limb-threatening ischemia of autologous vein bypass graft(s) of the right leg with ulceration
critical limb ischemia of autologous vein bypass graft(s) of the right leg with ulceration

Use additional code to identify severity of ulcer (L97.-)

I70.431   Atherosclerosis of autologous vein bypass graft(s) of the right leg with ulceration of thigh 🦠   A

I70.432   Atherosclerosis of autologous vein bypass graft(s) of the right leg with ulceration of calf 🦠   A

I70.433   Atherosclerosis of autologous vein bypass graft(s) of the right leg with ulceration of ankle 🦠   A

I70.434   Atherosclerosis of autologous vein bypass graft(s) of the right leg with ulceration of heel and midfoot 🦠   A
Atherosclerosis of autologous vein bypass graft(s) of right leg with ulceration of plantar surface of midfoot

I70.435   Atherosclerosis of autologous vein bypass graft(s) of the right leg with ulceration of other part of foot 🦠   A
Atherosclerosis of autologous vein bypass graft(s) of right leg with ulceration of toe

I70.438   Atherosclerosis of autologous vein bypass graft(s) of the right leg with ulceration of other part of lower leg 🦠   A

I70.439   Atherosclerosis of autologous vein bypass graft(s) of the right leg with ulceration of unspecified site 🦠   A

● **I70.44   Atherosclerosis of autologous vein bypass graft(s) of the left leg with ulceration**

Includes   any condition classifiable to I70.412 and I70.422
chronic limb-threatening ischemia of autologous vein bypass graft(s) of the left leg with ulceration
critical limb ischemia of autologous vein bypass graft(s) of the left leg with ulceration

Use additional code to identify severity of ulcer (L97.-)

I70.441   **Atherosclerosis of autologous vein bypass graft(s) of the left leg with ulceration of thigh** 🐾   A

I70.442   **Atherosclerosis of autologous vein bypass graft(s) of the left leg with ulceration of calf** 🐾   A

I70.443   **Atherosclerosis of autologous vein bypass graft(s) of the left leg with ulceration of ankle** 🐾   A

I70.444   **Atherosclerosis of autologous vein bypass graft(s) of the left leg with ulceration of heel and midfoot** 🐾   A
Atherosclerosis of autologous vein bypass graft(s) of left leg with ulceration of plantar surface of midfoot

I70.445   **Atherosclerosis of autologous vein bypass graft(s) of the left leg with ulceration of other part of foot** 🐾   A
Atherosclerosis of autologous vein bypass graft(s) of left leg with ulceration of toe

I70.448   **Atherosclerosis of autologous vein bypass graft(s) of the left leg with ulceration of other part of lower leg** 🐾   A

I70.449   **Atherosclerosis of autologous vein bypass graft(s) of the left leg with ulceration of unspecified site** 🐾   A

I70.45   **Atherosclerosis of autologous vein bypass graft(s) of other extremity with ulceration** 🐾   A

Includes   any condition classifiable to I70.418, I70.428, and I70.438

Use additional code to identify severity of ulcer (L98.49-)

● **I70.46   Atherosclerosis of autologous vein bypass graft(s) of the extremities with gangrene**

Includes   any condition classifiable to I70.41-, I70.42-, and I70.43-, I70.44-, I70.45
chronic limb-threatening ischemia of autologous vein bypass graft(s) of the extremities with gangrene
critical limb ischemia of autologous vein bypass graft(s) of the extremities with gangrene

Use additional code to identify the severity of any ulcer (L97.-, L98.49-), if applicable

I70.461   **Atherosclerosis of autologous vein bypass graft(s) of the extremities with gangrene, right leg**   A

I70.462   **Atherosclerosis of autologous vein bypass graft(s) of the extremities with gangrene, left leg** 🐾   A

I70.463   **Atherosclerosis of autologous vein bypass graft(s) of the extremities with gangrene, bilateral legs** 🐾   A

I70.468   **Atherosclerosis of autologous vein bypass graft(s) of the extremities with gangrene, other extremity** 🐾   A

I70.469   **Atherosclerosis of autologous vein bypass graft(s) of the extremities with gangrene, unspecified extremity** 🐾   A

● **I70.49   Other atherosclerosis of autologous vein bypass graft(s) of the extremities**

I70.491   **Other atherosclerosis of autologous vein bypass graft(s) of the extremities, right leg** 🐾   A

I70.492   **Other atherosclerosis of autologous vein bypass graft(s) of the extremities, left leg** 🐾   A

I70.493   **Other atherosclerosis of autologous vein bypass graft(s) of the extremities, bilateral legs** 🐾   A

I70.498   **Other atherosclerosis of autologous vein bypass graft(s) of the extremities, other extremity** 🐾   A

I70.499   **Other atherosclerosis of autologous vein bypass graft(s) of the extremities, unspecified extremity** 🐾   A

● **I70.5   Atherosclerosis of nonautologous biological bypass graft(s) of the extremities**

Use additional code, if applicable, to identify chronic total occlusion of artery of extremity (I70.92)

● **I70.50   Unspecified atherosclerosis of nonautologous biological bypass graft(s) of the extremities**

I70.501   **Unspecified atherosclerosis of nonautologous biological bypass graft(s) of the extremities, right leg** 🐾   A

I70.502   **Unspecified atherosclerosis of nonautologous biological bypass graft(s) of the extremities, left leg** 🐾   A

I70.503   **Unspecified atherosclerosis of nonautologous biological bypass graft(s) of the extremities, bilateral legs** 🐾   A

I70.508   **Unspecified atherosclerosis of nonautologous biological bypass graft(s) of the extremities, other extremity** 🐾   A

I70.509   **Unspecified atherosclerosis of nonautologous biological bypass graft(s) of the extremities, unspecified extremity** 🐾   A

● **I70.51   Atherosclerosis of nonautologous biological bypass graft(s) of the extremities intermittent claudication**

I70.511   **Atherosclerosis of nonautologous biological bypass graft(s) of the extremities with intermittent claudication, right leg** 🐾   A

I70.512   **Atherosclerosis of nonautologous biological bypass graft(s) of the extremities with intermittent claudication, left leg** 🐾   A

I70.513   **Atherosclerosis of nonautologous biological bypass graft(s) of the extremities with intermittent claudication, bilateral legs** 🐾   A

I70.518   **Atherosclerosis of nonautologous biological bypass graft(s) of the extremities with intermittent claudication, other extremity** 🐾   A

I70.519   **Atherosclerosis of nonautologous biological bypass graft(s) of the extremities with intermittent claudication, unspecified extremity** 🐾   A

▶ New   ➡ Revised   ~~deleted~~ Deleted   Excludes 1   Excludes 2   Includes   Use additional   Code first   Code also   Key words

OGCR Official Guidelines   X Assign placeholder X   ● Use Additional Character(s)   ▶ Manifestation Code   🐾 Hierarchical Condition Category   Coding Clinic

● **I70.52**   **Atherosclerosis of nonautologous biological bypass graft(s) of the extremities with rest pain**

     Includes   any condition classifiable to I70.51-

         chronic limb-threatening ischemia NOS of nonautologous biological bypass graft(s) of the extremities

         chronic limb-threatening ischemia of nonautologous biological bypass graft(s) of the extremities with rest pain

         critical limb ischemia NOS of nonautologous biological bypass graft(s) of the extremities

         critical limb ischemia of nonautologous biological bypass graft(s) of the extremities with rest pain

     I70.521   **Atherosclerosis of nonautologous biological bypass graft(s) of the extremities with rest pain, right leg** 🔗   A

     I70.522   **Atherosclerosis of nonautologous biological bypass graft(s) of the extremities with rest pain, left leg** 🔗 A

     I70.523   **Atherosclerosis of nonautologous biological bypass graft(s) of the extremities with rest pain, bilateral legs** 🔗   A

     I70.528   **Atherosclerosis of nonautologous biological bypass graft(s) of the extremities with rest pain, other extremity** 🔗   A

     I70.529   **Atherosclerosis of nonautologous biological bypass graft(s) of the extremities with rest pain, unspecified extremity** 🔗   A

● **I70.53**   **Atherosclerosis of nonautologous biological bypass graft(s) of the right leg with ulceration**

     Includes   any condition classifiable to I70.511 and I70.521

         chronic limb-threatening ischemia of nonautologous biological bypass graft(s) of the right leg with ulceration

         critical limb ischemia of nonautologous biological bypass graft(s) of the right leg with ulceration

     Use additional code to identify severity of ulcer (L97.-)

     I70.531   **Atherosclerosis of nonautologous biological bypass graft(s) of the right leg with ulceration of thigh** 🔗   A

     I70.532   **Atherosclerosis of nonautologous biological bypass graft(s) of the right leg with ulceration of calf** 🔗   A

     I70.533   **Atherosclerosis of nonautologous biological bypass graft(s) of the right leg with ulceration of ankle** 🔗   A

     I70.534   **Atherosclerosis of nonautologous biological bypass graft(s) of the right leg with ulceration of heel and midfoot** 🔗   A

         Atherosclerosis of nonautologous biological bypass graft(s) of right leg with ulceration of plantar surface of midfoot

     I70.535   **Atherosclerosis of nonautologous biological bypass graft(s) of the right leg with ulceration of other part of foot** 🔗   A

         Atherosclerosis of nonautologous biological bypass graft(s) of the right leg with ulceration of toe

     I70.538   **Atherosclerosis of nonautologous biological bypass graft(s) of the right leg with ulceration of other part of lower leg** 🔗   A

     I70.539   **Atherosclerosis of nonautologous biological bypass graft(s) of the right leg with ulceration of unspecified site** 🔗   A

● **I70.54**   **Atherosclerosis of nonautologous biological bypass graft(s) of the left leg with ulceration**

     Includes   any condition classifiable to I70.512 and I70.522

         chronic limb-threatening ischemia of nonautologous biological bypass graft(s) of the left leg with ulceration

         critical limb ischemia of nonautologous biological bypass graft(s) of the left leg with ulceration

     Use additional code to identify severity of ulcer (L97.-)

     I70.541   **Atherosclerosis of nonautologous biological bypass graft(s) of the left leg with ulceration of thigh** 🔗   A

     I70.542   **Atherosclerosis of nonautologous biological bypass graft(s) of the left leg with ulceration of calf** 🔗   A

     I70.543   **Atherosclerosis of nonautologous biological bypass graft(s) of the left leg with ulceration of ankle** 🔗   A

     I70.544   **Atherosclerosis of nonautologous biological bypass graft(s) of the left leg with ulceration of heel and midfoot** 🔗   A

         Atherosclerosis of nonautologous biological bypass graft(s) of left leg with ulceration of plantar surface of midfoot

     I70.545   **Atherosclerosis of nonautologous biological bypass graft(s) of the left leg with ulceration of other part of foot** 🔗   A

         Atherosclerosis of nonautologous biological bypass graft(s) of the left leg with ulceration of toe

     I70.548   **Atherosclerosis of nonautologous biological bypass graft(s) of the left leg with ulceration of other part of lower leg** 🔗   A

     I70.549   **Atherosclerosis of nonautologous biological bypass graft(s) of the left leg with ulceration of unspecified site** 🔗   A

I70.55   **Atherosclerosis of nonautologous biological bypass graft(s) of other extremity with ulceration** 🔗   A

     Includes   any condition classifiable to I70.518, I70.528, and I70.538

     Use additional code to identify severity of ulcer (L98.49)

CHAPTER 9 (I00-I99)

● **I70.56** **Atherosclerosis of nonautologous biological bypass graft(s) of the extremities with gangrene**

    Includes   any condition classifiable to I70.51-, I70.52-, and I70.53-, I70.54-, I70.55

             chronic limb-threatening ischemia of nonautologous biological bypass graft(s) of the extremities with gangrene

             critical limb ischemia of nonautologous biological bypass graft(s) of the extremities with gangrene

     Use additional code to identify the severity of any ulcer (L97.-, L98.49-), if applicable

     I70.561 **Atherosclerosis of nonautologous biological bypass graft(s) of the extremities with gangrene, right leg** 🐾   A

     I70.562 **Atherosclerosis of nonautologous biological bypass graft(s) of the extremities with gangrene, left leg** 🐾 A

     I70.563 **Atherosclerosis of nonautologous biological bypass graft(s) of the extremities with gangrene, bilateral legs** 🐾   A

     I70.568 **Atherosclerosis of nonautologous biological bypass graft(s) of the extremities with gangrene, other extremity** 🐾   A

     I70.569 **Atherosclerosis of nonautologous biological bypass graft(s) of the extremities with gangrene, unspecified extremity** 🐾   A

● **I70.59** **Other atherosclerosis of nonautologous biological bypass graft(s) of the extremities**

     I70.591 **Other atherosclerosis of nonautologous biological bypass graft(s) of the extremities, right leg** 🐾   A

     I70.592 **Other atherosclerosis of nonautologous biological bypass graft(s) of the extremities, left leg** 🐾   A

     I70.593 **Other atherosclerosis of nonautologous biological bypass graft(s) of the extremities, bilateral legs** 🐾   A

     I70.598 **Other atherosclerosis of nonautologous biological bypass graft(s) of the extremities, other extremity** 🐾   A

     I70.599 **Other atherosclerosis of nonautologous biological bypass graft(s) of the extremities, unspecified extremity** 🐾 A

● **I70.6** **Atherosclerosis of nonbiological bypass graft(s) of the extremities**

     Use additional code, if applicable, to identify chronic total occlusion of artery of extremity (I70.92)

● **I70.60** **Unspecified atherosclerosis of nonbiological bypass graft(s) of the extremities**

     I70.601 **Unspecified atherosclerosis of nonbiological bypass graft(s) of the extremities, right leg** 🐾   A

     I70.602 **Unspecified atherosclerosis of nonbiological bypass graft(s) of the extremities, left leg** 🐾   A

     I70.603 **Unspecified atherosclerosis of nonbiological bypass graft(s) of the extremities, bilateral legs** 🐾   A

     I70.608 **Unspecified atherosclerosis of nonbiological bypass graft(s) of the extremities, other extremity** 🐾   A

     I70.609 **Unspecified atherosclerosis of nonbiological bypass graft(s) of the extremities, unspecified extremity** 🐾 A

● **I70.61** **Atherosclerosis of nonbiological bypass graft(s) of the extremities with intermittent claudication**

     I70.611 **Atherosclerosis of nonbiological bypass graft(s) of the extremities with intermittent claudication, right leg** 🐾   A

     I70.612 **Atherosclerosis of nonbiological bypass graft(s) of the extremities with intermittent claudication, left leg** 🐾 A

     I70.613 **Atherosclerosis of nonbiological bypass graft(s) of the extremities with intermittent claudication, bilateral legs** 🐾   A

     I70.618 **Atherosclerosis of nonbiological bypass graft(s) of the extremities with intermittent claudication, other extremity** 🐾   A

     I70.619 **Atherosclerosis of nonbiological bypass graft(s) of the extremities with intermittent claudication, unspecified extremity** 🐾   A

● **I70.62** **Atherosclerosis of nonbiological bypass graft(s) of the extremities with rest pain**

    Includes   any condition classifiable to I70.61-

             chronic limb-threatening ischemia NOS of nonbiological bypass graft(s) of the extremities

             chronic limb-threatening ischemia of nonbiological bypass graft(s) of the extremities with rest pain

             critical limb ischemia NOS of nonbiological bypass graft(s) of the extremities

             critical limb ischemia of nonbiological bypass graft(s) of the extremities with rest pain

     I70.621 **Atherosclerosis of nonbiological bypass graft(s) of the extremities with rest pain, right leg** 🐾   A

     I70.622 **Atherosclerosis of nonbiological bypass graft(s) of the extremities with rest pain, left leg** 🐾   A

     I70.623 **Atherosclerosis of nonbiological bypass graft(s) of the extremities with rest pain, bilateral legs** 🐾   A

     I70.628 **Atherosclerosis of nonbiological bypass graft(s) of the extremities with rest pain, other extremity** 🐾   A

     I70.629 **Atherosclerosis of nonbiological bypass graft(s) of the extremities with rest pain, unspecified extremity** 🐾   A

● **I70.63** **Atherosclerosis of nonbiological bypass graft(s) of the right leg with ulceration**

    Includes   any condition classifiable to I70.611 and I70.621

             chronic limb-threatening ischemia of nonbiological bypass graft(s) of the right leg with ulceration

             critical limb ischemia of nonbiological bypass graft(s) of the right leg with ulceration

     Use additional code to identify severity of ulcer (L97.-)

     I70.631 **Atherosclerosis of nonbiological bypass graft(s) of the right leg with ulceration of thigh** 🐾   A

     I70.632 **Atherosclerosis of nonbiological bypass graft(s) of the right leg with ulceration of calf** 🐾   A

▶ New   ⇒ Revised   ~~deleted~~ Deleted   Excludes 1   Excludes 2   Includes   Use additional   Code first   Code also   Key words

OGCR Official Guidelines   X Assign placeholder X   ● Use Additional Character(s)   ▷ Manifestation Code   🐾 Hierarchical Condition Category   **Coding Clinic**

I70.633 **Atherosclerosis of nonbiological bypass graft(s) of the right leg with ulceration of ankle** 🔎   A

I70.634 **Atherosclerosis of nonbiological bypass graft(s) of the right leg with ulceration of heel and midfoot** 🔎   A
Atherosclerosis of nonbiological bypass graft(s) of right leg with ulceration of plantar surface of midfoot

I70.635 **Atherosclerosis of nonbiological bypass graft(s) of the right leg with ulceration of other part of foot** 🔎   A
Atherosclerosis of nonbiological bypass graft(s) of the right leg with ulceration of toe

I70.638 **Atherosclerosis of nonbiological bypass graft(s) of the right leg with ulceration of other part of lower leg** 🔎   A

I70.639 **Atherosclerosis of nonbiological bypass graft(s) of the right leg with ulceration of unspecified site** 🔎   A

● **I70.64** **Atherosclerosis of nonbiological bypass graft(s) of the left leg with ulceration**

> **Includes**   any condition classifiable to I70.612 and I70.622
> chronic limb-threatening ischemia of nonbiological bypass graft(s) of the left leg with ulceration
> critical limb ischemia of nonbiological bypass graft(s) of the left leg with ulceration

Use additional code to identify severity of ulcer (L97.-)

I70.641 **Atherosclerosis of nonbiological bypass graft(s) of the left leg with ulceration of thigh** 🔎   A

I70.642 **Atherosclerosis of nonbiological bypass graft(s) of the left leg with ulceration of calf** 🔎   A

I70.643 **Atherosclerosis of nonbiological bypass graft(s) of the left leg with ulceration of ankle** 🔎   A

I70.644 **Atherosclerosis of nonbiological bypass graft(s) of the left leg with ulceration of heel and midfoot** 🔎   A
Atherosclerosis of nonbiological bypass graft(s) of left leg with ulceration of plantar surface of midfoot

I70.645 **Atherosclerosis of nonbiological bypass graft(s) of the left leg with ulceration of other part of foot** 🔎   A
Atherosclerosis of nonbiological bypass graft(s) of the left leg with ulceration of toe

I70.648 **Atherosclerosis of nonbiological bypass graft(s) of the left leg with ulceration of other part of lower leg** 🔎   A

I70.649 **Atherosclerosis of nonbiological bypass graft(s) of the left leg with ulceration of unspecified site** 🔎   A

I70.65 **Atherosclerosis of nonbiological bypass graft(s) of other extremity with ulceration** 🔎   A

> **Includes**   any condition classifiable to I70.618 and I70.628

Use additional code to identify severity of ulcer (L98.49-)

● **I70.66** **Atherosclerosis of nonbiological bypass graft(s) of the extremities with gangrene**

> **Includes**   any condition classifiable to I70.61-, I70.62-, I70.63-, I70.64-, I70.65
> chronic limb-threatening ischemia of nonbiological bypass graft(s) of the extremities with gangrene
> critical limb ischemia of nonbiological bypass graft(s) of the extremities with gangrene

Use additional code to identify the severity of any ulcer (L97.-, L98.49-), if applicable

I70.661 **Atherosclerosis of nonbiological bypass graft(s) of the extremities with gangrene, right leg** 🔎   A

I70.662 **Atherosclerosis of nonbiological bypass graft(s) of the extremities with gangrene, left leg** 🔎   A

I70.663 **Atherosclerosis of nonbiological bypass graft(s) of the extremities with gangrene, bilateral legs** 🔎   A

I70.668 **Atherosclerosis of nonbiological bypass graft(s) of the extremities with gangrene, other extremity** 🔎   A

I70.669 **Atherosclerosis of nonbiological bypass graft(s) of the extremities with gangrene, unspecified extremity** 🔎   A

● **I70.69** **Other atherosclerosis of nonbiological bypass graft(s) of the extremities**

I70.691 **Other atherosclerosis of nonbiological bypass graft(s) of the extremities, right leg** 🔎   A

I70.692 **Other atherosclerosis of nonbiological bypass graft(s) of the extremities, left leg** 🔎   A

I70.693 **Other atherosclerosis of nonbiological bypass graft(s) of the extremities, bilateral legs** 🔎   A

I70.698 **Other atherosclerosis of nonbiological bypass graft(s) of the extremities, other extremity** 🔎   A

I70.699 **Other atherosclerosis of nonbiological bypass graft(s) of the extremities, unspecified extremity** 🔎   A

● **I70.7** **Atherosclerosis of other type of bypass graft(s) of the extremities**

Use additional code, if applicable, to identify chronic total occlusion of artery of extremity (I70.92)

● **I70.70** **Unspecified atherosclerosis of other type of bypass graft(s) of the extremities**

I70.701 **Unspecified atherosclerosis of other type of bypass graft(s) of the extremities, right leg** 🔎   A

I70.702 **Unspecified atherosclerosis of other type of bypass graft(s) of the extremities, left leg** 🔎   A

I70.703 **Unspecified atherosclerosis of other type of bypass graft(s) of the extremities, bilateral legs** 🔎   A

I70.708 **Unspecified atherosclerosis of other type of bypass graft(s) of the extremities, other extremity** 🔎   A

I70.709 **Unspecified atherosclerosis of other type of bypass graft(s) of the extremities, unspecified extremity** 🔎   A

CHAPTER 9 (I00-I99)

CHAPTER 9 (I00-I99)

● **I70.71** **Atherosclerosis of other type of bypass graft(s) of the extremities with intermittent claudication**

I70.711 Atherosclerosis of other type of bypass graft(s) of the extremities with intermittent claudication, right leg 🦴   A

I70.712 Atherosclerosis of other type of bypass graft(s) of the extremities with intermittent claudication, left leg 🦴   A

I70.713 Atherosclerosis of other type of bypass graft(s) of the extremities with intermittent claudication, bilateral legs 🦴   A

I70.718 Atherosclerosis of other type of bypass graft(s) of the extremities with intermittent claudication, other extremity 🦴   A

I70.719 Atherosclerosis of other type of bypass graft(s) of the extremities with intermittent claudication, unspecified extremity 🦴   A

● **I70.72** **Atherosclerosis of other type of bypass graft(s) of the extremities with rest pain**

> **Includes**   any condition classifiable to I70.71-
> chronic limb-threatening ischemia NOS of other type of bypass graft(s) of the extremities
> chronic limb-threatening ischemia of other type of bypass graft(s) of the extremities with rest pain
> critical limb ischemia NOS of other type of bypass graft(s) of the extremities
> critical limb ischemia of other type of bypass graft(s) of the extremities with rest pain

I70.721 Atherosclerosis of other type of bypass graft(s) of the extremities with rest pain, right leg 🦴   A

I70.722 Atherosclerosis of other type of bypass graft(s) of the extremities with rest pain, left leg 🦴   A

I70.723 Atherosclerosis of other type of bypass graft(s) of the extremities with rest pain, bilateral legs 🦴   A

I70.728 Atherosclerosis of other type of bypass graft(s) of the extremities with rest pain, other extremity 🦴   A

I70.729 Atherosclerosis of other type of bypass graft(s) of the extremities with rest pain, unspecified extremity 🦴   A

● **I70.73** **Atherosclerosis of other type of bypass graft(s) of the right leg with ulceration**

> **Includes**   any condition classifiable to I70.711 and I70.721
> chronic limb-threatening ischemia of other type of bypass graft(s) of the right leg with ulceration
> critical limb ischemia of other type of bypass graft(s) of the right leg with ulceration

Use additional code to identify severity of ulcer (L97.-)

I70.731 Atherosclerosis of other type of bypass graft(s) of the right leg with ulceration of thigh 🦴   A

I70.732 Atherosclerosis of other type of bypass graft(s) of the right leg with ulceration of calf 🦴   A

I70.733 Atherosclerosis of other type of bypass graft(s) of the right leg with ulceration of ankle 🦴   A

I70.734 Atherosclerosis of other type of bypass graft(s) of the right leg with ulceration of heel and midfoot 🦴   A
> Atherosclerosis of other type of bypass graft(s) of right leg with ulceration of plantar surface of midfoot

I70.735 Atherosclerosis of other type of bypass graft(s) of the right leg with ulceration of other part of foot 🦴   A
> Atherosclerosis of other type of bypass graft(s) of right leg with ulceration of toe

I70.738 Atherosclerosis of other type of bypass graft(s) of the right leg with ulceration of other part of lower leg 🦴   A

I70.739 Atherosclerosis of other type of bypass graft(s) of the right leg with ulceration of unspecified site 🦴   A

● **I70.74** **Atherosclerosis of other type of bypass graft(s) of the left leg with ulceration**

> **Includes**   any condition classifiable to I70.712 and I70.722
> chronic limb-threatening ischemia of other type of bypass graft(s) of the left leg with ulceration
> critical limb ischemia of other type of bypass graft(s) of the left leg with ulceration

Use additional code to identify severity of ulcer (L97.-)

I70.741 Atherosclerosis of other type of bypass graft(s) of the left leg with ulceration of thigh 🦴   A

I70.742 Atherosclerosis of other type of bypass graft(s) of the left leg with ulceration of calf 🦴   A

I70.743 Atherosclerosis of other type of bypass graft(s) of the left leg with ulceration of ankle 🦴   A

I70.744 Atherosclerosis of other type of bypass graft(s) of the left leg with ulceration of heel and midfoot 🦴   A
> Atherosclerosis of other type of bypass graft(s) of left leg with ulceration of plantar surface of midfoot

I70.745 Atherosclerosis of other type of bypass graft(s) of the left leg with ulceration of other part of foot 🦴   A
> Atherosclerosis of other type of bypass graft(s) of left leg with ulceration of toe

I70.748 Atherosclerosis of other type of bypass graft(s) of the left leg with ulceration of other part of lower leg 🦴   A

I70.749 Atherosclerosis of other type of bypass graft(s) of the left leg with ulceration of unspecified site 🦴   A

▶ New   ⇒ Revised   ~~deleted~~ Deleted   Excludes 1   Excludes 2   Includes   Use additional   Code first   Code also   Key words

OGCR Official Guidelines   X Assign placeholder X   ● Use Additional Character(s)   ▷ Manifestation Code   🦴 Hierarchical Condition Category   **Coding Clinic**

I70.75 Atherosclerosis of other type of bypass graft(s) of other extremity with ulceration 🔲 A
    Includes   any condition classifiable to I70.718 and I70.728
    Use additional code to identify severity of ulcer (L98.49)

● **I70.76** Atherosclerosis of other type of bypass graft(s) of the extremities with gangrene
    Includes   any condition classifiable to I70.71-, I70.72-, I70.73-, I70.74-, I70.75
        chronic limb-threatening ischemia of other type of bypass graft(s) of the extremities with gangrene
        critical limb ischemia of other type of bypass graft(s) of the extremities with gangrene
    Use additional code to identify the severity of any ulcer (L97.-, L98.49-), if applicable

    I70.761 Atherosclerosis of other type of bypass graft(s) of the extremities with gangrene, right leg 🔲 A

    I70.762 Atherosclerosis of other type of bypass graft(s) of the extremities with gangrene, left leg 🔲 A

    I70.763 Atherosclerosis of other type of bypass graft(s) of the extremities with gangrene, bilateral legs 🔲 A

    I70.768 Atherosclerosis of other type of bypass graft(s) of the extremities with gangrene, other extremity 🔲 A

    I70.769 Atherosclerosis of other type of bypass graft(s) of the extremities with gangrene, unspecified extremity 🔲 A

● **I70.79** Other atherosclerosis of other type of bypass graft(s) of the extremities

    I70.791 Other atherosclerosis of other type of bypass graft(s) of the extremities, right leg 🔲 A

    I70.792 Other atherosclerosis of other type of bypass graft(s) of the extremities, left leg 🔲 A

    I70.793 Other atherosclerosis of other type of bypass graft(s) of the extremities, bilateral legs 🔲 A

    I70.798 Other atherosclerosis of other type of bypass graft(s) of the extremities, other extremity 🔲 A

    I70.799 Other atherosclerosis of other type of bypass graft(s) of the extremities, unspecified extremity 🔲 A

I70.8 Atherosclerosis of other arteries A

● **I70.9** Other and unspecified atherosclerosis
    I70.90 Unspecified atherosclerosis A
    I70.91 Generalized atherosclerosis A
    I70.92 Chronic total occlusion of artery of the extremities 🔲 A
        Complete occlusion of artery of the extremities
        Total occlusion of artery of the extremities
        Code first atherosclerosis of arteries of the extremities (I70.2-, I70.3-, I70.4-, I70.5-, I70.6-, I70.7-)

● **I71** **Aortic aneurysm and dissection**
    ~~Excludes1~~ ~~aortic ectasia (I77.81-)~~
        ~~syphilitic aortic aneurysm (A52.01)~~
        ~~traumatic aortic aneurysm (S25.09, S35.09)~~
  ▶ *Code first, if applicable:*
  ▶ syphilitic aortic aneurysm (A52.01)
  ▶ traumatic aortic aneurysm (S25.09, S35.09)

● **I71.0** **Dissection of aorta**
    I71.00 Dissection of unspecified site of aorta 🔲
  ● **I71.01** Dissection of thoracic aorta 🔲
    ▶ **I71.010** Dissection of ascending aorta 🔲
    ▶ **I71.011** Dissection of aortic arch 🔲
    ▶ **I71.012** Dissection of descending thoracic aorta
    ▶ **I71.019** Dissection of thoracic aorta, unspecified
    I71.02 Dissection of abdominal aorta 🔲
    I71.03 Dissection of thoracoabdominal aorta 🔲

● **I71.1** **Thoracic aortic aneurysm, ruptured** 🔲
  ▶ **I71.10** Thoracic aortic aneurysm, ruptured, unspecified
  ▶ **I71.11** Aneurysm of the ascending aorta, ruptured
  ▶ **I71.12** Aneurysm of the aortic arch, ruptured
  ▶ **I71.13** Aneurysm of the descending thoracic aorta, ruptured

● **I71.2** **Thoracic aortic aneurysm, without rupture** 🔲
  ▶ **I71.20** Thoracic aortic aneurysm, without rupture, unspecified
  ▶ **I71.21** Aneurysm of the ascending aorta, without rupture
  ▶ **I71.22** Aneurysm of the aortic arch, without rupture
  ▶ **I71.23** Aneurysm of the descending thoracic aorta, without rupture

● **I71.3** **Abdominal aortic aneurysm, ruptured** 🔲
  ▶ **I71.30** Abdominal aortic aneurysm, ruptured, unspecified
  ▶ **I71.31** Pararenal abdominal aortic aneurysm, ruptured
  ▶ **I71.32** Juxtarenal abdominal aortic aneurysm, ruptured
  ▶ **I71.33** Infrarenal abdominal aortic aneurysm, ruptured

● **I71.4** **Abdominal aortic aneurysm, without rupture** 🔲
  ▶ **I71.40** Abdominal aortic aneurysm, without rupture, unspecified
  ▶ **I71.41** Pararenal abdominal aortic aneurysm, without rupture
  ▶ **I71.42** Juxtarenal abdominal aortic aneurysm, without rupture
  ▶ **I71.43** Infrarenal abdominal aortic aneurysm, without rupture

● **I71.5** **Thoracoabdominal aortic aneurysm, ruptured** 🔲
  ▶ **I71.50** Thoracoabdominal aortic aneurysm, ruptured, unspecified
  ▶ **I71.51** Supraceliac aneurysm of the abdominal aorta, ruptured
  ▶ **I71.52** Paravisceral aneurysm of the abdominal aorta, ruptured

● **I71.6** **Thoracoabdominal aortic aneurysm, without rupture** 🔲
  ▶ **I71.60** Thoracoabdominal aortic aneurysm, without rupture, unspecified
  ▶ **I71.61** Supraceliac aneurysm of the abdominal aorta, without rupture
  ▶ **I71.62** Paravisceral aneurysm of the abdominal aorta, without rupture

I71.8 Aortic aneurysm of unspecified site, ruptured 🔲
    Rupture of aorta NOS

I71.9 Aortic aneurysm of unspecified site, without rupture 🔲
    Aneurysm of aorta
    Dilatation of aorta
    Hyaline necrosis of aorta

● I72   Other aneurysm
        Includes   aneurysm (cirsoid) (false) (ruptured)
        Excludes2 acquired aneurysm (I77.0)
                       aneurysm (of) aorta (I71.-)
                       aneurysm (of) arteriovenous NOS (Q27.3-)
                       carotid artery dissection (I77.71)
                       cerebral (nonruptured) aneurysm (I67.1)
                       coronary aneurysm (I25.4)
                       coronary artery dissection (I25.42)
                       dissection of artery NEC (I77.79)
                       dissection of precerebral artery, congenital
                            (nonruptured) (Q28.1)
                       heart aneurysm (I25.3)
                       iliac artery dissection (I77.72)
                       precerebral artery, congential (nonruptured) (Q28.1)
                       pulmonary artery aneurysm (I28.1)
                       renal artery dissection (I77.73)
                       retinal aneurysm (H35.0)
                       ruptured cerebral aneurysm (I60.7)
                       varicose aneurysm (I77.0)
                       vertebral artery dissection (I77.74)

    I72.0   **Aneurysm of carotid artery** 🐾
            Aneurysm of common carotid artery
            Aneurysm of external carotid artery
            Aneurysm of internal carotid artery, extracranial
                portion
            Excludes1 aneurysm of internal carotid artery,
                            intracranial portion (I67.1)
                           aneurysm of internal carotid artery NOS
                            (I67.1)

    I72.1   **Aneurysm of artery of upper extremity** 🐾
    I72.2   **Aneurysm of renal artery** 🐾
    I72.3   **Aneurysm of iliac artery** 🐾
    I72.4   **Aneurysm of artery of lower extremity** 🐾
            Coding Clinic: 2019, Q2, P22
    I72.5   **Aneurysm of other precerebral arteries** 🐾
            Aneurysm of basilar artery (trunk)
            Excludes2 aneurysm of carotid artery (I72.0)
                           aneurysm of vertebral artery (I72.6)
                           dissection of carotid artery (I77.71)
                           dissection of other precerebral arteries
                            (I77.75)
                           dissection of vertebral artery (I77.74)
            Coding Clinic 2016, Q4, P28
    I72.6   **Aneurysm of vertebral artery** 🐾
            Excludes2 dissection of vertebral artery (I77.74)
            Coding Clinic 2016, Q4, P28
    I72.8   **Aneurysm of other specified arteries** 🐾
    I72.9   **Aneurysm of unspecified site** 🐾

● I73   Other peripheral vascular diseases
        Excludes2 chilblains (T69.1)
                       frostbite (T33-T34)
                       immersion hand or foot (T69.0-)
                       spasm of cerebral artery (G45.9)
        Coding Clinic: 2018, Q4, P87-88
   ● I73.0 **Raynaud's syndrome**
            Diminishing oxygen supply to fingers, toes, nose, and ears
                when exposed to temperature changes or stress
            Raynaud's disease
            Raynaud's phenomenon (secondary)
            I73.00   **Raynaud's syndrome without gangrene**
            I73.01   **Raynaud's syndrome with gangrene** 🐾
    I73.1   **Thromboangiitis obliterans [Buerger's disease]** 🐾
            Inflammatory occlusive disease resulting in poor circulation
                to the legs, feet, and sometimes the hands due to
                progressive inflammatory narrowing and eventually
                obliteration of the small arteries

Figure 9-5   Raynaud's syndrome. (From Hallett: Comprehensive Vascular and Endovascular Surgery, ed 2, Philadelphia, Mosby Ltd., 2010)

   ● I73.8 **Other specified peripheral vascular diseases**
            Excludes1 diabetic (peripheral) angiopathy
                            (E08-E13 with .51-.52)
            I73.81   **Erythromelalgia** 🐾
            I73.89   **Other specified peripheral vascular diseases** 🐾
                     Acrocyanosis
                     Erythrocyanosis
                     Simple acroparesthesia [Schultze's type]
                     Vasomotor acroparesthesia [Nothnagel's type]
    I73.9   **Peripheral vascular disease, unspecified** 🐾
            Intermittent claudication
            Peripheral angiopathy NOS
            Spasm of artery
            Excludes1 atherosclerosis of the extremities
                            (I70.2—I70.7-)
            Coding Clinic: 2018, Q4, P87

● I74   Arterial embolism and thrombosis
        Includes   embolic infarction
                       embolic occlusion
                       thrombotic infarction
                       thrombotic occlusion
        Code first embolism and thrombosis complicating abortion or
            ectopic or molar pregnancy (O00-O07, O08.2)
            embolism and thrombosis complicating pregnancy, childbirth
            and the puerperium (O88.-)
        Excludes2 atheroembolism (I75.-)
                       basilar embolism and thrombosis (I63.0-I63.2, I65.1)
                       carotid embolism and thrombosis (I63.0-I63.2, I65.2)
                       cerebral embolism and thrombosis (I63.3-I63.5,
                            I66.-)
                       coronary embolism and thrombosis (I21-I25)
                       mesenteric embolism and thrombosis (K55.0-)
                       ophthalmic embolism and thrombosis (H34.-)
                       precerebral embolism and thrombosis NOS
                            (I63.0-I63.2, I65.9)
                       pulmonary embolism and thrombosis (I26.-)
                       renal embolism and thrombosis (N28.0)
                       retinal embolism and thrombosis (H34.-)
                       septic embolism and thrombosis (I76)
                       vertebral embolism and thrombosis (I63.0-I63.2,
                            I65.0)
   ● I74.0 **Embolism and thrombosis of abdominal aorta**
            I74.01   **Saddle embolus of abdominal aorta** 🐾
            I74.09   **Other arterial embolism and thrombosis of
                     abdominal aorta** 🐾
                     Aortic bifurcation syndrome
                     Aortoiliac obstruction
                     Leriche's syndrome

▶ New   ⇒ Revised   ~~deleted~~ Deleted   Excludes 1   Excludes 2   Includes   Use additional   Code first   Code also   Key words
OGCR Official Guidelines   X Assign placeholder X   ● Use Additional Character(s)   ▷ Manifestation Code   🐾 Hierarchical Condition Category   Coding Clinic

● **I74.1** **Embolism and thrombosis of other and unspecified parts of aorta**

     I74.10 Embolism and thrombosis of unspecified parts of aorta 🔖

     I74.11 Embolism and thrombosis of thoracic aorta 🔖

     I74.19 Embolism and thrombosis of other parts of aorta 🔖

   I74.2 Embolism and thrombosis of arteries of the upper extremities 🔖

   I74.3 Embolism and thrombosis of arteries of the lower extremities 🔖

   I74.4 Embolism and thrombosis of arteries of extremities, unspecified 🔖

     Peripheral arterial embolism NOS

   I74.5 Embolism and thrombosis of iliac artery 🔖

   I74.8 Embolism and thrombosis of other arteries 🔖

   I74.9 Embolism and thrombosis of unspecified artery 🔖

● **I75** **Atheroembolism**

   Includes atherothrombotic microembolism
             cholesterol embolism

● **I75.0** **Atheroembolism of extremities**

   ● **I75.01** Atheroembolism of upper extremity

     I75.011 Atheroembolism of right upper extremity 🔖

     I75.012 Atheroembolism of left upper extremity 🔖

     I75.013 Atheroembolism of bilateral upper extremities 🔖

     I75.019 Atheroembolism of unspecified upper extremity 🔖

   ● **I75.02** Atheroembolism of lower extremity

     I75.021 Atheroembolism of right lower extremity 🔖

     I75.022 Atheroembolism of left lower extremity 🔖

     I75.023 Atheroembolism of bilateral lower extremities 🔖

     I75.029 Atheroembolism of unspecified lower extremity 🔖

● **I75.8** **Atheroembolism of other sites**

   I75.81 Atheroembolism of kidney 🔖

     Use additional code for any associated acute kidney failure and chronic kidney disease (N17.-, N18.-)

   I75.89 Atheroembolism of other site 🔖

I76 **Septic arterial embolism** 🔖

   Code first underlying infection, such as:
     infective endocarditis (I33.0)
     lung abscess (J85.-)
   Use additional code to identify the site of the embolism (I74.-)
   Excludes2 septic pulmonary embolism (I26.01, I26.90)

Item 9–9 An **embolus** is a mass of undissolved matter present in the blood that is transported by the blood current. A **thrombus** is a blood clot that occludes or shuts off a vessel. When a thrombus is dislodged, it becomes an embolus.

Embolus

Figure 9-6 An arterial embolus.

● **I77** **Other disorders of arteries and arterioles**

   Excludes2 collagen (vascular) diseases (M30-M36)
                hypersensitivity angiitis (M31.0)
                pulmonary artery (I28.-)

   I77.0 **Arteriovenous fistula, acquired** 🔖

     Aneurysmal varix
     Arteriovenous aneurysm, acquired

     Excludes1 arteriovenous aneurysm NOS (Q27.3-)
               presence of arteriovenous shunt (fistula) for dialysis (Z99.2)
               traumatic - see injury of blood vessel by body region

     Excludes2 cerebral (I67.1)
               coronary (I25.4)

   I77.1 **Stricture of artery** 🔖
     Narrowing of artery
     Coding Clinic: 2021, Q3, P13

   I77.2 **Rupture of artery** 🔖
     Erosion of artery
     Fistula of artery
     Ulcer of artery

     Excludes1 traumatic rupture of artery - see injury of blood vessel by body region

   I77.3 **Arterial fibromuscular dysplasia** 🔖
     Fibromuscular hyperplasia (of) carotid artery
     Fibromuscular hyperplasia (of) renal artery

   I77.4 **Celiac artery compression syndrome** 🔖
     Coding Clinic: 2021, Q3, P12-13

   I77.5 **Necrosis of artery** 🔖

   I77.6 **Arteritis, unspecified** 🔖
     Aortitis NOS
     Endarteritis NOS

     Excludes1 arteritis or endarteritis:
               aortic arch (M31.4)
               cerebral NEC (I67.7)
               coronary (I25.89)
               deformans (I70.-)
               giant cell (M31.5, M31.6)
               obliterans (I70.-)
               senile (I70.-)

● **I77.7** **Other arterial dissection**

     Excludes2 dissection of aorta (I71.0-)
               dissection of coronary artery (I25.42)

   I77.70 Dissection of unspecified artery 🔖
     Coding Clinic 2016, Q4, P28

   I77.71 Dissection of carotid artery 🔖

   I77.72 Dissection of iliac artery 🔖

   I77.73 Dissection of renal artery 🔖

   I77.74 Dissection of vertebral artery 🔖

     Excludes2 aneurysm of vertebral artery (I72.6)

   I77.75 Dissection of other precerebral arteries 🔖
     Dissection of basilar artery (trunk)

     Excludes2 aneurysm of carotid artery (I72.0)
               aneurysm of other precerebral arteries (I72.5)
               aneurysm of vertebral artery (I72.6)
               dissection of carotid artery (I77.71)
               dissection of vertebral artery (I77.74)

     Coding Clinic 2016, Q4, P28

   I77.76 Dissection of artery of upper extremity 🔖
     Coding Clinic 2016, Q4, P28

   I77.77 Dissection of artery of lower extremity 🔖
     Coding Clinic 2016, Q4, P28

   I77.79 Dissection of other specified artery 🔖
     Coding Clinic 2016, Q4, P28

CHAPTER 9 (I00-I99)

● **I77.8**   **Other specified disorders of arteries and arterioles**

    I77.81   **Aortic ectasia**
       Ectasis aorta

⟹   **Excludes1**   aortic aneurysm and dissection (I71.-)

       I77.810   **Thoracic aortic ectasia** 🔖
       I77.811   **Abdominal aortic ectasia** 🔖
       I77.812   **Thoracoabdominal aortic ectasia** 🔖
       I77.819   **Aortic ectasia, unspecified site** 🔖

▷ **I77.82**   **Antineutrophilic cytoplasmic antibody [ANCA] vasculitis**
     ▶ ANCA associated vasculitis
     ▶ ANCA positive vasculitis

     ▶ **Excludes2**   eosinophilic granulomatosis with polyangiitis (M30.1)
       ▶ granulomatosis with polyangiitis (M31.3-)
       ▶ microscopic polyangiitis (M31.7)

    I77.89   **Other specified disorders of arteries and arterioles** 🔖
       Coding Clinic 2021, Q1, P23

    I77.9   **Disorder of arteries and arterioles, unspecified** 🔖
       Coding Clinic 2021, Q1, P4

● **I78**   **Diseases of capillaries**

    I78.0   **Hereditary hemorrhagic telangiectasia** 🔖
       Rendu-Osler-Weber disease

    I78.1   **Nevus, non-neoplastic**
       Araneus nevus   Spider nevus
       Senile nevus   Stellar nevus

     Excludes1   nevus NOS (D22.-)
       vascular NOS (Q82.5)

     Excludes2   blue nevus (D22.-)
       flammeus nevus (Q82.5)
       hairy nevus (D22.-)
       melanocytic nevus (D22.-)
       pigmented nevus (D22.-)
       portwine nevus (Q82.5)
       sanguineous nevus (Q82.5)
       strawberry nevus (Q82.5)
       verrucous nevus (Q82.5)
       Coding Clinic: 2019, Q1, P21

    I78.8   **Other diseases of capillaries**
    I78.9   **Disease of capillaries, unspecified**

● **I79**   **Disorders of arteries, arterioles and capillaries in diseases classified elsewhere**

 ▷ *I79.0*   *Aneurysm of aorta in diseases classified elsewhere* 🔖
       Code first underlying disease
     Excludes1   syphilitic aneurysm (A52.01)

 ▷ *I79.1*   *Aortitis in diseases classified elsewhere* 🔖
       Code first underlying disease
     Excludes1   syphilitic aortitis (A52.02)

 ▷ *I79.8*   *Other disorders of arteries, arterioles and capillaries in diseases classified elsewhere* 🔖
       Code first underlying disease, such as:
       amyloidosis (E85.-)
     Excludes1   diabetic (peripheral) angiopathy (E08-E13 with .51-.52)
       syphilitic endarteritis (A52.09)
       tuberculous endarteritis (A18.89)

DISEASES OF VEINS, LYMPHATIC VESSELS AND LYMPH NODES, NOT ELSEWHERE CLASSIFIED (I80-I89)

● **I80**   **Phlebitis and thrombophlebitis**
     Inflammation of a vein with infiltration of walls (phlebitis)

    Includes   endophlebitis
       inflammation, vein
       periphlebitis
       suppurative phlebitis

    Code first phlebitis and thrombophlebitis complicating abortion, ectopic or molar pregnancy (O00-O07, O08.7)
       phlebitis and thrombophlebitis complicating pregnancy, childbirth and the puerperium (O22.-, O87.-)

    Excludes1   venous embolism and thrombosis of lower extremities (I82.4-, I82.5-, I82.81-)

● **I80.0**   **Phlebitis and thrombophlebitis of superficial vessels of lower extremities**
       Phlebitis and thrombophlebitis of femoropopliteal vein

    I80.00   **Phlebitis and thrombophlebitis of superficial vessels of unspecified lower extremity**
    I80.01   **Phlebitis and thrombophlebitis of superficial vessels of right lower extremity**
    I80.02   **Phlebitis and thrombophlebitis of superficial vessels of left lower extremity**
    I80.03   **Phlebitis and thrombophlebitis of superficial vessels of lower extremities, bilateral**

● **I80.1**   **Phlebitis and thrombophlebitis of femoral vein**
       Phlebitis and thrombophlebitis of common femoral vein
       Phlebitis and thrombophlebitis of deep femoral vein

    I80.10   **Phlebitis and thrombophlebitis of unspecified femoral vein** 🔖
    I80.11   **Phlebitis and thrombophlebitis of right femoral vein** 🔖
    I80.12   **Phlebitis and thrombophlebitis of left femoral vein** 🔖
    I80.13   **Phlebitis and thrombophlebitis of femoral vein, bilateral** 🔖

● **I80.2**   **Phlebitis and thrombophlebitis of other and unspecified deep vessels of lower extremities**

 ● **I80.20**   **Phlebitis and thrombophlebitis of unspecified deep vessels of lower extremities**
       I80.201   **Phlebitis and thrombophlebitis of unspecified deep vessels of right lower extremity** 🔖
       I80.202   **Phlebitis and thrombophlebitis of unspecified deep vessels of left lower extremity** 🔖
       I80.203   **Phlebitis and thrombophlebitis of unspecified deep vessels of lower extremities, bilateral** 🔖
       I80.209   **Phlebitis and thrombophlebitis of unspecified deep vessels of unspecified lower extremity** 🔖

 ● **I80.21**   **Phlebitis and thrombophlebitis of iliac vein**
       Phlebitis and thrombophlebitis of common iliac vein
       Phlebitis and thrombophlebitis of external iliac vein
       Phlebitis and thrombophlebitis of internal iliac vein
       I80.211   **Phlebitis and thrombophlebitis of right iliac vein** 🔖
       I80.212   **Phlebitis and thrombophlebitis of left iliac vein** 🔖
       I80.213   **Phlebitis and thrombophlebitis of iliac vein, bilateral** 🔖
       I80.219   **Phlebitis and thrombophlebitis of unspecified iliac vein** 🔖

▶ New   ⟹ Revised   ~~deleted~~ Deleted   Excludes 1   Excludes 2   Includes   Use additional   Code first   Code also   Key words
OGCR Official Guidelines   X Assign placeholder X   ● Use Additional Character(s)   ▷ Manifestation Code   🔖 Hierarchical Condition Category   Coding Clinic

CHAPTER 9 (I00-I99)

● **I80.22**   Phlebitis and thrombophlebitis of popliteal vein

    I80.221   Phlebitis and thrombophlebitis of right popliteal vein 🔖

    I80.222   Phlebitis and thrombophlebitis of left popliteal vein 🔖

    I80.223   Phlebitis and thrombophlebitis of popliteal vein, bilateral 🔖

    I80.229   Phlebitis and thrombophlebitis of unspecified popliteal vein 🔖

● **I80.23**   Phlebitis and thrombophlebitis of tibial vein
Phlebitis and thrombophlebitis of anterior tibial vein
Phlebitis and thrombophlebitis of posterior tibial vein

    I80.231   Phlebitis and thrombophlebitis of right tibial vein 🔖

    I80.232   Phlebitis and thrombophlebitis of left tibial vein 🔖

    I80.233   Phlebitis and thrombophlebitis of tibial vein, bilateral 🔖

    I80.239   Phlebitis and thrombophlebitis of unspecified tibial vein 🔖

● **I80.24**   Phlebitis and thrombophlebitis of peroneal vein

    I80.241   Phlebitis and thrombophlebitis of right peroneal vein

    I80.242   Phlebitis and thrombophlebitis of left peroneal vein

    I80.243   Phlebitis and thrombophlebitis of peroneal vein, bilateral

    I80.249   Phlebitis and thrombophlebitis of unspecified peroneal vein

● **I80.25**   Phlebitis and thrombophlebitis of calf muscular vein
Phlebitis and thrombophlebitis of calf muscular vein, NOS
Phlebitis and thrombophlebitis of gastrocnemial vein
Phlebitis and thrombophlebitis of soleal vein

    I80.251   Phlebitis and thrombophlebitis of right calf muscular vein

    I80.252   Phlebitis and thrombophlebitis of left calf muscular vein

    I80.253   Phlebitis and thrombophlebitis of calf muscular vein, bilateral

    I80.259   Phlebitis and thrombophlebitis of unspecified calf muscular vein

● **I80.29**   Phlebitis and thrombophlebitis of other deep vessels of lower extremities

    I80.291   Phlebitis and thrombophlebitis of other deep vessels of right lower extremity 🔖

    I80.292   Phlebitis and thrombophlebitis of other deep vessels of left lower extremity 🔖

    I80.293   Phlebitis and thrombophlebitis of other deep vessels of lower extremity, bilateral 🔖

    I80.299   Phlebitis and thrombophlebitis of other deep vessels of unspecified lower extremity 🔖

I80.3   Phlebitis and thrombophlebitis of lower extremities, unspecified

I80.8   Phlebitis and thrombophlebitis of other sites

I80.9   Phlebitis and thrombophlebitis of unspecified site

I81   Portal vein thrombosis
Portal (vein) obstruction

    Excludes2   hepatic vein thrombosis (I82.0)
               phlebitis of portal vein (K75.1)

    Coding Clinic: 2019, Q4, P68

● **I82**   Other venous embolism and thrombosis
Code first venous embolism and thrombosis complicating:
abortion, ectopic or molar pregnancy (O00-O07, O08.7)
pregnancy, childbirth and the puerperium (O22.-, O87.-)

    Excludes2   venous embolism and thrombosis (of):
               cerebral (I63.6, I67.6)
               coronary (I21-I25)
               intracranial and intraspinal, septic or NOS (G08)
               intracranial, nonpyogenic (I67.6)
               intraspinal, nonpyogenic (G95.1)
               mesenteric (K55.0-)
               portal (I81)
               pulmonary (I26.-)

    I82.0   Budd-Chiari syndrome 🔖
Hepatic vein thrombosis

    I82.1   Thrombophlebitis migrans
"White leg" is the other term to describe a migrating thrombus.

● **I82.2**   Embolism and thrombosis of vena cava and other thoracic veins

    ● **I82.21**   Embolism and thrombosis of superior vena cava

       I82.210   **Acute embolism and thrombosis of superior vena cava** 🔖
Embolism and thrombosis of superior vena cava NOS

       I82.211   Chronic embolism and thrombosis of superior vena cava 🔖

    ● **I82.22**   Embolism and thrombosis of inferior vena cava

       I82.220   **Acute embolism and thrombosis of inferior vena cava** 🔖
Embolism and thrombosis of inferior vena cava NOS

       I82.221   Chronic embolism and thrombosis of inferior vena cava 🔖

    ● **I82.29**   Embolism and thrombosis of other thoracic veins
Embolism and thrombosis of brachiocephalic (innominate) vein

       I82.290   Acute embolism and thrombosis of other thoracic veins 🔖

       I82.291   Chronic embolism and thrombosis of other thoracic veins 🔖

    I82.3   Embolism and thrombosis of renal vein 🔖

● **I82.4**   Acute embolism and thrombosis of deep veins of lower extremity

    I82.40   Acute embolism and thrombosis of unspecified deep veins of lower extremity
Deep vein thrombosis NOS
DVT NOS

       Excludes1   acute embolism and thrombosis of unspecified deep veins of distal lower extremity (I82.4Z-)
               acute embolism and thrombosis of unspecified deep veins of proximal lower extremity (I82.4Y-)

       I82.401   Acute embolism and thrombosis of unspecified deep veins of right lower extremity 🔖

       I82.402   Acute embolism and thrombosis of unspecified deep veins of left lower extremity 🔖

CHAPTER 9 (I00-I99)

CHAPTER 9 (I00-I99)

I82.403   Acute embolism and thrombosis of unspecified deep veins of lower extremity, bilateral 🦠

I82.409   Acute embolism and thrombosis of unspecified deep veins of unspecified lower extremity 🦠

● I82.41   Acute embolism and thrombosis of femoral vein
     Acute embolism and thrombosis of common femoral vein
     Acute embolism and thrombosis of deep femoral vein

     I82.411   Acute embolism and thrombosis of right femoral vein 🦠

     I82.412   Acute embolism and thrombosis of left femoral vein 🦠

     I82.413   Acute embolism and thrombosis of femoral vein, bilateral 🦠

     I82.419   Acute embolism and thrombosis of unspecified femoral vein 🦠

● I82.42   Acute embolism and thrombosis of iliac vein
     Acute embolism and thrombosis of common iliac vein
     Acute embolism and thrombosis of external iliac vein
     Acute embolism and thrombosis of internal iliac vein

     I82.421   Acute embolism and thrombosis of right iliac vein 🦠

     I82.422   Acute embolism and thrombosis of left iliac vein 🦠

     I82.423   Acute embolism and thrombosis of iliac vein, bilateral 🦠

     I82.429   Acute embolism and thrombosis of unspecified iliac vein 🦠

● I82.43   Acute embolism and thrombosis of popliteal vein

     I82.431   Acute embolism and thrombosis of right popliteal vein 🦠

     I82.432   Acute embolism and thrombosis of left popliteal vein 🦠

     I82.433   Acute embolism and thrombosis of popliteal vein, bilateral 🦠

     I82.439   Acute embolism and thrombosis of unspecified popliteal vein 🦠

● I82.44   Acute embolism and thrombosis of tibial vein
     Acute embolism and thrombosis of anterior tibial vein
     Acute embolism and thrombosis of posterior tibial vein

     I82.441   Acute embolism and thrombosis of right tibial vein 🦠

     I82.442   Acute embolism and thrombosis of left tibial vein 🦠

     I82.443   Acute embolism and thrombosis of tibial vein, bilateral 🦠

     I82.449   Acute embolism and thrombosis of unspecified tibial vein 🦠

● I82.45   Acute embolism and thrombosis of peroneal vein

     I82.451   Acute embolism and thrombosis of right peroneal vein

     I82.452   Acute embolism and thrombosis of left peroneal vein

     I82.453   Acute embolism and thrombosis of peroneal vein, bilateral

     I82.459   Acute embolism and thrombosis of unspecified peroneal vein

● I82.46   Acute embolism and thrombosis of calf muscular vein
     Acute embolism and thrombosis of calf muscular vein, NOS
     Acute embolism and thrombosis of gastrocnemial vein
     Acute embolism and thrombosis of soleal vein

     I82.461   Acute embolism and thrombosis of right calf muscular vein

     I82.462   Acute embolism and thrombosis of left calf muscular vein

     I82.463   Acute embolism and thrombosis of calf muscular vein, bilateral

     I82.469   Acute embolism and thrombosis of unspecified calf muscular vein

● I82.49   Acute embolism and thrombosis of other specified deep vein of lower extremity

     I82.491   Acute embolism and thrombosis of other specified deep vein of right lower extremity 🦠

     I82.492   Acute embolism and thrombosis of other specified deep vein of left lower extremity 🦠

     I82.493   Acute embolism and thrombosis of other specified deep vein of lower extremity, bilateral 🦠

     I82.499   Acute embolism and thrombosis of other specified deep vein of unspecified lower extremity 🦠

● I82.4Y   Acute embolism and thrombosis of unspecified deep veins of proximal lower extremity
     Acute embolism and thrombosis of deep vein of thigh NOS
     Acute embolism and thrombosis of deep vein of upper leg NOS

     I82.4Y1   Acute embolism and thrombosis of unspecified deep veins of right proximal lower extremity 🦠

     I82.4Y2   Acute embolism and thrombosis of unspecified deep veins of left proximal lower extremity 🦠

     I82.4Y3   Acute embolism and thrombosis of unspecified deep veins of proximal lower extremity, bilateral 🦠

     I82.4Y9   Acute embolism and thrombosis of unspecified deep veins of unspecified proximal lower extremity 🦠

● I82.4Z   Acute embolism and thrombosis of unspecified deep veins of distal lower extremity
     Acute embolism and thrombosis of deep vein of calf NOS
     Acute embolism and thrombosis of deep vein of lower leg NOS

     I82.4Z1   Acute embolism and thrombosis of unspecified deep veins of right distal lower extremity 🦠

     I82.4Z2   Acute embolism and thrombosis of unspecified deep veins of left distal lower extremity 🦠

     I82.4Z3   Acute embolism and thrombosis of unspecified deep veins of distal lower extremity, bilateral 🦠

     I82.4Z9   Acute embolism and thrombosis of unspecified deep veins of unspecified distal lower extremity 🦠

▶ New   ⇒ Revised   ~~deleted~~ Deleted   Excludes 1   Excludes 2   Includes   Use additional   Code first   Code also   Key words

OGCR Official Guidelines   X Assign placeholder X   ● Use Additional Character(s)   ▶ Manifestation Code   🦠 Hierarchical Condition Category   **Coding Clinic**

● **I82.5 Chronic embolism and thrombosis of deep veins of lower extremity**

> Use additional code, if applicable, for associated long-term (current) use of anticoagulants (Z79.01)

> **Excludes1** personal history of venous embolism and thrombosis (Z86.718)

● **I82.50 Chronic embolism and thrombosis of unspecified deep veins of lower extremity**

> **Excludes1** chronic embolism and thrombosis of unspecified deep veins of distal lower extremity (I82.5Z-)
> chronic embolism and thrombosis of unspecified deep veins of proximal lower extremity (I82.5Y-)

I82.501 **Chronic embolism and thrombosis of unspecified deep veins of right lower extremity**

I82.502 **Chronic embolism and thrombosis of unspecified deep veins of left lower extremity**

I82.503 **Chronic embolism and thrombosis of unspecified deep veins of lower extremity, bilateral**

I82.509 **Chronic embolism and thrombosis of unspecified deep veins of unspecified lower extremity**

● **I82.51 Chronic embolism and thrombosis of femoral vein**

> Chronic embolism and thrombosis of common femoral vein
> Chronic embolism and thrombosis of deep femoral vein

I82.511 **Chronic embolism and thrombosis of right femoral vein**

I82.512 **Chronic embolism and thrombosis of left femoral vein**

I82.513 **Chronic embolism and thrombosis of femoral vein, bilateral**

I82.519 **Chronic embolism and thrombosis of unspecified femoral vein**

● **I82.52 Chronic embolism and thrombosis of iliac vein**

> Chronic embolism and thrombosis of common iliac vein
> Chronic embolism and thrombosis of external iliac vein
> Chronic embolism and thrombosis of internal iliac vein

I82.521 **Chronic embolism and thrombosis of right iliac vein**

I82.522 **Chronic embolism and thrombosis of left iliac vein**

I82.523 **Chronic embolism and thrombosis of iliac vein, bilateral**

I82.529 **Chronic embolism and thrombosis of unspecified iliac vein**

● **I82.53 Chronic embolism and thrombosis of popliteal vein**

I82.531 **Chronic embolism and thrombosis of right popliteal vein**

I82.532 **Chronic embolism and thrombosis of left popliteal vein**

I82.533 **Chronic embolism and thrombosis of popliteal vein, bilateral**

I82.539 **Chronic embolism and thrombosis of unspecified popliteal vein**

Item 9–10 Varicose/Varicosities (varix = singular, varices = plural): Enlarged, engorged, tortuous, twisted vascular vessels (veins, arteries, lymphatics). As such, the condition can present in various parts of the body, although the most familiar locations are the lower extremities. A common complication of varices is thrombophlebitis. Varicosities of the anus and rectum are called hemorrhoids.

Figure 9-7 Varicose veins of the legs. (Getty Image)

● **I82.54 Chronic embolism and thrombosis of tibial vein**

> Chronic embolism and thrombosis of anterior tibial vein
> Chronic embolism and thrombosis of posterior tibial vein

I82.541 **Chronic embolism and thrombosis of right tibial vein**

I82.542 **Chronic embolism and thrombosis of left tibial vein**

I82.543 **Chronic embolism and thrombosis of tibial vein, bilateral**

I82.549 **Chronic embolism and thrombosis of unspecified tibial vein**

● **I82.55 Chronic embolism and thrombosis of peroneal vein**

I82.551 **Chronic embolism and thrombosis of right peroneal vein**

I82.552 **Chronic embolism and thrombosis of left peroneal vein**

I82.553 **Chronic embolism and thrombosis of peroneal vein, bilateral**

I82.559 **Chronic embolism and thrombosis of unspecified peroneal vein**

● **I82.56 Chronic embolism and thrombosis of calf muscular vein**

> Chronic embolism and thrombosis of calf muscular vein NOS
> Chronic embolism and thrombosis of gastrocnemial vein
> Chronic embolism and thrombosis of soleal vein

I82.561 **Chronic embolism and thrombosis of right calf muscular vein**

I82.562 **Chronic embolism and thrombosis of left calf muscular vein**

I82.563 **Chronic embolism and thrombosis of calf muscular vein, bilateral**

I82.569 **Chronic embolism and thrombosis of unspecified calf muscular vein**

● **I82.59 Chronic embolism and thrombosis of other specified deep vein of lower extremity**

I82.591 **Chronic embolism and thrombosis of other specified deep vein of right lower extremity**

I82.592 **Chronic embolism and thrombosis of other specified deep vein of left lower extremity**

I82.593 **Chronic embolism and thrombosis of other specified deep vein of lower extremity, bilateral**

I82.599 **Chronic embolism and thrombosis of other specified deep vein of unspecified lower extremity**

● **I82.5Y** **Chronic embolism and thrombosis of unspecified deep veins of proximal lower extremity**
Chronic embolism and thrombosis of deep veins of thigh NOS
Chronic embolism and thrombosis of deep veins of upper leg NOS

    I82.5Y1 **Chronic embolism and thrombosis of unspecified deep veins of right proximal lower extremity** 🐾

    I82.5Y2 **Chronic embolism and thrombosis of unspecified deep veins of left proximal lower extremity** 🐾

    I82.5Y3 **Chronic embolism and thrombosis of unspecified deep veins of proximal lower extremity, bilateral** 🐾

    I82.5Y9 **Chronic embolism and thrombosis of unspecified deep veins of unspecified proximal lower extremity** 🐾

● **I82.5Z** **Chronic embolism and thrombosis of unspecified deep veins of distal lower extremity**
Chronic embolism and thrombosis of deep veins of calf NOS
Chronic embolism and thrombosis of deep veins of lower leg NOS

    I82.5Z1 **Chronic embolism and thrombosis of unspecified deep veins of right distal lower extremity** 🐾

    I82.5Z2 **Chronic embolism and thrombosis of unspecified deep veins of left distal lower extremity** 🐾

    I82.5Z3 **Chronic embolism and thrombosis of unspecified deep veins of distal lower extremity, bilateral** 🐾

    I82.5Z9 **Chronic embolism and thrombosis of unspecified deep veins of unspecified distal lower extremity** 🐾

● **I82.6** **Acute embolism and thrombosis of veins of upper extremity**

  ● **I82.60** **Acute embolism and thrombosis of unspecified veins of upper extremity**

    I82.601 **Acute embolism and thrombosis of unspecified veins of right upper extremity**

    I82.602 **Acute embolism and thrombosis of unspecified veins of left upper extremity**

    I82.603 **Acute embolism and thrombosis of unspecified veins of upper extremity, bilateral**

    I82.609 **Acute embolism and thrombosis of unspecified veins of unspecified upper extremity**

  ● **I82.61** **Acute embolism and thrombosis of superficial veins of upper extremity**
Acute embolism and thrombosis of antecubital vein
Acute embolism and thrombosis of basilic vein
Acute embolism and thrombosis of cephalic vein

    I82.611 **Acute embolism and thrombosis of superficial veins of right upper extremity**

    I82.612 **Acute embolism and thrombosis of superficial veins of left upper extremity**

    I82.613 **Acute embolism and thrombosis of superficial veins of upper extremity, bilateral**

    I82.619 **Acute embolism and thrombosis of superficial veins of unspecified upper extremity**

● **I82.62** **Acute embolism and thrombosis of deep veins of upper extremity**
Acute embolism and thrombosis of brachial vein
Acute embolism and thrombosis of radial vein
Acute embolism and thrombosis of ulnar vein

    I82.621 **Acute embolism and thrombosis of deep veins of right upper extremity** 🐾

    I82.622 **Acute embolism and thrombosis of deep veins of left upper extremity** 🐾

    I82.623 **Acute embolism and thrombosis of deep veins of upper extremity, bilateral** 🐾

    I82.629 **Acute embolism and thrombosis of deep veins of unspecified upper extremity** 🐾

● **I82.7** **Chronic embolism and thrombosis of veins of upper extremity**
Use additional code, if applicable, for associated long-term (current) use of anticoagulants (Z79.01)

Excludes1 personal history of venous embolism and thrombosis (Z86.718)

  ● **I82.70** **Chronic embolism and thrombosis of unspecified veins of upper extremity**

    I82.701 **Chronic embolism and thrombosis of unspecified veins of right upper extremity**

    I82.702 **Chronic embolism and thrombosis of unspecified veins of left upper extremity**

    I82.703 **Chronic embolism and thrombosis of unspecified veins of upper extremity, bilateral**

    I82.709 **Chronic embolism and thrombosis of unspecified veins of unspecified upper extremity**

  ● **I82.71** **Chronic embolism and thrombosis of superficial veins of upper extremity**
Chronic embolism and thrombosis of antecubital vein
Chronic embolism and thrombosis of basilic vein
Chronic embolism and thrombosis of cephalic vein

    I82.711 **Chronic embolism and thrombosis of superficial veins of right upper extremity**

    I82.712 **Chronic embolism and thrombosis of superficial veins of left upper extremity**

    I82.713 **Chronic embolism and thrombosis of superficial veins of upper extremity, bilateral**

    I82.719 **Chronic embolism and thrombosis of superficial veins of unspecified upper extremity**

  ● **I82.72** **Chronic embolism and thrombosis of deep veins of upper extremity**
Chronic embolism and thrombosis of brachial vein
Chronic embolism and thrombosis of radial vein
Chronic embolism and thrombosis of ulnar vein

    I82.721 **Chronic embolism and thrombosis of deep veins of right upper extremity** 🐾

    I82.722 **Chronic embolism and thrombosis of deep veins of left upper extremity** 🐾

▶ New   ⇒ Revised   ~~deleted~~ Deleted   Excludes 1   Excludes 2   Includes   Use additional   Code first   Code also   Key words
OGCR Official Guidelines   X Assign placeholder X   ● Use Additional Character(s)   ▶ Manifestation Code   🐾 Hierarchical Condition Category   **Coding Clinic**

● **I82.723**   Chronic embolism and thrombosis of deep veins of upper extremity, bilateral 🔖

         I82.729   Chronic embolism and thrombosis of deep veins of unspecified upper extremity 🔖

● **I82.A**   Embolism and thrombosis of axillary vein

   ● **I82.A1**   Acute embolism and thrombosis of axillary vein

         I82.A11   Acute embolism and thrombosis of right axillary vein 🔖

         I82.A12   Acute embolism and thrombosis of left axillary vein 🔖

         I82.A13   Acute embolism and thrombosis of axillary vein, bilateral 🔖

         I82.A19   Acute embolism and thrombosis of unspecified axillary vein 🔖

   ● **I82.A2**   Chronic embolism and thrombosis of axillary vein

         I82.A21   Chronic embolism and thrombosis of right axillary vein 🔖

         I82.A22   Chronic embolism and thrombosis of left axillary vein 🔖

         I82.A23   Chronic embolism and thrombosis of axillary vein, bilateral 🔖

         I82.A29   Chronic embolism and thrombosis of unspecified axillary vein 🔖

● **I82.B**   Embolism and thrombosis of subclavian vein

   ● **I82.B1**   Acute embolism and thrombosis of subclavian vein

         I82.B11   Acute embolism and thrombosis of right subclavian vein 🔖

         I82.B12   Acute embolism and thrombosis of left subclavian vein 🔖

         I82.B13   Acute embolism and thrombosis of subclavian vein, bilateral 🔖

         I82.B19   Acute embolism and thrombosis of unspecified subclavian vein 🔖

   ● **I82.B2**   Chronic embolism and thrombosis of subclavian vein

         I82.B21   Chronic embolism and thrombosis of right subclavian vein 🔖

         I82.B22   Chronic embolism and thrombosis of left subclavian vein 🔖

         I82.B23   Chronic embolism and thrombosis of subclavian vein, bilateral 🔖

         I82.B29   Chronic embolism and thrombosis of unspecified subclavian vein 🔖

● **I82.C**   Embolism and thrombosis of internal jugular vein

   ● **I82.C1**   Acute embolism and thrombosis of internal jugular vein

         I82.C11   Acute embolism and thrombosis of right internal jugular vein 🔖

         I82.C12   Acute embolism and thrombosis of left internal jugular vein 🔖

         I82.C13   Acute embolism and thrombosis of internal jugular vein, bilateral 🔖

         I82.C19   Acute embolism and thrombosis of unspecified internal jugular vein 🔖

   ● **I82.C2**   Chronic embolism and thrombosis of internal jugular vein

         I82.C21   Chronic embolism and thrombosis of right internal jugular vein 🔖

         I82.C22   Chronic embolism and thrombosis of left internal jugular vein 🔖

         I82.C23   Chronic embolism and thrombosis of internal jugular vein, bilateral 🔖

         I82.C29   Chronic embolism and thrombosis of unspecified internal jugular vein 🔖

● **I82.8**   Embolism and thrombosis of other specified veins

     Use additional code, if applicable, for associated long-term (current) use of anticoagulants (Z79.01)

   ● **I82.81**   Embolism and thrombosis of superficial veins of lower extremities

         Embolism and thrombosis of saphenous vein (greater) (lesser)

         I82.811   Embolism and thrombosis of superficial veins of right lower extremity

         I82.812   Embolism and thrombosis of superficial veins of left lower extremity

         I82.813   Embolism and thrombosis of superficial veins of lower extremities, bilateral

         I82.819   Embolism and thrombosis of superficial veins of unspecified lower extremity

   ● **I82.89**   Embolism and thrombosis of other specified veins

         I82.890   Acute embolism and thrombosis of other specified veins

         I82.891   Chronic embolism and thrombosis of other specified veins

● **I82.9**   Embolism and thrombosis of unspecified vein

         I82.90   Acute embolism and thrombosis of unspecified vein

           Embolism of vein NOS

           Thrombosis (vein) NOS

         I82.91   Chronic embolism and thrombosis of unspecified vein

● **I83**   Varicose veins of lower extremities

   Excludes2   varicose veins complicating pregnancy (O22.0-)
         varicose veins complicating the puerperium (O87.4)

● **I83.0**   Varicose veins of lower extremities with ulcer

     Use additional code to identify severity of ulcer (L97.-)

   ● **I83.00**   Varicose veins of unspecified lower extremity with ulcer

         I83.001   Varicose veins of unspecified lower extremity with ulcer of thigh 🔖   A

         I83.002   Varicose veins of unspecified lower extremity with ulcer of calf 🔖   A

         I83.003   Varicose veins of unspecified lower extremity with ulcer of ankle 🔖   A

         I83.004   Varicose veins of unspecified lower extremity with ulcer of heel and midfoot 🔖   A

           Varicose veins of unspecified lower extremity with ulcer of plantar surface of midfoot

         I83.005   Varicose veins of unspecified lower extremity with ulcer other part of foot 🔖   A

           Varicose veins of unspecified lower extremity with ulcer of toe

         I83.008   Varicose veins of unspecified lower extremity with ulcer other part of lower leg 🔖   A

         I83.009   Varicose veins of unspecified lower extremity with ulcer of unspecified site 🔖   A

   ● **I83.01**   Varicose veins of right lower extremity with ulcer

         I83.011   Varicose veins of right lower extremity with ulcer of thigh 🔖   A

         I83.012   Varicose veins of right lower extremity with ulcer of calf 🔖   A

I83.013   Varicose veins of right lower extremity with ulcer of ankle 🦠   A

I83.014   Varicose veins of right lower extremity with ulcer of heel and midfoot 🦠   A

     Varicose veins of right lower extremity with ulcer of plantar surface of midfoot

I83.015   Varicose veins of right lower extremity with ulcer other part of foot 🦠   A

     Varicose veins of right lower extremity with ulcer of toe

I83.018   Varicose veins of right lower extremity with ulcer other part of lower leg 🦠   A

I83.019   Varicose veins of right lower extremity with ulcer of unspecified site 🦠   A

● I83.02   Varicose veins of left lower extremity with ulcer

I83.021   Varicose veins of left lower extremity with ulcer of thigh 🦠   A

I83.022   Varicose veins of left lower extremity with ulcer of calf 🦠   A

I83.023   Varicose veins of left lower extremity with ulcer of ankle 🦠   A

I83.024   Varicose veins of left lower extremity with ulcer of heel and midfoot 🦠   A

     Varicose veins of left lower extremity with ulcer of plantar surface of midfoot

I83.025   Varicose veins of left lower extremity with ulcer other part of foot 🦠   A

     Varicose veins of left lower extremity with ulcer of toe

I83.028   Varicose veins of left lower extremity with ulcer other part of lower leg 🦠   A

I83.029   Varicose veins of left lower extremity with ulcer of unspecified site 🦠   A

● I83.1   Varicose veins of lower extremities with inflammation

I83.10   Varicose veins of unspecified lower extremity with inflammation   A

I83.11   Varicose veins of right lower extremity with inflammation   A

I83.12   Varicose veins of left lower extremity with inflammation   A

● I83.2   Varicose veins of lower extremities with both ulcer and inflammation

     Use additional code to identify severity of ulcer (L97.-)

● I83.20   Varicose veins of unspecified lower extremity with both ulcer and inflammation

I83.201   Varicose veins of unspecified lower extremity with both ulcer of thigh and inflammation 🦠   A

I83.202   Varicose veins of unspecified lower extremity with both ulcer of calf and inflammation 🦠   A

I83.203   Varicose veins of unspecified lower extremity with both ulcer of ankle and inflammation 🦠   A

I83.204   Varicose veins of unspecified lower extremity with both ulcer of heel and midfoot and inflammation 🦠   A

     Varicose veins of unspecified lower extremity with both ulcer of plantar surface of midfoot and inflammation

I83.205   Varicose veins of unspecified lower extremity with both ulcer other part of foot and inflammation 🦠   A

     Varicose veins of unspecified lower extremity with both ulcer of toe and inflammation

I83.208   Varicose veins of unspecified lower extremity with both ulcer of other part of lower extremity and inflammation 🦠   A

I83.209   Varicose veins of unspecified lower extremity with both ulcer of unspecified site and inflammation 🦠 A

● I83.21   Varicose veins of right lower extremity with both ulcer and inflammation

I83.211   Varicose veins of right lower extremity with both ulcer of thigh and inflammation 🦠   A

I83.212   Varicose veins of right lower extremity with both ulcer of calf and inflammation 🦠   A

I83.213   Varicose veins of right lower extremity with both ulcer of ankle and inflammation 🦠   A

I83.214   Varicose veins of right lower extremity with both ulcer of heel and midfoot and inflammation 🦠   A

     Varicose veins of right lower extremity with both ulcer of plantar surface of midfoot and inflammation

I83.215   Varicose veins of right lower extremity with both ulcer other part of foot and inflammation 🦠   A

     Varicose veins of right lower extremity with both ulcer of toe and inflammation

I83.218   Varicose veins of right lower extremity with both ulcer of other part of lower extremity and inflammation 🦠   A

I83.219   Varicose veins of right lower extremity with both ulcer of unspecified site and inflammation 🦠 A

● I83.22   Varicose veins of left lower extremity with both ulcer and inflammation

I83.221   Varicose veins of left lower extremity with both ulcer of thigh and inflammation 🦠   A

I83.222   Varicose veins of left lower extremity with both ulcer of calf and inflammation 🦠   A

I83.223   Varicose veins of left lower extremity with both ulcer of ankle and inflammation 🦠   A

I83.224   Varicose veins of left lower extremity with both ulcer of heel and midfoot and inflammation 🦠   A

     Varicose veins of left lower extremity with both ulcer of plantar surface of midfoot and inflammation

I83.225   Varicose veins of left lower extremity with both ulcer other part of foot and inflammation 🦠   A

     Varicose veins of left lower extremity with both ulcer of toe and inflammation

I83.228   Varicose veins of left lower extremity with both ulcer of other part of lower extremity and inflammation 🦠   A

I83.229   Varicose veins of left lower extremity with both ulcer of unspecified site and inflammation 🦠   A

▶ New   ⇒ Revised   ~~deleted~~ Deleted   Excludes 1   Excludes 2   Includes   Use additional   Code first   Code also   Key words

OGCR Official Guidelines   X Assign placeholder X   ● Use Additional Character(s)   ▶ Manifestation Code   🦠 Hierarchical Condition Category   Coding Clinic

● **I83.8** **Varicose veins of lower extremities with other complications**
   ● **I83.81** **Varicose veins of lower extremities with pain**
      I83.811 Varicose veins of right lower extremity with pain A
      I83.812 Varicose veins of left lower extremity with pain A
      I83.813 Varicose veins of bilateral lower extremities with pain A
      I83.819 Varicose veins of unspecified lower extremity with pain A
   ● **I83.89** **Varicose veins of lower extremities with other complications**
      Varicose veins of lower extremities with edema
      Varicose veins of lower extremities with swelling
      I83.891 Varicose veins of right lower extremity with other complications A
      I83.892 Varicose veins of left lower extremity with other complications A
      I83.893 Varicose veins of bilateral lower extremities with other complications A
      I83.899 Varicose veins of unspecified lower extremity with other complications A
● **I83.9** **Asymptomatic varicose veins of lower extremities**
   Phlebectasia of lower extremities
   Varicose veins of lower extremities
   Varix of lower extremities
      I83.90 **Asymptomatic varicose veins of unspecified lower extremity** A
      Varicose veins NOS
      I83.91 **Asymptomatic varicose veins of right lower extremity** A
      I83.92 **Asymptomatic varicose veins of left lower extremity** A
      I83.93 **Asymptomatic varicose veins of bilateral lower extremities** A

● **I85** **Esophageal varices**
   Use additional code to identify:
   alcohol abuse and dependence (F10.-)
   ● **I85.0** **Esophageal varices**
      Idiopathic esophageal varices
      Primary esophageal varices
      I85.00 **Esophageal varices without bleeding** 🔍
      Esophageal varices NOS
      I85.01 **Esophageal varices with bleeding** 🔍
   ● **I85.1** **Secondary esophageal varices**
      Esophageal varices secondary to alcoholic liver disease
      Esophageal varices secondary to cirrhosis of liver
      Esophageal varices secondary to schistosomiasis
      Esophageal varices secondary to toxic liver disease
      Code first underlying disease
      I85.10 **Secondary esophageal varices without bleeding** 🔍
      I85.11 **Secondary esophageal varices with bleeding** 🔍

● **I86** **Varicose veins of other sites**
   Excludes1 varicose veins of unspecified site (I83.9-)
   Excludes2 retinal varices (H35.0-)
   I86.0 **Sublingual varices**
   I86.1 **Scrotal varices** ♂
      Varicocele
   I86.2 **Pelvic varices**
   I86.3 **Vulval varices** ♀
      Excludes1 vulval varices complicating childbirth and the puerperium (O87.8)
      vulval varices complicating pregnancy (O22.1-)
   I86.4 **Gastric varices**
   I86.8 **Varicose veins of other specified sites** A
      Varicose ulcer of nasal septum

● **I87** **Other disorders of veins**
   ● **I87.0** **Postthrombotic syndrome**
      Chronic venous hypertension due to deep vein thrombosis
      Postphlebitic syndrome
      Excludes1 chronic venous hypertension without deep vein thrombosis (I87.3-)
   ● **I87.00** **Postthrombotic syndrome without complications**
      Asymptomatic Postthrombotic syndrome
      I87.001 Postthrombotic syndrome without complications of right lower extremity
      I87.002 Postthrombotic syndrome without complications of left lower extremity
      I87.003 Postthrombotic syndrome without complications of bilateral lower extremity
      I87.009 Postthrombotic syndrome without complications of unspecified extremity
      Postthrombotic syndrome NOS
   ● **I87.01** **Postthrombotic syndrome with ulcer**
      Use additional code to specify site and severity of ulcer (L97.-)
      I87.011 Postthrombotic syndrome with ulcer of right lower extremity 🔍
      I87.012 Postthrombotic syndrome with ulcer of left lower extremity 🔍
      I87.013 Postthrombotic syndrome with ulcer of bilateral lower extremity 🔍
      I87.019 Postthrombotic syndrome with ulcer of unspecified lower extremity 🔍
   ● **I87.02** **Postthrombotic syndrome with inflammation**
      I87.021 Postthrombotic syndrome with inflammation of right lower extremity
      I87.022 Postthrombotic syndrome with inflammation of left lower extremity
      I87.023 Postthrombotic syndrome with inflammation of bilateral lower extremity
      I87.029 Postthrombotic syndrome with inflammation of unspecified lower extremity
   ● **I87.03** **Postthrombotic syndrome with ulcer and inflammation**
      Use additional code to specify site and severity of ulcer (L97.-)
      I87.031 Postthrombotic syndrome with ulcer and inflammation of right lower extremity 🔍
      I87.032 Postthrombotic syndrome with ulcer and inflammation of left lower extremity 🔍
      I87.033 Postthrombotic syndrome with ulcer and inflammation of bilateral lower extremity 🔍
      I87.039 Postthrombotic syndrome with ulcer and inflammation of unspecified lower extremity 🔍
   ● **I87.09** **Postthrombotic syndrome with other complications**
      I87.091 Postthrombotic syndrome with other complications of right lower extremity
      I87.092 Postthrombotic syndrome with other complications of left lower extremity
      I87.093 Postthrombotic syndrome with other complications of bilateral lower extremity
      I87.099 Postthrombotic syndrome with other complications of unspecified lower extremity

I87.1 **Compression of vein**
　　Stricture of vein
　　Vena cava syndrome (inferior) (superior)
　　　Excludes2　compression of pulmonary vein (I28.8)

I87.2 **Venous insufficiency (chronic) (peripheral)**
　　Stasis dermatitis
　　　Excludes1　stasis dermatitis with varicose veins of lower extremities (I83.1-, I83.2-)

● **I87.3** **Chronic venous hypertension (idiopathic)**
　　Stasis edema
　　　Excludes1　chronic venous hypertension due to deep vein thrombosis (I87.0-)
　　　　　　　　　varicose veins of lower extremities (I83.-)

　● **I87.30** **Chronic venous hypertension (idiopathic) without complications**
　　　Asymptomatic chronic venous hypertension (idiopathic)
　　　I87.301　**Chronic venous hypertension (idiopathic) without complications of right lower extremity**
　　　I87.302　**Chronic venous hypertension (idiopathic) without complications of left lower extremity**
　　　I87.303　**Chronic venous hypertension (idiopathic) without complications of bilateral lower extremity**
　　　I87.309　**Chronic venous hypertension (idiopathic) without complications of unspecified lower extremity**
　　　　　Chronic venous hypertension NOS

　● **I87.31** **Chronic venous hypertension (idiopathic) with ulcer**
　　　Use additional code to specify site and severity of ulcer (L97.-)
　　　I87.311　**Chronic venous hypertension (idiopathic) with ulcer of right lower extremity** 🦠
　　　I87.312　**Chronic venous hypertension (idiopathic) with ulcer of left lower extremity** 🦠
　　　I87.313　**Chronic venous hypertension (idiopathic) with ulcer of bilateral lower extremity** 🦠
　　　I87.319　**Chronic venous hypertension (idiopathic) with ulcer of unspecified lower extremity** 🦠

　● **I87.32** **Chronic venous hypertension (idiopathic) with inflammation**
　　　I87.321　**Chronic venous hypertension (idiopathic) with inflammation of right lower extremity**
　　　I87.322　**Chronic venous hypertension (idiopathic) with inflammation of left lower extremity**
　　　I87.323　**Chronic venous hypertension (idiopathic) with inflammation of bilateral lower extremity**
　　　I87.329　**Chronic venous hypertension (idiopathic) with inflammation of unspecified lower extremity**

　● **I87.33** **Chronic venous hypertension (idiopathic) with ulcer and inflammation**
　　　Use additional code to specify site and severity of ulcer (L97.-)
　　　I87.331　**Chronic venous hypertension (idiopathic) with ulcer and inflammation of right lower extremity** 🦠
　　　I87.332　**Chronic venous hypertension (idiopathic) with ulcer and inflammation of left lower extremity** 🦠

　　　I87.333　**Chronic venous hypertension (idiopathic) with ulcer and inflammation of bilateral lower extremity** 🦠
　　　I87.339　**Chronic venous hypertension (idiopathic) with ulcer and inflammation of unspecified lower extremity** 🦠

　● **I87.39** **Chronic venous hypertension (idiopathic) with other complications**
　　　I87.391　**Chronic venous hypertension (idiopathic) with other complications of right lower extremity**
　　　I87.392　**Chronic venous hypertension (idiopathic) with other complications of left lower extremity**
　　　I87.393　**Chronic venous hypertension (idiopathic) with other complications of bilateral lower extremity**
　　　I87.399　**Chronic venous hypertension (idiopathic) with other complications of unspecified lower extremity**

I87.8 **Other specified disorders of veins**
　　Phlebosclerosis
　　Venofibrosis

I87.9 **Disorder of vein, unspecified**

● **I88** **Nonspecific lymphadenitis**
　　　Excludes1　acute lymphadenitis, except mesenteric (L04.-)
　　　　　　　　　enlarged lymph nodes NOS (R59.-)
　　　　　　　　　human immunodeficiency virus [HIV] disease resulting in generalized lymphadenopathy (B20)

I88.0 **Nonspecific mesenteric lymphadenitis**
　　Mesenteric lymphadenitis (acute)(chronic)

I88.1 **Chronic lymphadenitis, except mesenteric**
　　Adenitis
　　Lymphadenitis

I88.8 **Other nonspecific lymphadenitis**

I88.9 **Nonspecific lymphadenitis, unspecified**
　　Lymphadenitis NOS

● **I89** **Other noninfective disorders of lymphatic vessels and lymph nodes**
　　　Excludes1　chylocele, tunica vaginalis (nonfilarial) NOS (N50.89)
　　　　　　　　　enlarged lymph nodes NOS (R59.-)
　　　　　　　　　filarial chylocele (B74.-)
　　　　　　　　　hereditary lymphedema (Q82.0)

I89.0 **Lymphedema, not elsewhere classified**
　　Elephantiasis (nonfilarial) NOS
　　Lymphangiectasis
　　Obliteration, lymphatic vessel
　　Praecox lymphedema
　　Secondary lymphedema
　　　Excludes1　postmastectomy lymphedema (I97.2)

I89.1 **Lymphangitis**
　　Chronic lymphangitis
　　Lymphangitis NOS
　　Subacute lymphangitis
　　　Excludes1　acute lymphangitis (L03.-)

I89.8 **Other specified noninfective disorders of lymphatic vessels and lymph nodes**
　　Chylocele (nonfilarial)
　　Chylous ascites
　　Chylous cyst
　　Lipomelanotic reticulosis
　　Lymph node or vessel fistula
　　Lymph node or vessel infarction
　　Lymph node or vessel rupture

I89.9 **Noninfective disorder of lymphatic vessels and lymph nodes, unspecified**
　　Disease of lymphatic vessels NOS

▶ New　⇒ Revised　~~deleted~~ Deleted　Excludes 1　Excludes 2　Includes　Use additional　Code first　Code also　Key words

OGCR Official Guidelines　X Assign placeholder X　● Use Additional Character(s)　▶ Manifestation Code　🦠 Hierarchical Condition Category　**Coding Clinic**

OTHER AND UNSPECIFIED DISORDERS OF THE CIRCULATORY SYSTEM (I95-I99)

● **I95**   **Hypotension**
Subnormal arterial blood pressure

     Excludes1   cardiovascular collapse (R57.9)
                maternal hypotension syndrome (O26.5-)
                nonspecific low blood pressure reading NOS (R03.1)

     I95.0   **Idiopathic hypotension**

     I95.1   **Orthostatic hypotension**
          Hypotension, postural
          Moving from a sitting or reclining position to a standing position precipitates a sudden drop in blood pressure (hypotension).

          Excludes1   neurogenic orthostatic hypotension [Shy-Drager] (G90.3)
                   orthostatic hypotension due to drugs (I95.2)

     I95.2   **Hypotension due to drugs**
          Orthostatic hypotension due to drugs

          Use additional code for adverse effect, if applicable, to identify drug (T36-T50 with fifth or sixth character 5)

     I95.3   **Hypotension of hemodialysis**
          Intra-dialytic hypotension

●   **I95.8**   **Other hypotension**

          I95.81   **Postprocedural hypotension**

          I95.89   **Other hypotension**
                   Chronic hypotension

     I95.9   **Hypotension, unspecified**

I96   **Gangrene, not elsewhere classified** 🔖
     Gangrenous cellulitis

     Excludes1   gangrene in atherosclerosis of native arteries of the extremities (I70.26)
                gangrene of certain specified sites - *see* Alphabetical Index
                gangrene in hernia (K40.1, K40.4, K41.1, K41.4, K42.1, K43.1-, K44.1, K45.1, K46.1)
                gangrene in other peripheral vascular diseases (I73.-)
                gas gangrene (A48.0)
                pyoderma gangrenosum (L88)

     Excludes2   gangrene in diabetes mellitus (E08-E13 with .52)

     Coding Clinic: 2018, Q4, P87; 2017, Q3, P6; 2013, Q2, P35

● **I97**   **Intraoperative and postprocedural complications and disorders of circulatory system, not elsewhere classified**

     Excludes2   postprocedural shock (T81.1-)

     Coding Clinic: 2019, Q2, P22

     I97.0   **Postcardiotomy syndrome**

●   **I97.1**   **Other postprocedural cardiac functional disturbances**

          Excludes2   acute pulmonary insufficiency following thoracic surgery (J95.1)
                   intraoperative cardiac functional disturbances (I97.7-)

     ●   **I97.11**   **Postprocedural cardiac insufficiency**

          I97.110   **Postprocedural cardiac insufficiency following cardiac surgery**

          I97.111   **Postprocedural cardiac insufficiency following other surgery**

     ●   **I97.12**   **Postprocedural cardiac arrest**

          I97.120   **Postprocedural cardiac arrest following cardiac surgery**

          I97.121   **Postprocedural cardiac arrest following other surgery**

     ●   **I97.13**   **Postprocedural heart failure**

          Use additional code to identify the heart failure (I50.-)

          I97.130   **Postprocedural heart failure following cardiac surgery**

          I97.131   **Postprocedural heart failure following other surgery**

●   **I97.19**   **Other postprocedural cardiac functional disturbances**

          Use additional code, if applicable, to further specify disorder

          I97.190   **Other postprocedural cardiac functional disturbances following cardiac surgery**

                Use Additional code, if applicable, for type 4 or type 5 myocardial infarction, to further specify disorder

                Coding Clinic: 2019, Q2, P32-33

          I97.191   **Other postprocedural cardiac functional disturbances following other surgery**

     I97.2   **Postmastectomy lymphedema syndrome**   A
          Elephantiasis due to mastectomy
          Obliteration of lymphatic vessels

     I97.3   **Postprocedural hypertension**

●   **I97.4**   **Intraoperative hemorrhage and hematoma of a circulatory system organ or structure complicating a procedure**

          Excludes1   intraoperative hemorrhage and hematoma of a circulatory system organ or structure due to accidental puncture and laceration during a procedure (I97.5-)

          Excludes2   intraoperative cerebrovascular hemorrhage complicating a procedure (G97.3-)

     ●   **I97.41**   **Intraoperative hemorrhage and hematoma of a circulatory system organ or structure complicating a circulatory system procedure**

          I97.410   **Intraoperative hemorrhage and hematoma of a circulatory system organ or structure complicating a cardiac catheterization**

          I97.411   **Intraoperative hemorrhage and hematoma of a circulatory system organ or structure complicating a cardiac bypass**

          I97.418   **Intraoperative hemorrhage and hematoma of a circulatory system organ or structure complicating other circulatory system procedure**

          I97.42   **Intraoperative hemorrhage and hematoma of a circulatory system organ or structure complicating other procedure**
                Coding Clinic: 2020, Q1, P20; 2016, Q4, P100

●   **I97.5**   **Accidental puncture and laceration of a circulatory system organ or structure during a procedure**

          Excludes2   accidental puncture and laceration of brain during a procedure (G97.4-)

          I97.51   **Accidental puncture and laceration of a circulatory system organ or structure during a circulatory system procedure**
                Coding Clinic: 2019, Q2, P24

          I97.52   **Accidental puncture and laceration of a circulatory system organ or structure during other procedure**

●   **I97.6**   **Postprocedural hemorrhage, hematoma and seroma of a circulatory system organ or structure following a procedure**

          Excludes2   postprocedural cerebrovascular hemorrhage complicating a procedure (G97.5-)

          Coding Clinic: 2016, Q4, P10

     ●   **I97.61**   **Postprocedural hemorrhage of a circulatory system organ or structure following a circulatory system procedure**

          I97.610   **Postprocedural hemorrhage of a circulatory system organ or structure following a cardiac catheterization**

I97.611   Postprocedural hemorrhage of a circulatory system organ or structure following cardiac bypass

I97.618   Postprocedural hemorrhage of a circulatory system organ or structure following other circulatory system procedure

● I97.62   Postprocedural hemorrhage, hematoma and seroma of a circulatory system organ or structure following other procedure

I97.620   Postprocedural hemorrhage of a circulatory system organ or structure following other procedure

I97.621   Postprocedural hematoma of a circulatory system organ or structure following other procedure

I97.622   Postprocedural seroma of a circulatory system organ or structure following other procedure

● I97.63   Postprocedural hematoma of a circulatory system organ or structure following a circulatory system procedure

I97.630   Postprocedural hematoma of a circulatory system organ or structure following a cardiac catheterization

I97.631   Postprocedural hematoma of a circulatory system organ or structure following cardiac bypass

I97.638   Postprocedural hematoma of a circulatory system organ or structure following other circulatory system procedure

● I97.64   Postprocedural seroma of a circulatory system organ or structure following a circulatory system procedure

I97.640   Postprocedural seroma of a circulatory system organ or structure following a cardiac catheterization

I97.641   Postprocedural seroma of a circulatory system organ or structure following cardiac bypass

I97.648   Postprocedural seroma of a circulatory system organ or structure following other circulatory system procedure

● I97.7   Intraoperative cardiac functional disturbances

Excludes2   acute pulmonary insufficiency following thoracic surgery (J95.1)
postprocedural cardiac functional disturbances (I97.1-)

● I97.71   Intraoperative cardiac arrest

I97.710   Intraoperative cardiac arrest during cardiac surgery

I97.711   Intraoperative cardiac arrest during other surgery

● I97.79   Other intraoperative cardiac functional disturbances

Use additional code, if applicable, to further specify disorder

I97.790   Other intraoperative cardiac functional disturbances during cardiac surgery

I97.791   Other intraoperative cardiac functional disturbances during other surgery

● I97.8   Other intraoperative and postprocedural complications and disorders of the circulatory system, not elsewhere classified

Use additional code, if applicable, to further specify disorder

● I97.81   Intraoperative cerebrovascular infarction

I97.810   Intraoperative cerebrovascular infarction during cardiac surgery 🐾

I97.811   Intraoperative cerebrovascular infarction during other surgery 🐾

● I97.82   Postprocedural cerebrovascular infarction

I97.820   Postprocedural cerebrovascular infarction following cardiac surgery 🐾

I97.821   Postprocedural cerebrovascular infarction following other surgery 🐾

I97.88   Other intraoperative complications of the circulatory system, not elsewhere classified

I97.89   Other postprocedural complications and disorders of the circulatory system, not elsewhere classified
Coding Clinic: 2019, Q2, P32-33

● I99   Other and unspecified disorders of circulatory system

I99.8   Other disorder of circulatory system

I99.9   Unspecified disorder of circulatory system

CHAPTER 10

DISEASES OF THE RESPIRATORY SYSTEM
(J00-J99)

OGCR Chapter-Specific Coding Guidelines

10. **Chapter 10: Diseases of the Respiratory System (J00-J99)**

   a. **Chronic Obstructive Pulmonary Disease [COPD] and Asthma**

   1) **Acute exacerbation of chronic obstructive bronchitis and asthma**

   The codes in categories J44 and J45 distinguish between uncomplicated cases and those in acute exacerbation. An acute exacerbation is a worsening or a decompensation of a chronic condition. An acute exacerbation is not equivalent to an infection superimposed on a chronic condition, though an exacerbation may be triggered by an infection.

   b. **Acute Respiratory Failure**

   1) **Acute respiratory failure as principal diagnosis**

   A code from subcategory J96.0, Acute respiratory failure, or subcategory J96.2, Acute and chronic respiratory failure, may be assigned as a principal diagnosis when it is the condition established after study to be chiefly responsible for occasioning the admission to the hospital, and the selection is supported by the Alphabetic Index and Tabular List. However, chapter-specific coding guidelines (such as obstetrics, poisoning, HIV, newborn) that provide sequencing direction take precedence.

   2) **Acute respiratory failure as secondary diagnosis**

   Respiratory failure may be listed as a secondary diagnosis if it occurs after admission, or if it is present on admission, but does not meet the definition of principal diagnosis.

   3) **Sequencing of acute respiratory failure and another acute condition**

   When a patient is admitted with respiratory failure and another acute condition (e.g., myocardial infarction, cerebrovascular accident, aspiration pneumonia), the principal diagnosis will not be the same in every situation. This applies whether the other acute condition is a respiratory or nonrespiratory condition. Selection of the principal diagnosis will be dependent on the circumstances of admission. If both the respiratory failure and the other acute condition are equally responsible for occasioning the admission to the hospital, and there are no chapter-specific sequencing rules, the guideline regarding two or more diagnoses that equally meet the definition for principal diagnosis (*Section II, C.*) may be applied in these situations.

   If the documentation is not clear as to whether acute respiratory failure and another condition are equally responsible for occasioning the admission, query the provider for clarification.

   c. **Influenza due to certain identified influenza viruses**

   Code only confirmed cases of influenza due to certain identified influenza viruses (category J09), and due to other identified influenza virus (category J10). This is an exception to the hospital inpatient guideline Section II, H. (Uncertain Diagnosis).

   In this context, "confirmation" does not require documentation of positive laboratory testing specific for avian or other novel influenza A or other identified influenza virus. However, coding should be based on the provider's diagnostic statement that the patient has avian influenza, or other novel influenza A, for category J09, or has another particular identified strain of influenza, such as H1N1 or H3N2, but not identified as novel or variant, for category J10.

   If the provider records "suspected" or "possible" or "probable" avian influenza, or novel influenza, or other identified influenza, then the appropriate influenza code from category J11, Influenza due to unidentified influenza virus, should be assigned. A code from category J09, Influenza due to certain identified influenza viruses, should not be assigned nor should a code from category J10, Influenza due to other identified influenza virus.

   d. **Ventilator associated Pneumonia**

   1) **Documentation of Ventilator associated Pneumonia**

   As with all procedural or postprocedural complications, code assignment is based on the provider's documentation of the relationship between the condition and the procedure.

   Code J95.851, Ventilator associated pneumonia, should be assigned only when the provider has documented ventilator associated pneumonia (VAP). An additional code to identify the organism (e.g., Pseudomonas aeruginosa, code B96.5) should also be assigned. Do not assign an additional code from categories J12-J18 to identify the type of pneumonia.

   Code J95.851 should not be assigned for cases where the patient has pneumonia and is on a mechanical ventilator and the provider has not specifically stated that the pneumonia is ventilator associated pneumonia. If the documentation is unclear as to whether the patient has a pneumonia that is a complication attributable to the mechanical ventilator, query the provider.

   2) **Ventilator associated Pneumonia Develops after Admission**

   A patient may be admitted with one type of pneumonia (e.g., code J13, Pneumonia due to Streptococcus pneumonia) and subsequently develop VAP. In this instance, the principal diagnosis would be the appropriate code from categories J12-J18 for the pneumonia diagnosed at the time of admission. Code J95.851, Ventilator associated pneumonia, would be assigned as an additional diagnosis when the provider has also documented the presence of ventilator associated pneumonia.

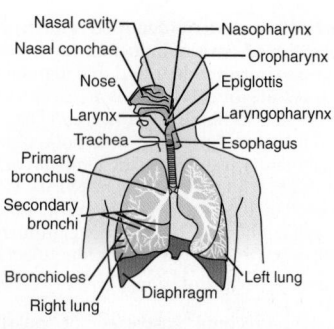

Figure 10-1 Respiratory system. (From Buck CJ: Step-by-Step Medical Coding, ed 2016, St. Louis, Elsevier, 2016)

Figure 10-2 Paranasal sinuses. (From Buck CJ: Step-by-Step Medical Coding, ed 2016, St. Louis, Elsevier, 2016)

Item 10-1 Pharyngitis is painful inflammation of the pharynx (sore throat). Ninety percent of the infections are caused by a virus with the remaining being bacterial and rarely a fungus (candidiasis). Other irritants such as pollutants, chemicals, or smoke may cause similar symptoms.

CHAPTER 10

DISEASES OF THE RESPIRATORY SYSTEM (J00-J99)

Note: When a respiratory condition is described as occurring in more than one site and is not specifically indexed, it should be classified to the lower anatomic site (e.g., tracheobronchitis to bronchitis in J40).

Use additional code, where applicable, to identify:
    exposure to environmental tobacco smoke (Z77.22)
    exposure to tobacco smoke in the perinatal period (P96.81)
    history of tobacco dependence (Z87.891)
    occupational exposure to environmental tobacco smoke (Z57.31)
    tobacco dependence (F17.-)
    tobacco use (Z72.0)

Excludes2   certain conditions originating in the perinatal period (P04-P96)
       certain infectious and parasitic diseases (A00-B99)
       complications of pregnancy, childbirth and the puerperium (O00-O99A)
       congenital malformations, deformations and chromosomal abnormalities (Q00-Q99)
       endocrine, nutritional and metabolic diseases (E00-E88)
       injury, poisoning and certain other consequences of external causes (S00-T88)
       neoplasms (C00-D49)
       smoke inhalation (T59.81-)
       symptoms, signs and abnormal clinical and laboratory findings, not elsewhere classified (R00-R94)

This chapter contains the following blocks:

J00-J06	Acute upper respiratory infections
J09-J18	Influenza and pneumonia
J20-J22	Other acute lower respiratory infections
J30-J39	Other diseases of upper respiratory tract
J40-J47	Chronic lower respiratory diseases
J60-J70	Lung diseases due to external agents
J80-J84	Other respiratory diseases principally affecting the interstitium
J85-J86	Suppurative and necrotic conditions of the lower respiratory tract
J90-J94	Other diseases of the pleura
J95	Intraoperative and postprocedural complications and disorders of respiratory system, not elsewhere classified
J96-J99	Other diseases of the respiratory system

ACUTE UPPER RESPIRATORY INFECTIONS (J00-J06)

Excludes1   chronic obstructive pulmonary disease with acute lower respiratory infection (J44.0)

J00   **Acute nasopharyngitis [common cold]**
    Acute rhinitis
    Coryza (acute)
    Infective nasopharyngitis NOS
    Infective rhinitis
    Nasal catarrh, acute
    Nasopharyngitis NOS

    Excludes1   acute pharyngitis (J02.-)
        acute sore throat NOS (J02.9)
        influenza virus with other respiratory manifestations (J09.X2, J10.1, J11.1)
        pharyngitis NOS (J02.9)
        rhinitis NOS (J31.0)
        sore throat NOS (J02.9)

    Excludes2   allergic rhinitis (J30.1-J30.9)
        chronic pharyngitis (J31.2)
        chronic rhinitis (J31.0)
        chronic sore throat (J31.2)
        nasopharyngitis, chronic (J31.1)
        vasomotor rhinitis (J30.0)

★ **(See Plate 27 of the Anatomy Illustrations.)**

● **J01**   **Acute sinusitis**

    Includes   acute abscess of sinus
        acute empyema of sinus
        acute infection of sinus
        acute inflammation of sinus
        acute suppuration of sinus

    Use additional code (B95-B97) to identify infectious agent.

    Excludes1   sinusitis NOS (J32.9)
    Excludes2   chronic sinusitis (J32.0-J32.8)

● **J01.0**   **Acute maxillary sinusitis**
    Acute antritis

    J01.00   Acute maxillary sinusitis, **unspecified**
    J01.01   Acute **recurrent** maxillary sinusitis

● **J01.1**   **Acute frontal sinusitis**
    J01.10   Acute frontal sinusitis, **unspecified**
    J01.11   Acute **recurrent** frontal sinusitis

● **J01.2**   **Acute ethmoidal sinusitis**
    J01.20   Acute ethmoidal sinusitis, **unspecified**
    J01.21   Acute **recurrent** ethmoidal sinusitis

● **J01.3**   **Acute sphenoidal sinusitis**
    J01.30   Acute sphenoidal sinusitis, **unspecified**
    J01.31   Acute **recurrent** sphenoidal sinusitis

● **J01.4**   **Acute pansinusitis**
    J01.40   Acute pansinusitis, **unspecified**
    J01.41   Acute **recurrent** pansinusitis

- **J01.8**   **Other acute sinusitis**
  - **J01.80**   **Other acute sinusitis**
    - Acute sinusitis involving more than one sinus but not pansinusitis
  - **J01.81**   **Other acute recurrent sinusitis**
    - Acute recurrent sinusitis involving more than one sinus but not pansinusitis
- **J01.9**   **Acute sinusitis, unspecified**
  - **J01.90**   **Acute sinusitis, unspecified**
  - **J01.91**   **Acute recurrent sinusitis, unspecified**

- **J02**   **Acute pharyngitis**
  - **Includes**   acute sore throat
  - **Excludes1**   acute laryngopharyngitis (J06.0)
    - peritonsillar abscess (J36)
    - pharyngeal abscess (J39.1)
    - retropharyngeal abscess (J39.0)
  - **Excludes2**   chronic pharyngitis (J31.2)
  - **J02.0**   **Streptococcal pharyngitis**
    - Septic pharyngitis
    - Streptococcal sore throat
    - **Excludes2**   scarlet fever (A38.-)
  - **J02.8**   **Acute pharyngitis due to other specified organisms**
    - Use additional code (B95-B97) to identify infectious agent
    - **Excludes1**   pharyngitis due to coxsackie virus (B08.5)
      - pharyngitis due to gonococcus (A54.5)
      - acute pharyngitis due to herpes [simplex] virus (B00.2)
      - acute pharyngitis due to infectious mononucleosis (B27.-)
      - enteroviral vesicular pharyngitis (B08.5)
  - **J02.9**   **Acute pharyngitis, unspecified**
    - Gangrenous pharyngitis (acute)
    - Infective pharyngitis (acute) NOS
    - Pharyngitis (acute) NOS
    - Sore throat (acute) NOS
    - Suppurative pharyngitis (acute)
    - Ulcerative pharyngitis (acute)
    - **Excludes1**   influenza virus with other respiratory manifestations (J09.X2, J10.1, J11.1)

- **J03**   **Acute tonsillitis**
  - *Inflammation of pharyngeal tonsils caused by virus or bacteria*
  - **Excludes1**   acute sore throat (J02.-)
    - hypertrophy of tonsils (J35.1)
    - peritonsillar abscess (J36)
    - sore throat NOS (J02.9)
    - streptococcal sore throat (J02.0)
  - **Excludes2**   chronic tonsillitis (J35.0)
  - **J03.0**   **Streptococcal tonsillitis**
    - **J03.00**   **Acute streptococcal tonsillitis, unspecified**
    - **J03.01**   **Acute recurrent streptococcal tonsillitis**
  - **J03.8**   **Acute tonsillitis due to other specified organisms**
    - Use additional code (B95-B97) to identify infectious agent.
    - **Excludes1**   diphtheritic tonsillitis (A36.0)
      - herpesviral pharyngotonsillitis (B00.2)
      - streptococcal tonsillitis (J03.0)
      - tuberculous tonsillitis (A15.8)
      - Vincent's tonsillitis (A69.1)
    - **J03.80**   **Acute tonsillitis due to other specified organisms**
    - **J03.81**   **Acute recurrent tonsillitis due to other specified organisms**

Item 10-2   **Laryngitis** is an inflammation of the larynx (voice box) resulting in hoarse voice or the complete loss of the voice. **Tracheitis** is an inflammation of the trachea (often following a URI) commonly caused by *staphylococcus aureus* resulting in inspiratory stridor (crowing sound on inspiration) and a crouplike cough.

- **J03.9**   **Acute tonsillitis, unspecified**
  - Follicular tonsillitis (acute)
  - Gangrenous tonsillitis (acute)
  - Infective tonsillitis (acute)
  - Tonsillitis (acute) NOS
  - Ulcerative tonsillitis (acute)
  - **Excludes1**   influenza virus with other respiratory manifestations (J09.X2, J10.1, J11.1)
  - **J03.90**   **Acute tonsillitis, unspecified**
  - **J03.91**   **Acute recurrent tonsillitis, unspecified**

- **J04**   **Acute laryngitis and tracheitis**
  - Use additional code (B95-B97) to identify infectious agent.
  - Code also influenza, if present, such as:
    - influenza due to identified novel influenza A virus with other respiratory manifestations (J09.X2)
    - influenza due to other identified influenza virus with other respiratory manifestations (J10.1)
    - influenza due to unidentified influenza virus with other respiratory manifestations (J11.1)
  - **Excludes1**   acute obstructive laryngitis [croup] and epiglottitis (J05.-)
  - **Excludes2**   laryngismus (stridulus) (J38.5)
  - **J04.0**   **Acute laryngitis**
    - Edematous laryngitis (acute)
    - Laryngitis (acute) NOS
    - Subglottic laryngitis (acute)
    - Suppurative laryngitis (acute)
    - Ulcerative laryngitis (acute)
    - **Excludes1**   acute obstructive laryngitis (J05.0)
    - **Excludes2**   chronic laryngitis (J37.0)
  - **J04.1**   **Acute tracheitis**
    - Acute viral tracheitis
    - Catarrhal tracheitis (acute)
    - Tracheitis (acute) NOS
    - **Excludes2**   chronic tracheitis (J42)
    - **J04.10**   **Acute tracheitis without obstruction**
    - **J04.11**   **Acute tracheitis with obstruction**
  - **J04.2**   **Acute laryngotracheitis**
    - Laryngotracheitis NOS
    - Tracheitis (acute) with laryngitis (acute)
    - **Excludes1**   acute obstructive laryngotracheitis (J05.0)
    - **Excludes2**   chronic laryngotracheitis (J37.1)
  - **J04.3**   **Supraglottitis, unspecified**
    - **J04.30**   **Supraglottitis, unspecified, without obstruction**
    - **J04.31**   **Supraglottitis, unspecified, with obstruction**

- **J05**   **Acute obstructive laryngitis [croup] and epiglottitis**
  - Use additional code (B95-B97) to identify infectious agent.
  - Code also influenza, if present, such as:
    - influenza due to identified novel influenza A virus with other respiratory manifestations (J09.X2)
    - influenza due to other identified influenza virus with other respiratory manifestations (J10.1)
    - influenza due to unidentified influenza virus with other respiratory manifestations (J11.1)
  - **J05.0**   **Acute obstructive laryngitis [croup]**
    - Obstructive laryngitis (acute) NOS
    - Obstructive laryngotracheitis NOS
  - **J05.1**   **Acute epiglottitis**
    - **Excludes2**   epiglottitis, chronic (J37.0)
    - **J05.10**   **Acute epiglottitis without obstruction**
      - Epiglottitis NOS
    - **J05.11**   **Acute epiglottitis with obstruction**

CHAPTER 10 (J00-J99)

● **J06**   **Acute upper respiratory infections of multiple and unspecified sites**

> **Excludes1**   acute respiratory infection NOS (J22)
> influenza virus with other respiratory manifestations (J09.X2, J10.1, J11.1)
> streptococcal pharyngitis (J02.0)
>
> Coding Clinic: 2020, Q1, P22

J06.0   **Acute laryngopharyngitis**

J06.9   **Acute upper respiratory infection, unspecified**
> Upper respiratory disease, acute
> Upper respiratory infection NOS
>
> Use additional code (B95-B97) to identify infectious agent, if known, such as:
> respiratory syncytial virus (RSV) (B97.4)

INFLUENZA AND PNEUMONIA (J09-J18)

> **Excludes2**   allergic or eosinophilic pneumonia (J82)
> aspiration pneumonia NOS (J69.0)
> meconium pneumonia (P24.01)
> neonatal aspiration pneumonia (P24.-)
> pneumonia due to solids and liquids (J69.-)
> congenital pneumonia (P23.9)
> lipid pneumonia (J69.1)
> rheumatic pneumonia (I00)
> ventilator associated pneumonia (J95.851)
>
> Coding Clinic: 2020, Q1, P22

● **J09**   **Influenza due to certain identified influenza viruses**

> **Excludes1**   influenza A/H1N1 (J10.-)
> influenza due to other influenza viruses (J10.-)
> influenza due to unidentified influenza virus (J11.-)
> seasonal influenza due to other identified influenza virus (J10.-)
> seasonal influenza due to unidentified influenza virus (J11.-)

● **J09.X**   **Influenza due to identified novel influenza A virus**
> Avian influenza
> Bird influenza
> Influenza A/H5N1
> Influenza of other animal origin, not bird or swine
> Swine influenza virus (viruses that normally cause infections in pigs)
> Coding Clinic: 2016, Q3, P11

J09.X1   **Influenza due to identified novel influenza A virus with pneumonia**
> Code also , if applicable, associated:
> lung abscess (J85.1)
> other specified type of pneumonia

J09.X2   **Influenza due to identified novel influenza A virus with other respiratory manifestations**
> Influenza due to identified novel influenza A virus NOS
> Influenza due to identified novel influenza A virus with laryngitis
> Influenza due to identified novel influenza A virus with pharyngitis
> Influenza due to identified novel influenza A virus with upper respiratory symptoms
>
> Use additional code, if applicable, for associated:
> pleural effusion (J91.8)
> sinusitis (J01.-)

J09.X3   **Influenza due to identified novel influenza A virus with gastrointestinal manifestations**
> Influenza due to identified novel influenza A virus gastroenteritis
>
> > **Excludes1**   'intestinal flu' [viral gastroenteritis] (A08.-)

J09.X9   **Influenza due to identified novel influenza A virus with other manifestations**
> Influenza due to identified novel influenza A virus with encephalopathy
> Influenza due to identified novel influenza A virus with myocarditis
> Influenza due to identified novel influenza A virus with otitis media
>
> Use additional code to identify manifestation

● **J10**   **Influenza due to other identified influenza virus**

> **Includes**   influenza A (non-novel)
> influenza B
> influenza C
>
> **Excludes1**   influenza due to avian influenza virus (J09.X-)
> influenza due to swine flu (J09.X-)
> influenza due to unidentified influenza virus (J11.-)

● **J10.0**   **Influenza due to other identified influenza virus with pneumonia**
> Code also associated lung abscess, if applicable (J85.1)

J10.00   **Influenza due to other identified influenza virus with unspecified type of pneumonia**

J10.01   **Influenza due to other identified influenza virus with the same other identified influenza virus pneumonia**

J10.08   **Influenza due to other identified influenza virus with other specified pneumonia**
> Code also other specified type of pneumonia
> Coding Clinic: 2017, Q4, P96

J10.1   **Influenza due to other identified influenza virus with other respiratory manifestations**
> Influenza due to other identified influenza virus NOS
> Influenza due to other identified influenza virus with laryngitis
> Influenza due to other identified influenza virus with pharyngitis
> Influenza due to other identified influenza virus with upper respiratory symptoms
>
> Use additional code for associated pleural effusion, if applicable (J91.8)
>
> Use additional code for associated sinusitis, if applicable (J01.-)
> Coding Clinic: 2016, Q3, P11

J10.2   **Influenza due to other identified influenza virus with gastrointestinal manifestations**
> Influenza due to other identified influenza virus gastroenteritis
>
> **Excludes1**   'intestinal flu' [viral gastroenteritis] (A08.-)

● **J10.8**   **Influenza due to other identified influenza virus with other manifestations**

J10.81   **Influenza due to other identified influenza virus with encephalopathy**

J10.82   **Influenza due to other identified influenza virus with myocarditis**

J10.83   **Influenza due to other identified influenza virus with otitis media**
> Use additional code for any associated perforated tympanic membrane (H72.-)

J10.89   **Influenza due to other identified influenza virus with other manifestations**
> Use additional codes to identify the manifestations

▶ New   ➡ Revised   ~~deleted~~ Deleted   Excludes 1   Excludes 2   Includes   Use additional   Code first   Code also   Key words

OGCR Official Guidelines   X Assign placeholder X   ● Use Additional Character(s)   ▶ Manifestation Code   🆁 Hierarchical Condition Category   **Coding Clinic**

● **J11   Influenza due to unidentified influenza virus**
  ● **J11.0   Influenza due to unidentified influenza virus with pneumonia**
     Code also associated lung abscess, if applicable (J85.1)
    J11.00   Influenza due to unidentified influenza virus with unspecified type of pneumonia
     Influenza with pneumonia NOS
     Coding Clinic: 2016, Q3, P12
    J11.08   Influenza due to unidentified influenza virus with specified pneumonia
     Code also other specified type of pneumonia
  J11.1   Influenza due to unidentified influenza virus with other respiratory manifestations
    Influenza NOS
    Influenzal laryngitis NOS
    Influenzal pharyngitis NOS
    Influenza with upper respiratory symptoms NOS
    Use additional code for associated pleural effusion, if applicable (J91.8)
    Use additional code for associated sinusitis, if applicable (J01.-)
  J11.2   Influenza due to unidentified influenza virus with gastrointestinal manifestations
    Influenza gastroenteritis NOS
    Excludes1   'intestinal flu' [viral gastroenteritis] (A08.-)
  ● **J11.8   Influenza due to unidentified influenza virus with other manifestations**
    J11.81   Influenza due to unidentified influenza virus with encephalopathy
     Influenzal encephalopathy NOS
    J11.82   Influenza due to unidentified influenza virus with myocarditis
     Influenzal myocarditis NOS
    J11.83   Influenza due to unidentified influenza virus with otitis media
     Influenzal otitis media NOS
     Use additional code for any associated perforated tympanic membrane (H72.-)
    J11.89   Influenza due to unidentified influenza virus with other manifestations
     Use additional codes to identify the manifestations

● **J12   Viral pneumonia, not elsewhere classified**
  Includes   bronchopneumonia due to viruses other than influenza viruses
  Code first associated influenza, if applicable (J09.X1, J10.0-, J11.0-)
  Code also associated abscess, if applicable (J85.1)
  Excludes1   aspiration pneumonia due to anesthesia during labor and delivery (O74.0)
    aspiration pneumonia due to anesthesia during pregnancy (O29)
    aspiration pneumonia due to anesthesia during puerperium (O89.0)
    aspiration pneumonia due to solids and liquids (J69.-)
    aspiration pneumonia NOS (J69.0)
    congenital pneumonia (P23.0)
    congenital rubella pneumonitis (P35.0)
    interstitial pneumonia NOS (J84.9)
    lipid pneumonia (J69.1)
    neonatal aspiration pneumonia (P24.-)
  Coding Clinic: 2021, Q1, P34
  J12.0   Adenoviral pneumonia
  J12.1   Respiratory syncytial virus pneumonia
    RSV pneumonia
  J12.2   Parainfluenza virus pneumonia
  J12.3   Human metapneumovirus pneumonia

Item 10-3 Pneumonia is an infection of the lungs, caused by a variety of microorganisms, including viruses, most commonly the Streptococcus pneumoniae (pneumococcus) bacteria, fungi, and parasites. Pneumonia occurs when the immune system is weakened, often by a URI or influenza.

  ● **J12.8   Other viral pneumonia**
    J12.81   Pneumonia due to SARS-associated coronavirus
     Severe acute respiratory syndrome NOS
    J12.82   Pneumonia due to coronavirus disease 2019
     Pneumonia due to 2019 novel coronavirus (SARS-CoV-2)
     Pneumonia due to COVID-19
     Code first COVID-19 (U07.1)
     Coding Clinic: 2021, Q1, P33-34, 42, 47, 49
    J12.89   Other viral pneumonia
     Coding Clinic: 2021, Q1, P33-34
  J12.9   Viral pneumonia, unspecified
J13   Pneumonia due to Streptococcus pneumoniae 🦠
  Bronchopneumonia due to S. pneumoniae
  Code first associated influenza, if applicable (J09.X1, J10.0-, J11.0-)
  Code also associated abscess, if applicable (J85.1)
  Excludes1   congenital pneumonia due to S. pneumoniae (P23.6)
    lobar pneumonia, unspecified organism (J18.1)
    pneumonia due to other streptococci (J15.3-J15.4)
J14   Pneumonia due to Hemophilus influenzae 🦠
  Bronchopneumonia due to H. influenzae
  Code first associated influenza, if applicable (J09.X1, J10.0-, J11.0-)
  Code also associated abscess, if applicable (J85.1)
  Excludes1   congenital pneumonia due to H. influenzae (P23.6)
● **J15   Bacterial pneumonia, not elsewhere classified**
  Includes   bronchopneumonia due to bacteria other than S. pneumoniae and H. influenzae
  Code first associated influenza, if applicable (J09.X1, J10.0-, J11.0-)
  Code also associated abscess, if applicable (J85.1)
  Excludes1   chlamydial pneumonia (J16.0)
    congenital pneumonia (P23.-)
    Legionnaires' disease (A48.1)
    spirochetal pneumonia (A69.8)
  J15.0   Pneumonia due to Klebsiella pneumoniae 🦠
  J15.1   Pneumonia due to Pseudomonas 🦠
  ● **J15.2   Pneumonia due to staphylococcus**
    J15.20   Pneumonia due to staphylococcus, unspecified
    ● **J15.21   Pneumonia due to staphylococcus aureus**
      J15.211   Pneumonia due to Methicillin susceptible Staphylococcus aureus 🦠
       MSSA pneumonia
       Pneumonia due to Staphylococcus aureus NOS
      J15.212   Pneumonia due to Methicillin resistant Staphylococcus aureus 🦠
    J15.29   Pneumonia due to other staphylococcus
  J15.3   Pneumonia due to streptococcus, group B 🦠
  J15.4   Pneumonia due to other streptococci 🦠
    Excludes1   pneumonia due to streptococcus, group B (J15.3)
     pneumonia due to Streptococcus pneumoniae (J13)
  J15.5   Pneumonia due to Escherichia coli 🦠
  J15.6   Pneumonia due to other Gram-negative bacteria 🦠
    Pneumonia due to other aerobic Gram-negative bacteria
    Pneumonia due to Serratia marcescens
  J15.7   Pneumonia due to Mycoplasma pneumoniae
  J15.8   Pneumonia due to other specified bacteria 🦠
  J15.9   Unspecified bacterial pneumonia
    Pneumonia due to gram-positive bacteria
    Coding Clinic: 2017, Q4, P96

CHAPTER 10 (J00-J99)

● **J16**   **Pneumonia due to other infectious organisms, not elsewhere classified**

Code first associated influenza, if applicable (J09.X1, J10.0-, J11.0-)

Code also associated abscess, if applicable (J85.1)

> **Excludes1**   congenital pneumonia (P23.-)
> ornithosis (A70)
> pneumocystosis (B59)
> pneumonia NOS (J18.9)

J16.0   **Chlamydial pneumonia**

J16.8   **Pneumonia due to other specified infectious organisms**

▶ **J17**   *Pneumonia in diseases classified elsewhere*

Code first underlying disease, such as:
> Q fever (A78)
> rheumatic fever (I00)
> schistosomiasis (B65.0-B65.9)

> **Excludes1**   candidial pneumonia (B37.1)
> chlamydial pneumonia (J16.0)
> gonorrheal pneumonia (A54.84)
> histoplasmosis pneumonia (B39.0-B39.2)
> measles pneumonia (B05.2)
> nocardiosis pneumonia (A43.0)
> pneumocystosis (B59)
> pneumonia due to Pneumocystis carinii (B59)
> pneumonia due to Pneumocystis jiroveci (B59)
> pneumonia in actinomycosis (A42.0)
> pneumonia in anthrax (A22.1)
> pneumonia in ascariasis (B77.81)
> pneumonia in aspergillosis (B44.0-B44.1)
> pneumonia in coccidioidomycosis (B38.0-B38.2)
> pneumonia in cytomegalovirus disease (B25.0)
> pneumonia in toxoplasmosis (B58.3)
> rubella pneumonia (B06.81)
> salmonella pneumonia (A02.22)
> spirochetal infection NEC with pneumonia (A69.8)
> tularemia pneumonia (A21.2)
> typhoid fever with pneumonia (A01.03)
> varicella pneumonia (B01.2)
> whooping cough with pneumonia (A37 with fifth-character 1)

● **J18**   **Pneumonia, unspecified organism**

Code first associated influenza, if applicable (J09.X1, J10.0-, J11.0-)

> **Excludes1**   abscess of lung with pneumonia (J85.1)
> aspiration pneumonia due to anesthesia during labor and delivery (O74.0)
> aspiration pneumonia due to anesthesia during pregnancy (O29)
> aspiration pneumonia due to anesthesia during puerperium (O89.0)
> aspiration pneumonia due to solids and liquids (J69.-)
> aspiration pneumonia NOS (J69.0)
> congenital pneumonia (P23.0)
> drug-induced interstitial lung disorder (J70.2-J70.4)
> interstitial pneumonia NOS (J84.9)
> lipid pneumonia (J69.1)
> neonatal aspiration pneumonia (P24.-)
> pneumonitis due to external agents (J67-J70)
> pneumonitis due to fumes and vapors (J68.0)
> usual interstitial pneumonia (J84.178)

J18.0   **Bronchopneumonia, unspecified organism**

> **Excludes1**   hypostatic bronchopneumonia (J18.2)
> lipid pneumonia (J69.1)

> **Excludes2**   acute bronchiolitis (J21.-)
> chronic bronchitis (J44.9)

J18.1   **Lobar pneumonia, unspecified organism** 🅗
     Coding Clinic: 2016, Q3, P15

J18.2   **Hypostatic pneumonia, unspecified organism**
     Hypostatic bronchopneumonia
     Passive pneumonia

J18.8   **Other pneumonia, unspecified organism**

J18.9   **Pneumonia, unspecified organism**
     Coding Clinic: Q3, P15; 2019, Q2, P28; Q1, P36; 2016, Q3, P15; 2012, Q4, P94

OTHER ACUTE LOWER RESPIRATORY INFECTIONS (J20-J22)

> **Excludes2**   chronic obstructive pulmonary disease with acute lower respiratory infection (J44.0)

● **J20**   **Acute bronchitis**

Inflammation/irritation of the bronchial tubes lasting 2-3 weeks, most commonly caused by a virus

> **Includes**   acute and subacute bronchitis (with) bronchospasm
> acute and subacute bronchitis (with) tracheitis
> acute and subacute bronchitis (with) tracheobronchitis, acute
> acute and subacute fibrinous bronchitis
> acute and subacute membranous bronchitis
> acute and subacute purulent bronchitis
> acute and subacute septic bronchitis

> **Excludes1**   bronchitis NOS (J40)
> tracheobronchitis NOS (J40)

> **Excludes2**   acute bronchitis with bronchiectasis (J47.0)
> acute bronchitis with chronic obstructive asthma (J44.0)
> acute bronchitis with chronic obstructive pulmonary disease (J44.0)
> allergic bronchitis NOS (J45.909-)
> bronchitis due to chemicals, fumes and vapors (J68.0)
> chronic bronchitis NOS (J42)
> chronic mucopurulent bronchitis (J41.1)
> chronic obstructive bronchitis (J44.-)
> chronic obstructive tracheobronchitis (J44.-)
> chronic simple bronchitis (J41.0)
> chronic tracheobronchitis (J42)

J20.0   **Acute bronchitis due to Mycoplasma pneumoniae**

J20.1   **Acute bronchitis due to Hemophilus influenzae**

J20.2   **Acute bronchitis due to streptococcus**

J20.3   **Acute bronchitis due to coxsackievirus**

J20.4   **Acute bronchitis due to parainfluenza virus**

J20.5   **Acute bronchitis due to respiratory syncytial virus**
     Acute bronchitis due to RSV

J20.6   **Acute bronchitis due to rhinovirus**
     Coding Clinic: 2016, Q3, P10

J20.7   **Acute bronchitis due to echovirus**

J20.8   **Acute bronchitis due to other specified organisms**
     Coding Clinic: 2016, Q3, P11

J20.9   **Acute bronchitis, unspecified**
     Coding Clinic: 2019, Q1, P35; 2016, Q3, P16

● **J21**   **Acute bronchiolitis**

Bronchiolitis obliterans with organizing pneumonia (BOOP) inflammation of bronchioles and surrounding tissue in lung

> **Includes**   acute bronchiolitis with bronchospasm

> **Excludes2**   respiratory bronchiolitis interstitial lung disease (J84.115)

J21.0   **Acute bronchiolitis due to respiratory syncytial virus**
     Acute bronchitis due to RSV

J21.1   **Acute bronchiolitis due to human metapneumovirus**

J21.8   **Acute bronchiolitis due to other specified organisms**

J21.9   **Acute bronchiolitis, unspecified**
     Bronchiolitis (acute)

> **Excludes1**   chronic bronchiolitis (J44.-)

J22   **Unspecified acute lower respiratory infection**
     Acute (lower) respiratory (tract) infection NOS

> **Excludes1**   upper respiratory infection (acute) (J06.9)

     Coding Clinic: 2020, Q1, P22-23

▶ New   ⇒ Revised   ~~deleted~~ Deleted   Excludes 1   Excludes 2   Includes   Use additional   Code first   Code also   Key words

OGCR Official Guidelines   X Assign placeholder X   ● Use Additional Character(s)   ▶ Manifestation Code   🅗 Hierarchical Condition Category   Coding Clinic

OTHER DISEASES OF UPPER RESPIRATORY TRACT (J30-J39)

● **J30   Vasomotor and allergic rhinitis**

    Includes   spasmodic rhinorrhea

    Excludes1   allergic rhinitis with asthma (bronchial) (J45.909)
                      rhinitis NOS (J31.0)

    J30.0   Vasomotor rhinitis

    J30.1   Allergic rhinitis due to pollen
              Allergy NOS due to pollen
              Hay fever
              Pollinosis

    J30.2   Other seasonal allergic rhinitis

    J30.5   Allergic rhinitis due to food

● **J30.8   Other allergic rhinitis**

        **J30.81   Allergic rhinitis due to animal (cat) (dog) hair
                    and dander**

        J30.89   Other allergic rhinitis
                    Perennial allergic rhinitis

    J30.9   Allergic rhinitis, unspecified

● **J31   Chronic rhinitis, nasopharyngitis and pharyngitis**
    Use additional code to identify:
        exposure to environmental tobacco smoke (Z77.22)
        exposure to tobacco smoke in the perinatal period (P96.81)
        history of tobacco dependence (Z87.891)
        occupational exposure to environmental tobacco smoke
            (Z57.31)
        tobacco dependence (F17.-)
        tobacco use (Z72.0)

    J31.0   Chronic rhinitis
              Atrophic rhinitis (chronic)
              Granulomatous rhinitis (chronic)
              Hypertrophic rhinitis (chronic)
              Obstructive rhinitis (chronic)
              Ozena
              Purulent rhinitis (chronic)
              Rhinitis (chronic) NOS
              Ulcerative rhinitis (chronic)

        Excludes1   allergic rhinitis (J30.1-J30.9)
                          vasomotor rhinitis (J30.0)

    J31.1   Chronic nasopharyngitis

        Excludes2   acute nasopharyngitis (J00)

    J31.2   Chronic pharyngitis
              Chronic sore throat
              Atrophic pharyngitis (chronic)
              Granular pharyngitis (chronic)
              Hypertrophic pharyngitis (chronic)

        Excludes2   acute pharyngitis (J02.9)

● **J32   Chronic sinusitis**

    Includes   sinus abscess
                    sinus empyema
                    sinus infection
                    sinus suppuration

    Use additional code to identify:
        exposure to environmental tobacco smoke (Z77.22)
        exposure to tobacco smoke in the perinatal period (P96.81)
        history of tobacco dependence (Z87.891)
        infectious agent (B95-B97)
        occupational exposure to environmental tobacco smoke
            (Z57.31)
        tobacco dependence (F17.-)
        tobacco use (Z72.0)

    Excludes2   acute sinusitis (J01.-)

    J32.0   Chronic maxillary sinusitis
              Antritis (chronic)
              Maxillary sinusitis NOS

    J32.1   Chronic frontal sinusitis
              Frontal sinusitis NOS

Item 10–4   Nasal polyps are an abnormal growth of tissue (tumor) projecting from a mucous membrane and attached to the surface by a narrow elongated stalk (pedunculated). Nasal polyps usually originate in the ethmoid sinus but also may occur in the maxillary sinus. Symptoms are nasal block, sinusitis, anosmia, and secondary infections.

    J32.2   Chronic ethmoidal sinusitis
              Ethmoidal sinusitis NOS

        Excludes1   Woakes' ethmoiditis (J33.1)

    J32.3   Chronic sphenoidal sinusitis
              Sphenoidal sinusitis NOS

    J32.4   Chronic pansinusitis
              Pansinusitis NOS

    J32.8   Other chronic sinusitis
              Sinusitis (chronic) involving more than one sinus but
                  not pansinusitis

    J32.9   Chronic sinusitis, unspecified
              Sinusitis (chronic) NOS

● **J33   Nasal polyp**
    Use additional code to identify:
        exposure to environmental tobacco smoke (Z77.22)
        exposure to tobacco smoke in the perinatal period (P96.81)
        history of tobacco dependence (Z87.891)
        occupational exposure to environmental tobacco smoke
            (Z57.31)
        tobacco dependence (F17.-)
        tobacco use (Z72.0)

    Excludes1   adenomatous polyps (D14.0)

    J33.0   Polyp of nasal cavity
              Choanal polyp
              Nasopharyngeal polyp

    J33.1   Polypoid sinus degeneration
              Woakes' syndrome or ethmoiditis

    J33.8   Other polyp of sinus
              Accessory polyp of sinus
              Ethmoidal polyp of sinus
              Maxillary polyp of sinus
              Sphenoidal polyp of sinus

    J33.9   Nasal polyp, unspecified

● **J34   Other and unspecified disorders of nose and nasal sinuses**

    Excludes2   varicose ulcer of nasal septum (I86.8)

    J34.0   Abscess, furuncle and carbuncle of nose
              Cellulitis of nose
              Necrosis of nose
              Ulceration of nose

    J34.1   Cyst and mucocele of nose and nasal sinus

    J34.2   Deviated nasal septum
              Deflection or deviation of septum (nasal) (acquired)

        Excludes1   congenital deviated nasal septum (Q67.4)

    J34.3   Hypertrophy of nasal turbinates

Deviated septal cartilage

Figure 10-3   Deviated nasal septum.

Item 10–5   A deviated nasal septum is the displacement of the septal cartilage that separates the nares. This displacement causes obstructed air flow through the nasal passages. A child can be born with this displacement (congenital), or the condition may be acquired through trauma, such as a sports injury. Symptoms include nasal block, sinusitis, and related secondary infections. Septoplasty is surgical repair of this condition.

CHAPTER 10 (J00-J99)

CHAPTER 10 (J00-J99)

● **J34.8   Other specified disorders of nose and nasal sinuses**
> **J34.81   Nasal mucositis (ulcerative)**
>> Code also type of associated therapy, such as:
>> antineoplastic and immunosuppressive drugs (T45.1X-)
>> radiological procedure and radiotherapy (Y84.2)
>>> **Excludes2**   gastrointestinal mucositis (ulcerative) (K92.81)
>>> mucositis (ulcerative) of vagina and vulva (N76.81)
>>> oral mucositis (ulcerative) (K12.3-)

> **J34.89   Other specified disorders of nose and nasal sinuses**
>> Perforation of nasal septum NOS
>> Rhinolith

J34.9   Unspecified disorder of nose and nasal sinuses

● **J35   Chronic diseases of tonsils and adenoids**
> Use additional code to identify:
> exposure to environmental tobacco smoke (Z77.22)
> exposure to tobacco smoke in the perinatal period (P96.81)
> history of tobacco dependence (Z87.891)
> occupational exposure to environmental tobacco smoke (Z57.31)
> tobacco dependence (F17.-)
> tobacco use (Z72.0)

● **J35.0   Chronic tonsillitis and adenoiditis**
>> **Excludes2**   acute tonsillitis (J03.-)
> **J35.01   Chronic tonsillitis**
> **J35.02   Chronic adenoiditis**
> **J35.03   Chronic tonsillitis and adenoiditis**

J35.1   Hypertrophy of tonsils
> Enlargement of tonsils
>> **Excludes1**   hypertrophy of tonsils with tonsillitis (J35.0-)

J35.2   Hypertrophy of adenoids
> Enlargement of adenoids
>> **Excludes1**   hypertrophy of adenoids with adenoiditis (J35.0-)

J35.3   Hypertrophy of tonsils with hypertrophy of adenoids
>> **Excludes1**   hypertrophy of tonsils and adenoids with tonsillitis and adenoiditis (J35.03)

J35.8   Other chronic diseases of tonsils and adenoids
> Adenoid vegetations
> Amygdalolith
> Calculus, tonsil
> Cicatrix of tonsil (and adenoid)
> Tonsillar tag
> Ulcer of tonsil

J35.9   Chronic disease of tonsils and adenoids, unspecified
> Disease (chronic) of tonsils and adenoids NOS

J36   Peritonsillar abscess
> **Includes**   abscess of tonsil
> peritonsillar cellulitis
> quinsy
> Use additional code (B95-B97) to identify infectious agent.
>> **Excludes1**   acute tonsillitis (J03.-)
>> chronic tonsillitis (J35.0)
>> retropharyngeal abscess (J39.0)
>> tonsillitis NOS (J03.9-)

● **J37   Chronic laryngitis and laryngotracheitis**
> Use additional code to identify:
> exposure to environmental tobacco smoke (Z77.22)
> exposure to tobacco smoke in the perinatal period (P96.81)
> history of tobacco dependence (Z87.891)
> infectious agent (B95-B97)
> occupational exposure to environmental tobacco smoke (Z57.31)
> tobacco dependence (F17.-)
> tobacco use (Z72.0)

> **J37.0   Chronic laryngitis**
>> Catarrhal laryngitis
>> Hypertrophic laryngitis
>> Sicca laryngitis
>>> **Excludes2**   acute laryngitis (J04.0)
>>> obstructive (acute) laryngitis (J05.0)

> **J37.1   Chronic laryngotracheitis**
>> Laryngitis, chronic, with tracheitis (chronic)
>> Tracheitis, chronic, with laryngitis
>>> **Excludes1**   chronic tracheitis (J42)
>>> **Excludes2**   acute laryngotracheitis (J04.2)
>>> acute tracheitis (J04.1)

● **J38   Diseases of vocal cords and larynx, not elsewhere classified**
> Use additional code to identify:
> exposure to environmental tobacco smoke (Z77.22)
> exposure to tobacco smoke in the perinatal period (P96.81)
> history of tobacco dependence (Z87.891)
> occupational exposure to environmental tobacco smoke (Z57.31)
> tobacco dependence (F17.-)
> tobacco use (Z72.0)
>> **Excludes1**   congenital laryngeal stridor (P28.89)
>> obstructive laryngitis (acute) (J05.0)
>> postprocedural subglottic stenosis (J95.5)
>> stridor (R06.1)
>> ulcerative laryngitis (J04.0)

● **J38.0   Paralysis of vocal cords and larynx**
>> Laryngoplegia
>> Paralysis of glottis
> **J38.00   Paralysis of vocal cords and larynx, unspecified**
> **J38.01   Paralysis of vocal cords and larynx, unilateral**
> **J38.02   Paralysis of vocal cords and larynx, bilateral**

J38.1   Polyp of vocal cord and larynx
>> **Excludes1**   adenomatous polyps (D14.1)

J38.2   Nodules of vocal cords
> Chorditis (fibrinous)(nodosa)(tuberosa)
> Singer's nodes
> Teacher's nodes

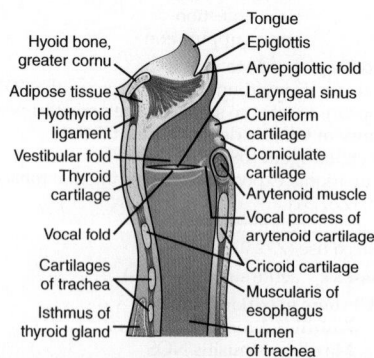

Figure 10-4   Coronal section of the larynx.

Item 10–6   The **larynx** extends from the tongue to the trachea and is divided into an upper and lower portion separated by folds. The framework of the larynx is cartilage composed of the single cricoid, thyroid, and epiglottic cartilages, and the paired arytenoid, cuneiform, and corniculate cartilages.

▶ New   ➡ Revised   ~~deleted~~ Deleted   Excludes 1   Excludes 2   Includes   Use additional   Code first   Code also   Key words
OGCR Official Guidelines   X Assign placeholder X   ● Use Additional Character(s)   ▮ Manifestation Code   🔖 Hierarchical Condition Category   **Coding Clinic**

J38.3   **Other diseases of vocal cords**
Abscess of vocal cords
Cellulitis of vocal cords
Granuloma of vocal cords
Leukokeratosis of vocal cords
Leukoplakia of vocal cords

J38.4   **Edema of larynx**
Edema (of) glottis
Subglottic edema
Supraglottic edema

> **Excludes1**   acute obstructive laryngitis [croup] (J05.0)
> edematous laryngitis (J04.0)

J38.5   **Laryngeal spasm**
Laryngismus (stridulus)

J38.6   **Stenosis of larynx**

J38.7   **Other diseases of larynx**
Abscess of larynx
Cellulitis of larynx
Disease of larynx NOS
Necrosis of larynx
Pachyderma of larynx
Perichondritis of larynx
Ulcer of larynx

● **J39**   **Other diseases of upper respiratory tract**

> **Excludes1**   acute respiratory infection NOS (J22)
> acute upper respiratory infection (J06.9)
> upper respiratory inflammation due to chemicals,
> gases, fumes or vapors (J68.2)

J39.0   **Retropharyngeal and parapharyngeal abscess**
Peripharyngeal abscess

> **Excludes1**   peritonsillar abscess (J36)

J39.1   **Other abscess of pharynx**
Cellulitis of pharynx
Nasopharyngeal abscess

J39.2   **Other diseases of pharynx**
Cyst of pharynx
Edema of pharynx

> **Excludes2**   chronic pharyngitis (J31.2)
> ulcerative pharyngitis (J02.9)

J39.3   **Upper respiratory tract hypersensitivity reaction, site unspecified**

> **Excludes1**   hypersensitivity reaction of upper
> respiratory tract, such as:
> extrinsic allergic alveolitis (J67.9)
> pneumoconiosis (J60-J67.9)

J39.8   **Other specified diseases of upper respiratory tract**

J39.9   **Disease of upper respiratory tract, unspecified**

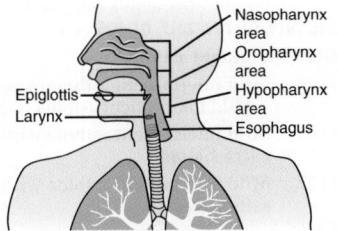

Figure 10-5   The pharynx.

Item 10-7   The **pharynx** is the passage for both food and air between the mouth and the esophagus and is divided into three areas: nasopharynx, oropharynx, and hypopharynx. The hypopharynx branches into the esophagus and the voice box.

Item 10-8   **Chronic bronchitis** is usually defined as being present in any patient who has persistent cough with sputum production for at least three months in at least two consecutive years. **Simple chronic bronchitis** is marked by a productive cough but no pathological airflow obstruction. **Chronic obstructive pulmonary disease (COPD)** is a group of conditions—bronchitis, emphysema, asthma, bronchiectasis, allergic alveolitis—marked by dyspnea. **Catarrhal** bronchitis is an acute form of bronchitis marked by profuse mucus and pus production (**mucopurulent** discharge). **Croupous** bronchitis, also known as pseudomembranous, fibrinous, plastic, exudative, or membranous, is marked by a violent cough and dyspnea.

CHRONIC LOWER RESPIRATORY DISEASES (J40-J47)

> **Excludes1**   bronchitis due to chemicals, gases, fumes and
> vapors (J68.0)

> **Excludes2**   cystic fibrosis (E84.-)

J40   **Bronchitis, not specified as acute or chronic**
Bronchitis NOS
Catarrhal bronchitis
Bronchitis with tracheitis NOS
Tracheobronchitis NOS
Use additional code to identify:
   exposure to environmental tobacco smoke (Z77.22)
   exposure to tobacco smoke in the perinatal period (P96.81)
   history of tobacco dependence (Z87.891)
   occupational exposure to environmental tobacco smoke
     (Z57.31)
   tobacco dependence (F17.-)
   tobacco use (Z72.0)

> **Excludes1**   acute bronchitis (J20.-)
> allergic bronchitis NOS (J45.909-)
> asthmatic bronchitis NOS (J45.9-)
> bronchitis due to chemicals, gases, fumes and
> vapors (J68.0)

● **J41**   **Simple and mucopurulent chronic bronchitis**
Use additional code to identify:
   exposure to environmental tobacco smoke (Z77.22)
   exposure to tobacco smoke in the perinatal period (P96.81)
   history of tobacco dependence (Z87.891)
   occupational exposure to environmental tobacco smoke
     (Z57.31)
   tobacco dependence (F17.-)
   tobacco use (Z72.0)

> **Excludes1**   chronic bronchitis NOS (J42)
> chronic obstructive bronchitis (J44.-)

J41.0   **Simple chronic bronchitis** 🔍

J41.1   **Mucopurulent chronic bronchitis** 🔍

J41.8   **Mixed simple and mucopurulent chronic bronchitis** 🔍

J42   **Unspecified chronic bronchitis** 🔍
Chronic bronchitis NOS
Chronic tracheitis
Chronic tracheobronchitis
Use additional code to identify:
   exposure to environmental tobacco smoke (Z77.22)
   exposure to tobacco smoke in the perinatal period (P96.81)
   history of tobacco dependence (Z87.891)
   occupational exposure to environmental tobacco smoke
     (Z57.31)
   tobacco dependence (F17.-)
   tobacco use (Z72.0)

> **Excludes1**   chronic asthmatic bronchitis (J44.-)
> chronic bronchitis with airways obstruction (J44.-)
> chronic emphysematous bronchitis (J44.-)
> chronic obstructive pulmonary disease NOS
> (J44.9)
> simple and mucopurulent chronic bronchitis
> (J41.-)

● **J43   Emphysema**

Use additional code to identify:
exposure to environmental tobacco smoke (Z77.22)
history of tobacco dependence (Z87.891)
occupational exposure to environmental tobacco smoke (Z57.31)
tobacco dependence (F17.-)
tobacco use (Z72.0)

Excludes1   compensatory emphysema (J98.3)
emphysema due to inhalation of chemicals, gases, fumes or vapors (J68.4)
emphysema with chronic (obstructive) bronchitis (J44.-)
emphysematous (obstructive) bronchitis (J44.-)
interstitial emphysema (J98.2)
mediastinal emphysema (J98.2)
neonatal interstitial emphysema (P25.0)
surgical (subcutaneous) emphysema (T81.82)

Excludes2   traumatic subcutaneous emphysema (T79.7)

J43.0   Unilateral pulmonary emphysema [MacLeod's syndrome]🐾
Swyer-James syndrome
Unilateral emphysema
Unilateral hyperlucent lung
Unilateral pulmonary artery functional hypoplasia
Unilateral transparency of lung

J43.1   Panlobular emphysema 🐾
Panacinar emphysema

J43.2   Centrilobular emphysema 🐾

J43.8   Other emphysema 🐾

J43.9   Emphysema, unspecified 🐾
Bullous emphysema (lung)(pulmonary)
Emphysema (lung)(pulmonary) NOS
Emphysematous bleb
Vesicular emphysema (lung)(pulmonary)
Coding Clinic: 2019, Q1, P35-37; 2017, Q4, P97-98

● **J44   Other chronic obstructive pulmonary disease**

Includes   asthma with chronic obstructive pulmonary disease
chronic asthmatic (obstructive) bronchitis
chronic bronchitis with airway obstruction
chronic bronchitis with emphysema
chronic emphysematous bronchitis
chronic obstructive asthma
chronic obstructive bronchitis
chronic obstructive tracheobronchitis

Code also type of asthma, if applicable (J45.-)

Use additional code to identify:
exposure to environmental tobacco smoke (Z77.22)
history of tobacco dependence (Z87.891)
occupational exposure to environmental tobacco smoke (Z57.31)
tobacco dependence (F17.-)
tobacco use (Z72.0)

Excludes1   bronchiectasis (J47.-)
chronic bronchitis NOS (J42)
chronic simple and mucopurulent bronchitis (J41.-)
chronic tracheitis (J42)
chronic tracheobronchitis (J42)
emphysema without chronic bronchitis (J43.-)
Coding Clinic: 2019, Q1, P34-36; 2017, Q4, P97; 2017, Q1, P25; 2016, Q3, P16

J44.0   Chronic obstructive pulmonary disease with (acute) lower respiratory infection 🐾
Code also to identify the infection
Coding Clinic: 2019, Q1, P35-36; 2017, Q4, P96; 2017, Q2, P30, Q1, P24-25; 2016, Q3, P15-16

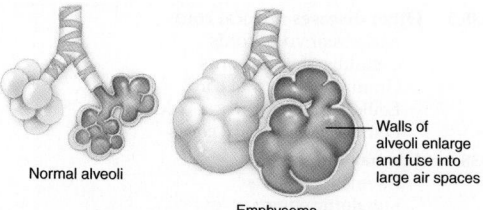

Figure 10-6   Emphysema. (From Shiland, BJ: Medical Terminology & Anatomy for ICD-10 Coding, ed 2, Mosby, 2015)

J44.1   Chronic obstructive pulmonary disease with (acute) exacerbation 🐾
Decompensated COPD
Decompensated COPD with (acute) exacerbation

Excludes2   chronic obstructive pulmonary disease [COPD] with acute bronchitis (J44.0)
lung diseases due to external agents (J60-J70)
Coding Clinic: 2019, Q1, P34-35; 2017, Q4, P96; 2017, Q1, P26; 2016, Q3, P15-16, Q1, P36

J44.9   Chronic obstructive pulmonary disease, unspecified 🐾
Chronic obstructive airway disease NOS
Chronic obstructive lung disease NOS

Excludes2   lung diseases due to external agents (J60-J70)
Coding Clinic: 2019, Q1, P36; 2017, Q4, P96-97; 2017, Q1, P24-25; 2016, Q1, P37

● **J45   Asthma**
Allergic (predominantly) asthma
Allergic bronchitis NOS
Allergic rhinitis with asthma
Atopic asthma
Extrinsic allergic asthma
Hay fever with asthma
Idiosyncratic asthma
Intrinsic nonallergic asthma
Nonallergic asthma

Use additional code to identify:
eosinophilic asthma (J82.83)
exposure to environmental tobacco smoke (Z77.22)
exposure to tobacco smoke in the perinatal period (P96.81)
history of tobacco dependence (Z87.891)
occupational exposure to environmental tobacco smoke (Z57.31)
tobacco dependence (F17.-)
tobacco use (Z72.0)

Excludes1   detergent asthma (J69.8)
eosinophilic asthma (J82)
miner's asthma (J60)
wheezing NOS (R06.2)
wood asthma (J67.8)

Excludes2   asthma with chronic obstructive pulmonary disease (J44.9)
chronic asthmatic (obstructive) bronchitis (J44.9)
chronic obstructive asthma (J44.9)
Coding Clinic: 2019, Q1, P37; 2017, Q1, P25

● **J45.2   Mild intermittent asthma**

J45.20   Mild intermittent asthma, uncomplicated
Mild intermittent asthma NOS

J45.21   Mild intermittent asthma with (acute) exacerbation

J45.22   Mild intermittent asthma with status asthmaticus

Item 10–9   Asthma is a bronchial condition marked by airway obstruction, hyper-responsiveness, and inflammation. **Extrinsic** asthma, also known as allergic asthma, is characterized by the same symptoms that occur with exposure to allergens and is divided into the following types: **atopic, occupational,** and **allergic bronchopulmonary aspergillosis. Intrinsic** asthma occurs in patients who have no history of allergy or sensitivities to allergens and is divided into the following types: **nonreaginic** and **pharmacologic. Status asthmaticus** is the most severe form of asthma attack and can last for days or weeks.

▶ New   ⇒ Revised   ~~deleted~~ Deleted   Excludes 1   Excludes 2   Includes   Use additional   Code first   Code also   Key words
OGCR Official Guidelines   X Assign placeholder X   ● Use Additional Character(s)   ▶ Manifestation Code   🐾 Hierarchical Condition Category   **Coding Clinic**

Figure 10-7   Factors causing expiratory obstruction in asthma. **A.** Cross section of a bronchiole occluded by muscle spasm, swollen mucosa, and mucus. **B.** Longitudinal section of an obstructed bronchiole. **C.** Cross section of a clear bronchiole. (From Shiland: Mastering Healthcare Terminology, ed 1, St. Louis, Mosby, 2003)

● **J45.3**   **Mild persistent asthma**

    J45.30   **Mild persistent asthma, uncomplicated**
         Mild persistent asthma NOS

    J45.31   **Mild persistent asthma with (acute) exacerbation**
         Coding Clinic: 2016, Q1, P35

    J45.32   **Mild persistent asthma with status asthmaticus**

● **J45.4**   **Moderate persistent asthma**

    J45.40   **Moderate persistent asthma, uncomplicated**
         Moderate persistent asthma NOS

    J45.41   **Moderate persistent asthma with (acute) exacerbation**
         Coding Clinic: 2017, Q1, P26

    J45.42   **Moderate persistent asthma with status asthmaticus**

● **J45.5**   **Severe persistent asthma**

    J45.50   **Severe persistent asthma, uncomplicated**
         Severe persistent asthma NOS

    J45.51   **Severe persistent asthma with (acute) exacerbation**

    J45.52   **Severe persistent asthma with status asthmaticus**

● **J45.9**   **Other and unspecified asthma**

    ● **J45.90**   **Unspecified asthma**
         Asthmatic bronchitis NOS
         Childhood asthma NOS
         Late onset asthma

       J45.901   **Unspecified asthma with (acute) exacerbation**
            Coding Clinic: 2017, Q4, P96

       J45.902   **Unspecified asthma with status asthmaticus**

       J45.909   **Unspecified asthma, uncomplicated**
            Asthma NOS

            Excludes2   lung diseases due to external agents (J60-J70)
            Coding Clinic: 2017, Q4, P96; 2017, Q1, P25

    ● **J45.99**   **Other asthma**

       J45.990   **Exercise induced bronchospasm**

       J45.991   **Cough variant asthma**

       J45.998   **Other asthma**

● **J47**   **Bronchiectasis**

    Includes   bronchiolectasis

    Use additional code to identify:
       exposure to environmental tobacco smoke (Z77.22)
       exposure to tobacco smoke in the perinatal period (P96.81)
       history of tobacco dependence (Z87.891)
       occupational exposure to environmental tobacco smoke (Z57.31)
       tobacco dependence (F17.-)
       tobacco use (Z72.0)

    Excludes1   congenital bronchiectasis (Q33.4)
              tuberculous bronchiectasis (current disease) (A15.0)

    J47.0   **Bronchiectasis with acute lower respiratory infection** 🖥
        Bronchiectasis with acute bronchitis
        Code also to identify infection, if applicable

    J47.1   **Bronchiectasis with (acute) exacerbation** 🖥
        Coding Clinic: 2021, Q1, P24

    J47.9   **Bronchiectasis, uncomplicated** 🖥
        Bronchiectasis NOS

LUNG DISEASES DUE TO EXTERNAL AGENTS (J60-J70)

    Excludes2   asthma (J45.-)
              malignant neoplasm of bronchus and lung (C34.-)

J60   **Coalworker's pneumoconiosis** 🖥   A
    Anthracosilicosis
    Anthracosis
    Black lung disease
    Coalworker's lung

    Excludes1   coalworker pneumoconiosis with tuberculosis, any type in A15 (J65)

J61   **Pneumoconiosis due to asbestos and other mineral fibers** 🖥   A
    Asbestosis

    Excludes1   pleural plaque with asbestosis (J92.0)
              pneumoconiosis with tuberculosis, any type in A15 (J65)

● **J62**   **Pneumoconiosis due to dust containing silica**

    Includes   silicotic fibrosis (massive) of lung

    Excludes1   pneumoconiosis with tuberculosis, any type in A15 (J65)

    J62.0   **Pneumoconiosis due to talc dust** 🖥

    J62.8   **Pneumoconiosis due to other dust containing silica** 🖥
        Silicosis NOS

● **J63**   **Pneumoconiosis due to other inorganic dusts**

    Excludes1   pneumoconiosis with tuberculosis, any type in A15 (J65)
    Coding Clinic: 2019, Q3, P8

    J63.0   **Aluminosis (of lung)** 🖥

    J63.1   **Bauxite fibrosis (of lung)** 🖥

    J63.2   **Berylliosis** 🖥

    J63.3   **Graphite fibrosis (of lung)** 🖥

    J63.4   **Siderosis** 🖥
        Coding Clinic: 2019, Q3, P8

Figure 10-8   Progressive massive fibrosis superimposed on coal workers' pneumoconiosis. The large, blackened scars are located principally in the upper lobe. (From Frazier MS, Drzymkowski JW: Essentials of Human Diseases and Conditions, St. Louis, MO, Saunders, 2004)

Item 10–10 Pneumoconiosis refers to a lung condition resulting from exposure to inorganic or organic airborne particles, such as coal dust or moldy hay, as well as chemical fumes and vapors, such as insecticides. In this condition, the lungs retain the airborne particles.

CHAPTER 10 (J00-J99)

J63.5 Stannosis 🦠

J63.6 Pneumoconiosis due to other specified inorganic dusts 🦠

J64   Unspecified pneumoconiosis 🦠

> **Excludes1** pneumonoconiosis with tuberculosis, any type in A15 (J65)

J65   Pneumoconiosis associated with tuberculosis 🦠
> Any condition in J60-J64 with tuberculosis, any type in A15
> Silicotuberculosis

● **J66   Airway disease due to specific organic dust**
> **Excludes2** allergic alveolitis (J67.-)
> asbestosis (J61)
> bagassosis (J67.1)
> farmer's lung (J67.0)
> hypersensitivity pneumonitis due to organic dust (J67.-)
> reactive airways dysfunction syndrome (J68.3)

J66.0 Byssinosis 🦠
> Airway disease due to cotton dust

J66.1 Flax-dressers' disease 🦠

J66.2 Cannabinosis 🦠

J66.8 Airway disease due to other specific organic dusts 🦠

● **J67   Hypersensitivity pneumonitis due to organic dust**
> **Includes** allergic alveolitis and pneumonitis due to inhaled organic dust and particles of fungal, actinomycetic or other origin

> **Excludes1** pneumonitis due to inhalation of chemicals, gases, fumes or vapors (J68.0)

J67.0 Farmer's lung 🦠
> Harvester's lung
> Haymaker's lung
> Moldy hay disease

J67.1 Bagassosis 🦠
> Bagasse disease
> Bagasse pneumonitis

J67.2 Bird fancier's lung 🦠
> Budgerigar fancier's disease or lung
> Pigeon fancier's disease or lung

J67.3 Suberosis 🦠
> Corkhandler's disease or lung
> Corkworker's disease or lung

J67.4 Maltworker's lung 🦠
> Alveolitis due to Aspergillus clavatus

J67.5 Mushroom-worker's lung 🦠

J67.6 Maple-bark-stripper's lung 🦠
> Alveolitis due to Cryptostroma corticale
> Cryptostromosis

J67.7 Air conditioner and humidifier lung 🦠
> Allergic alveolitis due to fungal, thermophilic actinomycetes and other organisms growing in ventilation [air conditioning] systems

J67.8 Hypersensitivity pneumonitis due to other organic dusts 🦠
> Cheese-washer's lung
> Coffee-worker's lung
> Fish-meal worker's lung
> Furrier's lung
> Sequoiosis

J67.9 Hypersensitivity pneumonitis due to unspecified organic dust 🦠
> Allergic alveolitis (extrinsic) NOS
> Hypersensitivity pneumonitis NOS

● **J68   Respiratory conditions due to inhalation of chemicals, gases, fumes and vapors**
> *Code first (T51-T65) to identify cause*
> Use additional code to identify associated respiratory conditions, such as:
> acute respiratory failure (J96.0-)

J68.0 Bronchitis and pneumonitis due to chemicals, gases, fumes and vapors
> Chemical bronchitis (acute)
> **Coding Clinic: 2019, Q2, P31-32**

J68.1 Pulmonary edema due to chemicals, gases, fumes and vapors 🦠
> Chemical pulmonary edema (acute) (chronic)
> **Excludes1** pulmonary edema (acute) (chronic) NOS (J81.-)

J68.2 Upper respiratory inflammation due to chemicals, gases, fumes and vapors, not elsewhere classified 🦠

J68.3 Other acute and subacute respiratory conditions due to chemicals, gases, fumes and vapors 🦠
> Reactive airways dysfunction syndrome

J68.4 Chronic respiratory conditions due to chemicals, gases, fumes and vapors 🦠
> Emphysema (diffuse) (chronic) due to inhalation of chemicals, gases, fumes and vapors
> Obliterative bronchiolitis (chronic) (subacute) due to inhalation of chemicals, gases, fumes and vapors
> Pulmonary fibrosis (chronic) due to inhalation of chemicals, gases, fumes and vapors
> **Excludes1** chronic pulmonary edema due to chemicals, gases, fumes and vapors (J68.1)

J68.8 Other respiratory conditions due to chemicals, gases, fumes and vapors 🦠

J68.9 Unspecified respiratory condition due to chemicals, gases, fumes and vapors 🦠

● **J69   Pneumonitis due to solids and liquids**
> **Excludes1** neonatal aspiration syndromes (P24.-)
> postprocedural pneumonitis (J95.4)

J69.0 Pneumonitis due to inhalation of food and vomit 🦠
> Aspiration pneumonia NOS
> Aspiration pneumonia (due to) food (regurgitated)
> Aspiration pneumonia (due to) gastric secretions
> Aspiration pneumonia (due to) milk
> Aspiration pneumonia (due to) vomit
> Code also any associated foreign body in respiratory tract (T17.-)
> **Excludes1** chemical pneumonitis due to anesthesia (J95.4)
> obstetric aspiration pneumonitis (O74.0)
> **Coding Clinic: 2021, Q1, P34; 2019, Q2, P7, 31-32; 2017, Q1, P24**

J69.1 Pneumonitis due to inhalation of oils and essences 🦠
> Exogenous lipoid pneumonia
> Lipid pneumonia NOS
> *Code first (T51-T65) to identify substance*
> **Excludes1** endogenous lipoid pneumonia (J84.89)

J69.8 Pneumonitis due to inhalation of other solids and liquids 🦠
> Pneumonitis due to aspiration of blood
> Pneumonitis due to aspiration of detergent
> *Code first (T51-T65) to identify substance*

● **J70   Respiratory conditions due to other external agents**

J70.0 Acute pulmonary manifestations due to radiation 🦠
> Radiation pneumonitis
> Use additional code (W88-W90, X39.0-) to identify the external cause

J70.1 Chronic and other pulmonary manifestations due to radiation 🦠
> Fibrosis of lung following radiation
> Use additional code (W88-W90, X39.0-) to identify the external cause

CHAPTER 10 (J00-J99)

J70.2   **Acute drug-induced interstitial lung disorders**
Use additional code for adverse effect, if applicable, to identify drug (T36-T50 with fifth or sixth character 5)
> **Excludes1**   interstitial pneumonia NOS (J84.9)
> lymphoid interstitial pneumonia (J84.2)

Coding Clinic: 2019, Q2, P28

J70.3   **Chronic drug-induced interstitial lung disorders**
Use additional code for adverse effect, if applicable, to identify drug (T36-T50 with fifth or sixth character 5)
> **Excludes1**   interstitial pneumonia NOS (J84.9)
> lymphoid interstitial pneumonia (J84.2)

J70.4   **Drug-induced interstitial lung disorders, unspecified**
Use additional code for adverse effect, if applicable, to identify drug (T36-T50 with fifth or sixth character 5)
> **Excludes1**   interstitial pneumonia NOS (J84.9)
> lymphoid interstitial pneumonia (J84.2)

Coding Clinic: 2019, Q2, P28

J70.5   **Respiratory conditions due to smoke inhalation**
Code first smoke inhalation (T59.81-)
> **Excludes2**   smoke inhalation due to chemicals, gases, fumes and vapors (J68.9)

J70.8   **Respiratory conditions due to other specified external agents**
Code first (T51-T65) to identify the external agent

J70.9   **Respiratory conditions due to unspecified external agent**
Code first (T51-T65) to identify the external agent

OTHER RESPIRATORY DISEASES PRINCIPALLY AFFECTING THE INTERSTITIUM (J80-J84)

J80   **Acute respiratory distress syndrome**
Acute respiratory distress syndrome in adult or child
Adult hyaline membrane disease
> **Excludes1**   respiratory distress syndrome in newborn (perinatal) (P22.0)

Coding Clinic: 2017, Q1, P26-27

J81   **Pulmonary edema**
Use additional code to identify:
exposure to environmental tobacco smoke (Z77.22)
history of tobacco dependence (Z87.891)
occupational exposure to environmental tobacco smoke (Z57.31)
tobacco dependence (F17.-)
tobacco use (Z72.0)
> **Excludes1**   chemical (acute) pulmonary edema (J68.1)
> hypostatic pneumonia (J18.2)
> passive pneumonia (J18.2)
> pulmonary edema due to external agents (J60-J70)
> pulmonary edema with heart disease NOS (I50.1)
> pulmonary edema with heart failure (I50.1)

J81.0   **Acute pulmonary edema**
Acute edema of lung
Coding Clinic: 2017, Q1, P26

J81.1   **Chronic pulmonary edema**
Pulmonary congestion (chronic) (passive)
Pulmonary edema NOS

Figure 10-9 Bullous emphysema with large subpleural bullae *(upper left)*. (From Kumar: Robbins and Cotran: Pathologic Basis of Disease, ed 8, Saunders, An Imprint of Elsevier, 2009)

J82   **Pulmonary eosinophilia, not elsewhere classified**
> **Excludes2**   pulmonary eosinophilia due to aspergillosis (B44.-)
> pulmonary eosinophilia due to drugs (J70.2-J70.4)
> pulmonary eosinophilia due to specified parasitic infection (B50-B83)
> pulmonary eosinophilia due to systemic connective tissue disorders (M30-M36)
> pulmonary infiltrate NOS (R91.8)

● **J82.8**   **Pulmonary eosinophilia, not elsewhere classified**

    J82.81   **Chronic eosinophilic pneumonia**
Eosinophilic pneumonia, NOS

    J82.82   **Acute eosinophilic pneumonia**

    J82.83   **Eosinophilic asthma**
Code first asthma, by type, such as:
mild intermittent asthma (J45.2-)
mild persistent asthma (J45.3-)
moderate persistent asthma (J45.4-)
severe persistent asthma (J45.5-)

    J82.89   **Other pulmonary eosinophilia, not elsewhere classified**
Allergic pneumonia
Löffler's pneumonia
Tropical (pulmonary) eosinophilia NOS

● **J84**   **Other interstitial pulmonary diseases**
> **Excludes1**   drug-induced interstitial lung disorders (J70.2-J70.4)
> interstitial emphysema (J98.2)
> **Excludes2**   lung diseases due to external agents (J60-J70)

Coding Clinic: 2019, Q2, P28

● **J84.0**   **Alveolar and parieto-alveolar conditions**

    J84.01   **Alveolar proteinosis**

    J84.02   **Pulmonary alveolar microlithiasis**

    J84.03   *Idiopathic pulmonary hemosiderosis*
Essential brown induration of lung
Code first underlying disease, such as:
disorders of iron metabolism (E83.1-)
> **Excludes1**   acute idiopathic pulmonary hemorrhage in infants [AIPHI] (R04.81)

    J84.09   **Other alveolar and parieto-alveolar conditions**

● **J84.1**   **Other interstitial pulmonary diseases with fibrosis**
> **Excludes1**   pulmonary fibrosis (chronic) due to inhalation of chemicals, gases, fumes or vapors (J68.4)
> pulmonary fibrosis (chronic) following radiation (J70.1)

    J84.10   **Pulmonary fibrosis, unspecified**
Capillary fibrosis of lung
Cirrhosis of lung NOS
Fibrosis of lung (atrophic) (chronic) (confluent) (massive) (perialveolar) (peribronchial) NOS
Induration of lung (chronic) NOS
Postinflammatory pulmonary fibrosis

● **J84.11**   **Idiopathic interstitial pneumonia**
> **Excludes1**   lymphoid interstitial pneumonia (J84.2)
> pneumocystis pneumonia (B59)

    J84.111   **Idiopathic interstitial pneumonia, not otherwise specified**

    J84.112   **Idiopathic pulmonary fibrosis**
Cryptogenic fibrosing alveolitis
Idiopathic fibrosing alveolitis

CHAPTER 10 (J00-J99)

CHAPTER 10 (J00-J99)

J84.113   **Idiopathic non-specific interstitial pneumonitis** 🔖

    Excludes1 non-specific interstitial pneumonia NOS, or due to known underlying cause (J84.89)

J84.114   **Acute interstitial pneumonitis** 🔖
Hamman-Rich syndrome

    Excludes1 pneumocystis pneumonia (B59)

J84.115   **Respiratory bronchiolitis interstitial lung disease** 🔖

J84.116   **Cryptogenic organizing pneumonia** 🔖

    Excludes1 organizing pneumonia NOS, or due to known underlying cause (J84.89)

J84.117   **Desquamative interstitial pneumonia** 🔖

●▶ **J84.17**   *Other interstitial pulmonary diseases with fibrosis in diseases classified elsewhere* 🔖

▶ **J84.170**   *Interstitial lung disease with progressive fibrotic phenotype in diseases classified elsewhere*
Progressive fibrotic interstitial lung disease

Code first underlying disease, such as:
lung diseases due to external agents (J60-J70)
rheumatoid arthritis (M05.00-M06.9)
sarcoidosis (D86)
systemic connective tissue disorders (M30-M36)

▶ **J84.178**   *Other interstitial pulmonary diseases with fibrosis in diseases classified elsewhere*
Interstitial pneumonia (nonspecific) (usual) due to collagen vascular disease
Interstitial pneumonia (nonspecific) (usual) in diseases classified elsewhere
Organizing pneumonia due to collagen vascular disease
Organizing pneumonia in diseases classified elsewhere

Code first underlying disease, such as:
progressive systemic sclerosis (M34.0)
rheumatoid arthritis (M05.00-M06.9)
systemic lupus erythematosis (M32.0-M32.9)

J84.2   **Lymphoid interstitial pneumonia** 🔖
Lymphoid interstitial pneumonitis

● **J84.8**   **Other specified interstitial pulmonary diseases**

    Excludes1 exogenous lipoid pneumonia (J69.1)
unspecified lipoid pneumonia (J69.1)

J84.81   **Lymphangioleiomyomatosis** 🔖
Lymphangiomyomatosis

J84.82   **Adult pulmonary Langerhans cell histiocytosis** 🔖
Adult PLCH

J84.83   **Surfactant mutations of the lung** 🔖

● **J84.84**   **Other interstitial lung diseases of childhood**

J84.841   **Neuroendocrine cell hyperplasia of infancy** 🔖

J84.842   **Pulmonary interstitial glycogenosis** 🔖

J84.843   **Alveolar capillary dysplasia with vein misalignment** 🔖

J84.848   **Other interstitial lung diseases of childhood** 🔖

J84.89   **Other specified interstitial pulmonary diseases** 🔖
Endogenous lipoid pneumonia
Interstitial pneumonitis
Non-specific interstitial pneumonitis NOS
Organizing pneumonia NOS

Code first, if applicable:
poisoning due to drug or toxin (T51-T65 with fifth or sixth character to indicate intent), for toxic pneumonopathy underlying cause of pneumonopathy, if known

Use additional code, for adverse effect, to identify drug (T36-T50 with fifth or sixth character 5), if drug-induced

    Excludes1 cryptogenic organizing pneumonia (J84.116)
idiopathic non-specific interstitial pneumonitis (J84.113)
lipoid pneumonia, exogenous or unspecified (J69.1)
lymphoid interstitial pneumonia (J84.2)

Coding Clinic: 2021, Q4, P106-107; 2021, Q1, P48; 2019, Q2, P28

J84.9   **Interstitial pulmonary disease, unspecified** 🔖
Interstitial pneumonia NOS

SUPPURATIVE AND NECROTIC CONDITIONS OF THE LOWER RESPIRATORY TRACT (J85-J86)

● **J85**   **Abscess of lung and mediastinum**
Use additional code (B95-B97) to identify infectious agent.

J85.0   **Gangrene and necrosis of lung** 🔖

J85.1   **Abscess of lung with pneumonia** 🔖
Code also the type of pneumonia

J85.2   **Abscess of lung without pneumonia** 🔖
Abscess of lung NOS

J85.3   **Abscess of mediastinum** 🔖

● **J86**   **Pyothorax**
Use additional code (B95-B97) to identify infectious agent.

    Excludes1 abscess of lung (J85.-)
pyothorax due to tuberculosis (A15.6)

J86.0   **Pyothorax with fistula** 🔖
Bronchocutaneous fistula
Bronchopleural fistula
Hepatopleural fistula
Mediastinal fistula
Pleural fistula
Thoracic fistula
Any condition classifiable to J86.9 with fistula

J86.9   **Pyothorax without fistula** 🔖
Abscess of pleura
Abscess of thorax
Empyema (chest) (lung) (pleura)
Fibrinopurulent pleurisy
Purulent pleurisy
Pyopneumothorax
Septic pleurisy
Seropurulent pleurisy
Suppurative pleurisy

Item 10-11 **Empyema** is a condition in which pus accumulates in a body cavity. Empyema **with fistula** occurs when the pus passes from one cavity to another organ or structure.

▶ New   ⇒ Revised   ~~deleted~~ Deleted   Excludes 1   Excludes 2   Includes   Use additional   Code first   Code also   Key words
OGCR Official Guidelines   X Assign placeholder X   ● Use Additional Character(s)   ▶ Manifestation Code   🔖 Hierarchical Condition Category   Coding Clinic

OTHER DISEASES OF THE PLEURA (J90-J94)

J90   Pleural effusion, not elsewhere classified
Encysted pleurisy
Pleural effusion NOS
Pleurisy with effusion (exudative) (serous)

> **Excludes1**   chylous (pleural) effusion (J94.0)
>   malignant pleural effusion (J91.0))
>   pleurisy NOS (R09.1)
>   tuberculous pleural effusion (A15.6)

     Coding Clinic: 2015, Q2, P16

J91   Pleural effusion in conditions classified elsewhere

> **Excludes2**   pleural effusion in heart failure (I50.-)
>   pleural effusion in systemic lupus erythematosus
>   (M32.13)

> *J91.0*   *Malignant pleural effusion*
>   ➡ *Code first underlying neoplasm (C00-D49)*

> *J91.8*   *Pleural effusion in other conditions classified elsewhere*
>   *Code first underlying disease, such as:*
>   filariasis (B74.0-B74.9)
>   influenza (J09.X2, J10.1, J11.1)
>   Coding Clinic: 2015, Q2, P16

J92   Pleural plaque

> **Includes**   pleural thickening

> **J92.0**   **Pleural plaque with presence of asbestos**

> **J92.9**   **Pleural plaque without asbestos**
>   Pleural plaque NOS

J93   Pneumothorax and air leak
Collapsed lung

> **Excludes1**   congenital or perinatal pneumothorax (P25.1)
>   postprocedural air leak (J95.812)
>   postprocedural pneumothorax (J95.811)
>   traumatic pneumothorax (S27.0)
>   tuberculous (current disease) pneumothorax
>   (A15.-)
>   pyopneumothorax (J86.-)

> **J93.0**   **Spontaneous tension pneumothorax**
>   *Tension pneumothorax (most serious type) occurs when air*
>   *(positive pressure) collects in the pleural space*

> **J93.1**   **Other spontaneous pneumothorax**

> > **J93.11**   **Primary spontaneous pneumothorax**

> > **J93.12**   **Secondary spontaneous pneumothorax**
> >   *Code first underlying condition, such as:*
> >   ➡ catamenial pneumothorax due to
> >   endometriosis (N80.B-)
> >   cystic fibrosis (E84.-)
> >   eosinophilic pneumonia (J82)
> >   lymphangioleiomyomatosis (J84.81)
> >   malignant neoplasm of bronchus and lung
> >   (C34.-)
> >   Marfan's syndrome (Q87.4)
> >   pneumonia due to Pneumocystis carinii
> >   (B59)
> >   secondary malignant neoplasm of lung
> >   (C78.0-)
> >   spontaneous rupture of the esophagus
> >   (K22.3)

> **J93.8**   **Other pneumothorax and air leak**

> > **J93.81**   **Chronic pneumothorax**

> > **J93.82**   **Other air leak**
> >   Persistent air leak

> > **J93.83**   **Other pneumothorax**
> >   Acute pneumothorax
> >   Spontaneous pneumothorax NOS

> **J93.9**   **Pneumothorax, unspecified**
>   Pneumothorax NOS

J94   Other pleural conditions

> **Excludes1**   pleurisy NOS (R09.1)
>   traumatic hemopneumothorax (S27.2)
>   traumatic hemothorax (S27.1)
>   tuberculous pleural conditions (current disease)
>   (A15.-)

> **J94.0**   **Chylous effusion**
>   Chyliform effusion

> **J94.1**   **Fibrothorax**

> **J94.2**   **Hemothorax**
>   Hemopneumothorax

> **J94.8**   **Other specified pleural conditions**
>   Hydropneumothorax
>   Hydrothorax
>   Coding Clinic: 2021, Q1, P49

> **J94.9**   **Pleural condition, unspecified**

INTRAOPERATIVE AND POSTPROCEDURAL COMPLICATIONS AND DISORDERS OF RESPIRATORY SYSTEM, NOT ELSEWHERE CLASSIFIED (J95)

J95   Intraoperative and postprocedural complications and disorders of respiratory system, not elsewhere classified

> **Excludes2**   aspiration pneumonia (J69.-)
>   emphysema (subcutaneous) resulting from a
>   procedure (T81.82)
>   hypostatic pneumonia (J18.2)
>   pulmonary manifestations due to radiation
>   (J70.0- J70.1)

> **J95.0**   **Tracheostomy complications**

> > **J95.00**   **Unspecified tracheostomy complication** 🔗

> > **J95.01**   **Hemorrhage from tracheostomy stoma** 🔗

> > **J95.02**   **Infection of tracheostomy stoma** 🔗
> >   Use additional code to identify type of
> >   infection, such as:
> >   cellulitis of neck (L03.221)
> >   sepsis (A40, A41.-)

> > **J95.03**   **Malfunction of tracheostomy stoma** 🔗
> >   Mechanical complication of tracheostomy
> >   stoma
> >   Obstruction of tracheostomy airway
> >   Tracheal stenosis due to tracheostomy

> > **J95.04**   **Tracheo-esophageal fistula following tracheostomy** 🔗

> > **J95.09**   **Other tracheostomy complication** 🔗

> **J95.1**   **Acute pulmonary insufficiency following thoracic surgery** 🔗

> > **Excludes2**   functional disturbances following cardiac
> >   surgery (I97.0, I97.1-)

> **J95.2**   **Acute pulmonary insufficiency following nonthoracic surgery** 🔗

> > **Excludes2**   functional disturbances following cardiac
> >   surgery (I97.0, I97.1-)

> **J95.3**   **Chronic pulmonary insufficiency following surgery** 🔗

> > **Excludes2**   functional disturbances following cardiac
> >   surgery (I97.0, I97.1-)

> **J95.4**   **Chemical pneumonitis due to anesthesia**
>   Mendelson's syndrome
>   Postprocedural aspiration pneumonia
>   Use additional code for adverse effect, if applicable, to
>   identify drug (T41.- with fifth or sixth character 5)

> > **Excludes1**   aspiration pneumonitis due to anesthesia
> >   complicating labor and delivery
> >   (O74.0)
> >   aspiration pneumonitis due to anesthesia
> >   complicating pregnancy (O29)
> >   aspiration pneumonitis due to anesthesia
> >   complicating the puerperium
> >   (O89.01)

CHAPTER 10 (J00-J99)

J95.5   Postprocedural subglottic stenosis

● J95.6   Intraoperative hemorrhage and hematoma of a respiratory system organ or structure complicating a procedure

> **Excludes1**   intraoperative hemorrhage and hematoma of a respiratory system organ or structure due to accidental puncture and laceration during procedure (J95.7-)

J95.61   Intraoperative hemorrhage and hematoma of a respiratory system organ or structure complicating a respiratory system procedure

J95.62   Intraoperative hemorrhage and hematoma of a respiratory system organ or structure complicating other procedure

● J95.7   Accidental puncture and laceration of a respiratory system organ or structure during a procedure

> **Excludes2**   postprocedural pneumothorax (J95.811)

J95.71   Accidental puncture and laceration of a respiratory system organ or structure during a respiratory system procedure

J95.72   Accidental puncture and laceration of a respiratory system organ or structure during other procedure

● J95.8   Other intraoperative and postprocedural complications and disorders of respiratory system, not elsewhere classified
> Coding Clinic: 2016, Q4, P10

● J95.81   Postprocedural pneumothorax and air leak

J95.811   Postprocedural pneumothorax
> Coding Clinic: 2021, Q1, P49

J95.812   Postprocedural air leak

● J95.82   Postprocedural respiratory failure

> **Excludes1**   Respiratory failure in other conditions (J96.-)

J95.821   **Acute postprocedural respiratory failure** 🔖
> Postprocedural respiratory failure NOS

J95.822   **Acute and chronic postprocedural respiratory failure** 🔖

● J95.83   Postprocedural hemorrhage of a respiratory system organ or structure following a procedure

J95.830   Postprocedural hemorrhage of a respiratory system organ or structure following a respiratory system procedure

J95.831   Postprocedural hemorrhage of a respiratory system organ or structure following other procedure

J95.84   Transfusion-related acute lung injury (TRALI)

● J95.85   Complication of respirator [ventilator]

J95.850   **Mechanical complication of respirator** 🔖

> **Excludes1**   encounter for respirator [ventilator] dependence during power failure (Z99.12)

J95.851   **Ventilator associated pneumonia** 🔖
> Ventilator associated pneumonitis
> Use additional code to identify the organism, if known (B95.-, B96.-, B97.-)

> **Excludes1**   ventilator lung in newborn (P27.8)

> Coding Clinic: 2017, Q1, P25

J95.859   **Other complication of respirator [ventilator]** 🔖
> Coding Clinic: 2021, Q1, P49

● J95.86   Postprocedural hematoma and seroma of a respiratory system organ or structure following a procedure

J95.860   Postprocedural hematoma of a respiratory system organ or structure following a respiratory system procedure

J95.861   Postprocedural hematoma of a respiratory system organ or structure following other procedure

J95.862   Postprocedural seroma of a respiratory system organ or structure following a respiratory system procedure

J95.863   Postprocedural seroma of a respiratory system organ or structure following other procedure

▶ J95.87   Transfusion-associated dyspnea (TAD)

> ▶ **Excludes1**   transfusion associated circulatory overload (TACO) (E87.71)
> ▶ transfusion-related acute lung injury (TRALI) (J95.84)

J95.88   Other intraoperative complications of respiratory system, not elsewhere classified

J95.89   Other postprocedural complications and disorders of respiratory system, not elsewhere classified

> Use additional code to identify disorder, such as:
> aspiration pneumonia (J69.-)
> bacterial or viral pneumonia (J12-J18)

> **Excludes2**   acute pulmonary insufficiency following thoracic surgery (J95.1)
> postprocedural subglottic stenosis (J95.5)

OTHER DISEASES OF THE RESPIRATORY SYSTEM (J96-J99)

● J96   Respiratory failure, not elsewhere classified

> **Excludes1**   acute respiratory distress syndrome (J80)
> cardiorespiratory failure (R09.2)
> newborn respiratory distress syndrome (P22.0)
> postprocedural respiratory failure (J95.82-)
> respiratory arrest (R09.2)
> respiratory arrest of newborn (P28.81)
> respiratory failure of newborn (P28.5)

● J96.0   Acute respiratory failure

J96.00   **Acute respiratory failure, unspecified whether with hypoxia or hypercapnia** 🔖
> Coding Clinic: 2016, Q3, P14

J96.01   **Acute respiratory failure with hypoxia** 🔖

J96.02   **Acute respiratory failure with hypercapnia** 🔖
> ▶ Acute respiratory acidosis

● J96.1   Chronic respiratory failure

J96.10   **Chronic respiratory failure, unspecified whether with hypoxia or hypercapnia** 🔖
> Coding Clinic: 2021, Q4, P105-106; 2021, Q1, P46; 2016, Q1, P38; 2015, Q1, P21

J96.11   **Chronic respiratory failure with hypoxia** 🔖

J96.12   **Chronic respiratory failure with hypercapnia** 🔖
> ▶ Chronic respiratory acidosis

● J96.2   Acute and chronic respiratory failure
> Acute on chronic respiratory failure

J96.20   **Acute and chronic respiratory failure, unspecified whether with hypoxia or hypercapnia**

J96.21   **Acute and chronic respiratory failure with hypoxia** 🔖

J96.22   **Acute and chronic respiratory failure with hypercapnia** 🔖

▶ New   ⇒ Revised   ~~deleted~~ Deleted   Excludes 1   Excludes 2   Includes   Use additional   Code first   Code also   Key words

OGCR Official Guidelines   X Assign placeholder X   ● Use Additional Character(s)   ▶ Manifestation Code   🔖 Hierarchical Condition Category   Coding Clinic

● **J96.9**   **Respiratory failure, unspecified**

     J96.90   **Respiratory failure, unspecified, unspecified whether with hypoxia or hypercapnia** 🔗
         Coding Clinic: 2021, Q1, P44

     J96.91   **Respiratory failure, unspecified with hypoxia** 🔗

     J96.92   **Respiratory failure, unspecified with hypercapnia** 🔗

● **J98**   **Other respiratory disorders**

     Use additional code to identify:
       exposure to environmental tobacco smoke (Z77.22)
       exposure to tobacco smoke in the perinatal period (P96.81)
       history of tobacco dependence (Z87.891)
       occupational exposure to environmental tobacco smoke (Z57.31)
       tobacco dependence (F17.-)
       tobacco use (Z72.0)

     Excludes1   newborn apnea (P28.4-)
               newborn sleep apnea (P28.3-)

     Excludes2   apnea NOS (R06.81)
               sleep apnea (G47.3-)

● **J98.0**   **Diseases of bronchus, not elsewhere classified**

     J98.01   **Acute bronchospasm**

         Excludes1   acute bronchiolitis with bronchospasm (J21.-)
                       acute bronchitis with bronchospasm (J20.-)
                       asthma (J45.-)
                       exercise induced bronchospasm (J45.990)

     J98.09   **Other diseases of bronchus, not elsewhere classified**
         Broncholithiasis
         Calcification of bronchus
         Stenosis of bronchus
         Tracheobronchial collapse
         Tracheobronchial dyskinesia
         Ulcer of bronchus

● **J98.1**   **Pulmonary collapse**

     Excludes1   therapeutic collapse of lung status (Z98.3)

     J98.11   **Atelectasis**

         Excludes1   newborn atelectasis
                       tuberculous atelectasis (current disease) (A15)

     J98.19   **Other pulmonary collapse**

J98.2   **Interstitial emphysema** 🔗
     Mediastinal emphysema

     Excludes1   emphysema NOS (J43.9)
               emphysema in newborn (P25.0)
               surgical emphysema (subcutaneous) (T81.82)
               traumatic subcutaneous emphysema (T79.7)

J98.3   **Compensatory emphysema** 🔗

J98.4   **Other disorders of lung**
     Calcification of lung
     Cystic lung disease (acquired)
     Lung disease NOS
     Pulmolithiasis

     Excludes1   acute interstitial pneumonitis (J84.114)
               pulmonary insufficiency following surgery (J95.1-J95.2)

● **J98.5**   **Diseases of mediastinum, not elsewhere classified**

     Excludes2   abscess of mediastinum (J85.3)
     Coding Clinic: 2016, Q4, P29

     J98.51   **Mediastinitis**

         Code first underlying condition, if applicable, such as postoperative mediastinitis (T81.-)

     J98.59   **Other diseases of mediastinum, not elsewhere classified**
         Fibrosis of mediastinum
         Hernia of mediastinum
         Retraction of mediastinum

J98.6   **Disorders of diaphragm**
     Diaphragmatitis
     Paralysis of diaphragm
     Relaxation of diaphragm

     Excludes1   congenital malformation of diaphragm NEC (Q79.1)
               congenital diaphragmatic hernia (Q79.0)

     Excludes2   diaphragmatic hernia (K44.-)

J98.8   **Other specified respiratory disorders**

J98.9   **Respiratory disorder, unspecified**
     Respiratory disease (chronic) NOS

◗ *J99*   *Respiratory disorders in diseases classified elsewhere* 🔗

     Code first underlying disease, such as:
       amyloidosis (E85.-)
       ankylosing spondylitis (M45)
       congenital syphilis (A50.5)
       cryoglobulinemia (D89.1)
       early congenital syphilis (A50.0)
       plasminogen deficiency (E88.02)
       schistosomiasis (B65.0-B65.9)

     Excludes1   respiratory disorders in:
               amebiasis (A06.5)
               blastomycosis (B40.0-B40.2)
               candidiasis (B37.1)
               coccidioidomycosis (B38.0-B38.2)
               cystic fibrosis with pulmonary manifestations (E84.0)
               dermatomyositis (M33.01, M33.11)
               histoplasmosis (B39.0-B39.2)
               late syphilis (A52.72, A52.73)
               polymyositis (M33.21)
               Sjögren syndrome (M35.02)
               systemic lupus erythematosus (M32.13)
               systemic sclerosis (M34.81)
               Wegener's granulomatosis (M31.30-M31.31)

CHAPTER 10 (J00–J99)

CHAPTER 11

DISEASES OF THE DIGESTIVE SYSTEM (K00-K95)

OGCR Chapter-Specific Coding Guidelines

> 11. Chapter 11: Diseases of the Digestive System (K00-K95)
> Reserved for future guideline expansion

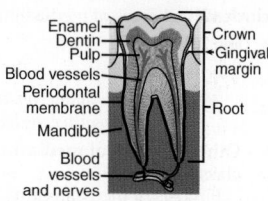

Figure 11-1 Anatomy of a tooth.

Item 11-1 **Anodontia** is the congenital absence of teeth. **Hypodontia** is partial anodontia. **Oligodontia** is the congenital absence of some teeth, whereas **supernumerary** is having more teeth than the normal number. **Mesiodens** are small extra teeth that often appear in pairs, although single small teeth are not uncommon.

CHAPTER 11

DISEASES OF THE DIGESTIVE SYSTEM (K00-K95)

Excludes2   certain conditions originating in the perinatal period (P04-P96)
certain infectious and parasitic diseases (A00-B99)
complications of pregnancy, childbirth and the puerperium (O00-O9A)
congenital malformations, deformations and chromosomal abnormalities (Q00-Q99)
endocrine, nutritional and metabolic diseases (E00-E88)
injury, poisoning and certain other consequences of external causes (S00-T88)
neoplasms (C00-D49)
symptoms, signs and abnormal clinical and laboratory findings, not elsewhere classified (R00-R94)

This chapter contains the following blocks:

K00-K14	Diseases of oral cavity and salivary glands
K20-K31	Diseases of esophagus, stomach and duodenum
K35-K38	Diseases of appendix
K40-K46	Hernia
K50-K52	Noninfective enteritis and colitis
K55-K64	Other diseases of intestines
K65-K68	Diseases of peritoneum and retroperitoneum
K70-K77	Diseases of liver
K80-K87	Disorders of gallbladder, biliary tract and pancreas
K90-K95	Other diseases of the digestive system

DISEASES OF ORAL CAVITY AND SALIVARY GLANDS (K00-K14)

● **K00**   **Disorders of tooth development and eruption**
     Excludes2   embedded and impacted teeth (K01.-)
     K00.0   **Anodontia**
         Hypodontia
         Oligodontia
         Excludes1   acquired absence of teeth (K08.1-)
     K00.1   **Supernumerary teeth**
         Distomolar
         Fourth molar
         Mesiodens
         Paramolar
         Supplementary teeth
         Excludes2   supernumerary roots (K00.2)

K00.2   **Abnormalities of size and form of teeth**
     Concrescence of teeth
     Fusion of teeth
     Gemination of teeth
     Dens evaginatus
     Dens in dente
     Dens invaginatus
     Enamel pearls
     Macrodontia
     Microdontia
     Peg-shaped [conical] teeth
     Supernumerary roots
     Taurodontism
     Tuberculum paramolare
     Excludes1   abnormalities of teeth due to congenital syphilis (A50.5)
         tuberculum Carabelli, which is regarded as a normal variation and should not be coded

K00.3   **Mottled teeth**
     Dental fluorosis
     Mottling of enamel
     Nonfluoride enamel opacities
     Excludes2   deposits [accretions] on teeth (K03.6)

K00.4   **Disturbances in tooth formation**
     Aplasia and hypoplasia of cementum
     Dilaceration of tooth
     Enamel hypoplasia (neonatal) (postnatal) (prenatal)
     Regional odontodysplasia
     Turner's tooth
     Excludes1   Hutchinson's teeth and mulberry molars in congenital syphilis (A50.5)
     Excludes2   mottled teeth (K00.3)

K00.5   **Hereditary disturbances in tooth structure, not elsewhere classified**
     Amelogenesis imperfecta
     Dentinogenesis imperfecta
     Odontogenesis imperfecta
     Dentinal dysplasia
     Shell teeth

K00.6   **Disturbances in tooth eruption**
     Dentia praecox
     Natal tooth
     Neonatal tooth
     Premature eruption of tooth
     Premature shedding of primary [deciduous] tooth
     Prenatal teeth
     Retained [persistent] primary tooth
     Excludes2   embedded and impacted teeth (K01.-)

K00.7   **Teething syndrome**

K00.8   **Other disorders of tooth development**
     Color changes during tooth formation
     Intrinsic staining of teeth NOS
     Excludes2   posteruptive color changes (K03.7)

K00.9   **Disorder of tooth development, unspecified**
     Disorder of odontogenesis NOS

● **K01**   **Embedded and impacted teeth**
     Excludes1   abnormal position of fully erupted teeth (M26.3-)
     K01.0   **Embedded teeth**
     K01.1   **Impacted teeth**

▶ New   ⇒ Revised   ~~deleted~~ Deleted   Excludes 1   Excludes 2   Includes   Use additional   Code first   Code also   Key words
OGCR Official Guidelines   X Assign placeholder X   ● Use Additional Character(s)   ▮ Manifestation Code   ✿ Hierarchical Condition Category   **Coding Clinic**

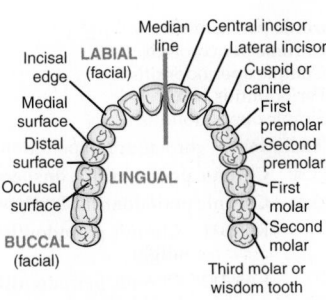

Figure 11-2 The permanent teeth within the dental arch.

Item 11-2 Each dental arch (jaw) normally contains 16 teeth. Tooth decay or **dental caries** is a disease of the enamel, dentin, and cementum of the tooth and can result in a cavity.

● **K02   Dental caries**

    Includes   caries of dentine
                   dental cavities
                   early childhood caries
                   pre-eruptive caries
                   recurrent caries (dentino enamel junction)
                     (enamel) (to the pulp)
                   tooth decay

    K02.3   Arrested dental caries
           Arrested coronal and root caries

●   **K02.5   Dental caries on pit and fissure surface**
           Dental caries on chewing surface of tooth

        K02.51   Dental caries on pit and fissure surface limited to enamel
               White spot lesions [initial caries] on pit and fissure surface of tooth

        K02.52   Dental caries on pit and fissure surface penetrating into dentin
               Primary dental caries, cervical origin

        K02.53   Dental caries on pit and fissure surface penetrating into pulp

●   **K02.6   Dental caries on smooth surface**

        K02.61   Dental caries on smooth surface limited to enamel
               White spot lesions [initial caries] on smooth surface of tooth

        K02.62   Dental caries on smooth surface penetrating into dentin

        K02.63   Dental caries on smooth surface penetrating into pulp

    K02.7   Dental root caries

    K02.9   Dental caries, unspecified

● **K03   Other diseases of hard tissues of teeth**

    Excludes2   bruxism (F45.8)
                    dental caries (K02.-)
                    teeth-grinding NOS (F45.8)

    K03.0   Excessive attrition of teeth
           Approximal wear of teeth
           Occlusal wear of teeth

    K03.1   Abrasion of teeth
           Dentifrice abrasion of teeth
           Habitual abrasion of teeth
           Occupational abrasion of teeth
           Ritual abrasion of teeth
           Traditional abrasion of teeth
           Wedge defect NOS

    K03.2   Erosion of teeth
           Erosion of teeth due to diet
           Erosion of teeth due to drugs and medicaments
           Erosion of teeth due to persistent vomiting
           Erosion of teeth NOS
           Idiopathic erosion of teeth
           Occupational erosion of teeth

    K03.3   Pathological resorption of teeth
           Internal granuloma of pulp
           Resorption of teeth (external)

    K03.4   Hypercementosis
           Cementation hyperplasia

    K03.5   Ankylosis of teeth

    K03.6   Deposits [accretions] on teeth
           Betel deposits [accretions] on teeth
           Black deposits [accretions] on teeth
           Extrinsic staining of teeth NOS
           Green deposits [accretions] on teeth
           Materia alba deposits [accretions] on teeth
           Orange deposits [accretions] on teeth
           Staining of teeth NOS
           Subgingival dental calculus
           Supragingival dental calculus
           Tobacco deposits [accretions] on teeth

    K03.7   Posteruptive color changes of dental hard tissues
        Excludes2   deposits [accretions] on teeth (K03.6)

●   **K03.8   Other specified diseases of hard tissues of teeth**
        K03.81   Cracked tooth
              Excludes1 asymptomatic craze lines in enamel - omit code
                                 broken or fractured tooth due to trauma (S02.5)

        K03.89   Other specified diseases of hard tissues of teeth

    K03.9   Disease of hard tissues of teeth, unspecified

K04   Diseases of pulp and periapical tissues
    Coding Clinic: 2016, Q4, P29

●   **K04.0   Pulpitis**
           Acute pulpitis
           Chronic (hyperplastic) (ulcerative) pulpitis

        K04.01   Reversible pulpitis

        K04.02   Irreversible pulpitis

    K04.1   Necrosis of pulp
           Pulpal gangrene

    K04.2   Pulp degeneration
           Denticles
           Pulpal calcifications
           Pulpal stones

    K04.3   Abnormal hard tissue formation in pulp
           Secondary or irregular dentine

    K04.4   Acute apical periodontitis of pulpal origin
           Acute apical periodontitis NOS
         Excludes1   acute periodontitis (K05.2-)

    K04.5   Chronic apical periodontitis
           Apical or periapical granuloma
           Apical periodontitis NOS
         Excludes1   chronic periodontitis (K05.3-)

    K04.6   Periapical abscess with sinus
           Dental abscess with sinus
           Dentoalveolar abscess with sinus

    K04.7   Periapical abscess without sinus
           Dental abscess without sinus
           Dentoalveolar abscess without sinus

    K04.8   Radicular cyst
           Apical (periodontal) cyst
           Periapical cyst
           Residual radicular cyst
         Excludes2   lateral periodontal cyst (K09.0)

●   **K04.9   Other and unspecified diseases of pulp and periapical tissues**
        K04.90   Unspecified diseases of pulp and periapical tissues

        K04.99   Other diseases of pulp and periapical tissues

CHAPTER 11 (K00-K95)

Item 11–3 Acute gingivitis, also known as orilitis or ulitis, is the short-term, severe inflammation of the gums (gingiva) caused by bacteria. **Chronic gingivitis** is persistent inflammation of the gums. When the gingivitis moves into the periodontium it is called periodontitis, also known as paradentitis.

● **K05 Gingivitis and periodontal diseases**
    Use additional code to identify:
        alcohol abuse and dependence (F10.-)
        exposure to environmental tobacco smoke (Z77.22)
        exposure to tobacco smoke in the perinatal period (P96.81)
        history of tobacco dependence (Z87.891)
        occupational exposure to environmental tobacco smoke (Z57.31)
        tobacco dependence (F17.-)
        tobacco use (Z72.0)
    Coding Clinic: 2016, Q4, P29

● **K05.0 Acute gingivitis**
    Excludes1 acute necrotizing ulcerative gingivitis (A69.1)
                 herpesviral [herpes simplex] gingivostomatitis (B00.2)

    K05.00 Acute gingivitis, plaque induced
        Acute gingivitis NOS
        Plaque induced gingival disease

    K05.01 Acute gingivitis, non-plaque induced

● **K05.1 Chronic gingivitis**
    Desquamative gingivitis (chronic)
    Gingivitis (chronic) NOS
    Hyperplastic gingivitis (chronic)
    Pregnancy associated gingivitis
    Simple marginal gingivitis (chronic)
    Ulcerative gingivitis (chronic)
    Code first, if applicable, diseases of the digestive system complicating pregnancy (O99.61-)

    K05.10 Chronic gingivitis, plaque induced
        Chronic gingivitis NOS
        Gingivitis NOS

    K05.11 Chronic gingivitis, non-plaque induced

● **K05.2 Aggressive periodontitis**
    Acute pericoronitis
    Excludes1 acute apical periodontitis (K04.4)
                 periapical abscess (K04.7)
                 periapical abscess with sinus (K04.6)

    K05.20 Aggressive periodontitis, unspecified
    K05.21 Aggressive periodontitis, localized
        Periodontal abscess
        K05.211 Aggressive periodontitis, localized, slight
        K05.212 Aggressive periodontitis, localized, moderate
        K05.213 Aggressive periodontitis, localized, severe
        K05.219 Aggressive periodontitis, localized, unspecified severity
    K05.22 Aggressive periodontitis, generalized
        K05.221 Aggressive periodontitis, generalized, slight
        K05.222 Aggressive periodontitis, generalized, moderate
        K05.223 Aggressive periodontitis, generalized, severe
        K05.229 Aggressive periodontitis, generalized, unspecified severity

● **K05.3 Chronic periodontitis**
    Chronic pericoronitis
    Complex periodontitis
    Periodontitis NOS
    Simplex periodontitis
    Excludes1 chronic apical periodontitis (K04.5)

    K05.30 Chronic periodontitis, unspecified
    K05.31 Chronic periodontitis, localized
        K05.311 Chronic periodontitis, localized, slight
        K05.312 Chronic periodontitis, localized, moderate
        K05.313 Chronic periodontitis, localized, severe
        K05.319 Chronic periodontitis, localized, unspecified severity
    K05.32 Chronic periodontitis, generalized
        K05.321 Chronic periodontitis, generalized, slight
        K05.322 Chronic periodontitis, generalized, moderate
        K05.323 Chronic periodontitis, generalized, severe
        K05.329 Chronic periodontitis, generalized, unspecified severity

K05.4 Periodontosis
    Juvenile periodontosis

K05.5 Other periodontal diseases
    Combined periodontic-endodontic lesion
    Narrow gingival width (of periodontal soft tissue)
    Excludes2 leukoplakia of gingiva (K13.21)

K05.6 Periodontal disease, unspecified

● **K06 Other disorders of gingiva and edentulous alveolar ridge**
    Excludes2 acute gingivitis (K05.0)
                 atrophy of edentulous alveolar ridge (K08.2)
                 chronic gingivitis (K05.1)
                 gingivitis NOS (K05.1)
    Coding Clinic: 2016, Q4, P29

● **K06.0 Gingival recession**
    Gingival recession (postinfective) (postprocedural)
    ● **K06.01 Gingival recession, localized**
        K06.010 Localized gingival recession, unspecified
            Localized gingival recession, NOS
        K06.011 Localized gingival recession, minimal
        K06.012 Localized gingival recession, moderate
        K06.013 Localized gingival recession, severe
    ● **K06.02 Gingival recession, generalized**
        K06.020 Generalized gingival recession, unspecified
            Generalized gingival recession, NOS
        K06.021 Generalized gingival recession, minimal
        K06.022 Generalized gingival recession, moderate
        K06.023 Generalized gingival recession, severe

K06.1 Gingival enlargement
    Gingival fibromatosis

K06.2 Gingival and edentulous alveolar ridge lesions associated with trauma
    Irritative hyperplasia of edentulous ridge [denture hyperplasia]
    Use additional code (Chapter 20) to identify external cause or denture status (Z97.2)

K06.3 Horizontal alveolar bone loss

▶ New ⇒ Revised ~~deleted~~ Deleted Excludes 1 Excludes 2 Includes Use additional Code first Code also Key words
OGCR Official Guidelines X Assign placeholder X ● Use Additional Character(s) ▶ Manifestation Code ⬟ Hierarchical Condition Category **Coding Clinic**

K06.8   **Other specified disorders of gingiva and edentulous alveolar ridge**
     Fibrous epulis
     Flabby alveolar ridge
     Giant cell epulis
     Peripheral giant cell granuloma of gingiva
     Pyogenic granuloma of gingiva
     Vertical ridge deficiency
     Excludes2   gingival cyst (K09.0)

K06.9   **Disorder of gingiva and edentulous alveolar ridge, unspecified**

K08   **Other disorders of teeth and supporting structures**
     Excludes2   dentofacial anomalies [including malocclusion] (M26.-)
                disorders of jaw (M27.-)
     Coding Clinic: 2016, Q4, P29

K08.0   **Exfoliation of teeth due to systemic causes**
     Code also underlying systemic condition

K08.1   **Complete loss of teeth**
     Acquired loss of teeth, complete
     Excludes1   congenital absence of teeth (K00.0)
                exfoliation of teeth due to systemic causes (K08.0)
                partial loss of teeth (K08.4-)

     K08.10   **Complete loss of teeth, unspecified cause**
         K08.101   Complete loss of teeth, unspecified cause, class I
         K08.102   Complete loss of teeth, unspecified cause, class II
         K08.103   Complete loss of teeth, unspecified cause, class III
         K08.104   Complete loss of teeth, unspecified cause, class IV
         K08.109   Complete loss of teeth, unspecified cause, unspecified class
            Edentulism NOS

     K08.11   **Complete loss of teeth due to trauma**
         K08.111   Complete loss of teeth due to trauma, class I
         K08.112   Complete loss of teeth due to trauma, class II
         K08.113   Complete loss of teeth due to trauma, class III
         K08.114   Complete loss of teeth due to trauma, class IV
         K08.119   Complete loss of teeth due to trauma, unspecified class

     K08.12   **Complete loss of teeth due to periodontal diseases**
         K08.121   Complete loss of teeth due to periodontal diseases, class I
         K08.122   Complete loss of teeth due to periodontal diseases, class II
         K08.123   Complete loss of teeth due to periodontal diseases, class III
         K08.124   Complete loss of teeth due to periodontal diseases, class IV
         K08.129   Complete loss of teeth due to periodontal diseases, unspecified class

     K08.13   **Complete loss of teeth due to caries**
         K08.131   Complete loss of teeth due to caries, class I
         K08.132   Complete loss of teeth due to caries, class II
         K08.133   Complete loss of teeth due to caries, class III
         K08.134   Complete loss of teeth due to caries, class IV
         K08.139   Complete loss of teeth due to caries, unspecified class

     K08.19   **Complete loss of teeth due to other specified cause**
         K08.191   Complete loss of teeth due to other specified cause, class I
         K08.192   Complete loss of teeth due to other specified cause, class II
         K08.193   Complete loss of teeth due to other specified cause, class III
         K08.194   Complete loss of teeth due to other specified cause, class IV
         K08.199   Complete loss of teeth due to other specified cause, unspecified class

K08.2   **Atrophy of edentulous alveolar ridge**
     K08.20   **Unspecified atrophy of edentulous alveolar ridge**
            Atrophy of the mandible NOS
            Atrophy of the maxilla NOS
     K08.21   **Minimal atrophy of the mandible**
            Minimal atrophy of the edentulous mandible
     K08.22   **Moderate atrophy of the mandible**
            Moderate atrophy of the edentulous mandible
     K08.23   **Severe atrophy of the mandible**
            Severe atrophy of the edentulous mandible
     K08.24   **Minimal atrophy of maxilla**
            Minimal atrophy of the edentulous maxilla
     K08.25   **Moderate atrophy of the maxilla**
            Moderate atrophy of the edentulous maxilla
     K08.26   **Severe atrophy of the maxilla**
            Severe atrophy of the edentulous maxilla

K08.3   **Retained dental root**

K08.4   **Partial loss of teeth**
     Acquired loss of teeth, partial
     Excludes1   complete loss of teeth (K08.1-)
                congenital absence of teeth (K00.0)
     Excludes2   exfoliation of teeth due to systemic causes (K08.0)

     K08.40   **Partial loss of teeth, unspecified cause**
         K08.401   Partial loss of teeth, unspecified cause, class I
         K08.402   Partial loss of teeth, unspecified cause, class II
         K08.403   Partial loss of teeth, unspecified cause, class III
         K08.404   Partial loss of teeth, unspecified cause, class IV
         K08.409   Partial loss of teeth, unspecified cause, unspecified class
            Tooth extraction status NOS

     K08.41   **Partial loss of teeth due to trauma**
         K08.411   Partial loss of teeth due to trauma, class I
         K08.412   Partial loss of teeth due to trauma, class II
         K08.413   Partial loss of teeth due to trauma, class III
         K08.414   Partial loss of teeth due to trauma, class IV
         K08.419   Partial loss of teeth due to trauma, unspecified class

     K08.42   **Partial loss of teeth due to periodontal diseases**
         K08.421   Partial loss of teeth due to periodontal diseases, class I
         K08.422   Partial loss of teeth due to periodontal diseases, class II
         K08.423   Partial loss of teeth due to periodontal diseases, class III
         K08.424   Partial loss of teeth due to periodontal diseases, class IV
         K08.429   Partial loss of teeth due to periodontal diseases, unspecified class

CHAPTER 11 (K00-K95)

● **K08.43 Partial loss of teeth due to caries**

     K08.431 Partial loss of teeth due to caries, class I

     K08.432 Partial loss of teeth due to caries, class II

     K08.433 Partial loss of teeth due to caries, class III

     K08.434 Partial loss of teeth due to caries, class IV

     K08.439 Partial loss of teeth due to caries, unspecified class

● **K08.49 Partial loss of teeth due to other specified cause**

     K08.491 Partial loss of teeth due to other specified cause, class I

     K08.492 Partial loss of teeth due to other specified cause, class II

     K08.493 Partial loss of teeth due to other specified cause, class III

     K08.494 Partial loss of teeth due to other specified cause, class IV

     K08.499 Partial loss of teeth due to other specified cause, unspecified class

● **K08.5 Unsatisfactory restoration of tooth**
    Defective bridge, crown, filling
    Defective dental restoration

    Excludes1   dental restoration status (Z98.811)

    Excludes2   endosseous dental implant failure (M27.6-)
              unsatisfactory endodontic treatment (M27.5-)

    K08.50 Unsatisfactory restoration of tooth, unspecified
       Defective dental restoration NOS

    K08.51 Open restoration margins of tooth
       Dental restoration failure of marginal integrity
       Open margin on tooth restoration
       Poor gingival margin to tooth restoration

    K08.52 Unrepairable overhanging of dental restorative materials
       Overhanging of tooth restoration

●   **K08.53 Fractured dental restorative material**

       Excludes1   cracked tooth (K03.81)
                 traumatic fracture of tooth (S02.5)

       K08.530 Fractured dental restorative material without loss of material

       K08.531 Fractured dental restorative material with loss of material

       K08.539 Fractured dental restorative material, unspecified

    K08.54 Contour of existing restoration of tooth biologically incompatible with oral health
       Dental restoration failure of periodontal anatomical integrity
       Unacceptable contours of existing restoration of tooth
       Unacceptable morphology of existing restoration of tooth

    K08.55 Allergy to existing dental restorative material
       Use additional code to identify the specific type of allergy

    K08.56 Poor aesthetic of existing restoration of tooth
       Dental restoration aesthetically inadequate or displeasing

    K08.59 Other unsatisfactory restoration of tooth
       Other defective dental restoration

● **K08.8 Other specified disorders of teeth and supporting structures**

    K08.81 Primary occlusal trauma

    K08.82 Secondary occlusal trauma

    K08.89 Other specified disorders of teeth and supporting structures
       Enlargement of alveolar ridge NOS
       Insufficient anatomic crown height
       Insufficient clinical crown length
       Irregular alveolar process
       Toothache NOS

K08.9 Disorder of teeth and supporting structures, unspecified

● **K09 Cysts of oral region, not elsewhere classified**

    Includes   lesions showing histological features both of aneurysmal cyst and of another fibro-osseous lesion

    Excludes2   cysts of jaw (M27.0-, M27.4-)
              radicular cyst (K04.8)

    K09.0 Developmental odontogenic cysts
       Dentigerous cyst
       Eruption cyst
       Follicular cyst
       Gingival cyst
       Lateral periodontal cyst
       Primordial cyst

       Excludes2   keratocysts (D16.4, D16.5)
                 odontogenic keratocystic tumors (D16.4, D16.5)

    K09.1 Developmental (nonodontogenic) cysts of oral region
       Cyst (of) incisive canal
       Cyst (of) palatine of papilla
       Globulomaxillary cyst
       Median palatal cyst
       Nasoalveolar cyst
       Nasolabial cyst
       Nasopalatine duct cyst

    K09.8 Other cysts of oral region, not elsewhere classified
       Dermoid cyst
       Epidermoid cyst
       Lymphoepithelial cyst
       Epstein's pearl

    K09.9 Cyst of oral region, unspecified

★ **(See Plate 28 of the Anatomy Illustrations.)**

● **K11 Diseases of salivary glands**
    Use additional code to identify:
       alcohol abuse and dependence (F10.-)
       exposure to environmental tobacco smoke (Z77.22)
       exposure to tobacco smoke in the perinatal period (P96.81)
       history of tobacco dependence (Z87.891)
       occupational exposure to environmental tobacco smoke (Z57.31)
       tobacco dependence (F17.-)
       tobacco use (Z72.0)

    K11.0 Atrophy of salivary gland

    K11.1 Hypertrophy of salivary gland

Item 11–4 Atrophy is wasting away of a tissue or organ, whereas **hypertrophy** is overdevelopment or enlargement of a tissue or organ. **Sialoadenitis** is salivary gland inflammation. **Parotitis** is the inflammation of the parotid gland. In the epidemic form, parotitis is also known as mumps. **Sialolithiasis** is the formation of calculus within a salivary gland. **Mucocele** is a polyp composed of mucus.

Figure 11-3   Major salivary glands.

Parotid gland
Sublingual gland
Submandibular gland

▶ New   ⇒ Revised   ~~deleted~~ Deleted   Excludes 1   Excludes 2   Includes   Use additional   Code first   Code also   Key words
OGCR Official Guidelines   X Assign placeholder X   ● Use Additional Character(s)   ▶ Manifestation Code   ⚕ Hierarchical Condition Category   **Coding Clinic**

● **K11.2**   **Sialoadenitis**
Parotitis
> **Excludes1**   epidemic parotitis (B26.-)
> mumps (B26.-)
> uveoparotid fever [Heerfordt] (D86.89)

    K11.20   **Sialoadenitis, unspecified**
    K11.21   **Acute sialoadenitis**
> **Excludes1**   acute recurrent sialoadenitis
> (K11.22)

    K11.22   **Acute recurrent sialoadenitis**
    K11.23   **Chronic sialoadenitis**

K11.3   **Abscess of salivary gland**

K11.4   **Fistula of salivary gland**
> **Excludes1**   congenital fistula of salivary gland
> (Q38.4)

K11.5   **Sialolithiasis**
Calculus of salivary gland or duct
Stone of salivary gland or duct

K11.6   **Mucocele of salivary gland**
Mucous extravasation cyst of salivary gland
Mucous retention cyst of salivary gland
Ranula

K11.7   **Disturbances of salivary secretion**
Hypoptyalism
Ptyalism
Xerostomia
> **Excludes2**   dry mouth NOS (R68.2)

K11.8   **Other diseases of salivary glands**
Benign lymphoepithelial lesion of salivary gland
Mikulicz' disease
Necrotizing sialometaplasia
Sialectasia
Stenosis of salivary duct
Stricture of salivary duct
> **Excludes1**   Sjögren syndrome (M35.0-)

K11.9   **Disease of salivary gland, unspecified**
Sialoadenopathy NOS

● **K12**   **Stomatitis and related lesions**
Use additional code to identify:
alcohol abuse and dependence (F10.-)
exposure to environmental tobacco smoke (Z77.22)
exposure to tobacco smoke in the perinatal period (P96.81)
history of tobacco dependence (Z87.891)
occupational exposure to environmental tobacco smoke (Z57.31)
tobacco dependence (F17.-)
tobacco use (Z72.0)
> **Excludes1**   cancrum oris (A69.0)
> cheilitis (K13.0)
> gangrenous stomatitis (A69.0)
> herpesviral [herpes simplex] gingivostomatitis
> (B00.2)
> noma (A69.0)

K12.0   **Recurrent oral aphthae**
Aphthous stomatitis (major) (minor)
Bednar's aphthae
Periadenitis mucosa necrotica recurrens
Recurrent aphthous ulcer
Stomatitis herpetiformis

K12.1   **Other forms of stomatitis**
Stomatitis NOS
Denture stomatitis
Ulcerative stomatitis
Vesicular stomatitis
> **Excludes1**   acute necrotizing ulcerative stomatitis
> (A69.1)
> Vincent's stomatitis (A69.1)

> **Item 11-5**   **Stomatitis** is the inflammation of the oral mucosa. **Mucositis** is the inflammation of the mucous membranes lining the digestive tract from the mouth to the anus. It is a common side effect of chemotherapy and of radiotherapy that involves any part of the digestive tract.

    K12.2   **Cellulitis and abscess of mouth**
Cellulitis of mouth (floor)
Submandibular abscess
> **Excludes2**   abscess of salivary gland (K11.3)
> abscess of tongue (K14.0)
> periapical abscess (K04.6-K04.7)
> periodontal abscess (K05.21)
> peritonsillar abscess (J36)

● **K12.3**   **Oral mucositis (ulcerative)**
Mucositis (oral) (oropharyneal)
> **Excludes2**   gastrointestinal mucositis (ulcerative)
> (K92.81)
> mucositis (ulcerative) of vagina and vulva
> (N76.81)
> nasal mucositis (ulcerative) (J34.81)

    K12.30   **Oral mucositis (ulcerative), unspecified**
    K12.31   **Oral mucositis (ulcerative) due to antineoplastic therapy**
> Use additional code for adverse effect, if
> applicable, to identify antineoplastic and
> immunosuppressive drugs (T45.1X5)
> Use additional code for other antineoplastic
> therapy, such as:
> radiological procedure and radiotherapy
> (Y84.2)

    K12.32   **Oral mucositis (ulcerative) due to other drugs**
> Use additional code for adverse effect, if
> applicable, to identify drug (T36-T50 with
> fifth or sixth character 5)

    K12.33   **Oral mucositis (ulcerative) due to radiation**
> Use additional external cause code (W88-W90,
> X39.0-) to identify cause

    K12.39   **Other oral mucositis (ulcerative)**
Viral oral mucositis (ulcerative)

● **K13**   **Other diseases of lip and oral mucosa**
> **Includes**   epithelial disturbances of tongue

Use additional code to identify:
alcohol abuse and dependence (F10.-)
exposure to environmental tobacco smoke (Z77.22)
exposure to tobacco smoke in the perinatal period (P96.81)
history of tobacco dependence (Z87.891)
occupational exposure to environmental tobacco smoke
(Z57.31)
tobacco dependence (F17.-)
tobacco use (Z72.0)
> **Excludes2**   certain disorders of gingiva and edentulous
> alveolar ridge (K05-K06)
> cysts of oral region (K09.-)
> diseases of tongue (K14.-)
> stomatitis and related lesions (K12.-)

    K13.0   **Diseases of lips**

Abscess of lips	Exfoliative cheilitis
Angular cheilitis	Fistula of lips
Cellulitis of lips	Glandular cheilitis
Cheilitis NOS	Hypertrophy of lips
Cheilodynia	Perlèche NEC
Cheilosis	

> **Excludes1**   ariboflavinosis (E53.0)
> cheilitis due to radiation-related disorders
> (L55-L59)
> congenital fistula of lips (Q38.0)
> congenital hypertrophy of lips (Q18.6)
> Perlèche due to candidiasis (B37.83)
> Perlèche due to riboflavin deficiency
> (E53.0)

    K13.1   **Cheek and lip biting**

CHAPTER 11 (KØØ-K95)

Figure 11-4 Oral leukoplakia and associated. (From Swartz MH: Textbook of Physical Diagnosis: History and Examination, Philadelphia, PA, Saunders/Elsevier, 2010)

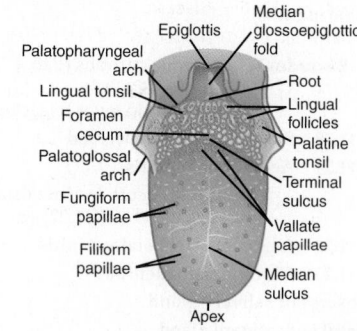

Figure 11-5 Structure of the tongue.

● **K13.2** **Leukoplakia and other disturbances of oral epithelium, including tongue**
> **Excludes1**   carcinoma in situ of oral epithelium (D00.0-)
> hairy leukoplakia (K13.3)

   K13.21 **Leukoplakia of oral mucosa, including tongue**
     Considered precancerous and evidenced by thickened white patches of epithelium on mucous membranes
     Leukokeratosis of oral mucosa
     Leukoplakia of gingiva, lips, tongue
> **Excludes1**   hairy leukoplakia (K13.3)
> leukokeratosis nicotina palati (K13.24)

   K13.22 **Minimal keratinized residual ridge mucosa**
     Minimal keratinization of alveolar ridge mucosa

   K13.23 **Excessive keratinized residual ridge mucosa**
     Excessive keratinization of alveolar ridge mucosa

   K13.24 **Leukokeratosis nicotina palati**
     Smoker's palate

   K13.29 **Other disturbances of oral epithelium, including tongue**
     Erythroplakia of mouth or tongue
     Focal epithelial hyperplasia of mouth or tongue
     Leukoedema of mouth or tongue
     Other oral epithelium disturbances

K13.3 **Hairy leukoplakia**

K13.4 **Granuloma and granuloma-like lesions of oral mucosa**
   Eosinophilic granuloma
   Granuloma pyogenicum
   Verrucous xanthoma

K13.5 **Oral submucous fibrosis**
   Submucous fibrosis of tongue

K13.6 **Irritative hyperplasia of oral mucosa**
> **Excludes2**   irritative hyperplasia of edentulous ridge [denture hyperplasia] (K06.2)

● **K13.7** **Other and unspecified lesions of oral mucosa**
   K13.70 **Unspecified lesions of oral mucosa**
   K13.79 **Other lesions of oral mucosa**
     Focal oral mucinosis
   Coding Clinic: 2022, Q2, P8

★ **(See Plate 26 of the Anatomy Illustrations.)**

● **K14** **Diseases of tongue**
   Use additional code to identify:
     alcohol abuse and dependence (F10.-)
     exposure to environmental tobacco smoke (Z77.22)
     history of tobacco dependence (Z87.891)
     occupational exposure to environmental tobacco smoke (Z57.31)
     tobacco dependence (F17.-)
     tobacco use (Z72.0)
> **Excludes2**   erythroplakia (K13.29)
> focal epithelial hyperplasia (K13.29)
> leukedema of tongue (K13.29)
> leukoplakia of tongue (K13.21)
> hairy leukoplakia (K13.3)
> macroglossia (congenital) (Q38.2)
> submucous fibrosis of tongue (K13.5)

K14.0 **Glossitis**
   Abscess of tongue
   Ulceration (traumatic) of tongue
> **Excludes1**   atrophic glossitis (K14.4)

K14.1 **Geographic tongue**
   Benign migratory glossitis
   Glossitis areata exfoliativa

K14.2 **Median rhomboid glossitis**

K14.3 **Hypertrophy of tongue papillae**
   Black hairy tongue
   Coated tongue
   Hypertrophy of foliate papillae
   Lingua villosa nigra

K14.4 **Atrophy of tongue papillae**
   Atrophic glossitis

K14.5 **Plicated tongue**
   Fissured tongue   Scrotal tongue
   Furrowed tongue
> **Excludes1**   fissured tongue, congenital (Q38.3)

K14.6 **Glossodynia**
   Glossopyrosis   Painful tongue

K14.8 **Other diseases of tongue**
   Atrophy of tongue   Glossocele
   Crenated tongue   Glossoptosis
   Enlargement of tongue   Hypertrophy of tongue

K14.9 **Disease of tongue, unspecified**
   Glossopathy NOS

DISEASES OF ESOPHAGUS, STOMACH AND DUODENUM (K20-K31)
> **Excludes2**   hiatus hernia (K44.-)

● **K20** **Esophagitis**
   Use additional code to identify:
     alcohol abuse and dependence (F10.-)
> **Excludes1**   erosion of esophagus (K22.1-)
> esophagitis with gastro-esophageal reflux disease (K21.0-)
> reflux esophagitis (K21.0-)
> ulcerative esophagitis (K22.1-)
> **Excludes2**   eosinophilic gastritis or gastroenteritis (K52.81)

   K20.0 **Eosinophilic esophagitis**
● **K20.8** **Other esophagitis**
   K20.80 **Other esophagitis without bleeding**
     Abscess of esophagus
     Other esophagitis NOS
   K20.81 **Other esophagitis with bleeding**
● **K20.9** **Esophagitis, unspecified**
   K20.90 **Esophagitis, unspecified without bleeding**
     Esophagitis NOS
   K20.91 **Esophagitis, unspecified with bleeding**

CHAPTER 11 (K00-K95)

● **K21   Gastro-esophageal reflux disease**

    Excludes1   newborn esophageal reflux (P78.83)

   ● **K21.0   Gastro-esophageal reflux disease with esophagitis**

     K21.00   Gastro-esophageal reflux disease with esophagitis, without bleeding
       Reflux esophagitis

     K21.01   Gastro-esophageal reflux disease with esophagitis, with bleeding

    K21.9   Gastro-esophageal reflux disease without esophagitis
      Esophageal reflux NOS
      Coding Clinic: 2016, Q1, P18

● **K22   Other diseases of esophagus**

    Excludes2   esophageal varices (I85.-)

   K22.0   Achalasia of cardia
     Achalasia NOS
     Cardiospasm

     Excludes1   congenital cardiospasm (Q39.5)

   ● **K22.1   Ulcer of esophagus**
     Barrett's ulcer
     Erosion of esophagus
     Fungal ulcer of esophagus
     Peptic ulcer of esophagus
     Ulcer of esophagus due to ingestion of chemicals
     Ulcer of esophagus due to ingestion of drugs and medicaments
     Ulcerative esophagitis

     Code first poisoning due to drug or toxin, if applicable (T36-T65 with fifth or sixth character 1-4 or 6)

     Use additional code for adverse effect, if applicable, to identify drug (T36-T50 with fifth or sixth character 5)

     Excludes1   Barrett's esophagus (K22.87-)

    K22.10   Ulcer of esophagus without bleeding
      Ulcer of esophagus NOS

    K22.11   Ulcer of esophagus with bleeding

     Excludes2   bleeding esophageal varices (I85.01, I85.11)

   K22.2   Esophageal obstruction
     Compression of esophagus
     Constriction of esophagus
     Stenosis of esophagus
     Stricture of esophagus

     Excludes1   congenital stenosis or stricture of esophagus (Q39.3)

   K22.3   Perforation of esophagus
     Rupture of esophagus

     Excludes1   traumatic perforation of (thoracic) esophagus (S27.8-)

   K22.4   Dyskinesia of esophagus
     Difficulty in moving
     Corkscrew esophagus
     Diffuse esophageal spasm
     Spasm of esophagus

     Excludes1   cardiospasm (K22.0)

   K22.5   Diverticulum of esophagus, acquired
     Esophageal pouch, acquired

     Excludes1   diverticulum of esophagus (congenital) (Q39.6)

   K22.6   Gastro-esophageal laceration-hemorrhage syndrome
     Mallory-Weiss syndrome

Item 11-6   Esophageal reflux is the return flow of the contents of the stomach to the esophagus and is referred to as GERD and/or "heartburn." **Gastroesophageal reflux** is the return flow of the contents of the stomach and duodenum to the esophagus. **Esophageal leukoplakia** are white areas on the mucous membrane of the esophagus for which no specific cause can be identified.

Figure 11-6   The esophagus is the muscular tube that connects the pharynx and the stomach. The 10-inch (25 cm) long esophagus is divided into three parts: **cervical, thoracic,** and **abdominal.**

Item 11-7   Achalasia is a condition in which the smooth muscle fibers of the esophagus do not relax. Most frequently, this condition occurs at the esophagogastric sphincter. **Cardiospasm,** also known as **megaesophagus,** is achalasia of the thoracic esophagus.

   ● **K22.7   Barrett's esophagus**
     Barrett's disease
     Barrett's syndrome

     Excludes1   Barrett's ulcer (K22.1)
         malignant neoplasm of esophagus (C15.-)

    K22.70   Barrett's esophagus without dysplasia
      Barrett's esophagus NOS

   ● **K22.71   Barrett's esophagus with dysplasia**

     K22.710   Barrett's esophagus with low grade dysplasia

     K22.711   Barrett's esophagus with high grade dysplasia

     K22.719   Barrett's esophagus with dysplasia, unspecified

   ● **K22.8   Other specified diseases of esophagus**

     K22.81   Esophageal polyp

       Excludes1   benign neoplasm of esophagus (D13.0)

     K22.82 Esophagogastric junction polyp

       Excludes1   benign neoplasm of stomach (D13.1)

     K22.89   Other specified disease of esophagus
       Hemorrhage of esophagus NOS

       Excludes2   esophageal varices (I85.-)
         Paterson-Kelly syndrome (D50.1)
       Coding Clinic: 2020, Q1, P16

   K22.9   Disease of esophagus, unspecified

▷ **K23   Disorders of esophagus in diseases classified elsewhere**

     Code first underlying disease, such as:
     congenital syphilis (A50.5)

     Excludes1   late syphilis (A52.79)
       megaesophagus due to Chagas' disease (B57.31)
       tuberculosis (A18.83)

● **K25   Gastric ulcer**

     Includes   erosion (acute) of stomach
         pylorus ulcer (peptic)
         stomach ulcer (peptic)

     Use additional code to identify:
     alcohol abuse and dependence (F10.-)

     Excludes1   acute gastritis (K29.0-)
       peptic ulcer NOS (K27.-)

   K25.0   Acute gastric ulcer with hemorrhage

   K25.1   Acute gastric ulcer with perforation 🔗

   K25.2   Acute gastric ulcer with both hemorrhage and perforation 🔗

   K25.3   Acute gastric ulcer without hemorrhage or perforation

   K25.4   Chronic or unspecified gastric ulcer with hemorrhage
      Coding Clinic: 2017, Q3, P27

A   B   C

Figure 11-7 **A.** Ulcer. **B.** Perforated ulcer. **C.** Laparoscopic view of a perforated duodenal ulcer *(arrow)* with fibrinous exudate on the adjacent peritoneum. (**C** from Feldman: Sleisenger & Fordtran's Gastrointestinal and Liver Disease, ed 8, Saunders, An Imprint of Elsevier, 2006)

Item 11–8   **Gastric ulcers** are lesions of the stomach that result in the death of the tissue and a defect of the surface. **Perforated ulcers** are those in which the lesion penetrates the gastric wall, leaving a hole. **Peptic ulcers** are lesions of the stomach or the duodenum. **Peptic** refers to the gastric juice, pepsin.

K25.5   Chronic or unspecified gastric ulcer with perforation 🖉
K25.6   Chronic or unspecified gastric ulcer with both hemorrhage and perforation 🖉
K25.7   Chronic gastric ulcer without hemorrhage or perforation
K25.9   Gastric ulcer, unspecified as acute or chronic, without hemorrhage or perforation
      Coding Clinic: 2021, Q1, P12

● K26   **Duodenal ulcer**
     Includes   erosion (acute) of duodenum
                duodenum ulcer (peptic)
                postpyloric ulcer (peptic)
     Use additional code to identify:
        alcohol abuse and dependence (F10.-)
     Excludes1   peptic ulcer NOS (K27.-)

K26.0   **Acute duodenal ulcer with** hemorrhage
K26.1   **Acute duodenal ulcer with** perforation 🖉
K26.2   **Acute duodenal ulcer with both hemorrhage and perforation** 🖉
K26.3   **Acute duodenal ulcer** without hemorrhage or perforation
K26.4   Chronic or unspecified duodenal ulcer with hemorrhage
      Coding Clinic: 2016, Q1, P14
K26.5   Chronic or unspecified duodenal ulcer with perforation 🖉
K26.6   Chronic or unspecified duodenal ulcer with both hemorrhage and perforation 🖉
K26.7   Chronic duodenal ulcer without hemorrhage or perforation
K26.9   Duodenal ulcer, unspecified as acute or chronic, without hemorrhage or perforation

● K27   **Peptic ulcer, site unspecified**
     Includes   gastroduodenal ulcer NOS
                peptic ulcer NOS
     Use additional code to identify:
        alcohol abuse and dependence (F10.-)
     Excludes1   peptic ulcer of newborn (P78.82)

K27.0   **Acute peptic ulcer, site unspecified, with** hemorrhage
K27.1   **Acute peptic ulcer, site unspecified, with** perforation 🖉
K27.2   **Acute peptic ulcer, site unspecified, with both hemorrhage and perforation** 🖉
K27.3   **Acute peptic ulcer, site unspecified, without hemorrhage or perforation**
K27.4   Chronic or unspecified peptic ulcer, site unspecified, with hemorrhage
K27.5   Chronic or unspecified peptic ulcer, site unspecified, with perforation 🖉
K27.6   Chronic or unspecified peptic ulcer, site unspecified, with both hemorrhage and perforation 🖉

K27.7   **Chronic peptic ulcer, site unspecified, without** hemorrhage or perforation
K27.9   **Peptic ulcer, site unspecified, unspecified as acute or chronic, without hemorrhage or perforation**

● K28   **Gastrojejunal ulcer**
     Includes   anastomotic ulcer (peptic) or erosion
                gastrocolic ulcer (peptic) or erosion
                gastrointestinal ulcer (peptic) or erosion
                gastrojejunal ulcer (peptic) or erosion
                jejunal ulcer (peptic) or erosion
                marginal ulcer (peptic) or erosion
                stomal ulcer (peptic) or erosion
     Use additional code to identify:
        alcohol abuse and dependence (F10.-)
     Excludes1   primary ulcer of small intestine (K63.3)

K28.0   **Acute gastrojejunal ulcer with** hemorrhage
K28.1   **Acute gastrojejunal ulcer with** perforation 🖉
K28.2   **Acute gastrojejunal ulcer with both hemorrhage and perforation** 🖉
K28.3   **Acute gastrojejunal ulcer without hemorrhage or perforation**
K28.4   **Chronic or unspecified gastrojejunal ulcer with hemorrhage**
K28.5   **Chronic or unspecified gastrojejunal ulcer with perforation** 🖉
K28.6   **Chronic or unspecified gastrojejunal ulcer with both hemorrhage and perforation** 🖉
K28.7   **Chronic gastrojejunal ulcer without hemorrhage or perforation**
K28.9   **Gastrojejunal ulcer, unspecified as acute or chronic, without hemorrhage or perforation**

● K29   **Gastritis and duodenitis**
     Excludes1   eosinophilic gastritis or gastroenteritis (K52.81)
                Zollinger-Ellison syndrome (E16.4)

● K29.0   **Acute gastritis**
     Use additional code to identify:
        alcohol abuse and dependence (F10.-)
     Excludes1   erosion (acute) of stomach (K25.-)
     K29.00   Acute gastritis without bleeding
     K29.01   Acute gastritis with bleeding

● K29.2   **Alcoholic gastritis**
     Use additional code to identify:
        alcohol abuse and dependence (F10.-)
     K29.20   Alcoholic gastritis without bleeding
     K29.21   Alcoholic gastritis with bleeding

● K29.3   **Chronic superficial gastritis**
     K29.30   Chronic superficial gastritis without bleeding
     K29.31   Chronic superficial gastritis with bleeding

● K29.4   **Chronic atrophic gastritis**
     Gastric atrophy
     K29.40   Chronic atrophic gastritis without bleeding
     K29.41   Chronic atrophic gastritis with bleeding

● K29.5   **Unspecified chronic gastritis**
     Chronic antral gastritis
     Chronic fundal gastritis
     K29.50   Unspecified chronic gastritis without bleeding
     K29.51   Unspecified chronic gastritis with bleeding

● K29.6   **Other gastritis**
     Giant hypertrophic gastritis
     Granulomatous gastritis
     Ménétrier's disease
     K29.60   Other gastritis without bleeding
     K29.61   Other gastritis with bleeding

● K29.7   **Gastritis, unspecified**
     K29.70   Gastritis, unspecified, without bleeding
     K29.71   Gastritis, unspecified, with bleeding

▶ New   ⇒ Revised   ~~deleted~~ Deleted   Excludes 1   Excludes 2   Includes   Use additional   Code first   Code also   Key words
  OGCR Official Guidelines   X Assign placeholder X   ● Use Additional Character(s)   ▶ Manifestation Code   🖉 Hierarchical Condition Category   **Coding Clinic**

Item 11–9 Gastritis is a severe inflammation of the stomach. **Atrophic gastritis** is a chronic inflammation of the stomach that results in destruction of the cells of the mucosa of the stomach. Duodenitis is an inflammation of the duodenum, the first section of the small intestine.

● **K29.8 Duodenitis**
  K29.80 Duodenitis without bleeding
  K29.81 Duodenitis with bleeding
● **K29.9 Gastroduodenitis, unspecified**
  K29.90 Gastroduodenitis, unspecified, without bleeding
  K29.91 Gastroduodenitis, unspecified, with bleeding

K30 Functional dyspepsia
  Indigestion
  Excludes1 dyspepsia NOS (R10.13)
    heartburn (R12)
    nervous dyspepsia (F45.8)
    neurotic dyspepsia (F45.8)
    psychogenic dyspepsia (F45.8)

● **K31 Other diseases of stomach and duodenum**
  Includes functional disorders of stomach
  Excludes2 diabetic gastroparesis (E08.43, E09.43, E10.43, E11.43, E13.43)
    diverticulum of duodenum (K57.00-K57.13)

  K31.0 Acute dilatation of stomach
    Acute distention of stomach
  K31.1 Adult hypertrophic pyloric stenosis   A
    Pyloric stenosis NOS
    Excludes1 congenital or infantile pyloric stenosis (Q40.0)
  K31.2 Hourglass stricture and stenosis of stomach
    Excludes1 congenital hourglass stomach (Q40.2)
      hourglass contraction of stomach (K31.89)
  K31.3 Pylorospasm, not elsewhere classified
    Excludes1 congenital or infantile pylorospasm (Q40.0)
      neurotic pylorospasm (F45.8)
      psychogenic pylorospasm (F45.8)
  K31.4 Gastric diverticulum
    Excludes1 congenital diverticulum of stomach (Q40.2)
  K31.5 Obstruction of duodenum
    Constriction of duodenum
    Duodenal ileus (chronic)
    Stenosis of duodenum
      Narrowing
    Stricture of duodenum
      Narrowing
    Volvulus of duodenum
      Twisting/knotting
    Excludes1 congenital stenosis of duodenum (Q41.0)
  K31.6 Fistula of stomach and duodenum
    Gastrocolic fistula
    Gastrojejunocolic fistula
  K31.7 Polyp of stomach and duodenum
    Excludes1 adenomatous polyp of stomach (D13.1)
    Coding Clinic: 2020, Q1, P16
● **K31.8 Other specified diseases of stomach and duodenum**
  ● **K31.81 Angiodysplasia of stomach and duodenum**
    K31.811 Angiodysplasia of stomach and duodenum with bleeding
    K31.819 Angiodysplasia of stomach and duodenum without bleeding
      Angiodysplasia of stomach and duodenum NOS

Item 11–10 Achlorhydria, also known as gastric anacidity, is the absence of gastric acid.

K31.82 Dieulafoy lesion (hemorrhagic) of stomach and duodenum
  Excludes2 Dieulafoy lesion of intestine (K63.81)
K31.83 Achlorhydria
K31.84 Gastroparesis
  Gastroparalysis
  Code first underlying disease, if known, such as:
    anorexia nervosa (F50.0-)
    diabetes mellitus (E08.43, E09.43, E10.43, E11.43, E13.43)
    scleroderma (M34.-)
K31.89 Other diseases of stomach and duodenum
  Coding Clinic: 2020, Q1, P16; 2017, Q1, P28
K31.9 Disease of stomach and duodenum, unspecified
● **K31.A Gastric intestinal metaplasia**
  K31.A0 Gastric intestinal metaplasia, unspecified
    Gastric intestinal metaplasia indefinite for dysplasia
    Gastric intestinal metaplasia NOS
  ● **K31.A1 Gastric intestinal metaplasia without dysplasia**
    K31.A11 Gastric intestinal metaplasia without dysplasia, involving the antrum
    K31.A12 Gastric intestinal metaplasia without dysplasia, involving the body(corpus)
    K31.A13 Gastric intestinal metaplasia without dysplasia, involving the fundus involving the cardia
    K31.A14 Gastric intestinal metaplasia without dysplasia, involving the cardia
    K31.A15 Gastric intestinal metaplasia without dysplasia, involving multiple sites
    K31.A19 Gastric intestinal metaplasia without dysplasia, unspecified site
  ● **K31.A2 Gastric intestinal metaplasia with dysplasia**
    K31.A21 Gastric intestinal metaplasia with low grade dysplasia
    K31.A22 Gastric intestinal metaplasia with high grade dysplasia
    K31.A29 Gastric intestinal metaplasia with dysplasia, unspecified

DISEASES OF APPENDIX (K35-K38)

● **K35 Acute appendicitis**
  ● **K35.2 Acute appendicitis with generalized peritonitis**
    Appendicitis (acute) with generalized (diffuse) peritonitis following rupture or perforation of appendix
    K35.20 Acute appendicitis with generalized peritonitis, without abscess (Acute) appendicitis with generalized peritonitis NOS
      Coding Clinic: 2018, Q4, P18
    K35.21 Acute appendicitis with generalized peritonitis, with abscess
  ● **K35.3 Acute appendicitis with localized peritonitis**
    K35.30 Acute appendicitis with localized peritonitis, without perforation or gangrene
      Acute appendicitis with localized peritonitis NOS
    K35.31 Acute appendicitis with localized peritonitis and gangrene, without perforation
    ➡ **K35.32 Acute appendicitis with perforation, localized peritonitis, and gangrene, without abscess**
      (Acute) appendicitis with perforation NOS
      Perforated appendix NOS
      Ruptured appendix (with localized peritonitis) NOS
      Coding Clinic: 2020, Q1, P16; 2018, Q4, P18
    ➡ **K35.33 Acute appendicitis with perforation, localized peritonitis, and gangrene, with abscess**
      (Acute) appendicitis with (peritoneal) abscess NOS
      Ruptured appendix with localized peritonitis and abscess

CHAPTER 11 (K00-K95)

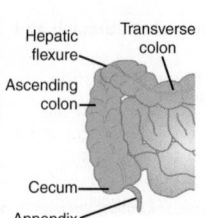

Figure 11-8 Acute appendicitis is the inflammation of the appendix, usually associated with obstruction. Most often this is a disease of adolescents and young adults.

● **K35.8** **Other and unspecified acute appendicitis**
  K35.80 **Unspecified acute appendicitis**
    Acute appendicitis NOS
    Acute appendicitis without (localized) (generalized) peritonitis
  ● **K35.89** **Other acute appendicitis**
    K35.890 **Other acute appendicitis without perforation or gangrene**
    K35.891 **Other acute appendicitis without perforation, with gangrene**
      (Acute) appendicitis with gangrene NOS

K36 **Other appendicitis**
  Chronic appendicitis
  Recurrent appendicitis

K37 **Unspecified appendicitis**
  Excludes1 unspecified appendicitis with peritonitis (K35.2-, K35.3)

● **K38** **Other diseases of appendix**
  K38.0 **Hyperplasia of appendix**
  K38.1 **Appendicular concretions**
    Fecalith of appendix
    Stercolith of appendix
  K38.2 **Diverticulum of appendix**
  K38.3 **Fistula of appendix**
  K38.8 **Other specified diseases of appendix**
    Intussusception of appendix
  K38.9 **Disease of appendix, unspecified**

HERNIA (K40-K46)

Note: Hernia with both gangrene and obstruction is classified to hernia with gangrene.
  Includes acquired hernia
    congenital [except diaphragmatic or hiatus] hernia
    recurrent hernia

● **K40** **Inguinal hernia**
  Includes bubonocele
    direct inguinal hernia
    double inguinal hernia
    indirect inguinal hernia
    inguinal hernia NOS
    oblique inguinal hernia
    scrotal hernia

  ● **K40.0** **Bilateral inguinal hernia, with obstruction, without gangrene**
    Inguinal hernia (bilateral) causing obstruction without gangrene
    Incarcerated inguinal hernia (bilateral) without gangrene
    Irreducible inguinal hernia (bilateral) without gangrene
    Strangulated inguinal hernia (bilateral) without gangrene
    K40.00 **Bilateral inguinal hernia, with obstruction, without gangrene, not specified as recurrent**
      Bilateral inguinal hernia, with obstruction, without gangrene NOS
    K40.01 **Bilateral inguinal hernia, with obstruction, without gangrene, recurrent**
  ● **K40.1** **Bilateral inguinal hernia, with gangrene**
    K40.10 **Bilateral inguinal hernia, with gangrene, not specified as recurrent**
      Bilateral inguinal hernia, with gangrene NOS
    K40.11 **Bilateral inguinal hernia, with gangrene, recurrent**

Item 11–11 **Hernias** of the groin are the most common type, accounting for 80 percent of all hernias. There are two major types of inguinal hernias: indirect (oblique) affecting men only and direct. **Indirect inguinal hernias** result when the intestines emerge through the abdominal wall in an indirect fashion through the inguinal canal. **Direct inguinal hernias** penetrate through the abdominal wall in a direct fashion. **Femoral hernias** occur at the femoral ring where the femoral vessels enter the thigh and is most common in women. An abdominal wall hernia is also called a ventral or epigastric hernia and occurs in both sexes. Classification is based on location of the hernia and whether there is obstruction or gangrene.

  Ventral, epigastric, or incisional hernia occurs on the abdominal surface caused by musculature weakness or a tear at a previous surgical site and is evidenced by a bulge that changes in size, becoming larger with exertion. An **incarcerated** hernia is one in which the intestines become trapped in the hernia. A **strangulated** hernia is one in which the blood supply to the intestines is lost. **Hiatal hernia** occurs when a loop of the stomach protrudes upward through the small opening in the diaphragm through which the esophagus passes, leaving the abdominal cavity and entering the chest. It occurs in both sexes.

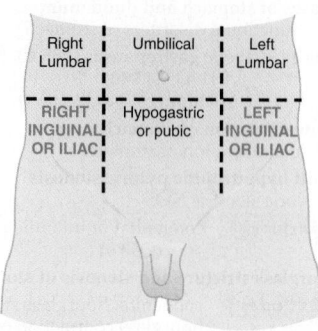

Figure 11-9 Inguinal hernias are those that are located in the inguinal or iliac areas of the abdomen.

  ● **K40.2** **Bilateral inguinal hernia, without obstruction or gangrene**
    K40.20 **Bilateral inguinal hernia, without obstruction or gangrene, not specified as recurrent**
      Bilateral inguinal hernia NOS
    K40.21 **Bilateral inguinal hernia, without obstruction or gangrene, recurrent**
  ● **K40.3** **Unilateral inguinal hernia, with obstruction, without gangrene**
    Inguinal hernia (unilateral) causing obstruction without gangrene
    Incarcerated inguinal hernia (unilateral) without gangrene
    Irreducible inguinal hernia (unilateral) without gangrene
    Strangulated inguinal hernia (unilateral) without gangrene
    K40.30 **Unilateral inguinal hernia, with obstruction, without gangrene, not specified as recurrent**
      Inguinal hernia, with obstruction NOS
      Unilateral inguinal hernia, with obstruction, without gangrene NOS
    K40.31 **Unilateral inguinal hernia, with obstruction, without gangrene, recurrent**
  ● **K40.4** **Unilateral inguinal hernia, with gangrene**
    K40.40 **Unilateral inguinal hernia, with gangrene, not specified as recurrent**
      Inguinal hernia with gangrene NOS
      Unilateral inguinal hernia with gangrene NOS
    K40.41 **Unilateral inguinal hernia, with gangrene, recurrent**

▶ New ⇒ Revised ~~deleted~~ Deleted Excludes 1 Excludes 2 Includes Use additional Code first Code also Key words
OGCR Official Guidelines X Assign placeholder X ● Use Additional Character(s) ▷ Manifestation Code ☜ Hierarchical Condition Category Coding Clinic

● **K40.9**   **Unilateral inguinal hernia, without obstruction or gangrene**

     K40.90   **Unilateral inguinal hernia, without obstruction or gangrene, not specified as recurrent**
         Inguinal hernia NOS
         Unilateral inguinal hernia NOS
         Coding Clinic: 2021, Q3, P31

     K40.91   **Unilateral inguinal hernia, without obstruction or gangrene, recurrent**
         Coding Clinic: 2021, Q3, P31

● **K41**   **Femoral hernia**

● **K41.0**   **Bilateral femoral hernia, with obstruction, without gangrene**
     Femoral hernia (bilateral) causing obstruction, without gangrene
     Incarcerated femoral hernia (bilateral), without gangrene
     Irreducible femoral hernia (bilateral), without gangrene
     Strangulated femoral hernia (bilateral), without gangrene

     K41.00   **Bilateral femoral hernia, with obstruction, without gangrene, not specified as recurrent**
         Bilateral femoral hernia, with obstruction, without gangrene NOS

     K41.01   **Bilateral femoral hernia, with obstruction, without gangrene, recurrent**

● **K41.1**   **Bilateral femoral hernia, with gangrene**

     K41.10   **Bilateral femoral hernia, with gangrene, not specified as recurrent**
         Bilateral femoral hernia, with gangrene NOS

     K41.11   **Bilateral femoral hernia, with gangrene, recurrent**

● **K41.2**   **Bilateral femoral hernia, without obstruction or gangrene**

     K41.20   **Bilateral femoral hernia, without obstruction or gangrene, not specified as recurrent**
         Bilateral femoral hernia NOS

     K41.21   **Bilateral femoral hernia, without obstruction or gangrene, recurrent**

● **K41.3**   **Unilateral femoral hernia, with obstruction, without gangrene**
     Femoral hernia (unilateral) causing obstruction, without gangrene
     Incarcerated femoral hernia (unilateral), without gangrene
     Irreducible femoral hernia (unilateral), without gangrene
     Strangulated femoral hernia (unilateral), without gangrene

     K41.30   **Unilateral femoral hernia, with obstruction, without gangrene, not specified as recurrent**
         Femoral hernia, with obstruction NOS
         Unilateral femoral hernia, with obstruction NOS

     K41.31   **Unilateral femoral hernia, with obstruction, without gangrene, recurrent**
         Coding Clinic: 2021, Q3, P30

● **K41.4**   **Unilateral femoral hernia, with gangrene**

     K41.40   **Unilateral femoral hernia, with gangrene, not specified as recurrent**
         Femoral hernia, with gangrene NOS
         Unilateral femoral hernia, with gangrene NOS

     K41.41   **Unilateral femoral hernia, with gangrene, recurrent**

● **K41.9**   **Unilateral femoral hernia, without obstruction or gangrene**

     K41.90   **Unilateral femoral hernia, without obstruction or gangrene, not specified as recurrent**
         Femoral hernia NOS
         Unilateral femoral hernia NOS
         Coding Clinic: 2021, Q3, P30-31

     K41.91   **Unilateral femoral hernia, without obstruction or gangrene, recurrent**

● **K42**   **Umbilical hernia**
     Includes   paraumbilical hernia
     Excludes1   omphalocele (Q79.2)

     K42.0   **Umbilical hernia with obstruction, without gangrene**
         Umbilical hernia causing obstruction, without gangrene
         Incarcerated umbilical hernia, without gangrene
         Irreducible umbilical hernia, without gangrene
         Strangulated umbilical hernia, without gangrene

     K42.1   **Umbilical hernia with gangrene**
         Gangrenous umbilical hernia

     K42.9   **Umbilical hernia without obstruction or gangrene**
         Umbilical hernia NOS

● **K43**   **Ventral hernia**

     K43.0   **Incisional hernia with obstruction, without gangrene**
         Incisional hernia causing obstruction, without gangrene
         Incarcerated incisional hernia, without gangrene
         Irreducible incisional hernia, without gangrene
         Strangulated incisional hernia, without gangrene

     K43.1   **Incisional hernia with gangrene**
         Gangrenous incisional hernia

     K43.2   **Incisional hernia without obstruction or gangrene**
         Incisional hernia NOS

     K43.3   **Parastomal hernia with obstruction, without gangrene**
         Incarcerated parastomal hernia, without gangrene
         Irreducible parastomal hernia, without gangrene
         Parastomal hernia causing obstruction, without gangrene
         Strangulated parastomal hernia, without gangrene

     K43.4   **Parastomal hernia with gangrene**
         Gangrenous parastomal hernia

     K43.5   **Parastomal hernia without obstruction or gangrene**
         Parastomal hernia NOS

     K43.6   **Other and unspecified ventral hernia with obstruction, without gangrene**
         Epigastric hernia causing obstruction, without gangrene
         Hypogastric hernia causing obstruction, without gangrene
         Incarcerated epigastric hernia without gangrene
         Incarcerated hypogastric hernia without gangrene
         Incarcerated midline hernia without gangrene
         Incarcerated spigelian hernia without gangrene
         Incarcerated subxiphoid hernia without gangrene
         Irreducible epigastric hernia without gangrene
         Irreducible hypogastric hernia without gangrene
         Irreducible midline hernia without gangrene
         Irreducible spigelian hernia without gangrene
         Irreducible subxiphoid hernia without gangrene
         Midline hernia causing obstruction, without gangrene
         Spigelian hernia causing obstruction, without gangrene
         Strangulated epigastric hernia without gangrene
         Strangulated hypogastric hernia without gangrene
         Strangulated midline hernia without gangrene
         Strangulated spigelian hernia without gangrene
         Strangulated subxiphoid hernia without gangrene
         Subxiphoid hernia causing obstruction, without gangrene

     K43.7   **Other and unspecified ventral hernia with gangrene**
         Any condition listed under K43.6 specified as gangrenous

     K43.9   **Ventral hernia without obstruction or gangrene**
         Epigastric hernia
         Ventral hernia NOS

● **K44 Diaphragmatic hernia**

　　Includes hiatus hernia (esophageal) (sliding)
　　　　　　　paraesophageal hernia

　　Excludes1 congenital diaphragmatic hernia (Q79.0)
　　　　　　　congenital hiatus hernia (Q40.1)

　　K44.0 Diaphragmatic hernia with obstruction, without gangrene

　　　　Diaphragmatic hernia causing obstruction
　　　　Incarcerated diaphragmatic hernia
　　　　Irreducible diaphragmatic hernia
　　　　Strangulated diaphragmatic hernia
　　　　Coding Clinic: 2022, Q2, P14

　　K44.1 Diaphragmatic hernia with gangrene
　　　　Gangrenous diaphragmatic hernia

　　K44.9 Diaphragmatic hernia without obstruction or gangrene
　　　　Diaphragmatic hernia NOS
　　　　Coding Clinic: 2017, Q1, P7

● **K45 Other abdominal hernia**

　　Includes abdominal hernia, specified site NEC
　　　　　　　lumbar hernia
　　　　　　　obturator hernia
　　　　　　　pudendal hernia
　　　　　　　retroperitoneal hernia
　　　　　　　sciatic hernia

　　K45.0 Other specified abdominal hernia with obstruction, without gangrene
　　　　Other specified abdominal hernia causing obstruction
　　　　Other specified incarcerated abdominal hernia
　　　　Other specified irreducible abdominal hernia
　　　　Other specified strangulated abdominal hernia

　　K45.1 Other specified abdominal hernia with gangrene
　　　　Any condition listed under K45 specified as gangrenous

　　K45.8 Other specified abdominal hernia without obstruction or gangrene

● **K46 Unspecified abdominal hernia**

　　Includes enterocele
　　　　　　　epiplocele
　　　　　　　hernia NOS
　　　　　　　interstitial hernia
　　　　　　　intestinal hernia
　　　　　　　intra-abdominal hernia

　　Excludes1 vaginal enterocele (N81.5)

　　K46.0 Unspecified abdominal hernia with obstruction, without gangrene
　　　　Unspecified abdominal hernia causing obstruction
　　　　Unspecified incarcerated abdominal hernia
　　　　Unspecified irreducible abdominal hernia
　　　　Unspecified strangulated abdominal hernia

　　K46.1 Unspecified abdominal hernia with gangrene
　　　　Any condition listed under K46 specified as gangrenous

　　K46.9 Unspecified abdominal hernia without obstruction or gangrene
　　　　Abdominal hernia NOS

★**(See Plate 32 of the Anatomy Illustrations.)**

NONINFECTIVE ENTERITIS AND COLITIS (K50-K52)

　　Includes noninfective inflammatory bowel disease
　　Excludes1 irritable bowel syndrome (K58.-)
　　　　　　　megacolon (K59.3-)

● **K50 Crohn's disease [regional enteritis]**

　　Includes granulomatous enteritis
　　Use additional code to identify manifestations, such as:
　　　　pyoderma gangrenosum (L88)
　　Excludes1 ulcerative colitis (K51.-)

Item 11-12 Crohn's disease, also known as **regional enteritis,** is a chronic inflammatory disease of the intestines. Classification is based on location in the small (duodenum, ileum, jejunum) or large (cecum, colon, rectum, anal canal) intestine.

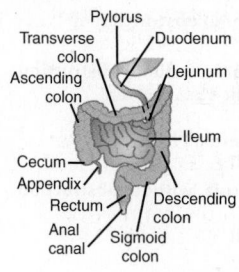

Figure 11-10 Small and large intestines.

● **K50.0 Crohn's disease of small intestine**
　　　Crohn's disease [regional enteritis] of duodenum
　　　Crohn's disease [regional enteritis] of ileum
　　　Crohn's disease [regional enteritis] of jejunum
　　　Regional ileitis
　　　Terminal ileitis

　　Excludes1 Crohn's disease of both small and large intestine (K50.8-)

　　K50.00 Crohn's disease of small intestine without complications 🦠

　　● **K50.01 Crohn's disease of small intestine with complications** 🦠

　　　　K50.011 Crohn's disease of small intestine with rectal bleeding 🦠

　　　　K50.012 Crohn's disease of small intestine with intestinal obstruction 🦠

　　　　K50.013 Crohn's disease of small intestine with fistula 🦠

　　　　K50.014 Crohn's disease of small intestine with abscess 🦠
　　　　　　Coding Clinic: 2012, Q4, P104

　　　　K50.018 Crohn's disease of small intestine with other complication 🦠

　　　　K50.019 Crohn's disease of small intestine with unspecified complications 🦠

● **K50.1 Crohn's disease of large intestine**
　　　Crohn's disease [regional enteritis] of colon
　　　Crohn's disease [regional enteritis] of large bowel
　　　Crohn's disease [regional enteritis] of rectum
　　　Granulomatous colitis
　　　Regional colitis

　　Excludes1 Crohn's disease of both small and large intestine (K50.8)

　　K50.10 Crohn's disease of large intestine without complications 🦠

　　● **K50.11 Crohn's disease of large intestine with complications** 🦠

　　　　K50.111 Crohn's disease of large intestine with rectal bleeding 🦠

　　　　K50.112 Crohn's disease of large intestine with intestinal obstruction 🦠

　　　　K50.113 Crohn's disease of large intestine with fistula 🦠

　　　　K50.114 Crohn's disease of large intestine with abscess 🦠
　　　　　　Coding Clinic: 2012, Q4, P104

　　　　K50.118 Crohn's disease of large intestine with other complication 🦠

　　　　K50.119 Crohn's disease of large intestine with unspecified complications 🦠

● **K50.8 Crohn's disease of both small and large intestine**

　　K50.80 Crohn's disease of both small and large intestine without complications 🦠

　　● **K50.81 Crohn's disease of both small and large intestine with complications** 🦠

　　　　K50.811 Crohn's disease of both small and large intestine with rectal bleeding 🦠

　　　　K50.812 Crohn's disease of both small and large intestine with intestinal obstruction 🦠

▶ New　　⮫ Revised　　~~deleted~~ Deleted　　Excludes 1　　Excludes 2　　Includes　　Use additional　　Code first　　Code also　　Key words
OGCR Official Guidelines　　X Assign placeholder X　　● Use Additional Character(s)　　▶ Manifestation Code　　🦠 Hierarchical Condition Category　　Coding Clinic

K50.813 Crohn's disease of both small and large intestine with fistula 🔍

K50.814 Crohn's disease of both small and large intestine with abscess 🔍
Coding Clinic: 2012, Q4, P104

K50.818 Crohn's disease of both small and large intestine with other complication 🔍

K50.819 Crohn's disease of both small and large intestine with unspecified complications 🔍

● K50.9 Crohn's disease, unspecified

K50.90 Crohn's disease, unspecified, without complications 🔍
Crohn's disease NOS
Regional enteritis NOS

● K50.91 Crohn's disease, unspecified, with complications

K50.911 Crohn's disease, unspecified, with rectal bleeding 🔍

K50.912 Crohn's disease, unspecified, with intestinal obstruction 🔍

K50.913 Crohn's disease, unspecified, with fistula 🔍

K50.914 Crohn's disease, unspecified, with abscess 🔍
Coding Clinic: 2012, Q4, P104

K50.918 Crohn's disease, unspecified, with other complication 🔍

K50.919 Crohn's disease, unspecified, with unspecified complications 🔍

● K51 **Ulcerative colitis**
Use additional code to identify manifestations, such as: pyoderma gangrenosum (L88)
Excludes1 Crohn's disease [regional enteritis] (K50.-)

● K51.0 Ulcerative (chronic) pancolitis
Backwash ileitis

K51.00 Ulcerative (chronic) pancolitis without complications 🔍
Ulcerative (chronic) pancolitis NOS

● K51.01 Ulcerative (chronic) pancolitis with complications

K51.011 Ulcerative (chronic) pancolitis with rectal bleeding 🔍

K51.012 Ulcerative (chronic) pancolitis with intestinal obstruction 🔍

K51.013 Ulcerative (chronic) pancolitis with fistula 🔍

K51.014 Ulcerative (chronic) pancolitis with abscess 🔍

K51.018 Ulcerative (chronic) pancolitis with other complication 🔍

K51.019 Ulcerative (chronic) pancolitis with unspecified complications 🔍

● K51.2 Ulcerative (chronic) proctitis

K51.20 Ulcerative (chronic) proctitis without complications 🔍
Ulcerative (chronic) proctitis NOS

● K51.21 Ulcerative (chronic) proctitis with complications

K51.211 Ulcerative (chronic) proctitis with rectal bleeding 🔍

K51.212 Ulcerative (chronic) proctitis with intestinal obstruction 🔍

K51.213 Ulcerative (chronic) proctitis with fistula 🔍

K51.214 Ulcerative (chronic) proctitis with abscess 🔍

K51.218 Ulcerative (chronic) proctitis with other complication 🔍

K51.219 Ulcerative (chronic) proctitis with unspecified complications 🔍

● K51.3 Ulcerative (chronic) rectosigmoiditis

K51.30 Ulcerative (chronic) rectosigmoiditis without complications 🔍
Ulcerative (chronic) rectosigmoiditis NOS

● K51.31 Ulcerative (chronic) rectosigmoiditis with complications

K51.311 Ulcerative (chronic) rectosigmoiditis with rectal bleeding 🔍

K51.312 Ulcerative (chronic) rectosigmoiditis with intestinal obstruction 🔍

K51.313 Ulcerative (chronic) rectosigmoiditis with fistula 🔍

K51.314 Ulcerative (chronic) rectosigmoiditis with abscess 🔍

K51.318 Ulcerative (chronic) rectosigmoiditis with other complication 🔍

K51.319 Ulcerative (chronic) rectosigmoiditis with unspecified complications 🔍

● K51.4 Inflammatory polyps of colon
Excludes1 adenomatous polyp of colon (D12.6)
polyposis of colon (D12.6)
polyps of colon NOS (K63.5)

K51.40 Inflammatory polyps of colon without complications 🔍
Inflammatory polyps of colon NOS

● K51.41 Inflammatory polyps of colon with complications

K51.411 Inflammatory polyps of colon with rectal bleeding 🔍

K51.412 Inflammatory polyps of colon with intestinal obstruction 🔍

K51.413 Inflammatory polyps of colon with fistula 🔍

K51.414 Inflammatory polyps of colon with abscess 🔍

K51.418 Inflammatory polyps of colon with other complication 🔍

K51.419 Inflammatory polyps of colon with unspecified complications 🔍

● K51.5 Left sided colitis
Left hemicolitis

K51.50 Left sided colitis without complications 🔍
Left sided colitis NOS

● K51.51 Left sided colitis with complications

K51.511 Left sided colitis with rectal bleeding 🔍

K51.512 Left sided colitis with intestinal obstruction 🔍

K51.513 Left sided colitis with fistula 🔍

K51.514 Left sided colitis with abscess 🔍

K51.518 Left sided colitis with other complication 🔍

K51.519 Left sided colitis with unspecified complications 🔍

● K51.8 Other ulcerative colitis

K51.80 Other ulcerative colitis without complications 🔍

● K51.81 Other ulcerative colitis with complications

K51.811 Other ulcerative colitis with rectal bleeding 🔍

K51.812 Other ulcerative colitis with intestinal obstruction 🔍

Item 11–13 Ulcerative colitis attacks the colonic mucosa and forms abscesses. The disease involves the intestines. Classification is based on the location:
• Enterocolitis: large and small intestine
• Ileocolitis: ileum and colon
• Proctitis: rectum
• Proctosigmoiditis: sigmoid colon and rectum

CHAPTER 11 (K00-K95)

K51.813   Other ulcerative colitis with fistula 🐷

K51.814   Other ulcerative colitis with abscess 🐷

K51.818   Other ulcerative colitis with other complication 🐷

K51.819   Other ulcerative colitis with unspecified complications 🐷

● K51.9   Ulcerative colitis, unspecified

K51.90   Ulcerative colitis, unspecified, without complications 🐷

● K51.91   Ulcerative colitis, unspecified, with complications

K51.911   Ulcerative colitis, unspecified with rectal bleeding 🐷

K51.912   Ulcerative colitis, unspecified with intestinal obstruction 🐷

K51.913   Ulcerative colitis, unspecified with fistula 🐷

K51.914   Ulcerative colitis, unspecified with abscess 🐷

K51.918   Ulcerative colitis, unspecified with other complication 🐷

K51.919   Ulcerative colitis, unspecified with unspecified complications 🐷

● K52   Other and unspecified noninfective gastroenteritis and colitis

K52.0   Gastroenteritis and colitis due to radiation

K52.1   Toxic gastroenteritis and colitis
Drug-induced gastroenteritis and colitis
Code first (T51-T65) to identify toxic agent
Use additional code for adverse effect, if applicable, to identify drug (T36-T50 with fifth or sixth character 5)
Coding Clinic: 2019, Q1, P17

● K52.2   Allergic and dietetic gastroenteritis and colitis
Food hypersensitivity gastroenteritis or colitis
Use additional code to identify type of food allergy (Z91.01-, Z91.02-)

Excludes2   allergic eosinophilic colitis (K52.82)
allergic eosinophilic esophagitis (K20.0)
allergic eosinophilic gastritis (K52.81)
allergic eosinophilic gastroenteritis (K52.81)
Coding Clinic: 2016, Q4, P30-31

K52.21   Food protein-induced enterocolitis syndrome
FPIES
Use additional code for hypovolemic shock, if present (R57.1)

K52.22   Food protein-induced enteropathy

K52.29   Other allergic and dietetic gastroenteritis and colitis
Allergic proctocolitis
Food hypersensitivity gastroenteritis or colitis
Food-induced eosinophilic proctocolitis
Food protein-induced proctocolitis
Immediate gastrointestinal hypersensitivity
Milk protein-induced proctocolitis

K52.3   Indeterminate colitis
Colonic inflammatory bowel disease unclassified (IBDU)
Excludes1   unspecified colitis (K52.9)

● K52.8   Other specified noninfective gastroenteritis and colitis

K52.81   Eosinophilic gastritis or gastroenteritis
Eosinophilic enteritis
Excludes2   eosinophilic esophagitis (K20.0)

K52.82   Eosinophilic colitis
Excludes2   allergic proctocolitis (K52.29)
food-induced eosinophilic proctocolitis (K52.29)
food protein-induced enterocolitis syndrome (FPIES) (K52.21)
food protein-induced proctocolitis (K52.29)
milk protein-induced proctocolitis (K52.29)

● K52.83   Microscopic colitis
Coding Clinic: 2016, Q4, P30-31

K52.831   Collagenous colitis

K52.832   Lymphocytic colitis

K52.838   Other microscopic colitis

K52.839   Microscopic colitis, unspecified

K52.89   Other specified noninfective gastroenteritis and colitis
Coding Clinic: 2019, Q1, P21

K52.9   Noninfective gastroenteritis and colitis, unspecified
Colitis NOS   Ileitis NOS
Enteritis NOS   Jejunitis NOS
Gastroenteritis NOS   Sigmoiditis NOS

Excludes1   diarrhea NOS (R19.7)
functional diarrhea (K59.1)
infectious gastroenteritis and colitis NOS (A09)
neonatal diarrhea (noninfective) (P78.3)
psychogenic diarrhea (F45.8)
Coding Clinic: 2021, Q3, P3-4

OTHER DISEASES OF INTESTINES (K55-K64)

● K55   Vascular disorders of intestine
Excludes1   necrotizing enterocolitis of newborn (P77.-)

● K55.0   Acute vascular disorders of intestine
Infarction of appendices epiploicae
Mesenteric (artery) (vein) embolism
Mesenteric (artery) (vein) infarction
Mesenteric (artery) (vein) thrombosis
Coding Clinic: 2019, Q4, P68

● K55.01   Acute (reversible) ischemia of small intestine
Coding Clinic: 2016, Q4, P32

K55.011   Focal (segmental) acute (reversible) ischemia of small intestine 🐷

K55.012   Diffuse acute (reversible) ischemia of small intestine 🐷

K55.019   Acute (reversible) ischemia of small intestine, extent unspecified 🐷

● K55.02   Acute infarction of small intestine
Gangrene of small intestine
Necrosis of small intestine
Coding Clinic: 2016, Q4, P32

K55.021   Focal (segmental) acute infarction of small intestine 🐷

K55.022   Diffuse acute infarction of small intestine 🐷

K55.029   Acute infarction of small intestine, extent unspecified 🐷

● K55.03   Acute (reversible) ischemia of large intestine
Acute fulminant ischemic colitis
Subacute ischemic colitis
Coding Clinic: 2016, Q4, P32

K55.031   Focal (segmental) acute (reversible) ischemia of large intestine 🐷

K55.032   Diffuse acute (reversible) ischemia of large intestine 🐷

K55.039   Acute (reversible) ischemia of large intestine, extent unspecified 🐷
Coding Clinic: 2019, Q4, P68

● K55.04   Acute infarction of large intestine
Gangrene of large intestine
Necrosis of large intestine
Coding Clinic: 2016, Q4, P32

K55.041   Focal (segmental) acute infarction of large intestine 🐷

K55.042   Diffuse acute infarction of large intestine 🐷

K55.049   Acute infarction of large intestine, extent unspecified 🐷

● K55.05   Acute (reversible) ischemia of intestine, part unspecified

     K55.051   Focal (segmental) acute (reversible) ischemia of intestine, part unspecified

     K55.052   Diffuse acute (reversible) ischemia of intestine, part unspecified

     K55.059   Acute (reversible) ischemia of intestine, part and extent unspecified

● K55.06   Acute infarction of intestine, part unspecified
     Acute intestinal infarction
     Gangrene of intestine
     Necrosis of intestine

     K55.061   Focal (segmental) acute infarction of intestine, part unspecified

     K55.062   Diffuse acute infarction of intestine, part unspecified

     K55.069   Acute infarction of intestine, part and extent unspecified

K55.1   Chronic vascular disorders of intestine
     Chronic ischemic colitis
     Chronic ischemic enteritis
     Chronic ischemic enterocolitis
     Ischemic stricture of intestine
     Mesenteric atherosclerosis
     Mesenteric vascular insufficiency

● K55.2   Angiodysplasia of colon

     K55.20   Angiodysplasia of colon without hemorrhage

     K55.21   Angiodysplasia of colon with hemorrhage

● K55.3   Necrotizing enterocolitis

     Excludes1   necrotizing enterocolitis of newborn (P77.-)

     Excludes2   necrotizing enterocolitis due to Clostridium difficile (A04.7-)

     K55.30   Necrotizing enterocolitis, unspecified
         Necrotizing enterocolitis, NOS

     K55.31   Stage 1 necrotizing enterocolitis
         Necrotizing enterocolitis without pneumatosis, without perforation
         Coding Clinic: 2016, Q4, P32

     K55.32   Stage 2 necrotizing enterocolitis
         Necrotizing enterocolitis with pneumatosis, without perforation
         Coding Clinic: 2016, Q4, P32

     K55.33   Stage 3 necrotizing enterocolitis
         Necrotizing enterocolitis with perforation
         Necrotizing enterocolitis with pneumatosis and perforation
         Coding Clinic: 2016, Q4, P32

K55.8   Other vascular disorders of intestine

K55.9   Vascular disorder of intestine, unspecified
     Ischemic colitis
     Ischemic enteritis
     Ischemic enterocolitis

● K56   Paralytic ileus and intestinal obstruction without hernia

     Excludes1   congenital stricture or stenosis of intestine (Q41-Q42)
         cystic fibrosis with meconium ileus (E84.11)
         ischemic stricture of intestine (K55.1)
         meconium ileus NOS (P76.0)
         neonatal intestinal obstructions classifiable to P76.-
         obstruction of duodenum (K31.5)
         postprocedural intestinal obstruction (K91.3-)

     Excludes2   stenosis of anus or rectum (K62.4)

K56.0   Paralytic ileus
     Paralysis of bowel
     Paralysis of colon
     Paralysis of intestine

     Excludes1   gallstone ileus (K56.3)
         ileus NOS (K56.7)
         obstructive ileus NOS (K56.69-)

Figure 11-11   Types of intussusception.

Item 11-14   Intussusception is the prolapse (telescoping) of a part of the intestine into another adjacent part of the intestine. Intussusception may be enteric (ileoileal, jejunoileal, jejunojejunal), colic (colocolic), or intracolic (ileocecal, ileocolic).

Item 11-15   Volvulus is the twisting of a segment of the intestine, resulting in obstruction. Paralytic ileus is paralysis of the intestine. It need not be a complete paralysis, but it must prohibit the passage of food through the intestine and lead to intestinal blockage. It is a common aftermath of some types of surgery.

K56.1   Intussusception
     Intussusception or invagination of bowel
     Intussusception or invagination of colon
     Intussusception or invagination of intestine
     Intussusception or invagination of rectum

     Excludes2   intussusception of appendix (K38.8)

K56.2   Volvulus
     Strangulation of colon or intestine
     Torsion of colon or intestine
     Twist of colon or intestine

     Excludes2   volvulus of duodenum (K31.5)

K56.3   Gallstone ileus
     Obstruction of intestine by gallstone

● K56.4   Other impaction of intestine

     K56.41   Fecal impaction

         Excludes1   constipation (K59.0-)
             incomplete defecation (R15.0)

     K56.49   Other impaction of intestine

● K56.5   Intestinal adhesions [bands] with obstruction (postinfection)
     Abdominal hernia due to adhesions with obstruction
     Peritoneal adhesions [bands] with intestinal obstruction (postinfection)

     K56.50   Intestinal adhesions [bands], unspecified as to partial versus complete obstruction
         Intestinal adhesions with obstruction NOS

     K56.51   Intestinal adhesions [bands], with partial obstruction
         Intestinal adhesions with incomplete obstruction

     K56.52   Intestinal adhesions [bands] with complete obstruction

● K56.6   Other and unspecified intestinal obstruction

     ● K56.60   Unspecified intestinal obstruction
         Coding Clinic: 2017, Q2, P12

         K56.600   Partial intestinal obstruction, unspecified as to cause
             Incomplete intestinal obstruction, NOS

         K56.601   Complete intestinal obstruction, unspecified as to cause

CHAPTER 11 (K00-K95)

CHAPTER 11 (K00-K95)

K56.609   Unspecified intestinal obstruction, unspecified as to partial versus complete obstruction ⓗ
Intestinal obstruction NOS

● **K56.69   Other intestinal obstruction**
Enterostenosis NOS
Obstructive ileus NOS
Occlusion of colon or intestine NOS
Stenosis of colon or intestine NOS
Stricture of colon or intestine NOS
Excludes1   intestinal obstruction due to specified condition-code to condition
Coding Clinic: 2017, Q2, P12

K56.690   Other partial intestinal obstruction ⓗ
Other incomplete intestinal obstruction

K56.691   Other complete intestinal obstruction ⓗ

K56.699   Other intestinal obstruction unspecified as to partial versus complete obstruction ⓗ
Other intestinal obstruction, NEC

K56.7   Ileus, unspecified ⓗ
Excludes1   obstructive ileus (K56.69-)
Excludes2   intestinal obstruction with hernia (K40-K46)
Coding Clinic: 2017, Q1, P41

● **K57   Diverticular disease of intestine**
Code also if applicable peritonitis K65.-
Excludes1   congenital diverticulum of intestine (Q43.8)
Meckel's diverticulum (Q43.0)
Excludes2   diverticulum of appendix (K38.2)
Coding Clinic: 2022, Q1, P26

● **K57.0   Diverticulitis of small intestine with perforation and abscess**
Excludes1   diverticulitis of both small and large intestine with perforation and abscess (K57.4-)

K57.00   Diverticulitis of small intestine with perforation and abscess without bleeding

K57.01   Diverticulitis of small intestine with perforation and abscess with bleeding

● **K57.1   Diverticular disease of small intestine without perforation or abscess**
Excludes1   diverticular disease of both small and large intestine without perforation or abscess (K57.5-)

K57.10   Diverticulosis of small intestine without perforation or abscess without bleeding
Diverticular disease of small intestine NOS

K57.11   Diverticulosis of small intestine without perforation or abscess with bleeding

K57.12   Diverticulitis of small intestine without perforation or abscess without bleeding

K57.13   Diverticulitis of small intestine without perforation or abscess with bleeding

● **K57.2   Diverticulitis of large intestine with perforation and abscess**
Excludes1   diverticulitis of both small and large intestine with perforation and abscess (K57.4-)
Coding Clinic: 2022, Q1, P27

K57.20   Diverticulitis of large intestine with perforation and abscess without bleeding
Coding Clinic: 2022, Q1, P26

K57.21   Diverticulitis of large intestine with perforation and abscess with bleeding

Figure 11-12   Diverticulosis. (From Shiland: Mastering Healthcare Terminology, ed 4, St. Louis, Mosby, 2012)

Item 11-16   Diverticula of the intestines are acquired herniations of the mucosa. Diverticulum (singular): Pocket or pouch that bulges outward through a weak spot (herniation) in the colon. Diverticula (plural). **Diverticulosis** is the condition of having diverticula. **Diverticulitis** is inflammation of these pouches or herniations. Classification is based on location (small intestine or colon) and whether it occurs with or without hemorrhage.

● **K57.3   Diverticular disease of large intestine without perforation or abscess**
Excludes1   diverticular disease of both small and large intestine without perforation or abscess (K57.5-)

K57.30   Diverticulosis of large intestine without perforation or abscess without bleeding
Diverticular disease of colon NOS

K57.31   Diverticulosis of large intestine without perforation or abscess with bleeding

K57.32   Diverticulitis of large intestine without perforation or abscess without bleeding

K57.33   Diverticulitis of large intestine without perforation or abscess with bleeding

● **K57.4   Diverticulitis of both small and large intestine with perforation and abscess**

K57.40   Diverticulitis of both small and large intestine with perforation and abscess without bleeding

K57.41   Diverticulitis of both small and large intestine with perforation and abscess with bleeding

● **K57.5   Diverticular disease of both small and large intestine without perforation or abscess**

K57.50   Diverticulosis of both small and large intestine without perforation or abscess without bleeding
Diverticular disease of both small and large intestine NOS

K57.51   Diverticulosis of both small and large intestine without perforation or abscess with bleeding

K57.52   Diverticulitis of both small and large intestine without perforation or abscess without bleeding

K57.53   Diverticulitis of both small and large intestine without perforation or abscess with bleeding

● **K57.8   Diverticulitis of intestine, part unspecified, with perforation and abscess**

K57.80   Diverticulitis of intestine, part unspecified, with perforation and abscess without bleeding

K57.81   Diverticulitis of intestine, part unspecified, with perforation and abscess with bleeding

▶ New   ➡ Revised   deleted Deleted   Excludes 1   Excludes 2   Includes   Use additional   Code first   Code also   Key words
OGCR Official Guidelines   X Assign placeholder X   ● Use Additional Character(s)   ▌ Manifestation Code   ⓗ Hierarchical Condition Category   Coding Clinic

● **K57.9   Diverticular disease of intestine, part unspecified, without perforation or abscess**

    K57.90   Diverticulosis of intestine, part unspecified, without perforation or abscess without bleeding
       Diverticular disease of intestine NOS
       Coding Clinic: 2021, Q1, P12

    K57.91   Diverticulosis of intestine, part unspecified, without perforation or abscess with bleeding

    K57.92   Diverticulitis of intestine, part unspecified, without perforation or abscess without bleeding

    K57.93   Diverticulitis of intestine, part unspecified, without perforation or abscess with bleeding

● **K58   Irritable bowel syndrome**

    Includes   irritable colon
                 spastic colon

    K58.0   Irritable bowel syndrome with diarrhea

    K58.1   Irritable bowel syndrome with constipation
       Coding Clinic: 2016, Q4, P32

    K58.2   Mixed irritable bowel syndrome
       Coding Clinic: 2016, Q4, P32

    K58.8   Other irritable bowel syndrome
       Coding Clinic: 2016, Q4, P32

    K58.9   Irritable bowel syndrome without diarrhea
       Irritable bowel syndrome NOS

● **K59   Other functional intestinal disorders**

    Excludes1   change in bowel habit NOS (R19.4)
                intestinal malabsorption (K90.-)
                psychogenic intestinal disorders (F45.8)

    Excludes2   functional disorders of stomach (K31.-)

● **K59.0   Constipation**

    Excludes1   fecal impaction (K56.41)
                incomplete defecation (R15.0)

    K59.00   Constipation, unspecified

    K59.01   Slow transit constipation

    K59.02   Outlet dysfunction constipation

    K59.03   Drug induced constipation
       Use additional code for adverse effect, if applicable, to identify drug (T36-T50 with fifth or sixth character 5)
       Coding Clinic: 2016, Q4, P33

    K59.04   Chronic idiopathic constipation
       Functional constipation
       Coding Clinic: 2016, Q4, P33

    K59.09   Other constipation
       Chronic constipation

    K59.1   Functional diarrhea

    Excludes1   diarrhea NOS (R19.7)
                irritable bowel syndrome with diarrhea (K58.0)

    K59.2   Neurogenic bowel, not elsewhere classified

● **K59.3   Megacolon, not elsewhere classified**
       Dilatation of colon
       Code first, if applicable (T51-T65) to identify toxic agent

    Excludes1   congenital megacolon (aganglionic) (Q43.1)
                megacolon (due to) (in) Chagas' disease (B57.32)
                megacolon (due to) (in) Clostridium difficile (A04.7-)
                megacolon (due to) (in) Hirschsprung's disease (Q43.1)
       Coding Clinic: 2016, Q4, P33

    K59.31   Toxic megacolon ⊚

    K59.39   Other megacolon
       Megacolon NOS

Item 11–17   A **fissure** is a groove in the surface, whereas a **fistula** is an abnormal passage. An **abscess** is an accumulation of pus in a tissue cavity resulting from a bacterial or parasitic infection.

    K59.4   Anal spasm
       Proctalgia fugax

● **K59.8   Other specified functional intestinal disorders**

    K59.81 Ogilvie syndrome
       Acute colonic pseudo-obstruction (ACPO)

    K59.89 Other specified functional intestinal disorders
       Atony of colon
       Pseudo-obstruction (acute) (chronic) of intestine

    K59.9   Functional intestinal disorder, unspecified

● **K60   Fissure and fistula of anal and rectal regions**

    Excludes1   fissure and fistula of anal and rectal regions with abscess or cellulitis (K61.-)

    Excludes2   anal sphincter tear (healed) (nontraumatic) (old) (K62.81)

    K60.0   Acute anal fissure

    K60.1   Chronic anal fissure

    K60.2   Anal fissure, unspecified

    K60.3   Anal fistula

    K60.4   Rectal fistula
       Fistula of rectum to skin

    Excludes1   rectovaginal fistula (N82.3)
                vesicorectal fistula (N32.1)

    K60.5   Anorectal fistula

● **K61   Abscess of anal and rectal regions**

    Includes   abscess of anal and rectal regions
                 cellulitis of anal and rectal regions

    K61.0   Anal abscess
       Perianal abscess

    Excludes2   intrasphincteric abscess (K61.4)

    K61.1   Rectal abscess
       Perirectal abscess

    Excludes1   ischiorectal abscess (K61.39)
       Coding Clinic: 2012, Q4, P104

    K61.2   Anorectal abscess

    K61.3   Ischiorectal abscess

       K61.31   Horseshoe abscess

       K61.39   Other ischiorectal abscess
          Abscess of ischiorectal fossa
          Ischiorectal abscess, NOS

    K61.4   Intrasphincteric abscess
       Intersphincteric abscess

    K61.5   Supralevator abscess

● **K62   Other diseases of anus and rectum**

    Includes   anal canal

    Excludes2   colostomy and enterostomy malfunction (K94.0-, K91.4-)
                fecal incontinence (R15.-)
                hemorrhoids (K64.-)

    K62.0   Anal polyp
       Coding Clinic: 2018, Q1, P7

    K62.1   Rectal polyp

    Excludes1   adenomatous polyp (D12.8)
       Coding Clinic: 2018, Q1, P7

    K62.2   Anal prolapse
       Prolapse of anal canal

    K62.3   Rectal prolapse
       Prolapse of rectal mucosa

    K62.4   Stenosis of anus and rectum
       Stricture of anus (sphincter)
       Coding Clinic: 2019, Q2, P13

K62.5   Hemorrhage of anus and rectum
> **Excludes1**   gastrointestinal bleeding NOS (K92.2)
> melena (K92.1)
> neonatal rectal hemorrhage (P54.2)

K62.6   Ulcer of anus and rectum
Solitary ulcer of anus and rectum
Stercoral ulcer of anus and rectum
> **Excludes1**   fissure and fistula of anus and rectum
> (K60.-)
> ulcerative colitis (K51.-)

K62.7   Radiation proctitis
Use additional code to identify the type of radiation
(W88.-) or radiation therapy (Y84.2)
Coding Clinic: 2019, Q1, P21

● **K62.8   Other specified diseases of anus and rectum**
> **Excludes2**   ulcerative proctitis (K51.2)

K62.81   Anal sphincter tear (healed) (nontraumatic) (old)
Tear of anus, nontraumatic
Use additional code for any associated fecal
incontinence (R15.-)
> **Excludes2**   anal fissure (K60.-)
> anal sphincter tear (healed)
> (old) complicating delivery
> (O34.7-)
> traumatic tear of anal sphincter
> (S31.831)

K62.82   Dysplasia of anus
Anal intraepithelial neoplasia I and II (AIN I
and II) (histologically confirmed)
Dysplasia of anus NOS
Mild and moderate dysplasia of anus
(histologically confirmed)
> **Excludes1**   abnormal results from anal
> cytologic examination
> without histologic
> confirmation (R85.61-)
> anal intraepithelial neoplasia III
> (D01.3)
> carcinoma in situ of anus (D01.3)
> HGSIL of anus (R85.613)
> severe dysplasia of anus (D01.3)

K62.89   Other specified diseases of anus and rectum
Proctitis NOS
Use additional code for any associated fecal
incontinence (R15.-)

K62.9   Disease of anus and rectum, unspecified

● **K63   Other diseases of intestine**

K63.0   Abscess of intestine
> **Excludes1**   abscess of intestine with Crohn's disease
> (K50.014, K50.114, K50.814, K50.914)
> abscess of intestine with diverticular
> disease (K57.0, K57.2, K57.4, K57.8)
> abscess of intestine with ulcerative colitis
> (K51.014, K51.214, K51.314, K51.414,
> K51.514, K51.814, K51.914)
> **Excludes2**   abscess of anal and rectal regions (K61.-)
> abscess of appendix (K35.3-)

K63.1   Perforation of intestine (nontraumatic) 🔾
Perforation (nontraumatic) of rectum
> **Excludes1**   perforation (nontraumatic) of duodenum
> (K26.-)
> perforation (nontraumatic) of intestine
> with diverticular disease (K57.0,
> K57.2, K57.4, K57.8)
> **Excludes2**   perforation (nontraumatic) of appendix
> (K35.2-, K35.3)

K63.2   Fistula of intestine
> **Excludes1**   fistula of duodenum (K31.6)
> fistula of intestine with Crohn's disease
> (K50.013, K50.113, K50.813, K50.913)
> fistula of intestine with ulcerative colitis
> (K51.013, K51.213, K51.313, K51.413,
> K51.513, K51.813, K51.913)
> **Excludes2**   fistula of anal and rectal regions (K60.-)
> fistula of appendix (K38.3)
> intestinal-genital fistula, female
> (N82.2-N82.4)
> vesicointestinal fistula (N32.1)
Coding Clinic: 2017, Q3, P4

K63.3   Ulcer of intestine
Primary ulcer of small intestine
> **Excludes1**   duodenal ulcer (K26.-)
> gastrointestinal ulcer (K28.-)
> gastrojejunal ulcer (K28.-)
> jejunal ulcer (K28.-)
> peptic ulcer, site unspecified (K27.-)
> ulcer of intestine with perforation (K63.1)
> ulcer of anus or rectum (K62.6)
> ulcerative colitis (K51.-)

K63.4   Enteroptosis

K63.5   Polyp of colon
> **Excludes1**   adenomatous polyp of colon (D12.-)
> inflammatory polyp of colon (K51.4-)
> polyposis of colon (D12.6)
Coding Clinic: 2019, Q1, P33; 2017, Q1, P15-16; 2015, Q2, P14

● **K63.8   Other specified diseases of intestine**

K63.81   Dieulafoy lesion of intestine
> **Excludes2**   Dieulafoy lesion of stomach and
> duodenum (K31.82)

K63.89   Other specified diseases of intestine
Coding Clinic: 2013, Q2, P31

K63.9   Disease of intestine, unspecified

● **K64   Hemorrhoids and perianal venous thrombosis**
> **Includes**   piles
> **Excludes1**   hemorrhoids complicating childbirth and the
> puerperium (O87.2)
> hemorrhoids complicating pregnancy (O22.4)

K64.0   First degree hemorrhoids
Grade/stage I hemorrhoids
Hemorrhoids (bleeding) without prolapse outside of
anal canal

K64.1   Second degree hemorrhoids
Grade/stage II hemorrhoids
Hemorrhoids (bleeding) that prolapse with straining,
but retract spontaneously

K64.2   Third degree hemorrhoids
Grade/stage III hemorrhoids
Hemorrhoids (bleeding) that prolapse with straining
and require manual replacement back inside anal
canal

K64.3   Fourth degree hemorrhoids
Grade/stage IV hemorrhoids
Hemorrhoids (bleeding) with prolapsed tissue that
cannot be manually replaced

K64.4   Residual hemorrhoidal skin tags
External hemorrhoids, NOS
Skin tags of anus

K64.5   Perianal venous thrombosis
External hemorrhoids with thrombosis
Perianal hematoma
Thrombosed hemorrhoids NOS

K64.8   Other hemorrhoids
Internal hemorrhoids, without mention of degree
Prolapsed hemorrhoids, degree not specified

K64.9   Unspecified hemorrhoids
Hemorrhoids (bleeding) NOS
Hemorrhoids (bleeding) without mention of degree

DISEASES OF PERITONEUM AND RETROPERITONEUM (K65-K68)

● **K65   Peritonitis**

Use additional code (B95-B97), to identify infectious agent, if known

Code also if applicable diverticular disease of intestine (K57.-)

Excludes1 acute appendicitis with generalized peritonitis (K35.2-)
aseptic peritonitis (T81.6)
benign paroxysmal peritonitis (E85.0)
chemical peritonitis (T81.6)
gonococcal peritonitis (A54.85)
neonatal peritonitis (P78.0-P78.1)
pelvic peritonitis, female (N73.3-N73.5)
periodic familial peritonitis (E85.0)
peritonitis due to talc or other foreign substance (T81.6)
peritonitis in chlamydia (A74.81)
peritonitis in diphtheria (A36.89)
peritonitis in syphilis (late) (A52.74)
peritonitis in tuberculosis (A18.31)
peritonitis with or following abortion or ectopic or molar pregnancy (O00-O07, O08.0)
peritonitis with or following appendicitis (K35.-)
puerperal peritonitis (O85)
retroperitoneal infections (K68.-)

Coding Clinic: 2022, Q1, P26

K65.0   Generalized (acute) peritonitis 🔾
Pelvic peritonitis (acute), male
Subphrenic peritonitis (acute)
Suppurative peritonitis (acute)

K65.1   Peritoneal abscess 🔾
Abdominopelvic abscess
Abscess (of) omentum
Abscess (of) peritoneum
Mesenteric abscess
Retrocecal abscess
Subdiaphragmatic abscess
Subhepatic abscess
Subphrenic abscess
Coding Clinic: 2022, Q1, P26; 2019, Q1, P15

K65.2   Spontaneous bacterial peritonitis 🔾
Excludes1 bacterial peritonitis NOS (K65.9)

K65.3   Choleperitonitis 🔾
Peritonitis due to bile

K65.4   Sclerosing mesenteritis 🔾
Fat necrosis of peritoneum
(Idiopathic) sclerosing mesenteric fibrosis
Mesenteric lipodystrophy
Mesenteric panniculitis
Retractile mesenteritis

K65.8   Other peritonitis 🔾
Chronic proliferative peritonitis
Peritonitis due to urine

K65.9   Peritonitis, unspecified 🔾
Bacterial peritonitis NOS
Coding Clinic: 2013, Q2, P31

● **K66   Other disorders of peritoneum**
Excludes2 ascites (R18.-)
peritoneal effusion (chronic) (R18.8)

K66.0   Peritoneal adhesions (postprocedural) (postinfection)
Adhesions (of) abdominal (wall)
Adhesions (of) diaphragm
Adhesions (of) intestine
Adhesions (of) male pelvis
Adhesions (of) omentum
Adhesions (of) stomach
Adhesive bands
Mesenteric adhesions
Excludes1 female pelvic adhesions [bands] (N73.6)
peritoneal adhesions with intestinal obstruction (K56.5-)

Item 11–18   Peritonitis is an inflammation of the lining (peritoneum) of the abdominal cavity and surface of the intestines.

Item 11-19   Retroperitoneal infections occur between the posterior parietal peritoneum and posterior abdominal wall where the kidneys, adrenal glands, ureters, duodenum, ascending colon, descending colon, pancreas, and the large vessels and nerves are located.

K66.1   Hemoperitoneum
Excludes1 traumatic hemoperitoneum (S36.8-)
Coding Clinic: 2022, Q1, P22-23

K66.8   Other specified disorders of peritoneum

K66.9   Disorder of peritoneum, unspecified

▶ **K67   Disorders of peritoneum in infectious diseases classified elsewhere** 🔾

Code first underlying disease, such as:
congenital syphilis (A50.0)
helminthiasis (B65.0-B83.9)
Excludes1 peritonitis in chlamydia (A74.81)
peritonitis in diphtheria (A36.89)
peritonitis in gonococcal (A54.85)
peritonitis in syphilis (late) (A52.74)
peritonitis in tuberculosis (A18.31)

● **K68   Disorders of retroperitoneum**
● **K68.1   Retroperitoneal abscess**

K68.11   Postprocedural retroperitoneal abscess
Excludes2 infection following procedure (T81.44)

K68.12   Psoas muscle abscess 🔾

K68.19   Other retroperitoneal abscess 🔾
Coding Clinic: 2019, Q1, P15

K68.9   Other disorders of retroperitoneum

DISEASES OF LIVER (K70-K77)

Excludes1 jaundice NOS (R17)

Excludes2 hemochromatosis (E83.11-)
Reye's syndrome (G93.7)
viral hepatitis (B15-B19)
Wilson's disease (E83.0)

● **K70   Alcoholic liver disease**
Use additional code to identify:
alcohol abuse and dependence (F10.-)

K70.0   Alcoholic fatty liver   A
● **K70.1   Alcoholic hepatitis**
K70.10   Alcoholic hepatitis without ascites   A
K70.11   Alcoholic hepatitis with ascites   A
K70.2   Alcoholic fibrosis and sclerosis of liver   A
● **K70.3   Alcoholic cirrhosis of liver**
Alcoholic cirrhosis NOS
K70.30   Alcoholic cirrhosis of liver without ascites 🔾 A
K70.31   Alcoholic cirrhosis of liver with ascites 🔾   A
Coding Clinic: 2018, Q1, P5
● **K70.4   Alcoholic hepatic failure**
Acute alcoholic hepatic failure
Alcoholic hepatic failure NOS
Chronic alcoholic hepatic failure
Subacute alcoholic hepatic failure
K70.40   Alcoholic hepatic failure without coma 🔾 A
K70.41   Alcoholic hepatic failure with coma 🔾   A
K70.9   Alcoholic liver disease, unspecified 🔾   A

CHAPTER 11 (K00-K95)

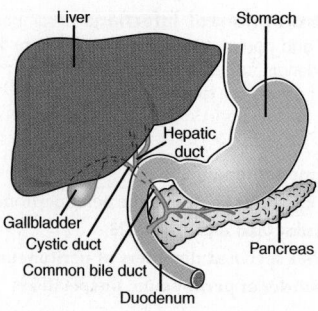

Figure 11-13 Liver and bile ducts.

Item 11–20 Cirrhosis is the progressive fibrosis of the liver resulting in loss of liver function. The main causes of cirrhosis of the liver are alcohol abuse, chronic hepatitis (inflammation of the liver), biliary disease, and excessive amounts of iron. **Alcoholic cirrhosis of the liver** is also called portal, Laënnec's, or fatty nutritional cirrhosis.

● **K71 Toxic liver disease**
   Includes drug-induced idiosyncratic (unpredictable) liver disease
     drug-induced toxic (predictable) liver disease
  Code first poisoning due to drug or toxin, if applicable (T36-T65 with fifth or sixth character 1-4 or 6)
  Use additional code for adverse effect, if applicable, to identify drug (T36-T50 with fifth or sixth character 5)
   Excludes2 alcoholic liver disease (K70.-)
     Budd-Chiari syndrome (I82.0)

  K71.0 Toxic liver disease with cholestasis
    Cholestasis with hepatocyte injury
    'Pure' cholestasis
● **K71.1 Toxic liver disease with hepatic necrosis**
    Hepatic failure (acute) (chronic) due to drugs
    K71.10 Toxic liver disease with hepatic necrosis, without coma
    K71.11 Toxic liver disease with hepatic necrosis, with coma ▶
  K71.2 Toxic liver disease with acute hepatitis
  K71.3 Toxic liver disease with chronic persistent hepatitis
  K71.4 Toxic liver disease with chronic lobular hepatitis
● **K71.5 Toxic liver disease with chronic active hepatitis**
    Toxic liver disease with lupoid hepatitis
    K71.50 Toxic liver disease with chronic active hepatitis without ascites
    K71.51 Toxic liver disease with chronic active hepatitis with ascites
      Coding Clinic: 2018, Q1, P4
  K71.6 Toxic liver disease with hepatitis, not elsewhere classified
  K71.7 Toxic liver disease with fibrosis and cirrhosis of liver
  K71.8 Toxic liver disease with other disorders of liver
    Toxic liver disease with focal nodular hyperplasia
    Toxic liver disease with hepatic granulomas
    Toxic liver disease with peliosis hepatis
    Toxic liver disease with veno-occlusive disease of liver
  K71.9 Toxic liver disease, unspecified

● **K72 Hepatic failure, not elsewhere classified**
   Includes fulminant hepatitis NEC, with hepatic failure
    ~~hepatic encephalopathy NOS~~
    liver (cell) necrosis with hepatic failure
    malignant hepatitis NEC, with hepatic failure
    yellow liver atrophy or dystrophy
   Excludes1 alcoholic hepatic failure (K70.4)
    hepatic failure with toxic liver disease (K71.1-)
    icterus of newborn (P55-P59)
    postprocedural hepatic failure (K91.82)
   Excludes2 hepatic failure complicating abortion or ectopic or molar pregnancy (O00-O07, O08.8)
    hepatic failure complicating pregnancy, childbirth and the puerperium (O26.6-)
    viral hepatitis with hepatic coma (B15-B19)
● **K72.0 Acute and subacute hepatic failure**
    Acute non-viral hepatitis NOS
    Coding Clinic: 2015, Q2, P17
    K72.00 Acute and subacute hepatic failure without coma
      Coding Clinic: 2021, Q1, P13; 2015, Q2, P17
    K72.01 Acute and subacute hepatic failure with coma ▶
● **K72.1 Chronic hepatic failure**
    End stage liver disease
    K72.10 Chronic hepatic failure without coma ▶
      Coding Clinic: 2021, Q1, P13; 2017, Q1, P41
    K72.11 Chronic hepatic failure with coma ▶
      Coding Clinic: 2020, Q1, P15
● **K72.9 Hepatic failure, unspecified**
    K72.90 Hepatic failure, unspecified without coma ▶
      Coding Clinic: 2022, Q1, P53; 2018, Q4, P21
    K72.91 Hepatic failure, unspecified with coma ▶
     Hepatic coma NOS
      Coding Clinic: 2016, Q2, P35

● **K73 Chronic hepatitis, not elsewhere classified**
   Excludes1 alcoholic hepatitis (chronic) (K70.1-)
    drug-induced hepatitis (chronic) (K71.-)
    granulomatous hepatitis (chronic) NEC (K75.3)
    reactive, nonspecific hepatitis (chronic) (K75.2)
    viral hepatitis (chronic) (B15-B19)
  K73.0 Chronic persistent hepatitis, not elsewhere classified ▶
  K73.1 Chronic lobular hepatitis, not elsewhere classified ▶
  K73.2 Chronic active hepatitis, not elsewhere classified ▶
  K73.8 Other chronic hepatitis, not elsewhere classified ▶
  K73.9 Chronic hepatitis, unspecified ▶

● **K74 Fibrosis and cirrhosis of liver**
  Code also, if applicable, viral hepatitis (acute) (chronic) (B15-B19)
   Excludes1 alcoholic cirrhosis (of liver) (K70.3)
    alcoholic fibrosis of liver (K70.2)
    cardiac sclerosis of liver (K76.1)
    cirrhosis (of liver) with toxic liver disease (K71.7)
    congenital cirrhosis (of liver) (P78.81)
    pigmentary cirrhosis (of liver) (E83.110)
● **K74.0 Hepatic fibrosis**
    Code first underlying liver disease, such as:
    nonalcoholic steatohepatitis (NASH) (K75.81)
    K74.00 Hepatic fibrosis, unspecified
    K74.01 Hepatic fibrosis, early fibrosis
     Hepatic fibrosis, stage F1 or stage F2
    K74.02 Hepatic fibrosis, advanced fibrosis
     Hepatic fibrosis, stage F3
      Excludes1 cirrhosis of liver (K74.6-)
       hepatic fibrosis, stage F4 (K74.6-)

CHAPTER 11 (K00-K95)

▶ New ⟹ Revised ~~deleted~~ Deleted Excludes 1 Excludes 2 Includes Use additional Code first Code also Key words
OGCR Official Guidelines X Assign placeholder X ● Use Additional Character(s) ▷ Manifestation Code 🐾 Hierarchical Condition Category Coding Clinic

K74.1   **Hepatic sclerosis**

K74.2   **Hepatic fibrosis with hepatic sclerosis**

K74.3   **Primary biliary cirrhosis** 🐞
    Chronic nonsuppurative destructive cholangitis
    Primary biliary cholangitis
    Excludes2   primary sclerosing cholangitis (K83.01)

K74.4   **Secondary biliary cirrhosis** 🐞

K74.5   **Biliary cirrhosis, unspecified** 🐞

● **K74.6**   **Other and unspecified cirrhosis of liver**

    K74.60   **Unspecified cirrhosis of liver** 🐞
        Cirrhosis (of liver) NOS
        Coding Clinic: 2018, Q1, P4

    K74.69   **Other cirrhosis of liver** 🐞
        Cryptogenic cirrhosis (of liver)
        Macronodular cirrhosis (of liver)
        Micronodular cirrhosis (of liver)
        Mixed type cirrhosis (of liver)
        Portal cirrhosis (of liver)
        Postnecrotic cirrhosis (of liver)

● **K75**   **Other inflammatory liver diseases**
    Excludes2   toxic liver disease (K71.-)

K75.0   **Abscess of liver**
    Cholangitic hepatic abscess
    Hematogenic hepatic abscess
    Hepatic abscess NOS
    Lymphogenic hepatic abscess
    Pylephlebitic hepatic abscess
    Excludes1   amebic liver abscess (A06.4)
             cholangitis without liver abscess (K83.09)
             pylephlebitis without liver abscess (K75.1)
    Excludes2   acute or subacute hepatitis NOS (B17.9)
             acute or subacute non-viral hepatitis (K72.0)
             chronic hepatitis NEC (K73.8)

K75.1   **Phlebitis of portal vein**
    Pylephlebitis
    Excludes1   pylephlebitic liver abscess (K75.0)

K75.2   **Nonspecific reactive hepatitis**
    Excludes1   acute or subacute hepatitis (K72.0-)
             chronic hepatitis NEC (K73.-)
             viral hepatitis (B15-B19)

K75.3   **Granulomatous hepatitis, not elsewhere classified**
    Excludes1   acute or subacute hepatitis (K72.0-)
             chronic hepatitis NEC (K73.-)
             viral hepatitis (B15-B19)

K75.4   **Autoimmune hepatitis** 🐞
    Lupoid hepatitis NEC

● **K75.8**   **Other specified inflammatory liver diseases**

    K75.81   **Nonalcoholic steatohepatitis (NASH)**
        Use additional code, if applicable, hepatic fibrosis (K74.0-)

    K75.89   **Other specified inflammatory liver diseases**

K75.9   **Inflammatory liver disease, unspecified**
    Hepatitis NOS
    Excludes1   acute or subacute hepatitis (K72.0-)
             chronic hepatitis NEC (K73.-)
             viral hepatitis (B15-B19)
    Coding Clinic: 2015, Q2, P17

● **K76**   **Other diseases of liver**
    Excludes2   alcoholic liver disease (K70.-)
             amyloid degeneration of liver (E85.-)
             cystic disease of liver (congenital) (Q44.6)
             hepatic vein thrombosis (I82.0)
             hepatomegaly NOS (R16.0)
             pigmentary cirrhosis (of liver) (E83.110)
             portal vein thrombosis (I81)
             toxic liver disease (K71.-)

K76.0   **Fatty (change of) liver, not elsewhere classified**
    Nonalcoholic fatty liver disease (NAFLD)
    Excludes1   nonalcoholic steatohepatitis (NASH) (K75.81)

K76.1   **Chronic passive congestion of liver**
    Cardiac cirrhosis
    Cardiac sclerosis

K76.2   **Central hemorrhagic necrosis of liver**
    Excludes1   liver necrosis with hepatic failure (K72.-)

K76.3   **Infarction of liver**

K76.4   **Peliosis hepatis**
    Hepatic angiomatosis

K76.5   **Hepatic veno-occlusive disease**
    Excludes1   Budd-Chiari syndrome (I82.0)

K76.6   **Portal hypertension** 🐞
    Use additional code for any associated complications, such as:
        portal hypertensive gastropathy (K31.89)
    Coding Clinic: 2020, Q1, P15

K76.7   **Hepatorenal syndrome** 🐞
    Excludes1   hepatorenal syndrome following labor and delivery (O90.4)
             postprocedural hepatorenal syndrome (K91.83)

● **K76.8**   **Other specified diseases of liver**

    K76.81   **Hepatopulmonary syndrome** 🐞
        Code first underlying liver disease, such as:
            alcoholic cirrhosis of liver (K70.3-)
            cirrhosis of liver without mention of alcohol (K74.6-)

    ▶ **K76.82**   **Hepatic encephalopathy**
        ▶ Hepatic encephalopathy, NOS
        ▶ Hepatic encephalopathy without coma
        ▶ Hepatocerebral intoxication
        ▶ Portal-systemic encephalopathy
        ▶ Code also underlying liver disease, such as:
            ▶ acute and subacute hepatic failure without coma (K72.00)
            ▶ alcoholic hepatic failure without coma (K70.40)
            ▶ chronic hepatic failure without coma (K72.10)
            ▶ hepatic failure with toxic liver disease without coma (K71.10)
            ▶ hepatic failure without coma (K72.90)
            ▶ icterus of newborn (P55-P59)
            ▶ postprocedural hepatic failure (K91.82)
            ▶ viral hepatitis without hepatic coma (B15.9, B16.1, B16.9, B17.10, B19.10, B19.20, B19.9)

        ▶ **Excludes1**   acute and subacute hepatic failure with coma (K72.01)
            ▶ alcoholic hepatic failure with coma (K70.41)
            ▶ chronic hepatic failure with coma (K72.11)
            ▶ hepatic failure with coma (K72.91)

    K76.89   **Other specified diseases of liver**
        Cyst (simple) of liver
        Focal nodular hyperplasia of liver
        Hepatoptosis

K76.9   **Liver disease, unspecified**

CHAPTER 11 (K00-K95)

▶ **K77** *Liver disorders in diseases classified elsewhere*
> *Code first underlying disease, such as:*
>> amyloidosis (E85.-)
>> congenital syphilis (A50.0, A50.5)
>> congenital toxoplasmosis (P37.1)
>> ➡ infectious mononucleosis with liver disease (B27.0-B27.9
>>> with fifth character 9)
>> schistosomiasis (B65.0-B65.9)

> **Excludes1** alcoholic hepatitis (K70.1-)
>> alcoholic liver disease (K70.-)
>> cytomegaloviral hepatitis (B25.1)
>> herpesviral [herpes simplex] hepatitis (B00.81)
>> mumps hepatitis (B26.81)
>> sarcoidosis with liver disease (D86.89)
>> secondary syphilis with liver disease (A51.45)
>> syphilis (late) with liver disease (A52.74)
>> toxoplasmosis (acquired) hepatitis (B58.1)
>> tuberculosis with liver disease (A18.83)

DISORDERS OF GALLBLADDER, BILIARY TRACT AND PANCREAS (K80–K87)

● **K80** **Cholelithiasis**
> *Presence or formation of gallstones*
> **Excludes1** retained cholelithiasis following cholecystectomy
>> (K91.86)

● **K80.0** **Calculus of gallbladder with acute cholecystitis**
> Any condition listed in K80.2 with acute cholecystitis
> Use additional code if applicable for associated
>> gangrene of gallbladder (K82.A1), or perforation of
>> gallbladder (K82.A2)
> *Check documentation for acute/chronic gallbladder/common
>> bile duct either with or without obstruction.*

> **K80.00** **Calculus of gallbladder with acute cholecystitis without obstruction**
>> Coding Clinic: 2018, Q4, P20

> **K80.01** **Calculus of gallbladder with acute cholecystitis with obstruction**

● **K80.1** **Calculus of gallbladder with other cholecystitis**
> Use additional code if applicable for associated
>> gangrene of gallbladder (K82.A1), or perforation of
>> gallbladder (K82.A2)

> **K80.10** **Calculus of gallbladder with chronic cholecystitis without obstruction**
>> Cholelithiasis with cholecystitis NOS

> **K80.11** **Calculus of gallbladder with chronic cholecystitis with obstruction**

> **K80.12** **Calculus of gallbladder with acute and chronic cholecystitis without obstruction**

> **K80.13** **Calculus of gallbladder with acute and chronic cholecystitis with obstruction**

> **K80.18** **Calculus of gallbladder with other cholecystitis without obstruction**

> **K80.19** **Calculus of gallbladder with other cholecystitis with obstruction**

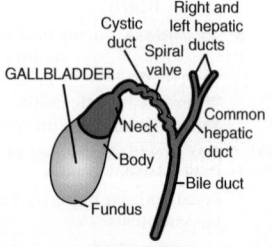

Figure 11-14 Gallbladder and bile ducts.

● **K80.2** **Calculus of gallbladder without cholecystitis**
> Cholecystolithiasis without cholecystitis
> Cholelithiasis (without cholecystitis)
> Colic (recurrent) of gallbladder (without cholecystitis)
> Gallstone (impacted) of cystic duct (without
>> cholecystitis)
> Gallstone (impacted) of gallbladder (without
>> cholecystitis)

> **K80.20** **Calculus of gallbladder without cholecystitis without obstruction**

> **K80.21** **Calculus of gallbladder without cholecystitis with obstruction**

● **K80.3** **Calculus of bile duct with cholangitis**
> Any condition listed in K80.5 with cholangitis

> **K80.30** **Calculus of bile duct with cholangitis, unspecified, without obstruction**

> **K80.31** **Calculus of bile duct with cholangitis, unspecified, with obstruction**

> **K80.32** **Calculus of bile duct with acute cholangitis without obstruction**

> **K80.33** **Calculus of bile duct with acute cholangitis with obstruction**

> **K80.34** **Calculus of bile duct with chronic cholangitis without obstruction**

> **K80.35** **Calculus of bile duct with chronic cholangitis with obstruction**

> **K80.36** **Calculus of bile duct with acute and chronic cholangitis without obstruction**

> **K80.37** **Calculus of bile duct with acute and chronic cholangitis with obstruction**

● **K80.4** **Calculus of bile duct with cholecystitis**
> Any condition listed in K80.5 with cholecystitis (with
>> cholangitis)
> ~~Code also fistula of bile duct (K83.3)~~
> ▶ Code also fistula of bile duct (K83.3)
> Use additional code if applicable for associated
>> gangrene of gallbladder (K82.A1), or perforation of
>> gallbladder (K82.A2)

> **K80.40** **Calculus of bile duct with cholecystitis, unspecified, without obstruction**

> **K80.41** **Calculus of bile duct with cholecystitis, unspecified, with obstruction**
>> Coding Clinic: 2019, Q1, P18

> **K80.42** **Calculus of bile duct with acute cholecystitis without obstruction**

> **K80.43** **Calculus of bile duct with acute cholecystitis with obstruction**

> **K80.44** **Calculus of bile duct with chronic cholecystitis without obstruction**

> **K80.45** **Calculus of bile duct with chronic cholecystitis with obstruction**

> **K80.46** **Calculus of bile duct with acute and chronic cholecystitis without obstruction**

> **K80.47** **Calculus of bile duct with acute and chronic cholecystitis with obstruction**

● **K80.5** **Calculus of bile duct without cholangitis or cholecystitis**
> Choledocholithiasis (without cholangitis or cholecystitis)
> Gallstone (impacted) of bile duct NOS (without
>> cholangitis or cholecystitis)
> Gallstone (impacted) of common duct (without
>> cholangitis or cholecystitis)
> Gallstone (impacted) of hepatic duct (without cholangitis
>> or cholecystitis)
> Hepatic cholelithiasis (without cholangitis or cholecystitis)
> Hepatic colic (recurrent) (without cholangitis or
>> cholecystitis)

> **K80.50** **Calculus of bile duct without cholangitis or cholecystitis without obstruction**

> **K80.51** **Calculus of bile duct without cholangitis or cholecystitis with obstruction**

● **K80.6**   **Calculus of gallbladder and bile duct with cholecystitis**

> Use additional code if applicable for associated gangrene of gallbladder (K82.A1), or perforation of gallbladder (K82.A2)

     K80.60   **Calculus of gallbladder and bile duct with cholecystitis, unspecified, without obstruction**

     K80.61   **Calculus of gallbladder and bile duct with cholecystitis, unspecified, with obstruction**

     K80.62   **Calculus of gallbladder and bile duct with acute cholecystitis without obstruction**

     K80.63   **Calculus of gallbladder and bile duct with acute cholecystitis with obstruction**

     K80.64   **Calculus of gallbladder and bile duct with chronic cholecystitis without obstruction**

     K80.65   **Calculus of gallbladder and bile duct with chronic cholecystitis with obstruction**

     K80.66   **Calculus of gallbladder and bile duct with acute and chronic cholecystitis without obstruction**

     K80.67   **Calculus of gallbladder and bile duct with acute and chronic cholecystitis with obstruction**

● **K80.7**   **Calculus of gallbladder and bile duct without cholecystitis**

     K80.70   **Calculus of gallbladder and bile duct without cholecystitis without obstruction**

     K80.71   **Calculus of gallbladder and bile duct without cholecystitis with obstruction**

● **K80.8**   **Other cholelithiasis**

     K80.80   **Other cholelithiasis without obstruction**

     K80.81   **Other cholelithiasis with obstruction**

● **K81**   **Cholecystitis**

> *Chronic or acute inflammation of the gallbladder*

> Use additional code if applicable for associated gangrene of gallbladder (K82.A1), or perforation of gallbladder (K82.A2)

> **Excludes1**   cholecystitis with cholelithiasis (K80.-)

     K81.0   **Acute cholecystitis**
         Abscess of gallbladder
         Angiocholecystitis
         Emphysematous (acute) cholecystitis
         Empyema of gallbladder
         Gangrene of gallbladder
         Gangrenous cholecystitis
         Suppurative cholecystitis

     K81.1   **Chronic cholecystitis**

     K81.2   **Acute cholecystitis with chronic cholecystitis**

     K81.9   **Cholecystitis, unspecified**

● **K82**   **Other diseases of gallbladder**

> **Excludes1**   nonvisualization of gallbladder (R93.2)
> postcholecystectomy syndrome (K91.5)

     K82.0   **Obstruction of gallbladder**
         Occlusion of cystic duct or gallbladder without cholelithiasis
         Stenosis of cystic duct or gallbladder without cholelithiasis
         Stricture of cystic duct or gallbladder without cholelithiasis

> **Excludes1**   obstruction of gallbladder with cholelithiasis (K80.-)

     K82.1   **Hydrops of gallbladder**
         Mucocele of gallbladder

     K82.2   **Perforation of gallbladder**
         Rupture of cystic duct or gallbladder

> **Excludes1**   Perforation of gallbladder in cholecystitis (K82.A2)

     K82.3   **Fistula of gallbladder**
         Cholecystocolic fistula
         Cholecystoduodenal fistula
         Coding Clinic: 2019, Q1, P18

     K82.4   **Cholesterolosis of gallbladder**
         Strawberry gallbladder

> **Excludes1**   cholesterolosis of gallbladder with cholecystitis (K81.-)
> cholesterolosis of gallbladder with cholelithiasis (K80.-)

     K82.8   **Other specified diseases of gallbladder**
         Adhesions of cystic duct or gallbladder
         Atrophy of cystic duct or gallbladder
         Cyst of cystic duct or gallbladder
         Dyskinesia of cystic duct or gallbladder
         Hypertrophy of cystic duct or gallbladder
         Nonfunctioning of cystic duct or gallbladder
         Ulcer of cystic duct or gallbladder

     K82.9   **Disease of gallbladder, unspecified**

● **K82.A**   **Disorders of gallbladder in diseases classified elsewhere**

> *Code first the type of cholecystitis (K81.-), or cholelithiasis with cholecystitis (K80.00-K80.19, K80.40-K80.47, K80.60-K80.67)*

     ▶ *K82.A1*   *Gangrene of gallbladder in cholecystitis*
         Coding Clinic: 2018, Q4, P20

     ● **K82.A2**   **Perforation of gallbladder in cholecystitis**
         Coding Clinic: 2018, Q4, P20

● **K83**   **Other diseases of biliary tract**

> **Excludes1**   postcholecystectomy syndrome (K91.5)
> **Excludes2**   conditions involving the gallbladder (K81-K82)
> conditions involving the cystic duct (K81-K82)

● **K83.0**   **Cholangitis**

> **Excludes1**   cholangitic liver abscess (K75.0)
> cholangitis with choledocholithiasis (K80.3-, K80.4-)

> **Excludes2**   chronic nonsuppurative destructive cholangitis (K74.3)
> primary biliary cholangitis (K74.3)
> primary biliary cirrhosis (K74.3)

     K83.01   **Primary sclerosing cholangitis**
         Coding Clinic: 2018, Q4, P21

     K83.09   **Other cholangitis**
         Ascending cholangitis
         Cholangitis NOS
         Primary cholangitis
         Recurrent cholangitis
         Sclerosing cholangitis
         Secondary cholangitis
         Stenosing cholangitis
         Suppurative cholangitis

     K83.1   **Obstruction of bile duct**
         Occlusion of bile duct without cholelithiasis
         Stenosis of bile duct without cholelithiasis
         Stricture of bile duct without cholelithiasis

> **Excludes1**   congenital obstruction of bile duct (Q44.3)
> obstruction of bile duct with cholelithiasis (K80.-)

         Coding Clinic: 2016, Q1, P18

     K83.2   **Perforation of bile duct**
         Rupture of bile duct

     K83.3   **Fistula of bile duct**
         Choledochoduodenal fistula

     K83.4   **Spasm of sphincter of Oddi**

     K83.5   **Biliary cyst**

     K83.8   **Other specified diseases of biliary tract**
         Adhesions of biliary tract
         Atrophy of biliary tract
         Hypertrophy of biliary tract
         Ulcer of biliary tract

CHAPTER 11 (K00-K95)

CHAPTER 11 (K00-K95)

K83.9   Disease of biliary tract, unspecified

Figure 11-15   Pancreatic ductal system.

● **K85**   **Acute pancreatitis**
Inflammatory process in which pancreatic enzymes autodigest the gland

    Includes   acute (recurrent) pancreatitis
                    subacute pancreatitis
    Coding Clinic: 2016, Q4, P34

  ● **K85.0**   **Idiopathic acute pancreatitis**

      K85.00   **Idiopathic acute pancreatitis without necrosis or infection**

      K85.01   **Idiopathic acute pancreatitis with uninfected necrosis**

      K85.02   **Idiopathic acute pancreatitis with infected necrosis**

  ● **K85.1**   **Biliary acute pancreatitis**
         Gallstone pancreatitis

      K85.10   **Biliary acute pancreatitis without necrosis or infection**

      K85.11   **Biliary acute pancreatitis with uninfected necrosis**

      K85.12   **Biliary acute pancreatitis with infected necrosis**

  ● **K85.2**   **Alcohol induced acute pancreatitis**

      Excludes2   alcohol induced chronic pancreatitis (K86.0)

      K85.20   **Alcohol induced acute pancreatitis without necrosis or infection**
               Coding Clinic: 2020, Q1, P9

      K85.21   **Alcohol induced acute pancreatitis with uninfected necrosis**

      K85.22   **Alcohol induced acute pancreatitis with infected necrosis**

  ● **K85.3**   **Drug induced acute pancreatitis**
         Use additional code for adverse effect, if applicable, to identify drug (T36-T50 with fifth or sixth character 5)
         Use additional code to identify drug abuse and dependence (F11.-F17.-)

      K85.30   **Drug induced acute pancreatitis without necrosis or infection**

      K85.31   **Drug induced acute pancreatitis with uninfected necrosis**

      K85.32   **Drug induced acute pancreatitis with infected necrosis**

  ● **K85.8**   **Other acute pancreatitis**

      K85.80   **Other acute pancreatitis without necrosis or infection**

      K85.81   **Other acute pancreatitis with uninfected necrosis**

      K85.82   **Other acute pancreatitis with infected necrosis**

  ● **K85.9**   **Acute pancreatitis, unspecified**
         Pancreatitis NOS

      K85.90   **Acute pancreatitis without necrosis or infection, unspecified**

      K85.91   **Acute pancreatitis with uninfected necrosis, unspecified**

      K85.92   **Acute pancreatitis with infected necrosis, unspecified**

● **K86**   **Other diseases of pancreas**

      Excludes2   fibrocystic disease of pancreas (E84.-)
                       islet cell tumor (of pancreas) (D13.7)
                       pancreatic steatorrhea (K90.3)

   K86.0   **Alcohol-induced chronic pancreatitis** 🄷
         Use additional code to identify:
            alcohol abuse and dependence (F10.-)

      Code also exocrine pancreatic insufficiency (K86.81)

      Excludes2   alcohol induced acute pancreatitis (K85.2-)

   K86.1   **Other chronic pancreatitis** 🄷
         Chronic pancreatitis NOS
         Infectious chronic pancreatitis
         Recurrent chronic pancreatitis
         Relapsing chronic pancreatitis
      Code also exocrine pancreatic insufficiency (K86.81)

   K86.2   **Cyst of pancreas**

   K86.3   **Pseudocyst of pancreas**

● **K86.8**   **Other specified diseases of pancreas**
         Coding Clinic: 2016, Q4, P34

      K86.81   **Exocrine pancreatic insufficiency**

      K86.89   **Other specified diseases of pancreas**
            Aseptic pancreatic necrosis, unrelated to acute pancreatitis
            Atrophy of pancreas
            Calculus of pancreas
            Cirrhosis of pancreas
            Fibrosis of pancreas
            Pancreatic fat necrosis, unrelated to acute pancreatitis
            Pancreatic infantilism
            Pancreatic necrosis NOS, unrelated to acute pancreatitis

   K86.9   **Disease of pancreas, unspecified**

▷ **K87**   *Disorders of gallbladder, biliary tract and pancreas in diseases classified elsewhere*

      Code first underlying disease

      Excludes1   cytomegaloviral pancreatitis (B25.2)
                     mumps pancreatitis (B26.3)
                     syphilitic gallbladder (A52.74)
                     syphilitic pancreas (A52.74)
                     tuberculosis of gallbladder (A18.83)
                     tuberculosis of pancreas (A18.83)

OTHER DISEASES OF THE DIGESTIVE SYSTEM (K90-K95)

● **K90**   **Intestinal malabsorption**

      Excludes1   intestinal malabsorption following gastrointestinal surgery (K91.2)

   K90.0   **Celiac disease**
         Celiac disease with steatorrhea
         Celiac gluten-sensitive enteropathy
         Nontropical sprue
      Use additional code for associated disorders including:
         dermatitis herpetiformis (L13.0)
         gluten ataxia (G32.81)
      Code also exocrine pancreatic insufficiency (K86.81)

   K90.1   **Tropical sprue**
         Sprue NOS
         Tropical steatorrhea

   K90.2   **Blind loop syndrome, not elsewhere classified**
         Blind loop syndrome NOS

      Excludes1   congenital blind loop syndrome (Q43.8)
                     postsurgical blind loop syndrome (K91.2)

   K90.3   **Pancreatic steatorrhea**

▶ New   ⇒ Revised   ~~deleted~~ Deleted   Excludes 1   Excludes 2   Includes   Use additional   Code first   Code also   Key words

OGCR Official Guidelines   X Assign placeholder X   ● Use Additional Character(s)   ▷ Manifestation Code   🄷 Hierarchical Condition Category   Coding Clinic

● K90.4 **Other malabsorption due to intolerance**
>>> **Excludes2** celiac gluten-sensitive enteropathy (K90.0)
>>> lactose intolerance (E73.-)
>>> Coding Clinic: 2016, Q4, P35-36

K90.41 **Non-celiac gluten sensitivity**
>> Gluten sensitivity NOS
>> Non-celiac gluten sensitive enteropathy

K90.49 **Malabsorption due to intolerance, not elsewhere classified**
>> Malabsorption due to intolerance to carbohydrate
>> Malabsorption due to intolerance to fat
>> Malabsorption due to intolerance to protein
>> Malabsorption due to intolerance to starch

● K90.8 **Other intestinal malabsorption**

K90.81 **Whipple's disease**

K90.89 **Other intestinal malabsorption**

K90.9 **Intestinal malabsorption, unspecified**
>> Coding Clinic: 2017, Q4, P108-109

● K91 **Intraoperative and postprocedural complications and disorders of digestive system, not elsewhere classified**
>> **Excludes2** complications of artificial opening of digestive system (K94.-)
>> complications of bariatric procedures (K95.-)
>> gastrojejunal ulcer (K28.-)
>> postprocedural (radiation) retroperitoneal abscess (K68.11)
>> radiation colitis (K52.0)
>> radiation gastroenteritis (K52.0)
>> radiation proctitis (K62.7)
> Coding Clinic: 2016, Q4, P10

K91.0 **Vomiting following gastrointestinal surgery**

K91.1 **Postgastric surgery syndromes**
>> Dumping syndrome
>> Postgastrectomy syndrome
>> Postvagotomy syndrome

K91.2 **Postsurgical malabsorption, not elsewhere classified**
>> Postsurgical blind loop syndrome
>> **Excludes1** malabsorption osteomalacia in adults (M83.2)
>> malabsorption osteoporosis, postsurgical (M80.8-, M81.8)

● K91.3 **Postprocedural intestinal obstruction**
>> Coding Clinic: 2017, Q1, P40-41

K91.30 **Postprocedural intestinal obstruction, unspecified as to partial versus complete**
>> Postprocedural intestinal obstruction NOS

K91.31 **Postprocedural partial intestinal obstruction**
>> Postprocedural incomplete intestinal obstruction

K91.32 **Postprocedural complete intestinal obstruction**

K91.5 **Postcholecystectomy syndrome**

● K91.6 **Intraoperative hemorrhage and hematoma of a digestive system organ or structure complicating a procedure**
>> **Excludes1** intraoperative hemorrhage and hematoma of a digestive system organ or structure due to accidental puncture and laceration during a procedure (K91.7-)

K91.61 **Intraoperative hemorrhage and hematoma of a digestive system organ or structure complicating a digestive system procedure**
>> Coding Clinic: 2020, Q1, P20

K91.62 **Intraoperative hemorrhage and hematoma of a digestive system organ or structure complicating other procedure**

● K91.7 **Accidental puncture and laceration of a digestive system organ or structure during a procedure**

K91.71 **Accidental puncture and laceration of a digestive system organ or structure during a digestive system procedure**
>> Coding Clinic: 2022, Q1, P51-52; 2021, Q2, P12

K91.72 **Accidental puncture and laceration of a digestive system organ or structure during other procedure**
>> Coding Clinic: 2022, Q1, P51; 2019, Q2, P24

● K91.8 **Other intraoperative and postprocedural complications and disorders of digestive system**

K91.81 **Other intraoperative complications of digestive system**

K91.82 **Postprocedural hepatic failure**

K91.83 **Postprocedural hepatorenal syndrome**

● K91.84 **Postprocedural hemorrhage of a digestive system organ or structure following a procedure**

K91.840 **Postprocedural hemorrhage of a digestive system organ or structure following a digestive system procedure**
>> Coding Clinic: 2016, Q1, P15

K91.841 **Postprocedural hemorrhage of a digestive system organ or structure following other procedure**

● K91.85 **Complications of intestinal pouch**

K91.850 **Pouchitis** ⚕
>> Inflammation of internal ileoanal pouch

K91.858 **Other complications of intestinal pouch** ⚕
>> Coding Clinic: 2019, Q2, P13

K91.86 **Retained cholelithiasis following cholecystectomy**

● K91.87 **Postprocedural hematoma and seroma of a digestive system organ or structure following a procedure**

K91.870 **Postprocedural hematoma of a digestive system organ or structure following a digestive system procedure**
>> Coding Clinic: 2022, Q1, P24

K91.871 **Postprocedural hematoma of a digestive system organ or structure following other procedure**

K91.872 **Postprocedural seroma of a digestive system organ or structure following a digestive system procedure**

K91.873 **Postprocedural seroma of a digestive system organ or structure following other procedure**

K91.89 **Other postprocedural complications and disorders of digestive system**
>> Use additional code, if applicable, to further specify disorder
>> **Excludes2** postprocedural retroperitoneal abscess (K68.11)
>> Coding Clinic: 2017, Q1, P41

CHAPTER 11 (K00-K95)

● **K92**   **Other diseases of digestive system**

     Excludes1   neonatal gastrointestinal hemorrhage (P54.0-P54.3)

   K92.0   **Hematemesis**

   K92.1   **Melena**

       Excludes1   occult blood in feces (R19.5)

   K92.2   **Gastrointestinal hemorrhage, unspecified**

       Gastric hemorrhage NOS

       Intestinal hemorrhage NOS

       Excludes1   acute hemorrhagic gastritis (K29.01)

                hemorrhage of anus and rectum (K62.5)

                angiodysplasia of stomach with hemorrhage (K31.811)

                diverticular disease with hemorrhage (K57.-)

                gastritis and duodenitis with hemorrhage (K29.-)

                peptic ulcer with hemorrhage (K25-K28)

       Coding Clinic: 2021, Q1, P12

● **K92.8**   **Other specified diseases of the digestive system**

     K92.81   **Gastrointestinal mucositis (ulcerative)**

       Code also type of associated therapy, such as:

          antineoplastic and immunosuppressive drugs (T45.1X-)

          radiological procedure and radiotherapy (Y84.2)

         Excludes2   mucositis (ulcerative) of vagina and vulva (N76.81)

                 nasal mucositis (ulcerative) (J34.81)

                 oral mucositis (ulcerative) (K12.3-)

     K92.89   **Other specified diseases of the digestive system**

   K92.9   **Disease of digestive system, unspecified**

● **K94**   **Complications of artificial openings of the digestive system**

   ● **K94.0**   **Colostomy complications**

     K94.00   **Colostomy complication, unspecified** 🐾

     K94.01   **Colostomy hemorrhage** 🐾

     K94.02   **Colostomy infection** 🐾

       Use additional code to specify type of infection, such as:

         cellulitis of abdominal wall (L03.311)

         sepsis (A40.-, A41.-)

     K94.03   **Colostomy malfunction** 🐾

       Mechanical complication of colostomy

     K94.09   **Other complications of colostomy** 🐾

   ● **K94.1**   **Enterostomy complications**

     K94.10   **Enterostomy complication, unspecified** 🐾

     K94.11   **Enterostomy hemorrhage** 🐾

     K94.12   **Enterostomy infection** 🐾

       Use additional code to specify type of infection, such as:

         cellulitis of abdominal wall (L03.311)

         sepsis (A40.-, A41.-)

     K94.13   **Enterostomy malfunction** 🐾

       Mechanical complication of enterostomy

       Coding Clinic: 2021, Q4, P18

     K94.19   **Other complications of enterostomy** 🐾

   ● **K94.2**   **Gastrostomy complications**

     K94.20   **Gastrostomy complication, unspecified** 🐾

     K94.21   **Gastrostomy hemorrhage** 🐾

     K94.22   **Gastrostomy infection** 🐾

       Use additional code to specify type of infection, such as:

         cellulitis of abdominal wall (L03.311)

         sepsis (A40.-, A41.-)

     K94.23   **Gastrostomy malfunction** 🐾

       Mechanical complication of gastrostomy

     K94.29   **Other complications of gastrostomy** 🐾

   ● **K94.3**   **Esophagostomy complications**

     K94.30   **Esophagostomy complications, unspecified** 🐾

     K94.31   **Esophagostomy hemorrhage** 🐾

     K94.32   **Esophagostomy infection** 🐾

       Use additional code to identify the infection

     K94.33   **Esophagostomy malfunction** 🐾

       Mechanical complication of esophagostomy

     K94.39   **Other complications of esophagostomy** 🐾

● **K95**   **Complications of bariatric procedures**

   ● **K95.0**   **Complications of gastric band procedure**

     K95.01   **Infection due to gastric band procedure**

       Use additional code to specify type of infection or organism, such as:

         bacterial and viral infectious agents (B95.-, B96.-)

         cellulitis of abdominal wall (L03.311)

         sepsis (A40.-, A41.-)

     K95.09   **Other complications of gastric band procedure**

       Use additional code, if applicable, to further specify complication

   ● **K95.8**   **Complications of other bariatric procedure**

     Excludes1   complications of gastric band surgery (K95.0-)

     K95.81   **Infection due to other bariatric procedure**

       Use additional code to specify type of infection or organism, such as:

         bacterial and viral infectious agents (B95.-, B96.-)

         cellulitis of abdominal wall (L03.311)

         sepsis (A40.-, A41.-)

     K95.89   **Other complications of other bariatric procedure**

       Use additional code, if applicable, to further specify complication

▶ New   ⇒ Revised   ~~deleted~~ Deleted   Excludes 1   Excludes 2   Includes   Use additional   Code first   Code also   Key words

OGCR Official Guidelines   X Assign placeholder X   ● Use Additional Character(s)   ▷ Manifestation Code   🐾 Hierarchical Condition Category   Coding Clinic

---

CHAPTER 12

DISEASES OF THE SKIN AND SUBCUTANEOUS TISSUE (L00-L99)

OGCR Chapter-Specific Coding Guidelines

12. Chapter 12: Diseases of the Skin and Subcutaneous Tissue (L00-L99)

a. Pressure ulcer stage codes

1) Pressure ulcer stages

Codes from category L89, Pressure ulcer, identify the site of the pressure ulcer as well as the stage of the ulcer.

The ICD-10-CM classifies pressure ulcer stages based on severity, which is designated by stages 1-4, unspecified stage and unstageable.

Assign as many codes from category L89 as needed to identify all the pressure ulcers the patient has, if applicable.

See Section I.B.14 for pressure ulcer stage documentation by clinicians other than patient's provider.

2) Unstageable pressure ulcers

Assignment of the code for unstageable pressure ulcer (L89.--0) should be based on the clinical documentation. These codes are used for pressure ulcers whose stage cannot be clinically determined (e.g., the ulcer is covered by eschar or has been treated with a skin or muscle graft) and pressure ulcers that are documented as deep tissue injury but not documented as due to trauma. This code should not be confused with the codes for unspecified stage (L89.--9). When there is no documentation regarding the stage of the pressure ulcer, assign the appropriate code for unspecified stage (L89.--9).

3) Documented pressure ulcer stage

Assignment of the pressure ulcer stage code should be guided by clinical documentation of the stage or documentation of the terms found in the Alphabetic Index. For clinical terms describing the stage that are not found in the Alphabetic Index, and there is no documentation of the stage, the provider should be queried.

4) Patients admitted with pressure ulcers documented as healed

No code is assigned if the documentation states that the pressure ulcer is completely healed.

5) Patients admitted with pressure ulcers documented as healing

Pressure ulcers described as healing should be assigned the appropriate pressure ulcer stage code based on the documentation in the medical record. If the documentation does not provide information about the stage of the healing pressure ulcer, assign the appropriate code for unspecified stage.

If the documentation is unclear as to whether the patient has a current (new) pressure ulcer or if the patient is being treated for a healing pressure ulcer, query the provider.

For ulcers that were present on admission but healed at the time of discharge, assign the code for the site and stage of the pressure ulcer at the time of admission.

6) Patient admitted with pressure ulcer evolving into another stage during the admission

If a patient is admitted to an inpatient hospital with a pressure ulcer at one stage and it progresses to a higher stage, two separate codes should be assigned: one code for the site and stage of the ulcer on admission and a second code for the same ulcer site and the highest stage reported during the stay.

b. Non-Pressure Chronic Ulcers

1) Patients admitted with non-pressure ulcers documented as healed

No code is assigned if the documentation states that the non-pressure ulcer is completely healed.

2) Patients admitted with non-pressure ulcers documented as healing

Non-pressure ulcers described as healing should be assigned the appropriate non-pressure ulcer code based on the documentation in the medical record. If the documentation does not provide information about the severity of the healing non-pressure ulcer, assign the appropriate code for unspecified severity.

If the documentation is unclear as to whether the patient has a current (new) non-pressure ulcer or if the patient is being treated for a healing non-pressure ulcer, query the provider.

For ulcers that were present on admission but healed at the time of discharge, assign the code for the site and severity of the non-pressure ulcer at the time of admission.

3) Patient admitted with non-pressure ulcer that progresses to another severity level during the admission

If a patient is admitted to an inpatient hospital with a non-pressure ulcer at one severity level and it progresses to a higher severity level, two separate codes should be assigned: one code for the site and severity level of the ulcer on admission and a second code for the same ulcer site and the highest severity level reported during the stay.

See Section I.B.14 for pressure ulcer stage documentation by clinicians other than patient's provider.

Figure 12-1 Furuncle, also known as a boil, is a staphylococcal infection. The organism enters the body through a hair follicle and so furuncles usually appear in hairy areas of the body. A cluster of furuncles is known as a carbuncle and involves infection into the deep subcutaneous fascia. These usually appear on the back and neck. (**B** from Habif TP, Binnick AN, Meyerson LB: Clinical Dermatology: A Color Guide to Diagnosis and Therapy, S.I., Mosby Elsevier, 2010)

CHAPTER 12

DISEASES OF THE SKIN AND SUBCUTANEOUS TISSUE (L00-L99)

Excludes2   certain conditions originating in the perinatal period (P04-P96)
certain infectious and parasitic diseases (A00-B99)
complications of pregnancy, childbirth and the puerperium (O00-O9A)
congenital malformations, deformations, and chromosomal abnormalities (Q00-Q99)
endocrine, nutritional and metabolic diseases (E00-E88)
lipomelanotic reticulosis (I89.8)
neoplasms (C00-D49)
symptoms, signs and abnormal clinical and laboratory findings, not elsewhere classified (R00-R94)
systemic connective tissue disorders (M30-M36)
viral warts (B07.-)

This chapter contains the following blocks:

L00-L08	Infections of the skin and subcutaneous tissue
L10-L14	Bullous disorders
L20-L30	Dermatitis and eczema
L40-L45	Papulosquamous disorders
L49-L54	Urticaria and erythema
L55-L59	Radiation-related disorders of the skin and subcutaneous tissue
L60-L75	Disorders of skin appendages
L76	Intraoperative and postprocedural complications of skin and subcutaneous tissue
L80-L99	Other disorders of the skin and subcutaneous tissue

CHAPTER 12 (L00-L99)

INFECTIONS OF THE SKIN AND SUBCUTANEOUS TISSUE (L00-L08)

Use additional code (B95-B97) to identify infectious agent.

Excludes2   hordeolum (H00.0)
infective dermatitis (L30.3)
local infections of skin classified in Chapter 1
lupus panniculitis (L93.2)
panniculitis NOS (M79.3)
panniculitis of neck and back (M54.0-)
Perlèche NOS (K13.0)
Perlèche due to candidiasis (B37.0)
Perlèche due to riboflavin deficiency (E53.0)
pyogenic granuloma (L98.0)
relapsing panniculitis [Weber-Christian] (M35.6)
viral warts (B07.-)
zoster (B02.-)

L00   Staphylococcal scalded skin syndrome
Ritter's disease

Use additional code to identify percentage of skin exfoliation
(L49.-)

Excludes1   bullous impetigo (L01.03)
pemphigus neonatorum (L01.03)
toxic epidermal necrolysis [Lyell] (L51.2)

● **L01   Impetigo**
Contagious skin infection caused by a streptococcus or staphylococcus aureus, common skin infections among children

Excludes1   impetigo herpetiformis (L40.1)

● **L01.0   Impetigo**
Impetigo contagiosa
Impetigo vulgaris

L01.00   Impetigo, unspecified
Impetigo NOS

L01.01   Non-bullous impetigo

L01.02   Bockhart's impetigo
Impetigo follicularis
Perifolliculitis NOS
Superficial pustular perifolliculitis

L01.03   Bullous impetigo
Impetigo neonatorum
Pemphigus neonatorum
Neonate = newborn

L01.09   Other impetigo
Ulcerative impetigo

L01.1   Impetiginization of other dermatoses

● **L02   Cutaneous abscess, furuncle and carbuncle**
Use additional code to identify organism (B95-B96)

Excludes2   abscess of anus and rectal regions (K61.-)
abscess of female genital organs (external) (N76.4)
abscess of male genital organs (external) (N48.2, N49.-)

● **L02.0   Cutaneous abscess, furuncle and carbuncle of face**

Excludes2   abscess of ear, external (H60.0)
abscess of eyelid (H00.0)
abscess of head [any part, except face] (L02.8)
abscess of lacrimal gland (H04.0)
abscess of lacrimal passages (H04.3)
abscess of mouth (K12.2)
abscess of nose (J34.0)
abscess of orbit (H05.0)
submandibular abscess (K12.2)

L02.01   Cutaneous abscess of face

L02.02   Furuncle of face
Boil of face
Folliculitis of face

L02.03   Carbuncle of face

● **L02.1   Cutaneous abscess, furuncle and carbuncle of neck**

L02.11   Cutaneous abscess of neck

L02.12   Furuncle of neck
Boil of neck
Folliculitis of neck

L02.13   Carbuncle of neck

● **L02.2   Cutaneous abscess, furuncle and carbuncle of trunk**

Excludes1   non-newborn omphalitis (L08.82)
omphalitis of newborn (P38.-)

Excludes2   abscess of breast (N61.1)
abscess of buttocks (L02.3)
abscess of female external genital organs (N76.4)
abscess of male external genital organs (N48.2, N49.-)
abscess of hip (L02.4)

● **L02.21   Cutaneous abscess of trunk**

L02.211   Cutaneous abscess of abdominal wall

L02.212   Cutaneous abscess of back [any part, except buttock]

L02.213   Cutaneous abscess of chest wall

L02.214   Cutaneous abscess of groin

L02.215   Cutaneous abscess of perineum

L02.216   Cutaneous abscess of umbilicus

L02.219   Cutaneous abscess of trunk, unspecified

● **L02.22   Furuncle of trunk**
Boil of trunk
Folliculitis of trunk

L02.221   Furuncle of abdominal wall

L02.222   Furuncle of back [any part, except buttock]

L02.223   Furuncle of chest wall

L02.224   Furuncle of groin

L02.225   Furuncle of perineum

L02.226   Furuncle of umbilicus

L02.229   Furuncle of trunk, unspecified

● **L02.23   Carbuncle of trunk**

L02.231   Carbuncle of abdominal wall

L02.232   Carbuncle of back [any part, except buttock]

L02.233   Carbuncle of chest wall

L02.234   Carbuncle of groin

L02.235   Carbuncle of perineum

L02.236   Carbuncle of umbilicus

L02.239   Carbuncle of trunk, unspecified

● **L02.3   Cutaneous abscess, furuncle and carbuncle of buttock**

Excludes1   pilonidal cyst with abscess (L05.01)

L02.31   Cutaneous abscess of buttock
Cutaneous abscess of gluteal region

L02.32   Furuncle of buttock
Boil of buttock
Folliculitis of buttock
Furuncle of gluteal region

L02.33   Carbuncle of buttock
Carbuncle of gluteal region

● **L02.4   Cutaneous abscess, furuncle and carbuncle of limb**

Excludes2   Cutaneous abscess, furuncle and carbuncle of groin (L02.214, L02.224, L02.234)
Cutaneous abscess, furuncle and carbuncle of hand (L02.5-)
Cutaneous abscess, furuncle and carbuncle of foot (L02.6-)

Figure 12-2 Impetigo. A thick, honey-yellow adherent crust covers the entire eroded surface. (From James WD, Elston DM, Berger TG, Andrews GC: Andrews' Diseases of the Skin: Clinical Dermatology, London, Saunders/Elsevier, 2011)

▶ New   ⇒ Revised   ~~deleted~~ Deleted   Excludes 1   Excludes 2   Includes   Use additional   Code first   Code also   Key words

OGCR Official Guidelines   X Assign placeholder X   ● Use Additional Character(s)   ▌ Manifestation Code   🗄 Hierarchical Condition Category   **Coding Clinic**

- L02.41   Cutaneous abscess of limb
    - L02.411   Cutaneous abscess of right axilla
    - L02.412   Cutaneous abscess of left axilla
    - L02.413   Cutaneous abscess of right upper limb
    - L02.414   Cutaneous abscess of left upper limb
    - L02.415   Cutaneous abscess of right lower limb
    - L02.416   Cutaneous abscess of left lower limb
    - L02.419   Cutaneous abscess of limb, unspecified
- L02.42   Furuncle of limb
    - Boil of limb
    - Folliculitis of limb
    - L02.421   Furuncle of right axilla
    - L02.422   Furuncle of left axilla
    - L02.423   Furuncle of right upper limb
    - L02.424   Furuncle of left upper limb
    - L02.425   Furuncle of right lower limb
    - L02.426   Furuncle of left lower limb
    - L02.429   Furuncle of limb, unspecified
- L02.43   Carbuncle of limb
    - L02.431   Carbuncle of right axilla
    - L02.432   Carbuncle of left axilla
    - L02.433   Carbuncle of right upper limb
    - L02.434   Carbuncle of left upper limb
    - L02.435   Carbuncle of right lower limb
    - L02.436   Carbuncle of left lower limb
    - L02.439   Carbuncle of limb, unspecified
- L02.5   Cutaneous abscess, furuncle and carbuncle of hand
    - L02.51   Cutaneous abscess of hand
        - L02.511   Cutaneous abscess of right hand
        - L02.512   Cutaneous abscess of left hand
        - L02.519   Cutaneous abscess of unspecified hand
    - L02.52   Furuncle hand
        - Boil of hand
        - Folliculitis of hand
        - L02.521   Furuncle right hand
        - L02.522   Furuncle left hand
        - L02.529   Furuncle unspecified hand
    - L02.53   Carbuncle of hand
        - L02.531   Carbuncle of right hand
        - L02.532   Carbuncle of left hand
        - L02.539   Carbuncle of unspecified hand
- L02.6   Cutaneous abscess, furuncle and carbuncle of foot
    - L02.61   Cutaneous abscess of foot
        - L02.611   Cutaneous abscess of right foot
        - L02.612   Cutaneous abscess of left foot
        - L02.619   Cutaneous abscess of unspecified foot
    - L02.62   Furuncle of foot
        - Boil of foot
        - Folliculitis of foot
        - L02.621   Furuncle of right foot
        - L02.622   Furuncle of left foot
        - L02.629   Furuncle of unspecified foot
    - L02.63   Carbuncle of foot
        - L02.631   Carbuncle of right foot
        - L02.632   Carbuncle of left foot
        - L02.639   Carbuncle of unspecified foot

- L02.8   Cutaneous abscess, furuncle and carbuncle of other sites
    - L02.81   Cutaneous abscess of other sites
        - L02.811   Cutaneous abscess of head [any part, except face]
        - L02.818   Cutaneous abscess of other sites
    - L02.82   Furuncle of other sites
        - Boil of other sites
        - Folliculitis of other sites
        - L02.821   Furuncle of head [any part, except face]
        - L02.828   Furuncle of other sites
    - L02.83   Carbuncle of other sites
        - L02.831   Carbuncle of head [any part, except face]
        - L02.838   Carbuncle of other sites
- L02.9   Cutaneous abscess, furuncle and carbuncle, unspecified
    - L02.91   Cutaneous abscess, unspecified
    - L02.92   Furuncle, unspecified
        - Boil NOS
        - Furunculosis NOS
    - L02.93   Carbuncle, unspecified
- L03   Cellulitis and acute lymphangitis
    - **Excludes2**   cellulitis of anal and rectal region (K61.-)
      cellulitis of external auditory canal (H60.1)
      cellulitis of eyelid (H00.0)
      cellulitis of female external genital organs (N76.4)
      cellulitis of lacrimal apparatus (H04.3)
      cellulitis of male external genital organs (N48.2, N49.-)
      cellulitis of mouth (K12.2)
      cellulitis of nose (J34.0)
      eosinophilic cellulitis [Wells] (L98.3)
      febrile neutrophilic dermatosis [Sweet] (L98.2)
      lymphangitis (chronic) (subacute) (I89.1)
    - L03.0   Cellulitis and acute lymphangitis of finger and toe
        - Infection of nail
        - Onychia
        - Paronychia
        - Perionychia
        - L03.01   Cellulitis of finger
            - Felon
            - Whitlow
            - **Excludes1**   herpetic whitlow (B00.89)
            - L03.011   Cellulitis of right finger
            - L03.012   Cellulitis of left finger
            - L03.019   Cellulitis of unspecified finger
        - L03.02   Acute lymphangitis of finger
            - Hangnail with lymphangitis of finger
            - L03.021   Acute lymphangitis of right finger
            - L03.022   Acute lymphangitis of left finger
            - L03.029   Acute lymphangitis of unspecified finger
        - L03.03   Cellulitis of toe
            - L03.031   Cellulitis of right toe
            - L03.032   Cellulitis of left toe
            - L03.039   Cellulitis of unspecified toe
        - L03.04   Acute lymphangitis of toe
            - Hangnail with lymphangitis of toe
            - L03.041   Acute lymphangitis of right toe
            - L03.042   Acute lymphangitis of left toe
            - L03.049   Acute lymphangitis of unspecified toe

Item 12-1   Onychia is an inflammation of the tissue surrounding the nail with pus accumulation and loss of the nail, resulting from microscopic pathogens entering through small wounds. **Paronychia** is a nail disease also known as felon or whitlow and is a bacterial or fungal infection.

Item 12-2 **Cellulitis** is an acute spreading bacterial infection below the surface of the skin characterized by redness (erythema), warmth, swelling, pain, fever, chills, and enlarged lymph nodes ("swollen glands").

● **L03.1**   **Cellulitis and acute lymphangitis of other parts of limb**
   ● **L03.11**   **Cellulitis of other parts of limb**
     Excludes2   cellulitis of fingers (L03.01-)
             cellulitis of toes (L03.03-)
             groin (L03.314)
     L03.111   **Cellulitis of right axilla**
     L03.112   **Cellulitis of left axilla**
     L03.113   **Cellulitis of right upper limb**
     L03.114   **Cellulitis of left upper limb**
          Coding Clinic: 2019, Q1, P13
     L03.115   **Cellulitis of right lower limb**
     L03.116   **Cellulitis of left lower limb**
     L03.119   **Cellulitis of unspecified part of limb**
   ● **L03.12**   **Acute lymphangitis of other parts of limb**
     Excludes2   acute lymphangitis of fingers (L03.2-)
             acute lymphangitis of toes (L03.04-)
             acute lymphangitis of groin (L03.324)
     L03.121   **Acute lymphangitis of right axilla**
     L03.122   **Acute lymphangitis of left axilla**
     L03.123   **Acute lymphangitis of right upper limb**
     L03.124   **Acute lymphangitis of left upper limb**
     L03.125   **Acute lymphangitis of right lower limb**
     L03.126   **Acute lymphangitis of left lower limb**
     L03.129   **Acute lymphangitis of unspecified part of limb**
● **L03.2**   **Cellulitis and acute lymphangitis of face and neck**
   ● **L03.21**   **Cellulitis and acute lymphangitis of face**
     L03.211   **Cellulitis of face**
       Excludes2   abscess of orbit (H05.01-)
               cellulitis of ear (H60.1-)
               cellulitis of eyelid (H00.0-)
               cellulitis of head (L03.81)
               cellulitis of lacrimal apparatus (H04.3)
               cellulitis of lip (K13.0)
               cellulitis of mouth (K12.2)
               cellulitis of nose (internal) (J34.0)
               cellulitis of orbit (H05.01-)
               cellulitis of scalp (L03.81)
     L03.212   **Acute lymphangitis of face**
     L03.213   **Periorbital cellulitis**
          Preseptal cellulitis
          Coding Clinic: 2016, Q4, P36
   ● **L03.22**   **Cellulitis and acute lymphangitis of neck**
     L03.221   **Cellulitis of neck**
     L03.222   **Acute lymphangitis of neck**

● **L03.3**   **Cellulitis and acute lymphangitis of trunk**
   ● **L03.31**   **Cellulitis of trunk**
     Excludes2   cellulitis of anal and rectal regions (K61.-)
             cellulitis of breast NOS (N61.0)
             cellulitis of female external genital organs (N76.4)
             cellulitis of male external genital organs (N48.2, N49.-)
             omphalitis of newborn (P38.-)
             puerperal cellulitis of breast (O91.2)
     L03.311   **Cellulitis of abdominal wall**
       Excludes2   cellulitis of umbilicus (L03.316)
               cellulitis of groin (L03.314)
     L03.312   **Cellulitis of back [any part except buttock]**
     L03.313   **Cellulitis of chest wall**
     L03.314   **Cellulitis of groin**
     L03.315   **Cellulitis of perineum**
     L03.316   **Cellulitis of umbilicus**
     L03.317   **Cellulitis of buttock**
     L03.319   **Cellulitis of trunk, unspecified**
   ● **L03.32**   **Acute lymphangitis of trunk**
     L03.321   **Acute lymphangitis of abdominal wall**
     L03.322   **Acute lymphangitis of back [any part except buttock]**
     L03.323   **Acute lymphangitis of chest wall**
     L03.324   **Acute lymphangitis of groin**
     L03.325   **Acute lymphangitis of perineum**
     L03.326   **Acute lymphangitis of umbilicus**
     L03.327   **Acute lymphangitis of buttock**
     L03.329   **Acute lymphangitis of trunk, unspecified**
● **L03.8**   **Cellulitis and acute lymphangitis of other sites**
   ● **L03.81**   **Cellulitis of other sites**
     L03.811   **Cellulitis of head [any part, except face]**
          Cellulitis of scalp
       Excludes2   cellulitis of face (L03.211)
     L03.818   **Cellulitis of other sites**
   ● **L03.89**   **Acute lymphangitis of other sites**
     L03.891   **Acute lymphangitis of head [any part, except face]**
     L03.898   **Acute lymphangitis of other sites**
● **L03.9**   **Cellulitis and acute lymphangitis, unspecified**
     L03.90   **Cellulitis, unspecified**
     L03.91   **Acute lymphangitis, unspecified**
       Excludes1   lymphangitis NOS (I89.1)

▶ New   ⇒ Revised   ~~deleted~~ Deleted   Excludes 1   Excludes 2   Includes   Use additional   Code first   Code also   Key words
OGCR Official Guidelines   X Assign placeholder X   ● Use Additional Character(s)   ▌Manifestation Code   ⓗ Hierarchical Condition Category   **Coding Clinic**

Item 12–3   **Abscess** is a localized collection of pus in tissues or organs and is a sign of infection, resulting in swelling and inflammation.

Item 12–4   **Pilonidal cyst,** also called a coccygeal cyst, is the result of a disorder called pilonidal disease. The cyst usually contains hair and pus.

● **L04**   **Acute lymphadenitis**
     Short-term inflammation of lymph nodes which can be regionalized to involve a given area of the lymph system or systemic involving much of the body

     Includes   abscess (acute) of lymph nodes, except mesenteric
                    acute lymphadenitis, except mesenteric

     Excludes1   chronic or subacute lymphadenitis, except mesenteric (I88.1)
                    enlarged lymph nodes (R59.-)
                    human immunodeficiency virus [HIV] disease resulting in generalized lymphadenopathy (B20)
                    lymphadenitis NOS (I88.9)
                    nonspecific mesenteric lymphadenitis (I88.0)

     L04.0   **Acute lymphadenitis of face, head and neck**
     L04.1   **Acute lymphadenitis of trunk**
     L04.2   **Acute lymphadenitis of upper limb**
          Acute lymphadenitis of axilla
          Acute lymphadenitis of shoulder
     L04.3   **Acute lymphadenitis of lower limb**
          Acute lymphadenitis of hip
          Excludes2   acute lymphadenitis of groin (L04.1)
     L04.8   **Acute lymphadenitis of other sites**
     L04.9   **Acute lymphadenitis, unspecified**

● **L05**   **Pilonidal cyst and sinus**
   ● **L05.0**   **Pilonidal cyst and sinus with abscess**
     L05.01   **Pilonidal cyst with abscess**
          Pilonidal abscess
          Pilonidal dimple with abscess
          Postanal dimple with abscess
          Excludes2   congenital sacral dimple (Q82.6)
                    parasacral dimple (Q82.6)
     L05.02   **Pilonidal sinus with abscess**
          Coccygeal fistula with abscess
          Coccygeal sinus with abscess
          Pilonidal fistula with abscess
   ● **L05.9**   **Pilonidal cyst and sinus without abscess**
     L05.91   **Pilonidal cyst without abscess**
          Pilonidal dimple
          Postanal dimple
          Pilonidal cyst NOS
          Excludes2   congenital sacral dimple (Q82.6)
                    parasacral dimple (Q82.6)
     L05.92   **Pilonidal sinus without abscess**
          Coccygeal fistula
          Coccygeal sinus without abscess
          Pilonidal fistula

● **L08**   **Other local infections of skin and subcutaneous tissue**
     L08.0   **Pyoderma**
          Dermatitis gangrenosa
          Purulent dermatitis
          Septic dermatitis
          Suppurative dermatitis
          Excludes1   pyoderma gangrenosum (L88)
                    pyoderma vegetans (L08.81)
     L08.1   **Erythrasma**

● **L08.8**   **Other specified local infections of the skin and subcutaneous tissue**
     L08.81   **Pyoderma vegetans**
          Excludes1   pyoderma gangrenosum (L88)
                    pyoderma NOS (L08.0)
     L08.82   **Omphalitis not of newborn**
          Excludes1   omphalitis of newborn (P38.-)
     L08.89   **Other specified local infections of the skin and subcutaneous tissue**
     L08.9   **Local infection of the skin and subcutaneous tissue, unspecified**

BULLOUS DISORDERS (L10-L14)

     Excludes1   benign familial pemphigus [Hailey-Hailey] (Q82.8)
                    staphylococcal scalded skin syndrome (L00)
                    toxic epidermal necrolysis [Lyell] (L51.2)

● **L10**   **Pemphigus**
     Excludes1   pemphigus neonatorum (L01.03)
     L10.0   **Pemphigus vulgaris**
     L10.1   **Pemphigus vegetans**
     L10.2   **Pemphigus foliaceous**
     L10.3   **Brazilian pemphigus [fogo selvagem]**
     L10.4   **Pemphigus erythematosus**
          Senear-Usher syndrome
     L10.5   **Drug-induced pemphigus**
          Use additional code for adverse effect, if applicable, to identify drug (T36-T50 with fifth or sixth character 5)
   ● **L10.8**   **Other pemphigus**
     L10.81   **Paraneoplastic pemphigus**
     L10.89   **Other pemphigus**
     L10.9   **Pemphigus, unspecified**

● **L11**   **Other acantholytic disorders**
     L11.0   **Acquired keratosis follicularis**
          Excludes1   keratosis follicularis (congenital) [Darier-White] (Q82.8)
     L11.1   **Transient acantholytic dermatosis [Grover]**
     L11.8   **Other specified acantholytic disorders**
     L11.9   **Acantholytic disorder, unspecified**

● **L12**   **Pemphigoid**
     Excludes1   herpes gestationis (O26.4-)
                    impetigo herpetiformis (L40.1)
     L12.0   **Bullous pemphigoid**
     L12.1   **Cicatricial pemphigoid**
          Benign mucous membrane pemphigoid
     L12.2   **Chronic bullous disease of childhood**   P
          Juvenile dermatitis herpetiformis
   ● **L12.3**   **Acquired epidermolysis bullosa**
          Excludes1   epidermolysis bullosa (congenital) (Q81.-)
     L12.30   **Acquired epidermolysis bullosa, unspecified** 🔖
     L12.31   **Epidermolysis bullosa due to drug** 🔖
          Use additional code for adverse effect, if applicable, to identify drug (T36-T50 with fifth or sixth character 5)
     L12.35   **Other acquired epidermolysis bullosa** 🔖
     L12.8   **Other pemphigoid**
     L12.9   **Pemphigoid, unspecified**

CHAPTER 12 (L00-L99)

Item 12–5 Dermatitis herpetiformis, also known as Duhring's disease, is a systemic disease characterized by small blisters (3 to 5 mm) and occasionally large bullae (> 5 mm).

Figure 12-3 Dermatitis herpetiformis. (From Terhorst D: BASICS Dermatologie, München, Elsevier, Urban & Fischer, 2011)

● **L13   Other bullous disorders**

    L13.0   Dermatitis herpetiformis
       Duhring's disease
       Hydroa herpetiformis
       Excludes1   juvenile dermatitis herpetiformis (L12.2)
                          senile dermatitis herpetiformis (L12.0)

    L13.1   Subcorneal pustular dermatitis
       Sneddon-Wilkinson disease

    L13.8   Other specified bullous disorders

    L13.9   Bullous disorder, unspecified

▷ *L14   Bullous disorders in diseases classified elsewhere*
      Code first underlying disease

DERMATITIS AND ECZEMA (L20-L30)

   Note: In this block the terms dermatitis and eczema are used synonymously and interchangeably.

    Excludes2   chronic (childhood) granulomatous disease (D71)
                     dermatitis gangrenosa (L08.0)
                     dermatitis herpetiformis (L13.0)
                     dry skin dermatitis (L85.3)
                     factitial dermatitis (L98.1)
                     perioral dermatitis (L71.0)
                     radiation-related disorders of the skin and
                          subcutaneous tissue (L55-L59)
                     stasis dermatitis (I87.2)

● **L20   Atopic dermatitis**

    L20.0   Besnier's prurigo

   ● **L20.8   Other atopic dermatitis**
       Excludes2   circumscribed neurodermatitis (L28.0)

       L20.81   Atopic neurodermatitis
             Diffuse neurodermatitis

       L20.82   Flexural eczema

       L20.83   Infantile (acute) (chronic) eczema   P

       L20.84   Intrinsic (allergic) eczema

       L20.89   Other atopic dermatitis

    L20.9   Atopic dermatitis, unspecified

● **L21   Seborrheic dermatitis**
    Excludes2   infective dermatitis (L30.3)
                     seborrheic keratosis (L82.-)

    L21.0   Seborrhea capitis
       Cradle cap
       Coding Clinic: 2018, Q1, P6

    L21.1   Seborrheic infantile dermatitis   P

    L21.8   Other seborrheic dermatitis

    L21.9   Seborrheic dermatitis, unspecified
       Seborrhea NOS

  L22   Diaper dermatitis
       Diaper erythema
       Diaper rash
       Psoriasiform diaper rash
       Coding Clinic: 2021, Q4, P18

Item 12–6 Seborrheic dermatitis is characterized by greasy, scaly, red patches and is associated with oily skin and scalp.

Figure 12-4 Seborrheic dermatitis. (Getty Image)

Item 12–7 Atopic dermatitis, also known as atopic eczema, infantile eczema, disseminated neuro dermatitis, flexural eczema, and *prurigo diathesique* (Besnier), is characterized by intense itching and is often hereditary.

Figure 12-5 Atopic dermatitis. (From Chabner D-E: The Language of Medicine, St. Louis, MO, Saunders/Elsevier, 2007)

● **L23   Allergic contact dermatitis**

    Excludes1   allergy NOS (T78.40)
                   contact dermatitis NOS (L25.9)
                   dermatitis NOS (L30.9)

    Excludes2   dermatitis due to substances taken internally (L27.-)
                   dermatitis of eyelid (H01.1-)
                   diaper dermatitis (L22)
                   eczema of external ear (H60.5-)
                   irritant contact dermatitis (L24.-)
                   perioral dermatitis (L71.0)
                   radiation-related disorders of the skin and
                      subcutaneous tissue (L55-L59)

    L23.0   Allergic contact dermatitis due to metals
       Allergic contact dermatitis due to chromium
       Allergic contact dermatitis due to nickel

    L23.1   Allergic contact dermatitis due to adhesives

    L23.2   Allergic contact dermatitis due to cosmetics

    L23.3   Allergic contact dermatitis due to drugs in contact with skin

       Use additional code for adverse effect, if applicable, to
          identify drug (T36-T50 with fifth or sixth character 5)
       Excludes2   dermatitis due to ingested drugs and
                       medicaments (L27.0-L27.1)

    L23.4   Allergic contact dermatitis due to dyes

    L23.5   Allergic contact dermatitis due to other chemical products
       Allergic contact dermatitis due to cement
       Allergic contact dermatitis due to insecticide
       Allergic contact dermatitis due to plastic
       Allergic contact dermatitis due to rubber

    L23.6   Allergic contact dermatitis due to food in contact with the skin
       Excludes2   dermatitis due to ingested food (L27.2)

    L23.7   Allergic contact dermatitis due to plants, except food
       Excludes2   allergy NOS due to pollen (J30.1)

   ● **L23.8   Allergic contact dermatitis due to other agents**

       L23.81   Allergic contact dermatitis due to animal (cat) (dog) dander
             Allergic contact dermatitis due to animal (cat)
                 (dog) hair

       L23.89   Allergic contact dermatitis due to other agents

    L23.9   Allergic contact dermatitis, unspecified cause
       Allergic contact eczema NOS

● **L24   Irritant contact dermatitis**

    Excludes1   allergy NOS (T78.40)
                   contact dermatitis NOS (L25.9)
                   dermatitis NOS (L30.9)

    Excludes2   allergic contact dermatitis (L23.-)
                   dermatitis due to substances taken internally (L27.-)
                   dermatitis of eyelid (H01.1-)
                   diaper dermatitis (L22)
                   eczema of external ear (H60.5-)
                   perioral dermatitis (L71.0)
                   radiation-related disorders of the skin and
                      subcutaneous tissue (L55-L59)

    L24.0   Irritant contact dermatitis due to detergents

    L24.1   Irritant contact dermatitis due to oils and greases

▶ New   ⇒ Revised   ~~deleted~~ Deleted   Excludes 1   Excludes 2   Includes   Use additional   Code first   Code also   Key words

OGCR Official Guidelines   **X** Assign placeholder X   ● Use Additional Character(s)   ▷ Manifestation Code   🔎 Hierarchical Condition Category   **Coding Clinic**

L24.2   **Irritant contact dermatitis due to solvents**
Irritant contact dermatitis due to chlorocompound
Irritant contact dermatitis due to cyclohexane
Irritant contact dermatitis due to ester
Irritant contact dermatitis due to glycol
Irritant contact dermatitis due to hydrocarbon
Irritant contact dermatitis due to ketone

L24.3   **Irritant contact dermatitis due to cosmetics**

L24.4   **Irritant contact dermatitis due to drugs in contact with skin**

Use additional code for adverse effect, if applicable, to identify drug (T36-T50 with fifth or sixth character 5)

L24.5   **Irritant contact dermatitis due to other chemical products**
Irritant contact dermatitis due to cement
Irritant contact dermatitis due to insecticide
Irritant contact dermatitis due to plastic
Irritant contact dermatitis due to rubber

L24.6   **Irritant contact dermatitis due to food in contact with skin**

> **Excludes2**   dermatitis due to ingested food (L27.2)

L24.7   **Irritant contact dermatitis due to plants, except food**

> **Excludes2**   allergy NOS to pollen (J30.1)

● **L24.8**   **Irritant contact dermatitis due to other agents**

    L24.81   **Irritant contact dermatitis due to metals**
Irritant contact dermatitis due to chromium
Irritant contact dermatitis due to nickel

    L24.89   **Irritant contact dermatitis due to other agents**
Irritant contact dermatitis due to dyes

L24.9   **Irritant contact dermatitis, unspecified cause**
Irritant contact eczema NOS

● **L24.A**   **Irritant contact dermatitis due to friction or contact with body fluids**

> **Excludes1**   virritant contact dermatitis related to stoma or fistula (L24.B-)
> **Excludes2**   erythema intertrigo (L30.4)

    L24.A0   **Irritant contact dermatitis due to friction or contact with body fluids, unspecified**

    L24.A1   **Irritant contact dermatitis due to saliva**

    L24.A2   **Irritant contact dermatitis due to fecal, urinary or dual incontinence**

> **Excludes1**   diaper dermatitis (L22)

      Coding Clinic: 2021, Q4, P18

    L24.A9   **Irritant contact dermatitis due friction or contact with other specified body fluids**
Irritant contact dermatitis related to endotracheal tube
Wound fluids, exudate

● **L24.B**   **Irritant contact dermatitis related to stoma or fistula**

Use additional code to identify any artificial opening status (Z93.-), if applicable, for contact dermatitis related to stoma secretions

    L24.B0   **Irritant contact dermatitis related to unspecified stoma or fistula**
Irritant contact dermatitis related to fistula NOS
Irritant contact dermatitis related to stoma NOS

    L24.B1   **Irritant contact dermatitis related to digestive stoma or fistula**
Irritant contact dermatitis related to gastrostomy
Irritant contact dermatitis related to jejunostomy
Irritant contact dermatitis related to saliva or spit fistula

    L24.B2   **Irritant contact dermatitis related to respiratory stoma or fistula**
Irritant contact dermatitis related to tracheostomy

    L24.B3   **Irritant contact dermatitis related to fecal or urinary stoma or fistula**
Irritant contact dermatitis related to colostomy
Irritant contact dermatitis related to enterocutaneous fistula
Irritant contact dermatitis related to ileostomy

      Coding Clinic: 2021, Q4, P17,19

● **L25**   **Unspecified contact dermatitis**

> **Excludes1**   allergic contact dermatitis (L23.-)
> allergy NOS (T78.40)
> dermatitis NOS (L30.9)
> irritant contact dermatitis (L24.-)

> **Excludes2**   dermatitis due to ingested substances (L27.-)
> dermatitis of eyelid (H01.1-)
> eczema of external ear (H60.5-)
> perioral dermatitis (L71.0)
> radiation-related disorders of the skin and subcutaneous tissue (L55-L59)

L25.0   **Unspecified contact dermatitis due to cosmetics**

L25.1   **Unspecified contact dermatitis due to drugs in contact with skin**

Use additional code for adverse effect, if applicable, to identify drug (T36-T50 with fifth or sixth character 5)

> **Excludes2**   dermatitis due to ingested drugs and medicaments (L27.0-L27.1)

L25.2   **Unspecified contact dermatitis due to dyes**

L25.3   **Unspecified contact dermatitis due to other chemical products**
Unspecified contact dermatitis due to cement
Unspecified contact dermatitis due to insecticide

L25.4   **Unspecified contact dermatitis due to food in contact with skin**

> **Excludes2**   dermatitis due to ingested food (L27.2)

L25.5   **Unspecified contact dermatitis due to plants, except food**

> **Excludes1**   nettle rash (L50.9)
> **Excludes2**   allergy NOS due to pollen (J30.1)

L25.8   **Unspecified contact dermatitis due to other agents**

L25.9   **Unspecified contact dermatitis, unspecified cause**
Contact dermatitis (occupational) NOS
Contact eczema (occupational) NOS

L26   **Exfoliative dermatitis**
Hebra's pityriasis

> **Excludes1**   Ritter's disease (L00)

● **L27**   **Dermatitis due to substances taken internally**

> **Excludes1**   allergy NOS (T78.40)

> **Excludes2**   adverse food reaction, except dermatitis (T78.0-T78.1)
> contact dermatitis (L23-L25)
> drug photoallergic response (L56.1)
> drug phototoxic response (L56.0)
> urticaria (L50.-)

L27.0   **Generalized skin eruption due to drugs and medicaments taken internally**

Use additional code for adverse effect, if applicable, to identify drug (T36-T50 with fifth or sixth character 5)

L27.1   **Localized skin eruption due to drugs and medicaments taken internally**

Use additional code for adverse effect, if applicable, to identify drug (T36-T50 with fifth or sixth character 5)

L27.2   **Dermatitis due to ingested food**

> **Excludes2**   dermatitis due to food in contact with skin (L23.6, L24.6, L25.4)

L27.8   **Dermatitis due to other substances taken internally**

L27.9   **Dermatitis due to unspecified substance taken internally**

● **L28**   **Lichen simplex chronicus and prurigo**

L28.0   **Lichen simplex chronicus**
Circumscribed neurodermatitis
Lichen NOS

L28.1   **Prurigo nodularis**

L28.2   **Other prurigo**
Prurigo NOS   Prurigo mitis
Prurigo Hebra   Urticaria papulosa

● **L29**   **Pruritus**

> **Excludes1**   neurotic excoriation (L98.1)
> psychogenic pruritus (F45.8)

   L29.0   **Pruritus ani**

   L29.1   **Pruritus scroti** ♂

   L29.2   **Pruritus vulvae** ♀

   L29.3   **Anogenital pruritus, unspecified**

   L29.8   **Other pruritus**

   L29.9   **Pruritus, unspecified**
       Itch NOS

● **L30**   **Other and unspecified dermatitis**

> **Excludes2**   contact dermatitis (L23-L25)
> dry skin dermatitis (L85.3)
> small plaque parapsoriasis (L41.3)
> stasis dermatitis (I87.2)

   L30.0   **Nummular dermatitis**

   L30.1   **Dyshidrosis [pompholyx]**

   L30.2   **Cutaneous autosensitization**
       Candidid [levurid]   Eczematid
       Dermatophytid

   L30.3   **Infective dermatitis**
       Infectious eczematoid dermatitis

   L30.4   **Erythema intertrigo**

   L30.5   **Pityriasis alba**
       Coding Clinic: 2018, Q1, P6

   L30.8   **Other specified dermatitis**

   L30.9   **Dermatitis, unspecified**
       Eczema NOS

PAPULOSQUAMOUS DISORDERS (L40-L45)

● **L40**   **Psoriasis**

   L40.0   **Psoriasis vulgaris**
       Nummular psoriasis   Plaque psoriasis

   L40.1   **Generalized pustular psoriasis**
       Impetigo herpetiformis   Von Zumbusch's disease

   L40.2   **Acrodermatitis continua**

   L40.3   **Pustulosis palmaris et plantaris**

   L40.4   **Guttate psoriasis**

   ● **L40.5**   **Arthropathic psoriasis**

      L40.50   **Arthropathic psoriasis, unspecified** 🅗

      L40.51   **Distal interphalangeal psoriatic arthropathy** 🅗

      L40.52   **Psoriatic arthritis mutilans** 🅗

      L40.53   **Psoriatic spondylitis** 🅗

      L40.54   **Psoriatic juvenile arthropathy** 🅗

      L40.59   **Other psoriatic arthropathy** 🅗

   L40.8   **Other psoriasis**
       Flexural psoriasis

   L40.9   **Psoriasis, unspecified**

● **L41**   **Parapsoriasis**

> **Excludes1**   poikiloderma vasculare atrophicans (L94.5)

   L41.0   **Pityriasis lichenoides et varioliformis acuta**
       Mucha-Habermann disease

   L41.1   **Pityriasis lichenoides chronica**

   L41.3   **Small plaque parapsoriasis**

   L41.4   **Large plaque parapsoriasis**

   L41.5   **Retiform parapsoriasis**

   L41.8   **Other parapsoriasis**

   L41.9   **Parapsoriasis, unspecified**

  L42   **Pityriasis rosea**

● **L43**   **Lichen planus**

> **Excludes1**   lichen planopilaris (L66.1)

   L43.0   **Hypertrophic lichen planus**

   L43.1   **Bullous lichen planus**

   L43.2   **Lichenoid drug reaction**
       Use additional code for adverse effect, if applicable, to identify drug (T36-T50 with fifth or sixth character 5)

   L43.3   **Subacute (active) lichen planus**
       Lichen planus tropicus

   L43.8   **Other lichen planus**

   L43.9   **Lichen planus, unspecified**

● **L44**   **Other papulosquamous disorders**

   L44.0   **Pityriasis rubra pilaris**

   L44.1   **Lichen nitidus**

   L44.2   **Lichen striatus**

   L44.3   **Lichen ruber moniliformis**

   L44.4   **Infantile papular acrodermatitis [Gianotti-Crosti]**   P

   L44.8   **Other specified papulosquamous disorders**

   L44.9   **Papulosquamous disorder, unspecified**

▷ *L45*   *Papulosquamous disorders in diseases classified elsewhere*
     Code first underlying disease

URTICARIA AND ERYTHEMA (L49-L54)

> **Excludes1**   Lyme disease (A69.2-)
> rosacea (L71.-)

● **L49**   **Exfoliation due to erythematous conditions according to extent of body surface involved**

   Code first erythematous condition causing exfoliation, such as:
     Ritter's disease (L00)
     (Staphylococcal) scalded skin syndrome (L00)
     Stevens-Johnson syndrome (L51.1)
     Stevens-Johnson syndrome-toxic epidermal necrolysis overlap syndrome (L51.3)
     Toxic epidermal necrolysis (L51.2)

   L49.0   **Exfoliation due to erythematous condition involving less than 10 percent of body surface**
       Exfoliation due to erythematous condition NOS

   L49.1   **Exfoliation due to erythematous condition involving 10-19 percent of body surface**

   L49.2   **Exfoliation due to erythematous condition involving 20-29 percent of body surface**

   L49.3   **Exfoliation due to erythematous condition involving 30-39 percent of body surface**

   L49.4   **Exfoliation due to erythematous condition involving 40-49 percent of body surface**

   L49.5   **Exfoliation due to erythematous condition involving 50-59 percent of body surface**

   L49.6   **Exfoliation due to erythematous condition involving 60-69 percent of body surface**

   L49.7   **Exfoliation due to erythematous condition involving 70-79 percent of body surface**

Figure 12-6   Erythematous plaques with silvery scales in a patient with psoriasis. (Getty Image)

Item 12–8 Psoriasis is a chronic, recurrent inflammatory skin disease characterized by small patches covered with thick, silvery scales. **Parapsoriasis** is a treatment-resistant erythroderma. **Pityriasis rosea** is characterized by a herald patch that is a single large lesion and that usually appears on the trunk and is followed by scattered, smaller lesions.

▶ New   ⇒ Revised   ~~deleted~~ Deleted   Excludes 1   Excludes 2   Includes   Use additional   Code first   Code also   Key words

OGCR Official Guidelines   X Assign placeholder X   ● Use Additional Character(s)   ▷ Manifestation Code   🅗 Hierarchical Condition Category   **Coding Clinic**

Figure 12-7 Urticaria (hives). *(Courtesy of David Effron, MD.)* *(Getty Image)*

Item 12–9 **Urticaria** is a vascular reaction in which wheals surrounded by a red halo appear and cause severe itching. The causes of urticaria or hives are extensive and varied (e.g., food, heat, cold, drugs, stress, infections).

L49.8 **Exfoliation due to erythematous condition involving 80-89 percent of body surface**

L49.9 **Exfoliation due to erythematous condition involving 90 or more percent of body surface**

● **L50** **Urticaria**
     Excludes1   allergic contact dermatitis (L23.-)
         angioneurotic edema (T78.3)
         giant urticaria (T78.3)
         hereditary angio-edema (D84.1)
         Quincke's edema (T78.3)
         serum urticaria (T80.6-)
         solar urticaria (L56.3)
         urticaria neonatorum (P83.8)
         urticaria papulosa (L28.2)
         urticaria pigmentosa (D47.01)

L50.0 **Allergic urticaria**
L50.1 **Idiopathic urticaria**
L50.2 **Urticaria due to cold and heat**
     Excludes2   familial cold urticaria (M04.2)
L50.3 **Dermatographic urticaria**
L50.4 **Vibratory urticaria**
L50.5 **Cholinergic urticaria**
L50.6 **Contact urticaria**
L50.8 **Other urticaria**
     Chronic urticaria
     Recurrent periodic urticaria
L50.9 **Urticaria, unspecified**

● **L51** **Erythema multiforme**
     Use additional code for adverse effect, if applicable, to identify drug (T36-T50 with fifth or sixth character 5)
     Use additional code to identify associated manifestations, such as:
     arthropathy associated with dermatological disorders (M14.8-)
     conjunctival edema (H11.42)
     conjunctivitis (H10.22-)
     corneal scars and opacities (H17.-)
     corneal ulcer (H16.0-)
     edema of eyelid (H02.84-)
     inflammation of eyelid (H01.8)
     keratoconjunctivitis sicca (H16.22-)
     mechanical lagophthalmos (H02.22-)
     stomatitis (K12.-)
     symblepharon (H11.23-)
     Use additional code to identify percentage of skin exfoliation (L49.-)
     Excludes1   staphylococcal scalded skin syndrome (L00)
         Ritter's disease (L00)

L51.0 **Nonbullous erythema multiforme**
L51.1 **Stevens-Johnson syndrome** 🔖
L51.2 **Toxic epidermal necrolysis [Lyell]** 🔖
L51.3 **Stevens-Johnson syndrome-toxic epidermal necrolysis overlap syndrome** 🔖
     SJS-TEN overlap syndrome
L51.8 **Other erythema multiforme**
L51.9 **Erythema multiforme, unspecified**
     Erythema iris
     Erythema multiforme major NOS
     Erythema multiforme minor NOS
     Herpes iris

L52 **Erythema nodosum**
     Excludes1   tuberculous erythema nodosum (A18.4)

● **L53** **Other erythematous conditions**
     Excludes1   erythema ab igne (L59.0)
         erythema due to external agents in contact with skin (L23-L25)
         erythema intertrigo (L30.4)

L53.0 **Toxic erythema**
     Code first poisoning due to drug or toxin, if applicable (T36-T65 with fifth or sixth character 1-4 or 6)
     Use additional code for adverse effect, if applicable, to identify drug (T36-T50 with fifth or sixth character 5)
     Excludes1   neonatal erythema toxicum (P83.1)
L53.1 **Erythema annulare centrifugum**
L53.2 **Erythema marginatum**
L53.3 **Other chronic figurate erythema**
L53.8 **Other specified erythematous conditions**
L53.9 **Erythematous condition, unspecified**
     Erythema NOS
     Erythroderma NOS

▷ **L54** *Erythema in diseases classified elsewhere*
     Code first underlying disease

RADIATION-RELATED DISORDERS OF THE SKIN AND SUBCUTANEOUS TISSUE (L55-L59)

● **L55** **Sunburn**
L55.0 **Sunburn of first degree**
L55.1 **Sunburn of second degree**
L55.2 **Sunburn of third degree**
L55.9 **Sunburn, unspecified**

● **L56** **Other acute skin changes due to ultraviolet radiation**
     Use additional code to identify the source of the ultraviolet radiation (W89, X32)
L56.0 **Drug phototoxic response**
     Use additional code for adverse effect, if applicable, to identify drug (T36-T50 with fifth or sixth character 5)
L56.1 **Drug photoallergic response**
     Use additional code for adverse effect, if applicable, to identify drug (T36-T50 with fifth or sixth character 5)
L56.2 **Photocontact dermatitis [berloque dermatitis]**
L56.3 **Solar urticaria**
L56.4 **Polymorphous light eruption**
L56.5 **Disseminated superficial actinic porokeratosis (DSAP)**
L56.8 **Other specified acute skin changes due to ultraviolet radiation**
L56.9 **Acute skin change due to ultraviolet radiation, unspecified**

● **L57** **Skin changes due to chronic exposure to nonionizing radiation**
     Use additional code to identify the source of the ultraviolet radiation (W89), or other nonionizing radiation (W90)
L57.0 **Actinic keratosis**
     Keratosis NOS   Solar keratosis
     Senile keratosis
L57.1 **Actinic reticuloid**
L57.2 **Cutis rhomboidalis nuchae**
L57.3 **Poikiloderma of Civatte**
L57.4 **Cutis laxa senilis**
     Elastosis senilis
L57.5 **Actinic granuloma**
L57.8 **Other skin changes due to chronic exposure to nonionizing radiation**
     Farmer's skin   Solar dermatitis
     Sailor's skin
L57.9 **Skin changes due to chronic exposure to nonionizing radiation, unspecified**

CHAPTER 12 (L00-L99)

● **L58**   **Radiodermatitis**
     Use additional code to identify the source of the radiation (W88, W90)
     L58.0   **Acute** radiodermatitis
     L58.1   **Chronic** radiodermatitis
     L58.9   Radiodermatitis, **unspecified**

● **L59**   **Other disorders of skin and subcutaneous tissue related to radiation**
     L59.0   Erythema ab igne [dermatitis ab igne]
     L59.8   **Other specified disorders of the skin and subcutaneous tissue related to radiation**
         Coding Clinic: 2017, Q1, P34
     L59.9   **Disorder of the skin and subcutaneous tissue related to radiation, unspecified**

DISORDERS OF SKIN APPENDAGES (L60-L75)

     Excludes1   congenital malformations of integument (Q84.-)

● **L60**   **Nail disorders**
     Excludes2   clubbing of nails (R68.3)
                 onychia and paronychia (L03.0-)
     L60.0   **Ingrowing nail**
     L60.1   **Onycholysis**
     L60.2   **Onychogryphosis**
     L60.3   **Nail dystrophy**
     L60.4   **Beau's lines**
     L60.5   **Yellow nail syndrome**
     L60.8   **Other nail disorders**
     L60.9   Nail disorder, **unspecified**

▶ **L62**   *Nail disorders in diseases classified elsewhere*
     Code first underlying disease, such as:
         pachydermoperiostosis (M89.4-)

● **L63**   **Alopecia areata**
     L63.0   Alopecia (capitis) **totalis**
     L63.1   Alopecia **universalis**
     L63.2   **Ophiasis**
     L63.8   **Other** alopecia areata
     L63.9   Alopecia areata, **unspecified**

Item 12-10   **Alopecia** is lack of hair and takes many forms. The most common is male pattern alopecia, also known as **androgenetic alopecia. Telogen effluvium** is early and excessive loss of hair resulting from a trauma to the hair follicle (fever, drugs, surgery, etc.).

Figure 12-8   Male pattern alopecia.

● **L64**   **Androgenic alopecia**
     Includes   male-pattern baldness
     L64.0   **Drug-induced androgenic alopecia**
         Use additional code for adverse effect, if applicable, to identify drug (T36-T50 with fifth or sixth character 5)
     L64.8   **Other androgenic alopecia**
     L64.9   Androgenic alopecia, **unspecified**

● **L65**   **Other nonscarring hair loss**
     Use additional code for adverse effect, if applicable, to identify drug (T36-T50 with fifth or sixth character 5)
     Excludes1   trichotillomania (F63.3)
     L65.0   **Telogen effluvium**
     L65.1   **Anagen effluvium**
     L65.2   **Alopecia mucinosa**
     L65.8   **Other specified nonscarring hair loss**
     L65.9   Nonscarring hair loss, **unspecified**
         Alopecia NOS

● **L66**   **Cicatricial alopecia [scarring hair loss]**
     L66.0   **Pseudopelade**
     L66.1   **Lichen planopilaris**
         Follicular lichen planus
     L66.2   **Folliculitis decalvans**
     L66.3   **Perifolliculitis capitis abscedens**
     L66.4   **Folliculitis ulerythematosa reticulata**
     L66.8   **Other cicatricial alopecia**
         Coding Clinic: 2015, Q1, P19
     L66.9   Cicatricial alopecia, **unspecified**

● **L67**   **Hair color and hair shaft abnormalities**
     Excludes1   monilethrix (Q84.1)
                pili annulati (Q84.1)
                telogen effluvium (L65.0)
     L67.0   **Trichorrhexis nodosa**
     L67.1   **Variations in hair color**
         Canities
         Greyness, hair (premature)
         Heterochromia of hair
         Poliosis circumscripta, acquired
         Poliosis NOS
     L67.8   **Other hair color and hair shaft abnormalities**
         Fragilitas crinium
     L67.9   Hair color and hair shaft abnormality, **unspecified**

● **L68**   **Hypertrichosis**
     Includes   excess hair
     Excludes1   congenital hypertrichosis (Q84.2)
                persistent lanugo (Q84.2)
     L68.0   **Hirsutism**
         Excessive growth of hair
     L68.1   **Acquired hypertrichosis lanuginosa**
     L68.2   **Localized hypertrichosis**
     L68.3   **Polytrichia**
     L68.8   **Other hypertrichosis**
     L68.9   Hypertrichosis, **unspecified**

● **L70**   **Acne**
     Excludes2   acne keloid (L73.0)
     L70.0   **Acne vulgaris**
     L70.1   **Acne conglobata**
     L70.2   **Acne varioliformis**
         Acne necrotica miliaris

CHAPTER 12 (L00-L99)

▶ New   ⇒ Revised   ~~deleted~~ Deleted   Excludes 1   Excludes 2   Includes   Use additional   Code first   Code also   Key words

OGCR Official Guidelines   X Assign placeholder X   ● Use Additional Character(s)   ▶ Manifestation Code   ⚙ Hierarchical Condition Category   **Coding Clinic**

● **L70.3**   Acne tropica

L70.4   Infantile acne   P

L70.5   Acné excoriée
       Acné excoriée des jeunes filles
       Picker's acne

L70.8   Other acne

L70.9   Acne, unspecified

● **L71**   Rosacea

       Use additional code for adverse effect, if applicable, to identify
       drug (T36-T50 with fifth or sixth character 5)

L71.0   Perioral dermatitis

L71.1   Rhinophyma

L71.8   Other rosacea
       Coding Clinic: 2018, Q4, P15

L71.9   Rosacea, unspecified

● **L72**   Follicular cysts of skin and subcutaneous tissue

L72.0   Epidermal cyst

● **L72.1**   Pilar and trichodermal cyst

     L72.11   Pilar cyst

     L72.12   Trichodermal cyst
           Trichilemmal (proliferating) cyst

L72.3   Sebaceous cyst

     Excludes2   pilar cyst (L72.11)
                   trichilemmal (proliferating) cyst (L72.12)

L72.2   Steatocystoma multiplex

L72.8   Other follicular cysts of the skin and subcutaneous
       tissue

L72.9   Follicular cyst of the skin and subcutaneous tissue,
       unspecified

● **L73**   Other follicular disorders

L73.0   Acne keloid

L73.1   Pseudofolliculitis barbae

L73.2   Hidradenitis suppurativa

L73.8   Other specified follicular disorders
       Sycosis barbae

L73.9   Follicular disorder, unspecified

● **L74**   Eccrine sweat disorders

     Excludes2   generalized hyperhidrosis (R61)

L74.0   Miliaria rubra

L74.1   Miliaria crystallina

L74.2   Miliaria profunda
       Miliaria tropicalis

L74.3   Miliaria, unspecified

L74.4   Anhidrosis
       Hypohidrosis

● **L74.5**   Focal hyperhidrosis

   ● **L74.51**   Primary focal hyperhidrosis

        L74.510   Primary focal hyperhidrosis, axilla

        L74.511   Primary focal hyperhidrosis, face

        L74.512   Primary focal hyperhidrosis, palms

        L74.513   Primary focal hyperhidrosis, soles

        L74.519   Primary focal hyperhidrosis,
                unspecified

     L74.52   Secondary focal hyperhidrosis
           Frey's syndrome

L74.8   Other eccrine sweat disorders

L74.9   Eccrine sweat disorder, unspecified
       Sweat gland disorder NOS

● **L75**   Apocrine sweat disorders

     Excludes1   dyshidrosis (L30.1)
                 hidradenitis suppurativa (L73.2)

L75.0   Bromhidrosis

L75.1   Chromhidrosis

L75.2   Apocrine miliaria
       Fox-Fordyce disease

L75.8   Other apocrine sweat disorders

L75.9   Apocrine sweat disorder, unspecified
       Intraoperative and postprocedural complications of
       skin and subcutaneous tissue (L76)

INTRAOPERATIVE AND POSTPROCEDURAL COMPLICATIONS OF SKIN AND SUBCUTANEOUS TISSUE (L76)

● **L76**   Intraoperative and postprocedural complications of skin and
subcutaneous tissue
       Coding Clinic: 2016, Q4, P10

 ● **L76.0**   Intraoperative hemorrhage and hematoma of skin and
subcutaneous tissue complicating a procedure

     Excludes1   intraoperative hemorrhage and
                 hematoma of skin and subcutaneous
                 tissue due to accidental puncture
                 and laceration during a procedure
                 (L76.1-)

     L76.01   Intraoperative hemorrhage and hematoma of
           skin and subcutaneous tissue complicating a
           dermatologic procedure

     L76.02   Intraoperative hemorrhage and hematoma of
           skin and subcutaneous tissue complicating
           other procedure

 ● **L76.1**   Accidental puncture and laceration of skin and
subcutaneous tissue during a procedure

     L76.11   Accidental puncture and laceration of skin and
           subcutaneous tissue during a dermatologic
           procedure

     L76.12   Accidental puncture and laceration of skin and
           subcutaneous tissue during other procedure

 ● **L76.2**   Postprocedural hemorrhage of skin and subcutaneous
tissue following a procedure

     L76.21   Postprocedural hemorrhage of skin and
           subcutaneous tissue following a dermatologic
           procedure

     L76.22   Postprocedural hemorrhage of skin and
           subcutaneous tissue following other procedure

● **L76.3**   Postprocedural hematoma and seroma of skin and
subcutaneous tissue following a procedure

     L76.31   Postprocedural hematoma of skin and
           subcutaneous tissue following a dermatologic
           procedure

     L76.32   Postprocedural hematoma of skin and
           subcutaneous tissue following other procedure

     L76.33   Postprocedural seroma of skin and
           subcutaneous tissue following a dermatologic
           procedure

     L76.34   Postprocedural seroma of skin and
           subcutaneous tissue following other procedure

 ● **L76.8**   Other intraoperative and postprocedural complications
of skin and subcutaneous tissue

       Use additional code, if applicable, to further specify
       disorder

     L76.81   Other intraoperative complications of skin and
           subcutaneous tissue

     L76.82   Other postprocedural complications of skin and
           subcutaneous tissue
           Coding Clinic: 2017, Q3, P6

CHAPTER 12 (L00-L99)

OTHER DISORDERS OF THE SKIN AND SUBCUTANEOUS TISSUE (L80-L99)

L80   Vitiligo
> **Excludes2**   vitiligo of eyelids (H02.73-)
> vitiligo of vulva (N90.89)

● **L81   Other disorders of pigmentation**
> **Excludes1**   birthmark NOS (Q82.5)
> ➠Peutz-Jeghers syndrome (Q85.89)
> **Excludes2**   nevus - see Alphabetical Index

L81.0   Postinflammatory hyperpigmentation
L81.1   Chloasma
L81.2   Freckles
L81.3   Café au lait spots
L81.4   Other melanin hyperpigmentation
> Lentigo

L81.5   Leukoderma, not elsewhere classified
L81.6   Other disorders of diminished melanin formation
L81.7   Pigmented purpuric dermatosis
> Angioma serpiginosum

L81.8   Other specified disorders of pigmentation
> Iron pigmentation
> Tattoo pigmentation

L81.9   Disorder of pigmentation, unspecified

● **L82   Seborrheic keratosis**
> **Includes**   basal cell papilloma
> dermatosis papulosa nigra
> Leser-Trélat disease
> **Excludes2**   seborrheic dermatitis (L21.-)

L82.0   Inflamed seborrheic keratosis
> Coding Clinic: 2021, Q3, P11

L82.1   Other seborrheic keratosis
> Seborrheic keratosis NOS

L83   Acanthosis nigricans
> Confluent and reticulated papillomatosis

L84   Corns and callosities
> Callus
> Clavus

● **L85   Other epidermal thickening**
> **Excludes2**   hypertrophic disorders of the skin (L91.-)

L85.0   Acquired ichthyosis
> **Excludes1**   congenital ichthyosis (Q80.-)

L85.1   Acquired keratosis [keratoderma] palmaris et plantaris
> **Excludes1**   inherited keratosis palmaris et plantaris (Q82.8)

L85.2   Keratosis punctata (palmaris et plantaris)
L85.3   Xerosis cutis
> Dry skin dermatitis

L85.8   Other specified epidermal thickening
> Cutaneous horn

L85.9   Epidermal thickening, unspecified

▷ *L86   Keratoderma in diseases classified elsewhere*
> *Firm horny papules that have a cobblestone appearance*
> *Code first underlying disease, such as:*
> Reiter's disease (M02.3-)
> **Excludes1**   gonococcal keratoderma (A54.89)
> gonococcal keratosis (A54.89)
> keratoderma due to vitamin A deficiency (E50.8)
> keratosis due to vitamin A deficiency (E50.8)
> xeroderma due to vitamin A deficiency (E50.8)

L87   Transepidermal elimination disorders
> **Excludes1**   granuloma annulare (perforating) (L92.0)

L87.0   Keratosis follicularis et parafollicularis in cutem penetrans
> Kyrle disease
> Hyperkeratosis follicularis penetrans

L87.1   Reactive perforating collagenosis

L87.2   Elastosis perforans serpiginosa
L87.8   Other transepidermal elimination disorders
L87.9   Transepidermal elimination disorder, unspecified

L88   Pyoderma gangrenosum
> Phagedenic pyoderma
> **Excludes1**   dermatitis gangrenosa (L08.0)

OGCR   Section I.B.14.

General Coding Guidelines

Documentation for BMI, *Depth of* Non-pressure ulcers, Pressure Ulcer Stages, **Coma Scale, and *NIH Stroke Scale***

For the Body Mass Index (BMI), depth of non-pressure chronic ulcers, pressure ulcer stage, **coma scale, and NIH stroke scale (NIHSS) codes,** code assignment may be based on medical record documentation from clinicians who are not the patient's provider (i.e., physician or other qualified healthcare practitioner legally accountable for establishing the patient's diagnosis), since this information is typically documented by other clinicians involved in the care of the patient (e.g., a dietitian often documents the BMI, a nurse often documents the pressure ulcer stages, **and an emergency medical technician often documents the coma scale**). However, the associated diagnosis (such as overweight, obesity, **acute stroke,** or pressure ulcer) must be documented by the patient's provider. If there is conflicting medical record documentation, either from the same clinician or different clinicians, the patient's attending provider should be queried for clarification.

The BMI, **coma scale, and NHSS** codes should only be reported as secondary diagnoses.

● **L89   Pressure ulcer**
> **Includes**   bed sore   pressure area
> decubitus ulcer   pressure sore
> plaster ulcer
> *Code first any associated gangrene (I96)*
> **Excludes2**   decubitus (trophic) ulcer of cervix (uteri) (N86)
> diabetic ulcers (E08.621, E08.622, E09.621, E09.622, E10.621, E10.622, E11.621, E11.622, E13.621, E13.622)
> non-pressure chronic ulcer of skin (L97.-)
> skin infections (L00-L08)
> varicose ulcer (I83.0, I83.2)
> Coding Clinic: 2019, Q4, P11; 2018, Q2, P22; 2016, Q4, P124

● **L89.0   Pressure ulcer of elbow**
> ● **L89.00   Pressure ulcer of unspecified elbow**

L89.000   Pressure ulcer of unspecified elbow, unstageable 🄷

L89.001   Pressure ulcer of unspecified elbow, stage 1
> Healing pressure ulcer of unspecified elbow, stage 1
> Pressure pre-ulcer skin changes limited to persistent focal edema, unspecified elbow

L89.002   Pressure ulcer of unspecified elbow, stage 2
> Healing pressure ulcer of unspecified elbow, stage 2
> Pressure ulcer with abrasion, blister, partial thickness skin loss involving epidermis and/or dermis, unspecified elbow

L89.003   Pressure ulcer of unspecified elbow, stage 3 🄷
> Healing pressure ulcer of unspecified elbow, stage 3
> Pressure ulcer with full thickness skin loss involving damage or necrosis of subcutaneous tissue, unspecified elbow

▶ New   ⇒ Revised   ~~deleted~~ Deleted   Excludes 1   Excludes 2   Includes   Use additional   Code first   Code also   Key words
OGCR Official Guidelines   X Assign placeholder X   ● Use Additional Character(s)   ▷ Manifestation Code   🄷 Hierarchical Condition Category   **Coding Clinic**

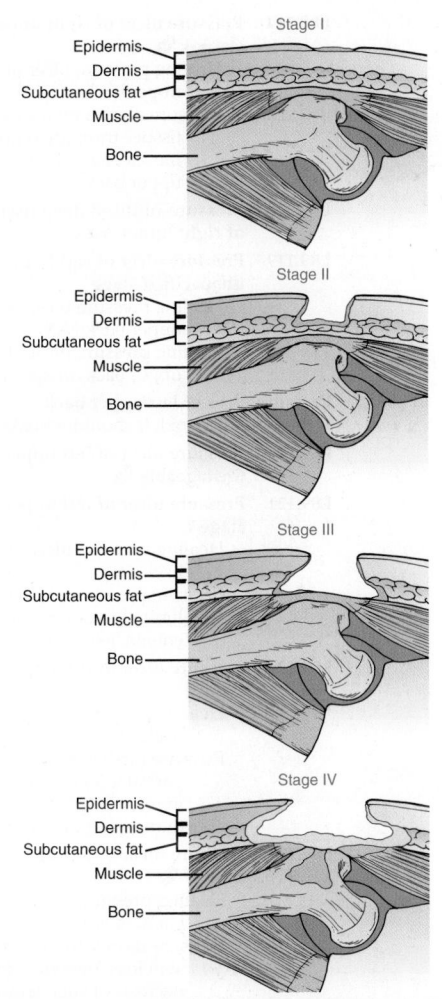

Figure 12-9   Stage I, II, III, and IV of pressure ulcers.

L89.004   **Pressure ulcer of unspecified elbow, stage 4** 🔖
     Healing pressure ulcer of unspecified elbow, stage 4
     Pressure ulcer with necrosis of soft tissues through to underlying muscle, tendon, or bone, unspecified elbow

L89.006   **Pressure-induced deep tissue damage of unspecified elbow**

L89.009   **Pressure ulcer of unspecified elbow, unspecified stage**
     Healing pressure ulcer of elbow NOS
     Healing pressure ulcer of unspecified elbow, unspecified stage

● **L89.01**   **Pressure ulcer of right elbow**

L89.010   **Pressure ulcer of right elbow, unstageable** 🔖

L89.011   **Pressure ulcer of right elbow, stage 1**
     Healing pressure ulcer of right elbow, stage 1
     Pressure pre-ulcer skin changes limited to persistent focal edema, right elbow

L89.012   **Pressure ulcer of right elbow, stage 2**
     Healing pressure ulcer of right elbow, stage 2
     Pressure ulcer with abrasion, blister, partial thickness skin loss involving epidermis and/or dermis, right elbow

L89.013   **Pressure ulcer of right elbow, stage 3** 🔖
     Healing pressure ulcer of right elbow, stage 3
     Pressure ulcer with full thickness skin loss involving damage or necrosis of subcutaneous tissue, right elbow

L89.014   **Pressure ulcer of right elbow, stage 4** 🔖
     Healing pressure ulcer of right elbow, stage 4
     Pressure ulcer with necrosis of soft tissues through to underlying muscle, tendon, or bone, right elbow

L89.016   **Pressure-induced deep tissue damage of right elbow**

L89.019   **Pressure ulcer of right elbow, unspecified stage**
     Healing pressure ulcer of right elbow NOS

● **L89.02**   **Pressure ulcer of left elbow**

L89.020   **Pressure ulcer of left elbow, unstageable** 🔖

L89.021   **Pressure ulcer of left elbow, stage 1**
     Healing pressure ulcer of left elbow, stage 1
     Pressure pre-ulcer skin changes limited to persistent focal edema, left elbow

L89.022   **Pressure ulcer of left elbow, stage 2**
     Healing pressure ulcer of left elbow, stage 2
     Pressure ulcer with abrasion, blister, partial thickness skin loss involving epidermis and/or dermis, left elbow

L89.023   **Pressure ulcer of left elbow, stage 3** 🔖
     Healing pressure ulcer of left elbow, stage 3
     Pressure ulcer with full thickness skin loss involving damage or necrosis of subcutaneous tissue, left elbow

L89.024   **Pressure ulcer of left elbow, stage 4** 🔖
     Healing pressure ulcer of left elbow, stage 4
     Pressure ulcer with necrosis of soft tissues through to underlying muscle, tendon, or bone, left elbow

L89.026   **Pressure-induced deep tissue damage of left elbow**

L89.029   **Pressure ulcer of left elbow, unspecified stage**
     Healing pressure ulcer of left elbow NOS

CHAPTER 12 (L00-L99)

CHAPTER 12 (L00-L99)

● **L89.1**   **Pressure ulcer of back**
  ● **L89.10**   **Pressure ulcer of unspecified part of back**
    L89.100   **Pressure ulcer of unspecified part of back, unstageable** 🐾
    L89.101   **Pressure ulcer of unspecified part of back, stage 1**
      Healing pressure ulcer of unspecified part of back, stage 1
      Pressure pre-ulcer skin changes limited to persistent focal edema, unspecified part of back
    L89.102   **Pressure ulcer of unspecified part of back, stage 2**
      Healing pressure ulcer of unspecified part of back, stage 2
      Pressure ulcer with abrasion, blister, partial thickness skin loss involving epidermis and/or dermis, unspecified part of back
    L89.103   **Pressure ulcer of unspecified part of back, stage 3** 🐾
      Healing pressure ulcer of unspecified part of back, stage 3
      Pressure ulcer with full thickness skin loss involving damage or necrosis of subcutaneous tissue, unspecified part of back
    L89.104   **Pressure ulcer of unspecified part of back, stage 4** 🐾
      Healing pressure ulcer of unspecified part of back, stage 4
      Pressure ulcer with necrosis of soft tissues through to underlying muscle, tendon, or bone, unspecified part of back
    L89.106   **Pressure-induced deep tissue damage of unspecified part of back**
    L89.109   **Pressure ulcer of unspecified part of back, unspecified stage**
      Healing pressure ulcer of unspecified part of back NOS
      Healing pressure ulcer of unspecified part of back, unspecified stage
  ● **L89.11**   **Pressure ulcer of right upper back**
    Pressure ulcer of right shoulder blade
    L89.110   **Pressure ulcer of right upper back, unstageable** 🐾
    L89.111   **Pressure ulcer of right upper back, stage 1**
      Healing pressure ulcer of right upper back, stage 1
      Pressure pre-ulcer skin changes limited to persistent focal edema, right upper back
    L89.112   **Pressure ulcer of right upper back, stage 2**
      Healing pressure ulcer of right upper back, stage 2
      Pressure ulcer with abrasion, blister, partial thickness skin loss involving epidermis and/or dermis, right upper back
    L89.113   **Pressure ulcer of right upper back, stage 3** 🐾
      Healing pressure ulcer of right upper back, stage 3
      Pressure ulcer with full thickness skin loss involving damage or necrosis of subcutaneous tissue, right upper back

    L89.114   **Pressure ulcer of right upper back, stage 4** 🐾
      Healing pressure ulcer of right upper back, stage 4
      Pressure ulcer with necrosis of soft tissues through to underlying muscle, tendon, or bone, right upper back
    L89.116   **Pressure-induced deep tissue damage of right upper back**
    L89.119   **Pressure ulcer of right upper back, unspecified stage**
      Healing pressure ulcer of right upper back NOS
      Healing pressure ulcer of right upper back, unspecified stage
  ● **L89.12**   **Pressure ulcer of left upper back**
    Pressure ulcer of left shoulder blade
    L89.120   **Pressure ulcer of left upper back, unstageable** 🐾
    L89.121   **Pressure ulcer of left upper back, stage 1**
      Healing pressure ulcer of left upper back, stage 1
      Pressure pre-ulcer skin changes limited to persistent focal edema, left upper back
    L89.122   **Pressure ulcer of left upper back, stage 2**
      Healing pressure ulcer of left upper back, stage 2
      Pressure ulcer with abrasion, blister, partial thickness skin loss involving epidermis and/or dermis, left upper back
    L89.123   **Pressure ulcer of left upper back, stage 3** 🐾
      Healing pressure ulcer of left upper back, stage 3
      Pressure ulcer with full thickness skin loss involving damage or necrosis of subcutaneous tissue, left upper back
    L89.124   **Pressure ulcer of left upper back, stage 4** 🐾
      Healing pressure ulcer of left upper back, stage 4
      Pressure ulcer with necrosis of soft tissues through to underlying muscle, tendon, or bone, left upper back
    L89.126   **Pressure-induced deep tissue damage of left upper back**
    L89.129   **Pressure ulcer of left upper back, unspecified stage**
      Healing pressure ulcer of left upper back NOS
      Healing pressure ulcer of left upper back, unspecified stage
  ● **L89.13**   **Pressure ulcer of right lower back**
    L89.130   **Pressure ulcer of right lower back, unstageable** 🐾
    L89.131   **Pressure ulcer of right lower back, stage 1**
      Healing pressure ulcer of right lower back, stage 1
      Pressure pre-ulcer skin changes limited to persistent focal edema, right lower back

▶ New   ⇒ Revised   ~~deleted~~ Deleted   Excludes 1   Excludes 2   Includes   Use additional   Code first   Code also   Key words   OGCR Official Guidelines   X Assign placeholder X   ● Use Additional Character(s)   ▶ Manifestation Code   🐾 Hierarchical Condition Category   Coding Clinic

L89.132   **Pressure ulcer of right lower back, stage 2**
> Healing pressure ulcer of right lower back, stage 2
> Pressure ulcer with abrasion, blister, partial thickness skin loss involving epidermis and/or dermis, right lower back

L89.133   **Pressure ulcer of right lower back, stage 3** 🔖
> Healing pressure ulcer of right lower back, stage 3
> Pressure ulcer with full thickness skin loss involving damage or necrosis of subcutaneous tissue, right lower back

L89.134   **Pressure ulcer of right lower back, stage 4** 🔖
> Healing pressure ulcer of right lower back, stage 4
> Pressure ulcer with necrosis of soft tissues through to underlying muscle, tendon, or bone, right lower back

L89.136   **Pressure-induced deep tissue damage of right lower back**

L89.139   **Pressure ulcer of right lower back, unspecified stage**
> Healing pressure ulcer of right lower back NOS
> Healing pressure ulcer of right lower back, unspecified stage

● **L89.14**   **Pressure ulcer of left lower back**

L89.140   **Pressure ulcer of left lower back, unstageable** 🔖

L89.141   **Pressure ulcer of left lower back, stage 1**
> Healing pressure ulcer of left lower back, stage 1
> Pressure pre-ulcer skin changes limited to persistent focal edema, left lower back

L89.142   **Pressure ulcer of left lower back, stage 2**
> Healing pressure ulcer of left lower back, stage 2
> Pressure ulcer with abrasion, blister, partial thickness skin loss involving epidermis and/or dermis, left lower back

L89.143   **Pressure ulcer of left lower back, stage 3** 🔖
> Healing pressure ulcer of left lower back, stage 3
> Pressure ulcer with full thickness skin loss involving damage or necrosis of subcutaneous tissue, left lower back

L89.144   **Pressure ulcer of left lower back, stage 4** 🔖
> Healing pressure ulcer of left lower back, stage 4
> Pressure ulcer with necrosis of soft tissues through to underlying muscle, tendon, or bone, left lower back

L89.146   **Pressure-induced deep tissue damage of left lower back**

L89.149   **Pressure ulcer of left lower back, unspecified stage**
> Healing pressure ulcer of left lower back NOS
> Healing pressure ulcer of left lower back, unspecified stage

● **L89.15**   **Pressure ulcer of sacral region**
> Pressure ulcer of coccyx
> Pressure ulcer of tailbone
> Coding Clinic: 2021, Q3, P10

L89.150   **Pressure ulcer of sacral region, unstageable** 🔖

L89.151   **Pressure ulcer of sacral region, stage 1**
> Healing pressure ulcer of sacral region, stage 1
> Pressure pre-ulcer skin changes limited to persistent focal edema, sacral region

L89.152   **Pressure ulcer of sacral region, stage 2**
> Healing pressure ulcer of sacral region, stage 2
> Pressure ulcer with abrasion, blister, partial thickness skin loss involving epidermis and/or dermis, sacral region

L89.153   **Pressure ulcer of sacral region, stage 3** 🔖
> Healing pressure ulcer of sacral region, stage 3
> Pressure ulcer with full thickness skin loss involving damage or necrosis of subcutaneous tissue, sacral region
> Coding Clinic: 2021, Q3, P10

L89.154   **Pressure ulcer of sacral region, stage 4** 🔖
> Healing pressure ulcer of sacral region, stage 4
> Pressure ulcer with necrosis of soft tissues through to underlying muscle, tendon, or bone, sacral region
> Coding Clinic: 2022, Q2, P9; 2021, Q1, P24

L89.156   **Pressure-induced deep tissue damage of sacral region**

L89.159   **Pressure ulcer of sacral region, unspecified stage**
> Healing pressure ulcer of sacral region NOS
> Healing pressure ulcer of sacral region, unspecified stage

● **L89.2**   **Pressure ulcer of hip**

  ● **L89.20**   **Pressure ulcer of unspecified hip**

L89.200   **Pressure ulcer of unspecified hip, unstageable** 🔖

L89.201   **Pressure ulcer of unspecified hip, stage 1**
> Healing pressure ulcer of unspecified hip back, stage 1
> Pressure pre-ulcer skin changes limited to persistent focal edema, unspecified hip

L89.202   **Pressure ulcer of unspecified hip, stage 2**
> Healing pressure ulcer of unspecified hip, stage 2
> Pressure ulcer with abrasion, blister, partial thickness skin loss involving epidermis and/or dermis, unspecified hip

L89.203   **Pressure ulcer of unspecified hip, stage 3** 🔖
> Healing pressure ulcer of unspecified hip, stage 3
> Pressure ulcer with full thickness skin loss involving damage or necrosis of subcutaneous tissue, unspecified hip

L89.204   **Pressure ulcer of unspecified hip, stage 4** 🦠
          Healing pressure ulcer of unspecified hip, stage 4
          Pressure ulcer with necrosis of soft tissues through to underlying muscle, tendon, or bone, unspecified hip

L89.206   **Pressure-induced deep tissue damage of unspecified hip**

L89.209   **Pressure ulcer of unspecified hip, unspecified stage**
          Healing pressure ulcer of unspecified hip NOS
          Healing pressure ulcer of unspecified hip, unspecified stage

● **L89.21   Pressure ulcer of right hip**

L89.210   **Pressure ulcer of right hip, unstageable** 🦠

L89.211   **Pressure ulcer of right hip, stage 1**
          Healing pressure ulcer of right hip back, stage 1
          Pressure pre-ulcer skin changes limited to persistent focal edema, right hip

L89.212   **Pressure ulcer of right hip, stage 2**
          Healing pressure ulcer of right hip, stage 2
          Pressure ulcer with abrasion, blister, partial thickness skin loss involving epidermis and/or dermis, right hip

L89.213   **Pressure ulcer of right hip, stage 3** 🦠
          Healing pressure ulcer of right hip, stage 3
          Pressure ulcer with full thickness skin loss involving damage or necrosis of subcutaneous tissue, right hip

L89.214   **Pressure ulcer of right hip, stage 4** 🦠
          Healing pressure ulcer of right hip, stage 4
          Pressure ulcer with necrosis of soft tissues through to underlying muscle, tendon, or bone, right hip

L89.216   **Pressure-induced deep tissue damage of right hip**

L89.219   **Pressure ulcer of right hip, unspecified stage**
          Healing pressure ulcer of right hip NOS
          Healing pressure ulcer of right hip, unspecified stage

● **L89.22   Pressure ulcer of left hip**

L89.220   **Pressure ulcer of left hip, unstageable** 🦠

L89.221   **Pressure ulcer of left hip, stage 1**
          Healing pressure ulcer of left hip back, stage 1
          Pressure pre-ulcer skin changes limited to persistent focal edema, left hip

L89.222   **Pressure ulcer of left hip, stage 2**
          Healing pressure ulcer of left hip, stage 2
          Pressure ulcer with abrasion, blister, partial thickness skin loss involving epidermis and/or dermis, left hip

L89.223   **Pressure ulcer of left hip, stage 3** 🦠
          Healing pressure ulcer of left hip, stage 3
          Pressure ulcer with full thickness skin loss involving damage or necrosis of subcutaneous tissue, left hip

L89.224   **Pressure ulcer of left hip, stage 4** 🦠
          Healing pressure ulcer of left hip, stage 4
          Pressure ulcer with necrosis of soft tissues through to underlying muscle, tendon, or bone, left hip

L89.226   **Pressure-induced deep tissue damage of left hip**

L89.229   **Pressure ulcer of left hip, unspecified stage**
          Healing pressure ulcer of left hip NOS
          Healing pressure ulcer of left hip, unspecified stage

● **L89.3   Pressure ulcer of buttock**

● **L89.30   Pressure ulcer of unspecified buttock**

L89.300   **Pressure ulcer of unspecified buttock, unstageable** 🦠

L89.301   **Pressure ulcer of unspecified buttock, stage 1**
          Healing pressure ulcer of unspecified buttock, stage 1
          Pressure pre-ulcer skin changes limited to persistent focal edema, unspecified buttock

L89.302   **Pressure ulcer of unspecified buttock, stage 2**
          Healing pressure ulcer of unspecified buttock, stage 2
          Pressure ulcer with abrasion, blister, partial thickness skin loss involving epidermis and/or dermis, unspecified buttock

L89.303   **Pressure ulcer of unspecified buttock, stage 3** 🦠
          Healing pressure ulcer of unspecified buttock, stage 3
          Pressure ulcer with full thickness skin loss involving damage or necrosis of subcutaneous tissue, unspecified buttock

L89.304   **Pressure ulcer of unspecified buttock, stage 4** 🦠
          Healing pressure ulcer of unspecified buttock, stage 4
          Pressure ulcer with necrosis of soft tissues through to underlying muscle, tendon, or bone, unspecified buttock

L89.306   **Pressure-induced deep tissue damage of unspecified buttock**

L89.309   **Pressure ulcer of unspecified buttock, unspecified stage**
          Healing pressure ulcer of unspecified buttock NOS
          Healing pressure ulcer of unspecified buttock, unspecified stage

● **L89.31   Pressure ulcer of right buttock**

L89.310   **Pressure ulcer of right buttock, unstageable** 🦠

L89.311   **Pressure ulcer of right buttock, stage 1**
          Healing pressure ulcer of right buttock, stage 1
          Pressure pre-ulcer skin changes limited to persistent focal edema, right buttock

▶ New   ⇒ Revised   ~~deleted~~ Deleted   Excludes 1   Excludes 2   Includes   Use additional   Code first   Code also   Key words
OGCR Official Guidelines   X Assign placeholder X   ● Use Additional Character(s)   ▶ Manifestation Code   🦠 Hierarchical Condition Category   **Coding Clinic**

L89.312   Pressure ulcer of right buttock, stage 2
Healing pressure ulcer of right buttock, stage 2
Pressure ulcer with abrasion, blister, partial thickness skin loss involving epidermis and/or dermis, right buttock

L89.313   Pressure ulcer of right buttock, stage 3 🔊
Healing pressure ulcer of right buttock, stage 3
Pressure ulcer with full thickness skin loss involving damage or necrosis of subcutaneous tissue, right buttock

L89.314   Pressure ulcer of right buttock, stage 4 🔊
Healing pressure ulcer of right buttock, stage 4
Pressure ulcer with necrosis of soft tissues through to underlying muscle, tendon, or bone, right buttock

L89.316   Pressure-induced deep tissue damage of right buttock

L89.319   Pressure ulcer of right buttock, unspecified stage
Healing pressure ulcer of right buttock NOS
Healing pressure ulcer of right buttock, unspecified stage

● L89.32   Pressure ulcer of left buttock

L89.320   Pressure ulcer of left buttock, unstageable 🔊

L89.321   Pressure ulcer of left buttock, stage 1
Healing pressure ulcer of left buttock, stage 1
Pressure pre-ulcer skin changes limited to persistent focal edema, left buttock

L89.322   Pressure ulcer of left buttock, stage 2
Healing pressure ulcer of left buttock, stage 2
Pressure ulcer with abrasion, blister, partial thickness skin loss involving epidermis and/or dermis, left buttock

L89.323   Pressure ulcer of left buttock, stage 3 🔊
Healing pressure ulcer of left buttock, stage 3
Pressure ulcer with full thickness skin loss involving damage or necrosis of subcutaneous tissue, left buttock

L89.324   Pressure ulcer of left buttock, stage 4 🔊
Healing pressure ulcer of left buttock, stage 4
Pressure ulcer with necrosis of soft tissues through to underlying muscle, tendon, or bone, left buttock

L89.326   Pressure-induced deep tissue damage of left buttock

L89.329   Pressure ulcer of left buttock, unspecified stage
Healing pressure ulcer of left buttock NOS
Healing pressure ulcer of left buttock, unspecified stage

● L89.4   Pressure ulcer of contiguous site of back, buttock and hip

L89.40   Pressure ulcer of contiguous site of back, buttock and hip, unspecified stage
Healing pressure ulcer of contiguous site of back, buttock and hip NOS
Healing pressure ulcer of contiguous site of back, buttock and hip, unspecified stage

L89.41   Pressure ulcer of contiguous site of back, buttock and hip, stage 1
Healing pressure ulcer of contiguous site of back, buttock and hip, stage 1
Pressure pre-ulcer skin changes limited to persistent focal edema, contiguous site of back, buttock and hip

L89.42   Pressure ulcer of contiguous site of back, buttock and hip, stage 2
Healing pressure ulcer of contiguous site of back, buttock and hip, stage 2
Pressure ulcer with abrasion, blister, partial thickness skin loss involving epidermis and/or dermis, contiguous site of back, buttock and hip

L89.43   Pressure ulcer of contiguous site of back, buttock and hip, stage 3 🔊
Healing pressure ulcer of contiguous site of back, buttock and hip, stage 3
Pressure ulcer with full thickness skin loss involving damage or necrosis of subcutaneous tissue, contiguous site of back, buttock and hip

L89.44   Pressure ulcer of contiguous site of back, buttock and hip, stage 4 🔊
Healing pressure ulcer of contiguous site of back, buttock and hip, stage 4
Pressure ulcer with necrosis of soft tissues through to underlying muscle, tendon, or bone, contiguous site of back, buttock and hip

L89.45   Pressure ulcer of contiguous site of back, buttock and hip, unstageable 🔊

L89.46   Pressure-induced deep tissue damage of contiguous site of back, buttock and hip

● L89.5   Pressure ulcer of ankle

● L89.50   Pressure ulcer of unspecified ankle

L89.500   Pressure ulcer of unspecified ankle, unstageable 🔊

L89.501   Pressure ulcer of unspecified ankle, stage 1
Healing pressure ulcer of unspecified ankle, stage 1
Pressure pre-ulcer skin changes limited to persistent focal edema, unspecified ankle

L89.502   Pressure ulcer of unspecified ankle, stage 2
Healing pressure ulcer of unspecified ankle, stage 2
Pressure ulcer with abrasion, blister, partial thickness skin loss involving epidermis and/or dermis, unspecified ankle

L89.503   Pressure ulcer of unspecified ankle, stage 3 🔊
Healing pressure ulcer of unspecified ankle, stage 3
Pressure ulcer with full thickness skin loss involving damage or necrosis of subcutaneous tissue, unspecified ankle

CHAPTER 12 (L00-L99)

CHAPTER 12 (L00-L99)

L89.504   **Pressure ulcer of unspecified ankle, stage 4** 🐾
Healing pressure ulcer of unspecified ankle, stage 4
Pressure ulcer with necrosis of soft tissues through to underlying muscle, tendon, or bone, unspecified ankle

L89.506   **Pressure-induced deep tissue damage of unspecified ankle**

L89.509   **Pressure ulcer of unspecified ankle, unspecified stage**
Healing pressure ulcer of unspecified ankle NOS
Healing pressure ulcer of unspecified ankle, unspecified stage

● **L89.51**   **Pressure ulcer of right ankle**

L89.510   **Pressure ulcer of right ankle, unstageable** 🐾

L89.511   **Pressure ulcer of right ankle, stage 1**
Healing pressure ulcer of right ankle, stage 1
Pressure pre-ulcer skin changes limited to persistent focal edema, right ankle

L89.512   **Pressure ulcer of right ankle, stage 2**
Healing pressure ulcer of right ankle, stage 2
Pressure ulcer with abrasion, blister, partial thickness skin loss involving epidermis and/or dermis, right ankle

L89.513   **Pressure ulcer of right ankle, stage 3** 🐾
Healing pressure ulcer of right ankle, stage 3
Pressure ulcer with full thickness skin loss involving damage or necrosis of subcutaneous tissue, right ankle

L89.514   **Pressure ulcer of right ankle, stage 4** 🐾
Healing pressure ulcer of right ankle, stage 4
Pressure ulcer with necrosis of soft tissues through to underlying muscle, tendon, or bone, right ankle

L89.516   **Pressure-induced deep tissue damage of right ankle**

L89.519   **Pressure ulcer of right ankle, unspecified stage**
Healing pressure ulcer of right ankle NOS
Healing pressure ulcer of right ankle, unspecified stage

● **L89.52**   **Pressure ulcer of left ankle**

L89.520   **Pressure ulcer of left ankle, unstageable**

L89.521   **Pressure ulcer of left ankle, stage 1**
Healing pressure ulcer of left ankle, stage 1
Pressure pre-ulcer skin changes limited to persistent focal edema, left ankle

L89.522   **Pressure ulcer of left ankle, stage 2**
Healing pressure ulcer of left ankle, stage 2
Pressure ulcer with abrasion, blister, partial thickness skin loss involving epidermis and/or dermis, left ankle

L89.523   **Pressure ulcer of left ankle, stage 3** 🐾
Healing pressure ulcer of left ankle, stage 3
Pressure ulcer with full thickness skin loss involving damage or necrosis of subcutaneous tissue, left ankle

L89.524   **Pressure ulcer of left ankle, stage 4** 🐾
Healing pressure ulcer of left ankle, stage 4
Pressure ulcer with necrosis of soft tissues through to underlying muscle, tendon, or bone, left ankle

L89.526   **Pressure-induced deep tissue damage of left ankle**

L89.529   **Pressure ulcer of left ankle, unspecified stage**
Healing pressure ulcer of left ankle NOS
Healing pressure ulcer of left ankle, unspecified stage

● **L89.6**   **Pressure ulcer of heel**

● **L89.60**   **Pressure ulcer of unspecified heel**

L89.600   **Pressure ulcer of unspecified heel, unstageable** 🐾

L89.601   **Pressure ulcer of unspecified heel, stage 1**
Healing pressure ulcer of unspecified heel, stage 1
Pressure pre-ulcer skin changes limited to persistent focal edema, unspecified heel

L89.602   **Pressure ulcer of unspecified heel, stage 2**
Healing pressure ulcer of unspecified heel, stage 2
Pressure ulcer with abrasion, blister, partial thickness skin loss involving epidermis and/or dermis, unspecified heel

L89.603   **Pressure ulcer of unspecified heel, stage 3** 🐾
Healing pressure ulcer of unspecified heel, stage 3
Pressure ulcer with full thickness skin loss involving damage or necrosis of subcutaneous tissue, unspecified heel

L89.604   **Pressure ulcer of unspecified heel, stage 4** 🐾
Healing pressure ulcer of unspecified heel, stage 4
Pressure ulcer with necrosis of soft tissues through to underlying muscle, tendon, or bone, unspecified heel

L89.606   **Pressure-induced deep tissue damage of unspecified heel**

L89.609   **Pressure ulcer of unspecified heel, unspecified stage**
Healing pressure ulcer of unspecified heel NOS
Healing pressure ulcer of unspecified heel, unspecified stage

● **L89.61**   **Pressure ulcer of right heel**

L89.610   **Pressure ulcer of right heel, unstageable** 🐾

L89.611   **Pressure ulcer of right heel, stage 1**
Healing pressure ulcer of right heel, stage 1
Pressure pre-ulcer skin changes limited to persistent focal edema, right heel

▶ New   ⇒ Revised   ~~deleted~~ Deleted   Excludes 1   Excludes 2   Includes   Use additional   Code first   Code also   Key words

OGCR Official Guidelines   X Assign placeholder X   ● Use Additional Character(s)   ▌ Manifestation Code   🐾 Hierarchical Condition Category   **Coding Clinic**

L89.612   **Pressure ulcer of right heel, stage 2**
Healing pressure ulcer of right heel, stage 2
Pressure ulcer with abrasion, blister, partial thickness skin loss involving epidermis and/or dermis, right heel

L89.613   **Pressure ulcer of right heel, stage 3** 🔖
Healing pressure ulcer of right heel, stage 3
Pressure ulcer with full thickness skin loss involving damage or necrosis of subcutaneous tissue, right heel

L89.614   **Pressure ulcer of right heel, stage 4** 🔖
Healing pressure ulcer of right heel, stage 4
Pressure ulcer with necrosis of soft tissues through to underlying muscle, tendon, or bone, right heel

L89.616   **Pressure-induced deep tissue damage of right heel**

L89.619   **Pressure ulcer of right heel, unspecified stage**
Healing pressure ulcer of right heel NOS
Healing pressure ulcer of right heel, unspecified stage

⬤ **L89.62**   **Pressure ulcer of left heel**

L89.620   **Pressure ulcer of left heel, unstageable** 🔖

L89.621   **Pressure ulcer of left heel, stage 1**
Healing pressure ulcer of left heel, stage 1
Pressure pre-ulcer skin changes limited to persistent focal edema, left heel

L89.622   **Pressure ulcer of left heel, stage 2**
Healing pressure ulcer of left heel, stage 2
Pressure ulcer with abrasion, blister, partial thickness skin loss involving epidermis and/or dermis, left heel
Coding Clinic: 2016, Q4, P142

L89.623   **Pressure ulcer of left heel, stage 3** 🔖
Healing pressure ulcer of left heel, stage 3
Pressure ulcer with full thickness skin loss involving damage or necrosis of subcutaneous tissue, left heel
Coding Clinic: 2016, Q4, P142

L89.624   **Pressure ulcer of left heel, stage 4** 🔖
Healing pressure ulcer of left heel, stage 4
Pressure ulcer with necrosis of soft tissues through to underlying muscle, tendon, or bone, left heel

L89.626   **Pressure-induced deep tissue damage of left heel**

L89.629   **Pressure ulcer of left heel, unspecified stage**
Healing pressure ulcer of left heel NOS
Healing pressure ulcer of left heel, unspecified stage

⬤ **L89.8**   **Pressure ulcer of other site**

⬤ **L89.81**   **Pressure ulcer of head**
Pressure ulcer of face

L89.810   **Pressure ulcer of head, unstageable** 🔖

L89.811   **Pressure ulcer of head, stage 1**
Healing pressure ulcer of head, stage 1
Pressure pre-ulcer skin changes limited to persistent focal edema, head

L89.812   **Pressure ulcer of head, stage 2**
Healing pressure ulcer of head, stage 2
Pressure ulcer with abrasion, blister, partial thickness skin loss involving epidermis and/or dermis, head

L89.813   **Pressure ulcer of head, stage 3** 🔖
Healing pressure ulcer of head, stage 3
Pressure ulcer with full thickness skin loss involving damage or necrosis of subcutaneous tissue, head

L89.814   **Pressure ulcer of head, stage 4** 🔖
Healing pressure ulcer of head, stage 4
Pressure ulcer with necrosis of soft tissues through to underlying muscle, tendon, or bone, head

L89.816   **Pressure-induced deep tissue damage of head**

L89.819   **Pressure ulcer of head, unspecified stage**
Healing pressure ulcer of head NOS
Healing pressure ulcer of head, unspecified stage

⬤ **L89.89**   **Pressure ulcer of other site**

L89.890   **Pressure ulcer of other site, unstageable** 🔖

L89.891   **Pressure ulcer of other site, stage 1**
Healing pressure ulcer of other site, stage 1
Pressure pre-ulcer skin changes limited to persistent focal edema, other site

L89.892   **Pressure ulcer of other site, stage 2**
Healing pressure ulcer of other site, stage 2
Pressure ulcer with abrasion, blister, partial thickness skin loss involving epidermis and/or dermis, other site

L89.893   **Pressure ulcer of other site, stage 3** 🔖
Healing pressure ulcer of other site, stage 3
Pressure ulcer with full thickness skin loss involving damage or necrosis of subcutaneous tissue, other site

L89.894   **Pressure ulcer of other site, stage 4** 🔖
Healing pressure ulcer of other site, stage 4
Pressure ulcer with necrosis of soft tissues through to underlying muscle, tendon, or bone, other site

L89.899   **Pressure ulcer of other site, unspecified stage**
Healing pressure ulcer of other site NOS
Healing pressure ulcer of other site, unspecified stage

CHAPTER 12 (L00-L99)

● **L89.9   Pressure ulcer of unspecified site**
    L89.90   Pressure ulcer of unspecified site, unspecified stage
       Healing pressure ulcer of unspecified site NOS
       Healing pressure ulcer of unspecified site, unspecified stage
    L89.91   Pressure ulcer of unspecified site, stage 1
       Healing pressure ulcer of unspecified site, stage 1
       Pressure pre-ulcer skin changes limited to persistent focal edema, unspecified site
    L89.92   Pressure ulcer of unspecified site, stage 2
       Healing pressure ulcer of unspecified site, stage 2
       Pressure ulcer with abrasion, blister, partial thickness skin loss involving epidermis and/or dermis, unspecified site
    L89.93   Pressure ulcer of unspecified site, stage 3 🅗
       Healing pressure ulcer of unspecified site, stage 3
       Pressure ulcer with full thickness skin loss involving damage or necrosis of subcutaneous tissue, unspecified site
    L89.94   Pressure ulcer of unspecified site, stage 4 🅗
       Healing pressure ulcer of unspecified site, stage 4
       Pressure ulcer with necrosis of soft tissues through to underlying muscle, tendon, or bone, unspecified site
    L89.95   Pressure ulcer of unspecified site, unstageable 🅗
    L89.96   Pressure-induced deep tissue damage of unspecified site

● **L90   Atrophic disorders of skin**
    L90.0   Lichen sclerosus et atrophicus
       Excludes2   lichen sclerosus of external female genital organs (N90.4)
                lichen sclerosus of external male genital organs (N48.0)
    L90.1   Anetoderma of Schweninger-Buzzi
    L90.2   Anetoderma of Jadassohn-Pellizzari
    L90.3   Atrophoderma of Pasini and Pierini
    L90.4   Acrodermatitis chronica atrophicans
    L90.5   Scar conditions and fibrosis of skin
       Adherent scar (skin)
       Cicatrix
       Disfigurement of skin due to scar
       Fibrosis of skin NOS
       Scar NOS
       Excludes2   hypertrophic scar (L91.0)
                keloid scar (L91.0)
       Coding Clinic: 2016, Q2, P5; 2015, Q1, P19
    L90.6   Striae atrophicae
    L90.8   Other atrophic disorders of skin
    L90.9   Atrophic disorder of skin, unspecified

● **L91   Hypertrophic disorders of skin**
    L91.0   Keloid scar
       Hypertrophic scar
       Keloid
       Excludes2   acne keloid (L73.0)
                scar NOS (L90.5)
    L91.8   Other hypertrophic disorders of the skin
    L91.9   Hypertrophic disorder of the skin, unspecified

Item 12–11   Scleroderma means hard skin. It is a group of diseases that causes abnormal growth of connective tissues that support the skin and organs. There are two types: localized scleroderma affecting the skin and systemic scleroderma affecting blood vessels and internal organs and the skin.

● **L92   Granulomatous disorders of skin and subcutaneous tissue**
    Excludes2   actinic granuloma (L57.5)
    L92.0   Granuloma annulare
       Perforating granuloma annulare
    L92.1   Necrobiosis lipoidica, not elsewhere classified
       Excludes1   necrobiosis lipoidica associated with diabetes mellitus (E08-E13 with .620)
    L92.2   Granuloma faciale [eosinophilic granuloma of skin]
    L92.3   Foreign body granuloma of the skin and subcutaneous tissue
       Use additional code to identify the type of retained foreign body (Z18.-)
    L92.8   Other granulomatous disorders of the skin and subcutaneous tissue
    L92.9   Granulomatous disorder of the skin and subcutaneous tissue, unspecified
       Excludes2   umbilical granuloma (P83.81)

● **L93   Lupus erythematosus**
    Use additional code for adverse effect, if applicable, to identify drug (T36-T50 with fifth or sixth character 5)
    Excludes1   lupus exedens (A18.4)
                lupus vulgaris (A18.4)
                scleroderma (M34.-)
                systemic lupus erythematosus (M32.-)
    L93.0   Discoid lupus erythematosus
       Lupus erythematosus NOS
    L93.1   Subacute cutaneous lupus erythematosus
    L93.2   Other local lupus erythematosus
       Lupus erythematosus profundus
       Lupus panniculitis

● **L94   Other localized connective tissue disorders**
    Excludes1   systemic connective tissue disorders (M30-M36)
    L94.0   Localized scleroderma [morphea]
       Circumscribed scleroderma
    L94.1   Linear scleroderma
       En coup de sabre lesion
    L94.2   Calcinosis cutis
    L94.3   Sclerodactyly
    L94.4   Gottron's papules
    L94.5   Poikiloderma vasculare atrophicans
    L94.6   Ainhum
    L94.8   Other specified localized connective tissue disorders
    L94.9   Localized connective tissue disorder, unspecified

● **L95   Vasculitis limited to skin, not elsewhere classified**
    Excludes1   angioma serpiginosum (L81.7)
                Henoch(-Schönlein) purpura (D69.0)
                hypersensitivity angiitis (M31.0)
                lupus panniculitis (L93.2)
                panniculitis NOS (M79.3)
                panniculitis of neck and back (M54.0-)
                polyarteritis nodosa (M30.0)
                relapsing panniculitis (M35.6)
                rheumatoid vasculitis (M05.2)
                serum sickness (T80.6-)
                urticaria (L50.-)
                Wegener's granulomatosis (M31.3-)
    L95.0   Livedoid vasculitis
       Atrophie blanche (en plaque)
    L95.1   Erythema elevatum diutinum
    L95.8   Other vasculitis limited to the skin
    L95.9   Vasculitis limited to the skin, unspecified

▶ New   ⟰ Revised   ~~deleted~~ Deleted   Excludes 1   Excludes 2   Includes   Use additional   Code first   Code also   Key words

OGCR Official Guidelines   X Assign placeholder X   ● Use Additional Character(s)   ▶ Manifestation Code   🅗 Hierarchical Condition Category   Coding Clinic

● **L97**   **Non-pressure chronic ulcer of lower limb, not elsewhere classified**

    Includes   chronic ulcer of skin of lower limb NOS
                    non-healing ulcer of skin
                    non-infected sinus of skin
                    trophic ulcer NOS
                    tropical ulcer NOS
                    ulcer of skin of lower limb NOS

    Code first any associated underlying condition, such as:
       any associated gangrene (I96)
       atherosclerosis of the lower extremities (I70.23-, I70.24-, I70.33-, I70.34-, I70.43-, I70.44-, I70.53-, I70.54-, I70.63-, I70.64-, I70.73-, I70.74-)
       chronic venous hypertension (I87.31-, I87.33-)
       diabetic ulcers (E08.621, E08.622, E09.621, E09.622, E10.621, E10.622, E11.621, E11.622, E13.621, E13.622)
       postphlebitic syndrome (I87.01-, I87.03-)
       postthrombotic syndrome (I87.01-, I87.03-)
       varicose ulcer (I83.0-, I83.2-)

    Excludes2   pressure ulcer (pressure area) (L89.-)
                    skin infections (L00-L08)
                    specific infections classified to A00-B99

● **L97.1**   **Non-pressure chronic ulcer of thigh**

   ● **L97.10**   **Non-pressure chronic ulcer of unspecified thigh**

      L97.101   Non-pressure chronic ulcer of unspecified thigh limited to breakdown of skin 🔖

      L97.102   Non-pressure chronic ulcer of unspecified thigh with fat layer exposed 🔖

      L97.103   Non-pressure chronic ulcer of unspecified thigh with necrosis of muscle 🔖

      L97.104   Non-pressure chronic ulcer of unspecified thigh with necrosis of bone 🔖

      L97.105   Non-pressure chronic ulcer of unspecified thigh with muscle involvement without evidence of necrosis 🔖

      L97.106   Non-pressure chronic ulcer of unspecified thigh with bone involvement without evidence of necrosis 🔖

      L97.108   Non-pressure chronic ulcer of unspecified thigh with other specified severity 🔖

      L97.109   Non-pressure chronic ulcer of unspecified thigh with unspecified severity 🔖

   ● **L97.11**   **Non-pressure chronic ulcer of right thigh**

      L97.111   Non-pressure chronic ulcer of right thigh limited to breakdown of skin 🔖

      L97.112   Non-pressure chronic ulcer of right thigh with fat layer exposed 🔖

      L97.113   Non-pressure chronic ulcer of right thigh with necrosis of muscle 🔖

      L97.114   Non-pressure chronic ulcer of right thigh with necrosis of bone 🔖

      L97.115   Non-pressure chronic ulcer of right thigh with muscle involvement without evidence of necrosis 🔖

      L97.116   Non-pressure chronic ulcer of right thigh with bone involvement without evidence of necrosis 🔖

      L97.118   Non-pressure chronic ulcer of right thigh with other specified severity 🔖

      L97.119   Non-pressure chronic ulcer of right thigh with unspecified severity 🔖

● **L97.12**   **Non-pressure chronic ulcer of left thigh**

      L97.121   Non-pressure chronic ulcer of left thigh limited to breakdown of skin 🔖

      L97.122   Non-pressure chronic ulcer of left thigh with fat layer exposed 🔖

      L97.123   Non-pressure chronic ulcer of left thigh with necrosis of muscle 🔖

      L97.124   Non-pressure chronic ulcer of left thigh with necrosis of bone 🔖

      L97.125   Non-pressure chronic ulcer of left thigh with muscle involvement without evidence of necrosis 🔖

      L97.126   Non-pressure chronic ulcer of left thigh with bone involvement without evidence of necrosis 🔖

      L97.128   Non-pressure chronic ulcer of left thigh with other specified severity 🔖

      L97.129   Non-pressure chronic ulcer of left thigh with unspecified severity 🔖

● **L97.2**   **Non-pressure chronic ulcer of calf**

   ● **L97.20**   **Non-pressure chronic ulcer of unspecified calf**

      L97.201   Non-pressure chronic ulcer of unspecified calf limited to breakdown of skin 🔖

      L97.202   Non-pressure chronic ulcer of unspecified calf with fat layer exposed 🔖

      L97.203   Non-pressure chronic ulcer of unspecified calf with necrosis of muscle 🔖

      L97.204   Non-pressure chronic ulcer of unspecified calf with necrosis of bone 🔖

      L97.205   Non-pressure chronic ulcer of unspecified calf with muscle involvement without evidence of necrosis 🔖

      L97.206   Non-pressure chronic ulcer of unspecified calf with bone involvement without evidence of necrosis 🔖

      L97.208   Non-pressure chronic ulcer of unspecified calf with other specified severity 🔖

      L97.209   Non-pressure chronic ulcer of unspecified calf with unspecified severity 🔖

   ● **L97.21**   **Non-pressure chronic ulcer of right calf**

      L97.211   Non-pressure chronic ulcer of right calf limited to breakdown of skin 🔖

      L97.212   Non-pressure chronic ulcer of right calf with fat layer exposed 🔖

      L97.213   Non-pressure chronic ulcer of right calf with necrosis of muscle 🔖

      L97.214   Non-pressure chronic ulcer of right calf with necrosis of bone 🔖

      L97.215   Non-pressure chronic ulcer of right calf with muscle involvement without evidence of necrosis 🔖

      L97.216   Non-pressure chronic ulcer of right calf with bone involvement without evidence of necrosis 🔖

      L97.218   Non-pressure chronic ulcer of right calf with other specified severity 🔖

      L97.219   Non-pressure chronic ulcer of right calf with unspecified severity 🔖

   ● **L97.22**   **Non-pressure chronic ulcer of left calf**

      L97.221   Non-pressure chronic ulcer of left calf limited to breakdown of skin 🔖

      L97.222   Non-pressure chronic ulcer of left calf with fat layer exposed 🔖

L97.223   Non-pressure chronic ulcer of left calf with necrosis of muscle 🐾

L97.224   Non-pressure chronic ulcer of left calf with necrosis of bone 🐾

L97.225   Non-pressure chronic ulcer of left calf with muscle involvement without evidence of necrosis 🐾

L97.226   Non-pressure chronic ulcer of left calf with bone involvement without evidence of necrosis 🐾

L97.228   Non-pressure chronic ulcer of left calf with other specified severity 🐾

L97.229   Non-pressure chronic ulcer of left calf with unspecified severity 🐾

● L97.3   Non-pressure chronic ulcer of ankle

● L97.30   Non-pressure chronic ulcer of unspecified ankle

L97.301   Non-pressure chronic ulcer of unspecified ankle limited to breakdown of skin 🐾

L97.302   Non-pressure chronic ulcer of unspecified ankle with fat layer exposed 🐾

L97.303   Non-pressure chronic ulcer of unspecified ankle with necrosis of muscle 🐾

L97.304   Non-pressure chronic ulcer of unspecified ankle with necrosis of bone 🐾

L97.305   Non-pressure chronic ulcer of unspecified ankle with muscle involvement without evidence of necrosis 🐾

L97.306   Non-pressure chronic ulcer of unspecified ankle with bone involvement without evidence of necrosis 🐾

L97.308   Non-pressure chronic ulcer of unspecified ankle with other specified severity 🐾

L97.309   Non-pressure chronic ulcer of unspecified ankle with unspecified severity 🐾

● L97.31   Non-pressure chronic ulcer of right ankle

L97.311   Non-pressure chronic ulcer of right ankle limited to breakdown of skin 🐾

L97.312   Non-pressure chronic ulcer of right ankle with fat layer exposed 🐾

L97.313   Non-pressure chronic ulcer of right ankle with necrosis of muscle 🐾

L97.314   Non-pressure chronic ulcer of right ankle with necrosis of bone 🐾

L97.315   Non-pressure chronic ulcer of right ankle with muscle involvement without evidence of necrosis 🐾
          Coding Clinic: 2017, Q4, P17

L97.316   Non-pressure chronic ulcer of right ankle with bone involvement without evidence of necrosis 🐾

L97.318   Non-pressure chronic ulcer of right ankle with other specified severity 🐾

L97.319   Non-pressure chronic ulcer of right ankle with unspecified severity 🐾

● L97.32   Non-pressure chronic ulcer of left ankle

L97.321   Non-pressure chronic ulcer of left ankle limited to breakdown of skin 🐾

L97.322   Non-pressure chronic ulcer of left ankle with fat layer exposed 🐾
          Coding Clinic: 2021, Q1, P8

L97.323   Non-pressure chronic ulcer of left ankle with necrosis of muscle 🐾

L97.324   Non-pressure chronic ulcer of left ankle with necrosis of bone 🐾

L97.325   Non-pressure chronic ulcer of left ankle with muscle involvement without evidence of necrosis 🐾

L97.326   Non-pressure chronic ulcer of left ankle with bone involvement without evidence of necrosis 🐾

L97.328   Non-pressure chronic ulcer of left ankle with other specified severity 🐾

L97.329   Non-pressure chronic ulcer of left ankle with unspecified severity 🐾

● L97.4   Non-pressure chronic ulcer of heel and midfoot
          Non-pressure chronic ulcer of plantar surface of midfoot

● L97.40   Non-pressure chronic ulcer of unspecified heel and midfoot

L97.401   Non-pressure chronic ulcer of unspecified heel and midfoot limited to breakdown of skin 🐾

L97.402   Non-pressure chronic ulcer of unspecified heel and midfoot with fat layer exposed 🐾

L97.403   Non-pressure chronic ulcer of unspecified heel and midfoot with necrosis of muscle 🐾

L97.404   Non-pressure chronic ulcer of unspecified heel and midfoot with necrosis of bone 🐾

L97.405   Non-pressure chronic ulcer of unspecified heel and midfoot with muscle involvement without evidence of necrosis 🐾

L97.406   Non-pressure chronic ulcer of unspecified heel and midfoot with bone involvement without evidence of necrosis 🐾

L97.408   Non-pressure chronic ulcer of unspecified heel and midfoot with other specified severity 🐾

L97.409   Non-pressure chronic ulcer of unspecified heel and midfoot with unspecified severity 🐾

● L97.41   Non-pressure chronic ulcer of right heel and midfoot

L97.411   Non-pressure chronic ulcer of right heel and midfoot limited to breakdown of skin 🐾

L97.412   Non-pressure chronic ulcer of right heel and midfoot with fat layer exposed 🐾

L97.413   Non-pressure chronic ulcer of right heel and midfoot with necrosis of muscle 🐾

L97.414   Non-pressure chronic ulcer of right heel and midfoot with necrosis of bone 🐾

L97.415   Non-pressure chronic ulcer of right heel and midfoot with muscle involvement without evidence of necrosis 🐾

L97.416   Non-pressure chronic ulcer of right heel and midfoot with bone involvement without evidence of necrosis 🐾

L97.418   Non-pressure chronic ulcer of right heel and midfoot with other specified severity 🐾

L97.419   Non-pressure chronic ulcer of right heel and midfoot with unspecified severity 🐾

▶ New   ⇒ Revised   ~~deleted~~ Deleted   Excludes 1   Excludes 2   Includes   Use additional   Code first   Code also   Key words

OGCR Official Guidelines   X Assign placeholder X   ● Use Additional Character(s)   ◗ Manifestation Code   🐾 Hierarchical Condition Category   Coding Clinic

● **L97.42**   Non-pressure chronic ulcer of left heel and midfoot

     L97.421   Non-pressure chronic ulcer of left heel and midfoot limited to breakdown of skin 🔖
           Coding Clinic: 2016, Q1, P13

     L97.422   Non-pressure chronic ulcer of left heel and midfoot with fat layer exposed 🔖

     L97.423   Non-pressure chronic ulcer of left heel and midfoot with necrosis of muscle 🔖

     L97.424   Non-pressure chronic ulcer of left heel and midfoot with necrosis of bone 🔖

     L97.425   Non-pressure chronic ulcer of left heel and midfoot with muscle involvement without evidence of necrosis 🔖

     L97.426   Non-pressure chronic ulcer of left heel and midfoot with bone involvement without evidence of necrosis 🔖

     L97.428   Non-pressure chronic ulcer of left heel and midfoot with other specified severity 🔖

     L97.429   Non-pressure chronic ulcer of left heel and midfoot with unspecified severity 🔖

● **L97.5**   Non-pressure chronic ulcer of other part of foot
     Non-pressure chronic ulcer of toe

 ● **L97.50**   Non-pressure chronic ulcer of other part of unspecified foot

     L97.501   Non-pressure chronic ulcer of other part of unspecified foot limited to breakdown of skin 🔖

     L97.502   Non-pressure chronic ulcer of other part of unspecified foot with fat layer exposed 🔖

     L97.503   Non-pressure chronic ulcer of other part of unspecified foot with necrosis of muscle 🔖

     L97.504   Non-pressure chronic ulcer of other part of unspecified foot with necrosis of bone 🔖

     L97.505   Non-pressure chronic ulcer of other part of unspecified foot with muscle involvement without evidence of necrosis 🔖

     L97.506   Non-pressure chronic ulcer of other part of unspecified foot with bone involvement without evidence of necrosis 🔖

     L97.508   Non-pressure chronic ulcer of other part of unspecified foot with other specified severity 🔖

     L97.509   Non-pressure chronic ulcer of other part of unspecified foot with unspecified severity 🔖

 ● **L97.51**   Non-pressure chronic ulcer of other part of right foot

     L97.511   Non-pressure chronic ulcer of other part of right foot limited to breakdown of skin 🔖
           Coding Clinic: 2020, Q1, P12

     L97.512   Non-pressure chronic ulcer of other part of right foot with fat layer exposed 🔖

     L97.513   Non-pressure chronic ulcer of other part of right foot with necrosis of muscle 🔖

     L97.514   Non-pressure chronic ulcer of other part of right foot with necrosis of bone 🔖

     L97.515   Non-pressure chronic ulcer of other part of right foot with muscle involvement without evidence of necrosis 🔖

     L97.516   Non-pressure chronic ulcer of other part of right foot with bone involvement without evidence of necrosis 🔖

     L97.518   Non-pressure chronic ulcer of other part of right foot with other specified severity 🔖

     L97.519   Non-pressure chronic ulcer of other part of right foot with unspecified severity 🔖

● **L97.52**   Non-pressure chronic ulcer of other part of left foot

     L97.521   Non-pressure chronic ulcer of other part of left foot limited to breakdown of skin 🔖

     L97.522   Non-pressure chronic ulcer of other part of left foot with fat layer exposed 🔖

     L97.523   Non-pressure chronic ulcer of other part of left foot with necrosis of muscle 🔖

     L97.524   Non-pressure chronic ulcer of other part of left foot with necrosis of bone 🔖

     L97.525   Non-pressure chronic ulcer of other part of left foot with muscle involvement without evidence of necrosis 🔖

     L97.526   Non-pressure chronic ulcer of other part of left foot with bone involvement without evidence of necrosis 🔖

     L97.528   Non-pressure chronic ulcer of other part of left foot with other specified severity 🔖

     L97.529   Non-pressure chronic ulcer of other part of left foot with unspecified severity 🔖

● **L97.8**   Non-pressure chronic ulcer of other part of lower leg

 ● **L97.80**   Non-pressure chronic ulcer of other part of unspecified lower leg

     L97.801   Non-pressure chronic ulcer of other part of unspecified lower leg limited to breakdown of skin 🔖

     L97.802   Non-pressure chronic ulcer of other part of unspecified lower leg with fat layer exposed 🔖

     L97.803   Non-pressure chronic ulcer of other part of unspecified lower leg with necrosis of muscle 🔖

     L97.804   Non-pressure chronic ulcer of other part of unspecified lower leg with necrosis of bone 🔖

     L97.805   Non-pressure chronic ulcer of other part of unspecified lower leg with muscle involvement without evidence of necrosis 🔖

     L97.806   Non-pressure chronic ulcer of other part of unspecified lower leg with bone involvement without evidence of necrosis 🔖

     L97.808   Non-pressure chronic ulcer of other part of unspecified lower leg with other specified severity 🔖

     L97.809   Non-pressure chronic ulcer of other part of unspecified lower leg with unspecified severity 🔖

CHAPTER 12 (L00-L99)

CHAPTER 12 (L00-L99)

● **L97.81**   Non-pressure chronic ulcer of other part of right lower leg

    L97.811   Non-pressure chronic ulcer of other part of right lower leg limited to breakdown of skin 🔖

    L97.812   Non-pressure chronic ulcer of other part of right lower leg with fat layer exposed 🔖

    L97.813   Non-pressure chronic ulcer of other part of right lower leg with necrosis of muscle 🔖

    L97.814   Non-pressure chronic ulcer of other part of right lower leg with necrosis of bone 🔖

    L97.815   Non-pressure chronic ulcer of other part of right lower leg with muscle involvement without evidence of necrosis 🔖

    L97.816   Non-pressure chronic ulcer of other part of right lower leg with bone involvement without evidence of necrosis 🔖

    L97.818   Non-pressure chronic ulcer of other part of right lower leg with other specified severity 🔖

    L97.819   Non-pressure chronic ulcer of other part of right lower leg with unspecified severity 🔖

● **L97.82**   Non-pressure chronic ulcer of other part of left lower leg

    L97.821   Non-pressure chronic ulcer of other part of left lower leg limited to breakdown of skin 🔖

    L97.822   Non-pressure chronic ulcer of other part of left lower leg with fat layer exposed 🔖

    L97.823   Non-pressure chronic ulcer of other part of left lower leg with necrosis of muscle 🔖

    L97.824   Non-pressure chronic ulcer of other part of left lower leg with necrosis of bone 🔖

    L97.825   Non-pressure chronic ulcer of other part of left lower leg with muscle involvement without evidence of necrosis 🔖

    L97.826   Non-pressure chronic ulcer of other part of left lower leg with bone involvement without evidence of necrosis 🔖

    L97.828   Non-pressure chronic ulcer of other part of left lower leg with other specified severity 🔖

    L97.829   Non-pressure chronic ulcer of other part of left lower leg with unspecified severity 🔖

● **L97.9**   Non-pressure chronic ulcer of unspecified part of lower leg

 ● **L97.90**   Non-pressure chronic ulcer of unspecified part of unspecified lower leg

    L97.901   Non-pressure chronic ulcer of unspecified part of unspecified lower leg limited to breakdown of skin 🔖

    L97.902   Non-pressure chronic ulcer of unspecified part of unspecified lower leg with fat layer exposed 🔖

    L97.903   Non-pressure chronic ulcer of unspecified part of unspecified lower leg with necrosis of muscle 🔖

    L97.904   Non-pressure chronic ulcer of unspecified part of unspecified lower leg with necrosis of bone 🔖

    L97.905   Non-pressure chronic ulcer of unspecified part of unspecified lower leg with muscle involvement without evidence of necrosis 🔖

    L97.906   Non-pressure chronic ulcer of unspecified part of unspecified lower leg with bone involvement without evidence of necrosis 🔖

    L97.908   Non-pressure chronic ulcer of unspecified part of unspecified lower leg with other specified severity 🔖

    L97.909   Non-pressure chronic ulcer of unspecified part of unspecified lower leg with unspecified severity 🔖

● **L97.91**   Non-pressure chronic ulcer of unspecified part of right lower leg

    L97.911   Non-pressure chronic ulcer of unspecified part of right lower leg limited to breakdown of skin 🔖

    L97.912   Non-pressure chronic ulcer of unspecified part of right lower leg with fat layer exposed 🔖

    L97.913   Non-pressure chronic ulcer of unspecified part of right lower leg with necrosis of muscle 🔖

    L97.914   Non-pressure chronic ulcer of unspecified part of right lower leg with necrosis of bone 🔖

    L97.915   Non-pressure chronic ulcer of unspecified part of right lower leg with muscle involvement without evidence of necrosis 🔖

    L97.916   Non-pressure chronic ulcer of unspecified part of right lower leg with bone involvement without evidence of necrosis 🔖

    L97.918   Non-pressure chronic ulcer of unspecified part of right lower leg with other specified severity 🔖

    L97.919   Non-pressure chronic ulcer of unspecified part of right lower leg with unspecified severity 🔖

● **L97.92**   Non-pressure chronic ulcer of unspecified part of left lower leg

    L97.921   Non-pressure chronic ulcer of unspecified part of left lower leg limited to breakdown of skin 🔖

    L97.922   Non-pressure chronic ulcer of unspecified part of left lower leg with fat layer exposed 🔖

    L97.923   Non-pressure chronic ulcer of unspecified part of left lower leg with necrosis of muscle 🔖

    L97.924   Non-pressure chronic ulcer of unspecified part of left lower leg with necrosis of bone 🔖

    L97.925   Non-pressure chronic ulcer of unspecified part of left lower leg with muscle involvement without evidence of necrosis 🔖

    L97.926   Non-pressure chronic ulcer of unspecified part of left lower leg with bone involvement without evidence of necrosis 🔖

    L97.928   Non-pressure chronic ulcer of unspecified part of left lower leg with other specified severity 🔖

    L97.929   Non-pressure chronic ulcer of unspecified part of left lower leg with unspecified severity 🔖

▶ New   ⟹ Revised   ~~deleted~~ Deleted   Excludes 1   Excludes 2   Includes   Use additional   Code first   Code also   Key words

OGCR Official Guidelines   X Assign placeholder X   ● Use Additional Character(s)   ▶ Manifestation Code   🔖 Hierarchical Condition Category   **Coding Clinic**

● **L98**   **Other disorders of skin and subcutaneous tissue, not elsewhere classified**

   L98.0   **Pyogenic granuloma**

     Excludes2   pyogenic granuloma of gingiva (K06.8)
pyogenic granuloma of maxillary alveolar ridge (K04.5)
pyogenic granuloma of oral mucosa (K13.4)

   L98.1   **Factitial dermatitis**
Neurotic excoriation

     Excludes1   Excoriation (skin-picking) disorder (F42.4)

     Coding Clinic: 2016, Q4, P15

   L98.2   **Febrile neutrophilic dermatosis [Sweet]**

   L98.3   **Eosinophilic cellulitis [Wells]**

● **L98.4**   **Non-pressure chronic ulcer of skin, not elsewhere classified**
Chronic ulcer of skin NOS
Tropical ulcer NOS
Ulcer of skin NOS

     Excludes2   pressure ulcer (pressure area) (L89.-)
gangrene (I96) 🐾
skin infections (L00-L08)
specific infections classified to A00-B99
ulcer of lower limb NEC (L97.-)
varicose ulcer (I83.0-I83.93)

    ● **L98.41**   **Non-pressure chronic ulcer of buttock**

       L98.411   Non-pressure chronic ulcer of buttock limited to breakdown of skin 🐾

       L98.412   Non-pressure chronic ulcer of buttock with fat layer exposed 🐾

       L98.413   Non-pressure chronic ulcer of buttock with necrosis of muscle 🐾

       L98.414   Non-pressure chronic ulcer of buttock with necrosis of bone 🐾

       L98.415   Non-pressure chronic ulcer of buttock with muscle involvement without evidence of necrosis 🐾

       L98.416   Non-pressure chronic ulcer of buttock with bone involvement without evidence of necrosis 🐾

       L98.418   Non-pressure chronic ulcer of buttock with other specified severity 🐾

       L98.419   Non-pressure chronic ulcer of buttock with unspecified severity 🐾

    ● **L98.42**   **Non-pressure chronic ulcer of back**

       L98.421   Non-pressure chronic ulcer of back limited to breakdown of skin 🐾

       L98.422   Non-pressure chronic ulcer of back with fat layer exposed 🐾

       L98.423   Non-pressure chronic ulcer of back with necrosis of muscle 🐾

       L98.424   Non-pressure chronic ulcer of back with necrosis of bone 🐾

       L98.425   Non-pressure chronic ulcer of back with muscle involvement without evidence of necrosis 🐾

       L98.426   Non-pressure chronic ulcer of back with bone involvement without evidence of necrosis 🐾

       L98.428   Non-pressure chronic ulcer of back with other specified severity 🐾

       L98.429   Non-pressure chronic ulcer of back with unspecified severity 🐾

    ● **L98.49**   **Non-pressure chronic ulcer of skin of other sites**
Non-pressure chronic ulcer of skin NOS

       L98.491   Non-pressure chronic ulcer of skin of other sites limited to breakdown of skin 🐾

       L98.492   Non-pressure chronic ulcer of skin of other sites with fat layer exposed 🐾

       L98.493   Non-pressure chronic ulcer of skin of other sites with necrosis of muscle 🐾

       L98.494   Non-pressure chronic ulcer of skin of other sites with necrosis of bone 🐾

       L98.495   Non-pressure chronic ulcer of skin of other sites with muscle involvement without evidence of necrosis 🐾

       L98.496   Non-pressure chronic ulcer of skin of other sites with bone involvement without evidence of necrosis 🐾

       L98.498   Non-pressure chronic ulcer of skin of other sites with other specified severity 🐾

       L98.499   Non-pressure chronic ulcer of skin of other sites with unspecified severity 🐾

   L98.5   **Mucinosis of the skin**
Focal mucinosis
Lichen myxedematosus
Reticular erythematous mucinosis

     Excludes1   focal oral mucinosis (K13.79)
myxedema (E03.9)

   L98.6   **Other infiltrative disorders of the skin and subcutaneous tissue**

     Excludes1   hyalinosis cutis et mucosae (E78.89)

   L98.7   **Excessive and redundant skin and subcutaneous tissue**
Loose or sagging skin following bariatric surgery weight loss
Loose or sagging skin following dietary weight loss
Loose or sagging skin, NOS

     Excludes2   acquired excess or redundant skin of eyelid (H02.3-)
congenital excess or redundant skin of eyelid (Q10.3)
skin changes due to chronic exposure to nonionizing radiation (L57.-)

     Coding Clinic: 2016, Q4, P36

   L98.8   **Other specified disorders of the skin and subcutaneous tissue**

     Coding Clinic: 2013, Q2, P32

   L98.9   **Disorder of the skin and subcutaneous tissue, unspecified**

▷ *L99*   *Other disorders of skin and subcutaneous tissue in diseases classified elsewhere*

     Code first underlying disease, such as:
amyloidosis (E85.-)

     Excludes1   skin disorders in diabetes (E08-E13 with .62-)
skin disorders in gonorrhea (A54.89)
skin disorders in syphilis (A51.31, A52.79)

CHAPTER 13

DISEASES OF THE MUSCULOSKELETAL SYSTEM AND CONNECTIVE TISSUE (M00-M99)

OGCR Chapter-Specific Coding Guidelines

13. **Chapter 13: Diseases of the Musculoskeletal System and Connective Tissue (M00-M99)**

   a. Site and laterality

   Most of the codes within Chapter 13 have site and laterality designations. The site represents the bone, joint or the muscle involved. For some conditions where more than one bone, joint or muscle is usually involved, such as osteoarthritis, there is a "multiple sites" code available. For categories where no multiple site code is provided and more than one bone, joint or muscle is involved, multiple codes should be used to indicate the different sites involved.

   1) Bone versus joint

   For certain conditions, the bone may be affected at the upper or lower end (e.g., avascular necrosis of bone, M87, Osteoporosis, M80, M81). Though the portion of the bone affected may be at the joint, the site designation will be the bone, not the joint.

   b. Acute traumatic versus chronic or recurrent musculoskeletal conditions

   Many musculoskeletal conditions are a result of previous injury or trauma to a site, or are recurrent conditions. Bone, joint or muscle conditions that are the result of a healed injury are usually found in Chapter 13. Recurrent bone, joint or muscle conditions are also usually found in Chapter 13. Any current, acute injury should be coded to the appropriate injury code from Chapter 19. Chronic or recurrent conditions should generally be coded with a code from Chapter 13. If it is difficult to determine from the documentation in the record which code is best to describe a condition, query the provider.

   c. Coding of Pathologic Fractures

   7th character A is for use as long as the patient is receiving active treatment for the fracture. While the patient may be seen by a new or different provider over the course of treatment for a pathological fracture, assignment of the 7th character is based on whether the patient is undergoing active treatment and not whether the provider is seeing the patient for the first time.

   7th character, D is to be used for encounters after the patient has completed active treatment for the fracture and is receiving routine care for the fracture during the healing or recovery phase. The other 7th characters, listed under each subcategory in the Tabular List, are to be used for subsequent encounters for treatment of problems associated with the healing, such as malunions, nonunions, and sequelae.

   Care for complications of surgical treatment for fracture repairs during the healing or recovery phase should be coded with the appropriate complication codes.

   See Section I.C.19. Coding of traumatic fractures.

   d. Osteoporosis

   Osteoporosis is a systemic condition, meaning that all bones of the musculoskeletal system are affected. Therefore, site is not a component of the codes under category M81, Osteoporosis without current pathological fracture. The site codes under category M80, Osteoporosis with current pathological fracture, identify the site of the fracture, not the osteoporosis.

   1) Osteoporosis without pathological fracture

   Category M81, Osteoporosis without current pathological fracture, is for use for patients with osteoporosis who do not currently have a pathologic fracture due to the osteoporosis, even if they have had a fracture in the past. For patients with a history of osteoporosis fractures, status code Z87.310, Personal history of (healed) osteoporosis fracture, should follow the code from M81.

   2) Osteoporosis with current pathological fracture

   Category M80, Osteoporosis with current pathological fracture, is for patients who have a current pathologic fracture at the time of an encounter. The codes under M80 identify the site of the fracture. A code from category M80, not a traumatic fracture code, should be used for any patient with known osteoporosis who suffers a fracture, even if the patient had a minor fall or trauma, if that fall or trauma would not usually break a normal, healthy bone.

CHAPTER 13

DISEASES OF THE MUSCULOSKELETAL SYSTEM AND CONNECTIVE TISSUE (M00-M99)

Note: Use an external cause code following the code for the musculoskeletal condition, if applicable, to identify the cause of the musculoskeletal condition

Excludes2   arthropathic psoriasis (L40.5-)
certain conditions originating in the perinatal period (P04-P96)
certain infectious and parasitic diseases (A00-B99)
compartment syndrome (traumatic) (T79.A-)
complications of pregnancy, childbirth and the puerperium (O00-O9A)
congenital malformations, deformations, and chromosomal abnormalities (Q00-Q99)
endocrine, nutritional and metabolic diseases (E00-E88)
injury, poisoning and certain other consequences of external causes (S00-T88)
neoplasms (C00-D49)
symptoms, signs and abnormal clinical and laboratory findings, not elsewhere classified (R00-R94)

This chapter contains the following blocks:

M00-M02	Infectious arthropathies
M04	Autoinflammatory syndromes
M05-M14	Inflammatory polyarthropathies
M15-M19	Osteoarthritis
M20-M25	Other joint disorders
M26-M27	Dentofacial anomalies [including malocclusion] and other disorders of jaw
M30-M36	Systemic connective tissue disorders
M40-M43	Deforming dorsopathies
M45-M49	Spondylopathies
M50-M54	Other dorsopathies
M60-M63	Disorders of muscles
M65-M67	Disorders of synovium and tendon
M70-M79	Other soft tissue disorders
M80-M85	Disorders of bone density and structure
M86-M90	Other osteopathies
M91-M94	Chondropathies
M95	Other disorders of the musculoskeletal system and connective tissue
M96	Intraoperative and postprocedural complications and disorders of musculoskeletal system, not elsewhere classified
M97	Periprosthetic fracture around internal prosthetic joint
M99	Biomechanical lesions, not elsewhere classified

Coding Clinic: 2016, Q4, P124

ARTHROPATHIES (M00-M25)

Includes   Disorders affecting predominantly peripheral (limb) joints

INFECTIOUS ARTHROPATHIES (M00-M02)

Note: This block comprises arthropathies due to microbiological agents.

Distinction is made between the following types of etiological relationship:

a) direct infection of joint, where organisms invade synovial tissue and microbial antigen is present in the joint;

b) indirect infection, which may be of two types: a reactive arthropathy, where microbial infection of the body is established but neither organisms nor antigens can be identified in the joint, and a postinfective arthropathy, where microbial antigen is present but recovery of an organism is inconstant and evidence of local multiplication is lacking.

▶ New   ⇒ Revised   ~~deleted~~ Deleted   Excludes 1   Excludes 2   Includes   Use additional   Code first   Code also   Key words
OGCR Official Guidelines   X Assign placeholder X   ● Use Additional Character(s)   ▶ Manifestation Code   🝱 Hierarchical Condition Category   Coding Clinic

● **M00   Pyogenic arthritis**
     Excludes2   infection and inflammatory reaction due to internal joint prosthesis (T84.5-)

● **M00.0   Staphylococcal arthritis and polyarthritis**
     Use additional code (B95.61-B95.8) to identify bacterial agent
     M00.00   Staphylococcal arthritis, unspecified joint 🔊
●   **M00.01   Staphylococcal arthritis, shoulder**
     M00.011   Staphylococcal arthritis, right shoulder 🔊
     M00.012   Staphylococcal arthritis, left shoulder 🔊
     M00.019   Staphylococcal arthritis, unspecified shoulder 🔊
●   **M00.02   Staphylococcal arthritis, elbow**
     M00.021   Staphylococcal arthritis, right elbow 🔊
     M00.022   Staphylococcal arthritis, left elbow 🔊
     M00.029   Staphylococcal arthritis, unspecified elbow 🔊
●   **M00.03   Staphylococcal arthritis, wrist**
     Staphylococcal arthritis of carpal bones
     M00.031   Staphylococcal arthritis, right wrist 🔊
     M00.032   Staphylococcal arthritis, left wrist 🔊
     M00.039   Staphylococcal arthritis, unspecified wrist 🔊
●   **M00.04   Staphylococcal arthritis, hand**
     Staphylococcal arthritis of metacarpus and phalanges
     M00.041   Staphylococcal arthritis, right hand 🔊
     M00.042   Staphylococcal arthritis, left hand 🔊
     M00.049   Staphylococcal arthritis, unspecified hand 🔊
●   **M00.05   Staphylococcal arthritis, hip**
     M00.051   Staphylococcal arthritis, right hip 🔊
     M00.052   Staphylococcal arthritis, left hip 🔊
     M00.059   Staphylococcal arthritis, unspecified hip 🔊
●   **M00.06   Staphylococcal arthritis, knee**
     M00.061   Staphylococcal arthritis, right knee 🔊
     M00.062   Staphylococcal arthritis, left knee 🔊
     M00.069   Staphylococcal arthritis, unspecified knee 🔊
●   **M00.07   Staphylococcal arthritis, ankle and foot**
     Staphylococcal arthritis, tarsus, metatarsus and phalanges
     M00.071   Staphylococcal arthritis, right ankle and foot 🔊
     M00.072   Staphylococcal arthritis, left ankle and foot 🔊
     M00.079   Staphylococcal arthritis, unspecified ankle and foot 🔊
     M00.08   Staphylococcal arthritis, vertebrae 🔊
     M00.09   Staphylococcal polyarthritis 🔊
● **M00.1   Pneumococcal arthritis and polyarthritis**
     M00.10   Pneumococcal arthritis, unspecified joint 🔊
●   **M00.11   Pneumococcal arthritis, shoulder**
     M00.111   Pneumococcal arthritis, right shoulder 🔊
     M00.112   Pneumococcal arthritis, left shoulder 🔊
     M00.119   Pneumococcal arthritis, unspecified shoulder 🔊

●   **M00.12   Pneumococcal arthritis, elbow**
     M00.121   Pneumococcal arthritis, right elbow 🔊
     M00.122   Pneumococcal arthritis, left elbow 🔊
     M00.129   Pneumococcal arthritis, unspecified elbow 🔊
●   **M00.13   Pneumococcal arthritis, wrist**
     Pneumococcal arthritis of carpal bones
     M00.131   Pneumococcal arthritis, right wrist 🔊
     M00.132   Pneumococcal arthritis, left wrist 🔊
     M00.139   Pneumococcal arthritis, unspecified wrist 🔊
●   **M00.14   Pneumococcal arthritis, hand**
     Pneumococcal arthritis of metacarpus and phalanges
     M00.141   Pneumococcal arthritis, right hand 🔊
     M00.142   Pneumococcal arthritis, left hand 🔊
     M00.149   Pneumococcal arthritis, unspecified hand 🔊
●   **M00.15   Pneumococcal arthritis, hip**
     M00.151   Pneumococcal arthritis, right hip 🔊
     M00.152   Pneumococcal arthritis, left hip 🔊
     M00.159   Pneumococcal arthritis, unspecified hip 🔊
●   **M00.16   Pneumococcal arthritis, knee**
     M00.161   Pneumococcal arthritis, right knee 🔊
     M00.162   Pneumococcal arthritis, left knee 🔊
     M00.169   Pneumococcal arthritis, unspecified knee 🔊
●   **M00.17   Pneumococcal arthritis, ankle and foot**
     Pneumococcal arthritis, tarsus, metatarsus and phalanges
     M00.171   Pneumococcal arthritis, right ankle and foot 🔊
     M00.172   Pneumococcal arthritis, left ankle and foot 🔊
     M00.179   Pneumococcal arthritis, unspecified ankle and foot 🔊
     M00.18   Pneumococcal arthritis, vertebrae 🔊
     M00.19   Pneumococcal polyarthritis 🔊
● **M00.2   Other streptococcal arthritis and polyarthritis**
     Use additional code (B95.0-B95.2, B95.4-B95.5) to identify bacterial agent
     M00.20   Other streptococcal arthritis, unspecified joint 🔊
●   **M00.21   Other streptococcal arthritis, shoulder**
     M00.211   Other streptococcal arthritis, right shoulder 🔊
     M00.212   Other streptococcal arthritis, left shoulder 🔊
     M00.219   Other streptococcal arthritis, unspecified shoulder 🔊
●   **M00.22   Other streptococcal arthritis, elbow**
     M00.221   Other streptococcal arthritis, right elbow 🔊
     M00.222   Other streptococcal arthritis, left elbow 🔊
     M00.229   Other streptococcal arthritis, unspecified elbow 🔊
●   **M00.23   Other streptococcal arthritis, wrist**
     Other streptococcal arthritis of carpal bones
     M00.231   Other streptococcal arthritis, right wrist 🔊
     M00.232   Other streptococcal arthritis, left wrist 🔊
     M00.239   Other streptococcal arthritis, unspecified wrist 🔊

CHAPTER 13 (M00-M99)

● **M00.24**   **Other streptococcal arthritis, hand**
Other streptococcal arthritis metacarpus and phalanges

   M00.241   Other streptococcal arthritis, right hand 🦠

   M00.242   Other streptococcal arthritis, left hand 🦠

   M00.249   Other streptococcal arthritis, unspecified hand 🦠

● **M00.25**   **Other streptococcal arthritis, hip**

   M00.251   Other streptococcal arthritis, right hip 🦠

   M00.252   Other streptococcal arthritis, left hip 🦠

   M00.259   Other streptococcal arthritis, unspecified hip 🦠

● **M00.26**   **Other streptococcal arthritis, knee**

   M00.261   Other streptococcal arthritis, right knee 🦠

   M00.262   Other streptococcal arthritis, left knee 🦠

   M00.269   Other streptococcal arthritis, unspecified knee 🦠

● **M00.27**   **Other streptococcal arthritis, ankle and foot**
Other streptococcal arthritis, tarsus, metatarsus and phalanges

   M00.271   Other streptococcal arthritis, right ankle and foot 🦠

   M00.272   Other streptococcal arthritis, left ankle and foot 🦠

   M00.279   Other streptococcal arthritis, unspecified ankle and foot 🦠

   M00.28   Other streptococcal arthritis, vertebrae 🦠

   M00.29   Other streptococcal polyarthritis 🦠

● **M00.8**   **Arthritis and polyarthritis due to other bacteria**
Use additional code (B96) to identify bacteria

   M00.80   Arthritis due to other bacteria, unspecified joint 🦠

● **M00.81**   **Arthritis due to other bacteria, shoulder**

   M00.811   Arthritis due to other bacteria, right shoulder 🦠

   M00.812   Arthritis due to other bacteria, left shoulder 🦠

   M00.819   Arthritis due to other bacteria, unspecified shoulder 🦠

● **M00.82**   **Arthritis due to other bacteria, elbow**

   M00.821   Arthritis due to other bacteria, right elbow 🦠

   M00.822   Arthritis due to other bacteria, left elbow 🦠

   M00.829   Arthritis due to other bacteria, unspecified elbow 🦠

● **M00.83**   **Arthritis due to other bacteria, wrist**
Arthritis due to other bacteria, carpal bones

   M00.831   Arthritis due to other bacteria, right wrist 🦠

   M00.832   Arthritis due to other bacteria, left wrist 🦠

   M00.839   Arthritis due to other bacteria, unspecified wrist 🦠

● **M00.84**   **Arthritis due to other bacteria, hand**
Arthritis due to other bacteria, metacarpus and phalanges

   M00.841   Arthritis due to other bacteria, right hand 🦠

   M00.842   Arthritis due to other bacteria, left hand 🦠

   M00.849   Arthritis due to other bacteria, unspecified hand 🦠

● **M00.85**   **Arthritis due to other bacteria, hip**

   M00.851   Arthritis due to other bacteria, right hip 🦠

   M00.852   Arthritis due to other bacteria, left hip 🦠

   M00.859   Arthritis due to other bacteria, unspecified hip 🦠

● **M00.86**   **Arthritis due to other bacteria, knee**

   M00.861   Arthritis due to other bacteria, right knee 🦠

   M00.862   Arthritis due to other bacteria, left knee 🦠
        Coding Clinic: 2019, Q3, P16

   M00.869   Arthritis due to other bacteria, unspecified knee 🦠

● **M00.87**   **Arthritis due to other bacteria, ankle and foot**
Arthritis due to other bacteria, tarsus, metatarsus, and phalanges

   M00.871   Arthritis due to other bacteria, right ankle and foot 🦠

   M00.872   Arthritis due to other bacteria, left ankle and foot 🦠

   M00.879   Arthritis due to other bacteria, unspecified ankle and foot 🦠

   M00.88   Arthritis due to other bacteria, vertebrae 🦠

   M00.89   Polyarthritis due to other bacteria 🦠

● **M00.9**   **Pyogenic arthritis, unspecified** 🦠
Infective arthritis NOS

● **M01**   **Direct infections of joint in infectious and parasitic diseases classified elsewhere**

> *Code first* underlying disease, such as:
> leprosy [Hansen's disease] (A30.-)
> mycoses (B35-B49)
> O'nyong-nyong fever (A92.1)
> paratyphoid fever (A01.1-A01.4)

Excludes1   arthropathy in Lyme disease (A69.23)
       gonococcal arthritis (A54.42)
       meningococcal arthritis (A39.83)
       mumps arthritis (B26.85)
       postinfective arthropathy (M02.-)
       postmeningococcal arthritis (A39.84)
       reactive arthritis (M02.3)
       rubella arthritis (B06.82)
       sarcoidosis arthritis (D86.86)
       typhoid fever arthritis (A01.04)
       tuberculosis arthritis (A18.01-A18.02)

● **M01.X**   **Direct infection of joint in infectious and parasitic diseases classified elsewhere**

▷ *M01.X0*   *Direct infection of unspecified joint in infectious and parasitic diseases classified elsewhere* 🦠

● *M01.X1*   *Direct infection of shoulder joint in infectious and parasitic diseases classified elsewhere*

▷ *M01.X11*   *Direct infection of right shoulder in infectious and parasitic diseases classified elsewhere* 🦠

▷ *M01.X12*   *Direct infection of left shoulder in infectious and parasitic diseases classified elsewhere* 🦠

▷ *M01.X19*   *Direct infection of unspecified shoulder in infectious and parasitic diseases classified elsewhere* 🦠

● *M01.X2*   *Direct infection of elbow in infectious and parasitic diseases classified elsewhere*

▷ *M01.X21*   *Direct infection of right elbow in infectious and parasitic diseases classified elsewhere* 🦠

▷ *M01.X22*   *Direct infection of left elbow in infectious and parasitic diseases classified elsewhere* 🦠

▷ *M01.X29*   *Direct infection of unspecified elbow in infectious and parasitic diseases classified elsewhere* 🦠

▶ New   ⇒ Revised   ~~deleted~~ Deleted   Excludes 1   Excludes 2   Includes   Use additional   Code first   Code also   Key words

OGCR Official Guidelines   X Assign placeholder X   ● Use Additional Character(s)   ▷ Manifestation Code   🦠 Hierarchical Condition Category   Coding Clinic

● **M01.X3** **Direct infection of wrist in infectious and parasitic diseases classified elsewhere**
 Direct infection of carpal bones in infectious and parasitic diseases classified elsewhere

▸ *M01.X31* *Direct infection of right wrist in infectious and parasitic diseases classified elsewhere* 🔲

▸ *M01.X32* *Direct infection of left wrist in infectious and parasitic diseases classified elsewhere* 🔲

▸ *M01.X39* *Direct infection of unspecified wrist in infectious and parasitic diseases classified elsewhere* 🔲

● **M01.X4** **Direct infection of hand in infectious and parasitic diseases classified elsewhere**
 Direct infection of metacarpus and phalanges in infectious and parasitic diseases classified elsewhere

▸ *M01.X41* *Direct infection of right hand in infectious and parasitic diseases classified elsewhere* 🔲

▸ *M01.X42* *Direct infection of left hand in infectious and parasitic diseases classified elsewhere* 🔲

▸ *M01.X49* *Direct infection of unspecified hand in infectious and parasitic diseases classified elsewhere* 🔲

● **M01.X5** **Direct infection of hip in infectious and parasitic diseases classified elsewhere**

▸ *M01.X51* *Direct infection of right hip in infectious and parasitic diseases classified elsewhere* 🔲

▸ *M01.X52* *Direct infection of left hip in infectious and parasitic diseases classified elsewhere* 🔲

▸ *M01.X59* *Direct infection of unspecified hip in infectious and parasitic diseases classified elsewhere* 🔲

● **M01.X6** **Direct infection of knee in infectious and parasitic diseases classified elsewhere**

▸ *M01.X61* *Direct infection of right knee in infectious and parasitic diseases classified elsewhere* 🔲

▸ *M01.X62* *Direct infection of left knee in infectious and parasitic diseases classified elsewhere* 🔲

▸ *M01.X69* *Direct infection of unspecified knee in infectious and parasitic diseases classified elsewhere* 🔲

● **M01.X7** **Direct infection of ankle and foot in infectious and parasitic diseases classified elsewhere**
 Direct infection of tarsus, metatarsus and phalanges in infectious and parasitic diseases classified elsewhere

▸ *M01.X71* *Direct infection of right ankle and foot in infectious and parasitic diseases classified elsewhere* 🔲

▸ *M01.X72* *Direct infection of left ankle and foot in infectious and parasitic diseases classified elsewhere* 🔲

▸ *M01.X79* *Direct infection of unspecified ankle and foot in infectious and parasitic diseases classified elsewhere* 🔲

▸ *M01.X8* *Direct infection of vertebrae in infectious and parasitic diseases classified elsewhere* 🔲

▸ *M01.X9* *Direct infection of multiple joints in infectious and parasitic diseases classified elsewhere* 🔲

● **M02** **Postinfective and reactive arthropathies**
 Code first underlying disease, such as:
 congenital syphilis [Clutton's joints] (A50.5)
 enteritis due to Yersinia enterocolitica (A04.6)
 infective endocarditis (I33.0)
 viral hepatitis (B15-B19)

 Excludes1 Behçet's disease (M35.2)
 direct infections of joint in infectious and parasitic diseases classified elsewhere (M01.-)
 postmeningococcal arthritis (A39.84)
 mumps arthritis (B26.85)
 rubella arthritis (B06.82)
 syphilis arthritis (late) (A52.77)
 rheumatic fever (I00)
 tabetic arthropathy [Charcôt's] (A52.16)

● **M02.0** **Arthropathy following intestinal bypass**

 M02.00 **Arthropathy following intestinal bypass, unspecified site**

● **M02.01** **Arthropathy following intestinal bypass, shoulder**

 M02.011 **Arthropathy following intestinal bypass, right shoulder**

 M02.012 **Arthropathy following intestinal bypass, left shoulder**

 M02.019 **Arthropathy following intestinal bypass, unspecified shoulder**

● **M02.02** **Arthropathy following intestinal bypass, elbow**

 M02.021 **Arthropathy following intestinal bypass, right elbow**

 M02.022 **Arthropathy following intestinal bypass, left elbow**

 M02.029 **Arthropathy following intestinal bypass, unspecified elbow**

● **M02.03** **Arthropathy following intestinal bypass, wrist**
 Arthropathy following intestinal bypass, carpal bones

 M02.031 **Arthropathy following intestinal bypass, right wrist**

 M02.032 **Arthropathy following intestinal bypass, left wrist**

 M02.039 **Arthropathy following intestinal bypass, unspecified wrist**

● **M02.04** **Arthropathy following intestinal bypass, hand**
 Arthropathy following intestinal bypass, metacarpals and phalanges

 M02.041 **Arthropathy following intestinal bypass, right hand**

 M02.042 **Arthropathy following intestinal bypass, left hand**

 M02.049 **Arthropathy following intestinal bypass, unspecified hand**

● **M02.05** **Arthropathy following intestinal bypass, hip**

 M02.051 **Arthropathy following intestinal bypass, right hip**

 M02.052 **Arthropathy following intestinal bypass, left hip**

 M02.059 **Arthropathy following intestinal bypass, unspecified hip**

● **M02.06** **Arthropathy following intestinal bypass, knee**

 M02.061 **Arthropathy following intestinal bypass, right knee**

 M02.062 **Arthropathy following intestinal bypass, left knee**

 M02.069 **Arthropathy following intestinal bypass, unspecified knee**

CHAPTER 13 (M00-M99)

● M02.07 **Arthropathy following intestinal bypass, ankle and foot**
Arthropathy following intestinal bypass, tarsus, metatarsus and phalanges

   M02.071 Arthropathy following intestinal bypass, right ankle and foot

   M02.072 Arthropathy following intestinal bypass, left ankle and foot

   M02.079 Arthropathy following intestinal bypass, unspecified ankle and foot

M02.08 **Arthropathy following intestinal bypass, vertebrae**

M02.09 **Arthropathy following intestinal bypass, multiple sites**

● M02.1 **Postdysenteric arthropathy**

   M02.10 Postdysenteric arthropathy, unspecified site ℞

● M02.11 Postdysenteric arthropathy, shoulder

   M02.111 Postdysenteric arthropathy, right shoulder ℞

   M02.112 Postdysenteric arthropathy, left shoulder ℞

   M02.119 Postdysenteric arthropathy, unspecified shoulder ℞

● M02.12 Postdysenteric arthropathy, elbow

   M02.121 Postdysenteric arthropathy, right elbow ℞

   M02.122 Postdysenteric arthropathy, left elbow ℞

   M02.129 Postdysenteric arthropathy, unspecified elbow ℞

● M02.13 Postdysenteric arthropathy, wrist
Postdysenteric arthropathy, carpal bones

   M02.131 Postdysenteric arthropathy, right wrist ℞

   M02.132 Postdysenteric arthropathy, left wrist ℞

   M02.139 Postdysenteric arthropathy, unspecified wrist ℞

● M02.14 Postdysenteric arthropathy, hand
Postdysenteric arthropathy, metacarpus and phalanges

   M02.141 Postdysenteric arthropathy, right hand ℞

   M02.142 Postdysenteric arthropathy, left hand ℞

   M02.149 Postdysenteric arthropathy, unspecified hand ℞

● M02.15 Postdysenteric arthropathy, hip

   M02.151 Postdysenteric arthropathy, right hip ℞

   M02.152 Postdysenteric arthropathy, left hip ℞

   M02.159 Postdysenteric arthropathy, unspecified hip ℞

● M02.16 Postdysenteric arthropathy, knee

   M02.161 Postdysenteric arthropathy, right knee ℞

   M02.162 Postdysenteric arthropathy, left knee ℞

   M02.169 Postdysenteric arthropathy, unspecified knee ℞

● M02.17 Postdysenteric arthropathy, ankle and foot
Postdysenteric arthropathy, tarsus, metatarsus and phalanges

   M02.171 Postdysenteric arthropathy, right ankle and foot ℞

   M02.172 Postdysenteric arthropathy, left ankle and foot ℞

   M02.179 Postdysenteric arthropathy, unspecified ankle and foot ℞

M02.18 Postdysenteric arthropathy, vertebrae ℞

M02.19 Postdysenteric arthropathy, multiple sites ℞

● M02.2 **Postimmunization arthropathy**

   M02.20 Postimmunization arthropathy, unspecified site

● M02.21 Postimmunization arthropathy, shoulder

   M02.211 Postimmunization arthropathy, right shoulder

   M02.212 Postimmunization arthropathy, left shoulder

   M02.219 Postimmunization arthropathy, unspecified shoulder

● M02.22 Postimmunization arthropathy, elbow

   M02.221 Postimmunization arthropathy, right elbow

   M02.222 Postimmunization arthropathy, left elbow

   M02.229 Postimmunization arthropathy, unspecified elbow

● M02.23 Postimmunization arthropathy, wrist
Postimmunization arthropathy, carpal bones

   M02.231 Postimmunization arthropathy, right wrist

   M02.232 Postimmunization arthropathy, left wrist

   M02.239 Postimmunization arthropathy, unspecified wrist

● M02.24 Postimmunization arthropathy, hand
Postimmunization arthropathy, metacarpus and phalanges

   M02.241 Postimmunization arthropathy, right hand

   M02.242 Postimmunization arthropathy, left hand

   M02.249 Postimmunization arthropathy, unspecified hand

● M02.25 Postimmunization arthropathy, hip

   M02.251 Postimmunization arthropathy, right hip

   M02.252 Postimmunization arthropathy, left hip

   M02.259 Postimmunization arthropathy, unspecified hip

● M02.26 Postimmunization arthropathy, knee

   M02.261 Postimmunization arthropathy, right knee

   M02.262 Postimmunization arthropathy, left knee

   M02.269 Postimmunization arthropathy, unspecified knee

● M02.27 Postimmunization arthropathy, ankle and foot
Postimmunization arthropathy, tarsus, metatarsus and phalanges

   M02.271 Postimmunization arthropathy, right ankle and foot

   M02.272 Postimmunization arthropathy, left ankle and foot

   M02.279 Postimmunization arthropathy, unspecified ankle and foot

M02.28 Postimmunization arthropathy, vertebrae

M02.29 Postimmunization arthropathy, multiple sites

● M02.3 **Reiter's disease**
Reactive arthritis

   M02.30 Reiter's disease, unspecified site ℞

● M02.31 Reiter's disease, shoulder

   M02.311 Reiter's disease, right shoulder ℞

   M02.312 Reiter's disease, left shoulder ℞

   M02.319 Reiter's disease, unspecified shoulder ℞

▶ New ⇒ Revised ~~deleted~~ Deleted | Excludes 1 | | Excludes 2 | | Includes | | Use additional | | Code first | | Code also | | Key words |

OGCR Official Guidelines X Assign placeholder X ● Use Additional Character(s) ❱ Manifestation Code ℞ Hierarchical Condition Category **Coding Clinic**

● **M02.32 Reiter's disease, elbow**
    M02.321 Reiter's disease, right elbow 🔗
    M02.322 Reiter's disease, left elbow 🔗
    M02.329 Reiter's disease, unspecified elbow 🔗

● **M02.33 Reiter's disease, wrist**
    Reiter's disease, carpal bones
    M02.331 Reiter's disease, right wrist 🔗
    M02.332 Reiter's disease, left wrist 🔗
    M02.339 Reiter's disease, unspecified wrist 🔗

● **M02.34 Reiter's disease, hand**
    Reiter's disease, metacarpus and phalanges
    M02.341 Reiter's disease, right hand 🔗
    M02.342 Reiter's disease, left hand 🔗
    M02.349 Reiter's disease, unspecified hand 🔗

● **M02.35 Reiter's disease, hip**
    M02.351 Reiter's disease, right hip 🔗
    M02.352 Reiter's disease, left hip 🔗
    M02.359 Reiter's disease, unspecified hip 🔗

● **M02.36 Reiter's disease, knee**
    M02.361 Reiter's disease, right knee 🔗
    M02.362 Reiter's disease, left knee 🔗
    M02.369 Reiter's disease, unspecified knee 🔗

● **M02.37 Reiter's disease, ankle and foot**
    Reiter's disease, tarsus, metatarsus and phalanges
    M02.371 Reiter's disease, right ankle and foot 🔗
    M02.372 Reiter's disease, left ankle and foot 🔗
    M02.379 Reiter's disease, unspecified ankle and foot 🔗

    M02.38 Reiter's disease, vertebrae 🔗
    M02.39 Reiter's disease, multiple sites 🔗

● **M02.8 Other reactive arthropathies**
  ▸ *M02.80 Other reactive arthropathies, unspecified site* 🔗
  ● **M02.81 Other reactive arthropathies, shoulder**
    ▸ *M02.811 Other reactive arthropathies, right shoulder* 🔗
    ▸ *M02.812 Other reactive arthropathies, left shoulder* 🔗
    ▸ *M02.819 Other reactive arthropathies, unspecified shoulder* 🔗
  ● **M02.82 Other reactive arthropathies, elbow**
    ▸ *M02.821 Other reactive arthropathies, right elbow* 🔗
    ▸ *M02.822 Other reactive arthropathies, left elbow* 🔗
    ▸ *M02.829 Other reactive arthropathies, unspecified elbow* 🔗
  ● **M02.83 Other reactive arthropathies, wrist**
    Other reactive arthropathies, carpal bones
    ▸ *M02.831 Other reactive arthropathies, right wrist* 🔗
    ▸ *M02.832 Other reactive arthropathies, left wrist* 🔗
    ▸ *M02.839 Other reactive arthropathies, unspecified wrist* 🔗
  ● **M02.84 Other reactive arthropathies, hand**
    Other reactive arthropathies, metacarpus and phalanges
    ▸ *M02.841 Other reactive arthropathies, right hand* 🔗
    ▸ *M02.842 Other reactive arthropathies, left hand* 🔗
    ▸ *M02.849 Other reactive arthropathies, unspecified hand* 🔗

● **M02.85 Other reactive arthropathies, hip**
    ▸ *M02.851 Other reactive arthropathies, right hip* 🔗
    ▸ *M02.852 Other reactive arthropathies, left hip* 🔗
    ▸ *M02.859 Other reactive arthropathies, unspecified hip* 🔗
● **M02.86 Other reactive arthropathies, knee**
    ▸ *M02.861 Other reactive arthropathies, right knee* 🔗
    ▸ *M02.862 Other reactive arthropathies, left knee* 🔗
    ▸ *M02.869 Other reactive arthropathies, unspecified knee* 🔗
● **M02.87 Other reactive arthropathies, ankle and foot**
    Other reactive arthropathies, tarsus, metatarsus and phalanges
    ▸ *M02.871 Other reactive arthropathies, right ankle and foot* 🔗
    ▸ *M02.872 Other reactive arthropathies, left ankle and foot* 🔗
    ▸ *M02.879 Other reactive arthropathies, unspecified ankle and foot* 🔗
  ▸ *M02.88 Other reactive arthropathies, vertebrae* 🔗
  ▸ *M02.89 Other reactive arthropathies, multiple sites* 🔗
▸ *M02.9 Reactive arthropathy, unspecified* 🔗

AUTOINFLAMMATORY SYNDROMES (M04)

● **M04 Autoinflammatory syndromes**
  Excludes2 Crohn's disease (K50.-)
  Coding Clinic: 2016, Q4, P37
  M04.1 Periodic fever syndromes 🔗
    Familial Mediterranean fever
    Hyperimmunoglobin D syndrome
    Mevalonate kinase deficiency
    Tumor necrosis factor receptor associated periodic syndrome [TRAPS]
  M04.2 Cryopyrin-associated periodic syndromes 🔗
    Chronic infantile neurological, cutaneous and articular syndrome [CINCA]
    Familial cold autoinflammatory syndrome
    Familial cold urticaria
    Muckle-Wells syndrome
    Neonatal onset multisystemic inflammatory disorder [NOMID]
  M04.8 Other autoinflammatory syndromes 🔗
    Blau syndrome
    Deficiency of interleukin 1 receptor antagonist [DIRA]
    Majeed syndrome
    Periodic fever, aphthous stomatitis, pharyngitis, and adenopathy syndrome [PFAPA]
    Pyogenic arthritis, pyoderma gangrenosum, and acne syndrome [PAPA]
  M04.9 Autoinflammatory syndrome, unspecified 🔗

INFLAMMATORY POLYARTHROPATHIES (M05-M14)

● **M05 Rheumatoid arthritis with rheumatoid factor**
  Excludes1 rheumatic fever (I00)
    juvenile rheumatoid arthritis (M08.-)
    rheumatoid arthritis of spine (M45.-)
  ● **M05.0 Felty's syndrome**
    Rheumatoid arthritis with splenoadenomegaly and leukopenia
    M05.00 Felty's syndrome, unspecified site 🔗

Item 13-1 Rheumatoid arthritis (RA) is a chronic systemic inflammatory autoimmune disease of undetermined etiology involving primarily the synovial membranes and articular structures of multiple joints. It can also affect other organs, including the eyes, blood vessels, heart, and lungs. The disease is often progressive. In late stages, deformity, ankylosis, and other **inflammatory polyarthropathies** develop.

● **M05.01** Felty's syndrome, shoulder
     M05.011 Felty's syndrome, right shoulder ℞
     M05.012 Felty's syndrome, left shoulder ℞
     M05.019 Felty's syndrome, unspecified shoulder ℞
● **M05.02** Felty's syndrome, elbow
     M05.021 Felty's syndrome, right elbow ℞
     M05.022 Felty's syndrome, left elbow ℞
     M05.029 Felty's syndrome, unspecified elbow ℞
● **M05.03** Felty's syndrome, wrist
     Felty's syndrome, carpal bones
     M05.031 Felty's syndrome, right wrist ℞
     M05.032 Felty's syndrome, left wrist ℞
     M05.039 Felty's syndrome, unspecified wrist ℞
● **M05.04** Felty's syndrome, hand
     Felty's syndrome, metacarpus and phalanges
     M05.041 Felty's syndrome, right hand ℞
     M05.042 Felty's syndrome, left hand ℞
     M05.049 Felty's syndrome, unspecified hand ℞
● **M05.05** Felty's syndrome, hip
     M05.051 Felty's syndrome, right hip ℞
     M05.052 Felty's syndrome, left hip ℞
     M05.059 Felty's syndrome, unspecified hip ℞
● **M05.06** Felty's syndrome, knee
     M05.061 Felty's syndrome, right knee ℞
     M05.062 Felty's syndrome, left knee ℞
     M05.069 Felty's syndrome, unspecified knee ℞
● **M05.07** Felty's syndrome, ankle and foot
     Felty's syndrome, tarsus, metatarsus and phalanges
     M05.071 Felty's syndrome, right ankle and foot ℞
     M05.072 Felty's syndrome, left ankle and foot ℞
     M05.079 Felty's syndrome, unspecified ankle and foot ℞
     M05.09 Felty's syndrome, multiple sites ℞
● **M05.1** Rheumatoid lung disease with rheumatoid arthritis
     M05.10 Rheumatoid lung disease with rheumatoid arthritis of unspecified site ℞
● **M05.11** Rheumatoid lung disease with rheumatoid arthritis of shoulder
     M05.111 Rheumatoid lung disease with rheumatoid arthritis of right shoulder ℞
     M05.112 Rheumatoid lung disease with rheumatoid arthritis of left shoulder ℞
     M05.119 Rheumatoid lung disease with rheumatoid arthritis of unspecified shoulder ℞
● **M05.12** Rheumatoid lung disease with rheumatoid arthritis of elbow
     M05.121 Rheumatoid lung disease with rheumatoid arthritis of right elbow ℞
     M05.122 Rheumatoid lung disease with rheumatoid arthritis of left elbow ℞
     M05.129 Rheumatoid lung disease with rheumatoid arthritis of unspecified elbow ℞
● **M05.13** Rheumatoid lung disease with rheumatoid arthritis of wrist
     Rheumatoid lung disease with rheumatoid arthritis, carpal bones
     M05.131 Rheumatoid lung disease with rheumatoid arthritis of right wrist ℞
     M05.132 Rheumatoid lung disease with rheumatoid arthritis of left wrist ℞
     M05.139 Rheumatoid lung disease with rheumatoid arthritis of unspecified wrist ℞

● **M05.14** Rheumatoid lung disease with rheumatoid arthritis of hand
     Rheumatoid lung disease with rheumatoid arthritis, metacarpus and phalanges
     M05.141 Rheumatoid lung disease with rheumatoid arthritis of right hand ℞
     M05.142 Rheumatoid lung disease with rheumatoid arthritis of left hand ℞
     M05.149 Rheumatoid lung disease with rheumatoid arthritis of unspecified hand ℞
● **M05.15** Rheumatoid lung disease with rheumatoid arthritis of hip
     M05.151 Rheumatoid lung disease with rheumatoid arthritis of right hip ℞
     M05.152 Rheumatoid lung disease with rheumatoid arthritis of left hip ℞
     M05.159 Rheumatoid lung disease with rheumatoid arthritis of unspecified hip ℞
● **M05.16** Rheumatoid lung disease with rheumatoid arthritis of knee
     M05.161 Rheumatoid lung disease with rheumatoid arthritis of right knee ℞
     M05.162 Rheumatoid lung disease with rheumatoid arthritis of left knee ℞
     M05.169 Rheumatoid lung disease with rheumatoid arthritis of unspecified knee ℞
● **M05.17** Rheumatoid lung disease with rheumatoid arthritis of ankle and foot
     Rheumatoid lung disease with rheumatoid arthritis, tarsus, metatarsus and phalanges
     M05.171 Rheumatoid lung disease with rheumatoid arthritis of right ankle and foot ℞
     M05.172 Rheumatoid lung disease with rheumatoid arthritis of left ankle and foot ℞
     M05.179 Rheumatoid lung disease with rheumatoid arthritis of unspecified ankle and foot ℞
     M05.19 Rheumatoid lung disease with rheumatoid arthritis of multiple sites ℞
● **M05.2** Rheumatoid vasculitis with rheumatoid arthritis
     M05.20 Rheumatoid vasculitis with rheumatoid arthritis of unspecified site ℞
● **M05.21** Rheumatoid vasculitis with rheumatoid arthritis of shoulder
     M05.211 Rheumatoid vasculitis with rheumatoid arthritis of right shoulder ℞
     M05.212 Rheumatoid vasculitis with rheumatoid arthritis of left shoulder ℞
     M05.219 Rheumatoid vasculitis with rheumatoid arthritis of unspecified shoulder ℞
● **M05.22** Rheumatoid vasculitis with rheumatoid arthritis of elbow
     M05.221 Rheumatoid vasculitis with rheumatoid arthritis of right elbow ℞
     M05.222 Rheumatoid vasculitis with rheumatoid arthritis of left elbow ℞
     M05.229 Rheumatoid vasculitis with rheumatoid arthritis of unspecified elbow ℞

▶ New   ⇒ Revised   ~~deleted~~ Deleted   Excludes 1   Excludes 2   Includes   Use additional   Code first   Code also   Key words
OGCR Official Guidelines   X Assign placeholder X   ● Use Additional Character(s)   ▷ Manifestation Code   ℞ Hierarchical Condition Category   Coding Clinic

● **M05.23**   Rheumatoid vasculitis with rheumatoid arthritis of wrist
> Rheumatoid vasculitis with rheumatoid arthritis, carpal bones

     M05.231   Rheumatoid vasculitis with rheumatoid arthritis of right wrist 🔖

     M05.232   Rheumatoid vasculitis with rheumatoid arthritis of left wrist 🔖

     M05.239   Rheumatoid vasculitis with rheumatoid arthritis of unspecified wrist 🔖

● **M05.24**   Rheumatoid vasculitis with rheumatoid arthritis of hand
> Rheumatoid vasculitis with rheumatoid arthritis, metacarpus and phalanges

     M05.241   Rheumatoid vasculitis with rheumatoid arthritis of right hand 🔖

     M05.242   Rheumatoid vasculitis with rheumatoid arthritis of left hand 🔖

     M05.249   Rheumatoid vasculitis with rheumatoid arthritis of unspecified hand 🔖

● **M05.25**   Rheumatoid vasculitis with rheumatoid arthritis of hip

     M05.251   Rheumatoid vasculitis with rheumatoid arthritis of right hip 🔖

     M05.252   Rheumatoid vasculitis with rheumatoid arthritis of left hip 🔖

     M05.259   Rheumatoid vasculitis with rheumatoid arthritis of unspecified hip 🔖

● **M05.26**   Rheumatoid vasculitis with rheumatoid arthritis of knee

     M05.261   Rheumatoid vasculitis with rheumatoid arthritis of right knee 🔖

     M05.262   Rheumatoid vasculitis with rheumatoid arthritis of left knee 🔖

     M05.269   Rheumatoid vasculitis with rheumatoid arthritis of unspecified knee 🔖

● **M05.27**   Rheumatoid vasculitis with rheumatoid arthritis of ankle and foot
> Rheumatoid vasculitis with rheumatoid arthritis, tarsus, metatarsus and phalanges

     M05.271   Rheumatoid vasculitis with rheumatoid arthritis of right ankle and foot 🔖

     M05.272   Rheumatoid vasculitis with rheumatoid arthritis of left ankle and foot 🔖

     M05.279   Rheumatoid vasculitis with rheumatoid arthritis of unspecified ankle and foot 🔖

     M05.29   Rheumatoid vasculitis with rheumatoid arthritis of multiple sites 🔖

● **M05.3**   Rheumatoid heart disease with rheumatoid arthritis
> Rheumatoid carditis
> Rheumatoid endocarditis
> Rheumatoid myocarditis
> Rheumatoid pericarditis

     M05.30   Rheumatoid heart disease with rheumatoid arthritis of unspecified site 🔖

● **M05.31**   Rheumatoid heart disease with rheumatoid arthritis of shoulder

     M05.311   Rheumatoid heart disease with rheumatoid arthritis of right shoulder 🔖

     M05.312   Rheumatoid heart disease with rheumatoid arthritis of left shoulder 🔖

     M05.319   Rheumatoid heart disease with rheumatoid arthritis of unspecified shoulder 🔖

● **M05.32**   Rheumatoid heart disease with rheumatoid arthritis of elbow

     M05.321   Rheumatoid heart disease with rheumatoid arthritis of right elbow 🔖

     M05.322   Rheumatoid heart disease with rheumatoid arthritis of left elbow 🔖

     M05.329   Rheumatoid heart disease with rheumatoid arthritis of unspecified elbow 🔖

● **M05.33**   Rheumatoid heart disease with rheumatoid arthritis of wrist
> Rheumatoid heart disease with rheumatoid arthritis, carpal bones

     M05.331   Rheumatoid heart disease with rheumatoid arthritis of right wrist 🔖

     M05.332   Rheumatoid heart disease with rheumatoid arthritis of left wrist 🔖

     M05.339   Rheumatoid heart disease with rheumatoid arthritis of unspecified wrist 🔖

● **M05.34**   Rheumatoid heart disease with rheumatoid arthritis of hand
> Rheumatoid heart disease with rheumatoid arthritis, metacarpus and phalanges

     M05.341   Rheumatoid heart disease with rheumatoid arthritis of right hand 🔖

     M05.342   Rheumatoid heart disease with rheumatoid arthritis of left hand 🔖

     M05.349   Rheumatoid heart disease with rheumatoid arthritis of unspecified hand 🔖

● **M05.35**   Rheumatoid heart disease with rheumatoid arthritis of hip

     M05.351   Rheumatoid heart disease with rheumatoid arthritis of right hip 🔖

     M05.352   Rheumatoid heart disease with rheumatoid arthritis of left hip 🔖

     M05.359   Rheumatoid heart disease with rheumatoid arthritis of unspecified hip 🔖

● **M05.36**   Rheumatoid heart disease with rheumatoid arthritis of knee

     M05.361   Rheumatoid heart disease with rheumatoid arthritis of right knee 🔖

     M05.362   Rheumatoid heart disease with rheumatoid arthritis of left knee 🔖

     M05.369   Rheumatoid heart disease with rheumatoid arthritis of unspecified knee 🔖

● **M05.37**   Rheumatoid heart disease with rheumatoid arthritis of ankle and foot
> Rheumatoid heart disease with rheumatoid arthritis, tarsus, metatarsus and phalanges

     M05.371   Rheumatoid heart disease with rheumatoid arthritis of right ankle and foot 🔖

     M05.372   Rheumatoid heart disease with rheumatoid arthritis of left ankle and foot 🔖

     M05.379   Rheumatoid heart disease with rheumatoid arthritis of unspecified ankle and foot 🔖

     M05.39   Rheumatoid heart disease with rheumatoid arthritis of multiple sites 🔖

● **M05.4**   Rheumatoid myopathy with rheumatoid arthritis

     M05.40   Rheumatoid myopathy with rheumatoid arthritis of unspecified site 🔖

● **M05.41**   Rheumatoid myopathy with rheumatoid arthritis of shoulder

     M05.411   Rheumatoid myopathy with rheumatoid arthritis of right shoulder 🔖

CHAPTER 13 (M00-M99)

M05.412   Rheumatoid myopathy with rheumatoid arthritis of left shoulder 🐾

M05.419   Rheumatoid myopathy with rheumatoid arthritis of unspecified shoulder 🐾

● M05.42   Rheumatoid myopathy with rheumatoid arthritis of elbow

M05.421   Rheumatoid myopathy with rheumatoid arthritis of right elbow 🐾

M05.422   Rheumatoid myopathy with rheumatoid arthritis of left elbow 🐾

M05.429   Rheumatoid myopathy with rheumatoid arthritis of unspecified elbow 🐾

● M05.43   Rheumatoid myopathy with rheumatoid arthritis of wrist
> Rheumatoid myopathy with rheumatoid arthritis, carpal bones

M05.431   Rheumatoid myopathy with rheumatoid arthritis of right wrist 🐾

M05.432   Rheumatoid myopathy with rheumatoid arthritis of left wrist 🐾

M05.439   Rheumatoid myopathy with rheumatoid arthritis of unspecified wrist 🐾

● M05.44   Rheumatoid myopathy with rheumatoid arthritis of hand
> Rheumatoid myopathy with rheumatoid arthritis, metacarpus and phalanges

M05.441   Rheumatoid myopathy with rheumatoid arthritis of right hand 🐾

M05.442   Rheumatoid myopathy with rheumatoid arthritis of left hand 🐾

M05.449   Rheumatoid myopathy with rheumatoid arthritis of unspecified hand 🐾

● M05.45   Rheumatoid myopathy with rheumatoid arthritis of hip

M05.451   Rheumatoid myopathy with rheumatoid arthritis of right hip 🐾

M05.452   Rheumatoid myopathy with rheumatoid arthritis of left hip 🐾

M05.459   Rheumatoid myopathy with rheumatoid arthritis of unspecified hip 🐾

● M05.46   Rheumatoid myopathy with rheumatoid arthritis of knee

M05.461   Rheumatoid myopathy with rheumatoid arthritis of right knee 🐾

M05.462   Rheumatoid myopathy with rheumatoid arthritis of left knee 🐾

M05.469   Rheumatoid myopathy with rheumatoid arthritis of unspecified knee 🐾

● M05.47   Rheumatoid myopathy with rheumatoid arthritis of ankle and foot
> Rheumatoid myopathy with rheumatoid arthritis, tarsus, metatarsus and phalanges

M05.471   Rheumatoid myopathy with rheumatoid arthritis of right ankle and foot 🐾

M05.472   Rheumatoid myopathy with rheumatoid arthritis of left ankle and foot 🐾

M05.479   Rheumatoid myopathy with rheumatoid arthritis of unspecified ankle and foot 🐾

M05.49   Rheumatoid myopathy with rheumatoid arthritis of multiple sites 🐾

● M05.5   Rheumatoid polyneuropathy with rheumatoid arthritis

M05.50   Rheumatoid polyneuropathy with rheumatoid arthritis of unspecified site 🐾

● M05.51   Rheumatoid polyneuropathy with rheumatoid arthritis of shoulder

M05.511   Rheumatoid polyneuropathy with rheumatoid arthritis of right shoulder 🐾

M05.512   Rheumatoid polyneuropathy with rheumatoid arthritis of left shoulder 🐾

M05.519   Rheumatoid polyneuropathy with rheumatoid arthritis of unspecified shoulder 🐾

● M05.52   Rheumatoid polyneuropathy with rheumatoid arthritis of elbow

M05.521   Rheumatoid polyneuropathy with rheumatoid arthritis of right elbow 🐾

M05.522   Rheumatoid polyneuropathy with rheumatoid arthritis of left elbow 🐾

M05.529   Rheumatoid polyneuropathy with rheumatoid arthritis of unspecified elbow 🐾

● M05.53   Rheumatoid polyneuropathy with rheumatoid arthritis of wrist
> Rheumatoid polyneuropathy with rheumatoid arthritis, carpal bones

M05.531   Rheumatoid polyneuropathy with rheumatoid arthritis of right wrist 🐾

M05.532   Rheumatoid polyneuropathy with rheumatoid arthritis of left wrist 🐾

M05.539   Rheumatoid polyneuropathy with rheumatoid arthritis of unspecified wrist 🐾

● M05.54   Rheumatoid polyneuropathy with rheumatoid arthritis of hand
> Rheumatoid polyneuropathy with rheumatoid arthritis, metacarpus and phalanges

M05.541   Rheumatoid polyneuropathy with rheumatoid arthritis of right hand 🐾

M05.542   Rheumatoid polyneuropathy with rheumatoid arthritis of left hand 🐾

M05.549   Rheumatoid polyneuropathy with rheumatoid arthritis of unspecified hand 🐾

● M05.55   Rheumatoid polyneuropathy with rheumatoid arthritis of hip

M05.551   Rheumatoid polyneuropathy with rheumatoid arthritis of right hip 🐾

M05.552   Rheumatoid polyneuropathy with rheumatoid arthritis of left hip 🐾

M05.559   Rheumatoid polyneuropathy with rheumatoid arthritis of unspecified hip 🐾

● M05.56   Rheumatoid polyneuropathy with rheumatoid arthritis of knee

M05.561   Rheumatoid polyneuropathy with rheumatoid arthritis of right knee 🐾

M05.562   Rheumatoid polyneuropathy with rheumatoid arthritis of left knee 🐾

M05.569   Rheumatoid polyneuropathy with rheumatoid arthritis of unspecified knee 🐾

▶ New   ⇒ Revised   ~~deleted~~ Deleted   Excludes 1   Excludes 2   Includes   Use additional   Code first   Code also   Key words

OGCR Official Guidelines   X Assign placeholder X   ● Use Additional Character(s)   ▌ Manifestation Code   🐾 Hierarchical Condition Category   **Coding Clinic**

- M05.57 **Rheumatoid polyneuropathy with rheumatoid arthritis of ankle and foot**
  Rheumatoid polyneuropathy with rheumatoid arthritis, tarsus, metatarsus and phalanges
  - M05.571 **Rheumatoid polyneuropathy with rheumatoid arthritis of right ankle and foot** 🔍
  - M05.572 **Rheumatoid polyneuropathy with rheumatoid arthritis of left ankle and foot** 🔍
  - M05.579 **Rheumatoid polyneuropathy with rheumatoid arthritis of unspecified ankle and foot** 🔍
  - M05.59 **Rheumatoid polyneuropathy with rheumatoid arthritis of multiple sites** 🔍
- M05.6 **Rheumatoid arthritis with involvement of other organs and systems**
  - M05.60 **Rheumatoid arthritis of unspecified site with involvement of other organs and systems** 🔍
- M05.61 **Rheumatoid arthritis of shoulder with involvement of other organs and systems**
  - M05.611 **Rheumatoid arthritis of right shoulder with involvement of other organs and systems** 🔍
  - M05.612 **Rheumatoid arthritis of left shoulder with involvement of other organs and systems** 🔍
  - M05.619 **Rheumatoid arthritis of unspecified shoulder with involvement of other organs and systems** 🔍
- M05.62 **Rheumatoid arthritis of elbow with involvement of other organs and systems**
  - M05.621 **Rheumatoid arthritis of right elbow with involvement of other organs and systems** 🔍
  - M05.622 **Rheumatoid arthritis of left elbow with involvement of other organs and systems** 🔍
  - M05.629 **Rheumatoid arthritis of unspecified elbow with involvement of other organs and systems** 🔍
- M05.63 **Rheumatoid arthritis of wrist with involvement of other organs and systems**
  Rheumatoid arthritis of carpal bones with involvement of other organs and systems
  - M05.631 **Rheumatoid arthritis of right wrist with involvement of other organs and systems** 🔍
  - M05.632 **Rheumatoid arthritis of left wrist with involvement of other organs and systems** 🔍
  - M05.639 **Rheumatoid arthritis of unspecified wrist with involvement of other organs and systems** 🔍
- M05.64 **Rheumatoid arthritis of hand with involvement of other organs and systems**
  Rheumatoid arthritis of metacarpus and phalanges with involvement of other organs and systems
  - M05.641 **Rheumatoid arthritis of right hand with involvement of other organs and systems** 🔍
  - M05.642 **Rheumatoid arthritis of left hand with involvement of other organs and systems** 🔍
  - M05.649 **Rheumatoid arthritis of unspecified hand with involvement of other organs and systems** 🔍

- M05.65 **Rheumatoid arthritis of hip with involvement of other organs and systems**
  - M05.651 **Rheumatoid arthritis of right hip with involvement of other organs and systems** 🔍
  - M05.652 **Rheumatoid arthritis of left hip with involvement of other organs and systems** 🔍
  - M05.659 **Rheumatoid arthritis of unspecified hip with involvement of other organs and systems** 🔍
- M05.66 **Rheumatoid arthritis of knee with involvement of other organs and systems**
  - M05.661 **Rheumatoid arthritis of right knee with involvement of other organs and systems** 🔍
  - M05.662 **Rheumatoid arthritis of left knee with involvement of other organs and systems** 🔍
  - M05.669 **Rheumatoid arthritis of unspecified knee with involvement of other organs and systems** 🔍
- M05.67 **Rheumatoid arthritis of ankle and foot with involvement of other organs and systems**
  Rheumatoid arthritis of tarsus, metatarsus and phalanges with involvement of other organs and systems
  - M05.671 **Rheumatoid arthritis of right ankle and foot with involvement of other organs and systems** 🔍
  - M05.672 **Rheumatoid arthritis of left ankle and foot with involvement of other organs and systems** 🔍
  - M05.679 **Rheumatoid arthritis of unspecified ankle and foot with involvement of other organs and systems** 🔍
  - M05.69 **Rheumatoid arthritis of multiple sites with involvement of other organs and systems** 🔍
- M05.7 **Rheumatoid arthritis with rheumatoid factor without organ or systems involvement**
  - M05.70 **Rheumatoid arthritis with rheumatoid factor of unspecified site without organ or systems involvement** 🔍
- M05.71 **Rheumatoid arthritis with rheumatoid factor of shoulder without organ or systems involvement**
  - M05.711 **Rheumatoid arthritis with rheumatoid factor of right shoulder without organ or systems involvement** 🔍
  - M05.712 **Rheumatoid arthritis with rheumatoid factor of left shoulder without organ or systems involvement** 🔍
  - M05.719 **Rheumatoid arthritis with rheumatoid factor of unspecified shoulder without organ or systems involvement** 🔍
- M05.72 **Rheumatoid arthritis with rheumatoid factor of elbow without organ or systems involvement**
  - M05.721 **Rheumatoid arthritis with rheumatoid factor of right elbow without organ or systems involvement** 🔍
  - M05.722 **Rheumatoid arthritis with rheumatoid factor of left elbow without organ or systems involvement** 🔍
  - M05.729 **Rheumatoid arthritis with rheumatoid factor of unspecified elbow without organ or systems involvement** 🔍

CHAPTER 13 (M00-M99)

● M05.73 Rheumatoid arthritis with rheumatoid factor of wrist without organ or systems involvement

    M05.731 Rheumatoid arthritis with rheumatoid factor of right wrist without organ or systems involvement 🦠

    M05.732 Rheumatoid arthritis with rheumatoid factor of left wrist without organ or systems involvement 🦠

    M05.739 Rheumatoid arthritis with rheumatoid factor of unspecified wrist without organ or systems involvement 🦠

● M05.74 Rheumatoid arthritis with rheumatoid factor of hand without organ or systems involvement

    M05.741 Rheumatoid arthritis with rheumatoid factor of right hand without organ or systems involvement 🦠

    M05.742 Rheumatoid arthritis with rheumatoid factor of left hand without organ or systems involvement 🦠

    M05.749 Rheumatoid arthritis with rheumatoid factor of unspecified hand without organ or systems involvement 🦠

● M05.75 Rheumatoid arthritis with rheumatoid factor of hip without organ or systems involvement

    M05.751 Rheumatoid arthritis with rheumatoid factor of right hip without organ or systems involvement 🦠

    M05.752 Rheumatoid arthritis with rheumatoid factor of left hip without organ or systems involvement 🦠

    M05.759 Rheumatoid arthritis with rheumatoid factor of unspecified hip without organ or systems involvement 🦠

● M05.76 Rheumatoid arthritis with rheumatoid factor of knee without organ or systems involvement

    M05.761 Rheumatoid arthritis with rheumatoid factor of right knee without organ or systems involvement 🦠

    M05.762 Rheumatoid arthritis with rheumatoid factor of left knee without organ or systems involvement 🦠

    M05.769 Rheumatoid arthritis with rheumatoid factor of unspecified knee without organ or systems involvement 🦠

● M05.77 Rheumatoid arthritis with rheumatoid factor of ankle and foot without organ or systems involvement

    M05.771 Rheumatoid arthritis with rheumatoid factor of right ankle and foot without organ or systems involvement 🦠

    M05.772 Rheumatoid arthritis with rheumatoid factor of left ankle and foot without organ or systems involvement 🦠

    M05.779 Rheumatoid arthritis with rheumatoid factor of unspecified ankle and foot without organ or systems involvement 🦠

M05.79 Rheumatoid arthritis with rheumatoid factor of multiple sites without organ or systems involvement 🦠

M05.7A Rheumatoid arthritis with rheumatoid factor of other specified site without organ or systems involvement

● M05.8 Other rheumatoid arthritis with rheumatoid factor

    M05.80 Other rheumatoid arthritis with rheumatoid factor of unspecified site 🦠

● M05.81 Other rheumatoid arthritis with rheumatoid factor of shoulder

    M05.811 Other rheumatoid arthritis with rheumatoid factor of right shoulder 🦠

    M05.812 Other rheumatoid arthritis with rheumatoid factor of left shoulder 🦠

    M05.819 Other rheumatoid arthritis with rheumatoid factor of unspecified shoulder 🦠

● M05.82 Other rheumatoid arthritis with rheumatoid factor of elbow

    M05.821 Other rheumatoid arthritis with rheumatoid factor of right elbow 🦠

    M05.822 Other rheumatoid arthritis with rheumatoid factor of left elbow 🦠

    M05.829 Other rheumatoid arthritis with rheumatoid factor of unspecified elbow 🦠

● M05.83 Other rheumatoid arthritis with rheumatoid factor of wrist

    M05.831 Other rheumatoid arthritis with rheumatoid factor of right wrist 🦠

    M05.832 Other rheumatoid arthritis with rheumatoid factor of left wrist 🦠

    M05.839 Other rheumatoid arthritis with rheumatoid factor of unspecified wrist 🦠

● M05.84 Other rheumatoid arthritis with rheumatoid factor of hand

    M05.841 Other rheumatoid arthritis with rheumatoid factor of right hand 🦠

    M05.842 Other rheumatoid arthritis with rheumatoid factor of left hand 🦠

    M05.849 Other rheumatoid arthritis with rheumatoid factor of unspecified hand 🦠

● M05.85 Other rheumatoid arthritis with rheumatoid factor of hip

    M05.851 Other rheumatoid arthritis with rheumatoid factor of right hip 🦠

    M05.852 Other rheumatoid arthritis with rheumatoid factor of left hip 🦠

    M05.859 Other rheumatoid arthritis with rheumatoid factor of unspecified hip 🦠

● M05.86 Other rheumatoid arthritis with rheumatoid factor of knee

    M05.861 Other rheumatoid arthritis with rheumatoid factor of right knee 🦠

    M05.862 Other rheumatoid arthritis with rheumatoid factor of left knee 🦠

    M05.869 Other rheumatoid arthritis with rheumatoid factor of unspecified knee 🦠

● **M05.87** Other rheumatoid arthritis with rheumatoid factor of ankle and foot
　　　M05.871 Other rheumatoid arthritis with rheumatoid factor of right ankle and foot 🔎
　　　M05.872 Other rheumatoid arthritis with rheumatoid factor of left ankle and foot 🔎
　　　M05.879 Other rheumatoid arthritis with rheumatoid factor of unspecified ankle and foot 🔎
　　M05.89 Other rheumatoid arthritis with rheumatoid factor of multiple sites 🔎
　　M05.8A Other rheumatoid arthritis with rheumatoid factor of other specified site
　M05.9 Rheumatoid arthritis with rheumatoid factor, unspecified 🔎

● **M06** Other rheumatoid arthritis
　● **M06.0** Rheumatoid arthritis without rheumatoid factor
　　M06.00 Rheumatoid arthritis without rheumatoid factor, unspecified site 🔎
　　● **M06.01** Rheumatoid arthritis without rheumatoid factor, shoulder
　　　M06.011 Rheumatoid arthritis without rheumatoid factor, right shoulder 🔎
　　　M06.012 Rheumatoid arthritis without rheumatoid factor, left shoulder 🔎
　　　M06.019 Rheumatoid arthritis without rheumatoid factor, unspecified shoulder 🔎
　　● **M06.02** Rheumatoid arthritis without rheumatoid factor, elbow
　　　M06.021 Rheumatoid arthritis without rheumatoid factor, right elbow 🔎
　　　M06.022 Rheumatoid arthritis without rheumatoid factor, left elbow 🔎
　　　M06.029 Rheumatoid arthritis without rheumatoid factor, unspecified elbow 🔎
　　● **M06.03** Rheumatoid arthritis without rheumatoid factor, wrist
　　　M06.031 Rheumatoid arthritis without rheumatoid factor, right wrist 🔎
　　　M06.032 Rheumatoid arthritis without rheumatoid factor, left wrist 🔎
　　　M06.039 Rheumatoid arthritis without rheumatoid factor, unspecified wrist 🔎
　　● **M06.04** Rheumatoid arthritis without rheumatoid factor, hand
　　　M06.041 Rheumatoid arthritis without rheumatoid factor, right hand 🔎
　　　M06.042 Rheumatoid arthritis without rheumatoid factor, left hand 🔎
　　　M06.049 Rheumatoid arthritis without rheumatoid factor, unspecified hand 🔎
　　● **M06.05** Rheumatoid arthritis without rheumatoid factor, hip
　　　M06.051 Rheumatoid arthritis without rheumatoid factor, right hip 🔎
　　　M06.052 Rheumatoid arthritis without rheumatoid factor, left hip 🔎
　　　M06.059 Rheumatoid arthritis without rheumatoid factor, unspecified hip 🔎

　　● **M06.06** Rheumatoid arthritis without rheumatoid factor, knee
　　　M06.061 Rheumatoid arthritis without rheumatoid factor, right knee 🔎
　　　M06.062 Rheumatoid arthritis without rheumatoid factor, left knee 🔎
　　　M06.069 Rheumatoid arthritis without rheumatoid factor, unspecified knee 🔎
　　● **M06.07** Rheumatoid arthritis without rheumatoid factor, ankle and foot
　　　M06.071 Rheumatoid arthritis without rheumatoid factor, right ankle and foot 🔎
　　　M06.072 Rheumatoid arthritis without rheumatoid factor, left ankle and foot 🔎
　　　M06.079 Rheumatoid arthritis without rheumatoid factor, unspecified ankle and foot 🔎
　　M06.08 Rheumatoid arthritis without rheumatoid factor, vertebrae 🔎
　　M06.09 Rheumatoid arthritis without rheumatoid factor, multiple sites 🔎
　　M06.0A Rheumatoid arthritis without rheumatoid factor, other specified site
　M06.1 Adult-onset Still's disease 🔎　　　　　　　　A
　　　Excludes1　Still's disease NOS (M08.2-)
　● **M06.2** Rheumatoid bursitis
　　M06.20 Rheumatoid bursitis, unspecified site 🔎
　　● **M06.21** Rheumatoid bursitis, shoulder
　　　M06.211 Rheumatoid bursitis, right shoulder 🔎
　　　M06.212 Rheumatoid bursitis, left shoulder 🔎
　　　M06.219 Rheumatoid bursitis, unspecified shoulder 🔎
　　● **M06.22** Rheumatoid bursitis, elbow
　　　M06.221 Rheumatoid bursitis, right elbow 🔎
　　　M06.222 Rheumatoid bursitis, left elbow 🔎
　　　M06.229 Rheumatoid bursitis, unspecified elbow 🔎
　　● **M06.23** Rheumatoid bursitis, wrist
　　　M06.231 Rheumatoid bursitis, right wrist 🔎
　　　M06.232 Rheumatoid bursitis, left wrist 🔎
　　　M06.239 Rheumatoid bursitis, unspecified wrist 🔎
　　● **M06.24** Rheumatoid bursitis, hand
　　　M06.241 Rheumatoid bursitis, right hand 🔎
　　　M06.242 Rheumatoid bursitis, left hand 🔎
　　　M06.249 Rheumatoid bursitis, unspecified hand 🔎
　　● **M06.25** Rheumatoid bursitis, hip
　　　M06.251 Rheumatoid bursitis, right hip 🔎
　　　M06.252 Rheumatoid bursitis, left hip 🔎
　　　M06.259 Rheumatoid bursitis, unspecified hip 🔎
　　● **M06.26** Rheumatoid bursitis, knee
　　　M06.261 Rheumatoid bursitis, right knee 🔎
　　　M06.262 Rheumatoid bursitis, left knee 🔎
　　　M06.269 Rheumatoid bursitis, unspecified knee 🔎

CHAPTER 13 (M00–M99)

CHAPTER 13 (M00–M99)

● M06.27   Rheumatoid bursitis, ankle and foot

    M06.271   Rheumatoid bursitis, right ankle and foot 🐾

    M06.272   Rheumatoid bursitis, left ankle and foot 🐾

    M06.279   Rheumatoid bursitis, unspecified ankle and foot 🐾

  M06.28   Rheumatoid bursitis, vertebrae 🐾

  M06.29   Rheumatoid bursitis, multiple sites 🐾

● M06.3   Rheumatoid nodule

  M06.30   Rheumatoid nodule, unspecified site 🐾

● M06.31   Rheumatoid nodule, shoulder

    M06.311   Rheumatoid nodule, right shoulder 🐾

    M06.312   Rheumatoid nodule, left shoulder 🐾

    M06.319   Rheumatoid nodule, unspecified shoulder 🐾

● M06.32   Rheumatoid nodule, elbow

    M06.321   Rheumatoid nodule, right elbow 🐾

    M06.322   Rheumatoid nodule, left elbow 🐾

    M06.329   Rheumatoid nodule, unspecified elbow 🐾

● M06.33   Rheumatoid nodule, wrist

    M06.331   Rheumatoid nodule, right wrist 🐾

    M06.332   Rheumatoid nodule, left wrist 🐾

    M06.339   Rheumatoid nodule, unspecified wrist 🐾

● M06.34   Rheumatoid nodule, hand

    M06.341   Rheumatoid nodule, right hand 🐾

    M06.342   Rheumatoid nodule, left hand 🐾

    M06.349   Rheumatoid nodule, unspecified hand 🐾

● M06.35   Rheumatoid nodule, hip

    M06.351   Rheumatoid nodule, right hip 🐾

    M06.352   Rheumatoid nodule, left hip 🐾

    M06.359   Rheumatoid nodule, unspecified hip 🐾

● M06.36   Rheumatoid nodule, knee

    M06.361   Rheumatoid nodule, right knee 🐾

    M06.362   Rheumatoid nodule, left knee 🐾

    M06.369   Rheumatoid nodule, unspecified knee 🐾

● M06.37   Rheumatoid nodule, ankle and foot

    M06.371   Rheumatoid nodule, right ankle and foot 🐾

    M06.372   Rheumatoid nodule, left ankle and foot 🐾

    M06.379   Rheumatoid nodule, unspecified ankle and foot 🐾

  M06.38   Rheumatoid nodule, vertebrae 🐾

  M06.39   Rheumatoid nodule, multiple sites 🐾

  M06.4   Inflammatory polyarthropathy 🐾

    Excludes1   polyarthritis NOS (M13.0)

● M06.8   Other specified rheumatoid arthritis

  M06.80   Other specified rheumatoid arthritis, unspecified site 🐾

● M06.81   Other specified rheumatoid arthritis, shoulder

    M06.811   Other specified rheumatoid arthritis, right shoulder 🐾

    M06.812   Other specified rheumatoid arthritis, left shoulder 🐾

    M06.819   Other specified rheumatoid arthritis, unspecified shoulder 🐾

● M06.82   Other specified rheumatoid arthritis, elbow

    M06.821   Other specified rheumatoid arthritis, right elbow 🐾

    M06.822   Other specified rheumatoid arthritis, left elbow 🐾

    M06.829   Other specified rheumatoid arthritis, unspecified elbow 🐾

● M06.83   Other specified rheumatoid arthritis, wrist

    M06.831   Other specified rheumatoid arthritis, right wrist 🐾

    M06.832   Other specified rheumatoid arthritis, left wrist 🐾

    M06.839   Other specified rheumatoid arthritis, unspecified wrist 🐾

● M06.84   Other specified rheumatoid arthritis, hand

    M06.841   Other specified rheumatoid arthritis, right hand 🐾

    M06.842   Other specified rheumatoid arthritis, left hand 🐾

    M06.849   Other specified rheumatoid arthritis, unspecified hand 🐾

● M06.85   Other specified rheumatoid arthritis, hip

    M06.851   Other specified rheumatoid arthritis, right hip 🐾

    M06.852   Other specified rheumatoid arthritis, left hip 🐾

    M06.859   Other specified rheumatoid arthritis, unspecified hip 🐾

● M06.86   Other specified rheumatoid arthritis, knee

    M06.861   Other specified rheumatoid arthritis, right knee 🐾

    M06.862   Other specified rheumatoid arthritis, left knee 🐾

    M06.869   Other specified rheumatoid arthritis, unspecified knee 🐾

● M06.87   Other specified rheumatoid arthritis, ankle and foot

    M06.871   Other specified rheumatoid arthritis, right ankle and foot 🐾

    M06.872   Other specified rheumatoid arthritis, left ankle and foot 🐾

    M06.879   Other specified rheumatoid arthritis, unspecified ankle and foot 🐾

  M06.88   Other specified rheumatoid arthritis, vertebrae 🐾

  M06.89   Other specified rheumatoid arthritis, multiple sites 🐾

  M06.8A   Other specified rheumatoid arthritis, other specified site

  M06.9   Rheumatoid arthritis, unspecified 🐾

● M07   Enteropathic arthropathies

  Code also associated enteropathy, such as:
    regional enteritis [Crohn's disease] (K50.-)
    ulcerative colitis (K51.-)

    Excludes1   psoriatic arthropathies (L40.5-)

● M07.6   Enteropathic arthropathies

  M07.60   Enteropathic arthropathies, unspecified site

● M07.61   Enteropathic arthropathies, shoulder

    M07.611   Enteropathic arthropathies, right shoulder

    M07.612   Enteropathic arthropathies, left shoulder

    M07.619   Enteropathic arthropathies, unspecified shoulder

▶ New   ⇒ Revised   ~~deleted~~ Deleted   Excludes 1   Excludes 2   Includes   Use additional   Code first   Code also   Key words

OGCR Official Guidelines   X Assign placeholder X   ● Use Additional Character(s)   ▶ Manifestation Code   🐾 Hierarchical Condition Category   **Coding Clinic**

● M07.62　Enteropathic arthropathies, elbow

　　M07.621　Enteropathic arthropathies, right elbow

　　M07.622　Enteropathic arthropathies, left elbow

　　M07.629　Enteropathic arthropathies, unspecified elbow

● M07.63　Enteropathic arthropathies, wrist

　　M07.631　Enteropathic arthropathies, right wrist

　　M07.632　Enteropathic arthropathies, left wrist

　　M07.639　Enteropathic arthropathies, unspecified wrist

● M07.64　Enteropathic arthropathies, hand

　　M07.641　Enteropathic arthropathies, right hand

　　M07.642　Enteropathic arthropathies, left hand

　　M07.649　Enteropathic arthropathies, unspecified hand

● M07.65　Enteropathic arthropathies, hip

　　M07.651　Enteropathic arthropathies, right hip

　　M07.652　Enteropathic arthropathies, left hip

　　M07.659　Enteropathic arthropathies, unspecified hip

● M07.66　Enteropathic arthropathies, knee

　　M07.661　Enteropathic arthropathies, right knee

　　M07.662　Enteropathic arthropathies, left knee

　　M07.669　Enteropathic arthropathies, unspecified knee

● M07.67　Enteropathic arthropathies, ankle and foot

　　M07.671　Enteropathic arthropathies, right ankle and foot

　　M07.672　Enteropathic arthropathies, left ankle and foot

　　M07.679　Enteropathic arthropathies, unspecified ankle and foot

　M07.68　Enteropathic arthropathies, vertebrae

　M07.69　Enteropathic arthropathies, multiple sites

● M08　Juvenile arthritis

　Code also any associated underlying condition, such as:
　　regional enteritis [Crohn's disease] (K50.-)
　　ulcerative colitis (K51.-)

　Excludes1　arthropathy in Whipple's disease (M14.8)
　　　　　　　Felty's syndrome (M05.0)
　　　　　　　juvenile dermatomyositis (M33.0-)
　　　　　　　psoriatic juvenile arthropathy (L40.54)

● M08.0　Unspecified juvenile rheumatoid arthritis
　　Juvenile rheumatoid arthritis with or without rheumatoid factor

　　M08.00　Unspecified juvenile rheumatoid arthritis of unspecified site 🔗

　● M08.01　Unspecified juvenile rheumatoid arthritis, shoulder

　　　M08.011　Unspecified juvenile rheumatoid arthritis, right shoulder 🔗

　　　M08.012　Unspecified juvenile rheumatoid arthritis, left shoulder 🔗

　　　M08.019　Unspecified juvenile rheumatoid arthritis, unspecified shoulder 🔗

　● M08.02　Unspecified juvenile rheumatoid arthritis of elbow

　　　M08.021　Unspecified juvenile rheumatoid arthritis, right elbow 🔗

　　　M08.022　Unspecified juvenile rheumatoid arthritis, left elbow 🔗

　　　M08.029　Unspecified juvenile rheumatoid arthritis, unspecified elbow 🔗

● M08.03　Unspecified juvenile rheumatoid arthritis, wrist

　　M08.031　Unspecified juvenile rheumatoid arthritis, right wrist 🔗

　　M08.032　Unspecified juvenile rheumatoid arthritis, left wrist 🔗

　　M08.039　Unspecified juvenile rheumatoid arthritis, unspecified wrist 🔗

● M08.04　Unspecified juvenile rheumatoid arthritis, hand

　　M08.041　Unspecified juvenile rheumatoid arthritis, right hand 🔗

　　M08.042　Unspecified juvenile rheumatoid arthritis, left hand 🔗

　　M08.049　Unspecified juvenile rheumatoid arthritis, unspecified hand 🔗

● M08.05　Unspecified juvenile rheumatoid arthritis, hip

　　M08.051　Unspecified juvenile rheumatoid arthritis, right hip 🔗

　　M08.052　Unspecified juvenile rheumatoid arthritis, left hip 🔗

　　M08.059　Unspecified juvenile rheumatoid arthritis, unspecified hip 🔗

● M08.06　Unspecified juvenile rheumatoid arthritis, knee

　　M08.061　Unspecified juvenile rheumatoid arthritis, right knee 🔗

　　M08.062　Unspecified juvenile rheumatoid arthritis, left knee 🔗

　　M08.069　Unspecified juvenile rheumatoid arthritis, unspecified knee 🔗

● M08.07　Unspecified juvenile rheumatoid arthritis, ankle and foot

　　M08.071　Unspecified juvenile rheumatoid arthritis, right ankle and foot 🔗

　　M08.072　Unspecified juvenile rheumatoid arthritis, left ankle and foot 🔗

　　M08.079　Unspecified juvenile rheumatoid arthritis, unspecified ankle and foot 🔗

　M08.08　Unspecified juvenile rheumatoid arthritis, vertebrae 🔗

　M08.09　Unspecified juvenile rheumatoid arthritis, multiple sites 🔗

　M08.0A　Unspecified juvenile rheumatoid arthritis, other specified site

M08.1　Juvenile ankylosing spondylitis 🔗

　Excludes1　ankylosing spondylitis in adults (M45.0-)

● M08.2　Juvenile rheumatoid arthritis with systemic onset
　　Still's disease NOS

　Excludes1　adult-onset Still's disease (M06.1-)

　　M08.20　Juvenile rheumatoid arthritis with systemic onset, unspecified site 🔗

　● M08.21　Juvenile rheumatoid arthritis with systemic onset, shoulder

　　　M08.211　Juvenile rheumatoid arthritis with systemic onset, right shoulder 🔗

　　　M08.212　Juvenile rheumatoid arthritis with systemic onset, left shoulder 🔗

　　　M08.219　Juvenile rheumatoid arthritis with systemic onset, unspecified shoulder 🔗

　● M08.22　Juvenile rheumatoid arthritis with systemic onset, elbow

　　　M08.221　Juvenile rheumatoid arthritis with systemic onset, right elbow 🔗

　　　M08.222　Juvenile rheumatoid arthritis with systemic onset, left elbow 🔗

　　　M08.229　Juvenile rheumatoid arthritis with systemic onset, unspecified elbow 🔗

CHAPTER 13 (M00-M99)

● **M08.23** Juvenile rheumatoid arthritis with systemic onset, wrist

    M08.231 Juvenile rheumatoid arthritis with systemic onset, right wrist 🐾

    M08.232 Juvenile rheumatoid arthritis with systemic onset, left wrist 🐾

    M08.239 Juvenile rheumatoid arthritis with systemic onset, unspecified wrist 🐾

● **M08.24** Juvenile rheumatoid arthritis with systemic onset, hand

    M08.241 Juvenile rheumatoid arthritis with systemic onset, right hand 🐾

    M08.242 Juvenile rheumatoid arthritis with systemic onset, left hand 🐾

    M08.249 Juvenile rheumatoid arthritis with systemic onset, unspecified hand 🐾

● **M08.25** Juvenile rheumatoid arthritis with systemic onset, hip

    M08.251 Juvenile rheumatoid arthritis with systemic onset, right hip 🐾

    M08.252 Juvenile rheumatoid arthritis with systemic onset, left hip 🐾

    M08.259 Juvenile rheumatoid arthritis with systemic onset, unspecified hip 🐾

● **M08.26** Juvenile rheumatoid arthritis with systemic onset, knee

    M08.261 Juvenile rheumatoid arthritis with systemic onset, right knee 🐾

    M08.262 Juvenile rheumatoid arthritis with systemic onset, left knee 🐾

    M08.269 Juvenile rheumatoid arthritis with systemic onset, unspecified knee 🐾

● **M08.27** Juvenile rheumatoid arthritis with systemic onset, ankle and foot

    M08.271 Juvenile rheumatoid arthritis with systemic onset, right ankle and foot 🐾

    M08.272 Juvenile rheumatoid arthritis with systemic onset, left ankle and foot 🐾

    M08.279 Juvenile rheumatoid arthritis with systemic onset, unspecified ankle and foot 🐾

  M08.28 Juvenile rheumatoid arthritis with systemic onset, vertebrae 🐾

  M08.29 Juvenile rheumatoid arthritis with systemic onset, multiple sites 🐾

  M08.2A Juvenile rheumatoid arthritis with systemic onset, other specified site

  M08.3 Juvenile rheumatoid polyarthritis (seronegative)

● **M08.4** Pauciarticular juvenile rheumatoid arthritis

  M08.40 Pauciarticular juvenile rheumatoid arthritis, unspecified site 🐾

● **M08.41** Pauciarticular juvenile rheumatoid arthritis, shoulder

    M08.411 Pauciarticular juvenile rheumatoid arthritis, right shoulder 🐾

    M08.412 Pauciarticular juvenile rheumatoid arthritis, left shoulder 🐾

    M08.419 Pauciarticular juvenile rheumatoid arthritis, unspecified shoulder 🐾

● **M08.42** Pauciarticular juvenile rheumatoid arthritis, elbow

    M08.421 Pauciarticular juvenile rheumatoid arthritis, right elbow 🐾

    M08.422 Pauciarticular juvenile rheumatoid arthritis, left elbow 🐾

    M08.429 Pauciarticular juvenile rheumatoid arthritis, unspecified elbow 🐾

● **M08.43** Pauciarticular juvenile rheumatoid arthritis, wrist

    M08.431 Pauciarticular juvenile rheumatoid arthritis, right wrist 🐾

    M08.432 Pauciarticular juvenile rheumatoid arthritis, left wrist 🐾

    M08.439 Pauciarticular juvenile rheumatoid arthritis, unspecified wrist 🐾

● **M08.44** Pauciarticular juvenile rheumatoid arthritis, hand

    M08.441 Pauciarticular juvenile rheumatoid arthritis, right hand 🐾

    M08.442 Pauciarticular juvenile rheumatoid arthritis, left hand 🐾

    M08.449 Pauciarticular juvenile rheumatoid arthritis, unspecified hand 🐾

● **M08.45** Pauciarticular juvenile rheumatoid arthritis, hip

    M08.451 Pauciarticular juvenile rheumatoid arthritis, right hip 🐾

    M08.452 Pauciarticular juvenile rheumatoid arthritis, left hip 🐾

    M08.459 Pauciarticular juvenile rheumatoid arthritis, unspecified hip 🐾

● **M08.46** Pauciarticular juvenile rheumatoid arthritis, knee

    M08.461 Pauciarticular juvenile rheumatoid arthritis, right knee 🐾

    M08.462 Pauciarticular juvenile rheumatoid arthritis, left knee 🐾

    M08.469 Pauciarticular juvenile rheumatoid arthritis, unspecified knee 🐾

● **M08.47** Pauciarticular juvenile rheumatoid arthritis, ankle and foot

    M08.471 Pauciarticular juvenile rheumatoid arthritis, right ankle and foot 🐾

    M08.472 Pauciarticular juvenile rheumatoid arthritis, left ankle and foot 🐾

    M08.479 Pauciarticular juvenile rheumatoid arthritis, unspecified ankle and foot 🐾

  M08.48 Pauciarticular juvenile rheumatoid arthritis, vertebrae 🐾

  M08.4A Pauciarticular juvenile rheumatoid arthritis, other specified site

● **M08.8** Other juvenile arthritis

  M08.80 Other juvenile arthritis, unspecified site 🐾

● **M08.81** Other juvenile arthritis, shoulder

    M08.811 Other juvenile arthritis, right shoulder 🐾

    M08.812 Other juvenile arthritis, left shoulder 🐾

    M08.819 Other juvenile arthritis, unspecified shoulder 🐾

● **M08.82** Other juvenile arthritis, elbow

    M08.821 Other juvenile arthritis, right elbow 🐾

    M08.822 Other juvenile arthritis, left elbow 🐾

    M08.829 Other juvenile arthritis, unspecified elbow 🐾

● **M08.83** Other juvenile arthritis, wrist

    M08.831 Other juvenile arthritis, right wrist 🐾

    M08.832 Other juvenile arthritis, left wrist 🐾

    M08.839 Other juvenile arthritis, unspecified wrist 🐾

▶ New   ⇒ Revised   ~~deleted~~ Deleted   Excludes 1   Excludes 2   Includes   Use additional   Code first   Code also   Key words

OGCR Official Guidelines   X Assign placeholder X   ● Use Additional Character(s)   ▶ Manifestation Code   🐾 Hierarchical Condition Category   **Coding Clinic**

● M08.84   Other juvenile arthritis, hand
     M08.841   Other juvenile arthritis, right hand 🐾
     M08.842   Other juvenile arthritis, left hand 🐾
     M08.849   Other juvenile arthritis, unspecified hand 🐾

● M08.85   Other juvenile arthritis, hip
     M08.851   Other juvenile arthritis, right hip 🐾
     M08.852   Other juvenile arthritis, left hip 🐾
     M08.859   Other juvenile arthritis, unspecified hip 🐾

● M08.86   Other juvenile arthritis, knee
     M08.861   Other juvenile arthritis, right knee 🐾
     M08.862   Other juvenile arthritis, left knee 🐾
     M08.869   Other juvenile arthritis, unspecified knee 🐾

● M08.87   Other juvenile arthritis, ankle and foot
     M08.871   Other juvenile arthritis, right ankle and foot 🐾
     M08.872   Other juvenile arthritis, left ankle and foot 🐾
     M08.879   Other juvenile arthritis, unspecified ankle and foot 🐾

     M08.88   Other juvenile arthritis, other specified site 🐾
                Other juvenile arthritis, vertebrae

     M08.89   Other juvenile arthritis, multiple sites 🐾

● M08.9   Juvenile arthritis, unspecified

> **Excludes1**   juvenile rheumatoid arthritis, unspecified (M08.0-)

     M08.90   Juvenile arthritis, unspecified, unspecified site 🐾

● M08.91   Juvenile arthritis, unspecified, shoulder
     M08.911   Juvenile arthritis, unspecified, right shoulder 🐾
     M08.912   Juvenile arthritis, unspecified, left shoulder 🐾
     M08.919   Juvenile arthritis, unspecified, unspecified shoulder 🐾

● M08.92   Juvenile arthritis, unspecified, elbow
     M08.921   Juvenile arthritis, unspecified, right elbow 🐾
     M08.922   Juvenile arthritis, unspecified, left elbow 🐾
     M08.929   Juvenile arthritis, unspecified, unspecified elbow 🐾

● M08.93   Juvenile arthritis, unspecified, wrist
     M08.931   Juvenile arthritis, unspecified, right wrist 🐾
     M08.932   Juvenile arthritis, unspecified, left wrist 🐾
     M08.939   Juvenile arthritis, unspecified, unspecified wrist 🐾

● M08.94   Juvenile arthritis, unspecified, hand
     M08.941   Juvenile arthritis, unspecified, right hand 🐾
     M08.942   Juvenile arthritis, unspecified, left hand 🐾
     M08.949   Juvenile arthritis, unspecified, unspecified hand 🐾

● M08.95   Juvenile arthritis, unspecified, hip
     M08.951   Juvenile arthritis, unspecified, right hip 🐾
     M08.952   Juvenile arthritis, unspecified, left hip 🐾
     M08.959   Juvenile arthritis, unspecified, unspecified hip 🐾

● M08.96   Juvenile arthritis, unspecified, knee
     M08.961   Juvenile arthritis, unspecified, right knee 🐾
     M08.962   Juvenile arthritis, unspecified, left knee 🐾
     M08.969   Juvenile arthritis, unspecified, unspecified knee 🐾

● M08.97   Juvenile arthritis, unspecified, ankle and foot
     M08.971   Juvenile arthritis, unspecified, right ankle and foot 🐾
     M08.972   Juvenile arthritis, unspecified, left ankle and foot 🐾
     M08.979   Juvenile arthritis, unspecified, unspecified ankle and foot 🐾

     M08.98   Juvenile arthritis, unspecified, vertebrae 🐾

     M08.99   Juvenile arthritis, unspecified, multiple sites 🐾

     M08.9A   Juvenile arthritis, unspecified, other specified site

● M1A   **Chronic gout**

Use additional code to identify:
     Autonomic neuropathy in diseases classified elsewhere (G99.0)
     Calculus of urinary tract in diseases classified elsewhere (N22)
     Cardiomyopathy in diseases classified elsewhere (I43)
     Disorders of external ear in diseases classified elsewhere (H61.1-, H62.8-)
     Disorders of iris and ciliary body in diseases classified elsewhere (H22)
     Glomerular disorders in diseases classified elsewhere (N08)

> **Excludes1**   gout NOS (M10.-)

> **Excludes2**   acute gout (M10.-)

The appropriate 7th character is to be added to each code from category M1A

0	without tophus (tophi)
1	with tophus (tophi)

● M1A.0   **Idiopathic chronic gout**
     Chronic gouty bursitis
     Primary chronic gout

X ● M1A.00   Idiopathic chronic gout, unspecified site

● M1A.01   Idiopathic chronic gout, shoulder
     ● M1A.011   Idiopathic chronic gout, right shoulder
     ● M1A.012   Idiopathic chronic gout, left shoulder
     ● M1A.019   Idiopathic chronic gout, unspecified shoulder

● M1A.02   Idiopathic chronic gout, elbow
     ● M1A.021   Idiopathic chronic gout, right elbow
     ● M1A.022   Idiopathic chronic gout, left elbow
     ● M1A.029   Idiopathic chronic gout, unspecified elbow

● M1A.03   Idiopathic chronic gout, wrist
     ● M1A.031   Idiopathic chronic gout, right wrist
     ● M1A.032   Idiopathic chronic gout, left wrist
     ● M1A.039   Idiopathic chronic gout, unspecified wrist

● M1A.04   Idiopathic chronic gout, hand
     ● M1A.041   Idiopathic chronic gout, right hand
     ● M1A.042   Idiopathic chronic gout, left hand
     ● M1A.049   Idiopathic chronic gout, unspecified hand

● M1A.05   Idiopathic chronic gout, hip
     ● M1A.051   Idiopathic chronic gout, right hip
     ● M1A.052   Idiopathic chronic gout, left hip
     ● M1A.059   Idiopathic chronic gout, unspecified hip

● M1A.06 Idiopathic chronic gout, knee
    ● M1A.061 Idiopathic chronic gout, right knee
    ● M1A.062 Idiopathic chronic gout, left knee
    ● M1A.069 Idiopathic chronic gout, unspecified knee
● M1A.07 Idiopathic chronic gout, ankle and foot
    ● M1A.071 Idiopathic chronic gout, right ankle and foot
    ● M1A.072 Idiopathic chronic gout, left ankle and foot
    ● M1A.079 Idiopathic chronic gout, unspecified ankle and foot
X ● M1A.08 Idiopathic chronic gout, vertebrae
X ● M1A.09 Idiopathic chronic gout, multiple sites

● M1A.1 Lead-induced chronic gout
Code first toxic effects of lead and its compounds (T56.0-)
X ● M1A.10 Lead-induced chronic gout, unspecified site
● M1A.11 Lead-induced chronic gout, shoulder
    ● M1A.111 Lead-induced chronic gout, right shoulder
    ● M1A.112 Lead-induced chronic gout, left shoulder
    ● M1A.119 Lead-induced chronic gout, unspecified shoulder
● M1A.12 Lead-induced chronic gout, elbow
    ● M1A.121 Lead-induced chronic gout, right elbow
    ● M1A.122 Lead-induced chronic gout, left elbow
    ● M1A.129 Lead-induced chronic gout, unspecified elbow
● M1A.13 Lead-induced chronic gout, wrist
    ● M1A.131 Lead-induced chronic gout, right wrist
    ● M1A.132 Lead-induced chronic gout, left wrist
    ● M1A.139 Lead-induced chronic gout, unspecified wrist
● M1A.14 Lead-induced chronic gout, hand
    ● M1A.141 Lead-induced chronic gout, right hand
    ● M1A.142 Lead-induced chronic gout, left hand
    ● M1A.149 Lead-induced chronic gout, unspecified hand
● M1A.15 Lead-induced chronic gout, hip
    ● M1A.151 Lead-induced chronic gout, right hip
    ● M1A.152 Lead-induced chronic gout, left hip
    ● M1A.159 Lead-induced chronic gout, unspecified hip
● M1A.16 Lead-induced chronic gout, knee
    ● M1A.161 Lead-induced chronic gout, right knee
    ● M1A.162 Lead-induced chronic gout, left knee
    ● M1A.169 Lead-induced chronic gout, unspecified knee
● M1A.17 Lead-induced chronic gout, ankle and foot
    ● M1A.171 Lead-induced chronic gout, right ankle and foot
    ● M1A.172 Lead-induced chronic gout, left ankle and foot
    ● M1A.179 Lead-induced chronic gout, unspecified ankle and foot
X ● M1A.18 Lead-induced chronic gout, vertebrae
X ● M1A.19 Lead-induced chronic gout, multiple sites

● M1A.2 Drug-induced chronic gout
Use additional code for adverse effect, if applicable, to identify drug (T36-T50 with fifth or sixth character 5)
X ● M1A.20 Drug-induced chronic gout, unspecified site
● M1A.21 Drug-induced chronic gout, shoulder
    ● M1A.211 Drug-induced chronic gout, right shoulder
    ● M1A.212 Drug-induced chronic gout, left shoulder
    ● M1A.219 Drug-induced chronic gout, unspecified shoulder
● M1A.22 Drug-induced chronic gout, elbow
    ● M1A.221 Drug-induced chronic gout, right elbow
    ● M1A.222 Drug-induced chronic gout, left elbow
    ● M1A.229 Drug-induced chronic gout, unspecified elbow
● M1A.23 Drug-induced chronic gout, wrist
    ● M1A.231 Drug-induced chronic gout, right wrist
    ● M1A.232 Drug-induced chronic gout, left wrist
    ● M1A.239 Drug-induced chronic gout, unspecified wrist
● M1A.24 Drug-induced chronic gout, hand
    ● M1A.241 Drug-induced chronic gout, right hand
    ● M1A.242 Drug-induced chronic gout, left hand
    ● M1A.249 Drug-induced chronic gout, unspecified hand
● M1A.25 Drug-induced chronic gout, hip
    ● M1A.251 Drug-induced chronic gout, right hip
    ● M1A.252 Drug-induced chronic gout, left hip
    ● M1A.259 Drug-induced chronic gout, unspecified hip
● M1A.26 Drug-induced chronic gout, knee
    ● M1A.261 Drug-induced chronic gout, right knee
    ● M1A.262 Drug-induced chronic gout, left knee
    ● M1A.269 Drug-induced chronic gout, unspecified knee
● M1A.27 Drug-induced chronic gout, ankle and foot
    ● M1A.271 Drug-induced chronic gout, right ankle and foot
    ● M1A.272 Drug-induced chronic gout, left ankle and foot
    ● M1A.279 Drug-induced chronic gout, unspecified ankle and foot
X ● M1A.28 Drug-induced chronic gout, vertebrae
X ● M1A.29 Drug-induced chronic gout, multiple sites

● M1A.3 Chronic gout due to renal impairment
Code first associated renal disease
X ● M1A.30 Chronic gout due to renal impairment, unspecified site
● M1A.31 Chronic gout due to renal impairment, shoulder
    ● M1A.311 Chronic gout due to renal impairment, right shoulder
    ● M1A.312 Chronic gout due to renal impairment, left shoulder
    ● M1A.319 Chronic gout due to renal impairment, unspecified shoulder

► New   ⇒ Revised   ~~deleted~~ Deleted   Excludes 1   Excludes 2   Includes   Use additional   Code first   Code also   Key words

OGCR Official Guidelines   X Assign placeholder X   ● Use Additional Character(s)   ▶ Manifestation Code   🍂 Hierarchical Condition Category   Coding Clinic

● M1A.32 Chronic gout due to renal impairment, elbow
　● M1A.321 Chronic gout due to renal impairment, right elbow
　● M1A.322 Chronic gout due to renal impairment, left elbow
　● M1A.329 Chronic gout due to renal impairment, unspecified elbow
● M1A.33 Chronic gout due to renal impairment, wrist
　● M1A.331 Chronic gout due to renal impairment, right wrist
　● M1A.332 Chronic gout due to renal impairment, left wrist
　● M1A.339 Chronic gout due to renal impairment, unspecified wrist
● M1A.34 Chronic gout due to renal impairment, hand
　● M1A.341 Chronic gout due to renal impairment, right hand
　● M1A.342 Chronic gout due to renal impairment, left hand
　● M1A.349 Chronic gout due to renal impairment, unspecified hand
● M1A.35 Chronic gout due to renal impairment, hip
　● M1A.351 Chronic gout due to renal impairment, right hip
　● M1A.352 Chronic gout due to renal impairment, left hip
　● M1A.359 Chronic gout due to renal impairment, unspecified hip
● M1A.36 Chronic gout due to renal impairment, knee
　● M1A.361 Chronic gout due to renal impairment, right knee
　● M1A.362 Chronic gout due to renal impairment, left knee
　● M1A.369 Chronic gout due to renal impairment, unspecified knee
● M1A.37 Chronic gout due to renal impairment, ankle and foot
　● M1A.371 Chronic gout due to renal impairment, right ankle and foot
　● M1A.372 Chronic gout due to renal impairment, left ankle and foot
　● M1A.379 Chronic gout due to renal impairment, unspecified ankle and foot
X ● M1A.38 Chronic gout due to renal impairment, vertebrae
X ● M1A.39 Chronic gout due to renal impairment, multiple sites
● M1A.4 Other secondary chronic gout
　Code first associated condition
X ● M1A.40 Other secondary chronic gout, unspecified site
● M1A.41 Other secondary chronic gout, shoulder
　● M1A.411 Other secondary chronic gout, right shoulder
　● M1A.412 Other secondary chronic gout, left shoulder
　● M1A.419 Other secondary chronic gout, unspecified shoulder
● M1A.42 Other secondary chronic gout, elbow
　● M1A.421 Other secondary chronic gout, right elbow
　● M1A.422 Other secondary chronic gout, left elbow
　● M1A.429 Other secondary chronic gout, unspecified elbow

● M1A.43 Other secondary chronic gout, wrist
　● M1A.431 Other secondary chronic gout, right wrist
　● M1A.432 Other secondary chronic gout, left wrist
　● M1A.439 Other secondary chronic gout, unspecified wrist
● M1A.44 Other secondary chronic gout, hand
　● M1A.441 Other secondary chronic gout, right hand
　● M1A.442 Other secondary chronic gout, left hand
　● M1A.449 Other secondary chronic gout, unspecified hand
● M1A.45 Other secondary chronic gout, hip
　● M1A.451 Other secondary chronic gout, right hip
　● M1A.452 Other secondary chronic gout, left hip
　● M1A.459 Other secondary chronic gout, unspecified hip
● M1A.46 Other secondary chronic gout, knee
　● M1A.461 Other secondary chronic gout, right knee
　● M1A.462 Other secondary chronic gout, left knee
　● M1A.469 Other secondary chronic gout, unspecified knee
● M1A.47 Other secondary chronic gout, ankle and foot
　● M1A.471 Other secondary chronic gout, right ankle and foot
　● M1A.472 Other secondary chronic gout, left ankle and foot
　● M1A.479 Other secondary chronic gout, unspecified ankle and foot
X ● M1A.48 Other secondary chronic gout, vertebrae
X ● M1A.49 Other secondary chronic gout, multiple sites
X ● M1A.9 Chronic gout, unspecified

● M10 Gout
　Accumulation of uric acid that results in swollen, red, hot, painful, stiff joints
　Acute gout
　Gout attack
　Gout flare
　Podagra
　Use additional code to identify:
　　Autonomic neuropathy in diseases classified elsewhere (G99.0)
　　Calculus of urinary tract in diseases classified elsewhere (N22)
　　Cardiomyopathy in diseases classified elsewhere (I43)
　　Disorders of external ear in diseases classified elsewhere (H61.1-, H62.8-)
　　Disorders of iris and ciliary body in diseases classified elsewhere (H22)
　　Glomerular disorders in diseases classified elsewhere (N08)
　Excludes2　chronic gout (M1A.-)
● M10.0 Idiopathic gout
　Gouty bursitis
　Primary gout
　M10.00 Idiopathic gout, unspecified site
● M10.01 Idiopathic gout, shoulder
　　M10.011 Idiopathic gout, right shoulder
　　M10.012 Idiopathic gout, left shoulder
　　M10.019 Idiopathic gout, unspecified shoulder
● M10.02 Idiopathic gout, elbow
　　M10.021 Idiopathic gout, right elbow
　　M10.022 Idiopathic gout, left elbow
　　M10.029 Idiopathic gout, unspecified elbow

CHAPTER 13 (M00-M99)

● M10.03   Idiopathic gout, wrist
     M10.031   Idiopathic gout, right wrist
     M10.032   Idiopathic gout, left wrist
     M10.039   Idiopathic gout, unspecified wrist
● M10.04   Idiopathic gout, hand
     M10.041   Idiopathic gout, right hand
     M10.042   Idiopathic gout, left hand
     M10.049   Idiopathic gout, unspecified hand
● M10.05   Idiopathic gout, hip
     M10.051   Idiopathic gout, right hip
     M10.052   Idiopathic gout, left hip
     M10.059   Idiopathic gout, unspecified hip
● M10.06   Idiopathic gout, knee
     M10.061   Idiopathic gout, right knee
     M10.062   Idiopathic gout, left knee
     M10.069   Idiopathic gout, unspecified knee
● M10.07   Idiopathic gout, ankle and foot
     M10.071   Idiopathic gout, right ankle and foot
     M10.072   Idiopathic gout, left ankle and foot
     M10.079   Idiopathic gout, unspecified ankle and foot
   M10.08   Idiopathic gout, vertebrae
   M10.09   Idiopathic gout, multiple sites
● M10.1   Lead-induced gout
     Code first toxic effects of lead and its compounds (T56.0-)
   M10.10   Lead-induced gout, unspecified site
● M10.11   Lead-induced gout, shoulder
     M10.111   Lead-induced gout, right shoulder
     M10.112   Lead-induced gout, left shoulder
     M10.119   Lead-induced gout, unspecified shoulder
● M10.12   Lead-induced gout, elbow
     M10.121   Lead-induced gout, right elbow
     M10.122   Lead-induced gout, left elbow
     M10.129   Lead-induced gout, unspecified elbow
● M10.13   Lead-induced gout, wrist
     M10.131   Lead-induced gout, right wrist
     M10.132   Lead-induced gout, left wrist
     M10.139   Lead-induced gout, unspecified wrist
● M10.14   Lead-induced gout, hand
     M10.141   Lead-induced gout, right hand
     M10.142   Lead-induced gout, left hand
     M10.149   Lead-induced gout, unspecified hand
● M10.15   Lead-induced gout, hip
     M10.151   Lead-induced gout, right hip
     M10.152   Lead-induced gout, left hip
     M10.159   Lead-induced gout, unspecified hip
● M10.16   Lead-induced gout, knee
     M10.161   Lead-induced gout, right knee
     M10.162   Lead-induced gout, left knee
     M10.169   Lead-induced gout, unspecified knee
● M10.17   Lead-induced gout, ankle and foot
     M10.171   Lead-induced gout, right ankle and foot
     M10.172   Lead-induced gout, left ankle and foot
     M10.179   Lead-induced gout, unspecified ankle and foot
   M10.18   Lead-induced gout, vertebrae
   M10.19   Lead-induced gout, multiple sites

● M10.2   Drug-induced gout
     Use additional code for adverse effect, if applicable, to identify drug (T36-T50 with fifth or sixth character 5)
   M10.20   Drug-induced gout, unspecified site
● M10.21   Drug-induced gout, shoulder
     M10.211   Drug-induced gout, right shoulder
     M10.212   Drug-induced gout, left shoulder
     M10.219   Drug-induced gout, unspecified shoulder
● M10.22   Drug-induced gout, elbow
     M10.221   Drug-induced gout, right elbow
     M10.222   Drug-induced gout, left elbow
     M10.229   Drug-induced gout, unspecified elbow
● M10.23   Drug-induced gout, wrist
     M10.231   Drug-induced gout, right wrist
     M10.232   Drug-induced gout, left wrist
     M10.239   Drug-induced gout, unspecified wrist
● M10.24   Drug-induced gout, hand
     M10.241   Drug-induced gout, right hand
     M10.242   Drug-induced gout, left hand
     M10.249   Drug-induced gout, unspecified hand
● M10.25   Drug-induced gout, hip
     M10.251   Drug-induced gout, right hip
     M10.252   Drug-induced gout, left hip
     M10.259   Drug-induced gout, unspecified hip
● M10.26   Drug-induced gout, knee
     M10.261   Drug-induced gout, right knee
     M10.262   Drug-induced gout, left knee
     M10.269   Drug-induced gout, unspecified knee
● M10.27   Drug-induced gout, ankle and foot
     M10.271   Drug-induced gout, right ankle and foot
     M10.272   Drug-induced gout, left ankle and foot
     M10.279   Drug-induced gout, unspecified ankle and foot
   M10.28   Drug-induced gout, vertebrae
   M10.29   Drug-induced gout, multiple sites
● M10.3   Gout due to renal impairment
     Code also associated renal disease
   M10.30   Gout due to renal impairment, unspecified site
● M10.31   Gout due to renal impairment, shoulder
     M10.311   Gout due to renal impairment, right shoulder
     M10.312   Gout due to renal impairment, left shoulder
     M10.319   Gout due to renal impairment, unspecified shoulder
● M10.32   Gout due to renal impairment, elbow
     M10.321   Gout due to renal impairment, right elbow
     M10.322   Gout due to renal impairment, left elbow
     M10.329   Gout due to renal impairment, unspecified elbow
● M10.33   Gout due to renal impairment, wrist
     M10.331   Gout due to renal impairment, right wrist
     M10.332   Gout due to renal impairment, left wrist
     M10.339   Gout due to renal impairment, unspecified wrist

▶ New   ⟹ Revised   ~~deleted~~ Deleted   Excludes 1   Excludes 2   Includes   Use additional   Code first   Code also   Key words
OGCR Official Guidelines   X Assign placeholder X   ● Use Additional Character(s)   ▶ Manifestation Code   🩺 Hierarchical Condition Category   **Coding Clinic**

● M10.34 Gout due to renal impairment, hand
    M10.341 Gout due to renal impairment, right hand
    M10.342 Gout due to renal impairment, left hand
    M10.349 Gout due to renal impairment, unspecified hand
● M10.35 Gout due to renal impairment, hip
    M10.351 Gout due to renal impairment, right hip
    M10.352 Gout due to renal impairment, left hip
    M10.359 Gout due to renal impairment, unspecified hip
● M10.36 Gout due to renal impairment, knee
    M10.361 Gout due to renal impairment, right knee
    M10.362 Gout due to renal impairment, left knee
    M10.369 Gout due to renal impairment, unspecified knee
● M10.37 Gout due to renal impairment, ankle and foot
    M10.371 Gout due to renal impairment, right ankle and foot
    M10.372 Gout due to renal impairment, left ankle and foot
    M10.379 Gout due to renal impairment, unspecified ankle and foot
  M10.38 Gout due to renal impairment, vertebrae
  M10.39 Gout due to renal impairment, multiple sites
● M10.4 Other secondary gout
    Code first associated condition
  M10.40 Other secondary gout, unspecified site
● M10.41 Other secondary gout, shoulder
    M10.411 Other secondary gout, right shoulder
    M10.412 Other secondary gout, left shoulder
    M10.419 Other secondary gout, unspecified shoulder
● M10.42 Other secondary gout, elbow
    M10.421 Other secondary gout, right elbow
    M10.422 Other secondary gout, left elbow
    M10.429 Other secondary gout, unspecified elbow
● M10.43 Other secondary gout, wrist
    M10.431 Other secondary gout, right wrist
    M10.432 Other secondary gout, left wrist
    M10.439 Other secondary gout, unspecified wrist
● M10.44 Other secondary gout, hand
    M10.441 Other secondary gout, right hand
    M10.442 Other secondary gout, left hand
    M10.449 Other secondary gout, unspecified hand
● M10.45 Other secondary gout, hip
    M10.451 Other secondary gout, right hip
    M10.452 Other secondary gout, left hip
    M10.459 Other secondary gout, unspecified hip
● M10.46 Other secondary gout, knee
    M10.461 Other secondary gout, right knee
    M10.462 Other secondary gout, left knee
    M10.469 Other secondary gout, unspecified knee

● M10.47 Other secondary gout, ankle and foot
    M10.471 Other secondary gout, right ankle and foot
    M10.472 Other secondary gout, left ankle and foot
    M10.479 Other secondary gout, unspecified ankle and foot
  M10.48 Other secondary gout, vertebrae
  M10.49 Other secondary gout, multiple sites
M10.9 Gout, unspecified
    Gout NOS

● M11 Other crystal arthropathies
  ● M11.0 Hydroxyapatite deposition disease
    M11.00 Hydroxyapatite deposition disease, unspecified site
  ● M11.01 Hydroxyapatite deposition disease, shoulder
    M11.011 Hydroxyapatite deposition disease, right shoulder
    M11.012 Hydroxyapatite deposition disease, left shoulder
    M11.019 Hydroxyapatite deposition disease, unspecified shoulder
  ● M11.02 Hydroxyapatite deposition disease, elbow
    M11.021 Hydroxyapatite deposition disease, right elbow
    M11.022 Hydroxyapatite deposition disease, left elbow
    M11.029 Hydroxyapatite deposition disease, unspecified elbow
  ● M11.03 Hydroxyapatite deposition disease, wrist
    M11.031 Hydroxyapatite deposition disease, right wrist
    M11.032 Hydroxyapatite deposition disease, left wrist
    M11.039 Hydroxyapatite deposition disease, unspecified wrist
  ● M11.04 Hydroxyapatite deposition disease, hand
    M11.041 Hydroxyapatite deposition disease, right hand
    M11.042 Hydroxyapatite deposition disease, left hand
    M11.049 Hydroxyapatite deposition disease, unspecified hand
  ● M11.05 Hydroxyapatite deposition disease, hip
    M11.051 Hydroxyapatite deposition disease, right hip
    M11.052 Hydroxyapatite deposition disease, left hip
    M11.059 Hydroxyapatite deposition disease, unspecified hip
  ● M11.06 Hydroxyapatite deposition disease, knee
    M11.061 Hydroxyapatite deposition disease, right knee
    M11.062 Hydroxyapatite deposition disease, left knee
    M11.069 Hydroxyapatite deposition disease, unspecified knee
  ● M11.07 Hydroxyapatite deposition disease, ankle and foot
    M11.071 Hydroxyapatite deposition disease, right ankle and foot
    M11.072 Hydroxyapatite deposition disease, left ankle and foot
    M11.079 Hydroxyapatite deposition disease, unspecified ankle and foot
  M11.08 Hydroxyapatite deposition disease, vertebrae
  M11.09 Hydroxyapatite deposition disease, multiple sites

CHAPTER 13 (M00-M99)

● M11.1   Familial chondrocalcinosis
    M11.10   Familial chondrocalcinosis, unspecified site
   ● M11.11   Familial chondrocalcinosis, shoulder
       M11.111   Familial chondrocalcinosis, right shoulder
       M11.112   Familial chondrocalcinosis, left shoulder
       M11.119   Familial chondrocalcinosis, unspecified shoulder
   ● M11.12   Familial chondrocalcinosis, elbow
       M11.121   Familial chondrocalcinosis, right elbow
       M11.122   Familial chondrocalcinosis, left elbow
       M11.129   Familial chondrocalcinosis, unspecified elbow
   ● M11.13   Familial chondrocalcinosis, wrist
       M11.131   Familial chondrocalcinosis, right wrist
       M11.132   Familial chondrocalcinosis, left wrist
       M11.139   Familial chondrocalcinosis, unspecified wrist
   ● M11.14   Familial chondrocalcinosis, hand
       M11.141   Familial chondrocalcinosis, right hand
       M11.142   Familial chondrocalcinosis, left hand
       M11.149   Familial chondrocalcinosis, unspecified hand
   ● M11.15   Familial chondrocalcinosis, hip
       M11.151   Familial chondrocalcinosis, right hip
       M11.152   Familial chondrocalcinosis, left hip
       M11.159   Familial chondrocalcinosis, unspecified hip
   ● M11.16   Familial chondrocalcinosis, knee
       M11.161   Familial chondrocalcinosis, right knee
       M11.162   Familial chondrocalcinosis, left knee
       M11.169   Familial chondrocalcinosis, unspecified knee
   ● M11.17   Familial chondrocalcinosis, ankle and foot
       M11.171   Familial chondrocalcinosis, right ankle and foot
       M11.172   Familial chondrocalcinosis, left ankle and foot
       M11.179   Familial chondrocalcinosis, unspecified ankle and foot
    M11.18   Familial chondrocalcinosis, vertebrae
    M11.19   Familial chondrocalcinosis, multiple sites
● M11.2   Other chondrocalcinosis
      Chondrocalcinosis NOS
    M11.20   Other chondrocalcinosis, unspecified site
   ● M11.21   Other chondrocalcinosis, shoulder
       M11.211   Other chondrocalcinosis, right shoulder
       M11.212   Other chondrocalcinosis, left shoulder
       M11.219   Other chondrocalcinosis, unspecified shoulder
   ● M11.22   Other chondrocalcinosis, elbow
       M11.221   Other chondrocalcinosis, right elbow
       M11.222   Other chondrocalcinosis, left elbow
       M11.229   Other chondrocalcinosis, unspecified elbow
   ● M11.23   Other chondrocalcinosis, wrist
       M11.231   Other chondrocalcinosis, right wrist
       M11.232   Other chondrocalcinosis, left wrist
       M11.239   Other chondrocalcinosis, unspecified wrist

   ● M11.24   Other chondrocalcinosis, hand
       M11.241   Other chondrocalcinosis, right hand
       M11.242   Other chondrocalcinosis, left hand
       M11.249   Other chondrocalcinosis, unspecified hand
   ● M11.25   Other chondrocalcinosis, hip
       M11.251   Other chondrocalcinosis, right hip
       M11.252   Other chondrocalcinosis, left hip
       M11.259   Other chondrocalcinosis, unspecified hip
   ● M11.26   Other chondrocalcinosis, knee
       M11.261   Other chondrocalcinosis, right knee
       M11.262   Other chondrocalcinosis, left knee
       M11.269   Other chondrocalcinosis, unspecified knee
   ● M11.27   Other chondrocalcinosis, ankle and foot
       M11.271   Other chondrocalcinosis, right ankle and foot
       M11.272   Other chondrocalcinosis, left ankle and foot
       M11.279   Other chondrocalcinosis, unspecified ankle and foot
    M11.28   Other chondrocalcinosis, vertebrae
    M11.29   Other chondrocalcinosis, multiple sites
● M11.8   Other specified crystal arthropathies
    M11.80   Other specified crystal arthropathies, unspecified site
   ● M11.81   Other specified crystal arthropathies, shoulder
       M11.811   Other specified crystal arthropathies, right shoulder
       M11.812   Other specified crystal arthropathies, left shoulder
       M11.819   Other specified crystal arthropathies, unspecified shoulder
   ● M11.82   Other specified crystal arthropathies, elbow
       M11.821   Other specified crystal arthropathies, right elbow
       M11.822   Other specified crystal arthropathies, left elbow
       M11.829   Other specified crystal arthropathies, unspecified elbow
   ● M11.83   Other specified crystal arthropathies, wrist
       M11.831   Other specified crystal arthropathies, right wrist
       M11.832   Other specified crystal arthropathies, left wrist
       M11.839   Other specified crystal arthropathies, unspecified wrist
   ● M11.84   Other specified crystal arthropathies, hand
       M11.841   Other specified crystal arthropathies, right hand
       M11.842   Other specified crystal arthropathies, left hand
       M11.849   Other specified crystal arthropathies, unspecified hand
   ● M11.85   Other specified crystal arthropathies, hip
       M11.851   Other specified crystal arthropathies, right hip
       M11.852   Other specified crystal arthropathies, left hip
       M11.859   Other specified crystal arthropathies, unspecified hip

▶ New   ⇒ Revised   ~~deleted~~ Deleted   Excludes 1   Excludes 2   Includes   Use additional   Code first   Code also   Key words
OGCR Official Guidelines   X Assign placeholder X   ● Use Additional Character(s)   ▷ Manifestation Code   ⬥ Hierarchical Condition Category   **Coding Clinic**

● M11.86   Other specified crystal arthropathies, knee

     M11.861   Other specified crystal arthropathies, right knee

     M11.862   Other specified crystal arthropathies, left knee

     M11.869   Other specified crystal arthropathies, unspecified knee

● M11.87   Other specified crystal arthropathies, ankle and foot

     M11.871   Other specified crystal arthropathies, right ankle and foot

     M11.872   Other specified crystal arthropathies, left ankle and foot

     M11.879   Other specified crystal arthropathies, unspecified ankle and foot

     M11.88   Other specified crystal arthropathies, vertebrae

     M11.89   Other specified crystal arthropathies, multiple sites

M11.9   Crystal arthropathy, unspecified

● M12   **Other and unspecified arthropathy**

     Excludes1   arthrosis (M15-M19)

               cricoarytenoid arthropathy (J38.7)

● M12.0   Chronic postrheumatic arthropathy [Jaccoud]

     M12.00   Chronic postrheumatic arthropathy [Jaccoud], unspecified site 🔵

● M12.01   Chronic postrheumatic arthropathy [Jaccoud], shoulder

     M12.011   Chronic postrheumatic arthropathy [Jaccoud], right shoulder 🔵

     M12.012   Chronic postrheumatic arthropathy [Jaccoud], left shoulder 🔵

     M12.019   Chronic postrheumatic arthropathy [Jaccoud], unspecified shoulder 🔵

● M12.02   Chronic postrheumatic arthropathy [Jaccoud], elbow

     M12.021   Chronic postrheumatic arthropathy [Jaccoud], right elbow 🔵

     M12.022   Chronic postrheumatic arthropathy [Jaccoud], left elbow 🔵

     M12.029   Chronic postrheumatic arthropathy [Jaccoud], unspecified elbow 🔵

● M12.03   Chronic postrheumatic arthropathy [Jaccoud], wrist

     M12.031   Chronic postrheumatic arthropathy [Jaccoud], right wrist 🔵

     M12.032   Chronic postrheumatic arthropathy [Jaccoud], left wrist 🔵

     M12.039   Chronic postrheumatic arthropathy [Jaccoud], unspecified wrist 🔵

● M12.04   Chronic postrheumatic arthropathy [Jaccoud], hand

     M12.041   Chronic postrheumatic arthropathy [Jaccoud], right hand 🔵

     M12.042   Chronic postrheumatic arthropathy [Jaccoud], left hand 🔵

     M12.049   Chronic postrheumatic arthropathy [Jaccoud], unspecified hand 🔵

● M12.05   Chronic postrheumatic arthropathy [Jaccoud], hip

     M12.051   Chronic postrheumatic arthropathy [Jaccoud], right hip 🔵

     M12.052   Chronic postrheumatic arthropathy [Jaccoud], left hip 🔵

     M12.059   Chronic postrheumatic arthropathy [Jaccoud], unspecified hip 🔵

● M12.06   Chronic postrheumatic arthropathy [Jaccoud], knee

     M12.061   Chronic postrheumatic arthropathy [Jaccoud], right knee 🔵

     M12.062   Chronic postrheumatic arthropathy [Jaccoud], left knee 🔵

     M12.069   Chronic postrheumatic arthropathy [Jaccoud], unspecified knee 🔵

● M12.07   Chronic postrheumatic arthropathy [Jaccoud], ankle and foot

     M12.071   Chronic postrheumatic arthropathy [Jaccoud], right ankle and foot 🔵

     M12.072   Chronic postrheumatic arthropathy [Jaccoud], left ankle and foot 🔵

     M12.079   Chronic postrheumatic arthropathy [Jaccoud], unspecified ankle and foot 🔵

     M12.08   Chronic postrheumatic arthropathy [Jaccoud], other specified site 🔵

           Chronic postrheumatic arthropathy [Jaccoud], vertebrae

     M12.09   Chronic postrheumatic arthropathy [Jaccoud], multiple sites 🔵

● M12.1   Kaschin-Beck disease

         Osteochondroarthrosis deformans endemica

     M12.10   Kaschin-Beck disease, unspecified site

● M12.11   Kaschin-Beck disease, shoulder

     M12.111   Kaschin-Beck disease, right shoulder

     M12.112   Kaschin-Beck disease, left shoulder

     M12.119   Kaschin-Beck disease, unspecified shoulder

● M12.12   Kaschin-Beck disease, elbow

     M12.121   Kaschin-Beck disease, right elbow

     M12.122   Kaschin-Beck disease, left elbow

     M12.129   Kaschin-Beck disease, unspecified elbow

● M12.13   Kaschin-Beck disease, wrist

     M12.131   Kaschin-Beck disease, right wrist

     M12.132   Kaschin-Beck disease, left wrist

     M12.139   Kaschin-Beck disease, unspecified wrist

● M12.14   Kaschin-Beck disease, hand

     M12.141   Kaschin-Beck disease, right hand

     M12.142   Kaschin-Beck disease, left hand

     M12.149   Kaschin-Beck disease, unspecified hand

● M12.15   Kaschin-Beck disease, hip

     M12.151   Kaschin-Beck disease, right hip

     M12.152   Kaschin-Beck disease, left hip

     M12.159   Kaschin-Beck disease, unspecified hip

● M12.16   Kaschin-Beck disease, knee

     M12.161   Kaschin-Beck disease, right knee

     M12.162   Kaschin-Beck disease, left knee

     M12.169   Kaschin-Beck disease, unspecified knee

● M12.17   Kaschin-Beck disease, ankle and foot

     M12.171   Kaschin-Beck disease, right ankle and foot

     M12.172   Kaschin-Beck disease, left ankle and foot

     M12.179   Kaschin-Beck disease, unspecified ankle and foot

     M12.18   Kaschin-Beck disease, vertebrae

     M12.19   Kaschin-Beck disease, multiple sites

CHAPTER 13 (M00-M99)

● M12.2   Villonodular synovitis (pigmented)
    M12.20   Villonodular synovitis (pigmented), unspecified site
● M12.21   Villonodular synovitis (pigmented), shoulder
    M12.211   Villonodular synovitis (pigmented), right shoulder
    M12.212   Villonodular synovitis (pigmented), left shoulder
    M12.219   Villonodular synovitis (pigmented), unspecified shoulder
● M12.22   Villonodular synovitis (pigmented), elbow
    M12.221   Villonodular synovitis (pigmented), right elbow
    M12.222   Villonodular synovitis (pigmented), left elbow
    M12.229   Villonodular synovitis (pigmented), unspecified elbow
● M12.23   Villonodular synovitis (pigmented), wrist
    M12.231   Villonodular synovitis (pigmented), right wrist
    M12.232   Villonodular synovitis (pigmented), left wrist
    M12.239   Villonodular synovitis (pigmented), unspecified wrist
● M12.24   Villonodular synovitis (pigmented), hand
    M12.241   Villonodular synovitis (pigmented), right hand
    M12.242   Villonodular synovitis (pigmented), left hand
    M12.249   Villonodular synovitis (pigmented), unspecified hand
● M12.25   Villonodular synovitis (pigmented), hip
    M12.251   Villonodular synovitis (pigmented), right hip
    M12.252   Villonodular synovitis (pigmented), left hip
    M12.259   Villonodular synovitis (pigmented), unspecified hip
● M12.26   Villonodular synovitis (pigmented), knee
    M12.261   Villonodular synovitis (pigmented), right knee
    M12.262   Villonodular synovitis (pigmented), left knee
    M12.269   Villonodular synovitis (pigmented), unspecified knee
● M12.27   Villonodular synovitis (pigmented), ankle and foot
    M12.271   Villonodular synovitis (pigmented), right ankle and foot
    M12.272   Villonodular synovitis (pigmented), left ankle and foot
    M12.279   Villonodular synovitis (pigmented), unspecified ankle and foot
    M12.28   Villonodular synovitis (pigmented), other specified site
              Villonodular synovitis (pigmented), vertebrae
    M12.29   Villonodular synovitis (pigmented), multiple sites
● M12.3   Palindromic rheumatism
    M12.30   Palindromic rheumatism, unspecified site
● M12.31   Palindromic rheumatism, shoulder
    M12.311   Palindromic rheumatism, right shoulder
    M12.312   Palindromic rheumatism, left shoulder
    M12.319   Palindromic rheumatism, unspecified shoulder
● M12.32   Palindromic rheumatism, elbow
    M12.321   Palindromic rheumatism, right elbow
    M12.322   Palindromic rheumatism, left elbow
    M12.329   Palindromic rheumatism, unspecified elbow
● M12.33   Palindromic rheumatism, wrist
    M12.331   Palindromic rheumatism, right wrist
    M12.332   Palindromic rheumatism, left wrist
    M12.339   Palindromic rheumatism, unspecified wrist
● M12.34   Palindromic rheumatism, hand
    M12.341   Palindromic rheumatism, right hand
    M12.342   Palindromic rheumatism, left hand
    M12.349   Palindromic rheumatism, unspecified hand
● M12.35   Palindromic rheumatism, hip
    M12.351   Palindromic rheumatism, right hip
    M12.352   Palindromic rheumatism, left hip
    M12.359   Palindromic rheumatism, unspecified hip
● M12.36   Palindromic rheumatism, knee
    M12.361   Palindromic rheumatism, right knee
    M12.362   Palindromic rheumatism, left knee
    M12.369   Palindromic rheumatism, unspecified knee
● M12.37   Palindromic rheumatism, ankle and foot
    M12.371   Palindromic rheumatism, right ankle and foot
    M12.372   Palindromic rheumatism, left ankle and foot
    M12.379   Palindromic rheumatism, unspecified ankle and foot
    M12.38   Palindromic rheumatism, other specified site
              Palindromic rheumatism, vertebrae
    M12.39   Palindromic rheumatism, multiple sites
● M12.4   Intermittent hydrarthrosis
    M12.40   Intermittent hydrarthrosis, unspecified site
● M12.41   Intermittent hydrarthrosis, shoulder
    M12.411   Intermittent hydrarthrosis, right shoulder
    M12.412   Intermittent hydrarthrosis, left shoulder
    M12.419   Intermittent hydrarthrosis, unspecified shoulder
● M12.42   Intermittent hydrarthrosis, elbow
    M12.421   Intermittent hydrarthrosis, right elbow
    M12.422   Intermittent hydrarthrosis, left elbow
    M12.429   Intermittent hydrarthrosis, unspecified elbow
● M12.43   Intermittent hydrarthrosis, wrist
    M12.431   Intermittent hydrarthrosis, right wrist
    M12.432   Intermittent hydrarthrosis, left wrist
    M12.439   Intermittent hydrarthrosis, unspecified wrist
● M12.44   Intermittent hydrarthrosis, hand
    M12.441   Intermittent hydrarthrosis, right hand
    M12.442   Intermittent hydrarthrosis, left hand
    M12.449   Intermittent hydrarthrosis, unspecified hand
● M12.45   Intermittent hydrarthrosis, hip
    M12.451   Intermittent hydrarthrosis, right hip
    M12.452   Intermittent hydrarthrosis, left hip
    M12.459   Intermittent hydrarthrosis, unspecified hip

▶ New   ⇒ Revised   ~~deleted~~ Deleted   Excludes 1   Excludes 2   Includes   Use additional   Code first   Code also   Key words
OGCR Official Guidelines   X Assign placeholder X   ● Use Additional Character(s)   ▶ Manifestation Code   🦘 Hierarchical Condition Category   Coding Clinic

● M12.46 Intermittent hydrarthrosis, knee
     M12.461 Intermittent hydrarthrosis, right knee
     M12.462 Intermittent hydrarthrosis, left knee
     M12.469 Intermittent hydrarthrosis, unspecified knee
● M12.47 Intermittent hydrarthrosis, ankle and foot
     M12.471 Intermittent hydrarthrosis, right ankle and foot
     M12.472 Intermittent hydrarthrosis, left ankle and foot
     M12.479 Intermittent hydrarthrosis, unspecified ankle and foot
   M12.48 Intermittent hydrarthrosis, other site
   M12.49 Intermittent hydrarthrosis, multiple sites
● M12.5 Traumatic arthropathy
     Excludes1   current injury-see Alphabetic Index
                 post-traumatic osteoarthritis of first carpometacarpal joint (M18.2-M18.3)
                 post-traumatic osteoarthritis of hip (M16.4-M16.5)
                 post-traumatic osteoarthritis of knee (M17.2-M17.3)
                 post-traumatic osteoarthritis NOS (M19.1-)
                 post-traumatic osteoarthritis of other single joints (M19.1-)
   M12.50 Traumatic arthropathy, unspecified site
● M12.51 Traumatic arthropathy, shoulder
     M12.511 Traumatic arthropathy, right shoulder
     M12.512 Traumatic arthropathy, left shoulder
     M12.519 Traumatic arthropathy, unspecified shoulder
● M12.52 Traumatic arthropathy, elbow
     M12.521 Traumatic arthropathy, right elbow
     M12.522 Traumatic arthropathy, left elbow
     M12.529 Traumatic arthropathy, unspecified elbow
● M12.53 Traumatic arthropathy, wrist
     M12.531 Traumatic arthropathy, right wrist
     M12.532 Traumatic arthropathy, left wrist
     M12.539 Traumatic arthropathy, unspecified wrist
● M12.54 Traumatic arthropathy, hand
     M12.541 Traumatic arthropathy, right hand
     M12.542 Traumatic arthropathy, left hand
     M12.549 Traumatic arthropathy, unspecified hand
● M12.55 Traumatic arthropathy, hip
     M12.551 Traumatic arthropathy, right hip
     M12.552 Traumatic arthropathy, left hip
         Coding Clinic: 2015, Q1, P17
     M12.559 Traumatic arthropathy, unspecified hip
● M12.56 Traumatic arthropathy, knee
     M12.561 Traumatic arthropathy, right knee
     M12.562 Traumatic arthropathy, left knee
     M12.569 Traumatic arthropathy, unspecified knee
● M12.57 Traumatic arthropathy, ankle and foot
     M12.571 Traumatic arthropathy, right ankle and foot
     M12.572 Traumatic arthropathy, left ankle and foot
     M12.579 Traumatic arthropathy, unspecified ankle and foot

   M12.58 Traumatic arthropathy, other specified site
     Traumatic arthropathy, vertebrae
   M12.59 Traumatic arthropathy, multiple sites
● M12.8 Other specific arthropathies, not elsewhere classified
     Transient arthropathy
   M12.80 Other specific arthropathies, not elsewhere classified, unspecified site
● M12.81 Other specific arthropathies, not elsewhere classified, shoulder
     M12.811 Other specific arthropathies, not elsewhere classified, right shoulder
     M12.812 Other specific arthropathies, not elsewhere classified, left shoulder
     M12.819 Other specific arthropathies, not elsewhere classified, unspecified shoulder
● M12.82 Other specific arthropathies, not elsewhere classified, elbow
     M12.821 Other specific arthropathies, not elsewhere classified, right elbow
     M12.822 Other specific arthropathies, not elsewhere classified, left elbow
     M12.829 Other specific arthropathies, not elsewhere classified, unspecified elbow
● M12.83 Other specific arthropathies, not elsewhere classified, wrist
     M12.831 Other specific arthropathies, not elsewhere classified, right wrist
     M12.832 Other specific arthropathies, not elsewhere classified, left wrist
     M12.839 Other specific arthropathies, not elsewhere classified, unspecified wrist
● M12.84 Other specific arthropathies, not elsewhere classified, hand
     M12.841 Other specific arthropathies, not elsewhere classified, right hand
     M12.842 Other specific arthropathies, not elsewhere classified, left hand
     M12.849 Other specific arthropathies, not elsewhere classified, unspecified hand
● M12.85 Other specific arthropathies, not elsewhere classified, hip
     M12.851 Other specific arthropathies, not elsewhere classified, right hip
     M12.852 Other specific arthropathies, not elsewhere classified, left hip
     M12.859 Other specific arthropathies, not elsewhere classified, unspecified hip
● M12.86 Other specific arthropathies, not elsewhere classified, knee
     M12.861 Other specific arthropathies, not elsewhere classified, right knee
     M12.862 Other specific arthropathies, not elsewhere classified, left knee
     M12.869 Other specific arthropathies, not elsewhere classified, unspecified knee
● M12.87 Other specific arthropathies, not elsewhere classified, ankle and foot
     M12.871 Other specific arthropathies, not elsewhere classified, right ankle and foot
     M12.872 Other specific arthropathies, not elsewhere classified, left ankle and foot
     M12.879 Other specific arthropathies, not elsewhere classified, unspecified ankle and foot

M12.88 Other specific arthropathies, not elsewhere classified, **other specified site**
> Other specific arthropathies, not elsewhere classified, vertebrae

M12.89 Other specific arthropathies, not elsewhere classified, **multiple sites**

M12.9 Arthropathy, **unspecified**

● M13 Other arthritis
> **Excludes1** arthrosis (M15-M19)
> osteoarthritis (M15-M19)

M13.0 Polyarthritis, **unspecified**

● M13.1 Monoarthritis, not elsewhere classified
> M13.10 Monoarthritis, not elsewhere classified, **unspecified site**
> ● M13.11 Monoarthritis, not elsewhere classified, **shoulder**
> > M13.111 Monoarthritis, not elsewhere classified, **right shoulder**
> > M13.112 Monoarthritis, not elsewhere classified, **left shoulder**
> > M13.119 Monoarthritis, not elsewhere classified, **unspecified shoulder**
> ● M13.12 Monoarthritis, not elsewhere classified, **elbow**
> > M13.121 Monoarthritis, not elsewhere classified, **right elbow**
> > M13.122 Monoarthritis, not elsewhere classified, **left elbow**
> > M13.129 Monoarthritis, not elsewhere classified, **unspecified elbow**
> ● M13.13 Monoarthritis, not elsewhere classified, **wrist**
> > M13.131 Monoarthritis, not elsewhere classified, **right wrist**
> > M13.132 Monoarthritis, not elsewhere classified, **left wrist**
> > M13.139 Monoarthritis, not elsewhere classified, **unspecified wrist**
> ● M13.14 Monoarthritis, not elsewhere classified, **hand**
> > M13.141 Monoarthritis, not elsewhere classified, **right hand**
> > M13.142 Monoarthritis, not elsewhere classified, **left hand**
> > M13.149 Monoarthritis, not elsewhere classified, **unspecified hand**
> ● M13.15 Monoarthritis, not elsewhere classified, **hip**
> > M13.151 Monoarthritis, not elsewhere classified, **right hip**
> > M13.152 Monoarthritis, not elsewhere classified, **left hip**
> > M13.159 Monoarthritis, not elsewhere classified, **unspecified hip**
> ● M13.16 Monoarthritis, not elsewhere classified, **knee**
> > M13.161 Monoarthritis, not elsewhere classified, **right knee**
> > M13.162 Monoarthritis, not elsewhere classified, **left knee**
> > M13.169 Monoarthritis, not elsewhere classified, **unspecified knee**
> ● M13.17 Monoarthritis, not elsewhere classified, **ankle and foot**
> > M13.171 Monoarthritis, not elsewhere classified, **right ankle and foot**
> > M13.172 Monoarthritis, not elsewhere classified, **left ankle and foot**
> > M13.179 Monoarthritis, not elsewhere classified, **unspecified ankle and foot**

● M13.8 Other specified arthritis
> Allergic arthritis
> **Excludes1** osteoarthritis (M15-M19)
> M13.80 Other specified arthritis, **unspecified site**
> ● M13.81 Other specified arthritis, **shoulder**
> > M13.811 Other specified arthritis, **right shoulder**
> > M13.812 Other specified arthritis, **left shoulder**
> > M13.819 Other specified arthritis, **unspecified shoulder**
> ● M13.82 Other specified arthritis, **elbow**
> > M13.821 Other specified arthritis, **right elbow**
> > M13.822 Other specified arthritis, **left elbow**
> > M13.829 Other specified arthritis, **unspecified elbow**
> ● M13.83 Other specified arthritis, **wrist**
> > M13.831 Other specified arthritis, **right wrist**
> > M13.832 Other specified arthritis, **left wrist**
> > M13.839 Other specified arthritis, **unspecified wrist**
> ● M13.84 Other specified arthritis, **hand**
> > M13.841 Other specified arthritis, **right hand**
> > M13.842 Other specified arthritis, **left hand**
> > M13.849 Other specified arthritis, **unspecified hand**
> ● M13.85 Other specified arthritis, **hip**
> > M13.851 Other specified arthritis, **right hip**
> > M13.852 Other specified arthritis, **left hip**
> > M13.859 Other specified arthritis, **unspecified hip**
> ● M13.86 Other specified arthritis, **knee**
> > M13.861 Other specified arthritis, **right knee**
> > M13.862 Other specified arthritis, **left knee**
> > M13.869 Other specified arthritis, **unspecified knee**
> ● M13.87 Other specified arthritis, **ankle and foot**
> > M13.871 Other specified arthritis, **right ankle and foot**
> > M13.872 Other specified arthritis, **left ankle and foot**
> > M13.879 Other specified arthritis, **unspecified ankle and foot**
> M13.88 Other specified arthritis, **other site**
> M13.89 Other specified arthritis, **multiple sites**

● M14 Arthropathies in other diseases classified elsewhere
> **Excludes1** arthropathy in:
> > diabetes mellitus (E08-E13 with .61-)
> > hematological disorders (M36.2-M36.3)
> > hypersensitivity reactions (M36.4)
> > neoplastic disease (M36.1)
> > neurosyphillis (A52.16)
> > sarcoidosis (D86.86)
> > enteropathic arthropathies (M07.0-)
> > juvenile psoriatic arthropathy (L40.54)
> > lipoid dermatoarthritis (E78.81)

● M14.6 Charcôt's joint
> Neuropathic arthropathy
> **Excludes1** Charcôt's joint in diabetes mellitus (E08-E13 with .610)
> > Charcôt's joint in tabes dorsalis (A52.16)
> M14.60 Charcôt's joint, **unspecified site**
> ● M14.61 Charcôt's joint, **shoulder**
> > M14.611 Charcôt's joint, **right shoulder**
> > M14.612 Charcôt's joint, **left shoulder**
> > M14.619 Charcôt's joint, **unspecified shoulder**

CHAPTER 13 (M00-M99)

- M14.62   Charcôt's joint, elbow
  - M14.621   Charcôt's joint, right elbow
  - M14.622   Charcôt's joint, left elbow
  - M14.629   Charcôt's joint, unspecified elbow
- M14.63   Charcôt's joint, wrist
  - M14.631   Charcôt's joint, right wrist
  - M14.632   Charcôt's joint, left wrist
  - M14.639   Charcôt's joint, unspecified wrist
- M14.64   Charcôt's joint, hand
  - M14.641   Charcôt's joint, right hand
  - M14.642   Charcôt's joint, left hand
  - M14.649   Charcôt's joint, unspecified hand
- M14.65   Charcôt's joint, hip
  - M14.651   Charcôt's joint, right hip
  - M14.652   Charcôt's joint, left hip
  - M14.659   Charcôt's joint, unspecified hip
- M14.66   Charcôt's joint, knee
  - M14.661   Charcôt's joint, right knee
  - M14.662   Charcôt's joint, left knee
  - M14.669   Charcôt's joint, unspecified knee
- M14.67   Charcôt's joint, ankle and foot
  - M14.671   Charcôt's joint, right ankle and foot
  - M14.672   Charcôt's joint, left ankle and foot
  - M14.679   Charcôt's joint, unspecified ankle and foot
- M14.68   Charcôt's joint, vertebrae
- M14.69   Charcôt's joint, multiple sites
- M14.8   Arthropathies in other specified diseases classified elsewhere

  Code first underlying disease, such as:
  amyloidosis (E85.-)
  erythema multiforme (L51.-)
  erythema nodosum (L52)
  hemochromatosis (E83.11-)
  hyperparathyroidism (E21.-)
  hypothyroidism (E00-E03)
  sickle-cell disorders (D57.-)
  thyrotoxicosis [hyperthyroidism] (E05.-)
  Whipple's disease (K90.81)

  - *M14.80*   *Arthropathies in other specified diseases classified elsewhere, unspecified site*
- M14.81   Arthropathies in other specified diseases classified elsewhere, shoulder
  - *M14.811*   *Arthropathies in other specified diseases classified elsewhere, right shoulder*
  - *M14.812*   *Arthropathies in other specified diseases classified elsewhere, left shoulder*
  - *M14.819*   *Arthropathies in other specified diseases classified elsewhere, unspecified shoulder*
- M14.82   Arthropathies in other specified diseases classified elsewhere, elbow
  - *M14.821*   *Arthropathies in other specified diseases classified elsewhere, right elbow*
  - *M14.822*   *Arthropathies in other specified diseases classified elsewhere, left elbow*
  - *M14.829*   *Arthropathies in other specified diseases classified elsewhere, unspecified elbow*
- M14.83   Arthropathies in other specified diseases classified elsewhere, wrist
  - *M14.831*   *Arthropathies in other specified diseases classified elsewhere, right wrist*
  - *M14.832*   *Arthropathies in other specified diseases classified elsewhere, left wrist*
  - *M14.839*   *Arthropathies in other specified diseases classified elsewhere, unspecified wrist*
- M14.84   Arthropathies in other specified diseases classified elsewhere, hand
  - *M14.841*   *Arthropathies in other specified diseases classified elsewhere, right hand*
  - *M14.842*   *Arthropathies in other specified diseases classified elsewhere, left hand*
  - *M14.849*   *Arthropathies in other specified diseases classified elsewhere, unspecified hand*
- M14.85   Arthropathies in other specified diseases classified elsewhere, hip
  - *M14.851*   *Arthropathies in other specified diseases classified elsewhere, right hip*
  - *M14.852*   *Arthropathies in other specified diseases classified elsewhere, left hip*
  - *M14.859*   *Arthropathies in other specified diseases classified elsewhere, unspecified hip*
- M14.86   Arthropathies in other specified diseases classified elsewhere, knee
  - *M14.861*   *Arthropathies in other specified diseases classified elsewhere, right knee*
  - *M14.862*   *Arthropathies in other specified diseases classified elsewhere, left knee*
  - *M14.869*   *Arthropathies in other specified diseases classified elsewhere, unspecified knee*
- M14.87   Arthropathies in other specified diseases classified elsewhere, ankle and foot
  - *M14.871*   *Arthropathies in other specified diseases classified elsewhere, right ankle and foot*
  - *M14.872*   *Arthropathies in other specified diseases classified elsewhere, left ankle and foot*
  - *M14.879*   *Arthropathies in other specified diseases classified elsewhere, unspecified ankle and foot*
  - *M14.88*   *Arthropathies in other specified diseases classified elsewhere, vertebrae*
  - *M14.89*   *Arthropathies in other specified diseases classified elsewhere, multiple sites*

OSTEOARTHRITIS (M15-M19)

Osteoarthritis is the most common degenerative joint disease and form of arthritis that breaks down the cartilage causing pain, swelling, and reduced motion in the joints.

    Excludes2   osteoarthritis of spine (M47.-)

- M15   Polyosteoarthritis
  - **Includes**   arthritis of multiple sites
  - **Excludes1**   bilateral involvement of single joint (M16-M19)
  - M15.0   Primary generalized (osteo)arthritis
  - M15.1   Heberden's nodes (with arthropathy)
    Interphalangeal distal osteoarthritis
  - M15.2   Bouchard's nodes (with arthropathy)
    Juxtaphalangeal distal osteoarthritis
  - M15.3   Secondary multiple arthritis
    Post-traumatic polyosteoarthritis
  - M15.4   Erosive (osteo)arthritis
  - M15.8   Other polyosteoarthritis
  - M15.9   Polyosteoarthritis, unspecified
    Generalized osteoarthritis NOS

CHAPTER 13 (M00-M99)

● M16   Osteoarthritis of hip

    M16.0   **Bilateral primary osteoarthritis of hip**
       Coding Clinic: 2018, Q2, P15; 2016, Q4, P146

   ● M16.1   **Unilateral primary osteoarthritis of hip**
       Primary osteoarthritis of hip NOS

       M16.10   Unilateral primary osteoarthritis, unspecified hip

       M16.11   Unilateral primary osteoarthritis, right hip

       M16.12   Unilateral primary osteoarthritis, left hip

    M16.2   **Bilateral osteoarthritis resulting from hip dysplasia**

   ● M16.3   **Unilateral osteoarthritis resulting from hip dysplasia**
       Dysplastic osteoarthritis of hip NOS

       M16.30   Unilateral osteoarthritis resulting from hip dysplasia, unspecified hip

       M16.31   Unilateral osteoarthritis resulting from hip dysplasia, right hip

       M16.32   Unilateral osteoarthritis resulting from hip dysplasia, left hip

    M16.4   **Bilateral post-traumatic osteoarthritis of hip**

   ● M16.5   **Unilateral post-traumatic osteoarthritis of hip**
       Post-traumatic osteoarthritis of hip NOS

       M16.50   Unilateral post-traumatic osteoarthritis, unspecified hip

       M16.51   Unilateral post-traumatic osteoarthritis, right hip

       M16.52   Unilateral post-traumatic osteoarthritis, left hip

    M16.6   **Other bilateral secondary osteoarthritis of hip**

    M16.7   **Other unilateral secondary osteoarthritis of hip**
       Secondary osteoarthritis of hip NOS

    M16.9   **Osteoarthritis of hip, unspecified**

● M17   Osteoarthritis of knee

    M17.0   **Bilateral primary osteoarthritis of knee**

   ● M17.1   **Unilateral primary osteoarthritis of knee**
       Primary osteoarthritis of knee NOS

       M17.10   Unilateral primary osteoarthritis, unspecified knee
         Coding Clinic: 2016, Q4, P147

       M17.11   Unilateral primary osteoarthritis, right knee

       M17.12   Unilateral primary osteoarthritis, left knee
         Coding Clinic: 2016, Q4, P146

    M17.2   **Bilateral post-traumatic osteoarthritis of knee**

   ● M17.3   **Unilateral post-traumatic osteoarthritis of knee**
       Post-traumatic osteoarthritis of knee NOS

       M17.30   Unilateral post-traumatic osteoarthritis, unspecified knee

       M17.31   Unilateral post-traumatic osteoarthritis, right knee

       M17.32   Unilateral post-traumatic osteoarthritis, left knee

    M17.4   **Other bilateral secondary osteoarthritis of knee**

    M17.5   **Other unilateral secondary osteoarthritis of knee**
       Secondary osteoarthritis of knee NOS

    M17.9   **Osteoarthritis of knee, unspecified**
       Coding Clinic: 2016, Q4, P146

● M18   Osteoarthritis of first carpometacarpal joint

    M18.0   **Bilateral primary osteoarthritis of first carpometacarpal joints**

   ● M18.1   **Unilateral primary osteoarthritis of first carpometacarpal joint**
       Primary osteoarthritis of first carpometacarpal joint NOS

       M18.10   Unilateral primary osteoarthritis of first carpometacarpal joint, unspecified hand

       M18.11   Unilateral primary osteoarthritis of first carpometacarpal joint, right hand

       M18.12   Unilateral primary osteoarthritis of first carpometacarpal joint, left hand

    M18.2   **Bilateral post-traumatic osteoarthritis of first carpometacarpal joints**

   ● M18.3   **Unilateral post-traumatic osteoarthritis of first carpometacarpal joint**
       Post-traumatic osteoarthritis of first carpometacarpal joint NOS

       M18.30   Unilateral post-traumatic osteoarthritis of first carpometacarpal joint, unspecified hand

       M18.31   Unilateral post-traumatic osteoarthritis of first carpometacarpal joint, right hand

       M18.32   Unilateral post-traumatic osteoarthritis of first carpometacarpal joint, left hand

    M18.4   **Other bilateral secondary osteoarthritis of first carpometacarpal joints**

   ● M18.5   **Other unilateral secondary osteoarthritis of first carpometacarpal joint**
       Secondary osteoarthritis of first carpometacarpal joint NOS

       M18.50   Other unilateral secondary osteoarthritis of first carpometacarpal joint, unspecified hand

       M18.51   Other unilateral secondary osteoarthritis of first carpometacarpal joint, right hand

       M18.52   Other unilateral secondary osteoarthritis of first carpometacarpal joint, left hand

    M18.9   **Osteoarthritis of first carpometacarpal joint, unspecified**

● M19   Other and unspecified osteoarthritis

     Excludes1   polyarthritis (M15.-)

     Excludes2   arthrosis of spine (M47.-)
               hallux rigidus (M20.2)
               osteoarthritis of spine (M47.-)

   ● M19.0   **Primary osteoarthritis of other joints**

     ● M19.01   **Primary osteoarthritis, shoulder**

       M19.011   Primary osteoarthritis, right shoulder
         Coding Clinic: 2016, Q4, P145

       M19.012   Primary osteoarthritis, left shoulder

       M19.019   Primary osteoarthritis, unspecified shoulder

     ● M19.02   **Primary osteoarthritis, elbow**

       M19.021   Primary osteoarthritis, right elbow

       M19.022   Primary osteoarthritis, left elbow

       M19.029   Primary osteoarthritis, unspecified elbow

     ● M19.03   **Primary osteoarthritis, wrist**

       M19.031   Primary osteoarthritis, right wrist

       M19.032   Primary osteoarthritis, left wrist

       M19.039   Primary osteoarthritis, unspecified wrist

     ● M19.04   **Primary osteoarthritis, hand**

       Excludes2   primary osteoarthritis of first carpometacarpal joint (M18.0-, M18.1-)

       M19.041   Primary osteoarthritis, right hand

       M19.042   Primary osteoarthritis, left hand

       M19.049   Primary osteoarthritis, unspecified hand

     ● M19.07   **Primary osteoarthritis ankle and foot**

       M19.071   Primary osteoarthritis, right ankle and foot

       M19.072   Primary osteoarthritis, left ankle and foot

       M19.079   Primary osteoarthritis, unspecified ankle and foot

      M19.09   Primary osteoarthritis, other specified site

▶ New   ⇒ Revised   ~~deleted~~ Deleted   Excludes 1   Excludes 2   Includes   Use additional   Code first   Code also   Key words

OGCR Official Guidelines   X Assign placeholder X   ● Use Additional Character(s)   ▷ Manifestation Code   🖤 Hierarchical Condition Category   **Coding Clinic**

- **M19.1** Post-traumatic osteoarthritis of other joints
  - **M19.11** Post-traumatic osteoarthritis, shoulder
    - M19.111 Post-traumatic osteoarthritis, right shoulder
    - M19.112 Post-traumatic osteoarthritis, left shoulder
    - M19.119 Post-traumatic osteoarthritis, unspecified shoulder
  - **M19.12** Post-traumatic osteoarthritis, elbow
    - M19.121 Post-traumatic osteoarthritis, right elbow
    - M19.122 Post-traumatic osteoarthritis, left elbow
    - M19.129 Post-traumatic osteoarthritis, unspecified elbow
  - **M19.13** Post-traumatic osteoarthritis, wrist
    - M19.131 Post-traumatic osteoarthritis, right wrist
    - M19.132 Post-traumatic osteoarthritis, left wrist
    - M19.139 Post-traumatic osteoarthritis, unspecified wrist
  - **M19.14** Post-traumatic osteoarthritis, hand
    - **Excludes2** post-traumatic osteoarthritis of first carpometacarpal joint (M18.2-, M18.3-)
    - M19.141 Post-traumatic osteoarthritis, right hand
    - M19.142 Post-traumatic osteoarthritis, left hand
    - M19.149 Post-traumatic osteoarthritis, unspecified hand
  - **M19.17** Post-traumatic osteoarthritis, ankle and foot
    - M19.171 Post-traumatic osteoarthritis, right ankle and foot
    - M19.172 Post-traumatic osteoarthritis, left ankle and foot
    - M19.179 Post-traumatic osteoarthritis, unspecified ankle and foot
    - M19.19 Post-traumatic osteoarthritis, other specified site
- **M19.2** Secondary osteoarthritis of other joints
  - **M19.21** Secondary osteoarthritis, shoulder
    - M19.211 Secondary osteoarthritis, right shoulder
    - M19.212 Secondary osteoarthritis, left shoulder
    - M19.219 Secondary osteoarthritis, unspecified shoulder
  - **M19.22** Secondary osteoarthritis, elbow
    - M19.221 Secondary osteoarthritis, right elbow
    - M19.222 Secondary osteoarthritis, left elbow
    - M19.229 Secondary osteoarthritis, unspecified elbow
  - **M19.23** Secondary osteoarthritis, wrist
    - M19.231 Secondary osteoarthritis, right wrist
    - M19.232 Secondary osteoarthritis, left wrist
    - M19.239 Secondary osteoarthritis, unspecified wrist
  - **M19.24** Secondary osteoarthritis, hand
    - M19.241 Secondary osteoarthritis, right hand
    - M19.242 Secondary osteoarthritis, left hand
    - M19.249 Secondary osteoarthritis, unspecified hand

- **M19.27** Secondary osteoarthritis, ankle and foot
  - M19.271 Secondary osteoarthritis, right ankle and foot
  - M19.272 Secondary osteoarthritis, left ankle and foot
  - M19.279 Secondary osteoarthritis, unspecified ankle and foot
  - M19.29 Secondary osteoarthritis, other specified site
- **M19.9** Osteoarthritis, unspecified site
  - M19.90 Unspecified osteoarthritis, unspecified site
    - Arthrosis NOS
    - Arthritis NOS
    - Osteoarthritis NOS
    - **Coding Clinic: 2016, Q4, P147**
  - M19.91 Primary osteoarthritis, unspecified site
    - Primary osteoarthritis NOS
  - M19.92 Post-traumatic osteoarthritis, unspecified site
    - Post-traumatic osteoarthritis NOS
  - M19.93 Secondary osteoarthritis, unspecified site
    - Secondary osteoarthritis NOS

OTHER JOINT DISORDERS (M20-M25)

Excludes2   joints of the spine (M40-M54)

- **M20** Acquired deformities of fingers and toes
  - **Excludes1**   acquired absence of fingers and toes (Z89.-)
    - congenital absence of fingers and toes (Q71.3-, Q72.3-)
    - congenital deformities and malformations of fingers and toes (Q66.-, Q68-Q70, Q74.-)
  - **M20.0** Deformity of finger(s)
    - **Excludes1**   clubbing of fingers (R68.3)
      - palmar fascial fibromatosis [Dupuytren] (M72.0)
      - trigger finger (M65.3)
    - **M20.00** Unspecified deformity of finger(s)
      - M20.001 Unspecified deformity of right finger(s)
      - M20.002 Unspecified deformity of left finger(s)
      - M20.009 Unspecified deformity of unspecified finger(s)
    - **M20.01** Mallet finger
      - M20.011 Mallet finger of right finger(s)
      - M20.012 Mallet finger of left finger(s)
      - M20.019 Mallet finger of unspecified finger(s)
    - **M20.02** Boutonnière deformity
      - M20.021 Boutonnière deformity of right finger(s)
      - M20.022 Boutonnière deformity of left finger(s)
      - M20.029 Boutonnière deformity of unspecified finger(s)
    - **M20.03** Swan-neck deformity
      - M20.031 Swan-neck deformity of right finger(s)
      - M20.032 Swan-neck deformity of left finger(s)
      - M20.039 Swan-neck deformity of unspecified finger(s)
    - **M20.09** Other deformity of finger(s)
      - M20.091 Other deformity of right finger(s)
      - M20.092 Other deformity of left finger(s)
      - M20.099 Other deformity of finger(s), unspecified finger(s)

Figure 13-1   Hallux valgus.

Item 13-2 Hallux valgus is a sometimes painful structural deformity caused by an inflammation of the bursal sac at the base of the metatarsophalangeal joint (big toe). **Hallus varus** is a deviation of the great toe to the inner side of the foot or away from the next toe.

● M20.1   Hallux valgus (acquired)
    Excludes2 bunion (M21.6-)
    Coding Clinic: 2016, Q4, P38
    M20.10 Hallux valgus (acquired), unspecified foot
    M20.11 Hallux valgus (acquired), right foot
    M20.12 Hallux valgus (acquired), left foot
● M20.2   Hallux rigidus
    M20.20 Hallux rigidus, unspecified foot
    M20.21 Hallux rigidus, right foot
    M20.22 Hallux rigidus, left foot
● M20.3   Hallux varus (acquired)
    M20.30 Hallux varus (acquired), unspecified foot
    M20.31 Hallux varus (acquired), right foot
    M20.32 Hallux varus (acquired), left foot
● M20.4   Other hammer toe(s) (acquired)
    M20.40 Other hammer toe(s) (acquired), unspecified foot
    M20.41 Other hammer toe(s) (acquired), right foot
    M20.42 Other hammer toe(s) (acquired), left foot
● M20.5   Other deformities of toe(s) (acquired)
    ● M20.5X Other deformities of toe(s) (acquired)
        M20.5X1 Other deformities of toe(s) (acquired), right foot
        M20.5X2 Other deformities of toe(s) (acquired), left foot
        M20.5X9 Other deformities of toe(s) (acquired), unspecified foot
● M20.6   Acquired deformities of toe(s), unspecified
    M20.60 Acquired deformities of toe(s), unspecified, unspecified foot
    M20.61 Acquired deformities of toe(s), unspecified, right foot
    M20.62 Acquired deformities of toe(s), unspecified, left foot

Item 13-3 Cubitus valgus is a deformity of the elbow resulting in an increased carrying angle in which the arm extends at the side and the palm faces forward, which results in the forearm and hand extended at greater than 15 degrees.

Item 13-4 Cubitus varus is a deformity of the elbow resulting in the arm extended at the side and the palm facing forward so that the forearm and hand are held at less than 5 degrees, decreasing the carrying angle.

● M21   Other acquired deformities of limbs
    Excludes1 acquired absence of limb (Z89.-)
        congenital absence of limbs (Q71-Q73)
        congenital deformities and malformations of limbs (Q65-Q66, Q68-Q74)
    Excludes2 acquired deformities of fingers or toes (M20.-)
        coxa plana (M91.2)
    ● M21.0   Valgus deformity, not elsewhere classified
        Excludes1 metatarsus valgus (Q66.6)
            talipes calcaneovalgus (Q66.4-)
        M21.00 Valgus deformity, not elsewhere classified, unspecified site
        ● M21.02 Valgus deformity, not elsewhere classified, elbow
            Cubitus valgus
            M21.021 Valgus deformity, not elsewhere classified, right elbow
            M21.022 Valgus deformity, not elsewhere classified, left elbow
            M21.029 Valgus deformity, not elsewhere classified, unspecified elbow
        ● M21.05 Valgus deformity, not elsewhere classified, hip
            M21.051 Valgus deformity, not elsewhere classified, right hip
            M21.052 Valgus deformity, not elsewhere classified, left hip
            M21.059 Valgus deformity, not elsewhere classified, unspecified hip
        ● M21.06 Valgus deformity, not elsewhere classified, knee
            Genu valgum
            Knock knee
            M21.061 Valgus deformity, not elsewhere classified, right knee
            M21.062 Valgus deformity, not elsewhere classified, left knee
            M21.069 Valgus deformity, not elsewhere classified, unspecified knee
        ● M21.07 Valgus deformity, not elsewhere classified, ankle
            M21.071 Valgus deformity, not elsewhere classified, right ankle
            M21.072 Valgus deformity, not elsewhere classified, left ankle
            M21.079 Valgus deformity, not elsewhere classified, unspecified ankle
    ● M21.1   Varus deformity, not elsewhere classified
        Excludes1 metatarsus varus (Q66.22-)
            tibia vara (M92.51-)
        M21.10 Varus deformity, not elsewhere classified, unspecified site
        ● M21.12 Varus deformity, not elsewhere classified, elbow
            Cubitus varus, elbow
            M21.121 Varus deformity, not elsewhere classified, right elbow
            M21.122 Varus deformity, not elsewhere classified, left elbow
            M21.129 Varus deformity, not elsewhere classified, unspecified elbow

CHAPTER 13 (M00-M99)

▶ New   ⇛ Revised   ~~deleted~~ Deleted   Excludes 1   Excludes 2   Includes   Use additional   Code first   Code also   Key words
OGCR Official Guidelines   X Assign placeholder X   ● Use Additional Character(s)   ▶ Manifestation Code   🦥 Hierarchical Condition Category   Coding Clinic

● M21.15   Varus deformity, not elsewhere classified, hip
    M21.151   Varus deformity, not elsewhere classified, right hip
    M21.152   Varus deformity, not elsewhere classified, left hip
    M21.159   Varus deformity, not elsewhere classified, unspecified

● M21.16   Varus deformity, not elsewhere classified, knee
    Bow leg
    Genu varum
    M21.161   Varus deformity, not elsewhere classified, right knee
    M21.162   Varus deformity, not elsewhere classified, left knee
    M21.169   Varus deformity, not elsewhere classified, unspecified knee

● M21.17   Varus deformity, not elsewhere classified, ankle
    M21.171   Varus deformity, not elsewhere classified, right ankle
    M21.172   Varus deformity, not elsewhere classified, left ankle
    M21.179   Varus deformity, not elsewhere classified, unspecified ankle

● M21.2   Flexion deformity
    M21.20   Flexion deformity, unspecified site

● M21.21   Flexion deformity, shoulder
    M21.211   Flexion deformity, right shoulder
    M21.212   Flexion deformity, left shoulder
    M21.219   Flexion deformity, unspecified shoulder

● M21.22   Flexion deformity, elbow
    M21.221   Flexion deformity, right elbow
    M21.222   Flexion deformity, left elbow
    M21.229   Flexion deformity, unspecified elbow

● M21.23   Flexion deformity, wrist
    M21.231   Flexion deformity, right wrist
    M21.232   Flexion deformity, left wrist
    M21.239   Flexion deformity, unspecified wrist

● M21.24   Flexion deformity, finger joints
    M21.241   Flexion deformity, right finger joints
    M21.242   Flexion deformity, left finger joints
    M21.249   Flexion deformity, unspecified finger joints

● M21.25   Flexion deformity, hip
    M21.251   Flexion deformity, right hip
    M21.252   Flexion deformity, left hip
    M21.259   Flexion deformity, unspecified hip

● M21.26   Flexion deformity, knee
    M21.261   Flexion deformity, right knee
    M21.262   Flexion deformity, left knee
    M21.269   Flexion deformity, unspecified knee

● M21.27   Flexion deformity, ankle and toes
    M21.271   Flexion deformity, right ankle and toes
    M21.272   Flexion deformity, left ankle and toes
    M21.279   Flexion deformity, unspecified ankle and toes

● M21.3   Wrist or foot drop (acquired)
   ● M21.33   Wrist drop (acquired)
    M21.331   Wrist drop, right wrist
    M21.332   Wrist drop, left wrist
    M21.339   Wrist drop, unspecified wrist

   ● M21.37   Foot drop (acquired)
    M21.371   Foot drop, right foot
    M21.372   Foot drop, left foot
    M21.379   Foot drop, unspecified foot

● M21.4   Flat foot [pes planus] (acquired)
    Excludes1   congenital pes planus (Q66.5-)
    M21.40   Flat foot [pes planus] (acquired), unspecified foot
    M21.41   Flat foot [pes planus] (acquired), right foot
    M21.42   Flat foot [pes planus] (acquired), left foot

● M21.5   Acquired clawhand, clubhand, clawfoot and clubfoot
    Excludes1   clubfoot, not specified as acquired (Q66.89)
   ● M21.51   Acquired clawhand
    M21.511   Acquired clawhand, right hand
    M21.512   Acquired clawhand, left hand
    M21.519   Acquired clawhand, unspecified hand

   ● M21.52   Acquired clubhand
    M21.521   Acquired clubhand, right hand
    M21.522   Acquired clubhand, left hand
    M21.529   Acquired clubhand, unspecified hand

   ● M21.53   Acquired clawfoot
    M21.531   Acquired clawfoot, right foot
    M21.532   Acquired clawfoot, left foot
    M21.539   Acquired clawfoot, unspecified foot

   ● M21.54   Acquired clubfoot
    M21.541   Acquired clubfoot, right foot
    M21.542   Acquired clubfoot, left foot
    M21.549   Acquired clubfoot, unspecified foot

● M21.6   Other acquired deformities of foot
    Excludes2   deformities of toe (acquired) (M20.1-M20.6-)
   ● M21.61   Bunion
    Coding Clinic: 2016, Q4, P38
    M21.611   Bunion of right foot
    M21.612   Bunion of left foot
    M21.619   Bunion of unspecified foot

   ● M21.62   Bunionette
    Coding Clinic: 2016, Q4, P38
    M21.621   Bunionette of right foot
    M21.622   Bunionette of left foot
    M21.629   Bunionette of unspecified foot

   ● M21.6X   Other acquired deformities of foot
    M21.6X1   Other acquired deformities of right foot
    M21.6X2   Other acquired deformities of left foot
    M21.6X9   Other acquired deformities of unspecified foot

● M21.7   Unequal limb length (acquired)
    Note: The site used should correspond to the shorter limb.
    M21.70   Unequal limb length (acquired), unspecified site

   ● M21.72   Unequal limb length (acquired), humerus
    M21.721   Unequal limb length (acquired), right humerus
    M21.722   Unequal limb length (acquired), left humerus
    M21.729   Unequal limb length (acquired), unspecified humerus

   ● M21.73   Unequal limb length (acquired), ulna and radius
    M21.731   Unequal limb length (acquired), right ulna
    M21.732   Unequal limb length (acquired), left ulna
    M21.733   Unequal limb length (acquired), right radius
    M21.734   Unequal limb length (acquired), left radius
    M21.739   Unequal limb length (acquired), unspecified ulna and radius

CHAPTER 13 (M00-M99)

● **M21.75** Unequal limb length (acquired), femur

    M21.751 Unequal limb length (acquired), right femur

    M21.752 Unequal limb length (acquired), left femur

    M21.759 Unequal limb length (acquired), unspecified femur

● **M21.76** Unequal limb length (acquired), tibia and fibula

    M21.761 Unequal limb length (acquired), right tibia

    M21.762 Unequal limb length (acquired), left tibia

    M21.763 Unequal limb length (acquired), right fibula

    M21.764 Unequal limb length (acquired), left fibula

    M21.769 Unequal limb length (acquired), unspecified tibia and fibula

● **M21.8** Other specified acquired deformities of limbs

    Excludes2   coxa plana (M91.2)

    M21.80 Other specified acquired deformities of unspecified limb

● **M21.82** Other specified acquired deformities of upper arm

    M21.821 Other specified acquired deformities of right upper arm

    M21.822 Other specified acquired deformities of left upper arm

    M21.829 Other specified acquired deformities of unspecified upper arm

● **M21.83** Other specified acquired deformities of forearm

    M21.831 Other specified acquired deformities of right forearm

    M21.832 Other specified acquired deformities of left forearm

    M21.839 Other specified acquired deformities of unspecified forearm

● **M21.85** Other specified acquired deformities of thigh

    M21.851 Other specified acquired deformities of right thigh

    M21.852 Other specified acquired deformities of left thigh

    M21.859 Other specified acquired deformities of unspecified thigh

● **M21.86** Other specified acquired deformities of lower leg

    M21.861 Other specified acquired deformities of right lower leg

    M21.862 Other specified acquired deformities of left lower leg

    M21.869 Other specified acquired deformities of unspecified lower leg

● **M21.9** Unspecified acquired deformity of limb and hand

    M21.90 Unspecified acquired deformity of unspecified limb

● **M21.92** Unspecified acquired deformity of upper arm

    M21.921 Unspecified acquired deformity of right upper arm

    M21.922 Unspecified acquired deformity of left upper arm

    M21.929 Unspecified acquired deformity of unspecified upper arm

● **M21.93** Unspecified acquired deformity of forearm

    M21.931 Unspecified acquired deformity of right forearm

    M21.932 Unspecified acquired deformity of left forearm

    M21.939 Unspecified acquired deformity of unspecified forearm

● **M21.94** Unspecified acquired deformity of hand

    M21.941 Unspecified acquired deformity of hand, right hand

    M21.942 Unspecified acquired deformity of hand, left hand

    M21.949 Unspecified acquired deformity of hand, unspecified hand

● **M21.95** Unspecified acquired deformity of thigh

    M21.951 Unspecified acquired deformity of right thigh

    M21.952 Unspecified acquired deformity of left thigh

    M21.959 Unspecified acquired deformity of unspecified thigh

● **M21.96** Unspecified acquired deformity of lower leg

    M21.961 Unspecified acquired deformity of right lower leg

    M21.962 Unspecified acquired deformity of left lower leg

    M21.969 Unspecified acquired deformity of unspecified lower leg

● **M22** Disorder of patella

    Excludes2   traumatic dislocation of patella (S83.0-)

● **M22.0** Recurrent dislocation of patella

    M22.00 Recurrent dislocation of patella, unspecified knee

    M22.01 Recurrent dislocation of patella, right knee

    M22.02 Recurrent dislocation of patella, left knee

● **M22.1** Recurrent subluxation of patella

    Incomplete dislocation of patella

    M22.10 Recurrent subluxation of patella, unspecified knee

    M22.11 Recurrent subluxation of patella, right knee

    M22.12 Recurrent subluxation of patella, left knee

● **M22.2** Patellofemoral disorders

    ● **M22.2X** Patellofemoral disorders

        M22.2X1 Patellofemoral disorders, right knee

        M22.2X2 Patellofemoral disorders, left knee

        M22.2X9 Patellofemoral disorders, unspecified knee

● **M22.3** Other derangements of patella

    ● **M22.3X** Other derangements of patella

        M22.3X1 Other derangements of patella, right knee

        M22.3X2 Other derangements of patella, left knee

        M22.3X9 Other derangements of patella, unspecified knee

● **M22.4** Chondromalacia patellae

    M22.40 Chondromalacia patellae, unspecified knee

    M22.41 Chondromalacia patellae, right knee

    M22.42 Chondromalacia patellae, left knee

● **M22.8** Other disorders of patella

    ● **M22.8X** Other disorders of patella

        M22.8X1 Other disorders of patella, right knee

        M22.8X2 Other disorders of patella, left knee

        M22.8X9 Other disorders of patella, unspecified knee

● **M22.9** Unspecified disorder of patella

    M22.90 Unspecified disorder of patella, unspecified knee

    M22.91 Unspecified disorder of patella, right knee

    M22.92 Unspecified disorder of patella, left knee

● **M23**   **Internal derangement of knee**
> **Excludes1**   ankylosis (M24.66)
> deformity of knee (M21.-)
> osteochondritis dissecans (M93.2)
>
> **Excludes2**   current injury - see injury of knee and lower leg (S80-S89)
> recurrent dislocation or subluxation of joints (M24.4)
> recurrent dislocation or subluxation of patella (M22.0-M22.1)
>
> Coding Clinic: 2019, Q2, P26

● **M23.0**   **Cystic meniscus**
> ● **M23.00**   Cystic meniscus, unspecified meniscus
> > Cystic meniscus, unspecified lateral meniscus
> > Cystic meniscus, unspecified medial meniscus
> >
> > M23.000   Cystic meniscus, unspecified lateral meniscus, right knee
> > M23.001   Cystic meniscus, unspecified lateral meniscus, left knee
> > M23.002   Cystic meniscus, unspecified lateral meniscus, unspecified knee
> > M23.003   Cystic meniscus, unspecified medial meniscus, right knee
> > M23.004   Cystic meniscus, unspecified medial meniscus, left knee
> > M23.005   Cystic meniscus, unspecified medial meniscus, unspecified knee
> > M23.006   Cystic meniscus, unspecified meniscus, right knee
> > M23.007   Cystic meniscus, unspecified meniscus, left knee
> > M23.009   Cystic meniscus, unspecified meniscus, unspecified knee
>
> ● **M23.01**   Cystic meniscus, anterior horn of medial meniscus
> > M23.011   Cystic meniscus, anterior horn of medial meniscus, right knee
> > M23.012   Cystic meniscus, anterior horn of medial meniscus, left knee
> > M23.019   Cystic meniscus, anterior horn of medial meniscus, unspecified knee
>
> ● **M23.02**   Cystic meniscus, posterior horn of medial meniscus
> > M23.021   Cystic meniscus, posterior horn of medial meniscus, right knee
> > M23.022   Cystic meniscus, posterior horn of medial meniscus, left knee
> > M23.029   Cystic meniscus, posterior horn of medial meniscus, unspecified knee
>
> ● **M23.03**   Cystic meniscus, other medial meniscus
> > M23.031   Cystic meniscus, other medial meniscus, right knee
> > M23.032   Cystic meniscus, other medial meniscus, left knee
> > M23.039   Cystic meniscus, other medial meniscus, unspecified knee
>
> ● **M23.04**   Cystic meniscus, anterior horn of lateral meniscus
> > M23.041   Cystic meniscus, anterior horn of lateral meniscus, right knee
> > M23.042   Cystic meniscus, anterior horn of lateral meniscus, left knee
> > M23.049   Cystic meniscus, anterior horn of lateral meniscus, unspecified knee

● **M23.05**   Cystic meniscus, posterior horn of lateral meniscus
> M23.051   Cystic meniscus, posterior horn of lateral meniscus, right knee
> M23.052   Cystic meniscus, posterior horn of lateral meniscus, left knee
> M23.059   Cystic meniscus, posterior horn of lateral meniscus, unspecified knee

● **M23.06**   Cystic meniscus, other lateral meniscus
> M23.061   Cystic meniscus, other lateral meniscus, right knee
> M23.062   Cystic meniscus, other lateral meniscus, left knee
> M23.069   Cystic meniscus, other lateral meniscus, unspecified knee

★ **(See Plate 34 of the Anatomy Illustrations.)**
> ● **M23.2**   Derangement of meniscus due to old tear or injury
> > Old bucket-handle tear
> >
> > ● **M23.20**   Derangement of unspecified meniscus due to old tear or injury
> > > Derangement of unspecified lateral meniscus due to old tear or injury
> > > Derangement of unspecified medial meniscus due to old tear or injury
> > >
> > > M23.200   Derangement of unspecified lateral meniscus due to old tear or injury, right knee
> > > M23.201   Derangement of unspecified lateral meniscus due to old tear or injury, left knee
> > > M23.202   Derangement of unspecified lateral meniscus due to old tear or injury, unspecified knee
> > > M23.203   Derangement of unspecified medial meniscus due to old tear or injury, right knee
> > > M23.204   Derangement of unspecified medial meniscus due to old tear or injury, left knee
> > > M23.205   Derangement of unspecified medial meniscus due to old tear or injury, unspecified knee
> > > M23.206   Derangement of unspecified meniscus due to old tear or injury, right knee
> > > M23.207   Derangement of unspecified meniscus due to old tear or injury, left knee
> > > M23.209   Derangement of unspecified meniscus due to old tear or injury, unspecified knee
> >
> > ● **M23.21**   Derangement of anterior horn of medial meniscus due to old tear or injury
> > > M23.211   Derangement of anterior horn of medial meniscus due to old tear or injury, right knee
> > > M23.212   Derangement of anterior horn of medial meniscus due to old tear or injury, left knee
> > > M23.219   Derangement of anterior horn of medial meniscus due to old tear or injury, unspecified knee
> >
> > ● **M23.22**   Derangement of posterior horn of medial meniscus due to old tear or injury
> > > M23.221   Derangement of posterior horn of medial meniscus due to old tear or injury, right knee
> > > M23.222   Derangement of posterior horn of medial meniscus due to old tear or injury, left knee
> > > M23.229   Derangement of posterior horn of medial meniscus due to old tear or injury, unspecified knee

● M23.23 Derangement of other medial meniscus due to old tear or injury

M23.231 Derangement of other medial meniscus due to old tear or injury, right knee

M23.232 Derangement of other medial meniscus due to old tear or injury, left knee

M23.239 Derangement of other medial meniscus due to old tear or injury, unspecified knee

● M23.24 Derangement of anterior horn of lateral meniscus due to old tear or injury

M23.241 Derangement of anterior horn of lateral meniscus due to old tear or injury, right knee

M23.242 Derangement of anterior horn of lateral meniscus due to old tear or injury, left knee

M23.249 Derangement of anterior horn of lateral meniscus due to old tear or injury, unspecified knee

● M23.25 Derangement of posterior horn of lateral meniscus due to old tear or injury

M23.251 Derangement of posterior horn of lateral meniscus due to old tear or injury, right knee

M23.252 Derangement of posterior horn of lateral meniscus due to old tear or injury, left knee

M23.259 Derangement of posterior horn of lateral meniscus due to old tear or injury, unspecified knee

● M23.26 Derangement of other lateral meniscus due to old tear or injury

M23.261 Derangement of other lateral meniscus due to old tear or injury, right knee

M23.262 Derangement of other lateral meniscus due to old tear or injury, left knee

M23.269 Derangement of other lateral meniscus due to old tear or injury, unspecified knee

● M23.3 Other meniscus derangements
Degenerate meniscus
Detached meniscus
Retained meniscus

● M23.30 Other meniscus derangements, unspecified meniscus
Other meniscus derangements, unspecified lateral meniscus
Other meniscus derangements, unspecified medial meniscus

M23.300 Other meniscus derangements, unspecified lateral meniscus, right knee

M23.301 Other meniscus derangements, unspecified lateral meniscus, left knee

M23.302 Other meniscus derangements, unspecified lateral meniscus, unspecified knee

M23.303 Other meniscus derangements, unspecified medial meniscus, right knee

M23.304 Other meniscus derangements, unspecified medial meniscus, left knee

M23.305 Other meniscus derangements, unspecified medial meniscus, unspecified knee

M23.306 Other meniscus derangements, unspecified meniscus, right knee

M23.307 Other meniscus derangements, unspecified meniscus, left knee

M23.309 Other meniscus derangements, unspecified meniscus, unspecified knee

● M23.31 Other meniscus derangements, anterior horn of medial meniscus

M23.311 Other meniscus derangements, anterior horn of medial meniscus, right knee

M23.312 Other meniscus derangements, anterior horn of medial meniscus, left knee

M23.319 Other meniscus derangements, anterior horn of medial meniscus, unspecified knee

● M23.32 Other meniscus derangements, posterior horn of medial meniscus

M23.321 Other meniscus derangements, posterior horn of medial meniscus, right knee

M23.322 Other meniscus derangements, posterior horn of medial meniscus, left knee

M23.329 Other meniscus derangements, posterior horn of medial meniscus, unspecified knee

● M23.33 Other meniscus derangements, other medial meniscus

M23.331 Other meniscus derangements, other medial meniscus, right knee

M23.332 Other meniscus derangements, other medial meniscus, left knee

M23.339 Other meniscus derangements, other medial meniscus, unspecified knee

● M23.34 Other meniscus derangements, anterior horn of lateral meniscus

M23.341 Other meniscus derangements, anterior horn of lateral meniscus, right knee

M23.342 Other meniscus derangements, anterior horn of lateral meniscus, left knee

M23.349 Other meniscus derangements, anterior horn of lateral meniscus, unspecified knee

● M23.35 Other meniscus derangements, posterior horn of lateral meniscus

M23.351 Other meniscus derangements, posterior horn of lateral meniscus, right knee

M23.352 Other meniscus derangements, posterior horn of lateral meniscus, left knee

M23.359 Other meniscus derangements, posterior horn of lateral meniscus, unspecified knee

● M23.36 Other meniscus derangements, other lateral meniscus

M23.361 Other meniscus derangements, other lateral meniscus, right knee

M23.362 Other meniscus derangements, other lateral meniscus, left knee

M23.369 Other meniscus derangements, other lateral meniscus, unspecified knee

▶ New   ⇛ Revised   ~~deleted~~ Deleted   Excludes 1   Excludes 2   Includes   Use additional   Code first   Code also   Key words

OGCR Official Guidelines   X Assign placeholder X   ● Use Additional Character(s)   ▷ Manifestation Code   🐱 Hierarchical Condition Category   Coding Clinic

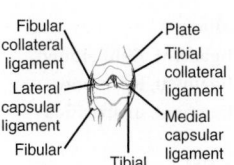

Figure 13-2 Collateral and cruciate ligament of knee. (From DeLee: DeLee and Drez's Orthopaedic Sports Medicine, ed 3, Saunders, 2009)

● M23.4   Loose body in knee
    M23.40   Loose body in knee, unspecified knee
    M23.41   Loose body in knee, right knee
    M23.42   Loose body in knee, left knee
● M23.5   Chronic instability of knee
    M23.50   Chronic instability of knee, unspecified knee
    M23.51   Chronic instability of knee, right knee
    M23.52   Chronic instability of knee, left knee
● M23.6   Other spontaneous disruption of ligament(s) of knee
    ● M23.60   Other spontaneous disruption of unspecified ligament of knee
       M23.601   Other spontaneous disruption of unspecified ligament of right knee
       M23.602   Other spontaneous disruption of unspecified ligament of left knee
       M23.609   Other spontaneous disruption of unspecified ligament of unspecified knee
    ● M23.61   Other spontaneous disruption of anterior cruciate ligament of knee
       M23.611   Other spontaneous disruption of anterior cruciate ligament of right knee
       M23.612   Other spontaneous disruption of anterior cruciate ligament of left knee
       M23.619   Other spontaneous disruption of anterior cruciate ligament of unspecified knee
    ● M23.62   Other spontaneous disruption of posterior cruciate ligament of knee
       M23.621   Other spontaneous disruption of posterior cruciate ligament of right knee
       M23.622   Other spontaneous disruption of posterior cruciate ligament of left knee
       M23.629   Other spontaneous disruption of posterior cruciate ligament of unspecified knee
    ● M23.63   Other spontaneous disruption of medial collateral ligament of knee
       M23.631   Other spontaneous disruption of medial collateral ligament of right knee
       M23.632   Other spontaneous disruption of medial collateral ligament of left knee
       M23.639   Other spontaneous disruption of medial collateral ligament of unspecified knee
    ● M23.64   Other spontaneous disruption of lateral collateral ligament of knee
       M23.641   Other spontaneous disruption of lateral collateral ligament of right knee
       M23.642   Other spontaneous disruption of lateral collateral ligament of left knee
       M23.649   Other spontaneous disruption of lateral collateral ligament of unspecified knee

    ● M23.67   Other spontaneous disruption of capsular ligament of knee
       M23.671   Other spontaneous disruption of capsular ligament of right knee
       M23.672   Other spontaneous disruption of capsular ligament of left knee
       M23.679   Other spontaneous disruption of capsular ligament of unspecified knee
● M23.8   Other internal derangements of knee
    Laxity of ligament of knee
    Snapping knee
    ● M23.8X   Other internal derangements of knee
       M23.8X1   Other internal derangements of right knee
       M23.8X2   Other internal derangements of left knee
       M23.8X9   Other internal derangements of unspecified knee
● M23.9   Unspecified internal derangement of knee
    M23.90   Unspecified internal derangement of unspecified knee
    M23.91   Unspecified internal derangement of right knee
    M23.92   Unspecified internal derangement of left knee
● M24   Other specific joint derangements
    Excludes1   current injury - see injury of joint by body region
    Excludes2   ganglion (M67.4)
                snapping knee (M23.8-)
                temporomandibular joint disorders (M26.6-)
    ● M24.0   Loose body in joint
       Excludes2   loose body in knee (M23.4)
       M24.00   Loose body in unspecified joint
       ● M24.01   Loose body in shoulder
          M24.011   Loose body in right shoulder
          M24.012   Loose body in left shoulder
          M24.019   Loose body in unspecified shoulder
       ● M24.02   Loose body in elbow
          M24.021   Loose body in right elbow
          M24.022   Loose body in left elbow
          M24.029   Loose body in unspecified elbow
       ● M24.03   Loose body in wrist
          M24.031   Loose body in right wrist
          M24.032   Loose body in left wrist
          M24.039   Loose body in unspecified wrist
       ● M24.04   Loose body in finger joints
          M24.041   Loose body in right finger joint(s)
          M24.042   Loose body in left finger joint(s)
          M24.049   Loose body in unspecified finger joint(s)
       ● M24.05   Loose body in hip
          M24.051   Loose body in right hip
          M24.052   Loose body in left hip
          M24.059   Loose body in unspecified hip
       ● M24.07   Loose body in ankle and toe joints
          M24.071   Loose body in right ankle
          M24.072   Loose body in left ankle
          M24.073   Loose body in unspecified ankle
          M24.074   Loose body in right toe joint(s)
          M24.075   Loose body in left toe joint(s)
          M24.076   Loose body in unspecified toe joints
       M24.08   Loose body, other site

CHAPTER 13 (M00-M99)

● **M24.1** Other articular cartilage disorders

Excludes2 chondrocalcinosis (M11.1, M11.2-)
internal derangement of knee (M23.-)
metastatic calcification (E83.5)
ochronosis (E70.2)

M24.10 Other articular cartilage disorders, unspecified site

● M24.11 Other articular cartilage disorders, shoulder

M24.111 Other articular cartilage disorders, right shoulder

M24.112 Other articular cartilage disorders, left shoulder

M24.119 Other articular cartilage disorders, unspecified shoulder

● M24.12 Other articular cartilage disorders, elbow

M24.121 Other articular cartilage disorders, right elbow

M24.122 Other articular cartilage disorders, left elbow

M24.129 Other articular cartilage disorders, unspecified elbow

● M24.13 Other articular cartilage disorders, wrist

M24.131 Other articular cartilage disorders, right wrist

M24.132 Other articular cartilage disorders, left wrist

M24.139 Other articular cartilage disorders, unspecified wrist

● M24.14 Other articular cartilage disorders, hand

M24.141 Other articular cartilage disorders, right hand

M24.142 Other articular cartilage disorders, left hand

M24.149 Other articular cartilage disorders, unspecified hand

● M24.15 Other articular cartilage disorders, hip

M24.151 Other articular cartilage disorders, right hip

M24.152 Other articular cartilage disorders, left hip

M24.159 Other articular cartilage disorders, unspecified hip

● M24.17 Other articular cartilage disorders, ankle and foot

M24.171 Other articular cartilage disorders, right ankle

M24.172 Other articular cartilage disorders, left ankle

M24.173 Other articular cartilage disorders, unspecified ankle

M24.174 Other articular cartilage disorders, right foot

M24.175 Other articular cartilage disorders, left foot

M24.176 Other articular cartilage disorders, unspecified foot

M24.19 Other articular cartilage disorders, other specified site

● **M24.2** Disorder of ligament

Instability secondary to old ligament injury
Ligamentous laxity NOS

Excludes1 familial ligamentous laxity (M35.7)
Excludes2 internal derangement of knee (M23.5-M23.8X9)

M24.20 Disorder of ligament, unspecified site

● M24.21 Disorder of ligament, shoulder

M24.211 Disorder of ligament, right shoulder

M24.212 Disorder of ligament, left shoulder

M24.219 Disorder of ligament, unspecified shoulder

● M24.22 Disorder of ligament, elbow

M24.221 Disorder of ligament, right elbow

M24.222 Disorder of ligament, left elbow

M24.229 Disorder of ligament, unspecified elbow

● M24.23 Disorder of ligament, wrist

M24.231 Disorder of ligament, right wrist

M24.232 Disorder of ligament, left wrist

M24.239 Disorder of ligament, unspecified wrist

● M24.24 Disorder of ligament, hand

M24.241 Disorder of ligament, right hand

M24.242 Disorder of ligament, left hand

M24.249 Disorder of ligament, unspecified hand

● M24.25 Disorder of ligament, hip

M24.251 Disorder of ligament, right hip

M24.252 Disorder of ligament, left hip

M24.259 Disorder of ligament, unspecified hip

● M24.27 Disorder of ligament, ankle and foot

M24.271 Disorder of ligament, right ankle

M24.272 Disorder of ligament, left ankle

M24.273 Disorder of ligament, unspecified ankle

M24.274 Disorder of ligament, right foot

M24.275 Disorder of ligament, left foot

M24.276 Disorder of ligament, unspecified foot

M24.28 Disorder of ligament, vertebrae

M24.29 Disorder of ligament, other specified site

● **M24.3** Pathological dislocation of joint, not elsewhere classified

Excludes1 congenital dislocation or displacement of joint - see congenital malformations and deformations of the musculoskeletal system (Q65-Q79)
current injury - see injury of joints and ligaments by body region
recurrent dislocation of joint (M24.4-)

M24.30 Pathological dislocation of unspecified joint, not elsewhere classified

● M24.31 Pathological dislocation of shoulder, not elsewhere classified

M24.311 Pathological dislocation of right shoulder, not elsewhere classified

M24.312 Pathological dislocation of left shoulder, not elsewhere classified

M24.319 Pathological dislocation of unspecified shoulder, not elsewhere classified

● M24.32 Pathological dislocation of elbow, not elsewhere classified

M24.321 Pathological dislocation of right elbow, not elsewhere classified

M24.322 Pathological dislocation of left elbow, not elsewhere classified

M24.329 Pathological dislocation of unspecified elbow, not elsewhere classified

● M24.33 Pathological dislocation of wrist, not elsewhere classified

M24.331 Pathological dislocation of right wrist, not elsewhere classified

M24.332 Pathological dislocation of left wrist, not elsewhere classified

M24.339 Pathological dislocation of unspecified wrist, not elsewhere classified

▶ New   ⇒ Revised   ~~deleted~~ Deleted   Excludes 1   Excludes 2   Includes   Use additional   Code first   Code also   Key words

OGCR Official Guidelines   X Assign placeholder X   ● Use Additional Character(s)   ▶ Manifestation Code   🔲 Hierarchical Condition Category   **Coding Clinic**

● M24.34 Pathological dislocation of hand, not elsewhere classified
   M24.341 Pathological dislocation of right hand, not elsewhere classified
   M24.342 Pathological dislocation of left hand, not elsewhere classified
   M24.349 Pathological dislocation of unspecified hand, not elsewhere classified
● M24.35 Pathological dislocation of hip, not elsewhere classified
   M24.351 Pathological dislocation of right hip, not elsewhere classified
     Coding Clinic: 2022, Q1, P32
   M24.352 Pathological dislocation of left hip, not elsewhere classified
     Coding Clinic: 2022, Q1, P32
   M24.359 Pathological dislocation of unspecified hip, not elsewhere classified
● M24.36 Pathological dislocation of knee, not elsewhere classified
   M24.361 Pathological dislocation of right knee, not elsewhere classified
   M24.362 Pathological dislocation of left knee, not elsewhere classified
   M24.369 Pathological dislocation of unspecified knee, not elsewhere classified
● M24.37 Pathological dislocation of ankle and foot, not elsewhere classified
   M24.371 Pathological dislocation of right ankle, not elsewhere classified
   M24.372 Pathological dislocation of left ankle, not elsewhere classified
   M24.373 Pathological dislocation of unspecified ankle, not elsewhere classified
   M24.374 Pathological dislocation of right foot, not elsewhere classified
   M24.375 Pathological dislocation of left foot, not elsewhere classified
   M24.376 Pathological dislocation of unspecified foot, not elsewhere classified
   M24.39 Pathological dislocation of other specified joint, not elsewhere classified
● M24.4 Recurrent dislocation of joint
   Recurrent subluxation of joint
   Excludes2 recurrent dislocation of patella (M22.0-M22.1)
     recurrent vertebral dislocation (M43.3-, M43.4, M43.5-)
   M24.40 Recurrent dislocation, unspecified joint
● M24.41 Recurrent dislocation, shoulder
   M24.411 Recurrent dislocation, right shoulder
   M24.412 Recurrent dislocation, left shoulder
   M24.419 Recurrent dislocation, unspecified shoulder
● M24.42 Recurrent dislocation, elbow
   M24.421 Recurrent dislocation, right elbow
   M24.422 Recurrent dislocation, left elbow
   M24.429 Recurrent dislocation, unspecified elbow
● M24.43 Recurrent dislocation, wrist
   M24.431 Recurrent dislocation, right wrist
   M24.432 Recurrent dislocation, left wrist
   M24.439 Recurrent dislocation, unspecified wrist

● M24.44 Recurrent dislocation, hand and finger(s)
   M24.441 Recurrent dislocation, right hand
   M24.442 Recurrent dislocation, left hand
   M24.443 Recurrent dislocation, unspecified hand
   M24.444 Recurrent dislocation, right finger
   M24.445 Recurrent dislocation, left finger
   M24.446 Recurrent dislocation, unspecified finger
● M24.45 Recurrent dislocation, hip
   M24.451 Recurrent dislocation, right hip
   M24.452 Recurrent dislocation, left hip
   M24.459 Recurrent dislocation, unspecified hip
● M24.46 Recurrent dislocation, knee
   M24.461 Recurrent dislocation, right knee
   M24.462 Recurrent dislocation, left knee
   M24.469 Recurrent dislocation, unspecified knee
● M24.47 Recurrent dislocation, ankle, foot and toes
   M24.471 Recurrent dislocation, right ankle
   M24.472 Recurrent dislocation, left ankle
   M24.473 Recurrent dislocation, unspecified ankle
   M24.474 Recurrent dislocation, right foot
   M24.475 Recurrent dislocation, left foot
   M24.476 Recurrent dislocation, unspecified foot
   M24.477 Recurrent dislocation, right toe(s)
   M24.478 Recurrent dislocation, left toe(s)
   M24.479 Recurrent dislocation, unspecified toe(s)
   M24.49 Recurrent dislocation, other specified joint
● M24.5 Contracture of joint
   Excludes1 contracture of muscle without contracture of joint (M62.4-)
     contracture of tendon (sheath) without contracture of joint (M62.4-)
     Dupuytren's contracture (M72.0)
   Excludes2 acquired deformities of limbs (M20-M21)
   M24.50 Contracture, unspecified joint
● M24.51 Contracture, shoulder
   M24.511 Contracture, right shoulder
   M24.512 Contracture, left shoulder
   M24.519 Contracture, unspecified shoulder
● M24.52 Contracture, elbow
   M24.521 Contracture, right elbow
   M24.522 Contracture, left elbow
   M24.529 Contracture, unspecified elbow
● M24.53 Contracture, wrist
   M24.531 Contracture, right wrist
   M24.532 Contracture, left wrist
   M24.539 Contracture, unspecified wrist
● M24.54 Contracture, hand
   M24.541 Contracture, right hand
   M24.542 Contracture, left hand
   M24.549 Contracture, unspecified hand
● M24.55 Contracture, hip
   M24.551 Contracture, right hip
     Coding Clinic: 2016, Q2, P6
   M24.552 Contracture, left hip
     Coding Clinic: 2016, Q2, P6
   M24.559 Contracture, unspecified hip

CHAPTER 13 (M00-M99)

Item 13–5 **Ankylosis** or arthrokleisis is a consolidation of a joint due to disease, injury, or surgical procedure. Spondylosis is the degeneration of the vertebral processes and formation of osteophytes and commonly occurs with age. **Spondylitis** or ankylosing spondylitis is a type of arthritis that affects the spine or backbone, causing back pain and stiffness.

- M24.56 Contracture, knee
  - M24.561 Contracture, right knee
    - Coding Clinic: 2016, Q2, P6
  - M24.562 Contracture, left knee
    - Coding Clinic: 2016, Q2, P6
  - M24.569 Contracture, unspecified knee
- M24.57 Contracture, ankle and foot
  - M24.571 Contracture, right ankle
  - M24.572 Contracture, left ankle
  - M24.573 Contracture, unspecified ankle
  - M24.574 Contracture, right foot
  - M24.575 Contracture, left foot
  - M24.576 Contracture, unspecified foot
- M24.59 Contracture, other specified joint
- M24.6 Ankylosis of joint
  - Excludes1 stiffness of joint without ankylosis (M25.6-)
  - Excludes2 spine (M43.2-)
  - M24.60 Ankylosis, unspecified joint
- M24.61 Ankylosis, shoulder
  - M24.611 Ankylosis, right shoulder
  - M24.612 Ankylosis, left shoulder
  - M24.619 Ankylosis, unspecified shoulder
- M24.62 Ankylosis, elbow
  - M24.621 Ankylosis, right elbow
  - M24.622 Ankylosis, left elbow
  - M24.629 Ankylosis, unspecified elbow
- M24.63 Ankylosis, wrist
  - M24.631 Ankylosis, right wrist
  - M24.632 Ankylosis, left wrist
  - M24.639 Ankylosis, unspecified wrist
- M24.64 Ankylosis, hand
  - M24.641 Ankylosis, right hand
  - M24.642 Ankylosis, left hand
  - M24.649 Ankylosis, unspecified hand
- M24.65 Ankylosis, hip
  - M24.651 Ankylosis, right hip
  - M24.652 Ankylosis, left hip
  - M24.659 Ankylosis, unspecified hip
- M24.66 Ankylosis, knee
  - M24.661 Ankylosis, right knee
  - M24.662 Ankylosis, left knee
  - M24.669 Ankylosis, unspecified knee
- M24.67 Ankylosis, ankle and foot
  - M24.671 Ankylosis, right ankle
  - M24.672 Ankylosis, left ankle
  - M24.673 Ankylosis, unspecified ankle
  - M24.674 Ankylosis, right foot
  - M24.675 Ankylosis, left foot
  - M24.676 Ankylosis, unspecified foot
- M24.69 Ankylosis, other specified joint
- M24.7 Protrusio acetabuli

- M24.8 Other specific joint derangements, not elsewhere classified
  - Excludes2 iliotibial band syndrome (M76.3)
  - M24.80 Other specific joint derangements of unspecified joint, not elsewhere classified
- M24.81 Other specific joint derangements of shoulder, not elsewhere classified
  - M24.811 Other specific joint derangements of right shoulder, not elsewhere classified
  - M24.812 Other specific joint derangements of left shoulder, not elsewhere classified
  - M24.819 Other specific joint derangements of unspecified shoulder, not elsewhere classified
- M24.82 Other specific joint derangements of elbow, not elsewhere classified
  - M24.821 Other specific joint derangements of right elbow, not elsewhere classified
  - M24.822 Other specific joint derangements of left elbow, not elsewhere classified
  - M24.829 Other specific joint derangements of unspecified elbow, not elsewhere classified
- M24.83 Other specific joint derangements of wrist, not elsewhere classified
  - M24.831 Other specific joint derangements of right wrist, not elsewhere classified
  - M24.832 Other specific joint derangements of left wrist, not elsewhere classified
  - M24.839 Other specific joint derangements of unspecified wrist, not elsewhere classified
- M24.84 Other specific joint derangements of hand, not elsewhere classified
  - M24.841 Other specific joint derangements of right hand, not elsewhere classified
  - M24.842 Other specific joint derangements of left hand, not elsewhere classified
  - M24.849 Other specific joint derangements of unspecified hand, not elsewhere classified
- M24.85 Other specific joint derangements of hip, not elsewhere classified
  - Irritable hip
  - M24.851 Other specific joint derangements of right hip, not elsewhere classified
  - M24.852 Other specific joint derangements of left hip, not elsewhere classified
  - M24.859 Other specific joint derangements of unspecified hip, not elsewhere classified
- M24.87 Other specific joint derangements of ankle and foot, not elsewhere classified
  - M24.871 Other specific joint derangements of right ankle, not elsewhere classified
  - M24.872 Other specific joint derangements of left ankle, not elsewhere classified
  - M24.873 Other specific joint derangements of unspecified ankle, not elsewhere classified
  - M24.874 Other specific joint derangements of right foot, not elsewhere classified
  - M24.875 Other specific joint derangements left foot, not elsewhere classified
  - M24.876 Other specific joint derangements of unspecified foot, not elsewhere classified
  - M24.89 Other specific joint derangement of other specified joint, not elsewhere classified
- M24.9 Joint derangement, unspecified

CHAPTER 13 (M00-M99)

● **M25 Other joint disorder, not elsewhere classified**

  Excludes2   abnormality of gait and mobility (R26.-)
            acquired deformities of limb (M20-M21)
            calcification of bursa (M71.4-)
            calcification of shoulder (joint) (M75.3)
            calcification of tendon (M65.2-)
            difficulty in walking (R26.2)
            temporomandibular joint disorder (M26.6-)

● **M25.0 Hemarthrosis**

  Excludes1   current injury - see injury of joint by body
            region
            hemophilic arthropathy (M36.2)

  M25.00 Hemarthrosis, unspecified joint
● M25.01 Hemarthrosis, shoulder
    M25.011 Hemarthrosis, right shoulder
    M25.012 Hemarthrosis, left shoulder
    M25.019 Hemarthrosis, unspecified shoulder
● M25.02 Hemarthrosis, elbow
    M25.021 Hemarthrosis, right elbow
    M25.022 Hemarthrosis, left elbow
    M25.029 Hemarthrosis, unspecified elbow
● M25.03 Hemarthrosis, wrist
    M25.031 Hemarthrosis, right wrist
    M25.032 Hemarthrosis, left wrist
    M25.039 Hemarthrosis, unspecified wrist
● M25.04 Hemarthrosis, hand
    M25.041 Hemarthrosis, right hand
    M25.042 Hemarthrosis, left hand
    M25.049 Hemarthrosis, unspecified hand
● M25.05 Hemarthrosis, hip
    M25.051 Hemarthrosis, right hip
    M25.052 Hemarthrosis, left hip
    M25.059 Hemarthrosis, unspecified hip
● M25.06 Hemarthrosis, knee
    M25.061 Hemarthrosis, right knee
    M25.062 Hemarthrosis, left knee
    M25.069 Hemarthrosis, unspecified knee
● M25.07 Hemarthrosis, ankle and foot
    M25.071 Hemarthrosis, right ankle
    M25.072 Hemarthrosis, left ankle
    M25.073 Hemarthrosis, unspecified ankle
    M25.074 Hemarthrosis, right foot
    M25.075 Hemarthrosis, left foot
    M25.076 Hemarthrosis, unspecified foot
  M25.08 Hemarthrosis, other specified site
            Hemarthrosis, vertebrae
● **M25.1 Fistula of joint**
  M25.10 Fistula, unspecified joint
● M25.11 Fistula, shoulder
    M25.111 Fistula, right shoulder
    M25.112 Fistula, left shoulder
    M25.119 Fistula, unspecified shoulder
● M25.12 Fistula, elbow
    M25.121 Fistula, right elbow
    M25.122 Fistula, left elbow
    M25.129 Fistula, unspecified elbow
● M25.13 Fistula, wrist
    M25.131 Fistula, right wrist
    M25.132 Fistula, left wrist
    M25.139 Fistula, unspecified wrist
● M25.14 Fistula, hand
    M25.141 Fistula, right hand
    M25.142 Fistula, left hand
    M25.149 Fistula, unspecified hand

● M25.15 Fistula, hip
    M25.151 Fistula, right hip
    M25.152 Fistula, left hip
    M25.159 Fistula, unspecified hip
● M25.16 Fistula, knee
    M25.161 Fistula, right knee
    M25.162 Fistula, left knee
    M25.169 Fistula, unspecified knee
● M25.17 Fistula, ankle and foot
    M25.171 Fistula, right ankle
    M25.172 Fistula, left ankle
    M25.173 Fistula, unspecified ankle
    M25.174 Fistula, right foot
    M25.175 Fistula, left foot
    M25.176 Fistula, unspecified foot
  M25.18 Fistula, other specified site
            Fistula, vertebrae
● **M25.2 Flail joint**
  M25.20 Flail joint, unspecified joint
● M25.21 Flail joint, shoulder
    M25.211 Flail joint, right shoulder
    M25.212 Flail joint, left shoulder
    M25.219 Flail joint, unspecified shoulder
● M25.22 Flail joint, elbow
    M25.221 Flail joint, right elbow
    M25.222 Flail joint, left elbow
    M25.229 Flail joint, unspecified elbow
● M25.23 Flail joint, wrist
    M25.231 Flail joint, right wrist
    M25.232 Flail joint, left wrist
    M25.239 Flail joint, unspecified wrist
● M25.24 Flail joint, hand
    M25.241 Flail joint, right hand
    M25.242 Flail joint, left hand
    M25.249 Flail joint, unspecified hand
● M25.25 Flail joint, hip
    M25.251 Flail joint, right hip
    M25.252 Flail joint, left hip
    M25.259 Flail joint, unspecified hip
● M25.26 Flail joint, knee
    M25.261 Flail joint, right knee
    M25.262 Flail joint, left knee
    M25.269 Flail joint, unspecified knee
● M25.27 Flail joint, ankle and foot
    M25.271 Flail joint, right ankle and foot
    M25.272 Flail joint, left ankle and foot
    M25.279 Flail joint, unspecified ankle and foot
  M25.28 Flail joint, other site
● **M25.3 Other instability of joint**

  Excludes1   instability of joint secondary to old
            ligament injury (M24.2-)
            instability of joint secondary to removal
            of joint prosthesis (M96.8-)

  Excludes2   spinal instabilities (M53.2-)

  M25.30 Other instability, unspecified joint
● M25.31 Other instability, shoulder
    M25.311 Other instability, right shoulder
    M25.312 Other instability, left shoulder
    M25.319 Other instability, unspecified
            shoulder
● M25.32 Other instability, elbow
    M25.321 Other instability, right elbow
    M25.322 Other instability, left elbow
    M25.329 Other instability, unspecified elbow

CHAPTER 13 (M00-M99)

CHAPTER 13 (M00-M99)

● M25.33 Other instability, wrist
  M25.331 Other instability, right wrist
  M25.332 Other instability, left wrist
  M25.339 Other instability, unspecified wrist
● M25.34 Other instability, hand
  M25.341 Other instability, right hand
  M25.342 Other instability, left hand
  M25.349 Other instability, unspecified hand
● M25.35 Other instability, hip
  M25.351 Other instability, right hip
  M25.352 Other instability, left hip
  M25.359 Other instability, unspecified hip
● M25.36 Other instability, knee
  M25.361 Other instability, right knee
  M25.362 Other instability, left knee
  M25.369 Other instability, unspecified knee
● M25.37 Other instability, ankle and foot
  M25.371 Other instability, right ankle
  M25.372 Other instability, left ankle
  M25.373 Other instability, unspecified ankle
  M25.374 Other instability, right foot
  M25.375 Other instability, left foot
  M25.376 Other instability, unspecified foot
M25.39 Other instability of joint
● M25.4 Effusion of joint
  Excludes1 hydrarthrosis in yaws (A66.6)
    intermittent hydrarthrosis (M12.4-)
    other infective (teno)synovitis (M65.1-)
M25.40 Effusion, unspecified joint
● M25.41 Effusion, shoulder
  M25.411 Effusion, right shoulder
  M25.412 Effusion, left shoulder
  M25.419 Effusion, unspecified shoulder
● M25.42 Effusion, elbow
  M25.421 Effusion, right elbow
  M25.422 Effusion, left elbow
  M25.429 Effusion, unspecified elbow
● M25.43 Effusion, wrist
  M25.431 Effusion, right wrist
  M25.432 Effusion, left wrist
  M25.439 Effusion, unspecified wrist
● M25.44 Effusion, hand
  M25.441 Effusion, right hand
  M25.442 Effusion, left hand
  M25.449 Effusion, unspecified hand
● M25.45 Effusion, hip
  M25.451 Effusion, right hip
  M25.452 Effusion, left hip
  M25.459 Effusion, unspecified hip
● M25.46 Effusion, knee
  M25.461 Effusion, right knee
  M25.462 Effusion, left knee
  M25.469 Effusion, unspecified knee
● M25.47 Effusion, ankle and foot
  M25.471 Effusion, right ankle
  M25.472 Effusion, left ankle
  M25.473 Effusion, unspecified ankle
  M25.474 Effusion, right foot
  M25.475 Effusion, left foot
  M25.476 Effusion, unspecified foot
M25.48 Effusion, other site

● M25.5 Pain in joint
  Excludes2 pain in hand (M79.64-)
    pain in fingers (M79.64-)
    pain in foot (M79.67-)
    pain in limb (M79.6-)
    pain in toes (M79.67-)
M25.50 Pain in unspecified joint
● M25.51 Pain in shoulder
  M25.511 Pain in right shoulder
  M25.512 Pain in left shoulder
  M25.519 Pain in unspecified shoulder
● M25.52 Pain in elbow
  M25.521 Pain in right elbow
  M25.522 Pain in left elbow
  M25.529 Pain in unspecified elbow
● M25.53 Pain in wrist
  M25.531 Pain in right wrist
  M25.532 Pain in left wrist
  M25.539 Pain in unspecified wrist
● M25.54 Pain in joints of hand
  Coding Clinic: 2016, Q4, P38
  M25.541 Pain in joints of right hand
  M25.542 Pain in joints of left hand
  M25.549 Pain in joints of unspecified hand
    Pain in joints of hand NOS
● M25.55 Pain in hip
  M25.551 Pain in right hip
  M25.552 Pain in left hip
  M25.559 Pain in unspecified hip
● M25.56 Pain in knee
  M25.561 Pain in right knee
  M25.562 Pain in left knee
  M25.569 Pain in unspecified knee
● M25.57 Pain in ankle and joints of foot
  M25.571 Pain in right ankle and joints of right foot
  M25.572 Pain in left ankle and joints of left foot
  M25.579 Pain in unspecified ankle and joints of unspecified foot
M25.59 Pain in other specified joint
● M25.6 Stiffness of joint, not elsewhere classified
  Excludes1 ankylosis of joint (M24.6-)
    contracture of joint (M24.5-)
M25.60 Stiffness of unspecified joint, not elsewhere classified
● M25.61 Stiffness of shoulder, not elsewhere classified
  M25.611 Stiffness of right shoulder, not elsewhere classified
  M25.612 Stiffness of left shoulder, not elsewhere classified
  M25.619 Stiffness of unspecified shoulder, not elsewhere classified
● M25.62 Stiffness of elbow, not elsewhere classified
  M25.621 Stiffness of right elbow, not elsewhere classified
  M25.622 Stiffness of left elbow, not elsewhere classified
  M25.629 Stiffness of unspecified elbow, not elsewhere classified
● M25.63 Stiffness of wrist, not elsewhere classified
  M25.631 Stiffness of right wrist, not elsewhere classified
  M25.632 Stiffness of left wrist, not elsewhere classified
  M25.639 Stiffness of unspecified wrist, not elsewhere classified

New   Revised   ~~deleted~~ Deleted   Excludes 1   Excludes 2   Includes   Use additional   Code first   Code also   Key words
OGCR Official Guidelines   X Assign placeholder X   ● Use Additional Character(s)   ▸ Manifestation Code   🐾 Hierarchical Condition Category   Coding Clinic

● M25.64   Stiffness of hand, not elsewhere classified
    M25.641   Stiffness of right hand, not elsewhere classified
    M25.642   Stiffness of left hand, not elsewhere classified
    M25.649   Stiffness of unspecified hand, not elsewhere classified
● M25.65   Stiffness of hip, not elsewhere classified
    M25.651   Stiffness of right hip, not elsewhere classified
    M25.652   Stiffness of left hip, not elsewhere classified
    M25.659   Stiffness of unspecified hip, not elsewhere classified
● M25.66   Stiffness of knee, not elsewhere classified
    M25.661   Stiffness of right knee, not elsewhere classified
    M25.662   Stiffness of left knee, not elsewhere classified
    M25.669   Stiffness of unspecified knee, not elsewhere classified
● M25.67   Stiffness of ankle and foot, not elsewhere classified
    M25.671   Stiffness of right ankle, not elsewhere classified
    M25.672   Stiffness of left ankle, not elsewhere classified
    M25.673   Stiffness of unspecified ankle, not elsewhere classified
    M25.674   Stiffness of right foot, not elsewhere classified
    M25.675   Stiffness of left foot, not elsewhere classified
    M25.676   Stiffness of unspecified foot, not elsewhere classified
   M25.69   Stiffness of other specified joint, not elsewhere classified
● M25.7   Osteophyte
   M25.70   Osteophyte, unspecified joint
● M25.71   Osteophyte, shoulder
    M25.711   Osteophyte, right shoulder
    M25.712   Osteophyte, left shoulder
    M25.719   Osteophyte, unspecified shoulder
● M25.72   Osteophyte, elbow
    M25.721   Osteophyte, right elbow
    M25.722   Osteophyte, left elbow
    M25.729   Osteophyte, unspecified elbow
● M25.73   Osteophyte, wrist
    M25.731   Osteophyte, right wrist
    M25.732   Osteophyte, left wrist
    M25.739   Osteophyte, unspecified wrist
● M25.74   Osteophyte, hand
    M25.741   Osteophyte, right hand
    M25.742   Osteophyte, left hand
    M25.749   Osteophyte, unspecified hand
● M25.75   Osteophyte, hip
    M25.751   Osteophyte, right hip
    M25.752   Osteophyte, left hip
    M25.759   Osteophyte, unspecified hip
● M25.76   Osteophyte, knee
    M25.761   Osteophyte, right knee
    M25.762   Osteophyte, left knee
    M25.769   Osteophyte, unspecified knee

● M25.77   Osteophyte, ankle and foot
    M25.771   Osteophyte, right ankle
    M25.772   Osteophyte, left ankle
    M25.773   Osteophyte, unspecified ankle
    M25.774   Osteophyte, right foot
    M25.775   Osteophyte, left foot
    M25.776   Osteophyte, unspecified foot
   M25.78   Osteophyte, vertebrae
● M25.8   Other specified joint disorders
   M25.80   Other specified joint disorders, unspecified joint
● M25.81   Other specified joint disorders, shoulder
    M25.811   Other specified joint disorders, right shoulder
    M25.812   Other specified joint disorders, left shoulder
    M25.819   Other specified joint disorders, unspecified shoulder
● M25.82   Other specified joint disorders, elbow
    M25.821   Other specified joint disorders, right elbow
    M25.822   Other specified joint disorders, left elbow
    M25.829   Other specified joint disorders, unspecified elbow
● M25.83   Other specified joint disorders, wrist
    M25.831   Other specified joint disorders, right wrist
    M25.832   Other specified joint disorders, left wrist
    M25.839   Other specified joint disorders, unspecified wrist
● M25.84   Other specified joint disorders, hand
    M25.841   Other specified joint disorders, right hand
    M25.842   Other specified joint disorders, left hand
    M25.849   Other specified joint disorders, unspecified hand
● M25.85   Other specified joint disorders, hip
    M25.851   Other specified joint disorders, right hip
    M25.852   Other specified joint disorders, left hip
    M25.859   Other specified joint disorders, unspecified hip
● M25.86   Other specified joint disorders, knee
    M25.861   Other specified joint disorders, right knee
    M25.862   Other specified joint disorders, left knee
    M25.869   Other specified joint disorders, unspecified knee
● M25.87   Other specified joint disorders, ankle and foot
    M25.871   Other specified joint disorders, right ankle and foot
    M25.872   Other specified joint disorders, left ankle and foot
    M25.879   Other specified joint disorders, unspecified ankle and foot

   M25.9   Joint disorder, unspecified

CHAPTER 13 (M00-M99)

Figure 13-3   Dentofacial malocclusion.

Item 13–6 Hyperplasia is a condition of overdevelopment, whereas **hypoplasia** is a condition of underdevelopment. **Macrogenia** is overdevelopment of the chin, whereas **microgenia** is underdevelopment of the chin.

DENTOFACIAL ANOMALIES [INCLUDING MALOCCLUSION] AND OTHER DISORDERS OF JAW (M26-M27)

> **Excludes1**   hemifacial atrophy or hypertrophy (Q67.4)
> unilateral condylar hyperplasia or hypoplasia (M27.8)

● **M26**   **Dentofacial anomalies [including malocclusion]**

   ● **M26.0**   **Major anomalies of jaw size**

> **Excludes1**   acromegaly (E22.0)
> Robin's syndrome (Q87.0)

     M26.00   Unspecified anomaly of jaw size

     M26.01   Maxillary hyperplasia

     M26.02   Maxillary hypoplasia

     M26.03   Mandibular hyperplasia

     M26.04   Mandibular hypoplasia

     M26.05   Macrogenia

     M26.06   Microgenia

     M26.07   Excessive tuberosity of jaw
         Entire maxillary tuberosity

     M26.09   Other specified anomalies of jaw size

   ● **M26.1**   **Anomalies of jaw-cranial base relationship**

     M26.10   Unspecified anomaly of jaw-cranial base relationship

     M26.11   Maxillary asymmetry

     M26.12   Other jaw asymmetry

     M26.19   Other specified anomalies of jaw-cranial base relationship
         Coding Clinic: 2020, Q1, P21

   ● **M26.2**   **Anomalies of dental arch relationship**

     M26.20   Unspecified anomaly of dental arch relationship

     ● **M26.21**   Malocclusion, Angle's class

        M26.211   Malocclusion, Angle's class I
            Neutro-occlusion

        M26.212   Malocclusion, Angle's class II
            Disto-occlusion Division I
            Disto-occlusion Division II

        M26.213   Malocclusion, Angle's class III
            Mesio-occlusion

        M26.219   Malocclusion, Angle's class, unspecified

     ● **M26.22**   Open occlusal relationship

        M26.220   Open anterior occlusal relationship
            Anterior open bite

        M26.221   Open posterior occlusal relationship
            Posterior open bite

     M26.23   Excessive horizontal overlap
         Excessive horizontal overjet

     M26.24   Reverse articulation
         Crossbite (anterior) (posterior)

     M26.25   Anomalies of interarch distance

     M26.29   Other anomalies of dental arch relationship
         Midline deviation of dental arch
         Overbite (excessive) deep
         Overbite (excessive) horizontal
         Overbite (excessive) vertical
         Posterior lingual occlusion of mandibular teeth

   ● **M26.3**   **Anomalies of tooth position of fully erupted tooth or teeth**

> **Excludes2**   embedded and impacted teeth (K01.-)

     M26.30   Unspecified anomaly of tooth position of fully erupted tooth or teeth
         Abnormal spacing of fully erupted tooth or teeth NOS
         Displacement of fully erupted tooth or teeth NOS
         Transposition of fully erupted tooth or teeth NOS

     M26.31   Crowding of fully erupted teeth

     M26.32   Excessive spacing of fully erupted teeth
         Diastema of fully erupted tooth or teeth NOS

     M26.33   Horizontal displacement of fully erupted tooth or teeth
         Tipped tooth or teeth
         Tipping of fully erupted tooth

     M26.34   Vertical displacement of fully erupted tooth or teeth
         Extruded tooth
         Infraeruption of tooth or teeth
         Supraeruption of tooth or teeth

     M26.35   Rotation of fully erupted tooth or teeth

     M26.36   Insufficient interocclusal distance of fully erupted teeth (ridge)
         Lack of adequate intermaxillary vertical dimension of fully erupted teeth

     M26.37   Excessive interocclusal distance of fully erupted teeth
         Excessive intermaxillary vertical dimension of fully erupted teeth
         Loss of occlusal vertical dimension of fully erupted teeth

     M26.39   Other anomalies of tooth position of fully erupted tooth or teeth

   M26.4   **Malocclusion, unspecified**

   ● **M26.5**   **Dentofacial functional abnormalities**

> **Excludes1**   bruxism (F45.8)
> teeth-grinding NOS (F45.8)

     M26.50   Dentofacial functional abnormalities, unspecified

     M26.51   Abnormal jaw closure

     M26.52   Limited mandibular range of motion

     M26.53   Deviation in opening and closing of the mandible

     M26.54   Insufficient anterior guidance
         Insufficient anterior occlusal guidance

     M26.55   Centric occlusion maximum intercuspation discrepancy

> **Excludes1**   centric occlusion NOS (M26.59)

     M26.56   Non-working side interference
         Balancing side interference

     M26.57   Lack of posterior occlusal support

     M26.59   Other dentofacial functional abnormalities
         Centric occlusion (of teeth) NOS
         Malocclusion due to abnormal swallowing
         Malocclusion due to mouth breathing
         Malocclusion due to tongue, lip or finger habits

▶ New   ⟹ Revised   ~~deleted~~ Deleted   Excludes 1   Excludes 2   Includes   Use additional   Code first   Code also   Key words

OGCR Official Guidelines   X Assign placeholder X   ● Use Additional Character(s)   ▸ Manifestation Code   🏷 Hierarchical Condition Category   **Coding Clinic**

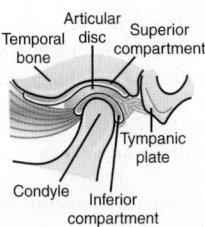

Figure 13-4   Temporomandibular joint.

Item 13–7 Dysfunction of the temporomandibular joint is termed **temporomandibular joint (TMJ) syndrome** and is characterized by pain and tenderness/spasm of the muscles of mastication, joint noise, and in the later stages, limited mandibular movement.

● M26.6   Temporomandibular joint disorders
　　Excludes2   current temporomandibular joint dislocation (S03.0)
　　　　　current temporomandibular joint sprain (S03.4)
　　Coding Clinic: 2016, Q4, P38-39
● M26.60   Temporomandibular joint disorder, unspecified
　　M26.601   Right temporomandibular joint disorder, unspecified
　　M26.602   Left temporomandibular joint disorder, unspecified
　　M26.603   Bilateral temporomandibular joint disorder, unspecified
　　M26.609   Unspecified temporomandibular joint disorder, unspecified side
　　　　　Temporomandibular joint disorder NOS
● M26.61   Adhesions and ankylosis of temporomandibular joint
　　M26.611   Adhesions and ankylosis of right temporomandibular joint
　　M26.612   Adhesions and ankylosis of left temporomandibular joint
　　M26.613   Adhesions and ankylosis of bilateral temporomandibular joint
　　M26.619   Adhesions and ankylosis of temporomandibular joint, unspecified side
● M26.62   Arthralgia of temporomandibular joint
　　M26.621   Arthralgia of right temporomandibular joint
　　M26.622   Arthralgia of left temporomandibular joint
　　M26.623   Arthralgia of bilateral temporomandibular joint
　　M26.629   Arthralgia of temporomandibular joint, unspecified side
● M26.63   Articular disc disorder of temporomandibular joint
　　M26.631   Articular disc disorder of right temporomandibular joint
　　M26.632   Articular disc disorder of left temporomandibular joint
　　M26.633   Articular disc disorder of bilateral temporomandibular joint
　　M26.639   Articular disc disorder of temporomandibular joint, unspecified side

● M26.64   Arthritis of temporomandibular joint
　　M26.641   Arthritis of right temporomandibular joint
　　M26.642   Arthritis of left temporomandibular joint
　　M26.643   Arthritis of bilateral temporomandibular joint
　　M26.649   Arthritis of unspecified temporomandibular joint
● M26.65   Arthropathy of temporomandibular joint
　　M26.651   Arthropathy of right temporomandibular joint
　　M26.652   Arthropathy of left temporomandibular joint
　　M26.653   Arthropathy of bilateral temporomandibular joint
　　M26.659   Arthropathy of unspecified temporomandibular joint
　　M26.69   Other specified disorders of temporomandibular joint
● M26.7   Dental alveolar anomalies
　　M26.70   Unspecified alveolar anomaly
　　M26.71   Alveolar maxillary hyperplasia
　　M26.72   Alveolar mandibular hyperplasia
　　M26.73   Alveolar maxillary hypoplasia
　　M26.74   Alveolar mandibular hypoplasia
　　M26.79   Other specified alveolar anomalies
● M26.8   Other dentofacial anomalies
　　M26.81   Anterior soft tissue impingement
　　　　　Anterior soft tissue impingement on teeth
　　M26.82   Posterior soft tissue impingement
　　　　　Posterior soft tissue impingement on teeth
　　M26.89   Other dentofacial anomalies
　　M26.9   Dentofacial anomaly, unspecified
● M27   Other diseases of jaws
　　M27.0   Developmental disorders of jaws
　　　　　Latent bone cyst of jaw
　　　　　Stafne's cyst
　　　　　Torus mandibularis
　　　　　Torus palatinus
　　M27.1   Giant cell granuloma, central
　　　　　Giant cell granuloma NOS
　　　　　Excludes1   peripheral giant cell granuloma (K06.8)
　　M27.2   Inflammatory conditions of jaws
　　　　　Osteitis of jaw(s)
　　　　　Osteomyelitis (neonatal) jaw(s)
　　　　　Osteoradionecrosis jaw(s)
　　　　　Periostitis jaw(s)
　　　　　Sequestrum of jaw bone
　　　　　Use additional code (W88-W90, X39.0) to identify radiation, if radiation-induced
　　　　　Excludes2   osteonecrosis of jaw due to drug (M87.180)
　　M27.3   Alveolitis of jaws
　　　　　Alveolar osteitis
　　　　　Dry socket
● M27.4   Other and unspecified cysts of jaw
　　　　　Excludes1   cysts of oral region (K09.-)
　　　　　　latent bone cyst of jaw (M27.0)
　　　　　　Stafne's cyst (M27.0)
　　M27.40   Unspecified cyst of jaw
　　　　　Cyst of jaw NOS
　　M27.49   Other cysts of jaw
　　　　　Aneurysmal cyst of jaw
　　　　　Hemorrhagic cyst of jaw
　　　　　Traumatic cyst of jaw

CHAPTER 13 (M00-M99)

● **M27.5** **Periradicular pathology associated with previous endodontic treatment**

     M27.51 **Perforation of root canal space due to endodontic treatment**

     M27.52 **Endodontic overfill**

     M27.53 **Endodontic underfill**

     M27.59 **Other periradicular pathology associated with previous endodontic treatment**

● **M27.6** **Endosseous dental implant failure**

     M27.61 **Osseointegration failure of dental implant**
         Hemorrhagic complications of dental implant placement
         Iatrogenic osseointegration failure of dental implant
         Osseointegration failure of dental implant due to complications of systemic disease
         Osseointegration failure of dental implant due to poor bone quality
         Pre-integration failure of dental implant NOS
         Pre-osseointegration failure of dental implant

     M27.62 **Post-osseointegration biological failure of dental implant**
         Failure of dental implant due to lack of attached gingiva
         Failure of dental implant due to occlusal trauma (caused by poor prosthetic design)
         Failure of dental implant due to parafunctional habits
         Failure of dental implant due to periodontal infection (peri–implantitis)
         Failure of dental implant due to poor oral hygiene
         Iatrogenic post-osseointegration failure of dental implant
         Post-osseointegration failure of dental implant due to complications of systemic disease

     M27.63 **Post-osseointegration mechanical failure of dental implant**
         Failure of dental prosthesis causing loss of dental implant
         Fracture of dental implant

         Excludes2   cracked tooth (K03.81)
                     fractured dental restorative material with loss of material (K08.531)
                     fractured dental restorative material without loss of material (K08.530)
                     fractured tooth (S02.5)

     M27.69 **Other endosseous dental implant failure**
         Dental implant failure NOS

M27.8 **Other specified diseases of jaws**
     Cherubism
     Exostosis
     Fibrous dysplasia
     Unilateral condylar hyperplasia
     Unilateral condylar hypoplasia

     Excludes1   jaw pain (R68.84)

M27.9 **Disease of jaws, unspecified**

SYSTEMIC CONNECTIVE TISSUE DISORDERS (M30-M36)

Includes   autoimmune disease NOS
            collagen (vascular) disease NOS
            systemic autoimmune disease
            systemic collagen (vascular) disease

Excludes1   autoimmune disease, single organ or single cell-type - code to relevant condition category

● **M30** **Polyarteritis nodosa and related conditions**

     Excludes1   microscopic polyarteritis (M31.7)

M30.0 **Polyarteritis nodosa** 🐾

M30.1 **Polyarteritis with lung involvement [Churg-Strauss]** 🐾
     Allergic granulomatous angiitis
     Eosinophilic granulomatosis with polyangiitis [EGPA]
     Coding Clinic: 2021, Q1, P23

M30.2 **Juvenile polyarteritis** 🐾

M30.3 **Mucocutaneous lymph node syndrome [Kawasaki]** 🐾

M30.8 **Other conditions related to polyarteritis nodosa** 🐾
     Polyangiitis overlap syndrome

● **M31** **Other necrotizing vasculopathies**

     M31.0 **Hypersensitivity angiitis** 🐾
         Goodpasture's syndrome

●   **M31.1** **Thrombotic microangiopathy** 🐾

     M31.10 **Thrombotic microangiopathy, unspecified**

     M31.11 **Hematopoietic stem cell transplantation-associated thrombotic microangiopathy [HSCT-TMA]**
         Transplant-associated thrombotic microangiopathy [TA-TMA]
         Code first if applicable:
            complications of bone marrow transplant (T86.0-)
            complications of stem cell transplant (T86.5)
         Use Additional code to identify specific organ dysfunction, such as:
            acute kidney failure (N17.-)
            acute respiratory distress syndrome (J80)
            capillary leak syndrome (I78.8)
            diffuse alveolar hemorrhage (R04.89)
            encephalopathy (metabolic) (septic) (G93.41)
            fluid overload, unspecified (E87.70)
            graft versus host disease (D89.81-)
            ▥hemolytic uremic syndrome (D59.3-)
            hepatic failure (K72.-)
            hepatic veno-occlusive disease (K76.5)
            idiopathic interstitial pneumonia (J84.11-)
            sinusoidal obstruction syndrome (K76.5)

     M31.19 **Other thrombotic microangiopathy**
         Thrombotic thrombocytopenic purpura

M31.2 **Lethal midline granuloma** 🐾

●   **M31.3** **Wegener's granulomatosis**
     Granulomatosis with polyangiitis
     Necrotizing respiratory granulomatosis
     Coding Clinic: 2021, Q1, P23

     M31.30 **Wegener's granulomatosis without renal involvement** 🐾
         Wegener's granulomatosis NOS
         Coding Clinic: 2021, Q2, P10

     M31.31 **Wegener's granulomatosis with renal involvement** 🐾

M31.4 **Aortic arch syndrome [Takayasu]** 🐾

M31.5 **Giant cell arteritis with polymyalgia rheumatica** 🐾

M31.6 **Other giant cell arteritis** 🐾

M31.7 **Microscopic polyangiitis** 🐾
     Microscopic polyarteritis

     Excludes1   polyarteritis nodosa (M30.0)
     Coding Clinic: 2021, Q1, P23

M31.8 **Other specified necrotizing vasculopathies** 🐾
     Hypocomplementemic vasculitis
     Septic vasculitis

M31.9 **Necrotizing vasculopathy, unspecified** 🐾

● **M32** **Systemic lupus erythematosus (SLE)**
     Autoimmune inflammatory connective tissue disease of unknown cause that occurs most often in women

     Excludes1   lupus erythematosus (discoid) (NOS) (L93.0)

     M32.0 **Drug-induced systemic lupus erythematosus** 🐾
         Use additional code for adverse effect, if applicable, to identify drug (T36-T50 with fifth or sixth character 5)

▶ New   ⇒ Revised   ~~deleted~~ Deleted   Excludes 1   Excludes 2   Includes   Use additional   Code first   Code also   Key words

OGCR Official Guidelines   X Assign placeholder X   ● Use Additional Character(s)   ▌ Manifestation Code   🐾 Hierarchical Condition Category   **Coding Clinic**

● M32.1　Systemic lupus erythematosus with organ or system involvement

　　M32.10　Systemic lupus erythematosus, organ or system involvement unspecified 🐾

　　M32.11　Endocarditis in systemic lupus erythematosus 🐾
　　　　　　Libman-Sacks disease

　　M32.12　Pericarditis in systemic lupus erythematosus 🐾
　　　　　　Lupus pericarditis

　　M32.13　Lung involvement in systemic lupus erythematosus 🐾
　　　　　　Pleural effusion due to systemic lupus erythematosus

　　M32.14　Glomerular disease in systemic lupus erythematosus 🐾
　　　　　　Lupus renal disease NOS

　　M32.15　Tubulo-interstitial nephropathy in systemic lupus erythematosus 🐾

　　M32.19　Other organ or system involvement in systemic lupus erythematosus 🐾

　M32.8　Other forms of systemic lupus erythematosus 🐾

　M32.9　Systemic lupus erythematosus, unspecified 🐾
　　　　SLE NOS
　　　　Systemic lupus erythematosus NOS
　　　　Systemic lupus erythematosus without organ involvement

● M33　Dermatopolymyositis
　● M33.0　Juvenile dermatomyositis
　　　M33.00　Juvenile dermatomyositis, organ involvement unspecified 🐾
　　　M33.01　Juvenile dermatomyositis with respiratory involvement 🐾
　　　M33.02　Juvenile dermatomyositis with myopathy 🐾
　　　M33.03　Juvenile dermatomyositis without myopathy 🐾
　　　M33.09　Juvenile dermatomyositis with other organ involvement 🐾

　● M33.1　Other dermatomyositis
　　　　Adult dermatomyositis
　　　M33.10　Other dermatomyositis, organ involvement unspecified 🐾
　　　M33.11　Other dermatomyositis with respiratory involvement 🐾
　　　M33.12　Other dermatomyositis with myopathy 🐾
　　　M33.13　Other dermatomyositis without myopathy 🐾
　　　　　　Dermatomyositis NOS
　　　M33.19　Other dermatomyositis with other organ involvement 🐾

　● M33.2　Polymyositis
　　　M33.20　Polymyositis, organ involvement unspecified 🐾
　　　M33.21　Polymyositis with respiratory involvement 🐾
　　　M33.22　Polymyositis with myopathy 🐾
　　　M33.29　Polymyositis with other organ involvement 🐾

　● M33.9　Dermatopolymyositis, unspecified
　　　M33.90　Dermatopolymyositis, unspecified, organ involvement unspecified 🐾
　　　M33.91　Dermatopolymyositis, unspecified with respiratory involvement 🐾
　　　M33.92　Dermatopolymyositis, unspecified with myopathy 🐾
　　　M33.93　Dermatopolymyositis, unspecified without myopathy 🐾
　　　M33.99　Dermatopolymyositis, unspecified with other organ involvement 🐾

Item 13–8　Polymyalgia rheumatica is a syndrome characterized by aching and morning stiffness and is related to aging and hereditary predisposition.

● M34　Systemic sclerosis [scleroderma]
　　Excludes1　circumscribed scleroderma (L94.0)
　　　　　　　　neonatal scleroderma (P83.88)

　M34.0　Progressive systemic sclerosis
　M34.1　CR(E)ST syndrome 🐾
　　　　Combination of calcinosis, Raynaud's phenomenon, esophageal dysfunction, sclerodactyly, telangiectasia
　M34.2　Systemic sclerosis induced by drug and chemical 🐾
　　　　Code first poisoning due to drug or toxin, if applicable (T36-T65 with fifth or sixth character 1-4 or 6)
　　　　Use additional code for adverse effect, if applicable, to identify drug (T36-T50 with fifth or sixth character 5)

　● M34.8　Other forms of systemic sclerosis
　　　M34.81　Systemic sclerosis with lung involvement 🐾
　　　　　　Code also if applicable:
　　　　　　　other interstitial pulmonary diseases (J84.89)
　　　　　　　secondary pulmonary arterial hypertension (I27.21)
　　　M34.82　Systemic sclerosis with myopathy 🐾
　　　M34.83　Systemic sclerosis with polyneuropathy 🐾
　　　M34.89　Other systemic sclerosis 🐾

　M34.9　Systemic sclerosis, unspecified 🐾

● M35　Other systemic involvement of connective tissue
　　Excludes1　reactive perforating collagenosis (L87.1)
　● M35.0　Sjögren syndrome
　　　　Sicca syndrome
　　　　Use Additional code to identify associated manifestations
　　　　Excludes1　dry mouth, unspecified (R68.2)
　　　M35.00　Sjögren syndrome, unspecified 🐾
　　　M35.01　Sjögren syndrome with keratoconjunctivitis 🐾
　　　M35.02　Sjögren syndrome with lung involvement 🐾
　　　M35.03　Sjögren syndrome with myopathy 🐾
　　　M35.04　Sjögren syndrome with tubulo-interstitial nephropathy 🐾
　　　　　　Renal tubular acidosis in sicca syndrome
　　　M35.05　Sjögren syndrome with inflammatory arthritis
　　　M35.06　Sjögren syndrome with peripheral nervous system involvement
　　　M35.07　Sjögren syndrome with central nervous system involvement
　　　M35.08　Sjögren syndrome with gastrointestinal involvement
　　　M35.09　Sjögren syndrome with other organ involvement
　　　M35.0A　Sjögren syndrome with glomerular disease
　　　M35.0B　Sjögren syndrome with vasculitis
　　　M35.0C　Sjögren syndrome with dental involvement

　M35.1　Other overlap syndromes 🐾
　　　　Mixed connective tissue disease
　　　　Excludes1　polyangiitis overlap syndrome (M30.8)

　M35.2　Behçet's disease
　M35.3　Polymyalgia rheumatica 🐾
　　　　Excludes1　polymyalgia rheumatica with giant cell arteritis (M31.5)

　M35.4　Diffuse (eosinophilic) fasciitis
　M35.5　Multifocal fibrosclerosis 🐾
　M35.6　Relapsing panniculitis [Weber-Christian]
　　　　Excludes1　lupus panniculitis (L93.2)
　　　　　　　　panniculitis NOS (M79.3-)

M35.7 **Hypermobility syndrome**
Familial ligamentous laxity
> **Excludes1** ligamentous laxity, NOS (M24.2-)

> **Excludes2** Ehlers-Danlos syndromes (Q79.6-)

● M35.8 **Other specified systemic involvement of connective tissue** 🅗
Coding Clinic: 2021, Q4, P102; 2021, Q1, P36

M35.81 **Multisystem inflammatory syndrome**
MIS-A
MIS-C
Multisystem inflammatory syndrome in adults
Multisystem inflammatory syndrome in children
Pediatric inflammatory multisystem syndrome
PIMS
Code first, if applicable, COVID-19 (U07.1)
Code also any associated complications such as:
acute hepatic failure (K72.0-)
acute kidney failure (N17.-)
acute myocarditis (I40.-)
acute respiratory distress syndrome (J80)
cardiac arrhythmia (I47-I49.-)
pneumonia due to COVID-19 (J12.82)
severe sepsis (R65.2-)
viral cardiomyopathy (B33.24)
viral pericarditis (B33.23)
Use additional code, if applicable, for:
exposure to COVID-19 or SARS-C
personal history of COVID-19 (Z86.16)
post COVID-19 condition (U09.9)
Coding Clinic: 2021, Q4, P102; 2021, Q1, P36, 42

M35.89 **Other specified systemic involvement of connective tissue**

M35.9 **Systemic involvement of connective tissue, unspecified** 🅗
Autoimmune disease (systemic) NOS
Collagen (vascular) disease NOS

● M36 **Systemic disorders of connective tissue in diseases classified elsewhere**
> **Excludes2** arthropathies in diseases classified elsewhere (M14.-)

▸ *M36.0 Dermato(poly)myositis in neoplastic disease* 🅗
Code first underlying neoplasm (C00-D49)

▸ *M36.1 Arthropathy in neoplastic disease*
Code first underlying neoplasm, such as:
leukemia (C91-C95)
malignant histiocytosis (C96.A)
multiple myeloma (C90.0)

▸ *M36.2 Hemophilic arthropathy*
Hemarthrosis in hemophilic arthropathy
Code first underlying disease, such as:
factor VIII deficiency (D66)
➡with vascular defect (D68.0-)
factor IX deficiency (D67)
hemophilia (classical) (D66)
hemophilia B (D67)
hemophilia C (D68.1)

▸ *M36.3 Arthropathy in other blood disorders*

▸ *M36.4 Arthropathy in hypersensitivity reactions classified elsewhere*
Code first underlying disease, such as:
Henoch (-Schönlein) purpura (D69.0)
serum sickness (T80.6-)

▸ *M36.8 Systemic disorders of connective tissue in other diseases classified elsewhere* 🅗
Code first underlying disease, such as:
alkaptonuria (E70.2)
hypogammaglobulinemia (D80.-)
ochronosis (E70.2)

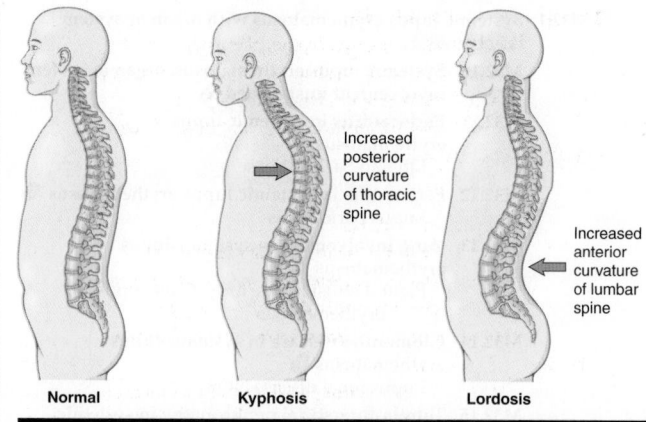

Figure 13-5 Kyphosis, Lordosis, Scoliosis. (From Chabner: The Language of Medicine, ed 8, St. Louis, Saunders, 2007)

Item 13-9 Kyphosis is an abnormal curvature of the spine. **Senile kyphosis** is a result of disc degeneration causing ossification (turning to bone). **Adolescent** or **juvenile** kyphosis is also known as **Scheuermann's disease,** a condition in which the discs of the lower thoracic spine herniate, causing the disc space to narrow and the spine to tilt forward. This condition is attributed to poor posture. **Lordosis or swayback** is an abnormal curvature of the spine resulting in an inward curve of the lumbar spine just above the buttocks. **Scoliosis** causes a sideways curve to the spine. The curves are S- or C-shaped, and it is most commonly acquired in late childhood and early teen years, when growth is fast.

DORSOPATHIES (M40-M54)

DEFORMING DORSOPATHIES (M40-M43)

● M40 **Kyphosis and lordosis**
> **Excludes1** congenital kyphosis and lordosis (Q76.4)
kyphoscoliosis (M41.-)
postprocedural kyphosis and lordosis (M96.-)
Code first underlying disease

● M40.0 **Postural kyphosis**
> **Excludes1** osteochondrosis of spine (M42.-)

M40.00 Postural kyphosis, site unspecified
M40.03 Postural kyphosis, cervicothoracic region
M40.04 Postural kyphosis, thoracic region
M40.05 Postural kyphosis, thoracolumbar region

● M40.1 **Other secondary kyphosis**
M40.10 Other secondary kyphosis, site unspecified
M40.12 Other secondary kyphosis, cervical region
M40.13 Other secondary kyphosis, cervicothoracic region
M40.14 Other secondary kyphosis, thoracic region
M40.15 Other secondary kyphosis, thoracolumbar region

● M40.2 **Other and unspecified kyphosis**
● M40.20 **Unspecified kyphosis**
M40.202 Unspecified kyphosis, cervical region
M40.203 Unspecified kyphosis, cervicothoracic region
M40.204 Unspecified kyphosis, thoracic region
M40.205 Unspecified kyphosis, thoracolumbar region
M40.209 Unspecified kyphosis, site unspecified
● M40.29 **Other kyphosis**
M40.292 Other kyphosis, cervical region
M40.293 Other kyphosis, cervicothoracic region
M40.294 Other kyphosis, thoracic region
M40.295 Other kyphosis, thoracolumbar region
M40.299 Other kyphosis, site unspecified

▶ New ⇒ Revised ~~deleted~~ Deleted Excludes 1 Excludes 2 Includes Use additional Code first Code also Key words
OGCR Official Guidelines X Assign placeholder X ● Use Additional Character(s) ▸ Manifestation Code 🅗 Hierarchical Condition Category Coding Clinic

CHAPTER 13 (M00-M99)

● **M40.3 Flatback** syndrome
    M40.30   Flatback syndrome, site unspecified
    M40.35   Flatback syndrome, thoracolumbar region
    M40.36   Flatback syndrome, lumbar region
    M40.37   Flatback syndrome, lumbosacral region
● **M40.4 Postural lordosis**
    Abnormal increase in the normal curvature of the lumbar spine (sway back)
    Acquired lordosis
    M40.40   Postural lordosis, site unspecified
    M40.45   Postural lordosis, thoracolumbar region
    M40.46   Postural lordosis, lumbar region
    M40.47   Postural lordosis, lumbosacral region
● **M40.5 Lordosis, unspecified**
    M40.50   Lordosis, unspecified, site unspecified
    M40.55   Lordosis, unspecified, thoracolumbar region
    M40.56   Lordosis, unspecified, lumbar region
    M40.57   Lordosis, unspecified, lumbosacral region

● **M41 Scoliosis**
    Includes   kyphoscoliosis
    Excludes1   congenital scoliosis NOS (Q67.5)
        congenital scoliosis due to bony malformation (Q76.3)
        postural congenital scoliosis (Q67.5)
        kyphoscoliotic heart disease (I27.1)
    Excludes2   postprocedural scoliosis (M96.-)
● **M41.0 Infantile idiopathic scoliosis**
    M41.00   Infantile idiopathic scoliosis, site unspecified
    M41.02   Infantile idiopathic scoliosis, cervical region
    M41.03   Infantile idiopathic scoliosis, cervicothoracic region
    M41.04   Infantile idiopathic scoliosis, thoracic region
    M41.05   Infantile idiopathic scoliosis, thoracolumbar region
    M41.06   Infantile idiopathic scoliosis, lumbar region
    M41.07   Infantile idiopathic scoliosis, lumbosacral region
    M41.08   Infantile idiopathic scoliosis, sacral and sacrococcygeal region
● **M41.1 Juvenile and adolescent idiopathic scoliosis**
  ● **M41.11 Juvenile idiopathic scoliosis**
    M41.112   Juvenile idiopathic scoliosis, cervical region
    M41.113   Juvenile idiopathic scoliosis, cervicothoracic region
    M41.114   Juvenile idiopathic scoliosis, thoracic region
    M41.115   Juvenile idiopathic scoliosis, thoracolumbar region
    M41.116   Juvenile idiopathic scoliosis, lumbar region
    M41.117   Juvenile idiopathic scoliosis, lumbosacral region
    M41.119   Juvenile idiopathic scoliosis, site unspecified
  ● **M41.12 Adolescent scoliosis**
    M41.122   Adolescent idiopathic scoliosis, cervical region
    M41.123   Adolescent idiopathic scoliosis, cervicothoracic region
    M41.124   Adolescent idiopathic scoliosis, thoracic region
    M41.125   Adolescent idiopathic scoliosis, thoracolumbar region
    M41.126   Adolescent idiopathic scoliosis, lumbar region
    M41.127   Adolescent idiopathic scoliosis, lumbosacral region
    M41.129   Adolescent idiopathic scoliosis, site unspecified
● **M41.2 Other idiopathic scoliosis**
    M41.20   Other idiopathic scoliosis, site unspecified
    M41.22   Other idiopathic scoliosis, cervical region
    M41.23   Other idiopathic scoliosis, cervicothoracic region
    M41.24   Other idiopathic scoliosis, thoracic region
    M41.25   Other idiopathic scoliosis, thoracolumbar region
    M41.26   Other idiopathic scoliosis, lumbar region
    M41.27   Other idiopathic scoliosis, lumbosacral region
● **M41.3 Thoracogenic scoliosis**
    M41.30   Thoracogenic scoliosis, site unspecified
    M41.34   Thoracogenic scoliosis, thoracic region
    M41.35   Thoracogenic scoliosis, thoracolumbar region
● **M41.4 Neuromuscular scoliosis**
    Scoliosis secondary to cerebral palsy, Friedreich's ataxia, poliomyelitis and other neuromuscular disorders
    Code also underlying condition
    M41.40   Neuromuscular scoliosis, site unspecified
    M41.41   Neuromuscular scoliosis, occipito-atlanto-axial region
    M41.42   Neuromuscular scoliosis, cervical region
    M41.43   Neuromuscular scoliosis, cervicothoracic region
    M41.44   Neuromuscular scoliosis, thoracic region
    M41.45   Neuromuscular scoliosis, thoracolumbar region
    M41.46   Neuromuscular scoliosis, lumbar region
    M41.47   Neuromuscular scoliosis, lumbosacral region
● **M41.5 Other secondary scoliosis**
    Coding Clinic: 2019, Q1, P19
    Code first underlying disease
    M41.50   Other secondary scoliosis, site unspecified
    M41.52   Other secondary scoliosis, cervical region
    M41.53   Other secondary scoliosis, cervicothoracic region
    M41.54   Other secondary scoliosis, thoracic region
    M41.55   Other secondary scoliosis, thoracolumbar region
    M41.56   Other secondary scoliosis, lumbar region
    M41.57   Other secondary scoliosis, lumbosacral region
● **M41.8 Other forms of scoliosis**
    Coding Clinic: 2022, Q1, P30
    M41.80   Other forms of scoliosis, site unspecified
    M41.82   Other forms of scoliosis, cervical region
    M41.83   Other forms of scoliosis, cervicothoracic region
    M41.84   Other forms of scoliosis, thoracic region
    M41.85   Other forms of scoliosis, thoracolumbar region
    M41.86   Other forms of scoliosis, lumbar region
    M41.87   Other forms of scoliosis, lumbosacral region
    M41.9   Scoliosis, unspecified
    Coding Clinic: 2022, Q1, P30
● **M42 Spinal osteochondrosis**
  ● **M42.0 Juvenile osteochondrosis of spine**
    Calvé's disease
    Scheuermann's disease
    Excludes1   postural kyphosis (M40.0)
    M42.00   Juvenile osteochondrosis of spine, site unspecified
    M42.01   Juvenile osteochondrosis of spine, occipito-atlanto-axial region
    M42.02   Juvenile osteochondrosis of spine, cervical region
    M42.03   Juvenile osteochondrosis of spine, cervicothoracic region

CHAPTER 13 (M00-M99)

Item 13–10   **Spondylolisthesis** is a condition caused by the slipping forward of one disc over another.

M42.04	Juvenile osteochondrosis of spine, thoracic region	
M42.05	Juvenile osteochondrosis of spine, thoracolumbar region	
M42.06	Juvenile osteochondrosis of spine, lumbar region	
M42.07	Juvenile osteochondrosis of spine, lumbosacral region	
M42.08	Juvenile osteochondrosis of spine, sacral and sacrococcygeal region	
M42.09	Juvenile osteochondrosis of spine, multiple sites in spine	

● M42.1   Adult osteochondrosis of spine

M42.10	Adult osteochondrosis of spine, site unspecified	A
M42.11	Adult osteochondrosis of spine, occipitoatlanto-axial region	A
M42.12	Adult osteochondrosis of spine, cervical region	A
M42.13	Adult osteochondrosis of spine, cervicothoracic region	A
M42.14	Adult osteochondrosis of spine, thoracic region	A
M42.15	Adult osteochondrosis of spine, thoracolumbar region	A
M42.16	Adult osteochondrosis of spine, lumbar region	A
M42.17	Adult osteochondrosis of spine, lumbosacral region	A
M42.18	Adult osteochondrosis of spine, sacral and sacrococcygeal region	A
M42.19	Adult osteochondrosis of spine, multiple sites in spine	A

M42.9   Spinal osteochondrosis, unspecified

● M43   Other deforming dorsopathies

> **Excludes1**   congenital spondylolysis and spondylolisthesis (Q76.2)
> hemivertebra (Q76.3-Q76.4)
> Klippel-Feil syndrome (Q76.1)
> lumbarization and sacralization (Q76.4)
> platyspondylisis (Q76.4)
> spina bifida occulta (Q76.0)
> spinal curvature in osteoporosis (M80.-)
> spinal curvature in Paget's disease of bone [osteitis deformans] (M88.-)

● M43.0   Spondylolysis

> **Excludes1**   congenital spondylolysis (Q76.2)
> spondylolisthesis (M43.1)

M43.00	Spondylolysis, site unspecified
M43.01	Spondylolysis, occipito-atlanto-axial region
M43.02	Spondylolysis, cervical region
M43.03	Spondylolysis, cervicothoracic region
M43.04	Spondylolysis, thoracic region
M43.05	Spondylolysis, thoracolumbar region
M43.06	Spondylolysis, lumbar region
M43.07	Spondylolysis, lumbosacral region
M43.08	Spondylolysis, sacral and sacrococcygeal region
M43.09	Spondylolysis, multiple sites in spine

● M43.1   Spondylolisthesis

> **Excludes1**   acute traumatic of lumbosacral region (S33.1)
> acute traumatic of sites other than lumbosacral - code to Fracture, vertebra, by region
> congenital spondylolisthesis (Q76.2)

M43.10	Spondylolisthesis, site unspecified
M43.11	Spondylolisthesis, occipito-atlanto-axial region
M43.12	Spondylolisthesis, cervical region
M43.13	Spondylolisthesis, cervicothoracic region
M43.14	Spondylolisthesis, thoracic region
M43.15	Spondylolisthesis, thoracolumbar region
M43.16	Spondylolisthesis, lumbar region
M43.17	Spondylolisthesis, lumbosacral region
M43.18	Spondylolisthesis, sacral and sacrococcygeal region
M43.19	Spondylolisthesis, multiple sites in spine

● M43.2   Fusion of spine

Ankylosis of spinal joint

> **Excludes1**   ankylosing spondylitis (M45.0-)
> congenital fusion of spine (Q76.4)

> **Excludes2**   arthrodesis status (Z98.1)
> pseudoarthrosis after fusion or arthrodesis (M96.0)

M43.20	Fusion of spine, site unspecified
M43.21	Fusion of spine, occipito-atlanto-axial region
M43.22	Fusion of spine, cervical region
M43.23	Fusion of spine, cervicothoracic region
M43.24	Fusion of spine, thoracic region
M43.25	Fusion of spine, thoracolumbar region
M43.26	Fusion of spine, lumbar region
M43.27	Fusion of spine, lumbosacral region
M43.28	Fusion of spine, sacral and sacrococcygeal region

M43.3   Recurrent atlantoaxial dislocation with myelopathy

M43.4   Other recurrent atlantoaxial dislocation

● M43.5   Other recurrent vertebral dislocation

> **Excludes1**   biomechanical lesions NEC (M99.-)

● M43.5X   Other recurrent vertebral dislocation

M43.5X2	Other recurrent vertebral dislocation, cervical region
M43.5X3	Other recurrent vertebral dislocation, cervicothoracic region
M43.5X4	Other recurrent vertebral dislocation, thoracic region
M43.5X5	Other recurrent vertebral dislocation, thoracolumbar region
M43.5X6	Other recurrent vertebral dislocation, lumbar region
M43.5X7	Other recurrent vertebral dislocation, lumbosacral region
M43.5X8	Other recurrent vertebral dislocation, sacral and sacrococcygeal region
M43.5X9	Other recurrent vertebral dislocation, site unspecified

M43.6   Torticollis

> **Excludes1**   congenital (sternomastoid) torticollis (Q68.0)
> current injury - see Injury, of spine, by body region ocular torticollis (R29.891)
> psychogenic torticollis (F45.8)
> spasmodic torticollis (G24.3)
> torticollis due to birth injury (P15.2)

● M43.8   Other specified deforming dorsopathies

> **Excludes2**   kyphosis and lordosis (M40.-)
> scoliosis (M41.-)

● M43.8X   Other specified deforming dorsopathies

M43.8X1	Other specified deforming dorsopathies, occipito-atlanto-axial region
M43.8X2	Other specified deforming dorsopathies, cervical region
M43.8X3	Other specified deforming dorsopathies, cervicothoracic region
M43.8X4	Other specified deforming dorsopathies, thoracic region
M43.8X5	Other specified deforming dorsopathies, thoracolumbar region
M43.8X6	Other specified deforming dorsopathies, lumbar region
M43.8X7	Other specified deforming dorsopathies, lumbosacral region

▶ New   ⇒ Revised   ~~deleted~~ Deleted   Excludes 1   Excludes 2   Includes   Use additional   Code first   Code also   Key words

OGCR Official Guidelines   X Assign placeholder X   ● Use Additional Character(s)   ▶ Manifestation Code   🔖 Hierarchical Condition Category   **Coding Clinic**

M43.8X8 Other specified deforming dorsopathies, sacral and sacrococcygeal region

M43.8X9 Other specified deforming dorsopathies, site unspecified

M43.9 Deforming dorsopathy, unspecified
Curvature of spine NOS

SPONDYLOPATHIES (M45-M49)

● M45 Ankylosing spondylitis
Rheumatoid arthritis of spine

Excludes1 arthropathy in Reiter's disease (M02.3-)
juvenile (ankylosing) spondylitis (M08.1)

Excludes2 Behçet's disease (M35.2)

M45.0 Ankylosing spondylitis of multiple sites in spine

M45.1 Ankylosing spondylitis of occipito-atlanto-axial region

M45.2 Ankylosing spondylitis of cervical region

M45.3 Ankylosing spondylitis of cervicothoracic region

M45.4 Ankylosing spondylitis of thoracic region

M45.5 Ankylosing spondylitis of thoracolumbar region

M45.6 Ankylosing spondylitis lumbar region

M45.7 Ankylosing spondylitis of lumbosacral region

M45.8 Ankylosing spondylitis sacral and sacrococcygeal region

M45.9 Ankylosing spondylitis of unspecified sites in spine

● M45.A Non-radiographic axial spondyloarthritis

M45.A0 Non-radiographic axial spondyloarthritis of unspecified sites in spine

M45.A1 Non-radiographic axial spondyloarthritis of occipito-atlanto-axial region

M45.A2 Non-radiographic axial spondyloarthritis of cervical region

M45.A3 Non-radiographic axial spondyloarthritis of cervicothoracic region

M45.A4 Non-radiographic axial spondyloarthritis of thoracic region

M45.A5 Non-radiographic axial spondyloarthritis of thoracolumbar region

M45.A6 Non-radiographic axial spondyloarthritis of lumbar region

M45.A7 Non-radiographic axial spondyloarthritis of lumbosacral region

M45.A8 Non-radiographic axial spondyloarthritis of sacral and sacrococcygeal region

M45.AB Non-radiographic axial spondyloarthritis of multiple sites in spine

● M46 Other inflammatory spondylopathies

● M46.0 Spinal enthesopathy
Disorder of ligamentous or muscular attachments of spine

M46.00 Spinal enthesopathy, site unspecified

M46.01 Spinal enthesopathy, occipito-atlanto-axial region

M46.02 Spinal enthesopathy, cervical region

M46.03 Spinal enthesopathy, cervicothoracic region

M46.04 Spinal enthesopathy, thoracic region

M46.05 Spinal enthesopathy, thoracolumbar region

M46.06 Spinal enthesopathy, lumbar region

M46.07 Spinal enthesopathy, lumbosacral region

M46.08 Spinal enthesopathy, sacral and sacrococcygeal region

M46.09 Spinal enthesopathy, multiple sites in spine

M46.1 Sacroiliitis, not elsewhere classified

● M46.2 Osteomyelitis of vertebra

M46.20 Osteomyelitis of vertebra, site unspecified

M46.21 Osteomyelitis of vertebra, occipito-atlanto-axial region

M46.22 Osteomyelitis of vertebra, cervical region

M46.23 Osteomyelitis of vertebra, cervicothoracic region

M46.24 Osteomyelitis of vertebra, thoracic region

M46.25 Osteomyelitis of vertebra, thoracolumbar region

M46.26 Osteomyelitis of vertebra, lumbar region

M46.27 Osteomyelitis of vertebra, lumbosacral region

M46.28 Osteomyelitis of vertebra, sacral and sacrococcygeal region

● M46.3 Infection of intervertebral disc (pyogenic)
Use additional code (B95-B97) to identify infectious agent

M46.30 Infection of intervertebral disc (pyogenic), site unspecified

M46.31 Infection of intervertebral disc (pyogenic), occipito-atlanto-axial region

M46.32 Infection of intervertebral disc (pyogenic), cervical region

M46.33 Infection of intervertebral disc (pyogenic), cervicothoracic region

M46.34 Infection of intervertebral disc (pyogenic), thoracic region

M46.35 Infection of intervertebral disc (pyogenic), thoracolumbar region

M46.36 Infection of intervertebral disc (pyogenic), lumbar region

M46.37 Infection of intervertebral disc (pyogenic), lumbosacral region

M46.38 Infection of intervertebral disc (pyogenic), sacral and sacrococcygeal region

M46.39 Infection of intervertebral disc (pyogenic), multiple sites in spine

● M46.4 Discitis, unspecified

M46.40 Discitis, unspecified, site unspecified

M46.41 Discitis, unspecified, occipito-atlanto-axial region

M46.42 Discitis, unspecified, cervical region

M46.43 Discitis, unspecified, cervicothoracic region

M46.44 Discitis, unspecified, thoracic region

M46.45 Discitis, unspecified, thoracolumbar region

M46.46 Discitis, unspecified, lumbar region

M46.47 Discitis, unspecified, lumbosacral region

M46.48 Discitis, unspecified, sacral and sacrococcygeal region

M46.49 Discitis, unspecified, multiple sites in spine

● M46.5 Other infective spondylopathies

M46.50 Other infective spondylopathies, site unspecified

M46.51 Other infective spondylopathies, occipitoatlanto-axial region

M46.52 Other infective spondylopathies, cervical region

M46.53 Other infective spondylopathies, cervicothoracic region

M46.54 Other infective spondylopathies, thoracic region

M46.55 Other infective spondylopathies, thoracolumbar region

M46.56 Other infective spondylopathies, lumbar region

M46.57 Other infective spondylopathies, lumbosacral region

M46.58 Other infective spondylopathies, sacral and sacrococcygeal region

M46.59 Other infective spondylopathies, multiple sites in spine

CHAPTER 13 (M00-M99)

CHAPTER 13 (M00-M99)

● M46.8   Other specified inflammatory spondylopathies

     M46.80   Other specified inflammatory spondylopathies, site unspecified 🦠

     M46.81   Other specified inflammatory spondylopathies, occipito-atlanto-axial region 🦠

     M46.82   Other specified inflammatory spondylopathies, cervical region 🦠

     M46.83   Other specified inflammatory spondylopathies, cervicothoracic region 🦠

     M46.84   Other specified inflammatory spondylopathies, thoracic region 🦠

     M46.85   Other specified inflammatory spondylopathies, thoracolumbar region 🦠

     M46.86   Other specified inflammatory spondylopathies, lumbar region 🦠

     M46.87   Other specified inflammatory spondylopathies, lumbosacral region 🦠

     M46.88   Other specified inflammatory spondylopathies, sacral and sacrococcygeal region 🦠

     M46.89   Other specified inflammatory spondylopathies, multiple sites in spine 🦠

● M46.9   Unspecified inflammatory spondylopathy

     M46.90   Unspecified inflammatory spondylopathy, site unspecified 🦠

     M46.91   Unspecified inflammatory spondylopathy, occipito-atlanto-axial region 🦠

     M46.92   Unspecified inflammatory spondylopathy, cervical region 🦠
         Coding Clinic: 2019, Q3, P10

     M46.93   Unspecified inflammatory spondylopathy, cervicothoracic region 🦠

     M46.94   Unspecified inflammatory spondylopathy, thoracic region 🦠

     M46.95   Unspecified inflammatory spondylopathy, thoracolumbar region 🦠

     M46.96   Unspecified inflammatory spondylopathy, lumbar region 🦠

     M46.97   Unspecified inflammatory spondylopathy, lumbosacral region 🦠

     M46.98   Unspecified inflammatory spondylopathy, sacral and sacrococcygeal region 🦠

     M46.99   Unspecified inflammatory spondylopathy, multiple sites in spine 🦠

● M47   Spondylosis

     Includes   arthrosis or osteoarthritis of spine
                 degeneration of facet joints

● M47.0   Anterior spinal and vertebral artery compression syndromes
     Coding Clinic: 2019, Q3, P10

   ● M47.01   Anterior spinal artery compression syndromes

     M47.011   Anterior spinal artery compression syndromes, occipito-atlanto-axial region

     M47.012   Anterior spinal artery compression syndromes, cervical region

     M47.013   Anterior spinal artery compression syndromes, cervicothoracic region

     M47.014   Anterior spinal artery compression syndromes, thoracic region

     M47.015   Anterior spinal artery compression syndromes, thoracolumbar region

     M47.016   Anterior spinal artery compression syndromes, lumbar region

     M47.019   Anterior spinal artery compression syndromes, site unspecified

   ● M47.02   Vertebral artery compression syndromes

     M47.021   Vertebral artery compression syndromes, occipito-atlanto-axial region

     M47.022   Vertebral artery compression syndromes, cervical region

     M47.029   Vertebral artery compression syndromes, site unspecified

● M47.1   Other spondylosis with myelopathy
     Spondylogenic compression of spinal cord

     Excludes1   vertebral subluxation (M43.3-M43.5X9)

     M47.10   Other spondylosis with myelopathy, site unspecified

     M47.11   Other spondylosis with myelopathy, occipito-atlanto-axial region

     M47.12   Other spondylosis with myelopathy, cervical region
         Coding Clinic: 2020, Q1, P17

     M47.13   Other spondylosis with myelopathy, cervicothoracic region

     M47.14   Other spondylosis with myelopathy, thoracic region

     M47.15   Other spondylosis with myelopathy, thoracolumbar region

     M47.16   Other spondylosis with myelopathy, lumbar region

● M47.2   Other spondylosis with radiculopathy

     M47.20   Other spondylosis with radiculopathy, site unspecified

     M47.21   Other spondylosis with radiculopathy, occipito-atlanto-axial region

     M47.22   Other spondylosis with radiculopathy, cervical region
         Coding Clinic: 2020, Q1, P17

     M47.23   Other spondylosis with radiculopathy, cervicothoracic region

     M47.24   Other spondylosis with radiculopathy, thoracic region

     M47.25   Other spondylosis with radiculopathy, thoracolumbar region

     M47.26   Other spondylosis with radiculopathy, lumbar region

     M47.27   Other spondylosis with radiculopathy, lumbosacral region

     M47.28   Other spondylosis with radiculopathy, sacral and sacrococcygeal region

● M47.8   Other spondylosis

   ● M47.81   Spondylosis without myelopathy or radiculopathy

     M47.811   Spondylosis without myelopathy or radiculopathy, occipito-atlanto-axial region

     M47.812   Spondylosis without myelopathy or radiculopathy, cervical region
         Coding Clinic: 2019, Q3, P10-11; 2018, Q2, P15

     M47.813   Spondylosis without myelopathy or radiculopathy, cervicothoracic region

     M47.814   Spondylosis without myelopathy or radiculopathy, thoracic region

     M47.815   Spondylosis without myelopathy or radiculopathy, thoracolumbar region

     M47.816   Spondylosis without myelopathy or radiculopathy, lumbar region

     M47.817   Spondylosis without myelopathy or radiculopathy, lumbosacral region

     M47.818   Spondylosis without myelopathy or radiculopathy, sacral and sacrococcygeal region

     M47.819   Spondylosis without myelopathy or radiculopathy, site unspecified

   ● M47.89   Other spondylosis

     M47.891   Other spondylosis, occipito-atlanto-axial region

     M47.892   Other spondylosis, cervical region

▶ New   ⇒ Revised   ~~deleted~~ Deleted   Excludes 1   Excludes 2   Includes   Use additional   Code first   Code also   Key words

  OGCR Official Guidelines   X Assign placeholder X   ● Use Additional Character(s)   ▶ Manifestation Code   🦠 Hierarchical Condition Category   **Coding Clinic**

         M47.893   Other spondylosis, cervicothoracic region

         M47.894   Other spondylosis, thoracic region

         M47.895   Other spondylosis, thoracolumbar region

         M47.896   Other spondylosis, lumbar region

         M47.897   Other spondylosis, lumbosacral region

         M47.898   Other spondylosis, sacral and sacrococcygeal region

         M47.899   Other spondylosis, site unspecified

     M47.9   Spondylosis, unspecified

● **M48**   **Other spondylopathies**

    ● M48.0   Spinal stenosis

       Caudal stenosis

         M48.00   Spinal stenosis, site unspecified

         M48.01   Spinal stenosis, occipito-atlanto-axial region

         M48.02   Spinal stenosis, cervical region
            Coding Clinic: 2020, Q1, P17

         M48.03   Spinal stenosis, cervicothoracic region

         M48.04   Spinal stenosis, thoracic region

         M48.05   Spinal stenosis, thoracolumbar region

    ● M48.06   Spinal stenosis, lumbar region
            Coding Clinic: 2017, Q3, P24

            M48.061   Spinal stenosis, lumbar region without neurogenic claudication
                Spinal stenosis, lumbar region NOS

            M48.062   Spinal stenosis, lumbar region with neurogenic claudication
                Coding Clinic: 2017, Q4, P19

         M48.07   Spinal stenosis, lumbosacral region

         M48.08   Spinal stenosis, sacral and sacrococcygeal region

    ● M48.1   Ankylosing hyperostosis [Forestier]
       Diffuse idiopathic skeletal hyperostosis [DISH]

         M48.10   Ankylosing hyperostosis [Forestier], site unspecified

         M48.11   Ankylosing hyperostosis [Forestier], occipito-atlanto-axial region

         M48.12   Ankylosing hyperostosis [Forestier], cervical region

         M48.13   Ankylosing hyperostosis [Forestier], cervicothoracic region

         M48.14   Ankylosing hyperostosis [Forestier], thoracic region

         M48.15   Ankylosing hyperostosis [Forestier], thoracolumbar region

         M48.16   Ankylosing hyperostosis [Forestier], lumbar region

         M48.17   Ankylosing hyperostosis [Forestier], lumbosacral region

         M48.18   Ankylosing hyperostosis [Forestier], sacral and sacrococcygeal region

         M48.19   Ankylosing hyperostosis [Forestier], multiple sites in spine

    ● M48.2   Kissing spine

         M48.20   Kissing spine, site unspecified

         M48.21   Kissing spine, occipito-atlanto-axial region

         M48.22   Kissing spine, cervical region

         M48.23   Kissing spine, cervicothoracic region

         M48.24   Kissing spine, thoracic region

         M48.25   Kissing spine, thoracolumbar region

         M48.26   Kissing spine, lumbar region

         M48.27   Kissing spine, lumbosacral region

    ● M48.3   Traumatic spondylopathy

         M48.30   Traumatic spondylopathy, site unspecified

         M48.31   Traumatic spondylopathy, occipito-atlanto-axial region

         M48.32   Traumatic spondylopathy, cervical region

         M48.33   Traumatic spondylopathy, cervicothoracic region

         M48.34   Traumatic spondylopathy, thoracic region

         M48.35   Traumatic spondylopathy, thoracolumbar region

         M48.36   Traumatic spondylopathy, lumbar region

         M48.37   Traumatic spondylopathy, lumbosacral region

         M48.38   Traumatic spondylopathy, sacral and sacrococcygeal region

    ● M48.4   Fatigue fracture of vertebra
       Stress fracture of vertebra

       Excludes1   pathological fracture NOS (M84.4-)
                pathological fracture of vertebra due to neoplasm (M84.58)
                pathological fracture of vertebra due to other diagnosis (M84.68)
                pathological fracture of vertebra due to osteoporosis (M80.-)
                traumatic fracture of vertebrae (S12.0-S12.3-, S22.0-, S32.0-)

       The appropriate 7th character is to be added to each code from subcategory M48.4:

A	initial encounter for fracture
D	subsequent encounter for fracture with routine healing
G	subsequent encounter for fracture with delayed healing
S	sequela of fracture

   X ● M48.40   Fatigue fracture of vertebra, site unspecified

   X ● M48.41   Fatigue fracture of vertebra, occipitoatlanto-axial region

   X ● M48.42   Fatigue fracture of vertebra, cervical region

   X ● M48.43   Fatigue fracture of vertebra, cervicothoracic region

   X ● M48.44   Fatigue fracture of vertebra, thoracic region

   X ● M48.45   Fatigue fracture of vertebra, thoracolumbar region

   X ● M48.46   Fatigue fracture of vertebra, lumbar region

   X ● M48.47   Fatigue fracture of vertebra, lumbosacral region

   X ● M48.48   Fatigue fracture of vertebra, sacral and sacrococcygeal region

    ● M48.5   Collapsed vertebra, not elsewhere classified
       Collapsed vertebra NOS
       Compression fracture of vertebra NOS
       Wedging of vertebra NOS

       Excludes1   current injury - see Injury of spine, by body region
                fatigue fracture of vertebra (M48.4)
                pathological fracture of vertebra due to neoplasm (M84.58)
                pathological fracture of vertebra due to other diagnosis (M84.68)
                pathological fracture of vertebra due to osteoporosis (M80.-)
                pathological fracture NOS (M84.4-)
                stress fracture of vertebra (M48.4-)
                traumatic fracture of vertebra (S12.-, S22.-, S32.-)

       The appropriate 7th character is to be added to each code from subcategory M48.5:

A	initial encounter for fracture
D	subsequent encounter for fracture with routine healing
G	subsequent encounter for fracture with delayed healing
S	sequela of fracture

CHAPTER 13 (M00-M99)

CHAPTER 13 (M00-M99)

X ● **M48.50** Collapsed vertebra, not elsewhere classified, site unspecified A 🦌

X ● **M48.51** Collapsed vertebra, not elsewhere classified, occipito-atlanto-axial region A 🦌

X ● **M48.52** Collapsed vertebra, not elsewhere classified, cervical region A 🦌

X ● **M48.53** Collapsed vertebra, not elsewhere classified, cervicothoracic region A 🦌

X ● **M48.54** Collapsed vertebra, not elsewhere classified, thoracic region A 🦌

X ● **M48.55** Collapsed vertebra, not elsewhere classified, thoracolumbar region A 🦌

X ● **M48.56** Collapsed vertebra, not elsewhere classified, lumbar region A 🦌

X ● **M48.57** Collapsed vertebra, not elsewhere classified, lumbosacral region A 🦌

X ● **M48.58** Collapsed vertebra, not elsewhere classified, sacral and sacrococcygeal region A 🦌

● **M48.8** Other specified spondylopathies
          Ossification of posterior longitudinal ligament

  ● **M48.8X** Other specified spondylopathies

       M48.8X1 Other specified spondylopathies, occipito-atlanto-axial region 🦌

       M48.8X2 Other specified spondylopathies, cervical region 🦌

       M48.8X3 Other specified spondylopathies, cervicothoracic region 🦌

       M48.8X4 Other specified spondylopathies, thoracic region 🦌

       M48.8X5 Other specified spondylopathies, thoracolumbar region 🦌

       M48.8X6 Other specified spondylopathies, lumbar region 🦌

       M48.8X7 Other specified spondylopathies, lumbosacral region 🦌

       M48.8X8 Other specified spondylopathies, sacral and sacrococcygeal region 🦌

       M48.8X9 Other specified spondylopathies, site unspecified 🦌

   M48.9 Spondylopathy, unspecified

● **M49** Spondylopathies in diseases classified elsewhere

     Includes   curvature of spine in diseases classified elsewhere
                   deformity of spine in diseases classified elsewhere
                   kyphosis in diseases classified elsewhere
                   scoliosis in diseases classified elsewhere
                   spondylopathy in diseases classified elsewhere

     Code first underlying disease, such as:
         brucellosis (A23.-)
         Charcot-Marie-Tooth disease (G60.0)
         enterobacterial infections (A01-A04)
         osteitis fibrosa cystica (E21.0)

     Excludes1   curvature of spine in tuberculosis [Pott's] (A18.01)
                   enteropathic arthropathies (M07.-)
                   gonococcal spondylitis (A54.41)
                   neuropathic [tabes dorsalis] spondylitis (A52.11)
                   neuropathic spondylopathy in syringomyelia (G95.0)
                   neuropathic spondylopathy in tabes dorsalis (A52.11)
                   nonsyphilitic neuropathic spondylopathy NEC (G98.0)
                   spondylitis in syphilis (acquired) (A52.77)
                   tuberculous spondylitis (A18.01)
                   typhoid fever spondylitis (A01.05)

  ● **M49.8** Spondylopathy in diseases classified elsewhere

    ▌ *M49.80* *Spondylopathy in diseases classified elsewhere, site unspecified* 🦌

    ▌ *M49.81* *Spondylopathy in diseases classified elsewhere, occipito-atlanto-axial region* 🦌

    ▌ *M49.82* *Spondylopathy in diseases classified elsewhere, cervical region* 🦌

    ▌ *M49.83* *Spondylopathy in diseases classified elsewhere, cervicothoracic region* 🦌

    ▌ *M49.84* *Spondylopathy in diseases classified elsewhere, thoracic region* 🦌

    ▌ *M49.85* *Spondylopathy in diseases classified elsewhere, thoracolumbar region* 🦌

    ▌ *M49.86* *Spondylopathy in diseases classified elsewhere, lumbar region* 🦌

    ▌ *M49.87* *Spondylopathy in diseases classified elsewhere, lumbosacral region* 🦌

    ▌ *M49.88* *Spondylopathy in diseases classified elsewhere, sacral and sacrococcygeal region* 🦌

    ▌ *M49.89* *Spondylopathy in diseases classified elsewhere, multiple sites in spine* 🦌

OTHER DORSOPATHIES (M50-M54)

     Excludes1   current injury - see injury of spine by body region
                   discitis NOS (M46.4-)

● **M50** Cervical disc disorders

   ~~Note: Code to the most superior level of disorder.~~

     Includes   cervicothoracic disc disorders with cervicalgia
                   cervicothoracic disc disorders

     Coding Clinic: 2016, Q1, P17

  ● **M50.0** Cervical disc disorder with myelopathy

     M50.00 Cervical disc disorder with myelopathy, unspecified cervical region

     M50.01 Cervical disc disorder with myelopathy, high cervical region
           C2-C3 disc disorder with myelopathy
           C3-C4 disc disorder with myelopathy
           Coding Clinic: 2016, Q1, P17

    ● **M50.02** Cervical disc disorder with myelopathy, mid-cervical region
           Coding Clinic: 2016, Q4, P39-40

       M50.020 Cervical disc disorder with myelopathy, mid-cervical region, unspecified level

       M50.021 Cervical disc disorder at C4-C5 level with myelopathy
            C4-C5 disc disorder with myelopathy

       M50.022 Cervical disc disorder at C5-C6 level with myelopathy
            C5-C6 disc disorder with myelopathy

       M50.023 Cervical disc disorder at C6-C7 level with myelopathy
            C6-C7 disc disorder with myelopathy

     M50.03 Cervical disc disorder with myelopathy, cervicothoracic region
           C7-T1 disc disorder with myelopathy

  ● **M50.1** Cervical disc disorder with radiculopathy

     Excludes2   brachial radiculitis NOS (M54.13)

     M50.10 Cervical disc disorder with radiculopathy, unspecified cervical region

     M50.11 Cervical disc disorder with radiculopathy, high cervical region
           C2-C3 disc disorder with radiculopathy
           C3 radiculopathy due to disc disorder
           C3-C4 disc disorder with radiculopathy
           C4 radiculopathy due to disc disorder

    ● **M50.12** Cervical disc disorder with radiculopathy, mid-cervical region
           Coding Clinic: 2016, Q4, P39-40

       M50.120 Mid-cervical disc disorder, unspecified level

       M50.121 Cervical disc disorder at C4-C5 level with radiculopathy
            C4-C5 disc disorder with radiculopathy
            C5 radiculopathy due to disc disorder

▶ New   ⇒ Revised   ~~deleted~~ Deleted   Excludes 1   Excludes 2   Includes   Use additional   Code first   Code also   Key words

OGCR Official Guidelines   X Assign placeholder X   ● Use Additional Character(s)   ▌ Manifestation Code   🦌 Hierarchical Condition Category   **Coding Clinic**

M50.122 Cervical disc disorder at C5-C6 level with radiculopathy
C5-C6 disc disorder with radiculopathy
C6 radiculopathy due to disc disorder

M50.123 Cervical disc disorder at C6-C7 level with radiculopathy
C6-C7 disc disorder with radiculopathy
C7 radiculopathy due to disc disorder

M50.13 Cervical disc disorder with radiculopathy, cervicothoracic region
C7-T1 disc disorder with radiculopathy
C8 radiculopathy due to disc disorder

● **M50.2 Other cervical disc displacement**
Coding Clinic: 2016, Q4, P40

M50.20 Other cervical disc displacement, unspecified cervical region

M50.21 Other cervical disc displacement, high cervical region
Other C2-C3 cervical disc displacement
Other C3-C4 cervical disc displacement
Coding Clinic: 2021, Q4, P12

● **M50.22 Other cervical disc displacement, mid-cervical region**

M50.220 Other cervical disc displacement, mid-cervical region, unspecified level

M50.221 Other cervical disc displacement at C4-C5 level
Other C4-C5 cervical disc displacement

M50.222 Other cervical disc displacement at C5-C6 level
Other C5-C6 cervical disc displacement

M50.223 Other cervical disc displacement at C6-C7 level
Other C6-C7 cervical disc displacement

M50.23 Other cervical disc displacement, cervicothoracic region
Other C7-T1 cervical disc displacement

● **M50.3 Other cervical disc degeneration**
Coding Clinic: 2016, Q4, P40

M50.30 Other cervical disc degeneration, unspecified cervical region

M50.31 Other cervical disc degeneration, high cervical region
Other C2-C3 cervical disc degeneration
Other C3-C4 cervical disc degeneration

● **M50.32 Other cervical disc degeneration, mid-cervical region**

M50.320 Other cervical disc degeneration, mid-cervical region, unspecified level

M50.321 Other cervical disc degeneration at C4-C5 level
Other C4-C5 cervical disc degeneration

M50.322 Other cervical disc degeneration at C5-C6 level
Other C5-C6 cervical disc degeneration

M50.323 Other cervical disc degeneration at C6-C7 level
Other C6-C7 cervical disc degeneration

M50.33 Other cervical disc degeneration, cervicothoracic region
Other C7-T1 cervical disc degeneration

● **M50.8 Other cervical disc disorders**
Coding Clinic: 2016, Q4, P40

M50.80 Other cervical disc disorders, unspecified cervical region

M50.81 Other cervical disc disorders, high cervical region
Other C2-C3 cervical disc disorders
Other C3-C4 cervical disc disorders

● **M50.82 Other cervical disc disorders, mid-cervical region**

M50.820 Other cervical disc disorders, mid-cervical region, unspecified level

M50.821 Other cervical disc disorders at C4-C5 level
Other C4-C5 cervical disc disorders

M50.822 Other cervical disc disorders at C5-C6 level
Other C5-C6 cervical disc disorders

M50.823 Other cervical disc disorders at C6-C7 level
Other C6-C7 cervical disc disorders

M50.83 Other cervical disc disorders, cervicothoracic region
Other C7-T1 cervical disc disorders

● **M50.9 Cervical disc disorder, unspecified**
Coding Clinic: 2016, Q4, P40

M50.90 Cervical disc disorder, unspecified, unspecified cervical region

M50.91 Cervical disc disorder, unspecified, high cervical region
C2-C3 cervical disc disorder, unspecified
C3-C4 cervical disc disorder, unspecified

● **M50.92 Cervical disc disorder, unspecified, mid-cervical region**

M50.920 Unspecified cervical disc disorder, mid-cervical region, unspecified level

M50.921 Unspecified cervical disc disorder at C4-C5 level
Unspecified C4-C5 cervical disc disorder

M50.922 Unspecified cervical disc disorder at C5-C6 level
Unspecified C5-C6 cervical disc disorder

M50.923 Unspecified cervical disc disorder at C6-C7 level
Unspecified C6-C7 cervical disc disorder

M50.93 Cervical disc disorder, unspecified, cervicothoracic region
C7-T1 cervical disc disorder, unspecified

● **M51 Thoracic, thoracolumbar, and lumbosacral intervertebral disc disorders**
Excludes2 cervical and cervicothoracic disc disorders (M50.-)
sacral and sacrococcygeal disorders (M53.3)

● **M51.0 Thoracic, thoracolumbar and lumbosacral intervertebral disc disorders with myelopathy**

M51.04 Intervertebral disc disorders with myelopathy, thoracic region

M51.05 Intervertebral disc disorders with myelopathy, thoracolumbar region

M51.06 Intervertebral disc disorders with myelopathy, lumbar region

CHAPTER 13 (M00-M99)

● **M51.1 Thoracic, thoracolumbar and lumbosacral intervertebral disc disorders with radiculopathy**
Sciatica due to intervertebral disc disorder
> **Excludes1**   lumbar radiculitis NOS (M54.16)
>   sciatica NOS (M54.3)

     M51.14 Intervertebral disc disorders with radiculopathy, thoracic region

     M51.15 Intervertebral disc disorders with radiculopathy, thoracolumbar region

     M51.16 Intervertebral disc disorders with radiculopathy, lumbar region

     M51.17 Intervertebral disc disorders with radiculopathy, lumbosacral region

● **M51.2 Other thoracic, thoracolumbar and lumbosacral intervertebral disc displacement**
Lumbago due to displacement of intervertebral disc

     M51.24 Other intervertebral disc displacement, thoracic region

     M51.25 Other intervertebral disc displacement, thoracolumbar region

     M51.26 Other intervertebral disc displacement, lumbar region

     M51.27 Other intervertebral disc displacement, lumbosacral region

● **M51.3 Other thoracic, thoracolumbar and lumbosacral intervertebral disc degeneration**
Coding Clinic: 2013, Q3, P22

     M51.34 Other intervertebral disc degeneration, thoracic region

     M51.35 Other intervertebral disc degeneration, thoracolumbar region

     M51.36 Other intervertebral disc degeneration, lumbar region
         Coding Clinic: 2018, Q2, P15

     M51.37 Other intervertebral disc degeneration, lumbosacral region
         Coding Clinic: 2022, Q1, P26

● **M51.4 Schmorl's nodes**

     M51.44 Schmorl's nodes, thoracic region

     M51.45 Schmorl's nodes, thoracolumbar region

     M51.46 Schmorl's nodes, lumbar region

     M51.47 Schmorl's nodes, lumbosacral region

● **M51.8 Other thoracic, thoracolumbar and lumbosacral intervertebral disc disorders**

     M51.84 Other intervertebral disc disorders, thoracic region

     M51.85 Other intervertebral disc disorders, thoracolumbar region

     M51.86 Other intervertebral disc disorders, lumbar region

     M51.87 Other intervertebral disc disorders, lumbosacral region

   M51.9 Unspecified thoracic, thoracolumbar and lumbosacral intervertebral disc disorder

▶ ● **M51.A Other lumbar and lumbosacral annulus fibrosus disc defects**

     ▶ **M51.A0 Intervertebral annulus fibrosus defect, lumbar region, unspecified size**
> ▶ *Code first, if applicable, lumbar disc herniation (M51.06, M51.16, M51.26)*

     ▶ **M51.A1 Intervertebral annulus fibrosus defect, small, lumbar region**
> ▶ *Code first, if applicable, lumbar disc herniation (M51.06, M51.16, M51.26)*

     ▶ **M51.A2 Intervertebral annulus fibrosus defect, large, lumbar region**
> ▶ *Code first, if applicable, lumbar disc herniation (M51.06, M51.16, M51.26)*

     ▶ **M51.A3 Intervertebral annulus fibrosus defect, lumbosacral region, unspecified size**
> ▶ *Code first, if applicable, lumbosacral disc herniation (M51.17, M51.27)*

     ▶ **M51.A4 Intervertebral annulus fibrosus defect, small, lumbosacral region**
> ▶ *Code first, if applicable, lumbosacral disc herniation (M51.17, M51.27)*

     ▶ **M51.A5 Intervertebral annulus fibrosus defect, large, lumbosacral region**
> ▶ *Code first, if applicable, lumbosacral disc herniation (M51.17, M51.27)*

● **M3 Other and unspecified dorsopathies, not elsewhere classified**

   M53.0 Cervicocranial syndrome
Posterior cervical sympathetic syndrome

   M53.1 Cervicobrachial syndrome
> **Excludes2**   cervical disc disorder (M50.-)
>   thoracic outlet syndrome (G54.0)

● **M53.2 Spinal instabilities**

   ● **M53.2X Spinal instabilities**

       M53.2X1 Spinal instabilities, occipito-atlanto-axial region

       M53.2X2 Spinal instabilities, cervical region

       M53.2X3 Spinal instabilities, cervicothoracic region

       M53.2X4 Spinal instabilities, thoracic region

       M53.2X5 Spinal instabilities, thoracolumbar region

       M53.2X6 Spinal instabilities, lumbar region

       M53.2X7 Spinal instabilities, lumbosacral region

       M53.2X8 Spinal instabilities, sacral and sacrococcygeal region

       M53.2X9 Spinal instabilities, site unspecified

   M53.3 Sacrococcygeal disorders, not elsewhere classified
Coccygodynia

● **M53.8 Other specified dorsopathies**

     M53.80 Other specified dorsopathies, site unspecified

     M53.81 Other specified dorsopathies, occipito-atlanto-axial region

     M53.82 Other specified dorsopathies, cervical region

     M53.83 Other specified dorsopathies, cervicothoracic region

     M53.84 Other specified dorsopathies, thoracic region

     M53.85 Other specified dorsopathies, thoracolumbar region

     M53.86 Other specified dorsopathies, lumbar region

     M53.87 Other specified dorsopathies, lumbosacral region

     M53.88 Other specified dorsopathies, sacral and sacrococcygeal region

   M53.9 Dorsopathy, unspecified

● **M54 Dorsalgia**
> **Excludes1**   psychogenic dorsalgia (F45.41)

● **M54.0 Panniculitis affecting regions of neck and back**
> **Excludes1**   lupus panniculitis (L93.2)
>   panniculitis NOS (M79.3)
>   relapsing [Weber-Christian] panniculitis (M35.6)

     M54.00 Panniculitis affecting regions of neck and back, site unspecified

     M54.01 Panniculitis affecting regions of neck and back, occipito-atlanto-axial region

     M54.02 Panniculitis affecting regions of neck and back, cervical region

     M54.03 Panniculitis affecting regions of neck and back, cervicothoracic region

     M54.04 Panniculitis affecting regions of neck and back, thoracic region

     M54.05 Panniculitis affecting regions of neck and back, thoracolumbar region

▶ New   ⇨ Revised   ~~deleted~~ Deleted   Excludes 1   Excludes 2   Includes   Use additional   Code first   Code also   Key words

OGCR Official Guidelines   X Assign placeholder X   ● Use Additional Character(s)   ▶ Manifestation Code   🐾 Hierarchical Condition Category   **Coding Clinic**

M54.06 Panniculitis affecting regions of neck and back, lumbar region

M54.07 Panniculitis affecting regions of neck and back, lumbosacral region

M54.08 Panniculitis affecting regions of neck and back, sacral and sacrococcygeal region

M54.09 Panniculitis affecting regions, neck and back, multiple sites in spine

● **M54.1 Radiculopathy**
Brachial neuritis or radiculitis NOS
Lumbar neuritis or radiculitis NOS
Lumbosacral neuritis or radiculitis NOS
Thoracic neuritis or radiculitis NOS
Radiculitis NOS

Excludes1   neuralgia and neuritis NOS (M79.2)
radiculopathy with cervical disc disorder (M50.1)
radiculopathy with lumbar and other intervertebral disc disorder (M51.1-)
radiculopathy with spondylosis (M47.2-)

M54.10 Radiculopathy, site unspecified

M54.11 Radiculopathy, occipito-atlanto-axial region

M54.12 Radiculopathy, cervical region

M54.13 Radiculopathy, cervicothoracic region

M54.14 Radiculopathy, thoracic region

M54.15 Radiculopathy, thoracolumbar region

M54.16 Radiculopathy, lumbar region

M54.17 Radiculopathy, lumbosacral region

M54.18 Radiculopathy, sacral and sacrococcygeal region

M54.2 Cervicalgia

Excludes1   cervicalgia due to intervertebral cervical disc disorder (M50.-)

● **M54.3 Sciatica**

Excludes1   lesion of sciatic nerve (G57.0)
sciatica due to intervertebral disc disorder (M51.1-)
sciatica with lumbago (M54.4-)

M54.30 Sciatica, unspecified side

M54.31 Sciatica, right side

M54.32 Sciatica, left side

● **M54.4 Lumbago with sciatica**

Excludes1   lumbago with sciatica due to intervertebral disc disorder (M51.1-)

M54.40 Lumbago with sciatica, unspecified side

M54.41 Lumbago with sciatica, right side

M54.42 Lumbago with sciatica, left side
Coding Clinic: 2016, Q2, P7

● **M54.5 Low back pain**

Excludes1   low back strain (S39.012)
lumbago due to intervertebral disc displacement (M51.2-)
lumbago with sciatica (M54.4-)

M54.50 Low back pain, unspecified
Loin pain
Lumbago NOS

M54.51 Vertebrogenic low back pain
Low back vertebral endplate pain
Coding Clinic: 2021, Q4, P22

M54.59 Other low back pain

M54.6 Pain in thoracic spine

Excludes1   pain in thoracic spine due to intervertebral disc disorder (M51.)

● **M54.8 Other dorsalgia**

Excludes1   dorsalgia in thoracic region (M54.6)
low back pain (M54.5-)

M54.81 Occipital neuralgia

M54.89 Other dorsalgia

M54.9 Dorsalgia, unspecified
Backache NOS
Back pain NOS

SOFT TISSUE DISORDERS (M60-M79)

DISORDERS OF MUSCLES (M60-M63)

Excludes1   dermatopolymyositis (M33.-)
muscular dystrophies and myopathies (G71-G72)
myopathy in amyloidosis (E85.-)
myopathy in polyarteritis nodosa (M30.0)
myopathy in rheumatoid arthritis (M05.32)
myopathy in scleroderma (M34.-)
myopathy in Sjögren's syndrome (M35.03)
myopathy in systemic lupus erythematosus (M32.-)

● **M60 Myositis**

Excludes2   inclusion body myositis [IBM] (G72.41)

● **M60.0 Infective myositis**
Tropical pyomyositis
Use additional code (B95-B97) to identify infectious agent

● **M60.00 Infective myositis, unspecified site**

M60.000 Infective myositis, unspecified right arm
Infective myositis, right upper limb NOS

M60.001 Infective myositis, unspecified left arm
Infective myositis, left upper limb NOS

M60.002 Infective myositis, unspecified arm
Infective myositis, upper limb NOS

M60.003 Infective myositis, unspecified right leg
Infective myositis, right lower limb NOS

M60.004 Infective myositis, unspecified left leg
Infective myositis, left lower limb NOS

M60.005 Infective myositis, unspecified leg
Infective myositis, lower limb NOS

M60.009 Infective myositis, unspecified site

● **M60.01 Infective myositis, shoulder**

M60.011 Infective myositis, right shoulder

M60.012 Infective myositis, left shoulder

M60.019 Infective myositis, unspecified shoulder

● **M60.02 Infective myositis, upper arm**

M60.021 Infective myositis, right upper arm

M60.022 Infective myositis, left upper arm

M60.029 Infective myositis, unspecified upper arm

● **M60.03 Infective myositis, forearm**

M60.031 Infective myositis, right forearm

M60.032 Infective myositis, left forearm

M60.039 Infective myositis, unspecified forearm

● **M60.04 Infective myositis, hand and fingers**

M60.041 Infective myositis, right hand

M60.042 Infective myositis, left hand

M60.043 Infective myositis, unspecified hand

M60.044 Infective myositis, right finger(s)

M60.045 Infective myositis, left finger(s)

M60.046 Infective myositis, unspecified finger(s)

● **M60.05 Infective myositis, thigh**

M60.051 Infective myositis, right thigh

M60.052 Infective myositis, left thigh

M60.059 Infective myositis, unspecified thigh

● **M60.06 Infective myositis, lower leg**

M60.061 Infective myositis, right lower leg

M60.062 Infective myositis, left lower leg

M60.069 Infective myositis, unspecified lower leg

CHAPTER 13 (M00-M99)

CHAPTER 13 (M00-M99)

● M60.07   Infective myositis, ankle, foot and toes
     M60.070   Infective myositis, right ankle
     M60.071   Infective myositis, left ankle
     M60.072   Infective myositis, unspecified ankle
     M60.073   Infective myositis, right foot
     M60.074   Infective myositis, left foot
     M60.075   Infective myositis, unspecified foot
     M60.076   Infective myositis, right toe(s)
     M60.077   Infective myositis, left toe(s)
     M60.078   Infective myositis, unspecified toe(s)
  M60.08   Infective myositis, other site
  M60.09   Infective myositis, multiple sites
● M60.1   Interstitial myositis
  M60.10   Interstitial myositis of unspecified site
● M60.11   Interstitial myositis, shoulder
     M60.111   Interstitial myositis, right shoulder
     M60.112   Interstitial myositis, left shoulder
     M60.119   Interstitial myositis, unspecified shoulder
● M60.12   Interstitial myositis, upper arm
     M60.121   Interstitial myositis, right upper arm
     M60.122   Interstitial myositis, left upper arm
     M60.129   Interstitial myositis, unspecified upper arm
● M60.13   Interstitial myositis, forearm
     M60.131   Interstitial myositis, right forearm
     M60.132   Interstitial myositis, left forearm
     M60.139   Interstitial myositis, unspecified forearm
● M60.14   Interstitial myositis, hand
     M60.141   Interstitial myositis, right hand
     M60.142   Interstitial myositis, left hand
     M60.149   Interstitial myositis, unspecified hand
● M60.15   Interstitial myositis, thigh
     M60.151   Interstitial myositis, right thigh
     M60.152   Interstitial myositis, left thigh
     M60.159   Interstitial myositis, unspecified thigh
● M60.16   Interstitial myositis, lower leg
     M60.161   Interstitial myositis, right lower leg
     M60.162   Interstitial myositis, left lower leg
     M60.169   Interstitial myositis, unspecified lower leg
● M60.17   Interstitial myositis, ankle and foot
     M60.171   Interstitial myositis, right ankle and foot
     M60.172   Interstitial myositis, left ankle and foot
     M60.179   Interstitial myositis, unspecified ankle and foot
  M60.18   Interstitial myositis, other site
  M60.19   Interstitial myositis, multiple sites
● M60.2   Foreign body granuloma of soft tissue, not elsewhere classified

     Use additional code to identify the type of retained foreign body (Z18.-)

     Excludes1   foreign body granuloma of skin and subcutaneous tissue (L92.3)

  M60.20   Foreign body granuloma of soft tissue, not elsewhere classified, unspecified site
● M60.21   Foreign body granuloma of soft tissue, not elsewhere classified, shoulder
     M60.211   Foreign body granuloma of soft tissue, not elsewhere classified, right shoulder

     M60.212   Foreign body granuloma of soft tissue, not elsewhere classified, left shoulder
     M60.219   Foreign body granuloma of soft tissue, not elsewhere classified, unspecified shoulder
● M60.22   Foreign body granuloma of soft tissue, not elsewhere classified, upper arm
     M60.221   Foreign body granuloma of soft tissue, not elsewhere classified, right upper arm
     M60.222   Foreign body granuloma of soft tissue, not elsewhere classified, left upper arm
     M60.229   Foreign body granuloma of soft tissue, not elsewhere classified, unspecified upper arm
● M60.23   Foreign body granuloma of soft tissue, not elsewhere classified, forearm
     M60.231   Foreign body granuloma of soft tissue, not elsewhere classified, right forearm
     M60.232   Foreign body granuloma of soft tissue, not elsewhere classified, left forearm
     M60.239   Foreign body granuloma of soft tissue, not elsewhere classified, unspecified forearm
● M60.24   Foreign body granuloma of soft tissue, not elsewhere classified, hand
     M60.241   Foreign body granuloma of soft tissue, not elsewhere classified, right hand
     M60.242   Foreign body granuloma of soft tissue, not elsewhere classified, left hand
     M60.249   Foreign body granuloma of soft tissue, not elsewhere classified, unspecified hand
● M60.25   Foreign body granuloma of soft tissue, not elsewhere classified, thigh
     M60.251   Foreign body granuloma of soft tissue, not elsewhere classified, right thigh
     M60.252   Foreign body granuloma of soft tissue, not elsewhere classified, left thigh
     M60.259   Foreign body granuloma of soft tissue, not elsewhere classified, unspecified thigh
● M60.26   Foreign body granuloma of soft tissue, not elsewhere classified, lower leg
     M60.261   Foreign body granuloma of soft tissue, not elsewhere classified, right lower leg
     M60.262   Foreign body granuloma of soft tissue, not elsewhere classified, left lower leg
     M60.269   Foreign body granuloma of soft tissue, not elsewhere classified, unspecified lower leg
● M60.27   Foreign body granuloma of soft tissue, not elsewhere classified, ankle and foot
     M60.271   Foreign body granuloma of soft tissue, not elsewhere classified, right ankle and foot
     M60.272   Foreign body granuloma of soft tissue, not elsewhere classified, left ankle and foot
     M60.279   Foreign body granuloma of soft tissue, not elsewhere classified, unspecified ankle and foot
  M60.28   Foreign body granuloma of soft tissue, not elsewhere classified, other site

● **M60.8   Other myositis**
     M60.80   Other myositis, unspecified site
   ● M60.81   Other myositis shoulder
         M60.811   Other myositis, right shoulder
         M60.812   Other myositis, left shoulder
         M60.819   Other myositis, unspecified shoulder
   ● M60.82   Other myositis, upper arm
         M60.821   Other myositis, right upper arm
         M60.822   Other myositis, left upper arm
         M60.829   Other myositis, unspecified upper arm
   ● M60.83   Other myositis, forearm
         M60.831   Other myositis, right forearm
         M60.832   Other myositis, left forearm
         M60.839   Other myositis, unspecified forearm
   ● M60.84   Other myositis, hand
         M60.841   Other myositis, right hand
         M60.842   Other myositis, left hand
         M60.849   Other myositis, unspecified hand
   ● M60.85   Other myositis, thigh
         M60.851   Other myositis, right thigh
         M60.852   Other myositis, left thigh
         M60.859   Other myositis, unspecified thigh
   ● M60.86   Other myositis, lower leg
         M60.861   Other myositis, right lower leg
         M60.862   Other myositis, left lower leg
         M60.869   Other myositis, unspecified lower leg
   ● M60.87   Other myositis, ankle and foot
         M60.871   Other myositis, right ankle and foot
         M60.872   Other myositis, left ankle and foot
         M60.879   Other myositis, unspecified ankle and foot
     M60.88   Other myositis, other site
     M60.89   Other myositis, multiple sites
  M60.9   Myositis, unspecified

● **M61   Calcification and ossification of muscle**
   ● M61.0   Myositis ossificans traumatica
     M61.00   Myositis ossificans traumatica, unspecified site
   ● M61.01   Myositis ossificans traumatica, shoulder
         M61.011   Myositis ossificans traumatica, right shoulder
         M61.012   Myositis ossificans traumatica, left shoulder
         M61.019   Myositis ossificans traumatica, unspecified shoulder
   ● M61.02   Myositis ossificans traumatica, upper arm
         M61.021   Myositis ossificans traumatica, right upper arm
         M61.022   Myositis ossificans traumatica, left upper arm
         M61.029   Myositis ossificans traumatica, unspecified upper arm
   ● M61.03   Myositis ossificans traumatica, forearm
         M61.031   Myositis ossificans traumatica, right forearm
         M61.032   Myositis ossificans traumatica, left forearm
         M61.039   Myositis ossificans traumatica, unspecified forearm
   ● M61.04   Myositis ossificans traumatica, hand
         M61.041   Myositis ossificans traumatica, right hand
         M61.042   Myositis ossificans traumatica, left hand
         M61.049   Myositis ossificans traumatica, unspecified hand

   ● M61.05   Myositis ossificans traumatica, thigh
         M61.051   Myositis ossificans traumatica, right thigh
         M61.052   Myositis ossificans traumatica, left thigh
         M61.059   Myositis ossificans traumatica, unspecified thigh
   ● M61.06   Myositis ossificans traumatica, lower leg
         M61.061   Myositis ossificans traumatica, right lower leg
         M61.062   Myositis ossificans traumatica, left lower leg
         M61.069   Myositis ossificans traumatica, unspecified lower leg
   ● M61.07   Myositis ossificans traumatica, ankle and foot
         M61.071   Myositis ossificans traumatica, right ankle and foot
         M61.072   Myositis ossificans traumatica, left ankle and foot
         M61.079   Myositis ossificans traumatica, unspecified ankle and foot
     M61.08   Myositis ossificans traumatica, other site
     M61.09   Myositis ossificans traumatica, multiple sites
   ● M61.1   Myositis ossificans progressiva
       Fibrodysplasia ossificans progressiva
     M61.10   Myositis ossificans progressiva, unspecified site
   ● M61.11   Myositis ossificans progressiva, shoulder
         M61.111   Myositis ossificans progressiva, right shoulder
         M61.112   Myositis ossificans progressiva, left shoulder
         M61.119   Myositis ossificans progressiva, unspecified shoulder
   ● M61.12   Myositis ossificans progressiva, upper arm
         M61.121   Myositis ossificans progressiva, right upper arm
         M61.122   Myositis ossificans progressiva, left upper arm
         M61.129   Myositis ossificans progressiva, unspecified arm
   ● M61.13   Myositis ossificans progressiva, forearm
         M61.131   Myositis ossificans progressiva, right forearm
         M61.132   Myositis ossificans progressiva, left forearm
         M61.139   Myositis ossificans progressiva, unspecified forearm
   ● M61.14   Myositis ossificans progressiva, hand and finger(s)
         M61.141   Myositis ossificans progressiva, right hand
         M61.142   Myositis ossificans progressiva, left hand
         M61.143   Myositis ossificans progressiva, unspecified hand
         M61.144   Myositis ossificans progressiva, right finger(s)
         M61.145   Myositis ossificans progressiva, left finger(s)
         M61.146   Myositis ossificans progressiva, unspecified finger(s)
   ● M61.15   Myositis ossificans progressiva, thigh
         M61.151   Myositis ossificans progressiva, right thigh
         M61.152   Myositis ossificans progressiva, left thigh
         M61.159   Myositis ossificans progressiva, unspecified thigh

CHAPTER 13 (M00-M99)

● M61.16   Myositis ossificans progressiva, lower leg
    M61.161   Myositis ossificans progressiva, right lower leg
    M61.162   Myositis ossificans progressiva, left lower leg
    M61.169   Myositis ossificans progressiva, unspecified lower leg

● M61.17   Myositis ossificans progressiva, ankle, foot and toe(s)
    M61.171   Myositis ossificans progressiva, right ankle
    M61.172   Myositis ossificans progressiva, left ankle
    M61.173   Myositis ossificans progressiva, unspecified ankle
    M61.174   Myositis ossificans progressiva, right foot
    M61.175   Myositis ossificans progressiva, left foot
    M61.176   Myositis ossificans progressiva, unspecified foot
    M61.177   Myositis ossificans progressiva, right toe(s)
    M61.178   Myositis ossificans progressiva, left toe(s)
    M61.179   Myositis ossificans progressiva, unspecified toe(s)

M61.18   Myositis ossificans progressiva, other site
M61.19   Myositis ossificans progressiva, multiple sites

● M61.2   Paralytic calcification and ossification of muscle
    Myositis ossificans associated with quadriplegia or paraplegia

M61.20   Paralytic calcification and ossification of muscle, unspecified site

● M61.21   Paralytic calcification and ossification of muscle, shoulder
    M61.211   Paralytic calcification and ossification of muscle, right shoulder
    M61.212   Paralytic calcification and ossification of muscle, left shoulder
    M61.219   Paralytic calcification and ossification of muscle, unspecified shoulder

● M61.22   Paralytic calcification and ossification of muscle, upper arm
    M61.221   Paralytic calcification and ossification of muscle, right upper arm
    M61.222   Paralytic calcification and ossification of muscle, left upper arm
    M61.229   Paralytic calcification and ossification of muscle, unspecified upper arm

● M61.23   Paralytic calcification and ossification of muscle, forearm
    M61.231   Paralytic calcification and ossification of muscle, right forearm
    M61.232   Paralytic calcification and ossification of muscle, left forearm
    M61.239   Paralytic calcification and ossification of muscle, unspecified forearm

● M61.24   Paralytic calcification and ossification of muscle, hand
    M61.241   Paralytic calcification and ossification of muscle, right hand
    M61.242   Paralytic calcification and ossification of muscle, left hand
    M61.249   Paralytic calcification and ossification of muscle, unspecified hand

● M61.25   Paralytic calcification and ossification of muscle, thigh
    M61.251   Paralytic calcification and ossification of muscle, right thigh
    M61.252   Paralytic calcification and ossification of muscle, left thigh
    M61.259   Paralytic calcification and ossification of muscle, unspecified thigh

● M61.26   Paralytic calcification and ossification of muscle, lower leg
    M61.261   Paralytic calcification and ossification of muscle, right lower leg
    M61.262   Paralytic calcification and ossification of muscle, left lower leg
    M61.269   Paralytic calcification and ossification of muscle, unspecified lower leg

● M61.27   Paralytic calcification and ossification of muscle, ankle and foot
    M61.271   Paralytic calcification and ossification of muscle, right ankle and foot
    M61.272   Paralytic calcification and ossification of muscle, left ankle and foot
    M61.279   Paralytic calcification and ossification of muscle, unspecified ankle and foot

M61.28   Paralytic calcification and ossification of muscle, other site
M61.29   Paralytic calcification and ossification of muscle, multiple sites

● M61.3   Calcification and ossification of muscles associated with burns
    Myositis ossificans associated with burns

M61.30   Calcification and ossification of muscles associated with burns, unspecified site

● M61.31   Calcification and ossification of muscles associated with burns, shoulder
    M61.311   Calcification and ossification of muscles associated with burns, right shoulder
    M61.312   Calcification and ossification of muscles associated with burns, left shoulder
    M61.319   Calcification and ossification of muscles associated with burns, unspecified shoulder

● M61.32   Calcification and ossification of muscles associated with burns, upper arm
    M61.321   Calcification and ossification of muscles associated with burns, right upper arm
    M61.322   Calcification and ossification of muscles associated with burns, left upper arm
    M61.329   Calcification and ossification of muscles associated with burns, unspecified upper arm

● M61.33   Calcification and ossification of muscles associated with burns, forearm
    M61.331   Calcification and ossification of muscles associated with burns, right forearm
    M61.332   Calcification and ossification of muscles associated with burns, left forearm
    M61.339   Calcification and ossification of muscles associated with burns, unspecified forearm

▶ New   ⇒ Revised   ~~deleted~~ Deleted   Excludes 1   Excludes 2   Includes   Use additional   Code first   Code also   Key words

OGCR Official Guidelines   X Assign placeholder X   ● Use Additional Character(s)   ▶ Manifestation Code   🝆 Hierarchical Condition Category   Coding Clinic

● M61.34   Calcification and ossification of muscles associated with burns, hand

     M61.341   Calcification and ossification of muscles associated with burns, right hand

     M61.342   Calcification and ossification of muscles associated with burns, left hand

     M61.349   Calcification and ossification of muscles associated with burns, unspecified hand

● M61.35   Calcification and ossification of muscles associated with burns, thigh

     M61.351   Calcification and ossification of muscles associated with burns, right thigh

     M61.352   Calcification and ossification of muscles associated with burns, left thigh

     M61.359   Calcification and ossification of muscles associated with burns, unspecified thigh

● M61.36   Calcification and ossification of muscles associated with burns, lower leg

     M61.361   Calcification and ossification of muscles associated with burns, right lower leg

     M61.362   Calcification and ossification of muscles associated with burns, left lower leg

     M61.369   Calcification and ossification of muscles associated with burns, unspecified lower leg

● M61.37   Calcification and ossification of muscles associated with burns, ankle and foot

     M61.371   Calcification and ossification of muscles associated with burns, right ankle and foot

     M61.372   Calcification and ossification of muscles associated with burns, left ankle and foot

     M61.379   Calcification and ossification of muscles associated with burns, unspecified ankle and foot

     M61.38   Calcification and ossification of muscles associated with burns, other site

     M61.39   Calcification and ossification of muscles associated with burns, multiple sites

● M61.4   **Other calcification of muscle**

     Excludes1   calcific tendinitis NOS (M65.2-)
                   calcific tendinitis of shoulder (M75.3)

     M61.40   Other calcification of muscle, unspecified site

● M61.41   Other calcification of muscle, shoulder

     M61.411   Other calcification of muscle, right shoulder

     M61.412   Other calcification of muscle, left shoulder

     M61.419   Other calcification of muscle, unspecified shoulder

● M61.42   Other calcification of muscle, upper arm

     M61.421   Other calcification of muscle, right upper arm

     M61.422   Other calcification of muscle, left upper arm

     M61.429   Other calcification of muscle, unspecified upper arm

● M61.43   Other calcification of muscle, forearm

     M61.431   Other calcification of muscle, right forearm

     M61.432   Other calcification of muscle, left forearm

     M61.439   Other calcification of muscle, unspecified forearm

● M61.44   Other calcification of muscle, hand

     M61.441   Other calcification of muscle, right hand

     M61.442   Other calcification of muscle, left hand

     M61.449   Other calcification of muscle, unspecified hand

● M61.45   Other calcification of muscle, thigh

     M61.451   Other calcification of muscle, right thigh

     M61.452   Other calcification of muscle, left thigh

     M61.459   Other calcification of muscle, unspecified thigh

● M61.46   Other calcification of muscle, lower leg

     M61.461   Other calcification of muscle, right lower leg

     M61.462   Other calcification of muscle, left lower leg

     M61.469   Other calcification of muscle, unspecified lower leg

● M61.47   Other calcification of muscle, ankle and foot

     M61.471   Other calcification of muscle, right ankle and foot

     M61.472   Other calcification of muscle, left ankle and foot

     M61.479   Other calcification of muscle, unspecified ankle and foot

     M61.48   Other calcification of muscle, other site

     M61.49   Other calcification of muscle, multiple sites

● M61.5   **Other ossification of muscle**

     M61.50   Other ossification of muscle, unspecified site

● M61.51   Other ossification of muscle, shoulder

     M61.511   Other ossification of muscle, right shoulder

     M61.512   Other ossification of muscle, left shoulder

     M61.519   Other ossification of muscle, unspecified shoulder

● M61.52   Other ossification of muscle, upper arm

     M61.521   Other ossification of muscle, right upper arm

     M61.522   Other ossification of muscle, left upper arm

     M61.529   Other ossification of muscle, unspecified upper arm

● M61.53   Other ossification of muscle, forearm

     M61.531   Other ossification of muscle, right forearm

     M61.532   Other ossification of muscle, left forearm

     M61.539   Other ossification of muscle, unspecified forearm

● M61.54   Other ossification of muscle, hand

     M61.541   Other ossification of muscle, right hand

     M61.542   Other ossification of muscle, left hand

     M61.549   Other ossification of muscle, unspecified hand

CHAPTER 13 (M00-M99)

● M61.55   Other ossification of muscle, thigh

     M61.551   Other ossification of muscle, right thigh

     M61.552   Other ossification of muscle, left thigh

     M61.559   Other ossification of muscle, unspecified thigh

● M61.56   Other ossification of muscle, lower leg

     M61.561   Other ossification of muscle, right lower leg

     M61.562   Other ossification of muscle, left lower leg

     M61.569   Other ossification of muscle, unspecified lower leg

● M61.57   Other ossification of muscle, ankle and foot

     M61.571   Other ossification of muscle, right ankle and foot

     M61.572   Other ossification of muscle, left ankle and foot

     M61.579   Other ossification of muscle, unspecified ankle and foot

   M61.58   Other ossification of muscle, other site

   M61.59   Other ossification of muscle, multiple sites

  M61.9   Calcification and ossification of muscle, unspecified

● M62   Other disorders of muscle

   Excludes1   alcoholic myopathy (G72.1)
                cramp and spasm (R25.2)
                drug-induced myopathy (G72.0)
                myalgia (M79.1-)
                stiff-man syndrome (G25.82)

   Excludes2   nontraumatic hematoma of muscle (M79.81)

● M62.0   Separation of muscle (nontraumatic)
        Diastasis of muscle

     Excludes1   diastasis recti complicating pregnancy, labor and delivery (O71.8)
                      traumatic separation of muscle - see strain of muscle by body region

   M62.00   Separation of muscle (nontraumatic), unspecified site

● M62.01   Separation of muscle (nontraumatic), shoulder

     M62.011   Separation of muscle (nontraumatic), right shoulder

     M62.012   Separation of muscle (nontraumatic), left shoulder

     M62.019   Separation of muscle (nontraumatic), unspecified shoulder

● M62.02   Separation of muscle (nontraumatic), upper arm

     M62.021   Separation of muscle (nontraumatic), right upper arm

     M62.022   Separation of muscle (nontraumatic), left upper arm

     M62.029   Separation of muscle (nontraumatic), unspecified upper arm

● M62.03   Separation of muscle (nontraumatic), forearm

     M62.031   Separation of muscle (nontraumatic), right forearm

     M62.032   Separation of muscle (nontraumatic), left forearm

     M62.039   Separation of muscle (nontraumatic), unspecified forearm

● M62.04   Separation of muscle (nontraumatic), hand

     M62.041   Separation of muscle (nontraumatic), right hand

     M62.042   Separation of muscle (nontraumatic), left hand

     M62.049   Separation of muscle (nontraumatic), unspecified hand

● M62.05   Separation of muscle (nontraumatic), thigh

     M62.051   Separation of muscle (nontraumatic), right thigh

     M62.052   Separation of muscle (nontraumatic), left thigh

     M62.059   Separation of muscle (nontraumatic), unspecified thigh

● M62.06   Separation of muscle (nontraumatic), lower leg

     M62.061   Separation of muscle (nontraumatic), right lower leg

     M62.062   Separation of muscle (nontraumatic), left lower leg

     M62.069   Separation of muscle (nontraumatic), unspecified lower leg

● M62.07   Separation of muscle (nontraumatic), ankle and foot

     M62.071   Separation of muscle (nontraumatic), right ankle and foot

     M62.072   Separation of muscle (nontraumatic), left ankle and foot

     M62.079   Separation of muscle (nontraumatic), unspecified ankle and foot

   M62.08   Separation of muscle (nontraumatic), other site

● M62.1   Other rupture of muscle (nontraumatic)

     Excludes1   traumatic rupture of muscle - see strain of muscle by body region

     Excludes2   rupture of tendon (M66.-)

   M62.10   Other rupture of muscle (nontraumatic), unspecified site

● M62.11   Other rupture of muscle (nontraumatic), shoulder

     M62.111   Other rupture of muscle (nontraumatic), right shoulder

     M62.112   Other rupture of muscle (nontraumatic), left shoulder

     M62.119   Other rupture of muscle (nontraumatic), unspecified shoulder

● M62.12   Other rupture of muscle (nontraumatic), upper arm

     M62.121   Other rupture of muscle (nontraumatic), right upper arm

     M62.122   Other rupture of muscle (nontraumatic), left upper arm

     M62.129   Other rupture of muscle (nontraumatic), unspecified upper arm

● M62.13   Other rupture of muscle (nontraumatic), forearm

     M62.131   Other rupture of muscle (nontraumatic), right forearm

     M62.132   Other rupture of muscle (nontraumatic), left forearm

     M62.139   Other rupture of muscle (nontraumatic), unspecified forearm

● M62.14   Other rupture of muscle (nontraumatic), hand

     M62.141   Other rupture of muscle (nontraumatic), right hand

     M62.142   Other rupture of muscle (nontraumatic), left hand

     M62.149   Other rupture of muscle (nontraumatic), unspecified hand

● M62.15   Other rupture of muscle (nontraumatic), thigh

     M62.151   Other rupture of muscle (nontraumatic), right thigh

     M62.152   Other rupture of muscle (nontraumatic), left thigh

     M62.159   Other rupture of muscle (nontraumatic), unspecified thigh

● **M62.16** Other rupture of muscle (nontraumatic), lower leg

     M62.161 Other rupture of muscle (nontraumatic), right lower leg

     M62.162 Other rupture of muscle (nontraumatic), left lower leg

     M62.169 Other rupture of muscle (nontraumatic), unspecified lower leg

● **M62.17** Other rupture of muscle (nontraumatic), ankle and foot

     M62.171 Other rupture of muscle (nontraumatic), right ankle and foot

     M62.172 Other rupture of muscle (nontraumatic), left ankle and foot

     M62.179 Other rupture of muscle (nontraumatic), unspecified ankle and foot

     M62.18 Other rupture of muscle (nontraumatic), other site

● **M62.2** Nontraumatic ischemic infarction of muscle

     Excludes1   compartment syndrome (traumatic) (T79.A-)

                nontraumatic compartment syndrome (M79.A-)

                traumatic ischemia of muscle (T79.6)

                rhabdomyolysis (M62.82)

                Volkmann's ischemic contracture (T79.6)

     M62.20 Nontraumatic ischemic infarction of muscle, unspecified site

● **M62.21** Nontraumatic ischemic infarction of muscle, shoulder

     M62.211 Nontraumatic ischemic infarction of muscle, right shoulder

     M62.212 Nontraumatic ischemic infarction of muscle, left shoulder

     M62.219 Nontraumatic ischemic infarction of muscle, unspecified shoulder

● **M62.22** Nontraumatic ischemic infarction of muscle, upper arm

     M62.221 Nontraumatic ischemic infarction of muscle, right upper arm

     M62.222 Nontraumatic ischemic infarction of muscle, left upper arm

     M62.229 Nontraumatic ischemic infarction of muscle, unspecified upper arm

● **M62.23** Nontraumatic ischemic infarction of muscle, forearm

     M62.231 Nontraumatic ischemic infarction of muscle, right forearm

     M62.232 Nontraumatic ischemic infarction of muscle, left forearm

     M62.239 Nontraumatic ischemic infarction of muscle, unspecified forearm

● **M62.24** Nontraumatic ischemic infarction of muscle, hand

     M62.241 Nontraumatic ischemic infarction of muscle, right hand

     M62.242 Nontraumatic ischemic infarction of muscle, left hand

     M62.249 Nontraumatic ischemic infarction of muscle, unspecified hand

● **M62.25** Nontraumatic ischemic infarction of muscle, thigh

     M62.251 Nontraumatic ischemic infarction of muscle, right thigh

     M62.252 Nontraumatic ischemic infarction of muscle, left thigh

     M62.259 Nontraumatic ischemic infarction of muscle, unspecified thigh

● **M62.26** Nontraumatic ischemic infarction of muscle, lower leg

     M62.261 Nontraumatic ischemic infarction of muscle, right lower leg

     M62.262 Nontraumatic ischemic infarction of muscle, left lower leg

     M62.269 Nontraumatic ischemic infarction of muscle, unspecified lower leg

● **M62.27** Nontraumatic ischemic infarction of muscle, ankle and foot

     M62.271 Nontraumatic ischemic infarction of muscle, right ankle and foot

     M62.272 Nontraumatic ischemic infarction of muscle, left ankle and foot

     M62.279 Nontraumatic ischemic infarction of muscle, unspecified ankle and foot

     M62.28 Nontraumatic ischemic infarction of muscle, other site

     M62.3 Immobility syndrome (paraplegic)

     M62.4 Contracture of muscle

         Contracture of tendon (sheath)

         Excludes1   contracture of joint (M24.5-)

     M62.40 Contracture of muscle, unspecified site

● **M62.41** Contracture of muscle, shoulder

     M62.411 Contracture of muscle, right shoulder

     M62.412 Contracture of muscle, left shoulder

     M62.419 Contracture of muscle, unspecified shoulder

● **M62.42** Contracture of muscle, upper arm

     M62.421 Contracture of muscle, right upper arm

     M62.422 Contracture of muscle, left upper arm

     M62.429 Contracture of muscle, unspecified upper arm

● **M62.43** Contracture of muscle, forearm

     M62.431 Contracture of muscle, right forearm

     M62.432 Contracture of muscle, left forearm

     M62.439 Contracture of muscle, unspecified forearm

● **M62.44** Contracture of muscle, hand

     M62.441 Contracture of muscle, right hand

     M62.442 Contracture of muscle, left hand

     M62.449 Contracture of muscle, unspecified hand

● **M62.45** Contracture of muscle, thigh

     M62.451 Contracture of muscle, right thigh

     M62.452 Contracture of muscle, left thigh

     M62.459 Contracture of muscle, unspecified thigh

● **M62.46** Contracture of muscle, lower leg

     M62.461 Contracture of muscle, right lower leg

     M62.462 Contracture of muscle, left lower leg

     M62.469 Contracture of muscle, unspecified lower leg

● **M62.47** Contracture of muscle, ankle and foot

     M62.471 Contracture of muscle, right ankle and foot

     M62.472 Contracture of muscle, left ankle and foot

     M62.479 Contracture of muscle, unspecified ankle and foot

     M62.48 Contracture of muscle, other site

     M62.49 Contracture of muscle, multiple sites

CHAPTER 13 (M00–M99)

● **M62.5 Muscle wasting and atrophy, not elsewhere classified**
    Disuse atrophy NEC

    Excludes1   neuralgic amyotrophy (G54.5)
                   progressive muscular atrophy (G12.21)
                   sarcopenia (M62.84)

    Excludes2   pelvic muscle wasting (N81.84)

  M62.50 Muscle wasting and atrophy, not elsewhere classified, unspecified site

● M62.51 Muscle wasting and atrophy, not elsewhere classified, shoulder

    M62.511 Muscle wasting and atrophy, not elsewhere classified, right shoulder

    M62.512 Muscle wasting and atrophy, not elsewhere classified, left shoulder

    M62.519 Muscle wasting and atrophy, not elsewhere classified, unspecified shoulder

● M62.52 Muscle wasting and atrophy, not elsewhere classified, upper arm

    M62.521 Muscle wasting and atrophy, not elsewhere classified, right upper arm

    M62.522 Muscle wasting and atrophy, not elsewhere classified, left upper arm

    M62.529 Muscle wasting and atrophy, not elsewhere classified, unspecified upper arm

● M62.53 Muscle wasting and atrophy, not elsewhere classified, forearm

    M62.531 Muscle wasting and atrophy, not elsewhere classified, right forearm

    M62.532 Muscle wasting and atrophy, not elsewhere classified, left forearm

    M62.539 Muscle wasting and atrophy, not elsewhere classified, unspecified forearm

● M62.54 Muscle wasting and atrophy, not elsewhere classified, hand

    M62.541 Muscle wasting and atrophy, not elsewhere classified, right hand

    M62.542 Muscle wasting and atrophy, not elsewhere classified, left hand

    M62.549 Muscle wasting and atrophy, not elsewhere classified, unspecified hand

● M62.55 Muscle wasting and atrophy, not elsewhere classified, thigh

    M62.551 Muscle wasting and atrophy, not elsewhere classified, right thigh

    M62.552 Muscle wasting and atrophy, not elsewhere classified, left thigh

    M62.559 Muscle wasting and atrophy, not elsewhere classified, unspecified thigh

● M62.56 Muscle wasting and atrophy, not elsewhere classified, lower leg

    M62.561 Muscle wasting and atrophy, not elsewhere classified, right lower leg

    M62.562 Muscle wasting and atrophy, not elsewhere classified, left lower leg

    M62.569 Muscle wasting and atrophy, not elsewhere classified, unspecified lower leg

● M62.57 Muscle wasting and atrophy, not elsewhere classified, ankle and foot

    M62.571 Muscle wasting and atrophy, not elsewhere classified, right ankle and foot

    M62.572 Muscle wasting and atrophy, not elsewhere classified, left ankle and foot

    M62.579 Muscle wasting and atrophy, not elsewhere classified, unspecified ankle and foot

  M62.58 Muscle wasting and atrophy, not elsewhere classified, other site

  M62.59 Muscle wasting and atrophy, not elsewhere classified, multiple sites

▶● M62.5A Muscle wasting and atrophy, not elsewhere classified, back

    ▶M62.5A0 Muscle wasting and atrophy, not elsewhere classified, back, cervical

    ▶M62.5A1 Muscle wasting and atrophy, not elsewhere classified, back, thoracic

    ▶M62.5A2 Muscle wasting and atrophy, not elsewhere classified, back, lumbosacral

    ▶M62.5A9 Muscle wasting and atrophy, not elsewhere classified, back, unspecified level

● **M62.8 Other specified disorders of muscle**

    Excludes2   nontraumatic hematoma of muscle (M79.81)

  M62.81 Muscle weakness (generalized)

    Excludes1   muscle weakness in sarcopenia (M62.84)

  M62.82 Rhabdomyolysis

    Excludes1   traumatic rhabdomyolysis (T79.6)

    Coding Clinic: 2019, Q2, P12

● M62.83 Muscle spasm

    M62.830 Muscle spasm of back

    M62.831 Muscle spasm of calf
              Charley-horse

    M62.838 Other muscle spasm

  M62.84 Sarcopenia
    Age-related sarcopenia

    Code first underlying disease, if applicable, such as:
      disorders of myoneural junction and muscle disease in diseases classified elsewhere (G73.-)
      other and unspecified myopathies (G72.-)
      primary disorders of muscles (G71.-)

    Coding Clinic: 2016, Q4, P41

  M62.89 Other specified disorders of muscle
    Muscle (sheath) hernia

  M62.9 Disorder of muscle, unspecified

● **M63 Disorders of muscle in diseases classified elsewhere**

    Code first underlying disease, such as:
    leprosy (A30.-)
    neoplasm (C49.-, C79.89, D21.-, D48.1)
    schistosomiasis (B65.-)
    trichinellosis (B75.)

    Excludes1   myopathy in cysticercosis (B69.81)
               myopathy in endocrine diseases (G73.7)
               myopathy in metabolic diseases (G73.7)
               myopathy in sarcoidosis (D86.87)
               myopathy in secondary syphilis (A51.49)
               myopathy in syphilis (late) (A52.78)
               myopathy in toxoplasmosis (B58.82)
               myopathy in tuberculosis (A18.09)

● M63.8 Disorders of muscle in diseases classified elsewhere

    ▷ *M63.80 Disorders of muscle in diseases classified elsewhere, unspecified site*

  ● M63.81 Disorders of muscle in diseases classified elsewhere, shoulder

    ▷ *M63.811 Disorders of muscle in diseases classified elsewhere, right shoulder*

▶ New   ⇛ Revised   ~~deleted~~ Deleted   Excludes 1   Excludes 2   Includes   Use additional   Code first   Code also   Key words

OGCR Official Guidelines   X Assign placeholder X   ● Use Additional Character(s)   ▷ Manifestation Code   🅱 Hierarchical Condition Category   **Coding Clinic**

> *M63.812*   *Disorders of muscle in diseases classified elsewhere, left shoulder*

> *M63.819*   *Disorders of muscle in diseases classified elsewhere, unspecified shoulder*

● M63.82   Disorders of muscle in diseases classified elsewhere, upper arm

> *M63.821*   *Disorders of muscle in diseases classified elsewhere, right upper arm*

> *M63.822*   *Disorders of muscle in diseases classified elsewhere, left upper arm*

> *M63.829*   *Disorders of muscle in diseases classified elsewhere, unspecified upper arm*

● M63.83   Disorders of muscle in diseases classified elsewhere, forearm

> *M63.831*   *Disorders of muscle in diseases classified elsewhere, right forearm*

> *M63.832*   *Disorders of muscle in diseases classified elsewhere, left forearm*

> *M63.839*   *Disorders of muscle in diseases classified elsewhere, unspecified forearm*

● M63.84   Disorders of muscle in diseases classified elsewhere, hand

> *M63.841*   *Disorders of muscle in diseases classified elsewhere, right hand*

> *M63.842*   *Disorders of muscle in diseases classified elsewhere, left hand*

> *M63.849*   *Disorders of muscle in diseases classified elsewhere, unspecified hand*

● M63.85   Disorders of muscle in diseases classified elsewhere, thigh

> *M63.851*   *Disorders of muscle in diseases classified elsewhere, right thigh*

> *M63.852*   *Disorders of muscle in diseases classified elsewhere, left thigh*

> *M63.859*   *Disorders of muscle in diseases classified elsewhere, unspecified thigh*

● M63.86   Disorders of muscle in diseases classified elsewhere, lower leg

> *M63.861*   *Disorders of muscle in diseases classified elsewhere, right lower leg*

> *M63.862*   *Disorders of muscle in diseases classified elsewhere, left lower leg*

> *M63.869*   *Disorders of muscle in diseases classified elsewhere, unspecified lower leg*

● M63.87   Disorders of muscle in diseases classified elsewhere, ankle and foot

> *M63.871*   *Disorders of muscle in diseases classified elsewhere, right ankle and foot*

> *M63.872*   *Disorders of muscle in diseases classified elsewhere, left ankle and foot*

> *M63.879*   *Disorders of muscle in diseases classified elsewhere, unspecified ankle and foot*

> *M63.88*   *Disorders of muscle in diseases classified elsewhere, other site*

> *M63.89*   *Disorders of muscle in diseases classified elsewhere, multiple sites*

DISORDERS OF SYNOVIUM AND TENDON (M65-M67)

● M65   Synovitis and tenosynovitis

   Excludes1   chronic crepitant synovitis of hand and wrist (M70.0-)

              current injury - see injury of ligament or tendon by body region

              soft tissue disorders related to use, overuse and pressure (M70.-)

Item 13–11   **Synovitis** is an inflammation of a synovial membrane resulting in pain on motion and is characterized by fluctuating swelling due to effusion in a synovial sac. **Tenosynovitis** is an inflammation of a tendon sheath and occurs most commonly in the wrists, hands, and feet. Bursitis is inflammation of a bursa (fluid-filled sac) caused by repetitive use, trauma, infection, or systemic inflammatory disease. Bursae act as protectors and facilitate movement between bones and overlapping muscles (deep bursae) or between bones and tendons/skin (superficial bursae).

● M65.0   Abscess of tendon sheath

     Use additional code (B95-B96) to identify bacterial agent

     M65.00   Abscess of tendon sheath, unspecified site

● M65.01   Abscess of tendon sheath, shoulder

     M65.011   Abscess of tendon sheath, right shoulder

     M65.012   Abscess of tendon sheath, left shoulder

     M65.019   Abscess of tendon sheath, unspecified shoulder

● M65.02   Abscess of tendon sheath, upper arm

     M65.021   Abscess of tendon sheath, right upper arm

     M65.022   Abscess of tendon sheath, left upper arm

     M65.029   Abscess of tendon sheath, unspecified upper arm

● M65.03   Abscess of tendon sheath, forearm

     M65.031   Abscess of tendon sheath, right forearm

     M65.032   Abscess of tendon sheath, left forearm

     M65.039   Abscess of tendon sheath, unspecified forearm

● M65.04   Abscess of tendon sheath, hand

     M65.041   Abscess of tendon sheath, right hand

     M65.042   Abscess of tendon sheath, left hand

     M65.049   Abscess of tendon sheath, unspecified hand

● M65.05   Abscess of tendon sheath, thigh

     M65.051   Abscess of tendon sheath, right thigh

     M65.052   Abscess of tendon sheath, left thigh

     M65.059   Abscess of tendon sheath, unspecified thigh

● M65.06   Abscess of tendon sheath, lower leg

     M65.061   Abscess of tendon sheath, right lower leg

     M65.062   Abscess of tendon sheath, left lower leg

     M65.069   Abscess of tendon sheath, unspecified lower leg

● M65.07   Abscess of tendon sheath, ankle and foot

     M65.071   Abscess of tendon sheath, right ankle and foot

     M65.072   Abscess of tendon sheath, left ankle and foot

     M65.079   Abscess of tendon sheath, unspecified ankle and foot

     M65.08   Abscess of tendon sheath, other site

● M65.1   Other infective (teno)synovitis

     M65.10   Other infective (teno)synovitis, unspecified site

● M65.11   Other infective (teno)synovitis, shoulder

     M65.111   Other infective (teno)synovitis, right shoulder

     M65.112   Other infective (teno)synovitis, left shoulder

     M65.119   Other infective (teno)synovitis, unspecified shoulder

---

CHAPTER 13 (M00-M99)

● M65.12   Other infective (teno)synovitis, elbow
    M65.121   Other infective (teno)synovitis, right elbow
    M65.122   Other infective (teno)synovitis, left elbow
    M65.129   Other infective (teno)synovitis, unspecified elbow

● M65.13   Other infective (teno)synovitis, wrist
    M65.131   Other infective (teno)synovitis, right wrist
    M65.132   Other infective (teno)synovitis, left wrist
    M65.139   Other infective (teno)synovitis, unspecified wrist

● M65.14   Other infective (teno)synovitis, hand
    M65.141   Other infective (teno)synovitis, right hand
    M65.142   Other infective (teno)synovitis, left hand
    M65.149   Other infective (teno)synovitis, unspecified hand

● M65.15   Other infective (teno)synovitis, hip
    M65.151   Other infective (teno)synovitis, right hip
    M65.152   Other infective (teno)synovitis, left hip
    M65.159   Other infective (teno)synovitis, unspecified hip

● M65.16   Other infective (teno)synovitis, knee
    M65.161   Other infective (teno)synovitis, right knee
    M65.162   Other infective (teno)synovitis, left knee
    M65.169   Other infective (teno)synovitis, unspecified knee

● M65.17   Other infective (teno)synovitis, ankle and foot
    M65.171   Other infective (teno)synovitis, right ankle and foot
    M65.172   Other infective (teno)synovitis, left ankle and foot
    M65.179   Other infective (teno)synovitis, unspecified ankle and foot

    M65.18   Other infective (teno)synovitis, other site
    M65.19   Other infective (teno)synovitis, multiple sites

● M65.2   Calcific tendinitis
    Excludes1   tendinitis as classified in M75-M77
                 calcified tendinitis of shoulder (M75.3)

    M65.20   Calcific tendinitis, unspecified site
● M65.22   Calcific tendinitis, upper arm
    M65.221   Calcific tendinitis, right upper arm
    M65.222   Calcific tendinitis, left upper arm
    M65.229   Calcific tendinitis, unspecified upper arm

● M65.23   Calcific tendinitis, forearm
    M65.231   Calcific tendinitis, right forearm
    M65.232   Calcific tendinitis, left forearm
    M65.239   Calcific tendinitis, unspecified forearm

● M65.24   Calcific tendinitis, hand
    M65.241   Calcific tendinitis, right hand
    M65.242   Calcific tendinitis, left hand
    M65.249   Calcific tendinitis, unspecified hand

● M65.25   Calcific tendinitis, thigh
    M65.251   Calcific tendinitis, right thigh
    M65.252   Calcific tendinitis, left thigh
    M65.259   Calcific tendinitis, unspecified thigh

● M65.26   Calcific tendinitis, lower leg
    M65.261   Calcific tendinitis, right lower leg
    M65.262   Calcific tendinitis, left lower leg
    M65.269   Calcific tendinitis, unspecified lower leg

● M65.27   Calcific tendinitis, ankle and foot
    M65.271   Calcific tendinitis, right ankle and foot
    M65.272   Calcific tendinitis, left ankle and foot
    M65.279   Calcific tendinitis, unspecified ankle and foot

    M65.28   Calcific tendinitis, other site
    M65.29   Calcific tendinitis, multiple sites

● M65.3   Trigger finger
    Nodular tendinous disease
    M65.30   Trigger finger, unspecified finger
● M65.31   Trigger thumb
    M65.311   Trigger thumb, right thumb
    M65.312   Trigger thumb, left thumb
    M65.319   Trigger thumb, unspecified thumb

● M65.32   Trigger finger, index finger
    M65.321   Trigger finger, right index finger
    M65.322   Trigger finger, left index finger
    M65.329   Trigger finger, unspecified index finger

● M65.33   Trigger finger, middle finger
    M65.331   Trigger finger, right middle finger
    M65.332   Trigger finger, left middle finger
    M65.339   Trigger finger, unspecified middle finger

● M65.34   Trigger finger, ring finger
    M65.341   Trigger finger, right ring finger
    M65.342   Trigger finger, left ring finger
    M65.349   Trigger finger, unspecified ring finger

● M65.35   Trigger finger, little finger
    M65.351   Trigger finger, right little finger
    M65.352   Trigger finger, left little finger
    M65.359   Trigger finger, unspecified little finger

    M65.4   Radial styloid tenosynovitis [de Quervain]
● M65.8   Other synovitis and tenosynovitis
    M65.80   Other synovitis and tenosynovitis, unspecified site
● M65.81   Other synovitis and tenosynovitis, shoulder
    M65.811   Other synovitis and tenosynovitis, right shoulder
    M65.812   Other synovitis and tenosynovitis, left shoulder
    M65.819   Other synovitis and tenosynovitis, unspecified shoulder

● M65.82   Other synovitis and tenosynovitis, upper arm
    M65.821   Other synovitis and tenosynovitis, right upper arm
    M65.822   Other synovitis and tenosynovitis, left upper arm
    M65.829   Other synovitis and tenosynovitis, unspecified upper arm

● M65.83   Other synovitis and tenosynovitis, forearm
    M65.831   Other synovitis and tenosynovitis, right forearm
    M65.832   Other synovitis and tenosynovitis, left forearm
    M65.839   Other synovitis and tenosynovitis, unspecified forearm

▶ New   ⇒ Revised   ~~deleted~~ Deleted   Excludes 1   Excludes 2   Includes   Use additional   Code first   Code also   Key words
OGCR Official Guidelines   X Assign placeholder X   ● Use Additional Character(s)   ▶ Manifestation Code   🔗 Hierarchical Condition Category   **Coding Clinic**

● M65.84   Other synovitis and tenosynovitis, hand
     M65.841   Other synovitis and tenosynovitis, right hand
     M65.842   Other synovitis and tenosynovitis, left hand
     M65.849   Other synovitis and tenosynovitis, unspecified hand
● M65.85   Other synovitis and tenosynovitis, thigh
     M65.851   Other synovitis and tenosynovitis, right thigh
     M65.852   Other synovitis and tenosynovitis, left thigh
     M65.859   Other synovitis and tenosynovitis, unspecified thigh
● M65.86   Other synovitis and tenosynovitis, lower leg
     M65.861   Other synovitis and tenosynovitis, right lower leg
     M65.862   Other synovitis and tenosynovitis, left lower leg
     M65.869   Other synovitis and tenosynovitis, unspecified lower leg
● M65.87   Other synovitis and tenosynovitis, ankle and foot
     M65.871   Other synovitis and tenosynovitis, right ankle and foot
     M65.872   Other synovitis and tenosynovitis, left ankle and foot
     M65.879   Other synovitis and tenosynovitis, unspecified ankle and foot
   M65.88   Other synovitis and tenosynovitis, other site
   M65.89   Other synovitis and tenosynovitis, multiple sites
  M65.9   Synovitis and tenosynovitis, unspecified

● M66   **Spontaneous rupture of synovium and tendon**

     Includes   rupture that occurs when a normal force is applied to tissues that are inferred to have less than normal strength

     Excludes2   rotator cuff syndrome (M75.1-)
                 rupture where an abnormal force is applied to normal tissue - see injury of tendon by body region

  M66.0   Rupture of popliteal cyst
● M66.1   Rupture of synovium
     Rupture of synovial cyst
     Excludes2   rupture of popliteal cyst (M66.0)
     M66.10   Rupture of synovium, unspecified joint
   ● M66.11   Rupture of synovium, shoulder
     M66.111   Rupture of synovium, right shoulder
     M66.112   Rupture of synovium, left shoulder
     M66.119   Rupture of synovium, unspecified shoulder
   ● M66.12   Rupture of synovium, elbow
     M66.121   Rupture of synovium, right elbow
     M66.122   Rupture of synovium, left elbow
     M66.129   Rupture of synovium, unspecified elbow
   ● M66.13   Rupture of synovium, wrist
     M66.131   Rupture of synovium, right wrist
     M66.132   Rupture of synovium, left wrist
     M66.139   Rupture of synovium, unspecified wrist

   ● M66.14   Rupture of synovium, hand and fingers
     M66.141   Rupture of synovium, right hand
     M66.142   Rupture of synovium, left hand
     M66.143   Rupture of synovium, unspecified hand
     M66.144   Rupture of synovium, right finger(s)
     M66.145   Rupture of synovium, left finger(s)
     M66.146   Rupture of synovium, unspecified finger(s)
   ● M66.15   Rupture of synovium, hip
     M66.151   Rupture of synovium, right hip
     M66.152   Rupture of synovium, left hip
     M66.159   Rupture of synovium, unspecified hip
   ● M66.17   Rupture of synovium, ankle, foot and toes
     M66.171   Rupture of synovium, right ankle
     M66.172   Rupture of synovium, left ankle
     M66.173   Rupture of synovium, unspecified ankle
     M66.174   Rupture of synovium, right foot
     M66.175   Rupture of synovium, left foot
     M66.176   Rupture of synovium, unspecified foot
     M66.177   Rupture of synovium, right toe(s)
     M66.178   Rupture of synovium, left toe(s)
     M66.179   Rupture of synovium, unspecified toe(s)
   M66.18   Rupture of synovium, other site
● M66.2   Spontaneous rupture of extensor tendons
     M66.20   Spontaneous rupture of extensor tendons, unspecified site
   ● M66.21   Spontaneous rupture of extensor tendons, shoulder
     M66.211   Spontaneous rupture of extensor tendons, right shoulder
     M66.212   Spontaneous rupture of extensor tendons, left shoulder
     M66.219   Spontaneous rupture of extensor tendons, unspecified shoulder
   ● M66.22   Spontaneous rupture of extensor tendons, upper arm
     M66.221   Spontaneous rupture of extensor tendons, right upper arm
     M66.222   Spontaneous rupture of extensor tendons, left upper arm
     M66.229   Spontaneous rupture of extensor tendons, unspecified upper arm
   ● M66.23   Spontaneous rupture of extensor tendons, forearm
     M66.231   Spontaneous rupture of extensor tendons, right forearm
     M66.232   Spontaneous rupture of extensor tendons, left forearm
     M66.239   Spontaneous rupture of extensor tendons, unspecified forearm
   ● M66.24   Spontaneous rupture of extensor tendons, hand
     M66.241   Spontaneous rupture of extensor tendons, right hand
     M66.242   Spontaneous rupture of extensor tendons, left hand
     M66.249   Spontaneous rupture of extensor tendons, unspecified hand

CHAPTER 13 (M00-M99)

● **M66.25** Spontaneous rupture of extensor tendons, thigh
    M66.251 Spontaneous rupture of extensor tendons, right thigh
    M66.252 Spontaneous rupture of extensor tendons, left thigh
    M66.259 Spontaneous rupture of extensor tendons, unspecified thigh
● **M66.26** Spontaneous rupture of extensor tendons, lower leg
    M66.261 Spontaneous rupture of extensor tendons, right lower leg
    M66.262 Spontaneous rupture of extensor tendons, left lower leg
    M66.269 Spontaneous rupture of extensor tendons, unspecified lower leg
● **M66.27** Spontaneous rupture of extensor tendons, ankle and foot
    M66.271 Spontaneous rupture of extensor tendons, right ankle and foot
    M66.272 Spontaneous rupture of extensor tendons, left ankle and foot
    M66.279 Spontaneous rupture of extensor tendons, unspecified ankle and foot
  M66.28 Spontaneous rupture of extensor tendons, other site
  M66.29 Spontaneous rupture of extensor tendons, multiple sites
● **M66.3** Spontaneous rupture of flexor tendons
  M66.30 Spontaneous rupture of flexor tendons, unspecified site
● **M66.31** Spontaneous rupture of flexor tendons, shoulder
    M66.311 Spontaneous rupture of flexor tendons, right shoulder
    M66.312 Spontaneous rupture of flexor tendons, left shoulder
    M66.319 Spontaneous rupture of flexor tendons, unspecified shoulder
● **M66.32** Spontaneous rupture of flexor tendons, upper arm
    M66.321 Spontaneous rupture of flexor tendons, right upper arm
    M66.322 Spontaneous rupture of flexor tendons, left upper arm
    M66.329 Spontaneous rupture of flexor tendons, unspecified upper arm
● **M66.33** Spontaneous rupture of flexor tendons, forearm
    M66.331 Spontaneous rupture of flexor tendons, right forearm
    M66.332 Spontaneous rupture of flexor tendons, left forearm
    M66.339 Spontaneous rupture of flexor tendons, unspecified forearm
● **M66.34** Spontaneous rupture of flexor tendons, hand
    M66.341 Spontaneous rupture of flexor tendons, right hand
    M66.342 Spontaneous rupture of flexor tendons, left hand
    M66.349 Spontaneous rupture of flexor tendons, unspecified hand
● **M66.35** Spontaneous rupture of flexor tendons, thigh
    M66.351 Spontaneous rupture of flexor tendons, right thigh
    M66.352 Spontaneous rupture of flexor tendons, left thigh
    M66.359 Spontaneous rupture of flexor tendons, unspecified thigh

● **M66.36** Spontaneous rupture of flexor tendons, lower leg
    M66.361 Spontaneous rupture of flexor tendons, right lower leg
    M66.362 Spontaneous rupture of flexor tendons, left lower leg
    M66.369 Spontaneous rupture of flexor tendons, unspecified lower leg
● **M66.37** Spontaneous rupture of flexor tendons, ankle and foot
    M66.371 Spontaneous rupture of flexor tendons, right ankle and foot
    M66.372 Spontaneous rupture of flexor tendons, left ankle and foot
    M66.379 Spontaneous rupture of flexor tendons, unspecified ankle and foot
  M66.38 Spontaneous rupture of flexor tendons, other site
  M66.39 Spontaneous rupture of flexor tendons, multiple sites
● **M66.8** Spontaneous rupture of other tendons
  M66.80 Spontaneous rupture of other tendons, unspecified site
● **M66.81** Spontaneous rupture of other tendons, shoulder
    M66.811 Spontaneous rupture of other tendons, right shoulder
    M66.812 Spontaneous rupture of other tendons, left shoulder
    M66.819 Spontaneous rupture of other tendons, unspecified shoulder
● **M66.82** Spontaneous rupture of other tendons, upper arm
    M66.821 Spontaneous rupture of other tendons, right upper arm
    M66.822 Spontaneous rupture of other tendons, left upper arm
    M66.829 Spontaneous rupture of other tendons, unspecified upper arm
● **M66.83** Spontaneous rupture of other tendons, forearm
    M66.831 Spontaneous rupture of other tendons, right forearm
    M66.832 Spontaneous rupture of other tendons, left forearm
    M66.839 Spontaneous rupture of other tendons, unspecified forearm
● **M66.84** Spontaneous rupture of other tendons, hand
    M66.841 Spontaneous rupture of other tendons, right hand
    M66.842 Spontaneous rupture of other tendons, left hand
    M66.849 Spontaneous rupture of other tendons, unspecified hand
● **M66.85** Spontaneous rupture of other tendons, thigh
    M66.851 Spontaneous rupture of other tendons, right thigh
    M66.852 Spontaneous rupture of other tendons, left thigh
    M66.859 Spontaneous rupture of other tendons, unspecified thigh
● **M66.86** Spontaneous rupture of other tendons, lower leg
    M66.861 Spontaneous rupture of other tendons, right lower leg
    M66.862 Spontaneous rupture of other tendons, left lower leg
    M66.869 Spontaneous rupture of other tendons, unspecified lower leg

▶ New   ⇒ Revised   ~~deleted~~ Deleted   Excludes 1   Excludes 2   Includes   Use additional   Code first   Code also   Key words
OGCR Official Guidelines   X Assign placeholder X   ● Use Additional Character(s)   ▷ Manifestation Code   🏷 Hierarchical Condition Category   **Coding Clinic**

● M66.87 **Spontaneous rupture of other tendons, ankle and foot**
    M66.871 **Spontaneous rupture of other tendons, right ankle and foot**
    M66.872 **Spontaneous rupture of other tendons, left ankle and foot**
    M66.879 **Spontaneous rupture of other tendons, unspecified ankle and foot**
  M66.88 **Spontaneous rupture of other tendons, other sites**
  M66.89 **Spontaneous rupture of other tendons, multiple sites**
 M66.9 **Spontaneous rupture of unspecified tendon**
    Rupture at musculotendinous junction, nontraumatic

● M67 **Other disorders of synovium and tendon**
  Excludes1 palmar fascial fibromatosis [Dupuytren] (M72.0)
         tendinitis NOS (M77.9-)
         xanthomatosis localized to tendons (E78.2)
● M67.0 **Short Achilles tendon (acquired)**
  M67.00 **Short Achilles tendon (acquired), unspecified ankle**
  M67.01 **Short Achilles tendon (acquired), right ankle**
  M67.02 **Short Achilles tendon (acquired), left ankle**
● M67.2 **Synovial hypertrophy, not elsewhere classified**
  Excludes1 villonodular synovitis (pigmented) (M12.2-)
  M67.20 **Synovial hypertrophy, not elsewhere classified, unspecified site**
 ● M67.21 **Synovial hypertrophy, not elsewhere classified, shoulder**
    M67.211 **Synovial hypertrophy, not elsewhere classified, right shoulder**
    M67.212 **Synovial hypertrophy, not elsewhere classified, left shoulder**
    M67.219 **Synovial hypertrophy, not elsewhere classified, unspecified shoulder**
 ● M67.22 **Synovial hypertrophy, not elsewhere classified, upper arm**
    M67.221 **Synovial hypertrophy, not elsewhere classified, right upper arm**
    M67.222 **Synovial hypertrophy, not elsewhere classified, left upper arm**
    M67.229 **Synovial hypertrophy, not elsewhere classified, unspecified upper arm**
 ● M67.23 **Synovial hypertrophy, not elsewhere classified, forearm**
    M67.231 **Synovial hypertrophy, not elsewhere classified, right forearm**
    M67.232 **Synovial hypertrophy, not elsewhere classified, left forearm**
    M67.239 **Synovial hypertrophy, not elsewhere classified, unspecified forearm**
 ● M67.24 **Synovial hypertrophy, not elsewhere classified, hand**
    M67.241 **Synovial hypertrophy, not elsewhere classified, right hand**
    M67.242 **Synovial hypertrophy, not elsewhere classified, left hand**
    M67.249 **Synovial hypertrophy, not elsewhere classified, unspecified hand**
 ● M67.25 **Synovial hypertrophy, not elsewhere classified, thigh**
    M67.251 **Synovial hypertrophy, not elsewhere classified, right thigh**
    M67.252 **Synovial hypertrophy, not elsewhere classified, left thigh**
    M67.259 **Synovial hypertrophy, not elsewhere classified, unspecified thigh**

● M67.26 **Synovial hypertrophy, not elsewhere classified, lower leg**
    M67.261 **Synovial hypertrophy, not elsewhere classified, right lower leg**
    M67.262 **Synovial hypertrophy, not elsewhere classified, left lower leg**
    M67.269 **Synovial hypertrophy, not elsewhere classified, unspecified lower leg**
● M67.27 **Synovial hypertrophy, not elsewhere classified, ankle and foot**
    M67.271 **Synovial hypertrophy, not elsewhere classified, right ankle and foot**
    M67.272 **Synovial hypertrophy, not elsewhere classified, left ankle and foot**
    M67.279 **Synovial hypertrophy, not elsewhere classified, unspecified ankle and foot**
  M67.28 **Synovial hypertrophy, not elsewhere classified, other site**
  M67.29 **Synovial hypertrophy, not elsewhere classified, multiple sites**
● M67.3 **Transient synovitis**
    Toxic synovitis
  Excludes1 palindromic rheumatism (M12.3-)
  M67.30 **Transient synovitis, unspecified site**
 ● M67.31 **Transient synovitis, shoulder**
    M67.311 **Transient synovitis, right shoulder**
    M67.312 **Transient synovitis, left shoulder**
    M67.319 **Transient synovitis, unspecified shoulder**
 ● M67.32 **Transient synovitis, elbow**
    M67.321 **Transient synovitis, right elbow**
    M67.322 **Transient synovitis, left elbow**
    M67.329 **Transient synovitis, unspecified elbow**
 ● M67.33 **Transient synovitis, wrist**
    M67.331 **Transient synovitis, right wrist**
    M67.332 **Transient synovitis, left wrist**
    M67.339 **Transient synovitis, unspecified wrist**
 ● M67.34 **Transient synovitis, hand**
    M67.341 **Transient synovitis, right hand**
    M67.342 **Transient synovitis, left hand**
    M67.349 **Transient synovitis, unspecified hand**
 ● M67.35 **Transient synovitis, hip**
    M67.351 **Transient synovitis, right hip**
    M67.352 **Transient synovitis, left hip**
    M67.359 **Transient synovitis, unspecified hip**
 ● M67.36 **Transient synovitis, knee**
    M67.361 **Transient synovitis, right knee**
    M67.362 **Transient synovitis, left knee**
    M67.369 **Transient synovitis, unspecified knee**
 ● M67.37 **Transient synovitis, ankle and foot**
    M67.371 **Transient synovitis, right ankle and foot**
    M67.372 **Transient synovitis, left ankle and foot**
    M67.379 **Transient synovitis, unspecified ankle and foot**
  M67.38 **Transient synovitis, other site**
  M67.39 **Transient synovitis, multiple sites**

CHAPTER 13 (M00-M99)

● **M67.4   Ganglion**
     Ganglion of joint or tendon (sheath)
     Excludes1   ganglion in yaws (A66.6)
     Excludes2   cyst of bursa (M71.2-M71.3)
               cyst of synovium (M71.2-M71.3)
     M67.40   Ganglion, unspecified site
●   M67.41   Ganglion, shoulder
       M67.411   Ganglion, right shoulder
       M67.412   Ganglion, left shoulder
       M67.419   Ganglion, unspecified shoulder
●   M67.42   Ganglion, elbow
       M67.421   Ganglion, right elbow
       M67.422   Ganglion, left elbow
       M67.429   Ganglion, unspecified elbow
●   M67.43   Ganglion, wrist
       M67.431   Ganglion, right wrist
       M67.432   Ganglion, left wrist
       M67.439   Ganglion, unspecified wrist
●   M67.44   Ganglion, hand
       M67.441   Ganglion, right hand
       M67.442   Ganglion, left hand
       M67.449   Ganglion, unspecified hand
●   M67.45   Ganglion, hip
       M67.451   Ganglion, right hip
       M67.452   Ganglion, left hip
       M67.459   Ganglion, unspecified hip
●   M67.46   Ganglion, knee
       M67.461   Ganglion, right knee
       M67.462   Ganglion, left knee
       M67.469   Ganglion, unspecified knee
●   M67.47   Ganglion, ankle and foot
       M67.471   Ganglion, right ankle and foot
       M67.472   Ganglion, left ankle and foot
       M67.479   Ganglion, unspecified ankle and foot
     M67.48   Ganglion, other site
     M67.49   Ganglion, multiple sites
● **M67.5   Plica syndrome**
     Plica knee
     M67.50   Plica syndrome, unspecified knee
     M67.51   Plica syndrome, right knee
     M67.52   Plica syndrome, left knee
● **M67.8   Other specified disorders of synovium and tendon**
     M67.80   Other specified disorders of synovium and tendon, unspecified site
●   M67.81   Other specified disorders of synovium and tendon, shoulder
       M67.811   Other specified disorders of synovium, right shoulder
       M67.812   Other specified disorders of synovium, left shoulder
       M67.813   Other specified disorders of tendon, right shoulder
       M67.814   Other specified disorders of tendon, left shoulder
       M67.819   Other specified disorders of synovium and tendon, unspecified shoulder

●   M67.82   Other specified disorders of synovium and tendon, elbow
       M67.821   Other specified disorders of synovium, right elbow
       M67.822   Other specified disorders of synovium, left elbow
       M67.823   Other specified disorders of tendon, right elbow
       M67.824   Other specified disorders of tendon, left elbow
       M67.829   Other specified disorders of synovium and tendon, unspecified elbow
●   M67.83   Other specified disorders of synovium and tendon, wrist
       M67.831   Other specified disorders of synovium, right wrist
       M67.832   Other specified disorders of synovium, left wrist
       M67.833   Other specified disorders of tendon, right wrist
       M67.834   Other specified disorders of tendon, left wrist
       M67.839   Other specified disorders of synovium and tendon, unspecified wrist
●   M67.84   Other specified disorders of synovium and tendon, hand
       M67.841   Other specified disorders of synovium, right hand
       M67.842   Other specified disorders of synovium, left hand
       M67.843   Other specified disorders of tendon, right hand
       M67.844   Other specified disorders of tendon, left hand
       M67.849   Other specified disorders of synovium and tendon, unspecified hand
●   M67.85   Other specified disorders of synovium and tendon, hip
       M67.851   Other specified disorders of synovium, right hip
       M67.852   Other specified disorders of synovium, left hip
       M67.853   Other specified disorders of tendon, right hip
       M67.854   Other specified disorders of tendon, left hip
       M67.859   Other specified disorders of synovium and tendon, unspecified hip
●   M67.86   Other specified disorders of synovium and tendon, knee
       M67.861   Other specified disorders of synovium, right knee
       M67.862   Other specified disorders of synovium, left knee
       M67.863   Other specified disorders of tendon, right knee
       M67.864   Other specified disorders of tendon, left knee
       M67.869   Other specified disorders of synovium and tendon, unspecified knee

▶ New   ⇒ Revised   ~~deleted~~ Deleted   Excludes 1   Excludes 2   Includes   Use additional   Code first   Code also   Key words
OGCR Official Guidelines   X Assign placeholder X   ● Use Additional Character(s)   ▶ Manifestation Code   🎯 Hierarchical Condition Category   **Coding Clinic**

● **M67.87** Other specified disorders of synovium and tendon, ankle and foot
  M67.871 Other specified disorders of synovium, right ankle and foot
  M67.872 Other specified disorders of synovium, left ankle and foot
  M67.873 Other specified disorders of tendon, right ankle and foot
  M67.874 Other specified disorders of tendon, left ankle and foot
  M67.879 Other specified disorders of synovium and tendon, unspecified ankle and foot
 M67.88 Other specified disorders of synovium and tendon, other site
 M67.89 Other specified disorders of synovium and tendon, multiple sites
● **M67.9** Unspecified disorder of synovium and tendon
 M67.90 Unspecified disorder of synovium and tendon, unspecified site
● **M67.91** Unspecified disorder of synovium and tendon, shoulder
  M67.911 Unspecified disorder of synovium and tendon, right shoulder
  M67.912 Unspecified disorder of synovium and tendon, left shoulder
  M67.919 Unspecified disorder of synovium and tendon, unspecified shoulder
● **M67.92** Unspecified disorder of synovium and tendon, upper arm
  M67.921 Unspecified disorder of synovium and tendon, right upper arm
  M67.922 Unspecified disorder of synovium and tendon, left upper arm
  M67.929 Unspecified disorder of synovium and tendon, unspecified upper arm
● **M67.93** Unspecified disorder of synovium and tendon, forearm
  M67.931 Unspecified disorder of synovium and tendon, right forearm
  M67.932 Unspecified disorder of synovium and tendon, left forearm
  M67.939 Unspecified disorder of synovium and tendon, unspecified forearm
● **M67.94** Unspecified disorder of synovium and tendon, hand
  M67.941 Unspecified disorder of synovium and tendon, right hand
  M67.942 Unspecified disorder of synovium and tendon, left hand
  M67.949 Unspecified disorder of synovium and tendon, unspecified hand
● **M67.95** Unspecified disorder of synovium and tendon, thigh
  M67.951 Unspecified disorder of synovium and tendon, right thigh
  M67.952 Unspecified disorder of synovium and tendon, left thigh
  M67.959 Unspecified disorder of synovium and tendon, unspecified thigh
● **M67.96** Unspecified disorder of synovium and tendon, lower leg
  M67.961 Unspecified disorder of synovium and tendon, right lower leg
  M67.962 Unspecified disorder of synovium and tendon, left lower leg
  M67.969 Unspecified disorder of synovium and tendon, unspecified lower leg

● **M67.97** Unspecified disorder of synovium and tendon, ankle and foot
  M67.971 Unspecified disorder of synovium and tendon, right ankle and foot
  M67.972 Unspecified disorder of synovium and tendon, left ankle and foot
  M67.979 Unspecified disorder of synovium and tendon, unspecified ankle and foot
 M67.98 Unspecified disorder of synovium and tendon, other site
 M67.99 Unspecified disorder of synovium and tendon, multiple sites

OTHER SOFT TISSUE DISORDERS (M70-M79)

● **M70** Soft tissue disorders related to use, overuse and pressure
  Includes   soft tissue disorders of occupational origin
  Use additional external cause code to identify activity causing disorder (Y93.-)
  Excludes1 bursitis NOS (M71.9-)
  Excludes2 bursitis of shoulder (M75.5)
         enthesopathies (M76-M77)
         pressure ulcer (pressure area) (L89.-)
● **M70.0** Crepitant synovitis (acute) (chronic) of hand and wrist
 ● **M70.03** Crepitant synovitis (acute) (chronic), wrist
   M70.031 Crepitant synovitis (acute) (chronic), right wrist
   M70.032 Crepitant synovitis (acute) (chronic), left wrist
   M70.039 Crepitant synovitis (acute) (chronic), unspecified wrist
 ● **M70.04** Crepitant synovitis (acute) (chronic), hand
   M70.041 Crepitant synovitis (acute) (chronic), right hand
   M70.042 Crepitant synovitis (acute) (chronic), left hand
   M70.049 Crepitant synovitis (acute) (chronic), unspecified hand
● **M70.1** Bursitis of hand
 M70.10 Bursitis, unspecified hand
 M70.11 Bursitis, right hand
 M70.12 Bursitis, left hand
● **M70.2** Olecranon bursitis
 M70.20 Olecranon bursitis, unspecified elbow
 M70.21 Olecranon bursitis, right elbow
 M70.22 Olecranon bursitis, left elbow
● **M70.3** Other bursitis of elbow
 M70.30 Other bursitis of elbow, unspecified elbow
 M70.31 Other bursitis of elbow, right elbow
 M70.32 Other bursitis of elbow, left elbow
● **M70.4** Prepatellar bursitis
 M70.40 Prepatellar bursitis, unspecified knee
 M70.41 Prepatellar bursitis, right knee
 M70.42 Prepatellar bursitis, left knee
● **M70.5** Other bursitis of knee
 M70.50 Other bursitis of knee, unspecified knee
 M70.51 Other bursitis of knee, right knee
 M70.52 Other bursitis of knee, left knee
● **M70.6** Trochanteric bursitis
  Trochanteric tendinitis
 M70.60 Trochanteric bursitis, unspecified hip
 M70.61 Trochanteric bursitis, right hip
 M70.62 Trochanteric bursitis, left hip

● **M70.7**   Other bursitis of hip
        Ischial bursitis

    M70.70   Other bursitis of hip, unspecified hip

    M70.71   Other bursitis of hip, right hip

    M70.72   Other bursitis of hip, left hip

● **M70.8**   Other soft tissue disorders related to use, overuse and pressure

    M70.80   Other soft tissue disorders related to use, overuse and pressure of unspecified site

    ● **M70.81**   Other soft tissue disorders related to use, overuse and pressure of shoulder

        M70.811   Other soft tissue disorders related to use, overuse and pressure, right shoulder

        M70.812   Other soft tissue disorders related to use, overuse and pressure, left shoulder

        M70.819   Other soft tissue disorders related to use, overuse and pressure, unspecified shoulder

    ● **M70.82**   Other soft tissue disorders related to use, overuse and pressure of upper arm

        M70.821   Other soft tissue disorders related to use, overuse and pressure, right upper arm

        M70.822   Other soft tissue disorders related to use, overuse and pressure, left upper arm

        M70.829   Other soft tissue disorders related to use, overuse and pressure, unspecified upper arms

    ● **M70.83**   Other soft tissue disorders related to use, overuse and pressure of forearm

        M70.831   Other soft tissue disorders related to use, overuse and pressure, right forearm

        M70.832   Other soft tissue disorders related to use, overuse and pressure, left forearm

        M70.839   Other soft tissue disorders related to use, overuse and pressure, unspecified forearm

    ● **M70.84**   Other soft tissue disorders related to use, overuse and pressure of hand

        M70.841   Other soft tissue disorders related to use, overuse and pressure, right hand

        M70.842   Other soft tissue disorders related to use, overuse and pressure, left hand

        M70.849   Other soft tissue disorders related to use, overuse and pressure, unspecified hand

    ● **M70.85**   Other soft tissue disorders related to use, overuse and pressure of thigh

        M70.851   Other soft tissue disorders related to use, overuse and pressure, right thigh

        M70.852   Other soft tissue disorders related to use, overuse and pressure, left thigh

        M70.859   Other soft tissue disorders related to use, overuse and pressure, unspecified thigh

    ● **M70.86**   Other soft tissue disorders related to use, overuse and pressure lower leg

        M70.861   Other soft tissue disorders related to use, overuse and pressure, right lower leg

        M70.862   Other soft tissue disorders related to use, overuse and pressure, left lower leg

        M70.869   Other soft tissue disorders related to use, overuse and pressure, unspecified leg

● **M70.87**   Other soft tissue disorders related to use, overuse and pressure of ankle and foot

    M70.871   Other soft tissue disorders related to use, overuse and pressure, right ankle and foot

    M70.872   Other soft tissue disorders related to use, overuse and pressure, left ankle and foot

    M70.879   Other soft tissue disorders related to use, overuse and pressure, unspecified ankle and foot

M70.88   Other soft tissue disorders related to use, overuse and pressure other site

M70.89   Other soft tissue disorders related to use, overuse and pressure multiple sites

● **M70.9**   Unspecified soft tissue disorder related to use, overuse and pressure

    M70.90   Unspecified soft tissue disorder related to use, overuse and pressure of unspecified site

    ● **M70.91**   Unspecified soft tissue disorder related to use, overuse and pressure of shoulder

        M70.911   Unspecified soft tissue disorder related to use, overuse and pressure, right shoulder

        M70.912   Unspecified soft tissue disorder related to use, overuse and pressure, left shoulder

        M70.919   Unspecified soft tissue disorder related to use, overuse and pressure, unspecified shoulder

    ● **M70.92**   Unspecified soft tissue disorder related to use, overuse and pressure of upper arm

        M70.921   Unspecified soft tissue disorder related to use, overuse and pressure, right upper arm

        M70.922   Unspecified soft tissue disorder related to use, overuse and pressure, left upper arm

        M70.929   Unspecified soft tissue disorder related to use, overuse and pressure, unspecified upper arm

    ● **M70.93**   Unspecified soft tissue disorder related to use, overuse and pressure of forearm

        M70.931   Unspecified soft tissue disorder related to use, overuse and pressure, right forearm

        M70.932   Unspecified soft tissue disorder related to use, overuse and pressure, left forearm

        M70.939   Unspecified soft tissue disorder related to use, overuse and pressure, unspecified forearm

    ● **M70.94**   Unspecified soft tissue disorder related to use, overuse and pressure of hand

        M70.941   Unspecified soft tissue disorder related to use, overuse and pressure, right hand

        M70.942   Unspecified soft tissue disorder related to use, overuse and pressure, left hand

        M70.949   Unspecified soft tissue disorder related to use, overuse and pressure, unspecified hand

▶ New   ⇛ Revised   ~~deleted~~ Deleted   Excludes 1   Excludes 2   Includes   Use additional   Code first   Code also   Key words

OGCR Official Guidelines   X Assign placeholder X   ● Use Additional Character(s)   ▶ Manifestation Code   Hierarchical Condition Category   Coding Clinic

● **M70.95** Unspecified soft tissue disorder related to use, overuse and pressure of thigh

     M70.951   Unspecified soft tissue disorder related to use, overuse and pressure, right thigh

     M70.952   Unspecified soft tissue disorder related to use, overuse and pressure, left thigh

     M70.959   Unspecified soft tissue disorder related to use, overuse and pressure, unspecified thigh

● **M70.96** Unspecified soft tissue disorder related to use, overuse and pressure lower leg

     M70.961   Unspecified soft tissue disorder related to use, overuse and pressure, right lower leg

     M70.962   Unspecified soft tissue disorder related to use, overuse and pressure, left lower leg

     M70.969   Unspecified soft tissue disorder related to use, overuse and pressure, unspecified lower leg

● **M70.97** Unspecified soft tissue disorder related to use, overuse and pressure of ankle and foot

     M70.971   Unspecified soft tissue disorder related to use, overuse and pressure, right ankle and foot

     M70.972   Unspecified soft tissue disorder related to use, overuse and pressure, left ankle and foot

     M70.979   Unspecified soft tissue disorder related to use, overuse and pressure, unspecified ankle and foot

   M70.98   Unspecified soft tissue disorder related to use, overuse and pressure other

   M70.99   Unspecified soft tissue disorder related to use, overuse and pressure multiple sites

● **M71 Other bursopathies**

   Excludes1   bunion (M20.1)
              bursitis related to use, overuse or pressure (M70.-)
              enthesopathies (M76-M77)

● **M71.0 Abscess of bursa**

     Use additional code (B95.-, B96.-) to identify causative organism

   M71.00   Abscess of bursa, unspecified site

● **M71.01** Abscess of bursa, shoulder

     M71.011   Abscess of bursa, right shoulder
     M71.012   Abscess of bursa, left shoulder
     M71.019   Abscess of bursa, unspecified shoulder

● **M71.02** Abscess of bursa, elbow

     M71.021   Abscess of bursa, right elbow
     M71.022   Abscess of bursa, left elbow
     M71.029   Abscess of bursa, unspecified elbow

● **M71.03** Abscess of bursa, wrist

     M71.031   Abscess of bursa, right wrist
     M71.032   Abscess of bursa, left wrist
     M71.039   Abscess of bursa, unspecified wrist

● **M71.04** Abscess of bursa, hand

     M71.041   Abscess of bursa, right hand
     M71.042   Abscess of bursa, left hand
     M71.049   Abscess of bursa, unspecified hand

● **M71.05** Abscess of bursa, hip

     M71.051   Abscess of bursa, right hip
     M71.052   Abscess of bursa, left hip
     M71.059   Abscess of bursa, unspecified hip

● **M71.06** Abscess of bursa, knee

     M71.061   Abscess of bursa, right knee
     M71.062   Abscess of bursa, left knee
     M71.069   Abscess of bursa, unspecified knee

● **M71.07** Abscess of bursa, ankle and foot

     M71.071   Abscess of bursa, right ankle and foot
     M71.072   Abscess of bursa, left ankle and foot
     M71.079   Abscess of bursa, unspecified ankle and foot

   M71.08   Abscess of bursa, other site
   M71.09   Abscess of bursa, multiple sites

● **M71.1 Other infective bursitis**

     Use additional code (B95.-, B96.-) to identify causative organism

   M71.10   Other infective bursitis, unspecified site

● **M71.11** Other infective bursitis, shoulder

     M71.111   Other infective bursitis, right shoulder
     M71.112   Other infective bursitis, left shoulder
     M71.119   Other infective bursitis, unspecified shoulder

● **M71.12** Other infective bursitis, elbow

     M71.121   Other infective bursitis, right elbow
     M71.122   Other infective bursitis, left elbow
     M71.129   Other infective bursitis, unspecified elbow

● **M71.13** Other infective bursitis, wrist

     M71.131   Other infective bursitis, right wrist
     M71.132   Other infective bursitis, left wrist
     M71.139   Other infective bursitis, unspecified wrist

● **M71.14** Other infective bursitis, hand

     M71.141   Other infective bursitis, right hand
     M71.142   Other infective bursitis, left hand
     M71.149   Other infective bursitis, unspecified hand

● **M71.15** Other infective bursitis, hip

     M71.151   Other infective bursitis, right hip
     M71.152   Other infective bursitis, left hip
     M71.159   Other infective bursitis, unspecified hip

● **M71.16** Other infective bursitis, knee

     M71.161   Other infective bursitis, right knee
     M71.162   Other infective bursitis, left knee
     M71.169   Other infective bursitis, unspecified knee

● **M71.17** Other infective bursitis, ankle and foot

     M71.171   Other infective bursitis, right ankle and foot
     M71.172   Other infective bursitis, left ankle and foot
     M71.179   Other infective bursitis, unspecified ankle and foot

   M71.18   Other infective bursitis, other site
   M71.19   Other infective bursitis, multiple sites

● **M71.2**   **Synovial cyst of popliteal space [Baker]**
Popliteal space = popliteal cavity, popliteal fossa. Depression in the posterior aspect of the knee (behind the knee).

> **Excludes1**   synovial cyst of popliteal space with rupture (M66.0)

     M71.20   Synovial cyst of popliteal space [Baker], **unspecified knee**

     M71.21   Synovial cyst of popliteal space [Baker], **right knee**

     M71.22   Synovial cyst of popliteal space [Baker], **left knee**

● **M71.3**   **Other bursal cyst**
Synovial cyst NOS

> **Excludes1**   synovial cyst with rupture (M66.1-)

     M71.30   Other bursal cyst, **unspecified site**

●   **M71.31**   Other bursal cyst, **shoulder**

       M71.311   Other bursal cyst, **right shoulder**

       M71.312   Other bursal cyst, **left shoulder**

       M71.319   Other bursal cyst, **unspecified shoulder**

●   **M71.32**   Other bursal cyst, **elbow**

       M71.321   Other bursal cyst, **right elbow**

       M71.322   Other bursal cyst, **left elbow**

       M71.329   Other bursal cyst, **unspecified elbow**

●   **M71.33**   Other bursal cyst, **wrist**

       M71.331   Other bursal cyst, **right wrist**

       M71.332   Other bursal cyst, **left wrist**

       M71.339   Other bursal cyst, **unspecified wrist**

●   **M71.34**   Other bursal cyst, **hand**

       M71.341   Other bursal cyst, **right hand**

       M71.342   Other bursal cyst, **left hand**

       M71.349   Other bursal cyst, **unspecified hand**

●   **M71.35**   Other bursal cyst, **hip**

       M71.351   Other bursal cyst, **right hip**

       M71.352   Other bursal cyst, **left hip**

       M71.359   Other bursal cyst, **unspecified hip**

●   **M71.37**   Other bursal cyst, **ankle and foot**

       M71.371   Other bursal cyst, **right ankle and foot**

       M71.372   Other bursal cyst, **left ankle and foot**

       M71.379   Other bursal cyst, **unspecified ankle and foot**

     M71.38   Other bursal cyst, **other site**

     M71.39   Other bursal cyst, **multiple sites**

● **M71.4**   **Calcium deposit in bursa**

> **Excludes2**   calcium deposit in bursa of shoulder (M75.3)

     M71.40   Calcium deposit in bursa, **unspecified site**

●   **M71.42**   Calcium deposit in bursa, **elbow**

       M71.421   Calcium deposit in bursa, **right elbow**

       M71.422   Calcium deposit in bursa, **left elbow**

       M71.429   Calcium deposit in bursa, **unspecified elbow**

●   **M71.43**   Calcium deposit in bursa, **wrist**

       M71.431   Calcium deposit in bursa, **right wrist**

       M71.432   Calcium deposit in bursa, **left wrist**

       M71.439   Calcium deposit in bursa, **unspecified wrist**

●   **M71.44**   Calcium deposit in bursa, **hand**

       M71.441   Calcium deposit in bursa, **right hand**

       M71.442   Calcium deposit in bursa, **left hand**

       M71.449   Calcium deposit in bursa, **unspecified hand**

●   **M71.45**   Calcium deposit in bursa, **hip**

       M71.451   Calcium deposit in bursa, **right hip**

       M71.452   Calcium deposit in bursa, **left hip**

       M71.459   Calcium deposit in bursa, **unspecified hip**

●   **M71.46**   Calcium deposit in bursa, **knee**

       M71.461   Calcium deposit in bursa, **right knee**

       M71.462   Calcium deposit in bursa, **left knee**

       M71.469   Calcium deposit in bursa, **unspecified knee**

●   **M71.47**   Calcium deposit in bursa, **ankle and foot**

       M71.471   Calcium deposit in bursa, **right ankle and foot**

       M71.472   Calcium deposit in bursa, **left ankle and foot**

       M71.479   Calcium deposit in bursa, **unspecified ankle and foot**

     M71.48   Calcium deposit in bursa, **other site**

     M71.49   Calcium deposit in bursa, **multiple sites**

● **M71.5**   **Other bursitis, not elsewhere classified**

> **Excludes1**   bursitis NOS (M71.9-)
> **Excludes2**   bursitis of shoulder (M75.5)
> bursitis of tibial collateral [Pellegrini-Stieda] (M76.4-)

     M71.50   Other bursitis, not elsewhere classified, **unspecified site**

●   **M71.52**   Other bursitis, not elsewhere classified, **elbow**

       M71.521   Other bursitis, not elsewhere classified, **right elbow**

       M71.522   Other bursitis, not elsewhere classified, **left elbow**

       M71.529   Other bursitis, not elsewhere classified, **unspecified elbow**

●   **M71.53**   Other bursitis, not elsewhere classified, **wrist**

       M71.531   Other bursitis, not elsewhere classified, **right wrist**

       M71.532   Other bursitis, not elsewhere classified, **left wrist**

       M71.539   Other bursitis, not elsewhere classified, **unspecified wrist**

●   **M71.54**   Other bursitis, not elsewhere classified, **hand**

       M71.541   Other bursitis, not elsewhere classified, **right hand**

       M71.542   Other bursitis, not elsewhere classified, **left hand**

       M71.549   Other bursitis, not elsewhere classified, **unspecified hand**

●   **M71.55**   Other bursitis, not elsewhere classified, **hip**

       M71.551   Other bursitis, not elsewhere classified, **right hip**

       M71.552   Other bursitis, not elsewhere classified, **left hip**

       M71.559   Other bursitis, not elsewhere classified, **unspecified hip**

●   **M71.56**   Other bursitis, not elsewhere classified, **knee**

       M71.561   Other bursitis, not elsewhere classified, **right knee**

       M71.562   Other bursitis, not elsewhere classified, **left knee**

       M71.569   Other bursitis, not elsewhere classified, **unspecified knee**

● M71.57   Other bursitis, not elsewhere classified, ankle and foot
   M71.571   Other bursitis, not elsewhere classified, right ankle and foot
   M71.572   Other bursitis, not elsewhere classified, left ankle and foot
   M71.579   Other bursitis, not elsewhere classified, unspecified ankle and foot
  M71.58   Other bursitis, not elsewhere classified, other site

● M71.8   Other specified bursopathies
  M71.80   Other specified bursopathies, unspecified site
● M71.81   Other specified bursopathies, shoulder
   M71.811   Other specified bursopathies, right shoulder
   M71.812   Other specified bursopathies, left shoulder
   M71.819   Other specified bursopathies, unspecified shoulder
● M71.82   Other specified bursopathies, elbow
   M71.821   Other specified bursopathies, right elbow
   M71.822   Other specified bursopathies, left elbow
   M71.829   Other specified bursopathies, unspecified elbow
● M71.83   Other specified bursopathies, wrist
   M71.831   Other specified bursopathies, right wrist
   M71.832   Other specified bursopathies, left wrist
   M71.839   Other specified bursopathies, unspecified wrist
● M71.84   Other specified bursopathies, hand
   M71.841   Other specified bursopathies, right hand
   M71.842   Other specified bursopathies, left hand
   M71.849   Other specified bursopathies, unspecified hand
● M71.85   Other specified bursopathies, hip
   M71.851   Other specified bursopathies, right hip
   M71.852   Other specified bursopathies, left hip
   M71.859   Other specified bursopathies, unspecified hip
● M71.86   Other specified bursopathies, knee
   M71.861   Other specified bursopathies, right knee
   M71.862   Other specified bursopathies, left knee
   M71.869   Other specified bursopathies, unspecified knee
● M71.87   Other specified bursopathies, ankle and foot
   M71.871   Other specified bursopathies, right ankle and foot
   M71.872   Other specified bursopathies, left ankle and foot
   M71.879   Other specified bursopathies, unspecified ankle and foot
  M71.88   Other specified bursopathies, other site
  M71.89   Other specified bursopathies, multiple sites
M71.9   Bursopathy, unspecified
  Bursitis NOS

● M72   Fibroblastic disorders
  Excludes2   retroperitoneal fibromatosis (D48.3)
  M72.0   Palmar fascial fibromatosis [Dupuytren]   A
  M72.1   Knuckle pads
  M72.2   Plantar fascial fibromatosis
   Plantar fasciitis
  M72.4   Pseudosarcomatous fibromatosis
   Nodular fasciitis
  M72.6   Necrotizing fasciitis
   Use additional code (B95.-, B96.-) to identify causative organism
  M72.8   Other fibroblastic disorders
   Abscess of fascia
   Fasciitis NEC
   Other infective fasciitis
   Use additional code to (B95.-, B96.-) identify causative organism
   Excludes1   diffuse (eosinophilic) fasciitis (M35.4)
    necrotizing fasciitis (M72.6)
    nodular fasciitis (M72.4)
    perirenal fasciitis NOS (N13.5)
    perirenal fasciitis with infection (N13.6)
    plantar fasciitis (M72.2)
  M72.9   Fibroblastic disorder, unspecified
   Fasciitis NOS
   Fibromatosis NOS

● M75   Shoulder lesions
  Excludes2   shoulder-hand syndrome (M89.0-)
● M75.0   Adhesive capsulitis of shoulder
   Frozen shoulder
   Periarthritis of shoulder
  M75.00   Adhesive capsulitis of unspecified shoulder
  M75.01   Adhesive capsulitis of right shoulder
  M75.02   Adhesive capsulitis of left shoulder
   Coding Clinic: 2015, Q2, P23
● M75.1   Rotator cuff tear or rupture, not specified as traumatic
   Rotator cuff syndrome
   Supraspinatus syndrome
   Supraspinatus tear or rupture, not specified as traumatic
   Excludes1   tear of rotator cuff, traumatic (S46.01-)
   Gradual onset due to repetitive stress to rotator cuff
● M75.10   Unspecified rotator cuff tear or rupture, not specified as traumatic
   M75.100   Unspecified rotator cuff tear or rupture of unspecified shoulder, not specified as traumatic
   M75.101   Unspecified rotator cuff tear or rupture of right shoulder, not specified as traumatic
   M75.102   Unspecified rotator cuff tear or rupture of left shoulder, not specified as traumatic
● M75.11   Incomplete rotator cuff tear or rupture not specified as traumatic
   M75.110   Incomplete rotator cuff tear or rupture of unspecified shoulder, not specified as traumatic
   M75.111   Incomplete rotator cuff tear or rupture of right shoulder, not specified as traumatic
   M75.112   Incomplete rotator cuff tear or rupture of left shoulder, not specified as traumatic

CHAPTER 13 (M00-M99)

- M75.12 Complete rotator cuff tear or rupture not specified as traumatic
    - M75.120 Complete rotator cuff tear or rupture of unspecified shoulder, not specified as traumatic
    - M75.121 Complete rotator cuff tear or rupture of right shoulder, not specified as traumatic
    - M75.122 Complete rotator cuff tear or rupture of left shoulder, not specified as traumatic
- M75.2 Bicipital tendinitis
    - M75.20 Bicipital tendinitis, unspecified shoulder
    - M75.21 Bicipital tendinitis, right shoulder
    - M75.22 Bicipital tendinitis, left shoulder
- M75.3 Calcific tendinitis of shoulder
    Calcified bursa of shoulder
    - M75.30 Calcific tendinitis of unspecified shoulder
    - M75.31 Calcific tendinitis of right shoulder
    - M75.32 Calcific tendinitis of left shoulder
- M75.4 Impingement syndrome of shoulder
    - M75.40 Impingement syndrome of unspecified shoulder
    - M75.41 Impingement syndrome of right shoulder
    - M75.42 Impingement syndrome of left shoulder
- M75.5 Bursitis of shoulder
    - M75.50 Bursitis of unspecified shoulder
    - M75.51 Bursitis of right shoulder
    - M75.52 Bursitis of left shoulder
- M75.8 Other shoulder lesions
    - M75.80 Other shoulder lesions, unspecified shoulder
    - M75.81 Other shoulder lesions, right shoulder
    - M75.82 Other shoulder lesions, left shoulder
- M75.9 Shoulder lesion, unspecified
    - M75.90 Shoulder lesion, unspecified, unspecified shoulder
    - M75.91 Shoulder lesion, unspecified, right shoulder
    - M75.92 Shoulder lesion, unspecified, left shoulder

- M76 Enthesopathies, lower limb, excluding foot
    - **Excludes2**   bursitis due to use, overuse and pressure (M70.-)
        enthesopathies of ankle and foot (M77.5-)
- M76.0 Gluteal tendinitis
    - M76.00 Gluteal tendinitis, unspecified hip
    - M76.01 Gluteal tendinitis, right hip
    - M76.02 Gluteal tendinitis, left hip
- M76.1 Psoas tendinitis
    - M76.10 Psoas tendinitis, unspecified hip
    - M76.11 Psoas tendinitis, right hip
    - M76.12 Psoas tendinitis, left hip
- M76.2 Iliac crest spur
    - M76.20 Iliac crest spur, unspecified hip
    - M76.21 Iliac crest spur, right hip
    - M76.22 Iliac crest spur, left hip
- M76.3 Iliotibial band syndrome
    - M76.30 Iliotibial band syndrome, unspecified leg
    - M76.31 Iliotibial band syndrome, right leg
    - M76.32 Iliotibial band syndrome, left leg
- M76.4 Tibial collateral bursitis [Pellegrini-Stieda]
    - M76.40 Tibial collateral bursitis [Pellegrini-Stieda], unspecified leg
    - M76.41 Tibial collateral bursitis [Pellegrini-Stieda], right leg
    - M76.42 Tibial collateral bursitis [Pellegrini-Stieda], left leg

- M76.5 Patellar tendinitis
    - M76.50 Patellar tendinitis, unspecified knee
    - M76.51 Patellar tendinitis, right knee
    - M76.52 Patellar tendinitis, left knee
- M76.6 Achilles tendinitis
    Achilles bursitis
    - M76.60 Achilles tendinitis, unspecified leg
    - M76.61 Achilles tendinitis, right leg
    - M76.62 Achilles tendinitis, left leg
- M76.7 Peroneal tendinitis
    - M76.70 Peroneal tendinitis, unspecified leg
    - M76.71 Peroneal tendinitis, right leg
    - M76.72 Peroneal tendinitis, left leg
- M76.8 Other specified enthesopathies of lower limb, excluding foot
    - M76.81 Anterior tibial syndrome
        - M76.811 Anterior tibial syndrome, right leg
        - M76.812 Anterior tibial syndrome, left leg
        - M76.819 Anterior tibial syndrome, unspecified leg
    - M76.82 Posterior tibial tendinitis
        - M76.821 Posterior tibial tendinitis, right leg
        - M76.822 Posterior tibial tendinitis, left leg
        - M76.829 Posterior tibial tendinitis, unspecified leg
    - M76.89 Other specified enthesopathies of lower limb, excluding foot
        - M76.891 Other specified enthesopathies of right lower limb, excluding foot
        - M76.892 Other specified enthesopathies of left lower limb, excluding foot
        - M76.899 Other specified enthesopathies of unspecified lower limb, excluding foot
    - M76.9 Unspecified enthesopathy, lower limb, excluding foot

- M77 Other enthesopathies
    - **Excludes1**   bursitis NOS (M71.9-)
    - **Excludes2**   bursitis due to use, overuse and pressure (M70.-)
        osteophyte (M25.7)
        spinal enthesopathy (M46.0-)
- M77.0 Medial epicondylitis
    - M77.00 Medial epicondylitis, unspecified elbow
    - M77.01 Medial epicondylitis, right elbow
    - M77.02 Medial epicondylitis, left elbow
- M77.1 Lateral epicondylitis
    Tennis elbow
    - M77.10 Lateral epicondylitis, unspecified elbow
    - M77.11 Lateral epicondylitis, right elbow
    - M77.12 Lateral epicondylitis, left elbow
- M77.2 Periarthritis of wrist
    - M77.20 Periarthritis, unspecified wrist
    - M77.21 Periarthritis, right wrist
    - M77.22 Periarthritis, left wrist
- M77.3 Calcaneal spur
    - M77.30 Calcaneal spur, unspecified foot
    - M77.31 Calcaneal spur, right foot
    - M77.32 Calcaneal spur, left foot
- M77.4 Metatarsalgia
    - **Excludes1**   Morton's metatarsalgia (G57.6)
    - M77.40 Metatarsalgia, unspecified foot
    - M77.41 Metatarsalgia, right foot
    - M77.42 Metatarsalgia, left foot

▶ New   ⇒ Revised   ~~deleted~~ Deleted   Excludes 1   Excludes 2   Includes   Use additional   Code first   Code also   Key words

OGCR Official Guidelines   X Assign placeholder X   ● Use Additional Character(s)   ▶ Manifestation Code   🏷 Hierarchical Condition Category   **Coding Clinic**

● M77.5   Other enthesopathy of foot and ankle
     M77.50   Other enthesopathy of unspecified foot and ankle
     M77.51   Other enthesopathy of right foot and ankle
     M77.52   Other enthesopathy of left foot and ankle

   M77.8   Other enthesopathies, not elsewhere classified

   M77.9   Enthesopathy, unspecified
       Bone spur NOS
       Capsulitis NOS
       Periarthritis NOS
       Tendinitis NOS

● M79   Other and unspecified soft tissue disorders, not elsewhere classified

     Excludes1   psychogenic rheumatism (F45.8)
               soft tissue pain, psychogenic (F45.41)

   M79.0   Rheumatism, unspecified
     Excludes1   fibromyalgia (M79.7)
               palindromic rheumatism (M12.3-)

● M79.1   Myalgia
       Myofascial pain syndrome
     M79.10   Myalgia, unspecified site
     M79.11   Myalgia of mastication muscle
     M79.12   Myalgia of auxiliary muscles, head and neck
     M79.18   Myalgia, other site
         Excludes1   fibromyalgia (M79.7)
                  myositis (M60.-)

   M79.2   Neuralgia and neuritis, unspecified
     Excludes1   brachial radiculitis NOS (M54.1)
               lumbosacral radiculitis NOS (M54.1)
               mononeuropathies (G56-G58)
               radiculitis NOS (M54.1)
               sciatica (M54.3-M54.4)

   M79.3   Panniculitis, unspecified
     Excludes1   lupus panniculitis (L93.2)
               neck and back panniculitis (M54.0-)
               relapsing [Weber-Christian] panniculitis (M35.6)

   M79.4   Hypertrophy of (infrapatellar) fat pad

   M79.5   Residual foreign body in soft tissue
     Excludes1   foreign body granuloma of skin and subcutaneous tissue (L92.3)
               foreign body granuloma of soft tissue (M60.2-)

● M79.6   Pain in limb, hand, foot, fingers and toes
     Excludes2   pain in joint (M25.5-)
   ● M79.60   Pain in limb, unspecified
     M79.601   Pain in right arm
         Pain in right upper limb NOS
     M79.602   Pain in left arm
         Pain in left upper limb NOS
     M79.603   Pain in arm, unspecified
         Pain in upper limb NOS
     M79.604   Pain in right leg
         Pain in right lower limb NOS
     M79.605   Pain in left leg
         Pain in left lower limb NOS
     M79.606   Pain in leg, unspecified
         Pain in lower limb NOS
     M79.609   Pain in unspecified limb
         Pain in limb NOS

   ● M79.62   Pain in upper arm
       Pain in axillary region
     M79.621   Pain in right upper arm
     M79.622   Pain in left upper arm
     M79.629   Pain in unspecified upper arm

   ● M79.63   Pain in forearm
     M79.631   Pain in right forearm
     M79.632   Pain in left forearm
     M79.639   Pain in unspecified forearm

● M79.64   Pain in hand and fingers
     M79.641   Pain in right hand
     M79.642   Pain in left hand
     M79.643   Pain in unspecified hand
     M79.644   Pain in right finger(s)
     M79.645   Pain in left finger(s)
     M79.646   Pain in unspecified finger(s)

● M79.65   Pain in thigh
     M79.651   Pain in right thigh
     M79.652   Pain in left thigh
     M79.659   Pain in unspecified thigh

● M79.66   Pain in lower leg
     M79.661   Pain in right lower leg
     M79.662   Pain in left lower leg
     M79.669   Pain in unspecified lower leg

● M79.67   Pain in foot and toes
     M79.671   Pain in right foot
     M79.672   Pain in left foot
     M79.673   Pain in unspecified foot
     M79.674   Pain in right toe(s)
     M79.675   Pain in left toe(s)
     M79.676   Pain in unspecified toe(s)

   M79.7   Fibromyalgia
       Fibromyositis
       Fibrositis
       Myofibrositis

● M79.A   Nontraumatic compartment syndrome
     Code first, if applicable, associated postprocedural complication
     Excludes1   compartment syndrome NOS (T79.A-)
               fibromyalgia (M79.7) nontraumatic ischemic infarction of muscle (M62.2-)
               traumatic compartment syndrome (T79.A-)

   ● M79.A1   Nontraumatic compartment syndrome of upper extremity
       Nontraumatic compartment syndrome of shoulder, arm, forearm, wrist, hand, and fingers
     M79.A11   Nontraumatic compartment syndrome of right upper extremity
     M79.A12   Nontraumatic compartment syndrome of left upper extremity
     M79.A19   Nontraumatic compartment syndrome of unspecified upper extremity

   ● M79.A2   Nontraumatic compartment syndrome of lower extremity
       Nontraumatic compartment syndrome of hip, buttock, thigh, leg, foot, and toes
     M79.A21   Nontraumatic compartment syndrome of right lower extremity
     M79.A22   Nontraumatic compartment syndrome of left lower extremity
     M79.A29   Nontraumatic compartment syndrome of unspecified lower extremity

     M79.A3   Nontraumatic compartment syndrome of abdomen

     M79.A9   Nontraumatic compartment syndrome of other sites

● M79.8   Other specified soft tissue disorders
     M79.81   Nontraumatic hematoma of soft tissue
         Nontraumatic hematoma of muscle
         Nontraumatic seroma of muscle and soft tissue
     M79.89   Other specified soft tissue disorders
         Polyalgia

   M79.9   Soft tissue disorder, unspecified

CHAPTER 13 (M00-M99)

OGCR See Section I.C., Chapter 13.d.

Osteoporosis

Osteoporosis is a systemic condition, meaning that all bones of the musculoskeletal system are affected. Therefore, site is not a component of the codes under category M81, Osteoporosis without current pathological fracture. The site codes under category M80, Osteoporosis with current pathological fracture, identify the site of the fracture, not the osteoporosis.

1) Osteoporosis without pathological fracture

Category M81, Osteoporosis without current pathological fracture, is for use for patients with osteoporosis who do not currently have a pathologic fracture due to the osteoporosis, even if they have had a fracture in the past. For patients with a history of osteoporosis fractures, status code Z87.310, Personal history of (healed) osteoporosis fracture, should follow the code from M81.

2) Osteoporosis with current pathological fracture

Category M80, Osteoporosis with current pathological fracture, is for patients who have a current pathologic fracture at the time of an encounter. The codes under M80 identify the site of the fracture. A code from category M80, not a traumatic fracture code, should be used for any patient with known osteoporosis who suffers a fracture, even if the patient had a minor fall or trauma, if that fall or trauma would not usually break a normal, healthy bone.

OSTEOPATHIES AND CHONDROPATHIES (M80-M94)

DISORDERS OF BONE DENSITY AND STRUCTURE (M80-M85)

M80   Osteoporosis with current pathological fracture
Excessive skeletal fragility (porous bone) resulting in bone fractures

Includes   osteoporosis with current fragility fracture

Use additional code to identify major osseous defect, if applicable (M89.7-)

Excludes1   collapsed vertebra NOS (M48.5)
pathological fracture NOS (M84.4)
wedging of vertebra NOS (M48.5)

Excludes2   personal history of (healed) osteoporosis fracture
(Z87.310)

Coding Clinic: 2018, Q2, P12

The appropriate 7th character is to be added to each code from category M80:

A	initial encounter for fracture
	All encounters involving diagnosis and treatment
D	subsequent encounter for fracture with routine healing
G	subsequent encounter for fracture with delayed healing
	Encounters for attention to casting or fixation devices, medication, and follow-up visits during the healing phase
K	subsequent encounter for fracture with nonunion
	Total failure of fracture healing
P	subsequent encounter for fracture with malunion
	Fracture ends do not heal together correctly.
S	sequela

● **M80.0   Age-related osteoporosis with current pathological fracture**
Involutional osteoporosis with current pathological fracture
Osteoporosis NOS with current pathological fracture
Postmenopausal osteoporosis with current pathological fracture
Senile osteoporosis with current pathological fracture

X ● **M80.00   Age-related osteoporosis with current pathological fracture, unspecified site**
A

● **M80.01   Age-related osteoporosis with current pathological fracture, shoulder**
● **M80.011   Age-related osteoporosis with current pathological fracture, right shoulder** A

● **M80.012   Age-related osteoporosis with current pathological fracture, left shoulder** A

● **M80.019   Age-related osteoporosis with current pathological fracture, unspecified shoulder** A

● **M80.02   Age-related osteoporosis with current pathological fracture, humerus**
● **M80.021   Age-related osteoporosis with current pathological fracture, right humerus** A

● **M80.022   Age-related osteoporosis with current pathological fracture, left humerus** A

● **M80.029   Age-related osteoporosis with current pathological fracture, unspecified humerus** A

● **M80.03   Age-related osteoporosis with current pathological fracture, forearm**
Age-related osteoporosis with current pathological fracture of wrist
● **M80.031   Age-related osteoporosis with current pathological fracture, right forearm** A

● **M80.032   Age-related osteoporosis with current pathological fracture, left forearm** A

● **M80.039   Age-related osteoporosis with current pathological fracture, unspecified forearm** A

● **M80.04   Age-related osteoporosis with current pathological fracture, hand**
● **M80.041   Age-related osteoporosis with current pathological fracture, right hand** A

● **M80.042   Age-related osteoporosis with current pathological fracture, left hand** A

● **M80.049   Age-related osteoporosis with current pathological fracture, unspecified hand** A

● **M80.05   Age-related osteoporosis with current pathological fracture, femur**
Age-related osteoporosis with current pathological fracture of hip
● **M80.051   Age-related osteoporosis with current pathological fracture, right femur** A 🐾 A

● **M80.052   Age-related osteoporosis with current pathological fracture, left femur** A 🐾 A
Coding Clinic: 2018, Q2, P12

● **M80.059   Age-related osteoporosis with current pathological fracture, unspecified femur** A 🐾 A

● **M80.06   Age-related osteoporosis with current pathological fracture, lower leg**
● **M80.061   Age-related osteoporosis with current pathological fracture, right lower leg** A

● **M80.062   Age-related osteoporosis with current pathological fracture, left lower leg** A

● **M80.069   Age-related osteoporosis with current pathological fracture, unspecified lower leg** A

● **M80.07   Age-related osteoporosis with current pathological fracture, ankle and foot**
● **M80.071   Age-related osteoporosis with current pathological fracture, right ankle and foot** A

● **M80.072   Age-related osteoporosis with current pathological fracture, left ankle and foot** A

● **M80.079   Age-related osteoporosis with current pathological fracture, unspecified ankle and foot** A

X ● **M80.08   Age-related osteoporosis with current pathological fracture, vertebra(e)** A 🐾 A

M80.0A   Age-related osteoporosis with current pathological fracture, other site A

▶ New   ⇒ Revised   ~~deleted~~ Deleted   Excludes 1   Excludes 2   Includes   Use additional   Code first   Code also   Key words
OGCR Official Guidelines   X Assign placeholder X   ● Use Additional Character(s)   ▶ Manifestation Code   🐾 Hierarchical Condition Category   Coding Clinic

● **M80.8   Other osteoporosis with current pathological fracture**
  Drug-induced osteoporosis with current pathological fracture
  Idiopathic osteoporosis with current pathological fracture
  Osteoporosis of disuse with current pathological fracture
  Postoophorectomy osteoporosis with current pathological fracture
  Postsurgical malabsorption osteoporosis with current pathological fracture
  Post-traumatic osteoporosis with current pathological fracture
  Use additional code for adverse effect, if applicable, to identify drug (T36-T50 with fifth or sixth character 5)

   X ● **M80.80   Other osteoporosis with current pathological fracture, unspecified site**   A

   ● **M80.81   Other osteoporosis with pathological fracture, shoulder**
     ● **M80.811   Other osteoporosis with current pathological fracture, right shoulder**
     ● **M80.812   Other osteoporosis with current pathological fracture, left shoulder**
     ● **M80.819   Other osteoporosis with current pathological fracture, unspecified shoulder**

   ● **M80.82   Other osteoporosis with current pathological fracture, humerus**
     ● **M80.821   Other osteoporosis with current pathological fracture, right humerus**
     ● **M80.822   Other osteoporosis with current pathological fracture, left humerus**
     ● **M80.829   Other osteoporosis with current pathological fracture, unspecified humerus**

   ● **M80.83   Other osteoporosis with current pathological fracture, forearm**
  Other osteoporosis with current pathological fracture of wrist
     ● **M80.831   Other osteoporosis with current pathological fracture, right forearm**
     ● **M80.832   Other osteoporosis with current pathological fracture, left forearm**
     ● **M80.839   Other osteoporosis with current pathological fracture, unspecified forearm**

   M80.8A   Other osteoporosis with current pathological fracture, other site

   ● **M80.84   Other osteoporosis with current pathological fracture, hand**
     ● **M80.841   Other osteoporosis with current pathological fracture, right hand**
     ● **M80.842   Other osteoporosis with current pathological fracture, left hand**
     ● **M80.849   Other osteoporosis with current pathological fracture, unspecified hand**

   ● **M80.85   Other osteoporosis with current pathological fracture, femur**
  Other osteoporosis with current pathological fracture of hip
     ● **M80.851   Other osteoporosis with current pathological fracture, right femur** A 🔬
     ● **M80.852   Other osteoporosis with current pathological fracture, left femur** A 🔬
     ● **M80.859   Other osteoporosis with current pathological fracture, unspecified femur** A 🔬

   ● **M80.86   Other osteoporosis with current pathological fracture, lower leg**
     ● **M80.861   Other osteoporosis with current pathological fracture, right lower leg**
     ● **M80.862   Other osteoporosis with current pathological fracture, left lower leg**
     ● **M80.869   Other osteoporosis with current pathological fracture, unspecified lower leg**

   ● **M80.87   Other osteoporosis with current pathological fracture, ankle and foot**
     ● **M80.871   Other osteoporosis with current pathological fracture, right ankle and foot**
     ● **M80.872   Other osteoporosis with current pathological fracture, left ankle and foot**
     ● **M80.879   Other osteoporosis with current pathological fracture, unspecified ankle and foot**

   X ● **M80.88   Other osteoporosis with current pathological fracture, vertebra(e)** A 🔬

● **M81   Osteoporosis without current pathological fracture**
  Use additional code to identify:
  major osseous defect, if applicable (M89.7-)
  personal history of (healed) osteoporosis fracture, if applicable (Z87.310)
   Excludes1   osteoporosis with current pathological fracture (M80.-)
           Sudeck's atrophy (M89.0)

   M81.0   Age-related osteoporosis without current pathological fracture   A
  Involutional osteoporosis without current pathological fracture
  Osteoporosis NOS
  Postmenopausal osteoporosis without current pathological fracture
  Senile osteoporosis without current pathological fracture

   M81.6   Localized osteoporosis [Lequesne]
     Excludes1   Sudeck's atrophy (M89.0)

   M81.8   Other osteoporosis without current pathological fracture
  Drug-induced osteoporosis without current pathological fracture
  Idiopathic osteoporosis without current pathological fracture
  Osteoporosis of disuse without current pathological fracture
  Postoophorectomy osteoporosis without current pathological fracture
  Postsurgical malabsorption osteoporosis without current pathological fracture
  Post-traumatic osteoporosis without current pathological fracture
  Use additional code for adverse effect, if applicable, to identify drug (T36-T50 with fifth or sixth character 5)

● **M83   Adult osteomalacia**
   Excludes1   infantile and juvenile osteomalacia (E55.0)
           renal osteodystrophy (N25.0)
           rickets (active) (E55.0)
           rickets (active) sequelae (E64.3)
           vitamin D-resistant osteomalacia (E83.3)
           vitamin D-resistant rickets (active) (E83.3)

   M83.0   Puerperal osteomalacia ♀   M
   M83.1   Senile osteomalacia   A
   M83.2   Adult osteomalacia due to malabsorption   A
  Postsurgical malabsorption osteomalacia in adults
   M83.3   Adult osteomalacia due to malnutrition   A
   M83.4   Aluminum bone disease

M83.5 Other drug-induced osteomalacia in adults   A
> Use additional code for adverse effect, if applicable, to identify drug (T36-T50 with fifth or sixth character 5)

M83.8 Other adult osteomalacia   A

M83.9 Adult osteomalacia, unspecified   A

● **M84 Disorder of continuity of bone**
> **Excludes2**   traumatic fracture of bone-see fracture, by site

● **M84.3 Stress fracture**
> Fatigue fracture
> March fracture
> Stress fracture NOS
> Stress reaction
> Use additional external cause code(s) to identify the cause of the stress fracture

> **Excludes1**   pathological fracture NOS (M84.4.-)
> pathological fracture due to osteoporosis (M80.-)
> traumatic fracture (S12.-, S22.-, S32.-, S42.-, S52.-, S62.-, S72.-, S82.-, S92.-)

> **Excludes2**   personal history of (healed) stress (fatigue) fracture (Z87.312)
> stress fracture of vertebra (M48.4-)

> The appropriate 7th character is to be added to each code from subcategory M84.3:

A	initial encounter for fracture
D	subsequent encounter for fracture with routine healing
G	subsequent encounter for fracture with delayed healing
K	subsequent encounter for fracture with nonunion
P	subsequent encounter for fracture with malunion
S	sequela

X ● **M84.30 Stress fracture, unspecified site**

● **M84.31 Stress fracture, shoulder**
> ● M84.311 Stress fracture, right shoulder
> ● M84.312 Stress fracture, left shoulder
> ● M84.319 Stress fracture, unspecified shoulder

● **M84.32 Stress fracture, humerus**
> ● M84.321 Stress fracture, right humerus
> ● M84.322 Stress fracture, left humerus
> ● M84.329 Stress fracture, unspecified humerus

● **M84.33 Stress fracture, ulna and radius**
> ● M84.331 Stress fracture, right ulna
> ● M84.332 Stress fracture, left ulna
> ● M84.333 Stress fracture, right radius
> ● M84.334 Stress fracture, left radius
> ● M84.339 Stress fracture, unspecified ulna and radius

● **M84.34 Stress fracture, hand and fingers**
> ● M84.341 Stress fracture, right hand
> ● M84.342 Stress fracture, left hand
> ● M84.343 Stress fracture, unspecified hand
> ● M84.344 Stress fracture, right finger(s)
> ● M84.345 Stress fracture, left finger(s)
> ● M84.346 Stress fracture, unspecified finger(s)

● **M84.35 Stress fracture, pelvis and femur**
> Stress fracture, hip
> ● M84.350 Stress fracture, pelvis
> ● M84.351 Stress fracture, right femur
> ● M84.352 Stress fracture, left femur
> ● M84.353 Stress fracture, unspecified femur
> ● M84.359 Stress fracture, hip, unspecified

● **M84.36 Stress fracture, tibia and fibula**
> ● M84.361 Stress fracture, right tibia
> ● M84.362 Stress fracture, left tibia

● M84.363 Stress fracture, right fibula
● M84.364 Stress fracture, left fibula
● M84.369 Stress fracture, unspecified tibia and fibula

● **M84.37 Stress fracture, ankle, foot and toes**
> ● M84.371 Stress fracture, right ankle
> ● M84.372 Stress fracture, left ankle
> ● M84.373 Stress fracture, unspecified ankle
> ● M84.374 Stress fracture, right foot
> ● M84.375 Stress fracture, left foot
> ● M84.376 Stress fracture, unspecified foot
> ● M84.377 Stress fracture, right toe(s)
> ● M84.378 Stress fracture, left toe(s)
> ● M84.379 Stress fracture, unspecified toe(s)

X ● **M84.38 Stress fracture, other site**
> **Excludes2**   stress fracture of vertebra (M48.4-)

● **M84.4 Pathological fracture, not elsewhere classified**
> Chronic fracture
> Pathological fracture NOS

> **Excludes1**   collapsed vertebra NEC (M48.5)
> pathological fracture in neoplastic disease (M84.5-)
> pathological fracture in osteoporosis (M80.-)
> pathological fracture in other disease (M84.6-)
> stress fracture (M84.3-)
> traumatic fracture (S12.-, S22.-, S32.-, S42.-, S52.-, S62.-, S72.-, S82.-, S92.-)

> **Excludes2**   personal history of (healed) pathological fracture (Z87.311)

> The appropriate 7th character is to be added to each code from subcategory M84.4:

A	initial encounter for fracture
D	subsequent encounter for fracture with routine healing
G	subsequent encounter for fracture with delayed healing
K	subsequent encounter for fracture with nonunion
P	subsequent encounter for fracture with malunion
S	sequela

X ● **M84.40 Pathological fracture, unspecified site**

● **M84.41 Pathological fracture, shoulder**
> ● M84.411 Pathological fracture, right shoulder
> ● M84.412 Pathological fracture, left shoulder
> ● M84.419 Pathological fracture, unspecified shoulder

● **M84.42 Pathological fracture, humerus**
> ● M84.421 Pathological fracture, right humerus
> ● M84.422 Pathological fracture, left humerus
> ● M84.429 Pathological fracture, unspecified humerus

● **M84.43 Pathological fracture, ulna and radius**
> ● M84.431 Pathological fracture, right ulna
> ● M84.432 Pathological fracture, left ulna
> ● M84.433 Pathological fracture, right radius
> ● M84.434 Pathological fracture, left radius
> ● M84.439 Pathological fracture, unspecified ulna and radius

● **M84.44 Pathological fracture, hand and fingers**
> ● M84.441 Pathological fracture, right hand
> ● M84.442 Pathological fracture, left hand
> ● M84.443 Pathological fracture, unspecified hand

▶ New   ⇒ Revised   ~~deleted~~ Deleted   Excludes 1   Excludes 2   Includes   Use additional   Code first   Code also   Key words
OGCR Official Guidelines   X Assign placeholder X   ● Use Additional Character(s)   ▌ Manifestation Code   ✿ Hierarchical Condition Category   **Coding Clinic**

● M84.444   Pathological fracture, right finger(s)

● M84.445   Pathological fracture, left finger(s)

● M84.446   Pathological fracture, unspecified finger(s)

● M84.45   Pathological fracture, femur and pelvis

    ● M84.451   Pathological fracture, right femur A 🔄

    ● M84.452   Pathological fracture, left femur A 🔄

    ● M84.453   Pathological fracture, unspecified femur A 🔄

    ● M84.454   Pathological fracture, pelvis A 🔄
            Coding Clinic: 2016, Q4, P43

    ● M84.459   Pathological fracture, hip, unspecified A 🔄

● M84.46   Pathological fracture, tibia and fibula

    ● M84.461   Pathological fracture, right tibia

    ● M84.462   Pathological fracture, left tibia

    ● M84.463   Pathological fracture, right fibula

    ● M84.464   Pathological fracture, left fibula

    ● M84.469   Pathological fracture, unspecified tibia and fibula

● M84.47   Pathological fracture, ankle, foot and toes

    ● M84.471   Pathological fracture, right ankle

    ● M84.472   Pathological fracture, left ankle

    ● M84.473   Pathological fracture, unspecified ankle

    ● M84.474   Pathological fracture, right foot

    ● M84.475   Pathological fracture, left foot

    ● M84.476   Pathological fracture, unspecified foot

    ● M84.477   Pathological fracture, right toe(s)

    ● M84.478   Pathological fracture, left toe(s)

    ● M84.479   Pathological fracture, unspecified toe(s)

X ● M84.48   Pathological fracture, other site

OGCR Section I.C. 13.C.

Coding of Pathologic Fractures

7th character A is for use as long as the patient is receiving active treatment for the fracture. While the patient may be seen by a new or different provider over the course of treatment for a pathological fracture, assignment of the 7th character is based on whether the patient is undergoing active treatment and not whether the provider is seeing the patient for the first time.

7th character, D is to be used for encounters after the patient has completed active treatment for the fracture and is receiving routine care for the fracture during the healing or recovery phase. The other 7th characters, listed under each subcategory in the Tabular List, are to be used for subsequent encounters for treatment of problems associated with the healing, such as malunions, nonunions, and sequelae.

Care for complications of surgical treatment for fracture repairs during the healing or recovery phase should be coded with the appropriate complication codes.

See Section I.C.19. Coding of traumatic fractures.

● M84.5   Pathological fracture in neoplastic disease

    Code also underlying neoplasm

    The appropriate 7th character is to be added to each code from subcategory M84.5:

A	initial encounter for fracture
D	subsequent encounter for fracture with routine healing
G	subsequent encounter for fracture with delayed healing
K	subsequent encounter for fracture with nonunion
P	subsequent encounter for fracture with malunion
S	sequela

X ● M84.50   Pathological fracture in neoplastic disease, unspecified site

● M84.51   Pathological fracture in neoplastic disease, shoulder

    ● M84.511   Pathological fracture in neoplastic disease, right shoulder

    ● M84.512   Pathological fracture in neoplastic disease, left shoulder

    ● M84.519   Pathological fracture in neoplastic disease, unspecified shoulder

● M84.52   Pathological fracture in neoplastic disease, humerus

    ● M84.521   Pathological fracture in neoplastic disease, right humerus

    ● M84.522   Pathological fracture in neoplastic disease, left humerus

    ● M84.529   Pathological fracture in neoplastic disease, unspecified humerus

● M84.53   Pathological fracture in neoplastic disease, ulna and radius

    ● M84.531   Pathological fracture in neoplastic disease, right ulna

    ● M84.532   Pathological fracture in neoplastic disease, left ulna

    ● M84.533   Pathological fracture in neoplastic disease, right radius

    ● M84.534   Pathological fracture in neoplastic disease, left radius

    ● M84.539   Pathological fracture in neoplastic disease, unspecified ulna and radius

● M84.54   Pathological fracture in neoplastic disease, hand

    ● M84.541   Pathological fracture in neoplastic disease, right hand

    ● M84.542   Pathological fracture in neoplastic disease, left hand

    ● M84.549   Pathological fracture in neoplastic disease, unspecified hand

● M84.55   Pathological fracture in neoplastic disease, pelvis and femur

    ● M84.550   Pathological fracture in neoplastic disease, pelvis

    ● M84.551   Pathological fracture in neoplastic disease, right femur A 🔄

    ● M84.552   Pathological fracture in neoplastic disease, left femur A 🔄

    ● M84.553   Pathological fracture in neoplastic disease, unspecified femur A 🔄

    ● M84.559   Pathological fracture in neoplastic disease, hip, unspecified A 🔄

● M84.56   Pathological fracture in neoplastic disease, tibia and fibula

    ● M84.561   Pathological fracture in neoplastic disease, right tibia

    ● M84.562   Pathological fracture in neoplastic disease, left tibia

    ● M84.563   Pathological fracture in neoplastic disease, right fibula

    ● M84.564   Pathological fracture in neoplastic disease, left fibula

    ● M84.569   Pathological fracture in neoplastic disease, unspecified tibia and fibula

● M84.57   Pathological fracture in neoplastic disease, ankle and foot

    ● M84.571   Pathological fracture in neoplastic disease, right ankle

    ● M84.572   Pathological fracture in neoplastic disease, left ankle

    ● M84.573   Pathological fracture in neoplastic disease, unspecified ankle

    ● M84.574   Pathological fracture in neoplastic disease, right foot

CHAPTER 13 (M00-M99)

● M84.575 Pathological fracture in neoplastic disease, left foot
● M84.576 Pathological fracture in neoplastic disease, unspecified foot
X● M84.58 Pathological fracture in neoplastic disease, other specified site
    Pathological fracture in neoplastic disease, vertebrae
● M84.6 Pathological fracture in other disease
    Code also underlying condition

    Excludes1 pathological fracture in osteoporosis (M80.-)

    The appropriate 7th character is to be added to each code from subcategory M84.6:

A	initial encounter for fracture
D	subsequent encounter for fracture with routine healing
G	subsequent encounter for fracture with delayed healing
K	subsequent encounter for fracture with nonunion
P	subsequent encounter for fracture with malunion
S	sequela

X● M84.60 Pathological fracture in other disease, unspecified site
● M84.61 Pathological fracture in other disease, shoulder
  ● M84.611 Pathological fracture in other disease, right shoulder
  ● M84.612 Pathological fracture in other disease, left shoulder
  ● M84.619 Pathological fracture in other disease, unspecified shoulder
● M84.62 Pathological fracture in other disease, humerus
  ● M84.621 Pathological fracture in other disease, right humerus
  ● M84.622 Pathological fracture in other disease, left humerus
  ● M84.629 Pathological fracture in other disease, unspecified humerus
● M84.63 Pathological fracture in other disease, ulna and radius
  ● M84.631 Pathological fracture in other disease, right ulna
  ● M84.632 Pathological fracture in other disease, left ulna
  ● M84.633 Pathological fracture in other disease, right radius
  ● M84.634 Pathological fracture in other disease, left radius
  ● M84.639 Pathological fracture in other disease, unspecified ulna and radius
● M84.64 Pathological fracture in other disease, hand
  ● M84.641 Pathological fracture in other disease, right hand
  ● M84.642 Pathological fracture in other disease, left hand
  ● M84.649 Pathological fracture in other disease, unspecified hand
● M84.65 Pathological fracture in other disease, pelvis and femur
  ● M84.650 Pathological fracture in other disease, pelvis
  ● M84.651 Pathological fracture in other disease, right femur A 🐾
  ● M84.652 Pathological fracture in other disease, left femur A 🐾

● M84.653 Pathological fracture in other disease, unspecified femur A 🐾
● M84.659 Pathological fracture in other disease, hip, unspecified A 🐾
● M84.66 Pathological fracture in other disease, tibia and fibula
  ● M84.661 Pathological fracture in other disease, right tibia
  ● M84.662 Pathological fracture in other disease, left tibia
  ● M84.663 Pathological fracture in other disease, right fibula
  ● M84.664 Pathological fracture in other disease, left fibula
  ● M84.669 Pathological fracture in other disease, unspecified tibia and fibula
● M84.67 Pathological fracture in other disease, ankle and foot
  ● M84.671 Pathological fracture in other disease, right ankle
  ● M84.672 Pathological fracture in other disease, left ankle
  ● M84.673 Pathological fracture in other disease, unspecified ankle
  ● M84.674 Pathological fracture in other disease, right foot
  ● M84.675 Pathological fracture in other disease, left foot
  ● M84.676 Pathological fracture in other disease, unspecified foot
X● M84.68 Pathological fracture in other disease, other site
● M84.7 Nontraumatic fracture, not elsewhere classified
  ● M84.75 Atypical femoral fracture

    The appropriate 7th character is to be added to each code from M84.75:

A	initial encounter for fracture
D	subsequent encounter for fracture with routine healing
G	subsequent encounter for fracture with delayed healing
K	subsequent encounter for fracture with nonunion
P	subsequent encounter for fracture with malunion
S	sequela

    Coding Clinic: 2016, Q4, P41

  ● M84.750 Atypical femoral fracture, unspecified
  ● M84.751 Incomplete atypical femoral fracture, right leg
  ● M84.752 Incomplete atypical femoral fracture, left leg
  ● M84.753 Incomplete atypical femoral fracture, unspecified leg
  ● M84.754 Complete transverse atypical femoral fracture, right leg A 🐾
  ● M84.755 Complete transverse atypical femoral fracture, left leg A 🐾
  ● M84.756 Complete transverse atypical femoral fracture, unspecified leg A 🐾
  ● M84.757 Complete oblique atypical femoral fracture, right leg A 🐾
  ● M84.758 Complete oblique atypical femoral fracture, left leg A 🐾
  ● M84.759 Complete oblique atypical femoral fracture, unspecified leg , A 🐾

CHAPTER 13 (M00-M99)

● M84.8 Other disorders of continuity of bone

   M84.80 Other disorders of continuity of bone, unspecified site

● M84.81 Other disorders of continuity of bone, shoulder

   M84.811 Other disorders of continuity of bone, right shoulder

   M84.812 Other disorders of continuity of bone, left shoulder

   M84.819 Other disorders of continuity of bone, unspecified shoulder

● M84.82 Other disorders of continuity of bone, humerus

   M84.821 Other disorders of continuity of bone, right humerus

   M84.822 Other disorders of continuity of bone, left humerus

   M84.829 Other disorders of continuity of bone, unspecified humerus

● M84.83 Other disorders of continuity of bone, ulna and radius

   M84.831 Other disorders of continuity of bone, right ulna

   M84.832 Other disorders of continuity of bone, left ulna

   M84.833 Other disorders of continuity of bone, right radius

   M84.834 Other disorders of continuity of bone, left radius

   M84.839 Other disorders of continuity of bone, unspecified ulna and radius

● M84.84 Other disorders of continuity of bone, hand

   M84.841 Other disorders of continuity of bone, right hand

   M84.842 Other disorders of continuity of bone, left hand

   M84.849 Other disorders of continuity of bone, unspecified hand

● M84.85 Other disorders of continuity of bone, pelvic region and thigh

   M84.851 Other disorders of continuity of bone, right pelvic region and thigh

   M84.852 Other disorders of continuity of bone, left pelvic region and thigh

   M84.859 Other disorders of continuity of bone, unspecified pelvic region and thigh

● M84.86 Other disorders of continuity of bone, tibia and fibula

   M84.861 Other disorders of continuity of bone, right tibia

   M84.862 Other disorders of continuity of bone, left tibia

   M84.863 Other disorders of continuity of bone, right fibula

   M84.864 Other disorders of continuity of bone, left fibula

   M84.869 Other disorders of continuity of bone, unspecified tibia and fibula

● M84.87 Other disorders of continuity of bone, ankle and foot

   M84.871 Other disorders of continuity of bone, right ankle and foot

   M84.872 Other disorders of continuity of bone, left ankle and foot

   M84.879 Other disorders of continuity of bone, unspecified ankle and foot

   M84.88 Other disorders of continuity of bone, other site

M84.9 Disorder of continuity of bone, unspecified

● M85 Other disorders of bone density and structure

   Excludes1 osteogenesis imperfecta (Q78.0)
           osteopetrosis (Q78.2)
           osteopoikilosis (Q78.8)
           polyostotic fibrous dysplasia (Q78.1)

● M85.0 Fibrous dysplasia (monostotic)

   Excludes2 fibrous dysplasia of jaw (M27.8)

   M85.00 Fibrous dysplasia (monostotic), unspecified site

● M85.01 Fibrous dysplasia (monostotic), shoulder

   M85.011 Fibrous dysplasia (monostotic), right shoulder

   M85.012 Fibrous dysplasia (monostotic), left shoulder

   M85.019 Fibrous dysplasia (monostotic), unspecified shoulder

● M85.02 Fibrous dysplasia (monostotic), upper arm

   M85.021 Fibrous dysplasia (monostotic), right upper arm

   M85.022 Fibrous dysplasia (monostotic), left upper arm

   M85.029 Fibrous dysplasia (monostotic), unspecified upper arm

● M85.03 Fibrous dysplasia (monostotic), forearm

   M85.031 Fibrous dysplasia (monostotic), right forearm

   M85.032 Fibrous dysplasia (monostotic), left forearm

   M85.039 Fibrous dysplasia (monostotic), unspecified forearm

● M85.04 Fibrous dysplasia (monostotic), hand

   M85.041 Fibrous dysplasia (monostotic), right hand

   M85.042 Fibrous dysplasia (monostotic), left hand

   M85.049 Fibrous dysplasia (monostotic), unspecified hand

● M85.05 Fibrous dysplasia (monostotic), thigh

   M85.051 Fibrous dysplasia (monostotic), right thigh

   M85.052 Fibrous dysplasia (monostotic), left thigh

   M85.059 Fibrous dysplasia (monostotic), unspecified thigh

● M85.06 Fibrous dysplasia (monostotic), lower leg

   M85.061 Fibrous dysplasia (monostotic), right lower leg

   M85.062 Fibrous dysplasia (monostotic), left lower leg

   M85.069 Fibrous dysplasia (monostotic), unspecified lower leg

● M85.07 Fibrous dysplasia (monostotic), ankle and foot

   M85.071 Fibrous dysplasia (monostotic), right ankle and foot

   M85.072 Fibrous dysplasia (monostotic), left ankle and foot

   M85.079 Fibrous dysplasia (monostotic), unspecified ankle and foot

   M85.08 Fibrous dysplasia (monostotic), other site

   M85.09 Fibrous dysplasia (monostotic), multiple sites

● M85.1 Skeletal fluorosis

   M85.10 Skeletal fluorosis, unspecified site

● M85.11 Skeletal fluorosis, shoulder

   M85.111 Skeletal fluorosis, right shoulder

   M85.112 Skeletal fluorosis, left shoulder

   M85.119 Skeletal fluorosis, unspecified shoulder

CHAPTER 13 (M00-M99)

● M85.12   Skeletal fluorosis, upper arm
    M85.121   Skeletal fluorosis, right upper arm
    M85.122   Skeletal fluorosis, left upper arm
    M85.129   Skeletal fluorosis, unspecified upper arm

● M85.13   Skeletal fluorosis, forearm
    M85.131   Skeletal fluorosis, right forearm
    M85.132   Skeletal fluorosis, left forearm
    M85.139   Skeletal fluorosis, unspecified forearm

● M85.14   Skeletal fluorosis, hand
    M85.141   Skeletal fluorosis, right hand
    M85.142   Skeletal fluorosis, left hand
    M85.149   Skeletal fluorosis, unspecified hand

● M85.15   Skeletal fluorosis, thigh
    M85.151   Skeletal fluorosis, right thigh
    M85.152   Skeletal fluorosis, left thigh
    M85.159   Skeletal fluorosis, unspecified thigh

● M85.16   Skeletal fluorosis, lower leg
    M85.161   Skeletal fluorosis, right lower leg
    M85.162   Skeletal fluorosis, left lower leg
    M85.169   Skeletal fluorosis, unspecified lower leg

● M85.17   Skeletal fluorosis, ankle and foot
    M85.171   Skeletal fluorosis, right ankle and foot
    M85.172   Skeletal fluorosis, left ankle and foot
    M85.179   Skeletal fluorosis, unspecified ankle and foot

   M85.18   Skeletal fluorosis, other site
   M85.19   Skeletal fluorosis, multiple sites

M85.2   Hyperostosis of skull

● M85.3   Osteitis condensans
   M85.30   Osteitis condensans, unspecified site

● M85.31   Osteitis condensans, shoulder
    M85.311   Osteitis condensans, right shoulder
    M85.312   Osteitis condensans, left shoulder
    M85.319   Osteitis condensans, unspecified shoulder

● M85.32   Osteitis condensans, upper arm
    M85.321   Osteitis condensans, right upper arm
    M85.322   Osteitis condensans, left upper arm
    M85.329   Osteitis condensans, unspecified upper arm

● M85.33   Osteitis condensans, forearm
    M85.331   Osteitis condensans, right forearm
    M85.332   Osteitis condensans, left forearm
    M85.339   Osteitis condensans, unspecified forearm

● M85.34   Osteitis condensans, hand
    M85.341   Osteitis condensans, right hand
    M85.342   Osteitis condensans, left hand
    M85.349   Osteitis condensans, unspecified hand

● M85.35   Osteitis condensans, thigh
    M85.351   Osteitis condensans, right thigh
    M85.352   Osteitis condensans, left thigh
    M85.359   Osteitis condensans, unspecified thigh

● M85.36   Osteitis condensans, lower leg
    M85.361   Osteitis condensans, right lower leg
    M85.362   Osteitis condensans, left lower leg
    M85.369   Osteitis condensans, unspecified lower leg

● M85.37   Osteitis condensans, ankle and foot
    M85.371   Osteitis condensans, right ankle and foot
    M85.372   Osteitis condensans, left ankle and foot
    M85.379   Osteitis condensans, unspecified ankle and foot

   M85.38   Osteitis condensans, other site
   M85.39   Osteitis condensans, multiple sites

● M85.4   Solitary bone cyst
    Excludes2   solitary cyst of jaw (M27.4)
   M85.40   Solitary bone cyst, unspecified site

● M85.41   Solitary bone cyst, shoulder
    M85.411   Solitary bone cyst, right shoulder
    M85.412   Solitary bone cyst, left shoulder
    M85.419   Solitary bone cyst, unspecified shoulder

● M85.42   Solitary bone cyst, humerus
    M85.421   Solitary bone cyst, right humerus
    M85.422   Solitary bone cyst, left humerus
    M85.429   Solitary bone cyst, unspecified humerus

● M85.43   Solitary bone cyst, ulna and radius
    M85.431   Solitary bone cyst, right ulna and radius
    M85.432   Solitary bone cyst, left ulna and radius
    M85.439   Solitary bone cyst, unspecified ulna and radius

● M85.44   Solitary bone cyst, hand
    M85.441   Solitary bone cyst, right hand
    M85.442   Solitary bone cyst, left hand
    M85.449   Solitary bone cyst, unspecified hand

● M85.45   Solitary bone cyst, pelvis
    M85.451   Solitary bone cyst, right pelvis
    M85.452   Solitary bone cyst, left pelvis
    M85.459   Solitary bone cyst, unspecified pelvis

● M85.46   Solitary bone cyst, tibia and fibula
    M85.461   Solitary bone cyst, right tibia and fibula
    M85.462   Solitary bone cyst, left tibia and fibula
    M85.469   Solitary bone cyst, unspecified tibia and fibula

● M85.47   Solitary bone cyst, ankle and foot
    M85.471   Solitary bone cyst, right ankle and foot
    M85.472   Solitary bone cyst, left ankle and foot
    M85.479   Solitary bone cyst, unspecified ankle and foot

   M85.48   Solitary bone cyst, other site

● M85.5   Aneurysmal bone cyst
    Excludes2   aneurysmal cyst of jaw (M27.4)
   M85.50   Aneurysmal bone cyst, unspecified site

● M85.51   Aneurysmal bone cyst, shoulder
    M85.511   Aneurysmal bone cyst, right shoulder
    M85.512   Aneurysmal bone cyst, left shoulder
    M85.519   Aneurysmal bone cyst, unspecified shoulder

● M85.52   Aneurysmal bone cyst, upper arm
    M85.521   Aneurysmal bone cyst, right upper arm
    M85.522   Aneurysmal bone cyst, left upper arm
    M85.529   Aneurysmal bone cyst, unspecified upper arm

▶ New   ⇒ Revised   ~~deleted~~ Deleted   Excludes 1   Excludes 2   Includes   Use additional   Code first   Code also   Key words
OGCR Official Guidelines   X Assign placeholder X   ● Use Additional Character(s)   ▶ Manifestation Code   🔃 Hierarchical Condition Category   Coding Clinic

● M85.53 Aneurysmal bone cyst, forearm
  M85.531 Aneurysmal bone cyst, right forearm
  M85.532 Aneurysmal bone cyst, left forearm
  M85.539 Aneurysmal bone cyst, unspecified forearm
● M85.54 Aneurysmal bone cyst, hand
  M85.541 Aneurysmal bone cyst, right hand
  M85.542 Aneurysmal bone cyst, left hand
  M85.549 Aneurysmal bone cyst, unspecified hand
● M85.55 Aneurysmal bone cyst, thigh
  M85.551 Aneurysmal bone cyst, right thigh
  M85.552 Aneurysmal bone cyst, left thigh
  M85.559 Aneurysmal bone cyst, unspecified thigh
● M85.56 Aneurysmal bone cyst, lower leg
  M85.561 Aneurysmal bone cyst, right lower leg
  M85.562 Aneurysmal bone cyst, left lower leg
  M85.569 Aneurysmal bone cyst, unspecified lower leg
● M85.57 Aneurysmal bone cyst, ankle and foot
  M85.571 Aneurysmal bone cyst, right ankle and foot
  M85.572 Aneurysmal bone cyst, left ankle and foot
  M85.579 Aneurysmal bone cyst, unspecified ankle and foot
  M85.58 Aneurysmal bone cyst, other site
  M85.59 Aneurysmal bone cyst, multiple sites
● M85.6 Other cyst of bone
  Excludes1 cyst of jaw NEC (M27.4)
             osteitis fibrosa cystica generalisata [von Recklinghausen's disease of bone] (E21.0)
  M85.60 Other cyst of bone, unspecified site
● M85.61 Other cyst of bone, shoulder
  M85.611 Other cyst of bone, right shoulder
  M85.612 Other cyst of bone, left shoulder
  M85.619 Other cyst of bone, unspecified shoulder
● M85.62 Other cyst of bone, upper arm
  M85.621 Other cyst of bone, right upper arm
  M85.622 Other cyst of bone, left upper arm
  M85.629 Other cyst of bone, unspecified upper arm
● M85.63 Other cyst of bone, forearm
  M85.631 Other cyst of bone, right forearm
  M85.632 Other cyst of bone, left forearm
  M85.639 Other cyst of bone, unspecified forearm
● M85.64 Other cyst of bone, hand
  M85.641 Other cyst of bone, right hand
  M85.642 Other cyst of bone, left hand
  M85.649 Other cyst of bone, unspecified hand
● M85.65 Other cyst of bone, thigh
  M85.651 Other cyst of bone, right thigh
  M85.652 Other cyst of bone, left thigh
  M85.659 Other cyst of bone, unspecified thigh
● M85.66 Other cyst of bone, lower leg
  M85.661 Other cyst of bone, right lower leg
  M85.662 Other cyst of bone, left lower leg
  M85.669 Other cyst of bone, unspecified lower leg

● M85.67 Other cyst of bone, ankle and foot
  M85.671 Other cyst of bone, right ankle and foot
  M85.672 Other cyst of bone, left ankle and foot
  M85.679 Other cyst of bone, unspecified ankle and foot
  M85.68 Other cyst of bone, other site
  M85.69 Other cyst of bone, multiple sites
● M85.8 Other specified disorders of bone density and structure
  Hyperostosis of bones, except skull
  Osteosclerosis, acquired
  Excludes1 diffuse idiopathic skeletal hyperostosis [DISH] (M48.1)
             osteosclerosis congenita (Q77.4)
             osteosclerosis fragilitas (generalista) (Q78.2)
             osteosclerosis myelofibrosis (D75.81)
  M85.80 Other specified disorders of bone density and structure, unspecified site
● M85.81 Other specified disorders of bone density and structure, shoulder
  M85.811 Other specified disorders of bone density and structure, right shoulder
  M85.812 Other specified disorders of bone density and structure, left shoulder
  M85.819 Other specified disorders of bone density and structure, unspecified shoulder
● M85.82 Other specified disorders of bone density and structure, upper arm
  M85.821 Other specified disorders of bone density and structure, right upper arm
  M85.822 Other specified disorders of bone density and structure, left upper arm
  M85.829 Other specified disorders of bone density and structure, unspecified upper arm
● M85.83 Other specified disorders of bone density and structure, forearm
  M85.831 Other specified disorders of bone density and structure, right forearm
  M85.832 Other specified disorders of bone density and structure, left forearm
  M85.839 Other specified disorders of bone density and structure, unspecified forearm
● M85.84 Other specified disorders of bone density and structure, hand
  M85.841 Other specified disorders of bone density and structure, right hand
  M85.842 Other specified disorders of bone density and structure, left hand
  M85.849 Other specified disorders of bone density and structure, unspecified hand
● M85.85 Other specified disorders of bone density and structure, thigh
  M85.851 Other specified disorders of bone density and structure, right thigh
  M85.852 Other specified disorders of bone density and structure, left thigh
  M85.859 Other specified disorders of bone density and structure, unspecified thigh

● **M85.86**   Other specified disorders of bone density and structure, lower leg

    M85.861   Other specified disorders of bone density and structure, right lower leg

    M85.862   Other specified disorders of bone density and structure, left lower leg

    M85.869   Other specified disorders of bone density and structure, unspecified lower leg

● **M85.87**   Other specified disorders of bone density and structure, ankle and foot

    M85.871   Other specified disorders of bone density and structure, right ankle and foot

    M85.872   Other specified disorders of bone density and structure, left ankle and foot

    M85.879   Other specified disorders of bone density and structure, unspecified ankle and foot

  M85.88   Other specified disorders of bone density and structure, other site

  M85.89   Other specified disorders of bone density and structure, multiple sites

M85.9   Disorder of bone density and structure, unspecified
    Coding Clinic: 2021, Q3, P11

OTHER OSTEOPATHIES (M86-M90)

Excludes1   postprocedural osteopathies (M96.-)

● **M86**   Osteomyelitis

    Use additional code (B95-B97) to identify infectious agent

    Use additional code to identify major osseous defect, if applicable (M89.7-)

    Excludes1   osteomyelitis due to:
              echinococcus (B67.2)
              gonococcus (A54.43)
              salmonella (A02.24)

    Excludes2   ostemyelitis of:
              orbit (H05.0-)
              petrous bone (H70.2-)
              vertebra (M46.2-)

  ● **M86.0**   Acute hematogenous osteomyelitis

    M86.00   Acute hematogenous osteomyelitis, unspecified site 🐾

    ● **M86.01**   Acute hematogenous osteomyelitis, shoulder

       M86.011   Acute hematogenous osteomyelitis, right shoulder 🐾

       M86.012   Acute hematogenous osteomyelitis, left shoulder 🐾

       M86.019   Acute hematogenous osteomyelitis, unspecified shoulder 🐾

    ● **M86.02**   Acute hematogenous osteomyelitis, humerus

       M86.021   Acute hematogenous osteomyelitis, right humerus 🐾

       M86.022   Acute hematogenous osteomyelitis, left humerus 🐾

       M86.029   Acute hematogenous osteomyelitis, unspecified humerus 🐾

    ● **M86.03**   Acute hematogenous osteomyelitis, radius and ulna

       M86.031   Acute hematogenous osteomyelitis, right radius and ulna 🐾

       M86.032   Acute hematogenous osteomyelitis, left radius and ulna 🐾

       M86.039   Acute hematogenous osteomyelitis, unspecified radius and ulna 🐾

Figure 13-6   Osteomyelitis of the spine. A lateral view of the lower thoracic spine demonstrates destruction of the disk space *(arrow)* as well as destruction of the adjoining vertebral bodies. (From Mettler: Essentials of Radiology, ed 2, Saunders, An Imprint of Elsevier, 2005)

Item 13–12 Osteomyelitis is an inflammation of the bone. **Acute osteomyelitis** is a rapidly destructive, pus-producing infection capable of causing severe bone destruction. **Chronic osteomyelitis** can remain long after the initial acute episode has passed and may lead to a recurrence of the acute phase. **Brodie's abscess** is an encapsulated focal abscess that must be surgically drained. **Periostitis** is an inflammation of the periosteum, a dense membrane composed of fibrous connective tissue that closely wraps all bone, except those with articulating surfaces in joints, which are covered by synovial membranes.

  ● **M86.04**   Acute hematogenous osteomyelitis, hand

       M86.041   Acute hematogenous osteomyelitis, right hand 🐾

       M86.042   Acute hematogenous osteomyelitis, left hand 🐾

       M86.049   Acute hematogenous osteomyelitis, unspecified hand 🐾

  ● **M86.05**   Acute hematogenous osteomyelitis, femur

       M86.051   Acute hematogenous osteomyelitis, right femur 🐾

       M86.052   Acute hematogenous osteomyelitis, left femur 🐾

       M86.059   Acute hematogenous osteomyelitis, unspecified femur 🐾

  ● **M86.06**   Acute hematogenous osteomyelitis, tibia and fibula

       M86.061   Acute hematogenous osteomyelitis, right tibia and fibula 🐾

       M86.062   Acute hematogenous osteomyelitis, left tibia and fibula 🐾

       M86.069   Acute hematogenous osteomyelitis, unspecified tibia and fibula 🐾

  ● **M86.07**   Acute hematogenous osteomyelitis, ankle and foot

       M86.071   Acute hematogenous osteomyelitis, right ankle and foot 🐾

       M86.072   Acute hematogenous osteomyelitis, left ankle and foot 🐾

       M86.079   Acute hematogenous osteomyelitis, unspecified ankle and foot 🐾

    M86.08   Acute hematogenous osteomyelitis, other sites 🐾

    M86.09   Acute hematogenous osteomyelitis, multiple sites 🐾

  ● **M86.1**   Other acute osteomyelitis

    M86.10   Other acute osteomyelitis, unspecified site 🐾

    ● **M86.11**   Other acute osteomyelitis, shoulder

       M86.111   Other acute osteomyelitis, right shoulder 🐾

       M86.112   Other acute osteomyelitis, left shoulder 🐾

M86.119   Other acute osteomyelitis, unspecified shoulder 🦴

● M86.12   Other acute osteomyelitis, humerus
M86.121   Other acute osteomyelitis, right humerus 🦴
M86.122   Other acute osteomyelitis, left humerus 🦴
M86.129   Other acute osteomyelitis, unspecified humerus 🦴

● M86.13   Other acute osteomyelitis, radius and ulna
M86.131   Other acute osteomyelitis, right radius and ulna 🦴
M86.132   Other acute osteomyelitis, left radius and ulna 🦴
M86.139   Other acute osteomyelitis, unspecified radius and ulna 🦴

● M86.14   Other acute osteomyelitis, hand
M86.141   Other acute osteomyelitis, right hand 🦴
M86.142   Other acute osteomyelitis, left hand 🦴
M86.149   Other acute osteomyelitis, unspecified hand 🦴

● M86.15   Other acute osteomyelitis, femur
M86.151   Other acute osteomyelitis, right femur 🦴
M86.152   Other acute osteomyelitis, left femur 🦴
M86.159   Other acute osteomyelitis, unspecified femur 🦴

● M86.16   Other acute osteomyelitis, tibia and fibula
M86.161   Other acute osteomyelitis, right tibia and fibula 🦴
M86.162   Other acute osteomyelitis, left tibia and fibula 🦴
M86.169   Other acute osteomyelitis, unspecified tibia and fibula 🦴

● M86.17   Other acute osteomyelitis, ankle and foot
M86.171   Other acute osteomyelitis, right ankle and foot 🦴
Coding Clinic: 2020, Q1, P12
M86.172   Other acute osteomyelitis, left ankle and foot 🦴
M86.179   Other acute osteomyelitis, unspecified ankle and foot 🦴

M86.18   Other acute osteomyelitis, other site 🦴
M86.19   Other acute osteomyelitis, multiple sites 🦴

● M86.2   Subacute osteomyelitis
M86.20   Subacute osteomyelitis, unspecified site 🦴

● M86.21   Subacute osteomyelitis, shoulder
M86.211   Subacute osteomyelitis, right shoulder 🦴
M86.212   Subacute osteomyelitis, left shoulder 🦴
M86.219   Subacute osteomyelitis, unspecified shoulder 🦴

● M86.22   Subacute osteomyelitis, humerus
M86.221   Subacute osteomyelitis, right humerus 🦴
M86.222   Subacute osteomyelitis, left humerus 🦴
M86.229   Subacute osteomyelitis, unspecified humerus 🦴

● M86.23   Subacute osteomyelitis, radius and ulna
M86.231   Subacute osteomyelitis, right radius and ulna 🦴
M86.232   Subacute osteomyelitis, left radius and ulna 🦴
M86.239   Subacute osteomyelitis, unspecified radius and ulna 🦴

● M86.24   Subacute osteomyelitis, hand
M86.241   Subacute osteomyelitis, right hand 🦴
M86.242   Subacute osteomyelitis, left hand 🦴
M86.249   Subacute osteomyelitis, unspecified hand 🦴

● M86.25   Subacute osteomyelitis, femur
M86.251   Subacute osteomyelitis, right femur 🦴
M86.252   Subacute osteomyelitis, left femur 🦴
M86.259   Subacute osteomyelitis, unspecified femur 🦴

● M86.26   Subacute osteomyelitis, tibia and fibula
M86.261   Subacute osteomyelitis, right tibia and fibula 🦴
M86.262   Subacute osteomyelitis, left tibia and fibula 🦴
M86.269   Subacute osteomyelitis, unspecified tibia and fibula 🦴

● M86.27   Subacute osteomyelitis, ankle and foot
M86.271   Subacute osteomyelitis, right ankle and foot 🦴
M86.272   Subacute osteomyelitis, left ankle and foot 🦴
M86.279   Subacute osteomyelitis, unspecified ankle and foot 🦴

M86.28   Subacute osteomyelitis, other site 🦴
M86.29   Subacute osteomyelitis, multiple sites 🦴

● M86.3   Chronic multifocal osteomyelitis
M86.30   Chronic multifocal osteomyelitis, unspecified site 🦴

● M86.31   Chronic multifocal osteomyelitis, shoulder
M86.311   Chronic multifocal osteomyelitis, right shoulder 🦴
M86.312   Chronic multifocal osteomyelitis, left shoulder 🦴
M86.319   Chronic multifocal osteomyelitis, unspecified shoulder 🦴

● M86.32   Chronic multifocal osteomyelitis, humerus
M86.321   Chronic multifocal osteomyelitis, right humerus 🦴
M86.322   Chronic multifocal osteomyelitis, left humerus 🦴
M86.329   Chronic multifocal osteomyelitis, unspecified humerus 🦴

● M86.33   Chronic multifocal osteomyelitis, radius and ulna
M86.331   Chronic multifocal osteomyelitis, right radius and ulna 🦴
M86.332   Chronic multifocal osteomyelitis, left radius and ulna 🦴
M86.339   Chronic multifocal osteomyelitis, unspecified radius and ulna 🦴

● M86.34   Chronic multifocal osteomyelitis, hand
M86.341   Chronic multifocal osteomyelitis, right hand 🦴
M86.342   Chronic multifocal osteomyelitis, left hand 🦴
M86.349   Chronic multifocal osteomyelitis, unspecified hand 🦴

CHAPTER 13 (M00-M99)

CHAPTER 13 (M00-M99)

● M86.35 Chronic multifocal osteomyelitis, femur
  M86.351 Chronic multifocal osteomyelitis, right femur
  M86.352 Chronic multifocal osteomyelitis, left femur
  M86.359 Chronic multifocal osteomyelitis, unspecified femur
● M86.36 Chronic multifocal osteomyelitis, tibia and fibula
  M86.361 Chronic multifocal osteomyelitis, right tibia and fibula
  M86.362 Chronic multifocal osteomyelitis, left tibia and fibula
  M86.369 Chronic multifocal osteomyelitis, unspecified tibia and fibula
● M86.37 Chronic multifocal osteomyelitis, ankle and foot
  M86.371 Chronic multifocal osteomyelitis, right ankle and foot
  M86.372 Chronic multifocal osteomyelitis, left ankle and foot
  M86.379 Chronic multifocal osteomyelitis, unspecified ankle and foot
  M86.38 Chronic multifocal osteomyelitis, other site
  M86.39 Chronic multifocal osteomyelitis, multiple sites
● M86.4 Chronic osteomyelitis with draining sinus
  M86.40 Chronic osteomyelitis with draining sinus, unspecified site
● M86.41 Chronic osteomyelitis with draining sinus, shoulder
  M86.411 Chronic osteomyelitis with draining sinus, right shoulder
  M86.412 Chronic osteomyelitis with draining sinus, left shoulder
  M86.419 Chronic osteomyelitis with draining sinus, unspecified shoulder
● M86.42 Chronic osteomyelitis with draining sinus, humerus
  M86.421 Chronic osteomyelitis with draining sinus, right humerus
  M86.422 Chronic osteomyelitis with draining sinus, left humerus
  M86.429 Chronic osteomyelitis with draining sinus, unspecified humerus
● M86.43 Chronic osteomyelitis with draining sinus, radius and ulna
  M86.431 Chronic osteomyelitis with draining sinus, right radius and ulna
  M86.432 Chronic osteomyelitis with draining sinus, left radius and ulna
  M86.439 Chronic osteomyelitis with draining sinus, unspecified radius and ulna
● M86.44 Chronic osteomyelitis with draining sinus, hand
  M86.441 Chronic osteomyelitis with draining sinus, right hand
  M86.442 Chronic osteomyelitis with draining sinus, left hand
  M86.449 Chronic osteomyelitis with draining sinus, unspecified hand
● M86.45 Chronic osteomyelitis with draining sinus, femur
  M86.451 Chronic osteomyelitis with draining sinus, right femur
  M86.452 Chronic osteomyelitis with draining sinus, left femur
  M86.459 Chronic osteomyelitis with draining sinus, unspecified femur

● M86.46 Chronic osteomyelitis with draining sinus, tibia and fibula
  M86.461 Chronic osteomyelitis with draining sinus, right tibia and fibula
  M86.462 Chronic osteomyelitis with draining sinus, left tibia and fibula
  M86.469 Chronic osteomyelitis with draining sinus, unspecified tibia and fibula
● M86.47 Chronic osteomyelitis with draining sinus, ankle and foot
  M86.471 Chronic osteomyelitis with draining sinus, right ankle and foot
  M86.472 Chronic osteomyelitis with draining sinus, left ankle and foot
  M86.479 Chronic osteomyelitis with draining sinus, unspecified ankle and foot
  M86.48 Chronic osteomyelitis with draining sinus, other site
  M86.49 Chronic osteomyelitis with draining sinus, multiple sites
● M86.5 Other chronic hematogenous osteomyelitis
  M86.50 Other chronic hematogenous osteomyelitis, unspecified site
● M86.51 Other chronic hematogenous osteomyelitis, shoulder
  M86.511 Other chronic hematogenous osteomyelitis, right shoulder
  M86.512 Other chronic hematogenous osteomyelitis, left shoulder
  M86.519 Other chronic hematogenous osteomyelitis, unspecified shoulder
● M86.52 Other chronic hematogenous osteomyelitis, humerus
  M86.521 Other chronic hematogenous osteomyelitis, right humerus
  M86.522 Other chronic hematogenous osteomyelitis, left humerus
  M86.529 Other chronic hematogenous osteomyelitis, unspecified humerus
● M86.53 Other chronic hematogenous osteomyelitis, radius and ulna
  M86.531 Other chronic hematogenous osteomyelitis, right radius and ulna
  M86.532 Other chronic hematogenous osteomyelitis, left radius and ulna
  M86.539 Other chronic hematogenous osteomyelitis, unspecified radius and ulna
● M86.54 Other chronic hematogenous osteomyelitis, hand
  M86.541 Other chronic hematogenous osteomyelitis, right hand
  M86.542 Other chronic hematogenous osteomyelitis, left hand
  M86.549 Other chronic hematogenous osteomyelitis, unspecified hand
● M86.55 Other chronic hematogenous osteomyelitis, femur
  M86.551 Other chronic hematogenous osteomyelitis, right femur
  M86.552 Other chronic hematogenous osteomyelitis, left femur
  M86.559 Other chronic hematogenous osteomyelitis, unspecified femur

- M86.56 Other chronic hematogenous osteomyelitis, tibia and fibula
  - M86.561 Other chronic hematogenous osteomyelitis, right tibia and fibula 🔍
  - M86.562 Other chronic hematogenous osteomyelitis, left tibia and fibula 🔍
  - M86.569 Other chronic hematogenous osteomyelitis, unspecified tibia and fibula 🔍
- M86.57 Other chronic hematogenous osteomyelitis, ankle and foot
  - M86.571 Other chronic hematogenous osteomyelitis, right ankle and foot 🔍
  - M86.572 Other chronic hematogenous osteomyelitis, left ankle and foot 🔍
  - M86.579 Other chronic hematogenous osteomyelitis, unspecified ankle and foot 🔍
  - M86.58 Other chronic hematogenous osteomyelitis, other site 🔍
  - M86.59 Other chronic hematogenous osteomyelitis, multiple sites 🔍
- M86.6 Other chronic osteomyelitis
  - M86.60 Other chronic osteomyelitis, unspecified site 🔍
- M86.61 Other chronic osteomyelitis, shoulder
  - M86.611 Other chronic osteomyelitis, right shoulder 🔍
  - M86.612 Other chronic osteomyelitis, left shoulder 🔍
  - M86.619 Other chronic osteomyelitis, unspecified shoulder 🔍
- M86.62 Other chronic osteomyelitis, humerus
  - M86.621 Other chronic osteomyelitis, right humerus 🔍
  - M86.622 Other chronic osteomyelitis, left humerus 🔍
  - M86.629 Other chronic osteomyelitis, unspecified humerus 🔍
- M86.63 Other chronic osteomyelitis, radius and ulna
  - M86.631 Other chronic osteomyelitis, right radius and ulna 🔍
  - M86.632 Other chronic osteomyelitis, left radius and ulna 🔍
  - M86.639 Other chronic osteomyelitis, unspecified radius and ulna 🔍
- M86.64 Other chronic osteomyelitis, hand
  - M86.641 Other chronic osteomyelitis, right hand 🔍
  - M86.642 Other chronic osteomyelitis, left hand 🔍
  - M86.649 Other chronic osteomyelitis, unspecified hand 🔍
- M86.65 Other chronic osteomyelitis, thigh
  - M86.651 Other chronic osteomyelitis, right thigh 🔍
  - M86.652 Other chronic osteomyelitis, left thigh 🔍
  - M86.659 Other chronic osteomyelitis, unspecified thigh 🔍
- M86.66 Other chronic osteomyelitis, tibia and fibula
  - M86.661 Other chronic osteomyelitis, right tibia and fibula 🔍
  - M86.662 Other chronic osteomyelitis, left tibia and fibula 🔍
  - M86.669 Other chronic osteomyelitis, unspecified tibia and fibula 🔍

- M86.67 Other chronic osteomyelitis, ankle and foot
  - M86.671 Other chronic osteomyelitis, right ankle and foot 🔍
    Coding Clinic: 2016, Q1, P13
  - M86.672 Other chronic osteomyelitis, left ankle and foot 🔍
  - M86.679 Other chronic osteomyelitis, unspecified ankle and foot 🔍
  - M86.68 Other chronic osteomyelitis, other site 🔍
  - M86.69 Other chronic osteomyelitis, multiple sites 🔍
- M86.8 Other osteomyelitis
  Brodie's abscess
  - M86.8X Other osteomyelitis
    - M86.8X0 Other osteomyelitis, multiple sites 🔍
    - M86.8X1 Other osteomyelitis, shoulder 🔍
    - M86.8X2 Other osteomyelitis, upper arm 🔍
    - M86.8X3 Other osteomyelitis, forearm 🔍
    - M86.8X4 Other osteomyelitis, hand 🔍
    - M86.8X5 Other osteomyelitis, thigh 🔍
    - M86.8X6 Other osteomyelitis, lower leg 🔍
    - M86.8X7 Other osteomyelitis, ankle and foot 🔍
    - M86.8X8 Other osteomyelitis, other site 🔍
      Coding Clinic: 2022, Q1, P31
    - M86.8X9 Other osteomyelitis, unspecified sites 🔍
  - M86.9 Osteomyelitis, unspecified 🔍
    Infection of bone NOS
    Periostitis without osteomyelitis

- M87 Osteonecrosis
  Includes   avascular necrosis of bone
  Use additional code to identify major osseous defect, if applicable (M89.7-)
  Excludes1   juvenile osteonecrosis (M91-M92)
  osteochondropathies (M90-M93)
  - M87.0 Idiopathic aseptic necrosis of bone
    - M87.00 Idiopathic aseptic necrosis of unspecified bone 🔍
    - M87.01 Idiopathic aseptic necrosis of shoulder
      Idiopathic aseptic necrosis of clavicle and scapula
      - M87.011 Idiopathic aseptic necrosis of right shoulder 🔍
      - M87.012 Idiopathic aseptic necrosis of left shoulder 🔍
      - M87.019 Idiopathic aseptic necrosis of unspecified shoulder 🔍
    - M87.02 Idiopathic aseptic necrosis of humerus
      - M87.021 Idiopathic aseptic necrosis of right humerus 🔍
      - M87.022 Idiopathic aseptic necrosis of left humerus 🔍
      - M87.029 Idiopathic aseptic necrosis of unspecified humerus 🔍
    - M87.03 Idiopathic aseptic necrosis of radius, ulna and carpus
      - M87.031 Idiopathic aseptic necrosis of right radius 🔍
      - M87.032 Idiopathic aseptic necrosis of left radius 🔍
      - M87.033 Idiopathic aseptic necrosis of unspecified radius 🔍
      - M87.034 Idiopathic aseptic necrosis of right ulna 🔍
      - M87.035 Idiopathic aseptic necrosis of left ulna 🔍

CHAPTER 13 (M00-M99)

CHAPTER 13 (M00-M99)

M87.036   Idiopathic aseptic necrosis of unspecified ulna 🐾

M87.037   Idiopathic aseptic necrosis of right carpus 🐾

M87.038   Idiopathic aseptic necrosis of left carpus 🐾

M87.039   Idiopathic aseptic necrosis of unspecified carpus 🐾

● M87.04   **Idiopathic aseptic necrosis of hand and fingers**
    Idiopathic aseptic necrosis of metacarpals and phalanges of hands

M87.041   Idiopathic aseptic necrosis of right hand 🐾

M87.042   Idiopathic aseptic necrosis of left hand 🐾

M87.043   Idiopathic aseptic necrosis of unspecified hand 🐾

M87.044   Idiopathic aseptic necrosis of right finger(s) 🐾

M87.045   Idiopathic aseptic necrosis of left finger(s) 🐾

M87.046   Idiopathic aseptic necrosis of unspecified finger(s) 🐾

● M87.05   **Idiopathic aseptic necrosis of pelvis and femur**

M87.050   Idiopathic aseptic necrosis of pelvis 🐾

M87.051   Idiopathic aseptic necrosis of right femur 🐾

M87.052   Idiopathic aseptic necrosis of left femur 🐾

M87.059   Idiopathic aseptic necrosis of unspecified femur 🐾
     Idiopathic aseptic necrosis of hip NOS

● M87.06   **Idiopathic aseptic necrosis of tibia and fibula**

M87.061   Idiopathic aseptic necrosis of right tibia 🐾

M87.062   Idiopathic aseptic necrosis of left tibia 🐾

M87.063   Idiopathic aseptic necrosis of unspecified tibia 🐾

M87.064   Idiopathic aseptic necrosis of right fibula 🐾

M87.065   Idiopathic aseptic necrosis of left fibula 🐾

M87.066   Idiopathic aseptic necrosis of unspecified fibula 🐾

● M87.07   **Idiopathic aseptic necrosis of ankle, foot and toes**
    Idiopathic aseptic necrosis of metatarsus, tarsus, and phalanges of toes

M87.071   Idiopathic aseptic necrosis of right ankle 🐾

M87.072   Idiopathic aseptic necrosis of left ankle 🐾

M87.073   Idiopathic aseptic necrosis of unspecified ankle 🐾

M87.074   Idiopathic aseptic necrosis of right foot 🐾

M87.075   Idiopathic aseptic necrosis of left foot 🐾

M87.076   Idiopathic aseptic necrosis of unspecified foot 🐾

M87.077   Idiopathic aseptic necrosis of right toe(s) 🐾

M87.078   Idiopathic aseptic necrosis of left toe(s) 🐾

M87.079   Idiopathic aseptic necrosis of unspecified toe(s) 🐾

M87.08   Idiopathic aseptic necrosis of bone, other site 🐾

M87.09   Idiopathic aseptic necrosis of bone, multiple sites 🐾

● M87.1   **Osteonecrosis due to drugs**
    Use additional code for adverse effect, if applicable, to identify drug (T36-T50 with fifth or sixth character 5)

M87.10   Osteonecrosis due to drugs, unspecified bone 🐾

● M87.11   **Osteonecrosis due to drugs, shoulder**

M87.111   Osteonecrosis due to drugs, right shoulder 🐾

M87.112   Osteonecrosis due to drugs, left shoulder 🐾

M87.119   Osteonecrosis due to drugs, unspecified shoulder 🐾

● M87.12   **Osteonecrosis due to drugs, humerus**

M87.121   Osteonecrosis due to drugs, right humerus 🐾

M87.122   Osteonecrosis due to drugs, left humerus 🐾

M87.129   Osteonecrosis due to drugs, unspecified humerus 🐾

● M87.13   **Osteonecrosis due to drugs of radius, ulna and carpus**

M87.131   Osteonecrosis due to drugs of right radius 🐾

M87.132   Osteonecrosis due to drugs of left radius 🐾

M87.133   Osteonecrosis due to drugs of unspecified radius 🐾

M87.134   Osteonecrosis due to drugs of right ulna 🐾

M87.135   Osteonecrosis due to drugs of left ulna 🐾

M87.136   Osteonecrosis due to drugs of unspecified ulna 🐾

M87.137   Osteonecrosis due to drugs of right carpus 🐾

M87.138   Osteonecrosis due to drugs of left carpus 🐾

M87.139   Osteonecrosis due to drugs of unspecified carpus 🐾

● M87.14   **Osteonecrosis due to drugs, hand and fingers**

M87.141   Osteonecrosis due to drugs, right hand 🐾

M87.142   Osteonecrosis due to drugs, left hand 🐾

M87.143   Osteonecrosis due to drugs, unspecified hand 🐾

M87.144   Osteonecrosis due to drugs, right finger(s) 🐾

M87.145   Osteonecrosis due to drugs, left finger(s) 🐾

M87.146   Osteonecrosis due to drugs, unspecified finger(s) 🐾

● M87.15   **Osteonecrosis due to drugs, pelvis and femur**

M87.150   Osteonecrosis due to drugs, pelvis 🐾

M87.151   Osteonecrosis due to drugs, right femur 🐾

M87.152   Osteonecrosis due to drugs, left femur 🐾

M87.159   Osteonecrosis due to drugs, unspecified femur 🐾

▶ New   ⇒ Revised   ~~deleted~~ Deleted   Excludes 1   Excludes 2   Includes   Use additional   Code first   Code also   Key words

OGCR Official Guidelines   X Assign placeholder X   ● Use Additional Character(s)   ▌ Manifestation Code   🐾 Hierarchical Condition Category   Coding Clinic

● M87.16 Osteonecrosis due to drugs, tibia and fibula
    M87.161 Osteonecrosis due to drugs, right tibia 🖉
    M87.162 Osteonecrosis due to drugs, left tibia 🖉
    M87.163 Osteonecrosis due to drugs, unspecified tibia 🖉
    M87.164 Osteonecrosis due to drugs, right fibula 🖉
    M87.165 Osteonecrosis due to drugs, left fibula 🖉
    M87.166 Osteonecrosis due to drugs, unspecified fibula 🖉

● M87.17 Osteonecrosis due to drugs, ankle, foot and toes
    M87.171 Osteonecrosis due to drugs, right ankle 🖉
    M87.172 Osteonecrosis due to drugs, left ankle 🖉
    M87.173 Osteonecrosis due to drugs, unspecified ankle 🖉
    M87.174 Osteonecrosis due to drugs, right foot 🖉
    M87.175 Osteonecrosis due to drugs, left foot 🖉
    M87.176 Osteonecrosis due to drugs, unspecified foot 🖉
    M87.177 Osteonecrosis due to drugs, right toe(s) 🖉
    M87.178 Osteonecrosis due to drugs, left toe(s) 🖉
    M87.179 Osteonecrosis due to drugs, unspecified toe(s) 🖉

● M87.18 Osteonecrosis due to drugs, other site
    M87.180 Osteonecrosis due to drugs, jaw 🖉
    M87.188 Osteonecrosis due to drugs, other site 🖉

  M87.19 Osteonecrosis due to drugs, multiple sites 🖉

● M87.2 Osteonecrosis due to previous trauma
  M87.20 Osteonecrosis due to previous trauma, unspecified bone 🖉

● M87.21 Osteonecrosis due to previous trauma, shoulder
    M87.211 Osteonecrosis due to previous trauma, right shoulder 🖉
    M87.212 Osteonecrosis due to previous trauma, left shoulder 🖉
    M87.219 Osteonecrosis due to previous trauma, unspecified shoulder 🖉

● M87.22 Osteonecrosis due to previous trauma, humerus
    M87.221 Osteonecrosis due to previous trauma, right humerus 🖉
    M87.222 Osteonecrosis due to previous trauma, left humerus 🖉
    M87.229 Osteonecrosis due to previous trauma, unspecified humerus 🖉

● M87.23 Osteonecrosis due to previous trauma of radius, ulna and carpus
    M87.231 Osteonecrosis due to previous trauma of right radius 🖉
    M87.232 Osteonecrosis due to previous trauma of left radius 🖉
    M87.233 Osteonecrosis due to previous trauma of unspecified radius 🖉
    M87.234 Osteonecrosis due to previous trauma of right ulna 🖉
    M87.235 Osteonecrosis due to previous trauma of left ulna 🖉
    M87.236 Osteonecrosis due to previous trauma of unspecified ulna 🖉
    M87.237 Osteonecrosis due to previous trauma of right carpus 🖉
    M87.238 Osteonecrosis due to previous trauma of left carpus 🖉
    M87.239 Osteonecrosis due to previous trauma of unspecified carpus 🖉

● M87.24 Osteonecrosis due to previous trauma, hand and fingers
    M87.241 Osteonecrosis due to previous trauma, right hand 🖉
    M87.242 Osteonecrosis due to previous trauma, left hand 🖉
    M87.243 Osteonecrosis due to previous trauma, unspecified hand 🖉
    M87.244 Osteonecrosis due to previous trauma, right finger(s) 🖉
    M87.245 Osteonecrosis due to previous trauma, left finger(s) 🖉
    M87.246 Osteonecrosis due to previous trauma, unspecified finger(s) 🖉

● M87.25 Osteonecrosis due to previous trauma, pelvis and femur
    M87.250 Osteonecrosis due to previous trauma, pelvis 🖉
    M87.251 Osteonecrosis due to previous trauma, right femur 🖉
    M87.252 Osteonecrosis due to previous trauma, left femur 🖉
    M87.256 Osteonecrosis due to previous trauma, unspecified femur 🖉

● M87.26 Osteonecrosis due to previous trauma, tibia and fibula
    M87.261 Osteonecrosis due to previous trauma, right tibia 🖉
    M87.262 Osteonecrosis due to previous trauma, left tibia 🖉
    M87.263 Osteonecrosis due to previous trauma, unspecified tibia 🖉
    M87.264 Osteonecrosis due to previous trauma, right fibula 🖉
    M87.265 Osteonecrosis due to previous trauma, left fibula 🖉
    M87.266 Osteonecrosis due to previous trauma, unspecified fibula 🖉

● M87.27 Osteonecrosis due to previous trauma, ankle, foot and toes
    M87.271 Osteonecrosis due to previous trauma, right ankle 🖉
    M87.272 Osteonecrosis due to previous trauma, left ankle 🖉
    M87.273 Osteonecrosis due to previous trauma, unspecified ankle 🖉
    M87.274 Osteonecrosis due to previous trauma, right foot 🖉
    M87.275 Osteonecrosis due to previous trauma, left foot 🖉
    M87.276 Osteonecrosis due to previous trauma, unspecified foot 🖉
    M87.277 Osteonecrosis due to previous trauma, right toe(s) 🖉
    M87.278 Osteonecrosis due to previous trauma, left toe(s) 🖉
    M87.279 Osteonecrosis due to previous trauma, unspecified toe(s) 🖉

  M87.28 Osteonecrosis due to previous trauma, other site 🖉

  M87.29 Osteonecrosis due to previous trauma, multiple sites 🖉

CHAPTER 13 (M00-M99)

CHAPTER 13 (M00-M99)

● M87.3   Other secondary osteonecrosis

     M87.30   Other secondary osteonecrosis, unspecified bone 🦠

     ● M87.31   Other secondary osteonecrosis, shoulder

         M87.311   Other secondary osteonecrosis, right shoulder 🦠

         M87.312   Other secondary osteonecrosis, left shoulder 🦠

         M87.319   Other secondary osteonecrosis, unspecified shoulder 🦠

     ● M87.32   Other secondary osteonecrosis, humerus

         M87.321   Other secondary osteonecrosis, right humerus 🦠

         M87.322   Other secondary osteonecrosis, left humerus 🦠

         M87.329   Other secondary osteonecrosis, unspecified humerus 🦠

     ● M87.33   Other secondary osteonecrosis of radius, ulna and carpus

         M87.331   Other secondary osteonecrosis of right radius 🦠

         M87.332   Other secondary osteonecrosis of left radius 🦠

         M87.333   Other secondary osteonecrosis of unspecified radius 🦠

         M87.334   Other secondary osteonecrosis of right ulna 🦠

         M87.335   Other secondary osteonecrosis of left ulna 🦠

         M87.336   Other secondary osteonecrosis of unspecified ulna 🦠

         M87.337   Other secondary osteonecrosis of right carpus 🦠

         M87.338   Other secondary osteonecrosis of left carpus 🦠

         M87.339   Other secondary osteonecrosis of unspecified carpus 🦠

     ● M87.34   Other secondary osteonecrosis, hand and fingers

         M87.341   Other secondary osteonecrosis, right hand 🦠

         M87.342   Other secondary osteonecrosis, left hand 🦠

         M87.343   Other secondary osteonecrosis, unspecified hand 🦠

         M87.344   Other secondary osteonecrosis, right finger(s) 🦠

         M87.345   Other secondary osteonecrosis, left finger(s) 🦠

         M87.346   Other secondary osteonecrosis, unspecified finger(s) 🦠

     ● M87.35   Other secondary osteonecrosis, pelvis and femur

         M87.350   Other secondary osteonecrosis, pelvis 🦠

         M87.351   Other secondary osteonecrosis, right femur 🦠

         M87.352   Other secondary osteonecrosis, left femur 🦠

         M87.353   Other secondary osteonecrosis, unspecified femur 🦠

     ● M87.36   Other secondary osteonecrosis, tibia and fibula

         M87.361   Other secondary osteonecrosis, right tibia 🦠

         M87.362   Other secondary osteonecrosis, left tibia 🦠

         M87.363   Other secondary osteonecrosis, unspecified tibia 🦠

         M87.364   Other secondary osteonecrosis, right fibula 🦠

         M87.365   Other secondary osteonecrosis, left fibula 🦠

         M87.366   Other secondary osteonecrosis, unspecified fibula 🦠

     ● M87.37   Other secondary osteonecrosis, ankle and foot

         M87.371   Other secondary osteonecrosis, right ankle 🦠

         M87.372   Other secondary osteonecrosis, left ankle 🦠

         M87.373   Other secondary osteonecrosis, unspecified ankle 🦠

         M87.374   Other secondary osteonecrosis, right foot 🦠

         M87.375   Other secondary osteonecrosis, left foot 🦠

         M87.376   Other secondary osteonecrosis, unspecified foot 🦠

         M87.377   Other secondary osteonecrosis, right toe(s) 🦠

         M87.378   Other secondary osteonecrosis, left toe(s) 🦠

         M87.379   Other secondary osteonecrosis, unspecified toe(s) 🦠

     M87.38   Other secondary osteonecrosis, other site 🦠

     M87.39   Other secondary osteonecrosis, multiple sites 🦠

● M87.8   Other osteonecrosis

     M87.80   Other osteonecrosis, unspecified bone 🦠

     ● M87.81   Other osteonecrosis, shoulder

         M87.811   Other osteonecrosis, right shoulder 🦠

         M87.812   Other osteonecrosis, left shoulder 🦠

         M87.819   Other osteonecrosis, unspecified shoulder 🦠

     ● M87.82   Other osteonecrosis, humerus

         M87.821   Other osteonecrosis, right humerus 🦠

         M87.822   Other osteonecrosis, left humerus 🦠

         M87.829   Other osteonecrosis, unspecified humerus 🦠

     ● M87.83   Other osteonecrosis of radius, ulna and carpus

         M87.831   Other osteonecrosis of right radius 🦠

         M87.832   Other osteonecrosis of left radius 🦠

         M87.833   Other osteonecrosis of unspecified radius 🦠

         M87.834   Other osteonecrosis of right ulna 🦠

         M87.835   Other osteonecrosis of left ulna 🦠

         M87.836   Other osteonecrosis of unspecified ulna 🦠

         M87.837   Other osteonecrosis of right carpus 🦠

         M87.838   Other osteonecrosis of left carpus 🦠

         M87.839   Other osteonecrosis of unspecified carpus 🦠

     ● M87.84   Other osteonecrosis, hand and fingers

         M87.841   Other osteonecrosis, right hand 🦠

         M87.842   Other osteonecrosis, left hand 🦠

         M87.843   Other osteonecrosis, unspecified hand 🦠

         M87.844   Other osteonecrosis, right finger(s) 🦠

         M87.845   Other osteonecrosis, left finger(s) 🦠

         M87.849   Other osteonecrosis, unspecified finger(s) 🦠

     ● M87.85   Other osteonecrosis, pelvis and femur

         M87.850   Other osteonecrosis, pelvis 🦠

         M87.851   Other osteonecrosis, right femur 🦠

         M87.852   Other osteonecrosis, left femur 🦠

         M87.859   Other osteonecrosis, unspecified femur 🦠

▶ New   ⇒ Revised   ~~deleted~~ Deleted   Excludes 1   Excludes 2   Includes   Use additional   Code first   Code also   Key words

OGCR Official Guidelines   X Assign placeholder X   ● Use Additional Character(s)   ▶ Manifestation Code   🦠 Hierarchical Condition Category   **Coding Clinic**

- M87.86   Other osteonecrosis, tibia and fibula
  - M87.861   Other osteonecrosis, right tibia
  - M87.862   Other osteonecrosis, left tibia
  - M87.863   Other osteonecrosis, unspecified tibia
  - M87.864   Other osteonecrosis, right fibula
  - M87.865   Other osteonecrosis, left fibula
  - M87.869   Other osteonecrosis, unspecified fibula
- M87.87   Other osteonecrosis, ankle, foot and toes
  - M87.871   Other osteonecrosis, right ankle
  - M87.872   Other osteonecrosis, left ankle
  - M87.873   Other osteonecrosis, unspecified ankle
  - M87.874   Other osteonecrosis, right foot
  - M87.875   Other osteonecrosis, left foot
  - M87.876   Other osteonecrosis, unspecified foot
  - M87.877   Other osteonecrosis, right toe(s)
  - M87.878   Other osteonecrosis, left toe(s)
  - M87.879   Other osteonecrosis, unspecified toe(s)
  - M87.88   Other osteonecrosis, other site
  - M87.89   Other osteonecrosis, multiple sites
- M87.9   Osteonecrosis, unspecified
  Necrosis of bone NOS

- M88   **Osteitis deformans [Paget's disease of bone]**
  Chronic disorder that results in enlarged and deformed bones. The excessive breakdown and formation of bone tissue causes bones to weaken and results in bone pain, arthritis, deformities, and fractures.
  Excludes1   osteitis deformans in neoplastic disease (M90.6)
  - M88.0   Osteitis deformans of skull
  - M88.1   Osteitis deformans of vertebrae
  - M88.8   Osteitis deformans of other bones
    - M88.81   Osteitis deformans of shoulder
      - M88.811   Osteitis deformans of right shoulder
      - M88.812   Osteitis deformans of left shoulder
      - M88.819   Osteitis deformans of unspecified shoulder
    - M88.82   Osteitis deformans of upper arm
      - M88.821   Osteitis deformans of right upper arm
      - M88.822   Osteitis deformans of left upper arm
      - M88.829   Osteitis deformans of unspecified upper arm
    - M88.83   Osteitis deformans of forearm
      - M88.831   Osteitis deformans of right forearm
      - M88.832   Osteitis deformans of left forearm
      - M88.839   Osteitis deformans of unspecified forearm
    - M88.84   Osteitis deformans of hand
      - M88.841   Osteitis deformans of right hand
      - M88.842   Osteitis deformans of left hand
      - M88.849   Osteitis deformans of unspecified hand
    - M88.85   Osteitis deformans of thigh
      - M88.851   Osteitis deformans of right thigh
      - M88.852   Osteitis deformans of left thigh
      - M88.859   Osteitis deformans of unspecified thigh
    - M88.86   Osteitis deformans of lower leg
      - M88.861   Osteitis deformans of right lower leg
      - M88.862   Osteitis deformans of left lower leg
      - M88.869   Osteitis deformans of unspecified lower leg

- M88.87   Osteitis deformans of ankle and foot
  - M88.871   Osteitis deformans of right ankle and foot
  - M88.872   Osteitis deformans of left ankle and foot
  - M88.879   Osteitis deformans of unspecified ankle and foot
- M88.88   Osteitis deformans of other bones
  Excludes2   osteitis deformans of skull (M88.0)
  osteitis deformans of vertebrae (M88.1)
  - M88.89   Osteitis deformans of multiple sites
- M88.9   Osteitis deformans of unspecified bone

- M89   **Other disorders of bone**
  - M89.0   Algoneurodystrophy
    Shoulder-hand syndrome
    Sudeck's atrophy
    Excludes1   causalgia, lower limb (G57.7-)
    causalgia, upper limb (G56.4-)
    complex regional pain syndrome II, lower limb (G57.7-)
    complex regional pain syndrome II, upper limb (G56.4-)
    reflex sympathetic dystrophy (G90.5-)
    - M89.00   Algoneurodystrophy, unspecified site
    - M89.01   Algoneurodystrophy, shoulder
      - M89.011   Algoneurodystrophy, right shoulder
      - M89.012   Algoneurodystrophy, left shoulder
      - M89.019   Algoneurodystrophy, unspecified shoulder
    - M89.02   Algoneurodystrophy, upper arm
      - M89.021   Algoneurodystrophy, right upper arm
      - M89.022   Algoneurodystrophy, left upper arm
      - M89.029   Algoneurodystrophy, unspecified upper arm
    - M89.03   Algoneurodystrophy, forearm
      - M89.031   Algoneurodystrophy, right forearm
      - M89.032   Algoneurodystrophy, left forearm
      - M89.039   Algoneurodystrophy, unspecified forearm
    - M89.04   Algoneurodystrophy, hand
      - M89.041   Algoneurodystrophy, right hand
      - M89.042   Algoneurodystrophy, left hand
      - M89.049   Algoneurodystrophy, unspecified hand
    - M89.05   Algoneurodystrophy, thigh
      - M89.051   Algoneurodystrophy, right thigh
      - M89.052   Algoneurodystrophy, left thigh
      - M89.059   Algoneurodystrophy, unspecified thigh
    - M89.06   Algoneurodystrophy, lower leg
      - M89.061   Algoneurodystrophy, right lower leg
      - M89.062   Algoneurodystrophy, left lower leg
      - M89.069   Algoneurodystrophy, unspecified lower leg
    - M89.07   Algoneurodystrophy, ankle and foot
      - M89.071   Algoneurodystrophy, right ankle and foot
      - M89.072   Algoneurodystrophy, left ankle and foot
      - M89.079   Algoneurodystrophy, unspecified ankle and foot
    - M89.08   Algoneurodystrophy, other site
    - M89.09   Algoneurodystrophy, multiple sites

● **M89.1 Physeal arrest**
   Arrest of growth plate
   Epiphyseal arrest
   Growth plate arrest
   ● **M89.12 Physeal arrest, humerus**
      **M89.121 Complete physeal arrest, right
                  proximal humerus**
      **M89.122 Complete physeal arrest, left proximal
                  humerus**
      **M89.123 Partial physeal arrest, right proximal
                  humerus**
      **M89.124 Partial physeal arrest, left proximal
                  humerus**
      **M89.125 Complete physeal arrest, right distal
                  humerus**
      **M89.126 Complete physeal arrest, left distal
                  humerus**
      **M89.127 Partial physeal arrest, right distal
                  humerus**
      **M89.128 Partial physeal arrest, left distal
                  humerus**
      M89.129 Physeal arrest, humerus, unspecified
   ● **M89.13 Physeal arrest, forearm**
      **M89.131 Complete physeal arrest, right distal
                  radius**
      **M89.132 Complete physeal arrest, left distal
                  radius**
      **M89.133 Partial physeal arrest, right distal
                  radius**
      **M89.134 Partial physeal arrest, left distal
                  radius**
      M89.138 Other physeal arrest of forearm
      M89.139 Physeal arrest, forearm, unspecified
   ● **M89.15 Physeal arrest, femur**
      **M89.151 Complete physeal arrest, right
                  proximal femur**
      **M89.152 Complete physeal arrest, left proximal
                  femur**
      **M89.153 Partial physeal arrest, right proximal
                  femur**
      **M89.154 Partial physeal arrest, left proximal
                  femur**
      **M89.155 Complete physeal arrest, right distal
                  femur**
      **M89.156 Complete physeal arrest, left distal
                  femur**
      **M89.157 Partial physeal arrest, right distal
                  femur**
      M89.158 Partial physeal arrest, left distal femur
      M89.159 Physeal arrest, femur, unspecified
   ● **M89.16 Physeal arrest, lower leg**
      **M89.160 Complete physeal arrest, right
                  proximal tibia**
      **M89.161 Complete physeal arrest, left proximal
                  tibia**
      **M89.162 Partial physeal arrest, right proximal
                  tibia**
      **M89.163 Partial physeal arrest, left proximal
                  tibia**
      **M89.164 Complete physeal arrest, right distal
                  tibia**
      **M89.165 Complete physeal arrest, left distal
                  tibia**
      **M89.166 Partial physeal arrest, right distal
                  tibia**
      M89.167 Partial physeal arrest, left distal tibia
      M89.168 Other physeal arrest of lower leg
      M89.169 Physeal arrest, lower leg, unspecified
   M89.18 Physeal arrest, other site

● **M89.2 Other disorders of bone development and growth**
   **M89.20 Other disorders of bone development and
              growth, unspecified site**
   ● **M89.21 Other disorders of bone development and
              growth, shoulder**
      **M89.211 Other disorders of bone development
                  and growth, right shoulder**
      **M89.212 Other disorders of bone development
                  and growth, left shoulder**
      **M89.219 Other disorders of bone development
                  and growth, unspecified shoulder**
   ● **M89.22 Other disorders of bone development and
              growth, humerus**
      **M89.221 Other disorders of bone development
                  and growth, right humerus**
      **M89.222 Other disorders of bone development
                  and growth, left humerus**
      **M89.229 Other disorders of bone development
                  and growth, unspecified humerus**
   ● **M89.23 Other disorders of bone development and
              growth, ulna and radius**
      **M89.231 Other disorders of bone development
                  and growth, right ulna**
      **M89.232 Other disorders of bone development
                  and growth, left ulna**
      **M89.233 Other disorders of bone development
                  and growth, right radius**
      **M89.234 Other disorders of bone development
                  and growth, left radius**
      **M89.239 Other disorders of bone development
                  and growth, unspecified ulna and
                  radius**
   ● **M89.24 Other disorders of bone development and
              growth, hand**
      **M89.241 Other disorders of bone development
                  and growth, right hand**
      **M89.242 Other disorders of bone development
                  and growth, left hand**
      **M89.249 Other disorders of bone development
                  and growth, unspecified hand**
   ● **M89.25 Other disorders of bone development and
              growth, femur**
      **M89.251 Other disorders of bone development
                  and growth, right femur**
      **M89.252 Other disorders of bone development
                  and growth, left femur**
      **M89.259 Other disorders of bone development
                  and growth, unspecified femur**
   ● **M89.26 Other disorders of bone development and
              growth, tibia and fibula**
      **M89.261 Other disorders of bone development
                  and growth, right tibia**
      **M89.262 Other disorders of bone development
                  and growth, left tibia**
      **M89.263 Other disorders of bone development
                  and growth, right fibula**
      **M89.264 Other disorders of bone development
                  and growth, left fibula**
      **M89.269 Other disorders of bone development
                  and growth, unspecified lower leg**
   ● **M89.27 Other disorders of bone development and
              growth, ankle and foot**
      **M89.271 Other disorders of bone development
                  and growth, right ankle and foot**
      **M89.272 Other disorders of bone development
                  and growth, left ankle and foot**
      **M89.279 Other disorders of bone development
                  and growth, unspecified ankle and
                  foot**

CHAPTER 13 (M00-M99)

▶ New   ⇒ Revised   ~~deleted~~ Deleted   Excludes 1   Excludes 2   Includes   Use additional   Code first   Code also   Key words

OGCR Official Guidelines   X Assign placeholder X   ● Use Additional Character(s)   �ష Manifestation Code   🗐 Hierarchical Condition Category   **Coding Clinic**

M89.28   Other disorders of bone development and growth, other site

M89.29   Other disorders of bone development and growth, multiple sites

● M89.3   **Hypertrophy of bone**

M89.30   Hypertrophy of bone, unspecified site

● M89.31   Hypertrophy of bone, shoulder

     M89.311   Hypertrophy of bone, right shoulder

     M89.312   Hypertrophy of bone, left shoulder

     M89.319   Hypertrophy of bone, unspecified shoulder

● M89.32   Hypertrophy of bone, humerus

     M89.321   Hypertrophy of bone, right humerus

     M89.322   Hypertrophy of bone, left humerus

     M89.329   Hypertrophy of bone, unspecified humerus

● M89.33   Hypertrophy of bone, ulna and radius

     M89.331   Hypertrophy of bone, right ulna

     M89.332   Hypertrophy of bone, left ulna

     M89.333   Hypertrophy of bone, right radius

     M89.334   Hypertrophy of bone, left radius

     M89.339   Hypertrophy of bone, unspecified ulna and radius

● M89.34   Hypertrophy of bone, hand

     M89.341   Hypertrophy of bone, right hand

     M89.342   Hypertrophy of bone, left hand

     M89.349   Hypertrophy of bone, unspecified hand

● M89.35   Hypertrophy of bone, femur

     M89.351   Hypertrophy of bone, right femur

     M89.352   Hypertrophy of bone, left femur

     M89.359   Hypertrophy of bone, unspecified femur

● M89.36   Hypertrophy of bone, tibia and fibula

     M89.361   Hypertrophy of bone, right tibia

     M89.362   Hypertrophy of bone, left tibia

     M89.363   Hypertrophy of bone, right fibula

     M89.364   Hypertrophy of bone, left fibula

     M89.369   Hypertrophy of bone, unspecified tibia and fibula

● M89.37   Hypertrophy of bone, ankle and foot

     M89.371   Hypertrophy of bone, right ankle and foot

     M89.372   Hypertrophy of bone, left ankle and foot

     M89.379   Hypertrophy of bone, unspecified ankle and foot

M89.38   Hypertrophy of bone, other site

M89.39   Hypertrophy of bone, multiple sites

● M89.4   **Other hypertrophic osteoarthropathy**
Marie-Bamberger disease
Pachydermoperiostosis

M89.40   Other hypertrophic osteoarthropathy, unspecified site

● M89.41   Other hypertrophic osteoarthropathy, shoulder

     M89.411   Other hypertrophic osteoarthropathy, right shoulder

     M89.412   Other hypertrophic osteoarthropathy, left shoulder

     M89.419   Other hypertrophic osteoarthropathy, unspecified shoulder

● M89.42   Other hypertrophic osteoarthropathy, upper arm

     M89.421   Other hypertrophic osteoarthropathy, right upper arm

     M89.422   Other hypertrophic osteoarthropathy, left upper arm

     M89.429   Other hypertrophic osteoarthropathy, unspecified upper arm

● M89.43   Other hypertrophic osteoarthropathy, forearm

     M89.431   Other hypertrophic osteoarthropathy, right forearm

     M89.432   Other hypertrophic osteoarthropathy, left forearm

     M89.439   Other hypertrophic osteoarthropathy, unspecified forearm

● M89.44   Other hypertrophic osteoarthropathy, hand

     M89.441   Other hypertrophic osteoarthropathy, right hand

     M89.442   Other hypertrophic osteoarthropathy, left hand

     M89.449   Other hypertrophic osteoarthropathy, unspecified hand

● M89.45   Other hypertrophic osteoarthropathy, thigh

     M89.451   Other hypertrophic osteoarthropathy, right thigh

     M89.452   Other hypertrophic osteoarthropathy, left thigh

     M89.459   Other hypertrophic osteoarthropathy, unspecified thigh

● M89.46   Other hypertrophic osteoarthropathy, lower leg

     M89.461   Other hypertrophic osteoarthropathy, right lower leg

     M89.462   Other hypertrophic osteoarthropathy, left lower leg

     M89.469   Other hypertrophic osteoarthropathy, unspecified lower leg

● M89.47   Other hypertrophic osteoarthropathy, ankle and foot

     M89.471   Other hypertrophic osteoarthropathy, right ankle and foot

     M89.472   Other hypertrophic osteoarthropathy, left ankle and foot

     M89.479   Other hypertrophic osteoarthropathy, unspecified ankle and foot

M89.48   Other hypertrophic osteoarthropathy, other site

M89.49   Other hypertrophic osteoarthropathy, multiple sites

● M89.5   **Osteolysis**

Use additional code to identify major osseous defect, if applicable (M89.7-)

Excludes2   periprosthetic osteolysis of internal prosthetic joint (T84.05-)

M89.50   Osteolysis, unspecified site

● M89.51   Osteolysis, shoulder

     M89.511   Osteolysis, right shoulder

     M89.512   Osteolysis, left shoulder

     M89.519   Osteolysis, unspecified shoulder

● M89.52   Osteolysis, upper arm

     M89.521   Osteolysis, right upper arm

     M89.522   Osteolysis, left upper arm

     M89.529   Osteolysis, unspecified upper arm

● M89.53   Osteolysis, forearm

     M89.531   Osteolysis, right forearm

     M89.532   Osteolysis, left forearm

     M89.539   Osteolysis, unspecified forearm

● M89.54   Osteolysis, hand

     M89.541   Osteolysis, right hand

     M89.542   Osteolysis, left hand

     M89.549   Osteolysis, unspecified hand

CHAPTER 13 (M00-M99)

● M89.55 Osteolysis, thigh
    M89.551 Osteolysis, right thigh
    M89.552 Osteolysis, left thigh
    M89.559 Osteolysis, unspecified thigh
● M89.56 Osteolysis, lower leg
    M89.561 Osteolysis, right lower leg
    M89.562 Osteolysis, left lower leg
    M89.569 Osteolysis, unspecified lower leg
● M89.57 Osteolysis, ankle and foot
    M89.571 Osteolysis, right ankle and foot
    M89.572 Osteolysis, left ankle and foot
    M89.579 Osteolysis, unspecified ankle and foot
M89.58 Osteolysis, other site
M89.59 Osteolysis, multiple sites

● M89.6 Osteopathy after poliomyelitis
    Use additional code (B91) to identify previous
    poliomyelitis
    Excludes1 postpolio syndrome (G14)
    M89.60 Osteopathy after poliomyelitis, unspecified
    site 🦠
● M89.61 Osteopathy after poliomyelitis, shoulder
    M89.611 Osteopathy after poliomyelitis, right
        shoulder 🦠
    M89.612 Osteopathy after poliomyelitis, left
        shoulder 🦠
    M89.619 Osteopathy after poliomyelitis,
        unspecified shoulder 🦠
● M89.62 Osteopathy after poliomyelitis, upper arm
    M89.621 Osteopathy after poliomyelitis, right
        upper arm 🦠
    M89.622 Osteopathy after poliomyelitis, left
        upper arm 🦠
    M89.629 Osteopathy after poliomyelitis,
        unspecified upper arm 🦠
● M89.63 Osteopathy after poliomyelitis, forearm
    M89.631 Osteopathy after poliomyelitis, right
        forearm 🦠
    M89.632 Osteopathy after poliomyelitis, left
        forearm 🦠
    M89.639 Osteopathy after poliomyelitis,
        unspecified forearm 🦠
● M89.64 Osteopathy after poliomyelitis, hand
    M89.641 Osteopathy after poliomyelitis, right
        hand 🦠
    M89.642 Osteopathy after poliomyelitis, left
        hand 🦠
    M89.649 Osteopathy after poliomyelitis,
        unspecified hand 🦠
● M89.65 Osteopathy after poliomyelitis, thigh
    M89.651 Osteopathy after poliomyelitis, right
        thigh 🦠
    M89.652 Osteopathy after poliomyelitis, left
        thigh 🦠
    M89.659 Osteopathy after poliomyelitis,
        unspecified thigh 🦠
● M89.66 Osteopathy after poliomyelitis, lower leg
    M89.661 Osteopathy after poliomyelitis, right
        lower leg 🦠
    M89.662 Osteopathy after poliomyelitis, left
        lower leg 🦠
    M89.669 Osteopathy after poliomyelitis,
        unspecified lower leg 🦠
● M89.67 Osteopathy after poliomyelitis, ankle and foot
    M89.671 Osteopathy after poliomyelitis, right
        ankle and foot 🦠

    M89.672 Osteopathy after poliomyelitis, left
        ankle and foot 🦠
    M89.679 Osteopathy after poliomyelitis,
        unspecified ankle and foot 🦠
M89.68 Osteopathy after poliomyelitis, other site 🦠
M89.69 Osteopathy after poliomyelitis, multiple
    sites 🦠

● M89.7 Major osseous defect
    Code first underlying disease, if known, such as:
      aseptic necrosis of bone (M87.-)
      malignant neoplasm of bone (C40.-)
      osteolysis (M89.5)
      osteomyelitis (M86.-)
      osteonecrosis (M87.-)
      osteoporosis (M80.-, M81.-)
      periprosthetic osteolysis (T84.05-)
M89.70 Major osseous defect, unspecified site
● M89.71 Major osseous defect, shoulder region
    Major osseous defect clavicle or scapula
    M89.711 Major osseous defect, right shoulder
        region
    M89.712 Major osseous defect, left shoulder
        region
    M89.719 Major osseous defect, unspecified
        shoulder region
● M89.72 Major osseous defect, humerus
    M89.721 Major osseous defect, right humerus
    M89.722 Major osseous defect, left humerus
    M89.729 Major osseous defect, unspecified
        humerus
● M89.73 Major osseous defect, forearm
    Major osseous defect of radius and ulna
    M89.731 Major osseous defect, right forearm
    M89.732 Major osseous defect, left forearm
    M89.739 Major osseous defect, unspecified
        forearm
● M89.74 Major osseous defect, hand
    Major osseous defect of carpus, fingers,
      metacarpus
    M89.741 Major osseous defect, right hand
    M89.742 Major osseous defect, left hand
    M89.749 Major osseous defect, unspecified
        hand
● M89.75 Major osseous defect, pelvic region and thigh
    Major osseous defect of femur and pelvis
    M89.751 Major osseous defect, right pelvic
        region and thigh
    M89.752 Major osseous defect, left pelvic
        region and thigh
    M89.759 Major osseous defect, unspecified
        pelvic region and thigh
● M89.76 Major osseous defect, lower leg
    Major osseous defect of fibula and tibia
    M89.761 Major osseous defect, right lower leg
    M89.762 Major osseous defect, left lower leg
    M89.769 Major osseous defect, unspecified
        lower leg
● M89.77 Major osseous defect, ankle and foot
    Major osseous defect of metatarsus, tarsus, toes
    M89.771 Major osseous defect, right ankle and
        foot
    M89.772 Major osseous defect, left ankle and
        foot
    M89.779 Major osseous defect, unspecified
        ankle and foot
M89.78 Major osseous defect, other site
M89.79 Major osseous defect, multiple sites

CHAPTER 13 (M00-M99)

▶ New   ⇒ Revised   ~~deleted~~ Deleted   Excludes 1   Excludes 2   Includes   Use additional   Code first   Code also   Key words

OGCR Official Guidelines   X Assign placeholder X   ● Use Additional Character(s)   ▶ Manifestation Code   🦠 Hierarchical Condition Category   **Coding Clinic**

● **M89.8 Other specified disorders of bone**
Infantile cortical hyperostoses
Post-traumatic subperiosteal ossification
Coding Clinic: 2022, Q2, P10
  ● **M89.8X Other specified disorders of bone**
      M89.8X0 Other specified disorders of bone, multiple sites
      M89.8X1 Other specified disorders of bone, shoulder
      M89.8X2 Other specified disorders of bone, upper arm
      M89.8X3 Other specified disorders of bone, forearm
      Coding Clinic: 2019, Q3, P10
      M89.8X4 Other specified disorders of bone, hand
      M89.8X5 Other specified disorders of bone, thigh
      M89.8X6 Other specified disorders of bone, lower leg
      M89.8X7 Other specified disorders of bone, ankle and foot
      M89.8X8 Other specified disorders of bone, other site
      M89.8X9 Other specified disorders of bone, unspecified site

  M89.9 Disorder of bone, unspecified

● **M90 Osteopathies in diseases classified elsewhere**
  Excludes1 osteochondritis, osteomyelitis, and osteopathy (in):
      cryptococcosis (B45.3)
      diabetes mellitus (E08-E13 with .69-)
      gonococcal (A54.43)
      neurogenic syphilis (A52.11)
      renal osteodystrophy (N25.0)
      salmonellosis (A02.24)
      secondary syphilis (A51.46)
      syphilis (late) (A52.77)

● **M90.5 Osteonecrosis in diseases classified elsewhere**
  Code first underlying disease, such as:
      caisson disease (T70.3)
      hemoglobinopathy (D50-D64)
  ▷ *M90.50 Osteonecrosis in diseases classified elsewhere, unspecified site*
  ● **M90.51 Osteonecrosis in diseases classified elsewhere, shoulder**
      ▷ *M90.511 Osteonecrosis in diseases classified elsewhere, right shoulder*
      ▷ *M90.512 Osteonecrosis in diseases classified elsewhere, left shoulder*
      ▷ *M90.519 Osteonecrosis in diseases classified elsewhere, unspecified shoulder*
  ● **M90.52 Osteonecrosis in diseases classified elsewhere, upper arm**
      ▷ *M90.521 Osteonecrosis in diseases classified elsewhere, right upper arm*
      ▷ *M90.522 Osteonecrosis in diseases classified elsewhere, left upper arm*
      ▷ *M90.529 Osteonecrosis in diseases classified elsewhere, unspecified upper arm*
  ● **M90.53 Osteonecrosis in diseases classified elsewhere, forearm**
      ▷ *M90.531 Osteonecrosis in diseases classified elsewhere, right forearm*
      ▷ *M90.532 Osteonecrosis in diseases classified elsewhere, left forearm*
      ▷ *M90.539 Osteonecrosis in diseases classified elsewhere, unspecified forearm*

● **M90.54 Osteonecrosis in diseases classified elsewhere, hand**
  ▷ *M90.541 Osteonecrosis in diseases classified elsewhere, right hand*
  ▷ *M90.542 Osteonecrosis in diseases classified elsewhere, left hand*
  ▷ *M90.549 Osteonecrosis in diseases classified elsewhere, unspecified hand*
● **M90.55 Osteonecrosis in diseases classified elsewhere, thigh**
  ▷ *M90.551 Osteonecrosis in diseases classified elsewhere, right thigh*
  ▷ *M90.552 Osteonecrosis in diseases classified elsewhere, left thigh*
  ▷ *M90.559 Osteonecrosis in diseases classified elsewhere, unspecified thigh*
● **M90.56 Osteonecrosis in diseases classified elsewhere, lower leg**
  ▷ *M90.561 Osteonecrosis in diseases classified elsewhere, right lower leg*
  ▷ *M90.562 Osteonecrosis in diseases classified elsewhere, left lower leg*
  ▷ *M90.569 Osteonecrosis in diseases classified elsewhere, unspecified lower leg*
● **M90.57 Osteonecrosis in diseases classified elsewhere, ankle and foot**
  ▷ *M90.571 Osteonecrosis in diseases classified elsewhere, right ankle and foot*
  ▷ *M90.572 Osteonecrosis in diseases classified elsewhere, left ankle and foot*
  ▷ *M90.579 Osteonecrosis in diseases classified elsewhere, unspecified ankle and foot*
  ▷ *M90.58 Osteonecrosis in diseases classified elsewhere, other site*
  ▷ *M90.59 Osteonecrosis in diseases classified elsewhere, multiple sites*
● **M90.6 Osteitis deformans in neoplastic diseases**
  Osteitis deformans in malignant neoplasm of bone
  Code first the neoplasm (C40.-, C41.-)
  Excludes1 osteitis deformans [Paget's disease of bone] (M88.-)
  ▷ *M90.60 Osteitis deformans in neoplastic diseases, unspecified site*
  ● **M90.61 Osteitis deformans in neoplastic diseases, shoulder**
      ▷ *M90.611 Osteitis deformans in neoplastic diseases, right shoulder*
      ▷ *M90.612 Osteitis deformans in neoplastic diseases, left shoulder*
      ▷ *M90.619 Osteitis deformans in neoplastic diseases, unspecified shoulder*
  ● **M90.62 Osteitis deformans in neoplastic diseases, upper arm**
      ▷ *M90.621 Osteitis deformans in neoplastic diseases, right upper arm*
      ▷ *M90.622 Osteitis deformans in neoplastic diseases, left upper arm*
      ▷ *M90.629 Osteitis deformans in neoplastic diseases, unspecified upper arm*
  ● **M90.63 Osteitis deformans in neoplastic diseases, forearm**
      ▷ *M90.631 Osteitis deformans in neoplastic diseases, right forearm*
      ▷ *M90.632 Osteitis deformans in neoplastic diseases, left forearm*
      ▷ *M90.639 Osteitis deformans in neoplastic diseases, unspecified forearm*

CHAPTER 13 (M00-M99)

● **M90.64** Osteitis deformans in neoplastic diseases, hand

▶ *M90.641* *Osteitis deformans in neoplastic diseases, right hand*

▶ *M90.642* *Osteitis deformans in neoplastic diseases, left hand*

▶ *M90.649* *Osteitis deformans in neoplastic diseases, unspecified hand*

● **M90.65** Osteitis deformans in neoplastic diseases, thigh

▶ *M90.651* *Osteitis deformans in neoplastic diseases, right thigh*

▶ *M90.652* *Osteitis deformans in neoplastic diseases, left thigh*

▶ *M90.659* *Osteitis deformans in neoplastic diseases, unspecified thigh*

● **M90.66** Osteitis deformans in neoplastic diseases, lower leg

▶ *M90.661* *Osteitis deformans in neoplastic diseases, right lower leg*

▶ *M90.662* *Osteitis deformans in neoplastic diseases, left lower leg*

▶ *M90.669* *Osteitis deformans in neoplastic diseases, unspecified lower leg*

● **M90.67** Osteitis deformans in neoplastic diseases, ankle and foot

▶ *M90.671* *Osteitis deformans in neoplastic diseases, right ankle and foot*

▶ *M90.672* *Osteitis deformans in neoplastic diseases, left ankle and foot*

▶ *M90.679* *Osteitis deformans in neoplastic diseases, unspecified ankle and foot*

▶ *M90.68* *Osteitis deformans in neoplastic diseases, other site*

▶ *M90.69* *Osteitis deformans in neoplastic diseases, multiple sites*

● **M90.8** Osteopathy in diseases classified elsewhere

Code first underlying disease, such as:
rickets (E55.0)
vitamin-D-resistant rickets (E83.3)

▶ *M90.80* *Osteopathy in diseases classified elsewhere, unspecified site*

● **M90.81** Osteopathy in diseases classified elsewhere, shoulder

▶ *M90.811* *Osteopathy in diseases classified elsewhere, right shoulder*

▶ *M90.812* *Osteopathy in diseases classified elsewhere, left shoulder*

▶ *M90.819* *Osteopathy in diseases classified elsewhere, unspecified shoulder*

● **M90.82** Osteopathy in diseases classified elsewhere, upper arm

▶ *M90.821* *Osteopathy in diseases classified elsewhere, right upper arm*

▶ *M90.822* *Osteopathy in diseases classified elsewhere, left upper arm*

▶ *M90.829* *Osteopathy in diseases classified elsewhere, unspecified upper arm*

● **M90.83** Osteopathy in diseases classified elsewhere, forearm

▶ *M90.831* *Osteopathy in diseases classified elsewhere, right forearm*

▶ *M90.832* *Osteopathy in diseases classified elsewhere, left forearm*

▶ *M90.839* *Osteopathy in diseases classified elsewhere, unspecified forearm*

● **M90.84** Osteopathy in diseases classified elsewhere, hand

▶ *M90.841* *Osteopathy in diseases classified elsewhere, right hand*

▶ *M90.842* *Osteopathy in diseases classified elsewhere, left hand*

▶ *M90.849* *Osteopathy in diseases classified elsewhere, unspecified hand*

● **M90.85** Osteopathy in diseases classified elsewhere, thigh

▶ *M90.851* *Osteopathy in diseases classified elsewhere, right thigh*

▶ *M90.852* *Osteopathy in diseases classified elsewhere, left thigh*

▶ *M90.859* *Osteopathy in diseases classified elsewhere, unspecified thigh*

● **M90.86** Osteopathy in diseases classified elsewhere, lower leg

▶ *M90.861* *Osteopathy in diseases classified elsewhere, right lower leg*

▶ *M90.862* *Osteopathy in diseases classified elsewhere, left lower leg*

▶ *M90.869* *Osteopathy in diseases classified elsewhere, unspecified lower leg*

● **M90.87** Osteopathy in diseases classified elsewhere, ankle and foot

▶ *M90.871* *Osteopathy in diseases classified elsewhere, right ankle and foot*

▶ *M90.872* *Osteopathy in diseases classified elsewhere, left ankle and foot*

▶ *M90.879* *Osteopathy in diseases classified elsewhere, unspecified ankle and foot*

▶ *M90.88* *Osteopathy in diseases classified elsewhere, other site*

▶ *M90.89* *Osteopathy in diseases classified elsewhere, multiple sites*

CHONDROPATHIES (M91-M94)

Excludes1   postprocedural chondropathies (M96.-)

● **M91** Juvenile osteochondrosis of hip and pelvis

⇒ **Excludes1**   slipped upper femoral epiphysis (nontraumatic) (M93.0-)

M91.0 Juvenile osteochondrosis of pelvis
Osteochondrosis (juvenile) of acetabulum
Osteochondrosis (juvenile) of iliac crest [Buchanan]
Osteochondrosis (juvenile) of ischiopubic synchondrosis [van Neck]
Osteochondrosis (juvenile) of symphysis pubis [Pierson]

● **M91.1** Juvenile osteochondrosis of head of femur [Legg-Calvé-Perthes]

M91.10 Juvenile osteochondrosis of head of femur [Legg-Calvé-Perthes], unspecified leg

M91.11 Juvenile osteochondrosis of head of femur [Legg-Calvé-Perthes], right leg

M91.12 Juvenile osteochondrosis of head of femur [Legg-Calvé-Perthes], left leg

● **M91.2** Coxa plana
Hip deformity due to previous juvenile osteochondrosis

M91.20 Coxa plana, unspecified hip

M91.21 Coxa plana, right hip

M91.22 Coxa plana, left hip

● **M91.3** Pseudocoxalgia

M91.30 Pseudocoxalgia, unspecified hip

M91.31 Pseudocoxalgia, right hip

M91.32 Pseudocoxalgia, left hip

● **M91.4** Coxa magna

M91.40 Coxa magna, unspecified hip

M91.41 Coxa magna, right hip

M91.42 Coxa magna, left hip

▶ New   ⇒ Revised   ~~deleted~~ Deleted   Excludes 1   Excludes 2   Includes   Use additional   Code first   Code also   Key words

OGCR Official Guidelines   X Assign placeholder X   ● Use Additional Character(s)   ▶ Manifestation Code   🅗 Hierarchical Condition Category   **Coding Clinic**

● **M91.8** Other juvenile osteochondrosis of hip and pelvis
Juvenile osteochondrosis after reduction of congenital dislocation of hip

   M91.80 Other juvenile osteochondrosis of hip and pelvis, unspecified leg

   M91.81 Other juvenile osteochondrosis of hip and pelvis, right leg

   M91.82 Other juvenile osteochondrosis of hip and pelvis, left leg

● **M91.9** Juvenile osteochondrosis of hip and pelvis, unspecified

   M91.90 Juvenile osteochondrosis of hip and pelvis, unspecified, unspecified leg

   M91.91 Juvenile osteochondrosis of hip and pelvis, unspecified, right leg

   M91.92 Juvenile osteochondrosis of hip and pelvis, unspecified, left leg

● **M92** Other juvenile osteochondrosis

 ● **M92.0** Juvenile osteochondrosis of humerus
Osteochondrosis (juvenile) of capitulum of humerus [Panner]
Osteochondrosis (juvenile) of head of humerus [Haas]

   M92.00 Juvenile osteochondrosis of humerus, unspecified arm

   M92.01 Juvenile osteochondrosis of humerus, right arm

   M92.02 Juvenile osteochondrosis of humerus, left arm

 ● **M92.1** Juvenile osteochondrosis of radius and ulna
Osteochondrosis (juvenile) of lower ulna [Burns]
Osteochondrosis (juvenile) of radial head [Brailsford]

   M92.10 Juvenile osteochondrosis of radius and ulna, unspecified arm

   M92.11 Juvenile osteochondrosis of radius and ulna, right arm

   M92.12 Juvenile osteochondrosis of radius and ulna, left arm

 ● **M92.2** Juvenile osteochondrosis, hand

  ● **M92.20** Unspecified juvenile osteochondrosis, hand

    M92.201 Unspecified juvenile osteochondrosis, right hand

    M92.202 Unspecified juvenile osteochondrosis, left hand

    M92.209 Unspecified juvenile osteochondrosis, unspecified hand

  ● **M92.21** Osteochondrosis (juvenile) of carpal lunate [Kienböck]

    M92.211 Osteochondrosis (juvenile) of carpal lunate [Kienböck], right hand

    M92.212 Osteochondrosis (juvenile) of carpal lunate [Kienböck], left hand

    M92.219 Osteochondrosis (juvenile) of carpal lunate [Kienböck], unspecified hand

  ● **M92.22** Osteochondrosis (juvenile) of metacarpal heads [Mauclaire]

    M92.221 Osteochondrosis (juvenile) of metacarpal heads [Mauclaire], right hand

    M92.222 Osteochondrosis (juvenile) of metacarpal heads [Mauclaire], left hand

    M92.229 Osteochondrosis (juvenile) of metacarpal heads [Mauclaire], unspecified hand

  ● **M92.29** Other juvenile osteochondrosis, hand

    M92.291 Other juvenile osteochondrosis, right hand

    M92.292 Other juvenile osteochondrosis, left hand

    M92.299 Other juvenile osteochondrosis, unspecified hand

● **M92.3** Other juvenile osteochondrosis, upper limb

   M92.30 Other juvenile osteochondrosis, unspecified upper limb

   M92.31 Other juvenile osteochondrosis, right upper limb

   M92.32 Other juvenile osteochondrosis, left upper limb

● **M92.4** Juvenile osteochondrosis of patella
Osteochondrosis (juvenile) of primary patellar center [Köhler]
Osteochondrosis (juvenile) of secondary patellar center [Sinding Larsen]

   M92.40 Juvenile osteochondrosis of patella, unspecified knee

   M92.41 Juvenile osteochondrosis of patella, right knee

   M92.42 Juvenile osteochondrosis of patella, left knee

● **M92.5** Juvenile osteochondrosis of tibia and fibula

 ● **M92.50** Unspecified juvenile osteochondrosis of tibia and fibula

    M92.501 Unspecified juvenile osteochondrosis, right leg

    M92.502 Unspecified juvenile osteochondrosis, left leg

    M92.503 Unspecified juvenile osteochondrosis, bilateral leg

    M92.509 Unspecified juvenile osteochondrosis, unspecified leg

 ● **M92.51** Juvenile osteochondrosis of proximal tibia
Blount disease
Tibia vara

    M92.511 Juvenile osteochondrosis of proximal tibia, right leg

    M92.512 Juvenile osteochondrosis of proximal tibia, left leg

    M92.513 Juvenile osteochondrosis of proximal tibia, bilateral

    M92.519 Juvenile osteochondrosis of proximal tibia, unspecified leg

 ● **M92.52** Juvenile osteochondrosis of tibia tubercle
Osgood-Schlatter disease

    M92.521 Juvenile osteochondrosis of tibia tubercle, right leg

    M92.522 Juvenile osteochondrosis of tibia tubercle, left leg

    M92.523 Juvenile osteochondrosis of tibia tubercle, bilateral

    M92.529 Juvenile osteochondrosis of tibia tubercle, unspecified leg

   M92.59 Other juvenile osteochondrosis of tibia and fibula

    M92.591 Other juvenile osteochondrosis of tibia and fibula, right leg

    M92.592 Other juvenile osteochondrosis of tibia and fibula, left leg

    M92.593 Other juvenile osteochondrosis of tibia and fibula, bilateral

    M92.599 Other juvenile osteochondrosis of tibia and fibula, unspecified leg

● **M92.6** Juvenile osteochondrosis of tarsus
Osteochondrosis (juvenile) of calcaneum [Sever]
Osteochondrosis (juvenile) of os tibiale externum [Haglund]
Osteochondrosis (juvenile) of talus [Diaz]
Osteochondrosis (juvenile) of tarsal navicular [Köhler]

   M92.60 Juvenile osteochondrosis of tarsus, unspecified ankle

   M92.61 Juvenile osteochondrosis of tarsus, right ankle

   M92.62 Juvenile osteochondrosis of tarsus, left ankle

CHAPTER 13 (M00-M99)

● M92.7   Juvenile osteochondrosis of metatarsus
     Osteochondrosis (juvenile) of fifth metatarsus [Iselin]
     Osteochondrosis (juvenile) of second metatarsus [Freiberg]

     M92.70   Juvenile osteochondrosis of metatarsus, **unspecified** foot

     M92.71   Juvenile osteochondrosis of metatarsus, **right** foot

     M92.72   Juvenile osteochondrosis of metatarsus, **left** foot

   M92.8   Other specified juvenile osteochondrosis
     Calcaneal apophysitis

   M92.9   Juvenile osteochondrosis, **unspecified**
     Juvenile apophysitis NOS
     Juvenile epiphysitis NOS
     Juvenile osteochondritis NOS
     Juvenile osteochondrosis NOS

● M93   Other osteochondropathies
     Excludes2   osteochondrosis of spine (M42.-)

● M93.0   Slipped upper femoral epiphysis (nontraumatic)
     ▶ Slipped capital femoral epiphysis (SCFE)
     ▶ Slipped upper femoral epiphysis (SUFE)
     Use additional code for associated chondrolysis (M94.3)

● M93.00   **Unspecified** slipped upper femoral epiphysis (nontraumatic)

     M93.001   Unspecified slipped upper femoral epiphysis (nontraumatic), **right** hip

     M93.002   Unspecified slipped upper femoral epiphysis (nontraumatic), **left** hip

     M93.003   Unspecified slipped upper femoral epiphysis (nontraumatic), **unspecified** hip

     ▶ M93.004   Unspecified slipped upper femoral epiphysis (nontraumatic), bilateral hips

⇒ ● M93.01   Acute slipped upper femoral epiphysis, stable (nontraumatic)

     ⇒ M93.011   Acute slipped upper femoral epiphysis, stable (nontraumatic), **right** hip

     ⇒ M93.012   Acute slipped upper femoral epiphysis, stable (nontraumatic), **left** hip

     ⇒ M93.013   Acute slipped upper femoral epiphysis, stable (nontraumatic), **unspecified** hip

     ▶ M93.014   Acute slipped upper femoral epiphysis, stable (nontraumatic), bilateral hips

⇒ ● M93.02   Chronic slipped upper femoral epiphysis, stable (nontraumatic)

     ⇒ M93.021   Chronic slipped upper femoral epiphysis, stable (nontraumatic), **right** hip

     ⇒ M93.022   Chronic slipped upper femoral epiphysis, stable (nontraumatic), **left** hip

     ⇒ M93.023   Chronic slipped upper femoral epiphysis, stable (nontraumatic), **unspecified** hip

     ▶ M93.024   Chronic slipped upper femoral epiphysis, stable (nontraumatic), bilateral hips

⇒ ● M93.03   Acute on chronic slipped upper femoral epiphysis, stable (nontraumatic)

     ⇒ M93.031   Acute on chronic slipped upper femoral epiphysis, stable (nontraumatic), **right** hip

     ⇒ M93.032   Acute on chronic slipped upper femoral epiphysis, stable (nontraumatic), **left** hip

⇒ M93.033   Acute on chronic slipped upper femoral epiphysis, stable (nontraumatic), **unspecified** hip

▶ M93.034   Acute on chronic slipped upper femoral epiphysis, stable (nontraumatic), bilateral hips

▶ ● M93.04   Acute slipped upper femoral epiphysis, unstable (nontraumatic)

     ▶ M93.041   Acute slipped upper femoral epiphysis, unstable (nontraumatic), right hip

     ▶ M93.042   Acute slipped upper femoral epiphysis, unstable (nontraumatic), left hip

     ▶ M93.043   Acute slipped upper femoral epiphysis, unstable (nontraumatic), unspecified hip

     ▶ M93.044   Acute slipped upper femoral epiphysis, unstable (nontraumatic), bilateral hips

▶ ● M93.05   Acute on chronic slipped upper femoral epiphysis, unstable (nontraumatic)

     ▶ M93.051   Acute on chronic slipped upper femoral epiphysis, unstable (nontraumatic), right hip

     ▶ M93.052   Acute on chronic slipped upper femoral epiphysis, unstable (nontraumatic), left hip

     ▶ M93.053   Acute on chronic slipped upper femoral epiphysis, unstable (nontraumatic), unspecified hip

     ▶ M93.054   Acute on chronic slipped upper femoral epiphysis, unstable (nontraumatic), bilateral hips

▶ ● M93.06   Acute slipped upper femoral epiphysis, unspecified stability (nontraumatic)

     ▶ M93.061   Acute slipped upper femoral epiphysis, unspecified stability (nontraumatic), right hip

     ▶ M93.062   Acute slipped upper femoral epiphysis, unspecified stability (nontraumatic), left hip

     ▶ M93.063   Acute slipped upper femoral epiphysis, unspecified stability (nontraumatic), unspecified hip

     ▶ M93.064   Acute slipped upper femoral epiphysis, unspecified stability (nontraumatic), bilateral hips

▶ ● M93.07   Acute on chronic slipped upper femoral epiphysis, unspecified stability (nontraumatic)

     ▶ M93.071   Acute on chronic slipped upper femoral epiphysis, unspecified stability (nontraumatic), right hip

     ▶ M93.072   Acute on chronic slipped upper femoral epiphysis, unspecified stability (nontraumatic), left hip

     ▶ M93.073   Acute on chronic slipped upper femoral epiphysis, unspecified stability (nontraumatic), unspecified hip

     ▶ M93.074   Acute on chronic slipped upper femoral epiphysis, unspecified stability (nontraumatic), bilateral hips

   M93.1   Kienböck's disease of adults   A
     Adult osteochondrosis of carpal lunates

● M93.2   Osteochondritis dissecans

     M93.20   Osteochondritis dissecans of **unspecified** site

   ● M93.21   Osteochondritis dissecans of **shoulder**

     M93.211   Osteochondritis dissecans, **right** shoulder

● M93.212 Osteochondritis dissecans, left shoulder

M93.219 Osteochondritis dissecans, unspecified shoulder

● M93.22 Osteochondritis dissecans of elbow

M93.221 Osteochondritis dissecans, right elbow

M93.222 Osteochondritis dissecans, left elbow

M93.229 Osteochondritis dissecans, unspecified elbow

● M93.23 Osteochondritis dissecans of wrist

M93.231 Osteochondritis dissecans, right wrist

M93.232 Osteochondritis dissecans, left wrist

M93.239 Osteochondritis dissecans, unspecified wrist

● M93.24 Osteochondritis dissecans of joints of hand

M93.241 Osteochondritis dissecans, joints of right hand

M93.242 Osteochondritis dissecans, joints of left hand

M93.249 Osteochondritis dissecans, joints of unspecified hand

● M93.25 Osteochondritis dissecans of hip

M93.251 Osteochondritis dissecans, right hip

M93.252 Osteochondritis dissecans, left hip

M93.259 Osteochondritis dissecans, unspecified hip

● M93.26 Osteochondritis dissecans knee

M93.261 Osteochondritis dissecans, right knee

M93.262 Osteochondritis dissecans, left knee

M93.269 Osteochondritis dissecans, unspecified knee

● M93.27 Osteochondritis dissecans of ankle and joints of foot

M93.271 Osteochondritis dissecans, right ankle and joints of right foot

M93.272 Osteochondritis dissecans, left ankle and joints of left foot

M93.279 Osteochondritis dissecans, unspecified ankle and joints of foot

M93.28 Osteochondritis dissecans other site

M93.29 Osteochondritis dissecans multiple sites

● M93.8 Other specified osteochondropathies

M93.80 Other specified osteochondropathies of unspecified site

● M93.81 Other specified osteochondropathies of shoulder

M93.811 Other specified osteochondropathies, right shoulder

M93.812 Other specified osteochondropathies, left shoulder

M93.819 Other specified osteochondropathies, unspecified shoulder

● M93.82 Other specified osteochondropathies of upper arm

M93.821 Other specified osteochondropathies, right upper arm

M93.822 Other specified osteochondropathies, left upper arm

M93.829 Other specified osteochondropathies, unspecified upper arm

● M93.83 Other specified osteochondropathies of forearm

M93.831 Other specified osteochondropathies, right forearm

M93.832 Other specified osteochondropathies, left forearm

M93.839 Other specified osteochondropathies, unspecified forearm

● M93.84 Other specified osteochondropathies of hand

M93.841 Other specified osteochondropathies, right hand

M93.842 Other specified osteochondropathies, left hand

M93.849 Other specified osteochondropathies, unspecified hand

● M93.85 Other specified osteochondropathies of thigh

M93.851 Other specified osteochondropathies, right thigh

M93.852 Other specified osteochondropathies, left thigh

M93.859 Other specified osteochondropathies, unspecified thigh

● M93.86 Other specified osteochondropathies lower leg

M93.861 Other specified osteochondropathies, right lower leg

M93.862 Other specified osteochondropathies, left lower leg

M93.869 Other specified osteochondropathies, unspecified lower leg

● M93.87 Other specified osteochondropathies of ankle and foot

M93.871 Other specified osteochondropathies, right ankle and foot

M93.872 Other specified osteochondropathies, left ankle and foot

M93.879 Other specified osteochondropathies, unspecified ankle and foot

M93.88 Other specified osteochondropathies other

M93.89 Other specified osteochondropathies multiple sites

M93.9 Osteochondropathy, unspecified
Apophysitis NOS
Epiphysitis NOS
Osteochondritis NOS
Osteochondrosis NOS

M93.90 Osteochondropathy, unspecified of unspecified site

● M93.91 Osteochondropathy, unspecified of shoulder

M93.911 Osteochondropathy, unspecified, right shoulder

M93.912 Osteochondropathy, unspecified, left shoulder

M93.919 Osteochondropathy, unspecified, unspecified shoulder

● M93.92 Osteochondropathy, unspecified of upper arm

M93.921 Osteochondropathy, unspecified, right upper arm

M93.922 Osteochondropathy, unspecified, left upper arm

M93.929 Osteochondropathy, unspecified, unspecified upper arm

● M93.93 Osteochondropathy, unspecified of forearm

M93.931 Osteochondropathy, unspecified, right forearm

M93.932 Osteochondropathy, unspecified, left forearm

M93.939 Osteochondropathy, unspecified, unspecified forearm

● M93.94 Osteochondropathy, unspecified of hand

M93.941 Osteochondropathy, unspecified, right hand

M93.942 Osteochondropathy, unspecified, left hand

M93.949 Osteochondropathy, unspecified, unspecified hand

CHAPTER 13 (M00-M99)

● M93.95   Osteochondropathy, unspecified of thigh

     M93.951   Osteochondropathy, unspecified, right thigh

     M93.952   Osteochondropathy, unspecified, left thigh

     M93.959   Osteochondropathy, unspecified, unspecified thigh

● M93.96   Osteochondropathy, unspecified lower leg

     M93.961   Osteochondropathy, unspecified, right lower leg

     M93.962   Osteochondropathy, unspecified, left lower leg

     M93.969   Osteochondropathy, unspecified, unspecified lower leg

● M93.97   Osteochondropathy, unspecified of ankle and foot

     M93.971   Osteochondropathy, unspecified, right ankle and foot

     M93.972   Osteochondropathy, unspecified, left ankle and foot

     M93.979   Osteochondropathy, unspecified, unspecified ankle and foot

   M93.98   Osteochondropathy, unspecified other

   M93.99   Osteochondropathy, unspecified multiple sites

● M94   Other disorders of cartilage

   M94.0   Chondrocostal junction syndrome [Tietze]
      Costochondritis

   M94.1   Relapsing polychondritis

● M94.2   Chondromalacia

     Excludes1   chondromalacia patellae (M22.4)

   M94.20   Chondromalacia, unspecified site

● M94.21   Chondromalacia, shoulder

     M94.211   Chondromalacia, right shoulder

     M94.212   Chondromalacia, left shoulder

     M94.219   Chondromalacia, unspecified shoulder

● M94.22   Chondromalacia, elbow

     M94.221   Chondromalacia, right elbow

     M94.222   Chondromalacia, left elbow

     M94.229   Chondromalacia, unspecified elbow

● M94.23   Chondromalacia, wrist

     M94.231   Chondromalacia, right wrist

     M94.232   Chondromalacia, left wrist

     M94.239   Chondromalacia, unspecified wrist

● M94.24   Chondromalacia, joints of hand

     M94.241   Chondromalacia, joints of right hand

     M94.242   Chondromalacia, joints of left hand

     M94.249   Chondromalacia, joints of unspecified hand

● M94.25   Chondromalacia, hip

     M94.251   Chondromalacia, right hip

     M94.252   Chondromalacia, left hip

     M94.259   Chondromalacia, unspecified hip

● M94.26   Chondromalacia, knee

     M94.261   Chondromalacia, right knee

     M94.262   Chondromalacia, left knee

     M94.269   Chondromalacia, unspecified knee

● M94.27   Chondromalacia, ankle and joints of foot

     M94.271   Chondromalacia, right ankle and joints of right foot

     M94.272   Chondromalacia, left ankle and joints of left foot

     M94.279   Chondromalacia, unspecified ankle and joints of foot

   M94.28   Chondromalacia, other site

   M94.29   Chondromalacia, multiple sites

● M94.3   Chondrolysis

     Code first any associated slipped upper femoral epiphysis (nontraumatic) (M93.0-)

● M94.35   Chondrolysis, hip

     M94.351   Chondrolysis, right hip

     M94.352   Chondrolysis, left hip

     M94.359   Chondrolysis, unspecified hip

● M94.8   Other specified disorders of cartilage

● M94.8X   Other specified disorders of cartilage

     M94.8X0   Other specified disorders of cartilage, multiple sites

     M94.8X1   Other specified disorders of cartilage, shoulder

     M94.8X2   Other specified disorders of cartilage, upper arm

     M94.8X3   Other specified disorders of cartilage, forearm

     M94.8X4   Other specified disorders of cartilage, hand

     M94.8X5   Other specified disorders of cartilage, thigh

     M94.8X6   Other specified disorders of cartilage, lower leg

     M94.8X7   Other specified disorders of cartilage, ankle and foot

     M94.8X8   Other specified disorders of cartilage, other site

     M94.8X9   Other specified disorders of cartilage, unspecified sites

   M94.9   Disorder of cartilage, unspecified

OTHER DISORDERS OF THE MUSCULOSKELETAL SYSTEM AND CONNECTIVE TISSUE (M95)

● M95   Other acquired deformities of musculoskeletal system and connective tissue

     Excludes2   acquired absence of limbs and organs (Z89-Z90)
         acquired deformities of limbs (M20-M21)
         congenital malformations and deformations of the musculoskeletal system (Q65-Q79)
         deforming dorsopathies (M40-M43)
         dentofacial anomalies [including malocclusion] (M26.-)
         postprocedural musculoskeletal disorders (M96.-)

   M95.0   Acquired deformity of nose

     Excludes2   deviated nasal septum (J34.2)

● M95.1   Cauliflower ear

     Excludes2   other acquired deformities of ear (H61.1)

   M95.10   Cauliflower ear, unspecified ear

   M95.11   Cauliflower ear, right ear

   M95.12   Cauliflower ear, left ear

   M95.2   Other acquired deformity of head

   M95.3   Acquired deformity of neck

   M95.4   Acquired deformity of chest and rib

   M95.5   Acquired deformity of pelvis

     Excludes1   maternal care for known or suspected disproportion (O33.-)

   M95.8   Other specified acquired deformities of musculoskeletal system

   M95.9   Acquired deformity of musculoskeletal system, unspecified

▶ New   ⇛ Revised   ~~deleted~~ Deleted   Excludes 1   Excludes 2   Includes   Use additional   Code first   Code also   Key words

OGCR Official Guidelines   X Assign placeholder X   ● Use Additional Character(s)   ▌ Manifestation Code   🏷 Hierarchical Condition Category   **Coding Clinic**

INTRAOPERATIVE AND POSTPROCEDURAL COMPLICATIONS AND DISORDERS OF MUSCULOSKELETAL SYSTEM, NOT ELSEWHERE CLASSIFIED (M96)

● **M96**   Intraoperative and postprocedural complications and disorders of musculoskeletal system, not elsewhere classified

> **Excludes2**   arthropathy following intestinal bypass (M02.0-)
> complications of internal orthopedic prosthetic devices, implants and grafts (T84.-)
> disorders associated with osteoporosis (M80)
> periprosthetic fracture around internal prosthetic joint (M97.-)
> presence of functional implants and other devices (Z96-Z97)

M96.0   Pseudarthrosis after fusion or arthrodesis

M96.1   Postlaminectomy syndrome, not elsewhere classified

M96.2   Postradiation kyphosis

M96.3   Postlaminectomy kyphosis

M96.4   Postsurgical lordosis

M96.5   Postradiation scoliosis

● **M96.6**   Fracture of bone following insertion of orthopedic implant, joint prosthesis, or bone plate
> Intraoperative fracture of bone during insertion of orthopedic implant, joint prosthesis, or bone plate
>> **Excludes2**   complication of internal orthopedic devices, implants or grafts (T84.-)

  ● **M96.62**   Fracture of humerus following insertion of orthopedic implant, joint prosthesis, or bone plate

     M96.621   Fracture of humerus following insertion of orthopedic implant, joint prosthesis, or bone plate, right arm 🔧

     M96.622   Fracture of humerus following insertion of orthopedic implant, joint prosthesis, or bone plate, left arm 🔧

     M96.629   Fracture of humerus following insertion of orthopedic implant, joint prosthesis, or bone plate, unspecified arm 🔧

  ● **M96.63**   Fracture of radius or ulna following insertion of orthopedic implant, joint prosthesis, or bone plate

     M96.631   Fracture of radius or ulna following insertion of orthopedic implant, joint prosthesis, or bone plate, right arm 🔧

     M96.632   Fracture of radius or ulna following insertion of orthopedic implant, joint prosthesis, or bone plate, left arm 🔧

     M96.639   Fracture of radius or ulna following insertion of orthopedic implant, joint prosthesis, or bone plate, unspecified arm 🔧

  M96.65   Fracture of pelvis following insertion of orthopedic implant, joint prosthesis, or bone plate 🔧

  ● **M96.66**   Fracture of femur following insertion of orthopedic implant, joint prosthesis, or bone plate

     M96.661   Fracture of femur following insertion of orthopedic implant, joint prosthesis, or bone plate, right leg 🔧

     M96.662   Fracture of femur following insertion of orthopedic implant, joint prosthesis, or bone plate, left leg 🔧

     M96.669   Fracture of femur following insertion of orthopedic implant, joint prosthesis, or bone plate, unspecified leg 🔧

● **M96.67**   Fracture of tibia or fibula following insertion of orthopedic implant, joint prosthesis, or bone plate

     M96.671   Fracture of tibia or fibula following insertion of orthopedic implant, joint prosthesis, or bone plate, right leg 🔧

     M96.672   Fracture of tibia or fibula following insertion of orthopedic implant, joint prosthesis, or bone plate, left leg 🔧

     M96.679   Fracture of tibia or fibula following insertion of orthopedic implant, joint prosthesis, or bone plate, unspecified leg 🔧

  M96.69   Fracture of other bone following insertion of orthopedic implant, joint prosthesis, or bone plate 🔧

● **M96.8**   Other intraoperative and postprocedural complications and disorders of musculoskeletal system, not elsewhere classified
> Coding Clinic: 2016, Q4, P10

  ● **M96.81**   Intraoperative hemorrhage and hematoma of a musculoskeletal structure complicating a procedure
>> **Excludes1**   intraoperative hemorrhage and hematoma of a musculoskeletal structure due to accidental puncture and laceration during a procedure (M96.82-)

     M96.810   Intraoperative hemorrhage and hematoma of a musculoskeletal structure complicating a musculoskeletal system procedure

     M96.811   Intraoperative hemorrhage and hematoma of a musculoskeletal structure complicating other procedure

  ● **M96.82**   Accidental puncture and laceration of a musculoskeletal structure during a procedure

     M96.820   Accidental puncture and laceration of a musculoskeletal structure during a musculoskeletal system procedure

     M96.821   Accidental puncture and laceration of a musculoskeletal structure during other procedure

  ● **M96.83**   Postprocedural hemorrhage of a musculoskeletal structure following a procedure

     M96.830   Postprocedural hemorrhage of a musculoskeletal structure following a musculoskeletal system procedure

     M96.831   Postprocedural hemorrhage of a musculoskeletal structure following other procedure

  ● **M96.84**   Postprocedural hematoma and seroma of a musculoskeletal structure following a procedure

     M96.840   Postprocedural hematoma of a musculoskeletal structure following a musculoskeletal system procedure

     M96.841   Postprocedural hematoma of a musculoskeletal structure following other procedure
> Coding Clinic: 2016, Q4, P10

     M96.842   Postprocedural seroma of a musculoskeletal structure following a musculoskeletal system procedure

     M96.843   Postprocedural seroma of a musculoskeletal structure following other procedure

M96.89 **Other intraoperative and postprocedural complications and disorders of the musculoskeletal system**
Instability of joint secondary to removal of joint prosthesis
Use additional code, if applicable, to further specify disorder
Coding Clinic: 2022, Q2, P14; 2021, Q1, P5

▶ M96.A **Fracture of ribs, sternum and thorax associated with compression of the chest and cardiopulmonary resuscitation**

M96.A1 **Fracture of sternum associated with chest compression and cardiopulmonary resuscitation**
▶ Fracture of xiphoid process associated with chest compression and cardiopulmonary resuscitation

▶ M96.A2 **Fracture of one rib associated with chest compression and cardiopulmonary resuscitation**

▶ M96.A3 **Multiple fractures of ribs associated with chest compression and cardiopulmonary resuscitation**

▶ M96.A4 **Flail chest associated with chest compression and cardiopulmonary resuscitation**

▶ M96.A9 **Other fracture associated with chest compression and cardiopulmonary resuscitation**

PERIPROSTHETIC FRACTURE AROUND INTERNAL PROSTHETIC JOINT (M97)

● M97 **Periprosthetic fracture around internal prosthetic joint**
Excludes2 fracture of bone following insertion of orthopedic implant, joint prosthesis or bone plate (M96.6-)
breakage (fracture) of prosthetic joint (T84.01-)
Coding Clinic: 2016, Q4, P42

The appropriate 7th character is to be added to each code from category M97:

A	initial encounter
D	subsequent encounter
S	sequela

● M97.0 **Periprosthetic fracture around internal prosthetic hip joint**
X ● M97.01 **Periprosthetic fracture around internal prosthetic right hip joint** 🐾
Coding Clinic: 2016, Q4, P43

X ● M97.02 **Periprosthetic fracture around internal prosthetic left hip joint** 🐾

● M97.1 **Periprosthetic fracture around internal prosthetic knee joint**
X ● M97.11 **Periprosthetic fracture around internal prosthetic right knee joint**

X ● M97.12 **Periprosthetic fracture around internal prosthetic left knee joint**

● M97.2 **Periprosthetic fracture around internal prosthetic ankle joint**
X ● M97.21 **Periprosthetic fracture around internal prosthetic right ankle joint**

X ● M97.22 **Periprosthetic fracture around internal prosthetic left ankle joint**

● M97.3 **Periprosthetic fracture around internal prosthetic shoulder joint**
X ● M97.31 **Periprosthetic fracture around internal prosthetic right shoulder joint**

X ● M97.32 **Periprosthetic fracture around internal prosthetic left shoulder joint**

● M97.4 **Periprosthetic fracture around internal prosthetic elbow joint**
X ● M97.41 **Periprosthetic fracture around internal prosthetic right elbow joint**

X ● M97.42 **Periprosthetic fracture around internal prosthetic left elbow joint**

X ● M97.8 **Periprosthetic fracture around other internal prosthetic joint**
Periprosthetic fracture around internal prosthetic finger joint
Periprosthetic fracture around internal prosthetic spinal joint
Periprosthetic fracture around internal prosthetic toe joint
Periprosthetic fracture around internal prosthetic wrist joint
Use additional code to identify the joint (Z96.6-)

X ● M97.9 **Periprosthetic fracture around unspecified internal prosthetic joint**

BIOMECHANICAL LESIONS, NOT ELSEWHERE CLASSIFIED (M99)

● M99 **Biomechanical lesions, not elsewhere classified**
Note: This category should not be used if the condition can be classified elsewhere.

● M99.0 **Segmental and somatic dysfunction**
M99.00 **Segmental and somatic dysfunction of head region**
M99.01 **Segmental and somatic dysfunction of cervical region**
M99.02 **Segmental and somatic dysfunction of thoracic region**
M99.03 **Segmental and somatic dysfunction of lumbar region**
M99.04 **Segmental and somatic dysfunction of sacral region**
M99.05 **Segmental and somatic dysfunction of pelvic region**
M99.06 **Segmental and somatic dysfunction of lower extremity**
M99.07 **Segmental and somatic dysfunction of upper extremity**
M99.08 **Segmental and somatic dysfunction of rib cage**
M99.09 **Segmental and somatic dysfunction of abdomen and other regions**

● M99.1 **Subluxation complex (vertebral)**
M99.10 **Subluxation complex (vertebral) of head region**
M99.11 **Subluxation complex (vertebral) of cervical region**
M99.12 **Subluxation complex (vertebral) of thoracic region**
M99.13 **Subluxation complex (vertebral) of lumbar region**
M99.14 **Subluxation complex (vertebral) of sacral region**
M99.15 **Subluxation complex (vertebral) of pelvic region**
M99.16 **Subluxation complex (vertebral) of lower extremity**
M99.17 **Subluxation complex (vertebral) of upper extremity**
M99.18 **Subluxation complex (vertebral) of rib cage**
M99.19 **Subluxation complex (vertebral) of abdomen and other regions**

● M99.2 **Subluxation stenosis of neural canal**
M99.20 **Subluxation stenosis of neural canal of head region**
M99.21 **Subluxation stenosis of neural canal of cervical region**
M99.22 **Subluxation stenosis of neural canal of thoracic region**

M99.23 Subluxation stenosis of neural canal of lumbar region
M99.24 Subluxation stenosis of neural canal of sacral region
M99.25 Subluxation stenosis of neural canal of pelvic region
M99.26 Subluxation stenosis of neural canal of lower extremity
M99.27 Subluxation stenosis of neural canal of upper extremity
M99.28 Subluxation stenosis of neural canal of rib cage
M99.29 Subluxation stenosis of neural canal of abdomen and other regions

● M99.3 Osseous stenosis of neural canal
M99.30 Osseous stenosis of neural canal of head region
M99.31 Osseous stenosis of neural canal of cervical region
M99.32 Osseous stenosis of neural canal of thoracic region
M99.33 Osseous stenosis of neural canal of lumbar region
M99.34 Osseous stenosis of neural canal of sacral region
M99.35 Osseous stenosis of neural canal of pelvic region
M99.36 Osseous stenosis of neural canal of lower extremity
M99.37 Osseous stenosis of neural canal of upper extremity
M99.38 Osseous stenosis of neural canal of rib cage
M99.39 Osseous stenosis of neural canal of abdomen and other regions

● M99.4 Connective tissue stenosis of neural canal
M99.40 Connective tissue stenosis of neural canal of head region
M99.41 Connective tissue stenosis of neural canal of cervical region
M99.42 Connective tissue stenosis of neural canal of thoracic region
M99.43 Connective tissue stenosis of neural canal of lumbar region
M99.44 Connective tissue stenosis of neural canal of sacral region
M99.45 Connective tissue stenosis of neural canal of pelvic region
M99.46 Connective tissue stenosis of neural canal of lower extremity
M99.47 Connective tissue stenosis of neural canal of upper extremity
M99.48 Connective tissue stenosis of neural canal of rib cage
M99.49 Connective tissue stenosis of neural canal of abdomen and other regions

● M99.5 Intervertebral disc stenosis of neural canal
M99.50 Intervertebral disc stenosis of neural canal of head region
M99.51 Intervertebral disc stenosis of neural canal of cervical region
M99.52 Intervertebral disc stenosis of neural canal of thoracic region
M99.53 Intervertebral disc stenosis of neural canal of lumbar region
M99.54 Intervertebral disc stenosis of neural canal of sacral region
M99.55 Intervertebral disc stenosis of neural canal of pelvic region
M99.56 Intervertebral disc stenosis of neural canal of lower extremity
M99.57 Intervertebral disc stenosis of neural canal of upper extremity
M99.58 Intervertebral disc stenosis of neural canal of rib cage
M99.59 Intervertebral disc stenosis of neural canal of abdomen and other regions

● M99.6 Osseous and subluxation stenosis of intervertebral foramina
M99.60 Osseous and subluxation stenosis of intervertebral foramina of head region
M99.61 Osseous and subluxation stenosis of intervertebral foramina of cervical region
M99.62 Osseous and subluxation stenosis of intervertebral foramina of thoracic region
M99.63 Osseous and subluxation stenosis of intervertebral foramina of lumbar region
M99.64 Osseous and subluxation stenosis of intervertebral foramina of sacral region
M99.65 Osseous and subluxation stenosis of intervertebral foramina of pelvic region
M99.66 Osseous and subluxation stenosis of intervertebral foramina of lower extremity
M99.67 Osseous and subluxation stenosis of intervertebral foramina of upper extremity
M99.68 Osseous and subluxation stenosis of intervertebral foramina of rib cage
M99.69 Osseous and subluxation stenosis of intervertebral foramina of abdomen and other regions

● M99.7 Connective tissue and disc stenosis of intervertebral foramina
M99.70 Connective tissue and disc stenosis of intervertebral foramina of head region
M99.71 Connective tissue and disc stenosis of intervertebral foramina of cervical region
M99.72 Connective tissue and disc stenosis of intervertebral foramina of thoracic region
M99.73 Connective tissue and disc stenosis of intervertebral foramina of lumbar region
M99.74 Connective tissue and disc stenosis of intervertebral foramina of sacral region
M99.75 Connective tissue and disc stenosis of intervertebral foramina of pelvic region
M99.76 Connective tissue and disc stenosis of intervertebral foramina of lower extremity
M99.77 Connective tissue and disc stenosis of intervertebral foramina of upper extremity
M99.78 Connective tissue and disc stenosis of intervertebral foramina of rib cage
M99.79 Connective tissue and disc stenosis of intervertebral foramina of abdomen and other regions

● M99.8 Other biomechanical lesions
M99.80 Other biomechanical lesions of head region
M99.81 Other biomechanical lesions of cervical region
M99.82 Other biomechanical lesions of thoracic region
M99.83 Other biomechanical lesions of lumbar region
M99.84 Other biomechanical lesions of sacral region
M99.85 Other biomechanical lesions of pelvic region
M99.86 Other biomechanical lesions of lower extremity
M99.87 Other biomechanical lesions of upper extremity
M99.88 Other biomechanical lesions of rib cage
M99.89 Other biomechanical lesions of abdomen and other regions

M99.9 Biomechanical lesion, unspecified

CHAPTER 13 (M00-M99)

CHAPTER 14

DISEASES OF THE GENITOURINARY SYSTEM (N00-N99)

OGCR Chapter-Specific Coding Guidelines

14. Chapter 14: Diseases of Genitourinary System (N00-N99)
 a. Chronic kidney disease
  1) **Stages of chronic kidney disease (CKD)**
The ICD-10-CM classifies CKD based on severity. The severity of CKD is designated by stages 1-5. Stage 2, code N18.2, equates to mild CKD; stage 3, code N18.3, equates to moderate CKD; and stage 4, code N18.4, equates to severe CKD. Code N18.6, End stage renal disease (ESRD), is assigned when the provider has documented end-stage-renal disease (ESRD).
 If both a stage of CKD and ESRD are documented, assign code N18.6 only.

  2) **Chronic kidney disease and kidney transplant status**
Patients who have undergone kidney transplant may still have some form of chronic kidney disease CKD because the kidney transplant may not fully restore kidney function. Therefore, the presence of CKD alone does not constitute a transplant complication. Assign the appropriate N18 code for the patient's stage of CKD and code Z94.0, Kidney transplant status. If a transplant complication such as failure or rejection or other transplant complication is documented, see Section I.C.19.g for information on coding complications of a kidney transplant. If the documentation is unclear as to whether the patient has a complication of the transplant, query the provider.

  3) **Chronic kidney disease with other conditions**
Patients with CKD may also suffer from other serious conditions, most commonly diabetes mellitus and hypertension. The sequencing of the CKD code in relationship to codes for other contributing conditions is based on the conventions in the Tabular List.
 See I.C.9. Hypertensive chronic kidney disease.
 See I.C.19. Chronic kidney disease and kidney transplant complications.

Item 14–1 Nephritis (inflammation) or **nephropathy** (disease) **with lesion of proliferative glomerulonephritis** results from a streptococcal infection.

Nephritis (inflammation) or **nephropathy** (disease) **with lesion of membranous glomerulonephritis** is characterized by deposits along the epithelial side of the basement membrane.

Nephritis (inflammation) or **nephropathy** (disease) **with lesion of membranoproliferative glomerulonephritis** is characterized by alterations in the basement membranes of the kidney and the glomerular cells.

Nephritis (inflammation) or **nephropathy** (disease) **with lesion of rapidly progressive glomerulonephritis** is characterized by rapid and progressive decline in renal function.

Nephritis (inflammation) or **nephropathy** (disease) **with lesion of renal cortical necrosis** is characterized by death of the cortical tissues.

Nephritis (inflammation) or **nephropathy** (disease) **with lesion of renal medullary necrosis** is characterized by death of the tissues that collect urine.

Figure 14-1 Kidneys within the urinary system.

Item 14–2 Glomerulonephritis is nephritis accompanied by inflammation of the glomeruli of the kidney, resulting in the degeneration of the glomeruli and the nephrons.

Acute glomerulonephritis primarily affects children and young adults and is usually a result of a streptococcal infection.

Proliferative glomerulonephritis is the acute form of the disease resulting from a streptococcal infection.

Rapidly progressive glomerulonephritis, also known as **crescentic** or **malignant glomerulonephritis**, is the acute form of the disease, which leads quickly to rapid and progressive decline in renal function.

CHAPTER 14

DISEASES OF THE GENITOURINARY SYSTEM (N00-N99)

Excludes2 certain conditions originating in the perinatal period (P04-P96)
certain infectious and parasitic diseases (A00-B99)
complications of pregnancy, childbirth and the puerperium (O00-O9A)
congenital malformations, deformations and chromosomal abnormalities (Q00-Q99)
endocrine, nutritional and metabolic diseases (E00-E88)
injury, poisoning and certain other consequences of external causes (S00-T88)
neoplasms (C00-D49)
symptoms, signs and abnormal clinical and laboratory findings, not elsewhere classified (R00-R94)

This chapter contains the following blocks:

N00-N08	Glomerular diseases
N10-N16	Renal tubulo-interstitial diseases
N17-N19	Acute kidney failure and chronic kidney disease
N20-N23	Urolithiasis
N25-N29	Other disorders of kidney and ureter
N30-N39	Other diseases of the urinary system
N40-N53	Diseases of male genital organs
N60-N65	Disorders of breast
N70-N77	Inflammatory diseases of female pelvic organs
N80-N98	Noninflammatory disorders of female genital tract
N99	Intraoperative and postprocedural complications and disorders of genitourinary system, not elsewhere classified

GLOMERULAR DISEASES (N00-N08)

Code also any associated kidney failure (N17-N19)
Excludes1 hypertensive chronic kidney disease (I12.-)

● **N00 Acute nephritic syndrome**
Includes acute glomerular disease
acute glomerulonephritis
acute nephritis
Excludes1 acute tubulo-interstitial nephritis (N10)
nephritic syndrome NOS (N05.-)

N00.0 **Acute nephritic syndrome with minor glomerular abnormality**
Acute nephritic syndrome with minimal change lesion

N00.1 **Acute nephritic syndrome with focal and segmental glomerular lesions**
Acute nephritic syndrome with focal and segmental hyalinosis
Acute nephritic syndrome with focal and segmental sclerosis
Acute nephritic syndrome with focal glomerulonephritis

N00.2 **Acute nephritic syndrome with diffuse membranous glomerulonephritis**

N00.3 **Acute nephritic syndrome with diffuse mesangial proliferative glomerulonephritis**

N00.4 **Acute nephritic syndrome with diffuse endocapillary proliferative glomerulonephritis**

N00.5 Acute nephritic syndrome with diffuse mesangiocapillary glomerulonephritis
Acute nephritic syndrome with membranoproliferative glomerulonephritis, types 1 and 3, or NOS
> **Excludes1** Acute nephritic syndrome with C3 glomerulonephritis (N00.A)
> Acute nephritic syndrome with C3 glomerulopathy (N00.A)

N00.6 Acute nephritic syndrome with dense deposit disease
Acute nephritic syndrome with C3 glomerulopathy with dense deposit disease
Acute nephritic syndrome with membranoproliferative glomerulonephritis, type 2

N00.7 Acute nephritic syndrome with diffuse crescentic glomerulonephritis
Acute nephritic syndrome with extracapillary glomerulonephritis

N00.8 Acute nephritic syndrome with other morphologic changes
Acute nephritic syndrome with proliferative glomerulonephritis NOS

N00.9 Acute nephritic syndrome with unspecified morphologic changes

N00.A Acute nephritic syndrome with C3 glomerulonephritis
Acute nephritic syndrome with C3 glomerulopathy, NOS
> **Excludes1** Acute nephritic syndrome (with C3 glomerulopathy) with dense deposit disease(N00.6)

● **N01 Rapidly progressive nephritic syndrome**
> **Includes** rapidly progressive glomerular disease
> rapidly progressive glomerulonephritis
> rapidly progressive nephritis
> **Excludes1** nephritic syndrome NOS (N05.-)

N01.0 Rapidly progressive nephritic syndrome with minor glomerular abnormality
Rapidly progressive nephritic syndrome with minimal change lesion

N01.1 Rapidly progressive nephritic syndrome with focal and segmental glomerular lesions
Rapidly progressive nephritic syndrome with focal and segmental hyalinosis
Rapidly progressive nephritic syndrome with focal and segmental sclerosis
Rapidly progressive nephritic syndrome with focal glomerulonephritis

N01.2 Rapidly progressive nephritic syndrome with diffuse membranous glomerulonephritis

N01.3 Rapidly progressive nephritic syndrome with diffuse mesangial proliferative glomerulonephritis

N01.4 Rapidly progressive nephritic syndrome with diffuse endocapillary proliferative glomerulonephritis

N01.5 Rapidly progressive nephritic syndrome with diffuse mesangiocapillary glomerulonephritis
Rapidly progressive nephritic syndrome with membranoproliferative glomerulonephritis, types 1 and 3, or NOS
> **Excludes1** Rapidly progressive nephritic syndrome with C3 glomerulonephritis (N01.A)
> Rapidly progressive nephritic syndrome with C3 glomerulopathy (N01.A)

N01.6 Rapidly progressive nephritic syndrome with dense deposit disease
Rapidly progressive nephritic syndrome with C3 glomerulopathy with dense deposit disease
Rapidly progressive nephritic syndrome with membranoproliferative glomerulonephritis, type 2

N01.7 Rapidly progressive nephritic syndrome with diffuse crescentic glomerulonephritis
Rapidly progressive nephritic syndrome with extracapillary glomerulonephritis

N01.8 Rapidly progressive nephritic syndrome with other morphologic changes
Rapidly progressive nephritic syndrome with proliferative glomerulonephritis NOS

N01.9 Rapidly progressive nephritic syndrome with unspecified morphologic changes

N01.A Rapidly progressive nephritic syndrome with C3 glomerulonephritis
Rapidly progressive nephritic syndrome with C3 glomerulopathy, NOS
> **Excludes1** Rapidly progressive nephritic syndrome (with C3 glomerulopathy) with dense deposit disease (N01.6)

● **N02 Recurrent and persistent hematuria**
> **Excludes1** acute cystitis with hematuria (N30.01)
> hematuria NOS (R31.9)
> hematuria not associated with specified morphologic lesions (R31.-)

N02.0 Recurrent and persistent hematuria with minor glomerular abnormality
Recurrent and persistent hematuria with minimal change lesion

N02.1 Recurrent and persistent hematuria with focal and segmental glomerular lesions
Recurrent and persistent hematuria with focal and segmental hyalinosis
Recurrent and persistent hematuria with focal and segmental sclerosis
Recurrent and persistent hematuria with focal glomerulonephritis

N02.2 Recurrent and persistent hematuria with diffuse membranous glomerulonephritis

N02.3 Recurrent and persistent hematuria with diffuse mesangial proliferative glomerulonephritis

N02.4 Recurrent and persistent hematuria with diffuse endocapillary proliferative glomerulonephritis

N02.5 Recurrent and persistent hematuria with diffuse mesangiocapillary glomerulonephritis
Recurrent and persistent hematuria with membranoproliferative glomerulonephritis, types 1 and 3, or NOS
> **Excludes1** Recurrent and persistent hematuria with C3 glomerulonephritis (N02.A)
> Recurrent and persistent hematuria with C3 glomerulopathy (N02.A)

N02.6 Recurrent and persistent hematuria with dense deposit disease
Recurrent and persistent hematuria with C3 glomerulopathy with dense deposit disease
Recurrent and persistent hematuria with membranoproliferative glomerulonephritis, type 2

N02.7 Recurrent and persistent hematuria with diffuse crescentic glomerulonephritis
Recurrent and persistent hematuria with extracapillary glomerulonephritis

N02.8 Recurrent and persistent hematuria with other morphologic changes
Recurrent and persistent hematuria with proliferative glomerulonephritis NOS

N02.9 Recurrent and persistent hematuria with unspecified morphologic changes
Coding Clinic: 2017, Q2, P5

N02.A Recurrent and persistent hematuria with C3 glomerulonephritis
Recurrent and persistent hematuria with C3 glomerulopathy
> **Excludes1** Recurrent and persistent hematuria (with C3 glomerulopathy) with dense deposit disease (N02.6)

CHAPTER 14 (N00-N99)

Item 14–3 Chronic glomerulonephritis (GN) persists over a period of years, with remissions and exacerbation.

Chronic GN with lesion of proliferative glomerulonephritis results from a streptococcal infection.

Chronic GN with lesion of membranous glomerulonephritis, also known as membranous nephropathy, is characterized by deposits along the epithelial side of the basement membrane.

Chronic GN with lesion of membrano-proliferative glomerulonephritis (MPGN) is a group of disorders characterized by alterations in the basement membranes of the kidney and the glomerular cells.

Chronic GN with lesion of rapidly progressive glomerulonephritis is characterized by necrosis, endothelial proliferation, and mesangial proliferation. The condition is marked by rapid and progressive decline in renal function.

● **N03   Chronic nephritic syndrome**

    Includes   chronic glomerular disease
                     chronic glomerulonephritis
                     chronic nephritis

    Excludes1   chronic tubulo-interstitial nephritis (N11.-)
                     diffuse sclerosing glomerulonephritis (N05.8-)
                     nephritic syndrome NOS (N05.-)

N03.0   Chronic nephritic syndrome with minor glomerular abnormality
       Chronic nephritic syndrome with minimal change lesion

N03.1   Chronic nephritic syndrome with focal and segmental glomerular lesions
       Chronic nephritic syndrome with focal and segmental hyalinosis
       Chronic nephritic syndrome with focal and segmental sclerosis
       Chronic nephritic syndrome with focal glomerulonephritis

N03.2   Chronic nephritic syndrome with diffuse membranous glomerulonephritis

N03.3   Chronic nephritic syndrome with diffuse mesangial proliferative glomerulonephritis

N03.4   Chronic nephritic syndrome with diffuse endocapillary proliferative glomerulonephritis

N03.5   Chronic nephritic syndrome with diffuse mesangiocapillary glomerulonephritis
       Chronic nephritic syndrome with membranoproliferative glomerulonephritis, types 1 and 3, or NOS

       Excludes1   Chronic nephritic syndrome with C3 glomerulonephritis (N03.A)
                     Chronic nephritic syndrome with C3 glomerulopathy (N03.A)

N03.6   Chronic nephritic syndrome with dense deposit disease
       Chronic nephritic syndrome with C3 glomerulopathy with dense deposit disease
       Chronic nephritic syndrome with membranoproliferative glomerulonephritis, type 2

N03.7   Chronic nephritic syndrome with diffuse crescentic glomerulonephritis
       Chronic nephritic syndrome with extracapillary glomerulonephritis

N03.8   Chronic nephritic syndrome with other morphologic changes
       Chronic nephritic syndrome with proliferative glomerulonephritis NOS

N03.9   Chronic nephritic syndrome with unspecified morphologic changes

N03.A   Chronic nephritic syndrome with C3 glomerulonephritis
       Chronic nephritic syndrome with C3 glomerulopathy

       Excludes1   Chronic nephritic syndrome (with C3 glomerulopathy) with dense deposit disease(N03.6)

● **N04   Nephrotic syndrome**

    Includes   congenital nephrotic syndrome
                     lipoid nephrosis

N04.0   Nephrotic syndrome with minor glomerular abnormality
       Nephrotic syndrome with minimal change lesion

N04.1   Nephrotic syndrome with focal and segmental glomerular lesions
       Nephrotic syndrome with focal and segmental hyalinosis
       Nephrotic syndrome with focal and segmental sclerosis
       Nephrotic syndrome with focal glomerulonephritis

N04.2   Nephrotic syndrome with diffuse membranous glomerulonephritis

N04.3   Nephrotic syndrome with diffuse mesangial proliferative glomerulonephritis

N04.4   Nephrotic syndrome with diffuse endocapillary proliferative glomerulonephritis

N04.5   Nephrotic syndrome with diffuse mesangiocapillary glomerulonephritis
       Nephrotic syndrome with membranoproliferative glomerulonephritis, types 1 and 3, or NOS

       Excludes1   Nephrotic syndrome with C3 glomerulonephritis (N04.A)
                     Nephrotic syndrome with C3 glomerulopathy (N04.A)

N04.6   Nephrotic syndrome with dense deposit disease
       Nephrotic syndrome with C3 glomerulopathy with dense deposit disease
       Nephrotic syndrome with membranoproliferative glomerulonephritis, type 2

N04.7   Nephrotic syndrome with diffuse crescentic glomerulonephritis
       Nephrotic syndrome with extracapillary glomerulonephritis

N04.8   Nephrotic syndrome with other morphologic changes
       Nephrotic syndrome with proliferative glomerulonephritis NOS

N04.9   Nephrotic syndrome with unspecified morphologic changes

N04.A   Nephrotic syndrome with C3 glomerulonephritis
       Nephrotic syndrome with C3 glomerulopathy

       Excludes1   Nephrotic syndrome (with C3 glomerulopathy) with dense deposit disease (N04.6)

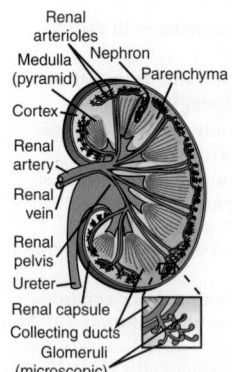

Renal arterioles
Medulla (pyramid)
Nephron
Parenchyma
Cortex
Renal artery
Renal vein
Renal pelvis
Ureter
Renal capsule
Collecting ducts
Glomeruli (microscopic)

Figure 14-2   Kidney cross section.

Item 14–4 Nephrotic syndrome (NS) is marked by massive proteinuria (protein in the urine) and water retention. Patients with NS are particularly vulnerable to staphylococcal and pneumococcal infections. NS with lesion of proliferative glomerulonephritis results from a streptococcal infection. NS with lesion of membranous glomerulonephritis results in thickening of the capillary walls. NS with lesion of minimal change glomerulonephritis is usually a benign disorder that occurs mostly in children and requires electron microscopy (biopsy) to verify changes in the glomeruli.

▶ New   ⇒ Revised   ~~deleted~~ Deleted   Excludes 1   Excludes 2   Includes   Use additional   Code first   Code also   Key words
OGCR Official Guidelines   X Assign placeholder X   ● Use Additional Character(s)   ▶ Manifestation Code   🝡 Hierarchical Condition Category   **Coding Clinic**

● **N05** **Unspecified nephritic syndrome**

Includes   glomerular disease NOS
glomerulonephritis NOS
nephritis NOS
nephropathy NOS and renal disease NOS with
morphological lesion specified in .0-.8

Excludes1   nephropathy NOS with no stated morphological
lesion (N28.9)
renal disease NOS with no stated morphological
lesion (N28.9)
tubulo-interstitial nephritis NOS (N12)

N05.0 **Unspecified nephritic syndrome with** minor glomerular abnormality
Unspecified nephritic syndrome with minimal change
lesion

N05.1 **Unspecified nephritic syndrome with** focal and segmental glomerular lesions
Unspecified nephritic syndrome with focal and
segmental hyalinosis
Unspecified nephritic syndrome with focal and
segmental sclerosis
Unspecified nephritic syndrome with focal
glomerulonephritis

N05.2 **Unspecified nephritic syndrome with** diffuse membranous glomerulonephritis

N05.3 **Unspecified nephritic syndrome with** diffuse mesangial proliferative glomerulonephritis

N05.4 **Unspecified nephritic syndrome with** diffuse endocapillary proliferative glomerulonephritis

N05.5 **Unspecified nephritic syndrome with** diffuse mesangiocapillary glomerulonephritis
Unspecified nephritic syndrome with
membranoproliferative glomerulonephritis, types
1 and 3, or NOS

   Excludes1   Unspecified nephritic syndrome with C3
glomerulonephritis (N05.A)
Unspecified nephritic syndrome with C3
glomerulopathy (N05.A)

N05.6 **Unspecified nephritic syndrome with** dense deposit disease
Unspecified nephritic syndrome with C3
glomerulopathy with dense deposit disease
Unspecified nephritic syndrome with
membranoproliferative glomerulonephritis, type 2

N05.7 **Unspecified nephritic syndrome with** diffuse crescentic glomerulonephritis
Unspecified nephritic syndrome with extracapillary
glomerulonephritis

N05.8 **Unspecified nephritic syndrome with** other morphologic changes
Unspecified nephritic syndrome with proliferative
glomerulonephritis NOS

N05.9 **Unspecified nephritic syndrome with** unspecified morphologic changes

N05.A **Unspecified nephritic syndrome with C3 glomerulonephritis**
Unspecified nephritic syndrome with C3
glomerulopathy

   Excludes1   Unspecified nephritic syndrome (with C3
glomerulopathy) with dense deposit
disease(N05.6)

● **N06** **Isolated proteinuria with specified morphological lesion**

Excludes1   proteinuria not associated with specific
morphologic lesions (R80.0)

N06.0 **Isolated proteinuria with** minor glomerular abnormality
Isolated proteinuria with minimal change lesion

N06.1 **Isolated proteinuria with** focal and segmental glomerular lesions
Isolated proteinuria with focal and segmental hyalinosis
Isolated proteinuria with focal and segmental sclerosis
Isolated proteinuria with focal glomerulonephritis

N06.2 **Isolated proteinuria with** diffuse membranous glomerulonephritis

N06.3 **Isolated proteinuria with** diffuse mesangial proliferative glomerulonephritis

N06.4 **Isolated proteinuria with** diffuse endocapillary proliferative glomerulonephritis

N06.5 **Isolated proteinuria with** diffuse mesangiocapillary glomerulonephritis
Isolated proteinuria with membranoproliferative
glomerulonephritis, types 1 and 3, or NOS

   Excludes1   Isolated proteinuria with C3
glomerulonephritis (N06.A)
Isolated proteinuria with C3
glomerulopathy (N06.A)

N06.6 **Isolated proteinuria with** dense deposit disease
Isolated proteinuria with C3 glomerulopathy with
dense deposit disease
Isolated proteinuria with membranoproliferative
glomerulonephritis, type 2

N06.7 **Isolated proteinuria with** diffuse crescentic glomerulonephritis
Isolated proteinuria with extracapillary
glomerulonephritis

N06.8 **Isolated proteinuria with** other morphologic lesion
Isolated proteinuria with proliferative
glomerulonephritis NOS

N06.9 **Isolated proteinuria with** unspecified morphologic lesion

N06.A **Isolated proteinuria with C3 glomerulonephritis**
Isolated proteinuria with C3 glomerulopathy

   Excludes1   Isolated proteinuria (with C3
glomerulopathy) with dense
deposit disease (N06.6)

● **N07** **Hereditary nephropathy, not elsewhere classified**

Excludes2   Alport's syndrome (Q87.81-)
hereditary amyloid nephropathy (E85.-)
nail patella syndrome (Q87.2)
non-neuropathic heredofamilial amyloidosis
(E85.-)

N07.0 **Hereditary nephropathy, not elsewhere classified with minor glomerular abnormality**
Hereditary nephropathy, not elsewhere classified with
minimal change lesion

N07.1 **Hereditary nephropathy, not elsewhere classified with focal and segmental glomerular lesions**
Hereditary nephropathy, not elsewhere classified with
focal and segmental hyalinosis
Hereditary nephropathy, not elsewhere classified with
focal and segmental sclerosis
Hereditary nephropathy, not elsewhere classified with
focal glomerulonephritis

CHAPTER 14 (N00-N99)

N07.2 Hereditary nephropathy, not elsewhere classified with diffuse membranous glomerulonephritis

N07.3 Hereditary nephropathy, not elsewhere classified with diffuse mesangial proliferative glomerulonephritis

N07.4 Hereditary nephropathy, not elsewhere classified with diffuse endocapillary proliferative glomerulonephritis

N07.5 Hereditary nephropathy, not elsewhere classified with diffuse mesangiocapillary glomerulonephritis

Hereditary nephropathy, not elsewhere classified with membranoproliferative glomerulonephritis, types 1 and 3, or NOS

> **Excludes1**   Hereditary nephropathy, not elsewhere classified with C3 glomerulonephritis (N07.A)
> Hereditary nephropathy, not elsewhere classified with C3 glomerulopathy (N07.A)

N07.6 Hereditary nephropathy, not elsewhere classified with dense deposit disease

Hereditary nephropathy, not elsewhere classified with C3 glomerulopathy with dense deposit disease
Hereditary nephropathy, not elsewhere classified with membranoproliferative glomerulonephritis, type 2

N07.7 Hereditary nephropathy, not elsewhere classified with diffuse crescentic glomerulonephritis

Hereditary nephropathy, not elsewhere classified with extracapillary glomerulonephritis

N07.8 Hereditary nephropathy, not elsewhere classified with other morphologic lesions

Hereditary nephropathy, not elsewhere classified with proliferative glomerulonephritis NOS

N07.9 Hereditary nephropathy, not elsewhere classified with unspecified morphologic lesions

N07.A Hereditary nephropathy, not elsewhere classified with C3 glomerulonephritis

Hereditary nephropathy, not elsewhere classified with C3 glomerulopathy

> **Excludes1**   Hereditary nephropathy, not elsewhere classified (with C3 glomerulopathy) with dense deposit disease (N07.6)

▶ *N08 Glomerular disorders in diseases classified elsewhere*

Glomerulonephritis
Nephritis
Nephropathy

Code first underlying disease, such as:
amyloidosis (E85.-)
congenital syphilis (A50.5)
cryoglobulinemia (D89.1)
disseminated intravascular coagulation (D65)
gout (M1A.-, M10.-)
microscopic polyangiitis (M31.7)
multiple myeloma (C90.0-)
sepsis (A40.0-A41.9)
sickle-cell disease (D57.0-D57.8)

> **Excludes1**   glomerulonephritis, nephritis and nephropathy (in):
> antiglomerular basement membrane disease (M31.0)
> diabetes (E08-E13 with .21)
> gonococcal (A54.21)
> Goodpasture's syndrome (M31.0)
> hemolytic-uremic syndrome (D59.3)
> lupus (M32.14)
> mumps (B26.83)
> syphilis (A52.75)
> systemic lupus erythematosus (M32.14)
> Wegener's granulomatosis (M31.31)
> pyelonephritis in diseases classified elsewhere (N16)
> renal tubulo-interstitial disorders classified elsewhere (N16)

Figure 14-3   Acute pyelonephritis. Cortical surface exhibits grayish white areas of inflammation and abscess formation. (From Frazier MS, Drzymkowski JW: Essentials of Human Diseases and Conditions, St. Louis, Saunders/Elsevier, 2009)

Item 14-5 Pyelonephritis is an infection of the kidneys and ureters and may be chronic or acute in one or both kidneys.

RENAL TUBULO-INTERSTITIAL DISEASES (N10-N16)

> **Includes**   pyelonephritis
> **Excludes1**   pyeloureteritis cystica (N28.85)

N10 Acute pyelonephritis

Acute infectious interstitial nephritis
Acute pyelitis
Acute tubulo-interstitial nephritis
Hemoglobin nephrosis
Myoglobin nephrosis

Use additional code (B95-B97), to identify infectious agent
Coding Clinic: 2019, Q3, P13-14

● **N11 Chronic tubulo-interstitial nephritis**

> **Includes**   chronic infectious interstitial nephritis
> chronic pyelitis
> chronic pyelonephritis

Use additional code (B95-B97), to identify infectious agent

N11.0 Nonobstructive reflux-associated chronic pyelonephritis

Pyelonephritis (chronic) associated with (vesicoureteral) reflux

> **Excludes1**   vesicoureteral reflux NOS (N13.70)

N11.1 Chronic obstructive pyelonephritis

Pyelonephritis (chronic) associated with anomaly of pelviureteric junction
Pyelonephritis (chronic) associated with anomaly of pyeloureteric junction
Pyelonephritis (chronic) associated with crossing of vessel
Pyelonephritis (chronic) associated with kinking of ureter
Pyelonephritis (chronic) associated with obstruction of ureter
Pyelonephritis (chronic) associated with stricture of pelviureteric junction
Pyelonephritis (chronic) associated with stricture of ureter

> **Excludes1**   calculous pyelonephritis (N20.9)
> obstructive uropathy (N13.-)

N11.8 Other chronic tubulo-interstitial nephritis

Nonobstructive chronic pyelonephritis NOS

N11.9 Chronic tubulo-interstitial nephritis, unspecified

Chronic interstitial nephritis NOS
Chronic pyelitis NOS
Chronic pyelonephritis NOS

N12 Tubulo-interstitial nephritis, not specified as acute or chronic

Interstitial nephritis NOS
Pyelitis NOS
Pyelonephritis NOS

> **Excludes1**   calculous pyelonephritis (N20.9)

▶ New   ⇒ Revised   ~~deleted~~ Deleted   Excludes 1   Excludes 2   Includes   Use additional   Code first   Code also   Key words
OGCR Official Guidelines   X Assign placeholder X   ● Use Additional Character(s)   ▶ Manifestation Code   🏵 Hierarchical Condition Category   **Coding Clinic**

Figure 14-4   Hydronephrosis of the kidney, with marked dilatation of pelvis and calyces and thinning of renal parenchyma. (From Kumar: Robbins and Cotran: Pathologic Basis of Disease, ed 8, Saunders, An Imprint of Elsevier, 2009)

● **N13**   **Obstructive and reflux uropathy**

> **Excludes2**   calculus of kidney and ureter without hydronephrosis (N20.-)
> congenital obstructive defects of renal pelvis and ureter (Q62.0-Q62.3)
> hydronephrosis with ureteropelvic junction obstruction (Q62.11)
> obstructive pyelonephritis (N11.1)

N13.0   **Hydronephrosis with ureteropelvic junction obstruction**
> Hydronephrosis due to acquired occlusion of ureteropelvic junction
>> **Excludes2**   Hydronephrosis with ureteropelvic junction obstruction due to calculus (N13.2)
>> *Coding Clinic: 2016, Q4, P43*

N13.1   **Hydronephrosis with ureteral stricture, not elsewhere classified**
>> **Excludes1**   hydronephrosis with ureteral stricture with infection (N13.6)

N13.2   **Hydronephrosis with renal and ureteral calculous obstruction**
>> **Excludes1**   hydronephrosis with renal and ureteral calculous obstruction with infection (N13.6)

● **N13.3**   **Other and unspecified hydronephrosis**
>> **Excludes1**   hydronephrosis with infection (N13.6)
>
> **N13.30**   Unspecified hydronephrosis
> **N13.39**   Other hydronephrosis

N13.4   **Hydroureter**
>> **Excludes1**   congenital hydroureter (Q62.3-)
>> hydroureter with infection (N13.6)
>> vesicoureteral-reflux with hydroureter (N13.73-)

N13.5   **Crossing vessel and stricture of ureter without hydronephrosis**
> Kinking and stricture of ureter without hydronephrosis
>> **Excludes1**   crossing vessel and stricture of ureter without hydronephrosis with infection (N13.6)
>> *Coding Clinic: 2016, Q4, P43*

N13.6   **Pyonephrosis**
> Conditions in N13.0-N13.5 with infection
> Obstructive uropathy with infection
>> Use additional code (B95-B97), to identify infectious agent
>> *Coding Clinic: 2018, Q2, P21*

● **N13.7**   **Vesicoureteral-reflux**
>> **Excludes1**   reflux-associated pyelonephritis (N11.0)
>
> **N13.70**   **Vesicoureteral-reflux, unspecified**
>> *Occurs when urine flows from bladder back into ureters*
>> Vesicoureteral-reflux NOS
>
> **N13.71**   **Vesicoureteral-reflux without reflux nephropathy**

● **N13.72**   **Vesicoureteral-reflux with reflux nephropathy without hydroureter**
> **N13.721**   Vesicoureteral-reflux with reflux nephropathy without hydroureter, unilateral
> **N13.722**   Vesicoureteral-reflux with reflux nephropathy without hydroureter, bilateral
> **N13.729**   Vesicoureteral-reflux with reflux nephropathy without hydroureter, unspecified

● **N13.73**   **Vesicoureteral-reflux with reflux nephropathy with hydroureter**
> **N13.731**   Vesicoureteral-reflux with reflux nephropathy with hydroureter, unilateral
> **N13.732**   Vesicoureteral-reflux with reflux nephropathy with hydroureter, bilateral
> **N13.739**   Vesicoureteral-reflux with reflux nephropathy with hydroureter, unspecified

N13.8   **Other obstructive and reflux uropathy**
> Urinary tract obstruction due to specified cause
> *Code first, if applicable, any causal condition first, such as:*
> enlarged prostate (N40.1)

N13.9   **Obstructive and reflux uropathy, unspecified**
> Urinary tract obstruction NOS

● **N14**   **Drug- and heavy-metal-induced tubulo-interstitial and tubular conditions**
> *Code first poisoning due to drug or toxin, if applicable (T36-T65 with fifth or sixth character 1-4 or 6)*
> Use additional code for adverse effect, if applicable, to identify drug (T36-T50 with fifth or sixth character 5)

N14.0   **Analgesic nephropathy**

● **N14.1**   **Nephropathy induced by other drugs, medicaments and biological substances**
> *Coding Clinic: 2021, Q3, P9-10*
>
> ▶ **N14.11**   **Contrast-induced nephropathy**
>> Contrast medium, radiography nephropathy
>>> ▶ **Excludes2**   acute kidney failure (N17.-)
>
> ▶ **N14.19**   **Nephropathy induced by other drugs, medicaments and biological substances**

N14.2   **Nephropathy induced by unspecified drug, medicament or biological substance**

N14.3   **Nephropathy induced by heavy metals**

N14.4   **Toxic nephropathy, not elsewhere classified**

● **N15**   **Other renal tubulo-interstitial diseases**

N15.0   **Balkan nephropathy**
> Balkan endemic nephropathy

N15.1   **Renal and perinephric abscess**

N15.8   **Other specified renal tubulo-interstitial diseases**

N15.9   **Renal tubulo-interstitial disease, unspecified**
> Infection of kidney NOS
>> **Excludes1**   urinary tract infection NOS (N39.0)

CHAPTER 14 (N00-N99)

▶ **N16**   *Renal tubulo-interstitial disorders in diseases classified elsewhere*
Pyelonephritis
Tubulo-interstitial nephritis
Code first underlying disease, such as:
brucellosis (A23.0-A23.9)
cryoglobulinemia (D89.1)
glycogen storage disease (E74.0)
leukemia (C91-C95)
lymphoma (C81.0-C85.9, C96.0-C96.9)
multiple myeloma (C90.0-)
sepsis (A40.0-A41.9)
Wilson's disease (E83.0)

Excludes1   diphtheritic pyelonephritis and tubulo-interstitial
nephritis (A36.84)
pyelonephritis and tubulo-interstitial nephritis in
candidiasis (B37.49)
pyelonephritis and tubulo-interstitial nephritis in
cystinosis (E72.04)
pyelonephritis and tubulo-interstitial nephritis in
salmonella infection (A02.25)
pyelonephritis and tubulo-interstitial nephritis in
sarcoidosis (D86.84)
pyelonephritis and tubulo-interstitial nephritis in
Sjögren syndrome (M35.04)
pyelonephritis and tubulo-interstitial nephritis in
systemic lupus erythematosus (M32.15)
pyelonephritis and tubulo-interstitial nephritis in
toxoplasmosis (B58.83)
renal tubular degeneration in diabetes (E08-E13
with .29)
syphilitic pyelonephritis and tubulo-interstitial
nephritis (A52.75)

ACUTE KIDNEY FAILURE AND CHRONIC KIDNEY DISEASE (N17-N19)

Excludes2   congenital renal failure (P96.0)
drug- and heavy-metal-induced tubulo-
interstitial and tubular conditions (N14.-)
extrarenal uremia (R39.2)
hemolytic-uremic syndrome (D59.3-)
hepatorenal syndrome (K76.7)
postpartum hepatorenal syndrome (O90.4)
posttraumatic renal failure (T79.5)
prerenal uremia (R39.2)
renal failure complicating abortion or ectopic or
molar pregnancy (O00-O07, O08.4)
renal failure following labor and delivery (O90.4)
renal failure postprocedural (N99.0)

● **N17**   **Acute kidney failure**
Code also associated underlying condition
Excludes1   posttraumatic renal failure (T79.5)

N17.0   **Acute kidney failure with tubular necrosis** 🐾
Acute tubular necrosis
Renal tubular necrosis
Tubular necrosis NOS
Coding Clinic: 2021, Q3, P10

N17.1   **Acute kidney failure with acute cortical necrosis** 🐾
Acute cortical necrosis
Cortical necrosis NOS
Renal cortical necrosis

N17.2   **Acute kidney failure with medullary necrosis** 🐾
Medullary [papillary] necrosis NOS
Acute medullary [papillary] necrosis
Renal medullary [papillary] necrosis

N17.8   **Other acute kidney failure** 🐾

N17.9   **Acute kidney failure, unspecified** 🐾
Acute kidney injury (nontraumatic)
Excludes2   traumatic kidney injury (S37.0-)
Coding Clinic: 2019, Q2, P7,25

Item 14–6 Decreased blood flow is the usual cause of **acute renal failure**
that offers a good prognosis for recovery.
    Chronic renal failure is usually the result of long-standing kidney disease
and is a very serious condition that generally results in death.

● **N18**   **Chronic kidney disease (CKD)**
Code first any associated:
diabetic chronic kidney disease (E08.22, E09.22, E10.22,
E11.22, E13.22)
hypertensive chronic kidney disease (I12.-, I13.-)
Use additional code to identify kidney transplant status, if
applicable, (Z94.0)
Coding Clinic: 2018, Q4, P89; 2016, Q4, P123

N18.1   **Chronic kidney disease, stage 1**
N18.2   **Chronic kidney disease, stage 2 (mild)**
● **N18.3**   **Chronic kidney disease, stage 3 (moderate)**
    N18.30   **Chronic kidney disease, stage 3 unspecified**
    N18.31   **Chronic kidney disease, stage 3a**
    N18.32   **Chronic kidney disease, stage 3b**
N18.4   **Chronic kidney disease, stage 4 (severe)** 🐾
    Coding Clinic: 2013, Q1, P24
N18.5   **Chronic kidney disease, stage 5** 🐾
Excludes1   chronic kidney disease, stage 5 requiring
chronic dialysis (N18.6)
N18.6   **End stage renal disease** 🐾
Chronic kidney disease requiring chronic dialysis
Use additional code to identify dialysis status (Z99.2)
Coding Clinic: 2016, Q3, P23, Q1, P13
N18.9   **Chronic kidney disease, unspecified**
Chronic renal disease
Chronic renal failure NOS
Chronic renal insufficiency
Chronic uremia NOS
Diffuse sclerosing glomerulonephritis NOS
Coding Clinic: 2018, Q4, P88

N19   **Unspecified kidney failure**
Uremia NOS
Excludes1   acute kidney failure (N17.-)
chronic kidney disease (N18.-)
chronic uremia (N18.9)
extrarenal uremia (R39.2)
prerenal uremia (R39.2)
renal insufficiency (acute) (N28.9)
uremia of newborn (P96.0)

UROLITHIASIS (N20-N23)

● **N20**   **Calculus of kidney and ureter**
Calculous pyelonephritis
Excludes1   nephrocalcinosis (E83.5)
that with hydronephrosis (N13.2)
Coding Clinic: 2019, Q3, P14

N20.0   **Calculus of kidney**
Nephrolithiasis NOS   Staghorn calculus
Renal calculus   Stone in kidney
Renal stone
Coding Clinic: 2019, Q3, P13; 2017, Q1, P5

N20.1   **Calculus of ureter**
Calculus of the ureteropelvic junction
Ureteric stone
Coding Clinic: 2016, Q3, P24

N20.2   **Calculus of kidney with calculus of ureter**
N20.9   **Urinary calculus, unspecified**

Figure 14-5   Multiple urinary calculi.

Multiple
calculi

▶ New   ⟹ Revised   ~~deleted~~ Deleted   Excludes 1   Excludes 2   Includes   Use additional   Code first   Code also   Key words
OGCR Official Guidelines   X Assign placeholder X   ● Use Additional Character(s)   ▶ Manifestation Code   🐾 Hierarchical Condition Category   Coding Clinic

● **N21**   **Calculus of lower urinary tract**
     Includes   calculus of lower urinary tract with cystitis and urethritis
     N21.0   **Calculus in bladder**
        Calculus in diverticulum of bladder
        Urinary bladder stone
        Excludes2   staghorn calculus (N20.0)
        Coding Clinic: 2015, Q2, P9
     N21.1   **Calculus in urethra**
        Excludes2   calculus of prostate (N42.0)
     N21.8   **Other lower urinary tract calculus**
     N21.9   **Calculus of lower urinary tract, unspecified**
        Excludes1   calculus of urinary tract NOS (N20.9)

▷ **N22**   *Calculus of urinary tract in diseases classified elsewhere*
     Code first underlying disease, such as:
        gout (M1A.-, M10.-)
        schistosomiasis (B65.0-B65.9)

N23   **Unspecified renal colic**

OTHER DISORDERS OF KIDNEY AND URETER (N25-N29)

     Excludes2   disorders of kidney and ureter with urolithiasis (N20-N23)

● **N25**   **Disorders resulting from impaired renal tubular function**
     N25.0   **Renal osteodystrophy**
        Azotemic osteodystrophy
        Phosphate-losing tubular disorders
        Renal rickets
        Renal short stature
        Excludes2   metabolic disorders classifiable to E70-E88
     N25.1   **Nephrogenic diabetes insipidus** 🐾
        Excludes1   diabetes insipidus NOS (E23.2)
●   **N25.8**   **Other disorders resulting from impaired renal tubular function**
        N25.81   **Secondary hyperparathyroidism of renal origin** 🐾
           Excludes1   secondary hyperparathyroidism, non-renal (E21.1)
           Excludes2   metabolic disorders classifiable to E70-E88
        N25.89   **Other disorders resulting from impaired renal tubular function**
           Hypokalemic nephropathy
           Lightwood-Albright syndrome
           Renal tubular acidosis NOS
     N25.9   **Disorder resulting from impaired renal tubular function, unspecified**

● **N26**   **Unspecified contracted kidney**
     Excludes1   contracted kidney due to hypertension (I12.-)
        diffuse sclerosing glomerulonephritis (N05.8.-)
        hypertensive nephrosclerosis (arteriolar) (arteriosclerotic) (I12.-)
        small kidney of unknown cause (N27.-)
     N26.1   **Atrophy of kidney (terminal)**
     N26.2   **Page kidney**
     N26.9   **Renal sclerosis, unspecified**

● **N27**   **Small kidney of unknown cause**
     Includes   oligonephronia
     N27.0   **Small kidney, unilateral**
     N27.1   **Small kidney, bilateral**
     N27.9   **Small kidney, unspecified**

● **N28**   **Other disorders of kidney and ureter, not elsewhere classified**
     N28.0   **Ischemia and infarction of kidney** 🐾
        Renal artery embolism
        Renal artery obstruction
        Renal artery occlusion
        Renal artery thrombosis
        Renal infarct
        Excludes1   atherosclerosis of renal artery (extrarenal part) (I70.1)
           congenital stenosis of renal artery (Q27.1)
           Goldblatt's kidney (I70.1)
     N28.1   **Cyst of kidney, acquired**
        Cyst (multiple) (solitary) of kidney, (acquired)
        Excludes1   cystic kidney disease (congenital) (Q61.-)
● **N28.8**   **Other specified disorders of kidney and ureter**
        Excludes1   hydroureter (N13.4)
           ureteric stricture with hydronephrosis (N13.1)
           ureteric stricture without hydronephrosis (N13.5)
        N28.81   **Hypertrophy of kidney**
        N28.82   **Megaloureter**
        N28.83   **Nephroptosis**
        N28.84   **Pyelitis cystica**
        N28.85   **Pyeloureteritis cystica**
        N28.86   **Ureteritis cystica**
        N28.89   **Other specified disorders of kidney and ureter**
     N28.9   **Disorder of kidney and ureter, unspecified**
        Nephropathy NOS
        Renal disease (acute) NOS
        Renal insufficiency (acute)
        Excludes1   chronic renal insufficiency (N18.9)
           unspecified nephritic syndrome (N05.-)
        Coding Clinic: 2016, Q1, P13

▷ **N29**   *Other disorders of kidney and ureter in diseases classified elsewhere*
     Code first underlying disease, such as:
        amyloidosis (E85.-)
        nephrocalcinosis (E83.5)
        schistosomiasis (B65.0-B65.9)
     Excludes1   disorders of kidney and ureter in:
        cystinosis (E72.0)
        gonorrhea (A54.21)
        syphilis (A52.75)
        tuberculosis (A18.11)

OTHER DISEASES OF THE URINARY SYSTEM (N30-N39)

     Excludes2   urinary infection (complicating):
        abortion or ectopic or molar pregnancy (O00-O07, O08.8)
        pregnancy, childbirth and the puerperium (O23.-, O75.3, O86.2-)

● **N30**   **Cystitis**
     Infection of bladder and irritation in lower urinary tract
     Use additional code to identify infectious agent (B95-B97)
     Excludes1   prostatocystitis (N41.3)
● **N30.0**   **Acute cystitis**
        Excludes1   irradiation cystitis (N30.4-)
           trigonitis (N30.3-)
        N30.00   **Acute cystitis without hematuria**
        N30.01   **Acute cystitis with hematuria**
● **N30.1**   **Interstitial cystitis (chronic)**
        Ongoing infection of kidney glomeruli and tubules
        N30.10   **Interstitial cystitis (chronic) without hematuria**
        N30.11   **Interstitial cystitis (chronic) with hematuria**

CHAPTER 14 (N00-N99)

● **N30.2** **Other chronic cystitis**
  N30.20 **Other chronic cystitis without hematuria**
  N30.21 **Other chronic cystitis with hematuria**
● **N30.3** **Trigonitis**
  Inflammation of triangular area of bladder (where the ureters and urethra come together)
  Urethrotrigonitis
  N30.30 **Trigonitis without hematuria**
  N30.31 **Trigonitis with hematuria**
● **N30.4** **Irradiation cystitis**
  N30.40 **Irradiation cystitis without hematuria**
  N30.41 **Irradiation cystitis with hematuria**
● **N30.8** **Other cystitis**
  Abscess of bladder
  N30.80 **Other cystitis without hematuria**
  N30.81 **Other cystitis with hematuria**
● **N30.9** **Cystitis, unspecified**
  N30.90 **Cystitis, unspecified without hematuria**
  N30.91 **Cystitis, unspecified with hematuria**
● **N31** **Neuromuscular dysfunction of bladder, not elsewhere classified**
  Use additional code to identify any associated urinary incontinence (N39.3-N39.4-)
  Excludes1 cord bladder NOS (G95.89)
  neurogenic bladder due to cauda equina syndrome (G83.4)
  neuromuscular dysfunction due to spinal cord lesion (G95.89)
  N31.0 **Uninhibited neuropathic bladder, not elsewhere classified**
  N31.1 **Reflex neuropathic bladder, not elsewhere classified**
  N31.2 **Flaccid neuropathic bladder, not elsewhere classified**
  Atonic (motor) (sensory) neuropathic bladder
  Diminished tone of bladder muscle
  Autonomous neuropathic bladder
  Nonreflex neuropathic bladder
  N31.8 **Other neuromuscular dysfunction of bladder**
  N31.9 **Neuromuscular dysfunction of bladder, unspecified**
  Neurogenic bladder dysfunction NOS
● **N32** **Other disorders of bladder**
  Excludes2 calculus of bladder (N21.0)
  cystocele (N81.1-)
  hernia or prolapse of bladder, female (N81.1-)
  N32.0 **Bladder-neck obstruction**
  Bladder-neck stenosis (acquired)
  Excludes1 congenital bladder-neck obstruction (Q64.3-)
  N32.1 **Vesicointestinal fistula**
  Vesicorectal fistula
  N32.2 **Vesical fistula, not elsewhere classified**
  Excludes1 fistula between bladder and female genital tract (N82.0-N82.1)
  N32.3 **Diverticulum of bladder**
  Formation of sac from a herniation of wall of bladder
  Excludes1 congenital diverticulum of bladder (Q64.6)
  diverticulitis of bladder (N30.8-)
● **N32.8** **Other specified disorders of bladder**
  N32.81 **Overactive bladder**
  Detrusor muscle hyperactivity
  Excludes1 frequent urination due to specified bladder condition-code to condition
  N32.89 **Other specified disorders of bladder**
  Bladder hemorrhage
  Bladder hypertrophy
  Calcified bladder
  Contracted bladder
  N32.9 **Bladder disorder, unspecified**

▷ **N33** *Bladder disorders in diseases classified elsewhere*
  Code first underlying disease, such as:
  schistosomiasis (B65.0-B65.9)
  Excludes1 bladder disorder in syphilis (A52.76)
  bladder disorder in tuberculosis (A18.12)
  candidal cystitis (B37.41)
  chlamydial cystitis(A56.01)
  cystitis in gonorrhea (A54.01)
  cystitis in neurogenic bladder (N31.-)
  diphtheritic cystitis (A36.85)
  syphilitic cystitis (A52.76)
  trichomonal cystitis (A59.03)
● **N34** **Urethritis and urethral syndrome**
  Use additional code (B95-B97), to identify infectious agent
  Excludes2 Reiter's disease (M02.3-)
  urethritis in diseases with a predominantly sexual mode of transmission (A50-A64)
  urethrotrigonitis (N30.3-)
  N34.0 **Urethral abscess**
  Abscess (of) Cowper's gland
  Abscess (of) Littré's gland
  Abscess (of) urethral (gland)
  Periurethral abscess
  Excludes1 urethral caruncle (N36.2)
  N34.1 **Nonspecific urethritis**
  Nongonococcal urethritis
  Nonvenereal urethritis
  N34.2 **Other urethritis**
  Inflammation of urethra
  Meatitis, urethral
  Postmenopausal urethritis
  Ulcer of urethra (meatus)
  Urethritis NOS
  N34.3 **Urethral syndrome, unspecified**
● **N35** **Urethral stricture**
  Narrowing of lumen of urethra caused by scarring due to infection or injury
  Excludes1 congenital urethral stricture (Q64.3-)
  postprocedural urethral stricture (N99.1-)
● **N35.0** **Post-traumatic urethral stricture**
  Urethral stricture due to injury
  Excludes1 postprocedural urethral stricture (N99.1-)
  ● **N35.01** **Post-traumatic urethral stricture, male**
    N35.010 **Post-traumatic urethral stricture, male, meatal** ♂
    N35.011 **Post-traumatic bulbous urethral stricture** ♂
    N35.012 **Post-traumatic membranous urethral stricture** ♂
    N35.013 **Post-traumatic anterior urethral stricture** ♂
    N35.014 **Post-traumatic urethral stricture, male, unspecified** ♂
    N35.016 **Post-traumatic urethral stricture, male, overlapping sites** ♂
  ● **N35.02** **Post-traumatic urethral stricture, female**
    N35.021 **Urethral stricture due to childbirth** ♀
    N35.028 **Other post-traumatic urethral stricture, female** ♀
● **N35.1** **Postinfective urethral stricture, not elsewhere classified**
  Excludes1 urethral stricture associated with schistosomiasis (B65.-, N29)
  gonococcal urethral stricture (A54.01)
  syphilitic urethral stricture (A52.76)
  ● **N35.11** **Postinfective urethral stricture, not elsewhere classified, male**
    N35.111 **Postinfective urethral stricture, not elsewhere classified, male, meatal** ♂
    N35.112 **Postinfective bulbous urethral stricture, not elsewhere classified, male** ♂

▶ New   ⇒ Revised   ~~deleted~~ Deleted   Excludes 1   Excludes 2   Includes   Use additional   Code first   Code also   Key words
OGCR Official Guidelines   X Assign placeholder X   ● Use Additional Character(s)   ▷ Manifestation Code   🐱 Hierarchical Condition Category   **Coding Clinic**

N35.113   Postinfective membranous urethral stricture, not elsewhere classified, male ♂

N35.114   Postinfective anterior urethral stricture, not elsewhere classified, male ♂

N35.116   Postinfective urethral stricture, not elsewhere classified, male, overlapping sites ♂

N35.119   Postinfective urethral stricture, not elsewhere classified, male, unspecified ♂

N35.12   Postinfective urethral stricture, not elsewhere classified, female ♀

● N35.8   **Other urethral stricture**
> **Excludes1**   postprocedural urethral stricture (N99.1-)

● N35.81   **Other urethral stricture, male**

N35.811   Other urethral stricture, male, meatal ♂

N35.812   Other urethral bulbous stricture, male ♂

N35.813   Other membranous urethral stricture, male ♂

N35.814   Other anterior urethral stricture, male ♂

N35.816   Other urethral stricture, male, overlapping sites ♂

N35.819   Other urethral stricture, male, unspecified site ♂

N35.82   Other urethral stricture, female ♀

● N35.9   **Urethral stricture, unspecified**

● N35.91   **Urethral stricture, unspecified, male**

N35.911   Unspecified urethral stricture, male, meatal ♂

N35.912   Unspecified bulbous urethral stricture, male ♂

N35.913   Unspecified membranous urethral stricture, male ♂

N35.914   Unspecified anterior urethral stricture, male ♂

N35.916   Unspecified urethral stricture, male, overlapping sites ♂

N35.919   Unspecified urethral stricture, male, unspecified site ♂
> Pinhole meatus NOS
> Urethral stricture NOS

N35.92   Unspecified urethral stricture, female ♀

● N36   **Other disorders of urethra**

N36.0   **Urethral fistula**
> Urethroperineal fistula
> Urethrorectal fistula
> Urinary fistula NOS
> **Excludes1**   urethroscrotal fistula (N50.89)
>   urethrovaginal fistula (N82.1)
>   urethrovesicovaginal fistula (N82.1)

N36.1   **Urethral diverticulum**

N36.2   **Urethral caruncle**

● N36.4   **Urethral functional and muscular disorders**
> Use additional code to identify associated urinary stress incontinence (N39.3)

N36.41   **Hypermobility of urethra**

N36.42   **Intrinsic sphincter deficiency (ISD)**

N36.43   **Combined hypermobility of urethra and intrinsic sphincter deficiency**

N36.44   **Muscular disorders of urethra**
> Bladder sphincter dyssynergy

N36.5   **Urethral false passage**

N36.8   **Other specified disorders of urethra**
> **Excludes1**   congenital urethrocele (Q64.7)
>   female urethrocele (N81.0)

N36.9   **Urethral disorder, unspecified**

▷ N37   *Urethral disorders in diseases classified elsewhere*
> *Code first underlying disease*
> **Excludes1**   urethritis (in):
>   candidal infection (B37.41)
>   chlamydial (A56.01)
>   gonorrhea (A54.01)
>   syphilis (A52.76)
>   trichomonal infection (A59.03)
>   tuberculosis (A18.13)

● N39   **Other disorders of urinary system**
> **Excludes2**   hematuria NOS (R31.-)
>   recurrent or persistent hematuria (N02.-)
>   recurrent or persistent hematuria with specified morphological lesion (N02.-)
>   proteinuria NOS (R80.-)

N39.0   **Urinary tract infection, site not specified**
> Use additional code (B95-B97), to identify infectious agent
> **Excludes1**   candidiasis of urinary tract (B37.4-)
>   neonatal urinary tract infection (P39.3)
>   pyuria (R82.81)
>   urinary tract infection of specified site, such as:
>   cystitis (N30.-)
>   urethritis (N34.-)
> **Coding Clinic: 2018, Q2, P22; Q1, P16; 2012, Q4, P94**

N39.3   **Stress incontinence (female) (male)**
> Code also any associated overactive bladder (N32.81)
> **Excludes1**   mixed incontinence (N39.46)
> **Coding Clinic: 2021, Q4, P18**

● N39.4   **Other specified urinary incontinence**
> Code also any associated overactive bladder (N32.81)
> **Excludes1**   enuresis NOS (R32)
>   functional urinary incontinence (R39.81)
>   urinary incontinence associated with cognitive impairment (R39.81)
>   urinary incontinence NOS (R32)
>   urinary incontinence of nonorganic origin (F98.0)

N39.41   **Urge incontinence**
> **Excludes1**   mixed incontinence (N39.46)

N39.42   **Incontinence without sensory awareness**
> Insensible (urinary) incontinence

N39.43   **Post-void dribbling**

Figure 14-6   Benign prostatic hyperplasia. (From Shiland: Mastering Healthcare Terminology, ed 3, St. Louis, Mosby, 2010)

CHAPTER 14 (N00-N99)

N39.44 Nocturnal enuresis
        Excludes2   nocturnal polyuria (R35.81)

N39.45 Continuous leakage

N39.46 Mixed incontinence
        Urge and stress incontinence

● N39.49 Other specified urinary incontinence
        N39.490 Overflow incontinence
        N39.491 Coital incontinence
                 Coding Clinic: 2016, Q4, P44
        N39.492 Postural (urinary) incontinence
                 Coding Clinic: 2016, Q4, P44
        N39.498 Other specified urinary incontinence
                 Reflex incontinence
                 Total incontinence

N39.8   Other specified disorders of urinary system

N39.9   Disorder of urinary system, unspecified

DISEASES OF MALE GENITAL ORGANS (N40-N53)

★ **(See Plate 5 of the Anatomy Illustrations.)**

● N40 Benign prostatic hyperplasia
        Includes   adenofibromatous hypertrophy of prostate
                       benign hypertrophy of the prostate
                       *Enlargement of prostate gland usually occurring
                       with age and causing obstructed urine flow*
                       benign prostatic hypertrophy
                       BPH
                       enlarged prostate
                       nodular prostate
                       polyp of prostate
        Excludes1 benign neoplasms of prostate (adenoma, benign)
                       (fibroadenoma) (fibroma) (myoma) (D29.1)
                       malignant neoplasm of prostate (C61)

N40.0   Benign prostatic hyperplasia **without lower urinary tract
        symptoms** ♂   A
        Enlarged prostate without LUTS
        Enlarged prostate NOS

N40.1   Benign prostatic hyperplasia **with lower urinary tract
        symptoms** ♂   A
        Enlarged prostate with LUTS

        Use additional code for associated symptoms, when
             specified:
        incomplete bladder emptying (R39.14)
        nocturia (R35.1)
        straining on urination (R39.16)
        urinary frequency (R35.0)
        urinary hesitancy (R39.11)
        urinary incontinence (N39.4-)
        urinary obstruction (N13.8)
        urinary retention (R33.8)
        urinary urgency (R39.15)
        weak urinary stream (R39.12)
        Coding Clinic: 2018, Q4, P55

N40.2   Nodular prostate **without lower urinary tract
        symptoms** ♂   A
        Nodular prostate without LUTS

N40.3   Nodular prostate **with lower urinary tract symptoms** ♂ A
        Use additional code for associated symptoms, when
             specified:
        incomplete bladder emptying (R39.14)
        nocturia (R35.1)
        straining on urination (R39.16)
        urinary frequency (R35.0)
        urinary hesitancy (R39.11)
        urinary incontinence (N39.4-)
        urinary obstruction (N13.8)
        urinary retention (R33.8)
        urinary urgency (R39.15)
        weak urinary stream (R39.12)

● N41 Inflammatory diseases of prostate
        Use additional code (B95-B97), to identify infectious agent
        N41.0 Acute prostatitis ♂   A
        N41.1 Chronic prostatitis ♂   A
        N41.2 Abscess of prostate ♂   A
        N41.3 Prostatocystitis ♂   A
        N41.4 Granulomatous prostatitis ♂   A
        N41.8 Other inflammatory diseases of prostate ♂   A
        N41.9 Inflammatory disease of prostate, unspecified ♂   A
               Prostatitis NOS

● N42 Other and unspecified disorders of prostate
        N42.0 Calculus of prostate ♂   A
               Prostatic stone
        N42.1 Congestion and hemorrhage of prostate ♂   A
               Excludes1 enlarged prostate (N40.-)
                             hematuria (R31.-)
                             hyperplasia of prostate (N40.-)
                             inflammatory diseases of prostate (N41.-)
      ● N42.3 Dysplasia of prostate
               Coding Clinic: 2016, Q4, P44
               N42.30 Unspecified dysplasia of prostate ♂
               N42.31 Prostatic intraepithelial neoplasia ♂
                       PIN
                       Prostatic intraepithelial neoplasia I (PIN I)
                       Prostatic intraepithelial neoplasia II (PIN II)
                       Excludes1 prostatic intraepithelial neoplasia
                                     III (PIN III) (D07.5)
               N42.32 Atypical small acinar proliferation of prostate ♂
               N42.39 Other dysplasia of prostate ♂
      ● N42.8 Other specified disorders of prostate
               N42.81 Prostatodynia syndrome ♂   A
                       Painful prostate syndrome
               N42.82 Prostatosis syndrome ♂   A
               N42.83 Cyst of prostate ♂   A
               N42.89 Other specified disorders of prostate ♂ A
        N42.9 Disorder of prostate, unspecified ♂   A

● N43 Hydrocele and spermatocele
        Includes   hydrocele of spermatic cord, testis or tunica
                       vaginalis
        Excludes1 congenital hydrocele (P83.5)
        N43.0 Encysted hydrocele ♂
        N43.1 Infected hydrocele ♂
               Use additional code (B95-B97), to identify infectious
                    agent
        N43.2 Other hydrocele ♂
        N43.3 Hydrocele, unspecified ♂
      ● N43.4 Spermatocele of epididymis
               Spermatic cyst
               N43.40 Spermatocele of epididymis, unspecified ♂
               N43.41 Spermatocele of epididymis, single ♂
               N43.42 Spermatocele of epididymis, multiple ♂

Item 14–7   Hydrocele is a sac of fluid accumulating in the testes membrane.

Figure 14-7   A. Hydrocele. **B.** Newborn with large right hydrocele.
(**B** from Nelson WE, Kliegman R: Nelson Textbook of Pediatrics,
Philadelphia, Saunders Elsevier, 2011)

Item 14–8 Male infertility is the inability of the female sex partner to conceive after one year of unprotected intercourse.

Azoospermia is no sperm ejaculated and **oligospermia** is few sperm ejaculated—both resulting in infertility. Extratesticular causes such as injury, infections, radiation, and chemotherapy may also cause male infertility.

● **N44　Noninflammatory disorders of testis**
　● **N44.0　Torsion of testis**
　　　　N44.00　Torsion of testis, unspecified ♂
　　　　N44.01　Extravaginal torsion of spermatic cord ♂
　　　　N44.02　Intravaginal torsion of spermatic cord ♂
　　　　　　　Torsion of spermatic cord NOS
　　　　N44.03　Torsion of appendix testis ♂
　　　　N44.04　Torsion of appendix epididymis ♂
　　N44.1　Cyst of tunica albuginea testis ♂
　　N44.2　Benign cyst of testis ♂
　　N44.8　Other noninflammatory disorders of the testis ♂

● **N45　Orchitis and epididymitis**
　　　Orchitis is inflammation of one or both of the testes as a result of mumps or other infection, trauma, or metastasis. Epididymitis is inflammation of the tubular structure that connects the testicle with the vas deferens.
　　　Use additional code (B95-B97), to identify infectious agent
　　N45.1　Epididymitis ♂
　　N45.2　Orchitis ♂
　　N45.3　Epididymo-orchitis ♂
　　N45.4　Abscess of epididymis or testis ♂

● **N46　Male infertility**
　　　Excludes1　vasectomy status (Z98.52)
　● **N46.0　Azoospermia**
　　　　Absolute male infertility
　　　　Male infertility due to germinal (cell) aplasia
　　　　Male infertility due to spermatogenic arrest (complete)
　　　　N46.01　Organic azoospermia ♂　　　　　A
　　　　　　　Azoospermia NOS
　　● **N46.02　Azoospermia due to extratesticular causes**
　　　　　　Code also associated cause
　　　　N46.021　Azoospermia due to drug therapy ♂　A
　　　　N46.022　Azoospermia due to infection ♂　A
　　　　N46.023　Azoospermia due to obstruction of efferent ducts ♂　A
　　　　N46.024　Azoospermia due to radiation ♂　A
　　　　N46.025　Azoospermia due to systemic disease ♂　A
　　　　N46.029　Azoospermia due to other extratesticular causes ♂　A
　● **N46.1　Oligospermia**
　　　　Male infertility due to germinal cell desquamation
　　　　Male infertility due to hypospermatogenesis
　　　　Male infertility due to incomplete spermatogenic arrest
　　　　N46.11　Organic oligospermia ♂　　　　A
　　　　　　　Oligospermia NOS
　　● **N46.12　Oligospermia due to extratesticular causes**
　　　　　　Code also associated cause
　　　　N46.121　Oligospermia due to drug therapy ♂　A
　　　　N46.122　Oligospermia due to infection ♂　A
　　　　N46.123　Oligospermia due to obstruction of efferent ducts ♂　A
　　　　N46.124　Oligospermia due to radiation ♂　A
　　　　N46.125　Oligospermia due to systemic disease ♂　A
　　　　N46.129　Oligospermia due to other extratesticular causes ♂　A
　　N46.8　Other male infertility ♂　　　　A
　　N46.9　Male infertility, unspecified ♂　　A

● **N47　Disorders of prepuce**
　　N47.0　Adherent prepuce, newborn ♂　　　　　　　　N
　　N47.1　Phimosis ♂
　　N47.2　Paraphimosis ♂
　　N47.3　Deficient foreskin ♂
　　N47.4　Benign cyst of prepuce ♂
　　N47.5　Adhesions of prepuce and glans penis ♂
　　N47.6　Balanoposthitis ♂
　　　　　Use additional code (B95-B97), to identify infectious agent
　　　　　Excludes1　balanitis (N48.1)
　　N47.7　Other inflammatory diseases of prepuce ♂
　　　　　Use additional code (B95-B97), to identify infectious agent
　　N47.8　Other disorders of prepuce ♂

● **N48　Other disorders of penis**
　　N48.0　Leukoplakia of penis ♂
　　　　　Balanitis xerotica obliterans
　　　　　Kraurosis of penis
　　　　　Lichen sclerosus of external male genital organs
　　　　　Excludes1　carcinoma in situ of penis (D07.4)
　　N48.1　Balanitis ♂
　　　　　Use additional code (B95-B97), to identify infectious agent
　　　　　Excludes1　amebic balanitis (A06.8)
　　　　　　　　balanitis xerotica obliterans (N48.0)
　　　　　　　　candidal balanitis (B37.42)
　　　　　　　　gonococcal balanitis (A54.23)
　　　　　　　　herpesviral [herpes simplex] balanitis (A60.01)
　● **N48.2　Other inflammatory disorders of penis**
　　　　　Use additional code (B95-B97), to identify infectious agent
　　　　　Excludes1　balanitis (N48.1)
　　　　　　　　balanitis xerotica obliterans (N48.0)
　　　　　　　　balanoposthitis (N47.6)
　　　　N48.21　Abscess of corpus cavernosum and penis ♂
　　　　N48.22　Cellulitis of corpus cavernosum and penis ♂
　　　　N48.29　Other inflammatory disorders of penis ♂
　● **N48.3　Priapism**
　　　　　Painful erection
　　　　　Code first underlying cause
　　　　N48.30　Priapism, unspecified ♂
　　　　N48.31　Priapism due to trauma ♂
　　　▷**N48.32　*Priapism due to disease classified elsewhere* ♂**
　　　　N48.33　Priapism, drug-induced ♂
　　　　N48.39　Other priapism ♂
　　N48.5　Ulcer of penis ♂
　　N48.6　Induration penis plastica ♂
　　　　　Peyronie's disease
　　　　　Plastic induration of penis
　● **N48.8　Other specified disorders of penis**
　　　　N48.81　Thrombosis of superficial vein of penis ♂
　　　　N48.82　Acquired torsion of penis ♂
　　　　　　　Acquired torsion of penis NOS
　　　　　　　Excludes1　congenital torsion of penis (Q55.63)
　　　　N48.83　Acquired buried penis ♂
　　　　　　　Excludes1　congenital hidden penis (Q55.64)
　　　　N48.89　Other specified disorders of penis ♂
　　N48.9　Disorder of penis, unspecified ♂

CHAPTER 14 (N00-N99)

Item 14–9 Seminal vesiculitis is an inflammation of the seminal vesicle. **Spermatocele** is a benign cystic accumulation of sperm arising from the head of the epididymis. **Torsion of the testis** is a medical emergency occurring most commonly in boys 7 to 12 years of age and results from a congenital abnormality of the covering of the testis allowing the testis to twist within its sac and cutting off the blood supply to the testis.

Figure 14-8 A. Torsion of testis. **B.** Torsion of the testis. (**B** from Kliegman R, Nelson WE: Nelson Textbook of Pediatrics, Philadelphia, Saunders, 2007)

● **N49   Inflammatory disorders of male genital organs, not elsewhere classified**

    Use additional code (B95-B97), to identify infectious agent

    Excludes1   inflammation of penis (N48.1, N48.2-)
                    orchitis and epididymitis (N45.-)

    N49.0   Inflammatory disorders of seminal vesicle ♂
           Vesiculitis NOS

    N49.1   Inflammatory disorders of spermatic cord, tunica vaginalis and vas deferens ♂
           Vasitis

    N49.2   Inflammatory disorders of scrotum ♂

    N49.3   Fournier gangrene ♂

    N49.8   Inflammatory disorders of other specified male genital organs ♂
           Inflammation of multiple sites in male genital organs

    N49.9   Inflammatory disorder of unspecified male genital organ ♂
           Abscess of unspecified male genital organ
           Boil of unspecified male genital organ
           Carbuncle of unspecified male genital organ
           Cellulitis of unspecified male genital organ

● **N50   Other and unspecified disorders of male genital organs**

    Excludes2   torsion of testis (N44.0-)

    N50.0   Atrophy of testis ♂

    N50.1   Vascular disorders of male genital organs ♂
           Hematocele, NOS, of male genital organs
           Hemorrhage of male genital organs
           Thrombosis of male genital organs

    N50.3   Cyst of epididymis ♂

●   **N50.8   Other specified disorders of male genital organs**
        Coding Clinic: 2016, Q4, P45

    ● **N50.81   Testicular pain**
        N50.811   Right testicular pain ♂
        N50.812   Left testicular pain ♂
        N50.819   Testicular pain, unspecified ♂

        N50.82   Scrotal pain ♂

    N50.89   Other specified disorders of the male genital organs ♂
           Atrophy of scrotum, seminal vesicle, spermatic cord, tunica vaginalis and vas deferens
           Chylocele, tunica vaginalis (nonfilarial) NOS
           Edema of scrotum, seminal vesicle, spermatic cord, tunica vaginalis and vas deferens
           Hypertrophy of scrotum, seminal vesicle, spermatic cord, tunica vaginalis and vas deferens
           Stricture of spermatic cord, tunica vaginalis, and vas deferens
           Ulcer of scrotum, seminal vesicle, spermatic cord, testis, tunica vaginalis and vas deferens
           Urethroscrotal fistula

    N50.9   Disorder of male genital organs, unspecified ♂

▷ *N51   Disorders of male genital organs in diseases classified elsewhere* ♂

    Code first underlying disease, such as:
        filariasis (B74.0-B74.9)

    Excludes1   amebic balanitis (A06.8)
                  candidal balanitis (B37.42)
                  gonococcal balanitis (A54.23)
                  gonococcal prostatitis (A54.22)
                  herpesviral [herpes simplex] balanitis (A60.01)
                  trichomonal prostatitis (A59.02)
                  tuberculous prostatitis (A18.14)

● **N52   Male erectile dysfunction**

    Excludes1   psychogenic impotence (F52.21)

  ● **N52.0   Vasculogenic erectile dysfunction**

        N52.01   Erectile dysfunction due to arterial insufficiency ♂   A

        N52.02   Corporo-venous occlusive erectile dysfunction ♂   A

        N52.03   Combined arterial insufficiency and corporo-venous occlusive erectile dysfunction ♂   A

▷ *N52.1   Erectile dysfunction due to diseases classified elsewhere* ♂   A

        Code first underlying disease

    N52.2   Drug-induced erectile dysfunction ♂   A

  ● **N52.3   Postprocedural erectile dysfunction**

        N52.31   Erectile dysfunction following radical prostatectomy ♂   A

        N52.32   Erectile dysfunction following radical cystectomy ♂   A

        N52.33   Erectile dysfunction following urethral surgery ♂   A

        N52.34   Erectile dysfunction following simple prostatectomy ♂   A

        N52.35   Erectile dysfunction following radiation therapy ♂   A
           Coding Clinic: 2016, Q4, P45

        N52.36   Erectile dysfunction following interstitial seed therapy ♂   A
           Coding Clinic: 2016, Q4, P45

        N52.37   Erectile dysfunction following prostate ablative therapy ♂   A
           Erectile dysfunction following cryotherapy
           Erectile dysfunction following other prostate ablative therapies
           Erectile dysfunction following ultrasound ablative therapies
           Coding Clinic: 2016, Q4, P45

        N52.39   Other and unspecified postprocedural erectile dysfunction ♂   A

    N52.8   Other male erectile dysfunction ♂   A

    N52.9   Male erectile dysfunction, unspecified ♂   A
           Impotence NOS

CHAPTER 14 (N00-N99)

● **N53   Other male sexual dysfunction**
> **Excludes1**   psychogenic sexual dysfunction (F52.-)

● **N53.1   Ejaculatory dysfunction**
> **Excludes1**   premature ejaculation (F52.4)

   N53.11   Retarded ejaculation ♂

   N53.12   Painful ejaculation ♂

   N53.13   Anejaculatory orgasm ♂

   N53.14   Retrograde ejaculation ♂

   N53.19   Other ejaculatory dysfunction ♂
       Ejaculatory dysfunction NOS

  N53.8   Other male sexual dysfunction ♂

  N53.9   Unspecified male sexual dysfunction ♂

DISORDERS OF BREAST (N60–N65)

> **Excludes1**   disorders of breast associated with childbirth (O91-O92)

● **N60   Benign mammary dysplasia**
Benign lumpiness of breast
> **Includes**   fibrocystic mastopathy

● **N60.0   Solitary cyst of breast**
Cyst of breast

   N60.01   Solitary cyst of right breast

   N60.02   Solitary cyst of left breast

   N60.09   Solitary cyst of unspecified breast

● **N60.1   Diffuse cystic mastopathy**
Cystic breast
Fibrocystic disease of breast
> **Excludes1**   diffuse cystic mastopathy with epithelial proliferation (N60.3-)

   N60.11   Diffuse cystic mastopathy of right breast   A

   N60.12   Diffuse cystic mastopathy of left breast   A

   N60.19   Diffuse cystic mastopathy of unspecified breast   A

● **N60.2   Fibroadenosis of breast**
Adenofibrosis of breast
> **Excludes2**   fibroadenoma of breast (D24.-)

   N60.21   Fibroadenosis of right breast

   N60.22   Fibroadenosis of left breast

   N60.29   Fibroadenosis of unspecified breast

● **N60.3   Fibrosclerosis of breast**
Cystic mastopathy with epithelial proliferation

   N60.31   Fibrosclerosis of right breast

   N60.32   Fibrosclerosis of left breast

   N60.39   Fibrosclerosis of unspecified breast

● **N60.4   Mammary duct ectasia**

   N60.41   Mammary duct ectasia of right breast

   N60.42   Mammary duct ectasia of left breast

   N60.49   Mammary duct ectasia of unspecified breast

● **N60.8   Other benign mammary dysplasias**

   N60.81   Other benign mammary dysplasias of right breast

   N60.82   Other benign mammary dysplasias of left breast

   N60.89   Other benign mammary dysplasias of unspecified breast

● **N60.9   Unspecified benign mammary dysplasia**

   N60.91   Unspecified benign mammary dysplasia of right breast

   N60.92   Unspecified benign mammary dysplasia of left breast

   N60.99   Unspecified benign mammary dysplasia of unspecified breast

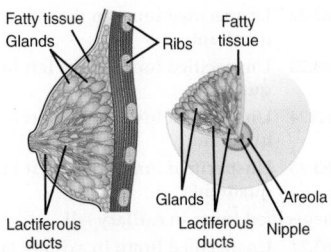

Figure 14-9   Breast.

● **N61   Inflammatory disorders of breast**
> **Excludes1**   inflammatory carcinoma of breast (C50.9)
> inflammatory disorder of breast associated with childbirth (O91.-)
> neonatal infective mastitis (P39.0)
> thrombophlebitis of breast [Mondor's disease] (I80.8)

  N61.0   Mastitis without abscess
Infective mastitis (acute) (nonpuerperal) (subacute)
Mastitis (acute) (nonpuerperal) (subacute) NOS
Cellulitis (acute) (nonpuerperal) (subacute) of breast NOS
Cellulitis (acute) (nonpuerperal) (subacute) of nipple NOS

  N61.1   Abscess of the breast and nipple
Abscess (acute) (chronic) (nonpuerperal) of areola
Abscess (acute) (chronic) (nonpuerperal) of breast
Carbuncle of breast
Mastitis with abscess

● **N61.2   Granulomatous mastitis**

   N61.20   Granulomatous mastitis, unspecified breast

   N61.21   Granulomatous mastitis, right breast

   N61.22   Granulomatous mastitis, left breast

   N61.23   Granulomatous mastitis, bilateral breast

N62   Hypertrophy of breast
Gynecomastia
Hypertrophy of breast NOS
Massive pubertal hypertrophy of breast
> **Excludes1**   breast engorgement of newborn (P83.4)
> disproportion of reconstructed breast (N65.1)

● **N63   Unspecified lump in breast**
Nodule(s) NOS in breast

  N63.0   Unspecified lump in unspecified breast

● **N63.1   Unspecified lump in the right breast**

   N63.10   Unspecified lump in the right breast, unspecified quadrant

   N63.11   Unspecified lump in the right breast, upper outer quadrant
       Coding Clinic: 2017, Q4, P19

   N63.12   Unspecified lump in the right breast, upper inner quadrant

   N63.13   Unspecified lump in the right breast, lower outer quadrant

   N63.14   Unspecified lump in the right breast, lower inner quadrant

   N63.15   Unspecified lump in the right breast, overlapping quadrants

● **N63.2   Unspecified lump in the left breast**

   N63.20   Unspecified lump in the left breast, unspecified quadrant

   N63.21   Unspecified lump in the left breast, upper outer quadrant

CHAPTER 14 (N00-N99)

N63.22 Unspecified lump in the left breast, upper inner quadrant

N63.23 Unspecified lump in the left breast, lower outer quadrant

N63.24 Unspecified lump in the left breast, lower inner quadrant

N63.25 Unspecified lump in the left breast, overlapping quadrants

● **N63.3** Unspecified lump in axillary tail

N63.31 Unspecified lump in axillary tail of the right breast

N63.32 Unspecified lump in axillary tail of the left breast

● **N63.4** Unspecified lump in breast, subareolar

N63.41 Unspecified lump in right breast, subareolar

N63.42 Unspecified lump in left breast, subareolar

● **N64** Other disorders of breast

Excludes2 mechanical complication of breast prosthesis and implant (T85.4-)

N64.0 Fissure and fistula of nipple

N64.1 Fat necrosis of breast
Fat necrosis (segmental) of breast
Code first breast necrosis due to breast graft (T85.898)

N64.2 Atrophy of breast

N64.3 Galactorrhea not associated with childbirth
Excessive or spontaneous flow of milk

N64.4 Mastodynia

● **N64.5** Other signs and symptoms in breast

Excludes2 abnormal findings on diagnostic imaging of breast (R92.-)

N64.51 Induration of breast

N64.52 Nipple discharge

Excludes1 abnormal findings in nipple discharge (R89.-)

N64.53 Retraction of nipple

N64.59 Other signs and symptoms in breast

● **N64.8** Other specified disorders of breast

N64.81 Ptosis of breast   A

Excludes1 ptosis of native breast in relation to reconstructed breast (N65.1)

N64.82 Hypoplasia of breast   A
Micromastia

Excludes1 congenital absence of breast (Q83.0)
hypoplasia of native breast in relation to reconstructed breast (N65.1)

N64.89 Other specified disorders of breast
Galactocele
Subinvolution of breast (postlactational)
Coding Clinic: 2019, Q1, P32; 2018, Q1, P4

N64.9 Disorder of breast, unspecified
Coding Clinic: 2018, Q1, P4

● **N65** Deformity and disproportion of reconstructed breast

N65.0 Deformity of reconstructed breast   A
Contour irregularity in reconstructed breast
Excess tissue in reconstructed breast
Misshapen reconstructed breast

N65.1 Disproportion of reconstructed breast   A
Breast asymmetry between native breast and reconstructed breast
Disproportion between native breast and reconstructed breast

INFLAMMATORY DISEASES OF FEMALE PELVIC ORGANS (N70-N77)

Excludes1 inflammatory diseases of female pelvic organs complicating:
abortion or ectopic or molar pregnancy (O00-O07, O08.0)
pregnancy, childbirth and the puerperium (O23.-, O75.3, O85, O86.-)

★**(See Plate 35 of the Anatomy Illustrations.)**

● **N70** Salpingitis and oophoritis
Oophoritis = inflammation of ovary
Salpingitis = inflammation of falloplan tube

Includes abscess (of) fallopian tube
abscess (of) ovary
pyosalpinx
salpingo-oophoritis
tubo-ovarian abscess
tubo-ovarian inflammatory disease

Use additional code (B95-B97), to identify infectious agent

Excludes1 gonococcal infection (A54.24)
tuberculous infection (A18.17)

● **N70.0** Acute salpingitis and oophoritis

N70.01 Acute salpingitis ♀

N70.02 Acute oophoritis ♀

N70.03 Acute salpingitis and oophoritis ♀

● **N70.1** Chronic salpingitis and oophoritis
Hydrosalpinx

N70.11 Chronic salpingitis ♀

N70.12 Chronic oophoritis ♀

N70.13 Chronic salpingitis and oophoritis ♀

● **N70.9** Salpingitis and oophoritis, unspecified

N70.91 Salpingitis, unspecified ♀

N70.92 Oophoritis, unspecified ♀

N70.93 Salpingitis and oophoritis, unspecified ♀

● **N71** Inflammatory disease of uterus, except cervix

Includes endo (myo) metritis
metritis
myometritis
pyometra
uterine abscess

Use additional code (B95-B97), to identify infectious agent

Excludes1 hyperplastic endometritis (N85.0-)
infection of uterus following delivery (O85, O86.-)

N71.0 Acute inflammatory disease of uterus ♀

N71.1 Chronic inflammatory disease of uterus ♀

N71.9 Inflammatory disease of uterus, unspecified ♀

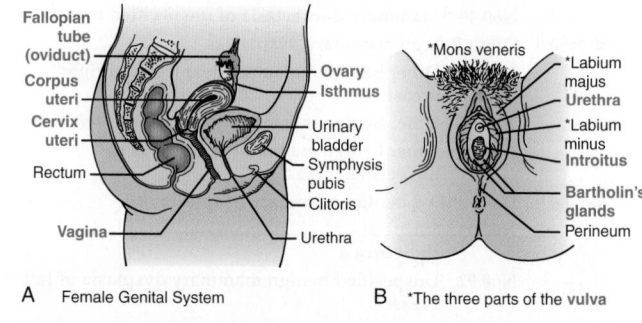

Figure 14-10 A. Female genital system. **B.** External female genital system. (From Buck CJ: Step-by-Step Medical Coding, ed 2016, St. Louis, Elsevier, 2016)

Item 14–10 Salpingitis is an infection of one or both fallopian tubes. **Oophoritis** is an infection of one or both ovaries.

▶ New   ➡ Revised   ~~deleted~~ Deleted   Excludes 1   Excludes 2   Includes   Use additional   Code first   Code also   Key words

OGCR Official Guidelines   X Assign placeholder X   ● Use Additional Character(s)   ▶ Manifestation Code   Hierarchical Condition Category   **Coding Clinic**

N72   **Inflammatory disease of cervix uteri** ♀

Includes	cervicitis (with or without erosion or ectropion)
	endocervicitis (with or without erosion or ectropion)
	exocervicitis (with or without erosion or ectropion)

Use additional code (B95-B97), to identify infectious agent

Excludes1	erosion and ectropion of cervix without cervicitis (N86)

● N73   **Other female pelvic inflammatory diseases**

Use additional code (B95-B97), to identify infectious agent

N73.0   **Acute parametritis and pelvic cellulitis** ♀
Abscess of broad ligament
Abscess of parametrium
Pelvic cellulitis, female

N73.1   **Chronic parametritis and pelvic cellulitis** ♀
Any condition in N73.0 specified as chronic

Excludes1	tuberculous parametritis and pelvic cellultis (A18.17)

N73.2   **Unspecified parametritis and pelvic cellulitis** ♀
Any condition in N73.0 unspecified whether acute or chronic

N73.3   **Female acute pelvic peritonitis** ♀
N73.4   **Female chronic pelvic peritonitis** ♀

Excludes1	tuberculous pelvic (female) peritonitis (A18.17)

N73.5   **Female pelvic peritonitis, unspecified** ♀
N73.6   **Female pelvic peritoneal adhesions (postinfective)** ♀

Excludes2	postprocedural pelvic peritoneal adhesions (N99.4)

N73.8   **Other specified female pelvic inflammatory diseases** ♀
N73.9   **Female pelvic inflammatory disease, unspecified** ♀
Female pelvic infection or inflammation NOS

▷ N74   *Female pelvic inflammatory disorders in diseases classified elsewhere* ♀

Code first underlying disease

Excludes1	chlamydial cervicitis (A56.02)
	chlamydial pelvic inflammatory disease (A56.11)
	gonococcal cervicitis (A54.03)
	gonococcal pelvic inflammatory disease (A54.24)
	herpesviral [herpes simplex] cervicitis (A60.03)
	herpesviral [herpes simplex] pelvic inflammatory disease (A60.09)
	syphilitic cervicitis (A52.76)
	syphilitic pelvic inflammatory disease (A52.76)
	trichomonal cervicitis (A59.09)
	tuberculous cervicitis (A18.16)
	tuberculous pelvic inflammatory disease (A18.17)

● N75   **Diseases of Bartholin's gland**

N75.0   **Cyst of Bartholin's gland** ♀
Cysts filled with liquid or semisolid material

N75.1   **Abscess of Bartholin's gland** ♀
Localized collection of pus

N75.8   **Other diseases of Bartholin's gland** ♀
Bartholinitis

N75.9   **Disease of Bartholin's gland, unspecified** ♀

● N76   **Other inflammation of vagina and vulva**

Use additional code (B95-B97), to identify infectious agent

Excludes2	senile (atrophic) vaginitis (N95.2)
	vulvar vestibulitis (N94.810)

N76.0   **Acute vaginitis** ♀
Acute vulvovaginitis
Vaginitis NOS
Vulvovaginitis NOS

N76.1   **Subacute and chronic vaginitis** ♀
Chronic vulvovaginitis
Subacute vulvovaginitis

N76.2   **Acute vulvitis** ♀
Vulvitis NOS

N76.3   **Subacute and chronic vulvitis** ♀

N76.4   **Abscess of vulva** ♀
Furuncle of vulva

N76.5   **Ulceration of vagina** ♀

N76.6   **Ulceration of vulva** ♀

● N76.8   **Other specified inflammation of vagina and vulva**

N76.81   **Mucositis (ulcerative) of vagina and vulva** ♀

Code also type of associated therapy, such as:
antineoplastic and immunosuppressive drugs (T45.1X-)
radiological procedure and radiotherapy (Y84.2)

Excludes2	gastrointestinal mucositis (ulcerative) (K92.81)
	nasal mucositis (ulcerative) (J34.81)
	oral mucositis (ulcerative) (K12.3-)

▷ N76.82   **Fournier disease of vagina and vulva** ♀
▷ Fournier gangrene of vagina and vulva

▷ Code also, if applicable, diabetes mellitus (E08-E13 with .9)

▷ **Excludes1**	gangrene in diabetes mellitus (E08-E13 with .52)

N76.89   **Other specified inflammation of vagina and vulva** ♀

● N77   **Vulvovaginal ulceration and inflammation in diseases classified elsewhere**

▷ N77.0   *Ulceration of vulva in diseases classified elsewhere* ♀

Code first underlying disease, such as:
Behçet's disease (M35.2)

Excludes1	ulceration of vulva in gonococcal infection (A54.02)
	ulceration of vulva in herpesviral [herpes simplex] infection (A60.04)
	ulceration of vulva in syphilis (A51.0)
	ulceration of vulva in tuberculosis (A18.18)

▷ N77.1   *Vaginitis, vulvitis and vulvovaginitis in diseases classified elsewhere* ♀

Code first underlying disease, such as:
pinworm (B80)

⇒ **Excludes1**	candidial vulvovaginitis (B37.3-)
	chlamydial vulvovaginitis (A56.02)
	gonococcal vulvovaginitis (A54.02)
	herpesviral [herpes simplex] vulvovaginitis (A60.04)
	trichomonal vulvovaginitis (A59.01)
	tuberculous vulvovaginitis (A18.18)
	vulvovaginitis in early syphilis (A51.0)
	vulvovaginitis in late syphilis (A52.76)

NONINFLAMMATORY DISORDERS OF FEMALE GENITAL TRACT (N80-N98)

● N80   **Endometriosis**

● N80.0   **Endometriosis of uterus** ♀
~~Adenomyosis~~
▷ Endometriosis of the cervix

Excludes1	stromal endometriosis (D39.0)

▷ N80.00   **Endometriosis of the uterus, unspecified** ♀
▷ N80.01   **Superficial endometriosis of the uterus** ♀
▷ N80.02   **Deep endometriosis of the uterus** ♀
▷ Deep retrocervical endometriosis
▷ N80.03   **Adenomyosis of the uterus** ♀
▷ Adenomyosis NOS

● N80.1   **Endometriosis of ovary** ♀
▷ ● N80.10   **Endometriosis of ovary, unspecified depth** ♀
▷ N80.101   **Endometriosis of right ovary, unspecified depth** ♀
▷ N80.102   **Endometriosis of left ovary, unspecified depth** ♀
▷ N80.103   **Endometriosis of bilateral ovaries, unspecified depth** ♀
▷ N80.109   **Endometriosis of ovary, unspecified side, unspecified depth** ♀
Endometriosis of ovary NOS

CHAPTER 14 (N00-N99)

▶ ● N80.11   Superficial endometriosis of the ovary ♀
    ▶ N80.111   Superficial endometriosis of right ovary ♀
    ▶ N80.112   Superficial endometriosis of left ovary ♀
    ▶ N80.113   Superficial endometriosis of bilateral ovaries ♀
    ▶ N80.119   Superficial endometriosis of ovary, unspecified ovary ♀

▶ ● N80.12   Deep endometriosis of ovary ♀
    ▶ Deep ovarian endometriosis
       Endometrioma
    ▶ N80.121   Deep endometriosis of right ovary ♀
    ▶ N80.122   Deep endometriosis of left ovary ♀
    ▶ N80.123   Deep endometriosis of bilateral ovaries ♀
    ▶ N80.129   Deep endometriosis of ovary, unspecified ovary ♀

● N80.2   Endometriosis of fallopian tube ♀
  ▶ ● N80.20   Endometriosis of fallopian tube, unspecified depth ♀
    ▶ N80.201   Endometriosis of right fallopian tube, unspecified depth ♀
    ▶ N80.202   Endometriosis of left fallopian tube, unspecified depth ♀
    ▶ N80.203   Endometriosis of bilateral fallopian tubes, unspecified depth ♀
    ▶ N80.209   Endometriosis of unspecified fallopian tube, unspecified depth ♀
       ▶ Endometriosis fallopian tube NOS

  ▶ ● N80.21   Superficial endometriosis of fallopian tube ♀
    ▶ N80.211   Superficial endometriosis of right fallopian tube ♀
    ▶ N80.212   Superficial endometriosis of left fallopian tube ♀
    ▶ N80.213   Superficial endometriosis of bilateral fallopian tubes ♀
    ▶ N80.219   Superficial endometriosis of unspecified fallopian tube ♀

  ▶ ● N80.22   Deep endometriosis of the fallopian tube ♀
    ▶ Deep endometriosis involving muscular wall of fallopian tube
    ▶ N80.221   Deep endometriosis of right fallopian tube ♀
    ▶ N80.222   Deep endometriosis of left fallopian tube ♀
    ▶ N80.223   Deep endometriosis of bilateral fallopian tubes ♀
    ▶ N80.229   Deep endometriosis of unspecified fallopian tube ♀

● N80.3   Endometriosis of pelvic peritoneum ♀
  ▶ N80.30   Endometriosis of pelvic peritoneum, unspecified ♀
    ▶ Endometriosis of the retroperitoneum NOS

  ▶ ● N80.31   Endometriosis of the anterior cul-de-sac ♀
    ▶ N80.311   Superficial endometriosis of the anterior cul-de-sac ♀
    ▶ N80.312   Deep endometriosis of the anterior cul-de-sac ♀
    ▶ N80.319   Endometriosis of the anterior cul-de-sac, unspecified depth ♀
       ▶ Endometriosis of the anterior cul-de-sac NOS

▶ ● N80.32   Endometriosis of the posterior cul-de-sac ♀
    ▶ N80.321   Superficial endometriosis of the posterior cul-de-sac ♀
    ▶ N80.322   Deep endometriosis of the posterior cul-de-sac ♀
    ▶ N80.329   Endometriosis of the posterior cul-de-sac, unspecified depth ♀
       ▶ Endometriosis of the posterior cul-de-sac NOS

▶ ● N80.33   Superficial endometriosis of the pelvic sidewall ♀
    ▶ N80.331   Superficial endometriosis of the right pelvic sidewall ♀
    ▶ N80.332   Superficial endometriosis of the left pelvic sidewall ♀
    ▶ N80.333   Superficial endometriosis of bilateral pelvic sidewall ♀
    ▶ N80.339   Superficial endometriosis of pelvic sidewall, unspecified side ♀

▶ ● N80.34   Deep endometriosis of the pelvic sidewall ♀
    ▶ N80.341   Deep endometriosis of the right pelvic sidewall ♀
    ▶ N80.342   Deep endometriosis of the left pelvic sidewall ♀
    ▶ N80.343   Deep endometriosis of the bilateral pelvic sidewall ♀
    ▶ N80.349   Deep endometriosis of the pelvic sidewall, unspecified side ♀

▶ ● N80.35   Endometriosis of the pelvic sidewall, unspecified depth ♀
    ▶ N80.351   Endometriosis of the right pelvic sidewall, unspecified depth ♀
    ▶ N80.352   Endometriosis of the left pelvic sidewall, unspecified depth ♀
    ▶ N80.353   Endometriosis of bilateral pelvic sidewall, unspecified depth ♀
    ▶ N80.359   Endometriosis of pelvic sidewall, unspecified side, unspecified depth ♀
       ▶ Endometriosis of the pelvic sidewall NOS

▶ ● N80.36   Superficial endometriosis of the pelvic brim ♀
    ▶ N80.361   Superficial endometriosis of the right pelvic brim ♀
    ▶ N80.362   Superficial endometriosis of the left pelvic brim ♀
    ▶ N80.363   Superficial endometriosis of bilateral pelvic brim ♀
    ▶ N80.369   Superficial endometriosis of the pelvic brim, unspecified side ♀

▶ ● N80.37   Deep endometriosis of the pelvic brim ♀
    ▶ N80.371   Deep endometriosis of the right pelvic brim ♀
    ▶ N80.372   Deep endometriosis of the left pelvic brim ♀
    ▶ N80.373   Deep endometriosis of bilateral pelvic brim ♀
    ▶ N80.379   Deep endometriosis of the pelvic brim, unspecified side ♀

▶ ● N80.38   Endometriosis of the pelvic brim, unspecified depth ♀
    ▶ N80.381   Endometriosis of the right pelvic brim, unspecified depth ♀
    ▶ N80.382   Endometriosis of the left pelvic brim, unspecified depth ♀
    ▶ N80.383   Endometriosis of bilateral pelvic brim, unspecified depth ♀
    ▶ N80.389   Endometriosis of the pelvic brim, unspecified side, unspecified depth ♀
       ▶ Endometriosis of the pelvic brim NOS

▶ New   ⇒ Revised   ~~deleted~~ Deleted   Excludes 1   Excludes 2   Includes   Use additional   Code first   Code also   Key words
OGCR Official Guidelines   X Assign placeholder X   ● Use Additional Character(s)   ▷ Manifestation Code   ℞ Hierarchical Condition Category   Coding Clinic

▶● **N80.39**   Endometriosis of other pelvic peritoneum ♀
    ▶ **N80.391**   Superficial endometriosis of the pelvic peritoneum, other specified sites ♀
    ▶ **N80.392**   Deep endometriosis of the pelvic peritoneum, other specified sites ♀
    ▶ **N80.399**   Endometriosis of the pelvic peritoneum, other specified sites, unspecified depth ♀
▶● **N80.3A**   Superficial endometriosis of the uterosacral ligament(s) ♀
    ▶ **N80.3A1**   Superficial endometriosis of the right uterosacral ligament ♀
    ▶ **N80.3A2**   Superficial endometriosis of the left uterosacral ligament ♀
    ▶ **N80.3A3**   Superficial endometriosis of the bilateral uterosacral ligament(s) ♀
    ▶ **N80.3A9**   Superficial endometriosis of the uterosacral ligament(s), unspecified side ♀
▶● **N80.3B**   Deep endometriosis of the uterosacral ligament(s) ♀
    ▶ **N80.3B1**   Deep endometriosis of the right uterosacral ligament ♀
    ▶ **N80.3B2**   Deep endometriosis of the left uterosacral ligament ♀
    ▶ **N80.3B3**   Deep endometriosis of bilateral uterosacral ligament(s) ♀
    ▶ **N80.3B9**   Deep endometriosis of the uterosacral ligament(s), unspecified side ♀
▶● **N80.3C**   Endometriosis of the uterosacral ligament(s), unspecified depth ♀
    ▶ **N80.3C1**   Endometriosis of the right uterosacral ligament, unspecified depth ♀
    ▶ **N80.3C2**   Endometriosis of the left uterosacral ligament, unspecified depth ♀
    ▶ **N80.3C3**   Endometriosis of bilateral uterosacral ligament(s), unspecified depth ♀
    ▶ **N80.3C9**   Endometriosis of the uterosacral ligament(s), unspecified side, unspecified depth ♀
        ▶ Endometriosis of the uterosacral ligament(s) NOS
● **N80.4**   Endometriosis of rectovaginal septum and vagina ♀
    ▶ **N80.40**   Endometriosis of rectovaginal septum, unspecified involvement of vagina ♀
        ▶ Endometriosis of the rectovaginal septum, NOS
    ▶ **N80.41**   Endometriosis of rectovaginal septum without involvement of vagina ♀
    ▶ **N80.42**   Endometriosis of rectovaginal septum with involvement of vagina ♀
● **N80.5**   Endometriosis of intestine ♀
    ▶ **N80.50**   Endometriosis of intestine, unspecified ♀
    ▶● **N80.51**   Endometriosis of the rectum ♀
        ▶ **N80.511**   Superficial endometriosis of the rectum ♀
        ▶ **N80.512**   Deep endometriosis of the rectum ♀
            ▶ Deep endometriosis of the rectum, multifocal
        ▶ **N80.519**   Endometriosis of the rectum, unspecified depth ♀
            ▶ Endometriosis of the rectum NOS
    ▶● **N80.52**   Endometriosis of the sigmoid colon ♀
        ▶ **N80.521**   Superficial endometriosis of the sigmoid colon ♀
        ▶ **N80.522**   Deep endometriosis of the sigmoid colon ♀
        ▶ **N80.529**   Endometriosis of the sigmoid colon, unspecified depth ♀
            ▶ Endometriosis of the sigmoid colon NOS

▶● **N80.53**   Endometriosis of the cecum ♀
    ▶ **N80.531**   Superficial endometriosis of the cecum ♀
    ▶ **N80.532**   Deep endometriosis of the cecum ♀
    ▶ **N80.539**   Endometriosis of the cecum, unspecified depth ♀
        ▶ Endometriosis of the cecum NOS
▶● **N80.54**   Endometriosis of the appendix ♀
    ▶ **N80.541**   Superficial endometriosis of the appendix ♀
    ▶ **N80.542**   Deep endometriosis of the appendix ♀
    ▶ **N80.549**   Endometriosis of the appendix, unspecified depth ♀
        ▶ Endometriosis of the appendix NOS
▶● **N80.55**   Endometriosis of other parts of the colon ♀
    ▶ Endometriosis of descending colon
    ▶ Endometriosis of transverse colon
    ▶ **N80.551**   Superficial endometriosis of other parts of the colon ♀
    ▶ **N80.552**   Deep endometriosis of other parts of the colon ♀
    ▶ **N80.559**   Endometriosis of other parts of the colon, unspecified depth ♀
        ▶ Endometriosis of colon NOS

N80.6   Endometriosis in cutaneous scar ♀
N80.8   Other endometriosis ♀
    ▷ Endometriosis of other sites
N80.9   Endometriosis, unspecified ♀
▶● **N80.A**   Endometriosis of bladder and ureters ♀
    ▶ **N80.A0**   Endometriosis of bladder, unspecified depth ♀
        ▶ Endometriosis of bladder NOS
    ▶ **N80.A1**   Superficial endometriosis of bladder ♀
    ▶ **N80.A2**   Deep endometriosis of bladder ♀
    ▶● **N80.A4**   Superficial endometriosis of ureter ♀
        ▶ Extrinsic endometriosis of ureter
        ▶ Code also, if applicable, obstructive and reflux uropathy (N13.-)
        ▶ **N80.A41**   Superficial endometriosis of right ureter ♀
        ▶ **N80.A42**   Superficial endometriosis of left ureter ♀
        ▶ **N80.A43**   Superficial endometriosis of bilateral ureters ♀
        ▶ **N80.A49**   Superficial endometriosis of unspecified ureter ♀
    ▶● **N80.A5**   Deep endometriosis of ureter ♀
        ▶ Intrinsic endometriosis of ureter
        ▶ Code also, if applicable, obstructive and reflux uropathy (N13.-)
        ▶ **N80.A51**   Deep endometriosis of right ureter ♀
        ▶ **N80.A52**   Deep endometriosis of left ureter ♀
        ▶ **N80.A53**   Deep endometriosis of bilateral ureters ♀
        ▶ **N80.A59**   Deep endometriosis of unspecified ureter ♀
    ▶● **N80.A6**   Endometriosis of ureter, unspecified depth ♀
        ▶ Code also, if applicable, obstructive and reflux uropathy (N13.-)
        ▶ **N80.A61**   Endometriosis of right ureter, unspecified depth ♀
        ▶ **N80.A62**   Endometriosis of left ureter, unspecified depth ♀
        ▶ **N80.A63**   Endometriosis of bilateral ureters, unspecified depth ♀
        ▶ **N80.A69**   Endometriosis of unspecified ureter, unspecified depth ♀

CHAPTER 14 (N00-N99)

Item 14–11 Endometriosis is a condition for which no clear cause has been identified. Endometrial tissue is expelled from the uterus into the abdominal cavity and can implant onto a variety of organs. Classification is based on the site of implant of the endometrial tissue.

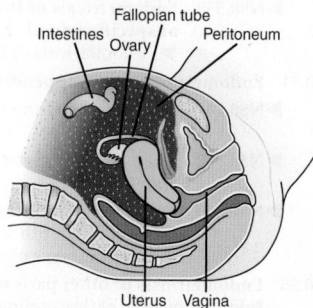

Figure 14-11   Sites of potential endometrial implants.

Figure 14-12   Three stages of uterine prolapse. **A.** Uterus is prolapsed. **B.** Vagina and uterus are prolapsed (incomplete uterovaginal prolapse). **C.** Vagina and uterus are completely prolapsed and are exposed through the external genitalia (complete uterovaginal prolapse).

▶● **N80.B**   **Endometriosis of cardiothoracic space** ♀
  ▶ Endometriosis of thorax
  ▶ Code also, if applicable:
    ▶ catamenial hemothorax (J94.2)
    ▶ catamenial pneumothorax (J93.12)
  ▶ **N80.B1**   **Endometriosis of pleura** ♀
  ▶ **N80.B2**   **Endometriosis of lung** ♀
▶● **N80.B3**   **Endometriosis of diaphragm** ♀
    ▶ **N80.B31**   **Superficial endometriosis of diaphragm** ♀
    ▶ **N80.B32**   **Deep endometriosis of diaphragm** ♀
    ▶ **N80.B39**   **Endometriosis of diaphragm, unspecified depth** ♀
        ▶ Endometriosis of the diaphragm NOS
  ▶ **N80.B4**   **Endometriosis of the pericardial space** ♀
  ▶ **N80.B5**   **Endometriosis of the mediastinal space** ♀
  ▶ **N80.B6**   **Endometriosis of cardiothoracic space** ♀
▶ **N80.C**   **Endometriosis of the abdomen**
  ▶ **N80.C0**   **Endometriosis of the abdomen, unspecified** ♀
        ▶ Endometriosis of the abdomen NOS
  ▶● **N80.C1**   **Endometriosis of the anterior abdominal wall** ♀
    ▶ **N80.C10**   **Endometriosis of the anterior abdominal wall, subcutaneous tissue** ♀
    ▶ **N80.C11**   **Endometriosis of the anterior abdominal wall, fascia and muscular layers** ♀
    ▶ **N80.C19**   **Endometriosis of the anterior abdominal wall, unspecified depth** ♀
        ▶ Endometriosis of the anterior abdominal wall NOS
  ▶ **N80.C2**   **Endometriosis of the umbilicus** ♀
  ▶ **N80.C3**   **Endometriosis of the inguinal canal** ♀
  ▶ **N80.C4**   **Endometriosis of extra-pelvic abdominal peritoneum** ♀
  ▶ **N80.C9**   **Endometriosis of other site of abdomen** ♀
▶● **N80.D**   **Endometriosis of the pelvic nerves** ♀
    ▶ Endometriosis of the nerves of the retroperitoneum
  ▶ **N80.D0**   **Endometriosis of the pelvic nerves, unspecified** ♀
        ▶ Endometriosis of nerve of the retroperitoneum, NOS
  ▶ **N80.D1**   **Endometriosis of the sacral splanchnic nerves** ♀
        ▶ Endometriosis of the pelvic splanchnic nerves
  ▶ **N80.D2**   **Endometriosis of the sacral nerve roots** ♀
  ▶ **N80.D3**   **Endometriosis of the obturator nerve** ♀
  ▶ **N80.D4**   **Endometriosis of the sciatic nerve** ♀
  ▶ **N80.D5**   **Endometriosis of the pudendal nerve** ♀

  ▶ **N80.D6**   **Endometriosis of the femoral nerve** ♀
  ▶ **N80.D9**   **Endometriosis of other pelvic nerve** ♀
        ▶ Endometriosis of the other nerves of the retroperitoneum
● **N81**   **Female genital prolapse**
    Excludes1   genital prolapse complicating pregnancy, labor or delivery (O34.5-)
        prolapse and hernia of ovary and fallopian tube (N83.4-)
        prolapse of vaginal vault after hysterectomy (N99.3)
  N81.0   **Urethrocele** ♀
        Excludes1   urethrocele with cystocele (N81.1-)
        urethrocele with prolapse of uterus (N81.2-N81.4)
● **N81.1**   **Cystocele**
        Cystocele with urethrocele
        Cystourethrocele
        Excludes1   cystocele with prolapse of uterus (N81.2-N81.4)
    N81.10   **Cystocele, unspecified** ♀
            Prolapse of (anterior) vaginal wall NOS
    N81.11   **Cystocele, midline** ♀
    N81.12   **Cystocele, lateral** ♀
            Paravaginal cystocele
  N81.2   **Incomplete uterovaginal prolapse** ♀
        First degree uterine prolapse
        Prolapse of cervix NOS
        Second degree uterine prolapse
        Excludes1   cervical stump prolapse (N81.85)
  N81.3   **Complete uterovaginal prolapse** ♀
        Procidentia (uteri) NOS
        Third degree uterine prolapse
  N81.4   **Uterovaginal prolapse, unspecified** ♀
        Prolapse of uterus NOS
  N81.5   **Vaginal enterocele** ♀
        Excludes1   enterocele with prolapse of uterus (N81.2-N81.4)
  N81.6   **Rectocele** ♀
        Prolapse of posterior vaginal wall
        Use additional code for any associated fecal incontinence, if applicable (R15.-)
        Excludes2   perineocele (N81.81)
        rectal prolapse (K62.3)
        rectocele with prolapse of uterus (N81.2-N81.4)
● **N81.8**   **Other female genital prolapse**
    N81.81   **Perineocele** ♀
    N81.82   **Incompetence or weakening of pubocervical tissue** ♀
    N81.83   **Incompetence or weakening of rectovaginal tissue** ♀
    N81.84   **Pelvic muscle wasting** ♀
            Disuse atrophy of pelvic muscles and anal sphincter

▶ New   ⇒ Revised   ~~deleted~~ Deleted   Excludes 1   Excludes 2   Includes   Use additional   Code first   Code also   Key words

OGCR Official Guidelines   X Assign placeholder X   ● Use Additional Character(s)   ▶ Manifestation Code   🔖 Hierarchical Condition Category   **Coding Clinic**

N81.85   **Cervical stump prolapse** ♀

N81.89   **Other female genital prolapse** ♀
Deficient perineum
Old laceration of muscles of pelvic floor

N81.9   **Female genital prolapse, unspecified** ♀

● **N82   Fistulae involving female genital tract**
Excludes1   vesicointestinal fistulae (N32.1)

N82.0   **Vesicovaginal fistula** ♀

N82.1   **Other female urinary-genital tract fistulae** ♀
Cervicovesical fistula
Ureterovaginal fistula
Urethrovaginal fistula
Uteroureteric fistula
Uterovesical fistula
Coding Clinic: 2017, Q3, P4

N82.2   **Fistula of vagina to small intestine** ♀

N82.3   **Fistula of vagina to large intestine** ♀
Rectovaginal fistula

N82.4   **Other female intestinal-genital tract fistulae** ♀
Intestinouterine fistula

N82.5   **Female genital tract-skin fistulae** ♀
Uterus to abdominal wall fistula
Vaginoperineal fistula

N82.8   **Other female genital tract fistulae** ♀

N82.9   **Female genital tract fistula, unspecified** ♀

● **N83   Noninflammatory disorders of ovary, fallopian tube and broad ligament**
Excludes2   hydrosalpinx (N70.1-)

● N83.0   **Follicular cyst of ovary**
Cyst of graafian follicle
Hemorrhagic follicular cyst (of ovary)
Coding Clinic: 2016, Q4, P46

N83.00   **Follicular cyst of ovary, unspecified side** ♀

N83.01   **Follicular cyst of right ovary** ♀

N83.02   **Follicular cyst of left ovary** ♀

● N83.1   **Corpus luteum cyst**
Hemorrhagic corpus luteum cyst
Coding Clinic: 2016, Q4, P46

N83.10   **Corpus luteum cyst of ovary, unspecified side** ♀

N83.11   **Corpus luteum cyst of right ovary** ♀

N83.12   **Corpus luteum cyst of left ovary** ♀
Coding Clinic: 2022, Q1, P23

● N83.2   **Other and unspecified ovarian cysts**
Excludes1   developmental ovarian cyst (Q50.1)
neoplastic ovarian cyst (D27.-)
polycystic ovarian syndrome (E28.2)
Stein-Leventhal syndrome (E28.2)
Coding Clinic: 2016, Q4, P46

● N83.20   **Unspecified ovarian cysts**
Coding Clinic: 2022, Q1, P23

N83.201   **Unspecified ovarian cyst, right side** ♀

N83.202   **Unspecified ovarian cyst, left side** ♀
Coding Clinic: 2022, Q1, P23

N83.209   **Unspecified ovarian cyst, unspecified side** ♀
Ovarian cyst, NOS

● N83.29   **Other ovarian cysts**
Retention cyst of ovary
Simple cyst of ovary

N83.291   **Other ovarian cyst, right side** ♀

N83.292   **Other ovarian cyst, left side** ♀

N83.299   **Other ovarian cyst, unspecified side** ♀

● N83.3   **Acquired atrophy of ovary and fallopian tube**
Coding Clinic: 2016, Q4, P46

● N83.31   **Acquired atrophy of ovary**

N83.311   **Acquired atrophy of right ovary** ♀

N83.312   **Acquired atrophy of left ovary** ♀

N83.319   **Acquired atrophy of ovary, unspecified side** ♀
Acquired atrophy of ovary, NOS

● N83.32   **Acquired atrophy of fallopian tube**

N83.321   **Acquired atrophy of right fallopian tube** ♀

N83.322   **Acquired atrophy of left fallopian tube** ♀

N83.329   **Acquired atrophy of fallopian tube, unspecified side** ♀
Acquired atrophy of fallopian tube, NOS

● N83.33   **Acquired atrophy of ovary and fallopian tube**

N83.331   **Acquired atrophy of right ovary and fallopian tube** ♀

N83.332   **Acquired atrophy of left ovary and fallopian tube** ♀

N83.339   **Acquired atrophy of ovary and fallopian tube, unspecified side** ♀
Acquired atrophy of ovary and fallopian tube, NOS

● N83.4   **Prolapse and hernia of ovary and fallopian tube**
Coding Clinic: 2016, Q4, P46

N83.40   **Prolapse and hernia of ovary and fallopian tube, unspecified side** ♀
Prolapse and hernia of ovary and fallopian tube, NOS

N83.41   **Prolapse and hernia of right ovary and fallopian tube** ♀

N83.42   **Prolapse and hernia of left ovary and fallopian tube** ♀

● N83.5   **Torsion of ovary, ovarian pedicle and fallopian tube**
Torsion of accessory tube
Coding Clinic: 2016, Q4, P46

● N83.51   **Torsion of ovary and ovarian pedicle**

N83.511   **Torsion of right ovary and ovarian pedicle** ♀

N83.512   **Torsion of left ovary and ovarian pedicle** ♀

N83.519   **Torsion of ovary and ovarian pedicle, unspecified side** ♀
Torsion of ovary and ovarian pedicle, NOS

● N83.52   **Torsion of fallopian tube**
Torsion of hydatid of Morgagni

N83.521   **Torsion of right fallopian tube** ♀

N83.522   **Torsion of left fallopian tube** ♀

N83.529   **Torsion of fallopian tube, unspecified side** ♀
Torsion of fallopian tube, NOS

N83.53   **Torsion of ovary, ovarian pedicle and fallopian tube** ♀

N83.6   **Hematosalpinx** ♀
Excludes1   hematosalpinx (with) (in):
hematocolpos (N89.7)
hematometra (N85.7)
tubal pregnancy (O00.1-)

N83.7   **Hematoma of broad ligament** ♀

N83.8   **Other noninflammatory disorders of ovary, fallopian tube and broad ligament** ♀
Broad ligament laceration syndrome [Allen-Masters]

N83.9   **Noninflammatory disorder of ovary, fallopian tube and broad ligament, unspecified** ♀

● **N84   Polyp of female genital tract**
Excludes1   adenomatous polyp (D28.-)
placental polyp (O90.89)

N84.0   **Polyp of corpus uteri** ♀
Polyp of endometrium
Polyp of uterus NOS
Excludes1   polypoid endometrial hyperplasia (N85.0-)

N84.1   **Polyp of cervix uteri** ♀
Mucous polyp of cervix

CHAPTER 14 (N00-N99)

N84.2　**Polyp of** vagina ♀

N84.3　**Polyp of** vulva ♀
　　　　Polyp of labia

N84.8　**Polyp of other parts of female genital tract** ♀

N84.9　**Polyp of female genital tract,** unspecified ♀

● N85　**Other noninflammatory disorders of uterus, except cervix**
　　　Excludes1　endometriosis (N80.-)
　　　　　　　　　inflammatory diseases of uterus (N71.-)
　　　　　　　　　noninflammatory disorders of cervix, except
　　　　　　　　　　malposition (N86-N88)
　　　　　　　　　polyp of corpus uteri (N84.0)
　　　　　　　　　uterine prolapse (N81.-)

● N85.0　**Endometrial hyperplasia**

　N85.00　**Endometrial hyperplasia,** unspecified ♀
　　　　　　Hyperplasia (adenomatous) (cystic)
　　　　　　　(glandular) of endometrium
　　　　　　Hyperplastic endometritis

　N85.01　**Benign endometrial hyperplasia** ♀
　　　　　　Endometrial hyperplasia (complex) (simple)
　　　　　　　without atypia

　N85.02　**Endometrial intraepithelial neoplasia [EIN]** ♀
　　　　　　Endometrial hyperplasia with atypia
　　　　　　Excludes1　malignant neoplasm of
　　　　　　　　　　　　endometrium (with
　　　　　　　　　　　　endometrial intraepithelial
　　　　　　　　　　　　neoplasia [EIN]) (C54.1)

　N85.2　**Hypertrophy of uterus** ♀
　　　　　Bulky or enlarged uterus
　　　　　Excludes1　puerperal hypertrophy of uterus (O90.89)

　N85.3　**Subinvolution of uterus** ♀
　　　　　Excludes1　puerperal subinvolution of uterus
　　　　　　　　　　　　(O90.89)

　N85.4　**Malposition of uterus** ♀
　　　　　Anteversion of uterus
　　　　　Retroflexion of uterus
　　　　　Retroversion of uterus
　　　　　Excludes1　malposition of uterus complicating
　　　　　　　　　　　　pregnancy, labor or delivery (O34.5-,
　　　　　　　　　　　　O65.5)

　N85.5　**Inversion of uterus** ♀
　　　　　Excludes1　current obstetric trauma (O71.2)
　　　　　　　　　　　　postpartum inversion of uterus (O71.2)

　N85.6　**Intrauterine synechiae** ♀

　N85.7　**Hematometra** ♀
　　　　　Hematosalpinx with hematometra
　　　　　Excludes1　hematometra with hematocolpos (N89.7)

　N85.8　**Other specified noninflammatory disorders of uterus** ♀
　　　　　Atrophy of uterus, acquired
　　　　　Fibrosis of uterus NOS

　N85.9　**Noninflammatory disorder of uterus,** unspecified ♀
　　　　　Disorder of uterus NOS

▶ N85.A　**Isthmocele** ♀
　　　　▶ Isthmocele (non-pregnant state)
　　　　▶ Code also any associated conditions such as:
　　　　　▶ abnormal uterine and vaginal bleeding, unspecified
　　　　　　(N93.9)
　　　　　▶ female infertility of uterine origin (N97.2)
　　　　　▶ pelvic and perineal pain (R10.2)
　　　　▶ **Excludes1**　maternal care for cesarean scar defect
　　　　　　　　　　　　(isthmocele) (O34.22)

N86　**Erosion and ectropion of cervix uteri** ♀
　　　Decubitus (trophic) ulcer of cervix
　　　Eversion of cervix
　　　Excludes1　erosion and ectropion of cervix with cervicitis
　　　　　　　　　　(N72)

● N87　**Dysplasia of cervix uteri**
　　　Excludes1　abnormal results from cervical cytologic
　　　　　　　　　　examination without histologic confirmation
　　　　　　　　　　(R87.61-)
　　　　　　　　　carcinoma in situ of cervix uteri (D06.-)
　　　　　　　　　cervical intraepithelial neoplasia III [CIN III]
　　　　　　　　　　(D06.-)
　　　　　　　　　HGSIL of cervix (R87.613)
　　　　　　　　　severe dysplasia of cervix uteri (D06.-)

　N87.0　**Mild cervical dysplasia** ♀
　　　　　Cervical intraepithelial neoplasia I [CIN I]

　N87.1　**Moderate cervical dysplasia** ♀
　　　　　Cervical intraepithelial neoplasia II [CIN II]

　N87.9　**Dysplasia of cervix uteri,** unspecified ♀
　　　　　Anaplasia of cervix
　　　　　Cervical atypism
　　　　　Cervical dysplasia NOS

● N88　**Other noninflammatory disorders of cervix uteri**
　　　Excludes2　inflammatory disease of cervix (N72)
　　　　　　　　　　polyp of cervix (N84.1)

　N88.0　**Leukoplakia of cervix uteri** ♀

　N88.1　**Old laceration of cervix uteri** ♀
　　　　　Adhesions of cervix
　　　　　Excludes1　current obstetric trauma (O71.3)

　N88.2　**Stricture and stenosis of cervix uteri** ♀
　　　　　Excludes1　stricture and stenosis of cervix uteri
　　　　　　　　　　　　complicating labor (O65.5)

　N88.3　**Incompetence of cervix uteri** ♀
　　　　　Investigation and management of (suspected) cervical
　　　　　　incompetence in a nonpregnant woman
　　　　　Excludes1　cervical incompetence complicating
　　　　　　　　　　　　pregnancy (O34.3-)

　N88.4　**Hypertrophic elongation of cervix uteri** ♀

　N88.8　**Other specified noninflammatory disorders of cervix
　　　　　uteri** ♀
　　　　　Excludes1　current obstetric trauma (O71.3)

　N88.9　**Noninflammatory disorder of cervix uteri,** unspecified ♀

● N89　**Other noninflammatory disorders of vagina**
　　　Excludes1　abnormal results from vaginal cytologic
　　　　　　　　　　examination without histologic confirmation
　　　　　　　　　　(R87.62-)
　　　　　　　　　carcinoma in situ of vagina (D07.2)
　　　　　　　　　HGSIL of vagina (R87.623)
　　　　　　　　　inflammation of vagina (N76.-)
　　　　　　　　　senile (atrophic) vaginitis (N95.2)
　　　　　　　　　severe dysplasia of vagina (D07.2)
　　　　　　　　　trichomonal leukorrhea (A59.00)
　　　　　　　　　vaginal intraepithelial neoplasia [VAIN], grade
　　　　　　　　　　III (D07.2)

　N89.0　**Mild vaginal dysplasia** ♀
　　　　　Vaginal intraepithelial neoplasia [VAIN], grade I

　N89.1　**Moderate vaginal dysplasia** ♀
　　　　　Vaginal intraepithelial neoplasia [VAIN], grade II

　N89.3　**Dysplasia of vagina,** unspecified ♀

　N89.4　**Leukoplakia of vagina** ♀

　N89.5　**Stricture and atresia of vagina** ♀
　　　　　Vaginal adhesions　　　　Vaginal stenosis
　　　　　Excludes1　congenital atresia or stricture (Q52.4)
　　　　　　　　　　　　postprocedural adhesions of vagina
　　　　　　　　　　　　(N99.2)

　N89.6　**Tight hymenal ring** ♀
　　　　　Rigid hymen　　　　Tight introitus
　　　　　Excludes1　imperforate hymen (Q52.3)

　N89.7　**Hematocolpos** ♀
　　　　　Hematocolpos with hematometra or hematosalpinx
　　　　　Coding Clinic: 2016, Q4, P59

N89.8   **Other specified noninflammatory disorders of vagina** ♀
     Leukorrhea NOS
     Old vaginal laceration
     Pessary ulcer of vagina
     Excludes1   current obstetric trauma (O70.-, O71.4,
            O71.7-O71.8)
         old laceration involving muscles of pelvic
            floor (N81.8)

N89.9   **Noninflammatory disorder of vagina, unspecified** ♀

● **N90**   **Other noninflammatory disorders of vulva and perineum**
     Excludes1   anogenital (venereal) warts (A63.0)
         carcinoma in situ of vulva (D07.1)
         condyloma acuminatum (A63.0)
         current obstetric trauma (O70.-, O71.7-O71.8)
         inflammation of vulva (N76.-)
         severe dysplasia of vulva (D07.1)
         vulvar intraepithelial neoplasm III [VIN III]
            (D07.1)

N90.0   **Mild vulvar dysplasia** ♀
     Vulvar intraepithelial neoplasia [VIN], grade I

N90.1   **Moderate vulvar dysplasia** ♀
     Vulvar intraepithelial neoplasia [VIN], grade II

N90.3   **Dysplasia of vulva, unspecified** ♀

N90.4   **Leukoplakia of vulva** ♀
     Dystrophy of vulva
     Kraurosis of vulva
     Lichen sclerosus of external female genital organs

N90.5   **Atrophy of vulva** ♀
     Stenosis of vulva

● **N90.6**   **Hypertrophy of vulva**
     Coding Clinic: 2016, Q4, P46

     N90.60   **Unspecified hypertrophy of vulva** ♀
         Unspecified hypertrophy of labia

     N90.61   **Childhood asymmetric labium majus enlargement** ♀
         CALME

     N90.69   **Other specified hypertrophy of vulva** ♀
         Other specified hypertrophy of labia

N90.7   **Vulvar cyst** ♀

● **N90.8**   **Other specified noninflammatory disorders of vulva and perineum**

     ● **N90.81**   **Female genital mutilation status**
         Female genital cutting status

         N90.810   **Female genital mutilation status, unspecified** ♀
            Female genital cutting status, unspecified
            Female genital mutilation status NOS

         N90.811   **Female genital mutilation Type I status** ♀
            Clitorectomy status
            Female genital cutting Type I status

         N90.812   **Female genital mutilation Type II status** ♀
            Clitorectomy with excision of labia minora status
            Female genital cutting Type II status

         N90.813   **Female genital mutilation Type III status** ♀
            Female genital cutting Type III status
            Infibulation status

         N90.818   **Other female genital mutilation status** ♀
            Female genital cutting Type IV status
            Female genital mutilation Type IV status
            Other female genital cutting status

N90.89   **Other specified noninflammatory disorders of vulva and perineum** ♀
     Adhesions of vulva
     Hypertrophy of clitoris

N90.9   **Noninflammatory disorder of vulva and perineum, unspecified** ♀

● **N91**   **Absent, scanty and rare menstruation**
     Excludes1   ovarian dysfunction (E28.-)

N91.0   **Primary amenorrhea** ♀

N91.1   **Secondary amenorrhea** ♀

N91.2   **Amenorrhea, unspecified** ♀

N91.3   **Primary oligomenorrhea** ♀

N91.4   **Secondary oligomenorrhea** ♀

N91.5   **Oligomenorrhea, unspecified** ♀
     Hypomenorrhea NOS

● **N92**   **Excessive, frequent and irregular menstruation**
     Excludes1   postmenopausal bleeding (N95.0)
         precocious puberty (menstruation) (E30.1)

N92.0   **Excessive and frequent menstruation with regular cycle** ♀
     Heavy periods NOS   Polymenorrhea
     Menorrhagia NOS

N92.1   **Excessive and frequent menstruation with irregular cycle** ♀
     Irregular intermenstrual bleeding
     Irregular, shortened intervals between menstrual bleeding
     Menometrorrhagia
     Metrorrhagia

N92.2   **Excessive menstruation at puberty** ♀   P
     Excessive bleeding associated with onset of menstrual periods
     Pubertal menorrhagia
     Puberty bleeding

N92.3   **Ovulation bleeding** ♀
     Regular intermenstrual bleeding

N92.4   **Excessive bleeding in the premenopausal period** ♀
     Climacteric menorrhagia or metrorrhagia
     Menopausal menorrhagia or metrorrhagia
     Perimenopausal bleeding
     Perimenopausal menorrhagia or metrorrhagia
     Preclimacteric menorrhagia or metrorrhagia
     Premenopausal menorrhagia or metrorrhagia

N92.5   **Other specified irregular menstruation** ♀

N92.6   **Irregular menstruation, unspecified** ♀
     Irregular bleeding NOS
     Irregular periods NOS
     Excludes1   irregular menstruation with:
         lengthened intervals or scanty bleeding
            (N91.3-N91.5)
         shortened intervals or excessive
            bleeding (N92.1)

● **N93**   **Other abnormal uterine and vaginal bleeding**
     Excludes1   neonatal vaginal hemorrhage (P54.6)
         precocious puberty (menstruation) (E30.1)
         pseudomenses (P54.6)

N93.0   **Postcoital and contact bleeding** ♀

N93.1   **Pre-pubertal vaginal bleeding** ♀
     Coding Clinic: 2016, Q4, P47

N93.8   **Other specified abnormal uterine and vaginal bleeding** ♀
     Dysfunctional or functional uterine or vaginal bleeding NOS

N93.9   **Abnormal uterine and vaginal bleeding, unspecified** ♀

CHAPTER 14 (N00-N99)

● **N94   Pain and other conditions associated with female genital organs and menstrual cycle**

     N94.0   Mittelschmerz ♀
         Ovulation pain

●   **N94.1   Dyspareunia**
         Painful intercourse/coitus
         Excludes1   psychogenic dyspareunia (F52.6)
         Coding Clinic: 2016, Q4, P47

         N94.10   Unspecified dyspareunia ♀
         N94.11   Superficial (introital) dyspareunia ♀
         N94.12   Deep dyspareunia ♀
         N94.19   Other specified dyspareunia ♀

     N94.2   Vaginismus ♀
         Vagina tightness
         Excludes1   psychogenic vaginismus (F52.5)

     N94.3   Premenstrual tension syndrome ♀
         AKA: PMS
         Code also associated menstrual migraine (G43.82-, G43.83-)
         Excludes1   Premenstrual dysphoric disorder (F32.81)
         Coding Clinic: 2016, Q4, P14

     N94.4   Primary dysmenorrhea ♀
         Lifelong painful menstruation

     N94.5   Secondary dysmenorrhea ♀
         Later onset of painful menstruation

     N94.6   Dysmenorrhea, unspecified ♀
         Excludes1   psychogenic dysmenorrhea (F45.8)

●   **N94.8   Other specified conditions associated with female genital organs and menstrual cycle**

●   **N94.81   Vulvodynia**
         N94.810   Vulvar vestibulitis ♀
         N94.818   Other vulvodynia ♀
         N94.819   Vulvodynia, unspecified ♀
                 Vulvodynia NOS

       N94.89   Other specified conditions associated with female genital organs and menstrual cycle ♀

     N94.9   Unspecified condition associated with female genital organs and menstrual cycle ♀

● **N95   Menopausal and other perimenopausal disorders**
     Menopausal and other perimenopausal disorders due to naturally occurring (age-related) menopause and perimenopause

     Excludes1   excessive bleeding in the premenopausal period (N92.4)
                menopausal and perimenopausal disorders due to artificial or premature menopause (E89.4-, E28.31-)
                premature menopause (E28.31-)

     Excludes2   postmenopausal osteoporosis (M81.0-)
                postmenopausal osteoporosis with current pathological fracture (M80.0-)
                postmenopausal urethritis (N34.2)

     N95.0   Postmenopausal bleeding ♀

     N95.1   Menopausal and female climacteric states ♀
         Symptoms such as flushing, sleeplessness, headache, lack of concentration, associated with natural (age-related) menopause
         Use additional code for associated symptoms
         Excludes1   asymptomatic menopausal state (Z78.0)
                  symptoms associated with artificial menopause (E89.41)
                  symptoms associated with premature menopause (E28.310)

     N95.2   Postmenopausal atrophic vaginitis ♀
         Senile (atrophic) vaginitis

     N95.8   Other specified menopausal and perimenopausal disorders ♀

     N95.9   Unspecified menopausal and perimenopausal disorder ♀

N96   Recurrent pregnancy loss ♀
     Investigation or care in a nonpregnant woman with history of recurrent pregnancy loss
     Excludes1   recurrent pregnancy loss with current pregnancy (O26.2-)

● **N97   Female infertility**
     Includes   inability to achieve a pregnancy
               sterility, female NOS
     Excludes2   female infertility associated with:
                hypopituitarism (E23.0)
                Stein-Leventhal syndrome (E28.2)
                incompetence of cervix uteri (N88.3)

     N97.0   Female infertility associated with anovulation ♀

     N97.1   Female infertility of tubal origin ♀
         Female infertility associated with congenital anomaly of tube
         Female infertility due to tubal block
         Female infertility due to tubal occlusion
         Female infertility due to tubal stenosis

     N97.2   Female infertility of uterine origin ♀
         Female infertility associated with congenital anomaly of uterus
         Female infertility due to nonimplantation of ovum

     N97.8   Female infertility of other origin ♀

     N97.9   Female infertility, unspecified ♀

● **N98   Complications associated with artificial fertilization**

     N98.0   Infection associated with artificial insemination ♀

     N98.1   Hyperstimulation of ovaries ♀
         Hyperstimulation of ovaries NOS
         Hyperstimulation of ovaries associated with induced ovulation

     N98.2   Complications of attempted introduction of fertilized ovum following in vitro fertilization ♀

     N98.3   Complications of attempted introduction of embryo in embryo transfer ♀

     N98.8   Other complications associated with artificial fertilization ♀

     N98.9   Complication associated with artificial fertilization, unspecified ♀

INTRAOPERATIVE AND POSTPROCEDURAL COMPLICATIONS AND DISORDERS OF GENITOURINARY SYSTEM, NOT ELSEWHERE CLASSIFIED (N99)

● **N99   Intraoperative and postprocedural complications and disorders of genitourinary system, not elsewhere classified**
     Excludes2   irradiation cystitis (N30.4-)
                postoophorectomy osteoporosis with current pathological fracture (M80.8-)
                postoophorectomy osteoporosis without current pathological fracture (M81.8)

     N99.0   Postprocedural (acute) (chronic) kidney failure
         Use additional code to type of kidney disease

●   **N99.1   Postprocedural urethral stricture**
         Postcatheterization urethral stricture

●   **N99.11   Postprocedural urethral stricture, male**
         N99.110   Postprocedural urethral stricture, male, meatal ♂
         N99.111   Postprocedural bulbous urethral stricture, male ♂
         N99.112   Postprocedural membranous urethral stricture, male ♂

▶ New   ⟹ Revised   ~~deleted~~ Deleted   Excludes 1   Excludes 2   Includes   Use additional   Code first   Code also   Key words

1126   **OGCR** Official Guidelines   **X** Assign placeholder X   ● Use Additional Character(s)   ▶ Manifestation Code   Hierarchical Condition Category   **Coding Clinic**

N99.113   Postprocedural anterior bulbous urethral stricture, male ♂
     Coding Clinic: 2016, Q4, P48

N99.114   Postprocedural urethral stricture, male, unspecified ♂

N99.115   Postprocedural fossa navicularis urethral stricture ♂
     Coding Clinic: 2016, Q4, P47

N99.116   Postprocedural urethral stricture, male, overlapping sites ♂

N99.12   Postprocedural urethral stricture, female ♀

N99.2   Postprocedural adhesions of vagina ♀

N99.3   Prolapse of vaginal vault after hysterectomy ♀

N99.4   Postprocedural pelvic peritoneal adhesions
     Excludes2   pelvic peritoneal adhesions NOS (N73.6)
         postinfective pelvic peritoneal adhesions (N73.6)

● N99.5   Complications of stoma of urinary tract
     Excludes2   mechanical complication of urinary catheter (T83.0-)

   ● N99.51   Complication of cystostomy

     N99.510   Cystostomy hemorrhage 🦠

     N99.511   Cystostomy infection 🦠

     N99.512   Cystostomy malfunction 🦠

     N99.518   Other cystostomy complication 🦠

   ● N99.52   Complication of incontinent external stoma of urinary tract

     N99.520   Hemorrhage of incontinent external stoma of urinary tract 🦠

     N99.521   Infection of incontinent external stoma of urinary tract 🦠
         Coding Clinic: 2016, Q4, P48

     N99.522   Malfunction of incontinent external stoma of urinary tract 🦠

     N99.523   Herniation of incontinent stoma of urinary tract 🦠
         Coding Clinic: 2016, Q4, P48

     N99.524   Stenosis of incontinent stoma of urinary tract 🦠
         Coding Clinic: 2016, Q4, P48

     N99.528   Other complication of incontinent external stoma of urinary tract 🦠

   ● N99.53   Complication of continent stoma of urinary tract

     N99.530   Hemorrhage of continent stoma of urinary tract 🦠

     N99.531   Infection of continent stoma of urinary tract 🦠

     N99.532   Malfunction of continent stoma of urinary tract 🦠

     N99.533   Herniation of continent stoma of urinary tract 🦠
         Coding Clinic: 2016, Q4, P48

     N99.534   Stenosis of continent stoma of urinary tract 🦠
         Coding Clinic: 2016, Q4, P48

     N99.538   Other complication of continent stoma of urinary tract 🦠

● N99.6   Intraoperative hemorrhage and hematoma of a genitourinary system organ or structure complicating a procedure
     Excludes1   intraoperative hemorrhage and hematoma of a genitourinary system organ or structure due to accidental puncture or laceration during a procedure (N99.7-)

   N99.61   Intraoperative hemorrhage and hematoma of a genitourinary system organ or structure complicating a genitourinary system procedure

   N99.62   Intraoperative hemorrhage and hematoma of a genitourinary system organ or structure complicating other procedure

● N99.7   Accidental puncture and laceration of a genitourinary system organ or structure during a procedure

   N99.71   Accidental puncture and laceration of a genitourinary system organ or structure during a genitourinary system procedure

   N99.72   Accidental puncture and laceration of a genitourinary system organ or structure during other procedure

● N99.8   Other intraoperative and postprocedural complications and disorders of genitourinary system
     Coding Clinic: 2016, Q4, P10

   N99.81   Other intraoperative complications of genitourinary system

   ● N99.82   Postprocedural hemorrhage of a genitourinary system organ or structure following a procedure

     N99.820   Postprocedural hemorrhage of a genitourinary system organ or structure following a genitourinary system procedure

     N99.821   Postprocedural hemorrhage of a genitourinary system organ or structure following other procedure

   N99.83   Residual ovary syndrome ♀

   ● N99.84   Postprocedural hematoma and seroma of a genitourinary system organ or structure following a procedure

     N99.840   Postprocedural hematoma of a genitourinary system organ or structure following a genitourinary system procedure

     N99.841   Postprocedural hematoma of a genitourinary system organ or structure following other procedure

     N99.842   Postprocedural seroma of a genitourinary system organ or structure following a genitourinary system procedure

     N99.843   Postprocedural seroma of a genitourinary system organ or structure following other procedure

   N99.85   Post endometrial ablation syndrome
     Coding Clinic: 2019, Q4, P12

   N99.89   Other postprocedural complications and disorders of genitourinary system

CHAPTER 14 (N00-N99)

CHAPTER 15

PREGNANCY, CHILDBIRTH, AND THE PUERPERIUM (O00–O9A)

OGCR Chapter-Specific Coding Guidelines

15. Chapter 15: Pregnancy, Childbirth, and the Puerperium (O00–O9A)

a. General Rules for Obstetric Cases

1) Codes from Chapter 15 and sequencing priority
Obstetric cases require codes from Chapter 15, codes in the range O00–O9A, Pregnancy, Childbirth, and the Puerperium. Chapter 15 codes have sequencing priority over codes from other chapters. Additional codes from other chapters may be used in conjunction with Chapter 15 codes to further specify conditions. Should the provider document that the pregnancy is incidental to the encounter, then code Z33.1, Pregnant state, incidental, should be used in place of any Chapter 15 codes. It is the provider's responsibility to state that the condition being treated is not affecting the pregnancy.

2) Chapter 15 codes used only on the maternal record
Chapter 15 codes are to be used only on the maternal record, never on the record of the newborn.

3) Final character for trimester
The majority of codes in Chapter 15 have a final character indicating the trimester of pregnancy. The timeframes for the trimesters are indicated at the beginning of the chapter. If trimester is not a component of a code it is because the condition always occurs in a specific trimester, or the concept of trimester of pregnancy is not applicable. Certain codes have characters for only certain trimesters because the condition does not occur in all trimesters, but it may occur in more than just one.

Assignment of the final character for trimester should be based on the provider's documentation of the trimester (or number of weeks) for the current admission/encounter. This applies to the assignment of trimester for pre-existing conditions as well as those that develop during or are due to the pregnancy. The provider's documentation of the number of weeks may be used to assign the appropriate code identifying the trimester.

Whenever delivery occurs during the current admission, and there is an "in childbirth" option for the obstetric complication being coded, the "in childbirth" code should be assigned.

4) Selection of trimester for inpatient admissions that encompass more than one trimester
In instances when a patient is admitted to a hospital for complications of pregnancy during one trimester and remains in the hospital into a subsequent trimester, the trimester character for the antepartum complication code should be assigned on the basis of the trimester when the complication developed, not the trimester of the discharge. If the condition developed prior to the current admission/encounter or represents a pre-existing condition, the trimester character for the trimester at the time of the admission/encounter should be assigned.

5) Unspecified trimester
Each category that includes codes for trimester has a code for "unspecified trimester." The "unspecified trimester" code should rarely be used, such as when the documentation in the record is insufficient to determine the trimester and it is not possible to obtain clarification.

6) 7th character for Fetus Identification
Where applicable, a 7th character is to be assigned for certain categories (O31, O32, O33.3 - O33.6, O35, O36, O40, O41, O60.1, O60.2, O64, and O69) to identify the fetus for which the complication code applies.

Assign 7th character "0":
- For single gestations
- When the documentation in the record is insufficient to determine the fetus affected and it is not possible to obtain clarification.
- When it is not possible to clinically determine which fetus is affected.

b. Selection of OB Principal or First-listed Diagnosis

1) Routine outpatient prenatal visits
For routine outpatient prenatal visits when no complications are present, a code from category Z34, Encounter for supervision of normal pregnancy, should be used as the first-listed diagnosis. These codes should not be used in conjunction with Chapter 15 codes.

2) Supervision of High-Risk Pregnancy
Codes from category O09, Supervision of high-risk pregnancy, are intended for use only during the prenatal period. For complications during the labor or delivery episode as a result of a high-risk pregnancy, assign the applicable complication codes from Chapter 15. If there are no complications during the labor or delivery episode, assign code O80, Encounter for full-term uncomplicated delivery.

For routine prenatal outpatient visits for patients with high-risk pregnancies, a code from category O09, Supervision of high-risk pregnancy, should be used as the first-listed diagnosis. Secondary Chapter 15 codes may be used in conjunction with these codes if appropriate.

3) Episodes when no delivery occurs
In episodes when no delivery occurs, the principal diagnosis should correspond to the principal complication of the pregnancy which necessitated the encounter. Should more than one complication exist, all of which are treated or monitored, any of the complications codes may be sequenced first.

4) When a delivery occurs
When an obstetric patient is admitted and delivers during that admission, the condition that prompted the admission should be sequenced as the principal diagnosis. If multiple conditions prompted the admission, sequence the one most related to the delivery as the principal diagnosis. A code for any complication of the delivery should be assigned as an additional diagnosis. In cases of cesarean delivery, if the patient was admitted with a condition that resulted in the performance of a cesarean procedure, that condition should be selected as the principal diagnosis. If the reason for the admission was unrelated to the condition resulting in the cesarean delivery, the condition related to the reason for the admission should be selected as the principal diagnosis.

5) Outcome of delivery
A code from category Z37, Outcome of delivery, should be included on every maternal record when a delivery has occurred. These codes are not to be used on subsequent records or on the newborn record.

c. Pre-existing conditions versus conditions due to the pregnancy
Certain categories in Chapter 15 distinguish between conditions of the mother that existed prior to pregnancy (pre-existing) and those that are a direct result of pregnancy. When assigning codes from Chapter 15, it is important to assess if a condition was pre-existing prior to pregnancy or developed during or due to the pregnancy in order to assign the correct code.

Categories that do not distinguish between pre-existing and pregnancy-related conditions may be used for either. It is acceptable to use codes specifically for the puerperium with codes complicating pregnancy and childbirth if a condition arises postpartum during the delivery encounter.

d. Pre-existing hypertension in pregnancy
Category O10, Pre-existing hypertension complicating pregnancy, childbirth and the puerperium, includes codes for hypertensive heart and hypertensive chronic kidney disease. When assigning one of the O10 codes that includes hypertensive heart disease or hypertensive chronic kidney disease, it is necessary to add a secondary code from the appropriate hypertension category to specify the type of heart failure or chronic kidney disease.
See Section I.C.9. Hypertension.

e. Fetal Conditions Affecting the Management of the Mother

1) Codes from categories O35 and O36
Codes from categories O35, Maternal care for known or suspected fetal abnormality and damage, and O36, Maternal care for other fetal problems, are assigned only when the fetal condition is actually responsible for modifying the management of the mother, i.e., by requiring diagnostic studies, additional observation, special care, or termination of pregnancy. The fact that the fetal condition exists does not justify assigning a code from this series to the mother's record.

2) In utero surgery
In cases when surgery is performed on the fetus, a diagnosis code from category O35, Maternal care for known or suspected fetal abnormality and damage, should be assigned identifying the fetal condition. Assign the appropriate procedure code for the procedure performed.

No code from Chapter 16, the perinatal codes, should be used on the mother's record to identify fetal conditions. Surgery performed in utero on a fetus is still to be coded as an obstetric encounter.

f. HIV Infection in Pregnancy, Childbirth, and the Puerperium
During pregnancy, childbirth or the puerperium, a patient admitted because of an HIV-related illness should receive a principal diagnosis from subcategory O98.7-, Human immunodeficiency [HIV] disease complicating pregnancy, childbirth and the puerperium, followed by the code(s) for the HIV-related illness(es).

Patients with asymptomatic HIV infection status admitted during pregnancy, childbirth, or the puerperium should receive codes of O98.7- and Z21, Asymptomatic human immunodeficiency virus [HIV] infection status.

g. Diabetes mellitus in pregnancy
Diabetes mellitus is a significant complicating factor in pregnancy. Pregnant women who are diabetic should be assigned a code from category O24, Diabetes mellitus in pregnancy, childbirth, and the puerperium, first, followed by the appropriate diabetes code(s) (E08-E13) from Chapter 4.

h. Long-term use of insulin and oral hypoglycemics
See Section I.C.4.a.3 for information on the long-term use of insulin and oral hypoglycemic.

i. Gestational (pregnancy induced) diabetes
Gestational (pregnancy induced) diabetes can occur during the second and third trimester of pregnancy in women who were not diabetic prior to pregnancy. Gestational diabetes can cause complications in the pregnancy similar to those of pre-existing diabetes mellitus. It also puts the woman at greater risk of developing diabetes after the pregnancy. Codes for gestational diabetes are in subcategory O24.4, Gestational diabetes mellitus. No other code from category O24, Diabetes mellitus in pregnancy, childbirth, and the puerperium, should be used with a code from O24.4.

The codes under subcategory O24.4 include diet controlled, insulin controlled, and controlled by oral hypoglycemic drugs. If a patient with gestational diabetes is treated with both diet and insulin, only the code for insulin-controlled is required. If a patient with gestational diabetes is treated with both diet and oral hypoglycemic medications, only the code for "controlled by oral hypoglycemic drugs" is required. Code Z79.4, Long-term (current) use of insulin or code Z79.84, Long-term (current) use of oral hypoglycemic drugs, should not be assigned with codes from subcategory O24.4.

An abnormal glucose tolerance in pregnancy is assigned a code from subcategory O99.81, Abnormal glucose complicating pregnancy, childbirth, and the puerperium.

j. Sepsis and septic shock complicating abortion, pregnancy, childbirth and the puerperium
When assigning a Chapter 15 code for sepsis complicating abortion, pregnancy, childbirth, and the puerperium, a code for the specific type of infection should be assigned as an additional diagnosis. If severe sepsis is present, a code from subcategory R65.2, Severe sepsis, and code(s) for associated organ dysfunction(s) should also be assigned as additional diagnoses.

k. Puerperal sepsis
Code O85, Puerperal sepsis, should be assigned with a secondary code to identify the causal organism (e.g., for a bacterial infection, assign a code from category B95-B96, Bacterial infections in conditions classified elsewhere). A code from category A40, Streptococcal sepsis, or A41, Other sepsis, should not be used for puerperal sepsis. If applicable, use additional codes to identify severe sepsis (R65.2-) and any associated acute organ dysfunction.

l. Alcohol, tobacco and drug use during pregnancy, childbirth and the puerperium

1) Alcohol use during pregnancy, childbirth and the puerperium
Codes under subcategory O99.31, Alcohol use complicating pregnancy, childbirth, and the puerperium, should be assigned for any pregnancy case when a mother uses alcohol during the pregnancy or postpartum. A secondary code from category F10, Alcohol-related disorders, should also be assigned to identify manifestations of the alcohol use.

2) Tobacco use during pregnancy, childbirth, and the puerperium
Codes under subcategory O99.33, Smoking (tobacco) complicating pregnancy, childbirth, and the puerperium, should be assigned for any pregnancy case when a mother uses any type of tobacco product during the pregnancy or postpartum. A secondary code from category F17, Nicotine dependence, should also be assigned to identify the type of nicotine dependence.

3) Drug use during pregnancy, childbirth and the puerperium
Codes under subcategory O99.32, Drug use complicating pregnancy, childbirth, and the puerperium, should be assigned for any pregnancy case when a mother uses drugs during the pregnancy or postpartum. This can involve illegal drugs, or inappropriate use or abuse of prescription drugs. Secondary code(s) from categories F11-F16 and F18F19 should also be assigned to identify manifestations of the drug use.

m. Poisoning, toxic effects, adverse effects and underdosing in a pregnant patient
A code from subcategory O9A.2, Injury, poisoning and certain other consequences of external causes complicating pregnancy, childbirth, and the puerperium, should be sequenced first, followed by the appropriate injury, poisoning, toxic effect, adverse effect or underdosing code, and then the additional code(s) that specifies the condition caused by the poisoning, toxic effect, adverse effect or underdosing.
See Section I.C.19. Adverse effects, poisoning, underdosing and toxic effects.

n. Normal Delivery, Code O80

1) Encounter for full-term uncomplicated delivery
Code O80 should be assigned when a woman is admitted for a full-term normal delivery and delivers a single, healthy infant without any complications antepartum, during the delivery, or postpartum during the delivery episode. Code O80 is always a principal diagnosis. It is not to be used if any other code from Chapter 15 is needed to describe a current complication of the antenatal, delivery, or perinatal period. Additional codes from other chapters may be used with code O80 if they are not related to or are in any way complicating the pregnancy.

2) Uncomplicated delivery with resolved antepartum complication
Code O80 may be used if the patient had a complication at some point during the pregnancy, but the complication is not present at the time of the admission for delivery.

3) Outcome of delivery for O80
Z37.0, Single live birth, is the only outcome of delivery code appropriate for use with O80.

o. The Peripartum and Postpartum Periods

1) Peripartum and Postpartum periods
The postpartum period begins immediately after delivery and continues for six weeks following delivery. The peripartum period is defined as the last month of pregnancy to five months postpartum.

2) Peripartum and postpartum complication
A postpartum complication is any complication occurring within the six-week period.

3) Pregnancy-related complications after 6 week period
Chapter 15 codes may also be used to describe pregnancy-related complications after the peripartum or postpartum period if the provider documents that a condition is pregnancy related.

4) Admission for routine postpartum care following delivery outside hospital
When the mother delivers outside the hospital prior to admission and is admitted for routine postpartum care and no complications are noted, code Z39.0, Encounter for care and examination of mother immediately after delivery, should be assigned as the principal diagnosis.

5) Pregnancy associated cardiomyopathy
Pregnancy associated cardiomyopathy, code O90.3, is unique in that it may be diagnosed in the third trimester of pregnancy but may continue to progress months after delivery. For this reason, it is referred to as peripartum cardiomyopathy. Code O90.3 is only for use when the cardiomyopathy develops as a result of pregnancy in a woman who did not have pre-existing heart disease.

p. Code O94, Sequelae of complication of pregnancy, childbirth, and the puerperium

1) Code O94
Code O94, Sequelae of complication of pregnancy, childbirth, and the puerperium, is for use in those cases when an initial complication of a pregnancy develops a sequelae requiring care or treatment at a future date.

2) After the initial postpartum period
This code may be used at any time after the initial postpartum period.

3) Sequencing of Code O94
This code, like all sequela codes, is to be sequenced following the code describing the sequelae of the complication.

q. Termination of Pregnancy and Spontaneous abortions

1) Abortion with Liveborn Fetus
When an attempted termination of pregnancy results in a liveborn fetus assign code Z33.2, Encounter for elective termination of pregnancy and a code from category Z37, Outcome of Delivery.

2) Retained Products of Conception following an abortion
Subsequent encounters for retained products of conception following a spontaneous abortion or elective termination of pregnancy, without complications are assigned O03.4, Incomplete spontaneous, abortion without complication, or codes O07.4, Failed attempted termination of pregnancy without complication. This advice is appropriate even when the patient was discharged previously with a discharge diagnosis of complete abortion. If the patient has a specific complication associated with the spontaneous abortion or elective termination of pregnancy in addition to retained products of conception, assign the appropriate complication in category O03 or O07 instead of code O03.4 or O07.4

3) Complications leading to abortion
Codes from Chapter 15 may be used as additional codes to identify any documented complications of the pregnancy in conjunction with codes in categories in O04, O07 and O08.

r. Abuse in a pregnant patient
For suspected or confirmed cases of abuse of a pregnant patient, a code(s) from subcategories O9A.3, Physical abuse complicating pregnancy, childbirth, and the puerperium, O9A.4, Sexual abuse complicating pregnancy, childbirth, and the puerperium, and O9A.5, Psychological abuse complicating pregnancy, childbirth, and the puerperium, should be sequenced first, followed by the appropriate codes (if applicable) to identify any associated current injury due to physical abuse, sexual abuse, and the perpetrator of abuse.
See Section I.C.19. Adult and child abuse, neglect and other maltreatment.

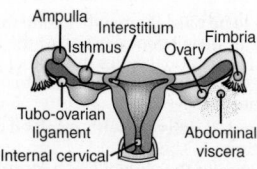

Figure 15-1 Implantation sites of ectopic pregnancy.

Item 15-1 Ectopic pregnancy most often occurs in the fallopian tube. Pregnancy outside the uterus may end in a lifethreatening rupture.

★**(See Plate 4 of the Anatomy Illustrations.)**

CHAPTER 15

PREGNANCY, CHILDBIRTH, AND THE PUERPERIUM (O00-O9A)

Note: CODES FROM THIS CHAPTER ARE FOR USE ONLY ON MATERNAL RECORDS, NEVER ON NEWBORN RECORDS

Codes from this chapter are for use for conditions related to or aggravated by the pregnancy, childbirth, or by the puerperium (maternal causes or obstetric causes)

Trimesters are counted from the first day of the last menstrual period. They are defined as follows:

1st trimester - less than 14 weeks 0 days

2nd trimester - 14 weeks 0 days to less than 28 weeks 0 days

3rd trimester - 28 weeks 0 days until delivery

Use additional code from category Z3A, Weeks of gestation, to identify the specific week of the pregnancy, if known.

Excludes1 supervision of normal pregnancy (Z34.-)

Excludes2 mental and behavioral disorders associated with the puerperium (F53.-)
obstetrical tetanus (A34)
postpartum necrosis of pituitary gland (E23.0)
puerperal osteomalacia (M83.0)

This chapter contains the following blocks:

O00-O08	Pregnancy with abortive outcome
O09	Supervision of high risk pregnancy
O10-O16	Edema, proteinuria and hypertensive disorders in pregnancy, childbirth and the puerperium
O20-O29	Other maternal disorders predominantly related to pregnancy
O30-O48	Maternal care related to the fetus and amniotic cavity and possible delivery problems
O60-O77	Complications of labor and delivery
O80, O82	Encounter for delivery
O85-O92	Complications predominantly related to the puerperium
O94-O9A	Other obstetric conditions, not elsewhere classified

PREGNANCY WITH ABORTIVE OUTCOME (O00-O08)

Excludes1 continuing pregnancy in multiple gestation after abortion of one fetus or more (O31.1-, O31.3-)
Coding Clinic: 2016, Q4, P130

● **O00**   **Ectopic pregnancy**
    Includes   ruptured ectopic pregnancy
    Use additional code from category O08 to identify any associated complication

● **O00.0** **Abdominal pregnancy**
    Excludes1 maternal care for viable fetus in abdominal pregnancy (O36.7-)
    Coding Clinic: 2016, Q4, P49

    O00.00 **Abdominal pregnancy without intrauterine pregnancy** ♀   M
         Abdominal pregnancy NOS

    O00.01 **Abdominal pregnancy with intrauterine pregnancy** ♀   M

● **O00.1** **Tubal pregnancy**
    Fallopian pregnancy
    Rupture of (fallopian) tube due to pregnancy
    Tubal abortion
    Coding Clinic: 2016, Q4, P49

 ● **O00.10** **Tubal pregnancy without intrauterine pregnancy**
      Tubal pregnancy NOS

    O00.101 **Right tubal pregnancy without intrauterine pregnancy** ♀   M

    O00.102 **Left tubal pregnancy without intrauterine pregnancy** ♀   M

    O00.109 **Unspecified tubal pregnancy without intrauterine pregnancy** ♀   M

 ● **O00.11** **Tubal pregnancy with intrauterine pregnancy**

    O00.111 **Right tubal pregnancy with intrauterine pregnancy** ♀   M

    O00.112 **Left tubal pregnancy with intrauterine pregnancy** ♀   M

    O00.119 **Unspecified tubal pregnancy with intrauterine pregnancy** ♀   M

● **O00.2** **Ovarian pregnancy**
    Coding Clinic: 2016, Q4, P49

 ● **O00.20** **Ovarian pregnancy without intrauterine pregnancy**
      Ovarian pregnancy NOS

    O00.201 **Right ovarian pregnancy without intrauterine pregnancy** ♀   M

    O00.202 **Left ovarian pregnancy without intrauterine pregnancy** ♀   M

    O00.209 **Unspecified ovarian pregnancy without intrauterine pregnancy** ♀   M

 ● **O00.21** **Ovarian pregnancy with intrauterine pregnancy**

    O00.211 **Right ovarian pregnancy with intrauterine pregnancy** ♀   M

    O00.212 **Left ovarian pregnancy with intrauterine pregnancy** ♀   M

    O00.219 **Unspecified ovarian pregnancy with intrauterine pregnancy** ♀   M

● **O00.8** **Other ectopic pregnancy**
    Cervical pregnancy
    Cornual pregnancy
    Intraligamentous pregnancy
    Mural pregnancy
    Coding Clinic: 2016, Q4, P49

    O00.80 **Other ectopic pregnancy without intrauterine pregnancy** ♀   M
         Other ectopic pregnancy NOS

    O00.81 **Other ectopic pregnancy with intrauterine pregnancy** ♀   M

● **O00.9 Ectopic pregnancy, unspecified**
   Coding Clinic: 2016, Q4, P49
   **O00.90 Unspecified ectopic pregnancy without
   intrauterine pregnancy** ♀   M
      Ectopic pregnancy NOS
   **O00.91 Unspecified ectopic pregnancy with
   intrauterine pregnancy** ♀   M

● **O01 Hydatidiform mole**
   Use additional code from category O08 to identify any
   associated complication
   Excludes1 chorioadenoma (destruens) (D39.2)
            malignant hydatidiform mole (D39.2)
   O01.0 Classical hydatidiform mole ♀   M
      Complete hydatidiform mole
   O01.1 Incomplete and partial hydatidiform mole ♀ M
   O01.9 Hydatidiform mole, unspecified ♀   M
      Trophoblastic disease NOS
      Vesicular mole NOS

● **O02 Other abnormal products of conception**
   Use additional code from category O08 to identify any
   associated complication
   Excludes1 papyraceous fetus (O31.0-)
   O02.0 Blighted ovum and nonhydatidiform mole ♀ M
      Carneous mole   Molar pregnancy NEC
      Fleshy mole   Pathological ovum
      Intrauterine mole NOS
   O02.1 Missed abortion ♀   M
      Early fetal death, before completion of 20 weeks of
         gestation, with retention of dead fetus
      Excludes1 failed induced abortion (O07.-)
               fetal death (intrauterine) (late) (O36.4)
               missed abortion with blighted ovum
                  (O02.0)
               missed abortion with hydatidiform mole
                  (O01.-)
               missed abortion with nonhydatidiform
                  (O02.0)
               missed abortion with other abnormal
                  products of conception (O02.8-)
               missed delivery (O36.4)
               stillbirth (P95)
      Coding Clinic: 2022, Q2, P3-4; 2019, Q3, P12
● **O02.8 Other specified abnormal products of conception**
      Excludes1 abnormal products of conception with
                  blighted ovum (O02.0)
               abnormal products of conception with
                  hydatidiform mole (O01.-)
               abnormal products of conception with
                  nonhydatidiform mole (O02.0)
      **O02.81 Inappropriate change in quantitative human
      chorionic gonadotropin (hCG) in early
      pregnancy** ♀   M
         Biochemical pregnancy
         Chemical pregnancy
         Inappropriate level of quantitative human
            chorionic gonadotropin (hCG) for
            gestational age in early pregnancy
      O02.89 Other abnormal products of conception ♀ M
   O02.9 Abnormal product of conception, unspecified ♀ M

● **O03 Spontaneous abortion**
   Note: Incomplete abortion includes retained products of
      conception following spontaneous abortion.
   Includes miscarriage
   **O03.0 Genital tract and pelvic infection following incomplete
   spontaneous abortion** ♀   M
      Endometritis following incomplete spontaneous
         abortion
      Oophoritis following incomplete spontaneous abortion
      Parametritis following incomplete spontaneous
         abortion
      Pelvic peritonitis following incomplete spontaneous
         abortion
      Salpingitis following incomplete spontaneous abortion
      Salpingo-oophoritis following incomplete spontaneous
         abortion
      Excludes1 sepsis following incomplete spontaneous
                  abortion (O03.37)
               urinary tract infection following
                  incomplete spontaneous abortion
                  (O03.38)
   **O03.1 Delayed or excessive hemorrhage following incomplete
   spontaneous abortion** ♀   M
      Afibrinogenemia following incomplete spontaneous
         abortion
      Defibrination syndrome following incomplete
         spontaneous abortion
      Hemolysis following incomplete spontaneous abortion
      Intravascular coagulation following incomplete
         spontaneous abortion
   **O03.2 Embolism following incomplete spontaneous
   abortion** ♀   M
      Air embolism following incomplete spontaneous
         abortion
      Amniotic fluid embolism following incomplete
         spontaneous abortion
      Blood-clot embolism following incomplete spontaneous
         abortion
      Embolism NOS following incomplete spontaneous
         abortion
      Fat embolism following incomplete spontaneous
         abortion
      Pulmonary embolism following incomplete
         spontaneous abortion
      Pyemic embolism following incomplete spontaneous
         abortion
      Septic or septicopyemic embolism following incomplete
         spontaneous abortion
      Soap embolism following incomplete spontaneous
         abortion
● **O03.3 Other and unspecified complications following
   incomplete spontaneous abortion**
   **O03.30 Unspecified complication following incomplete
      spontaneous abortion** ♀   M
   **O03.31 Shock following incomplete spontaneous
      abortion** ♀   M
      Circulatory collapse following incomplete
         spontaneous abortion
      Shock (postprocedural) following incomplete
         spontaneous abortion
      Excludes1 shock due to infection following
                  incomplete spontaneous
                  abortion (O03.37)
   **O03.32 Renal failure following incomplete
      spontaneous abortion** ♀   M
      Kidney failure (acute) following incomplete
         spontaneous abortion
      Oliguria following incomplete spontaneous
         abortion
      Renal shutdown following incomplete
         spontaneous abortion
      Renal tubular necrosis following incomplete
         spontaneous abortion
      Uremia following incomplete spontaneous
         abortion

CHAPTER 15 (O00-O9A)

Item 15-2 A **hydatidiform** mole is an overproduction of placental tissue. The tumor secretes a hormone, chorionic gonadotropic hormone (CGH), that indicates a positive pregnancy test. There is no viable fetus. More than 80% of hydatidiform moles are noncancerous.

O03.33 **Metabolic disorder** following incomplete
spontaneous abortion ♀   M

O03.34 **Damage to pelvic organs** following incomplete
spontaneous abortion ♀   M

Laceration, perforation, tear or chemical
damage of bladder following incomplete
spontaneous abortion

Laceration, perforation, tear or chemical
damage of bowel following incomplete
spontaneous abortion

Laceration, perforation, tear or chemical
damage of broad ligament following
incomplete spontaneous abortion

Laceration, perforation, tear or chemical
damage of cervix following incomplete
spontaneous abortion

Laceration, perforation, tear or chemical
damage of periurethral tissue following
incomplete spontaneous abortion

Laceration, perforation, tear or chemical
damage of uterus following incomplete
spontaneous abortion

Laceration, perforation, tear or chemical
damage of vagina following incomplete
spontaneous abortion

O03.35 **Other venous complications** following
incomplete spontaneous abortion ♀   M

O03.36 **Cardiac arrest** following incomplete
spontaneous abortion ♀   M

O03.37 **Sepsis** following incomplete spontaneous
abortion ♀   M

Use additional code to identify infectious
agent (B95-B97)

Use additional code to identify severe sepsis, if
applicable (R65.2-)

Excludes1 septic or septicopyemic
embolism following
incomplete spontaneous
abortion (O03.2)

O03.38 **Urinary tract infection** following incomplete
spontaneous abortion ♀   M

Cystitis following incomplete spontaneous
abortion

O03.39 **Incomplete spontaneous abortion with other
complications** ♀   M

O03.4 **Incomplete spontaneous abortion without
complication** ♀   M

O03.5 **Genital tract and pelvic infection** following **complete or
unspecified spontaneous abortion** ♀   M

Endometritis following complete or unspecified
spontaneous abortion

Oophoritis following complete or unspecified
spontaneous abortion

Parametritis following complete or unspecified
spontaneous abortion

Pelvic peritonitis following complete or unspecified
spontaneous abortion

Salpingitis following complete or unspecified
spontaneous abortion

Salpingo-oophoritis following complete or unspecified
spontaneous abortion

Excludes1 sepsis following complete or unspecified
spontaneous abortion (O03.87)
urinary tract infection following complete
or unspecified spontaneous abortion
(O03.88)

O03.6 **Delayed or excessive hemorrhage** following **complete or
unspecified spontaneous abortion** ♀   M

Afibrinogenemia following complete or unspecified
spontaneous abortion

Defibrination syndrome following complete or
unspecified spontaneous abortion

Hemolysis following complete or unspecified
spontaneous abortion

Intravascular coagulation following complete or
unspecified spontaneous abortion

Coding Clinic: 2022, Q1, P19

O03.7 **Embolism** following **complete or unspecified
spontaneous abortion** ♀   M

Air embolism following complete or unspecified
spontaneous abortion

Amniotic fluid embolism following complete or
unspecified spontaneous abortion

Blood-clot embolism following complete or unspecified
spontaneous abortion

Embolism NOS following complete or unspecified
spontaneous abortion

Fat embolism following complete or unspecified
spontaneous abortion

Pulmonary embolism following complete or
unspecified spontaneous abortion

Pyemic embolism following complete or unspecified
spontaneous abortion

Septic or septicopyemic embolism following complete
or unspecified spontaneous abortion

Soap embolism following complete or unspecified
spontaneous abortion

● **O03.8** **Other and unspecified complications** following
complete or unspecified spontaneous abortion

O03.80 **Unspecified complication** following complete
or unspecified spontaneous abortion ♀   M

O03.81 **Shock** following complete or **unspecified
spontaneous abortion** ♀   M

Circulatory collapse following complete or
unspecified spontaneous abortion

Shock (postprocedural) following complete or
unspecified spontaneous abortion

Excludes1 shock due to infection following
complete or unspecified
spontaneous abortion
(O03.87)

O03.82 **Renal failure** following **complete or unspecified
spontaneous abortion** ♀   M

Kidney failure (acute) following complete or
unspecified spontaneous abortion

Oliguria following complete or unspecified
spontaneous abortion

Renal shutdown following complete or
unspecified spontaneous abortion

Renal tubular necrosis following complete or
unspecified spontaneous abortion

Uremia following complete or unspecified
spontaneous abortion

O03.83 **Metabolic disorder** following **complete or
unspecified spontaneous abortion** ♀   M

O03.84 **Damage to pelvic organs** following **complete or
unspecified spontaneous abortion** ♀   M

Laceration, perforation, tear or chemical
damage of bladder following complete or
unspecified spontaneous abortion

Laceration, perforation, tear or chemical
damage of bowel following complete or
unspecified spontaneous abortion

Laceration, perforation, tear or chemical
damage of broad ligament following
complete or unspecified spontaneous
abortion

Laceration, perforation, tear or chemical
damage of cervix following complete or
unspecified spontaneous abortion

Laceration, perforation, tear or chemical
damage of periurethral tissue following
complete or unspecified spontaneous
abortion

Laceration, perforation, tear or chemical
damage of uterus following complete or
unspecified spontaneous abortion

Laceration, perforation, tear or chemical
damage of vagina following complete or
unspecified spontaneous abortion

▶ New   ⇒ Revised   ~~deleted~~ Deleted   Excludes 1   Excludes 2   Includes   Use additional   Code first   Code also   Key words

OGCR Official Guidelines   X Assign placeholder X   ● Use Additional Character(s)   ▷ Manifestation Code   🦌 Hierarchical Condition Category   Coding Clinic

O03.85 **Other venous complications following complete or unspecified spontaneous abortion** ♀ M

O03.86 **Cardiac arrest following complete or unspecified spontaneous abortion** ♀ M

O03.87 **Sepsis following complete or unspecified spontaneous abortion** ♀ M

Use additional code to identify infectious agent (B95-B97)

Use additional code to identify severe sepsis, if applicable (R65.2-)

Excludes1 septic or septicopyemic embolism following complete or unspecified spontaneous abortion (O03.7)

O03.88 **Urinary tract infection following complete or unspecified spontaneous abortion** ♀ M

Cystitis following complete or unspecified spontaneous abortion

O03.89 **Complete or unspecified spontaneous abortion with other complications** ♀ M

O03.9 **Complete or unspecified spontaneous abortion without complication** ♀ M

Miscarriage NOS

Spontaneous abortion NOS

● O04 **Complications following (induced) termination of pregnancy**

Includes complications following (induced) termination of pregnancy

Excludes1 encounter for elective termination of pregnancy, uncomplicated (Z33.2)

failed attempted termination of pregnancy (O07.-)

O04.5 **Genital tract and pelvic infection following (induced) termination of pregnancy** ♀ M

Endometritis following (induced) termination of pregnancy

Oophoritis following (induced) termination of pregnancy

Parametritis following (induced) termination of pregnancy

Pelvic peritonitis following (induced) termination of pregnancy

Salpingitis following (induced) termination of pregnancy

Salpingo-oophoritis following (induced) termination of pregnancy

Excludes1 sepsis following (induced) termination of pregnancy (O04.87)

urinary tract infection following (induced) termination of pregnancy (O04.88)

O04.6 **Delayed or excessive hemorrhage following (induced) termination of pregnancy** ♀ M

Afibrinogenemia following (induced) termination of pregnancy

Defibrination syndrome following (induced) termination of pregnancy

Hemolysis following (induced) termination of pregnancy

Intravascular coagulation following (induced) termination of pregnancy

Coding Clinic: 2019, Q3, P12

O04.7 **Embolism following (induced) termination of pregnancy** ♀ M

Air embolism following (induced) termination of pregnancy

Amniotic fluid embolism following (induced) termination of pregnancy

Blood-clot embolism following (induced) termination of pregnancy

Embolism NOS following (induced) termination of pregnancy

Fat embolism following (induced) termination of pregnancy

Pulmonary embolism following (induced) termination of pregnancy

Pyemic embolism following (induced) termination of pregnancy

Septic or septicopyemic embolism following (induced) termination of pregnancy

Soap embolism following (induced) termination of pregnancy

● O04.8 **(Induced) termination of pregnancy with other and unspecified complications**

O04.80 **(Induced) termination of pregnancy with unspecified complications** ♀ M

O04.81 **Shock following (induced) termination of pregnancy** ♀ M

Circulatory collapse following (induced) termination of pregnancy

Shock (postprocedural) following (induced) termination of pregnancy

Excludes1 shock due to infection following (induced) termination of pregnancy (O04.87)

O04.82 **Renal failure following (induced) termination of pregnancy** ♀ M

Kidney failure (acute) following (induced) termination of pregnancy

Oliguria following (induced) termination of pregnancy

Renal shutdown following (induced) termination of pregnancy

Renal tubular necrosis following (induced) termination of pregnancy

Uremia following (induced) termination of pregnancy

O04.83 **Metabolic disorder following (induced) termination of pregnancy** ♀ M

O04.84 **Damage to pelvic organs following (induced) termination of pregnancy** ♀ M

Laceration, perforation, tear or chemical damage of bladder following (induced) termination of pregnancy

Laceration, perforation, tear or chemical damage of bowel following (induced) termination of pregnancy

Laceration, perforation, tear or chemical damage of broad ligament following (induced) termination of pregnancy

Laceration, perforation, tear or chemical damage of cervix following (induced) termination of pregnancy

Laceration, perforation, tear or chemical damage of periurethral tissue following (induced) termination of pregnancy

Laceration, perforation, tear or chemical damage of uterus following (induced) termination of pregnancy

Laceration, perforation, tear or chemical damage of vagina following (induced) termination of pregnancy

O04.85 **Other venous complications following (induced) termination of pregnancy** ♀ M

O04.86 **Cardiac arrest following (induced) termination of pregnancy** ♀ M

CHAPTER 15 (O00-O9A)

O04.87   **Sepsis following (induced) termination of pregnancy** ♀   M

> Use additional code to identify infectious agent (B95-B97)
>
> Use additional code to identify severe sepsis, if applicable (R65.2-)
>
> **Excludes1**   septic or septicopyemic embolism following (induced) termination of pregnancy (O04.7)

O04.88   **Urinary tract infection following (induced) termination of pregnancy** ♀   M

> Cystitis following (induced) termination of pregnancy

O04.89   **(Induced) termination of pregnancy with other complications** ♀   M

● **O07**   **Failed attempted termination of pregnancy**

> **Includes**   failure of attempted induction of termination of pregnancy
> incomplete elective abortion
>
> **Excludes1**   incomplete spontaneous abortion (O03.0-)

O07.0   **Genital tract and pelvic infection following failed attempted termination of pregnancy** ♀   M

> Endometritis following failed attempted termination of pregnancy
> Oophoritis following failed attempted termination of pregnancy
> Parametritis following failed attempted termination of pregnancy
> Pelvic peritonitis following failed attempted termination of pregnancy
> Salpingitis following failed attempted termination of pregnancy
> Salpingo-oophoritis following failed attempted termination of pregnancy
>
> **Excludes1**   sepsis following failed attempted termination of pregnancy (O07.37)
> urinary tract infection following failed attempted termination of pregnancy (O07.38)

O07.1   **Delayed or excessive hemorrhage following failed attempted termination of pregnancy** ♀   M

> Afibrinogenemia following failed attempted termination of pregnancy
> Defibrination syndrome following failed attempted termination of pregnancy
> Hemolysis following failed attempted termination of pregnancy
> Intravascular coagulation following failed attempted termination of pregnancy

O07.2   **Embolism following failed attempted termination of pregnancy** ♀   M

> Air embolism following failed attempted termination of pregnancy
> Amniotic fluid embolism following failed attempted termination of pregnancy
> Blood-clot embolism following failed attempted termination of pregnancy
> Embolism NOS following failed attempted termination of pregnancy
> Fat embolism following failed attempted termination of pregnancy
> Pulmonary embolism following failed attempted termination of pregnancy
> Pyemic embolism following failed attempted termination of pregnancy
> Septic or septicopyemic embolism following failed attempted termination of pregnancy
> Soap embolism following failed attempted termination of pregnancy

● **O07.3**   **Failed attempted termination of pregnancy with other and unspecified complications**

O07.30   **Failed attempted termination of pregnancy with unspecified complications** ♀   M

O07.31   **Shock following failed attempted termination of pregnancy** ♀   M

> Circulatory collapse following failed attempted termination of pregnancy
> Shock (postprocedural) following failed attempted termination of pregnancy
>
> **Excludes1**   shock due to infection following failed attempted termination of pregnancy (O07.37)

O07.32   **Renal failure following failed attempted termination of pregnancy** ♀   M

> Kidney failure (acute) following failed attempted termination of pregnancy
> Oliguria following failed attempted termination of pregnancy
> Renal shutdown following failed attempted termination of pregnancy
> Renal tubular necrosis following failed attempted termination of pregnancy
> Uremia following failed attempted termination of pregnancy

O07.33   **Metabolic disorder following failed attempted termination of pregnancy** ♀   M

O07.34   **Damage to pelvic organs following failed attempted termination of pregnancy** ♀   M

> Laceration, perforation, tear or chemical damage of bladder following failed attempted termination of pregnancy
> Laceration, perforation, tear or chemical damage of bowel following failed attempted termination of pregnancy
> Laceration, perforation, tear or chemical damage of broad ligament following failed attempted termination of pregnancy
> Laceration, perforation, tear or chemical damage of cervix following failed attempted termination of pregnancy
> Laceration, perforation, tear or chemical damage of periurethral tissue following failed attempted termination of pregnancy
> Laceration, perforation, tear or chemical damage of uterus following failed attempted termination of pregnancy
> Laceration, perforation, tear or chemical damage of vagina following failed attempted termination of pregnancy

O07.35   **Other venous complications following failed attempted termination of pregnancy** ♀   M

O07.36   **Cardiac arrest following failed attempted termination of pregnancy** ♀   M

O07.37   **Sepsis following failed attempted termination of pregnancy** ♀   M

> Use additional code (B95-B97), to identify infectious agent
>
> Use additional code (R65.2-) to identify severe sepsis, if applicable
>
> **Excludes1**   septic or septicopyemic embolism following failed attempted termination of pregnancy (O07.2)

O07.38   **Urinary tract infection following failed attempted termination of pregnancy** ♀   M

> Cystitis following failed attempted termination of pregnancy

O07.39   **Failed attempted termination of pregnancy with other complications** ♀   M

O07.4   **Failed attempted termination of pregnancy without complication** ♀   M

● **O08**   **Complications following ectopic and molar pregnancy**

> This category is for use with categories O00-O02 to identify any associated complications.

▶ New   ⇒ Revised   ~~deleted~~ Deleted   Excludes 1   Excludes 2   Includes   Use additional   Code first   Code also   Key words

OGCR Official Guidelines   X Assign placeholder X   ● Use Additional Character(s)   ▶ Manifestation Code   ◐ Hierarchical Condition Category   **Coding Clinic**

O08.0   **Genital tract and pelvic infection** following ectopic and molar pregnancy ♀   M
> Endometritis following ectopic and molar pregnancy
> Oophoritis following ectopic and molar pregnancy
> Parametritis following ectopic and molar pregnancy
> Pelvic peritonitis following ectopic and molar pregnancy
> Salpingitis following ectopic and molar pregnancy
> Salpingo-oophoritis following ectopic and molar pregnancy
>
> **Excludes1**   sepsis following ectopic and molar pregnancy (O08.82)
> urinary tract infection (O08.83)

O08.1   **Delayed or excessive hemorrhage** following ectopic and molar pregnancy ♀   M
> Afibrinogenemia following ectopic and molar pregnancy
> Defibrination syndrome following ectopic and molar pregnancy
> Hemolysis following ectopic and molar pregnancy
> Intravascular coagulation following ectopic and molar pregnancy
>
> **Excludes1**   delayed or excessive hemorrhage due to incomplete abortion (O03.1)

O08.2   **Embolism following ectopic and molar pregnancy** ♀   M
> Air embolism following ectopic and molar pregnancy
> Amniotic fluid embolism following ectopic and molar pregnancy
> Blood-clot embolism following ectopic and molar pregnancy
> Embolism NOS following ectopic and molar pregnancy
> Fat embolism following ectopic and molar pregnancy
> Pulmonary embolism following ectopic and molar pregnancy
> Pyemic embolism following ectopic and molar pregnancy
> Septic or septicopyemic embolism following ectopic and molar pregnancy
> Soap embolism following ectopic and molar pregnancy

O08.3   **Shock following ectopic and molar pregnancy** ♀   M
> Circulatory collapse following ectopic and molar pregnancy
> Shock (postprocedural) following ectopic and molar pregnancy
>
> **Excludes1**   shock due to infection following ectopic and molar pregnancy (O08.82)

O08.4   **Renal failure following ectopic and molar pregnancy** ♀   M
> Kidney failure (acute) following ectopic and molar pregnancy
> Oliguria following ectopic and molar pregnancy
> Renal shutdown following ectopic and molar pregnancy
> Renal tubular necrosis following ectopic and molar pregnancy
> Uremia following ectopic and molar pregnancy

O08.5   **Metabolic disorders** following an ectopic and molar pregnancy ♀   M

O08.6   **Damage to pelvic organs and tissues** following an ectopic and molar pregnancy ♀   M
> Laceration, perforation, tear or chemical damage of bladder following an ectopic and molar pregnancy
> Laceration, perforation, tear or chemical damage of bowel following an ectopic and molar pregnancy
> Laceration, perforation, tear or chemical damage of broad ligament following an ectopic and molar pregnancy
> Laceration, perforation, tear or chemical damage of cervix following an ectopic and molar pregnancy
> Laceration, perforation, tear or chemical damage of periurethral tissue following an ectopic and molar pregnancy
> Laceration, perforation, tear or chemical damage of uterus following an ectopic and molar pregnancy
> Laceration, perforation, tear or chemical damage of vagina following an ectopic and molar pregnancy

O08.7   **Other venous complications** following an ectopic and molar pregnancy ♀   M

● **O08.8**   **Other** complications following an ectopic and molar pregnancy

   O08.81   **Cardiac arrest** following an ectopic and molar pregnancy ♀   M

   O08.82   **Sepsis** following ectopic and molar pregnancy ♀   M
> Use additional code (B95-B97), to identify infectious agent
> Use additional code (R65.2-) to identify severe sepsis, if applicable
>
> **Excludes1**   septic or septicopyemic embolism following ectopic and molar pregnancy (O08.2)

   O08.83   **Urinary tract infection** following an ectopic and molar pregnancy ♀   M
> Cystitis following an ectopic and molar pregnancy

   O08.89   **Other complications** following an ectopic and molar pregnancy ♀   M

O08.9   **Unspecified complication** following an ectopic and molar pregnancy ♀   M

SUPERVISION OF HIGH RISK PREGNANCY (O09)

● **O09**   **Supervision of high risk pregnancy**
> Coding Clinic: 2016, Q4, P125, 150

 ● **O09.0**   **Supervision of pregnancy with history of infertility**

   O09.00   Supervision of pregnancy with history of infertility, unspecified trimester ♀   M

   O09.01   Supervision of pregnancy with history of infertility, first trimester ♀   M

   O09.02   Supervision of pregnancy with history of infertility, second trimester ♀   M

   O09.03   Supervision of pregnancy with history of infertility, third trimester ♀   M

 ● **O09.1**   **Supervision of pregnancy with history of ectopic pregnancy**
> Coding Clinic: 2016, Q4, P49-50

   O09.10   Supervision of pregnancy with history of ectopic pregnancy, unspecified trimester ♀   M

   O09.11   Supervision of pregnancy with history of ectopic pregnancy, first trimester ♀   M

   O09.12   Supervision of pregnancy with history of ectopic pregnancy, second trimester ♀   M

   O09.13   Supervision of pregnancy with history of ectopic pregnancy, third trimester ♀   M

 ● **O09.A**   **Supervision of pregnancy with history of molar pregnancy**
> Coding Clinic: 2016, Q4, P50

   O09.A0   Supervision of pregnancy with history of molar pregnancy, unspecified trimester ♀   M

   O09.A1   Supervision of pregnancy with history of molar pregnancy, first trimester ♀   M

   O09.A2   Supervision of pregnancy with history of molar pregnancy, second trimester ♀   M

   O09.A3   Supervision of pregnancy with history of molar pregnancy, third trimester ♀   M

 ● **O09.2**   **Supervision of pregnancy with other poor reproductive or obstetric history**
> **Excludes2**   pregnancy care for patient with history of recurrent pregnancy loss (O26.2-)

  ● **O09.21**   **Supervision of pregnancy with history of pre-term labor**

    O09.211   Supervision of pregnancy with history of pre-term labor, first trimester ♀   M

    O09.212   Supervision of pregnancy with history of pre-term labor, second trimester ♀ M

O09.213 Supervision of pregnancy with history of pre-term labor, third trimester ♀ M

O09.219 Supervision of pregnancy with history of pre-term labor, unspecified trimester ♀ M

● **O09.29** Supervision of pregnancy with other poor reproductive or obstetric history
Supervision of pregnancy with history of neonatal death
Supervision of pregnancy with history of stillbirth

O09.291 Supervision of pregnancy with other poor reproductive or obstetric history, first trimester ♀ M

O09.292 Supervision of pregnancy with other poor reproductive or obstetric history, second trimester ♀ M

O09.293 Supervision of pregnancy with other poor reproductive or obstetric history, third trimester ♀ M

O09.299 Supervision of pregnancy with other poor reproductive or obstetric history, unspecified trimester ♀ M

● **O09.3** Supervision of pregnancy with insufficient antenatal care
Supervision of concealed pregnancy
Supervision of hidden pregnancy

O09.30 Supervision of pregnancy with insufficient antenatal care, unspecified trimester ♀

O09.31 Supervision of pregnancy with insufficient antenatal care, first trimester ♀ M

O09.32 Supervision of pregnancy with insufficient antenatal care, second trimester ♀ M

O09.33 Supervision of pregnancy with insufficient antenatal care, third trimester ♀ M

● **O09.4** Supervision of pregnancy with grand multiparity

O09.40 Supervision of pregnancy with grand multiparity, unspecified trimester ♀ M

O09.41 Supervision of pregnancy with grand multiparity, first trimester ♀ M

O09.42 Supervision of pregnancy with grand multiparity, second trimester ♀ M

O09.43 Supervision of pregnancy with grand multiparity, third trimester ♀ M

● **O09.5** Supervision of elderly primigravida and multigravida
Pregnancy for a female 35 years and older at expected date of delivery

● **O09.51** Supervision of elderly primigravida

O09.511 Supervision of elderly primigravida, first trimester ♀ M

O09.512 Supervision of elderly primigravida, second trimester ♀ M

O09.513 Supervision of elderly primigravida, third trimester ♀ M

O09.519 Supervision of elderly primigravida, unspecified trimester ♀ M

● **O09.52** Supervision of elderly multigravida

O09.521 Supervision of elderly multigravida, first trimester ♀ M

O09.522 Supervision of elderly multigravida, second trimester ♀ M

O09.523 Supervision of elderly multigravida, third trimester ♀ M
Coding Clinic: 2016, Q4, P150

O09.529 Supervision of elderly multigravida, unspecified trimester ♀ M

● **O09.6** Supervision of young primigravida and multigravida
Supervision of pregnancy for a female less than 16 years old at expected date of delivery

● **O09.61** Supervision of young primigravida

O09.611 Supervision of young primigravida, first trimester ♀ M

O09.612 Supervision of young primigravida, second trimester ♀ M

O09.613 Supervision of young primigravida, third trimester ♀ M

O09.619 Supervision of young primigravida, unspecified trimester ♀ M

● **O09.62** Supervision of young multigravida

O09.621 Supervision of young multigravida, first trimester ♀ M

O09.622 Supervision of young multigravida, second trimester ♀ M

O09.623 Supervision of young multigravida, third trimester ♀ M

O09.629 Supervision of young multigravida, unspecified trimester ♀ M

● **O09.7** Supervision of high risk pregnancy due to social problems

O09.70 Supervision of high risk pregnancy due to social problems, unspecified trimester ♀ M

O09.71 Supervision of high risk pregnancy due to social problems, first trimester ♀ M

O09.72 Supervision of high risk pregnancy due to social problems, second trimester ♀ M

O09.73 Supervision of high risk pregnancy due to social problems, third trimester ♀ M

● **O09.8** Supervision of other high risk pregnancies

● **O09.81** Supervision of pregnancy resulting from assisted reproductive technology
Supervision of pregnancy resulting from in-vitro fertilization

Excludes2 gestational carrier status (Z33.3)

O09.811 Supervision of pregnancy resulting from assisted reproductive technology, first trimester ♀ M

O09.812 Supervision of pregnancy resulting from assisted reproductive technology, second trimester ♀ M

O09.813 Supervision of pregnancy resulting from assisted reproductive technology, third trimester ♀ M

O09.819 Supervision of pregnancy resulting from assisted reproductive technology, unspecified trimester ♀ M

● **O09.82** Supervision of pregnancy with history of in utero procedure during previous pregnancy

O09.821 Supervision of pregnancy with history of in utero procedure during previous pregnancy, first trimester ♀ M

O09.822 Supervision of pregnancy with history of in utero procedure during previous pregnancy, second trimester ♀ M

O09.823 Supervision of pregnancy with history of in utero procedure during previous pregnancy, third trimester ♀ M

O09.829   Supervision of pregnancy with history of in utero procedure during previous pregnancy, unspecified trimester ♀   M

     Excludes1   supervision of pregnancy affected by in utero procedure during current pregnancy (O35.7)

● O09.89   Supervision of other high risk pregnancies

O09.891   Supervision of other high risk pregnancies, first trimester ♀   M

O09.892   Supervision of other high risk pregnancies, second trimester ♀   M

O09.893   Supervision of other high risk pregnancies, third trimester ♀   M

O09.899   Supervision of other high risk pregnancies, unspecified trimester ♀   M

● O09.9   Supervision of high risk pregnancy, unspecified

O09.90   Supervision of high risk pregnancy, unspecified, unspecified trimester ♀   M

O09.91   Supervision of high risk pregnancy, unspecified, first trimester ♀   M

O09.92   Supervision of high risk pregnancy, unspecified, second trimester ♀   M

O09.93   Supervision of high risk pregnancy, unspecified, third trimester ♀   M

EDEMA, PROTEINURIA AND HYPERTENSIVE DISORDERS IN PREGNANCY, CHILDBIRTH AND THE PUERPERIUM (O10-O16)

● O10   Pre-existing hypertension complicating pregnancy, childbirth and the puerperium

     Includes   pre-existing hypertension with pre-existing proteinuria complicating pregnancy, childbirth and the puerperium

     Excludes2   pre-existing hypertension with superimposed pre-eclampsia complicating pregnancy, childbirth and the puerperium (O11.-)

     Coding Clinic: 2016, Q4, P50

● O10.0   Pre-existing essential hypertension complicating pregnancy, childbirth and the puerperium

     Any condition in I10 specified as a reason for obstetric care during pregnancy, childbirth or the puerperium

● O10.01   Pre-existing essential hypertension complicating pregnancy

O10.011   Pre-existing essential hypertension complicating pregnancy, first trimester ♀   M

O10.012   Pre-existing essential hypertension complicating pregnancy, second trimester ♀   M

O10.013   Pre-existing essential hypertension complicating pregnancy, third trimester ♀   M

O10.019   Pre-existing essential hypertension complicating pregnancy, unspecified trimester ♀   M

O10.02   Pre-existing essential hypertension complicating childbirth ♀   M

O10.03   Pre-existing essential hypertension complicating the puerperium ♀   M

● O10.1   Pre-existing hypertensive heart disease complicating pregnancy, childbirth and the puerperium

     Any condition in I11 specified as a reason for obstetric care during pregnancy, childbirth or the puerperium

     Use additional code from I11 to identify the type of hypertensive heart disease

● O10.11   Pre-existing hypertensive heart disease complicating pregnancy

O10.111   Pre-existing hypertensive heart disease complicating pregnancy, first trimester ♀   M

O10.112   Pre-existing hypertensive heart disease complicating pregnancy, second trimester ♀   M

O10.113   Pre-existing hypertensive heart disease complicating pregnancy, third trimester ♀   M

O10.119   Pre-existing hypertensive heart disease complicating pregnancy, unspecified trimester ♀   M

O10.12   Pre-existing hypertensive heart disease complicating childbirth ♀   M

O10.13   Pre-existing hypertensive heart disease complicating the puerperium ♀   M

● O10.2   Pre-existing hypertensive chronic kidney disease complicating pregnancy, childbirth and the puerperium

     Any condition in I12 specified as a reason for obstetric care during pregnancy, childbirth or the puerperium

     Use additional code from I12 to identify the type of hypertensive chronic kidney disease

● O10.21   Pre-existing hypertensive chronic kidney disease complicating pregnancy

O10.211   Pre-existing hypertensive chronic kidney disease complicating pregnancy, first trimester ♀   M

O10.212   Pre-existing hypertensive chronic kidney disease complicating pregnancy, second trimester ♀   M

O10.213   Pre-existing hypertensive chronic kidney disease complicating pregnancy, third trimester ♀   M

O10.219   Pre-existing hypertensive chronic kidney disease complicating pregnancy, unspecified trimester ♀   M

O10.22   Pre-existing hypertensive chronic kidney disease complicating childbirth ♀   M

O10.23   Pre-existing hypertensive chronic kidney disease complicating the puerperium ♀   M

● O10.3   Pre-existing hypertensive heart and chronic kidney disease complicating pregnancy, childbirth and the puerperium

     Any condition in I13 specified as a reason for obstetric care during pregnancy, childbirth or the puerperium

     Use additional code from I13 to identify the type of hypertensive heart and chronic kidney disease

● O10.31   Pre-existing hypertensive heart and chronic kidney disease complicating pregnancy

O10.311   Pre-existing hypertensive heart and chronic kidney disease complicating pregnancy, first trimester ♀   M

O10.312   Pre-existing hypertensive heart and chronic kidney disease complicating pregnancy, second trimester ♀   M

O10.313   Pre-existing hypertensive heart and chronic kidney disease complicating pregnancy, third trimester ♀   M

O10.319   Pre-existing hypertensive heart and chronic kidney disease complicating pregnancy, unspecified trimester ♀   M

O10.32   Pre-existing hypertensive heart and chronic kidney disease complicating childbirth ♀ M

O10.33   Pre-existing hypertensive heart and chronic kidney disease complicating the puerperium ♀ M

● O10.4   **Pre-existing secondary hypertension complicating pregnancy, childbirth and the puerperium**

Any condition in I15 specified as a reason for obstetric care during pregnancy, childbirth or the puerperium

Use additional code from I15 to identify the type of secondary hypertension

● O10.41   Pre-existing secondary hypertension complicating pregnancy

O10.411   Pre-existing secondary hypertension complicating pregnancy, first trimester ♀ M

O10.412   Pre-existing secondary hypertension complicating pregnancy, second trimester ♀ M

O10.413   Pre-existing secondary hypertension complicating pregnancy, third trimester ♀ M

O10.419   Pre-existing secondary hypertension complicating pregnancy, unspecified trimester ♀ M

O10.42   Pre-existing secondary hypertension complicating childbirth ♀ M

O10.43   Pre-existing secondary hypertension complicating the puerperium ♀ M

● O10.9   Unspecified pre-existing hypertension complicating pregnancy, childbirth and the puerperium

● O10.91   Unspecified pre-existing hypertension complicating pregnancy

O10.911   Unspecified pre-existing hypertension complicating pregnancy, first trimester ♀ M

O10.912   Unspecified pre-existing hypertension complicating pregnancy, second trimester ♀ M

O10.913   Unspecified pre-existing hypertension complicating pregnancy, third trimester ♀ M

O10.919   Unspecified pre-existing hypertension complicating pregnancy, unspecified trimester ♀ M

O10.92   Unspecified pre-existing hypertension complicating childbirth ♀ M

O10.93   Unspecified pre-existing hypertension complicating the puerperium ♀ M

● O11   **Pre-existing hypertension with pre-eclampsia**

Includes   conditions in O10 complicated by pre-eclampsia
pre-eclampsia superimposed pre-existing hypertension

Use additional code from O10 to identify the type of hypertension

Coding Clinic: 2016, Q4, P50

O11.1   Pre-existing hypertension with pre-eclampsia, first trimester ♀ M

O11.2   Pre-existing hypertension with pre-eclampsia, second trimester ♀ M

O11.3   Pre-existing hypertension with pre-eclampsia, third trimester ♀ M

O11.4   Pre-existing hypertension with pre-eclampsia, complicating childbirth ♀ M

O11.5   Pre-existing hypertension with pre-eclampsia, complicating the puerperium ♀ M

O11.9   Pre-existing hypertension with pre-eclampsia, unspecified trimester ♀ M

● O12   **Gestational [pregnancy-induced] edema and proteinuria without hypertension**

Coding Clinic: 2016, Q4, P50

● O12.0   Gestational edema

O12.00   Gestational edema, unspecified trimester ♀ M

O12.01   Gestational edema, first trimester ♀ M

O12.02   Gestational edema, second trimester ♀ M

O12.03   Gestational edema, third trimester ♀ M

O12.04   Gestational edema, complicating childbirth ♀ M

O12.05   Gestational edema, complicating the puerperium ♀ M

● O12.1   Gestational proteinuria

O12.10   Gestational proteinuria, unspecified trimester ♀ M

O12.11   Gestational proteinuria, first trimester ♀ M

O12.12   Gestational proteinuria, second trimester ♀ M

O12.13   Gestational proteinuria, third trimester ♀ M

O12.14   Gestational proteinuria, complicating childbirth ♀ M

O12.15   Gestational proteinuria, complicating the puerperium ♀ M

● O12.2   Gestational edema with proteinuria

O12.20   Gestational edema with proteinuria, unspecified trimester ♀ M

O12.21   Gestational edema with proteinuria, first trimester ♀ M

O12.22   Gestational edema with proteinuria, second trimester ♀ M

O12.23   Gestational edema with proteinuria, third trimester ♀ M

O12.24   Gestational edema with proteinuria, complicating childbirth ♀ M

O12.25   Gestational edema with proteinuria, complicating the puerperium ♀ M

● O13   **Gestational [pregnancy-induced] hypertension without significant proteinuria**

Includes   gestational hypertension NOS
transient hypertension of pregnancy ♀

Coding Clinic: 2016, Q4, P50

O13.1   Gestational [pregnancy-induced] hypertension without significant proteinuria, first trimester ♀ M

O13.2   Gestational [pregnancy-induced] hypertension without significant proteinuria, second trimester ♀ M

O13.3   Gestational [pregnancy-induced] hypertension without significant proteinuria, third trimester ♀ M

O13.4   Gestational [pregnancy-induced] hypertension without significant proteinuria, complicating childbirth ♀ M

O13.5   Gestational [pregnancy-induced] hypertension without significant proteinuria, complicating the puerperium ♀ M

O13.9   Gestational [pregnancy-induced] hypertension without significant proteinuria, unspecified trimester ♀ M

● O14   **Pre-eclampsia**

Excludes 1   pre-existing hypertension with pre-eclampsia (O11)

Coding Clinic: 2016, Q4, P50

● O14.0   Mild to moderate pre-eclampsia

O14.00   Mild to moderate pre-eclampsia, unspecified trimester ♀ M

O14.02   Mild to moderate pre-eclampsia, second trimester ♀ M

O14.03   Mild to moderate pre-eclampsia, third trimester ♀ M

O14.04   Mild to moderate pre-eclampsia, complicating childbirth ♀
Coding Clinic: 2019, Q2, P8   M

O14.05   Mild to moderate pre-eclampsia, complicating the puerperium ♀ M

● **O14.1**   **Severe pre-eclampsia**

     Excludes1   HELLP syndrome (O14.2-)

     H=hemolysis, EL=elevated liver enzymes, LP=low platelet count

     Coding Clinic: 2019, Q3, P12

     O14.10   Severe pre-eclampsia, unspecified trimester ♀   M

     O14.12   Severe pre-eclampsia, second trimester ♀   M

     O14.13   Severe pre-eclampsia, third trimester ♀   M

     O14.14   Severe pre-eclampsia complicating childbirth ♀   M

     O14.15   Severe pre-eclampsia, complicating the puerperium ♀   M

● **O14.2**   **HELLP syndrome**

     Severe pre-eclampsia with hemolysis, elevated liver enzymes and low platelet count (HELLP)

     O14.20   HELLP syndrome (HELLP), unspecified trimester ♀   M

     O14.22   HELLP syndrome (HELLP), second trimester ♀   M

     O14.23   HELLP syndrome (HELLP), third trimester ♀   M

     O14.24   HELLP syndrome, complicating childbirth ♀   M

     O14.25   HELLP syndrome, complicating the puerperium ♀   M

● **O14.9**   **Unspecified pre-eclampsia**

     O14.90   Unspecified pre-eclampsia, unspecified trimester ♀   M

     O14.92   Unspecified pre-eclampsia, second trimester ♀   M

     O14.93   Unspecified pre-eclampsia, third trimester ♀   M

     O14.94   Unspecified pre-eclampsia, complicating childbirth ♀   M

     O14.95   Unspecified pre-eclampsia, complicating the puerperium ♀   M

● **O15**   **Eclampsia**

     Includes   convulsions following conditions in O10-O14 and O16

   ● **O15.0**   **Eclampsia complicating pregnancy**

     Coding Clinic: 2016, Q4, P50

     O15.00   Eclampsia complicating pregnancy, unspecified trimester ♀   M

     O15.02   Eclampsia complicating pregnancy, second trimester ♀   M

     O15.03   Eclampsia complicating pregnancy, third trimester ♀   M

     O15.1   Eclampsia complicating labor ♀   M

     O15.2   Eclampsia complicating the puerperium ♀   M

     O15.9   Eclampsia, unspecified as to time period ♀   M

       Eclampsia NOS

● **O16**   **Unspecified maternal hypertension**

     Coding Clinic: 2016, Q4, P50

     O16.1   Unspecified maternal hypertension, first trimester ♀   M

     O16.2   Unspecified maternal hypertension, second trimester ♀   M

     O16.3   Unspecified maternal hypertension, third trimester ♀   M

     O16.4   Unspecified maternal hypertension, complicating childbirth ♀   M

     O16.5   Unspecified maternal hypertension, complicating the puerperium ♀   M

     O16.9   Unspecified maternal hypertension, unspecified trimester ♀   M

OTHER MATERNAL DISORDERS PREDOMINANTLY RELATED TO PREGNANCY (O20-O29)

     Excludes2   maternal care related to the fetus and amniotic cavity and possible delivery problems (O30-O48)

         maternal diseases classifiable elsewhere but complicating pregnancy, labor and delivery, and the puerperium (O98-O99)

● **O20**   **Hemorrhage in early pregnancy**

     Includes   hemorrhage before completion of 20 weeks gestation

     Excludes1   pregnancy with abortive outcome (O00-O08)

     O20.0   Threatened abortion ♀   M

       Hemorrhage specified as due to threatened abortion

     O20.8   Other hemorrhage in early pregnancy ♀   M

     O20.9   Hemorrhage in early pregnancy, unspecified ♀   M

● **O21**   **Excessive vomiting in pregnancy**

     O21.0   Mild hyperemesis gravidarum ♀   M

       Hyperemesis gravidarum, mild or unspecified, starting before the end of the 20th week of gestation

     O21.1   Hyperemesis gravidarum with metabolic disturbance ♀   M

       Hyperemesis gravidarum, starting before the end of the 20th week of gestation, with metabolic disturbance such as carbohydrate depletion

       Hyperemesis gravidarum, starting before the end of the 20th week of gestation, with metabolic disturbance such as dehydration

       Hyperemesis gravidarum, starting before the end of the 20th week of gestation, with metabolic disturbance such as electrolyte imbalance

     O21.2   Late vomiting of pregnancy ♀   M

       Excessive vomiting starting after 20 completed weeks of gestation

     O21.8   Other vomiting complicating pregnancy ♀   M

       Vomiting due to diseases classified elsewhere, complicating pregnancy

       Use additional code, to identify cause

     O21.9   Vomiting of pregnancy, unspecified ♀   M

● **O22**   **Venous complications and hemorrhoids in pregnancy**

     Excludes1   venous complications of:

         abortion NOS (O03.9)

         ectopic or molar pregnancy (O08.7)

         failed attempted abortion (O07.35)

         induced abortion (O04.85)

         spontaneous abortion (O03.89)

     Excludes2   obstetric pulmonary embolism (O88.-)

         venous complications and hemorrhoids of childbirth and the puerperium (O87.-)

   ● **O22.0**   **Varicose veins of lower extremity in pregnancy**

     Varicose veins NOS in pregnancy

     O22.00   Varicose veins of lower extremity in pregnancy, unspecified trimester ♀   M

     O22.01   Varicose veins of lower extremity in pregnancy, first trimester ♀   M

     O22.02   Varicose veins of lower extremity in pregnancy, second trimester ♀   M

     O22.03   Varicose veins of lower extremity in pregnancy, third trimester ♀   M

   ● **O22.1**   **Genital varices in pregnancy**

     Perineal varices in pregnancy

     Vaginal varices in pregnancy

     Vulval varices in pregnancy

     O22.10   Genital varices in pregnancy, unspecified trimester ♀   M

     O22.11   Genital varices in pregnancy, first trimester ♀   M

     O22.12   Genital varices in pregnancy, second trimester ♀   M

     O22.13   Genital varices in pregnancy, third trimester ♀ M

CHAPTER 15 (O00-O9A)

CHAPTER 15 (O00-O9A)

● **O22.2 Superficial thrombophlebitis in pregnancy**
Phlebitis in pregnancy NOS
Thrombophlebitis of legs in pregnancy
Thrombosis in pregnancy NOS
Use additional code to identify the superficial
thrombophlebitis (I80.0-)

     O22.20 Superficial thrombophlebitis in pregnancy, unspecified trimester ♀   M

     O22.21 Superficial thrombophlebitis in pregnancy, first trimester ♀   M

     O22.22 Superficial thrombophlebitis in pregnancy, second trimester ♀   M

     O22.23 Superficial thrombophlebitis in pregnancy, third trimester ♀   M

● **O22.3 Deep phlebothrombosis in pregnancy**
Deep vein thrombosis, antepartum
Use additional code to identify the deep vein
thrombosis (I82.4-, I82.5-, I82.62-, I82.72-)
Use additional code, if applicable, for associated long-
term (current) use of anticoagulants (Z79.01)

     O22.30 Deep phlebothrombosis in pregnancy, unspecified trimester ♀   M

     O22.31 Deep phlebothrombosis in pregnancy, first trimester ♀   M

     O22.32 Deep phlebothrombosis in pregnancy, second trimester ♀   M

     O22.33 Deep phlebothrombosis in pregnancy, third trimester ♀   M

● **O22.4 Hemorrhoids in pregnancy**

     O22.40 Hemorrhoids in pregnancy, unspecified trimester ♀   M

     O22.41 Hemorrhoids in pregnancy, first trimester ♀   M

     O22.42 Hemorrhoids in pregnancy, second trimester ♀   M

     O22.43 Hemorrhoids in pregnancy, third trimester ♀   M

● **O22.5 Cerebral venous thrombosis in pregnancy**
Cerebrovenous sinus thrombosis in pregnancy

     O22.50 Cerebral venous thrombosis in pregnancy, unspecified trimester ♀   M

     O22.51 Cerebral venous thrombosis in pregnancy, first trimester ♀   M

     O22.52 Cerebral venous thrombosis in pregnancy, second trimester ♀   M

     O22.53 Cerebral venous thrombosis in pregnancy, third trimester ♀   M

● **O22.8 Other venous complications in pregnancy**

  ● **O22.8X Other venous complications in pregnancy**

     O22.8X1 Other venous complications in pregnancy, first trimester ♀   M

     O22.8X2 Other venous complications in pregnancy, second trimester ♀   M

     O22.8X3 Other venous complications in pregnancy, third trimester ♀   M

     O22.8X9 Other venous complications in pregnancy, unspecified trimester ♀   M

● **O22.9 Venous complication in pregnancy, unspecified**
Gestational phlebitis NOS
Gestational phlebopathy NOS
Gestational thrombosis NOS

     O22.90 Venous complication in pregnancy, unspecified, unspecified trimester ♀   M

     O22.91 Venous complication in pregnancy, unspecified, first trimester ♀   M

     O22.92 Venous complication in pregnancy, unspecified, second trimester ♀   M

     O22.93 Venous complication in pregnancy, unspecified, third trimester ♀   M

● **O23 Infections of genitourinary tract in pregnancy**
Use additional code to identify organism (B95.-, B96.-)

    Excludes2   gonococcal infections complicating pregnancy, childbirth and the puerperium (O98.2)
infections with a predominantly sexual mode of transmission NOS complicating pregnancy, childbirth and the puerperium (O98.3)
syphilis complicating pregnancy, childbirth and the puerperium (O98.1)
tuberculosis of genitourinary system complicating pregnancy, childbirth and the puerperium (O98.0)
venereal disease NOS complicating pregnancy, childbirth and the puerperium (O98.3)

● **O23.0 Infections of kidney in pregnancy**
Pyelonephritis in pregnancy

     O23.00 Infections of kidney in pregnancy, unspecified trimester ♀   M

     O23.01 Infections of kidney in pregnancy, first trimester ♀   M

     O23.02 Infections of kidney in pregnancy, second trimester ♀   M

     O23.03 Infections of kidney in pregnancy, third trimester ♀   M

● **O23.1 Infections of bladder in pregnancy**

     O23.10 Infections of bladder in pregnancy, unspecified trimester ♀   M

     O23.11 Infections of bladder in pregnancy, first trimester ♀   M

     O23.12 Infections of bladder in pregnancy, second trimester ♀   M

     O23.13 Infections of bladder in pregnancy, third trimester ♀   M

● **O23.2 Infections of urethra in pregnancy**

     O23.20 Infections of urethra in pregnancy, unspecified trimester ♀   M

     O23.21 Infections of urethra in pregnancy, first trimester ♀   M

     O23.22 Infections of urethra in pregnancy, second trimester ♀   M

     O23.23 Infections of urethra in pregnancy, third trimester ♀   M

● **O23.3 Infections of other parts of urinary tract in pregnancy**

     O23.30 Infections of other parts of urinary tract in pregnancy, unspecified trimester ♀   M

     O23.31 Infections of other parts of urinary tract in pregnancy, first trimester ♀   M

     O23.32 Infections of other parts of urinary tract in pregnancy, second trimester ♀   M

     O23.33 Infections of other parts of urinary tract in pregnancy, third trimester ♀   M

● **O23.4 Unspecified infection of urinary tract in pregnancy**

     O23.40 Unspecified infection of urinary tract in pregnancy, unspecified trimester ♀   M

     O23.41 Unspecified infection of urinary tract in pregnancy, first trimester ♀   M

     O23.42 Unspecified infection of urinary tract in pregnancy, second trimester ♀   M

     O23.43 Unspecified infection of urinary tract in pregnancy, third trimester ♀   M

● **O23.5 Infections of the genital tract in pregnancy**

  ● **O23.51 Infection of cervix in pregnancy**

     O23.511 Infections of cervix in pregnancy, first trimester ♀   M

     O23.512 Infections of cervix in pregnancy, second trimester ♀   M

     O23.513 Infections of cervix in pregnancy, third trimester ♀   M

     O23.519 Infections of cervix in pregnancy, unspecified trimester ♀   M

● **O23.52   Salpingo-oophoritis in pregnancy**
Oophoritis = inflammation of ovary
Salpingitis = inflammation of fallopian tube
Oophoritis in pregnancy
Salpingitis in pregnancy

　　O23.521   **Salpingo-oophoritis in pregnancy, first trimester** ♀   M

　　O23.522   **Salpingo-oophoritis in pregnancy, second trimester** ♀   M

　　O23.523   **Salpingo-oophoritis in pregnancy, third trimester** ♀   M

　　O23.529   **Salpingo-oophoritis in pregnancy, unspecified trimester** ♀   M

● **O23.59   Infection of other part of genital tract in pregnancy**
　　Coding Clinic: 2022, Q1, P20

　　O23.591   **Infection of other part of genital tract in pregnancy, first trimester** ♀   M

　　O23.592   **Infection of other part of genital tract in pregnancy, second trimester** ♀   M

　　O23.593   **Infection of other part of genital tract in pregnancy, third trimester** ♀   M
　　　　Coding Clinic: 2022, Q1, P20

　　O23.599   **Infection of other part of genital tract in pregnancy, unspecified trimester** ♀   M

● **O23.9   Unspecified genitourinary tract infection in pregnancy**
Genitourinary tract infection in pregnancy NOS

　　O23.90   **Unspecified genitourinary tract infection in pregnancy, unspecified trimester** ♀   M

　　O23.91   **Unspecified genitourinary tract infection in pregnancy, first trimester** ♀   M

　　O23.92   **Unspecified genitourinary tract infection in pregnancy, second trimester** ♀   M

　　O23.93   **Unspecified genitourinary tract infection in pregnancy, third trimester** ♀   M

OGCR Section I.C.15.g.

Diabetes mellitus in pregnancy

Diabetes mellitus is a significant complicating factor in pregnancy. Pregnant women who are diabetic should be assigned a code from category O24, Diabetes mellitus in pregnancy, childbirth, and the puerperium, first, followed by the appropriate diabetes code(s) (E08-E13) from Chapter 4.

● **O24   Diabetes mellitus in pregnancy, childbirth, and the puerperium**

● **O24.0   Pre-existing type 1 diabetes mellitus, in pregnancy, childbirth and the puerperium**
Juvenile onset diabetes mellitus, in pregnancy, childbirth and the puerperium
Ketosis-prone diabetes mellitus in pregnancy, childbirth and the puerperium
Use additional code from category E10 to further identify any manifestations

● **O24.01   Pre-existing type 1 diabetes mellitus, in pregnancy**

　　O24.011   **Pre-existing type 1 diabetes mellitus, in pregnancy, first trimester** ♀   M

　　O24.012   **Pre-existing type 1 diabetes mellitus, in pregnancy, second trimester** ♀   M

　　O24.013   **Pre-existing type 1 diabetes mellitus, in pregnancy, third trimester** ♀   M

　　O24.019   **Pre-existing type 1 diabetes mellitus, in pregnancy, unspecified trimester** ♀   M

　　O24.02   **Pre-existing type 1 diabetes mellitus, in childbirth** ♀   M

　　O24.03   **Pre-existing type 1 diabetes mellitus, in the puerperium** ♀   M

● **O24.1   Pre-existing type 2 diabetes mellitus, in pregnancy, childbirth and the puerperium**
Insulin-resistant diabetes mellitus in pregnancy, childbirth and the puerperium
Use additional code (for):
from category E11 to further identify any manifestations
long-term (current) use of insulin (Z79.4)

● **O24.11   Pre-existing type 2 diabetes mellitus, in pregnancy**

　　O24.111   **Pre-existing type 2 diabetes mellitus, in pregnancy, first trimester** ♀   M

　　O24.112   **Pre-existing type 2 diabetes mellitus, in pregnancy, second trimester** ♀   M

　　O24.113   **Pre-existing type 2 diabetes mellitus, in pregnancy, third trimester** ♀   M

　　O24.119   **Pre-existing type 2 diabetes mellitus, in pregnancy, unspecified trimester** ♀   M

　　O24.12   **Pre-existing type 2 diabetes mellitus, in childbirth** ♀   M

　　O24.13   **Pre-existing type 2 diabetes mellitus, in the puerperium** ♀   M

● **O24.3   Unspecified pre-existing diabetes mellitus in pregnancy, childbirth and the puerperium**
Use additional code (for):
from category E11 to further identify any manifestation
long-term (current) use of insulin (Z79.4)

● **O24.31   Unspecified pre-existing diabetes mellitus in pregnancy**

　　O24.311   **Unspecified pre-existing diabetes mellitus in pregnancy, first trimester** ♀   M

　　O24.312   **Unspecified pre-existing diabetes mellitus in pregnancy, second trimester** ♀   M

　　O24.313   **Unspecified pre-existing diabetes mellitus in pregnancy, third trimester** ♀   M

　　O24.319   **Unspecified pre-existing diabetes mellitus in pregnancy, unspecified trimester** ♀   M

　　O24.32   **Unspecified pre-existing diabetes mellitus in childbirth** ♀   M

　　O24.33   **Unspecified pre-existing diabetes mellitus in the puerperium** ♀   M

● **O24.4   Gestational diabetes mellitus**
Diabetes mellitus arising in pregnancy
Gestational diabetes mellitus NOS
Coding Clinic: 2016, Q4, P50, 126

● **O24.41   Gestational diabetes mellitus in pregnancy**

　　O24.410   **Gestational diabetes mellitus in pregnancy, diet controlled** ♀   M

　　O24.414   **Gestational diabetes mellitus in pregnancy, insulin controlled** ♀   M

　　O24.415   **Gestational diabetes mellitus in pregnancy, controlled by oral hypoglycemic drugs** ♀   M
　　　　Gestational diabetes mellitus in pregnancy, controlled by oral antidiabetic drugs
　　　　Coding Clinic: 2016, Q4, P50

　　O24.419   **Gestational diabetes mellitus in pregnancy, unspecified control** ♀   M
　　　　Coding Clinic: 2015, Q4, P34

● **O24.42   Gestational diabetes mellitus in childbirth**

　　O24.420   **Gestational diabetes mellitus in childbirth, diet controlled** ♀   M

　　O24.424   **Gestational diabetes mellitus in childbirth, insulin controlled** ♀   M

CHAPTER 15 (O00-O9A)

CHAPTER 15 (O00-O9A)

O24.425   Gestational diabetes mellitus in childbirth, controlled by oral hypoglycemic drugs ♀   M
  Gestational diabetes mellitus in childbirth, controlled by oral antidiabetic drugs
  Coding Clinic: 2016, Q4, P50

O24.429   Gestational diabetes mellitus in childbirth, unspecified control ♀   M

OGCR Section I.C.15.i.

Gestational (pregnancy induced) diabetes

Gestational (pregnancy induced) diabetes can occur during the second and third trimester of pregnancy in women who were not diabetic prior to pregnancy. Gestational diabetes can cause complications in the pregnancy similar to those of pre-existing diabetes mellitus. It also puts the woman at greater risk of developing diabetes after the pregnancy. Codes for gestational diabetes are in subcategory O24.4, Gestational diabetes mellitus. No other code from category O24, Diabetes mellitus in pregnancy, childbirth, and the puerperium, should be used with a code from O24.4

The codes under subcategory O24.4 include diet controlled, insulin controlled, **and controlled by oral hypoglycemic drugs.** If a patient with gestational diabetes is treated with both diet and insulin, only the code for insulin-controlled is required. **If a patient with gestational diabetes is treated with both diet and oral hypoglycemic medications, only the code for "controlled by oral hypoglycemic drugs" is required.** Code Z79.4, Long-term (current) use of insulin or code Z79.84, Long-term (current) use of oral hypoglycemic drugs, should not be assigned with codes from subcategory O24.4.

An abnormal glucose tolerance in pregnancy is assigned a code from subcategory O99.81, Abnormal glucose complicating pregnancy, childbirth, and the puerperium.

● O24.43   Gestational diabetes mellitus in the puerperium
  O24.430   Gestational diabetes mellitus in the puerperium, diet controlled ♀   M
  O24.434   Gestational diabetes mellitus in the puerperium, insulin controlled ♀   M
  O24.435   Gestational diabetes mellitus in puerperium, controlled by oral hypoglycemic drugs ♀   M
    Gestational diabetes mellitus in puerperium, controlled by oral antidiabetic drugs
    Coding Clinic: 2016, Q4, P50
  O24.439   Gestational diabetes mellitus in the puerperium, unspecified control ♀   M

● O24.8   Other pre-existing diabetes mellitus in pregnancy, childbirth, and the puerperium
  Use additional code (for):
    from categories E08, E09 and E13 to further identify any manifestation
    long-term (current) use of insulin (Z79.4)
  ● O24.81   Other pre-existing diabetes mellitus in pregnancy
    O24.811   Other pre-existing diabetes mellitus in pregnancy, first trimester ♀   M
    O24.812   Other pre-existing diabetes mellitus in pregnancy, second trimester ♀   M
    O24.813   Other pre-existing diabetes mellitus in pregnancy, third trimester ♀   M
    O24.819   Other pre-existing diabetes mellitus in pregnancy, unspecified trimester ♀   M
  O24.82   Other pre-existing diabetes mellitus in childbirth ♀   M
  O24.83   Other pre-existing diabetes mellitus in the puerperium ♀   M

● O24.9   Unspecified diabetes mellitus in pregnancy, childbirth and the puerperium
  Use additional code for long-term (current) use of insulin (Z79.4)
  Unknown whether patient was diabetic before pregnancy occurred
  ● O24.91   Unspecified diabetes mellitus in pregnancy
    O24.911   Unspecified diabetes mellitus in pregnancy, first trimester ♀   M
    O24.912   Unspecified diabetes mellitus in pregnancy, second trimester ♀   M
    O24.913   Unspecified diabetes mellitus in pregnancy, third trimester ♀   M
    O24.919   Unspecified diabetes mellitus in pregnancy, unspecified trimester ♀   M
  O24.92   Unspecified diabetes mellitus in childbirth ♀   M
  O24.93   Unspecified diabetes mellitus in the puerperium ♀   M

● O25   Malnutrition in pregnancy, childbirth and the puerperium
  ● O25.1   Malnutrition in pregnancy
    O25.10   Malnutrition in pregnancy, unspecified trimester ♀   M
    O25.11   Malnutrition in pregnancy, first trimester ♀   M
    O25.12   Malnutrition in pregnancy, second trimester ♀ M
    O25.13   Malnutrition in pregnancy, third trimester ♀   M
  O25.2   Malnutrition in childbirth ♀   M
  O25.3   Malnutrition in the puerperium ♀   M

● O26   Maternal care for other conditions predominantly related to pregnancy
  ● O26.0   Excessive weight gain in pregnancy
    Excludes2   gestational edema (O12.0, O12.2)
    O26.00   Excessive weight gain in pregnancy, unspecified trimester ♀   M
    O26.01   Excessive weight gain in pregnancy, first trimester ♀   M
    O26.02   Excessive weight gain in pregnancy, second trimester ♀   M
    O26.03   Excessive weight gain in pregnancy, third trimester ♀   M
  ● O26.1   Low weight gain in pregnancy
    O26.10   Low weight gain in pregnancy, unspecified trimester ♀   M
    O26.11   Low weight gain in pregnancy, first trimester ♀   M
    O26.12   Low weight gain in pregnancy, second trimester ♀   M
    O26.13   Low weight gain in pregnancy, third trimester ♀   M
  ● O26.2   Pregnancy care for patient with recurrent pregnancy loss
    O26.20   Pregnancy care for patient with recurrent pregnancy loss, unspecified trimester ♀   M
    O26.21   Pregnancy care for patient with recurrent pregnancy loss, first trimester ♀   M
    O26.22   Pregnancy care for patient with recurrent pregnancy loss, second trimester ♀   M
    O26.23   Pregnancy care for patient with recurrent pregnancy loss, third trimester ♀   M
  ● O26.3   Retained intrauterine contraceptive device in pregnancy
    O26.30   Retained intrauterine contraceptive device in pregnancy, unspecified trimester ♀   M
    O26.31   Retained intrauterine contraceptive device in pregnancy, first trimester ♀   M
    O26.32   Retained intrauterine contraceptive device in pregnancy, second trimester ♀   M
    O26.33   Retained intrauterine contraceptive device in pregnancy, third trimester ♀   M

▶ New   ⇒ Revised   ~~deleted~~ Deleted   Excludes 1   Excludes 2   Includes   Use additional   Code first   Code also   Key words
OGCR Official Guidelines   X Assign placeholder X   ● Use Additional Character(s)   ⟩ Manifestation Code   ⓗ Hierarchical Condition Category   **Coding Clinic**

● O26.4 Herpes gestationis
    O26.40 Herpes gestationis, unspecified trimester ♀   M
    O26.41 Herpes gestationis, first trimester ♀   M
    O26.42 Herpes gestationis, second trimester ♀   M
    O26.43 Herpes gestationis, third trimester ♀   M

● O26.5 Maternal hypotension syndrome
    Supine hypotensive syndrome
    O26.50 Maternal hypotension syndrome, unspecified trimester ♀   M
    O26.51 Maternal hypotension syndrome, first trimester ♀   M
    O26.52 Maternal hypotension syndrome, second trimester ♀   M
    O26.53 Maternal hypotension syndrome, third trimester ♀   M

● O26.6 Liver and biliary tract disorders in pregnancy, childbirth and the puerperium
    Use additional code to identify the specific disorder
    Excludes2 hepatorenal syndrome following labor and delivery (O90.4)

  ● O26.61 Liver and biliary tract disorders in pregnancy
    O26.611 Liver and biliary tract disorders in pregnancy, first trimester ♀   M
    O26.612 Liver and biliary tract disorders in pregnancy, second trimester ♀   M
    O26.613 Liver and biliary tract disorders in pregnancy, third trimester ♀   M
    O26.619 Liver and biliary tract disorders in pregnancy, unspecified trimester ♀ M
    O26.62 Liver and biliary tract disorders in childbirth ♀   M
    O26.63 Liver and biliary tract disorders in the puerperium ♀   M

● O26.7 Subluxation of symphysis (pubis) in pregnancy, childbirth and the puerperium
    Excludes1 traumatic separation of symphysis (pubis) during childbirth (O71.6)

  ● O26.71 Subluxation of symphysis (pubis) in pregnancy
    O26.711 Subluxation of symphysis (pubis) in pregnancy, first trimester ♀   M
    O26.712 Subluxation of symphysis (pubis) in pregnancy, second trimester ♀   M
    O26.713 Subluxation of symphysis (pubis) in pregnancy, third trimester ♀   M
    O26.719 Subluxation of symphysis (pubis) in pregnancy, unspecified trimester ♀ M
    O26.72 Subluxation of symphysis (pubis) in childbirth ♀   M
    O26.73 Subluxation of symphysis (pubis) in the puerperium ♀   M

● O26.8 Other specified pregnancy related conditions
  ● O26.81 Pregnancy related exhaustion and fatigue
    O26.811 Pregnancy related exhaustion and fatigue, first trimester ♀   M
    O26.812 Pregnancy related exhaustion and fatigue, second trimester ♀   M
    O26.813 Pregnancy related exhaustion and fatigue, third trimester ♀   M
    O26.819 Pregnancy related exhaustion and fatigue, unspecified trimester ♀ M

  ● O26.82 Pregnancy related peripheral neuritis
    O26.821 Pregnancy related peripheral neuritis, first trimester ♀   M
    O26.822 Pregnancy related peripheral neuritis, second trimester ♀   M
    O26.823 Pregnancy related peripheral neuritis, third trimester ♀   M
    O26.829 Pregnancy related peripheral neuritis, unspecified trimester ♀ M

● O26.83 Pregnancy related renal disease
    Use additional code to identify the specific disorder
    O26.831 Pregnancy related renal disease, first trimester ♀   M
    O26.832 Pregnancy related renal disease, second trimester ♀   M
    O26.833 Pregnancy related renal disease, third trimester ♀   M
    O26.839 Pregnancy related renal disease, unspecified trimester ♀ M

● O26.84 Uterine size-date discrepancy complicating pregnancy
    Excludes1 encounter for suspected problem with fetal growth ruled out (Z03.74)
    O26.841 Uterine size-date discrepancy, first trimester ♀   M
    O26.842 Uterine size-date discrepancy, second trimester ♀   M
    O26.843 Uterine size-date discrepancy, third trimester ♀   M
    O26.849 Uterine size-date discrepancy, unspecified trimester ♀ M

● O26.85 Spotting complicating pregnancy
    O26.851 Spotting complicating pregnancy, first trimester ♀   M
    O26.852 Spotting complicating pregnancy, second trimester ♀   M
    O26.853 Spotting complicating pregnancy, third trimester ♀   M
    O26.859 Spotting complicating pregnancy, unspecified trimester ♀ M

    O26.86 Pruritic urticarial papules and plaques of pregnancy (PUPPP) ♀   M
    Polymorphic eruption of pregnancy

● O26.87 Cervical shortening
    Excludes1 encounter for suspected cervical shortening ruled out (Z03.75)
    O26.872 Cervical shortening, second trimester ♀   M
    O26.873 Cervical shortening, third trimester ♀   M
    O26.879 Cervical shortening, unspecified trimester ♀ M

● O26.89 Other specified pregnancy related conditions
    O26.891 Other specified pregnancy related conditions, first trimester ♀   M
    O26.892 Other specified pregnancy related conditions, second trimester ♀   M
    O26.893 Other specified pregnancy related conditions, third trimester ♀   M
    Coding Clinic: 2015, Q3, P40
    O26.899 Other specified pregnancy related conditions, unspecified trimester ♀ M

● O26.9 Pregnancy related conditions, unspecified
    O26.90 Pregnancy related conditions, unspecified, unspecified trimester ♀   M
    O26.91 Pregnancy related conditions, unspecified, first trimester ♀   M
    O26.92 Pregnancy related conditions, unspecified, second trimester ♀   M
    O26.93 Pregnancy related conditions, unspecified, third trimester ♀   M

CHAPTER 15 (O00-O9A)

● **O28**   **Abnormal findings on antenatal screening of mother**
> **Excludes1**   diagnostic findings classified elsewhere - see Alphabetical Index

O28.0   Abnormal hematological finding on antenatal screening of mother ♀   M

O28.1   Abnormal biochemical finding on antenatal screening of mother ♀   M

O28.2   Abnormal cytological finding on antenatal screening of mother ♀   M

O28.3   Abnormal ultrasonic finding on antenatal screening of mother ♀   M
> Coding Clinic: 2016, Q4, P5

O28.4   Abnormal radiological finding on antenatal screening of mother ♀   M

O28.5   Abnormal chromosomal and genetic finding on antenatal screening of mother ♀   M

O28.8   Other abnormal findings on antenatal screening of mother ♀   M

O28.9   Unspecified abnormal findings on antenatal screening of mother ♀   M

● **O29**   **Complications of anesthesia during pregnancy**
> **Includes**   maternal complications arising from the administration of a general, regional or local anesthetic, analgesic or other sedation during pregnancy
> Use additional code, if necessary, to identify the complication
> **Excludes2**   complications of anesthesia during labor and delivery (O74.-)
> complications of anesthesia during the puerperium (O89.-)

● **O29.0**   **Pulmonary complications of anesthesia during pregnancy**

   ● **O29.01**   **Aspiration pneumonitis due to anesthesia during pregnancy**
> Inhalation of stomach contents or secretions NOS due to anesthesia during pregnancy
> Mendelson's syndrome due to anesthesia during pregnancy

     O29.011   Aspiration pneumonitis due to anesthesia during pregnancy, first trimester ♀   M

     O29.012   Aspiration pneumonitis due to anesthesia during pregnancy, second trimester ♀   M

     O29.013   Aspiration pneumonitis due to anesthesia during pregnancy, third trimester ♀   M

     O29.019   Aspiration pneumonitis due to anesthesia during pregnancy, unspecified trimester ♀   M

   ● **O29.02**   **Pressure collapse of lung due to anesthesia during pregnancy**

     O29.021   Pressure collapse of lung due to anesthesia during pregnancy, first trimester ♀   M

     O29.022   Pressure collapse of lung due to anesthesia during pregnancy, second trimester ♀   M

     O29.023   Pressure collapse of lung due to anesthesia during pregnancy, third trimester ♀   M

     O29.029   Pressure collapse of lung due to anesthesia during pregnancy, unspecified trimester ♀   M

   ● **O29.09**   **Other pulmonary complications of anesthesia during pregnancy**

     O29.091   Other pulmonary complications of anesthesia during pregnancy, first trimester ♀   M

     O29.092   Other pulmonary complications of anesthesia during pregnancy, second trimester ♀   M

     O29.093   Other pulmonary complications of anesthesia during pregnancy, third trimester ♀   M

     O29.099   Other pulmonary complications of anesthesia during pregnancy, unspecified trimester ♀   M

● **O29.1**   **Cardiac complications of anesthesia during pregnancy**

   ● **O29.11**   **Cardiac arrest due to anesthesia during pregnancy**

     O29.111   Cardiac arrest due to anesthesia during pregnancy, first trimester ♀   M

     O29.112   Cardiac arrest due to anesthesia during pregnancy, second trimester ♀   M

     O29.113   Cardiac arrest due to anesthesia during pregnancy, third trimester ♀   M

     O29.119   Cardiac arrest due to anesthesia during pregnancy, unspecified trimester ♀   M

   ● **O29.12**   **Cardiac failure due to anesthesia during pregnancy**

     O29.121   Cardiac failure due to anesthesia during pregnancy, first trimester ♀   M

     O29.122   Cardiac failure due to anesthesia during pregnancy, second trimester ♀   M

     O29.123   Cardiac failure due to anesthesia during pregnancy, third trimester ♀   M

     O29.129   Cardiac failure due to anesthesia during pregnancy, unspecified trimester ♀   M

   ● **O29.19**   **Other cardiac complications of anesthesia during pregnancy**

     O29.191   Other cardiac complications of anesthesia during pregnancy, first trimester ♀   M

     O29.192   Other cardiac complications of anesthesia during pregnancy, second trimester ♀   M

     O29.193   Other cardiac complications of anesthesia during pregnancy, third trimester ♀   M

     O29.199   Other cardiac complications of anesthesia during pregnancy, unspecified trimester ♀   M

● **O29.2**   **Central nervous system complications of anesthesia during pregnancy**

   ● **O29.21**   **Cerebral anoxia due to anesthesia during pregnancy**

     O29.211   Cerebral anoxia due to anesthesia during pregnancy, first trimester ♀   M

     O29.212   Cerebral anoxia due to anesthesia during pregnancy, second trimester ♀   M

     O29.213   Cerebral anoxia due to anesthesia during pregnancy, third trimester ♀   M

     O29.219   Cerebral anoxia due to anesthesia during pregnancy, unspecified trimester ♀   M

   ● **O29.29**   **Other central nervous system complications of anesthesia during pregnancy**

     O29.291   Other central nervous system complications of anesthesia during pregnancy, first trimester ♀   M

     O29.292   Other central nervous system complications of anesthesia during pregnancy, second trimester ♀   M

O29.293 Other central nervous system complications of anesthesia during pregnancy, third trimester ♀ M

O29.299 Other central nervous system complications of anesthesia during pregnancy, unspecified trimester ♀ M

● O29.3 Toxic reaction to local anesthesia during pregnancy

● O29.3X Toxic reaction to local anesthesia during pregnancy

O29.3X1 Toxic reaction to local anesthesia during pregnancy, first trimester ♀ M

O29.3X2 Toxic reaction to local anesthesia during pregnancy, second trimester ♀ M

O29.3X3 Toxic reaction to local anesthesia during pregnancy, third trimester ♀ M

O29.3X9 Toxic reaction to local anesthesia during pregnancy, unspecified trimester ♀ M

● O29.4 Spinal and epidural anesthesia induced headache during pregnancy

O29.40 Spinal and epidural anesthesia induced headache during pregnancy, unspecified trimester ♀ M

O29.41 Spinal and epidural anesthesia induced headache during pregnancy, first trimester ♀ M

O29.42 Spinal and epidural anesthesia induced headache during pregnancy, second trimester ♀ M

O29.43 Spinal and epidural anesthesia induced headache during pregnancy, third trimester ♀ M

● O29.5 Other complications of spinal and epidural anesthesia during pregnancy

● O29.5X Other complications of spinal and epidural anesthesia during pregnancy

O29.5X1 Other complications of spinal and epidural anesthesia during pregnancy, first trimester ♀ M

O29.5X2 Other complications of spinal and epidural anesthesia during pregnancy, second trimester ♀ M

O29.5X3 Other complications of spinal and epidural anesthesia during pregnancy, third trimester ♀ M

O29.5X9 Other complications of spinal and epidural anesthesia during pregnancy, unspecified trimester ♀ M

● O29.6 Failed or difficult intubation for anesthesia during pregnancy

O29.60 Failed or difficult intubation for anesthesia during pregnancy, unspecified trimester ♀ M

O29.61 Failed or difficult intubation for anesthesia during pregnancy, first trimester ♀ M

O29.62 Failed or difficult intubation for anesthesia during pregnancy, second trimester ♀ M

O29.63 Failed or difficult intubation for anesthesia during pregnancy, third trimester ♀ M

● O29.8 Other complications of anesthesia during pregnancy

● O29.8X Other complications of anesthesia during pregnancy

O29.8X1 Other complications of anesthesia during pregnancy, first trimester ♀ M

O29.8X2 Other complications of anesthesia during pregnancy, second trimester ♀ M

O29.8X3 Other complications of anesthesia during pregnancy, third trimester ♀ M

O29.8X9 Other complications of anesthesia during pregnancy, unspecified trimester ♀ M

● O29.9 Unspecified complication of anesthesia during pregnancy

O29.90 Unspecified complication of anesthesia during pregnancy, unspecified trimester ♀ M

O29.91 Unspecified complication of anesthesia during pregnancy, first trimester ♀ M

O29.92 Unspecified complication of anesthesia during pregnancy, second trimester ♀ M

O29.93 Unspecified complication of anesthesia during pregnancy, third trimester ♀ M

MATERNAL CARE RELATED TO THE FETUS AND AMNIOTIC CAVITY AND POSSIBLE DELIVERY PROBLEMS (O30-O48)

● O30 Multiple gestation

Code also any complications specific to multiple gestation

Coding Clinic: 2016, Q4, P51

● O30.0 Twin pregnancy

● O30.00 Twin pregnancy, unspecified number of placenta and unspecified number of amniotic sacs

O30.001 Twin pregnancy, unspecified number of placenta and unspecified number of amniotic sacs, first trimester ♀ M

O30.002 Twin pregnancy, unspecified number of placenta and unspecified number of amniotic sacs, second trimester ♀ M

O30.003 Twin pregnancy, unspecified number of placenta and unspecified number of amniotic sacs, third trimester ♀ M

O30.009 Twin pregnancy, unspecified number of placenta and unspecified number of amniotic sacs, unspecified trimester ♀ M

● O30.01 Twin pregnancy, monochorionic/monoamniotic
Twin pregnancy, one placenta, one amniotic sac

Excludes1 conjoined twins (O30.02-)

O30.011 Twin pregnancy, monochorionic/monoamniotic, first trimester ♀ M

O30.012 Twin pregnancy, monochorionic/monoamniotic, second trimester ♀ M

O30.013 Twin pregnancy, monochorionic/monoamniotic, third trimester ♀ M

O30.019 Twin pregnancy, monochorionic/monoamniotic, unspecified trimester ♀ M

● O30.02 Conjoined twin pregnancy

O30.021 Conjoined twin pregnancy, first trimester ♀ M

O30.022 Conjoined twin pregnancy, second trimester ♀ M

O30.023 Conjoined twin pregnancy, third trimester ♀ M

O30.029 Conjoined twin pregnancy, unspecified trimester ♀ M

● O30.03 Twin pregnancy, monochorionic/diamniotic
Twin pregnancy, one placenta, two amniotic sacs

O30.031 Twin pregnancy, monochorionic/diamniotic, first trimester ♀ M

O30.032 Twin pregnancy, monochorionic/diamniotic, second trimester ♀ M

O30.033   Twin pregnancy, monochorionic/
            diamniotic, third trimester ♀   M

O30.039   Twin pregnancy, monochorionic/
            diamniotic, unspecified trimester ♀ M

● O30.04   **Twin pregnancy, dichorionic/diamniotic**
            Twin pregnancy, two placentae, two amniotic
            sacs

O30.041   Twin pregnancy, dichorionic/
            diamniotic, first trimester ♀   M

O30.042   Twin pregnancy, dichorionic/
            diamniotic, second trimester ♀   M

O30.043   Twin pregnancy, dichorionic/
            diamniotic, third trimester ♀   M

O30.049   Twin pregnancy, dichorionic/
            diamniotic, unspecified trimester ♀ M

● O30.09   **Twin pregnancy, unable to determine number
            of placenta and number of amniotic sacs**

O30.091   Twin pregnancy, unable to determine
            number of placenta and number of
            amniotic sacs, first trimester ♀   M

O30.092   Twin pregnancy, unable to determine
            number of placenta and number of
            amniotic sacs, second trimester ♀ M

O30.093   Twin pregnancy, unable to determine
            number of placenta and number of
            amniotic sacs, third trimester ♀   M

O30.099   Twin pregnancy, unable to determine
            number of placenta and number
            of amniotic sacs, unspecified
            trimester ♀   M

● O30.1   **Triplet pregnancy**

● O30.10   **Triplet pregnancy, unspecified number of
            placenta and unspecified number of amniotic
            sacs**

O30.101   Triplet pregnancy, unspecified
            number of placenta and unspecified
            number of amniotic sacs, first
            trimester ♀   M

O30.102   Triplet pregnancy, unspecified
            number of placenta and unspecified
            number of amniotic sacs, second
            trimester ♀   M

O30.103   Triplet pregnancy, unspecified
            number of placenta and unspecified
            number of amniotic sacs, third
            trimester ♀   M
            Coding Clinic: 2016, Q2, P8

O30.109   Triplet pregnancy, unspecified
            number of placenta and unspecified
            number of amniotic sacs, unspecified
            trimester ♀   M

● O30.11   **Triplet pregnancy with two or more
            monochorionic fetuses**

O30.111   Triplet pregnancy with two or
            more monochorionic fetuses, first
            trimester ♀   M

O30.112   Triplet pregnancy with two or more
            monochorionic fetuses, second
            trimester ♀   M

O30.113   Triplet pregnancy with two or
            more monochorionic fetuses, third
            trimester ♀   M

O30.119   Triplet pregnancy with two or more
            monochorionic fetuses, unspecified
            trimester ♀   M

● O30.12   **Triplet pregnancy with two or more
            monoamniotic fetuses**

O30.121   Triplet pregnancy with two or
            more monoamniotic fetuses, first
            trimester ♀   M

O30.122   Triplet pregnancy with two or more
            monoamniotic fetuses, second
            trimester ♀   M

O30.123   Triplet pregnancy with two or
            more monoamniotic fetuses, third
            trimester ♀   M

O30.129   Triplet pregnancy with two or more
            monoamniotic fetuses, unspecified
            trimester ♀   M

● O30.13   **Triplet pregnancy, trichorionic/triamniotic**

O30.131   Triplet pregnancy, trichorionic/
            triamniotic, first trimester ♀   M

O30.132   Triplet pregnancy, trichorionic/
            triamniotic, second trimester ♀   M

O30.133   Triplet pregnancy, trichorionic/
            triamniotic, third trimester ♀   M

O30.139   Triplet pregnancy, trichorionic/
            triamniotic, unspecified trimester ♀ M

● O30.19   **Triplet pregnancy, unable to determine number
            of placenta and number of amniotic sacs**

O30.191   Triplet pregnancy, unable to
            determine number of placenta
            and number of amniotic sacs, first
            trimester ♀   M

O30.192   Triplet pregnancy, unable to
            determine number of placenta and
            number of amniotic sacs, second
            trimester ♀   M

O30.193   Triplet pregnancy, unable to
            determine number of placenta and
            number of amniotic sacs, third
            trimester ♀   M

O30.199   Triplet pregnancy, unable to
            determine number of placenta and
            number of amniotic sacs, unspecified
            trimester ♀   M

● O30.2   **Quadruplet pregnancy**

● O30.20   **Quadruplet pregnancy, unspecified number of
            placenta and unspecified number of amniotic
            sacs**

O30.201   Quadruplet pregnancy, unspecified
            number of placenta and unspecified
            number of amniotic sacs, first
            trimester ♀   M

O30.202   Quadruplet pregnancy, unspecified
            number of placenta and unspecified
            number of amniotic sacs, second
            trimester ♀   M

O30.203   Quadruplet pregnancy, unspecified
            number of placenta and unspecified
            number of amniotic sacs, third
            trimester ♀   M

O30.209   Quadruplet pregnancy, unspecified
            number of placenta and unspecified
            number of amniotic sacs, unspecified
            trimester ♀   M

● O30.21   **Quadruplet pregnancy with two or more
            monochorionic fetuses**

O30.211   Quadruplet pregnancy with two or
            more monochorionic fetuses, first
            trimester ♀   M

O30.212   Quadruplet pregnancy with two or
            more monochorionic fetuses, second
            trimester ♀   M

O30.213   Quadruplet pregnancy with two or
            more monochorionic fetuses, third
            trimester ♀   M

O30.219   Quadruplet pregnancy with two
            or more monochorionic fetuses,
            unspecified trimester ♀   M

▶ New   ⇒ Revised   ~~deleted~~ Deleted   Excludes 1   Excludes 2   Includes   Use additional   Code first   Code also   Key words

OGCR Official Guidelines   X Assign placeholder X   ● Use Additional Character(s)   ▶ Manifestation Code   🔖 Hierarchical Condition Category   **Coding Clinic**

● **O30.22** Quadruplet pregnancy with two or more monoamniotic fetuses

  O30.221 Quadruplet pregnancy with two or more monoamniotic fetuses, first trimester ♀   M

  O30.222 Quadruplet pregnancy with two or more monoamniotic fetuses, second trimester ♀   M

  O30.223 Quadruplet pregnancy with two or more monoamniotic fetuses, third trimester ♀   M

  O30.229 Quadruplet pregnancy with two or more monoamniotic fetuses, unspecified trimester ♀   M

● **O30.23** Quadruplet pregnancy, quadrachorionic/quadra-amniotic

  O30.231 Quadruplet pregnancy, quadrachorionic/quadra-amniotic, first trimester ♀   M

  O30.232 Quadruplet pregnancy, quadrachorionic/quadra-amniotic, second trimester ♀   M

  O30.233 Quadruplet pregnancy, quadrachorionic/quadra-amniotic, third trimester ♀   M

  O30.239 Quadruplet pregnancy, quadrachorionic/quadra-amniotic, unspecifiedtrimester ♀   M

● **O30.29** Quadruplet pregnancy, unable to determine number of placenta and number of amniotic sacs

  O30.291 Quadruplet pregnancy, unable to determine number of placenta and number of amniotic sacs, first trimester ♀   M

  O30.292 Quadruplet pregnancy, unable to determine number of placenta and number of amniotic sacs, second trimester ♀   M

  O30.293 Quadruplet pregnancy, unable to determine number of placenta and number of amniotic sacs, third trimester ♀   M

  O30.299 Quadruplet pregnancy, unable to determine number of placenta and number of amniotic sacs, unspecified trimester ♀   M

● **O30.8** Other specified multiple gestation
  Multiple gestation pregnancy greater then quadruplets

● **O30.80** Other specified multiple gestation, unspecified number of placenta and unspecified number of amniotic sacs

  O30.801 Other specified multiple gestation, unspecified number of placenta and unspecified number of amniotic sacs, first trimester ♀   M

  O30.802 Other specified multiple gestation, unspecified number of placenta and unspecified number of amniotic sacs, second trimester ♀   M

  O30.803 Other specified multiple gestation, unspecified number of placenta and unspecified number of amniotic sacs, third trimester ♀   M

  O30.809 Other specified multiple gestation, unspecified number of placenta and unspecified number of amniotic sacs, unspecified trimester ♀   M

● **O30.81** Other specified multiple gestation with two or more monochorionic fetuses

  O30.811 Other specified multiple gestation with two or more monochorionic fetuses, first trimester ♀   M

  O30.812 Other specified multiple gestation with two or more monochorionic fetuses, second trimester ♀   M

  O30.813 Other specified multiple gestation with two or more monochorionic fetuses, third trimester ♀   M

  O30.819 Other specified multiple gestation with two or more monochorionic fetuses, unspecified trimester ♀   M

● **O30.82** Other specified multiple gestation with two or more monoamniotic fetuses

  O30.821 Other specified multiple gestation with two or more monoamniotic fetuses, first trimester ♀   M

  O30.822 Other specified multiple gestation with two or more monoamniotic fetuses, second trimester ♀   M

  O30.823 Other specified multiple gestation with two or more monoamniotic fetuses, third trimester ♀   M

  O30.829 Other specified multiple gestation with two or more monoamniotic fetuses, unspecified trimester ♀   M

● **O30.83** Other specified multiple gestation, number of chorions and amnions are both equalto the number of fetuses
  Pentachorionic, penta-amniotic pregnancy (quintuplets)
  Hexachorionic, hexa-amniotic pregnancy (sextuplets)
  Heptachorionic, hepta-amniotic pregnancy (septuplets)

  O30.831 Other specified multiple gestation, number of chorions and amnions are both equal to the number of fetuses, first trimester ♀   M

  O30.832 Other specified multiple gestation, number of chorions and amnions are both equal to the number of fetuses, second trimester ♀   M

  O30.833 Other specified multiple gestation, number of chorions and amnions are both equal to the number of fetuses, third trimester ♀   M

  O30.839 Other specified multiple gestation, number of chorions and amnions are both equal to the number of fetuses, unspecified trimester ♀   M

● **O30.89** Other specified multiple gestation, unable to determine number of placenta and number of amniotic sacs

  O30.891 Other specified multiple gestation, unable to determine number of placenta and number of amniotic sacs, first trimester ♀   M

  O30.892 Other specified multiple gestation, unable to determine number of placenta and number of amniotic sacs, second trimester ♀   M

  O30.893 Other specified multiple gestation, unable to determine number of placenta and number of amniotic sacs, third trimester ♀   M

  O30.899 Other specified multiple gestation, unable to determine number of placenta and number of amniotic sacs, unspecified trimester ♀   M

CHAPTER 15 (O00-O9A)

● **O30.9 Multiple gestation, unspecified**
Multiple pregnancy NOS

    O30.90 Multiple gestation, unspecified, unspecified trimester ♀   M

    O30.91 Multiple gestation, unspecified, first trimester ♀   M

    O30.92 Multiple gestation, unspecified, second trimester ♀   M

    O30.93 Multiple gestation, unspecified, third trimester ♀   M

● **O31 Complications specific to multiple gestation**

  Excludes2 delayed delivery of second twin, triplet, etc. (O63.2)
       malpresentation of one fetus or more (O32.9)
       placental transfusion syndromes (O43.0-)

Coding Clinic: 2012, Q4, P107

One of the following 7th characters is to be assigned to each code under category O31. 7th character 0 is for single gestations and multiple gestations where the fetus is unspecified. 7th characters 1 through 9 are for cases of multiple gestations to identify the fetus for which the code applies. The appropriate code from category O30, Multiple gestation, must also be assigned when assigning a code from category O31 that has a 7th character of 1 through 9.

0	not applicable or unspecified
1	fetus 1
2	fetus 2
3	fetus 3
4	fetus 4
5	fetus 5
9	other fetus

● **O31.0 Papyraceous fetus**
Fetus compressus

  X● **O31.00 Papyraceous fetus, unspecified trimester** ♀   M
  X● **O31.01 Papyraceous fetus, first trimester** ♀   M
  X● **O31.02 Papyraceous fetus, second trimester** ♀   M
  X● **O31.03 Papyraceous fetus, third trimester** ♀   M

● **O31.1 Continuing pregnancy after spontaneous abortion of one fetus or more**

  X● **O31.10 Continuing pregnancy after spontaneous abortion of one fetus or more, unspecified trimester** ♀   M
  X● **O31.11 Continuing pregnancy after spontaneous abortion of one fetus or more, first trimester** ♀ M
  X● **O31.12 Continuing pregnancy after spontaneous abortion of one fetus or more, second trimester** ♀   M
  X● **O31.13 Continuing pregnancy after spontaneous abortion of one fetus or more, third trimester** ♀   M

● **O31.2 Continuing pregnancy after intrauterine death of one fetus or more**

  X● **O31.20 Continuing pregnancy after intrauterine death of one fetus or more, unspecified trimester** ♀ M
  X● **O31.21 Continuing pregnancy after intrauterine death of one fetus or more, first trimester** ♀   M
  X● **O31.22 Continuing pregnancy after intrauterine death of one fetus or more, second trimester** ♀
  X● **O31.23 Continuing pregnancy after intrauterine death of one fetus or more, third trimester** ♀   M

● **O31.3 Continuing pregnancy after elective fetal reduction of one fetus or more**
Continuing pregnancy after selective termination of one fetus or more

  X● **O31.30 Continuing pregnancy after elective fetal reduction of one fetus or more, unspecified trimester** ♀   M

  X● **O31.31 Continuing pregnancy after elective fetal reduction of one fetus or more, first trimester** ♀   M
  X● **O31.32 Continuing pregnancy after elective fetal reduction of one fetus or more, second trimester** ♀   M
  X● **O31.33 Continuing pregnancy after elective fetal reduction of one fetus or more, third trimester** ♀   M

● **O31.8 Other complications specific to multiple gestation**
  ● **O31.8X Other complications specific to multiple gestation**
    ● **O31.8X1 Other complications specific to multiple gestation, first trimester** ♀ M
    ● **O31.8X2 Other complications specific to multiple gestation, second trimester** ♀   M
    ● **O31.8X3 Other complications specific to multiple gestation, third trimester** ♀ M
    ● **O31.8X9 Other complications specific to multiple gestation, unspecified trimester** ♀   M

● **O32 Maternal care for malpresentation of fetus**

  Includes the listed conditions as a reason for observation, hospitalization or other obstetric care of the mother, or for cesarean delivery before onset of labor

  Excludes1 malpresentation of fetus with obstructed labor (O64.-)

Coding Clinic: 2012, Q4, P107

One of the following 7th characters is to be assigned to each code under category O32. 7th character 0 is for single gestations and multiple gestations where the fetus is unspecified. 7th characters 1 through 9 are for cases of multiple gestations to identify the fetus for which the code applies. The appropriate code from category O30, Multiple gestation, must also be assigned when assigning a code from category O32 that has a 7th character of 1 through 9.

0	not applicable or unspecified
1	fetus 1
2	fetus 2
3	fetus 3
4	fetus 4
5	fetus 5
9	other fetus

X● **O32.0 Maternal care for unstable lie** ♀   M
X● **O32.1 Maternal care for breech presentation** ♀   M
  Maternal care for buttocks presentation
  Maternal care for complete breech
  Maternal care for frank breech
  Excludes1 footling presentation (O32.8)
       incomplete breech (O32.8)
X● **O32.2 Maternal care for transverse and oblique lie** ♀   M
  Maternal care for oblique presentation
  Maternal care for transverse presentation
X● **O32.3 Maternal care for face, brow and chin presentation** ♀   M
X● **O32.4 Maternal care for high head at term** ♀   M
  Maternal care for failure of head to enter pelvic brim
X● **O32.6 Maternal care for compound presentation** ♀   M
X● **O32.8 Maternal care for other malpresentation of fetus** ♀   M
  Maternal care for footling presentation
  Maternal care for incomplete breech
X● **O32.9 Maternal care for malpresentation of fetus, unspecified** ♀   M

CHAPTER 15 (O00-O9A)

▶ New   ⇒ Revised   ~~deleted~~ Deleted   Excludes 1   Excludes 2   Includes   Use additional   Code first   Code also   Key words
OGCR Official Guidelines   X Assign placeholder X   ● Use Additional Character(s)   ▶ Manifestation Code   🗞 Hierarchical Condition Category   Coding Clinic

● **O33**   **Maternal care for disproportion**

> **Includes**   the listed conditions as a reason for observation, hospitalization or other obstetric care of the mother, or for cesarean delivery before onset of labor

> **Excludes1**   disproportion with obstructed labor (O65-O66)

O33.0   **Maternal care for disproportion due to deformity of maternal pelvic bones** ♀   M

> Maternal care for disproportion due to pelvic deformity causing disproportion NOS

O33.1   **Maternal care for disproportion due to generally contracted pelvis** ♀   M

> Maternal care for disproportion due to contracted pelvis NOS causing disproportion

O33.2   **Maternal care for disproportion due to inlet contraction of pelvis** ♀   M

> Maternal care for disproportion due to inlet contraction (pelvis) causing disproportion

X ● **O33.3**   **Maternal care for disproportion due to outlet contraction of pelvis** ♀   M

> Maternal care for disproportion due to mid-cavity contraction (pelvis)
>
> Maternal care for disproportion due to outlet contraction (pelvis)
>
> One of the following 7th characters is to be assigned to code O33.3. 7th character 0 is for single gestations and multiple gestations where the fetus is unspecified. 7th characters 1 through 9 are for cases of multiple gestations to identify the fetus for which the code applies. The appropriate code from category O30, Multiple gestation, must also be assigned when assigning code O33.3 with a 7th character of 1 through 9.

> | 0 | not applicable or unspecified |
> |---|---|
> | 1 | fetus 1 |
> | 2 | fetus 2 |
> | 3 | fetus 3 |
> | 4 | fetus 4 |
> | 5 | fetus 5 |
> | 9 | other fetus |

X ● **O33.4**   **Maternal care for disproportion of mixed maternal and fetal origin** ♀   M

> One of the following 7th characters is to be assigned to code O33.4. 7th character 0 is for single gestations and multiple gestations where the fetus is unspecified. 7th characters 1 through 9 are for cases of multiple gestations to identify the fetus for which the code applies. The appropriate code from category O30, Multiple gestation, must also be assigned when assigning code O33.4 with a 7th character of 1 through 9.

> | 0 | not applicable or unspecified |
> |---|---|
> | 1 | fetus 1 |
> | 2 | fetus 2 |
> | 3 | fetus 3 |
> | 4 | fetus 4 |
> | 5 | fetus 5 |
> | 9 | other fetus |

X ● **O33.5**   **Maternal care for disproportion due to unusually large fetus** ♀   M

> Maternal care for disproportion due to disproportion of fetal origin with normally formed fetus
>
> Maternal care for disproportion due to fetal disproportion NOS
>
> One of the following 7th characters is to be assigned to code O33.5. 7th character 0 is for single gestations and multiple gestations where the fetus is unspecified. 7th characters 1 through 9 are for cases of multiple gestations to identify the fetus for which the code applies. The appropriate code from category O30, Multiple gestation, must also be assigned when assigning code O33.5 with a 7th character of 1 through 9.

> | 0 | not applicable or unspecified |
> |---|---|
> | 1 | fetus 1 |
> | 2 | fetus 2 |
> | 3 | fetus 3 |
> | 4 | fetus 4 |
> | 5 | fetus 5 |
> | 9 | other fetus |

X ● **O33.6**   **Maternal care for disproportion due to hydrocephalic fetus** ♀   M

> One of the following 7th characters is to be assigned to code O33.6. 7th character 0 is for single gestations and multiple gestations where the fetus is unspecified. 7th characters 1 through 9 are for cases of multiple gestations to identify the fetus for which the code applies. The appropriate code from category O30, Multiple gestation, must also be assigned when assigning code O33.6 with a 7th character of 1 through 9.

> | 0 | not applicable or unspecified |
> |---|---|
> | 1 | fetus 1 |
> | 2 | fetus 2 |
> | 3 | fetus 3 |
> | 4 | fetus 4 |
> | 5 | fetus 5 |
> | 9 | other fetus |

X ● **O33.7**   **Maternal care for disproportion due to other fetal deformities** ♀   M

> Maternal care for disproportion due to fetal ascites
>
> Maternal care for disproportion due to fetal hydrops
>
> Maternal care for disproportion due to fetal meningomyelocele
>
> Maternal care for disproportion due to fetal sacral teratoma
>
> Maternal care for disproportion due to fetal tumor

> **Excludes1**   obstructed labor due to other fetal deformities (O66.3)

> **Coding Clinic: 2016, Q4, P51**

> One of the following 7th characters is to be assigned to code O33.7. 7th character 0 is for single gestations and multiple gestations where the fetus is unspecified. 7th characters 1 through 9 are for cases of multiple gestations to identify the fetus for which the code applies. The appropriate code from category O30, Multiple gestation, must also be assigned when assigning code O33.7 with a 7th character of 1 through 9.

> | 0 | not applicable or unspecified |
> |---|---|
> | 1 | fetus 1 |
> | 2 | fetus 2 |
> | 3 | fetus 3 |
> | 4 | fetus 4 |
> | 5 | fetus 5 |
> | 9 | other fetus |

CHAPTER 15 (O00-O9A)

O33.8　Maternal care for disproportion of other origin ♀　M

O33.9　Maternal care for disproportion, unspecified ♀　M
　　　Maternal care for disproportion due to cephalopelvic disproportion NOS
　　　Maternal care for disproportion due to fetopelvic disproportion NOS

● O34　Maternal care for abnormality of pelvic organs

　　Includes　the listed conditions as a reason for hospitalization or other obstetric care of the mother, or for cesarean delivery before onset of labor

　Code first any associated obstructed labor (O65.5)
　Use additional code for specific condition

　● O34.0　Maternal care for congenital malformation of uterus
　　　Maternal care for double uterus
　　　Maternal care for uterus bicornis

　　　O34.00　Maternal care for unspecified congenital malformation of uterus, unspecified trimester ♀　M

　　　O34.01　Maternal care for unspecified congenital malformation of uterus, first trimester ♀　M

　　　O34.02　Maternal care for unspecified congenital malformation of uterus, second trimester ♀　M

　　　O34.03　Maternal care for unspecified congenital malformation of uterus, third trimester ♀　M

　● O34.1　Maternal care for benign tumor of corpus uteri

　　　Excludes2　maternal care for benign tumor of cervix (O34.4-)
　　　　　maternal care for malignant neoplasm of uterus (O9A.1-)

　　　O34.10　Maternal care for benign tumor of corpus uteri, unspecified trimester ♀　M

　　　O34.11　Maternal care for benign tumor of corpus uteri, first trimester ♀　M

　　　O34.12　Maternal care for benign tumor of corpus uteri, second trimester ♀　M

　　　O34.13　Maternal care for benign tumor of corpus uteri, third trimester ♀　M

　● O34.2　Maternal care due to uterine scar from previous surgery
　　　Coding Clinic: 2016, Q4, P76

　　　● O34.21　Maternal care for scar from previous cesarean delivery
　　　　　Coding Clinic: 2016, Q4, P51

　　　　　O34.211　Maternal care for low transverse scar from previous cesarean delivery ♀　M

　　　　　O34.212　Maternal care for vertical scar from previous cesarean delivery ♀　M
　　　　　　Maternal care for classical scar from previous cesarean delivery

　　　　　O34.218　Maternal care for other type scar from previous cesarean delivery ♀　M
　　　　　　Mid-transverse T incision

　　　　　O34.219　Maternal care for unspecified type scar from previous cesarean delivery ♀　M

　　　O34.22　Maternal care for cesarean scar defect (isthmocele) ♀　M

　　　O34.29　Maternal care due to uterine scar from other previous surgery ♀　M
　　　　　Maternal care due to uterine scar from other transmural uterine incision

　● O34.3　Maternal care for cervical incompetence
　　　Maternal care for cerclage with or without cervical incompetence
　　　Maternal care for Shirodkar suture with or without cervical incompetence

　　　O34.30　Maternal care for cervical incompetence, unspecified trimester ♀　M

　　　O34.31　Maternal care for cervical incompetence, first trimester ♀　M

　　　O34.32　Maternal care for cervical incompetence, second trimester ♀　M

　　　O34.33　Maternal care for cervical incompetence, third trimester ♀　M

　● O34.4　Maternal care for other abnormalities of cervix

　　　O34.40　Maternal care for other abnormalities of cervix, unspecified trimester ♀　M

　　　O34.41　Maternal care for other abnormalities of cervix, first trimester ♀　M

　　　O34.42　Maternal care for other abnormalities of cervix, second trimester ♀　M

　　　O34.43　Maternal care for other abnormalities of cervix, third trimester ♀　M

　● O34.5　Maternal care for other abnormalities of gravid uterus

　　　● O34.51　Maternal care for incarceration of gravid uterus

　　　　　O34.511　Maternal care for incarceration of gravid uterus, first trimester ♀　M

　　　　　O34.512　Maternal care for incarceration of gravid uterus, second trimester ♀　M

　　　　　O34.513　Maternal care for incarceration of gravid uterus, third trimester ♀　M

　　　　　O34.519　Maternal care for incarceration of gravid uterus, unspecified trimester ♀　M

　　　● O34.52　Maternal care for prolapse of gravid uterus

　　　　　O34.521　Maternal care for prolapse of gravid uterus, first trimester ♀　M

　　　　　O34.522　Maternal care for prolapse of gravid uterus, second trimester ♀　M

　　　　　O34.523　Maternal care for prolapse of gravid uterus, third trimester ♀　M

　　　　　O34.529　Maternal care for prolapse of gravid uterus, unspecified trimester ♀　M

　　　● O34.53　Maternal care for retroversion of gravid uterus

　　　　　O34.531　Maternal care for retroversion of gravid uterus, first trimester ♀　M

　　　　　O34.532　Maternal care for retroversion of gravid uterus, second trimester ♀　M

　　　　　O34.533　Maternal care for retroversion of gravid uterus, third trimester ♀　M

　　　　　O34.539　Maternal care for retroversion of gravid uterus, unspecified trimester ♀　M

　　　● O34.59　Maternal care for other abnormalities of gravid uterus

　　　　　O34.591　Maternal care for other abnormalities of gravid uterus, first trimester ♀　M

　　　　　O34.592　Maternal care for other abnormalities of gravid uterus, second trimester ♀　M

　　　　　O34.593　Maternal care for other abnormalities of gravid uterus, third trimester ♀　M

　　　　　O34.599　Maternal care for other abnormalities of gravid uterus, unspecified trimester ♀　M

　● O34.6　Maternal care for abnormality of vagina

　　　Excludes2　maternal care for vaginal varices in pregnancy (O22.1-)

　　　O34.60　Maternal care for abnormality of vagina, unspecified trimester ♀　M

　　　O34.61　Maternal care for abnormality of vagina, first trimester ♀　M

　　　O34.62　Maternal care for abnormality of vagina, second trimester ♀　M

　　　O34.63　Maternal care for abnormality of vagina, third trimester ♀　M

▶ New　⟫ Revised　~~deleted~~ Deleted　Excludes 1　Excludes 2　Includes　Use additional　Code first　Code also　Key words
OGCR Official Guidelines　X Assign placeholder X　● Use Additional Character(s)　▷ Manifestation Code　🄷 Hierarchical Condition Category　Coding Clinic

● O34.7 Maternal care for abnormality of vulva and perineum

   Excludes2   maternal care for perineal and vulval varices in pregnancy (O22.1-)

   O34.70 Maternal care for abnormality of vulva and perineum, unspecified trimester ♀   M

   O34.71 Maternal care for abnormality of vulva and perineum, first trimester ♀   M

   O34.72 Maternal care for abnormality of vulva and perineum, second trimester ♀   M

   O34.73 Maternal care for abnormality of vulva and perineum, third trimester ♀   M

● O34.8 Maternal care for other abnormalities of pelvic organs

   O34.80 Maternal care for other abnormalities of pelvic organs, unspecified trimester ♀   M

   O34.81 Maternal care for other abnormalities of pelvic organs, first trimester ♀   M

   O34.82 Maternal care for other abnormalities of pelvic organs, second trimester ♀   M

   O34.83 Maternal care for other abnormalities of pelvic organs, third trimester ♀   M

● O34.9 Maternal care for abnormality of pelvic organ, unspecified

   O34.90 Maternal care for abnormality of pelvic organ, unspecified, unspecified trimester ♀   M

   O34.91 Maternal care for abnormality of pelvic organ, unspecified, first trimester ♀   M

   O34.92 Maternal care for abnormality of pelvic organ, unspecified, second trimester ♀   M

   O34.93 Maternal care for abnormality of pelvic organ, unspecified, third trimester ♀   M

● O35 Maternal care for known or suspected fetal abnormality and damage

   Includes   the listed conditions in the fetus as a reason for hospitalization or other obstetric care to the mother, or for termination of pregnancy

   Code also any associated maternal condition

   Excludes1   encounter for suspected maternal and fetal conditions ruled out (Z03.7-)

   One of the following 7th characters is to be assigned to each code under category O35. 7th character 0 is for single gestations and multiple gestations where the fetus is unspecified. 7th characters 1 through 9 are for cases of multiple gestations to identify the fetus for which the code applies. The appropriate code from category O30, Multiple gestation, must also be assigned when assigning a code from category O35 that has a 7th character of 1 through 9.

0	not applicable or unspecified
1	fetus 1
2	fetus 2
3	fetus 3
4	fetus 4
5	fetus 5
9	other fetus

X● O35.0 Maternal care for (suspected) central nervous system malformation in fetus ♀   M

   ~~Maternal care for fetal anencephaly~~
   ~~Maternal care for fetal hydrocephalus~~
   ~~Maternal care for fetal spina bifida~~

   ➠ **Excludes2**   chromosomal abnormality in fetus (O35.1-)

   ▶X● O35.00 Maternal care for (suspected) central nervous system malformation or damage in fetus, unspecified ♀   M

   ▶X● O35.01 Maternal care for (suspected) central nervous system malformation or damage in fetus, agenesis of the corpus callosum ♀   M

   ▶X● O35.02 Maternal care for (suspected) central nervous system malformation or damage in fetus, anencephaly ♀   M

   ▶X● O35.03 Maternal care for (suspected) central nervous system malformation or damage in fetus, choroid plexus cysts ♀   M

   ▶X● O35.04 Maternal care for (suspected) central nervous system malformation or damage in fetus, encephalocele ♀   M

   ▶X● O35.05 Maternal care for (suspected) central nervous system malformation or damage in fetus, holoprosencephaly ♀   M

   ▶X● O35.06 Maternal care for (suspected) central nervous system malformation or damage in fetus, hydrocephaly ♀   M
   ▶ Maternal care for fetal hydrocephalus

   ▶X● O35.07 Maternal care for (suspected) central nervous system malformation or damage in fetus, microcephaly ♀   M

   ▶X● O35.08 Maternal care for (suspected) central nervous system malformation or damage in fetus, spina bifida ♀   M

   ▶X● O35.09 Maternal care for (suspected) other central nervous system malformation or damage in Fetus ♀   M

X● O35.1 Maternal care for (suspected) chromosomal abnormality in fetus ♀   M

   ▶X● O35.10 Maternal care for (suspected) chromosomal abnormality in fetus, unspecified ♀   M

   ▶X● O35.11 Maternal care for (suspected) chromosomal abnormality in fetus, Trisomy 13 ♀   M

   ▶X● O35.12 Maternal care for (suspected) chromosomal abnormality in fetus, Trisomy 18 ♀   M

   ▶X● O35.13 Maternal care for (suspected) chromosomal abnormality in fetus, Trisomy 21 ♀   M

   ▶X● O35.14 Maternal care for (suspected) chromosomal abnormality in fetus, Turner Syndrome ♀   M

   ▶X● O35.15 Maternal care for (suspected) chromosomal abnormality in fetus, sex chromosome Abnormality ♀   M

   ▶X● O35.19 Maternal care for (suspected) chromosomal abnormality in fetus, other chromosomal abnormality ♀   M

X● O35.2 Maternal care for (suspected) hereditary disease in fetus ♀   M

   ➠ **Excludes2**   chromosomal abnormality in fetus (O35.1-)

X● O35.3 Maternal care for (suspected) damage to fetus from viral disease in mother ♀   M

   Maternal care for damage to fetus from maternal cytomegalovirus infection
   Maternal care for damage to fetus from maternal rubella
   Coding Clinic: 2016, Q4, P6

X● O35.4 Maternal care for (suspected) damage to fetus from alcohol ♀   M

X● O35.5 Maternal care for (suspected) damage to fetus by drugs ♀   M
   Maternal care for damage to fetus from drug addiction

X● O35.6 Maternal care for (suspected) damage to fetus by radiation ♀   M

X● O35.7 Maternal care for (suspected) damage to fetus by other medical procedures ♀   M
   Maternal care for damage to fetus by amniocentesis
   Maternal care for damage to fetus by biopsy procedures
   Maternal care for damage to fetus by hematological investigation
   Maternal care for damage to fetus by intrauterine contraceptive device
   Maternal care for damage to fetus by intrauterine surgery

X● O35.8 Maternal care for other (suspected) fetal abnormality and damage ♀   M
   Maternal care for damage to fetus from maternal listeriosis
   Maternal care for damage to fetus from maternal toxoplasmosis

X● O35.9 Maternal care for (suspected) fetal abnormality and damage, unspecified ♀   M

CHAPTER 15 (O00–O9A)

▶X● **O35.A** Maternal care for other (suspected) fetal abnormality and damage, fetal facial anomalies ♀   M

▶X● **O35.B** Maternal care for other (suspected) fetal abnormality and damage, fetal cardiac anomalies ♀   M

▶X● **O35.C** Maternal care for other (suspected) fetal abnormality and damage, fetal pulmonary anomalies ♀   M

▶X● **O35.D** Maternal care for other (suspected) fetal abnormality and damage, fetal gastrointestinal anomalies ♀   M

▶X● **O35.E** Maternal care for other (suspected) fetal abnormality and damage, fetal genitourinary anomalies ♀   M

▶X● **O35.F** Maternal care for other (suspected) fetal abnormality and damage, fetal musculoskeletal anomalies of trunk ♀   M

     ▶ **Excludes2**   maternal care for other (suspected) fetal abnormality and damage, fetal lower extremities anomalies (O35.H)

         ▶ maternal care for other (suspected) fetal abnormality and damage, fetal upper extremities anomalies (O35.G)

▶X● **O35.G** Maternal care for other (suspected) fetal abnormality and damage, fetal upper extremities anomalies ♀   M

▶X● **O35.H** Maternal care for other (suspected) fetal abnormality and damage, fetal lower extremities Anomalies ♀   M

OGCR Section I.C.15.e.l.

Fetal Conditions Affecting the Management of the Mother

1) Code from categories O35 and O36

Codes from categories O35, Maternal care for known or suspected fetal abnormality and damage, and O36, Maternal care for other fetal problems, are assigned only when the fetal condition is actually responsible for modifying the management of the mother, i.e., by requiring diagnostic studies, additional observation, special care, or termination of pregnancy. The fact that the fetal condition exists does not justify assigning a code from this series to the mother's record.

2) In utero surgery

In cases when surgery is performed on the fetus, a diagnosis code from category O35, Maternal care for known or suspected fetal abnormality and damage, should be assigned identifying the fetal condition. Assign the appropriate procedure code for the procedure performed.

No code from Chapter 16, the perinatal codes, should be used on the mother's record to identify fetal conditions. Surgery performed in utero on a fetus is still to be coded as an obstetric encounter.

● **O36** Maternal care for other fetal problems

     Includes   the listed conditions in the fetus as a reason for hospitalization or other obstetric care of the mother, or for termination of pregnancy

     Excludes1   encounter for suspected maternal and fetal conditions ruled out (Z03.7-)
         placental transfusion syndromes (O43.0-)

     Excludes2   labor and delivery complicated by fetal stress (O77.-)

One of the following 7th characters is to be assigned to each code under category O36. 7th character 0 is for single gestations and multiple gestations where the fetus is unspecified. 7th characters 1 through 9 are for cases of multiple gestations to identify the fetus for which the code applies. The appropriate code from category O30, Multiple gestation, must also be assigned when assigning a code from category O36 that has a 7th character of 1 through 9.

0	not applicable or unspecified
1	fetus 1
2	fetus 2
3	fetus 3
4	fetus 4
5	fetus 5
9	other fetus

Coding Clinic: 2015, Q3, P40

● **O36.0** Maternal care for rhesus isoimmunization

     Maternal care for Rh incompatibility (with hydrops fetalis)

     ● **O36.01** Maternal care for anti-D [Rh] antibodies

         ● **O36.011** Maternal care for anti-D [Rh] antibodies, first trimester ♀   M

         ● **O36.012** Maternal care for anti-D [Rh] antibodies, second trimester ♀   M

         ● **O36.013** Maternal care for anti-D [Rh] antibodies, third trimester ♀   M

         ● **O36.019** Maternal care for anti-D [Rh] antibodies, unspecified trimester ♀   M

     ● **O36.09** Maternal care for other rhesus isoimmunization

         ● **O36.091** Maternal care for other rhesus isoimmunization, first trimester ♀   M

         ● **O36.092** Maternal care for other rhesus isoimmunization, second trimester ♀   M

         ● **O36.093** Maternal care for other rhesus isoimmunization, third trimester ♀   M
             Coding Clinic: 2015, Q3, P40

         ● **O36.099** Maternal care for other rhesus isoimmunization, unspecified trimester ♀   M

● **O36.1** Maternal care for other isoimmunization

     Maternal care for ABO isoimmunization

     ● **O36.11** Maternal care for Anti-A sensitization

         Maternal care for isoimmunization NOS (with hydrops fetalis)

         ● **O36.111** Maternal care for Anti-A sensitization, first trimester ♀   M

         ● **O36.112** Maternal care for Anti-A sensitization, second trimester ♀   M

         ● **O36.113** Maternal care for Anti-A sensitization, third trimester ♀   M

         ● **O36.119** Maternal care for Anti-A sensitization, unspecified trimester ♀   M

     ● **O36.19** Maternal care for other isoimmunization

         Maternal care for Anti-B sensitization

         ● **O36.191** Maternal care for other isoimmunization, first trimester ♀   M

         ● **O36.192** Maternal care for other isoimmunization, second trimester ♀   M

         ● **O36.193** Maternal care for other isoimmunization, third trimester ♀   M

         ● **O36.199** Maternal care for other isoimmunization, unspecified trimester ♀   M

● **O36.2** Maternal care for hydrops fetalis

     Maternal care for hydrops fetalis NOS

     Maternal care for hydrops fetalis not associated with isoimmunization

     Excludes1   hydrops fetalis associated with ABO isoimmunization (O36.1-)
         hydrops fetalis associated with rhesus isoimmunization (O36.0-)

     ● **O36.20** Maternal care for hydrops fetalis, unspecified trimester ♀   M

     ● **O36.21** Maternal care for hydrops fetalis, first trimester ♀   M

     ● **O36.22** Maternal care for hydrops fetalis, second trimester ♀   M

     ● **O36.23** Maternal care for hydrops fetalis, third trimester ♀   M

● **O36.4** Maternal care for intrauterine death ♀   M

     Maternal care for intrauterine fetal death NOS

     Maternal care for intrauterine fetal death after completion of 20 weeks of gestation

     Maternal care for late fetal death

     Maternal care for missed delivery

     Excludes1   missed abortion (O02.1)
         stillbirth (P95)

     Coding Clinic: 2022, Q2, P3-4

CHAPTER 15 (O00-O9A)

▶ New   ⇒ Revised   ~~deleted~~ Deleted   Excludes 1   Excludes 2   Includes   Use additional   Code first   Code also   Key words

OGCR Official Guidelines   X Assign placeholder X   ● Use Additional Character(s)   ▶ Manifestation Code   🔖 Hierarchical Condition Category   **Coding Clinic**

- O36.5   Maternal care for known or suspected poor fetal growth
  - O36.51   Maternal care for known or suspected placental insufficiency
    - O36.511   Maternal care for known or suspected placental insufficiency, first trimester ♀   M
    - O36.512   Maternal care for known or suspected placental insufficiency, second trimester ♀   M
    - O36.513   Maternal care for known or suspected placental insufficiency, third trimester ♀   M
    - O36.519   Maternal care for known or suspected placental insufficiency, unspecified trimester ♀   M
  - O36.59   Maternal care for other known or suspected poor fetal growth
    Maternal care for known or suspected light-for-dates NOS
    Maternal care for known or suspected small-for-dates NOS
    - O36.591   Maternal care for other known or suspected poor fetal growth, first trimester ♀   M
    - O36.592   Maternal care for other known or suspected poor fetal growth, second trimester ♀   M
    - O36.593   Maternal care for other known or suspected poor fetal growth, third trimester ♀   M
    - O36.599   Maternal care for other known or suspected poor fetal growth, unspecified trimester ♀   M
- O36.6   Maternal care for excessive fetal growth
  Maternal care for known or suspected large-for-dates
  - X O36.60   Maternal care for excessive fetal growth, unspecified trimester ♀   M
  - X O36.61   Maternal care for excessive fetal growth, first trimester ♀   M
  - X O36.62   Maternal care for excessive fetal growth, second trimester ♀   M
  - X O36.63   Maternal care for excessive fetal growth, third trimester ♀   M
- O36.7   Maternal care for viable fetus in abdominal pregnancy
  - X O36.70   Maternal care for viable fetus in abdominal pregnancy, unspecified trimester ♀   M
  - X O36.71   Maternal care for viable fetus in abdominal pregnancy, first trimester ♀   M
  - X O36.72   Maternal care for viable fetus in abdominal pregnancy, second trimester ♀   M
  - X O36.73   Maternal care for viable fetus in abdominal pregnancy, third trimester ♀   M
- O36.8   Maternal care for other specified fetal problems
  - X O36.80   Pregnancy with inconclusive fetal viability ♀   M
    Encounter to determine fetal viability of pregnancy
    Coding Clinic: 2019, Q2, P29
  - O36.81   Decreased fetal movements
    - O36.812   Decreased fetal movements, second trimester ♀   M
    - O36.813   Decreased fetal movements, third trimester ♀   M
    - O36.819   Decreased fetal movements, unspecified trimester ♀   M
  - O36.82   Fetal anemia and thrombocytopenia
    - O36.821   Fetal anemia and thrombocytopenia, first trimester ♀   M
    - O36.822   Fetal anemia and thrombocytopenia, second trimester ♀   M
    - O36.823   Fetal anemia and thrombocytopenia, third trimester ♀   M
    - O36.829   Fetal anemia and thrombocytopenia, unspecified trimester ♀   M
  - O36.83   Maternal care for abnormalities of the fetal heart rate or rhythm
    Maternal care for depressed fetal heart rate tones
    Maternal care for fetal bradycardia
    Maternal care for fetal heart rate abnormal variability
    Maternal care for fetal heart rate decelerations
    Maternal care for fetal heart rate irregularity
    Maternal care for fetal tachycardia
    Maternal care for non-reassuring fetal heart rate or rhythm
    - O36.831   Maternal care for abnormalities of the fetal heart rate or rhythm, first trimester ♀   M
    - O36.832   Maternal care for abnormalities of the fetal heart rate or rhythm, second trimester ♀   M
    - O36.833   Maternal care for abnormalities of the fetal heart rate or rhythm, third trimester ♀   M
    - O36.839   Maternal care for abnormalities of the fetal heart rate or rhythm, unspecified trimester ♀   M
  - O36.89   Maternal care for other specified fetal problems
    - O36.891   Maternal care for other specified fetal problems, first trimester ♀   M
    - O36.892   Maternal care for other specified fetal problems, second trimester ♀   M
    - O36.893   Maternal care for other specified fetal problems, third trimester ♀   M
    - O36.899   Maternal care for other specified fetal problems, unspecified trimester ♀   M
- O36.9   Maternal care for fetal problem, unspecified
  - X O36.90   Maternal care for fetal problem, unspecified, unspecified trimester ♀   M
  - X O36.91   Maternal care for fetal problem, unspecified, first trimester ♀   M
  - X O36.92   Maternal care for fetal problem, unspecified, second trimester ♀   M
  - X O36.93   Maternal care for fetal problem, unspecified, third trimester ♀   M

- O40   Polyhydramnios
  Overabundance of amniotic fluid

Includes	hydramnios
Excludes1	encounter for suspected maternal and fetal conditions ruled out (Z03.7-)

  One of the following 7th characters is to be assigned to each code under category O40. 7th character 0 is for single gestations and multiple gestations where the fetus is unspecified. 7th characters 1 through 9 are for cases of multiple gestations to identify the fetus for which the code applies. The appropriate code from category O30, Multiple gestation, must also be assigned when assigning a code from category O40 that has a 7th character of 1 through 9.

0	not applicable or unspecified
1	fetus 1
2	fetus 2
3	fetus 3
4	fetus 4
5	fetus 5
9	other fetus

  - X O40.1   Polyhydramnios, first trimester ♀   M
  - X O40.2   Polyhydramnios, second trimester ♀   M
  - X O40.3   Polyhydramnios, third trimester ♀   M
  - X O40.9   Polyhydramnios, unspecified trimester ♀   M

CHAPTER 15 (O00-O9A)

● O41   Other disorders of amniotic fluid and membranes

Excludes1   encounter for suspected maternal and fetal
conditions ruled out (Z03.7-)

One of the following 7th characters is to be assigned to each
code under category O41. 7th character 0 is for single
gestations and multiple gestations where the fetus is
unspecified. 7th characters 1 through 9 are for cases of
multiple gestations to identify the fetus for which the code
applies. The appropriate code from category O30, Multiple
gestation, must also be assigned when assigning a code
from category O41 that has a 7th character of 1 through 9.

0	not applicable or unspecified
1	fetus 1
2	fetus 2
3	fetus 3
4	fetus 4
5	fetus 5
9	other fetus

● O41.0   Oligohydramnios
Scant volume of amniotic fluid
Oligohydramnios without rupture of membranes
X ● O41.00   Oligohydramnios, unspecified trimester ♀   M
X ● O41.01   Oligohydramnios, first trimester ♀   M
X ● O41.02   Oligohydramnios, second trimester ♀   M
X ● O41.03   Oligohydramnios, third trimester ♀   M
● O41.1   Infection of amniotic sac and membranes
● O41.10   Infection of amniotic sac and membranes,
unspecified
● O41.101   Infection of amniotic sac and
membranes, unspecified, first
trimester ♀   M
● O41.102   Infection of amniotic sac and
membranes, unspecified, second
trimester ♀   M
● O41.103   Infection of amniotic sac and
membranes, unspecified, third
trimester ♀   M
● O41.109   Infection of amniotic sac and
membranes, unspecified, unspecified
trimester ♀   M
● O41.12   Chorioamnionitis
Coding Clinic: 2019, Q2, P34-35
● O41.121   Chorioamnionitis, first trimester ♀   M
● O41.122   Chorioamnionitis, second
trimester ♀   M
● O41.123   Chorioamnionitis, third trimester ♀   M
● O41.129   Chorioamnionitis, unspecified
trimester ♀   M
● O41.14   Placentitis
● O41.141   Placentitis, first trimester ♀   M
● O41.142   Placentitis, second trimester ♀   M
● O41.143   Placentitis, third trimester ♀   M
● O41.149   Placentitis, unspecified trimester ♀   M
● O41.8   Other specified disorders of amniotic fluid and
membranes
● O41.8X   Other specified disorders of amniotic fluid and
membranes
● O41.8X1   Other specified disorders of
amniotic fluid and membranes, first
trimester ♀   M
● O41.8X2   Other specified disorders of amniotic
fluid and membranes, second
trimester ♀   M
● O41.8X3   Other specified disorders of
amniotic fluid and membranes, third
trimester ♀   M
● O41.8X9   Other specified disorders of amniotic
fluid and membranes, unspecified
trimester ♀   M

● O41.9   Disorder of amniotic fluid and membranes, unspecified
X ● O41.90   Disorder of amniotic fluid and membranes,
unspecified, unspecified trimester ♀   M
X ● O41.91   Disorder of amniotic fluid and membranes,
unspecified, first trimester ♀   M
X ● O41.92   Disorder of amniotic fluid and membranes,
unspecified, second trimester ♀   M
X ● O41.93   Disorder of amniotic fluid and membranes,
unspecified, third trimester ♀   M
● O42   Premature rupture of membranes
● O42.0   Premature rupture of membranes, onset of labor within
24 hours of rupture
O42.00   Premature rupture of membranes, onset of
labor within 24 hours of rupture, unspecified
weeks of gestation ♀   M
● O42.01   Preterm premature rupture of membranes,
onset of labor within 24 hours of rupture
Premature rupture of membranes before 37
completed weeks of gestation
O42.011   Preterm premature rupture of
membranes, onset of labor within 24
hours of rupture, first trimester ♀   M
O42.012   Preterm premature rupture of
membranes, onset of labor within 24
hours of rupture, second trimester ♀ M
O42.013   Preterm premature rupture of
membranes, onset of labor within 24
hours of rupture, third trimester ♀   M
O42.019   Preterm premature rupture of
membranes, onset of labor within
24 hours of rupture, unspecified
trimester ♀   M
O42.02   Full-term premature rupture of membranes,
onset of labor within 24 hours of rupture ♀   M
Premature rupture of membranes at or after
37 completed weeks of gestation, onset of
labor within 24 hours of rupture
● O42.1   Premature rupture of membranes, onset of labor more
than 24 hours following rupture
O42.10   Premature rupture of membranes, onset of
labor more than 24 hours following rupture,
unspecified weeks of gestation ♀   M
● O42.11   Preterm premature rupture of membranes,
onset of labor more than 24 hours following
rupture
Premature rupture of membranes before 37
completed weeks of gestation
O42.111   Preterm premature rupture of
membranes, onset of labor more
than 24 hours following rupture, first
trimester ♀   M
O42.112   Preterm premature rupture of
membranes, onset of labor more than
24 hours following rupture, second
trimester ♀   M
O42.113   Preterm premature rupture of
membranes, onset of labor more than
24 hours following rupture, third
trimester ♀   M
O42.119   Preterm premature rupture of
membranes, onset of labor more
than 24 hours following rupture,
unspecified trimester ♀   M
O42.12   Full-term premature rupture of membranes,
onset of labor more than 24 hours following
rupture ♀   M
Premature rupture of membranes at or after
37 completed weeks of gestation, onset
of labor more than 24 hours following
rupture

▶ New   ⇒ Revised   ~~deleted~~ Deleted   Excludes 1   Excludes 2   Includes   Use additional   Code first   Code also   Key words

OGCR Official Guidelines   X Assign placeholder X   ● Use Additional Character(s)   ▶ Manifestation Code   🜲 Hierarchical Condition Category   **Coding Clinic**

● **O42.9** **Premature rupture of membranes, unspecified as to length of time between rupture and onset of labor**

    O42.90 Premature rupture of membranes, unspecified as to length of time between rupture and onset of labor, unspecified weeks of gestation ♀   M

  ● **O42.91** **Preterm premature rupture of membranes, unspecified as to length of time between rupture and onset of labor**
      Premature rupture of membranes before 37 completed weeks of gestation

    O42.911 Preterm premature rupture of membranes, unspecified as to length of time between rupture and onset of labor, first trimester ♀   M

    O42.912 Preterm premature rupture of membranes, unspecified as to length of time between rupture and onset of labor, second trimester ♀   M

    O42.913 Preterm premature rupture of membranes, unspecified as to length of time between rupture and onset of labor, third trimester ♀   M

    O42.919 Preterm premature rupture of membranes, unspecified as to length of time between rupture and onset of labor, unspecified trimester ♀   M

    O42.92 Full-term premature rupture of membranes, unspecified as to length of time between rupture and onset of labor ♀   M
      Premature rupture of membranes at or after 37 completed weeks of gestation, unspecified as to length of time between rupture and onset of labor

● **O43** **Placental disorders**

  Excludes2   maternal care for poor fetal growth due to placental insufficiency (O36.5-)
      placenta previa (O44.-)
      placental polyp (O90.89)
      placentitis (O41.14-)
      premature separation of placenta [abruptio placentae] (O45.-)

● **O43.0** **Placental transfusion syndromes**

  ● **O43.01** **Fetomaternal placental transfusion syndrome**
      Maternofetal placental transfusion syndrome

    O43.011 Fetomaternal placental transfusion syndrome, first trimester ♀   M

    O43.012 Fetomaternal placental transfusion syndrome, second trimester ♀   M

    O43.013 Fetomaternal placental transfusion syndrome, third trimester ♀   M

    O43.019 Fetomaternal placental transfusion syndrome, unspecified trimester ♀   M

  ● **O43.02** **Fetus-to-fetus placental transfusion syndrome**

    O43.021 Fetus-to-fetus placental transfusion syndrome, first trimester ♀   M

    O43.022 Fetus-to-fetus placental transfusion syndrome, second trimester ♀   M

    O43.023 Fetus-to-fetus placental transfusion syndrome, third trimester ♀   M

    O43.029 Fetus-to-fetus placental transfusion syndrome, unspecified trimester ♀   M

● **O43.1** **Malformation of placenta**

  ● **O43.10** **Malformation of placenta, unspecified**
      Abnormal placenta NOS

    O43.101 Malformation of placenta, unspecified, first trimester ♀   M

    O43.102 Malformation of placenta, unspecified, second trimester ♀   M

    O43.103 Malformation of placenta, unspecified, third trimester ♀   M

    O43.109 Malformation of placenta, unspecified, unspecified trimester ♀   M

● **O43.11** **Circumvallate placenta**

    O43.111 Circumvallate placenta, first trimester ♀   M

    O43.112 Circumvallate placenta, second trimester ♀   M

    O43.113 Circumvallate placenta, third trimester ♀   M

    O43.119 Circumvallate placenta, unspecified trimester ♀   M

● **O43.12** **Velamentous insertion of umbilical cord**

    O43.121 Velamentous insertion of umbilical cord, first trimester ♀   M

    O43.122 Velamentous insertion of umbilical cord, second trimester ♀   M

    O43.123 Velamentous insertion of umbilical cord, third trimester ♀   M

    O43.129 Velamentous insertion of umbilical cord, unspecified trimester ♀   M

● **O43.19** **Other malformation of placenta**

    O43.191 Other malformation of placenta, first trimester ♀   M

    O43.192 Other malformation of placenta, second trimester ♀   M

    O43.193 Other malformation of placenta, third trimester ♀   M

    O43.199 Other malformation of placenta, unspecified trimester ♀   M

● **O43.2** **Morbidly adherent placenta**
    Code also associated third stage postpartum hemorrhage, if applicable (O72.0)
    Excludes1   retained placenta (O73.-)

  ● **O43.21** **Placenta accreta**
    O43.211 Placenta accreta, first trimester ♀ M
    O43.212 Placenta accreta, second trimester ♀ M
    O43.213 Placenta accreta, third trimester ♀ M
    O43.219 Placenta accreta, unspecified trimester ♀ M

  ● **O43.22** **Placenta increta**
    O43.221 Placenta increta, first trimester ♀ M
    O43.222 Placenta increta, second trimester ♀ M
      Coding Clinic: 2022, Q1, P21
    O43.223 Placenta increta, third trimester ♀
    O43.229 Placenta increta, unspecified trimester ♀

  ● **O43.23** **Placenta percreta**
    O43.231 Placenta percreta, first trimester ♀ M
    O43.232 Placenta percreta, second trimester ♀ M
    O43.233 Placenta percreta, third trimester ♀ M
    O43.239 Placenta percreta, unspecified trimester ♀ M

● **O43.8** **Other placental disorders**

  ● **O43.81** **Placental infarction**
    O43.811 Placental infarction, first trimester ♀ M
    O43.812 Placental infarction, second trimester ♀ M
    O43.813 Placental infarction, third trimester ♀ M
    O43.819 Placental infarction, unspecified trimester ♀ M

  ● **O43.89** **Other placental disorders**
      Placental dysfunction
    O43.891 Other placental disorders, first trimester ♀ M
    O43.892 Other placental disorders, second trimester ♀ M
    O43.893 Other placental disorders, third trimester ♀ M
    O43.899 Other placental disorders, unspecified trimester ♀

CHAPTER 15 (O00–O9A)

Figure 15-2 A. Marginal placento previa. **B.** Partial placenta previa. **C.** Total placento previa.

Item 15–3 Placenta previa is a condition in which the opening of the cervix is obstructed by the displaced placenta. The three types, marginal, partial, and total, are varying degrees of placenta displacement. Placenta abruption is the premature breaking away of the placenta from the site of the uterine implant before the delivery of the fetus.

● O43.9 Unspecified placental disorder
  O43.90 Unspecified placental disorder, unspecified trimester ♀ M
  O43.91 Unspecified placental disorder, first trimester ♀ M
  O43.92 Unspecified placental disorder, second trimester ♀ M
  O43.93 Unspecified placental disorder, third trimester ♀ M

● O44 Placenta previa
  Coding Clinic: 2016, Q4, P52
  ● O44.0 Complete placenta previa NOS or without hemorrhage
    Placenta previa NOS
    O44.00 Complete placenta previa NOS or without hemorrhage, unspecified trimester ♀ M
    O44.01 Complete placenta previa NOS or without hemorrhage, first trimester ♀ M
    O44.02 Complete placenta previa NOS or without hemorrhage, second trimester ♀ M
    O44.03 Complete placenta previa NOS or without hemorrhage, third trimester ♀ M
  ● O44.1 Complete placenta previa with hemorrhage
    Excludes1 labor and delivery complicated by hemorrhage from vasa previa (O69.4)
    O44.10 Complete placenta previa with hemorrhage, unspecified trimester ♀ M
    O44.11 Complete placenta previa with hemorrhage, first trimester ♀ M
    O44.12 Complete placenta previa with hemorrhage, second trimester ♀ M
    O44.13 Complete placenta previa with hemorrhage, third trimester ♀ M
  ● O44.2 Partial placenta previa without hemorrhage
    Marginal placenta previa, NOS or without hemorrhage
    O44.20 Partial placenta previa NOS or without hemorrhage, unspecified trimester ♀ M
    O44.21 Partial placenta previa NOS or without hemorrhage, first trimester ♀ M
    O44.22 Partial placenta previa NOS or without hemorrhage, second trimester ♀ M
    O44.23 Partial placenta previa NOS or without hemorrhage, third trimester ♀ M
  ● O44.3 Partial placenta previa with hemorrhage
    Marginal placenta previa with hemorrhage
    O44.30 Partial placenta previa with hemorrhage, unspecified trimester ♀ M
    O44.31 Partial placenta previa with hemorrhage, first trimester ♀ M
    O44.32 Partial placenta previa with hemorrhage, second trimester ♀ M
    O44.33 Partial placenta previa with hemorrhage, third trimester ♀ M

Figure 15-3 Abruptio placentae is classified according to the grade of separation of the placenta from the uterine wall. **A.** Mild separation in which hemorrhage is internal. **B.** Moderate separation in which there is external hemorrhage. **C.** Severe separation in which there is external hemorrhage and extreme separation.

● O44.4 Low lying placenta NOS or without hemorrhage
    Low implantation of placenta NOS or without hemorrhage
    O44.40 Low lying placenta NOS or without hemorrhage, unspecified trimester ♀ M
    O44.41 Low lying placenta NOS or without hemorrhage, first trimester ♀ M
    O44.42 Low lying placenta NOS or without hemorrhage, second trimester ♀ M
    O44.43 Low lying placenta NOS or without hemorrhage, third trimester ♀ M
● O44.5 Low lying placenta with hemorrhage
    Low implantation of placenta with hemorrhage
    O44.50 Low lying placenta with hemorrhage, unspecified trimester ♀ M
    O44.51 Low lying placenta with hemorrhage, first trimester ♀ M
    O44.52 Low lying placenta with hemorrhage, second trimester ♀ M
    O44.53 Low lying placenta with hemorrhage, third trimester ♀ M

● O45 Premature separation of placenta [abruptio placentae]
  ● O45.0 Premature separation of placenta with coagulation defect
    ● O45.00 Premature separation of placenta with coagulation defect, unspecified
      O45.001 Premature separation of placenta with coagulation defect, unspecified, first trimester ♀ M
      O45.002 Premature separation of placenta with coagulation defect, unspecified, second trimester ♀ M
      O45.003 Premature separation of placenta with coagulation defect, unspecified, third trimester ♀ M
      O45.009 Premature separation of placenta with coagulation defect, unspecified, unspecified trimester ♀ M
    ● O45.01 Premature separation of placenta with afibrinogenemia
      Premature separation of placenta with hypofibrinogenemia
      O45.011 Premature separation of placenta with afibrinogenemia, first trimester ♀ M
      O45.012 Premature separation of placenta with afibrinogenemia, second trimester ♀ M
      O45.013 Premature separation of placenta with afibrinogenemia, third trimester ♀ M
      O45.019 Premature separation of placenta with afibrinogenemia, unspecified trimester ♀ M
    ● O45.02 Premature separation of placenta with disseminated intravascular coagulation
      O45.021 Premature separation of placenta with disseminated intravascular coagulation, first trimester ♀ M

▶ New   ⇒ Revised   ~~deleted~~ Deleted   Excludes 1   Excludes 2   Includes   Use additional   Code first   Code also   Key words
OGCR Official Guidelines   X Assign placeholder X   ● Use Additional Character(s)   ▶ Manifestation Code   🔵 Hierarchical Condition Category   **Coding Clinic**

O45.022   Premature separation of placenta with disseminated intravascular coagulation, second trimester ♀   M

O45.023   Premature separation of placenta with disseminated intravascular coagulation, third trimester ♀   M

O45.029   Premature separation of placenta with disseminated intravascular coagulation, unspecified trimester ♀ M

● O45.09   Premature separation of placenta with other coagulation defect

O45.091   Premature separation of placenta with other coagulation defect, first trimester ♀   M

O45.092   Premature separation of placenta with other coagulation defect, second trimester ♀   M

O45.093   Premature separation of placenta with other coagulation defect, third trimester ♀   M

O45.099   Premature separation of placenta with other coagulation defect, unspecified trimester ♀   M

● O45.8   Other premature separation of placenta

● O45.8X   Other premature separation of placenta

O45.8X1   Other premature separation of placenta, first trimester ♀   M

O45.8X2   Other premature separation of placenta, second trimester ♀   M

O45.8X3   Other premature separation of placenta, third trimester ♀   M

O45.8X9   Other premature separation of placenta, unspecified trimester ♀   M

● O45.9   Premature separation of placenta, unspecified
Abruptio placentae NOS

O45.90   Premature separation of placenta, unspecified, unspecified trimester ♀   M

O45.91   Premature separation of placenta, unspecified, first trimester ♀   M

O45.92   Premature separation of placenta, unspecified, second trimester ♀   M

O45.93   Premature separation of placenta, unspecified, third trimester ♀   M

● O46   Antepartum hemorrhage, not elsewhere classified

Excludes1   hemorrhage in early pregnancy (O20.-)
intrapartum hemorrhage NEC (O67.-)
placenta previa (O44.-)
premature separation of placenta [abruptio placentae] (O45.-)

● O46.0   Antepartum hemorrhage with coagulation defect

● O46.00   Antepartum hemorrhage with coagulation defect, unspecified

O46.001   Antepartum hemorrhage with coagulation defect, unspecified, first trimester ♀   M

O46.002   Antepartum hemorrhage with coagulation defect, unspecified, second trimester ♀   M

O46.003   Antepartum hemorrhage with coagulation defect, unspecified, third trimester ♀   M

O46.009   Antepartum hemorrhage with coagulation defect, unspecified, unspecified trimester ♀   M

● O46.01   Antepartum hemorrhage with afibrinogenemia
Antepartum hemorrhage with hypofibrinogenemia

O46.011   Antepartum hemorrhage with afibrinogenemia, first trimester ♀   M

O46.012   Antepartum hemorrhage with afibrinogenemia, second trimester ♀ M

O46.013   Antepartum hemorrhage with afibrinogenemia, third trimester ♀   M

O46.019   Antepartum hemorrhage with afibrinogenemia, unspecified trimester ♀   M

● O46.02   Antepartum hemorrhage with disseminated intravascular coagulation

O46.021   Antepartum hemorrhage with disseminated intravascular coagulation, first trimester ♀   M

O46.022   Antepartum hemorrhage with disseminated intravascular coagulation, second trimester ♀   M

O46.023   Antepartum hemorrhage with disseminated intravascular coagulation, third trimester ♀   M

O46.029   Antepartum hemorrhage with disseminated intravascular coagulation, unspecified trimester ♀ M

● O46.09   Antepartum hemorrhage with other coagulation defect

O46.091   Antepartum hemorrhage with other coagulation defect, first trimester ♀ M

O46.092   Antepartum hemorrhage with other coagulation defect, second trimester ♀

O46.093   Antepartum hemorrhage with other coagulation defect, third trimester ♀ M

O46.099   Antepartum hemorrhage with other coagulation defect, unspecified trimester ♀   M

● O46.8   Other antepartum hemorrhage

● O46.8x   Other antepartum hemorrhage

O46.8x1   Other antepartum hemorrhage, first trimester ♀   M

O46.8x2   Other antepartum hemorrhage, second trimester ♀   M

O46.8x3   Other antepartum hemorrhage, third trimester ♀   M

O46.8x9   Other antepartum hemorrhage, unspecified trimester ♀   M

● O46.9   Antepartum hemorrhage, unspecified

O46.90   Antepartum hemorrhage, unspecified, unspecified trimester ♀   M

O46.91   Antepartum hemorrhage, unspecified, first trimester ♀   M

O46.92   Antepartum hemorrhage, unspecified, second trimester ♀   M

O46.93   Antepartum hemorrhage, unspecified, third trimester ♀   M

● O47   False labor

Includes   Braxton Hicks contractions
threatened labor

Excludes1   preterm labor (O60.-)

● O47.0   False labor before 37 completed weeks of gestation

O47.00   False labor before 37 completed weeks of gestation, unspecified trimester ♀   M

O47.02   False labor before 37 completed weeks of gestation, second trimester ♀   M

O47.03   False labor before 37 completed weeks of gestation, third trimester ♀   M

O47.1   False labor at or after 37 completed weeks of gestation ♀   M
Coding Clinic: 2022, Q2, P3-4; 2021, Q1, P10

O47.9   False labor, unspecified ♀   M

● O48   Late pregnancy

O48.0   Post-term pregnancy ♀   M
Pregnancy over 40 completed weeks to 42 completed weeks gestation

O48.1   Prolonged pregnancy ♀   M
Pregnancy which has advanced beyond 42 completed weeks gestation
Coding Clinic: 2022, Q2 P3-4

CHAPTER 15 (O00-O9A)

COMPLICATIONS OF LABOR AND DELIVERY (O60-O77)

● O60   **Preterm labor**

     Includes   onset (spontaneous) of labor before 37 completed weeks of gestation

     Excludes1   false labor (O47.0-)
                 threatened labor NOS (O47.0-)

● O60.0   **Preterm labor without delivery**

     O60.00   **Preterm labor without delivery, unspecified trimester** ♀   M

     O60.02   **Preterm labor without delivery, second trimester** ♀   M

     O60.03   **Preterm labor without delivery, third trimester** ♀   M

● O60.1   **Preterm labor with preterm delivery**

     One of the following 7th characters is to be assigned to each code under subcategory O60.1. 7th character 0 is for single gestations and multiple gestations where the fetus is unspecified. 7th characters 1 through 9 are for cases of multiple gestations to identify the fetus for which the code applies. The appropriate code from category O30, Multiple gestation, must also be assigned when assigning a code from subcategory O60.1 that has a 7th character of 1 through 9.

0	not applicable or unspecified
1	fetus 1
2	fetus 2
3	fetus 3
4	fetus 4
5	fetus 5
9	other fetus

Coding Clinic: 2016, Q2, P11

X ● O60.10   **Preterm labor with preterm delivery, unspecified trimester** ♀   M
              Preterm labor with delivery NOS

X ● O60.12   **Preterm labor second trimester with preterm delivery second trimester** ♀   M

X ● O60.13   **Preterm labor second trimester with preterm delivery third trimester** ♀   M

X ● O60.14   **Preterm labor third trimester with preterm delivery third trimester** ♀   M
          Coding Clinic: 2016, Q2, P10

● O60.2   **Term delivery with preterm labor**

     One of the following 7th characters is to be assigned to each code under subcategory O60.2. 7th character 0 is for single gestations and multiple gestations where the fetus is unspecified. 7th characters 1 through 9 are for cases of multiple gestations to identify the fetus for which the code applies. The appropriate code from category O30, Multiple gestation, must also be assigned when assigning a code from subcategory O60.2 that has a 7th character of 1 through 9.

0	not applicable or unspecified
1	fetus 1
2	fetus 2
3	fetus 3
4	fetus 4
5	fetus 5
9	other fetus

X ● O60.20   **Term delivery with preterm labor, unspecified trimester** ♀   M

X ● O60.22   **Term delivery with preterm labor, second trimester** ♀   M

X ● O60.23   **Term delivery with preterm labor, third trimester** ♀   M

● O61   **Failed induction of labor**

     O61.0   **Failed medical induction of labor** ♀   M
          Failed induction (of labor) by oxytocin
          Failed induction (of labor) by prostaglandins

     O61.1   **Failed instrumental induction of labor** ♀   M
          Failed mechanical induction (of labor)
          Failed surgical induction (of labor)

     O61.8   **Other failed induction of labor** ♀   M

     O61.9   **Failed induction of labor, unspecified** ♀   M

● O62   **Abnormalities of forces of labor**

     O62.0   **Primary inadequate contractions** ♀   M
          Failure of cervical dilatation
          Primary hypotonic uterine dysfunction
          Uterine inertia during latent phase of labor

     O62.1   **Secondary uterine inertia** ♀   M
          Arrested active phase of labor
          Secondary hypotonic uterine dysfunction

     O62.2   **Other uterine inertia** ♀   M
          Atony of uterus without hemorrhage
          Atony of uterus NOS
          Desultory labor
          Hypotonic uterine dysfunction NOS
          Irregular labor
          Poor contractions
          Slow slope active phase of labor
          Uterine inertia NOS

         Excludes1   atony of uterus with hemorrhage (postpartum) (O72.1)
                  postpartum atony of uterus without hemorrhage (O75.89)

     O62.3   **Precipitate labor** ♀   M

     O62.4   **Hypertonic, incoordinate, and prolonged uterine contractions** ♀   M
          Cervical spasm
          Contraction ring dystocia
          Dyscoordinate labor
          Hour-glass contraction of uterus
          Hypertonic uterine dysfunction
          Incoordinate uterine action
          Tetanic contractions
          Uterine dystocia NOS
          Uterine spasm

         Excludes1   dystocia (fetal) (maternal) NOS (O66.9)

     O62.8   **Other abnormalities of forces of labor** ♀   M

     O62.9   **Abnormality of forces of labor, unspecified** ♀   M

● O63   **Long labor**

     O63.0   **Prolonged first stage (of labor)** ♀   M

     O63.1   **Prolonged second stage (of labor)** ♀   M

     O63.2   **Delayed delivery of second twin, triplet, etc.** ♀   M

     O63.9   **Long labor, unspecified** ♀   M
          Prolonged labor NOS

● O64   **Obstructed labor due to malposition and malpresentation of fetus**

     One of the following 7th characters is to be assigned to each code under category O64. 7th character 0 is for single gestations and multiple gestations where the fetus is unspecified. 7th characters 1 through 9 are for cases of multiple gestations to identify the fetus for which the code applies. The appropriate code from category O30, Multiple gestation, must also be assigned when assigning a code from category O64 that has a 7th character of 1 through 9.

0	not applicable or unspecified
1	fetus 1
2	fetus 2
3	fetus 3
4	fetus 4
5	fetus 5
9	other fetus

▶ New   ⇒ Revised   ~~deleted~~ Deleted   Excludes 1   Excludes 2   Includes   Use additional   Code first   Code also   Key words

OGCR Official Guidelines   X Assign placeholder X   ● Use Additional Character(s)   ▶ Manifestation Code   🔖 Hierarchical Condition Category   **Coding Clinic**

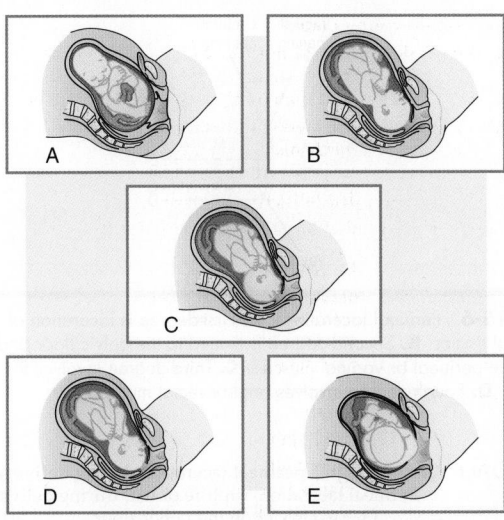

Figure 15-4 Five types of malposition and malpresentation of the fetus: **A.** Breech. **B.** Vertex. **C.** Face. **D.** Brow. **E.** Shoulder.

Figure 15-5 Hydrocephalic fetus causing disproportion.

X ● **O64.0 Obstructed labor due to incomplete rotation of fetal head** ♀   M
     Deep transverse arrest
     Obstructed labor due to persistent occipitoiliac (position)
     Obstructed labor due to persistent occipitoposterior (position)
     Obstructed labor due to persistent occipitosacral (position)
     Obstructed labor due to persistent occipitotransverse (position)

X ● **O64.1 Obstructed labor due to breech presentation** ♀   M
     Obstructed labor due to buttocks presentation
     Obstructed labor due to complete breech presentation
     Obstructed labor due to frank breech presentation

X ● **O64.2 Obstructed labor due to face presentation** ♀   M
     Obstructed labor due to chin presentation

X ● **O64.3 Obstructed labor due to brow presentation** ♀   M

X ● **O64.4 Obstructed labor due to shoulder presentation** ♀   M
     Prolapsed arm
     Excludes1   impacted shoulders (O66.0)
                    shoulder dystocia (O66.0)

X ● **O64.5 Obstructed labor due to compound presentation** ♀   M

X ● **O64.8 Obstructed labor due to other malposition and malpresentation** ♀   M
     Obstructed labor due to footling presentation
     Obstructed labor due to incomplete breech presentation

X ● **O64.9 Obstructed labor due to malposition and malpresentation, unspecified** ♀   M

● **O65 Obstructed labor due to maternal pelvic abnormality**

   O65.0 Obstructed labor due to deformed pelvis ♀   M

   O65.1 Obstructed labor due to generally contracted pelvis ♀   M

   O65.2 Obstructed labor due to pelvic inlet contraction ♀   M

   O65.3 Obstructed labor due to pelvic outlet and mid-cavity contraction ♀   M

   O65.4 Obstructed labor due to fetopelvic disproportion, unspecified ♀   M
     Excludes1   dystocia due to abnormality of fetus (O66.2-O66.3)

   O65.5 Obstructed labor due to abnormality of maternal pelvic organs ♀   M
     Obstructed labor due to conditions listed in O34.-
     Use additional code to identify abnormality of pelvic organs O34.-

   O65.8 Obstructed labor due to other maternal pelvic abnormalities ♀   M

   O65.9 Obstructed labor due to maternal pelvic abnormality, unspecified ♀   M

● **O66 Other obstructed labor**

   O66.0 Obstructed labor due to shoulder dystocia ♀   M
     Impacted shoulders

   O66.1 Obstructed labor due to locked twins ♀   M

   O66.2 Obstructed labor due to unusually large fetus ♀   M

   O66.3 Obstructed labor due to other abnormalities of fetus ♀   M
     Dystocia due to fetal ascites
     Dystocia due to fetal hydrops
     Dystocia due to fetal meningomyelocele
     Dystocia due to fetal sacral teratoma
     Dystocia due to fetal tumor
     Dystocia due to hydrocephalic fetus
     Use additional code to identify cause of obstruction

● **O66.4 Failed trial of labor**

     O66.40 Failed trial of labor, unspecified ♀   M

     O66.41 Failed attempted vaginal birth after previous cesarean delivery ♀   M
         Code first rupture of uterus, if applicable (O71.0-, O71.1)

   O66.5 Attempted application of vacuum extractor and forceps ♀   M
     Attempted application of vacuum or forceps, with subsequent delivery by forceps or cesarean delivery

   O66.6 Obstructed labor due to other multiple fetuses ♀   M

   O66.8 Other specified obstructed labor ♀   M
     Use additional code to identify cause of obstruction

   O66.9 Obstructed labor, unspecified ♀   M
     Dystocia NOS
     Fetal dystocia NOS
     Maternal dystocia NOS

● **O67 Labor and delivery complicated by intrapartum hemorrhage, not elsewhere classified**

     Excludes1   antepartum hemorrhage NEC (O46.-)
                    placenta previa (O44.-)
                    premature separation of placenta [abruptio placentae] (O45.-)

     Excludes2   postpartum hemorrhage (O72.-)

   O67.0 Intrapartum hemorrhage with coagulation defect ♀   M
     Intrapartum hemorrhage (excessive) associated with afibrinogenemia
     Intrapartum hemorrhage (excessive) associated with disseminated intravascular coagulation
     Intrapartum hemorrhage (excessive) associated with hyperfibrinolysis
     Intrapartum hemorrhage (excessive) associated with hypofibrinogenemia

   O67.8 Other intrapartum hemorrhage ♀   M
     Excessive intrapartum hemorrhage

   O67.9 Intrapartum hemorrhage, unspecified ♀   M

  O68 Labor and delivery complicated by abnormality of fetal acid-base balance ♀   M
     Fetal acidemia complicating labor and delivery
     Fetal acidosis complicating labor and delivery
     Fetal alkalosis complicating labor and delivery
     Fetal metabolic acidemia complicating labor and delivery

     Excludes1   fetal stress NOS (O77.9)
                    labor and delivery complicated by electrocardiographic evidence of fetal stress (O77.8)
                    labor and delivery complicated by ultrasonic evidence of fetal stress (O77.8)

     Excludes2   abnormality in fetal heart rate or rhythm (O76)
                    labor and delivery complicated by meconium in amniotic fluid (O77.0)

CHAPTER 15 (O00-O9A)

● O69 Labor and delivery complicated by umbilical cord complications

One of the following 7th characters is to be assigned to each code under category O69. 7th character 0 is for single gestations and multiple gestations where the fetus is unspecified. 7th characters 1 through 9 are for cases of multiple gestations to identify the fetus for which the code applies. The appropriate code from category O30, Multiple gestation, must also be assigned when assigning a code from category O69 that has a 7th character of 1 through 9.

0	not applicable or unspecified
1	fetus 1
2	fetus 2
3	fetus 3
4	fetus 4
5	fetus 5
9	other fetus

X ● **O69.0 Labor and delivery complicated by prolapse of cord** ♀   M

X ● **O69.1 Labor and delivery complicated by cord around neck, with compression** ♀   M

> **Excludes1** labor and delivery complicated by cord around neck, without compression (O69.81)

X ● **O69.2 Labor and delivery complicated by other cord entanglement, with compression** ♀   M
> Labor and delivery complicated by compression of cord NOS
> Labor and delivery complicated by entanglement of cords of twins in monoamniotic sac
> Labor and delivery complicated by knot in cord
>
> **Excludes1** labor and delivery complicated by other cord entanglement, without compression (O69.82)

X ● **O69.3 Labor and delivery complicated by short cord** ♀   M

X ● **O69.4 Labor and delivery complicated by vasa previa** ♀   M
> Labor and delivery complicated by hemorrhage from vasa previa

X ● **O69.5 Labor and delivery complicated by vascular lesion of cord** ♀   M
> Labor and delivery complicated by cord bruising
> Labor and delivery complicated by cord hematoma
> Labor and delivery complicated by thrombosis of umbilical vessels

● **O69.8 Labor and delivery complicated by other cord complications**

> X ● **O69.81 Labor and delivery complicated by cord around neck, without compression** ♀   M

> X ● **O69.82 Labor and delivery complicated by other cord entanglement, without compression** ♀   M

> X ● **O69.89 Labor and delivery complicated by other cord complications** ♀   M

X ● **O69.9 Labor and delivery complicated by cord complication, unspecified** ♀   M

● O70 Perineal laceration during delivery

> **Includes** episiotomy extended by laceration
> **Excludes1** obstetric high vaginal laceration alone (O71.4)

O70.0 First degree perineal laceration during delivery ♀   M
> Perineal laceration, rupture or tear involving fourchette during delivery
> Perineal laceration, rupture or tear involving labia during delivery
> Perineal laceration, rupture or tear involving skin during delivery
> Perineal laceration, rupture or tear involving vagina during delivery
> Perineal laceration, rupture or tear involving vulva during delivery
> Slight perineal laceration, rupture or tear during delivery

Figure 15-6 Perineal lacerations: **A.** First-degree is laceration of superficial tissues. **B.** Second-degree is limited to the pelvic floor and may involve the perineal or vaginal muscles. **C.** Third-degree involves the anal sphincter. **D.** Fourth-degree involves anal or rectal mucosa.

O70.1 Second degree perineal laceration during delivery ♀   M
> Perineal laceration, rupture or tear during delivery as in O70.0, also involving pelvic floor
> Perineal laceration, rupture or tear during delivery as in O70.0, also involving perineal muscles
> Perineal laceration, rupture or tear during delivery as in O70.0, also involving vaginal muscles
>
> **Excludes1** perineal laceration involving anal sphincter (O70.2)
>
> **Coding Clinic: 2016, CODING CIQ4, P53, Q2, P34**

● **O70.2 Third degree perineal laceration during delivery**
> Perineal laceration, rupture or tear during delivery as in O70.1, also involving anal sphincter
> Perineal laceration, rupture or tear during delivery as in O70.1, also involving rectovaginal septum
> Perineal laceration, rupture or tear during delivery as in O70.1, also involving sphincter NOS
>
> **Excludes1** anal sphincter tear during delivery without third degree perineal laceration (O70.4)
> perineal laceration involving anal or rectal mucosa (O70.3)

> **O70.20 Third degree perineal laceration during delivery, unspecified** ♀   M

> **O70.21 Third degree perineal laceration during delivery, IIIa** ♀   M
> > Third degree perineal laceration during delivery with less than 50% of external anal sphincter (EAS) thickness torn

> **O70.22 Third degree perineal laceration during delivery, IIIb** ♀   M
> > Third degree perineal laceration during delivery with more than 50% external anal sphincter (EAS) thickness torn

> **O70.23 Third degree perineal laceration during delivery, IIIc** ♀   M
> > Third degree perineal laceration during delivery with both external anal sphincter (EAS) and internal anal sphincter (IAS) torn

O70.3 Fourth degree perineal laceration during delivery ♀   M
> Perineal laceration, rupture or tear during delivery as in O70.2, also involving anal mucosa
> Perineal laceration, rupture or tear during delivery as in O70.2, also involving rectal mucosa

O70.4 Anal sphincter tear complicating delivery, not associated with third degree laceration ♀   M
> **Excludes1** anal sphincter tear with third degree perineal laceration (O70.2)

O70.9 Perineal laceration during delivery, unspecified ♀   M

CHAPTER 15 (O00-O9A)

▶ New   ⇒ Revised   ~~deleted~~ Deleted   Excludes 1   Excludes 2   Includes   Use additional   Code first   Code also   Key words

OGCR Official Guidelines   X Assign placeholder X   ● Use Additional Character(s)   ▶ Manifestation Code   🝔 Hierarchical Condition Category   **Coding Clinic**

● **O71   Other obstetric trauma**

     Includes   obstetric damage from instruments

 ● **O71.0   Rupture of uterus (spontaneous) before onset of labor**

       Excludes1   disruption of (current) cesarean delivery wound (O90.0)

                  laceration of uterus, NEC (O71.81)

       O71.00   Rupture of uterus before onset of labor, unspecified trimester ♀   M

       O71.02   Rupture of uterus before onset of labor, second trimester ♀   M

       O71.03   Rupture of uterus before onset of labor, third trimester ♀   M

    O71.1   Rupture of uterus during labor ♀   M

       Rupture of uterus not stated as occurring before onset of labor

       Excludes1   disruption of cesarean delivery wound (O90.0)

                  laceration of uterus, NEC (O71.81)

    O71.2   Postpartum inversion of uterus ♀   M

    O71.3   Obstetric laceration of cervix ♀   M

       Annular detachment of cervix

    O71.4   Obstetric high vaginal laceration alone ♀   M

       Laceration of vaginal wall without perineal laceration

       Excludes1   obstetric high vaginal laceration with perineal laceration (O70.-)

    O71.5   Other obstetric injury to pelvic organs ♀   M

       Obstetric injury to bladder

       Obstetric injury to urethra

       Excludes2   obstetric periurethral trauma (O71.82)

    O71.6   Obstetric damage to pelvic joints and ligaments ♀   M

       Obstetric avulsion of inner symphyseal cartilage

       Obstetric damage to coccyx

       Obstetric traumatic separation of symphysis (pubis)

    O71.7   Obstetric hematoma of pelvis ♀   M

       Obstetric hematoma of perineum

       Obstetric hematoma of vagina

       Obstetric hematoma of vulva

 ● **O71.8   Other specified obstetric trauma**

       O71.81   Laceration of uterus, not elsewhere classified ♀   M

       O71.82   Other specified trauma to perineum and vulva ♀   M

              ♀

              Obstetric periurethral trauma

       O71.89   Other specified obstetric trauma ♀   M

    O71.9   Obstetric trauma, unspecified ♀   M

● **O72   Postpartum hemorrhage**

     Includes   hemorrhage after delivery of fetus or infant

    O72.0   Third-stage hemorrhage ♀   M

       Hemorrhage associated with retained, trapped or adherent placenta

       Retained placenta NOS

       Code also type of adherent placenta (O43.2-)

    O72.1   Other immediate postpartum hemorrhage ♀   M

       Hemorrhage following delivery of placenta

       Postpartum hemorrhage (atonic) NOS

       Uterine atony with hemorrhage

       Excludes1   uterine atony NOS (O62.2)

                  uterine atony without hemorrhage (O62.2)

                  postpartum atony of uterus without hemorrhage (O75.89)

    O72.2   Delayed and secondary postpartum hemorrhage ♀   M

       Hemorrhage associated with retained portions of placenta or membranes after the first 24 hours following delivery of placenta

       Retained products of conception NOS, following delivery

    O72.3   Postpartum coagulation defects ♀   M

       Postpartum afibrinogenemia

       Postpartum fibrinolysis

● **O73   Retained placenta and membranes, without hemorrhage**

     Excludes1   placenta accreta (O43.21-)

               placenta increta (O43.22-)

               placenta percreta (O43.23-)

    O73.0   Retained placenta without hemorrhage ♀   M

       Adherent placenta, without hemorrhage

       Trapped placenta without hemorrhage

    O73.1   Retained portions of placenta and membranes, without hemorrhage ♀   M

       Retained products of conception following delivery, without hemorrhage

● **O74   Complications of anesthesia during labor and delivery**

     Includes   maternal complications arising from the administration of a general, regional or local anesthetic, analgesic or other sedation during labor and delivery

    Use additional code, if applicable, to identify specific complication

    O74.0   Aspiration pneumonitis due to anesthesia during labor and delivery ♀   M

       Inhalation of stomach contents or secretions NOS due to anesthesia during labor and delivery

       Mendelson's syndrome due to anesthesia during labor and delivery

    O74.1   Other pulmonary complications of anesthesia during labor and delivery ♀   M

    O74.2   Cardiac complications of anesthesia during labor and delivery ♀   M

    O74.3   Central nervous system complications of anesthesia during labor and delivery ♀   M

    O74.4   Toxic reaction to local anesthesia during labor and delivery ♀   M

    O74.5   Spinal and epidural anesthesia-induced headache during labor and delivery ♀   M

    O74.6   Other complications of spinal and epidural anesthesia during labor and delivery ♀   M

    O74.7   Failed or difficult intubation for anesthesia during labor and delivery ♀   M

    O74.8   Other complications of anesthesia during labor and delivery ♀   M

    O74.9   Complication of anesthesia during labor and delivery, unspecified ♀   M

● **O75   Other complications of labor and delivery, not elsewhere classified**

     Excludes2   puerperal (postpartum) infection (O86.-)

               puerperal (postpartum) sepsis (O85)

    O75.0   Maternal distress during labor and delivery ♀   M

    O75.1   Shock during or following labor and delivery ♀   M

       Obstetric shock following labor and delivery

    O75.2   Pyrexia during labor, not elsewhere classified ♀   M

    O75.3   Other infection during labor ♀   M

       Sepsis during labor

       Use additional code (B95-B97), to identify infectious agent

    O75.4   Other complications of obstetric surgery and procedures ♀   M

       Cardiac arrest following obstetric surgery or procedures

       Cardiac failure following obstetric surgery or procedures

       Cerebral anoxia following obstetric surgery or procedures

       Pulmonary edema following obstetric surgery or procedures

       Use additional code to identify specific complication

       Excludes2   complications of anesthesia during labor and delivery (O74.-)

                 disruption of obstetrical (surgical) wound (O90.0-O90.1)

                 hematoma of obstetrical (surgical) wound (O90.2)

                 infection of obstetrical (surgical) wound (O86.0-)

CHAPTER 15 (O00-O9A)

O75.5   **Delayed delivery after artificial rupture of membranes** ♀   M

● **O75.8**   **Other specified complications of labor and delivery**

     O75.81   **Maternal exhaustion complicating labor and delivery** ♀   M

     O75.82   **Onset (spontaneous) of labor after 37 completed weeks of gestation but before 39 completed weeks gestation, with delivery by (planned) cesarean section** ♀   M

         Delivery by (planned) cesarean section occurring after 37 completed weeks of gestation but before 39 completed weeks gestation due to (spontaneous) onset of labor

         Code first to specify reason for planned cesarean section such as:
            cephalopelvic disproportion (normally formed fetus) (O33.9)
            previous cesarean delivery (O34.21)
         Coding Clinic: 2022, Q2, P3-4

     O75.89   **Other specified complications of labor and delivery** ♀   M

   O75.9   **Complication of labor and delivery, unspecified** ♀   M

O76   **Abnormality in fetal heart rate and rhythm complicating labor and delivery** ♀   M

     Depressed fetal heart rate tones complicating labor and delivery
     Fetal bradycardia complicating labor and delivery
     Fetal heart rate decelerations complicating labor and delivery
     Fetal heart rate irregularity complicating labor and delivery
     Fetal heart rate abnormal variability complicating labor and delivery
     Fetal tachycardia complicating labor and delivery
     Non-reassuring fetal heart rate or rhythm complicating labor and delivery

     Excludes1   fetal stress NOS (O77.9)
            labor and delivery complicated by electrocardiographic evidence of fetal stress (O77.8)
            labor and delivery complicated by ultrasonic evidence of fetal stress (O77.8)

     Excludes2   fetal metabolic acidemia (O68)
            other fetal stress (O77.0-O77.1)

● **O77**   **Other fetal stress complicating labor and delivery**

   O77.0   **Labor and delivery complicated by meconium in amniotic fluid** ♀   M

   O77.1   **Fetal stress in labor or delivery due to drug administration** ♀   M
         Coding Clinic: 2022, Q2, P16

   O77.8   **Labor and delivery complicated by other evidence of fetal stress** ♀   M

     Labor and delivery complicated by electrocardiographic evidence of fetal stress
     Labor and delivery complicated by ultrasonic evidence of fetal stress

     Excludes1   abnormality of fetal acid-base balance (O68)
            abnormality in fetal heart rate or rhythm (O76)
            fetal metabolic acidemia (O68)

   O77.9   **Labor and delivery complicated by fetal stress, unspecified** ♀   M

     Excludes1   abnormality of fetal acid-base balance (O68)
            abnormality in fetal heart rate or rhythm (O76)
            fetal metabolic acidemia (O68)

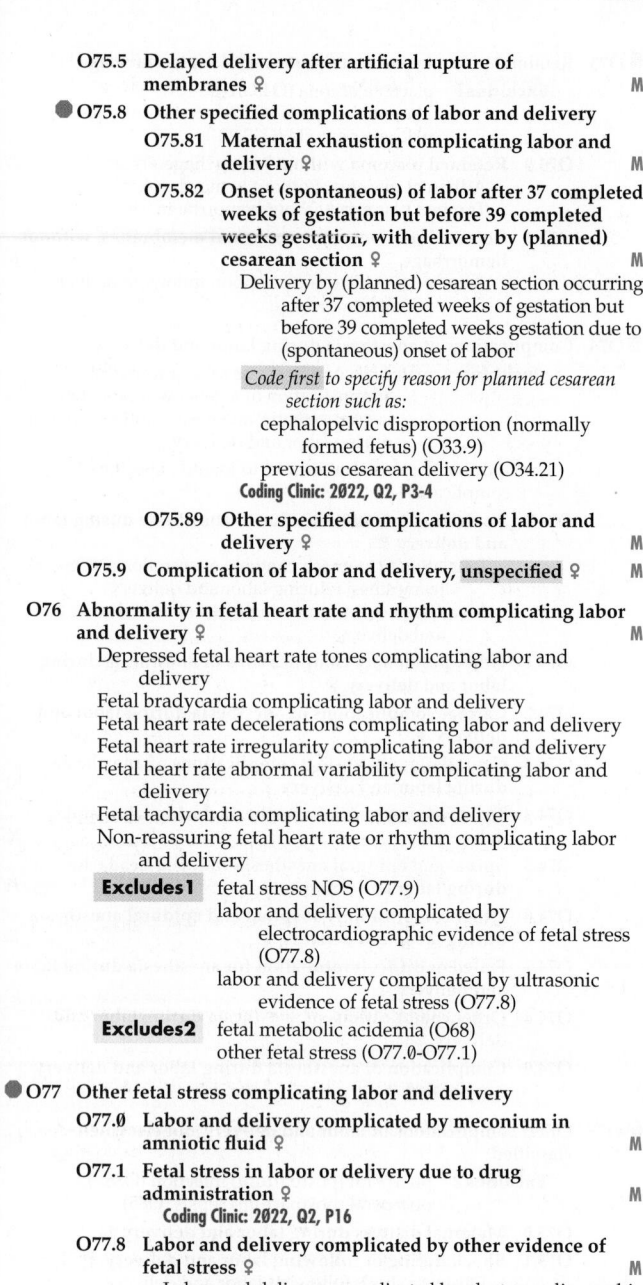

Figure 15-7   The four stages of normal delivery: **I.** Lightening, which occurs 2 to 4 weeks before birth, at which time the fetus turns with head toward the vagina. **II.** Regular contractions begin, the amniotic sac ruptures, and dilation is complete. **III.** Delivery of the head and rotation. **IV.** Expulsion of placenta.

OGCR Section I.C., Chapter 15.n.

Normal Delivery, Code O80

1) Encounter for full-term uncomplicated delivery

Code O80 should be assigned when a woman is admitted for a full-term normal delivery and delivers a single, healthy infant without any complications antepartum, during the delivery, or postpartum during the delivery episode. Code O80 is always a principal diagnosis. It is not to be used if any other code from Chapter 15 is needed to describe a current complication of the antenatal, delivery, or perinatal period. Additional codes from other chapters may be used with code O80 if they are not related to or are in any way complicating the pregnancy.

2) Uncomplicated delivery with resolved antepartum complication

Code O80 may be used if the patient had a complication at some point during the pregnancy, but the complication is not present at the time of the admission for delivery.

3) Outcome of delivery for O80

Z37.0, Single live brith, is the only outcome of delivery code appropriate for use with O80.

ENCOUNTER FOR DELIVERY (O80-O82)

O80   **Encounter for full-term uncomplicated delivery** ♀   M

     Delivery requiring minimal or no assistance, with or without episiotomy, without fetal manipulation [e.g., rotation version] or instrumentation [forceps] of a spontaneous, cephalic, vaginal, full-term, single, live-born infant. This code is for use as a single diagnosis code and is not to be used with any other code from Chapter 15.

     Use additional code to indicate outcome of delivery (Z37.0)
     Coding Clinic: 2016, Q4, P124, 150

O82   **Encounter for cesarean delivery without indication** ♀   M

     Use additional code to indicate outcome of delivery (Z37.0)

CHAPTER 15 (O00-O9A)

▶ New   ⏵ Revised   ~~deleted~~ Deleted   Excludes 1   Excludes 2   Includes   Use additional   Code first   Code also   Key words
OGCR Official Guidelines   X Assign placeholder X   ● Use Additional Character(s)   ▶ Manifestation Code   🝔 Hierarchical Condition Category   **Coding Clinic**

COMPLICATIONS PREDOMINANTLY RELATED TO THE PUERPERIUM (O85-O92)

Excludes2   mental and behavioral disorders associated with the puerperium (F53.-)
obstetrical tetanus (A34)
puerperal osteomalacia (M83.0)

O85 Puerperal sepsis ♀   M
Postpartum sepsis
Puerperal peritonitis
Puerperal pyemia
Use additional code (B95-B97), to identify infectious agent
Use additional code (R65.2-) to identify severe sepsis, if applicable

Excludes1   fever of unknown origin following delivery (O86.4)
genital tract infection following delivery (O86.1-)
obstetric pyemic and septic embolism (O88.3-)
puerperal septic thrombophlebitis (O86.81)
urinary tract infection following delivery (O86.2-)

Excludes2   sepsis during labor (O75.3)
Coding Clinic: 2022, Q2, P5; 2018, Q4, P23

● O86 Other puerperal infections
Use additional code (B95-B97), to identify infectious agent

Excludes2   infection during labor (O75.3)
obstetrical tetanus (A34)

● O86.0 Infection of obstetric surgical wound
Infected cesarean delivery wound following delivery
Infected perineal repair following delivery

Excludes1   complications of procedures, not elsewhere classified (T81.44)
postprocedural fever NOS (R50.82)
postprocedural retroperitoneal abscess (K68.11)

O86.00   Infection of obstetric surgical wound, unspecified ♀   M

O86.01   Infection of obstetric surgical wound, superficial incisional site ♀   M
Subcutaneous abscess following an obstetrical procedure
Stitch abscess following an obstetrical procedure

O86.02   Infection of obstetric surgical wound, deep incisional site ♀   M
Intramuscular abscess following an obstetrical procedure
Sub-fascial abscess following an obstetrical procedure
Coding Clinic: 2018, Q4, P23

O86.03   Infection of obstetric surgical wound, organ and space site ♀   M
Intraabdominal abscess following an obstetrical procedure
Subphrenic abscess following an obstetrical procedure

O86.04   Sepsis following an obstetrical procedure ♀   M
Use additional code to identify the sepsis

O86.09   Infection of obstetric surgical wound, other surgical site ♀   M

● O86.1 Other infection of genital tract following delivery
O86.11   Cervicitis following delivery ♀   M
O86.12   Endometritis following delivery ♀   M
O86.13   Vaginitis following delivery ♀   M
O86.19   Other infection of genital tract following delivery ♀   M

● O86.2 Urinary tract infection following delivery
O86.20   Urinary tract infection following delivery, unspecified ♀   M
Puerperal urinary tract infection NOS
Coding Clinic: 2022, Q2, P5
O86.21   Infection of kidney following delivery ♀   M

O86.22   Infection of bladder following delivery ♀   M
Infection of urethra following delivery
O86.29   Other urinary tract infection following delivery ♀   M

O86.4   Pyrexia of unknown origin following delivery ♀   M
Puerperal infection NOS following delivery
Puerperal pyrexia NOS following delivery
Excludes2   pyrexia during labor (O75.2)

● O86.8 Other specified puerperal infections
O86.81   Puerperal septic thrombophlebitis ♀   M
O86.89   Other specified puerperal infections ♀   M

● O87 Venous complications and hemorrhoids in the puerperium
Includes   venous complications in labor, delivery and the puerperium
Excludes2   obstetric embolism (O88.-)
puerperal septic thrombophlebitis (O86.81)
venous complications in pregnancy (O22.-)

O87.0   Superficial thrombophlebitis in the puerperium ♀   M
Puerperal phlebitis NOS
Puerperal thrombosis NOS

O87.1   Deep phlebothrombosis in the puerperium ♀   M
Deep vein thrombosis, postpartum
Pelvic thrombophlebitis, postpartum
Use additional code to identify the deep vein thrombosis (I82.4-, I82.5-, I82.62-, I82.72-)
Use additional code, if applicable, for associated long-term (current) use of anticoagulants (Z79.01)

O87.2   Hemorrhoids in the puerperium   M
O87.3   Cerebral venous thrombosis in the puerperium ♀   M
Cerebrovenous sinus thrombosis in the puerperium
O87.4   Varicose veins of lower extremity in the puerperium ♀   M
O87.8   Other venous complications in the puerperium ♀   M
Genital varices in the puerperium
O87.9   Venous complication in the puerperium, unspecified ♀   M
Puerperal phlebopathy NOS

O88 Obstetric embolism
Excludes1   embolism complicating abortion NOS (O03.2)
embolism complicating ectopic or molar pregnancy (O08.2)
embolism complicating failed attempted abortion (O07.2)
embolism complicating induced abortion (O04.7)
embolism complicating spontaneous abortion (O03.2, O03.7)

● O88.0 Obstetric air embolism
● O88.01 Obstetric air embolism in pregnancy
O88.011   Air embolism in pregnancy, first trimester ♀   M
O88.012   Air embolism in pregnancy, second trimester ♀   M
O88.013   Air embolism in pregnancy, third trimester ♀   M
O88.019   Air embolism in pregnancy, unspecified trimester ♀   M
O88.02   Air embolism in childbirth ♀   M
O88.03   Air embolism in the puerperium ♀   M

● O88.1 Amniotic fluid embolism
Anaphylactoid syndrome in pregnancy
● O88.11 Amniotic fluid embolism in pregnancy
O88.111   Amniotic fluid embolism in pregnancy, first trimester ♀   M
O88.112   Amniotic fluid embolism in pregnancy, second trimester ♀   M
O88.113   Amniotic fluid embolism in pregnancy, third trimester ♀   M
O88.119   Amniotic fluid embolism in pregnancy, unspecified trimester ♀   M
O88.12   Amniotic fluid embolism in childbirth ♀   M
O88.13   Amniotic fluid embolism in the puerperium ♀   M

CHAPTER 15 (O00-O9A)

● **O88.2 Obstetric thromboembolism**
  ● **O88.21 Thromboembolism in pregnancy**
    Obstetric (pulmonary) embolism NOS
    O88.211 Thromboembolism in pregnancy, first trimester ♀   M
    O88.212 Thromboembolism in pregnancy, second trimester ♀   M
    O88.213 Thromboembolism in pregnancy, third trimester ♀   M
    O88.219 Thromboembolism in pregnancy, unspecified trimester ♀   M
  O88.22 Thromboembolism in childbirth ♀   M
  O88.23 Thromboembolism in the puerperium ♀   M
    Puerperal (pulmonary) embolism NOS

● **O88.3 Obstetric pyemic and septic embolism**
  ● **O88.31 Pyemic and septic embolism in pregnancy**
    O88.311 Pyemic and septic embolism in pregnancy, first trimester ♀   M
    O88.312 Pyemic and septic embolism in pregnancy, second trimester ♀   M
    O88.313 Pyemic and septic embolism in pregnancy, third trimester ♀   M
    O88.319 Pyemic and septic embolism in pregnancy, unspecified trimester ♀   M
  O88.32 Pyemic and septic embolism in childbirth ♀   M
  O88.33 Pyemic and septic embolism in the puerperium ♀   M

● **O88.8 Other obstetric embolism**
  Obstetric fat embolism
  ● **O88.81 Other embolism in pregnancy**
    O88.811 Other embolism in pregnancy, first trimester ♀   M
    O88.812 Other embolism in pregnancy, second trimester ♀   M
    O88.813 Other embolism in pregnancy, third trimester ♀   M
    O88.819 Other embolism in pregnancy, unspecified trimester ♀   M
  O88.82 Other embolism in childbirth ♀   M
  O88.83 Other embolism in the puerperium ♀   M

● **O89 Complications of anesthesia during the puerperium**
  Includes maternal complications arising from the administration of a general, regional or local anesthetic, analgesic or other sedation during the puerperium
  Use additional code, if applicable, to identify specific complication
  ● **O89.0 Pulmonary complications of anesthesia during the puerperium**
    O89.01 Aspiration pneumonitis due to anesthesia during the puerperium ♀   M
    Inhalation of stomach contents or secretions NOS due to anesthesia during the puerperium
    Mendelson's syndrome due to anesthesia during the puerperium
    O89.09 Other pulmonary complications of anesthesia during the puerperium ♀   M
  O89.1 Cardiac complications of anesthesia during the puerperium ♀   M
  O89.2 Central nervous system complications of anesthesia during the puerperium ♀   M
  O89.3 Toxic reaction to local anesthesia during the puerperium ♀   M
  O89.4 Spinal and epidural anesthesia-induced headache during the puerperium ♀   M
  O89.5 Other complications of spinal and epidural anesthesia during the puerperium ♀   M
  O89.6 Failed or difficult intubation for anesthesia during the puerperium ♀   M
  O89.8 Other complications of anesthesia during the puerperium ♀   M

O89.9 Complication of anesthesia during the puerperium, unspecified ♀   M

● **O90 Complications of the puerperium, not elsewhere classified**
  O90.0 Disruption of cesarean delivery wound ♀   M
    Dehiscence of cesarean delivery wound
    Excludes1 rupture of uterus (spontaneous) before onset of labor (O71.0-)
           rupture of uterus during labor (O71.1)
  O90.1 Disruption of perineal obstetric wound ♀   M
    Disruption of wound of episiotomy
    Disruption of wound of perineal laceration
    Secondary perineal tear
  O90.2 Hematoma of obstetric wound ♀   M
  O90.3 Peripartum cardiomyopathy ♀   M
    Conditions in I42.- arising during pregnancy and the puerperium
    Excludes1 pre-existing heart disease complicating pregnancy and the puerperium (O99.4-)
  O90.4 Postpartum acute kidney failure ♀   M
    Hepatorenal syndrome following labor and delivery
  O90.5 Postpartum thyroiditis ♀   M
  O90.6 Postpartum mood disturbance ♀   M
    Postpartum blues   Postpartum sadness
    Postpartum dysphoria
    Excludes1 postpartum depression (F53.0)
           puerperal psychosis (F53.1)
  ● **O90.8 Other complications of the puerperium, not elsewhere classified**
    O90.81 Anemia of the puerperium ♀   M
    Postpartum anemia NOS
    Excludes1 pre-existing anemia complicating the puerperium (O99.03)
    O90.89 Other complications of the puerperium, not elsewhere classified ♀   M
    Placental polyp
  O90.9 Complication of the puerperium, unspecified ♀   M

● **O91 Infections of breast associated with pregnancy, the puerperium and lactation**
  Use additional code to identify infection
  ● **O91.0 Infection of nipple associated with pregnancy, the puerperium and lactation**
    ● **O91.01 Infection of nipple associated with pregnancy**
      Gestational abscess of nipple
      O91.011 Infection of nipple associated with pregnancy, first trimester ♀   M
      O91.012 Infection of nipple associated with pregnancy, second trimester ♀   M
      O91.013 Infection of nipple associated with pregnancy, third trimester ♀   M
      O91.019 Infection of nipple associated with pregnancy, unspecified trimester ♀   M
    O91.02 Infection of nipple associated with the puerperium ♀   M
      Puerperal abscess of nipple
    O91.03 Infection of nipple associated with lactation ♀ M
      Abscess of nipple associated with lactation
  ● **O91.1 Abscess of breast associated with pregnancy, the puerperium and lactation**
    ● **O91.11 Abscess of breast associated with pregnancy**
      Gestational mammary abscess
      Gestational purulent mastitis
      Gestational subareolar abscess
      O91.111 Abscess of breast associated with pregnancy, first trimester ♀   M
      O91.112 Abscess of breast associated with pregnancy, second trimester ♀   M
      O91.113 Abscess of breast associated with pregnancy, third trimester ♀   M
      O91.119 Abscess of breast associated with pregnancy, unspecified trimester ♀   M

▶ New   ⇒ Revised   ~~deleted~~ Deleted   Excludes 1   Excludes 2   Includes   Use additional   Code first   Code also   Key words
OGCR Official Guidelines   **X** Assign placeholder X   ● Use Additional Character(s)   ▷ Manifestation Code   🔖 Hierarchical Condition Category   **Coding Clinic**

O91.12   Abscess of breast associated with the puerperium ♀   M
     Puerperal mammary abscess
     Puerperal purulent mastitis
     Puerperal subareolar abscess

O91.13   Abscess of breast associated with lactation ♀   M
     Mammary abscess associated with lactation
     Purulent mastitis associated with lactation
     Subareolar abscess associated with lactation

● **O91.2**   Nonpurulent mastitis associated with pregnancy, the puerperium and lactation

   ● **O91.21**   Nonpurulent mastitis associated with pregnancy
     Gestational interstitial mastitis
     Gestational lymphangitis of breast
     Gestational mastitis NOS
     Gestational parenchymatous mastitis

     O91.211   Nonpurulent mastitis associated with pregnancy, first trimester ♀   M

     O91.212   Nonpurulent mastitis associated with pregnancy, second trimester ♀   M

     O91.213   Nonpurulent mastitis associated with pregnancy, third trimester ♀   M

     O91.219   Nonpurulent mastitis associated with pregnancy, unspecified trimester ♀   M

   O91.22   Nonpurulent mastitis associated with the puerperium ♀   M
     Puerperal interstitial mastitis
     Puerperal lymphangitis of breast
     Puerperal mastitis NOS
     Puerperal parenchymatous mastitis

   O91.23   Nonpurulent mastitis associated with lactation ♀   M
     Interstitial mastitis associated with lactation
     Lymphangitis of breast associated with lactation
     Mastitis NOS associated with lactation
     Parenchymatous mastitis associated with lactation

● **O92**   Other disorders of breast and disorders of lactation associated with pregnancy and the puerperium

   ● **O92.0**   Retracted nipple associated with pregnancy, the puerperium, and lactation

     ● **O92.01**   Retracted nipple associated with pregnancy

       O92.011   Retracted nipple associated with pregnancy, first trimester ♀   M

       O92.012   Retracted nipple associated with pregnancy, second trimester ♀   M

       O92.013   Retracted nipple associated with pregnancy, third trimester ♀   M

       O92.019   Retracted nipple associated with pregnancy, unspecified trimester ♀   M

     O92.02   Retracted nipple associated with the puerperium ♀   M

     O92.03   Retracted nipple associated with lactation ♀   M

   ● **O92.1**   Cracked nipple associated with pregnancy, the puerperium, and lactation
     Fissure of nipple, gestational or puerperal

     ● **O92.11**   Cracked nipple associated with pregnancy

       O92.111   Cracked nipple associated with pregnancy, first trimester ♀   M

       O92.112   Cracked nipple associated with pregnancy, second trimester ♀   M

       O92.113   Cracked nipple associated with pregnancy, third trimester ♀   M

       O92.119   Cracked nipple associated with pregnancy, unspecified trimester ♀   M

     O92.12   Cracked nipple associated with the puerperium ♀   M

     O92.13   Cracked nipple associated with lactation ♀   M

● **O92.2**   Other and unspecified disorders of breast associated with pregnancy and the puerperium

     O92.20   Unspecified disorder of breast associated with pregnancy and the puerperium ♀   M

     O92.29   Other disorders of breast associated with pregnancy and the puerperium ♀   M

   O92.3   Agalactia ♀   M
     Primary agalactia

     Excludes1   elective agalactia (O92.5)
                secondary agalactia (O92.5)
                therapeutic agalactia (O92.5)

   O92.4   Hypogalactia ♀   M

   O92.5   Suppressed lactation ♀   M
     Elective agalactia   Therapeutic agalactia
     Secondary agalactia

     Excludes1   primary agalactia (O92.3)

   O92.6   Galactorrhea ♀   M

   ● **O92.7**   Other and unspecified disorders of lactation

     O92.70   Unspecified disorders of lactation ♀   M

     O92.79   Other disorders of lactation ♀   M
       Puerperal galactocele

OTHER OBSTETRIC CONDITIONS, NOT ELSEWHERE CLASSIFIED (O94–O9A)

O94   Sequelae of complication of pregnancy, childbirth, and the puerperium ♀   M

   Note: This category is to be used to indicate conditions in O00–O77.-, O85–O94 and O98–O9A.- as the cause of late effects. The "sequelae" include conditions specified as such, or as late effects, which may occur at any time after the puerperium.

   Code first condition resulting from (sequela) of complication of pregnancy, childbirth, and the puerperium

O98   Maternal infectious and parasitic diseases classifiable elsewhere but complicating pregnancy, childbirth and the puerperium

   Includes   the listed conditions when complicating the pregnant state, when aggravated by the pregnancy, or as a reason for obstetric care

   Use additional code (Chapter 1), to identify specific infectious or parasitic disease

   Excludes2   herpes gestationis (O26.4-)
               infectious carrier state (O99.82-, O99.83-)
               obstetrical tetanus (A34)
               puerperal infection (O86.-)
               puerperal sepsis (O85)
               when the reason for maternal care is that the disease is known or suspected to have affected the fetus (O35–O36)

   ● **O98.0**   Tuberculosis complicating pregnancy, childbirth and the puerperium
     Conditions in A15–A19

     ● **O98.01**   Tuberculosis complicating pregnancy

       O98.011   Tuberculosis complicating pregnancy, first trimester ♀   M

       O98.012   Tuberculosis complicating pregnancy, second trimester ♀   M

       O98.013   Tuberculosis complicating pregnancy, third trimester ♀   M

       O98.019   Tuberculosis complicating pregnancy, unspecified trimester ♀   M

     O98.02   Tuberculosis complicating childbirth ♀   M

     O98.03   Tuberculosis complicating the puerperium ♀   M

   ● **O98.1**   Syphilis complicating pregnancy, childbirth and the puerperium
     Conditions in A50–A53

     ● **O98.11**   Syphilis complicating pregnancy

       O98.111   Syphilis complicating pregnancy, first trimester ♀   M

       O98.112   Syphilis complicating pregnancy, second trimester ♀   M

CHAPTER 15 (O00–O9A)

O98.113   Syphilis complicating pregnancy, third trimester ♀   M

O98.119   Syphilis complicating pregnancy, unspecified trimester ♀   M

O98.12   Syphilis complicating childbirth ♀   M

O98.13   Syphilis complicating the puerperium ♀   M

● O98.2   **Gonorrhea complicating pregnancy, childbirth and the puerperium**
Conditions in A54.-

● O98.21   Gonorrhea complicating pregnancy

O98.211   Gonorrhea complicating pregnancy, first trimester ♀   M

O98.212   Gonorrhea complicating pregnancy, second trimester ♀   M

O98.213   Gonorrhea complicating pregnancy, third trimester ♀   M

O98.219   Gonorrhea complicating pregnancy, unspecified trimester ♀   M

O98.22   Gonorrhea complicating childbirth ♀   M

O98.23   Gonorrhea complicating the puerperium ♀   M

● O98.3   **Other infections with a predominantly sexual mode of transmission complicating pregnancy, childbirth and the puerperium**
Conditions in A55-A64

● O98.31   Other infections with a predominantly sexual mode of transmission complicating pregnancy

O98.311   Other infections with a predominantly sexual mode of transmission complicating pregnancy, first trimester ♀   M

O98.312   Other infections with a predominantly sexual mode of transmission complicating pregnancy, second trimester ♀   M

O98.313   Other infections with a predominantly sexual mode of transmission complicating pregnancy, third trimester ♀   M

O98.319   Other infections with a predominantly sexual mode of transmission complicating pregnancy, unspecified trimester ♀ M

O98.32   Other infections with a predominantly sexual mode of transmission complicating childbirth ♀   M
Coding Clinic: 2020, Q1, P20

O98.33   Other infections with a predominantly sexual mode of transmission complicating the puerperium ♀   M

● O98.4   **Viral hepatitis complicating pregnancy, childbirth and the puerperium**
Conditions in B15-B19

● O98.41   Viral hepatitis complicating pregnancy

O98.411   Viral hepatitis complicating pregnancy, first trimester ♀   M

O98.412   Viral hepatitis complicating pregnancy, second trimester ♀   M

O98.413   Viral hepatitis complicating pregnancy, third trimester ♀   M

O98.419   Viral hepatitis complicating pregnancy, unspecified trimester ♀   M

O98.42   Viral hepatitis complicating childbirth ♀   M

O98.43   Viral hepatitis complicating the puerperium ♀   M

● O98.5   **Other viral diseases complicating pregnancy, childbirth and the puerperium**
Conditions in A80-B09, B25-B34, R87.81-, R87.82-

Excludes:1   human immunodeficiency virus [HIV] disease complicating pregnancy, childbirth and the puerperium (O98.7-)

● O98.51   Other viral diseases complicating pregnancy

O98.511   Other viral diseases complicating pregnancy, first trimester ♀   M

O98.512   Other viral diseases complicating pregnancy, second trimester ♀   M
Coding Clinic: 2016, Q4, P5-6

O98.513   Other viral diseases complicating pregnancy, third trimester ♀   M
Coding Clinic: 2016, Q4, P6

O98.519   Other viral diseases complicating pregnancy, unspecified trimester ♀ M

O98.52   Other viral diseases complicating childbirth ♀   M

O98.53   Other viral diseases complicating the puerperium ♀   M

● O98.6   **Protozoal diseases complicating pregnancy, childbirth and the puerperium**
Conditions in B50-B64

● O98.61   Protozoal diseases complicating pregnancy

O98.611   Protozoal diseases complicating pregnancy, first trimester ♀   M

O98.612   Protozoal diseases complicating pregnancy, second trimester ♀   M

O98.613   Protozoal diseases complicating pregnancy, third trimester ♀   M

O98.619   Protozoal diseases complicating pregnancy, unspecified trimester ♀   M

O98.62   Protozoal diseases complicating childbirth ♀   M

O98.63   Protozoal diseases complicating the puerperium ♀   M

● O98.7   **Human immunodeficiency virus [HIV] disease complicating pregnancy, childbirth and the puerperium**
Use additional code to identify the type of HIV disease:
Acquired immune deficiency syndrome (AIDS) (B20)
Asymptomatic HIV status (Z21)
HIV positive NOS (Z21)
Symptomatic HIV disease (B20)

OGCR   Section I.C.15.f.

HIV Infection in Pregnancy, Childbirth and the Puerperium

During pregnancy, childbirth or the puerperium, a patient admitted because of an HIV-related illness should receive a principal diagnosis from subcategory O98.7-. Human immunodeficiency [HIV] disease complicating pregnancy, childbirth and the puerperium, followed by the code(s) for the HIV-related illness(es).

Patients with asymptomatic HIV infection status admitted during pregnancy, childbirth, or the puerperium should receive codes of O98.7- and Z21, Asymptomatic human immunodeficiency virus [HIV] infection status.

● O98.71   Human immunodeficiency virus [HIV] disease complicating pregnancy

O98.711   Human immunodeficiency virus [HIV] disease complicating pregnancy, first trimester ♀   M

O98.712   Human immunodeficiency virus [HIV] disease complicating pregnancy, second trimester ♀   M

O98.713   Human immunodeficiency virus [HIV] disease complicating pregnancy, third trimester ♀   M

O98.719   Human immunodeficiency virus [HIV] disease complicating pregnancy, unspecified trimester ♀ M

O98.72   Human immunodeficiency virus [HIV] disease complicating childbirth ♀   M

O98.73   Human immunodeficiency virus [HIV] disease complicating the puerperium ♀   M

▶ New   ⇒ Revised   ~~deleted~~ Deleted   Excludes 1   Excludes 2   Includes   Use additional   Code first   Code also   Key words
OGCR Official Guidelines   X Assign placeholder X   ● Use Additional Character(s)   ▷ Manifestation Code   🏷 Hierarchical Condition Category   Coding Clinic

- **O98.8 Other maternal infectious and parasitic diseases complicating pregnancy, childbirth and the puerperium**
  - **O98.81 Other maternal infectious and parasitic diseases complicating pregnancy**
    - O98.811 Other maternal infectious and parasitic diseases complicating pregnancy, first trimester ♀   M
    - O98.812 Other maternal infectious and parasitic diseases complicating pregnancy, second trimester ♀   M
    - O98.813 Other maternal infectious and parasitic diseases complicating pregnancy, third trimester ♀   M
    - O98.819 Other maternal infectious and parasitic diseases complicating pregnancy, unspecified trimester ♀   M
  - O98.82 Other maternal infectious and parasitic diseases complicating childbirth ♀   M
    - Coding Clinic: 2020, Q1, P10
  - O98.83 Other maternal infectious and parasitic diseases complicating the puerperium ♀   M
    - Coding Clinic: 2022, Q2, P5
- **O98.9 Unspecified maternal infectious and parasitic disease complicating pregnancy, childbirth and the puerperium**
  - **O98.91 Unspecified maternal infectious and parasitic disease complicating pregnancy**
    - O98.911 Unspecified maternal infectious and parasitic disease complicating pregnancy, first trimester ♀   M
    - O98.912 Unspecified maternal infectious and parasitic disease complicating pregnancy, second trimester ♀   M
    - O98.913 Unspecified maternal infectious and parasitic disease complicating pregnancy, third trimester ♀   M
    - O98.919 Unspecified maternal infectious and parasitic disease complicating pregnancy, unspecified trimester ♀   M
  - O98.92 Unspecified maternal infectious and parasitic disease complicating childbirth ♀   M
  - O98.93 Unspecified maternal infectious and parasitic disease complicating the puerperium ♀   M

- **O99 Other maternal diseases classifiable elsewhere but complicating pregnancy, childbirth and the puerperium**
  - **Includes:** conditions which complicate the pregnant state, are aggravated by the pregnancy or are a main reason for obstetric care
  - Use additional code to identify specific condition
  - **Excludes2** when the reason for maternal care is that the condition is known or suspected to have affected the fetus (O35-O36)
  - Coding Clinic: 2018, Q4, P8-9
- **O99.0 Anemia complicating pregnancy, childbirth and the puerperium**
  - Conditions in D50-D64
  - **Excludes1** anemia arising in the puerperium (O90.81)
    - postpartum anemia NOS (O90.81)
  - **O99.01 Anemia complicating pregnancy**
    - O99.011 Anemia complicating pregnancy, first trimester ♀   M
    - O99.012 Anemia complicating pregnancy, second trimester ♀   M
    - O99.013 Anemia complicating pregnancy, third trimester ♀   M
    - O99.019 Anemia complicating pregnancy, unspecified trimester ♀   M
  - O99.02 Anemia complicating childbirth ♀   M
  - O99.03 Anemia complicating the puerperium ♀   M
    - **Excludes1** postpartum anemia not pre-existing prior to delivery (O90.81)

- **O99.1 Other diseases of the blood and blood-forming organs and certain disorders involving the immune mechanism complicating pregnancy, childbirth and the puerperium**
  - Conditions in D65-D89
  - **Excludes1** hemorrhage with coagulation defects (O45.-, O46.0-, O67.0, O72.3)
  - **O99.11 Other diseases of the blood and blood-forming organs and certain disorders involving the immune mechanism complicating pregnancy**
    - O99.111 Other diseases of the blood and blood-forming organs and certain disorders involving the immune mechanism complicating pregnancy, first trimester ♀   M
    - O99.112 Other diseases of the blood and blood-forming organs and certain disorders involving the immune mechanism complicating pregnancy, second trimester ♀   M
    - O99.113 Other diseases of the blood and blood-forming organs and certain disorders involving the immune mechanism complicating pregnancy, third trimester ♀   M
    - O99.119 Other diseases of the blood and blood-forming organs and certain disorders involving the immune mechanism complicating pregnancy, unspecified trimester ♀   M
  - O99.12 Other diseases of the blood and blood-forming organs and certain disorders involving the immune mechanism complicating childbirth ♀   M
  - O99.13 Other diseases of the blood and blood-forming organs and certain disorders involving the immune mechanism complicating the puerperium ♀   M
- **O99.2 Endocrine, nutritional and metabolic diseases complicating pregnancy, childbirth and the puerperium**
  - Conditions in E00-E89
  - **Excludes2** diabetes mellitus (O24.-)
    - malnutrition (O25.-)
    - postpartum thyroiditis (O90.5)
  - **O99.21 Obesity complicating pregnancy, childbirth, and the puerperium**
    - Use additional code to identify the type of obesity (E66.-)
    - O99.210 Obesity complicating pregnancy, unspecified trimester ♀   M
    - O99.211 Obesity complicating pregnancy, first trimester ♀   M
    - O99.212 Obesity complicating pregnancy, second trimester ♀   M
    - O99.213 Obesity complicating pregnancy, third trimester ♀   M
    - O99.214 Obesity complicating childbirth ♀   M
      - Coding Clinic: 2021, Q2, P10-11; 2018, Q4, P80
    - O99.215 Obesity complicating the puerperium ♀   M
  - **O99.28 Other endocrine, nutritional and metabolic diseases complicating pregnancy, childbirth and the puerperium**
    - O99.280 Endocrine, nutritional and metabolic diseases complicating pregnancy, unspecified trimester ♀   M
    - O99.281 Endocrine, nutritional and metabolic diseases complicating pregnancy, first trimester ♀   M

CHAPTER 15 (O00-O9A)

O99.282 Endocrine, nutritional and metabolic diseases complicating pregnancy, second trimester ♀ M

O99.283 Endocrine, nutritional and metabolic diseases complicating pregnancy, third trimester ♀ M

O99.284 Endocrine, nutritional and metabolic diseases complicating childbirth ♀ M

O99.285 Endocrine, nutritional and metabolic diseases complicating the puerperium ♀ M
Coding Clinic: 2021, Q1, P9

● O99.3 **Mental disorders and diseases of the nervous system complicating pregnancy, childbirth and the puerperium**

● O99.31 **Alcohol** use complicating pregnancy, childbirth, and the puerperium
Use additional code(s) from F10 to identify manifestations of the alcohol use

O99.310 Alcohol use complicating pregnancy, unspecified trimester ♀ M

O99.311 Alcohol use complicating pregnancy, first trimester ♀ M

O99.312 Alcohol use complicating pregnancy, second trimester ♀ M

O99.313 Alcohol use complicating pregnancy, third trimester ♀ M

O99.314 Alcohol use complicating childbirth ♀ M

O99.315 Alcohol use complicating the puerperium ♀ M

● O99.32 **Drug use** complicating pregnancy, childbirth, and the puerperium
Use additional code(s) from F11-F16 and F18-F19 to identify manifestations of the drug use

O99.320 Drug use complicating pregnancy, unspecified trimester ♀ M

O99.321 Drug use complicating pregnancy, first trimester ♀ M

O99.322 Drug use complicating pregnancy, second trimester ♀ M

O99.323 Drug use complicating pregnancy, third trimester ♀ M

O99.324 Drug use complicating childbirth ♀ M

O99.325 Drug use complicating the puerperium ♀ M

● O99.33 **Tobacco use** disorder complicating pregnancy, childbirth, and the puerperium
Smoking complicating pregnancy, childbirth, and the puerperium
Use additional code from category F17 to identify type of tobacco nicotine dependence

O99.330 Smoking (tobacco) complicating pregnancy, unspecified trimester ♀ M

O99.331 Smoking (tobacco) complicating pregnancy, first trimester ♀ M

O99.332 Smoking (tobacco) complicating pregnancy, second trimester ♀ M

O99.333 Smoking (tobacco) complicating pregnancy, third trimester ♀ M

O99.334 Smoking (tobacco) complicating childbirth ♀ M

O99.335 Smoking (tobacco) complicating the puerperium ♀ M

● O99.34 **Other mental disorders** complicating pregnancy, childbirth, and the puerperium
Conditions in F01-F09, F20-F52 and F54-F99
Excludes2 postpartum mood disturbance (O90.6)
postnatal psychosis (F53.1)
puerperal psychosis (F53.1)
Coding Clinic: 2018, Q4, P9

O99.340 Other mental disorders complicating pregnancy, unspecified trimester ♀ M

O99.341 Other mental disorders complicating pregnancy, first trimester ♀ M

O99.342 Other mental disorders complicating pregnancy, second trimester ♀ M

O99.343 Other mental disorders complicating pregnancy, third trimester ♀ M

O99.344 Other mental disorders complicating childbirth ♀ M

O99.345 Other mental disorders complicating the puerperium ♀ M
Coding Clinic: 2018, Q4, P8-9

● O99.35 **Diseases of the nervous system** complicating pregnancy, childbirth, and the puerperium
Conditions in G00-G99
Excludes2 pregnancy related peripheral neuritis (O26.8-)

O99.350 Diseases of the nervous system complicating pregnancy, unspecified trimester ♀ M

O99.351 Diseases of the nervous system complicating pregnancy, first trimester ♀ M

O99.352 Diseases of the nervous system complicating pregnancy, second trimester ♀ M

O99.353 Diseases of the nervous system complicating pregnancy, third trimester ♀ M

O99.354 Diseases of the nervous system complicating childbirth ♀ M

O99.355 Diseases of the nervous system complicating the puerperium ♀ M

● O99.4 **Diseases of the circulatory system** complicating pregnancy, childbirth and the puerperium
Conditions in I00-I99
Excludes1 peripartum cardiomyopathy (O90.3)
Excludes2 hypertensive disorders (O10-O16)
obstetric embolism (O88.-)
venous complications and cerebrovenous sinus thrombosis in labor, childbirth and the puerperium (O87.-)
venous complications and cerebrovenous sinus thrombosis in pregnancy (O22.-)

● O99.41 Diseases of the circulatory system complicating pregnancy
Coding Clinic: 2016, Q2, P8

O99.411 Diseases of the circulatory system complicating pregnancy, first trimester ♀ M

O99.412 Diseases of the circulatory system complicating pregnancy, second trimester ♀ M

O99.413 Diseases of the circulatory system complicating pregnancy, third trimester ♀ M

O99.419 Diseases of the circulatory system complicating pregnancy, unspecified trimester ♀ M

O99.42 Diseases of the circulatory system complicating childbirth ♀ M

O99.43 Diseases of the circulatory system complicating the puerperium ♀ M

● **O99.5 Diseases of the respiratory system** complicating **pregnancy, childbirth and the puerperium**
Conditions in J00-J99

  ● **O99.51 Diseases of the respiratory system** complicating **pregnancy**

    O99.511 Diseases of the respiratory system complicating pregnancy, first trimester ♀   M

    O99.512 Diseases of the respiratory system complicating pregnancy, second trimester ♀   M

    O99.513 Diseases of the respiratory system complicating pregnancy, third trimester ♀   M

    O99.519 Diseases of the respiratory system complicating pregnancy, unspecified trimester ♀   M

  O99.52 Diseases of the respiratory system complicating childbirth ♀   M

  O99.53 Diseases of the respiratory system complicating the puerperium ♀   M

● **O99.6 Diseases of the digestive system** complicating **pregnancy, childbirth and the puerperium**
Conditions in K00-K93

  Excludes2   hemorrhoids in pregnancy (O22.4-)
       liver and biliary tract disorders in pregnancy, childbirth and the puerperium (O26.6-)

  ● **O99.61 Diseases of the digestive system complicating pregnancy**

    O99.611 Diseases of the digestive system complicating pregnancy, first trimester ♀   M

    O99.612 Diseases of the digestive system complicating pregnancy, second trimester ♀   M

    O99.613 Diseases of the digestive system complicating pregnancy, third trimester ♀   M

    O99.619 Diseases of the digestive system complicating pregnancy, unspecified trimester ♀   M

  O99.62 Diseases of the digestive system complicating childbirth ♀   M

  O99.63 Diseases of the digestive system complicating the puerperium ♀   M

● **O99.7 Diseases of the skin and subcutaneous tissue** complicating **pregnancy, childbirth and the puerperium**
Conditions in L00-L99

  Excludes2   herpes gestationis (O26.4)
       pruritic urticarial papules and plaques of pregnancy (PUPPP) (O26.86)

  ● **O99.71 Diseases of the skin and subcutaneous tissue complicating pregnancy**

    O99.711 Diseases of the skin and subcutaneous tissue complicating pregnancy, first trimester ♀   M

    O99.712 Diseases of the skin and subcutaneous tissue complicating pregnancy, second trimester ♀   M

    O99.713 Diseases of the skin and subcutaneous tissue complicating pregnancy, third trimester ♀   M

    O99.719 Diseases of the skin and subcutaneous tissue complicating pregnancy, unspecified trimester ♀   M

  O99.72 Diseases of the skin and subcutaneous tissue complicating childbirth ♀   M

  O99.73 Diseases of the skin and subcutaneous tissue complicating the puerperium ♀   M

● **O99.8 Other specified diseases and conditions** complicating **pregnancy, childbirth and the puerperium**
Conditions in D00-D48, H00-H95, M00-N99, and Q00-Q99

Use additional code to identify condition

  Excludes2   genitourinary infections in pregnancy (O23.-)
       infection of genitourinary tract following delivery (O86.1-O86.4)
       malignant neoplasm complicating pregnancy, childbirth and the puerperium (O9A.1-)
       maternal care for known or suspected abnormality of maternal pelvic organs (O34.-)
       postpartum acute kidney failure (O90.4)
       traumatic injuries in pregnancy (O9A.2-)

  ● **O99.81 Abnormal glucose complicating pregnancy, childbirth and the puerperium**

    Excludes1   gestational diabetes (O24.4-)

    O99.810 Abnormal glucose complicating pregnancy ♀   M

    O99.814 Abnormal glucose complicating childbirth ♀   M

    O99.815 Abnormal glucose complicating the puerperium ♀   M

  ● **O99.82 Streptococcus B carrier state complicating pregnancy, childbirth and the puerperium**

    Excludes1   Carrier of streptococcus group B (GBS) in a nonpregnant woman (Z22.330)

    O99.820 Streptococcus B carrier state complicating pregnancy ♀   M

    O99.824 Streptococcus B carrier state complicating childbirth ♀   M
       Coding Clinic: 2019, Q2, P9

    O99.825 Streptococcus B carrier state complicating the puerperium ♀   M

  ● **O99.83 Other infection carrier state complicating pregnancy, childbirth and the puerperium**

    Use additional code to identify the carrier state (Z22.-)

    O99.830 Other infection carrier state complicating pregnancy ♀   M

    O99.834 Other infection carrier state complicating childbirth ♀   M

    O99.835 Other infection carrier state complicating the puerperium ♀   M

  ● **O99.84 Bariatric surgery status complicating pregnancy, childbirth and the puerperium**
    Gastric banding status complicating pregnancy, childbirth and the puerperium
    Gastric bypass status for obesity complicating pregnancy, childbirth and the puerperium
    Obesity surgery status complicating pregnancy, childbirth and the puerperium

    O99.840 Bariatric surgery status complicating pregnancy, unspecified trimester ♀   M

    O99.841 Bariatric surgery status complicating pregnancy, first trimester ♀   M

    O99.842 Bariatric surgery status complicating pregnancy, second trimester ♀   M

    O99.843 Bariatric surgery status complicating pregnancy, third trimester ♀   M

    O99.844 Bariatric surgery status complicating childbirth ♀   M

    O99.845 Bariatric surgery status complicating the puerperium ♀   M

CHAPTER 15 (O00-O9A)

● O99.89   Other specified diseases and conditions complicating pregnancy, childbirth and the puerperium ♀   M

　　O99.891   Other specified diseases and conditions complicating pregnancy ♀   M

　　O99.892   Other specified diseases and conditions complicating childbirth ♀   M

　　O99.893   Other specified diseases and conditions complicating puerperium ♀   M

OGCR Section I.C.2.I.3.

> **Malignant neoplasm in a pregnant patient**
> When a pregnant woman has a malignant neoplasm, a code from subcategory O9A.1-, Malignant neoplasm complicating pregnancy, childbirth, and the puerperium, should be sequenced first, followed by the appropriate code from Chapter 2 to indicate the type of neoplasm.

● O9A   Maternal malignant neoplasms, traumatic injuries and abuse classifiable elsewhere but complicating pregnancy, childbirth and the puerperium

　● O9A.1   Malignant neoplasm complicating pregnancy, childbirth and the puerperium
　　　Conditions in C00-C96
　　　Use additional code to identify neoplasm
　　　Excludes2   maternal care for benign tumor of corpus uteri (O34.1-)
　　　　　maternal care for benign tumor of cervix (O34.4-)

　　● O9A.11   Malignant neoplasm complicating pregnancy

　　　　O9A.111   Malignant neoplasm complicating pregnancy, first trimester ♀   M

　　　　O9A.112   Malignant neoplasm complicating pregnancy, second trimester ♀   M

　　　　O9A.113   Malignant neoplasm complicating pregnancy, third trimester ♀   M

　　　　O9A.119   Malignant neoplasm complicating pregnancy, unspecified trimester ♀   M

　　　O9A.12   Malignant neoplasm complicating childbirth ♀   M

　　　O9A.13   Malignant neoplasm complicating the puerperium ♀   M
　　　　　Coding Clinic: 2015, Q3, P19

　● O9A.2   Injury, poisoning and certain other consequences of external causes complicating pregnancy, childbirth and the puerperium
　　　Conditions in S00-T88, except T74 and T76
　　　Use additional code(s) to identify the injury or poisoning
　　　Excludes2   physical, sexual and psychological abuse complicating pregnancy, childbirth and the puerperium (O9A.3-, O9A.4-, O9A.5-)

　　● O9A.21   Injury, poisoning and certain other consequences of external causes complicating pregnancy

　　　　O9A.211   Injury, poisoning and certain other consequences of external causes complicating pregnancy, first trimester ♀

　　　　O9A.212   Injury, poisoning and certain other consequences of external causes complicating pregnancy, second trimester ♀   M

　　　　O9A.213   Injury, poisoning and certain other consequences of external causes complicating pregnancy, third trimester ♀   M

　　　　O9A.219   Injury, poisoning and certain other consequences of external causes complicating pregnancy, unspecified trimester ♀   M

　　　O9A.22   Injury, poisoning and certain other consequences of external causes complicating childbirth ♀   M

　　　O9A.23   Injury, poisoning and certain other consequences of external causes complicating the puerperium ♀   M

　● O9A.3   Physical abuse complicating pregnancy, childbirth and the puerperium
　　　Conditions in T74.11 or T76.11
　　　Use additional code (if applicable):
　　　　to identify any associated current injury due to physical abuse
　　　　to identify the perpetrator of abuse (Y07.-)
　　　Excludes2   sexual abuse complicating pregnancy, childbirth and the puerperium (O9A.4)

　　● O9A.31   Physical abuse complicating pregnancy

　　　　O9A.311   Physical abuse complicating pregnancy, first trimester ♀   M

　　　　O9A.312   Physical abuse complicating pregnancy, second trimester ♀   M

　　　　O9A.313   Physical abuse complicating pregnancy, third trimester ♀   M

　　　　O9A.319   Physical abuse complicating pregnancy, unspecified trimester ♀   M

　　　O9A.32   Physical abuse complicating childbirth ♀   M

　　　O9A.33   Physical abuse complicating the puerperium ♀   M

　● O9A.4   Sexual abuse complicating pregnancy, childbirth and the puerperium
　　　Conditions in T74.21 or T76.21
　　　Use additional code (if applicable):
　　　　to identify any associated current injury due to sexual abuse
　　　　to identify the perpetrator of abuse (Y07.-)

　　● O9A.41   Sexual abuse complicating pregnancy

　　　　O9A.411   Sexual abuse complicating pregnancy, first trimester ♀   M

　　　　O9A.412   Sexual abuse complicating pregnancy, second trimester ♀   M

　　　　O9A.413   Sexual abuse complicating pregnancy, third trimester ♀   M

　　　　O9A.419   Sexual abuse complicating pregnancy, unspecified trimester ♀   M

　　　O9A.42   Sexual abuse complicating childbirth ♀   M

　　　O9A.43   Sexual abuse complicating the puerperium ♀   M

　● O9A.5   Psychological abuse complicating pregnancy, childbirth and the puerperium
　　　Conditions in T74.31 or T76.31
　　　Use additional code to identify the perpetrator of abuse (Y07.-)

　　● O9A.51   Psychological abuse complicating pregnancy

　　　　O9A.511   Psychological abuse complicating pregnancy, first trimester ♀   M

　　　　O9A.512   Psychological abuse complicating pregnancy, second trimester ♀   M

　　　　O9A.513   Psychological abuse complicating pregnancy, third trimester ♀   M

　　　　O9A.519   Psychological abuse complicating pregnancy, unspecified trimester ♀   M

　　　O9A.52   Psychological abuse complicating childbirth ♀M

　　　O9A.53   Psychological abuse complicating the puerperium ♀   M

▶ New   ⟹ Revised   ~~deleted~~ Deleted   Excludes 1   Excludes 2   Includes   Use additional   Code first   Code also   Key words
OGCR Official Guidelines   X Assign placeholder X   ● Use Additional Character(s)   ▷ Manifestation Code   🄗 Hierarchical Condition Category   **Coding Clinic**

CHAPTER 16

CERTAIN CONDITIONS ORIGINATING IN THE PERINATAL PERIOD (P00-P96)

OGCR Chapter-Specific Coding Guidelines

16. **Chapter 16: Certain Conditions Originating in the Perinatal Period (P00-P96)**

   For coding and reporting purposes the perinatal period is defined as before birth through the 28th day following birth. The following guidelines are provided for reporting purposes

   a. **General Perinatal Rules**

   1) **Use of Chapter 16 Codes**

   Codes in this chapter are <u>never</u> for use on the maternal record. Codes from Chapter 15, the obstetric chapter, are never permitted on the newborn record. Chapter 16 codes may be used throughout the life of the patient if the condition is still present.

   2) **Principal Diagnosis for Birth Record**

   When coding the birth episode in a newborn record, assign a code from category Z38, Liveborn infants according to place of birth and type of delivery, as the principal diagnosis. A code from category Z38 is assigned only once, to a newborn at the time of birth. If a newborn is transferred to another institution, a code from category Z38 should not be used at the receiving hospital.

   A code from category Z38 is used only on the newborn record, not on the mother's record.

   3) **Use of Codes from other Chapters with Codes from Chapter 16**

   Codes from other chapters may be used with codes from chapter 16 if the codes from the other chapters provide more specific detail. Codes for signs and symptoms may be assigned when a definitive diagnosis has not been established. If the reason for the encounter is a perinatal condition, the code from Chapter 16 should be sequenced first.

   4) **Use of Chapter 16 Codes after the Perinatal Period**

   Should a condition originate in the perinatal period, and continue throughout the life of the patient, the perinatal code should continue to be used regardless of the patient's age.

   5) **Birth process or community acquired conditions**

   If a newborn has a condition that may be either due to the birth process or community acquired and the documentation does not indicate which it is, the default is due to the birth process and the code from Chapter 16 should be used. If the condition is community-acquired, a code from Chapter 16 should not be assigned.

   6) **Code all clinically significant conditions**

   All clinically significant conditions noted on routine newborn examination should be coded. A condition is clinically significant if it requires:
   - clinical evaluation; or
   - therapeutic treatment; or
   - diagnostic procedures; or
   - extended length of hospital stay; or
   - increased nursing care and/or monitoring; or
   - has implications for future health care needs

   Note: The perinatal guidelines listed above are the same as the general coding guidelines for "additional diagnoses", except for the final point regarding implications for future health care needs. Codes should be assigned for conditions that have been specified by the provider as having implications for future health care needs.

   b. **Observation and Evaluation of Newborns for Suspected Conditions Not Found**

   1) **Use of Z05 codes**

   Assign a code from category Z05, Observation and evaluation of newborns and infants for suspected conditions ruled out, to identify those instances when a healthy newborn is evaluated for a suspected condition that is determined after study not to be present. Do not use a code from category Z05 when the patient has identified signs or symptoms of a suspected problem; in such cases code the sign or symptom.

   2) **Z05 on Other than the Birth Record**

   A code from category Z05 may also be assigned as a principal or first-listed code for readmissions or encounters when the code from category Z38 code no longer applies. Codes from category Z05 are for use only for healthy newborns and infants for which no condition after study is found to be present.

   3) **Z05 on a birth record**

   A code from category Z05 is to be used as a secondary code after the code from category Z38, Liveborn infants according to place of birth and type of delivery.

   c. **Coding Additional Perinatal Diagnoses**

   1) **Assigning codes for conditions that require treatment**

   Assign codes for conditions that require treatment or further investigation, prolong the length of stay, or require resource utilization.

   2) **Codes for conditions specified as having implications for future health care needs**

   Assign codes for conditions that have been specified by the provider as having implications for future health care needs.

   Note: This guideline should not be used for adult patients.

   d. **Prematurity and Fetal Growth Retardation**

   Providers utilize different criteria in determining prematurity. A code for prematurity should not be assigned unless it is documented. Assignment of codes in categories P05, Disorders of newborn related to slow fetal growth and fetal malnutrition, and P07, Disorders of newborn related to short gestation and low birth weight, not elsewhere classified, should be based on the recorded birth weight and estimated gestational age.

   When both birth weight and gestational age are available, two codes from category P07 should be assigned, with the code for birth weight sequenced before the code for gestational age.

   e. **Low birth weight and immaturity status**

   Codes from category P07, Disorders of newborn related to short gestation and low birth weight, not elsewhere classified, are for use for a child or adult who was premature or had a low birth weight as a newborn and this is affecting the patient's current health status.

   See Section I.C.21. Factors influencing health status and contact with health services, Status.

   f. **Bacterial Sepsis of Newborn**

   Category P36, Bacterial sepsis of newborn, includes congenital sepsis. If a perinate is documented as having sepsis without documentation of congenital or community acquired, the default is congenital and a code from category P36 should be assigned. If the P36 code includes the causal organism, an additional code from category B95, Streptococcus, Staphylococcus, and Enterococcus as the cause of diseases classified elsewhere, or B96, Other bacterial agents as the cause of diseases classified elsewhere, should not be assigned. If the P36 code does not include the causal organism, assign an additional code from category B96. If applicable, use additional codes to identify severe sepsis (R65.2-) and any associated acute organ dysfunction.

   g. **Stillbirth**

   Code P95, Stillbirth, is only for use in institutions that maintain separate records for stillbirths. No other code should be used with P95. Code P95 should not be used on the mother's record.

CHAPTER 16

CERTAIN CONDITIONS ORIGINATING IN THE PERINATAL PERIOD (P00-P96)

Note: Codes from this chapter are for use on newborn records only, never on maternal records.

> **Includes**   conditions that have their origin in the fetal or perinatal period (before birth through the first 28 days after birth) even if morbidity occurs later
>
> **Excludes2**   congenital malformations, deformations and chromosomal abnormalities (Q00-Q99)
> endocrine, nutritional and metabolic diseases (E00-E88)
> injury, poisoning and certain other consequences of external causes (S00-T88)
> neoplasms (C00-D49)
> tetanus neonatorum (A33)

This chapter contains the following blocks:

P00-P04	Newborn affected by maternal factors and by complications of pregnancy, labor, and delivery
P05-P08	Disorders of newborns related to length of gestation and fetal growth
P09	Abnormal findings on neonatal screening
P10-P15	Birth trauma
P19-P29	Respiratory and cardiovascular disorders specific to the perinatal period
P35-P39	Infections specific to the perinatal period
P50-P61	Hemorrhagic and hematological disorders of newborn
P70-P74	Transitory endocrine and metabolic disorders specific to newborn
P76-P78	Digestive system disorders of newborn
P80-P83	Conditions involving the integument and temperature regulation of newborn
P84	Other problems with newborn
P90-P96	Other disorders originating in the perinatal period

NEWBORN AFFECTED BY MATERNAL FACTORS AND BY COMPLICATIONS OF PREGNANCY, LABOR, AND DELIVERY (P00–P04)

Note: These codes are for use when the listed maternal conditions are specified as the cause of confirmed morbidity or potential morbidity which have their origin in the perinatal period (before birth through the first 28 days after birth).

● **P00**   **Newborn affected by maternal conditions that may be unrelated to present pregnancy**

Code first any current condition in newborn

> **Excludes2**   encounter for observation of newborn for suspected diseases and conditions ruled out (Z05.-)
> newborn affected by maternal complications of pregnancy (P01.-)
> newborn affected by maternal endocrine and metabolic disorders (P70–P74)
> newborn affected by noxious substances transmitted via placenta or breast milk (P04.-)

Coding Clinic: 2016, Q4, P54

P00.0   **Newborn affected by maternal hypertensive disorders**
Newborn affected by maternal conditions classifiable to O10-O11, O13-O16

P00.1   **Newborn affected by maternal renal and urinary tract diseases**
Newborn affected by maternal conditions classifiable to N00-N39

P00.2   **Newborn affected by maternal infectious and parasitic diseases**
Newborn affected by maternal infectious disease classifiable to A00-B99, J09 and J10

> **Excludes1**   maternal genital tract or other localized infections (P00.8)
>
> **Excludes2**   infections specific to the perinatal period (P35-P39)
> newborn affected by (positive) maternal group B streptococcus (GBS) colonization (P00.82)

Coding Clinic: 2019, Q2, P10; 2015, Q3, P21

P00.3   **Newborn affected by other maternal circulatory and respiratory diseases**
Newborn affected by maternal conditions classifiable to I00-I99, J00-J99, Q20-Q34 and not included in P00.0, P00.2

P00.4   **Newborn affected by maternal nutritional disorders**
Newborn affected by maternal disorders classifiable to E40-E64
Maternal malnutrition NOS

P00.5   **Newborn affected by maternal injury**
Newborn affected by maternal conditions classifiable to O9A.2-

P00.6   **Newborn affected by surgical procedure on mother**
Newborn affected by amniocentesis

> **Excludes1**   Cesarean delivery for present delivery (P03.4)
> damage to placenta from amniocentesis, cesarean delivery or surgical induction (P02.1)
> previous surgery to uterus or pelvic organs (P03.89)
>
> **Excludes2**   newborn affected by complication of (fetal) intrauterine procedure (P96.5)

P00.7   **Newborn affected by other medical procedures on mother, not elsewhere classified**
Newborn affected by radiation to mother

> **Excludes1**   damage to placenta from amniocentesis, cesarean delivery or surgical induction (P02.1)
> newborn affected by other complications of labor and delivery (P03.-)

● **P00.8**   **Newborn affected by other maternal conditions**

P00.81   **Newborn affected by periodontal disease in mother**

P00.82   **Newborn affected by (positive) maternal group B streptococcus (GBS) colonization**
Contact with positive maternal group B streptococcus
Coding Clinic: 2021, Q4, P23

P00.89   **Newborn affected by other maternal conditions**
Newborn affected by conditions classifiable to T80-T88
Newborn affected by maternal genital tract or other localized infections
Newborn affected by maternal systemic lupus erythematosus
Use additional code to identify infectious agent, if known

> **Excludes2**   newborn affected by positive maternal group B streptococcus (GBS) colonization (P00.82)

Coding Clinic: 2019, Q2, P9

P00.9   **Newborn affected by unspecified maternal condition**

● **P01**   **Newborn affected by maternal complications of pregnancy**

Code first any current condition in newborn

> **Excludes2**   encounter for observation of newborn for suspected diseases and conditions ruled out (Z05.-)

Coding Clinic: 2016, Q4, P54

P01.0   **Newborn affected by incompetent cervix**

P01.1   **Newborn affected by premature rupture of membranes**

▶ New   ⇒ Revised   ~~deleted~~ Deleted   Excludes 1   Excludes 2   Includes   Use additional   Code first   Code also   Key words
OGCR Official Guidelines   X Assign placeholder X   ● Use Additional Character(s)   ▌ Manifestation Code   🔖 Hierarchical Condition Category   Coding Clinic

P01.2   **Newborn affected by oligohydramnios**
       Excludes1   oligohydramnios due to premature rupture of membranes (P01.1)

P01.3   **Newborn affected by polyhydramnios**
       Excess of amniotic fluid, usually > 2000 mL
       Newborn affected by hydramnios

P01.4   **Newborn affected by ectopic pregnancy**
       Newborn affected by abdominal pregnancy

P01.5   **Newborn affected by multiple pregnancy**
       Newborn affected by triplet (pregnancy)
       Newborn affected by twin (pregnancy)

P01.6   **Newborn affected by maternal death**

P01.7   **Newborn affected by malpresentation before labor**
       Newborn affected by breech presentation before labor
       Newborn affected by external version before labor
       Newborn affected by face presentation before labor
       Newborn affected by transverse lie before labor
       Newborn affected by unstable lie before labor

P01.8   **Newborn affected by other maternal complications of pregnancy**

P01.9   **Newborn affected by maternal complication of pregnancy, unspecified**

● P02   **Newborn affected by complications of placenta, cord and membranes**
       Code first any current condition in newborn
       Excludes2   encounter for observation of newborn for suspected diseases and conditions ruled out (Z05.-)
       Coding Clinic: 2016, Q4, P54

P02.0   **Newborn affected by placenta previa**

P02.1   **Newborn affected by other forms of placental separation and hemorrhage**
       Newborn affected by abruptio placenta
       Newborn affected by accidental hemorrhage
       Newborn affected by antepartum hemorrhage
       Newborn affected by damage to placenta from amniocentesis, cesarean delivery or surgical induction
       Newborn affected by maternal blood loss
       Newborn affected by premature separation of placenta

● P02.2   **Newborn affected by other and unspecified morphological and functional abnormalities of placenta**

     P02.20   **Newborn affected by unspecified morphological and functional abnormalities of placenta**

     P02.29   **Newborn affected by other morphological and functional abnormalities of placenta**
         Newborn affected by placental dysfunction
         Newborn affected by placental infarction
         Newborn affected by placental insufficiency

P02.3   **Newborn affected by placental transfusion syndromes**
       Newborn affected by placental and cord abnormalities resulting in twin-to-twin or other transplacental transfusion

P02.4   **Newborn affected by prolapsed cord**

P02.5   **Newborn affected by other compression of umbilical cord**
       Newborn affected by umbilical cord (tightly) around neck
       Newborn affected by entanglement of umbilical cord
       Newborn affected by knot in umbilical cord
       Coding Clinic: 2022, Q1, P22

● P02.6   **Newborn affected by other and unspecified conditions of umbilical cord**

     P02.60   **Newborn affected by unspecified conditions of umbilical cord**

     P02.69   **Newborn affected by other conditions of umbilical cord**
         Newborn affected by short umbilical cord
         Newborn affected by vasa previa
         Excludes1   newborn affected by single umbilical artery (Q27.0)

● P02.7   **Newborn affected by chorioamnionitis**
       Inflammation of chorion and amnion

     P02.70   **Newborn affected by fetal inflammatory response syndrome** 🔒
         Newborn affected by FIRS

     P02.78   **Newborn affected by other conditions from chorioamnionitis**
         Newborn affected by amnionitis
         Newborn affected by membranitis
         Newborn affected by placentitis

P02.8   **Newborn affected by other abnormalities of membranes**

P02.9   **Newborn affected by abnormality of membranes, unspecified**

● P03   **Newborn affected by other complications of labor and delivery**
       Code first any current condition in newborn
       Excludes2   encounter for observation of newborn for suspected diseases and conditions ruled out (Z05.-)
       Coding Clinic: 2016, Q4, P54

P03.0   **Newborn affected by breech delivery and extraction**

P03.1   **Newborn affected by other malpresentation, malposition and disproportion during labor and delivery**
       Newborn affected by contracted pelvis
       Newborn affected by conditions classifiable to O64-O66
       Newborn affected by persistent occipitoposterior
       Newborn affected by transverse lie

P03.2   **Newborn affected by forceps delivery**

P03.3   **Newborn affected by delivery by vacuum extractor [ventouse]**

P03.4   **Newborn affected by Cesarean delivery**

P03.5   **Newborn affected by precipitate delivery**
       Newborn affected by rapid second stage

P03.6   **Newborn affected by abnormal uterine contractions**
       Newborn affected by conditions classifiable to O62.-, except O62.3
       Newborn affected by hypertonic labor
       Newborn affected by uterine inertia

● P03.8   **Newborn affected by other specified complications of labor and delivery**

   ● P03.81   **Newborn affected by abnormality in fetal (intrauterine) heart rate or rhythm**

       Excludes1   neonatal cardiac dysrhythmia (P29.1-)

     P03.810   **Newborn affected by abnormality in fetal (intrauterine) heart rate or rhythm before the onset of labor**

     P03.811   **Newborn affected by abnormality in fetal (intrauterine) heart rate or rhythm during labor**

     P03.819   **Newborn affected by abnormality in fetal (intrauterine) heart rate or rhythm, unspecified as to time of onset**

     P03.82   **Meconium passage during delivery**
       Excludes1   meconium aspiration (P24.00, P24.01)
                   meconium staining (P96.83)

     P03.89   **Newborn affected by other specified complications of labor and delivery**
         Newborn affected by abnormality of maternal soft tissues
         Newborn affected by conditions classifiable to O60-O75 and by procedures used in labor and delivery not included in P02.- and P03.0-P03.6
         Newborn affected by induction of labor

P03.9   **Newborn affected by complication of labor and delivery, unspecified**

CHAPTER 16 (P00-P96)

● **P04**   **Newborn affected by noxious substances transmitted via placenta or breast milk**

Code first any current condition in newborn, if applicable

Includes   nonteratogenic effects of substances transmitted via placenta

Excludes2   congenital malformations (Q00-Q99)

encounter for observation of newborn for suspected diseases and conditions ruled out (Z05.-)

neonatal jaundice from excessive hemolysis due to drugs or toxins transmitted from mother (P58.4)

newborn in contact with and (suspected) exposures hazardous to health not transmitted via placenta or breast milk (Z77.-)

Coding Clinic: 2016, Q4, P54

P04.0   **Newborn affected by maternal anesthesia and analgesia in pregnancy, labor and delivery**

Newborn affected by reactions and intoxications from maternal opiates and tranquilizers administered for procedures during pregnancy or labor and delivery

Excludes2   newborn affected by other maternal medication (P04.1-)

● **P04.1**   **Newborn affected by other maternal medication**

Code first withdrawal symptoms from maternal use of drugs of addiction, if applicable (P96.1)

Excludes1   dysmorphism due to warfarin (Q86.2)

fetal hydantoin syndrome (Q86.1)

Excludes2   maternal anesthesia and analgesia in pregnancy, labor and delivery (P04.0)

maternal use of drugs of addiction (P04.4-)

P04.11   **Newborn affected by maternal antineoplastic chemotherapy**

P04.12   **Newborn affected by maternal cytotoxic drugs**

P04.13   **Newborn affected by maternal use of anticonvulsants**

P04.14   **Newborn affected by maternal use of opiates**

P04.15   **Newborn affected by maternal use of antidepressants**

P04.16   **Newborn affected by maternal use of amphetamines**

P04.17   **Newborn affected by maternal use of sedative-hypnotics**

P04.1A   **Newborn affected by maternal use of anxiolytics**

P04.18   **Newborn affected by other maternal medication**

P04.19   **Newborn affected by maternal use of unspecified medication**

Coding Clinic: 2016, Q4, P55

P04.2   **Newborn affected by maternal use of tobacco**

Newborn affected by exposure in utero to tobacco smoke

Excludes2   newborn exposure to environmental tobacco smoke (P96.81)

P04.3   **Newborn affected by maternal use of alcohol**

Excludes1   fetal alcohol syndrome (Q86.0)

● **P04.4**   **Newborn affected by maternal use of drugs of addiction**

P04.40   **Newborn affected by maternal use of unspecified drugs of addiction**

P04.41   **Newborn affected by maternal use of cocaine**

P04.42   **Newborn affected by maternal use of hallucinogens**

Excludes2   newborn affected by other maternal medication (P04.1-)

P04.49   **Newborn affected by maternal use of other drugs of addiction**

Excludes2   newborn affected by maternal anesthesia and analgesia (P04.0)

withdrawal symptoms from maternal use of drugs of addiction (P96.1)

P04.5   **Newborn affected by maternal use of nutritional chemical substances**

P04.6   **Newborn affected by maternal exposure to environmental chemical substances**

● **P04.8**   **Newborn affected by other maternal noxious substances**

P04.81   **Newborn affected by maternal use of cannabis**

P04.89   **Newborn affected by other maternal noxious substances**

P04.9   **Newborn affected by maternal noxious substance, unspecified**

OGCR   Section I.C.16.d.

Prematurity and Fetal Growth Retardation

Providers utilize different criteria in determining prematurity. A code for prematurity should not be assigned unless it is documented. Assignment of codes in categories P05, Disorders of newborn related to slow fetal growth and fetal malnutrition, and P07, Disorders of newborn related to short gestation and low birth weight, not elsewhere classified, should be based on the recorded birth weight and estimated gestational age.

When both birth weight and gestational age are available, two codes from category P07 should be assigned, with the code for birth weight sequenced before the code for gestational age.

DISORDERS OF NEWBORN RELATED TO LENGTH OF GESTATION AND FETAL GROWTH (P05-P08)

● **P05**   **Disorders of newborn related to slow fetal growth and fetal malnutrition**

Coding Clinic: 2016, Q4, P56

● **P05.0**   **Newborn light for gestational age**

Newborn light-for-dates

Weight below but length above 10th percentile for gestational age

P05.00   **Newborn light for gestational age, unspecified weight**

P05.01   **Newborn light for gestational age, less than 500 grams**

P05.02   **Newborn light for gestational age, 500-749 grams**

P05.03   **Newborn light for gestational age, 750-999 grams**

P05.04   **Newborn light for gestational age, 1000-1249 grams**

P05.05   **Newborn light for gestational age, 1250-1499 grams**

P05.06   **Newborn light for gestational age, 1500-1749 grams**

P05.07   **Newborn light for gestational age, 1750-1999 grams**

P05.08   **Newborn light for gestational age, 2000-2499 grams**

P05.09   **Newborn light for gestational age, 2500 grams and over**

Newborn light for gestational age, other

Coding Clinic: 2016, Q4, P55

▶ New   ⇒ Revised   ~~deleted~~ Deleted   Excludes 1   Excludes 2   Includes   Use additional   Code first   Code also   Key words

OGCR Official Guidelines   X Assign placeholder X   ● Use Additional Character(s)   ▌ Manifestation Code   Hierarchical Condition Category   Coding Clinic

● **P05.1**   **Newborn small for gestational age**
Newborn small-and-light-for-dates
Newborn small-for-dates
Weight and length below 10th percentile for gestational age

   P05.10   **Newborn small for gestational age, unspecified weight**

   P05.11   **Newborn small for gestational age, less than 500 grams**

   P05.12   **Newborn small for gestational age, 500-749 grams**

   P05.13   **Newborn small for gestational age, 750-999 grams**

   P05.14   **Newborn small for gestational age, 1000-1249 grams**

   P05.15   **Newborn small for gestational age, 1250-1499 grams**

   P05.16   **Newborn small for gestational age, 1500-1749 grams**

   P05.17   **Newborn small for gestational age, 1750-1999 grams**

   P05.18   **Newborn small for gestational age, 2000-2499 grams**

   P05.19   **Newborn small for gestational age, other**
Newborn small for gestational age, 2500 grams and over
Coding Clinic: 2016, Q4, P55

P05.2   **Newborn affected by fetal (intrauterine) malnutrition not light or small for gestational age**
Infant, not light or small for gestational age, showing signs of fetal malnutrition, such as dry, peeling skin and loss of subcutaneous tissue

   Excludes1   newborn affected by fetal malnutrition with light for gestational age (P05.0-)
newborn affected by fetal malnutrition with small for gestational age (P05.1-)

P05.9   **Newborn affected by slow intrauterine growth, unspecified**
Newborn affected by fetal growth retardation NOS

● **P07**   **Disorders of newborn related to short gestation and low birth weight, not elsewhere classified**
Note: When both birth weight and gestational age of the newborn are available, both should be coded with birth weight sequenced before gestational age.

   Includes   the listed conditions, without further specification, as the cause of morbidity or additional care, in newborn

● **P07.0**   **Extremely low birth weight newborn**
Newborn birth weight 999 g. or less

   Excludes1   low birth weight due to slow fetal growth and fetal malnutrition (P05.-)

   P07.00   **Extremely low birth weight newborn, unspecified weight**

   P07.01   **Extremely low birth weight newborn, less than 500 grams**

   P07.02   **Extremely low birth weight newborn, 500-749 grams**

   P07.03   **Extremely low birth weight newborn, 750-999 grams**

● **P07.1**   **Other low birth weight newborn**
Newborn birth weight 1000-2499 g.

   Excludes1   low birth weight due to slow fetal growth and fetal malnutrition (P05.-)

   P07.10   **Other low birth weight newborn, unspecified weight**

   P07.14   **Other low birth weight newborn, 1000-1249 grams**

   P07.15   **Other low birth weight newborn, 1250-1499 grams**

   P07.16   **Other low birth weight newborn, 1500-1749 grams**

   P07.17   **Other low birth weight newborn, 1750-1999 grams**

   P07.18   **Other low birth weight newborn, 2000-2499 grams**

● **P07.2**   **Extreme immaturity of newborn**
Less than 28 completed weeks (less than 196 completed days) of gestation

   P07.20   **Extreme immaturity of newborn, unspecified weeks of gestation**
Gestational age less than 28 completed weeks NOS

   P07.21   **Extreme immaturity of newborn, gestational age less than 23 completed weeks**
Extreme immaturity of newborn, gestational age less than 23 weeks, 0 days

   P07.22   **Extreme immaturity of newborn, gestational age 23 completed weeks**
Extreme immaturity of newborn, gestational age 23 weeks, 0 days through 23 weeks, 6 days

   P07.23   **Extreme immaturity of newborn, gestational age 24 completed weeks**
Extreme immaturity of newborn, gestational age 24 weeks, 0 days through 24 weeks, 6 days

   P07.24   **Extreme immaturity of newborn, gestational age 25 completed weeks**
Extreme immaturity of newborn, gestational age 25 weeks, 0 days through 25 weeks, 6 days

   P07.25   **Extreme immaturity of newborn, gestational age 26 completed weeks**
Extreme immaturity of newborn, gestational age 26 weeks, 0 days through 26 weeks, 6 days

   P07.26   **Extreme immaturity of newborn, gestational age 27 completed weeks**
Extreme immaturity of newborn, gestational age 27 weeks, 0 days through 27 weeks, 6 days

● **P07.3**   **Preterm [premature] newborn [other]**
28 completed weeks or more but less than 37 completed weeks (196 completed days but less than 259 completed days) of gestation
Prematurity NOS

   P07.30   **Preterm newborn, unspecified weeks of gestation**

   P07.31   **Preterm newborn, gestational age 28 completed weeks**
Preterm newborn, gestational age 28 weeks, 0 days through 28 weeks, 6 days

   P07.32   **Preterm newborn, gestational age 29 completed weeks**
Preterm newborn, gestational age 29 weeks, 0 days through 29 weeks, 6 days

   P07.33   **Preterm newborn, gestational age 30 completed weeks**
Preterm newborn, gestational age 30 weeks, 0 days through 30 weeks, 6 days

   P07.34   **Preterm newborn, gestational age 31 completed weeks**
Preterm newborn, gestational age 31 weeks, 0 days through 31 weeks, 6 days

   P07.35   **Preterm newborn, gestational age 32 completed weeks**
Preterm newborn, gestational age 32 weeks, 0 days through 32 weeks, 6 days

   P07.36   **Preterm newborn, gestational age 33 completed weeks**
Preterm newborn, gestational age 33 weeks, 0 days through 33 weeks, 6 days

CHAPTER 16 (P00-P96)

CHAPTER 16 (P00-P96)

P07.37 **Preterm newborn, gestational age 34 completed weeks**
Preterm newborn, gestational age 34 weeks, 0 days through 34 weeks, 6 days
Coding Clinic: 2017, Q2, P7

P07.38 **Preterm newborn, gestational age 35 completed weeks**
Preterm newborn, gestational age 35 weeks, 0 days through 35 weeks, 6 days

P07.39 **Preterm newborn, gestational age 36 completed weeks**
Preterm newborn, gestational age 36 weeks, 0 days through 36 weeks, 6 days
Coding Clinic: 2017, Q3, P26

● **P08** **Disorders of newborn related to long gestation and high birth weight**
Note: When both birth weight and gestational age of the newborn are available, priority of assignment should be given to birth weight.
Includes the listed conditions, without further specification, as causes of morbidity or additional care, in newborn

P08.0 **Exceptionally large newborn baby**
Usually implies a birth weight of 4500 g. or more
Excludes1 syndrome of infant of diabetic mother (P70.1)
syndrome of infant of mother with gestational diabetes (P70.0)

P08.1 **Other heavy for gestational age newborn**
Other newborn heavy- or large-for-dates regardless of period of gestation
Usually implies a birth weight of 4000 g. to 4499 g.
Excludes1 newborn with a birth weight of 4500 or more (P08.0)
syndrome of infant of diabetic mother (P70.1)
syndrome of infant of mother with gestational diabetes (P70.0)

● **P08.2** **Late newborn, not heavy for gestational age**
P08.21 **Post-term newborn**
Newborn with gestation period over 40 completed weeks to 42 completed weeks

P08.22 **Prolonged gestation of newborn**
Newborn with gestation period over 42 completed weeks (294 days or more), not heavy- or large-for-dates
Postmaturity NOS

ABNORMAL FINDINGS ON NEONATAL SCREENING (P09)

● **P09** **Abnormal findings on neonatal screening**
Includes: Abnormal findings on state mandated newborn screens
Failed newborn screening
Excludes2 nonspecific serologic evidence of human immunodeficiency virus [HIV] (R75)

P09.1 **Abnormal findings on neonatal screening for inborn errors of metabolism**

P09.2 **Abnormal findings on neonatal screening for congenital endocrine disease**
Abnormal findings on neonatal screening for congenital adrenal hyperplasia
Abnormal findings on neonatal screening for hypothyroidism screen

P09.3 **Abnormal findings on neonatal screening for congenital hematologic disorders**
Abnormal findings for hemoglobinothies screen
Abnormal findings on red cell membrane defects screen
Abnormal findings on sickle cell screen

P09.4 **Abnormal findings on neonatal screening for cystic fibrosis**

P09.5 **Abnormal findings on neonatal screening for critical congenital heart disease**
Neonatal congenital heart disease screening failure

P09.6 **Abnormal findings on neonatal screening for neonatal hearing loss**
Excludes2 encounter for hearing examination following failed hearing screening (Z01.110)

P09.8 **Other abnormal findings on neonatal screening**

P09.9 **Abnormal findings on neonatal screening, unspecified**

BIRTH TRAUMA (P10-P15)

● **P10** **Intracranial laceration and hemorrhage due to birth injury**
Excludes1 intracranial hemorrhage of newborn NOS (P52.9)
intracranial hemorrhage of newborn due to anoxia or hypoxia (P52.-)
nontraumatic intracranial hemorrhage of newborn (P52.-)

P10.0 **Subdural hemorrhage due to birth injury**
Subdural hematoma (localized) due to birth injury
Excludes1 subdural hemorrhage accompanying tentorial tear (P10.4)

P10.1 **Cerebral hemorrhage due to birth injury**

P10.2 **Intraventricular hemorrhage due to birth injury**

P10.3 **Subarachnoid hemorrhage due to birth injury**

P10.4 **Tentorial tear due to birth injury**
Pertaining to tentorium of cerebellum (extension of dura mater that separates cerebellum from inferior portion of occipital lobes)

P10.8 **Other intracranial lacerations and hemorrhages due to birth injury**

P10.9 **Unspecified intracranial laceration and hemorrhage due to birth injury**

● **P11** **Other birth injuries to central nervous system**
P11.0 **Cerebral edema due to birth injury**
P11.1 **Other specified brain damage due to birth injury**
P11.2 **Unspecified brain damage due to birth injury**
P11.3 **Birth injury to facial nerve**
Facial palsy due to birth injury
P11.4 **Birth injury to other cranial nerves**
P11.5 **Birth injury to spine and spinal cord**
Fracture of spine due to birth injury
P11.9 **Birth injury to central nervous system, unspecified**

● **P12** **Birth injury to scalp**
P12.0 **Cephalhematoma due to birth injury**
P12.1 **Chignon (from vacuum extraction) due to birth injury**
P12.2 **Epicranial subaponeurotic hemorrhage due to birth injury**
Subgaleal hemorrhage
P12.3 **Bruising of scalp due to birth injury**
P12.4 **Injury of scalp of newborn due to monitoring equipment**
Sampling incision of scalp of newborn
Scalp clip (electrode) injury of newborn
● **P12.8** **Other birth injuries to scalp**
P12.81 **Caput succedaneum**
P12.89 **Other birth injuries to scalp**
P12.9 **Birth injury to scalp, unspecified**

● **P13** **Birth injury to skeleton**
Excludes2 birth injury to spine (P11.5)
P13.0 **Fracture of skull due to birth injury**
P13.1 **Other birth injuries to skull**
Excludes1 cephalhematoma (P12.0)

▶ New ➡ Revised ~~deleted~~ Deleted Excludes 1 Excludes 2 Includes Use additional Code first Code also Key words
OGCR Official Guidelines X Assign placeholder X ● Use Additional Character(s) ▷ Manifestation Code 🔗 Hierarchical Condition Category **Coding Clinic**

Item 16-1 The **peripheral nervous system** consists of 31 pairs of spinal nerves, 12 pairs of cranial nerves, and the autonomic nerves, which are divided into the parasympathetic and sympathetic nerves. The cranial nerves are: olfactory (I), optic (II), oculomotor (III), trochlear (IV), trigeminal (V), abducens (VI), facial (VII), vestibulocochlear (VIII), glossopharyngeal (IX), vagus (X), accessory (XI), and hypoglossal (XII).

Central Nervous System

• Brain
• Spinal cord

Peripheral Nervous System

• Cranial nerves (12)
• Spinal nerves
   cervical (8)
   thoracic (12)
   lumbar (5)
   sacral (5)
   coccyx (1)

Figure 16-1 The central nervous system consists of the brain and spinal cord. The peripheral nervous system consists of nerves that lie outside the skull and spinal cord. (From Stoy: Mosby's EMT-Basic Textbook, ed 2, St. Louis, Mosby, 2007)

P13.2   **Birth injury to femur**
P13.3   **Birth injury to other long bones**
P13.4   **Fracture of clavicle due to birth injury**
P13.8   **Birth injuries to other parts of skeleton**
P13.9   **Birth injury to skeleton, unspecified**

⬤ **P14**   **Birth injury to peripheral nervous system**
P14.0   **Erb's paralysis due to birth injury**
P14.1   **Klumpke's paralysis due to birth injury**
P14.2   **Phrenic nerve paralysis due to birth injury**
P14.3   **Other brachial plexus birth injuries**
P14.8   **Birth injuries to other parts of peripheral nervous system**
P14.9   **Birth injury to peripheral nervous system, unspecified**

⬤ **P15**   **Other birth injuries**
P15.0   **Birth injury to liver**
         Rupture of liver due to birth injury
P15.1   **Birth injury to spleen**
         Rupture of spleen due to birth injury
P15.2   **Sternomastoid injury due to birth injury**

P15.3   **Birth injury to eye**
         Subconjunctival hemorrhage due to birth injury
         Traumatic glaucoma due to birth injury
P15.4   **Birth injury to face**
         Facial congestion due to birth injury
P15.5   **Birth injury to external genitalia**
P15.6   **Subcutaneous fat necrosis due to birth injury**
P15.8   **Other specified birth injuries**
P15.9   **Birth injury, unspecified**

RESPIRATORY AND CARDIOVASCULAR DISORDERS SPECIFIC TO THE PERINATAL PERIOD (P19-P29)

⬤ **P19**   **Metabolic acidemia in newborn**
    Includes   metabolic acidemia in newborn
P19.0   **Metabolic acidemia in newborn first noted before onset of labor**
P19.1   **Metabolic acidemia in newborn first noted during labor**
P19.2   **Metabolic acidemia noted at birth**
P19.9   **Metabolic acidemia, unspecified**

⬤ **P22**   **Respiratory distress of newborn**
    Coding Clinic: 2019, Q2, P29
P22.0   **Respiratory distress syndrome of newborn**
         Cardiorespiratory distress syndrome of newborn
         Hyaline membrane disease
         Idiopathic respiratory distress syndrome [IRDS or RDS] of newborn
         Pulmonary hypoperfusion syndrome
         Respiratory distress syndrome, type I
      Excludes2   respiratory arrest of newborn (P28.81)
                 respiratory failure of newborn NOS (P28.5)
      Coding Clinic: 2019, Q2, P29
P22.1   **Transient tachypnea of newborn**
         Idiopathic tachypnea of newborn
         Respiratory distress syndrome, type II
         Wet lung syndrome
P22.8   **Other respiratory distress of newborn**
      Excludes1   respiratory arrest of newborn (P28.81)
                 respiratory failure of newborn NOS (P28.5)
P22.9   **Respiratory distress of newborn, unspecified**
      Excludes1   respiratory arrest of newborn (P28.81)
                 respiratory failure of newborn NOS (P28.5)

⬤ **P23**   **Congenital pneumonia**
    Includes   infective pneumonia acquired in utero or during birth
    Excludes1   neonatal pneumonia resulting from aspiration (P24.-)
P23.0   **Congenital pneumonia due to viral agent**
         Use additional code (B97) to identify organism
      Excludes1   congenital rubella pneumonitis (P35.0)
P23.1   **Congenital pneumonia due to Chlamydia**
P23.2   **Congenital pneumonia due to staphylococcus**
P23.3   **Congenital pneumonia due to streptococcus, group B**
P23.4   **Congenital pneumonia due to Escherichia coli**
P23.5   **Congenital pneumonia due to Pseudomonas**
P23.6   **Congenital pneumonia due to other bacterial agents**
         Congenital pneumonia due to Hemophilus influenzae
         Congenital pneumonia due to Klebsiella pneumoniae
         Congenital pneumonia due to Mycoplasma
         Congenital pneumonia due to Streptococcus, except group B
         Use additional code (B95-B96) to identify organism
P23.8   **Congenital pneumonia due to other organisms**
P23.9   **Congenital pneumonia, unspecified**

CHAPTER 16 (P00-P96)

CHAPTER 16 (P00-P96)

● P24   **Neonatal aspiration**
   Includes   aspiration in utero and during delivery
● P24.0   **Meconium aspiration**
   Excludes1   meconium passage (without aspiration) during delivery (P03.82)
                   meconium staining (P96.83)
   P24.00   **Meconium aspiration without respiratory symptoms**
            Meconium aspiration NOS
   P24.01   **Meconium aspiration with respiratory symptoms**
            Meconium aspiration pneumonia
            Meconium aspiration pneumonitis
            Meconium aspiration syndrome NOS
            Use additional code to identify any secondary pulmonary hypertension, if applicable (I27.2-)
● P24.1   **Neonatal aspiration of (clear) amniotic fluid and mucus**
            Neonatal aspiration of liquor (amnii)
   P24.10   **Neonatal aspiration of (clear) amniotic fluid and mucus without respiratory symptoms**
            Neonatal aspiration of amniotic fluid and mucus NOS
   P24.11   **Neonatal aspiration of (clear) amniotic fluid and mucus with respiratory symptoms**
            Neonatal aspiration of amniotic fluid and mucus with pneumonia
            Neonatal aspiration of amniotic fluid and mucus with pneumonitis
            Use additional code to identify any secondary pulmonary hypertension, if applicable (I27.2-)
● P24.2   **Neonatal aspiration of blood**
   P24.20   **Neonatal aspiration of blood without respiratory symptoms**
            Neonatal aspiration of blood NOS
   P24.21   **Neonatal aspiration of blood with respiratory symptoms**
            Neonatal aspiration of blood with pneumonia
            Neonatal aspiration of blood with pneumonitis
            Use additional code to identify any secondary pulmonary hypertension, if applicable (I27.2-)
● P24.3   **Neonatal aspiration of milk and regurgitated food**
            Neonatal aspiration of stomach contents
   P24.30   **Neonatal aspiration of milk and regurgitated food without respiratory symptoms**
            Neonatal aspiration of milk and regurgitated food NOS
   P24.31   **Neonatal aspiration of milk and regurgitated food with respiratory symptoms**
            Neonatal aspiration of milk and regurgitated food with pneumonia
            Neonatal aspiration of milk and regurgitated food with pneumonitis
            Use additional code to identify any secondary pulmonary hypertension, if applicable (I27.2-)
● P24.8   **Other neonatal aspiration**
   P24.80   **Other neonatal aspiration without respiratory symptoms**
            Neonatal aspiration NEC
   P24.81   **Other neonatal aspiration with respiratory symptoms**
            Neonatal aspiration pneumonia NEC
            Neonatal aspiration with pneumonitis NEC
            Neonatal aspiration with pneumonia NOS
            Neonatal aspiration with pneumonitis NOS
            Use additional code to identify any secondary pulmonary hypertension, if applicable (I27.2-)
   P24.9   **Neonatal aspiration, unspecified**

● P25   **Interstitial emphysema and related conditions originating in the perinatal period**
   P25.0   **Interstitial emphysema originating in the perinatal period**
   P25.1   **Pneumothorax originating in the perinatal period**
   P25.2   **Pneumomediastinum originating in the perinatal period**
   P25.3   **Pneumopericardium originating in the perinatal period**
   P25.8   **Other conditions related to interstitial emphysema originating in the perinatal period**
● P26   **Pulmonary hemorrhage originating in the perinatal period**
   Excludes1   acute idiopathic hemorrhage in infants over 28 days old (R04.81)
   P26.0   **Tracheobronchial hemorrhage originating in the perinatal period**
   P26.1   **Massive pulmonary hemorrhage originating in the perinatal period**
   P26.8   **Other pulmonary hemorrhages originating in the perinatal period**
   P26.9   **Unspecified pulmonary hemorrhage originating in the perinatal period**
● P27   **Chronic respiratory disease originating in the perinatal period**
   Excludes2   respiratory distress of newborn (P22.0-P22.9)
   P27.0   **Wilson-Mikity syndrome**
            Pulmonary dysmaturity
   P27.1   **Bronchopulmonary dysplasia originating in the perinatal period**
   P27.8   **Other chronic respiratory diseases originating in the perinatal period**
            Congenital pulmonary fibrosis
            Ventilator lung in newborn
   P27.9   **Unspecified chronic respiratory disease originating in the perinatal period**
● P28   **Other respiratory conditions originating in the perinatal period**
   ~~Excludes1   congenital malformations of the respiratory system (Q30-Q34)~~
   ▶ Code also, if applicable, congenital malformations of the respiratory system (Q30-Q34)
   P28.0   **Primary atelectasis of newborn**
            Failure of lungs to expand properly at birth
            Primary failure to expand terminal respiratory units
            Pulmonary hypoplasia associated with short gestation
            Pulmonary immaturity NOS
● P28.1   **Other and unspecified atelectasis of newborn**
   P28.10   **Unspecified atelectasis of newborn**
            Atelectasis of newborn NOS
   P28.11   **Resorption atelectasis without respiratory distress syndrome**
            Excludes1   resorption atelectasis with respiratory distress syndrome (P22.0)
   P28.19   **Other atelectasis of newborn**
            Partial atelectasis of newborn
            Secondary atelectasis of newborn
   P28.2   **Cyanotic attacks of newborn**
            ⇒ **Excludes1**   apnea of newborn (P28.3- - P28.4-)
● P28.3   **Primary sleep apnea of newborn**
            ~~Central sleep apnea of newborn~~
            ~~Obstructive sleep apnea of newborn~~
            Sleep apnea of newborn NOS
            ▶ **Excludes2**   other apnea of newborn (P28.4-)
   ▶P28.30   **Primary sleep apnea of newborn, unspecified**
            ▶Transient oxygen desaturation spells of newborn during sleep
   ▶P28.31   **Primary central sleep apnea of newborn**
   ▶P28.32   **Primary obstructive sleep apnea of newborn**
   ▶P28.33   **Primary mixed sleep apnea of newborn**
   ▶P28.39   **Other primary sleep apnea of newborn**

● **P28.4**   **Other apnea of newborn**
   ~~Apnea of prematurity~~
   ~~Obstructive apnea of newborn~~
   ~~Excludes1   obstructive sleep apnea of newborn (P28.3)~~

   ▶ **Excludes2**   primary sleep apnea of newborn (P28.3-)

   ▶**P28.40**   **Unspecified apnea of newborn**
     ▶Apnea of newborn, NOS
     ▶Transient oxygen desaturation spells of newborn

   ▶**P28.41**   **Central neonatal apnea of newborn**

   ▶**P28.42**   **Obstructive apnea of newborn**

   ▶**P28.43**   **Mixed neonatal apnea of newborn**

   ▶**P28.49**   **Other apnea of newborn**
     ▶Apnea of prematurity

P28.5   **Respiratory failure of newborn**
   Excludes1   respiratory arrest of newborn (P28.81)
         respiratory distress of newborn (P22.0-)
   Coding Clinic: 2019, Q2, P29

● **P28.8**   **Other specified respiratory conditions of newborn**

   P28.81   **Respiratory arrest of newborn**
     Coding Clinic: 2017, Q2, P6

   P28.89   **Other specified respiratory conditions of newborn**
     Congenital laryngeal stridor
     Sniffles in newborn
     Snuffles in newborn
     Excludes1   early congenital syphilitic rhinitis (A50.05)

P28.9   **Respiratory condition of newborn, unspecified**
   Respiratory depression in newborn

● **P29**   **Cardiovascular disorders originating in the perinatal period**
   Excludes2   congenital malformations of the circulatory system (Q20-Q28)

P29.0   **Neonatal cardiac failure**

● **P29.1**   **Neonatal cardiac dysrhythmia**

   P29.11   **Neonatal tachycardia**

   P29.12   **Neonatal bradycardia**

P29.2   **Neonatal hypertension**

● **P29.3**   **Persistent fetal circulation**

   P29.30   **Pulmonary hypertension of newborn**
     Persistent pulmonary hypertension of newborn

   P29.38   **Other persistent fetal circulation**
     Delayed closure of ductus arteriosus

P29.4   **Transient myocardial ischemia in newborn**

● **P29.8**   **Other cardiovascular disorders originating in the perinatal period**

   P29.81   **Cardiac arrest of newborn**

   P29.89   **Other cardiovascular disorders originating in the perinatal period**

P29.9   **Cardiovascular disorder originating in the perinatal period, unspecified**

INFECTIONS SPECIFIC TO THE PERINATAL PERIOD (P35-P39)

Infections acquired in utero, during birth via the umbilicus, or during the first 28 days after birth

   Excludes2   asymptomatic human immunodeficiency virus [HIV] infection status (Z21)
     congenital gonococcal infection (A54.-)
     congenital pneumonia (P23.-)
     congenital syphilis (A50.-)
     human immunodeficiency virus [HIV] disease (B20)
     infant botulism (A48.51)
     infectious diseases not specific to the perinatal period (A00-B99, J09, J10.-)
     intestinal infectious disease (A00-A09)
     laboratory evidence of human immunodeficiency virus [HIV] (R75)
     tetanus neonatorum (A33)

● **P35**   **Congenital viral diseases**
   Includes   infections acquired in utero or during birth

   P35.0   **Congenital rubella syndrome**
     Congenital rubella pneumonitis

   P35.1   **Congenital cytomegalovirus infection**
     Viruses transmitted by multiple routes that cause mild/ subclinical infection

   P35.2   **Congenital herpesviral [herpes simplex] infection**

   P35.3   **Congenital viral hepatitis**

   P35.4   **Congenital Zika virus disease**
     Use additional code to identify manifestations of congenital Zika virus disease
     Coding Clinic: 2018, Q4, P26

   P35.8   **Other congenital viral diseases**
     Congenital varicella [chickenpox]
     Coding Clinic: 2016, Q4, P7

   P35.9   **Congenital viral disease, unspecified**

● **P36**   **Bacterial sepsis of newborn**
   Includes   congenital sepsis
   Use additional code(s), if applicable, to identify severe sepsis (R65.2-) and associated acute organ dysfunction(s)

   P36.0   **Sepsis of newborn due to streptococcus, group B** 🔧

●   **P36.1**   **Sepsis of newborn due to other and unspecified streptococci**

     P36.10   **Sepsis of newborn due to unspecified streptococci** 🔧

     P36.19   **Sepsis of newborn due to other streptococci** 🔧

   P36.2   **Sepsis of newborn due to Staphylococcus aureus** 🔧

●   **P36.3**   **Sepsis of newborn due to other and unspecified staphylococci**

     P36.30   **Sepsis of newborn due to unspecified staphylococci** 🔧

     P36.39   **Sepsis of newborn due to other staphylococci** 🔧

   P36.4   **Sepsis of newborn due to Escherichia coli** 🔧

   P36.5   **Sepsis of newborn due to anaerobes** 🔧

   P36.8   **Other bacterial sepsis of newborn** 🔧
     Use additional code from category B96 to identify organism

   P36.9   **Bacterial sepsis of newborn, unspecified** 🔧

● **P37**   **Other congenital infectious and parasitic diseases**
   Excludes2   congenital syphilis (A50.-)
     infectious neonatal diarrhea (A00-A09)
     necrotizing enterocolitis in newborn (P77.-)
     noninfectious neonatal diarrhea (P78.3)
     ophthalmia neonatorum due to gonococcus (A54.31)
     tetanus neonatorum (A33)

   P37.0   **Congenital tuberculosis**

   P37.1   **Congenital toxoplasmosis**
     Parasitic infection, often causing mild flu-like illness
     Hydrocephalus due to congenital toxoplasmosis

   P37.2   **Neonatal (disseminated) listeriosis**
     Acquired transplacentally or during/after parturition in which symptoms are those of sepsis

   P37.3   **Congenital falciparum malaria**

   P37.4   **Other congenital malaria**

   P37.5   **Neonatal candidiasis**

   P37.8   **Other specified congenital infectious and parasitic diseases**

   P37.9   **Congenital infectious or parasitic disease, unspecified**

● **P38**   **Omphalitis of newborn**
   Inflammation of umbilicus
   Excludes1   omphalitis not of newborn (L08.82)
     tetanus omphalitis (A33)
     umbilical hemorrhage of newborn (P51.-)

   P38.1   **Omphalitis with mild hemorrhage**

   P38.9   **Omphalitis without hemorrhage**
     Omphalitis of newborn NOS

CHAPTER 16 (P00-P96)

- **P39 Other infections specific to the perinatal period**
  Use additional code to identify organism or specific infection
  - **P39.0 Neonatal infective mastitis**
    - **Excludes1** breast engorgement of newborn (P83.4)
      noninfective mastitis of newborn (P83.4)
  - **P39.1 Neonatal conjunctivitis and dacryocystitis**
    Neonatal chlamydial conjunctivitis
    Ophthalmia neonatorum NOS
    Neonate = newborn
    - **Excludes1** gonococcal conjunctivitis (A54.31)
  - **P39.2 Intra-amniotic infection affecting newborn, not elsewhere classified**
  - **P39.3 Neonatal urinary tract infection**
  - **P39.4 Neonatal skin infection**
    Neonatal pyoderma
    - **Excludes1** pemphigus neonatorum (L00)
      staphylococcal scalded skin syndrome (L00)
  - **P39.8 Other specified infections specific to the perinatal period**
  - **P39.9 Infection specific to the perinatal period, unspecified**

HEMORRHAGIC AND HEMATOLOGICAL DISORDERS OF NEWBORN (P50-P61)

- **Excludes1** congenital stenosis and stricture of bile ducts (Q44.3)
  Crigler-Najjar syndrome (E80.5)
  Dubin-Johnson syndrome (E80.6)
  Gilbert syndrome (E80.4)
  hereditary hemolytic anemias (D55-D58)

- **P50 Newborn affected by intrauterine (fetal) blood loss**
  - **Excludes1** congenital anemia from intrauterine (fetal) blood loss (P61.3)
  - **P50.0 Newborn affected by intrauterine (fetal) blood loss from vasa previa**
  - **P50.1 Newborn affected by intrauterine (fetal) blood loss from ruptured cord**
  - **P50.2 Newborn affected by intrauterine (fetal) blood loss from placenta**
  - **P50.3 Newborn affected by hemorrhage into co-twin**
  - **P50.4 Newborn affected by hemorrhage into maternal circulation**
  - **P50.5 Newborn affected by intrauterine (fetal) blood loss from cut end of co-twin's cord**
  - **P50.8 Newborn affected by other intrauterine (fetal) blood loss**
  - **P50.9 Newborn affected by intrauterine (fetal) blood loss, unspecified**
    Newborn affected by fetal hemorrhage NOS

- **P51 Umbilical hemorrhage of newborn**
  - **Excludes1** omphalitis with mild hemorrhage (P38.1)
    umbilical hemorrhage from cut end of co-twins cord (P50.5)
  - **P51.0 Massive umbilical hemorrhage of newborn**
  - **P51.8 Other umbilical hemorrhages of newborn**
    Slipped umbilical ligature NOS
  - **P51.9 Umbilical hemorrhage of newborn, unspecified**

- **P52 Intracranial nontraumatic hemorrhage of newborn**
  - **Includes** intracranial hemorrhage due to anoxia or hypoxia
  - **Excludes1** intracranial hemorrhage due to birth injury (P10.-)
    intracranial hemorrhage due to other injury (S06.-)
  - **P52.0 Intraventricular (nontraumatic) hemorrhage, grade 1, of newborn**
    Subependymal hemorrhage (without intraventricular extension)
    Bleeding into germinal matrix

- **P52.1 Intraventricular (nontraumatic) hemorrhage, grade 2, of newborn**
  Subependymal hemorrhage with intraventricular extension
  Bleeding into ventricle
- **P52.2 Intraventricular (nontraumatic) hemorrhage, grade 3 and grade 4, of newborn**
  - **P52.21 Intraventricular (nontraumatic) hemorrhage, grade 3, of newborn**
    Subependymal hemorrhage with intraventricular extension with enlargement of ventricle
  - **P52.22 Intraventricular (nontraumatic) hemorrhage, grade 4, of newborn**
    Bleeding into cerebral cortex
    Subependymal hemorrhage with intracerebral extension
- **P52.3 Unspecified intraventricular (nontraumatic) hemorrhage of newborn**
- **P52.4 Intracerebral (nontraumatic) hemorrhage of newborn**
- **P52.5 Subarachnoid (nontraumatic) hemorrhage of newborn**
- **P52.6 Cerebellar (nontraumatic) and posterior fossa hemorrhage of newborn**
- **P52.8 Other intracranial (nontraumatic) hemorrhages of newborn**
- **P52.9 Intracranial (nontraumatic) hemorrhage of newborn, unspecified**

- **P53 Hemorrhagic disease of newborn**
  Vitamin K deficiency of newborn
- **P54 Other neonatal hemorrhages**
  - **Excludes1** newborn affected by (intrauterine) blood loss (P50.-)
    pulmonary hemorrhage originating in the perinatal period (P26.-)
  - **P54.0 Neonatal hematemesis**
    Vomiting of blood
    - **Excludes1** neonatal hematemesis due to swallowed maternal blood (P78.2)
  - **P54.1 Neonatal melena**
    Dark-colored feces stained with blood pigments
    - **Excludes1** neonatal melena due to swallowed maternal blood (P78.2)
  - **P54.2 Neonatal rectal hemorrhage**
  - **P54.3 Other neonatal gastrointestinal hemorrhage**
  - **P54.4 Neonatal adrenal hemorrhage**
  - **P54.5 Neonatal cutaneous hemorrhage**
    Neonatal bruising
    Neonatal ecchymoses
    Neonatal petechiae
    Neonatal superficial hematomata
    - **Excludes2** bruising of scalp due to birth injury (P12.3)
      cephalhematoma due to birth injury (P12.0)
  - **P54.6 Neonatal vaginal hemorrhage ♀**
    Neonatal pseudomenses
  - **P54.8 Other specified neonatal hemorrhages**
  - **P54.9 Neonatal hemorrhage, unspecified**

- **P55 Hemolytic disease of newborn**
  AKA erythroblastosis fetalis and is due to Rh isoimmunization, result of Rh blood factor incompatibilities between mother (Rh negative) and fetus (Rh positive)
  - **P55.0 Rh isoimmunization of newborn**
  - **P55.1 ABO isoimmunization of newborn**
    Coding Clinic: 2015, Q3, P20
  - **P55.8 Other hemolytic diseases of newborn**
  - **P55.9 Hemolytic disease of newborn, unspecified**

▶ New ⇒ Revised ~~deleted~~ Deleted | Excludes 1 | Excludes 2 | Includes | Use additional | Code first | Code also | Key words
OGCR Official Guidelines X Assign placeholder X ● Use Additional Character(s) ▶ Manifestation Code ℞ Hierarchical Condition Category **Coding Clinic**

CHAPTER 16 (P00-P96)

● **P56**   **Hydrops fetalis due to hemolytic disease**
Caused by maternal sensitization to fetal blood group antigen
> **Excludes1**   hydrops fetalis NOS (P83.2)

    P56.0   Hydrops fetalis due to isoimmunization
● **P56.9**   Hydrops fetalis due to other and unspecified hemolytic disease
      P56.90   Hydrops fetalis due to unspecified hemolytic disease
      P56.99   Hydrops fetalis due to other hemolytic disease

● **P57**   **Kernicterus**
High levels of bilirubin in blood, with severe neural symptoms
    P57.0   Kernicterus due to isoimmunization
    P57.8   Other specified kernicterus
> **Excludes1**   Crigler-Najjar syndrome (E80.5)

    P57.9   Kernicterus, unspecified

● **P58**   **Neonatal jaundice due to other excessive hemolysis**
> **Excludes1**   jaundice due to isoimmunization (P55-P57)

    P58.0   Neonatal jaundice due to bruising
    P58.1   Neonatal jaundice due to bleeding
    P58.2   Neonatal jaundice due to infection
    P58.3   Neonatal jaundice due to polycythemia
● **P58.4**   Neonatal jaundice due to drugs or toxins transmitted from mother or given to newborn
> *Code first poisoning due to drug or toxin, if applicable (T36-T65 with fifth or sixth character 1-4 or 6)*
> Use additional code for adverse effect, if applicable, to identify drug (T36-T50 with fifth or sixth character 5)

      P58.41   Neonatal jaundice due to drugs or toxins transmitted from mother
      P58.42   Neonatal jaundice due to drugs or toxins given to newborn
    P58.5   Neonatal jaundice due to swallowed maternal blood
    P58.8   Neonatal jaundice due to other specified excessive hemolysis
    P58.9   Neonatal jaundice due to excessive hemolysis, unspecified

● **P59**   **Neonatal jaundice from other and unspecified causes**
> **Excludes1**   jaundice due to inborn errors of metabolism (E70-E88)
> kernicterus (P57.-)

    P59.0   Neonatal jaundice associated with preterm delivery
Hyperbilirubinemia of prematurity
Jaundice due to delayed conjugation associated with preterm delivery
    P59.1   Inspissated bile syndrome
● **P59.2**   Neonatal jaundice from other and unspecified hepatocellular damage
> **Excludes1**   congenital viral hepatitis (P35.3)

      P59.20   Neonatal jaundice from unspecified hepatocellular damage
      P59.29   Neonatal jaundice from other hepatocellular damage
Neonatal giant cell hepatitis
Neonatal (idiopathic) hepatitis
    P59.3   Neonatal jaundice from breast milk inhibitor
    P59.8   Neonatal jaundice from other specified causes
    P59.9   Neonatal jaundice, unspecified
Neonatal physiological jaundice (intense)(prolonged) NOS
Coding Clinic: 2015, Q3, P20

P60   **Disseminated intravascular coagulation of newborn**
Defibrination syndrome of newborn

● **P61**   **Other perinatal hematological disorders**
> **Excludes1**   transient hypogammaglobulinemia of infancy (D80.7)

    P61.0   Transient neonatal thrombocytopenia
Lack of sufficient numbers of circulating thrombocytes (platelets)
Neonatal thrombocytopenia due to exchange transfusion
Neonatal thrombocytopenia due to idiopathic maternal thrombocytopenia
Neonatal thrombocytopenia due to isoimmunization
    P61.1   Polycythemia neonatorum
Neonate = newborn
    P61.2   Anemia of prematurity
    P61.3   Congenital anemia from fetal blood loss
    P61.4   Other congenital anemias, not elsewhere classified
Congenital anemia NOS
    P61.5   Transient neonatal neutropenia
Low levels of granulocytic neutrophilic white blood cells
> **Excludes1**   congenital neutropenia (nontransient) (D70.0)

    P61.6   Other transient neonatal disorders of coagulation
    P61.8   Other specified perinatal hematological disorders
    P61.9   Perinatal hematological disorder, unspecified

TRANSITORY ENDOCRINE AND METABOLIC DISORDERS SPECIFIC TO NEWBORN (P70-P74)

> **Includes**   transitory endocrine and metabolic disturbances caused by the infant's response to maternal endocrine and metabolic factors, or its adjustment to extrauterine environment

● **P70**   **Transitory disorders of carbohydrate metabolism specific to newborn**
    P70.0   Syndrome of infant of mother with gestational diabetes
Newborn (with hypoglycemia) affected by maternal gestational diabetes
> **Excludes1**   newborn (with hypoglycemia) affected by maternal (pre-existing) diabetes mellitus (P70.1)
> syndrome of infant of a diabetic mother (P70.1)

    P70.1   Syndrome of infant of a diabetic mother
Newborn (with hypoglycemia) affected by maternal (pre-existing) diabetes mellitus
> **Excludes1**   newborn (with hypoglycemia) affected by maternal gestational diabetes (P70.0)
> syndrome of infant of mother with gestational diabetes (P70.0)

    P70.2   Neonatal diabetes mellitus
    P70.3   Iatrogenic neonatal hypoglycemia
    P70.4   Other neonatal hypoglycemia
Transitory neonatal hypoglycemia
    P70.8   Other transitory disorders of carbohydrate metabolism of newborn
    P70.9   Transitory disorder of carbohydrate metabolism of newborn, unspecified

● **P71**   **Transitory neonatal disorders of calcium and magnesium metabolism**
    P71.0   Cow's milk hypocalcemia in newborn
    P71.1   Other neonatal hypocalcemia
> **Excludes1**   neonatal hypoparathyroidism (P71.4)

    P71.2   Neonatal hypomagnesemia
    P71.3   Neonatal tetany without calcium or magnesium deficiency
Neonatal tetany NOS

CHAPTER 16 (P00-P96)

P71.4   Transitory neonatal hypoparathyroidism

P71.8   Other transitory neonatal disorders of calcium and magnesium metabolism
Coding Clinic: 2016, Q4, P55

P71.9   Transitory neonatal disorder of calcium and magnesium metabolism, unspecified

● **P72**   Other transitory neonatal endocrine disorders

> **Excludes1**   congenital hypothyroidism with or without goiter (E03.0-E03.1)
> dyshormogenetic goiter (E07.1)
> Pendred's syndrome (E07.1)

P72.0   Neonatal goiter, not elsewhere classified
Transitory congenital goiter with normal functioning

P72.1   Transitory neonatal hyperthyroidism
Neonatal thyrotoxicosis

P72.2   Other transitory neonatal disorders of thyroid function, not elsewhere classified
Transitory neonatal hypothyroidism

P72.8   Other specified transitory neonatal endocrine disorders

P72.9   Transitory neonatal endocrine disorder, unspecified

● **P74**   Other transitory neonatal electrolyte and metabolic disturbances

P74.0   Late metabolic acidosis of newborn

> **Excludes1**   (fetal) metabolic acidosis of newborn (P19)

P74.1   Dehydration of newborn

● **P74.2**   Disturbances of sodium balance of newborn
Coding Clinic: 2018, Q2, P6

P74.21   Hypernatremia of newborn

P74.22   Hyponatremia of newborn

● **P74.3**   Disturbances of potassium balance of newborn

P74.31   Hyperkalemia of newborn

P74.32   Hypokalemia of newborn

● **P74.4**   Other transitory electrolyte disturbances of newborn

P74.41   Alkalosis of newborn
Hyperbicarbonatemia

● **P74.42**   Disturbances of chlorine balance of newborn

P74.421   Hyperchloremia of newborn
Hyperchloremic metabolic acidosis

> **Excludes2**   late metabolic acidosis of the newborn (P74.0)

P74.422   Hypochloremia of newborn

P74.49   Other transitory electrolyte disturbance of newborn

P74.5   Transitory tyrosinemia of newborn

P74.6   Transitory hyperammonemia of newborn

P74.8   Other transitory metabolic disturbances of newborn
Amino-acid metabolic disorders described as transitory

P74.9   Transitory metabolic disturbance of newborn, unspecified

DIGESTIVE SYSTEM DISORDERS OF NEWBORN (P76-P78)

● **P76**   Other intestinal obstruction of newborn

P76.0   Meconium plug syndrome
Fetal stool obstruction in large intestine, present at birth; may be symptom of organic disease.
Meconium ileus NOS

> **Excludes1**   meconium ileus in cystic fibrosis (E84.11)

P76.1   Transitory ileus of newborn
Temporary obstruction of ileus (small intestine)

> **Excludes1**   Hirschsprung's disease (Q43.1)

P76.2   Intestinal obstruction due to inspissated milk
Being thickened, dried, or made less fluid

P76.8   Other specified intestinal obstruction of newborn

> **Excludes1**   intestinal obstruction classifiable to K56.-

P76.9   Intestinal obstruction of newborn, unspecified

● **P77**   Necrotizing enterocolitis of newborn

P77.1   Stage 1 necrotizing enterocolitis in newborn
Necrotizing enterocolitis without pneumatosis, without perforation

P77.2   Stage 2 necrotizing enterocolitis in newborn
Necrotizing enterocolitis with pneumatosis, without perforation

P77.3   Stage 3 necrotizing enterocolitis in newborn
Necrotizing enterocolitis with perforation
Necrotizing enterocolitis with pneumatosis and perforation

P77.9   Necrotizing enterocolitis in newborn, unspecified
Necrotizing enterocolitis in newborn, NOS

● **P78**   Other perinatal digestive system disorders

> **Excludes1**   cystic fibrosis (E84.0-E84.9)
> neonatal gastrointestinal hemorrhages (P54.0-P54.3)

P78.0   Perinatal intestinal perforation
Meconium peritonitis

P78.1   Other neonatal peritonitis
Neonatal peritonitis NOS

P78.2   Neonatal hematemesis and melena due to swallowed maternal blood

P78.3   Noninfective neonatal diarrhea
Neonatal diarrhea NOS

● **P78.8**   Other specified perinatal digestive system disorders

P78.81   Congenital cirrhosis (of liver)

P78.82   Peptic ulcer of newborn

P78.83   Newborn esophageal reflux
Neonatal esophageal reflux

P78.84   Gestational alloimmune liver disease
GALD
Neonatal hemochromatosis

> **Excludes1**   hemochromatosis (E83.11-)

P78.89   Other specified perinatal digestive system disorders

P78.9   Perinatal digestive system disorder, unspecified

CONDITIONS INVOLVING THE INTEGUMENT AND TEMPERATURE REGULATION OF NEWBORN (P80-P83)

● **P80**   Hypothermia of newborn

P80.0   Cold injury syndrome
Severe and usually chronic hypothermia associated with a pink flushed appearance, edema and neurological and biochemical abnormalities.

> **Excludes1**   mild hypothermia of newborn (P80.8)

P80.8   Other hypothermia of newborn
Mild hypothermia of newborn

P80.9   Hypothermia of newborn, unspecified

● **P81**   Other disturbances of temperature regulation of newborn

P81.0   Environmental hyperthermia of newborn

P81.8   Other specified disturbances of temperature regulation of newborn

P81.9   Disturbance of temperature regulation of newborn, unspecified
Fever of newborn NOS

▶ New   ⇒ Revised   ~~deleted~~ Deleted   Excludes 1   Excludes 2   Includes   Use additional   Code first   Code also   Key words
OGCR Official Guidelines   X Assign placeholder X   ● Use Additional Character(s)   ▶ Manifestation Code   🏷 Hierarchical Condition Category   Coding Clinic

● **P83**   **Other conditions of integument specific to newborn**

    Excludes1 congenital malformations of skin and integument
              (Q80–Q84)
           hydrops fetalis due to hemolytic disease (P56.-)
           neonatal skin infection (P39.4)
           staphylococcal scalded skin syndrome (L00)

    Excludes2 cradle cap (L21.0)
           diaper [napkin] dermatitis (L22)

  P83.0 **Sclerema neonatorum**
      Neonate = newborn

  P83.1 **Neonatal erythema toxicum**
      Benign, generalized, transient pustules that become firm
          vesicles

  P83.2 **Hydrops fetalis not due to hemolytic disease**
      Severe, life-threatening problem of severe edema (swelling)
          as a result of too much fluid leaving blood and entering
          tissue
      Hydrops fetalis NOS

● **P83.3** **Other and unspecified edema specific to newborn**
      P83.30 **Unspecified edema specific to newborn**
      P83.39 **Other edema specific to newborn**

  P83.4 **Breast engorgement of newborn**
      Noninfective mastitis of newborn

  P83.5 **Congenital hydrocele** ♂

  P83.6 **Umbilical polyp of newborn**

● **P83.8** **Other specified conditions of integument specific to
      newborn**
      P83.81 **Umbilical granuloma**
          Excludes2 Granulomatous disorder of the
                 skin and subcutaneous
                 tissue, unspecified (L92.9)

      P83.88 **Other specified conditions of integument
          specific to newborn**
          Bronze baby syndrome
          Neonatal scleroderma
          Urticaria neonatorum

  P83.9 **Condition of the integument specific to newborn,
      unspecified**

OTHER PROBLEMS WITH NEWBORN (P84)

P84 **Other problems with newborn**
    Acidemia of newborn
    Acidosis of newborn
    Anoxia of newborn NOS
    Asphyxia of newborn NOS
    Hypercapnia of newborn
    Hypoxemia of newborn
    Hypoxia of newborn NOS
    Mixed metabolic and respiratory acidosis of newborn

    Excludes1 intracranial hemorrhage due to anoxia or hypoxia
           (P52.-)
           hypoxic ischemic encephalopathy [HIE] (P91.6-)
           late metabolic acidosis of newborn (P74.0)

OTHER DISORDERS ORIGINATING IN THE PERINATAL PERIOD (P90-P96)

P90 **Convulsions of newborn**
    Excludes1 benign myoclonic epilepsy in infancy (G40.3-)
           benign neonatal convulsions (familial) (G40.3-)

● **P91** **Other disturbances of cerebral status of newborn**
  P91.0 **Neonatal cerebral ischemia**
      Excludes1 Neonatal cerebral infarction (P91.82-)

  P91.1 **Acquired periventricular cysts of newborn**

  P91.2 **Neonatal cerebral leukomalacia**
      Degeneration of white matter adjacent to cerebral ventricles
          following cerebral hypoxia or brain ischemia in neonates
      Periventricular leukomalacia

  P91.3 **Neonatal cerebral irritability**
  P91.4 **Neonatal cerebral depression**
  P91.5 **Neonatal coma**
● **P91.6** **Hypoxic ischemic encephalopathy [HIE]**
      Excludes1 Neonatal cerebral depression (P91.4)
             Neonatal cerebral irritability (P91.3)
             Neonatal coma (P91.5)

      P91.60 **Hypoxic ischemic encephalopathy [HIE],
          unspecified**
      P91.61 **Mild hypoxic ischemic encephalopathy
          [HIE]**
      P91.62 **Moderate hypoxic ischemic encephalopathy
          [HIE]**
      P91.63 **Severe hypoxic ischemic encephalopathy [HIE]**

● **P91.8** **Other specified disturbances of cerebral status of newborn**
    ● **P91.81** **Neonatal encephalopathy**
      ▶ *P91.811* *Neonatal encephalopathy in diseases
              classified elsewhere*
            Code first underlying condition, if known,
              such as:
             congenital cirrhosis (of liver) (P78.81)
             intracranial nontraumatic
               hemorrhage of newborn (P52.-)
             kernicterus (P57.-)
      P91.819 **Neonatal encephalopathy, unspecified**

    ● **P91.82** **Neonatal cerebral infarction**
      Neonatal stroke
      Perinatal arterial ischemic stroke
      Perinatal cerebral infarction
        Excludes1 cerebral infarction (I63.-)
        Excludes2 intracranial hemorrhage of
                newborn (P52.-)
      P91.821 **Neonatal cerebral infarction, right
          side of brain**
      P91.822 **Neonatal cerebral infarction, left side
          of brain**
      P91.823 **Neonatal cerebral infarction, bilateral**
      P91.829 **Neonatal cerebral infarction,
          unspecified side**

      P91.88 **Other specified disturbances of cerebral status
          of newborn**

  P91.9 **Disturbance of cerebral status of newborn, unspecified**

● **P92** **Feeding problems of newborn**
    Excludes2 feeding problems in child over 28 days old
           (R63.3)

    Coding Clinic: 2017, Q1, P28; 2016, Q3, P19

● **P92.0** **Vomiting of newborn**
      Excludes1 vomiting of child over 28 days old (R11.-)
      P92.01 **Bilious vomiting of newborn**
          Excludes1 bilious vomiting in child over
                28 days old (R11.14)
      P92.09 **Other vomiting of newborn**
          Excludes1 regurgitation of food in newborn
                (P92.1)

  P92.1 **Regurgitation and rumination of newborn**
  P92.2 **Slow feeding of newborn**
  P92.3 **Underfeeding of newborn**
  P92.4 **Overfeeding of newborn**
  P92.5 **Neonatal difficulty in feeding at breast**
      Coding Clinic: 2017, Q1, P28; 2016, Q3, P19
  P92.6 **Failure to thrive in newborn**
      Excludes1 failure to thrive in child over 28 days old
           (R62.51)

  P92.8 **Other feeding problems of newborn**
  P92.9 **Feeding problem of newborn, unspecified**

CHAPTER 16 (P00-P96)

● **P93** **Reactions and intoxications due to drugs administered to newborn**

> **Includes** reactions and intoxications due to drugs administered to fetus affecting newborn
>
> **Excludes1** jaundice due to drugs or toxins transmitted from mother or given to newborn (P58.4-)
> reactions and intoxications from maternal opiates, tranquilizers and other medication (P04.0-P04.1, P04.4-)
> withdrawal symptoms from maternal use of drugs of addiction (P96.1)
> withdrawal symptoms from therapeutic use of drugs in newborn (P96.2)

P93.0 **Grey baby syndrome**
Grey syndrome from chloramphenicol administration in newborn

P93.8 **Other reactions and intoxications due to drugs administered to newborn**
> Use additional code for adverse effect, if applicable, to identify drug (T36-T50 with fifth or sixth character 5)

● **P94** **Disorders of muscle tone of newborn**

P94.0 **Transient neonatal myasthenia gravis**
> **Excludes1** myasthenia gravis (G70.0)

P94.1 **Congenital hypertonia**

P94.2 **Congenital hypotonia**
Floppy baby syndrome, unspecified

P94.8 **Other disorders of muscle tone of newborn**

P94.9 **Disorder of muscle tone of newborn, unspecified**

OGCR Section I.C.16.g.

> Stillbirth
>
> Code P95, Stillbirth, is only for use for institutions that maintain separate records for stillbirths. No other code should be used with P95. Code P95 should not be used on the mother's record.

P95 **Stillbirth**
Deadborn fetus NOS
Fetal death of unspecified cause
Stillbirth NOS

> **Excludes1** maternal care for intrauterine death (O36.4)
> missed abortion (O02.1)
> outcome of delivery, stillbirth (Z37.1, Z37.3, Z37.4, Z37.7)

● **P96** **Other conditions originating in the perinatal period**

P96.0 **Congenital renal failure**
Uremia of newborn

P96.1 **Neonatal withdrawal symptoms from maternal use of drugs of addiction**
Drug withdrawal syndrome in infant of dependent mother
Neonatal abstinence syndrome

> **Excludes1** reactions and intoxications from maternal opiates and tranquilizers administered during labor and delivery (P04.0)

P96.2 **Withdrawal symptoms from therapeutic use of drugs in newborn**

P96.3 **Wide cranial sutures of newborn**
Neonatal craniotabes

P96.5 **Complication to newborn due to (fetal) intrauterine procedure**

> **Excludes2** newborn affected by amniocentesis (P00.6)

● **P96.8** **Other specified conditions originating in the perinatal period**

P96.81 **Exposure to (parental) (environmental) tobacco smoke in the perinatal period**

> **Excludes2** newborn affected by in utero exposure to tobacco (P04.2)
> exposure to environmental tobacco smoke after the perinatal period (Z77.22)

P96.82 **Delayed separation of umbilical cord**

P96.83 **Meconium staining**

> **Excludes1** meconium aspiration (P24.00, P24.01)
> meconium passage during delivery (P03.82)

P96.89 **Other specified conditions originating in the perinatal period**
> Use additional code to specify condition

P96.9 **Condition originating in the perinatal period, unspecified**
Congenital debility NOS

▶ New ⇒ Revised ~~deleted~~ Deleted | Excludes 1 | Excludes 2 | Includes | Use additional | Code first | Code also | Key words
OGCR Official Guidelines X Assign placeholder X ● Use Additional Character(s) ▸ Manifestation Code ◓ Hierarchical Condition Category **Coding Clinic**

CHAPTER 17

CONGENITAL MALFORMATIONS, DEFORMATIONS, AND CHROMOSOMAL ABNORMALITIES (Q00-Q99)

OGCR Chapter-Specific Coding Guidelines

17. **Chapter 17: Congenital malformations, deformations, and chromosomal abnormalities (Q00-Q99)**

Assign an appropriate code(s) from categories Q00-Q99, Congenital malformations, deformations, and chromosomal abnormalities when a malformation/deformation or chromosomal abnormality is documented. A malformation/deformation/ or chromosomal abnormality may be the principal/first-listed diagnosis on a record or a secondary diagnosis.

When a malformation/deformation/or chromosomal abnormality does not have a unique code assignment, assign additional code(s) for any manifestations that may be present.

When the code assignment specifically identifies the malformation/deformation/or chromosomal abnormality, manifestations that are an inherent component of the anomaly should not be coded separately. Additional codes should be assigned for manifestations that are not an inherent component.

Codes from Chapter 17 may be used throughout the life of the patient. If a congenital malformation or deformity has been corrected, a personal history code should be used to identify the history of the malformation or deformity. Although present at birth, malformation/deformation/or chromosomal abnormality may not be identified until later in life. Whenever the condition is diagnosed by the physician, it is appropriate to assign a code from codes Q00-Q99.

For the birth admission, the appropriate code from category Z38, Liveborn infants, according to place of birth and type of delivery, should be sequenced as the principal diagnosis, followed by any congenital anomaly codes, Q00-Q99.

CHAPTER 17

CONGENITAL MALFORMATIONS, DEFORMATIONS, AND CHROMOSOMAL ABNORMALITIES (Q00-Q99)

Note: Codes from this chapter are not for use on maternal records

Excludes2 inborn errors of metabolism (E70-E88)

This chapter contains the following blocks:

Q00-Q07	Congenital malformations of the nervous system
Q10-Q18	Congenital malformations of eye, ear, face and neck
Q20-Q28	Congenital malformations of the circulatory system
Q30-Q34	Congenital malformations of the respiratory system
Q35-Q37	Cleft lip and cleft palate
Q38-Q45	Other congenital malformations of the digestive system
Q50-Q56	Congenital malformations of genital organs
Q60-Q64	Congenital malformations of the urinary system
Q65-Q79	Congenital malformations and deformations of the musculoskeletal system
Q80-Q89	Other congenital malformations
Q90-Q99	Chromosomal abnormalities, not elsewhere classified

Figure 17-1 An infant with a large occipital encephalocele. The large skin-covered encephalocele is visible. (From Swaiman KF, Ashwal S, Ferriero DM: Pediatric Neurology: Principles and Practice, Philadelphia, Saunders, 2012)

CONGENITAL MALFORMATIONS OF THE NERVOUS SYSTEM (Q00–Q07)

● **Q00 Anencephaly and similar malformations**

Q00.0 Anencephaly 🔧
Absence of skull with cerebral hemispheres missing or reduced to small masses attached to base of cranium
Acephaly
Acrania
Amyelencephaly
Hemianencephaly
Hemicephaly

Q00.1 Craniorachischisis 🔧
Developmental anomaly consisting of fissure of cranium and vertebral column

Q00.2 Iniencephaly 🔧
Developmental anomaly characterized by enlargement of foramen magnum and absence of laminae and spinous processes of cervical, dorsal

● **Q01 Encephalocele**
Sac-like protrusions of brain and membranes visible through an opening in skull

    Includes   Arnold-Chiari syndrome, type III
                    encephalocystocele
                    encephalomyelocele
                    hydroencephalocele
                    hydromeningocele, cranial
                    meningocele, cerebral
                    meningoencephalocele

    Excludes1   Meckel-Gruber syndrome (Q61.9)

Q01.0 Frontal encephalocele 🔧
Q01.1 Nasofrontal encephalocele 🔧
Q01.2 Occipital encephalocele 🔧
Q01.8 Encephalocele of other sites 🔧
Q01.9 Encephalocele, unspecified 🔧

Q02 Microcephaly 🔧
Head size measures significantly below normal based on standardized charts

    Includes   hydromicrocephaly
                    micrencephalon

Code first, if applicable, congenital Zika virus disease

    Excludes1   Meckel-Gruber syndrome (Q61.9)

Coding Clinic: 2018, Q4, P26; 2016, Q4, P7

● **Q03 Congenital hydrocephalus**
Accumulation of cerebrospinal fluid in ventricles resulting in swelling and enlargement

    Includes   hydrocephalus in newborn
    Excludes1   Arnold-Chiari syndrome, type II (Q07.0-)
                    acquired hydrocephalus (G91.-)
                    hydrocephalus due to congenital toxoplasmosis (P37.1)
                    hydrocephalus with spina bifida (Q05.0-Q05.4)

Q03.0 Malformations of aqueduct of Sylvius 🔧
Anomaly of aqueduct of Sylvius
Obstruction of aqueduct of Sylvius, congenital
Stenosis of aqueduct of Sylvius

Q03.1 Atresia of foramina of Magendie and Luschka 🔧
Dandy-Walker syndrome

Q03.8 Other congenital hydrocephalus 🔧

Q03.9 Congenital hydrocephalus, unspecified 🔧

CHAPTER 17 (Q00-Q99)

● **Q04   Other congenital malformations of brain**

    Excludes1   cyclopia (Q87.0)
                   macrocephaly (Q75.3)

    Q04.0   Congenital malformations of corpus callosum 🐾
         Agenesis of corpus callosum

    Q04.1   Arhinencephaly 🐾
         Congenital absence of olfactory bulbs, tract, or nerves

    Q04.2   Holoprosencephaly 🐾
         Failure of cleavage of forebrain (prosencephalon) resulting in incomplete or absent cortical separation and deficits in midline facial development

    Q04.3   Other reduction deformities of brain 🐾
         Absence of part of brain
         Agenesis of part of brain
            Cerebral cortex are not fully formed, brain surface is smooth
         Agyria
         Aplasia of part of brain
         Hydranencephaly
         Hypoplasia of part of brain
         Lissencephaly
            Congenital malformation or absence of convolutions of cerebral cortex
         Microgyria
            Malformation of brain characterized by excessive number of small convolutions (gyri) on surface
         Pachygyria
            Reduction in number of sulci of cerebrum
         Excludes1   congenital malformations of corpus callosum (Q04.0)

    Q04.4   Septo-optic dysplasia of brain 🐾

    Q04.5   Megalencephaly 🐾
         Abnormally large brain

    Q04.6   Congenital cerebral cysts 🐾
         Porencephaly   Schizencephaly
         Excludes1   acquired porencephalic cyst (G93.0)

    Q04.8   Other specified congenital malformations of brain 🐾
         Arnold-Chiari syndrome, type IV
         Macrogyria

    Q04.9   Congenital malformation of brain, unspecified 🐾
         Congenital anomaly NOS of brain
         Congenital deformity NOS of brain
         Congenital disease or lesion NOS of brain
         Multiple anomalies NOS of brain, congenital

● **Q05   Spina bifida**
    Developmental anomaly characterized by defective closure of vertebral arch, through which spinal cord and meninges may protrude

    Includes   hydromeningocele (spinal)
               meningocele (spinal)
               meningomyelocele
               myelocele
               myelomeningocele
               rachischisis
               spina bifida (aperta)(cystica)
               syringomyelocele

    Use additional code for any associated paraplegia (paraparesis) (G82.2-)

    Excludes1   Arnold-Chiari syndrome, type II (Q07.0-)
                   spina bifida occulta (Q76.0)

    Q05.0   Cervical spina bifida with hydrocephalus 🐾

    Q05.1   Thoracic spina bifida with hydrocephalus 🐾
         Dorsal spina bifida with hydrocephalus
         Thoracolumbar spina bifida with hydrocephalus

    Q05.2   Lumbar spina bifida with hydrocephalus 🐾
         Lumbosacral spina bifida with hydrocephalus

    Q05.3   Sacral spina bifida with hydrocephalus 🐾

    Q05.4   Unspecified spina bifida with hydrocephalus 🐾

    Q05.5   Cervical spina bifida without hydrocephalus 🐾

    Q05.6   Thoracic spina bifida without hydrocephalus 🐾
         Dorsal spina bifida NOS
         Thoracolumbar spina bifida NOS

    Q05.7   Lumbar spina bifida without hydrocephalus 🐾
         Lumbosacral spina bifida NOS

    Q05.8   Sacral spina bifida without hydrocephalus 🐾

    Q05.9   Spina bifida, unspecified 🐾

● **Q06   Other congenital malformations of spinal cord**

    Q06.0   Amyelia 🐾
         Congenital absence of spinal cord

    Q06.1   Hypoplasia and dysplasia of spinal cord 🐾
         Underdevelopment of spinal cord
         Atelomyelia
            Congenitally incomplete development of spinal cord
         Myelatelia
         Myelodysplasia of spinal cord
            Defective development of spinal cord, especially lower segments

    Q06.2   Diastematomyelia 🐾
         Congenital anomaly, associated with spina bifida, in which spinal cord is split into halves and surrounded by dural sac

    Q06.3   Other congenital cauda equina malformations 🐾

    Q06.4   Hydromyelia 🐾
         Dilation of central canal of spinal cord with increased fluid accumulation
         Hydrorachis

    Q06.8   Other specified congenital malformations of spinal cord 🐾

    Q06.9   Congenital malformation of spinal cord, unspecified 🐾
         Congenital anomaly NOS of spinal cord
         Congenital deformity NOS of spinal cord
         Congenital disease or lesion NOS of spinal cord

● **Q07   Other congenital malformations of nervous system**

    Excludes2   congenital central alveolar hypoventilation syndrome (G47.35)
                   familial dysautonomia [Riley-Day] (G90.1)
                   neurofibromatosis (nonmalignant) (Q85.0-)

● **Q07.0   Arnold-Chiari syndrome**
         Herniation of cerebellar tonsils and vermis through foramen magnum into spinal canal
         Arnold-Chiari syndrome, type II
         Excludes1   Arnold-Chiari syndrome, type III (Q01.-)
                        Arnold-Chiari syndrome, type IV (Q04.8)

    Q07.00   Arnold-Chiari syndrome without spina bifida or hydrocephalus 🐾

    Q07.01   Arnold-Chiari syndrome with spina bifida 🐾

    Q07.02   Arnold-Chiari syndrome with hydrocephalus 🐾

    Q07.03   Arnold-Chiari syndrome with spina bifida and hydrocephalus 🐾

    Q07.8   Other specified congenital malformations of nervous system 🐾
         Agenesis of nerve
         Displacement of brachial plexus
         Jaw-winking syndrome
         Marcus Gunn's syndrome

    Q07.9   Congenital malformation of nervous system, unspecified 🐾
         Congenital anomaly NOS of nervous system
         Congenital deformity NOS of nervous system
         Congenital disease or lesion NOS of nervous system

CONGENITAL MALFORMATIONS OF EYE, EAR, FACE AND NECK (Q10-Q18)

> **Excludes2**   cleft lip and cleft palate (Q35-Q37)
> congenital malformation of cervical spine (Q05.0, Q05.5, Q67.5, Q76.0-Q76.4)
> congenital malformation of larynx (Q31.-)
> congenital malformation of lip NEC (Q38.0)
> congenital malformation of nose (Q30.-)
> congenital malformation of parathyroid gland (Q89.2)
> congenital malformation of thyroid gland (Q89.2)

● **Q10   Congenital malformations of eyelid, lacrimal apparatus and orbit**

> **Excludes1**   cryptophthalmos NOS (Q11.2)
> cryptophthalmos syndrome (Q87.0)

Q10.0   Congenital ptosis
> *Prolapse or drooping of upper eyelid from paralysis of third nerve or from sympathetic innervations*

Q10.1   Congenital ectropion
> *Outward turning of eyelid*

Q10.2   Congenital entropion
> *Inward turning of eyelid*

Q10.3   Other congenital malformations of eyelid
> Ablepharon
> Blepharophimosis, congenital
> Coloboma of eyelid
> Congenital absence or agenesis of cilia
> Congenital absence or agenesis of eyelid
> Congenital accessory eyelid
> Congenital accessory eye muscle
> Congenital malformation of eyelid NOS

Q10.4   Absence and agenesis of lacrimal apparatus
> Congenital absence of punctum lacrimale

Q10.5   Congenital stenosis and stricture of lacrimal duct

Q10.6   Other congenital malformations of lacrimal apparatus
> Congenital malformation of lacrimal apparatus NOS

Q10.7   Congenital malformation of orbit

● **Q11   Anophthalmos, microphthalmos and macrophthalmos**
> *Absence of eye and optic pit*

Q11.0   Cystic eyeball

Q11.1   Other anophthalmos
> Anophthalmos NOS
> Agenesis of eye
> > *Absence of eye*
> Aplasia of eye

Q11.2   Microphthalmos
> *Partial absence of eye and optic pit*
> Cryptophthalmos NOS
> Dysplasia of eye
> Hypoplasia of eye
> Rudimentary eye
> > **Excludes1**   cryptophthalmos syndrome (Q87.0)

Q11.3   Macrophthalmos
> *Congenital enlargement of eyes*
> > **Excludes1**   macrophthalmos in congenital glaucoma (Q15.0)

● **Q12   Congenital lens malformations**

Q12.0   Congenital cataract

Q12.1   Congenital displaced lens

Q12.2   Coloboma of lens

Q12.3   Congenital aphakia

Q12.4   Spherophakia
> *Smaller, more spherical optic lens than normal*

Q12.8   Other congenital lens malformations
> Microphakia

Q12.9   Congenital lens malformation, unspecified

Figure 17-2   Bilateral congenital **hydrophthalmia,** in which the eyes are very large in comparison to the other facial features due to glaucoma.

● **Q13   Congenital malformations of anterior segment of eye**

Q13.0   Coloboma of iris
> Coloboma NOS

Q13.1   Absence of iris
> Aniridia
> Use additional code for associated glaucoma (H42)

Q13.2   Other congenital malformations of iris
> Anisocoria, congenital
> Atresia of pupil
> Congenital malformation of iris NOS
> Corectopia

Q13.3   Congenital corneal opacity

Q13.4   Other congenital corneal malformations
> Congenital malformation of cornea NOS
> Microcornea
> Peter's anomaly

Q13.5   Blue sclera
> *Condition of unusual blueness of sclera; not harmful*

● **Q13.8   Other congenital malformations of anterior segment of eye**

> **Q13.81   Rieger's anomaly**
> > Use additional code for associated glaucoma (H42)

> **Q13.89   Other congenital malformations of anterior segment of eye**

Q13.9   Congenital malformation of anterior segment of eye, unspecified

● **Q14   Congenital malformations of posterior segment of eye**

> **Excludes2**   optic nerve hypoplasia (H47.03-)

Q14.0   Congenital malformation of vitreous humor
> Congenital vitreous opacity

Q14.1   Congenital malformation of retina
> Congenital retinal aneurysm

Q14.2   Congenital malformation of optic disc
> Coloboma of optic disc

Q14.3   Congenital malformation of choroid

Q14.8   Other congenital malformations of posterior segment of eye
> Coloboma of the fundus

Q14.9   Congenital malformation of posterior segment of eye, unspecified

● **Q15   Other congenital malformations of eye**

> **Excludes1**   congenital nystagmus (H55.01)
> ocular albinism (E70.31-)
> optic nerve hypoplasia (H47.03-)
> retinitis pigmentosa (H35.52)

Q15.0   Congenital glaucoma
> Axenfeld's anomaly
> Buphthalmos
> > *Congenital syndrome characterized by enlargement of the eye with symptoms of glaucoma.*
> Glaucoma of childhood
> Glaucoma of newborn
> Hydrophthalmos
> Keratoglobus, congenital, with glaucoma
> Macrocornea with glaucoma
> Macrophthalmos in congenital glaucoma
> Megalocornea with glaucoma

CHAPTER 17 (Q00–Q99)

Q15.8   **Other specified congenital malformations of eye**

Q15.9   **Congenital malformation of eye, unspecified**
Congenital anomaly of eye
Congenital deformity of eye

● **Q16**   **Congenital malformations of ear causing impairment of hearing**
Excludes1   congenital deafness (H90.-)

Q16.0   **Congenital absence of (ear) auricle**

Q16.1   **Congenital absence, atresia and stricture of auditory canal (external)**
Congenital atresia or stricture of osseous meatus

Q16.2   **Absence of eustachian tube**

Q16.3   **Congenital malformation of ear ossicles**
Congenital fusion of ear ossicles

Q16.4   **Other congenital malformations of middle ear**
Congenital malformation of middle ear NOS

Q16.5   **Congenital malformation of inner ear**
Congenital anomaly of membranous labyrinth
Congenital anomaly of organ of Corti

Q16.9   **Congenital malformation of ear causing impairment of hearing, unspecified**
Congenital absence of ear NOS

● **Q17**   **Other congenital malformations of ear**
Excludes1   congenital malformations of ear with impairment of hearing (Q16.0-Q16.9)
preauricular sinus (Q18.1)

Q17.0   **Accessory auricle**
Accessory tragus
Polyotia
Preauricular appendage or tag
Supernumerary ear
Supernumerary lobule

Q17.1   **Macrotia**
Enlarged ears

Q17.2   **Microtia**
An abnormally small or underdeveloped external ear

Q17.3   **Other misshapen ear**
Pointed ear

Q17.4   **Misplaced ear**
Low-set ears
Excludes1   cervical auricle (Q18.2)

Q17.5   **Prominent ear**
Bat ear

Q17.8   **Other specified congenital malformations of ear**
Congenital absence of lobe of ear

Q17.9   **Congenital malformation of ear, unspecified**
Congenital anomaly of ear NOS

● **Q18**   **Other congenital malformations of face and neck**
Excludes1   cleft lip and cleft palate (Q35-Q37)
conditions classified to Q67.0-Q67.4
congenital malformations of skull and face bones (Q75.-)
cyclopia (Q87.0)
dentofacial anomalies [including malocclusion] (M26.-)
malformation syndromes affecting facial appearance (Q87.0)
persistent thyroglossal duct (Q89.2)

Q18.0   **Sinus, fistula and cyst of branchial cleft**
Branchial vestige
Branchial remnants (cysts, fistula, skin tags) that are developmental anomalies

Q18.1   **Preauricular sinus and cyst**
Fistula of auricle, congenital
Cervicoaural fistula
Abnormal passage in neck originating from first branchial cleft

Q18.2   **Other branchial cleft malformations**
Branchial cleft malformation NOS
Cervical auricle
Otocephaly

Q18.3   **Webbing of neck**
Pterygium colli
Thick fold of skin on side of neck

Q18.4   **Macrostomia**
Results from failure of union of maxillary and mandibular processes, results in abnormally large mouth

Q18.5   **Microstomia**

Q18.6   **Macrocheilia**
Excessive size of lips
Hypertrophy of lip, congenital

Q18.7   **Microcheilia**
Abnormal smallness of lips

Q18.8   **Other specified congenital malformations of face and neck**
Medial cyst of face and neck
Medial fistula of face and neck
Medial sinus of face and neck

Q18.9   **Congenital malformation of face and neck, unspecified**
Congenital anomaly NOS of face and neck

CONGENITAL MALFORMATIONS OF THE CIRCULATORY SYSTEM (Q20-Q28)

● **Q20**   **Congenital malformations of cardiac chambers and connections**
Excludes1   dextrocardia with situs inversus (Q89.3)
mirror-image atrial arrangement with situs inversus (Q89.3)

Q20.0   **Common arterial trunk**
Persistent truncus arteriosus
Excludes1   aortic septal defect (Q21.4)

Q20.1   **Double outlet right ventricle**
Taussig-Bing syndrome

Q20.2   **Double outlet left ventricle**

Q20.3   **Discordant ventriculoarterial connection**
Dextrotransposition of aorta
Transposition of great vessels (complete)

Q20.4   **Double inlet ventricle**
Common ventricle
Cor triloculare biatriatum
Single ventricle

Q20.5   **Discordant atrioventricular connection**
Corrected transposition
Levotransposition
Ventricular inversion

Q20.6   **Isomerism of atrial appendages**
Isomerism of atrial appendages with asplenia or polysplenia

Q20.8   **Other congenital malformations of cardiac chambers and connections**
Cor binoculare

Q20.9   **Congenital malformation of cardiac chambers and connections, unspecified**

● **Q21**   **Congenital malformations of cardiac septa**
Excludes1   acquired cardiac septal defect (I51.0)

Q21.0   **Ventricular septal defect**
Roger's disease

Q21.1   **Atrial septal defect**
~~Coronary sinus defect~~
~~Patent or persistent foramen ovale~~
~~Patent or persistent ostium secundum defect (type II)~~
~~Patent or persistent sinus venosus defect~~
▶ **Excludes 2**   ostium primum atrial septal defect (type I) (Q21.20)

▶ **Q21.10**   **Atrial septal defect, unspecified**

▶ **Q21.11**   **Secundum atrial septal defect**
▶ Fenestrated atrial septum
▶ Patent or persistent ostium secundum defect (type II)

▶ **Q21.12**   **Patent foramen ovale**
▶ Persistent foramen ovale

▶ **Q21.13**   **Coronary sinus atrial septal defect**
▶ Coronary sinus defect
▶ Unroofed coronary sinus

▶ **Q21.14**   **Superior sinus venosus atrial septal defect**
▶ Superior vena cava type atrial septal defect

▶ New   ⇒ Revised   ~~deleted~~ Deleted   Excludes 1   Excludes 2   Includes   Use additional   Code first   Code also   Key words
OGCR Official Guidelines   X Assign placeholder X   ● Use Additional Character(s)   ▌ Manifestation Code   🐾 Hierarchical Condition Category   **Coding Clinic**

▶**Q21.15** **Inferior sinus venosus atrial septal defect**
  ▶Inferior vena cava type atrial septal defect

▶**Q21.16** **Sinus venosus atrial septal defect, unspecified**
  ▶Sinus venosus defect, NOS

▶**Q21.19** **Other specified atrial septal defect**
  ▶Common atrium
  ▶Other specified atrial septal abnormality

Q21.2 **Atrioventricular septal defect**
  ~~Common atrioventricular canal~~
  ▶Atrioventricular canal defect
  Endocardial cushion defect
  Ostium primum atrial septal defect (type I)

▶**Q21.20** **Atrioventricular septal defect, unspecified as to partial or complete**
  ▶Atrioventricular canal, NOS
  ▶Endocardial cushion defect NOS
  ▶Ostium primum atrial septal defect (type I) NOS

▶**Q21.21** **Partial atrioventricular septal defect**
  ▶Incomplete atrioventricular canal
  ▶Incomplete atrioventricular septal defect
  ▶Incomplete endocardial cushion defect
  ▶Ostium primum atrial septal defect (type I) with separate atrioventricular valves
  ▶Partial atrioventricular canal
  ▶Partial endocardial cushion defect

▶**Q21.22** **Transitional atrioventricular septal defect**
  ▶Intermediate atrioventricular canal
  ▶Intermediate atrioventricular septal defect
  ▶Intermediate endocardial cushion defect
  ▶Ostium primum atrial septal defect (type I) with separate atrioventricular valves and a small or restrictive inlet VSD
  ▶Transitional atrioventricular canal
  ▶Transitional endocardial cushion defect

▶**Q21.23** **Complete atrioventricular septal defect**
  ▶Common atrioventricular canal
  ▶Common atrioventricular septal defect
  ▶Common endocardial cushion defect
  ▶Ostium primum atrial septal defect (type I) with common atrioventricular valve and a moderate or larger inlet VSD

Q21.3 **Tetralogy of Fallot**
  Ventricular septal defect with pulmonary stenosis or atresia, dextroposition of aorta and hypertrophy of right ventricle.

Q21.4 **Aortopulmonary septal defect**
  Aortic septal defect
  Aortopulmonary window

Q21.8 **Other congenital malformations of cardiac septa**
  Eisenmenger's defect
  Pentalogy of Fallot
  Code also, if applicable:
    Eisenmenger's complex (I27.83)
    Eisenmenger's syndrome (I27.83)

Q21.9 **Congenital malformation of cardiac septum, unspecified**
  Septal (heart) defect NOS

● **Q22** **Congenital malformations of pulmonary and tricuspid valves**

Q22.0 **Pulmonary valve atresia**

Q22.1 **Congenital pulmonary valve stenosis**

Q22.2 **Congenital pulmonary valve insufficiency**
  Congenital pulmonary valve regurgitation

Q22.3 **Other congenital malformations of pulmonary valve**
  Congenital malformation of pulmonary valve NOS
  Supernumerary cusps of pulmonary valve

Q22.4 **Congenital tricuspid stenosis**
  Congenital tricuspid atresia

Q22.5 **Ebstein's anomaly**
  Malformation of tricuspid valve

Q22.6 **Hypoplastic right heart syndrome**

Q22.8 **Other congenital malformations of tricuspid valve**

Q22.9 **Congenital malformation of tricuspid valve, unspecified**

● **Q23** **Congenital malformations of aortic and mitral valves**

Q23.0 **Congenital stenosis of aortic valve**
  Congenital aortic atresia
  Congenital aortic stenosis NOS

  Excludes1 congenital stenosis of aortic valve in hypoplastic left heart syndrome (Q23.4)
    congenital subaortic stenosis (Q24.4)
    supravalvular aortic stenosis (congenital) (Q25.3)

Q23.1 **Congenital insufficiency of aortic valve**
  Bicuspid aortic valve
  Congenital aortic insufficiency

Q23.2 **Congenital mitral stenosis**
  Congenital mitral atresia

Q23.3 **Congenital mitral insufficiency**

Q23.4 **Hypoplastic left heart syndrome**

Q23.8 **Other congenital malformations of aortic and mitral valves**

Q23.9 **Congenital malformation of aortic and mitral valves, unspecified**

● **Q24** **Other congenital malformations of heart**
  Excludes1 endocardial fibroelastosis (I42.4)

Q24.0 **Dextrocardia**
  Heart is located in right hemithorax

  Excludes1 dextrocardia with situs inversus (Q89.3)
    isomerism of atrial appendages (with asplenia or polysplenia) (Q20.6)
    mirror-image atrial arrangement with situs inversus (Q89.3)

Q24.1 **Levocardia**
  Normal position of heart but related structures on wrong side

Q24.2 **Cor triatriatum**
  Congenital heart defect; left atrium is subdivided

Q24.3 **Pulmonary infundibular stenosis**
  Subvalvular pulmonic stenosis

Q24.4 **Congenital subaortic stenosis**

Q24.5 **Malformation of coronary vessels**
  Congenital coronary (artery) aneurysm

Q24.6 **Congenital heart block**

Q24.8 **Other specified congenital malformations of heart**
  Congenital diverticulum of left ventricle
  Congenital malformation of myocardium
  Congenital malformation of pericardium
  Malposition of heart
  Uhl's disease

Q24.9 **Congenital malformation of heart, unspecified**
  Congenital anomaly of heart
  Congenital disease of heart

● **Q25** **Congenital malformations of great arteries**

Q25.0 **Patent ductus arteriosus**
  Fetal blood vessel connecting left pulmonary artery directly to descending aorta
  Patent ductus Botallo
  Persistent ductus arteriosus

Q25.1 **Coarctation of aorta**
  Coarctation of aorta (preductal) (postductal)
  Stenosis of aorta
  Coding Clinic: 2016, Q4, P56-57

● **Q25.2** **Atresia of aorta**
  Coding Clinic: 2016, Q4, P56

  Q25.21 **Interruption of aortic arch**
    Atresia of aortic arch

  Q25.29 **Other atresia of aorta**
    Atresia of aorta

Q25.3 **Supravalvular aortic stenosis**

  Excludes1 congenital aortic stenosis NOS (Q23.0)
    congenital stenosis of aortic valve (Q23.0)

CHAPTER 17 (Q00-Q99)

● **Q25.4 Other congenital malformations of aorta**

Excludes1   hypoplasia of aorta in hypoplastic left
heart syndrome (Q23.4)

Coding Clinic: 2016, Q4, P57

**Q25.40 Congenital malformation of aorta
unspecified**

Q25.41 Absence and aplasia of aorta

Q25.42 Hypoplasia of aorta

Q25.43 Congenital aneurysm of aorta
Congenital aneurysm of aortic root
Congenital aneurysm of aortic sinus

Q25.44 Congenital dilation of aorta

Q25.45 Double aortic arch
Vascular ring of aorta

Q25.46 Tortuous aortic arch
Persistent convolutions of aortic arch

Q25.47 Right aortic arch
Persistent right aortic arch

Q25.48 Anomalous origin of subclavian artery

Q25.49 Other congenital malformations of aorta
Aortic arch
Bovine arch

Q25.5 Atresia of pulmonary artery

Q25.6 Stenosis of pulmonary artery
Supravalvular pulmonary stenosis

● **Q25.7 Other congenital malformations of pulmonary artery**

Q25.71 Coarctation of pulmonary artery

**Q25.72 Congenital pulmonary arteriovenous
malformation**
Congenital pulmonary arteriovenous
aneurysm

**Q25.79 Other congenital malformations of pulmonary
artery**
Aberrant pulmonary artery
Agenesis of pulmonary artery
Congenital aneurysm of pulmonary artery
Congenital anomaly of pulmonary artery
Hypoplasia of pulmonary artery

Q25.8 Other congenital malformations of other great arteries

Q25.9 Congenital malformation of great arteries, unspecified

● **Q26 Congenital malformations of great veins**

Q26.0 Congenital stenosis of vena cava
Congenital stenosis of vena cava (inferior)(superior)

Q26.1 Persistent left superior vena cava

Q26.2 Total anomalous pulmonary venous connection
Total anomalous pulmonary venous return [TAPVR],
subdiaphragmatic
Total anomalous pulmonary venous return [TAPVR],
supradiaphragmatic

Q26.3 Partial anomalous pulmonary venous connection
Partial anomalous pulmonary venous return

Q26.4 Anomalous pulmonary venous connection, unspecified

Q26.5 Anomalous portal venous connection

Q26.6 Portal vein-hepatic artery fistula

Q26.8 Other congenital malformations of great veins
Absence of vena cava (inferior) (superior)
Azygos continuation of inferior vena cava
Persistent left posterior cardinal vein
Scimitar syndrome

Q26.9 Congenital malformation of great vein, unspecified
Congenital anomaly of vena cava (inferior) (superior)
NOS

● **Q27 Other congenital malformations of peripheral vascular system**

Excludes2   anomalies of cerebral and precerebral vessels
(Q28.0-Q28.3)
anomalies of coronary vessels (Q24.5)
anomalies of pulmonary artery (Q25.5-Q25.7)
congenital retinal aneurysm (Q14.1)
hemangioma and lymphangioma (D18.-)

Q27.0 Congenital absence and hypoplasia of umbilical artery
Single umbilical artery

Q27.1 Congenital renal artery stenosis

Q27.2 Other congenital malformations of renal artery
Congenital malformation of renal artery NOS
Multiple renal arteries

● **Q27.3 Arteriovenous malformation (peripheral)**
Arteriovenous aneurysm

Excludes1   acquired arteriovenous aneurysm (I77.0)
Excludes2   arteriovenous malformation of cerebral
vessels (Q28.2)
arteriovenous malformation of
precerebral vessels (Q28.0)

Q27.30 Arteriovenous malformation, site unspecified

**Q27.31 Arteriovenous malformation of vessel of upper
limb**

**Q27.32 Arteriovenous malformation of vessel of lower
limb**

**Q27.33 Arteriovenous malformation of digestive
system vessel**

Q27.34 Arteriovenous malformation of renal vessel

Q27.39 Arteriovenous malformation, other site

Q27.4 Congenital phlebectasia

**Q27.8 Other specified congenital malformations of peripheral
vascular system**
Absence of peripheral vascular system
Atresia of peripheral vascular system
Congenital aneurysm (peripheral)
Congenital stricture, artery
Congenital varix

Excludes1   arteriovenous malformation (Q27.3-)

**Q27.9 Congenital malformation of peripheral vascular system,
unspecified**
Anomaly of artery or vein NOS

● **Q28 Other congenital malformations of circulatory system**

Excludes1   congenital aneurysm NOS (Q27.8)
congenital coronary aneurysm (Q24.5)
ruptured cerebral arteriovenous malformation
(I60.8)
ruptured malformation of precerebral vessels
(I72.0)

Excludes2   congenital peripheral aneurysm (Q27.8)
congenital pulmonary aneurysm (Q25.79)
congenital retinal aneurysm (Q14.1)

Q28.0 Arteriovenous malformation of precerebral vessels
Congenital arteriovenous precerebral aneurysm
(nonruptured)

Q28.1 Other malformations of precerebral vessels
Congenital malformation of precerebral vessels NOS
Congenital precerebral aneurysm (nonruptured)

Q28.2 Arteriovenous malformation of cerebral vessels
Arteriovenous malformation of brain NOS
Congenital arteriovenous cerebral aneurysm
(nonruptured)

Q28.3 Other malformations of cerebral vessels
Congenital cerebral aneurysm (nonruptured)
Congenital malformation of cerebral vessels NOS
Developmental venous anomaly

**Q28.8 Other specified congenital malformations of circulatory
system**
Congenital aneurysm, specified site NEC
Spinal vessel anomaly

**Q28.9 Congenital malformation of circulatory system,
unspecified**

▶ New   ➡ Revised   ~~deleted~~ Deleted   Excludes 1   Excludes 2   Includes   Use additional   Code first   Code also   Key words
OGCR Official Guidelines   X Assign placeholder X   ● Use Additional Character(s)   ❙ Manifestation Code   ℞ Hierarchical Condition Category   **Coding Clinic**

CONGENITAL MALFORMATIONS OF THE RESPIRATORY SYSTEM (Q30–Q34)

● **Q30 Congenital malformations of nose**

    Excludes1 congenital deviation of nasal septum (Q67.4)

    Q30.0 Choanal atresia
        Atresia of nares (anterior) (posterior)
        Congenital stenosis of nares (anterior) (posterior)

    Q30.1 Agenesis and underdevelopment of nose
        Congenital absent of nose

    Q30.2 Fissured, notched and cleft nose

    Q30.3 Congenital perforated nasal septum

    Q30.8 Other congenital malformations of nose
        Accessory nose
        Congenital anomaly of nasal sinus wall
        Coding Clinic: 2022, Q2, P17

    Q30.9 Congenital malformation of nose, unspecified

● **Q31 Congenital malformations of larynx**

    Excludes1 congenital laryngeal stridor NOS (P28.89)

    Q31.0 Web of larynx
        Glottic web of larynx
        Subglottic web of larynx
        Web of larynx NOS

    Q31.1 Congenital subglottic stenosis

    Q31.2 Laryngeal hypoplasia

    Q31.3 Laryngocele

    Q31.5 Congenital laryngomalacia

    Q31.8 Other congenital malformations of larynx
        Absence of larynx
        Agenesis of larynx
        Atresia of larynx
        Congenital cleft thyroid cartilage
        Congenital fissure of epiglottis
        Congenital stenosis of larynx NEC
        Posterior cleft of cricoid cartilage

    Q31.9 Congenital malformation of larynx, unspecified

● **Q32 Congenital malformations of trachea and bronchus**

    Excludes1 congenital bronchiectasis (Q33.4)

    Q32.0 Congenital tracheomalacia

    Q32.1 Other congenital malformations of trachea
        Atresia of trachea
        Congenital anomaly of tracheal cartilage
        Congenital dilatation of trachea
        Congenital malformation of trachea
        Congenital stenosis of trachea
        Congenital tracheocele

    Q32.2 Congenital bronchomalacia

    Q32.3 Congenital stenosis of bronchus

    Q32.4 Other congenital malformations of bronchus
        Absence of bronchus
        Agenesis of bronchus
        Atresia of bronchus
        Congenital diverticulum of bronchus
        Congenital malformation of bronchus NOS

● **Q33 Congenital malformations of lung**

    Q33.0 Congenital cystic lung
        Congenital cystic lung disease
        Congenital honeycomb lung
        Congenital polycystic lung disease
        Excludes1 cystic fibrosis (E84.0)
                    cystic lung disease, acquired or
                         unspecified (J98.4)

    Q33.1 Accessory lobe of lung
        Azygos lobe (fissured), lung

    Q33.2 Sequestration of lung

    Q33.3 Agenesis of lung
        Congenital absence of lung (lobe)

    Q33.4 Congenital bronchiectasis

    Q33.5 Ectopic tissue in lung

    Q33.6 Congenital hypoplasia and dysplasia of lung
        Excludes1 pulmonary hypoplasia associated with
                  short gestation (P28.0)

    Q33.8 Other congenital malformations of lung

    Q33.9 Congenital malformation of lung, unspecified

● **Q34 Other congenital malformations of respiratory system**

    Excludes2 congenital central alveolar hypoventilation
                  syndrome (G47.35)

    Q34.0 Anomaly of pleura

    Q34.1 Congenital cyst of mediastinum

    Q34.8 Other specified congenital malformations of respiratory system
        Atresia of nasopharynx

    Q34.9 Congenital malformation of respiratory system, unspecified
        Congenital absence of respiratory system
        Congenital anomaly of respiratory system NOS

CLEFT LIP AND CLEFT PALATE (Q35-Q37)

Use additional code to identify associated malformation of the nose (Q30.2)

    Excludes2 Robin's syndrome (Q87.0)

● **Q35 Cleft palate**

    Includes fissure of palate
              palatoschisis

    Excludes1 cleft palate with cleft lip (Q37.-)

    Q35.1 Cleft hard palate

    Q35.3 Cleft soft palate

    Q35.5 Cleft hard palate with cleft soft palate

    Q35.7 Cleft uvula

    Q35.9 Cleft palate, unspecified
        Cleft palate NOS

● **Q36 Cleft lip**

    Includes cheiloschisis
              congenital fissure of lip
              harelip
              labium leporinum

    Excludes1 cleft lip with cleft palate (Q37.-)

    Q36.0 Cleft lip, bilateral

    Q36.1 Cleft lip, median

    Q36.9 Cleft lip, unilateral
        Cleft lip NOS

● **Q37 Cleft palate with cleft lip**

    Includes cheilopalatoschisis

    Q37.0 Cleft hard palate with bilateral cleft lip

    Q37.1 Cleft hard palate with unilateral cleft lip
        Cleft hard palate with cleft lip NOS

    Q37.2 Cleft soft palate with bilateral cleft lip

    Q37.3 Cleft soft palate with unilateral cleft lip
        Cleft soft palate with cleft lip NOS

    Q37.4 Cleft hard and soft palate with bilateral cleft lip

    Q37.5 Cleft hard and soft palate with unilateral cleft lip
        Cleft hard and soft palate with cleft lip NOS

    Q37.8 Unspecified cleft palate with bilateral cleft lip

    Q37.9 Unspecified cleft palate with unilateral cleft lip
        Cleft palate with cleft lip NOS

Figure 17-3 Cleft palate.

CHAPTER 17 (Q00-Q99)

CHAPTER 17 (Q00-Q99)

OTHER CONGENITAL MALFORMATIONS OF THE DIGESTIVE SYSTEM (Q38-Q45)

● **Q38   Other congenital malformations of tongue, mouth and pharynx**

   Excludes1   dentofacial anomalies (M26.-)
                   macrostomia (Q18.4)
                   microstomia (Q18.5)

   Q38.0   Congenital malformations of lips, not elsewhere classified
   Congenital fistula of lip
   Congenital malformation of lip NOS
   Van der Woude's syndrome

   Excludes1   cleft lip (Q36.-)
                   cleft lip with cleft palate (Q37.-)
                   macrocheilia (Q18.6)
                   microcheilia (Q18.7)

   Q38.1   Ankyloglossia
   Restricted movement of tongue resulting in speech difficulty
   Tongue tie

   Q38.2   Macroglossia
   Excessive size of tongue
   Congenital hypertrophy of tongue

   Q38.3   Other congenital malformations of tongue
   Aglossia
   Bifid tongue
   Congenital adhesion of tongue
   Congenital fissure of tongue
   Congenital malformation of tongue NOS
   Double tongue
   Hypoglossia
   Hypoplasia of tongue
   Microglossia

   Q38.4   Congenital malformations of salivary glands and ducts
   Atresia of salivary glands and ducts
   Congenital absence of salivary glands and ducts
   Congenital accessory salivary glands and ducts
   Congenital fistula of salivary gland

   Q38.5   Congenital malformations of palate, not elsewhere classified
   Congenital absence of uvula
   Congenital malformation of palate NOS
   Congenital high arched palate

   Excludes1   cleft palate (Q35.-)
                   cleft palate with cleft lip (Q37.-)

   Q38.6   Other congenital malformations of mouth
   Congenital malformation of mouth NOS

   Q38.7   Congenital pharyngeal pouch
   Congenital diverticulum of pharynx

   Excludes1   pharyngeal pouch syndrome (D82.1)

   Q38.8   Other congenital malformations of pharynx
   Congenital malformation of pharynx NOS
   Imperforate pharynx

● **Q39   Congenital malformations of esophagus**

   Q39.0   Atresia of esophagus without fistula
   Atresia of esophagus NOS

   Q39.1   Atresia of esophagus with tracheo-esophageal fistula
   Atresia of esophagus with broncho-esophageal fistula

   Q39.2   Congenital tracheo-esophageal fistula without atresia
   Congenital tracheo-esophageal fistula NOS

   Q39.3   Congenital stenosis and stricture of esophagus

   Q39.4   Esophageal web

   Q39.5   Congenital dilatation of esophagus
   Congenital cardiospasm

   Q39.6   Congenital diverticulum of esophagus
   Congenital esophageal pouch

   Q39.8   Other congenital malformations of esophagus
   Congenital absence of esophagus
   Congenital displacement of esophagus
   Congenital duplication of esophagus

   Q39.9   Congenital malformation of esophagus, unspecified

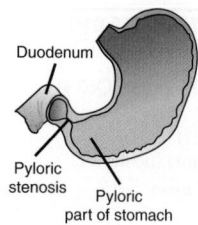

Duodenum

Pyloric
stenosis   Pyloric
               part of stomach

Figure 17-4 Pyloric stenosis.

● **Q40   Other congenital malformations of upper alimentary tract**

   Q40.0   Congenital hypertrophic pyloric stenosis
   Congenital or infantile constriction
   Congenital or infantile hypertrophy
   Congenital or infantile spasm
   Congenital or infantile stenosis
   Congenital or infantile stricture

   Q40.1   Congenital hiatus hernia
   Congenital displacement of cardia through esophageal hiatus

   Excludes1   congenital diaphragmatic hernia (Q79.0)

   Q40.2   Other specified congenital malformations of stomach
   Congenital displacement of stomach
   Congenital diverticulum of stomach
   Congenital hourglass stomach
   Congenital duplication of stomach
   Megalogastria
   Microgastria

   Q40.3   Congenital malformation of stomach, unspecified

   Q40.8   Other specified congenital malformations of upper alimentary tract

   Q40.9   Congenital malformation of upper alimentary tract, unspecified
   Congenital anomaly of upper alimentary tract
   Congenital deformity of upper alimentary tract

● **Q41   Congenital absence, atresia and stenosis of small intestine**

   Includes   congenital obstruction, occlusion or stricture of
                   small intestine or intestine NOS

   Excludes1   cystic fibrosis with intestinal manifestation
                   (E84.11)
                   meconium ileus NOS (without cystic fibrosis)
                   (P76.0)

   Q41.0   Congenital absence, atresia and stenosis of duodenum

   Q41.1   Congenital absence, atresia and stenosis of jejunum
   Apple peel syndrome
   Imperforate jejunum

   Q41.2   Congenital absence, atresia and stenosis of ileum

   Q41.8   Congenital absence, atresia and stenosis of other specified parts of small intestine

   Q41.9   Congenital absence, atresia and stenosis of small intestine, part unspecified
   Congenital absence, atresia and stenosis of intestine NOS

● **Q42   Congenital absence, atresia and stenosis of large intestine**

   Includes   congenital obstruction, occlusion and stricture of
                   large intestine

   Q42.0   Congenital absence, atresia and stenosis of rectum with fistula

   Q42.1   Congenital absence, atresia and stenosis of rectum without fistula
   Imperforate rectum

   Q42.2   Congenital absence, atresia and stenosis of anus with fistula

   Q42.3   Congenital absence, atresia and stenosis of anus without fistula
   Imperforate anus

   Q42.8   Congenital absence, atresia and stenosis of other parts of large intestine

   Q42.9   Congenital absence, atresia and stenosis of large intestine, part unspecified

▶ New   �b Revised   ~~deleted~~ Deleted   Excludes 1   Excludes 2   Includes   Use additional   Code first   Code also   Key words

OGCR Official Guidelines   X Assign placeholder X   ● Use Additional Character(s)   ▶ Manifestation Code   ⚡ Hierarchical Condition Category   **Coding Clinic**

● **Q43   Other congenital malformations of intestine**

Q43.0   Meckel's diverticulum (displaced) (hypertrophic)
Congenital abnormality in which a pouch remains on the lower end of the small intestine
Persistent omphalomesenteric duct
Persistent vitelline duct

Q43.1   Hirschsprung's disease
Developmental disorder of enteric nervous system characterized by absence of ganglion cells in distal colon resulting in functional obstruction
Aganglionosis
Congenital (aganglionic) megacolon

Q43.2   Other congenital functional disorders of colon
Congenital dilatation of colon

Q43.3   Congenital malformations of intestinal fixation
Congenital omental, anomalous adhesions [bands]
Congenital peritoneal adhesions [bands]
Incomplete rotation of cecum and colon
Insufficient rotation of cecum and colon
Jackson's membrane
Malrotation of colon
Rotation failure of cecum and colon
Universal mesentery

Q43.4   Duplication of intestine

Q43.5   Ectopic anus
Anal opening in abnormal location

Q43.6   Congenital fistula of rectum and anus

> **Excludes1**   congenital fistula of anus with absence, atresia and stenosis (Q42.2)
> congenital fistula of rectum with absence, atresia and stenosis (Q42.0)
> congenital rectovaginal fistula (Q52.2)
> congenital urethrorectal fistula (Q64.73)
> pilonidal fistula or sinus (L05.-)

Q43.7   Persistent cloaca
Malformation in which rectum, vagina, and urinary tract form one channel; AKA congenital cloaca
Cloaca NOS

Q43.8   Other specified congenital malformations of intestine
Congenital blind loop syndrome
Congenital diverticulitis, colon
Congenital diverticulum, intestine
Dolichocolon
Megaloappendix
Megaloduodenum
Microcolon
Transposition of appendix
Transposition of colon
Transposition of intestine

Q43.9   Congenital malformation of intestine, unspecified

● **Q44   Congenital malformations of gallbladder, bile ducts and liver**

Q44.0   Agenesis, aplasia and hypoplasia of gallbladder
Congenital absence of gallbladder

Q44.1   Other congenital malformations of gallbladder
Congenital malformation of gallbladder NOS
Intrahepatic gallbladder

Q44.2   Atresia of bile ducts

Q44.3   Congenital stenosis and stricture of bile ducts

Q44.4   Choledochal cyst

Q44.5   Other congenital malformations of bile ducts
Accessory hepatic duct
Biliary duct duplication
Congenital malformation of bile duct NOS
Cystic duct duplication

Q44.6   Cystic disease of liver
Fibrocystic disease of liver

Q44.7   Other congenital malformations of liver
Accessory liver
Alagille's syndrome
Congenital absence of liver
Congenital hepatomegaly
Congenital malformation of liver NOS

● **Q45   Other congenital malformations of digestive system**

> **Excludes2**   congenital diaphragmatic hernia (Q79.0)
> congenital hiatus hernia (Q40.1)

Q45.0   Agenesis, aplasia and hypoplasia of pancreas
Congenital absence of pancreas

Q45.1   Annular pancreas

Q45.2   Congenital pancreatic cyst

Q45.3   Other congenital malformations of pancreas and pancreatic duct
Accessory pancreas
Congenital malformation of pancreas or pancreatic duct NOS

> **Excludes1**   congenital diabetes mellitus (E10.-)
> cystic fibrosis (E84.0-E84.9)
> fibrocystic disease of pancreas (E84.-)
> neonatal diabetes mellitus (P70.2)

Q45.8   Other specified congenital malformations of digestive system
Absence (complete) (partial) of alimentary tract NOS
Duplication of digestive system
Malposition, congenital of digestive system

Q45.9   Congenital malformation of digestive system, unspecified
Congenital anomaly of digestive system
Congenital deformity of digestive system

CONGENITAL MALFORMATIONS OF GENITAL ORGANS (Q50-Q56)

> **Excludes1**   androgen insensitivity syndrome (E34.5-)
> syndromes associated with anomalies in the number and form of chromosomes (Q90-Q99)

● **Q50   Congenital malformations of ovaries, fallopian tubes and broad ligaments**

● **Q50.0   Congenital absence of ovary**

> **Excludes1**   Turner's syndrome (Q96.-)

Q50.01   Congenital absence of ovary, unilateral ♀

Q50.02   Congenital absence of ovary, bilateral ♀

Q50.1   Developmental ovarian cyst ♀

Q50.2   Congenital torsion of ovary ♀

● **Q50.3   Other congenital malformations of ovary**

Q50.31   Accessory ovary ♀

Q50.32   Ovarian streak ♀
Inadequate ovaries with absent follicular and hormonal function
46, XX with streak gonads

Q50.39   Other congenital malformation of ovary ♀
Congenital malformation of ovary NOS

Q50.4   Embryonic cyst of fallopian tube ♀
Fimbrial cyst

Q50.5   Embryonic cyst of broad ligament ♀
Epoophoron cyst
Parovarian cyst

Q50.6   Other congenital malformations of fallopian tube and broad ligament ♀
Absence of fallopian tube and broad ligament
Accessory fallopian tube and broad ligament
Atresia of fallopian tube and broad ligament
Congenital malformation of fallopian tube or broad ligament NOS

● **Q51   Congenital malformations of uterus and cervix**

Q51.0   Agenesis and aplasia of uterus ♀
Congenital absence of uterus

● **Q51.1   Doubling of uterus with doubling of cervix and vagina**

Q51.10   Doubling of uterus with doubling of cervix and vagina without obstruction ♀
Doubling of uterus with doubling of cervix and vagina NOS

Q51.11   Doubling of uterus with doubling of cervix and vagina with obstruction ♀

- Q51.2   **Other doubling of uterus**
          Doubling of uterus NOS
          Septate uterus
     Q51.21   **Complete doubling of uterus** ♀
               Complete septate uterus
     Q51.22   **Partial doubling of uterus** ♀
               Partial septate uterus
     Q51.28   **Other and unspecified doubling of uterus** ♀
               Septate uterus NOS
  Q51.3   **Bicornate uterus** ♀
          Bicornate uterus, complete or partial
          Birth defect in which uterus has two separate "horns" that form top of uterus
  Q51.4   **Unicornate uterus** ♀
          Unicornate uterus with or without a separate uterine horn
          Uterus with only one functioning horn
          Uterus with half being undeveloped
  Q51.5   **Agenesis and aplasia of cervix** ♀
          Congenital absence of cervix
  Q51.6   **Embryonic cyst of cervix** ♀
  Q51.7   **Congenital fistulae between uterus and digestive and urinary tracts** ♀
- Q51.8   Other congenital malformations of uterus and cervix
  - Q51.81   **Other congenital malformations of uterus**
          Q51.810   **Arcuate uterus** ♀
                     Arcuatus uterus
          Q51.811   **Hypoplasia of uterus** ♀
          Q51.818   **Other congenital malformations of uterus** ♀
                     Müllerian anomaly of uterus NEC
  - Q51.82   **Other congenital malformations of cervix**
          Q51.820   **Cervical duplication** ♀
          Q51.821   **Hypoplasia of cervix** ♀
          Q51.828   **Other congenital malformations of cervix** ♀
  Q51.9   **Congenital malformation of uterus and cervix, unspecified** ♀

- Q52   Other congenital malformations of female genitalia
  Q52.0   **Congenital absence of vagina** ♀
          Vaginal agenesis, total or partial
- Q52.1   **Doubling of vagina**
     Excludes1   doubling of vagina with doubling of uterus and cervix (Q51.1-)
     Q52.10   **Doubling of vagina, unspecified** ♀
               Septate vagina NOS
     Q52.11   **Transverse vaginal septum** ♀
  - Q52.12   **Longitudinal vaginal septum**
               Coding Clinic: 2016, Q4, P58
          Q52.120   **Longitudinal vaginal septum, nonobstructing** ♀
          Q52.121   **Longitudinal vaginal septum, obstructing, right side** ♀
          Q52.122   **Longitudinal vaginal septum, obstructing, left side** ♀
          Q52.123   **Longitudinal vaginal septum, microperforate, right side** ♀
          Q52.124   **Longitudinal vaginal septum, microperforate, left side** ♀
                     Coding Clinic: 2016, Q4, P59
          Q52.129   **Other and unspecified longitudinal vaginal septum** ♀
  Q52.2   **Congenital rectovaginal fistula** ♀
          Excludes1   cloaca (Q43.7)

Item 17-1   Testes form in the abdomen of the male and only descend into the scrotum during normal embryonic development. "Ectopic" testes are out of their normal place or "retained" (left behind) in the abdomen. Crypto (hidden) orchism (testicle) is a major risk factor for testicular cancer.

ECTOPIC TESTES	CRYPTORCHID TESTES
Penile	Abdominal
Superficial inguinal	Inguinal
(most common)	Prepubic
Femoral	(most common)

Figure 17-5   Undescended testes and the positions of the testes in various types of cryptorchidism or abnormal paths of descent.

  Q52.3   **Imperforate hymen** ♀
          Membrane (hymen) completely closes vaginal orifice
  Q52.4   **Other congenital malformations of vagina** ♀
          Canal of Nuck cyst, congenital
          Congenital malformation of vagina NOS
          Embryonic vaginal cyst
          Gartner's duct cyst
          Coding Clinic: 2022, Q2, P16
  Q52.5   **Fusion of labia** ♀
  Q52.6   **Congenital malformation of clitoris** ♀
- Q52.7   **Other and unspecified congenital malformations of vulva**
     Q52.70   **Unspecified congenital malformations of vulva** ♀
               Congenital malformation of vulva NOS
     Q52.71   **Congenital absence of vulva** ♀
     Q52.79   **Other congenital malformations of vulva** ♀
               Congenital cyst of vulva
  Q52.8   **Other specified congenital malformations of female genitalia** ♀
  Q52.9   **Congenital malformation of female genitalia, unspecified** ♀

- Q53   Undescended and ectopic testicle
  - Q53.0   **Ectopic testis**
          Q53.00   Ectopic testis, unspecified ♂
          Q53.01   Ectopic testis, unilateral ♂
          Q53.02   Ectopic testes, bilateral ♂
  - Q53.1   **Undescended testicle, unilateral**
          Q53.10   **Unspecified undescended testicle, unilateral** ♂
     - Q53.11   **Abdominal testis, unilateral**
               Q53.111   Unilateral intraabdominal testis ♂
               Q53.112   Unilateral inguinal testis ♂
          Q53.12   Ectopic perineal testis, unilateral ♂
          Q53.13   Unilateral high scrotal testis ♂
  - Q53.2   **Undescended testicle, bilateral**
          Q53.20   Undescended testicle, unspecified, bilateral ♂
     - Q53.21   **Abdominal testis, bilateral**
               Q53.211   Bilateral intraabdominal testes ♂
               Q53.212   Bilateral inguinal testes ♂
          Q53.22   Ectopic perineal testis, bilateral ♂
          Q53.23   Bilateral high scrotal testes ♂
  Q53.9   **Undescended testicle, unspecified** ♂
          Cryptorchism NOS

▶ New   ⇒ Revised   ~~deleted~~ Deleted   Excludes 1   Excludes 2   Includes   Use additional   Code first   Code also   Key words
OGCR Official Guidelines   X Assign placeholder X   ● Use Additional Character(s)   ⟩ Manifestation Code   🔖 Hierarchical Condition Category   **Coding Clinic**

● **Q54 Hypospadias**
  Birth defect of male; urethra opens in abnormal location on shaft
   Excludes1 epispadias (Q64.0)
  Q54.0 Hypospadias, balanic ♂
    Hypospadias, coronal
    Hypospadias, glandular
  Q54.1 Hypospadias, penile ♂
  Q54.2 Hypospadias, penoscrotal ♂
  Q54.3 Hypospadias, perineal ♂
  Q54.4 Congenital chordee ♂
    Chordee without hypospadias
  Q54.8 Other hypospadias ♂
    Hypospadias with intersex state
  Q54.9 Hypospadias, unspecified ♂

● **Q55 Other congenital malformations of male genital organs**
   Excludes1 congenital hydrocele (P83.5)
         hypospadias (Q54.-)
  Q55.0 Absence and aplasia of testis ♂
    Monorchism
  Q55.1 Hypoplasia of testis and scrotum ♂
    Fusion of testes
  ● **Q55.2 Other and unspecified congenital malformations of testis and scrotum**
    Q55.20 Unspecified congenital malformations of testis and scrotum ♂
      Congenital malformation of testis or scrotum NOS
    Q55.21 Polyorchism ♂
      Developmental anomaly characterized by presence of more than two testes
    Q55.22 Retractile testis ♂
    Q55.23 Scrotal transposition ♂
    Q55.29 Other congenital malformations of testis and scrotum ♂
  Q55.3 Atresia of vas deferens ♂
    Code first any associated cystic fibrosis (E84.-)
  Q55.4 Other congenital malformations of vas deferens, epididymis, seminal vesicles and prostate ♂
    Absence or aplasia of prostate
    Absence or aplasia of spermatic cord
    Congenital malformation of vas deferens, epididymis, seminal vesicles or prostate NOS
  Q55.5 Congenital absence and aplasia of penis ♂
  ● **Q55.6 Other congenital malformations of penis**
    Q55.61 Curvature of penis (lateral) ♂
    Q55.62 Hypoplasia of penis ♂
      Underdevelopment penis
      Micropenis
    Q55.63 Congenital torsion of penis ♂
      Excludes1 acquired torsion of penis (N48.82)
    Q55.64 Hidden penis ♂
      Buried penis
      Concealed penis
      Excludes1 acquired buried penis (N48.83)
    Q55.69 Other congenital malformation of penis ♂
      Congenital malformation of penis NOS
  Q55.7 Congenital vasocutaneous fistula ♂
    Abnormal opening between vas deferens and skin
  Q55.8 Other specified congenital malformations of male genital organs ♂
  Q55.9 Congenital malformation of male genital organ, unspecified ♂
    Congenital anomaly of male genital organ
    Congenital deformity of male genital organ

● **Q56 Indeterminate sex and pseudohermaphroditism**
  Internal reproductive organs are opposite external physical characteristics.
   Excludes1 46,XX true hermaphrodite (Q99.1)
         androgen insensitivity syndrome (E34.5-)
         chimera 46,XX/46,XY true hermaphrodite (Q99.0)
         female pseudohermaphroditism with adrenocortical disorder (E25.-)
         pseudohermaphroditism with specified chromosomal anomaly (Q96-Q99)
         pure gonadal dysgenesis (Q99.1)
  Q56.0 Hermaphroditism, not elsewhere classified
    Ovotestis
  Q56.1 Male pseudohermaphroditism, not elsewhere classified ♂
    46, XY with streak gonads
    Male pseudohermaphroditism NOS
  Q56.2 Female pseudohermaphroditism, not elsewhere classified ♀
    Female pseudohermaphroditism NOS
  Q56.3 Pseudohermaphroditism, unspecified
  Q56.4 Indeterminate sex, unspecified
    Ambiguous genitalia

CONGENITAL MALFORMATIONS OF THE URINARY SYSTEM (Q60-Q64)

● **Q60 Renal agenesis and other reduction defects of kidney**
   Includes congenital absence of kidney
        congenital atrophy of kidney
        infantile atrophy of kidney
  Q60.0 Renal agenesis, unilateral
  Q60.1 Renal agenesis, bilateral
  Q60.2 Renal agenesis, unspecified
  Q60.3 Renal hypoplasia, unilateral
  Q60.4 Renal hypoplasia, bilateral
  Q60.5 Renal hypoplasia, unspecified
  Q60.6 Potter's syndrome

● **Q61 Cystic kidney disease**
  Cysts that develop in failing kidney due to end-stage renal disease
   Excludes1 acquired cyst of kidney (N28.1)
         Potter's syndrome (Q60.6)
  ● **Q61.0 Congenital renal cyst**
    Q61.00 Congenital renal cyst, unspecified
      Cyst of kidney NOS (congenital)
    Q61.01 Congenital single renal cyst
    Q61.02 Congenital multiple renal cysts
  ● **Q61.1 Polycystic kidney, infantile type**
    Polycystic kidney, autosomal recessive
    Q61.11 Cystic dilatation of collecting ducts
    Q61.19 Other polycystic kidney, infantile type
  Q61.2 Polycystic kidney, adult type
    Polycystic kidney, autosomal dominant
  Q61.3 Polycystic kidney, unspecified
    Coding Clinic: 2016, Q3, P23
  Q61.4 Renal dysplasia
    Multicystic dysplastic kidney
    Multicystic kidney (development)
    Multicystic kidney disease
    Multicystic renal dysplasia
    Excludes1 polycystic kidney disease (Q61.11-Q61.3)
  Q61.5 Medullary cystic kidney
    Nephronophthisis
    Sponge kidney NOS
  Q61.8 Other cystic kidney diseases
    Fibrocystic kidney
    Fibrocystic renal degeneration or disease
  Q61.9 Cystic kidney disease, unspecified
    Meckel-Gruber syndrome

CHAPTER 17 (Q00-Q99)

● **Q62 Congenital obstructive defects of renal pelvis and congenital malformations of ureter**

Q62.0 Congenital hydronephrosis

● **Q62.1 Congenital occlusion of ureter**
Atresia and stenosis of ureter

Q62.10 Congenital occlusion of ureter, unspecified

Q62.11 Congenital occlusion of ureteropelvic junction

Q62.12 Congenital occlusion of ureterovesical orifice

Q62.2 Congenital megaureter
Congenital dilatation of ureter

● **Q62.3 Other obstructive defects of renal pelvis and ureter**

Q62.31 Congenital ureterocele, orthotopic

Q62.32 Cecoureterocele
Ectopic ureterocele

Q62.39 Other obstructive defects of renal pelvis and ureter
Ureteropelvic junction obstruction NOS

Q62.4 Agenesis of ureter
Congenital absence ureter

Q62.5 Duplication of ureter
Accessory ureter
Double ureter

● **Q62.6 Malposition of ureter**

Q62.60 Malposition of ureter, unspecified

Q62.61 Deviation of ureter

Q62.62 Displacement of ureter

Q62.63 Anomalous implantation of ureter
Ectopia of ureter
Ectopic ureter

Q62.69 Other malposition of ureter

Q62.7 Congenital vesico-uretero-renal reflux

Q62.8 Other congenital malformations of ureter
Anomaly of ureter NOS

● **Q63 Other congenital malformations of kidney**

Excludes1 congenital nephrotic syndrome (N04.-)

Q63.0 Accessory kidney

Q63.1 Lobulated, fused and horseshoe kidney

Q63.2 Ectopic kidney
Congenital displaced kidney
Malrotation of kidney

Q63.3 Hyperplastic and giant kidney
Compensatory hypertrophy of kidney

Q63.8 Other specified congenital malformations of kidney
Congenital renal calculi

Q63.9 Congenital malformation of kidney, unspecified

● **Q64 Other congenital malformations of urinary system**

Q64.0 Epispadias
Urethral opening somewhere on dorsum of penis

Excludes1 hypospadias (Q54.-)

● **Q64.1 Exstrophy of urinary bladder**
Bladder is exposed, inside out, and protrudes through abdominal wall

Q64.10 Exstrophy of urinary bladder, unspecified
Ectopia vesicae

Q64.11 Supravesical fissure of urinary bladder

Q64.12 Cloacal exstrophy of urinary bladder

Q64.19 Other exstrophy of urinary bladder
Extroversion of bladder

Q64.2 Congenital posterior urethral valves

● **Q64.3 Other atresia and stenosis of urethra and bladder neck**

Q64.31 Congenital bladder neck obstruction
Congenital obstruction of vesicourethral orifice

Q64.32 Congenital stricture of urethra

Q64.33 Congenital stricture of urinary meatus

Q64.39 Other atresia and stenosis of urethra and bladder neck
Atresia and stenosis of urethra and bladder neck NOS

Q64.4 Malformation of urachus
Cyst of urachus
Patent urachus
Prolapse of urachus

Q64.5 Congenital absence of bladder and urethra

Q64.6 Congenital diverticulum of bladder

● **Q64.7 Other and unspecified congenital malformations of bladder and urethra**

Excludes1 congenital prolapse of bladder (mucosa) (Q79.4)

Q64.70 Unspecified congenital malformation of bladder and urethra
Malformation of bladder or urethra NOS

Q64.71 Congenital prolapse of urethra

Q64.72 Congenital prolapse of urinary meatus

Q64.73 Congenital urethrorectal fistula

Q64.74 Double urethra

Q64.75 Double urinary meatus

Q64.79 Other congenital malformations of bladder and urethra

Q64.8 Other specified congenital malformations of urinary system

Q64.9 Congenital malformation of urinary system, unspecified
Congenital anomaly NOS of urinary system
Congenital deformity NOS of urinary system

CONGENITAL MALFORMATIONS AND DEFORMATIONS OF THE MUSCULOSKELETAL SYSTEM (Q65-Q79)

● **Q65 Congenital deformities of hip**

Excludes1 clicking hip (R29.4)

● **Q65.0 Congenital dislocation of hip, unilateral**

Q65.00 Congenital dislocation of unspecified hip, unilateral

Q65.01 Congenital dislocation of right hip, unilateral

Q65.02 Congenital dislocation of left hip, unilateral

Q65.1 Congenital dislocation of hip, bilateral

Q65.2 Congenital dislocation of hip, unspecified

● **Q65.3 Congenital partial dislocation of hip, unilateral**

Q65.30 Congenital partial dislocation of unspecified hip, unilateral

Q65.31 Congenital partial dislocation of right hip, unilateral

Q65.32 Congenital partial dislocation of left hip, unilateral

Q65.4 Congenital partial dislocation of hip, bilateral

Q65.5 Congenital partial dislocation of hip, unspecified

Q65.6 Congenital unstable hip
Congenital dislocatable hip

● **Q65.8 Other congenital deformities of hip**

Q65.81 Congenital coxa valga

Q65.82 Congenital coxa vara

Q65.89 Other specified congenital deformities of hip
Anteversion of femoral neck
Congenital acetabular dysplasia

Q65.9 Congenital deformity of hip, unspecified

● **Q66 Congenital deformities of feet**

Excludes1 reduction defects of feet (Q72.-)
valgus deformities (acquired) (M21.0-)
varus deformities (acquired) (M21.1-)

● **Q66.0 Congenital talipes equinovarus**
Heel is turned inward from midline and foot is plantar flexed; AKA clubfoot

Q66.00 Congenital talipes equinovarus, unspecified foot

Q66.01 Congenital talipes equinovarus, right foot

Q66.02 Congenital talipes equinovarus, left foot

▶ New ⇒ Revised ~~deleted~~ Deleted Excludes 1 Excludes 2 Includes Use additional Code first Code also Key words
OGCR Official Guidelines X Assign placeholder X ● Use Additional Character(s) ⟩ Manifestation Code 🝏 Hierarchical Condition Category **Coding Clinic**

Item 17-2 Equinus foot is a term referring to the hoof of a horse. The deformity is usually congenital or spastic. **Talipes equinovarus** is referred to as clubfoot. The foot tends to be smaller than normal, with the heel pointing downward and the forefoot turning inward. The heel cord (Achilles tendon) is tight, causing the heel to be drawn up toward the leg.

Figure 17-6 Supination and cavus deformity of forefoot. (From Kliegman R, Nelson WE: Nelson Textbook of Pediatrics, Philadelphia, Saunders, 2007)

Talipes cavus　Talipes equinus　Talipes calcaneus

Talipes valgus　Talipes equinovalgus　Talipes calcaneovalgus

Talipes varus　Talipes cavovarus　Talipes equinovarus　Talipes calcaneocavus

Figure 17-7 Talipes. (From Dorland: Dorland's Illustrated Medical Dictionary, ed 31, Saunders, 2007, p 1893)

● **Q66.1** Congenital talipes calcaneovarus
  Deformity of foot in which heel is turned toward midline of body and anterior of foot is elevated

    Q66.10 Congenital talipes calcaneovarus, unspecified foot

    Q66.11 Congenital talipes calcaneovarus, right foot

    Q66.12 Congenital talipes calcaneovarus, left foot

● **Q66.2** Congenital metatarsus (primus) varus
  Angulation of first metatarsal bone toward midline of body
  Coding Clinic: 2016, Q4, P59

  ● **Q66.21** Congenital metatarsus primus varus

    Q66.211 Congenital metatarsus primus varus, right foot

    Q66.212 Congenital metatarsus primus varus, left foot

    Q66.219 Congenital metatarsus primus varus, unspecified foot

  ● **Q66.22** Congenital metatarsus adductus
  Congenital metatarsus varus

    Q66.221 Congenital metatarsus adductus, right foot

    Q66.222 Congenital metatarsus adductus, left foot

    Q66.229 Congenital metatarsus adductus, unspecified foot

● **Q66.3** Other congenital varus deformities of feet
  Hallux varus, congenital

    Q66.30 Other congenital varus deformities of feet, unspecified foot

    Q66.31 Other congenital varus deformities of feet, right foot

    Q66.32 Other congenital varus deformities of feet, left foot

● **Q66.4** Congenital talipes calcaneovalgus

    Q66.40 Congenital talipes calcaneovalgus, unspecified foot

    Q66.41 Congenital talipes calcaneovalgus, right foot

    Q66.42 Congenital talipes calcaneovalgus, left foot

● **Q66.5** Congenital pes planus
  Congenital flat foot
  Congenital rigid flat foot
  Congenital spastic (everted) flat foot
  Excludes1 pes planus, acquired (M21.4)

    Q66.50 Congenital pes planus, unspecified foot

    Q66.51 Congenital pes planus, right foot

    Q66.52 Congenital pes planus, left foot

Q66.6 Other congenital valgus deformities of feet
  Inward angulation
  Congenital metatarsus valgus

● **Q66.7** Congenital pes cavus

    Q66.70 Congenital pes cavus, unspecified foot

    Q66.71 Congenital pes cavus, right foot

    Q66.72 Congenital pes cavus, left foot

● **Q66.8** Other congenital deformities of feet

    Q66.80 Congenital vertical talus deformity, unspecified foot

    Q66.81 Congenital vertical talus deformity, right foot

    Q66.82 Congenital vertical talus deformity, left foot

    Q66.89 Other specified congenital deformities of feet
  Congenital asymmetric talipes
  Congenital clubfoot NOS
  Congenital talipes NOS
  Congenital tarsal coalition
  Hammer toe, congenital

● **Q66.9** Congenital deformity of feet, unspecified

    Q66.90 Congenital deformity of feet, unspecified, unspecified foot

    Q66.91 Congenital deformity of feet, unspecified, right foot

    Q66.92 Congenital deformity of feet, unspecified, left foot

● **Q67** Congenital musculoskeletal deformities of head, face, spine and chest
  Excludes1 congenital malformation syndromes classified to Q87.-
  Potter's syndrome (Q60.6)

Q67.0 Congenital facial asymmetry

Q67.1 Congenital compression facies

Q67.2 Dolichocephaly
  Long head dimension

Q67.3 Plagiocephaly
  Asymmetric shape of head resulting from irregular closure of cranial sutures

Q67.4 Other congenital deformities of skull, face and jaw
  Congenital depressions in skull
  Congenital hemifacial atrophy or hypertrophy
  Deviation of nasal septum, congenital
  Squashed or bent nose, congenital
  Excludes1 dentofacial anomalies [including malocclusion] (M26.-)
  syphilitic saddle nose (A50.5)

Q67.5 Congenital deformity of spine
  Congenital postural scoliosis
  Congenital scoliosis NOS
  Excludes1 infantile idiopathic scoliosis (M41.0)
  scoliosis due to congenital bony malformation (Q76.3)

CHAPTER 17 (Q00-Q99)

Figure 17-8 Mild to moderate inbowing of the lower leg. (From Lissauer T, Clayden G: Illustrated Textbook of Paediatrics, Edinburgh, Mosby, 2011)

Figure 17-9 Thumb and index finger. (From Chung K: Hand and Upper Extremity Reconstruction, 1e, Saunders, 2008)

Q67.6 **Pectus excavatum**
 Congenital funnel chest
 Funnel-shaped chest depression

Q67.7 **Pectus carinatum**
 Congenital pigeon chest

Q67.8 **Other congenital deformities of chest**
 Congenital deformity of chest wall NOS

● Q68 **Other congenital musculoskeletal deformities**
 Excludes1 reduction defects of limb(s) (Q71-Q73)
 Excludes2 congenital myotonic chondrodystrophy (G71.13)

Q68.0 **Congenital deformity of sternocleidomastoid muscle**
 Congenital contracture of sternocleidomastoid (muscle)
 Congenital (sternomastoid) torticollis
 Sternomastoid tumor (congenital)

Q68.1 **Congenital deformity of finger(s) and hand**
 Congenital clubfinger
 Spade-like hand (congenital)

Q68.2 **Congenital deformity of knee**
 Congenital dislocation of knee
 Congenital genu recurvatum
 Hyperextension of knee resulting from hypermobility

Q68.3 **Congenital bowing of femur**
 Excludes1 anteversion of femur (neck) (Q65.89)

Q68.4 **Congenital bowing of tibia and fibula**

Q68.5 **Congenital bowing of long bones of leg, unspecified**

Q68.6 **Discoid meniscus**

Q68.8 **Other specified congenital musculoskeletal deformities**
 Congenital deformity of clavicle
 Congenital deformity of elbow
 Congenital deformity of forearm
 Congenital deformity of scapula
 Congenital deformity of wrist
 Congenital dislocation of elbow
 Congenital dislocation of shoulder
 Congenital dislocation of wrist

● Q69 **Polydactyly**
 AKA hyperdactyly, consists of supernumerary fingers or toes

Q69.0 **Accessory finger(s)**

Q69.1 **Accessory thumb(s)**

Q69.2 **Accessory toe(s)**
 Accessory hallux

Q69.9 **Polydactyly, unspecified**
 Supernumerary digit(s) NOS

● Q70 **Syndactyly**
 Webbing between distal phalanges of adjacent digits

● Q70.0 **Fused fingers**
 Complex syndactyly of fingers with synostosis

Q70.00 **Fused fingers, unspecified hand**
Q70.01 **Fused fingers, right hand**
Q70.02 **Fused fingers, left hand**
Q70.03 **Fused fingers, bilateral**

● Q70.1 **Webbed fingers**
 Simple syndactyly of fingers without synostosis

Q70.10 **Webbed fingers, unspecified hand**
Q70.11 **Webbed fingers, right hand**
Q70.12 **Webbed fingers, left hand**
Q70.13 **Webbed fingers, bilateral**

● Q70.2 **Fused toes**
 Complex syndactyly of toes with synostosis

Q70.20 **Fused toes, unspecified foot**
Q70.21 **Fused toes, right foot**
Q70.22 **Fused toes, left foot**
Q70.23 **Fused toes, bilateral**

● Q70.3 **Webbed toes**
 Simple syndactyly of toes without synostosis

Q70.30 **Webbed toes, unspecified foot**
Q70.31 **Webbed toes, right foot**
Q70.32 **Webbed toes, left foot**
Q70.33 **Webbed toes, bilateral**

Q70.4 **Polysyndactyly, unspecified**
 Excludes1 specified syndactyly of hand and
  feet - code to specified conditions
  (Q70.0- -Q70.3-)
 Extra and webbed digits

Q70.9 **Syndactyly, unspecified**
 Symphalangy NOS

● Q71 **Reduction defects of upper limb**

● Q71.0 **Congenital complete absence of upper limb**

Q71.00 **Congenital complete absence of unspecified upper limb**
Q71.01 **Congenital complete absence of right upper limb**
Q71.02 **Congenital complete absence of left upper limb**
Q71.03 **Congenital complete absence of upper limb, bilateral**

● Q71.1 **Congenital absence of upper arm and forearm with hand present**

Q71.10 **Congenital absence of unspecified upper arm and forearm with hand present**
Q71.11 **Congenital absence of right upper arm and forearm with hand present**
Q71.12 **Congenital absence of left upper arm and forearm with hand present**
Q71.13 **Congenital absence of upper arm and forearm with hand present, bilateral**

● Q71.2 **Congenital absence of both forearm and hand**

Q71.20 **Congenital absence of both forearm and hand, unspecified upper limb**
Q71.21 **Congenital absence of both forearm and hand, right upper limb**
Q71.22 **Congenital absence of both forearm and hand, left upper limb**
Q71.23 **Congenital absence of both forearm and hand, bilateral**

● **Q71.3**   Congenital absence of hand and finger
   Q71.30   Congenital absence of unspecified hand and finger
   Q71.31   Congenital absence of right hand and finger
   Q71.32   Congenital absence of left hand and finger
   Q71.33   Congenital absence of hand and finger, bilateral

● **Q71.4**   Longitudinal reduction defect of radius
    Clubhand (congenital)
    Radial clubhand
   Q71.40   Longitudinal reduction defect of unspecified radius
   Q71.41   Longitudinal reduction defect of right radius
   Q71.42   Longitudinal reduction defect of left radius
   Q71.43   Longitudinal reduction defect of radius, bilateral

● **Q71.5**   Longitudinal reduction defect of ulna
   Q71.50   Longitudinal reduction defect of unspecified ulna
   Q71.51   Longitudinal reduction defect of right ulna
   Q71.52   Longitudinal reduction defect of left ulna
   Q71.53   Longitudinal reduction defect of ulna, bilateral

● **Q71.6**   Lobster-claw hand
   Q71.60   Lobster-claw hand, unspecified hand
   Q71.61   Lobster-claw right hand
   Q71.62   Lobster-claw left hand
   Q71.63   Lobster-claw hand, bilateral

● **Q71.8**   Other reduction defects of upper limb
 ● **Q71.81**   Congenital shortening of upper limb
    Q71.811   Congenital shortening of right upper limb
    Q71.812   Congenital shortening of left upper limb
    Q71.813   Congenital shortening of upper limb, bilateral
    Q71.819   Congenital shortening of unspecified upper limb
 ● **Q71.89**   Other reduction defects of upper limb
    Q71.891   Other reduction defects of right upper limb
    Q71.892   Other reduction defects of left upper limb
    Q71.893   Other reduction defects of upper limb, bilateral
    Q71.899   Other reduction defects of unspecified upper limb

● **Q71.9**   Unspecified reduction defect of upper limb
   Q71.90   Unspecified reduction defect of unspecified upper limb
   Q71.91   Unspecified reduction defect of right upper limb
   Q71.92   Unspecified reduction defect of left upper limb
   Q71.93   Unspecified reduction defect of upper limb, bilateral

● **Q72**   Reduction defects of lower limb
 ● **Q72.0**   Congenital complete absence of lower limb
   Q72.00   Congenital complete absence of unspecified lower limb
   Q72.01   Congenital complete absence of right lower limb
   Q72.02   Congenital complete absence of left lower limb
   Q72.03   Congenital complete absence of lower limb, bilateral
 ● **Q72.1**   Congenital absence of thigh and lower leg with foot present
   Q72.10   Congenital absence of unspecified thigh and lower leg with foot present
   Q72.11   Congenital absence of right thigh and lower leg with foot present

   Q72.12   Congenital absence of left thigh and lower leg with foot present
   Q72.13   Congenital absence of thigh and lower leg with foot present, bilateral

● **Q72.2**   Congenital absence of both lower leg and foot
   Q72.20   Congenital absence of both lower leg and foot, unspecified lower limb
   Q72.21   Congenital absence of both lower leg and foot, right lower limb
   Q72.22   Congenital absence of both left lower leg and foot, left lower limb
   Q72.23   Congenital absence of both lower leg and foot, bilateral

● **Q72.3**   Congenital absence of foot and toe(s)
   Q72.30   Congenital absence of unspecified foot and toe(s)
   Q72.31   Congenital absence of right foot and toe(s)
   Q72.32   Congenital absence of left foot and toe(s)
   Q72.33   Congenital absence of foot and toe(s), bilateral

● **Q72.4**   Longitudinal reduction defect of femur
    Proximal femoral focal deficiency
   Q72.40   Longitudinal reduction defect of unspecified femur
   Q72.41   Longitudinal reduction defect of right femur
   Q72.42   Longitudinal reduction defect of left femur
   Q72.43   Longitudinal reduction defect of femur, bilateral

● **Q72.5**   Longitudinal reduction defect of tibia
   Q72.50   Longitudinal reduction defect of unspecified tibia
   Q72.51   Longitudinal reduction defect of right tibia
   Q72.52   Longitudinal reduction defect of left tibia
   Q72.53   Longitudinal reduction defect of tibia, bilateral

● **Q72.6**   Longitudinal reduction defect of fibula
   Q72.60   Longitudinal reduction defect of unspecified fibula
   Q72.61   Longitudinal reduction defect of right fibula
   Q72.62   Longitudinal reduction defect of left fibula
   Q72.63   Longitudinal reduction defect of fibula, bilateral

● **Q72.7**   Split foot
   Q72.70   Split foot, unspecified lower limb
   Q72.71   Split foot, right lower limb
   Q72.72   Split foot, left lower limb
   Q72.73   Split foot, bilateral

● **Q72.8**   Other reduction defects of lower limb
 ● **Q72.81**   Congenital shortening of lower limb
    Q72.811   Congenital shortening of right lower limb
    Q72.812   Congenital shortening of left lower limb
    Q72.813   Congenital shortening of lower limb, bilateral
    Q72.819   Congenital shortening of unspecified lower limb
 ● **Q72.89**   Other reduction defects of lower limb
    Q72.891   Other reduction defects of right lower limb
    Q72.892   Other reduction defects of left lower limb
    Q72.893   Other reduction defects of lower limb, bilateral
    Q72.899   Other reduction defects of unspecified lower limb

CHAPTER 17 (Q00-Q99)

- Q72.9 **Unspecified reduction defect of lower limb**
  - Q72.90 **Unspecified reduction defect of unspecified lower limb**
  - Q72.91 **Unspecified reduction defect of right lower limb**
  - Q72.92 **Unspecified reduction defect of left lower limb**
  - Q72.93 **Unspecified reduction defect of lower limb, bilateral**

- Q73 **Reduction defects of unspecified limb**
  - Q73.0 **Congenital absence of unspecified limb(s)**
    - Amelia NOS
  - Q73.1 **Phocomelia, unspecified limb(s)**
    - Phocomelia NOS
      - *Absence/shortening of long bones primarily as a result of thalidomide*
  - Q73.8 **Other reduction defects of unspecified limb(s)**
    - Longitudinal reduction deformity of unspecified limb(s)
    - Ectromelia of limb NOS
      - *Gross hypoplasia or aplasia of one or more long bones of limb(s)*
    - Hemimelia of limb NOS
      - *Absence of one-half of long bone*
    - Reduction defect of limb NOS

- Q74 **Other congenital malformations of limb(s)**
  - Excludes1   polydactyly (Q69.-)
              reduction defect of limb (Q71-Q73)
              syndactyly (Q70.-)
  - Q74.0 **Other congenital malformations of upper limb(s), including shoulder girdle**
    - Accessory carpal bones
    - Cleidocranial dysostosis
    - Congenital pseudarthrosis of clavicle
    - Macrodactylia (fingers)
    - Madelung's deformity
    - Radioulnar synostosis
    - Sprengel's deformity
    - Triphalangeal thumb
  - Q74.1 **Congenital malformation of knee**
    - Congenital absence of patella
    - Congenital dislocation of patella
    - Congenital genu valgum
    - Congenital genu varum
    - Rudimentary patella
    - Excludes1   congenital dislocation of knee (Q68.2)
                congenital genu recurvatum (Q68.2)
                nail patella syndrome (Q87.2)
  - Q74.2 **Other congenital malformations of lower limb(s), including pelvic girdle**
    - Congenital fusion of sacroiliac joint
    - Congenital malformation of ankle joint
    - Congenital malformation of sacroiliac joint
    - Excludes1   anteversion of femur (neck) (Q65.89)
  - Q74.3 **Arthrogryposis multiplex congenita**
  - Q74.8 **Other specified congenital malformations of limb(s)**
  - Q74.9 **Unspecified congenital malformation of limb(s)**
    - Congenital anomaly of limb(s) NOS

- Q75 **Other congenital malformations of skull and face bones**
  - Excludes1   congenital malformation of face NOS (Q18.-)
              congenital malformation syndromes classified to Q87.-
              dentofacial anomalies [including malocclusion] (M26.-)
              musculoskeletal deformities of head and face (Q67.0-Q67.4)
              skull defects associated with congenital anomalies of brain such as:
              anencephaly (Q00.0)
              encephalocele (Q01.-)
              hydrocephalus (Q03.-)
              microcephaly (Q02)

Figure 17-10 Generalized craniosynostosis without symptoms or signs of increased intracranial pressure. (From Goetz C: Textbook of Clinical Neurology, St. Louis, MO, Elsevier, 2007)

Item 17-3 Anencephalus is a congenital deformity of the cranial vault. **Craniosynostosis,** also known as craniostenosis and stenocephaly, signifies any form of congenital deformity of the skull that results from the premature closing of the sutures of the skull. **Iniencephaly** is a deformity in which the head and neck are flexed backward to a great extent and the head is very large in comparison to the shortened body.

- Q75.0 **Craniosynostosis**
  - *Premature closure of sutures of skull*
  - Acrocephaly
  - Imperfect fusion of skull
  - Oxycephaly
  - Trigonocephaly
- Q75.1 **Craniofacial dysostosis**
  - *Congenital deformity of head*
  - Crouzon's disease
- Q75.2 **Hypertelorism**
- Q75.3 **Macrocephaly**
  - *Unusually large size of head; AKA megalocephaly*
- Q75.4 **Mandibulofacial dysostosis**
  - Franceschetti syndrome
  - Treacher Collins syndrome
- Q75.5 **Oculomandibular dysostosis**
  - *Ossification of occular and mandibular bones*
- Q75.8 **Other specified congenital malformations of skull and face bones**
  - Absence of skull bone, congenital
  - Congenital deformity of forehead
  - Platybasia
- Q75.9 **Congenital malformation of skull and face bones, unspecified**
  - Congenital anomaly of face bones NOS
  - Congenital anomaly of skull NOS

- Q76 **Congenital malformations of spine and bony thorax**
  - Excludes1   congenital musculoskeletal deformities of spine and chest (Q67.5-Q67.8)
  - Q76.0 **Spina bifida occulta**
    - Excludes1   meningocele (spinal) (Q05.-)
                spina bifida (aperta) (cystica) (Q05.-)
  - Q76.1 **Klippel-Feil syndrome**
    - Cervical fusion syndrome
  - Q76.2 **Congenital spondylolisthesis**
    - Congenital spondylolysis
    - Excludes1   spondylolisthesis (acquired) (M43.1-)
                spondylolysis (acquired) (M43.0-)
  - Q76.3 **Congenital scoliosis due to congenital bony malformation**
    - Hemivertebra fusion or failure of segmentation with scoliosis
  - Q76.4 **Other congenital malformations of spine, not associated with scoliosis**
    - Q76.41 **Congenital kyphosis**
      - *Abnormal increase in convexity curvature of thoracic spinal column; AKA humpback*
      - Q76.411 **Congenital kyphosis, occipito-atlanto-axial region**
      - Q76.412 **Congenital kyphosis, cervical region**
      - Q76.413 **Congenital kyphosis, cervicothoracic region**
      - Q76.414 **Congenital kyphosis, thoracic region**

▶ New   ⇛ Revised   ~~deleted~~ Deleted   Excludes 1   Excludes 2   Includes   Use additional   Code first   Code also   Key words
OGCR Official Guidelines   X Assign placeholder X   ● Use Additional Character(s)   ▶ Manifestation Code   ⬠ Hierarchical Condition Category   **Coding Clinic**

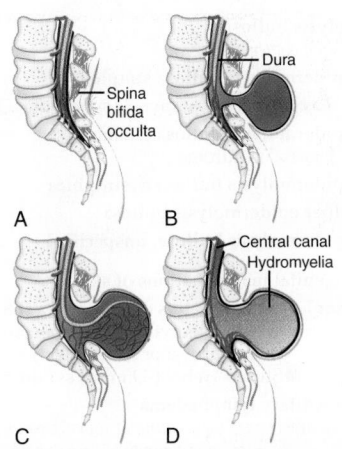

Figure 17-11 **A.** Spina bifida occulta. **B.** Meningocele. **C.** Myelomeningocele. **D.** Myelocystocele (syringomyelocele) or hydromyelia.

Item 17–4 **Spina bifida** is a midline spinal defect in which one or more vertebrae fail to fuse, leaving an opening in the vertebral canal. When the defect is not visible, it is called spina bifida occulta, and when it is visible, it is called spina bifida cystica.

         Q76.415   **Congenital kyphosis, thoracolumbar region**

         Q76.419   **Congenital kyphosis, unspecified region**

● Q76.42   **Congenital lordosis**
         An abnormal increase in curvature of lumbar spine (sway back)

         Q76.425   **Congenital lordosis, thoracolumbar region**

         Q76.426   **Congenital lordosis, lumbar region**

         Q76.427   **Congenital lordosis, lumbosacral region**

         Q76.428   **Congenital lordosis, sacral and sacrococcygeal region**

         Q76.429   **Congenital lordosis, unspecified region**

   Q76.49   **Other congenital malformations of spine, not associated with scoliosis**
         Congenital absence of vertebra NOS
         Congenital fusion of spine NOS
         Congenital malformation of lumbosacral (joint) (region) NOS
         Congenital malformation of spine NOS
         Hemivertebra NOS
         Malformation of spine NOS
         Platyspondylisis NOS
         Supernumerary vertebra NOS

Q76.5   **Cervical rib**
     Supernumerary rib in cervical region

Q76.6   **Other congenital malformations of ribs**
     Accessory rib
     Congenital absence of rib
     Congenital fusion of ribs
     Congenital malformation of ribs NOS
     Excludes1   short rib syndrome (Q77.2)

Q76.7   **Congenital malformation of sternum**
     Congenital absence of sternum
     Sternum bifidum

Q76.8   **Other congenital malformations of bony thorax**

Q76.9   **Congenital malformation of bony thorax, unspecified**

● **Q77**   **Osteochondrodysplasia with defects of growth of tubular bones and spine**
     Excludes1   mucopolysaccharidosis (E76.0-E76.3)
     Excludes2   congenital myotonic chondrodystrophy (G71.13)

Q77.0   **Achondrogenesis**
     Hypochondrogenesis

Q77.1   **Thanatophoric short stature**

Q77.2   **Short rib syndrome**
     Asphyxiating thoracic dysplasia [Jeune]

Q77.3   **Chondrodysplasia punctata**
     Benign cartilaginous neoplasms
     Excludes1   rhizomelic chondrodysplasia punctata (E71.43)

Q77.4   **Achondroplasia**
     Disturbance of epiphyseal chondroblastic growth and maturation, results in dwarfism
     Hypochondroplasia
     Osteosclerosis congenita

Q77.5   **Diastrophic dysplasia**

Q77.6   **Chondroectodermal dysplasia**
     Defective development of skin, hair, teeth, with polydactyly and defect of cardiac septum
     Ellis-van Creveld syndrome

Q77.7   **Spondyloepiphyseal dysplasia**

Q77.8   **Other osteochondrodysplasia with defects of growth of tubular bones and spine**

Q77.9   **Osteochondrodysplasia with defects of growth of tubular bones and spine, unspecified**

● **Q78**   **Other osteochondrodysplasias**
     Disorder of development of bone and cartilage; common cause of dwarfism
     Excludes2   congenital myotonic chondrodystrophy (G71.13)

Q78.0   **Osteogenesis imperfecta**
     Fragilitas ossium
     Osteopsathyrosis

Q78.1   **Polyostotic fibrous dysplasia**
     Albright(-McCune)(-Sternberg) syndrome

Q78.2   **Osteopetrosis**
     Abnormally dense bone; AKA marble bones disease, ivory bones
     Albers-Schönberg syndrome
     Osteosclerosis NOS

Q78.3   **Progressive diaphyseal dysplasia**
     Camurati-Engelmann syndrome

Q78.4   **Enchondromatosis**
     Thinning of overlying cortex of bone and distorted length
     Maffucci's syndrome
     Ollier's disease

Q78.5   **Metaphyseal dysplasia**
     Disturbance in enchondral bone growth, causing ends of shafts to remain larger than normal in circumference
     Pyle's syndrome

Q78.6   **Multiple congenital exostoses**
     Diaphyseal aclasis

Q78.8   **Other specified osteochondrodysplasias**
     Osteopoikilosis

Q78.9   **Osteochondrodysplasia, unspecified**
     Chondrodystrophy NOS
     AKA skeletal dysplasia (dwarfism) caused by genetic mutations affecting hyaline cartilage capping long bones and vertebrae
     Osteodystrophy NOS

CHAPTER 17 (Q00-Q99)

● **Q79** **Congenital malformations of musculoskeletal system, not elsewhere classified**

> **Excludes2**   congenital (sternomastoid) torticollis (Q68.0)

Q79.0 **Congenital diaphragmatic hernia**
> **Excludes1**   congenital hiatus hernia (Q40.1)

Q79.1 **Other congenital malformations of diaphragm**
Absence of diaphragm
Congenital malformation of diaphragm NOS
Eventration of diaphragm

Q79.2 **Exomphalos**
Abdominal hernia in which part of intestine protrudes at umbilicus; AKA exomphalos and exumbilication
Omphalocele
> **Excludes1**   umbilical hernia (K42.-)

Q79.3 **Gastroschisis**
Congenital fissure of anterior abdominal wall often with protrusion of small/large intestine

Q79.4 **Prune belly syndrome**
Congenital prolapse of bladder mucosa
Eagle-Barrett syndrome

● **Q79.5** **Other congenital malformations of abdominal wall**
> **Excludes1**   umbilical hernia (K42.-)

Q79.51 **Congenital hernia of bladder**

Q79.59 **Other congenital malformations of abdominal wall**

● **Q79.6** **Ehlers-Danlos syndromes**
Group of inherited disorders of connective tissue; AKA cutis hyperelastica

Q79.60 **Ehlers-Danlos syndrome, unspecified**

Q79.61 **Classical Ehlers-Danlos syndrome**
Classical EDS (cEDS)

Q79.62 **Hypermobile Ehlers-Danlos syndrome**
Hypermobile EDS (hEDS)

Q79.63 **Vascular Ehlers-Danlos syndrome**
Vascular EDS (vEDS)

Q79.69 **Other Ehlers-Danlos syndromes**

Q79.8 **Other congenital malformations of musculoskeletal system**
Absence of muscle
Absence of tendon
Accessory muscle
Amyotrophia congenita
Congenital constricting bands
Congenital shortening of tendon
Poland syndrome

Q79.9 **Congenital malformation of musculoskeletal system, unspecified**
Congenital anomaly of musculoskeletal system NOS
Congenital deformity of musculoskeletal system NOS

OTHER CONGENITAL MALFORMATIONS (Q80-Q89)

● **Q80** **Congenital ichthyosis**
Characterized by increased keratinization, resulting in noninflammatory scaling of skin
> **Excludes1**   Refsum's disease (G60.1)

Q80.0 **Ichthyosis vulgaris**

Q80.1 **X-linked ichthyosis**

Q80.2 **Lamellar ichthyosis**
Collodion baby

Q80.3 **Congenital bullous ichthyosiform erythroderma**

Q80.4 **Harlequin fetus**

Q80.8 **Other congenital ichthyosis**

Q80.9 **Congenital ichthyosis, unspecified**

● **Q81** **Epidermolysis bullosa**
Loosening of epidermis

Q81.0 **Epidermolysis bullosa simplex**
> **Excludes1**   Cockayne's syndrome (Q87.19)

Q81.1 **Epidermolysis bullosa letalis**
Herlitz' syndrome

Q81.2 **Epidermolysis bullosa dystrophica**

Q81.8 **Other epidermolysis bullosa**

Q81.9 **Epidermolysis bullosa, unspecified**

● **Q82** **Other congenital malformations of skin**
> **Excludes1**   acrodermatitis enteropathica (E83.2)
> congenital erythropoietic porphyria (E80.0)
> pilonidal cyst or sinus (L05.-)
> ▬▶Sturge-Weber (-Dimitri) syndrome (Q85.89)

Q82.0 **Hereditary lymphedema**
Characterized by swelling of subcutaneous tissue caused by obstruction of lymphatic vessels and resulting edema of lymph fluid

Q82.1 **Xeroderma pigmentosum**
Extreme sensitivity to ultraviolet rays that most commonly affects the eyes and skin, but may also involve the nervous system

Q82.2 **Congenital cutaneous mastocytosis**
Characterized by infiltrates of mast cells in tissues/organs
Congenital diffuse cutaneous mastocytosis
Congenital maculopapular cutaneous mastocytosis
Congenital urticaria pigmentosa
> **Excludes1**   cutaneous mastocytosis NOS (D47.01)
> diffuse cutaneous mastocytosis (with onset after newborn period) (D47.01)
> malignant mastocytosis (C96.2-)
> systemic mastocytosis (D47.02)
> urticaria pigmentosa (non-congenital) (with onset after newborn period) (D47.01)

Q82.3 **Incontinentia pigmenti**
Characterized by hypopigmented cutaneous in adults and early childhood

Q82.4 **Ectodermal dysplasia (anhidrotic)**
Absence/deficiency of tissues/structures, including teeth, hair, nails, and certain glands
> **Excludes1**   Ellis-van Creveld syndrome (Q77.6)

Q82.5 **Congenital non-neoplastic nevus**
Birthmark NOS
Flammeus Nevus
Portwine Nevus
Sanguineous Nevus
Strawberry Nevus
Vascular Nevus NOS
Verrucous Nevus
> **Excludes2**   Café au lait spots (L81.3)
> lentigo (L81.4)
> nevus NOS (D22.-)
> araneus nevus (I78.1)
> melanocytic nevus (D22.-)
> pigmented nevus (D22.-)
> spider nevus (I78.1)
> stellar nevus (I78.1)

Q82.6 **Congenital sacral dimple**
Parasacral dimple
> **Excludes2**   pilonidal cyst with abscess (L05.01)
> pilonidal cyst without abscess (L05.91)
> **Coding Clinic: 2016, Q4, P60**

▶ New   ▬▶ Revised   ~~deleted~~ Deleted   Excludes 1   Excludes 2   Includes   Use additional   Code first   Code also   Key words

OGCR Official Guidelines   X Assign placeholder X   ● Use Additional Character(s)   ▶ Manifestation Code   🅗 Hierarchical Condition Category   **Coding Clinic**

Q82.8   **Other specified congenital malformations of skin**
  Abnormal palmar creases
  Accessory skin tags
  Benign familial pemphigus [Hailey-Hailey]
  Congenital poikiloderma
  Cutis laxa (hyperelastica)
  Dermatoglyphic anomalies
  Inherited keratosis palmaris et plantaris
  Keratosis follicularis [Darier-White]
  Excludes1   Ehlers-Danlos syndromes (Q79.6-)
  Coding Clinic: 2016, Q1, P17

Q82.9   **Congenital malformation of skin, unspecified**

● **Q83**   **Congenital malformations of breast**
  Excludes2   absence of pectoral muscle (Q79.8)
      hypoplasia of breast (N64.82)
      micromastia (N64.82)

Q83.0   **Congenital absence of breast with absent nipple**

Q83.1   **Accessory breast**
  Supernumerary breast

Q83.2   **Absent nipple**

Q83.3   **Accessory nipple**
  Supernumerary nipple

Q83.8   **Other congenital malformations of breast**

Q83.9   **Congenital malformation of breast, unspecified**

● **Q84**   **Other congenital malformations of integument**

Q84.0   **Congenital alopecia**
  Congenital atrichosis

Q84.1   **Congenital morphological disturbances of hair, not elsewhere classified**
  Beaded hair
  Monilethrix
  Pili annulati
  Excludes1   Menkes' kinky hair syndrome (E83.0)

Q84.2   **Other congenital malformations of hair**
  Congenital hypertrichosis
  Congenital malformation of hair NOS
  Persistent lanugo

Q84.3   **Anonychia**
  Absence of nail
  Excludes1   nail patella syndrome (Q87.2)

Q84.4   **Congenital leukonychia**
  Opaque, whitish discoloration of nails; AKA leukopathia unguium

Q84.5   **Enlarged and hypertrophic nails**
  Congenital onychauxis
  Pachyonychia

Q84.6   **Other congenital malformations of nails**
  Congenital clubnail
  Congenital koilonychia
  Congenital malformation of nail NOS

Q84.8   **Other specified congenital malformations of integument**
  Aplasia cutis congenita

Q84.9   **Congenital malformation of integument, unspecified**
  Congenital anomaly of integument NOS
  Congenital deformity of integument NOS

● **Q85**   **Phakomatoses, not elsewhere classified**
  Excludes1   ataxia telangiectasia [Louis-Bar] (G11.3)
      familial dysautonomia [Riley-Day] (G90.1)

● **Q85.0**   **Neurofibromatosis (nonmalignant)**
  Developmental changes in nervous system and other structures, with formation of neurofibromas

Q85.00   **Neurofibromatosis, unspecified** 🐾

Q85.01   **Neurofibromatosis, type 1** 🐾
  Von Recklinghausen disease

Q85.02   **Neurofibromatosis, type 2** 🐾
  Acoustic neurofibromatosis

Q85.03   **Schwannomatosis** 🐾

Q85.09   **Other neurofibromatosis** 🐾

Q85.1   **Tuberous sclerosis** 🐾
  Bourneville's disease
  Epiloia

● **Q85.8**   **Other phakomatoses, not elsewhere classified** 🐾
  ~~Peutz-Jeghers Syndrome~~
  ~~Sturge-Weber(-Dimitri) syndrome~~
  ~~von Hippel-Lindau syndrome~~
  Excludes1   Meckel-Gruber syndrome (Q61.9)
  Coding Clinic: 2021, Q3, P12

▶ **Q85.81**   **PTEN tumor syndrome**
  ▶ PHTS
  ▶ PTEN hamartoma tumor syndrome
  ▶ PTEN related Cowden syndrome
  ▶ Code also, if applicable, genetic susceptibility to malignant neoplasm (Z15.0-)

▶ **Q85.82**   **Other Cowden syndrome**

▶ **Q85.83**   **Von Hippel-Lindau syndrome**
  ▶ Code also manifestations

▶ **Q85.89**   **Other phakomatoses, not elsewhere classified**
  ▶ Peutz-Jeghers syndrome
  ▶ Sturge-Weber(-Dimitri) syndrome

Q85.9   **Phakomatosis, unspecified** 🐾
  Hamartosis NOS

● **Q86**   **Congenital malformation syndromes due to known exogenous causes, not elsewhere classified**
  Excludes2   iodine-deficiency-related hypothyroidism (E00-E02)
      nonteratogenic effects of substances transmitted via placenta or breast milk (P04.-)

Q86.0   **Fetal alcohol syndrome (dysmorphic)**

Q86.1   **Fetal hydantoin syndrome**
  Meadow's syndrome

Q86.2   **Dysmorphism due to warfarin**

Q86.8   **Other congenital malformation syndromes due to known exogenous causes**

● **Q87**   **Other specified congenital malformation syndromes affecting multiple systems**
  Use additional code(s) to identify all associated manifestations

Q87.0   **Congenital malformation syndromes predominantly affecting facial appearance**
  Acrocephalopolysyndactyly
  Acrocephalosyndactyly [Apert]
  Cryptophthalmos syndrome
  Cyclopia
  Goldenhar syndrome
  Moebius syndrome
  Oro-facial-digital syndrome
  Robin syndrome
  Whistling face

● **Q87.1**   **Congenital malformation syndromes predominantly associated with short stature**

Q87.11   **Prader-Willi syndrome**

Q87.19   **Other congenital malformation syndromes predominantly associated with short stature**
  Aarskog syndrome
  Cockayne syndrome
  De Lange syndrome
  Dubowitz syndrome
  Noonan syndrome
  Robinow-Silverman-Smith syndrome
  Russell-Silver syndrome
  Seckel syndrome
  Excludes1   Ellis-van Creveld syndrome (Q77.6)
      Smith-Lemli-Opitz syndrome (E78.72)

Q87.2   Congenital malformation syndromes predominantly involving limbs
Holt-Oram syndrome
Klippel-Trenaunay-Weber syndrome
Nail patella syndrome
Rubinstein-Taybi syndrome
Sirenomelia syndrome
Thrombocytopenia with absent radius [TAR] syndrome
VATER syndrome

Q87.3   Congenital malformation syndromes involving early overgrowth
Beckwith-Wiedemann syndrome
Sotos' syndrome
Weaver syndrome

● **Q87.4   Marfan's syndrome**

   Q87.40   Marfan's syndrome, unspecified

● **Q87.41   Marfan's syndrome with cardiovascular manifestations**

      Q87.410   Marfan's syndrome with aortic dilation

      Q87.418   Marfan's syndrome with other cardiovascular manifestations

   Q87.42   Marfan's syndrome with ocular manifestations

   Q87.43   Marfan's syndrome with skeletal manifestation

Q87.5   Other congenital malformation syndromes with other skeletal changes

● **Q87.8   Other specified congenital malformation syndromes, not elsewhere classified**

   Excludes1   Zellweger syndrome (E71.510)

   Q87.81   Alport syndrome
   Progressive sensorineural hearing loss, progressive pyelonephritis or glomerulonephritis, and ocular defects

      Use additional code to identify stage of chronic kidney disease (N18.1-N18.6)

   Q87.82   Arterial tortuosity syndrome
   Coding Clinic: 2016, Q4, P60-61

   Q87.89   Other specified congenital malformation syndromes, not elsewhere classified
   Laurence-Moon (-Bardet)-Biedl syndrome

● **Q89   Other congenital malformations, not elsewhere classified**

● **Q89.0   Congenital absence and malformations of spleen**

   Excludes1   isomerism of atrial appendages (with asplenia or polysplenia) (Q20.6)

   Q89.01   Asplenia (congenital)

   Q89.09   Congenital malformations of spleen
   Congenital splenomegaly

Q89.1   Congenital malformations of adrenal gland

   Excludes1   adrenogenital disorders (E25.-)
   congenital adrenal hyperplasia (E25.0)

Q89.2   Congenital malformations of other endocrine glands
Congenital malformation of parathyroid or thyroid gland
Persistent thyroglossal duct
Thyroglossal cyst

   Excludes1   congenital goiter (E03.0)
   congenital hypothyroidism (E03.1)

Q89.3   Situs inversus
Lateral transposition of viscera of thorax and abdomen
Dextrocardia with situs inversus
Mirror-image atrial arrangement with situs inversus
Situs inversus or transversus abdominalis
Situs inversus or transversus thoracis
Transposition of abdominal viscera
Transposition of thoracic viscera

   Excludes1   dextrocardia NOS (Q24.0)

Q89.4   Conjoined twins
Craniopagus
Dicephaly
Pygopagus
Thoracopagus

Q89.7   Multiple congenital malformations, not elsewhere classified
Multiple congenital anomalies NOS
Multiple congenital deformities NOS

   Excludes1   congenital malformation syndromes affecting multiple systems (Q87.-)

Q89.8   Other specified congenital malformations
Use additional code(s) to identify all associated manifestations
Coding Clinic: 2021, Q3, P12

Q89.9   Congenital malformation, unspecified
Congenital anomaly NOS
Congenital deformity NOS

CHROMOSOMAL ABNORMALITIES, NOT ELSEWHERE CLASSIFIED (Q90-Q99)

   Excludes2   mitochondrial metabolic disorders (E88.4-)

● **Q90   Down syndrome**
Use additional code(s) to identify any associated physical conditions and degree of intellectual disabilities (F70-F79)

   Q90.0   Trisomy 21, nonmosaicism (meiotic nondisjunction)
   Trisomy 21, nondisjunction, accounts for 95% of Downs syndrome cases

   Q90.1   Trisomy 21, mosaicism (mitotic nondisjunction)

   Q90.2   Trisomy 21, translocation

   Q90.9   Down syndrome, unspecified
   Trisomy 21 NOS

● **Q91   Trisomy 18 and Trisomy 13**

   Q91.0   Trisomy 18, nonmosaicism (meiotic nondisjunction)

   Q91.1   Trisomy 18, mosaicism (mitotic nondisjunction)

   Q91.2   Trisomy 18, translocation

   Q91.3   Trisomy 18, unspecified

   Q91.4   Trisomy 13, nonmosaicism (meiotic nondisjunction)

   Q91.5   Trisomy 13, mosaicism (mitotic nondisjunction)

   Q91.6   Trisomy 13, translocation

   Q91.7   Trisomy 13, unspecified

● **Q92   Other trisomies and partial trisomies of the autosomes, not elsewhere classified**

   Includes   unbalanced translocations and insertions
   Excludes1   trisomies of chromosomes 13, 18, 21 (Q90-Q91)

   Q92.0   Whole chromosome trisomy, nonmosaicism (meiotic nondisjunction)

   Q92.1   Whole chromosome trisomy, mosaicism (mitotic nondisjunction)

   Q92.2   Partial trisomy
   Less than whole arm duplicated
   Whole arm or more duplicated

   Excludes1   partial trisomy due to unbalanced translocation (Q92.5)

   Q92.5   Duplications with other complex rearrangements
   Partial trisomy due to unbalanced translocations

   Code also any associated deletions due to unbalanced translocations, inversions and insertions (Q93.7)

● **Q92.6   Marker chromosomes**
   Trisomies due to dicentrics
   Trisomies due to extra rings
   Trisomies due to isochromosomes
   Individual with marker heterochromatin

   Q92.61   Marker chromosomes in normal individual

   Q92.62   Marker chromosomes in abnormal individual

   Q92.7   Triploidy and polyploidy

   Q92.8   Other specified trisomies and partial trisomies of autosomes
   Duplications identified by fluorescence in situ hybridization (FISH)
   Duplications identified by in situ hybridization (ISH)
   Duplications seen only at prometaphase

   Q92.9   Trisomy and partial trisomy of autosomes, unspecified

▶ New   ⇒ Revised   ~~deleted~~ Deleted   Excludes 1   Excludes 2   Includes   Use additional   Code first   Code also   Key words
OGCR Official Guidelines   X Assign placeholder X   ● Use Additional Character(s)   ❭ Manifestation Code   🐾 Hierarchical Condition Category   Coding Clinic

● **Q93**   **Monosomies and deletions from the autosomes, not elsewhere classified**

  Q93.0   Whole chromosome monosomy, nonmosaicism (meiotic nondisjunction)

  Q93.1   Whole chromosome monosomy, mosaicism (mitotic nondisjunction)

  Q93.2   Chromosome replaced with ring, dicentric or isochromosome

  Q93.3   Deletion of short arm of chromosome 4
        Wolff-Hirschorn syndrome

  Q93.4   Deletion of short arm of chromosome 5
        Cri-du-chat syndrome

● **Q93.5**   Other deletions of part of a chromosome

    Q93.51   Angelman syndrome

    Q93.59   Other deletions of part of a chromosome

  Q93.7   Deletions with other complex rearrangements
        Deletions due to unbalanced translocations, inversions and insertions
        Code also any associated duplications due to unbalanced translocations, inversions and insertions (Q92.5)

● **Q93.8**   Other deletions from the autosomes

    Q93.81   Velo-cardio-facial syndrome
          Deletion 22q11.2
          Coding Clinic: 2019, Q3, P14

    Q93.82   Williams syndrome

    Q93.88   Other microdeletions Miller-Dieker syndrome
          Smith-Magenis syndrome

    Q93.89   Other deletions from the autosomes
          Deletions identified by fluorescence in situ hybridization (FISH)
          Deletions identified by in situ hybridization (ISH)
          Deletions seen only at prometaphase

  Q93.9   Deletion from autosomes, unspecified

● **Q95**   **Balanced rearrangements and structural markers, not elsewhere classified**

    Includes   Robertsonian and balanced reciprocal translocations and insertions

  Q95.0   Balanced translocation and insertion in normal individual

  Q95.1   Chromosome inversion in normal individual

  Q95.2   Balanced autosomal rearrangement in abnormal individual

  Q95.3   Balanced sex/autosomal rearrangement in abnormal individual

  Q95.5   Individual with autosomal fragile site

  Q95.8   Other balanced rearrangements and structural markers

  Q95.9   Balanced rearrangement and structural marker, unspecified

● **Q96**   **Turner's syndrome**
    Caused by missing or incomplete X chromosome affecting growth and sexual development

    Excludes1   Noonan syndrome (Q87.19)

  Q96.0   Karyotype 45, X ♀

  Q96.1   Karyotype 46, X iso (Xq) ♀
        Karyotype 46, isochromosome Xq

  Q96.2   Karyotype 46, X with abnormal sex chromosome, except iso (Xq) ♀
        Karyotype 46, X with abnormal sex chromosome, except isochromosome Xq

  Q96.3   Mosaicism, 45, X/46, XX or XY ♀

  Q96.4   Mosaicism, 45, X/other cell line(s) with abnormal sex chromosome ♀

  Q96.8   Other variants of Turner's syndrome ♀

  Q96.9   Turner's syndrome, unspecified ♀

● **Q97**   **Other sex chromosome abnormalities, female phenotype, not elsewhere classified**

    Excludes1   Turner's syndrome (Q96.-)

  Q97.0   Karyotype 47, XXX ♀

  Q97.1   Female with more than three X chromosomes ♀

  Q97.2   Mosaicism, lines with various numbers of X chromosomes ♀

  Q97.3   Female with 46, XY karyotype ♀

  Q97.8   Other specified sex chromosome abnormalities, female phenotype ♀

  Q97.9   Sex chromosome abnormality, female phenotype, unspecified ♀

● **Q98**   **Other sex chromosome abnormalities, male phenotype, not elsewhere classified**

  Q98.0   Klinefelter syndrome karyotype 47, XXY ♂

  Q98.1   Klinefelter syndrome, male with more than two X chromosomes ♂

  Q98.3   Other male with 46, XX karyotype ♂

  Q98.4   Klinefelter syndrome, unspecified ♂

  Q98.5   Karyotype 47, XYY

  Q98.6   Male with structurally abnormal sex chromosome ♂

  Q98.7   Male with sex chromosome mosaicism ♂

  Q98.8   Other specified sex chromosome abnormalities, male phenotype ♂

  Q98.9   Sex chromosome abnormality, male phenotype, unspecified ♂

● **Q99**   **Other chromosome abnormalities, not elsewhere classified**

  Q99.0   Chimera 46, XX/46, XY
        Chimera 46, XX/46, XY true hermaphrodite

  Q99.1   46, XX true hermaphrodite
        46, XX with streak gonads
        46, XY with streak gonads
        Pure gonadal dysgenesis

  Q99.2   Fragile X chromosome
        Fragile X syndrome

  Q99.8   Other specified chromosome abnormalities

  Q99.9   Chromosomal abnormality, unspecified

CHAPTER 17 (Q00–Q99)

CHAPTER 18

SYMPTOMS, SIGNS, AND ABNORMAL CLINICAL AND LABORATORY FINDINGS, NOT ELSEWHERE CLASSIFIED (R00-R99)

OGCR Chapter-Specific Coding Guidelines

18. **Chapter 18: Symptoms, signs, and abnormal clinical and laboratory findings, not elsewhere classified (R00-R99)**
    Chapter 18 includes symptoms, signs, abnormal results of clinical or other investigative procedures, and ill-defined conditions regarding which no diagnosis classifiable elsewhere is recorded. Signs and symptoms that point to a specific diagnosis have been assigned to a category in other chapters of the classification.

    a. Use of symptom codes
    Codes that describe symptoms and signs are acceptable for reporting purposes when a related definitive diagnosis has not been established (confirmed) by the provider.

    b. Use of a symptom code with a definitive diagnosis code
    Codes for signs and symptoms may be reported in addition to a related definitive diagnosis when the sign or symptom is not routinely associated with that diagnosis, such as the various signs and symptoms associated with complex syndromes. The definitive diagnosis code should be sequenced before the symptom code.

    Signs or symptoms that are associated routinely with a disease process should not be assigned as additional codes, unless otherwise instructed by the classification.

    c. Combination codes that include symptoms
    ICD-10-CM contains a number of combination codes that identify both the definitive diagnosis and common symptoms of that diagnosis. When using one of these combination codes, an additional code should not be assigned for the symptom.

    d. Repeated falls
    Code R29.6, Repeated falls, is for use for encounters when a patient has recently fallen and the reason for the fall is being investigated.

    Code Z91.81, History of falling, is for use when a patient has fallen in the past and is at risk for future falls. When appropriate, both codes R29.6 and Z91.81 may be assigned together.

    e. Coma scale
    The coma scale codes (R40.2-) can be used in conjunction with traumatic brain injury codes, acute cerebrovascular disease or sequelae of cerebrovascular disease codes. These codes are primarily for use by trauma registries, but they may be used in any setting where this information is collected. The coma scale may also be used to assess the status of the central nervous system for other non-trauma conditions, such as monitoring patients in the intensive care unit regardless of medical condition. The coma scale codes should be sequenced after the diagnosis code(s).

    These codes, one from each subcategory, are needed to complete the scale. The 7th character indicates when the scale was recorded. The 7th character should match for all three codes.

At a minimum, report the initial score documented on presentation at your facility. This may be a score from the emergency medicine technician (EMT) or in the emergency department. If desired, a facility may choose to capture multiple coma scale scores.

Assign code R40.24, Glasgow coma scale, total score, when only the total score is documented in the medical record and not the individual score(s).

Do not report codes for individual or total Glasgow coma scale scores for a patient with a medically induced coma or a sedated patient.

See Section I.B.14 for coma scale documentation by clinicians other than patient's provider.

f. Functional quadriplegia
GUIDELINE HAS BEEN DELETED EFFECTIVE OCTOBER 1, 2017

g. SIRS due to Non-Infectious Process
The systemic inflammatory response syndrome (SIRS) can develop as a result of certain non-infectious disease processes, such as trauma, malignant neoplasm, or pancreatitis. When SIRS is documented with a noninfectious condition, and no subsequent infection is documented, the code for the underlying condition, such as an injury, should be assigned, followed by code R65.10, Systemic inflammatory response syndrome (SIRS) of non-infectious origin without acute organ dysfunction, or code R65.11, Systemic inflammatory response syndrome (SIRS) of non-infectious origin with acute organ dysfunction. If an associated acute organ dysfunction is documented, the appropriate code(s) for the specific type of organ dysfunction(s) should be assigned in addition to code R65.11. If acute organ dysfunction is documented, but it cannot be determined if the acute organ dysfunction is associated with SIRS or due to another condition (e.g., directly due to the trauma), the provider should be queried.

h. Death NOS
Code R99, Ill-defined and unknown cause of mortality, is only for use in the very limited circumstance when a patient who has already died is brought into an emergency department or other healthcare facility and is pronounced dead upon arrival. It does not represent the discharge disposition of death.

i. NIHSS Stroke Scale
The NIH stroke scale (NIHSS) codes (R29.7- -) can be used in conjunction with acute stroke codes (I63) to identify the patient's neurological status and the severity of the stroke. The stroke scale codes should be sequenced after the acute stroke diagnosis code(s).

At a minimum, report the initial score documented. If desired, a facility may choose to capture multiple stroke scale scores.

See Section I.B.14 for NIHSS stroke scale documentation by clinicians other than patient's provider.

OGCR Section I.B.4.

Signs and symptoms
Codes that describe symptoms and signs, as opposed to diagnoses, are acceptable for reporting purposes when a related definitive diagnosis has not been established (confirmed) by the provider. Chapter 18 of ICD-10-CM, Symptoms, Signs, and Abnormal Clinical and Laboratory Findings, Not Elsewhere Classified (codes R00.0-R99) contains many, but not all codes for symptoms.

CHAPTER 18

SYMPTOMS, SIGNS, AND ABNORMAL CLINICAL AND LABORATORY FINDINGS, NOT ELSEWHERE CLASSIFIED (R00-R99)

Note: This chapter includes symptoms, signs, abnormal results of clinical or other investigative procedures, and ill-defined conditions regarding which no diagnosis classifiable elsewhere is recorded.

Signs and symptoms that point rather definitely to a given diagnosis have been assigned to a category in other chapters of the classification. In general, categories in this chapter include the less well-defined conditions and symptoms that, without the necessary study of the case to establish a final diagnosis, point perhaps equally to two or more diseases or to two or more systems of the body. Practically all categories in the chapter could be designated "not otherwise specified", "unknown etiology" or "transient". The Alphabetical Index should be consulted to determine which symptoms and signs are to be allocated here and which to other chapters. The residual subcategories, numbered .8, are generally provided for other relevant symptoms that cannot be allocated elsewhere in the classification.

The conditions and signs or symptoms included in categories R00-R94 consist of:
(a) cases for which no more specific diagnosis can be made even after all the facts bearing on the case have been investigated;
(b) signs or symptoms existing at the time of initial encounter that proved to be transient and whose causes could not be determined;
(c) provisional diagnosis in a patient who failed to return for further investigation or care;
(d) cases referred elsewhere for investigation or treatment before the diagnosis was made;
(e) cases in which a more precise diagnosis was not available for any other reason;
(f) certain symptoms, for which supplementary information is provided, that represent important problems in medical care in their own right.

Excludes2 abnormal findings on antenatal screening of mother (O28.-)
certain conditions originating in the perinatal period (P04-P96)
signs and symptoms classified in the body system chapters
signs and symptoms of breast (N63, N64.5)

This chapter contains the following blocks:

R00-R09	Symptoms and signs involving the circulatory and respiratory systems
R10-R19	Symptoms and signs involving the digestive system and abdomen
R20-R23	Symptoms and signs involving the skin and subcutaneous tissue
R25-R29	Symptoms and signs involving the nervous and musculoskeletal systems
R30-R39	Symptoms and signs involving the genitourinary system
R40-R46	Symptoms and signs involving cognition, perception, emotional state and behavior
R47-R49	Symptoms and signs involving speech and voice
R50-R69	General symptoms and signs
R70-R79	Abnormal findings on examination of blood, without diagnosis
R80-R82	Abnormal findings on examination of urine, without diagnosis
R83-R89	Abnormal findings on examination of other body fluids, substances and tissues, without diagnosis
R90-R94	Abnormal findings on diagnostic imaging and in function studies, without diagnosis
R97	Abnormal tumor markers
R99	Ill-defined and unknown cause of mortality

SYMPTOMS AND SIGNS INVOLVING THE CIRCULATORY AND RESPIRATORY SYSTEMS (R00-R09)

● **R00**   **Abnormalities of heart beat**

    Excludes1   abnormalities originating in the perinatal period (P29.1-)

    Excludes2   specified arrhythmias (I47-I49)

   R00.0   **Tachycardia, unspecified**
      Rapid heart rate >100 beats
      Rapid heart beat
      Sinoauricular tachycardia NOS
      Sinus [sinusal] tachycardia NOS

      Excludes1   neonatal tachycardia (P29.11)
                paroxysmal tachycardia (I47.-)

   R00.1   **Bradycardia, unspecified**
      Slow heart rate, <60
      Sinoatrial bradycardia
      Sinus bradycardia
      Slow heart beat
      Vagal bradycardia

      Use additional code for adverse effect, if applicable, to identify drug (T36-T50 with fifth or sixth character 5)

      Excludes1   neonatal bradycardia (P29.12)

   R00.2   **Palpitations**
      Awareness of heart beat

   R00.8   **Other abnormalities of heart beat**

   R00.9   **Unspecified abnormalities of heart beat**

CHAPTER 18 (R00-R99)

● **R01**   **Cardiac murmurs and other cardiac sounds**

     Excludes1   cardiac murmurs and sounds originating in the perinatal period (P29.8)

     R01.0   **Benign and innocent cardiac murmurs**
         Functional cardiac murmur

     R01.1   **Cardiac murmur, unspecified**
         Cardiac bruit NOS
         Heart murmur NOS
         Systolic murmur NOS

     R01.2   **Other cardiac sounds**
         Cardiac dullness, increased or decreased
         Precordial friction

     OGCR   Section I.C.9.a.7.

     Hypertension, Transient

     Assign code R03.0, Elevated blood pressure reading without diagnosis of hypertension, unless patient has an established diagnosis of hypertension. Assign code O13.-, Gestational [pregnancy-induced] hypertension with significant proteinuria, or O14.-, Pre-eclampsia, for transient hypertension of pregnancy.

● **R03**   **Abnormal blood-pressure reading, without diagnosis**

     R03.0   **Elevated blood-pressure reading, without diagnosis of hypertension**

         Note: This category is to be used to record an episode of elevated blood pressure in a patient in whom no formal diagnosis of hypertension has been made, or as an isolated incidental finding.

     R03.1   **Nonspecific low blood-pressure reading**
         Excludes1   hypotension (I95.-)
                  maternal hypotension syndrome (O26.5-)
                  neurogenic orthostatic hypotension (G90.3)

● **R04**   **Hemorrhage from respiratory passages**

     R04.0   **Epistaxis**
         Hemorrhage from nose
         Nosebleed
         Coding Clinic: 2018, Q4, P38

     R04.1   **Hemorrhage from throat**
         Excludes2   hemoptysis (R04.2)

     R04.2   **Hemoptysis**
         Blood-stained sputum
         Cough with hemorrhage

●   **R04.8**   **Hemorrhage from other sites in respiratory passages**

         R04.81   **Acute idiopathic pulmonary hemorrhage in infants**   P
                  AIPHI
                  Acute idiopathic hemorrhage in infants over 28 days old
                  Excludes1   perinatal pulmonary hemorrhage (P26.-)
                           ⇒von Willebrand's disease (D68.0-)

         R04.89   **Hemorrhage from other sites in respiratory passages**
                  Pulmonary hemorrhage NOS

     R04.9   **Hemorrhage from respiratory passages, unspecified**

● **R05**   **Cough**

     Excludes1   paroxysmal cough due to Bordetella pertussis (A37.0-)
                  smoker's cough (J41.0)

     Excludes2   cough with hemorrhage (R04.2))

     R05.1   **Acute cough**

     R05.2   **Subacute cough**

     R05.3   **Chronic cough**
         Persistent cough
         Refractory cough
         Unexplained cough

     R05.4   **Cough syncope**
         Code first syncope and collapse (R55)

     R05.8   **Other specified cough**

     R05.9   **Cough, unspecified**

● **R06**   **Abnormalities of breathing**

     Excludes1   acute respiratory distress syndrome (J80)
                  respiratory arrest (R09.2)
                  respiratory arrest of newborn (P28.81)
                  respiratory distress syndrome of newborn (P22.-)
                  respiratory failure (J96.-)
                  respiratory failure of newborn (P28.5)

●   **R06.0**   **Dyspnea**

         Excludes1   tachypnea NOS (R06.82)
                      transient tachypnea of newborn (P22.1)

         R06.00   **Dyspnea, unspecified**
                  Coding Clinic: 2017, Q1, P26-27

         R06.01   **Orthopnea**

         R06.02   **Shortness of breath**

         R06.03   **Acute respiratory distress**

         R06.09   **Other forms of dyspnea**

     R06.1   **Stridor**
         Harsh, high-pitched breath sound
         Excludes1   congenital laryngeal stridor (P28.89)
                      laryngismus (stridulus) (J38.5)

     R06.2   **Wheezing**
         Excludes1   Asthma (J45.-)
         Coding Clinic: 2016, Q2, P34

     R06.3   **Periodic breathing**
         Cheyne-Stokes breathing
         An abnormal pattern of breathing with gradually increasing and decreasing tidal volume with some periods of apnea

     R06.4   **Hyperventilation**
         Excludes1   psychogenic hyperventilation (F45.8)

     R06.5   **Mouth breathing**
         Excludes2   dry mouth NOS (R68.2)

     R06.6   **Hiccough**
         Excludes1   psychogenic hiccough (F45.8)

     R06.7   **Sneezing**

●   **R06.8**   **Other abnormalities of breathing**

         R06.81   **Apnea, not elsewhere classified**
                  Apnea NOS
              ⇒ **Excludes1**   apnea (of) newborn (P28.4-)
                           sleep apnea (G47.3-)
                           ⇒sleep apnea of newborn (primary) (P28.3-)

         R06.82   **Tachypnea, not elsewhere classified**
                  Tachypnea NOS
                  Excludes1   transitory tachypnea of newborn (P22.1)

         R06.83   **Snoring**

         R06.89   **Other abnormalities of breathing**
                  Breath-holding (spells)
                  Sighing

     R06.9   **Unspecified abnormalities of breathing**

● **R07**   **Pain in throat and chest**

     Excludes1   epidemic myalgia (B33.0)
     Excludes2   jaw pain R68.84
                  pain in breast (N64.4)

     R07.0   **Pain in throat**
         Excludes1   chronic sore throat (J31.2)
                      sore throat (acute) NOS (J02.9)
         Excludes2   dysphagia (R13.1-)
                      pain in neck (M54.2)

     R07.1   **Chest pain on breathing**
         Painful respiration

     R07.2   **Precordial pain**

▶ New   ⇒ Revised   ~~deleted~~ Deleted   Excludes 1   Excludes 2   Includes   Use additional   Code first   Code also   Key words

OGCR Official Guidelines   X Assign placeholder X   ● Use Additional Character(s)   ▌ Manifestation Code   🖢 Hierarchical Condition Category   **Coding Clinic**

● **R07.8** **Other chest pain**

    R07.81 **Pleurodynia**

        Pleurodynia NOS

        Excludes1 epidemic pleurodynia (B33.0)

    R07.82 **Intercostal pain**

    R07.89 **Other chest pain**

        Anterior chest-wall pain NOS

        Coding Clinic: 2021, Q1, P42

  R07.9 **Chest pain, unspecified**

● **R09** **Other symptoms and signs involving the circulatory and respiratory system**

    Excludes1 acute respiratory distress syndrome (J80)

        respiratory arrest of newborn (P28.81)

        respiratory distress syndrome of newborn (P22.0)

        respiratory failure (J96.-)

        respiratory failure of newborn (P28.5)

● **R09.0** **Asphyxia and hypoxemia**

    Excludes1 asphyxia due to carbon monoxide (T58.-)

        asphyxia due to foreign body in respiratory tract (T17.-)

        birth (intrauterine) asphyxia (P84)

        hyperventilation (R06.4)

        traumatic asphyxia (T71.-)

    Excludes2 hypercapnia (R06.89)

    R09.01 **Asphyxia**

    R09.02 **Hypoxemia**

        Coding Clinic: 2019, Q3, P15

  R09.1 **Pleurisy**

    Occurs when double membrane (pleura) lining chest cavity and lung surface becomes inflamed, causing sharp pain on inspiration/expiration

    Excludes1 pleurisy with effusion (J90)

  R09.2 **Respiratory arrest** 🔗

    Cardiorespiratory failure

    Excludes1 cardiac arrest (I46.-)

        respiratory arrest of newborn (P28.81)

        respiratory distress of newborn (P22.0)

        respiratory failure (J96.-)

        respiratory failure of newborn (P28.5)

        respiratory insufficiency (R06.89)

        respiratory insufficiency of newborn (P28.5)

  R09.3 **Abnormal sputum**

    Abnormal amount of sputum

    Abnormal color of sputum

    Abnormal odor of sputum

    Excessive sputum

    Excludes1 blood-stained sputum (R04.2)

● **R09.8** **Other specified symptoms and signs involving the circulatory and respiratory systems**

    R09.81 **Nasal congestion**

    R09.82 **Postnasal drip**

    R09.89 **Other specified symptoms and signs involving the circulatory and respiratory systems**

        Bruit (arterial)

        Abnormal chest percussion

        Feeling of foreign body in throat

        Friction sounds in chest

        Chest tympany

        Choking sensation

        Rales

        Wet rattling, clicking, crackling sounds on auscultation

        Weak pulse

        Excludes2 foreign body in throat (T17.2-)

            wheezing (R06.2)

        Coding Clinic: 2021, Q1, P42

SYMPTOMS AND SIGNS INVOLVING THE DIGESTIVE SYSTEM AND ABDOMEN (R10-R19)

  Excludes2 congenital or infantile pylorospasm (Q40.0)

    gastrointestinal hemorrhage (K92.0-K92.2)

    intestinal obstruction (K56.-)

    newborn gastrointestinal hemorrhage (P54.0-P54.3)

    newborn intestinal obstruction (P76.-)

    pylorospasm (K31.3)

    signs and symptoms involving the urinary system (R30-R39)

    symptoms referable to female genital organs (N94.-)

    symptoms referable to male genital organs (N48-N50)

● **R10** **Abdominal and pelvic pain**

    Excludes1 renal colic (N23)

    Excludes2 dorsalgia (M54.-)

        flatulence and related conditions (R14.-)

  R10.0 **Acute abdomen**

    Severe abdominal pain (generalized) (with abdominal rigidity)

    Excludes1 abdominal rigidity NOS (R19.3)

        generalized abdominal pain NOS (R10.84)

        localized abdominal pain (R10.1-R10.3-)

● **R10.1** **Pain localized to upper abdomen**

    R10.10 **Upper abdominal pain, unspecified**

    R10.11 **Right upper quadrant pain**

    R10.12 **Left upper quadrant pain**

    R10.13 **Epigastric pain**

        Dyspepsia

        Excludes1 functional dyspepsia (K30)

  R10.2 **Pelvic and perineal pain**

    Excludes1 vulvodynia (N94.81)

● **R10.3** **Pain localized to other parts of lower abdomen**

    R10.30 **Lower abdominal pain, unspecified**

    R10.31 **Right lower quadrant pain**

    R10.32 **Left lower quadrant pain**

    R10.33 **Periumbilical pain**

● **R10.8** **Other abdominal pain**

  ● **R10.81** **Abdominal tenderness**

    Abdominal tenderness NOS

    R10.811 **Right upper quadrant abdominal tenderness**

    R10.812 **Left upper quadrant abdominal tenderness**

    R10.813 **Right lower quadrant abdominal tenderness**

    R10.814 **Left lower quadrant abdominal tenderness**

    R10.815 **Periumbilic abdominal tenderness**

    R10.816 **Epigastric abdominal tenderness**

    R10.817 **Generalized abdominal tenderness**

    R10.819 **Abdominal tenderness, unspecified site**

  ● **R10.82** **Rebound abdominal tenderness**

    R10.821 **Right upper quadrant rebound abdominal tenderness**

    R10.822 **Left upper quadrant rebound abdominal tenderness**

    R10.823 **Right lower quadrant rebound abdominal tenderness**

    R10.824 **Left lower quadrant rebound abdominal tenderness**

    R10.825 **Periumbilic rebound abdominal tenderness**

    R10.826 **Epigastric rebound abdominal tenderness**

CHAPTER 18 (R00-R99)

R10.827 Generalized rebound abdominal tenderness

R10.829 Rebound abdominal tenderness, unspecified site

R10.83 Colic　　　　　　　　　　　P
Colic NOS
Infantile colic

　　Excludes1　colic in adult and child over 12 months old (R10.84)

R10.84 Generalized abdominal pain

　　Excludes1　generalized abdominal pain associated with acute abdomen (R10.0)

R10.9 Unspecified abdominal pain

● **R11 Nausea and vomiting**

Excludes1　cyclical vomiting associated with migraine (G43.A-)
excessive vomiting in pregnancy (O21.-)
hematemesis (K92.0)
neonatal hematemesis (P54.0)
newborn vomiting (P92.0-)
psychogenic vomiting (F50.89)
vomiting associated with bulimia nervosa (F50.2)
vomiting following gastrointestinal surgery (K91.0)

Coding Clinic: 2017, Q1, P27

● **R11.0 Nausea**
Nausea NOS
Nausea without vomiting

● **R11.1 Vomiting**

R11.10 Vomiting, unspecified
Vomiting NOS

R11.11 Vomiting without nausea

R11.12 Projectile vomiting

R11.13 Vomiting of fecal matter

R11.14 Bilious vomiting
Bilious emesis

R11.15 Cyclical vomiting syndrome unrelated to migraine
Cyclic vomiting syndrome NOS
Persistent vomiting

　　Excludes1　cyclical vomiting in migraine (G43.A-)

　　Excludes2　bulimia nervosa (F50.2)
diabetes mellitus due to underlying condition (E08.-)

R11.2 Nausea with vomiting, unspecified
Persistent nausea with vomiting NOS
Coding Clinic: 2020, Q1, P8

R12 Heartburn

Excludes1　dyspepsia NOS (R10.13)
functional dyspepsia (K30)

● **R13 Aphagia and dysphagia**

R13.0 Aphagia
Inability to swallow

　　Excludes1　psychogenic aphagia (F50.9)

● **R13.1 Dysphagia**
Difficulty swallowing

Code first, if applicable, dysphagia following cerebrovascular disease (I69. with final characters -91)

Excludes1　psychogenic dysphagia (F45.8)

R13.10 Dysphagia, unspecified
Difficulty in swallowing NOS

R13.11 Dysphagia, oral phase

R13.12 Dysphagia, oropharyngeal phase

R13.13 Dysphagia, pharyngeal phase

R13.14 Dysphagia, pharyngoesophageal phase

R13.19 Other dysphagia
Cervical dysphagia
Neurogenic dysphagia

● **R14 Flatulence and related conditions**

Excludes1　psychogenic aerophagy (F45.8)

R14.0 Abdominal distension (gaseous)
Bloating
Tympanites (abdominal) (intestinal)

R14.1 Gas pain

R14.2 Eructation
Belching air from stomach through mouth

R14.3 Flatulence

● **R15 Fecal incontinence**

Includes　encopresis NOS

Excludes1　fecal incontinence of nonorganic origin (F98.1)

R15.0 Incomplete defecation

　　Excludes1　constipation (K59.0-)
fecal impaction (K56.41)

R15.1 Fecal smearing
Fecal soiling

R15.2 Fecal urgency

R15.9 Full incontinence of feces
Fecal incontinence NOS

● **R16 Hepatomegaly and splenomegaly, not elsewhere classified**
Enlargement of liver or spleen

R16.0 Hepatomegaly, not elsewhere classified
Hepatomegaly NOS

R16.1 Splenomegaly, not elsewhere classified
Splenomegaly NOS

R16.2 Hepatomegaly with splenomegaly, not elsewhere classified
Hepatosplenomegaly NOS

R17 Unspecified jaundice

Excludes1　neonatal jaundice (P55, P57-P59)

● **R18 Ascites**

Includes　fluid in peritoneal cavity

Excludes1　ascites in alcoholic cirrhosis (K70.31)
ascites in alcoholic hepatitis (K70.11)
ascites in toxic liver disease with chronic active hepatitis (K71.51)

R18.0 Malignant ascites
Code first malignancy, such as:
malignant neoplasm of ovary (C56.-)
secondary malignant neoplasm of retroperitoneum and peritoneum (C78.6)

R18.8 Other ascites
Ascites NOS
Peritoneal effusion (chronic)
Coding Clinic: 2018, Q1, P4

● **R19 Other symptoms and signs involving the digestive system and abdomen**

Excludes1　acute abdomen (R10.0)

● **R19.0 Intra-abdominal and pelvic swelling, mass and lump**

Excludes1　abdominal distension (gaseous) (R14.-)
ascites (R18.-)

R19.00 Intra-abdominal and pelvic swelling, mass and lump, unspecified site

R19.01 Right upper quadrant abdominal swelling, mass and lump

R19.02 Left upper quadrant abdominal swelling, mass and lump

R19.03 Right lower quadrant abdominal swelling, mass and lump

R19.04 Left lower quadrant abdominal swelling, mass and lump

R19.05 Periumbilic swelling, mass or lump
Diffuse or generalized umbilical swelling or mass

▶ New　⇒ Revised　~~deleted~~ Deleted　Excludes 1　Excludes 2　Includes　Use additional　Code first　Code also　Key words

OGCR Official Guidelines　X Assign placeholder X　● Use Additional Character(s)　▶ Manifestation Code　🐄 Hierarchical Condition Category　Coding Clinic

R19.06   **Epigastric swelling, mass or lump**

R19.07   **Generalized intra-abdominal and pelvic swelling, mass and lump**
     Diffuse or generalized intra-abdominal swelling or mass NOS
     Diffuse or generalized pelvic swelling or mass NOS

R19.09   **Other intra-abdominal and pelvic swelling, mass and lump**

● R19.1   **Abnormal bowel sounds**

R19.11   **Absent bowel sounds**

R19.12   **Hyperactive bowel sounds**

R19.15   **Other abnormal bowel sounds**
     Abnormal bowel sounds NOS

R19.2   **Visible peristalsis**
     Hyperperistalsis

● R19.3   **Abdominal rigidity**
     Excludes1   abdominal rigidity with severe abdominal pain (R10.0)

R19.30   **Abdominal rigidity, unspecified site**

R19.31   **Right upper quadrant abdominal rigidity**

R19.32   **Left upper quadrant abdominal rigidity**

R19.33   **Right lower quadrant abdominal rigidity**

R19.34   **Left lower quadrant abdominal rigidity**

R19.35   **Periumbilic abdominal rigidity**

R19.36   **Epigastric abdominal rigidity**

R19.37   **Generalized abdominal rigidity**

R19.4   **Change in bowel habit**
     Excludes1   constipation (K59.0-)
         functional diarrhea (K59.1)

R19.5   **Other fecal abnormalities**
     Abnormal stool color
     Bulky stools
     Mucus in stools
     Occult blood in feces
     Occult blood in stools
     Excludes1   melena (K92.1)
         neonatal melena (P54.1)
     Coding Clinic: 2021, Q1, P10; 2019, Q1, P32

R19.6   **Halitosis**

R19.7   **Diarrhea, unspecified**
     Diarrhea NOS
     Excludes1   functional diarrhea (K59.1)
         neonatal diarrhea (P78.3)
         psychogenic diarrhea (F45.8)
     Coding Clinic: 2021, Q3, P4

R19.8   **Other specified symptoms and signs involving the digestive system and abdomen**

SYMPTOMS AND SIGNS INVOLVING THE SKIN AND SUBCUTANEOUS TISSUE (R20-R23)

     Excludes2   symptoms relating to breast (N64.4-N64.5)

● R20   **Disturbances of skin sensation**
     Excludes1   dissociative anesthesia and sensory loss (F44.6)
         psychogenic disturbances (F45.8)

R20.0   **Anesthesia of skin**
     Loss of sensation

R20.1   **Hypoesthesia of skin**
     Unpleasant abnormal sensation

R20.2   **Paresthesia of skin**
     Abnormal touch sensation, including burning, prickling, often in absence of external stimulus
     Formication   Tingling skin
     Pins and needles
     Excludes1   acroparesthesia (I73.8)

R20.3   **Hyperesthesia**

R20.8   **Other disturbances of skin sensation**

R20.9   **Unspecified disturbances of skin sensation**

R21   **Rash and other nonspecific skin eruption**
     Includes   rash NOS
     Excludes1   specified type of rash- code to condition
         vesicular eruption (R23.8)

● R22   **Localized swelling, mass and lump of skin and subcutaneous tissue**
     Includes   subcutaneous nodules (localized) (superficial)
     Excludes1   abnormal findings on diagnostic imaging (R90-R93)
         edema (R60.-)
         enlarged lymph nodes (R59.-)
         localized adiposity (E65)
         swelling of joint (M25.4-)

R22.0   **Localized swelling, mass and lump, head**

R22.1   **Localized swelling, mass and lump, neck**

R22.2   **Localized swelling, mass and lump, trunk**
     Excludes1   intra-abdominal or pelvic mass and lump (R19.0-)
         intra-abdominal or pelvic swelling (R19.0-)
     Excludes2   breast mass and lump (N63)

● R22.3   **Localized swelling, mass and lump, upper limb**

R22.30   **Localized swelling, mass and lump, unspecified upper limb**

R22.31   **Localized swelling, mass and lump, right upper limb**

R22.32   **Localized swelling, mass and lump, left upper limb**

R22.33   **Localized swelling, mass and lump, upper limb, bilateral**

● R22.4   **Localized swelling, mass and lump, lower limb**

R22.40   **Localized swelling, mass and lump, unspecified lower limb**

R22.41   **Localized swelling, mass and lump, right lower limb**

R22.42   **Localized swelling, mass and lump, left lower limb**

R22.43   **Localized swelling, mass and lump, lower limb, bilateral**

R22.9   **Localized swelling, mass and lump, unspecified**

● R23   **Other skin changes**

R23.0   **Cyanosis**
     Excludes1   acrocyanosis (I73.8)
         cyanotic attacks of newborn (P28.2)

R23.1   **Pallor**
     Clammy skin

R23.2   **Flushing**
     Excessive blushing
     Code first, if applicable, menopausal and female climacteric states (N95.1)

R23.3   **Spontaneous ecchymoses**
     Small hemorrhagic spot of skin; AKA black and blue spot
     Petechiae
     Excludes1   ecchymoses of newborn (P54.5)
         purpura (D69.-)

R23.4   **Changes in skin texture**
     Desquamation of skin   Scaling of skin
     Induration of skin
     Excludes1   epidermal thickening NOS (L85.9)

R23.8   **Other skin changes**

R23.9   **Unspecified skin changes**

CHAPTER 18 (R00-R99)

SYMPTOMS AND SIGNS INVOLVING THE NERVOUS AND MUSCULOSKELETAL SYSTEMS (R25-R29)

● **R25** **Abnormal involuntary movements**
    Excludes1 specific movement disorders (G20-G26)
               stereotyped movement disorders (F98.4)
               tic disorders (F95.-)

  R25.0 **Abnormal head movements**

  R25.1 **Tremor, unspecified**
      Excludes1 chorea NOS (G25.5)
                essential tremor (G25.0)
                hysterical tremor (F44.4)
                intention tremor (G25.2)

  R25.2 **Cramp and spasm**
      Excludes2 carpopedal spasm (R29.0)
                charley-horse (M62.831)
                infantile spasms (G40.4-)
                muscle spasm of back (M62.830)
                muscle spasm of calf (M62.831)

  R25.3 **Fasciculation**
      Twitching NOS

  R25.8 **Other abnormal involuntary movements**

  R25.9 **Unspecified abnormal involuntary movements**

● **R26** **Abnormalities of gait and mobility**
    Excludes1 ataxia NOS (R27.0)
               hereditary ataxia (G11.-)
               locomotor (syphilitic) ataxia (A52.11)
               immobility syndrome (paraplegic) (M62.3)

  R26.0 **Ataxic gait**
      Staggering gait
      Coding Clinic: 2022, Q2, P12

  R26.1 **Paralytic gait**
      Spastic gait

  R26.2 **Difficulty in walking, not elsewhere classified**
      Excludes1 falling (R29.6)
                unsteadiness on feet (R26.81)
      Coding Clinic: 2016, Q2, P7

● **R26.8** **Other abnormalities of gait and mobility**
      R26.81   **Unsteadiness on feet**
      R26.89   **Other abnormalities of gait and mobility**

  R26.9 **Unspecified abnormalities of gait and mobility**

● **R27** **Other lack of coordination**
    Excludes1 ataxic gait (R26.0)
               hereditary ataxia (G11.-)
               vertigo NOS (R42)

  R27.0 **Ataxia, unspecified**
      Excludes1 ataxia following cerebrovascular disease
                     (I69. with final characters -93)

  R27.8 **Other lack of coordination**

  R27.9 **Unspecified lack of coordination**

● **R29** **Other symptoms and signs involving the nervous and musculoskeletal systems**

  R29.0 **Tetany**
      Hyperexcitability of nerves and muscles characterized by spasm, twitching, and cramps
      Carpopedal spasm
      Excludes1 hysterical tetany (F44.5)
                neonatal tetany (P71.3)
                parathyroid tetany (E20.9)
                post-thyroidectomy tetany (E89.2)

  R29.1 **Meningismus**

  R29.2 **Abnormal reflex**
      Excludes2 abnormal pupillary reflex (H57.0)
                hyperactive gag reflex (J39.2)
                vasovagal reaction or syncope (R55)

  R29.3 **Abnormal posture**

  R29.4 **Clicking hip**
      Excludes1 congenital deformities of hip (Q65.-)

  R29.5 **Transient paralysis**
      Code first any associated spinal cord injury (S14.0, S14.1-, S24.0, S24.1-, S34.0-, S34.1-)
      Excludes1 transient ischemic attack (G45.9)

  R29.6 **Repeated falls**
      Falling
      Tendency to fall
      Excludes2 at risk for falling (Z91.81)
                history of falling (Z91.81)

  OGCR Section I.C.18.d.

> Repeated falls
>
> Code R29.6, Repeated falls, is for use for encounters when a patient has recently fallen and the reason for the fall is being investigated.
>
> Code Z91.81, History of falling, is for use when a patient has fallen in the past and is at risk for future falls. When appropriate, both codes R29.6 and Z91.81 may be assigned together.

  Coding Clinic: 2016, Q2, P7

● **R29.7** **National Institutes of Health Stroke Scale (NIHSS) score**
      Code first the type of cerebral infarction (I63.-)
      Coding Clinic: 2016, Q4, P61, 127

● **R29.70** **NIHSS score 0-9**
      R29.700 **NIHSS score 0**
      R29.701 **NIHSS score 1**
      R29.702 **NIHSS score 2**
      R29.703 **NIHSS score 3**
      R29.704 **NIHSS score 4**
      R29.705 **NIHSS score 5**
      R29.706 **NIHSS score 6**
      R29.707 **NIHSS score 7**
      R29.708 **NIHSS score 8**
      R29.709 **NIHSS score 9**

● **R29.71** **NIHSS score 10-19**
      R29.710 **NIHSS score 10**
      R29.711 **NIHSS score 11**
      R29.712 **NIHSS score 12**
      R29.713 **NIHSS score 13**
      R29.714 **NIHSS score 14**
      R29.715 **NIHSS score 15**
      R29.716 **NIHSS score 16**
      R29.717 **NIHSS score 17**
      R29.718 **NIHSS score 18**
      R29.719 **NIHSS score 19**

● **R29.72** **NIHSS score 20-29**
      R29.720 **NIHSS score 20**
      R29.721 **NIHSS score 21**
      R29.722 **NIHSS score 22**
      R29.723 **NIHSS score 23**
      R29.724 **NIHSS score 24**
      R29.725 **NIHSS score 25**
      R29.726 **NIHSS score 26**
      R29.727 **NIHSS score 27**
      R29.728 **NIHSS score 28**
      R29.729 **NIHSS score 29**

  OGCR Section I.C.18.i.

> NIHSS Stroke Scale
>
> The NIH stroke scale (NIHSS) codes (R29.7- -) can be used in conjunction with acute stroke codes (I63) to identify the patient's neurological status and the severity of the stroke. The stroke scale codes should be sequenced after the acute stroke diagnosis code(s).
>
> At a minimum, report the initial score documented. If desired, a facility may choose to capture multiple stroke scale scores.

▶ New   ⇒ Revised   ~~deleted~~ Deleted   Excludes 1   Excludes 2   Includes   Use additional   Code first   Code also   Key words
OGCR Official Guidelines   X Assign placeholder X   ● Use Additional Character(s)   ▌ Manifestation Code   🔖 Hierarchical Condition Category   Coding Clinic

● **R29.73**   NIHSS score 30-39
     R29.730   NIHSS score 30
          Coding Clinic: 2016, Q4, P62
     R29.731   NIHSS score 31
     R29.732   NIHSS score 32
     R29.733   NIHSS score 33
     R29.734   NIHSS score 34
     R29.735   NIHSS score 35
     R29.736   NIHSS score 36
     R29.737   NIHSS score 37
     R29.738   NIHSS score 38
     R29.739   NIHSS score 39
● **R29.74**   NIHSS score 40-42
     R29.740   NIHSS score 40
     R29.741   NIHSS score 41
     R29.742   NIHSS score 42

● **R29.8**   Other symptoms and signs involving the nervous and musculoskeletal systems
  ● **R29.81**   Other symptoms and signs involving the nervous system
     R29.810   Facial weakness
         Facial droop
         Excludes1   Bell's palsy (G51.0)
                   facial weakness following cerebrovascular disease (I69. with final characters -92)
     R29.818   Other symptoms and signs involving the nervous system
  ● **R29.89**   Other symptoms and signs involving the musculoskeletal system
         Excludes2   pain in limb (M79.6-)
     R29.890   Loss of height
         Excludes1   osteoporosis (M80-M81)
     R29.891   Ocular torticollis
         Excludes1   congenital (sterno-mastoid) torticollis Q68.0
                   psychogenic torticollis (F45.8)
                   spasmodic torticollis (G24.3)
                   torticollis due to birth injury (P15.8)
                   torticollis NOS M43.6
     R29.898   Other symptoms and signs involving the musculoskeletal system

● **R29.9**   Unspecified symptoms and signs involving the nervous and musculoskeletal systems
     R29.90   Unspecified symptoms and signs involving the nervous system
     R29.91   Unspecified symptoms and signs involving the musculoskeletal system

SYMPTOMS AND SIGNS INVOLVING THE GENITOURINARY SYSTEM (R30-R39)

● **R30**   Pain associated with micturition
     Excludes1   psychogenic pain associated with micturition (F45.8)
   R30.0   Dysuria
      Painful urination
      Strangury
   R30.1   Vesical tenesmus
      Straining to urinate, with sensation of a full bladder even when empty
   R30.9   Painful micturition, unspecified
      Painful urination NOS

● **R31**   Hematuria
     Excludes1   hematuria included with underlying conditions, such as:
                   acute cystitis with hematuria (N30.01)
                   recurrent and persistent hematuria in glomerular diseases (N02.-)
   R31.0   Gross hematuria
      Coding Clinic: 2017, Q1, P17
   R31.1   Benign essential microscopic hematuria
 ● **R31.2**   Other microscopic hematuria
      Coding Clinic: 2016, Q4, P62
     R31.21   Asymptomatic microscopic hematuria
         AMH
     R31.29   Other microscopic hematuria
   R31.9   Hematuria, unspecified
      Coding Clinic: 2017, Q1, P6

● **R32**   Unspecified urinary incontinence
     Enuresis NOS
     Excludes1   functional urinary incontinence (R39.81)
              nonorganic enuresis (F98.0)
              stress incontinence and other specified urinary incontinence (N39.3-N39.4-)
              urinary incontinence associated with cognitive impairment (R39.81)
     Coding Clinic: 2021, Q4, P18

● **R33**   Retention of urine
     Excludes1   psychogenic retention of urine (F45.8)
   R33.0   Drug induced retention of urine
      Use additional code for adverse effect, if applicable, to identify drug (T36-T50 with fifth or sixth character 5)
   R33.8   Other retention of urine
      Code first, if applicable, any causal condition, such as:
      enlarged prostate (N40.1)
      Coding Clinic: 2018, Q4, P55
   R33.9   Retention of urine, unspecified

● **R34**   Anuria and oliguria
     Excludes1   anuria and oliguria complicating abortion or ectopic or molar pregnancy (O00-O07, O08.4)
              anuria and oliguria complicating pregnancy (O26.83-)
              anuria and oliguria complicating the puerperium (O90.4)

● **R35**   Polyuria
     Passage of excessive volume of urine
     Code first, if applicable, any causal condition, such as:
     enlarged prostate (N40.1)
     Excludes1   psychogenic polyuria (F45.8)
   R35.0   Frequency of micturition
      Discharge or passage of urine; AKA uresis
   R35.1   Nocturia
      Urinary frequency at night
 ● **R35.8**   Other polyuria
     R35.81   Nocturnal polyuria
         Excludes2   nocturnal enuresis (N39.44)
     R35.89   Other polyuria
         Polyuria NOS

● **R36**   Urethral discharge
   R36.0   Urethral discharge without blood
   R36.1   Hematospermia ♂
      Presence of blood in semen
   R36.9   Urethral discharge, unspecified
      Penile discharge NOS
      Urethrorrhea

R37   Sexual dysfunction, unspecified

CHAPTER 18 (R00-R99)

● **R39   Other and unspecified symptoms and signs involving the genitourinary system**

    R39.0   Extravasation of urine
        Leakage, discharge

●   **R39.1   Other difficulties with micturition**
        Code first, if applicable, any causal condition, such as:
        enlarged prostate (N40.1)

        R39.11   Hesitancy of micturition

        R39.12   Poor urinary stream
            Weak urinary steam

        R39.13   Splitting of urinary stream

        R39.14   Feeling of incomplete bladder emptying

        R39.15   Urgency of urination
            Excludes1   urge incontinence (N39.41, N39.46)

        R39.16   Straining to void

●   **R39.19   Other difficulties with micturition**
            Coding Clinic: 2016, Q4, P63

            R39.191   Need to immediately re-void

            R39.192   Position dependent micturition

            R39.198   Other difficulties with micturition

    R39.2   Extrarenal uremia
        Prerenal uremia
        Excludes1   uremia NOS (N19)

●   **R39.8   Other symptoms and signs involving the genitourinary system**

        R39.81   Functional urinary incontinence
            Urinary incontinence due to cognitive impairment, or severe physical disability or immobility
            Excludes1   stress incontinence and other specified urinary incontinence (N39.3-N39.4-)
                        urinary incontinence NOS (R32)

        R39.82   Chronic bladder pain
            Coding Clinic: 2016, Q4, P64

        R39.83   Unilateral non-palpable testicle ♂

        R39.84   Bilateral non-palpable testicles ♂

        R39.89   Other symptoms and signs involving the genitourinary system
            Coding Clinic: 2016, Q4, P64

    R39.9   Unspecified symptoms and signs involving the genitourinary system

---

SYMPTOMS AND SIGNS INVOLVING COGNITION, PERCEPTION, EMOTIONAL STATE AND BEHAVIOR (R40-R46)

    Excludes2   symptoms and signs constituting part of a pattern of mental disorder (F01-F99)
    Coding Clinic: 2015, Q4, P40

● **R40   Somnolence, stupor and coma**
    Excludes1   neonatal coma (P91.5)
              somnolence, stupor and coma in diabetes (E08-E13)
              somnolence, stupor and coma in hepatic failure (K72.-)
              somnolence, stupor and coma in hypoglycemia (nondiabetic) (E15)

    R40.0   Somnolence
        Drowsiness
        Excludes1   coma (R40.2-)

    R40.1   Stupor
        Lowered level of consciousness
        Catatonic stupor
        Semicoma
        Excludes1   catatonic schizophrenia (F20.2)
                 coma (R40.2-)
                 depressive stupor (F31-F33)
                 dissociative stupor (F44.2)
                 manic stupor (F30.2)

Coma scale

The coma scale codes (R40.2-) can be used in conjunction with traumatic brain injury codes, acute cerebrovascular disease or sequelae of cerebrovascular disease codes. These codes are primarily for use by trauma registries, but they may be used in any setting where this information is collected. The coma scale may also be used to assess the status of the central nervous system for other non-trauma conditions, such as monitoring patients in the intensive care unit regardless of medical condition. The coma scale codes should be sequenced after the diagnosis code(s).

These codes, one from each subcategory, are needed to complete the scale. The 7th character indicates when the scale was recorded. The 7th character should match for all three codes.

At a minimum, report the initial score documented on presentation at your facility. This may be a score from the emergency medicine technician (EMT) or in the emergency department. If desired, a facility may choose to capture multiple coma scale scores.

Assign code R40.24, Glasgow coma scale, total score, when only the total score is documented in the medical record and not the individual score(s).

● **R40.2   Coma**
    Code first any associated:
        fracture of skull (S02.-)
        intracranial injury (S06.-)
    Note: One code from each subcategory R40.21-R40-23 is required to complete the coma scale
    Coding Clinic: 2021, Q4, P112; 2016, Q4, P127

    R40.20   Unspecified coma 🅗
        Coma NOS
        Unconsciousness NOS
        Coding Clinic: 2021, Q4, P112

●   **R40.21   Coma scale, eyes open**
        The following appropriate 7th character is to be added to subcategory R40.21-:

0	unspecified time
1	in the field [EMT or ambulance]
2	at arrival to emergency department
3	at hospital admission
4	24 hours or more after hospital admission

        Coding Clinic: 2021, Q4, P112; 2017, Q4, P25; 2015, Q2, P18

●   **R40.211   Coma scale, eyes open, never** 🅗
            Coma scale eye opening score of 1

●   **R40.212   Coma scale, eyes open, to pain** 🅗
            Coma scale eye opening score of 2

●   **R40.213   Coma scale, eyes open, to sound**
            Coma scale eye opening score of 3

●   **R40.214   Coma scale, eyes open, spontaneous**
            Coma scale eye opening score of 4

●   **R40.22   Coma scale, best verbal response**
        The following appropriate 7th character is to be added to subcategory R40.22-:

0	unspecified time
1	in the field [EMT or ambulance]
2	at arrival to emergency department
3	at hospital admission
4	24 hours or more after hospital admission

        Coding Clinic: 2021, Q4, P112; 2017, Q4, P25; 2015, Q2, P18

●   **R40.221   Coma scale, best verbal response, none** 🅗
            Coma scale verbal score of 1

●   **R40.222   Coma scale, best verbal response, incomprehensible words** 🅗
            Coma scale verbal score of 2
            Incomprehensible sounds (2-5 years of age)
            Moans/grunts to pain; restless (< 2 years old)

Glasgow Coma Scale

Eye Opening Response	
• Spontaneous--open with blinking at baseline	4 points
• To verbal stimuli, command, speech	3 points
• To pain only (not applied to face)	2 points
• No response	1 point
Verbal Response	
• Oriented	5 points
• Confused conversation, but able to answer questions	4 points
• Inappropriate words	3 points
• Incomprehensible speech	2 points
• No response	1 point
Motor Response	
• Obeys commands for movement	6 points
• Purposeful movement to painful stimulus	5 points
• Withdraws in response to pain	4 points
• Flexion in response to pain (decorticate posturing)	3 points
• Extension response in response to pain (decerebrate posturing)	2 points
• No response	1 point
Categorization: Coma: No eye opening, no ability to follow commands, no word verbalizations (3-8)	
Head Injury Classification: Severe Head Injury--GCS score of 8 or less Moderate Head Injury--GCS score of 9 to 12 Mild head injury--GCS score of 13 to 15	
(Adapted from: Advanced Trauma Life Support: Course for Physicians, American College of Surgeons, 1993). http://www.bt.cdc.gov/masscasulatires/gscale.asp	

Figure 18-1

● R40.223 **Coma scale, best verbal response, inappropriate words**
Coma scale verbal score of 3
Inappropriate crying or screaming (< 2 years of age)
Screaming (2-5 years of age)

● R40.224 **Coma scale, best verbal response, confused conversation**
Coma scale verbal score of 4
Inappropriate words (2-5 years of age)
Irritable cries (< 2 years of age)

● R40.225 **Coma scale, best verbal response, oriented**
Coma scale verbal score of 5
Cooing or babbling or crying appropriately (< 2 years of age)
Uses appropriate words (2- 5 years of age)

● R40.23 Coma scale, **best motor response**
The following appropriate 7th character is to be added to subcategory R40.23-:

0	unspecified time
1	in the field [EMT or ambulance]
2	at arrival to emergency department
3	at hospital admission
4	24 hours or more after hospital admission

Coding Clinic: 2017, Q4, P25; 2015, Q2, P18

● R40.231 **Coma scale, best motor response, none** 🖥
Coma scale motor score of 1

● R40.232 **Coma scale, best motor response, extension** 🖥
Abnormal extensor posturing to pain or noxious stimuli (< 2 years of age)
Coma scale motor score of 2
Extensor posturing to pain or noxious stimuli (2-5 years of age)

● R40.233 **Coma scale, best motor response, abnormal flexion**
Coma scale motor score of 3
Abnormal flexure posturing to pain or noxious stimuli (2-5 years of age)
Flexion/decorticate posturing (< 2 years of age)

● R40.234 **Coma scale, best motor response, flexion withdrawal** 🖥
Coma scale motor score of 4
Withdraws from pain or noxious stimuli (2-5 years of age)

● R40.235 **Coma scale, best motor response, localizes pain**
Coma scale motor score of 5
Localizes pain (2-5 years of age)
Withdraws to touch (< 2 years of age)

● R40.236 **Coma scale, best motor response, obeys commands**
Coma scale motor score of 6
Normal or spontaneous movement (< 2 years of age)
Obeys commands (2-5 years of age)

● R40.24 **Glasgow coma scale, total score**
Note: Assign a code from subcategory R40.24, when only the total coma score is documented
The following appropriate 7th character is to be added to subcategory R40.24-:

0	unspecified time
1	in the field [EMT or ambulance]
2	at arrival to emergency department
3	at hospital admission
4	24 hours or more after hospital admission

Coding Clinic: 2016, Q4, P64; 2015, Q2, P18

● R40.241 Glasgow coma scale score **13-15**
● R40.242 Glasgow coma scale score **9-12**
● R40.243 Glasgow coma scale score **3-8** 🖥
● R40.244 **Other coma, without documented Glasgow coma scale score, or with partial score reported** 🖥

R40.3 **Persistent vegetative state** 🖥
R40.4 **Transient alteration of awareness**

● R41 **Other symptoms and signs involving cognitive functions and awareness**

Excludes1 dissociative [conversion] disorders (F44.-)
mild cognitive impairment, so stated (G31.84)

R41.0 **Disorientation, unspecified**
Confusion NOS   Delirium NOS
Coding Clinic: 2022, Q2, P11; 2019, Q2, P34; 2016, Q4, P71

R41.1 **Anterograde amnesia**
R41.2 **Retrograde amnesia**

CHAPTER 18 (R00-R99)

R41.3 **Other amnesia**
Amnesia NOS
Memory loss NOS

> **Excludes1** amnestic disorder due to known physiologic condition (F04)
> amnestic syndrome due to psychoactive substance use (F10-F19 with 5th character .6)
> mild memory disturbance due to known physiological condition (F06.8)
> transient global amnesia (G45.4)

R41.4 **Neurologic neglect syndrome**
Asomatognosia
Hemi-akinesia
Hemi-inattention
Hemispatial neglect
Left-sided neglect
Sensory neglect
Visuospatial neglect

> **Excludes1** visuospatial deficit (R41.842)

● R41.8 **Other symptoms and signs involving cognitive functions and awareness**

R41.81 **Age-related cognitive decline** A
Senility NOS

R41.82 **Altered mental status, unspecified**
Change in mental status NOS

> **Excludes1** altered level of consciousness (R40.-)
> altered mental status due to known condition - code to condition
> delirium NOS (R41.0)
> Coding Clinic: 2012, Q4, P98

R41.83 **Borderline intellectual functioning**
IQ level 71 to 84

> **Excludes1** intellectual disabilities (F70-F79)

● R41.84 **Other specified cognitive deficit**

> **Excludes1** cognitive deficits as sequelae of cerebrovascular disease (I69.01-, I69.11-, I69.21-, I69.31-, I69.81-, I69.91-)

R41.840 **Attention and concentration deficit**

> **Excludes1** attention-deficit hyperactivity disorders (F90.-)

R41.841 **Cognitive communication deficit**
R41.842 **Visuospatial deficit**
R41.843 **Psychomotor deficit**
R41.844 **Frontal lobe and executive function deficit**

R41.89 **Other symptoms and signs involving cognitive functions and awareness**
Anosognosia

R41.9 **Unspecified symptoms and signs involving cognitive functions and awareness**
Unspecified neurocognitive disorder

R42 **Dizziness and giddiness**
Light-headedness
Vertigo NOS

> **Excludes1** vertiginous syndromes (H81.-)
> vertigo from infrasound (T75.23)
> Coding Clinic: 2015, Q4, P40

● R43 **Disturbances of smell and taste**

R43.0 **Anosmia**
Absence of sense of smell; AKA anosphresia and olfactory anesthesia

R43.1 **Parosmia**

R43.2 **Parageusia**
Perversion of sense of taste or bad taste in mouth; AKA dysgeusia

R43.8 **Other disturbances of smell and taste**
Mixed disturbance of smell and taste

R43.9 **Unspecified disturbances of smell and taste**

● R44 **Other symptoms and signs involving general sensations and perceptions**

> **Excludes1** alcoholic hallucinations (F10.151, F10.251, F10.951)
> hallucinations in drug psychosis (F11-F19 with fifth to sixth characters 51)
> hallucinations in mood disorders with psychotic symptoms (F30.2, F31.5, F32.3, F33.3)
> hallucinations in schizophrenia, schizotypal and delusional disorders (F20-F29)

> **Excludes2** disturbances of skin sensation (R20.-)

R44.0 **Auditory hallucinations**
R44.1 **Visual hallucinations**
R44.2 **Other hallucinations**
R44.3 **Hallucinations, unspecified**
Coding Clinic: 2022, Q2, P11

R44.8 **Other symptoms and signs involving general sensations and perceptions**

R44.9 **Unspecified symptoms and signs involving general sensations and perceptions**

● R45 **Symptoms and signs involving emotional state**

R45.0 **Nervousness**
Nervous tension
R45.1 **Restlessness and agitation**
R45.2 **Unhappiness**
R45.3 **Demoralization and apathy**

> **Excludes1** anhedonia (R45.84)

R45.4 **Irritability and anger**
R45.5 **Hostility**
R45.6 **Violent behavior**
R45.7 **State of emotional shock and stress, unspecified**

● R45.8 **Other symptoms and signs involving emotional state**

R45.81 **Low self-esteem**
R45.82 **Worries**
R45.83 **Excessive crying of child, adolescent or adult**

> **Excludes1** excessive crying of infant (baby) R68.11

R45.84 **Anhedonia**
Total loss of feeling of pleasure in pleasurable acts

● R45.85 **Homicidal and suicidal ideations**

> **Excludes1** suicide attempt (T14.91)

R45.850 **Homicidal ideations**
R45.851 **Suicidal ideations**
Coding Clinic: 2022, Q1, P29

R45.86 **Emotional lability**
R45.87 **Impulsiveness**
R45.88 **Nonsuicidal self-harm**
Nonsuicidal self-injury
Nonsuicidal self-mutilation
Self-inflicted injury without suicidal intent

> Code also injury, if known
> Coding Clinic: 2021, Q4, P27

R45.89 **Other symptoms and signs involving emotional state**

● R46 **Symptoms and signs involving appearance and behavior**

> **Excludes1** appearance and behavior in schizophrenia, schizotypal and delusional disorders (F20-F29)
> mental and behavioral disorders (F01-F99)

R46.0 **Very low level of personal hygiene**
R46.1 **Bizarre personal appearance**
R46.2 **Strange and inexplicable behavior**
R46.3 **Overactivity**
R46.4 **Slowness and poor responsiveness**

> **Excludes1** stupor (R40.1)

R46.5 **Suspiciousness and marked evasiveness**
R46.6 **Undue concern and preoccupation with stressful events**
R46.7 **Verbosity and circumstantial detail obscuring reason for contact**

- **R46.8**   **Other symptoms and signs involving appearance and behavior**
  - **R46.81**   **Obsessive-compulsive behavior**
    - **Excludes1**   obsessive-compulsive disorder (F42.-)
  - **R46.89**   **Other symptoms and signs involving appearance and behavior**

SYMPTOMS AND SIGNS INVOLVING SPEECH AND VOICE (R47-R49)

- **R47**   **Speech disturbances, not elsewhere classified**
  - **Excludes1**   autism (F84.0)
    cluttering (F80.81)
    specific developmental disorders of speech and language (F80.-)
    stuttering (F80.81)
  - **R47.0**   **Dysphasia and aphasia**
    - **R47.01**   **Aphasia**
      - **Excludes1**   aphasia following cerebrovascular disease (I69. with final characters -20)
        progressive isolated aphasia (G31.01)
    - **R47.02**   **Dysphasia**
      Impairment in comprehension of speech, caused by left-sided brain damage
      - **Excludes1**   dysphasia following cerebrovascular disease (I69. with final characters -21)
  - **R47.1**   **Dysarthria and anarthria**
    Motor speech disorder
    - **Excludes1**   dysarthria following cerebrovascular disease (I69. with final characters -22)
  - **R47.8**   **Other speech disturbances**
    - **Excludes1**   dysarthria following cerebrovascular disease (I69. with final characters -28)
    - **R47.81**   **Slurred speech**
    - **R47.82**   *Fluency disorder in conditions classified elsewhere*
      Stuttering in conditions classified elsewhere
      Code first underlying disease or condition, such as:
      Parkinson's disease (G20)
      - **Excludes1**   adult onset fluency disorder (F98.5)
        childhood onset fluency disorder (F80.81)
        fluency disorder (stuttering) following cerebrovascular disease (I69. with final characters -23)
    - **R47.89**   **Other speech disturbances**
  - **R47.9**   **Unspecified speech disturbances**
- **R48**   **Dyslexia and other symbolic dysfunctions, not elsewhere classified**
  - **Excludes1**   specific developmental disorders of scholastic skills (F81.-)
  - **R48.0**   **Dyslexia and alexia**
  - **R48.1**   **Agnosia**
    Loss of ability to recognize objects, persons, sounds, shapes, or smells
    Astereognosia (astereognosis)
    Autotopagnosia
    - **Excludes1**   visual object agnosia (R48.3)
  - **R48.2**   **Apraxia**
    Loss of ability to execute or carry out learned purposeful movements
    - **Excludes1**   apraxia following cerebrovascular disease (I69. with final characters -90)

- **R48.3**   **Visual agnosia**
  Prosopagnosia
  Simultanagnosia (asimultagnosia)
- **R48.8**   **Other symbolic dysfunctions**
  Acalculia
  Difficulty performing simple mathematical tasks resulting from neurological injury
  Agraphia
  Coding Clinic: 2017, Q1, P27
- **R48.9**   **Unspecified symbolic dysfunctions**
- **R49**   **Voice and resonance disorders**
  - **Excludes1**   psychogenic voice and resonance disorders (F44.4)
  - **R49.0**   **Dysphonia**
    Hoarseness
  - **R49.1**   **Aphonia**
    Loss of voice
  - **R49.2**   **Hypernasality and hyponasality**
    - **R49.21**   **Hypernasality**
    - **R49.22**   **Hyponasality**
  - **R49.8**   **Other voice and resonance disorders**
  - **R49.9**   **Unspecified voice and resonance disorder**
    Change in voice NOS
    Resonance disorder NOS

GENERAL SYMPTOMS AND SIGNS (R50-R69)

- **R50**   **Fever of other and unknown origin**
  - **Excludes1**   chills without fever (R68.83)
    febrile convulsions (R56.0-)
    fever of unknown origin during labor (O75.2)
    fever of unknown origin in newborn (P81.9)
    hypothermia due to illness (R68.0)
    malignant hyperthermia due to anesthesia (T88.3)
    puerperal pyrexia NOS (O86.4)
  - **R50.2**   **Drug induced fever**
    Use additional code for adverse effect, if applicable, to identify drug (T36-T50 with fifth or sixth character 5)
    - **Excludes1**   postvaccination (postimmunization) fever (R50.83)
  - **R50.8**   **Other specified fever**
    - **R50.81**   *Fever presenting with conditions classified elsewhere*
      Code first underlying condition when associated fever is present, such as with:
      leukemia (C91-C95)
      neutropenia (D70.-)
      sickle-cell disease (D57.-)
      Coding Clinic: 2019, Q2, P25
    - **R50.82**   **Postprocedural fever**
      - **Excludes1**   postprocedural infection (T81.44)
        posttransfusion fever (R50.84)
        postvaccination (postimmunization) fever (R50.83)
    - **R50.83**   **Postvaccination fever**
      Postimmunization fever
    - **R50.84**   **Febrile nonhemolytic transfusion reaction**
      FNHTR
      Posttransfusion fever
  - **R50.9**   **Fever, unspecified**
    Fever NOS
    Fever of unknown origin [FUO]
    Fever with chills
    Fever with rigors
    Hyperpyrexia NOS
    Persistent fever
    Pyrexia NOS

CHAPTER 18 (R00-R99)

● **R51   Headache**

Excludes2   atypical face pain (G50.1)
migraine and other headache syndromes
(G43-G44)
trigeminal neuralgia (G50.0)

R51.0   Headache with orthostatic component, not elsewhere classified
Headache with positional component, not elsewhere classified

R51.9 Headache, unspecified
Facial pain NOS

R52   Pain, unspecified
Acute pain NOS
Generalized pain NOS

Excludes1   acute and chronic pain, not elsewhere classified (G89.-)
localized pain, unspecified type - code to pain by site, such as:
abdomen pain (R10.-)
back pain (M54.9)
breast pain (N64.4)
chest pain (R07.1-R07.9)
ear pain (H92.0-)
eye pain (H57.1)
headache (R51.9)
joint pain (M25.5-)
limb pain (M79.6-)
lumbar region pain (M54.5-)
pelvic and perineal pain (R10.2)
shoulder pain (M25.51-)
spine pain (M54.-)
throat pain (R07.0)
tongue pain (K14.6)
tooth pain (K08.8)
renal colic (N23)
pain disorders exclusively related to psychological factors (F45.41)

● **R53   Malaise and fatigue**

R53.0   Neoplastic (malignant) related fatigue
Code first associated neoplasm

R53.1   Weakness
Asthenia NOS

Excludes1   age-related weakness (R54)
muscle weakness (generalized) (M62.81)
sarcopenia (M62.84)
senile asthenia (R54)
Coding Clinic: 2021, Q4, P103; 2017, Q1, P7

R53.2   Functional quadriplegia 🗝
Complete immobility due to severe physical disability or frailty

Excludes1   frailty NOS (R54)
hysterical paralysis (F44.4)
immobility syndrome (M62.3)
neurologic quadriplegia (G82.5-)
quadriplegia (G82.50)
Coding Clinic: 2016, Q2, P6

● **R53.8   Other malaise and fatigue**

Excludes1   combat exhaustion and fatigue (F43.0)
congenital debility (P96.9)
exhaustion and fatigue due to excessive exertion (T73.3)
exhaustion and fatigue due to exposure (T73.2)
exhaustion and fatigue due to heat (T67.-)
exhaustion and fatigue due to pregnancy (O26.8-)
exhaustion and fatigue due to recurrent depressive episode (F33)
exhaustion and fatigue due to senile debility (R54)

R53.81   Other malaise
Chronic debility
Debility NOS
General physical deterioration
Malaise NOS
Nervous debility

Excludes1   age-related physical debility (R54)
Coding Clinic: 2021, Q1, P43

R53.82   Chronic fatigue, unspecified
~~Chronic fatigue syndrome NOS~~

Excludes1   ~~postviral fatigue syndrome (G93.3)~~
▶chronic fatigue syndrome (G93.32)
▶myalgic encephalomyelitis (G93.32)
▶post infection and related fatigue syndromes (G93.39)
▶postviral fatigue syndrome (G93.31)

R53.83   Other fatigue
Fatigue NOS   Lethargy
Lack of energy   Tiredness

Excludes2   exhaustion and fatigue due to depressive episode (F32.-)
Coding Clinic: 2017, Q1, P7

R54   Age-related physical debility   A
Frailty   Senile asthenia
Old age   Senile debility
Senescence

Excludes1   age-related cognitive decline (R41.81)
sarcopenia (M62.84)
senile psychosis (F03)
senility NOS (R41.81)

R55   Syncope and collapse
Blackout
Fainting
Vasovagal attack

Excludes1   cardiogenic shock (R57.0)
carotid sinus syncope (G90.01)
heat syncope (T67.1)
neurocirculatory asthenia (F45.8)
neurogenic orthostatic hypotension (G90.3)
orthostatic hypotension (I95.1)
postprocedural shock (T81.1-)
psychogenic syncope (F48.8)
shock NOS (R57.9)
shock complicating or following abortion or ectopic or molar pregnancy (O00-O07, O08.3)
shock complicating or following labor and delivery (O75.1)
Stokes-Adams attack (I45.9)
unconsciousness NOS (R40.2-)

● **R56   Convulsions, not elsewhere classified**

Excludes1   dissociative convulsions and seizures (F44.5)
epileptic convulsions and seizures (G40.-)
newborn convulsions and seizures (P90)

● **R56.0   Febrile convulsions**

R56.00   Simple febrile convulsions 🗝
Febrile convulsion NOS
Febrile seizure NOS

R56.01   Complex febrile convulsions 🗝
Atypical febrile seizure
Complex febrile seizure
Complicated febrile seizure

Excludes1   status epilepticus (G40.901)

▶ New   ⇒ Revised   ~~deleted~~ Deleted   Excludes 1   Excludes 2   Includes   Use additional   Code first   Code also   Key words
OGCR Official Guidelines   X Assign placeholder X   ● Use Additional Character(s)   ▶ Manifestation Code   🗝 Hierarchical Condition Category   Coding Clinic

R56.1   Post traumatic seizures 🦴
> **Excludes1**   post traumatic epilepsy (G40.-)

R56.9   Unser Unspecified convulsions🦴
> Convulsion disorder   Recurrent convulsions
> Fit NOS   Seizure(s) (convulsive) NOS
> **Coding Clinic: 2021, Q1, P3; 2019, Q4, P18**

● **R57**   Shock, not elsewhere classified
> **Excludes1**   anaphylactic shock NOS (T78.2)
> anaphylactic reaction or shock due to adverse food reaction (T78.0-)
> anaphylactic shock due to adverse effect of correct drug or medicament properly administered (T88.6)
> anaphylactic shock due to serum (T80.5-)
> electric shock (T75.4)
> obstetric shock (O75.1)
> postprocedural shock (T81.1-)
> psychic shock (F43.0)
> shock complicating or following ectopic or molar pregnancy (O00-O07, O08.3)
> shock due to anesthesia (T88.2)
> shock due to lightning (T75.01)
> traumatic shock (T79.4)
> toxic shock syndrome (A48.3)

R57.0   Cardiogenic shock 🦴
> **Excludes2**   septic shock (R65.21)

R57.1   Hypovolemic shock 🦴
> *Decreased blood volume (loss)*
> **Coding Clinic: 2019, Q2, P7-8**

R57.8   Other shock 🦴

R57.9   Shock, unspecified 🦴
> Failure of peripheral circulation NOS
> *Resulting in significant blood pressure drop*

R58   Hemorrhage, not elsewhere classified
> Hemorrhage NOS
> **Excludes1**   hemorrhage included with underlying conditions, such as:
> acute duodenal ulcer with hemorrhage (K26.0)
> acute gastritis with bleeding (K29.01)
> ulcerative enterocolitis with rectal bleeding (K51.01)

● **R59**   Enlarged lymph nodes
> **Includes**   swollen glands
> **Excludes1**   lymphadenitis NOS (I88.9)
> acute lymphadenitis (L04.-)
> chronic lymphadenitis (I88.1)
> mesenteric (acute) (chronic) lymphadenitis (I88.0)

R59.0   Localized enlarged lymph nodes

R59.1   Generalized enlarged lymph nodes
> Lymphadenopathy NOS

R59.9   Enlarged lymph nodes, unspecified

● **R60**   Edema, not elsewhere classified
> **Excludes1**   angioneurotic edema (T78.3)
> ascites (R18.-)
> cerebral edema (G93.6)
> cerebral edema due to birth injury (P11.0)
> edema of larynx (J38.4)
> edema of nasopharynx (J39.2)
> edema of pharynx (J39.2)
> gestational edema (O12.0-)
> hereditary edema (Q82.0)
> hydrops fetalis NOS (P83.2)
> hydrothorax (J94.8)
> hydrops fetalis NOS (P83.2)
> newborn edema (P83.3)
> pulmonary edema (J81.-)

R60.0   Localized edema

R60.1   Generalized edema
> **Excludes2**   nutritional edema (E40-E46)

R60.9   Edema, unspecified
> Fluid retention NOS

R61   Generalized hyperhidrosis
> Excessive sweating
> Night sweats
> Secondary hyperhidrosis
> *Code first, if applicable, menopausal and female climacteric states (N95.1)*
> **Excludes1**   focal (primary) (secondary) hyperhidrosis (L74.5-)
> Frey's syndrome (L74.52)
> localized (primary) (secondary) hyperhidrosis (L74.5-)

● **R62**   Lack of expected normal physiological development in childhood and adults
> **Excludes1**   delayed puberty (E30.0)
> gonadal dysgenesis (Q99.1)
> hypopituitarism (E23.0)

R62.0   Delayed milestone in childhood   P
> Delayed attainment of expected physiological developmental stage
> Late talker
> Late walker

● **R62.5**   Other and unspecified lack of expected normal physiological development in childhood
> **Excludes1**   HIV disease resulting in failure to thrive (B20)
> physical retardation due to malnutrition (E45)

R62.50   Unspecified lack of expected normal physiological development in childhood
> Infantilism NOS

R62.51   Failure to thrive (child)   P
> Failure to gain weight
> **Excludes1**   failure to thrive in child under 28 days old (P92.6)
> **Coding Clinic: 2018, Q4, P82**

R62.52   Short stature (child)
> Lack of growth   Short stature NOS
> Physical retardation
> ➡ **Excludes1**   short stature due to endocrine disorder (E34.3-)

R62.59   Other lack of expected normal physiological development in childhood

R62.7   Adult failure to thrive   A

● **R63**   Symptoms and signs concerning food and fluid intake
> **Excludes1**   bulimia NOS (F50.2)

R63.0   Anorexia
> Loss of appetite
> **Excludes1**   anorexia nervosa (F50.0-)
> loss of appetite of nonorganic origin (F50.89)

R63.1   Polydipsia
> Excessive thirst

R63.2   Polyphagia
> Excessive eating   Hyperalimentation NOS

● **R63.3**   Feeding difficulties
> **Excludes2**   eating disorders (F50.-)
> feeding problems of newborn (P92.-)
> infant feeding disorder of nonorganic origin (F98.2-)

R63.30   Feeding difficulties, unspecified   P

R63.31   Pediatric feeding disorder, acute
> Pediatric feeding dysfunction, acute
> Code also, if applicable, associated conditions such as:
> aspiration pneumonia (J69.0)
> dysphagia (R13.1-)
> gastro-esophageal reflux disease (K21.-)
> malnutrition (E40-E46)

CHAPTER 18 (R00-R99)

R63.32   Pediatric feeding disorder, chronic   P
Pediatric feeding dysfunction, chronic
Code also, if applicable, associated conditions
such as:
aspiration pneumonia (J69.0)
dysphagia (R13.1-)
gastro-esophageal reflux disease (K21.-)
malnutrition (E40-E46)

R63.39   Other feeding difficulties
Feeding problem (elderly) (infant) NOS
Picky eater
Coding Clinic: 2017, Q1, P27; 2016, Q3, P19

R63.4   Abnormal weight loss

R63.5   Abnormal weight gain
Excludes1   excessive weight gain in pregnancy
(O26.0-)
obesity (E66.-)

R63.6   Underweight
Use additional code to identify body mass index (BMI),
if known (Z68.-)
Excludes1   abnormal weight loss (R63.4)
anorexia nervosa (F50.0-)
malnutrition (E40-E46)

**R63.8   Other symptoms and signs concerning food and fluid
intake**

R64   Cachexia 🐾
Wasting syndrome
Code first underlying condition, if known
Excludes1   abnormal weight loss (R63.4)
nutritional marasmus (E41)
Coding Clinic: 2017, Q3, P25

● **R65   Symptoms and signs specifically associated with systemic
inflammation and infection**
● **R65.1   Systemic inflammatory response syndrome (SIRS) of
non-infectious origin**
Code first underlying condition, such as:
heatstroke (T67.0-)
injury and trauma (S00-T88)
Excludes1   sepsis - code to infection
severe sepsis (R65.2)
Coding Clinic: 2019, Q2, P38

**R65.10   Systemic inflammatory response syndrome
(SIRS) of non-infectious origin without acute
organ dysfunction** 🐾
Systemic inflammatory response syndrome
(SIRS) NOS
Coding Clinic: 2019, Q2, P25, 38

**R65.11   Systemic inflammatory response syndrome
(SIRS) of non-infectious origin with acute
organ dysfunction** 🐾
Use additional code to identify specific acute
organ dysfunction, such as:
acute kidney failure (N17.-)
acute respiratory failure (J96.0-)
critical illness myopathy (G72.81)
critical illness polyneuropathy (G62.81)
disseminated intravascular coagulopathy
[DIC] (D65)
encephalopathy (metabolic) (septic) (G93.41)
hepatic failure (K72.0-)

OGCR Section I.C.18.g.

SIRS due to Non-Infectious Process
The systemic inflammatory response syndrome (SIRS) can develop as
a result of certain non-infectious disease processes, such as trauma,
malignant neoplasm, or pancreatitis. When SIRS is documented
with a noninfectious condition, and no subsequent infection is
documented, the code for the underlying condition, such as an injury,
should be assigned, followed by code R65.10. Systemic inflammatory
response syndrome (SIRS) of non-infectious origin without
acute organ dysfunction, or code R65.11, Systemic inflammatory
response syndrome (SIRS) of non-infectious origin with acute organ
dysfunction. If an associated acute organ dysfunction is documented,
the appropriate code(s) for the specific type of organ dysfunction(s)
should be assigned in addition to code R65.11. If acute organ
dysfunction is documented, but it cannot be determined if the acute
organ dysfunction is associated with SIRS or due to another condition
(e.g., directly due to the trauma), the provider should be queried.

● **R65.2   Severe sepsis**
Infection with associated acute organ dysfunction
Sepsis with acute organ dysfunction
Sepsis with multiple organ dysfunction
Systemic inflammatory response syndrome due to
infectious process with acute organ dysfunction
Code first underlying infection, such as:
infection following a procedure (T81.44)
infections following infusion, transfusion and
therapeutic injection (T80.2-)
puerperal sepsis (O85)
sepsis following complete or unspecified
spontaneous abortion (O03.87)
sepsis following ectopic and molar pregnancy
(O08.82)
sepsis following incomplete spontaneous abortion
(O03.37)
sepsis following (induced) termination of pregnancy
(O04.87)
sepsis NOS (A41.9)
Use additional code to identify specific acute organ
dysfunction, such as:
acute kidney failure (N17.-)
acute respiratory failure (J96.0-)
critical illness myopathy (G72.81)
critical illness polyneuropathy (G62.81)
disseminated intravascular coagulopathy [DIC] (D65)
encephalopathy (metabolic) (septic) (G93.41)
hepatic failure (K72.0-)
Coding Clinic: 2017, Q4, P99; 2016, Q3, P8

R65.20   Severe sepsis without septic shock 🐾
Severe sepsis NOS
Coding Clinic: 2019, Q1, P14; 2018, Q4, P90; 2016, Q3, P14

R65.21   Severe sepsis with septic shock 🐾

● **R68   Other general symptoms and signs**
**R68.0   Hypothermia, not associated with low environmental
temperature**
Excludes1   hypothermia NOS (accidental) (T68)
hypothermia due to anesthesia (T88.51)
hypothermia due to low environmental
temperature (T68)
newborn hypothermia (P80.-)

● **R68.1   Nonspecific symptoms peculiar to infancy**
Excludes1   colic, infantile (R10.83)
neonatal cerebral irritability (P91.3)
teething syndrome (K00.7)

R68.11   Excessive crying of infant (baby)   P
Excludes1   excessive crying of child,
adolescent, or adult (R45.83)

R68.12   Fussy infant (baby)   P
Irritable infant

▶ New   ⇒ Revised   ~~deleted~~ Deleted   Excludes 1   Excludes 2   Includes   Use additional   Code first   Code also   Key words
OGCR Official Guidelines   X Assign placeholder X   ● Use Additional Character(s)   ▷ Manifestation Code   🐾 Hierarchical Condition Category   Coding Clinic

R68.13 Apparent life threatening event in infant (ALTE)   P
    Apparent life threatening event in newborn
    Brief resolved unexplained event (BRUE)
    Code first confirmed diagnosis, if known
    Use additional code(s) for associated signs and symptoms if no confirmed diagnosis established, or if signs and symptoms are not associated routinely with confirmed diagnosis, or provide additional information for cause of ALTE

R68.19 Other nonspecific symptoms peculiar to infancy   P

R68.2 Dry mouth, unspecified
   Excludes1   dry mouth due to dehydration (E86.0)
      dry mouth due to Sjögren syndrome (M35.0-)
      salivary gland hyposecretion (K11.7)

R68.3 Clubbing of fingers
   Clubbing of nails
   Excludes1   congenital clubfinger (Q68.1)

● **R68.8 Other general symptoms and signs**
   R68.81 Early satiety
   R68.82 Decreased libido   A
     Decreased sexual desire
   R68.83 Chills (without fever)
     Chills NOS
     Excludes1   chills with fever (R50.9)
   R68.84 Jaw pain
     Mandibular pain
     Maxilla pain
     Excludes1   temporomandibular joint arthralgia (M26.62-)
   R68.89 Other general symptoms and signs

R69 Illness, unspecified
   Unknown and unspecified cases of morbidity

ABNORMAL FINDINGS ON EXAMINATION OF BLOOD, WITHOUT DIAGNOSIS (R70-R79)

   Excludes2   abnormal findings on antenatal screening of mother (O28.-)
     abnormalities of lipids (E78.-)
     abnormalities of platelets and thrombocytes (D69.-)
     abnormalities of white blood cells classified elsewhere (D70-D72)
     coagulation hemorrhagic disorders (D65-D68)
     diagnostic abnormal findings classified elsewhere —*see* Alphabetical Index
     hemorrhagic and hematological disorders of newborn (P50-P61)

● **R70 Elevated erythrocyte sedimentation rate and abnormality of plasma viscosity**
   R70.0 Elevated erythrocyte sedimentation rate
   R70.1 Abnormal plasma viscosity

● **R71 Abnormality of red blood cells**
   Excludes1   anemias (D50-D64)
     anemia of premature infant (P61.2)
     benign (familial) polycythemia (D75.0)
     congenital anemias (P61.2-P61.4)
     newborn anemia due to isoimmunization (P55.-)
     polycythemia neonatorum (P61.1)
     polycythemia NOS (D75.1)
     polycythemia vera (D45)
     secondary polycythemia (D75.1)
   R71.0 Precipitous drop in hematocrit
     Drop (precipitous) in hemoglobin
     Drop in hematocrit
     Blood volume that has decreased red blood cells

R71.8 Other abnormality of red blood cells
   Abnormal red-cell morphology NOS
   Abnormal red-cell volume NOS
   Anisocytosis
     Red blood cells of unequal size
   Poikilocytosis
     Red blood cells of abnormal shape

● **R73 Elevated blood glucose level**
   Excludes1   diabetes mellitus (E08-E13)
     diabetes mellitus in pregnancy, childbirth and the puerperium (O24.-)
     neonatal disorders (P70.0-P70.2)
     postsurgical hypoinsulinemia (E89.1)
   ● **R73.0 Abnormal glucose**
     Excludes1   abnormal glucose in pregnancy (O99.81-)
      diabetes mellitus (E08-E13)
      dysmetabolic syndrome X (E88.81)
      gestational diabetes (O24.4-)
      glycosuria (R81)
      hypoglycemia (E16.2)
     R73.01 Impaired fasting glucose
      Elevated fasting glucose
     R73.02 Impaired glucose tolerance (oral)
      Elevated glucose tolerance
     R73.03 Prediabetes
      Latent diabetes
      Coding Clinic: 2016, Q4, P65
     R73.09 Other abnormal glucose
      Abnormal glucose NOS
      Abnormal non-fasting glucose tolerance
      Coding Clinic: 2016, Q4, P65
   R73.9 Hyperglycemia, unspecified

● **R74 Abnormal serum enzyme levels**
   ● **R74.0 Nonspecific elevation of levels of transaminase and lactic acid dehydrogenase [LDH]**
     R74.01 Elevation of levels of liver transaminase levels
      Elevation of levels of alanine transaminase (ALT)
      Elevation of levels of aspartate transaminase (AST)
     R74.02 Elevation of levels of lactic acid dehydrogenase [LDH]
   R74.8 Abnormal levels of other serum enzymes
     Abnormal level of acid phosphatase
     Abnormal level of alkaline phosphatase
     Abnormal level of amylase
     Abnormal level of lipase [triacylglycerol lipase]
     Coding Clinic: 2019, Q2, P6
   R74.9 Abnormal serum enzyme level, unspecified

R75 Inconclusive laboratory evidence of human immunodeficiency virus [HIV]
   Nonconclusive HIV-test finding in infants
   Excludes1   asymptomatic human immunodeficiency virus [HIV] infection status (Z21)
     human immunodeficiency virus [HIV] disease (B20)

OGCR Section I.C.1.e and f.

Patients with inconclusive HIV serology

e. Patients with inconclusive HIV serology, but no definitive diagnosis or manifestations of the illness, may be assigned code R75, Inconclusive laboratory evidence of human immunodeficiency virus [HIV].

f. Previously diagnosed HIV-related illness

Patients with any known prior diagnosis of an HIV-related illness should be coded to B20. Once a patient has developed an HIV-related illness, the patient should always be assigned code B20 on every subsequent admission/encounter. Patients previously diagnosed with any HIV illness (B20) should never be assigned to R75 or Z21, Asymptomatic human immunodeficiency virus [HIV] infection status.

CHAPTER 18 (R00-R99)

● R76   **Other abnormal immunological findings in serum**

    R76.0   **Raised antibody titer**

        Excludes1   isoimmunization in pregnancy (O36.0-O36.1)

                          isoimmunization affecting newborn (P55.-)

        Coding Clinic: 2021, Q1, P7

    ● R76.1   **Nonspecific reaction to test for tuberculosis**

        R76.11   **Nonspecific reaction to tuberculin skin test without active tuberculosis**

            Abnormal result of Mantoux test

            PPD positive

            Tuberculin (skin test) positive

            Tuberculin (skin test) reactor

            Excludes1   nonspecific reaction to cell mediated immunity measurement of gamma interferon antigen response without active tuberculosis (R76.12)

        R76.12   **Nonspecific reaction to cell mediated immunity measurement of gamma interferon antigen response without active tuberculosis**

            Nonspecific reaction to QuantiFERON-TB test (QFT) without active tuberculosis

            Excludes1   nonspecific reaction to tuberculin skin test without active tuberculosis (R76.11)

                            positive tuberculin skin test (R76.11)

    R76.8   **Other specified abnormal immunological findings in serum**

        Raised level of immunoglobulins NOS

        Coding Clinic: 2021, Q1, P7

    R76.9   **Abnormal immunological finding in serum, unspecified**

● R77   **Other abnormalities of plasma proteins**

        Excludes1   disorders of plasma-protein metabolism (E88.0-)

    R77.0   **Abnormality of albumin**

    R77.1   **Abnormality of globulin**

        Hyperglobulinemia NOS

    R77.2   **Abnormality of alphafetoprotein**

    R77.8   **Other specified abnormalities of plasma proteins**

        Coding Clinic: 2019, Q2, P6

    R77.9   **Abnormality of plasma protein, unspecified**

        Coding Clinic: 2019, Q2, P6

● R78   **Findings of drugs and other substances, not normally found in blood**

    Use additional code to identify any retained foreign body, if applicable (Z18.-)

        Excludes1   mental or behavioral disorders due to psychoactive substance use (F10-F19)

    R78.0   **Finding of alcohol in blood**

        Use additional external cause code (Y90.-), for detail regarding alcohol level.

    R78.1   **Finding of opiate drug in blood**

    R78.2   **Finding of cocaine in blood**

    R78.3   **Finding of hallucinogen in blood**

    R78.4   **Finding of other drugs of addictive potential in blood**

    R78.5   **Finding of other psychotropic drug in blood**

    R78.6   **Finding of steroid agent in blood**

    ● R78.7   **Finding of abnormal level of heavy metals in blood**

        R78.71   **Abnormal lead level in blood**

            Excludes1   lead poisoning (T56.0-)

        R78.79   **Finding of abnormal level of heavy metals in blood**

    ● R78.8   **Finding of other specified substances, not normally found in blood**

        R78.81   **Bacteremia**

            Blood poisoning/bacteremia

            Excludes1   sepsis-code to specified infection

        R78.89   **Finding of other specified substances, not normally found in blood**

            Finding of abnormal level of lithium in blood

    R78.9   **Finding of unspecified substance, not normally found in blood**

● R79   **Other abnormal findings of blood chemistry**

    Use additional code to identify any retained foreign body, if applicable (Z18.-)

        Excludes1   asymptomatic hyperuricemia (E79.0)

                    hyperglycemia NOS (R73.9)

                    hypoglycemia NOS (E16.2)

                    neonatal hypoglycemia (P70.3-P70.4)

                    specific findings indicating disorder of amino-acid metabolism (E70-E72)

                    specific findings indicating disorder of carbohydrate metabolism (E73-E74)

                    specific findings indicating disorder of lipid metabolism (E75.-)

    R79.0   **Abnormal level of blood mineral**

        Abnormal blood level of cobalt

        Abnormal blood level of copper

        Abnormal blood level of iron

        Abnormal blood level of magnesium

        Abnormal blood level of mineral NEC

        Abnormal blood level of zinc

        Excludes1   abnormal level of lithium (R78.89)

                    disorders of mineral metabolism (E83.-)

                    neonatal hypomagnesemia (P71.2)

                    nutritional mineral deficiency (E58-E61)

    R79.1   **Abnormal coagulation profile**

        Abnormal or prolonged bleeding time

        Abnormal or prolonged coagulation time

        Abnormal or prolonged partial thromboplastin time [PTT]

        Abnormal or prolonged prothrombin time [PT]

    ▶Low von Willebrand factor

        Excludes1   coagulation defects (D68.-)

        Excludes2   abnormality of fluid, electrolyte or acid-base balance (E86-E87)

    ● R79.8   **Other specified abnormal findings of blood chemistry**

        R79.81   **Abnormal blood-gas level**

        R79.82   **Elevated C-reactive protein (CRP)**

        R79.83   **Abnormal findings of blood amino-acid level**

            Homocysteinemia

            Excludes1   disorders of amino-acid metabolism (E70-E72)

            Coding Clinic: 2021, Q4, P28

        R79.89   **Other specified abnormal findings of blood chemistry**

            Coding Clinic: 2019, Q2, P6

    R79.9   **Abnormal finding of blood chemistry, unspecified**

ABNORMAL FINDINGS ON EXAMINATION OF URINE, WITHOUT DIAGNOSIS (R80-R82)

        Excludes1   abnormal findings on antenatal screening of mother (O28.-)

                    diagnostic abnormal findings classified elsewhere - see Alphabetical Index

                    specific findings indicating disorder of amino-acid metabolism (E70-E72)

                    specific findings indicating disorder of carbohydrate metabolism (E73-E74)

● R80   **Proteinuria**

        Excludes1   gestational proteinuria (O12.1-)

    R80.0   **Isolated proteinuria**

        Idiopathic proteinuria

        Excludes1   isolated proteinuria with specific morphological lesion (N06.-)

    R80.1   **Persistent proteinuria, unspecified**

    R80.2   **Orthostatic proteinuria, unspecified**

        Postural proteinuria

    R80.3   **Bence Jones proteinuria**

R80.8   **Other proteinuria**

R80.9   **Proteinuria, unspecified**
Albuminuria NOS

R81   **Glycosuria**
> **Excludes1**   renal glycosuria (E74.818)

● R82   **Other and unspecified abnormal findings in urine**
> **Includes**   chromoabnormalities in urine

Use additional code to identify any retained foreign body, if applicable (Z18.-)
> **Excludes2**   hematuria (R31.-)

R82.0   **Chyluria**
White milky urine
> **Excludes1**   filarial chyluria (B74.-)

R82.1   **Myoglobinuria**
Presence of myoglobin (iron containing protein) in urine

R82.2   **Biliuria**
Presence of bile pigments/salts in urine

R82.3   **Hemoglobinuria**
Presence of hemoglobin in urine
> **Excludes1**   hemoglobinuria due to hemolysis from external causes NEC (D59.6)
> hemoglobinuria due to paroxysmal nocturnal [Marchiafava-Micheli] (D59.5)

R82.4   **Acetonuria**
Ketonuria

R82.5   **Elevated urine levels of drugs, medicaments and biological substances**
Elevated urine levels of catecholamines
Elevated urine levels of indoleacetic acid
Elevated urine levels of 17-ketosteroids
Elevated urine levels of steroids

R82.6   **Abnormal urine levels of substances chiefly nonmedicinal as to source**
Abnormal urine level of heavy metals

● R82.7   **Abnormal findings on microbiological examination of urine**
> **Excludes1**   colonization status (Z22.-)
Coding Clinic: 2016, Q4, P65

R82.71   **Bacteriuria**

R82.79   **Other abnormal findings on microbiological examination of urine**
Positive culture findings of urine

● R82.8   **Abnormal findings on cytological and histological examination of urine**

R82.81   **Pyuria**
Sterile pyuria
Coding Clinic: 2019, Q4, P16

R82.89   **Other abnormal findings on cytological and histological examination of urine**

● R82.9   **Other and unspecified abnormal findings in urine**

R82.90   **Unspecified abnormal findings in urine**

R82.91   **Other chromoabnormalities of urine**
Chromoconversion (dipstick)
Idiopathic dipstick converts positive for blood with no cellular forms in sediment
> **Excludes1**   hemoglobinuria (R82.3)
> myoglobinuria (R82.1)

● R82.99   **Other abnormal findings in urine**

R82.991   **Hypocitraturia**

R82.992   **Hyperoxaluria**
> **Excludes1**   Primary hyperoxaluria (E72.53)

R82.993   **Hyperuricosuria**

R82.994   **Hypercalciuria**
Idiopathic hypercalciuria

R82.998   **Other abnormal findings in urine**
Cells and casts in urine
Crystalluria
Melanuria

ABNORMAL FINDINGS ON EXAMINATION OF OTHER BODY FLUIDS, SUBSTANCES AND TISSUES, WITHOUT DIAGNOSIS (R83-R89)

> **Excludes1**   abnormal findings on antenatal screening of mother (O28.-)
> diagnostic abnormal findings classified elsewhere - see Alphabetical Index

> **Excludes2**   abnormal findings on examination of blood, without diagnosis (R70-R79)
> abnormal findings on examination of urine, without diagnosis (R80-R82)
> abnormal tumor markers (R97.-)

● R83   **Abnormal findings in cerebrospinal fluid**

R83.0   **Abnormal level of enzymes in cerebrospinal fluid**

R83.1   **Abnormal level of hormones in cerebrospinal fluid**

R83.2   **Abnormal level of other drugs, medicaments and biological substances in cerebrospinal fluid**

R83.3   **Abnormal level of substances chiefly nonmedicinal as to source in cerebrospinal fluid**

R83.4   **Abnormal immunological findings in cerebrospinal fluid**

R83.5   **Abnormal microbiological findings in cerebrospinal fluid**
Positive culture findings in cerebrospinal fluid
> **Excludes1**   colonization status (Z22.-)

R83.6   **Abnormal cytological findings in cerebrospinal fluid**

R83.8   **Other abnormal findings in cerebrospinal fluid**
Abnormal chromosomal findings in cerebrospinal fluid

R83.9   **Unspecified abnormal finding in cerebrospinal fluid**

● R84   **Abnormal findings in specimens from respiratory organs and thorax**
> **Includes**   abnormal findings in bronchial washings
> abnormal findings in nasal secretions
> abnormal findings in pleural fluid
> abnormal findings in sputum
> abnormal findings in throat scrapings
> **Excludes1**   blood-stained sputum (R04.2)

R84.0   **Abnormal level of enzymes in specimens from respiratory organs and thorax**

R84.1   **Abnormal level of hormones in specimens from respiratory organs and thorax**

R84.2   **Abnormal level of other drugs, medicaments and biological substances in specimens from respiratory organs and thorax**

R84.3   **Abnormal level of substances chiefly nonmedicinal as to source in specimens from respiratory organs and thorax**

R84.4   **Abnormal immunological findings in specimens from respiratory organs and thorax**

R84.5   **Abnormal microbiological findings in specimens from respiratory organs and thorax**
Positive culture findings in specimens from respiratory organs and thorax
> **Excludes1**   colonization status (Z22.-)

R84.6   **Abnormal cytological findings in specimens from respiratory organs and thorax**

R84.7   **Abnormal histological findings in specimens from respiratory organs and thorax**

R84.8   **Other abnormal findings in specimens from respiratory organs and thorax**
Abnormal chromosomal findings in specimens from respiratory organs and thorax

R84.9   **Unspecified abnormal finding in specimens from respiratory organs and thorax**

CHAPTER 18 (R00-R99)

● R85   **Abnormal findings in specimens from digestive organs and abdominal cavity**

   Includes   abnormal findings in peritoneal fluid
                  abnormal findings in saliva

   Excludes1 cloudy peritoneal dialysis effluent (R88.0)
                  fecal abnormalities (R19.5)

R85.0   **Abnormal level of enzymes in specimens from digestive organs and abdominal cavity**

R85.1   **Abnormal level of hormones in specimens from digestive organs and abdominal cavity**

R85.2   **Abnormal level of other drugs, medicaments and biological substances in specimens from digestive organs and abdominal cavity**

R85.3   **Abnormal level of substances chiefly nonmedicinal as to source in specimens from digestive organs and abdominal cavity**

R85.4   **Abnormal immunological findings in specimens from digestive organs and abdominal cavity**

R85.5   **Abnormal microbiological findings in specimens from digestive organs and abdominal cavity**
        Positive culture findings in specimens from digestive organs and abdominal cavity

        Excludes1   colonization status (Z22.-)

● R85.6   **Abnormal cytological findings in specimens from digestive organs and abdominal cavity**

   ● R85.61   **Abnormal cytologic smear of anus**

        Excludes1   abnormal cytological findings in specimens from other digestive organs and abdominal cavity (R85.69)
                        carcinoma in situ of anus (histologically confirmed) (D01.3)
                        anal intraepithelial neoplasia I [AIN I] (K62.82)
                        anal intraepithelial neoplasia II [AIN II] (K62.82)
                        anal intraepithelial neoplasia III [AIN III] (D01.3)
                        dysplasia (mild) (moderate) of anus (histologically confirmed) (K62.82)
                        severe dysplasia of anus (histologically confirmed) (D01.3)

        Excludes2   anal high risk human papillomavirus (HPV) DNA test positive (R85.81)
                        anal low risk human papillomavirus (HPV) DNA test positive (R85.82)

      R85.610   **Atypical squamous cells of undetermined significance on cytologic smear of anus (ASC-US)**

      R85.611   **Atypical squamous cells cannot exclude high grade squamous intraepithelial lesion on cytologic smear of anus (ASC-H)**

      R85.612   **Low grade squamous intraepithelial lesion on cytologic smear of anus (LGSIL)**

      R85.613   **High grade squamous intraepithelial lesion on cytologic smear of anus (HGSIL)**

      R85.614   **Cytologic evidence of malignancy on smear of anus**

      R85.615   **Unsatisfactory cytologic smear of anus**
                Inadequate sample of cytologic smear of anus

      R85.616   **Satisfactory anal smear but lacking transformation zone**

      R85.618   **Other abnormal cytological findings on specimens from anus**

      R85.619   **Unspecified abnormal cytological findings in specimens from anus**
                Abnormal anal cytology NOS
                Atypical glandular cells of anus NOS

   R85.69   **Abnormal cytological findings in specimens from other digestive organs and abdominal cavity**

R85.7   **Abnormal histological findings in specimens from digestive organs and abdominal cavity**

● R85.8   **Other abnormal findings in specimens from digestive organs and abdominal cavity**

   R85.81   **Anal high risk human papillomavirus (HPV) DNA test positive**

        Excludes1   anogenital warts due to human papillomavirus (HPV) (A63.0)
                        condyloma acuminatum (A63.0)

   R85.82   **Anal low risk human papillomavirus (HPV) DNA test positive**
            Use additional code for associated human papillomavirus (B97.7)

   R85.89   **Other abnormal findings in specimens from digestive organs and abdominal cavity**
            Abnormal chromosomal findings in specimens from digestive organs and abdominal cavity

R85.9   **Unspecified abnormal finding in specimens from digestive organs and abdominal cavity**

● R86   **Abnormal findings in specimens from male genital organs**

   Includes   abnormal findings in prostatic secretions
                  abnormal findings in semen, seminal fluid
                  abnormal spermatozoa

   Excludes1 azoospermia (N46.0-)
                  oligospermia (N46.1-)

R86.0   **Abnormal level of enzymes in specimens from male genital organs** ♂

R86.1   **Abnormal level of hormones in specimens from male genital organs** ♂

R86.2   **Abnormal level of other drugs, medicaments and biological substances in specimens from male genital organs** ♂

R86.3   **Abnormal level of substances chiefly nonmedicinal as to source in specimens from male genital organs** ♂

R86.4   **Abnormal immunological findings in specimens from male genital organs** ♂

R86.5   **Abnormal microbiological findings in specimens from male genital organs** ♂
        Positive culture findings in specimens from male genital organs

        Excludes1   colonization status (Z22.-)

R86.6   **Abnormal cytological findings in specimens from male genital organs** ♂

R86.7   **Abnormal histological findings in specimens from male genital organs** ♂

R86.8   **Other abnormal findings in specimens from male genital organs** ♂
        Abnormal chromosomal findings in specimens from male genital organs

R86.9   **Unspecified abnormal finding in specimens from male genital organs** ♂

▶ New   ⇒ Revised   ~~deleted~~ Deleted   Excludes 1   Excludes 2   Includes   Use additional   Code first   Code also   Key words
OGCR Official Guidelines   X Assign placeholder X   ● Use Additional Character(s)   ▷ Manifestation Code   ⌘ Hierarchical Condition Category   **Coding Clinic**

● R87   Abnormal findings in specimens from female genital organs

Includes	abnormal findings in secretion and smears from cervix uteri
	abnormal findings in secretion and smears from vagina
	abnormal findings in secretion and smears from vulva

R87.0   Abnormal level of enzymes in specimens from female genital organs ♀

R87.1   Abnormal level of hormones in specimens from female genital organs ♀

R87.2   Abnormal level of other drugs, medicaments and biological substances in specimens from female genital organs ♀

R87.3   Abnormal level of substances chiefly nonmedicinal as to source in specimens from female genital organs ♀

R87.4   Abnormal immunological findings in specimens from female genital organs ♀

R87.5   Abnormal microbiological findings in specimens from female genital organs ♀

Positive culture findings in specimens from female genital organs

Excludes1	colonization status (Z22.-)

● R87.6   Abnormal cytological findings in specimens from female genital organs

● R87.61   Abnormal cytological findings in specimens from cervix uteri

Excludes1	abnormal cytological findings in specimens from other female genital organs (R87.69)
	abnormal cytological findings in specimens from vagina (R87.62-)
	carcinoma in situ of cervix uteri (histologically confirmed) (D06.-)
	cervical intraepithelial neoplasia I [CIN I] (N87.0)
	cervical intraepithelial neoplasia II [CIN II] (N87.1)
	cervical intraepithelial neoplasia III [CIN III] (D06.-)
	dysplasia (mild) (moderate) of cervix uteri (histologically confirmed) (N87.-)
	severe dysplasia of cervix uteri (histologically confirmed) (D06.-)

Excludes2	cervical high risk human papillomavirus (HPV) DNA test positive (R87.810)
	cervical low risk human papillomavirus (HPV) DNA test positive (R87.820)

R87.610   Atypical squamous cells of undetermined significance on cytologic smear of cervix (ASC-US) ♀

R87.611   Atypical squamous cells cannot exclude high grade squamous intraepithelial lesion on cytologic smear of cervix (ASC-H) ♀

R87.612   Low grade squamous intraepithelial lesion on cytologic smear of cervix (LGSIL) ♀

R87.613   High grade squamous intraepithelial lesion on cytologic smear of cervix (HGSIL) ♀

R87.614   Cytologic evidence of malignancy on smear of cervix ♀

R87.615   Unsatisfactory cytologic smear of cervix ♀

Inadequate sample of cytologic smear of cervix

R87.616   Satisfactory cervical smear but lacking transformation zone ♀

R87.618   Other abnormal cytological findings on specimens from cervix uteri ♀

R87.619   Unspecified abnormal cytological findings in specimens from cervix uteri ♀

Abnormal cervical cytology NOS

Abnormal Papanicolaou smear of cervix NOS

Abnormal thin preparation smear of cervix NOS

Atypical endocervial cells of cervix NOS

Atypical endometrial cells of cervix NOS

Atypical glandular cells of cervix NOS

● R87.62   Abnormal cytological findings in specimens from vagina

Use additional code to identify acquired absence of uterus and cervix, if applicable (Z90.71-)

Excludes1	abnormal cytological findings in specimens from cervix uteri (R87.61-)
	abnormal cytological findings in specimens from other female genital organs (R87.69)
	carcinoma in situ of vagina (histologically confirmed) (D07.2)
	vaginal intraepithelial neoplasia I [VAIN I] (N89.0)
	vaginal intraepithelial neoplasia II [VAIN II] (N89.1)
	vaginal intraepithelial neoplasia III [VAIN III] (D07.2)
	dysplasia (mild) (moderate) of vagina (histologically confirmed) (N89.-)
	severe dysplasia of vagina (histologically confirmed) (D07.2)

Excludes2	vaginal high risk human papillomavirus (HPV) DNA test positive (R87.811)
	vaginal low risk human papillomavirus (HPV) DNA test positive (R87.821)

R87.620   Atypical squamous cells of undetermined significance on cytologic smear of vagina (ASC-US) ♀

R87.621   Atypical squamous cells cannot exclude high grade squamous intraepithelial lesion on cytologic smear of vagina (ASC-H) ♀

R87.622   Low grade squamous intraepithelial lesion on cytologic smear of vagina (LGSIL) ♀

R87.623   High grade squamous intraepithelial lesion on cytologic smear of vagina (HGSIL) ♀

R87.624   Cytologic evidence of malignancy on smear of vagina ♀

R87.625   Unsatisfactory cytologic smear of vagina ♀

Inadequate sample of cytologic smear of vagina

R87.628   Other abnormal cytological findings on specimens from vagina ♀

CHAPTER 18 (R00-R99)

R87.629   **Unspecified abnormal cytological findings in specimens from vagina** ♀
Abnormal Papanicolaou smear of vagina NOS
Abnormal thin preparation smear of vagina NOS
Abnormal vaginal cytology NOS
Atypical endocervical cells of vagina NOS
Atypical endometrial cells of vagina NOS
Atypical glandular cells of vagina NOS

R87.69   **Abnormal cytological findings in specimens from other female genital organs** ♀
Abnormal cytological findings in specimens from female genital organs NOS
Excludes1   dysplasia of vulva (histologically confirmed) (N90.0-N90.3)

R87.7   **Abnormal histological findings in specimens from female genital organs** ♀
Excludes1   carcinoma in situ (histologically confirmed) of female genital organs (D06-D07.3)
cervical intraepithelial neoplasia I [CIN I] (N87.0)
cervical intraepithelial neoplasia II [CIN II] (N87.1)
cervical intraepithelial neoplasia III [CIN III] (D06.-)
dysplasia (mild) (moderate) of cervix uteri (histologically confirmed) (N87.-)
dysplasia (mild) (moderate) of vagina (histologically confirmed) (N89.-)
vaginal intraepithelial neoplasia I [VAIN I] (N89.0)
vaginal intraepithelial neoplasia II [VAIN II] (N89.1)
vaginal intraepithelial neoplasia III [VAIN III] (D07.2)
severe dysplasia of cervix uteri (histologically confirmed) (D06.-)
severe dysplasia of vagina (histologically confirmed) (D07.2)

● R87.8   **Other abnormal findings in specimens from female genital organs**
   ● R87.81   **High risk human papillomavirus (HPV) DNA test positive from female genital organs**
Excludes1   anogenital warts due to human papillomavirus (HPV) (A63.0)
condyloma acuminatum (A63.0)

R87.810   **Cervical high risk human papillomavirus (HPV) DNA test positive** ♀

R87.811   **Vaginal high risk human papillomavirus (HPV) DNA test positive** ♀

   ● R87.82   **Low risk human papillomavirus (HPV) DNA test positive from female genital organs**
Use additional code for associated human papillomavirus (B97.7)

R87.820   **Cervical low risk human papillomavirus (HPV) DNA test positive** ♀

R87.821   **Vaginal low risk human papillomavirus (HPV) DNA test positive** ♀

R87.89   **Other abnormal findings in specimens from female genital organs** ♀
Abnormal chromosomal findings in specimens from female genital organs

R87.9   **Unspecified abnormal finding in specimens from female genital organs** ♀

● R88   **Abnormal findings in other body fluids and substances**
R88.0   **Cloudy (hemodialysis) (peritoneal) dialysis effluent**
R88.8   **Abnormal findings in other body fluids and substances**

● R89   **Abnormal findings in specimens from other organs, systems and tissues**
Includes   abnormal findings in nipple discharge
abnormal findings in synovial fluid
abnormal findings in wound secretions

R89.0   **Abnormal level of enzymes in specimens from other organs, systems and tissues**

R89.1   **Abnormal level of hormones in specimens from other organs, systems and tissues**

R89.2   **Abnormal level of other drugs, medicaments and biological substances in specimens from other organs, systems and tissues**

R89.3   **Abnormal level of substances chiefly nonmedicinal as to source in specimens from other organs, systems and tissues**

R89.4   **Abnormal immunological findings in specimens from other organs, systems and tissues**

R89.5   **Abnormal microbiological findings in specimens from other organs, systems and tissues**
Positive culture findings in specimens from other organs, systems and tissues
Excludes1   colonization status (Z22.-)

R89.6   **Abnormal cytological findings in specimens from other organs, systems and tissues**

R89.7   **Abnormal histological findings in specimens from other organs, systems and tissues**

R89.8   **Other abnormal findings in specimens from other organs, systems and tissues**
Abnormal chromosomal findings in specimens from other organs, systems and tissues

R89.9   **Unspecified abnormal finding in specimens from other organs, systems and tissues**

ABNORMAL FINDINGS ON DIAGNOSTIC IMAGING AND IN FUNCTION STUDIES, WITHOUT DIAGNOSIS (R90-R94)

Includes   nonspecific abnormal findings on diagnostic imaging by computerized axial tomography [CAT scan]
nonspecific abnormal findings on diagnostic imaging by magnetic resonance imaging [MRI][NMR]
nonspecific abnormal findings on diagnostic imaging by positron emission tomography [PET scan]
nonspecific abnormal findings on diagnostic imaging by thermography
nonspecific abnormal findings on diagnostic imaging by ultrasound [echogram]
nonspecific abnormal findings on diagnostic imaging by X-ray examination

Excludes1   abnormal findings on antenatal screening of mother (O28.-)
diagnostic abnormal findings classified elsewhere - see Alphabetical Index

● R90   **Abnormal findings on diagnostic imaging of central nervous system**
R90.0   **Intracranial space-occupying lesion found on diagnostic imaging of central nervous system**

● R90.8   **Other abnormal findings on diagnostic imaging of central nervous system**
R90.81   **Abnormal echoencephalogram**
R90.82   **White matter disease, unspecified**
R90.89   **Other abnormal findings on diagnostic imaging of central nervous system**
Other cerebrovascular abnormality found on diagnostic imaging of central nervous system

▶ New   ⇛ Revised   ~~deleted~~ Deleted   Excludes 1   Excludes 2   Includes   Use additional   Code first   Code also   Key words
OGCR Official Guidelines   X Assign placeholder X   ● Use Additional Character(s)   ▶ Manifestation Code   🏷 Hierarchical Condition Category   **Coding Clinic**

● **R91 Abnormal findings on diagnostic imaging of lung**

    R91.1 Solitary pulmonary nodule
        Coin lesion lung
        Solitary pulmonary nodule, subsegmental branch of the bronchial tree

    R91.8 Other nonspecific abnormal finding of lung field
        Lung mass NOS found on diagnostic imaging of lung
        Pulmonary infiltrate NOS
        Shadow, lung

● **R92 Abnormal and inconclusive findings on diagnostic imaging of breast**

    R92.0 Mammographic microcalcification found on diagnostic imaging of breast
        Excludes2 mammographic calcification (calculus) found on diagnostic imaging of breast (R92.1)

    R92.1 Mammographic calcification found on diagnostic imaging of breast
        Mammographic calculus found on diagnostic imaging of breast

    R92.2 Inconclusive mammogram
        Dense breasts NOS
        Inconclusive mammogram NEC
        Inconclusive mammography due to dense breasts
        Inconclusive mammography NEC
        Coding Clinic: 2015, Q1, P24

    R92.8 Other abnormal and inconclusive findings on diagnostic imaging of breast

● **R93 Abnormal findings on diagnostic imaging of other body structures**

    R93.0 Abnormal findings on diagnostic imaging of skull and head, not elsewhere classified
        Excludes1 intracranial space-occupying lesion found on diagnostic imaging (R90.0)

    R93.1 Abnormal findings on diagnostic imaging of heart and coronary circulation
        Abnormal echocardiogram NOS
        Abnormal heart shadow

    R93.2 Abnormal findings on diagnostic imaging of liver and biliary tract
        Nonvisualization of gallbladder

    R93.3 Abnormal findings on diagnostic imaging of other parts of digestive tract

●   **R93.4 Abnormal findings on diagnostic imaging of urinary organs**
        Excludes2 hypertrophy of kidney (N28.81)
        Coding Clinic: 2016, Q4, P66

        R93.41 Abnormal radiologic findings on diagnostic imaging of renal pelvis, ureter, or bladder
            Filling defect of bladder found on diagnostic imaging
            Filling defect of renal pelvis found on diagnostic imaging
            Filling defect of ureter found on diagnostic imaging

●   **R93.42 Abnormal radiologic findings on diagnostic imaging of kidney**
            R93.421 Abnormal radiologic findings on diagnostic imaging of right kidney
            R93.422 Abnormal radiologic findings on diagnostic imaging of left kidney
            R93.429 Abnormal radiologic findings on diagnostic imaging of unspecified kidney

        R93.49 Abnormal radiologic findings on diagnostic imaging of other urinary organs

    R93.5 Abnormal findings on diagnostic imaging of other abdominal regions, including retroperitoneum

    R93.6 Abnormal findings on diagnostic imaging of limbs
        Excludes2 abnormal finding in skin and subcutaneous tissue (R93.8-)
        Coding Clinic: 2020, Q1, P14

    R93.7 Abnormal findings on diagnostic imaging of other parts of musculoskeletal system
        Excludes2 abnormal findings on diagnostic imaging of skull (R93.0)

● **R93.8 Abnormal findings on diagnostic imaging of other specified body structures**

   ● **R93.81 Abnormal radiologic findings on diagnostic imaging of testis**
        R93.811 Abnormal radiologic findings on diagnostic imaging of right testicle ♂
        R93.812 Abnormal radiologic findings on diagnostic imaging of left testicle ♂
        R93.813 Abnormal radiologic findings on diagnostic imaging of testicles, bilateral ♂
        R93.819 Abnormal radiologic findings on diagnostic imaging of unspecified testicle ♂

        R93.89 Abnormal findings on diagnostic imaging of other specified body structures
            Abnormal finding by radioisotope localization of placenta
            Abnormal radiological finding in skin and subcutaneous tissue
            Mediastinal shift

    R93.9 Diagnostic imaging inconclusive due to excess body fat of patient

● **R94 Abnormal results of function studies**
    Includes abnormal results of radionuclide [radioisotope] uptake studies
                abnormal results of scintigraphy

● **R94.0 Abnormal results of function studies of central nervous system**
    R94.01 Abnormal electroencephalogram [EEG]
    R94.02 Abnormal brain scan
    R94.09 Abnormal results of other function studies of central nervous system

● **R94.1 Abnormal results of function studies of peripheral nervous system and special senses**

   ● **R94.11 Abnormal results of function studies of eye**
        R94.110 Abnormal electro-oculogram [EOG]
        R94.111 Abnormal electroretinogram [ERG]
            Abnormal retinal function study
        R94.112 Abnormal visually evoked potential [VEP]
        R94.113 Abnormal oculomotor study
        R94.118 Abnormal results of other function studies of eye

   ● **R94.12 Abnormal results of function studies of ear and other special senses**
        R94.120 Abnormal auditory function study
            Coding Clinic: 2016, Q3, P17
        R94.121 Abnormal vestibular function study
        R94.128 Abnormal results of other function studies of ear and other special senses

Trochlear nerve (IV)

Optic nerve (II)

Olfactory nerve (I)

Abducens nerve (VI)

Oculomotor nerve (III)

Facial nerve (VII)

Trigeminal nerve (V)

Vestibulocochlear nerve (VIII)

Glossopharyngeal nerve (IX)

Vagus nerve (X)

Accessory nerve (XI)

Hypoglossal nerve (XII)

Figure 18-2 Cranial nerves. (From Patton and Thibodeau: Anatomy and physiology, ed 7, St. Louis, Mosby, 2009)

Item 18–1 The **peripheral nervous system** consists of 31 pairs of spinal nerves, 12 pairs of cranial nerves, and the autonomic nerves, which are divided into the parasympathetic and sympathetic nerves. The cranial nerves are: olfactory (I), optic (II), oculomotor (III), trochlear (IV), trigeminal (V), abducens (VI), facial (VII), vestibulocochlear (VIII), glossopharyngeal (IX), vagus (X), accessory (XI), and hypoglossal (XII).

● **R94.13** **Abnormal results of function studies of peripheral nervous system**

　　　　R94.130 **Abnormal response to nerve stimulation, unspecified**

　　　　R94.131 **Abnormal electromyogram [EMG]**
　　　　　　　　Excludes1 electromyogram of eye (R94.113)

　　　　R94.138 **Abnormal results of other function studies of peripheral nervous system**

　R94.2 **Abnormal results of pulmonary function studies**
　　　　Reduced ventilatory capacity
　　　　Reduced vital capacity

● **R94.3** **Abnormal results of cardiovascular function studies**

　　　　R94.30 **Abnormal result of cardiovascular function study, unspecified**

　　　　R94.31 **Abnormal electrocardiogram [ECG] [EKG]**
　　　　　　　　Excludes1 long QT syndrome (I45.81)

　　　　R94.39 **Abnormal result of other cardiovascular function study**
　　　　　　　　Abnormal electrophysiological intracardiac studies
　　　　　　　　Abnormal phonocardiogram
　　　　　　　　Abnormal vectorcardiogram

　R94.4 **Abnormal results of kidney function studies**
　　　　Abnormal renal function test

　R94.5 **Abnormal results of liver function studies**

　R94.6 **Abnormal results of thyroid function studies**

　R94.7 **Abnormal results of other endocrine function studies**
　　　　Excludes2 abnormal glucose (R73.0-)

　R94.8 **Abnormal results of function studies of other organs and systems**
　　　　Abnormal basal metabolic rate [BMR]
　　　　Abnormal bladder function test
　　　　Abnormal splenic function test

ABNORMAL TUMOR MARKERS (R97)

● **R97** **Abnormal tumor markers**
　　　Elevated tumor associated antigens [TAA]
　　　Elevated tumor specific antigens [TSA]

　　R97.0 **Elevated carcinoembryonic antigen [CEA]**

　　R97.1 **Elevated cancer antigen 125 [CA 125]**

● **R97.2** **Elevated prostate specific antigen [PSA]**
　　　　Coding Clinic: 2016, Q4, P66

　　　　R97.20 **Elevated prostate specific antigen [PSA]** ♂   A

　　　　R97.21 **Rising PSA following treatment for malignant neoplasm of prostate** ♂   A

　　R97.8 **Other abnormal tumor markers**

ILL-DEFINED AND UNKNOWN CAUSE OF MORTALITY (R99)

R99 **Ill-defined and unknown cause of mortality**
　　Death (unexplained) NOS
　　Unspecified cause of mortality

OGCR Section I.C.18.h.

Death NOS

Code R99, Ill-defined and unknown cause of mortality, is only for use in the very limited circumstance when a patient who has already died is brought into the emergency department or other healthcare facility and is pronounced dead upon arrival. It does not represent the discharge disposition of death.

▶ New　⇒ Revised　~~deleted~~ Deleted　Excludes 1　Excludes 2　Includes　Use additional　Code first　Code also　Key words

OGCR Official Guidelines　X Assign placeholder X　● Use Additional Character(s)　▶ Manifestation Code　🐱 Hierarchical Condition Category　**Coding Clinic**

CHAPTER 19

INJURY, POISONING AND CERTAIN OTHER CONSEQUENCES OF EXTERNAL CAUSES (S00-T88)

OGCR Chapter-Specific Coding Guidelines

19. **Chapter 19: Injury, poisoning, and certain other consequences of external causes (S00-T88)**

   a. **Application of 7th Characters in Chapter 19**
   Most categories in Chapter 19 have a 7th character requirement for each applicable code. Most categories in this chapter have three 7th character values (with the exception of fractures): A, initial encounter, D, subsequent encounter and S, sequela. Categories for traumatic fractures have additional 7th character values. While the patient may be seen by a new or different provider over the course of treatment for an injury, assignment of the 7th character is based on whether the patient is undergoing active treatment and not whether the provider is seeing the patient for the first time.

   For complication codes, active treatment refers to treatment for the condition described by the code, even though it may be related to an earlier precipitating problem. For example, code T84.50XA, Infection and inflammatory reaction due to unspecified internal joint prosthesis, initial encounter, is used when active treatment is provided for the infection, even though the condition relates to the prosthetic device, implant or graft that was placed at a previous encounter.

   7th character "A", initial encounter is used for each encounter where the patient is receiving active treatment for the condition.

   7th character "D" subsequent encounter is used for encounters after the patient has completed active treatment of the condition and is receiving routine care for the condition during the healing or recovery phase.

   The aftercare Z codes should not be used for aftercare for conditions such as injuries or poisonings, where 7th characters are provided to identify subsequent care. For example, for aftercare of an injury, assign the acute injury code with the 7th character "D" (subsequent encounter).

   7th character "S", sequela, is for use for complications or conditions that arise as a direct result of a condition, such as scar formation after a burn. The scars are sequelae of the burn. When using 7th character "S", it is necessary to use both the injury code that precipitated the sequela and the code for the sequela itself. The "S" is added only to the injury code, not the sequela code. The 7th character "S" identifies the injury responsible for the sequela. The specific type of sequela (e.g. scar) is sequenced first, followed by the injury code.
   See Section I.B.10. Sequelae, (Late Effects).

   b. **Coding of Injuries**
   When coding injuries, assign separate codes for each injury unless a combination code is provided, in which case the combination code is assigned. Codes from category T07, Unspecified multiple injuries should not be assigned in the inpatient setting unless information for a more specific code is not available. Traumatic injury codes (S00-T14.9) are not to be used for normal, healing surgical wounds or to identify complications of surgical wounds.

   The code for the most serious injury, as determined by the provider and the focus of treatment, is sequenced first.

   1) **Superficial injuries**
   Superficial injuries such as abrasions or contusions are not coded when associated with more severe injuries of the same site.

   2) **Primary injury with damage to nerves/blood vessels**
   When a primary injury results in minor damage to peripheral nerves or blood vessels, the primary injury is sequenced first with additional code(s) for injuries to nerves and spinal cord (such as category S04), and/or injury to blood vessels (such as category S15). When the primary injury is to the blood vessels or nerves, that injury should be sequenced first.

   c. **Coding of Traumatic Fractures**
   The principles of multiple coding of injuries should be followed in coding fractures. Fractures of specified sites are coded individually by site in accordance with both the provisions within

categories S02, S12, S22, S32, S42, S49, S52, S59, S62, S72, S79, S82, S89, S92 and the level of detail furnished by medical record content.

A fracture not indicated as open or closed should be coded to closed. A fracture not indicated whether displaced or not displaced should be coded to displaced.

More specific guidelines are as follows:

   1) **Initial vs. Subsequent Encounter for Fractures**
   Traumatic fractures are coded using the appropriate 7th character for initial encounter (A, B, C) for each encounter where the patient is receiving active treatment for the fracture. The appropriate 7th character for initial encounter should also be assigned for a patient who delayed seeking treatment for the fracture or nonunion.

   Fractures are coded using the appropriate 7th character for subsequent care for encounters after the patient has completed active treatment of the fracture and is receiving routine care for the fracture during the healing or recovery phase.

   Care for complications of surgical treatment for fracture repairs during the healing or recovery phase should be coded with the appropriate complication codes.

   Care of complications of fractures, such as malunion and nonunion, should be reported with the appropriate 7th character for subsequent care with nonunion (K, M, N,) or subsequent care with malunion (P, Q, R).

   Malunion/nonunion: The appropriate 7th character for initial encounter should also be assigned for a patient who delayed seeking treatment for the fracture or nonunion.

   The open fracture designations in the assignment of the 7th character for fractures of the forearm, femur and lower leg, including ankle are based on the Gustilo open fracture classification. When the Gustilo classification type is not specified for an open fracture, the 7th character for open fracture type I or II should be assigned (B, E, H, M, Q).

   A code from category M80, not a traumatic fracture code, should be used for any patient with known osteoporosis who suffers a fracture, even if the patient had a minor fall or trauma, if that fall or trauma would not usually break a normal, healthy bone.
   See Section I.C.13. Osteoporosis.

   The aftercare Z codes should not be used for aftercare for traumatic fractures. For aftercare of a traumatic fracture, assign the acute fracture code with the appropriate 7th character.

   2) **Multiple fractures sequencing**
   Multiple fractures are sequenced in accordance with the severity of the fracture.

   d. **Coding of Burns and Corrosions**
   The ICD-10-CM makes a distinction between burns and corrosions. The burn codes are for thermal burns, except sunburns, that come from a heat source, such as a fire or hot appliance. The burn codes are also for burns resulting from electricity and radiation. Corrosions are burns due to chemicals. The guidelines are the same for burns and corrosions.

   Current burns (T20-T25) are classified by depth, extent and by agent (X code). Burns are classified by depth as first degree (erythema), second degree (blistering), and third degree (full-thickness involvement). Burns of the eye and internal organs (T26-T28) are classified by site, but not by degree.

   1) **Sequencing of burn and related condition codes**
   Sequence first the code that reflects the highest degree of burn when more than one burn is present.

   a. When the reason for the admission or encounter is for treatment of external multiple burns, sequence first the code that reflects the burn of the highest degree.

   b. When a patient has both internal and external burns, the circumstances of admission govern the selection of the principal diagnosis or first-listed diagnosis.

   c. When a patient is admitted for burn injuries and other related conditions such as smoke inhalation and/or respiratory failure, the circumstances of admission govern the selection of the principal or first-listed diagnosis.

2) Burns of the same *anatomic* site
Classify burns of the same anatomic site and on the same side but of different degrees to the subcategory identifying the highest degree recorded in the diagnosis (e.g., for second- and third-degree burns of right thigh, assign only code T24.311-).

3) Non-healing burns
Non-healing burns are coded as acute burns.
Necrosis of burned skin should be coded as a non-healed burn.

4) Infected Burn
For any documented infected burn site, use an additional code for the infection.

5) Assign separate codes for each burn site
When coding burns, assign separate codes for each burn site. Category T30, Burn and corrosion, body region unspecified is extremely vague and should rarely be used.
Codes for burns of "multiple sites" should only be assigned when the medical record documentation does not specify the individual sites.

6) Burns and Corrosions Classified According to Extent of Body Surface Involved
Assign codes from category T31, Burns classified according to extent of body surface involved, or T32, Corrosions classified according to extent of body surface involved, when the site of the burn is not specified or when there is a need for additional data. It is advisable to use category T31 as additional coding when needed to provide data for evaluating burn mortality, such as that needed by burn units. It is also advisable to use category T31 as an additional code for reporting purposes when there is mention of a third-degree burn involving 20 percent or more of the body surface.
Categories T31 and T32 are based on the classic "rule of nines" in estimating body surface involved: head and neck are assigned nine percent, each arm nine percent, each leg 18 percent, the anterior trunk 18 percent, posterior trunk 18 percent, and genitalia one percent. Providers may change these percentage assignments where necessary to accommodate infants and children who have proportionally larger heads than adults, and patients who have large buttocks, thighs, or abdomen that involve burns.

7) Encounters for treatment of sequela of burns
Encounters for the treatment of the late effects of burns or corrosions (i.e., scars or joint contractures) should be coded with a burn or corrosion code with the 7th character "S" for sequela.

8) Sequelae with a late effect code and current burn
When appropriate, both a code for a current burn or corrosion with 7th character "A" or "D" and a burn or corrosion code with 7th character "S" may be assigned on the same record (when both a current burn and sequelae of an old burn exist). Burns and corrosions do not heal at the same rate and a current healing wound may still exist with sequela of a healed burn or corrosion.
See Section I.B.10. Sequela, (Late Effects).

9) Use of an external cause code with burns and corrosions
An external cause code should be used with burns and corrosions to identify the source and intent of the burn, as well as the place where it occurred.

e. Adverse Effects, Poisoning , Underdosing and Toxic Effects
Codes in categories T36-T65 are combination codes that include the substance that was taken as well as the intent. No additional external cause code is required for poisonings, toxic effects, adverse effects and underdosing codes.

1) Do not code directly from the Table of Drugs
Do not code directly from the Table of Drugs and Chemicals. Always refer back to the Tabular List.

2) Use as many codes as necessary to describe
Use as many codes as necessary to describe completely all drugs, medicinal or biological substances.

3) If the same code would describe the causative agent
If the same code would describe the causative agent for more than one adverse reaction, poisoning, toxic effect or underdosing, assign the code only once.

4) If two or more drugs, medicinal or biological substances
If two or more drugs, medicinal or biological substances are reported, code each individually unless a combination code is listed in the Table of Drugs and Chemicals.

5) The occurrence of drug toxicity is classified in ICD-10-CM as follows:

(a) Adverse Effect
When coding an adverse effect of a drug that has been correctly prescribed and properly administered, assign the appropriate code for the nature of the adverse effect followed by the appropriate code for the adverse effect of the drug (T36-T50). The code for the drug should have a 5th or 6th character "5" (for example T36.0X5-) Examples of the nature of an adverse effect are tachycardia, delirium, gastrointestinal hemorrhaging, vomiting, hypokalemia, hepatitis, renal failure, or respiratory failure.

(b) Poisoning
When coding a poisoning or reaction to the improper use of a medication (e.g., overdose, wrong substance given or taken in error, wrong route of administration), first assign the appropriate code from categories T36-T50. The poisoning codes have an associated intent as their 5th or 6th character (accidental, intentional self-harm, assault and undetermined). If the intent of the poisoning is unknown or unspecified, code the intent as accidental intent. The undetermined intent is only for use if the documentation in the record specifies that the intent cannot be determined. Use additional code(s) for all manifestations of poisonings.
If there is also a diagnosis of abuse or dependence of the substance, the abuse or dependence is assigned as an additional code.
Examples of poisoning include:

(i) Error was made in drug prescription
Errors made in drug prescription or in the administration of the drug by provider, nurse, patient, or other person.

(ii) Overdose of a drug intentionally taken If an overdose of a drug was intentionally taken or administered and resulted in drug toxicity, it would be coded as a poisoning.

(iii) Nonprescribed drug taken with correctly prescribed and properly administered drug. If a nonprescribed drug or medicinal agent was taken in combination with a correctly prescribed and properly administered drug, any drug toxicity or other reaction resulting from the interaction of the two drugs would be classified as a poisoning.

(iv) Interaction of drug(s) and alcohol. When a reaction results from the interaction of a drug(s) and alcohol, this would be classified as poisoning.
See Section I.C.4. if poisoning is the result of insulin pump malfunctions.

(c) Underdosing
Underdosing refers to taking less of a medication than is prescribed by a provider or a manufacturer's instruction. Discontinuing the use of a prescribed medication on the patient's own initiative (not directed by the patient's provider) is also classified as an underdosing. For underdosing, assign the code from categories T36-T50 (fifth or sixth character "6").

Codes for underdosing should never be assigned as principal or first-listed codes. If a patient has a relapse or exacerbation of the medical condition for which the drug is prescribed because of the reduction in dose, then the medical condition itself should be coded.

Noncompliance (Z91.12-, Z91.13- and Z91.14-) or complication of care (Y63.6-Y63.9) codes are to be used with an underdosing code to indicate intent, if known.

(d) Toxic Effects

When a harmful substance is ingested or comes in contact with a person, this is classified as a toxic effect. The toxic effect codes are in categories T51-T65.

Toxic effect codes have an associated intent: accidental, intentional self-harm, assault and undetermined.

f. Adult and child abuse, neglect and other maltreatment

Sequence first the appropriate code from categories T74 (Adult and child abuse, neglect and other maltreatment, confirmed) or T76 (Adult and child abuse, neglect and other maltreatment, suspected) for abuse, neglect and other maltreatment, followed by any accompanying mental health or injury code(s).

If the documentation in the medical record states abuse or neglect it is coded as confirmed (T74.-). It is coded as suspected if it is documented as suspected (T76.-).

For cases of confirmed abuse or neglect an external cause code from the assault section (X92-Y09) should be added to identify the cause of any physical injuries. A perpetrator code (Y07) should be added when the perpetrator of the abuse is known. For suspected cases of abuse or neglect, do not report external cause or perpetrator code.

If a suspected case of abuse, neglect or mistreatment is ruled out during an encounter code Z04.71, Encounter for examination and observation following alleged physical adult abuse, ruled out, or code Z04.72, Encounter for examination and observation following alleged child physical abuse, ruled out, should be used, not a code from T76.

If a suspected case of alleged rape or sexual abuse is ruled out during an encounter code Z04.41, Encounter for examination and observation following alleged adult rape or code Z04.42, Encounter for examination and observation following alleged child rape, should be used, not a code from T76.

If a suspected case of forced sexual exploitation or forced labor exploitation is ruled out during an encounter, code Z04.81, Encounter for examination and observation of victim following forced sexual exploitation, or code Z04.82, Encounter for examination and observation of victim following forced labor exploitation, should be used, not a code from T76.

See Section I.C.15. Abuse in a pregnant patient.

g. Complications of care

1) General guidelines for complications of care

(a) Documentation of complications of care

See Section I.B.16. for information on documentation of complications of care.

2) Pain due to medical devices

Pain associated with devices, implants or grafts left in a surgical site (for example painful hip prosthesis) is assigned to the appropriate code(s) found in Chapter 19, Injury, poisoning, and certain other consequences of external causes. Specific codes for pain due to medical devices are found in the T code section of the ICD-10-CM. Use additional code(s) from category G89 to identify acute or chronic pain due to presence of the device, implant or graft (G89.18 or G89.28).

3) Transplant complications

(a) Transplant complications other than kidney

Codes under category T86, Complications of transplanted organs and tissues, are for use for both complications and rejection of transplanted organs. A transplant complication code is only assigned if the complication affects the function of the transplanted organ. Two codes are required to fully describe a transplant complication: the appropriate code from category T86 and a secondary code that identifies the complication.

Pre-existing conditions or conditions that develop after the transplant are not coded as complications unless they affect the function of the transplanted organs.

See I.C.21. for transplant organ removal status.

See I.C.2. for malignant neoplasm associated with transplanted organ.

(b) Kidney transplant complications

Patients who have undergone kidney transplant may still have some form of chronic kidney disease (CKD) because the kidney transplant may not fully restore kidney function. Code T86.1- should be assigned for documented complications of a kidney transplant, such as transplant failure or rejection or other transplant complication. Code T86.1- should not be assigned for post kidney transplant patients who have chronic kidney (CKD) unless a transplant complication such as transplant failure or rejection is documented. If the documentation is unclear as to whether the patient has a complication of the transplant, query the provider.

Conditions that affect the function of the transplanted kidney, other than CKD, should be assigned a code from subcategory T86.1, Complications of transplanted organ, Kidney, and a secondary code that identifies the complication.

For patients with CKD following a kidney transplant, but who do not have a complication such as failure or rejection, *see Section I.C.14. Chronic kidney disease and kidney transplant status.*

4) Complication codes that include the external cause

As with certain other T codes, some of the complications of care codes have the external cause included in the code. The code includes the nature of the complication as well as the type of procedure that caused the complication. No external cause code indicating the type of procedure is necessary for these codes.

5) Complications of care codes within the body system chapters

Intraoperative and postprocedural complication codes are found within the body system chapters with codes specific to the organs and structures of that body system. These codes should be sequenced first, followed by a code(s) for the specific complication, if applicable.

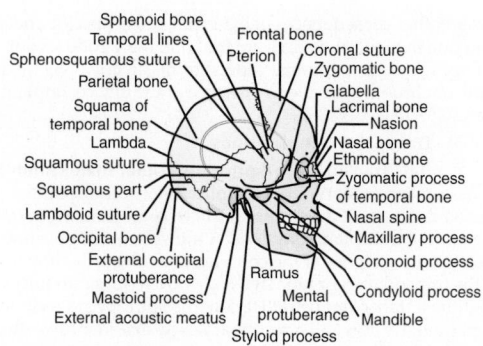

Figure 19-1 Lateral view of skull.

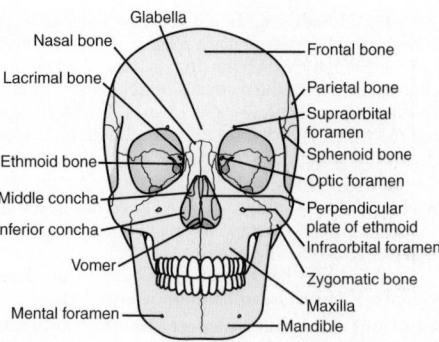

Figure 19-2 Frontal view of skull.

Figure 19-3 Anterior view of vertebral column.

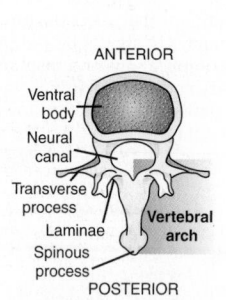

Figure 19-4 Vertebra viewed from above.

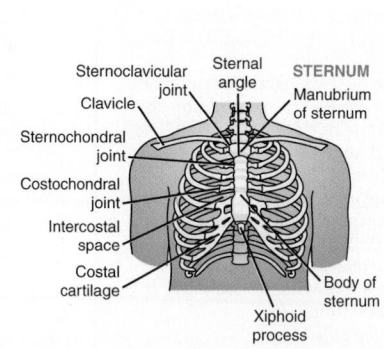

Figure 19-5 Anterior view of rib cage.

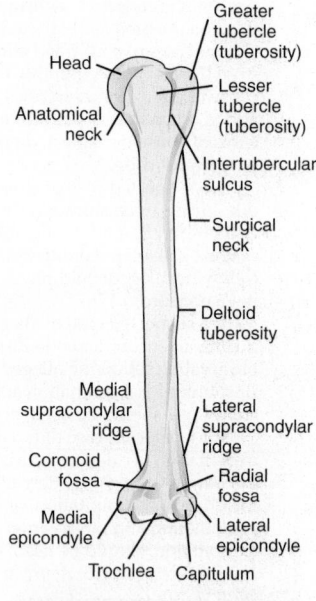

Figure 19-6 Anterior aspect of left humerus.

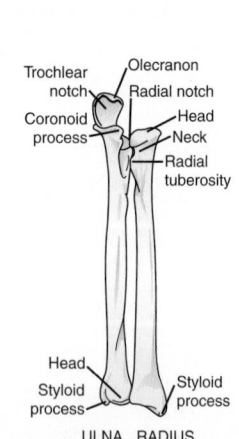

Figure 19-7 Anterior aspect of left radius and ulna.

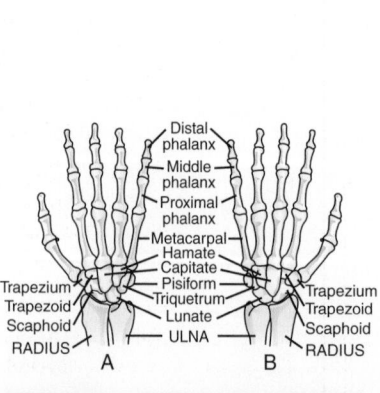

Figure 19-8 Right hand and wrist: **A.** Dorsal surface. **B.** Palmar surface.

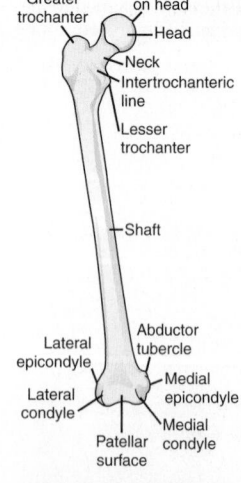

Figure 19-9 Anterior aspect of right femur.

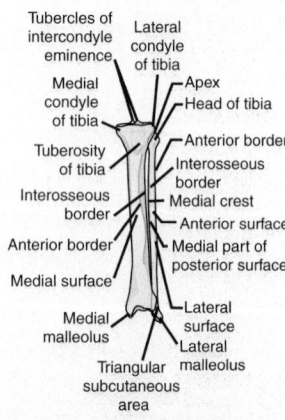

Figure 19-10 Anterior aspect of left tibia and fibula.

CHAPTER 19 (S00-T88)

▶ New ⟹ Revised ~~deleted~~ Deleted Excludes 1 Excludes 2 Includes Use additional Code first Code also Key words

OGCR Official Guidelines X Assign placeholder X ● Use Additional Character(s) ▸ Manifestation Code ⌖ Hierarchical Condition Category **Coding Clinic**

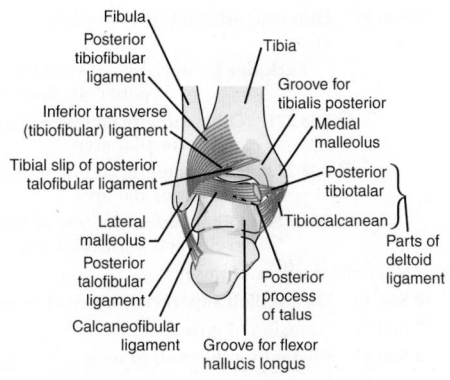

Figure 19-11 Posterior aspect of the left ankle joint.

Figure 19-12 Right foot viewed from above.

CHAPTER 19

INJURY, POISONING AND CERTAIN OTHER CONSEQUENCES OF EXTERNAL CAUSES (S00-T88)

Note: Use secondary code(s) from Chapter 20, External causes of morbidity, to indicate cause of injury. Codes within the T section that include the external cause do not require an additional external cause code.

Use additional code to identify any retained foreign body, if applicable (Z18.-)

Excludes1   birth trauma (P10-P15)
                obstetric trauma (O70-O71)

Note: The chapter uses the S-section for coding different types of injuries related to single body regions and the T-section to cover injuries to unspecified body regions as well as poisoning and certain other consequences of external causes.

This chapter contains the following blocks:

S00-S09	Injuries to the head
S10-S19	Injuries to the neck
S20-S29	Injuries to the thorax
S30-S39	Injuries to the abdomen, lower back, lumbar spine, pelvis and external genitals
S40-S49	Injuries to the shoulder and upper arm
S50-S59	Injuries to the elbow and forearm
S60-S69	Injuries to the wrist, hand, and fingers
S70-S79	Injuries to the hip and thigh
S80-S89	Injuries to the knee and lower leg
S90-S99	Injuries to the ankle and foot

T07	Injuries involving multiple body regions
T14	Injury of unspecified body region
T15-T19	Effects of foreign body entering through natural orifice
T20-T25	Burns and corrosions of external body surface, specified by site
T26-T28	Burns and corrosions confined to eye and internal organs
T30-T32	Burns and corrosions of multiple and unspecified body regions
T33-T34	Frostbite
T36-T50	Poisoning by, adverse effect of and underdosing of drugs, medicaments and biological substances
T51-T65	Toxic effects of substances chiefly nonmedicinal as to source
T66-T78	Other and unspecified effects of external causes
T79	Certain early complications of trauma
T80-T88	Complications of surgical and medical care, not elsewhere classified

INJURIES TO THE HEAD (S00-S09)

Includes   injuries of ear
              injuries of eye
              injuries of face [any part]
              injuries of gum
              injuries of jaw
              injuries of oral cavity
              injuries of palate
              injuries of periocular area
              injuries of scalp
              injuries of temporomandibular joint area
              injuries of tongue
              injuries of tooth

Code also for any associated infection

Excludes2   burns and corrosions (T20-T32)
              effects of foreign body in ear (T16)
              effects of foreign body in larynx (T17.3)
              effects of foreign body in mouth NOS (T18.0)
              effects of foreign body in nose (T17.0-T17.1)
              effects of foreign body in pharynx (T17.2)
              effects of foreign body on external eye (T15.-)
              frostbite (T33-T34)
              insect bite or sting, venomous (T63.4)

● S00   **Superficial injury of head**

Excludes1   diffuse cerebral contusion (S06.2-)
              focal cerebral contusion (S06.3-)
              injury of eye and orbit (S05.-)
              open wound of head (S01.-)

The appropriate 7th character is to be added to each code from category S00

A	initial encounter
	All encounters involving diagnosis and treatment
D	subsequent encounter
	Encounters during the healing phase
S	sequela

● S00.0   **Superficial injury of scalp**

X● S00.00   **Unspecified superficial injury of scalp**

X● S00.01   **Abrasion of scalp**

X● S00.02   **Blister (nonthermal) of scalp**

X● S00.03   **Contusion of scalp**
              Bruise of scalp
              Hematoma of scalp

X● S00.04   **External constriction of part of scalp**

X● S00.05   **Superficial foreign body of scalp**
              Splinter in the scalp

X● S00.06   **Insect bite (nonvenomous) of scalp**

X● S00.07   **Other superficial bite of scalp**
              Excludes1   open bite of scalp (S01.05)

● **S00.1**   **Contusion of eyelid and periocular area**
Black eye
> **Excludes2**   contusion of eyeball and orbital tissues (S05.1-)

X ● **S00.10**   Contusion of unspecified eyelid and periocular area

X ● **S00.11**   Contusion of right eyelid and periocular area

X ● **S00.12**   Contusion of left eyelid and periocular area

● **S00.2**   **Other and unspecified superficial injuries of eyelid and periocular area**
> **Excludes2**   superficial injury of conjunctiva and cornea (S05.0-)

● **S00.20**   Unspecified superficial injury of eyelid and periocular area

  ● **S00.201**   Unspecified superficial injury of right eyelid and periocular area

  ● **S00.202**   Unspecified superficial injury of left eyelid and periocular area

  ● **S00.209**   Unspecified superficial injury of unspecified eyelid and periocular area

● **S00.21**   Abrasion of eyelid and periocular area

  ● **S00.211**   Abrasion of right eyelid and periocular area

  ● **S00.212**   Abrasion of left eyelid and periocular area

  ● **S00.219**   Abrasion of unspecified eyelid and periocular area

● **S00.22**   Blister (nonthermal) of eyelid and periocular area

  ● **S00.221**   Blister (nonthermal) of right eyelid and periocular area

  ● **S00.222**   Blister (nonthermal) of left eyelid and periocular area

  ● **S00.229**   Blister (nonthermal) of unspecified eyelid and periocular area

● **S00.24**   External constriction of eyelid and periocular area

  ● **S00.241**   External constriction of right eyelid and periocular area

  ● **S00.242**   External constriction of left eyelid and periocular area

  ● **S00.249**   External constriction of unspecified eyelid and periocular area

● **S00.25**   Superficial foreign body of eyelid and periocular area
Splinter of eyelid and periocular area
> **Excludes2**   retained foreign body in eyelid (H02.81-)

  ● **S00.251**   Superficial foreign body of right eyelid and periocular area

  ● **S00.252**   Superficial foreign body of left eyelid and periocular area

  ● **S00.259**   Superficial foreign body of unspecified eyelid and periocular area

● **S00.26**   Insect bite (nonvenomous) of eyelid and periocular area

  ● **S00.261**   Insect bite (nonvenomous) of right eyelid and periocular area

  ● **S00.262**   Insect bite (nonvenomous) of left eyelid and periocular area

  ● **S00.269**   Insect bite (nonvenomous) of unspecified eyelid and periocular area

● **S00.27**   Other superficial bite of eyelid and periocular area
> **Excludes1**   open bite of eyelid and periocular area (S01.15)

  ● **S00.271**   Other superficial bite of right eyelid and periocular area

  ● **S00.272**   Other superficial bite of left eyelid and periocular area

  ● **S00.279**   Other superficial bite of unspecified eyelid and periocular area

● **S00.3**   **Superficial injury of nose**

X ● **S00.30**   Unspecified superficial injury of nose

X ● **S00.31**   Abrasion of nose

X ● **S00.32**   Blister (nonthermal) of nose

X ● **S00.33**   Contusion of nose
Bruise of nose
Hematoma of nose

X ● **S00.34**   External constriction of nose

X ● **S00.35**   Superficial foreign body of nose
Splinter in the nose

X ● **S00.36**   Insect bite (nonvenomous) of nose

X ● **S00.37**   Other superficial bite of nose
> **Excludes1**   open bite of nose (S01.25)

● **S00.4**   **Superficial injury of ear**

● **S00.40**   Unspecified superficial injury of ear

  ● **S00.401**   Unspecified superficial injury of right ear

  ● **S00.402**   Unspecified superficial injury of left ear

  ● **S00.409**   Unspecified superficial injury of unspecified ear

● **S00.41**   Abrasion of ear

  ● **S00.411**   Abrasion of right ear

  ● **S00.412**   Abrasion of left ear

  ● **S00.419**   Abrasion of unspecified ear

● **S00.42**   Blister (nonthermal) of ear

  ● **S00.421**   Blister (nonthermal) of right ear

  ● **S00.422**   Blister (nonthermal) of left ear

  ● **S00.429**   Blister (nonthermal) of unspecified ear

● **S00.43**   Contusion of ear
Bruise of ear
Hematoma of ear

  ● **S00.431**   Contusion of right ear

  ● **S00.432**   Contusion of left ear

  ● **S00.439**   Contusion of unspecified ear

● **S00.44**   External constriction of ear

  ● **S00.441**   External constriction of right ear

  ● **S00.442**   External constriction of left ear

  ● **S00.449**   External constriction of unspecified ear

● **S00.45**   Superficial foreign body of ear
Splinter in the ear

  ● **S00.451**   Superficial foreign body of right ear

  ● **S00.452**   Superficial foreign body of left ear

  ● **S00.459**   Superficial foreign body of unspecified ear

● **S00.46**   Insect bite (nonvenomous) of ear

  ● **S00.461**   Insect bite (nonvenomous) of right ear

  ● **S00.462**   Insect bite (nonvenomous) of left ear

  ● **S00.469**   Insect bite (nonvenomous) of unspecified ear

▶ New   ⇒ Revised   ~~deleted~~ Deleted   Excludes 1   Excludes 2   Includes   Use additional   Code first   Code also   Key words

OGCR Official Guidelines   X Assign placeholder X   ● Use Additional Character(s)   ▷ Manifestation Code   🔖 Hierarchical Condition Category   **Coding Clinic**

● **S00.47**   **Other superficial bite of ear**
     Excludes1   open bite of ear (S01.35)
   ● **S00.471**   Other superficial bite of right ear
   ● **S00.472**   Other superficial bite of left ear
   ● **S00.479**   Other superficial bite of unspecified ear

● **S00.5**   **Superficial injury of lip and oral cavity**
  ● **S00.50**   Unspecified superficial injury of lip and oral cavity
   ● **S00.501**   Unspecified superficial injury of lip
   ● **S00.502**   Unspecified superficial injury of oral cavity
  ● **S00.51**   Abrasion of lip and oral cavity
   ● **S00.511**   Abrasion of lip
   ● **S00.512**   Abrasion of oral cavity
  ● **S00.52**   Blister (nonthermal) of lip and oral cavity
   ● **S00.521**   Blister (nonthermal) of lip
   ● **S00.522**   Blister (nonthermal) of oral cavity
  ● **S00.53**   Contusion of lip and oral cavity
   ● **S00.531**   Contusion of lip
     Bruise of lip
     Hematoma of lip
   ● **S00.532**   Contusion of oral cavity
     Bruise of oral cavity
     Hematoma of oral cavity
  ● **S00.54**   External constriction of lip and oral cavity
   ● **S00.541**   External constriction of lip
   ● **S00.542**   External constriction of oral cavity
  ● **S00.55**   Superficial foreign body of lip and oral cavity
   ● **S00.551**   Superficial foreign body of lip
     Splinter of lip and oral cavity
   ● **S00.552**   Superficial foreign body of oral cavity
     Splinter of lip and oral cavity
  ● **S00.56**   Insect bite (nonvenomous) of lip and oral cavity
   ● **S00.561**   Insect bite (nonvenomous) of lip
   ● **S00.562**   Insect bite (nonvenomous) of oral cavity
  ● **S00.57**   Other superficial bite of lip and oral cavity
   ● **S00.571**   Other superficial bite of lip
     Excludes1   open bite of lip (S01.551)
   ● **S00.572**   Other superficial bite of oral cavity
     Excludes1   open bite of oral cavity (S01.552)

● **S00.8**   **Superficial injury of other parts of head**
   Superficial injuries of face [any part]
  X ● **S00.80**   Unspecified superficial injury of other part of head
  X ● **S00.81**   Abrasion of other part of head
  X ● **S00.82**   Blister (nonthermal) of other part of head
  X ● **S00.83**   Contusion of other part of head
     Bruise of other part of head
     Hematoma of other part of head
  X ● **S00.84**   External constriction of other part of head
  X ● **S00.85**   Superficial foreign body of other part of head
     Splinter in other part of head
  X ● **S00.86**   Insect bite (nonvenomous) of other part of head
  X ● **S00.87**   Other superficial bite of other part of head
     Excludes1   open bite of other part of head (S01.85)

● **S00.9**   **Superficial injury of unspecified part of head**
  X ● **S00.90**   Unspecified superficial injury of unspecified part of head
  X ● **S00.91**   Abrasion of unspecified part of head
  X ● **S00.92**   Blister (nonthermal) of unspecified part of head

  X ● **S00.93**   **Contusion of unspecified part of head**
     Bruise of head
     Hematoma of head
  X ● **S00.94**   **External constriction of unspecified part of head**
  X ● **S00.95**   **Superficial foreign body of unspecified part of head**
     Splinter of head
  X ● **S00.96**   **Insect bite (nonvenomous) of unspecified part of head**
  X ● **S00.97**   **Other superficial bite of unspecified part of head**
     Excludes1   open bite of head (S01.95)

● **S01**   **Open wound of head**
   Code also any associated:
     injury of cranial nerve (S04.-)
     injury of muscle and tendon of head (S09.1-)
     intracranial injury (S06.-)
     wound infection
   Excludes1   open skull fracture (S02.- with 7th character B)
   Excludes2   injury of eye and orbit (S05.-)
     traumatic amputation of part of head (S08.-)
   The appropriate 7th character is to be added to each code from category S01

     | | |
     A   initial encounter
     D   subsequent encounter
     S   sequela

● **S01.0**   **Open wound of scalp**
   Excludes1   avulsion of scalp (S08.0-)
  X ● **S01.00**   Unspecified open wound of scalp
  X ● **S01.01**   Laceration without foreign body of scalp
  X ● **S01.02**   Laceration with foreign body of scalp
     Coding Clinic: 2015, Q1, P5-7
  X ● **S01.03**   Puncture wound without foreign body of scalp
  X ● **S01.04**   Puncture wound with foreign body of scalp
  X ● **S01.05**   Open bite of scalp
     Bite of scalp NOS
     Excludes1   superficial bite of scalp (S00.06, S00.07-)

● **S01.1**   **Open wound of eyelid and periocular area**
   Open wound of eyelid and periocular area with or without involvement of lacrimal passages
  ● **S01.10**   Unspecified open wound of eyelid and periocular area
   ● **S01.101**   Unspecified open wound of right eyelid and periocular area
   ● **S01.102**   Unspecified open wound of left eyelid and periocular area
   ● **S01.109**   Unspecified open wound of unspecified eyelid and periocular area
  ● **S01.11**   Laceration without foreign body of eyelid and periocular area
   ● **S01.111**   Laceration without foreign body of right eyelid and periocular area
   ● **S01.112**   Laceration without foreign body of left eyelid and periocular area
   ● **S01.119**   Laceration without foreign body of unspecified eyelid and periocular area
  ● **S01.12**   Laceration with foreign body of eyelid and periocular area
   ● **S01.121**   Laceration with foreign body of right eyelid and periocular area
   ● **S01.122**   Laceration with foreign body of left eyelid and periocular area

CHAPTER 19 (S00-T88)

CHAPTER 19 (S00–T88)

- S01.129   Laceration with foreign body of unspecified eyelid and periocular area
- S01.13   Puncture wound without foreign body of eyelid and periocular area
  - S01.131   Puncture wound without foreign body of right eyelid and periocular area
  - S01.132   Puncture wound without foreign body of left eyelid and periocular area
  - S01.139   Puncture wound without foreign body of unspecified eyelid and periocular area
- S01.14   Puncture wound with foreign body of eyelid and periocular area
  - S01.141   Puncture wound with foreign body of right eyelid and periocular area
  - S01.142   Puncture wound with foreign body of left eyelid and periocular area
  - S01.149   Puncture wound with foreign body of unspecified eyelid and periocular area
- S01.15   Open bite of eyelid and periocular area
  Bite of eyelid and periocular area NOS
  Excludes1   superficial bite of eyelid and periocular area (S00.26, S00.27)
  - S01.151   Open bite of right eyelid and periocular area
  - S01.152   Open bite of left eyelid and periocular area
  - S01.159   Open bite of unspecified eyelid and periocular area
- S01.2   Open wound of nose
  - X S01.20   Unspecified open wound of nose
  - X S01.21   Laceration without foreign body of nose
    Coding Clinic: 2015, Q1, P5-6
  - X S01.22   Laceration with foreign body of nose
  - X S01.23   Puncture wound without foreign body of nose
  - X S01.24   Puncture wound with foreign body of nose
  - X S01.25   Open bite of nose
    Bite of nose NOS
    Excludes1   superficial bite of nose (S00.36, S00.37)
- S01.3   Open wound of ear
  - S01.30   Unspecified open wound of ear
    - S01.301   Unspecified open wound of right ear
    - S01.302   Unspecified open wound of left ear
    - S01.309   Unspecified open wound of unspecified ear
  - S01.31   Laceration without foreign body of ear
    - S01.311   Laceration without foreign body of right ear
    - S01.312   Laceration without foreign body of left ear
    - S01.319   Laceration without foreign body of unspecified ear
  - S01.32   Laceration with foreign body of ear
    - S01.321   Laceration with foreign body of right ear
    - S01.322   Laceration with foreign body of left ear
    - S01.329   Laceration with foreign body of unspecified ear

- S01.33   Puncture wound without foreign body of ear
  - S01.331   Puncture wound without foreign body of right ear
  - S01.332   Puncture wound without foreign body of left ear
  - S01.339   Puncture wound without foreign body of unspecified ear
- S01.34   Puncture wound with foreign body of ear
  - S01.341   Puncture wound with foreign body of right ear
  - S01.342   Puncture wound with foreign body of left ear
  - S01.349   Puncture wound with foreign body of unspecified ear
- S01.35   Open bite of ear
  Bite of ear NOS
  Excludes1   superficial bite of ear (S00.46, S00.47)
  - S01.351   Open bite of right ear
  - S01.352   Open bite of left ear
  - S01.359   Open bite of unspecified ear
- S01.4   Open wound of cheek and temporomandibular area
  - S01.40   Unspecified open wound of cheek and temporomandibular area
    - S01.401   Unspecified open wound of right cheek and temporomandibular area
    - S01.402   Unspecified open wound of left cheek and temporomandibular area
    - S01.409   Unspecified open wound of unspecified cheek and temporomandibular area
  - S01.41   Laceration without foreign body of cheek and temporomandibular area
    - S01.411   Laceration without foreign body of right cheek and temporomandibular area
      Coding Clinic: 2015, Q1, P5-7
    - S01.412   Laceration without foreign body of left cheek and temporomandibular area
    - S01.419   Laceration without foreign body of unspecified cheek and temporomandibular area
  - S01.42   Laceration with foreign body of cheek and temporomandibular area
    - S01.421   Laceration with foreign body of right cheek and temporomandibular area
    - S01.422   Laceration with foreign body of left cheek and temporomandibular area
    - S01.429   Laceration with foreign body of unspecified cheek and temporomandibular area
  - S01.43   Puncture wound without foreign body of cheek and temporomandibular area
    - S01.431   Puncture wound without foreign body of right cheek and temporomandibular area
    - S01.432   Puncture wound without foreign body of left cheek and temporomandibular area
    - S01.439   Puncture wound without foreign body of unspecified cheek and temporomandibular area

▶ New   ⇒ Revised   ~~deleted~~ Deleted   Excludes 1   Excludes 2   Includes   Use additional   Code first   Code also   Key words

OGCR Official Guidelines   X Assign placeholder X   ● Use Additional Character(s)   ▷ Manifestation Code   🔏 Hierarchical Condition Category   **Coding Clinic**

● **S01.44**   **Puncture wound with foreign body of cheek and temporomandibular area**

     ● **S01.441**   Puncture wound with foreign body of right cheek and temporomandibular area

     ● **S01.442**   Puncture wound with foreign body of left cheek and temporomandibular area

     ● **S01.449**   Puncture wound with foreign body of unspecified cheek and temporomandibular area

● **S01.45**   **Open bite of cheek and temporomandibular area**

     Bite of cheek and temporomandibular area NOS

     Excludes2   superficial bite of cheek and temporomandibular area (S00.86, S00.87)

     ● **S01.451**   Open bite of right cheek and temporomandibular area

     ● **S01.452**   Open bite of left cheek and temporomandibular area

     ● **S01.459**   Open bite of unspecified cheek and temporomandibular area

● **S01.5**   **Open wound of lip and oral cavity**

     Excludes2   tooth dislocation (S03.2)
                     tooth fracture (S02.5)

   ● **S01.50**   **Unspecified open wound of lip and oral cavity**

     ● **S01.501**   Unspecified open wound of lip

     ● **S01.502**   Unspecified open wound of oral cavity

   ● **S01.51**   **Laceration of lip and oral cavity without foreign body**

     ● **S01.511**   Laceration without foreign body of lip

     ● **S01.512**   Laceration without foreign body of oral cavity

   ● **S01.52**   **Laceration of lip and oral cavity with foreign body**

     ● **S01.521**   Laceration with foreign body of lip

     ● **S01.522**   Laceration with foreign body of oral cavity

   ● **S01.53**   **Puncture wound of lip and oral cavity without foreign body**

     ● **S01.531**   Puncture wound without foreign body of lip

     ● **S01.532**   Puncture wound without foreign body of oral cavity

   ● **S01.54**   **Puncture wound of lip and oral cavity with foreign body**

     ● **S01.541**   Puncture wound with foreign body of lip

     ● **S01.542**   Puncture wound with foreign body of oral cavity

   ● **S01.55**   **Open bite of lip and oral cavity**

     ● **S01.551**   Open bite of lip
                     Bite of lip NOS

         Excludes1   superficial bite of lip (S00.571)

     ● **S01.552**   Open bite of oral cavity
                     Bite of oral cavity NOS

         Excludes1   superficial bite of oral cavity (S00.572)

● **S01.8**   **Open wound of other parts of head**

   X ● **S01.80**   Unspecified open wound of other part of head

   X ● **S01.81**   Laceration without foreign body of other part of head

   X ● **S01.82**   Laceration with foreign body of other part of head

   X ● **S01.83**   Puncture wound without foreign body of other part of head

   X ● **S01.84**   Puncture wound with foreign body of other part of head

   X ● **S01.85**   Open bite of other part of head
                     Bite of other part of head NOS

         Excludes1   superficial bite of other part of head (S00.87)

● **S01.9**   **Open wound of unspecified part of head**

   X ● **S01.90**   Unspecified open wound of unspecified part of head

   X ● **S01.91**   Laceration without foreign body of unspecified part of head

   X ● **S01.92**   Laceration with foreign body of unspecified part of head

   X ● **S01.93**   Puncture wound without foreign body of unspecified part of head

   X ● **S01.94**   Puncture wound with foreign body of unspecified part of head

   X ● **S01.95**   Open bite of unspecified part of head
                     Bite of head NOS

         Excludes1   superficial bite of head NOS (S00.97)

● **S02**   **Fracture of skull and facial bones**

   Note: A fracture not indicated as open or closed should be coded to closed

        The appropriate 7th character is to be added to each code from category S02

A	initial encounter for closed fracture
B	initial encounter for open fracture
D	subsequent encounter for fracture with routine healing
G	subsequent encounter for fracture with delayed healing
K	subsequent encounter for fracture with nonunion
S	sequela

   Code also any associated intracranial injury (S06.-)

  X ● **S02.0**   **Fracture of vault of skull A, B, S** 🔖
               Fracture of frontal bone
               Fracture of parietal bone

● **S02.1**   **Fracture of base of skull**

     Excludes2   lateral orbital wall (S02.84-)
                     medial orbital wall (S02.83-)
                     orbital floor (S02.3-)

     Coding Clinic: 2016, Q4, P66

   ● **S02.10**   Unspecified fracture of base of skull

     ● **S02.101**   Fracture of base of skull, right side A, B, S 🔖

     ● **S02.102**   Fracture of base of skull, left side A, B, S 🔖

     ● **S02.109**   Fracture of base of skull, unspecified side A, B, S 🔖

   ● **S02.11**   Fracture of occiput

     ● **S02.110**   Type I occipital condyle fracture, unspecified side A, B, S 🔖

     ● **S02.111**   Type II occipital condyle fracture, unspecified side A, B, S 🔖

     ● **S02.112**   Type III occipital condyle fracture, unspecified side A, B, S 🔖

     ● **S02.113**   Unspecified occipital condyle fracture A, B, S 🔖

     ● **S02.118**   Other fracture of occiput, unspecified side A, B, S 🔖

     ● **S02.119**   Unspecified fracture of occiput A, B, S 🔖

CHAPTER 19 (S00-T88)

● S02.11A   Type I occipital condyle fracture, right side A, B, S 🐾

● S02.11B   Type I occipital condyle fracture, left side A, B, S 🐾

● S02.11C   Type II occipital condyle fracture, right side A, B, S 🐾

● S02.11D   Type II occipital condyle fracture, left side A, B, S 🐾

● S02.11E   Type III occipital condyle fracture, right side A, B, S 🐾

● S02.11F   Type III occipital condyle fracture, left side A, B, S 🐾

● S02.11G   Other fracture of occiput, right side A, B, S 🐾

● S02.11H   Other fracture of occiput, left side A, B, S 🐾

S02.12   Fracture of orbital roof

     S02.121   Fracture of orbital roof, right side

     S02.122   Fracture of orbital roof, left side

     S02.129   Fracture of orbital roof, unspecified side

X ● S02.19   Other fracture of base of skull A, B, S 🐾
     Fracture of anterior fossa of base of skull
     Fracture of ethmoid sinus
     Fracture of frontal sinus
     Fracture of middle fossa of base of skull
     Fracture of posterior fossa of base of skull
     Fracture of sphenoid
     Fracture of temporal bone

X ● S02.2   Fracture of nasal bones

● S02.3   Fracture of orbital floor
     Fracture of inferior orbital wall

     Excludes1   orbit NOS (S02.85)

     Excludes2   lateral orbital wall (S02.84-)
                medial orbital wall (S02.83-)
                orbital roof (S02.1-)
     Coding Clinic: 2016, Q4, P66

X ● S02.30   Fracture of orbital floor, unspecified side A, B, S 🐾

X ● S02.31   Fracture of orbital floor, right side A, B, S 🐾

X ● S02.32   Fracture of orbital floor, left side A, B, S 🐾

● S02.4   Fracture of malar, maxillary and zygoma bones
     Fracture of superior maxilla
     Fracture of upper jaw (bone)
     Fracture of zygomatic process of temporal bone
     Coding Clinic: 2016, Q4, P66

● S02.40   Fracture of malar, maxillary and zygoma bones, unspecified

     ● S02.400   Malar fracture unspecified side A, B, S 🐾

     ● S02.401   Maxillary fracture, unspecified side A, B, S 🐾

     ● S02.402   Zygomatic fracture, unspecified side A, B, S 🐾

     ● S02.40A   Malar fracture, right side A, B, S 🐾

     ● S02.40B   Malar fracture, left side A, B, S 🐾

     ● S02.40C   Maxillary fracture, right side A, B, S 🐾

     ● S02.40D   Maxillary fracture, left side A, B, S 🐾

     ● S02.40E   Zygomatic fracture, right side A, B, S 🐾

     ● S02.40F   Zygomatic fracture, left side A, B, S 🐾

● S02.41   LeFort fracture

     ● S02.411   LeFort I fracture A, B, S 🐾

     ● S02.412   LeFort II fracture A, B, S 🐾

     ● S02.413   LeFort III fracture A, B, S 🐾

X ● S02.42   Fracture of alveolus of maxilla A, B, S 🐾

X ● S02.5   Fracture of tooth (traumatic) Broken tooth

     Excludes1   cracked tooth (nontraumatic) (K03.81)

● S02.6   Fracture of mandible
     Fracture of lower jaw (bone)
     Coding Clinic: 2016, Q4, P66

● S02.60   Fracture of mandible of unspecified site

     ● S02.600   Fracture of unspecified part of body of mandible, unspecified side A, B, S 🐾

     ● S02.601   Fracture of unspecified part of body of right mandible A, B, S 🐾

     ● S02.602   Fracture of unspecified part of body of left mandible A, B, S 🐾

     ● S02.609   Fracture of mandible, unspecified A, B, S 🐾

● S02.61   Fracture of condylar process of mandible

     ● S02.610   Fracture of condylar process of mandible, unspecified side A, B, S 🐾

     ● S02.611   Fracture of condylar process of right mandible A, B, S 🐾
         Coding Clinic: 2021, Q1, P6

     ● S02.612   Fracture of condylar process of left mandible A, B, S 🐾

● S02.62   Fracture of subcondylar process of mandible

     ● S02.620   Fracture of subcondylar process of mandible, unspecified side A, B, S 🐾

     ● S02.621   Fracture of subcondylar process of right mandible A, B, S 🐾

     ● S02.622   Fracture of subcondylar process of left mandible A, B, S 🐾

● S02.63   Fracture of coronoid process of mandible

     ● S02.630   Fracture of coronoid process of mandible, unspecified side A, B, S 🐾

     ● S02.631   Fracture of coronoid process of right mandible A, B, S 🐾

     ● S02.632   Fracture of coronoid process of left mandible A, B, S 🐾

● S02.64   Fracture of ramus of mandible

     ● S02.640   Fracture of ramus of mandible, unspecified side A, B, S 🐾

     ● S02.641   Fracture of ramus of right mandible A, B, S 🐾

     ● S02.642   Fracture of ramus of left mandible A, B, S 🐾

● S02.65   Fracture of angle of mandible

     ● S02.650   Fracture of angle of mandible, unspecified side A, B, S 🐾

     ● S02.651   Fracture of angle of right mandible A, B, S 🐾

     ● S02.652   Fracture of angle of left mandible A, B, S 🐾

X ● S02.66   Fracture of symphysis of mandible A, B, S 🐾
     Coding Clinic: 2021, Q1, P6

● S02.67   Fracture of alveolus of mandible

     ● S02.670   Fracture of alveolus of mandible, unspecified side A, B, S 🐾

     ● S02.671   Fracture of alveolus of right mandible A, B, S 🐾

     ● S02.672   Fracture of alveolus of left mandible A, B, S 🐾

X ● S02.69   Fracture of mandible of other specified site A, B, S 🐾

▶ New   ⇒ Revised   ~~deleted~~ Deleted   Excludes 1   Excludes 2   Includes   Use additional   Code first   Code also   Key words

OGCR Official Guidelines   X Assign placeholder X   ● Use Additional Character(s)   ▶ Manifestation Code   🐾 Hierarchical Condition Category   Coding Clinic

● **S02.8**   **Fractures of other specified skull and facial bones**
      Fracture of palate
      Excludes2   lateral orbital wall (S02.84-)
                medial orbital wall (S02.83-)
      Coding Clinic: 2016, Q4, P66

  X● **S02.80**   Fracture of other specified skull and facial bones, unspecified side A, B, S 🐾

  X● **S02.81**   Fracture of other specified skull and facial bones, right side A, B, S 🐾

  X● **S02.82**   Fracture of other specified skull and facial bones, left side A, B, S 🐾

  ● **S02.83 Fracture of medial orbital wall**
      Excludes2   orbital floor (S02.3-)
                orbital roof (S02.12-)

    S02.831   Fracture of medial orbital wall, right side

    S02.832   Fracture of medial orbital wall, left side

    S02.839   Fracture of medial orbital wall, unspecified side

  ● **S02.84 Fracture of lateral orbital wall**
      Excludes2   orbital floor (S02.3-)
                orbital roof (S02.12-)

    S02.841   Fracture of lateral orbital wall, right side

    S02.842   Fracture of lateral orbital wall, left side

    S02.849   Fracture of lateral orbital wall, unspecified side

  S02.85 Fracture of orbit, unspecified
      Fracture of orbit NOS
      Fracture of orbit wall NOS
      Excludes1   lateral orbital wall (S02.84-)
                medial orbital wall (S02.83-)
                orbital floor (S02.3-)
                orbital roof (S02.12-)

● **S02.9**   **Fracture of unspecified skull and facial bones**

  X● **S02.91**   Unspecified fracture of skull A, B, S 🐾

  X● **S02.92**   Unspecified fracture of facial bones A, B, S 🐾

● **S03**   **Dislocation and sprain of joints and ligaments of head**
    Includes   avulsion of joint (capsule) or ligament of head
             laceration of cartilage, joint (capsule) or ligament of head
             sprain of cartilage, joint (capsule) or ligament of head
             traumatic hemarthrosis of joint or ligament of head
             traumatic rupture of joint or ligament of head
             traumatic subluxation of joint or ligament of head
             traumatic tear of joint or ligament of head

  Code also any associated open wound
    Excludes2   Strain of muscle or tendon of head (S09.1)
  The appropriate 7th character is to be added to each code from category S03

    | | |
    A   initial encounter
    D   subsequent encounter
    S   sequela

● **S03.0**   **Dislocation of jaw**
      Dislocation of jaw (cartilage) (meniscus)
      Dislocation of mandible
      Dislocation of temporomandibular (joint)
      Coding Clinic: 2016, Q4, P67

  X● **S03.00**   Dislocation of jaw, unspecified side
  X● **S03.01**   Dislocation of jaw, right side
  X● **S03.02**   Dislocation of jaw, left side
  X● **S03.03**   Dislocation of jaw, bilateral side

X● **S03.1**   Dislocation of septal cartilage of nose
X● **S03.2**   Dislocation of tooth

● **S03.4**   **Sprain of jaw**
      Sprain of temporomandibular (joint) (ligament)
      Coding Clinic: 2016, Q4, P67

  X● **S03.40**   Sprain of jaw, unspecified side
  X● **S03.41**   Sprain of jaw, right side
  X● **S03.42**   Sprain of jaw, left side
  X● **S03.43**   Sprain of jaw, bilateral side

  X● **S03.8**   Sprain of joints and ligaments of other parts of head
  X● **S03.9**   Sprain of joints and ligaments of unspecified parts of head

● **S04**   **Injury of cranial nerve**
    The selection of side should be based on the side of the body being affected
    Code first any associated intracranial injury (S06.-)
    Code also any associated:
      open wound of head (S01.-)
      skull fracture (S02.-)
    The appropriate 7th character is to be added to each code from category S04

    A   initial encounter
    D   subsequent encounter
    S   sequela

● **S04.0**   **Injury of optic nerve and pathways**
    Use additional code to identify any visual field defect or blindness (H53.4-, H54.-)

  ● **S04.01**   **Injury of optic nerve**
      Injury of 2nd cranial nerve

    ● **S04.011**   Injury of optic nerve, right eye
    ● **S04.012**   Injury of optic nerve, left eye
    ● **S04.019**   Injury of optic nerve, unspecified eye
      Injury of optic nerve NOS

  X● **S04.02**   Injury of optic chiasm

  ● **S04.03**   Injury of optic tract and pathways
      Injury of optic radiation

    ● **S04.031**   Injury of optic tract and pathways, right side
    ● **S04.032**   Injury of optic tract and pathways, left side
    ● **S04.039**   Injury of optic tract and pathways, unspecified side
      Injury of optic tract and pathways NOS

  ● **S04.04**   **Injury of visual cortex**
    ● **S04.041**   Injury of visual cortex, right side
    ● **S04.042**   Injury of visual cortex, left side
    ● **S04.049**   Injury of visual cortex, unspecified side
      Injury of visual cortex NOS

● **S04.1**   **Injury of oculomotor nerve**
    Injury of 3rd cranial nerve

  X● **S04.10**   Injury of oculomotor nerve, unspecified side
  X● **S04.11**   Injury of oculomotor nerve, right side
  X● **S04.12**   Injury of oculomotor nerve, left side

● **S04.2**   **Injury of trochlear nerve**
    Injury of 4th cranial nerve

  X● **S04.20**   Injury of trochlear nerve, unspecified side
  X● **S04.21**   Injury of trochlear nerve, right side
  X● **S04.22**   Injury of trochlear nerve, left side

● **S04.3**   **Injury of trigeminal nerve**
    Injury of 5th cranial nerve

  X● **S04.30**   Injury of trigeminal nerve, unspecified side
  X● **S04.31**   Injury of trigeminal nerve, right side
  X● **S04.32**   Injury of trigeminal nerve, left side

● **S04.4**   **Injury of abducent nerve**
    Injury of 6th cranial nerve

  X● **S04.40**   Injury of abducent nerve, unspecified side
  X● **S04.41**   Injury of abducent nerve, right side
  X● **S04.42**   Injury of abducent nerve, left side

CHAPTER 19 (S00–T88)

Figure 19-13 Cranial nerves. (From Patton and Thibodeau: Anatomy and physiology, ed 7, St. Louis, Mosby, 2009)

Trochlear nerve (IV)

Optic nerve (II)

Olfactory nerve (I)

Abducens nerve (VI)

Oculomotor nerve (III)

Facial nerve (VII)

Trigeminal nerve (V)

Vestibulocochlear nerve (VIII)

Glossopharyngeal nerve (IX)

Vagus nerve (X)

Accessory nerve (XI)

Hypoglossal nerve (XII)

● **S04.5   Injury of facial nerve**
　　　Injury of 7th cranial nerve
　X ● **S04.50   Injury of facial nerve, unspecified side**
　X ● **S04.51   Injury of facial nerve, right side**
　X ● **S04.52   Injury of facial nerve, left side**
● **S04.6   Injury of acoustic nerve**
　　　Injury of auditory nerve
　　　Injury of 8th cranial nerve
　X ● **S04.60   Injury of acoustic nerve, unspecified side**
　X ● **S04.61   Injury of acoustic nerve, right side**
　X ● **S04.62   Injury of acoustic nerve, left side**
● **S04.7   Injury of accessory nerve**
　　　Injury of 11th cranial nerve
　X ● **S04.70   Injury of accessory nerve, unspecified side**
　X ● **S04.71   Injury of accessory nerve, right side**
　X ● **S04.72   Injury of accessory nerve, left side**
● **S04.8   Injury of other cranial nerves**
　● **S04.81   Injury of olfactory [1st] nerve**
　　● **S04.811   Injury of olfactory [1st] nerve, right side**
　　● **S04.812   Injury of olfactory [1st] nerve, left side**
　　● **S04.819   Injury of olfactory [1st] nerve, unspecified side**
　● **S04.89   Injury of other cranial nerves**
　　　Injury of vagus [10th] nerve
　　● **S04.891   Injury of other cranial nerves, right side**
　　● **S04.892   Injury of other cranial nerves, left side**
　　● **S04.899   Injury of other cranial nerves, unspecified side**
　X ● **S04.9   Injury of unspecified cranial nerve**

● **S05   Injury of eye and orbit**

　Includes   open wound of eye and orbit
　Excludes2   2nd cranial [optic] nerve injury (S04.0-)
　　　　　　　3rd cranial [oculomotor] nerve injury (S04.1-)
　　　　　　　open wound of eyelid and periocular area (S01.1-)
　　　　　　　orbital bone fracture (S02.1-, S02.3-, S02.8-)
　　　　　　　superficial injury of eyelid (S00.1-S00.2)

The appropriate 7th character is to be added to each code from category S05

A	initial encounter
D	subsequent encounter
S	sequela

● **S05.0   Injury of conjunctiva and corneal abrasion without foreign body**
　Excludes1   foreign body in conjunctival sac (T15.1)
　　　　　　　foreign body in cornea (T15.0)
　X ● **S05.00   Injury of conjunctiva and corneal abrasion without foreign body, unspecified eye**
　X ● **S05.01   Injury of conjunctiva and corneal abrasion without foreign body, right eye**
　X ● **S05.02   Injury of conjunctiva and corneal abrasion without foreign body, left eye**
● **S05.1   Contusion of eyeball and orbital tissues**
　　　Traumatic hyphema
　Excludes2   black eye NOS (S00.1)
　　　　　　　contusion of eyelid and periocular area (S00.1)
　X ● **S05.10   Contusion of eyeball and orbital tissues, unspecified eye**
　X ● **S05.11   Contusion of eyeball and orbital tissues, right eye**
　X ● **S05.12   Contusion of eyeball and orbital tissues, left eye**

▶ New   ⇒ Revised   ~~deleted~~ Deleted   Excludes 1   Excludes 2   Includes   Use additional   Code first   Code also   Key words
OGCR Official Guidelines   X Assign placeholder X   ● Use Additional Character(s)   ▸ Manifestation Code   ⟲ Hierarchical Condition Category   **Coding Clinic**

● **S05.2**   Ocular laceration and rupture with prolapse or loss of intraocular tissue
- X● **S05.20**   Ocular laceration and rupture with prolapse or loss of intraocular tissue, unspecified eye
- X● **S05.21**   Ocular laceration and rupture with prolapse or loss of intraocular tissue, right eye
- X● **S05.22**   Ocular laceration and rupture with prolapse or loss of intraocular tissue, left eye

● **S05.3**   Ocular laceration without prolapse or loss of intraocular tissue
     Laceration of eye NOS
- X● **S05.30**   Ocular laceration without prolapse or loss of intraocular tissue, unspecified eye
- X● **S05.31**   Ocular laceration without prolapse or loss of intraocular tissue, right eye
- X● **S05.32**   Ocular laceration without prolapse or loss of intraocular tissue, left eye

● **S05.4**   Penetrating wound of orbit with or without foreign body
     Excludes2   retained (old) foreign body following penetrating wound in orbit (H05.5-)
- X● **S05.40**   Penetrating wound of orbit with or without foreign body, unspecified eye
- X● **S05.41**   Penetrating wound of orbit with or without foreign body, right eye
- X● **S05.42**   Penetrating wound of orbit with or without foreign body, left eye

● **S05.5**   Penetrating wound with foreign body of eyeball
     Excludes2   retained (old) intraocular foreign body (H44.6-, H44.7)
- X● **S05.50**   Penetrating wound with foreign body of unspecified eyeball
- X● **S05.51**   Penetrating wound with foreign body of right eyeball
- X● **S05.52**   Penetrating wound with foreign body of left eyeball

● **S05.6**   Penetrating wound without foreign body of eyeball
     Ocular penetration NOS
- X● **S05.60**   Penetrating wound without foreign body of unspecified eyeball
- X● **S05.61**   Penetrating wound without foreign body of right eyeball
- X● **S05.62**   Penetrating wound without foreign body of left eyeball

● **S05.7**   Avulsion of eye
     Traumatic enucleation
- X● **S05.70**   Avulsion of unspecified eye
- X● **S05.71**   Avulsion of right eye
- X● **S05.72**   Avulsion of left eye

● **S05.8**   Other injuries of eye and orbit
     Lacrimal duct injury
- ● **S05.8X**   Other injuries of eye and orbit
  - ● **S05.8X1**   Other injuries of right eye and orbit
  - ● **S05.8X2**   Other injuries of left eye and orbit
  - ● **S05.8X9**   Other injuries of unspecified eye and orbit

● **S05.9**   Unspecified injury of eye and orbit
     Injury of eye NOS
- X● **S05.90**   Unspecified injury of unspecified eye and orbit
- X● **S05.91**   Unspecified injury of right eye and orbit
- X● **S05.92**   Unspecified injury of left eye and orbit

● **S06**   Intracranial injury
     Includes   traumatic brain injury
     Code also any associated:
       open wound of head (S01.-)
       skull fracture (S02.-)
     Excludes1   head injury NOS (S09.90)

The appropriate 7th character is to be added to each code from category S06

A	initial encounter
D	subsequent encounter
S	sequela

Note: 7th characters D and S do not apply to codes in category S06 with 6th character 7 - death due to brain injury prior to regaining consciousness, or 8 - death due to other cause prior to regaining consciousness.
Coding Clinic: 2015, Q4, P40

● **S06.0**   Concussion
     Commotio cerebri
     ⇒ **Excludes1**   concussion with other intracranial injuries classified in subcategories S06.1- to S06.6- , and S06.81- to S06.82-, code to specified intracranial injury
     Coding Clinic: 2016, Q4, P67

- ● **S06.0X**   Concussion
  - ● **S06.0X0**   Concussion without loss of consciousness S 🦟
  - ● **S06.0X1**   Concussion with loss of consciousness of 30 minutes or less S 🦟
    - ▶ Concussion with brief loss of consciousness
  - ● **S06.0X9**   Concussion with loss of consciousness of unspecified duration S 🦟
    - ~~Concussion NOS~~
    - Coding Clinic: 2016, Q4, P68
  - ▶ ● **S06.0XA**   Concussion with loss of consciousness status unknown
    - ▶ Concussion NOS

● **S06.1**   Traumatic cerebral edema
     Diffuse traumatic cerebral edema
     Focal traumatic cerebral edema
     Coding Clinic: 2016, Q4, P67

- ● **S06.1X**   Traumatic cerebral edema
  - ● **S06.1X0**   Traumatic cerebral edema without loss of consciousness A, S 🦟
    - Coding Clinic: 2015, Q1, P12
  - ● **S06.1X1**   Traumatic cerebral edema with loss of consciousness of 30 minutes or less A, S 🦟
    - ▶ Traumatic cerebral edema with brief loss of consciousness
  - ● **S06.1X2**   Traumatic cerebral edema with loss of consciousness of 31 minutes to 59 minutes A, S 🦟
  - ● **S06.1X3**   Traumatic cerebral edema with loss of consciousness of 1 hour to 5 hours 59 minutes A, S 🦟
  - ● **S06.1X4**   Traumatic cerebral edema with loss of consciousness of 6 hours to 24 hours A, S 🦟
  - ● **S06.1X5**   Traumatic cerebral edema with loss of consciousness greater than 24 hours with return to pre-existing conscious level A, S 🦟
  - ● **S06.1X6**   Traumatic cerebral edema with loss of consciousness greater than 24 hours without return to pre-existing conscious level with patient surviving A, S 🦟

● **S06.1X7** **Traumatic cerebral edema with loss of consciousness of any duration with death due to brain injury prior to regaining consciousness**

● **S06.1X8** **Traumatic cerebral edema with loss of consciousness of any duration with death due to other cause prior to regaining consciousness**

● **S06.1X9** **Traumatic cerebral edema with loss of consciousness of unspecified duration** A, S 🐾

~~Traumatic cerebral edema NOS~~

▶ ● **S06.1XA** **Traumatic cerebral edema with loss of consciousness status unknown**
▶Traumatic cerebral edema NOS

● **S06.2** **Diffuse traumatic brain injury**
Diffuse axonal brain injury

Excludes1 traumatic diffuse cerebral edema (S06.1X-)

Use Additional code, if applicable, for traumatic brain compression or herniation (S06.A-)

● **S06.2X** **Diffuse traumatic brain injury**

● **S06.2X0** **Diffuse traumatic brain injury without loss of consciousness** A, S 🐾

● **S06.2X1** **Diffuse traumatic brain injury with loss of consciousness of 30 minutes or less** A, S 🐾
▶ Diffuse traumatic brain injury with brief loss of consciousness

● **S06.2X2** **Diffuse traumatic brain injury with loss of consciousness of 31 minutes to 59 minutes** A, S 🐾

● **S06.2X3** **Diffuse traumatic brain injury with loss of consciousness of 1 hour to 5 hours 59 minutes** A, S 🐾

● **S06.2X4** **Diffuse traumatic brain injury with loss of consciousness of 6 hours to 24 hours** A, S 🐾

● **S06.2X5** **Diffuse traumatic brain injury with loss of consciousness greater than 24 hours with return to pre-existing conscious levels** A, S 🐾

● **S06.2X6** **Diffuse traumatic brain injury with loss of consciousness greater than 24 hours without return to pre-existing conscious level with patient surviving** A, S 🐾

● **S06.2X7** **Diffuse traumatic brain injury with loss of consciousness of any duration with death due to brain injury prior to regaining consciousness**

● **S06.2X8** **Diffuse traumatic brain injury with loss of consciousness of any duration with death due to other cause prior to regaining consciousness**

● **S06.2X9** **Diffuse traumatic brain injury with loss of consciousness of unspecified duration** A, S 🐾
Diffuse traumatic brain injury NOS

▶ ● **S06.2XA** **Diffuse traumatic brain injury with loss of consciousness status unknown**
▶Diffuse traumatic brain injury NOS

● **S06.3** **Focal traumatic brain injury**

Excludes1 any condition classifiable to S06.4-S06.6

Excludes2 focal cerebral edema (S06.1)

Use Additional code, if applicable, for traumatic brain compression or herniation (S06.A-)

● **S06.30** **Unspecified focal traumatic brain injury**

● **S06.300** **Unspecified focal traumatic brain injury without loss of consciousness** A, S 🐾

● **S06.301** **Unspecified focal traumatic brain injury with loss of consciousness of 30 minutes or less** A, S 🐾
▶ Unspecified focal traumatic brain injury with brief loss of consciousness

● **S06.302** **Unspecified focal traumatic brain injury with loss of consciousness of 31 minutes to 59 minutes** A, S 🐾

● **S06.303** **Unspecified focal traumatic brain injury with loss of consciousness of 1 hour to 5 hours 59 minutes** A, S 🐾

● **S06.304** **Unspecified focal traumatic brain injury with loss of consciousness of 6 hours to 24 hours** A, S 🐾

● **S06.305** **Unspecified focal traumatic brain injury with loss of consciousness greater than 24 hours with return to pre-existing conscious level** A, S 🐾

● **S06.306** **Unspecified focal traumatic brain injury with loss of consciousness greater than 24 hours without return to pre-existing conscious level with patient surviving** A, S 🐾

● **S06.307** **Unspecified focal traumatic brain injury with loss of consciousness of any duration with death due to brain injury prior to regaining consciousness**

● **S06.308** **Unspecified focal traumatic brain injury with loss of consciousness of any duration with death due to other cause prior to regaining consciousness**

● **S06.309** **Unspecified focal traumatic brain injury with loss of consciousness of unspecified duration** A, S 🐾
~~Unspecified focal traumatic brain injury NOS~~

▶ ● **S06.30A** **Unspecified focal traumatic brain injury with loss of consciousness status unknown**
▶Unspecified focal traumatic brain injury NOS

● **S06.31** **Contusion and laceration of right cerebrum**

● **S06.310** **Contusion and laceration of right cerebrum without loss of consciousness** A, S 🐾

● **S06.311** **Contusion and laceration of right cerebrum with loss of consciousness of 30 minutes or less** A, S 🐾
▶ Contusion and laceration of right cerebrum with brief loss of consciousness

● **S06.312** **Contusion and laceration of right cerebrum with loss of consciousness of 31 minutes to 59 minutes** A, S 🐾

● **S06.313** **Contusion and laceration of right cerebrum with loss of consciousness of 1 hour to 5 hours 59 minutes** A, S 🐾

● **S06.314** **Contusion and laceration of right cerebrum with loss of consciousness of 6 hours to 24 hours** A, S 🐾

● **S06.315** **Contusion and laceration of right cerebrum with loss of consciousness greater than 24 hours with return to pre-existing conscious level** A, S 🐾

● **S06.316** **Contusion and laceration of right cerebrum with loss of consciousness greater than 24 hours without return to pre-existing conscious level with patient surviving** A, S 🐾

CHAPTER 19 (S00-T88)

● S06.317   Contusion and laceration of right
             cerebrum with loss of consciousness
             of any duration with death due
             to brain injury prior to regaining
             consciousness
● S06.318   Contusion and laceration of right
             cerebrum with loss of consciousness
             of any duration with death due
             to other cause prior to regaining
             consciousness
● S06.319   Contusion and laceration of right
             cerebrum with loss of consciousness
             of unspecified duration A, S 🔒
             ~~Contusion and laceration of right
             cerebrum NOS~~

▶ ● S06.31A   Contusion and laceration of right
             cerebrum with loss of consciousness
             status unknown
             ▶ Contusion and laceration of right
               cerebrum NOS

● S06.32   Contusion and laceration of left cerebrum
    ● S06.320   Contusion and laceration of left
                 cerebrum without loss of
                 consciousness A, S 🔒
    ● S06.321   Contusion and laceration of left
                 cerebrum with loss of consciousness
                 of 30 minutes or less A, S 🔒
                 ▶ Contusion and laceration of left
                   cerebrum with brief loss of
                   consciousness
    ● S06.322   Contusion and laceration of left
                 cerebrum with loss of consciousness
                 of 31 minutes to 59 minutes A, S 🔒
    ● S06.323   Contusion and laceration of left
                 cerebrum with loss of consciousness
                 of 1 hour to 5 hours 59 minutes
                 A, S 🔒
    ● S06.324   Contusion and laceration of left
                 cerebrum with loss of consciousness
                 of 6 hours to 24 hours A, S 🔒
    ● S06.325   Contusion and laceration of left
                 cerebrum with loss of consciousness
                 greater than 24 hours with return to
                 pre-existing conscious level A, S 🔒
    ● S06.326   Contusion and laceration of left
                 cerebrum with loss of consciousness
                 greater than 24 hours without return
                 to pre-existing conscious level with
                 patient surviving A, S 🔒
    ● S06.327   Contusion and laceration of left
                 cerebrum with loss of consciousness
                 of any duration with death due
                 to brain injury prior to regaining
                 consciousness
    ● S06.328   Contusion and laceration of left
                 cerebrum with loss of consciousness
                 of any duration with death due
                 to other cause prior to regaining
                 consciousness
    ● S06.329   Contusion and laceration of left
                 cerebrum with loss of consciousness
                 of unspecified duration A, S 🔒
                 ~~Contusion and laceration of left
                 cerebrum NOS~~

▶ ● S06.32A   Contusion and laceration of left
             cerebrum with loss of consciousness
             status unknown
             ▶ Contusion and laceration of left
               cerebrum NOS

● S06.33   Contusion and laceration of cerebrum,
            unspecified
    ● S06.330   Contusion and laceration of
                 cerebrum, unspecified, without loss of
                 consciousness A, S 🔒

● S06.331   Contusion and laceration of
             cerebrum, unspecified, with loss of
             consciousness of 30 minutes or less
             A, S 🔒
             ▶ Contusion and laceration of
               cerebrum, unspecified, with
               brief loss of consciousness
● S06.332   Contusion and laceration of
             cerebrum, unspecified, with loss of
             consciousness of 31 minutes to
             59 minutes A, S 🔒
● S06.333   Contusion and laceration of
             cerebrum, unspecified, with loss of
             consciousness of 1 hour to 5 hours
             59 minutes A, S 🔒
● S06.334   Contusion and laceration of
             cerebrum, unspecified, with loss of
             consciousness of 6 hours to 24 hours
             A, S 🔒
● S06.335   Contusion and laceration of
             cerebrum, unspecified, with loss of
             consciousness greater than 24 hours
             with return to pre-existing conscious
             level A, S 🔒
● S06.336   Contusion and laceration of
             cerebrum, unspecified, with loss of
             consciousness greater than 24 hours
             without return to pre-existing
             conscious level with patient surviving
             A, S 🔒
● S06.337   Contusion and laceration of
             cerebrum, unspecified, with loss of
             consciousness of any duration with
             death due to brain injury prior to
             regaining consciousness
● S06.338   Contusion and laceration of
             cerebrum, unspecified, with loss of
             consciousness of any duration with
             death due to other cause prior to
             regaining consciousness
● S06.339   Contusion and laceration of
             cerebrum, unspecified, with loss of
             consciousness of unspecified duration
             A, S 🔒
             ~~Contusion and laceration of
             cerebrum NOS~~

▶ ● S06.33A   Contusion and laceration of
             cerebrum, unspecified, with loss of
             consciousness status unknown
             ▶ Contusion and laceration of
               cerebrum NOS

● S06.34   Traumatic hemorrhage of right cerebrum
            Traumatic intracerebral hemorrhage and
            hematoma of right cerebrum
    ● S06.340   Traumatic hemorrhage of right
                 cerebrum without loss of
                 consciousness A, S 🔒
                 Coding Clinic: 2015, Q1, P12
    ● S06.341   Traumatic hemorrhage of right
                 cerebrum with loss of consciousness of
                 30 minutes or less A, S 🔒
                 ▶ Traumatic hemorrhage of right
                   cerebrum with loss of
                   consciousness
    ● S06.342   Traumatic hemorrhage of right
                 cerebrum with loss of consciousness of
                 31 minutes to 59 minutes A, S 🔒
    ● S06.343   Traumatic hemorrhage of right
                 cerebrum with loss of consciousness of
                 1 hours to 5 hours 59 minutes A, S 🔒
    ● S06.344   Traumatic hemorrhage of right
                 cerebrum with loss of consciousness of
                 6 hours to 24 hours A, S 🔒

CHAPTER 19 (S00-T88)

● **S06.345** Traumatic hemorrhage of right cerebrum with loss of consciousness greater than 24 hours with return to pre-existing conscious level A, S 🐾

● **S06.346** Traumatic hemorrhage of right cerebrum with loss of consciousness greater than 24 hours without return to pre-existing conscious level with patient surviving A, S 🐾

● **S06.347** Traumatic hemorrhage of right cerebrum with loss of consciousness of any duration with death due to brain injury prior to regaining consciousness

● **S06.348** Traumatic hemorrhage of right cerebrum with loss of consciousness of any duration with death due to other cause prior to regaining consciousness

● **S06.349** Traumatic hemorrhage of right cerebrum with loss of consciousness of unspecified duration A, S 🐾
~~Traumatic hemorrhage of right cerebrum NOS~~

▶● **S06.34A** Traumatic hemorrhage of right cerebrum with loss of consciousness status unknown
▶ Traumatic hemorrhage of right cerebrum NOS

● **S06.35** Traumatic hemorrhage of left cerebrum
Traumatic intracerebral hemorrhage and hematoma of left cerebrum

● **S06.350** Traumatic hemorrhage of left cerebrum without loss of consciousness A, S 🐾

● **S06.351** Traumatic hemorrhage of left cerebrum with loss of consciousness of 30 minutes or less A, S 🐾
▶ Traumatic hemorrhage of left cerebrum with brief loss of consciousness

● **S06.352** Traumatic hemorrhage of left cerebrum with loss of consciousness of 31 minutes to 59 minutes A, S 🐾

● **S06.353** Traumatic hemorrhage of left cerebrum with loss of consciousness of 1 hours to 5 hours 59 minutes A, S 🐾

● **S06.354** Traumatic hemorrhage of left cerebrum with loss of consciousness of 6 hours to 24 hours A, S 🐾

● **S06.355** Traumatic hemorrhage of left cerebrum with loss of consciousness greater than 24 hours with return to pre-existing conscious level A, S 🐾

● **S06.356** Traumatic hemorrhage of left cerebrum with loss of consciousness greater than 24 hours without return to pre-existing conscious level with patient surviving A, S 🐾

● **S06.357** Traumatic hemorrhage of left cerebrum with loss of consciousness of any duration with death due to brain injury prior to regaining consciousness

● **S06.358** Traumatic hemorrhage of left cerebrum with loss of consciousness of any duration with death due to other cause prior to regaining consciousness

● **S06.359** Traumatic hemorrhage of left cerebrum with loss of consciousness of unspecified duration A, S 🐾
~~Traumatic hemorrhage of left cerebrum NOS~~

▶● **S06.35A** Traumatic hemorrhage of left cerebrum with loss of consciousness status unknown
▶ Traumatic hemorrhage of left cerebrum NOS

● **S06.36** Traumatic hemorrhage of cerebrum, unspecified
Traumatic intracerebral hemorrhage and hematoma, unspecified

● **S06.360** Traumatic hemorrhage of cerebrum, unspecified, without loss of consciousness A, S 🐾

● **S06.361** Traumatic hemorrhage of cerebrum, unspecified, with loss of consciousness of 30 minutes or less A, S 🐾
▶ Traumatic hemorrhage of cerebrum, unspecified, with brief loss of consciousness

● **S06.362** Traumatic hemorrhage of cerebrum, unspecified, with loss of consciousness of 31 minutes to 59 minutes A, S 🐾

● **S06.363** Traumatic hemorrhage of cerebrum, unspecified, with loss of consciousness of 1 hours to 5 hours 59 minutes A, S 🐾

● **S06.364** Traumatic hemorrhage of cerebrum, unspecified, with loss of consciousness of 6 hours to 24 hours A, S 🐾

● **S06.365** Traumatic hemorrhage of cerebrum, unspecified, with loss of consciousness greater than 24 hours with return to pre-existing conscious level A, S 🐾

● **S06.366** Traumatic hemorrhage of cerebrum, unspecified, with loss of consciousness greater than 24 hours without return to pre-existing conscious level with patient surviving A, S 🐾

● **S06.367** Traumatic hemorrhage of cerebrum, unspecified, with loss of consciousness of any duration with death due to brain injury prior to regaining consciousness

● **S06.368** Traumatic hemorrhage of cerebrum, unspecified, with loss of consciousness of any duration with death due to other cause prior to regaining consciousness

● **S06.369** Traumatic hemorrhage of cerebrum, unspecified, with loss of consciousness of unspecified duration A, S 🐾
~~Traumatic hemorrhage of cerebrum NOS~~

▶● **S06.36A** Traumatic hemorrhage of cerebrum, unspecified, with loss of consciousness status unknown
▶ Traumatic hemorrhage of cerebrum NOS

● **S06.37** Contusion, laceration, and hemorrhage of cerebellum

● **S06.370** Contusion, laceration, and hemorrhage of cerebellum without loss of consciousness A, S 🐾

● **S06.371** Contusion, laceration, and hemorrhage of cerebellum with loss of consciousness of 30 minutes or less A, S 🐾
▶ Contusion, laceration, and hemorrhage of cerebellum with brief loss of consciousness

● S06.372   Contusion, laceration, and hemorrhage of cerebellum with loss of consciousness of 31 minutes to 59 minutes A, S 🔖

● S06.373   Contusion, laceration, and hemorrhage of cerebellum with loss of consciousness of 1 hour to 5 hours 59 minutes A, S 🔖

● S06.374   Contusion, laceration, and hemorrhage of cerebellum with loss of consciousness of 6 hours to 24 hours A, S 🔖

● S06.375   Contusion, laceration, and hemorrhage of cerebellum with loss of consciousness greater than 24 hours with return to pre-existing conscious level A, S 🔖

● S06.376   Contusion, laceration, and hemorrhage of cerebellum with loss of consciousness greater than 24 hours without return to pre-existing conscious level with patient surviving A, S 🔖

● S06.377   Contusion, laceration, and hemorrhage of cerebellum with loss of consciousness of any duration with death due to brain injury prior to regaining consciousness

● S06.378   Contusion, laceration, and hemorrhage of cerebellum with loss of consciousness of any duration with death due to other cause prior to regaining consciousness

● S06.379   Contusion, laceration, and hemorrhage of cerebellum with loss of consciousness of unspecified duration A, S 🔖
     ~~Contusion, laceration, and hemorrhage of cerebellum NOS~~

▶ ● S06.37A   Contusion, laceration, and hemorrhage of cerebellum with loss of consciousness status unknown
     Contusion, laceration, and hemorrhage of cerebellum NOS

● S06.38   Contusion, laceration, and hemorrhage of brainstem

● S06.380   Contusion, laceration, and hemorrhage of brainstem without loss of consciousness A, S 🔖

● S06.381   Contusion, laceration, and hemorrhage of brainstem with loss of consciousness of 30 minutes or less A, S 🔖
     ▶ Contusion, laceration, and hemorrhage of brainstem with brief loss of consciousness

● S06.382   Contusion, laceration, and hemorrhage of brainstem with loss of consciousness of 31 minutes to 59 minutes A, S 🔖

● S06.383   Contusion, laceration, and hemorrhage of brainstem with loss of consciousness of 1 hour to 5 hours 59 minutes A, S 🔖

● S06.384   Contusion, laceration, and hemorrhage of brainstem with loss of consciousness of 6 hours to 24 hours A, S 🔖

● S06.385   Contusion, laceration, and hemorrhage of brainstem with loss of consciousness greater than 24 hours with return to pre-existing conscious level A, S 🔖

● S06.386   Contusion, laceration, and hemorrhage of brainstem with loss of consciousness greater than 24 hours without return to pre-existing conscious level with patient surviving A, S 🔖

● S06.387   Contusion, laceration, and hemorrhage of brainstem with loss of consciousness of any duration with death due to brain injury prior to regaining consciousness

● S06.388   Contusion, laceration, and hemorrhage of brainstem with loss of consciousness of any duration with death due to other cause prior to regaining consciousness

● S06.389   Contusion, laceration, and hemorrhage of brainstem with loss of consciousness of unspecified duration A, S 🔖
     ~~Contusion, laceration, and hemorrhage of brainstem NOS~~

▶ ● S06.38A   Contusion, laceration, and hemorrhage of brainstem with loss of consciousness status unknown
     ▶ Contusion, laceration, and hemorrhage of brainstem NOS

● S06.4   **Epidural hemorrhage**
     Situated outside dura mater
     Extradural hemorrhage NOS
     Intracranial hemorrhage due to trauma
     Extradural hemorrhage (traumatic)

● S06.4X   Epidural hemorrhage

● S06.4X0   Epidural hemorrhage without loss of consciousness A, S 🔖

● S06.4X1   Epidural hemorrhage with loss of consciousness of 30 minutes or less A, S 🔖
     ▶ Epidural hemorrhage with brief loss of consciousness

● S06.4X2   Epidural hemorrhage with loss of consciousness of 31 minutes to 59 minutes A, S 🔖

● S06.4X3   Epidural hemorrhage with loss of consciousness of 1 hour to 5 hours 59 minutes A, S 🔖

● S06.4X4   Epidural hemorrhage with loss of consciousness of 6 hours to 24 hours A, S 🔖

● S06.4X5   Epidural hemorrhage with loss of consciousness greater than 24 hours with return to pre-existing conscious level A, S 🔖

● S06.4X6   Epidural hemorrhage with loss of consciousness greater than 24 hours without return to pre-existing conscious level with patient surviving A, S 🔖

● S06.4X7   Epidural hemorrhage with loss of consciousness of any duration with death due to brain injury prior to regaining consciousness

● S06.4X8   Epidural hemorrhage with loss of consciousness of any duration with death due to other causes prior to regaining consciousness

● S06.4X9   Epidural hemorrhage with loss of consciousness of unspecified duration A, S 🔖
     ~~Epidural hemorrhage NOS~~

▶ ● S06.4XA   Epidural hemorrhage with loss of consciousness status unknown
     ▶ Epidural hemorrhage NOS

CHAPTER 19 (S00–T88)

● **S06.5   Traumatic subdural hemorrhage**

> Use Additional code, if applicable, for traumatic brain compression or herniation (S06.A-)

● **S06.5X   Traumatic subdural hemorrhage**

● **S06.5X0   Traumatic subdural hemorrhage without loss of consciousness** A, S 🖤
> Coding Clinic: 2021, Q1, P4; 2018, Q2, P13; 2015, Q3, P37

● **S06.5X1   Traumatic subdural hemorrhage with loss of consciousness of 30 minutes or less** A, S 🖤
> ▶ Traumatic subdural hemorrhage with brief loss of consciousness

● **S06.5X2   Traumatic subdural hemorrhage with loss of consciousness of 31 minutes to 59 minutes** A, S 🖤

● **S06.5X3   Traumatic subdural hemorrhage with loss of consciousness of 1 hour to 5 hours 59 minutes** A, S 🖤

● **S06.5X4   Traumatic subdural hemorrhage with loss of consciousness of 6 hours to 24 hours** A, S 🖤

● **S06.5X5   Traumatic subdural hemorrhage with loss of consciousness greater than 24 hours with return to pre-existing conscious level** A, S 🖤

● **S06.5X6   Traumatic subdural hemorrhage with loss of consciousness greater than 24 hours without return to pre-existing conscious level with patient surviving** A, S 🖤
> Coding Clinic: 2021, Q2, P5

● **S06.5X7   Traumatic subdural hemorrhage with loss of consciousness of any duration with death due to brain injury before regaining consciousness**

● **S06.5X8   Traumatic subdural hemorrhage with loss of consciousness of any duration with death due to other cause before regaining consciousness**

● **S06.5X9   Traumatic subdural hemorrhage with loss of consciousness of unspecified duration** A, S 🖤
> ~~Traumatic subdural hemorrhage NOS~~

▶● **S06.5XA   Traumatic subdural hemorrhage with loss of consciousness status unknown**
> ▶Traumatic subdural hemorrhage NOS

● **S06.6   Traumatic subarachnoid hemorrhage**
> *Between arachnoid and pia mater*
> Use Additional code, if applicable, for traumatic brain compression or herniation (S06.A-)
> Coding Clinic: 2016, Q4, P67

● **S06.6X   Traumatic subarachnoid hemorrhage**

● **S06.6X0   Traumatic subarachnoid hemorrhage without loss of consciousness** A, S 🖤
> Coding Clinic: 2015, Q3, P37

● **S06.6X1   Traumatic subarachnoid hemorrhage with loss of consciousness of 30 minutes or less** A, S 🖤
> ▶ Traumatic subarachnoid hemorrhage with brief loss of consciousness

● **S06.6X2   Traumatic subarachnoid hemorrhage with loss of consciousness of 31 minutes to 59 minutes** A, S 🖤

● **S06.6X3   Traumatic subarachnoid hemorrhage with loss of consciousness of 1 hour to 5 hours 59 minutes** A, S 🖤

● **S06.6X4   Traumatic subarachnoid hemorrhage with loss of consciousness of 6 hours to 24 hours** A, S 🖤

● **S06.6X5   Traumatic subarachnoid hemorrhage with loss of consciousness greater than 24 hours with return to pre-existing conscious level** A, S 🖤

● **S06.6X6   Traumatic subarachnoid hemorrhage with loss of consciousness greater than 24 hours without return to pre-existing conscious level with patient surviving** A, S 🖤
> Coding Clinic: 2021, Q2, P5

● **S06.6X7   Traumatic subarachnoid hemorrhage with loss of consciousness of any duration with death due to brain injury prior to regaining consciousness**

● **S06.6X8   Traumatic subarachnoid hemorrhage with loss of consciousness of any duration with death due to other cause prior to regaining consciousness**

● **S06.6X9   Traumatic subarachnoid hemorrhage with loss of consciousness of unspecified duration** A, S 🖤
> ~~Traumatic subarachnoid hemorrhage NOS~~

▶● **S06.6XA   Traumatic subarachnoid hemorrhage with loss of consciousness status unknown**
> ▶Traumatic subarachnoid hemorrhage NOS

● **S06.8   Other specified intracranial injuries**

● **S06.81   Injury of right internal carotid artery, intracranial portion, not elsewhere classified**
> Coding Clinic: 2016, Q4, P67

● **S06.810   Injury of right internal carotid artery, intracranial portion, not elsewhere classified without loss of consciousness** A, S 🖤

● **S06.811   Injury of right internal carotid artery, intracranial portion, not elsewhere classified with loss of consciousness of 30 minutes or less** A, S 🖤
> ▶ Injury of right internal carotid artery, intracranial portion, not elsewhere classified with brief loss of consciousness

● **S06.812   Injury of right internal carotid artery, intracranial portion, not elsewhere classified with loss of consciousness of 31 minutes to 59 minutes** A, S 🖤

● **S06.813   Injury of right internal carotid artery, intracranial portion, not elsewhere classified with loss of consciousness of 1 hour to 5 hours 59 minutes** A, S 🖤

● **S06.814   Injury of right internal carotid artery, intracranial portion, not elsewhere classified with loss of consciousness of 6 hours to 24 hours** A, S 🖤

● **S06.815   Injury of right internal carotid artery, intracranial portion, not elsewhere classified with loss of consciousness greater than 24 hours with return to pre-existing conscious level** A, S 🖤

● **S06.816   Injury of right internal carotid artery, intracranial portion, not elsewhere classified with loss of consciousness greater than 24 hours without return to pre-existing conscious level with patient surviving** A, S 🖤

▶ New   ⇒ Revised   ~~deleted~~ Deleted   Excludes 1   Excludes 2   Includes   Use additional   Code first   Code also   Key words

OGCR Official Guidelines   X Assign placeholder X   ● Use Additional Character(s)   ▶ Manifestation Code   🖤 Hierarchical Condition Category   **Coding Clinic**

● S06.817　Injury of right internal carotid artery, intracranial portion, not elsewhere classified with loss of consciousness of any duration with death due to brain injury prior to regaining consciousness

● S06.818　Injury of right internal carotid artery, intracranial portion, not elsewhere classified with loss of consciousness of any duration with death due to other cause prior to regaining consciousness

● S06.819　Injury of right internal carotid artery, intracranial portion, not elsewhere classified with loss of consciousness of unspecified duration A, S 🐾

　　　　　Injury of right internal carotid artery, intracranial portion, not elsewhere classified NOS

▶ ● S06.81A　Injury of right internal carotid artery, intracranial portion, not elsewhere classified with loss of consciousness status unknown

　　　　　▶ Injury of right internal carotid artery, intracranial portion, not elsewhere classified NOS

● S06.82　Injury of left internal carotid artery, intracranial portion, not elsewhere classified
　　　　　Coding Clinic: 2016, Q4, P67

● S06.820　Injury of left internal carotid artery, intracranial portion, not elsewhere classified without loss of consciousness A, S 🐾

● S06.821　Injury of left internal carotid artery, intracranial portion, not elsewhere classified with loss of consciousness of 30 minutes or less A, S 🐾

　　　　　▶ Injury of left internal carotid artery, intracranial portion, not elsewhere classified with brief loss of consciousness

● S06.822　Injury of left internal carotid artery, intracranial portion, not elsewhere classified with loss of consciousness of 31 minutes to 59 minutes A, S 🐾

● S06.823　Injury of left internal carotid artery, intracranial portion, not elsewhere classified with loss of consciousness of 1 hour to 5 hours 59 minutes A, S 🐾

● S06.824　Injury of left internal carotid artery, intracranial portion, not elsewhere classified with loss of consciousness of 6 hours to 24 hours A, S 🐾

● S06.825　Injury of left internal carotid artery, intracranial portion, not elsewhere classified with loss of consciousness greater than 24 hours with return to pre-existing conscious level

● S06.826　Injury of left internal carotid artery, intracranial portion, not elsewhere classified with loss of consciousness greater than 24 hours without return to pre-existing conscious level with patient surviving A, S 🐾

● S06.827　Injury of left internal carotid artery, intracranial portion, not elsewhere classified with loss of consciousness of any duration with death due to brain injury prior to regaining consciousness

● S06.828　Injury of left internal carotid artery, intracranial portion, not elsewhere classified with loss of consciousness of any duration with death due to other cause prior to regaining consciousness

● S06.829　Injury of left internal carotid artery, intracranial portion, not elsewhere classified with loss of consciousness of unspecified duration A, S 🐾

　　　　　Injury of left internal carotid artery, intracranial portion, not elsewhere classified NOS

▶ ● S06.82A　Injury of left internal carotid artery, intracranial portion, not elsewhere classified with loss of consciousness status unknown

　　　　　▶ Injury of left internal carotid artery, intracranial portion, not elsewhere classified NOS

● S06.89　Other specified intracranial injury
　　　　　Excludes1　concussion (S06.0X-)

● S06.890　Other specified intracranial injury without loss of consciousness A, S 🐾

● S06.891　Other specified intracranial injury with loss of consciousness of 30 minutes or less A, S 🐾

　　　　　▶ Other specified intracranial injury with brief loss of consciousness

● S06.892　Other specified intracranial injury with loss of consciousness of 31 minutes to 59 minutes A, S 🐾

● S06.893　Other specified intracranial injury with loss of consciousness of 1 hour to 5 hours 59 minutes A, S 🐾

● S06.894　Other specified intracranial injury with loss of consciousness of 6 hours to 24 hours A, S 🐾

● S06.895　Other specified intracranial injury with loss of consciousness greater than 24 hours with return to pre-existing conscious level A, S 🐾

● S06.896　Other specified intracranial injury with loss of consciousness greater than 24 hours without return to pre-existing conscious level with patient surviving A, S 🐾

● S06.897　Other specified intracranial injury with loss of consciousness of any duration with death due to brain injury prior to regaining consciousness

● S06.898　Other specified intracranial injury with loss of consciousness of any duration with death due to other cause prior to regaining consciousness

● S06.899　Other specified intracranial injury with loss of consciousness of unspecified duration A, S 🐾

▶ ● S06.89A　Other specified intracranial injury with loss of consciousness status unknown

CHAPTER 19 (S00-T88)

CHAPTER 19 (S00-T88)

▶● **S06.8A Primary blast injury of brain, not elsewhere classified**

▶ Code also, if applicable, focal traumatic brain injury (S06.3-)

▶ **Excludes2** traumatic cerebral edema (S06.1)

▶● **S06.8A0 Primary blast injury of brain, not elsewhere classified without loss of consciousness**

▶● **S06.8A1 Primary blast injury of brain, not elsewhere classified with loss of consciousness of 30 minutes or less**
▶ Primary blast injury of brain, not elsewhere classified with brief loss of consciousness

▶● **S06.8A2 Primary blast injury of brain, not elsewhere classified with loss of consciousness of 31 minutes to 59 minutes**

▶● **S06.8A3 Primary blast injury of brain, not elsewhere classified with loss of consciousness of 1 hour to 5 hours 59 minutes**

▶● **S06.8A4 Primary blast injury of brain, not elsewhere classified with loss of consciousness of 6 hours to 24 hours**

▶● **S06.8A5 Primary blast injury of brain, not elsewhere classified with loss of consciousness greater than 24 hours with return to pre-existing conscious level**

▶● **S06.8A6 Primary blast injury of brain, not elsewhere classified with loss of consciousness greater than 24 hours without return to pre-existing conscious level with patient surviving**

▶● **S06.8A7 Primary blast injury of brain, not elsewhere classified with loss of consciousness of any duration with death due to brain injury prior to regaining consciousness**

▶● **S06.8A8 Primary blast injury of brain, not elsewhere classified with loss of consciousness of any duration with death due to other cause prior to regaining consciousness**

▶● **S06.8AA Primary blast injury of brain, not elsewhere classified with loss of consciousness status unknown**
▶ Primary blast injury of brain NOS

▶● **S06.8A9 Primary blast injury of brain, not elsewhere classified with loss of consciousness of unspecified duration**

● **S06.9 Unspecified intracranial injury**
Brain injury NOS
Head injury NOS with loss of consciousness
Traumatic brain injury NOS

Excludes1 conditions classifiable to S06.0- to S06.8- code to specified intracranial injury head injury NOS (S09.90)

● **S06.9X Unspecified intracranial injury**

● **S06.9X0 Unspecified intracranial injury without loss of consciousness** A, S 🐾

● **S06.9X1 Unspecified intracranial injury with loss of consciousness of 30 minutes or less** A, S 🐾
▶ Unspecified intracranial injury with brief loss of consciousness

● **S06.9X2 Unspecified intracranial injury with loss of consciousness of 31 minutes to 59 minutes** A, S 🐾

● **S06.9X3 Unspecified intracranial injury with loss of consciousness of 1 hour to 5 hours 59 minutes** A, S 🐾

● **S06.9X4 Unspecified intracranial injury with loss of consciousness of 6 hours to 24 hours** A, S 🐾

● **S06.9X5 Unspecified intracranial injury with loss of consciousness greater than 24 hours with return to pre-existing conscious level** A, S 🐾

● **S06.9X6 Unspecified intracranial injury with loss of consciousness greater than 24 hours without return to pre-existing conscious level with patient surviving** A, S 🐾

● **S06.9X7 Unspecified intracranial injury with loss of consciousness of any duration with death due to brain injury prior to regaining consciousness**

● **S06.9X8 Unspecified intracranial injury with loss of consciousness of any duration with death due to other cause prior to regaining consciousness**

● **S06.9X9 Unspecified intracranial injury with loss of consciousness of unspecified duration** A, S 🐾

▶● **S06.9XA Unspecified intracranial injury with loss of consciousness status unknown**

● **S06.A Traumatic brain compression and herniation**
Traumatic cerebral compression

Code first the underlying traumatic brain injury, such as:
diffuse traumatic brain injury (S06.2-)
focal traumatic brain injury (S06.3-)
traumatic subdural hemorrhage (S06.5-)
traumatic subarachnoid hemorrhage (S06.6-)

S06.A0 Traumatic brain compression without herniation
Traumatic brain compression NOS
Traumatic cerebral compression NOS

S06.A1 Traumatic brain compression with herniation
Traumatic brain herniation
Traumatic brainstem compression with herniation
Traumatic cerebellar compression with herniation
Traumatic cerebral compression with herniation

● **S07 Crushing injury of head**
Use additional code for all associated injuries, such as:
intracranial injuries (S06.-)
skull fractures (S02.-)

The appropriate 7th character is to be added to each code from category S07

A	initial encounter
D	subsequent encounter
S	sequela

X● **S07.0 Crushing injury of face**
X● **S07.1 Crushing injury of skull**
X● **S07.8 Crushing injury of other parts of head**
X● **S07.9 Crushing injury of head, part unspecified**

● **S08 Avulsion and traumatic amputation of part of head**
An amputation not identified as partial or complete should be coded to complete

The appropriate 7th character is to be added to each code from category S08

A	initial encounter
D	subsequent encounter
S	sequela

X● **S08.0 Avulsion of scalp**

● **S08.1**   Traumatic amputation of ear
   ● **S08.11**   Complete traumatic amputation of ear
     ● **S08.111**   Complete traumatic amputation of right ear
     ● **S08.112**   Complete traumatic amputation of left ear
     ● **S08.119**   Complete traumatic amputation of unspecified ear
   ● **S08.12**   Partial traumatic amputation of ear
     ● **S08.121**   Partial traumatic amputation of right ear
     ● **S08.122**   Partial traumatic amputation of left ear
     ● **S08.129**   Partial traumatic amputation of unspecified ear
● **S08.8**   Traumatic amputation of other parts of head
   ● **S08.81**   Traumatic amputation of nose
     ● **S08.811**   Complete traumatic amputation of nose
     ● **S08.812**   Partial traumatic amputation of nose
   X● **S08.89**   Traumatic amputation of other parts of head

● **S09**   Other and unspecified injuries of head

The appropriate 7th character is to be added to each code from category S09

A	initial encounter
D	subsequent encounter
S	sequela

   X● **S09.0**   Injury of blood vessels of head, not elsewhere classified
     Excludes1   injury of cerebral blood vessels (S06.-)
                 injury of precerebral blood vessels (S15.-)
   ● **S09.1**   Injury of muscle and tendon of head
     Code also any associated open wound (S01.-)
     Excludes2   sprain to joints and ligament of head (S03.9)
     X● **S09.10**   Unspecified injury of muscle and tendon of head
         Injury of muscle and tendon of head NOS
     X● **S09.11**   Strain of muscle and tendon of head
     X● **S09.12**   Laceration of muscle and tendon of head
     X● **S09.19**   Other specified injury of muscle and tendon of head
   ● **S09.2**   Traumatic rupture of ear drum
     Excludes1   traumatic rupture of ear drum due to blast injury (S09.31-)
     X● **S09.20**   Traumatic rupture of unspecified ear drum
     X● **S09.21**   Traumatic rupture of right ear drum
     X● **S09.22**   Traumatic rupture of left ear drum
   ● **S09.3**   Other specified and unspecified injury of middle and inner ear
     Excludes1   injury to ear NOS (S09.91-)
     Excludes2   injury to external ear (S00.4-, S01.3-, S08.1-)
     ● **S09.30**   Unspecified injury of middle and inner ear
       ● **S09.301**   Unspecified injury of right middle and inner ear
       ● **S09.302**   Unspecified injury of left middle and inner ear
       ● **S09.309**   Unspecified injury of unspecified middle and inner ear
     ● **S09.31**   Primary blast injury of ear
         Blast injury of ear NOS
       ● **S09.311**   Primary blast injury of right ear
       ● **S09.312**   Primary blast injury of left ear
       ● **S09.313**   Primary blast injury of ear, bilateral
       ● **S09.319**   Primary blast injury of unspecified ear

     ● **S09.39**   Other specified injury of middle and inner ear
         Secondary blast injury to ear
       ● **S09.391**   Other specified injury of right middle and inner ear
       ● **S09.392**   Other specified injury of left middle and inner ear
       ● **S09.399**   Other specified injury of unspecified middle and inner ear
   X● **S09.8**   Other specified injuries of head
   ● **S09.9**   Unspecified injury of face and head
     X● **S09.90**   Unspecified injury of head
         Head injury NOS
         Excludes1   brain injury NOS (S06.9-)
                     head injury NOS with loss of consciousness (S06.9-)
                     intracranial injury NOS (S06.9-)
     X● **S09.91**   Unspecified injury of ear
         Injury of ear NOS
     X● **S09.92**   Unspecified injury of nose
         Injury of nose NOS
     X● **S09.93**   Unspecified injury of face
         Injury of face NOS

INJURIES TO THE NECK (S10-S19)

Includes	injuries of nape
	injuries of supraclavicular region
	injuries of throat

Excludes2	burns and corrosions (T20-T32)
	effects of foreign body in esophagus (T18.1)
	effects of foreign body in larynx (T17.3)
	effects of foreign body in pharynx (T17.2)
	effects of foreign body in trachea (T17.4)
	frostbite (T33-T34)
	insect bite or sting, venomous (T63.4)

● **S10**   Superficial injury of neck

The appropriate 7th character is to be added to each code from category S10

A	initial encounter
D	subsequent encounter
S	sequela

   X● **S10.0**   Contusion of throat
     Contusion of cervical esophagus
     Contusion of larynx
     Contusion of pharynx
     Contusion of trachea
   ● **S10.1**   Other and unspecified superficial injuries of throat
     X● **S10.10**   Unspecified superficial injuries of throat
     X● **S10.11**   Abrasion of throat
     X● **S10.12**   Blister (nonthermal) of throat
     X● **S10.14**   External constriction of part of throat
     X● **S10.15**   Superficial foreign body of throat
         Splinter in the throat
     X● **S10.16**   Insect bite (nonvenomous) of throat
     X● **S10.17**   Other superficial bite of throat
         Excludes1   open bite of throat (S11.85)
   ● **S10.8**   Superficial injury of other specified parts of neck
     X● **S10.80**   Unspecified superficial injury of other specified part of neck
     X● **S10.81**   Abrasion of other specified part of neck
     X● **S10.82**   Blister (nonthermal) of other specified part of neck
     X● **S10.83**   Contusion of other specified part of neck
     X● **S10.84**   External constriction of other specified part of neck
     X● **S10.85**   Superficial foreign body of other specified part of neck
         Splinter in other part of neck

X ● **S10.86**   Insect bite of other specified part of neck

X ● **S10.87**   Other superficial bite of other specified part of neck

> **Excludes1**   open bite of other specified parts of neck (S11.85)

● **S10.9**   Superficial injury of unspecified part of neck

X ● **S10.90**   Unspecified superficial injury of unspecified part of neck

X ● **S10.91**   Abrasion of unspecified part of neck

X ● **S10.92**   Blister (nonthermal) of unspecified part of neck

X ● **S10.93**   Contusion of unspecified part of neck

X ● **S10.94**   External constriction of unspecified part of neck

X ● **S10.95**   Superficial foreign body of unspecified part of neck

X ● **S10.96**   Insect bite of unspecified part of neck

X ● **S10.97**   Other superficial bite of unspecified part of neck

● **S11**   **Open wound of neck**

Code also any associated:
     spinal cord injury (S14.0, S14.1-)
     wound infection

> **Excludes2**   open fracture of vertebra (S12.- with 7th character B)

The appropriate 7th character is to be added to each code from category S11

> A   initial encounter
> D   subsequent encounter
> S   sequela

● **S11.0**   Open wound of larynx and trachea

    ● **S11.01**   Open wound of larynx

> **Excludes2**   open wound of vocal cord (S11.03)

      ● **S11.011**   Laceration without foreign body of larynx

      ● **S11.012**   Laceration with foreign body of larynx

      ● **S11.013**   Puncture wound without foreign body of larynx

      ● **S11.014**   Puncture wound with foreign body of larynx

      ● **S11.015**   Open bite of larynx
          Bite of larynx NOS

      ● **S11.019**   Unspecified open wound of larynx

    ● **S11.02**   Open wound of trachea
       Open wound of cervical trachea
       Open wound of trachea NOS

> **Excludes2**   open wound of thoracic trachea (S27.5-)

      ● **S11.021**   Laceration without foreign body of trachea

      ● **S11.022**   Laceration with foreign body of trachea

      ● **S11.023**   Puncture wound without foreign body of trachea

      ● **S11.024**   Puncture wound with foreign body of trachea

      ● **S11.025**   Open bite of trachea
          Bite of trachea NOS

      ● **S11.029**   Unspecified open wound of trachea

    ● **S11.03**   Open wound of vocal cord

      ● **S11.031**   Laceration without foreign body of vocal cord

      ● **S11.032**   Laceration with foreign body of vocal cord

      ● **S11.033**   Puncture wound without foreign body of vocal cord

      ● **S11.034**   Puncture wound with foreign body of vocal cord

      ● **S11.035**   Open bite of vocal cord
          Bite of vocal cord NOS

      ● **S11.039**   Unspecified open wound of vocal cord

● **S11.1**   Open wound of thyroid gland

X ● **S11.10**   Unspecified open wound of thyroid gland

X ● **S11.11**   Laceration without foreign body of thyroid gland

X ● **S11.12**   Laceration with foreign body of thyroid gland

X ● **S11.13**   Puncture wound without foreign body of thyroid gland

X ● **S11.14**   Puncture wound with foreign body of thyroid gland

X ● **S11.15**   Open bite of thyroid gland
          Bite of thyroid gland NOS

● **S11.2**   Open wound of pharynx and cervical esophagus

> **Excludes1**   open wound of esophagus NOS (S27.8-)

X ● **S11.20**   Unspecified open wound of pharynx and cervical esophagus

X ● **S11.21**   Laceration without foreign body of pharynx and cervical esophagus

X ● **S11.22**   Laceration with foreign body of pharynx and cervical esophagus

X ● **S11.23**   Puncture wound without foreign body of pharynx and cervical esophagus

X ● **S11.24**   Puncture wound with foreign body of pharynx and cervical esophagus

X ● **S11.25**   Open bite of pharynx and cervical esophagus
          Bite of pharynx and cervical esophagus NOS

● **S11.8**   Open wound of other specified parts of neck

X ● **S11.80**   Unspecified open specified wound of other part of neck

X ● **S11.81**   Laceration without foreign body of other specified part of neck

X ● **S11.82**   Laceration with foreign body of other specified part of neck

X ● **S11.83**   Puncture wound without foreign body of other specified part of neck

X ● **S11.84**   Puncture wound with foreign body of other specified part of neck

X ● **S11.85**   Open bite of other specified part of neck
          Bite of other part of neck NOS

> **Excludes1**   superficial bite of other specified part of neck (S10.87)

X ● **S11.89**   Other open wound of other part of neck

● **S11.9**   Open wound of unspecified part of neck

X ● **S11.90**   Unspecified open wound of unspecified part of neck

X ● **S11.91**   Laceration without foreign body of unspecified part of neck

X ● **S11.92**   Laceration with foreign body of unspecified part of neck

X ● **S11.93**   Puncture wound without foreign body of unspecified part of neck

X ● **S11.94**   Puncture wound with foreign body of unspecified part of neck

X ● **S11.95**   Open bite of unspecified part of neck
          Bite of neck NOS

> **Excludes1**   superficial bite of neck (S10.97)

▶ New   ⇒ Revised   ~~deleted~~ Deleted   Excludes 1   Excludes 2   Includes   Use additional   Code first   Code also   Key words

OGCR Official Guidelines   X Assign placeholder X   ● Use Additional Character(s)   ▶ Manifestation Code   🔖 Hierarchical Condition Category   **Coding Clinic**

● **S12** **Fracture of cervical vertebra and other parts of neck**

  Note: A fracture not indicated as displaced or nondisplaced should be coded to displaced

  A fracture not indicated as open or closed should be coded to closed

  Includes fracture of cervical neural arch
  fracture of cervical spine
  fracture of cervical spinous process
  fracture of cervical transverse process
  fracture of cervical vertebral arch
  fracture of neck

  Code first any associated cervical spinal cord injury (S14.0, S14.1-)

  The appropriate 7th character is to be added to all codes from subcategories S12.0-S12.6

A	initial encounter for closed fracture
B	initial encounter for open fracture
D	subsequent encounter for fracture with routine healing
G	subsequent encounter for fracture with delayed healing
K	subsequent encounter for fracture with nonunion
S	sequela

● **S12.0** **Fracture of first cervical vertebra**
  Atlas

  ● **S12.00** **Unspecified fracture of first cervical vertebra**

    ● **S12.000** **Unspecified displaced fracture of first cervical vertebra** A, B 🖎

    ● **S12.001** **Unspecified nondisplaced fracture of first cervical vertebra** A, B 🖎

  X ● **S12.01** **Stable burst fracture of first cervical vertebra** A, B 🖎

  X ● **S12.02** **Unstable burst fracture of first cervical vertebra** A, B 🖎

  ● **S12.03** **Posterior arch fracture of first cervical vertebra**

    ● **S12.030** **Displaced posterior arch fracture of first cervical vertebra** A, B 🖎

    ● **S12.031** **Nondisplaced posterior arch fracture of first cervical vertebra** A, B 🖎

  ● **S12.04** **Lateral mass fracture of first cervical vertebra**

    ● **S12.040** **Displaced lateral mass fracture of first cervical vertebra** A, B 🖎

    ● **S12.041** **Nondisplaced lateral mass fracture of first cervical vertebra** A, B 🖎

  ● **S12.09** **Other fracture of first cervical vertebra**

    ● **S12.090** **Other displaced fracture of first cervical vertebra** A, B 🖎

    ● **S12.091** **Other nondisplaced fracture of first cervical vertebra** A, B 🖎

● **S12.1** **Fracture of second cervical vertebra**
  Axis

  ● **S12.10** **Unspecified fracture of second cervical vertebra**

    ● **S12.100** **Unspecified displaced fracture of second cervical vertebra** A, B 🖎

    ● **S12.101** **Unspecified nondisplaced fracture of second cervical vertebra** A, B 🖎

  ● **S12.11** **Type II dens fracture**

    ● **S12.110** **Anterior displaced Type II dens fracture** A, B 🖎

    ● **S12.111** **Posterior displaced Type II dens fracture** A, B 🖎

    ● **S12.112** **Nondisplaced Type II dens fracture** A, B 🖎

  ● **S12.12** **Other dens fracture**

    ● **S12.120** **Other displaced dens fracture** A, B 🖎

    ● **S12.121** **Other nondisplaced dens fracture** A, B 🖎

● **S12.13** **Unspecified traumatic spondylolisthesis of second cervical vertebra**

    ● **S12.130** **Unspecified traumatic displaced spondylolisthesis of second cervical vertebra** A, B 🖎

    ● **S12.131** **Unspecified traumatic nondisplaced spondylolisthesis of second cervical vertebra** A, B 🖎

  X ● **S12.14** **Type III traumatic spondylolisthesis of second cervical vertebra** A, B 🖎

  ● **S12.15** **Other traumatic spondylolisthesis of second cervical vertebra**

    ● **S12.150** **Other traumatic displaced spondylolisthesis of second cervical vertebra** A, B 🖎

    ● **S12.151** **Other traumatic nondisplaced spondylolisthesis of second cervical vertebra** A, B 🖎

  ● **S12.19** **Other fracture of second cervical vertebra**

    ● **S12.190** **Other displaced fracture of second cervical vertebra** A, B 🖎

    ● **S12.191** **Other nondisplaced fracture of second cervical vertebra** A, B 🖎

● **S12.2** **Fracture of third cervical vertebra**

  ● **S12.20** **Unspecified fracture of third cervical vertebra**

    ● **S12.200** **Unspecified displaced fracture of third cervical vertebra** A, B 🖎

    ● **S12.201** **Unspecified nondisplaced fracture of third cervical vertebra** A, B 🖎

  ● **S12.23** **Unspecified traumatic spondylolisthesis of third cervical vertebra**

    ● **S12.230** **Unspecified traumatic displaced spondylolisthesis of third cervical vertebra** A, B 🖎

    ● **S12.231** **Unspecified traumatic nondisplaced spondylolisthesis of third cervical vertebra** A, B 🖎

  X ● **S12.24** **Type III traumatic spondylolisthesis of third cervical vertebra** A, B 🖎

  ● **S12.25** **Other traumatic spondylolisthesis of third cervical vertebra**

    ● **S12.250** **Other traumatic displaced spondylolisthesis of third cervical vertebra** A, B 🖎

    ● **S12.251** **Other traumatic nondisplaced spondylolisthesis of third cervical vertebra** A, B 🖎

  ● **S12.29** **Other fracture of third cervical vertebra**

    ● **S12.290** **Other displaced fracture of third cervical vertebra** A, B 🖎

    ● **S12.291** **Other nondisplaced fracture of third cervical vertebra** A, B 🖎

● **S12.3** **Fracture of fourth cervical vertebra**

  ● **S12.30** **Unspecified fracture of fourth cervical vertebra**

    ● **S12.300** **Unspecified displaced fracture of fourth cervical vertebra** A, B 🖎

    ● **S12.301** **Unspecified nondisplaced fracture of fourth cervical vertebra** A, B 🖎

  ● **S12.33** **Unspecified traumatic spondylolisthesis of fourth cervical vertebra**

    ● **S12.330** **Unspecified traumatic displaced spondylolisthesis of fourth cervical vertebra** A, B 🖎

    ● **S12.331** **Unspecified traumatic nondisplaced spondylolisthesis of fourth cervical vertebra** A, B 🖎

  X ● **S12.34** **Type III traumatic spondylolisthesis of fourth cervical vertebra** A, B 🖎

  ● **S12.35** **Other traumatic spondylolisthesis of fourth cervical vertebra**

- S12.350   Other traumatic displaced spondylolisthesis of fourth cervical vertebra A, B 🐾
- S12.351   Other traumatic nondisplaced spondylolisthesis of fourth cervical vertebra A, B 🐾
- S12.39   Other fracture of fourth cervical vertebra
  - S12.390   Other displaced fracture of fourth cervical vertebra A, B 🐾
  - S12.391   Other nondisplaced fracture of fourth cervical vertebra A, B 🐾
- S12.4   Fracture of fifth cervical vertebra
  - S12.40   Unspecified fracture of fifth cervical vertebra
    - S12.400   Unspecified displaced fracture of fifth cervical vertebra A, B 🐾
    - S12.401   Unspecified nondisplaced fracture of fifth cervical vertebra A, B 🐾
  - S12.43   Unspecified traumatic spondylolisthesis of fifth cervical vertebra
    - S12.430   Unspecified traumatic displaced spondylolisthesis of fifth cervical vertebra A, B 🐾
    - S12.431   Unspecified traumatic nondisplaced spondylolisthesis of fifth cervical vertebra A, B 🐾
  - X● S12.44   Type III traumatic spondylolisthesis of fifth cervical vertebra A, B 🐾
  - S12.45   Other traumatic spondylolisthesis of fifth cervical vertebra
    - S12.450   Other traumatic displaced spondylolisthesis of fifth cervical vertebra A, B 🐾
    - S12.451   Other traumatic nondisplaced spondylolisthesis of fifth cervical vertebra A, B 🐾
  - S12.49   Other fracture of fifth cervical vertebra
    - S12.490   Other displaced fracture of fifth cervical vertebra A, B 🐾
    - S12.491   Other nondisplaced fracture of fifth cervical vertebra A, B 🐾
- S12.5   Fracture of sixth cervical vertebra
  - S12.50   Unspecified fracture of sixth cervical vertebra
    - S12.500   Unspecified displaced fracture of sixth cervical vertebra A, B 🐾
    - S12.501   Unspecified nondisplaced fracture of sixth cervical vertebra A, B 🐾
  - S12.53   Unspecified traumatic spondylolisthesis of sixth cervical vertebra
    - S12.530   Unspecified traumatic displaced spondylolisthesis of sixth cervical vertebra A, B 🐾
    - S12.531   Unspecified traumatic nondisplaced spondylolisthesis of sixth cervical vertebra A, B 🐾
  - X● S12.54   Type III traumatic spondylolisthesis of sixth cervical vertebra A, B 🐾
  - S12.55   Other traumatic spondylolisthesis of sixth cervical vertebra
    - S12.550   Other traumatic displaced spondylolisthesis of sixth cervical vertebra A, B 🐾
    - S12.551   Other traumatic nondisplaced spondylolisthesis of sixth cervical vertebra A, B 🐾
  - S12.59   Other fracture of sixth cervical vertebra
    - S12.590   Other displaced fracture of sixth cervical vertebra A, B 🐾
    - S12.591   Other nondisplaced fracture of sixth cervical vertebra A, B 🐾

- S12.6   Fracture of seventh cervical vertebra
  - S12.60   Unspecified fracture of seventh cervical vertebra
    - S12.600   Unspecified displaced fracture of seventh cervical vertebra A, B 🐾
    - S12.601   Unspecified nondisplaced fracture of seventh cervical vertebra A, B 🐾
  - S12.63   Unspecified traumatic spondylolisthesis of seventh cervical vertebra
    - S12.630   Unspecified traumatic displaced spondylolisthesis of seventh cervical vertebra A, B 🐾
    - S12.631   Unspecified traumatic nondisplaced spondylolisthesis of seventh cervical vertebra A, B 🐾
  - X● S12.64   Type III traumatic spondylolisthesis of seventh cervical vertebra A, B 🐾
  - S12.65   Other traumatic spondylolisthesis of seventh cervical vertebra
    - S12.650   Other traumatic displaced spondylolisthesis of seventh cervical vertebra A, B 🐾
    - S12.651   Other traumatic nondisplaced spondylolisthesis of seventh cervical vertebra A, B 🐾
  - S12.69   Other fracture of seventh cervical vertebra
    - S12.690   Other displaced fracture of seventh cervical vertebra A, B 🐾
    - S12.691   Other nondisplaced fracture of seventh cervical vertebra A, B 🐾
- X● S12.8   Fracture of other parts of neck A 🐾

  | Hyoid bone | Thyroid cartilage |
  | Larynx | Trachea |

  The appropriate 7th character is to be added to code S12.8

A	initial encounter
D	subsequent encounter
S	sequela

- X● S12.9   Fracture of neck, unspecified A 🐾

  Fracture of neck NOS
  Fracture of cervical spine NOS
  Fracture of cervical vertebra NOS

  The appropriate 7th character is to be added to code S12.9

A	initial encounter
D	subsequent encounter
S	sequela

- S13   Dislocation and sprain of joints and ligaments at neck level

  Includes   avulsion of joint or ligament at neck level
  laceration of cartilage, joint or ligament at neck level
  sprain of cartilage, joint or ligament at neck level
  traumatic hemarthrosis of joint or ligament at neck level
  traumatic rupture of joint or ligament at neck level
  traumatic subluxation of joint or ligament at neck level
  traumatic tear of joint or ligament at neck level

  Code also any associated open wound

  Excludes2   strain of muscle or tendon at neck level (S16.1)

  The appropriate 7th character is to be added to each code from category S13

A	initial encounter
D	subsequent encounter
S	sequela

▶ New   ⇒ Revised   ~~deleted~~ Deleted   Excludes 1   Excludes 2   Includes   Use additional   Code first   Code also   Key words

1252   **OGCR** Official Guidelines   X Assign placeholder X   ● Use Additional Character(s)   ▸ Manifestation Code   🐾 Hierarchical Condition Category   **Coding Clinic**

X● **S13.0**   **Traumatic rupture of cervical intervertebral disc**
> **Excludes1**   rupture or displacement (nontraumatic) of cervical intervertebral disc NOS (M50.-)

● **S13.1**   **Subluxation and dislocation of cervical vertebrae**
> Code also any associated:
> open wound of neck (S11.-)
> spinal cord injury (S14.1-)
>
> **Excludes2**   fracture of cervical vertebrae (S12.0-S12.3-)

  ● **S13.10**   **Subluxation and dislocation of unspecified cervical vertebrae**

    ● **S13.100**   **Subluxation of unspecified cervical vertebrae**

    ● **S13.101**   **Dislocation of unspecified cervical vertebrae**

  ● **S13.11**   **Subluxation and dislocation of C0/C1 cervical vertebrae**
> Subluxation and dislocation of atlantooccipital joint
> Subluxation and dislocation of atloidooccipital joint
> Subluxation and dislocation of occipitoatloid joint

    ● **S13.110**   **Subluxation of C0/C1 cervical vertebrae**

    ● **S13.111**   **Dislocation of C0/C1 cervical vertebrae**

  ● **S13.12**   **Subluxation and dislocation of C1/C2 cervical vertebrae**
> Subluxation and dislocation of atlantoaxial joint

    ● **S13.120**   **Subluxation of C1/C2 cervical vertebrae**

    ● **S13.121**   **Dislocation of C1/C2 cervical vertebrae**

  ● **S13.13**   **Subluxation and dislocation of C2/C3 cervical vertebrae**

    ● **S13.130**   **Subluxation of C2/C3 cervical vertebrae**

    ● **S13.131**   **Dislocation of C2/C3 cervical vertebrae**

  ● **S13.14**   **Subluxation and dislocation of C3/C4 cervical vertebrae**

    ● **S13.140**   **Subluxation of C3/C4 cervical vertebrae**

    ● **S13.141**   **Dislocation of C3/C4 cervical vertebrae**

  ● **S13.15**   **Subluxation and dislocation of C4/C5 cervical vertebrae**

    ● **S13.150**   **Subluxation of C4/C5 cervical vertebrae**

    ● **S13.151**   **Dislocation of C4/C5 cervical vertebrae**

  ● **S13.16**   **Subluxation and dislocation of C5/C6 cervical vertebrae**

    ● **S13.160**   **Subluxation of C5/C6 cervical vertebrae**

    ● **S13.161**   **Dislocation of C5/C6 cervical vertebrae**

  ● **S13.17**   **Subluxation and dislocation of C6/C7 cervical vertebrae**

    ● **S13.170**   **Subluxation of C6/C7 cervical vertebrae**

    ● **S13.171**   **Dislocation of C6/C7 cervical vertebrae**

  ● **S13.18**   **Subluxation and dislocation of C7/T1 cervical vertebrae**

    ● **S13.180**   **Subluxation of C7/T1 cervical vertebrae**

    ● **S13.181**   **Dislocation of C7/T1 cervical vertebrae**

● **S13.2**   **Dislocation of other and unspecified parts of neck**

  X● **S13.20**   **Dislocation of unspecified parts of neck**

  X● **S13.29**   **Dislocation of other parts of neck**

X● **S13.4**   **Sprain of ligaments of cervical spine**
> Sprain of anterior longitudinal (ligament), cervical
> Sprain of atlanto-axial (joints)
> Sprain of atlanto-occipital (joints)
> Whiplash injury of cervical spine

X● **S13.5**   **Sprain of thyroid region**
> Sprain of cricoarytenoid (joint) (ligament)
> Sprain of cricothyroid (joint) (ligament)
> Sprain of thyroid cartilage

X● **S13.8**   **Sprain of joints and ligaments of other parts of neck**

X● **S13.9**   **Sprain of joints and ligaments of unspecified parts of neck**

● **S14**   **Injury of nerves and spinal cord at neck level**
> **Note:** Code to highest level of cervical cord injury
>
> Code also any associated:
> fracture of cervical vertebra (S12.0--S12.6.-)
> open wound of neck (S11.-)
> transient paralysis (R29.5)
>
> The appropriate 7th character is to be added to each code from category S14

> | | |
> |---|---|
> | A | initial encounter |
> | D | subsequent encounter |
> | S | sequela |

X● **S14.0**   **Concussion and edema of cervical spinal cord** A, D, S 🔖

● **S14.1**   **Other and unspecified injuries of cervical spinal cord**

  ● **S14.10**   **Unspecified injury of cervical spinal cord**

    ● **S14.101**   **Unspecified injury at C1 level of cervical spinal cord** A, D, S 🔖

    ● **S14.102**   **Unspecified injury at C2 level of cervical spinal cord** A, D, S 🔖

    ● **S14.103**   **Unspecified injury at C3 level of cervical spinal cord** A, D, S 🔖

    ● **S14.104**   **Unspecified injury at C4 level of cervical spinal cord** A, D, S 🔖

    ● **S14.105**   **Unspecified injury at C5 level of cervical spinal cord** A, D, S 🔖

    ● **S14.106**   **Unspecified injury at C6 level of cervical spinal cord** A, D, S 🔖

    ● **S14.107**   **Unspecified injury at C7 level of cervical spinal cord** A, D, S 🔖

    ● **S14.108**   **Unspecified injury at C8 level of cervical spinal cord** A, D, S 🔖

    ● **S14.109**   **Unspecified injury at unspecified level of cervical spinal cord** A, D, S 🔖
> Injury of cervical spinal cord NOS

  ● **S14.11**   **Complete lesion of cervical spinal cord**

    ● **S14.111**   **Complete lesion at C1 level of cervical spinal cord** A, D, S 🔖

    ● **S14.112**   **Complete lesion at C2 level of cervical spinal cord** A, D, S 🔖

    ● **S14.113**   **Complete lesion at C3 level of cervical spinal cord** A, D, S 🔖

    ● **S14.114**   **Complete lesion at C4 level of cervical spinal cord** A, D, S 🔖

    ● **S14.115**   **Complete lesion at C5 level of cervical spinal cord** A, D, S 🔖

    ● **S14.116**   **Complete lesion at C6 level of cervical spinal cord** A, D, S 🔖

    ● **S14.117**   **Complete lesion at C7 level of cervical spinal cord** A, D, S 🔖

    ● **S14.118**   **Complete lesion at C8 level of cervical spinal cord** A, D, S 🔖

    ● **S14.119**   **Complete lesion at unspecified level of cervical spinal cord** A, D, S 🔖

● S14.12   Central cord syndrome of cervical spinal cord
  ● S14.121   Central cord syndrome at C1 level of cervical spinal cord A, D, S 🐾
  ● S14.122   Central cord syndrome at C2 level of cervical spinal cord A, D, S 🐾
  ● S14.123   Central cord syndrome at C3 level of cervical spinal cord A, D, S 🐾
  ● S14.124   Central cord syndrome at C4 level of cervical spinal cord A, D, S 🐾
  ● S14.125   Central cord syndrome at C5 level of cervical spinal cord A, D, S 🐾
  ● S14.126   Central cord syndrome at C6 level of cervical spinal cord A, D, S 🐾
  ● S14.127   Central cord syndrome at C7 level of cervical spinal cord A, D, S 🐾
  ● S14.128   Central cord syndrome at C8 level of cervical spinal cord A, D, S 🐾
  ● S14.129   Central cord syndrome at unspecified level of cervical spinal cord A, D, S 🐾

● S14.13   Anterior cord syndrome of cervical spinal cord
  ● S14.131   Anterior cord syndrome at C1 level of cervical spinal cord A, D, S 🐾
  ● S14.132   Anterior cord syndrome at C2 level of cervical spinal cord A, D, S 🐾
  ● S14.133   Anterior cord syndrome at C3 level of cervical spinal cord A, D, S 🐾
  ● S14.134   Anterior cord syndrome at C4 level of cervical spinal cord A, D, S 🐾
  ● S14.135   Anterior cord syndrome at C5 level of cervical spinal cord A, D, S 🐾
  ● S14.136   Anterior cord syndrome at C6 level of cervical spinal cord A, D, S 🐾
  ● S14.137   Anterior cord syndrome at C7 level of cervical spinal cord A, D, S 🐾
  ● S14.138   Anterior cord syndrome at C8 level of cervical spinal cord A, D, S 🐾
  ● S14.139   Anterior cord syndrome at unspecified level of cervical spinal cord A, D, S 🐾

● S14.14   Brown-Séquard syndrome of cervical spinal cord
  ● S14.141   Brown-Séquard syndrome at C1 level of cervical spinal cord A, D, S 🐾
  ● S14.142   Brown-Séquard syndrome at C2 level of cervical spinal cord A, D, S 🐾
  ● S14.143   Brown-Séquard syndrome at C3 level of cervical spinal cord A, D, S 🐾
  ● S14.144   Brown-Séquard syndrome at C4 level of cervical spinal cord A, D, S 🐾
  ● S14.145   Brown-Séquard syndrome at C5 level of cervical spinal cord A, D, S 🐾
  ● S14.146   Brown-Séquard syndrome at C6 level of cervical spinal cord A, D, S 🐾
  ● S14.147   Brown-Séquard syndrome at C7 level of cervical spinal cord A, D, S 🐾
  ● S14.148   Brown-Séquard syndrome at C8 level of cervical spinal cord A, D, S 🐾
  ● S14.149   Brown-Séquard syndrome at unspecified level of cervical spinal cord A, D, S 🐾

● S14.15   Other incomplete lesions of cervical spinal cord
Incomplete lesion of cervical spinal cord NOS
Posterior cord syndrome of cervical spinal cord
  ● S14.151   Other incomplete lesion at C1 level of cervical spinal cord A, D, S 🐾
  ● S14.152   Other incomplete lesion at C2 level of cervical spinal cord A, D, S 🐾
  ● S14.153   Other incomplete lesion at C3 level of cervical spinal cord A, D, S 🐾

  ● S14.154   Other incomplete lesion at C4 level of cervical spinal cord A, D, S 🐾
  ● S14.155   Other incomplete lesion at C5 level of cervical spinal cord A, D, S 🐾
  ● S14.156   Other incomplete lesion at C6 level of cervical spinal cord A, D, S 🐾
  ● S14.157   Other incomplete lesion at C7 level of cervical spinal cord A, D, S 🐾
  ● S14.158   Other incomplete lesion at C8 level of cervical spinal cord A, D, S 🐾
  ● S14.159   Other incomplete lesion at unspecified level of cervical spinal cord A, D, S 🐾

X ● S14.2   Injury of nerve root of cervical spine
X ● S14.3   Injury of brachial plexus
X ● S14.4   Injury of peripheral nerves of neck
X ● S14.5   Injury of cervical sympathetic nerves
X ● S14.8   Injury of other specified nerves of neck
X ● S14.9   Injury of unspecified nerves of neck

● S15   Injury of blood vessels at neck level
Code also any associated open wound (S11.-)
The appropriate 7th character is to be added to each code from category S15

A	initial encounter
D	subsequent encounter
S	sequela

● S15.0   Injury of carotid artery of neck
Injury of carotid artery (common) (external) (internal, extracranial portion)
Injury of carotid artery NOS

Excludes1   injury of internal carotid artery, intracranial portion (S06.8)

  ● S15.00   Unspecified injury of carotid artery
    ● S15.001   Unspecified injury of right carotid artery
    ● S15.002   Unspecified injury of left carotid artery
    ● S15.009   Unspecified injury of unspecified carotid artery

  ● S15.01   Minor laceration of carotid artery
Incomplete transection of carotid artery
Laceration of carotid artery NOS
Superficial laceration of carotid artery
    ● S15.011   Minor laceration of right carotid artery
    ● S15.012   Minor laceration of left carotid artery
    ● S15.019   Minor laceration of unspecified carotid artery

  ● S15.02   Major laceration of carotid artery
Complete transection of carotid artery
Traumatic rupture of carotid artery
    ● S15.021   Major laceration of right carotid artery
    ● S15.022   Major laceration of left carotid artery
    ● S15.029   Major laceration of unspecified carotid artery

  ● S15.09   Other specified injury of carotid artery
    ● S15.091   Other specified injury of right carotid artery
    ● S15.092   Other specified injury of left carotid artery
    ● S15.099   Other specified injury of unspecified carotid artery

CHAPTER 19 (S00-T88)

▶ New   ⇒ Revised   ~~deleted~~ Deleted   Excludes 1   Excludes 2   Includes   Use additional   Code first   Code also   Key words
OGCR Official Guidelines   X Assign placeholder X   ● Use Additional Character(s)   ▶ Manifestation Code   🐾 Hierarchical Condition Category   Coding Clinic

● S15.1   Injury of vertebral artery
   ● S15.10   Unspecified injury of vertebral artery
      ● S15.101   Unspecified injury of right vertebral artery
      ● S15.102   Unspecified injury of left vertebral artery
      ● S15.109   Unspecified injury of unspecified vertebral artery
   ● S15.11   Minor laceration of vertebral artery
      Incomplete transection of vertebral artery
      Laceration of vertebral artery NOS
      Superficial laceration of vertebral artery
      ● S15.111   Minor laceration of right vertebral artery
      ● S15.112   Minor laceration of left vertebral artery
      ● S15.119   Minor laceration of unspecified vertebral artery
   ● S15.12   Major laceration of vertebral artery
      Complete transection of vertebral artery
      Traumatic rupture of vertebral artery
      ● S15.121   Major laceration of right vertebral artery
      ● S15.122   Major laceration of left vertebral artery
      ● S15.129   Major laceration of unspecified vertebral artery
   ● S15.19   Other specified injury of vertebral artery
      ● S15.191   Other specified injury of right vertebral artery
      ● S15.192   Other specified injury of left vertebral artery
      ● S15.199   Other specified injury of unspecified vertebral artery
● S15.2   Injury of external jugular vein
   ● S15.20   Unspecified injury of external jugular vein
      ● S15.201   Unspecified injury of right external jugular vein
      ● S15.202   Unspecified injury of left external jugular vein
      ● S15.209   Unspecified injury of unspecified external jugular vein
   ● S15.21   Minor laceration of external jugular vein
      Incomplete transection of external jugular vein
      Laceration of external jugular vein NOS
      Superficial laceration of external jugular vein
      ● S15.211   Minor laceration of right external jugular vein
      ● S15.212   Minor laceration of left external jugular vein
      ● S15.219   Minor laceration of unspecified external jugular vein
   ● S15.22   Major laceration of external jugular vein
      Complete transection of external jugular vein
      Traumatic rupture of external jugular vein
      ● S15.221   Major laceration of right external jugular vein
      ● S15.222   Major laceration of left external jugular vein
      ● S15.229   Major laceration of unspecified external jugular vein
   ● S15.29   Other specified injury of external jugular vein
      ● S15.291   Other specified injury of right external jugular vein
      ● S15.292   Other specified injury of left external jugular vein
      ● S15.299   Other specified injury of unspecified external jugular vein

● S15.3   Injury of internal jugular vein
   ● S15.30   Unspecified injury of internal jugular vein
      ● S15.301   Unspecified injury of right internal jugular vein
      ● S15.302   Unspecified injury of left internal jugular vein
      ● S15.309   Unspecified injury of unspecified internal jugular vein
   ● S15.31   Minor laceration of internal jugular vein
      Incomplete transection of internal jugular vein
      Laceration of internal jugular vein NOS
      Superficial laceration of internal jugular vein
      ● S15.311   Minor laceration of right internal jugular vein
      ● S15.312   Minor laceration of left internal jugular vein
      ● S15.319   Minor laceration of unspecified internal jugular vein
   ● S15.32   Major laceration of internal jugular vein
      Complete transection of internal jugular vein
      Traumatic rupture of internal jugular vein
      ● S15.321   Major laceration of right internal jugular vein
      ● S15.322   Major laceration of left internal jugular vein
      ● S15.329   Major laceration of unspecified internal jugular vein
   ● S15.39   Other specified injury of internal jugular vein
      ● S15.391   Other specified injury of right internal jugular vein
      ● S15.392   Other specified injury of left internal jugular vein
      ● S15.399   Other specified injury of unspecified internal jugular vein
X ● S15.8   Injury of other specified blood vessels at neck level
X ● S15.9   Injury of unspecified blood vessel at neck level

● S16   Injury of muscle, fascia and tendon at neck level
   Code also any associated open wound (S11.-)
   Excludes2   sprain of joint or ligament at neck level (S13.9)
   The appropriate 7th character is to be added to each code from category S16

A	initial encounter
D	subsequent encounter
S	sequela

X ● S16.1   Strain of muscle, fascia and tendon at neck level
X ● S16.2   Laceration of muscle, fascia and tendon at neck level
X ● S16.8   Other specified injury of muscle, fascia and tendon at neck level
X ● S16.9   Unspecified injury of muscle, fascia and tendon at neck level

● S17   Crushing injury of neck
   Use additional code for all associated injuries, such as:
     injury of blood vessels (S15.-)
     open wound of neck (S11.-)
     spinal cord injury (S14.0, S14.1-)
     vertebral fracture (S12.0--S12.3-)
   The appropriate 7th character is to be added to each code from category S17

A	initial encounter
D	subsequent encounter
S	sequela

X ● S17.0   Crushing injury of larynx and trachea
X ● S17.8   Crushing injury of other specified parts of neck
X ● S17.9   Crushing injury of neck, part unspecified

CHAPTER 19 (S00-T88)

● **S19 Other and unspecified injuries of neck**

The appropriate 7th character is to be added to each code from category S19

> A   initial encounter
> D   subsequent encounter
> S   sequela

● **S19.8 Other specified injuries of neck**

X ● **S19.80** Other specified injuries of unspecified part of neck

X ● **S19.81** Other specified injuries of larynx

X ● **S19.82** Other specified injuries of cervical trachea

> **Excludes2**   other specified injury of thoracic trachea (S27.5-)

X ● **S19.83** Other specified injuries of vocal cord

X ● **S19.84** Other specified injuries of thyroid gland

X ● **S19.85** Other specified injuries of pharynx and cervical esophagus
> Coding Clinic: 2022, Q1, P27

X ● **S19.89** Other specified injuries of other specified part of neck

X ● **S19.9 Unspecified injury of neck**

INJURIES TO THE THORAX (S20-S29)

Includes   injuries of breast
injuries of chest (wall)
injuries of interscapular area

Excludes2   burns and corrosions (T20-T32)
effects of foreign body in bronchus (T17.5)
effects of foreign body in esophagus (T18.1)
effects of foreign body in lung (T17.8)
effects of foreign body in trachea (T17.4)
frostbite (T33-T34)
injuries of axilla
injuries of clavicle
injuries of scapular region
injuries of shoulder
insect bite or sting, venomous (T63.4)

● **S20 Superficial injury of thorax**

The appropriate 7th character is to be added to each code from category S20

> A   initial encounter
> D   subsequent encounter
> S   sequela

● **S20.0 Contusion of breast**

X ● **S20.00** Contusion of breast, unspecified breast

X ● **S20.01** Contusion of right breast

X ● **S20.02** Contusion of left breast

● **S20.1 Other and unspecified superficial injuries of breast**

● **S20.10** Unspecified superficial injuries of breast

● **S20.101** Unspecified superficial injuries of breast, right breast

● **S20.102** Unspecified superficial injuries of breast, left breast

● **S20.109** Unspecified superficial injuries of breast, unspecified breast

● **S20.11** Abrasion of breast

● **S20.111** Abrasion of breast, right breast

● **S20.112** Abrasion of breast, left breast

● **S20.119** Abrasion of breast, unspecified breast

● **S20.12** Blister (nonthermal) of breast

● **S20.121** Blister (nonthermal) of breast, right breast

● **S20.122** Blister (nonthermal) of breast, left breast

● **S20.129** Blister (nonthermal) of breast, unspecified breast

● **S20.14 External constriction of part of breast**

● **S20.141** External constriction of part of breast, right breast

● **S20.142** External constriction of part of breast, left breast

● **S20.149** External constriction of part of breast, unspecified breast

● **S20.15 Superficial foreign body of breast**
Splinter in the breast

● **S20.151** Superficial foreign body of breast, right breast

● **S20.152** Superficial foreign body of breast, left breast

● **S20.159** Superficial foreign body of breast, unspecified breast

● **S20.16 Insect bite (nonvenomous) of breast**

● **S20.161** Insect bite (nonvenomous) of breast, right breast

● **S20.162** Insect bite (nonvenomous) of breast, left breast

● **S20.169** Insect bite (nonvenomous) of breast, unspecified breast

● **S20.17 Other superficial bite of breast**

> **Excludes1**   open bite of breast (S21.05-)

● **S20.171** Other superficial bite of breast, right breast

● **S20.172** Other superficial bite of breast, left breast

● **S20.179** Other superficial bite of breast, unspecified breast

● **S20.2 Contusion of thorax**

X ● **S20.20** Contusion of thorax, unspecified

● **S20.21** Contusion of front wall of thorax

● **S20.211** Contusion of right front wall of thorax

● **S20.212** Contusion of left front wall of thorax

S20.213 Contusion of bilateral front wall of thorax

S20.214 Contusion of middle front wall of thorax

● **S20.219** Contusion of unspecified front wall of thorax

● **S20.22** Contusion of back wall of thorax

● **S20.221** Contusion of right back wall of thorax

● **S20.222** Contusion of left back wall of thorax

S20.223 Contusion of bilateral back wall of thorax

S20.224 Contusion of middle back wall of thorax

● **S20.229** Contusion of unspecified back wall of thorax

● **S20.3 Other and unspecified superficial injuries of front wall of thorax**

● **S20.30** Unspecified superficial injuries of front wall of thorax

● **S20.301** Unspecified superficial injuries of right front wall of thorax

● **S20.302** Unspecified superficial injuries of left front wall of thorax

S20.303 Unspecified superficial injuries of bilateral front wall of thorax

S20.304 Unspecified superficial injuries of middle front wall of thorax

● **S20.309** Unspecified superficial injuries of unspecified front wall of thorax

● **S20.31** Abrasion of front wall of thorax

● **S20.311** Abrasion of right front wall of thorax

● **S20.312** Abrasion of left front wall of thorax

S20.313 Abrasion of bilateral front wall of thorax

● S20.314   Abrasion of middle front wall of thorax

● S20.319   Abrasion of unspecified front wall of thorax

● S20.32   Blister (nonthermal) of front wall of thorax

  ● S20.321   Blister (nonthermal) of right front wall of thorax

  ● S20.322   Blister (nonthermal) of left front wall of thorax

    S20.323   Blister (nonthermal) of bilateral front wall of thorax

    S20.324   Blister (nonthermal) of middle front wall of thorax

  ● S20.329   Blister (nonthermal) of unspecified front wall of thorax

● S20.34   External constriction of front wall of thorax

  ● S20.341   External constriction of right front wall of thorax

  ● S20.342   External constriction of left front wall of thorax

    S20.343   External constriction of bilateral front wall of thorax

    S20.344   External constriction of middle front wall of thorax

  ● S20.349   External constriction of unspecified front wall of thorax

● S20.35   Superficial foreign body of front wall of thorax
    Splinter in front wall of thorax

  ● S20.351   Superficial foreign body of right front wall of thorax

  ● S20.352   Superficial foreign body of left front wall of thorax

    S20.353   Superficial foreign body of bilateral front wall of thorax

    S20.354   Superficial foreign body of middle front wall of thorax

  ● S20.359   Superficial foreign body of unspecified front wall of thorax

● S20.36   Insect bite (nonvenomous) of front wall of thorax

  ● S20.361   Insect bite (nonvenomous) of right front wall of thorax

  ● S20.362   Insect bite (nonvenomous) of left front wall of thorax

    S20.363   Insect bite (nonvenomous) of bilateral front wall of thorax

    S20.364   Insect bite (nonvenomous) of middle front wall of thorax

  ● S20.369   Insect bite (nonvenomous) of unspecified front wall of thorax

● S20.37   Other superficial bite of front wall of thorax
    Excludes1   open bite of front wall of thorax (S21.14)

  ● S20.371   Other superficial bite of right front wall of thorax

  ● S20.372   Other superficial bite of left front wall of thorax

    S20.373   Other superficial bite of bilateral front wall of thorax

    S20.374   Other superficial bite of middle front wall of thorax

  ● S20.379   Other superficial bite of unspecified front wall of thorax

● S20.4   Other and unspecified superficial injuries of back wall of thorax

  ● S20.40   Unspecified superficial injuries of back wall of thorax

    ● S20.401   Unspecified superficial injuries of right back wall of thorax

    ● S20.402   Unspecified superficial injuries of left back wall of thorax

    ● S20.409   Unspecified superficial injuries of unspecified back wall of thorax

  ● S20.41   Abrasion of back wall of thorax

    ● S20.411   Abrasion of right back wall of thorax

    ● S20.412   Abrasion of left back wall of thorax

    ● S20.419   Abrasion of unspecified back wall of thorax

  ● S20.42   Blister (nonthermal) of back wall of thorax

    ● S20.421   Blister (nonthermal) of right back wall of thorax

    ● S20.422   Blister (nonthermal) of left back wall of thorax

    ● S20.429   Blister (nonthermal) of unspecified back wall of thorax

  ● S20.44   External constriction of back wall of thorax

    ● S20.441   External constriction of right back wall of thorax

    ● S20.442   External constriction of left back wall of thorax

    ● S20.449   External constriction of unspecified back wall of thorax

  ● S20.45   Superficial foreign body of back wall of thorax
    Splinter of back wall of thorax

    ● S20.451   Superficial foreign body of right back wall of thorax

    ● S20.452   Superficial foreign body of left back wall of thorax

    ● S20.459   Superficial foreign body of unspecified back wall of thorax

  ● S20.46   Insect bite (nonvenomous) of back wall of thorax

    ● S20.461   Insect bite (nonvenomous) of right back wall of thorax

    ● S20.462   Insect bite (nonvenomous) of left back wall of thorax

    ● S20.469   Insect bite (nonvenomous) of unspecified back wall of thorax

  ● S20.47   Other superficial bite of back wall of thorax
    Excludes1   open bite of back wall of thorax (S21.24)

    ● S20.471   Other superficial bite of right back wall of thorax

    ● S20.472   Other superficial bite of left back wall of thorax

    ● S20.479   Other superficial bite of unspecified back wall of thorax

● S20.9   Superficial injury of unspecified parts of thorax
    Excludes1   contusion of thorax NOS (S20.20)

X ● S20.90   Unspecified superficial injury of unspecified parts of thorax
    Superficial injury of thoracic wall NOS

X ● S20.91   Abrasion of unspecified parts of thorax

X ● S20.92   Blister (nonthermal) of unspecified parts of thorax

X ● S20.94   External constriction of unspecified parts of thorax

X ● S20.95   Superficial foreign body of unspecified parts of thorax
    Splinter in thorax NOS

X ● S20.96   Insect bite (nonvenomous) of unspecified parts of thorax

X ● S20.97   Other superficial bite of unspecified parts of thorax
    Excludes1   open bite of thorax NOS (S21.95)

● **S21   Open wound of thorax**

> Code also any associated injury such as:
>   injury of heart (S26.-)
>   injury of intrathoracic organs (S27.-)
>   rib fracture (S22.3-, S22.4-)
>   spinal cord injury (S24.0-, S24.1-)
>   traumatic hemothorax (S27.1)
>   traumatic hemopneumothorax (S27.3)
>   traumatic pneumothorax (S27.0)
>   wound infection

> **Excludes1**   traumatic amputation (partial) of thorax (S28.1)

> The appropriate 7th character is to be added to each code from category S21

> | A | initial encounter |
> |---|---|
> | D | subsequent encounter |
> | S | sequela |

● **S21.0   Open wound of breast**

   ● **S21.00   Unspecified open wound of breast**

      ● **S21.001   Unspecified open wound of right breast**

      ● **S21.002   Unspecified open wound of left breast**

      ● **S21.009   Unspecified open wound of unspecified breast**

   ● **S21.01   Laceration without foreign body of breast**

      ● **S21.011   Laceration without foreign body of right breast**

      ● **S21.012   Laceration without foreign body of left breast**

      ● **S21.019   Laceration without foreign body of unspecified breast**

   ● **S21.02   Laceration with foreign body of breast**

      ● **S21.021   Laceration with foreign body of right breast**

      ● **S21.022   Laceration with foreign body of left breast**

      ● **S21.029   Laceration with foreign body of unspecified breast**

   ● **S21.03   Puncture wound without foreign body of breast**

      ● **S21.031   Puncture wound without foreign body of right breast**

      ● **S21.032   Puncture wound without foreign body of left breast**

      ● **S21.039   Puncture wound without foreign body of unspecified breast**

   ● **S21.04   Puncture wound with foreign body of breast**

      ● **S21.041   Puncture wound with foreign body of right breast**

      ● **S21.042   Puncture wound with foreign body of left breast**

      ● **S21.049   Puncture wound with foreign body of unspecified breast**

   ● **S21.05   Open bite of breast**
      Bite of breast NOS

      Excludes1   superficial bite of breast (S20.17)

      ● **S21.051   Open bite of right breast**

      ● **S21.052   Open bite of left breast**

      ● **S21.059   Open bite of unspecified breast**

Item 19–1 Pneumothorax is a collection of gas (positive air pressure) in the pleural space, resulting in the lung collapsing. A **tension pneumothorax** is life-threatening and is a result of air in the pleural space causing a displacement in the mediastinal structures and cardiopulmonary function compromise. A **traumatic pneumothorax** results from blunt or penetrating injury that disrupts the parietal/visceral pleura. **Hemothorax** is blood or bloody fluid in the pleural cavity as a result of traumatic blood vessel rupture or inflammation of the lungs from pneumonia.

● **S21.1   Open wound of front wall of thorax without penetration into thoracic cavity**
   Open wound of chest without penetration into thoracic cavity

   ● **S21.10   Unspecified open wound of front wall of thorax without penetration into thoracic cavity**

      ● **S21.101   Unspecified open wound of right front wall of thorax without penetration into thoracic cavity**

      ● **S21.102   Unspecified open wound of left front wall of thorax without penetration into thoracic cavity**

      ● **S21.109   Unspecified open wound of unspecified front wall of thorax without penetration into thoracic cavity**

   ● **S21.11   Laceration without foreign body of front wall of thorax without penetration into thoracic cavity**

      ● **S21.111   Laceration without foreign body of right front wall of thorax without penetration into thoracic cavity**

      ● **S21.112   Laceration without foreign body of left front wall of thorax without penetration into thoracic cavity**

      ● **S21.119   Laceration without foreign body of unspecified front wall of thorax without penetration into thoracic cavity**

   ● **S21.12   Laceration with foreign body of front wall of thorax without penetration into thoracic cavity**

      ● **S21.121   Laceration with foreign body of right front wall of thorax without penetration into thoracic cavity**

      ● **S21.122   Laceration with foreign body of left front wall of thorax without penetration into thoracic cavity**

      ● **S21.129   Laceration with foreign body of unspecified front wall of thorax without penetration into thoracic cavity**

   ● **S21.13   Puncture wound without foreign body of front wall of thorax without penetration into thoracic cavity**

      ● **S21.131   Puncture wound without foreign body of right front wall of thorax without penetration into thoracic cavity**

      ● **S21.132   Puncture wound without foreign body of left front wall of thorax without penetration into thoracic cavity**

      ● **S21.139   Puncture wound without foreign body of unspecified front wall of thorax without penetration into thoracic cavity**

   ● **S21.14   Puncture wound with foreign body of front wall of thorax without penetration into thoracic cavity**

      ● **S21.141   Puncture wound with foreign body of right front wall of thorax without penetration into thoracic cavity**

      ● **S21.142   Puncture wound with foreign body of left front wall of thorax without penetration into thoracic cavity**

      ● **S21.149   Puncture wound with foreign body of unspecified front wall of thorax without penetration into thoracic cavity**

▶ New   ⇒ Revised   ~~deleted~~ Deleted   Excludes 1   Excludes 2   Includes   Use additional   Code first   Code also   Key words

OGCR Official Guidelines   X Assign placeholder X   ● Use Additional Character(s)   ▷ Manifestation Code   🔗 Hierarchical Condition Category   **Coding Clinic**

● **S21.15**   Open bite of front wall of thorax without penetration into thoracic cavity
>> Bite of front wall of thorax NOS
>> **Excludes1**   superficial bite of front wall of thorax (S20.37)

   ● **S21.151**   Open bite of right front wall of thorax without penetration into thoracic cavity

   ● **S21.152**   Open bite of left front wall of thorax without penetration into thoracic cavity

   ● **S21.159**   Open bite of unspecified front wall of thorax without penetration into thoracic cavity

● **S21.2**   Open wound of back wall of thorax without penetration into thoracic cavity

  ● **S21.20**   Unspecified open wound of back wall of thorax without penetration into thoracic cavity

   ● **S21.201**   Unspecified open wound of right back wall of thorax without penetration into thoracic cavity

   ● **S21.202**   Unspecified open wound of left back wall of thorax without penetration into thoracic cavity

   ● **S21.209**   Unspecified open wound of unspecified back wall of thorax without penetration into thoracic cavity

  ● **S21.21**   Laceration without foreign body of back wall of thorax without penetration into thoracic cavity

   ● **S21.211**   Laceration without foreign body of right back wall of thorax without penetration into thoracic cavity

   ● **S21.212**   Laceration without foreign body of left back wall of thorax without penetration into thoracic cavity

   ● **S21.219**   Laceration without foreign body of unspecified back wall of thorax without penetration into thoracic cavity

  ● **S21.22**   Laceration with foreign body of back wall of thorax without penetration into thoracic cavity

   ● **S21.221**   Laceration with foreign body of right back wall of thorax without penetration into thoracic cavity

   ● **S21.222**   Laceration with foreign body of left back wall of thorax without penetration into thoracic cavity

   ● **S21.229**   Laceration with foreign body of unspecified back wall of thorax without penetration into thoracic cavity

  ● **S21.23**   Puncture wound without foreign body of back wall of thorax without penetration into thoracic cavity

   ● **S21.231**   Puncture wound without foreign body of right back wall of thorax without penetration into thoracic cavity

   ● **S21.232**   Puncture wound without foreign body of left back wall of thorax without penetration into thoracic cavity

   ● **S21.239**   Puncture wound without foreign body of unspecified back wall of thorax without penetration into thoracic cavity

  ● **S21.24**   Puncture wound with foreign body of back wall of thorax without penetration into thoracic cavity

   ● **S21.241**   Puncture wound with foreign body of right back wall of thorax without penetration into thoracic cavity

   ● **S21.242**   Puncture wound with foreign body of left back wall of thorax without penetration into thoracic cavity

   ● **S21.249**   Puncture wound with foreign body of unspecified back wall of thorax without penetration into thoracic cavity

● **S21.25**   Open bite of back wall of thorax without penetration into thoracic cavity
>> Bite of back wall of thorax NOS
>> **Excludes1**   superficial bite of back wall of thorax (S20.47)

   ● **S21.251**   Open bite of right back wall of thorax without penetration into thoracic cavity

   ● **S21.252**   Open bite of left back wall of thorax without penetration into thoracic cavity

   ● **S21.259**   Open bite of unspecified back wall of thorax without penetration into thoracic cavity

● **S21.3**   Open wound of front wall of thorax with penetration into thoracic cavity
>> Open wound of chest with penetration into thoracic cavity

  ● **S21.30**   Unspecified open wound of front wall of thorax with penetration into thoracic cavity

   ● **S21.301**   Unspecified open wound of right front wall of thorax with penetration into thoracic cavity

   ● **S21.302**   Unspecified open wound of left front wall of thorax with penetration into thoracic cavity

   ● **S21.309**   Unspecified open wound of unspecified front wall of thorax with penetration into thoracic cavity

  ● **S21.31**   Laceration without foreign body of front wall of thorax with penetration into thoracic cavity

   ● **S21.311**   Laceration without foreign body of right front wall of thorax with penetration into thoracic cavity

   ● **S21.312**   Laceration without foreign body of left front wall of thorax with penetration into thoracic cavity

   ● **S21.319**   Laceration without foreign body of unspecified front wall of thorax with penetration into thoracic cavity

  ● **S21.32**   Laceration with foreign body of front wall of thorax with penetration into thoracic cavity

   ● **S21.321**   Laceration with foreign body of right front wall of thorax with penetration into thoracic cavity

   ● **S21.322**   Laceration with foreign body of left front wall of thorax with penetration into thoracic cavity

   ● **S21.329**   Laceration with foreign body of unspecified front wall of thorax with penetration into thoracic cavity

  ● **S21.33**   Puncture wound without foreign body of front wall of thorax with penetration into thoracic cavity

   ● **S21.331**   Puncture wound without foreign body of right front wall of thorax with penetration into thoracic cavity

   ● **S21.332**   Puncture wound without foreign body of left front wall of thorax with penetration into thoracic cavity

   ● **S21.339**   Puncture wound without foreign body of unspecified front wall of thorax with penetration into thoracic cavity

CHAPTER 19 (S00-T88)

● S21.34   Puncture wound with foreign body of front wall of thorax with penetration into thoracic cavity

　　● S21.341   Puncture wound with foreign body of right front wall of thorax with penetration into thoracic cavity

　　● S21.342   Puncture wound with foreign body of left front wall of thorax with penetration into thoracic cavity

　　● S21.349   Puncture wound with foreign body of unspecified front wall of thorax with penetration into thoracic cavity

● S21.35   Open bite of front wall of thorax with penetration into thoracic cavity

　　Excludes1   superficial bite of front wall of thorax (S20.37)

　　● S21.351   Open bite of right front wall of thorax with penetration into thoracic cavity

　　● S21.352   Open bite of left front wall of thorax with penetration into thoracic cavity

　　● S21.359   Open bite of unspecified front wall of thorax with penetration into thoracic cavity

● S21.4   Open wound of back wall of thorax with penetration into thoracic cavity

　　● S21.40   Unspecified open wound of back wall of thorax with penetration into thoracic cavity

　　　　● S21.401   Unspecified open wound of right back wall of thorax with penetration into thoracic cavity

　　　　● S21.402   Unspecified open wound of left back wall of thorax with penetration into thoracic cavity

　　　　● S21.409   Unspecified open wound of unspecified back wall of thorax with penetration into thoracic cavity

　　● S21.41   Laceration without foreign body of back wall of thorax with penetration into thoracic cavity

　　　　● S21.411   Laceration without foreign body of right back wall of thorax with penetration into thoracic cavity

　　　　● S21.412   Laceration without foreign body of left back wall of thorax with penetration into thoracic cavity

　　　　● S21.419   Laceration without foreign body of unspecified back wall of thorax with penetration into thoracic cavity

　　● S21.42   Laceration with foreign body of back wall of thorax with penetration into thoracic cavity

　　　　● S21.421   Laceration with foreign body of right back wall of thorax with penetration into thoracic cavity

　　　　● S21.422   Laceration with foreign body of left back wall of thorax with penetration into thoracic cavity

　　　　● S21.429   Laceration with foreign body of unspecified back wall of thorax with penetration into thoracic cavity

　　● S21.43   Puncture wound without foreign body of back wall of thorax with penetration into thoracic cavity

　　　　● S21.431   Puncture wound without foreign body of right back wall of thorax with penetration into thoracic cavity

　　　　● S21.432   Puncture wound without foreign body of left back wall of thorax with penetration into thoracic cavity

　　　　● S21.439   Puncture wound without foreign body of unspecified back wall of thorax with penetration into thoracic cavity

● S21.44   Puncture wound with foreign body of back wall of thorax with penetration into thoracic cavity

　　● S21.441   Puncture wound with foreign body of right back wall of thorax with penetration into thoracic cavity

　　● S21.442   Puncture wound with foreign body of left back wall of thorax with penetration into thoracic cavity

　　● S21.449   Puncture wound with foreign body of unspecified back wall of thorax with penetration into thoracic cavity

● S21.45   Open bite of back wall of thorax with penetration into thoracic cavity
Bite of back wall of thorax NOS

　　Excludes1   superficial bite of back wall of thorax (S20.47)

　　● S21.451   Open bite of right back wall of thorax with penetration into thoracic cavity

　　● S21.452   Open bite of left back wall of thorax with penetration into thoracic cavity

　　● S21.459   Open bite of unspecified back wall of thorax with penetration into thoracic cavity

● S21.9   Open wound of unspecified part of thorax
Open wound of thoracic wall NOS

X ● S21.90   Unspecified open wound of unspecified part of thorax

X ● S21.91   Laceration without foreign body of unspecified part of thorax

X ● S21.92   Laceration with foreign body of unspecified part of thorax

X ● S21.93   Puncture wound without foreign body of unspecified part of thorax

X ● S21.94   Puncture wound with foreign body of unspecified part of thorax

X ● S21.95   Open bite of unspecified part of thorax

　　Excludes1   superficial bite of thorax (S20.97)

● S22   Fracture of rib(s), sternum and thoracic spine

Note: A fracture not indicated as displaced or nondisplaced should be coded to displaced

A fracture not indicated as open or closed should be coded to closed

Includes   fracture of thoracic neural arch
fracture of thoracic spinous process
fracture of thoracic transverse process
fracture of thoracic vertebra
fracture of thoracic vertebral arch

Code first any associated:
injury of intrathoracic organ (S27.-)
spinal cord injury (S24.0-, S24.1-)

Excludes1   transection of thorax (S28.1)
Excludes2   fracture of clavicle (S42.0-)
fracture of scapula (S42.1-)

The appropriate 7th character is to be added to each code from category S22

A	initial encounter for closed fracture
B	initial encounter for open fracture
D	subsequent encounter for fracture with routine healing
G	subsequent encounter for fracture with delayed healing
K	subsequent encounter for fracture with nonunion
S	sequela

● S22.0   Fracture of thoracic vertebra

　　● S22.00   Fracture of unspecified thoracic vertebra

　　　　● S22.000   Wedge compression fracture of unspecified thoracic vertebra A, B 🐾

　　　　● S22.001   Stable burst fracture of unspecified thoracic vertebra A, B 🐾

　　　　● S22.002   Unstable burst fracture of unspecified thoracic vertebra A, B 🐾

▶ New   ⇒ Revised   ~~deleted~~ Deleted   Excludes 1   Excludes 2   Includes   Use additional   Code first   Code also   Key words
OGCR Official Guidelines   X Assign placeholder X   ● Use Additional Character(s)   ▶ Manifestation Code   🐾 Hierarchical Condition Category   **Coding Clinic**

● S22.008   Other fracture of unspecified thoracic vertebra A, B 🔒

● S22.009   Unspecified fracture of unspecified thoracic vertebra A, B 🔒

● S22.01   Fracture of first thoracic vertebra

   ● S22.010   Wedge compression fracture of first thoracic vertebra A, B 🔒

   ● S22.011   Stable burst fracture of first thoracic vertebra A, B 🔒

   ● S22.012   Unstable burst fracture of first thoracic vertebra A, B 🔒

   ● S22.018   Other fracture of first thoracic vertebra A, B 🔒

   ● S22.019   Unspecified fracture of first thoracic vertebra A, B 🔒

● S22.02   Fracture of second thoracic vertebra

   ● S22.020   Wedge compression fracture of second thoracic vertebra A, B 🔒

   ● S22.021   Stable burst fracture of second thoracic vertebra A, B 🔒

   ● S22.022   Unstable burst fracture of second thoracic vertebra A, B 🔒

   ● S22.028   Other fracture of second thoracic vertebra A, B 🔒

   ● S22.029   Unspecified fracture of second thoracic vertebra A, B 🔒

● S22.03   Fracture of third thoracic vertebra

   ● S22.030   Wedge compression fracture of third thoracic vertebra A, B 🔒

   ● S22.031   Stable burst fracture of third thoracic vertebra A, B 🔒

   ● S22.032   Unstable burst fracture of third thoracic vertebra A, B 🔒

   ● S22.038   Other fracture of third thoracic vertebra A, B 🔒

   ● S22.039   Unspecified fracture of third thoracic vertebra A, B 🔒

● S22.04   Fracture of fourth thoracic vertebra

   ● S22.040   Wedge compression fracture of fourth thoracic vertebra A, B 🔒

   ● S22.041   Stable burst fracture of fourth thoracic vertebra A, B 🔒

   ● S22.042   Unstable burst fracture of fourth thoracic vertebra A, B 🔒

   ● S22.048   Other fracture of fourth thoracic vertebra A, B 🔒

   ● S22.049   Unspecified fracture of fourth thoracic vertebra A, B 🔒

● S22.05   Fracture of T5-T6 vertebra

   ● S22.050   Wedge compression fracture of T5-T6 vertebra A, B 🔒

   ● S22.051   Stable burst fracture of T5-T6 vertebra A, B 🔒

   ● S22.052   Unstable burst fracture of T5-T6 vertebra A, B 🔒

   ● S22.058   Other fracture of T5-T6 vertebra A, B 🔒

   ● S22.059   Unspecified fracture of T5-T6 vertebra A, B 🔒

● S22.06   Fracture of T7-T8 vertebra

   ● S22.060   Wedge compression fracture of T7-T8 vertebra A, B 🔒

   ● S22.061   Stable burst fracture of T7-T8 vertebra A, B 🔒

   ● S22.062   Unstable burst fracture of T7-T8 vertebra A, B 🔒

   ● S22.068   Other fracture of T7-T8 thoracic vertebra A, B 🔒

   ● S22.069   Unspecified fracture of T7-T8 vertebra A, B 🔒

● S22.07   Fracture of T9-T10 vertebra

   ● S22.070   Wedge compression fracture of T9-T10 vertebra A, B 🔒

   ● S22.071   Stable burst fracture of T9-T10 vertebra A, B 🔒

   ● S22.072   Unstable burst fracture of T9-T10 vertebra A, B 🔒

   ● S22.078   Other fracture of T9-T10 vertebra A, B 🔒

   ● S22.079   Unspecified fracture of T9-T10 vertebra A, B 🔒

● S22.08   Fracture of T11-T12 vertebra

   ● S22.080   Wedge compression fracture of T11-T12 vertebra A, B 🔒

   ● S22.081   Stable burst fracture of T11-T12 vertebra A, B 🔒

   ● S22.082   Unstable burst fracture of T11-T12 vertebra A, B 🔒

   ● S22.088   Other fracture of T11-T12 vertebra A, B 🔒

   ● S22.089   Unspecified fracture of T11-T12 vertebra A, B 🔒

● S22.2   Fracture of sternum

  X ● S22.20   Unspecified fracture of sternum

  X ● S22.21   Fracture of manubrium

  X ● S22.22   Fracture of body of sternum

  X ● S22.23   Sternal manubrial dissociation

  X ● S22.24   Fracture of xiphoid process

● S22.3 Fracture of one rib

  X ● S22.31   Fracture of one rib, right side

  X ● S22.32   Fracture of one rib, left side

  X ● S22.39   Fracture of one rib, unspecified side

● S22.4   Multiple fractures of ribs

    Fractures of two or more ribs

    Excludes1   flail chest (S22.5-)

  X ● S22.41   Multiple fractures of ribs, right side

  X ● S22.42   Multiple fractures of ribs, left side

  X ● S22.43   Multiple fractures of ribs, bilateral

  X ● S22.49   Multiple fractures of ribs, unspecified side

X ● S22.5   Flail chest

    Unstable chest due to sternum and/or rib fracture

X ● S22.9   Fracture of bony thorax, part unspecified

● S23   Dislocation and sprain of joints and ligaments of thorax

  Includes   avulsion of joint or ligament of thorax
    laceration of cartilage, joint or ligament of thorax
    sprain of cartilage, joint or ligament of thorax
    traumatic hemarthrosis of joint or ligament of thorax
    traumatic rupture of joint or ligament of thorax
    traumatic subluxation of joint or ligament of thorax
    traumatic tear of joint or ligament of thorax

Code also any associated: open wound

Excludes2   dislocation, sprain of sternoclavicular joint (S43.2, S43.6)
    strain of muscle or tendon of thorax (S29.01-)

The appropriate 7th character is to be added to each code from category S23

A	initial encounter
D	subsequent encounter
S	sequela

X ● S23.0   Traumatic rupture of thoracic intervertebral disc

  Excludes1   rupture or displacement (nontraumatic) of thoracic intervertebral disc NOS (M51.- with fifth character 4)

CHAPTER 19 (S00-T88)

● **S23.1**   **Subluxation and dislocation of thoracic vertebra**
    Code also any associated
      open wound of thorax (S21.-)
      spinal cord injury (S24.0-, S24.1-)
    Excludes2   fracture of thoracic vertebrae (S22.0-)

  ● **S23.10**   **Subluxation and dislocation of unspecified thoracic vertebra**
    ● **S23.100**   **Subluxation of unspecified thoracic vertebra**
    ● **S23.101**   **Dislocation of unspecified thoracic vertebra**

  ● **S23.11**   **Subluxation and dislocation of T1/T2 thoracic vertebra**
    ● **S23.110**   **Subluxation of T1/T2 thoracic vertebra**
    ● **S23.111**   **Dislocation of T1/T2 thoracic vertebra**

  ● **S23.12**   **Subluxation and dislocation of T2/T3-T3/T4 thoracic vertebra**
    ● **S23.120**   **Subluxation of T2/T3 thoracic vertebra**
    ● **S23.121**   **Dislocation of T2/T3 thoracic vertebra**
    ● **S23.122**   **Subluxation of T3/T4 thoracic vertebra**
    ● **S23.123**   **Dislocation of T3/T4 thoracic vertebra**

  ● **S23.13**   **Subluxation and dislocation of T4/T5-T5/T6 thoracic vertebra**
    ● **S23.130**   **Subluxation of T4/T5 thoracic vertebra**
    ● **S23.131**   **Dislocation of T4/T5 thoracic vertebra**
    ● **S23.132**   **Subluxation of T5/T6 thoracic vertebra**
    ● **S23.133**   **Dislocation of T5/T6 thoracic vertebra**

  ● **S23.14**   **Subluxation and dislocation of T6/T7-T7/T8 thoracic vertebra**
    ● **S23.140**   **Subluxation of T6/T7 thoracic vertebra**
    ● **S23.141**   **Dislocation of T6/T7 thoracic vertebra**
    ● **S23.142**   **Subluxation of T7/T8 thoracic vertebra**
    ● **S23.143**   **Dislocation of T7/T8 thoracic vertebra**

  ● **S23.15**   **Subluxation and dislocation of T8/T9-T9/T10 thoracic vertebra**
    ● **S23.150**   **Subluxation of T8/T9 thoracic vertebra**
    ● **S23.151**   **Dislocation of T8/T9 thoracic vertebra**
    ● **S23.152**   **Subluxation of T9/T10 thoracic vertebra**
    ● **S23.153**   **Dislocation of T9/T10 thoracic vertebra**

  ● **S23.16**   **Subluxation and dislocation of T10/T11-T11/T12 thoracic vertebra**
    ● **S23.160**   **Subluxation of T10/T11 thoracic vertebra**
    ● **S23.161**   **Dislocation of T10/T11 thoracic vertebra**
    ● **S23.162**   **Subluxation of T11/T12 thoracic vertebra**
    ● **S23.163**   **Dislocation of T11/T12 thoracic vertebra**

  ● **S23.17**   **Subluxation and dislocation of T12/L1 thoracic vertebra**
    ● **S23.170**   **Subluxation of T12/L1 thoracic vertebra**
    ● **S23.171**   **Dislocation of T12/L1 thoracic vertebra**

● **S23.2**   **Dislocation of other and unspecified parts of thorax**
  X ● **S23.20**   **Dislocation of unspecified part of thorax**
  X ● **S23.29**   **Dislocation of other parts of thorax**
X ● **S23.3**   **Sprain of ligaments of thoracic spine**

● **S23.4**   **Sprain of ribs and sternum**
  X ● **S23.41**   **Sprain of ribs**
  ● **S23.42**   **Sprain of sternum**
    ● **S23.420**   **Sprain of sternoclavicular (joint) (ligament)**
    ● **S23.421**   **Sprain of chondrosternal joint**
    ● **S23.428**   **Other sprain of sternum**
    ● **S23.429**   **Unspecified sprain of sternum**
X ● **S23.8**   **Sprain of other specified parts of thorax**
X ● **S23.9**   **Sprain of unspecified parts of thorax**

● **S24**   **Injury of nerves and spinal cord at thorax level**
  Note: Code to highest level of thoracic spinal cord injury.

    Injuries to the spinal cord (S24.0 and S24.1) refer to the cord level and not bone level injury, and can affect nerve roots at and below the level given.

  Code also any associated:
    fracture of thoracic vertebra (S22.0-)
    open wound of thorax (S21.-)
    transient paralysis (R29.5)
  Excludes2   injury of brachial plexus (S14.3)

  The appropriate 7th character is to be added to each code from category S24

    A   initial encounter
    D   subsequent encounter
    S   sequela

X ● **S24.0**   **Concussion and edema of thoracic spinal cord** A, D, S 🐾
● **S24.1**   **Other and unspecified injuries of thoracic spinal cord**
  ● **S24.10**   **Unspecified injury of thoracic spinal cord**
    ● **S24.101**   **Unspecified injury at T1 level of thoracic spinal cord** A, D, S 🐾
    ● **S24.102**   **Unspecified injury at T2-T6 level of thoracic spinal cord** A, D, S 🐾
    ● **S24.103**   **Unspecified injury at T7-T10 level of thoracic spinal cord** A, D, S 🐾
    ● **S24.104**   **Unspecified injury at T11-T12 level of thoracic spinal cord** A, D, S 🐾
    ● **S24.109**   **Unspecified injury at unspecified level of thoracic spinal cord** A, D, S 🐾
      Injury of thoracic spinal cord NOS

  ● **S24.11**   **Complete lesion of thoracic spinal cord**
    ● **S24.111**   **Complete lesion at T1 level of thoracic spinal cord** A, D, S 🐾
    ● **S24.112**   **Complete lesion at T2-T6 level of thoracic spinal cord** A, D, S 🐾
    ● **S24.113**   **Complete lesion at T7-T10 level of thoracic spinal cord** A, D, S 🐾
    ● **S24.114**   **Complete lesion at T11-T12 level of thoracic spinal cord** A, D, S 🐾
    ● **S24.119**   **Complete lesion at unspecified level of thoracic spinal cord** A, D, S 🐾

  ● **S24.13**   **Anterior cord syndrome of thoracic spinal cord**
    ● **S24.131**   **Anterior cord syndrome at T1 level of thoracic spinal cord** A, D, S 🐾
    ● **S24.132**   **Anterior cord syndrome at T2-T6 level of thoracic spinal cord** A, D, S 🐾
    ● **S24.133**   **Anterior cord syndrome at T7-T10 level of thoracic spinal cord** A, D, S 🐾
    ● **S24.134**   **Anterior cord syndrome at T11-T12 level of thoracic spinal cord** A, D, S 🐾
    ● **S24.139**   **Anterior cord syndrome at unspecified level of thoracic spinal cord** A, D, S 🐾

  ● **S24.14**   **Brown-Séquard syndrome of thoracic spinal cord**
    ● **S24.141**   **Brown-Séquard syndrome at T1 level of thoracic spinal cord** A, D, S 🐾

● S24.142   Brown-Séquard syndrome at T2-T6 level of thoracic spinal cord A, D, S 🐾

● S24.143   Brown-Séquard syndrome at T7-T10 level of thoracic spinal cord A, D, S 🐾

● S24.144   Brown-Séquard syndrome at T11-T12 level of thoracic spinal cord A, D, S 🐾

● S24.149   Brown-Séquard syndrome at unspecified level of thoracic spinal cord A, D, S 🐾

● S24.15   **Other incomplete lesions of thoracic spinal cord**
Incomplete lesion of thoracic spinal cord NOS
Posterior cord syndrome of thoracic spinal cord

● S24.151   Other incomplete lesion at T1 level of thoracic spinal cord A, D, S 🐾

● S24.152   Other incomplete lesion at T2-T6 level of thoracic spinal cord A, D, S 🐾

● S24.153   Other incomplete lesion at T7-T10 level of thoracic spinal cord A, D, S 🐾

● S24.154   Other incomplete lesion at T11-T12 level of thoracic spinal cord A, D, S 🐾

● S24.159   Other incomplete lesion at unspecified level of thoracic spinal cord A, D, S 🐾

X● S24.2   **Injury of nerve root of thoracic spine**

X● S24.3   **Injury of peripheral nerves of thorax**

X● S24.4   **Injury of thoracic sympathetic nervous system**
Injury of cardiac plexus
Injury of esophageal plexus
Injury of pulmonary plexus
Injury of stellate ganglion
Injury of thoracic sympathetic ganglion

X● S24.8   **Injury of other specified nerves of thorax**

X● S24.9   **Injury of unspecified nerve of thorax**

● S25   **Injury of blood vessels of thorax**
The appropriate 7th character is to be added to each code from category S25

> A   initial encounter
> D   subsequent encounter
> S   sequela

Code also any associated open wound (S21.-)

● S25.0   **Injury of thoracic aorta**
Injury of aorta NOS

X● S25.00   **Unspecified injury of thoracic aorta**

X● S25.01   **Minor laceration of thoracic aorta**
Incomplete transection of thoracic aorta
Laceration of thoracic aorta NOS
Superficial laceration of thoracic aorta

X● S25.02   **Major laceration of thoracic aorta**
Complete transection of thoracic aorta
Traumatic rupture of thoracic aorta

X● S25.09   **Other specified injury of thoracic aorta**

● S25.1   **Injury of innominate or subclavian artery**

● S25.10   **Unspecified injury of innominate or subclavian artery**

● S25.101   Unspecified injury of right innominate or subclavian artery

● S25.102   Unspecified injury of left innominate or subclavian artery

● S25.109   Unspecified injury of unspecified innominate or subclavian artery

● S25.11   **Minor laceration of innominate or subclavian artery**
Incomplete transection of innominate or subclavian artery
Laceration of innominate or subclavian artery NOS
Superficial laceration of innominate or subclavian artery

● S25.111   Minor laceration of right innominate or subclavian artery

● S25.112   Minor laceration of left innominate or subclavian artery

● S25.119   Minor laceration of unspecified innominate or subclavian artery

● S25.12   **Major laceration of innominate or subclavian artery**
Complete transection of innominate or subclavian artery
Traumatic rupture of innominate or subclavian artery

● S25.121   Major laceration of right innominate or subclavian artery

● S25.122   Major laceration of left innominate or subclavian artery

● S25.129   Major laceration of unspecified innominate or subclavian artery

● S25.19   **Other specified injury of innominate or subclavian artery**

● S25.191   Other specified injury of right innominate or subclavian artery

● S25.192   Other specified injury of left innominate or subclavian artery

● S25.199   Other specified injury of unspecified innominate or subclavian artery

● S25.2   **Injury of superior vena cava**
Injury of vena cava NOS

X● S25.20   **Unspecified injury of superior vena cava**

X● S25.21   **Minor laceration of superior vena cava**
Incomplete transection of superior vena cava
Laceration of superior vena cava NOS
Superficial laceration of superior vena cava

X● S25.22   **Major laceration of superior vena cava**
Complete transection of superior vena cava
Traumatic rupture of superior vena cava

X● S25.29   **Other specified injury of superior vena cava**

● S25.3   **Injury of innominate or subclavian vein**

● S25.30   **Unspecified injury of innominate or subclavian vein**

● S25.301   Unspecified injury of right innominate or subclavian vein

● S25.302   Unspecified injury of left innominate or subclavian vein

● S25.309   Unspecified injury of unspecified innominate or subclavian vein

● S25.31   **Minor laceration of innominate or subclavian vein**
Incomplete transection of innominate or subclavian vein
Laceration of innominate or subclavian vein NOS
Superficial laceration of innominate or subclavian vein

● S25.311   Minor laceration of right innominate or subclavian vein

● S25.312   Minor laceration of left innominate or subclavian vein

● S25.319   Minor laceration of unspecified innominate or subclavian vein

● S25.32   **Major laceration of innominate or subclavian vein**
Complete transection of innominate or subclavian vein
Traumatic rupture of innominate or subclavian vein

● S25.321   Major laceration of right innominate or subclavian vein

● S25.322   Major laceration of left innominate or subclavian vein

● S25.329   Major laceration of unspecified innominate or subclavian vein

CHAPTER 19 (S00-T88)

S25.39 Other specified injury of innominate or subclavian vein
- S25.391 Other specified injury of right innominate or subclavian vein
- S25.392 Other specified injury of left innominate or subclavian vein
- S25.399 Other specified injury of unspecified innominate or subclavian vein

S25.4 Injury of pulmonary blood vessels
- S25.40 Unspecified injury of pulmonary blood vessels
  - S25.401 Unspecified injury of right pulmonary blood vessels
  - S25.402 Unspecified injury of left pulmonary blood vessels
  - S25.409 Unspecified injury of unspecified pulmonary blood vessels
- S25.41 Minor laceration of pulmonary blood vessels
  - Incomplete transection of pulmonary blood vessels
  - Laceration of pulmonary blood vessels NOS
  - Superficial laceration of pulmonary blood vessels
    - S25.411 Minor laceration of right pulmonary blood vessels
    - S25.412 Minor laceration of left pulmonary blood vessels
    - S25.419 Minor laceration of unspecified pulmonary blood vessels
- S25.42 Major laceration of pulmonary blood vessels
  - Complete transection of pulmonary blood vessels
  - Traumatic rupture of pulmonary blood vessels
    - S25.421 Major laceration of right pulmonary blood vessels
    - S25.422 Major laceration of left pulmonary blood vessels
    - S25.429 Major laceration of unspecified pulmonary blood vessels
- S25.49 Other specified injury of pulmonary blood vessels
  - S25.491 Other specified injury of right pulmonary blood vessels
  - S25.492 Other specified injury of left pulmonary blood vessels
  - S25.499 Other specified injury of unspecified pulmonary blood vessels

S25.5 Injury of intercostal blood vessels
- S25.50 Unspecified injury of intercostal blood vessels
  - S25.501 Unspecified injury of intercostal blood vessels, right side
  - S25.502 Unspecified injury of intercostal blood vessels, left side
  - S25.509 Unspecified injury of intercostal blood vessels, unspecified side
- S25.51 Laceration of intercostal blood vessels
  - S25.511 Laceration of intercostal blood vessels, right side
  - S25.512 Laceration of intercostal blood vessels, left side
  - S25.519 Laceration of intercostal blood vessels, unspecified side
- S25.59 Other specified injury of intercostal blood vessels
  - S25.591 Other specified injury of intercostal blood vessels, right side
  - S25.592 Other specified injury of intercostal blood vessels, left side
  - S25.599 Other specified injury of intercostal blood vessels, unspecified side

S25.8 Injury of other blood vessels of thorax
- Injury of azygos vein
- Injury of mammary artery or vein
- S25.80 Unspecified injury of other blood vessels of thorax
  - S25.801 Unspecified injury of other blood vessels of thorax, right side
  - S25.802 Unspecified injury of other blood vessels of thorax, left side
  - S25.809 Unspecified injury of other blood vessels of thorax, unspecified side
- S25.81 Laceration of other blood vessels of thorax
  - S25.811 Laceration of other blood vessels of thorax, right side
  - S25.812 Laceration of other blood vessels of thorax, left side
  - S25.819 Laceration of other blood vessels of thorax, unspecified side
- S25.89 Other specified injury of other blood vessels of thorax
  - S25.891 Other specified injury of other blood vessels of thorax, right side
  - S25.892 Other specified injury of other blood vessels of thorax, left side
  - S25.899 Other specified injury of other blood vessels of thorax, unspecified side

S25.9 Injury of unspecified blood vessel of thorax
- X S25.90 Unspecified injury of unspecified blood vessel of thorax
- X S25.91 Laceration of unspecified blood vessel of thorax
- X S25.99 Other specified injury of unspecified blood vessel of thorax

S26 Injury of heart

The appropriate 7th character is to be added to each code from category S26

A	initial encounter
D	subsequent encounter
S	sequela

Code also any associated:
- open wound of thorax (S21.-)
- traumatic hemopneumothorax (S27.2)
- traumatic hemothorax (S27.1)
- traumatic pneumothorax (S27.0)

S26.0 Injury of heart with hemopericardium
- *Hemopericardium: effusion of blood within pericardium*
- X S26.00 Unspecified injury of heart with hemopericardium
- X S26.01 Contusion of heart with hemopericardium
- S26.02 Laceration of heart with hemopericardium
  - S26.020 Mild laceration of heart with hemopericardium
    - Laceration of heart without penetration of heart chamber
  - S26.021 Moderate laceration of heart with hemopericardium
    - Laceration of heart with penetration of heart chamber
  - S26.022 Major laceration of heart with hemopericardium
    - Laceration of heart with penetration of multiple heart chambers
- X S26.09 Other injury of heart with hemopericardium

S26.1 Injury of heart without hemopericardium
- *Hemopericardium: effusion of blood within pericardium*
- X S26.10 Unspecified injury of heart without hemopericardium
- X S26.11 Contusion of heart without hemopericardium

▶ New   ⇒ Revised   ~~deleted~~ Deleted   Excludes 1   Excludes 2   Includes   Use additional   Code first   Code also   Key words
OGCR Official Guidelines   X Assign placeholder X   ● Use Additional Character(s)   ▷ Manifestation Code   ⦿ Hierarchical Condition Category   **Coding Clinic**

X● S26.12   Laceration of heart without hemopericardium
X● S26.19   Other injury of heart without hemopericardium
● S26.9   Injury of heart, unspecified with or without hemopericardium
     Hemopericardium: effusion of blood within pericardium
X● S26.90   Unspecified injury of heart, unspecified with or without hemopericardium
X● S26.91   Contusion of heart, unspecified with or without hemopericardium
X● S26.92   Laceration of heart, unspecified with or without hemopericardium
     Laceration of heart NOS
X● S26.99   Other injury of heart, unspecified with or without hemopericardium

● S27   Injury of other and unspecified intrathoracic organs
     Code also any associated open wound of thorax (S21.-)
     Excludes2   injury of cervical esophagus (S10-S19)
               injury of trachea (cervical) (S10-S19)
     The appropriate 7th character is to be added to each code from category S27

A	initial encounter
D	subsequent encounter
S	sequela

X● S27.0   Traumatic pneumothorax
     Excludes1   spontaneous pneumothorax (J93.-)
X● S27.1   Traumatic hemothorax
X● S27.2   Traumatic hemopneumothorax
● S27.3   Other and unspecified injuries of lung
   ● S27.30   Unspecified injury of lung
     ● S27.301   Unspecified injury of lung, unilateral
     ● S27.302   Unspecified injury of lung, bilateral
     ● S27.309   Unspecified injury of lung, unspecified
   ● S27.31   Primary blast injury of lung
     Blast injury of lung NOS
     ● S27.311   Primary blast injury of lung, unilateral
     ● S27.312   Primary blast injury of lung, bilateral
     ● S27.319   Primary blast injury of lung, unspecified
   ● S27.32   Contusion of lung
     ● S27.321   Contusion of lung, unilateral
     ● S27.322   Contusion of lung, bilateral
     ● S27.329   Contusion of lung, unspecified
   ● S27.33   Laceration of lung
     ● S27.331   Laceration of lung, unilateral
     ● S27.332   Laceration of lung, bilateral
     ● S27.339   Laceration of lung, unspecified
   ● S27.39   Other injuries of lung
     Secondary blast injury of lung
     ● S27.391   Other injuries of lung, unilateral
     ● S27.392   Other injuries of lung, bilateral
     ● S27.399   Other injuries of lung, unspecified

● S27.4   Injury of bronchus
   ● S27.40   Unspecified injury of bronchus
     ● S27.401   Unspecified injury of bronchus, unilateral
     ● S27.402   Unspecified injury of bronchus, bilateral
     ● S27.409   Unspecified injury of bronchus, unspecified
   ● S27.41   Primary blast injury of bronchus
     Blast injury of bronchus NOS
     ● S27.411   Primary blast injury of bronchus, unilateral
     ● S27.412   Primary blast injury of bronchus, bilateral
     ● S27.419   Primary blast injury of bronchus, unspecified
   ● S27.42   Contusion of bronchus
     ● S27.421   Contusion of bronchus, unilateral
     ● S27.422   Contusion of bronchus, bilateral
     ● S27.429   Contusion of bronchus, unspecified
   ● S27.43   Laceration of bronchus
     ● S27.431   Laceration of bronchus, unilateral
     ● S27.432   Laceration of bronchus, bilateral
     ● S27.439   Laceration of bronchus, unspecified
   ● S27.49   Other injury of bronchus
     Secondary blast injury of bronchus
     ● S27.491   Other injury of bronchus, unilateral
     ● S27.492   Other injury of bronchus, bilateral
     ● S27.499   Other injury of bronchus, unspecified

● S27.5   Injury of thoracic trachea
   X● S27.50   Unspecified injury of thoracic trachea
   X● S27.51   Primary blast injury of thoracic trachea
     Blast injury of thoracic trachea NOS
   X● S27.52   Contusion of thoracic trachea
   X● S27.53   Laceration of thoracic trachea
   X● S27.59   Other injury of thoracic trachea
     Secondary blast injury of thoracic trachea

● S27.6   Injury of pleura
   X● S27.60   Unspecified injury of pleura
   X● S27.63   Laceration of pleura
   X● S27.69   Other injury of pleura

● S27.8   Injury of other specified intrathoracic organs
   ● S27.80   Injury of diaphragm
     ● S27.802   Contusion of diaphragm
     ● S27.803   Laceration of diaphragm
     ● S27.808   Other injury of diaphragm
     ● S27.809   Unspecified injury of diaphragm
   ● S27.81   Injury of esophagus (thoracic part)
     ● S27.812   Contusion of esophagus (thoracic part)
     ● S27.813   Laceration of esophagus (thoracic part)
     ● S27.818   Other injury of esophagus (thoracic part)
     ● S27.819   Unspecified injury of esophagus (thoracic part)
   ● S27.89   Injury of other specified intrathoracic organs
     Injury of lymphatic thoracic duct
     Injury of thymus gland
     ● S27.892   Contusion of other specified intrathoracic organs
     ● S27.893   Laceration of other specified intrathoracic organs
     ● S27.898   Other injury of other specified intrathoracic organs
     ● S27.899   Unspecified injury of other specified intrathoracic organs

X● S27.9   Injury of unspecified intrathoracic organ

Item 19–2 Pneumothorax is a collection of gas (positive air pressure) in the pleural space resulting in the lung collapsing. A **tension pneumothorax** is life-threatening and is a result of air in the pleural space causing a displacement in the mediastinal structures and cardiopulmonary function compromise. A **traumatic pneumothorax** results from blunt or penetrating injury that disrupts the parietal/visceral pleura. **Hemothorax** is blood or bloody fluid in the pleural cavity as a result of traumatic blood vessel rupture or inflammation of the lungs from pneumonia.

CHAPTER 19 (S00-T88)

S28 **Crushing injury of thorax, and traumatic amputation of part of thorax**

The appropriate 7th character is to be added to each code from category S28

A	initial encounter
D	subsequent encounter
S	sequela

X ● **S28.0** **Crushed chest**

Use additional code for all associated injuries

Excludes1 flail chest (S22.5)

X ● **S28.1** **Traumatic amputation (partial) of part of thorax, except breast**

● **S28.2** **Traumatic amputation of breast**

● **S28.21** **Complete traumatic amputation of breast**

Traumatic amputation of breast NOS

● **S28.211** **Complete traumatic amputation of right breast**

● **S28.212** **Complete traumatic amputation of left breast**

● **S28.219** **Complete traumatic amputation of unspecified breast**

● **S28.22** **Partial traumatic amputation of breast**

● **S28.221** **Partial traumatic amputation of right breast**

● **S28.222** **Partial traumatic amputation of left breast**

● **S28.229** **Partial traumatic amputation of unspecified breast**

● **S29** **Other and unspecified injuries of thorax**

Code also any associated open wound (S21.-)

The appropriate 7th character is to be added to each code from category S29

A	initial encounter
D	subsequent encounter
S	sequela

● **S29.0** **Injury of muscle and tendon at thorax level**

● **S29.00** **Unspecified injury of muscle and tendon of thorax**

● **S29.001** **Unspecified injury of muscle and tendon of front wall of thorax**

● **S29.002** **Unspecified injury of muscle and tendon of back wall of thorax**

● **S29.009** **Unspecified injury of muscle and tendon of unspecified wall of thorax**

● **S29.01** **Strain of muscle and tendon of thorax**

● **S29.011** **Strain of muscle and tendon of front wall of thorax**

● **S29.012** **Strain of muscle and tendon of back wall of thorax**

● **S29.019** **Strain of muscle and tendon of unspecified wall of thorax**

● **S29.02** **Laceration of muscle and tendon of thorax**

● **S29.021** **Laceration of muscle and tendon of front wall of thorax**

● **S29.022** **Laceration of muscle and tendon of back wall of thorax**

● **S29.029** **Laceration of muscle and tendon of unspecified wall of thorax**

● **S29.09** **Other injury of muscle and tendon of thorax**

● **S29.091** **Other injury of muscle and tendon of front wall of thorax**

● **S29.092** **Other injury of muscle and tendon of back wall of thorax**

● **S29.099** **Other injury of muscle and tendon of unspecified wall of thorax**

X ● **S29.8** **Other specified injuries of thorax**

X ● **S29.9** **Unspecified injury of thorax**

INJURIES TO THE ABDOMEN, LOWER BACK, LUMBAR SPINE PELVIS AND EXTERNAL GENITALS (S30-S39)

Includes injuries to the abdominal wall
injuries to the anus
injuries to the buttock
injuries to the external genitalia
injuries to the flank
injuries to the groin

Excludes2 burns and corrosions (T20-T32)
effects of foreign body in anus and rectum (T18.5)
effects of foreign body in genitourinary tract (T19.-)
effects of foreign body in stomach, small intestine and colon (T18.2-T18.4)
frostbite (T33-T34)
insect bite or sting, venomous (T63.4)

● **S30** **Superficial injury of abdomen, lower back, pelvis and external genitals**

Excludes2 superficial injury of hip (S70.-)

The appropriate 7th character is to be added to each code from category S30

A	initial encounter
D	subsequent encounter
S	sequela

X ● **S30.0** **Contusion of lower back and pelvis**

Contusion of buttock

X ● **S30.1** **Contusion of abdominal wall**

Contusion of flank
Contusion of groin

● **S30.2** **Contusion of external genital organs**

● **S30.20** **Contusion of unspecified external genital organ**

● **S30.201** **Contusion of unspecified external genital organ, male** ♂

● **S30.202** **Contusion of unspecified external genital organ, female** ♀

X ● **S30.21** **Contusion of penis** ♂

X ● **S30.22** **Contusion of scrotum and testes** ♂

X ● **S30.23** **Contusion of vagina and vulva** ♀

X ● **S30.3** **Contusion of anus**

● **S30.8** **Other superficial injuries of abdomen, lower back, pelvis and external genitals**

● **S30.81** **Abrasion of abdomen, lower back, pelvis and external genitals**

● **S30.810** **Abrasion of lower back and pelvis**

● **S30.811** **Abrasion of abdominal wall**

● **S30.812** **Abrasion of penis** ♂

● **S30.813** **Abrasion of scrotum and testes** ♂

● **S30.814** **Abrasion of vagina and vulva** ♀

● **S30.815** **Abrasion of unspecified external genital organs, male** ♂

● **S30.816** **Abrasion of unspecified external genital organs, female** ♀

● **S30.817** **Abrasion of anus**

● **S30.82** **Blister (nonthermal) of abdomen, lower back, pelvis and external genitals**

● **S30.820** **Blister (nonthermal) of lower back and pelvis**

● **S30.821** **Blister (nonthermal) of abdominal wall**

● **S30.822** **Blister (nonthermal) of penis** ♂

● **S30.823** **Blister (nonthermal) of scrotum and testes** ♂

● **S30.824** **Blister (nonthermal) of vagina and vulva** ♀

● **S30.825** **Blister (nonthermal) of unspecified external genital organs, male** ♂

▶ New   ⇒ Revised   ~~deleted~~ Deleted   Excludes 1   Excludes 2   Includes   Use additional   Code first   Code also   Key words

OGCR Official Guidelines   X Assign placeholder X   ● Use Additional Character(s)   ) Manifestation Code   🦠 Hierarchical Condition Category   **Coding Clinic**

● S30.826 Blister (nonthermal) of unspecified external genital organs, female ♀

● S30.827 Blister (nonthermal) of anus

● S30.84 **External constriction of abdomen, lower back, pelvis and external genitals**

  ● S30.840 External constriction of lower back and pelvis

  ● S30.841 External constriction of abdominal wall

  ● S30.842 External constriction of penis ♂
             Hair tourniquet syndrome of penis
             Use additional cause code to identify the constricting item (W49.0-)

  ● S30.843 External constriction of scrotum and testes ♂

  ● S30.844 External constriction of vagina and vulva ♀

  ● S30.845 External constriction of unspecified external genital organs, male ♂

  ● S30.846 External constriction of unspecified external genital organs, female ♀

● S30.85 **Superficial foreign body of abdomen, lower back, pelvis and external genitals**
          Splinter in the abdomen, lower back, pelvis and external genitals

  ● S30.850 Superficial foreign body of lower back and pelvis

  ● S30.851 Superficial foreign body of abdominal wall

  ● S30.852 Superficial foreign body of penis ♂

  ● S30.853 Superficial foreign body of scrotum and testes ♂

  ● S30.854 Superficial foreign body of vagina and vulva ♀

  ● S30.855 Superficial foreign body of unspecified external genital organs, male ♂

  ● S30.856 Superficial foreign body of unspecified external genital organs, female ♀

  ● S30.857 Superficial foreign body of anus

● S30.86 **Insect bite (nonvenomous) of abdomen, lower back, pelvis and external genitals**

  ● S30.860 Insect bite (nonvenomous) of lower back and pelvis

  ● S30.861 Insect bite (nonvenomous) of abdominal wall

  ● S30.862 Insect bite (nonvenomous) of penis ♂

  ● S30.863 Insect bite (nonvenomous) of scrotum and testes ♂

  ● S30.864 Insect bite (nonvenomous) of vagina and vulva ♀

  ● S30.865 Insect bite (nonvenomous) of unspecified external genital organs, male ♂

  ● S30.866 Insect bite (nonvenomous) of unspecified external genital organs, female ♀

  ● S30.867 Insect bite (nonvenomous) of anus

● S30.87 **Other superficial bite of abdomen, lower back, pelvis and external genitals**

  Excludes1   open bite of abdomen, lower back, pelvis and external genitals (S31.05, S31.15, S31.25, S31.35, S31.45, S31.55)

  ● S30.870 Other superficial bite of lower back and pelvis

  ● S30.871 Other superficial bite of abdominal wall

  ● S30.872 Other superficial bite of penis ♂

● S30.873 Other superficial bite of scrotum and testes ♂

● S30.874 Other superficial bite of vagina and vulva ♀

● S30.875 Other superficial bite of unspecified external genital organs, male ♂

● S30.876 Other superficial bite of unspecified external genital organs, female ♀

● S30.877 Other superficial bite of anus

● S30.9 **Unspecified superficial injury of abdomen, lower back, pelvis and external genitals**

  X ● S30.91 Unspecified superficial injury of lower back and pelvis

  X ● S30.92 Unspecified superficial injury of abdominal wall

  X ● S30.93 Unspecified superficial injury of penis ♂

  X ● S30.94 Unspecified superficial injury of scrotum and testes ♂

  X ● S30.95 Unspecified superficial injury of vagina and vulva ♀

  X ● S30.96 Unspecified superficial injury of unspecified external genital organs, male ♂

  X ● S30.97 Unspecified superficial injury of unspecified external genital organs, female ♀

  X ● S30.98 Unspecified superficial injury of anus

● S31 **Open wound of abdomen, lower back, pelvis and external genitals**

  Code also any associated:
     spinal cord injury (S24.0, S24.1-, S34.0-, S34.1-)
     wound infection

  Excludes1   traumatic amputation of part of abdomen, lower back and pelvis (S38.2-, S38.3)

  Excludes2   open wound of hip (S71.00-S71.02)
                  open fracture of pelvis (S32.1--S32.9 with 7th character B)

  The appropriate 7th character is to be added to each code from category S31

A	initial encounter
D	subsequent encounter
S	sequela

● S31.0 **Open wound of lower back and pelvis**

  ● S31.00 **Unspecified open wound of lower back and pelvis**

    ● S31.000 Unspecified open wound of lower back and pelvis without penetration into retroperitoneum
               Unspecified open wound of lower back and pelvis NOS

    ● S31.001 Unspecified open wound of lower back and pelvis with penetration into retroperitoneum

  ● S31.01 **Laceration without foreign body of lower back and pelvis**

    ● S31.010 Laceration without foreign body of lower back and pelvis without penetration into retroperitoneum
               Laceration without foreign body of lower back and pelvis NOS

    ● S31.011 Laceration without foreign body of lower back and pelvis with penetration into retroperitoneum

  ● S31.02 **Laceration with foreign body of lower back and pelvis**

    ● S31.020 Laceration with foreign body of lower back and pelvis without penetration into retroperitoneum
               Laceration with foreign body of lower back and pelvis NOS

    ● S31.021 Laceration with foreign body of lower back and pelvis with penetration into retroperitoneum

CHAPTER 19 (S00-T88)

● S31.Ø3   **Puncture wound without foreign body of lower back and pelvis**

   ● S31.Ø3Ø   **Puncture wound without foreign body of lower back and pelvis without penetration into retroperitoneum**
       Puncture wound without foreign body of lower back and pelvis NOS

   ● S31.Ø31   **Puncture wound without foreign body of lower back and pelvis with penetration into retroperitoneum**

● S31.Ø4   **Puncture wound with foreign body of lower back and pelvis**

   ● S31.Ø4Ø   **Puncture wound with foreign body of lower back and pelvis without penetration into retroperitoneum**
       Puncture wound with foreign body of lower back and pelvis NOS

   ● S31.Ø41   **Puncture wound with foreign body of lower back and pelvis with penetration into retroperitoneum**

● S31.Ø5   **Open bite of lower back and pelvis**
     Bite of lower back and pelvis NOS
     Excludes1 superficial bite of lower back and pelvis (S30.860, S30.870)

   ● S31.Ø5Ø   **Open bite of lower back and pelvis without penetration into retroperitoneum**
       Open bite of lower back and pelvis NOS

   ● S31.Ø51   **Open bite of lower back and pelvis with penetration into retroperitoneum**

● S31.1   **Open wound of abdominal wall without penetration into peritoneal cavity**
     Open wound of abdominal wall NOS
     Excludes2 open wound of abdominal wall with penetration into peritoneal cavity (S31.6-)

   ● S31.1Ø   **Unspecified open wound of abdominal wall without penetration into peritoneal cavity**

   ● S31.1ØØ   **Unspecified open wound of abdominal wall, right upper quadrant without penetration into peritoneal cavity**

   ● S31.1Ø1   **Unspecified open wound of abdominal wall, left upper quadrant without penetration into peritoneal cavity**

   ● S31.1Ø2   **Unspecified open wound of abdominal wall, epigastric region without penetration into peritoneal cavity**

   ● S31.1Ø3   **Unspecified open wound of abdominal wall, right lower quadrant without penetration into peritoneal cavity**

   ● S31.1Ø4   **Unspecified open wound of abdominal wall, left lower quadrant without penetration into peritoneal cavity**

   ● S31.1Ø5   **Unspecified open wound of abdominal wall, periumbilic region without penetration into peritoneal cavity**

   ● S31.1Ø9   **Unspecified open wound of abdominal wall, unspecified quadrant without penetration into peritoneal cavity**
       Unspecified open wound of abdominal wall NOS

● S31.11   **Laceration without foreign body of abdominal wall without penetration into peritoneal cavity**

   ● S31.11Ø   **Laceration without foreign body of abdominal wall, right upper quadrant without penetration into peritoneal cavity**

   ● S31.111   **Laceration without foreign body of abdominal wall, left upper quadrant without penetration into peritoneal cavity**

   ● S31.112   **Laceration without foreign body of abdominal wall, epigastric region without penetration into peritoneal cavity**

   ● S31.113   **Laceration without foreign body of abdominal wall, right lower quadrant without penetration into peritoneal cavity**

   ● S31.114   **Laceration without foreign body of abdominal wall, left lower quadrant without penetration into peritoneal cavity**

   ● S31.115   **Laceration without foreign body of abdominal wall, periumbilic region without penetration into peritoneal cavity**

   ● S31.119   **Laceration without foreign body of abdominal wall, unspecified quadrant without penetration into peritoneal cavity**

● S31.12   **Laceration with foreign body of abdominal wall without penetration into peritoneal cavity**

   ● S31.12Ø   **Laceration of abdominal wall with foreign body, right upper quadrant without penetration into peritoneal cavity**

   ● S31.121   **Laceration of abdominal wall with foreign body, left upper quadrant without penetration into peritoneal cavity**

   ● S31.122   **Laceration of abdominal wall with foreign body, epigastric region without penetration into peritoneal cavity**

   ● S31.123   **Laceration of abdominal wall with foreign body, right lower quadrant without penetration into peritoneal cavity**

   ● S31.124   **Laceration of abdominal wall with foreign body, left lower quadrant without penetration into peritoneal cavity**

   ● S31.125   **Laceration of abdominal wall with foreign body, periumbilic region without penetration into peritoneal cavity**

   ● S31.129   **Laceration of abdominal wall with foreign body, unspecified quadrant without penetration into peritoneal cavity**

● S31.13   **Puncture wound of abdominal wall without foreign body without penetration into peritoneal cavity**

   ● S31.13Ø   **Puncture wound of abdominal wall without foreign body, right upper quadrant without penetration into peritoneal cavity**

   ● S31.131   **Puncture wound of abdominal wall without foreign body, left upper quadrant without penetration into peritoneal cavity**

● S31.132   Puncture wound of abdominal wall without foreign body, epigastric region without penetration into peritoneal cavity

● S31.133   Puncture wound of abdominal wall without foreign body, right lower quadrant without penetration into peritoneal cavity

● S31.134   Puncture wound of abdominal wall without foreign body, left lower quadrant without penetration into peritoneal cavity

● S31.135   Puncture wound of abdominal wall without foreign body, periumbilic region without penetration into peritoneal cavity

● S31.139   Puncture wound of abdominal wall without foreign body, unspecified quadrant without penetration into peritoneal cavity

● S31.14   Puncture wound of abdominal wall with foreign body without penetration into peritoneal cavity

● S31.140   Puncture wound of abdominal wall with foreign body, right upper quadrant without penetration into peritoneal cavity

● S31.141   Puncture wound of abdominal wall with foreign body, left upper quadrant without penetration into peritoneal cavity

● S31.142   Puncture wound of abdominal wall with foreign body, epigastric region without penetration into peritoneal cavity

● S31.143   Puncture wound of abdominal wall with foreign body, right lower quadrant without penetration into peritoneal cavity

● S31.144   Puncture wound of abdominal wall with foreign body, left lower quadrant without penetration into peritoneal cavity

● S31.145   Puncture wound of abdominal wall with foreign body, periumbilic region without penetration into peritoneal cavity

● S31.149   Puncture wound of abdominal wall with foreign body, unspecified quadrant without penetration into peritoneal cavity

● S31.15   Open bite of abdominal wall without penetration into peritoneal cavity
Bite of abdominal wall NOS

Excludes1   superficial bite of abdominal wall (S30.871)

● S31.150   Open bite of abdominal wall, right upper quadrant without penetration into peritoneal cavity

● S31.151   Open bite of abdominal wall, left upper quadrant without penetration into peritoneal cavity

● S31.152   Open bite of abdominal wall, epigastric region without penetration into peritoneal cavity

● S31.153   Open bite of abdominal wall, right lower quadrant without penetration into peritoneal cavity

● S31.154   Open bite of abdominal wall, left lower quadrant without penetration into peritoneal cavity

● S31.155   Open bite of abdominal wall, periumbilic region without penetration into peritoneal cavity

● S31.159   Open bite of abdominal wall, unspecified quadrant without penetration into peritoneal cavity

● S31.2   Open wound of penis
X ● S31.20   Unspecified open wound of penis ♂
X ● S31.21   Laceration without foreign body of penis ♂
X ● S31.22   Laceration with foreign body of penis ♂
X ● S31.23   Puncture wound without foreign body of penis ♂
X ● S31.24   Puncture wound with foreign body of penis ♂
X ● S31.25   Open bite of penis ♂
Bite of penis NOS

Excludes1   superficial bite of penis (S30.862, S30.872)

● S31.3   Open wound of scrotum and testes
X ● S31.30   Unspecified open wound of scrotum and testes ♂
X ● S31.31   Laceration without foreign body of scrotum and testes ♂
X ● S31.32   Laceration with foreign body of scrotum and testes ♂
X ● S31.33   Puncture wound without foreign body of scrotum and testes ♂
X ● S31.34   Puncture wound with foreign body of scrotum and testes ♂
X ● S31.35   Open bite of scrotum and testes ♂
Bite of scrotum and testes NOS

Excludes1   superficial bite of scrotum and testes (S30.863, S30.873)

● S31.4   Open wound of vagina and vulva

Excludes1   injury to vagina and vulva during delivery (O70.-, O71.4)

X ● S31.40   Unspecified open wound of vagina and vulva ♀
X ● S31.41   Laceration without foreign body of vagina and vulva ♀
X ● S31.42   Laceration with foreign body of vagina and vulva ♀
X ● S31.43   Puncture wound without foreign body of vagina and vulva ♀
X ● S31.44   Puncture wound with foreign body of vagina and vulva ♀
X ● S31.45   Open bite of vagina and vulva ♀
Bite of vagina and vulva NOS

Excludes1   superficial bite of vagina and vulva (S30.864, S30.874)

● S31.5   Open wound of unspecified external genital organs

Excludes1   traumatic amputation of external genital organs (S38.21, S38.22)

● S31.50   Unspecified open wound of unspecified external genital organs

● S31.501   Unspecified open wound of unspecified external genital organs, male ♂

● S31.502   Unspecified open wound of unspecified external genital organs, female ♀

● S31.51   Laceration without foreign body of unspecified external genital organs

● S31.511   Laceration without foreign body of unspecified external genital organs, male ♂

● S31.512   Laceration without foreign body of unspecified external genital organs, female ♀

- ● S31.52   Laceration with foreign body of unspecified external genital organs
  - ● S31.521   Laceration with foreign body of unspecified external genital organs, male ♂
  - ● S31.522   Laceration with foreign body of unspecified external genital organs, female ♀
- ● S31.53   Puncture wound without foreign body of unspecified external genital organs
  - ● S31.531   Puncture wound without foreign body of unspecified external genital organs, male ♂
  - ● S31.532   Puncture wound without foreign body of unspecified external genital organs, female ♀
- ● S31.54   Puncture wound with foreign body of unspecified external genital organs
  - ● S31.541   Puncture wound with foreign body of unspecified external genital organs, male ♂
  - ● S31.542   Puncture wound with foreign body of unspecified external genital organs, female ♀
- ● S31.55   Open bite of unspecified external genital organs

  Bite of unspecified external genital organs NOS

  Excludes1   superficial bite of unspecified external genital organs (S30.865, S30.866, S30.875, S30.876)
  - ● S31.551   Open bite of unspecified external genital organs, male ♂
  - ● S31.552   Open bite of unspecified external genital organs, female ♀
- ● S31.6   Open wound of abdominal wall with penetration into peritoneal cavity
  - ● S31.60   Unspecified open wound of abdominal wall with penetration into peritoneal cavity
    - ● S31.600   Unspecified open wound of abdominal wall, right upper quadrant with penetration into peritoneal cavity
    - ● S31.601   Unspecified open wound of abdominal wall, left upper quadrant with penetration into peritoneal cavity
    - ● S31.602   Unspecified open wound of abdominal wall, epigastric region with penetration into peritoneal cavity
    - ● S31.603   Unspecified open wound of abdominal wall, right lower quadrant with penetration into peritoneal cavity
    - ● S31.604   Unspecified open wound of abdominal wall, left lower quadrant with penetration into peritoneal cavity
    - ● S31.605   Unspecified open wound of abdominal wall, periumbilic region with penetration into peritoneal cavity
    - ● S31.609   Unspecified open wound of abdominal wall, unspecified quadrant with penetration into peritoneal cavity

- ● S31.61   Laceration without foreign body of abdominal wall with penetration into peritoneal cavity
  - ● S31.610   Laceration without foreign body of abdominal wall, right upper quadrant with penetration into peritoneal cavity
  - ● S31.611   Laceration without foreign body of abdominal wall, left upper quadrant with penetration into peritoneal cavity
  - ● S31.612   Laceration without foreign body of abdominal wall, epigastric region with penetration into peritoneal cavity
  - ● S31.613   Laceration without foreign body of abdominal wall, right lower quadrant with penetration into peritoneal cavity

    Coding Clinic: 2015, Q4, P37
  - ● S31.614   Laceration without foreign body of abdominal wall, left lower quadrant with penetration into peritoneal cavity
  - ● S31.615   Laceration without foreign body of abdominal wall, periumbilic region with penetration into peritoneal cavity
  - ● S31.619   Laceration without foreign body of abdominal wall, unspecified quadrant with penetration into peritoneal cavity
- ● S31.62   Laceration with foreign body of abdominal wall with penetration into peritoneal cavity
  - ● S31.620   Laceration with foreign body of abdominal wall, right upper quadrant with penetration into peritoneal cavity
  - ● S31.621   Laceration with foreign body of abdominal wall, left upper quadrant with penetration into peritoneal cavity
  - ● S31.622   Laceration with foreign body of abdominal wall, epigastric region with penetration into peritoneal cavity
  - ● S31.623   Laceration with foreign body of abdominal wall, right lower quadrant with penetration into peritoneal cavity
  - ● S31.624   Laceration with foreign body of abdominal wall, left lower quadrant with penetration into peritoneal cavity
  - ● S31.625   Laceration with foreign body of abdominal wall, periumbilic region with penetration into peritoneal cavity
  - ● S31.629   Laceration with foreign body of abdominal wall, unspecified quadrant with penetration into peritoneal cavity
- ● S31.63   Puncture wound without foreign body of abdominal wall with penetration into peritoneal cavity
  - ● S31.630   Puncture wound without foreign body of abdominal wall, right upper quadrant with penetration into peritoneal cavity
  - ● S31.631   Puncture wound without foreign body of abdominal wall, left upper quadrant with penetration into peritoneal cavity

- S31.632   Puncture wound without foreign body of abdominal wall, epigastric region with penetration into peritoneal cavity
- S31.633   Puncture wound without foreign body of abdominal wall, right lower quadrant with penetration into peritoneal cavity
- S31.634   Puncture wound without foreign body of abdominal wall, left lower quadrant with penetration into peritoneal cavity
- S31.635   Puncture wound without foreign body of abdominal wall, periumbilic region with penetration into peritoneal cavity
- S31.639   Puncture wound without foreign body of abdominal wall, unspecified quadrant with penetration into peritoneal cavity
- S31.64   Puncture wound with foreign body of abdominal wall with penetration into peritoneal cavity
  - S31.640   Puncture wound with foreign body of abdominal wall, right upper quadrant with penetration into peritoneal cavity
  - S31.641   Puncture wound with foreign body of abdominal wall, left upper quadrant with penetration into peritoneal cavity
  - S31.642   Puncture wound with foreign body of abdominal wall, epigastric region with penetration into peritoneal cavity
  - S31.643   Puncture wound with foreign body of abdominal wall, right lower quadrant with penetration into peritoneal cavity
  - S31.644   Puncture wound with foreign body of abdominal wall, left lower quadrant with penetration into peritoneal cavity
  - S31.645   Puncture wound with foreign body of abdominal wall, periumbilic region with penetration into peritoneal cavity
  - S31.649   Puncture wound with foreign body of abdominal wall, unspecified quadrant with penetration into peritoneal cavity
- S31.65   Open bite of abdominal wall with penetration into peritoneal cavity

  Excludes1   superficial bite of abdominal wall (S30.861, S30.871)

  - S31.650   Open bite of abdominal wall, right upper quadrant with penetration into peritoneal cavity
  - S31.651   Open bite of abdominal wall, left upper quadrant with penetration into peritoneal cavity
  - S31.652   Open bite of abdominal wall, epigastric region with penetration into peritoneal cavity
  - S31.653   Open bite of abdominal wall, right lower quadrant with penetration into peritoneal cavity
  - S31.654   Open bite of abdominal wall, left lower quadrant with penetration into peritoneal cavity
  - S31.655   Open bite of abdominal wall, periumbilic region with penetration into peritoneal cavity
  - S31.659   Open bite of abdominal wall, unspecified quadrant with penetration into peritoneal cavity
- S31.8   **Open wound of other parts of abdomen, lower back and pelvis**
  - S31.80   Open wound of unspecified buttock
    - S31.801   Laceration without foreign body of unspecified buttock
    - S31.802   Laceration with foreign body of unspecified buttock
    - S31.803   Puncture wound without foreign body of unspecified buttock
    - S31.804   Puncture wound with foreign body of unspecified buttock
    - S31.805   Open bite of unspecified buttock
      Bite of buttock NOS

      Excludes1   superficial bite of buttock (S30.870)

    - S31.809   Unspecified open wound of unspecified buttock
  - S31.81   Open wound of right buttock
    - S31.811   Laceration without foreign body of right buttock
    - S31.812   Laceration with foreign body of right buttock
    - S31.813   Puncture wound without foreign body of right buttock
    - S31.814   Puncture wound with foreign body of right buttock
    - S31.815   Open bite of right buttock
      Bite of right buttock NOS

      Excludes1   superficial bite of buttock (S30.870)

    - S31.819   Unspecified open wound of right buttock
  - S31.82   Open wound of left buttock
    - S31.821   Laceration without foreign body of left buttock
    - S31.822   Laceration with foreign body of left buttock
    - S31.823   Puncture wound without foreign body of left buttock
    - S31.824   Puncture wound with foreign body of left buttock
    - S31.825   Open bite of left buttock
      Bite of left buttock NOS

      Excludes1   superficial bite of buttock (S30.870)

    - S31.829   Unspecified open wound of left buttock
  - S31.83   Open wound of anus
    - S31.831   Laceration without foreign body of anus
    - S31.832   Laceration with foreign body of anus
    - S31.833   Puncture wound without foreign body of anus
    - S31.834   Puncture wound with foreign body of anus
    - S31.835   Open bite of anus
      Bite of anus NOS

      Excludes1   superficial bite of anus (S30.877)

    - S31.839   Unspecified open wound of anus

● S32   Fracture of lumbar spine and pelvis

Note: A fracture not indicated as displaced or nondisplaced should be coded to displaced

A fracture not indicated as opened or closed should be coded to closed

Includes   fracture of lumbosacral neural arch
fracture of lumbosacral spinous process
fracture of lumbosacral transverse process
fracture of lumbosacral vertebra
fracture of lumbosacral vertebral arch

Code first any associated spinal cord and spinal nerve injury (S34.-)

Excludes1   transection of abdomen (S38.3)

Excludes2   fracture of hip NOS (S72.0-)

The appropriate 7th character is to be added to each code from category S32

A	initial encounter for closed fracture
B	initial encounter for open fracture
D	subsequent encounter for fracture with routine healing
G	subsequent encounter for fracture with delayed healing
K	subsequent encounter for fracture with nonunion
S	sequela

● S32.0   Fracture of lumbar vertebra
Fracture of lumbar spine NOS

     ● S32.00   Fracture of unspecified lumbar vertebra

         ● S32.000   Wedge compression fracture of unspecified lumbar vertebra A, B 🐾

         ● S32.001   Stable burst fracture of unspecified lumbar vertebra A, B 🐾

         ● S32.002   Unstable burst fracture of unspecified lumbar vertebra A, B 🐾

         ● S32.008   Other fracture of unspecified lumbar vertebra A, B 🐾

         ● S32.009   Unspecified fracture of unspecified lumbar vertebra A, B 🐾

     ● S32.01   Fracture of first lumbar vertebra

         ● S32.010   Wedge compression fracture of first lumbar vertebra A, B 🐾

         ● S32.011   Stable burst fracture of first lumbar vertebra A, B 🐾

         ● S32.012   Unstable burst fracture of first lumbar vertebra A, B 🐾

         ● S32.018   Other fracture of first lumbar vertebra A, B 🐾

         ● S32.019   Unspecified fracture of first lumbar vertebra A, B 🐾

     ● S32.02   Fracture of second lumbar vertebra

         ● S32.020   Wedge compression fracture of second lumbar vertebra A, B 🐾

         ● S32.021   Stable burst fracture of second lumbar vertebra A, B 🐾

         ● S32.022   Unstable burst fracture of second lumbar vertebra A, B 🐾

         ● S32.028   Other fracture of second lumbar vertebra A, B 🐾

         ● S32.029   Unspecified fracture of second lumbar vertebra A, B 🐾

     ● S32.03   Fracture of third lumbar vertebra

         ● S32.030   Wedge compression fracture of third lumbar vertebra A, B 🐾

         ● S32.031   Stable burst fracture of third lumbar vertebra A, B 🐾

         ● S32.032   Unstable burst fracture of third lumbar vertebra A, B 🐾

         ● S32.038   Other fracture of third lumbar vertebra A, B 🐾

         ● S32.039   Unspecified fracture of third lumbar vertebra A, B 🐾

● S32.04   Fracture of fourth lumbar vertebra

     ● S32.040   Wedge compression fracture of fourth lumbar vertebra A, B 🐾

     ● S32.041   Stable burst fracture of fourth lumbar vertebra A, B 🐾

     ● S32.042   Unstable burst fracture of fourth lumbar vertebra A, B 🐾

     ● S32.048   Other fracture of fourth lumbar vertebra A, B 🐾

     ● S32.049   Unspecified fracture of fourth lumbar vertebra A, B 🐾

● S32.05   Fracture of fifth lumbar vertebra

     ● S32.050   Wedge compression fracture of fifth lumbar vertebra A, B 🐾

     ● S32.051   Stable burst fracture of fifth lumbar vertebra A, B 🐾

     ● S32.052   Unstable burst fracture of fifth lumbar vertebra A, B 🐾

     ● S32.058   Other fracture of fifth lumbar vertebra A, B 🐾

     ● S32.059   Unspecified fracture of fifth lumbar vertebra A, B 🐾

● S32.1   Fracture of sacrum
For vertical fractures, code to most medial fracture extension
Use two codes if both a vertical and transverse fracture are present
Code also any associated fracture of pelvic ring (S32.8-)

X **● S32.10   Unspecified fracture of sacrum** A, B 🐾

● S32.11   Zone I fracture of sacrum
Vertical sacral ala fracture of sacrum

     ● S32.110   Nondisplaced Zone I fracture of sacrum A, B 🐾

     ● S32.111   Minimally displaced Zone I fracture of sacrum A, B 🐾

     ● S32.112   Severely displaced Zone I fracture of sacrum A, B 🐾

     ● S32.119   Unspecified Zone I fracture of sacrum A, B 🐾

● S32.12   Zone II fracture of sacrum
Vertical foraminal region fracture of sacrum

     ● S32.120   Nondisplaced Zone II fracture of sacrum A, B 🐾

     ● S32.121   Minimally displaced Zone II fracture of sacrum A, B 🐾

     ● S32.122   Severely displaced Zone II fracture of sacrum A, B 🐾

     ● S32.129   Unspecified Zone II fracture of sacrum A, B 🐾

● S32.13   Zone III fracture of sacrum
Vertical fracture into spinal canal region of sacrum

     ● S32.130   Nondisplaced Zone III fracture of sacrum A, B 🐾

     ● S32.131   Minimally displaced Zone III fracture of sacrum A, B 🐾

     ● S32.132   Severely displaced Zone III fracture of sacrum A, B 🐾

     ● S32.139   Unspecified Zone III fracture of sacrum A, B 🐾

X **● S32.14   Type 1 fracture of sacrum** A, B 🐾
Transverse flexion fracture of sacrum without displacement

X **● S32.15   Type 2 fracture of sacrum** A, B 🐾
Transverse flexion fracture of sacrum with posterior displacement

X **● S32.16   Type 3 fracture of sacrum** A, B 🐾
Transverse extension fracture of sacrum with anterior displacement

X ● **S32.17**   Type 4 fracture of sacrum A, B 🔖
           Transverse segmental comminution of upper sacrum

X ● **S32.19**   Other fracture of sacrum A, B 🔖

X ● **S32.2**   Fracture of coccyx A, B 🔖

● **S32.3**   Fracture of ilium

     Excludes1   fracture of ilium with associated disruption of pelvic ring (S32.8-)

   ● **S32.30**   Unspecified fracture of ilium

     ● **S32.301**   Unspecified fracture of right ilium A, B 🔖

     ● **S32.302**   Unspecified fracture of left ilium A, B 🔖

     ● **S32.309**   Unspecified fracture of unspecified ilium A, B 🔖

   ● **S32.31**   Avulsion fracture of ilium

     ● **S32.311**   Displaced avulsion fracture of right ilium A, B 🔖

     ● **S32.312**   Displaced avulsion fracture of left ilium A, B 🔖

     ● **S32.313**   Displaced avulsion fracture of unspecified ilium A, B 🔖

     ● **S32.314**   Nondisplaced avulsion fracture of right ilium A, B 🔖

     ● **S32.315**   Nondisplaced avulsion fracture of left ilium A, B 🔖

     ● **S32.316**   Nondisplaced avulsion fracture of unspecified ilium A, B 🔖

   ● **S32.39**   Other fracture of ilium

     ● **S32.391**   Other fracture of right ilium A, B 🔖

     ● **S32.392**   Other fracture of left ilium A, B 🔖

     ● **S32.399**   Other fracture of unspecified ilium A, B 🔖

● **S32.4**   Fracture of acetabulum

     Code also any associated fracture of pelvic ring (S32.8-)

   ● **S32.40**   Unspecified fracture of acetabulum

     ● **S32.401**   Unspecified fracture of right acetabulum A, B 🔖

     ● **S32.402**   Unspecified fracture of left acetabulum A, B 🔖

     ● **S32.409**   Unspecified fracture of unspecified acetabulum A, B 🔖

   ● **S32.41**   Fracture of anterior wall of acetabulum

     ● **S32.411**   Displaced fracture of anterior wall of right acetabulum A, B 🔖

     ● **S32.412**   Displaced fracture of anterior wall of left acetabulum A, B 🔖

     ● **S32.413**   Displaced fracture of anterior wall of unspecified acetabulum A, B 🔖

     ● **S32.414**   Nondisplaced fracture of anterior wall of right acetabulum A, B 🔖

     ● **S32.415**   Nondisplaced fracture of anterior wall of left acetabulum A, B 🔖

     ● **S32.416**   Nondisplaced fracture of anterior wall of unspecified acetabulum A, B 🔖

   ● **S32.42**   Fracture of posterior wall of acetabulum

     ● **S32.421**   Displaced fracture of posterior wall of right acetabulum A, B 🔖

     ● **S32.422**   Displaced fracture of posterior wall of left acetabulum A, B 🔖

     ● **S32.423**   Displaced fracture of posterior wall of unspecified acetabulum A, B 🔖

     ● **S32.424**   Nondisplaced fracture of posterior wall of right acetabulum A, B 🔖

     ● **S32.425**   Nondisplaced fracture of posterior wall of left acetabulum A, B 🔖

     ● **S32.426**   Nondisplaced fracture of posterior wall of unspecified acetabulum A, B 🔖

● **S32.43**   Fracture of anterior column [iliopubic] of acetabulum

     ● **S32.431**   Displaced fracture of anterior column [iliopubic] of right acetabulum A, B 🔖

     ● **S32.432**   Displaced fracture of anterior column [iliopubic] of left acetabulum A, B 🔖

     ● **S32.433**   Displaced fracture of anterior column [iliopubic] of unspecified acetabulum A, B 🔖

     ● **S32.434**   Nondisplaced fracture of anterior column [iliopubic] of right acetabulum A, B 🔖

     ● **S32.435**   Nondisplaced fracture of anterior column [iliopubic] of left acetabulum A, B 🔖

     ● **S32.436**   Nondisplaced fracture of anterior column [iliopubic] of unspecified acetabulum A, B 🔖

● **S32.44**   Fracture of posterior column [ilioischial] of acetabulum

     ● **S32.441**   Displaced fracture of posterior column [ilioischial] of right acetabulum A, B 🔖

     ● **S32.442**   Displaced fracture of posterior column [ilioischial] of left acetabulum A, B 🔖

     ● **S32.443**   Displaced fracture of posterior column [ilioischial] of unspecified acetabulum A, B 🔖

     ● **S32.444**   Nondisplaced fracture of posterior column [ilioischial] of right acetabulum A, B 🔖

     ● **S32.445**   Nondisplaced fracture of posterior column [ilioischial] of left acetabulum A, B 🔖

     ● **S32.446**   Nondisplaced fracture of posterior column [ilioischial] of unspecified acetabulum A, B 🔖

● **S32.45**   Transverse fracture of acetabulum

     ● **S32.451**   Displaced transverse fracture of right acetabulum A, B 🔖

     ● **S32.452**   Displaced transverse fracture of left acetabulum A, B 🔖

     ● **S32.453**   Displaced transverse fracture of unspecified acetabulum A, B 🔖

     ● **S32.454**   Nondisplaced transverse fracture of right acetabulum A, B 🔖

     ● **S32.455**   Nondisplaced transverse fracture of left acetabulum A, B 🔖

     ● **S32.456**   Nondisplaced transverse fracture of unspecified acetabulum A, B 🔖

● **S32.46**   Associated transverse-posterior fracture of acetabulum

     ● **S32.461**   Displaced associated transverse-posterior fracture of right acetabulum A, B 🔖

     ● **S32.462**   Displaced associated transverse-posterior fracture of left acetabulum A, B 🔖

     ● **S32.463**   Displaced associated transverse-posterior fracture of unspecified acetabulum A, B 🔖

     ● **S32.464**   Nondisplaced associated transverse-posterior fracture of right acetabulum A, B 🔖

     ● **S32.465**   Nondisplaced associated transverse-posterior fracture of left acetabulum A, B 🔖

     ● **S32.466**   Nondisplaced associated transverse-posterior fracture of unspecified acetabulum A, B 🔖

CHAPTER 19 (S00-T88)

- ● S32.47   Fracture of medial wall of acetabulum
  - ● S32.471   Displaced fracture of medial wall of right acetabulum A, B 🦠
  - ● S32.472   Displaced fracture of medial wall of left acetabulum A, B 🦠
  - ● S32.473   Displaced fracture of medial wall of unspecified acetabulum A, B 🦠
  - ● S32.474   Nondisplaced fracture of medial wall of right acetabulum A, B 🦠
  - ● S32.475   Nondisplaced fracture of medial wall of left acetabulum A, B 🦠
  - ● S32.476   Nondisplaced fracture of medial wall of unspecified acetabulum A, B 🦠
- ● S32.48   Dome fracture of acetabulum
  - ● S32.481   Displaced dome fracture of right acetabulum A, B 🦠
  - ● S32.482   Displaced dome fracture of left acetabulum A, B 🦠
  - ● S32.483   Displaced dome fracture of unspecified acetabulum A, B 🦠
  - ● S32.484   Nondisplaced dome fracture of right acetabulum A, B 🦠
  - ● S32.485   Nondisplaced dome fracture of left acetabulum A, B 🦠
  - ● S32.486   Nondisplaced dome fracture of unspecified acetabulum A, B 🦠
- ● S32.49   Other fracture of acetabulum
  - ● S32.491   Other fracture of right acetabulum A, B 🦠
  - ● S32.492   Other fracture of left acetabulum A, B 🦠
  - ● S32.499   Other fracture of unspecified acetabulum A, B 🦠
- ● S32.5   Fracture of pubis
  - **Excludes1**   fracture of pubis with associated disruption of pelvic ring (S32.8-)
  - ● S32.50   Unspecified fracture of pubis
    - ● S32.501   Unspecified fracture of right pubis A, B 🦠
    - ● S32.502   Unspecified fracture of left pubis A, B 🦠
    - ● S32.509   Unspecified fracture of unspecified pubis A, B 🦠
  - ● S32.51   Fracture of superior rim of pubis
    - ● S32.511   Fracture of superior rim of right pubis A, B 🦠
    - ● S32.512   Fracture of superior rim of left pubis A, B 🦠
    - ● S32.519   Fracture of superior rim of unspecified pubis A, B 🦠
  - ● S32.59   Other specified fracture of pubis
    - ● S32.591   Other specified fracture of right pubis A, B 🦠
    - ● S32.592   Other specified fracture of left pubis A, B 🦠
    - ● S32.599   Other specified fracture of unspecified pubis A, B 🦠
- ● S32.6   Fracture of ischium
  - **Excludes1**   fracture of ischium with associated disruption of pelvic ring (S32.8-)
  - ● S32.60   Unspecified fracture of ischium
    - ● S32.601   Unspecified fracture of right ischium A, B 🦠
    - ● S32.602   Unspecified fracture of left ischium A, B 🦠
    - ● S32.609   Unspecified fracture of unspecified ischium A, B 🦠
  - ● S32.61   Avulsion fracture of ischium
    - ● S32.611   Displaced avulsion fracture of right ischium A, B 🦠

- ● S32.612   Displaced avulsion fracture of left ischium A, B 🦠
- ● S32.613   Displaced avulsion fracture of unspecified ischium A, B 🦠
- ● S32.614   Nondisplaced avulsion fracture of right ischium A, B 🦠
- ● S32.615   Nondisplaced avulsion fracture of left ischium A, B 🦠
- ● S32.616   Nondisplaced avulsion fracture of unspecified ischium A, B 🦠
- ● S32.69   Other specified fracture of ischium
  - ● S32.691   Other specified fracture of right ischium A, B 🦠
  - ● S32.692   Other specified fracture of left ischium A, B 🦠
  - ● S32.699   Other specified fracture of unspecified ischium A, B 🦠
- ● S32.8   Fracture of other parts of pelvis
  - Code also any associated:
    - fracture of acetabulum (S32.4-)
    - sacral fracture (S32.1-)
  - ● S32.81   Multiple fractures of pelvis with disruption of pelvic ring
    - Multiple pelvic fractures with disruption of pelvic circle
    - ● S32.810   Multiple fractures of pelvis with stable disruption of pelvic ring A, B 🦠
    - ● S32.811   Multiple fractures of pelvis with unstable disruption of pelvic ring A, B 🦠
  - X ● S32.82   Multiple fractures of pelvis without disruption of pelvic ring A, B 🦠
    - Multiple pelvic fractures without disruption of pelvic circle
  - X ● S32.89   Fracture of other parts of pelvis A, B 🦠
- X ● S32.9   Fracture of unspecified parts of lumbosacral spine and pelvis A, B 🦠
  - Fracture of lumbosacral spine NOS
  - Fracture of pelvis NOS
  - **Coding Clinic: 2012, Q4, P93**

- ● S33   Dislocation and sprain of joints and ligaments of lumbar spine and pelvis
  - **Includes**   avulsion of joint or ligament of lumbar spine and pelvis
    - laceration of cartilage, joint or ligament of lumbar spine and pelvis
    - sprain of cartilage, joint or ligament of lumbar spine and pelvis
    - traumatic hemarthrosis of joint or ligament of lumbar spine and pelvis
    - traumatic rupture of joint or ligament of lumbar spine and pelvis
    - traumatic subluxation of joint or ligament of lumbar spine and pelvis
    - traumatic tear of joint or ligament of lumbar spine and pelvis
  - Code also any associated open wound
  - **Excludes1**   nontraumatic rupture or displacement of lumbar intervertebral disc NOS (M51.-)
    - obstetric damage to pelvic joints and ligaments (O71.6)
  - **Excludes2**   dislocation and sprain of joints and ligaments of hip (S73.-)
    - strain of muscle of lower back and pelvis (S39.01-)
  - The appropriate 7th character is to be added to each code from category S33

A	initial encounter
D	subsequent encounter
S	sequela

X ● **S33.0**   **Traumatic rupture of lumbar intervertebral disc**
    Excludes1   rupture or displacement (nontraumatic) of lumbar intervertebral disc NOS (M51.- with fifth character 6)

● **S33.1**   **Subluxation and dislocation of lumbar vertebra**
    Code also any associated:
       open wound of abdomen, lower back and pelvis (S31)
       spinal cord injury (S24.0, S24.1-, S34.0-, S34.1-)
    Excludes2   fracture of lumbar vertebrae (S32.0-)

   ● **S33.10**   **Subluxation and dislocation of unspecified lumbar vertebra**
     ● **S33.100**   **Subluxation of unspecified lumbar vertebra**
     ● **S33.101**   **Dislocation of unspecified lumbar vertebra**

   ● **S33.11**   **Subluxation and dislocation of L1/L2 lumbar vertebra**
     ● **S33.110**   **Subluxation of L1/L2 lumbar vertebra**
     ● **S33.111**   **Dislocation of L1/L2 lumbar vertebra**

   ● **S33.12**   **Subluxation and dislocation of L2/L3 lumbar vertebra**
     ● **S33.120**   **Subluxation of L2/L3 lumbar vertebra**
     ● **S33.121**   **Dislocation of L2/L3 lumbar vertebra**

   ● **S33.13**   **Subluxation and dislocation of L3/L4 lumbar vertebra**
     ● **S33.130**   **Subluxation of L3/L4 lumbar vertebra**
     ● **S33.131**   **Dislocation of L3/L4 lumbar vertebra**

   ● **S33.14**   **Subluxation and dislocation of L4/L5 lumbar vertebra**
     ● **S33.140**   **Subluxation of L4/L5 lumbar vertebra**
     ● **S33.141**   **Dislocation of L4/L5 lumbar vertebra**

X ● **S33.2**   **Dislocation of sacroiliac and sacrococcygeal joint**

● **S33.3**   **Dislocation of other and unspecified parts of lumbar spine and pelvis**
   X ● **S33.30**   **Dislocation of unspecified parts of lumbar spine and pelvis**
   X ● **S33.39**   **Dislocation of other parts of lumbar spine and pelvis**

X ● **S33.4**   **Traumatic rupture of symphysis pubis**
X ● **S33.5**   **Sprain of ligaments of lumbar spine**
X ● **S33.6**   **Sprain of sacroiliac joint**
X ● **S33.8**   **Sprain of other parts of lumbar spine and pelvis**
X ● **S33.9**   **Sprain of unspecified parts of lumbar spine and pelvis**

● **S34**   **Injury of lumbar and sacral spinal cord and nerves at abdomen, lower back and pelvis level**
    Note: Code to highest level of lumbar cord injury
       Injuries to the spinal cord (S34.0 and S34.1) refer to the cord level and not bone level injury, and can affect nerve roots at and below the level given.
    The appropriate 7th character is to be added to each code from category S34

> | | |
> |---|---|
> | A | initial encounter |
> | D | subsequent encounter |
> | S | sequela |

    Code also any associated:
       fracture of vertebra (S22.0-, S32.0-)
       open wound of abdomen, lower back and pelvis (S31.-)
       transient paralysis (R29.5)

   ● **S34.0**   **Concussion and edema of lumbar and sacral spinal cord**
    X ● **S34.01**   **Concussion and edema of lumbar spinal cord** A, D, S 🔖
    X ● **S34.02**   **Concussion and edema of sacral spinal cord** A, D, S 🔖
       Concussion and edema of conus medullaris

● **S34.1**   **Other and unspecified injury of lumbar and sacral spinal cord**
   ● **S34.10**   **Unspecified injury to lumbar spinal cord**
    ● **S34.101**   **Unspecified injury to L_1 level of lumbar spinal cord** A, D, S 🔖
       Unspecified injury to lumbar spinal cord level 1
    ● **S34.102**   **Unspecified injury to L_2 level of lumbar spinal cord** A, D, S 🔖
       Unspecified injury to lumbar spinal cord level 2
    ● **S34.103**   **Unspecified injury to L_3 level of lumbar spinal cord** A, D, S 🔖
       Unspecified injury to lumbar spinal cord level 3
    ● **S34.104**   **Unspecified injury to L_4 level of lumbar spinal cord** A, D, S 🔖
       Unspecified injury to lumbar spinal cord level 4
    ● **S34.105**   **Unspecified injury to L_5 level of lumbar spinal cord** A, D, S 🔖
       Unspecified injury to lumbar spinal cord level 5
    ● **S34.109**   **Unspecified injury to unspecified level of lumbar spinal cord** A, D, S 🔖

   ● **S34.11**   **Complete lesion of lumbar spinal cord**
    ● **S34.111**   **Complete lesion of L_1 level of lumbar spinal cord** A, D, S 🔖
       Complete lesion of lumbar spinal cord level 1
    ● **S34.112**   **Complete lesion of L_2 level of lumbar spinal cord** A, D, S 🔖
       Complete lesion of lumbar spinal cord level 2
    ● **S34.113**   **Complete lesion of L_3 level of lumbar spinal cord** A, D, S 🔖
       Complete lesion of lumbar spinal cord level 3
    ● **S34.114**   **Complete lesion of L_4 level of lumbar spinal cord** A, D, S 🔖
       Complete lesion of lumbar spinal cord level 4
    ● **S34.115**   **Complete lesion of L_5 level of lumbar spinal cord** A, D, S 🔖
       Complete lesion of lumbar spinal cord level 5
    ● **S34.119**   **Complete lesion of unspecified level of lumbar spinal cord** A, D, S 🔖

   ● **S34.12**   **Incomplete lesion of lumbar spinal cord**
    ● **S34.121**   **Incomplete lesion of L_1 level of lumbar spinal cord** A, D, S 🔖
       Incomplete lesion of lumbar spinal cord level 1
    ● **S34.122**   **Incomplete lesion of L_2 level of lumbar spinal cord** A, D, S 🔖
       Incomplete lesion of lumbar spinal cord level 2
    ● **S34.123**   **Incomplete lesion of L_3 level of lumbar spinal cord** A, D, S 🔖
       Incomplete lesion of lumbar spinal cord level 3
    ● **S34.124**   **Incomplete lesion of L_4 level of lumbar spinal cord** A, D, S 🔖
       Incomplete lesion of lumbar spinal cord level 4
    ● **S34.125**   **Incomplete lesion of L_5 level of lumbar spinal cord** A, D, S 🔖
       Incomplete lesion of lumbar spinal cord level 5
    ● **S34.129**   **Incomplete lesion of unspecified level of lumbar spinal cord** A, D, S 🔖

CHAPTER 19 (S00-T88)

- **S34.13** **Other and unspecified injury to sacral spinal cord**
  Other injury to conus medullaris
  - **S34.131** **Complete lesion of sacral spinal cord A, D, S** 🅷
    Complete lesion of conus medullaris
  - **S34.132** **Incomplete lesion of sacral spinal cord A, D, S** 🅷
    Incomplete lesion of conus medullaris
  - **S34.139** **Unspecified injury to sacral spinal cord A, D, S** 🅷
    Unspecified injury of conus medullaris
- **S34.2** **Injury of nerve root of lumbar and sacral spine**
  - X **S34.21** **Injury of nerve root of lumbar spine**
  - X **S34.22** **Injury of nerve root of sacral spine**
- X **S34.3** **Injury of cauda equina A, D, S** 🅷
- X **S34.4** **Injury of lumbosacral plexus**
- X **S34.5** **Injury of lumbar, sacral and pelvic sympathetic nerves**
  Injury of celiac ganglion or plexus
  Injury of hypogastric plexus
  Injury of mesenteric plexus (inferior) (superior)
  Injury of splanchnic nerve
- X **S34.6** **Injury of peripheral nerve(s) at abdomen, lower back and pelvis level**
- X **S34.8** **Injury of other nerves at abdomen, lower back and pelvis level**
- X **S34.9** **Injury of unspecified nerves at abdomen, lower back and pelvis level**

- **S35** **Injury of blood vessels at abdomen, lower back and pelvis level**

  The appropriate 7th character is to be added to each code from category S35

A	initial encounter
D	subsequent encounter
S	sequela

  Code also any associated open wound (S31.-)

- **S35.0** **Injury of abdominal aorta**

  Excludes1 injury of aorta NOS (S25.0)

  - X **S35.00** **Unspecified injury of abdominal aorta**
  - X **S35.01** **Minor laceration of abdominal aorta**
    Incomplete transection of abdominal aorta
    Laceration of abdominal aorta NOS
    Superficial laceration of abdominal aorta
  - X **S35.02** **Major laceration of abdominal aorta**
    Complete transection of abdominal aorta
    Traumatic rupture of abdominal aorta
  - X **S35.09** **Other injury of abdominal aorta**
- **S35.1** **Injury of inferior vena cava**
  Injury of hepatic vein

  Excludes1 injury of vena cava NOS (S25.2)

  - X **S35.10** **Unspecified injury of inferior vena cava**
  - X **S35.11** **Minor laceration of inferior vena cava**
    Incomplete transection of inferior vena cava
    Laceration of inferior vena cava NOS
    Superficial laceration of inferior vena cava
  - X **S35.12** **Major laceration of inferior vena cava**
    Complete transection of inferior vena cava
    Traumatic rupture of inferior vena cava
  - X **S35.19** **Other injury of inferior vena cava**
- **S35.2** **Injury of celiac or mesenteric artery and branches**
  - **S35.21** **Injury of celiac artery**
    - **S35.211** **Minor laceration of celiac artery**
      Incomplete transection of celiac artery
      Laceration of celiac artery NOS
      Superficial laceration of celiac artery

- **S35.212** **Major laceration of celiac artery**
  Complete transection of celiac artery
  Traumatic rupture of celiac artery
- **S35.218** **Other injury of celiac artery**
- **S35.219** **Unspecified injury of celiac artery**
- **S35.22** **Injury of superior mesenteric artery**
  - **S35.221** **Minor laceration of superior mesenteric artery**
    Incomplete transection of superior mesenteric artery
    Laceration of superior mesenteric artery NOS
    Superficial laceration of superior mesenteric artery
  - **S35.222** **Major laceration of superior mesenteric artery**
    Complete transection of superior mesenteric artery
    Traumatic rupture of superior mesenteric artery
  - **S35.228** **Other injury of superior mesenteric artery**
  - **S35.229** **Unspecified injury of superior mesenteric artery**
- **S35.23** **Injury of inferior mesenteric artery**
  - **S35.231** **Minor laceration of inferior mesenteric artery**
    Incomplete transection of inferior mesenteric artery
    Laceration of inferior mesenteric artery NOS
    Superficial laceration of inferior mesenteric artery
  - **S35.232** **Major laceration of inferior mesenteric artery**
    Complete transection of inferior mesenteric artery
    Traumatic rupture of inferior mesenteric artery
  - **S35.238** **Other injury of inferior mesenteric artery**
  - **S35.239** **Unspecified injury of inferior mesenteric artery**
- **S35.29** **Injury of branches of celiac and mesenteric artery**
  Injury of gastric artery
  Injury of gastroduodenal artery
  Injury of hepatic artery
  Injury of splenic artery
  - **S35.291** **Minor laceration of branches of celiac and mesenteric artery**
    Incomplete transection of branches of celiac and mesenteric artery
    Laceration of branches of celiac and mesenteric artery NOS
    Superficial laceration of branches of celiac and mesenteric artery
  - **S35.292** **Major laceration of branches of celiac and mesenteric artery**
    Complete transection of branches of celiac and mesenteric artery
    Traumatic rupture of branches of celiac and mesenteric artery
  - **S35.298** **Other injury of branches of celiac and mesenteric artery**
  - **S35.299** **Unspecified injury of branches of celiac and mesenteric artery**

▶ New　⇒ Revised　~~deleted~~ Deleted　Excludes 1　Excludes 2　Includes　Use additional　Code first　Code also　Key words
OGCR Official Guidelines　X Assign placeholder X　● Use Additional Character(s)　❭ Manifestation Code　🅷 Hierarchical Condition Category　**Coding Clinic**

- **S35.3** **Injury of portal or splenic vein and branches**
  - **S35.31** Injury of portal vein
    - **S35.311** Laceration of portal vein
    - **S35.318** Other specified injury of portal vein
    - **S35.319** Unspecified injury of portal vein
  - **S35.32** Injury of splenic vein
    - **S35.321** Laceration of splenic vein
    - **S35.328** Other specified injury of splenic vein
    - **S35.329** Unspecified injury of splenic vein
  - **S35.33** Injury of superior mesenteric vein
    - **S35.331** Laceration of superior mesenteric vein
    - **S35.338** Other specified injury of superior mesenteric vein
    - **S35.339** Unspecified injury of superior mesenteric vein
  - **S35.34** Injury of inferior mesenteric vein
    - **S35.341** Laceration of inferior mesenteric vein
    - **S35.348** Other specified injury of inferior mesenteric vein
    - **S35.349** Unspecified injury of inferior mesenteric vein
- **S35.4** **Injury of renal blood vessels**
  - **S35.40** Unspecified injury of renal blood vessel
    - **S35.401** Unspecified injury of right renal artery
    - **S35.402** Unspecified injury of left renal artery
    - **S35.403** Unspecified injury of unspecified renal artery
    - **S35.404** Unspecified injury of right renal vein
    - **S35.405** Unspecified injury of left renal vein
    - **S35.406** Unspecified injury of unspecified renal vein
  - **S35.41** Laceration of renal blood vessel
    - **S35.411** Laceration of right renal artery
    - **S35.412** Laceration of left renal artery
    - **S35.413** Laceration of unspecified renal artery
    - **S35.414** Laceration of right renal vein
    - **S35.415** Laceration of left renal vein
    - **S35.416** Laceration of unspecified renal vein
  - **S35.49** Other specified injury of renal blood vessel
    - **S35.491** Other specified injury of right renal artery
    - **S35.492** Other specified injury of left renal artery
    - **S35.493** Other specified injury of unspecified renal artery
    - **S35.494** Other specified injury of right renal vein
    - **S35.495** Other specified injury of left renal vein
    - **S35.496** Other specified injury of unspecified renal vein
- **S35.5** **Injury of iliac blood vessels**
  - X **S35.50** Injury of unspecified iliac blood vessel(s)
  - **S35.51** Injury of iliac artery or vein
    Injury of hypogastric artery or vein
    - **S35.511** Injury of right iliac artery
    - **S35.512** Injury of left iliac artery
    - **S35.513** Injury of unspecified iliac artery
    - **S35.514** Injury of right iliac vein
    - **S35.515** Injury of left iliac vein
    - **S35.516** Injury of unspecified iliac vein

- **S35.53** Injury of uterine artery or vein
  - **S35.531** Injury of right uterine artery ♀
  - **S35.532** Injury of left uterine artery ♀
  - **S35.533** Injury of unspecified uterine artery ♀
  - **S35.534** Injury of right uterine vein ♀
  - **S35.535** Injury of left uterine vein ♀
  - **S35.536** Injury of unspecified uterine vein ♀
  - X **S35.59** Injury of other iliac blood vessels
- **S35.8** **Injury of other blood vessels at abdomen, lower back and pelvis level**
  Injury of ovarian artery or vein
  - **S35.8X** Injury of other blood vessels at abdomen, lower back and pelvis level
    - **S35.8X1** Laceration of other blood vessels at abdomen, lower back and pelvis level
    - **S35.8X8** Other specified injury of other blood vessels at abdomen, lower back and pelvis level
    - **S35.8X9** Unspecified injury of other blood vessels at abdomen, lower back and pelvis level
- **S35.9** **Injury of unspecified blood vessel at abdomen, lower back and pelvis level**
  - X **S35.90** Unspecified injury of unspecified blood vessel at abdomen, lower back and pelvis level
  - X **S35.91** Laceration of unspecified blood vessel at abdomen, lower back and pelvis level
  - X **S35.99** Other specified injury of unspecified blood vessel at abdomen, lower back and pelvis level
- **S36** **Injury of intra-abdominal organs**
  The appropriate 7th character is to be added to each code from category S36

A	initial encounter
D	subsequent encounter
S	sequela

  Code also any associated open wound (S31.-)
  - **S36.0** **Injury of spleen**
    - X **S36.00** Unspecified injury of spleen
    - **S36.02** Contusion of spleen
      - **S36.020** Minor contusion of spleen
        Contusion of spleen less than 2 cm
      - **S36.021** Major contusion of spleen
        Contusion of spleen greater than 2 cm
      - **S36.029** Unspecified contusion of spleen
        Coding Clinic: 2015, Q2, P36, Q1, P11
    - **S36.03** Laceration of spleen
      - **S36.030** Superficial (capsular) laceration of spleen
        Laceration of spleen less than 1 cm
        Minor laceration of spleen
      - **S36.031** Moderate laceration of spleen
        Laceration of spleen 1 to 3 cm
        Coding Clinic: 2022, Q1, P23;
        2015, Q2, P36, Q1, P11
      - **S36.032** Major laceration of spleen
        Avulsion of spleen
        Laceration of spleen greater than 3 cm
        Massive laceration of spleen
        Multiple moderate lacerations of spleen
        Stellate laceration of spleen
      - **S36.039** Unspecified laceration of spleen
    - X **S36.09** Other injury of spleen

CHAPTER 19 (S00–T88)

- S36.1   Injury of liver and gallbladder and bile duct
  - S36.11   Injury of liver
    - S36.112   Contusion of liver
    - S36.113   Laceration of liver, unspecified degree
    - S36.114   Minor laceration of liver
      Laceration involving capsule only, or, without significant involvement of hepatic parenchyma [i.e., less than 1 cm deep]
    - S36.115   Moderate laceration of liver
      Laceration involving parenchyma but without major disruption of parenchyma [i.e., less than 10 cm long and less than 3 cm deep]
    - S36.116   Major laceration of liver
      Laceration with significant disruption of hepatic parenchyma [i.e., greater than 10 cm long and 3 cm deep]
      Multiple moderate lacerations, with or without hematoma
      Stellate laceration of liver
    - S36.118   Other injury of liver
    - S36.119   Unspecified injury of liver
      Coding Clinic: 2015, Q2, P17
  - S36.12   Injury of gallbladder
    - S36.122   Contusion of gallbladder
    - S36.123   Laceration of gallbladder
    - S36.128   Other injury of gallbladder
    - S36.129   Unspecified injury of gallbladder
  - X S36.13   Injury of bile duct
- S36.2   Injury of pancreas
  - S36.20   Unspecified injury of pancreas
    - S36.200   Unspecified injury of head of pancreas
    - S36.201   Unspecified injury of body of pancreas
    - S36.202   Unspecified injury of tail of pancreas
    - S36.209   Unspecified injury of unspecified part of pancreas
  - S36.22   Contusion of pancreas
    - S36.220   Contusion of head of pancreas
    - S36.221   Contusion of body of pancreas
    - S36.222   Contusion of tail of pancreas
    - S36.229   Contusion of unspecified part of pancreas
  - S36.23   Laceration of pancreas, unspecified degree
    - S36.230   Laceration of head of pancreas, unspecified degree
    - S36.231   Laceration of body of pancreas, unspecified degree
    - S36.232   Laceration of tail of pancreas, unspecified degree
    - S36.239   Laceration of unspecified part of pancreas, unspecified degree
  - S36.24   Minor laceration of pancreas
    - S36.240   Minor laceration of head of pancreas
    - S36.241   Minor laceration of body of pancreas
    - S36.242   Minor laceration of tail of pancreas
    - S36.249   Minor laceration of unspecified part of pancreas

- S36.25   Moderate laceration of pancreas
  - S36.250   Moderate laceration of head of pancreas
  - S36.251   Moderate laceration of body of pancreas
  - S36.252   Moderate laceration of tail of pancreas
  - S36.259   Moderate laceration of unspecified part of pancreas
- S36.26   Major laceration of pancreas
  - S36.260   Major laceration of head of pancreas
  - S36.261   Major laceration of body of pancreas
  - S36.262   Major laceration of tail of pancreas
  - S36.269   Major laceration of unspecified part of pancreas
- S36.29   Other injury of pancreas
  - S36.290   Other injury of head of pancreas
  - S36.291   Other injury of body of pancreas
  - S36.292   Other injury of tail of pancreas
  - S36.299   Other injury of unspecified part of pancreas
- S36.3   Injury of stomach
  - X S36.30   Unspecified injury of stomach
  - X S36.32   Contusion of stomach
  - X S36.33   Laceration of stomach
  - X S36.39   Other injury of stomach
- S36.4   Injury of small intestine
  - S36.40   Unspecified injury of small intestine
    - S36.400   Unspecified injury of duodenum
    - S36.408   Unspecified injury of other part of small intestine
    - S36.409   Unspecified injury of unspecified part of small intestine
  - S36.41   Primary blast injury of small intestine
    Blast injury of small intestine NOS
    - S36.410   Primary blast injury of duodenum
    - S36.418   Primary blast injury of other part of small intestine
    - S36.419   Primary blast injury of unspecified part of small intestine
  - S36.42   Contusion of small intestine
    - S36.420   Contusion of duodenum
    - S36.428   Contusion of other part of small intestine
    - S36.429   Contusion of unspecified part of small intestine
  - S36.43   Laceration of small intestine
    - S36.430   Laceration of duodenum
    - S36.438   Laceration of other part of small intestine
    - S36.439   Laceration of unspecified part of small intestine
  - S36.49   Other injury of small intestine
    - S36.490   Other injury of duodenum
    - S36.498   Other injury of other part of small intestine
    - S36.499   Other injury of unspecified part of small intestine

CHAPTER 19 (S00-T88)

● **S36.5   Injury of colon**
     Excludes2   injury of rectum (S36.6-)
   ● **S36.50   Unspecified injury of colon**
     ● **S36.500   Unspecified injury of ascending [right] colon**
     ● **S36.501   Unspecified injury of transverse colon**
     ● **S36.502   Unspecified injury of descending [left] colon**
     ● **S36.503   Unspecified injury of sigmoid colon**
     ● **S36.508   Unspecified injury of other part of colon**
     ● **S36.509   Unspecified injury of unspecified part of colon**
   ● **S36.51   Primary blast injury of colon**
     Blast injury of colon NOS
     ● **S36.510   Primary blast injury of ascending [right] colon**
     ● **S36.511   Primary blast injury of transverse colon**
     ● **S36.512   Primary blast injury of descending [left] colon**
     ● **S36.513   Primary blast injury of sigmoid colon**
     ● **S36.518   Primary blast injury of other part of colon**
     ● **S36.519   Primary blast injury of unspecified part of colon**
   ● **S36.52   Contusion of colon**
     ● **S36.520   Contusion of ascending [right] colon**
     ● **S36.521   Contusion of transverse colon**
     ● **S36.522   Contusion of descending [left] colon**
     ● **S36.523   Contusion of sigmoid colon**
     ● **S36.528   Contusion of other part of colon**
     ● **S36.529   Contusion of unspecified part of colon**
   ● **S36.53   Laceration of colon**
     ● **S36.530   Laceration of ascending [right] colon**
     ● **S36.531   Laceration of transverse colon**
     ● **S36.532   Laceration of descending [left] colon**
     ● **S36.533   Laceration of sigmoid colon**
     ● **S36.538   Laceration of other part of colon**
     S36.539   Laceration of unspecified part of colon
   ● **S36.59   Other injury of colon**
     Secondary blast injury of colon
     ● **S36.590   Other injury of ascending [right] colon**
     ● **S36.591   Other injury of transverse colon**
     ● **S36.592   Other injury of descending [left] colon**
     ● **S36.593   Other injury of sigmoid colon**
     ● **S36.598   Other injury of other part of colon**
     ● **S36.599   Other injury of unspecified part of colon**

● **S36.6   Injury of rectum**
   X● **S36.60   Unspecified injury of rectum**
   X● **S36.61   Primary blast injury of rectum**
     Blast injury of rectum NOS
   X● **S36.62   Contusion of rectum**
   X● **S36.63   Laceration of rectum**
   X● **S36.69   Other injury of rectum**
     Secondary blast injury of rectum

● **S36.8   Injury of other intra-abdominal organs**
   X● **S36.81   Injury of peritoneum**
   ● **S36.89   Injury of other intra-abdominal organs**
     Injury of retroperitoneum
     ● **S36.892   Contusion of other intra-abdominal organs**
     ● **S36.893   Laceration of other intra-abdominal organs**
     ● **S36.898   Other injury of other intra-abdominal organs**
     S36.899   Unspecified injury of other intra-abdominal organs

● **S36.9   Injury of unspecified intra-abdominal organ**
   X● **S36.90   Unspecified injury of unspecified intra-abdominal organ**
   X● **S36.92   Contusion of unspecified intra-abdominal organ**
   X● **S36.93   Laceration of unspecified intra-abdominal organ**
   X● **S36.99   Other injury of unspecified intra-abdominal organ**

● **S37   Injury of urinary and pelvic organs**
     Code also any associated open wound (S31.-)
     Excludes1   obstetric trauma to pelvic organs (O71.-)
     Excludes2   injury of peritoneum (S36.81)
                 injury of retroperitoneum (S36.89-)
     The appropriate 7th character is to be added to each code from category S37

A	initial encounter
D	subsequent encounter
S	sequela

● **S37.0   Injury of kidney**
     Excludes2   acute kidney injury (nontraumatic) (N17.9)
   ● **S37.00   Unspecified injury of kidney**
     ● **S37.001   Unspecified injury of right kidney**
     ● **S37.002   Unspecified injury of left kidney**
     ● **S37.009   Unspecified injury of unspecified kidney**
   ● **S37.01   Minor contusion of kidney**
     Contusion of kidney less than 2 cm
     Contusion of kidney NOS
     ● **S37.011   Minor contusion of right kidney**
     ● **S37.012   Minor contusion of left kidney**
     ● **S37.019   Minor contusion of unspecified kidney**
   ● **S37.02   Major contusion of kidney**
     Contusion of kidney greater than 2 cm
     ● **S37.021   Major contusion of right kidney**
     ● **S37.022   Major contusion of left kidney**
     ● **S37.029   Major contusion of unspecified kidney**
   ● **S37.03   Laceration of kidney, unspecified degree**
     ● **S37.031   Laceration of right kidney, unspecified degree**
     ● **S37.032   Laceration of left kidney, unspecified degree**
     ● **S37.039   Laceration of unspecified kidney, unspecified degree**
   ● **S37.04   Minor laceration of kidney**
     Laceration of kidney less than 1 cm
     ● **S37.041   Minor laceration of right kidney**
     ● **S37.042   Minor laceration of left kidney**
     ● **S37.049   Minor laceration of unspecified kidney**

CHAPTER 19 (S00–T88)

● S37.05   **Moderate laceration of kidney**
         Laceration of kidney 1 to 3 cm
   ● S37.051   **Moderate laceration of right kidney**
   ● S37.052   **Moderate laceration of left kidney**
   ● S37.059   **Moderate laceration of unspecified kidney**

● S37.06   **Major laceration of kidney**
         Avulsion of kidney
         Laceration of kidney greater than 3 cm
         Massive laceration of kidney
         Multiple moderate lacerations of kidney
         Stellate laceration of kidney
   ● S37.061   **Major laceration of right kidney**
   ● S37.062   **Major laceration of left kidney**
   ● S37.069   **Major laceration of unspecified kidney**

● S37.09   **Other injury of kidney**
   ● S37.091   **Other injury of right kidney**
   ● S37.092   **Other injury of left kidney**
   ● S37.099   **Other injury of unspecified kidney**

● S37.1   **Injury of ureter**
   X ● S37.10   **Unspecified injury of ureter**
   X ● S37.12   **Contusion of ureter**
   X ● S37.13   **Laceration of ureter**
   X ● S37.19   **Other injury of ureter**

● S37.2   **Injury of bladder**
   X ● S37.20   **Unspecified injury of bladder**
   X ● S37.22   **Contusion of bladder**
   X ● S37.23   **Laceration of bladder**
   X ● S37.29   **Other injury of bladder**

● S37.3   **Injury of urethra**
   X ● S37.30   **Unspecified injury of urethra**
   X ● S37.32   **Contusion of urethra**
   X ● S37.33   **Laceration of urethra**
   X ● S37.39   **Other injury of urethra**

● S37.4   **Injury of ovary**
   ● S37.40   **Unspecified injury of ovary**
     ● S37.401   **Unspecified injury of ovary, unilateral** ♀
     ● S37.402   **Unspecified injury of ovary, bilateral** ♀
     ● S37.409   **Unspecified injury of ovary, unspecified** ♀

   ● S37.42   **Contusion of ovary**
     ● S37.421   **Contusion of ovary, unilateral** ♀
     ● S37.422   **Contusion of ovary, bilateral** ♀
     ● S37.429   **Contusion of ovary, unspecified** ♀

   ● S37.43   **Laceration of ovary**
     ● S37.431   **Laceration of ovary, unilateral** ♀
     ● S37.432   **Laceration of ovary, bilateral** ♀
     ● S37.439   **Laceration of ovary, unspecified** ♀

   ● S37.49   **Other injury of ovary**
     ● S37.491   **Other injury of ovary, unilateral** ♀
     ● S37.492   **Other injury of ovary, bilateral** ♀
     ● S37.499   **Other injury of ovary, unspecified** ♀

● S37.5   **Injury of fallopian tube**
   ● S37.50   **Unspecified injury of fallopian tube**
     ● S37.501   **Unspecified injury of fallopian tube, unilateral** ♀
     ● S37.502   **Unspecified injury of fallopian tube, bilateral** ♀
     ● S37.509   **Unspecified injury of fallopian tube, unspecified** ♀

   ● S37.51   **Primary blast injury of fallopian tube**
         Blast injury of fallopian tube NOS
     ● S37.511   **Primary blast injury of fallopian tube, unilateral** ♀
     ● S37.512   **Primary blast injury of fallopian tube, bilateral** ♀
     ● S37.519   **Primary blast injury of fallopian tube, unspecified** ♀

   ● S37.52   **Contusion of fallopian tube**
     ● S37.521   **Contusion of fallopian tube, unilateral** ♀
     ● S37.522   **Contusion of fallopian tube, bilateral** ♀
     ● S37.529   **Contusion of fallopian tube, unspecified** ♀

   ● S37.53   **Laceration of fallopian tube**
     ● S37.531   **Laceration of fallopian tube, unilateral** ♀
     ● S37.532   **Laceration of fallopian tube, bilateral** ♀
     ● S37.539   **Laceration of fallopian tube, unspecified** ♀

   ● S37.59   **Other injury of fallopian tube**
         Secondary blast injury of fallopian tube
     ● S37.591   **Other injury of fallopian tube, unilateral** ♀
     ● S37.592   **Other injury of fallopian tube, bilateral** ♀
     ● S37.599   **Other injury of fallopian tube, unspecified** ♀

● S37.6   **Injury of uterus**
   Excludes1   injury to gravid uterus (O9A.2-)
               injury to uterus during delivery (O71.-)
   X ● S37.60   **Unspecified injury of uterus** ♀
   X ● S37.62   **Contusion of uterus** ♀
   X ● S37.63   **Laceration of uterus** ♀
   X ● S37.69   **Other injury of uterus** ♀

● S37.8   **Injury of other urinary and pelvic organs**
   ● S37.81   **Injury of adrenal gland**
     ● S37.812   **Contusion of adrenal gland**
     ● S37.813   **Laceration of adrenal gland**
     ● S37.818   **Other injury of adrenal gland**
     ● S37.819   **Unspecified injury of adrenal gland**

   ● S37.82   **Injury of prostate**
     ● S37.822   **Contusion of prostate** ♂
     ● S37.823   **Laceration of prostate** ♂
     ● S37.828   **Other injury of prostate** ♂
     ● S37.829   **Unspecified injury of prostate** ♂

   ● S37.89   **Injury of other urinary and pelvic organ**
     ● S37.892   **Contusion of other urinary and pelvic organ**
     ● S37.893   **Laceration of other urinary and pelvic organ**
     ● S37.898   **Other injury of other urinary and pelvic organ**
     ● S37.899   **Unspecified injury of other urinary and pelvic organ**

● S37.9   **Injury of unspecified urinary and pelvic organ**
   X ● S37.90   **Unspecified injury of unspecified urinary and pelvic organ**
   X ● S37.92   **Contusion of unspecified urinary and pelvic organ**
   X ● S37.93   **Laceration of unspecified urinary and pelvic organ**
   X ● S37.99   **Other injury of unspecified urinary and pelvic organ**

▶ New   ⇒ Revised   ~~deleted~~ Deleted   Excludes 1   Excludes 2   Includes   Use additional   Code first   Code also   Key words
OGCR Official Guidelines   X Assign placeholder X   ● Use Additional Character(s)   ▷ Manifestation Code   🔖 Hierarchical Condition Category   **Coding Clinic**

● **S38** **Crushing injury and traumatic amputation of abdomen, lower back, pelvis and external genitals**

An amputation not identified as partial or complete should be coded to complete

The appropriate 7th character is to be added to each code from category S38

A	initial encounter
D	subsequent encounter
S	sequela

● **S38.0** **Crushing injury of external genital organs**

Use additional code for any associated injuries

● **S38.00** **Crushing injury of unspecified external genital organs**

● **S38.001** Crushing injury of unspecified external genital organs, male ♂

● **S38.002** Crushing injury of unspecified external genital organs, female ♀

X● **S38.01** Crushing injury of penis ♂

X● **S38.02** Crushing injury of scrotum and testis ♂

X● **S38.03** Crushing injury of vulva ♀

X● **S38.1** **Crushing injury of abdomen, lower back, and pelvis**

Use additional code for all associated injuries, such as:
fracture of thoracic or lumbar spine and pelvis (S22.0-, S32.-)
injury to intra-abdominal organs (S36.-)
injury to urinary and pelvic organs (S37.-)
open wound of abdominal wall (S31.-)
spinal cord injury (S34.0, S34.1-)

Excludes2 crushing injury of external genital organs (S38.0-)

● **S38.2** **Traumatic amputation of external genital organs**

● **S38.21** **Traumatic amputation of female external genital organs**

Traumatic amputation of clitoris
Traumatic amputation of labium (majus) (minus)
Traumatic amputation of vulva

● **S38.211** Complete traumatic amputation of female external genital organs ♀

● **S38.212** Partial traumatic amputation of female external genital organs ♀

● **S38.22** **Traumatic amputation of penis**

● **S38.221** Complete traumatic amputation of penis ♂

● **S38.222** Partial traumatic amputation of penis ♂

● **S38.23** **Traumatic amputation of scrotum and testis**

● **S38.231** Complete traumatic amputation of scrotum and testis ♂

● **S38.232** Partial traumatic amputation of scrotum and testis ♂

X● **S38.3** **Transection (partial) of abdomen**

● **S39** **Other and unspecified injuries of abdomen, lower back, pelvis and external genitals**

Code also any associated open wound (S31.-)

Excludes2 sprain of joints and ligaments of lumbar spine and pelvis (S33.-)

The appropriate 7th character is to be added to each code from category S39

A	initial encounter
D	subsequent encounter
S	sequela

● **S39.0** **Injury of muscle, fascia and tendon of abdomen, lower back and pelvis**

● **S39.00** **Unspecified injury of muscle, fascia and tendon of abdomen, lower back and pelvis**

● **S39.001** Unspecified injury of muscle, fascia and tendon of abdomen

● **S39.002** Unspecified injury of muscle, fascia and tendon of lower back

● **S39.003** Unspecified injury of muscle, fascia and tendon of pelvis

● **S39.01** **Strain of muscle, fascia and tendon of abdomen, lower back and pelvis**

● **S39.011** Strain of muscle, fascia and tendon of abdomen

● **S39.012** Strain of muscle, fascia and tendon of lower back
Coding Clinic: 2016, Q4, P74

● **S39.013** Strain of muscle, fascia and tendon of pelvis

● **S39.02** **Laceration of muscle, fascia and tendon of abdomen, lower back and pelvis**

● **S39.021** Laceration of muscle, fascia and tendon of abdomen

● **S39.022** Laceration of muscle, fascia and tendon of lower back

● **S39.023** Laceration of muscle, fascia and tendon of pelvis

● **S39.09** **Other injury of muscle, fascia and tendon of abdomen, lower back and pelvis**

● **S39.091** Other injury of muscle, fascia and tendon of abdomen

● **S39.092** Other injury of muscle, fascia and tendon of lower back

● **S39.093** Other injury of muscle, fascia and tendon of pelvis

● **S39.8** **Other specified injuries of abdomen, lower back, pelvis and external genitals**

X● **S39.81** Other specified injuries of abdomen

X● **S39.82** Other specified injuries of lower back

X● **S39.83** Other specified injuries of pelvis

● **S39.84** **Other specified injuries of external genitals**

● **S39.840** Fracture of corpus cavernosum penis ♂

● **S39.848** Other specified injuries of external genitals

● **S39.9** **Unspecified injury of abdomen, lower back, pelvis and external genitals**

X● **S39.91** Unspecified injury of abdomen

X● **S39.92** Unspecified injury of lower back

X● **S39.93** Unspecified injury of pelvis

X● **S39.94** Unspecified injury of external genitals

INJURIES TO THE SHOULDER AND UPPER ARM (S40-S49)

Includes	injuries of axilla injuries of scapular region
Excludes2	burns and corrosions (T20-T32)
	frostbite (T33-T34)
	injuries of elbow (S50-S59)
	insect bite or sting, venomous (T63.4)

● **S40** **Superficial injury of shoulder and upper arm**

The appropriate 7th character is to be added to each code from category S40

A	initial encounter
D	subsequent encounter
S	sequela

● **S40.0** **Contusion of shoulder and upper arm**

● **S40.01** **Contusion of shoulder**

● **S40.011** Contusion of right shoulder

● **S40.012** Contusion of left shoulder

● **S40.019** Contusion of unspecified shoulder

● S40.02   Contusion of upper arm
- ● S40.021   Contusion of right upper arm
- ● S40.022   Contusion of left upper arm
- ● S40.029   Contusion of unspecified upper arm

● S40.2   Other superficial injuries of shoulder
- ● S40.21   Abrasion of shoulder
  - ● S40.211   Abrasion of right shoulder
  - ● S40.212   Abrasion of left shoulder
  - ● S40.219   Abrasion of unspecified shoulder
- ● S40.22   Blister (nonthermal) of shoulder
  - ● S40.221   Blister (nonthermal) of right shoulder
  - ● S40.222   Blister (nonthermal) of left shoulder
  - ● S40.229   Blister (nonthermal) of unspecified shoulder
- ● S40.24   External constriction of shoulder
  - ● S40.241   External constriction of right shoulder
  - ● S40.242   External constriction of left shoulder
  - ● S40.249   External constriction of unspecified shoulder
- ● S40.25   Superficial foreign body of shoulder
  Splinter in the shoulder
  - ● S40.251   Superficial foreign body of right shoulder
  - ● S40.252   Superficial foreign body of left shoulder
  - ● S40.259   Superficial foreign body of unspecified shoulder
- ● S40.26   Insect bite (nonvenomous) of shoulder
  - ● S40.261   Insect bite (nonvenomous) of right shoulder
  - ● S40.262   Insect bite (nonvenomous) of left shoulder
  - ● S40.269   Insect bite (nonvenomous) of unspecified shoulder
- ● S40.27   Other superficial bite of shoulder
  - Excludes1   open bite of shoulder (S41.05)
  - ● S40.271   Other superficial bite of right shoulder
  - ● S40.272   Other superficial bite of left shoulder
  - ● S40.279   Other superficial bite of unspecified shoulder

● S40.8   Other superficial injuries of upper arm
- ● S40.81   Abrasion of upper arm
  - ● S40.811   Abrasion of right upper arm
  - ● S40.812   Abrasion of left upper arm
  - ● S40.819   Abrasion of unspecified upper arm
- ● S40.82   Blister (nonthermal) of upper arm
  - ● S40.821   Blister (nonthermal) of right upper arm
  - ● S40.822   Blister (nonthermal) of left upper arm
  - ● S40.829   Blister (nonthermal) of unspecified upper arm
- ● S40.84   External constriction of upper arm
  - ● S40.841   External constriction of right upper arm
  - ● S40.842   External constriction of left upper arm
  - ● S40.849   External constriction of unspecified upper arm
- ● S40.85   Superficial foreign body of upper arm
  Splinter in the upper arm
  - ● S40.851   Superficial foreign body of right upper arm
  - ● S40.852   Superficial foreign body of left upper arm
  - ● S40.859   Superficial foreign body of unspecified upper arm

● S40.86   Insect bite (nonvenomous) of upper arm
- ● S40.861   Insect bite (nonvenomous) of right upper arm
- ● S40.862   Insect bite (nonvenomous) of left upper arm
- ● S40.869   Insect bite (nonvenomous) of unspecified upper arm

● S40.87   Other superficial bite of upper arm
- Excludes1   open bite of upper arm (S41.14)
- Excludes2   other superficial bite of shoulder (S40.27-)
- ● S40.871   Other superficial bite of right upper arm
- ● S40.872   Other superficial bite of left upper arm
- ● S40.879   Other superficial bite of unspecified upper arm

● S40.9   Unspecified superficial injury of shoulder and upper arm
- ● S40.91   Unspecified superficial injury of shoulder
  - ● S40.911   Unspecified superficial injury of right shoulder
  - ● S40.912   Unspecified superficial injury of left shoulder
  - ● S40.919   Unspecified superficial injury of unspecified shoulder
- ● S40.92   Unspecified superficial injury of upper arm
  - ● S40.921   Unspecified superficial injury of right upper arm
  - ● S40.922   Unspecified superficial injury of left upper arm
  - ● S40.929   Unspecified superficial injury of unspecified upper arm

● S41   Open wound of shoulder and upper arm

Code also any associated wound infection

Excludes1   traumatic amputation of shoulder and upper arm (S48.-)

Excludes2   open fracture of shoulder and upper arm (S42.- with 7th character B or C)

The appropriate 7th character is to be added to each code from category S41

A	initial encounter
D	subsequent encounter
S	sequela

● S41.0   Open wound of shoulder
- ● S41.00   Unspecified open wound of shoulder
  - ● S41.001   Unspecified open wound of right shoulder
  - ● S41.002   Unspecified open wound of left shoulder
  - ● S41.009   Unspecified open wound of unspecified shoulder
- ● S41.01   Laceration without foreign body of shoulder
  - ● S41.011   Laceration without foreign body of right shoulder
  - ● S41.012   Laceration without foreign body of left shoulder
  - ● S41.019   Laceration without foreign body of unspecified shoulder
- ● S41.02   Laceration with foreign body of shoulder
  - ● S41.021   Laceration with foreign body of right shoulder
  - ● S41.022   Laceration with foreign body of left shoulder
  - ● S41.029   Laceration with foreign body of unspecified shoulder

1282

▶ New   ➠ Revised   ~~deleted~~ Deleted   Excludes 1   Excludes 2   Includes   Use additional   Code first   Code also   Key words

OGCR Official Guidelines   X Assign placeholder X   ● Use Additional Character(s)   ▶ Manifestation Code   ✿ Hierarchical Condition Category   Coding Clinic

- **S41.03** **Puncture wound without foreign body of shoulder**
  - **S41.031** Puncture wound without foreign body of **right** shoulder
  - **S41.032** Puncture wound without foreign body of **left** shoulder
  - **S41.039** Puncture wound without foreign body of **unspecified** shoulder
- **S41.04** **Puncture wound with foreign body of shoulder**
  - **S41.041** Puncture wound with foreign body of **right** shoulder
  - **S41.042** Puncture wound with foreign body of **left** shoulder
  - **S41.049** Puncture wound with foreign body of **unspecified** shoulder
- **S41.05** **Open bite of shoulder**
  Bite of shoulder NOS
  > **Excludes1** superficial bite of shoulder (S40.27)
  - **S41.051** Open bite of **right** shoulder
  - **S41.052** Open bite of **left** shoulder
  - **S41.059** Open bite of **unspecified** shoulder
- **S41.1** **Open wound of upper arm**
  - **S41.10** **Unspecified open wound of upper arm**
    - **S41.101** Unspecified open wound of **right** upper arm
    - **S41.102** Unspecified open wound of **left** upper arm
    - **S41.109** Unspecified open wound of **unspecified** upper arm
  - **S41.11** **Laceration without foreign body of upper arm**
    - **S41.111** Laceration without foreign body of **right** upper arm
    - **S41.112** Laceration without foreign body of **left** upper arm
    - **S41.119** Laceration without foreign body of **unspecified** upper arm
  - **S41.12** **Laceration with foreign body of upper arm**
    - **S41.121** Laceration with foreign body of **right** upper arm
    - **S41.122** Laceration with foreign body of **left** upper arm
    - **S41.129** Laceration with foreign body of **unspecified** upper arm
  - **S41.13** **Puncture wound without foreign body of upper arm**
    - **S41.131** Puncture wound without foreign body of **right** upper arm
    - **S41.132** Puncture wound without foreign body of **left** upper arm
    - **S41.139** Puncture wound without foreign body of **unspecified** upper arm
  - **S41.14** **Puncture wound with foreign body of upper arm**
    - **S41.141** Puncture wound with foreign body of **right** upper arm
    - **S41.142** Puncture wound with foreign body of **left** upper arm
    - **S41.149** Puncture wound with foreign body of **unspecified** upper arm
  - **S41.15** **Open bite of upper arm**
    Bite of upper arm NOS
    > **Excludes1** superficial bite of upper arm (S40.87)
    - **S41.151** Open bite of **right** upper arm
    - **S41.152** Open bite of **left** upper arm
    - **S41.159** Open bite of **unspecified** upper arm

- **S42** **Fracture of shoulder and upper arm**
  Note: A fracture not indicated as displaced or nondisplaced should be coded to displaced
  A fracture not indicated as open or closed should be coded to closed
  > **Excludes1** traumatic amputation of shoulder and upper arm (S48.-)
  The appropriate 7th character is to be added to all codes from category S42

A	initial encounter for closed fracture
B	initial encounter for open fracture
D	subsequent encounter for fracture with routine healing
G	subsequent encounter for fracture with delayed healing
K	subsequent encounter for fracture with nonunion
P	subsequent encounter for fracture with malunion
S	sequela

  - **S42.0** **Fracture of clavicle**
    - **S42.00** **Fracture of unspecified part of clavicle**
      - **S42.001** Fracture of unspecified part of **right** clavicle
      - **S42.002** Fracture of unspecified part of **left** clavicle
      - **S42.009** Fracture of unspecified part of **unspecified** clavicle
        Coding Clinic: 2012, Q4, P3
    - **S42.01** **Fracture of sternal end of clavicle**
      - **S42.011** Anterior displaced fracture of sternal end of **right** clavicle
      - **S42.012** Anterior displaced fracture of sternal end of **left** clavicle
      - **S42.013** Anterior displaced fracture of sternal end of **unspecified** clavicle
        Displaced fracture of sternal end of clavicle NOS
      - **S42.014** Posterior displaced fracture of sternal end of **right** clavicle
      - **S42.015** Posterior displaced fracture of sternal end of **left** clavicle
      - **S42.016** Posterior displaced fracture of sternal end of **unspecified** clavicle
      - **S42.017** Nondisplaced fracture of sternal end of **right** clavicle
      - **S42.018** Nondisplaced fracture of sternal end of **left** clavicle
      - **S42.019** Nondisplaced fracture of sternal end of **unspecified** clavicle
    - **S42.02** **Fracture of shaft of clavicle**
      - **S42.021** Displaced fracture of shaft of **right** clavicle
      - **S42.022** Displaced fracture of shaft of **left** clavicle
      - **S42.023** Displaced fracture of shaft of **unspecified** clavicle
      - **S42.024** Nondisplaced fracture of shaft of **right** clavicle
      - **S42.025** Nondisplaced fracture of shaft of **left** clavicle
      - **S42.026** Nondisplaced fracture of shaft of **unspecified** clavicle
    - **S42.03** **Fracture of lateral end of clavicle**
      Fracture of acromial end of clavicle
      - **S42.031** Displaced fracture of lateral end of **right** clavicle
      - **S42.032** Displaced fracture of lateral end of **left** clavicle
      - **S42.033** Displaced fracture of lateral end of **unspecified** clavicle
      - **S42.034** Nondisplaced fracture of lateral end of **right** clavicle

CHAPTER 19 (S00-T88)

● S42.035   Nondisplaced fracture of lateral end of left clavicle

● S42.036   Nondisplaced fracture of lateral end of unspecified clavicle

● S42.1   Fracture of scapula

● S42.10   Fracture of unspecified part of scapula

● S42.101   Fracture of unspecified part of scapula, right shoulder

● S42.102   Fracture of unspecified part of scapula, left shoulder

● S42.109   Fracture of unspecified part of scapula, unspecified shoulder

● S42.11   Fracture of body of scapula

● S42.111   Displaced fracture of body of scapula, right shoulder

● S42.112   Displaced fracture of body of scapula, left shoulder

● S42.113   Displaced fracture of body of scapula, unspecified shoulder

● S42.114   Nondisplaced fracture of body of scapula, right shoulder

● S42.115   Nondisplaced fracture of body of scapula, left shoulder

● S42.116   Nondisplaced fracture of body of scapula, unspecified shoulder

● S42.12   Fracture of acromial process

● S42.121   Displaced fracture of acromial process, right shoulder

● S42.122   Displaced fracture of acromial process, left shoulder

● S42.123   Displaced fracture of acromial process, unspecified shoulder

● S42.124   Nondisplaced fracture of acromial process, right shoulder

● S42.125   Nondisplaced fracture of acromial process, left shoulder

● S42.126   Nondisplaced fracture, of acromial process, unspecified shoulder

● S42.13   Fracture of coracoid process

● S42.131   Displaced fracture of coracoid process, right shoulder

● S42.132   Displaced fracture of coracoid process, left shoulder

● S42.133   Displaced fracture of coracoid process, unspecified shoulder

● S42.134   Nondisplaced fracture of coracoid process, right shoulder

● S42.135   Nondisplaced fracture of coracoid process, left shoulder

● S42.136   Nondisplaced fracture of coracoid process, unspecified shoulder

● S42.14   Fracture of glenoid cavity of scapula

● S42.141   Displaced fracture of glenoid cavity of scapula, right shoulder

● S42.142   Displaced fracture of glenoid cavity of scapula, left shoulder

● S42.143   Displaced fracture of glenoid cavity of scapula, unspecified shoulder

● S42.144   Nondisplaced fracture of glenoid cavity of scapula, right shoulder

● S42.145   Nondisplaced fracture of glenoid cavity of scapula, left shoulder

● S42.146   Nondisplaced fracture of glenoid cavity of scapula, unspecified shoulder

● S42.15   Fracture of neck of scapula

● S42.151   Displaced fracture of neck of scapula, right shoulder

● S42.152   Displaced fracture of neck of scapula, left shoulder

● S42.153   Displaced fracture of neck of scapula, unspecified shoulder

● S42.154   Nondisplaced fracture of neck of scapula, right shoulder

● S42.155   Nondisplaced fracture of neck of scapula, left shoulder

● S42.156   Nondisplaced fracture of neck of scapula, unspecified shoulder

● S42.19   Fracture of other part of scapula

● S42.191   Fracture of other part of scapula, right shoulder

● S42.192   Fracture of other part of scapula, left shoulder

● S42.199   Fracture of other part of scapula, unspecified shoulder

● S42.2   Fracture of upper end of humerus
Fracture of proximal end of humerus

Excludes2   fracture of shaft of humerus (S42.3-)
physeal fracture of upper end of humerus (S49.0-)

● S42.20   Unspecified fracture of upper end of humerus

● S42.201   Unspecified fracture of upper end of right humerus

● S42.202   Unspecified fracture of upper end of left humerus

● S42.209   Unspecified fracture of upper end of unspecified humerus

● S42.21   Unspecified fracture of surgical neck of humerus
Fracture of neck of humerus NOS

● S42.211   Unspecified displaced fracture of surgical neck of right humerus

● S42.212   Unspecified displaced fracture of surgical neck of left humerus

● S42.213   Unspecified displaced fracture of surgical neck of unspecified humerus

● S42.214   Unspecified nondisplaced fracture of surgical neck of right humerus

● S42.215   Unspecified nondisplaced fracture of surgical neck of left humerus

● S42.216   Unspecified nondisplaced fracture of surgical neck of unspecified humerus

● S42.22 2-part fracture of surgical neck of humerus

● S42.221   2-part displaced fracture of surgical neck of right humerus

● S42.222   2-part displaced fracture of surgical neck of left humerus

● S42.223   2-part displaced fracture of surgical neck of unspecified humerus

● S42.224   2-part nondisplaced fracture of surgical neck of right humerus

● S42.225   2-part nondisplaced fracture of surgical neck of left humerus

● S42.226   2-part nondisplaced fracture of surgical neck of unspecified humerus

● S42.23   3-part fracture of surgical neck of humerus

● S42.231   3-part fracture of surgical neck of right humerus

● S42.232   3-part fracture of surgical neck of left humerus

● S42.239   3-part fracture of surgical neck of unspecified humerus

▶ New   ⇒ Revised   deleted Deleted   Excludes 1   Excludes 2   Includes   Use additional   Code first   Code also   Key words
OGCR Official Guidelines   X Assign placeholder X   ● Use Additional Character(s)   ▶ Manifestation Code   ⚘ Hierarchical Condition Category   **Coding Clinic**

- ● **S42.24** 4-part fracture of surgical neck of humerus
  - ● **S42.241** 4-part fracture of surgical neck of right humerus
  - ● **S42.242** 4-part fracture of surgical neck of left humerus
  - ● **S42.249** 4-part fracture of surgical neck of unspecified humerus
- ● **S42.25** Fracture of greater tuberosity of humerus
  - ● **S42.251** Displaced fracture of greater tuberosity of right humerus
  - ● **S42.252** Displaced fracture of greater tuberosity of left humerus
  - ● **S42.253** Displaced fracture of greater tuberosity of unspecified humerus
  - ● **S42.254** Nondisplaced fracture of greater tuberosity of right humerus
  - ● **S42.255** Nondisplaced fracture of greater tuberosity of left humerus
  - ● **S42.256** Nondisplaced fracture of greater tuberosity of unspecified humerus
- ● **S42.26** Fracture of lesser tuberosity of humerus
  - ● **S42.261** Displaced fracture of lesser tuberosity of right humerus
  - ● **S42.262** Displaced fracture of lesser tuberosity of left humerus
  - ● **S42.263** Displaced fracture of lesser tuberosity of unspecified humerus
  - ● **S42.264** Nondisplaced fracture of lesser tuberosity of right humerus
  - ● **S42.265** Nondisplaced fracture of lesser tuberosity of left humerus
  - ● **S42.266** Nondisplaced fracture of lesser tuberosity of unspecified humerus
- ● **S42.27** Torus fracture of upper end of humerus

  The appropriate 7th character is to be added to all codes in subcategory S42.27

A	initial encounter for closed fracture
D	subsequent encounter for fracture with routine healing
G	subsequent encounter for fracture with delayed healing
K	subsequent encounter for fracture with nonunion
P	subsequent encounter for fracture with malunion
S	sequela

  - ● **S42.271** Torus fracture of upper end of right humerus
  - ● **S42.272** Torus fracture of upper end of left humerus
  - ● **S42.279** Torus fracture of upper end of unspecified humerus
- ● **S42.29** Other fracture of upper end of humerus

  Fracture of anatomical neck of humerus
  Fracture of articular head of humerus
  - ● **S42.291** Other displaced fracture of upper end of right humerus
  - ● **S42.292** Other displaced fracture of upper end of left humerus
  - ● **S42.293** Other displaced fracture of upper end of unspecified humerus

- ● **S42.294** Other nondisplaced fracture of upper end of right humerus
- ● **S42.295** Other nondisplaced fracture of upper end of left humerus
  Coding Clinic: 2019, Q1, P19
- ● **S42.296** Other nondisplaced fracture of upper end of unspecified humerus
- ● **S42.3** Fracture of shaft of humerus

  Fracture of humerus NOS
  Fracture of upper arm NOS

  Excludes2 physeal fractures of upper end of humerus (S49.0-)
  physeal fractures of lower end of humerus (S49.1-)

  - ● **S42.30** Unspecified fracture of shaft of humerus
    - ● **S42.301** Unspecified fracture of shaft of humerus, right arm
    - ● **S42.302** Unspecified fracture of shaft of humerus, left arm
    - ● **S42.309** Unspecified fracture of shaft of humerus, unspecified arm
  - ● **S42.31** Greenstick fracture of shaft of humerus

    The appropriate 7th character is to be added to all codes in subcategory S42.3

A	initial encounter for closed fracture
D	subsequent encounter for fracture with routine healing
G	subsequent encounter for fracture with delayed healing
K	subsequent encounter for fracture with nonunion
P	subsequent encounter for fracture with malunion
S	sequela

    - ● **S42.311** Greenstick fracture of shaft of humerus, right arm
    - ● **S42.312** Greenstick fracture of shaft of humerus, left arm
    - ● **S42.319** Greenstick fracture of shaft of humerus, unspecified arm
  - ● **S42.32** Transverse fracture of shaft of humerus
    - ● **S42.321** Displaced transverse fracture of shaft of humerus, right arm
    - ● **S42.322** Displaced transverse fracture of shaft of humerus, left arm
    - ● **S42.323** Displaced transverse fracture of shaft of humerus, unspecified arm
    - ● **S42.324** Nondisplaced transverse fracture of shaft of humerus, right arm
    - ● **S42.325** Nondisplaced transverse fracture of shaft of humerus, left arm
    - ● **S42.326** Nondisplaced transverse fracture of shaft of humerus, unspecified arm
  - ● **S42.33** Oblique fracture of shaft of humerus
    - ● **S42.331** Displaced oblique fracture of shaft of humerus, right arm
    - ● **S42.332** Displaced oblique fracture of shaft of humerus, left arm
    - ● **S42.333** Displaced oblique fracture of shaft of humerus, unspecified arm
    - ● **S42.334** Nondisplaced oblique fracture of shaft of humerus, right arm
    - ● **S42.335** Nondisplaced oblique fracture of shaft of humerus, left arm
    - ● **S42.336** Nondisplaced oblique fracture of shaft of humerus, unspecified arm

CHAPTER 19 (S00-T88)

CHAPTER 19 (S00-T88)

● S42.34   Spiral fracture of shaft of humerus
> ● S42.341   Displaced spiral fracture of shaft of humerus, right arm
> ● S42.342   Displaced spiral fracture of shaft of humerus, left arm
> ● S42.343   Displaced spiral fracture of shaft of humerus, unspecified arm
> ● S42.344   Nondisplaced spiral fracture of shaft of humerus, right arm
> ● S42.345   Nondisplaced spiral fracture of shaft of humerus, left arm
> ● S42.346   Nondisplaced spiral fracture of shaft of humerus, unspecified arm

● S42.35   Comminuted fracture of shaft of humerus
> ● S42.351   Displaced comminuted fracture of shaft of humerus, right arm
> ● S42.352   Displaced comminuted fracture of shaft of humerus, left arm
> ● S42.353   Displaced comminuted fracture of shaft of humerus, unspecified arm
> ● S42.354   Nondisplaced comminuted fracture of shaft of humerus, right arm
> ● S42.355   Nondisplaced comminuted fracture of shaft of humerus, left arm
> ● S42.356   Nondisplaced comminuted fracture of shaft of humerus, unspecified arm

● S42.36   Segmental fracture of shaft of humerus
> ● S42.361   Displaced segmental fracture of shaft of humerus, right arm
> ● S42.362   Displaced segmental fracture of shaft of humerus, left arm
> ● S42.363   Displaced segmental fracture of shaft of humerus, unspecified arm
> ● S42.364   Nondisplaced segmental fracture of shaft of humerus, right arm
> ● S42.365   Nondisplaced segmental fracture of shaft of humerus, left arm
> ● S42.366   Nondisplaced segmental fracture of shaft of humerus, unspecified arm

● S42.39   Other fracture of shaft of humerus
> ● S42.391   Other fracture of shaft of right humerus
> ● S42.392   Other fracture of shaft of left humerus
> ● S42.399   Other fracture of shaft of unspecified humerus

● S42.4   Fracture of lower end of humerus
> Fracture of distal end of humerus
>> **Excludes2**   fracture of shaft of humerus (S42.3-)
>> physeal fracture of lower end of humerus (S49.1-)

● S42.40   Unspecified fracture of lower end of humerus
> Fracture of elbow NOS
> ● S42.401   Unspecified fracture of lower end of right humerus
> ● S42.402   Unspecified fracture of lower end of left humerus
> ● S42.409   Unspecified fracture of lower end of unspecified humerus

● S42.41   Simple supracondylar fracture without intercondylar fracture of humerus
> ● S42.411   Displaced simple supracondylar fracture without intercondylar fracture of right humerus
> ● S42.412   Displaced simple supracondylar fracture without intercondylar fracture of left humerus

> ● S42.413   Displaced simple supracondylar fracture without intercondylar fracture of unspecified humerus
> ● S42.414   Nondisplaced simple supracondylar fracture without intercondylar fracture of right humerus
> ● S42.415   Nondisplaced simple supracondylar fracture without intercondylar fracture of left humerus
> ● S42.416   Nondisplaced simple supracondylar fracture without intercondylar fracture of unspecified humerus

● S42.42   Comminuted supracondylar fracture without intercondylar fracture of humerus
> ● S42.421   Displaced comminuted supracondylar fracture without intercondylar fracture of right humerus
> ● S42.422   Displaced comminuted supracondylar fracture without intercondylar fracture of left humerus
> ● S42.423   Displaced comminuted supracondylar fracture without intercondylar fracture of unspecified humerus
> ● S42.424   Nondisplaced comminuted supracondylar fracture without intercondylar fracture of right humerus
> ● S42.425   Nondisplaced comminuted supracondylar fracture without intercondylar fracture of left humerus
> ● S42.426   Nondisplaced comminuted supracondylar fracture without intercondylar fracture of unspecified humerus

● S42.43   Fracture (avulsion) of lateral epicondyle of humerus
> ● S42.431   Displaced fracture (avulsion) of lateral epicondyle of right humerus
> ● S42.432   Displaced fracture (avulsion) of lateral epicondyle of left humerus
> ● S42.433   Displaced fracture (avulsion) of lateral epicondyle of unspecified humerus
> ● S42.434   Nondisplaced fracture (avulsion) of lateral epicondyle of right humerus
> ● S42.435   Nondisplaced fracture (avulsion) of lateral epicondyle of left humerus
> ● S42.436   Nondisplaced fracture (avulsion) of lateral epicondyle of unspecified humerus

● S42.44   Fracture (avulsion) of medial epicondyle of humerus
> ● S42.441   Displaced fracture (avulsion) of medial epicondyle of right humerus
> ● S42.442   Displaced fracture (avulsion) of medial epicondyle of left humerus
> ● S42.443   Displaced fracture (avulsion) of medial epicondyle of unspecified humerus
> ● S42.444   Nondisplaced fracture (avulsion) of medial epicondyle of right humerus
> ● S42.445   Nondisplaced fracture (avulsion) of medial epicondyle of left humerus
> ● S42.446   Nondisplaced fracture (avulsion) of medial epicondyle of unspecified humerus
> ● S42.447   Incarcerated fracture (avulsion) of medial epicondyle of right humerus

● S42.448   Incarcerated fracture (avulsion) of medial epicondyle of left humerus

● S42.449   Incarcerated fracture (avulsion) of medial epicondyle of unspecified humerus

● S42.45   Fracture of lateral condyle of humerus
Fracture of capitellum of humerus

● S42.451   Displaced fracture of lateral condyle of right humerus

● S42.452   Displaced fracture of lateral condyle of left humerus

● S42.453   Displaced fracture of lateral condyle of unspecified humerus

● S42.454   Nondisplaced fracture of lateral condyle of right humerus

● S42.455   Nondisplaced fracture of lateral condyle of left humerus

● S42.456   Nondisplaced fracture of lateral condyle of unspecified humerus

● S42.46   Fracture of medial condyle of humerus
Trochlea fracture of humerus

● S42.461   Displaced fracture of medial condyle of right humerus

● S42.462   Displaced fracture of medial condyle of left humerus

● S42.463   Displaced fracture of medial condyle of unspecified humerus

● S42.464   Nondisplaced fracture of medial condyle of right humerus

● S42.465   Nondisplaced fracture of medial condyle of left humerus

● S42.466   Nondisplaced fracture of medial condyle of unspecified humerus

● S42.47   Transcondylar fracture of humerus

● S42.471   Displaced transcondylar fracture of right humerus

● S42.472   Displaced transcondylar fracture of left humerus

● S42.473   Displaced transcondylar fracture of unspecified humerus

● S42.474   Nondisplaced transcondylar fracture of right humerus

● S42.475   Nondisplaced transcondylar fracture of left humerus

● S42.476   Nondisplaced transcondylar fracture of unspecified humerus

● S42.48   Torus fracture of lower end of humerus

The appropriate 7th character is to be added to all codes in subcategory S42.48

A	initial encounter for closed fracture
D	subsequent encounter for fracture with routine healing
G	subsequent encounter for fracture with delayed healing
K	subsequent encounter for fracture with nonunion
P	subsequent encounter for fracture with malunion
S	sequela

● S42.481   Torus fracture of lower end of right humerus

● S42.482   Torus fracture of lower end of left humerus

● S42.489   Torus fracture of lower end of unspecified humerus

● S42.49   Other fracture of lower end of humerus

● S42.491   Other displaced fracture of lower end of right humerus

● S42.492   Other displaced fracture of lower end of left humerus

● S42.493   Other displaced fracture of lower end of unspecified humerus

● S42.494   Other nondisplaced fracture of lower end of right humerus

● S42.495   Other nondisplaced fracture of lower end of left humerus

● S42.496   Other nondisplaced fracture of lower end of unspecified humerus

● S42.9   Fracture of shoulder girdle, part unspecified
Fracture of shoulder NOS

X ● S42.90   Fracture of unspecified shoulder girdle, part unspecified

X ● S42.91   Fracture of right shoulder girdle, part unspecified

X ● S42.92   Fracture of left shoulder girdle, part unspecified

● S43   Dislocation and sprain of joints and ligaments of shoulder girdle

Includes   avulsion of joint or ligament of shoulder girdle
laceration of cartilage, joint or ligament of shoulder girdle
sprain of cartilage, joint or ligament of shoulder girdle
traumatic hemarthrosis of joint or ligament of shoulder girdle
traumatic rupture of joint or ligament of shoulder girdle
traumatic subluxation of joint or ligament of shoulder girdle
traumatic tear of joint or ligament of shoulder girdle

Code also any associated open wound

Excludes2   strain of muscle, fascia and tendon of shoulder and upper arm (S46.-)

The appropriate 7th character is to be added to each code from category S43

A	initial encounter
D	subsequent encounter
S	sequela

● S43.0   Subluxation and dislocation of shoulder joint
Dislocation of glenohumeral joint
Subluxation of glenohumeral joint

● S43.00   Unspecified subluxation and dislocation of shoulder joint
Dislocation of humerus NOS
Subluxation of humerus NOS

● S43.001   Unspecified subluxation of right shoulder joint

● S43.002   Unspecified subluxation of left shoulder joint

● S43.003   Unspecified subluxation of unspecified shoulder joint

● S43.004   Unspecified dislocation of right shoulder joint

● S43.005   Unspecified dislocation of left shoulder joint

● S43.006   Unspecified dislocation of unspecified shoulder joint

● S43.01   Anterior subluxation and dislocation of
            humerus
    ● S43.011   Anterior subluxation of right
                humerus
    ● S43.012   Anterior subluxation of left humerus
    ● S43.013   Anterior subluxation of unspecified
                humerus
    ● S43.014   Anterior dislocation of right humerus
    ● S43.015   Anterior dislocation of left humerus
    ● S43.016   Anterior dislocation of unspecified
                humerus
● S43.02   Posterior subluxation and dislocation of
            humerus
    ● S43.021   Posterior subluxation of right
                humerus
    ● S43.022   Posterior subluxation of left humerus
    ● S43.023   Posterior subluxation of unspecified
                humerus
    ● S43.024   Posterior dislocation of right humerus
    ● S43.025   Posterior dislocation of left humerus
    ● S43.026   Posterior dislocation of unspecified
                humerus
● S43.03   Inferior subluxation and dislocation of
            humerus
    ● S43.031   Inferior subluxation of right humerus
    ● S43.032   Inferior subluxation of left humerus
    ● S43.033   Inferior subluxation of unspecified
                humerus
    ● S43.034   Inferior dislocation of right humerus
    ● S43.035   Inferior dislocation of left humerus
    ● S43.036   Inferior dislocation of unspecified
                humerus
● S43.08   Other subluxation and dislocation of shoulder
            joint
    ● S43.081   Other subluxation of right shoulder
                joint
    ● S43.082   Other subluxation of left shoulder
                joint
    ● S43.083   Other subluxation of unspecified
                shoulder joint
    ● S43.084   Other dislocation of right shoulder
                joint
    ● S43.085   Other dislocation of left shoulder
                joint
    ● S43.086   Other dislocation of unspecified
                shoulder joint
● S43.1   Subluxation and dislocation of acromioclavicular joint
    ● S43.10   Unspecified dislocation of acromioclavicular
                joint
        ● S43.101   Unspecified dislocation of right
                    acromioclavicular joint
        ● S43.102   Unspecified dislocation of left
                    acromioclavicular joint
        ● S43.109   Unspecified dislocation of unspecified
                    acromioclavicular joint
    ● S43.11   Subluxation of acromioclavicular joint
        ● S43.111   Subluxation of right
                    acromioclavicular joint
        ● S43.112   Subluxation of left acromioclavicular
                    joint
        ● S43.119   Subluxation of unspecified
                    acromioclavicular joint
    ● S43.12   Dislocation of acromioclavicular joint,
                100%-200% displacement
        ● S43.121   Dislocation of right acromioclavicular
                    joint, 100%-200% displacement
        ● S43.122   Dislocation of left acromioclavicular
                    joint, 100%-200% displacement

● S43.129   Dislocation of unspecified
            acromioclavicular joint, 100%-200%
            displacement
● S43.13   Dislocation of acromioclavicular joint, greater
            than 200% displacement
    ● S43.131   Dislocation of right acromioclavicular
                joint, greater than 200% displacement
    ● S43.132   Dislocation of left acromioclavicular
                joint, greater than 200% displacement
    ● S43.139   Dislocation of unspecified
                acromioclavicular joint, greater than
                200% displacement
● S43.14   Inferior dislocation of acromioclavicular joint
    ● S43.141   Inferior dislocation of right
                acromioclavicular joint
    ● S43.142   Inferior dislocation of left
                acromioclavicular joint
    ● S43.149   Inferior dislocation of unspecified
                acromioclavicular joint
● S43.15   Posterior dislocation of acromioclavicular joint
    ● S43.151   Posterior dislocation of right
                acromioclavicular joint
    ● S43.152   Posterior dislocation of left
                acromioclavicular joint
    ● S43.159   Posterior dislocation of unspecified
                acromioclavicular joint
● S43.2   Subluxation and dislocation of sternoclavicular joint
    ● S43.20   Unspecified subluxation and dislocation of
                sternoclavicular joint
        ● S43.201   Unspecified subluxation of right
                    sternoclavicular joint
        ● S43.202   Unspecified subluxation of left
                    sternoclavicular joint
        ● S43.203   Unspecified subluxation of
                    unspecified sternoclavicular joint
        ● S43.204   Unspecified dislocation of right
                    sternoclavicular joint
        ● S43.205   Unspecified dislocation of left
                    sternoclavicular joint
        ● S43.206   Unspecified dislocation of unspecified
                    sternoclavicular joint
    ● S43.21   Anterior subluxation and dislocation of
                sternoclavicular joint
        ● S43.211   Anterior subluxation of right
                    sternoclavicular joint
        ● S43.212   Anterior subluxation of left
                    sternoclavicular joint
        ● S43.213   Anterior subluxation of unspecified
                    sternoclavicular joint
        ● S43.214   Anterior dislocation of right
                    sternoclavicular joint
        ● S43.215   Anterior dislocation of left
                    sternoclavicular joint
        ● S43.216   Anterior dislocation of unspecified
                    sternoclavicular joint
    ● S43.22   Posterior subluxation and dislocation of
                sternoclavicular joint
        ● S43.221   Posterior subluxation of right
                    sternoclavicular joint
        ● S43.222   Posterior subluxation of left
                    sternoclavicular joint
        ● S43.223   Posterior subluxation of unspecified
                    sternoclavicular joint
        ● S43.224   Posterior dislocation of right
                    sternoclavicular joint
        ● S43.225   Posterior dislocation of left
                    sternoclavicular joint
        ● S43.226   Posterior dislocation of unspecified
                    sternoclavicular joint

▶ New   ⇒ Revised   d̶e̶l̶e̶t̶e̶d̶ Deleted   Excludes 1   Excludes 2   Includes   Use additional   Code first   Code also   Key words

OGCR Official Guidelines   X Assign placeholder X   ● Use Additional Character(s)   ▷ Manifestation Code   🅗 Hierarchical Condition Category   Coding Clinic

- ● S43.3   **Subluxation and dislocation of other and unspecified parts of shoulder girdle**
  - ● S43.30   **Subluxation and dislocation of unspecified parts of shoulder girdle**
    Dislocation of shoulder girdle NOS
    Subluxation of shoulder girdle NOS
    - ● S43.301   **Subluxation of unspecified parts of right shoulder girdle**
    - ● S43.302   **Subluxation of unspecified parts of left shoulder girdle**
    - ● S43.303   **Subluxation of unspecified parts of unspecified shoulder girdle**
    - ● S43.304   **Dislocation of unspecified parts of right shoulder girdle**
    - ● S43.305   **Dislocation of unspecified parts of left shoulder girdle**
    - ● S43.306   **Dislocation of unspecified parts of unspecified shoulder girdle**
  - ● S43.31   **Subluxation and dislocation of scapula**
    - ● S43.311   **Subluxation of right scapula**
    - ● S43.312   **Subluxation of left scapula**
    - ● S43.313   **Subluxation of unspecified scapula**
    - ● S43.314   **Dislocation of right scapula**
    - ● S43.315   **Dislocation of left scapula**
    - ● S43.316   **Dislocation of unspecified scapula**
  - ● S43.39   **Subluxation and dislocation of other parts of shoulder girdle**
    - ● S43.391   **Subluxation of other parts of right shoulder girdle**
    - ● S43.392   **Subluxation of other parts of left shoulder girdle**
    - ● S43.393   **Subluxation of other parts of unspecified shoulder girdle**
    - ● S43.394   **Dislocation of other parts of right shoulder girdle**
    - ● S43.395   **Dislocation of other parts of left shoulder girdle**
    - ● S43.396   **Dislocation of other parts of unspecified shoulder girdle**
- ● S43.4   **Sprain of shoulder joint**
  - ● S43.40   **Unspecified sprain of shoulder joint**
    - ● S43.401   **Unspecified sprain of right shoulder joint**
    - ● S43.402   **Unspecified sprain of left shoulder joint**
    - ● S43.409   **Unspecified sprain of unspecified shoulder joint**
  - ● S43.41   **Sprain of coracohumeral (ligament)**
    - ● S43.411   **Sprain of right coracohumeral (ligament)**
    - ● S43.412   **Sprain of left coracohumeral (ligament)**
    - ● S43.419   **Sprain of unspecified coracohumeral (ligament)**
  - ● S43.42   **Sprain of rotator cuff capsule**
    Encounters during the healing phase
    > **Excludes1**   rotator cuff syndrome (complete) (incomplete), not specified as traumatic (M75.1-)
    > **Excludes2**   injury of tendon of rotator cuff (S46.0-)
    - ● S43.421   **Sprain of right rotator cuff capsule**
    - ● S43.422   **Sprain of left rotator cuff capsule**
    - ● S43.429   **Sprain of unspecified rotator cuff capsule**

- ● S43.43   **Superior glenoid labrum lesion**
  SLAP lesion
  Coding Clinic: 2019, Q2, P27
  - ● S43.431   **Superior glenoid labrum lesion of right shoulder**
  - ● S43.432   **Superior glenoid labrum lesion of left shoulder**
  - ● S43.439   **Superior glenoid labrum lesion of unspecified shoulder**
- ● S43.49   **Other sprain of shoulder joint**
  - ● S43.491   **Other sprain of right shoulder joint**
  - ● S43.492   **Other sprain of left shoulder joint**
  - ● S43.499   **Other sprain of unspecified shoulder joint**
- ● S43.5   **Sprain of acromioclavicular joint**
  Sprain of acromioclavicular ligament
  - X ● S43.50   **Sprain of unspecified acromioclavicular joint**
  - X ● S43.51   **Sprain of right acromioclavicular joint**
  - X ● S43.52   **Sprain of left acromioclavicular joint**
- ● S43.6   **Sprain of sternoclavicular joint**
  - X ● S43.60   **Sprain of unspecified sternoclavicular joint**
  - X ● S43.61   **Sprain of right sternoclavicular joint**
  - X ● S43.62   **Sprain of left sternoclavicular joint**
- ● S43.8   **Sprain of other specified parts of shoulder girdle**
  - X ● S43.80   **Sprain of other specified parts of unspecified shoulder girdle**
  - X ● S43.81   **Sprain of other specified parts of right shoulder girdle**
  - X ● S43.82   **Sprain of other specified parts of left shoulder girdle**
- ● S43.9   **Sprain of unspecified parts of shoulder girdle**
  - X ● S43.90   **Sprain of unspecified parts of unspecified shoulder girdle**
    Sprain of shoulder girdle NOS
  - X ● S43.91   **Sprain of unspecified parts of right shoulder girdle**
  - X ● S43.92   **Sprain of unspecified parts of left shoulder girdle**
- ● S44   **Injury of nerves at shoulder and upper arm level**
  Code also any associated open wound (S41.-)
  > **Excludes2**   injury of brachial plexus (S14.3-)

  The appropriate 7th character is to be added to each code from category S44

A	initial encounter
D	subsequent encounter
S	sequela

  - ● S44.0   **Injury of ulnar nerve at upper arm level**
    > **Excludes1**   ulnar nerve NOS (S54.0)
    - X ● S44.00   **Injury of ulnar nerve at upper arm level, unspecified arm**
    - X ● S44.01   **Injury of ulnar nerve at upper arm level, right arm**
    - X ● S44.02   **Injury of ulnar nerve at upper arm level, left arm**
  - ● S44.1   **Injury of median nerve at upper arm level**
    > **Excludes1**   median nerve NOS (S54.1)
    - X ● S44.10   **Injury of median nerve at upper arm level, unspecified arm**
    - X ● S44.11   **Injury of median nerve at upper arm level, right arm**
    - X ● S44.12   **Injury of median nerve at upper arm level, left arm**

- S44.2 **Injury of radial nerve at upper arm level**
  - **Excludes1** radial nerve NOS (S54.2)
  - X ● S44.20 **Injury of radial nerve at upper arm level, unspecified arm**
  - X ● S44.21 **Injury of radial nerve at upper arm level, right arm**
  - X ● S44.22 **Injury of radial nerve at upper arm level, left arm**
- S44.3 **Injury of axillary nerve**
  - X ● S44.30 **Injury of axillary nerve, unspecified arm**
  - X ● S44.31 **Injury of axillary nerve, right arm**
  - X ● S44.32 **Injury of axillary nerve, left arm**
- S44.4 **Injury of musculocutaneous nerve**
  - X ● S44.40 **Injury of musculocutaneous nerve, unspecified arm**
  - X ● S44.41 **Injury of musculocutaneous nerve, right arm**
  - X ● S44.42 **Injury of musculocutaneous nerve, left arm**
- S44.5 **Injury of cutaneous sensory nerve at shoulder and upper arm level**
  - X ● S44.50 **Injury of cutaneous sensory nerve at shoulder and upper arm level, unspecified arm**
  - X ● S44.51 **Injury of cutaneous sensory nerve at shoulder and upper arm level, right arm**
  - X ● S44.52 **Injury of cutaneous sensory nerve at shoulder and upper arm level, left arm**
- S44.8 **Injury of other nerves at shoulder and upper arm level**
  - ● S44.8X **Injury of other nerves at shoulder and upper arm level**
    - ● S44.8X1 **Injury of other nerves at shoulder and upper arm level, right arm**
    - ● S44.8X2 **Injury of other nerves at shoulder and upper arm level, left arm**
    - ● S44.8X9 **Injury of other nerves at shoulder and upper arm level, unspecified arm**
- S44.9 **Injury of unspecified nerve at shoulder and upper arm level**
  - X ● S44.90 **Injury of unspecified nerve at shoulder and upper arm level, unspecified arm**
  - X ● S44.91 **Injury of unspecified nerve at shoulder and upper arm level, right arm**
  - X ● S44.92 **Injury of unspecified nerve at shoulder and upper arm level, left arm**

- S45 **Injury of blood vessels at shoulder and upper arm level**
  - Code also any associated open wound (S41.-)
  - **Excludes2** injury of subclavian artery (S25.1)
    injury of subclavian vein (S25.3)
  - The appropriate 7th character is to be added to each code from category S45

A	initial encounter
D	subsequent encounter
S	sequela

  - S45.0 **Injury of axillary artery**
    - ● S45.00 **Unspecified injury of axillary artery**
      - ● S45.001 **Unspecified injury of axillary artery, right side**
      - ● S45.002 **Unspecified injury of axillary artery, left side**
      - ● S45.009 **Unspecified injury of axillary artery, unspecified side**
    - ● S45.01 **Laceration of axillary artery**
      - ● S45.011 **Laceration of axillary artery, right side**
      - ● S45.012 **Laceration of axillary artery, left side**
      - ● S45.019 **Laceration of axillary artery, unspecified side**

- ● S45.09 **Other specified injury of axillary artery**
  - ● S45.091 **Other specified injury of axillary artery, right side**
  - ● S45.092 **Other specified injury of axillary artery, left side**
  - ● S45.099 **Other specified injury of axillary artery, unspecified side**
- S45.1 **Injury of brachial artery**
  - ● S45.10 **Unspecified injury of brachial artery**
    - ● S45.101 **Unspecified injury of brachial artery, right side**
    - ● S45.102 **Unspecified injury of brachial artery, left side**
    - ● S45.109 **Unspecified injury of brachial artery, unspecified side**
  - ● S45.11 **Laceration of brachial artery**
    - ● S45.111 **Laceration of brachial artery, right side**
    - ● S45.112 **Laceration of brachial artery, left side**
    - ● S45.119 **Laceration of brachial artery, unspecified side**
  - ● S45.19 **Other specified injury of brachial artery**
    - ● S45.191 **Other specified injury of brachial artery, right side**
    - ● S45.192 **Other specified injury of brachial artery, left side**
    - ● S45.199 **Other specified injury of brachial artery, unspecified side**
- S45.2 **Injury of axillary or brachial vein**
  - ● S45.20 **Unspecified injury of axillary or brachial vein**
    - ● S45.201 **Unspecified injury of axillary or brachial vein, right side**
    - ● S45.202 **Unspecified injury of axillary or brachial vein, left side**
    - ● S45.209 **Unspecified injury of axillary or brachial vein, unspecified side**
  - ● S45.21 **Laceration of axillary or brachial vein**
    - ● S45.211 **Laceration of axillary or brachial vein, right side**
    - ● S45.212 **Laceration of axillary or brachial vein, left side**
    - ● S45.219 **Laceration of axillary or brachial vein, unspecified side**
  - ● S45.29 **Other specified injury of axillary or brachial vein**
    - ● S45.291 **Other specified injury of axillary or brachial vein, right side**
    - ● S45.292 **Other specified injury of axillary or brachial vein, left side**
    - ● S45.299 **Other specified injury of axillary or brachial vein, unspecified side**
- S45.3 **Injury of superficial vein at shoulder and upper arm level**
  - ● S45.30 **Unspecified injury of superficial vein at shoulder and upper arm level**
    - ● S45.301 **Unspecified injury of superficial vein at shoulder and upper arm level, right arm**
    - ● S45.302 **Unspecified injury of superficial vein at shoulder and upper arm level, left arm**
    - ● S45.309 **Unspecified injury of superficial vein at shoulder and upper arm level, unspecified arm**

- **S45.31** Laceration of superficial vein at shoulder and upper arm level
  - **S45.311** Laceration of superficial vein at shoulder and upper arm level, right arm
  - **S45.312** Laceration of superficial vein at shoulder and upper arm level, left arm
  - **S45.319** Laceration of superficial vein at shoulder and upper arm level, unspecified arm
- **S45.39** Other specified injury of superficial vein at shoulder and upper arm level
  - **S45.391** Other specified injury of superficial vein at shoulder and upper arm level, right arm
  - **S45.392** Other specified injury of superficial vein at shoulder and upper arm level, left arm
  - **S45.399** Other specified injury of superficial vein at shoulder and upper arm level, unspecified arm
- **S45.8** Injury of other specified blood vessels at shoulder and upper arm level
  - **S45.80** Unspecified injury of other specified blood vessels at shoulder and upper arm level
    - **S45.801** Unspecified injury of other specified blood vessels at shoulder and upper arm level, right arm
    - **S45.802** Unspecified injury of other specified blood vessels at shoulder and upper arm level, left arm
    - **S45.809** Unspecified injury of other specified blood vessels at shoulder and upper arm level, unspecified arm
  - **S45.81** Laceration of other specified blood vessels at shoulder and upper arm level
    - **S45.811** Laceration of other specified blood vessels at shoulder and upper arm level, right arm
    - **S45.812** Laceration of other specified blood vessels at shoulder and upper arm level, left arm
    - **S45.819** Laceration of other specified blood vessels at shoulder and upper arm level, unspecified arm
  - **S45.89** Other specified injury of other specified blood vessels at shoulder and upper arm level
    - **S45.891** Other specified injury of other specified blood vessels at shoulder and upper arm level, right arm
    - **S45.892** Other specified injury of other specified blood vessels at shoulder and upper arm level, left arm
    - **S45.899** Other specified injury of other specified blood vessels at shoulder and upper arm level, unspecified arm
- **S45.9** Injury of unspecified blood vessel at shoulder and upper arm level
  - **S45.90** Unspecified injury of unspecified blood vessel at shoulder and upper arm level
    - **S45.901** Unspecified injury of unspecified blood vessel at shoulder and upper arm level, right arm
    - **S45.902** Unspecified injury of unspecified blood vessel at shoulder and upper arm level, left arm
    - **S45.909** Unspecified injury of unspecified blood vessel at shoulder and upper arm level, unspecified arm

- **S45.91** Laceration of unspecified blood vessel at shoulder and upper arm level
  - **S45.911** Laceration of unspecified blood vessel at shoulder and upper arm level, right arm
  - **S45.912** Laceration of unspecified blood vessel at shoulder and upper arm level, left arm
  - **S45.919** Laceration of unspecified blood vessel at shoulder and upper arm level, unspecified arm
- **S45.99** Other specified injury of unspecified blood vessel at shoulder and upper arm level
  - **S45.991** Other specified injury of unspecified blood vessel at shoulder and upper arm level, right arm
  - **S45.992** Other specified injury of unspecified blood vessel at shoulder and upper arm level, left arm
  - **S45.999** Other specified injury of unspecified blood vessel at shoulder and upper arm level, unspecified arm

- **S46** Injury of muscle, fascia and tendon at shoulder and upper arm level

  Code also any associated open wound (S41.-)

  Excludes2   injury of muscle, fascia and tendon at elbow (S56.-)

  sprain of joints and ligaments of shoulder girdle (S43.9)

  The appropriate 7th character is to be added to each code from category S46

A	initial encounter
D	subsequent encounter
S	sequela

  - **S46.0** Injury of muscle(s) and tendon(s) of the rotator cuff of shoulder
    - **S46.00** Unspecified injury of muscle(s) and tendon(s) of the rotator cuff of shoulder
      - **S46.001** Unspecified injury of muscle(s) and tendon(s) of the rotator cuff of right shoulder
      - **S46.002** Unspecified injury of muscle(s) and tendon(s) of the rotator cuff of left shoulder
      - **S46.009** Unspecified injury of muscle(s) and tendon(s) of the rotator cuff of unspecified shoulder
    - **S46.01** Strain of muscle(s) and tendon(s) of the rotator cuff of shoulder

      Acute onset due to trauma to rotator cuff muscle/ tendon
      - **S46.011** Strain of muscle(s) and tendon(s) of the rotator cuff of right shoulder
      - **S46.012** Strain of muscle(s) and tendon(s) of the rotator cuff of left shoulder
      - **S46.019** Strain of muscle(s) and tendon(s) of the rotator cuff of unspecified shoulder
    - **S46.02** Laceration of muscle(s) and tendon(s) of the rotator cuff of shoulder
      - **S46.021** Laceration of muscle(s) and tendon(s) of the rotator cuff of right shoulder
      - **S46.022** Laceration of muscle(s) and tendon(s) of the rotator cuff of left shoulder
      - **S46.029** Laceration of muscle(s) and tendon(s) of the rotator cuff of unspecified shoulder

CHAPTER 19 (S00-T88)

- S46.09   Other injury of muscle(s) and tendon(s) of the rotator cuff of shoulder
  - S46.091   Other injury of muscle(s) and tendon(s) of the rotator cuff of right shoulder
  - S46.092   Other injury of muscle(s) and tendon(s) of the rotator cuff of left shoulder
  - S46.099   Other injury of muscle(s) and tendon(s) of the rotator cuff of unspecified shoulder
- S46.1   Injury of muscle, fascia and tendon of long head of biceps
  - S46.10   Unspecified injury of muscle, fascia and tendon of long head of biceps
    - S46.101   Unspecified injury of muscle, fascia and tendon of long head of biceps, right arm
    - S46.102   Unspecified injury of muscle, fascia and tendon of long head of biceps, left arm
    - S46.109   Unspecified injury of muscle, fascia and tendon of long head of biceps, unspecified arm
  - S46.11   Strain of muscle, fascia and tendon of long head of biceps
    Coding Clinic: 2019, Q2, P27
    - S46.111   Strain of muscle, fascia and tendon of long head of biceps, right arm
    - S46.112   Strain of muscle, fascia and tendon of long head of biceps, left arm
    - S46.119   Strain of muscle, fascia and tendon of long head of biceps, unspecified arm
  - S46.12   Laceration of muscle, fascia and tendon of long head of biceps
    - S46.121   Laceration of muscle, fascia and tendon of long head of biceps, right arm
    - S46.122   Laceration of muscle, fascia and tendon of long head of biceps, left arm
    - S46.129   Laceration of muscle, fascia and tendon of long head of biceps, unspecified arm
  - S46.19   Other injury of muscle, fascia and tendon of long head of biceps
    - S46.191   Other injury of muscle, fascia and tendon of long head of biceps, right arm
    - S46.192   Other injury of muscle, fascia and tendon of long head of biceps, left arm
    - S46.199   Other injury of muscle, fascia and tendon of long head of biceps, unspecified arm
- S46.2   Injury of muscle, fascia and tendon of other parts of biceps
  - S46.20   Unspecified injury of muscle, fascia and tendon of other parts of biceps
    - S46.201   Unspecified injury of muscle, fascia and tendon of other parts of biceps, right arm
    - S46.202   Unspecified injury of muscle, fascia and tendon of other parts of biceps, left arm
    - S46.209   Unspecified injury of muscle, fascia and tendon of other parts of biceps, unspecified arm
- S46.21   Strain of muscle, fascia and tendon of other parts of biceps
  - S46.211   Strain of muscle, fascia and tendon of other parts of biceps, right arm
  - S46.212   Strain of muscle, fascia and tendon of other parts of biceps, left arm
  - S46.219   Strain of muscle, fascia and tendon of other parts of biceps, unspecified arm
- S46.22   Laceration of muscle, fascia and tendon of other parts of biceps
  - S46.221   Laceration of muscle, fascia and tendon of other parts of biceps, right arm
  - S46.222   Laceration of muscle, fascia and tendon of other parts of biceps, left arm
  - S46.229   Laceration of muscle, fascia and tendon of other parts of biceps, unspecified arm
- S46.29   Other injury of muscle, fascia and tendon of other parts of biceps
  - S46.291   Other injury of muscle, fascia and tendon of other parts of biceps, right arm
  - S46.292   Other injury of muscle, fascia and tendon of other parts of biceps, left arm
  - S46.299   Other injury of muscle, fascia and tendon of other parts of biceps, unspecified arm
- S46.3   Injury of muscle, fascia and tendon of triceps
  - S46.30   Unspecified injury of muscle, fascia and tendon of triceps
    - S46.301   Unspecified injury of muscle, fascia and tendon of triceps, right arm
    - S46.302   Unspecified injury of muscle, fascia and tendon of triceps, left arm
    - S46.309   Unspecified injury of muscle, fascia and tendon of triceps, unspecified arm
  - S46.31   Strain of muscle, fascia and tendon of triceps
    - S46.311   Strain of muscle, fascia and tendon of triceps, right arm
    - S46.312   Strain of muscle, fascia and tendon of triceps, left arm
    - S46.319   Strain of muscle, fascia and tendon of triceps, unspecified arm
  - S46.32   Laceration of muscle, fascia and tendon of triceps
    - S46.321   Laceration of muscle, fascia and tendon of triceps, right arm
    - S46.322   Laceration of muscle, fascia and tendon of triceps, left arm
    - S46.329   Laceration of muscle, fascia and tendon of triceps, unspecified arm
  - S46.39   Other injury of muscle, fascia and tendon of triceps
    - S46.391   Other injury of muscle, fascia and tendon of triceps, right arm
    - S46.392   Other injury of muscle, fascia and tendon of triceps, left arm
    - S46.399   Other injury of muscle, fascia and tendon of triceps, unspecified arm

▶ New   ⇒ Revised   ~~deleted~~ Deleted   Excludes 1   Excludes 2   Includes   Use additional   Code first   Code also   Key words

OGCR Official Guidelines   X Assign placeholder X   ● Use Additional Character(s)   ▷ Manifestation Code   ⬮ Hierarchical Condition Category   **Coding Clinic**

● S46.8   Injury of other muscles, fascia and tendons at shoulder and upper arm level
  ● S46.80   Unspecified injury of other muscles, fascia and tendons at shoulder and upper arm level
    ● S46.801   Unspecified injury of other muscles, fascia and tendons at shoulder and upper arm level, right arm
    ● S46.802   Unspecified injury of other muscles, fascia and tendons at shoulder and upper arm level, left arm
    ● S46.809   Unspecified injury of other muscles, fascia and tendons at shoulder and upper arm level, unspecified arm
  ● S46.81   Strain of other muscles, fascia and tendons at shoulder and upper arm level
    ● S46.811   Strain of other muscles, fascia and tendons at shoulder and upper arm level, right arm
    ● S46.812   Strain of other muscles, fascia and tendons at shoulder and upper arm level, left arm
    ● S46.819   Strain of other muscles, fascia and tendons at shoulder and upper arm level, unspecified arm
  ● S46.82   Laceration of other muscles, fascia and tendons at shoulder and upper arm level
    ● S46.821   Laceration of other muscles, fascia and tendons at shoulder and upper arm level, right arm
    ● S46.822   Laceration of other muscles, fascia and tendons at shoulder and upper arm level, left arm
    ● S46.829   Laceration of other muscles, fascia and tendons at shoulder and upper arm level, unspecified arm
  ● S46.89   Other injury of other muscles, fascia and tendons at shoulder and upper arm level
    ● S46.891   Other injury of other muscles, fascia and tendons at shoulder and upper arm level, right arm
    ● S46.892   Other injury of other muscles, fascia and tendons at shoulder and upper arm level, left arm
    ● S46.899   Other injury of other muscles, fascia and tendons at shoulder and upper arm level, unspecified arm
● S46.9   Injury of unspecified muscle, fascia and tendon at shoulder and upper arm level
  ● S46.90   Unspecified injury of unspecified muscle, fascia and tendon at shoulder and upper arm level
    ● S46.901   Unspecified injury of unspecified muscle, fascia and tendon at shoulder and upper arm level, right arm
    ● S46.902   Unspecified injury of unspecified muscle, fascia and tendon at shoulder and upper arm level, left arm
    ● S46.909   Unspecified injury of unspecified muscle, fascia and tendon at shoulder and upper arm level, unspecified arm
  ● S46.91   Strain of unspecified muscle, fascia and tendon at shoulder and upper arm level
    ● S46.911   Strain of unspecified muscle, fascia and tendon at shoulder and upper arm level, right arm
    ● S46.912   Strain of unspecified muscle, fascia and tendon at shoulder and upper arm level, left arm
    ● S46.919   Strain of unspecified muscle, fascia and tendon at shoulder and upper arm level, unspecified arm

● S46.92   Laceration of unspecified muscle, fascia and tendon at shoulder and upper arm level
    ● S46.921   Laceration of unspecified muscle, fascia and tendon at shoulder and upper arm level, right arm
    ● S46.922   Laceration of unspecified muscle, fascia and tendon at shoulder and upper arm level, left arm
    ● S46.929   Laceration of unspecified muscle, fascia and tendon at shoulder and upper arm level, unspecified arm
  ● S46.99   Other injury of unspecified muscle, fascia and tendon at shoulder and upper arm level
    ● S46.991   Other injury of unspecified muscle, fascia and tendon at shoulder and upper arm level, right arm
    ● S46.992   Other injury of unspecified muscle, fascia and tendon at shoulder and upper arm level, left arm
    ● S46.999   Other injury of unspecified muscle, fascia and tendon at shoulder and upper arm level, unspecified arm

● S47   Crushing injury of shoulder and upper arm
        Use additional code for all associated injuries
        Excludes2   crushing injury of elbow (S57.0-)
        The appropriate 7th character is to be added to each code from category S47

A	initial encounter
D	subsequent encounter
S	sequela

  X ● S47.1   Crushing injury of right shoulder and upper arm
  X ● S47.2   Crushing injury of left shoulder and upper arm
  X ● S47.9   Crushing injury of shoulder and upper arm, unspecified arm

● S48   Traumatic amputation of shoulder and upper arm
        An amputation not identified as partial or complete should be coded to complete
        Excludes1   traumatic amputation at elbow level (S58.0)
        The appropriate 7th character is to be added to each code from category S48

A	initial encounter
D	subsequent encounter
S	sequela

  ● S48.0   Traumatic amputation at shoulder joint
    ● S48.01   Complete traumatic amputation at shoulder joint
      ● S48.011   Complete traumatic amputation at right shoulder joint A, S ▨
      ● S48.012   Complete traumatic amputation at left shoulder joint A, S ▨
      ● S48.019   Complete traumatic amputation at unspecified shoulder joint A, S ▨
    ● S48.02   Partial traumatic amputation at shoulder joint
      ● S48.021   Partial traumatic amputation at right shoulder joint A, S ▨
      ● S48.022   Partial traumatic amputation at left shoulder joint A, S ▨
      ● S48.029   Partial traumatic amputation at unspecified shoulder joint A, S ▨
  ● S48.1   Traumatic amputation at level between shoulder and elbow
    ● S48.11   Complete traumatic amputation at level between shoulder and elbow
      ● S48.111   Complete traumatic amputation at level between right shoulder and elbow A, S ▨

CHAPTER 19 (S00-T88)

CHAPTER 19 (S00-T88)

- ● S48.112   Complete traumatic amputation at level between left shoulder and elbow A, S 🐾
- ● S48.119   Complete traumatic amputation at level between unspecified shoulder and elbow A, S 🐾
  - ● S48.12   **Partial** traumatic amputation at level between shoulder and elbow
    - ● S48.121   Partial traumatic amputation at level between right shoulder and elbow A, S 🐾
    - ● S48.122   Partial traumatic amputation at level between left shoulder and elbow A, S 🐾
    - ● S48.129   Partial traumatic amputation at level between unspecified shoulder and elbow A, S 🐾
- ● S48.9   Traumatic amputation of shoulder and upper arm, level unspecified
  - ● S48.91   **Complete** traumatic amputation of shoulder and upper arm, level unspecified
    - ● S48.911   Complete traumatic amputation of right shoulder and upper arm, level unspecified A, S 🐾
    - ● S48.912   Complete traumatic amputation of left shoulder and upper arm, level unspecified A, S 🐾
    - ● S48.919   Complete traumatic amputation of unspecified shoulder and upper arm, level unspecified A, S 🐾
  - ● S48.92   **Partial** traumatic amputation of shoulder and upper arm, level unspecified
    - ● S48.921   Partial traumatic amputation of right shoulder and upper arm, level unspecified A, S 🐾
    - ● S48.922   Partial traumatic amputation of left shoulder and upper arm, level unspecified A, S 🐾
    - ● S48.929   Partial traumatic amputation of unspecified shoulder and upper arm, level unspecified A, S 🐾

● S49   **Other and unspecified injuries of shoulder and upper arm**

The appropriate 7th character is to be added to each code from subcategories S49.0 and S49.1

A	initial encounter for closed fracture
D	subsequent encounter for fracture with routine healing
G	subsequent encounter for fracture with delayed healing
K	subsequent encounter for fracture with nonunion
P	subsequent encounter for fracture with malunion
S	sequela

- ● S49.0   **Physeal fracture of upper end of humerus**
  - ● S49.00   **Unspecified** physeal fracture of upper end of humerus
    - ● S49.001   Unspecified physeal fracture of upper end of humerus, right arm
    - ● S49.002   Unspecified physeal fracture of upper end of humerus, left arm
    - ● S49.009   Unspecified physeal fracture of upper end of humerus, unspecified arm
  - ● S49.01   Salter-Harris Type I physeal fracture of upper end of humerus
    - ● S49.011   Salter-Harris Type I physeal fracture of upper end of humerus, right arm
    - ● S49.012   Salter-Harris Type I physeal fracture of upper end of humerus, left arm
    - ● S49.019   Salter-Harris Type I physeal fracture of upper end of humerus, unspecified arm

Item 19–3   **SALTER-HARRIS TYPE 1:** epiphysis is completely separated from end of bone, or metaphysic growth plate remains attached to epiphysis

     SALTER-HARRIS TYPE 2: epiphysis and growth plate are partially separated from metaphysis, which is cracked—most common type

     SALTER-HARRIS TYPE 3: fracture occurring through epiphysis and separates part of epiphysis and growth plate from metaphysis fracture, usually at distal end of tibia

     SALTER-HARRIS TYPE 4: fracture runs through epiphysis, across growth plate, into metaphysic, surgery is required to restore joint surface to normal and align growth plate

- ● S49.02   Salter-Harris Type II physeal fracture of upper end of humerus
  - ● S49.021   Salter-Harris Type II physeal fracture of upper end of humerus, right arm
  - ● S49.022   Salter-Harris Type II physeal fracture of upper end of humerus, left arm
  - ● S49.029   Salter-Harris Type II physeal fracture of upper end of humerus, unspecified arm
- ● S49.03   Salter-Harris Type III physeal fracture of upper end of humerus
  - ● S49.031   Salter-Harris Type III physeal fracture of upper end of humerus, right arm
  - ● S49.032   Salter-Harris Type III physeal fracture of upper end of humerus, left arm
  - ● S49.039   Salter-Harris Type III physeal fracture of upper end of humerus, unspecified arm
- ● S49.04   Salter-Harris Type IV physeal fracture of upper end of humerus
  - ● S49.041   Salter-Harris Type IV physeal fracture of upper end of humerus, right arm
  - ● S49.042   Salter-Harris Type IV physeal fracture of upper end of humerus, left arm
  - ● S49.049   Salter-Harris Type IV physeal fracture of upper end of humerus, unspecified arm
- ● S49.09   Other physeal fracture of upper end of humerus
  - ● S49.091   Other physeal fracture of upper end of humerus, right arm
  - ● S49.092   Other physeal fracture of upper end of humerus, left arm
  - ● S49.099   Other physeal fracture of upper end of humerus, unspecified arm
- ● S49.1   **Physeal fracture of lower end of humerus**
  - ● S49.10   **Unspecified** physeal fracture of lower end of humerus
    - ● S49.101   Unspecified physeal fracture of lower end of humerus, right arm
    - ● S49.102   Unspecified physeal fracture of lower end of humerus, left arm
    - ● S49.109   Unspecified physeal fracture of lower end of humerus, unspecified arm
  - ● S49.11   Salter-Harris Type I physeal fracture of lower end of humerus
    - ● S49.111   Salter-Harris Type I physeal fracture of lower end of humerus, right arm
    - ● S49.112   Salter-Harris Type I physeal fracture of lower end of humerus, left arm
    - ● S49.119   Salter-Harris Type I physeal fracture of lower end of humerus, unspecified arm
  - ● S49.12   Salter-Harris Type II physeal fracture of lower end of humerus
    - ● S49.121   Salter-Harris Type II physeal fracture of lower end of humerus, right arm
    - ● S49.122   Salter-Harris Type II physeal fracture of lower end of humerus, left arm
    - ● S49.129   Salter-Harris Type II physeal fracture of lower end of humerus, unspecified arm

▶ New   ⇒ Revised   ~~deleted~~ Deleted   Excludes 1   Excludes 2   Includes   Use additional   Code first   Code also   Key words

OGCR Official Guidelines   X Assign placeholder X   ● Use Additional Character(s)   ▶ Manifestation Code   🐾 Hierarchical Condition Category   **Coding Clinic**

● S49.13   **Salter-Harris Type III** physeal fracture of lower end of humerus
     ● S49.131   Salter-Harris Type III physeal fracture of lower end of humerus, **right arm**
     ● S49.132   Salter-Harris Type III physeal fracture of lower end of humerus, **left arm**
     ● S49.139   Salter-Harris Type III physeal fracture of lower end of humerus, **unspecified arm**

● S49.14   **Salter-Harris Type IV** physeal fracture of lower end of humerus
     ● S49.141   Salter-Harris Type IV physeal fracture of lower end of humerus, **right arm**
     ● S49.142   Salter-Harris Type IV physeal fracture of lower end of humerus, **left arm**
     ● S49.149   Salter-Harris Type IV physeal fracture of lower end of humerus, **unspecified arm**

● S49.19   **Other** physeal fracture of lower end of humerus
     ● S49.191   Other physeal fracture of lower end of humerus, **right arm**
     ● S49.192   Other physeal fracture of lower end of humerus, **left arm**
     ● S49.199   Other physeal fracture of lower end of humerus, **unspecified arm**

● S49.8   **Other specified injuries** of shoulder and upper arm

The appropriate 7th character is to be added to each code in subcategory S49.8

A	initial encounter
D	subsequent encounter
S	sequela

X ● S49.80   Other specified injuries of shoulder and upper arm, **unspecified arm**
X ● S49.81   Other specified injuries of **right** shoulder and upper arm
X ● S49.82   Other specified injuries of **left** shoulder and upper arm

● S49.9   **Unspecified injury** of shoulder and upper arm

The appropriate 7th character is to be added to each code in subcategory S49.9

A	initial encounter
D	subsequent encounter
S	sequela

X ● S49.90   Unspecified injury of shoulder and upper arm, **unspecified arm**
X ● S49.91   Unspecified injury of **right** shoulder and upper arm
X ● S49.92   Unspecified injury of **left** shoulder and upper arm

INJURIES TO THE ELBOW AND FOREARM (S50-S59)

Excludes2   burns and corrosions (T20-T32)
         frostbite (T33-T34)
         injuries of wrist and hand (S60-S69)
         insect bite or sting, venomous (T63.4)

● S50   **Superficial injury of elbow and forearm**

Excludes2   superficial injury of wrist and hand (S60.-)

The appropriate 7th character is to be added to each code from category S50

A	initial encounter
D	subsequent encounter
S	sequela

● S50.0   **Contusion of elbow**
   X ● S50.00   Contusion of **unspecified** elbow
   X ● S50.01   Contusion of **right** elbow
   X ● S50.02   Contusion of **left** elbow

● S50.1   **Contusion of forearm**
   X ● S50.10   Contusion of **unspecified** forearm
   X ● S50.11   Contusion of **right** forearm
   X ● S50.12   Contusion of **left** forearm

● S50.3   **Other superficial injuries** of elbow
   ● S50.31   **Abrasion** of elbow
     ● S50.311   Abrasion of **right** elbow
     ● S50.312   Abrasion of **left** elbow
     ● S50.319   Abrasion of **unspecified** elbow
   ● S50.32   **Blister (nonthermal)** of elbow
     ● S50.321   Blister (nonthermal) of **right** elbow
     ● S50.322   Blister (nonthermal) of **left** elbow
     ● S50.329   Blister (nonthermal) of **unspecified** elbow
   ● S50.34   **External constriction** of elbow
     ● S50.341   External constriction of **right** elbow
     ● S50.342   External constriction of **left** elbow
     ● S50.349   External constriction of **unspecified** elbow
   ● S50.35   **Superficial foreign body** of elbow
     Splinter in the elbow
     ● S50.351   Superficial foreign body of **right** elbow
     ● S50.352   Superficial foreign body of **left** elbow
     ● S50.359   Superficial foreign body of **unspecified** elbow
   ● S50.36   **Insect bite (nonvenomous)** of elbow
     ● S50.361   Insect bite (nonvenomous) of **right** elbow
     ● S50.362   Insect bite (nonvenomous) of **left** elbow
     ● S50.369   Insect bite (nonvenomous) of **unspecified** elbow
   ● S50.37   **Other superficial bite** of elbow
     Excludes1   open bite of elbow (S51.04)
     ● S50.371   Other superficial bite of **right** elbow
     ● S50.372   Other superficial bite of **left** elbow
     ● S50.379   Other superficial bite of **unspecified** elbow

● S50.8   **Other superficial injuries** of forearm
   ● S50.81   **Abrasion** of forearm
     ● S50.811   Abrasion of **right** forearm
     ● S50.812   Abrasion of **left** forearm
     ● S50.819   Abrasion of **unspecified** forearm
   ● S50.82   **Blister (nonthermal)** of forearm
     ● S50.821   Blister (nonthermal) of **right** forearm
     ● S50.822   Blister (nonthermal) of **left** forearm
     ● S50.829   Blister (nonthermal) of **unspecified** forearm
   ● S50.84   **External constriction** of forearm
     ● S50.841   External constriction of **right** forearm
     ● S50.842   External constriction of **left** forearm
     ● S50.849   External constriction of **unspecified** forearm
   ● S50.85   **Superficial foreign body** of forearm
     Splinter in the forearm
     ● S50.851   Superficial foreign body of **right** forearm
     ● S50.852   Superficial foreign body of **left** forearm
     ● S50.859   Superficial foreign body of **unspecified** forearm

CHAPTER 19 (S00-T88)

- ● S50.86   Insect bite (nonvenomous) of forearm
  - ● S50.861   Insect bite (nonvenomous) of right forearm
  - ● S50.862   Insect bite (nonvenomous) of left forearm
  - ● S50.869   Insect bite (nonvenomous) of unspecified forearm
- ● S50.87   Other superficial bite of forearm
  - **Excludes1**   open bite of forearm (S51.84)
  - ● S50.871   Other superficial bite of right forearm
  - ● S50.872   Other superficial bite of left forearm
  - ● S50.879   Other superficial bite of unspecified forearm
- ● S50.9   Unspecified superficial injury of elbow and forearm
  - ● S50.90   Unspecified superficial injury of elbow
    - ● S50.901   Unspecified superficial injury of right elbow
    - ● S50.902   Unspecified superficial injury of left elbow
    - ● S50.909   Unspecified superficial injury of unspecified elbow
  - ● S50.91   Unspecified superficial injury of forearm
    - ● S50.911   Unspecified superficial injury of right forearm
    - ● S50.912   Unspecified superficial injury of left forearm
    - ● S50.919   Unspecified superficial injury of unspecified forearm

- ● S51   Open wound of elbow and forearm
  - Code also any associated wound infection
  - **Excludes1**   open fracture of elbow and forearm (S52.- with open fracture 7th character)
    - traumatic amputation of elbow and forearm (S58.-)
  - **Excludes2**   open wound of wrist and hand (S61.-)
  - The appropriate 7th character is to be added to each code from category S51

A	initial encounter
D	subsequent encounter
S	sequela

  - ● S51.0   Open wound of elbow
    - ● S51.00   Unspecified open wound of elbow
      - ● S51.001   Unspecified open wound of right elbow
        - **Coding Clinic: 2012, Q4, P108**
      - ● S51.002   Unspecified open wound of left elbow
      - ● S51.009   Unspecified open wound of unspecified elbow
        - Open wound of elbow NOS
    - ● S51.01   Laceration without foreign body of elbow
      - ● S51.011   Laceration without foreign body of right elbow
      - ● S51.012   Laceration without foreign body of left elbow
      - ● S51.019   Laceration without foreign body of unspecified elbow
    - ● S51.02   Laceration with foreign body of elbow
      - ● S51.021   Laceration with foreign body of right elbow
      - ● S51.022   Laceration with foreign body of left elbow
      - ● S51.029   Laceration with foreign body of unspecified elbow

  - ● S51.03   Puncture wound without foreign body of elbow
    - ● S51.031   Puncture wound without foreign body of right elbow
    - ● S51.032   Puncture wound without foreign body of left elbow
    - ● S51.039   Puncture wound without foreign body of unspecified elbow
  - ● S51.04   Puncture wound with foreign body of elbow
    - ● S51.041   Puncture wound with foreign body of right elbow
    - ● S51.042   Puncture wound with foreign body of left elbow
    - ● S51.049   Puncture wound with foreign body of unspecified elbow
  - ● S51.05   Open bite of elbow
    - Bite of elbow NOS
    - **Excludes1**   superficial bite of elbow (S50.36, S50.37)
    - ● S51.051   Open bite, right elbow
    - ● S51.052   Open bite, left elbow
    - ● S51.059   Open bite, unspecified elbow
- ● S51.8   Open wound of forearm
  - **Excludes2**   open wound of elbow (S51.0-)
  - ● S51.80   Unspecified open wound of forearm
    - ● S51.801   Unspecified open wound of right forearm
    - ● S51.802   Unspecified open wound of left forearm
    - ● S51.809   Unspecified open wound of unspecified forearm
      - Open wound of forearm NOS
  - ● S51.81   Laceration without foreign body of forearm
    - ● S51.811   Laceration without foreign body of right forearm
    - ● S51.812   Laceration without foreign body of left forearm
    - ● S51.819   Laceration without foreign body of unspecified forearm
  - ● S51.82   Laceration with foreign body of forearm
    - ● S51.821   Laceration with foreign body of right forearm
    - ● S51.822   Laceration with foreign body of left forearm
    - ● S51.829   Laceration with foreign body of unspecified forearm
  - ● S51.83   Puncture wound without foreign body of forearm
    - ● S51.831   Puncture wound without foreign body of right forearm
    - ● S51.832   Puncture wound without foreign body of left forearm
    - ● S51.839   Puncture wound without foreign body of unspecified forearm
  - ● S51.84   Puncture wound with foreign body of forearm
    - ● S51.841   Puncture wound with foreign body of right forearm
    - ● S51.842   Puncture wound with foreign body of left forearm
    - ● S51.849   Puncture wound with foreign body of unspecified forearm
  - ● S51.85   Open bite of forearm
    - Bite of forearm NOS
    - **Excludes1**   superficial bite of forearm (S50.86, S50.87)
    - ● S51.851   Open bite of right forearm
    - ● S51.852   Open bite of left forearm
    - ● S51.859   Open bite of unspecified forearm

▶ New   ⇒ Revised   deleted Deleted   Excludes 1   Excludes 2   Includes   Use additional   Code first   Code also   Key words
OGCR Official Guidelines   X Assign placeholder X   ● Use Additional Character(s)   ▶ Manifestation Code   🔖 Hierarchical Condition Category   Coding Clinic

● **S52** **Fracture of forearm**

Note: A fracture not identified as displaced or nondisplaced should be coded to displaced

A fracture not designated as open or closed should be coded to closed

The open fracture designations are based on the Gustilo open fracture classification

Excludes1 traumatic amputation of forearm (S58.-)

Excludes2 fracture at wrist and hand level (S62.-)

The appropriate 7th character is to be added to all codes from category S52

A	initial encounter for closed fracture
B	initial encounter for open fracture type I or II
	initial encounter for open fracture NOS
C	initial encounter for open fracture type IIIA, IIIB, or IIIC
D	subsequent encounter for closed fracture with routine healing
E	subsequent encounter for open fracture type I or II with routine healing
F	subsequent encounter for open fracture type IIIA, IIIB, or IIIC with routine healing
G	subsequent encounter for closed fracture with delayed healing
H	subsequent encounter for open fracture type I or II with delayed healing
J	subsequent encounter for open fracture type IIIA, IIIB, or IIIC with delayed healing
K	subsequent encounter for closed fracture with nonunion
M	subsequent encounter for open fracture type I or II with nonunion
N	subsequent encounter for open fracture type IIIA, IIIB, or IIIC with nonunion
P	subsequent encounter for closed fracture with malunion
Q	subsequent encounter for open fracture type I or II with malunion
R	subsequent encounter for open fracture type IIIA, IIIB, or IIIC with malunion
S	sequela

Coding Clinic: 2016, Q1, P33

● **S52.0** **Fracture of upper end of ulna**

Fracture of proximal end of ulna

Excludes2 fracture of elbow NOS (S42.40-)

fractures of shaft of ulna (S52.2-)

● **S52.00** **Unspecified fracture of upper end of ulna**

● **S52.001** Unspecified fracture of upper end of right ulna

● **S52.002** Unspecified fracture of upper end of left ulna

● **S52.009** Unspecified fracture of upper end of unspecified ulna

● **S52.01** **Torus fracture of upper end of ulna**

The appropriate 7th character is to be added to all codes in subcategory S52.01

A	initial encounter for closed fracture
D	subsequent encounter for fracture with routine healing
G	subsequent encounter for fracture with delayed healing
K	subsequent encounter for fracture with nonunion
P	subsequent encounter for fracture with malunion
S	sequela

● **S52.011** Torus fracture of upper end of right ulna

● **S52.012** Torus fracture of upper end of left ulna

● **S52.019** Torus fracture of upper end of unspecified ulna

● **S52.02** **Fracture of olecranon process without intraarticular extension of ulna**

● **S52.021** Displaced fracture of olecranon process without intraarticular extension of right ulna

● **S52.022** Displaced fracture of olecranon process without intraarticular extension of left ulna

● **S52.023** Displaced fracture of olecranon process without intraarticular extension of unspecified ulna

● **S52.024** Nondisplaced fracture of olecranon process without intraarticular extension of right ulna

● **S52.025** Nondisplaced fracture of olecranon process without intraarticular extension of left ulna

● **S52.026** Nondisplaced fracture of olecranon process without intraarticular extension of unspecified ulna

● **S52.03** **Fracture of olecranon process with intraarticular extension of ulna**

● **S52.031** Displaced fracture of olecranon process with intraarticular extension of right ulna

● **S52.032** Displaced fracture of olecranon process with intraarticular extension of left ulna

● **S52.033** Displaced fracture of olecranon process with intraarticular extension of unspecified ulna

● **S52.034** Nondisplaced fracture of olecranon process with intraarticular extension of right ulna

● **S52.035** Nondisplaced fracture of olecranon process with intraarticular extension of left ulna

● **S52.036** Nondisplaced fracture of olecranon process with intraarticular extension of unspecified ulna

● **S52.04** **Fracture of coronoid process of ulna**

● **S52.041** Displaced fracture of coronoid process of right ulna

● **S52.042** Displaced fracture of coronoid process of left ulna

● **S52.043** Displaced fracture of coronoid process of unspecified ulna

● **S52.044** Nondisplaced fracture of coronoid process of right ulna

● **S52.045** Nondisplaced fracture of coronoid process of left ulna

● **S52.046** Nondisplaced fracture of coronoid process of unspecified ulna

● **S52.09** **Other fracture of upper end of ulna**

● **S52.091** Other fracture of upper end of right ulna

● **S52.092** Other fracture of upper end of left ulna

● **S52.099** Other fracture of upper end of unspecified ulna

● **S52.1** **Fracture of upper end of radius**

Fracture of proximal end of radius

Excludes2 physeal fractures of upper end of radius (S59.2-)

fracture of shaft of radius (S52.3-)

● **S52.10** **Unspecified fracture of upper end of radius**

● **S52.101** Unspecified fracture of upper end of right radius

● **S52.102** Unspecified fracture of upper end of left radius

● **S52.109** Unspecified fracture of upper end of unspecified radius

CHAPTER 19 (S00-T88)

● S52.11   Torus fracture of upper end of radius

The appropriate 7th character is to be added to all codes in subcategory S52.11

A	initial encounter for closed fracture
D	subsequent encounter for fracture with routine healing
G	subsequent encounter for fracture with delayed healing
K	subsequent encounter for fracture with nonunion
P	subsequent encounter for fracture with malunion
S	sequela

   ● S52.111   Torus fracture of upper end of right radius
   ● S52.112   Torus fracture of upper end of left radius
   ● S52.119   Torus fracture of upper end of unspecified radius
● S52.12   Fracture of head of radius
   ● S52.121   Displaced fracture of head of right radius
   ● S52.122   Displaced fracture of head of left radius
   ● S52.123   Displaced fracture of head of unspecified radius
   ● S52.124   Nondisplaced fracture of head of right radius
   ● S52.125   Nondisplaced fracture of head of left radius
   ● S52.126   Nondisplaced fracture of head of unspecified radius
● S52.13   Fracture of neck of radius
   ● S52.131   Displaced fracture of neck of right radius
   ● S52.132   Displaced fracture of neck of left radius
   ● S52.133   Displaced fracture of neck of unspecified radius
   ● S52.134   Nondisplaced fracture of neck of right radius
   ● S52.135   Nondisplaced fracture of neck of left radius
   ● S52.136   Nondisplaced fracture of neck of unspecified radius
● S52.18   Other fracture of upper end of radius
   ● S52.181   Other fracture of upper end of right radius
   ● S52.182   Other fracture of upper end of left radius
   ● S52.189   Other fracture of upper end of unspecified radius
● S52.2   Fracture of shaft of ulna
   ● S52.20   Unspecified fracture of shaft of ulna
               Fracture of ulna NOS
      ● S52.201   Unspecified fracture of shaft of right ulna
      ● S52.202   Unspecified fracture of shaft of left ulna
      ● S52.209   Unspecified fracture of shaft of unspecified ulna

● S52.21   Greenstick fracture of shaft of ulna

The appropriate 7th character is to be added to all codes in subcategory S52.21

A	initial encounter for closed fracture
D	subsequent encounter for fracture with routine healing
G	subsequent encounter for fracture with delayed healing
K	subsequent encounter for fracture with nonunion
P	subsequent encounter for fracture with malunion
S	sequela

   ● S52.211   Greenstick fracture of shaft of right ulna
   ● S52.212   Greenstick fracture of shaft of left ulna
   ● S52.219   Greenstick fracture of shaft of unspecified ulna
● S52.22   Transverse fracture of shaft of ulna
   ● S52.221   Displaced transverse fracture of shaft of right ulna
   ● S52.222   Displaced transverse fracture of shaft of left ulna
   ● S52.223   Displaced transverse fracture of shaft of unspecified ulna
   ● S52.224   Nondisplaced transverse fracture of shaft of right ulna
   ● S52.225   Nondisplaced transverse fracture of shaft of left ulna
   ● S52.226   Nondisplaced transverse fracture of shaft of unspecified ulna
● S52.23   Oblique fracture of shaft of ulna
   ● S52.231   Displaced oblique fracture of shaft of right ulna
   ● S52.232   Displaced oblique fracture of shaft of left ulna
   ● S52.233   Displaced oblique fracture of shaft of unspecified ulna
   ● S52.234   Nondisplaced oblique fracture of shaft of right ulna
   ● S52.235   Nondisplaced oblique fracture of shaft of left ulna
   ● S52.236   Nondisplaced oblique fracture of shaft of unspecified ulna
● S52.24   Spiral fracture of shaft of ulna
   ● S52.241   Displaced spiral fracture of shaft of ulna, right arm
   ● S52.242   Displaced spiral fracture of shaft of ulna, left arm
   ● S52.243   Displaced spiral fracture of shaft of ulna, unspecified arm
   ● S52.244   Nondisplaced spiral fracture of shaft of ulna, right arm
   ● S52.245   Nondisplaced spiral fracture of shaft of ulna, left arm
   ● S52.246   Nondisplaced spiral fracture of shaft of ulna, unspecified arm
● S52.25   Comminuted fracture of shaft of ulna
   ● S52.251   Displaced comminuted fracture of shaft of ulna, right arm
   ● S52.252   Displaced comminuted fracture of shaft of ulna, left arm
   ● S52.253   Displaced comminuted fracture of shaft of ulna, unspecified arm

▶ New   ➡ Revised   ~~deleted~~ Deleted   Excludes 1   Excludes 2   Includes   Use additional   Code first   Code also   Key words
OGCR Official Guidelines   X Assign placeholder X   ● Use Additional Character(s)   ▶ Manifestation Code   🔖 Hierarchical Condition Category   Coding Clinic

● S52.254 Nondisplaced comminuted fracture of shaft of ulna, **right arm**
● S52.255 Nondisplaced comminuted fracture of shaft of ulna, **left arm**
● S52.256 Nondisplaced comminuted fracture of shaft of ulna, **unspecified arm**
● S52.26 Segmental fracture of shaft of ulna
  ● S52.261 Displaced segmental fracture of shaft of ulna, **right arm**
  ● S52.262 Displaced segmental fracture of shaft of ulna, **left arm**
  ● S52.263 Displaced segmental fracture of shaft of ulna, **unspecified arm**
  ● S52.264 Nondisplaced segmental fracture of shaft of ulna, **right arm**
  ● S52.265 Nondisplaced segmental fracture of shaft of ulna, **left arm**
  ● S52.266 Nondisplaced segmental fracture of shaft of ulna, **unspecified arm**
● S52.27 Monteggia's fracture of ulna
  Fracture of upper shaft of ulna with dislocation of radial head
  ● S52.271 Monteggia's fracture of **right** ulna
  ● S52.272 Monteggia's fracture of **left** ulna
  ● S52.279 Monteggia's fracture of **unspecified** ulna
● S52.28 Bent bone of ulna
  ● S52.281 Bent bone of **right** ulna
  ● S52.282 Bent bone of **left** ulna
  ● S52.283 Bent bone of **unspecified** ulna
● S52.29 Other fracture of shaft of ulna
  ● S52.291 Other fracture of shaft of **right** ulna
  ● S52.292 Other fracture of shaft of **left** ulna
  ● S52.299 Other fracture of shaft of **unspecified** ulna
● S52.3 Fracture of shaft of radius
  ● S52.30 Unspecified fracture of shaft of radius
    ● S52.301 Unspecified fracture of shaft of **right** radius
    ● S52.302 Unspecified fracture of shaft of **left** radius
    ● S52.309 Unspecified fracture of shaft of **unspecified** radius
  ● S52.31 Greenstick fracture of shaft of radius
    The appropriate 7th character is to be added to all codes in subcategory S52.31

A	initial encounter for closed fracture
D	subsequent encounter for fracture with routine healing
G	subsequent encounter for fracture with delayed healing
K	subsequent encounter for fracture with nonunion
P	subsequent encounter for fracture with malunion
S	sequela

    ● S52.311 Greenstick fracture of shaft of radius, **right arm**
    ● S52.312 Greenstick fracture of shaft of radius, **left arm**
    ● S52.319 Greenstick fracture of shaft of radius, **unspecified arm**

● S52.32 Transverse fracture of shaft of radius
  ● S52.321 Displaced transverse fracture of shaft of **right** radius
  ● S52.322 Displaced transverse fracture of shaft of **left** radius
  ● S52.323 Displaced transverse fracture of shaft of **unspecified** radius
  ● S52.324 Nondisplaced transverse fracture of shaft of **right** radius
  ● S52.325 Nondisplaced transverse fracture of shaft of **left** radius
  ● S52.326 Nondisplaced transverse fracture of shaft of **unspecified** radius
● S52.33 Oblique fracture of shaft of radius
  ● S52.331 Displaced oblique fracture of shaft of **right** radius
  ● S52.332 Displaced oblique fracture of shaft of **left** radius
  ● S52.333 Displaced oblique fracture of shaft of **unspecified** radius
  ● S52.334 Nondisplaced oblique fracture of shaft of **right** radius
  ● S52.335 Nondisplaced oblique fracture of shaft of **left** radius
  ● S52.336 Nondisplaced oblique fracture of shaft of **unspecified** radius
● S52.34 Spiral fracture of shaft of radius
  ● S52.341 Displaced spiral fracture of shaft of radius, **right arm**
  ● S52.342 Displaced spiral fracture of shaft of radius, **left arm**
  ● S52.343 Displaced spiral fracture of shaft of radius, **unspecified arm**
  ● S52.344 Nondisplaced spiral fracture of shaft of radius, **right arm**
  ● S52.345 Nondisplaced spiral fracture of shaft of radius, **left arm**
  ● S52.346 Nondisplaced spiral fracture of shaft of radius, **unspecified arm**
● S52.35 Comminuted fracture of shaft of radius
  ● S52.351 Displaced comminuted fracture of shaft of radius, **right arm**
  ● S52.352 Displaced comminuted fracture of shaft of radius, **left arm**
  ● S52.353 Displaced comminuted fracture of shaft of radius, **unspecified arm**
  ● S52.354 Nondisplaced comminuted fracture of shaft of radius, **right arm**
  ● S52.355 Nondisplaced comminuted fracture of shaft of radius, **left arm**
  ● S52.356 Nondisplaced comminuted fracture of shaft of radius, **unspecified arm**
● S52.36 Segmental fracture of shaft of radius
  ● S52.361 Displaced segmental fracture of shaft of radius, **right arm**
  ● S52.362 Displaced segmental fracture of shaft of radius, **left arm**
  ● S52.363 Displaced segmental fracture of shaft of radius, **unspecified arm**
  ● S52.364 Nondisplaced segmental fracture of shaft of radius, **right arm**
  ● S52.365 Nondisplaced segmental fracture of shaft of radius, **left arm**
  ● S52.366 Nondisplaced segmental fracture of shaft of radius, **unspecified arm**

CHAPTER 19 (S00-T88)

- **S52.37** **Galeazzi's fracture**
  Fracture of lower shaft of radius with
  radioulnar joint dislocation
  - **S52.371** Galeazzi's fracture of right radius
  - **S52.372** Galeazzi's fracture of left radius
  - **S52.379** Galeazzi's fracture of unspecified radius
- **S52.38** **Bent bone of radius**
  - **S52.381** Bent bone of right radius
  - **S52.382** Bent bone of left radius
  - **S52.389** Bent bone of unspecified radius
- **S52.39** **Other fracture of shaft of radius**
  - **S52.391** Other fracture of shaft of radius, right arm
  - **S52.392** Other fracture of shaft of radius, left arm
  - **S52.399** Other fracture of shaft of radius, unspecified arm
- **S52.5** **Fracture of lower end of radius**
  Fracture of distal end of radius
  Excludes2 physeal fractures of lower end of radius (S59.2-)
  - **S52.50** **Unspecified fracture of the lower end of radius**
    - **S52.501** Unspecified fracture of the lower end of right radius
    - **S52.502** Unspecified fracture of the lower end of left radius
    - **S52.509** Unspecified fracture of the lower end of unspecified radius
  - **S52.51** **Fracture of radial styloid process**
    - **S52.511** Displaced fracture of right radial styloid process
    - **S52.512** Displaced fracture of left radial styloid process
    - **S52.513** Displaced fracture of unspecified radial styloid process
    - **S52.514** Nondisplaced fracture of right radial styloid process
    - **S52.515** Nondisplaced fracture of left radial styloid process
    - **S52.516** Nondisplaced fracture of unspecified radial styloid process
  - **S52.52** **Torus fracture of lower end of radius**
    The appropriate 7th character is to be added to all codes in subcategory S52.52

A	initial encounter for closed fracture
D	subsequent encounter for fracture with routine healing
G	subsequent encounter for fracture with delayed healing
K	subsequent encounter for fracture with nonunion
P	subsequent encounter for fracture with malunion
S	sequela

    - **S52.521** Torus fracture of lower end of right radius
    - **S52.522** Torus fracture of lower end of left radius
    - **S52.529** Torus fracture of lower end of unspecified radius
  - **S52.53** **Colles' fracture**
    - **S52.531** Colles' fracture of right radius
    - **S52.532** Colles' fracture of left radius
      Coding Clinic: 2016, Q2, P5
    - **S52.539** Colles' fracture of unspecified radius

- **S52.54** **Smith's fracture**
  - **S52.541** Smith's fracture of right radius
  - **S52.542** Smith's fracture of left radius
  - **S52.549** Smith's fracture of unspecified radius
- **S52.55** **Other extraarticular fracture of lower end of radius**
  - **S52.551** Other extraarticular fracture of lower end of right radius
  - **S52.552** Other extraarticular fracture of lower end of left radius
  - **S52.559** Other extraarticular fracture of lower end of unspecified radius
- **S52.56** **Barton's fracture**
  - **S52.561** Barton's fracture of right radius
  - **S52.562** Barton's fracture of left radius
  - **S52.569** Barton's fracture of unspecified radius
- **S52.57** **Other intraarticular fracture of lower end of radius**
  - **S52.571** Other intraarticular fracture of lower end of right radius
  - **S52.572** Other intraarticular fracture of lower end of left radius
  - **S52.579** Other intraarticular fracture of lower end of unspecified radius
- **S52.59** **Other fractures of lower end of radius**
  - **S52.591** Other fractures of lower end of right radius
    Coding Clinic: 2019, Q3, P10
  - **S52.592** Other fractures of lower end of left radius
  - **S52.599** Other fractures of lower end of unspecified radius
- **S52.6** **Fracture of lower end of ulna**
  - **S52.60** **Unspecified fracture of lower end of ulna**
    - **S52.601** Unspecified fracture of lower end of right ulna
    - **S52.602** Unspecified fracture of lower end of left ulna
    - **S52.609** Unspecified fracture of lower end of unspecified ulna
  - **S52.61** **Fracture of ulna styloid process**
    - **S52.611** Displaced fracture of right ulna styloid process
    - **S52.612** Displaced fracture of left ulna styloid process
    - **S52.613** Displaced fracture of unspecified ulna styloid process
    - **S52.614** Nondisplaced fracture of right ulna styloid process
    - **S52.615** Nondisplaced fracture of left ulna styloid process
    - **S52.616** Nondisplaced fracture of unspecified ulna styloid process
  - **S52.62** **Torus fracture of lower end of ulna**
    The appropriate 7th character is to be added to all codes in subcategory S52.62

A	initial encounter for closed fracture
D	subsequent encounter for fracture with routine healing
G	subsequent encounter for fracture with delayed healing
K	subsequent encounter for fracture with nonunion
P	subsequent encounter for fracture with malunion
S	sequela

    - **S52.621** Torus fracture of lower end of right ulna

● S52.622   Torus fracture of lower end of left ulna

● S52.629   Torus fracture of lower end of unspecified ulna

● S52.69   Other fracture of lower end of ulna

    ● S52.691   Other fracture of lower end of right ulna
       Coding Clinic: 2019, Q3, P10

    ● S52.692   Other fracture of lower end of left ulna

    ● S52.699   Other fracture of lower end of unspecified ulna

● S52.9   Unspecified fracture of forearm

  X ● S52.90   Unspecified fracture of unspecified forearm

  X ● S52.91   Unspecified fracture of right forearm

  X ● S52.92   Unspecified fracture of left forearm

● **S53**   **Dislocation and sprain of joints and ligaments of elbow**

    Includes   avulsion of joint or ligament of elbow
       laceration of cartilage, joint or ligament of elbow
       sprain of cartilage, joint or ligament of elbow
       traumatic hemarthrosis of joint or ligament of elbow
       traumatic rupture of joint or ligament of elbow
       traumatic subluxation of joint or ligament of elbow
       traumatic tear of joint or ligament of elbow

    Code also any associated open wound

    Excludes2   strain of muscle, fascia and tendon at forearm level (S56.-)

    The appropriate 7th character is to be added to each code from category S53

    | | |
    A   initial encounter
    D   subsequent encounter
    S   sequela

● S53.0   Subluxation and dislocation of radial head
    Dislocation of radiohumeral joint
    Subluxation of radiohumeral joint

    Excludes1   Monteggia's fracture-dislocation (S52.27-)

  ● S53.00   Unspecified subluxation and dislocation of radial head

    ● S53.001   Unspecified subluxation of right radial head

    ● S53.002   Unspecified subluxation of left radial head

    ● S53.003   Unspecified subluxation of unspecified radial head

    ● S53.004   Unspecified dislocation of right radial head

    ● S53.005   Unspecified dislocation of left radial head

    ● S53.006   Unspecified dislocation of unspecified radial head

  ● S53.01   Anterior subluxation and dislocation of radial head
    Anteriomedial subluxation and dislocation of radial head

    ● S53.011   Anterior subluxation of right radial head

    ● S53.012   Anterior subluxation of left radial head

    ● S53.013   Anterior subluxation of unspecified radial head

    ● S53.014   Anterior dislocation of right radial head

    ● S53.015   Anterior dislocation of left radial head

    ● S53.016   Anterior dislocation of unspecified radial head

● S53.02   Posterior subluxation and dislocation of radial head
    Posteriolateral subluxation and dislocation of radial head

    ● S53.021   Posterior subluxation of right radial head

    ● S53.022   Posterior subluxation of left radial head

    ● S53.023   Posterior subluxation of unspecified radial head

    ● S53.024   Posterior dislocation of right radial head

    ● S53.025   Posterior dislocation of left radial head

    ● S53.026   Posterior dislocation of unspecified radial head

● S53.03   Nursemaid's elbow

    ● S53.031   Nursemaid's elbow, right elbow
       Coding Clinic: 2015, Q1, P7-8

    ● S53.032   Nursemaid's elbow, left elbow

    ● S53.033   Nursemaid's elbow, unspecified elbow

● S53.09   Other subluxation and dislocation of radial head

    ● S53.091   Other subluxation of right radial head

    ● S53.092   Other subluxation of left radial head

    ● S53.093   Other subluxation of unspecified radial head

    ● S53.094   Other dislocation of right radial head

    ● S53.095   Other dislocation of left radial head

    ● S53.096   Other dislocation of unspecified radial head

● S53.1   Subluxation and dislocation of ulnohumeral joint
    Subluxation and dislocation of elbow NOS

    Excludes1   dislocation of radial head alone (S53.0-)

  ● S53.10   Unspecified subluxation and dislocation of ulnohumeral joint

    ● S53.101   Unspecified subluxation of right ulnohumeral joint

    ● S53.102   Unspecified subluxation of left ulnohumeral joint

    ● S53.103   Unspecified subluxation of unspecified ulnohumeral joint

    ● S53.104   Unspecified dislocation of right ulnohumeral joint

    ● S53.105   Unspecified dislocation of left ulnohumeral joint

    ● S53.106   Unspecified dislocation of unspecified ulnohumeral joint

  ● S53.11   Anterior subluxation and dislocation of ulnohumeral joint

    ● S53.111   Anterior subluxation of right ulnohumeral joint

    ● S53.112   Anterior subluxation of left ulnohumeral joint

    ● S53.113   Anterior subluxation of unspecified ulnohumeral joint

    ● S53.114   Anterior dislocation of right ulnohumeral joint
       Coding Clinic: 2012, Q4, P108

    ● S53.115   Anterior dislocation of left ulnohumeral joint

    ● S53.116   Anterior dislocation of unspecified ulnohumeral joint

  ● S53.12   Posterior subluxation and dislocation of ulnohumeral joint

    ● S53.121   Posterior subluxation of right ulnohumeral joint

    ● S53.122   Posterior subluxation of left ulnohumeral joint

S53.123   Posterior subluxation of unspecified ulnohumeral joint

S53.124   Posterior dislocation of right ulnohumeral joint

S53.125   Posterior dislocation of left ulnohumeral joint

S53.126   Posterior dislocation of unspecified ulnohumeral joint

S53.13   Medial subluxation and dislocation of ulnohumeral joint

S53.131   Medial subluxation of right ulnohumeral joint

S53.132   Medial subluxation of left ulnohumeral joint

S53.133   Medial subluxation of unspecified ulnohumeral joint

S53.134   Medial dislocation of right ulnohumeral joint

S53.135   Medial dislocation of left ulnohumeral joint

S53.136   Medial dislocation of unspecified ulnohumeral joint

S53.14   Lateral subluxation and dislocation of ulnohumeral joint

S53.141   Lateral subluxation of right ulnohumeral joint

S53.142   Lateral subluxation of left ulnohumeral joint

S53.143   Lateral subluxation of unspecified ulnohumeral joint

S53.144   Lateral dislocation of right ulnohumeral joint

S53.145   Lateral dislocation of left ulnohumeral joint

S53.146   Lateral dislocation of unspecified ulnohumeral joint

S53.19   Other subluxation and dislocation of ulnohumeral joint

S53.191   Other subluxation of right ulnohumeral joint

S53.192   Other subluxation of left ulnohumeral joint

S53.193   Other subluxation of unspecified ulnohumeral joint

S53.194   Other dislocation of right ulnohumeral joint

S53.195   Other dislocation of left ulnohumeral joint

S53.196   Other dislocation of unspecified ulnohumeral joint

S53.2   Traumatic rupture of radial collateral ligament

   Excludes1   sprain of radial collateral ligament NOS (S53.43-)

X   S53.20   Traumatic rupture of unspecified radial collateral ligament

X   S53.21   Traumatic rupture of right radial collateral ligament

X   S53.22   Traumatic rupture of left radial collateral ligament

S53.3   Traumatic rupture of ulnar collateral ligament

   Excludes1   sprain of ulnar collateral ligament (S53.44-)

X   S53.30   Traumatic rupture of unspecified ulnar collateral ligament

X   S53.31   Traumatic rupture of right ulnar collateral ligament

X   S53.32   Traumatic rupture of left ulnar collateral ligament

S53.4   Sprain of elbow

   Excludes2   traumatic rupture of radial collateral ligament (S53.2-)

                   traumatic rupture of ulnar collateral ligament (S53.3-)

S53.40   Unspecified sprain of elbow

S53.401   Unspecified sprain of right elbow

S53.402   Unspecified sprain of left elbow

S53.409   Unspecified sprain of unspecified elbow

            Sprain of elbow NOS

S53.41   Radiohumeral (joint) sprain

S53.411   Radiohumeral (joint) sprain of right elbow

S53.412   Radiohumeral (joint) sprain of left elbow

S53.419   Radiohumeral (joint) sprain of unspecified elbow

S53.42   Ulnohumeral (joint) sprain

S53.421   Ulnohumeral (joint) sprain of right elbow

S53.422   Ulnohumeral (joint) sprain of left elbow

S53.429   Ulnohumeral (joint) sprain of unspecified elbow

S53.43   Radial collateral ligament sprain

S53.431   Radial collateral ligament sprain of right elbow

S53.432   Radial collateral ligament sprain of left elbow

S53.439   Radial collateral ligament sprain of unspecified elbow

S53.44   Ulnar collateral ligament sprain

S53.441   Ulnar collateral ligament sprain of right elbow

S53.442   Ulnar collateral ligament sprain of left elbow

S53.449   Ulnar collateral ligament sprain of unspecified elbow

S53.49   Other sprain of elbow

S53.491   Other sprain of right elbow

S53.492   Other sprain of left elbow

S53.499   Other sprain of unspecified elbow

S54   Injury of nerves at forearm level

   Code also any associated open wound (S51.-)

   Excludes2   injury of nerves at wrist and hand level (S64.-)

   The appropriate 7th character is to be added to each code from category S54

A	initial encounter
D	subsequent encounter
S	sequela

S54.0   Injury of ulnar nerve at forearm level

   Injury of ulnar nerve NOS

X   S54.00   Injury of ulnar nerve at forearm level, unspecified arm

X   S54.01   Injury of ulnar nerve at forearm level, right arm

X   S54.02   Injury of ulnar nerve at forearm level, left arm

S54.1   Injury of median nerve at forearm level

   Injury of median nerve NOS

X   S54.10   Injury of median nerve at forearm level, unspecified arm

X   S54.11   Injury of median nerve at forearm level, right arm

X   S54.12   Injury of median nerve at forearm level, left arm

● **S54.2**   **Injury of radial nerve at forearm level**
      Injury of radial nerve NOS
   X ● **S54.20**   Injury of radial nerve at forearm level, **unspecified** arm
   X ● **S54.21**   Injury of radial nerve at forearm level, **right** arm
   X ● **S54.22**   Injury of radial nerve at forearm level, **left** arm

● **S54.3**   **Injury of cutaneous sensory nerve at forearm level**
   X ● **S54.30**   Injury of cutaneous sensory nerve at forearm level, **unspecified** arm
   X ● **S54.31**   Injury of cutaneous sensory nerve at forearm level, **right** arm
   X ● **S54.32**   Injury of cutaneous sensory nerve at forearm level, **left** arm

● **S54.8**   **Injury of other nerves at forearm level**
   ● **S54.8X**   Injury of other nerves at forearm level
     ● **S54.8X1**   Injury of other nerves at forearm level, **right** arm
     ● **S54.8X2**   Injury of other nerves at forearm level, **left** arm
     ● **S54.8X9**   Injury of other nerves at forearm level, **unspecified** arm

● **S54.9**   **Injury of unspecified nerve at forearm level**
   X ● **S54.90**   Injury of unspecified nerve at forearm level, **unspecified** arm
   X ● **S54.91**   Injury of unspecified nerve at forearm level, **right** arm
   X ● **S54.92**   Injury of unspecified nerve at forearm level, **left** arm

● **S55**   **Injury of blood vessels at forearm level**
     Code also any associated open wound (S51.-)
     Excludes2   injury of blood vessels at wrist and hand level (S65.-)
                injury of brachial vessels (S45.1-S45.2)
     The appropriate 7th character is to be added to each code from category S55

A	initial encounter
D	subsequent encounter
S	sequela

● **S55.0**   **Injury of ulnar artery at forearm level**
   ● **S55.00**   Unspecified injury of ulnar artery at forearm level
     ● **S55.001**   Unspecified injury of ulnar artery at forearm level, **right** arm
     ● **S55.002**   Unspecified injury of ulnar artery at forearm level, **left** arm
     ● **S55.009**   Unspecified injury of ulnar artery at forearm level, **unspecified** arm
   ● **S55.01**   Laceration of ulnar artery at forearm level
     ● **S55.011**   Laceration of ulnar artery at forearm level, **right** arm
     ● **S55.012**   Laceration of ulnar artery at forearm level, **left** arm
     ● **S55.019**   Laceration of ulnar artery at forearm level, **unspecified** arm
   ● **S55.09**   Other specified injury of ulnar artery at forearm level
     ● **S55.091**   Other specified injury of ulnar artery at forearm level, **right** arm
     ● **S55.092**   Other specified injury of ulnar artery at forearm level, **left** arm
     ● **S55.099**   Other specified injury of ulnar artery at forearm level, **unspecified** arm

● **S55.1**   **Injury of radial artery at forearm level**
   ● **S55.10**   Unspecified injury of radial artery at forearm level
     ● **S55.101**   Unspecified injury of radial artery at forearm level, **right** arm

● **S55.102**   Unspecified injury of radial artery at forearm level, **left** arm
● **S55.109**   Unspecified injury of radial artery at forearm level, **unspecified** arm

 ● **S55.11**   Laceration of radial artery at forearm level
   ● **S55.111**   Laceration of radial artery at forearm level, **right** arm
   ● **S55.112**   Laceration of radial artery at forearm level, **left** arm
   ● **S55.119**   Laceration of radial artery at forearm level, **unspecified** arm

 ● **S55.19**   Other specified injury of radial artery at forearm level
   ● **S55.191**   Other specified injury of radial artery at forearm level, **right** arm
   ● **S55.192**   Other specified injury of radial artery at forearm level, **left** arm
   ● **S55.199**   Other specified injury of radial artery at forearm level, **unspecified** arm

● **S55.2**   **Injury of vein at forearm level**
 ● **S55.20**   Unspecified injury of vein at forearm level
   ● **S55.201**   Unspecified injury of vein at forearm level, **right** arm
   ● **S55.202**   Unspecified injury of vein at forearm level, **left** arm
   ● **S55.209**   Unspecified injury of vein at forearm level, **unspecified** arm
 ● **S55.21**   Laceration of vein at forearm level
   ● **S55.211**   Laceration of vein at forearm level, **right** arm
   ● **S55.212**   Laceration of vein at forearm level, **left** arm
   ● **S55.219**   Laceration of vein at forearm level, **unspecified** arm
 ● **S55.29**   Other specified injury of vein at forearm level
   ● **S55.291**   Other specified injury of vein at forearm level, **right** arm
   ● **S55.292**   Other specified injury of vein at forearm level, **left** arm
   ● **S55.299**   Other specified injury of vein at forearm level, **unspecified** arm

● **S55.8**   **Injury of other blood vessels at forearm level**
 ● **S55.80**   Unspecified injury of other blood vessels at forearm level
   ● **S55.801**   Unspecified injury of other blood vessels at forearm level, **right** arm
   ● **S55.802**   Unspecified injury of other blood vessels at forearm level, **left** arm
   ● **S55.809**   Unspecified injury of other blood vessels at forearm level, **unspecified** arm
 ● **S55.81**   Laceration of other blood vessels at forearm level
   ● **S55.811**   Laceration of other blood vessels at forearm level, **right** arm
   ● **S55.812**   Laceration of other blood vessels at forearm level, **left** arm
   ● **S55.819**   Laceration of other blood vessels at forearm level, **unspecified** arm
 ● **S55.89**   Other specified injury of other blood vessels at forearm level
   ● **S55.891**   Other specified injury of other blood vessels at forearm level, **right** arm
   ● **S55.892**   Other specified injury of other blood vessels at forearm level, **left** arm
   ● **S55.899**   Other specified injury of other blood vessels at forearm level, **unspecified** arm

CHAPTER 19 (S00-T88)

- S55.9   Injury of unspecified blood vessel at forearm level
  - S55.90   Unspecified injury of unspecified blood vessel at forearm level
    - S55.901   Unspecified injury of unspecified blood vessel at forearm level, right arm
    - S55.902   Unspecified injury of unspecified blood vessel at forearm level, left arm
    - S55.909   Unspecified injury of unspecified blood vessel at forearm level, unspecified arm
  - S55.91   Laceration of unspecified blood vessel at forearm level
    - S55.911   Laceration of unspecified blood vessel at forearm level, right arm
    - S55.912   Laceration of unspecified blood vessel at forearm level, left arm
    - S55.919   Laceration of unspecified blood vessel at forearm level, unspecified arm
  - S55.99   Other specified injury of unspecified blood vessel at forearm level
    - S55.991   Other specified injury of unspecified blood vessel at forearm level, right arm
    - S55.992   Other specified injury of unspecified blood vessel at forearm level, left arm
    - S55.999   Other specified injury of unspecified blood vessel at forearm level, unspecified arm

- S56   Injury of muscle, fascia and tendon at forearm level

  Code also any associated open wound (S51.-)

  Excludes2   injury of muscle, fascia and tendon at or below wrist (S66.-)

              sprain of joints and ligaments of elbow (S53.4-)

  The appropriate 7th character is to be added to each code from category S56

  > A   initial encounter
  > D   subsequent encounter
  > S   sequela

  - S56.0   Injury of flexor muscle, fascia and tendon of thumb at forearm level
    - S56.00   Unspecified injury of flexor muscle, fascia and tendon of thumb at forearm level
      - S56.001   Unspecified injury of flexor muscle, fascia and tendon of right thumb at forearm level
      - S56.002   Unspecified injury of flexor muscle, fascia and tendon of left thumb at forearm level
      - S56.009   Unspecified injury of flexor muscle, fascia and tendon of unspecified thumb at forearm level
    - S56.01   Strain of flexor muscle, fascia and tendon of thumb at forearm level
      - S56.011   Strain of flexor muscle, fascia and tendon of right thumb at forearm level
      - S56.012   Strain of flexor muscle, fascia and tendon of left thumb at forearm level
      - S56.019   Strain of flexor muscle, fascia and tendon of unspecified thumb at forearm level
    - S56.02   Laceration of flexor muscle, fascia and tendon of thumb at forearm level
      - S56.021   Laceration of flexor muscle, fascia and tendon of right thumb at forearm level
      - S56.022   Laceration of flexor muscle, fascia and tendon of left thumb at forearm level
      - S56.029   Laceration of flexor muscle, fascia and tendon of unspecified thumb at forearm level
    - S56.09   Other injury of flexor muscle, fascia and tendon of thumb at forearm level
      - S56.091   Other injury of flexor muscle, fascia and tendon of right thumb at forearm level
      - S56.092   Other injury of flexor muscle, fascia and tendon of left thumb at forearm level
      - S56.099   Other injury of flexor muscle, fascia and tendon of unspecified thumb at forearm level
  - S56.1   Injury of flexor muscle, fascia and tendon of other and unspecified finger at forearm level
    - S56.10   Unspecified injury of flexor muscle, fascia and tendon of other and unspecified finger at forearm level
      - S56.101   Unspecified injury of flexor muscle, fascia and tendon of right index finger at forearm level
      - S56.102   Unspecified injury of flexor muscle, fascia and tendon of left index finger at forearm level
      - S56.103   Unspecified injury of flexor muscle, fascia and tendon of right middle finger at forearm level
      - S56.104   Unspecified injury of flexor muscle, fascia and tendon of left middle finger at forearm level
      - S56.105   Unspecified injury of flexor muscle, fascia and tendon of right ring finger at forearm level
      - S56.106   Unspecified injury of flexor muscle, fascia and tendon of left ring finger at forearm level
      - S56.107   Unspecified injury of flexor muscle, fascia and tendon of right little finger at forearm level
      - S56.108   Unspecified injury of flexor muscle, fascia and tendon of left little finger at forearm level
      - S56.109   Unspecified injury of flexor muscle, fascia and tendon of unspecified finger at forearm level
    - S56.11   Strain of flexor muscle, fascia and tendon of other and unspecified finger at forearm level
      - S56.111   Strain of flexor muscle, fascia and tendon of right index finger at forearm level
      - S56.112   Strain of flexor muscle, fascia and tendon of left index finger at forearm level
      - S56.113   Strain of flexor muscle, fascia and tendon of right middle finger at forearm level
      - S56.114   Strain of flexor muscle, fascia and tendon of left middle finger at forearm level
      - S56.115   Strain of flexor muscle, fascia and tendon of right ring finger at forearm level

▶ New   ⇒ Revised   ~~deleted~~ Deleted   Excludes 1   Excludes 2   Includes   Use additional   Code first   Code also   Key words

OGCR Official Guidelines   X Assign placeholder X   ● Use Additional Character(s)   ▶ Manifestation Code   🦠 Hierarchical Condition Category   **Coding Clinic**

● S56.116 Strain of flexor muscle, fascia and tendon of left ring finger at forearm level

● S56.117 Strain of flexor muscle, fascia and tendon of right little finger at forearm level

● S56.118 Strain of flexor muscle, fascia and tendon of left little finger at forearm level

● S56.119 Strain of flexor muscle, fascia and tendon of finger of unspecified finger at forearm level

● S56.12 Laceration of flexor muscle, fascia and tendon of other and unspecified finger at forearm level

● S56.121 Laceration of flexor muscle, fascia and tendon of right index finger at forearm level

● S56.122 Laceration of flexor muscle, fascia and tendon of left index finger at forearm level

● S56.123 Laceration of flexor muscle, fascia and tendon of right middle finger at forearm level

● S56.124 Laceration of flexor muscle, fascia and tendon of left middle finger at forearm level

● S56.125 Laceration of flexor muscle, fascia and tendon of right ring finger at forearm level

● S56.126 Laceration of flexor muscle, fascia and tendon of left ring finger at forearm level

● S56.127 Laceration of flexor muscle, fascia and tendon of right little finger at forearm level

● S56.128 Laceration of flexor muscle, fascia and tendon of left little finger at forearm level

● S56.129 Laceration of flexor muscle, fascia and tendon of unspecified finger at forearm level

● S56.19 Other injury of flexor muscle, fascia and tendon of other and unspecified finger at forearm level

● S56.191 Other injury of flexor muscle, fascia and tendon of right index finger at forearm level

● S56.192 Other injury of flexor muscle, fascia and tendon of left index finger at forearm level

● S56.193 Other injury of flexor muscle, fascia and tendon of right middle finger at forearm level

● S56.194 Other injury of flexor muscle, fascia and tendon of left middle finger at forearm level

● S56.195 Other injury of flexor muscle, fascia and tendon of right ring finger at forearm level

● S56.196 Other injury of flexor muscle, fascia and tendon of left ring finger at forearm level

● S56.197 Other injury of flexor muscle, fascia and tendon of right little finger at forearm level

● S56.198 Other injury of flexor muscle, fascia and tendon of left little finger at forearm level

● S56.199 Other injury of flexor muscle, fascia and tendon of unspecified finger at forearm level

● S56.2 Injury of other flexor muscle, fascia and tendon at forearm level

● S56.20 Unspecified injury of other flexor muscle, fascia and tendon at forearm level

● S56.201 Unspecified injury of other flexor muscle, fascia and tendon at forearm level, right arm

● S56.202 Unspecified injury of other flexor muscle, fascia and tendon at forearm level, left arm

● S56.209 Unspecified injury of other flexor muscle, fascia and tendon at forearm level, unspecified arm

● S56.21 Strain of other flexor muscle, fascia and tendon at forearm level

● S56.211 Strain of other flexor muscle, fascia and tendon at forearm level, right arm

● S56.212 Strain of other flexor muscle, fascia and tendon at forearm level, left arm

● S56.219 Strain of other flexor muscle, fascia and tendon at forearm level, unspecified arm

● S56.22 Laceration of other flexor muscle, fascia and tendon at forearm level

● S56.221 Laceration of other flexor muscle, fascia and tendon at forearm level, right arm

● S56.222 Laceration of other flexor muscle, fascia and tendon at forearm level, left arm

● S56.229 Laceration of other flexor muscle, fascia and tendon at forearm level, unspecified arm

● S56.29 Other injury of other flexor muscle, fascia and tendon at forearm level

● S56.291 Other injury of other flexor muscle, fascia and tendon at forearm level, right arm

● S56.292 Other injury of other flexor muscle, fascia and tendon at forearm level, left arm

● S56.299 Other injury of other flexor muscle, fascia and tendon at forearm level, unspecified arm

● S56.3 Injury of extensor or abductor muscles, fascia and tendons of thumb at forearm level

● S56.30 Unspecified injury of extensor or abductor muscles, fascia and tendons of thumb at forearm level

● S56.301 Unspecified injury of extensor or abductor muscles, fascia and tendons of right thumb at forearm level

● S56.302 Unspecified injury of extensor or abductor muscles, fascia and tendons of left thumb at forearm level

● S56.309 Unspecified injury of extensor or abductor muscles, fascia and tendons of unspecified thumb at forearm level

● S56.31 Strain of extensor or abductor muscles, fascia and tendons of thumb at forearm level

● S56.311 Strain of extensor or abductor muscles, fascia and tendons of right thumb at forearm level

● S56.312 Strain of extensor or abductor muscles, fascia and tendons of left thumb at forearm level

● S56.319 Strain of extensor or abductor muscles, fascia and tendons of unspecified thumb at forearm level

CHAPTER 19 (S00-T88)

● S56.32   Laceration of extensor or abductor muscles, fascia and tendons of thumb at forearm level
- ● S56.321   Laceration of extensor or abductor muscles, fascia and tendons of right thumb at forearm level
- ● S56.322   Laceration of extensor or abductor muscles, fascia and tendons of left thumb at forearm level
- ● S56.329   Laceration of extensor or abductor muscles, fascia and tendons of unspecified thumb at forearm level

● S56.39   Other injury of extensor or abductor muscles, fascia and tendons of thumb at forearm level
- ● S56.391   Other injury of extensor or abductor muscles, fascia and tendons of right thumb at forearm level
- ● S56.392   Other injury of extensor or abductor muscles, fascia and tendons of left thumb at forearm level
- ● S56.399   Other injury of extensor or abductor muscles, fascia and tendons of unspecified thumb at forearm level

● S56.4   Injury of extensor muscle, fascia and tendon of other and unspecified finger at forearm level

● S56.40   Unspecified injury of extensor muscle, fascia and tendon of other and unspecified finger at forearm level
- ● S56.401   Unspecified injury of extensor muscle, fascia and tendon of right index finger at forearm level
- ● S56.402   Unspecified injury of extensor muscle, fascia and tendon of left index finger at forearm level
- ● S56.403   Unspecified injury of extensor muscle, fascia and tendon of right middle finger at forearm level
- ● S56.404   Unspecified injury of extensor muscle, fascia and tendon of left middle finger at forearm level
- ● S56.405   Unspecified injury of extensor muscle, fascia and tendon of right ring finger at forearm level
- ● S56.406   Unspecified injury of extensor muscle, fascia and tendon of left ring finger at forearm level
- ● S56.407   Unspecified injury of extensor muscle, fascia and tendon of right little finger at forearm level
- ● S56.408   Unspecified injury of extensor muscle, fascia and tendon of left little finger at forearm level
- ● S56.409   Unspecified injury of extensor muscle, fascia and tendon of unspecified finger at forearm level

● S56.41   Strain of extensor muscle, fascia and tendon of other and unspecified finger at forearm level
- ● S56.411   Strain of extensor muscle, fascia and tendon of right index finger at forearm level
- ● S56.412   Strain of extensor muscle, fascia and tendon of left index finger at forearm level
- ● S56.413   Strain of extensor muscle, fascia and tendon of right middle finger at forearm level
- ● S56.414   Strain of extensor muscle, fascia and tendon of left middle finger at forearm level
- ● S56.415   Strain of extensor muscle, fascia and tendon of right ring finger at forearm level

- ● S56.416   Strain of extensor muscle, fascia and tendon of left ring finger at forearm level
- ● S56.417   Strain of extensor muscle, fascia and tendon of right little finger at forearm level
- ● S56.418   Strain of extensor muscle, fascia and tendon of left little finger at forearm level
- ● S56.419   Strain of extensor muscle, fascia and tendon of finger, unspecified finger at forearm level

● S56.42   Laceration of extensor muscle, fascia and tendon of other and unspecified finger at forearm level
- ● S56.421   Laceration of extensor muscle, fascia and tendon of right index finger at forearm level
- ● S56.422   Laceration of extensor muscle, fascia and tendon of left index finger at forearm level
- ● S56.423   Laceration of extensor muscle, fascia and tendon of right middle finger at forearm level
- ● S56.424   Laceration of extensor muscle, fascia and tendon of left middle finger at forearm level
- ● S56.425   Laceration of extensor muscle, fascia and tendon of right ring finger at forearm level
- ● S56.426   Laceration of extensor muscle, fascia and tendon of left ring finger at forearm level
- ● S56.427   Laceration of extensor muscle, fascia and tendon of right little finger at forearm level
- ● S56.428   Laceration of extensor muscle, fascia and tendon of left little finger at forearm level
- ● S56.429   Laceration of extensor muscle, fascia and tendon of unspecified finger at forearm level

● S56.49   Other injury of extensor muscle, fascia and tendon of other and unspecified finger at forearm level
- ● S56.491   Other injury of extensor muscle, fascia and tendon of right index finger at forearm level
- ● S56.492   Other injury of extensor muscle, fascia and tendon of left index finger at forearm level
- ● S56.493   Other injury of extensor muscle, fascia and tendon of right middle finger at forearm level
- ● S56.494   Other injury of extensor muscle, fascia and tendon of left middle finger at forearm level
- ● S56.495   Other injury of extensor muscle, fascia and tendon of right ring finger at forearm level
- ● S56.496   Other injury of extensor muscle, fascia and tendon of left ring finger at forearm level
- ● S56.497   Other injury of extensor muscle, fascia and tendon of right little finger at forearm level
- ● S56.498   Other injury of extensor muscle, fascia and tendon of left little finger at forearm level
- ● S56.499   Other injury of extensor muscle, fascia and tendon of unspecified finger at forearm level

▶ New   ⇒ Revised   ~~deleted~~ Deleted   Excludes 1   Excludes 2   Includes   Use additional   Code first   Code also   Key words

OGCR Official Guidelines   X Assign placeholder X   ● Use Additional Character(s)   ▶ Manifestation Code   🐾 Hierarchical Condition Category   **Coding Clinic**

● S56.5　Injury of other extensor muscle, fascia and tendon at forearm level
　● S56.50　Unspecified injury of other extensor muscle, fascia and tendon at forearm level
　　● S56.501　Unspecified injury of other extensor muscle, fascia and tendon at forearm level, right arm
　　● S56.502　Unspecified injury of other extensor muscle, fascia and tendon at forearm level, left arm
　　● S56.509　Unspecified injury of other extensor muscle, fascia and tendon at forearm level, unspecified arm
　● S56.51　Strain of other extensor muscle, fascia and tendon at forearm level
　　● S56.511　Strain of other extensor muscle, fascia and tendon at forearm level, right arm
　　● S56.512　Strain of other extensor muscle, fascia and tendon at forearm level, left arm
　　● S56.519　Strain of other extensor muscle, fascia and tendon at forearm level, unspecified arm
　● S56.52　Laceration of other extensor muscle, fascia and tendon at forearm level
　　● S56.521　Laceration of other extensor muscle, fascia and tendon at forearm level, right arm
　　● S56.522　Laceration of other extensor muscle, fascia and tendon at forearm level, left arm
　　● S56.529　Laceration of other extensor muscle, fascia and tendon at forearm level, unspecified arm
　● S56.59　Other injury of other extensor muscle, fascia and tendon at forearm level
　　● S56.591　Other injury of other extensor muscle, fascia and tendon at forearm level, right arm
　　● S56.592　Other injury of other extensor muscle, fascia and tendon at forearm level, left arm
　　● S56.599　Other injury of other extensor muscle, fascia and tendon at forearm level, unspecified arm
● S56.8　Injury of other muscles, fascia and tendons at forearm level
　● S56.80　Unspecified injury of other muscles, fascia and tendons at forearm level
　　● S56.801　Unspecified injury of other muscles, fascia and tendons at forearm level, right arm
　　● S56.802　Unspecified injury of other muscles, fascia and tendons at forearm level, left arm
　　● S56.809　Unspecified injury of other muscles, fascia and tendons at forearm level, unspecified arm
　● S56.81　Strain of other muscles, fascia and tendons at forearm level
　　● S56.811　Strain of other muscles, fascia and tendons at forearm level, right arm
　　● S56.812　Strain of other muscles, fascia and tendons at forearm level, left arm
　　● S56.819　Strain of other muscles, fascia and tendons at forearm level, unspecified arm

● S56.82　Laceration of other muscles, fascia and tendons at forearm level
　　● S56.821　Laceration of other muscles, fascia and tendons at forearm level, right arm
　　● S56.822　Laceration of other muscles, fascia and tendons at forearm level, left arm
　　● S56.829　Laceration of other muscles, fascia and tendons at forearm level, unspecified arm
　● S56.89　Other injury of other muscles, fascia and tendons at forearm level
　　● S56.891　Other injury of other muscles, fascia and tendons at forearm level, right arm
　　● S56.892　Other injury of other muscles, fascia and tendons at forearm level, left arm
　　● S56.899　Other injury of other muscles, fascia and tendons at forearm level, unspecified arm
● S56.9　Injury of unspecified muscles, fascia and tendons at forearm level
　● S56.90　Unspecified injury of unspecified muscles, fascia and tendons at forearm level
　　● S56.901　Unspecified injury of unspecified muscles, fascia and tendons at forearm level, right arm
　　● S56.902　Unspecified injury of unspecified muscles, fascia and tendons at forearm level, left arm
　　● S56.909　Unspecified injury of unspecified muscles, fascia and tendons at forearm level, unspecified arm
　● S56.91　Strain of unspecified muscles, fascia and tendons at forearm level
　　● S56.911　Strain of unspecified muscles, fascia and tendons at forearm level, right arm
　　● S56.912　Strain of unspecified muscles, fascia and tendons at forearm level, left arm
　　● S56.919　Strain of unspecified muscles, fascia and tendons at forearm level, unspecified arm
　● S56.92　Laceration of unspecified muscles, fascia and tendons at forearm level
　　● S56.921　Laceration of unspecified muscles, fascia and tendons at forearm level, right arm
　　● S56.922　Laceration of unspecified muscles, fascia and tendons at forearm level, left arm
　　● S56.929　Laceration of unspecified muscles, fascia and tendons at forearm level, unspecified arm
　● S56.99　Other injury of unspecified muscles, fascia and tendons at forearm level
　　● S56.991　Other injury of unspecified muscles, fascia and tendons at forearm level, right arm
　　● S56.992　Other injury of unspecified muscles, fascia and tendons at forearm level, left arm
　　● S56.999　Other injury of unspecified muscles, fascia and tendons at forearm level, unspecified arm

CHAPTER 19 (S00-T88)

● S57   **Crushing injury of elbow and forearm**
Use additional code(s) for all associated injuries
Excludes2   crushing injury of wrist and hand (S67.-)
The appropriate 7th character is to be added to each code from category S57

> A   initial encounter
> D   subsequent encounter
> S   sequela

● S57.0   **Crushing injury of elbow**
X● S57.00   Crushing injury of unspecified elbow
X● S57.01   Crushing injury of right elbow
X● S57.02   Crushing injury of left elbow
● S57.8   **Crushing injury of forearm**
X● S57.80   Crushing injury of unspecified forearm
X● S57.81   Crushing injury of right forearm
X● S57.82   Crushing injury of left forearm

● S58   **Traumatic amputation of elbow and forearm**
An amputation not identified as partial or complete should be coded to complete
Excludes1   traumatic amputation of wrist and hand (S68.-)
The appropriate 7th character is to be added to each code from category S58

> A   initial encounter
> D   subsequent encounter
> S   sequela

● S58.0   **Traumatic amputation at elbow level**
● S58.01   **Complete traumatic amputation at elbow level**
● S58.011   Complete traumatic amputation at elbow level, right arm A, S 🐾
● S58.012   Complete traumatic amputation at elbow level, left arm A, S 🐾
● S58.019   Complete traumatic amputation at elbow level, unspecified arm A, S 🐾
● S58.02   **Partial traumatic amputation at elbow level**
● S58.021   Partial traumatic amputation at elbow level, right arm A, S 🐾
● S58.022   Partial traumatic amputation at elbow level, left arm A, S 🐾
● S58.029   Partial traumatic amputation at elbow level, unspecified arm A, S 🐾
● S58.1   **Traumatic amputation at level between elbow and wrist**
● S58.11   **Complete traumatic amputation at level between elbow and wrist**
● S58.111   Complete traumatic amputation at level between elbow and wrist, right arm A, S 🐾
● S58.112   Complete traumatic amputation at level between elbow and wrist, left arm A, S 🐾
● S58.119   Complete traumatic amputation at level between elbow and wrist, unspecified arm A, S 🐾
● S58.12   **Partial traumatic amputation at level between elbow and wrist**
● S58.121   Partial traumatic amputation at level between elbow and wrist, right arm A, S 🐾
● S58.122   Partial traumatic amputation at level between elbow and wrist, left arm A, S 🐾
● S58.129   Partial traumatic amputation at level between elbow and wrist, unspecified arm A, S 🐾

● S58.9   **Traumatic amputation of forearm, level unspecified**
Excludes1   traumatic amputation of wrist (S68.-)
● S58.91   **Complete traumatic amputation of forearm, level unspecified**
● S58.911   Complete traumatic amputation of right forearm, level unspecified A, S 🐾
● S58.912   Complete traumatic amputation of left forearm, level unspecified A, S 🐾
● S58.919   Complete traumatic amputation of unspecified forearm, level unspecified A, S 🐾
● S58.92   **Partial traumatic amputation of forearm, level unspecified**
● S58.921   Partial traumatic amputation of right forearm, level unspecified A, S 🐾
● S58.922   Partial traumatic amputation of left forearm, level unspecified A, S 🐾
● S58.929   Partial traumatic amputation of unspecified forearm, level unspecified A, S 🐾

● S59   **Other and unspecified injuries of elbow and forearm**
Excludes2   other and unspecified injuries of wrist and hand (S69.-)
The appropriate 7th character is to be added to each code from subcategories S59.0, S59.1, and S59.2

> A   initial encounter for closed fracture
> D   subsequent encounter for fracture with routine healing
> G   subsequent encounter for fracture with delayed healing
> K   subsequent encounter for fracture with nonunion
> P   subsequent encounter for fracture with malunion
> S   sequela

● S59.0   **Physeal fracture of lower end of ulna**
● S59.00   **Unspecified physeal fracture of lower end of ulna**
● S59.001   Unspecified physeal fracture of lower end of ulna, right arm
● S59.002   Unspecified physeal fracture of lower end of ulna, left arm
● S59.009   Unspecified physeal fracture of lower end of ulna, unspecified arm
● S59.01   **Salter-Harris Type I physeal fracture of lower end of ulna**
● S59.011   Salter-Harris Type I physeal fracture of lower end of ulna, right arm
● S59.012   Salter-Harris Type I physeal fracture of lower end of ulna, left arm
● S59.019   Salter-Harris Type I physeal fracture of lower end of ulna, unspecified arm

Item 19–4   SALTER-HARRIS TYPE 1: epiphysis is completely separated from end of bone, or metaphysic growth plate remains attached to epiphysis
SALTER-HARRIS TYPE 2: epiphysis and growth plate are partially separated from metaphysis, which is cracked—most common type
SALTER-HARRIS TYPE 3: fracture occurring through epiphysis and separates part of epiphysis and growth plate from metaphysis fracture, usually at distal end of tibia
SALTER-HARRIS TYPE 4: fracture runs through epiphysis, across growth plate, into metaphysic, surgery is required to restore joint surface to normal and align growth plate

▶ New   ⇒ Revised   ~~deleted~~ Deleted   Excludes 1   Excludes 2   Includes   Use additional   Code first   Code also   Key words
OGCR Official Guidelines   X Assign placeholder X   ● Use Additional Character(s)   ▶ Manifestation Code   🐾 Hierarchical Condition Category   **Coding Clinic**

● S59.02   Salter-Harris Type II physeal fracture of lower end of ulna

     ● S59.021   Salter-Harris Type II physeal fracture of lower end of ulna, right arm

     ● S59.022   Salter-Harris Type II physeal fracture of lower end of ulna, left arm

     ● S59.029   Salter-Harris Type II physeal fracture of lower end of ulna, unspecified arm

● S59.03   Salter-Harris Type III physeal fracture of lower end of ulna

     ● S59.031   Salter-Harris Type III physeal fracture of lower end of ulna, right arm

     ● S59.032   Salter-Harris Type III physeal fracture of lower end of ulna, left arm

     ● S59.039   Salter-Harris Type III physeal fracture of lower end of ulna, unspecified arm

● S59.04   Salter-Harris Type IV physeal fracture of lower end of ulna

     ● S59.041   Salter-Harris Type IV physeal fracture of lower end of ulna, right arm

     ● S59.042   Salter-Harris Type IV physeal fracture of lower end of ulna, left arm

     ● S59.049   Salter-Harris Type IV physeal fracture of lower end of ulna, unspecified arm

● S59.09   Other physeal fracture of lower end of ulna

     ● S59.091   Other physeal fracture of lower end of ulna, right arm

     ● S59.092   Other physeal fracture of lower end of ulna, left arm

     ● S59.099   Other physeal fracture of lower end of ulna, unspecified arm

● S59.1   Physeal fracture of upper end of radius

     ● S59.10   Unspecified physeal fracture of upper end of radius

         ● S59.101   Unspecified physeal fracture of upper end of radius, right arm

         ● S59.102   Unspecified physeal fracture of upper end of radius, left arm

         ● S59.109   Unspecified physeal fracture of upper end of radius, unspecified arm

     ● S59.11   Salter-Harris Type I physeal fracture of upper end of radius

         ● S59.111   Salter-Harris Type I physeal fracture of upper end of radius, right arm

         ● S59.112   Salter-Harris Type I physeal fracture of upper end of radius, left arm

         ● S59.119   Salter-Harris Type I physeal fracture of upper end of radius, unspecified arm

     ● S59.12   Salter-Harris Type II physeal fracture of upper end of radius

         ● S59.121   Salter-Harris Type II physeal fracture of upper end of radius, right arm

         ● S59.122   Salter-Harris Type II physeal fracture of upper end of radius, left arm

         ● S59.129   Salter-Harris Type II physeal fracture of upper end of radius, unspecified arm

     ● S59.13   Salter-Harris Type III physeal fracture of upper end of radius

         ● S59.131   Salter-Harris Type III physeal fracture of upper end of radius, right arm

         ● S59.132   Salter-Harris Type III physeal fracture of upper end of radius, left arm

         ● S59.139   Salter-Harris Type III physeal fracture of upper end of radius, unspecified arm

● S59.14   Salter-Harris Type IV physeal fracture of upper end of radius

     ● S59.141   Salter-Harris Type IV physeal fracture of upper end of radius, right arm

     ● S59.142   Salter-Harris Type IV physeal fracture of upper end of radius, left arm

     ● S59.149   Salter-Harris Type IV physeal fracture of upper end of radius, unspecified arm

● S59.19   Other physeal fracture of upper end of radius

     ● S59.191   Other physeal fracture of upper end of radius, right arm

     ● S59.192   Other physeal fracture of upper end of radius, left arm

     ● S59.199   Other physeal fracture of upper end of radius, unspecified arm

● S59.2   Physeal fracture of lower end of radius

     ● S59.20   Unspecified physeal fracture of lower end of radius

         ● S59.201   Unspecified physeal fracture of lower end of radius, right arm

         ● S59.202   Unspecified physeal fracture of lower end of radius, left arm

         ● S59.209   Unspecified physeal fracture of lower end of radius, unspecified arm

     ● S59.21   Salter-Harris Type I physeal fracture of lower end of radius

         ● S59.211   Salter-Harris Type I physeal fracture of lower end of radius, right arm

         ● S59.212   Salter-Harris Type I physeal fracture of lower end of radius, left arm

         ● S59.219   Salter-Harris Type I physeal fracture of lower end of radius, unspecified arm

     ● S59.22   Salter-Harris Type II physeal fracture of lower end of radius

         ● S59.221   Salter-Harris Type II physeal fracture of lower end of radius, right arm

         ● S59.222   Salter-Harris Type II physeal fracture of lower end of radius, left arm

         ● S59.229   Salter-Harris Type II physeal fracture of lower end of radius, unspecified arm

     ● S59.23   Salter-Harris Type III physeal fracture of lower end of radius

         ● S59.231   Salter-Harris Type III physeal fracture of lower end of radius, right arm

         ● S59.232   Salter-Harris Type III physeal fracture of lower end of radius, left arm

         ● S59.239   Salter-Harris Type III physeal fracture of lower end of radius, unspecified arm

     ● S59.24   Salter-Harris Type IV physeal fracture of lower end of radius

         ● S59.241   Salter-Harris Type IV physeal fracture of lower end of radius, right arm

         ● S59.242   Salter-Harris Type IV physeal fracture of lower end of radius, left arm

         ● S59.249   Salter-Harris Type IV physeal fracture of lower end of radius, unspecified arm

     ● S59.29   Other physeal fracture of lower end of radius

         ● S59.291   Other physeal fracture of lower end of radius, right arm

         ● S59.292   Other physeal fracture of lower end of radius, left arm

         ● S59.299   Other physeal fracture of lower end of radius, unspecified arm

CHAPTER 19 (S00–T88)

- **S59.8**   Other specified injuries of elbow and forearm

  The appropriate 7th character is to be added to each code in subcategory S59.8

A	initial encounter
D	subsequent encounter
S	sequela

  - **S59.80**   Other specified injuries of elbow
    - **S59.801**   Other specified injuries of right elbow
    - **S59.802**   Other specified injuries of left elbow
    - **S59.809**   Other specified injuries of unspecified elbow
  - **S59.81**   Other specified injuries of forearm
    - **S59.811**   Other specified injuries right forearm
    - **S59.812**   Other specified injuries left forearm
    - **S59.819**   Other specified injuries unspecified forearm

- **S59.9**   Unspecified injury of elbow and forearm

  The appropriate 7th character is to be added to each code in subcategory S59.9

A	initial encounter
D	subsequent encounter
S	sequela

  - **S59.90**   Unspecified injury of elbow
    - **S59.901**   Unspecified injury of right elbow
    - **S59.902**   Unspecified injury of left elbow
    - **S59.909**   Unspecified injury of unspecified elbow
  - **S59.91**   Unspecified injury of forearm
    - **S59.911**   Unspecified injury of right forearm
    - **S59.912**   Unspecified injury of left forearm
    - **S59.919**   Unspecified injury of unspecified forearm

INJURIES TO THE WRIST, HAND AND FINGERS (S60-S69)

Excludes2   burns and corrosions (T20-T32)
frostbite (T33-T34)
insect bite or sting, venomous (T63.4)

- **S60**   Superficial injury of wrist, hand and fingers

  The appropriate 7th character is to be added to each code from category S60

A	initial encounter
D	subsequent encounter
S	sequela

  - **S60.0**   Contusion of finger without damage to nail
    - **Excludes1**   contusion involving nail (matrix) (S60.1)
    - X **S60.00**   Contusion of unspecified finger without damage to nail
      Contusion of finger(s) NOS
    - **S60.01**   Contusion of thumb without damage to nail
      - **S60.011**   Contusion of right thumb without damage to nail
      - **S60.012**   Contusion of left thumb without damage to nail
      - **S60.019**   Contusion of unspecified thumb without damage to nail
    - **S60.02**   Contusion of index finger without damage to nail
      - **S60.021**   Contusion of right index finger without damage to nail
      - **S60.022**   Contusion of left index finger without damage to nail
      - **S60.029**   Contusion of unspecified index finger without damage to nail

  - **S60.03**   Contusion of middle finger without damage to nail
    - **S60.031**   Contusion of right middle finger without damage to nail
    - **S60.032**   Contusion of left middle finger without damage to nail
    - **S60.039**   Contusion of unspecified middle finger without damage to nail
  - **S60.04**   Contusion of ring finger without damage to nail
    - **S60.041**   Contusion of right ring finger without damage to nail
    - **S60.042**   Contusion of left ring finger without damage to nail
    - **S60.049**   Contusion of unspecified ring finger without damage to nail
  - **S60.05**   Contusion of little finger without damage to nail
    - **S60.051**   Contusion of right little finger without damage to nail
    - **S60.052**   Contusion of left little finger without damage to nail
    - **S60.059**   Contusion of unspecified little finger without damage to nail
  - **S60.1**   Contusion of finger with damage to nail
    - X **S60.10**   Contusion of unspecified finger with damage to nail
    - **S60.11**   Contusion of thumb with damage to nail
      - **S60.111**   Contusion of right thumb with damage to nail
      - **S60.112**   Contusion of left thumb with damage to nail
      - **S60.119**   Contusion of unspecified thumb with damage to nail
    - **S60.12**   Contusion of index finger with damage to nail
      - **S60.121**   Contusion of right index finger with damage to nail
      - **S60.122**   Contusion of left index finger with damage to nail
      - **S60.129**   Contusion of unspecified index finger with damage to nail
    - **S60.13**   Contusion of middle finger with damage to nail
      - **S60.131**   Contusion of right middle finger with damage to nail
      - **S60.132**   Contusion of left middle finger with damage to nail
      - **S60.139**   Contusion of unspecified middle finger with damage to nail
    - **S60.14**   Contusion of ring finger with damage to nail
      - **S60.141**   Contusion of right ring finger with damage to nail
      - **S60.142**   Contusion of left ring finger with damage to nail
      - **S60.149**   Contusion of unspecified ring finger with damage to nail
    - **S60.15**   Contusion of little finger with damage to nail
      - **S60.151**   Contusion of right little finger with damage to nail
      - **S60.152**   Contusion of left little finger with damage to nail
      - **S60.159**   Contusion of unspecified little finger with damage to nail
  - **S60.2**   Contusion of wrist and hand
    - **Excludes2**   contusion of fingers (S60.0-, S60.1-)
    - **S60.21**   Contusion of wrist
      - **S60.211**   Contusion of right wrist
      - **S60.212**   Contusion of left wrist
      - **S60.219**   Contusion of unspecified wrist

▶ New   ⇒ Revised   ~~deleted~~ Deleted   Excludes 1   Excludes 2   Includes   Use additional   Code first   Code also   Key words

OGCR Official Guidelines   X Assign placeholder X   ● Use Additional Character(s)   ▶ Manifestation Code   🏷 Hierarchical Condition Category   **Coding Clinic**

- ● S60.22   Contusion of hand
  - ● S60.221   Contusion of right hand
  - ● S60.222   Contusion of left hand
  - ● S60.229   Contusion of unspecified hand
- ● S60.3   Other superficial injuries of thumb
  - ● S60.31   Abrasion of thumb
    - ● S60.311   Abrasion of right thumb
    - ● S60.312   Abrasion of left thumb
    - ● S60.319   Abrasion of unspecified thumb
  - ● S60.32   Blister (nonthermal) of thumb
    - ● S60.321   Blister (nonthermal) of right thumb
    - ● S60.322   Blister (nonthermal) of left thumb
    - ● S60.329   Blister (nonthermal) of unspecified thumb
  - ● S60.34   External constriction of thumb
    Hair tourniquet syndrome of thumb
    Use additional cause code to identify the constricting item (W49.0-)
    - ● S60.341   External constriction of right thumb
    - ● S60.342   External constriction of left thumb
    - ● S60.349   External constriction of unspecified thumb
  - ● S60.35   Superficial foreign body of thumb
    Splinter in the thumb
    - ● S60.351   Superficial foreign body of right thumb
    - ● S60.352   Superficial foreign body of left thumb
    - ● S60.359   Superficial foreign body of unspecified thumb
  - ● S60.36   Insect bite (nonvenomous) of thumb
    - ● S60.361   Insect bite (nonvenomous) of right thumb
    - ● S60.362   Insect bite (nonvenomous) of left thumb
    - ● S60.369   Insect bite (nonvenomous) of unspecified thumb
  - ● S60.37   Other superficial bite of thumb
    - **Excludes1**   open bite of thumb (S61.05-, S61.15-)
    - ● S60.371   Other superficial bite of right thumb
    - ● S60.372   Other superficial bite of left thumb
    - ● S60.379   Other superficial bite of unspecified thumb
  - ● S60.39   Other superficial injuries of thumb
    - ● S60.391   Other superficial injuries of right thumb
    - ● S60.392   Other superficial injuries of left thumb
    - ● S60.399   Other superficial injuries of unspecified thumb
- ● S60.4   Other superficial injuries of other fingers
  - ● S60.41   Abrasion of fingers
    - ● S60.410   Abrasion of right index finger
    - ● S60.411   Abrasion of left index finger
    - ● S60.412   Abrasion of right middle finger
    - ● S60.413   Abrasion of left middle finger
    - ● S60.414   Abrasion of right ring finger
    - ● S60.415   Abrasion of left ring finger
    - ● S60.416   Abrasion of right little finger
    - ● S60.417   Abrasion of left little finger
    - ● S60.418   Abrasion of other finger
      Abrasion of specified finger with unspecified laterality
    - ● S60.419   Abrasion of unspecified finger

- ● S60.42   Blister (nonthermal) of fingers
  - ● S60.420   Blister (nonthermal) of right index finger
  - ● S60.421   Blister (nonthermal) of left index finger
  - ● S60.422   Blister (nonthermal) of right middle finger
  - ● S60.423   Blister (nonthermal) of left middle finger
  - ● S60.424   Blister (nonthermal) of right ring finger
  - ● S60.425   Blister (nonthermal) of left ring finger
  - ● S60.426   Blister (nonthermal) of right little finger
  - ● S60.427   Blister (nonthermal) of left little finger
  - ● S60.428   Blister (nonthermal) of other finger
    Blister (nonthermal) of specified finger with unspecified laterality
  - ● S60.429   Blister (nonthermal) of unspecified finger
- ● S60.44   External constriction of fingers
  Hair tourniquet syndrome of finger
  Use additional cause code to identify the constricting item (W49.0-)
  - ● S60.440   External constriction of right index finger
  - ● S60.441   External constriction of left index finger
  - ● S60.442   External constriction of right middle finger
  - ● S60.443   External constriction of left middle finger
  - ● S60.444   External constriction of right ring finger
  - ● S60.445   External constriction of left ring finger
  - ● S60.446   External constriction of right little finger
  - ● S60.447   External constriction of left little finger
  - ● S60.448   External constriction of other finger
    External constriction of specified finger with unspecified laterality
  - ● S60.449   External constriction of unspecified finger
- ● S60.45   Superficial foreign body of fingers
  Splinter in the finger(s)
  - ● S60.450   Superficial foreign body of right index finger
  - ● S60.451   Superficial foreign body of left index finger
  - ● S60.452   Superficial foreign body of right middle finger
  - ● S60.453   Superficial foreign body of left middle finger
  - ● S60.454   Superficial foreign body of right ring finger
  - ● S60.455   Superficial foreign body of left ring finger
  - ● S60.456   Superficial foreign body of right little finger
  - ● S60.457   Superficial foreign body of left little finger
  - ● S60.458   Superficial foreign body of other finger
    Superficial foreign body of specified finger with unspecified laterality
  - ● S60.459   Superficial foreign body of unspecified finger

CHAPTER 19 (S00–T88)

CHAPTER 19 (S00-T88)

- S60.46   Insect bite (nonvenomous) of fingers
  - S60.460   Insect bite (nonvenomous) of right index finger
  - S60.461   Insect bite (nonvenomous) of left index finger
  - S60.462   Insect bite (nonvenomous) of right middle finger
  - S60.463   Insect bite (nonvenomous) of left middle finger
  - S60.464   Insect bite (nonvenomous) of right ring finger
  - S60.465   Insect bite (nonvenomous) of left ring finger
  - S60.466   Insect bite (nonvenomous) of right little finger
  - S60.467   Insect bite (nonvenomous) of left little finger
  - S60.468   Insect bite (nonvenomous) of other finger
    - Insect bite (nonvenomous) of specified finger with unspecified laterality
  - S60.469   Insect bite (nonvenomous) of unspecified finger
- S60.47   Other superficial bite of fingers
  - **Excludes1**   open bite of fingers (S61.25-, S61.35-)
  - S60.470   Other superficial bite of right index finger
  - S60.471   Other superficial bite of left index finger
  - S60.472   Other superficial bite of right middle finger
  - S60.473   Other superficial bite of left middle finger
  - S60.474   Other superficial bite of right ring finger
  - S60.475   Other superficial bite of left ring finger
  - S60.476   Other superficial bite of right little finger
  - S60.477   Other superficial bite of left little finger
  - S60.478   Other superficial bite of other finger
    - Other superficial bite of specified finger with unspecified laterality
  - S60.479   Other superficial bite of unspecified finger
- S60.5   Other superficial injuries of hand
  - **Excludes2**   superficial injuries of fingers (S60.3-, S60.4-)
  - S60.51   Abrasion of hand
    - S60.511   Abrasion of right hand
    - S60.512   Abrasion of left hand
    - S60.519   Abrasion of unspecified hand
  - S60.52   Blister (nonthermal) of hand
    - S60.521   Blister (nonthermal) of right hand
    - S60.522   Blister (nonthermal) of left hand
    - S60.529   Blister (nonthermal) of unspecified hand
  - S60.54   External constriction of hand
    - S60.541   External constriction of right hand
    - S60.542   External constriction of left hand
    - S60.549   External constriction of unspecified hand

- S60.55   Superficial foreign body of hand
  - Splinter in the hand
  - S60.551   Superficial foreign body of right hand
  - S60.552   Superficial foreign body of left hand
  - S60.559   Superficial foreign body of unspecified hand
- S60.56   Insect bite (nonvenomous) of hand
  - S60.561   Insect bite (nonvenomous) of right hand
  - S60.562   Insect bite (nonvenomous) of left hand
  - S60.569   Insect bite (nonvenomous) of unspecified hand
- S60.57   Other superficial bite of hand
  - **Excludes1**   open bite of hand (S61.45-)
  - S60.571   Other superficial bite of hand of right hand
  - S60.572   Other superficial bite of hand of left hand
  - S60.579   Other superficial bite of hand of unspecified hand
- S60.8   Other superficial injuries of wrist
  - S60.81   Abrasion of wrist
    - S60.811   Abrasion of right wrist
    - S60.812   Abrasion of left wrist
    - S60.819   Abrasion of unspecified wrist
  - S60.82   Blister (nonthermal) of wrist
    - S60.821   Blister (nonthermal) of right wrist
    - S60.822   Blister (nonthermal) of left wrist
    - S60.829   Blister (nonthermal) of unspecified wrist
  - S60.84   External constriction of wrist
    - S60.841   External constriction of right wrist
    - S60.842   External constriction of left wrist
    - S60.849   External constriction of unspecified wrist
  - S60.85   Superficial foreign body of wrist
    - Splinter in the wrist
    - S60.851   Superficial foreign body of right wrist
    - S60.852   Superficial foreign body of left wrist
    - S60.859   Superficial foreign body of unspecified wrist
  - S60.86   Insect bite (nonvenomous) of wrist
    - S60.861   Insect bite (nonvenomous) of right wrist
    - S60.862   Insect bite (nonvenomous) of left wrist
    - S60.869   Insect bite (nonvenomous) of unspecified wrist
  - S60.87   Other superficial bite of wrist
    - **Excludes1**   open bite of wrist (S61.55)
    - S60.871   Other superficial bite of right wrist
    - S60.872   Other superficial bite of left wrist
    - S60.879   Other superficial bite of unspecified wrist
- S60.9   Unspecified superficial injury of wrist, hand and fingers
  - S60.91   Unspecified superficial injury of wrist
    - S60.911   Unspecified superficial injury of right wrist
    - S60.912   Unspecified superficial injury of left wrist
    - S60.919   Unspecified superficial injury of unspecified wrist

● S60.92 **Unspecified** superficial injury of **hand**
  ● S60.921   Unspecified superficial injury of **right** hand
  ● S60.922   Unspecified superficial injury of **left** hand
  ● S60.929   Unspecified superficial injury of **unspecified** hand

● S60.93 **Unspecified** superficial injury of **thumb**
  ● S60.931   Unspecified superficial injury of **right** thumb
  ● S60.932   Unspecified superficial injury of **left** thumb
  ● S60.939   Unspecified superficial injury of **unspecified** thumb

● S60.94 **Unspecified** superficial injury of **other fingers**
  ● S60.940   Unspecified superficial injury of **right** index finger
  ● S60.941   Unspecified superficial injury of **left** index finger
  ● S60.942   Unspecified superficial injury of **right** middle finger
  ● S60.943   Unspecified superficial injury of **left** middle finger
  ● S60.944   Unspecified superficial injury of **right** ring finger
  ● S60.945   Unspecified superficial injury of **left** ring finger
  ● S60.946   Unspecified superficial injury of **right** little finger
  ● S60.947   Unspecified superficial injury of **left** little finger
  ● S60.948   Unspecified superficial injury of **other** finger
             Unspecified superficial injury of specified finger with unspecified laterality
  ● S60.949   Unspecified superficial injury of **unspecified** finger

● **S61** **Open wound of wrist, hand and fingers**
    Code also any associated wound infection
    Excludes1   open fracture of wrist, hand and finger (S62.- with 7th character B)
               traumatic amputation of wrist and hand (S68.-)

    The appropriate 7th character is to be added to each code from category S61

A	initial encounter
D	subsequent encounter
S	sequela

● S61.0   **Open wound of thumb without damage to nail**
    Excludes1   open wound of thumb with damage to nail (S61.1-)
  ● S61.00 **Unspecified** open wound of thumb without damage to nail
    ● S61.001   Unspecified open wound of **right** thumb without damage to nail
    ● S61.002   Unspecified open wound of **left** thumb without damage to nail
    ● S61.009   Unspecified open wound of **unspecified** thumb without damage to nail
  ● S61.01 **Laceration without foreign body** of thumb without damage to nail
    ● S61.011   Laceration without foreign body of **right** thumb without damage to nail
    ● S61.012   Laceration without foreign body of **left** thumb without damage to nail
    ● S61.019   Laceration without foreign body of **unspecified** thumb without damage to nail

● S61.02 **Laceration with foreign body** of thumb without damage to nail
  ● S61.021   Laceration with foreign body of **right** thumb without damage to nail
  ● S61.022   Laceration with foreign body of **left** thumb without damage to nail
  ● S61.029   Laceration with foreign body of **unspecified** thumb without damage to nail

● S61.03 **Puncture wound without foreign body** of thumb without damage to nail
  ● S61.031   Puncture wound without foreign body of **right** thumb without damage to nail
  ● S61.032   Puncture wound without foreign body of **left** thumb without damage to nail
  ● S61.039   Puncture wound without foreign body of **unspecified** thumb without damage to nail

● S61.04 **Puncture wound with foreign body** of thumb without damage to nail
  ● S61.041   Puncture wound with foreign body of **right** thumb without damage to nail
  ● S61.042   Puncture wound with foreign body of **left** thumb without damage to nail
  ● S61.049   Puncture wound with foreign body of **unspecified** thumb without damage to nail

● S61.05 **Open bite of thumb without damage to nail**
    Bite of thumb NOS
    Excludes1   superficial bite of thumb (S60.36-, S60.37-)
  ● S61.051   Open bite of **right** thumb without damage to nail
  ● S61.052   Open bite of **left** thumb without damage to nail
  ● S61.059   Open bite of **unspecified** thumb without damage to nail

● S61.1   **Open wound of thumb with damage to nail**
  ● S61.10 **Unspecified** open wound of thumb with damage to nail
    ● S61.101   Unspecified open wound of **right** thumb with damage to nail
    ● S61.102   Unspecified open wound of **left** thumb with damage to nail
    ● S61.109   Unspecified open wound of **unspecified** thumb with damage to nail
  ● S61.11 **Laceration without foreign body** of thumb with damage to nail
    ● S61.111   Laceration without foreign body of **right** thumb with damage to nail
    ● S61.112   Laceration without foreign body of **left** thumb with damage to nail
    ● S61.119   Laceration without foreign body of **unspecified** thumb with damage to nail
  ● S61.12 **Laceration with foreign body** of thumb with damage to nail
    ● S61.121   Laceration with foreign body of **right** thumb with damage to nail
    ● S61.122   Laceration with foreign body of **left** thumb with damage to nail
    ● S61.129   Laceration with foreign body of **unspecified** thumb with damage to nail

● **S61.13** Puncture wound without foreign body of thumb with damage to nail

  ● **S61.131** Puncture wound without foreign body of right thumb with damage to nail

  ● **S61.132** Puncture wound without foreign body of left thumb with damage to nail

  ● **S61.139** Puncture wound without foreign body of unspecified thumb with damage to nail

● **S61.14** Puncture wound with foreign body of thumb with damage to nail

  ● **S61.141** Puncture wound with foreign body of right thumb with damage to nail

  ● **S61.142** Puncture wound with foreign body of left thumb with damage to nail

  ● **S61.149** Puncture wound with foreign body of unspecified thumb with damage to nail

● **S61.15** Open bite of thumb with damage to nail

Bite of thumb with damage to nail NOS

> **Excludes1** superficial bite of thumb (S60.36-, S60.37-)

  ● **S61.151** Open bite of right thumb with damage to nail

  ● **S61.152** Open bite of left thumb with damage to nail

  ● **S61.159** Open bite of unspecified thumb with damage to nail

● **S61.2** Open wound of other finger without damage to nail

> **Excludes1** open wound of finger involving nail (matrix) (S61.3-)

> **Excludes2** open wound of thumb without damage to nail (S61.0-)

● **S61.20** Unspecified open wound of other finger without damage to nail

  ● **S61.200** Unspecified open wound of right index finger without damage to nail

  ● **S61.201** Unspecified open wound of left index finger without damage to nail

  ● **S61.202** Unspecified open wound of right middle finger without damage to nail

  ● **S61.203** Unspecified open wound of left middle finger without damage to nail

  ● **S61.204** Unspecified open wound of right ring finger without damage to nail

  ● **S61.205** Unspecified open wound of left ring finger without damage to nail

  ● **S61.206** Unspecified open wound of right little finger without damage to nail

  ● **S61.207** Unspecified open wound of left little finger without damage to nail

  ● **S61.208** Unspecified open wound of other finger without damage to nail

Unspecified open wound of specified finger with unspecified laterality without damage to nail

  ● **S61.209** Unspecified open wound of unspecified finger without damage to nail

● **S61.21** Laceration without foreign body of finger without damage to nail

  ● **S61.210** Laceration without foreign body of right index finger without damage to nail

  ● **S61.211** Laceration without foreign body of left index finger without damage to nail

  ● **S61.212** Laceration without foreign body of right middle finger without damage to nail

  ● **S61.213** Laceration without foreign body of left middle finger without damage to nail

  ● **S61.214** Laceration without foreign body of right ring finger without damage to nail

  ● **S61.215** Laceration without foreign body of left ring finger without damage to nail

  ● **S61.216** Laceration without foreign body of right little finger without damage to nail

  ● **S61.217** Laceration without foreign body of left little finger without damage to nail

  ● **S61.218** Laceration without foreign body of other finger without damage to nail

Laceration without foreign body of specified finger with unspecified laterality without damage to nail

  ● **S61.219** Laceration without foreign body of unspecified finger without damage to nail

● **S61.22** Laceration with foreign body of finger without damage to nail

  ● **S61.220** Laceration with foreign body of right index finger without damage to nail

  ● **S61.221** Laceration with foreign body of left index finger without damage to nail

  ● **S61.222** Laceration with foreign body of right middle finger without damage to nail

  ● **S61.223** Laceration with foreign body of left middle finger without damage to nail

  ● **S61.224** Laceration with foreign body of right ring finger without damage to nail

  ● **S61.225** Laceration with foreign body of left ring finger without damage to nail

  ● **S61.226** Laceration with foreign body of right little finger without damage to nail

  ● **S61.227** Laceration with foreign body of left little finger without damage to nail

  ● **S61.228** Laceration with foreign body of other finger without damage to nail

Laceration with foreign body of specified finger with unspecified laterality without damage to nail

  ● **S61.229** Laceration with foreign body of unspecified finger without damage to nail

● **S61.23** Puncture wound without foreign body of finger without damage to nail

  ● **S61.230** Puncture wound without foreign body of right index finger without damage to nail

  ● **S61.231** Puncture wound without foreign body of left index finger without damage to nail

  ● **S61.232** Puncture wound without foreign body of right middle finger without damage to nail

  ● **S61.233** Puncture wound without foreign body of left middle finger without damage to nail

  ● **S61.234** Puncture wound without foreign body of right ring finger without damage to nail

  ● **S61.235** Puncture wound without foreign body of left ring finger without damage to nail

  ● **S61.236** Puncture wound without foreign body of right little finger without damage to nail

● S61.237 Puncture wound without foreign body of left little finger without damage to nail

● S61.238 Puncture wound without foreign body of other finger without damage to nail

Puncture wound without foreign body of specified finger with unspecified laterality without damage to nail

● S61.239 Puncture wound without foreign body of unspecified finger without damage to nail

● S61.24 Puncture wound with foreign body of finger without damage to nail

● S61.240 Puncture wound with foreign body of right index finger without damage to nail

● S61.241 Puncture wound with foreign body of left index finger without damage to nail

● S61.242 Puncture wound with foreign body of right middle finger without damage to nail

● S61.243 Puncture wound with foreign body of left middle finger without damage to nail

● S61.244 Puncture wound with foreign body of right ring finger without damage to nail

● S61.245 Puncture wound with foreign body of left ring finger without damage to nail

● S61.246 Puncture wound with foreign body of right little finger without damage to nail

● S61.247 Puncture wound with foreign body of left little finger without damage to nail

● S61.248 Puncture wound with foreign body of other finger without damage to nail

Puncture wound with foreign body of specified finger with unspecified laterality without damage to nail

● S61.249 Puncture wound with foreign body of unspecified finger without damage to nail

● S61.25 Open bite of finger without damage to nail

Bite of finger without damage to nail NOS

Excludes1 superficial bite of finger (S60.46-, S60.47-)

● S61.250 Open bite of right index finger without damage to nail

● S61.251 Open bite of left index finger without damage to nail

● S61.252 Open bite of right middle finger without damage to nail

● S61.253 Open bite of left middle finger without damage to nail

● S61.254 Open bite of right ring finger without damage to nail

● S61.255 Open bite of left ring finger without damage to nail

● S61.256 Open bite of right little finger without damage to nail

● S61.257 Open bite of left little finger without damage to nail

● S61.258 Open bite of other finger without damage to nail

Open bite of specified finger with unspecified laterality without damage to nail

● S61.259 Open bite of unspecified finger without damage to nail

● S61.3 Open wound of other finger with damage to nail

● S61.30 Unspecified open wound of finger with damage to nail

● S61.300 Unspecified open wound of right index finger with damage to nail

● S61.301 Unspecified open wound of left index finger with damage to nail

● S61.302 Unspecified open wound of right middle finger with damage to nail

● S61.303 Unspecified open wound of left middle finger with damage to nail

● S61.304 Unspecified open wound of right ring finger with damage to nail

● S61.305 Unspecified open wound of left ring finger with damage to nail

● S61.306 Unspecified open wound of right little finger with damage to nail

● S61.307 Unspecified open wound of left little finger with damage to nail

● S61.308 Unspecified open wound of other finger with damage to nail

Unspecified open wound of specified finger with unspecified laterality with damage to nail

● S61.309 Unspecified open wound of unspecified finger with damage to nail

● S61.31 Laceration without foreign body of finger with damage to nail

● S61.310 Laceration without foreign body of right index finger with damage to nail

● S61.311 Laceration without foreign body of left index finger with damage to nail

● S61.312 Laceration without foreign body of right middle finger with damage to nail

● S61.313 Laceration without foreign body of left middle finger with damage to nail

● S61.314 Laceration without foreign body of right ring finger with damage to nail

● S61.315 Laceration without foreign body of left ring finger with damage to nail

● S61.316 Laceration without foreign body of right little finger with damage to nail

● S61.317 Laceration without foreign body of left little finger with damage to nail

● S61.318 Laceration without foreign body of other finger with damage to nail

Laceration without foreign body of specified finger with unspecified laterality with damage to nail

● S61.319 Laceration without foreign body of unspecified finger with damage to nail

● S61.32 Laceration with foreign body of finger with damage to nail

● S61.320 Laceration with foreign body of right index finger with damage to nail

● S61.321 Laceration with foreign body of left index finger with damage to nail

● S61.322 Laceration with foreign body of right middle finger with damage to nail

CHAPTER 19 (S00-T88)

● S61.323   Laceration with foreign body of left middle finger with damage to nail

● S61.324   Laceration with foreign body of right ring finger with damage to nail

● S61.325   Laceration with foreign body of left ring finger with damage to nail

● S61.326   Laceration with foreign body of right little finger with damage to nail

● S61.327   Laceration with foreign body of left little finger with damage to nail

● S61.328   Laceration with foreign body of other finger with damage to nail

Laceration with foreign body of specified finger with unspecified laterality with damage to nail

● S61.329   Laceration with foreign body of unspecified finger with damage to nail

● S61.33   Puncture wound without foreign body of finger with damage to nail

● S61.330   Puncture wound without foreign body of right index finger with damage to nail

● S61.331   Puncture wound without foreign body of left index finger with damage to nail

● S61.332   Puncture wound without foreign body of right middle finger with damage to nail

● S61.333   Puncture wound without foreign body of left middle finger with damage to nail

● S61.334   Puncture wound without foreign body of right ring finger with damage to nail

● S61.335   Puncture wound without foreign body of left ring finger with damage to nail

● S61.336   Puncture wound without foreign body of right little finger with damage to nail

● S61.337   Puncture wound without foreign body of left little finger with damage to nail

● S61.338   Puncture wound without foreign body of other finger with damage to nail

Puncture wound without foreign body of specified finger with unspecified laterality with damage to nail

● S61.339   Puncture wound without foreign body of unspecified finger with damage to nail

● S61.34   Puncture wound with foreign body of finger with damage to nail

● S61.340   Puncture wound with foreign body of right index finger with damage to nail

● S61.341   Puncture wound with foreign body of left index finger with damage to nail

● S61.342   Puncture wound with foreign body of right middle finger with damage to nail

● S61.343   Puncture wound with foreign body of left middle finger with damage to nail

● S61.344   Puncture wound with foreign body of right ring finger with damage to nail

● S61.345   Puncture wound with foreign body of left ring finger with damage to nail

● S61.346   Puncture wound with foreign body of right little finger with damage to nail

● S61.347   Puncture wound with foreign body of left little finger with damage to nail

● S61.348   Puncture wound with foreign body of other finger with damage to nail

Puncture wound with foreign body of specified finger with unspecified laterality with damage to nail

● S61.349   Puncture wound with foreign body of unspecified finger with damage to nail

● S61.35   Open bite of finger with damage to nail

Bite of finger with damage to nail NOS

Excludes1   superficial bite of finger (S60.46-, S60.47-)

● S61.350   Open bite of right index finger with damage to nail

● S61.351   Open bite of left index finger with damage to nail

● S61.352   Open bite of right middle finger with damage to nail

● S61.353   Open bite of left middle finger with damage to nail

● S61.354   Open bite of right ring finger with damage to nail

● S61.355   Open bite of left ring finger with damage to nail

● S61.356   Open bite of right little finger with damage to nail

● S61.357   Open bite of left little finger with damage to nail

● S61.358   Open bite of other finger with damage to nail

Open bite of specified finger with unspecified laterality with damage to nail

● S61.359   Open bite of unspecified finger with damage to nail

● S61.4   Open wound of hand

● S61.40   Unspecified open wound of hand

● S61.401   Unspecified open wound of right hand

● S61.402   Unspecified open wound of left hand

● S61.409   Unspecified open wound of unspecified hand

● S61.41   Laceration without foreign body of hand

● S61.411   Laceration without foreign body of right hand

● S61.412   Laceration without foreign body of left hand

● S61.419   Laceration without foreign body of unspecified hand

● S61.42   Laceration with foreign body of hand

● S61.421   Laceration with foreign body of right hand

● S61.422   Laceration with foreign body of left hand

● S61.429   Laceration with foreign body of unspecified hand

●S61.43   **Puncture wound without foreign body** of hand
　　　●S61.431   Puncture wound without foreign body of **right** hand
　　　●S61.432   Puncture wound without foreign body of **left** hand
　　　●S61.439   Puncture wound without foreign body of **unspecified** hand
●S61.44   **Puncture wound with foreign body** of hand
　　　●S61.441   Puncture wound with foreign body of **right** hand
　　　●S61.442   Puncture wound with foreign body of **left** hand
　　　●S61.449   Puncture wound with foreign body of **unspecified** hand
●S61.45   **Open bite of hand**
　　　Bite of hand NOS
　　　　Excludes1   superficial bite of hand (S60.56-, S60.57-)
　　　●S61.451   Open bite of **right** hand
　　　●S61.452   Open bite of **left** hand
　　　●S61.459   Open bite of **unspecified** hand
●S61.5   **Open wound of wrist**
　　●S61.50   **Unspecified** open wound of wrist
　　　●S61.501   Unspecified open wound of **right** wrist
　　　●S61.502   Unspecified open wound of **left** wrist
　　　●S61.509   Unspecified open wound of **unspecified** wrist
　　●S61.51   **Laceration without foreign body** of wrist
　　　●S61.511   Laceration without foreign body of **right** wrist
　　　●S61.512   Laceration without foreign body of **left** wrist
　　　●S61.519   Laceration without foreign body of **unspecified** wrist
　　●S61.52   **Laceration with foreign body** of wrist
　　　●S61.521   Laceration with foreign body of **right** wrist
　　　●S61.522   Laceration with foreign body of **left** wrist
　　　●S61.529   Laceration with foreign body of **unspecified** wrist
　　●S61.53   **Puncture wound without foreign** body of wrist
　　　●S61.531   Puncture wound without foreign body of **right** wrist
　　　●S61.532   Puncture wound without foreign body of **left** wrist
　　　●S61.539   Puncture wound without foreign body of **unspecified** wrist
　　●S61.54   **Puncture wound with foreign body** of wrist
　　　●S61.541   Puncture wound with foreign body of **right** wrist
　　　●S61.542   Puncture wound with foreign body of **left** wrist
　　　●S61.549   Puncture wound with foreign body of **unspecified** wrist
　　●S61.55   **Open bite of wrist**
　　　Bite of wrist NOS
　　　　Excludes1   superficial bite of wrist (S60.86-, S60.87-)
　　　●S61.551   Open bite of **right** wrist
　　　●S61.552   Open bite of **left** wrist
　　　●S61.559   Open bite of **unspecified** wrist

●S62   **Fracture at wrist and hand level**
　　Note: A fracture not indicated as displaced or nondisplaced should be coded to displaced
　　　　A fracture not indicated as open or closed should be coded to closed
　　　Excludes1   traumatic amputation of wrist and hand (S68.-)
　　　Excludes2   fracture of distal parts of ulna and radius (S52.-)
　　The appropriate 7th character is to be added to each code from category S62

A	initial encounter for closed fracture
B	initial encounter for open fracture
D	subsequent encounter for fracture with routine healing
G	subsequent encounter for fracture with delayed healing
K	subsequent encounter for fracture with nonunion
P	subsequent encounter for fracture with malunion
S	sequela

●S62.0   **Fracture of navicular [scaphoid] bone** of wrist
　　●S62.00   **Unspecified** fracture of navicular [scaphoid] bone of wrist
　　　●S62.001   Unspecified fracture of navicular [scaphoid] bone of **right** wrist
　　　●S62.002   Unspecified fracture of navicular [scaphoid] bone of **left** wrist
　　　　Coding Clinic: 2012, Q4, P106
　　　●S62.009   Unspecified fracture of navicular [scaphoid] bone of **unspecified** wrist
　　●S62.01   **Fracture of distal pole** of navicular [scaphoid] bone of wrist
　　　Fracture of volar tuberosity of navicular [scaphoid] bone of wrist
　　　●S62.011   **Displaced** fracture of distal pole of navicular [scaphoid] bone of **right** wrist
　　　●S62.012   **Displaced** fracture of distal pole of navicular [scaphoid] bone of **left** wrist
　　　●S62.013   **Displaced** fracture of distal pole of navicular [scaphoid] bone of **unspecified** wrist
　　　●S62.014   **Nondisplaced** fracture of distal pole of navicular [scaphoid] bone of **right** wrist
　　　●S62.015   **Nondisplaced** fracture of distal pole of navicular [scaphoid] bone of **left** wrist
　　　●S62.016   **Nondisplaced** fracture of distal pole of navicular [scaphoid] bone of **unspecified** wrist
　　●S62.02   **Fracture of middle third** of navicular [scaphoid] bone of wrist
　　　●S62.021   **Displaced** fracture of middle third of navicular [scaphoid] bone of **right** wrist
　　　●S62.022   **Displaced** fracture of middle third of navicular [scaphoid] bone of **left** wrist
　　　●S62.023   **Displaced** fracture of middle third of navicular [scaphoid] bone of **unspecified** wrist
　　　●S62.024   **Nondisplaced** fracture of middle third of navicular [scaphoid] bone of **right** wrist
　　　●S62.025   **Nondisplaced** fracture of middle third of navicular [scaphoid] bone of **left** wrist
　　　●S62.026   **Nondisplaced** fracture of middle third of navicular [scaphoid] bone of **unspecified** wrist

CHAPTER 19 (S00-T88)

● S62.03   Fracture of proximal third of navicular [scaphoid] bone of wrist

     ● S62.031   Displaced fracture of proximal third of navicular [scaphoid] bone of right wrist

     ● S62.032   Displaced fracture of proximal third of navicular [scaphoid] bone of left wrist

     ● S62.033   Displaced fracture of proximal third of navicular [scaphoid] bone of unspecified wrist

     ● S62.034   Nondisplaced fracture of proximal third of navicular [scaphoid] bone of right wrist

     ● S62.035   Nondisplaced fracture of proximal third of navicular [scaphoid] bone of left wrist

     ● S62.036   Nondisplaced fracture of proximal third of navicular [scaphoid] bone of unspecified wrist

● S62.1   Fracture of other and unspecified carpal bone(s)

     Excludes2   fracture of scaphoid of wrist (S62.0-)

   ● S62.10   Fracture of unspecified carpal bone
         Fracture of wrist NOS

     ● S62.101   Fracture of unspecified carpal bone, right wrist

     ● S62.102   Fracture of unspecified carpal bone, left wrist

         Coding Clinic: 2012, Q4, P95

     ● S62.109   Fracture of unspecified carpal bone, unspecified wrist

   ● S62.11   Fracture of triquetrum [cuneiform] bone of wrist

     ● S62.111   Displaced fracture of triquetrum [cuneiform] bone, right wrist

     ● S62.112   Displaced fracture of triquetrum [cuneiform] bone, left wrist

     ● S62.113   Displaced fracture of triquetrum [cuneiform] bone, unspecified wrist

     ● S62.114   Nondisplaced fracture of triquetrum [cuneiform] bone, right wrist

     ● S62.115   Nondisplaced fracture of triquetrum [cuneiform] bone, left wrist

     ● S62.116   Nondisplaced fracture of triquetrum [cuneiform] bone, unspecified wrist

   ● S62.12   Fracture of lunate [semilunar]

     ● S62.121   Displaced fracture of lunate [semilunar], right wrist

     ● S62.122   Displaced fracture of lunate [semilunar], left wrist

     ● S62.123   Displaced fracture of lunate [semilunar], unspecified wrist

     ● S62.124   Nondisplaced fracture of lunate [semilunar], right wrist

     ● S62.125   Nondisplaced fracture of lunate [semilunar], left wrist

     ● S62.126   Nondisplaced fracture of lunate [semilunar], unspecified wrist

   ● S62.13   Fracture of capitate [os magnum] bone

     ● S62.131   Displaced fracture of capitate [os magnum] bone, right wrist

     ● S62.132   Displaced fracture of capitate [os magnum] bone, left wrist

     ● S62.133   Displaced fracture of capitate [os magnum] bone, unspecified wrist

     ● S62.134   Nondisplaced fracture of capitate [os magnum] bone, right wrist

     ● S62.135   Nondisplaced fracture of capitate [os magnum] bone, left wrist

     ● S62.136   Nondisplaced fracture of capitate [os magnum] bone, unspecified wrist

● S62.14   Fracture of body of hamate [unciform] bone
     Fracture of hamate [unciform] bone NOS

     ● S62.141   Displaced fracture of body of hamate [unciform] bone, right wrist

     ● S62.142   Displaced fracture of body of hamate [unciform] bone, left wrist

     ● S62.143   Displaced fracture of body of hamate [unciform] bone, unspecified wrist

     ● S62.144   Nondisplaced fracture of body of hamate [unciform] bone, right wrist

     ● S62.145   Nondisplaced fracture of body of hamate [unciform] bone, left wrist

     ● S62.146   Nondisplaced fracture of body of hamate [unciform] bone, unspecified wrist

● S62.15   Fracture of hook process of hamate [unciform] bone
     Fracture of unciform process of hamate [unciform] bone

     ● S62.151   Displaced fracture of hook process of hamate [unciform] bone, right wrist

     ● S62.152   Displaced fracture of hook process of hamate [unciform] bone, left wrist

     ● S62.153   Displaced fracture of hook process of hamate [unciform] bone, unspecified wrist

     ● S62.154   Nondisplaced fracture of hook process of hamate [unciform] bone, right wrist

     ● S62.155   Nondisplaced fracture of hook process of hamate [unciform] bone, left wrist

     ● S62.156   Nondisplaced fracture of hook process of hamate [unciform] bone, unspecified wrist

● S62.16   Fracture of pisiform

     ● S62.161   Displaced fracture of pisiform, right wrist

     ● S62.162   Displaced fracture of pisiform, left wrist

     ● S62.163   Displaced fracture of pisiform, unspecified wrist

     ● S62.164   Nondisplaced fracture of pisiform, right wrist

     ● S62.165   Nondisplaced fracture of pisiform, left wrist

     ● S62.166   Nondisplaced fracture of pisiform, unspecified wrist

● S62.17   Fracture of trapezium [larger multangular]

     ● S62.171   Displaced fracture of trapezium [larger multangular], right wrist

     ● S62.172   Displaced fracture of trapezium [larger multangular], left wrist

     ● S62.173   Displaced fracture of trapezium [larger multangular], unspecified wrist

     ● S62.174   Nondisplaced fracture of trapezium [larger multangular], right wrist

     ● S62.175   Nondisplaced fracture of trapezium [larger multangular], left wrist

     ● S62.176   Nondisplaced fracture of trapezium [larger multangular], unspecified wrist

● S62.18   Fracture of trapezoid [smaller multangular]

     ● S62.181   Displaced fracture of trapezoid [smaller multangular], right wrist

     ● S62.182   Displaced fracture of trapezoid [smaller multangular], left wrist

     ● S62.183   Displaced fracture of trapezoid [smaller multangular], unspecified wrist

     ● S62.184   Nondisplaced fracture of trapezoid [smaller multangular], right wrist

▶ New   ⇒ Revised   ~~deleted~~ Deleted   Excludes 1   Excludes 2   Includes   Use additional   Code first   Code also   Key words

OGCR Official Guidelines   X Assign placeholder X   ● Use Additional Character(s)   ▷ Manifestation Code   ⓠ Hierarchical Condition Category   **Coding Clinic**

- ● S62.185   Nondisplaced fracture of trapezoid [smaller multangular], left wrist
- ● S62.186   Nondisplaced fracture of trapezoid [smaller multangular], unspecified wrist
- ● S62.2   Fracture of first metacarpal bone
  - ● S62.20   Unspecified fracture of first metacarpal bone
    - ● S62.201   Unspecified fracture of first metacarpal bone, right hand
    - ● S62.202   Unspecified fracture of first metacarpal bone, left hand
    - ● S62.209   Unspecified fracture of first metacarpal bone, unspecified hand
  - ● S62.21   Bennett's fracture
    - ● S62.211   Bennett's fracture, right hand
    - ● S62.212   Bennett's fracture, left hand
    - ● S62.213   Bennett's fracture, unspecified hand
  - ● S62.22   Rolando's fracture
    - ● S62.221   Displaced Rolando's fracture, right hand
    - ● S62.222   Displaced Rolando's fracture, left hand
    - ● S62.223   Displaced Rolando's fracture, unspecified hand
    - ● S62.224   Nondisplaced Rolando's fracture, right hand
    - ● S62.225   Nondisplaced Rolando's fracture, left hand
    - ● S62.226   Nondisplaced Rolando's fracture, unspecified hand
  - ● S62.23   Other fracture of base of first metacarpal bone
    - ● S62.231   Other displaced fracture of base of first metacarpal bone, right hand
    - ● S62.232   Other displaced fracture of base of first metacarpal bone, left hand
    - ● S62.233   Other displaced fracture of base of first metacarpal bone, unspecified hand
    - ● S62.234   Other nondisplaced fracture of base of first metacarpal bone, right hand
    - ● S62.235   Other nondisplaced fracture of base of first metacarpal bone, left hand
    - ● S62.236   Other nondisplaced fracture of base of first metacarpal bone, unspecified hand
  - ● S62.24   Fracture of shaft of first metacarpal bone
    - ● S62.241   Displaced fracture of shaft of first metacarpal bone, right hand
    - ● S62.242   Displaced fracture of shaft of first metacarpal bone, left hand
    - ● S62.243   Displaced fracture of shaft of first metacarpal bone, unspecified hand
    - ● S62.244   Nondisplaced fracture of shaft of first metacarpal bone, right hand
    - ● S62.245   Nondisplaced fracture of shaft of first metacarpal bone, left hand
    - ● S62.246   Nondisplaced fracture of shaft of first metacarpal bone, unspecified hand
  - ● S62.25   Fracture of neck of first metacarpal bone
    - ● S62.251   Displaced fracture of neck of first metacarpal bone, right hand
    - ● S62.252   Displaced fracture of neck of first metacarpal bone, left hand
    - ● S62.253   Displaced fracture of neck of first metacarpal bone, unspecified hand
    - ● S62.254   Nondisplaced fracture of neck of first metacarpal bone, right hand
    - ● S62.255   Nondisplaced fracture of neck of first metacarpal bone, left hand
    - ● S62.256   Nondisplaced fracture of neck of first metacarpal bone, unspecified hand

- ● S62.29   Other fracture of first metacarpal bone
  - ● S62.291   Other fracture of first metacarpal bone, right hand
  - ● S62.292   Other fracture of first metacarpal bone, left hand
  - ● S62.299   Other fracture of first metacarpal bone, unspecified hand
- ● S62.3   Fracture of other and unspecified metacarpal bone
  > **Excludes2**   fracture of first metacarpal bone (S62.2-)
  - ● S62.30   Unspecified fracture of other metacarpal bone
    - ● S62.300   Unspecified fracture of second metacarpal bone, right hand
    - ● S62.301   Unspecified fracture of second metacarpal bone, left hand
    - ● S62.302   Unspecified fracture of third metacarpal bone, right hand
    - ● S62.303   Unspecified fracture of third metacarpal bone, left hand
    - ● S62.304   Unspecified fracture of fourth metacarpal bone, right hand
    - ● S62.305   Unspecified fracture of fourth metacarpal bone, left hand
    - ● S62.306   Unspecified fracture of fifth metacarpal bone, right hand
    - ● S62.307   Unspecified fracture of fifth metacarpal bone, left hand
    - ● S62.308   Unspecified fracture of other metacarpal bone
      Unspecified fracture of specified metacarpal bone with unspecified laterality
    - ● S62.309   Unspecified fracture of unspecified metacarpal bone
  - ● S62.31   Displaced fracture of base of other metacarpal bone
    - ● S62.310   Displaced fracture of base of second metacarpal bone, right hand
    - ● S62.311   Displaced fracture of base of second metacarpal bone, left hand
    - ● S62.312   Displaced fracture of base of third metacarpal bone, right hand
    - ● S62.313   Displaced fracture of base of third metacarpal bone, left hand
    - ● S62.314   Displaced fracture of base of fourth metacarpal bone, right hand
    - ● S62.315   Displaced fracture of base of fourth metacarpal bone, left hand
    - ● S62.316   Displaced fracture of base of fifth metacarpal bone, right hand
    - ● S62.317   Displaced fracture of base of fifth metacarpal bone, left hand
    - ● S62.318   Displaced fracture of base of other metacarpal bone
      Displaced fracture of base of specified metacarpal bone with unspecified laterality
    - ● S62.319   Displaced fracture of base of unspecified metacarpal bone
  - ● S62.32   Displaced fracture of shaft of other metacarpal bone
    - ● S62.320   Displaced fracture of shaft of second metacarpal bone, right hand
    - ● S62.321   Displaced fracture of shaft of second metacarpal bone, left hand
    - ● S62.322   Displaced fracture of shaft of third metacarpal bone, right hand
    - ● S62.323   Displaced fracture of shaft of third metacarpal bone, left hand
    - ● S62.324   Displaced fracture of shaft of fourth metacarpal bone, right hand

CHAPTER 19 (S00-T88)

● S62.325   Displaced fracture of shaft of fourth metacarpal bone, left hand

● S62.326   Displaced fracture of shaft of fifth metacarpal bone, right hand

● S62.327   Displaced fracture of shaft of fifth metacarpal bone, left hand

● S62.328   Displaced fracture of shaft of other metacarpal bone
Displaced fracture of shaft of specified metacarpal bone with unspecified laterality

● S62.329   Displaced fracture of shaft of unspecified metacarpal bone

● S62.33   Displaced fracture of neck of other metacarpal bone

● S62.330   Displaced fracture of neck of second metacarpal bone, right hand

● S62.331   Displaced fracture of neck of second metacarpal bone, left hand

● S62.332   Displaced fracture of neck of third metacarpal bone, right hand

● S62.333   Displaced fracture of neck of third metacarpal bone, left hand

● S62.334   Displaced fracture of neck of fourth metacarpal bone, right hand

● S62.335   Displaced fracture of neck of fourth metacarpal bone, left hand

● S62.336   Displaced fracture of neck of fifth metacarpal bone, right hand

● S62.337   Displaced fracture of neck of fifth metacarpal bone, left hand

● S62.338   Displaced fracture of neck of other metacarpal bone
Displaced fracture of neck of specified metacarpal bone with unspecified laterality

● S62.339   Displaced fracture of neck of unspecified metacarpal bone

● S62.34   Nondisplaced fracture of base of other metacarpal bone

● S62.340   Nondisplaced fracture of base of second metacarpal bone, right hand

● S62.341   Nondisplaced fracture of base of second metacarpal bone, left hand

● S62.342   Nondisplaced fracture of base of third metacarpal bone, right hand

● S62.343   Nondisplaced fracture of base of third metacarpal bone, left hand

● S62.344   Nondisplaced fracture of base of fourth metacarpal bone, right hand

● S62.345   Nondisplaced fracture of base of fourth metacarpal bone, left hand

● S62.346   Nondisplaced fracture of base of fifth metacarpal bone, right hand

● S62.347   Nondisplaced fracture of base of fifth metacarpal bone, left hand

● S62.348   Nondisplaced fracture of base of other metacarpal bone
Nondisplaced fracture of base of specified metacarpal bone with unspecified laterality

● S62.349   Nondisplaced fracture of base of unspecified metacarpal bone

● S62.35   Nondisplaced fracture of shaft of other metacarpal bone

● S62.350   Nondisplaced fracture of shaft of second metacarpal bone, right hand

● S62.351   Nondisplaced fracture of shaft of second metacarpal bone, left hand

● S62.352   Nondisplaced fracture of shaft of third metacarpal bone, right hand

● S62.353   Nondisplaced fracture of shaft of third metacarpal bone, left hand

● S62.354   Nondisplaced fracture of shaft of fourth metacarpal bone, right hand

● S62.355   Nondisplaced fracture of shaft of fourth metacarpal bone, left hand

● S62.356   Nondisplaced fracture of shaft of fifth metacarpal bone, right hand

● S62.357   Nondisplaced fracture of shaft of fifth metacarpal bone, left hand

● S62.358   Nondisplaced fracture of shaft of other metacarpal bone
Nondisplaced fracture of shaft of specified metacarpal bone with unspecified laterality

● S62.359   Nondisplaced fracture of shaft of unspecified metacarpal bone

● S62.36   Nondisplaced fracture of neck of other metacarpal bone

● S62.360   Nondisplaced fracture of neck of second metacarpal bone, right hand

● S62.361   Nondisplaced fracture of neck of second metacarpal bone, left hand

● S62.362   Nondisplaced fracture of neck of third metacarpal bone, right hand

● S62.363   Nondisplaced fracture of neck of third metacarpal bone, left hand

● S62.364   Nondisplaced fracture of neck of fourth metacarpal bone, right hand

● S62.365   Nondisplaced fracture of neck of fourth metacarpal bone, left hand

● S62.366   Nondisplaced fracture of neck of fifth metacarpal bone, right hand

● S62.367   Nondisplaced fracture of neck of fifth metacarpal bone, left hand

● S62.368   Nondisplaced fracture of neck of other metacarpal bone
Nondisplaced fracture of neck of specified metacarpal bone with unspecified laterality

● S62.369   Nondisplaced fracture of neck of unspecified metacarpal bone

● S62.39   Other fracture of other metacarpal bone

● S62.390   Other fracture of second metacarpal bone, right hand

● S62.391   Other fracture of second metacarpal bone, left hand

● S62.392   Other fracture of third metacarpal bone, right hand

● S62.393   Other fracture of third metacarpal bone, left hand

● S62.394   Other fracture of fourth metacarpal bone, right hand

● S62.395   Other fracture of fourth metacarpal bone, left hand

▶ New   ⇒ Revised   ~~deleted~~ Deleted   Excludes 1   Excludes 2   Includes   Use additional   Code first   Code also   Key words
OGCR Official Guidelines   X Assign placeholder X   ● Use Additional Character(s)   ▷ Manifestation Code   🍳 Hierarchical Condition Category   **Coding Clinic**

● S62.396 Other fracture of fifth metacarpal bone, right hand

● S62.397 Other fracture of fifth metacarpal bone, left hand

● S62.398 Other fracture of other metacarpal bone
　　Other fracture of specified metacarpal bone with unspecified laterality

● S62.399 Other fracture of unspecified metacarpal bone

● S62.5　Fracture of thumb

　● S62.50　Fracture of unspecified phalanx of thumb

　　● S62.501 Fracture of unspecified phalanx of right thumb

　　● S62.502 Fracture of unspecified phalanx of left thumb

　　● S62.509 Fracture of unspecified phalanx of unspecified thumb

　● S62.51　Fracture of proximal phalanx of thumb

　　● S62.511 Displaced fracture of proximal phalanx of right thumb

　　● S62.512 Displaced fracture of proximal phalanx of left thumb

　　● S62.513 Displaced fracture of proximal phalanx of unspecified thumb

　　● S62.514 Nondisplaced fracture of proximal phalanx of right thumb

　　● S62.515 Nondisplaced fracture of proximal phalanx of left thumb

　　● S62.516 Nondisplaced fracture of proximal phalanx of unspecified thumb

　● S62.52　Fracture of distal phalanx of thumb

　　● S62.521 Displaced fracture of distal phalanx of right thumb

　　● S62.522 Displaced fracture of distal phalanx of left thumb

　　● S62.523 Displaced fracture of distal phalanx of unspecified thumb

　　● S62.524 Nondisplaced fracture of distal phalanx of right thumb

　　● S62.525 Nondisplaced fracture of distal phalanx of left thumb

　　● S62.526 Nondisplaced fracture of distal phalanx of unspecified thumb

● S62.6　Fracture of other and unspecified finger(s)

　Excludes2　fracture of thumb (S62.5-)

　● S62.60　Fracture of unspecified phalanx of finger

　　● S62.600 Fracture of unspecified phalanx of right index finger

　　● S62.601 Fracture of unspecified phalanx of left index finger

　　● S62.602 Fracture of unspecified phalanx of right middle finger

　　● S62.603 Fracture of unspecified phalanx of left middle finger

　　● S62.604 Fracture of unspecified phalanx of right ring finger

　　● S62.605 Fracture of unspecified phalanx of left ring finger

　　● S62.606 Fracture of unspecified phalanx of right little finger

　　● S62.607 Fracture of unspecified phalanx of left little finger

　　● S62.608 Fracture of unspecified phalanx of other finger
　　　　Fracture of unspecified phalanx of specified finger with unspecified laterality

　　● S62.609 Fracture of unspecified phalanx of unspecified finger

　● S62.61　Displaced fracture of proximal phalanx of finger

　　● S62.610 Displaced fracture of proximal phalanx of right index finger

　　● S62.611 Displaced fracture of proximal phalanx of left index finger

　　● S62.612 Displaced fracture of proximal phalanx of right middle finger

　　● S62.613 Displaced fracture of proximal phalanx of left middle finger

　　● S62.614 Displaced fracture of proximal phalanx of right ring finger

　　● S62.615 Displaced fracture of proximal phalanx of left ring finger

　　● S62.616 Displaced fracture of proximal phalanx of right little finger

　　● S62.617 Displaced fracture of proximal phalanx of left little finger

　　● S62.618 Displaced fracture of proximal phalanx of other finger
　　　　Displaced fracture of proximal phalanx of specified finger with unspecified laterality

　　● S62.619 Displaced fracture of proximal phalanx of unspecified finger

　● S62.62　Displaced fracture of middle phalanx of finger

　　● S62.620 Displaced fracture of middle phalanx of right index finger

　　● S62.621 Displaced fracture of middle phalanx of left index finger

　　● S62.622 Displaced fracture of middle phalanx of right middle finger

　　● S62.623 Displaced fracture of middle phalanx of left middle finger

　　● S62.624 Displaced fracture of middle phalanx of right ring finger

　　● S62.625 Displaced fracture of middle phalanx of left ring finger

　　● S62.626 Displaced fracture of middle phalanx of right little finger

　　● S62.627 Displaced fracture of middle phalanx of left little finger

　　● S62.628 Displaced fracture of middle phalanx of other finger
　　　　Displaced fracture of middle phalanx of specified finger with unspecified laterality

　　● S62.629 Displaced fracture of middle phalanx of unspecified finger

　● S62.63　Displaced fracture of distal phalanx of finger

　　● S62.630 Displaced fracture of distal phalanx of right index finger

　　● S62.631 Displaced fracture of distal phalanx of left index finger

- ● S62.632   Displaced fracture of distal phalanx of right middle finger
- ● S62.633   Displaced fracture of distal phalanx of left middle finger
- ● S62.634   Displaced fracture of distal phalanx of right ring finger
- ● S62.635   Displaced fracture of distal phalanx of left ring finger
- ● S62.636   Displaced fracture of distal phalanx of right little finger
- ● S62.637   Displaced fracture of distal phalanx of left little finger
- ● S62.638   Displaced fracture of distal phalanx of other finger
  - Displaced fracture of distal phalanx of specified finger with unspecified laterality
- ● S62.639   Displaced fracture of distal phalanx of unspecified finger
- ● S62.64   **Nondisplaced fracture of proximal phalanx of finger**
  - ● S62.640   Nondisplaced fracture of proximal phalanx of right index finger
  - ● S62.641   Nondisplaced fracture of proximal phalanx of left index finger
  - ● S62.642   Nondisplaced fracture of proximal phalanx of right middle finger
  - ● S62.643   Nondisplaced fracture of proximal phalanx of left middle finger
  - ● S62.644   Nondisplaced fracture of proximal phalanx of right ring finger
  - ● S62.645   Nondisplaced fracture of proximal phalanx of left ring finger
  - ● S62.646   Nondisplaced fracture of proximal phalanx of right little finger
  - ● S62.647   Nondisplaced fracture of proximal phalanx of left little finger
  - ● S62.648   Nondisplaced fracture of proximal phalanx of other finger
    - Nondisplaced fracture of proximal phalanx of specified finger with unspecified laterality
  - ● S62.649   Nondisplaced fracture of proximal phalanx of unspecified finger
- ● S62.65   **Nondisplaced fracture of middle phalanx of finger**
  - ● S62.650   Nondisplaced fracture of middle phalanx of right index finger
  - ● S62.651   Nondisplaced fracture of middle phalanx of left index finger
  - ● S62.652   Nondisplaced fracture of middle phalanx of right middle finger
  - ● S62.653   Nondisplaced fracture of middle phalanx of left middle finger
  - ● S62.654   Nondisplaced fracture of middle phalanx of right ring finger
  - ● S62.655   Nondisplaced fracture of middle phalanx of left ring finger
  - ● S62.656   Nondisplaced fracture of middle phalanx of right little finger
  - ● S62.657   Nondisplaced fracture of middle phalanx of left little finger

Figure 19-14   Dorsal dislocation of the distal phalanx of the index finger. (From Hardy M, Snaith B: Musculoskeletal Trauma: A Guide to Assessment and Diagnosis, 1e, Elsevier, 2011)

- ● S62.658   Nondisplaced fracture of middle phalanx of other finger
  - Nondisplaced fracture of middle phalanx of specified finger with unspecified laterality
- ● S62.659   Nondisplaced fracture of middle phalanx of unspecified finger
- ● S62.66   **Nondisplaced fracture of distal phalanx of finger**
  - ● S62.660   Nondisplaced fracture of distal phalanx of right index finger
  - ● S62.661   Nondisplaced fracture of distal phalanx of left index finger
  - ● S62.662   Nondisplaced fracture of distal phalanx of right middle finger
  - ● S62.663   Nondisplaced fracture of distal phalanx of left middle finger
  - ● S62.664   Nondisplaced fracture of distal phalanx of right ring finger
  - ● S62.665   Nondisplaced fracture of distal phalanx of left ring finger
  - ● S62.666   Nondisplaced fracture of distal phalanx of right little finger
  - ● S62.667   Nondisplaced fracture of distal phalanx of left little finger
  - ● S62.668   Nondisplaced fracture of distal phalanx of other finger
    - Nondisplaced fracture of distal phalanx of specified finger with unspecified laterality
  - ● S62.669   Nondisplaced fracture of distal phalanx of unspecified finger
- ● S62.9   **Unspecified fracture of wrist and hand**
  - X ● S62.90   Unspecified fracture of unspecified wrist and hand
  - X ● S62.91   Unspecified fracture of right wrist and hand
  - X ● S62.92   Unspecified fracture of left wrist and hand

▶ New   ⇒ Revised   ~~deleted~~ Deleted   Excludes 1   Excludes 2   Includes   Use additional   Code first   Code also   Key words

OGCR Official Guidelines   X Assign placeholder X   ● Use Additional Character(s)   ▶ Manifestation Code   ℞ Hierarchical Condition Category   **Coding Clinic**

● S63 **Dislocation and sprain of joints and ligaments at wrist and hand level**

Includes avulsion of joint or ligament at wrist and hand level

laceration of cartilage, joint or ligament at wrist and hand level

sprain of cartilage, joint or ligament at wrist and hand level

traumatic hemarthrosis of joint or ligament at wrist and hand level

traumatic rupture of joint or ligament at wrist and hand level

traumatic subluxation of joint or ligament at wrist and hand level

traumatic tear of joint or ligament at wrist and hand level

Code also any associated open wound

Excludes2 strain of muscle, fascia and tendon of wrist and hand (S66.-)

The appropriate 7th character is to be added to each code from category S63

A	initial encounter
D	subsequent encounter
S	sequela

● S63.0 **Subluxation and dislocation of wrist and hand joints**

● S63.00 **Unspecified subluxation and dislocation of wrist and hand**

Dislocation of carpal bone NOS

Dislocation of distal end of radius NOS

Subluxation of carpal bone NOS

Subluxation of distal end of radius NOS

● S63.001 **Unspecified subluxation of right wrist and hand**

● S63.002 **Unspecified subluxation of left wrist and hand**

● S63.003 **Unspecified subluxation of unspecified wrist and hand**

● S63.004 **Unspecified dislocation of right wrist and hand**

● S63.005 **Unspecified dislocation of left wrist and hand**

● S63.006 **Unspecified dislocation of unspecified wrist and hand**

● S63.01 **Subluxation and dislocation of distal radioulnar joint**

● S63.011 **Subluxation of distal radioulnar joint of right wrist**

● S63.012 **Subluxation of distal radioulnar joint of left wrist**

● S63.013 **Subluxation of distal radioulnar joint of unspecified wrist**

● S63.014 **Dislocation of distal radioulnar joint of right wrist**

● S63.015 **Dislocation of distal radioulnar joint of left wrist**

● S63.016 **Dislocation of distal radioulnar joint of unspecified wrist**

● S63.02 **Subluxation and dislocation of radiocarpal joint**

● S63.021 **Subluxation of radiocarpal joint of right wrist**

● S63.022 **Subluxation of radiocarpal joint of left wrist**

● S63.023 **Subluxation of radiocarpal joint of unspecified wrist**

● S63.024 **Dislocation of radiocarpal joint of right wrist**

● S63.025 **Dislocation of radiocarpal joint of left wrist**

● S63.026 **Dislocation of radiocarpal joint of unspecified wrist**

● S63.03 **Subluxation and dislocation of midcarpal joint**

● S63.031 **Subluxation of midcarpal joint of right wrist**

● S63.032 **Subluxation of midcarpal joint of left wrist**

● S63.033 **Subluxation of midcarpal joint of unspecified wrist**

● S63.034 **Dislocation of midcarpal joint of right wrist**

● S63.035 **Dislocation of midcarpal joint of left wrist**

● S63.036 **Dislocation of midcarpal joint of unspecified wrist**

● S63.04 **Subluxation and dislocation of carpometacarpal joint of thumb**

Excludes2 interphalangeal subluxation and dislocation of thumb (S63.1-)

● S63.041 **Subluxation of carpometacarpal joint of right thumb**

● S63.042 **Subluxation of carpometacarpal joint of left thumb**

● S63.043 **Subluxation of carpometacarpal joint of unspecified thumb**

● S63.044 **Dislocation of carpometacarpal joint of right thumb**

● S63.045 **Dislocation of carpometacarpal joint of left thumb**

● S63.046 **Dislocation of carpometacarpal joint of unspecified thumb**

● S63.05 **Subluxation and dislocation of other carpometacarpal joint**

Excludes2 subluxation and dislocation of carpometacarpal joint of thumb (S63.04-)

● S63.051 **Subluxation of other carpometacarpal joint of right hand**

● S63.052 **Subluxation of other carpometacarpal joint of left hand**

● S63.053 **Subluxation of other carpometacarpal joint of unspecified hand**

● S63.054 **Dislocation of other carpometacarpal joint of right hand**

● S63.055 **Dislocation of other carpometacarpal joint of left hand**

● S63.056 **Dislocation of other carpometacarpal joint of unspecified hand**

● S63.06 **Subluxation and dislocation of metacarpal (bone), proximal end**

● S63.061 **Subluxation of metacarpal (bone), proximal end of right hand**

● S63.062 **Subluxation of metacarpal (bone), proximal end of left hand**

● S63.063 **Subluxation of metacarpal (bone), proximal end of unspecified hand**

● S63.064 **Dislocation of metacarpal (bone), proximal end of right hand**

● S63.065 **Dislocation of metacarpal (bone), proximal end of left hand**

● S63.066 **Dislocation of metacarpal (bone), proximal end of unspecified hand**

CHAPTER 19 (S00–T88)

● S63.07   Subluxation and dislocation of distal end of ulna
- ● S63.071   Subluxation of distal end of right ulna
- ● S63.072   Subluxation of distal end of left ulna
- ● S63.073   Subluxation of distal end of unspecified ulna
- ● S63.074   Dislocation of distal end of right ulna
- ● S63.075   Dislocation of distal end of left ulna
- ● S63.076   Dislocation of distal end of unspecified ulna

● S63.09   Other subluxation and dislocation of wrist and hand
- ● S63.091   Other subluxation of right wrist and hand
- ● S63.092   Other subluxation of left wrist and hand
- ● S63.093   Other subluxation of unspecified wrist and hand
- ● S63.094   Other dislocation of right wrist and hand
- ● S63.095   Other dislocation of left wrist and hand
- ● S63.096   Other dislocation of unspecified wrist and hand

● S63.1   Subluxation and dislocation of thumb
● S63.10   Unspecified subluxation and dislocation of thumb
- ● S63.101   Unspecified subluxation of right thumb
- ● S63.102   Unspecified subluxation of left thumb
- ● S63.103   Unspecified subluxation of unspecified thumb
- ● S63.104   Unspecified dislocation of right thumb
- ● S63.105   Unspecified dislocation of left thumb
- ● S63.106   Unspecified dislocation of unspecified thumb

● S63.11   Subluxation and dislocation of metacarpophalangeal joint of thumb
- ● S63.111   Subluxation of metacarpophalangeal joint of right thumb
- ● S63.112   Subluxation of metacarpophalangeal joint of left thumb
- ● S63.113   Subluxation of metacarpophalangeal joint of unspecified thumb
- ● S63.114   Dislocation of metacarpophalangeal joint of right thumb
- ● S63.115   Dislocation of metacarpophalangeal joint of left thumb
- ● S63.116   Dislocation of metacarpophalangeal joint of unspecified thumb

● S63.12   Subluxation and dislocation of interphalangeal joint of thumb
- ● S63.121   Subluxation of interphalangeal joint of right thumb
- ● S63.122   Subluxation of interphalangeal joint of left thumb
- ● S63.123   Subluxation of interphalangeal joint of unspecified thumb
- ● S63.124   Dislocation of interphalangeal joint of right thumb
- ● S63.125   Dislocation of interphalangeal joint of left thumb
- ● S63.126   Dislocation of interphalangeal joint of unspecified thumb

● S63.2   Subluxation and dislocation of other finger(s)
   Excludes2   subluxation and dislocation of thumb (S63.1-)
● S63.20   Unspecified subluxation of other finger
- ● S63.200   Unspecified subluxation of right index finger
- ● S63.201   Unspecified subluxation of left index finger
- ● S63.202   Unspecified subluxation of right middle finger
- ● S63.203   Unspecified subluxation of left middle finger
- ● S63.204   Unspecified subluxation of right ring finger
- ● S63.205   Unspecified subluxation of left ring finger
- ● S63.206   Unspecified subluxation of right little finger
- ● S63.207   Unspecified subluxation of left little finger
- ● S63.208   Unspecified subluxation of other finger
  Unspecified subluxation of specified finger with unspecified laterality
- ● S63.209   Unspecified subluxation of unspecified finger

● S63.21   Subluxation of metacarpophalangeal joint of finger
- ● S63.210   Subluxation of metacarpophalangeal joint of right index finger
- ● S63.211   Subluxation of metacarpophalangeal joint of left index finger
- ● S63.212   Subluxation of metacarpophalangeal joint of right middle finger
- ● S63.213   Subluxation of metacarpophalangeal joint of left middle finger
- ● S63.214   Subluxation of metacarpophalangeal joint of right ring finger
- ● S63.215   Subluxation of metacarpophalangeal joint of left ring finger
- ● S63.216   Subluxation of metacarpophalangeal joint of right little finger
- ● S63.217   Subluxation of metacarpophalangeal joint of left little finger
- ● S63.218   Subluxation of metacarpophalangeal joint of other finger
  Subluxation of metacarpophalangeal joint of specified finger with unspecified laterality
- ● S63.219   Subluxation of metacarpophalangeal joint of unspecified finger

● S63.22   Subluxation of unspecified interphalangeal joint of finger
- ● S63.220   Subluxation of unspecified interphalangeal joint of right index finger
- ● S63.221   Subluxation of unspecified interphalangeal joint of left index finger
- ● S63.222   Subluxation of unspecified interphalangeal joint of right middle finger
- ● S63.223   Subluxation of unspecified interphalangeal joint of left middle finger

● **S63.224**   Subluxation of unspecified
            interphalangeal joint of right ring
            finger
● **S63.225**   Subluxation of unspecified
            interphalangeal joint of left ring
            finger
● **S63.226**   Subluxation of unspecified
            interphalangeal joint of right little
            finger
● **S63.227**   Subluxation of unspecified
            interphalangeal joint of left little
            finger
● **S63.228**   Subluxation of unspecified
            interphalangeal joint of other finger
            Subluxation of unspecified
                interphalangeal joint
                of specified finger with
                unspecified laterality
● **S63.229**   Subluxation of unspecified
            interphalangeal joint of unspecified
            finger
● **S63.23**   Subluxation of proximal interphalangeal joint
          of finger
● **S63.230**   Subluxation of proximal
            interphalangeal joint of right index
            finger
● **S63.231**   Subluxation of proximal
            interphalangeal joint of left index
            finger
● **S63.232**   Subluxation of proximal
            interphalangeal joint of right middle
            finger
● **S63.233**   Subluxation of proximal
            interphalangeal joint of left middle
            finger
● **S63.234**   Subluxation of proximal
            interphalangeal joint of right ring
            finger
● **S63.235**   Subluxation of proximal
            interphalangeal joint of left ring
            finger
● **S63.236**   Subluxation of proximal
            interphalangeal joint of right little
            finger
● **S63.237**   Subluxation of proximal
            interphalangeal joint of left little
            finger
● **S63.238**   Subluxation of proximal
            interphalangeal joint of other finger
            Subluxation of proximal
                interphalangeal joint
                of specified finger with
                unspecified laterality
● **S63.239**   Subluxation of proximal
            interphalangeal joint of unspecified
            finger
● **S63.24**   Subluxation of distal interphalangeal joint of
          finger
● **S63.240**   Subluxation of distal interphalangeal
            joint of right index finger
● **S63.241**   Subluxation of distal interphalangeal
            joint of left index finger
● **S63.242**   Subluxation of distal interphalangeal
            joint of right middle finger
● **S63.243**   Subluxation of distal interphalangeal
            joint of left middle finger
● **S63.244**   Subluxation of distal interphalangeal
            joint of right ring finger

● **S63.245**   Subluxation of distal interphalangeal
            joint of left ring finger
● **S63.246**   Subluxation of distal interphalangeal
            joint of right little finger
● **S63.247**   Subluxation of distal interphalangeal
            joint of left little finger
● **S63.248**   Subluxation of distal interphalangeal
            joint of other finger
            Subluxation of distal interphalangeal
                joint of specified finger with
                unspecified laterality
● **S63.249**   Subluxation of distal interphalangeal
            joint of unspecified finger
● **S63.25**   Unspecified dislocation of other finger
● **S63.250**   Unspecified dislocation of right index
            finger
● **S63.251**   Unspecified dislocation of left index
            finger
● **S63.252**   Unspecified dislocation of right
            middle finger
● **S63.253**   Unspecified dislocation of left middle
            finger
● **S63.254**   Unspecified dislocation of right ring
            finger
● **S63.255**   Unspecified dislocation of left ring
            finger
● **S63.256**   Unspecified dislocation of right little
            finger
● **S63.257**   Unspecified dislocation of left little
            finger
● **S63.258**   Unspecified dislocation of other
            finger
            Unspecified dislocation of specified
                finger with unspecified
                laterality
● **S63.259**   Unspecified dislocation of unspecified
            finger
            Unspecified dislocation of
                unspecified finger with
                unspecified laterality
● **S63.26**   Dislocation of metacarpophalangeal joint of
          finger
● **S63.260**   Dislocation of metacarpophalangeal
            joint of right index finger
● **S63.261**   Dislocation of metacarpophalangeal
            joint of left index finger
● **S63.262**   Dislocation of metacarpophalangeal
            joint of right middle finger
● **S63.263**   Dislocation of metacarpophalangeal
            joint of left middle finger
● **S63.264**   Dislocation of metacarpophalangeal
            joint of right ring finger
● **S63.265**   Dislocation of metacarpophalangeal
            joint of left ring finger
● **S63.266**   Dislocation of metacarpophalangeal
            joint of right little finger
● **S63.267**   Dislocation of metacarpophalangeal
            joint of left little finger
● **S63.268**   Dislocation of metacarpophalangeal
            joint of other finger
            Dislocation of metacarpophalangeal
                joint of specified finger with
                unspecified laterality
● **S63.269**   Dislocation of metacarpophalangeal
            joint of unspecified finger

CHAPTER 19 (S00-T88)

S63.27 Dislocation of unspecified interphalangeal joint of finger

- **S63.270** Dislocation of unspecified interphalangeal joint of right index finger
- **S63.271** Dislocation of unspecified interphalangeal joint of left index finger
- **S63.272** Dislocation of unspecified interphalangeal joint of right middle finger
- **S63.273** Dislocation of unspecified interphalangeal joint of left middle finger
- **S63.274** Dislocation of unspecified interphalangeal joint of right ring finger
- **S63.275** Dislocation of unspecified interphalangeal joint of left ring finger
- **S63.276** Dislocation of unspecified interphalangeal joint of right little finger
- **S63.277** Dislocation of unspecified interphalangeal joint of left little finger
- **S63.278** Dislocation of unspecified interphalangeal joint of other finger
  - Dislocation of unspecified interphalangeal joint of specified finger with unspecified laterality
- **S63.279** Dislocation of unspecified interphalangeal joint of unspecified finger
  - Dislocation of unspecified interphalangeal joint of unspecified finger without specified laterality

S63.28 Dislocation of proximal interphalangeal joint of finger

- **S63.280** Dislocation of proximal interphalangeal joint of right index finger
- **S63.281** Dislocation of proximal interphalangeal joint of left index finger
- **S63.282** Dislocation of proximal interphalangeal joint of right middle finger
- **S63.283** Dislocation of proximal interphalangeal joint of left middle finger
- **S63.284** Dislocation of proximal interphalangeal joint of right ring finger
- **S63.285** Dislocation of proximal interphalangeal joint of left ring finger
- **S63.286** Dislocation of proximal interphalangeal joint of right little finger
- **S63.287** Dislocation of proximal interphalangeal joint of left little finger
- **S63.288** Dislocation of proximal interphalangeal joint of other finger
  - Dislocation of proximal interphalangeal joint of specified finger with unspecified laterality
- **S63.289** Dislocation of proximal interphalangeal joint of unspecified finger

S63.29 Dislocation of distal interphalangeal joint of finger

- **S63.290** Dislocation of distal interphalangeal joint of right index finger
- **S63.291** Dislocation of distal interphalangeal joint of left index finger
- **S63.292** Dislocation of distal interphalangeal joint of right middle finger
- **S63.293** Dislocation of distal interphalangeal joint of left middle finger
- **S63.294** Dislocation of distal interphalangeal joint of right ring finger
- **S63.295** Dislocation of distal interphalangeal joint of left ring finger
- **S63.296** Dislocation of distal interphalangeal joint of right little finger
- **S63.297** Dislocation of distal interphalangeal joint of left little finger
- **S63.298** Dislocation of distal interphalangeal joint of other finger
  - Dislocation of distal interphalangeal joint of specified finger with unspecified laterality
- **S63.299** Dislocation of distal interphalangeal joint of unspecified finger

S63.3 Traumatic rupture of ligament of wrist

S63.30 Traumatic rupture of unspecified ligament of wrist

- **S63.301** Traumatic rupture of unspecified ligament of right wrist
- **S63.302** Traumatic rupture of unspecified ligament of left wrist
- **S63.309** Traumatic rupture of unspecified ligament of unspecified wrist

S63.31 Traumatic rupture of collateral ligament of wrist

- **S63.311** Traumatic rupture of collateral ligament of right wrist
- **S63.312** Traumatic rupture of collateral ligament of left wrist
- **S63.319** Traumatic rupture of collateral ligament of unspecified wrist

S63.32 Traumatic rupture of radiocarpal ligament

- **S63.321** Traumatic rupture of right radiocarpal ligament
- **S63.322** Traumatic rupture of left radiocarpal ligament
- **S63.329** Traumatic rupture of unspecified radiocarpal ligament

S63.33 Traumatic rupture of ulnocarpal (palmar) ligament

- **S63.331** Traumatic rupture of right ulnocarpal (palmar) ligament
- **S63.332** Traumatic rupture of left ulnocarpal (palmar) ligament
- **S63.339** Traumatic rupture of unspecified ulnocarpal (palmar) ligament

S63.39 Traumatic rupture of other ligament of wrist

- **S63.391** Traumatic rupture of other ligament of right wrist
- **S63.392** Traumatic rupture of other ligament of left wrist
- **S63.399** Traumatic rupture of other ligament of unspecified wrist

▶ New   ⇛ Revised   ~~deleted~~ Deleted   Excludes 1   Excludes 2   Includes   Use additional   Code first   Code also   Key words

OGCR Official Guidelines   X Assign placeholder X   ● Use Additional Character(s)   ▶ Manifestation Code   ⬛ Hierarchical Condition Category   **Coding Clinic**

● **S63.4** Traumatic rupture of ligament of finger at metacarpophalangeal and interphalangeal joint(s)

　● **S63.40** Traumatic rupture of unspecified ligament of finger at metacarpophalangeal and interphalangeal joint

　　● **S63.400** Traumatic rupture of unspecified ligament of right index finger at metacarpophalangeal and interphalangeal joint

　　● **S63.401** Traumatic rupture of unspecified ligament of left index finger at metacarpophalangeal and interphalangeal joint

　　● **S63.402** Traumatic rupture of unspecified ligament of right middle finger at metacarpophalangeal and interphalangeal joint

　　● **S63.403** Traumatic rupture of unspecified ligament of left middle finger at metacarpophalangeal and interphalangeal joint

　　● **S63.404** Traumatic rupture of unspecified ligament of right ring finger at metacarpophalangeal and interphalangeal joint

　　● **S63.405** Traumatic rupture of unspecified ligament of left ring finger at metacarpophalangeal and interphalangeal joint

　　● **S63.406** Traumatic rupture of unspecified ligament of right little finger at metacarpophalangeal and interphalangeal joint

　　● **S63.407** Traumatic rupture of unspecified ligament of left little finger at metacarpophalangeal and interphalangeal joint

　　● **S63.408** Traumatic rupture of unspecified ligament of other finger at metacarpophalangeal and interphalangeal joint
　　　　Traumatic rupture of unspecified ligament of specified finger with unspecified laterality at metacarpophalangeal and interphalangeal joint

　　● **S63.409** Traumatic rupture of unspecified ligament of unspecified finger at metacarpophalangeal and interphalangeal joint

　● **S63.41** Traumatic rupture of collateral ligament of finger at metacarpophalangeal and interphalangeal joint

　　● **S63.410** Traumatic rupture of collateral ligament of right index finger at metacarpophalangeal and interphalangeal joint

　　● **S63.411** Traumatic rupture of collateral ligament of left index finger at metacarpophalangeal and interphalangeal joint

　　● **S63.412** Traumatic rupture of collateral ligament of right middle finger at metacarpophalangeal and interphalangeal joint

　　● **S63.413** Traumatic rupture of collateral ligament of left middle finger at metacarpophalangeal and interphalangeal joint

　　● **S63.414** Traumatic rupture of collateral ligament of right ring finger at metacarpophalangeal and interphalangeal joint

　　● **S63.415** Traumatic rupture of collateral ligament of left ring finger at metacarpophalangeal and interphalangeal joint

　　● **S63.416** Traumatic rupture of collateral ligament of right little finger at metacarpophalangeal and interphalangeal joint

　　● **S63.417** Traumatic rupture of collateral ligament of left little finger at metacarpophalangeal and interphalangeal joint

　　● **S63.418** Traumatic rupture of collateral ligament of other finger at metacarpophalangeal and interphalangeal joint
　　　　Traumatic rupture of collateral ligament of specified finger with unspecified laterality at metacarpophalangeal and interphalangeal joint

　　● **S63.419** Traumatic rupture of collateral ligament of unspecified finger at metacarpophalangeal and interphalangeal joint

　● **S63.42** Traumatic rupture of palmar ligament of finger at metacarpophalangeal and interphalangeal joint

　　● **S63.420** Traumatic rupture of palmar ligament of right index finger at metacarpophalangeal and interphalangeal joint

　　● **S63.421** Traumatic rupture of palmar ligament of left index finger at metacarpophalangeal and interphalangeal joint

　　● **S63.422** Traumatic rupture of palmar ligament of right middle finger at metacarpophalangeal and interphalangeal joint

　　● **S63.423** Traumatic rupture of palmar ligament of left middle finger at metacarpophalangeal and interphalangeal joint

　　● **S63.424** Traumatic rupture of palmar ligament of right ring finger at metacarpophalangeal and interphalangeal joint

　　● **S63.425** Traumatic rupture of palmar ligament of left ring finger at metacarpophalangeal and interphalangeal joint

　　● **S63.426** Traumatic rupture of palmar ligament of right little finger at metacarpophalangeal and interphalangeal joint

　　● **S63.427** Traumatic rupture of palmar ligament of left little finger at metacarpophalangeal and interphalangeal joint

　　● **S63.428** Traumatic rupture of palmar ligament of other finger at metacarpophalangeal and interphalangeal joint
　　　　Traumatic rupture of palmar ligament of specified finger with unspecified laterality at metacarpophalangeal and interphalangeal joint

　　● **S63.429** Traumatic rupture of palmar ligament of unspecified finger at metacarpophalangeal and interphalangeal joint

CHAPTER 19 (S00-T88)

- S63.43 Traumatic rupture of volar plate of finger at metacarpophalangeal and interphalangeal joint
  - S63.430 Traumatic rupture of volar plate of right index finger at metacarpophalangeal and interphalangeal joint
  - S63.431 Traumatic rupture of volar plate of left index finger at metacarpophalangeal and interphalangeal joint
  - S63.432 Traumatic rupture of volar plate of right middle finger at metacarpophalangeal and interphalangeal joint
  - S63.433 Traumatic rupture of volar plate of left middle finger at metacarpophalangeal and interphalangeal joint
  - S63.434 Traumatic rupture of volar plate of right ring finger at metacarpophalangeal and interphalangeal joint
  - S63.435 Traumatic rupture of volar plate of left ring finger at metacarpophalangeal and interphalangeal joint
  - S63.436 Traumatic rupture of volar plate of right little finger at metacarpophalangeal and interphalangeal joint
  - S63.437 Traumatic rupture of volar plate of left little finger at metacarpophalangeal and interphalangeal joint
  - S63.438 Traumatic rupture of volar plate of other finger at metacarpophalangeal and interphalangeal joint
    Traumatic rupture of volar plate of specified finger with unspecified laterality at metacarpophalangeal and interphalangeal joint
  - S63.439 Traumatic rupture of volar plate of unspecified finger at metacarpophalangeal and interphalangeal joint
- S63.49 Traumatic rupture of other ligament of finger at metacarpophalangeal and interphalangeal joint
  - S63.490 Traumatic rupture of other ligament of right index finger at metacarpophalangeal and interphalangeal joint
  - S63.491 Traumatic rupture of other ligament of left index finger at metacarpophalangeal and interphalangeal joint
  - S63.492 Traumatic rupture of other ligament of right middle finger at metacarpophalangeal and interphalangeal joint
  - S63.493 Traumatic rupture of other ligament of left middle finger at metacarpophalangeal and interphalangeal joint
  - S63.494 Traumatic rupture of other ligament of right ring finger at metacarpophalangeal and interphalangeal joint
  - S63.495 Traumatic rupture of other ligament of left ring finger at metacarpophalangeal and interphalangeal joint
  - S63.496 Traumatic rupture of other ligament of right little finger at metacarpophalangeal and interphalangeal joint
  - S63.497 Traumatic rupture of other ligament of left little finger at metacarpophalangeal and interphalangeal joint
  - S63.498 Traumatic rupture of other ligament of other finger at metacarpophalangeal and interphalangeal joint
    Traumatic rupture of ligament of specified finger with unspecified laterality at metacarpophalangeal and interphalangeal joint
  - S63.499 Traumatic rupture of other ligament of unspecified finger at metacarpophalangeal and interphalangeal joint
- S63.5 Other and unspecified sprain of wrist
  - S63.50 Unspecified sprain of wrist
    - S63.501 Unspecified sprain of right wrist
    - S63.502 Unspecified sprain of left wrist
    - S63.509 Unspecified sprain of unspecified wrist
  - S63.51 Sprain of carpal (joint)
    - S63.511 Sprain of carpal joint of right wrist
    - S63.512 Sprain of carpal joint of left wrist
    - S63.519 Sprain of carpal joint of unspecified wrist
  - S63.52 Sprain of radiocarpal joint
    - **Excludes 1** traumatic rupture of radiocarpal ligament (S63.32-)
    - S63.521 Sprain of radiocarpal joint of right wrist
    - S63.522 Sprain of radiocarpal joint of left wrist
    - S63.529 Sprain of radiocarpal joint of unspecified wrist
  - S63.59 Other specified sprain of wrist
    - S63.591 Other specified sprain of right wrist
    - S63.592 Other specified sprain of left wrist
    - S63.599 Other specified sprain of unspecified wrist
- S63.6 Other and unspecified sprain of finger(s)
  - **Excludes 1** traumatic rupture of ligament of finger at metacarpophalangeal and interphalangeal joint(s) (S63.4-)
  - S63.60 Unspecified sprain of thumb
    - S63.601 Unspecified sprain of right thumb
    - S63.602 Unspecified sprain of left thumb
    - S63.609 Unspecified sprain of unspecified thumb
  - S63.61 Unspecified sprain of other and unspecified finger(s)
    - S63.610 Unspecified sprain of right index finger
    - S63.611 Unspecified sprain of left index finger
    - S63.612 Unspecified sprain of right middle finger
    - S63.613 Unspecified sprain of left middle finger
    - S63.614 Unspecified sprain of right ring finger
    - S63.615 Unspecified sprain of left ring finger

● S63.616   Unspecified sprain of right little finger
● S63.617   Unspecified sprain of left little finger
● S63.618   Unspecified sprain of other finger
      Unspecified sprain of specified finger with unspecified laterality
● S63.619   Unspecified sprain of unspecified finger

● S63.62   Sprain of interphalangeal joint of thumb
● S63.621   Sprain of interphalangeal joint of right thumb
● S63.622   Sprain of interphalangeal joint of left thumb
● S63.629   Sprain of interphalangeal joint of unspecified thumb

● S63.63   Sprain of interphalangeal joint of other and unspecified finger(s)
● S63.630   Sprain of interphalangeal joint of right index finger
● S63.631   Sprain of interphalangeal joint of left index finger
● S63.632   Sprain of interphalangeal joint of right middle finger
● S63.633   Sprain of interphalangeal joint of left middle finger
● S63.634   Sprain of interphalangeal joint of right ring finger
● S63.635   Sprain of interphalangeal joint of left ring finger
● S63.636   Sprain of interphalangeal joint of right little finger
● S63.637   Sprain of interphalangeal joint of left little finger
● S63.638   Sprain of interphalangeal joint of other finger
● S63.639   Sprain of interphalangeal joint of unspecified finger

● S63.64   Sprain of metacarpophalangeal joint of thumb
● S63.641   Sprain of metacarpophalangeal joint of right thumb
● S63.642   Sprain of metacarpophalangeal joint of left thumb
● S63.649   Sprain of metacarpophalangeal joint of unspecified thumb

● S63.65   Sprain of metacarpophalangeal joint of other and unspecified finger(s)
● S63.650   Sprain of metacarpophalangeal joint of right index finger
● S63.651   Sprain of metacarpophalangeal joint of left index finger
● S63.652   Sprain of metacarpophalangeal joint of right middle finger
● S63.653   Sprain of metacarpophalangeal joint of left middle finger
● S63.654   Sprain of metacarpophalangeal joint of right ring finger
● S63.655   Sprain of metacarpophalangeal joint of left ring finger
● S63.656   Sprain of metacarpophalangeal joint of right little finger
● S63.657   Sprain of metacarpophalangeal joint of left little finger
● S63.658   Sprain of metacarpophalangeal joint of other finger
      Sprain of metacarpophalangeal joint of specified finger with unspecified laterality
● S63.659   Sprain of metacarpophalangeal joint of unspecified finger

● S63.68   Other sprain of thumb
● S63.681   Other sprain of right thumb
● S63.682   Other sprain of left thumb
● S63.689   Other sprain of unspecified thumb

● S63.69   Other sprain of other and unspecified finger(s)
● S63.690   Other sprain of right index finger
● S63.691   Other sprain of left index finger
● S63.692   Other sprain of right middle finger
● S63.693   Other sprain of left middle finger
● S63.694   Other sprain of right ring finger
● S63.695   Other sprain of left ring finger
● S63.696   Other sprain of right little finger
● S63.697   Other sprain of left little finger
● S63.698   Other sprain of other finger
      Other sprain of specified finger with unspecified laterality
● S63.699   Other sprain of unspecified finger

● S63.8   Sprain of other part of wrist and hand
● S63.8X   Sprain of other part of wrist and hand
● S63.8X1   Sprain of other part of right wrist and hand
● S63.8X2   Sprain of other part of left wrist and hand
● S63.8X9   Sprain of other part of unspecified wrist and hand

● S63.9   Sprain of unspecified part of wrist and hand
X ● S63.90   Sprain of unspecified part of unspecified wrist and hand
X ● S63.91   Sprain of unspecified part of right wrist and hand
X ● S63.92   Sprain of unspecified part of left wrist and hand

● S64   Injury of nerves at wrist and hand level
      The appropriate 7th character is to be added to each code from category S64

> A   initial encounter
> D   subsequent encounter
> S   sequela

      Code also any associated open wound (S61.-)

● S64.0   Injury of ulnar nerve at wrist and hand level
X ● S64.00   Injury of ulnar nerve at wrist and hand level of unspecified arm
X ● S64.01   Injury of ulnar nerve at wrist and hand level of right arm
X ● S64.02   Injury of ulnar nerve at wrist and hand level of left arm

● S64.1   Injury of median nerve at wrist and hand level
X ● S64.10   Injury of median nerve at wrist and hand level of unspecified arm
X ● S64.11   Injury of median nerve at wrist and hand level of right arm
X ● S64.12   Injury of median nerve at wrist and hand level of left arm

● S64.2   Injury of radial nerve at wrist and hand level
X ● S64.20   Injury of radial nerve at wrist and hand level of unspecified arm
X ● S64.21   Injury of radial nerve at wrist and hand level of right arm
X ● S64.22   Injury of radial nerve at wrist and hand level of left arm

● S64.3   Injury of digital nerve of thumb
X ● S64.30   Injury of digital nerve of unspecified thumb
X ● S64.31   Injury of digital nerve of right thumb
X ● S64.32   Injury of digital nerve of left thumb

● S64.4   Injury of digital nerve of other and unspecified finger
   X ● S64.40   Injury of digital nerve of unspecified finger
   ● S64.49   Injury of digital nerve of other finger
     ● S64.490   Injury of digital nerve of right index finger
     ● S64.491   Injury of digital nerve of left index finger
     ● S64.492   Injury of digital nerve of right middle finger
     ● S64.493   Injury of digital nerve of left middle finger
     ● S64.494   Injury of digital nerve of right ring finger
     ● S64.495   Injury of digital nerve of left ring finger
     ● S64.496   Injury of digital nerve of right little finger
     ● S64.497   Injury of digital nerve of left little finger
     ● S64.498   Injury of digital nerve of other finger
           Injury of digital nerve of specified finger with unspecified laterality

● S64.8   Injury of other nerves at wrist and hand level
   ● S64.8X   Injury of other nerves at wrist and hand level
     ● S64.8X1   Injury of other nerves at wrist and hand level of right arm
     ● S64.8X2   Injury of other nerves at wrist and hand level of left arm
     ● S64.8X9   Injury of other nerves at wrist and hand level of unspecified arm

● S64.9   Injury of unspecified nerve at wrist and hand level
   X ● S64.90   Injury of unspecified nerve at wrist and hand level of unspecified arm
   X ● S64.91   Injury of unspecified nerve at wrist and hand level of right arm
   X ● S64.92   Injury of unspecified nerve at wrist and hand level of left arm

● S65   Injury of blood vessels at wrist and hand level
    The appropriate 7th character is to be added to each code from category S65

     | | |
     A   initial encounter
     D   subsequent encounter
     S   sequela

    Code also any associated open wound (S61.-)

● S65.0   Injury of ulnar artery at wrist and hand level
   ● S65.00   Unspecified injury of ulnar artery at wrist and hand level
     ● S65.001   Unspecified injury of ulnar artery at wrist and hand level of right arm
     ● S65.002   Unspecified injury of ulnar artery at wrist and hand level of left arm
     ● S65.009   Unspecified injury of ulnar artery at wrist and hand level of unspecified arm
   ● S65.01   Laceration of ulnar artery at wrist and hand level
     ● S65.011   Laceration of ulnar artery at wrist and hand level of right arm
     ● S65.012   Laceration of ulnar artery at wrist and hand level of left arm
     ● S65.019   Laceration of ulnar artery at wrist and hand level of unspecified arm

● S65.09   Other specified injury of ulnar artery at wrist and hand level
     ● S65.091   Other specified injury of ulnar artery at wrist and hand level of right arm
     ● S65.092   Other specified injury of ulnar artery at wrist and hand level of left arm
     ● S65.099   Other specified injury of ulnar artery at wrist and hand level of unspecified arm

● S65.1   Injury of radial artery at wrist and hand level
   ● S65.10   Unspecified injury of radial artery at wrist and hand level
     ● S65.101   Unspecified injury of radial artery at wrist and hand level of right arm
     ● S65.102   Unspecified injury of radial artery at wrist and hand level of left arm
     ● S65.109   Unspecified injury of radial artery at wrist and hand level of unspecified arm
   ● S65.11   Laceration of radial artery at wrist and hand level
     ● S65.111   Laceration of radial artery at wrist and hand level of right arm
     ● S65.112   Laceration of radial artery at wrist and hand level of left arm
     ● S65.119   Laceration of radial artery at wrist and hand level of unspecified arm
   ● S65.19   Other specified injury of radial artery at wrist and hand level
     ● S65.191   Other specified injury of radial artery at wrist and hand level of right arm
     ● S65.192   Other specified injury of radial artery at wrist and hand level of left arm
     ● S65.199   Other specified injury of radial artery at wrist and hand level of unspecified arm

● S65.2   Injury of superficial palmar arch
   ● S65.20   Unspecified injury of superficial palmar arch
     ● S65.201   Unspecified injury of superficial palmar arch of right hand
     ● S65.202   Unspecified injury of superficial palmar arch of left hand
     ● S65.209   Unspecified injury of superficial palmar arch of unspecified hand
   ● S65.21   Laceration of superficial palmar arch
     ● S65.211   Laceration of superficial palmar arch of right hand
     ● S65.212   Laceration of superficial palmar arch of left hand
     ● S65.219   Laceration of superficial palmar arch of unspecified hand
   ● S65.29   Other specified injury of superficial palmar arch
     ● S65.291   Other specified injury of superficial palmar arch of right hand
     ● S65.292   Other specified injury of superficial palmar arch of left hand
     ● S65.299   Other specified injury of superficial palmar arch of unspecified hand

● S65.3   Injury of deep palmar arch
   ● S65.30   Unspecified injury of deep palmar arch
     ● S65.301   Unspecified injury of deep palmar arch of right hand
     ● S65.302   Unspecified injury of deep palmar arch of left hand
     ● S65.309   Unspecified injury of deep palmar arch of unspecified hand

▶ New   ➡ Revised   ~~deleted~~ Deleted   Excludes 1   Excludes 2   Includes   Use additional   Code first   Code also   Key words
OGCR Official Guidelines   X Assign placeholder X   ● Use Additional Character(s)   ▌ Manifestation Code   🔲 Hierarchical Condition Category   **Coding Clinic**

● S65.31   Laceration of deep palmar arch
  ● S65.311   Laceration of deep palmar arch of right hand
  ● S65.312   Laceration of deep palmar arch of left hand
  ● S65.319   Laceration of deep palmar arch of unspecified hand

● S65.39   Other specified injury of deep palmar arch
  ● S65.391   Other specified injury of deep palmar arch of right hand
  ● S65.392   Other specified injury of deep palmar arch of left hand
  ● S65.399   Other specified injury of deep palmar arch of unspecified hand

● S65.4   Injury of blood vessel of thumb
  ● S65.40   Unspecified injury of blood vessel of thumb
    ● S65.401   Unspecified injury of blood vessel of right thumb
    ● S65.402   Unspecified injury of blood vessel of left thumb
    ● S65.409   Unspecified injury of blood vessel of unspecified thumb

  ● S65.41   Laceration of blood vessel of thumb
    ● S65.411   Laceration of blood vessel of right thumb
    ● S65.412   Laceration of blood vessel of left thumb
    ● S65.419   Laceration of blood vessel of unspecified thumb

  ● S65.49   Other specified injury of blood vessel of thumb
    ● S65.491   Other specified injury of blood vessel of right thumb
    ● S65.492   Other specified injury of blood vessel of left thumb
    ● S65.499   Other specified injury of blood vessel of unspecified thumb

● S65.5   Injury of blood vessel of other and unspecified finger
  ● S65.50   Unspecified injury of blood vessel of other and unspecified finger
    ● S65.500   Unspecified injury of blood vessel of right index finger
    ● S65.501   Unspecified injury of blood vessel of left index finger
    ● S65.502   Unspecified injury of blood vessel of right middle finger
    ● S65.503   Unspecified injury of blood vessel of left middle finger
    ● S65.504   Unspecified injury of blood vessel of right ring finger
    ● S65.505   Unspecified injury of blood vessel of left ring finger
    ● S65.506   Unspecified injury of blood vessel of right little finger
    ● S65.507   Unspecified injury of blood vessel of left little finger
    ● S65.508   Unspecified injury of blood vessel of other finger
      Unspecified injury of blood vessel of specified finger with unspecified laterality
    ● S65.509   Unspecified injury of blood vessel of unspecified finger

● S65.51   Laceration of blood vessel of other and unspecified finger
  ● S65.510   Laceration of blood vessel of right index finger
  ● S65.511   Laceration of blood vessel of left index finger
  ● S65.512   Laceration of blood vessel of right middle finger
  ● S65.513   Laceration of blood vessel of left middle finger
  ● S65.514   Laceration of blood vessel of right ring finger
  ● S65.515   Laceration of blood vessel of left ring finger
  ● S65.516   Laceration of blood vessel of right little finger
  ● S65.517   Laceration of blood vessel of left little finger
  ● S65.518   Laceration of blood vessel of other finger
    Laceration of blood vessel of specified finger with unspecified laterality
  ● S65.519   Laceration of blood vessel of unspecified finger

● S65.59   Other specified injury of blood vessel of other and unspecified finger
  ● S65.590   Other specified injury of blood vessel of right index finger
  ● S65.591   Other specified injury of blood vessel of left index finger
  ● S65.592   Other specified injury of blood vessel of right middle finger
  ● S65.593   Other specified injury of blood vessel of left middle finger
  ● S65.594   Other specified injury of blood vessel of right ring finger
  ● S65.595   Other specified injury of blood vessel of left ring finger
  ● S65.596   Other specified injury of blood vessel of right little finger
  ● S65.597   Other specified injury of blood vessel of left little finger
  ● S65.598   Other specified injury of blood vessel of other finger
    Other specified injury of blood vessel of specified finger with unspecified laterality
  ● S65.599   Other specified injury of blood vessel of unspecified finger

● S65.8   Injury of other blood vessels at wrist and hand level
  ● S65.80   Unspecified injury of other blood vessels at wrist and hand level
    ● S65.801   Unspecified injury of other blood vessels at wrist and hand level of right arm
    ● S65.802   Unspecified injury of other blood vessels at wrist and hand level of left arm
    ● S65.809   Unspecified injury of other blood vessels at wrist and hand level of unspecified arm

  ● S65.81   Laceration of other blood vessels at wrist and hand level
    ● S65.811   Laceration of other blood vessels at wrist and hand level of right arm
    ● S65.812   Laceration of other blood vessels at wrist and hand level of left arm
    ● S65.819   Laceration of other blood vessels at wrist and hand level of unspecified arm

CHAPTER 19 (S00–T88)

● **S65.89** Other specified injury of other blood vessels at wrist and hand level
  ● **S65.891** Other specified injury of other blood vessels at wrist and hand level of right arm
  ● **S65.892** Other specified injury of other blood vessels at wrist and hand level of left arm
  ● **S65.899** Other specified injury of other blood vessels at wrist and hand level of unspecified arm
● **S65.9** Injury of unspecified blood vessel at wrist and hand level
 ● **S65.90** Unspecified injury of unspecified blood vessel at wrist and hand level
  ● **S65.901** Unspecified injury of unspecified blood vessel at wrist and hand level of right arm
  ● **S65.902** Unspecified injury of unspecified blood vessel at wrist and hand level of left arm
  ● **S65.909** Unspecified injury of unspecified blood vessel at wrist and hand level of unspecified arm
 ● **S65.91** Laceration of unspecified blood vessel at wrist and hand level
  ● **S65.911** Laceration of unspecified blood vessel at wrist and hand level of right arm
  ● **S65.912** Laceration of unspecified blood vessel at wrist and hand level of left arm
  ● **S65.919** Laceration of unspecified blood vessel at wrist and hand level of unspecified arm
 ● **S65.99** Other specified injury of unspecified blood vessel at wrist and hand level
  ● **S65.991** Other specified injury of unspecified blood vessel at wrist and hand of right arm
  ● **S65.992** Other specified injury of unspecified blood vessel at wrist and hand of left arm
  ● **S65.999** Other specified injury of unspecified blood vessel at wrist and hand of unspecified arm

● **S66** **Injury of muscle, fascia and tendon at wrist and hand level**
 Code also any associated open wound (S61.-)
 Excludes2 sprain of joints and ligaments of wrist and hand (S63.-)
 The appropriate 7th character is to be added to each code from category S66

A	initial encounter
D	subsequent encounter
S	sequela

 ● **S66.0** Injury of long flexor muscle, fascia and tendon of thumb at wrist and hand level
  ● **S66.00** Unspecified injury of long flexor muscle, fascia and tendon of thumb at wrist and hand level
   ● **S66.001** Unspecified injury of long flexor muscle, fascia and tendon of right thumb at wrist and hand level
   ● **S66.002** Unspecified injury of long flexor muscle, fascia and tendon of left thumb at wrist and hand level
   ● **S66.009** Unspecified injury of long flexor muscle, fascia and tendon of unspecified thumb at wrist and hand level

 ● **S66.01** Strain of long flexor muscle, fascia and tendon of thumb at wrist and hand level
  ● **S66.011** Strain of long flexor muscle, fascia and tendon of right thumb at wrist and hand level
  ● **S66.012** Strain of long flexor muscle, fascia and tendon of left thumb at wrist and hand level
  ● **S66.019** Strain of long flexor muscle, fascia and tendon of unspecified thumb at wrist and hand level
 ● **S66.02** Laceration of long flexor muscle, fascia and tendon of thumb at wrist and hand level
  ● **S66.021** Laceration of long flexor muscle, fascia and tendon of right thumb at wrist and hand level
  ● **S66.022** Laceration of long flexor muscle, fascia and tendon of left thumb at wrist and hand level
  ● **S66.029** Laceration of long flexor muscle, fascia and tendon of unspecified thumb at wrist and hand level
 ● **S66.09** Other specified injury of long flexor muscle, fascia and tendon of thumb at wrist and hand level
  ● **S66.091** Other specified injury of long flexor muscle, fascia and tendon of right thumb at wrist and hand level
  ● **S66.092** Other specified injury of long flexor muscle, fascia and tendon of left thumb at wrist and hand level
  ● **S66.099** Other specified injury of long flexor muscle, fascia and tendon of unspecified thumb at wrist and hand level
● **S66.1** Injury of flexor muscle, fascia and tendon of other and unspecified finger at wrist and hand level
 Excludes2 injury of long flexor muscle, fascia and tendon of thumb at wrist and hand level (S66.0-)
 ● **S66.10** Unspecified injury of flexor muscle, fascia and tendon of other and unspecified finger at wrist and hand level
  ● **S66.100** Unspecified injury of flexor muscle, fascia and tendon of right index finger at wrist and hand level
  ● **S66.101** Unspecified injury of flexor muscle, fascia and tendon of left index finger at wrist and hand level
  ● **S66.102** Unspecified injury of flexor muscle, fascia and tendon of right middle finger at wrist and hand level
  ● **S66.103** Unspecified injury of flexor muscle, fascia and tendon of left middle finger at wrist and hand level
  ● **S66.104** Unspecified injury of flexor muscle, fascia and tendon of right ring finger at wrist and hand level
  ● **S66.105** Unspecified injury of flexor muscle, fascia and tendon of left ring finger at wrist and hand level
  ● **S66.106** Unspecified injury of flexor muscle, fascia and tendon of right little finger at wrist and hand level
  ● **S66.107** Unspecified injury of flexor muscle, fascia and tendon of left little finger at wrist and hand level

▶ New ⟹ Revised ~~deleted~~ Deleted Excludes 1 Excludes 2 Includes Use additional Code first Code also Key words
OGCR Official Guidelines X Assign placeholder X ● Use Additional Character(s) ❱ Manifestation Code 🔖 Hierarchical Condition Category **Coding Clinic**

● S66.108   Unspecified injury of flexor muscle, fascia and tendon of other finger at wrist and hand level
             Unspecified injury of flexor muscle, fascia and tendon of specified finger with unspecified laterality at wrist and hand level

● S66.109   Unspecified injury of flexor muscle, fascia and tendon of unspecified finger at wrist and hand level

● S66.11   Strain of flexor muscle, fascia and tendon of other and unspecified finger at wrist and hand level

● S66.110   Strain of flexor muscle, fascia and tendon of right index finger at wrist and hand level

● S66.111   Strain of flexor muscle, fascia and tendon of left index finger at wrist and hand level

● S66.112   Strain of flexor muscle, fascia and tendon of right middle finger at wrist and hand level

● S66.113   Strain of flexor muscle, fascia and tendon of left middle finger at wrist and hand level

● S66.114   Strain of flexor muscle, fascia and tendon of right ring finger at wrist and hand level

● S66.115   Strain of flexor muscle, fascia and tendon of left ring finger at wrist and hand level

● S66.116   Strain of flexor muscle, fascia and tendon of right little finger at wrist and hand level

● S66.117   Strain of flexor muscle, fascia and tendon of left little finger at wrist and hand level

● S66.118   Strain of flexor muscle, fascia and tendon of other finger at wrist and hand level
             Strain of flexor muscle, fascia and tendon of specified finger with unspecified laterality at wrist and hand level

● S66.119   Strain of flexor muscle, fascia and tendon of unspecified finger at wrist and hand level

● S66.12   Laceration of flexor muscle, fascia and tendon of other and unspecified finger at wrist and hand level

● S66.120   Laceration of flexor muscle, fascia and tendon of right index finger at wrist and hand level

● S66.121   Laceration of flexor muscle, fascia and tendon of left index finger at wrist and hand level

● S66.122   Laceration of flexor muscle, fascia and tendon of right middle finger at wrist and hand level

● S66.123   Laceration of flexor muscle, fascia and tendon of left middle finger at wrist and hand level

● S66.124   Laceration of flexor muscle, fascia and tendon of right ring finger at wrist and hand level

● S66.125   Laceration of flexor muscle, fascia and tendon of left ring finger at wrist and hand level

● S66.126   Laceration of flexor muscle, fascia and tendon of right little finger at wrist and hand level

● S66.127   Laceration of flexor muscle, fascia and tendon of left little finger at wrist and hand level

● S66.128   Laceration of flexor muscle, fascia and tendon of other finger at wrist and hand level
             Laceration of flexor muscle, fascia and tendon of specified finger with unspecified laterality at wrist and hand level

● S66.129   Laceration of flexor muscle, fascia and tendon of unspecified finger at wrist and hand level

● S66.19   Other injury of flexor muscle, fascia and tendon of other and unspecified finger at wrist and hand level

● S66.190   Other injury of flexor muscle, fascia and tendon of right index finger at wrist and hand level

● S66.191   Other injury of flexor muscle, fascia and tendon of left index finger at wrist and hand level

● S66.192   Other injury of flexor muscle, fascia and tendon of right middle finger at wrist and hand level

● S66.193   Other injury of flexor muscle, fascia and tendon of left middle finger at wrist and hand level

● S66.194   Other injury of flexor muscle, fascia and tendon of right ring finger at wrist and hand level

● S66.195   Other injury of flexor muscle, fascia and tendon of left ring finger at wrist and hand level

● S66.196   Other injury of flexor muscle, fascia and tendon of right little finger at wrist and hand level

● S66.197   Other injury of flexor muscle, fascia and tendon of left little finger at wrist and hand level

● S66.198   Other injury of flexor muscle, fascia and tendon of other finger at wrist and hand level
             Other injury of flexor muscle, fascia and tendon of specified finger with unspecified laterality at wrist and hand level

● S66.199   Other injury of flexor muscle, fascia and tendon of unspecified finger at wrist and hand level

● S66.2   Injury of extensor muscle, fascia and tendon of thumb at wrist and hand level

● S66.20   Unspecified injury of extensor muscle, fascia and tendon of thumb at wrist and hand level

● S66.201   Unspecified injury of extensor muscle, fascia and tendon of right thumb at wrist and hand level

● S66.202   Unspecified injury of extensor muscle, fascia and tendon of left thumb at wrist and hand level

● S66.209   Unspecified injury of extensor muscle, fascia and tendon of unspecified thumb at wrist and hand level

● S66.21   Strain of extensor muscle, fascia and tendon of thumb at wrist and hand level

● S66.211   Strain of extensor muscle, fascia and tendon of right thumb at wrist and hand level

● S66.212   Strain of extensor muscle, fascia and tendon of left thumb at wrist and hand level

● S66.219   Strain of extensor muscle, fascia and tendon of unspecified thumb at wrist and hand level

CHAPTER 19 (S00-T88)

● **S66.22**   **Laceration** of extensor muscle, fascia and tendon of thumb at wrist and hand level

　　● S66.221   Laceration of extensor muscle, fascia and tendon of **right** thumb at wrist and hand level

　　● S66.222   Laceration of extensor muscle, fascia and tendon of **left** thumb at wrist and hand level

　　● S66.229   Laceration of extensor muscle, fascia and tendon of **unspecified** thumb at wrist and hand level

● **S66.29**   **Other** specified injury of extensor muscle, fascia and tendon of thumb at wrist and hand level

　　● S66.291   Other specified injury of extensor muscle, fascia and tendon of **right** thumb at wrist and hand level

　　● S66.292   Other specified injury of extensor muscle, fascia and tendon of **left** thumb at wrist and hand level

　　● S66.299   Other specified injury of extensor muscle, fascia and tendon of **unspecified** thumb at wrist and hand level

● **S66.3**   **Injury** of **extensor** muscle, fascia and tendon of other and unspecified **finger** at wrist and hand level

　　Excludes2   injury of extensor muscle, fascia and tendon of thumb at wrist and hand level (S66.2-)

● **S66.30**   **Unspecified** injury of extensor muscle, fascia and tendon of other and unspecified finger at wrist and hand level

　　● S66.300   Unspecified injury of extensor muscle, fascia and tendon of **right index** finger at wrist and hand level

　　● S66.301   Unspecified injury of extensor muscle, fascia and tendon of **left index** finger at wrist and hand level

　　● S66.302   Unspecified injury of extensor muscle, fascia and tendon of **right middle** finger at wrist and hand level

　　● S66.303   Unspecified injury of extensor muscle, fascia and tendon of **left middle** finger at wrist and hand level

　　● S66.304   Unspecified injury of extensor muscle, fascia and tendon of **right ring** finger at wrist and hand level

　　● S66.305   Unspecified injury of extensor muscle, fascia and tendon of **left ring** finger at wrist and hand level

　　● S66.306   Unspecified injury of extensor muscle, fascia and tendon of **right little** finger at wrist and hand level

　　● S66.307   Unspecified injury of extensor muscle, fascia and tendon of **left little** finger at wrist and hand level

　　● S66.308   Unspecified injury of extensor muscle, fascia and tendon of **other** finger at wrist and hand level

　　　　Unspecified injury of extensor muscle, fascia and tendon of specified finger with unspecified laterality at wrist and hand level

　　● S66.309   Unspecified injury of extensor muscle, fascia and tendon of **unspecified** finger at wrist and hand level

● **S66.31**   **Strain** of extensor muscle, fascia and tendon of other and unspecified finger at wrist and hand level

　　● S66.310   Strain of extensor muscle, fascia and tendon of **right index** finger at wrist and hand level

　　● S66.311   Strain of extensor muscle, fascia and tendon of **left index** finger at wrist and hand level

　　● S66.312   Strain of extensor muscle, fascia and tendon of **right middle** finger at wrist and hand level

　　● S66.313   Strain of extensor muscle, fascia and tendon of **left middle** finger at wrist and hand level

　　● S66.314   Strain of extensor muscle, fascia and tendon of **right ring** finger at wrist and hand level

　　● S66.315   Strain of extensor muscle, fascia and tendon of **left ring** finger at wrist and hand level

　　● S66.316   Strain of extensor muscle, fascia and tendon of **right little** finger at wrist and hand level

　　● S66.317   Strain of extensor muscle, fascia and tendon of **left little** finger at wrist and hand level

　　● S66.318   Strain of extensor muscle, fascia and tendon of **other** finger at wrist and hand level

　　　　Strain of extensor muscle, fascia and tendon of specified finger with unspecified laterality at wrist and hand level

　　● S66.319   Strain of extensor muscle, fascia and tendon of **unspecified** finger at wrist and hand level

● **S66.32**   **Laceration** of extensor muscle, fascia and tendon of other and unspecified finger at wrist and hand level

　　● S66.320   Laceration of extensor muscle, fascia and tendon of **right index** finger at wrist and hand level

　　● S66.321   Laceration of extensor muscle, fascia and tendon of **left index** finger at wrist and hand level

　　● S66.322   Laceration of extensor muscle, fascia and tendon of **right middle** finger at wrist and hand level

　　● S66.323   Laceration of extensor muscle, fascia and tendon of **left middle** finger at wrist and hand level

　　● S66.324   Laceration of extensor muscle, fascia and tendon of **right ring** finger at wrist and hand level

　　● S66.325   Laceration of extensor muscle, fascia and tendon of **left ring** finger at wrist and hand level

　　● S66.326   Laceration of extensor muscle, fascia and tendon of **right little** finger at wrist and hand level

　　● S66.327   Laceration of extensor muscle, fascia and tendon of **left little** finger at wrist and hand level

　　● S66.328   Laceration of extensor muscle, fascia and tendon of **other** finger at wrist and hand level

　　　　Laceration of extensor muscle, fascia and tendon of specified finger with unspecified laterality at wrist and hand level

　　● S66.329   Laceration of extensor muscle, fascia and tendon of **unspecified** finger at wrist and hand level

▶ New　⟹ Revised　~~deleted~~ Deleted　Excludes 1　Excludes 2　Includes　Use additional　Code first　Code also　Key words
OGCR Official Guidelines　X Assign placeholder X　● Use Additional Character(s)　⟩ Manifestation Code　🕸 Hierarchical Condition Category　**Coding Clinic**

● S66.39   Other injury of extensor muscle, fascia and tendon of other and unspecified finger at wrist and hand level
  ● S66.390   Other injury of extensor muscle, fascia and tendon of right index finger at wrist and hand level
  ● S66.391   Other injury of extensor muscle, fascia and tendon of left index finger at wrist and hand level
  ● S66.392   Other injury of extensor muscle, fascia and tendon of right middle finger at wrist and hand level
  ● S66.393   Other injury of extensor muscle, fascia and tendon of left middle finger at wrist and hand level
  ● S66.394   Other injury of extensor muscle, fascia and tendon of right ring finger at wrist and hand level
  ● S66.395   Other injury of extensor muscle, fascia and tendon of left ring finger at wrist and hand level
  ● S66.396   Other injury of extensor muscle, fascia and tendon of right little finger at wrist and hand level
  ● S66.397   Other injury of extensor muscle, fascia and tendon of left little finger at wrist and hand level
  ● S66.398   Other injury of extensor muscle, fascia and tendon of other finger at wrist and hand level
       Other injury of extensor muscle, fascia and tendon of specified finger with unspecified laterality at wrist and hand level
  ● S66.399   Other injury of extensor muscle, fascia and tendon of unspecified finger at wrist and hand level

● S66.4   Injury of intrinsic muscle, fascia and tendon of thumb at wrist and hand level
 ● S66.40   Unspecified injury of intrinsic muscle, fascia and tendon of thumb at wrist and hand level
  ● S66.401   Unspecified injury of intrinsic muscle, fascia and tendon of right thumb at wrist and hand level
  ● S66.402   Unspecified injury of intrinsic muscle, fascia and tendon of left thumb at wrist and hand level
  ● S66.409   Unspecified injury of intrinsic muscle, fascia and tendon of unspecified thumb at wrist and hand level
 ● S66.41   Strain of intrinsic muscle, fascia and tendon of thumb at wrist and hand level
  ● S66.411   Strain of intrinsic muscle, fascia and tendon of right thumb at wrist and hand level
  ● S66.412   Strain of intrinsic muscle, fascia and tendon of left thumb at wrist and hand level
  ● S66.419   Strain of intrinsic muscle, fascia and tendon of unspecified thumb at wrist and hand level
 ● S66.42   Laceration of intrinsic muscle, fascia and tendon of thumb at wrist and hand level
  ● S66.421   Laceration of intrinsic muscle, fascia and tendon of right thumb at wrist and hand level
  ● S66.422   Laceration of intrinsic muscle, fascia and tendon of left thumb at wrist and hand level
  ● S66.429   Laceration of intrinsic muscle, fascia and tendon of unspecified thumb at wrist and hand level

● S66.49   Other specified injury of intrinsic muscle, fascia and tendon of thumb at wrist and hand level
  ● S66.491   Other specified injury of intrinsic muscle, fascia and tendon of right thumb at wrist and hand level
  ● S66.492   Other specified injury of intrinsic muscle, fascia and tendon of left thumb at wrist and hand level
  ● S66.499   Other specified injury of intrinsic muscle, fascia and tendon of unspecified thumb at wrist and hand level

● S66.5   Injury of intrinsic muscle, fascia and tendon of other and unspecified finger at wrist and hand level
    Excludes2   injury of intrinsic muscle, fascia and tendon of thumb at wrist and hand level (S66.4-)
 ● S66.50   Unspecified injury of intrinsic muscle, fascia and tendon of other and unspecified finger at wrist and hand level
  ● S66.500   Unspecified injury of intrinsic muscle, fascia and tendon of right index finger at wrist and hand level
  ● S66.501   Unspecified injury of intrinsic muscle, fascia and tendon of left index finger at wrist and hand level
  ● S66.502   Unspecified injury of intrinsic muscle, fascia and tendon of right middle finger at wrist and hand level
  ● S66.503   Unspecified injury of intrinsic muscle, fascia and tendon of left middle finger at wrist and hand level
  ● S66.504   Unspecified injury of intrinsic muscle, fascia and tendon of right ring finger at wrist and hand level
  ● S66.505   Unspecified injury of intrinsic muscle, fascia and tendon of left ring finger at wrist and hand level
  ● S66.506   Unspecified injury of intrinsic muscle, fascia and tendon of right little finger at wrist and hand level
  ● S66.507   Unspecified injury of intrinsic muscle, fascia and tendon of left little finger at wrist and hand level
  ● S66.508   Unspecified injury of intrinsic muscle, fascia and tendon of other finger at wrist and hand level
       Unspecified injury of intrinsic muscle, fascia and tendon of specified finger with unspecified laterality at wrist and hand level
  ● S66.509   Unspecified injury of intrinsic muscle, fascia and tendon of unspecified finger at wrist and hand level
 ● S66.51   Strain of intrinsic muscle, fascia and tendon of other and unspecified finger at wrist and hand level
  ● S66.510   Strain of intrinsic muscle, fascia and tendon of right index finger at wrist and hand level
  ● S66.511   Strain of intrinsic muscle, fascia and tendon of left index finger at wrist and hand level
  ● S66.512   Strain of intrinsic muscle, fascia and tendon of right middle finger at wrist and hand level
  ● S66.513   Strain of intrinsic muscle, fascia and tendon of left middle finger at wrist and hand level
  ● S66.514   Strain of intrinsic muscle, fascia and tendon of right ring finger at wrist and hand level

CHAPTER 19 (S00-T88)

● S66.515   Strain of intrinsic muscle, fascia and tendon of left ring finger at wrist and hand level

● S66.516   Strain of intrinsic muscle, fascia and tendon of right little finger at wrist and hand level

● S66.517   Strain of intrinsic muscle, fascia and tendon of left little finger at wrist and hand level

● S66.518   Strain of intrinsic muscle, fascia and tendon of other finger at wrist and hand level

     Strain of intrinsic muscle, fascia and tendon of specified finger with unspecified laterality at wrist and hand level

● S66.519   Strain of intrinsic muscle, fascia and tendon of unspecified finger at wrist and hand level

● S66.52   Laceration of intrinsic muscle, fascia and tendon of other and unspecified finger at wrist and hand level

● S66.520   Laceration of intrinsic muscle, fascia and tendon of right index finger at wrist and hand level

● S66.521   Laceration of intrinsic muscle, fascia and tendon of left index finger at wrist and hand level

● S66.522   Laceration of intrinsic muscle, fascia and tendon of right middle finger at wrist and hand level

● S66.523   Laceration of intrinsic muscle, fascia and tendon of left middle finger at wrist and hand level

● S66.524   Laceration of intrinsic muscle, fascia and tendon of right ring finger at wrist and hand level

● S66.525   Laceration of intrinsic muscle, fascia and tendon of left ring finger at wrist and hand level

● S66.526   Laceration of intrinsic muscle, fascia and tendon of right little finger at wrist and hand level

● S66.527   Laceration of intrinsic muscle, fascia and tendon of left little finger at wrist and hand level

● S66.528   Laceration of intrinsic muscle, fascia and tendon of other finger at wrist and hand level

     Laceration of intrinsic muscle, fascia and tendon of specified finger with unspecified laterality at wrist and hand level

● S66.529   Laceration of intrinsic muscle, fascia and tendon of unspecified finger at wrist and hand level

● S66.59   Other injury of intrinsic muscle, fascia and tendon of other and unspecified finger at wrist and hand level

● S66.590   Other injury of intrinsic muscle, fascia and tendon of right index finger at wrist and hand level

● S66.591   Other injury of intrinsic muscle, fascia and tendon of left index finger at wrist and hand level

● S66.592   Other injury of intrinsic muscle, fascia and tendon of right middle finger at wrist and hand level

● S66.593   Other injury of intrinsic muscle, fascia and tendon of left middle finger at wrist and hand level

● S66.594   Other injury of intrinsic muscle, fascia and tendon of right ring finger at wrist and hand level

● S66.595   Other injury of intrinsic muscle, fascia and tendon of left ring finger at wrist and hand level

● S66.596   Other injury of intrinsic muscle, fascia and tendon of right little finger at wrist and hand level

● S66.597   Other injury of intrinsic muscle, fascia and tendon of left little finger at wrist and hand level

● S66.598   Other injury of intrinsic muscle, fascia and tendon of other finger at wrist and hand level

     Other injury of intrinsic muscle, fascia and tendon of specified finger with unspecified laterality at wrist and hand level

● S66.599   Other injury of intrinsic muscle, fascia and tendon of unspecified finger at wrist and hand level

● S66.8   Injury of other specified muscles, fascia and tendons at wrist and hand level

● S66.80   Unspecified injury of other specified muscles, fascia and tendons at wrist and hand level

● S66.801   Unspecified injury of other specified muscles, fascia and tendons at wrist and hand level, right hand

● S66.802   Unspecified injury of other specified muscles, fascia and tendons at wrist and hand level, left hand

● S66.809   Unspecified injury of other specified muscles, fascia and tendons at wrist and hand level, unspecified hand

● S66.81   Strain of other specified muscles, fascia and tendons at wrist and hand level

● S66.811   Strain of other specified muscles, fascia and tendons at wrist and hand level, right hand

● S66.812   Strain of other specified muscles, fascia and tendons at wrist and hand level, left hand

● S66.819   Strain of other specified muscles, fascia and tendons at wrist and hand level, unspecified hand

● S66.82   Laceration of other specified muscles, fascia and tendons at wrist and hand level

● S66.821   Laceration of other specified muscles, fascia and tendons at wrist and hand level, right hand

● S66.822   Laceration of other specified muscles, fascia and tendons at wrist and hand level, left hand

● S66.829   Laceration of other specified muscles, fascia and tendons at wrist and hand level, unspecified hand

● S66.89   Other injury of other specified muscles, fascia and tendons at wrist and hand level

● S66.891   Other injury of other specified muscles, fascia and tendons at wrist and hand level, right hand

● S66.892   Other injury of other specified muscles, fascia and tendons at wrist and hand level, left hand

● S66.899   Other injury of other specified muscles, fascia and tendons at wrist and hand level, unspecified hand

▶ New   ⇒ Revised   ~~deleted~~ Deleted   Excludes 1   Excludes 2   Includes   Use additional   Code first   Code also   Key words

OGCR Official Guidelines   X Assign placeholder X   ● Use Additional Character(s)   ▷ Manifestation Code   ✆ Hierarchical Condition Category   **Coding Clinic**

● **S66.9**   Injury of unspecified muscle, fascia and tendon at wrist and hand level

  ● **S66.90**   Unspecified injury of unspecified muscle, fascia and tendon at wrist and hand level

    ● **S66.901**   Unspecified injury of unspecified muscle, fascia and tendon at wrist and hand level, right hand

    ● **S66.902**   Unspecified injury of unspecified muscle, fascia and tendon at wrist and hand level, left hand

    ● **S66.909**   Unspecified injury of unspecified muscle, fascia and tendon at wrist and hand level, unspecified hand

  ● **S66.91**   Strain of unspecified muscle, fascia and tendon at wrist and hand level

    ● **S66.911**   Strain of unspecified muscle, fascia and tendon at wrist and hand level, right hand

    ● **S66.912**   Strain of unspecified muscle, fascia and tendon at wrist and hand level, left hand

    ● **S66.919**   Strain of unspecified muscle, fascia and tendon at wrist and hand level, unspecified hand

  ● **S66.92**   Laceration of unspecified muscle, fascia and tendon at wrist and hand level

    ● **S66.921**   Laceration of unspecified muscle, fascia and tendon at wrist and hand level, right hand

    ● **S66.922**   Laceration of unspecified muscle, fascia and tendon at wrist and hand level, left hand

    ● **S66.929**   Laceration of unspecified muscle, fascia and tendon at wrist and hand level, unspecified hand

  ● **S66.99**   Other injury of unspecified muscle, fascia and tendon at wrist and hand level

    ● **S66.991**   Other injury of unspecified muscle, fascia and tendon at wrist and hand level, right hand

    ● **S66.992**   Other injury of unspecified muscle, fascia and tendon at wrist and hand level, left hand

    ● **S66.999**   Other injury of unspecified muscle, fascia and tendon at wrist and hand level, unspecified hand

● **S67**   Crushing injury of wrist, hand and fingers

     Use additional code for all associated injuries, such as:
         fracture of wrist and hand (S62.-)
         open wound of wrist and hand (S61.-)

     The appropriate 7th character is to be added to each code from category S67

A	initial encounter
D	subsequent encounter
S	sequela

  ● **S67.0**   Crushing injury of thumb

    X ● **S67.00**   Crushing injury of unspecified thumb

    X ● **S67.01**   Crushing injury of right thumb

    X ● **S67.02**   Crushing injury of left thumb

  ● **S67.1**   Crushing injury of other and unspecified finger(s)

     Excludes2   crushing injury of thumb (S67.0-)

    X ● **S67.10**   Crushing injury of unspecified finger(s)

    ● **S67.19**   Crushing injury of other finger(s)

      ● **S67.190**   Crushing injury of right index finger

      ● **S67.191**   Crushing injury of left index finger

      ● **S67.192**   Crushing injury of right middle finger

      ● **S67.193**   Crushing injury of left middle finger

      ● **S67.194**   Crushing injury of right ring finger

      ● **S67.195**   Crushing injury of left ring finger

      ● **S67.196**   Crushing injury of right little finger

      ● **S67.197**   Crushing injury of left little finger

      ● **S67.198**   Crushing injury of other finger
            Crushing injury of specified finger with unspecified laterality

  ● **S67.2**   Crushing injury of hand

     Excludes2   crushing injury of fingers (S67.1-)
                 crushing injury of thumb (S67.0-)

    X ● **S67.20**   Crushing injury of unspecified hand

    X ● **S67.21**   Crushing injury of right hand

    X ● **S67.22**   Crushing injury of left hand

  ● **S67.3**   Crushing injury of wrist

    X ● **S67.30**   Crushing injury of unspecified wrist

    X ● **S67.31**   Crushing injury of right wrist

    X ● **S67.32**   Crushing injury of left wrist

  ● **S67.4**   Crushing injury of wrist and hand

     Excludes1   crushing injury of hand alone (S67.2-)
                 crushing injury of wrist alone (S67.3-)

     Excludes2   crushing injury of fingers (S67.1-)
                 crushing injury of thumb (S67.0-)

    X ● **S67.40**   Crushing injury of unspecified wrist and hand

    X ● **S67.41**   Crushing injury of right wrist and hand

    X ● **S67.42**   Crushing injury of left wrist and hand

  ● **S67.9**   Crushing injury of unspecified part(s) of wrist, hand and fingers

    X ● **S67.90**   Crushing injury of unspecified part(s) of unspecified wrist, hand and fingers

    X ● **S67.91**   Crushing injury of unspecified part(s) of right wrist, hand and fingers

    X ● **S67.92**   Crushing injury of unspecified part(s) of left wrist, hand and fingers

● **S68**   Traumatic amputation of wrist, hand and fingers

     An amputation not identified as partial or complete should be coded to complete

     The appropriate 7th character is to be added to each code from category S68

A	initial encounter
D	subsequent encounter
S	sequela

  ● **S68.0**   Traumatic metacarpophalangeal amputation of thumb
       Traumatic amputation of thumb NOS

    ● **S68.01**   Complete traumatic metacarpophalangeal amputation of thumb

      ● **S68.011**   Complete traumatic metacarpophalangeal amputation of right thumb S 🖐

      ● **S68.012**   Complete traumatic metacarpophalangeal amputation of left thumb S 🖐

      ● **S68.019**   Complete traumatic metacarpophalangeal amputation of unspecified thumb S 🖐

    ● **S68.02**   Partial traumatic metacarpophalangeal amputation of thumb

      ● **S68.021**   Partial traumatic metacarpophalangeal amputation of right thumb S 🖐

      ● **S68.022**   Partial traumatic metacarpophalangeal amputation of left thumb S 🖐

      ● **S68.029**   Partial traumatic metacarpophalangeal amputation of unspecified thumb S 🖐

● S68.1   Traumatic metacarpophalangeal amputation of other and
unspecified finger
    Traumatic amputation of finger NOS
    Excludes2   traumatic metacarpophalangeal
                     amputation of thumb (S68.0-)
    ● S68.11   Complete traumatic metacarpophalangeal
               amputation of other and unspecified finger
        ● S68.110   Complete traumatic
                     metacarpophalangeal amputation of
                     right index finger S 🐾
        ● S68.111   Complete traumatic
                     metacarpophalangeal amputation of
                     left index finger S 🐾
        ● S68.112   Complete traumatic
                     metacarpophalangeal amputation of
                     right middle finger S 🐾
        ● S68.113   Complete traumatic
                     metacarpophalangeal amputation of
                     left middle finger S 🐾
        ● S68.114   Complete traumatic
                     metacarpophalangeal amputation of
                     right ring finger S 🐾
        ● S68.115   Complete traumatic
                     metacarpophalangeal amputation of
                     left ring finger S 🐾
        ● S68.116   Complete traumatic
                     metacarpophalangeal amputation of
                     right little finger S 🐾
        ● S68.117   Complete traumatic
                     metacarpophalangeal amputation of
                     left little finger S 🐾
        ● S68.118   Complete traumatic
                     metacarpophalangeal amputation of
                     other finger S 🐾
                     Complete traumatic
                         metacarpophalangeal
                         amputation of specified finger
                         with unspecified laterality
        ● S68.119   Complete traumatic
                     metacarpophalangeal amputation of
                     unspecified finger S 🐾
    ● S68.12   Partial traumatic metacarpophalangeal
               amputation of other and unspecified finger
        ● S68.120   Partial traumatic
                     metacarpophalangeal amputation of
                     right index finger S 🐾
        ● S68.121   Partial traumatic
                     metacarpophalangeal amputation of
                     left index finger S 🐾
        ● S68.122   Partial traumatic
                     metacarpophalangeal amputation of
                     right middle finger S 🐾
        ● S68.123   Partial traumatic
                     metacarpophalangeal amputation of
                     left middle finger S 🐾
        ● S68.124   Partial traumatic
                     metacarpophalangeal amputation of
                     right ring finger S 🐾
        ● S68.125   Partial traumatic
                     metacarpophalangeal amputation of
                     left ring finger S 🐾
        ● S68.126   Partial traumatic
                     metacarpophalangeal amputation of
                     right little finger S 🐾
        ● S68.127   Partial traumatic
                     metacarpophalangeal amputation of
                     left little finger S 🐾

        ● S68.128   Partial traumatic
                     metacarpophalangeal amputation of
                     other finger S 🐾
                     Partial traumatic
                         metacarpophalangeal
                         amputation of specified finger
                         with unspecified laterality
        ● S68.129   Partial traumatic
                     metacarpophalangeal amputation of
                     unspecified finger S 🐾
● S68.4   Traumatic amputation of hand at wrist level
    Traumatic amputation of hand NOS
    Traumatic amputation of wrist
    ● S68.41   Complete traumatic amputation of hand at
               wrist level
        ● S68.411   Complete traumatic amputation of
                     right hand at wrist level A, S 🐾
        ● S68.412   Complete traumatic amputation of
                     left hand at wrist level A, S 🐾
        ● S68.419   Complete traumatic amputation of
                     unspecified hand at wrist level A, S 🐾
    ● S68.42   Partial traumatic amputation of hand at wrist
               level
        ● S68.421   Partial traumatic amputation of right
                     hand at wrist level A, S 🐾
        ● S68.422   Partial traumatic amputation of left
                     hand at wrist level A, S 🐾
        ● S68.429   Partial traumatic amputation of
                     unspecified hand at wrist level A, S 🐾
● S68.5   Traumatic transphalangeal amputation of thumb
    Traumatic interphalangeal joint amputation of thumb
    ● S68.51   Complete traumatic transphalangeal
               amputation of thumb
        ● S68.511   Complete traumatic transphalangeal
                     amputation of right thumb S 🐾
        ● S68.512   Complete traumatic transphalangeal
                     amputation of left thumb S 🐾
        ● S68.519   Complete traumatic transphalangeal
                     amputation of unspecified thumb S 🐾
    ● S68.52   Partial traumatic transphalangeal amputation of
               thumb
        ● S68.521   Partial traumatic transphalangeal
                     amputation of right thumb S 🐾
        ● S68.522   Partial traumatic transphalangeal
                     amputation of left thumb S 🐾
        ● S68.529   Partial traumatic transphalangeal
                     amputation of unspecified thumb S 🐾
● S68.6   Traumatic transphalangeal amputation of other and
          unspecified finger
    ● S68.61   Complete traumatic transphalangeal
               amputation of other and unspecified finger(s)
        ● S68.610   Complete traumatic transphalangeal
                     amputation of right index finger S 🐾
        ● S68.611   Complete traumatic transphalangeal
                     amputation of left index finger S 🐾
        ● S68.612   Complete traumatic transphalangeal
                     amputation of right middle
                     finger S 🐾
        ● S68.613   Complete traumatic transphalangeal
                     amputation of left middle finger S 🐾
        ● S68.614   Complete traumatic transphalangeal
                     amputation of right ring finger S 🐾
        ● S68.615   Complete traumatic transphalangeal
                     amputation of left ring finger S 🐾
        ● S68.616   Complete traumatic transphalangeal
                     amputation of right little finger S 🐾

▶ New   ⇒ Revised   ~~deleted~~ Deleted   Excludes 1   Excludes 2   Includes   Use additional   Code first   Code also   Key words

OGCR Official Guidelines   X Assign placeholder X   ● Use Additional Character(s)   ▷ Manifestation Code   🐾 Hierarchical Condition Category   **Coding Clinic**

● S68.617 Complete traumatic transphalangeal amputation of left little finger S 🐾

● S68.618 Complete traumatic transphalangeal amputation of other finger S 🐾

    Complete traumatic transphalangeal amputation of specified finger with unspecified laterality

● S68.619 Complete traumatic transphalangeal amputation of unspecified finger S 🐾

● S68.62 Partial traumatic transphalangeal amputation of other and unspecified finger

● S68.620 Partial traumatic transphalangeal amputation of right index finger S 🐾

● S68.621 Partial traumatic transphalangeal amputation of left index finger S 🐾

● S68.622 Partial traumatic transphalangeal amputation of right middle finger S 🐾

● S68.623 Partial traumatic transphalangeal amputation of left middle finger S 🐾

● S68.624 Partial traumatic transphalangeal amputation of right ring finger S 🐾

● S68.625 Partial traumatic transphalangeal amputation of left ring finger S 🐾

● S68.626 Partial traumatic transphalangeal amputation of right little finger S 🐾

● S68.627 Partial traumatic transphalangeal amputation of left little finger S 🐾

● S68.628 Partial traumatic transphalangeal amputation of other finger S 🐾

    Partial traumatic transphalangeal amputation of specified finger with unspecified laterality

● S68.629 Partial traumatic transphalangeal amputation of unspecified finger S 🐾

● S68.7 Traumatic transmetacarpal amputation of hand

● S68.71 Complete traumatic transmetacarpal amputation of hand

● S68.711 Complete traumatic transmetacarpal amputation of right hand A, S 🐾

● S68.712 Complete traumatic transmetacarpal amputation of left hand A, S 🐾

● S68.719 Complete traumatic transmetacarpal amputation of unspecified hand A, S 🐾

● S68.72 Partial traumatic transmetacarpal amputation of hand

● S68.721 Partial traumatic transmetacarpal amputation of right hand A, S 🐾

● S68.722 Partial traumatic transmetacarpal amputation of left hand A, S 🐾

● S68.729 Partial traumatic transmetacarpal amputation of unspecified hand A, S 🐾

● S69 Other and unspecified injuries of wrist, hand and finger(s)

The appropriate 7th character is to be added to each code from category S69

A	initial encounter
D	subsequent encounter
S	sequela

● S69.8 Other specified injuries of wrist, hand and finger(s)

X ● S69.80 Other specified injuries of unspecified wrist, hand and finger(s)

X ● S69.81 Other specified injuries of right wrist, hand and finger(s)

X ● S69.82 Other specified injuries of left wrist, hand and finger(s)

● S69.9 Unspecified injury of wrist, hand and finger(s)

X ● S69.90 Unspecified injury of unspecified wrist, hand and finger(s)

X ● S69.91 Unspecified injury of right wrist, hand and finger(s)

X ● S69.92 Unspecified injury of left wrist, hand and finger(s)

INJURIES TO THE HIP AND THIGH (S70-S79)

Excludes2 burns and corrosions (T20-T32)
              frostbite (T33-T34)
              snake bite (T63.0-)
              venomous insect bite or sting (T63.4-)

● S70 Superficial injury of hip and thigh

The appropriate 7th character is to be added to each code from category S70

A	initial encounter
D	subsequent encounter
S	sequela

● S70.0 Contusion of hip

X ● S70.00 Contusion of unspecified hip

X ● S70.01 Contusion of right hip

X ● S70.02 Contusion of left hip

● S70.1 Contusion of thigh

X ● S70.10 Contusion of unspecified thigh

X ● S70.11 Contusion of right thigh

X ● S70.12 Contusion of left thigh

● S70.2 Other superficial injuries of hip

● S70.21 Abrasion of hip

● S70.211 Abrasion, right hip

● S70.212 Abrasion, left hip

● S70.219 Abrasion, unspecified hip

● S70.22 Blister (nonthermal) of hip

● S70.221 Blister (nonthermal), right hip

● S70.222 Blister (nonthermal), left hip

● S70.229 Blister (nonthermal), unspecified hip

● S70.24 External constriction of hip

● S70.241 External constriction, right hip

● S70.242 External constriction, left hip

● S70.249 External constriction, unspecified hip

● S70.25 Superficial foreign body of hip

Splinter in the hip

● S70.251 Superficial foreign body, right hip

● S70.252 Superficial foreign body, left hip

● S70.259 Superficial foreign body, unspecified hip

● S70.26 Insect bite (nonvenomous) of hip

● S70.261 Insect bite (nonvenomous), right hip

● S70.262 Insect bite (nonvenomous), left hip

● S70.269 Insect bite (nonvenomous), unspecified hip

● S70.27 Other superficial bite of hip

Excludes1 open bite of hip (S71.05-)

● S70.271 Other superficial bite of hip, right hip

● S70.272 Other superficial bite of hip, left hip

● S70.279 Other superficial bite of hip, unspecified hip

● S70.3 Other superficial injuries of thigh

● S70.31 Abrasion of thigh

● S70.311 Abrasion, right thigh

● S70.312 Abrasion, left thigh

● S70.319 Abrasion, unspecified thigh

- S70.32 Blister (nonthermal) of thigh
  - S70.321 Blister (nonthermal), right thigh
  - S70.322 Blister (nonthermal), left thigh
  - S70.329 Blister (nonthermal), unspecified thigh
- S70.34 External constriction of thigh
  - S70.341 External constriction, right thigh
  - S70.342 External constriction, left thigh
  - S70.349 External constriction, unspecified thigh
- S70.35 Superficial foreign body of thigh
  Splinter in the thigh
  - S70.351 Superficial foreign body, right thigh
  - S70.352 Superficial foreign body, left thigh
  - S70.359 Superficial foreign body, unspecified thigh
- S70.36 Insect bite (nonvenomous) of thigh
  - S70.361 Insect bite (nonvenomous), right thigh
  - S70.362 Insect bite (nonvenomous), left thigh
  - S70.369 Insect bite (nonvenomous), unspecified thigh
- S70.37 Other superficial bite of thigh
  - **Excludes1** open bite of thigh (S71.15)
  - S70.371 Other superficial bite of right thigh
  - S70.372 Other superficial bite of left thigh
  - S70.379 Other superficial bite of unspecified thigh
- S70.9 Unspecified superficial injury of hip and thigh
  - S70.91 Unspecified superficial injury of hip
    - S70.911 Unspecified superficial injury of right hip
    - S70.912 Unspecified superficial injury of left hip
    - S70.919 Unspecified superficial injury of unspecified hip
  - S70.92 Unspecified superficial injury of thigh
    - S70.921 Unspecified superficial injury of right thigh
    - S70.922 Unspecified superficial injury of left thigh
    - S70.929 Unspecified superficial injury of unspecified thigh
- S71 Open wound of hip and thigh
  Code also any associated wound infection
  - **Excludes1** open fracture of hip and thigh (S72.-)
    traumatic amputation of hip and thigh (S78.-)
  - **Excludes2** bite of venomous animal (T63.-)
    open wound of ankle, foot and toes (S91.-)
    open wound of knee and lower leg (S81.-)

  The appropriate 7th character is to be added to each code from category S71

A	initial encounter
D	subsequent encounter
S	sequela

  - S71.0 Open wound of hip
    - S71.00 Unspecified open wound of hip
      - S71.001 Unspecified open wound, right hip
      - S71.002 Unspecified open wound, left hip
      - S71.009 Unspecified open wound, unspecified hip

- S71.01 Laceration without foreign body of hip
  - S71.011 Laceration without foreign body, right hip
  - S71.012 Laceration without foreign body, left hip
  - S71.019 Laceration without foreign body, unspecified hip
- S71.02 Laceration with foreign body of hip
  - S71.021 Laceration with foreign body, right hip
  - S71.022 Laceration with foreign body, left hip
  - S71.029 Laceration with foreign body, unspecified hip
- S71.03 Puncture wound without foreign body of hip
  - S71.031 Puncture wound without foreign body, right hip
  - S71.032 Puncture wound without foreign body, left hip
  - S71.039 Puncture wound without foreign body, unspecified hip
- S71.04 Puncture wound with foreign body of hip
  - S71.041 Puncture wound with foreign body, right hip
  - S71.042 Puncture wound with foreign body, left hip
  - S71.049 Puncture wound with foreign body, unspecified hip
- S71.05 Open bite of hip
  Bite of hip NOS
  - **Excludes1** superficial bite of hip (S70.26, S70.27)
  - S71.051 Open bite, right hip
  - S71.052 Open bite, left hip
  - S71.059 Open bite, unspecified hip
- S71.1 Open wound of thigh
  - S71.10 Unspecified open wound of thigh
    - S71.101 Unspecified open wound, right thigh
    - S71.102 Unspecified open wound, left thigh
    - S71.109 Unspecified open wound, unspecified thigh
  - S71.11 Laceration without foreign body of thigh
    - S71.111 Laceration without foreign body, right thigh
    - S71.112 Laceration without foreign body, left thigh
    - S71.119 Laceration without foreign body, unspecified thigh
  - S71.12 Laceration with foreign body of thigh
    - S71.121 Laceration with foreign body, right thigh
    - S71.122 Laceration with foreign body, left thigh
    - S71.129 Laceration with foreign body, unspecified thigh
  - S71.13 Puncture wound without foreign body of thigh
    - S71.131 Puncture wound without foreign body, right thigh
    - S71.132 Puncture wound without foreign body, left thigh
    - S71.139 Puncture wound without foreign body, unspecified thigh

▶ New   ⇒ Revised   ~~deleted~~ Deleted   Excludes 1   Excludes 2   Includes   Use additional   Code first   Code also   Key words
OGCR Official Guidelines   X Assign placeholder X   ● Use Additional Character(s)   ▷ Manifestation Code   🔖 Hierarchical Condition Category   Coding Clinic

● S71.14   **Puncture wound with foreign body of thigh**
   ● S71.141   **Puncture wound with foreign body, right thigh**
   ● S71.142   **Puncture wound with foreign body, left thigh**
   ● S71.149   **Puncture wound with foreign body, unspecified thigh**
● S71.15   **Open bite of thigh**
    Bite of thigh NOS
    Excludes1   superficial bite of thigh (S70.37-)
   ● S71.151   **Open bite, right thigh**
   ● S71.152   **Open bite, left thigh**
   ● S71.159   **Open bite, unspecified thigh**

● S72   **Fracture of femur**
   Note: A fracture not indicated as displaced or nondisplaced should be coded to displaced
    A fracture not indicated as open or closed should be coded to closed
    The open fracture designations are based on the Gustilo open fracture classification
   Excludes1   traumatic amputation of hip and thigh (S78.-)
   Excludes2   fracture of lower leg and ankle (S82.-)
            fracture of foot (S92.-)
            periprosthetic fracture of prosthetic implant of hip (M97.0-)
   The appropriate 7th character is to be added to all codes from category S72

A	initial encounter for closed fracture
B	initial encounter for open fracture type I or II initial encounter for open fracture NOS
C	initial encounter for open fracture type IIIA, IIIB, or IIIC
D	subsequent encounter for closed fracture with routine healing
E	subsequent encounter for open fracture type I or II with routine healing
F	subsequent encounter for open fracture type IIIA, IIIB, or IIIC with routine healing
G	subsequent encounter for closed fracture with delayed healing
H	subsequent encounter for open fracture type I or II with delayed healing
J	subsequent encounter for open fracture type IIIA, IIIB, or IIIC with delayed healing
K	subsequent encounter for closed fracture with nonunion
M	subsequent encounter for open fracture type I or II with nonunion
N	subsequent encounter for open fracture type IIIA, IIIB, or IIIC with nonunion
P	subsequent encounter for closed fracture with malunion
Q	subsequent encounter for open fracture type I or II with malunion
R	subsequent encounter for open fracture type IIIA, IIIB, or IIIC with malunion
S	sequela

● S72.0   **Fracture of head and neck of femur**
   Excludes2   physeal fracture of upper end of femur (S79.0-)
  ● S72.00   **Fracture of unspecified part of neck of femur**
    Fracture of hip NOS
    Fracture of neck of femur NOS
   ● S72.001   **Fracture of unspecified part of neck of right femur** A, B, C 🐾
   ● S72.002   **Fracture of unspecified part of neck of left femur** A, B, C 🐾
      Coding Clinic: 2015, Q4, P37, Q1, P17
   ● S72.009   **Fracture of unspecified part of neck of unspecified femur** A, B, C 🐾

● S72.01   **Unspecified intracapsular fracture of femur**
    Subcapital fracture of femur
   ● S72.011   **Unspecified intracapsular fracture of right femur** A, B, C 🐾
   ● S72.012   **Unspecified intracapsular fracture of left femur** A, B, C 🐾
   ● S72.019   **Unspecified intracapsular fracture of unspecified femur** A, B, C 🐾
● S72.02   **Fracture of epiphysis (separation) (upper) of femur**
    Transepiphyseal fracture of femur
    Fracture and separation across growth plate
    Excludes1   capital femoral epiphyseal fracture (pediatric) of femur (S79.01-)
            Salter-Harris Type I physeal fracture of upper end of femur (S79.01-)
   ● S72.021   **Displaced fracture of epiphysis (separation) (upper) of right femur** A, B, C 🐾
   ● S72.022   **Displaced fracture of epiphysis (separation) (upper) of left femur** A, B, C 🐾
   ● S72.023   **Displaced fracture of epiphysis (separation) (upper) of unspecified femur** A, B, C 🐾
   ● S72.024   **Nondisplaced fracture of epiphysis (separation) (upper) of right femur** A, B, C 🐾
   ● S72.025   **Nondisplaced fracture of epiphysis (separation) (upper) of left femur** A, B, C 🐾
   ● S72.026   **Nondisplaced fracture of epiphysis (separation) (upper) of unspecified femur** A, B, C 🐾
● S72.03   **Midcervical fracture of femur**
    Transcervical fracture of femur NOS
   ● S72.031   **Displaced midcervical fracture of right femur** A, B, C 🐾
   ● S72.032   **Displaced midcervical fracture of left femur** A, B, C 🐾
   ● S72.033   **Displaced midcervical fracture of unspecified femur** A, B, C 🐾
   ● S72.034   **Nondisplaced midcervical fracture of right femur** A, B, C 🐾
   ● S72.035   **Nondisplaced midcervical fracture of left femur** A, B, C 🐾
   ● S72.036   **Nondisplaced midcervical fracture of unspecified femur** A, B, C 🐾
● S72.04   **Fracture of base of neck of femur**
    Cervicotrochanteric fracture of femur
   ● S72.041   **Displaced fracture of base of neck of right femur** A, B, C 🐾
   ● S72.042   **Displaced fracture of base of neck of left femur** A, B, C 🐾
   ● S72.043   **Displaced fracture of base of neck of unspecified femur** A, B, C 🐾
   ● S72.044   **Nondisplaced fracture of base of neck of right femur** A, B, C 🐾
   ● S72.045   **Nondisplaced fracture of base of neck of left femur** A, B, C 🐾
   ● S72.046   **Nondisplaced fracture of base of neck of unspecified femur** A, B, C 🐾
● S72.05   **Unspecified fracture of head of femur**
    Fracture of head of femur NOS
   ● S72.051   **Unspecified fracture of head of right femur** A, B, C 🐾
   ● S72.052   **Unspecified fracture of head of left femur** A, B, C 🐾
   ● S72.059   **Unspecified fracture of head of unspecified femur** A, B, C 🐾

- S72.06 Articular fracture of head of femur
  - S72.061 Displaced articular fracture of head of right femur A, B, C 🖤
  - S72.062 Displaced articular fracture of head of left femur A, B, C 🖤
  - S72.063 Displaced articular fracture of head of unspecified femur A, B, C 🖤
  - S72.064 Nondisplaced articular fracture of head of right femur A, B, C 🖤
  - S72.065 Nondisplaced articular fracture of head of left femur A, B, C 🖤
  - S72.066 Nondisplaced articular fracture of head of unspecified femur A, B, C 🖤
- S72.09 Other fracture of head and neck of femur
  - S72.091 Other fracture of head and neck of right femur A, B, C 🖤
  - S72.092 Other fracture of head and neck of left femur A, B, C 🖤
  - S72.099 Other fracture of head and neck of unspecified femur A, B, C 🖤
- S72.1 Pertrochanteric fracture
  Fracture extending close to, but not into, joint
  - S72.10 Unspecified trochanteric fracture of femur
    Fracture of trochanter NOS
    - S72.101 Unspecified trochanteric fracture of right femur A, B, C 🖤
    - S72.102 Unspecified trochanteric fracture of left femur A, B, C 🖤
    - S72.109 Unspecified trochanteric fracture of unspecified femur A, B, C 🖤
  - S72.11 Fracture of greater trochanter of femur
    - S72.111 Displaced fracture of greater trochanter of right femur A, B, C 🖤
    - S72.112 Displaced fracture of greater trochanter of left femur A, B, C 🖤
    - S72.113 Displaced fracture of greater trochanter of unspecified femur A, B, C 🖤
    - S72.114 Nondisplaced fracture of greater trochanter of right femur A, B, C 🖤
    - S72.115 Nondisplaced fracture of greater trochanter of left femur A, B, C 🖤
    - S72.116 Nondisplaced fracture of greater trochanter of unspecified femur A, B, C 🖤
  - S72.12 Fracture of lesser trochanter of femur
    - S72.121 Displaced fracture of lesser trochanter of right femur A, B, C 🖤
    - S72.122 Displaced fracture of lesser trochanter of left femur A, B, C 🖤
    - S72.123 Displaced fracture of lesser trochanter of unspecified femur A, B, C 🖤
    - S72.124 Nondisplaced fracture of lesser trochanter of right femur A, B, C 🖤
    - S72.125 Nondisplaced fracture of lesser trochanter of left femur A, B, C 🖤
    - S72.126 Nondisplaced fracture of lesser trochanter of unspecified femur A, B, C 🖤
  - S72.13 Apophyseal fracture of femur
    Pertaining to articulations between articular facets of adjacent vertebrae
    Excludes1 chronic (nontraumatic) slipped upper femoral epiphysis (M93.0-)
    - S72.131 Displaced apophyseal fracture of right femur A, B, C 🖤
    - S72.132 Displaced apophyseal fracture of left femur A, B, C 🖤
    - S72.133 Displaced apophyseal fracture of unspecified femur A, B, C 🖤

- S72.134 Nondisplaced apophyseal fracture of right femur A, B, C 🖤
- S72.135 Nondisplaced apophyseal fracture of left femur A, B, C 🖤
- S72.136 Nondisplaced apophyseal fracture of unspecified femur A, B, C 🖤
- S72.14 Intertrochanteric fracture of femur
  - S72.141 Displaced intertrochanteric fracture of right femur A, B, C 🖤
    Coding Clinic: 2016, Q3, P17
  - S72.142 Displaced intertrochanteric fracture of left femur A, B, C 🖤
  - S72.143 Displaced intertrochanteric fracture of unspecified femur A, B, C 🖤
  - S72.144 Nondisplaced intertrochanteric fracture of right femur A, B, C 🖤
  - S72.145 Nondisplaced intertrochanteric fracture of left femur A, B, C 🖤
  - S72.146 Nondisplaced intertrochanteric fracture of unspecified femur A, B, C 🖤
- S72.2 Subtrochanteric fracture of femur
  Subtrochanteric: inferior to trochanter
  - X S72.21 Displaced subtrochanteric fracture of right femur A, B, C 🖤
  - X S72.22 Displaced subtrochanteric fracture of left femur A, B, C 🖤
  - X S72.23 Displaced subtrochanteric fracture of unspecified femur A, B, C 🖤
  - X S72.24 Nondisplaced subtrochanteric fracture of right femur A, B, C 🖤
  - X S72.25 Nondisplaced subtrochanteric fracture of left femur A, B, C 🖤
  - X S72.26 Nondisplaced subtrochanteric fracture of unspecified femur A, B, C 🖤
- S72.3 Fracture of shaft of femur
  - S72.30 Unspecified fracture of shaft of femur
    - S72.301 Unspecified fracture of shaft of right femur A, B, C 🖤
      Coding Clinic: 2018, Q2, P12
    - S72.302 Unspecified fracture of shaft of left femur A, B, C 🖤
    - S72.309 Unspecified fracture of shaft of unspecified femur A, B, C 🖤
  - S72.32 Transverse fracture of shaft of femur
    - S72.321 Displaced transverse fracture of shaft of right femur A, B, C 🖤
    - S72.322 Displaced transverse fracture of shaft of left femur A, B, C 🖤
    - S72.323 Displaced transverse fracture of shaft of unspecified femur A, B, C 🖤
    - S72.324 Nondisplaced transverse fracture of shaft of right femur A, B, C 🖤
    - S72.325 Nondisplaced transverse fracture of shaft of left femur A, B, C 🖤
    - S72.326 Nondisplaced transverse fracture of shaft of unspecified femur A, B, C 🖤
  - S72.33 Oblique fracture of shaft of femur
    - S72.331 Displaced oblique fracture of shaft of right femur A, B, C 🖤
    - S72.332 Displaced oblique fracture of shaft of left femur A, B, C 🖤
    - S72.333 Displaced oblique fracture of shaft of unspecified femur A, B, C 🖤
    - S72.334 Nondisplaced oblique fracture of shaft of right femur A, B, C 🖤
    - S72.335 Nondisplaced oblique fracture of shaft of left femur A, B, C 🖤
    - S72.336 Nondisplaced oblique fracture of shaft of unspecified femur A, B, C 🖤

▶ New   ⇒ Revised   ~~deleted~~ Deleted   Excludes 1   Excludes 2   Includes   Use additional   Code first   Code also   Key words
OGCR Official Guidelines   X Assign placeholder X   ● Use Additional Character(s)   ▶ Manifestation Code   🖤 Hierarchical Condition Category   Coding Clinic

● S72.34 Spiral fracture of shaft of femur
  ● S72.341 Displaced spiral fracture of shaft of right femur A, B, C 🔒
  ● S72.342 Displaced spiral fracture of shaft of left femur A, B, C 🔒
  ● S72.343 Displaced spiral fracture of shaft of unspecified femur A, B, C 🔒
  ● S72.344 Nondisplaced spiral fracture of shaft of right femur A, B, C 🔒
  ● S72.345 Nondisplaced spiral fracture of shaft of left femur A, B, C 🔒
  ● S72.346 Nondisplaced spiral fracture of shaft of unspecified femur A, B, C 🔒
● S72.35 Comminuted fracture of shaft of femur
  ● S72.351 Displaced comminuted fracture of shaft of right femur A, B, C 🔒
  ● S72.352 Displaced comminuted fracture of shaft of left femur A, B, C 🔒
  ● S72.353 Displaced comminuted fracture of shaft of unspecified femur A, B, C 🔒
  ● S72.354 Nondisplaced comminuted fracture of shaft of right femur A, B, C 🔒
  ● S72.355 Nondisplaced comminuted fracture of shaft of left femur A, B, C 🔒
  ● S72.356 Nondisplaced comminuted fracture of shaft of unspecified femur A, B, C 🔒
● S72.36 Segmental fracture of shaft of femur
  ● S72.361 Displaced segmental fracture of shaft of right femur A, B, C 🔒
  ● S72.362 Displaced segmental fracture of shaft of left femur A, B, C 🔒
  ● S72.363 Displaced segmental fracture of shaft of unspecified femur A, B, C 🔒
  ● S72.364 Nondisplaced segmental fracture of shaft of right femur A, B, C 🔒
  ● S72.365 Nondisplaced segmental fracture of shaft of left femur A, B, C 🔒
  ● S72.366 Nondisplaced segmental fracture of shaft of unspecified femur A, B, C 🔒
● S72.39 Other fracture of shaft of femur
  ● S72.391 Other fracture of shaft of right femur A, B, C 🔒
  ● S72.392 Other fracture of shaft of left femur A, B, C 🔒
  ● S72.399 Other fracture of shaft of unspecified femur A, B, C 🔒
● S72.4 Fracture of lower end of femur
    Fracture of distal end of femur
    Excludes2 fracture of shaft of femur (S72.3-)
              physeal fracture of lower end of femur (S79.1-)
  ● S72.40 Unspecified fracture of lower end of femur
    ● S72.401 Unspecified fracture of lower end of right femur A, B, C 🔒
              Coding Clinic: 2016, Q4, P43
    ● S72.402 Unspecified fracture of lower end of left femur A, B, C 🔒
    ● S72.409 Unspecified fracture of lower end of unspecified femur A, B, C 🔒
  ● S72.41 Unspecified condyle fracture of lower end of femur
              Condyle fracture of femur NOS
    ● S72.411 Displaced unspecified condyle fracture of lower end of right femur A, B, C 🔒
    ● S72.412 Displaced unspecified condyle fracture of lower end of left femur A, B, C 🔒
    ● S72.413 Displaced unspecified condyle fracture of lower end of unspecified femur A, B, C 🔒

● S72.414 Nondisplaced unspecified condyle fracture of lower end of right femur A, B, C 🔒
● S72.415 Nondisplaced unspecified condyle fracture of lower end of left femur A, B, C 🔒
● S72.416 Nondisplaced unspecified condyle fracture of lower end of unspecified femur A, B, C 🔒
● S72.42 Fracture of lateral condyle of femur
  ● S72.421 Displaced fracture of lateral condyle of right femur A, B, C 🔒
  ● S72.422 Displaced fracture of lateral condyle of left femur A, B, C 🔒
  ● S72.423 Displaced fracture of lateral condyle of unspecified femur A, B, C 🔒
  ● S72.424 Nondisplaced fracture of lateral condyle of right femur A, B, C 🔒
  ● S72.425 Nondisplaced fracture of lateral condyle of left femur A, B, C 🔒
  ● S72.426 Nondisplaced fracture of lateral condyle of unspecified femur A, B, C 🔒
● S72.43 Fracture of medial condyle of femur
  ● S72.431 Displaced fracture of medial condyle of right femur A, B, C 🔒
  ● S72.432 Displaced fracture of medial condyle of left femur A, B, C 🔒
  ● S72.433 Displaced fracture of medial condyle of unspecified femur A, B, C 🔒
  ● S72.434 Nondisplaced fracture of medial condyle of right femur A, B, C 🔒
  ● S72.435 Nondisplaced fracture of medial condyle of left femur A, B, C 🔒
  ● S72.436 Nondisplaced fracture of medial condyle of unspecified femur A, B, C 🔒
● S72.44 Fracture of lower epiphysis (separation) of femur
    Excludes1 Salter-Harris Type I physeal fracture of lower end of femur (S79.11-)
  ● S72.441 Displaced fracture of lower epiphysis (separation) of right femur A, B, C 🔒
  ● S72.442 Displaced fracture of lower epiphysis (separation) of left femur A, B, C 🔒
  ● S72.443 Displaced fracture of lower epiphysis (separation) of unspecified femur A, B, C 🔒
  ● S72.444 Nondisplaced fracture of lower epiphysis (separation) of right femur A, B, C 🔒
  ● S72.445 Nondisplaced fracture of lower epiphysis (separation) of left femur A, B, C 🔒
  ● S72.446 Nondisplaced fracture of lower epiphysis (separation) of unspecified femur A, B, C 🔒
● S72.45 Supracondylar fracture without intracondylar extension of lower end of femur
    Supracondylar fracture of lower end of femur NOS
    Excludes1 supracondylar fracture with intracondylar extension of lower end of femur (S72.46-)
  ● S72.451 Displaced supracondylar fracture without intracondylar extension of lower end of right femur A, B, C 🔒
  ● S72.452 Displaced supracondylar fracture without intracondylar extension of lower end of left femur A, B, C 🔒

CHAPTER 19 (S00-T88)

S72.453   Displaced supracondylar fracture without intracondylar extension of lower end of unspecified femur A, B, C 🐾

S72.454   Nondisplaced supracondylar fracture without intracondylar extension of lower end of right femur A, B, C 🐾

S72.455   Nondisplaced supracondylar fracture without intracondylar extension of lower end of left femur A, B, C 🐾

S72.456   Nondisplaced supracondylar fracture without intracondylar extension of lower end of unspecified femur A, B, C 🐾

S72.46   **Supracondylar fracture with intracondylar extension of lower end of femur**

Excludes1   supracondylar fracture without intracondylar extension of lower end of femur (S72.45-)

S72.461   Displaced supracondylar fracture with intracondylar extension of lower end of right femur A, B, C 🐾

S72.462   Displaced supracondylar fracture with intracondylar extension of lower end of left femur A, B, C 🐾

S72.463   Displaced supracondylar fracture with intracondylar extension of lower end of unspecified femur A, B, C 🐾

S72.464   Nondisplaced supracondylar fracture with intracondylar extension of lower end of right femur A, B, C 🐾

S72.465   Nondisplaced supracondylar fracture with intracondylar extension of lower end of left femur A, B, C 🐾

S72.466   Nondisplaced supracondylar fracture with intracondylar extension of lower end of unspecified femur A, B, C 🐾

S72.47   **Torus fracture of lower end of femur**

The appropriate 7th character is to be added to all codes in subcategory S72.47

A	initial encounter for closed fracture
D	subsequent encounter for fracture with routine healing
G	subsequent encounter for fracture with delayed healing
K	subsequent encounter for fracture with nonunion
P	subsequent encounter for fracture with malunion
S	sequela

S72.471   Torus fracture of lower end of right femur A 🐾

S72.472   Torus fracture of lower end of left femur A 🐾

S72.479   Torus fracture of lower end of unspecified femur A 🐾

S72.49   **Other fracture of lower end of femur**

S72.491   Other fracture of lower end of right femur A, B, C 🐾

S72.492   Other fracture of lower end of left femur A, B, C 🐾

S72.499   Other fracture of lower end of unspecified femur A, B, C 🐾

S72.8   **Other fracture of femur**

S72.8X   **Other fracture of femur**

S72.8X1   Other fracture of right femur A, B, C 🐾

S72.8X2   Other fracture of left femur A, B, C 🐾

S72.8X9   Other fracture of unspecified femur A, B, C 🐾

S72.9   **Unspecified fracture of femur**
Fracture of thigh NOS
Fracture of upper leg NOS

Excludes1   fracture of hip NOS (S72.00-, S72.01-)

X● S72.90   Unspecified fracture of unspecified femur A, B, C 🐾
Coding Clinic: 2012, Q4, P94

X● S72.91   Unspecified fracture of right femur A, B, C 🐾

X● S72.92   Unspecified fracture of left femur A, B, C 🐾

S73   **Dislocation and sprain of joint and ligaments of hip**

Includes   avulsion of joint or ligament of hip
laceration of cartilage, joint or ligament of hip
sprain of cartilage, joint or ligament of hip
traumatic hemarthrosis of joint or ligament of hip
traumatic rupture of joint or ligament of hip
traumatic subluxation of joint or ligament of hip
traumatic tear of joint or ligament of hip

Code also any associated open wound

Excludes2   strain of muscle, fascia and tendon of hip and thigh (S76.-)

The appropriate 7th character is to be added to each code from category S73

A	initial encounter
D	subsequent encounter
S	sequela

S73.0   **Subluxation and dislocation of hip**
Out of position

Excludes2   dislocation and subluxation of hip prosthesis (T84.020, T84.021)

S73.00   **Unspecified subluxation and dislocation of hip**
Dislocation of hip NOS
Subluxation of hip NOS

S73.001   Unspecified subluxation of right hip A 🐾

S73.002   Unspecified subluxation of left hip A 🐾

S73.003   Unspecified subluxation of unspecified hip A 🐾

S73.004   Unspecified dislocation of right hip A 🐾

S73.005   Unspecified dislocation of left hip A 🐾

S73.006   Unspecified dislocation of unspecified hip A 🐾

S73.01   **Posterior subluxation and dislocation of hip**

S73.011   Posterior subluxation of right hip A 🐾

S73.012   Posterior subluxation of left hip A 🐾

S73.013   Posterior subluxation of unspecified hip A 🐾

S73.014   Posterior dislocation of right hip A 🐾

S73.015   Posterior dislocation of left hip A 🐾

S73.016   Posterior dislocation of unspecified hip A 🐾

S73.02   **Obturator subluxation and dislocation of hip**

S73.021   Obturator subluxation of right hip A 🐾

S73.022   Obturator subluxation of left hip A 🐾

S73.023   Obturator subluxation of unspecified hip A 🐾

S73.024   Obturator dislocation of right hip A 🐾

S73.025   Obturator dislocation of left hip A 🐾

S73.026   Obturator dislocation of unspecified hip A 🐾

CHAPTER 19 (S00-T88)

▶ New   ⇒ Revised   ~~deleted~~ Deleted   Excludes 1   Excludes 2   Includes   Use additional   Code first   Code also   Key words
OGCR Official Guidelines   X Assign placeholder X   ● Use Additional Character(s)   ▌ Manifestation Code   🐾 Hierarchical Condition Category   Coding Clinic

- S73.03   Other anterior subluxation and dislocation of hip
  - S73.031   Other anterior subluxation of right hip A
  - S73.032   Other anterior subluxation of left hip A
  - S73.033   Other anterior subluxation of unspecified hip A
  - S73.034   Other anterior dislocation of right hip A
  - S73.035   Other anterior dislocation of left hip A
  - S73.036   Other anterior dislocation of unspecified hip A
- S73.04   Central subluxation and dislocation of hip
  - S73.041   Central subluxation of right hip A
  - S73.042   Central subluxation of left hip A
  - S73.043   Central subluxation of unspecified hip A
  - S73.044   Central dislocation of right hip A
  - S73.045   Central dislocation of left hip A
  - S73.046   Central dislocation of unspecified hip A
- S73.1   Sprain of hip
  - S73.10   Unspecified sprain of hip
    - S73.101   Unspecified sprain of right hip
    - S73.102   Unspecified sprain of left hip
    - S73.109   Unspecified sprain of unspecified hip
  - S73.11   Iliofemoral ligament sprain of hip
    - S73.111   Iliofemoral ligament sprain of right hip
    - S73.112   Iliofemoral ligament sprain of left hip
    - S73.119   Iliofemoral ligament sprain of unspecified hip
  - S73.12   Ischiocapsular (ligament) sprain of hip
    - S73.121   Ischiocapsular ligament sprain of right hip
    - S73.122   Ischiocapsular ligament sprain of left hip
    - S73.129   Ischiocapsular ligament sprain of unspecified hip
  - S73.19   Other sprain of hip
    - S73.191   Other sprain of right hip
    - S73.192   Other sprain of left hip
    - S73.199   Other sprain of unspecified hip

- S74   Injury of nerves at hip and thigh level

  Code also any associated open wound (S71.-)

  Excludes2   injury of nerves at ankle and foot level (S94.-)
  injury of nerves at lower leg level (S84.-)

  The appropriate 7th character is to be added to each code from category S74

A	initial encounter
D	subsequent encounter
S	sequela

  - S74.0   Injury of sciatic nerve at hip and thigh level
    - X S74.00   Injury of sciatic nerve at hip and thigh level, unspecified leg
    - X S74.01   Injury of sciatic nerve at hip and thigh level, right leg
    - X S74.02   Injury of sciatic nerve at hip and thigh level, left leg
  - S74.1   Injury of femoral nerve at hip and thigh level
    - X S74.10   Injury of femoral nerve at hip and thigh level, unspecified leg
    - X S74.11   Injury of femoral nerve at hip and thigh level, right leg

    - X S74.12   Injury of femoral nerve at hip and thigh level, left leg
  - S74.2   Injury of cutaneous sensory nerve at hip and thigh level
    - X S74.20   Injury of cutaneous sensory nerve at hip and thigh level, unspecified leg
    - X S74.21   Injury of cutaneous sensory nerve at hip and high level, right leg
    - X S74.22   Injury of cutaneous sensory nerve at hip and thigh level, left leg
  - S74.8   Injury of other nerves at hip and thigh level
    - S74.8X   Injury of other nerves at hip and thigh level
      - S74.8X1   Injury of other nerves at hip and thigh level, right leg
      - S74.8X2   Injury of other nerves at hip and thigh level, left leg
      - S74.8X9   Injury of other nerves at hip and thigh level, unspecified leg
  - S74.9   Injury of unspecified nerve at hip and thigh level
    - X S74.90   Injury of unspecified nerve at hip and thigh level, unspecified leg
    - X S74.91   Injury of unspecified nerve at hip and thigh level, right leg
    - X S74.92   Injury of unspecified nerve at hip and thigh level, left leg

- S75   Injury of blood vessels at hip and thigh level

  Code also any associated open wound (S71.-)

  Excludes2   injury of blood vessels at lower leg level (S85.-)
  injury of popliteal artery (S85.0)

  The appropriate 7th character is to be added to each code from category S75

A	initial encounter
D	subsequent encounter
S	sequela

  - S75.0   Injury of femoral artery
    - S75.00   Unspecified injury of femoral artery
      - S75.001   Unspecified injury of femoral artery, right leg
      - S75.002   Unspecified injury of femoral artery, left leg
      - S75.009   Unspecified injury of femoral artery, unspecified leg
    - S75.01   Minor laceration of femoral artery

      Incomplete transection of femoral artery
      Laceration of femoral artery NOS
      Superficial laceration of femoral artery

      - S75.011   Minor laceration of femoral artery, right leg
      - S75.012   Minor laceration of femoral artery, left leg
      - S75.019   Minor laceration of femoral artery, unspecified leg
    - S75.02   Major laceration of femoral artery

      Complete transection of femoral artery
      Traumatic rupture of femoral artery

      - S75.021   Major laceration of femoral artery, right leg
      - S75.022   Major laceration of femoral artery, left leg
      - S75.029   Major laceration of femoral artery, unspecified leg
    - S75.09   Other specified injury of femoral artery
      - S75.091   Other specified injury of femoral artery, right leg
      - S75.092   Other specified injury of femoral artery, left leg
      - S75.099   Other specified injury of femoral artery, unspecified leg

- S75.1 **Injury of femoral vein at hip and thigh level**
  - S75.10 **Unspecified injury of femoral vein at hip and thigh level**
    - S75.101 **Unspecified injury of femoral vein at hip and thigh level, right leg**
    - S75.102 **Unspecified injury of femoral vein at hip and thigh level, left leg**
    - S75.109 **Unspecified injury of femoral vein at hip and thigh level, unspecified leg**
  - S75.11 **Minor laceration of femoral vein at hip and thigh level**
    Incomplete transection of femoral vein at hip and thigh level
    Laceration of femoral vein at hip and thigh level NOS
    Superficial laceration of femoral vein at hip and thigh level
    - S75.111 **Minor laceration of femoral vein at hip and thigh level, right leg**
    - S75.112 **Minor laceration of femoral vein at hip and thigh level, left leg**
    - S75.119 **Minor laceration of femoral vein at hip and thigh level, unspecified leg**
  - S75.12 **Major laceration of femoral vein at hip and thigh level**
    Complete transection of femoral vein at hip and thigh level
    Traumatic rupture of femoral vein at hip and thigh level
    - S75.121 **Major laceration of femoral vein at hip and thigh level, right leg**
    - S75.122 **Major laceration of femoral vein at hip and thigh level, left leg**
    - S75.129 **Major laceration of femoral vein at hip and thigh level, unspecified leg**
  - S75.19 **Other specified injury of femoral vein at hip and thigh level**
    - S75.191 **Other specified injury of femoral vein at hip and thigh level, right leg**
    - S75.192 **Other specified injury of femoral vein at hip and thigh level, left leg**
    - S75.199 **Other specified injury of femoral vein at hip and thigh level, unspecified leg**
- S75.2 **Injury of greater saphenous vein at hip and thigh level**
  Excludes1 greater saphenous vein NOS (S85.3)
  - S75.20 **Unspecified injury of greater saphenous vein at hip and thigh level**
    - S75.201 **Unspecified injury of greater saphenous vein at hip and thigh level, right leg**
    - S75.202 **Unspecified injury of greater saphenous vein at hip and thigh level, left leg**
    - S75.209 **Unspecified injury of greater saphenous vein at hip and thigh level, unspecified leg**
  - S75.21 **Minor laceration of greater saphenous vein at hip and thigh level**
    Incomplete transection of greater saphenous vein at hip and thigh level
    Laceration of greater saphenous vein at hip and thigh level NOS
    Superficial laceration of greater saphenous vein at hip and thigh level
    - S75.211 **Minor laceration of greater saphenous vein at hip and thigh level, right leg**
    - S75.212 **Minor laceration of greater saphenous vein at hip and thigh level, left leg**
    - S75.219 **Minor laceration of greater saphenous vein at hip and thigh level, unspecified leg**

- S75.22 **Major laceration of greater saphenous vein at hip and thigh level**
  Complete transection of greater saphenous vein at hip and thigh level
  Traumatic rupture of greater saphenous vein at hip and thigh level
  - S75.221 **Major laceration of greater saphenous vein at hip and thigh level, right leg**
  - S75.222 **Major laceration of greater saphenous vein at hip and thigh level, left leg**
  - S75.229 **Major laceration of greater saphenous vein at hip and thigh level, unspecified leg**
  - S75.29 **Other specified injury of greater saphenous vein at hip and thigh level**
    - S75.291 **Other specified injury of greater saphenous vein at hip and thigh level, right leg**
    - S75.292 **Other specified injury of greater saphenous vein at hip and thigh level, left leg**
    - S75.299 **Other specified injury of greater saphenous vein at hip and thigh level, unspecified leg**
- S75.8 **Injury of other blood vessels at hip and thigh level**
  - S75.80 **Unspecified injury of other blood vessels at hip and thigh level**
    - S75.801 **Unspecified injury of other blood vessels at hip and thigh level, right leg**
    - S75.802 **Unspecified injury of other blood vessels at hip and thigh level, left leg**
    - S75.809 **Unspecified injury of other blood vessels at hip and thigh level, unspecified leg**
  - S75.81 **Laceration of other blood vessels at hip and thigh level**
    - S75.811 **Laceration of other blood vessels at hip and thigh level, right leg**
    - S75.812 **Laceration of other blood vessels at hip and thigh level, left leg**
    - S75.819 **Laceration of other blood vessels at hip and thigh level, unspecified leg**
  - S75.89 **Other specified injury of other blood vessels at hip and thigh level**
    - S75.891 **Other specified injury of other blood vessels at hip and thigh level, right leg**
    - S75.892 **Other specified injury of other blood vessels at hip and thigh level, left leg**
    - S75.899 **Other specified injury of other blood vessels at hip and thigh level, unspecified leg**
- S75.9 **Injury of unspecified blood vessel at hip and thigh level**
  - S75.90 **Unspecified injury of unspecified blood vessel at hip and thigh level**
    - S75.901 **Unspecified injury of unspecified blood vessel at hip and thigh level, right leg**
    - S75.902 **Unspecified injury of unspecified blood vessel at hip and thigh level, left leg**
    - S75.909 **Unspecified injury of unspecified blood vessel at hip and thigh level, unspecified leg**
  - S75.91 **Laceration of unspecified blood vessel at hip and thigh level**
    - S75.911 **Laceration of unspecified blood vessel at hip and thigh level, right leg**
    - S75.912 **Laceration of unspecified blood vessel at hip and thigh level, left leg**

CHAPTER 19 (S00-T88)

▶ New ⇒ Revised ~~deleted~~ Deleted Excludes 1 Excludes 2 Includes Use additional Code first Code also Key words
OGCR Official Guidelines X Assign placeholder X ● Use Additional Character(s) ▶ Manifestation Code 🔾 Hierarchical Condition Category **Coding Clinic**

● S75.919 Laceration of unspecified blood vessel at hip and thigh level, unspecified leg

● S75.99 Other specified injury of unspecified blood vessel at hip and thigh level

  ● S75.991 Other specified injury of unspecified blood vessel at hip and thigh level, right leg

  ● S75.992 Other specified injury of unspecified blood vessel at hip and thigh level, left leg

  ● S75.999 Other specified injury of unspecified blood vessel at hip and thigh level, unspecified leg

● S76 Injury of muscle, fascia and tendon at hip and thigh level

  Code also any associated open wound (S71.-)

  Excludes2 injury of muscle, fascia and tendon at lower leg level (S86)
  sprain of joint and ligament of hip (S73.1)

  The appropriate 7th character is to be added to each code from category S76

A	initial encounter
D	subsequent encounter
S	sequela

● S76.0 Injury of muscle, fascia and tendon of hip

  ● S76.00 Unspecified injury of muscle, fascia and tendon of hip

    ● S76.001 Unspecified injury of muscle, fascia and tendon of right hip

    ● S76.002 Unspecified injury of muscle, fascia and tendon of left hip

    ● S76.009 Unspecified injury of muscle, fascia and tendon of unspecified hip

  ● S76.01 Strain of muscle, fascia and tendon of hip

    ● S76.011 Strain of muscle, fascia and tendon of right hip

    ● S76.012 Strain of muscle, fascia and tendon of left hip

    ● S76.019 Strain of muscle, fascia and tendon of unspecified hip

  ● S76.02 Laceration of muscle, fascia and tendon of hip

    ● S76.021 Laceration of muscle, fascia and tendon of right hip

    ● S76.022 Laceration of muscle, fascia and tendon of left hip

    ● S76.029 Laceration of muscle, fascia and tendon of unspecified hip

  ● S76.09 Other specified injury of muscle, fascia and tendon of hip

    ● S76.091 Other specified injury of muscle, fascia and tendon of right hip

    ● S76.092 Other specified injury of muscle, fascia and tendon of left hip

    ● S76.099 Other specified injury of muscle, fascia and tendon of unspecified hip

● S76.1 Injury of quadriceps muscle, fascia and tendon
  Injury of patellar ligament (tendon)

  ● S76.10 Unspecified injury of quadriceps muscle, fascia and tendon

    ● S76.101 Unspecified injury of right quadriceps muscle, fascia and tendon

    ● S76.102 Unspecified injury of left quadriceps muscle, fascia and tendon

    ● S76.109 Unspecified injury of unspecified quadriceps muscle, fascia and tendon

  ● S76.11 Strain of quadriceps muscle, fascia and tendon

    ● S76.111 Strain of right quadriceps muscle, fascia and tendon

    ● S76.112 Strain of left quadriceps muscle, fascia and tendon

    ● S76.119 Strain of unspecified quadriceps muscle, fascia and tendon

  ● S76.12 Laceration of quadriceps muscle, fascia and tendon

    ● S76.121 Laceration of right quadriceps muscle, fascia and tendon

    ● S76.122 Laceration of left quadriceps muscle, fascia and tendon

    ● S76.129 Laceration of unspecified quadriceps muscle, fascia and tendon

  ● S76.19 Other specified injury of quadriceps muscle, fascia and tendon

    ● S76.191 Other specified injury of right quadriceps muscle, fascia and tendon

    ● S76.192 Other specified injury of left quadriceps muscle, fascia and tendon

    ● S76.199 Other specified injury of unspecified quadriceps muscle, fascia and tendon

● S76.2 Injury of adductor muscle, fascia and tendon of thigh

  ● S76.20 Unspecified injury of adductor muscle, fascia and tendon of thigh

    ● S76.201 Unspecified injury of adductor muscle, fascia and tendon of right thigh

    ● S76.202 Unspecified injury of adductor muscle, fascia and tendon of left thigh

    ● S76.209 Unspecified injury of adductor muscle, fascia and tendon of unspecified thigh

  ● S76.21 Strain of adductor muscle, fascia and tendon of thigh

    ● S76.211 Strain of adductor muscle, fascia and tendon of right thigh

    ● S76.212 Strain of adductor muscle, fascia and tendon of left thigh

    ● S76.219 Strain of adductor muscle, fascia and tendon of unspecified thigh

  ● S76.22 Laceration of adductor muscle, fascia and tendon of thigh

    ● S76.221 Laceration of adductor muscle, fascia and tendon of right thigh

    ● S76.222 Laceration of adductor muscle, fascia and tendon of left thigh

    ● S76.229 Laceration of adductor muscle, fascia and tendon of unspecified thigh

  ● S76.29 Other injury of adductor muscle, fascia and tendon of thigh

    ● S76.291 Other injury of adductor muscle, fascia and tendon of right thigh

    ● S76.292 Other injury of adductor muscle, fascia and tendon of left thigh

    ● S76.299 Other injury of adductor muscle, fascia and tendon of unspecified thigh

● S76.3 Injury of muscle, fascia and tendon of the posterior muscle group at thigh level

  ● S76.30 Unspecified injury of muscle, fascia and tendon of the posterior muscle group at thigh level

    ● S76.301 Unspecified injury of muscle, fascia and tendon of the posterior muscle group at thigh level, right thigh

    ● S76.302 Unspecified injury of muscle, fascia and tendon of the posterior muscle group at thigh level, left thigh

    ● S76.309 Unspecified injury of muscle, fascia and tendon of the posterior muscle group at thigh level, unspecified thigh

- S76.31 Strain of muscle, fascia and tendon of the posterior muscle group at thigh level
  - S76.311 Strain of muscle, fascia and tendon of the posterior muscle group at thigh level, right thigh
  - S76.312 Strain of muscle, fascia and tendon of the posterior muscle group at thigh level, left thigh
  - S76.319 Strain of muscle, fascia and tendon of the posterior muscle group at thigh level, unspecified thigh
- S76.32 Laceration of muscle, fascia and tendon of the posterior muscle group at thigh level
  - S76.321 Laceration of muscle, fascia and tendon of the posterior muscle group at thigh level, right thigh
  - S76.322 Laceration of muscle, fascia and tendon of the posterior muscle group at thigh level, left thigh
  - S76.329 Laceration of muscle, fascia and tendon of the posterior muscle group at thigh level, unspecified thigh
- S76.39 Other specified injury of muscle, fascia and tendon of the posterior muscle group at thigh level
  - S76.391 Other specified injury of muscle, fascia and tendon of the posterior muscle group at thigh level, right thigh
  - S76.392 Other specified injury of muscle, fascia and tendon of the posterior muscle group at thigh level, left thigh
  - S76.399 Other specified injury of muscle, fascia and tendon of the posterior muscle group at thigh level, unspecified thigh
- S76.8 Injury of other specified muscles, fascia and tendons at thigh level
  - S76.80 Unspecified injury of other specified muscles, fascia and tendons at thigh level
    - S76.801 Unspecified injury of other specified muscles, fascia and tendons at thigh level, right thigh
    - S76.802 Unspecified injury of other specified muscles, fascia and tendons at thigh level, left thigh
    - S76.809 Unspecified injury of other specified muscles, fascia and tendons at thigh level, unspecified thigh
  - S76.81 Strain of other specified specified muscles, fascia and tendons at thigh level
    - S76.811 Strain of other specified muscles, fascia and tendons at thigh level, right thigh
    - S76.812 Strain of other specified muscles, fascia and tendons at thigh level, left thigh
    - S76.819 Strain of other specified muscles, fascia and tendons at thigh level, unspecified thigh
  - S76.82 Laceration of other specified muscles, fascia and tendons at thigh level
    - S76.821 Laceration of other specified muscles, fascia and tendons at thigh level, right thigh
    - S76.822 Laceration of other specified muscles, fascia and tendons at thigh level, left thigh
    - S76.829 Laceration of other specified muscles, fascia and tendons at thigh level, unspecified thigh

- S76.89 Other injury of other specified muscles, fascia and tendons at thigh level
  - S76.891 Other injury of other specified muscles, fascia and tendons at thigh level, right thigh
  - S76.892 Other injury of other specified muscles, fascia and tendons at thigh level, left thigh
  - S76.899 Other injury of other specified muscles, fascia and tendons at thigh level, unspecified thigh
- S76.9 Injury of unspecified muscles, fascia and tendons at thigh level
  - S76.90 Unspecified injury of unspecified muscles, fascia and tendons at thigh level
    - S76.901 Unspecified injury of unspecified muscles, fascia and tendons at thigh level, right thigh
    - S76.902 Unspecified injury of unspecified muscles, fascia and tendons at thigh level, left thigh
    - S76.909 Unspecified injury of unspecified muscles, fascia and tendons at thigh level, unspecified thigh
  - S76.91 Strain of unspecified muscles, fascia and tendons at thigh level
    - S76.911 Strain of unspecified muscles, fascia and tendons at thigh level, right thigh
    - S76.912 Strain of unspecified muscles, fascia and tendons at thigh level, left thigh
    - S76.919 Strain of unspecified muscles fascia and tendons at thigh level, unspecified thigh
  - S76.92 Laceration of unspecified muscles, fascia and tendons at thigh level
    - S76.921 Laceration of unspecified muscles, fascia and tendons at thigh level, right thigh
    - S76.922 Laceration of unspecified muscles, fascia and tendons at thigh level, left thigh
    - S76.929 Laceration of unspecified muscles, fascia and tendons at thigh level, unspecified thigh
  - S76.99 Other specified injury of unspecified muscles, fascia and tendons at thigh level
    - S76.991 Other specified injury of unspecified muscles, fascia and tendons at thigh level, right thigh
    - S76.992 Other specified injury of unspecified muscles, fascia and tendons at thigh level, left thigh
    - S76.999 Other specified injury of unspecified muscles, fascia and tendons at thigh level, unspecified thigh

- S77 Crushing injury of hip and thigh

  Use additional code(s) for all associated injuries

  Excludes2 crushing injury of ankle and foot (S97.-)
  crushing injury of lower leg (S87.-)

  The appropriate 7th character is to be added to each code from category S77

A	initial encounter
D	subsequent encounter
S	sequela

  - S77.0 Crushing injury of hip
    - X S77.00 Crushing injury of unspecified hip
    - X S77.01 Crushing injury of right hip
    - X S77.02 Crushing injury of left hip

▶ New   ⇒ Revised   ~~deleted~~ Deleted   Excludes 1   Excludes 2   Includes   Use additional   Code first   Code also   Key words

OGCR Official Guidelines   X Assign placeholder X   ● Use Additional Character(s)   ▶ Manifestation Code   🐷 Hierarchical Condition Category   Coding Clinic

- **S77.1**   Crushing injury of thigh
  - X● **S77.10**   Crushing injury of unspecified thigh
  - X● **S77.11**   Crushing injury of right thigh
  - X● **S77.12**   Crushing injury of left thigh
- **S77.2**   Crushing injury of hip with thigh
  - X● **S77.20**   Crushing injury of unspecified hip with thigh
  - X● **S77.21**   Crushing injury of right hip with thigh
  - X● **S77.22**   Crushing injury of left hip with thigh
- ● **S78**   **Traumatic amputation of hip and thigh**

  An amputation not identified as partial or complete should be coded to complete

  > **Excludes1**   traumatic amputation of knee (S88.0-)

  The appropriate 7th character is to be added to each code from category S78

A	initial encounter
D	subsequent encounter
S	sequela

  - ● **S78.0**   Traumatic amputation at hip joint
    - ● **S78.01**   Complete traumatic amputation at hip joint
      - ● **S78.011**   Complete traumatic amputation at right hip joint A, D, S 🐾
      - ● **S78.012**   Complete traumatic amputation at left hip joint A, D, S 🐾
      - ● **S78.019**   Complete traumatic amputation at unspecified hip joint A, D, S 🐾
    - ● **S78.02**   Partial traumatic amputation at hip joint
      - ● **S78.021**   Partial traumatic amputation at right hip joint A, D, S 🐾
      - ● **S78.022**   Partial traumatic amputation at left hip joint A, D, S 🐾
      - ● **S78.029**   Partial traumatic amputation at unspecified hip joint A, D, S 🐾
  - ● **S78.1**   Traumatic amputation at level between hip and knee
    > **Excludes1**   traumatic amputation of knee (S88.0-)
    - ● **S78.11**   Complete traumatic amputation at level between hip and knee
      - ● **S78.111**   Complete traumatic amputation at level between right hip and knee A, D, S 🐾
      - ● **S78.112**   Complete traumatic amputation at level between left hip and knee A, D, S 🐾
      - ● **S78.119**   Complete traumatic amputation at level between unspecified hip and knee A, D, S 🐾
    - ● **S78.12**   Partial traumatic amputation at level between hip and knee
      - ● **S78.121**   Partial traumatic amputation at level between right hip and knee A, D, S 🐾
      - ● **S78.122**   Partial traumatic amputation at level between left hip and knee A, D, S 🐾
      - ● **S78.129**   Partial traumatic amputation at level between unspecified hip and knee A, D, S 🐾
  - ● **S78.9**   Traumatic amputation of hip and thigh, level unspecified
    - ● **S78.91**   Complete traumatic amputation of hip and thigh, level unspecified
      - ● **S78.911**   Complete traumatic amputation of right hip and thigh, level unspecified A, D, S 🐾
      - ● **S78.912**   Complete traumatic amputation of left hip and thigh, level unspecified A, D, S 🐾
      - ● **S78.919**   Complete traumatic amputation of unspecified hip and thigh, level unspecified A, D, S 🐾

- ● **S78.92**   Partial traumatic amputation of hip and thigh, level unspecified
  - ● **S78.921**   Partial traumatic amputation of right hip and thigh, level unspecified A, D, S 🐾
  - ● **S78.922**   Partial traumatic amputation of left hip and thigh, level unspecified A, D, S 🐾
  - ● **S78.929**   Partial traumatic amputation of unspecified hip and thigh, level unspecified A, D, S 🐾

- ● **S79**   **Other and unspecified injuries of hip and thigh**

  Note: A fracture not indicated as open or closed should be coded to closed

  The appropriate 7th character is to be added to each code from subcategories S79.0 and S79.1

A	initial encounter for closed fracture
D	subsequent encounter for fracture with routine healing
G	subsequent encounter for fracture with delayed healing
K	subsequent encounter for fracture with nonunion
P	subsequent encounter for fracture with malunion
S	sequela

  - ● **S79.0**   Physeal fracture of upper end of femur
    > **Excludes1**   apophyseal fracture of upper end of femur (S72.13-)
    > nontraumatic slipped upper femoral epiphysis (M93.0-)
    - ● **S79.00**   Unspecified physeal fracture of upper end of femur
      - ● **S79.001**   Unspecified physeal fracture of upper end of right femur A 🐾
      - ● **S79.002**   Unspecified physeal fracture of upper end of left femur A 🐾
      - ● **S79.009**   Unspecified physeal fracture of upper end of unspecified femur A 🐾
    - ● **S79.01**   Salter-Harris Type I physeal fracture of upper end of femur

      Acute on chronic slipped capital femoral epiphysis (traumatic)

      Acute slipped capital femoral epiphysis (traumatic)

      Capital femoral epiphyseal fracture

      > **Excludes1**   chronic slipped upper femoral epiphysis (nontraumatic) (M93.02-)
      - ● **S79.011**   Salter-Harris Type I physeal fracture of upper end of right femur A 🐾
      - ● **S79.012**   Salter-Harris Type I physeal fracture of upper end of left femur A 🐾
      - ● **S79.019**   Salter-Harris Type I physeal fracture of upper end of unspecified femur A 🐾
    - ● **S79.09**   Other physeal fracture of upper end of femur
      - ● **S79.091**   Other physeal fracture of upper end of right femur A 🐾
      - ● **S79.092**   Other physeal fracture of upper end of left femur A 🐾
      - ● **S79.099**   Other physeal fracture of upper end of unspecified femur A 🐾

Item 19–5   SALTER-HARRIS TYPE 1: epiphysis is completely separated from end of bone, or metaphysic growth plate remains attached to epiphysis

SALTER-HARRIS TYPE 2: epiphysis and growth plate are partially separated from metaphysis, which is cracked—most common type

SALTER-HARRIS TYPE 3: fracture occurring through epiphysis and separates part of epiphysis and growth plate from metaphysis fracture, usually at distal end of tibia

SALTER-HARRIS TYPE 4: fracture runs through epiphysis, across growth plate, into metaphysic; surgery is required to restore joint surface to normal and align growth plate

CHAPTER 19 (S00-T88)

● **S79.1**   Physeal fracture of lower end of femur
   ● **S79.10**   Unspecified physeal fracture of lower end of femur
     ● **S79.101**   Unspecified physeal fracture of lower end of right femur A 🐾
     ● **S79.102**   Unspecified physeal fracture of lower end of left femur A 🐾
     ● **S79.109**   Unspecified physeal fracture of lower end of unspecified femur A 🐾
   ● **S79.11**   Salter-Harris Type I physeal fracture of lower end of femur
     ● **S79.111**   Salter-Harris Type I physeal fracture of lower end of right femur A 🐾
     ● **S79.112**   Salter-Harris Type I physeal fracture of lower end of left femur A 🐾
     ● **S79.119**   Salter-Harris Type I physeal fracture of lower end of unspecified femur A 🐾
   ● **S79.12**   Salter-Harris Type II physeal fracture of lower end of femur
     ● **S79.121**   Salter-Harris Type II physeal fracture of lower end of right femur A 🐾
     ● **S79.122**   Salter-Harris Type II physeal fracture of lower end of left femur A 🐾
     ● **S79.129**   Salter-Harris Type II physeal fracture of lower end of unspecified femur A 🐾
   ● **S79.13**   Salter-Harris Type III physeal fracture of lower end of femur
     ● **S79.131**   Salter-Harris Type III physeal fracture of lower end of right femur A 🐾
     ● **S79.132**   Salter-Harris Type III physeal fracture of lower end of left femur A 🐾
     ● **S79.139**   Salter-Harris Type III physeal fracture of lower end of unspecified femur A 🐾
   ● **S79.14**   Salter-Harris Type IV physeal fracture of lower end of femur
     ● **S79.141**   Salter-Harris Type IV physeal fracture of lower end of right femur A 🐾
     ● **S79.142**   Salter-Harris Type IV physeal fracture of lower end of left femur A 🐾
     ● **S79.149**   Salter-Harris Type IV physeal fracture of lower end of unspecified femur A 🐾
   ● **S79.19**   Other physeal fracture of lower end of femur
     ● **S79.191**   Other physeal fracture of lower end of right femur A 🐾
     ● **S79.192**   Other physeal fracture of lower end of left femur A 🐾
     ● **S79.199**   Other physeal fracture of lower end of unspecified femur A 🐾

● **S79.8** Other specified injuries of hip and thigh
   The appropriate 7th character is to be added to each code in subcategory S79.8

> | | |
> |---|---|
> | A | initial encounter |
> | D | subsequent encounter |
> | S | sequela |

   ● **S79.81**   Other specified injuries of hip
     ● **S79.811**   Other specified injuries of right hip
     ● **S79.812**   Other specified injuries of left hip
     ● **S79.819**   Other specified injuries of unspecified hip
   ● **S79.82**   Other specified injuries of thigh
     ● **S79.821**   Other specified injuries of right thigh
     ● **S79.822**   Other specified injuries of left thigh
     ● **S79.829**   Other specified injuries of unspecified thigh

● **S79.9**   Unspecified injury of hip and thigh
   The appropriate 7th character is to be added to each code in subcategory S79.9

> | | |
> |---|---|
> | A | initial encounter |
> | D | subsequent encounter |
> | S | sequela |

   ● **S79.91**   Unspecified injury of hip
     ● **S79.911**   Unspecified injury of right hip
     ● **S79.912**   Unspecified injury of left hip
     ● **S79.919**   Unspecified injury of unspecified hip
   ● **S79.92**   Unspecified injury of thigh
     ● **S79.921**   Unspecified injury of right thigh
     ● **S79.922**   Unspecified injury of left thigh
     ● **S79.929**   Unspecified injury of unspecified thigh

INJURIES TO THE KNEE AND LOWER LEG (S80-S89)

Excludes2   burns and corrosions (T20-T32)
     frostbite (T33-T34)
     injuries of ankle and foot, except fracture of ankle and malleolus (S90-S99)
     insect bite or sting, venomous (T63.4)

● **S80**   Superficial injury of knee and lower leg
   Excludes2   superficial injury of ankle and foot (S90.-)
   The appropriate 7th character is to be added to each code from category S80

> | | |
> |---|---|
> | A | initial encounter |
> | D | subsequent encounter |
> | S | sequela |

   ● **S80.0**   Contusion of knee
    X ● **S80.00**   Contusion of unspecified knee
    X ● **S80.01**   Contusion of right knee
    X ● **S80.02**   Contusion of left knee
   ● **S80.1**   Contusion of lower leg
    X ● **S80.10**   Contusion of unspecified lower leg
    X ● **S80.11**   Contusion of right lower leg
    X ● **S80.12**   Contusion of left lower leg
   ● **S80.2**   Other superficial injuries of knee
     ● **S80.21**   Abrasion of knee
       ● **S80.211**   Abrasion, right knee
       ● **S80.212**   Abrasion, left knee
       ● **S80.219**   Abrasion, unspecified knee
     ● **S80.22**   Blister (nonthermal) of knee
       ● **S80.221**   Blister (nonthermal), right knee
       ● **S80.222**   Blister (nonthermal), left knee
       ● **S80.229**   Blister (nonthermal), unspecified knee
     ● **S80.24**   External constriction of knee
       ● **S80.241**   External constriction, right knee
       ● **S80.242**   External constriction, left knee
       ● **S80.249**   External constriction, unspecified knee
     ● **S80.25**   Superficial foreign body of knee
       Splinter in the knee
       ● **S80.251**   Superficial foreign body, right knee
       ● **S80.252**   Superficial foreign body, left knee
       ● **S80.259**   Superficial foreign body, unspecified knee
     ● **S80.26**   Insect bite (nonvenomous) of knee
       ● **S80.261**   Insect bite (nonvenomous), right knee
       ● **S80.262**   Insect bite (nonvenomous), left knee
       ● **S80.269**   Insect bite (nonvenomous), unspecified knee

- S80.27 Other superficial bite of knee
  Excludes1 open bite of knee (S81.05-)
  - S80.271 Other superficial bite of right knee
  - S80.272 Other superficial bite of left knee
  - S80.279 Other superficial bite of unspecified knee
- S80.8 Other superficial injuries of lower leg
  - S80.81 Abrasion of lower leg
    - S80.811 Abrasion, right lower leg
    - S80.812 Abrasion, left lower leg
    - S80.819 Abrasion, unspecified lower leg
  - S80.82 Blister (nonthermal) of lower leg
    - S80.821 Blister (nonthermal), right lower leg
    - S80.822 Blister (nonthermal), left lower leg
    - S80.829 Blister (nonthermal), unspecified lower leg
  - S80.84 External constriction of lower leg
    - S80.841 External constriction, right lower leg
    - S80.842 External constriction, left lower leg
    - S80.849 External constriction, unspecified lower leg
  - S80.85 Superficial foreign body of lower leg
    Splinter in the lower leg
    - S80.851 Superficial foreign body, right lower leg
    - S80.852 Superficial foreign body, left lower leg
    - S80.859 Superficial foreign body, unspecified lower leg
  - S80.86 Insect bite (nonvenomous) of lower leg
    - S80.861 Insect bite (nonvenomous), right lower leg
    - S80.862 Insect bite (nonvenomous), left lower leg
    - S80.869 Insect bite (nonvenomous), unspecified lower leg
  - S80.87 Other superficial bite of lower leg
    Excludes1 open bite of lower leg (S81.85-)
    - S80.871 Other superficial bite, right lower leg
    - S80.872 Other superficial bite, left lower leg
    - S80.879 Other superficial bite, unspecified lower leg
- S80.9 Unspecified superficial injury of knee and lower leg
  - S80.91 Unspecified superficial injury of knee
    - S80.911 Unspecified superficial injury of right knee
    - S80.912 Unspecified superficial injury of left knee
    - S80.919 Unspecified superficial injury of unspecified knee
  - S80.92 Unspecified superficial injury of lower leg
    - S80.921 Unspecified superficial injury of right lower leg
    - S80.922 Unspecified superficial injury of left lower leg
    - S80.929 Unspecified superficial injury of unspecified lower leg
- S81 Open wound of knee and lower leg
  Code also any associated wound infection
  Excludes1 open fracture of knee and lower leg (S82.-)
  traumatic amputation of lower leg (S88.-)
  Excludes2 open wound of ankle and foot (S91.-)
  The appropriate 7th character is to be added to each code from category S81

A	initial encounter
D	subsequent encounter
S	sequela

- S81.0 Open wound of knee
  - S81.00 Unspecified open wound of knee
    - S81.001 Unspecified open wound, right knee
    - S81.002 Unspecified open wound, left knee
    - S81.009 Unspecified open wound, unspecified knee
  - S81.01 Laceration without foreign body of knee
    - S81.011 Laceration without foreign body, right knee
    - S81.012 Laceration without foreign body, left knee
    - S81.019 Laceration without foreign body, unspecified knee
  - S81.02 Laceration with foreign body of knee
    - S81.021 Laceration with foreign body, right knee
    - S81.022 Laceration with foreign body, left knee
    - S81.029 Laceration with foreign body, unspecified knee
  - S81.03 Puncture wound without foreign body of knee
    - S81.031 Puncture wound without foreign body, right knee
    - S81.032 Puncture wound without foreign body, left knee
    - S81.039 Puncture wound without foreign body, unspecified knee
  - S81.04 Puncture wound with foreign body of knee
    - S81.041 Puncture wound with foreign body, right knee
    - S81.042 Puncture wound with foreign body, left knee
    - S81.049 Puncture wound with foreign body, unspecified knee
  - S81.05 Open bite of knee
    Bite of knee NOS
    Excludes1 superficial bite of knee (S80.27-)
    - S81.051 Open bite, right knee
    - S81.052 Open bite, left knee
    - S81.059 Open bite, unspecified knee
- S81.8 Open wound of lower leg
  - S81.80 Unspecified open wound of lower leg
    - S81.801 Unspecified open wound, right lower leg
    - S81.802 Unspecified open wound, left lower leg
    - S81.809 Unspecified open wound, unspecified lower leg
  - S81.81 Laceration without foreign body of lower leg
    - S81.811 Laceration without foreign body, right lower leg
    - S81.812 Laceration without foreign body, left lower leg
    - S81.819 Laceration without foreign body, unspecified lower leg
  - S81.82 Laceration with foreign body of lower leg
    - S81.821 Laceration with foreign body, right lower leg
    - S81.822 Laceration with foreign body, left lower leg
    - S81.829 Laceration with foreign body, unspecified lower leg
  - S81.83 Puncture wound without foreign body of lower leg
    - S81.831 Puncture wound without foreign body, right lower leg
    - S81.832 Puncture wound without foreign body, left lower leg
    - S81.839 Puncture wound without foreign body, unspecified lower leg

S81.84   **Puncture wound with foreign body of lower leg**

- S81.841   **Puncture wound with foreign body, right lower leg**
  Coding Clinic: 2016, Q3, P46
- S81.842   **Puncture wound with foreign body, left lower leg**
- S81.849   **Puncture wound with foreign body, unspecified lower leg**

S81.85   **Open bite of lower leg**
Bite of lower leg NOS

> **Excludes1**   superficial bite of lower leg (S80.86-, S80.87-)

- S81.851   **Open bite, right lower leg**
- S81.852   **Open bite, left lower leg**
- S81.859   **Open bite, unspecified lower leg**

● S82   **Fracture of lower leg, including ankle**

Note: A fracture not indicated as displaced or nondisplaced should be coded to displaced

A fracture not indicated as open or closed should be coded to closed

The open fracture designations are based on the Gustilo open fracture classification

Includes   fracture of malleolus

Excludes1   traumatic amputation of lower leg (S88.-)

Excludes2   fracture of foot, except ankle (S92.-)

periprosthetic fracture around internal of prosthetic implant of knee joint (M97.1-)

The appropriate 7th character is to be added to all codes from category S82

A	initial encounter for closed fracture
B	initial encounter for open fracture type I or II initial encounter for open fracture NOS
C	initial encounter for open fracture type IIIA, IIIB, or IIIC
D	subsequent encounter for closed fracture with routine healing
E	subsequent encounter for open fracture type I or II with routine healing
F	subsequent encounter for open fracture type IIIA, IIIB, or IIIC with routine healing
G	subsequent encounter for closed fracture with delayed healing
H	subsequent encounter for open fracture type I or II with delayed healing
J	subsequent encounter for open fracture type IIIA, IIIB, or IIIC with delayed healing
K	subsequent encounter for closed fracture with nonunion
M	subsequent encounter for open fracture type I or II with nonunion
N	subsequent encounter for open fracture type IIIA, IIIB, or IIIC with nonunion
P	subsequent encounter for closed fracture with malunion
Q	subsequent encounter for open fracture type I or II with malunion
R	subsequent encounter for open fracture type IIIA, IIIB, or IIIC with malunion
S	sequela

● S82.0   **Fracture of patella**
Knee cap

S82.00   **Unspecified fracture of patella**
- S82.001   Unspecified fracture of right patella
- S82.002   Unspecified fracture of left patella
- S82.009   Unspecified fracture of unspecified patella

S82.01   Osteochondral fracture of patella
- S82.011   **Displaced osteochondral fracture of right patella**
- S82.012   **Displaced osteochondral fracture of left patella**
- S82.013   **Displaced osteochondral fracture of unspecified patella**
- S82.014   **Nondisplaced osteochondral fracture of right patella**
- S82.015   **Nondisplaced osteochondral fracture of left patella**
- S82.016   **Nondisplaced osteochondral fracture of unspecified patella**

S82.02   Longitudinal fracture of patella
- S82.021   **Displaced longitudinal fracture of right patella**
- S82.022   **Displaced longitudinal fracture of left patella**
- S82.023   **Displaced longitudinal fracture of unspecified patella**
- S82.024   **Nondisplaced longitudinal fracture of right patella**
- S82.025   **Nondisplaced longitudinal fracture of left patella**
- S82.026   **Nondisplaced longitudinal fracture of unspecified patella**

S82.03   Transverse fracture of patella
- S82.031   **Displaced transverse fracture of right patella**
- S82.032   **Displaced transverse fracture of left patella**
- S82.033   **Displaced transverse fracture of unspecified patella**
- S82.034   **Nondisplaced transverse fracture of right patella**
- S82.035   **Nondisplaced transverse fracture of left patella**
- S82.036   **Nondisplaced transverse fracture of unspecified patella**

S82.04   **Comminuted fracture of patella**
- S82.041   **Displaced comminuted fracture of right patella**
- S82.042   **Displaced comminuted fracture of left patella**
- S82.043   **Displaced comminuted fracture of unspecified patella**
- S82.044   **Nondisplaced comminuted fracture of right patella**
- S82.045   **Nondisplaced comminuted fracture of left patella**
- S82.046   **Nondisplaced comminuted fracture of unspecified patella**

S82.09   **Other fracture of patella**
- S82.091   Other fracture of right patella
- S82.092   Other fracture of left patella
- S82.099   Other fracture of unspecified patella

● S82.1   **Fracture of upper end of tibia**
Fracture of proximal end of tibia

> **Excludes2**   fracture of shaft of tibia (S82.2-)
> physeal fracture of upper end of tibia (S89.0-)

S82.10   **Unspecified fracture of upper end of tibia**
- S82.101   Unspecified fracture of upper end of right tibia
- S82.102   Unspecified fracture of upper end of left tibia
- S82.109   Unspecified fracture of upper end of unspecified tibia

- S82.11   Fracture of tibial spine
  - S82.111   Displaced fracture of right tibial spine
  - S82.112   Displaced fracture of left tibial spine
  - S82.113   Displaced fracture of unspecified tibial spine
  - S82.114   Nondisplaced fracture of right tibial spine
  - S82.115   Nondisplaced fracture of left tibial spine
  - S82.116   Nondisplaced fracture of unspecified tibial spine
- S82.12   Fracture of lateral condyle of tibia
  - S82.121   Displaced fracture of lateral condyle of right tibia
  - S82.122   Displaced fracture of lateral condyle of left tibia
  - S82.123   Displaced fracture of lateral condyle of unspecified tibia
  - S82.124   Nondisplaced fracture of lateral condyle of right tibia
  - S82.125   Nondisplaced fracture of lateral condyle of left tibia
  - S82.126   Nondisplaced fracture of lateral condyle of unspecified tibia
- S82.13   Fracture of medial condyle of tibia
  - S82.131   Displaced fracture of medial condyle of right tibia
  - S82.132   Displaced fracture of medial condyle of left tibia
  - S82.133   Displaced fracture of medial condyle of unspecified tibia
  - S82.134   Nondisplaced fracture of medial condyle of right tibia
  - S82.135   Nondisplaced fracture of medial condyle of left tibia
  - S82.136   Nondisplaced fracture of medial condyle of unspecified tibia
- S82.14   Bicondylar fracture of tibia
  Fracture of tibial plateau NOS
  - S82.141   Displaced bicondylar fracture of right tibia
  - S82.142   Displaced bicondylar fracture of left tibia
  - S82.143   Displaced bicondylar fracture of unspecified tibia
  - S82.144   Nondisplaced bicondylar fracture of right tibia
  - S82.145   Nondisplaced bicondylar fracture of left tibia
  - S82.146   Nondisplaced bicondylar fracture of unspecified tibia
- S82.15   Fracture of tibial tuberosity
  - S82.151   Displaced fracture of right tibial tuberosity
  - S82.152   Displaced fracture of left tibial tuberosity
  - S82.153   Displaced fracture of unspecified tibial tuberosity
  - S82.154   Nondisplaced fracture of right tibial tuberosity
  - S82.155   Nondisplaced fracture of left tibial tuberosity
  - S82.156   Nondisplaced fracture of unspecified tibial tuberosity

- S82.16   Torus fracture of upper end of tibia

  The appropriate 7th character is to be added to all codes in subcategory S82.16

A	initial encounter for closed fracture
D	subsequent encounter for fracture with routine healing
G	subsequent encounter for fracture with delayed healing
K	subsequent encounter for fracture with nonunion
P	subsequent encounter for fracture with malunion
S	sequela

  - S82.161   Torus fracture of upper end of right tibia
  - S82.162   Torus fracture of upper end of left tibia
  - S82.169   Torus fracture of upper end of unspecified tibia
- S82.19   Other fracture of upper end of tibia
  - S82.191   Other fracture of upper end of right tibia
  - S82.192   Other fracture of upper end of left tibia
  - S82.199   Other fracture of upper end of unspecified tibia
- S82.2   Fracture of shaft of tibia
  - S82.20   Unspecified fracture of shaft of tibia
    Fracture of tibia NOS
    - S82.201   Unspecified fracture of shaft of right tibia
    - S82.202   Unspecified fracture of shaft of left tibia
    - S82.209   Unspecified fracture of shaft of unspecified tibia
  - S82.22   Transverse fracture of shaft of tibia
    - S82.221   Displaced transverse fracture of shaft of right tibia
    - S82.222   Displaced transverse fracture of shaft of left tibia
    - S82.223   Displaced transverse fracture of shaft of unspecified tibia
    - S82.224   Nondisplaced transverse fracture of shaft of right tibia
    - S82.225   Nondisplaced transverse fracture of shaft of left tibia
    - S82.226   Nondisplaced transverse fracture of shaft of unspecified tibia
  - S82.23   Oblique fracture of shaft of tibia
    - S82.231   Displaced oblique fracture of shaft of right tibia
    - S82.232   Displaced oblique fracture of shaft of left tibia
    - S82.233   Displaced oblique fracture of shaft of unspecified tibia
    - S82.234   Nondisplaced oblique fracture of shaft of right tibia
      Coding Clinic: 2015, Q1, P9-10
    - S82.235   Nondisplaced oblique fracture of shaft of left tibia
    - S82.236   Nondisplaced oblique fracture of shaft of unspecified tibia
  - S82.24   Spiral fracture of shaft of tibia
    Toddler fracture
    - S82.241   Displaced spiral fracture of shaft of right tibia
    - S82.242   Displaced spiral fracture of shaft of left tibia
    - S82.243   Displaced spiral fracture of shaft of unspecified tibia

S82.244　Nondisplaced spiral fracture of shaft of right tibia

S82.245　Nondisplaced spiral fracture of shaft of left tibia

S82.246　Nondisplaced spiral fracture of shaft of unspecified tibia

S82.25　Comminuted fracture of shaft of tibia

　S82.251　Displaced comminuted fracture of shaft of right tibia
　　Coding Clinic: 2015, Q2, P6

　S82.252　Displaced comminuted fracture of shaft of left tibia

　S82.253　Displaced comminuted fracture of shaft of unspecified tibia

　S82.254　Nondisplaced comminuted fracture of shaft of right tibia

　S82.255　Nondisplaced comminuted fracture of shaft of left tibia

　S82.256　Nondisplaced comminuted fracture of shaft of unspecified tibia

S82.26　Segmental fracture of shaft of tibia

　S82.261　Displaced segmental fracture of shaft of right tibia

　S82.262　Displaced segmental fracture of shaft of left tibia

　S82.263　Displaced segmental fracture of shaft of unspecified tibia

　S82.264　Nondisplaced segmental fracture of shaft of right tibia

　S82.265　Nondisplaced segmental fracture of shaft of left tibia

　S82.266　Nondisplaced segmental fracture of shaft of unspecified tibia

S82.29　Other fracture of shaft of tibia

　S82.291　Other fracture of shaft of right tibia

　S82.292　Other fracture of shaft of left tibia

　S82.299　Other fracture of shaft of unspecified tibia

S82.3　Fracture of lower end of tibia

　Excludes1　bimalleolar fracture of lower leg (S82.84-)
　　　　fracture of medial malleolus alone (S82.5-)
　　　　Maisonneuve's fracture (S82.86-)
　　　　pilon fracture of distal tibia (S82.87-)
　　　　trimalleolar fractures of lower leg (S82.85-)

S82.30　Unspecified fracture of lower end of tibia

　S82.301　Unspecified fracture of lower end of right tibia

　S82.302　Unspecified fracture of lower end of left tibia

　S82.309　Unspecified fracture of lower end of unspecified tibia

S82.31　Torus fracture of lower end of tibia

　The appropriate 7th character is to be added to all codes in subcategory S82.31

A	initial encounter for closed fracture
D	subsequent encounter for fracture with routine healing
G	subsequent encounter for fracture with delayed healing
K	subsequent encounter for fracture with nonunion
P	subsequent encounter for fracture with malunion
S	sequela

　S82.311　Torus fracture of lower end of right tibia

　S82.312　Torus fracture of lower end of left tibia

　S82.319　Torus fracture of lower end of unspecified tibia

S82.39　Other fracture of lower end of tibia

　S82.391　Other fracture of lower end of right tibia

　S82.392　Other fracture of lower end of left tibia
　　Coding Clinic: 2015, Q1, P25

　S82.399　Other fracture of lower end of unspecified tibia

S82.4　Fracture of shaft of fibula

　Excludes2　fracture of lateral malleolus alone (S82.6-)

S82.40　Unspecified fracture of shaft of fibula

　S82.401　Unspecified fracture of shaft of right fibula

　S82.402　Unspecified fracture of shaft of left fibula

　S82.409　Unspecified fracture of shaft of unspecified fibula

S82.42　Transverse fracture of shaft of fibula

　S82.421　Displaced transverse fracture of shaft of right fibula

　S82.422　Displaced transverse fracture of shaft of left fibula

　S82.423　Displaced transverse fracture of shaft of unspecified fibula

　S82.424　Nondisplaced transverse fracture of shaft of right fibula

　S82.425　Nondisplaced transverse fracture of shaft of left fibula

　S82.426　Nondisplaced transverse fracture of shaft of unspecified fibula

S82.43　Oblique fracture of shaft of fibula

　S82.431　Displaced oblique fracture of shaft of right fibula

　S82.432　Displaced oblique fracture of shaft of left fibula

　S82.433　Displaced oblique fracture of shaft of unspecified fibula

　S82.434　Nondisplaced oblique fracture of shaft of right fibula

　S82.435　Nondisplaced oblique fracture of shaft of left fibula

　S82.436　Nondisplaced oblique fracture of shaft of unspecified fibula

S82.44　Spiral fracture of shaft of fibula

　S82.441　Displaced spiral fracture of shaft of right fibula

　S82.442　Displaced spiral fracture of shaft of left fibula

　S82.443　Displaced spiral fracture of shaft of unspecified fibula

　S82.444　Nondisplaced spiral fracture of shaft of right fibula

　S82.445　Nondisplaced spiral fracture of shaft of left fibula

　S82.446　Nondisplaced spiral fracture of shaft of unspecified fibula

S82.45　Comminuted fracture of shaft of fibula

　S82.451　Displaced comminuted fracture of shaft of right fibula

　S82.452　Displaced comminuted fracture of shaft of left fibula

　S82.453　Displaced comminuted fracture of shaft of unspecified fibula

　S82.454　Nondisplaced comminuted fracture of shaft of right fibula

　S82.455　Nondisplaced comminuted fracture of shaft of left fibula

　S82.456　Nondisplaced comminuted fracture of shaft of unspecified fibula

▶ New　　⇒ Revised　　deleted Deleted　　Excludes 1　　Excludes 2　　Includes　　Use additional　　Code first　　Code also　　Key words
OGCR Official Guidelines　　X Assign placeholder X　　● Use Additional Character(s)　　▶ Manifestation Code　　🐾 Hierarchical Condition Category　　Coding Clinic

● S82.46   Segmental fracture of shaft of fibula
     ● S82.461   Displaced segmental fracture of shaft of right fibula
     ● S82.462   Displaced segmental fracture of shaft of left fibula
     ● S82.463   Displaced segmental fracture of shaft of unspecified fibula
     ● S82.464   Nondisplaced segmental fracture of shaft of right fibula
     ● S82.465   Nondisplaced segmental fracture of shaft of left fibula
     ● S82.466   Nondisplaced segmental fracture of shaft of unspecified fibula
● S82.49   Other fracture of shaft of fibula
     ● S82.491   Other fracture of shaft of right fibula
     ● S82.492   Other fracture of shaft of left fibula
     ● S82.499   Other fracture of shaft of unspecified fibula
● S82.5   **Fracture of medial malleolus**
     Excludes1   pilon fracture of distal tibia (S82.87-)
           Salter-Harris type III of lower end of tibia (S89.13-)
           Salter-Harris type IV of lower end of tibia (S89.14-)
X ● S82.51   Displaced fracture of medial malleolus of right tibia
X ● S82.52   Displaced fracture of medial malleolus of left tibia
X ● S82.53   Displaced fracture of medial malleolus of unspecified tibia
X ● S82.54   Nondisplaced fracture of medial malleolus of right tibia
X ● S82.55   Nondisplaced fracture of medial malleolus of left tibia
X ● S82.56   Nondisplaced fracture of medial malleolus of unspecified tibia
● S82.6   **Fracture of lateral malleolus**
     Excludes1   pilon fracture of distal tibia (S82.87-)
X ● S82.61   Displaced fracture of lateral malleolus of right fibula
X ● S82.62   Displaced fracture of lateral malleolus of left fibula
X ● S82.63   Displaced fracture of lateral malleolus of unspecified fibula
X ● S82.64   Nondisplaced fracture of lateral malleolus of right fibula
X ● S82.65   Nondisplaced fracture of lateral malleolus of left fibula
X ● S82.66   Nondisplaced fracture of lateral malleolus of unspecified fibula
● S82.8   **Other fractures of lower leg**
     ● S82.81   Torus fracture of upper end of fibula
         The appropriate 7th character is to be added to all codes in subcategory S82.81

A	initial encounter for closed fracture
D	subsequent encounter for fracture with routine healing
G	subsequent encounter for fracture with delayed healing
K	subsequent encounter for fracture with nonunion
P	subsequent encounter for fracture with malunion
S	sequela

     ● S82.811   Torus fracture of upper end of right fibula
     ● S82.812   Torus fracture of upper end of left fibula
     ● S82.819   Torus fracture of upper end of unspecified fibula

● S82.82   Torus fracture of lower end of fibula
     The appropriate 7th character is to be added to all codes in subcategory S82.82

A	initial encounter for closed fracture
D	subsequent encounter for fracture with routine healing
G	subsequent encounter for fracture with delayed healing
K	subsequent encounter for fracture with nonunion
P	subsequent encounter for fracture with malunion
S	sequela

     ● S82.821   Torus fracture of lower end of right fibula
     ● S82.822   Torus fracture of lower end of left fibula
     ● S82.829   Torus fracture of lower end of unspecified fibula
● S82.83   Other fracture of upper and lower end of fibula
     ● S82.831   Other fracture of upper and lower end of right fibula
     ● S82.832   Other fracture of upper and lower end of left fibula
         Coding Clinic: 2015, Q1, P9-10
     ● S82.839   Other fracture of upper and lower end of unspecified fibula
● S82.84   Bimalleolar fracture of lower leg
     ● S82.841   Displaced bimalleolar fracture of right lower leg
     ● S82.842   Displaced bimalleolar fracture of left lower leg
     ● S82.843   Displaced bimalleolar fracture of unspecified lower leg
     ● S82.844   Nondisplaced bimalleolar fracture of right lower leg
     ● S82.845   Nondisplaced bimalleolar fracture of left lower leg
     ● S82.846   Nondisplaced bimalleolar fracture of unspecified lower leg
● S82.85   Trimalleolar fracture of lower leg
     ● S82.851   Displaced trimalleolar fracture of right lower leg
     ● S82.852   Displaced trimalleolar fracture of left lower leg
     ● S82.853   Displaced trimalleolar fracture of unspecified lower leg
     ● S82.854   Nondisplaced trimalleolar fracture of right lower leg
     ● S82.855   Nondisplaced trimalleolar fracture of left lower leg
     ● S82.856   Nondisplaced trimalleolar fracture of unspecified lower leg
● S82.86   Maisonneuve's fracture
     ● S82.861   Displaced Maisonneuve's fracture of right leg
     ● S82.862   Displaced Maisonneuve's fracture of left leg
     ● S82.863   Displaced Maisonneuve's fracture of unspecified leg
     ● S82.864   Nondisplaced Maisonneuve's fracture of right leg
     ● S82.865   Nondisplaced Maisonneuve's fracture of left leg
     ● S82.866   Nondisplaced Maisonneuve's fracture of unspecified leg
● S82.87   Pilon fracture of tibia
     ● S82.871   Displaced pilon fracture of right tibia
     ● S82.872   Displaced pilon fracture of left tibia

CHAPTER 19 (S00-T88)

● S82.873   Displaced pilon fracture of
            unspecified tibia
● S82.874   Nondisplaced pilon fracture of right
            tibia
● S82.875   Nondisplaced pilon fracture of left
            tibia
● S82.876   Nondisplaced pilon fracture of
            unspecified tibia
S82.89   Other fractures of lower leg
         Fracture of ankle NOS
   ● S82.891   Other fracture of right lower leg
   ● S82.892   Other fracture of left lower leg
   ● S82.899   Other fracture of unspecified lower
               leg
■ S82.9   Unspecified fracture of lower leg
   X ● S82.90   Unspecified fracture of unspecified lower leg
   X ● S82.91   Unspecified fracture of right lower leg
   X ● S82.92   Unspecified fracture of left lower leg

● S83   Dislocation and sprain of joints and ligaments of knee
   Includes   avulsion of joint or ligament of knee
                  laceration of cartilage, joint or ligament of knee
                  sprain of cartilage, joint or ligament of knee
                  traumatic hemarthrosis of joint or ligament of
                     knee
                  traumatic rupture of joint or ligament of knee
                  traumatic subluxation of joint or ligament of knee
                  traumatic tear of joint or ligament of knee

   Code also any associated open wound
   Excludes2   derangement of patella (M22.0-M22.3)
                   injury of patellar ligament (tendon) (S76.1-)
                   internal derangement of knee (M23.-)
                   old dislocation of knee (M24.36)
                   pathological dislocation of knee (M24.36)
                   recurrent dislocation of knee (M22.0)
                   strain of muscle, fascia and tendon of lower leg
                      (S86.-)
   Coding Clinic: 2019, Q2, P26

   The appropriate 7th character is to be added to each code from
      category S83

A	initial encounter
D	subsequent encounter
S	sequela

■ S83.0   Subluxation and dislocation of patella
   ● S83.00   Unspecified subluxation and dislocation of
              patella
      ● S83.001   Unspecified subluxation of right
                  patella
      ● S83.002   Unspecified subluxation of left
                  patella
      ● S83.003   Unspecified subluxation of
                  unspecified patella
      ● S83.004   Unspecified dislocation of right
                  patella
      ● S83.005   Unspecified dislocation of left patella
      ● S83.006   Unspecified dislocation of unspecified
                  patella
   ● S83.01   Lateral subluxation and dislocation of patella
      ● S83.011   Lateral subluxation of right patella
      ● S83.012   Lateral subluxation of left patella
      ● S83.013   Lateral subluxation of unspecified
                  patella
      ● S83.014   Lateral dislocation of right patella
      ● S83.015   Lateral dislocation of left patella
      ● S83.016   Lateral dislocation of unspecified
                  patella
   ● S83.09   Other subluxation and dislocation of patella
      ● S83.091   Other subluxation of right patella
      ● S83.092   Other subluxation of left patella

● S83.093   Other subluxation of unspecified
            patella
● S83.094   Other dislocation of right patella
● S83.095   Other dislocation of left patella
● S83.096   Other dislocation of unspecified
            patella
■ S83.1   Subluxation and dislocation of knee
   Excludes2   instability of knee prosthesis (T84.022,
                   T84.023)
   ● S83.10   Unspecified subluxation and dislocation of
              knee
      ● S83.101   Unspecified subluxation of right knee
      ● S83.102   Unspecified subluxation of left knee
      ● S83.103   Unspecified subluxation of
                  unspecified knee
      ● S83.104   Unspecified dislocation of right knee
      ● S83.105   Unspecified dislocation of left knee
      ● S83.106   Unspecified dislocation of unspecified
                  knee
   ● S83.11   Anterior subluxation and dislocation of
              proximal end of tibia
              Posterior subluxation and dislocation of distal
                 end of femur
      ● S83.111   Anterior subluxation of proximal end
                  of tibia, right knee
      ● S83.112   Anterior subluxation of proximal end
                  of tibia, left knee
      ● S83.113   Anterior subluxation of proximal end
                  of tibia, unspecified knee
      ● S83.114   Anterior dislocation of proximal end
                  of tibia, right knee
      ● S83.115   Anterior dislocation of proximal end
                  of tibia, left knee
      ● S83.116   Anterior dislocation of proximal end
                  of tibia, unspecified knee
   ● S83.12   Posterior subluxation and dislocation of
              proximal end of tibia
              Anterior dislocation of distal end of femur
      ● S83.121   Posterior subluxation of proximal end
                  of tibia, right knee
      ● S83.122   Posterior subluxation of proximal end
                  of tibia, left knee
      ● S83.123   Posterior subluxation of proximal end
                  of tibia, unspecified knee
      ● S83.124   Posterior dislocation of proximal end
                  of tibia, right knee
      ● S83.125   Posterior dislocation of proximal end
                  of tibia, left knee
      ● S83.126   Posterior dislocation of proximal end
                  of tibia, unspecified knee
   ● S83.13   Medial subluxation and dislocation of proximal
              end of tibia
      ● S83.131   Medial subluxation of proximal end
                  of tibia, right knee
      ● S83.132   Medial subluxation of proximal end
                  of tibia, left knee
      ● S83.133   Medial subluxation of proximal end
                  of tibia, unspecified knee
      ● S83.134   Medial dislocation of proximal end of
                  tibia, right knee
      ● S83.135   Medial dislocation of proximal end of
                  tibia, left knee
      ● S83.136   Medial dislocation of proximal end of
                  tibia, unspecified knee
   ● S83.14   Lateral subluxation and dislocation of proximal
              end of tibia
      ● S83.141   Lateral subluxation of proximal end
                  of tibia, right knee
      ● S83.142   Lateral subluxation of proximal end
                  of tibia, left knee

▶ New   ⇒ Revised   ~~deleted~~ Deleted   Excludes 1   Excludes 2   Includes   Use additional   Code first   Code also   Key words
OGCR Official Guidelines   X Assign placeholder X   ● Use Additional Character(s)   ▌ Manifestation Code   🐾 Hierarchical Condition Category   **Coding Clinic**

● S83.143   Lateral subluxation of proximal end of tibia, unspecified knee
● S83.144   Lateral dislocation of proximal end of tibia, right knee
● S83.145   Lateral dislocation of proximal end of tibia, left knee
● S83.146   Lateral dislocation of proximal end of tibia, unspecified knee

● S83.19   Other subluxation and dislocation of knee
  ● S83.191   Other subluxation of right knee
  ● S83.192   Other subluxation of left knee
  ● S83.193   Other subluxation of unspecified knee
  ● S83.194   Other dislocation of right knee
  ● S83.195   Other dislocation of left knee
  ● S83.196   Other dislocation of unspecified knee

● S83.2   Tear of meniscus, current injury
  Excludes1   old bucket-handle tear (M23.2)

● S83.20   Tear of unspecified meniscus, current injury
  Tear of meniscus of knee NOS
  ● S83.200   Bucket-handle tear of unspecified meniscus, current injury, right knee
  ● S83.201   Bucket-handle tear of unspecified meniscus, current injury, left knee
  ● S83.202   Bucket-handle tear of unspecified meniscus, current injury, unspecified knee
  ● S83.203   Other tear of unspecified meniscus, current injury, right knee
  ● S83.204   Other tear of unspecified meniscus, current injury, left knee
  ● S83.205   Other tear of unspecified meniscus, current injury, unspecified knee
  ● S83.206   Unspecified tear of unspecified meniscus, current injury, right knee
  ● S83.207   Unspecified tear of unspecified meniscus, current injury, left knee
  ● S83.209   Unspecified tear of unspecified meniscus, current injury, unspecified knee

● S83.21   Bucket-handle tear of medial meniscus, current injury
  ● S83.211   Bucket-handle tear of medial meniscus, current injury, right knee
  ● S83.212   Bucket-handle tear of medial meniscus, current injury, left knee
  ● S83.219   Bucket-handle tear of medial meniscus, current injury, unspecified knee

● S83.22   Peripheral tear of medial meniscus, current injury
  ● S83.221   Peripheral tear of medial meniscus, current injury, right knee
  ● S83.222   Peripheral tear of medial meniscus, current injury, left knee
  ● S83.229   Peripheral tear of medial meniscus, current injury, unspecified knee

● S83.23   Complex tear of medial meniscus, current injury
  ● S83.231   Complex tear of medial meniscus, current injury, right knee
  ● S83.232   Complex tear of medial meniscus, current injury, left knee
    Coding Clinic: 2019, Q2, P26
  ● S83.239   Complex tear of medial meniscus, current injury, unspecified knee

● S83.24   Other tear of medial meniscus, current injury
  ● S83.241   Other tear of medial meniscus, current injury, right knee
  ● S83.242   Other tear of medial meniscus, current injury, left knee
  ● S83.249   Other tear of medial meniscus, current injury, unspecified knee

● S83.25   Bucket-handle tear of lateral meniscus, current injury
  ● S83.251   Bucket-handle tear of lateral meniscus, current injury, right knee
  ● S83.252   Bucket-handle tear of lateral meniscus, current injury, left knee
  ● S83.259   Bucket-handle tear of lateral meniscus, current injury, unspecified knee

● S83.26   Peripheral tear of lateral meniscus, current injury
  ● S83.261   Peripheral tear of lateral meniscus, current injury, right knee
  ● S83.262   Peripheral tear of lateral meniscus, current injury, left knee
  ● S83.269   Peripheral tear of lateral meniscus, current injury, unspecified knee

● S83.27   Complex tear of lateral meniscus, current injury
  ● S83.271   Complex tear of lateral meniscus, current injury, right knee
  ● S83.272   Complex tear of lateral meniscus, current injury, left knee
  ● S83.279   Complex tear of lateral meniscus, current injury, unspecified knee

● S83.28   Other tear of lateral meniscus, current injury
  ● S83.281   Other tear of lateral meniscus, current injury, right knee
  ● S83.282   Other tear of lateral meniscus, current injury, left knee
  ● S83.289   Other tear of lateral meniscus, current injury, unspecified knee

● S83.3   Tear of articular cartilage of knee, current
  X ● S83.30   Tear of articular cartilage of unspecified knee, current
  X ● S83.31   Tear of articular cartilage of right knee, current
  X ● S83.32   Tear of articular cartilage of left knee, current

● S83.4   Sprain of collateral ligament of knee
  ● S83.40   Sprain of unspecified collateral ligament of knee
  ● S83.401   Sprain of unspecified collateral ligament of right knee
  ● S83.402   Sprain of unspecified collateral ligament of left knee
  ● S83.409   Sprain of unspecified collateral ligament of unspecified knee

  ● S83.41   Sprain of medial collateral ligament of knee
    Sprain of tibial collateral ligament
  ● S83.411   Sprain of medial collateral ligament of right knee
  ● S83.412   Sprain of medial collateral ligament of left knee
  ● S83.419   Sprain of medial collateral ligament of unspecified knee

  ● S83.42   Sprain of lateral collateral ligament of knee
    Sprain of fibular collateral ligament
  ● S83.421   Sprain of lateral collateral ligament of right knee
  ● S83.422   Sprain of lateral collateral ligament of left knee
  ● S83.429   Sprain of lateral collateral ligament of unspecified knee

● S83.5   Sprain of cruciate ligament of knee
  ● S83.50   Sprain of unspecified cruciate ligament of knee
    ● S83.501   Sprain of unspecified cruciate ligament of right knee
    ● S83.502   Sprain of unspecified cruciate ligament of left knee
    ● S83.509   Sprain of unspecified cruciate ligament of unspecified knee
  ● S83.51   Sprain of anterior cruciate ligament of knee
    ● S83.511   Sprain of anterior cruciate ligament of right knee
         Coding Clinic: 2016, Q2, P4
    ● S83.512   Sprain of anterior cruciate ligament of left knee
    ● S83.519   Sprain of anterior cruciate ligament of unspecified knee
  ● S83.52   Sprain of posterior cruciate ligament of knee
    ● S83.521   Sprain of posterior cruciate ligament of right knee
    ● S83.522   Sprain of posterior cruciate ligament of left knee
    ● S83.529   Sprain of posterior cruciate ligament of unspecified knee
● S83.6   Sprain of the superior tibiofibular joint and ligament
  X ● S83.60   Sprain of the superior tibiofibular joint and ligament, unspecified knee
  X ● S83.61   Sprain of the superior tibiofibular joint and ligament, right knee
  X ● S83.62   Sprain of the superior tibiofibular joint and ligament, left knee
● S83.8   Sprain of other specified parts of knee
  ● S83.8X   Sprain of other specified parts of knee
    ● S83.8X1   Sprain of other specified parts of right knee
    ● S83.8X2   Sprain of other specified parts of left knee
    ● S83.8X9   Sprain of other specified parts of unspecified knee
● S83.9   Sprain of unspecified site of knee
  X ● S83.90   Sprain of unspecified site of unspecified knee
  X ● S83.91   Sprain of unspecified site of right knee
  X ● S83.92   Sprain of unspecified site of left knee

● S84   Injury of nerves at lower leg level
  Code also any associated open wound (S81.-)
  Excludes2   injury of nerves at ankle and foot level (S94.-)
  The appropriate 7th character is to be added to each code from category S84

A	initial encounter
D	subsequent encounter
S	sequela

● S84.0   Injury of tibial nerve at lower leg level
  X ● S84.00   Injury of tibial nerve at lower leg level, unspecified leg
  X ● S84.01   Injury of tibial nerve at lower leg level, right leg
  X ● S84.02   Injury of tibial nerve at lower leg level, left leg
● S84.1   Injury of peroneal nerve at lower leg level
  X ● S84.10   Injury of peroneal nerve at lower leg level, unspecified leg
  X ● S84.11   Injury of peroneal nerve at lower leg level, right leg
  X ● S84.12   Injury of peroneal nerve at lower leg level, left leg

● S84.2   Injury of cutaneous sensory nerve at lower leg level
  X ● S84.20   Injury of cutaneous sensory nerve at lower leg level, unspecified leg
  X ● S84.21   Injury of cutaneous sensory nerve at lower leg level, right leg
  X ● S84.22   Injury of cutaneous sensory nerve at lower leg level, left leg
● S84.8   Injury of other nerves at lower leg level
  ● S84.80   Injury of other nerves at lower leg level
    ● S84.801   Injury of other nerves at lower leg level, right leg
    ● S84.802   Injury of other nerves at lower leg level, left leg
    ● S84.809   Injury of other nerves at lower leg level, unspecified leg
● S84.9   Injury of unspecified nerve at lower leg level
  X ● S84.90   Injury of unspecified nerve at lower leg level, unspecified leg
  X ● S84.91   Injury of unspecified nerve at lower leg level, right leg
  X ● S84.92   Injury of unspecified nerve at lower leg level, left leg

● S85   Injury of blood vessels at lower leg level
  Code also any associated open wound (S81.-)
  Excludes2   injury of blood vessels at ankle and foot level (S95.-)
  The appropriate 7th character is to be added to each code from category S85

A	initial encounter
D	subsequent encounter
S	sequela

● S85.0   Injury of popliteal artery
  ● S85.00   Unspecified injury of popliteal artery
    ● S85.001   Unspecified injury of popliteal artery, right leg
    ● S85.002   Unspecified injury of popliteal artery, left leg
    ● S85.009   Unspecified injury of popliteal artery, unspecified leg
  ● S85.01   Laceration of popliteal artery
    ● S85.011   Laceration of popliteal artery, right leg
    ● S85.012   Laceration of popliteal artery, left leg
    ● S85.019   Laceration of popliteal artery, unspecified leg
  ● S85.09   Other specified injury of popliteal artery
    ● S85.091   Other specified injury of popliteal artery, right leg
    ● S85.092   Other specified injury of popliteal artery, left leg
    ● S85.099   Other specified injury of popliteal artery, unspecified leg
● S85.1   Injury of tibial artery
  ● S85.10   Unspecified injury of unspecified tibial artery
    Injury of tibial artery NOS
    ● S85.101   Unspecified injury of unspecified tibial artery, right leg
    ● S85.102   Unspecified injury of unspecified tibial artery, left leg
    ● S85.109   Unspecified injury of unspecified tibial artery, unspecified leg
  ● S85.11   Laceration of unspecified tibial artery
    ● S85.111   Laceration of unspecified tibial artery, right leg
    ● S85.112   Laceration of unspecified tibial artery, left leg
    ● S85.119   Laceration of unspecified tibial artery, unspecified leg

- S85.12   Other specified injury of unspecified tibial artery
  - S85.121   Other specified injury of unspecified tibial artery, right leg
  - S85.122   Other specified injury of unspecified tibial artery, left leg
  - S85.129   Other specified injury of unspecified tibial artery, unspecified leg
- S85.13   Unspecified injury of anterior tibial artery
  - S85.131   Unspecified injury of anterior tibial artery, right leg
  - S85.132   Unspecified injury of anterior tibial artery, left leg
  - S85.139   Unspecified injury of anterior tibial artery, unspecified leg
- S85.14   Laceration of anterior tibial artery
  - S85.141   Laceration of anterior tibial artery, right leg
  - S85.142   Laceration of anterior tibial artery, left leg
  - S85.149   Laceration of anterior tibial artery, unspecified leg
- S85.15   Other specified injury of anterior tibial artery
  - S85.151   Other specified injury of anterior tibial artery, right leg
  - S85.152   Other specified injury of anterior tibial artery, left leg
  - S85.159   Other specified injury of anterior tibial artery, unspecified leg
- S85.16   Unspecified injury of posterior tibial artery
  - S85.161   Unspecified injury of posterior tibial artery, right leg
  - S85.162   Unspecified injury of posterior tibial artery, left leg
  - S85.169   Unspecified injury of posterior tibial artery, unspecified leg
- S85.17   Laceration of posterior tibial artery
  - S85.171   Laceration of posterior tibial artery, right leg
  - S85.172   Laceration of posterior tibial artery, left leg
  - S85.179   Laceration of posterior tibial artery, unspecified leg
- S85.18   Other specified injury of posterior tibial artery
  - S85.181   Other specified injury of posterior tibial artery, right leg
  - S85.182   Other specified injury of posterior tibial artery, left leg
  - S85.189   Other specified injury of posterior tibial artery, unspecified leg
- S85.2   Injury of peroneal artery
  - S85.20   Unspecified injury of peroneal artery
    - S85.201   Unspecified injury of peroneal artery, right leg
    - S85.202   Unspecified injury of peroneal artery, left leg
    - S85.209   Unspecified injury of peroneal artery, unspecified leg
  - S85.21   Laceration of peroneal artery
    - S85.211   Laceration of peroneal artery, right leg
    - S85.212   Laceration of peroneal artery, left leg
    - S85.219   Laceration of peroneal artery, unspecified leg
  - S85.29   Other specified injury of peroneal artery
    - S85.291   Other specified injury of peroneal artery, right leg
    - S85.292   Other specified injury of peroneal artery, left leg
    - S85.299   Other specified injury of peroneal artery, unspecified leg

- S85.3   Injury of greater saphenous vein at lower leg level
  Injury of greater saphenous vein NOS
  Injury of saphenous vein NOS
  - S85.30   Unspecified injury of greater saphenous vein at lower leg level
    - S85.301   Unspecified injury of greater saphenous vein at lower leg level, right leg
    - S85.302   Unspecified injury of greater saphenous vein at lower leg level, left leg
    - S85.309   Unspecified injury of greater saphenous vein at lower leg level, unspecified leg
  - S85.31   Laceration of greater saphenous vein at lower leg level
    - S85.311   Laceration of greater saphenous vein at lower leg level, right leg
    - S85.312   Laceration of greater saphenous vein at lower leg level, left leg
    - S85.319   Laceration of greater saphenous vein at lower leg level, unspecified leg
  - S85.39   Other specified injury of greater saphenous vein at lower leg level
    - S85.391   Other specified injury of greater saphenous vein at lower leg level, right leg
    - S85.392   Other specified injury of greater saphenous vein at lower leg level, left leg
    - S85.399   Other specified injury of greater saphenous vein at lower leg level, unspecified leg
- S85.4   Injury of lesser saphenous vein at lower leg level
  - S85.40   Unspecified injury of lesser saphenous vein at lower leg level
    - S85.401   Unspecified injury of lesser saphenous vein at lower leg level, right leg
    - S85.402   Unspecified injury of lesser saphenous vein at lower leg level, left leg
    - S85.409   Unspecified injury of lesser saphenous vein at lower leg level, unspecified leg
  - S85.41   Laceration of lesser saphenous vein at lower leg level
    - S85.411   Laceration of lesser saphenous vein at lower leg level, right leg
    - S85.412   Laceration of lesser saphenous vein at lower leg level, left leg
    - S85.419   Laceration of lesser saphenous vein at lower leg level, unspecified leg
  - S85.49   Other specified injury of lesser saphenous vein at lower leg level
    - S85.491   Other specified injury of lesser saphenous vein at lower leg level, right leg
    - S85.492   Other specified injury of lesser saphenous vein at lower leg level, left leg
    - S85.499   Other specified injury of lesser saphenous vein at lower leg level, unspecified leg
- S85.5   Injury of popliteal vein
  - S85.50   Unspecified injury of popliteal vein
    - S85.501   Unspecified injury of popliteal vein, right leg
    - S85.502   Unspecified injury of popliteal vein, left leg
    - S85.509   Unspecified injury of popliteal vein, unspecified leg

● S85.51   Laceration of popliteal vein
  ● S85.511   Laceration of popliteal vein, right leg
  ● S85.512   Laceration of popliteal vein, left leg
  ● S85.519   Laceration of popliteal vein, unspecified leg
● S85.59   Other specified injury of popliteal vein
  ● S85.591   Other specified injury of popliteal vein, right leg
  ● S85.592   Other specified injury of popliteal vein, left leg
  ● S85.599   Other specified injury of popliteal vein, unspecified leg

● S85.8   Injury of other blood vessels at lower leg level
  ● S85.80   Unspecified injury of other blood vessels at lower leg level
    ● S85.801   Unspecified injury of other blood vessels at lower leg level, right leg
    ● S85.802   Unspecified injury of other blood vessels at lower leg level, left leg
    ● S85.809   Unspecified injury of other blood vessels at lower leg level, unspecified leg
  ● S85.81   Laceration of other blood vessels at lower leg level
    ● S85.811   Laceration of other blood vessels at lower leg level, right leg
    ● S85.812   Laceration of other blood vessels at lower leg level, left leg
    ● S85.819   Laceration of other blood vessels at lower leg level, unspecified leg
  ● S85.89   Other specified injury of other blood vessels at lower leg level
    ● S85.891   Other specified injury of other blood vessels at lower leg level, right leg
    ● S85.892   Other specified injury of other blood vessels at lower leg level, left leg
    ● S85.899   Other specified injury of other blood vessels at lower leg level, unspecified leg

● S85.9   Injury of unspecified blood vessel at lower leg level
  ● S85.90   Unspecified injury of unspecified blood vessel at lower leg level
    ● S85.901   Unspecified injury of unspecified blood vessel at lower leg level, right leg
    ● S85.902   Unspecified injury of unspecified blood vessel at lower leg level, left leg
    ● S85.909   Unspecified injury of unspecified blood vessel at lower leg level, unspecified leg
  ● S85.91   Laceration of unspecified blood vessel at lower leg level
    ● S85.911   Laceration of unspecified blood vessel at lower leg level, right leg
    ● S85.912   Laceration of unspecified blood vessel at lower leg level, left leg
    ● S85.919   Laceration of unspecified blood vessel at lower leg level, unspecified leg
  ● S85.99   Other specified injury of unspecified blood vessel at lower leg level
    ● S85.991   Other specified injury of unspecified blood vessel at lower leg level, right leg
    ● S85.992   Other specified injury of unspecified blood vessel at lower leg level, left leg
    ● S85.999   Other specified injury of unspecified blood vessel at lower leg level, unspecified leg

● S86   Injury of muscle, fascia and tendon at lower leg level
Code also any associated open wound (S81.-)

Excludes2   injury of muscle, fascia and tendon at ankle (S96.-)
injury of patellar ligament (tendon) (S76.1-)
sprain of joints and ligaments of knee (S83.-)

The appropriate 7th character is to be added to each code from category S86

A	initial encounter
D	subsequent encounter
S	sequela

● S86.0   Injury of Achilles tendon
  ● S86.00   Unspecified injury of Achilles tendon
    ● S86.001   Unspecified injury of right Achilles tendon
    ● S86.002   Unspecified injury of left Achilles tendon
    ● S86.009   Unspecified injury of unspecified Achilles tendon
  ● S86.01   Strain of Achilles tendon
    ● S86.011   Strain of right Achilles tendon
    ● S86.012   Strain of left Achilles tendon
    ● S86.019   Strain of unspecified Achilles tendon
  ● S86.02   Laceration of Achilles tendon
    ● S86.021   Laceration of right Achilles tendon
    ● S86.022   Laceration of left Achilles tendon
    ● S86.029   Laceration of unspecified Achilles tendon
  ● S86.09   Other specified injury of Achilles tendon
    ● S86.091   Other specified injury of right Achilles tendon
    ● S86.092   Other specified injury of left Achilles tendon
    ● S86.099   Other specified injury of unspecified Achilles tendon

● S86.1   Injury of other muscle(s) and tendon(s) of posterior muscle group at lower leg level
  ● S86.10   Unspecified injury of other muscle(s) and tendon(s) of posterior muscle group at lower leg level
    ● S86.101   Unspecified injury of other muscle(s) and tendon(s) of posterior muscle group at lower leg level, right leg
    ● S86.102   Unspecified injury of other muscle(s) and tendon(s) of posterior muscle group at lower leg level, left leg
    ● S86.109   Unspecified injury of other muscle(s) and tendon(s) of posterior muscle group at lower leg level, unspecified leg
  ● S86.11   Strain of other muscle(s) and tendon(s) of posterior muscle group at lower leg level
    ● S86.111   Strain of other muscle(s) and tendon(s) of posterior muscle group at lower leg level, right leg
    ● S86.112   Strain of other muscle(s) and tendon(s) of posterior muscle group at lower leg level, left leg
    ● S86.119   Strain of other muscle(s) and tendon(s) of posterior muscle group at lower leg level, unspecified leg

▶ New   ⇛ Revised   ~~deleted~~ Deleted   Excludes 1   Excludes 2   Includes   Use additional   Code first   Code also   Key words
OGCR Official Guidelines   X Assign placeholder X   ● Use Additional Character(s)   ▶ Manifestation Code   🆀 Hierarchical Condition Category   Coding Clinic

● S86.12 Laceration of other muscle(s) and tendon(s) of posterior muscle group at lower leg level

    ● S86.121 Laceration of other muscle(s) and tendon(s) of posterior muscle group at lower leg level, right leg

    ● S86.122 Laceration of other muscle(s) and tendon(s) of posterior muscle group at lower leg level, left leg

    ● S86.129 Laceration of other muscle(s) and tendon(s) of posterior muscle group at lower leg level, unspecified leg

● S86.19 Other injury of other muscle(s) and tendon(s) of posterior muscle group at lower leg level

    ● S86.191 Other injury of other muscle(s) and tendon(s) of posterior muscle group at lower leg level, right leg

    ● S86.192 Other injury of other muscle(s) and tendon(s) of posterior muscle group at lower leg level, left leg

    ● S86.199 Other injury of other muscle(s) and tendon(s) of posterior muscle group at lower leg level, unspecified leg

● S86.2 Injury of muscle(s) and tendon(s) of anterior muscle group at lower leg level

  ● S86.20 Unspecified injury of muscle(s) and tendon(s) of anterior muscle group at lower leg level

    ● S86.201 Unspecified injury of muscle(s) and tendon(s) of anterior muscle group at lower leg level, right leg

    ● S86.202 Unspecified injury of muscle(s) and tendon(s) of anterior muscle group at lower leg level, left leg

    ● S86.209 Unspecified injury of muscle(s) and tendon(s) of anterior muscle group at lower leg level, unspecified leg

  ● S86.21 Strain of muscle(s) and tendon(s) of anterior muscle group at lower leg level

    ● S86.211 Strain of muscle(s) and tendon(s) of anterior muscle group at lower leg level, right leg

    ● S86.212 Strain of muscle(s) and tendon(s) of anterior muscle group at lower leg level, left leg

    ● S86.219 Strain of muscle(s) and tendon(s) of anterior muscle group at lower leg level, unspecified leg

  ● S86.22 Laceration of muscle(s) and tendon(s) of anterior muscle group at lower leg level

    ● S86.221 Laceration of muscle(s) and tendon(s) of anterior muscle group at lower leg level, right leg

    ● S86.222 Laceration of muscle(s) and tendon(s) of anterior muscle group at lower leg level, left leg

    ● S86.229 Laceration of muscle(s) and tendon(s) of anterior muscle group at lower leg level, unspecified leg

  ● S86.29 Other injury of muscle(s) and tendon(s) of anterior muscle group at lower leg level

    ● S86.291 Other injury of muscle(s) and tendon(s) of anterior muscle group at lower leg level, right leg

    ● S86.292 Other injury of muscle(s) and tendon(s) of anterior muscle group at lower leg level, left leg

    ● S86.299 Other injury of muscle(s) and tendon(s) of anterior muscle group at lower leg level, unspecified leg

● S86.3 Injury of muscle(s) and tendon(s) of peroneal muscle group at lower leg level

  ● S86.30 Unspecified injury of muscle(s) and tendon(s) of peroneal muscle group at lower leg level

    ● S86.301 Unspecified injury of muscle(s) and tendon(s) of peroneal muscle group at lower leg level, right leg

    ● S86.302 Unspecified injury of muscle(s) and tendon(s) of peroneal muscle group at lower leg level, left leg

    ● S86.309 Unspecified injury of muscle(s) and tendon(s) of peroneal muscle group at lower leg level, unspecified leg

  ● S86.31 Strain of muscle(s) and tendon(s) of peroneal muscle group at lower leg level

    ● S86.311 Strain of muscle(s) and tendon(s) of peroneal muscle group at lower leg level, right leg

    ● S86.312 Strain of muscle(s) and tendon(s) of peroneal muscle group at lower leg level, left leg

    ● S86.319 Strain of muscle(s) and tendon(s) of peroneal muscle group at lower leg level, unspecified leg

  ● S86.32 Laceration of muscle(s) and tendon(s) of peroneal muscle group at lower leg level

    ● S86.321 Laceration of muscle(s) and tendon(s) of peroneal muscle group at lower leg level, right leg

    ● S86.322 Laceration of muscle(s) and tendon(s) of peroneal muscle group at lower leg level, left leg

    ● S86.329 Laceration of muscle(s) and tendon(s) of peroneal muscle group at lower leg level, unspecified leg

  ● S86.39 Other injury of muscle(s) and tendon(s) of peroneal muscle group at lower leg level

    ● S86.391 Other injury of muscle(s) and tendon(s) of peroneal muscle group at lower leg level, right leg

    ● S86.392 Other injury of muscle(s) and tendon(s) of peroneal muscle group at lower leg level, left leg

    ● S86.399 Other injury of muscle(s) and tendon(s) of peroneal muscle group at lower leg level, unspecified leg

● S86.8 Injury of other muscles and tendons at lower leg level

  ● S86.80 Unspecified injury of other muscles and tendons at lower leg level

    ● S86.801 Unspecified injury of other muscle(s) and tendon(s) at lower leg level, right leg

    ● S86.802 Unspecified injury of other muscle(s) and tendon(s) at lower leg level, left leg

    ● S86.809 Unspecified injury of other muscle(s) and tendon(s) at lower leg level, unspecified leg

  ● S86.81 Strain of other muscles and tendons at lower leg level

    ● S86.811 Strain of other muscle(s) and tendon(s) at lower leg level, right leg

    ● S86.812 Strain of other muscle(s) and tendon(s) at lower leg level, left leg

    ● S86.819 Strain of other muscle(s) and tendon(s) at lower leg level, unspecified leg

CHAPTER 19 (S00–T88)

● S86.82   Laceration of other muscles and tendons at lower leg level

    ● S86.821   Laceration of other muscle(s) and tendon(s) at lower leg level, right leg

    ● S86.822   Laceration of other muscle(s) and tendon(s) at lower leg level, left leg

    ● S86.829   Laceration of other muscle(s) and tendon(s) at lower leg level, unspecified leg

 ● S86.89   Other injury of other muscles and tendons at lower leg level

    ● S86.891   Other injury of other muscle(s) and tendon(s) at lower leg level, right leg

    ● S86.892   Other injury of other muscle(s) and tendon(s) at lower leg level, left leg

    ● S86.899   Other injury of other muscle(s) and tendon(s) at lower leg level, unspecified leg

● S86.9   Injury of unspecified muscle and tendon at lower leg level

 ● S86.90   Unspecified injury of unspecified muscle and tendon at lower leg level

    ● S86.901   Unspecified injury of unspecified muscle(s) and tendon(s) at lower leg level, right leg

    ● S86.902   Unspecified injury of unspecified muscle(s) and tendon(s) at lower leg level, left leg

    ● S86.909   Unspecified injury of unspecified muscle(s) and tendon(s) at lower leg level, unspecified leg

 ● S86.91   Strain of unspecified muscle and tendon at lower leg level

    ● S86.911   Strain of unspecified muscle(s) and tendon(s) at lower leg level, right leg

    ● S86.912   Strain of unspecified muscle(s) and tendon(s) at lower leg level, left leg

    ● S86.919   Strain of unspecified muscle(s) and tendon(s) at lower leg level, unspecified leg

 ● S86.92   Laceration of unspecified muscle and tendon at lower leg level

    ● S86.921   Laceration of unspecified muscle(s) and tendon(s) at lower leg level, right leg

    ● S86.922   Laceration of unspecified muscle(s) and tendon(s) at lower leg level, left leg

    ● S86.929   Laceration of unspecified muscle(s) and tendon(s) at lower leg level, unspecified leg

 ● S86.99   Other injury of unspecified muscle and tendon at lower leg level

    ● S86.991   Other injury of unspecified muscle(s) and tendon(s) at lower leg level, right leg

    ● S86.992   Other injury of unspecified muscle(s) and tendon(s) at lower leg level, left leg

    ● S86.999   Other injury of unspecified muscle(s) and tendon(s) at lower leg level, unspecified leg

● S87   Crushing injury of lower leg

    Use additional code(s) for all associated injuries

    Excludes2   crushing injury of ankle and foot (S97.-)

    The appropriate 7th character is to be added to each code from category S87

      | | |
      A   initial encounter
      D   subsequent encounter
      S   sequela

● S87.0   Crushing injury of knee

   X ● S87.00   Crushing injury of unspecified knee

   X ● S87.01   Crushing injury of right knee

   X ● S87.02   Crushing injury of left knee

● S87.8   Crushing injury of lower leg

   X ● S87.80   Crushing injury of unspecified lower leg

   X ● S87.81   Crushing injury of right lower leg

   X ● S87.82   Crushing injury of left lower leg

● S88   Traumatic amputation of lower leg

    An amputation not identified as partial or complete should be coded to complete

    Excludes1   traumatic amputation of ankle and foot (S98.-)

    The appropriate 7th character is to be added to each code from category S88

      A   initial encounter
      D   subsequent encounter
      S   sequela

● S88.0   Traumatic amputation at knee level

 ● S88.01   Complete traumatic amputation at knee level

    ● S88.011   Complete traumatic amputation at knee level, right lower leg A, D, S 🐖

    ● S88.012   Complete traumatic amputation at knee level, left lower leg A, D, S 🐖

    ● S88.019   Complete traumatic amputation at knee level, unspecified lower leg A, D, S 🐖

 ● S88.02   Partial traumatic amputation at knee level

    ● S88.021   Partial traumatic amputation at knee level, right lower leg A, D, S 🐖

    ● S88.022   Partial traumatic amputation at knee level, left lower leg A, D, S 🐖

    ● S88.029   Partial traumatic amputation at knee level, unspecified lower leg A, D, S 🐖

● S88.1   Traumatic amputation at level between knee and ankle

 ● S88.11   Complete traumatic amputation at level between knee and ankle

    ● S88.111   Complete traumatic amputation at level between knee and ankle, right lower leg A, D, S 🐖

    ● S88.112   Complete traumatic amputation at level between knee and ankle, left lower leg A, D, S 🐖

    ● S88.119   Complete traumatic amputation at level between knee and ankle, unspecified lower leg A, D, S 🐖

 ● S88.12   Partial traumatic amputation at level between knee and ankle

    ● S88.121   Partial traumatic amputation at level between knee and ankle, right lower leg A, D, S 🐖

    ● S88.122   Partial traumatic amputation at level between knee and ankle, left lower leg A, D, S 🐖

    ● S88.129   Partial traumatic amputation at level between knee and ankle, unspecified lower leg A, D, S 🐖

● S88.9   Traumatic amputation of lower leg, level unspecified

 ● S88.91   Complete traumatic amputation of lower leg, level unspecified

    ● S88.911   Complete traumatic amputation of right lower leg, level unspecified A, D, S 🐖

    ● S88.912   Complete traumatic amputation of left lower leg, level unspecified A, D, S 🐖

    ● S88.919   Complete traumatic amputation of unspecified lower leg, level unspecified A, D, S 🐖

▶ New   ⇒ Revised   ~~deleted~~ Deleted   Excludes 1   Excludes 2   Includes   Use additional   Code first   Code also   Key words

OGCR Official Guidelines   X Assign placeholder X   ● Use Additional Character(s)   ▌ Manifestation Code   🐖 Hierarchical Condition Category   **Coding Clinic**

● S88.92   Partial traumatic amputation of lower leg, level unspecified

   ● S88.921   Partial traumatic amputation of right lower leg, level unspecified A, D, S 🔖

   ● S88.922   Partial traumatic amputation of left lower leg, level unspecified A, D, S 🔖

   ● S88.929   Partial traumatic amputation of unspecified lower leg, level unspecified A, D, S 🔖

● S89   Other and unspecified injuries of lower leg

   Note: A fracture not indicated as open or closed should be coded to closed

   Excludes2   other and unspecified injuries of ankle and foot (S99.-)

   The appropriate 7th character is to be added to each code from subcategories S89.0, S89.1, S89.2, and S89.3

A	initial encounter for closed fracture
D	subsequent encounter for fracture with routine healing
G	subsequent encounter for fracture with delayed healing
K	subsequent encounter for fracture with nonunion
P	subsequent encounter for fracture with malunion
S	sequela

● S89.0   Physeal fracture of upper end of tibia

  ● S89.00   Unspecified physeal fracture of upper end of tibia

   ● S89.001   Unspecified physeal fracture of upper end of right tibia

   ● S89.002   Unspecified physeal fracture of upper end of left tibia

   ● S89.009   Unspecified physeal fracture of upper end of unspecified tibia

  ● S89.01   Salter-Harris Type I physeal fracture of upper end of tibia

   ● S89.011   Salter-Harris Type I physeal fracture of upper end of right tibia

   ● S89.012   Salter-Harris Type I physeal fracture of upper end of left tibia

   ● S89.019   Salter-Harris Type I physeal fracture of upper end of unspecified tibia

  ● S89.02   Salter-Harris Type II physeal fracture of upper end of tibia

   ● S89.021   Salter-Harris Type II physeal fracture of upper end of right tibia

   ● S89.022   Salter-Harris Type II physeal fracture of upper end of left tibia

   ● S89.029   Salter-Harris Type II physeal fracture of upper end of unspecified tibia

  ● S89.03   Salter-Harris Type III physeal fracture of upper end of tibia

   ● S89.031   Salter-Harris Type III physeal fracture of upper end of right tibia

   ● S89.032   Salter-Harris Type III physeal fracture of upper end of left tibia

   ● S89.039   Salter-Harris Type III physeal fracture of upper end of unspecified tibia

  ● S89.04   Salter-Harris Type IV physeal fracture of upper end of tibia

   ● S89.041   Salter-Harris Type IV physeal fracture of upper end of right tibia

   ● S89.042   Salter-Harris Type IV physeal fracture of upper end of left tibia

   ● S89.049   Salter-Harris Type IV physeal fracture of upper end of unspecified tibia

  ● S89.09   Other physeal fracture of upper end of tibia

   ● S89.091   Other physeal fracture of upper end of right tibia

   ● S89.092   Other physeal fracture of upper end of left tibia

   ● S89.099   Other physeal fracture of upper end of unspecified tibia

● S89.1   Physeal fracture of lower end of tibia

  ● S89.10   Unspecified physeal fracture of lower end of tibia

   ● S89.101   Unspecified physeal fracture of lower end of right tibia

   ● S89.102   Unspecified physeal fracture of lower end of left tibia

   ● S89.109   Unspecified physeal fracture of lower end of unspecified tibia

  ● S89.11   Salter-Harris Type I physeal fracture of lower end of tibia

   ● S89.111   Salter-Harris Type I physeal fracture of lower end of right tibia

   ● S89.112   Salter-Harris Type I physeal fracture of lower end of left tibia

   ● S89.119   Salter-Harris Type I physeal fracture of lower end of unspecified tibia

  ● S89.12   Salter-Harris Type II physeal fracture of lower end of tibia

   ● S89.121   Salter-Harris Type II physeal fracture of lower end of right tibia

   ● S89.122   Salter-Harris Type II physeal fracture of lower end of left tibia

   ● S89.129   Salter-Harris Type II physeal fracture of lower end of unspecified tibia

  ● S89.13   Salter-Harris Type III physeal fracture of lower end of tibia

    Excludes1   fracture of medial malleolus (adult) (S82.5-)

   ● S89.131   Salter-Harris Type III physeal fracture of lower end of right tibia

   ● S89.132   Salter-Harris Type III physeal fracture of lower end of left tibia

   ● S89.139   Salter-Harris Type III physeal fracture of lower end of unspecified tibia

  ● S89.14   Salter-Harris Type IV physeal fracture of lower end of tibia

    Excludes1   fracture of medial malleolus (adult) (S82.5-)

   ● S89.141   Salter-Harris Type IV physeal fracture of lower end of right tibia

   ● S89.142   Salter-Harris Type IV physeal fracture of lower end of left tibia

   ● S89.149   Salter-Harris Type IV physeal fracture of lower end of unspecified tibia

  ● S89.19   Other physeal fracture of lower end of tibia

   ● S89.191   Other physeal fracture of lower end of right tibia

   ● S89.192   Other physeal fracture of lower end of left tibia

   ● S89.199   Other physeal fracture of lower end of unspecified tibia

● S89.2   Physeal fracture of upper end of fibula

  ● S89.20   Unspecified physeal fracture of upper end of fibula

   ● S89.201   Unspecified physeal fracture of upper end of right fibula

   ● S89.202   Unspecified physeal fracture of upper end of left fibula

   ● S89.209   Unspecified physeal fracture of upper end of unspecified fibula

  ● S89.21   Salter-Harris Type I physeal fracture of upper end of fibula

   ● S89.211   Salter-Harris Type I physeal fracture of upper end of right fibula

   ● S89.212   Salter-Harris Type I physeal fracture of upper end of left fibula

   ● S89.219   Salter-Harris Type I physeal fracture of upper end of unspecified fibula

CHAPTER 19 (S00-T88)

● **S89.22**   Salter-Harris Type II physeal fracture of upper end of fibula

  ● **S89.221**   Salter-Harris Type II physeal fracture of upper end of right fibula

  ● **S89.222**   Salter-Harris Type II physeal fracture of upper end of left fibula

  ● **S89.229**   Salter-Harris Type II physeal fracture of upper end of unspecified fibula

● **S89.29**   Other physeal fracture of upper end of fibula

  ● **S89.291**   Other physeal fracture of upper end of right fibula

  ● **S89.292**   Other physeal fracture of upper end of left fibula

  ● **S89.299**   Other physeal fracture of upper end of unspecified fibula

● **S89.3**   Physeal fracture of lower end of fibula

● **S89.30**   Unspecified physeal fracture of lower end of fibula

  ● **S89.301**   Unspecified physeal fracture of lower end of right fibula

  ● **S89.302**   Unspecified physeal fracture of lower end of left fibula

  ● **S89.309**   Unspecified physeal fracture of lower end of unspecified fibula

● **S89.31**   Salter-Harris Type I physeal fracture of lower end of fibula

  ● **S89.311**   Salter-Harris Type I physeal fracture of lower end of right fibula

  ● **S89.312**   Salter-Harris Type I physeal fracture of lower end of left fibula

  ● **S89.319**   Salter-Harris Type I physeal fracture of lower end of unspecified fibula

● **S89.32**   Salter-Harris Type II physeal fracture of lower end of fibula

  ● **S89.321**   Salter-Harris Type II physeal fracture of lower end of right fibula

  ● **S89.322**   Salter-Harris Type II physeal fracture of lower end of left fibula

  ● **S89.329**   Salter-Harris Type II physeal fracture of lower end of unspecified fibula

● **S89.39**   Other physeal fracture of lower end of fibula

  ● **S89.391**   Other physeal fracture of lower end of right fibula

  ● **S89.392**   Other physeal fracture of lower end of left fibula

  ● **S89.399**   Other physeal fracture of lower end of unspecified fibula

● **S89.8**   Other specified injuries of lower leg

The appropriate 7th character is to be added to each code in subcategory S89.8

A	initial encounter
D	subsequent encounter
S	sequela

X ● **S89.80**   Other specified injuries of unspecified lower leg

X ● **S89.81**   Other specified injuries of right lower leg

X ● **S89.82**   Other specified injuries of left lower leg

● **S89.9**   Unspecified injury of lower leg

The appropriate 7th character is to be added to each code in subcategory S89.9

A	initial encounter
D	subsequent encounter
S	sequela

X ● **S89.90**   Unspecified injury of unspecified lower leg

X ● **S89.91**   Unspecified injury of right lower leg

X ● **S89.92**   Unspecified injury of left lower leg

INJURIES TO THE ANKLE AND FOOT (S90-S99)

Excludes2   burns and corrosions (T20-T32)
fracture of ankle and malleolus (S82.-)
frostbite (T33-T34)
insect bite or sting, venomous (T63.4)

● **S90**   Superficial injury of ankle, foot and toes

The appropriate 7th character is to be added to each code from category S90

A	initial encounter
D	subsequent encounter
S	sequela

● **S90.0**   Contusion of ankle

X ● **S90.00**   Contusion of unspecified ankle

X ● **S90.01**   Contusion of right ankle

X ● **S90.02**   Contusion of left ankle

● **S90.1**   Contusion of toe without damage to nail

  ● **S90.11**   Contusion of great toe without damage to nail

    ● **S90.111**   Contusion of right great toe without damage to nail

    ● **S90.112**   Contusion of left great toe without damage to nail

    ● **S90.119**   Contusion of unspecified great toe without damage to nail

  ● **S90.12**   Contusion of lesser toe without damage to nail

    ● **S90.121**   Contusion of right lesser toe(s) without damage to nail

    ● **S90.122**   Contusion of left lesser toe(s) without damage to nail

    ● **S90.129**   Contusion of unspecified lesser toe(s) without damage to nail
       Contusion of toe NOS

● **S90.2**   Contusion of toe with damage to nail

  ● **S90.21**   Contusion of great toe with damage to nail

    ● **S90.211**   Contusion of right great toe with damage to nail

    ● **S90.212**   Contusion of left great toe with damage to nail

    ● **S90.219**   Contusion of unspecified great toe with damage to nail

  ● **S90.22**   Contusion of lesser toe with damage to nail

    ● **S90.221**   Contusion of right lesser toe(s) with damage to nail

    ● **S90.222**   Contusion of left lesser toe(s) with damage to nail

    ● **S90.229**   Contusion of unspecified lesser toe(s) with damage to nail

● **S90.3**   Contusion of foot

Excludes2   contusion of toes (S90.1-, S90.2-)

X ● **S90.30**   Contusion of unspecified foot
       Contusion of foot NOS

X ● **S90.31**   Contusion of right foot

X ● **S90.32**   Contusion of left foot

● **S90.4**   Other superficial injuries of toe

  ● **S90.41**   Abrasion of toe

    ● **S90.411**   Abrasion, right great toe

    ● **S90.412**   Abrasion, left great toe

    ● **S90.413**   Abrasion, unspecified great toe

    ● **S90.414**   Abrasion, right lesser toe(s)

    ● **S90.415**   Abrasion, left lesser toe(s)

    ● **S90.416**   Abrasion, unspecified lesser toe(s)

  ● **S90.42**   Blister (nonthermal) of toe

    ● **S90.421**   Blister (nonthermal), right great toe

    ● **S90.422**   Blister (nonthermal), left great toe

    ● **S90.423**   Blister (nonthermal), unspecified great toe

    ● **S90.424**   Blister (nonthermal), right lesser toe(s)

▶ New   ⇒ Revised   ~~deleted~~ Deleted   Excludes 1   Excludes 2   Includes   Use additional   Code first   Code also   Key words

OGCR Official Guidelines   X Assign placeholder X   ● Use Additional Character(s)   ▶ Manifestation Code   🔍 Hierarchical Condition Category   Coding Clinic

- S90.425   Blister (nonthermal), left lesser toe(s)
- S90.426   Blister (nonthermal), unspecified lesser toe(s)
- S90.44   **External constriction of toe**
  Hair tourniquet syndrome of toe
  - S90.441   External constriction, right great toe
  - S90.442   External constriction, left great toe
  - S90.443   External constriction, unspecified great toe
  - S90.444   External constriction, right lesser toe(s)
  - S90.445   External constriction, left lesser toe(s)
  - S90.446   External constriction, unspecified lesser toe(s)
- S90.45   **Superficial foreign body of toe**
  Splinter in the toe
  - S90.451   Superficial foreign body, right great toe
  - S90.452   Superficial foreign body, left great toe
  - S90.453   Superficial foreign body, unspecified great toe
  - S90.454   Superficial foreign body, right lesser toe(s)
  - S90.455   Superficial foreign body, left lesser toe(s)
  - S90.456   Superficial foreign body, unspecified lesser toe(s)
- S90.46   **Insect bite (nonvenomous) of toe**
  - S90.461   Insect bite (nonvenomous), right great toe
  - S90.462   Insect bite (nonvenomous), left great toe
  - S90.463   Insect bite (nonvenomous), unspecified great toe
  - S90.464   Insect bite (nonvenomous), right lesser toe(s)
  - S90.465   Insect bite (nonvenomous), left lesser toe(s)
  - S90.466   Insect bite (nonvenomous), unspecified lesser toe(s)
- S90.47   **Other superficial bite of toe**
  Excludes1   open bite of toe (S91.15-, S91.25-)
  - S90.471   Other superficial bite of right great toe
  - S90.472   Other superficial bite of left great toe
  - S90.473   Other superficial bite of unspecified great toe
  - S90.474   Other superficial bite of right lesser toe(s)
  - S90.475   Other superficial bite of left lesser toe(s)
  - S90.476   Other superficial bite of unspecified lesser toe(s)
- S90.5   **Other superficial injuries of ankle**
  - S90.51   **Abrasion of ankle**
    - S90.511   Abrasion, right ankle
    - S90.512   Abrasion, left ankle
    - S90.519   Abrasion, unspecified ankle
  - S90.52   **Blister (nonthermal) of ankle**
    - S90.521   Blister (nonthermal), right ankle
    - S90.522   Blister (nonthermal), left ankle
    - S90.529   Blister (nonthermal), unspecified ankle
  - S90.54   **External constriction of ankle**
    - S90.541   External constriction, right ankle
    - S90.542   External constriction, left ankle
    - S90.549   External constriction, unspecified ankle

- S90.55   **Superficial foreign body of ankle**
  Splinter in the ankle
  - S90.551   Superficial foreign body, right ankle
  - S90.552   Superficial foreign body, left ankle
  - S90.559   Superficial foreign body, unspecified ankle
- S90.56   **Insect bite (nonvenomous) of ankle**
  - S90.561   Insect bite (nonvenomous), right ankle
  - S90.562   Insect bite (nonvenomous), left ankle
  - S90.569   Insect bite (nonvenomous), unspecified ankle
- S90.57   **Other superficial bite of ankle**
  Excludes1   open bite of ankle (S91.05-)
  - S90.571   Other superficial bite of ankle, right ankle
  - S90.572   Other superficial bite of ankle, left ankle
  - S90.579   Other superficial bite of ankle, unspecified ankle
- S90.8   **Other superficial injuries of foot**
  - S90.81   **Abrasion of foot**
    - S90.811   Abrasion, right foot
    - S90.812   Abrasion, left foot
    - S90.819   Abrasion, unspecified foot
  - S90.82   **Blister (nonthermal) of foot**
    - S90.821   Blister (nonthermal), right foot
    - S90.822   Blister (nonthermal), left foot
    - S90.829   Blister (nonthermal), unspecified foot
  - S90.84   **External constriction of foot**
    - S90.841   External constriction, right foot
    - S90.842   External constriction, left foot
    - S90.849   External constriction, unspecified foot
  - S90.85   **Superficial foreign body of foot**
    Splinter in the foot
    - S90.851   Superficial foreign body, right foot
    - S90.852   Superficial foreign body, left foot
    - S90.859   Superficial foreign body, unspecified foot
  - S90.86   **Insect bite (nonvenomous) of foot**
    - S90.861   Insect bite (nonvenomous), right foot
    - S90.862   Insect bite (nonvenomous), left foot
    - S90.869   Insect bite (nonvenomous), unspecified foot
  - S90.87   **Other superficial bite of foot**
    Excludes1   open bite of foot (S91.35-)
    - S90.871   Other superficial bite of right foot
    - S90.872   Other superficial bite of left foot
    - S90.879   Other superficial bite of unspecified foot
- S90.9   **Unspecified superficial injury of ankle, foot and toe**
  - S90.91   **Unspecified superficial injury of ankle**
    - S90.911   Unspecified superficial injury of right ankle
    - S90.912   Unspecified superficial injury of left ankle
    - S90.919   Unspecified superficial injury of unspecified ankle
  - S90.92   **Unspecified superficial injury of foot**
    - S90.921   Unspecified superficial injury of right foot
    - S90.922   Unspecified superficial injury of left foot
    - S90.929   Unspecified superficial injury of unspecified foot

CHAPTER 19 (S00-T88)

S90.93   Unspecified superficial injury of toes

● S90.931   Unspecified superficial injury of right great toe

● S90.932   Unspecified superficial injury of left great toe

● S90.933   Unspecified superficial injury of unspecified great toe

● S90.934   Unspecified superficial injury of right lesser toe(s)

● S90.935   Unspecified superficial injury of left lesser toe(s)

● S90.936   Unspecified superficial injury of unspecified lesser toe(s)

● S91   Open wound of ankle, foot and toes

Code also any associated wound infection

Excludes1   open fracture of ankle, foot and toes (S92.-with 7th character B)

traumatic amputation of ankle and foot (S98.-)

The appropriate 7th character is to be added to each code from category S91

A	initial encounter
D	subsequent encounter
S	sequela

● S91.0   Open wound of ankle

● S91.00   Unspecified open wound of ankle

● S91.001   Unspecified open wound, right ankle

● S91.002   Unspecified open wound, left ankle

● S91.009   Unspecified open wound, unspecified ankle

● S91.01   Laceration without foreign body of ankle

● S91.011   Laceration without foreign body, right ankle

● S91.012   Laceration without foreign body, left ankle

Coding Clinic: 2021, Q1, P8

● S91.019   Laceration without foreign body, unspecified ankle

● S91.02   Laceration with foreign body of ankle

● S91.021   Laceration with foreign body, right ankle

● S91.022   Laceration with foreign body, left ankle

● S91.029   Laceration with foreign body, unspecified ankle

● S91.03   Puncture wound without foreign body of ankle

● S91.031   Puncture wound without foreign body, right ankle

● S91.032   Puncture wound without foreign body, left ankle

● S91.039   Puncture wound without foreign body, unspecified ankle

● S91.04   Puncture wound with foreign body of ankle

● S91.041   Puncture wound with foreign body, right ankle

● S91.042   Puncture wound with foreign body, left ankle

● S91.049   Puncture wound with foreign body, unspecified ankle

● S91.05   Open bite of ankle

Excludes1   superficial bite of ankle (S90.56-, S90.57-)

● S91.051   Open bite, right ankle

● S91.052   Open bite, left ankle

● S91.059   Open bite, unspecified ankle

● S91.1   Open wound of toe without damage to nail

● S91.10   Unspecified open wound of toe without damage to nail

● S91.101   Unspecified open wound of right great toe without damage to nail

● S91.102   Unspecified open wound of left great toe without damage to nail

● S91.103   Unspecified open wound of unspecified great toe without damage to nail

● S91.104   Unspecified open wound of right lesser toe(s) without damage to nail

● S91.105   Unspecified open wound of left lesser toe(s) without damage to nail

● S91.106   Unspecified open wound of unspecified lesser toe(s) without damage to nail

● S91.109   Unspecified open wound of unspecified toe(s) without damage to nail

● S91.11   Laceration without foreign body of toe without damage to nail

● S91.111   Laceration without foreign body of right great toe without damage to nail

● S91.112   Laceration without foreign body of left great toe without damage to nail

● S91.113   Laceration without foreign body of unspecified great toe without damage to nail

● S91.114   Laceration without foreign body of right lesser toe(s) without damage to nail

● S91.115   Laceration without foreign body of left lesser toe(s) without damage to nail

● S91.116   Laceration without foreign body of unspecified lesser toe(s) without damage to nail

● S91.119   Laceration without foreign body of unspecified toe without damage to nail

● S91.12   Laceration with foreign body of toe without damage to nail

● S91.121   Laceration with foreign body of right great toe without damage to nail

● S91.122   Laceration with foreign body of left great toe without damage to nail

● S91.123   Laceration with foreign body of unspecified great toe without damage to nail

● S91.124   Laceration with foreign body of right lesser toe(s) without damage to nail

● S91.125   Laceration with foreign body of left lesser toe(s) without damage to nail

● S91.126   Laceration with foreign body of unspecified lesser toe(s) without damage to nail

● S91.129   Laceration with foreign body of unspecified toe(s) without damage to nail

● S91.13   Puncture wound without foreign body of toe without damage to nail

● S91.131   Puncture wound without foreign body of right great toe without damage to nail

● S91.132   Puncture wound without foreign body of left great toe without damage to nail

● S91.133   Puncture wound without foreign body of unspecified great toe without damage to nail

▶ New   ⇨ Revised   ~~deleted~~ Deleted   Excludes 1   Excludes 2   Includes   Use additional   Code first   Code also   Key words

OGCR Official Guidelines   X Assign placeholder X   ● Use Additional Character(s)   ▶ Manifestation Code   ❀ Hierarchical Condition Category   Coding Clinic

● S91.134   Puncture wound without foreign body of right lesser toe(s) without damage to nail

● S91.135   Puncture wound without foreign body of left lesser toe(s) without damage to nail

● S91.136   Puncture wound without foreign body of unspecified lesser toe(s) without damage to nail

● S91.139   Puncture wound without foreign body of unspecified toe(s) without damage to nail

● S91.14   Puncture wound with foreign body of toe without damage to nail

● S91.141   Puncture wound with foreign body of right great toe without damage to nail

● S91.142   Puncture wound with foreign body of left great toe without damage to nail

● S91.143   Puncture wound with foreign body of unspecified great toe without damage to nail

● S91.144   Puncture wound with foreign body of right lesser toe(s) without damage to nail

● S91.145   Puncture wound with foreign body of left lesser toe(s) without damage to nail

● S91.146   Puncture wound with foreign body of unspecified lesser toe(s) without damage to nail

● S91.149   Puncture wound with foreign body of unspecified toe(s) without damage to nail

● S91.15   Open bite of toe without damage to nail
Bite of toe NOS

Excludes1   superficial bite of toe (S90.46-, S90.47-)

● S91.151   Open bite of right great toe without damage to nail

● S91.152   Open bite of left great toe without damage to nail

● S91.153   Open bite of unspecified great toe without damage to nail

● S91.154   Open bite of right lesser toe(s) without damage to nail

● S91.155   Open bite of left lesser toe(s) without damage to nail

● S91.156   Open bite of unspecified lesser toe(s) without damage to nail

● S91.159   Open bite of unspecified toe(s) without damage to nail

● S91.2   Open wound of toe with damage to nail

● S91.20   Unspecified open wound of toe with damage to nail

● S91.201   Unspecified open wound of right great toe with damage to nail

● S91.202   Unspecified open wound of left great toe with damage to nail

● S91.203   Unspecified open wound of unspecified great toe with damage to nail

● S91.204   Unspecified open wound of right lesser toe(s) with damage to nail

● S91.205   Unspecified open wound of left lesser toe(s) with damage to nail

● S91.206   Unspecified open wound of unspecified lesser toe(s) with damage to nail

● S91.209   Unspecified open wound of unspecified toe(s) with damage to nail

● S91.21   Laceration without foreign body of toe with damage to nail

● S91.211   Laceration without foreign body of right great toe with damage to nail

● S91.212   Laceration without foreign body of left great toe with damage to nail

● S91.213   Laceration without foreign body of unspecified great toe with damage to nail

● S91.214   Laceration without foreign body of right lesser toe(s) with damage to nail

● S91.215   Laceration without foreign body of left lesser toe(s) with damage to nail

● S91.216   Laceration without foreign body of unspecified lesser toe(s) with damage to nail

● S91.219   Laceration without foreign body of unspecified toe(s) with damage to nail

● S91.22   Laceration with foreign body of toe with damage to nail

● S91.221   Laceration with foreign body of right great toe with damage to nail

● S91.222   Laceration with foreign body of left great toe with damage to nail

● S91.223   Laceration with foreign body of unspecified great toe with damage to nail

● S91.224   Laceration with foreign body of right lesser toe(s) with damage to nail

● S91.225   Laceration with foreign body of left lesser toe(s) with damage to nail

● S91.226   Laceration with foreign body of unspecified lesser toe(s) with damage to nail

● S91.229   Laceration with foreign body of unspecified toe(s) with damage to nail

● S91.23   Puncture wound without foreign body of toe with damage to nail

● S91.231   Puncture wound without foreign body of right great toe with damage to nail

● S91.232   Puncture wound without foreign body of left great toe with damage to nail

● S91.233   Puncture wound without foreign body of unspecified great toe with damage to nail

● S91.234   Puncture wound without foreign body of right lesser toe(s) with damage to nail

● S91.235   Puncture wound without foreign body of left lesser toe(s) with damage to nail

● S91.236   Puncture wound without foreign body of unspecified lesser toe(s) with damage to nail

● S91.239   Puncture wound without foreign body of unspecified toe(s) with damage to nail

● S91.24   Puncture wound with foreign body of toe with damage to nail

● S91.241   Puncture wound with foreign body of right great toe with damage to nail

● S91.242   Puncture wound with foreign body of left great toe with damage to nail

● S91.243   Puncture wound with foreign body of unspecified great toe with damage to nail

● S91.244   Puncture wound with foreign body of right lesser toe(s) with damage to nail

- S91.245 Puncture wound with foreign body of left lesser toe(s) with damage to nail
- S91.246 Puncture wound with foreign body of unspecified lesser toe(s) with damage to nail
- S91.249 Puncture wound with foreign body of unspecified toe(s) with damage to nail
- S91.25 Open bite of toe with damage to nail
  Bite of toe with damage to nail NOS
  > **Excludes1** superficial bite of toe (S90.46-, S90.47-)
  - S91.251 Open bite of right great toe with damage to nail
  - S91.252 Open bite of left great toe with damage to nail
  - S91.253 Open bite of unspecified great toe with damage to nail
  - S91.254 Open bite of right lesser toe(s) with damage to nail
  - S91.255 Open bite of left lesser toe(s) with damage to nail
  - S91.256 Open bite of unspecified lesser toe(s) with damage to nail
  - S91.259 Open bite of unspecified toe(s) with damage to nail
- S91.3 Open wound of foot
  - S91.30 Unspecified open wound of foot
    - S91.301 Unspecified open wound, right foot
    - S91.302 Unspecified open wound, left foot
    - S91.309 Unspecified open wound, unspecified foot
  - S91.31 Laceration without foreign body of foot
    - S91.311 Laceration without foreign body, right foot
    - S91.312 Laceration without foreign body, left foot
    - S91.319 Laceration without foreign body, unspecified foot
  - S91.32 Laceration with foreign body of foot
    - S91.321 Laceration with foreign body, right foot
    - S91.322 Laceration with foreign body, left foot
    - S91.329 Laceration with foreign body, unspecified foot
  - S91.33 Puncture wound without foreign body of foot
    - S91.331 Puncture wound without foreign body, right foot
    - S91.332 Puncture wound without foreign body, left foot
    - S91.339 Puncture wound without foreign body, unspecified foot
  - S91.34 Puncture wound with foreign body of foot
    - S91.341 Puncture wound with foreign body, right foot
    - S91.342 Puncture wound with foreign body, left foot
    - S91.349 Puncture wound with foreign body, unspecified foot
  - S91.35 Open bite of foot
    > **Excludes1** superficial bite of foot (S90.86-, S90.87-)
    - S91.351 Open bite, right foot
    - S91.352 Open bite, left foot
    - S91.359 Open bite, unspecified foot

- S92 Fracture of foot and toe, except ankle
  Note: A fracture not indicated as displaced or nondisplaced should be coded to displaced
  A fracture not indicated as open or closed should be coded to closed
  > **Excludes2** fracture of ankle (S82.-)
  > fracture of malleolus (S82.-)
  > traumatic amputation of ankle and foot (S98.-)

  The appropriate 7th character is to be added to each code from category S92

A	initial encounter for closed fracture
B	initial encounter for open fracture
D	subsequent encounter for fracture with routine healing
G	subsequent encounter for fracture with delayed healing
K	subsequent encounter for fracture with nonunion
P	subsequent encounter for fracture with malunion
S	sequela

  - S92.0 Fracture of calcaneus
    Heel bone   Os calcis
    > **Excludes2** Physeal fracture of calcaneus (S99.0-)
    - S92.00 Unspecified fracture of calcaneus
      - S92.001 Unspecified fracture of right calcaneus
      - S92.002 Unspecified fracture of left calcaneus
      - S92.009 Unspecified fracture of unspecified calcaneus
    - S92.01 Fracture of body of calcaneus
      - S92.011 Displaced fracture of body of right calcaneus
      - S92.012 Displaced fracture of body of left calcaneus
      - S92.013 Displaced fracture of body of unspecified calcaneus
      - S92.014 Nondisplaced fracture of body of right calcaneus
      - S92.015 Nondisplaced fracture of body of left calcaneus
      - S92.016 Nondisplaced fracture of body of unspecified calcaneus
    - S92.02 Fracture of anterior process of calcaneus
      - S92.021 Displaced fracture of anterior process of right calcaneus
      - S92.022 Displaced fracture of anterior process of left calcaneus
      - S92.023 Displaced fracture of anterior process of unspecified calcaneus
      - S92.024 Nondisplaced fracture of anterior process of right calcaneus
      - S92.025 Nondisplaced fracture of anterior process of left calcaneus
      - S92.026 Nondisplaced fracture of anterior process of unspecified calcaneus
    - S92.03 Avulsion fracture of tuberosity of calcaneus
      - S92.031 Displaced avulsion fracture of tuberosity of right calcaneus
      - S92.032 Displaced avulsion fracture of tuberosity of left calcaneus
      - S92.033 Displaced avulsion fracture of tuberosity of unspecified calcaneus
      - S92.034 Nondisplaced avulsion fracture of tuberosity of right calcaneus
      - S92.035 Nondisplaced avulsion fracture of tuberosity of left calcaneus
      - S92.036 Nondisplaced avulsion fracture of tuberosity of unspecified calcaneus

- ● S92.04   Other fracture of tuberosity of calcaneus
  - ● S92.041   Displaced other fracture of tuberosity of right calcaneus
  - ● S92.042   Displaced other fracture of tuberosity of left calcaneus
  - ● S92.043   Displaced other fracture of tuberosity of unspecified calcaneus
  - ● S92.044   Nondisplaced other fracture of tuberosity of right calcaneus
  - ● S92.045   Nondisplaced other fracture of tuberosity of left calcaneus
  - ● S92.046   Nondisplaced other fracture of tuberosity of unspecified calcaneus
- ● S92.05   Other extraarticular fracture of calcaneus
  - ● S92.051   Displaced other extraarticular fracture of right calcaneus
  - ● S92.052   Displaced other extraarticular fracture of left calcaneus
  - ● S92.053   Displaced other extraarticular fracture of unspecified calcaneus
  - ● S92.054   Nondisplaced other extraarticular fracture of right calcaneus
  - ● S92.055   Nondisplaced other extraarticular fracture of left calcaneus
  - ● S92.056   Nondisplaced other extraarticular fracture of unspecified calcaneus
- ● S92.06   Intraarticular fracture of calcaneus
  - ● S92.061   Displaced intraarticular fracture of right calcaneus
  - ● S92.062   Displaced intraarticular fracture of left calcaneus
  - ● S92.063   Displaced intraarticular fracture of unspecified calcaneus
  - ● S92.064   Nondisplaced intraarticular fracture of right calcaneus
  - ● S92.065   Nondisplaced intraarticular fracture of left calcaneus
  - ● S92.066   Nondisplaced intraarticular fracture of unspecified calcaneus
- ● S92.1   Fracture of talus
  - Astragalus
  - ● S92.10   Unspecified fracture of talus
    - ● S92.101   Unspecified fracture of right talus
    - ● S92.102   Unspecified fracture of left talus
    - ● S92.109   Unspecified fracture of unspecified talus
  - ● S92.11   Fracture of neck of talus
    - ● S92.111   Displaced fracture of neck of right talus
    - ● S92.112   Displaced fracture of neck of left talus
    - ● S92.113   Displaced fracture of neck of unspecified talus
    - ● S92.114   Nondisplaced fracture of neck of right talus
    - ● S92.115   Nondisplaced fracture of neck of left talus
    - ● S92.116   Nondisplaced fracture of neck of unspecified talus
  - ● S92.12   Fracture of body of talus
    - ● S92.121   Displaced fracture of body of right talus
    - ● S92.122   Displaced fracture of body of left talus
    - ● S92.123   Displaced fracture of body of unspecified talus
    - ● S92.124   Nondisplaced fracture of body of right talus

- ● S92.125   Nondisplaced fracture of body of left talus
- ● S92.126   Nondisplaced fracture of body of unspecified talus
- ● S92.13   Fracture of posterior process of talus
  - ● S92.131   Displaced fracture of posterior process of right talus
  - ● S92.132   Displaced fracture of posterior process of left talus
  - ● S92.133   Displaced fracture of posterior process of unspecified talus
  - ● S92.134   Nondisplaced fracture of posterior process of right talus
  - ● S92.135   Nondisplaced fracture of posterior process of left talus
  - ● S92.136   Nondisplaced fracture of posterior process of unspecified talus
- ● S92.14   Dome fracture of talus
  - **Excludes1**   osteochondritis dissecans (M93.2)
  - ● S92.141   Displaced dome fracture of right talus
  - ● S92.142   Displaced dome fracture of left talus
  - ● S92.143   Displaced dome fracture of unspecified talus
  - ● S92.144   Nondisplaced dome fracture of right talus
  - ● S92.145   Nondisplaced dome fracture of left talus
  - ● S92.146   Nondisplaced dome fracture of unspecified talus
- ● S92.15   Avulsion fracture (chip fracture) of talus
  - ● S92.151   Displaced avulsion fracture (chip fracture) of right talus
  - ● S92.152   Displaced avulsion fracture (chip fracture) of left talus
  - ● S92.153   Displaced avulsion fracture (chip fracture) of unspecified talus
  - ● S92.154   Nondisplaced avulsion fracture (chip fracture) of right talus
  - ● S92.155   Nondisplaced avulsion fracture (chip fracture) of left talus
  - ● S92.156   Nondisplaced avulsion fracture (chip fracture) of unspecified talus
- ● S92.19   Other fracture of talus
  - ● S92.191   Other fracture of right talus
  - ● S92.192   Other fracture of left talus
  - ● S92.199   Other fracture of unspecified talus
- ● S92.2   Fracture of other and unspecified tarsal bone(s)
  - ● S92.20   Fracture of unspecified tarsal bone(s)
    - ● S92.201   Fracture of unspecified tarsal bone(s) of right foot
    - ● S92.202   Fracture of unspecified tarsal bone(s) of left foot
    - ● S92.209   Fracture of unspecified tarsal bone(s) of unspecified foot
  - ● S92.21   Fracture of cuboid bone
    - ● S92.211   Displaced fracture of cuboid bone of right foot
    - ● S92.212   Displaced fracture of cuboid bone of left foot
    - ● S92.213   Displaced fracture of cuboid bone of unspecified foot
    - ● S92.214   Nondisplaced fracture of cuboid bone of right foot
    - ● S92.215   Nondisplaced fracture of cuboid bone of left foot
    - ● S92.216   Nondisplaced fracture of cuboid bone of unspecified foot

CHAPTER 19 (S00-T88)

● **S92.22** Fracture of lateral cuneiform
- ● **S92.221** Displaced fracture of lateral cuneiform of right foot
- ● **S92.222** Displaced fracture of lateral cuneiform of left foot
- ● **S92.223** Displaced fracture of lateral cuneiform of unspecified foot
- ● **S92.224** Nondisplaced fracture of lateral cuneiform of right foot
- ● **S92.225** Nondisplaced fracture of lateral cuneiform of left foot
- ● **S92.226** Nondisplaced fracture of lateral cuneiform of unspecified foot

● **S92.23** Fracture of intermediate cuneiform
- ● **S92.231** Displaced fracture of intermediate cuneiform of right foot
- ● **S92.232** Displaced fracture of intermediate cuneiform of left foot
- ● **S92.233** Displaced fracture of intermediate cuneiform of unspecified foot
- ● **S92.234** Nondisplaced fracture of intermediate cuneiform of right foot
- ● **S92.235** Nondisplaced fracture of intermediate cuneiform of left foot
- ● **S92.236** Nondisplaced fracture of intermediate cuneiform of unspecified foot

● **S92.24** Fracture of medial cuneiform
- ● **S92.241** Displaced fracture of medial cuneiform of right foot
- ● **S92.242** Displaced fracture of medial cuneiform of left foot
- ● **S92.243** Displaced fracture of medial cuneiform of unspecified foot
- ● **S92.244** Nondisplaced fracture of medial cuneiform of right foot
- ● **S92.245** Nondisplaced fracture of medial cuneiform of left foot
- ● **S92.246** Nondisplaced fracture of medial cuneiform of unspecified foot

● **S92.25** Fracture of navicular [scaphoid] of foot
- ● **S92.251** Displaced fracture of navicular [scaphoid] of right foot
- ● **S92.252** Displaced fracture of navicular [scaphoid] of left foot
- ● **S92.253** Displaced fracture of navicular [scaphoid] of unspecified foot
- ● **S92.254** Nondisplaced fracture of navicular [scaphoid] of right foot
- ● **S92.255** Nondisplaced fracture of navicular [scaphoid] of left foot
- ● **S92.256** Nondisplaced fracture of navicular [scaphoid] of unspecified foot

● **S92.3** Fracture of metatarsal bone(s)
> **Excludes2**   Physeal fracture of metatarsal (S99.1-)

● **S92.30** Fracture of unspecified metatarsal bone(s)
- ● **S92.301** Fracture of unspecified metatarsal bone(s), right foot
- ● **S92.302** Fracture of unspecified metatarsal bone(s), left foot
- ● **S92.309** Fracture of unspecified metatarsal bone(s), unspecified foot

● **S92.31** Fracture of first metatarsal bone
- ● **S92.311** Displaced fracture of first metatarsal bone, right foot
- ● **S92.312** Displaced fracture of first metatarsal bone, left foot
- ● **S92.313** Displaced fracture of first metatarsal bone, unspecified foot
- ● **S92.314** Nondisplaced fracture of first metatarsal bone, right foot

- ● **S92.315** Nondisplaced fracture of first metatarsal bone, left foot
- ● **S92.316** Nondisplaced fracture of first metatarsal bone, unspecified foot

● **S92.32** Fracture of second metatarsal bone
- ● **S92.321** Displaced fracture of second metatarsal bone, right foot
- ● **S92.322** Displaced fracture of second metatarsal bone, left foot
- ● **S92.323** Displaced fracture of second metatarsal bone, unspecified foot
- ● **S92.324** Nondisplaced fracture of second metatarsal bone, right foot
- ● **S92.325** Nondisplaced fracture of second metatarsal bone, left foot
- ● **S92.326** Nondisplaced fracture of second metatarsal bone, unspecified foot

● **S92.33** Fracture of third metatarsal bone
Coding Clinic: 2018, Q1, P3
- ● **S92.331** Displaced fracture of third metatarsal bone, right foot
- ● **S92.332** Displaced fracture of third metatarsal bone, left foot
- ● **S92.333** Displaced fracture of third metatarsal bone, unspecified foot
- ● **S92.334** Nondisplaced fracture of third metatarsal bone, right foot
- ● **S92.335** Nondisplaced fracture of third metatarsal bone, left foot
- ● **S92.336** Nondisplaced fracture of third metatarsal bone, unspecified foot

● **S92.34** Fracture of fourth metatarsal bone
- ● **S92.341** Displaced fracture of fourth metatarsal bone, right foot
- ● **S92.342** Displaced fracture of fourth metatarsal bone, left foot
- ● **S92.343** Displaced fracture of fourth metatarsal bone, unspecified foot
- ● **S92.344** Nondisplaced fracture of fourth metatarsal bone, right foot
- ● **S92.345** Nondisplaced fracture of fourth metatarsal bone, left foot
- ● **S92.346** Nondisplaced fracture of fourth metatarsal bone, unspecified foot

● **S92.35** Fracture of fifth metatarsal bone
- ● **S92.351** Displaced fracture of fifth metatarsal bone, right foot
- ● **S92.352** Displaced fracture of fifth metatarsal bone, left foot
- ● **S92.353** Displaced fracture of fifth metatarsal bone, unspecified foot
- ● **S92.354** Nondisplaced fracture of fifth metatarsal bone, right foot
- ● **S92.355** Nondisplaced fracture of fifth metatarsal bone, left foot
- ● **S92.356** Nondisplaced fracture of fifth metatarsal bone, unspecified foot

● **S92.4** Fracture of great toe
> **Excludes2**   Physeal fracture of phalanx of toe (S99.2-)

● **S92.40** Unspecified fracture of great toe
- ● **S92.401** Displaced unspecified fracture of right great toe
- ● **S92.402** Displaced unspecified fracture of left great toe
- ● **S92.403** Displaced unspecified fracture of unspecified great toe
- ● **S92.404** Nondisplaced unspecified fracture of right great toe

▶ New   ⇒ Revised   ~~deleted~~ Deleted   Excludes 1   Excludes 2   Includes   Use additional   Code first   Code also   Key words
OGCR Official Guidelines   X Assign placeholder X   ● Use Additional Character(s)   ▷ Manifestation Code   ⚘ Hierarchical Condition Category   **Coding Clinic**

● S92.405   Nondisplaced unspecified fracture of left great toe

● S92.406   Nondisplaced unspecified fracture of unspecified great toe

● S92.41   Fracture of proximal phalanx of great toe

● S92.411   Displaced fracture of proximal phalanx of right great toe

● S92.412   Displaced fracture of proximal phalanx of left great toe

● S92.413   Displaced fracture of proximal phalanx of unspecified great toe

● S92.414   Nondisplaced fracture of proximal phalanx of right great toe

● S92.415   Nondisplaced fracture of proximal phalanx of left great toe

● S92.416   Nondisplaced fracture of proximal phalanx of unspecified great toe

● S92.42   Fracture of distal phalanx of great toe

● S92.421   Displaced fracture of distal phalanx of right great toe

● S92.422   Displaced fracture of distal phalanx of left great toe

● S92.423   Displaced fracture of distal phalanx of unspecified great toe

● S92.424   Nondisplaced fracture of distal phalanx of right great toe

● S92.425   Nondisplaced fracture of distal phalanx of left great toe

● S92.426   Nondisplaced fracture of distal phalanx of unspecified great toe

● S92.49   Other fracture of great toe

● S92.491   Other fracture of right great toe

● S92.492   Other fracture of left great toe

● S92.499   Other fracture of unspecified great toe

● S92.5   Fracture of lesser toe(s)

    Excludes2   Physeal fracture of phalanx of toe (S99.2-)

● S92.50   Unspecified fracture of lesser toe(s)

● S92.501   Displaced unspecified fracture of right lesser toe(s)

● S92.502   Displaced unspecified fracture of left lesser toe(s)

● S92.503   Displaced unspecified fracture of unspecified lesser toe(s)

● S92.504   Nondisplaced unspecified fracture of right lesser toe(s)

● S92.505   Nondisplaced unspecified fracture of left lesser toe(s)

● S92.506   Nondisplaced unspecified fracture of unspecified lesser toe(s)

● S92.51   Fracture of proximal phalanx of lesser toe(s)

● S92.511   Displaced fracture of proximal phalanx of right lesser toe(s)

● S92.512   Displaced fracture of proximal phalanx of left lesser toe(s)

● S92.513   Displaced fracture of proximal phalanx of unspecified lesser toe(s)

● S92.514   Nondisplaced fracture of proximal phalanx of right lesser toe(s)

● S92.515   Nondisplaced fracture of proximal phalanx of left lesser toe(s)

● S92.516   Nondisplaced fracture of proximal phalanx of unspecified lesser toe(s)

● S92.52   Fracture of middle phalanx of lesser toe(s)

● S92.521   Displaced fracture of middle phalanx of right lesser toe(s)

● S92.522   Displaced fracture of middle phalanx of left lesser toe(s)

● S92.523   Displaced fracture of middle phalanx of unspecified lesser toe(s)

● S92.524   Nondisplaced fracture of middle phalanx of right lesser toe(s)

● S92.525   Nondisplaced fracture of middle phalanx of left lesser toe(s)

● S92.526   Nondisplaced fracture of middle phalanx of unspecified lesser toe(s)

● S92.53   Fracture of distal phalanx of lesser toe(s)

● S92.531   Displaced fracture of distal phalanx of right lesser toe(s)

● S92.532   Displaced fracture of distal phalanx of left lesser toe(s)

● S92.533   Displaced fracture of distal phalanx of unspecified lesser toe(s)

● S92.534   Nondisplaced fracture of distal phalanx of right lesser toe(s)

● S92.535   Nondisplaced fracture of distal phalanx of left lesser toe(s)

● S92.536   Nondisplaced fracture of distal phalanx of unspecified lesser toe(s)

● S92.59   Other fracture of lesser toe(s)

● S92.591   Other fracture of right lesser toe(s)

● S92.592   Other fracture of left lesser toe(s)

● S92.599   Other fracture of unspecified lesser toe(s)

● S92.8   Other fracture of foot, except ankle

● S92.81   Other fracture of foot

    Sesamoid fracture of foot

    Coding Clinic: 2016, Q4, P68

● S92.811   Other fracture of right foot

● S92.812   Other fracture of left foot

● S92.819   Other fracture of unspecified foot

● S92.9   Unspecified fracture of foot and toe

● S92.90   Unspecified fracture of foot

● S92.901   Unspecified fracture of right foot

● S92.902   Unspecified fracture of left foot

● S92.909   Unspecified fracture of unspecified foot

● S92.91   Unspecified fracture of toe

● S92.911   Unspecified fracture of right toe(s)

● S92.912   Unspecified fracture of left toe(s)

● S92.919   Unspecified fracture of unspecified toe(s)

● S93   Dislocation and sprain of joints and ligaments at ankle, foot and toe level

    Includes   avulsion of joint or ligament of ankle, foot and toe

    laceration of cartilage, joint or ligament of ankle, foot and toe

    sprain of cartilage, joint or ligament of ankle, foot and toe

    traumatic hemarthrosis of joint or ligament of ankle, foot and toe

    traumatic rupture of joint or ligament of ankle, foot and toe

    traumatic subluxation of joint or ligament of ankle, foot and toe

    traumatic tear of joint or ligament of ankle, foot and toe

    Code also any associated open wound

    Excludes2   strain of muscle and tendon of ankle and foot (S96.-)

    The appropriate 7th character is to be added to each code from category S93

    | A | initial encounter |
    | D | subsequent encounter |
    | S | sequela |

CHAPTER 19 (S00-T88)

● **S93.0**   **Subluxation and dislocation of ankle joint**
     Subluxation and dislocation of astragalus
     Subluxation and dislocation of fibula, lower end
     Subluxation and dislocation of talus
     Subluxation and dislocation of tibia, lower end
   X● **S93.01**   Subluxation of right ankle joint
   X● **S93.02**   Subluxation of left ankle joint
   X● **S93.03**   Subluxation of unspecified ankle joint
   X● **S93.04**   Dislocation of right ankle joint
   X● **S93.05**   Dislocation of left ankle joint
   X● **S93.06**   Dislocation of unspecified ankle joint

● **S93.1**   **Subluxation and dislocation of toe**
   ● **S93.10**   Unspecified subluxation and dislocation of toe
      Dislocation of toe NOS
      Subluxation of toe NOS
     ● **S93.101**   Unspecified subluxation of right toe(s)
     ● **S93.102**   Unspecified subluxation of left toe(s)
     ● **S93.103**   Unspecified subluxation of unspecified toe(s)
     ● **S93.104**   Unspecified dislocation of right toe(s)
     ● **S93.105**   Unspecified dislocation of left toe(s)
     ● **S93.106**   Unspecified dislocation of unspecified toe(s)
   ● **S93.11**   Dislocation of interphalangeal joint
     ● **S93.111**   Dislocation of interphalangeal joint of right great toe
     ● **S93.112**   Dislocation of interphalangeal joint of left great toe
     ● **S93.113**   Dislocation of interphalangeal joint of unspecified great toe
     ● **S93.114**   Dislocation of interphalangeal joint of right lesser toe(s)
     ● **S93.115**   Dislocation of interphalangeal joint of left lesser toe(s)
     ● **S93.116**   Dislocation of interphalangeal joint of unspecified lesser toe(s)
     ● **S93.119**   Dislocation of interphalangeal joint of unspecified toe(s)
   ● **S93.12**   Dislocation of metatarsophalangeal joint
     ● **S93.121**   Dislocation of metatarsophalangeal joint of right great toe
     ● **S93.122**   Dislocation of metatarsophalangeal joint of left great toe
     ● **S93.123**   Dislocation of metatarsophalangeal joint of unspecified great toe
     ● **S93.124**   Dislocation of metatarsophalangeal joint of right lesser toe(s)
     ● **S93.125**   Dislocation of metatarsophalangeal joint of left lesser toe(s)
     ● **S93.126**   Dislocation of metatarsophalangeal joint of unspecified lesser toe(s)
     ● **S93.129**   Dislocation of metatarsophalangeal joint of unspecified toe(s)
   ● **S93.13**   Subluxation of interphalangeal joint
     ● **S93.131**   Subluxation of interphalangeal joint of right great toe
     ● **S93.132**   Subluxation of interphalangeal joint of left great toe
     ● **S93.133**   Subluxation of interphalangeal joint of unspecified great toe
     ● **S93.134**   Subluxation of interphalangeal joint of right lesser toe(s)
     ● **S93.135**   Subluxation of interphalangeal joint of left lesser toe(s)

     ● **S93.136**   Subluxation of interphalangeal joint of unspecified lesser toe(s)
     ● **S93.139**   Subluxation of interphalangeal joint of unspecified toe(s)
   ● **S93.14**   Subluxation of metatarsophalangeal joint
     ● **S93.141**   Subluxation of metatarsophalangeal joint of right great toe
     ● **S93.142**   Subluxation of metatarsophalangeal joint of left great toe
     ● **S93.143**   Subluxation of metatarsophalangeal joint of unspecified great toe
     ● **S93.144**   Subluxation of metatarsophalangeal joint of right lesser toe(s)
     ● **S93.145**   Subluxation of metatarsophalangeal joint of left lesser toe(s)
     ● **S93.146**   Subluxation of metatarsophalangeal joint of unspecified lesser toe(s)
     ● **S93.149**   Subluxation of metatarsophalangeal joint of unspecified toe(s)

● **S93.3**   **Subluxation and dislocation of foot**
   Excludes2   dislocation of toe (S93.1-)
   ● **S93.30**   Unspecified subluxation and dislocation of foot
      Dislocation of foot NOS
      Subluxation of foot NOS
     ● **S93.301**   Unspecified subluxation of right foot
     ● **S93.302**   Unspecified subluxation of left foot
     ● **S93.303**   Unspecified subluxation of unspecified foot
     ● **S93.304**   Unspecified dislocation of right foot
     ● **S93.305**   Unspecified dislocation of left foot
     ● **S93.306**   Unspecified dislocation of unspecified foot
   ● **S93.31**   Subluxation and dislocation of tarsal joint
     ● **S93.311**   Subluxation of tarsal joint of right foot
     ● **S93.312**   Subluxation of tarsal joint of left foot
     ● **S93.313**   Subluxation of tarsal joint of unspecified foot
     ● **S93.314**   Dislocation of tarsal joint of right foot
     ● **S93.315**   Dislocation of tarsal joint of left foot
     ● **S93.316**   Dislocation of tarsal joint of unspecified foot
   ● **S93.32**   Subluxation and dislocation of tarsometatarsal joint
     ● **S93.321**   Subluxation of tarsometatarsal joint of right foot
     ● **S93.322**   Subluxation of tarsometatarsal joint of left foot
     ● **S93.323**   Subluxation of tarsometatarsal joint of unspecified foot
     ● **S93.324**   Dislocation of tarsometatarsal joint of right foot
     ● **S93.325**   Dislocation of tarsometatarsal joint of left foot
     ● **S93.326**   Dislocation of tarsometatarsal joint of unspecified foot
   ● **S93.33**   Other subluxation and dislocation of foot
     ● **S93.331**   Other subluxation of right foot
     ● **S93.332**   Other subluxation of left foot
     ● **S93.333**   Other subluxation of unspecified foot
     ● **S93.334**   Other dislocation of right foot
     ● **S93.335**   Other dislocation of left foot
     ● **S93.336**   Other dislocation of unspecified foot

CHAPTER 19 (S00-T88)

▶ New   ⟹ Revised   ~~deleted~~ Deleted   Excludes 1   Excludes 2   Includes   Use additional   Code first   Code also   Key words
OGCR Official Guidelines   X Assign placeholder X   ● Use Additional Character(s)   ▶ Manifestation Code   🏥 Hierarchical Condition Category   **Coding Clinic**

● **S93.4   Sprain of ankle**
Injury to ligaments when one or more is stretched/torn
Excludes2   injury of Achilles tendon (S86.0-)
● **S93.40   Sprain of unspecified ligament of ankle**
Sprain of ankle NOS
Sprained ankle NOS
● S93.401   Sprain of unspecified ligament of right ankle
● S93.402   Sprain of unspecified ligament of left ankle
● S93.409   Sprain of unspecified ligament of unspecified ankle
● **S93.41   Sprain of calcaneofibular ligament**
● S93.411   Sprain of calcaneofibular ligament of right ankle
● S93.412   Sprain of calcaneofibular ligament of left ankle
● S93.419   Sprain of calcaneofibular ligament of unspecified ankle
● **S93.42   Sprain of deltoid ligament**
● S93.421   Sprain of deltoid ligament of right ankle
● S93.422   Sprain of deltoid ligament of left ankle
● S93.429   Sprain of deltoid ligament of unspecified ankle
● **S93.43   Sprain of tibiofibular ligament**
● S93.431   Sprain of tibiofibular ligament of right ankle
● S93.432   Sprain of tibiofibular ligament of left ankle
● S93.439   Sprain of tibiofibular ligament of unspecified ankle
● **S93.49   Sprain of other ligament of ankle**
Sprain of internal collateral ligament
Sprain of talofibular ligament
● S93.491   Sprain of other ligament of right ankle
● S93.492   Sprain of other ligament of left ankle
● S93.499   Sprain of other ligament of unspecified ankle
● **S93.5   Sprain of toe**
● **S93.50   Unspecified sprain of toe**
● S93.501   Unspecified sprain of right great toe
● S93.502   Unspecified sprain of left great toe
● S93.503   Unspecified sprain of unspecified great toe
● S93.504   Unspecified sprain of right lesser toe(s)
● S93.505   Unspecified sprain of left lesser toe(s)
● S93.506   Unspecified sprain of unspecified lesser toe(s)
● S93.509   Unspecified sprain of unspecified toe(s)
● **S93.51   Sprain of interphalangeal joint of toe**
● S93.511   Sprain of interphalangeal joint of right great toe
● S93.512   Sprain of interphalangeal joint of left great toe
● S93.513   Sprain of interphalangeal joint of unspecified great toe
● S93.514   Sprain of interphalangeal joint of right lesser toe(s)
● S93.515   Sprain of interphalangeal joint of left lesser toe(s)
● S93.516   Sprain of interphalangeal joint of unspecified lesser toe(s)
● S93.519   Sprain of interphalangeal joint of unspecified toe(s)

● **S93.52   Sprain of metatarsophalangeal joint of toe**
● S93.521   Sprain of metatarsophalangeal joint of right great toe
● S93.522   Sprain of metatarsophalangeal joint of left great toe
● S93.523   Sprain of metatarsophalangeal joint of unspecified great toe
● S93.524   Sprain of metatarsophalangeal joint of right lesser toe(s)
● S93.525   Sprain of metatarsophalangeal joint of left lesser toe(s)
● S93.526   Sprain of metatarsophalangeal joint of unspecified lesser toe(s)
● S93.529   Sprain of metatarsophalangeal joint of unspecified toe(s)
● **S93.6   Sprain of foot**
Excludes2   sprain of metatarsophalangeal joint of toe (S93.52-)
sprain of toe (S93.5-)
● **S93.60   Unspecified sprain of foot**
● S93.601   Unspecified sprain of right foot
● S93.602   Unspecified sprain of left foot
● S93.609   Unspecified sprain of unspecified foot
● **S93.61   Sprain of tarsal ligament of foot**
● S93.611   Sprain of tarsal ligament of right foot
● S93.612   Sprain of tarsal ligament of left foot
● S93.619   Sprain of tarsal ligament of unspecified foot
● **S93.62   Sprain of tarsometatarsal ligament of foot**
● S93.621   Sprain of tarsometatarsal ligament of right foot
● S93.622   Sprain of tarsometatarsal ligament of left foot
● S93.629   Sprain of tarsometatarsal ligament of unspecified foot
● **S93.69   Other sprain of foot**
● S93.691   Other sprain of right foot
● S93.692   Other sprain of left foot
● S93.699   Other sprain of unspecified foot
● **S94   Injury of nerves at ankle and foot level**
The appropriate 7th character is to be added to each code from category S94

A	initial encounter
D	subsequent encounter
S	sequela

Code also any associated open wound (S91.-)
● **S94.0   Injury of lateral plantar nerve**
X ● S94.00   Injury of lateral plantar nerve, unspecified leg
X ● S94.01   Injury of lateral plantar nerve, right leg
X ● S94.02   Injury of lateral plantar nerve, left leg
● **S94.1   Injury of medial plantar nerve**
X ● S94.10   Injury of medial plantar nerve, unspecified leg
X ● S94.11   Injury of medial plantar nerve, right leg
X ● S94.12   Injury of medial plantar nerve, left leg
● **S94.2   Injury of deep peroneal nerve at ankle and foot level**
Injury of terminal, lateral branch of deep peroneal nerve
X ● S94.20   Injury of deep peroneal nerve at ankle and foot level, unspecified leg
X ● S94.21   Injury of deep peroneal nerve at ankle and foot level, right leg
X ● S94.22   Injury of deep peroneal nerve at ankle and foot level, left leg

CHAPTER 19 (S00-T88)

CHAPTER 19 (S00-T88)

● S94.3 Injury of cutaneous sensory nerve at ankle and foot level
  X ● S94.30 Injury of cutaneous sensory nerve at ankle and foot level, unspecified leg
  X ● S94.31 Injury of cutaneous sensory nerve at ankle and foot level, right leg
  X ● S94.32 Injury of cutaneous sensory nerve at ankle and foot level, left leg
● S94.8 Injury of other nerves at ankle and foot level
  ● S94.8X Injury of other nerves at ankle and foot level
    ● S94.8X1 Injury of other nerves at ankle and foot level, right leg
    ● S94.8X2 Injury of other nerves at ankle and foot level, left leg
    ● S94.8X9 Injury of other nerves at ankle and foot level, unspecified leg
● S94.9 Injury of unspecified nerve at ankle and foot level
  X ● S94.90 Injury of unspecified nerve at ankle and foot level, unspecified leg
  X ● S94.91 Injury of unspecified nerve at ankle and foot level, right leg
  X ● S94.92 Injury of unspecified nerve at ankle and foot level, left leg

● S95 Injury of blood vessels at ankle and foot level
  Code also any associated open wound (S91.-)
  Excludes2 injury of posterior tibial artery and vein (S85.1-, S85.8-)

  The appropriate 7th character is to be added to each code from category S95

A	initial encounter
D	subsequent encounter
S	sequela

● S95.0 Injury of dorsal artery of foot
  ● S95.00 Unspecified injury of dorsal artery of foot
    ● S95.001 Unspecified injury of dorsal artery of right foot
    ● S95.002 Unspecified injury of dorsal artery of left foot
    ● S95.009 Unspecified injury of dorsal artery of unspecified foot
  ● S95.01 Laceration of dorsal artery of foot
    ● S95.011 Laceration of dorsal artery of right foot
    ● S95.012 Laceration of dorsal artery of left foot
    ● S95.019 Laceration of dorsal artery of unspecified foot
  ● S95.09 Other specified injury of dorsal artery of foot
    ● S95.091 Other specified injury of dorsal artery of right foot
    ● S95.092 Other specified injury of dorsal artery of left foot
    ● S95.099 Other specified injury of dorsal artery of unspecified foot
● S95.1 Injury of plantar artery of foot
  ● S95.10 Unspecified injury of plantar artery of foot
    ● S95.101 Unspecified injury of plantar artery of right foot
    ● S95.102 Unspecified injury of plantar artery of left foot
    ● S95.109 Unspecified injury of plantar artery of unspecified foot
  ● S95.11 Laceration of plantar artery of foot
    ● S95.111 Laceration of plantar artery of right foot
    ● S95.112 Laceration of plantar artery of left foot
    ● S95.119 Laceration of plantar artery of unspecified foot

● S95.19 Other specified injury of plantar artery of foot
  ● S95.191 Other specified injury of plantar artery of right foot
  ● S95.192 Other specified injury of plantar artery of left foot
  ● S95.199 Other specified injury of plantar artery of unspecified foot
● S95.2 Injury of dorsal vein of foot
  ● S95.20 Unspecified injury of dorsal vein of foot
    ● S95.201 Unspecified injury of dorsal vein of right foot
    ● S95.202 Unspecified injury of dorsal vein of left foot
    ● S95.209 Unspecified injury of dorsal vein of unspecified foot
  ● S95.21 Laceration of dorsal vein of foot
    ● S95.211 Laceration of dorsal vein of right foot
    ● S95.212 Laceration of dorsal vein of left foot
    ● S95.219 Laceration of dorsal vein of unspecified foot
  ● S95.29 Other specified injury of dorsal vein of foot
    ● S95.291 Other specified injury of dorsal vein of right foot
    ● S95.292 Other specified injury of dorsal vein of left foot
    ● S95.299 Other specified injury of dorsal vein of unspecified foot
● S95.8 Injury of other blood vessels at ankle and foot level
  ● S95.80 Unspecified injury of other blood vessels at ankle and foot level
    ● S95.801 Unspecified injury of other blood vessels at ankle and foot level, right leg
    ● S95.802 Unspecified injury of other blood vessels at ankle and foot level, left leg
    ● S95.809 Unspecified injury of other blood vessels at ankle and foot level, unspecified leg
  ● S95.81 Laceration of other blood vessels at ankle and foot level
    ● S95.811 Laceration of other blood vessels at ankle and foot level, right leg
    ● S95.812 Laceration of other blood vessels at ankle and foot level, left leg
    ● S95.819 Laceration of other blood vessels at ankle and foot level, unspecified leg
  ● S95.89 Other specified injury of other blood vessels at ankle and foot level
    ● S95.891 Other specified injury of other blood vessels at ankle and foot level, right leg
    ● S95.892 Other specified injury of other blood vessels at ankle and foot level, left leg
    ● S95.899 Other specified injury of other blood vessels at ankle and foot level, unspecified leg
● S95.9 Injury of unspecified blood vessel at ankle and foot level
  ● S95.90 Unspecified injury of unspecified blood vessel at ankle and foot level
    ● S95.901 Unspecified injury of unspecified blood vessel at ankle and foot level, right leg
    ● S95.902 Unspecified injury of unspecified blood vessel at ankle and foot level, left leg
    ● S95.909 Unspecified injury of unspecified blood vessel at ankle and foot level, unspecified leg

▶ New ⇒ Revised ~~deleted~~ Deleted Excludes 1 Excludes 2 Includes Use additional Code first Code also Key words
OGCR Official Guidelines X Assign placeholder X ● Use Additional Character(s) ▶ Manifestation Code 🔖 Hierarchical Condition Category **Coding Clinic**

● S95.91   Laceration of unspecified blood vessel at ankle and foot level

  ● S95.911   Laceration of unspecified blood vessel at ankle and foot level, right leg

  ● S95.912   Laceration of unspecified blood vessel at ankle and foot level, left leg

  ● S95.919   Laceration of unspecified blood vessel at ankle and foot level, unspecified leg

● S95.99   Other specified injury of unspecified blood vessel at ankle and foot level

  ● S95.991   Other specified injury of unspecified blood vessel at ankle and foot level, right leg

  ● S95.992   Other specified injury of unspecified blood vessel at ankle and foot level, left leg

  ● S95.999   Other specified injury of unspecified blood vessel at ankle and foot level, unspecified leg

● S96   Injury of muscle and tendon at ankle and foot level

Code also any associated open wound (S91.-)

Excludes2   injury of Achilles tendon (S86.0-)
           sprain of joints and ligaments of ankle and foot (S93.-)

The appropriate 7th character is to be added to each code from category S96

A	initial encounter
D	subsequent encounter
S	sequela

● S96.0   Injury of muscle and tendon of long flexor muscle of toe at ankle and foot level

  ● S96.00   Unspecified injury of muscle and tendon of long flexor muscle of toe at ankle and foot level

    ● S96.001   Unspecified injury of muscle and tendon of long flexor muscle of toe at ankle and foot level, right foot

    ● S96.002   Unspecified injury of muscle and tendon of long flexor muscle of toe at ankle and foot level, left foot

    ● S96.009   Unspecified injury of muscle and tendon of long flexor muscle of toe at ankle and foot level, unspecified foot

  ● S96.01   Strain of muscle and tendon of long flexor muscle of toe at ankle and foot level

    ● S96.011   Strain of muscle and tendon of long flexor muscle of toe at ankle and foot level, right foot

    ● S96.012   Strain of muscle and tendon of long flexor muscle of toe at ankle and foot level, left foot

    ● S96.019   Strain of muscle and tendon of long flexor muscle of toe at ankle and foot level, unspecified foot

  ● S96.02   Laceration of muscle and tendon of long flexor muscle of toe at ankle and foot level

    ● S96.021   Laceration of muscle and tendon of long flexor muscle of toe at ankle and foot level, right foot

    ● S96.022   Laceration of muscle and tendon of long flexor muscle of toe at ankle and foot level, left foot

    ● S96.029   Laceration of muscle and tendon of long flexor muscle of toe at ankle and foot level, unspecified foot

  ● S96.09   Other injury of muscle and tendon of long flexor muscle of toe at ankle and foot level

    ● S96.091   Other injury of muscle and tendon of long flexor muscle of toe at ankle and foot level, right foot

    ● S96.092   Other injury of muscle and tendon of long flexor muscle of toe at ankle and foot level, left foot

    ● S96.099   Other injury of muscle and tendon of long flexor muscle of toe at ankle and foot level, unspecified foot

● S96.1   Injury of muscle and tendon of long extensor muscle of toe at ankle and foot level

  ● S96.10   Unspecified injury of muscle and tendon of long extensor muscle of toe at ankle and foot level

    ● S96.101   Unspecified injury of muscle and tendon of long extensor muscle of toe at ankle and foot level, right foot

    ● S96.102   Unspecified injury of muscle and tendon of long extensor muscle of toe at ankle and foot level, left foot

    ● S96.109   Unspecified injury of muscle and tendon of long extensor muscle of toe at ankle and foot level, unspecified foot

  ● S96.11   Strain of muscle and tendon of long extensor muscle of toe at ankle and foot level

    ● S96.111   Strain of muscle and tendon of long extensor muscle of toe at ankle and foot level, right foot

    ● S96.112   Strain of muscle and tendon of long extensor muscle of toe at ankle and foot level, left foot

    ● S96.119   Strain of muscle and tendon of long extensor muscle of toe at ankle and foot level, unspecified foot

  ● S96.12   Laceration of muscle and tendon of long extensor muscle of toe at ankle and foot level

    ● S96.121   Laceration of muscle and tendon of long extensor muscle of toe at ankle and foot level, right foot

    ● S96.122   Laceration of muscle and tendon of long extensor muscle of toe at ankle and foot level, left foot

    ● S96.129   Laceration of muscle and tendon of long extensor muscle of toe at ankle and foot level, unspecified foot

  ● S96.19   Other specified injury of muscle and tendon of long extensor muscle of toe at ankle and foot level

    ● S96.191   Other specified injury of muscle and tendon of long extensor muscle of toe at ankle and foot level, right foot

    ● S96.192   Other specified injury of muscle and tendon of long extensor muscle of toe at ankle and foot level, left foot

    ● S96.199   Other specified injury of muscle and tendon of long extensor muscle of toe at ankle and foot level, unspecified foot

● S96.2   Injury of intrinsic muscle and tendon at ankle and foot level

  ● S96.20   Unspecified injury of intrinsic muscle and tendon at ankle and foot level

    ● S96.201   Unspecified injury of intrinsic muscle and tendon at ankle and foot level, right foot

    ● S96.202   Unspecified injury of intrinsic muscle and tendon at ankle and foot level, left foot

    ● S96.209   Unspecified injury of intrinsic muscle and tendon at ankle and foot level, unspecified foot

- ● S96.21   **Strain** of intrinsic muscle and tendon at ankle and foot level
  - ● S96.211   Strain of intrinsic muscle and tendon at ankle and foot level, **right** foot
  - ● S96.212   Strain of intrinsic muscle and tendon at ankle and foot level, **left** foot
  - ● S96.219   Strain of intrinsic muscle and tendon at ankle and foot level, **unspecified** foot
- ● S96.22   **Laceration** of intrinsic muscle and tendon at ankle and foot level
  - ● S96.221   Laceration of intrinsic muscle and tendon at ankle and foot level, **right** foot
  - ● S96.222   Laceration of intrinsic muscle and tendon at left ankle and foot level, **left** foot
  - ● S96.229   Laceration of intrinsic muscle and tendon at ankle and foot level, **unspecified** foot
- ● S96.29   **Other** specified injury of intrinsic muscle and tendon at ankle and foot level
  - ● S96.291   Other specified injury of intrinsic muscle and tendon at ankle and foot level, **right** foot
  - ● S96.292   Other specified injury of intrinsic muscle and tendon at ankle and foot level, **left** foot
  - ● S96.299   Other specified injury of intrinsic muscle and tendon at ankle and foot level, **unspecified** foot
- ● S96.8   **Injury** of **other** specified muscles and tendons at ankle and foot level
  - ● S96.80   **Unspecified** injury of other specified muscles and tendons at ankle and foot level
    - ● S96.801   Unspecified injury of other specified muscles and tendons at ankle and foot level, **right** foot
    - ● S96.802   Unspecified injury of other specified muscles and tendons at ankle and foot level, **left** foot
    - ● S96.809   Unspecified injury of other specified muscles and tendons at ankle and foot level, **unspecified** foot
  - ● S96.81   **Strain** of other specified muscles and tendons at ankle and foot level
    - ● S96.811   Strain of other specified muscles and tendons at ankle and foot level, **right** foot
    - ● S96.812   Strain of other specified muscles and tendons at ankle and foot level, **left** foot
    - ● S96.819   Strain of other specified muscles and tendons at ankle and foot level, **unspecified** foot
  - ● S96.82   **Laceration** of other specified muscles and tendons at ankle and foot level
    - ● S96.821   Laceration of other specified muscles and tendons at ankle and foot level, **right** foot
    - ● S96.822   Laceration of other specified muscles and tendons at ankle and foot level, **left** foot
    - ● S96.829   Laceration of other specified muscles and tendons at ankle and foot level, **unspecified** foot

- ● S96.89   **Other** specified injury of other specified muscles and tendons at ankle and foot level
  - ● S96.891   Other specified injury of other specified muscles and tendons at ankle and foot level, **right** foot
  - ● S96.892   Other specified injury of other specified muscles and tendons at ankle and foot level, **left** foot
  - ● S96.899   Other specified injury of other specified muscles and tendons at ankle and foot level, **unspecified** foot
- ● S96.9   **Injury** of **unspecified** muscle and tendon at ankle and foot level
  - ● S96.90   **Unspecified** injury of unspecified muscle and tendon at ankle and foot level
    - ● S96.901   Unspecified injury of unspecified muscle and tendon at ankle and foot level, **right** foot
    - ● S96.902   Unspecified injury of unspecified muscle and tendon at ankle and foot level, **left** foot
    - ● S96.909   Unspecified injury of unspecified muscle and tendon at ankle and foot level, **unspecified** foot
  - ● S96.91   **Strain** of unspecified muscle and tendon at ankle and foot level
    - ● S96.911   Strain of unspecified muscle and tendon at ankle and foot level, **right** foot
    - ● S96.912   Strain of unspecified muscle and tendon at ankle and foot level, **left** foot
    - ● S96.919   Strain of unspecified muscle and tendon at ankle and foot level, **unspecified** foot
  - ● S96.92   **Laceration** of unspecified muscle and tendon at ankle and foot level
    - ● S96.921   Laceration of unspecified muscle and tendon at ankle and foot level, **right** foot
    - ● S96.922   Laceration of unspecified muscle and tendon at ankle and foot level, **left** foot
    - ● S96.929   Laceration of unspecified muscle and tendon at ankle and foot level, **unspecified** foot
  - ● S96.99   **Other** specified injury of unspecified muscle and tendon at ankle and foot level
    - ● S96.991   Other specified injury of unspecified muscle and tendon at ankle and foot level, **right** foot
    - ● S96.992   Other specified injury of unspecified muscle and tendon at ankle and foot level, **left** foot
    - ● S96.999   Other specified injury of unspecified muscle and tendon at ankle and foot level, **unspecified** foot

- ● S97   **Crushing injury of ankle and foot**

  Use additional code(s) for all associated injuries

  The appropriate 7th character is to be added to each code from category S97

A	initial encounter
D	subsequent encounter
S	sequela

  - ● S97.0   **Crushing injury of ankle**
    - X ● S97.00   Crushing injury of **unspecified** ankle
    - X ● S97.01   Crushing injury of **right** ankle
    - X ● S97.02   Crushing injury of **left** ankle

▶ New   ⟹ Revised   ~~deleted~~ Deleted   Excludes 1   Excludes 2   Includes   Use additional   Code first   Code also   Key words

OGCR Official Guidelines   X Assign placeholder X   ● Use Additional Character(s)   ▶ Manifestation Code   🔖 Hierarchical Condition Category   **Coding Clinic**

● S97.1   Crushing injury of toe
   ● S97.10   Crushing injury of unspecified toe(s)
     ● S97.101   Crushing injury of unspecified right toe(s)
     ● S97.102   Crushing injury of unspecified left toe(s)
     ● S97.109   Crushing injury of unspecified toe(s)
        Crushing injury of toe NOS
   ● S97.11   Crushing injury of great toe
     ● S97.111   Crushing injury of right great toe
     ● S97.112   Crushing injury of left great toe
     ● S97.119   Crushing injury of unspecified great toe
   ● S97.12   Crushing injury of lesser toe(s)
     ● S97.121   Crushing injury of right lesser toe(s)
     ● S97.122   Crushing injury of left lesser toe(s)
     ● S97.129   Crushing injury of lesser toe(s), unspecified toe(s)

● S97.8   Crushing injury of foot
   X ● S97.80   Crushing injury of foot, unspecified side
        Crushing injury of foot NOS
   X ● S97.81   Crushing injury of right foot
   X ● S97.82   Crushing injury of left foot

● S98   Traumatic amputation of ankle and foot
   An amputation not identified as partial or complete should be coded to complete
   The appropriate 7th character is to be added to each code from category S98

> A   initial encounter
> D   subsequent encounter
> S   sequela

● S98.0   Traumatic amputation of foot at ankle level
   ● S98.01   Complete traumatic amputation of foot at ankle level
     ● S98.011   Complete traumatic amputation of right foot at ankle level A, D, S ✪
     ● S98.012   Complete traumatic amputation of left foot at ankle level A, D, S ✪
     ● S98.019   Complete traumatic amputation of unspecified foot at ankle level A, D, S ✪
   ● S98.02   Partial traumatic amputation of foot at ankle level
     ● S98.021   Partial traumatic amputation of right foot at ankle level A, D, S ✪
     ● S98.022   Partial traumatic amputation of left foot at ankle level A, D, S ✪
     ● S98.029   Partial traumatic amputation of unspecified foot at ankle level A, D, S ✪

● S98.1   Traumatic amputation of one toe
   ● S98.11   Complete traumatic amputation of great toe
     ● S98.111   Complete traumatic amputation of right great toe A, D, S ✪
     ● S98.112   Complete traumatic amputation of left great toe A, D, S ✪
     ● S98.119   Complete traumatic amputation of unspecified great toe A, D, S ✪
   ● S98.12   Partial traumatic amputation of great toe
     ● S98.121   Partial traumatic amputation of right great toe A, D, S ✪
     ● S98.122   Partial traumatic amputation of left great toe A, D, S ✪
     ● S98.129   Partial traumatic amputation of unspecified great toe A, D, S ✪

● S98.13   Complete traumatic amputation of one lesser toe
        Traumatic amputation of toe NOS
     ● S98.131   Complete traumatic amputation of one right lesser toe A, D, S ✪
     ● S98.132   Complete traumatic amputation of one left lesser toe A, D, S ✪
     ● S98.139   Complete traumatic amputation of one unspecified lesser toe A, D, S ✪
   ● S98.14   Partial traumatic amputation of one lesser toe
     ● S98.141   Partial traumatic amputation of one right lesser toe A, D, S ✪
     ● S98.142   Partial traumatic amputation of one left lesser toe A, D, S ✪
     ● S98.149   Partial traumatic amputation of one unspecified lesser toe A, D, S ✪

● S98.2   Traumatic amputation of two or more lesser toes
   ● S98.21   Complete traumatic amputation of two or more lesser toes
     ● S98.211   Complete traumatic amputation of two or more right lesser toes A, D, S ✪
     ● S98.212   Complete traumatic amputation of two or more left lesser toes A, D, S ✪
     ● S98.219   Complete traumatic amputation of two or more unspecified lesser toes A, D, S ✪
   ● S98.22   Partial traumatic amputation of two or more lesser toes
     ● S98.221   Partial traumatic amputation of two or more right lesser toes A, D, S ✪
     ● S98.222   Partial traumatic amputation of two or more left lesser toes A, D, S ✪
     ● S98.229   Partial traumatic amputation of two or more unspecified lesser toes A, D, S ✪

● S98.3   Traumatic amputation of midfoot
   ● S98.31   Complete traumatic amputation of midfoot
     ● S98.311   Complete traumatic amputation of right midfoot A, D, S ✪
     ● S98.312   Complete traumatic amputation of left midfoot A, D, S ✪
     ● S98.319   Complete traumatic amputation of unspecified midfoot A, D, S ✪
   ● S98.32   Partial traumatic amputation of midfoot
     ● S98.321   Partial traumatic amputation of right midfoot A, D, S ✪
     ● S98.322   Partial traumatic amputation of left midfoot A, D, S ✪
     ● S98.329   Partial traumatic amputation of unspecified midfoot A, D, S ✪

● S98.9   Traumatic amputation of foot, level unspecified
   ● S98.91   Complete traumatic amputation of foot, level unspecified
     ● S98.911   Complete traumatic amputation of right foot, level unspecified A, D, S ✪
     ● S98.912   Complete traumatic amputation of left foot, level unspecified A, D, S ✪
     ● S98.919   Complete traumatic amputation of unspecified foot, level unspecified A, D, S ✪
   ● S98.92   Partial traumatic amputation of foot, level unspecified
     ● S98.921   Partial traumatic amputation of right foot, level unspecified A, D, S ✪
     ● S98.922   Partial traumatic amputation of left foot, level unspecified A, D, S ✪
     ● S98.929   Partial traumatic amputation of unspecified foot, level unspecified A, D, S ✪

CHAPTER 19 (S00–T88)

● **S99**   **Other and unspecified injuries of ankle and foot**
      Coding Clinic: 2016, Q4, P68

  ● **S99.0**   **Physeal fracture of calcaneus**

      The appropriate 7th character is to be added to each
      code from subcategories S99.0

A	initial encounter for closed fracture
B	initial encounter for open fracture
D	subsequent encounter for fracture with routine healing
G	subsequent encounter for fracture with delayed healing
K	subsequent encounter for fracture with nonunion
P	subsequent encounter for fracture with malunion
S	sequela

    ● **S99.00**   **Unspecified physeal fracture of calcaneus**

      ● **S99.001**   Unspecified physeal fracture of **right** calcaneus

      ● **S99.002**   Unspecified physeal fracture of **left** calcaneus

      ● **S99.009**   Unspecified physeal fracture of **unspecified** calcaneus

    ● **S99.01**   **Salter-Harris Type I physeal fracture of calcaneus**
         Coding Clinic: 2016, Q4, P69

      ● **S99.011**   Salter-Harris Type I physeal fracture of **right** calcaneus

      ● **S99.012**   Salter-Harris Type I physeal fracture of **left** calcaneus

      ● **S99.019**   Salter-Harris Type I physeal fracture of **unspecified** calcaneus

    ● **S99.02**   **Salter-Harris Type II physeal fracture of calcaneus**
         Coding Clinic: 2016, Q4, P69

      ● **S99.021**   Salter-Harris Type II physeal fracture of **right** calcaneus

      ● **S99.022**   Salter-Harris Type II physeal fracture of **left** calcaneus

      ● **S99.029**   Salter-Harris Type II physeal fracture of **unspecified** calcaneus

    ● **S99.03**   **Salter-Harris Type III physeal fracture of calcaneus**
         Coding Clinic: 2016, Q4, P69

      ● **S99.031**   Salter-Harris Type III physeal fracture of **right** calcaneus

      ● **S99.032**   Salter-Harris Type III physeal fracture of **left** calcaneus

      ● **S99.039**   Salter-Harris Type III physeal fracture of **unspecified** calcaneus

    ● **S99.04**   **Salter-Harris Type IV physeal fracture of calcaneus**
         Coding Clinic: 2016, Q4, P69

      ● **S99.041**   Salter-Harris Type IV physeal fracture of **right** calcaneus

      ● **S99.042**   Salter-Harris Type IV physeal fracture of **left** calcaneus

      ● **S99.049**   Salter-Harris Type IV physeal fracture of **unspecified** calcaneus

    ● **S99.09**   **Other physeal fracture of calcaneus**
         Coding Clinic: 2016, Q4, P69

      ● **S99.091**   Other physeal fracture of **right** calcaneus

      ● **S99.092**   Other physeal fracture of **left** calcaneus

      ● **S99.099**   Other physeal fracture of **unspecified** calcaneus

  ● **S99.1**   **Physeal fracture of metatarsal**

      The appropriate 7th character is to be added to each
      code from subcategories S99.1

A	initial encounter for closed fracture
B	initial encounter for open fracture
D	subsequent encounter for fracture with routine healing
G	subsequent encounter for fracture with delayed healing
K	subsequent encounter for fracture with nonunion
P	subsequent encounter for fracture with malunion
S	sequela

    ● **S99.10**   **Unspecified physeal fracture of metatarsal**

      ● **S99.101**   Unspecified physeal fracture of **right** metatarsal

      ● **S99.102**   Unspecified physeal fracture of **left** metatarsal

      ● **S99.109**   Unspecified physeal fracture of **unspecified** metatarsal

    ● **S99.11**   **Salter-Harris Type I physeal fracture of metatarsal**
         Coding Clinic: 2016, Q4, P69

      ● **S99.111**   Salter-Harris Type I physeal fracture of **right** metatarsal

      ● **S99.112**   Salter-Harris Type I physeal fracture of **left** metatarsal
           Coding Clinic: 2018, Q1, P3

      ● **S99.119**   Salter-Harris Type I physeal fracture of **unspecified** metatarsal

    ● **S99.12**   **Salter-Harris Type II physeal fracture of metatarsal**
         Coding Clinic: 2016, Q4, P69

      ● **S99.121**   Salter-Harris Type II physeal fracture of **right** metatarsal

      ● **S99.122**   Salter-Harris Type II physeal fracture of **left** metatarsal

      ● **S99.129**   Salter-Harris Type II physeal fracture of **unspecified** metatarsal

    ● **S99.13**   **Salter-Harris Type III physeal fracture of metatarsal**
         Coding Clinic: 2016, Q4, P69

      ● **S99.131**   Salter-Harris Type III physeal fracture of **right** metatarsal

      ● **S99.132**   Salter-Harris Type III physeal fracture of **left** metatarsal

      ● **S99.139**   Salter-Harris Type III physeal fracture of **unspecified** metatarsal

    ● **S99.14**   **Salter-Harris Type IV physeal fracture of metatarsal**
         Coding Clinic: 2016, Q4, P69

      ● **S99.141**   Salter-Harris Type IV physeal fracture of **right** metatarsal

      ● **S99.142**   Salter-Harris Type IV physeal fracture of **left** metatarsal

      ● **S99.149**   Salter-Harris Type IV physeal fracture of **unspecified** metatarsal

    ● **S99.19**   **Other physeal fracture of metatarsal**
         Coding Clinic: 2016, Q4, P69

      ● **S99.191**   Other physeal fracture of **right** metatarsal

      ● **S99.192**   Other physeal fracture of **left** metatarsal

      ● **S99.199**   Other physeal fracture of **unspecified** metatarsal

▶ New   ⇒ Revised   ~~deleted~~ Deleted   Excludes 1   Excludes 2   Includes   Use additional   Code first   Code also   Key words

OGCR Official Guidelines   X Assign placeholder X   ● Use Additional Character(s)   ▸ Manifestation Code   🔖 Hierarchical Condition Category   **Coding Clinic**

● **S99.2   Physeal fracture of phalanx of toe**

The appropriate 7th character is to be added to each code from subcategories S99.2

A	initial encounter for closed fracture
B	initial encounter for open fracture
D	subsequent encounter for fracture with routine healing
G	subsequent encounter for fracture with delayed healing
K	subsequent encounter for fracture with nonunion
P	subsequent encounter for fracture with malunion
S	sequela

● **S99.20   Unspecified physeal fracture of phalanx of toe**

● S99.201   Unspecified physeal fracture of phalanx of right toe

● S99.202   Unspecified physeal fracture of phalanx of right toe

● S99.209   Unspecified physeal fracture of phalanx of unspecified toe

● **S99.21   Salter-Harris Type I physeal fracture of phalanx of toe**
Coding Clinic: 2016, Q4, P69

● S99.211   Salter-Harris Type I physeal fracture of phalanx of right toe

● S99.212   Salter-Harris Type I physeal fracture of phalanx of left toe

● S99.219   Salter-Harris Type I physeal fracture of phalanx of unspecified toe

● **S99.22   Salter-Harris Type II physeal fracture of phalanx of toe**
Coding Clinic: 2016, Q4, P69

● S99.221   Salter-Harris Type II physeal fracture of phalanx of right toe

● S99.222   Salter-Harris Type II physeal fracture of phalanx of left toe

● S99.229   Salter-Harris Type II physeal fracture of phalanx of unspecified toe

● **S99.23   Salter-Harris Type III physeal fracture of phalanx of toe**
Coding Clinic: 2016, Q4, P69

● S99.231   Salter-Harris Type III physeal fracture of phalanx of right toe

● S99.232   Salter-Harris Type III physeal fracture of phalanx of left toe

● S99.239   Salter-Harris Type III physeal fracture of phalanx of unspecified toe

● **S99.24   Salter-Harris Type IV physeal fracture of phalanx of toe**
Coding Clinic: 2016, Q4, P69

● S99.241   Salter-Harris Type IV physeal fracture of phalanx of right toe

● S99.242   Salter-Harris Type IV physeal fracture of phalanx of left toe

● S99.249   Salter-Harris Type IV physeal fracture of phalanx of unspecified toe

● **S99.29   Other physeal fracture of phalanx of toe**
Coding Clinic: 2016, Q4, P69

● S99.291   Other physeal fracture of phalanx of right toe

● S99.292   Other physeal fracture of phalanx of left toe

● S99.299   Other physeal fracture of phalanx of unspecified toe

● **S99.8   Other specified injuries of ankle and foot**

The appropriate 7th character is to be added to each code from subcategory S99.8

A	initial encounter
D	subsequent encounter
S	sequela

● **S99.81   Other specified injuries of ankle**
● S99.811   Other specified injuries of right ankle
● S99.812   Other specified injuries of left ankle
● S99.819   Other specified injuries of unspecified ankle

● **S99.82   Other specified injuries of foot**
● S99.821   Other specified injuries of right foot
● S99.822   Other specified injuries of left foot
● S99.829   Other specified injuries of unspecified foot

● **S99.9   Unspecified injury of ankle and foot**

The appropriate 7th character is to be added to each code from subcategory S99.9

A	initial encounter
D	subsequent encounter
S	sequela

● **S99.91   Unspecified injury of ankle**
● S99.911   Unspecified injury of right ankle
● S99.912   Unspecified injury of left ankle
● S99.919   Unspecified injury of unspecified ankle

● **S99.92   Unspecified injury of foot**
● S99.921   Unspecified injury of right foot
● S99.922   Unspecified injury of left foot
● S99.929   Unspecified injury of unspecified foot

INJURY, POISONING AND CERTAIN OTHER CONSEQUENCES OF EXTERNAL CAUSES (T07-T88)

INJURIES INVOLVING MULTIPLE BODY REGIONS (T07)

Excludes1   burns and corrosions (T20-T32)
frostbite (T33-T34)
insect bite or sting, venomous (T63.4)
sunburn (L55.-)

X ● **T07   Unspecified multiple injuries**

The appropriate 7th character is to be added to code T07

A	initial encounter
D	subsequent encounter
S	sequela

Excludes1   injury NOS (T14.90)

INJURY OF UNSPECIFIED BODY REGION (T14)

● **T14   Injury of unspecified body region**

The appropriate 7th character is to be added to each code from category T14

A	initial encounter
D	subsequent encounter
S	sequela

Excludes1   multiple unspecified injuries (T07)

X ● **T14.8   Other injury of unspecified body region**

Abrasion NOS	Skin injury NOS
Contusion NOS	Vascular injury NOS
Crush injury NOS	Wound NOS
Fracture NOS	

● **T14.9   Unspecified injury**

X ● **T14.90   Injury, unspecified**
Injury NOS

X ● **T14.91   Suicide attempt** A, D, S 🔧
Attempted suicide NOS

CHAPTER 19 (S00-T88)

EFFECTS OF FOREIGN BODY ENTERING THROUGH NATURAL ORIFICE (T15-T19)

Excludes2   foreign body accidentally left in operation wound (T81.5-)
foreign body in penetrating wound - see open wound by body region
residual foreign body in soft tissue (M79.5)
splinter, without open wound - see superficial injury by body region

● **T15**   **Foreign body on external eye**

Excludes2   foreign body in penetrating wound of orbit and eye ball (S05.4-, S05.5-)
open wound of eyelid and periocular area (S01.1-)
retained foreign body in eyelid (H02.8-)
retained (old) foreign body in penetrating wound of orbit and eye ball (H05.5-, H44.6-, H44.7-)
superficial foreign body of eyelid and periocular area (S00.25-)

The appropriate 7th character is to be added to each code from category T15

> A   initial encounter
> D   subsequent encounter
> S   sequela

● **T15.0**   **Foreign body in cornea**
   X● **T15.00**   **Foreign body in cornea, unspecified eye**
   X● **T15.01**   **Foreign body in cornea, right eye**
   X● **T15.02**   **Foreign body in cornea, left eye**
● **T15.1**   **Foreign body in conjunctival sac**
   X● **T15.10**   **Foreign body in conjunctival sac, unspecified eye**
   X● **T15.11**   **Foreign body in conjunctival sac, right eye**
   X● **T15.12**   **Foreign body in conjunctival sac, left eye**
● **T15.8**   **Foreign body in other and multiple parts of external eye**
     Foreign body in lacrimal punctum
   X● **T15.80**   **Foreign body in other and multiple parts of external eye, unspecified eye**
   X● **T15.81**   **Foreign body in other and multiple parts of external eye, right eye**
   X● **T15.82**   **Foreign body in other and multiple parts of external eye, left eye**
● **T15.9**   **Foreign body on external eye, part unspecified**
   X● **T15.90**   **Foreign body on external eye, part unspecified, unspecified eye**
   X● **T15.91**   **Foreign body on external eye, part unspecified, right eye**
   X● **T15.92**   **Foreign body on external eye, part unspecified, left eye**

● **T16**   **Foreign body in ear**

Includes   foreign body in auditory canal

The appropriate 7th character is to be added to each code from category T16

> A   initial encounter
> D   subsequent encounter
> S   sequela

   X● **T16.1**   **Foreign body in right ear**
   X● **T16.2**   **Foreign body in left ear**
   X● **T16.9**   **Foreign body in ear, unspecified ear**

● **T17**   **Foreign body in respiratory tract**

The appropriate 7th character is to be added to each code from category T17

> A   initial encounter
> D   subsequent encounter
> S   sequela

   X● **T17.0**   **Foreign body in nasal sinus**
   X● **T17.1**   **Foreign body in nostril**
     Foreign body in nose NOS
● **T17.2**   **Foreign body in pharynx**
     Foreign body in nasopharynx
     Foreign body in throat NOS
   ● **T17.20**   **Unspecified foreign body in pharynx**
     ● **T17.200**   **Unspecified foreign body in pharynx causing asphyxiation**
     ● **T17.208**   **Unspecified foreign body in pharynx causing other injury**
   ● **T17.21**   **Gastric contents in pharynx**
     Aspiration of gastric contents into pharynx
     Vomitus in pharynx
     ● **T17.210**   **Gastric contents in pharynx causing asphyxiation**
     ● **T17.218**   **Gastric contents in pharynx causing other injury**
   ● **T17.22**   **Food in pharynx**
     Bones in pharynx
     Seeds in pharynx
     ● **T17.220**   **Food in pharynx causing asphyxiation**
     ● **T17.228**   **Food in pharynx causing other injury**
   ● **T17.29**   **Other foreign object in pharynx**
     ● **T17.290**   **Other foreign object in pharynx causing asphyxiation**
     ● **T17.298**   **Other foreign object in pharynx causing other injury**
● **T17.3**   **Foreign body in larynx**
   ● **T17.30**   **Unspecified foreign body in larynx**
     ● **T17.300**   **Unspecified foreign body in larynx causing asphyxiation**
     ● **T17.308**   **Unspecified foreign body in larynx causing other injury**
   ● **T17.31**   **Gastric contents in larynx**
     Aspiration of gastric contents into larynx
     Vomitus in larynx
     ● **T17.310**   **Gastric contents in larynx causing asphyxiation**
     ● **T17.318**   **Gastric contents in larynx causing other injury**
   ● **T17.32**   **Food in larynx**
     Bones in larynx
     Seeds in larynx
     ● **T17.320**   **Food in larynx causing asphyxiation**
     ● **T17.328**   **Food in larynx causing other injury**
   ● **T17.39**   **Other foreign object in larynx**
     ● **T17.390**   **Other foreign object in larynx causing asphyxiation**
     ● **T17.398**   **Other foreign object in larynx causing other injury**
● **T17.4**   **Foreign body in trachea**
   ● **T17.40**   **Unspecified foreign body in trachea**
     ● **T17.400**   **Unspecified foreign body in trachea causing asphyxiation**
     ● **T17.408**   **Unspecified foreign body in trachea causing other injury**

●T17.41   Gastric contents in trachea
          Aspiration of gastric contents into trachea
          Vomitus in trachea
    ●T17.410   Gastric contents in trachea causing
               asphyxiation
    ●T17.418   Gastric contents in trachea causing
               other injury
●T17.42   Food in trachea
          Bones in trachea
          Seeds in trachea
    ●T17.420   Food in trachea causing asphyxiation
    ●T17.428   Food in trachea causing other injury
●T17.49   Other foreign object in trachea
    ●T17.490   Other foreign object in trachea
               causing asphyxiation
    ●T17.498   Other foreign object in trachea
               causing other injury
●T17.5 Foreign body in bronchus
  ●T17.50   Unspecified foreign body in bronchus
    ●T17.500   Unspecified foreign body in bronchus
               causing asphyxiation
    ●T17.508   Unspecified foreign body in bronchus
               causing other injury
  ●T17.51   Gastric contents in bronchus
            Aspiration of gastric contents into bronchus
            Vomitus in bronchus
    ●T17.510   Gastric contents in bronchus causing
               asphyxiation
    ●T17.518   Gastric contents in bronchus causing
               other injury
  ●T17.52   Food in bronchus
            Bones in bronchus
            Seeds in bronchus
    ●T17.520   Food in bronchus causing
               asphyxiation
    ●T17.528   Food in bronchus causing other
               injury
  ●T17.59   Other foreign object in bronchus
    ●T17.590   Other foreign object in bronchus
               causing asphyxiation
    ●T17.598   Other foreign object in bronchus
               causing other injury
●T17.8 Foreign body in other parts of respiratory tract
        Foreign body in bronchioles
        Foreign body in lung
  ●T17.80   Unspecified foreign body in other parts of
            respiratory tract
    ●T17.800   Unspecified foreign body in other
               parts of respiratory tract causing
               asphyxiation
    ●T17.808   Unspecified foreign body in other
               parts of respiratory tract causing other
               injury
  ●T17.81   Gastric contents in other parts of respiratory
            tract
            Aspiration of gastric contents into other parts
               of respiratory tract
            Vomitus in other parts of respiratory tract
    ●T17.810   Gastric contents in other parts of
               respiratory tract causing asphyxiation
    ●T17.818   Gastric contents in other parts of
               respiratory tract causing other injury
  ●T17.82   Food in other parts of respiratory tract
            Bones in other parts of respiratory tract
            Seeds in other parts of respiratory tract
    ●T17.820   Food in other parts of respiratory tract
               causing asphyxiation
    ●T17.828   Food in other parts of respiratory tract
               causing other injury

●T17.89   Other foreign object in other parts of
          respiratory tract
    ●T17.890   Other foreign object in other parts of
               respiratory tract causing asphyxiation
    ●T17.898   Other foreign object in other parts of
               respiratory tract causing other injury
●T17.9 Foreign body in respiratory tract, part unspecified
  ●T17.90   Unspecified foreign body in respiratory tract,
            part unspecified
    ●T17.900   Unspecified foreign body in
               respiratory tract, part unspecified
               causing asphyxiation
    ●T17.908   Unspecified foreign body in
               respiratory tract, part unspecified
               causing other injury
  ●T17.91   Gastric contents in respiratory tract, part
            unspecified
            Aspiration of gastric contents into respiratory
               tract, part unspecified
            Vomitus in trachea respiratory tract, part
               unspecified
    ●T17.910   Gastric contents in respiratory tract,
               part unspecified causing asphyxiation
    ●T17.918   Gastric contents in respiratory tract,
               part unspecified causing other injury
  ●T17.92   Food in respiratory tract, part unspecified
            Bones in respiratory tract, part unspecified
            Seeds in respiratory tract, part unspecified
    ●T17.920   Food in respiratory tract, part
               unspecified causing asphyxiation
    ●T17.928   Food in respiratory tract, part
               unspecified causing other injury
  ●T17.99   Other foreign object in respiratory tract, part
            unspecified
    ●T17.990   Other foreign object in respiratory
               tract, part unspecified in causing
               asphyxiation
               Coding Clinic: 2019, Q3, P15
    ●T17.998   Other foreign object in respiratory
               tract, part unspecified causing other
               injury

●T18   Foreign body in alimentary tract
       Excludes2   foreign body in pharynx (T17.2-)
       The appropriate 7th character is to be added to each code from
          category T18

       | A   initial encounter |
       | D   subsequent encounter |
       | S   sequela |

X●T18.0   Foreign body in mouth
X●T18.1   Foreign body in esophagus
         Excludes2   foreign body in respiratory tract (T17.-)
  ●T18.10   Unspecified foreign body in esophagus
    ●T18.100   Unspecified foreign body in
               esophagus causing compression of
               trachea
               Unspecified foreign body in
                  esophagus causing obstruction
                  of respiration
    ●T18.108   Unspecified foreign body in
               esophagus causing other injury
  ●T18.11   Gastric contents in esophagus
            Vomitus in esophagus
    ●T18.110   Gastric contents in esophagus causing
               compression of trachea
               Gastric contents in esophagus
                  causing obstruction of
                  respiration
    ●T18.118   Gastric contents in esophagus causing
               other injury

CHAPTER 19 (S00–T88)

CHAPTER 19 (S00-T88)

● **T18.12** **Food in esophagus**
　　　Bones in esophagus
　　　Seeds in esophagus

　　● **T18.120** **Food in esophagus causing compression of trachea**
　　　　　Food in esophagus causing obstruction of respiration

　　● **T18.128** **Food in esophagus causing other injury**

● **T18.19** **Other foreign object in esophagus**

　　● **T18.190** **Other foreign object in esophagus causing compression of trachea**
　　　　　Other foreign body in esophagus causing obstruction of respiration
　　　　　Coding Clinic: 2015, Q1, P24

　　● **T18.198** **Other foreign object in esophagus causing other injury**
　　　　　Coding Clinic: 2015, Q1, P24

X● **T18.2** **Foreign body in stomach**
X● **T18.3** **Foreign body in small intestine**
X● **T18.4** **Foreign body in colon**
X● **T18.5** **Foreign body in anus and rectum**
　　　Foreign body in rectosigmoid (junction)
X● **T18.8** **Foreign body in other parts of alimentary tract**
X● **T18.9** **Foreign body of alimentary tract, part unspecified**
　　　Foreign body in digestive system NOS
　　　Swallowed foreign body NOS

● **T19** **Foreign body in genitourinary tract**
　　Excludes2 complications due to implanted mesh (T83.7-)
　　　　　mechanical complications of contraceptive device (intrauterine) (vaginal) (T83.3-)
　　　　　presence of contraceptive device (intrauterine) (vaginal) (Z97.5)

The appropriate 7th character is to be added to each code from category T19

A	initial encounter
D	subsequent encounter
S	sequela

X● **T19.0** **Foreign body in urethra**
X● **T19.1** **Foreign body in bladder**
X● **T19.2** **Foreign body in vulva and vagina ♀**
X● **T19.3** **Foreign body in uterus ♀**
X● **T19.4** **Foreign body in penis ♂**
X● **T19.8** **Foreign body in other parts of genitourinary tract**
X● **T19.9** **Foreign body in genitourinary tract, part unspecified**

BURNS AND CORROSIONS (T20-T32)

Includes burns (thermal) from electrical heating appliances
　　　　burns (thermal) from electricity
　　　　burns (thermal) from flame
　　　　burns (thermal) from friction
　　　　burns (thermal) from hot air and hot gases
　　　　burns (thermal) from hot objects
　　　　burns (thermal) from lightning
　　　　burns (thermal) from radiation chemical
　　　　burn [corrosion] (external) (internal) scalds

Excludes2 erythema [dermatitis] ab igne (L59.0)
　　　　radiation-related disorders of the skin and subcutaneous tissue (L55-L59)
　　　　sunburn (L55.-)

OGCR Section I.C.19.d.

Burns and Corrosions

The ICD-10-CM makes a distinction between burn and corrosions. The burn codes are for thermal burns, except sunburns, that come from a heat source, such as a fire or hot appliance. The burn codes are also for burns resulting from electricity and radiation. Corrosions are burns due to chemicals. The guidelines for burns and corrosions are the same.

Current burns (T20-T25) are classified by depth, extent and by agent (X code). Burns are classified by depth as first degree (erythema), second degree (blistering), and third degree (full-thickness involvement). Burns of the eye and internal organs (T26-T28) are classified by site, but not by degree.

1) Sequencing of burn and related condition codes

Sequence first the code that reflects the highest degree of burn when more than one burn is present.

a. When the reason for the admission or encounter is for treatment of external multiple burns, sequence first the code that reflects the burn of the highest degree.

b. When a patient has both internal and external burns, the circumstances of admission govern the selection of the principal diagnosis or first-listed diagnosis.

c. When a patient is admitted for burn injuries and other related conditions such as smoke inhalation and/or respiratory failure, the circumstances of admission govern the selection of the principal or first-listed diagnosis.

2) Burns of the same local site

Classify burns of the same local site (three-character category level, T20-T28) but of different degrees to the subcategory identifying the highest degree recorded in the diagnosis.

BURNS AND CORROSIONS OF EXTERNAL BODY SURFACE, SPECIFIED BY SITE (T20-T25)

Includes burns and corrosions of first degree [erythema]
　　　　burns and corrosions of second degree [blisters] [epidermal loss]
　　　　burns and corrosions of third degree [deep necrosis of underlying tissue] [full-thickness skin loss]

Use additional code from category T31 or T32 to identify extent of body surface involved

● **T20** **Burn and corrosion of head, face, and neck**
　　Excludes2 burn and corrosion of ear drum (T28.41, T28.91)
　　　　　burn and corrosion of eye and adnexa (T26.-)
　　　　　burn and corrosion of mouth and pharynx (T28.0)

The appropriate 7th character is to be added to each code from category T20

A	initial encounter
D	subsequent encounter
S	sequela

● **T20.0** **Burn of unspecified degree of head, face, and neck**
　　　Use additional external cause code to identify the source, place and intent of the burn (X00-X19, X75-X77, X96-X98, Y92)

X● **T20.00** **Burn of unspecified degree of head, face, and neck, unspecified site**

● **T20.01** **Burn of unspecified degree of ear [any part, except ear drum]**
　　　Excludes2 burn of ear drum (T28.41-)

● **T20.011** **Burn of unspecified degree of right ear [any part, except ear drum]**

● **T20.012** **Burn of unspecified degree of left ear [any part, except ear drum]**

● **T20.019** **Burn of unspecified degree of unspecified ear [any part, except ear drum]**

Figure 19-15 **A.** Second-degree burn. **B.** Third-degree burn. (A. From Black J, Hawks J: Medical-Surgical Nursing: Clinical Management for Positive Outcomes, 8e, Saunders, 2008. B. From Marx J, Hockberger R, Walls R: Rosen's Emergency Medicine - Concepts and Clinical Practice, 7e, Mosby, 2009)

X ● **T20.02** Burn of unspecified degree of lip(s)

X ● **T20.03** Burn of unspecified degree of chin

X ● **T20.04** Burn of unspecified degree of nose (septum)

X ● **T20.05** Burn of unspecified degree of scalp [any part]

X ● **T20.06** Burn of unspecified degree of forehead and cheek

X ● **T20.07** Burn of unspecified degree of neck

X ● **T20.09** Burn of unspecified degree of multiple sites of head, face, and neck

● **T20.1** Burn of first degree of head, face, and neck

　　　Use additional external cause code to identify the source, place and intent of the burn (X00-X19, X75-X77, X96-X98, Y92)

X ● **T20.10** Burn of first degree of head, face, and neck, unspecified site

● **T20.11** Burn of first degree of ear [any part, except ear drum]

　　　　Excludes2   burn of ear drum (T28.41-)

● **T20.111** Burn of first degree of right ear [any part, except ear drum]

● **T20.112** Burn of first degree of left ear [any part, except ear drum]

● **T20.119** Burn of first degree of unspecified ear [any part, except ear drum]

X ● **T20.12** Burn of first degree of lip(s)

X ● **T20.13** Burn of first degree of chin

X ● **T20.14** Burn of first degree of nose (septum)

X ● **T20.15** Burn of first degree of scalp [any part]

X ● **T20.16** Burn of first degree of forehead and cheek

X ● **T20.17** Burn of first degree of neck

X ● **T20.19** Burn of first degree of multiple sites of head, face, and neck

● **T20.2** Burn of second degree of head, face, and neck

　　　Use additional external cause code to identify the source, place and intent of the burn (X00-X19, X75-X77, X96-X98, Y92)

X ● **T20.20** Burn of second degree of head, face, and neck, unspecified site

● **T20.21** Burn of second degree of ear [any part, except ear drum]

　　　　Excludes2   burn of ear drum (T28.41-)

● **T20.211** Burn of second degree of right ear [any part, except ear drum]

● **T20.212** Burn of second degree of left ear [any part, except ear drum]

● **T20.219** Burn of second degree of unspecified ear [any part, except ear drum]

X ● **T20.22** Burn of second degree of lip(s)

X ● **T20.23** Burn of second degree of chin

X ● **T20.24** Burn of second degree of nose (septum)

X ● **T20.25** Burn of second degree of scalp [any part]
　　　　Coding Clinic: 2015, Q1, P19

X ● **T20.26** Burn of second degree of forehead and cheek

X ● **T20.27** Burn of second degree of neck

X ● **T20.29** Burn of second degree of multiple sites of head, face, and neck

● **T20.3** Burn of third degree of head, face, and neck

　　　Use additional external cause code to identify the source, place and intent of the burn (X00-X19, X75-X77, X96-X98, Y92)

X ● **T20.30** Burn of third degree of head, face, and neck, unspecified site

● **T20.31** Burn of third degree of ear [any part, except ear drum]

　　　　Excludes2   burn of ear drum (T28.41-)

● **T20.311** Burn of third degree of right ear [any part, except ear drum]

● **T20.312** Burn of third degree of left ear [any part, except ear drum]
　　　　Coding Clinic: 2015, Q1, P18

● **T20.319** Burn of third degree of unspecified ear [any part, except ear drum]

X ● **T20.32** Burn of third degree of lip(s)

X ● **T20.33** Burn of third degree of chin

X ● **T20.34** Burn of third degree of nose (septum)

X ● **T20.35** Burn of third degree of scalp [any part]

X ● **T20.36** Burn of third degree of forehead and cheek

X ● **T20.37** Burn of third degree of neck

X ● **T20.39** Burn of third degree of multiple sites of head, face, and neck

● **T20.4** Corrosion of unspecified degree of head, face, and neck

　　　Code first (T51-T65) to identify chemical and intent

　　　Use additional external cause code to identify place (Y92)

X ● **T20.40** Corrosion of unspecified degree of head, face, and neck, unspecified site

● **T20.41** Corrosion of unspecified degree of ear [any part, except ear drum]

　　　　Excludes2   corrosion of ear drum (T28.91-)

● **T20.411** Corrosion of unspecified degree of right ear [any part, except ear drum]

● **T20.412** Corrosion of unspecified degree of left ear [any part, except ear drum]

● **T20.419** Corrosion of unspecified degree of unspecified ear [any part, except ear drum]

X ● **T20.42** Corrosion of unspecified degree of lip(s)

X ● **T20.43** Corrosion of unspecified degree of chin

X ● **T20.44** Corrosion of unspecified degree of nose (septum)

X ● **T20.45** Corrosion of unspecified degree of scalp [any part]

X ● **T20.46** Corrosion of unspecified degree of forehead and cheek

X ● **T20.47** Corrosion of unspecified degree of neck

X ● **T20.49** Corrosion of unspecified degree of multiple sites of head, face, and neck

● **T20.5** Corrosion of first degree of head, face, and neck

　　　Code first (T51-T65) to identify chemical and intent

　　　Use additional external cause code to identify place (Y92)

X ● **T20.50** Corrosion of first degree of head, face, and neck, unspecified site

● **T20.51** Corrosion of first degree of ear [any part, except ear drum]

　　　　Excludes2   corrosion of ear drum (T28.91-)

CHAPTER 19 (S00-T88)

● **T20.511** Corrosion of first degree of **right ear** [any part, except ear drum]

● **T20.512** Corrosion of first degree of **left ear** [any part, except ear drum]

● **T20.519** Corrosion of first degree of **unspecified ear** [any part, except ear drum]

X● **T20.52** Corrosion of first degree of **lip(s)**

X● **T20.53** Corrosion of first degree of **chin**

X● **T20.54** Corrosion of first degree of **nose (septum)**

X● **T20.55** Corrosion of first degree of **scalp** [any part]

X● **T20.56** Corrosion of first degree of **forehead and cheek**

X● **T20.57** Corrosion of first degree of **neck**

X● **T20.59** Corrosion of first degree of **multiple sites of head, face, and neck**

● **T20.6** Corrosion of **second degree** of head, face, and neck

Code first (T51-T65) *to identify chemical and intent*

Use additional external cause code to identify place (Y92)

X● **T20.60** Corrosion of second degree of head, face, and neck, **unspecified site**

● **T20.61** Corrosion of second degree of **ear** [any part, except ear drum]

     Excludes2   corrosion of ear drum (T28.91-)

● **T20.611** Corrosion of second degree of **right ear** [any part, except ear drum]

● **T20.612** Corrosion of second degree of **left ear** [any part, except ear drum]

● **T20.619** Corrosion of second degree of **unspecified ear** [any part, except ear drum]

X● **T20.62** Corrosion of second degree of **lip(s)**

X● **T20.63** Corrosion of second degree of **chin**

X● **T20.64** Corrosion of second degree of **nose (septum)**

X● **T20.65** Corrosion of second degree of **scalp** [any part]

X● **T20.66** Corrosion of second degree of **forehead and cheek**

X● **T20.67** Corrosion of second degree of **neck**

X● **T20.69** Corrosion of second degree of **multiple sites of head, face, and neck**

● **T20.7** Corrosion of **third degree** of head, face, and neck

Code first (T51-T65) *to identify chemical and intent*

Use additional external cause code to identify place (Y92)

X● **T20.70** Corrosion of third degree of head, face, and neck, **unspecified site**

● **T20.71** Corrosion of third degree of **ear** [any part, except ear drum]

     Excludes2   corrosion of ear drum (T28.91-)

● **T20.711** Corrosion of third degree of **right ear** [any part, except ear drum]

● **T20.712** Corrosion of third degree of **left ear** [any part, except ear drum]

● **T20.719** Corrosion of third degree of **unspecified ear** [any part, except ear drum]

X● **T20.72** Corrosion of third degree of **lip(s)**

X● **T20.73** Corrosion of third degree of **chin**

X● **T20.74** Corrosion of third degree of **nose (septum)**

X● **T20.75** Corrosion of third degree of **scalp** [any part]

X● **T20.76** Corrosion of third degree of **forehead and cheek**

X● **T20.77** Corrosion of third degree of **neck**

X● **T20.79** Corrosion of third degree of **multiple sites of head, face, and neck**

● **T21** Burn and corrosion of trunk

    Includes   burns and corrosion of hip region

    Excludes2   burns and corrosion of axilla (T22.- with fifth character 4)

burns and corrosion of scapular region (T22.- with fifth character 6)

burns and corrosion of shoulder (T22.- with fifth character 5)

The appropriate 7th character is to be added to each code from category T21

A	initial encounter
D	subsequent encounter
S	sequela

● **T21.0** Burn of **unspecified degree of trunk**

Use additional external cause code to identify the source, place and intent of the burn (X00-X19, X75-X77, X96-X98, Y92)

X● **T21.00** Burn of unspecified degree of trunk, **unspecified site**

X● **T21.01** Burn of unspecified degree of **chest wall**

Burn of unspecified degree of breast

X● **T21.02** Burn of unspecified degree of **abdominal wall**

Burn of unspecified degree of flank

Burn of unspecified degree of groin

X● **T21.03** Burn of unspecified degree of **upper back**

Burn of unspecified degree of interscapular region

X● **T21.04** Burn of unspecified degree of **lower back**

X● **T21.05** Burn of unspecified degree of **buttock**

Burn of unspecified degree of anus

X● **T21.06** Burn of unspecified degree of **male genital region** ♂

Burn of unspecified degree of penis

Burn of unspecified degree of scrotum

Burn of unspecified degree of testis

X● **T21.07** Burn of unspecified degree of **female genital region** ♀

Burn of unspecified degree of labium (majus) (minus)

Burn of unspecified degree of perineum

Burn of unspecified degree of vulva

     Excludes2   burn of vagina (T28.3)

X● **T21.09** Burn of unspecified degree of **other site of trunk**

● **T21.1** Burn of **first degree of trunk**

Use additional external cause code to identify the source, place and intent of the burn (X00-X19, X75-X77, X96-X98, Y92)

X● **T21.10** Burn of first degree of trunk, **unspecified site**

X● **T21.11** Burn of first degree of **chest wall**

Burn of first degree of breast

X● **T21.12** Burn of first degree of **abdominal wall**

Burn of first degree of flank

Burn of first degree of groin

X● **T21.13** Burn of first degree of **upper back**

Burn of first degree of interscapular region

X● **T21.14** Burn of first degree of **lower back**

X● **T21.15** Burn of first degree of **buttock**

Burn of first degree of anus

X● **T21.16** Burn of first degree of **male genital region** ♂

Burn of first degree of penis

Burn of first degree of scrotum

Burn of first degree of testis

X● **T21.17** Burn of first degree of **female genital region** ♀

Burn of first degree of labium (majus) (minus)

Burn of first degree of perineum

Burn of first degree of vulva

     Excludes2   burn of vagina (T28.3)

X● **T21.19** Burn of first degree of **other site of trunk**

● **T21.2**   **Burn of second degree of trunk**
     Use additional external cause code to identify the
       source, place and intent of the burn (X00-X19,
       X75-X77, X96-X98, Y92)

X● **T21.20**   **Burn of second degree of trunk, unspecified site**

X● **T21.21**   **Burn of second degree of chest wall**
     Burn of second degree of breast

X● **T21.22**   **Burn of second degree of abdominal wall**
     Burn of second degree of flank
     Burn of second degree of groin

X● **T21.23**   **Burn of second degree of upper back**
     Burn of second degree of interscapular region

X● **T21.24**   **Burn of second degree of lower back**

X● **T21.25**   **Burn of second degree of buttock**
     Burn of second degree of anus

X● **T21.26**   **Burn of second degree of male genital region** ♂
     Burn of second degree of penis
     Burn of second degree of scrotum
     Burn of second degree of testis

X● **T21.27**   **Burn of second degree of female genital region** ♀
     Burn of second degree of labium (majus)
       (minus)
     Burn of second degree of perineum
     Burn of second degree of vulva
     Excludes2   burn of vagina (T28.3)

X● **T21.29**   **Burn of second degree of other site of trunk**

● **T21.3**   **Burn of third degree of trunk**
     Use additional external cause code to identify the
       source, place and intent of the burn (X00-X19,
       X75-X77, X96-X98, Y92)

X● **T21.30**   **Burn of third degree of trunk, unspecified site**

X● **T21.31**   **Burn of third degree of chest wall**
     Burn of third degree of breast
     Coding Clinic: 2016, Q2, P6

X● **T21.32**   **Burn of third degree of abdominal wall**
     Burn of third degree of flank
     Burn of third degree of groin

X● **T21.33**   **Burn of third degree of upper back**
     Burn of third degree of interscapular region

X● **T21.34**   **Burn of third degree of lower back**

X● **T21.35**   **Burn of third degree of buttock**
     Burn of third degree of anus

X● **T21.36**   **Burn of third degree of male genital region** ♂
     Burn of third degree of penis
     Burn of third degree of scrotum
     Burn of third degree of testis

X● **T21.37**   **Burn of third degree of female genital region** ♀
     Burn of third degree of labium (majus) (minus)
     Burn of third degree of perineum
     Burn of third degree of vulva
     Excludes2   burn of vagina (T28.3)

X● **T21.39**   **Burn of third degree of other site of trunk**

● **T21.4**   **Corrosion of unspecified degree of trunk**
     Code first (T51-T65) to identify chemical and intent
     Use additional external cause code to identify
       place (Y92)

X● **T21.40**   **Corrosion of unspecified degree of trunk, unspecified site**

X● **T21.41**   **Corrosion of unspecified degree of chest wall**
     Corrosion of unspecified degree of breast

X● **T21.42**   **Corrosion of unspecified degree of abdominal wall**
     Corrosion of unspecified degree of flank
     Corrosion of unspecified degree of groin

X● **T21.43**   **Corrosion of unspecified degree of upper back**
     Corrosion of unspecified degree of
       interscapular region

X● **T21.44**   **Corrosion of unspecified degree of lower back**

X● **T21.45**   **Corrosion of unspecified degree of buttock**
     Corrosion of unspecified degree of anus

X● **T21.46**   **Corrosion of unspecified degree of male genital region** ♂
     Corrosion of unspecified degree of penis
     Corrosion of unspecified degree of scrotum
     Corrosion of unspecified degree of testis

X● **T21.47**   **Corrosion of unspecified degree of female genital region** ♀
     Corrosion of unspecified degree of labium
       (majus) (minus)
     Corrosion of unspecified degree of perineum
     Corrosion of unspecified degree of vulva
     Excludes2   corrosion of vagina (T28.8)

X● **T21.49**   **Corrosion of unspecified degree of other site of trunk**

● **T21.5**   **Corrosion of first degree of trunk**
     Code first (T51-T65) to identify chemical and intent
     Use additional external cause code to identify
       place (Y92)

X● **T21.50**   **Corrosion of first degree of trunk, unspecified site**

X● **T21.51**   **Corrosion of first degree of chest wall**
     Corrosion of first degree of breast

X● **T21.52**   **Corrosion of first degree of abdominal wall**
     Corrosion of first degree of flank
     Corrosion of first degree of groin

X● **T21.53**   **Corrosion of first degree of upper back**
     Corrosion of first degree of interscapular
       region

X● **T21.54**   **Corrosion of first degree of lower back**

X● **T21.55**   **Corrosion of first degree of buttock**
     Corrosion of first degree of anus

X● **T21.56**   **Corrosion of first degree of male genital region** ♂
     Corrosion of first degree of penis
     Corrosion of first degree of scrotum
     Corrosion of first degree of testis

X● **T21.57**   **Corrosion of first degree of female genital region** ♀
     Corrosion of first degree of labium (majus)
       (minus)
     Corrosion of first degree of perineum
     Corrosion of first degree of vulva
     Excludes2   corrosion of vagina (T28.8)

X● **T21.59**   **Corrosion of first degree of other site of trunk**

● **T21.6**   **Corrosion of second degree of trunk**
     Code first (T51-T65) to identify chemical and intent
     Use additional external cause code to identify
       place (Y92)

X● **T21.60**   **Corrosion of second degree of trunk, unspecified site**

X● **T21.61**   **Corrosion of second degree of chest wall**
     Corrosion of second degree of breast

X● **T21.62**   **Corrosion of second degree of abdominal wall**
     Corrosion of second degree of flank
     Corrosion of second degree of groin

CHAPTER 19 (S00-T88)

X ● **T21.63** **Corrosion of second degree of upper back**
Corrosion of second degree of interscapular region

X ● **T21.64** **Corrosion of second degree of lower back**

X ● **T21.65** **Corrosion of second degree of buttock**
Corrosion of second degree of anus

X ● **T21.66** **Corrosion of second degree of male genital region** ♂
Corrosion of second degree of penis
Corrosion of second degree of scrotum
Corrosion of second degree of testis

X ● **T21.67** **Corrosion of second degree of female genital region** ♀
Corrosion of second degree of labium (majus) (minus)
Corrosion of second degree of perineum
Corrosion of second degree of vulva
Excludes2   corrosion of vagina (T28.8)

X ● **T21.69** **Corrosion of second degree of other site of trunk**

● **T21.7** **Corrosion of third degree of trunk**
Code first (T51-T65) to identify chemical and intent
Use additional external cause code to identify place (Y92)

X ● **T21.70** **Corrosion of third degree of trunk, unspecified site**

X ● **T21.71** **Corrosion of third degree of chest wall**
Corrosion of third degree of breast

X ● **T21.72** **Corrosion of third degree of abdominal wall**
Corrosion of third degree of flank
Corrosion of third degree of groin

X ● **T21.73** **Corrosion of third degree of upper back**
Corrosion of third degree of interscapular region

X ● **T21.74** **Corrosion of third degree of lower back**

X ● **T21.75** **Corrosion of third degree of buttock**
Corrosion of third degree of anus

X ● **T21.76** **Corrosion of third degree of male genital region** ♂
Corrosion of third degree of penis
Corrosion of third degree of scrotum
Corrosion of third degree of testis

X ● **T21.77** **Corrosion of third degree of female genital region** ♀
Corrosion of third degree of labium (majus) (minus)
Corrosion of third degree of perineum
Corrosion of third degree of vulva
Excludes2   corrosion of vagina (T28.8)

X ● **T21.79** **Corrosion of third degree of other site of trunk**

● **T22** **Burn and corrosion of shoulder and upper limb, except wrist and hand**
Excludes2   burn and corrosion of interscapular region (T21.-)
burn and corrosion of wrist and hand (T23.-)

The appropriate 7th character is to be added to each code from category T22

A	initial encounter
D	subsequent encounter
S	sequela

● **T22.0** **Burn of unspecified degree of shoulder and upper limb, except wrist and hand**
Use additional external cause code to identify the source, place and intent of the burn (X00-X19, X75-X77, X96-X98, Y92)

X ● **T22.00** **Burn of unspecified degree of shoulder and upper limb, except wrist and hand, unspecified site**

● **T22.01** **Burn of unspecified degree of forearm**

● **T22.011** **Burn of unspecified degree of right forearm**

● **T22.012** **Burn of unspecified degree of left forearm**

● **T22.019** **Burn of unspecified degree of unspecified forearm**

● **T22.02** **Burn of unspecified degree of elbow**

● **T22.021** **Burn of unspecified degree of right elbow**

● **T22.022** **Burn of unspecified degree of left elbow**

● **T22.029** **Burn of unspecified degree of unspecified elbow**

● **T22.03** **Burn of unspecified degree of upper arm**

● **T22.031** **Burn of unspecified degree of right upper arm**

● **T22.032** **Burn of unspecified degree of left upper arm**

● **T22.039** **Burn of unspecified degree of unspecified upper arm**

● **T22.04** **Burn of unspecified degree of axilla**

● **T22.041** **Burn of unspecified degree of right axilla**

● **T22.042** **Burn of unspecified degree of left axilla**

● **T22.049** **Burn of unspecified degree of unspecified axilla**

● **T22.05** **Burn of unspecified degree of shoulder**

● **T22.051** **Burn of unspecified degree of right shoulder**

● **T22.052** **Burn of unspecified degree of left shoulder**

● **T22.059** **Burn of unspecified degree of unspecified shoulder**

● **T22.06** **Burn of unspecified degree of scapular region**

● **T22.061** **Burn of unspecified degree of right scapular region**

● **T22.062** **Burn of unspecified degree of left scapular region**

● **T22.069** **Burn of unspecified degree of unspecified scapular region**

● **T22.09** **Burn of unspecified degree of multiple sites of shoulder and upper limb, except wrist and hand**

● **T22.091** **Burn of unspecified degree of multiple sites of right shoulder and upper limb, except wrist and hand**

● **T22.092** **Burn of unspecified degree of multiple sites of left shoulder and upper limb, except wrist and hand**

● **T22.099** **Burn of unspecified degree of multiple sites of unspecified shoulder and upper limb, except wrist and hand**

▶ New   ⫸ Revised   ~~deleted~~ Deleted   Excludes 1   Excludes 2   Includes   Use additional   Code first   Code also   Key words
OGCR Official Guidelines   X Assign placeholder X   ● Use Additional Character(s)   ▶ Manifestation Code   🔗 Hierarchical Condition Category   **Coding Clinic**

● T22.1   Burn of first degree of shoulder and upper limb, except wrist and hand

> Use additional external cause code to identify the source, place and intent of the burn (X00-X19, X75-X77, X96-X98, Y92)

X ● T22.10   Burn of first degree of shoulder and upper limb, except wrist and hand, unspecified site

● T22.11   Burn of first degree of forearm

   ● T22.111   Burn of first degree of right forearm

   ● T22.112   Burn of first degree of left forearm

   ● T22.119   Burn of first degree of unspecified forearm

● T22.12   Burn of first degree of elbow

   ● T22.121   Burn of first degree of right elbow

   ● T22.122   Burn of first degree of left elbow

   ● T22.129   Burn of first degree of unspecified elbow

● T22.13   Burn of first degree of upper arm

   ● T22.131   Burn of first degree of right upper arm

   ● T22.132   Burn of first degree of left upper arm

   ● T22.139   Burn of first degree of unspecified upper arm

● T22.14   Burn of first degree of axilla

   ● T22.141   Burn of first degree of right axilla

   ● T22.142   Burn of first degree of left axilla

   ● T22.149   Burn of first degree of unspecified axilla

● T22.15   Burn of first degree of shoulder

   ● T22.151   Burn of first degree of right shoulder

   ● T22.152   Burn of first degree of left shoulder

   ● T22.159   Burn of first degree of unspecified shoulder

● T22.16   Burn of first degree of scapular region

   ● T22.161   Burn of first degree of right scapular region

   ● T22.162   Burn of first degree of left scapular region

   ● T22.169   Burn of first degree of unspecified scapular region

● T22.19   Burn of first degree of multiple sites of shoulder and upper limb, except wrist and hand

   ● T22.191   Burn of first degree of multiple sites of right shoulder and upper limb, except wrist and hand

   ● T22.192   Burn of first degree of multiple sites of left shoulder and upper limb, except wrist and hand

   ● T22.199   Burn of first degree of multiple sites of unspecified shoulder and upper limb, except wrist and hand

● T22.2   Burn of second degree of shoulder and upper limb, except wrist and hand

> Use additional external cause code to identify the source, place and intent of the burn (X00-X19, X75-X77, X96-X98, Y92)

X ● T22.20   Burn of second degree of shoulder and upper limb, except wrist and hand, unspecified site

● T22.21   Burn of second degree of forearm

   ● T22.211   Burn of second degree of right forearm

   ● T22.212   Burn of second degree of left forearm

   ● T22.219   Burn of second degree of unspecified forearm

● T22.22   Burn of second degree of elbow

   ● T22.221   Burn of second degree of right elbow

   ● T22.222   Burn of second degree of left elbow

   ● T22.229   Burn of second degree of unspecified elbow

● T22.23   Burn of second degree of upper arm

   ● T22.231   Burn of second degree of right upper arm

   ● T22.232   Burn of second degree of left upper arm

   ● T22.239   Burn of second degree of unspecified upper arm

● T22.24   Burn of second degree of axilla

   ● T22.241   Burn of second degree of right axilla

   ● T22.242   Burn of second degree of left axilla

   ● T22.249   Burn of second degree of unspecified axilla

● T22.25   Burn of second degree of shoulder

   ● T22.251   Burn of second degree of right shoulder

   ● T22.252   Burn of second degree of left shoulder

   ● T22.259   Burn of second degree of unspecified shoulder

● T22.26   Burn of second degree of scapular region

   ● T22.261   Burn of second degree of right scapular region

   ● T22.262   Burn of second degree of left scapular region

   ● T22.269   Burn of second degree of unspecified scapular region

● T22.29   Burn of second degree of multiple sites of shoulder and upper limb, except wrist and hand

   ● T22.291   Burn of second degree of multiple sites of right shoulder and upper limb, except wrist and hand

   ● T22.292   Burn of second degree of multiple sites of left shoulder and upper limb, except wrist and hand

   ● T22.299   Burn of second degree of multiple sites of unspecified shoulder and upper limb, except wrist and hand

● T22.3   Burn of third degree of shoulder and upper limb, except wrist and hand

> Use additional external cause code to identify the source, place and intent of the burn (X00-X19, X75-X77, X96-X98, Y92)

X ● T22.30   Burn of third degree of shoulder and upper limb, except wrist and hand, unspecified site

● T22.31   Burn of third degree of forearm

   ● T22.311   Burn of third degree of right forearm

   ● T22.312   Burn of third degree of left forearm

   ● T22.319   Burn of third degree of unspecified forearm

● T22.32   Burn of third degree of elbow

   ● T22.321   Burn of third degree of right elbow

   ● T22.322   Burn of third degree of left elbow

   ● T22.329   Burn of third degree of unspecified elbow

● T22.33   Burn of third degree of upper arm

   ● T22.331   Burn of third degree of right upper arm

   ● T22.332   Burn of third degree of left upper arm

   ● T22.339   Burn of third degree of unspecified upper arm

● **T22.34**   **Burn of third degree of axilla**
    ● **T22.341**   Burn of third degree of right axilla
    ● **T22.342**   Burn of third degree of left axilla
    ● **T22.349**   Burn of third degree of unspecified axilla

● **T22.35**   **Burn of third degree of shoulder**
    ● **T22.351**   Burn of third degree of right shoulder
    ● **T22.352**   Burn of third degree of left shoulder
    ● **T22.359**   Burn of third degree of unspecified shoulder

● **T22.36**   **Burn of third degree of scapular region**
    ● **T22.361**   Burn of third degree of right scapular region
    ● **T22.362**   Burn of third degree of left scapular region
    ● **T22.369**   Burn of third degree of unspecified scapular region

● **T22.39**   **Burn of third degree of multiple sites of shoulder and upper limb, except wrist and hand**
    ● **T22.391**   Burn of third degree of multiple sites of right shoulder and upper limb, except wrist and hand
    ● **T22.392**   Burn of third degree of multiple sites of left shoulder and upper limb, except wrist and hand
    ● **T22.399**   Burn of third degree of multiple sites of unspecified shoulder and upper limb, except wrist and hand

● **T22.4**   **Corrosion of unspecified degree of shoulder and upper limb, except wrist and hand**
    Code first (T51-T65) to identify chemical and intent
    Use additional external cause code to identify place (Y92)
    X ● **T22.40**   Corrosion of unspecified degree of shoulder and upper limb, except wrist and hand, unspecified site
    ● **T22.41**   Corrosion of unspecified degree of forearm
      ● **T22.411**   Corrosion of unspecified degree of right forearm
      ● **T22.412**   Corrosion of unspecified degree of left forearm
      ● **T22.419**   Corrosion of unspecified degree of unspecified forearm
    ● **T22.42**   Corrosion of unspecified degree of elbow
      ● **T22.421**   Corrosion of unspecified degree of right elbow
      ● **T22.422**   Corrosion of unspecified degree of left elbow
      ● **T22.429**   Corrosion of unspecified degree of unspecified elbow
    ● **T22.43**   Corrosion of unspecified degree of upper arm
      ● **T22.431**   Corrosion of unspecified degree of right upper arm
      ● **T22.432**   Corrosion of unspecified degree of left upper arm
      ● **T22.439**   Corrosion of unspecified degree of unspecified upper arm
    ● **T22.44**   Corrosion of unspecified degree of axilla
      ● **T22.441**   Corrosion of unspecified degree of right axilla
      ● **T22.442**   Corrosion of unspecified degree of left axilla
      ● **T22.449**   Corrosion of unspecified degree of unspecified axilla

● **T22.45**   **Corrosion of unspecified degree of shoulder**
    ● **T22.451**   Corrosion of unspecified degree of right shoulder
    ● **T22.452**   Corrosion of unspecified degree of left shoulder
    ● **T22.459**   Corrosion of unspecified degree of unspecified shoulder

● **T22.46**   **Corrosion of unspecified degree of scapular region**
    ● **T22.461**   Corrosion of unspecified degree of right scapular region
    ● **T22.462**   Corrosion of unspecified degree of left scapular region
    ● **T22.469**   Corrosion of unspecified degree of unspecified scapular region

● **T22.49**   **Corrosion of unspecified degree of multiple sites of shoulder and upper limb, except wrist and hand**
    ● **T22.491**   Corrosion of unspecified degree of multiple sites of right shoulder and upper limb, except wrist and hand
    ● **T22.492**   Corrosion of unspecified degree of multiple sites of left shoulder and upper limb, except wrist and hand
    ● **T22.499**   Corrosion of unspecified degree of multiple sites of unspecified shoulder and upper limb, except wrist and hand

● **T22.5**   **Corrosion of first degree of shoulder and upper limb, except wrist and hand**
    Code first (T51-T65) to identify chemical and intent
    Use additional external cause code to identify place (Y92)
    X ● **T22.50**   Corrosion of first degree of shoulder and upper limb, except wrist and hand unspecified site
    ● **T22.51**   Corrosion of first degree of forearm
      ● **T22.511**   Corrosion of first degree of right forearm
      ● **T22.512**   Corrosion of first degree of left forearm
      ● **T22.519**   Corrosion of first degree of unspecified forearm
    ● **T22.52**   Corrosion of first degree of elbow
      ● **T22.521**   Corrosion of first degree of right elbow
      ● **T22.522**   Corrosion of first degree of left elbow
      ● **T22.529**   Corrosion of first degree of unspecified elbow
    ● **T22.53**   Corrosion of first degree of upper arm
      ● **T22.531**   Corrosion of first degree of right upper arm
      ● **T22.532**   Corrosion of first degree of left upper arm
      ● **T22.539**   Corrosion of first degree of unspecified upper arm
    ● **T22.54**   Corrosion of first degree of axilla
      ● **T22.541**   Corrosion of first degree of right axilla
      ● **T22.542**   Corrosion of first degree of left axilla
      ● **T22.549**   Corrosion of first degree of unspecified axilla
    ● **T22.55**   Corrosion of first degree of shoulder
      ● **T22.551**   Corrosion of first degree of right shoulder
      ● **T22.552**   Corrosion of first degree of left shoulder
      ● **T22.559**   Corrosion of first degree of unspecified shoulder

▶ New   ⇒ Revised   ~~deleted~~ Deleted   Excludes 1   Excludes 2   Includes   Use additional   Code first   Code also   Key words
OGCR Official Guidelines   X Assign placeholder X   ● Use Additional Character(s)   ▶ Manifestation Code   Hierarchical Condition Category   **Coding Clinic**

● T22.56   Corrosion of first degree of scapular region
  ● T22.561   Corrosion of first degree of right scapular region
  ● T22.562   Corrosion of first degree of left scapular region
  ● T22.569   Corrosion of first degree of unspecified scapular region
● T22.59   Corrosion of first degree of multiple sites of shoulder and upper limb, except wrist and hand
  ● T22.591   Corrosion of first degree of multiple sites of right shoulder and upper limb, except wrist and hand
  ● T22.592   Corrosion of first degree of multiple sites of left shoulder and upper limb, except wrist and hand
  ● T22.599   Corrosion of first degree of multiple sites of unspecified shoulder and upper limb, except wrist and hand
● T22.6   Corrosion of second degree of shoulder and upper limb, except wrist and hand

  Code first (T51-T65) *to identify chemical and intent*
  Use additional external cause code to identify place (Y92)

  X ● T22.60   Corrosion of second degree of shoulder and upper limb, except wrist and hand, unspecified site
  ● T22.61   Corrosion of second degree of forearm
    ● T22.611   Corrosion of second degree of right forearm
    ● T22.612   Corrosion of second degree of left forearm
    ● T22.619   Corrosion of second degree of unspecified forearm
  ● T22.62   Corrosion of second degree of elbow
    ● T22.621   Corrosion of second degree of right elbow
    ● T22.622   Corrosion of second degree of left elbow
    ● T22.629   Corrosion of second degree of unspecified elbow
  ● T22.63   Corrosion of second degree of upper arm
    ● T22.631   Corrosion of second degree of right upper arm
    ● T22.632   Corrosion of second degree of left upper arm
    ● T22.639   Corrosion of second degree of unspecified upper arm
  ● T22.64   Corrosion of second degree of axilla
    ● T22.641   Corrosion of second degree of right axilla
    ● T22.642   Corrosion of second degree of left axilla
    ● T22.649   Corrosion of second degree of unspecified axilla
  ● T22.65   Corrosion of second degree of shoulder
    ● T22.651   Corrosion of second degree of right shoulder
    ● T22.652   Corrosion of second degree of left shoulder
    ● T22.659   Corrosion of second degree of unspecified shoulder

● T22.66   Corrosion of second degree of scapular region
  ● T22.661   Corrosion of second degree of right scapular region
  ● T22.662   Corrosion of second degree of left scapular region
  ● T22.669   Corrosion of second degree of unspecified scapular region
● T22.69   Corrosion of second degree of multiple sites of shoulder and upper limb, except wrist and hand
  ● T22.691   Corrosion of second degree of multiple sites of right shoulder and upper limb, except wrist and hand
  ● T22.692   Corrosion of second degree of multiple sites of left shoulder and upper limb, except wrist and hand
  ● T22.699   Corrosion of second degree of multiple sites of unspecified shoulder and upper limb, except wrist and hand
● T22.7   Corrosion of third degree of shoulder and upper limb, except wrist and hand

  Code first (T51-T65) *to identify chemical and intent*
  Use additional external cause code to identify place (Y92)

  X ● T22.70   Corrosion of third degree of shoulder and upper limb, except wrist and hand, unspecified site
  ● T22.71   Corrosion of third degree of forearm
    ● T22.711   Corrosion of third degree of right forearm
    ● T22.712   Corrosion of third degree of left forearm
    ● T22.719   Corrosion of third degree of unspecified forearm
  ● T22.72   Corrosion of third degree of elbow
    ● T22.721   Corrosion of third degree of right elbow
    ● T22.722   Corrosion of third degree of left elbow
    ● T22.729   Corrosion of third degree of unspecified elbow
  ● T22.73   Corrosion of third degree of upper arm
    ● T22.731   Corrosion of third degree of right upper arm
    ● T22.732   Corrosion of third degree of left upper arm
    ● T22.739   Corrosion of third degree of unspecified upper arm
  ● T22.74   Corrosion of third degree of axilla
    ● T22.741   Corrosion of third degree of right axilla
    ● T22.742   Corrosion of third degree of left axilla
    ● T22.749   Corrosion of third degree of unspecified axilla
  ● T22.75   Corrosion of third degree of shoulder
    ● T22.751   Corrosion of third degree of right shoulder
    ● T22.752   Corrosion of third degree of left shoulder
    ● T22.759   Corrosion of third degree of unspecified shoulder

CHAPTER 19 (S00-T88)

- T22.76 Corrosion of third degree of scapular region
  - T22.761 Corrosion of third degree of right scapular region
  - T22.762 Corrosion of third degree of left scapular region
  - T22.769 Corrosion of third degree of unspecified scapular region
- T22.79 Corrosion of third degree of multiple sites of shoulder and upper limb, except wrist and hand
  - T22.791 Corrosion of third degree of multiple sites of right shoulder and upper limb, except wrist and hand
  - T22.792 Corrosion of third degree of multiple sites of left shoulder and upper limb, except wrist and hand
  - T22.799 Corrosion of third degree of multiple sites of unspecified shoulder and upper limb, except wrist and hand

- T23 Burn and corrosion of wrist and hand

  The appropriate 7th character is to be added to each code from category T23

A	initial encounter
D	subsequent encounter
S	sequela

- T23.0 Burn of unspecified degree of wrist and hand

  Use additional external cause code to identify the source, place and intent of the burn (X00-X19, X75-X77, X96-X98, Y92)

  - T23.00 Burn of unspecified degree of hand, unspecified site
    - T23.001 Burn of unspecified degree of right hand, unspecified site
    - T23.002 Burn of unspecified degree of left hand, unspecified site
    - T23.009 Burn of unspecified degree of unspecified hand, unspecified site
  - T23.01 Burn of unspecified degree of thumb (nail)
    - T23.011 Burn of unspecified degree of right thumb (nail)
    - T23.012 Burn of unspecified degree of left thumb (nail)
    - T23.019 Burn of unspecified degree of unspecified thumb (nail)
  - T23.02 Burn of unspecified degree of single finger (nail) except thumb
    - T23.021 Burn of unspecified degree of single right finger (nail) except thumb
    - T23.022 Burn of unspecified degree of single left finger (nail) except thumb
    - T23.029 Burn of unspecified degree of unspecified single finger (nail) except thumb
  - T23.03 Burn of unspecified degree of multiple fingers (nail), not including thumb
    - T23.031 Burn of unspecified degree of multiple right fingers (nail), not including thumb
    - T23.032 Burn of unspecified degree of multiple left fingers (nail), not including thumb
    - T23.039 Burn of unspecified degree of unspecified multiple fingers (nail), not including thumb

- T23.04 Burn of unspecified degree of multiple fingers (nail), including thumb
  - T23.041 Burn of unspecified degree of multiple right fingers (nail), including thumb
  - T23.042 Burn of unspecified degree of multiple left fingers (nail), including thumb
  - T23.049 Burn of unspecified degree of unspecified multiple fingers (nail), including thumb
- T23.05 Burn of unspecified degree of palm
  - T23.051 Burn of unspecified degree of right palm
  - T23.052 Burn of unspecified degree of left palm
  - T23.059 Burn of unspecified degree of unspecified palm
- T23.06 Burn of unspecified degree of back of hand
  - T23.061 Burn of unspecified degree of back of right hand
  - T23.062 Burn of unspecified degree of back of left hand
  - T23.069 Burn of unspecified degree of back of unspecified hand
- T23.07 Burn of unspecified degree of wrist
  - T23.071 Burn of unspecified degree of right wrist
  - T23.072 Burn of unspecified degree of left wrist
  - T23.079 Burn of unspecified degree of unspecified wrist
- T23.09 Burn of unspecified degree of multiple sites of wrist and hand
  - T23.091 Burn of unspecified degree of multiple sites of right wrist and hand
  - T23.092 Burn of unspecified degree of multiple sites of left wrist and hand
  - T23.099 Burn of unspecified degree of multiple sites of unspecified wrist and hand

- T23.1 Burn of first degree of wrist and hand

  Use additional external cause code to identify the source, place and intent of the burn (X00-X19, X75-X77, X96-X98, Y92)

  - T23.10 Burn of first degree of hand, unspecified site
    - T23.101 Burn of first degree of right hand, unspecified site
    - T23.102 Burn of first degree of left hand, unspecified site
    - T23.109 Burn of first degree of unspecified hand, unspecified site
  - T23.11 Burn of first degree of thumb (nail)
    - T23.111 Burn of first degree of right thumb (nail)
    - T23.112 Burn of first degree of left thumb (nail)
    - T23.119 Burn of first degree of unspecified thumb (nail)
  - T23.12 Burn of first degree of single finger (nail) except thumb
    - T23.121 Burn of first degree of single right finger (nail) except thumb
    - T23.122 Burn of first degree of single left finger (nail) except thumb
    - T23.129 Burn of first degree of unspecified single finger (nail) except thumb

▶ New   ⇒ Revised   ~~deleted~~ Deleted   Excludes 1   Excludes 2   Includes   Use additional   Code first   Code also   Key words

OGCR Official Guidelines   X Assign placeholder X   ● Use Additional Character(s)   ▶ Manifestation Code   🐷 Hierarchical Condition Category   **Coding Clinic**

● T23.13   Burn of first degree of multiple fingers (nail), not including thumb

    ● T23.131   Burn of first degree of multiple right fingers (nail), not including thumb

    ● T23.132   Burn of first degree of multiple left fingers (nail), not including thumb

    ● T23.139   Burn of first degree of unspecified multiple fingers (nail), not including thumb

● T23.14   Burn of first degree of multiple fingers (nail), including thumb

    ● T23.141   Burn of first degree of multiple right fingers (nail), including thumb

    ● T23.142   Burn of first degree of multiple left fingers (nail), including thumb

    ● T23.149   Burn of first degree of unspecified multiple fingers (nail), including thumb

● T23.15   Burn of first degree of palm

    ● T23.151   Burn of first degree of right palm

    ● T23.152   Burn of first degree of left palm

    ● T23.159   Burn of first degree of unspecified palm

● T23.16   Burn of first degree of back of hand

    ● T23.161   Burn of first degree of back of right hand

    ● T23.162   Burn of first degree of back of left hand

    ● T23.169   Burn of first degree of back of unspecified hand

● T23.17   Burn of first degree of wrist

    ● T23.171   Burn of first degree of right wrist

    ● T23.172   Burn of first degree of left wrist

    ● T23.179   Burn of first degree of unspecified wrist

● T23.19   Burn of first degree of multiple sites of wrist and hand

    ● T23.191   Burn of first degree of multiple sites of right wrist and hand

    ● T23.192   Burn of first degree of multiple sites of left wrist and hand

    ● T23.199   Burn of first degree of multiple sites of unspecified wrist and hand

● T23.2   Burn of second degree of wrist and hand

Use additional external cause code to identify the source, place and intent of the burn (X00-X19, X75-X77, X96-X98, Y92)

● T23.20   Burn of second degree of hand, unspecified site

    ● T23.201   Burn of second degree of right hand, unspecified site

    ● T23.202   Burn of second degree of left hand, unspecified site

    ● T23.209   Burn of second degree of unspecified hand, unspecified site

● T23.21   Burn of second degree of thumb (nail)

    ● T23.211   Burn of second degree of right thumb (nail)

    ● T23.212   Burn of second degree of left thumb (nail)

    ● T23.219   Burn of second degree of unspecified thumb (nail)

● T23.22   Burn of second degree of single finger (nail) except thumb

    ● T23.221   Burn of second degree of single right finger (nail) except thumb

    ● T23.222   Burn of second degree of single left finger (nail) except thumb

    ● T23.229   Burn of second degree of unspecified single finger (nail) except thumb

● T23.23   Burn of second degree of multiple fingers (nail), not including thumb

    ● T23.231   Burn of second degree of multiple right fingers (nail), not including thumb

    ● T23.232   Burn of second degree of multiple left fingers (nail), not including thumb

    ● T23.239   Burn of second degree of unspecified multiple fingers (nail), not including thumb

● T23.24   Burn of second degree of multiple fingers (nail), including thumb

    ● T23.241   Burn of second degree of multiple right fingers (nail), including thumb

    ● T23.242   Burn of second degree of multiple left fingers (nail), including thumb

    ● T23.249   Burn of second degree of unspecified multiple fingers (nail), including thumb

● T23.25   Burn of second degree of palm

    ● T23.251   Burn of second degree of right palm

    ● T23.252   Burn of second degree of left palm

    ● T23.259   Burn of second degree of unspecified palm

● T23.26   Burn of second degree of back of hand

    ● T23.261   Burn of second degree of back of right hand

    ● T23.262   Burn of second degree of back of left hand

    ● T23.269   Burn of second degree of back of unspecified hand

● T23.27   Burn of second degree of wrist

    ● T23.271   Burn of second degree of right wrist

    ● T23.272   Burn of second degree of left wrist

    ● T23.279   Burn of second degree of unspecified wrist

● T23.29   Burn of second degree of multiple sites of wrist and hand

    ● T23.291   Burn of second degree of multiple sites of right wrist and hand

    ● T23.292   Burn of second degree of multiple sites of left wrist and hand

    ● T23.299   Burn of second degree of multiple sites of unspecified wrist and hand

● T23.3   Burn of third degree of wrist and hand

Use additional external cause code to identify the source, place and intent of the burn (X00-X19, X75-X77, X96-X98, Y92)

● T23.30   Burn of third degree of hand, unspecified site

    ● T23.301   Burn of third degree of right hand, unspecified site
        Coding Clinic: 2015, Q1, P19

    ● T23.302   Burn of third degree of left hand, unspecified site
        Coding Clinic: 2016, Q2, P5

    ● T23.309   Burn of third degree of unspecified hand, unspecified site

CHAPTER 19 (S00-T88)

● T23.31   Burn of third degree of thumb (nail)
- ● T23.311   Burn of third degree of right thumb (nail)
- ● T23.312   Burn of third degree of left thumb (nail)
- ● T23.319   Burn of third degree of unspecified thumb (nail)

● T23.32   Burn of third degree of single finger (nail) except thumb
- ● T23.321   Burn of third degree of single right finger (nail) except thumb
- ● T23.322   Burn of third degree of single left finger (nail) except thumb
- ● T23.329   Burn of third degree of unspecified single finger (nail) except thumb

● T23.33   Burn of third degree of multiple fingers (nail), not including thumb
- ● T23.331   Burn of third degree of multiple right fingers (nail), not including thumb
- ● T23.332   Burn of third degree of multiple left fingers (nail), not including thumb
- ● T23.339   Burn of third degree of unspecified multiple fingers (nail), not including thumb

● T23.34   Burn of third degree of multiple fingers (nail), including thumb
- ● T23.341   Burn of third degree of multiple right fingers (nail), including thumb
- ● T23.342   Burn of third degree of multiple left fingers (nail), including thumb
- ● T23.349   Burn of third degree of unspecified multiple fingers (nail), including thumb

● T23.35   Burn of third degree of palm
- ● T23.351   Burn of third degree of right palm
- ● T23.352   Burn of third degree of left palm
- ● T23.359   Burn of third degree of unspecified palm

● T23.36   Burn of third degree of back of hand
- ● T23.361   Burn of third degree of back of right hand
- ● T23.362   Burn of third degree of back of left hand
- ● T23.369   Burn of third degree of back of unspecified hand

● T23.37   Burn of third degree of wrist
- ● T23.371   Burn of third degree of right wrist
- ● T23.372   Burn of third degree of left wrist
- ● T23.379   Burn of third degree of unspecified wrist

● T23.39   Burn of third degree of multiple sites of wrist and hand
- ● T23.391   Burn of third degree of multiple sites of right wrist and hand
- ● T23.392   Burn of third degree of multiple sites of left wrist and hand
- ● T23.399   Burn of third degree of multiple sites of unspecified wrist and hand

● T23.4   Corrosion of unspecified degree of wrist and hand
Code first (T51-T65) to identify chemical and intent
Use additional external cause code to identify place (Y92)

● T23.40   Corrosion of unspecified degree of hand, unspecified site
- ● T23.401   Corrosion of unspecified degree of right hand, unspecified site
- ● T23.402   Corrosion of unspecified degree of left hand, unspecified site
- ● T23.409   Corrosion of unspecified degree of unspecified hand, unspecified site

● T23.41   Corrosion of unspecified degree of thumb (nail)
- ● T23.411   Corrosion of unspecified degree of right thumb (nail)
- ● T23.412   Corrosion of unspecified degree of left thumb (nail)
- ● T23.419   Corrosion of unspecified degree of unspecified thumb (nail)

● T23.42   Corrosion of unspecified degree of single finger (nail) except thumb
- ● T23.421   Corrosion of unspecified degree of single right finger (nail) except thumb
- ● T23.422   Corrosion of unspecified degree of single left finger (nail) except thumb
- ● T23.429   Corrosion of unspecified degree of unspecified single finger (nail) except thumb

● T23.43   Corrosion of unspecified degree of multiple fingers (nail), not including thumb
- ● T23.431   Corrosion of unspecified degree of multiple right fingers (nail), not including thumb
- ● T23.432   Corrosion of unspecified degree of multiple left fingers (nail), not including thumb
- ● T23.439   Corrosion of unspecified degree of unspecified multiple fingers (nail), not including thumb

● T23.44   Corrosion of unspecified degree of multiple fingers (nail), including thumb
- ● T23.441   Corrosion of unspecified degree of multiple right fingers (nail), including thumb
- ● T23.442   Corrosion of unspecified degree of multiple left fingers (nail), including thumb
- ● T23.449   Corrosion of unspecified degree of unspecified multiple fingers (nail), including thumb

● T23.45   Corrosion of unspecified degree of palm
- ● T23.451   Corrosion of unspecified degree of right palm
- ● T23.452   Corrosion of unspecified degree of left palm
- ● T23.459   Corrosion of unspecified degree of unspecified palm

● T23.46   Corrosion of unspecified degree of back of hand
- ● T23.461   Corrosion of unspecified degree of back of right hand
- ● T23.462   Corrosion of unspecified degree of back of left hand
- ● T23.469   Corrosion of unspecified degree of back of unspecified hand

▶ New   ➡ Revised   ~~deleted~~ Deleted   Excludes 1   Excludes 2   Includes   Use additional   Code first   Code also   Key words

OGCR Official Guidelines   X Assign placeholder X   ● Use Additional Character(s)   ⟩ Manifestation Code   🐝 Hierarchical Condition Category   **Coding Clinic**

● **T23.47** Corrosion of unspecified degree of wrist

   ● **T23.471** Corrosion of unspecified degree of right wrist

   ● **T23.472** Corrosion of unspecified degree of left wrist

   ● **T23.479** Corrosion of unspecified degree of unspecified wrist

● **T23.49** Corrosion of unspecified degree of multiple sites of wrist and hand

   ● **T23.491** Corrosion of unspecified degree of multiple sites of right wrist and hand

   ● **T23.492** Corrosion of unspecified degree of multiple sites of left wrist and hand

   ● **T23.499** Corrosion of unspecified degree of multiple sites of unspecified wrist and hand

● **T23.5** Corrosion of first degree of wrist and hand

   Code first (T51-T65) *to identify chemical and intent*

   Use additional external cause code to identify place (Y92)

   ● **T23.50** Corrosion of first degree of hand, unspecified site

      ● **T23.501** Corrosion of first degree of right hand, unspecified site

      ● **T23.502** Corrosion of first degree of left hand, unspecified site

      ● **T23.509** Corrosion of first degree of unspecified hand, unspecified site

   ● **T23.51** Corrosion of first degree of thumb (nail)

      ● **T23.511** Corrosion of first degree of right thumb (nail)

      ● **T23.512** Corrosion of first degree of left thumb (nail)

      ● **T23.519** Corrosion of first degree of unspecified thumb (nail)

   ● **T23.52** Corrosion of first degree of single finger (nail) except thumb

      ● **T23.521** Corrosion of first degree of single right finger (nail) except thumb

      ● **T23.522** Corrosion of first degree of single left finger (nail) except thumb

      ● **T23.529** Corrosion of first degree of unspecified single finger (nail) except thumb

   ● **T23.53** Corrosion of first degree of multiple fingers (nail), not including thumb

      ● **T23.531** Corrosion of first degree of multiple right fingers (nail), not including thumb

      ● **T23.532** Corrosion of first degree of multiple left fingers (nail), not including thumb

      ● **T23.539** Corrosion of first degree of unspecified multiple fingers (nail), not including thumb

   ● **T23.54** Corrosion of first degree of multiple fingers (nail), including thumb

      ● **T23.541** Corrosion of first degree of multiple right fingers (nail), including thumb

      ● **T23.542** Corrosion of first degree of multiple left fingers (nail), including thumb

      ● **T23.549** Corrosion of first degree of unspecified multiple fingers (nail), including thumb

   ● **T23.55** Corrosion of first degree of palm

      ● **T23.551** Corrosion of first degree of right palm

      ● **T23.552** Corrosion of first degree of left palm

      ● **T23.559** Corrosion of first degree of unspecified palm

● **T23.56** Corrosion of first degree of back of hand

   ● **T23.561** Corrosion of first degree of back of right hand

   ● **T23.562** Corrosion of first degree of back of left hand

   ● **T23.569** Corrosion of first degree of back of unspecified hand

● **T23.57** Corrosion of first degree of wrist

   ● **T23.571** Corrosion of first degree of right wrist

   ● **T23.572** Corrosion of first degree of left wrist

   ● **T23.579** Corrosion of first degree of unspecified wrist

● **T23.59** Corrosion of first degree of multiple sites of wrist and hand

   ● **T23.591** Corrosion of first degree of multiple sites of right wrist and hand

   ● **T23.592** Corrosion of first degree of multiple sites of left wrist and hand

   ● **T23.599** Corrosion of first degree of multiple sites of unspecified wrist and hand

● **T23.6** Corrosion of second degree of wrist and hand

   Code first (T51-T65) *to identify chemical and intent*

   Use additional external cause code to identify place (Y92)

   ● **T23.60** Corrosion of second degree of hand, unspecified site

      ● **T23.601** Corrosion of second degree of right hand, unspecified site

      ● **T23.602** Corrosion of second degree of left hand, unspecified site

      ● **T23.609** Corrosion of second degree of unspecified hand, unspecified site

   ● **T23.61** Corrosion of second degree of thumb (nail)

      ● **T23.611** Corrosion of second degree of right thumb (nail)

      ● **T23.612** Corrosion of second degree of left thumb (nail)

      ● **T23.619** Corrosion of second degree of unspecified thumb (nail)

   ● **T23.62** Corrosion of second degree of single finger (nail) except thumb

      ● **T23.621** Corrosion of second degree of single right finger (nail) except thumb

      ● **T23.622** Corrosion of second degree of single left finger (nail) except thumb

      ● **T23.629** Corrosion of second degree of unspecified single finger (nail) except thumb

   ● **T23.63** Corrosion of second degree of multiple fingers (nail), not including thumb

      ● **T23.631** Corrosion of second degree of multiple right fingers (nail), not including thumb

      ● **T23.632** Corrosion of second degree of multiple left fingers (nail), not including thumb

      ● **T23.639** Corrosion of second degree of unspecified multiple fingers (nail), not including thumb

   ● **T23.64** Corrosion of second degree of multiple fingers (nail), including thumb

      ● **T23.641** Corrosion of second degree of multiple right fingers (nail), including thumb

      ● **T23.642** Corrosion of second degree of multiple left fingers (nail), including thumb

      ● **T23.649** Corrosion of second degree of unspecified multiple fingers (nail), including thumb

CHAPTER 19 (S00-T88)

CHAPTER 19 (S00-T88)

● T23.65   Corrosion of second degree of palm
  ● T23.651   Corrosion of second degree of right palm
  ● T23.652   Corrosion of second degree of left palm
  ● T23.659   Corrosion of second degree of unspecified palm
● T23.66   Corrosion of second degree of back of hand
  ● T23.661   Corrosion of second degree back of right hand
  ● T23.662   Corrosion of second degree back of left hand
  ● T23.669   Corrosion of second degree back of unspecified hand
● T23.67   Corrosion of second degree of wrist
  ● T23.671   Corrosion of second degree of right wrist
  ● T23.672   Corrosion of second degree of left wrist
  ● T23.679   Corrosion of second degree of unspecified wrist
● T23.69   Corrosion of second degree of multiple sites of wrist and hand
  ● T23.691   Corrosion of second degree of multiple sites of right wrist and hand
  ● T23.692   Corrosion of second degree of multiple sites of left wrist and hand
  ● T23.699   Corrosion of second degree of multiple sites of unspecified wrist and hand

● T23.7   Corrosion of third degree of wrist and hand
    Code first (T51-T65) to identify chemical and intent
    Use additional external cause code to identify place (Y92)
  ● T23.70   Corrosion of third degree of hand, unspecified site
    ● T23.701   Corrosion of third degree of right hand, unspecified site
    ● T23.702   Corrosion of third degree of left hand, unspecified site
    ● T23.709   Corrosion of third degree of unspecified hand, unspecified site
  ● T23.71   Corrosion of third degree of thumb (nail)
    ● T23.711   Corrosion of third degree of right thumb (nail)
    ● T23.712   Corrosion of third degree of left thumb (nail)
    ● T23.719   Corrosion of third degree of unspecified thumb (nail)
  ● T23.72   Corrosion of third degree of single finger (nail) except thumb
    ● T23.721   Corrosion of third degree of single right finger (nail) except thumb
    ● T23.722   Corrosion of third degree of single left finger (nail) except thumb
    ● T23.729   Corrosion of third degree of unspecified single finger (nail) except thumb
  ● T23.73   Corrosion of third degree of multiple fingers (nail), not including thumb
    ● T23.731   Corrosion of third degree of multiple right fingers (nail), not including thumb
    ● T23.732   Corrosion of third degree of multiple left fingers (nail), not including thumb
    ● T23.739   Corrosion of third degree of unspecified multiple fingers (nail), not including thumb

● T23.74   Corrosion of third degree of multiple fingers (nail), including thumb
  ● T23.741   Corrosion of third degree of multiple right fingers (nail), including thumb
  ● T23.742   Corrosion of third degree of multiple left fingers (nail), including thumb
  ● T23.749   Corrosion of third degree of unspecified multiple fingers (nail), including thumb
● T23.75   Corrosion of third degree of palm
  ● T23.751   Corrosion of third degree of right palm
  ● T23.752   Corrosion of third degree of left palm
  ● T23.759   Corrosion of third degree of unspecified palm
● T23.76   Corrosion of third degree of back of hand
  ● T23.761   Corrosion of third degree of back of right hand
  ● T23.762   Corrosion of third degree of back of left hand
  ● T23.769   Corrosion of third degree of back of unspecified hand
● T23.77   Corrosion of third degree of wrist
  ● T23.771   Corrosion of third degree of right wrist
  ● T23.772   Corrosion of third degree of left wrist
  ● T23.779   Corrosion of third degree of unspecified wrist
● T23.79   Corrosion of third degree of multiple sites of wrist and hand
  ● T23.791   Corrosion of third degree of multiple sites of right wrist and hand
  ● T23.792   Corrosion of third degree of multiple sites of left wrist and hand
  ● T23.799   Corrosion of third degree of multiple sites of unspecified wrist and hand

● T24   Burn and corrosion of lower limb, except ankle and foot
    Excludes2   burn and corrosion of ankle and foot (T25.-)
                    burn and corrosion of hip region (T21.-)
    The appropriate 7th character is to be added to each code from category T24

A	initial encounter
D	subsequent encounter
S	sequela

  ● T24.0   Burn of unspecified degree of lower limb, except ankle and foot
      Use additional external cause code to identify the source, place and intent of the burn (X00-X19, X75-X77, X96-X98, Y92)
    ● T24.00   Burn of unspecified degree of unspecified site of lower limb, except ankle and foot
      ● T24.001   Burn of unspecified degree of unspecified site of right lower limb, except ankle and foot
      ● T24.002   Burn of unspecified degree of unspecified site of left lower limb, except ankle and foot
      ● T24.009   Burn of unspecified degree of unspecified site of unspecified lower limb, except ankle and foot
    ● T24.01   Burn of unspecified degree of thigh
      ● T24.011   Burn of unspecified degree of right thigh
      ● T24.012   Burn of unspecified degree of left thigh
      ● T24.019   Burn of unspecified degree of unspecified thigh

● T24.02   Burn of unspecified degree of knee
  ● T24.021   Burn of unspecified degree of right knee
  ● T24.022   Burn of unspecified degree of left knee
  ● T24.029   Burn of unspecified degree of unspecified knee
● T24.03   Burn of unspecified degree of lower leg
  ● T24.031   Burn of unspecified degree of right lower leg
  ● T24.032   Burn of unspecified degree of left lower leg
  ● T24.039   Burn of unspecified degree of unspecified lower leg
● T24.09   Burn of unspecified degree of multiple sites of lower limb, except ankle and foot
  ● T24.091   Burn of unspecified degree of multiple sites of right lower limb, except ankle and foot
  ● T24.092   Burn of unspecified degree of multiple sites of left lower limb, except ankle and foot
  ● T24.099   Burn of unspecified degree of multiple sites of unspecified lower limb, except ankle and foot
● T24.1   Burn of first degree of lower limb, except ankle and foot
    Use additional external cause code to identify the source, place and intent of the burn (X00-X19, X75-X77, X96-X98, Y92)
  ● T24.10   Burn of first degree of unspecified site of lower limb, except ankle and foot
    ● T24.101   Burn of first degree of unspecified site of right lower limb, except ankle and foot
    ● T24.102   Burn of first degree of unspecified site of left lower limb, except ankle and foot
    ● T24.109   Burn of first degree of unspecified site of unspecified lower limb, except ankle and foot
  ● T24.11   Burn of first degree of thigh
    ● T24.111   Burn of first degree of right thigh
    ● T24.112   Burn of first degree of left thigh
    ● T24.119   Burn of first degree of unspecified thigh
  ● T24.12   Burn of first degree of knee
    ● T24.121   Burn of first degree of right knee
    ● T24.122   Burn of first degree of left knee
    ● T24.129   Burn of first degree of unspecified knee
  ● T24.13   Burn of first degree of lower leg
    ● T24.131   Burn of first degree of right lower leg
    ● T24.132   Burn of first degree of left lower leg
    ● T24.139   Burn of first degree of unspecified lower leg
  ● T24.19   Burn of first degree of multiple sites of lower limb, except ankle and foot
    ● T24.191   Burn of first degree of multiple sites of right lower limb, except ankle and foot
    ● T24.192   Burn of first degree of multiple sites of left lower limb, except ankle and foot
    ● T24.199   Burn of first degree of multiple sites of unspecified lower limb, except ankle and foot

● T24.2   Burn of second degree of lower limb, except ankle and foot
    Use additional external cause code to identify the source, place and intent of the burn (X00-X19, X75-X77, X96-X98, Y92)
  ● T24.20   Burn of second degree of unspecified site of lower limb, except ankle and foot
    ● T24.201   Burn of second degree of unspecified site of right lower limb, except ankle and foot
    ● T24.202   Burn of second degree of unspecified site of left lower limb, except ankle and foot
    ● T24.209   Burn of second degree of unspecified site of unspecified lower limb, except ankle and foot
  ● T24.21   Burn of second degree of thigh
    ● T24.211   Burn of second degree of right thigh
    ● T24.212   Burn of second degree of left thigh
    ● T24.219   Burn of second degree of unspecified thigh
  ● T24.22   Burn of second degree of knee
    ● T24.221   Burn of second degree of right knee
    ● T24.222   Burn of second degree of left knee
    ● T24.229   Burn of second degree of unspecified knee
  ● T24.23   Burn of second degree of lower leg
    ● T24.231   Burn of second degree of right lower leg
    ● T24.232   Burn of second degree of left lower leg
    ● T24.239   Burn of second degree of unspecified lower leg
  ● T24.29   Burn of second degree of multiple sites of lower limb, except ankle and foot
    ● T24.291   Burn of second degree of multiple sites of right lower limb, except ankle and foot
    ● T24.292   Burn of second degree of multiple sites of left lower limb, except ankle and foot
    ● T24.299   Burn of second degree of multiple sites of unspecified lower limb, except ankle and foot
● T24.3   Burn of third degree of lower limb, except ankle and foot
    Use additional external cause code to identify the source, place and intent of the burn (X00-X19, X75-X77, X96-X98, Y92)
  ● T24.30   Burn of third degree of unspecified site of lower limb, except ankle and foot
    ● T24.301   Burn of third degree of unspecified site of right lower limb, except ankle and foot
    ● T24.302   Burn of third degree of unspecified site of left lower limb, except ankle and foot
    ● T24.309   Burn of third degree of unspecified site of unspecified lower limb, except ankle and foot
  ● T24.31   Burn of third degree of thigh
    ● T24.311   Burn of third degree of right thigh
    ● T24.312   Burn of third degree of left thigh
    ● T24.319   Burn of third degree of unspecified thigh

● T24.32   Burn of third degree of knee
  ● T24.321   Burn of third degree of right knee
  ● T24.322   Burn of third degree of left knee
  ● T24.329   Burn of third degree of unspecified knee
● T24.33   Burn of third degree of lower leg
  ● T24.331   Burn of third degree of right lower leg
  ● T24.332   Burn of third degree of left lower leg
  ● T24.339   Burn of third degree of unspecified lower leg
● T24.39   Burn of third degree of multiple sites of lower limb, except ankle and foot
  ● T24.391   Burn of third degree of multiple sites of right lower limb, except ankle and foot
          Coding Clinic: 2016, Q2, P5
  ● T24.392   Burn of third degree of multiple sites of left lower limb, except ankle and foot
  ● T24.399   Burn of third degree of multiple sites of unspecified lower limb, except ankle and foot
● T24.4   Corrosion of unspecified degree of lower limb, except ankle and foot
        Code first (T51-T65) *to identify chemical and intent*
        Use additional external cause code to identify place (Y92)
  ● T24.40   Corrosion of unspecified degree of unspecified site of lower limb, except ankle and foot
    ● T24.401   Corrosion of unspecified degree of unspecified site of right lower limb, except ankle and foot
    ● T24.402   Corrosion of unspecified degree of unspecified site of left lower limb, except ankle and foot
    ● T24.409   Corrosion of unspecified degree of unspecified site of unspecified lower limb, except ankle and foot
  ● T24.41   Corrosion of unspecified degree of thigh
    ● T24.411   Corrosion of unspecified degree of right thigh
    ● T24.412   Corrosion of unspecified degree of left thigh
    ● T24.419   Corrosion of unspecified degree of unspecified thigh
  ● T24.42   Corrosion of unspecified degree of knee
    ● T24.421   Corrosion of unspecified degree of right knee
    ● T24.422   Corrosion of unspecified degree of left knee
    ● T24.429   Corrosion of unspecified degree of unspecified knee
  ● T24.43   Corrosion of unspecified degree of lower leg
    ● T24.431   Corrosion of unspecified degree of right lower leg
    ● T24.432   Corrosion of unspecified degree of left lower leg
    ● T24.439   Corrosion of unspecified degree of unspecified lower leg
  ● T24.49   Corrosion of unspecified degree of multiple sites of lower limb, except ankle and foot
    ● T24.491   Corrosion of unspecified degree of multiple sites of right lower limb, except ankle and foot
    ● T24.492   Corrosion of unspecified degree of multiple sites of left lower limb, except ankle and foot
    ● T24.499   Corrosion of unspecified degree of multiple sites of unspecified lower limb, except ankle and foot

● T24.5   Corrosion of first degree of lower limb, except ankle and foot
        Code first (T51-T65) *to identify chemical and intent*
        Use additional external cause code to identify place (Y92)
  ● T24.50   Corrosion of first degree of unspecified site of lower limb, except ankle and foot
    ● T24.501   Corrosion of first degree of unspecified site of right lower limb, except ankle and foot
    ● T24.502   Corrosion of first degree of unspecified site of left lower limb, except ankle and foot
    ● T24.509   Corrosion of first degree of unspecified site of unspecified lower limb, except ankle and foot
  ● T24.51   Corrosion of first degree of thigh
    ● T24.511   Corrosion of first degree of right thigh
    ● T24.512   Corrosion of first degree of left thigh
    ● T24.519   Corrosion of first degree of unspecified thigh
  ● T24.52   Corrosion of first degree of knee
    ● T24.521   Corrosion of first degree of right knee
    ● T24.522   Corrosion of first degree of left knee
    ● T24.529   Corrosion of first degree of unspecified knee
  ● T24.53   Corrosion of first degree of lower leg
    ● T24.531   Corrosion of first degree of right lower leg
    ● T24.532   Corrosion of first degree of left lower leg
    ● T24.539   Corrosion of first degree of unspecified lower leg
  ● T24.59   Corrosion of first degree of multiple sites of lower limb, except ankle and foot
    ● T24.591   Corrosion of first degree of multiple sites of right lower limb, except ankle and foot
    ● T24.592   Corrosion of first degree of multiple sites of left lower limb, except ankle and foot
    ● T24.599   Corrosion of first degree of multiple sites of unspecified lower limb, except ankle and foot
● T24.6   Corrosion of second degree of lower limb, except ankle and foot
        Code first (T51-T65) *to identify chemical and intent*
        Use additional external cause code to identify place (Y92)
  ● T24.60   Corrosion of second degree of unspecified site of lower limb, except ankle and foot
    ● T24.601   Corrosion of second degree of unspecified site of right lower limb, except ankle and foot
    ● T24.602   Corrosion of second degree of unspecified site of left lower limb, except ankle and foot
    ● T24.609   Corrosion of second degree of unspecified site of unspecified lower limb, except ankle and foot
  ● T24.61   Corrosion of second degree of thigh
    ● T24.611   Corrosion of second degree of right thigh
    ● T24.612   Corrosion of second degree of left thigh
    ● T24.619   Corrosion of second degree of unspecified thigh

▶ New   ⇒ Revised   ~~deleted~~ Deleted   Excludes 1   Excludes 2   Includes   Use additional   Code first   Code also   Key words
OGCR Official Guidelines   X Assign placeholder X   ● Use Additional Character(s)   ▌ Manifestation Code   🔖 Hierarchical Condition Category   Coding Clinic

● **T24.62** Corrosion of second degree of knee
  ● **T24.621** Corrosion of second degree of right knee
  ● **T24.622** Corrosion of second degree of left knee
  ● **T24.629** Corrosion of second degree of unspecified knee
● **T24.63** Corrosion of second degree of lower leg
  ● **T24.631** Corrosion of second degree of right lower leg
  ● **T24.632** Corrosion of second degree of left lower leg
  ● **T24.639** Corrosion of second degree of unspecified lower leg
● **T24.69** Corrosion of second degree of multiple sites of lower limb, except ankle and foot
  ● **T24.691** Corrosion of second degree of multiple sites of right lower limb, except ankle and foot
  ● **T24.692** Corrosion of second degree of multiple sites of left lower limb, except ankle and foot
  ● **T24.699** Corrosion of second degree of multiple sites of unspecified lower limb, except ankle and foot
● **T24.7** Corrosion of third degree of lower limb, except ankle and foot

  Code first (T51-T65) to identify chemical and intent

  Use additional external cause code to identify place (Y92)

  ● **T24.70** Corrosion of third degree of unspecified site of lower limb, except ankle and foot
    ● **T24.701** Corrosion of third degree of unspecified site of right lower limb, except ankle and foot
    ● **T24.702** Corrosion of third degree of unspecified site of left lower limb, except ankle and foot
    ● **T24.709** Corrosion of third degree of unspecified site of unspecified lower limb, except ankle and foot
  ● **T24.71** Corrosion of third degree of thigh
    ● **T24.711** Corrosion of third degree of right thigh
    ● **T24.712** Corrosion of third degree of left thigh
    ● **T24.719** Corrosion of third degree of unspecified thigh
  ● **T24.72** Corrosion of third degree of knee
    ● **T24.721** Corrosion of third degree of right knee
    ● **T24.722** Corrosion of third degree of left knee
    ● **T24.729** Corrosion of third degree of unspecified knee
  ● **T24.73** Corrosion of third degree of lower leg
    ● **T24.731** Corrosion of third degree of right lower leg
    ● **T24.732** Corrosion of third degree of left lower leg
    ● **T24.739** Corrosion of third degree of unspecified lower leg
  ● **T24.79** Corrosion of third degree of multiple sites of lower limb, except ankle and foot
    ● **T24.791** Corrosion of third degree of multiple sites of right lower limb, except ankle and foot
    ● **T24.792** Corrosion of third degree of multiple sites of left lower limb, except ankle and foot
    ● **T24.799** Corrosion of third degree of multiple sites of unspecified lower limb, except ankle and foot

● **T25** Burn and corrosion of ankle and foot

  The appropriate 7th character is to be added to each code from category T25

A	initial encounter
D	subsequent encounter
S	sequela

  ● **T25.0** Burn of unspecified degree of ankle and foot

  Use additional external cause code to identify the source, place and intent of the burn (X00-X19, X75-X77, X96-X98, Y92)

    ● **T25.01** Burn of unspecified degree of ankle
      ● **T25.011** Burn of unspecified degree of right ankle
      ● **T25.012** Burn of unspecified degree of left ankle
      ● **T25.019** Burn of unspecified degree of unspecified ankle
    ● **T25.02** Burn of unspecified degree of foot

      Excludes2 burn of unspecified degree of toe(s) (nail) (T25.03-)

      ● **T25.021** Burn of unspecified degree of right foot
      ● **T25.022** Burn of unspecified degree of left foot
      ● **T25.029** Burn of unspecified degree of unspecified foot
    ● **T25.03** Burn of unspecified degree of toe(s) (nail)
      ● **T25.031** Burn of unspecified degree of right toe(s) (nail)
      ● **T25.032** Burn of unspecified degree of left toe(s) (nail)
      ● **T25.039** Burn of unspecified degree of unspecified toe(s) (nail)
    ● **T25.09** Burn of unspecified degree of multiple sites of ankle and foot
      ● **T25.091** Burn of unspecified degree of multiple sites of right ankle and foot
      ● **T25.092** Burn of unspecified degree of multiple sites of left ankle and foot
      ● **T25.099** Burn of unspecified degree of multiple sites of unspecified ankle and foot
  ● **T25.1** Burn of first degree of ankle and foot

  Use additional external cause code to identify the source, place and intent of the burn (X00-X19, X75-X77, X96-X98, Y92)

    ● **T25.11** Burn of first degree of ankle
      ● **T25.111** Burn of first degree of right ankle
      ● **T25.112** Burn of first degree of left ankle
      ● **T25.119** Burn of first degree of unspecified ankle
    ● **T25.12** Burn of first degree of foot

      Excludes2 burn of first degree of toe(s) (nail) (T25.13-)

      ● **T25.121** Burn of first degree of right foot
      ● **T25.122** Burn of first degree of left foot
      ● **T25.129** Burn of first degree of unspecified foot
    ● **T25.13** Burn of first degree of toe(s) (nail)
      ● **T25.131** Burn of first degree of right toe(s) (nail)
      ● **T25.132** Burn of first degree of left toe(s) (nail)
      ● **T25.139** Burn of first degree of unspecified toe(s) (nail)

CHAPTER 19 (S00-T88)

● T25.19   Burn of first degree of multiple sites of ankle and foot
- ● T25.191   Burn of first degree of multiple sites of right ankle and foot
- ● T25.192   Burn of first degree of multiple sites of left ankle and foot
- ● T25.199   Burn of first degree of multiple sites of unspecified ankle and foot

● T25.2   Burn of second degree of ankle and foot

Use additional external cause code to identify the source, place and intent of the burn (X00-X19, X75-X77, X96-X98, Y92)

- ● T25.21   Burn of second degree of ankle
  - ● T25.211   Burn of second degree of right ankle
  - ● T25.212   Burn of second degree of left ankle
  - ● T25.219   Burn of second degree of unspecified ankle
- ● T25.22   Burn of second degree of foot

  Excludes2   burn of second degree of toe(s) (nail) (T25.23-)

  - ● T25.221   Burn of second degree of right foot
  - ● T25.222   Burn of second degree of left foot
  - ● T25.229   Burn of second degree of unspecified foot
- ● T25.23   Burn of second degree of toe(s) (nail)
  - ● T25.231   Burn of second degree of right toe(s) (nail)
  - ● T25.232   Burn of second degree of left toe(s) (nail)
  - ● T25.239   Burn of second degree of unspecified toe(s) (nail)
- ● T25.29   Burn of second degree of multiple sites of ankle and foot
  - ● T25.291   Burn of second degree of multiple sites of right ankle and foot
  - ● T25.292   Burn of second degree of multiple sites of left ankle and foot
  - ● T25.299   Burn of second degree of multiple sites of unspecified ankle and foot

● T25.3   Burn of third degree of ankle and foot

Use additional external cause code to identify the source, place and intent of the burn (X00-X19, X75-X77, X96-X98, Y92)

- ● T25.31   Burn of third degree of ankle
  - ● T25.311   Burn of third degree of right ankle
  - ● T25.312   Burn of third degree of left ankle
  - ● T25.319   Burn of third degree of unspecified ankle
- ● T25.32   Burn of third degree of foot

  Excludes2   burn of third degree of toe(s) (nail) (T25.33-)

  - ● T25.321   Burn of third degree of right foot
  - ● T25.322   Burn of third degree of left foot
  - ● T25.329   Burn of third degree of unspecified foot
- ● T25.33   Burn of third degree of toe(s) (nail)
  - ● T25.331   Burn of third degree of right toe(s) (nail)
  - ● T25.332   Burn of third degree of left toe(s) (nail)
  - ● T25.339   Burn of third degree of unspecified toe(s) (nail)

● T25.39   Burn of third degree of multiple sites of ankle and foot
- ● T25.391   Burn of third degree of multiple sites of right ankle and foot
- ● T25.392   Burn of third degree of multiple sites of left ankle and foot
- ● T25.399   Burn of third degree of multiple sites of unspecified ankle and foot

● T25.4   Corrosion of unspecified degree of ankle and foot

Code first (T51-T65) to identify chemical and intent

Use additional external cause code to identify place (Y92)

- ● T25.41   Corrosion of unspecified degree of ankle
  - ● T25.411   Corrosion of unspecified degree of right ankle
  - ● T25.412   Corrosion of unspecified degree of left ankle
  - ● T25.419   Corrosion of unspecified degree of unspecified ankle
- ● T25.42   Corrosion of unspecified degree of foot

  Excludes2   corrosion of unspecified degree of toe(s) (nail) (T25.43-)

  - ● T25.421   Corrosion of unspecified degree of right foot
  - ● T25.422   Corrosion of unspecified degree of left foot
  - ● T25.429   Corrosion of unspecified degree of unspecified foot
- ● T25.43   Corrosion of unspecified degree of toe(s) (nail)
  - ● T25.431   Corrosion of unspecified degree of right toe(s) (nail)
  - ● T25.432   Corrosion of unspecified degree of left toe(s) (nail)
  - ● T25.439   Corrosion of unspecified degree of unspecified toe(s) (nail)
- ● T25.49   Corrosion of unspecified degree of multiple sites of ankle and foot
  - ● T25.491   Corrosion of unspecified degree of multiple sites of right ankle and foot
  - ● T25.492   Corrosion of unspecified degree of multiple sites of left ankle and foot
  - ● T25.499   Corrosion of unspecified degree of multiple sites of unspecified ankle and foot

● T25.5   Corrosion of first degree of ankle and foot

Code first (T51-T65) to identify chemical and intent

Use additional external cause code to identify place (Y92)

- ● T25.51   Corrosion of first degree of ankle
  - ● T25.511   Corrosion of first degree of right ankle
  - ● T25.512   Corrosion of first degree of left ankle
  - ● T25.519   Corrosion of first degree of unspecified ankle
- ● T25.52   Corrosion of first degree of foot

  Excludes2   corrosion of first degree of toe(s) (nail) (T25.53-)

  - ● T25.521   Corrosion of first degree of right foot
  - ● T25.522   Corrosion of first degree of left foot
  - ● T25.529   Corrosion of first degree of unspecified foot

● **T25.53**   Corrosion of first degree of toe(s) (nail)
- ● **T25.531**   Corrosion of first degree of right toe(s) (nail)
- ● **T25.532**   Corrosion of first degree of left toe(s) (nail)
- ● **T25.539**   Corrosion of first degree of unspecified toe(s) (nail)

● **T25.59**   Corrosion of first degree of multiple sites of ankle and foot
- ● **T25.591**   Corrosion of first degree of multiple sites of right ankle and foot
- ● **T25.592**   Corrosion of first degree of multiple sites of left ankle and foot
- ● **T25.599**   Corrosion of first degree of multiple sites of unspecified ankle and foot

● **T25.6**   Corrosion of second degree of ankle and foot

Code first (T51-T65) *to identify chemical and intent*

Use additional external cause code to identify place (Y92)

● **T25.61**   Corrosion of second degree of ankle
- ● **T25.611**   Corrosion of second degree of right ankle
- ● **T25.612**   Corrosion of second degree of left ankle
- ● **T25.619**   Corrosion of second degree of unspecified ankle

● **T25.62**   Corrosion of second degree of foot

Excludes2   corrosion of second degree of toe(s) (nail) (T25.63-)

- ● **T25.621**   Corrosion of second degree of right foot
- ● **T25.622**   Corrosion of second degree of left foot
- ● **T25.629**   Corrosion of second degree of unspecified foot

● **T25.63**   Corrosion of second degree of toe(s) (nail)
- ● **T25.631**   Corrosion of second degree of right toe(s) (nail)
- ● **T25.632**   Corrosion of second degree of left toe(s) (nail)
- ● **T25.639**   Corrosion of second degree of unspecified toe(s) (nail)

● **T25.69**   Corrosion of second degree of multiple sites of ankle and foot
- ● **T25.691**   Corrosion of second degree of right ankle and foot
- ● **T25.692**   Corrosion of second degree of left ankle and foot
- ● **T25.699**   Corrosion of second degree of unspecified ankle and foot

● **T25.7**   Corrosion of third degree of ankle and foot

Code first (T51-T65) *to identify chemical and intent*

Use additional external cause code to identify place (Y92)

● **T25.71**   Corrosion of third degree of ankle
- ● **T25.711**   Corrosion of third degree of right ankle
- ● **T25.712**   Corrosion of third degree of left ankle
- ● **T25.719**   Corrosion of third degree of unspecified ankle

● **T25.72**   Corrosion of third degree of foot

Excludes2   corrosion of third degree of toe(s) (nail) (T25.73-)

- ● **T25.721**   Corrosion of third degree of right foot
- ● **T25.722**   Corrosion of third degree of left foot
- ● **T25.729**   Corrosion of third degree of unspecified foot

● **T25.73**   Corrosion of third degree of toe(s) (nail)
- ● **T25.731**   Corrosion of third degree of right toe(s) (nail)
- ● **T25.732**   Corrosion of third degree of left toe(s) (nail)
- ● **T25.739**   Corrosion of third degree of unspecified toe(s) (nail)

● **T25.79**   Corrosion of third degree of multiple sites of ankle and foot
- ● **T25.791**   Corrosion of third degree of multiple sites of right ankle and foot
- ● **T25.792**   Corrosion of third degree of multiple sites of left ankle and foot
- ● **T25.799**   Corrosion of third degree of multiple sites of unspecified ankle and foot

BURNS AND CORROSIONS CONFINED TO EYE AND INTERNAL ORGANS (T26-T28)

● **T26**   Burn and corrosion confined to eye and adnexa

The appropriate 7th character is to be added to each code from category T26

A	initial encounter
D	subsequent encounter
S	sequela

● **T26.0**   Burn of eyelid and periocular area

Use additional external cause code to identify the source, place and intent of the burn (X00-X19, X75-X77, X96-X98, Y92)

- X ● **T26.00**   Burn of unspecified eyelid and periocular area
- X ● **T26.01**   Burn of right eyelid and periocular area
- X ● **T26.02**   Burn of left eyelid and periocular area

● **T26.1**   Burn of cornea and conjunctival sac

Use additional external cause code to identify the source, place and intent of the burn (X00-X19, X75-X77, X96-X98, Y92)

- X ● **T26.10**   Burn of cornea and conjunctival sac, unspecified eye
- X ● **T26.11**   Burn of cornea and conjunctival sac, right eye
- X ● **T26.12**   Burn of cornea and conjunctival sac, left eye

● **T26.2**   Burn with resulting rupture and destruction of eyeball

Use additional external cause code to identify the source, place and intent of the burn (X00-X19, X75-X77, X96-X98, Y92)

- X ● **T26.20**   Burn with resulting rupture and destruction of unspecified eyeball
- X ● **T26.21**   Burn with resulting rupture and destruction of right eyeball
- X ● **T26.22**   Burn with resulting rupture and destruction of left eyeball

● **T26.3**   Burns of other specified parts of eye and adnexa

Use additional external cause code to identify the source, place and intent of the burn (X00-X19, X75-X77, X96-X98, Y92)

- X ● **T26.30**   Burns of other specified parts of unspecified eye and adnexa
- X ● **T26.31**   Burns of other specified parts of right eye and adnexa
- X ● **T26.32**   Burns of other specified parts of left eye and adnexa

● **T26.4**   Burn of eye and adnexa, part unspecified

Use additional external cause code to identify the source, place and intent of the burn (X00-X19, X75-X77, X96-X98, Y92)

- X ● **T26.40**   Burn of unspecified eye and adnexa, part unspecified
- X ● **T26.41**   Burn of right eye and adnexa, part unspecified
- X ● **T26.42**   Burn of left eye and adnexa, part unspecified

CHAPTER 19 (S00-T88)

● **T26.5**   Corrosion of eyelid and periocular area

> *Code first* (T51-T65) *to identify chemical and intent*
>
> Use additional external cause code to identify place (Y92)

X ● **T26.50**   Corrosion of unspecified eyelid and periocular area

X ● **T26.51**   Corrosion of right eyelid and periocular area

X ● **T26.52**   Corrosion of left eyelid and periocular area

● **T26.6**   Corrosion of cornea and conjunctival sac

> *Code first* (T51-T65) *to identify chemical and intent*
>
> Use additional external cause code to identify place (Y92)

X ● **T26.60**   Corrosion of cornea and conjunctival sac, unspecified eye

X ● **T26.61**   Corrosion of cornea and conjunctival sac, right eye

X ● **T26.62**   Corrosion of cornea and conjunctival sac, left eye

● **T26.7**   Corrosion with resulting rupture and destruction of eyeball

> *Code first* (T51-T65) *to identify chemical and intent*
>
> Use additional external cause code to identify place (Y92)

X ● **T26.70**   Corrosion with resulting rupture and destruction of unspecified eyeball

X ● **T26.71**   Corrosion with resulting rupture and destruction of right eyeball

X ● **T26.72**   Corrosion with resulting rupture and destruction of left eyeball

● **T26.8**   Corrosions of other specified parts of eye and adnexa

> *Code first* (T51-T65) *to identify chemical and intent*
>
> Use additional external cause code to identify place (Y92)

X ● **T26.80**   Corrosions of other specified parts of unspecified eye and adnexa

X ● **T26.81**   Corrosions of other specified parts of right eye and adnexa

X ● **T26.82**   Corrosions of other specified parts of left eye and adnexa

● **T26.9**   Corrosion of eye and adnexa, part unspecified

> *Code first* (T51-T65) *to identify chemical and intent*
>
> Use additional external cause code to identify place (Y92)

X ● **T26.90**   Corrosion of unspecified eye and adnexa, part unspecified

X ● **T26.91**   Corrosion of right eye and adnexa, part unspecified

X ● **T26.92**   Corrosion of left eye and adnexa, part unspecified

● **T27**   Burn and corrosion of respiratory tract

> Use additional external cause code to identify the source and intent of the burn (X00-X19, X75-X77, X96-X98)
>
> Use additional external cause code to identify place (Y92)
>
> The appropriate 7th character is to be added to each code from category T27

A	initial encounter
D	subsequent encounter
S	sequela

X ● **T27.0**   Burn of larynx and trachea

X ● **T27.1**   Burn involving larynx and trachea with lung

X ● **T27.2**   Burn of other parts of respiratory tract

> Burn of thoracic cavity

X ● **T27.3**   Burn of respiratory tract, part unspecified

X ● **T27.4**   Corrosion of larynx and trachea

> *Code first* (T51-T65) *to identify chemical and intent*

X ● **T27.5**   Corrosion involving larynx and trachea with lung

> *Code first* (T51-T65) *to identify chemical and intent*

X ● **T27.6**   Corrosion of other parts of respiratory tract

> *Code first* (T51-T65) *to identify chemical and intent*

X ● **T27.7**   Corrosion of respiratory tract, part unspecified

> *Code first* (T51-T65) *to identify chemical and intent*

● **T28**   Burn and corrosion of other internal organs

> Use additional external cause code to identify the source and intent of the burn (X00-X19, X75-X77, X96-X98)
>
> Use additional external cause code to identify place (Y92)
>
> The appropriate 7th character is to be added to each code from category T28

A	initial encounter
D	subsequent encounter
S	sequela

X ● **T28.0**   Burn of mouth and pharynx

X ● **T28.1**   Burn of esophagus

X ● **T28.2**   Burn of other parts of alimentary tract

X ● **T28.3**   Burn of internal genitourinary organs

X ● **T28.4**   Burns of other and unspecified internal organs

X ● **T28.40**   Burn of unspecified internal organ

● **T28.41**   Burn of ear drum

● **T28.411**   Burn of right ear drum

● **T28.412**   Burn of left ear drum

● **T28.419**   Burn of unspecified ear drum

X ● **T28.49**   Burn of other internal organ

X ● **T28.5**   Corrosion of mouth and pharynx

> *Code first* (T51-T65) *to identify chemical and intent*

X ● **T28.6**   Corrosion of esophagus

> *Code first* (T51-T65) *to identify chemical and intent*

X ● **T28.7**   Corrosion of other parts of alimentary tract

> *Code first* (T51-T65) *to identify chemical and intent*

X ● **T28.8**   Corrosion of internal genitourinary organs

> *Code first* (T51-T65) *to identify chemical and intent*

● **T28.9**   Corrosions of other and unspecified internal organs

> *Code first* (T51-T65) *to identify chemical and intent*

X ● **T28.90**   Corrosions of unspecified internal organs

● **T28.91**   Corrosions of ear drum

● **T28.911**   Corrosions of right ear drum

● **T28.912**   Corrosions of left ear drum

● **T28.919**   Corrosions of unspecified ear drum

X ● **T28.99**   Corrosions of other internal organs

OGCR Section I.C.19.d.5.

> Assign separate code for each burn site
>
> When coding burns, assign separate codes for each burn site. Category T30, Burn and corrosion, body region unspecified is extremely vague and should rarely be used.

BURNS AND CORROSIONS OF MULTIPLE AND UNSPECIFIED BODY REGIONS (T30-T32)

● **T30**   Burn and corrosion, body region unspecified

T30.0   Burn of unspecified body region, unspecified degree

> This code is not for inpatient use. Code to specified site and degree of burns
>
> Burn NOS
>
> Multiple burns NOS

T30.4   Corrosion of unspecified body region, unspecified degree

> This code is not for inpatient use. Code to specified site and degree of corrosion
>
> Corrosion NOS
>
> Multiple corrosion NOS

▶ New   ⯈ Revised   ~~deleted~~ Deleted   Excludes 1   Excludes 2   Includes   Use additional   Code first   Code also   Key words

OGCR Official Guidelines   X Assign placeholder X   ● Use Additional Character(s)   ⯈ Manifestation Code   ⬭ Hierarchical Condition Category   **Coding Clinic**

● **T31**   **Burns** classified according to **extent of body surface involved**

> **Note:** This category is to be used as the primary code only when the site of the burn is unspecified. It should be used as a supplementary code with categories T20-T25 when the site is specified.

T31.0   Burns involving **less than 10%** of body surface

● **T31.1**   Burns involving **10-19%** of body surface

     T31.10   Burns involving **10-19%** of body surface with **0% to 9% third degree burns**
> Burns involving 10-19% of body surface NOS

     T31.11   Burns involving **10-19%** of body surface with **10-19% third degree burns** 🔲

● **T31.2**   Burns involving **20-29%** of body surface

     T31.20   Burns involving **20-29%** of body surface with **0% to 9% third degree burns**
> Burns involving 20-29% of body surface NOS

     T31.21   Burns involving **20-29%** of body surface with **10-19% third degree burns** 🔲

     T31.22   Burns involving **20-29%** of body surface with **20-29% third degree burns** 🔲

● **T31.3**   Burns involving **30-39%** of body surface

     T31.30   Burns involving **30-39%** of body surface with **0% to 9% third degree burns**
> Burns involving 30-39% of body surface NOS

     T31.31   Burns involving **30-39%** of body surface with **10-19% third degree burns** 🔲

     T31.32   Burns involving **30-39%** of body surface with **20-29% third degree burns** 🔲

     T31.33   Burns involving **30-39%** of body surface with **30-39% third degree burns** 🔲

● **T31.4**   Burns involving **40-49%** of body surface

     T31.40   Burns involving **40-49%** of body surface with **0% to 9% third degree burns**
> Burns involving 40-49% of body surface NOS

     T31.41   Burns involving **40-49%** of body surface with **10-19% third degree burns** 🔲

     T31.42   Burns involving **40-49%** of body surface with **20-29% third degree burns** 🔲

     T31.43   Burns involving **40-49%** of body surface with **30-39% third degree burns** 🔲

     T31.44   Burns involving **40-49%** of body surface with **40-49% third degree burns** 🔲

● **T31.5**   Burns involving **50-59%** of body surface

     T31.50   Burns involving **50-59%** of body surface with **0% to 9% third degree burns**
> Burns involving 50-59% of body surface NOS

     T31.51   Burns involving **50-59%** of body surface with **10-19% third degree burns** 🔲

     T31.52   Burns involving **50-59%** of body surface with **20-29% third degree burns** 🔲

     T31.53   Burns involving **50-59%** of body surface with **30-39% third degree burns** 🔲

     T31.54   Burns involving **50-59%** of body surface with **40-49% third degree burns** 🔲

     T31.55   Burns involving **50-59%** of body surface with **50-59% third degree burns** 🔲

● **T31.6**   Burns involving **60-69%** of body surface

     T31.60   Burns involving **60-69%** of body surface with **0% to 9% third degree burns**
> Burns involving 60-69% of body surface NOS

     T31.61   Burns involving **60-69%** of body surface with **10-19% third degree burns** 🔲

     T31.62   Burns involving **60-69%** of body surface with **20-29% third degree burns** 🔲

     T31.63   Burns involving **60-69%** of body surface with **30-39% third degree burns** 🔲

     T31.64   Burns involving **60-69%** of body surface with **40-49% third degree burns** 🔲

     T31.65   Burns involving **60-69%** of body surface with **50-59% third degree burns** 🔲

     T31.66   Burns involving **60-69%** of body surface with **60-69% third degree burns** 🔲

● **T31.7**   Burns involving **70-79%** of body surface

     T31.70   Burns involving **70-79%** of body surface with **0% to 9% third degree burns**
> Burns involving 70-79% of body surface NOS

     T31.71   Burns involving **70-79%** of body surface with **10-19% third degree burns** 🔲

     T31.72   Burns involving **70-79%** of body surface with **20-29% third degree burns** 🔲

     T31.73   Burns involving **70-79%** of body surface with **30-39% third degree burns** 🔲

     T31.74   Burns involving **70-79%** of body surface with **40-49% third degree burns** 🔲

     T31.75   Burns involving **70-79%** of body surface with **50-59% third degree burns** 🔲

     T31.76   Burns involving **70-79%** of body surface with **60-69% third degree burns** 🔲

     T31.77   Burns involving **70-79%** of body surface with **70-79% third degree burns** 🔲

● **T31.8**   Burns involving **80-89%** of body surface

     T31.80   Burns involving **80-89%** of body surface with **0% to 9% third degree burns**
> Burns involving 80-89% of body surface NOS

     T31.81   Burns involving **80-89%** of body surface with **10-19% third degree burns** 🔲

     T31.82   Burns involving **80-89%** of body surface with **20-29% third degree burns** 🔲

     T31.83   Burns involving **80-89%** of body surface with **30-39% third degree burns** 🔲

     T31.84   Burns involving **80-89%** of body surface with **40-49% third degree burns** 🔲

     T31.85   Burns involving **80-89%** of body surface with **50-59% third degree burns** 🔲

     T31.86   Burns involving **80-89%** of body surface with **60-69% third degree burns** 🔲

     T31.87   Burns involving **80-89%** of body surface with **70-79% third degree burns** 🔲

     T31.88   Burns involving **80-89%** of body surface with **80-89% third degree burns** 🔲

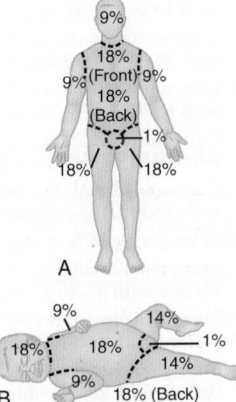

Figure 19-16   Rule of nines: percentages of total body area. (From Marx: Rosen's Emergency Medicine: Concepts and Clinical Practice, ed 6, Mosby, 2006)

● **T31.9** Burns involving 90% or more of body surface

     T31.90 Burns involving 90% or more of body surface with 0% to 9% third degree burns
         Burns involving 90% or more of body surface NOS

     T31.91 Burns involving 90% or more of body surface with 10-19% third degree burns 🐌

     T31.92 Burns involving 90% or more of body surface with 20-29% third degree burns 🐌

     T31.93 Burns involving 90% or more of body surface with 30-39% third degree burns 🐌

     T31.94 Burns involving 90% or more of body surface with 40-49% third degree burns 🐌

     T31.95 Burns involving 90% or more of body surface with 50-59% third degree burns 🐌

     T31.96 Burns involving 90% or more of body surface with 60-69% third degree burns 🐌

     T31.97 Burns involving 90% or more of body surface with 70-79% third degree burns 🐌

     T31.98 Burns involving 90% or more of body surface with 80-89% third degree burns 🐌

     T31.99 Burns involving 90% or more of body surface with 90% or more third degree burns 🐌

● **T32** Corrosions classified according to extent of body surface involved

     Note: This category is to be used as the primary code only when the site of the corrosion is unspecified. It may be used as a supplementary code with categories T20-T25 when the site is specified.

   T32.0 Corrosions involving less than 10% of body surface

● **T32.1** Corrosions involving 10-19% of body surface

     T32.10 Corrosions involving 10-19% of body surface with 0% to 9% third degree corrosion
         Corrosions involving 10-19% of body surface NOS

     T32.11 Corrosions involving 10-19% of body surface with 10-19% third degree corrosion 🐌

● **T32.2** Corrosions involving 20-29% of body surface

     T32.20 Corrosions involving 20-29% of body surface with 0% to 9% third degree corrosion

     T32.21 Corrosions involving 20-29% of body surface with 10-19% third degree corrosion 🐌

     T32.22 Corrosions involving 20-29% of body surface with 20-29% third degree corrosion 🐌

● **T32.3** Corrosions involving 30-39% of body surface

     T32.30 Corrosions involving 30-39% of body surface with 0% to 9% third degree corrosion

     T32.31 Corrosions involving 30-39% of body surface with 10-19% third degree corrosion 🐌

     T32.32 Corrosions involving 30-39% of body surface with 20-29% third degree corrosion 🐌

     T32.33 Corrosions involving 30-39% of body surface with 30-39% third degree corrosion 🐌

● **T32.4** Corrosions involving 40-49% of body surface

     T32.40 Corrosions involving 40-49% of body surface with 0% to 9% third degree corrosion

     T32.41 Corrosions involving 40-49% of body surface with 10-19% third degree corrosion 🐌

     T32.42 Corrosions involving 40-49% of body surface with 20-29% third degree corrosion 🐌

     T32.43 Corrosions involving 40-49% of body surface with 30-39% third degree corrosion 🐌

     T32.44 Corrosions involving 40-49% of body surface with 40-49% third degree corrosion 🐌

● **T32.5** Corrosions involving 50-59% of body surface

     T32.50 Corrosions involving 50-59% of body surface with 0% to 9% third degree corrosion

     T32.51 Corrosions involving 50-59% of body surface with 10-19% third degree corrosion 🐌

     T32.52 Corrosions involving 50-59% of body surface with 20-29% third degree corrosion 🐌

     T32.53 Corrosions involving 50-59% of body surface with 30-39% third degree corrosion 🐌

     T32.54 Corrosions involving 50-59% of body surface with 40-49% third degree corrosion 🐌

     T32.55 Corrosions involving 50-59% of body surface with 50-59% third degree corrosion 🐌

● **T32.6** Corrosions involving 60-69% of body surface

     T32.60 Corrosions involving 60-69% of body surface with 0% to 9% third degree corrosion

     T32.61 Corrosions involving 60-69% of body surface with 10-19% third degree corrosion 🐌

     T32.62 Corrosions involving 60-69% of body surface with 20-29% third degree corrosion 🐌

     T32.63 Corrosions involving 60-69% of body surface with 30-39% third degree corrosion 🐌

     T32.64 Corrosions involving 60-69% of body surface with 40-49% third degree corrosion 🐌

     T32.65 Corrosions involving 60-69% of body surface with 50-59% third degree corrosion 🐌

     T32.66 Corrosions involving 60-69% of body surface with 60-69% third degree corrosion 🐌

● **T32.7** Corrosions involving 70-79% of body surface

     T32.70 Corrosions involving 70-79% of body surface with 0% to 9% third degree corrosion

     T32.71 Corrosions involving 70-79% of body surface with 10-19% third degree corrosion 🐌

     T32.72 Corrosions involving 70-79% of body surface with 20-29% third degree corrosion 🐌

     T32.73 Corrosions involving 70-79% of body surface with 30-39% third degree corrosion 🐌

     T32.74 Corrosions involving 70-79% of body surface with 40-49% third degree corrosion 🐌

     T32.75 Corrosions involving 70-79% of body surface with 50-59% third degree corrosion 🐌

     T32.76 Corrosions involving 70-79% of body surface with 60-69% third degree corrosion 🐌

     T32.77 Corrosions involving 70-79% of body surface with 70-79% third degree corrosion 🐌

● **T32.8** Corrosions involving 80-89% of body surface

     T32.80 Corrosions involving 80-89% of body surface with 0% to 9% third degree corrosion

     T32.81 Corrosions involving 80-89% of body surface with 10-19% third degree corrosion 🐌

     T32.82 Corrosions involving 80-89% of body surface with 20-29% third degree corrosion 🐌

     T32.83 Corrosions involving 80-89% of body surface with 30-39% third degree corrosion 🐌

     T32.84 Corrosions involving 80-89% of body surface with 40-49% third degree corrosion 🐌

     T32.85 Corrosions involving 80-89% of body surface with 50-59% third degree corrosion 🐌

     T32.86 Corrosions involving 80-89% of body surface with 60-69% third degree corrosion 🐌

     T32.87 Corrosions involving 80-89% of body surface with 70-79% third degree corrosion 🐌

     T32.88 Corrosions involving 80-89% of body surface with 80-89% third degree corrosion 🐌

● **T32.9** Corrosions involving 90% or more of body surface

     T32.90 Corrosions involving 90% or more of body surface with 0% to 9% third degree corrosion

     T32.91 Corrosions involving 90% or more of body surface with 10-19% third degree corrosion 🐌

     T32.92 Corrosions involving 90% or more of body surface with 20-29% third degree corrosion 🐌

     T32.93 Corrosions involving 90% or more of body surface with 30-39% third degree corrosion 🐌

▶ New   ⟹ Revised   ~~deleted~~ Deleted   Excludes 1   Excludes 2   Includes   Use additional   Code first   Code also   Key words

OGCR Official Guidelines   X Assign placeholder X   ● Use Additional Character(s)   ▌ Manifestation Code   🐌 Hierarchical Condition Category   **Coding Clinic**

T32.94   Corrosions involving 90% or more of body surface with 40-49% third degree corrosion ⚫

T32.95   Corrosions involving 90% or more of body surface with 50-59% third degree corrosion ⚫

T32.96   Corrosions involving 90% or more of body surface with 60-69% third degree corrosion ⚫

T32.97   Corrosions involving 90% or more of body surface with 70-79% third degree corrosion ⚫

T32.98   Corrosions involving 90% or more of body surface with 80-89% third degree corrosion ⚫

T32.99   Corrosions involving 90% or more of body surface with 90% or more third degree corrosion ⚫

FROSTBITE (T33-T34)

Excludes2   hypothermia and other effects of reduced temperature (T68, T69.-)

⚫T33   Superficial frostbite

Includes   frostbite with partial thickness skin loss

The appropriate 7th character is to be added to each code from category T33

A	initial encounter
D	subsequent encounter
S	sequela

⚫T33.0   Superficial frostbite of head

  ⚫T33.01   Superficial frostbite of ear

    ⚫T33.011   Superficial frostbite of right ear

    ⚫T33.012   Superficial frostbite of left ear

    ⚫T33.019   Superficial frostbite of unspecified ear

  X⚫T33.02   Superficial frostbite of nose

  X⚫T33.09   Superficial frostbite of other part of head

X⚫T33.1   Superficial frostbite of neck

X⚫T33.2   Superficial frostbite of thorax

X⚫T33.3   Superficial frostbite of abdominal wall, lower back and pelvis

⚫T33.4   Superficial frostbite of arm

  Excludes2   superficial frostbite of wrist and hand (T33.5-)

  X⚫T33.40   Superficial frostbite of unspecified arm

  X⚫T33.41   Superficial frostbite of right arm

  X⚫T33.42   Superficial frostbite of left arm

⚫T33.5   Superficial frostbite of wrist, hand, and fingers

  ⚫T33.51   Superficial frostbite of wrist

    ⚫T33.511   Superficial frostbite of right wrist

    ⚫T33.512   Superficial frostbite of left wrist

    ⚫T33.519   Superficial frostbite of unspecified wrist

  ⚫T33.52   Superficial frostbite of hand

    Excludes2   superficial frostbite of fingers (T33.53-)

    ⚫T33.521   Superficial frostbite of right hand

    ⚫T33.522   Superficial frostbite of left hand

    ⚫T33.529   Superficial frostbite of unspecified hand

  ⚫T33.53   Superficial frostbite of finger(s)

    ⚫T33.531   Superficial frostbite of right finger(s)

    ⚫T33.532   Superficial frostbite of left finger(s)

    ⚫T33.539   Superficial frostbite of unspecified finger(s)

⚫T33.6   Superficial frostbite of hip and thigh

  X⚫T33.60   Superficial frostbite of unspecified hip and thigh

  X⚫T33.61   Superficial frostbite of right hip and thigh

  X⚫T33.62   Superficial frostbite of left hip and thigh

⚫T33.7   Superficial frostbite of knee and lower leg

  Excludes2   superficial frostbite of ankle and foot (T33.8-)

  X⚫T33.70   Superficial frostbite of unspecified knee and lower leg

  X⚫T33.71   Superficial frostbite of right knee and lower leg

  X⚫T33.72   Superficial frostbite of left knee and lower leg

⚫T33.8   Superficial frostbite of ankle, foot, and toe(s)

  ⚫T33.81   Superficial frostbite of ankle

    ⚫T33.811   Superficial frostbite of right ankle

    ⚫T33.812   Superficial frostbite of left ankle

    ⚫T33.819   Superficial frostbite of unspecified ankle

  ⚫T33.82   Superficial frostbite of foot

    ⚫T33.821   Superficial frostbite of right foot

    ⚫T33.822   Superficial frostbite of left foot

    ⚫T33.829   Superficial frostbite of unspecified foot

  ⚫T33.83   Superficial frostbite of toe(s)

    ⚫T33.831   Superficial frostbite of right toe(s)

    ⚫T33.832   Superficial frostbite of left toe(s)

    ⚫T33.839   Superficial frostbite of unspecified toe(s)

⚫T33.9   Superficial frostbite of other and unspecified sites

  X⚫T33.90   Superficial frostbite of unspecified sites
    Superficial frostbite NOS

  X⚫T33.99   Superficial frostbite of other sites
    Superficial frostbite of leg NOS
    Superficial frostbite of trunk NOS

⚫T34   Frostbite with tissue necrosis

The appropriate 7th character is to be added to each code from category T34

A	initial encounter
D	subsequent encounter
S	sequela

⚫T34.0   Frostbite with tissue necrosis of head

  ⚫T34.01   Frostbite with tissue necrosis of ear

    ⚫T34.011   Frostbite with tissue necrosis of right ear

    ⚫T34.012   Frostbite with tissue necrosis of left ear

    ⚫T34.019   Frostbite with tissue necrosis of unspecified ear

  X⚫T34.02   Frostbite with tissue necrosis of nose

  X⚫T34.09   Frostbite with tissue necrosis of other part of head

X⚫T34.1   Frostbite with tissue necrosis of neck

X⚫T34.2   Frostbite with tissue necrosis of thorax

X⚫T34.3   Frostbite with tissue necrosis of abdominal wall, lower back and pelvis

⚫T34.4   Frostbite with tissue necrosis of arm

  Excludes2   frostbite with tissue necrosis of wrist and hand (T34.5-)

  X⚫T34.40   Frostbite with tissue necrosis of unspecified arm

  X⚫T34.41   Frostbite with tissue necrosis of right arm

  X⚫T34.42   Frostbite with tissue necrosis of left arm

- T34.5   Frostbite with tissue necrosis of wrist, hand, and finger(s)
  - T34.51   Frostbite with tissue necrosis of wrist
    - T34.511   Frostbite with tissue necrosis of right wrist
    - T34.512   Frostbite with tissue necrosis of left wrist
    - T34.519   Frostbite with tissue necrosis of unspecified wrist
  - T34.52   Frostbite with tissue necrosis of hand
    - **Excludes2**   frostbite with tissue necrosis of finger(s) (T34.53-)
    - T34.521   Frostbite with tissue necrosis of right hand
    - T34.522   Frostbite with tissue necrosis of left hand
    - T34.529   Frostbite with tissue necrosis of unspecified hand
  - T34.53   Frostbite with tissue necrosis of finger(s)
    - T34.531   Frostbite with tissue necrosis of right finger(s)
    - T34.532   Frostbite with tissue necrosis of left finger(s)
    - T34.539   Frostbite with tissue necrosis of unspecified finger(s)
- T34.6   Frostbite with tissue necrosis of hip and thigh
  - X T34.60   Frostbite with tissue necrosis of unspecified hip and thigh
  - X T34.61   Frostbite with tissue necrosis of right hip and thigh
  - X T34.62   Frostbite with tissue necrosis of left hip and thigh
- T34.7   Frostbite with tissue necrosis of knee and lower leg
  - **Excludes2**   frostbite with tissue necrosis of ankle and foot (T34.8-)
  - X T34.70   Frostbite with tissue necrosis of unspecified knee and lower leg
  - X T34.71   Frostbite with tissue necrosis of right knee and lower leg
  - X T34.72   Frostbite with tissue necrosis of left knee and lower leg
- T34.8   Frostbite with tissue necrosis of ankle, foot, and toe(s)
  - T34.81   Frostbite with tissue necrosis of ankle
    - T34.811   Frostbite with tissue necrosis of right ankle
    - T34.812   Frostbite with tissue necrosis of left ankle
    - T34.819   Frostbite with tissue necrosis of unspecified ankle
  - T34.82   Frostbite with tissue necrosis of foot
    - T34.821   Frostbite with tissue necrosis of right foot
    - T34.822   Frostbite with tissue necrosis of left foot
    - T34.829   Frostbite with tissue necrosis of unspecified foot
  - T34.83   Frostbite with tissue necrosis of toe(s)
    - T34.831   Frostbite with tissue necrosis of right toe(s)
    - T34.832   Frostbite with tissue necrosis of left toe(s)
    - T34.839   Frostbite with tissue necrosis of unspecified toe(s)

- T34.9   Frostbite with tissue necrosis of other and unspecified sites
  - X T34.90   Frostbite with tissue necrosis of unspecified sites
    - Frostbite with tissue necrosis NOS
  - X T34.99   Frostbite with tissue necrosis of other sites
    - Frostbite with tissue necrosis of leg NOS
    - Frostbite with tissue necrosis of trunk NOS

OGCR See Section I.C.19.e.

Adverse Effects, Poisoning, Underdosing and Toxic Effects

Codes in categories T36-T65 are combination codes that include the substance that was taken as well as the intent. No additional external cause code is required for poisonings, toxic effects, adverse effects and underdosing codes.

POISONING BY, ADVERSE EFFECTS OF AND UNDERDOSING OF DRUGS MEDICAMENTS AND BIOLOGICAL SUBSTANCES (T36-T50)

Includes   adverse effect of correct substance properly administered
poisoning by overdose of substance
poisoning by wrong substance given or taken in error
underdosing by (inadvertently) (deliberately) taking less substance than prescribed or instructed

Code first, for adverse effects, the nature of the adverse effect, such as:
adverse effect NOS (T88.7)
aspirin gastritis (K29.-)
blood disorders (D56-D76)
contact dermatitis (L23-L25)
dermatitis due to substances taken internally (L27.-)
nephropathy (N14.0-N14.2)

Note: The drug giving rise to the adverse effect should be identified by use of codes from categories T36-T50 with fifth or sixth character 5.

Use additional code(s) to specify:
manifestations of poisoning
underdosing or failure in dosage during medical and surgical care (Y63.6, Y63.8-Y63.9)
underdosing of medication regimen (Z91.12-, Z91.13-)

Excludes1   toxic reaction to local anesthesia in pregnancy (O29.3-)

Excludes2   abuse and dependence of psychoactive substances (F10-F19)
abuse of non-dependence-producing substances (F55.-)
drug reaction and poisoning affecting newborn (P00-P96)
immunodeficiency due to drugs (D84.821)
pathological drug intoxication (inebriation) (F10-F19)

- T36   **Poisoning by, adverse effect of and underdosing of systemic antibiotics**
  - **Excludes1**   antineoplastic antibiotics (T45.1-)
    locally applied antibiotic NEC (T49.0)
    topically used antibiotic for ear, nose and throat (T49.6)
    topically used antibiotic for eye (T49.5)
  - The appropriate 7th character is to be added to each code from category T36

A	initial encounter
D	subsequent encounter
S	sequela

▶ New   ⇒ Revised   ~~deleted~~ Deleted   Excludes 1   Excludes 2   Includes   Use additional   Code first   Code also   Key words
OGCR Official Guidelines   X Assign placeholder X   ● Use Additional Character(s)   ▶ Manifestation Code   Hierarchical Condition Category   **Coding Clinic**

● **T36.0** Poisoning by, adverse effect of and underdosing of penicillins

  ● **T36.0X** Poisoning by, adverse effect of and underdosing of penicillins

    ● **T36.0X1** Poisoning by penicillins, accidental (unintentional)
        Poisoning by penicillins NOS

    ● **T36.0X2** Poisoning by penicillins, intentional self-harm A, S 🐾

    ● **T36.0X3** Poisoning by penicillins, assault

    ● **T36.0X4** Poisoning by penicillins, undetermined

    ● **T36.0X5** Adverse effect of penicillins

    ● **T36.0X6** Underdosing of penicillins

● **T36.1** Poisoning by, adverse effect of and underdosing of cephalosporins and other betalactam antibiotics

  ● **T36.1X** Poisoning by, adverse effect of and underdosing of cephalosporins and other beta-lactam antibiotics

    ● **T36.1X1** Poisoning by cephalosporins and other beta-lactam antibiotics, accidental (unintentional)
        Poisoning by cephalosporins and other beta-lactam antibiotics NOS

    ● **T36.1X2** Poisoning by cephalosporins and other beta-lactam antibiotics, intentional self-harm A, S 🐾

    ● **T36.1X3** Poisoning by cephalosporins and other beta-lactam antibiotics, assault

    ● **T36.1X4** Poisoning by cephalosporins and other beta-lactam antibiotics, undetermined

    ● **T36.1X5** Adverse effect of cephalosporins and other beta-lactam antibiotics

    ● **T36.1X6** Underdosing of cephalosporins and other beta-lactam antibiotics

● **T36.2** Poisoning by, adverse effect of and underdosing of chloramphenicol group

  ● **T36.2X** Poisoning by, adverse effect of and underdosing of chloramphenicol group

    ● **T36.2X1** Poisoning by chloramphenicol group, accidental (unintentional)
        Poisoning by chloramphenicol group NOS

    ● **T36.2X2** Poisoning by chloramphenicol group, intentional self-harm A, S 🐾

    ● **T36.2X3** Poisoning by chloramphenicol group, assault

    ● **T36.2X4** Poisoning by chloramphenicol group, undetermined

    ● **T36.2X5** Adverse effect of chloramphenicol group

    ● **T36.2X6** Underdosing of chloramphenicol group

● **T36.3** Poisoning by, adverse effect of and underdosing of macrolides

  ● **T36.3X** Poisoning by, adverse effect of and underdosing of macrolides

    ● **T36.3X1** Poisoning by macrolides, accidental (unintentional)
        Poisoning by macrolides NOS

    ● **T36.3X2** Poisoning by macrolides, intentional self-harm A, S 🐾

    ● **T36.3X3** Poisoning by macrolides, assault

    ● **T36.3X4** Poisoning by macrolides, undetermined

    ● **T36.3X5** Adverse effect of macrolides

    ● **T36.3X6** Underdosing of macrolides

● **T36.4** Poisoning by, adverse effect of and underdosing of tetracyclines

  ● **T36.4X** Poisoning by, adverse effect of and underdosing of tetracyclines

    ● **T36.4X1** Poisoning by tetracyclines, accidental (unintentional)
        Poisoning by tetracyclines NOS

    ● **T36.4X2** Poisoning by tetracyclines, intentional self-harm A, S 🐾

    ● **T36.4X3** Poisoning by tetracyclines, assault

    ● **T36.4X4** Poisoning by tetracyclines, undetermined

    ● **T36.4X5** Adverse effect of tetracyclines

    ● **T36.4X6** Underdosing of tetracyclines

● **T36.5** Poisoning by, adverse effect of and underdosing of aminoglycosides
    Poisoning by, adverse effect of and underdosing of streptomycin

  ● **T36.5X** Poisoning by, adverse effect of and underdosing of aminoglycosides

    ● **T36.5X1** Poisoning by aminoglycosides, accidental (unintentional)
        Poisoning by aminoglycosides NOS

    ● **T36.5X2** Poisoning by aminoglycosides, intentional self-harm A, S 🐾

    ● **T36.5X3** Poisoning by aminoglycosides, assault

    ● **T36.5X4** Poisoning by aminoglycosides, undetermined

    ● **T36.5X5** Adverse effect of aminoglycosides

    ● **T36.5X6** Underdosing of aminoglycosides

● **T36.6** Poisoning by, adverse effect of and underdosing of rifampicins

  ● **T36.6X** Poisoning by, adverse effect of and underdosing of rifampicins

    ● **T36.6X1** Poisoning by rifampicins, accidental (unintentional)
        Poisoning by rifampicins NOS

    ● **T36.6X2** Poisoning by rifampicins, intentional self-harm A, S 🐾

    ● **T36.6X3** Poisoning by rifampicins, assault

    ● **T36.6X4** Poisoning by rifampicins, undetermined

    ● **T36.6X5** Adverse effect of rifampicins

    ● **T36.6X6** Underdosing of rifampicins

● **T36.7** Poisoning by, adverse effect of and underdosing of antifungal antibiotics, systemically used

  ● **T36.7X** Poisoning by, adverse effect of and underdosing of antifungal antibiotics, systemically used

    ● **T36.7X1** Poisoning by antifungal antibiotics, systemically used, accidental (unintentional)
        Poisoning by antifungal antibiotics, systemically used NOS

    ● **T36.7X2** Poisoning by antifungal antibiotics, systemically used, intentional self-harm A, S 🐾

    ● **T36.7X3** Poisoning by antifungal antibiotics, systemically used, assault

    ● **T36.7X4** Poisoning by antifungal antibiotics, systemically used, undetermined

    ● **T36.7X5** Adverse effect of antifungal antibiotics, systemically used

    ● **T36.7X6** Underdosing of antifungal antibiotics, systemically used

CHAPTER 19 (S00-T88)

CHAPTER 19 (S00-T88)

- **T36.8** Poisoning by, adverse effect of and underdosing of other systemic antibiotics
  - **T36.8X** Poisoning by, adverse effect of and underdosing of other systemic antibiotics
    - **T36.8X1** Poisoning by other systemic antibiotics, accidental (unintentional)
      Poisoning by other systemic antibiotics NOS
    - **T36.8X2** Poisoning by other systemic antibiotics, intentional self-harm A, S
    - **T36.8X3** Poisoning by other systemic antibiotics, assault
    - **T36.8X4** Poisoning by other systemic antibiotics, undetermined
    - **T36.8X5** Adverse effect of other systemic antibiotics
      Coding Clinic: 2017, Q1, P39
    - **T36.8X6** Underdosing of other systemic antibiotics
- **T36.9** Poisoning by, adverse effect of and underdosing of unspecified systemic antibiotic
  - X **T36.91** Poisoning by unspecified systemic antibiotic, accidental (unintentional)
    Poisoning by systemic antibiotic NOS
  - X **T36.92** Poisoning by unspecified systemic antibiotic, intentional self-harm A, S
  - X **T36.93** Poisoning by unspecified systemic antibiotic, assault
  - X **T36.94** Poisoning by unspecified systemic antibiotic, undetermined
  - X **T36.95** Adverse effect of unspecified systemic antibiotic
  - X **T36.96** Underdosing of unspecified systemic antibiotic
- **T37** Poisoning by, adverse effect of and underdosing of other systemic anti-infectives and antiparasitics
  - **Excludes1** anti-infectives topically used for ear, nose and throat (T49.6-)
    anti-infectives topically used for eye (T49.5-)
    locally applied anti-infectives NEC (T49.0-)

  The appropriate 7th character is to be added to each code from category T37

A	initial encounter
D	subsequent encounter
S	sequela

  - **T37.0** Poisoning by, adverse effect of and underdosing of sulfonamides
    - **T37.0X** Poisoning by, adverse effect of and underdosing of sulfonamides
      - **T37.0X1** Poisoning by sulfonamides, accidental (unintentional)
        Poisoning by sulfonamides NOS
      - **T37.0X2** Poisoning by sulfonamides, intentional self-harm A, S
      - **T37.0X3** Poisoning by sulfonamides, assault
      - **T37.0X4** Poisoning by sulfonamides, undetermined
      - **T37.0X5** Adverse effect of sulfonamides
      - **T37.0X6** Underdosing of sulfonamides
  - **T37.1** Poisoning by, adverse effect of and underdosing of antimycobacterial drugs
    - **Excludes1** rifampicins (T36.6-) streptomycin (T36.5-)
    - **T37.1X** Poisoning by, adverse effect of and underdosing of antimycobacterial drugs
      - **T37.1X1** Poisoning by antimycobacterial drugs, accidental (unintentional)
        Poisoning by antimycobacterial drugs NOS
      - **T37.1X2** Poisoning by antimycobacterial drugs, intentional self-harm A, S

- **T37.1X3** Poisoning by antimycobacterial drugs, assault
- **T37.1X4** Poisoning by antimycobacterial drugs, undetermined
- **T37.1X5** Adverse effect of antimycobacterial drugs
- **T37.1X6** Underdosing of antimycobacterial drugs
- **T37.2** Poisoning by, adverse effect of and underdosing of antimalarials and drugs acting on other blood protozoa
  - **Excludes1** hydroxyquinoline derivatives (T37.8-)
  - **T37.2X** Poisoning by, adverse effect of and underdosing of antimalarials and drugs acting on other blood protozoa
    - **T37.2X1** Poisoning by antimalarials and drugs acting on other blood protozoa, accidental (unintentional)
      Poisoning by antimalarials and drugs acting on other blood protozoa NOS
    - **T37.2X2** Poisoning by antimalarials and drugs acting on other blood protozoa, intentional self-harm A, S
    - **T37.2X3** Poisoning by antimalarials and drugs acting on other blood protozoa, assault
    - **T37.2X4** Poisoning by antimalarials and drugs acting on other blood protozoa, undetermined
    - **T37.2X5** Adverse effect of antimalarials and drugs acting on other blood protozoa
    - **T37.2X6** Underdosing of antimalarials and drugs acting on other blood protozoa
- **T37.3** Poisoning by, adverse effect of and underdosing of other antiprotozoal drugs
  - **T37.3X** Poisoning by, adverse effect of and underdosing of other antiprotozoal drugs
    - **T37.3X1** Poisoning by other antiprotozoal drugs, accidental (unintentional)
      Poisoning by other antiprotozoal drugs NOS
    - **T37.3X2** Poisoning by other antiprotozoal drugs, intentional self-harm A, S
    - **T37.3X3** Poisoning by other antiprotozoal drugs, assault
    - **T37.3X4** Poisoning by other antiprotozoal drugs, undetermined
    - **T37.3X5** Adverse effect of other antiprotozoal drugs
    - **T37.3X6** Underdosing of other antiprotozoal drugs
- **T37.4** Poisoning by, adverse effect of and underdosing of anthelminthics
  - **T37.4X** Poisoning by, adverse effect of and underdosing of anthelminthics
    - **T37.4X1** Poisoning by anthelminthics, accidental (unintentional)
      Poisoning by anthelminthics NOS
    - **T37.4X2** Poisoning by anthelminthics, intentional self-harm A, S
    - **T37.4X3** Poisoning by anthelminthics, assault
    - **T37.4X4** Poisoning by anthelminthics, undetermined
    - **T37.4X5** Adverse effect of anthelminthics
    - **T37.4X6** Underdosing of anthelminthics

▶ New   ⇒ Revised   ~~deleted~~ Deleted   Excludes 1   Excludes 2   Includes   Use additional   Code first   Code also   Key words
OGCR Official Guidelines   X Assign placeholder X   ● Use Additional Character(s)   ▶ Manifestation Code   🖫 Hierarchical Condition Category   **Coding Clinic**

● **T37.5 Poisoning by, adverse effect of and underdosing of antiviral drugs**
    Excludes1 amantadine (T42.8-)
                cytarabine (T45.1-)

● **T37.5X Poisoning by, adverse effect of and underdosing of antiviral drugs**
  ● **T37.5X1 Poisoning by antiviral drugs, accidental (unintentional)**
      Poisoning by antiviral drugs NOS
  ● **T37.5X2 Poisoning by antiviral drugs, intentional self-harm A, S**
  ● **T37.5X3 Poisoning by antiviral drugs, assault**
  ● **T37.5X4 Poisoning by antiviral drugs, undetermined**
  ● **T37.5X5 Adverse effect of antiviral drugs**
  ● **T37.5X6 Underdosing of antiviral drugs**

● **T37.8 Poisoning by, adverse effect of and underdosing of other specified systemic anti-infectives and antiparasitics**
  Poisoning by, adverse effect of and underdosing of hydroxyquinoline derivatives
  Excludes1 antimalarial drugs (T37.2-)

● **T37.8X Poisoning by, adverse effect of and underdosing of other specified systemic anti-infectives and antiparasitics**
  ● **T37.8X1 Poisoning by other specified systemic anti-infectives and antiparasitics, accidental (unintentional)**
      Poisoning by other specified systemic anti-infectives and antiparasitics NOS
  ● **T37.8X2 Poisoning by other specified systemic anti-infectives and antiparasitics, intentional self-harm A, S**
  ● **T37.8X3 Poisoning by other specified systemic anti-infectives and antiparasitics, assault**
  ● **T37.8X4 Poisoning by other specified systemic anti-infectives and antiparasitics, undetermined**
  ● **T37.8X5 Adverse effect of other specified systemic anti-infectives and antiparasitics**
  ● **T37.8X6 Underdosing of other specified systemic anti-infectives and antiparasitics**

● **T37.9 Poisoning by, adverse effect of and underdosing of unspecified systemic anti-infective and antiparasitics**
  X● **T37.91 Poisoning by unspecified systemic anti-infective and antiparasitics, accidental (unintentional)**
      Poisoning by, adverse effect of and underdosing of systemic anti-infective and antiparasitics NOS
  X● **T37.92 Poisoning by unspecified systemic anti-infective and antiparasitics, intentional self-harm A, S**
  X● **T37.93 Poisoning by unspecified systemic anti-infective and antiparasitics, assault**
  X● **T37.94 Poisoning by unspecified systemic anti-infective and antiparasitics, undetermined**
  X● **T37.95 Adverse effect of unspecified systemic anti-infective and antiparasitic**
  X● **T37.96 Underdosing of unspecified systemic anti-infectives and antiparasitics**

● **T38 Poisoning by, adverse effect of and underdosing of hormones and their synthetic substitutes and antagonists, not elsewhere classified**
  Excludes1 mineralocorticoids and their antagonists (T50.0-)
          oxytocic hormones (T48.0-)
          parathyroid hormones and derivatives (T50.9-)

The appropriate 7th character is to be added to each code from category T38

A	initial encounter
D	subsequent encounter
S	sequela

● **T38.0 Poisoning by, adverse effect of and underdosing of glucocorticoids and synthetic analogues**
  Excludes1 glucocorticoids, topically used (T49.-)
● **T38.0X Poisoning by, adverse effect of and underdosing of glucocorticoids and synthetic analogues**
  ● **T38.0X1 Poisoning by glucocorticoids and synthetic analogues, accidental (unintentional)**
      Poisoning by glucocorticoids and synthetic analogues NOS
  ● **T38.0X2 Poisoning by glucocorticoids and synthetic analogues, intentional self-harm A, S**
  ● **T38.0X3 Poisoning by glucocorticoids and synthetic analogues, assault**
  ● **T38.0X4 Poisoning by glucocorticoids and synthetic analogues, undetermined**
  ● **T38.0X5 Adverse effect of glucocorticoids and synthetic analogues**
  ● **T38.0X6 Underdosing of glucocorticoids and synthetic analogues**

● **T38.1 Poisoning by, adverse effect of and underdosing of thyroid hormones and substitutes**
● **T38.1X Poisoning by, adverse effect of and underdosing of thyroid hormones and substitutes**
  ● **T38.1X1 Poisoning by thyroid hormones and substitutes, accidental (unintentional)**
      Poisoning by thyroid hormones and substitutes NOS
  ● **T38.1X2 Poisoning by thyroid hormones and substitutes, intentional self-harm A, S**
  ● **T38.1X3 Poisoning by thyroid hormones and substitutes, assault**
  ● **T38.1X4 Poisoning by thyroid hormones and substitutes, undetermined**
  ● **T38.1X5 Adverse effect of thyroid hormones and substitutes**
  ● **T38.1X6 Underdosing of thyroid hormones and substitutes**

● **T38.2 Poisoning by, adverse effect of and underdosing of antithyroid drugs**
● **T38.2X Poisoning by, adverse effect of and underdosing of antithyroid drugs**
  ● **T38.2X1 Poisoning by antithyroid drugs, accidental (unintentional)**
      Poisoning by antithyroid drugs NOS
  ● **T38.2X2 Poisoning by antithyroid drugs, intentional self-harm A, S**
  ● **T38.2X3 Poisoning by antithyroid drugs, assault**

● T38.2X4   Poisoning by antithyroid drugs,
            undetermined
● T38.2X5   Adverse effect of antithyroid drugs
● T38.2X6   Underdosing of antithyroid drugs

● T38.3   Poisoning by, adverse effect of and underdosing of
          insulin and oral hypoglycemic [antidiabetic] drugs
    ● T38.3X   Poisoning by, adverse effect of and
               underdosing of insulin and oral hypoglycemic
               [antidiabetic] drugs
        ● T38.3X1   Poisoning by insulin and oral
                    hypoglycemic [antidiabetic] drugs,
                    accidental (unintentional)
                        Poisoning by insulin and oral
                        hypoglycemic [antidiabetic]
                        drugs NOS
        ● T38.3X2   Poisoning by insulin and oral
                    hypoglycemic [antidiabetic] drugs,
                    intentional self-harm
        ● T38.3X3   Poisoning by insulin and oral
                    hypoglycemic [antidiabetic] drugs,
                    assault A, S 🐾
        ● T38.3X4   Poisoning by insulin and oral
                    hypoglycemic [antidiabetic] drugs,
                    undetermined
        ● T38.3X5   Adverse effect of insulin and oral
                    hypoglycemic [antidiabetic] drugs
        ● T38.3X6   Underdosing of insulin and oral
                    hypoglycemic [antidiabetic] drugs

● T38.4   Poisoning by, adverse effect of and underdosing of oral
          contraceptives
              Poisoning by, adverse effect of and underdosing of
              multiple- and single-ingredient oral contraceptive
              preparations
    ● T38.4X   Poisoning by, adverse effect of and
               underdosing of oral contraceptives
        ● T38.4X1   Poisoning by oral contraceptives,
                    accidental (unintentional)
                        Poisoning by oral contraceptives
                        NOS
        ● T38.4X2   Poisoning by oral contraceptives,
                    intentional self-harm A, S 🐾
        ● T38.4X3   Poisoning by oral contraceptives,
                    assault
        ● T38.4X4   Poisoning by oral contraceptives,
                    undetermined
        ● T38.4X5   Adverse effect of oral contraceptives
        ● T38.4X6   Underdosing of oral contraceptives

● T38.5   Poisoning by, adverse effect of and underdosing of other
          estrogens and progestogens
              Poisoning by, adverse effect of and underdosing
              of estrogens and progestogens mixtures and
              substitutes
    ● T38.5X   Poisoning by, adverse effect of and underdosing
               of other estrogens and progestogens
        ● T38.5X1   Poisoning by other estrogens
                    and progestogens, accidental
                    (unintentional)
                        Poisoning by other estrogens and
                        progestogens NOS
        ● T38.5X2   Poisoning by other estrogens and
                    progestogens, intentional self-harm
                    A, S 🐾
        ● T38.5X3   Poisoning by other estrogens and
                    progestogens, assault
        ● T38.5X4   Poisoning by other estrogens and
                    progestogens, undetermined

● T38.5X5   Adverse effect of other estrogens and
            progestogens
● T38.5X6   Underdosing of other estrogens and
            progestogens

● T38.6   Poisoning by, adverse effect of and underdosing of
          antigonadotrophins, antiestrogens, antiandrogens, not
          elsewhere classified
              Poisoning by, adverse effect of and underdosing of
              tamoxifen
    ● T38.6X   Poisoning by, adverse effect of and
               underdosing of antigonadotrophins,
               antiestrogens, antiandrogens, not elsewhere
               classified
        ● T38.6X1   Poisoning by antigonadotrophins,
                    antiestrogens, antiandrogens, not
                    elsewhere classified, accidental
                    (unintentional)
                        Poisoning by antigonadotrophins,
                        antiestrogens, antiandrogens,
                        not elsewhere classified NOS
        ● T38.6X2   Poisoning by antigonadotrophins,
                    antiestrogens, antiandrogens, not
                    elsewhere classified, intentional
                    self-harm A, S 🐾
        ● T38.6X3   Poisoning by antigonadotrophins,
                    antiestrogens, antiandrogens, not
                    elsewhere classified, assault
        ● T38.6X4   Poisoning by antigonadotrophins,
                    antiestrogens, antiandrogens, not
                    elsewhere classified, undetermined
        ● T38.6X5   Adverse effect of antigonadotrophins,
                    antiestrogens, antiandrogens, not
                    elsewhere classified
        ● T38.6X6   Underdosing of antigonadotrophins,
                    antiestrogens, antiandrogens, not
                    elsewhere classified

● T38.7   Poisoning by, adverse effect of and underdosing of
          androgens and anabolic congeners
    ● T38.7X   Poisoning by, adverse effect of and
               underdosing of androgens and anabolic
               congeners
        ● T38.7X1   Poisoning by androgens and anabolic
                    congeners, accidental (unintentional)
                        Poisoning by androgens and
                        anabolic congeners NOS
        ● T38.7X2   Poisoning by androgens and anabolic
                    congeners, intentional self-harm
                    A, S 🐾
        ● T38.7X3   Poisoning by androgens and anabolic
                    congeners, assault
        ● T38.7X4   Poisoning by androgens and anabolic
                    congeners, undetermined
        ● T38.7X5   Adverse effect of androgens and
                    anabolic congeners
        ● T38.7X6   Underdosing of androgens and
                    anabolic congeners

● T38.8   Poisoning by, adverse effect of and underdosing of other
          and unspecified hormones and synthetic substitutes
    ● T38.80   Poisoning by, adverse effect of and
               underdosing of unspecified hormones and
               synthetic substitutes
        ● T38.801   Poisoning by unspecified hormones
                    and synthetic substitutes, accidental
                    (unintentional)
                        Poisoning by unspecified hormones
                        and synthetic substitutes NOS
        ● T38.802   Poisoning by unspecified hormones
                    and synthetic substitutes, intentional
                    self-harm A, S 🐾

▶ New   ⇒ Revised   deleted Deleted   Excludes 1   Excludes 2   Includes   Use additional   Code first   Code also   Key words
OGCR Official Guidelines   X Assign placeholder X   ● Use Additional Character(s)   ▶ Manifestation Code   🐾 Hierarchical Condition Category   Coding Clinic

● **T38.803**   Poisoning by unspecified hormones and synthetic substitutes, assault

● **T38.804**   Poisoning by unspecified hormones and synthetic substitutes, undetermined

● **T38.805**   Adverse effect of unspecified hormones and synthetic substitutes

● **T38.806**   Underdosing of unspecified hormones and synthetic substitutes

● **T38.81**   Poisoning by, adverse effect of and underdosing of anterior pituitary [adenohypophyseal] hormones

     ● **T38.811**   Poisoning by anterior pituitary [adenohypophyseal] hormones, accidental (unintentional)
         Poisoning by anterior pituitary [adenohypophyseal] hormones NOS

     ● **T38.812**   Poisoning by anterior pituitary [adenohypophyseal] hormones, intentional self-harm A, S 🔖

     ● **T38.813**   Poisoning by anterior pituitary [adenohypophyseal] hormones, assault

     ● **T38.814**   Poisoning by anterior pituitary [adenohypophyseal] hormones, undetermined

     ● **T38.815**   Adverse effect of anterior pituitary [adenohypophyseal] hormones

     ● **T38.816**   Underdosing of anterior pituitary [adenohypophyseal] hormones

● **T38.89**   Poisoning by, adverse effect of and underdosing of other hormones and synthetic substitutes

     ● **T38.891**   Poisoning by other hormones and synthetic substitutes, accidental (unintentional)
         Poisoning by other hormones and synthetic substitutes NOS

     ● **T38.892**   Poisoning by other hormones and synthetic substitutes, intentional self-harm A, S 🔖

     ● **T38.893**   Poisoning by other hormones and synthetic substitutes, assault

     ● **T38.894**   Poisoning by other hormones and synthetic substitutes, undetermined

     ● **T38.895**   Adverse effect of other hormones and synthetic substitutes

     ● **T38.896**   Underdosing of other hormones and synthetic substitutes

● **T38.9**   Poisoning by, adverse effect of and underdosing of other and unspecified hormone antagonists

● **T38.90**   Poisoning by, adverse effect of and underdosing of unspecified hormone antagonists

     ● **T38.901**   Poisoning by unspecified hormone antagonists, accidental (unintentional)
         Poisoning by unspecified hormone antagonists NOS

     ● **T38.902**   Poisoning by unspecified hormone antagonists, intentional self-harm A, S 🔖

     ● **T38.903**   Poisoning by unspecified hormone antagonists, assault

     ● **T38.904**   Poisoning by unspecified hormone antagonists, undetermined

     ● **T38.905**   Adverse effect of unspecified hormone antagonists

     ● **T38.906**   Underdosing of unspecified hormone antagonists

● **T38.99**   Poisoning by, adverse effect of and underdosing of other hormone antagonists

     ● **T38.991**   Poisoning by other hormone antagonists, accidental (unintentional)
         Poisoning by other hormone antagonists NOS

     ● **T38.992**   Poisoning by other hormone antagonists, intentional self-harm A, S 🔖

     ● **T38.993**   Poisoning by other hormone antagonists, assault

     ● **T38.994**   Poisoning by other hormone antagonists, undetermined

     ● **T38.995**   Adverse effect of other hormone antagonists

     ● **T38.996**   Underdosing of other hormone antagonists

● **T39**   Poisoning by, adverse effect of and underdosing of nonopioid analgesics, antipyretics and antirheumatics

     The appropriate 7th character is to be added to each code from category T39

> A   initial encounter
> D   subsequent encounter
> S   sequela

● **T39.0**   Poisoning by, adverse effect of and underdosing of salicylates

● **T39.01**   Poisoning by, adverse effect of and underdosing of aspirin
     Poisoning by, adverse effect of and underdosing of acetylsalicylic acid

     ● **T39.011**   Poisoning by aspirin, accidental (unintentional)

     ● **T39.012**   Poisoning by aspirin, intentional self-harm A, S 🔖

     ● **T39.013**   Poisoning by aspirin, assault

     ● **T39.014**   Poisoning by aspirin, undetermined

     ● **T39.015**   Adverse effect of aspirin
         Coding Clinic: 2016, Q1, P15

     ● **T39.016**   Underdosing of aspirin

● **T39.09**   Poisoning by, adverse effect of and underdosing of other salicylates

     ● **T39.091**   Poisoning by salicylates, accidental (unintentional)
         Poisoning by salicylates NOS

     ● **T39.092**   Poisoning by salicylates, intentional self-harm A, S 🔖

     ● **T39.093**   Poisoning by salicylates, assault

     ● **T39.094**   Poisoning by salicylates, undetermined

     ● **T39.095**   Adverse effect of salicylates

     ● **T39.096**   Underdosing of salicylates

● **T39.1**   Poisoning by, adverse effect of and underdosing of 4-Aminophenol derivatives

● **T39.1X**   Poisoning by, adverse effect of and underdosing of 4-Aminophenol derivatives

     ● **T39.1X1**   Poisoning by 4-Aminophenol derivatives, accidental (unintentional)
         Poisoning by 4-Aminophenol derivatives NOS

     ● **T39.1X2**   Poisoning by 4-Aminophenol derivatives, intentional self-harm A, S 🔖

CHAPTER 19 (S00-T88)

● T39.1X3　Poisoning by 4-Aminophenol derivatives, assault

● T39.1X4　Poisoning by 4-Aminophenol derivatives, undetermined

● T39.1X5　Adverse effect of 4-Aminophenol derivatives

● T39.1X6　Underdosing of 4-Aminophenol derivatives

● T39.2　Poisoning by, adverse effect of and underdosing of pyrazolone derivatives

● T39.2X　Poisoning by, adverse effect of and underdosing of pyrazolone derivatives

● T39.2X1　Poisoning by pyrazolone derivatives, accidental (unintentional)
　　　　　　Poisoning by pyrazolone derivatives NOS

● T39.2X2　Poisoning by pyrazolone derivatives, intentional self-harm A, S 🕭

● T39.2X3　Poisoning by pyrazolone derivatives, assault

● T39.2X4　Poisoning by pyrazolone derivatives, undetermined

● T39.2X5　Adverse effect of pyrazolone derivatives

● T39.2X6　Underdosing of pyrazolone derivatives

● T39.3　Poisoning by, adverse effect of and underdosing of other nonsteroidal anti-inflammatory drugs [NSAID]

● T39.31　Poisoning by, adverse effect of and underdosing of propionic acid derivatives
　　　　Poisoning by, adverse effect of and underdosing of fenoprofen
　　　　Poisoning by, adverse effect of and underdosing of flurbiprofen
　　　　Poisoning by, adverse effect of and underdosing of ibuprofen
　　　　Poisoning by, adverse effect of and underdosing of ketoprofen
　　　　Poisoning by, adverse effect of and underdosing of naproxen
　　　　Poisoning by, adverse effect of and underdosing of oxaprozin

● T39.311　Poisoning by propionic acid derivatives, accidental (unintentional)

● T39.312　Poisoning by propionic acid derivatives, intentional self-harm A, S 🕭

● T39.313　Poisoning by propionic acid derivatives, assault

● T39.314　Poisoning by propionic acid derivatives, undetermined

● T39.315　Adverse effect of propionic acid derivatives

● T39.316　Underdosing of propionic acid derivatives

● T39.39　Poisoning by, adverse effect of and underdosing of other nonsteroidal anti-inflammatory drugs [NSAID]

● T39.391　Poisoning by other nonsteroidal anti-inflammatory drugs [NSAID], accidental (unintentional)
　　　　　　Poisoning by other nonsteroidal anti-inflammatory drugs NOS

● T39.392　Poisoning by other nonsteroidal anti-inflammatory drugs [NSAID], intentional self-harm A, S 🕭

● T39.393　Poisoning by other nonsteroidal anti-inflammatory drugs [NSAID], assault

● T39.394　Poisoning by other nonsteroidal anti-inflammatory drugs [NSAID], undetermined

● T39.395　Adverse effect of other nonsteroidal anti-inflammatory drugs [NSAID]

● T39.396　Underdosing of other nonsteroidal anti-inflammatory drugs [NSAID]

● T39.4　Poisoning by, adverse effect of and underdosing of antirheumatics, not elsewhere classified

Excludes1　poisoning by, adverse effect of and underdosing of glucocorticoids (T38.0-)
　　　　　　poisoning by, adverse effect of and underdosing of salicylates (T39.0-)

● T39.4X　Poisoning by, adverse effect of and underdosing of antirheumatics, not elsewhere classified

● T39.4X1　Poisoning by antirheumatics, not elsewhere classified, accidental (unintentional)
　　　　　　Poisoning by antirheumatics, not elsewhere classified NOS

● T39.4X2　Poisoning by antirheumatics, not elsewhere classified, intentional self-harm A, S 🕭

● T39.4X3　Poisoning by antirheumatics, not elsewhere classified, assault

● T39.4X4　Poisoning by antirheumatics, not elsewhere classified, undetermined

● T39.4X5　Adverse effect of antirheumatics, not elsewhere classified

● T39.4X6　Underdosing of antirheumatics, not elsewhere classified

● T39.8　Poisoning by, adverse effect of and underdosing of other nonopioid analgesics and antipyretics, not elsewhere classified

● T39.8X　Poisoning by, adverse effect of and underdosing of other nonopioid analgesics and antipyretics, not elsewhere classified

● T39.8X1　Poisoning by other nonopioid analgesics and antipyretics, not elsewhere classified, accidental (unintentional)
　　　　　　Poisoning by other nonopioid analgesics and antipyretics, not elsewhere classified NOS

● T39.8X2　Poisoning by other nonopioid analgesics and antipyretics, not elsewhere classified, intentional self-harm A, S 🕭

● T39.8X3　Poisoning by other nonopioid analgesics and antipyretics, not elsewhere classified, assault

● T39.8X4　Poisoning by other nonopioid analgesics and antipyretics, not elsewhere classified, undetermined

● T39.8X5　Adverse effect of other nonopioid analgesics and antipyretics, not elsewhere classified

● T39.8X6　Underdosing of other nonopioid analgesics and antipyretics, not elsewhere classified

▶ New　⇒ Revised　~~deleted~~ Deleted　Excludes 1　Excludes 2　Includes　Use additional　Code first　Code also　Key words
OGCR Official Guidelines　X Assign placeholder X　● Use Additional Character(s)　▷ Manifestation Code　🕭 Hierarchical Condition Category　**Coding Clinic**

● T39.9 Poisoning by, adverse effect of and underdosing of unspecified nonopioid analgesic, antipyretic and antirheumatic

　X ● T39.91 Poisoning by unspecified nonopioid analgesic, antipyretic and antirheumatic, accidental (unintentional)
　　　　Poisoning by nonopioid analgesic, antipyretic and antirheumatic NOS

　X ● T39.92 Poisoning by unspecified nonopioid analgesic, antipyretic and antirheumatic, intentional self-harm A, S 🔬

　X ● T39.93 Poisoning by unspecified nonopioid analgesic, antipyretic and antirheumatic, assault

　X ● T39.94 Poisoning by unspecified nonopioid analgesic, antipyretic and antirheumatic, undetermined

　X ● T39.95 Adverse effect of unspecified nonopioid analgesic, antipyretic and antirheumatic

　X ● T39.96 Underdosing of unspecified nonopioid analgesic, antipyretic and antirheumatic

● T40 Poisoning by, adverse effect of and underdosing of narcotics and psychodysleptics [hallucinogens]

　Excludes2 drug dependence and related mental and behavioral disorders due to psychoactive substance use (F10.-F19.-)

　The appropriate 7th character is to be added to each code from category T40

　┌─────────────────────────────┐
　│ A   initial encounter   │
　│ D   subsequent encounter   │
　│ S   sequela   │
　└─────────────────────────────┘

● T40.0 Poisoning by, adverse effect of and underdosing of opium

　● T40.0X Poisoning by, adverse effect of and underdosing of opium

　　● T40.0X1 Poisoning by opium, accidental (unintentional)
　　　　Poisoning by opium NOS

　　● T40.0X2 Poisoning by opium, intentional self-harm A, S 🔬

　　● T40.0X3 Poisoning by opium, assault

　　● T40.0X4 Poisoning by opium, undetermined

　　● T40.0X5 Adverse effect of opium

　　● T40.0X6 Underdosing of opium

● T40.1 Poisoning by and adverse effect of heroin

　● T40.1X Poisoning by and adverse effect of heroin

　　● T40.1X1 Poisoning by heroin, accidental (unintentional)
　　　　Poisoning by heroin NOS

　　● T40.1X2 Poisoning by heroin, intentional self-harm A, S 🔬

　　● T40.1X3 Poisoning by heroin, assault

　　● T40.1X4 Poisoning by heroin, undetermined

● T40.2 Poisoning by, adverse effect of and underdosing of other opioids

　● T40.2X Poisoning by, adverse effect of and underdosing of other opioids

　　● T40.2X1 Poisoning by other opioids, accidental (unintentional)
　　　　Poisoning by other opioids NOS

　　● T40.2X2 Poisoning by other opioids, intentional self-harm A, S 🔬

　　● T40.2X3 Poisoning by other opioids, assault

　　● T40.2X4 Poisoning by other opioids, undetermined

　　● T40.2X5 Adverse effect of other opioids

　　● T40.2X6 Underdosing of other opioids

● T40.3 Poisoning by, adverse effect of and underdosing of methadone

　● T40.3X Poisoning by, adverse effect of and underdosing of methadone

　　● T40.3X1 Poisoning by methadone, accidental (unintentional)
　　　　Poisoning by methadone NOS

　　● T40.3X2 Poisoning by methadone, intentional self-harm A, S 🔬

　　● T40.3X3 Poisoning by methadone, assault

　　● T40.3X4 Poisoning by methadone, undetermined

　　● T40.3X5 Adverse effect of methadone

　　● T40.3X6 Underdosing of methadone

● T40.4 Poisoning by, adverse effect of and underdosing of other synthetic narcotics

　● T40.41 Poisoning by, adverse effect of and underdosing of fentanyl or fentanyl analogs

　　T40.411 Poisoning by fentanyl or fentanyl analogs, accidental (unintentional)

　　T40.412 Poisoning by fentanyl or fentanyl analogs, intentional self-harm

　　T40.413 Poisoning by fentanyl or fentanyl analogs, assault

　　T40.414 Poisoning by fentanyl or fentanyl analogs, undetermined

　　T40.415 Adverse effect of fentanyl or fentanyl analogs

　　T40.416 Underdosing of fentanyl or fentanyl analogs

　● T40.42 Poisoning by, adverse effect of and underdosing of tramadol

　　T40.421 Poisoning by tramadol, accidental (unintentional)

　　T40.422 Poisoning by tramadol, intentional self-harm

　　T40.423 Poisoning by tramadol, assault

　　T40.424 Poisoning by tramadol, undetermined

　　T40.425 Adverse effect of tramadol

　　T40.426 Underdosing of tramadol

　● T40.49 Poisoning by, adverse effect of and underdosing of other synthetic narcotics

　　T40.491 Poisoning by other synthetic narcotics, accidental (unintentional)

　　T40.492 Poisoning by other synthetic narcotics, intentional self-harm

　　T40.493 Poisoning by other synthetic narcotics, assault

　　T40.494 Poisoning by other synthetic narcotics, undetermined

　　T40.495 Adverse effect of other synthetic narcotics

　　T40.496 Underdosing of other synthetic narcotics

● T40.5 Poisoning by, adverse effect of and underdosing of cocaine

　● T40.5X Poisoning by, adverse effect of and underdosing of cocaine

　　● T40.5X1 Poisoning by cocaine, accidental (unintentional)
　　　　Poisoning by cocaine NOS
　　　　Coding Clinic: 2016, Q2, P9

　　● T40.5X2 Poisoning by cocaine, intentional self-harm A, S 🔬

　　● T40.5X3 Poisoning by cocaine, assault

　　● T40.5X4 Poisoning by cocaine, undetermined

　　● T40.5X5 Adverse effect of cocaine

　　● T40.5X6 Underdosing of cocaine

CHAPTER 19 (S00-T88)

- T40.6   Poisoning by, adverse effect of and underdosing of other and unspecified narcotics
  - T40.60   Poisoning by, adverse effect of and underdosing of unspecified narcotics
    - T40.601   Poisoning by unspecified narcotics, accidental (unintentional)
      Poisoning by narcotics NOS
    - T40.602   Poisoning by unspecified narcotics, intentional self-harm A, S 🐾
    - T40.603   Poisoning by unspecified narcotics, assault
    - T40.604   Poisoning by unspecified narcotics, undetermined
    - T40.605   Adverse effect of unspecified narcotics
    - T40.606   Underdosing of unspecified narcotics
  - T40.69   Poisoning by, adverse effect of and underdosing of other narcotics
    - T40.691   Poisoning by other narcotics, accidental (unintentional)
      Poisoning by other narcotics NOS
    - T40.692   Poisoning by other narcotics, intentional self-harm A, S 🐾
    - T40.693   Poisoning by other narcotics, assault
    - T40.694   Poisoning by other narcotics, undetermined
    - T40.695   Adverse effect of other narcotics
    - T40.696   Underdosing of other narcotics
- T40.7   Poisoning by, adverse effect of and underdosing of cannabis (derivatives)
  - T40.71   Poisoning by, adverse effect of and underdosing of cannabis (derivatives)
    - T40.711   Poisoning by cannabis, accidental (unintentional)
    - T40.712   Poisoning by cannabis, intentional self-harm
    - T40.713   Poisoning by cannabis, assault
    - T40.714   Poisoning by cannabis, undetermined
    - T40.715   Adverse effect of cannabis
    - T40.716   Underdosing of cannabis
  - T40.72   Poisoning by, adverse effect of and underdosing of synthetic cannabinoids
    - T40.721   Poisoning by synthetic cannabinoids, accidental (unintentional)
    - T40.722   Poisoning by synthetic cannabinoids, intentional self-harm
    - T40.723   Poisoning by synthetic cannabinoids, assault
    - T40.724   Poisoning by synthetic cannabinoids, undetermined
    - T40.725   Adverse effect of synthetic cannabinoids
    - T40.726   Underdosing of synthetic cannabinoids
- T40.8   Poisoning by and adverse effect of lysergide [LSD]
  - T40.8X   Poisoning by and adverse effect of lysergide [LSD]
    - T40.8X1   Poisoning by lysergide [LSD], accidental (unintentional)
      Poisoning by lysergide [LSD] NOS
    - T40.8X2   Poisoning by lysergide [LSD], intentional self-harm A, S 🐾
    - T40.8X3   Poisoning by lysergide [LSD], assault
    - T40.8X4   Poisoning by lysergide [LSD], undetermined

- T40.9   Poisoning by, adverse effect of and underdosing of other and unspecified psychodysleptics [hallucinogens]
  - T40.90   Poisoning by, adverse effect of and underdosing of unspecified psychodysleptics [hallucinogens]
    - T40.901   Poisoning by unspecified psychodysleptics [hallucinogens], accidental (unintentional)
    - T40.902   Poisoning by unspecified psychodysleptics [hallucinogens], intentional self-harm A, S 🐾
    - T40.903   Poisoning by unspecified psychodysleptics [hallucinogens], assault
    - T40.904   Poisoning by unspecified psychodysleptics [hallucinogens], undetermined
    - T40.905   Adverse effect of unspecified psychodysleptics [hallucinogens]
    - T40.906   Underdosing of unspecified psychodysleptics [hallucinogens]
  - T40.99   Poisoning by, adverse effect of and underdosing of other psychodysleptics [hallucinogens]
    - T40.991   Poisoning by other psychodysleptics [hallucinogens], accidental (unintentional)
      Poisoning by other psychodysleptics [hallucinogens] NOS
    - T40.992   Poisoning by other psychodysleptics [hallucinogens], intentional self-harm A, S 🐾
    - T40.993   Poisoning by other psychodysleptics [hallucinogens], assault
    - T40.994   Poisoning by other psychodysleptics [hallucinogens], undetermined
    - T40.995   Adverse effect of other psychodysleptics [hallucinogens]
    - T40.996   Underdosing of other psychodysleptics [hallucinogens]
- T41   Poisoning by, adverse effect of and underdosing of anesthetics and therapeutic gases

  Excludes1   benzodiazepines (T42.4-)
  cocaine (T40.5-)
  complications of anesthesia during pregnancy (O29.-)
  complications of anesthesia during labor and delivery (O74.-)
  complications of anesthesia during the puerperium (O89.-) opioids (T40.0-T40.2-)

  The appropriate 7th character is to be added to each code from category T41

A	initial encounter
D	subsequent encounter
S	sequela

- T41.0   Poisoning by, adverse effect of and underdosing of inhaled anesthetics

  Excludes1   oxygen (T41.5-)
  - T41.0X   Poisoning by, adverse effect of and underdosing of inhaled anesthetics
    - T41.0X1   Poisoning by inhaled anesthetics, accidental (unintentional)
      Poisoning by inhaled anesthetics NOS
    - T41.0X2   Poisoning by inhaled anesthetics, intentional self-harm A, S 🐾
    - T41.0X3   Poisoning by inhaled anesthetics, assault
    - T41.0X4   Poisoning by inhaled anesthetics, undetermined
    - T41.0X5   Adverse effect of inhaled anesthetics
    - T41.0X6   Underdosing of inhaled anesthetics

- ● **T41.1**   **Poisoning by, adverse effect of and underdosing of intravenous anesthetics**
  Poisoning by, adverse effect of and underdosing of thiobarbiturates
  - ● **T41.1X**   Poisoning by, adverse effect of and underdosing of intravenous anesthetics
    - ● **T41.1X1**   Poisoning by intravenous anesthetics, accidental (unintentional)
      Poisoning by intravenous anesthetics NOS
    - ● **T41.1X2**   Poisoning by intravenous anesthetics, intentional self-harm A, S 🐞
    - ● **T41.1X3**   Poisoning by intravenous anesthetics, assault
    - ● **T41.1X4**   Poisoning by intravenous anesthetics, undetermined
    - ● **T41.1X5**   Adverse effect of intravenous anesthetics
    - ● **T41.1X6**   Underdosing of intravenous anesthetics
- ● **T41.2**   **Poisoning by, adverse effect of and underdosing of other and unspecified general anesthetics**
  - ● **T41.20**   Poisoning by, adverse effect of and underdosing of unspecified general anesthetics
    - ● **T41.201**   Poisoning by unspecified general anesthetics, accidental (unintentional)
      Poisoning by general anesthetics NOS
    - ● **T41.202**   Poisoning by unspecified general anesthetics, intentional self-harm A, S 🐞
    - ● **T41.203**   Poisoning by unspecified general anesthetics, assault
    - ● **T41.204**   Poisoning by unspecified general anesthetics, undetermined
    - ● **T41.205**   Adverse effect of unspecified general anesthetics
      Coding Clinic: 2016, Q4, P73
    - ● **T41.206**   Underdosing of unspecified general anesthetics
  - ● **T41.29**   Poisoning by, adverse effect of and underdosing of other general anesthetics
    - ● **T41.291**   Poisoning by other general anesthetics, accidental (unintentional)
      Poisoning by other general anesthetics NOS
    - ● **T41.292**   Poisoning by other general anesthetics, intentional self-harm A, S 🐞
    - ● **T41.293**   Poisoning by other general anesthetics, assault
    - ● **T41.294**   Poisoning by other general anesthetics, undetermined
    - ● **T41.295**   Adverse effect of other general anesthetics
    - ● **T41.296**   Underdosing of other general anesthetics
- ● **T41.3**   **Poisoning by, adverse effect of and underdosing of local anesthetics**
  Cocaine (topical)
  Excludes2   poisoning by cocaine used as a central nervous system stimulant (T40.5X1-T40.5X4)
  - ● **T41.3X**   Poisoning by, adverse effect of and underdosing of local anesthetics
    - ● **T41.3X1**   Poisoning by local anesthetics, accidental (unintentional)
      Poisoning by local anesthetics NOS
    - ● **T41.3X2**   Poisoning by local anesthetics, intentional self-harm A, S 🐞
    - ● **T41.3X3**   Poisoning by local anesthetics, assault
    - ● **T41.3X4**   Poisoning by local anesthetics, undetermined
    - ● **T41.3X5**   Adverse effect of local anesthetics
    - ● **T41.3X6**   Underdosing of local anesthetics

- ● **T41.4**   **Poisoning by, adverse effect of and underdosing of unspecified anesthetic**
  - X ● **T41.41**   Poisoning by unspecified anesthetic, accidental (unintentional)
    Poisoning by anesthetic NOS
  - X ● **T41.42**   Poisoning by unspecified anesthetic, intentional self-harm A, S 🐞
  - X ● **T41.43**   Poisoning by unspecified anesthetic, assault
  - X ● **T41.44**   Poisoning by unspecified anesthetic, undetermined
  - X ● **T41.45**   Adverse effect of unspecified anesthetic
  - X ● **T41.46**   Underdosing of unspecified anesthetics
- ● **T41.5**   **Poisoning by, adverse effect of and underdosing of therapeutic gases**
  - ● **T41.5X**   Poisoning by, adverse effect of and underdosing of therapeutic gases
    - ● **T41.5X1**   Poisoning by therapeutic gases, accidental (unintentional)
      Poisoning by therapeutic gases NOS
    - ● **T41.5X2**   Poisoning by therapeutic gases, intentional self-harm A, S 🐞
    - ● **T41.5X3**   Poisoning by therapeutic gases, assault
    - ● **T41.5X4**   Poisoning by therapeutic gases, undetermined
    - ● **T41.5X5**   Adverse effect of therapeutic gases
    - ● **T41.5X6**   Underdosing of therapeutic gases
- ● **T42**   **Poisoning by, adverse effect of and underdosing of antiepileptic, sedative-hypnotic and antiparkinsonism drugs**
  Excludes2   drug dependence and related mental and behavioral disorders due to psychoactive substance use (F10.--F19.-)

  The appropriate 7th character is to be added to each code from category T42

A	initial encounter
D	subsequent encounter
S	sequela

  - ● **T42.0**   Poisoning by, adverse effect of and underdosing of hydantoin derivatives
    - ● **T42.0X**   Poisoning by, adverse effect of and underdosing of hydantoin derivatives
      - ● **T42.0X1**   Poisoning by hydantoin derivatives, accidental (unintentional)
        Poisoning by hydantoin derivatives NOS
      - ● **T42.0X2**   Poisoning by hydantoin derivatives, intentional self-harm A, S 🐞
      - ● **T42.0X3**   Poisoning by hydantoin derivatives, assault
      - ● **T42.0X4**   Poisoning by hydantoin derivatives, undetermined
      - ● **T42.0X5**   Adverse effect of hydantoin derivatives
      - ● **T42.0X6**   Underdosing of hydantoin derivatives
  - ● **T42.1**   Poisoning by, adverse effect of and underdosing of iminostilbenes
    Poisoning by, adverse effect of and underdosing of carbamazepine
    - ● **T42.1X**   Poisoning by, adverse effect of and underdosing of iminostilbenes
      - ● **T42.1X1**   Poisoning by iminostilbenes, accidental (unintentional)
        Poisoning by iminostilbenes NOS
      - ● **T42.1X2**   Poisoning by iminostilbenes, intentional self-harm A, S 🐞
      - ● **T42.1X3**   Poisoning by iminostilbenes, assault
      - ● **T42.1X4**   Poisoning by iminostilbenes, undetermined
      - ● **T42.1X5**   Adverse effect of iminostilbenes
      - ● **T42.1X6**   Underdosing of iminostilbenes

CHAPTER 19 (S00-T88)

- T42.2 Poisoning by, adverse effect of and underdosing of succinimides and oxazolidinediones
  - T42.2X Poisoning by, adverse effect of and underdosing of succinimides and oxazolidinediones
    - T42.2X1 Poisoning by succinimides and oxazolidinediones, accidental (unintentional)
      Poisoning by succinimides and oxazolidinediones NOS
    - T42.2X2 Poisoning by succinimides and oxazolidinediones, intentional self-harm A, S
    - T42.2X3 Poisoning by succinimides and oxazolidinediones, assault
    - T42.2X4 Poisoning by succinimides and oxazolidinediones, undetermined
    - T42.2X5 Adverse effect of succinimides and oxazolidinediones
    - T42.2X6 Underdosing of succinimides and oxazolidinediones
- T42.3 Poisoning by, adverse effect of and underdosing of barbiturates
  - Excludes1 poisoning by, adverse effect of and underdosing of thiobarbiturates (T41.1-)
  - T42.3X Poisoning by, adverse effect of and underdosing of barbiturates
    - T42.3X1 Poisoning by barbiturates, accidental (unintentional)
      Poisoning by barbiturates NOS
    - T42.3X2 Poisoning by barbiturates, intentional self-harm A, S
    - T42.3X3 Poisoning by barbiturates, assault
    - T42.3X4 Poisoning by barbiturates, undetermined
    - T42.3X5 Adverse effect of barbiturates
    - T42.3X6 Underdosing of barbiturates
- T42.4 Poisoning by, adverse effect of and underdosing of benzodiazepines
  - T42.4X Poisoning by, adverse effect of and underdosing of benzodiazepines
    - T42.4X1 Poisoning by benzodiazepines, accidental (unintentional)
      Poisoning by benzodiazepines NOS
    - T42.4X2 Poisoning by benzodiazepines, intentional self-harm A, S
    - T42.4X3 Poisoning by benzodiazepines, assault
    - T42.4X4 Poisoning by benzodiazepines, undetermined
    - T42.4X5 Adverse effect of benzodiazepines
    - T42.4X6 Underdosing of benzodiazepines
- T42.5 Poisoning by, adverse effect of and underdosing of mixed antiepileptics
  - T42.5X Poisoning by, adverse effect of and underdosing of antiepileptics
    - T42.5X1 Poisoning by mixed antiepileptics, accidental (unintentional)
      Poisoning by mixed antiepileptics NOS
    - T42.5X2 Poisoning by mixed antiepileptics, intentional self-harm A, S
    - T42.5X3 Poisoning by mixed antiepileptics, assault
    - T42.5X4 Poisoning by mixed antiepileptics, undetermined
    - T42.5X5 Adverse effect of mixed antiepileptics
    - T42.5X6 Underdosing of mixed antiepileptics

- T42.6 Poisoning by, adverse effect of and underdosing of other antiepileptic and sedative-hypnotic drugs
  Poisoning by, adverse effect of and underdosing of methaqualone
  Poisoning by, adverse effect of and underdosing of valproic acid
  - Excludes1 poisoning by, adverse effect of and underdosing of carbamazepine (T42.1-)
  - T42.6X Poisoning by, adverse effect of and underdosing of other antiepileptic and sedative-hypnotic drugs
    - T42.6X1 Poisoning by other antiepileptic and sedative-hypnotic drugs, accidental (unintentional)
      Poisoning by other antiepileptic and sedative-hypnotic drugs NOS
    - T42.6X2 Poisoning by other antiepileptic and sedative-hypnotic drugs, intentional self-harm A, S
    - T42.6X3 Poisoning by other antiepileptic and sedative-hypnotic drugs, assault
    - T42.6X4 Poisoning by other antiepileptic and sedative-hypnotic drugs, undetermined
    - T42.6X5 Adverse effect of other antiepileptic and sedative-hypnotic drugs
    - T42.6X6 Underdosing of other antiepileptic and sedative-hypnotic drugs
- T42.7 Poisoning by, adverse effect of and underdosing of unspecified antiepileptic and sedative-hypnotic drugs
  - X T42.71 Poisoning by unspecified antiepileptic and sedative-hypnotic drugs, accidental (unintentional)
    Poisoning by antiepileptic and sedative-hypnotic drugs NOS
  - X T42.72 Poisoning by unspecified antiepileptic and sedative-hypnotic drugs, intentional self-harm A, S
  - X T42.73 Poisoning by unspecified antiepileptic and sedative-hypnotic drugs, assault
  - X T42.74 Poisoning by unspecified antiepileptic and sedative-hypnotic drugs, undetermined
  - X T42.75 Adverse effect of unspecified antiepileptic and sedative-hypnotic drugs
  - X T42.76 Underdosing of unspecified antiepileptic and sedative-hypnotic drugs
- T42.8 Poisoning by, adverse effect of and underdosing of antiparkinsonism drugs and other central muscle-tone depressants
  Poisoning by, adverse effect of and underdosing of amantadine
  - T42.8X Poisoning by, adverse effect of and underdosing of antiparkinsonism drugs and other central muscle-tone depressants
    - T42.8X1 Poisoning by antiparkinsonism drugs and other central muscle-tone depressants, accidental (unintentional)
      Poisoning by antiparkinsonism drugs and other central muscle-tone depressants NOS
    - T42.8X2 Poisoning by antiparkinsonism drugs and other central muscle-tone depressants, intentional self-harm A, S
    - T42.8X3 Poisoning by antiparkinsonism drugs and other central muscle-tone depressants, assault
    - T42.8X4 Poisoning by antiparkinsonism drugs and other central muscle-tone depressants, undetermined

▶ New   ⇒ Revised   ~~deleted~~ Deleted   Excludes 1   Excludes 2   Includes   Use additional   Code first   Code also   Key words

OGCR Official Guidelines   X Assign placeholder X   ● Use Additional Character(s)   ▌ Manifestation Code   🐾 Hierarchical Condition Category   **Coding Clinic**

● T42.8X5 Adverse effect of antiparkinsonism drugs and other central muscle-tone depressants

● T42.8X6 Underdosing of antiparkinsonism drugs and other central muscle-tone depressants

● T43   Poisoning by, adverse effect of and underdosing of psychotropic drugs, not elsewhere classified

    Excludes1   appetite depressants (T50.5-)
                barbiturates (T42.3-)
                benzodiazepines (T42.4-)
                methaqualone (T42.6-)
                psychodysleptics [hallucinogens] (T40.7-T40.9-)

    Excludes2   drug dependence and related mental and behavioral disorders due to psychoactive substance use (F10.--F19.-)

The appropriate 7th character is to be added to each code from category T43

A	initial encounter
D	subsequent encounter
S	sequela

● T43.0   Poisoning by, adverse effect of and underdosing of tricyclic and tetracyclic antidepressants

   ● T43.01   Poisoning by, adverse effect of and underdosing of tricyclic antidepressants

     ● T43.011   Poisoning by tricyclic antidepressants, accidental (unintentional)
             Poisoning by tricyclic antidepressants NOS

     ● T43.012   Poisoning by tricyclic antidepressants, intentional self-harm A, S 🔗

     ● T43.013   Poisoning by tricyclic antidepressants, assault

     ● T43.014   Poisoning by tricyclic antidepressants, undetermined

     ● T43.015   Adverse effect of tricyclic antidepressants

     ● T43.016   Underdosing of tricyclic antidepressants

   ● T43.02   Poisoning by, adverse effect of and underdosing of tetracyclic antidepressants

     ● T43.021   Poisoning by tetracyclic antidepressants, accidental (unintentional)
             Poisoning by tetracyclic antidepressants NOS

     ● T43.022   Poisoning by tetracyclic antidepressants, intentional self-harm A, S 🔗

     ● T43.023   Poisoning by tetracyclic antidepressants, assault

     ● T43.024   Poisoning by tetracyclic antidepressants, undetermined

     ● T43.025   Adverse effect of tetracyclic antidepressants

     ● T43.026   Underdosing of tetracyclic antidepressants

● T43.1   Poisoning by, adverse effect of and underdosing of monoamine-oxidase-inhibitor antidepressants

   ● T43.1X   Poisoning by, adverse effect of and underdosing of monoamine-oxidase-inhibitor antidepressants

     ● T43.1X1   Poisoning by monoamine-oxidase-inhibitor antidepressants, accidental (unintentional)
             Poisoning by monoamine-oxidase-inhibitor antidepressants NOS

     ● T43.1X2   Poisoning by monoamine-oxidase-inhibitor antidepressants, intentional self-harm A, S 🔗

     ● T43.1X3   Poisoning by monoamine-oxidase-inhibitor antidepressants, assault

     ● T43.1X4   Poisoning by monoamine-oxidase-inhibitor antidepressants, undetermined

     ● T43.1X5   Adverse effect of monoamine-oxidase-inhibitor antidepressants

     ● T43.1X6   Underdosing of monoamine-oxidase-inhibitor antidepressants

● T43.2   Poisoning by, adverse effect of and underdosing of other and unspecified antidepressants

   ● T43.20   Poisoning by, adverse effect of and underdosing of unspecified antidepressants

     ● T43.201   Poisoning by unspecified antidepressants, accidental (unintentional)
             Poisoning by antidepressants NOS

     ● T43.202   Poisoning by unspecified antidepressants, intentional self-harm A, S 🔗

     ● T43.203   Poisoning by unspecified antidepressants, assault

     ● T43.204   Poisoning by unspecified antidepressants, undetermined

     ● T43.205   Adverse effect of unspecified antidepressants
             Antidepressant discontinuation syndrome

     ● T43.206   Underdosing of unspecified antidepressants

   ● T43.21   Poisoning by, adverse effect of and underdosing of selective serotonin and norepinephrine reuptake inhibitors
        Poisoning by, adverse effect of and underdosing of SSNRI antidepressants

     ● T43.211   Poisoning by selective serotonin and norepinephrine reuptake inhibitors, accidental (unintentional)

     ● T43.212   Poisoning by selective serotonin and norepinephrine reuptake inhibitors, intentional self-harm A, S 🔗

     ● T43.213   Poisoning by selective serotonin and norepinephrine reuptake inhibitors, assault

     ● T43.214   Poisoning by selective serotonin and norepinephrine reuptake inhibitors, undetermined

     ● T43.215   Adverse effect of selective serotonin and norepinephrine reuptake inhibitors

     ● T43.216   Underdosing of selective serotonin and norepinephrine reuptake inhibitors

   ● T43.22   Poisoning by, adverse effect of and underdosing of selective serotonin reuptake inhibitors
        Poisoning by, adverse effect of and underdosing of SSRI antidepressants

     ● T43.221   Poisoning by selective serotonin reuptake inhibitors, accidental (unintentional)

     ● T43.222   Poisoning by selective serotonin reuptake inhibitors, intentional self-harm A, S 🔗

     ● T43.223   Poisoning by selective serotonin reuptake inhibitors, assault

     ● T43.224   Poisoning by selective serotonin reuptake inhibitors, undetermined

     ● T43.225   Adverse effect of selective serotonin reuptake inhibitors
          Coding Clinic: 2022, Q2, P11

     ● T43.226   Underdosing of selective serotonin reuptake inhibitors

CHAPTER 19 (S00-T88)

● **T43.29**   Poisoning by, adverse effect of and underdosing of other antidepressants

    ● **T43.291**   Poisoning by other antidepressants, accidental (unintentional)
        Poisoning by other antidepressants NOS

    ● **T43.292**   Poisoning by other antidepressants, intentional self-harm A, S 🐾

    ● **T43.293**   Poisoning by other antidepressants, assault

    ● **T43.294**   Poisoning by other antidepressants, undetermined

    ● **T43.295**   Adverse effect of other antidepressants

    ● **T43.296**   Underdosing of other antidepressants

● **T43.3**   Poisoning by, adverse effect of and underdosing of phenothiazine antipsychotics and neuroleptics

   ● **T43.3X**   Poisoning by, adverse effect of and underdosing of phenothiazine antipsychotics and neuroleptics

    ● **T43.3X1**   Poisoning by phenothiazine antipsychotics and neuroleptics, accidental (unintentional)
        Poisoning by phenothiazine antipsychotics and neuroleptics NOS

    ● **T43.3X2**   Poisoning by phenothiazine antipsychotics and neuroleptics, intentional self-harm A, S 🐾

    ● **T43.3X3**   Poisoning by phenothiazine antipsychotics and neuroleptics, assault

    ● **T43.3X4**   Poisoning by phenothiazine antipsychotics and neuroleptics, undetermined

    ● **T43.3X5**   Adverse effect of phenothiazine antipsychotics and neuroleptics

    ● **T43.3X6**   Underdosing of phenothiazine antipsychotics and neuroleptics

● **T43.4**   Poisoning by, adverse effect of and underdosing of butyrophenone and thiothixene neuroleptics

   ● **T43.4X**   Poisoning by, adverse effect of and underdosing of butyrophenone and thiothixene neuroleptics

    ● **T43.4X1**   Poisoning by butyrophenone and thiothixene neuroleptics, accidental (unintentional)
        Poisoning by butyrophenone and thiothixene neuroleptics NOS

    ● **T43.4X2**   Poisoning by butyrophenone and thiothixene neuroleptics, intentional self-harm A, S 🐾

    ● **T43.4X3**   Poisoning by butyrophenone and thiothixene neuroleptics, assault

    ● **T43.4X4**   Poisoning by butyrophenone and thiothixene neuroleptics, undetermined

    ● **T43.4X5**   Adverse effect of butyrophenone and thiothixene neuroleptics

    ● **T43.4X6**   Underdosing of butyrophenone and thiothixene neuroleptics

● **T43.5**   Poisoning by, adverse effect of and underdosing of other and unspecified antipsychotics and neuroleptics

    Excludes1   poisoning by, adverse effect of and underdosing of rauwolfia (T46.5-)

   ● **T43.50**   Poisoning by, adverse effect of and underdosing of unspecified antipsychotics and neuroleptics

    ● **T43.501**   Poisoning by unspecified antipsychotics and neuroleptics, accidental (unintentional)
        Poisoning by antipsychotics and neuroleptics NOS

    ● **T43.502**   Poisoning by unspecified antipsychotics and neuroleptics, intentional self-harm A, S 🐾

    ● **T43.503**   Poisoning by unspecified antipsychotics and neuroleptics, assault

    ● **T43.504**   Poisoning by unspecified antipsychotics and neuroleptics, undetermined

    ● **T43.505**   Adverse effect of unspecified antipsychotics and neuroleptics

    ● **T43.506**   Underdosing of unspecified antipsychotics and neuroleptics

   ● **T43.59**   Poisoning by, adverse effect of and underdosing of other antipsychotics and neuroleptics

    ● **T43.591**   Poisoning by other antipsychotics and neuroleptics, accidental (unintentional)
        Poisoning by other antipsychotics and neuroleptics NOS

    ● **T43.592**   Poisoning by other antipsychotics and neuroleptics, intentional self-harm A, S 🐾
        Coding Clinic: 2017, Q1, P40

    ● **T43.593**   Poisoning by other antipsychotics and neuroleptics, assault

    ● **T43.594**   Poisoning by other antipsychotics and neuroleptics, undetermined

    ● **T43.595**   Adverse effect of other antipsychotics and neuroleptics
        Coding Clinic: 2022, Q2, P11

    ● **T43.596**   Underdosing of other antipsychotics and neuroleptics

● **T43.6**   Poisoning by, adverse effect of and underdosing of psychostimulants

    Excludes1   poisoning by, adverse effect of and underdosing of cocaine (T40.5-)

   ● **T43.60**   Poisoning by, adverse effect of and underdosing of unspecified psychostimulant

    ● **T43.601**   Poisoning by unspecified psychostimulants, accidental (unintentional)
        Poisoning by psychostimulants NOS

    ● **T43.602**   Poisoning by unspecified psychostimulants, intentional self-harm A, S 🐾

    ● **T43.603**   Poisoning by unspecified psychostimulants, assault

    ● **T43.604**   Poisoning by unspecified psychostimulants, undetermined

    ● **T43.605**   Adverse effect of unspecified psychostimulants

    ● **T43.606**   Underdosing of unspecified psychostimulants

▶ New   ⇒ Revised   ~~deleted~~ Deleted   Excludes 1   Excludes 2   Includes   Use additional   Code first   Code also   Key words
OGCR Official Guidelines   X Assign placeholder X   ● Use Additional Character(s)   ▌ Manifestation Code   🐾 Hierarchical Condition Category   Coding Clinic

● **T43.61**   Poisoning by, adverse effect of and underdosing of caffeine
    ● **T43.611**   Poisoning by caffeine, accidental (unintentional)
       Poisoning by caffeine NOS
    ● **T43.612**   Poisoning by caffeine, intentional self-harm A, S 🔗
    ● **T43.613**   Poisoning by caffeine, assault
    ● **T43.614**   Poisoning by caffeine, undetermined
    ● **T43.615**   Adverse effect of caffeine
    ● **T43.616**   Underdosing of caffeine

● **T43.62**   Poisoning by, adverse effect of and underdosing of amphetamines
    ~~Poisoning by, adverse effect of and underdosing of methamphetamines~~
    ● **T43.621**   Poisoning by amphetamines, accidental (unintentional)
       Poisoning by amphetamines NOS
       Coding Clinic: 2021, Q3, P8
    ● **T43.622**   Poisoning by amphetamines, intentional self-harm A, S 🔗
    ● **T43.623**   Poisoning by amphetamines, assault
    ● **T43.624**   Poisoning by amphetamines, undetermined
    ● **T43.625**   Adverse effect of amphetamines
    ● **T43.626**   Underdosing of amphetamines

● **T43.63**   Poisoning by, adverse effect of and underdosing of methylphenidate
    ● **T43.631**   Poisoning by methylphenidate, accidental (unintentional)
       Poisoning by methylphenidate NOS
    ● **T43.632**   Poisoning by methylphenidate, intentional self-harm A, S 🔗
    ● **T43.633**   Poisoning by methylphenidate, assault
    ● **T43.634**   Poisoning by methylphenidate, undetermined
    ● **T43.635**   Adverse effect of methylphenidate
    ● **T43.636**   Underdosing of methylphenidate

● **T43.64**   Poisoning by ecstasy
    Poisoning by MDMA
    Poisoning by 3,4-methylenedioxymethamphetamine
    ● **T43.641**   Poisoning by ecstasy, accidental (unintentional)
       Poisoning by ecstasy NOS
       Coding Clinic: 2018, Q4, P31
    ● **T43.642**   Poisoning by ecstasy, intentional self-harm A, S 🔗
    ● **T43.643**   Poisoning by ecstasy, assault
    ● **T43.644**   Poisoning by ecstasy, undetermined

▶● **T43.65**   Poisoning by, adverse effect of and underdosing of methamphetamines
    ▶● **T43.651**   Poisoning by methamphetamines accidental (unintentional)
       ▶ Poisoning by methamphetamines NOS
    ▶● **T43.652**   Poisoning by methamphetamines intentional self-harm
    ▶● **T43.653**   Poisoning by methamphetamines, assault
    ▶● **T43.654**   Poisoning by methamphetamines, undetermined
    ▶● **T43.655**   Adverse effect of methamphetamines
    ▶● **T43.656**   Underdosing of methamphetamines

● **T43.69**   Poisoning by, adverse effect of and underdosing of other psychostimulants
    ● **T43.691**   Poisoning by other psychostimulants, accidental (unintentional)
       Poisoning by other psychostimulants NOS
    ● **T43.692**   Poisoning by other psychostimulants, intentional self-harm A, S 🔗
    ● **T43.693**   Poisoning by other psychostimulants, assault
    ● **T43.694**   Poisoning by other psychostimulants, undetermined
    ● **T43.695**   Adverse effect of other psychostimulants
    ● **T43.696**   Underdosing of other psychostimulants

● **T43.8**   Poisoning by, adverse effect of and underdosing of other psychotropic drugs
    ● **T43.8X**   Poisoning by, adverse effect of and underdosing of other psychotropic drugs
    ● **T43.8X1**   Poisoning by other psychotropic drugs, accidental (unintentional)
       Poisoning by other psychotropic drugs NOS
    ● **T43.8X2**   Poisoning by other psychotropic drugs, intentional self-harm A, S 🔗
    ● **T43.8X3**   Poisoning by other psychotropic drugs, assault
    ● **T43.8X4**   Poisoning by other psychotropic drugs, undetermined
    ● **T43.8X5**   Adverse effect of other psychotropic drugs
    ● **T43.8X6**   Underdosing of other psychotropic drugs

● **T43.9**   Poisoning by, adverse effect of and underdosing of unspecified psychotropic drug
    X ● **T43.91**   Poisoning by unspecified psychotropic drug, accidental (unintentional)
       Poisoning by psychotropic drug NOS
    X ● **T43.92**   Poisoning by unspecified psychotropic drug, intentional self-harm A, S 🔗
    X ● **T43.93**   Poisoning by unspecified psychotropic drug, assault
    X ● **T43.94**   Poisoning by unspecified psychotropic drug, undetermined
    X ● **T43.95**   Adverse effect of unspecified psychotropic drug
    X ● **T43.96**   Underdosing of unspecified psychotropic drug

● **T44**   Poisoning by, adverse effect of and underdosing of drugs primarily affecting the autonomic nervous system
    The appropriate 7th character is to be added to each code from category T44

A	initial encounter
D	subsequent encounter
S	sequela

● **T44.0**   Poisoning by, adverse effect of and underdosing of anticholinesterase agents
    ● **T44.0X**   Poisoning by, adverse effect of and underdosing of anticholinesterase agents
    ● **T44.0X1**   Poisoning by anticholinesterase agents, accidental (unintentional)
       Poisoning by anticholinesterase agents NOS
    ● **T44.0X2**   Poisoning by anticholinesterase agents, intentional self-harm A, S 🔗
    ● **T44.0X3**   Poisoning by anticholinesterase agents, assault

● T44.0X4 Poisoning by anticholinesterase agents, undetermined
● T44.0X5 Adverse effect of anticholinesterase agents
● T44.0X6 Underdosing of anticholinesterase agents

● T44.1 Poisoning by, adverse effect of and underdosing of other parasympathomimetics [cholinergics]
  ● T44.1X Poisoning by, adverse effect of and underdosing of other parasympathomimetics [cholinergics]
    ● T44.1X1 Poisoning by other parasympathomimetics [cholinergics], accidental (unintentional)
             Poisoning by other parasympathomimetics [cholinergics] NOS
    ● T44.1X2 Poisoning by other parasympathomimetics [cholinergics], intentional self-harm A, S 🏵
    ● T44.1X3 Poisoning by other parasympathomimetics [cholinergics], assault
    ● T44.1X4 Poisoning by other parasympathomimetics [cholinergics], undetermined
    ● T44.1X5 Adverse effect of other parasympathomimetics [cholinergics]
    ● T44.1X6 Underdosing of other parasympathomimetics [cholinergics]

● T44.2 Poisoning by, adverse effect of and underdosing of ganglionic blocking drugs
  ● T44.2X Poisoning by, adverse effect of and underdosing of ganglionic blocking drugs
    ● T44.2X1 Poisoning by ganglionic blocking drugs, accidental (unintentional)
             Poisoning by ganglionic blocking drugs NOS
    ● T44.2X2 Poisoning by ganglionic blocking drugs, intentional self-harm A, S 🏵
    ● T44.2X3 Poisoning by ganglionic blocking drugs, assault
    ● T44.2X4 Poisoning by ganglionic blocking drugs, undetermined
    ● T44.2X5 Adverse effect of ganglionic blocking drugs
    ● T44.2X6 Underdosing of ganglionic blocking drugs

● T44.3 Poisoning by, adverse effect of and underdosing of other parasympatholytics [anticholinergics and antimuscarinics] and spasmolytics
             Poisoning by, adverse effect of and underdosing of papaverine
  ● T44.3X Poisoning by, adverse effect of and underdosing of other parasympatholytics [anticholinergics and antimuscarinics] and spasmolytics
    ● T44.3X1 Poisoning by other parasympatholytics [anticholinergics and antimuscarinics] and spasmolytics, accidental (unintentional)
             Poisoning by other parasympatholytics [anticholinergics and antimuscarinics] and spasmolytics NOS

● T44.3X2 Poisoning by other parasympatholytics [anticholinergics and antimuscarinics] and spasmolytics, intentional self-harm A, S 🏵
● T44.3X3 Poisoning by other parasympatholytics [anticholinergics and antimuscarinics] and spasmolytics, assault
● T44.3X4 Poisoning by other parasympatholytics [anticholinergics and antimuscarinics] and spasmolytics, undetermined
● T44.3X5 Adverse effect of other parasympatholytics [anticholinergics and antimuscarinics] and spasmolytics
● T44.3X6 Underdosing of other parasympatholytics [anticholinergics and antimuscarinics] and spasmolytics

● T44.4 Poisoning by, adverse effect of and underdosing of predominantly alpha-adrenoreceptor agonists
             Poisoning by, adverse effect of and underdosing of metaraminol
  ● T44.4X Poisoning by, adverse effect of and underdosing of predominantly alpha-adrenoreceptor agonists
    ● T44.4X1 Poisoning by predominantly alpha-adrenoreceptor agonists, accidental (unintentional)
             Poisoning by predominantly alpha-adrenoreceptor agonists NOS
    ● T44.4X2 Poisoning by predominantly alpha-adrenoreceptor agonists, intentional self-harm A, S 🏵
    ● T44.4X3 Poisoning by predominantly alpha-adrenoreceptor agonists, assault
    ● T44.4X4 Poisoning by predominantly alpha-adrenoreceptor agonists, undetermined
    ● T44.4X5 Adverse effect of predominantly alpha-adrenoreceptor agonists
    ● T44.4X6 Underdosing of predominantly alpha-adrenoreceptor agonists

● T44.5 Poisoning by, adverse effect of and underdosing of predominantly beta-adrenoreceptor agonists
  Excludes1 poisoning by, adverse effect of and underdosing of beta-adrenoreceptor agonists used in asthma therapy (T48.6-)
  ● T44.5X Poisoning by, adverse effect of and underdosing of predominantly beta-adrenoreceptor agonists
    ● T44.5X1 Poisoning by predominantly beta-adrenoreceptor agonists, accidental (unintentional)
             Poisoning by predominantly beta-adrenoreceptor agonists NOS
    ● T44.5X2 Poisoning by predominantly beta-adrenoreceptor agonists, intentional self-harm A, S 🏵
    ● T44.5X3 Poisoning by predominantly beta-adrenoreceptor agonists, assault
    ● T44.5X4 Poisoning by predominantly beta-adrenoreceptor agonists, undetermined
    ● T44.5X5 Adverse effect of predominantly beta-adrenoreceptor agonists
    ● T44.5X6 Underdosing of predominantly beta-adrenoreceptor agonists

▶ New   ⇒ Revised   ~~deleted~~ Deleted   Excludes 1   Excludes 2   Includes   Use additional   Code first   Code also   Key words
OGCR Official Guidelines   X Assign placeholder X   ● Use Additional Character(s)   ▷ Manifestation Code   🏵 Hierarchical Condition Category   Coding Clinic

● T44.6   **Poisoning by, adverse effect of and underdosing of alpha-adrenoreceptor antagonists**

> **Excludes1**   poisoning by, adverse effect of and underdosing of ergot alkaloids (T48.0)

   ● T44.6X   **Poisoning by, adverse effect of and underdosing of alpha-adrenoreceptor antagonists**

     ● T44.6X1   **Poisoning by alpha-adrenoreceptor antagonists, accidental (unintentional)**

> Poisoning by alpha-adrenoreceptor antagonists NOS

     ● T44.6X2   **Poisoning by alpha-adrenoreceptor antagonists, intentional self-harm** A, S 🔏

     ● T44.6X3   **Poisoning by alpha-adrenoreceptor antagonists, assault**

     ● T44.6X4   **Poisoning by alpha-adrenoreceptor antagonists, undetermined**

     ● T44.6X5   **Adverse effect of alpha-adrenoreceptor antagonists**

     ● T44.6X6   **Underdosing of alpha-adrenoreceptor antagonists**

● T44.7   **Poisoning by, adverse effect of and underdosing of beta-adrenoreceptor antagonists**

   ● T44.7X   **Poisoning by, adverse effect of and underdosing of beta-adrenoreceptor antagonists**

     ● T44.7X1   **Poisoning by beta-adrenoreceptor antagonists, accidental (unintentional)**

> Poisoning by beta-adrenoreceptor antagonists NOS

     ● T44.7X2   **Poisoning by beta-adrenoreceptor antagonists, intentional self-harm** A, S 🔏

     ● T44.7X3   **Poisoning by beta-adrenoreceptor antagonists, assault**

     ● T44.7X4   **Poisoning by beta-adrenoreceptor antagonists, undetermined**

     ● T44.7X5   **Adverse effect of beta-adrenoreceptor antagonists**

     ● T44.7X6   **Underdosing of beta-adrenoreceptor antagonists**

● T44.8   **Poisoning by, adverse effect of and underdosing of centrally-acting and adrenergic-neuron-blocking agents**

> **Excludes2**   poisoning by, adverse effect of and underdosing of clonidine (T46.5)
> poisoning by, adverse effect of and underdosing of guanethidine (T46.5)

   ● T44.8X   **Poisoning by, adverse effect of and underdosing of centrally-acting and adrenergic-neuron-blocking agents**

     ● T44.8X1   **Poisoning by centrally-acting and adrenergic-neuron-blocking agents, accidental (unintentional)**

> Poisoning by centrally-acting and adrenergic-neuron-blocking agents NOS

     ● T44.8X2   **Poisoning by centrally-acting and adrenergic-neuron-blocking agents, intentional self-harm** A, S 🔏

     ● T44.8X3   **Poisoning by centrally-acting and adrenergic-neuron-blocking agents, assault**

     ● T44.8X4   **Poisoning by centrally-acting and adrenergic-neuron-blocking agents, undetermined**

     ● T44.8X5   **Adverse effect of centrally-acting and adrenergic-neuron-blocking agents**

     ● T44.8X6   **Underdosing of centrally-acting and adrenergic-neuron-blocking agents**

● T44.9   **Poisoning by, adverse effect of and underdosing of other and unspecified drugs primarily affecting the autonomic nervous system**

> Poisoning by, adverse effect of and underdosing of drug stimulating both alpha and beta-adrenoreceptors

   ● T44.90   **Poisoning by, adverse effect of and underdosing of unspecified drugs primarily affecting the autonomic nervous system**

     ● T44.901   **Poisoning by unspecified drugs primarily affecting the autonomic nervous system, accidental (unintentional)**

> Poisoning by unspecified drugs primarily affecting the autonomic nervous system NOS

     ● T44.902   **Poisoning by unspecified drugs primarily affecting the autonomic nervous system, intentional self-harm** A, S 🔏

     ● T44.903   **Poisoning by unspecified drugs primarily affecting the autonomic nervous system, assault**

     ● T44.904   **Poisoning by unspecified drugs primarily affecting the autonomic nervous system, undetermined**

     ● T44.905   **Adverse effect of unspecified drugs primarily affecting the autonomic nervous system**

     ● T44.906   **Underdosing of unspecified drugs primarily affecting the autonomic nervous system**

   ● T44.99   **Poisoning by, adverse effect of and underdosing of other drugs primarily affecting the autonomic nervous system**

     ● T44.991   **Poisoning by other drug primarily affecting the autonomic nervous system, accidental (unintentional)**

> Poisoning by other drugs primarily affecting the autonomic nervous system NOS

     ● T44.992   **Poisoning by other drug primarily affecting the autonomic nervous system, intentional self-harm** A, S 🔏

     ● T44.993   **Poisoning by other drug primarily affecting the autonomic nervous system, assault**

     ● T44.994   **Poisoning by other drug primarily affecting the autonomic nervous system, undetermined**

     ● T44.995   **Adverse effect of other drug primarily affecting the autonomic nervous system**

     ● T44.996   **Underdosing of other drug primarily affecting the autonomic nervous system**

CHAPTER 19 (S00-T88)

CHAPTER 19 (S00-T88)

● T45 **Poisoning by, adverse effect of and underdosing of primarily systemic and hematological agents, not elsewhere classified**

The appropriate 7th character is to be added to each code from category T45

> A   initial encounter
> D   subsequent encounter
> S   sequela

● T45.0 **Poisoning by, adverse effect of and underdosing of antiallergic and antiemetic drugs**

    Excludes1 poisoning by, adverse effect of and underdosing of phenothiazine-based neuroleptics (T43.3)

  ● T45.0X **Poisoning by, adverse effect of and underdosing of antiallergic and antiemetic drugs**

    ● T45.0X1 **Poisoning by antiallergic and antiemetic drugs, accidental (unintentional)**
        Poisoning by antiallergic and antiemetic drugs NOS

    ● T45.0X2 **Poisoning by antiallergic and antiemetic drugs, intentional self-harm A, S** 🔲

    ● T45.0X3 **Poisoning by antiallergic and antiemetic drugs, assault**

    ● T45.0X4 **Poisoning by antiallergic and antiemetic drugs, undetermined**

    ● T45.0X5 **Adverse effect of antiallergic and antiemetic drugs**

    ● T45.0X6 **Underdosing of antiallergic and antiemetic drugs**

● T45.1 **Poisoning by, adverse effect of and underdosing of antineoplastic and immunosuppressive drugs**

    Excludes1 poisoning by, adverse effect of and underdosing of tamoxifen (T38.6)

  ● T45.1X **Poisoning by, adverse effect of and underdosing of antineoplastic and immunosuppressive drugs**

    ● T45.1X1 **Poisoning by antineoplastic and immunosuppressive drugs, accidental (unintentional)**
        Poisoning by antineoplastic and immunosuppressive drugs NOS

    ● T45.1X2 **Poisoning by antineoplastic and immunosuppressive drugs, intentional self-harm A, S** 🔲

    ● T45.1X3 **Poisoning by antineoplastic and immunosuppressive drugs, assault**

    ● T45.1X4 **Poisoning by antineoplastic and immunosuppressive drugs, undetermined**

    ● T45.1X5 **Adverse effect of antineoplastic and immunosuppressive drugs**
        Coding Clinic: 2021, Q3, P4; 2019, Q2, P25, 28; Q1, P17, 21

    ● T45.1X6 **Underdosing of antineoplastic and immunosuppressive drugs**

● T45.2 **Poisoning by, adverse effect of and underdosing of vitamins**

    Excludes2 poisoning by, adverse effect of and underdosing of nicotinic acid (derivatives) (T46.7)
        poisoning by, adverse effect of and underdosing of iron (T45.4)
        poisoning by, adverse effect of and underdosing of vitamin K (T45.7)

  ● T45.2X **Poisoning by, adverse effect of and underdosing of vitamins**

    ● T45.2X1 **Poisoning by vitamins, accidental (unintentional)**
        Poisoning by vitamins NOS

    ● T45.2X2 **Poisoning by vitamins, intentional self-harm A, S** 🔲

    ● T45.2X3 **Poisoning by vitamins, assault**

    ● T45.2X4 **Poisoning by vitamins, undetermined**

    ● T45.2X5 **Adverse effect of vitamins**

    ● T45.2X6 **Underdosing of vitamins**
        Excludes1 vitamin deficiencies (E50-E56)

● T45.3 **Poisoning by, adverse effect of and underdosing of enzymes**

  ● T45.3X **Poisoning by, adverse effect of and underdosing of enzymes**

    ● T45.3X1 **Poisoning by enzymes, accidental (unintentional)**
        Poisoning by enzymes NOS

    ● T45.3X2 **Poisoning by enzymes, intentional self-harm A, S** 🔲

    ● T45.3X3 **Poisoning by enzymes, assault**

    ● T45.3X4 **Poisoning by enzymes, undetermined**

    ● T45.3X5 **Adverse effect of enzymes**

    ● T45.3X6 **Underdosing of enzymes**

● T45.4 **Poisoning by, adverse effect of and underdosing of iron and its compounds**

  ● T45.4X **Poisoning by, adverse effect of and underdosing of iron and its compounds**

    ● T45.4X1 **Poisoning by iron and its compounds, accidental (unintentional)**
        Poisoning by iron and its compounds NOS

    ● T45.4X2 **Poisoning by iron and its compounds, intentional self-harm A, S** 🔲

    ● T45.4X3 **Poisoning by iron and its compounds, assault**

    ● T45.4X4 **Poisoning by iron and its compounds, undetermined**

    ● T45.4X5 **Adverse effect of iron and its compounds**

    ● T45.4X6 **Underdosing of iron and its compounds**
        Excludes1 iron deficiency (E61.1)

● T45.5 **Poisoning by, adverse effect of and underdosing of anticoagulants and antithrombotic drugs**

  ● T45.51 **Poisoning by, adverse effect of and underdosing of anticoagulants**

    ● T45.511 **Poisoning by anticoagulants, accidental (unintentional)**
        Poisoning by anticoagulants NOS

    ● T45.512 **Poisoning by anticoagulants, intentional self-harm A, S** 🔲

    ● T45.513 **Poisoning by anticoagulants, assault**

▶ New   ⇒ Revised   ~~deleted~~ Deleted   Excludes 1   Excludes 2   Includes   Use additional   Code first   Code also   Key words

OGCR Official Guidelines   X Assign placeholder X   ● Use Additional Character(s)   ▶ Manifestation Code   🔲 Hierarchical Condition Category   **Coding Clinic**

- T45.514   Poisoning by anticoagulants, undetermined
- T45.515   Adverse effect of anticoagulants
  Coding Clinic: 2021, Q1, P5; 2016, Q1, P14; 2013, Q2, P35
- T45.516   Underdosing of anticoagulants
- T45.52   Poisoning by, adverse effect of and underdosing of antithrombotic drugs
  Poisoning by, adverse effect of and underdosing of antiplatelet drugs

  Excludes2   poisoning by, adverse effect of and underdosing of aspirin (T39.01-)
  poisoning by, adverse effect of and underdosing of acetylsalicylic acid (T39.01-)

  - T45.521   Poisoning by antithrombotic drugs, accidental (unintentional)
    Poisoning by antithrombotic drug NOS
  - T45.522   Poisoning by antithrombotic drugs, intentional self-harm A, S
  - T45.523   Poisoning by antithrombotic drugs, assault
  - T45.524   Poisoning by antithrombotic drugs, undetermined
  - T45.525   Adverse effect of antithrombotic drugs
    Coding Clinic: 2016, Q1, P15
  - T45.526   Underdosing of antithrombotic drugs
- T45.6   Poisoning by, adverse effect of and underdosing of fibrinolysis-affecting drugs
  - T45.60   Poisoning by, adverse effect of and underdosing of unspecified fibrinolysis-affecting drugs
    - T45.601   Poisoning by unspecified fibrinolysis-affecting drugs, accidental (unintentional)
      Poisoning by fibrinolysis-affecting drug NOS
    - T45.602   Poisoning by unspecified fibrinolysis-affecting drugs, intentional self-harm A, S
    - T45.603   Poisoning by unspecified fibrinolysis-affecting drugs, assault
    - T45.604   Poisoning by unspecified fibrinolysis-affecting drugs, undetermined
    - T45.605   Adverse effect of unspecified fibrinolysis-affecting drugs
    - T45.606   Underdosing of unspecified fibrinolysis-affecting drugs
  - T45.61   Poisoning by, adverse effect of and underdosing of thrombolytic drugs
    - T45.611   Poisoning by thrombolytic drug, accidental (unintentional)
      Poisoning by thrombolytic drug NOS
    - T45.612   Poisoning by thrombolytic drug, intentional self-harm A, S
    - T45.613   Poisoning by thrombolytic drug, assault
    - T45.614   Poisoning by thrombolytic drug, undetermined
    - T45.615   Adverse effect of thrombolytic drugs
      Coding Clinic: 2017, Q2, P10
    - T45.616   Underdosing of thrombolytic drugs

- T45.62   Poisoning by, adverse effect of and underdosing of hemostatic drugs
  - T45.621   Poisoning by hemostatic drug, accidental (unintentional)
    Poisoning by hemostatic drug NOS
  - T45.622   Poisoning by hemostatic drug, intentional self-harm A, S
  - T45.623   Poisoning by hemostatic drug, assault
  - T45.624   Poisoning by hemostatic drug, undetermined
  - T45.625   Adverse effect of hemostatic drug
  - T45.626   Underdosing of hemostatic drugs
- T45.69   Poisoning by, adverse effect of and underdosing of other fibrinolysis-affecting drugs
  - T45.691   Poisoning by other fibrinolysis-affecting drugs, accidental (unintentional)
    Poisoning by other fibrinolysis-affecting drug NOS
  - T45.692   Poisoning by other fibrinolysis-affecting drugs, intentional self-harm A, S
  - T45.693   Poisoning by other fibrinolysis-affecting drugs, assault
  - T45.694   Poisoning by other fibrinolysis-affecting drugs, undetermined
  - T45.695   Adverse effect of other fibrinolysis-affecting drugs
  - T45.696   Underdosing of other fibrinolysis-affecting drugs
- T45.7   Poisoning by, adverse effect of and underdosing of anticoagulant antagonists, vitamin K and other coagulants
  - T45.7X   Poisoning by, adverse effect of and underdosing of anticoagulant antagonists, vitamin K and other coagulants
    - T45.7X1   Poisoning by anticoagulant antagonists, vitamin K and other coagulants, accidental (unintentional)
      Poisoning by anticoagulant antagonists, vitamin K and other coagulants NOS
    - T45.7X2   Poisoning by anticoagulant antagonists, vitamin K and other coagulants, intentional self-harm A, S
    - T45.7X3   Poisoning by anticoagulant antagonists, vitamin K and other coagulants, assault
    - T45.7X4   Poisoning by anticoagulant antagonists, vitamin K and other coagulants, undetermined
    - T45.7X5   Adverse effect of anticoagulant antagonists, vitamin K and other coagulants
    - T45.7X6   Underdosing of anticoagulant antagonist, vitamin K and other coagulants

      Excludes1   vitamin K deficiency (E56.1)

● **T45.8** **Poisoning by, adverse effect of and underdosing of other primarily systemic and hematological agents**
Poisoning by, adverse effect of and underdosing of liver preparations and other antianemic agents
Poisoning by, adverse effect of and underdosing of natural blood and blood products
Poisoning by, adverse effect of and underdosing of plasma substitute

Excludes2 poisoning by, adverse effect of and underdosing of immunoglobulin (T50.Z1)
poisoning by, adverse effect of and underdosing of iron (T45.4)
transfusion reactions (T80.-)

● **T45.8X** **Poisoning by, adverse effect of and underdosing of other primarily systemic and hematological agents**

● **T45.8X1** **Poisoning by other primarily systemic and hematological agents, accidental (unintentional)**
Poisoning by other primarily systemic and hematological agents NOS

● **T45.8X2** **Poisoning by other primarily systemic and hematological agents, intentional self-harm** A, S

● **T45.8X3** **Poisoning by other primarily systemic and hematological agents, assault**

● **T45.8X4** **Poisoning by other primarily systemic and hematological agents, undetermined**

● **T45.8X5** **Adverse effect of other primarily systemic and hematological agents**
Coding Clinic: 2016, Q4, P42

● **T45.8X6** **Underdosing of other primarily systemic and hematological agents**

● **T45.9** **Poisoning by, adverse effect of and underdosing of unspecified primarily systemic and hematological agent**

X● **T45.91** **Poisoning by unspecified primarily systemic and hematological agent, accidental (unintentional)**
Poisoning by primarily systemic and hematological agent NOS

X● **T45.92** **Poisoning by unspecified primarily systemic and hematological agent, intentional self-harm** A, S

X● **T45.93** **Poisoning by unspecified primarily systemic and hematological agent, assault**

X● **T45.94** **Poisoning by unspecified primarily systemic and hematological agent, undetermined**

X● **T45.95** **Adverse effect of unspecified primarily systemic and hematological agent**

X● **T45.96** **Underdosing of unspecified primarily systemic and hematological agent**

● **T46** **Poisoning by, adverse effect of and underdosing of agents primarily affecting the cardiovascular system**

Excludes1 poisoning by, adverse effect of and underdosing of metaraminol (T44.4)

The appropriate 7th character is to be added to each code from category T46

A	initial encounter
D	subsequent encounter
S	sequela

● **T46.0** **Poisoning by, adverse effect of and underdosing of cardiac-stimulant glycosides and drugs of similar action**

● **T46.0X** **Poisoning by, adverse effect of and underdosing of cardiac-stimulant glycosides and drugs of similar action**

● **T46.0X1** **Poisoning by cardiac-stimulant glycosides and drugs of similar action, accidental (unintentional)**

Poisoning by cardiac-stimulant glycosides and drugs of similar action NOS

● **T46.0X2** **Poisoning by cardiac-stimulant glycosides and drugs of similar action, intentional self-harm** A, S

● **T46.0X3** **Poisoning by cardiac-stimulant glycosides and drugs of similar action, assault**

● **T46.0X4** **Poisoning by cardiac-stimulant glycosides and drugs of similar action, undetermined**

● **T46.0X5** **Adverse effect of cardiac-stimulant glycosides and drugs of similar action**

● **T46.0X6** **Underdosing of cardiac-stimulant glycosides and drugs of similar action**

● **T46.1** **Poisoning by, adverse effect of and underdosing of calcium-channel blockers**

● **T46.1X** **Poisoning by, adverse effect of and underdosing of calcium-channel blockers**

● **T46.1X1** **Poisoning by calcium-channel blockers, accidental (unintentional)**
Poisoning by calcium-channel blockers NOS

● **T46.1X2** **Poisoning by calcium-channel blockers, intentional self-harm** A, S

● **T46.1X3** **Poisoning by calcium-channel blockers, assault**

● **T46.1X4** **Poisoning by calcium-channel blockers, undetermined**

● **T46.1X5** **Adverse effect of calcium-channel blockers**

● **T46.1X6** **Underdosing of calcium-channel blockers**

● **T46.2** **Poisoning by, adverse effect of and underdosing of other antidysrhythmic drugs, not elsewhere classified**

Excludes1 poisoning by, adverse effect of and underdosing of beta-adrenoreceptor antagonists (T44.7-)

● **T46.2X** **Poisoning by, adverse effect of and underdosing of other antidysrhythmic drugs**

● **T46.2X1** **Poisoning by other antidysrhythmic drugs, accidental (unintentional)**
Poisoning by other antidysrhythmic drugs NOS

● **T46.2X2** **Poisoning by other antidysrhythmic drugs, intentional self-harm** A, S

● **T46.2X3** **Poisoning by other antidysrhythmic drugs, assault**

● **T46.2X4** **Poisoning by other antidysrhythmic drugs, undetermined**

● **T46.2X5** **Adverse effect of other antidysrhythmic drugs**

● **T46.2X6** **Underdosing of other antidysrhythmic drugs**

● **T46.3** **Poisoning by, adverse effect of and underdosing of coronary vasodilators**
Poisoning by, adverse effect of and underdosing of dipyridamole

Excludes1 poisoning by, adverse effect of and underdosing of calcium-channel blockers (T46.1)

● **T46.3X** **Poisoning by, adverse effect of and underdosing of coronary vasodilators**

● **T46.3X1** **Poisoning by coronary vasodilators, accidental (unintentional)**
Poisoning by coronary vasodilators NOS

● **T46.3X2** **Poisoning by coronary vasodilators, intentional self-harm** A, S

● T46.3X3   Poisoning by coronary vasodilators, **assault**

● T46.3X4   Poisoning by coronary vasodilators, **undetermined**

● T46.3X5   **Adverse effect** of coronary vasodilators

● T46.3X6   **Underdosing** of coronary vasodilators

● T46.4   Poisoning by, adverse effect of and underdosing of angiotensin-converting-enzyme inhibitors

● T46.4X   Poisoning by, adverse effect of and underdosing of angiotensin-converting-enzyme inhibitors

● T46.4X1   Poisoning by angiotensin-converting-enzyme inhibitors, **accidental (unintentional)**

     Poisoning by angiotensin-converting-enzyme inhibitors NOS

● T46.4X2   Poisoning by angiotensin-converting-enzyme inhibitors, **intentional self-harm A, S** 🔖

● T46.4X3   Poisoning by angiotensin-converting-enzyme inhibitors, **assault**

● T46.4X4   Poisoning by angiotensin-converting-enzyme inhibitors, **undetermined**

● T46.4X5   **Adverse effect** of angiotensin-converting-enzyme inhibitors

● T46.4X6   **Underdosing** of angiotensin-converting-enzyme inhibitors

● T46.5   Poisoning by, adverse effect of and underdosing of other antihypertensive drugs

Excludes2   poisoning by, adverse effect of and underdosing of beta-adrenoreceptor antagonists (T44.7)
poisoning by, adverse effect of and underdosing of calcium-channel blockers (T46.1)
poisoning by, adverse effect of and underdosing of diuretics (T50.0-T50.2)

● T46.5X   Poisoning by, adverse effect of and underdosing of **other antihypertensive drugs**

● T46.5X1   Poisoning by other antihypertensive drugs, **accidental (unintentional)**

     Poisoning by other antihypertensive drugs NOS

● T46.5X2   Poisoning by other antihypertensive drugs, **intentional self-harm A, S** 🔖

● T46.5X3   Poisoning by other antihypertensive drugs, **assault**

● T46.5X4   Poisoning by other antihypertensive drugs, **undetermined**

● T46.5X5   **Adverse effect** of other antihypertensive drugs

● T46.5X6   **Underdosing** of other antihypertensive drugs

     Coding Clinic: 2022, Q1, P36

● T46.6   Poisoning by, adverse effect of and underdosing of antihyperlipidemic and antiarteriosclerotic drugs

● T46.6X   Poisoning by, adverse effect of and underdosing of **antihyperlipidemic and antiarteriosclerotic drugs**

● T46.6X1   Poisoning by antihyperlipidemic and antiarteriosclerotic drugs, **accidental (unintentional)**

     Poisoning by antihyperlipidemic and antiarteriosclerotic drugs NOS

● T46.6X2   Poisoning by antihyperlipidemic and antiarteriosclerotic drugs, **intentional self-harm A, S** 🔖

● T46.6X3   Poisoning by antihyperlipidemic and antiarteriosclerotic drugs, **assault**

● T46.6X4   Poisoning by antihyperlipidemic and antiarteriosclerotic drugs, **undetermined**

● T46.6X5   **Adverse effect** of antihyperlipidemic and antiarteriosclerotic drugs

● T46.6X6   **Underdosing** of antihyperlipidemic and antiarteriosclerotic drugs

● T46.7   Poisoning by, adverse effect of and underdosing of peripheral vasodilators

     Poisoning by, adverse effect of and underdosing of nicotinic acid (derivatives)

     Excludes1   poisoning by, adverse effect of and underdosing of papaverine (T44.3)

● T46.7X   Poisoning by, adverse effect of and underdosing of **peripheral vasodilators**

● T46.7X1   Poisoning by peripheral vasodilators, **accidental (unintentional)**

     Poisoning by peripheral vasodilators NOS

● T46.7X2   Poisoning by peripheral vasodilators, **intentional self-harm A, S** 🔖

● T46.7X3   Poisoning by peripheral vasodilators, **assault**

● T46.7X4   Poisoning by peripheral vasodilators, **undetermined**

● T46.7X5   **Adverse effect** of peripheral vasodilators

● T46.7X6   **Underdosing** of peripheral vasodilators

● T46.8   Poisoning by, adverse effect of and underdosing of antivaricose drugs, including sclerosing agents

● T46.8X   Poisoning by, adverse effect of and underdosing of **antivaricose drugs, including sclerosing agents**

● T46.8X1   Poisoning by antivaricose drugs, including sclerosing agents, **accidental (unintentional)**

     Poisoning by antivaricose drugs, including sclerosing agents NOS

● T46.8X2   Poisoning by antivaricose drugs, including sclerosing agents, **intentional self-harm A, S** 🔖

● T46.8X3   Poisoning by antivaricose drugs, including sclerosing agents, **assault**

● T46.8X4   Poisoning by antivaricose drugs, including sclerosing agents, **undetermined**

● T46.8X5   **Adverse effect** of antivaricose drugs, including sclerosing agents

● T46.8X6   **Underdosing** of antivaricose drugs, including sclerosing agents

● T46.9   Poisoning by, adverse effect of and underdosing of other and unspecified agents primarily affecting the cardiovascular system

● T46.90   Poisoning by, adverse effect of and underdosing of **unspecified agents primarily affecting the cardiovascular system**

● T46.901   Poisoning by unspecified agents primarily affecting the cardiovascular system, **accidental (unintentional)**

● T46.902   Poisoning by unspecified agents primarily affecting the cardiovascular system, **intentional self-harm A, S** 🔖

● T46.903   Poisoning by unspecified agents primarily affecting the cardiovascular system, **assault**

● T46.904   Poisoning by unspecified agents primarily affecting the cardiovascular system, **undetermined**

CHAPTER 19 (S00-T88)

● T46.905 Adverse effect of unspecified agents primarily affecting the cardiovascular system

● T46.906 Underdosing of unspecified agents primarily affecting the cardiovascular system

● T46.99 Poisoning by, adverse effect of and underdosing of other agents primarily affecting the cardiovascular system

● T46.991 Poisoning by other agents primarily affecting the cardiovascular system, accidental (unintentional)

● T46.992 Poisoning by other agents primarily affecting the cardiovascular system, intentional self-harm A, S 🦠

● T46.993 Poisoning by other agents primarily affecting the cardiovascular system, assault

● T46.994 Poisoning by other agents primarily affecting the cardiovascular system, undetermined

● T46.995 Adverse effect of other agents primarily affecting the cardiovascular system

● T46.996 Underdosing of other agents primarily affecting the cardiovascular system

● T47 Poisoning by, adverse effect of and underdosing of agents primarily affecting the gastrointestinal system

The appropriate 7th character is to be added to each code from category T47

A	initial encounter
D	subsequent encounter
S	sequela

● T47.0 Poisoning by, adverse effect of and underdosing of histamine H2-receptor blockers

● T47.0X Poisoning by, adverse effect of and underdosing of histamine H2-receptor blockers

● T47.0X1 Poisoning by histamine H2-receptor blockers, accidental (unintentional)
Poisoning by histamine H2-receptor blockers NOS

● T47.0X2 Poisoning by histamine H2-receptor blockers, intentional self-harm A, S 🦠

● T47.0X3 Poisoning by histamine H2-receptor blockers, assault

● T47.0X4 Poisoning by histamine H2-receptor blockers, undetermined

● T47.0X5 Adverse effect of histamine H2-receptor blockers

● T47.0X6 Underdosing of histamine H2-receptor blockers

● T47.1 Poisoning by, adverse effect of and underdosing of other antacids and anti-gastric-secretion drugs

● T47.1X Poisoning by, adverse effect of and underdosing of other antacids and anti-gastric-secretion drugs

● T47.1X1 Poisoning by other antacids and anti-gastric-secretion drugs, accidental (unintentional)
Poisoning by other antacids and anti-gastric-secretion drugs NOS

● T47.1X2 Poisoning by other antacids and anti-gastric-secretion drugs, intentional self-harm A, S 🦠

● T47.1X3 Poisoning by other antacids and anti-gastric-secretion drugs, assault

● T47.1X4 Poisoning by other antacids and anti-gastric-secretion drugs, undetermined

● T47.1X5 Adverse effect of other antacids and anti-gastric-secretion drugs

● T47.1X6 Underdosing of other antacids and anti-gastric-secretion drugs

● T47.2 Poisoning by, adverse effect of and underdosing of stimulant laxatives

● T47.2X Poisoning by, adverse effect of and underdosing of stimulant laxatives

● T47.2X1 Poisoning by stimulant laxatives, accidental (unintentional)
Poisoning by stimulant laxatives NOS

● T47.2X2 Poisoning by stimulant laxatives, intentional self-harm A, S 🦠

● T47.2X3 Poisoning by stimulant laxatives, assault

● T47.2X4 Poisoning by stimulant laxatives, undetermined

● T47.2X5 Adverse effect of stimulant laxatives

● T47.2X6 Underdosing of stimulant laxatives

● T47.3 Poisoning by, adverse effect of and underdosing of saline and osmotic laxatives

● T47.3X Poisoning by and adverse effect of saline and osmotic laxatives

● T47.3X1 Poisoning by saline and osmotic laxatives, accidental (unintentional)
Poisoning by saline and osmotic laxatives NOS

● T47.3X2 Poisoning by saline and osmotic laxatives, intentional self-harm

● T47.3X3 Poisoning by saline and osmotic laxatives, assault A, S 🦠

● T47.3X4 Poisoning by saline and osmotic laxatives, undetermined

● T47.3X5 Adverse effect of saline and osmotic laxatives

● T47.3X6 Underdosing of saline and osmotic laxatives

● T47.4 Poisoning by, adverse effect of and underdosing of other laxatives

● T47.4X Poisoning by, adverse effect of and underdosing of other laxatives

● T47.4X1 Poisoning by other laxatives, accidental (unintentional)
Poisoning by other laxatives NOS

● T47.4X2 Poisoning by other laxatives, intentional self-harm A, S 🦠

● T47.4X3 Poisoning by other laxatives, assault

● T47.4X4 Poisoning by other laxatives, undetermined

● T47.4X5 Adverse effect of other laxatives

● T47.4X6 Underdosing of other laxatives

● T47.5 Poisoning by, adverse effect of and underdosing of digestants

● T47.5X Poisoning by, adverse effect of and underdosing of digestants

● T47.5X1 Poisoning by digestants, accidental (unintentional)
Poisoning by digestants NOS

● T47.5X2 Poisoning by digestants, intentional self-harm A, S 🦠

● T47.5X3 Poisoning by digestants, assault

● T47.5X4 Poisoning by digestants, undetermined

● T47.5X5 Adverse effect of digestants

● T47.5X6 Underdosing of digestants

▶ New   ⇒ Revised   deleted Deleted   Excludes 1   Excludes 2   Includes   Use additional   Code first   Code also   Key words

OGCR Official Guidelines   X Assign placeholder X   ● Use Additional Character(s)   ▶ Manifestation Code   🦠 Hierarchical Condition Category   Coding Clinic

● **T47.6** Poisoning by, adverse effect of and underdosing of antidiarrheal drugs

   Excludes2 poisoning by, adverse effect of and underdosing of systemic antibiotics and other anti-infectives (T36-T37)

  ● **T47.6X** Poisoning by, adverse effect of and underdosing of antidiarrheal drugs

    ● **T47.6X1** Poisoning by antidiarrheal drugs, accidental (unintentional)
       Poisoning by antidiarrheal drugs NOS

    ● **T47.6X2** Poisoning by antidiarrheal drugs, intentional self-harm A, S 🔖

    ● **T47.6X3** Poisoning by antidiarrheal drugs, assault

    ● **T47.6X4** Poisoning by antidiarrheal drugs, undetermined

    ● **T47.6X5** Adverse effect of antidiarrheal drugs

    ● **T47.6X6** Underdosing of antidiarrheal drugs

● **T47.7** Poisoning by, adverse effect of and underdosing of emetics

  ● **T47.7X** Poisoning by, adverse effect of and underdosing of emetics

    ● **T47.7X1** Poisoning by emetics, accidental (unintentional)
       Poisoning by emetics NOS

    ● **T47.7X2** Poisoning by emetics, intentional self-harm A, S 🔖

    ● **T47.7X3** Poisoning by emetics, assault

    ● **T47.7X4** Poisoning by emetics, undetermined

    ● **T47.7X5** Adverse effect of emetics

    ● **T47.7X6** Underdosing of emetics

● **T47.8** Poisoning by, adverse effect of and underdosing of other agents primarily affecting gastrointestinal system

  ● **T47.8X** Poisoning by, adverse effect of and underdosing of other agents primarily affecting gastrointestinal system

    ● **T47.8X1** Poisoning by other agents primarily affecting gastrointestinal system, accidental (unintentional)
       Poisoning by other agents primarily affecting gastrointestinal system NOS

    ● **T47.8X2** Poisoning by other agents primarily affecting gastrointestinal system, intentional self-harm A, S 🔖

    ● **T47.8X3** Poisoning by other agents primarily affecting gastrointestinal system, assault

    ● **T47.8X4** Poisoning by other agents primarily affecting gastrointestinal system, undetermined

    ● **T47.8X5** Adverse effect of other agents primarily affecting gastrointestinal system

    ● **T47.8X6** Underdosing of other agents primarily affecting gastrointestinal system

● **T47.9** Poisoning by, adverse effect of and underdosing of unspecified agents primarily affecting the gastrointestinal system

  X● **T47.91** Poisoning by unspecified agents primarily affecting the gastrointestinal system, accidental (unintentional)
       Poisoning by agents primarily affecting the gastrointestinal system NOS

  X● **T47.92** Poisoning by unspecified agents primarily affecting the gastrointestinal system, intentional self-harm A, S 🔖

  X● **T47.93** Poisoning by unspecified agents primarily affecting the gastrointestinal system, assault

  X● **T47.94** Poisoning by unspecified agents primarily affecting the gastrointestinal system, undetermined

  X● **T47.95** Adverse effect of unspecified agents primarily affecting the gastrointestinal system

  X● **T47.96** Underdosing of unspecified agents primarily affecting the gastrointestinal system

● **T48** Poisoning by, adverse effect of and underdosing of agents primarily acting on smooth and skeletal muscles and the respiratory system

  The appropriate 7th character is to be added to each code from category T48

    A initial encounter
    D subsequent encounter
    S sequela

● **T48.0** Poisoning by, adverse effect of and underdosing of oxytocic drugs

   Excludes1 poisoning by, adverse effect of and underdosing of estrogens, progestogens and antagonists (T38.4-T38.6)

  ● **T48.0X** Poisoning by, adverse effect of and underdosing of oxytocic drugs

    ● **T48.0X1** Poisoning by oxytocic drugs, accidental (unintentional)
       Poisoning by oxytocic drugs NOS

    ● **T48.0X2** Poisoning by oxytocic drugs, intentional self-harm A, S 🔖

    ● **T48.0X3** Poisoning by oxytocic drugs, assault

    ● **T48.0X4** Poisoning by oxytocic drugs, undetermined

    ● **T48.0X5** Adverse effect of oxytocic drugs

    ● **T48.0X6** Underdosing of oxytocic drugs

● **T48.1** Poisoning by, adverse effect of and underdosing of skeletal muscle relaxants [neuromuscular blocking agents]

  ● **T48.1X** Poisoning by, adverse effect of and underdosing of skeletal muscle relaxants [neuromuscular blocking agents]

    ● **T48.1X1** Poisoning by skeletal muscle relaxants [neuromuscular blocking agents], accidental (unintentional)
       Poisoning by skeletal muscle relaxants [neuromuscular blocking agents] NOS

    ● **T48.1X2** Poisoning by skeletal muscle relaxants [neuromuscular blocking agents], intentional self-harm A, S 🔖

    ● **T48.1X3** Poisoning by skeletal muscle relaxants [neuromuscular blocking agents], assault

    ● **T48.1X4** Poisoning by skeletal muscle relaxants [neuromuscular blocking agents], undetermined

    ● **T48.1X5** Adverse effect of skeletal muscle relaxants [neuromuscular blocking agents]

    ● **T48.1X6** Underdosing of skeletal muscle relaxants [neuromuscular blocking agents]

● **T48.2** Poisoning by, adverse effect of and underdosing of other and unspecified drugs acting on muscles

  ● **T48.20** Poisoning by, adverse effect of and underdosing of unspecified drugs acting on muscles

    ● **T48.201** Poisoning by unspecified drugs acting on muscles, accidental (unintentional)
       Poisoning by unspecified drugs acting on muscles NOS

    ● **T48.202** Poisoning by unspecified drugs acting on muscles, intentional self-harm A, S 🔖

- T48.203 Poisoning by unspecified drugs acting on muscles, assault
- T48.204 Poisoning by unspecified drugs acting on muscles, undetermined
- T48.205 Adverse effect of unspecified drugs acting on muscles
- T48.206 Underdosing of unspecified drugs acting on muscles
- T48.29 Poisoning by, adverse effect of and underdosing of other drugs acting on muscles
  - T48.291 Poisoning by other drugs acting on muscles, accidental (unintentional)
    Poisoning by other drugs acting on muscles NOS
  - T48.292 Poisoning by other drugs acting on muscles, intentional self-harm A, S 🐾
  - T48.293 Poisoning by other drugs acting on muscles, assault
  - T48.294 Poisoning by other drugs acting on muscles, undetermined
  - T48.295 Adverse effect of other drugs acting on muscles
  - T48.296 Underdosing of other drugs acting on muscles
- T48.3 Poisoning by, adverse effect of and underdosing of antitussives
  - T48.3X Poisoning by, adverse effect of and underdosing of antitussives
    - T48.3X1 Poisoning by antitussives, accidental (unintentional)
      Poisoning by antitussives NOS
    - T48.3X2 Poisoning by antitussives, intentional self-harm A, S 🐾
    - T48.3X3 Poisoning by antitussives, assault
    - T48.3X4 Poisoning by antitussives, undetermined
    - T48.3X5 Adverse effect of antitussives
    - T48.3X6 Underdosing of antitussives
- T48.4 Poisoning by, adverse effect of and underdosing of expectorants
  - T48.4X Poisoning by, adverse effect of and underdosing of expectorants
    - T48.4X1 Poisoning by expectorants, accidental (unintentional)
      Poisoning by expectorants NOS
    - T48.4X2 Poisoning by expectorants, intentional self-harm A, S 🐾
    - T48.4X3 Poisoning by expectorants, assault
    - T48.4X4 Poisoning by expectorants, undetermined
    - T48.4X5 Adverse effect of expectorants
    - T48.4X6 Underdosing of expectorants
- T48.5 Poisoning by, adverse effect of and underdosing of other anti-common-cold drugs
  Poisoning by, adverse effect of and underdosing of decongestants

  Excludes2   poisoning by, adverse effect of and underdosing of antipyretics, NEC (T39.9-)
  poisoning by, adverse effect of and underdosing of non-steroidal antiinflammatory drugs (T39.3-)
  poisoning by, adverse effect of and underdosing of salicylates (T39.0-)
  - T48.5X Poisoning by, adverse effect of and underdosing of other anti-common-cold drugs
    - T48.5X1 Poisoning by other anti-common-cold drugs, accidental (unintentional)
      Poisoning by other anti-common-cold drugs NOS
    - T48.5X2 Poisoning by other anti-common-cold drugs, intentional self-harm A, S 🐾

- T48.5X3 Poisoning by other anti-common-cold drugs, assault
- T48.5X4 Poisoning by other anti-common-cold drugs, undetermined
- T48.5X5 Adverse effect of other anti-common-cold drugs
- T48.5X6 Underdosing of other anti-common-cold drugs
- T48.6 Poisoning by, adverse effect of and underdosing of antiasthmatics, not elsewhere classified
  Poisoning by, adverse effect of and underdosing of beta-adrenoreceptor agonists used in asthma therapy

  Excludes1   poisoning by, adverse effect of and underdosing of beta-adrenoreceptor agonists not used in asthma therapy (T44.5)
  poisoning by, adverse effect of and underdosing of anterior pituitary [adenohypophyseal] hormones (T38.8)
  - T48.6X Poisoning by, adverse effect of and underdosing of antiasthmatics
    - T48.6X1 Poisoning by antiasthmatics, accidental (unintentional)
      Poisoning by antiasthmatics NOS
    - T48.6X2 Poisoning by antiasthmatics, intentional self-harm A, S 🐾
    - T48.6X3 Poisoning by antiasthmatics, assault
    - T48.6X4 Poisoning by antiasthmatics, undetermined
    - T48.6X5 Adverse effect of antiasthmatics
    - T48.6X6 Underdosing of antiasthmatics
- T48.9 Poisoning by, adverse effect of and underdosing of other and unspecified agents primarily acting on the respiratory system
  - T48.90 Poisoning by, adverse effect of and underdosing of unspecified agents primarily acting on the respiratory system
    - T48.901 Poisoning by unspecified agents primarily acting on the respiratory system, accidental (unintentional)
    - T48.902 Poisoning by unspecified agents primarily acting on the respiratory system, intentional self-harm A, S 🐾
    - T48.903 Poisoning by unspecified agents primarily acting on the respiratory system, assault
    - T48.904 Poisoning by unspecified agents primarily acting on the respiratory system, undetermined
    - T48.905 Adverse effect of unspecified agents primarily acting on the respiratory system
    - T48.906 Underdosing of unspecified agents primarily acting on the respiratory system
  - T48.99 Poisoning by, adverse effect of and underdosing of other agents primarily acting on the respiratory system
    - T48.991 Poisoning by other agents primarily acting on the respiratory system, accidental (unintentional)
    - T48.992 Poisoning by other agents primarily acting on the respiratory system, intentional self-harm A, S 🐾
    - T48.993 Poisoning by other agents primarily acting on the respiratory system, assault
    - T48.994 Poisoning by other agents primarily acting on the respiratory system, undetermined

▶ New   ⇒ Revised   ~~deleted~~ Deleted   Excludes 1   Excludes 2   Includes   Use additional   Code first   Code also   Key words
OGCR Official Guidelines   X Assign placeholder X   ● Use Additional Character(s)   ) Manifestation Code   🐾 Hierarchical Condition Category   Coding Clinic

● **T48.995** Adverse effect of other agents primarily acting on the respiratory system
● **T48.996** Underdosing of other agents primarily acting on the respiratory system

● **T49** Poisoning by, adverse effect of and underdosing of topical agents primarily affecting skin and mucous membrane and by ophthalmological, otorhinolaryngological and dental drugs

Includes   poisoning by, adverse effect of and underdosing of glucocorticoids, topically used

The appropriate 7th character is to be added to each code from category T49

A   initial encounter
D   subsequent encounter
S   sequela

● **T49.0** Poisoning by, adverse effect of and underdosing of local antifungal, anti-infective and anti-inflammatory drugs
● **T49.0X** Poisoning by, adverse effect of and underdosing of local antifungal, anti-infective and anti-inflammatory drugs
● **T49.0X1** Poisoning by local antifungal, anti-infective and anti-inflammatory drugs, accidental (unintentional)
  Poisoning by local antifungal, anti-infective and anti-inflammatory drugs NOS
● **T49.0X2** Poisoning by local antifungal, anti-infective and anti-inflammatory drugs, intentional self-harm A, S
● **T49.0X3** Poisoning by local antifungal, anti-infective and anti-inflammatory drugs, assault
● **T49.0X4** Poisoning by local antifungal, anti-infective and anti-inflammatory drugs, undetermined
● **T49.0X5** Adverse effect of local antifungal, anti-infective and anti-inflammatory drugs
● **T49.0X6** Underdosing of local antifungal, anti-infective and anti-inflammatory drugs

● **T49.1** Poisoning by, adverse effect of and underdosing of antipruritics
● **T49.1X** Poisoning by, adverse effect of and underdosing of antipruritics
● **T49.1X1** Poisoning by antipruritics, accidental (unintentional)
  Poisoning by antipruritics NOS
● **T49.1X2** Poisoning by antipruritics, intentional self-harm A, S
● **T49.1X3** Poisoning by antipruritics, assault
● **T49.1X4** Poisoning by antipruritics, undetermined
● **T49.1X5** Adverse effect of antipruritics
● **T49.1X6** Underdosing of antipruritics

● **T49.2** Poisoning by, adverse effect of and underdosing of local astringents and local detergents
● **T49.2X** Poisoning by, adverse effect of and underdosing of local astringents and local detergents
● **T49.2X1** Poisoning by local astringents and local detergents, accidental (unintentional)
  Poisoning by local astringents and local detergents NOS
● **T49.2X2** Poisoning by local astringents and local detergents, intentional self-harm A, S
● **T49.2X3** Poisoning by local astringents and local detergents, assault

● **T49.2X4** Poisoning by local astringents and local detergents, undetermined
● **T49.2X5** Adverse effect of local astringents and local detergents
● **T49.2X6** Underdosing of local astringents and local detergents

● **T49.3** Poisoning by, adverse effect of and underdosing of emollients, demulcents and protectants
● **T49.3X** Poisoning by, adverse effect of and underdosing of emollients, demulcents and protectants
● **T49.3X1** Poisoning by emollients, demulcents and protectants, accidental (unintentional)
  Poisoning by emollients, demulcents and protectants NOS
● **T49.3X2** Poisoning by emollients, demulcents and protectants, intentional self-harm A, S
● **T49.3X3** Poisoning by emollients, demulcents and protectants, assault
● **T49.3X4** Poisoning by emollients, demulcents and protectants, undetermined
● **T49.3X5** Adverse effect of emollients, demulcents and protectants
● **T49.3X6** Underdosing of emollients, demulcents and protectants

● **T49.4** Poisoning by, adverse effect of and underdosing of keratolytics, keratoplastics, and other hair treatment drugs and preparations
● **T49.4X** Poisoning by, adverse effect of and underdosing of keratolytics, keratoplastics, and other hair treatment drugs and preparations
● **T49.4X1** Poisoning by keratolytics, keratoplastics, and other hair treatment drugs and preparations, accidental (unintentional)
  Poisoning by keratolytics, keratoplastics, and other hair treatment drugs and preparations NOS
● **T49.4X2** Poisoning by keratolytics, keratoplastics, and other hair treatment drugs and preparations, intentional self-harm A, S
● **T49.4X3** Poisoning by keratolytics, keratoplastics, and other hair treatment drugs and preparations, assault
● **T49.4X4** Poisoning by keratolytics, keratoplastics, and other hair treatment drugs and preparations, undetermined
● **T49.4X5** Adverse effect of keratolytics, keratoplastics, and other hair treatment drugs and preparations
● **T49.4X6** Underdosing of keratolytics, keratoplastics, and other hair treatment drugs and preparations

● **T49.5** Poisoning by, adverse effect of and underdosing of ophthalmological drugs and preparations
● **T49.5X** Poisoning by, adverse effect of and underdosing of ophthalmological drugs and preparations
● **T49.5X1** Poisoning by ophthalmological drugs and preparations, accidental (unintentional)
  Poisoning by ophthalmological drugs and preparations NOS
● **T49.5X2** Poisoning by ophthalmological drugs and preparations, intentional self-harm A, S
● **T49.5X3** Poisoning by ophthalmological drugs and preparations, assault

- T49.5X4   Poisoning by ophthalmological drugs and preparations, undetermined
- T49.5X5   Adverse effect of ophthalmological drugs and preparations
- T49.5X6   Underdosing of ophthalmological drugs and preparations
- T49.6   Poisoning by, adverse effect of and underdosing of otorhinolaryngological drugs and preparations
  - T49.6X   Poisoning by, adverse effect of and underdosing of otorhinolaryngological drugs and preparations
    - T49.6X1   Poisoning by otorhinolaryngological drugs and preparations, accidental (unintentional)
      Poisoning by otorhinolaryngological drugs and preparations NOS
    - T49.6X2   Poisoning by otorhinolaryngological drugs and preparations, intentional self-harm A, S 🐾
    - T49.6X3   Poisoning by otorhinolaryngological drugs and preparations, assault
    - T49.6X4   Poisoning by otorhinolaryngological drugs and preparations, undetermined
    - T49.6X5   Adverse effect of otorhinolaryngological drugs and preparations
    - T49.6X6   Underdosing of otorhinolaryngological drugs and preparations
- T49.7   Poisoning by, adverse effect of and underdosing of dental drugs, topically applied
  - T49.7X   Poisoning by, adverse effect of and underdosing of dental drugs, topically applied
    - T49.7X1   Poisoning by dental drugs, topically applied, accidental (unintentional)
      Poisoning by dental drugs, topically applied NOS
    - T49.7X2   Poisoning by dental drugs, topically applied, intentional self-harm A, S 🐾
    - T49.7X3   Poisoning by dental drugs, topically applied, assault
    - T49.7X4   Poisoning by dental drugs, topically applied, undetermined
    - T49.7X5   Adverse effect of dental drugs, topically applied
    - T49.7X6   Underdosing of dental drugs, topically applied
- T49.8   Poisoning by, adverse effect of and underdosing of other topical agents
    Poisoning by, adverse effect of and underdosing of spermicides
  - T49.8X   Poisoning by, adverse effect of and underdosing of other topical agents
    - T49.8X1   Poisoning by other topical agents, accidental (unintentional)
      Poisoning by other topical agents NOS
    - T49.8X2   Poisoning by other topical agents, intentional self-harm A, S 🐾
    - T49.8X3   Poisoning by other topical agents, assault
    - T49.8X4   Poisoning by other topical agents, undetermined
    - T49.8X5   Adverse effect of other topical agents
    - T49.8X6   Underdosing of other topical agents

- T49.9   Poisoning by, adverse effect of and underdosing of unspecified topical agent
  - X T49.91   Poisoning by unspecified topical agent, accidental (unintentional)
  - X T49.92   Poisoning by unspecified topical agent, intentional self-harm A, S 🐾
  - X T49.93   Poisoning by unspecified topical agent, assault
  - X T49.94   Poisoning by unspecified topical agent, undetermined
  - X T49.95   Adverse effect of unspecified topical agent
  - X T49.96   Underdosing of unspecified topical agent
- T50   Poisoning by, adverse effect of and underdosing of diuretics and other and unspecified drugs, medicaments and biological substances

    The appropriate 7th character is to be added to each code from category T50

A	initial encounter
D	subsequent encounter
S	sequela

  - T50.0   Poisoning by, adverse effect of and underdosing of mineralocorticoids and their antagonists
    - T50.0X   Poisoning by, adverse effect of and underdosing of mineralocorticoids and their antagonists
      - T50.0X1   Poisoning by mineralocorticoids and their antagonists, accidental (unintentional)
        Poisoning by mineralocorticoids and their antagonists NOS
      - T50.0X2   Poisoning by mineralocorticoids and their antagonists, intentional self-harm A, S 🐾
      - T50.0X3   Poisoning by mineralocorticoids and their antagonists, assault
      - T50.0X4   Poisoning by mineralocorticoids and their antagonists, undetermined
      - T50.0X5   Adverse effect of mineralocorticoids and their antagonists
      - T50.0X6   Underdosing of mineralocorticoids and their antagonists
  - T50.1   Poisoning by, adverse effect of and underdosing of loop [high-ceiling] diuretics
    - T50.1X   Poisoning by, adverse effect of and underdosing of loop [high-ceiling] diuretics
      - T50.1X1   Poisoning by loop [high-ceiling] diuretics, accidental (unintentional)
        Poisoning by loop [high-ceiling] diuretics NOS
      - T50.1X2   Poisoning by loop [high-ceiling] diuretics, intentional self-harm A, S 🐾
      - T50.1X3   Poisoning by loop [high-ceiling] diuretics, assault
      - T50.1X4   Poisoning by loop [high-ceiling] diuretics, undetermined
      - T50.1X5   Adverse effect of loop [high-ceiling] diuretics
      - T50.1X6   Underdosing of loop [high-ceiling] diuretics

▶ New   ⇒ Revised   ~~deleted~~ Deleted   Excludes 1   Excludes 2   Includes   Use additional   Code first   Code also   Key words
OGCR Official Guidelines   X Assign placeholder X   ● Use Additional Character(s)   ▌ Manifestation Code   🐾 Hierarchical Condition Category   **Coding Clinic**

● **T50.2** Poisoning by, adverse effect of and underdosing of carbonic-anhydrase inhibitors, benzothiadiazides and other diuretics
> Poisoning by, adverse effect of and underdosing of acetazolamide

● **T50.2X** Poisoning by, adverse effect of and underdosing of carbonic-anhydrase inhibitors, benzothiadiazides and other diuretics

● **T50.2X1** Poisoning by carbonic-anhydrase inhibitors, benzothiadiazides and other diuretics, accidental (unintentional)
> Poisoning by carbonic-anhydrase inhibitors, benzothiadiazides and other diuretics NOS

● **T50.2X2** Poisoning by carbonic-anhydrase inhibitors, benzothiadiazides and other diuretics, intentional self-harm A, S 🔖

● **T50.2X3** Poisoning by carbonic-anhydrase inhibitors, benzothiadiazides and other diuretics, assault

● **T50.2X4** Poisoning by carbonic-anhydrase inhibitors, benzothiadiazides and other diuretics, undetermined

● **T50.2X5** Adverse effect of carbonic-anhydrase inhibitors, benzothiadiazides and other diuretics

● **T50.2X6** Underdosing of carbonic-anhydrase inhibitors, benzothiadiazides and other diuretics

● **T50.3** Poisoning by, adverse effect of and underdosing of electrolytic, caloric and water-balance agents
> Poisoning by, adverse effect of and underdosing of oral rehydration salts

● **T50.3X** Poisoning by, adverse effect of and underdosing of electrolytic, caloric and water-balance agents

● **T50.3X1** Poisoning by electrolytic, caloric and water-balance agents, accidental (unintentional)
> Poisoning by electrolytic, caloric and water-balance agents NOS

● **T50.3X2** Poisoning by electrolytic, caloric and water-balance agents, intentional self-harm A, S 🔖

● **T50.3X3** Poisoning by electrolytic, caloric and water-balance agents, assault

● **T50.3X4** Poisoning by electrolytic, caloric and water-balance agents, undetermined

● **T50.3X5** Adverse effect of electrolytic, caloric and water-balance agents
> **Coding Clinic: 2022, Q2, P11**

● **T50.3X6** Underdosing of electrolytic, caloric and water-balance agents

● **T50.4** Poisoning by, adverse effect of and underdosing of drugs affecting uric acid metabolism

● **T50.4X** Poisoning by, adverse effect of and underdosing of drugs affecting uric acid metabolism

● **T50.4X1** Poisoning by drugs affecting uric acid metabolism, accidental (unintentional)
> Poisoning by drugs affecting uric acid metabolism NOS

● **T50.4X2** Poisoning by drugs affecting uric acid metabolism, intentional self-harm A, S 🔖

● **T50.4X3** Poisoning by drugs affecting uric acid metabolism, assault

● **T50.4X4** Poisoning by drugs affecting uric acid metabolism, undetermined

● **T50.4X5** Adverse effect of drugs affecting uric acid metabolism

● **T50.4X6** Underdosing of drugs affecting uric acid metabolism

● **T50.5** Poisoning by, adverse effect of and underdosing of appetite depressants

● **T50.5X** Poisoning by, adverse effect of and underdosing of appetite depressants

● **T50.5X1** Poisoning by appetite depressants, accidental (unintentional)
> Poisoning by appetite depressants NOS

● **T50.5X2** Poisoning by appetite depressants, intentional self-harm A, S 🔖

● **T50.5X3** Poisoning by appetite depressants, assault

● **T50.5X4** Poisoning by appetite depressants, undetermined

● **T50.5X5** Adverse effect of appetite depressants

● **T50.5X6** Underdosing of appetite depressants

● **T50.6** Poisoning by, adverse effect of and underdosing of antidotes and chelating agents
> Poisoning by, adverse effect of and underdosing of alcohol deterrents

● **T50.6X** Poisoning by, adverse effect of and underdosing of antidotes and chelating agents

● **T50.6X1** Poisoning by antidotes and chelating agents, accidental (unintentional)
> Poisoning by antidotes and chelating agents NOS

● **T50.6X2** Poisoning by antidotes and chelating agents, intentional self-harm A, S 🔖

● **T50.6X3** Poisoning by antidotes and chelating agents, assault

● **T50.6X4** Poisoning by antidotes and chelating agents, undetermined

● **T50.6X5** Adverse effect of antidotes and chelating agents

● **T50.6X6** Underdosing of antidotes and chelating agents

● **T50.7** Poisoning by, adverse effect of and underdosing of analeptics and opioid receptor antagonists

● **T50.7X** Poisoning by, adverse effect of and underdosing of analeptics and opioid receptor antagonists

● **T50.7X1** Poisoning by analeptics and opioid receptor antagonists, accidental (unintentional)
> Poisoning by analeptics and opioid receptor antagonists NOS

● **T50.7X2** Poisoning by analeptics and opioid receptor antagonists, intentional self-harm A, S 🔖

● **T50.7X3** Poisoning by analeptics and opioid receptor antagonists, assault

● **T50.7X4** Poisoning by analeptics and opioid receptor antagonists, undetermined

● **T50.7X5** Adverse effect of analeptics and opioid receptor antagonists

● **T50.7X6** Underdosing of analeptics and opioid receptor antagonists

● **T50.8** Poisoning by, adverse effect of and underdosing of diagnostic agents

● **T50.8X** Poisoning by, adverse effect of and underdosing of diagnostic agents

● **T50.8X1** Poisoning by diagnostic agents, accidental (unintentional)
> Poisoning by diagnostic agents NOS

● **T50.8X2** Poisoning by diagnostic agents, intentional self-harm A, S 🔖

CHAPTER 19 (S00-T88)

CHAPTER 19 (S00-T88)

- **T50.8X3** Poisoning by diagnostic agents, assault
- **T50.8X4** Poisoning by diagnostic agents, undetermined
- **T50.8X5** Adverse effect of diagnostic agents
  Coding Clinic: 2021, Q3, P9-10
- **T50.8X6** Underdosing of diagnostic agents
- **T50.A** Poisoning by, adverse effect of and underdosing of bacterial vaccines
  - **T50.A1** Poisoning by, adverse effect of and underdosing of pertussis vaccine, including combinations with a pertussis component
    - **T50.A11** Poisoning by pertussis vaccine, including combinations with a pertussis component, accidental (unintentional)
    - **T50.A12** Poisoning by pertussis vaccine, including combinations with a pertussis component, intentional self-harm A, S 🐾
    - **T50.A13** Poisoning by pertussis vaccine, including combinations with a pertussis component, assault
    - **T50.A14** Poisoning by pertussis vaccine, including combinations with a pertussis component, undetermined
    - **T50.A15** Adverse effect of pertussis vaccine, including combinations with a pertussis component
    - **T50.A16** Underdosing of pertussis vaccine, including combinations with a pertussis component
  - **T50.A2** Poisoning by, adverse effect of and underdosing of mixed bacterial vaccines without a pertussis component
    - **T50.A21** Poisoning by mixed bacterial vaccines without a pertussis component, accidental (unintentional)
    - **T50.A22** Poisoning by mixed bacterial vaccines without a pertussis component, intentional self-harm A, S 🐾
    - **T50.A23** Poisoning by mixed bacterial vaccines without a pertussis component, assault
    - **T50.A24** Poisoning by mixed bacterial vaccines without a pertussis component, undetermined
    - **T50.A25** Adverse effect of mixed bacterial vaccines without a pertussis component
    - **T50.A26** Underdosing of mixed bacterial vaccines without a pertussis component
  - **T50.A9** Poisoning by, adverse effect of and underdosing of other bacterial vaccines
    - **T50.A91** Poisoning by other bacterial vaccines, accidental (unintentional)
    - **T50.A92** Poisoning by other bacterial vaccines, intentional self-harm A, S 🐾
    - **T50.A93** Poisoning by other bacterial vaccines, assault
    - **T50.A94** Poisoning by other bacterial vaccines, undetermined
    - **T50.A95** Adverse effect of other bacterial vaccines
    - **T50.A96** Underdosing of other bacterial vaccines

- **T50.B** Poisoning by, adverse effect of and underdosing of viral vaccines
  - **T50.B1** Poisoning by, adverse effect of and underdosing of smallpox vaccines
    - **T50.B11** Poisoning by smallpox vaccines, accidental (unintentional)
    - **T50.B12** Poisoning by smallpox vaccines, intentional self-harm A, S 🐾
    - **T50.B13** Poisoning by smallpox vaccines, assault
    - **T50.B14** Poisoning by smallpox vaccines, undetermined
    - **T50.B15** Adverse effect of smallpox vaccines
    - **T50.B16** Underdosing of smallpox vaccines
  - **T50.B9** Poisoning by, adverse effect of and underdosing of other viral vaccines
    - **T50.B91** Poisoning by other viral vaccines, accidental (unintentional)
    - **T50.B92** Poisoning by other viral vaccines, intentional self-harm A, S 🐾
    - **T50.B93** Poisoning by other viral vaccines, assault
    - **T50.B94** Poisoning by other viral vaccines, undetermined
    - **T50.B95** Adverse effect of other viral vaccines
      Coding Clinic: 2021, Q1, P43-44
    - **T50.B96** Underdosing of other viral vaccines
- **T50.Z** Poisoning by, adverse effect of and underdosing of other vaccines and biological substances
  - **T50.Z1** Poisoning by, adverse effect of and underdosing of immunoglobulin
    - **T50.Z11** Poisoning by immunoglobulin, accidental (unintentional)
    - **T50.Z12** Poisoning by immunoglobulin, intentional self-harm A, S 🐾
    - **T50.Z13** Poisoning by immunoglobulin, assault
    - **T50.Z14** Poisoning by immunoglobulin, undetermined
    - **T50.Z15** Adverse effect of immunoglobulin
    - **T50.Z16** Underdosing of immunoglobulin
  - **T50.Z9** Poisoning by, adverse effect of and underdosing of other vaccines and biological substances
    - **T50.Z91** Poisoning by other vaccines and biological substances, accidental (unintentional)
    - **T50.Z92** Poisoning by other vaccines and biological substances, intentional self-harm A, S 🐾
    - **T50.Z93** Poisoning by other vaccines and biological substances, assault
    - **T50.Z94** Poisoning by other vaccines and biological substances, undetermined
    - **T50.Z95** Adverse effect of other vaccines and biological substances
      Coding Clinic: 2020, Q1, P19
    - **T50.Z96** Underdosing of other vaccines and biological substances

● T50.9   Poisoning by, adverse effect of and underdosing of other and unspecified drugs, medicaments and biological substances

   ● T50.90   Poisoning by, adverse effect of and underdosing of unspecified drugs, medicaments and biological substances

      ● T50.901   Poisoning by unspecified drugs, medicaments and biological substances, accidental (unintentional)
                  Coding Clinic: 2015, Q1, P21

      ● T50.902   Poisoning by unspecified drugs, medicaments and biological substances, intentional self-harm A, S 🕮

      ● T50.903   Poisoning by unspecified drugs, medicaments and biological substances, assault

      ● T50.904   Poisoning by unspecified drugs, medicaments and biological substances, undetermined

      ● T50.905   Adverse effect of unspecified drugs, medicaments and biological substances

      ● T50.906   Underdosing of unspecified drugs, medicaments and biological substances

   ● T50.91   Poisoning by, adverse effect of and underdosing of multiple unspecified drugs, medicaments and biological substances
              Multiple drug ingestion NOS
              Code also any specific drugs, medicaments and biological substances

      ● T50.911   Poisoning by multiple unspecified drugs, medicaments and biological substances, accidental (unintentional)

      ● T50.912   Poisoning by multiple unspecified drugs, medicaments and biological substances, intentional self-harm

      ● T50.913   Poisoning by multiple unspecified drugs, medicaments and biological substances, assault

      ● T50.914   Poisoning by multiple unspecified drugs, medicaments and biological substances, undetermined

      ● T50.915   Adverse effect of multiple unspecified drugs, medicaments and biological substances

      ● T50.916   Underdosing of multiple unspecified drugs, medicaments and biological substances

   ● T50.99   Poisoning by, adverse effect of and underdosing of other drugs, medicaments and biological substances

      ● T50.991   Poisoning by other drugs, medicaments and biological substances, accidental (unintentional)

      ● T50.992   Poisoning by other drugs, medicaments and biological substances, intentional self-harm A, S 🕮

      ● T50.993   Poisoning by other drugs, medicaments and biological substances, assault

      ● T50.994   Poisoning by other drugs, medicaments and biological substances, undetermined

      ● T50.995   Adverse effect of other drugs, medicaments and biological substances

      ● T50.996   Underdosing of other drugs, medicaments and biological substances

TOXIC EFFECTS OF SUBSTANCES CHIEFLY NONMEDICINAL AS TO SOURCE (T51-T65)

Note: When no intent is indicated code to accidental. Undetermined intent is only for use when there is specific documentation in the record that the intent of the toxic effect cannot be determined.

Use additional code(s): for all associated manifestations of toxic effect, such as:
   respiratory conditions due to external agents (J60-J70)
   personal history of foreign body fully removed (Z87.821)
   to identify any retained foreign body, if applicable (Z18.-)

Excludes1   contact with and (suspected) exposure to toxic substances (Z77.-)

● T51   Toxic effect of alcohol

   The appropriate 7th character is to be added to each code from category T51

A	initial encounter
D	subsequent encounter
S	sequela

   ● T51.0   Toxic effect of ethanol
             Toxic effect of ethyl alcohol

      Excludes2   acute alcohol intoxication or 'hangover' effects (F10.129, F10.229, F10.929)
                      drunkenness (F10.129, F10.229, F10.929)
                      pathological alcohol intoxication (F10.129, F10.229, F10.929)

      ● T51.0X   Toxic effect of ethanol

         ● T51.0X1   Toxic effect of ethanol, accidental (unintentional)
                     Toxic effect of ethanol NOS

         ● T51.0X2   Toxic effect of ethanol, intentional self-harm A, S 🕮

         ● T51.0X3   Toxic effect of ethanol, assault

         ● T51.0X4   Toxic effect of ethanol, undetermined

   ● T51.1   Toxic effect of methanol
             Toxic effect of methyl alcohol

      ● T51.1X   Toxic effect of methanol

         ● T51.1X1   Toxic effect of methanol, accidental (unintentional)
                     Toxic effect of methanol NOS

         ● T51.1X2   Toxic effect of methanol, intentional self-harm A, S 🕮

         ● T51.1X3   Toxic effect of methanol, assault

         ● T51.1X4   Toxic effect of methanol, undetermined

   ● T51.2   Toxic effect of 2-Propanol
             Toxic effect of isopropyl alcohol

      ● T51.2X   Toxic effect of 2-Propanol

         ● T51.2X1   Toxic effect of 2-Propanol, accidental (unintentional)
                     Toxic effect of 2-Propanol NOS

         ● T51.2X2   Toxic effect of 2-Propanol, intentional self-harm A, S 🕮

         ● T51.2X3   Toxic effect of 2-Propanol, assault

         ● T51.2X4   Toxic effect of 2-Propanol, undetermined

   ● T51.3   Toxic effect of fusel oil
             Toxic effect of amyl alcohol
             Toxic effect of butyl [1-butanol] alcohol
             Toxic effect of propyl [1-propanol] alcohol

      ● T51.3X   Toxic effect of fusel oil

         ● T51.3X1   Toxic effect of fusel oil, accidental (unintentional)
                     Toxic effect of fusel oil NOS

         ● T51.3X2   Toxic effect of fusel oil, intentional self-harm A, S 🕮

         ● T51.3X3   Toxic effect of fusel oil, assault

         ● T51.3X4   Toxic effect of fusel oil, undetermined

CHAPTER 19 (S00-T88)

CHAPTER 19 (S00–T88)

● T51.8   Toxic effect of other alcohols
  ● T51.8X   Toxic effect of other alcohols
    ● T51.8X1   Toxic effect of other alcohols,
      accidental (unintentional)
        Toxic effect of other alcohols NOS
    ● T51.8X2   Toxic effect of other alcohols,
      intentional self-harm A, S 🐾
    ● T51.8X3   Toxic effect of other alcohols, assault
    ● T51.8X4   Toxic effect of other alcohols,
      undetermined

● T51.9   Toxic effect of unspecified alcohol
  X ● T51.91   Toxic effect of unspecified alcohol, accidental
    (unintentional)
  X ● T51.92   Toxic effect of unspecified alcohol, intentional
    self-harm A, S 🐾
  X ● T51.93   Toxic effect of unspecified alcohol, assault
  X ● T51.94   Toxic effect of unspecified alcohol,
    undetermined

● T52   Toxic effect of organic solvents

  Excludes1   halogen derivatives of aliphatic and aromatic
    hydrocarbons (T53.-)

  The appropriate 7th character is to be added to each code from
  category T52

A	initial encounter
D	subsequent encounter
S	sequela

  ● T52.0   Toxic effects of petroleum products
    Toxic effects of gasoline [petrol]
    Toxic effects of kerosene [paraffin oil]
    Toxic effects of paraffin wax
    Toxic effects of ether petroleum
    Toxic effects of naphtha petroleum
    Toxic effects of spirit petroleum
    ● T52.0X   Toxic effects of petroleum products
      ● T52.0X1   Toxic effect of petroleum products,
        accidental (unintentional)
          Toxic effects of petroleum products
          NOS
      ● T52.0X2   Toxic effect of petroleum products,
        intentional self-harm A, S 🐾
      ● T52.0X3   Toxic effect of petroleum products,
        assault
      ● T52.0X4   Toxic effect of petroleum products,
        undetermined

  ● T52.1   Toxic effects of benzene

    Excludes1   homologues of benzene (T52.2)
      nitroderivatives and aminoderivatives of
      benzene and its homologues (T65.3)

    ● T52.1X   Toxic effects of benzene
      ● T52.1X1   Toxic effect of benzene, accidental
        (unintentional)
          Toxic effects of benzene NOS
      ● T52.1X2   Toxic effect of benzene, intentional
        self-harm A, S 🐾
      ● T52.1X3   Toxic effect of benzene, assault
      ● T52.1X4   Toxic effect of benzene, undetermined

  ● T52.2   Toxic effects of homologues of benzene
    Toxic effects of toluene [methylbenzene]
    Toxic effects of xylene [dimethylbenzene]
    ● T52.2X   Toxic effects of homologues of benzene
      ● T52.2X1   Toxic effect of homologues of
        benzene, accidental (unintentional)
          Toxic effects of homologues of
          benzene NOS
      ● T52.2X2   Toxic effect of homologues of
        benzene, intentional self-harm A, S 🐾

● T52.2X3   Toxic effect of homologues of
  benzene, assault
● T52.2X4   Toxic effect of homologues of
  benzene, undetermined

● T52.3   Toxic effects of glycols
  ● T52.3X   Toxic effects of glycols
    ● T52.3X1   Toxic effect of glycols, accidental
      (unintentional)
        Toxic effects of glycols NOS
    ● T52.3X2   Toxic effect of glycols, intentional
      self-harm A, S 🐾
    ● T52.3X3   Toxic effect of glycols, assault
    ● T52.3X4   Toxic effect of glycols, undetermined

● T52.4   Toxic effects of ketones
  ● T52.4X   Toxic effects of ketones
    ● T52.4X1   Toxic effect of ketones, accidental
      (unintentional)
        Toxic effects of ketones NOS
    ● T52.4X2   Toxic effect of ketones, intentional
      self-harm A, S 🐾
    ● T52.4X3   Toxic effect of ketones, assault
    ● T52.4X4   Toxic effect of ketones, undetermined

● T52.8   Toxic effects of other organic solvents
  ● T52.8X   Toxic effects of other organic solvents
    ● T52.8X1   Toxic effect of other organic solvents,
      accidental (unintentional)
        Toxic effects of other organic
        solvents NOS
    ● T52.8X2   Toxic effect of other organic solvents,
      intentional self-harm A, S 🐾
    ● T52.8X3   Toxic effect of other organic solvents,
      assault
    ● T52.8X4   Toxic effect of other organic solvents,
      undetermined

● T52.9   Toxic effects of unspecified organic solvent
  X ● T52.91   Toxic effect of unspecified organic solvent,
    accidental (unintentional)
  X ● T52.92   Toxic effect of unspecified organic solvent,
    intentional self-harm A, S 🐾
  X ● T52.93   Toxic effect of unspecified organic solvent,
    assault
  X ● T52.94   Toxic effect of unspecified organic solvent,
    undetermined

● T53   Toxic effect of halogen derivatives of aliphatic and aromatic
  hydrocarbons

  The appropriate 7th character is to be added to each code from
  category T53

A	initial encounter
D	subsequent encounter
S	sequela

  ● T53.0   Toxic effects of carbon tetrachloride
    Toxic effects of tetrachloromethane
    ● T53.0X   Toxic effects of carbon tetrachloride
      ● T53.0X1   Toxic effect of carbon tetrachloride,
        accidental (unintentional)
          Toxic effects of carbon tetrachloride
          NOS
      ● T53.0X2   Toxic effect of carbon tetrachloride,
        intentional self-harm A, S 🐾
      ● T53.0X3   Toxic effect of carbon tetrachloride,
        assault
      ● T53.0X4   Toxic effect of carbon tetrachloride,
        undetermined

▶ New   ⟹ Revised   ~~deleted~~ Deleted | Excludes 1 | | Excludes 2 | | Includes | | Use additional | | Code first | | Code also | | Key words |

OGCR Official Guidelines   X Assign placeholder X   ● Use Additional Character(s)   ⟩ Manifestation Code   🐾 Hierarchical Condition Category   **Coding Clinic**

● **T53.1 Toxic effects of chloroform**
Toxic effects of trichloromethane

   ● **T53.1X Toxic effects of chloroform**

     ● **T53.1X1 Toxic effect of chloroform, accidental (unintentional)**
Toxic effects of chloroform NOS

     ● **T53.1X2 Toxic effect of chloroform, intentional self-harm A, S** 🔗

     ● **T53.1X3 Toxic effect of chloroform, assault**

     ● **T53.1X4 Toxic effect of chloroform, undetermined**

● **T53.2 Toxic effects of trichloroethylene**
Toxic effects of trichloroethene

   ● **T53.2X Toxic effects of trichloroethylene**

     ● **T53.2X1 Toxic effect of trichloroethylene, accidental (unintentional)**
Toxic effects of trichloroethylene NOS

     ● **T53.2X2 Toxic effect of trichloroethylene, intentional self-harm A, S** 🔗

     ● **T53.2X3 Toxic effect of trichloroethylene, assault**

     ● **T53.2X4 Toxic effect of trichloroethylene, undetermined**

● **T53.3 Toxic effects of tetrachloroethylene**
Toxic effects of perchloroethylene
Toxic effect of tetrachloroethene

   ● **T53.3X Toxic effects of tetrachloroethylene**

     ● **T53.3X1 Toxic effect of tetrachloroethylene, accidental (unintentional)**
Toxic effects of tetrachloroethylene NOS

     ● **T53.3X2 Toxic effect of tetrachloroethylene, intentional self-harm A, S** 🔗

     ● **T53.3X3 Toxic effect of tetrachloroethylene, assault**

     ● **T53.3X4 Toxic effect of tetrachloroethylene, undetermined**

● **T53.4 Toxic effects of dichloromethane**
Toxic effects of methylene chloride

   ● **T53.4X Toxic effects of dichloromethane**

     ● **T53.4X1 Toxic effect of dichloromethane, accidental (unintentional)**
Toxic effects of dichloromethane NOS

     ● **T53.4X2 Toxic effect of dichloromethane, intentional self-harm A, S** 🔗

     ● **T53.4X3 Toxic effect of dichloromethane, assault**

     ● **T53.4X4 Toxic effect of dichloromethane, undetermined**

● **T53.5 Toxic effects of chlorofluorocarbons**

   ● **T53.5X Toxic effects of chlorofluorocarbons**

     ● **T53.5X1 Toxic effect of chlorofluorocarbons, accidental (unintentional)**
Toxic effects of chlorofluorocarbons NOS

     ● **T53.5X2 Toxic effect of chlorofluorocarbons, intentional self-harm A, S** 🔗

     ● **T53.5X3 Toxic effect of chlorofluorocarbons, assault**

     ● **T53.5X4 Toxic effect of chlorofluorocarbons, undetermined**

● **T53.6 Toxic effects of other halogen derivatives of aliphatic hydrocarbons**

   ● **T53.6X Toxic effects of other halogen derivatives of aliphatic hydrocarbons**

     ● **T53.6X1 Toxic effect of other halogen derivatives of aliphatic hydrocarbons, accidental (unintentional)**
Toxic effects of other halogen derivatives of aliphatic hydrocarbons NOS

     ● **T53.6X2 Toxic effect of other halogen derivatives of aliphatic hydrocarbons, intentional self-harm A, S** 🔗

     ● **T53.6X3 Toxic effect of other halogen derivatives of aliphatic hydrocarbons, assault**

     ● **T53.6X4 Toxic effect of other halogen derivatives of aliphatic hydrocarbons, undetermined**

● **T53.7 Toxic effects of other halogen derivatives of aromatic hydrocarbons**

   ● **T53.7X Toxic effects of other halogen derivatives of aromatic hydrocarbons**

     ● **T53.7X1 Toxic effect of other halogen derivatives of aromatic hydrocarbons, accidental (unintentional)**
Toxic effects of other halogen derivatives of aromatic hydrocarbons NOS

     ● **T53.7X2 Toxic effect of other halogen derivatives of aromatic hydrocarbons, intentional self-harm A, S** 🔗

     ● **T53.7X3 Toxic effect of other halogen derivatives of aromatic hydrocarbons, assault**

     ● **T53.7X4 Toxic effect of other halogen derivatives of aromatic hydrocarbons, undetermined**

● **T53.9 Toxic effects of unspecified halogen derivatives of aliphatic and aromatic hydrocarbons**

   X ● **T53.91 Toxic effect of unspecified halogen derivatives of aliphatic and aromatic hydrocarbons, accidental (unintentional)**

   X ● **T53.92 Toxic effect of unspecified halogen derivatives of aliphatic and aromatic hydrocarbons, intentional self-harm A, S** 🔗

   X ● **T53.93 Toxic effect of unspecified halogen derivatives of aliphatic and aromatic hydrocarbons, assault**

   X ● **T53.94 Toxic effect of unspecified halogen derivatives of aliphatic and aromatic hydrocarbons, undetermined**

● **T54 Toxic effect of corrosive substances**
The appropriate 7th character is to be added to each code from category T54.

> | | |
> |---|---|
> | A | initial encounter |
> | D | subsequent encounter |
> | S | sequela |

● **T54.0 Toxic effects of phenol and phenol homologues**

   ● **T54.0X Toxic effects of phenol and phenol homologues**

     ● **T54.0X1 Toxic effect of phenol and phenol homologues, accidental (unintentional)**
Toxic effects of phenol and phenol homologues NOS

     ● **T54.0X2 Toxic effect of phenol and phenol homologues, intentional self-harm A, S** 🔗

     ● **T54.0X3 Toxic effect of phenol and phenol homologues, assault**

     ● **T54.0X4 Toxic effect of phenol and phenol homologues, undetermined**

CHAPTER 19 (S00-T88)

CHAPTER 19 (S00-T88)

● **T54.1** Toxic effects of other corrosive organic compounds
  ● **T54.1X** Toxic effects of other corrosive organic compounds
    ● **T54.1X1** Toxic effect of other corrosive organic compounds, accidental (unintentional)
      Toxic effects of other corrosive organic compounds NOS
    ● **T54.1X2** Toxic effect of other corrosive organic compounds, intentional self-harm A, S 🐾
    ● **T54.1X3** Toxic effect of other corrosive organic compounds, assault
    ● **T54.1X4** Toxic effect of other corrosive organic compounds, undetermined
● **T54.2** Toxic effects of corrosive acids and acid-like substances
    Toxic effects of hydrochloric acid
    Toxic effects of sulfuric acid
  ● **T54.2X** Toxic effects of corrosive acids and acid-like substances
    ● **T54.2X1** Toxic effect of corrosive acids and acid-like substances, accidental (unintentional)
      Toxic effects of corrosive acids and acid-like substances NOS
    ● **T54.2X2** Toxic effect of corrosive acids and acid-like substances, intentional self-harm A, S 🐾
    ● **T54.2X3** Toxic effect of corrosive acids and acid-like substances, assault
    ● **T54.2X4** Toxic effect of corrosive acids and acid-like substances, undetermined
● **T54.3** Toxic effects of corrosive alkalis and alkali-like substances
    Toxic effects of potassium hydroxide
    Toxic effects of sodium hydroxide
  ● **T54.3X** Toxic effects of corrosive alkalis and alkali-like substances
    ● **T54.3X1** Toxic effect of corrosive alkalis and alkali-like substances, accidental (unintentional)
      Toxic effects of corrosive alkalis and alkali-like substances NOS
    ● **T54.3X2** Toxic effect of corrosive alkalis and alkali-like substances, intentional self-harm A, S 🐾
    ● **T54.3X3** Toxic effect of corrosive alkalis and alkali-like substances, assault
    ● **T54.3X4** Toxic effect of corrosive alkalis and alkali-like substances, undetermined
● **T54.9** Toxic effects of unspecified corrosive substance
  X● **T54.91** Toxic effect of unspecified corrosive substance, accidental (unintentional)
  X● **T54.92** Toxic effect of unspecified corrosive substance, intentional self-harm A, S 🐾
  X● **T54.93** Toxic effect of unspecified corrosive substance, assault
  X● **T54.94** Toxic effect of unspecified corrosive substance, undetermined

● **T55** Toxic effect of soaps and detergents
    The appropriate 7th character is to be added to each code from category T55

A	initial encounter
D	subsequent encounter
S	sequela

● **T55.0** Toxic effect of soaps
  ● **T55.0X** Toxic effect of soaps
    ● **T55.0X1** Toxic effect of soaps, accidental (unintentional)
      Toxic effect of soaps NOS

● **T55.0X2** Toxic effect of soaps, intentional self-harm A, S 🐾
● **T55.0X3** Toxic effect of soaps, assault
● **T55.0X4** Toxic effect of soaps, undetermined
● **T55.1** Toxic effect of detergents
  ● **T55.1X** Toxic effect of detergents
    ● **T55.1X1** Toxic effect of detergents, accidental (unintentional)
      Toxic effect of detergents NOS
    ● **T55.1X2** Toxic effect of detergents, intentional self-harm A, S 🐾
    ● **T55.1X3** Toxic effect of detergents, assault
    ● **T55.1X4** Toxic effect of detergents, undetermined
● **T56** Toxic effect of metals

  Includes   toxic effects of fumes and vapors of metals
           toxic effects of metals from all sources, except medicinal substances

  Use additional code to identify any retained metal foreign body, if applicable (Z18.0-, T18.1-)

  Excludes1   arsenic and its compounds (T57.0)
           manganese and its compounds (T57.2)

  The appropriate 7th character is to be added to each code from category T56

A	initial encounter
D	subsequent encounter
S	sequela

● **T56.0** Toxic effects of lead and its compounds
  ● **T56.0X** Toxic effects of lead and its compounds
    ● **T56.0X1** Toxic effect of lead and its compounds, accidental (unintentional)
      Toxic effects of lead and its compounds NOS
    ● **T56.0X2** Toxic effect of lead and its compounds, intentional self-harm A, S 🐾
    ● **T56.0X3** Toxic effect of lead and its compounds, assault
    ● **T56.0X4** Toxic effect of lead and its compounds, undetermined
● **T56.1** Toxic effects of mercury and its compounds
  ● **T56.1X** Toxic effects of mercury and its compounds
    ● **T56.1X1** Toxic effect of mercury and its compounds, accidental (unintentional)
      Toxic effects of mercury and its compounds NOS
    ● **T56.1X2** Toxic effect of mercury and its compounds, intentional self-harm A, S 🐾
    ● **T56.1X3** Toxic effect of mercury and its compounds, assault
    ● **T56.1X4** Toxic effect of mercury and its compounds, undetermined
● **T56.2** Toxic effects of chromium and its compounds
  ● **T56.2X** Toxic effects of chromium and its compounds
    ● **T56.2X1** Toxic effect of chromium and its compounds, accidental (unintentional)
      Toxic effects of chromium and its compounds NOS
    ● **T56.2X2** Toxic effect of chromium and its compounds, intentional self-harm A, S 🐾
    ● **T56.2X3** Toxic effect of chromium and its compounds, assault
    ● **T56.2X4** Toxic effect of chromium and its compounds, undetermined

▶ New   ⇒ Revised   ~~deleted~~ Deleted   Excludes 1   Excludes 2   Includes   Use additional   Code first   Code also   Key words
OGCR Official Guidelines   X Assign placeholder X   ● Use Additional Character(s)   ▶ Manifestation Code   🐾 Hierarchical Condition Category   **Coding Clinic**

● **T56.3**   Toxic effects of cadmium and its compounds
   ● **T56.3X**   Toxic effects of cadmium and its compounds
     ● **T56.3X1**   Toxic effect of cadmium and its compounds, **accidental (unintentional)**
         Toxic effects of cadmium and its compounds NOS
     ● **T56.3X2**   Toxic effect of cadmium and its compounds, **intentional self-harm** A, S 🐾
     ● **T56.3X3**   Toxic effect of cadmium and its compounds, **assault**
     ● **T56.3X4**   Toxic effect of cadmium and its compounds, **undetermined**

● **T56.4**   Toxic effects of copper and its compounds
   ● **T56.4X**   Toxic effects of copper and its compounds
     ● **T56.4X1**   Toxic effect of copper and its compounds, **accidental (unintentional)**
         Toxic effects of copper and its compounds NOS
     ● **T56.4X2**   Toxic effect of copper and its compounds, **intentional self-harm** A, S 🐾
     ● **T56.4X3**   Toxic effect of copper and its compounds, **assault**
     ● **T56.4X4**   Toxic effect of copper and its compounds, **undetermined**

● **T56.5**   Toxic effects of zinc and its compounds
   ● **T56.5X**   Toxic effects of zinc and its compounds
     ● **T56.5X1**   Toxic effect of zinc and its compounds, **accidental (unintentional)**
         Toxic effects of zinc and its compounds NOS
     ● **T56.5X2**   Toxic effect of zinc and its compounds, **intentional self-harm** A, S 🐾
     ● **T56.5X3**   Toxic effect of zinc and its compounds, **assault**
     ● **T56.5X4**   Toxic effect of zinc and its compounds, **undetermined**

● **T56.6**   Toxic effects of tin and its compounds
   ● **T56.6X**   Toxic effects of tin and its compounds
     ● **T56.6X1**   Toxic effect of tin and its compounds, **accidental (unintentional)**
         Toxic effects of tin and its compounds NOS
     ● **T56.6X2**   Toxic effect of tin and its compounds, **intentional self-harm** A, S 🐾
     ● **T56.6X3**   Toxic effect of tin and its compounds, **assault**
     ● **T56.6X4**   Toxic effect of tin and its compounds, **undetermined**

● **T56.7**   Toxic effects of beryllium and its compounds
   ● **T56.7X**   Toxic effects of beryllium and its compounds
     ● **T56.7X1**   Toxic effect of beryllium and its compounds, **accidental (unintentional)**
         Toxic effects of beryllium and its compounds NOS
     ● **T56.7X2**   Toxic effect of beryllium and its compounds, **intentional self-harm** A, S 🐾
     ● **T56.7X3**   Toxic effect of beryllium and its compounds, **assault**
     ● **T56.7X4**   Toxic effect of beryllium and its compounds, **undetermined**

● **T56.8**   Toxic effects of other metals
   ● **T56.81**   Toxic effect of thallium
     ● **T56.811**   Toxic effect of thallium, **accidental (unintentional)**
         Toxic effect of thallium NOS
     ● **T56.812**   Toxic effect of thallium, **intentional self-harm** A, S 🐾
     ● **T56.813**   Toxic effect of thallium, **assault**
     ● **T56.814**   Toxic effect of thallium, **undetermined**
   ● **T56.89**   Toxic effects of other metals
     ● **T56.891**   Toxic effect of other metals, **accidental (unintentional)**
         Toxic effects of other metals NOS
     ● **T56.892**   Toxic effect of other metals, **intentional self-harm** A, S 🐾
     ● **T56.893**   Toxic effect of other metals, **assault**
     ● **T56.894**   Toxic effect of other metals, **undetermined**

● **T56.9**   Toxic effects of unspecified metal
   X ● **T56.91**   Toxic effect of unspecified metal, **accidental (unintentional)**
   X ● **T56.92**   Toxic effect of unspecified metal, **intentional self-harm** A, S 🐾
   X ● **T56.93**   Toxic effect of unspecified metal, **assault**
   X ● **T56.94**   Toxic effect of unspecified metal, **undetermined**

● **T57**   Toxic effect of other inorganic substances
   The appropriate 7th character is to be added to each code from category T57

> | | |
> |---|---|
> | A | initial encounter |
> | D | subsequent encounter |
> | S | sequela |

● **T57.0**   Toxic effect of arsenic and its compounds
   ● **T57.0X**   Toxic effect of arsenic and its compounds
     ● **T57.0X1**   Toxic effect of arsenic and its compounds, **accidental (unintentional)**
         Toxic effect of arsenic and its compounds NOS
     ● **T57.0X2**   Toxic effect of arsenic and its compounds, **intentional self-harm** A, S 🐾
     ● **T57.0X3**   Toxic effect of arsenic and its compounds, **assault**
     ● **T57.0X4**   Toxic effect of arsenic and its compounds, **undetermined**

● **T57.1**   Toxic effect of phosphorus and its compounds
   Excludes 1   organophosphate insecticides (T60.0)
   ● **T57.1X**   Toxic effect of phosphorus and its compounds
     ● **T57.1X1**   Toxic effect of phosphorus and its compounds, **accidental (unintentional)**
         Toxic effect of phosphorus and its compounds NOS
     ● **T57.1X2**   Toxic effect of phosphorus and its compounds, **intentional self-harm** A, S 🐾
     ● **T57.1X3**   Toxic effect of phosphorus and its compounds, **assault**
     ● **T57.1X4**   Toxic effect of phosphorus and its compounds, **undetermined**

● **T57.2**   Toxic effect of manganese and its compounds
   ● **T57.2X**   Toxic effect of manganese and its compounds
     ● **T57.2X1**   Toxic effect of manganese and its compounds, **accidental (unintentional)**
         Toxic effect of manganese and its compounds NOS

CHAPTER 19 (S00-T88)

CHAPTER 19 (S00-T88)

● T57.2X2   Toxic effect of manganese and its compounds, intentional self-harm A, S 🦠

● T57.2X3   Toxic effect of manganese and its compounds, assault

● T57.2X4   Toxic effect of manganese and its compounds, undetermined

● T57.3   Toxic effect of hydrogen cyanide

  ● T57.3X   Toxic effect of hydrogen cyanide

    ● T57.3X1   Toxic effect of hydrogen cyanide, accidental (unintentional)

        Toxic effect of hydrogen cyanide NOS

    ● T57.3X2   Toxic effect of hydrogen cyanide, intentional self-harm A, S 🦠

    ● T57.3X3   Toxic effect of hydrogen cyanide, assault

    ● T57.3X4   Toxic effect of hydrogen cyanide, undetermined

● T57.8   Toxic effect of other specified inorganic substances

  ● T57.8X   Toxic effect of other specified inorganic substances

    ● T57.8X1   Toxic effect of other specified inorganic substances, accidental (unintentional)

        Toxic effect of other specified inorganic substances NOS

    ● T57.8X2   Toxic effect of other specified inorganic substances, intentional self-harm A, S 🦠

    ● T57.8X3   Toxic effect of other specified inorganic substances, assault

    ● T57.8X4   Toxic effect of other specified inorganic substances, undetermined

● T57.9   Toxic effect of unspecified inorganic substance

  X ● T57.91   Toxic effect of unspecified inorganic substance, accidental (unintentional)

  X ● T57.92   Toxic effect of unspecified inorganic substance, intentional self-harm A, S 🦠

  X ● T57.93   Toxic effect of unspecified inorganic substance, assault

  X ● T57.94   Toxic effect of unspecified inorganic substance, undetermined

● T58   Toxic effect of carbon monoxide

Includes	asphyxiation from carbon monoxide
	toxic effect of carbon monoxide from all sources

The appropriate 7th character is to be added to each code from category T58

A	initial encounter
D	subsequent encounter
S	sequela

● T58.0   Toxic effect of carbon monoxide from motor vehicle exhaust

    Toxic effect of exhaust gas from gas engine

    Toxic effect of exhaust gas from motor pump

  X ● T58.01   Toxic effect of carbon monoxide from motor vehicle exhaust, accidental (unintentional)

  X ● T58.02   Toxic effect of carbon monoxide from motor vehicle exhaust, intentional self-harm A, S 🦠

  X ● T58.03   Toxic effect of carbon monoxide from motor vehicle exhaust, assault

  X ● T58.04   Toxic effect of carbon monoxide from motor vehicle exhaust, undetermined

● T58.1   Toxic effect of carbon monoxide from utility gas

    Toxic effect of acetylene

    Toxic effect of gas NOS used for lighting, heating, cooking

    Toxic effect of water gas

  X ● T58.11   Toxic effect of carbon monoxide from utility gas, accidental (unintentional)

  X ● T58.12   Toxic effect of carbon monoxide from utility gas, intentional self-harm A, S 🦠

  X ● T58.13   Toxic effect of carbon monoxide from utility gas, assault

  X ● T58.14   Toxic effect of carbon monoxide from utility gas, undetermined

● T58.2   Toxic effect of carbon monoxide from incomplete combustion of other domestic fuels

    Toxic effect of carbon monoxide from incomplete combustion of coal, coke, kerosene, wood

  ● T58.2X   Toxic effect of carbon monoxide from incomplete combustion of other domestic fuels

    ● T58.2X1   Toxic effect of carbon monoxide from incomplete combustion of other domestic fuels, accidental (unintentional)

    ● T58.2X2   Toxic effect of carbon monoxide from incomplete combustion of other domestic fuels, intentional self-harm A, S 🦠

    ● T58.2X3   Toxic effect of carbon monoxide from incomplete combustion of other domestic fuels, assault

    ● T58.2X4   Toxic effect of carbon monoxide from incomplete combustion of other domestic fuels, undetermined

● T58.8   Toxic effect of carbon monoxide from other source

    Toxic effect of carbon monoxide from blast furnace gas

    Toxic effect of carbon monoxide from fuels in industrial use

    Toxic effect of carbon monoxide from kiln vapor

  ● T58.8X   Toxic effect of carbon monoxide from other source

    ● T58.8X1   Toxic effect of carbon monoxide from other source, accidental (unintentional)

    ● T58.8X2   Toxic effect of carbon monoxide from other source, intentional self-harm A, S 🦠

    ● T58.8X3   Toxic effect of carbon monoxide from other source, assault

    ● T58.8X4   Toxic effect of carbon monoxide from other source, undetermined

● T58.9   Toxic effect of carbon monoxide from unspecified source

  X ● T58.91   Toxic effect of carbon monoxide from unspecified source, accidental (unintentional)

  X ● T58.92   Toxic effect of carbon monoxide from unspecified source, intentional self-harm A, S 🦠

  X ● T58.93   Toxic effect of carbon monoxide from unspecified source, assault

  X ● T58.94   Toxic effect of carbon monoxide from unspecified source, undetermined

▶ New   ⇒ Revised   ~~deleted~~ Deleted   Excludes 1   Excludes 2   Includes   Use additional   Code first   Code also   Key words

OGCR Official Guidelines   X Assign placeholder X   ● Use Additional Character(s)   ▶ Manifestation Code   🦠 Hierarchical Condition Category   Coding Clinic

● **T59**   **Toxic effect of other gases, fumes and vapors**

     Includes   aerosol propellants

     Excludes1   chlorofluorocarbons (T53.5)

     The appropriate 7th character is to be added to each code from category T59

       A   initial encounter
       D   subsequent encounter
       S   sequela

● **T59.0**   **Toxic effect of nitrogen oxides**

   ● **T59.0X**   Toxic effect of nitrogen oxides

     ● **T59.0X1**   Toxic effect of nitrogen oxides, accidental (unintentional)
            Toxic effect of nitrogen oxides NOS

     ● **T59.0X2**   Toxic effect of nitrogen oxides, intentional self-harm A, S 🔒

     ● **T59.0X3**   Toxic effect of nitrogen oxides, assault

     ● **T59.0X4**   Toxic effect of nitrogen oxides, undetermined

● **T59.1**   **Toxic effect of sulfur dioxide**

   ● **T59.1X**   Toxic effect of sulfur dioxide

     ● **T59.1X1**   Toxic effect of sulfur dioxide, accidental (unintentional)
            Toxic effect of sulfur dioxide NOS

     ● **T59.1X2**   Toxic effect of sulfur dioxide, intentional self-harm A, S 🔒

     ● **T59.1X3**   Toxic effect of sulfur dioxide, assault

     ● **T59.1X4**   Toxic effect of sulfur dioxide, undetermined

● **T59.2**   **Toxic effect of formaldehyde**

   ● **T59.2X**   Toxic effect of formaldehyde

     ● **T59.2X1**   Toxic effect of formaldehyde, accidental (unintentional)
            Toxic effect of formaldehyde NOS

     ● **T59.2X2**   Toxic effect of formaldehyde, intentional self-harm A, S 🔒

     ● **T59.2X3**   Toxic effect of formaldehyde, assault

     ● **T59.2X4**   Toxic effect of formaldehyde, undetermined

● **T59.3**   **Toxic effect of lacrimogenic gas**
     Toxic effect of tear gas

   ● **T59.3X**   Toxic effect of lacrimogenic gas

     ● **T59.3X1**   Toxic effect of lacrimogenic gas, accidental (unintentional)
            Toxic effect of lacrimogenic gas NOS

     ● **T59.3X2**   Toxic effect of lacrimogenic gas, intentional self-harm A, S 🔒

     ● **T59.3X3**   Toxic effect of lacrimogenic gas, assault

     ● **T59.3X4**   Toxic effect of lacrimogenic gas, undetermined

● **T59.4**   **Toxic effect of chlorine gas**

   ● **T59.4X**   Toxic effect of chlorine gas

     ● **T59.4X1**   Toxic effect of chlorine gas, accidental (unintentional)
            Toxic effect of chlorine gas NOS

     ● **T59.4X2**   Toxic effect of chlorine gas, intentional self-harm A, S 🔒

     ● **T59.4X3**   Toxic effect of chlorine gas, assault

     ● **T59.4X4**   Toxic effect of chlorine gas, undetermined

● **T59.5**   **Toxic effect of fluorine gas and hydrogen fluoride**

   ● **T59.5X**   Toxic effect of fluorine gas and hydrogen fluoride

     ● **T59.5X1**   Toxic effect of fluorine gas and hydrogen fluoride, accidental (unintentional)
            Toxic effect of fluorine gas and hydrogen fluoride NOS

     ● **T59.5X2**   Toxic effect of fluorine gas and hydrogen fluoride, intentional self-harm A, S 🔒

     ● **T59.5X3**   Toxic effect of fluorine gas and hydrogen fluoride, assault

     ● **T59.5X4**   Toxic effect of fluorine gas and hydrogen fluoride, undetermined

● **T59.6**   **Toxic effect of hydrogen sulfide**

   ● **T59.6X**   Toxic effect of hydrogen sulfide

     ● **T59.6X1**   Toxic effect of hydrogen sulfide, accidental (unintentional)
            Toxic effect of hydrogen sulfide NOS

     ● **T59.6X2**   Toxic effect of hydrogen sulfide, intentional self-harm A, S 🔒

     ● **T59.6X3**   Toxic effect of hydrogen sulfide, assault

     ● **T59.6X4**   Toxic effect of hydrogen sulfide, undetermined

● **T59.7**   **Toxic effect of carbon dioxide**

   ● **T59.7X**   Toxic effect of carbon dioxide

     ● **T59.7X1**   Toxic effect of carbon dioxide, accidental (unintentional)
            Toxic effect of carbon dioxide NOS

     ● **T59.7X2**   Toxic effect of carbon dioxide, intentional self-harm A, S 🔒

     ● **T59.7X3**   Toxic effect of carbon dioxide, assault

     ● **T59.7X4**   Toxic effect of carbon dioxide, undetermined

● **T59.8**   **Toxic effect of other specified gases, fumes and vapors**

   ● **T59.81**   Toxic effect of smoke
      Smoke inhalation

      Excludes2   toxic effect of cigarette (tobacco) smoke (T65.22-)

     ● **T59.811**   Toxic effect of smoke, accidental (unintentional)
            Toxic effect of smoke NOS

     ● **T59.812**   Toxic effect of smoke, intentional self-harm A, S 🔒

     ● **T59.813**   Toxic effect of smoke, assault

     ● **T59.814**   Toxic effect of smoke, undetermined

   ● **T59.89**   Toxic effect of other specified gases, fumes and vapors

     ● **T59.891**   Toxic effect of other specified gases, fumes and vapors, accidental (unintentional)

     ● **T59.892**   Toxic effect of other specified gases, fumes and vapors, intentional self-harm A, S 🔒

     ● **T59.893**   Toxic effect of other specified gases, fumes and vapors, assault

     ● **T59.894**   Toxic effect of other specified gases, fumes and vapors, undetermined

CHAPTER 19 (S00-T88)

- T59.9   Toxic effect of unspecified gases, fumes and vapors
  - X ● T59.91   Toxic effect of unspecified gases, fumes and vapors, accidental (unintentional)
  - X ● T59.92   Toxic effect of unspecified gases, fumes and vapors, intentional self-harm A, S 🐾
  - X ● T59.93   Toxic effect of unspecified gases, fumes and vapors, assault
  - X ● T59.94   Toxic effect of unspecified gases, fumes and vapors, undetermined
- T60   Toxic effect of pesticides

  Includes   toxic effect of wood preservatives

  The appropriate 7th character is to be added to each code from category T60

A	initial encounter
D	subsequent encounter
S	sequela

  - T60.0   Toxic effect of organophosphate and carbamate insecticides
    - T60.0X   Toxic effect of organophosphate and carbamate insecticides
      - ● T60.0X1   Toxic effect of organophosphate and carbamate insecticides, accidental (unintentional)
        Toxic effect of organophosphate and carbamate insecticides NOS
      - ● T60.0X2   Toxic effect of organophosphate and carbamate insecticides, intentional self-harm A, S 🐾
      - ● T60.0X3   Toxic effect of organophosphate and carbamate insecticides, assault
      - ● T60.0X4   Toxic effect of organophosphate and carbamate insecticides, undetermined
  - T60.1   Toxic effect of halogenated insecticides

    Excludes1   chlorinated hydrocarbon (T53.-)
    - T60.1X   Toxic effect of halogenated insecticides
      - ● T60.1X1   Toxic effect of halogenated insecticides, accidental (unintentional)
        Toxic effect of halogenated insecticides NOS
      - ● T60.1X2   Toxic effect of halogenated insecticides, intentional self-harm A, S 🐾
      - ● T60.1X3   Toxic effect of halogenated insecticides, assault
      - ● T60.1X4   Toxic effect of halogenated insecticides, undetermined
  - T60.2   Toxic effect of other insecticides
    - T60.2X   Toxic effect of other insecticides
      - ● T60.2X1   Toxic effect of other insecticides, accidental (unintentional)
        Toxic effect of other insecticides NOS
      - ● T60.2X2   Toxic effect of other insecticides, intentional self-harm A, S 🐾
      - ● T60.2X3   Toxic effect of other insecticides, assault
      - ● T60.2X4   Toxic effect of other insecticides, undetermined
  - T60.3   Toxic effect of herbicides and fungicides
    - T60.3X   Toxic effect of herbicides and fungicides
      - ● T60.3X1   Toxic effect of herbicides and fungicides, accidental (unintentional)
        Toxic effect of herbicides and fungicides NOS
      - ● T60.3X2   Toxic effect of herbicides and fungicides, intentional self-harm A, S 🐾
      - ● T60.3X3   Toxic effect of herbicides and fungicides, assault
      - ● T60.3X4   Toxic effect of herbicides and fungicides, undetermined

- T60.4   Toxic effect of rodenticides

  Excludes1   strychnine and its salts (T65.1)
        thallium (T56.81-)
  - T60.4X   Toxic effect of rodenticides
    - ● T60.4X1   Toxic effect of rodenticides, accidental (unintentional)
      Toxic effect of rodenticides NOS
    - ● T60.4X2   Toxic effect of rodenticides, intentional self-harm A, S 🐾
    - ● T60.4X3   Toxic effect of rodenticides, assault
    - ● T60.4X4   Toxic effect of rodenticides, undetermined
- T60.8   Toxic effect of other pesticides
  - T60.8X   Toxic effect of other pesticides
    - ● T60.8X1   Toxic effect of other pesticides, accidental (unintentional)
      Toxic effect of other pesticides NOS
    - ● T60.8X2   Toxic effect of other pesticides, intentional self-harm A, S 🐾
    - ● T60.8X3   Toxic effect of other pesticides, assault
    - ● T60.8X4   Toxic effect of other pesticides, undetermined
- T60.9   Toxic effect of unspecified pesticide
  - X ● T60.91   Toxic effect of unspecified pesticide, accidental (unintentional)
  - X ● T60.92   Toxic effect of unspecified pesticide, intentional self-harm A, S 🐾
  - X ● T60.93   Toxic effect of unspecified pesticide, assault
  - X ● T60.94   Toxic effect of unspecified pesticide, undetermined
- T61   Toxic effect of noxious substances eaten as seafood

  Excludes1   allergic reaction to food, such as:
       anaphylactic reaction or shock due to adverse food reaction (T78.0-)
       bacterial foodborne intoxications (A05.-)
       dermatitis (L23.6, L25.4, L27.2)
       food protein-induced enterocolitis syndrome (K52.21)
       food protein-induced enteropathy (K52.22)
       gastroenteritis (noninfective) (K52.29)
       toxic effect of aflatoxin and other mycotoxins (T64)
       toxic effect of cyanides (T65.0-)
       toxic effect of harmful algae bloom (T65.82-)
       toxic effect of hydrogen cyanide (T57.3-)
       toxic effect of mercury (T56.1-)
       toxic effect of red tide (T65.82-)

  The appropriate 7th character is to be added to each code from category T61

A	initial encounter
D	subsequent encounter
S	sequela

  - T61.0   Ciguatera fish poisoning
    - X ● T61.01   Ciguatera fish poisoning, accidental (unintentional)
    - X ● T61.02   Ciguatera fish poisoning, intentional self-harm A, S 🐾
    - X ● T61.03   Ciguatera fish poisoning, assault
    - X ● T61.04   Ciguatera fish poisoning, undetermined
  - T61.1   Scombroid fish poisoning
    Histamine-like syndrome
    - X ● T61.11   Scombroid fish poisoning, accidental (unintentional)
    - X ● T61.12   Scombroid fish poisoning, intentional self-harm A, S 🐾
    - X ● T61.13   Scombroid fish poisoning, assault
    - X ● T61.14   Scombroid fish poisoning, undetermined

▶ New   ⟹ Revised   ~~deleted~~ Deleted   Excludes 1   Excludes 2   Includes   Use additional   Code first   Code also   Key words

OGCR Official Guidelines   X Assign placeholder X   ● Use Additional Character(s)   ▶ Manifestation Code   🐾 Hierarchical Condition Category   **Coding Clinic**

● **T61.7**   **Other fish and shellfish poisoning**
   ● **T61.77**   **Other fish poisoning**
      ● **T61.771**   Other fish poisoning, accidental (unintentional)
      ● **T61.772**   Other fish poisoning, intentional self-harm A, S 🐞
      ● **T61.773**   Other fish poisoning, assault
      ● **T61.774**   Other fish poisoning, undetermined
   ● **T61.78**   **Other shellfish poisoning**
      ● **T61.781**   Other shellfish poisoning, accidental (unintentional)
      ● **T61.782**   Other shellfish poisoning, intentional self-harm A, S 🐞
      ● **T61.783**   Other shellfish poisoning, assault
      ● **T61.784**   Other shellfish poisoning, undetermined
● **T61.8**   **Toxic effect of other seafood**
   ● **T61.8X**   **Toxic effect of other seafood**
      ● **T61.8X1**   Toxic effect of other seafood, accidental (unintentional)
      ● **T61.8X2**   Toxic effect of other seafood, intentional self-harm A, S 🐞
      ● **T61.8X3**   Toxic effect of other seafood, assault
      ● **T61.8X4**   Toxic effect of other seafood, undetermined
● **T61.9**   **Toxic effect of unspecified seafood**
   X ● **T61.91**   Toxic effect of unspecified seafood, accidental (unintentional)
   X ● **T61.92**   Toxic effect of unspecified seafood, intentional self-harm A, S 🐞
   X ● **T61.93**   Toxic effect of unspecified seafood, assault
   X ● **T61.94**   Toxic effect of unspecified seafood, undetermined

● **T62**   **Toxic effect of other noxious substances eaten as food**

   Excludes1   allergic reaction to food, such as:
      anaphylactic shock (reaction) due to adverse food reaction (T78.0-)
      dermatitis (L23.6, L25.4, L27.2)
      food protein-induced enterocolitis syndrome (K52.21)
      food protein-induced enteropathy (K52.22)
      gastroenteritis (noninfective) (K52.29)
      bacterial food borne intoxications (A05.-)
      toxic effect of aflatoxin and other mycotoxins (T64)
      toxic effect of cyanides (T65.0-)
      toxic effect of hydrogen cyanide (T57.3-)
      toxic effect of mercury (T56.1-)

   The appropriate 7th character is to be added to each code from category T62

A	initial encounter
D	subsequent encounter
S	sequela

● **T62.0**   **Toxic effect of ingested mushrooms**
   ● **T62.0X**   **Toxic effect of ingested mushrooms**
      ● **T62.0X1**   Toxic effect of ingested mushrooms, accidental (unintentional)
         Toxic effect of ingested mushrooms NOS
      ● **T62.0X2**   Toxic effect of ingested mushrooms, intentional self-harm A, S 🐞
      ● **T62.0X3**   Toxic effect of ingested mushrooms, assault
      ● **T62.0X4**   Toxic effect of ingested mushrooms, undetermined

● **T62.1**   **Toxic effect of ingested berries**
   ● **T62.1X**   **Toxic effect of ingested berries**
      ● **T62.1X1**   Toxic effect of ingested berries, accidental (unintentional)
         Toxic effect of ingested berries NOS
      ● **T62.1X2**   Toxic effect of ingested berries, intentional self-harm A, S 🐞
      ● **T62.1X3**   Toxic effect of ingested berries, assault
      ● **T62.1X4**   Toxic effect of ingested berries, undetermined
● **T62.2**   **Toxic effect of other ingested (parts of) plant(s)**
   ● **T62.2X**   **Toxic effect of other ingested (parts of) plant(s)**
      ● **T62.2X1**   Toxic effect of other ingested (parts of) plant(s), accidental (unintentional)
         Toxic effect of other ingested (parts of) plant(s) NOS
      ● **T62.2X2**   Toxic effect of other ingested (parts of) plant(s), intentional self-harm A, S 🐞
      ● **T62.2X3**   Toxic effect of other ingested (parts of) plant(s), assault
      ● **T62.2X4**   Toxic effect of other ingested (parts of) plant(s), undetermined
● **T62.8**   **Toxic effect of other specified noxious substances eaten as food**
   ● **T62.8X**   **Toxic effect of other specified noxious substances eaten as food**
      ● **T62.8X1**   Toxic effect of other specified noxious substances eaten as food, accidental (unintentional)
         Toxic effect of other specified noxious substances eaten as food NOS
      ● **T62.8X2**   Toxic effect of other specified noxious substances eaten as food, intentional self-harm A, S 🐞
      ● **T62.8X3**   Toxic effect of other specified noxious substances eaten as food, assault
      ● **T62.8X4**   Toxic effect of other specified noxious substances eaten as food, undetermined
● **T62.9**   **Toxic effect of unspecified noxious substance eaten as food**
   X ● **T62.91**   Toxic effect of unspecified noxious substance eaten as food, accidental (unintentional)
         Toxic effect of unspecified noxious substance eaten as food NOS
   X ● **T62.92**   Toxic effect of unspecified noxious substance eaten as food, intentional self-harm A, S 🐞
   X ● **T62.93**   Toxic effect of unspecified noxious substance eaten as food, assault
   X ● **T62.94**   Toxic effect of unspecified noxious substance eaten as food, undetermined

● **T63**   **Toxic effect of contact with venomous animals and plants**

   Includes   bite or touch of venomous animal
      pricked or stuck by thorn or leaf

   Excludes2   ingestion of toxic animal or plant (T61.-, T62.-)

   The appropriate 7th character is to be added to each code from category T63

A	initial encounter
D	subsequent encounter
S	sequela

● **T63.0**   **Toxic effect of snake venom**
   ● **T63.00**   **Toxic effect of unspecified snake venom**
      ● **T63.001**   Toxic effect of unspecified snake venom, accidental (unintentional)
         Toxic effect of unspecified snake venom NOS

● T63.002   Toxic effect of unspecified snake
             venom, intentional self-harm A, S 🐾

● T63.003   Toxic effect of unspecified snake
             venom, assault

● T63.004   Toxic effect of unspecified snake
             venom, undetermined

● T63.01 Toxic effect of rattlesnake venom

● T63.011   Toxic effect of rattlesnake venom,
             accidental (unintentional)
                Toxic effect of rattlesnake venom
                NOS

● T63.012   Toxic effect of rattlesnake venom,
             intentional self-harm A, S 🐾

● T63.013   Toxic effect of rattlesnake venom,
             assault

● T63.014   Toxic effect of rattlesnake venom,
             undetermined

● T63.02 Toxic effect of coral snake venom

● T63.021   Toxic effect of coral snake venom,
             accidental (unintentional)
                Toxic effect of coral snake venom
                NOS

● T63.022   Toxic effect of coral snake venom,
             intentional self-harm A, S 🐾

● T63.023   Toxic effect of coral snake venom,
             assault

● T63.024   Toxic effect of coral snake venom,
             undetermined

● T63.03 Toxic effect of taipan venom

● T63.031   Toxic effect of taipan venom,
             accidental (unintentional)
                Toxic effect of taipan venom NOS

● T63.032   Toxic effect of taipan venom,
             intentional self-harm A, S 🐾

● T63.033   Toxic effect of taipan venom, assault

● T63.034   Toxic effect of taipan venom,
             undetermined

● T63.04 Toxic effect of cobra venom

● T63.041   Toxic effect of cobra venom,
             accidental (unintentional)
                Toxic effect of cobra venom NOS

● T63.042   Toxic effect of cobra venom,
             intentional self-harm A, S 🐾

● T63.043   Toxic effect of cobra venom, assault

● T63.044   Toxic effect of cobra venom,
             undetermined

● T63.06 Toxic effect of venom of other North and South
          American snake

● T63.061   Toxic effect of venom of other North
             and South American snake, accidental
             (unintentional)
                Toxic effect of venom of other North
                and South American snake
                NOS

● T63.062   Toxic effect of venom of other North
             and South American snake,
             intentional self-harm A, S 🐾

● T63.063   Toxic effect of venom of other North
             and South American snake, assault

● T63.064   Toxic effect of venom of other
             North and South American snake,
             undetermined

● T63.07 Toxic effect of venom of other Australian snake

● T63.071   Toxic effect of venom of other
             Australian snake, accidental
             (unintentional)
                Toxic effect of venom of other
                Australian snake NOS

● T63.072   Toxic effect of venom of other
             Australian snake, intentional
             self-harm A, S 🐾

● T63.073   Toxic effect of venom of other
             Australian snake, assault

● T63.074   Toxic effect of venom of other
             Australian snake, undetermined

● T63.08 Toxic effect of venom of other African and
          Asian snake

● T63.081   Toxic effect of venom of other
             African and Asian snake, accidental
             (unintentional)
                Toxic effect of venom of other
                African and Asian snake NOS

● T63.082   Toxic effect of venom of other African
             and Asian snake, intentional
             self-harm A, S 🐾

● T63.083   Toxic effect of venom of other African
             and Asian snake, assault

● T63.084   Toxic effect of venom of other African
             and Asian snake, undetermined

● T63.09 Toxic effect of venom of other snake

● T63.091   Toxic effect of venom of other snake,
             accidental (unintentional)
                Toxic effect of venom of other snake
                NOS

● T63.092   Toxic effect of venom of other snake,
             intentional self-harm A, S 🐾

● T63.093   Toxic effect of venom of other snake,
             assault

● T63.094   Toxic effect of venom of other snake,
             undetermined

● T63.1 Toxic effect of venom of other reptiles

● T63.11 Toxic effect of venom of gila monster

● T63.111   Toxic effect of venom of gila monster,
             accidental (unintentional)
                Toxic effect of venom of gila monster
                NOS

● T63.112   Toxic effect of venom of gila monster,
             intentional self-harm A, S 🐾

● T63.113   Toxic effect of venom of gila monster,
             assault

● T63.114   Toxic effect of venom of gila monster,
             undetermined

● T63.12 Toxic effect of venom of other venomous lizard

● T63.121   Toxic effect of venom of other
             venomous lizard, accidental
             (unintentional)
                Toxic effect of venom of other
                venomous lizard NOS

● T63.122   Toxic effect of venom of other
             venomous lizard, intentional
             self-harm A, S 🐾

● T63.123   Toxic effect of venom of other
             venomous lizard, assault

● T63.124   Toxic effect of venom of other
             venomous lizard, undetermined

● T63.19 Toxic effect of venom of other reptiles

● T63.191   Toxic effect of venom of other
             reptiles, accidental (unintentional)
                Toxic effect of venom of other
                reptiles NOS

● T63.192   Toxic effect of venom of other
             reptiles, intentional self-harm A, S 🐾

● T63.193   Toxic effect of venom of other
             reptiles, assault

● T63.194   Toxic effect of venom of other
             reptiles, undetermined

● T63.2 Toxic effect of venom of scorpion

● T63.2X Toxic effect of venom of scorpion

● T63.2X1   Toxic effect of venom of scorpion,
             accidental (unintentional)
                Toxic effect of venom of scorpion
                NOS

▶ New   ⇒ Revised   ~~deleted~~ Deleted   Excludes 1   Excludes 2   Includes   Use additional   Code first   Code also   Key words

OGCR Official Guidelines   X Assign placeholder X   ● Use Additional Character(s)   ⟩ Manifestation Code   🐾 Hierarchical Condition Category   Coding Clinic

● T63.2X2 Toxic effect of venom of scorpion, intentional self-harm A, S 🔖

● T63.2X3 Toxic effect of venom of scorpion, assault

● T63.2X4 Toxic effect of venom of scorpion, undetermined

● T63.3 Toxic effect of venom of spider

  ● T63.30 Toxic effect of unspecified spider venom

    ● T63.301 Toxic effect of unspecified spider venom, accidental (unintentional)

    ● T63.302 Toxic effect of unspecified spider venom, intentional self-harm A, S 🔖

    ● T63.303 Toxic effect of unspecified spider venom, assault

    ● T63.304 Toxic effect of unspecified spider venom, undetermined

  ● T63.31 Toxic effect of venom of black widow spider

    ● T63.311 Toxic effect of venom of black widow spider, accidental (unintentional)

    ● T63.312 Toxic effect of venom of black widow spider, intentional self-harm A, S 🔖

    ● T63.313 Toxic effect of venom of black widow spider, assault

    ● T63.314 Toxic effect of venom of black widow spider, undetermined

  ● T63.32 Toxic effect of venom of tarantula

    ● T63.321 Toxic effect of venom of tarantula, accidental (unintentional)

    ● T63.322 Toxic effect of venom of tarantula, intentional self-harm A, S 🔖

    ● T63.323 Toxic effect of venom of tarantula, assault

    ● T63.324 Toxic effect of venom of tarantula, undetermined

  ● T63.33 Toxic effect of venom of brown recluse spider

    ● T63.331 Toxic effect of venom of brown recluse spider, accidental (unintentional)

    ● T63.332 Toxic effect of venom of brown recluse spider, intentional self-harm A, S 🔖

    ● T63.333 Toxic effect of venom of brown recluse spider, assault

    ● T63.334 Toxic effect of venom of brown recluse spider, undetermined

  ● T63.39 Toxic effect of venom of other spider

    ● T63.391 Toxic effect of venom of other spider, accidental (unintentional)

    ● T63.392 Toxic effect of venom of other spider, intentional self-harm A, S 🔖

    ● T63.393 Toxic effect of venom of other spider, assault

    ● T63.394 Toxic effect of venom of other spider, undetermined

● T63.4 Toxic effect of venom of other arthropods

  ● T63.41 Toxic effect of venom of centipedes and venomous millipedes

    ● T63.411 Toxic effect of venom of centipedes and venomous millipedes, accidental (unintentional)

    ● T63.412 Toxic effect of venom of centipedes and venomous millipedes, intentional self-harm A, S 🔖

    ● T63.413 Toxic effect of venom of centipedes and venomous millipedes, assault

    ● T63.414 Toxic effect of venom of centipedes and venomous millipedes, undetermined

● T63.42 Toxic effect of venom of ants

    ● T63.421 Toxic effect of venom of ants, accidental (unintentional)

    ● T63.422 Toxic effect of venom of ants, intentional self-harm A, S 🔖

    ● T63.423 Toxic effect of venom of ants, assault

    ● T63.424 Toxic effect of venom of ants, undetermined

● T63.43 Toxic effect of venom of caterpillars

    ● T63.431 Toxic effect of venom of caterpillars, accidental (unintentional)

    ● T63.432 Toxic effect of venom of caterpillars, intentional self-harm A, S 🔖

    ● T63.433 Toxic effect of venom of caterpillars, assault

    ● T63.434 Toxic effect of venom of caterpillars, undetermined

● T63.44 Toxic effect of venom of bees

    ● T63.441 Toxic effect of venom of bees, accidental (unintentional)

    ● T63.442 Toxic effect of venom of bees, intentional self-harm A, S 🔖

    ● T63.443 Toxic effect of venom of bees, assault

    ● T63.444 Toxic effect of venom of bees, undetermined

● T63.45 Toxic effect of venom of hornets

    ● T63.451 Toxic effect of venom of hornets, accidental (unintentional)

    ● T63.452 Toxic effect of venom of hornets, intentional self-harm A, S 🔖

    ● T63.453 Toxic effect of venom of hornets, assault

    ● T63.454 Toxic effect of venom of hornets, undetermined

● T63.46 Toxic effect of venom of wasps
    Toxic effect of yellow jacket

    ● T63.461 Toxic effect of venom of wasps, accidental (unintentional)

    ● T63.462 Toxic effect of venom of wasps, intentional self-harm A, S 🔖

    ● T63.463 Toxic effect of venom of wasps, assault

    ● T63.464 Toxic effect of venom of wasps, undetermined

● T63.48 Toxic effect of venom of other arthropod

    ● T63.481 Toxic effect of venom of other arthropod, accidental (unintentional)

    ● T63.482 Toxic effect of venom of other arthropod, intentional self-harm A, S 🔖

    ● T63.483 Toxic effect of venom of other arthropod, assault

    ● T63.484 Toxic effect of venom of other arthropod, undetermined

● T63.5 Toxic effect of contact with venomous fish

  Excludes2 poisoning by ingestion of fish (T61.-)

  ● T63.51 Toxic effect of contact with stingray

    ● T63.511 Toxic effect of contact with stingray, accidental (unintentional)

    ● T63.512 Toxic effect of contact with stingray, intentional self-harm A, S 🔖

    ● T63.513 Toxic effect of contact with stingray, assault

    ● T63.514 Toxic effect of contact with stingray, undetermined

CHAPTER 19 (S00–T88)

● T63.59   Toxic effect of contact with other venomous fish
- ● T63.591   Toxic effect of contact with other venomous fish, accidental (unintentional)
- ● T63.592   Toxic effect of contact with other venomous fish, intentional self-harm A, S 🝙
- ● T63.593   Toxic effect of contact with other venomous fish, assault
- ● T63.594   Toxic effect of contact with other venomous fish, undetermined

● T63.6   Toxic effect of contact with other venomous marine animals

> **Excludes1**   sea-snake venom (T63.09)
>
> **Excludes2**   poisoning by ingestion of shellfish (T61.78-)

● T63.61   Toxic effect of contact with Portuguese Man-o-war
> Toxic effect of contact with bluebottle
- ● T63.611   Toxic effect of contact with Portuguese Man-o-war, accidental (unintentional)
- ● T63.612   Toxic effect of contact with Portuguese Man-o-war, intentional self-harm A, S 🝙
- ● T63.613   Toxic effect of contact with Portuguese Man-o-war, assault
- ● T63.614   Toxic effect of contact with Portuguese Man-o-war, undetermined

● T63.62   Toxic effect of contact with other jellyfish
- ● T63.621   Toxic effect of contact with other jellyfish, accidental (unintentional)
- ● T63.622   Toxic effect of contact with other jellyfish, intentional self-harm A, S 🝙
- ● T63.623   Toxic effect of contact with other jellyfish, assault
- ● T63.624   Toxic effect of contact with other jellyfish, undetermined

● T63.63   Toxic effect of contact with sea anemone
- ● T63.631   Toxic effect of contact with sea anemone, accidental (unintentional)
- ● T63.632   Toxic effect of contact with sea anemone, intentional self-harm A, S 🝙
- ● T63.633   Toxic effect of contact with sea anemone, assault
- ● T63.634   Toxic effect of contact with sea anemone, undetermined

● T63.69   Toxic effect of contact with other venomous marine animals
- ● T63.691   Toxic effect of contact with other venomous marine animals, accidental (unintentional)
- ● T63.692   Toxic effect of contact with other venomous marine animals, intentional self-harm A, S 🝙
- ● T63.693   Toxic effect of contact with other venomous marine animals, assault
- ● T63.694   Toxic effect of contact with other venomous marine animals, undetermined

● T63.7   Toxic effect of contact with venomous plant
- ● T63.71   Toxic effect of contact with venomous marine plant
  - ● T63.711   Toxic effect of contact with venomous marine plant, accidental (unintentional)
  - ● T63.712   Toxic effect of contact with venomous marine plant, intentional self-harm A, S 🝙
  - ● T63.713   Toxic effect of contact with venomous marine plant, assault
  - ● T63.714   Toxic effect of contact with venomous marine plant, undetermined

● T63.79   Toxic effect of contact with other venomous plant
- ● T63.791   Toxic effect of contact with other venomous plant, accidental (unintentional)
- ● T63.792   Toxic effect of contact with other venomous plant, intentional self-harm A, S 🝙
- ● T63.793   Toxic effect of contact with other venomous plant, assault
- ● T63.794   Toxic effect of contact with other venomous plant, undetermined

● T63.8   Toxic effect of contact with other venomous animals
- ● T63.81   Toxic effect of contact with venomous frog
  > **Excludes1**   contact with nonvenomous frog (W62.0)
  - ● T63.811   Toxic effect of contact with venomous frog, accidental (unintentional)
  - ● T63.812   Toxic effect of contact with venomous frog, intentional self-harm A, S 🝙
  - ● T63.813   Toxic effect of contact with venomous frog, assault
  - ● T63.814   Toxic effect of contact with venomous frog, undetermined
- ● T63.82   Toxic effect of contact with venomous toad
  > **Excludes1**   contact with nonvenomous toad (W62.1)
  - ● T63.821   Toxic effect of contact with venomous toad, accidental (unintentional)
  - ● T63.822   Toxic effect of contact with venomous toad, intentional self-harm A, S 🝙
  - ● T63.823   Toxic effect of contact with venomous toad, assault
  - ● T63.824   Toxic effect of contact with venomous toad, undetermined
- ● T63.83   Toxic effect of contact with other venomous amphibian
  > **Excludes1**   contact with nonvenomous amphibian (W62.9)
  - ● T63.831   Toxic effect of contact with other venomous amphibian, accidental (unintentional)
  - ● T63.832   Toxic effect of contact with other venomous amphibian, intentional self-harm A, S 🝙
  - ● T63.833   Toxic effect of contact with other venomous amphibian, assault
  - ● T63.834   Toxic effect of contact with other venomous amphibian, undetermined
- ● T63.89   Toxic effect of contact with other venomous animals
  - ● T63.891   Toxic effect of contact with other venomous animals, accidental (unintentional)
  - ● T63.892   Toxic effect of contact with other venomous animals, intentional self-harm A, S 🝙
  - ● T63.893   Toxic effect of contact with other venomous animals, assault
  - ● T63.894   Toxic effect of contact with other venomous animals, undetermined

● T63.9   Toxic effect of contact with unspecified venomous animal
- X ● T63.91   Toxic effect of contact with unspecified venomous animal, accidental (unintentional)
- X ● T63.92   Toxic effect of contact with unspecified venomous animal, intentional self-harm A, S 🝙
- X ● T63.93   Toxic effect of contact with unspecified venomous animal, assault
- X ● T63.94   Toxic effect of contact with unspecified venomous animal, undetermined

▶ New   ⇒ Revised   ~~deleted~~ Deleted   Excludes 1   Excludes 2   Includes   Use additional   Code first   Code also   Key words

OGCR Official Guidelines   X Assign placeholder X   ● Use Additional Character(s)   ⟩ Manifestation Code   🝙 Hierarchical Condition Category   **Coding Clinic**

● **T64** **Toxic effect of aflatoxin and other mycotoxin food contaminants**

  The appropriate 7th character is to be added to each code from category T64

A	initial encounter
D	subsequent encounter
S	sequela

 ● **T64.0** **Toxic effect of aflatoxin**

  X ● **T64.01** Toxic effect of aflatoxin, accidental (unintentional)

  X ● **T64.02** Toxic effect of aflatoxin, intentional self-harm A, S 🔖

  X ● **T64.03** Toxic effect of aflatoxin, assault

  X ● **T64.04** Toxic effect of aflatoxin, undetermined

 ● **T64.8** **Toxic effect of other mycotoxin food contaminants**

  X ● **T64.81** Toxic effect of other mycotoxin food contaminants, accidental (unintentional)

  X ● **T64.82** Toxic effect of other mycotoxin food contaminants, intentional self-harm A, S 🔖

  X ● **T64.83** Toxic effect of other mycotoxin food contaminants, assault

  X ● **T64.84** Toxic effect of other mycotoxin food contaminants, undetermined

● **T65** **Toxic effect of other and unspecified substances**

  The appropriate 7th character is to be added to each code from category T65

A	initial encounter
D	subsequent encounter
S	sequela

 ● **T65.0** **Toxic effect of cyanides**

  Excludes1 hydrogen cyanide (T57.3-)

  ● **T65.0X** **Toxic effect of cyanides**

   ● **T65.0X1** Toxic effect of cyanides, accidental (unintentional)
     Toxic effect of cyanides NOS

   ● **T65.0X2** Toxic effect of cyanides, intentional self-harm A, S 🔖

   ● **T65.0X3** Toxic effect of cyanides, assault

   ● **T65.0X4** Toxic effect of cyanides, undetermined

 ● **T65.1** **Toxic effect of strychnine and its salts**

  ● **T65.1X** **Toxic effect of strychnine and its salts**

   ● **T65.1X1** Toxic effect of strychnine and its salts, accidental (unintentional)
     Toxic effect of strychnine and its salts NOS

   ● **T65.1X2** Toxic effect of strychnine and its salts, intentional self-harm A, S 🔖

   ● **T65.1X3** Toxic effect of strychnine and its salts, assault

   ● **T65.1X4** Toxic effect of strychnine and its salts, undetermined

 ● **T65.2** **Toxic effect of tobacco and nicotine**

  Excludes2 nicotine dependence (F17.-)

  ● **T65.21** **Toxic effect of chewing tobacco**

   ● **T65.211** Toxic effect of chewing tobacco, accidental (unintentional)
     Toxic effect of chewing tobacco NOS

   ● **T65.212** Toxic effect of chewing tobacco, intentional self-harm A, S 🔖

   ● **T65.213** Toxic effect of chewing tobacco, assault

   ● **T65.214** Toxic effect of chewing tobacco, undetermined

● **T65.22** **Toxic effect of tobacco cigarettes**
  Toxic effect of tobacco smoke

  Use additional code for exposure to second hand tobacco smoke (Z57.31, Z77.22)

 ● **T65.221** Toxic effect of tobacco cigarettes, accidental (unintentional)
   Toxic effect of tobacco cigarettes NOS

 ● **T65.222** Toxic effect of tobacco cigarettes, intentional self-harm A, S 🔖

 ● **T65.223** Toxic effect of tobacco cigarettes, assault

 ● **T65.224** Toxic effect of tobacco cigarettes, undetermined

● **T65.29** **Toxic effect of other tobacco and nicotine**

 ● **T65.291** Toxic effect of other tobacco and nicotine, accidental (unintentional)
   Toxic effect of other tobacco and nicotine NOS

 ● **T65.292** Toxic effect of other tobacco and nicotine, intentional self-harm A, S 🔖

 ● **T65.293** Toxic effect of other tobacco and nicotine, assault

 ● **T65.294** Toxic effect of other tobacco and nicotine, undetermined

● **T65.3** **Toxic effect of nitroderivatives and aminoderivatives of benzene and its homologues**
  Toxic effect of anilin [benzenamine]
  Toxic effect of nitrobenzene
  Toxic effect of trinitrotoluene

 ● **T65.3X** **Toxic effect of nitroderivatives and aminoderivatives of benzene and its homologues**

  ● **T65.3X1** Toxic effect of nitroderivatives and aminoderivatives of benzene and its homologues, accidental (unintentional)
    Toxic effect of nitroderivatives and aminoderivatives of benzene and its homologues NOS

  ● **T65.3X2** Toxic effect of nitroderivatives and aminoderivatives of benzene and its homologues, intentional self-harm A, S 🔖

  ● **T65.3X3** Toxic effect of nitroderivatives and aminoderivatives of benzene and its homologues, assault

  ● **T65.3X4** Toxic effect of nitroderivatives and aminoderivatives of benzene and its homologues, undetermined

● **T65.4** **Toxic effect of carbon disulfide**

 ● **T65.4X** **Toxic effect of carbon disulfide**

  ● **T65.4X1** Toxic effect of carbon disulfide, accidental (unintentional)
    Toxic effect of carbon disulfide NOS

  ● **T65.4X2** Toxic effect of carbon disulfide, intentional self-harm A, S 🔖

  ● **T65.4X3** Toxic effect of carbon disulfide, assault

  ● **T65.4X4** Toxic effect of carbon disulfide, undetermined

CHAPTER 19 (S00-T88)

● **T65.5**   **Toxic effect of nitroglycerin and other nitric acids and esters**
  Toxic effect of 1,2,3-Propanetriol trinitrate

   ● **T65.5X**   **Toxic effect of nitroglycerin and other nitric acids and esters**

     ● **T65.5X1**   **Toxic effect of nitroglycerin and other nitric acids and esters, accidental (unintentional)**
        Toxic effect of nitroglycerin and other nitric acids and esters NOS

     ● **T65.5X2**   **Toxic effect of nitroglycerin and other nitric acids and esters, intentional self-harm A, S** 🝠

     ● **T65.5X3**   **Toxic effect of nitroglycerin and other nitric acids and esters, assault**

     ● **T65.5X4**   **Toxic effect of nitroglycerin and other nitric acids and esters, undetermined**

● **T65.6**   **Toxic effect of paints and dyes, not elsewhere classified**

   ● **T65.6X**   **Toxic effect of paints and dyes, not elsewhere classified**

     ● **T65.6X1**   **Toxic effect of paints and dyes, not elsewhere classified, accidental (unintentional)**
        Toxic effect of paints and dyes NOS

     ● **T65.6X2**   **Toxic effect of paints and dyes, not elsewhere classified, intentional self-harm A, S** 🝠

     ● **T65.6X3**   **Toxic effect of paints and dyes, not elsewhere classified, assault**

     ● **T65.6X4**   **Toxic effect of paints and dyes, not elsewhere classified, undetermined**

● **T65.8**   **Toxic effect of other specified substances**

   ● **T65.81**   **Toxic effect of latex**

     ● **T65.811**   **Toxic effect of latex, accidental (unintentional)**
        Toxic effect of latex NOS

     ● **T65.812**   **Toxic effect of latex, intentional self-harm A, S** 🝠

     ● **T65.813**   **Toxic effect of latex, assault**

     ● **T65.814**   **Toxic effect of latex, undetermined**

   ● **T65.82**   **Toxic effect of harmful algae and algae toxins**
      Toxic effect of (harmful) algae bloom NOS
      Toxic effect of blue-green algae bloom
      Toxic effect of brown tide
      Toxic effect of cyanobacteria bloom
      Toxic effect of Florida red tide
      Toxic effect of pfiesteria piscicida
      Toxic effect of red tide

     ● **T65.821**   **Toxic effect of harmful algae and algae toxins, accidental (unintentional)**
        Toxic effect of harmful algae and algae toxins NOS

     ● **T65.822**   **Toxic effect of harmful algae and algae toxins, intentional self-harm A, S** 🝠

     ● **T65.823**   **Toxic effect of harmful algae and algae toxins, assault**

     ● **T65.824**   **Toxic effect of harmful algae and algae toxins, undetermined**

   ● **T65.83**   **Toxic effect of fiberglass**

     ● **T65.831**   **Toxic effect of fiberglass, accidental (unintentional)**
        Toxic effect of fiberglass NOS

     ● **T65.832**   **Toxic effect of fiberglass, intentional self-harm A, S** 🝠

     ● **T65.833**   **Toxic effect of fiberglass, assault**

     ● **T65.834**   **Toxic effect of fiberglass, undetermined**

● **T65.89**   **Toxic effect of other specified substances**

   ● **T65.891**   **Toxic effect of other specified substances, accidental (unintentional)**
      Toxic effect of other specified substances NOS
      Coding Clinic: 2018, Q1, P5

   ● **T65.892**   **Toxic effect of other specified substances, intentional self-harm A, S** 🝠

   ● **T65.893**   **Toxic effect of other specified substances, assault**

   ● **T65.894**   **Toxic effect of other specified substances, undetermined**

● **T65.9**   **Toxic effect of unspecified substance**

   X ● **T65.91**   **Toxic effect of unspecified substance, accidental (unintentional)**
      Poisoning NOS

   X ● **T65.92**   **Toxic effect of unspecified substance, intentional self-harm A, S** 🝠

   X ● **T65.93**   **Toxic effect of unspecified substance, assault**

   X ● **T65.94**   **Toxic effect of unspecified substance, undetermined**

OTHER AND UNSPECIFIED EFFECTS OF EXTERNAL CAUSES (T66-T78)

● **T66**   **Radiation sickness, unspecified**

   Excludes1   specified adverse effects of radiation, such as:
          burns (T20-T31)
          leukemia (C91-C95)
          radiation gastroenteritis and colitis (K52.0)
          radiation pneumonitis (J70.0)
          radiation related disorders of the skin and
            subcutaneous tissue (L55-L59)
          sunburn (L55.-)

   The appropriate 7th character is to be added to code T66

     | | |
     A   initial encounter
     D   subsequent encounter
     S   sequela

● **T67**   **Effects of heat and light**

   Excludes1   erythema [dermatitis] ab igne (L59.0)
          malignant hyperpyrexia due to anesthesia (T88.3)
          radiation-related disorders of the skin and
            subcutaneous tissue (L55-L59)

   Excludes2   burns (T20-T31)
          sunburn (L55.-)
          sweat disorder due to heat (L74-L75)

   The appropriate 7th character is to be added to each code from
     category T67

     A   initial encounter
     D   subsequent encounter
     S   sequela

   X ● **T67.0**   **Heatstroke and sunstroke**
      Use additional code(s) to identify any associated
        complications of heatstroke, such as:
      coma and stupor (R40.-)
      rhabdomyolysis (M62.82)
      systemic inflammatory response syndrome (R65.1-)
      Coding Clinic: 2019, Q4, P18

     X ● **T67.01**   **Heatstroke and sunstroke**
        Heat apoplexy
        Heat pyrexia
        Siriasis
        Thermoplegia

     X ● **T67.02**   **Exertional heatstroke**
        Coding Clinic: 2019, Q4, P18

     X ● **T67.09**   **Other heatstroke and sunstroke**

   X ● **T67.1**   **Heat syncope**
      Heat collapse

   X ● **T67.2**   **Heat cramp**

▶ New   ⇒ Revised   ~~deleted~~ Deleted   Excludes 1   Excludes 2   Includes   Use additional   Code first   Code also   Key words

OGCR Official Guidelines   X Assign placeholder X   ● Use Additional Character(s)   ▶ Manifestation Code   🝠 Hierarchical Condition Category   Coding Clinic

X● **T67.3**   **Heat exhaustion, anhydrotic**
     Heat prostration due to water depletion
       Excludes1   heat exhaustion due to salt depletion
                     (T67.4)

X● **T67.4**   **Heat exhaustion due to salt depletion**
     Heat prostration due to salt (and water) depletion

X● **T67.5**   **Heat exhaustion, unspecified**
     Heat prostration NOS

X● **T67.6**   **Heat fatigue, transient**

X● **T67.7**   **Heat edema**

X● **T67.8**   **Other effects of heat and light**

X● **T67.9**   **Effect of heat and light, unspecified**

X● **T68**   **Hypothermia**
     Accidental hypothermia
     Hypothermia NOS
     Use additional code to identify source of exposure:
       Exposure to excessive cold of man-made origin (W93)
       Exposure to excessive cold of natural origin (X31)
       Excludes1   hypothermia following anesthesia (T88.51)
                  hypothermia not associated with low
                     environmental temperature (R68.0)
                  hypothermia of newborn (P80.-)
       Excludes2   frostbite (T33-T34)
     The appropriate 7th character is to be added to code T68

       | | |
       A   initial encounter
       D   subsequent encounter
       S   sequela

● **T69**   **Other effects of reduced temperature**
     Use additional code to identify source of exposure:
       Exposure to excessive cold of man-made origin (W93)
       Exposure to excessive cold of natural origin (X31)
       Excludes2   frostbite (T33-T34)
     The appropriate 7th character is to be added to each code from
       category T69

       A   initial encounter
       D   subsequent encounter
       S   sequela

● **T69.0**   **Immersion hand and foot**

● **T69.01**   **Immersion hand**

● **T69.011**   **Immersion hand, right hand**

● **T69.012**   **Immersion hand, left hand**

● **T69.019**   **Immersion hand, unspecified hand**

● **T69.02**   **Immersion foot**
     Trench foot

● **T69.021**   **Immersion foot, right foot**

● **T69.022**   **Immersion foot, left foot**

● **T69.029**   **Immersion foot, unspecified foot**

X● **T69.1**   **Chilblains**

X● **T69.8**   **Other specified effects of reduced temperature**

X● **T69.9**   **Effect of reduced temperature, unspecified**

● **T70**   **Effects of air pressure and water pressure**
     The appropriate 7th character is to be added to each code from
       category T70

       A   initial encounter
       D   subsequent encounter
       S   sequela

X● **T70.0**   **Otitic barotrauma**
     Aero-otitis media
     Effects of change in ambient atmospheric pressure or
       water pressure on ears

X● **T70.1**   **Sinus barotrauma**
     Aerosinusitis
     Effects of change in ambient atmospheric pressure on
       sinuses

● **T70.2**   **Other and unspecified effects of high altitude**
       Excludes2   polycythemia due to high altitude (D75.1)

X● **T70.20**   **Unspecified effects of high altitude**

X● **T70.29**   **Other effects of high altitude**
     Alpine sickness
     Anoxia due to high altitude
     Barotrauma NOS
     Hypobaropathy
     Mountain sickness

X● **T70.3**   **Caisson disease [decompression sickness]**
     Compressed-air disease
     Diver's palsy or paralysis

X● **T70.4**   **Effects of high-pressure fluids**
     Hydraulic jet injection (industrial)
     Pneumatic jet injection (industrial)
     Traumatic jet injection (industrial)

X● **T70.8**   **Other effects of air pressure and water pressure**

X● **T70.9**   **Effect of air pressure and water pressure, unspecified**

● **T71**   **Asphyxiation**
     Mechanical suffocation
     Traumatic suffocation
       Excludes1   acute respiratory distress (syndrome) (J80)
                  anoxia due to high altitude (T70.2)
                  asphyxia NOS (R09.01)
                  asphyxia from carbon monoxide (T58.-)
                  asphyxia from inhalation of food or foreign body
                     (T17.-)
                  asphyxia from other gases, fumes and vapors
                     (T59.-)
                  respiratory distress (syndrome) in newborn
                     (P22.-)
     The appropriate 7th character is to be added to each code from
       category T71

       A   initial encounter
       D   subsequent encounter
       S   sequela

● **T71.1**   **Asphyxiation due to mechanical threat to breathing**
     Suffocation due to mechanical threat to breathing

● **T71.11**   **Asphyxiation due to smothering under pillow**

● **T71.111**   **Asphyxiation due to smothering under pillow, accidental**
     Asphyxiation due to smothering under pillow NOS

● **T71.112**   **Asphyxiation due to smothering under pillow, intentional self-harm A, S** 🔒

● **T71.113**   **Asphyxiation due to smothering under pillow, assault**

● **T71.114**   **Asphyxiation due to smothering under pillow, undetermined**

● **T71.12**   **Asphyxiation due to plastic bag**

● **T71.121**   **Asphyxiation due to plastic bag, accidental**
     Asphyxiation due to plastic bag NOS

● **T71.122**   **Asphyxiation due to plastic bag, intentional self-harm A, S** 🔒

● **T71.123**   **Asphyxiation due to plastic bag, assault**

● **T71.124**   **Asphyxiation due to plastic bag, undetermined**

● **T71.13**   **Asphyxiation due to being trapped in bed linens**

● **T71.131**   **Asphyxiation due to being trapped in bed linens, accidental**
     Asphyxiation due to being trapped in bed linens NOS

● **T71.132**   **Asphyxiation due to being trapped in bed linens, intentional self-harm A, S** 🔒

CHAPTER 19 (S00-T88)

● T71.133 Asphyxiation due to being trapped in bed linens, assault

● T71.134 Asphyxiation due to being trapped in bed linens, undetermined

● T71.14 Asphyxiation due to smothering under another person's body (in bed)

   ● T71.141 Asphyxiation due to smothering under another person's body (in bed), accidental

      Asphyxiation due to smothering under another person's body (in bed) NOS

   ● T71.143 Asphyxiation due to smothering under another person's body (in bed), assault

   ● T71.144 Asphyxiation due to smothering under another person's body (in bed), undetermined

● T71.15 Asphyxiation due to smothering in furniture

   ● T71.151 Asphyxiation due to smothering in furniture, accidental

      Asphyxiation due to smothering in furniture NOS

   ● T71.152 Asphyxiation due to smothering in furniture, intentional self-harm A, S 🦀

   ● T71.153 Asphyxiation due to smothering in furniture, assault

   ● T71.154 Asphyxiation due to smothering in furniture, undetermined

● T71.16 Asphyxiation due to hanging

   Hanging by window shade cord

   Use additional code for any associated injuries, such as:

      crushing injury of neck (S17.-)

      fracture of cervical vertebrae (S12.0-S12.2-)

      open wound of neck (S11.-)

   ● T71.161 Asphyxiation due to hanging, accidental

      Asphyxiation due to hanging NOS

      Hanging NOS

   ● T71.162 Asphyxiation due to hanging, intentional self-harm A, S 🦀

   ● T71.163 Asphyxiation due to hanging, assault

   ● T71.164 Asphyxiation due to hanging, undetermined

● T71.19 Asphyxiation due to mechanical

   Threat to breathing due to other causes

   ● T71.191 Asphyxiation due to mechanical threat to breathing due to other causes, accidental

      Asphyxiation due to other causes NOS

      Coding Clinic: 2016, Q4, P76

   ● T71.192 Asphyxiation due to mechanical threat to breathing due to other causes, intentional self-harm A, S 🦀

   ● T71.193 Asphyxiation due to mechanical threat to breathing due to other causes, assault

   ● T71.194 Asphyxiation due to mechanical threat to breathing due to other causes, undetermined

● T71.2 Asphyxiation due to systemic oxygen deficiency due to low oxygen content in ambient air

   Suffocation due to systemic oxygen deficiency due to low oxygen content in ambient air

   X ● T71.20 Asphyxiation due to systemic oxygen deficiency due to low oxygen content in ambient air due to unspecified cause

   X ● T71.21 Asphyxiation due to cave-in or falling earth

      Use additional code for any associated cataclysm (X34-X38)

● T71.22 Asphyxiation due to being trapped in a car trunk

   ● T71.221 Asphyxiation due to being trapped in a car trunk, accidental

   ● T71.222 Asphyxiation due to being trapped in a car trunk, intentional self-harm A, S 🦀

   ● T71.223 Asphyxiation due to being trapped in a car trunk, assault

   ● T71.224 Asphyxiation due to being trapped in a car trunk, undetermined

● T71.23 Asphyxiation due to being trapped in a (discarded) refrigerator

   ● T71.231 Asphyxiation due to being trapped in a (discarded) refrigerator, accidental

   ● T71.232 Asphyxiation due to being trapped in a (discarded) refrigerator, intentional self-harm A, S 🦀

   ● T71.233 Asphyxiation due to being trapped in a (discarded) refrigerator, assault

   ● T71.234 Asphyxiation due to being trapped in a (discarded) refrigerator, undetermined

X ● T71.29 Asphyxiation due to being trapped in other low oxygen environment

X ● T71.9 Asphyxiation due to unspecified cause

   Suffocation (by strangulation) due to unspecified cause

   Suffocation NOS

   Systemic oxygen deficiency due to low oxygen content in ambient air due to unspecified cause

   Systemic oxygen deficiency due to mechanical threat to breathing due to unspecified cause

   Traumatic asphyxia NOS

● **T73 Effects of other deprivation**

   The appropriate 7th character is to be added to each code from category T73

A	initial encounter
D	subsequent encounter
S	sequela

X ● T73.0 **Starvation**

   Deprivation of food

X ● T73.1 **Deprivation of water**

X ● T73.2 **Exhaustion due to exposure**

X ● T73.3 **Exhaustion due to excessive exertion**

   Exhaustion due to overexertion

X ● T73.8 **Other effects of deprivation**

X ● T73.9 **Effect of deprivation, unspecified**

● **T74 Adult and child abuse, neglect and other maltreatment, confirmed**

   Use additional code, if applicable, to identify any associated current injury

   Use additional external cause code to identify perpetrator, if known (Y07.-)

   Excludes1 abuse and maltreatment in pregnancy (O9A.3-, O9A.4-, O9A.5-)

      adult and child maltreatment, suspected (T76.-)

   The appropriate 7th character is to be added to each code from category T74

A	initial encounter
D	subsequent encounter
S	sequela

● T74.0 **Neglect or abandonment, confirmed**

   X ● T74.01 **Adult neglect or abandonment, confirmed** A

   X ● T74.02 **Child neglect or abandonment, confirmed** P

▶ New   ➡ Revised   ~~deleted~~ Deleted   Excludes 1   Excludes 2   Includes   Use additional   Code first   Code also   Key words

OGCR Official Guidelines   X Assign placeholder X   ● Use Additional Character(s)   ❱ Manifestation Code   🦀 Hierarchical Condition Category   Coding Clinic

● **T74.1   Physical abuse, confirmed**
    Excludes2   sexual abuse (T74.2-)
  X● **T74.11   Adult physical abuse, confirmed**   A
  X● **T74.12   Child physical abuse, confirmed**   P
      Excludes2   shaken infant syndrome (T74.4)
● **T74.2   Sexual abuse, confirmed**
    Rape, confirmed
    Sexual assault, confirmed
  X● **T74.21   Adult sexual abuse, confirmed**   A
  X● **T74.22   Child sexual abuse, confirmed**   P
● **T74.3   Psychological abuse, confirmed**
    Bullying and intimidation, confirmed
    Intimidation through social media, confirmed
  X● **T74.31   Adult psychological abuse, confirmed**   A
  X● **T74.32   Child psychological abuse, confirmed**   P
X● **T74.4   Shaken infant syndrome**   P
● **T74.5   Forced sexual exploitation, confirmed**
  X● **T74.51   Adult forced sexual exploitation, confirmed**   P
  X● **T74.52   Child sexual exploitation, confirmed**   P
● **T74.6   Forced labor exploitation, confirmed**
  X● **T74.61   Adult forced labor exploitation, confirmed**   P
  X● **T74.62   Child forced labor exploitation, confirmed**   P
● **T74.9   Unspecified maltreatment, confirmed**
  X● **T74.91   Unspecified adult maltreatment, confirmed**   A
  X● **T74.92   Unspecified child maltreatment, confirmed**   P

● **T75   Other and unspecified effects of other external causes**
    Excludes1   adverse effects NEC (T78.-)
    Excludes2   burns (electric) (T20-T31)
    The appropriate 7th character is to be added to each code from category T75

A	initial encounter
D	subsequent encounter
S	sequela

● **T75.0   Effects of lightning**
    Struck by lightning
  X● **T75.00   Unspecified effects of lightning**
      Struck by lightning NOS
  X● **T75.01   Shock due to being struck by lightning**
  X● **T75.09   Other effects of lightning**
      Use additional code for other effects of lightning
X● **T75.1   Unspecified effects of drowning and nonfatal submersion**
    Immersion
      Excludes1   specified effects of drowning code to effects
● **T75.2   Effects of vibration**
  X● **T75.20   Unspecified effects of vibration**
  X● **T75.21   Pneumatic hammer syndrome**
  X● **T75.22   Traumatic vasospastic syndrome**
  X● **T75.23   Vertigo from infrasound**
      Excludes1   vertigo NOS (R42)
  X● **T75.29   Other effects of vibration**
X● **T75.3   Motion sickness**
    Airsickness   Travel sickness
    Seasickness
    Use additional external cause code to identify vehicle or type of motion (Y92.81-, Y93.5-)
X● **T75.4   Electrocution**
    Shock from electric current
    Shock from electroshock gun (taser)
● **T75.8   Other specified effects of external causes**
  X● **T75.81   Effects of abnormal gravitation [G] forces**
  X● **T75.82   Effects of weightlessness**
  X● **T75.89   Other specified effects of external causes**

● **T76   Adult and child abuse, neglect and other maltreatment, suspected**
    Use additional code, if applicable, to identify any associated current injury
    Excludes1   adult and child maltreatment, confirmed (T74.-)
      suspected abuse and maltreatment in pregnancy (O9A.3-, O9A.4-, O9A.5-)
      suspected adult physical abuse, ruled out (Z04.71)
      suspected adult sexual abuse, ruled out (Z04.41)
      suspected child physical abuse, ruled out (Z04.72)
      suspected child sexual abuse, ruled out (Z04.42)
    The appropriate 7th character is to be added to each code from category T76

A	initial encounter
D	subsequent encounter
S	sequela

Coding Clinic: 2016, Q4, P129
● **T76.0   Neglect or abandonment, suspected**
  X● **T76.01   Adult neglect or abandonment, suspected**   A
  X● **T76.02   Child neglect or abandonment, suspected**   P
● **T76.1   Physical abuse, suspected**
  X● **T76.11   Adult physical abuse, suspected**   A
  X● **T76.12   Child physical abuse, suspected**   P
      Coding Clinic: 2019, Q2, P12
● **T76.2   Sexual abuse, suspected**
    Rape, suspected
      Excludes1   alleged abuse, ruled out (Z04.7)
  X● **T76.21   Adult sexual abuse, suspected**   A
  X● **T76.22   Child sexual abuse, suspected**   P
● **T76.3   Psychological abuse, suspected**
    Bullying and intimidation, suspected
    Intimidation through social media, suspected
  X● **T76.31   Adult psychological abuse, suspected**   A
  X● **T76.32   Child psychological abuse, suspected**   P
● **T76.5   Forced sexual exploitation, suspected**
  X● **T76.51   Adult forced sexual exploitation, suspected**   P
  X● **T76.52   Child sexual exploitation, suspected**   P
● **T76.6   Forced labor exploitation, suspected**
  X● **T76.61   Adult forced labor exploitation, suspected**   P
  X● **T76.62   Child forced labor exploitation, suspected**   P
● **T76.9   Unspecified maltreatment, suspected**
  X● **T76.91   Unspecified adult maltreatment, suspected**   A
  X● **T76.92   Unspecified child maltreatment, suspected**   P

● **T78   Adverse effects, not elsewhere classified**
    Excludes2   complications of surgical and medical care NEC (T80-T88)
    The appropriate 7th character is to be added to each code from category T78

A	initial encounter
D	subsequent encounter
S	sequela

● **T78.0   Anaphylactic reaction due to food**
    Anaphylactic reaction due to adverse food reaction
    Anaphylactic shock or reaction due to nonpoisonous foods
    Anaphylactoid reaction due to food
  X● **T78.00   Anaphylactic reaction due to unspecified food**
  X● **T78.01   Anaphylactic reaction due to peanuts**
  X● **T78.02   Anaphylactic reaction due to shellfish (crustaceans)**
  X● **T78.03   Anaphylactic reaction due to other fish**
  X● **T78.04   Anaphylactic reaction due to fruits and vegetables**

CHAPTER 19 (S00-T88)

X⬤ **T78.05** **Anaphylactic reaction due to** tree nuts and seeds

    Excludes2   anaphylactic reaction due to peanuts (T78.01)

X⬤ **T78.06** **Anaphylactic reaction due to** food additives

X⬤ **T78.07** **Anaphylactic reaction due to** milk and dairy products

X⬤ **T78.08** **Anaphylactic reaction due to** eggs

X⬤ **T78.09** **Anaphylactic reaction due to** other food products

X⬤ **T78.1** **Other adverse food reactions, not elsewhere classified**

Use additional code to identify the type of reaction, if applicable

    Excludes1   anaphylactic reaction or shock due to adverse food reaction (T78.0-)
anaphylactic reaction due to food (T78.0-)
bacterial food borne intoxications (A05.-)

    Excludes2   allergic and dietetic gastroenteritis and colitis (K52.29)
allergic rhinitis due to food (J30.5)
dermatitis due to food in contact with skin (L23.6, L24.6, L25.4)
dermatitis due to ingested food (L27.2)
food protein-induced enterocolitis syndrome (K52.21)
food protein-induced enteropathy (K52.22)

X⬤ **T78.2** **Anaphylactic shock,** unspecified

Occurs when allergic response triggers large quantities of histamines, prostaglandins, leukotrienes resulting in systemic vasodilation

Allergic shock
Anaphylactic reaction
Anaphylaxis

    Excludes1   anaphylactic reaction or shock due to adverse effect of correct medicinal substance properly administered (T88.6)
anaphylactic reaction or shock due to adverse food reaction (T78.0-)
anaphylactic reaction or shock due to serum (T80.5-)

X⬤ **T78.3** **Angioneurotic edema**

Allergic angioedema
Giant urticaria
Vascular disorder resulting from abnormalities of autonomic nervous system fibers supplying blood vessels
Quincke's edema

    Excludes1   serum urticaria (T80.6-)
urticaria (L50.-)

⬤ **T78.4** **Other and unspecified allergy**

    Excludes1   specified types of allergic reaction such as:
allergic diarrhea (K52.29)
allergic gastroenteritis and colitis (K52.29)
dermatitis (L23-L25, L27.-)
food protein-induced enterocolitis syndrome (K52.21)
food protein-induced enteropathy (K52.22)
hay fever (J30.1)

X⬤ **T78.40** **Allergy,** unspecified
Allergic reaction NOS
Hypersensitivity NOS

X⬤ **T78.41** **Arthus phenomenon**
Arthus reaction

X⬤ **T78.49** **Other allergy**
Coding Clinic: 2021, Q1, P42

X⬤ **T78.8** **Other adverse effects, not elsewhere classified**

CERTAIN EARLY COMPLICATIONS OF TRAUMA (T79)

⬤ **T79** **Certain early complications of trauma, not elsewhere classified**

    Excludes2   acute respiratory distress syndrome (J80)
complications occurring during or following medical procedures (T80-T88)
complications of surgical and medical care NEC (T80-T88)
newborn respiratory distress syndrome (P22.0)

The appropriate 7th character is to be added to each code from category T79

A	initial encounter
D	subsequent encounter
S	sequela

X⬤ **T79.0** **Air embolism (traumatic)** A 🐾

    Excludes1   air embolism complicating abortion or ectopic or molar pregnancy (O00-O07, O08.2)
air embolism complicating pregnancy, childbirth and the puerperium (O88.0)
air embolism following infusion, transfusion, and therapeutic injection (T80.0)
air embolism following procedure NEC (T81.7-)

X⬤ **T79.1** **Fat embolism (traumatic)** A 🐾

    Excludes1   fat embolism complicating:
abortion or ectopic or molar pregnancy (O00-O07, O08.2)
pregnancy, childbirth and the puerperium (O88.8)

X⬤ **T79.2** **Traumatic secondary and recurrent hemorrhage and seroma** A 🐾

X⬤ **T79.4** **Traumatic shock** A 🐾
Shock (immediate) (delayed) following injury

    Excludes1   anaphylactic shock due to adverse food reaction (T78.0-)
anaphylactic shock due to correct medicinal substance properly administered (T88.6)
anaphylactic shock due to serum (T80.5-)
anaphylactic shock NOS (T78.2)
electric shock (T75.4)
nontraumatic shock NEC (R57.-)
obstetric shock (O75.1)
postprocedural shock (T81.1-)
septic shock (R65.21)
shock complicating abortion or ectopic or molar pregnancy (O00-O07, O08.3)
shock due to anesthesia (T88.2)
shock due to lightning (T75.01)
shock NOS (R57.9)

X⬤ **T79.5** **Traumatic anuria** A 🐾
Crush syndrome
Renal failure following crushing

X⬤ **T79.6** **Traumatic ischemia of muscle** A 🐾
Traumatic rhabdomyolysis
Volkmann's ischemic contracture

    Excludes2   anterior tibial syndrome (M76.8)
compartment syndrome (traumatic) (T79.A-)
nontraumatic ischemia of muscle (M62.2-)

X⬤ **T79.7** **Traumatic subcutaneous emphysema** A 🐾

    Excludes2   emphysema NOS (J43)
emphysema (subcutaneous) resulting from a procedure (T81.82)

⬤ **T79.A** **Traumatic compartment syndrome**

    Excludes1   fibromyalgia (M79.7)
nontraumatic compartment syndrome (M79.A-)

    Excludes2   traumatic ischemic infarction of muscle (T79.6)

▶ New   ⇒ Revised   ~~deleted~~ Deleted   Excludes 1   Excludes 2   Includes   Use additional   Code first   Code also   Key words
OGCR Official Guidelines   X Assign placeholder X   ⬤ Use Additional Character(s)   ▎ Manifestation Code   🐾 Hierarchical Condition Category   **Coding Clinic**

X ● **T79.A0 Compartment syndrome, unspecified**
     Compartment syndrome NOS

● **T79.A1 Traumatic compartment syndrome of upper extremity**
     Traumatic compartment syndrome of shoulder, arm, forearm, wrist, hand, and fingers

● **T79.A11 Traumatic compartment syndrome of right upper extremity A** 🐾

● **T79.A12 Traumatic compartment syndrome of left upper extremity A** 🐾

● **T79.A19 Traumatic compartment syndrome of unspecified upper extremity A** 🐾

● **T79.A2 Traumatic compartment syndrome of lower extremity**
     Traumatic compartment syndrome of hip, buttock, thigh, leg, foot, and toes

● **T79.A21 Traumatic compartment syndrome of right lower extremity A** 🐾

● **T79.A22 Traumatic compartment syndrome of left lower extremity A** 🐾

● **T79.A29 Traumatic compartment syndrome of unspecified lower extremity**

X ● **T79.A3 Traumatic compartment syndrome of abdomen A** 🐾

X ● **T79.A9 Traumatic compartment syndrome of other sites A** 🐾

X ● **T79.8 Other early complications of trauma A** 🐾

X ● **T79.9 Unspecified early complication of trauma A** 🐾

COMPLICATIONS OF SURGICAL AND MEDICAL CARE NOT ELSEWHERE CLASSIFIED (T80-T88)

Use additional code for adverse effect, if applicable, to identify drug (T36-T50 with fifth or sixth character 5)

Use additional code(s) to identify the specified condition resulting from the complication.

Use additional code to identify devices involved and details of circumstances (Y62-Y82)

Excludes2 any encounters with medical care for postprocedural conditions in which no complications are present, such as:
     artificial opening status (Z93.-)
     closure of external stoma (Z43.-)
     fitting and adjustment of external prosthetic device (Z44.-)
   burns and corrosions from local applications and irradiation (T20-T32)
   complications of surgical procedures during pregnancy, childbirth and the puerperium (O00-O9A)
   mechanical complication of respirator [ventilator] (J95.850)
   poisoning and toxic effects of drugs and chemicals (T36-T65 with fifth or sixth character 1-4 or 6)
   postprocedural fever (R50.82)
   specified complications classified elsewhere, such as:
     cerebrospinal fluid leak from spinal puncture (G97.0)
     colostomy malfunction (K94.0-)
     disorders of fluid and electrolyte imbalance (E86-E87)
     functional disturbances following cardiac surgery (I97.0-I97.1)
     intraoperative and postprocedural complications of specified body systems (D78.-, E36.-, E89.-, G97.3-, G97.4, H59.3-, H59.-, H95.2-, H95.3, I97.4-, I97.5, J95.6-, J95.7, K91.6-, L76.-, M96.-, N99.-)
     ostomy complications (J95.0-, K94.-, N99.5-)
     postgastric surgery syndromes (K91.1)
     postlaminectomy syndrome NEC (M96.1)
     postmastectomy lymphedema syndrome (I97.2)
     postsurgical blind-loop syndrome (K91.2)
     ventilator associated pneumonia (J95.851)

● **T80 Complications following infusion, transfusion and therapeutic injection**

     Includes   complications following perfusion

     Excludes2 bone marrow transplant rejection (T86.01)
                 febrile nonhemolytic transfusion reaction (R50.84)
                 fluid overload due to transfusion (E87.71)
                 posttransfusion purpura (D69.51)
                 transfusion associated circulatory overload (TACO) (E87.71)
                 transfusion (red blood cell) associated hemochromatosis (E83.111)
                 transfusion related acute lung injury (TRALI) (J95.84)

The appropriate 7th character is to be added to each code from category T80

A	initial encounter
D	subsequent encounter
S	sequela

X ● **T80.0 Air embolism following infusion, transfusion and therapeutic injection**

X ● **T80.1 Vascular complications following infusion, transfusion and therapeutic injection**
     Use additional code to identify the vascular complication

     Excludes2 extravasation of vesicant agent (T80.81-)
                 infiltration of vesicant agent (T80.81-)
                 vascular complications specified as due to prosthetic devices, implants and grafts (T82.8- T83.8-, T84.8-, T85.8-)
                 postprocedural vascular complications (T81.7-)

● **T80.2 Infections following infusion, transfusion and therapeutic injection**
     Use additional code to identify the specific infection, such as:
       sepsis (A41.9)
     Use additional code (R65.2-) to identify severe sepsis, if applicable

     Excludes2 infections specified as due to prosthetic devices, implants and grafts (T82.6-T82.7, T83.5-T83.6, T84.5-T84.7, T85.7)
                 postprocedural infections (T81.44)

     Coding Clinic: 2018, Q4, P89

● **T80.21 Infection due to central venous catheter**
     Infection due to pulmonary artery catheter (Swan-Ganz catheter)
     Coding Clinic: 2019, Q1, P13-14; 2018, Q4, P89

● **T80.211 Bloodstream infection due to central venous catheter**
     Catheter-related bloodstream infection (CRBSI) NOS
     Central line-associated bloodstream infection (CLABSI)
     Bloodstream infection due to Hickman catheter
     Bloodstream infection due to peripherally inserted central catheter (PICC)
     Bloodstream infection due to portacath (port-a-cath)
     Bloodstream infection due to pulmonary artery catheter
     Bloodstream infection due to triple lumen catheter
     Bloodstream infection due to umbilical venous catheter
     Coding Clinic: 2018, Q4, P89

● **T80.212** **Local infection due to central venous catheter**
  Exit or insertion site infection
  Local infection due to Hickman catheter
  Local infection due to peripherally inserted central catheter (PICC)
  Local infection due to portacath (port-a-cath)
  Local infection due to pulmonary artery catheter
  Local infection due to triple lumen catheter
  Local infection due to umbilical venous catheter
  Port or reservoir infection
  Tunnel infection

● **T80.218** **Other infection due to central venous catheter**
  Other central line-associated infection
  Other infection due to Hickman catheter
  Other infection due to peripherally inserted central catheter (PICC)
  Other infection due to portacath (port-a-cath)
  Other infection due to pulmonary artery catheter
  Other infection due to triple lumen catheter
  Other infection due to umbilical venous catheter

● **T80.219** **Unspecified infection due to central venous catheter**
  Central line-associated infection NOS
  Unspecified infection due to Hickman catheter
  Unspecified infection due to peripherally inserted central catheter (PICC)
  Unspecified infection due to portacath (port-a-cath)
  Unspecified infection due to pulmonary artery catheter
  Unspecified infection due to triple lumen catheter
  Unspecified infection due to umbilical venous catheter

X● **T80.22** **Acute infection following transfusion, infusion, or injection of blood and blood products**

X● **T80.29** **Infection following other infusion, transfusion and therapeutic injection**

● **T80.3** **ABO incompatibility reaction due to transfusion of blood or blood products**

  Excludes1 minor blood group antigens reactions (Duffy) (E) (K) (Kell) (Kidd) (Lewis) (M) (N) (P) (S) (T80.A-)

X● **T80.30** **ABO incompatibility reaction due to transfusion of blood or blood products, unspecified**
  ABO incompatibility blood transfusion NOS
  Reaction to ABO incompatibility from transfusion NOS

● **T80.31** **ABO incompatibility with hemolytic transfusion reaction**

● **T80.310** **ABO incompatibility with acute hemolytic transfusion reaction**
  ABO incompatibility with hemolytic transfusion reaction less than 24 hours after transfusion
  Acute hemolytic transfusion reaction (AHTR) due to ABO incompatibility

● **T80.311** **ABO incompatibility with delayed hemolytic transfusion reaction**
  ABO incompatibility with hemolytic transfusion reaction 24 hours or more after transfusion
  Delayed hemolytic transfusion reaction (DHTR) due to ABO incompatibility

● **T80.319** **ABO incompatibility with hemolytic transfusion reaction, unspecified**
  ABO incompatibility with hemolytic transfusion reaction at unspecified time after transfusion
  Hemolytic transfusion reaction (HTR) due to ABO incompatibility NOS

X● **T80.39** **Other ABO incompatibility reaction due to transfusion of blood or blood products**
  Delayed serologic transfusion reaction (DSTR) from ABO incompatibility
  Other ABO incompatible blood transfusion
  Other reaction to ABO incompatible blood transfusion

● **T80.4** **Rh incompatibility reaction due to transfusion of blood or blood products**
  Reaction due to incompatibility of Rh antigens (C) (c) (D) (E) (e)

X● **T80.40** **Rh incompatibility reaction due to transfusion of blood or blood products, unspecified**
  Reaction due to Rh factor in transfusion NOS
  Rh incompatible blood transfusion NOS

● **T80.41** **Rh incompatibility with hemolytic transfusion reaction**

● **T80.410** **Rh incompatibility with acute hemolytic transfusion reaction**
  Acute hemolytic transfusion reaction (AHTR) due to Rh incompatibility
  Rh incompatibility with hemolytic transfusion reaction less than 24 hours after transfusion

● **T80.411** **Rh incompatibility with delayed hemolytic transfusion reaction**
  Delayed hemolytic transfusion reaction (DHTR) due to Rh incompatibility
  Rh incompatibility with hemolytic transfusion reaction 24 hours or more after transfusion

● **T80.419** **Rh incompatibility with hemolytic transfusion reaction, unspecified**
  Rh incompatibility with hemolytic transfusion reaction at unspecified time after transfusion
  Hemolytic transfusion reaction (HTR) due to Rh incompatibility NOS

X● **T80.49** **Other Rh incompatibility reaction due to transfusion of blood or blood products**
  Delayed serologic transfusion reaction (DSTR) from Rh incompatibility
  Other reaction to Rh incompatible blood transfusion

▶ New   ⇒ Revised   ~~deleted~~ Deleted   Excludes 1   Excludes 2   Includes   Use additional   Code first   Code also   Key words
OGCR Official Guidelines   X Assign placeholder X   ● Use Additional Character(s)   ▶ Manifestation Code   🐾 Hierarchical Condition Category   Coding Clinic

● **T80.A   Non-ABO incompatibility reaction due to transfusion of blood or blood products**
Reaction due to incompatibility of minor antigens (Duffy) (Kell) (Kidd) (Lewis) (M) (N) (P) (S)

X● **T80.A0   Non-ABO incompatibility reaction due to transfusion of blood or blood products, unspecified**
Non-ABO antigen incompatibility reaction from transfusion NOS

● **T80.A1   Non-ABO incompatibility with hemolytic transfusion reaction**

● **T80.A10   Non-ABO incompatibility with acute hemolytic transfusion reaction**
Acute hemolytic transfusion reaction (AHTR) due to non-ABO incompatibility
Non-ABO incompatibility with hemolytic transfusion reaction less than 24 hours after transfusion

● **T80.A11   Non-ABO incompatibility with delayed hemolytic transfusion reaction**
Delayed hemolytic transfusion reaction (DHTR) due to non-ABO incompatibility
Non-ABO incompatibility with hemolytic transfusion reaction 24 or more hours after transfusion

● **T80.A19   Non-ABO incompatibility with hemolytic transfusion reaction, unspecified**
Hemolytic transfusion reaction (HTR) due to non-ABO incompatibility NOS
Non-ABO incompatibility with hemolytic transfusion reaction at unspecified time after transfusion

X● **T80.A9   Other non-ABO incompatibility reaction due to transfusion of blood or blood products**
Delayed serologic transfusion reaction (DSTR) from non-ABO incompatibility
Other reaction to non-ABO incompatible blood transfusion

● **T80.5   Anaphylactic reaction due to serum**
Allergic reaction due to serum
Anaphylactic shock due to serum
Anaphylactoid reaction due to serum
Anaphylaxis due to serum

Excludes1   ABO incompatibility reaction due to transfusion of blood or blood products (T80.3-)
allergic reaction or shock NOS (T78.2)
anaphylactic reaction or shock NOS (T78.2)
anaphylactic reaction or shock due to adverse effect of correct medicinal substance properly administered (T88.6)
other serum reaction (T80.6-)

X● **T80.51   Anaphylactic reaction due to administration of blood and blood products**

X● **T80.52   Anaphylactic reaction due to vaccination**
Coding Clinic: 2021, Q1, P43

X● **T80.59   Anaphylactic reaction due to other serum**

● **T80.6   Other serum reactions**
Intoxication by serum   Serum sickness
Protein sickness   Serum urticaria
Serum rash

Excludes2   serum hepatitis (B16-B19)

X● **T80.61   Other serum reaction due to administration of blood and blood products**

X● **T80.62   Other serum reaction due to vaccination**
Coding Clinic: 2021, Q1, P42

X● **T80.69   Other serum reaction due to other serum**
Code also, if applicable, arthropathy in hypersensitivity reactions classified elsewhere (M36.4)

● **T80.8   Other complications following infusion, transfusion and therapeutic injection**

● **T80.81   Extravasation of vesicant agent**
Infiltration of vesicant agent

● **T80.810   Extravasation of vesicant antineoplastic chemotherapy**
Infiltration of vesicant antineoplastic chemotherapy

● **T80.818   Extravasation of other vesicant agent**
Infiltration of other vesicant agent

T80.82 Complication of immune effector cellular therapy
Complication of chimeric antigen receptor (CAR-T) cell therapy
Complication of IEC therapy

Excludes2   complication of bone marrow transplant (T86.0)
complication of stem cell transplant (T86.5)

Use additional code to identify the specific complication, such as:
cytokine release syndrome (D89.83-)
immune effector cell-associated neurotoxicity syndrome (G92.0-)

X● **T80.89   Other complications following infusion, transfusion and therapeutic injection**
Delayed serologic transfusion reaction (DSTR), unspecified incompatibility
Use additional code to identify graft-versus-host reaction, if applicable, (D89.81-)

● **T80.9   Unspecified complication following infusion, transfusion and therapeutic injection**

X● **T80.90   Unspecified complication following infusion and therapeutic injection**

● **T80.91   Hemolytic transfusion reaction, unspecified incompatibility**

Excludes1   ABO incompatibility with hemolytic transfusion reaction (T80.31-)
Non-ABO incompatibility with hemolytic transfusion reaction (T80.A1-)
Rh incompatibility with hemolytic transfusion reaction (T80.41-)

● **T80.910   Acute hemolytic transfusion reaction, unspecified incompatibility**

● **T80.911   Delayed hemolytic transfusion reaction, unspecified incompatibility**

● **T80.919   Hemolytic transfusion reaction, unspecified incompatibility, unspecified as acute or delayed**
Hemolytic transfusion reaction NOS

X● **T80.92   Unspecified transfusion reaction**
Transfusion reaction NOS

CHAPTER 19 (S00-T88)

● T81   Complications of procedures, not elsewhere classified

Use additional code for adverse effect, if applicable, to identify drug (T36-T50 with fifth or sixth character 5)

Excludes2   complications following immunization (T88.0-T88.1)

complications following infusion, transfusion and therapeutic injection (T80.-)

complications of transplanted organs and tissue (T86.-)

poisoning and toxic effects of drugs and chemicals (T36-T65 with fifth or sixth character 1-4 or 6)

specified complications classified elsewhere, such as:

complication of prosthetic devices, implants and grafts (T82-T85)

dermatitis due to drugs and medicaments (L23.3, L24.4, L25.1, L27.0-L27.1)

endosseous dental implant failure (M27.6-)

floppy iris syndrome (IFIS) (intraoperative) H21.81

intraoperative and postprocedural complications of specific body system (D78.-, E36.-, E89.-, G97.3-, G97.4, H59.3-, H59.-, H95.2-, H95.3, I97.4-, I97.5, J95, K91.-, L76.-, M96.-, N99.-)

ostomy complications (J95.0-, K94.-, N99.5-)

plateau iris syndrome (post-iridectomy) (postprocedural) H21.82

Coding Clinic: 2019, Q2, P21-22; 2016, Q4, P29

The appropriate 7th character is to be added to each code from category T81

> A   initial encounter
> D   subsequent encounter
> S   sequela

● T81.1   Postprocedural shock

Shock during or resulting from a procedure, not elsewhere classified

Excludes1   anaphylactic shock NOS (T78.2)

anaphylactic shock due to correct substance properly administered (T88.6)

anaphylactic shock due to serum (T80.5-)

electric shock (T75.4)

obstetric shock (O75.1)

septic shock (R65.21)

shock due to anesthesia (T88.2)

shock following abortion or ectopic or molar pregnancy (O00-O07, O08.3)

traumatic shock (T79.4)

X ● T81.10   Postprocedural shock unspecified

Collapse NOS during or resulting from a procedure, not elsewhere classified

Postprocedural failure of peripheral circulation

Postprocedural shock NOS

X ● T81.11   Postprocedural cardiogenic shock A 🐾

X ● T81.12   Postprocedural septic shock A 🐾

Postprocedural endotoxic shock resulting from a procedure, not elsewhere classified

Postprocedural gram-negative shock resulting from a procedure, not elsewhere classified

Code first underlying infection

Use additional code, to identify any associated acute organ dysfunction, if applicable

X ● T81.19   Other postprocedural shock

Postprocedural hypovolemic shock

Coding Clinic: 2021, Q1, P14

● T81.3   Disruption of wound, not elsewhere classified

Disruption of any suture materials or other closure methods

Excludes1   breakdown (mechanical) of permanent sutures (T85.612)

displacement of permanent sutures (T85.622)

disruption of cesarean delivery wound (O90.0)

disruption of perineal obstetric wound (O90.1)

mechanical complication of permanent sutures NEC (T85.692)

X ● T81.30   Disruption of wound, unspecified

Disruption of wound NOS

X ● T81.31   Disruption of external operation (surgical) wound, not elsewhere classified

Excludes1   dehiscence of amputation stump (T87.81)

Dehiscence of operation wound NOS

Disruption of operation wound NOS

Disruption or dehiscence of closure of cornea

Disruption or dehiscence of closure of mucosa

Disruption or dehiscence of closure of skin and subcutaneous tissue

Full-thickness skin disruption or dehiscence

Superficial disruption or dehiscence of operation wound

Coding Clinic: 2015, Q1, P20

X ● T81.32   Disruption of internal operation (surgical) wound, not elsewhere classified

Deep disruption or dehiscence of operation wound NOS

Disruption or dehiscence of closure of internal organ or other internal tissue

Disruption or dehiscence of closure of muscle or muscle flap

Disruption or dehiscence of closure of ribs or rib cage

Disruption or dehiscence of closure of skull or craniotomy

Disruption or dehiscence of closure of sternum or sternotomy

Disruption or dehiscence of closure of tendon or ligament

Disruption or dehiscence of closure of superficial or muscular fascia

Coding Clinic: 2017, Q3, P4

X ● T81.33   Disruption of traumatic injury wound repair

Disruption or dehiscence of closure of traumatic laceration (external) (internal)

● T81.4   Infection following a procedure

Use additional code to identify infection

Use additional code (R65.2-) to identify severe sepsis, if applicable

Excludes2   bleb associated endophthalmitis (H59.4-)

infection due to infusion, transfusion and therapeutic injection (T80.2-)

infection due to prosthetic devices, implants and grafts (T82.6-T82.7, T83.5-T83.6, T84.5-T84.7, T85.7)

obstetric surgical wound infection (O86.0-)

postprocedural fever NOS (R50.82)

postprocedural retroperitoneal abscess (K68.11)

X ● T81.40   Infection following a procedure, unspecified

X ● T81.41   Infection following a procedure, superficial incisional surgical site

Subcutaneous abscess following a procedure

Stitch abscess following a procedure

Coding Clinic: 2018, Q4, P34

X ● T81.42   Infection following a procedure, deep incisional surgical site

Intra-muscular abscess following a procedure

CHAPTER 19 (S00-T88)

X ● **T81.43**   **Infection following a procedure, organ and space surgical site**
     Intra-abdominal abscess following a procedure
     Subphrenic abscess following a procedure

X ● **T81.44**   **Sepsis following a procedure** A 🔄
     Use additional code to identify the sepsis

X ● **T81.49**   **Infection following a procedure, other surgical site**
     Coding Clinic: 2015, Q4, P37

● **T81.5**   **Complications of foreign body accidentally left in body following procedure**

   ● **T81.50**   **Unspecified complication of foreign body accidentally left in body following procedure**

     ● **T81.500**   Unspecified complication of foreign body accidentally left in body following surgical operation

     ● **T81.501**   Unspecified complication of foreign body accidentally left in body following infusion or transfusion

     ● **T81.502**   Unspecified complication of foreign body accidentally left in body following kidney dialysis A, D, S 🔄

     ● **T81.503**   Unspecified complication of foreign body accidentally left in body following injection or immunization

     ● **T81.504**   Unspecified complication of foreign body accidentally left in body following endoscopic examination

     ● **T81.505**   Unspecified complication of foreign body accidentally left in body following heart catheterization

     ● **T81.506**   Unspecified complication of foreign body accidentally left in body following aspiration, puncture or other catheterization

     ● **T81.507**   Unspecified complication of foreign body accidentally left in body following removal of catheter or packing

     ● **T81.508**   Unspecified complication of foreign body accidentally left in body following other procedure

     ● **T81.509**   Unspecified complication of foreign body accidentally left in body following unspecified procedure

   ● **T81.51**   **Adhesions due to foreign body accidentally left in body following procedure**

     ● **T81.510**   Adhesions due to foreign body accidentally left in body following surgical operation

     ● **T81.511**   Adhesions due to foreign body accidentally left in body following infusion or transfusion

     ● **T81.512**   Adhesions due to foreign body accidentally left in body following kidney dialysis A, D, S 🔄

     ● **T81.513**   Adhesions due to foreign body accidentally left in body following injection or immunization

     ● **T81.514**   Adhesions due to foreign body accidentally left in body following endoscopic examination

     ● **T81.515**   Adhesions due to foreign body accidentally left in body following heart catheterization

     ● **T81.516**   Adhesions due to foreign body accidentally left in body following aspiration, puncture or other catheterization

     ● **T81.517**   Adhesions due to foreign body accidentally left in body following removal of catheter or packing

     ● **T81.518**   Adhesions due to foreign body accidentally left in body following other procedure

     ● **T81.519**   Adhesions due to foreign body accidentally left in body following unspecified procedure

   ● **T81.52**   **Obstruction due to foreign body accidentally left in body following procedure**

     ● **T81.520**   Obstruction due to foreign body accidentally left in body following surgical operation

     ● **T81.521**   Obstruction due to foreign body accidentally left in body following infusion or transfusion

     ● **T81.522**   Obstruction due to foreign body accidentally left in body following kidney dialysis A, D, S 🔄

     ● **T81.523**   Obstruction due to foreign body accidentally left in body following injection or immunization

     ● **T81.524**   Obstruction due to foreign body accidentally left in body following endoscopic examination

     ● **T81.525**   Obstruction due to foreign body accidentally left in body following heart catheterization

     ● **T81.526**   Obstruction due to foreign body accidentally left in body following aspiration, puncture or other catheterization

     ● **T81.527**   Obstruction due to foreign body accidentally left in body following removal of catheter or packing

     ● **T81.528**   Obstruction due to foreign body accidentally left in body following other procedure

     ● **T81.529**   Obstruction due to foreign body accidentally left in body following unspecified procedure

   ● **T81.53**   **Perforation due to foreign body accidentally left in body following procedure**

     ● **T81.530**   Perforation due to foreign body accidentally left in body following surgical operation

     ● **T81.531**   Perforation due to foreign body accidentally left in body following infusion or transfusion

     ● **T81.532**   Perforation due to foreign body accidentally left in body following kidney dialysis A, D, S 🔄

     ● **T81.533**   Perforation due to foreign body accidentally left in body following injection or immunization

     ● **T81.534**   Perforation due to foreign body accidentally left in body following endoscopic examination

     ● **T81.535**   Perforation due to foreign body accidentally left in body following heart catheterization

     ● **T81.536**   Perforation due to foreign body accidentally left in body following aspiration, puncture or other catheterization

     ● **T81.537**   Perforation due to foreign body accidentally left in body following removal of catheter or packing

     ● **T81.538**   Perforation due to foreign body accidentally left in body following other procedure

     ● **T81.539**   Perforation due to foreign body accidentally left in body following unspecified procedure

CHAPTER 19 (S00-T88)

● T81.59   Other complications of foreign body accidentally left in body following procedure

> **Excludes2**   obstruction or perforation due to prosthetic devices and implants intentionally left in body (T82.0-T82.5, T83.0-T83.4, T83.7, T84.0-T84.4, T85.0-T85.6)

● T81.590   Other complications of foreign body accidentally left in body following surgical operation

● T81.591   Other complications of foreign body accidentally left in body following infusion or transfusion

● T81.592   Other complications of foreign body accidentally left in body following kidney dialysis A, D, S 🅒

● T81.593   Other complications of foreign body accidentally left in body following injection or immunization

● T81.594   Other complications of foreign body accidentally left in body following endoscopic examination

● T81.595   Other complications of foreign body accidentally left in body following heart catheterization

● T81.596   Other complications of foreign body accidentally left in body following aspiration, puncture or other catheterization

● T81.597   Other complications of foreign body accidentally left in body following removal of catheter or packing

● T81.598   Other complications of foreign body accidentally left in body following other procedure

● T81.599   Other complications of foreign body accidentally left in body following unspecified procedure

● T81.6   Acute reaction to foreign substance accidentally left during a procedure

> **Excludes2**   complications of foreign body accidentally left in body cavity or operation wound following procedure (T81.5-)

X ● T81.60   Unspecified acute reaction to foreign substance accidentally left during a procedure

X ● T81.61   Aseptic peritonitis due to foreign substance accidentally left during a procedure
    Chemical peritonitis

X ● T81.69   Other acute reaction to foreign substance accidentally left during a procedure

● T81.7   Vascular complications following a procedure, not elsewhere classified
    Air embolism following procedure NEC
    Phlebitis or thrombophlebitis resulting from a procedure

> **Excludes1**   embolism complicating abortion or ectopic or molar pregnancy (O00-O07, O08.2)
    embolism complicating pregnancy, childbirth and the puerperium (O88.-)
    traumatic embolism (T79.0)

> **Excludes2**   embolism due to prosthetic devices, implants and grafts (T82.8, T83.81, T84.8-, T85.1-)
    embolism following infusion, transfusion and therapeutic injection (T80.0)

    Coding Clinic: 2019, Q2, P23

● T81.71   Complication of artery following a procedure, not elsewhere classified
    Coding Clinic: 2019, Q2, P22

● T81.710   Complication of mesenteric artery following a procedure, not elsewhere classified

● T81.711   Complication of renal artery following a procedure, not elsewhere classified

● T81.718   Complication of other artery following a procedure, not elsewhere classified
    Coding Clinic: 2019, Q2, P22-23

● T81.719   Complication of unspecified artery following a procedure, not elsewhere classified

X ● T81.72   Complication of vein following a procedure, not elsewhere classified
    Coding Clinic: 2019, Q2, P22

● T81.8   Other complications of procedures, not elsewhere classified

> **Excludes2**   hypothermia following anesthesia (T88.51)
    malignant hyperpyrexia due to anesthesia (T88.3)

X ● T81.81   Complication of inhalation therapy

X ● T81.82   Emphysema (subcutaneous) resulting from a procedure

X ● T81.83   Persistent postprocedural fistula
    Coding Clinic: 2017, Q3, P3-5

X ● T81.89   Other complications of procedures, not elsewhere classified
    Use additional code to specify complication, such as:
    postprocedural delirium (F05)

X ● T81.9   Unspecified complication of procedure

● T82   Complications of cardiac and vascular prosthetic devices, implants and grafts

> **Excludes2**   failure and rejection of transplanted organs and tissue (T86.-)

The appropriate 7th character is to be added to each code from category T82

> | A | initial encounter |
> |---|---|
> | D | subsequent encounter |
> | S | sequela |

● T82.0   Mechanical complication of heart valve prosthesis
    Mechanical complication of artificial heart valve

> **Excludes1**   mechanical complication of biological heart valve graft (T82.22-)

X ● T82.01   Breakdown (mechanical) of heart valve prosthesis

X ● T82.02   Displacement of heart valve prosthesis
    Malposition of heart valve prosthesis

X ● T82.03   Leakage of heart valve prosthesis

X ● T82.09   Other mechanical complication of heart valve prosthesis
    Obstruction (mechanical) of heart valve prosthesis
    Perforation of heart valve prosthesis
    Protrusion of heart valve prosthesis

● T82.1   Mechanical complication of cardiac electronic device

● T82.11   Breakdown (mechanical) of cardiac electronic device

● T82.110   Breakdown (mechanical) of cardiac electrode

● T82.111   Breakdown (mechanical) of cardiac pulse generator (battery)

● T82.118   Breakdown (mechanical) of other cardiac electronic device

● T82.119   Breakdown (mechanical) of unspecified cardiac electronic device

● T82.12   Displacement of cardiac electronic device
Malposition of cardiac electronic device

● T82.120   Displacement of cardiac electrode

● T82.121   Displacement of cardiac pulse generator (battery)

● T82.128   Displacement of other cardiac electronic device

● T82.129   Displacement of unspecified cardiac electronic device

● T82.19   Other mechanical complication of cardiac electronic device
Leakage of cardiac electronic device
Obstruction of cardiac electronic device
Perforation of cardiac electronic device
Protrusion of cardiac electronic device

● T82.190   Other mechanical complication of cardiac electrode

● T82.191   Other mechanical complication of cardiac pulse generator (battery)

● T82.198   Other mechanical complication of other cardiac electronic device

● T82.199   Other mechanical complication of unspecified cardiac device

● T82.2   Mechanical complication of coronary artery bypass graft and biological heart valve graft
Excludes1   mechanical complication of artificial heart valve prosthesis (T82.0-)

● T82.21   Mechanical complication of coronary artery bypass graft

● T82.211   Breakdown (mechanical) of coronary artery bypass graft

● T82.212   Displacement of coronary artery bypass graft
Malposition of coronary artery bypass graft

● T82.213   Leakage of coronary artery bypass graft

● T82.218   Other mechanical complication of coronary artery bypass graft
Obstruction, mechanical of coronary artery bypass graft
Perforation of coronary artery bypass graft
Protrusion of coronary artery bypass graft

● T82.22   Mechanical complication of biological heart valve graft

● T82.221   Breakdown (mechanical) of biological heart valve graft

● T82.222   Displacement of biological heart valve graft
Malposition of biological heart valve graft

● T82.223   Leakage of biological heart valve graft

● T82.228   Other mechanical complication of biological heart valve graft
Obstruction of biological heart valve graft
Perforation of biological heart valve graft
Protrusion of biological heart valve graft

● T82.3   Mechanical complication of other vascular grafts

● T82.31   Breakdown (mechanical) of other vascular grafts

● T82.310   Breakdown (mechanical) of aortic (bifurcation) graft (replacement) A 🐾

● T82.311   Breakdown (mechanical) of carotid arterial graft (bypass) A 🐾

● T82.312   Breakdown (mechanical) of femoral arterial graft (bypass) A 🐾

● T82.318   Breakdown (mechanical) of other vascular grafts A 🐾

● T82.319   Breakdown (mechanical) of unspecified vascular grafts A 🐾

● T82.32   Displacement of other vascular grafts
Malposition of other vascular grafts

● T82.320   Displacement of aortic (bifurcation) graft (replacement) A 🐾

● T82.321   Displacement of carotid arterial graft (bypass) A 🐾

● T82.322   Displacement of femoral arterial graft (bypass) A 🐾

● T82.328   Displacement of other vascular grafts A 🐾

● T82.329   Displacement of unspecified vascular grafts A 🐾

● T82.33   Leakage of other vascular grafts

● T82.330   Leakage of aortic (bifurcation) graft (replacement) A 🐾

● T82.331   Leakage of carotid arterial graft (bypass) A 🐾

● T82.332   Leakage of femoral arterial graft (bypass) A 🐾

● T82.338   Leakage of other vascular grafts A 🐾

● T82.339   Leakage of unspecified vascular graft A 🐾

● T82.39   Other mechanical complication of other vascular grafts
Obstruction (mechanical) of other vascular grafts
Perforation of other vascular grafts
Protrusion of other vascular grafts

● T82.390   Other mechanical complication of aortic (bifurcation) graft (replacement) A 🐾

● T82.391   Other mechanical complication of carotid arterial graft (bypass) A 🐾

● T82.392   Other mechanical complication of femoral arterial graft (bypass) A 🐾

● T82.398   Other mechanical complication of other vascular grafts A 🐾

● T82.399   Other mechanical complication of unspecified vascular grafts A 🐾

● T82.4   Mechanical complication of vascular dialysis catheter
Mechanical complication of hemodialysis catheter
Excludes1   mechanical complication of intraperitoneal dialysis catheter (T85.62)

X ● T82.41   Breakdown (mechanical) of vascular dialysis catheter A, D, S

X ● T82.42   Displacement of vascular dialysis catheter A, D, S 🐾
Malposition of vascular dialysis catheter

X ● T82.43   Leakage of vascular dialysis catheter A, D, S 🐾

X ● T82.49   Other complication of vascular dialysis catheter A, D, S 🐾
Obstruction (mechanical) of vascular dialysis catheter
Perforation of vascular dialysis catheter
Protrusion of vascular dialysis catheter

CHAPTER 19 (SØØ-T88)

● **T82.5   Mechanical complication of other cardiac and vascular devices and implants**

    Excludes2 mechanical complication of epidural and subdural infusion catheter (T85.61)

  ● **T82.51   Breakdown (mechanical) of other cardiac and vascular devices and implants**

    ● **T82.510** Breakdown (mechanical) of surgically created arteriovenous fistula A 🐾

    ● **T82.511** Breakdown (mechanical) of surgically created arteriovenous shunt A 🐾

    ● **T82.512** Breakdown (mechanical) of artificial heart

    ● **T82.513** Breakdown (mechanical) of balloon (counterpulsation) device A 🐾

    ● **T82.514** Breakdown (mechanical) of infusion catheter A 🐾

    ● **T82.515** Breakdown (mechanical) of umbrella device A 🐾

    ● **T82.518** Breakdown (mechanical) of other cardiac and vascular devices and implants A 🐾

    ● **T82.519** Breakdown (mechanical) of unspecified cardiac and vascular devices and implants

  ● **T82.52   Displacement of other cardiac and vascular devices and implants**

    Malposition of other cardiac and vascular devices and implants

    ● **T82.520** Displacement of surgically created arteriovenous fistula A 🐾

    ● **T82.521** Displacement of surgically created arteriovenous shunt A 🐾

    ● **T82.522** Displacement of artificial heart

    ● **T82.523** Displacement of balloon (counterpulsation) device A 🐾

    ● **T82.524** Displacement of infusion catheter A 🐾
        Coding Clinic: 2019, Q3, P15

    ● **T82.525** Displacement of umbrella device A 🐾

    ● **T82.528** Displacement of other cardiac and vascular devices and implants A 🐾

    ● **T82.529** Displacement of unspecified cardiac and vascular devices and implants

  ● **T82.53   Leakage of other cardiac and vascular devices and implants**

    ● **T82.530** Leakage of surgically created arteriovenous fistula A 🐾

    ● **T82.531** Leakage of surgically created arteriovenous shunt A 🐾

    ● **T82.532** Leakage of artificial heart

    ● **T82.533** Leakage of balloon (counterpulsation) device A 🐾

    ● **T82.534** Leakage of infusion catheter A 🐾

    ● **T82.535** Leakage of umbrella device A 🐾

    ● **T82.538** Leakage of other cardiac and vascular devices and implants A 🐾

    ● **T82.539** Leakage of unspecified cardiac and vascular devices and implants

  ● **T82.59   Other mechanical complication of other cardiac and vascular devices and implants**

    Obstruction (mechanical) of other cardiac and vascular devices and implants

    Perforation of other cardiac and vascular devices and implants

    Protrusion of other cardiac and vascular devices and implants

    ● **T82.590** Other mechanical complication of surgically created arteriovenous fistula A 🐾

    ● **T82.591** Other mechanical complication of surgically created arteriovenous shunt A 🐾

    ● **T82.592** Other mechanical complication of artificial heart

    ● **T82.593** Other mechanical complication of balloon (counterpulsation) device A 🐾

    ● **T82.594** Other mechanical complication of infusion catheter A 🐾

    ● **T82.595** Other mechanical complication of umbrella device A 🐾

    ● **T82.598** Other mechanical complication of other cardiac and vascular devices and implants A 🐾

    ● **T82.599** Other mechanical complication of unspecified cardiac and vascular devices and implants

X ● **T82.6   Infection and inflammatory reaction due to cardiac valve prosthesis A 🐾**

    Use additional code to identify infection

X ● **T82.7   Infection and inflammatory reaction due to other cardiac and vascular devices, implants and grafts A 🐾**

    Use additional code to identify infection
    Coding Clinic: 2019, Q1, P13-14; 2018, Q4, P89

● **T82.8   Other specified complications of cardiac and vascular prosthetic devices, implants and grafts**

  ● **T82.81   Embolism due to cardiac and vascular prosthetic devices, implants and grafts**
    Coding Clinic: 2016, Q4, P70

    ● **T82.817** Embolism due to cardiac prosthetic devices, implants and grafts
        Coding Clinic: 2016, Q4, P70; 2015, Q1, P20

    ● **T82.818** Embolism due to vascular prosthetic devices, implants and grafts A 🐾

  ◐ **T82.82   Fibrosis due to cardiac and vascular prosthetic devices, implants and grafts**
    Coding Clinic: 2016, Q4, P70

    ● **T82.827** Fibrosis due to cardiac prosthetic devices, implants and grafts

    ● **T82.828** Fibrosis due to vascular prosthetic devices, implants and grafts A 🐾

  ● **T82.83   Hemorrhage due to cardiac and vascular prosthetic devices, implants and grafts**
    Coding Clinic: 2016, Q4, P70

    ● **T82.837** Hemorrhage due to cardiac prosthetic devices, implants and grafts

    ● **T82.838** Hemorrhage due to vascular prosthetic devices, implants and grafts A 🐾

  ● **T82.84   Pain due to cardiac and vascular prosthetic devices, implants and grafts**
    Coding Clinic: 2016, Q4, P70

    ● **T82.847** Pain due to cardiac prosthetic devices, implants and grafts

    ● **T82.848** Pain due to vascular prosthetic devices, implants and grafts A 🐾

  ● **T82.85   Stenosis due to cardiac and vascular prosthetic devices, implants and grafts**

    ● **T82.855** Stenosis of coronary artery stent
        In-stent stenosis (restenosis) of coronary artery stent
        Restenosis of coronary artery stent
        Coding Clinic: 2021, Q3, P6-7; 2016, Q4, P70

    ● **T82.856** Stenosis of peripheral vascular stent A 🐾
        In-stent stenosis (restenosis) of peripheral vascular stent
        Restenosis of peripheral vascular stent
        Coding Clinic: 2016, Q4, P70

CHAPTER 19 (S00-T88)

▶ New   ⇒ Revised   ~~deleted~~ Deleted   Excludes 1   Excludes 2   Includes   Use additional   Code first   Code also   Key words
OGCR Official Guidelines   X Assign placeholder X   ● Use Additional Character(s)   ) Manifestation Code   🐾 Hierarchical Condition Category   **Coding Clinic**

● **T82.857** Stenosis of other cardiac prosthetic devices, implants and grafts
Coding Clinic: 2016, Q4, P70

● **T82.858** Stenosis of other vascular prosthetic devices, implants and grafts A ⬡
Coding Clinic: 2016, Q4, P70

● **T82.86** Thrombosis of cardiac and vascular prosthetic devices, implants and grafts

● **T82.867** Thrombosis due to cardiac prosthetic devices, implants and grafts

● **T82.868** Thrombosis due to vascular prosthetic devices, implants and grafts A ⬡

● **T82.89** Other specified complication of cardiac and vascular prosthetic devices, implants and grafts

● **T82.897** Other specified complication of cardiac prosthetic devices, implants and grafts
Coding Clinic: 2019, Q2, P32-33

● **T82.898** Other specified complication of vascular prosthetic devices, implants and grafts A ⬡

X ● **T82.9** Unspecified complication of cardiac and vascular prosthetic device, implant and graft

● **T83** Complications of genitourinary prosthetic devices, implants and grafts

Excludes2 failure and rejection of transplanted organs and tissue (T86.-)

The appropriate 7th character is to be added to each code from category T83

A	initial encounter
D	subsequent encounter
S	sequela

Coding Clinic: 2016, Q4, P70-71

● **T83.0** Mechanical complication of urinary catheter

Excludes2 complications of stoma of urinary tract (N99.5-)
Coding Clinic: 2016, Q4, P70

● **T83.01** Breakdown (mechanical) of urinary catheter

● **T83.010** Breakdown (mechanical) of cystostomy catheter A ⬡

● **T83.011** Breakdown (mechanical) of indwelling urethral catheter A ⬡

● **T83.012** Breakdown (mechanical) of nephrostomy catheter A ⬡

● **T83.018** Breakdown (mechanical) of other urinary catheter A ⬡
Breakdown (mechanical) of Hopkins catheter
Breakdown (mechanical) of ileostomy catheter
Breakdown (mechanical) urostomy catheter

● **T83.02** Displacement of urinary catheter
Malposition of urinary catheter

● **T83.020** Displacement of cystostomy catheter A ⬡

● **T83.021** Displacement of indwelling urethral catheter A ⬡

● **T83.022** Displacement of nephrostomy catheter A ⬡

● **T83.028** Displacement of other urinary catheter A ⬡
Displacement of Hopkins catheter
Displacement of ileostomy catheter
Displacement of urostomy catheter

● **T83.03** Leakage of urinary catheter

● **T83.030** Leakage of cystostomy catheter A ⬡
Coding Clinic: 2021, Q4, P19

● **T83.031** Leakage of indwelling urethral catheter A ⬡

● **T83.032** Leakage of nephrostomy catheter A ⬡

● **T83.038** Leakage of other urinary catheter A ⬡
Leakage of Hopkins catheter
Leakage of ileostomy catheter
Leakage of urostomy catheter

● **T83.09** Other mechanical complication of urinary catheter
Obstruction (mechanical) of urinary catheter
Perforation of urinary catheter
Protrusion of urinary catheter

● **T83.090** Other mechanical complication of cystostomy catheter A ⬡

● **T83.091** Other mechanical complication of indwelling urethral catheter A ⬡

● **T83.092** Other mechanical complication of nephrostomy catheter A ⬡

● **T83.098** Other mechanical complication of other urinary catheter A ⬡
Other mechanical complication of Hopkins catheter
Other mechanical complication of ileostomy catheter
Other mechanical complication of urostomy catheter

● **T83.1** Mechanical complication of other urinary devices and implants
Coding Clinic: 2016, Q4, P70

● **T83.11** Breakdown (mechanical) of other urinary devices and implants

● **T83.110** Breakdown (mechanical) of urinary electronic stimulator device A ⬡

Excludes2 Breakdown (mechanical) of electrode (lead) for sacral nerve neurostimulator (T85.111)
Breakdown (mechanical) of implanted electronic sacral neurostimulator, pulse generator or receiver (T85.113)

● **T83.111** Breakdown (mechanical) of implanted urinary sphincter A ⬡

● **T83.112** Breakdown (mechanical) of indwelling ureteral stent A ⬡

● **T83.113** Breakdown (mechanical) of other urinary stents A ⬡
Breakdown (mechanical) of ileal conduit stent
Breakdown (mechanical) of nephroureteral stent

● **T83.118** Breakdown (mechanical) of other urinary devices and implants A ⬡

● **T83.12** Displacement of other urinary devices and implants
Malposition of other urinary devices and implants

● **T83.120** Displacement of urinary electronic stimulator device A ⬡

Excludes2 Displacement of electrode (lead) for sacral nerve neurostimulator (T85.121)
Displacement of implanted electronic sacral neurostimulator, pulse generator or receiver (T85.123)

● T83.121   **Displacement of** implanted urinary sphincter A 🦠

● T83.122   **Displacement of** indwelling ureteral stent A 🦠

● T83.123   **Displacement of** other urinary stents A 🦠
     Displacement of ileal conduit stent
     Displacement of nephroureteral stent

● T83.128   **Displacement of** other urinary devices and implants A 🦠

● T83.19   Other mechanical complication of other urinary devices and implants
     Leakage of other urinary devices and implants
     Obstruction (mechanical) of other urinary devices and implants
     Perforation of other urinary devices and implants
     Protrusion of other urinary devices and implants

● T83.190   **Other mechanical complication of urinary** electronic stimulator device A 🦠

     Excludes2   Other mechanical complication of electrode (lead) for sacral nerve neurostimulator (T85.191)
                 Other mechanical complication of implanted electronic sacral neurostimulator, pulse generator or receiver (T85.193)

● T83.191   **Other mechanical complication of** implanted urinary sphincter A 🦠

● T83.192   **Other mechanical complication of** indwelling ureteral stent A 🦠

● T83.193   **Other mechanical complication of other urinary stent** A 🦠
     Other mechanical complication of ileal conduit stent
     Other mechanical complication of nephroureteral stent

● T83.198   **Other mechanical complication of other urinary devices and implants** A 🦠

● T83.2   Mechanical complication of graft of urinary organ
     Coding Clinic: 2016, Q4, P70

X ● T83.21   **Breakdown (mechanical) of graft of urinary organ** A 🦠

X ● T83.22   **Displacement of graft of urinary organ** A 🦠
     Malposition of graft of urinary organ

X ● T83.23   **Leakage of graft of urinary organ** A 🦠

X ● T83.24   **Erosion of graft of urinary organ** A 🦠
     Coding Clinic: 2016, Q4, P70

X ● T83.25   **Exposure of graft of urinary organ** A 🦠
     Coding Clinic: 2016, Q4, P70

X ● T83.29   Other mechanical complication of graft of urinary organ A 🦠
     Obstruction (mechanical) of graft of urinary organ
     Perforation of graft of urinary organ
     Protrusion of graft of urinary organ

● T83.3   Mechanical complication of intrauterine contraceptive device

X ● T83.31   **Breakdown (mechanical) of intrauterine contraceptive device** ♀

X ● T83.32   **Displacement of intrauterine contraceptive device** ♀
     Malposition of intrauterine contraceptive device
     Missing string of intrauterine contraceptive device

X ● T83.39   Other mechanical complication of intrauterine contraceptive device ♀
     Leakage of intrauterine contraceptive device
     Obstruction (mechanical) of intrauterine contraceptive device
     Perforation of intrauterine contraceptive device
     Protrusion of intrauterine contraceptive device

● T83.4   Mechanical complication of other prosthetic devices, implants and grafts of genital tract
     Coding Clinic: 2016, Q4, P71

● T83.41   Breakdown (mechanical) of other prosthetic devices, implants and grafts of genital tract

● T83.410   **Breakdown (mechanical) of implanted penile prosthesis** ♂ A 🦠
     Breakdown (mechanical) of penile prosthesis cylinder
     Breakdown (mechanical) of penile prosthesis pump
     Breakdown (mechanical) of penile prosthesis reservoir

● T83.411   **Breakdown (mechanical) of implanted testicular prosthesis** A 🦠

● T83.418   **Breakdown (mechanical) of other prosthetic devices, implants and grafts of genital tract** A 🦠

● T83.42   Displacement of other prosthetic devices, implants and grafts of genital tract
     Malposition of other prosthetic devices, implants and grafts of genital tract

● T83.420   **Displacement of implanted penile prosthesis** ♂ A 🦠
     Displacement of penile prosthesis cylinder
     Displacement of penile prosthesis pump
     Displacement of penile prosthesis reservoir

● T83.421   **Displacement of implanted testicular prosthesis** A 🦠

● T83.428   **Displacement of other prosthetic devices, implants and grafts of genital tract** A 🦠
     Coding Clinic: 2018, Q1, P6

● T83.49   Other mechanical complication of other prosthetic devices, implants and grafts of genital tract
     Leakage of other prosthetic devices, implants and grafts of genital tract
     Obstruction, mechanical of other prosthetic devices, implants and grafts of genital tract
     Perforation of other prosthetic devices, implants and grafts of genital tract
     Protrusion of other prosthetic devices, implants and grafts of genital tract

● T83.490   **Other mechanical complication of implanted penile prosthesis** ♂ A 🦠
     Other mechanical complication of penile prosthesis cylinder
     Other mechanical complication of penile prosthesis pump
     Other mechanical complication of penile prosthesis reservoir

●T83.491 Other mechanical complication of implanted testicular prosthesis A 🦎

●T83.498 Other mechanical complication of other prosthetic devices, implants and grafts of genital tract A 🦎

●T83.5 Infection and inflammatory reaction due to prosthetic device, implant and graft in urinary system
   Use additional code to identify infection
   Coding Clinic: 2016, Q4, P71

●T83.51 Infection and inflammatory reaction due to urinary catheter
   Excludes2   complications of stoma of urinary tract (N99.5-)

●T83.510 Infection and inflammatory reaction due to cystostomy catheter A 🦎

●T83.511 Infection and inflammatory reaction due to indwelling urethral catheter A 🦎
   Coding Clinic: 2022, Q2, P7

●T83.512 Infection and inflammatory reaction due to nephrostomy catheter A 🦎

●T83.518 Infection and inflammatory reaction due to other urinary catheter A 🦎
   Infection and inflammatory reaction due to Hopkins catheter
   Infection and inflammatory reaction due to ileostomy catheter
   Infection and inflammatory reaction due to urostomy catheter

●T83.59 Infection and inflammatory reaction due to prosthetic device, implant and graft in urinary system

●T83.590 Infection and inflammatory reaction due to implanted urinary neurostimulation device A 🦎
   Excludes2   Infection and inflammatory reaction due to electrode lead of sacral nerve neurostimulator (T85.732)
   Infection and inflammatory reaction due to pulse generator or receiver of sacral nerve neurostimulator (T85.734)

●T83.591 Infection and inflammatory reaction due to implanted urinary sphincter A 🦎

●T83.592 Infection and inflammatory reaction due to indwelling ureteral stent A 🦎

●T83.593 Infection and inflammatory reaction due to other urinary stents A 🦎
   Infection and inflammatory reaction due to ileal conduit stents
   Infection and inflammatory reaction due to nephroureteral stent

●T83.598 Infection and inflammatory reaction due to other prosthetic device, implant and graft in urinary system A 🦎

●T83.6 Infection and inflammatory reaction due to prosthetic device, implant and graft in genital tract
   Use additional code to identify infection
   Coding Clinic: 2016, Q4, P71

●T83.61 Infection and inflammatory reaction due to implanted penile prosthesis A 🦎
   Infection and inflammatory reaction due to penile prosthesis cylinder
   Infection and inflammatory reaction due to penile prosthesis pump
   Infection and inflammatory reaction due to penile prosthesis reservoir

●T83.62 Infection and inflammatory reaction due to implanted testicular prosthesis A 🦎

●T83.69 Infection and inflammatory reaction due to other prosthetic device, implant and graft in genital tract A 🦎

●T83.7 Complications due to implanted mesh and other prosthetic materials
   Coding Clinic: 2016, Q4, P71

●T83.71 Erosion of implanted mesh and other prosthetic materials to surrounding organ or tissue
   Coding Clinic: 2016, Q4, P71

●T83.711 Erosion of implanted vaginal mesh to surrounding organ or tissue ♀ A 🦎
   Erosion of implanted vaginal mesh into pelvic floor muscles
   Coding Clinic: 2016, Q4, P71

●T83.712 Erosion of implanted urethral mesh to surrounding organ or tissue A 🦎
   Erosion of implanted female urethral sling
   Erosion of implanted male urethral sling
   Erosion of implanted urethral mesh into pelvic floor muscles

●T83.713 Erosion of implanted urethral bulking agent to surrounding organ or tissue A 🦎

●T83.714 Erosion of implanted ureteral bulking agent to surrounding organ or tissue A 🦎

●T83.718 Erosion of other implanted mesh to organ or tissue A 🦎
   Coding Clinic: 2016, Q4, P71

●T83.719 Erosion of other prosthetic materials to surrounding organ or tissue A 🦎
   Coding Clinic: 2016, Q4, P71

●T83.72 Exposure of implanted mesh and other prosthetic materials into surrounding organ or tissue
   Extrusion of implanted mesh
   Coding Clinic: 2016, Q4, P71

●T83.721 Exposure of implanted vaginal mesh into vagina ♀ A 🦎
   Exposure of implanted vaginal mesh through vaginal wall

●T83.722 Exposure of implanted urethral mesh into urethra A 🦎
   Exposure of implanted female urethral sling
   Exposure of implanted male urethral sling
   Exposure of implanted urethral mesh through urethral wall

●T83.723 Exposure of implanted urethral bulking agent into urethra A 🦎

CHAPTER 19 (S00–T88)

- T83.724   Exposure of implanted ureteral bulking agent into ureter A ⬡
- T83.728   Exposure of other implanted mesh into organ or tissue A ⬡
  - Coding Clinic: 2016, Q4, P71
- T83.729   Exposure of other prosthetic materials into organ or tissue A ⬡
  - Coding Clinic: 2016, Q4, P71
- X● T83.79   Other specified complications due to other genitourinary prosthetic materials A ⬡
- T83.8   Other specified complications of genitourinary prosthetic devices, implants and grafts
  - X● T83.81   Embolism due to genitourinary prosthetic devices, implants and grafts A ⬡
  - X● T83.82   Fibrosis due to genitourinary prosthetic devices, implants and grafts A ⬡
  - X● T83.83   Hemorrhage due to genitourinary prosthetic devices, implants and grafts A ⬡
  - X● T83.84   Pain due to genitourinary prosthetic devices, implants and grafts A ⬡
  - X● T83.85   Stenosis due to genitourinary prosthetic devices, implants and grafts A ⬡
  - X● T83.86   Thrombosis due to genitourinary prosthetic devices, implants and grafts A ⬡
  - X● T83.89   Other specified complication of genitourinary prosthetic devices, implants and grafts A ⬡
- X● T83.9   Unspecified complication of genitourinary prosthetic device, implant and graft A ⬡

● T84   Complications of internal orthopedic prosthetic devices, implants and grafts
  - **Excludes2**   failure and rejection of transplanted organs and tissues (T86.-)
    - fracture of bone following insertion of orthopedic implant, joint prosthesis or bone plate (M96.6)
  - The appropriate 7th character is to be added to each code from category T84

A	initial encounter
D	subsequent encounter
S	sequela

- T84.0   Mechanical complication of internal joint prosthesis
  - T84.01   Broken internal joint prosthesis
    - Breakage (fracture) of prosthetic joint
    - Broken prosthetic joint implant
    - **Excludes1**   periprosthetic joint implant fracture (M97.-)
    - Coding Clinic: 2016, Q4, P42
    - T84.010   Broken internal right hip prosthesis A ⬡
    - T84.011   Broken internal left hip prosthesis A ⬡
    - T84.012   Broken internal right knee prosthesis A ⬡
    - T84.013   Broken internal left knee prosthesis A ⬡
    - T84.018   Broken internal joint prosthesis, other site A ⬡
      - Use additional code to identify the joint (Z96.6-)
    - T84.019   Broken internal joint prosthesis, unspecified site A ⬡
  - T84.02   Dislocation of internal joint prosthesis
    - Instability of internal joint prosthesis
    - Subluxation of internal joint prosthesis
    - T84.020   Dislocation of internal right hip prosthesis A ⬡
    - T84.021   Dislocation of internal left hip prosthesis A ⬡
      - Coding Clinic: 2019, Q2, P27
    - T84.022   Instability of internal right knee prosthesis A ⬡

- T84.023   Instability of internal left knee prosthesis A ⬡
- T84.028   Dislocation of other internal joint prosthesis A ⬡
  - Use additional code to identify the joint (Z96.6-)
- T84.029   Dislocation of unspecified internal joint prosthesis A ⬡
- T84.03   Mechanical loosening of internal prosthetic joint
  - Aseptic loosening of prosthetic joint
  - T84.030   Mechanical loosening of internal right hip prosthetic joint A ⬡
  - T84.031   Mechanical loosening of internal left hip prosthetic joint A ⬡
  - T84.032   Mechanical loosening of internal right knee prosthetic joint A ⬡
  - T84.033   Mechanical loosening of internal left knee prosthetic joint A ⬡
  - T84.038   Mechanical loosening of other internal prosthetic joint A ⬡
    - Use additional code to identify the joint (Z96.6-)
  - T84.039   Mechanical loosening of unspecified internal prosthetic joint A ⬡
- T84.05   Periprosthetic osteolysis of internal prosthetic joint
  - Use additional code to identify major osseous defect, if applicable (M89.7-)
  - T84.050   Periprosthetic osteolysis of internal prosthetic right hip joint A ⬡
  - T84.051   Periprosthetic osteolysis of internal prosthetic left hip joint A ⬡
  - T84.052   Periprosthetic osteolysis of internal prosthetic right knee joint A ⬡
  - T84.053   Periprosthetic osteolysis of internal prosthetic left knee joint A ⬡
  - T84.058   Periprosthetic osteolysis of other internal prosthetic joint A ⬡
    - Use additional code to identify the joint (Z96.6-)
  - T84.059   Periprosthetic osteolysis of unspecified internal prosthetic joint A ⬡
- T84.06   Wear of articular bearing surface of internal prosthetic joint
  - T84.060   Wear of articular bearing surface of internal prosthetic right hip joint A ⬡
  - T84.061   Wear of articular bearing surface of internal prosthetic left hip joint A ⬡
  - T84.062   Wear of articular bearing surface of internal prosthetic right knee joint A ⬡
  - T84.063   Wear of articular bearing surface of internal prosthetic left knee joint A ⬡
  - T84.068   Wear of articular bearing surface of other internal prosthetic joint A ⬡
    - Use additional code to identify the joint (Z96.6-)
  - T84.069   Wear of articular bearing surface of unspecified internal prosthetic joint A ⬡
- T84.09   Other mechanical complication of internal joint prosthesis
  - Prosthetic joint implant failure NOS
  - T84.090   Other mechanical complication of internal right hip prosthesis A ⬡
    - Coding Clinic: 2019, Q1, P20
  - T84.091   Other mechanical complication of internal left hip prosthesis A ⬡
  - T84.092   Other mechanical complication of internal right knee prosthesis A ⬡

● T84.093   Other mechanical complication of internal left knee prosthesis A 🔖

● T84.098   Other mechanical complication of other internal joint prosthesis A 🔖

      Use additional code to identify the joint (Z96.6-)

● T84.099   Other mechanical complication of unspecified internal joint prosthesis A 🔖

● T84.1   Mechanical complication of internal fixation device of bones of limb

    Excludes2   mechanical complication of internal fixation device of bones of feet (T84.2-)

                  mechanical complication of internal fixation device of bones of fingers (T84.2-)

                  mechanical complication of internal fixation device of bones of hands (T84.2-)

                  mechanical complication of internal fixation device of bones of toes (T84.2-)

● T84.11   Breakdown (mechanical) of internal fixation device of bones of limb

   ● T84.110   Breakdown (mechanical) of internal fixation device of right humerus A 🔖

   ● T84.111   Breakdown (mechanical) of internal fixation device of left humerus A 🔖

   ● T84.112   Breakdown (mechanical) of internal fixation device of bone of right forearm A 🔖

   ● T84.113   Breakdown (mechanical) of internal fixation device of bone of left forearm A 🔖

   ● T84.114   Breakdown (mechanical) of internal fixation device of right femur A 🔖

   ● T84.115   Breakdown (mechanical) of internal fixation device of left femur A 🔖

   ● T84.116   Breakdown (mechanical) of internal fixation device of bone of right lower leg A 🔖

   ● T84.117   Breakdown (mechanical) of internal fixation device of bone of left lower leg A 🔖

   ● T84.119   Breakdown (mechanical) of internal fixation device of unspecified bone of limb A 🔖

● T84.12   Displacement of internal fixation device of bones of limb

     Malposition of internal fixation device of bones of limb

   ● T84.120   Displacement of internal fixation device of right humerus A 🔖

   ● T84.121   Displacement of internal fixation device of left humerus A 🔖

   ● T84.122   Displacement of internal fixation device of bone of right forearm A 🔖

   ● T84.123   Displacement of internal fixation device of bone of left forearm A 🔖

   ● T84.124   Displacement of internal fixation device of right femur A 🔖

   ● T84.125   Displacement of internal fixation device of left femur A 🔖

   ● T84.126   Displacement of internal fixation device of bone of right lower leg A 🔖

   ● T84.127   Displacement of internal fixation device of bone of left lower leg A 🔖

   ● T84.129   Displacement of internal fixation device of unspecified bone of limb A 🔖

● T84.19   Other mechanical complication of internal fixation device of bones of limb

     Obstruction (mechanical) of internal fixation device of bones of limb

     Perforation of internal fixation device of bones of limb

     Protrusion of internal fixation device of bones of limb

   ● T84.190   Other mechanical complication of internal fixation device of right humerus A 🔖

   ● T84.191   Other mechanical complication of internal fixation device of left humerus A 🔖

   ● T84.192   Other mechanical complication of internal fixation device of bone of right forearm A 🔖

   ● T84.193   Other mechanical complication of internal fixation device of bone of left forearm A 🔖

   ● T84.194   Other mechanical complication of internal fixation device of right femur A 🔖

   ● T84.195   Other mechanical complication of internal fixation device of left femur A 🔖

   ● T84.196   Other mechanical complication of internal fixation device of bone of right lower leg A 🔖

   ● T84.197   Other mechanical complication of internal fixation device of bone of left lower leg A 🔖

   ● T84.199   Other mechanical complication of internal fixation device of unspecified bone of limb A 🔖

● T84.2   Mechanical complication of internal fixation device of other bones

   ● T84.21   Breakdown (mechanical) of internal fixation device of other bones

     ● T84.210   Breakdown (mechanical) of internal fixation device of bones of hand and fingers A 🔖

     ● T84.213   Breakdown (mechanical) of internal fixation device of bones of foot and toes A 🔖

     ● T84.216   Breakdown (mechanical) of internal fixation device of vertebrae A 🔖

     ● T84.218   Breakdown (mechanical) of internal fixation device of other bones A 🔖

   ● T84.22   Displacement of internal fixation device of other bones

     Malposition of internal fixation device of other bones

     ● T84.220   Displacement of internal fixation device of bones of hand and fingers A 🔖

     ● T84.223   Displacement of internal fixation device of bones of foot and toes A 🔖

     ● T84.226   Displacement of internal fixation device of vertebrae A 🔖

     ● T84.228   Displacement of internal fixation device of other bones A 🔖

   ● T84.29   Other mechanical complication of internal fixation device of other bones

     Obstruction (mechanical) of internal fixation device of other bones

     Perforation of internal fixation device of other bones

     Protrusion of internal fixation device of other bones

     ● T84.290   Other mechanical complication of internal fixation device of bones of hand and fingers A 🔖

CHAPTER 19 (S00-T88)

● T84.293   Other mechanical complication of internal fixation device of bones of foot and toes A 🐾

● T84.296   Other mechanical complication of internal fixation device of vertebrae A 🐾

● T84.298   Other mechanical complication of internal fixation device of other bones A 🐾

● T84.3   Mechanical complication of other bone devices, implants and grafts

   Excludes2   other complications of bone graft (T86.83-)

● T84.31   Breakdown (mechanical) of other bone devices, implants and grafts

● T84.310   Breakdown (mechanical) of electronic bone stimulator A 🐾

● T84.318   Breakdown (mechanical) of other bone devices, implants and grafts A 🐾

● T84.32   Displacement of other bone devices, implants and grafts

    Malposition of other bone devices, implants and grafts

● T84.320   Displacement of electronic bone stimulator A 🐾

● T84.328   Displacement of other bone devices, implants and grafts A 🐾

● T84.39   Other mechanical complication of other bone devices, implants and grafts

    Obstruction (mechanical) of other bone devices, implants and grafts

    Perforation of other bone devices, implants and grafts

    Protrusion of other bone devices, implants and grafts

● T84.390   Other mechanical complication of electronic bone stimulator A 🐾

● T84.398   Other mechanical complication of other bone devices, implants and grafts A 🐾

● T84.4   Mechanical complication of other internal orthopedic devices, implants and grafts

● T84.41   Breakdown (mechanical) of other internal orthopedic devices, implants and grafts

● T84.410   Breakdown (mechanical) of muscle and tendon graft A 🐾

● T84.418   Breakdown (mechanical) of other internal orthopedic devices, implants and grafts A 🐾

● T84.42   Displacement of other internal orthopedic devices, implants and grafts

    Malposition of other internal orthopedic devices, implants and grafts

● T84.420   Displacement of muscle and tendon graft A 🐾

● T84.428   Displacement of other internal orthopedic devices, implants and grafts A 🐾

● T84.49   Other mechanical complication of other internal orthopedic devices, implants and grafts

    Mechanical complication of other internal orthopedic devices, implants and grafts NOS

    Obstruction (mechanical) of other internal orthopedic devices, implants and grafts

    Perforation of other internal orthopedic devices, implants and grafts

    Protrusion of other internal orthopedic devices, implants and grafts

● T84.490   Other mechanical complication of muscle and tendon graft A 🐾

● T84.498   Other mechanical complication of other internal orthopedic devices, implants and grafts A 🐾

● T84.5   Infection and inflammatory reaction due to internal joint prosthesis

    Use additional code to identify infection

    Coding Clinic: 2015, Q1, P16

X ● T84.50   Infection and inflammatory reaction due to unspecified internal joint prosthesis A 🐾
    Coding Clinic: 2015, Q1, P3

X ● T84.51   Infection and inflammatory reaction due to internal right hip prosthesis A 🐾
    Coding Clinic: 2015, Q4, P36

X ● T84.52   Infection and inflammatory reaction due to internal left hip prosthesis A 🐾
    Coding Clinic: 2015, Q1, P16-17

X ● T84.53   Infection and inflammatory reaction due to internal right knee prosthesis A 🐾

X ● T84.54   Infection and inflammatory reaction due to internal left knee prosthesis A 🐾
    Coding Clinic: 2019, Q3, P16

X ● T84.59   Infection and inflammatory reaction due to other internal joint prosthesis A 🐾

● T84.6   Infection and inflammatory reaction due to internal fixation device

    Use additional code to identify infection

X ● T84.60   Infection and inflammatory reaction due to internal fixation device of unspecified site A 🐾

● T84.61   Infection and inflammatory reaction due to internal fixation device of arm

● T84.610   Infection and inflammatory reaction due to internal fixation device of right humerus A 🐾

● T84.611   Infection and inflammatory reaction due to internal fixation device of left humerus A 🐾

● T84.612   Infection and inflammatory reaction due to internal fixation device of right radius A 🐾

● T84.613   Infection and inflammatory reaction due to internal fixation device of left radius A 🐾

● T84.614   Infection and inflammatory reaction due to internal fixation device of right ulna A 🐾

● T84.615   Infection and inflammatory reaction due to internal fixation device of left ulna A 🐾

● T84.619   Infection and inflammatory reaction due to internal fixation device of unspecified bone of arm A 🐾

● T84.62   Infection and inflammatory reaction due to internal fixation device of leg

● T84.620   Infection and inflammatory reaction due to internal fixation device of right femur A 🐾

● T84.621   Infection and inflammatory reaction due to internal fixation device of left femur A 🐾

● T84.622   Infection and inflammatory reaction due to internal fixation device of right tibia A 🐾

● T84.623   Infection and inflammatory reaction due to internal fixation device of left tibia A 🐾

● T84.624   Infection and inflammatory reaction due to internal fixation device of right fibula A 🐾

● T84.625   Infection and inflammatory reaction due to internal fixation device of left fibula A 🐾

● T84.629   Infection and inflammatory reaction due to internal fixation device of unspecified bone of leg A 🐾

X● **T84.63** Infection and inflammatory reaction due to internal fixation device of spine A 🐾

X● **T84.69** Infection and inflammatory reaction due to internal fixation device of other site A 🐾

● **T84.7** Infection and inflammatory reaction due to other internal orthopedic prosthetic devices, implants and grafts A 🐾

Use additional code to identify infection

● **T84.8** Other specified complications of internal orthopedic prosthetic devices, implants and grafts

X● **T84.81** Embolism due to internal orthopedic prosthetic devices, implants and grafts A 🐾

X● **T84.82** Fibrosis due to internal orthopedic prosthetic devices, implants and grafts A 🐾

X● **T84.83** Hemorrhage due to internal orthopedic prosthetic devices, implants and grafts A 🐾

X● **T84.84** Pain due to internal orthopedic prosthetic devices, implants and grafts A 🐾

X● **T84.85** Stenosis due to internal orthopedic prosthetic devices, implants and grafts A 🐾

X● **T84.86** Thrombosis due to internal orthopedic prosthetic devices, implants and grafts A 🐾

X● **T84.89** Other specified complication of internal orthopedic prosthetic devices, implants and grafts A 🐾

X● **T84.9** Unspecified complication of internal orthopedic prosthetic device, implant and graft A 🐾

● **T85** Complications of other internal prosthetic devices, implants and grafts

Excludes2   failure and rejection of transplanted organs and tissue (T86.-)

The appropriate 7th character is to be added to each code from category T85

A	initial encounter
D	subsequent encounter
S	sequela

Coding Clinic: 2016, Q4, P71

● **T85.0** Mechanical complication of ventricular intracranial (communicating) shunt

X● **T85.01** Breakdown (mechanical) of ventricular intracranial (communicating) shunt A 🐾

X● **T85.02** Displacement of ventricular intracranial (communicating) shunt A 🐾
Malposition of ventricular intracranial (communicating) shunt

X● **T85.03** Leakage of ventricular intracranial (communicating) shunt A 🐾

X● **T85.09** Other mechanical complication of ventricular intracranial (communicating) shunt A 🐾
Obstruction (mechanical) of ventricular intracranial (communicating) shunt
Perforation of ventricular intracranial (communicating) shunt
Protrusion of ventricular intracranial (communicating) shunt

● **T85.1** Mechanical complication of implanted electronic stimulator of nervous system
Coding Clinic: 2016, Q4, P71

● **T85.11** Breakdown (mechanical) of implanted electronic stimulator of nervous system

● **T85.110** Breakdown (mechanical) of implanted electronic neurostimulator of brain electrode (lead) A 🐾

● **T85.111** Breakdown (mechanical) of implanted electronic neurostimulator of peripheral nerve electrode (lead) A 🐾
Breakdown of electrode (lead) for cranial nerve neurostimulators
Breakdown of electrode (lead) for gastric neurostimulator
Breakdown of electrode (lead) for sacral nerve neurostimulator
Breakdown of electrode (lead) for vagal nerve neurostimulators

● **T85.112** Breakdown (mechanical) of implanted electronic neurostimulator of spinal cord electrode (lead) A 🐾

● **T85.113** Breakdown (mechanical) of implanted electronic neurostimulator, generator A 🐾
Breakdown (mechanical) of implanted electronic neurostimulator generator, brain, peripheral, gastric, spinal
Breakdown (mechanical) of implanted electronic sacral neurostimulator, pulse generator or receiver

● **T85.118** Breakdown (mechanical) of other implanted electronic stimulator of nervous system A 🐾

● **T85.12** Displacement of implanted electronic stimulator of nervous system
Malposition of implanted electronic stimulator of nervous system

● **T85.120** Displacement of implanted electronic neurostimulator of brain electrode (lead) A 🐾

● **T85.121** Displacement of implanted electronic neurostimulator of peripheral nerve electrode (lead) A 🐾
Displacement of electrode (lead) for cranial nerve neurostimulators
Displacement of electrode (lead) for gastric neurostimulator
Displacement of electrode (lead) for sacral nerve neurostimulator
Displacement of electrode (lead) for vagal nerve neurostimulators

● **T85.122** Displacement of implanted electronic neurostimulator of spinal cord electrode (lead) A 🐾

● **T85.123** Displacement of implanted electronic neurostimulator, generator A 🐾
Displacement of implanted electronic neurostimulator generator, brain, peripheral, gastric, spinal
Displacement of implanted electronic sacral neurostimulator, pulse generator or receiver

● **T85.128** Displacement of other implanted electronic stimulator of nervous system A 🐾

● **T85.19** Other mechanical complication of implanted electronic stimulator of nervous system
Leakage of implanted electronic stimulator of nervous system
Obstruction (mechanical) of implanted electronic stimulator of nervous system
Perforation of implanted electronic stimulator of nervous system
Protrusion of implanted electronic stimulator of nervous system

CHAPTER 19 (S00–T88)

● **T85.190** Other mechanical complication of implanted electronic neurostimulator of brain electrode (lead) A 🦟

● **T85.191** Other mechanical complication of implanted electronic neurostimulator of peripheral nerve electrode (lead) A 🦟

Other mechanical complication of electrode (lead) for cranial nerve neurostimulators

Other mechanical complication of electrode (lead) for gastric neurostimulator

Other mechanical complication of electrode (lead) for sacral nerve neurostimulator

Other mechanical complication of electrode (lead) for vagal nerve neurostimulators

● **T85.192** Other mechanical complication of implanted electronic neurostimulator of spinal cord electrode (lead) A 🦟

● **T85.193** Other mechanical complication of implanted electronic neurostimulator, generator A 🦟

Other mechanical complication of implanted electronic neurostimulator generator, brain, peripheral, gastric, spinal

Other mechanical complication of implanted electronic sacral neurostimulator, pulse generator or receiver

● **T85.199** Other mechanical complication of other implanted electronic stimulator of nervous system A 🦟

● **T85.2** Mechanical complication of intraocular lens

X ● **T85.21** Breakdown (mechanical) of intraocular lens

X ● **T85.22** Displacement of intraocular lens
Malposition of intraocular lens

X ● **T85.29** Other mechanical complication of intraocular lens
Obstruction (mechanical) of intraocular lens
Perforation of intraocular lens
Protrusion of intraocular lens

● **T85.3** Mechanical complication of other ocular prosthetic devices, implants and grafts

Excludes2   other complications of corneal graft (T86.84-)

● **T85.31** Breakdown (mechanical) of other ocular prosthetic devices, implants and grafts

● **T85.310** Breakdown (mechanical) of prosthetic orbit of right eye

● **T85.311** Breakdown (mechanical) of prosthetic orbit of left eye

● **T85.318** Breakdown (mechanical) of other ocular prosthetic devices, implants and grafts

● **T85.32** Displacement of other ocular prosthetic devices, implants and grafts
Malposition of other ocular prosthetic devices, implants and grafts

● **T85.320** Displacement of prosthetic orbit of right eye

● **T85.321** Displacement of prosthetic orbit of left eye

● **T85.328** Displacement of other ocular prosthetic devices, implants and grafts

● **T85.39** Other mechanical complication of other ocular prosthetic devices, implants and grafts
Obstruction (mechanical) of other ocular prosthetic devices, implants and grafts
Perforation of other ocular prosthetic devices, implants and grafts
Protrusion of other ocular prosthetic devices, implants and grafts

● **T85.390** Other mechanical complication of prosthetic orbit of right eye

● **T85.391** Other mechanical complication of prosthetic orbit of left eye

● **T85.398** Other mechanical complication of other ocular prosthetic devices, implants and grafts

● **T85.4** Mechanical complication of breast prosthesis and implant

X ● **T85.41** Breakdown (mechanical) of breast prosthesis and implant

X ● **T85.42** Displacement of breast prosthesis and implant
Malposition of breast prosthesis and implant

X ● **T85.43** Leakage of breast prosthesis and implant

X ● **T85.44** Capsular contracture of breast implant

X ● **T85.49** Other mechanical complication of breast prosthesis and implant
Obstruction (mechanical) of breast prosthesis and implant
Perforation of breast prosthesis and implant
Protrusion of breast prosthesis and implant

● **T85.5** Mechanical complication of gastrointestinal prosthetic devices, implants and grafts

● **T85.51** Breakdown (mechanical) of gastrointestinal prosthetic devices, implants and grafts

● **T85.510** Breakdown (mechanical) of bile duct prosthesis

● **T85.511** Breakdown (mechanical) of esophageal anti-reflux device

● **T85.518** Breakdown (mechanical) of other gastrointestinal prosthetic devices, implants and grafts

● **T85.52** Displacement of gastrointestinal prosthetic devices, implants and grafts
Malposition of gastrointestinal prosthetic devices, implants and grafts

● **T85.520** Displacement of bile duct prosthesis

● **T85.521** Displacement of esophageal anti-reflux device

● **T85.528** Displacement of other gastrointestinal prosthetic devices, implants and grafts

● **T85.59** Other mechanical complication of gastrointestinal prosthetic devices, implants and
Obstruction, mechanical of gastrointestinal prosthetic devices, implants and grafts
Perforation of gastrointestinal prosthetic devices, implants and grafts
Protrusion of gastrointestinal prosthetic devices, implants and grafts

● **T85.590** Other mechanical complication of bile duct prosthesis

● **T85.591** Other mechanical complication of esophageal anti-reflux device

● **T85.598** Other mechanical complication of other gastrointestinal prosthetic devices, implants and grafts

● **T85.6　Mechanical complication of other specified internal and external prosthetic devices, implants and grafts**
　　Coding Clinic: 2016, Q4, P71

● **T85.61　Breakdown (mechanical) of other specified internal prosthetic devices, implants and grafts**

● **T85.610　Breakdown (mechanical) of cranial or spinal infusion catheter**
　　Breakdown (mechanical) of epidural infusion catheter
　　Breakdown (mechanical) of intrathecal infusion catheter
　　Breakdown (mechanical) of subarachnoid infusion catheter
　　Breakdown (mechanical) of subdural infusion catheter

● **T85.611　Breakdown (mechanical) of intraperitoneal dialysis catheter A, D, S 🔒**
　　　Excludes1　mechanical complication of vascular dialysis catheter (T82.4-)

● **T85.612　Breakdown (mechanical) of permanent sutures**
　　　Excludes1　mechanical complication of permanent (wire) suture used in bone repair (T84.1-T84.2)

● **T85.613　Breakdown (mechanical) of artificial skin graft and decellularized allodermis**
　　Failure of artificial skin graft and decellularized allodermis
　　Non-adherence of artificial skin graft and decellularized allodermis
　　Poor incorporation of artificial skin graft and decellularized allodermis
　　Shearing of artificial skin graft and decellularized allodermis

● **T85.614　Breakdown (mechanical) of insulin pump**

● **T85.615　Breakdown (mechanical) of other nervous system device, implant or graft A 🔒**
　　Breakdown (mechanical) of intrathecal infusion pump

● **T85.618　Breakdown (mechanical) of other specified internal prosthetic devices, implants and grafts**

● **T85.62　Displacement of other specified internal prosthetic devices, implants and grafts**
　　Malposition of other specified internal prosthetic devices, implants and grafts

● **T85.620　Displacement of cranial or spinal infusion catheter**
　　Displacement of epidural infusion catheter
　　Displacement of intrathecal infusion catheter
　　Displacement of subarachnoid infusion catheter
　　Displacement of subdural infusion catheter

● **T85.621　Displacement of intraperitoneal dialysis catheter A, D, S 🔒**
　　　Excludes1　mechanical complication of vascular dialysis catheter (T82.4-)

● **T85.622　Displacement of permanent sutures**
　　　Excludes1　mechanical complication of permanent (wire) suture used in bone repair (T84.1-T84.2)

● **T85.623　Displacement of artificial skin graft and decellularized allodermis**
　　Dislodgement of artificial skin graft and decellularized allodermis

● **T85.624　Displacement of insulin pump**

● **T85.625　Displacement of other nervous system device, implant or graft A 🔒**
　　Displacement of intrathecal infusion pump

● **T85.628　Displacement of other specified internal prosthetic devices, implants and grafts**
　　Coding Clinic: 2015, Q1, P15

● **T85.63　Leakage of other specified internal prosthetic devices, implants and grafts**

● **T85.630　Leakage of cranial or spinal infusion catheter**
　　Leakage of epidural infusion catheter
　　Leakage of intrathecal infusion catheter
　　Leakage of subdural infusion catheter
　　Leakage of subarachnoid infusion catheter

● **T85.631　Leakage of intraperitoneal dialysis catheter A, D, S 🔒**
　　　Excludes1　mechanical complication of vascular dialysis catheter (T82.4)

● **T85.633　Leakage of insulin pump**

● **T85.635　Leakage of other nervous system device, implant or graft A 🔒**
　　Leakage of intrathecal infusion pump

● **T85.638　Leakage of other specified internal prosthetic devices, implants and grafts**

● **T85.69　Other mechanical complication of other specified internal prosthetic devices, implants and grafts**
　　Obstruction, mechanical of other specified internal prosthetic devices, implants and grafts
　　Perforation of other specified internal prosthetic devices, implants and grafts
　　Protrusion of other specified internal prosthetic devices, implants and grafts

● **T85.690　Other mechanical complication of cranial or spinal infusion catheter**
　　Other mechanical complication of epidural infusion catheter
　　Other mechanical complication of intrathecal infusion catheter
　　Other mechanical complication of subarachnoid infusion catheter
　　Other mechanical complication of subdural infusion catheter

CHAPTER 19 (S00-T88)

● **T85.691** **Other mechanical complication of intraperitoneal dialysis catheter** A, D, S 🐾

> **Excludes1**   mechanical complication of vascular dialysis catheter (T82.4)

● **T85.692** **Other mechanical complication of permanent sutures**

> **Excludes1**   mechanical complication of permanent (wire) suture used in bone repair (T84.1-T84.2)

● **T85.693** **Other mechanical complication of artificial skin graft and decellularized allodermis**

● **T85.694** **Other mechanical complication of insulin pump**

● **T85.695** **Other mechanical complication of other nervous system device, implant or graft** A 🐾

> Other mechanical complication of intrathecal infusion pump

● **T85.698** **Other mechanical complication of other specified internal prosthetic devices, implants and grafts**

> Mechanical complication of nonabsorbable surgical material NOS

● **T85.7** **Infection and inflammatory reaction due to other internal prosthetic devices, implants and grafts**

> Use additional code to identify infection
>
> Coding Clinic: 2016, Q4, P72

X ● **T85.71** **Infection and inflammatory reaction due to peritoneal dialysis catheter** A, D, S 🐾

X ● **T85.72** **Infection and inflammatory reaction due to insulin pump** A 🐾

● **T85.73** **Infection and inflammatory reaction due to nervous system devices, implants and graft**

● **T85.730** **Infection and inflammatory reaction due to ventricular intracranial (communicating) shunt** A 🐾

● **T85.731** **Infection and inflammatory reaction due to implanted electronic neurostimulator of brain, electrode (lead)** A 🐾

● **T85.732** **Infection and inflammatory reaction due to implanted electronic neurostimulator of peripheral nerve, electrode (lead)** A 🐾

> Infection and inflammatory reaction due to electrode (lead) for cranial nerve neurostimulators
> Infection and inflammatory reaction due to electrode (lead) for gastric neurostimulator
> Infection and inflammatory reaction due to electrode (lead) for sacral nerve neurostimulator
> Infection and inflammatory reaction due to electrode (lead) for vagal nerve neurostimulators

● **T85.733** **Infection and inflammatory reaction due to implanted electronic neurostimulator of spinal cord, electrode (lead)** A 🐾

● **T85.734** **Infection and inflammatory reaction due to implanted electronic neurostimulator, generator** A 🐾

> Generator pocket infection

● **T85.735** **Infection and inflammatory reaction due to cranial or spinal infusion catheter** A 🐾

> Infection and inflammatory reaction due to epidural catheter
> Infection and inflammatory reaction due to intrathecal infusion catheter
> Infection and inflammatory reaction due to subarachnoid catheter
> Infection and inflammatory reaction due to subdural catheter

● **T85.738** **Infection and inflammatory reaction due to other nervous system device, implant or graft** A 🐾

> Infection and inflammatory reaction due to intrathecal infusion pump

X ● **T85.79** **Infection and inflammatory reaction due to other internal prosthetic devices, implants and grafts** A 🐾

> Coding Clinic: 2022, Q2, P8; 2016, Q4, P72

● **T85.8** **Other specified complications of internal prosthetic devices, implants and grafts, not elsewhere classified**

> Coding Clinic: 2016, Q4, P72

● **T85.81** **Embolism due to internal prosthetic devices, implants and grafts, not elsewhere classified**

● **T85.810** **Embolism due to nervous system prosthetic devices, implants and grafts** A 🐾

● **T85.818** **Embolism due to other internal prosthetic devices, implants and grafts**

● **T85.82** **Fibrosis due to internal prosthetic devices, implants and grafts, not elsewhere classified**

● **T85.820** **Fibrosis due to nervous system prosthetic devices, implants and grafts** A 🐾

● **T85.828** **Fibrosis due to other internal prosthetic devices, implants and grafts**

● **T85.83** **Hemorrhage due to internal prosthetic devices, implants and grafts, not elsewhere classified**

● **T85.830** **Hemorrhage due to nervous system prosthetic devices, implants and grafts** A 🐾

● **T85.838** **Hemorrhage due to other internal prosthetic devices, implants and grafts**

● **T85.84** **Pain due to internal prosthetic devices, implants and grafts, not elsewhere classified**

● **T85.840** **Pain due to nervous system prosthetic devices, implants and grafts** A 🐾

● **T85.848** **Pain due to other internal prosthetic devices, implants and grafts**

● **T85.85** **Stenosis due to internal prosthetic devices, implants and grafts, not elsewhere classified**

● **T85.850** **Stenosis due to nervous system prosthetic devices, implants and grafts** A 🐾

● **T85.858** **Stenosis due to other internal prosthetic devices, implants and grafts**

● **T85.86** **Thrombosis due to internal prosthetic devices, implants and grafts, not elsewhere classified**

● **T85.860** **Thrombosis due to nervous system prosthetic devices, implants and grafts** A 🐾

● **T85.868** **Thrombosis due to other internal prosthetic devices, implants and grafts**

▶ New   ⇒ Revised   ~~deleted~~ Deleted   Excludes 1   Excludes 2   Includes   Use additional   Code first   Code also   Key words

OGCR Official Guidelines   X Assign placeholder X   ● Use Additional Character(s)   ▷ Manifestation Code   🐾 Hierarchical Condition Category   Coding Clinic

● **T85.89** **Other specified complication of internal prosthetic devices, implants and grafts, not elsewhere classified**
Coding Clinic: 2016, Q4, P72

     ● **T85.890** **Other specified complication of nervous system prosthetic devices, implants and grafts** A 🔍

     ● **T85.898** **Other specified complication of other internal prosthetic devices, implants and grafts**

X ● **T85.9** **Unspecified complication of internal prosthetic device, implant and graft**
     Complication of internal prosthetic device, implant and graft NOS

OGCR Section I.C.19.g.3.

Organ Transplant Complications

Transplant Complications

(a) Transplant complications other than kidney

Codes under category T86, Complications of transplanted organs and tissues, are for use for both complications and rejection of transplanted organs. A transplant complication code is only assigned if the complication affects the function of the transplanted organ. Two codes are required to fully describe a transplant complication: the appropriate code from category T86 and a secondary code that identifies the complication.

Pre-existing conditions or conditions that develop after the transplant are not coded as complications unless they affect the function of the transplanted organs.

See I.C.21 for transplant organ removal status.

See I.C.2 for malignant neoplasm associated with transplanted organ.

● **T86** **Complications of transplanted organs and tissue**
     Use additional code to identify other transplant complications, such as:
         graft-versus-host disease (D89.81-)
         malignancy associated with organ transplant (C80.2)
         post-transplant lymphoproliferative disorders (PTLD) (D47.Z1)

   ● **T86.0** **Complications of bone marrow transplant**

     T86.00 **Unspecified complication of bone marrow transplant** 🔍

     T86.01 **Bone marrow transplant rejection** 🔍

     T86.02 **Bone marrow transplant failure** 🔍

     T86.03 **Bone marrow transplant infection** 🔍

     T86.09 **Other complications of bone marrow transplant** 🔍

   ● **T86.1** **Complications of kidney transplant**

     T86.10 **Unspecified complication of kidney transplant**

     T86.11 **Kidney transplant rejection**

     T86.12 **Kidney transplant failure**
         Coding Clinic: 2013, Q1, P24

     T86.13 **Kidney transplant infection**
         Use additional code to specify infection

     T86.19 **Other complication of kidney transplant**
         Coding Clinic: 2019, Q2, P7

   ● **T86.2** **Complications of heart transplant**
     Excludes1   complication of:
         artificial heart device (T82.5-)
         heart-lung transplant (T86.3-)

     T86.20 **Unspecified complication of heart transplant** 🔍

     T86.21 **Heart transplant rejection** 🔍

     T86.22 **Heart transplant failure** 🔍

     T86.23 **Heart transplant infection** 🔍
         Use additional code to specify infection

   ● **T86.29** **Other complications of heart transplant**

     T86.290 **Cardiac allograft vasculopathy** 🔍
         Excludes1   atherosclerosis of coronary arteries (I25.75-, I25.76-, I25.81-)

     T86.298 **Other complications of heart transplant** 🔍

   ● **T86.3** **Complications of heart-lung transplant**

     T86.30 **Unspecified complication of heart-lung transplant** 🔍

     T86.31 **Heart-lung transplant rejection** 🔍

     T86.32 **Heart-lung transplant failure** 🔍

     T86.33 **Heart-lung transplant infection** 🔍
         Use additional code to specify infection

     T86.39 **Other complications of heart-lung transplant** 🔍

   ● **T86.4** **Complications of liver transplant**

     T86.40 **Unspecified complication of liver transplant** 🔍

     T86.41 **Liver transplant rejection** 🔍

     T86.42 **Liver transplant failure** 🔍

     T86.43 **Liver transplant infection** 🔍
         Use additional code to identify infection, such as:
         Cytomegalovirus (CMV) infection (B25.-)

     T86.49 **Other complications of liver transplant** 🔍

   ● **T86.5** **Complications of stem cell transplant** 🔍
     Complications from stem cells from peripheral blood
     Complications from stem cells from umbilical cord

   ● **T86.8** **Complications of other transplanted organs and tissues**

     ● **T86.81** **Complications of lung transplant**
         Excludes1   complication of heart-lung transplant (T86.3-)

         T86.810 **Lung transplant rejection** 🔍

         T86.811 **Lung transplant failure** 🔍

         T86.812 **Lung transplant infection** 🔍
         Use additional code to specify infection

         T86.818 **Other complications of lung transplant** 🔍
         Coding Clinic: 2019, Q2, P7

         T86.819 **Unspecified complication of lung transplant** 🔍

     ● **T86.82** **Complications of skin graft (allograft) (autograft)**
         Excludes2   complication of artificial skin graft (T85.693)

         T86.820 **Skin graft (allograft) rejection**

         T86.821 **Skin graft (allograft) (autograft) failure**

         T86.822 **Skin graft (allograft) (autograft) infection**
         Use additional code to specify infection

         T86.828 **Other complications of skin graft (allograft) (autograft)**

         T86.829 **Unspecified complication of skin graft (allograft) (autograft)**

     ● **T86.83** **Complications of bone graft**
         Excludes2   mechanical complications of bone graft (T84.3-)

         T86.830 **Bone graft rejection**

         T86.831 **Bone graft failure**

         T86.832 **Bone graft infection**
         Use additional code to specify infection

         T86.838 **Other complications of bone graft**

         T86.839 **Unspecified complication of bone graft**

CHAPTER 19 (S00-T88)

● **T86.84**   **Complications of corneal transplant**
        Excludes2   mechanical complications of corneal graft (T85.3-)

   ● **T86.840**   **Corneal transplant rejection**

       T86.8401   Corneal transplant rejection, right eye

       T86.8402   Corneal transplant rejection, left eye

       T86.8403   Corneal transplant rejection, bilateral

       T86.8409   Corneal transplant rejection, unspecified eye

   ● **T86.841**   **Corneal transplant failure**

       T86.8411   Corneal transplant failure, right eye

       T86.8412   Corneal transplant failure, left eye

       T86.8413   Corneal transplant failure, bilateral

       T86.8419   Corneal transplant failure, unspecified eye

   ● **T86.842**   **Corneal transplant infection** 🗞
       Use additional code to specify infection

       T86.8421   Corneal transplant infection, right eye

       T86.8422   Corneal transplant infection, left eye

       T86.8423   Corneal transplant infection, bilateral

       T86.8429   Corneal transplant infection, unspecified eye

   ● **T86.848**   **Other complications of corneal transplant**

       T86.8481   Other complications of corneal transplant, right eye

       T86.8482   Other complications of corneal transplant, left eye

       T86.8483   Other complications of corneal transplant, bilateral

       T86.8489   Other complications of corneal transplant, unspecified eye

   ● **T86.849**   **Unspecified complication of corneal transplant**

       T86.8491   Unspecified complication of corneal transplant, right eye

       T86.8492   Unspecified complication of corneal transplant, left eye

       T86.8493   Unspecified complication of corneal transplant, bilateral

       T86.8499   Unspecified complication of corneal transplant, unspecified eye

● **T86.85**   **Complication of intestine transplant**

   T86.850   Intestine transplant rejection 🗞

   T86.851   Intestine transplant failure 🗞

   T86.852   Intestine transplant infection 🗞
       Use additional code to specify infection

   T86.858   Other complications of intestine transplant 🗞

   T86.859   Unspecified complication of intestine transplant 🗞

● **T86.89**   **Complications of other transplanted tissue**
Transplant failure or rejection of pancreas

   T86.890   Other transplanted tissue rejection

   T86.891   Other transplanted tissue failure

   T86.892   Other transplanted tissue infection
       Use additional code to specify infection

   T86.898   Other complications of other transplanted tissue

   T86.899   Unspecified complication of other transplanted tissue

● **T86.9**   **Complication of unspecified transplanted organ and tissue**

   T86.90   Unspecified complication of unspecified transplanted organ and tissue

   T86.91   Unspecified transplanted organ and tissue rejection

   T86.92   Unspecified transplanted organ and tissue failure

   T86.93   Unspecified transplanted organ and tissue infection
       Use additional code to specify infection

   T86.99   Other complications of unspecified transplanted organ and tissue

● **T87**   **Complications peculiar to reattachment and amputation**

   ● **T87.0**   **Complications of reattached (part of) upper extremity**

     ● **T87.0X**   **Complications of reattached (part of) upper extremity**

       T87.0X1   Complications of reattached (part of) right upper extremity 🗞

       T87.0X2   Complications of reattached (part of) left upper extremity 🗞

       T87.0X9   Complications of reattached (part of) unspecified upper extremity 🗞

   ● **T87.1**   **Complications of reattached (part of) lower extremity**

     ● **T87.1X**   **Complications of reattached (part of) lower extremity**

       T87.1X1   Complications of reattached (part of) right lower extremity 🗞

       T87.1X2   Complications of reattached (part of) left lower extremity 🗞

       T87.1X9   Complications of reattached (part of) unspecified lower extremity 🗞

   T87.2   **Complications of other reattached body part** 🗞

   ● **T87.3**   **Neuroma of amputation stump**

     T87.30   Neuroma of amputation stump, unspecified extremity 🗞

     T87.31   Neuroma of amputation stump, right upper extremity 🗞

     T87.32   Neuroma of amputation stump, left upper extremity 🗞

     T87.33   Neuroma of amputation stump, right lower extremity 🗞

     T87.34   Neuroma of amputation stump, left lower extremity 🗞

   ● **T87.4**   **Infection of amputation stump**

     T87.40   Infection of amputation stump, unspecified extremity 🗞

     T87.41   Infection of amputation stump, right upper extremity 🗞

     T87.42   Infection of amputation stump, left upper extremity 🗞

     T87.43   Infection of amputation stump, right lower extremity 🗞

     T87.44   Infection of amputation stump, left lower extremity 🗞

▶ New   ➡ Revised   ~~deleted~~ Deleted   Excludes 1   Excludes 2   Includes   Use additional   Code first   Code also   Key words

OGCR Official Guidelines   X Assign placeholder X   ● Use Additional Character(s)   ▶ Manifestation Code   🗞 Hierarchical Condition Category   **Coding Clinic**

● **T87.5**   **Necrosis of amputation stump**

     T87.50   **Necrosis of amputation stump, unspecified extremity** 🔁

     T87.51   **Necrosis of amputation stump, right upper extremity** 🔁

     T87.52   **Necrosis of amputation stump, left upper extremity** 🔁

     T87.53   **Necrosis of amputation stump, right lower extremity** 🔁

     T87.54   **Necrosis of amputation stump, left lower extremity** 🔁

● **T87.8**   **Other complications of amputation stump**

     T87.81   **Dehiscence of amputation stump** 🔁

     T87.89   **Other complications of amputation stump** 🔁

         Amputation stump contracture

         Amputation stump contracture of next proximal joint

         Amputation stump flexion

         Amputation stump edema

         Amputation stump hematoma

         Excludes2   phantom limb syndrome (G54.6-G54.7)

     T87.9   **Unspecified complications of amputation stump** 🔁

● **T88**   **Other complications of surgical and medical care, not elsewhere classified**

     Excludes2   complication following infusion, transfusion and therapeutic injection (T80.-)
         complication following procedure NEC (T81.-)
         complications of anesthesia in labor and delivery (O74.-)
         complications of anesthesia in pregnancy (O29.-)
         complications of anesthesia in puerperium (O89.-)
         complications of devices, implants and grafts (T82-T85)
         complications of obstetric surgery and procedure (O75.4)
         dermatitis due to drugs and medicaments (L23.3, L24.4, L25.1, L27.0-L27.1)
         poisoning and toxic effects of drugs and chemicals (T36-T65 with fifth or sixth character 1-4 or 6)
         specified complications classified elsewhere

     The appropriate 7th character is to be added to each code from category T88

A	initial encounter
D	subsequent encounter
S	sequela

X ● **T88.0**   **Infection following immunization**

     Sepsis following immunization

     Coding Clinic: 2022, Q2, P8; 2019, Q1, P14; 2018, Q4, P90

X ● **T88.1**   **Other complications following immunization, not elsewhere classified**

     Generalized vaccinia

     Rash following immunization

     Excludes1   vaccinia not from vaccine (B08.011)

     Excludes2   anaphylactic shock due to serum (T80.5-)
         other serum reactions (T80.6-)
         postimmunization arthropathy (M02.2)
         postimmunization encephalitis (G04.02)
         postimmunization fever (R50.83)

X ● **T88.2**   **Shock due to anesthesia**

     Use additional code for adverse effect, if applicable, to identify drug (T41.- with fifth or sixth character 5)

     Excludes1   complications of anesthesia (in):
         labor and delivery (O74.-)
         pregnancy (O29.-)
         puerperium (O89.-)
         postprocedural shock NOS (T81.1-)

X ● **T88.3**   **Malignant hyperthermia due to anesthesia**

     Use additional code for adverse effect, if applicable, to identify drug (T41.- with fifth or sixth character 5)

X ● **T88.4**   **Failed or difficult intubation**

● **T88.5**   **Other complications of anesthesia**

     Use additional code for adverse effect, if applicable, to identify drug (T41.- with fifth or sixth character 5)

     Coding Clinic: 2016, Q4, P72

     X ● **T88.51**   **Hypothermia following anesthesia**

     X ● **T88.52**   **Failed moderate sedation during procedure**

         Failed conscious sedation during procedure

         Excludes2   personal history of failed moderate sedation (Z92.83)

     X ● **T88.53**   **Unintended awareness under general anesthesia during procedure**

         Excludes2   personal history of unintended awareness under general anesthesia (Z92.84)

         Coding Clinic: 2016, Q4, P72-73

     X ● **T88.59**   **Other complications of anesthesia**

X ● **T88.6**   **Anaphylactic reaction due to adverse effect of correct drug or medicament properly administered**

     Anaphylactic shock due to adverse effect of correct drug or medicament properly administered

     Anaphylactoid reaction NOS

     Use additional code for adverse effect, if applicable, to identify drug (T36-T50 with fifth or sixth character 5)

     Excludes1   anaphylactic reaction due to serum (T80.5-)
         anaphylactic shock or reaction due to adverse food reaction (T78.0-)

     Coding Clinic: 2020, Q1, P18

X ● **T88.7**   **Unspecified adverse effect of drug or medicament**

     Drug hypersensitivity NOS

     Drug reaction NOS

     Use additional code for adverse effect, if applicable, to identify drug (T36-T50 with fifth or sixth character 5)

     Excludes1   specified adverse effects of drugs and medicaments (A00-R94 and T80-T88.6, T88.8)

X ● **T88.8**   **Other specified complications of surgical and medical care, not elsewhere classified**

     Use additional code to identify the complication

X ● **T88.9**   **Complication of surgical and medical care, unspecified**

CHAPTER 20

EXTERNAL CAUSES OF MORBIDITY (V00-Y99)

20. Chapter 20: External Causes of Morbidity (V00-Y99)

The external causes of morbidity codes should never be sequenced as the first-listed or principal diagnosis.

External cause codes are intended to provide data for injury research and evaluation of injury prevention strategies. These codes capture how the injury or health condition happened (cause), the intent (unintentional or accidental; or intentional, such as suicide or assault), the place where the event occurred the activity of the patient at the time of the event, and the person's status (e.g., civilian, military).

There is no national requirement for mandatory ICD-10-CM external cause code reporting. Unless a provider is subject to a state-based external cause code reporting mandate or these codes are required by a particular payer, reporting of ICD-10-CM codes in Chapter 20, External Causes of Morbidity, is not required. In the absence of a mandatory reporting requirement, providers are encouraged to voluntarily report external cause codes, as they provide valuable data for injury research and evaluation of injury prevention strategies.

a. General External Cause Coding Guidelines

1) Used with any code in the range of A00.0-T88.9, Z00-Z99

An external cause code may be used with any code in the range of A00.0-T88.9, Z00-Z99, classification that represents a health condition due to an external cause. Though they are most applicable to injuries, they are also valid for use with such things as infections or diseases due to an external source, and other health conditions, such as a heart attack that occurs during strenuous physical activity.

2) External cause code used for length of treatment

Assign the external cause code, with the appropriate 7th character (initial encounter, subsequent encounter or sequela) for each encounter for which the injury or condition is being treated.

Most categories in Chapter 20 have a 7th character requirement for each applicable code. Most categories in this chapter have three 7th character values: A, initial encounter, D, subsequent encounter and S, sequela. While the patient may be seen by a new or different provider over the course of treatment for an injury or condition, assignment of the 7th character for external cause should match the 7th character of the code assigned for the associated injury or condition for the encounter.

3) Use the full range of external cause codes

Use the full range of external cause codes to completely describe the cause, the intent, the place of occurrence and if applicable, the activity of the patient at the time of the event, and the patient's status, for all injuries, and other health conditions due to an external cause.

4) Assign as many external cause codes as necessary

Assign as many external cause codes as necessary to fully explain each cause. If only one external code can be recorded, assign the code most related to the principal diagnosis.

5) The selection of the appropriate external cause code

The selection of the appropriate external cause code is guided by the Alphabetic Index of External Causes and by Inclusion and Exclusion notes in the Tabular List.

6) External cause code can never be a principal diagnosis

An external cause code can never be a principal (first-listed) diagnosis.

7) Combination external cause codes

Certain of the external cause codes are combination codes that identify sequential events that result in an injury, such as a fall which results in striking against an object. The injury may be due to either event or both. The combination external cause code used should correspond to the sequence of events regardless of which caused the most serious injury.

8) No external cause code needed in certain circumstances

No external cause code from Chapter 20 is needed if the external cause and intent are included in a code from another chapter (e.g., T36.0X1- Poisoning by penicillins, accidental (unintentional)).

b. Place of Occurrence Guideline

Codes from category Y92, Place of occurrence of the external cause, are secondary codes for use after other external cause codes to identify the location of the patient at the time of injury or other condition.

Generally, a place of occurrence code is assigned only once, at the initial encounter for treatment. However, in the rare instance that a new injury occurs during hospitalization, an additional place of occurrence code may be assigned. No 7th characters are used for Y92. Only one code from Y92 should be recorded on a medical record.

Do not use place of occurrence code Y92.9 if the place is not stated or is not applicable.

c. Activity Code

Assign a code from category Y93, Activity code, to describe the activity of the patient at the time the injury or other health condition occurred.

An activity code is used only once, at the initial encounter for treatment. Only one code from Y93 should be recorded on a medical record.

The activity codes are not applicable to poisonings, adverse effects, misadventures or sequela.

Do not assign Y93.9, Unspecified activity, if the activity is not stated.

A code from category Y93 is appropriate for use with external cause and intent codes if identifying the activity provides additional information about the event.

d. Place of Occurrence, Activity, and Status Codes Used with Other External Cause Code

When applicable, place of occurrence, activity, and external cause status codes are sequenced after the main external cause code(s). Regardless of the number of external cause codes assigned, there should be only one place of occurrence code, one activity code, and one external cause status code assigned to an encounter.

e. If the Reporting Format Limits the Number of External Cause Codes

If the reporting format limits the number of external cause codes that can be used in reporting clinical data, report the code for the cause/intent most related to the principal diagnosis. If the format permits capture of additional external cause codes, the cause/intent, including medical misadventures, of the additional events should be reported rather than the codes for place, activity, or external status.

f. Multiple External Cause Coding Guidelines

More than one external cause code is required to fully describe the external cause of an illness or injury. The assignment of external cause codes should be sequenced in the following priority:

If two or more events cause separate injuries, an external cause code should be assigned for each cause. The first-listed external cause code will be selected in the following order:

External codes for child and adult abuse take priority over all other external cause codes.

See Section I.C.19., Child and Adult abuse guidelines.

External codes for terrorism events take priority over all other external cause codes except child and adult abuse.

External cause codes for cataclysmic events take priority over all other external cause codes except child and adult abuse and terrorism.

External cause codes for transport accidents take priority over all other external cause codes except cataclysmic events, child and adult abuse and terrorism.

Activity and external cause status codes are assigned following all causal (intent) external cause codes.

The first-listed external cause code should correspond to the cause of the most serious diagnosis due to an assault, accident, or self-harm, following the order of hierarchy listed above.

g. Child and Adult Abuse Guideline

Adult and child abuse, neglect and maltreatment are classified as assault. Any of the assault codes may be used to indicate the external cause of any injury resulting from the confirmed abuse.

For confirmed cases of abuse, neglect and maltreatment, when the perpetrator is known, a code from Y07, Perpetrator of maltreatment and neglect, should accompany any other assault codes.

See Section I.C.19. Adult and child abuse, neglect and other maltreatment

h. Unknown or Undetermined Intent Guideline

If the intent (accident, self-harm, assault) of the cause of an injury or other condition is unknown or unspecified, code the intent as accidental intent. All transport accident categories assume accidental intent.

1) Use of undetermined intent

External cause codes for events of undetermined intent are only for use if the documentation in the record specifies that the intent cannot be determined.

i. Sequelae (Late Effects) of External Cause Guidelines

1) Sequelae external cause codes

Sequela are reported using the external cause code with the 7th character "S" for sequela. These codes should be used with any report of a late effect or sequela resulting from a previous injury.

See Section I.B.10. Sequela, (Late Effects).

2) Sequela external cause code with a related current injury

A sequela external cause code should never be used with a related current nature of injury code.

3) Use of sequela external cause codes for subsequent visits

Use a late effect external cause code for subsequent visits when a late effect of the initial injury is being treated. Do not use a late effect external cause code for subsequent visits for follow-up care (e.g., to assess healing, to receive rehabilitative therapy) of the injury when no late effect of the injury has been documented.

j. Terrorism Guidelines

1) Cause of injury identified by the Federal Government (FBI) as terrorism

When the cause of an injury is identified by the Federal Government (FBI) as terrorism, the first-listed external cause code should be a code from category Y38, Terrorism. The definition of terrorism employed by the FBI is found at the inclusion note at the beginning of category Y38. Use additional code for place of occurrence (Y92.-). More than one Y38 code may be assigned if the injury is the result of more than one mechanism of terrorism.

2) Cause of an injury is suspected to be the result of terrorism

When the cause of an injury is suspected to be the result of terrorism a code from category Y38 should not be assigned. Suspected cases should be classified as assault.

3) Code Y38.9, Terrorism, secondary effects

Assign code Y38.9, Terrorism, secondary effects, for conditions occurring subsequent to the terrorist event. This code should not be assigned for conditions that are due to the initial terrorist act.

It is acceptable to assign code Y38.9 with another code from Y38 if there is an injury due to the initial terrorist event and an injury that is a subsequent result of the terrorist event.

k. External cause status

A code from category Y99, External cause status, should be assigned whenever any other external cause code is assigned for an encounter, including an Activity code, except for the events noted below. Assign a code from category Y99, External cause status, to indicate the work status of the person at the time the event occurred. The status code indicates whether the event occurred during military activity, whether a non-military person was at work, whether an individual including a student or volunteer was involved in a non-work activity at the time of the causal event.

A code from Y99, External cause status, should be assigned, when applicable, with other external cause codes, such as transport accidents and falls. The external cause status codes are not applicable to poisonings, adverse effects, misadventures or late effects.

Do not assign a code from category Y99 if no other external cause codes (cause, activity) are applicable for the encounter.

An external cause status code is used only once, at the initial encounter for treatment. Only one code from Y99 should be recorded on a medical record.

Do not assign code Y99.9, Unspecified external cause status, if the status is not stated.

CHAPTER 20

EXTERNAL CAUSES OF MORBIDITY (V00-Y99)

Note: This chapter permits the classification of environmental events and circumstances as the cause of injury, and other adverse effects. Where a code from this section is applicable, it is intended that it shall be used secondary to a code from another chapter of the Classification indicating the nature of the condition. Most often, the condition will be classifiable to Chapter 19, Injury, poisoning and certain other consequences of external causes (S00-T88). Other conditions that may be stated to be due to external causes are classified in Chapters 1 to 18. For these conditions, codes from Chapter 20 should be used to provide additional information as to the cause of the condition.

This chapter contains the following blocks:

V00-X58	Accidents
V00-V99	Transport accidents
V00-V09	Pedestrian injured in transport accident
V10-V19	Pedal cycle rider injured in transport accident
V20-V29	Motorcycle rider injured in transport accident
V30-V39	Occupant of three-wheeled motor vehicle injured in transport accident
V40-V49	Car occupant injured in transport accident
V50-V59	Occupant of pick-up truck or van injured in transport accident
V60-V69	Occupant of heavy transport vehicle injured in transport accident
V70-V79	Bus occupant injured in transport accident
V80-V89	Other land transport accidents
V90-V94	Water transport accidents
V95-V97	Air and space transport accidents
V98-V99	Other and unspecified transport accidents
W00-X58	Other external causes of accidental injury
W00-W19	Slipping, tripping, stumbling and falls
W20-W49	Exposure to inanimate mechanical forces
W50-W64	Exposure to animate mechanical forces
W65-W74	Accidental non-transport drowning and submersion
W85-W99	Exposure to electric current, radiation and extreme ambient air temperature and pressure
X00-X08	Exposure to smoke, fire and flames
X10-X19	Contact with heat and hot substances
X30-X39	Exposure to forces of nature
X50	Overexertion and strenuous or repetitive movements
X52, X58	Accidental exposure to other specified factors
X71-X83	Intentional self-harm
X92-Y09	Assault
Y21-Y33	Event of undetermined intent
Y35-Y38	Legal intervention, operations of war, military operations, and terrorism
Y62-Y84	Complications of medical and surgical care
Y62-Y69	Misadventures to patients during surgical and medical care
Y70-Y82	Medical devices associated with adverse incidents in diagnostic and therapeutic use
Y83-Y84	Surgical and other medical procedures as the cause of abnormal reaction of the patient, or of later complication, without mention of misadventure at the time of the procedure
Y90-Y99	Supplementary factors related to causes of morbidity classified elsewhere

ACCIDENTS (V00-X58)

TRANSPORT ACCIDENTS (V00-V99)

Note: This section is structured in 12 groups. Those relating to land transport accidents (V00-V89) reflect the victim's mode of transport and are subdivided to identify the victim's 'counterpart' or the type of event. The vehicle of which the injured person is an occupant is identified in the first two characters since it is seen as the most important factor to identify for prevention purposes. A transport accident is one in which the vehicle involved must be moving or running or in use for transport purposes at the time of the accident.

Use additional code to identify:
Airbag injury (W22.1)
Type of street or road (Y92.4-)
Use of cellular telephone and other electronic equipment at the time of the transport accident (Y93.C-)

Excludes1 agricultural vehicles in stationary use or maintenance (W31.-)
assault by crashing of motor vehicle (Y03.-)
automobile or motor cycle in stationary use or maintenance - code to type of accident
crashing of motor vehicle, undetermined intent (Y32)
intentional self-harm by crashing of motor vehicle (X82)

Excludes2 transport accidents due to cataclysm (X34-X38)

Note: Definitions related to transport accidents:

(a) A transport accident (V00-V99) is any accident involving a device designed primarily for, or used at the time primarily for, conveying persons or good from one place to another.

(b) A public highway [trafficway] or street is the entire width between property lines (or other boundary lines) of land open to the public as a matter of right or custom for purposes of moving persons or property from one place to another. A roadway is that part of the public highway designed, improved and customarily used for vehicular traffic.

(c) A traffic accident is any vehicle accident occurring on the public highway [i.e., originating on, terminating on, or involving a vehicle partially on the highway]. A vehicle accident is assumed to have occurred on the public highway unless another place is specified, except in the case of accidents involving only off-road motor vehicles, which are classified as nontraffic accidents unless the contrary is stated.

(d) A nontraffic accident is any vehicle accident that occurs entirely in any place other than a public highway.

(e) A pedestrian is any person involved in an accident who was not at the time of the accident riding in or on a motor vehicle, railway train, streetcar or animal-drawn or other vehicle, or on a pedal cycle or animal. This includes, a person changing a tire, working on a parked car, or a person on foot. It also includes the user of a pedestrian conveyance such as a baby stroller, ice-skates, skis, sled, roller skates, a skateboard, nonmotorized or motorized wheelchair, motorized mobility scooter, or nonmotorized scooter.

(f) A driver is an occupant of a transport vehicle who is operating or intending to operate it.

(g) A passenger is any occupant of a transport vehicle other than the driver, except a person traveling on the outside of the vehicle.

(h) A person on the outside of a vehicle is any person being transported by a vehicle but not occupying the space normally reserved for the driver or passengers, or the space intended for the transport of property. This includes a person travelling on the bodywork, bumper, fender, roof, running board or step of a vehicle, as well as, hanging on the outside of the vehicle.

(i) A pedal cycle is any land transport vehicle operated solely by nonmotorized pedals including a bicycle or tricycle.

(j) A pedal cyclist is any person riding a pedal cycle or in a sidecar or trailer attached to a pedal cycle.

▶ New ⇒ Revised ~~deleted~~ Deleted Excludes 1 Excludes 2 Includes Use additional Code first Code also Key words
OGCR Official Guidelines X Assign placeholder X ● Use Additional Character(s) ▶ Manifestation Code 🏷 Hierarchical Condition Category Coding Clinic

(k) A motorcycle is a two-wheeled motor vehicle with one or two riding saddles and sometimes with a third wheel for the support of a sidecar. The sidecar is considered part of the motorcycle. This includes a moped, motor scooter, or motorized bicycle.

(l) A motorcycle rider is any person riding a motorcycle or in a sidecar or trailer attached to the motorcycle.

(m) A three-wheeled motor vehicle is a motorized tricycle designed primarily for on-road use. This includes a motor-driven tricycle, a motorized rickshaw, or a three-wheeled motor car.

(n) A car [automobile] is a four-wheeled motor vehicle designed primarily for carrying up to 7 persons. A trailer being towed by the car is considered part of the car. It does not include a van or minivan—see definition (o)

(o) A pick-up truck or van is a four or six-wheeled motor vehicle designed for carrying passengers as well as property or cargo weighing less than the local limit for classification as a heavy goods vehicle, and not requiring a special driver's license. This includes a minivan and a sport-utility vehicle (SUV).

(p) A heavy transport vehicle is a motor vehicle designed primarily for carrying property, meeting local criteria for classification as a heavy goods vehicle in terms of weight and requiring a special driver's license.

(q) A bus (coach) is a motor vehicle designed or adapted primarily for carrying more than 10 passengers, and requiring a special driver's license.

(r) A railway train or railway vehicle is any device, with or without freight or passenger cars coupled to it, designed for traffic on a railway track. This includes subterranean (subways) or elevated trains.

(s) A streetcar is a device designed and used primarily for transporting passengers within a municipality, running on rails, usually subject to normal traffic control signals, and operated principally on a right-of-way that forms part of the roadway. This includes a tram or trolley that runs on rails. A trailer being towed by a streetcar is considered part of the streetcar.

(t) A special vehicle mainly used on industrial premises is a motor vehicle designed primarily for use within the buildings and premises of industrial or commercial establishments. This includes battery-powered airport passenger vehicles or baggage/mail trucks, forklifts, coal-cars in a coal mine, logging cars and trucks used in mines or quarries.

(u) A special vehicle mainly used in agriculture is a motor vehicle designed specifically for use in farming and agriculture (horticulture), to work the land, tend and harvest crops and transport materials on the farm. This includes harvesters, farm machinery and tractor and trailers.

(v) A special construction vehicle is a motor vehicle designed specifically for use on construction and demolition sites. This includes bulldozers, diggers, earth levellers, dump trucks, backhoes, front-end loaders, pavers, and mechanical shovels.

(w) A special all-terrain vehicle is a motor vehicle of special design to enable it to negotiate over rough or soft terrain, snow or sand. Examples of special design are high construction, special wheels and tires, tracks, and support on a cushion of air. This includes snow mobiles, all-terrain vehicles (ATV), and dune buggies. It does not include passenger vehicle designated as sport utility vehicles (SUV).

(x) A watercraft is any device designed for transporting passengers or goods on water. This includes motor or sail boats, ships, and hovercraft.

(y) An aircraft is any device for transporting passengers or goods in the air. This includes hot-air balloons, gliders, helicopters, and airplanes.

(z) A military vehicle is any motorized vehicle operating on a public roadway owned by the military and being operated by a member of the military.

PEDESTRIAN INJURED IN TRANSPORT ACCIDENT (V00-V09)

Includes   person changing tire on transport vehicle
               person examining engine of vehicle broken down in (on side of) road

Excludes1   fall due to non-transport collision with other person (W03)
               pedestrian on foot falling (slipping) on ice and snow (W00.-)
               struck or bumped by another person (W51)

● **V00**   **Pedestrian conveyance accident**

Use additional place of occurrence and activity external cause codes, if known (Y92.-, Y93.-)

Excludes1   collision with another person without fall (W51)
               fall due to person on foot colliding with another person on foot (W03)
               fall from non-moving wheelchair, nonmotorized scooter and motorized mobility scooter without collision (W05.-)
               pedestrian (conveyance) collision with other land transport vehicle (V01-V09)
               pedestrian on foot falling (slipping) on ice and snow (W00.-)

The appropriate 7th character is to be added to each code from category V00

> A   initial encounter
> D   subsequent encounter
> S   sequela

● **V00.0** **Pedestrian on foot injured in collision with pedestrian conveyance**

  X ● **V00.01** **Pedestrian on foot injured in collision with roller-skater**

  X ● **V00.02** **Pedestrian on foot injured in collision with skateboarder**

  ● **V00.03** **Pedestrian on foot injured in collision with standing micro-mobility pedestrian conveyance**

      V00.031 **Pedestrian on foot injured in collision with rider of standing electric scooter**

      V00.038 **Pedestrian on foot injured in collision with rider of other standing micro-mobility pedestrian conveyance**
             Pedestrian on foot injured in collision with rider of hoverboard
             Pedestrian on foot injured in collision with rider of segway

  X ● **V00.09** **Pedestrian on foot injured in collision with other pedestrian conveyance**

● **V00.1** **Rolling-type pedestrian conveyance accident**

  Excludes1   accident with baby stroller (V00.82-)
               accident with wheelchair (powered) (V00.81-)
               accident with motorized mobility scooter (V00.83-)

  ● **V00.11** **In-line roller-skate accident**

    ● **V00.111** **Fall from in-line roller-skates**

    ● **V00.112** **In-line roller-skater colliding with stationary object**

    ● **V00.118** **Other in-line roller-skate accident**

      Excludes1   roller-skater collision with other land transport vehicle (V01-V09 with 5th character 1)

CHAPTER 20 (V00-Y99)

CHAPTER 20 (V00–Y99)

● **V00.12   Non-in-line roller-skate accident**
    ● **V00.121   Fall from non-in-line roller-skates**
    ● **V00.122   Non-in-line roller-skater colliding with stationary object**
    ● **V00.128   Other non-in-line roller-skating accident**
         Excludes1   roller-skater collision with other land transport vehicle (V01–V09 with 5th character 1)

● **V00.13   Skateboard accident**
    ● **V00.131   Fall from skateboard**
    ● **V00.132   Skateboarder colliding with stationary object**
    ● **V00.138   Other skateboard accident**
         Excludes1   skateboarder collision with other land transport vehicle (V01–V09 with 5th character 2)

● **V00.14   Scooter (nonmotorized) accident**
         Excludes1   motor scooter accident (V20–V29)
    ● **V00.141   Fall from scooter (nonmotorized)**
    ● **V00.142   Scooter (nonmotorized) colliding with stationary object**
    ● **V00.148   Other scooter (nonmotorized) accident**
         Excludes1   scooter (non-motorized) collision with other land transport vehicle (V01–V09 with fifth character 9)

● **V00.15   Heelies accident**
     Rolling shoe
     Wheeled shoe
     Wheelies accident
    ● **V00.151   Fall from heelies**
    ● **V00.152   Heelies colliding with stationary object**
    ● **V00.158   Other heelies accident**

● **V00.18   Accident on other rolling-type pedestrian conveyance**
    ● **V00.181   Fall from other rolling-type pedestrian conveyance**
    ● **V00.182   Pedestrian on other rolling-type pedestrian conveyance colliding with stationary object**
    ● **V00.188   Other accident on other rolling-type pedestrian conveyance**

● **V00.2   Gliding-type pedestrian conveyance accident**
    ● **V00.21   Ice-skates accident**
        ● **V00.211   Fall from ice-skates**
        ● **V00.212   Ice-skater colliding with stationary object**
        ● **V00.218   Other ice-skates accident**
             Excludes1   ice-skater collision with other land transport vehicle (V01–V09 with 5th character 9)

    ● **V00.22   Sled accident**
        ● **V00.221   Fall from sled**
        ● **V00.222   Sledder colliding with stationary object**
        ● **V00.228   Other sled accident**
             Excludes1   sled collision with other land transport vehicle (V01–V09 with 5th character 9)

● **V00.28   Other gliding-type pedestrian conveyance accident**
    ● **V00.281   Fall from other gliding-type pedestrian conveyance**
    ● **V00.282   Pedestrian on other gliding-type pedestrian conveyance colliding with stationary object**
    ● **V00.288   Other accident on other gliding-type pedestrian conveyance**
         Excludes1   gliding-type pedestrian conveyance collision with other land transport vehicle (V01–V09 with 5th character 9)

● **V00.3   Flat-bottomed pedestrian conveyance accident**
    ● **V00.31   Snowboard accident**
        ● **V00.311   Fall from snowboard**
        ● **V00.312   Snowboarder colliding with stationary object**
        ● **V00.318   Other snowboard accident**
             Excludes1   snowboarder collision with other land transport vehicle (V01–V09 with 5th character 9)

    ● **V00.32   Snow-ski accident**
        ● **V00.321   Fall from snow-skis**
             Coding Clinic: 2015, Q1, P12
        ● **V00.322   Snow-skier colliding with stationary object**
        ● **V00.328   Other snow-ski accident**
             Excludes1   snow-skier collision with other land transport vehicle (V01–V09 with 5th character 9)

    ● **V00.38   Other flat-bottomed pedestrian conveyance accident**
        ● **V00.381   Fall from other flat-bottomed pedestrian conveyance**
        ● **V00.382   Pedestrian on other flat-bottomed pedestrian conveyance colliding with stationary object**
        ● **V00.388   Other accident on other flat-bottomed pedestrian conveyance**

● **V00.8   Accident on other pedestrian conveyance**
    ● **V00.81   Accident with wheelchair (powered)**
        ● **V00.811   Fall from moving wheelchair (powered)**
             Excludes1   fall from non-moving wheelchair (W05.0)
        ● **V00.812   Wheelchair (powered) colliding with stationary object**
        ● **V00.818   Other accident with wheelchair (powered)**

    ● **V00.82   Accident with baby stroller**
        ● **V00.821   Fall from baby stroller**
        ● **V00.822   Baby stroller colliding with stationary object**
        ● **V00.828   Other accident with baby stroller**

▶ New   ⟹ Revised   ~~deleted~~ Deleted   Excludes 1   Excludes 2   Includes   Use additional   Code first   Code also   Key words
OGCR Official Guidelines   X Assign placeholder X   ● Use Additional Character(s)   ▶ Manifestation Code   🜲 Hierarchical Condition Category   Coding Clinic

● **V00.83** **Accident with** motorized mobility scooter
　　● **V00.831** **Fall from motorized mobility scooter**
　　　　Excludes1　fall from non-moving motorized mobility scooter (W05.2)
　　● **V00.832** **Motorized mobility scooter** colliding with stationary object
　　● **V00.838** **Other accident with motorized mobility scooter**
● **V00.84** **Accident with standing micro-mobility pedestrian conveyance**
　　V00.841 **Fall from standing electric scooter**
　　V00.842 **Pedestrian on standing electric scooter colliding with stationary object**
　　V00.848 **Other accident with standing micro-mobility pedestrian conveyance**
　　　　Accident with hoverboard
　　　　Accident with segway
● **V00.89** **Accident on** other pedestrian conveyance
　　● **V00.891** **Fall from other pedestrian conveyance**
　　● **V00.892** **Pedestrian on other pedestrian conveyance** colliding with stationary object
　　● **V00.898** **Other accident on other pedestrian conveyance**
　　　　Excludes1　other pedestrian (conveyance) collision with other land transport vehicle (V01-V09 with 5th character 9)

● **V01** **Pedestrian injured in collision with pedal cycle**
　　The appropriate 7th character is to be added to each code from category V01

A	initial encounter
D	subsequent encounter
S	sequela

● **V01.0** **Pedestrian injured in collision with pedal cycle in** nontraffic accident
　X● **V01.00** **Pedestrian on** foot **injured in collision with pedal cycle in nontraffic accident**
　　　　Pedestrian NOS injured in collision with pedal cycle in nontraffic accident
　X● **V01.01** **Pedestrian on** roller-skates **injured in collision with pedal cycle in nontraffic accident**
　X● **V01.02** **Pedestrian on** skateboard **injured in collision with pedal cycle in nontraffic accident**
　● **V01.03** **Pedestrian on standing micro-mobility pedestrian conveyance injured in collision with pedal cycle in nontraffic accident**
　　　V01.031 **Pedestrian on standing electric scooter injured in collision with pedal cycle in nontraffic accident**
　　　V01.038 **Pedestrian on other standing micro-mobility pedestrian conveyance injured in collision with pedal cycle in nontraffic accident**
　　　　　Pedestrian on hoverboard injured in collision with pedal cycle in nontraffic accident
　　　　　Pedestrian on segway injured in collision with pedal cycle in nontraffic accident

　X● **V01.09** **Pedestrian with** other conveyance **injured in collision with pedal cycle in nontraffic accident**
　　　　Pedestrian with baby stroller injured in collision with pedal cycle in nontraffic accident
　　　　Pedestrian in wheelchair (powered) injured in collision with pedal cycle in nontraffic accident
　　　　Pedestrian in motorized mobility scooter injured in collision with pedal cycle in nontraffic accident
　　　　Pedestrian on ice-skates injured in collision with pedal cycle in nontraffic accident
　　　　Pedestrian on nonmotorized scooter injured in collision with pedal cycle in nontraffic accident
　　　　Pedestrian on sled injured in collision with pedal cycle in nontraffic accident
　　　　Pedestrian on snowboard injured in collision with pedal cycle in nontraffic accident
　　　　Pedestrian on snow-skis injured in collision with pedal cycle in nontraffic accident
● **V01.1** **Pedestrian injured in collision with pedal cycle in** traffic accident
　X● **V01.10** **Pedestrian on** foot **injured in collision with pedal cycle in traffic accident**
　　　　Pedestrian NOS injured in collision with pedal cycle in traffic accident
　X● **V01.11** **Pedestrian on** roller-skates **injured in collision with pedal cycle in traffic accident**
　X● **V01.12** **Pedestrian on** skateboard **injured in collision with pedal cycle in traffic accident**
　● **V01.13** **Pedestrian on standing micro-mobility pedestrian conveyance injured in collision with pedal cycle in traffic accident**
　　　V01.131 **Pedestrian on standing electric scooter injured in collision with pedal cycle in traffic accident**
　　　V01.138 **Pedestrian on other standing micro-mobility pedestrian conveyance injured in collision with pedal cycle in traffic accident**
　　　　　Pedestrian on hoverboard injured in collision with pedal cycle in traffic accident
　　　　　Pedestrian on segway injured in collision with pedal cycle in traffic accident
　X● **V01.19** **Pedestrian with** other conveyance **injured in collision with pedal cycle in traffic accident**
　　　　Pedestrian with baby stroller injured in collision with pedal cycle in traffic accident
　　　　Pedestrian in wheelchair (powered) injured in collision with pedal cycle in traffic accident
　　　　Pedestrian in motorized mobility scooter injured in collision with pedal cycle in traffic accident
　　　　Pedestrian on ice-skates injured in collision with pedal cycle in traffic accident
　　　　Pedestrian on nonmotorized scooter injured in collision with pedal cycle in traffic accident
　　　　Pedestrian on sled injured in collision with pedal cycle in traffic accident
　　　　Pedestrian on snowboard injured in collision with pedal cycle in traffic accident
　　　　Pedestrian on snow-skis injured in collision with pedal cycle in traffic accident

● **V01.9**   **Pedestrian injured in collision with pedal cycle, unspecified whether traffic or nontraffic accident**

X ● **V01.90**   **Pedestrian on foot injured in collision with pedal cycle, unspecified whether traffic or nontraffic accident**

Pedestrian NOS injured in collision with pedal cycle, unspecified whether traffic or nontraffic accident

X ● **V01.91**   **Pedestrian on roller-skates injured in collision with pedal cycle, unspecified whether traffic or nontraffic accident**

X ● **V01.92**   **Pedestrian on skateboard injured in collision with pedal cycle, unspecified whether traffic or nontraffic accident**

● **V01.93**   **Pedestrian on standing micro-mobility pedestrian conveyance injured in collision with pedal cycle, unspecified whether traffic or nontraffic accident**

V01.931   **Pedestrian on standing electric scooter injured in collision with pedal cycle, unspecified whether traffic or nontraffic accident**

V01.938   **Pedestrian on other standing micro-mobility pedestrian conveyance injured in collision with pedal cycle, unspecified whether traffic or nontraffic accident**

Pedestrian on hoverboard injured in collision with pedal cycle, unspecified whether traffic or nontraffic accident

Pedestrian on segway injured in collision with pedal cycle, unspecified whether traffic or nontraffic accident

X ● **V01.99**   **Pedestrian with other conveyance injured in collision with pedal cycle, unspecified whether traffic or nontraffic accident**

Pedestrian with baby stroller injured in collision with pedal cycle, unspecified whether traffic or nontraffic accident

Pedestrian in wheelchair (powered) injured in collision with pedal cycle, unspecified whether traffic or nontraffic accident

Pedestrian in motorized mobility scooter injured in collision with pedal cycle, unspecified whether traffic or nontraffic accident

Pedestrian on ice-skates injured in collision with pedal cycle unspecified, whether traffic or nontraffic accident

Pedestrian on nonmotorized scooter injured in collision with pedal cycle, unspecified whether traffic or nontraffic accident

Pedestrian on sled injured in collision with pedal cycle unspecified, whether traffic or nontraffic accident

Pedestrian on snowboard injured in collision with pedal cycle, unspecified whether traffic or nontraffic accident

Pedestrian on snow-skis injured in collision with pedal cycle, unspecified whether traffic or nontraffic accident

● **V02**   **Pedestrian injured in collision with two- or three-wheeled motor vehicle**

The appropriate 7th character is to be added to each code from category V02

A	initial encounter
D	subsequent encounter
S	sequela

● **V02.0**   **Pedestrian injured in collision with two- or three-wheeled motor vehicle in nontraffic accident**

X ● **V02.00**   **Pedestrian on foot injured in collision with two- or three-wheeled motor vehicle in nontraffic accident**

Pedestrian NOS injured in collision with two- or three-wheeled motor vehicle in nontraffic accident

X ● **V02.01**   **Pedestrian on roller-skates injured in collision with two- or three-wheeled motor vehicle in nontraffic accident**

X ● **V02.02**   **Pedestrian on skateboard injured in collision with two- or three-wheeled motor vehicle in nontraffic accident**

● **V02.03**   **Pedestrian on standing micro-mobility pedestrian conveyance injured in collision with two- or three-wheeled motor vehicle in nontraffic accident**

V02.031   **Pedestrian on standing electric scooter injured in collision with two- or three-wheeled motor vehicle in nontraffic accident**

V02.038   **Pedestrian on other standing micro-mobility pedestrian conveyance injured in collision with two- or three-wheeled motor vehicle in nontraffic accident**

Pedestrian on hoverboard injured in collision with two-or three wheeled motor vehicle in nontraffic accident

Pedestrian on segway injured in collision with two- or three-wheeled motor vehicle in nontraffic accident

X ● **V02.09**   **Pedestrian with other conveyance injured in collision with two- or three-wheeled motor vehicle in nontraffic accident**

Pedestrian with baby stroller injured in collision with two- or three-wheeled motor vehicle in nontraffic accident

Pedestrian on ice-skates injured in collision with two- or three-wheeled motor vehicle in nontraffic accident

Pedestrian in wheelchair (powered) injured in collision with two- or three-wheeled motor vehicle in nontraffic accident

Pedestrian in motorized mobility scooter injured in collision with two- or three-wheeled motor vehicle in nontraffic accident

Pedestrian on nonmotorized scooter injured in collision with two- or three-wheeled motor vehicle in nontraffic accident

Pedestrian on sled injured in collision with two- or three-wheeled motor vehicle in nontraffic accident

Pedestrian on snowboard injured in collision with two- or three-wheeled motor vehicle in nontraffic accident

Pedestrian on snow-skis injured in collision with two- or three-wheeled motor vehicle in nontraffic accident

● **V02.1 Pedestrian injured in collision with two- or three-wheeled motor vehicle in traffic accident**

X ● **V02.10** Pedestrian on foot injured in collision with two- or three-wheeled motor vehicle in traffic accident

Pedestrian NOS injured in collision with two- or three-wheeled motor vehicle in traffic accident

X ● **V02.11** Pedestrian on roller-skates injured in collision with two- or three-wheeled motor vehicle in traffic accident

X ● **V02.12** Pedestrian on skateboard injured in collision with two- or three-wheeled motor vehicle in traffic accident

● **V02.13** Pedestrian on standing micro-mobility pedestrian conveyance injured in collision with two- or three-wheeled motor vehicle in traffic accident

V02.131 Pedestrian on standing electric scooter injured in collision with two- or three-wheeled motor vehicle in traffic accident

V02.138 Pedestrian on other standing micro-mobility pedestrian conveyance injured in collision with two- or three-wheeled motor vehicle in traffic accident

Pedestrian on hoverboard injured in collision with two-or three wheeled motor vehicle in traffic accident

Pedestrian on segway injured in collision with two- or three-wheeled motor vehicle in traffic accident

X ● **V02.19** Pedestrian with other conveyance injured in collision with two- or three-wheeled motor vehicle in traffic accident

Pedestrian with baby stroller injured in collision with two- or three-wheeled motor vehicle in traffic accident

Pedestrian in wheelchair (powered) injured in collision with two- or three-wheeled motor vehicle in traffic accident

Pedestrian in motorized mobility scooter injured in collision with two- or three-wheeled motor vehicle in traffic accident

Pedestrian on ice-skates injured in collision with two- or three-wheeled motor vehicle in traffic accident

Pedestrian on nonmotorized scooter injured in collision with two- or three-wheeled motor vehicle in traffic accident

Pedestrian on sled injured in collision with two- or three-wheeled motor vehicle in traffic accident

Pedestrian on snowboard injured in collision with two- or three-wheeled motor vehicle in traffic accident

Pedestrian on snow-skis injured in collision with two- or three-wheeled motor vehicle in traffic accident

● **V02.9 Pedestrian injured in collision with two- or three-wheeled motor vehicle, unspecified whether traffic or nontraffic accident**

X ● **V02.90** Pedestrian on foot injured in collision with two- or three-wheeled motor vehicle, unspecified whether traffic or nontraffic accident

Pedestrian NOS injured in collision with two- or three-wheeled motor vehicle, unspecified whether traffic or nontraffic accident

X ● **V02.91** Pedestrian on roller-skates injured in collision with two- or three-wheeled motor vehicle, unspecified whether traffic or nontraffic accident

X ● **V02.92** Pedestrian on skateboard injured in collision with two- or three-wheeled motor vehicle, unspecified whether traffic or nontraffic accident

● **V02.93** Pedestrian on standing micro-mobility pedestrian conveyance injured in collision with two-or three-wheeled motor vehicle, unspecified whether traffic or nontraffic accident

V02.931 Pedestrian on standing electric scooter injured in collision with two- or three wheeled motor vehicle, unspecified whether traffic or nontraffic accident

V02.938 Pedestrian on other standing micro-mobility pedestrian conveyance injured in collision with two- or three wheeled motor vehicle, unspecified whether traffic or nontraffic accident

Pedestrian on hoverboard injured in collision with two-three-wheeled motor vehicle, unspecified whether traffic or nontraffic accident

Pedestrian on segway injured in collision with two- or three wheeled motor vehicle, unspecified whether traffic or nontraffic accident

X ● **V02.99** Pedestrian with other conveyance injured in collision with two- or three-wheeled motor vehicle, unspecified whether traffic or nontraffic accident

Pedestrian with baby stroller injured in collision with two- or three-wheeled motor vehicle, unspecified whether traffic or nontraffic accident

Pedestrian in wheelchair (powered) injured in collision with two- or three-wheeled motor vehicle, unspecified whether traffic or nontraffic accident

Pedestrian in motorized mobility scooter injured in collision with two- or three-wheeled motor vehicle, unspecified whether traffic or nontraffic accident

Pedestrian on ice-skates injured in collision with two- or three-wheeled motor vehicle, unspecified whether traffic or nontraffic accident

Pedestrian on nonmotorized scooter injured in collision with two- or three-wheeled motor vehicle, unspecified whether traffic or nontraffic accident

Pedestrian on sled injured in collision with two- or three-wheeled motor vehicle, unspecified whether traffic or nontraffic accident

Pedestrian on snowboard injured in collision with two- or three-wheeled motor vehicle, unspecified whether traffic or nontraffic accident

Pedestrian on snow-skis injured in collision with two- or three-wheeled motor vehicle, unspecified whether traffic or nontraffic accident

CHAPTER 20 (V00-Y99)

● V03 **Pedestrian injured in collision with car, pick-up truck or van**

The appropriate 7th character is to be added to each code from
— category V03

A	initial encounter
D	subsequent encounter
S	sequela

● V03.0 **Pedestrian injured in collision with car, pick-up truck or van in** nontraffic accident

X ● V03.00 **Pedestrian on** foot **injured in collision with car, pick-up truck or van in nontraffic accident**

Pedestrian NOS injured in collision with car, pick-up truck or van in nontraffic accident

X ● V03.01 **Pedestrian on** roller-skates **injured in collision with car, pick-up truck or van in nontraffic accident**

X ● V03.02 **Pedestrian on** skateboard **injured in collision with car, pick-up truck or van in nontraffic accident**

● V03.03 **Pedestrian on standing micro-mobility pedestrian conveyance injured in collision with car, pick-up or van in nontraffic accident**

V03.031 **Pedestrian on standing electric scooter injured in collision with car, pick-up or van in nontraffic accident**

V03.038 **Pedestrian on other standing micro-mobility pedestrian conveyance injured in collision with car, pick-up or van in nontraffic accident**

Pedestrian on hoverboard injured in collision with car, pick-up or van in nontraffic accident

Pedestrian on segway injured in collision with car, pick-up or van in nontraffic accident

X ● V03.09 **Pedestrian with** other **conveyance injured in collision with car, pick-up truck or van in nontraffic accident**

Pedestrian with baby stroller injured in collision with car, pick-up truck or van in nontraffic accident

Pedestrian in wheelchair (powered) injured in collision with car, pick-up truck or van in nontraffic accident

Pedestrian in motorized mobility scooter injured in collision with car, pick-up truck or van in nontraffic accident

Pedestrian on ice-skates injured in collision with car, pick-up truck or van in nontraffic accident

Pedestrian on nonmotorized scooter injured in collision with car, pick-up truck or van in nontraffic accident

Pedestrian on sled injured in collision with car, pick-up truck or van in nontraffic accident

Pedestrian on snowboard injured in collision with car, pick-up truck or van in nontraffic accident

Pedestrian on snow-skis injured in collision with car, pick-up truck or van in nontraffic accident

● V03.1 **Pedestrian injured in collision with car, pick-up truck or van in** traffic accident

X ● V03.10 **Pedestrian on** foot **injured in collision with car, pick-up truck or van in traffic accident**

Pedestrian NOS injured in collision with car, pick-up truck or van in traffic accident

X ● V03.11 **Pedestrian on** roller-skates **injured in collision with car, pick-up truck or van in traffic accident**

X ● V03.12 **Pedestrian on** skateboard **injured in collision with car, pick-up truck or van in traffic accident**

● V03.13 **Pedestrian on standing micro-mobility pedestrian conveyance injured in collision with car, pick-up or van in traffic accident**

V03.131 **Pedestrian on standing electric scooter injured in collision with car, pick-up or van in traffic accident**

V03.138 **Pedestrian on other standing micro-mobility pedestrian conveyance injured in collision with car, pick-up or van in traffic accident**

Pedestrian on hoverboard injured in collision with car, pick-up or van in traffic accident

Pedestrian on segway injured in collision with car, pick-up or van in traffic accident

X ● V03.19 **Pedestrian with** other **conveyance injured in collision with car, pick-up truck or van in traffic accident**

Pedestrian with baby stroller injured in collision with car, pick-up truck or van in traffic accident

Pedestrian in wheelchair (powered) injured in collision with car, pick-up truck or van in traffic accident

Pedestrian in motorized mobility scooter injured in collision with car, pick-up truck or van in traffic accident

Pedestrian on ice-skates injured in collision with car, pick-up truck or van in traffic accident

Pedestrian on nonmotorized scooter injured in collision with car, pick-up truck or van in traffic accident

Pedestrian on sled injured in collision with car, pick-up truck or van in traffic accident

Pedestrian on snowboard injured in collision with car, pick-up truck or van in traffic accident

Pedestrian on snow-skis injured in collision with car, pick-up truck or van in traffic accident

● V03.9 **Pedestrian injured in collision with car, pick-up truck or van,** unspecified whether traffic or nontraffic accident

X ● V03.90 **Pedestrian on** foot **injured in collision with car, pick-up truck or van, unspecified whether traffic or nontraffic accident**

Pedestrian NOS injured in collision with car, pick-up truck or van, unspecified whether traffic or nontraffic accident

X ● V03.91 **Pedestrian on** roller-skates **injured in collision with car, pick-up truck or van, unspecified whether traffic or nontraffic accident**

X ● V03.92 **Pedestrian on** skateboard **injured in collision with car, pick-up truck or van, unspecified whether traffic or nontraffic accident**

▶ New   ⇒ Revised   ~~deleted~~ Deleted   Excludes 1   Excludes 2   Includes   Use additional   Code first   Code also   Key words

OGCR Official Guidelines   X Assign placeholder X   ● Use Additional Character(s)   ▶ Manifestation Code   🏷 Hierarchical Condition Category   Coding Clinic

● V03.93 **Pedestrian on standing micro-mobility pedestrian conveyance injured in collision with car, pick-up or van, unspecified whether traffic or nontraffic accident**

    V03.931 Pedestrian on standing electric scooter injured in collision with car, pick-up or van, unspecified whether traffic or nontraffic accident

    V03.938 Pedestrian on other standing micro-mobility pedestrian conveyance injured in collision with car, pick-up or van, unspecified whether traffic or nontraffic accident

        Pedestrian on hoverboard injured in collision with car, pick-up or van, unspecified whether traffic or nontraffic accident

        Pedestrian on segway injured in collision with car, pick-up or van, unspecified whether traffic or nontraffic accident

X ● V03.99 **Pedestrian with other conveyance injured in collision with car, pick-up truck or van, unspecified whether traffic or nontraffic accident**

    Pedestrian with baby stroller injured in collision with car, pick-up truck or van, unspecified whether traffic or nontraffic accident

    Pedestrian in wheelchair (powered) injured in collision with car, pick-up truck or van, unspecified whether traffic or nontraffic accident

    Pedestrian in motorized mobility scooter injured in collision with car, pick-up truck or van, unspecified whether traffic or nontraffic accident

    Pedestrian on ice-skates injured in collision with car, pick-up truck or van, unspecified whether traffic or nontraffic accident

    Pedestrian on nonmotorized scooter injured in collision with car, pick-up truck or van, unspecified whether traffic or nontraffic accident

    Pedestrian on sled injured in collision with car, pick-up truck or van in nontraffic accident

    Pedestrian on snowboard injured in collision with car, pick-up truck or van, unspecified whether traffic or nontraffic accident

    Pedestrian on snow-skis injured in collision with car, pick-up truck or van, unspecified whether traffic or nontraffic accident

● V04 **Pedestrian injured in collision with heavy transport vehicle or bus**

    Excludes1   pedestrian injured in collision with military vehicle (V09.01, V09.21)

    The appropriate 7th character is to be added to each code from category V04

A	initial encounter
D	subsequent encounter
S	sequela

● V04.0 **Pedestrian injured in collision with heavy transport vehicle or bus in nontraffic accident**

X ● V04.00 **Pedestrian on foot injured in collision with heavy transport vehicle or bus in nontraffic accident**

    Pedestrian NOS injured in collision with heavy transport vehicle or bus in nontraffic accident

X ● V04.01 **Pedestrian on roller-skates injured in collision with heavy transport vehicle or bus in nontraffic accident**

X ● V04.02 **Pedestrian on skateboard injured in collision with heavy transport vehicle or bus in nontraffic accident**

● V04.03 **Pedestrian on standing micro-mobility pedestrian conveyance injured in collision with heavy transport vehicle or bus in nontraffic accident**

    V04.031 Pedestrian on standing electric scooter injured in collision with heavy transport vehicle or bus in nontraffic accident

    V04.038 Pedestrian on other standing micro-mobility pedestrian conveyance injured in collision with heavy transport vehicle or bus in nontraffic accident

        Pedestrian on hoverboard injured in collision with heavy transport vehicle or bus in nontraffic accident

        Pedestrian on segway injured in collision with heavy transport vehicle or bus in nontraffic accident

X ● V04.09 **Pedestrian with other conveyance injured in collision with heavy transport vehicle or bus in nontraffic accident**

    Pedestrian with baby stroller injured in collision with heavy transport vehicle or bus in nontraffic accident

    Pedestrian in wheelchair (powered) injured in collision with heavy transport vehicle or bus in nontraffic accident

    Pedestrian in motorized mobility scooter injured in collision with heavy transport vehicle or bus in nontraffic accident

    Pedestrian on ice-skates injured in collision with heavy transport vehicle or bus in nontraffic accident

    Pedestrian on nonmotorized scooter injured in collision with heavy transport vehicle or bus in nontraffic accident

    Pedestrian on sled injured in collision with heavy transport vehicle or bus in nontraffic accident

    Pedestrian on snowboard injured in collision with heavy transport vehicle or bus in nontraffic accident

    Pedestrian on snow-skis injured in collision with heavy transport vehicle or bus in nontraffic accident

● V04.1 **Pedestrian injured in collision with heavy transport vehicle or bus in traffic accident**

X ● V04.10 **Pedestrian on foot injured in collision with heavy transport vehicle or bus in traffic accident**

    Pedestrian NOS injured in collision with heavy transport vehicle or bus in traffic accident

X ● V04.11 **Pedestrian on roller-skates injured in collision with heavy transport vehicle or bus in traffic accident**

X ● V04.12 **Pedestrian on skateboard injured in collision with heavy transport vehicle or bus in traffic accident**

● V04.13 **Pedestrian on standing micro-mobility pedestrian conveyance injured in collision with heavy transport vehicle or bus in traffic accident**

    V04.131 Pedestrian on standing electric scooter injured in collision with heavy transport vehicle or bus in traffic accident

V04.138 Pedestrian on other standing micro-mobility pedestrian conveyance injured in collision with heavy transport vehicle or bus in traffic accident

> Pedestrian on hoverboard injured in collision with heavy transport vehicle or bus in traffic accident
> Pedestrian on segway injured in collision with heavy transport vehicle or bus in traffic accident

X● **V04.19** Pedestrian with other conveyance injured in collision with heavy transport vehicle or bus in traffic accident

> Pedestrian with baby stroller injured in collision with heavy transport vehicle or bus in traffic accident
> Pedestrian in wheelchair (powered) injured in collision with heavy transport vehicle or bus in traffic accident
> Pedestrian in motorized mobility scooter injured in collision with heavy transport vehicle or bus in traffic accident
> Pedestrian on ice-skates injured in collision with heavy transport vehicle or bus in traffic accident
> Pedestrian on nonmotorized scooter injured in collision with heavy transport vehicle or bus in traffic accident
> Pedestrian on sled injured in collision with heavy transport vehicle or bus in traffic accident
> Pedestrian on snowboard injured in collision with heavy transport vehicle or bus in traffic accident
> Pedestrian on snow-skis injured in collision with heavy transport vehicle or bus in traffic accident

● **V04.9** Pedestrian injured in collision with heavy transport vehicle or bus, unspecified whether traffic or nontraffic accident

X● **V04.90** Pedestrian on foot injured in collision with heavy transport vehicle or bus, unspecified whether traffic or nontraffic accident

> Pedestrian NOS injured in collision with heavy transport vehicle or bus, unspecified whether traffic or nontraffic accident

X● **V04.91** Pedestrian on roller-skates injured in collision with heavy transport vehicle or bus, unspecified whether traffic or nontraffic accident

X● **V04.92** Pedestrian on skateboard injured in collision with heavy transport vehicle or bus, unspecified whether traffic or nontraffic accident

● **V04.93** Pedestrian on standing micro-mobility pedestrian conveyance injured in collision with heavy transport vehicle or bus, unspecified whether traffic or nontraffic accident

V04.931 Pedestrian on standing electric scooter injured in collision with heavy transport vehicle or bus, unspecified whether traffic or nontraffic accident

V04.938 Pedestrian on other standing micro-mobility pedestrian conveyance injured in collision with heavy transport vehicle or bus, unspecified whether traffic or nontraffic accident

> Pedestrian on hoverboard injured in collision with heavy transport vehicle or bus, unspecified whether traffic or nontraffic accident
> Pedestrian on segway injured in collision with heavy transport vehicle or bus, unspecified whether traffic or nontraffic accident

X● **V04.99** Pedestrian with other conveyance injured in collision with heavy transport vehicle or bus, unspecified whether traffic or nontraffic accident

> Pedestrian with baby stroller injured in collision with heavy transport vehicle or bus, unspecified whether traffic or nontraffic accident
> Pedestrian in wheelchair (powered) injured in collision with heavy transport vehicle or bus, unspecified whether traffic or nontraffic accident
> Pedestrian in motorized mobility scooter injured in collision with heavy transport vehicle or bus, unspecified whether traffic or nontraffic accident
> Pedestrian on ice-skates injured in collision with heavy transport vehicle or bus, unspecified whether traffic or nontraffic accident
> Pedestrian on nonmotorized scooter injured in collision with heavy transport vehicle or bus, unspecified whether traffic or nontraffic accident
> Pedestrian on sled injured in collision with heavy transport vehicle or bus, unspecified whether traffic or nontraffic accident
> Pedestrian on snowboard injured in collision with heavy transport vehicle or bus, unspecified whether traffic or nontraffic accident
> Pedestrian on snow-skis injured in collision with heavy transport vehicle or bus, unspecified whether traffic or nontraffic accident

● **V05** Pedestrian injured in collision with railway train or railway vehicle

> The appropriate 7th character is to be added to each code from category V05

A	initial encounter
D	subsequent encounter
S	sequela

● **V05.0** Pedestrian injured in collision with railway train or railway vehicle in nontraffic accident

X● **V05.00** Pedestrian on foot injured in collision with railway train or railway vehicle in nontraffic accident

> Pedestrian NOS injured in collision with railway train or railway vehicle in nontraffic accident

X● **V05.01** Pedestrian on roller-skates injured in collision with railway train or railway vehicle in nontraffic accident

X● **V05.02** Pedestrian on skateboard injured in collision with railway train or railway vehicle in nontraffic accident

● **V05.03** Pedestrian on standing micro-mobility pedestrian conveyance injured in collision with railway train or railway vehicle in nontraffic accident

V05.031 Pedestrian on standing electric scooter injured in collision with railway train or railway vehicle in nontraffic accident

V05.038 Pedestrian on other standing micro-mobility pedestrian conveyance injured in collision with railway train or railway vehicle in nontraffic accident

> Pedestrian on hoverboard injured in collision with railway train or railway vehicle in nontraffic accident
> Pedestrian on segway injured in collision with railway train or railway vehicle in nontraffic accident

▶ New ⇒ Revised ~~deleted~~ Deleted Excludes 1 Excludes 2 Includes Use additional Code first Code also Key words
OGCR Official Guidelines X Assign placeholder X ● Use Additional Character(s) ▶ Manifestation Code ⬥ Hierarchical Condition Category Coding Clinic

X ● **V05.09** **Pedestrian with other conveyance injured in collision with railway train or railway vehicle in nontraffic accident**

Pedestrian with baby stroller injured in collision with railway train or railway vehicle in nontraffic accident

Pedestrian in wheelchair (powered) injured in collision with railway train or railway vehicle in nontraffic accident

Pedestrian in motorized mobility scooter injured in collision with railway train or railway vehicle in nontraffic accident

Pedestrian on ice-skates injured in collision with railway train or railway vehicle in nontraffic accident

Pedestrian on nonmotorized scooter injured in collision with railway train or railway vehicle in nontraffic accident

Pedestrian on sled injured in collision with railway train or railway vehicle in nontraffic accident

Pedestrian on snowboard injured in collision with railway train or railway vehicle in nontraffic accident

Pedestrian on snow-skis injured in collision with railway train or railway vehicle in nontraffic accident

● **V05.1** **Pedestrian injured in collision with railway train or railway vehicle in traffic accident**

X ● **V05.10** **Pedestrian on foot injured in collision with railway train or railway vehicle in traffic accident**

Pedestrian NOS injured in collision with railway train or railway vehicle in traffic accident

X ● **V05.11** **Pedestrian on roller-skates injured in collision with railway train or railway vehicle in traffic accident**

X ● **V05.12** **Pedestrian on skateboard injured in collision with railway train or railway vehicle in traffic accident**

● **V05.13** **Pedestrian on standing micro-mobility pedestrian conveyance injured in collision with railway train or railway vehicle in traffic accident**

V05.131 **Pedestrian on standing electric scooter injured in collision with railway train or railway vehicle in traffic accident**

V05.138 **Pedestrian on other standing micro-mobility pedestrian conveyance injured in collision with railway train or railway vehicle in traffic accident**

Pedestrian on hoverboard injured in collision with railway train or railway vehicle in traffic accident

Pedestrian on segway injured in collision with railway train or railway vehicle in traffic accident

X ● **V05.19** **Pedestrian with other conveyance injured in collision with railway train or railway vehicle in traffic accident**

Pedestrian with baby stroller injured in collision with railway train or railway vehicle in traffic accident

Pedestrian in wheelchair (powered) injured in collision with railway train or railway vehicle in traffic accident

Pedestrian in motorized mobility scooter injured in collision with railway train or railway vehicle in traffic accident

Pedestrian on ice-skates injured in collision with railway train or railway vehicle in traffic accident

Pedestrian on nonmotorized scooter injured in collision with railway train or railway vehicle in traffic accident

Pedestrian on sled injured in collision with railway train or railway vehicle in traffic accident

Pedestrian on snowboard injured in collision with railway train or railway vehicle in traffic accident

Pedestrian on snow-skis injured in collision with railway train or railway vehicle in traffic accident

● **V05.9** **Pedestrian injured in collision with railway train or railway vehicle, unspecified whether traffic or nontraffic accident**

X ● **V05.90** **Pedestrian on foot injured in collision with railway train or railway vehicle, unspecified whether traffic or nontraffic accident**

Pedestrian NOS injured in collision with railway train or railway vehicle, unspecified whether traffic or nontraffic accident

X ● **V05.91** **Pedestrian on roller-skates injured in collision with railway train or railway vehicle, unspecified whether traffic or nontraffic accident**

X ● **V05.92** **Pedestrian on skateboard injured in collision with railway train or railway vehicle, unspecified whether traffic or nontraffic accident**

● **V05.93** **Pedestrian on standing micro-mobility pedestrian conveyance injured in collision with railway train or railway vehicle, unspecified whether traffic or nontraffic accident**

V05.931 **Pedestrian on standing electric scooter injured in collision with railway train or railway vehicle, unspecified whether traffic or nontraffic accident**

V05.938 **Pedestrian on other standing micro-mobility pedestrian conveyance injured in collision with railway train or railway vehicle, unspecified whether traffic or nontraffic accident**

Pedestrian on hoverboard injured in collision with railway train or railway vehicle, unspecified whether traffic or nontraffic accident

Pedestrian on segway injured in collision with railway train or railway vehicle, unspecified whether traffic or nontraffic accident

X● **V05.99** **Pedestrian with other conveyance injured in collision with railway train or railway vehicle, unspecified whether traffic or nontraffic accident**

    Pedestrian with baby stroller injured in collision with railway train or railway vehicle, unspecified whether traffic or nontraffic

    Pedestrian in wheelchair (powered) injured in collision with railway train or railway vehicle, unspecified whether traffic or nontraffic

    Pedestrian in motorized mobility scooter injured in collision with railway train or railway vehicle, unspecified whether traffic or nontraffic

    Pedestrian on ice-skates injured in collision with railway train or railway vehicle, unspecified whether traffic or nontraffic

    Pedestrian on nonmotorized scooter injured in collision with railway train or railway vehicle, unspecified whether traffic or nontraffic

    Pedestrian on sled injured in collision with railway train or railway vehicle, unspecified whether traffic or nontraffic

    Pedestrian on snowboard injured in collision with railway train or railway vehicle, unspecified whether traffic or nontraffic

    Pedestrian on snow-skis injured in collision with railway train or railway vehicle, unspecified whether traffic or nontraffic

●**V06** **Pedestrian injured in collision with other nonmotor vehicle**

  Includes   collision with animal-drawn vehicle, animal being ridden, nonpowered streetcar

  Excludes1   pedestrian injured in collision with pedestrian conveyance (V00.0-)

The appropriate 7th character is to be added to each code from category V06

> A   initial encounter
> D   subsequent encounter
> S   sequela

●**V06.0** **Pedestrian injured in collision with other nonmotor vehicle in nontraffic accident**

X● **V06.00** **Pedestrian on foot injured in collision with other nonmotor vehicle in nontraffic accident**

    Pedestrian NOS injured in collision with other nonmotor vehicle in nontraffic accident

X● **V06.01** **Pedestrian on roller-skates injured in collision with other nonmotor vehicle in nontraffic accident**

X● **V06.02** **Pedestrian on skateboard injured in collision with other nonmotor vehicle in nontraffic accident**

●**V06.03** **Pedestrian on standing micro-mobility pedestrian conveyance injured in collision with other nonmotor vehicle in nontraffic accident**

V06.031 **Pedestrian on standing electric scooter injured in collision with other nonmotor vehicle in nontraffic accident**

V06.038 **Pedestrian on other standing micro-mobility pedestrian conveyance injured in collision with other nonmotor vehicle in nontraffic accident**

    Pedestrian on hoverboard injured in collision with other nonmotor vehicle in nontraffic accident

    Pedestrian on segway injured in collision with other nonmotor vehicle in nontraffic accident

X● **V06.09** **Pedestrian with other conveyance injured in collision with other nonmotor vehicle in nontraffic accident**

    Pedestrian with baby stroller injured in collision with other nonmotor vehicle in nontraffic accident

    Pedestrian in wheelchair (powered) injured in collision with other nonmotor vehicle in nontraffic accident

    Pedestrian in motorized mobility scooter injured in collision with other nonmotor vehicle in nontraffic accident

    Pedestrian on ice-skates injured in collision with other nonmotor vehicle in nontraffic accident

    Pedestrian on nonmotorized scooter injured in collision with other nonmotor vehicle in nontraffic accident

    Pedestrian on sled injured in collision with other nonmotor vehicle in nontraffic accident

    Pedestrian on snowboard injured in collision with other nonmotor vehicle in nontraffic accident

    Pedestrian on snow-skis injured in collision with other nonmotor vehicle in nontraffic accident

●**V06.1** **Pedestrian injured in collision with other nonmotor vehicle in traffic accident**

X● **V06.10** **Pedestrian on foot injured in collision with other nonmotor vehicle in traffic accident**

    Pedestrian NOS injured in collision with other nonmotor vehicle in traffic accident

X● **V06.11** **Pedestrian on roller-skates injured in collision with other nonmotor vehicle in traffic accident**

X● **V06.12** **Pedestrian on skateboard injured in collision with other nonmotor vehicle in traffic accident**

●**V06.13** **Pedestrian on standing micro-mobility pedestrian conveyance injured in collision with other nonmotor vehicle in traffic accident**

V06.131 **Pedestrian on standing electric scooter injured in collision with other nonmotor vehicle in traffic accident**

V06.138 **Pedestrian on other standing micro-mobility pedestrian conveyance injured in collision with other nonmotor vehicle in traffic accident**

    Pedestrian on hoverboard injured in collision with other nonmotor vehicle in traffic accident

    Pedestrian on segway injured in collision with other nonmotor vehicle in traffic accident

X● **V06.19** **Pedestrian with other conveyance injured in collision with other nonmotor vehicle in traffic accident**

    Pedestrian with baby stroller injured in collision with other nonmotor vehicle in nontraffic accident

    Pedestrian in wheelchair (powered) injured in collision with other nonmotor vehicle in traffic accident

    Pedestrian in motorized mobility scooter injured in collision with other nonmotor vehicle in traffic accident

    Pedestrian on ice-skates injured in collision with other nonmotor vehicle in traffic accident

    Pedestrian on nonmotorized scooter injured in collision with other nonmotor vehicle in traffic accident

    Pedestrian on sled injured in collision with other nonmotor vehicle in traffic accident

    Pedestrian on snowboard injured in collision with other nonmotor vehicle in traffic accident

    Pedestrian on snow-skis injured in collision with other nonmotor vehicle in traffic accident

● **V06.9 Pedestrian injured in collision with other nonmotor vehicle, unspecified whether traffic or nontraffic accident**

X ● **V06.90 Pedestrian on foot injured in collision with other nonmotor vehicle, unspecified whether traffic or nontraffic accident**

Pedestrian NOS injured in collision with other nonmotor vehicle, unspecified whether traffic or nontraffic accident

X ● **V06.91 Pedestrian on roller-skates injured in collision with other nonmotor vehicle, unspecified whether traffic or nontraffic accident**

X ● **V06.92 Pedestrian on skateboard injured in collision with other nonmotor vehicle, unspecified whether traffic or nontraffic accident**

● **V06.93 Pedestrian on standing micro-mobility pedestrian conveyance injured in collision with other nonmotor vehicle, unspecified whether traffic or nontraffic accident**

V06.931 Pedestrian on standing electric scooter injured in collision with other nonmotor vehicle, unspecified whether traffic or nontraffic accident

V06.938 Pedestrian on other standing micro-mobility pedestrian conveyance injured in collision with other nonmotor vehicle, unspecified whether traffic or nontraffic accident

Pedestrian on hoverboard injured in collision with other nonmotor, unspecified whether traffic or nontraffic accident

Pedestrian on segway injured in collision with other nonmotor vehicle, unspecified whether traffic or nontraffic accident

X ● **V06.99 Pedestrian with other conveyance injured in collision with other nonmotor vehicle, unspecified whether traffic or nontraffic accident**

Pedestrian with baby stroller injured in collision with other nonmotor vehicle, unspecified whether traffic or nontraffic accident

Pedestrian in wheelchair (powered) injured in collision with other nonmotor vehicle, unspecified whether traffic or nontraffic accident

Pedestrian in motorized mobility scooter injured in collision with other nonmotor vehicle, unspecified whether traffic or nontraffic accident

Pedestrian on ice-skates injured in collision with other nonmotor vehicle, unspecified whether traffic or nontraffic accident

Pedestrian on nonmotorized scooter injured in collision with other nonmotor vehicle, unspecified whether traffic or nontraffic accident

Pedestrian on sled injured in collision with other nonmotor vehicle, unspecified whether traffic or nontraffic accident

Pedestrian on snowboard injured in collision with other nonmotor vehicle, unspecified whether traffic or nontraffic accident

Pedestrian on snow-skis injured in collision with other nonmotor vehicle, unspecified whether traffic or nontraffic accident

● **V09 Pedestrian injured in other and unspecified transport accidents**

The appropriate 7th character is to be added to each code from category V09

A	initial encounter
D	subsequent encounter
S	sequela

● **V09.0 Pedestrian injured in nontraffic accident involving other and unspecified motor vehicles**

X ● **V09.00 Pedestrian injured in nontraffic accident involving unspecified motor vehicles**

X ● **V09.01 Pedestrian injured in nontraffic accident involving military vehicle**

X ● **V09.09 Pedestrian injured in nontraffic accident involving other motor vehicles**

Pedestrian injured in nontraffic accident by special vehicle

X ● **V09.1 Pedestrian injured in unspecified nontraffic accident**

● **V09.2 Pedestrian injured in traffic accident involving other and unspecified motor vehicles**

X ● **V09.20 Pedestrian injured in traffic accident involving unspecified motor vehicles**

X ● **V09.21 Pedestrian injured in traffic accident involving military vehicle**

X ● **V09.29 Pedestrian injured in traffic accident involving other motor vehicles**

X ● **V09.3 Pedestrian injured in unspecified traffic accident**

X ● **V09.9 Pedestrian injured in unspecified transport accident**

PEDAL CYCLE RIDER INJURED IN TRANSPORT ACCIDENT (V10-V19)

Includes   any non-motorized vehicle, excluding an animal-drawn vehicle, or a sidecar or trailer attached to the pedal cycle

Excludes2   rupture of pedal cycle tire (W37.0)

● **V10 Pedal cycle rider injured in collision with pedestrian or animal**

Excludes1   pedal cycle rider collision with animal-drawn vehicle or animal being ridden (V16.-)

The appropriate 7th character is to be added to each code from category V10

A	initial encounter
D	subsequent encounter
S	sequela

X ● **V10.0 Pedal cycle driver injured in collision with pedestrian or animal in nontraffic accident**

X ● **V10.1 Pedal cycle passenger injured in collision with pedestrian or animal in nontraffic accident**

X ● **V10.2 Unspecified pedal cyclist injured in collision with pedestrian or animal in nontraffic accident**

X ● **V10.3 Person boarding or alighting a pedal cycle injured in collision with pedestrian or animal**

X ● **V10.4 Pedal cycle driver injured in collision with pedestrian or animal in traffic accident**

X ● **V10.5 Pedal cycle passenger injured in collision with pedestrian or animal in traffic accident**

X ● **V10.9 Unspecified pedal cyclist injured in collision with pedestrian or animal in traffic accident**

CHAPTER 20 (V00-Y99)

● **V11 Pedal cycle rider injured in collision with other pedal cycle**

The appropriate 7th character is to be added to each code from category V11

> A initial encounter
> D subsequent encounter
> S sequela

X● **V11.0** Pedal cycle driver injured in collision with other pedal cycle in nontraffic accident

X● **V11.1** Pedal cycle passenger injured in collision with other pedal cycle in nontraffic accident

X● **V11.2** Unspecified pedal cyclist injured in collision with other pedal cycle in nontraffic accident

X● **V11.3** Person boarding or alighting a pedal cycle injured in collision with other pedal cycle

X● **V11.4** Pedal cycle driver injured in collision with other pedal cycle in traffic accident

X● **V11.5** Pedal cycle passenger injured in collision with other pedal cycle in traffic accident

X● **V11.9** Unspecified pedal cyclist injured in collision with other pedal cycle in traffic accident

● **V12 Pedal cycle rider injured in collision with two- or three-wheeled motor vehicle**

The appropriate 7th character is to be added to each code from category V12

> A initial encounter
> D subsequent encounter
> S sequela

X● **V12.0** Pedal cycle driver injured in collision with two- or three-wheeled motor vehicle in nontraffic accident

X● **V12.1** Pedal cycle passenger injured in collision with two- or three-wheeled motor vehicle in nontraffic accident

X● **V12.2** Unspecified pedal cyclist injured in collision with two- or three-wheeled motor vehicle in nontraffic accident

X● **V12.3** Person boarding or alighting a pedal cycle injured in collision with two- or three-wheeled motor vehicle

X● **V12.4** Pedal cycle driver injured in collision with two- or three-wheeled motor vehicle in traffic accident

X● **V12.5** Pedal cycle passenger injured in collision with two- or three-wheeled motor vehicle in traffic accident

X● **V12.9** Unspecified pedal cyclist injured in collision with two- or three-wheeled motor vehicle in traffic accident

● **V13 Pedal cycle rider injured in collision with car, pick-up truck or van**

The appropriate 7th character is to be added to each code from category V13

> A initial encounter
> D subsequent encounter
> S sequela

X● **V13.0** Pedal cycle driver injured in collision with car, pick-up truck or van in nontraffic accident

X● **V13.1** Pedal cycle passenger injured in collision with car, pick-up truck or van in nontraffic accident

X● **V13.2** Unspecified pedal cyclist injured in collision with car, pick-up truck or van in nontraffic accident

X● **V13.3** Person boarding or alighting a pedal cycle injured in collision with car, pick-up truck or van

X● **V13.4** Pedal cycle driver injured in collision with car, pick-up truck or van in traffic accident

X● **V13.5** Pedal cycle passenger injured in collision with car, pick-up truck or van in traffic accident

X● **V13.9** Unspecified pedal cyclist injured in collision with car, pick-up truck or van in traffic accident

● **V14 Pedal cycle rider injured in collision with heavy transport vehicle or bus**

> **Excludes1** pedal cycle rider injured in collision with military vehicle (V19.81)

The appropriate 7th character is to be added to each code from category V14

> A initial encounter
> D subsequent encounter
> S sequela

X● **V14.0** Pedal cycle driver injured in collision with heavy transport vehicle or bus in nontraffic accident

X● **V14.1** Pedal cycle passenger injured in collision with heavy transport vehicle or bus in nontraffic accident

X● **V14.2** Unspecified pedal cyclist injured in collision with heavy transport vehicle or bus in nontraffic accident

X● **V14.3** Person boarding or alighting a pedal cycle injured in collision with heavy transport vehicle or bus

X● **V14.4** Pedal cycle driver injured in collision with heavy transport vehicle or bus in traffic accident

X● **V14.5** Pedal cycle passenger injured in collision with heavy transport vehicle or bus in traffic accident

X● **V14.9** Unspecified pedal cyclist injured in collision with heavy transport vehicle or bus in traffic accident

● **V15 Pedal cycle rider injured in collision with railway train or railway vehicle**

The appropriate 7th character is to be added to each code from category V15

> A initial encounter
> D subsequent encounter
> S sequela

X● **V15.0** Pedal cycle driver injured in collision with railway train or railway vehicle in nontraffic accident

X● **V15.1** Pedal cycle passenger injured in collision with railway train or railway vehicle in nontraffic accident

X● **V15.2** Unspecified pedal cyclist injured in collision with railway train or railway vehicle in nontraffic accident

X● **V15.3** Person boarding or alighting a pedal cycle injured in collision with railway train or railway vehicle

X● **V15.4** Pedal cycle driver injured in collision with railway train or railway vehicle in traffic accident

X● **V15.5** Pedal cycle passenger injured in collision with railway train or railway vehicle in traffic accident

X● **V15.9** Unspecified pedal cyclist injured in collision with railway train or railway vehicle in traffic accident

● **V16 Pedal cycle rider injured in collision with other nonmotor vehicle**

> **Includes** collision with animal-drawn vehicle, animal being ridden, streetcar

The appropriate 7th character is to be added to each code from category V16

> A initial encounter
> D subsequent encounter
> S sequela

X● **V16.0** Pedal cycle driver injured in collision with other nonmotor vehicle in nontraffic accident

X● **V16.1** Pedal cycle passenger injured in collision with other nonmotor vehicle in nontraffic accident

X● **V16.2** Unspecified pedal cyclist injured in collision with other nonmotor vehicle in nontraffic accident

X● **V16.3** Person boarding or alighting a pedal cycle injured in collision with other nonmotor vehicle in nontraffic accident

X● **V16.4** Pedal cycle driver injured in collision with other nonmotor vehicle in traffic accident

X ● **V16.5** Pedal cycle passenger injured in collision with other nonmotor vehicle in traffic accident

X ● **V16.9** Unspecified pedal cyclist injured in collision with other nonmotor vehicle in traffic accident

● **V17** Pedal cycle rider injured in collision with fixed or stationary object

The appropriate 7th character is to be added to each code from category V17

A	initial encounter
D	subsequent encounter
S	sequela

X ● **V17.0** Pedal cycle driver injured in collision with fixed or stationary object in nontraffic accident

X ● **V17.1** Pedal cycle passenger injured in collision with fixed or stationary object in nontraffic accident

X ● **V17.2** Unspecified pedal cyclist injured in collision with fixed or stationary object in nontraffic accident

X ● **V17.3** Person boarding or alighting a pedal cycle injured in collision with fixed or stationary object

X ● **V17.4** Pedal cycle driver injured in collision with fixed or stationary object in traffic accident

X ● **V17.5** Pedal cycle passenger injured in collision with fixed or stationary object in traffic accident

X ● **V17.9** Unspecified pedal cyclist injured in collision with fixed or stationary object in traffic accident

● **V18** Pedal cycle rider injured in noncollision transport accident

Includes   fall or thrown from pedal cycle (without antecedent collision)
overturning pedal cycle NOS
overturning pedal cycle without collision

The appropriate 7th character is to be added to each code from category V18

A	initial encounter
D	subsequent encounter
S	sequela

X ● **V18.0** Pedal cycle driver injured in noncollision transport accident in nontraffic accident

X ● **V18.1** Pedal cycle passenger injured in noncollision transport accident in nontraffic accident

X ● **V18.2** Unspecified pedal cyclist injured in noncollision transport accident in nontraffic accident

X ● **V18.3** Person boarding or alighting a pedal cycle injured in noncollision transport accident

X ● **V18.4** Pedal cycle driver injured in noncollision transport accident in traffic accident

X ● **V18.5** Pedal cycle passenger injured in noncollision transport accident in traffic accident

X ● **V18.9** Unspecified pedal cyclist injured in noncollision transport accident in traffic accident

● **V19** Pedal cycle rider injured in other and unspecified transport accidents

The appropriate 7th character is to be added to each code from category V19

A	initial encounter
D	subsequent encounter
S	sequela

● **V19.0** Pedal cycle driver injured in collision with other and unspecified motor vehicles in nontraffic accident

X ● **V19.00** Pedal cycle driver injured in collision with unspecified motor vehicles in nontraffic accident

X ● **V19.09** Pedal cycle driver injured in collision with other motor vehicles in nontraffic accident

● **V19.1** Pedal cycle passenger injured in collision with other and unspecified motor vehicles in nontraffic accident

X ● **V19.10** Pedal cycle passenger injured in collision with unspecified motor vehicles in nontraffic accident

X ● **V19.19** Pedal cycle passenger injured in collision with other motor vehicles in nontraffic accident

● **V19.2** Unspecified pedal cyclist injured in collision with other and unspecified motor vehicles in nontraffic accident

X ● **V19.20** Unspecified pedal cyclist injured in collision with unspecified motor vehicles in nontraffic accident
Pedal cycle collision NOS, nontraffic

X ● **V19.29** Unspecified pedal cyclist injured in collision with other motor vehicles in nontraffic accident

X ● **V19.3** Pedal cyclist (driver) (passenger) injured in unspecified nontraffic accident
Pedal cycle accident NOS, nontraffic
Pedal cyclist injured in nontraffic accident NOS

● **V19.4** Pedal cycle driver injured in collision with other and unspecified motor vehicles in traffic accident

X ● **V19.40** Pedal cycle driver injured in collision with unspecified motor vehicles in traffic accident

X ● **V19.49** Pedal cycle driver injured in collision with other motor vehicles in traffic accident

● **V19.5** Pedal cycle passenger injured in collision with other and unspecified motor vehicles in traffic accident

X ● **V19.50** Pedal cycle passenger injured in collision with unspecified motor vehicles in traffic accident

X ● **V19.59** Pedal cycle passenger injured in collision with other motor vehicles in traffic accident

● **V19.6** Unspecified pedal cyclist injured in collision with other and unspecified motor vehicles in traffic accident

X ● **V19.60** Unspecified pedal cyclist injured in collision with unspecified motor vehicles in traffic accident
Pedal cycle collision NOS (traffic)

X ● **V19.69** Unspecified pedal cyclist injured in collision with other motor vehicles in traffic accident

● **V19.8** Pedal cyclist (driver) (passenger) injured in other specified transport accidents

X ● **V19.81** Pedal cyclist (driver) (passenger) injured in transport accident with military vehicle

X ● **V19.88** Pedal cyclist (driver) (passenger) injured in other specified transport accidents

X ● **V19.9** Pedal cyclist (driver) (passenger) injured in unspecified traffic accident
Pedal cycle accident NOS

MOTORCYCLE RIDER INJURED IN TRANSPORT ACCIDENT (V20-V29)

▶ **Includes**   electric bicycle
▶ e-bike
▶ e-bicycle
moped motorcycle with sidecar motorized bicycle
motor scooter

Excludes 1   three-wheeled motor vehicle (V30-V39)

● **V20** Motorcycle rider injured in collision with pedestrian or animal

Excludes 1   motorcycle rider collision with animal-drawn vehicle or animal being ridden (V26.-)

The appropriate 7th character is to be added to each code from category V20

A	initial encounter
D	subsequent encounter
S	sequela

X ● **V20.0** Motorcycle driver injured in collision with pedestrian or animal in nontraffic accident

▶ X ● **V20.01** Electric (assisted) bicycle driver injured in collision with pedestrian or animal in nontraffic accident

▶ X ● **V20.09** Other motorcycle driver injured in collision with pedestrian or animal in nontraffic accident

X● **V20.1** Motorcycle passenger injured in collision with pedestrian or animal in nontraffic accident

▶X● **V20.11** Electric (assisted) bicycle passenger injured in collision with pedestrian or animal in nontraffic accident

▶X● **V20.19** Other motorcycle passenger injured in collision with pedestrian or animal in nontraffic accident

X● **V20.2** Unspecified motorcycle rider injured in collision with pedestrian or animal in nontraffic accident

▶X● **V20.21** Unspecified electric (assisted) bicycle rider injured in collision with pedestrian or animal in nontraffic accident

▶X● **V20.29** Unspecified rider of other motorcycle injured in collision with pedestrian or animal in nontraffic accident

X● **V20.3** Person boarding or alighting a motorcycle injured in collision with pedestrian or animal

▶X● **V20.31** Person boarding or alighting an electric (assisted) bicycle injured in collision with pedestrian or animal

▶X● **V20.39** Person boarding or alighting other motorcycle injured in collision with pedestrian or animal

X● **V20.4** Motorcycle driver injured in collision with pedestrian or animal in traffic accident

▶X● **V20.41** Electric (assisted) bicycle driver injured in collision with pedestrian or animal in traffic accident

▶X● **V20.49** Other motorcycle driver injured in collision with pedestrian or animal in traffic accident

X● **V20.5** Motorcycle passenger injured in collision with pedestrian or animal in traffic accident

▶X● **V20.51** Electric (assisted) bicycle passenger injured in collision with pedestrian or animal in traffic accident

▶X● **V20.59** Other motorcycle passenger injured in collision with pedestrian or animal in traffic accident

X● **V20.9** Unspecified motorcycle rider injured in collision with pedestrian or animal in traffic accident

▶X● **V20.91** Unspecified electric (assisted) bicycle rider injured in collision with pedestrian or animal in traffic accident

▶X● **V20.99** Unspecified rider of other motorcycle injured in collision with pedestrian or animal in traffic accident

● **V21** Motorcycle rider injured in collision with pedal cycle

The appropriate 7th character is to be added to each code from category V21

A	initial encounter
D	subsequent encounter
S	sequela

X● **V21.0** Motorcycle driver injured in collision with pedal cycle in nontraffic accident

▶X● **V21.01** Electric (assisted) bicycle driver injured in collision with pedal cycle in nontraffic accident

▶X● **V21.09** Other motorcycle driver injured in collision with pedal cycle in nontraffic accident

X● **V21.1** Motorcycle passenger injured in collision with pedal cycle in nontraffic accident

▶X● **V21.11** Electric (assisted) bicycle passenger injured in collision with pedal cycle in nontraffic accident

▶X● **V21.19** Other motorcycle passenger injured in collision with pedal cycle in nontraffic accident

X● **V21.2** Unspecified motorcycle rider injured in collision with pedal cycle in nontraffic accident

▶X● **V21.21** Unspecified electric (assisted) bicycle rider injured in collision with pedal cycle in nontraffic accident

▶X● **V21.29** Unspecified rider of other motorcycle injured in collision with pedal cycle in nontraffic accident

X● **V21.3** Person boarding or alighting a motorcycle injured in collision with pedal cycle

▶X● **V21.31** Person boarding or alighting an electric (assisted) bicycle injured in collision with pedal cycle

▶X● **V21.39** Person boarding or alighting other motorcycle injured in collision with pedal cycle

X● **V21.4** Motorcycle driver injured in collision with pedal cycle in traffic accident

▶X● **V21.41** Electric (assisted) bicycle driver injured in collision with pedal cycle in traffic accident

▶X● **V21.49** Other motorcycle driver injured in collision with pedal cycle in traffic accident

X● **V21.5** Motorcycle passenger injured in collision with pedal cycle in traffic accident

▶X● **V21.51** Electric (assisted) bicycle passenger injured in collision with pedal cycle in traffic accident

▶X● **V21.59** Other motorcycle passenger injured in collision with pedal cycle in traffic accident

X● **V21.9** Unspecified motorcycle rider injured in collision with pedal cycle in traffic accident

▶X● **V21.91** Unspecified electric (assisted) bicycle rider injured in collision with pedal cycle in traffic accident

▶X● **V21.99** Unspecified rider of other motorcycle injured in collision with pedal cycle in traffic accident

● **V22** Motorcycle rider injured in collision with two- or three-wheeled motor vehicle

The appropriate 7th character is to be added to each code from category V22

A	initial encounter
D	subsequent encounter
S	sequela

X● **V22.0** Motorcycle driver injured in collision with two- or three-wheeled motor vehicle in nontraffic accident

▶X● **V22.01** Electric (assisted) bicycle driver injured in collision with two- or three-wheeled motor vehicle in nontraffic accident

▶X● **V22.09** Other motorcycle driver injured in collision with two- or three-wheeled motor vehicle in nontraffic accident

X● **V22.1** Motorcycle passenger injured in collision with two- or three-wheeled motor vehicle in nontraffic accident

▶X● **V22.11** Electric (assisted) bicycle passenger injured in collision with two- or three-wheeled motor vehicle in nontraffic accident

▶X● **V22.19** Other motorcycle passenger injured in collision with two- or three-wheeled motor vehicle in nontraffic accident

X● **V22.2** Unspecified motorcycle rider injured in collision with two- or three-wheeled motor vehicle in nontraffic accident

▶X● **V22.21** Unspecified electric (assisted) bicycle rider injured in collision with two- or three-wheeled motor vehicle in nontraffic accident

▶X● **V22.29** Unspecified rider of other motorcycle injured in collision with two- or three-wheeled motor vehicle in nontraffic accident

X● **V22.3** Person boarding or alighting a motorcycle injured in collision with two- or three-wheeled motor vehicle

▶X● **V22.31** Person boarding or alighting an electric (assisted) bicycle injured in collision with two- or three-wheeled motor vehicle

▶X● **V22.39** Person boarding or alighting other motorcycle injured in collision with two- or three-wheeled motor vehicle

▶ New   ⇒ Revised   ~~deleted~~ Deleted   Excludes 1   Excludes 2   Includes   Use additional   Code first   Code also   Key words

OGCR Official Guidelines   X Assign placeholder X   ● Use Additional Character(s)   ▶ Manifestation Code   🐾 Hierarchical Condition Category   **Coding Clinic**

X ● **V22.4** Motorcycle driver injured in collision with two- or three-wheeled motor vehicle in traffic accident

▶ X ● **V22.41** Electric (assisted) bicycle driver injured in collision with two- or three-wheeled motor vehicle in traffic accident

▶ X ● **V22.49** Other motorcycle driver injured in collision with two- or three-wheeled motor vehicle in traffic accident

X ● **V22.5** Motorcycle passenger injured in collision with two- or three-wheeled motor vehicle in traffic accident

▶ X ● **V22.51** Electric (assisted) bicycle passenger injured in collision with two- or three-wheeled motor vehicle in traffic accident

▶ X ● **V22.59** Other motorcycle passenger injured in collision with two- or three-wheeled motor vehicle in traffic accident

X ● **V22.9** Unspecified motorcycle rider injured in collision with two- or three-wheeled motor vehicle in traffic accident

▶ X ● **V22.91** Unspecified electric (assisted) bicycle rider injured in collision with two- or three-wheeled motor vehicle in traffic accident

▶ X ● **V22.99** Unspecified rider of other motorcycle injured in collision with two- or three-wheeled motor vehicle in traffic accident

● **V23** Motorcycle rider injured in collision with car, pick-up truck or van

The appropriate 7th character is to be added to each code from category V23

A	initial encounter
D	subsequent encounter
S	sequela

X ● **V23.0** Motorcycle driver injured in collision with car, pick-up truck or van in nontraffic accident

▶ X ● **V23.01** Electric (assisted) bicycle driver injured in collision with car, pick-up truck or van in nontraffic accident

▶ X ● **V23.09** Other motorcycle driver injured in collision with car, pick-up truck or van in nontraffic accident

X ● **V23.1** Motorcycle passenger injured in collision with car, pick-up truck or van in nontraffic accident

▶ X ● **V23.11** Electric (assisted) bicycle passenger injured in collision with car, pick-up truck or van in nontraffic accident

▶ X ● **V23.19** Other motorcycle passenger injured in collision with car, pick-up truck or van in nontraffic accident

X ● **V23.2** Unspecified motorcycle rider injured in collision with car, pick-up truck or van in nontraffic accident

▶ X ● **V23.21** Unspecified electric (assisted) bicycle rider injured in collision with car, pick-up truck or van in nontraffic accident

▶ X ● **V23.29** Unspecified rider of other motorcycle injured in collision with car, pick-up truck or van in nontraffic accident

X ● **V23.3** Person boarding or alighting a motorcycle injured in collision with car, pick-up truck or van

▶ X ● **V23.31** Person boarding or alighting an electric (assisted) bicycle injured in collision with car, pick-up truck or van

▶ X ● **V23.39** Person boarding or alighting other motorcycle injured in collision with car, pick-up truck or van

X ● **V23.4** Motorcycle driver injured in collision with car, pick-up truck or van in traffic accident

▶ X ● **V23.41** Electric (assisted) bicycle driver injured in collision with car, pick-up truck or van in traffic accident

▶ X ● **V23.49** Other motorcycle driver injured in collision with car, pick-up truck or van in traffic accident

X ● **V23.5** Motorcycle passenger injured in collision with car, pick-up truck or van in traffic accident

▶ X ● **V23.51** Electric (assisted) bicycle passenger injured in collision with car, pick-up truck or van in traffic accident

▶ X ● **V23.59** Other motorcycle passenger injured in collision with car, pick-up truck or van in traffic accident

X ● **V23.9** Unspecified motorcycle rider injured in collision with car, pick-up truck or van in traffic accident

▶ X ● **V23.91** Unspecified electric (assisted) bicycle rider injured in collision with car, pick-up truck or van in traffic accident

▶ X ● **V23.99** Unspecified rider of other motorcycle injured in collision with car, pick-up truck or van in traffic accident

● **V24** Motorcycle rider injured in collision with heavy transport vehicle or bus

➡ **Excludes1**   motorcycle rider injured in collision with military vehicle (V29.818)

The appropriate 7th character is to be added to each code from category V24

A	initial encounter
D	subsequent encounter
S	sequela

X ● **V24.0** Motorcycle driver injured in collision with heavy transport vehicle or bus in nontraffic accident

▶ X ● **V24.01** Electric (assisted) bicycle driver injured in collision with heavy transport vehicle or bus in nontraffic accident

▶ X ● **V24.09** Other motorcycle driver injured in collision with heavy transport vehicle or bus in nontraffic accident

X ● **V24.1** Motorcycle passenger injured in collision with heavy transport vehicle or bus in nontraffic accident

▶ X ● **V24.11** Electric (assisted) bicycle passenger injured in collision with heavy transport vehicle or bus in nontraffic accident

▶ X ● **V24.19** Other motorcycle passenger injured in collision with heavy transport vehicle or bus in nontraffic accident

X ● **V24.2** Unspecified motorcycle rider injured in collision with heavy transport vehicle or bus in nontraffic accident

▶ X ● **V24.21** Unspecified electric (assisted) bicycle rider injured in collision with heavy transport vehicle or bus in nontraffic accident

▶ X ● **V24.29** Unspecified rider of other motorcycle injured in collision with heavy transport vehicle or bus in nontraffic accident

X ● **V24.3** Person boarding or alighting a motorcycle injured in collision with heavy transport vehicle or bus

▶ X ● **V24.31** Person boarding or alighting an electric (assisted) bicycle injured in collision with heavy transport vehicle or bus

▶ X ● **V24.39** Person boarding or alighting other motorcycle injured in collision with heavy transport vehicle or bus

X ● **V24.4** Motorcycle driver injured in collision with heavy transport vehicle or bus in traffic accident

▶ X ● **V24.41** Electric (assisted) bicycle driver injured in collision with heavy transport vehicle or bus in traffic accident

▶ X ● **V24.49** Other motorcycle driver injured in collision with heavy transport vehicle or bus in traffic accident

X ● **V24.5** Motorcycle passenger injured in collision with heavy transport vehicle or bus in traffic accident

▶ X ● **V24.51** Electric (assisted) bicycle passenger injured in collision with heavy transport vehicle or bus in traffic accident

▶ X ● **V24.59** Other motorcycle passenger injured in collision with heavy transport vehicle or bus in traffic accident

CHAPTER 20 (V00-Y99)

X ● **V24.9**   **Unspecified** motorcycle rider injured in collision with heavy transport vehicle or bus in traffic accident

▶ X ● **V24.91**   Unspecified electric (assisted) bicycle rider injured in collision with heavy transport vehicle or bus in traffic accident

▶ X ● **V24.99**   Unspecified rider of other motorcycle injured in collision with heavy transport vehicle or bus in traffic accident

● **V25**   Motorcycle rider injured in collision with railway train or railway vehicle

The appropriate 7th character is to be added to each code from category V25

> A   initial encounter
> D   subsequent encounter
> S   sequela

X ● **V25.0**   Motorcycle driver injured in collision with railway train or railway vehicle in nontraffic accident

▶ X ● **V25.01**   Electric (assisted) bicycle driver injured in collision with railway train or railway vehicle in nontraffic accident

▶ X ● **V25.09**   Other motorcycle driver injured in collision with railway train or railway vehicle in nontraffic accident

X ● **V25.1**   Motorcycle passenger injured in collision with railway train or railway vehicle in nontraffic accident

▶ X ● **V25.11**   Electric (assisted) bicycle passenger injured in collision with railway train or railway vehicle in nontraffic accident

▶ X ● **V25.19**   Other motorcycle passenger injured in collision with railway train or railway vehicle in nontraffic accident

X ● **V25.2**   Unspecified motorcycle rider injured in collision with railway train or railway vehicle in nontraffic accident

▶ X ● **V25.21**   Unspecified electric (assisted) bicycle rider injured in collision with railway train or railway vehicle in nontraffic accident

▶ X ● **V25.29**   Unspecified rider of other motorcycle injured in collision with railway train or railway vehicle in nontraffic accident

X ● **V25.3**   Person boarding or alighting a motorcycle injured in collision with railway train or railway vehicle

▶ X ● **V25.31**   Person boarding or alighting an electric (assisted) bicycle injured in collision with railway train or railway vehicle

▶ X ● **V25.39**   Person boarding or alighting other motorcycle injured in collision with railway train or railway vehicle

X ● **V25.4**   Motorcycle driver injured in collision with railway train or railway vehicle in traffic accident

▶ X ● **V25.41**   Electric (assisted) bicycle driver injured in collision with railway train or railway vehicle in traffic accident

▶ X ● **V25.49**   Other motorcycle driver injured in collision with railway train or railway vehicle in traffic accident

X ● **V25.5**   Motorcycle passenger injured in collision with railway train or railway vehicle in traffic accident

▶ X ● **V25.51**   Electric (assisted) bicycle passenger injured in collision with railway train or railway vehicle in traffic accident

▶ X ● **V25.59**   Other motorcycle passenger injured in collision with railway train or railway vehicle in traffic accident

X ● **V25.9**   Unspecified motorcycle rider injured in collision with railway train or railway vehicle in traffic accident

▶ X ● **V25.91**   Unspecified electric (assisted) bicycle rider injured in collision with railway train or railway vehicle in traffic accident

▶ X ● **V25.99**   Unspecified rider of other motorcycle injured in collision with railway train or railway vehicle in traffic accident

● **V26**   Motorcycle rider injured in collision with other nonmotor vehicle

> **Includes**   collision with animal-drawn vehicle, animal being ridden, streetcar

The appropriate 7th character is to be added to each code from category V26

> A   initial encounter
> D   subsequent encounter
> S   sequela

X ● **V26.0**   Motorcycle driver injured in collision with other nonmotor vehicle in nontraffic accident

▶ X ● **V26.01**   Electric (assisted) bicycle driver injured in collision with other nonmotor vehicle in nontraffic accident

▶ X ● **V26.09**   Other motorcycle driver injured in collision with other nonmotor vehicle in nontraffic accident

X ● **V26.1**   Motorcycle passenger injured in collision with other nonmotor vehicle in nontraffic accident

▶ X ● **V26.11**   Electric (assisted) bicycle passenger injured in collision with other nonmotor vehicle in nontraffic accident

▶ X ● **V26.19**   Other motorcycle passenger injured in collision with other nonmotor vehicle in nontraffic accident

X ● **V26.2**   Unspecified motorcycle rider injured in collision with other nonmotor vehicle in nontraffic accident

▶ X ● **V26.21**   Unspecified electric (assisted) bicycle rider injured in collision with other nonmotor vehicle in nontraffic accident

▶ X ● **V26.29**   Unspecified rider of other motorcycle injured in collision with other nonmotor vehicle in nontraffic accident

X ● **V26.3**   Person boarding or alighting a motorcycle injured in collision with other nonmotor vehicle

▶ X ● **V26.31**   Person boarding or alighting an electric (assisted) bicycle injured in collision with other nonmotor vehicle

▶ X ● **V26.39**   Person boarding or alighting other motorcycle injured in collision with other nonmotor vehicle

X ● **V26.4**   Motorcycle driver injured in collision with other nonmotor vehicle in traffic accident

▶ X ● **V26.41**   Electric (assisted) bicycle driver injured in collision with other nonmotor vehicle in traffic accident

▶ X ● **V26.49**   Other motorcycle driver injured in collision with other nonmotor vehicle in traffic accident

X ● **V26.5**   Motorcycle passenger injured in collision with other nonmotor vehicle in traffic accident

▶ X ● **V26.51**   Electric (assisted) bicycle passenger injured in collision with other nonmotor vehicle in traffic accident

▶ X ● **V26.59**   Other motorcycle passenger injured in collision with other nonmotor vehicle in traffic accident

X ● **V26.9**   Unspecified motorcycle rider injured in collision with other nonmotor vehicle in traffic accident

▶ X ● **V26.91**   Unspecified electric (assisted) bicycle rider injured in collision with other nonmotor vehicle in traffic accident

▶ X ● **V26.99**   Unspecified rider of other motorcycle injured in collision with other nonmotor vehicle in traffic accident

● **V27**   **Motorcycle rider injured in collision with fixed or stationary object**

> The appropriate 7th character is to be added to each code from category V27

A	initial encounter
D	subsequent encounter
S	sequela

X● **V27.0**   Motorcycle driver injured in collision with fixed or stationary object in nontraffic accident

▶X● **V27.01**   Electric (assisted) bicycle driver injured in collision with fixed or stationary object in nontraffic accident

▶X● **V27.09**   Other motorcycle driver injured in collision with fixed or stationary object in nontraffic accident

X● **V27.1**   Motorcycle passenger injured in collision with fixed or stationary object in nontraffic accident

▶X● **V27.11**   Electric (assisted) bicycle passenger injured in collision with fixed or stationary object in nontraffic accident

▶X● **V27.19**   Other motorcycle passenger injured in collision with fixed or stationary object in nontraffic accident

X● **V27.2**   Unspecified motorcycle rider injured in collision with fixed or stationary object in nontraffic accident

▶X● **V27.21**   Unspecified electric (assisted) bicycle rider injured in collision with fixed or stationary object in nontraffic accident

▶X● **V27.29**   Unspecified rider of other motorcycle injured in collision with fixed or stationary object in nontraffic accident

X● **V27.3**   Person boarding or alighting a motorcycle injured in collision with fixed or stationary object

▶X● **V27.31**   Person boarding or alighting an electric (assisted) bicycle injured in collision with fixed or stationary object

▶X● **V27.39**   Person boarding or alighting other motorcycle injured in collision with fixed or stationary object

X● **V27.4**   Motorcycle driver injured in collision with fixed or stationary object in traffic accident

▶X● **V27.41**   Electric (assisted) bicycle driver injured in collision with fixed or stationary object in traffic accident

▶X● **V27.49**   Other motorcycle driver injured in collision with fixed or stationary object in traffic accident

X● **V27.5**   Motorcycle passenger injured in collision with fixed or stationary object in traffic accident

▶X● **V27.51**   Electric (assisted) bicycle passenger injured in collision with fixed or stationary object in traffic accident

▶X● **V27.59**   Other motorcycle passenger injured in collision with fixed or stationary object in traffic accident

X● **V27.9**   Unspecified motorcycle rider injured in collision with fixed or stationary object in traffic accident

▶X● **V27.91**   Unspecified electric (assisted) bicycle rider injured in collision with fixed or stationary object in traffic accident

▶X● **V27.99**   Unspecified rider of other motorcycle injured in collision with fixed or stationary object in traffic accident

● **V28**   **Motorcycle rider injured in noncollision transport accident**

Includes   fall or thrown from motorcycle (without antecedent collision)
overturning motorcycle NOS
overturning motorcycle without collision

> The appropriate 7th character is to be added to each code from category V28

A	initial encounter
D	subsequent encounter
S	sequela

X● **V28.0**   Motorcycle driver injured in noncollision transport accident in nontraffic accident

▶X● **V28.01**   Electric (assisted) bicycle driver injured in noncollision transport accident in nontraffic accident

▶X● **V28.09**   Other motorcycle driver injured in noncollision transport accident in nontraffic accident

X● **V28.1**   Motorcycle passenger injured in noncollision transport accident in nontraffic accident

▶X● **V28.11**   Electric (assisted) bicycle passenger injured in noncollision transport accident in nontraffic accident

▶X● **V28.19**   Other motorcycle passenger injured in noncollision transport accident in nontraffic accident

X● **V28.2**   Unspecified motorcycle rider injured in noncollision transport accident in nontraffic accident

▶X● **V28.21**   Unspecified electric (assisted) bicycle rider injured in noncollision transport accident in nontraffic accident

▶X● **V28.29**   Unspecified rider of other motorcycle injured in noncollision transport accident in nontraffic accident

X● **V28.3**   Person boarding or alighting a motorcycle injured in noncollision transport accident

▶X● **V28.31**   Person boarding or alighting an electric (assisted) bicycle injured in noncollision transport accident

▶X● **V28.39**   Person boarding or alighting other motorcycle injured in noncollision transport accident

X● **V28.4**   Motorcycle driver injured in noncollision transport accident in traffic accident

▶X● **V28.41**   Electric (assisted) bicycle driver injured in noncollision transport accident in traffic accident

▶X● **V28.49**   Other motorcycle driver injured in noncollision transport accident in traffic accident

X● **V28.5**   Motorcycle passenger injured in noncollision transport accident in traffic accident

▶X● **V28.51**   Electric (assisted) bicycle passenger injured in noncollision transport accident in traffic accident

▶X● **V28.59**   Other motorcycle passenger injured in noncollision transport accident in traffic accident

X● **V28.9**   Unspecified motorcycle rider injured in noncollision transport accident in traffic accident

▶X● **V28.91**   Unspecified electric (assisted) bicycle rider injured in noncollision transport accident in traffic accident

▶X● **V28.99**   Unspecified rider of other motorcycle injured in noncollision transport accident in traffic accident

CHAPTER 20 (V00-Y99)

V29   Motorcycle rider injured in other and unspecified transport accidents

The appropriate 7th character is to be added to each code from category V29

A	initial encounter
D	subsequent encounter
S	sequela

Coding Clinic: 2015, Q3, P20

V29.0   Motorcycle driver injured in collision with other and unspecified motor vehicles in nontraffic accident

X **V29.00   Motorcycle driver injured in collision with unspecified motor vehicles in nontraffic accident**

▶ X **V29.001   Electric (assisted) bicycle driver injured in collision with unspecified motor vehicles in nontraffic accident**

▶ X **V29.008   Other motorcycle driver injured in collision with unspecified motor vehicles in nontraffic accident**

X **V29.09   Motorcycle driver injured in collision with other motor vehicles in nontraffic accident**

▶ X **V29.091   Electric (assisted) bicycle driver injured in collision with other motor vehicles in nontraffic accident**

▶ X **V29.098   Other motorcycle driver injured in collision with other motor vehicles in nontraffic accident**

V29.1   Motorcycle passenger injured in collision with other and unspecified motor vehicles in nontraffic accident

X **V29.10   Motorcycle passenger injured in collision with unspecified motor vehicles in nontraffic accident**

▶ X **V29.101   Electric (assisted) bicycle passenger injured in collision with unspecified motor vehicles in nontraffic accident**

▶ X **V29.108   Other motorcycle passenger injured in collision with unspecified motor vehicles in nontraffic accident**

X **V29.19   Motorcycle passenger injured in collision with other motor vehicles in nontraffic accident**

▶ X **V29.191   Electric (assisted) bicycle passenger injured in collision with other motor vehicles in nontraffic accident**

▶ X **V29.198   Other motorcycle passenger injured in collision with other motor vehicles in nontraffic accident**

V29.2   Unspecified motorcycle rider injured in collision with other and unspecified motor vehicles in nontraffic accident

X **V29.20   Unspecified motorcycle rider injured in collision with unspecified motor vehicles in nontraffic accident**
▶Motorcycle collision NOS, nontraffic

▶ X **V29.201   Unspecified electric (assisted) bicycle rider injured in collision with unspecified motor vehicles in nontraffic accident**

▶ X **V29.208   Unspecified rider of other motorcycle injured in collision with unspecified motor vehicles in nontraffic accident**
▶Motorcycle collision NOS, nontraffic

X **V29.29   Unspecified motorcycle rider injured in collision with other motor vehicles in nontraffic accident**

▶ X **V29.291   Unspecified electric (assisted) bicycle rider injured in collision with other motor vehicles in nontraffic accident**

▶ X **V29.298   Unspecified rider of other motorcycle injured in collision with other motor vehicles in nontraffic accident**

X **V29.3   Motorcycle rider (driver) (passenger) injured in unspecified nontraffic accident**
Motorcycle accident NOS, nontraffic
Motorcycle rider injured in nontraffic accident NOS

▶ X **V29.31   Electric (assisted) bicycle (driver) (passenger) injured in unspecified nontraffic accident**

▶ X **V29.39   Other motorcycle (driver) (passenger) injured in unspecified nontraffic accident**
▶Motorcycle accident NOS, nontraffic
▶Motorcycle rider injured in nontraffic accident NOS

V29.4   Motorcycle driver injured in collision with other and unspecified motor vehicles in traffic accident

X **V29.40   Motorcycle driver injured in collision with unspecified motor vehicles in traffic accident**

▶ X **V29.401   Electric (assisted) bicycle driver injured in collision with unspecified motor vehicles in traffic accident**

▶ X **V29.408   Other motorcycle driver injured in collision with unspecified motor vehicles in traffic accident**

X **V29.49   Motorcycle driver injured in collision with other motor vehicles in traffic accident**

▶ X **V29.491   Electric (assisted) bicycle driver injured in collision with other motor vehicles in traffic accident**

▶ X **V29.498   Other motorcycle driver injured in collision with other motor vehicles in traffic accident**

V29.5   Motorcycle passenger injured in collision with other and unspecified motor vehicles in traffic accident

X **V29.50   Motorcycle passenger injured in collision with unspecified motor vehicles in traffic accident**

▶ X **V29.501   Electric (assisted) bicycle passenger injured in collision with unspecified motor vehicles in traffic accident**

▶ X **V29.508   Other motorcycle passenger injured in collision with unspecified motor vehicles in traffic accident**

X **V29.59   Motorcycle passenger injured in collision with other motor vehicles in traffic accident**

▶ X **V29.591   Electric (assisted) bicycle passenger injured in collision with other motor vehicles in traffic accident**

▶ X **V29.598   Other motorcycle passenger injured in collision with other motor vehicles in traffic accident**

V29.6   Unspecified motorcycle rider injured in collision with other and unspecified motor vehicles in traffic accident

X **V29.60   Unspecified motorcycle rider injured in collision with unspecified motor vehicles in traffic accident**
Motorcycle collision NOS (traffic)

▶ X **V29.601   Unspecified electric (assisted) bicycle rider injured in collision with unspecified motor vehicles in traffic accident**

▶ X **V29.608   Unspecified rider of other motorcycle injured in collision with unspecified motor vehicles in traffic accident**
▶Motorcycle collision NOS (traffic)

X **V29.69   Unspecified motorcycle rider injured in collision with other motor vehicles in traffic accident**

▶ X **V29.691   Unspecified electric (assisted) bicycle rider injured in collision with other motor vehicles in traffic accident**

▶ X **V29.698   Unspecified rider of other motorcycle injured in collision with other motor vehicles in traffic accident**

CHAPTER 20 (V00-Y99)

▶ New   ⇒ Revised   ~~deleted~~ Deleted   Excludes 1   Excludes 2   Includes   Use additional   Code first   Code also   Key words

OGCR Official Guidelines   X Assign placeholder X   ● Use Additional Character(s)   ▶ Manifestation Code   ⬧ Hierarchical Condition Category   Coding Clinic

● V29.8   Motorcycle rider (driver) (passenger) injured in other specified transport accidents

   X● V29.81   Motorcycle rider (driver) (passenger) injured in transport accident with military vehicle

     ▶X● V29.811   Electric (assisted) bicycle rider (driver) (passenger) injured in transport accident with military vehicle

     ▶X● V29.818   Rider (driver) (passenger) of other motorcycle injured in transport accident with military vehicle

   X● V29.88   Motorcycle rider (driver) (passenger) injured in other specified transport accidents

     ▶X● V29.881   Electric (assisted) bicycle rider (driver) (passenger) injured in other specified transport accidents

     ▶X● V29.888   Rider (driver) (passenger) of other motorcycle injured in other specified transport accidents

  X● V29.9   Motorcycle rider (driver) (passenger) injured in unspecified traffic accident

     Motorcycle accident NOS

   ▶X● V29.91   Electric (assisted) bicycle rider (driver) (passenger) injured in unspecified traffic accident

   ▶X● V29.99   Rider (driver) (passenger) of other motorcycle injured in unspecified traffic accident

     ▶ Motorcycle accident NOS

OCCUPANT OF THREE-WHEELED MOTOR VEHICLE INJURED IN TRANSPORT ACCIDENT (V30-V39)

Includes   motorized tricycle
             motorized rickshaw
             three-wheeled motor car

Excludes1   all-terrain vehicles (V86.-)
             motorcycle with sidecar (V20-V29)
             vehicle designed primarily for off-road use (V86.-)

● V30   Occupant of three-wheeled motor vehicle injured in collision with pedestrian or animal

    Excludes1   three-wheeled motor vehicle collision with animal-drawn vehicle or animal being ridden (V36.-)

The appropriate 7th character is to be added to each code from category V30

A	initial encounter
D	subsequent encounter
S	sequela

  X● V30.0   Driver of three-wheeled motor vehicle injured in collision with pedestrian or animal in nontraffic accident

  X● V30.1   Passenger in three-wheeled motor vehicle injured in collision with pedestrian or animal in nontraffic accident

  X● V30.2   Person on outside of three-wheeled motor vehicle injured in collision with pedestrian or animal in nontraffic accident

  X● V30.3   Unspecified occupant of three-wheeled motor vehicle injured in collision with pedestrian or animal in nontraffic accident

  X● V30.4   Person boarding or alighting a three-wheeled motor vehicle injured in collision with pedestrian or animal

  X● V30.5   Driver of three-wheeled motor vehicle injured in collision with pedestrian or animal in traffic accident

  X● V30.6   Passenger in three-wheeled motor vehicle injured in collision with pedestrian or animal in traffic accident

  X● V30.7   Person on outside of three-wheeled motor vehicle injured in collision with pedestrian or animal in traffic accident

  X● V30.9   Unspecified occupant of three-wheeled motor vehicle injured in collision with pedestrian or animal in traffic accident

● V31   Occupant of three-wheeled motor vehicle injured in collision with pedal cycle

The appropriate 7th character is to be added to each code from category V31

A	initial encounter
D	subsequent encounter
S	sequela

  X● V31.0   Driver of three-wheeled motor vehicle injured in collision with pedal cycle in nontraffic accident

  X● V31.1   Passenger in three-wheeled motor vehicle injured in collision with pedal cycle in nontraffic accident

  X● V31.2   Person on outside of three-wheeled motor vehicle injured in collision with pedal cycle in nontraffic accident

  X● V31.3   Unspecified occupant of three-wheeled motor vehicle injured in collision with pedal cycle in nontraffic accident

  X● V31.4   Person boarding or alighting a three-wheeled motor vehicle injured in collision with pedal cycle

  X● V31.5   Driver of three-wheeled motor vehicle injured in collision with pedal cycle in traffic accident

  X● V31.6   Passenger in three-wheeled motor vehicle injured in collision with pedal cycle in traffic accident

  X● V31.7   Person on outside of three-wheeled motor vehicle injured in collision with pedal cycle in traffic accident

  X● V31.9   Unspecified occupant of three-wheeled motor vehicle injured in collision with pedal cycle in traffic accident

● V32   Occupant of three-wheeled motor vehicle injured in collision with two- or three-wheeled motor vehicle

The appropriate 7th character is to be added to each code from category V32

A	initial encounter
D	subsequent encounter
S	sequela

  X● V32.0   Driver of three-wheeled motor vehicle injured in collision with two- or three-wheeled motor vehicle in nontraffic accident

  X● V32.1   Passenger in three-wheeled motor vehicle injured in collision with two- or three-wheeled motor vehicle in nontraffic accident

  X● V32.2   Person on outside of three-wheeled motor vehicle injured in collision with two- or three-wheeled motor vehicle in nontraffic accident

  X● V32.3   Unspecified occupant of three-wheeled motor vehicle injured in collision with two- or three-wheeled motor vehicle in nontraffic accident

  X● V32.4   Person boarding or alighting a three-wheeled motor vehicle injured in collision with two- or three-wheeled motor vehicle

  X● V32.5   Driver of three-wheeled motor vehicle injured in collision with two- or three-wheeled motor vehicle in traffic accident

  X● V32.6   Passenger in three-wheeled motor vehicle injured in collision with two- or three-wheeled motor vehicle in traffic accident

  X● V32.7   Person on outside of three-wheeled motor vehicle injured in collision with two- or three-wheeled motor vehicle in traffic accident

  X● V32.9   Unspecified occupant of three-wheeled motor vehicle injured in collision with two- or three-wheeled motor vehicle in traffic accident

● **V33 Occupant of three-wheeled motor vehicle injured in collision with car, pick-up truck or van**

> The appropriate 7th character is to be added to each code from category V33

> | | |
> |---|---|
> | A | initial encounter |
> | D | subsequent encounter |
> | S | sequela |

X ● **V33.0** Driver of three-wheeled motor vehicle injured in collision with car, pick-up truck or van in nontraffic accident

X ● **V33.1** Passenger in three-wheeled motor vehicle injured in collision with car, pick-up truck or van in nontraffic accident

X ● **V33.2** Person on outside of three-wheeled motor vehicle injured in collision with car, pick-up truck or van in nontraffic accident

X ● **V33.3** Unspecified occupant of three-wheeled motor vehicle injured in collision with car, pick-up truck or van in nontraffic accident

X ● **V33.4** Person boarding or alighting a three-wheeled motor vehicle injured in collision with car, pick-up truck or van

X ● **V33.5** Driver of three-wheeled motor vehicle injured in collision with car, pick-up truck or van in traffic accident

X ● **V33.6** Passenger in three-wheeled motor vehicle injured in collision with car, pick-up truck or van in traffic accident

X ● **V33.7** Person on outside of three-wheeled motor vehicle injured in collision with car, pick-up truck or van in traffic accident

X ● **V33.9** Unspecified occupant of three-wheeled motor vehicle injured in collision with car, pick-up truck or van in traffic accident

● **V34 Occupant of three-wheeled motor vehicle injured in collision with heavy transport vehicle or bus**

> **Excludes1**   occupant of three-wheeled motor vehicle injured in collision with military vehicle (V39.81)

> The appropriate 7th character is to be added to each code from category V34

> | | |
> |---|---|
> | A | initial encounter |
> | D | subsequent encounter |
> | S | sequela |

X ● **V34.0** Driver of three-wheeled motor vehicle injured in collision with heavy transport vehicle or bus in nontraffic accident

X ● **V34.1** Passenger in three-wheeled motor vehicle injured in collision with heavy transport vehicle or bus in nontraffic accident

X ● **V34.2** Person on outside of three-wheeled motor vehicle injured in collision with heavy transport vehicle or bus in nontraffic accident

X ● **V34.3** Unspecified occupant of three-wheeled motor vehicle injured in collision with heavy transport vehicle or bus in nontraffic accident

X ● **V34.4** Person boarding or alighting a three-wheeled motor vehicle injured in collision with heavy transport vehicle or bus

X ● **V34.5** Driver of three-wheeled motor vehicle injured in collision with heavy transport vehicle or bus in traffic accident

X ● **V34.6** Passenger in three-wheeled motor vehicle injured in collision with heavy transport vehicle or bus in traffic accident

X ● **V34.7** Person on outside of three-wheeled motor vehicle injured in collision with heavy transport vehicle or bus in traffic accident

X ● **V34.9** Unspecified occupant of three-wheeled motor vehicle injured in collision with heavy transport vehicle or bus in traffic accident

● **V35 Occupant of three-wheeled motor vehicle injured in collision with railway train or railway vehicle**

> The appropriate 7th character is to be added to each code from category V35

> | | |
> |---|---|
> | A | initial encounter |
> | D | subsequent encounter |
> | S | sequela |

X ● **V35.0** Driver of three-wheeled motor vehicle injured in collision with railway train or railway vehicle in nontraffic accident

X ● **V35.1** Passenger in three-wheeled motor vehicle injured in collision with railway train or railway vehicle in nontraffic accident

X ● **V35.2** Person on outside of three-wheeled motor vehicle injured in collision with railway train or railway vehicle in nontraffic accident

X ● **V35.3** Unspecified occupant of three-wheeled motor vehicle injured in collision with railway train or railway vehicle in nontraffic accident

X ● **V35.4** Person boarding or alighting a three-wheeled motor vehicle injured in collision with railway train or railway vehicle

X ● **V35.5** Driver of three-wheeled motor vehicle injured in collision with railway train or railway vehicle in traffic accident

X ● **V35.6** Passenger in three-wheeled motor vehicle injured in collision with railway train or railway vehicle in traffic accident

X ● **V35.7** Person on outside of three-wheeled motor vehicle injured in collision with railway train or railway vehicle in traffic accident

X ● **V35.9** Unspecified occupant of three-wheeled motor vehicle injured in collision with railway train or railway vehicle in traffic accident

● **V36 Occupant of three-wheeled motor vehicle injured in collision with other nonmotor vehicle**

> **Includes**   collision with animal-drawn vehicle, animal being ridden, streetcar

> The appropriate 7th character is to be added to each code from category V36

> | | |
> |---|---|
> | A | initial encounter |
> | D | subsequent encounter |
> | S | sequela |

X ● **V36.0** Driver of three-wheeled motor vehicle injured in collision with other nonmotor vehicle in nontraffic accident

X ● **V36.1** Passenger in three-wheeled motor vehicle injured in collision with other nonmotor vehicle in nontraffic accident

X ● **V36.2** Person on outside of three-wheeled motor vehicle injured in collision with other nonmotor vehicle in nontraffic accident

X ● **V36.3** Unspecified occupant of three-wheeled motor vehicle injured in collision with other nonmotor vehicle in nontraffic accident

X ● **V36.4** Person boarding or alighting a three-wheeled motor vehicle injured in collision with other nonmotor vehicle

X ● **V36.5** Driver of three-wheeled motor vehicle injured in collision with other nonmotor vehicle in traffic accident

X ● **V36.6** Passenger in three-wheeled motor vehicle injured in collision with other nonmotor vehicle in traffic accident

X ● **V36.7** Person on outside of three-wheeled motor vehicle injured in collision with other nonmotor vehicle in traffic accident

X ● **V36.9** Unspecified occupant of three-wheeled motor vehicle injured in collision with other nonmotor vehicle in traffic accident

▶ New   ⇒ Revised   ~~deleted~~ Deleted   Excludes 1   Excludes 2   Includes   Use additional   Code first   Code also   Key words

OGCR Official Guidelines   X Assign placeholder X   ● Use Additional Character(s)   ❙ Manifestation Code   ✎ Hierarchical Condition Category   **Coding Clinic**

● **V37**   **Occupant of three-wheeled motor vehicle injured in collision with fixed or stationary object**

The appropriate 7th character is to be added to each code from category V37

A	initial encounter
D	subsequent encounter
S	sequela

X● **V37.0**   Driver of three-wheeled motor vehicle injured in collision with fixed or stationary object in nontraffic accident

X● **V37.1**   Passenger in three-wheeled motor vehicle injured in collision with fixed or stationary object in nontraffic accident

X● **V37.2**   Person on outside of three-wheeled motor vehicle injured in collision with fixed or stationary object in nontraffic accident

X● **V37.3**   Unspecified occupant of three-wheeled motor vehicle injured in collision with fixed or stationary object in nontraffic accident

X● **V37.4**   Person boarding or alighting a three-wheeled motor vehicle injured in collision with fixed or stationary object

X● **V37.5**   Driver of three-wheeled motor vehicle injured in collision with fixed or stationary object in traffic accident

X● **V37.6**   Passenger in three-wheeled motor vehicle injured in collision with fixed or stationary object in traffic accident

X● **V37.7**   Person on outside of three-wheeled motor vehicle injured in collision with fixed or stationary object in traffic accident

X● **V37.9**   Unspecified occupant of three-wheeled motor vehicle injured in collision with fixed or stationary object in traffic accident

● **V38**   **Occupant of three-wheeled motor vehicle injured in noncollision transport accident**

Includes	fall or thrown from three-wheeled motor vehicle
	overturning of three-wheeled motor vehicle NOS
	overturning of three-wheeled motor vehicle without collision

The appropriate 7th character is to be added to each code from category V38

A	initial encounter
D	subsequent encounter
S	sequela

X● **V38.0**   Driver of three-wheeled motor vehicle injured in noncollision transport accident in nontraffic accident

X● **V38.1**   Passenger in three-wheeled motor vehicle injured in noncollision transport accident in nontraffic accident

X● **V38.2**   Person on outside of three-wheeled motor vehicle injured in noncollision transport accident in nontraffic accident

X● **V38.3**   Unspecified occupant of three-wheeled motor vehicle injured in noncollision transport accident in nontraffic accident

X● **V38.4**   Person boarding or alighting a three-wheeled motor vehicle injured in noncollision transport accident

X● **V38.5**   Driver of three-wheeled motor vehicle injured in noncollision transport accident in traffic accident

X● **V38.6**   Passenger in three-wheeled motor vehicle injured in noncollision transport accident in traffic accident

X● **V38.7**   Person on outside of three-wheeled motor vehicle injured in noncollision transport accident in traffic accident

X● **V38.9**   Unspecified occupant of three-wheeled motor vehicle injured in noncollision transport accident in traffic accident

● **V39**   **Occupant of three-wheeled motor vehicle injured in other and unspecified transport accidents**

The appropriate 7th character is to be added to each code from category V39

A	initial encounter
D	subsequent encounter
S	sequela

● **V39.0**   Driver of three-wheeled motor vehicle injured in collision with other and unspecified motor vehicles in nontraffic accident

X● **V39.00**   Driver of three-wheeled motor vehicle injured in collision with unspecified motor vehicles in nontraffic accident

X● **V39.09**   Driver of three-wheeled motor vehicle injured in collision with other motor vehicles in nontraffic accident

● **V39.1**   Passenger in three-wheeled motor vehicle injured in collision with other and unspecified motor vehicles in nontraffic accident

X● **V39.10**   Passenger in three-wheeled motor vehicle injured in collision with unspecified motor vehicles in nontraffic accident

X● **V39.19**   Passenger in three-wheeled motor vehicle injured in collision with other motor vehicles in nontraffic accident

● **V39.2**   Unspecified occupant of three-wheeled motor vehicle injured in collision with other and unspecified motor vehicles in nontraffic accident

X● **V39.20**   Unspecified occupant of three-wheeled motor vehicle injured in collision with unspecified motor vehicles in nontraffic accident

Collision NOS involving three-wheeled motor vehicle, nontraffic

X● **V39.29**   Unspecified occupant of three-wheeled motor vehicle injured in collision with other motor vehicles in nontraffic accident

● **V39.3**   Occupant (driver) (passenger) of three-wheeled motor vehicle injured in unspecified nontraffic accident

Accident NOS involving three-wheeled motor vehicle, nontraffic

Occupant of three-wheeled motor vehicle injured in nontraffic accident NOS

● **V39.4**   Driver of three-wheeled motor vehicle injured in collision with other and unspecified motor vehicles in traffic accident

X● **V39.40**   Driver of three-wheeled motor vehicle injured in collision with unspecified motor vehicles in traffic accident

X● **V39.49**   Driver of three-wheeled motor vehicle injured in collision with other motor vehicles in traffic accident

● **V39.5**   Passenger in three-wheeled motor vehicle injured in collision with other and unspecified motor vehicles in traffic accident

X● **V39.50**   Passenger in three-wheeled motor vehicle injured in collision with unspecified motor vehicles in traffic accident

X● **V39.59**   Passenger in three-wheeled motor vehicle injured in collision with other motor vehicles in traffic accident

● **V39.6**   Unspecified occupant of three-wheeled motor vehicle injured in collision with other and unspecified motor vehicles in traffic accident

X● **V39.60**   Unspecified occupant of three-wheeled motor vehicle injured in collision with unspecified motor vehicles in traffic accident

Collision NOS involving three-wheeled motor vehicle (traffic)

X● **V39.69**   Unspecified occupant of three-wheeled motor vehicle injured in collision with other motor vehicles in traffic accident

CHAPTER 20 (V00-Y99)

● **V39.8**   Occupant (driver) (passenger) of three-wheeled motor vehicle injured in other specified transport accidents

X● **V39.81**   Occupant (driver) (passenger) of three-wheeled motor vehicle injured in transport accident with military vehicle

X● **V39.89**   Occupant (driver) (passenger) of three-wheeled motor vehicle injured in other specified transport accidents

X● **V39.9**   Occupant (driver) (passenger) of three-wheeled motor vehicle injured in unspecified traffic accident

Accident NOS involving three-wheeled motor vehicle

CAR OCCUPANT INJURED IN TRANSPORT ACCIDENT (V40-V49)

Includes   a four-wheeled motor vehicle designed primarily for carrying passengers

automobile (pulling a trailer or camper)

Excludes1   bus (V50-V59)

minibus (V50-V59)

minivan (V50-V59)

motorcoach (V70-V79)

pick-up truck (V50-V59)

sport utility vehicle (SUV) (V50-V59)

● **V40**   Car occupant injured in collision with pedestrian or animal

Excludes1   car collision with animal-drawn vehicle or animal being ridden (V46.-)

The appropriate 7th character is to be added to each code from category V40

> A   initial encounter
> D   subsequent encounter
> S   sequela

X● **V40.0**   Car driver injured in collision with pedestrian or animal in nontraffic accident

X● **V40.1**   Car passenger injured in collision with pedestrian or animal in nontraffic accident

X● **V40.2**   Person on outside of car injured in collision with pedestrian or animal in nontraffic accident

X● **V40.3**   Unspecified car occupant injured in collision with pedestrian or animal in nontraffic accident

X● **V40.4**   Person boarding or alighting a car injured in collision with pedestrian or animal

X● **V40.5**   Car driver injured in collision with pedestrian or animal in traffic accident

X● **V40.6**   Car passenger injured in collision with pedestrian or animal in traffic accident

X● **V40.7**   Person on outside of car injured in collision with pedestrian or animal in traffic accident

X● **V40.9**   Unspecified car occupant injured in collision with pedestrian or animal in traffic accident

● **V41**   Car occupant injured in collision with pedal cycle

The appropriate 7th character is to be added to each code from category V41

> A   initial encounter
> D   subsequent encounter
> S   sequela

X● **V41.0**   Car driver injured in collision with pedal cycle in nontraffic accident

X● **V41.1**   Car passenger injured in collision with pedal cycle in nontraffic accident

X● **V41.2**   Person on outside of car injured in collision with pedal cycle in nontraffic accident

X● **V41.3**   Unspecified car occupant injured in collision with pedal cycle in nontraffic accident

X● **V41.4**   Person boarding or alighting a car injured in collision with pedal cycle

X● **V41.5**   Car driver injured in collision with pedal cycle in traffic accident

X● **V41.6**   Car passenger injured in collision with pedal cycle in traffic accident

X● **V41.7**   Person on outside of car injured in collision with pedal cycle in traffic accident

X● **V41.9**   Unspecified car occupant injured in collision with pedal cycle in traffic accident

● **V42**   Car occupant injured in collision with two- or three-wheeled motor vehicle

The appropriate 7th character is to be added to each code from category V42

> A   initial encounter
> D   subsequent encounter
> S   sequela

X● **V42.0**   Car driver injured in collision with two- or three-wheeled motor vehicle in nontraffic accident

X● **V42.1**   Car passenger injured in collision with two- or three-wheeled motor vehicle in nontraffic accident

X● **V42.2**   Person on outside of car injured in collision with two- or three-wheeled motor vehicle in nontraffic accident

X● **V42.3**   Unspecified car occupant injured in collision with two- or three-wheeled motor vehicle in nontraffic accident

X● **V42.4**   Person boarding or alighting a car injured in collision with two- or three-wheeled motor vehicle

X● **V42.5**   Car driver injured in collision with two- or three-wheeled motor vehicle in traffic accident

X● **V42.6**   Car passenger injured in collision with two- or three-wheeled motor vehicle in traffic accident

X● **V42.7**   Person on outside of car injured in collision with two- or three-wheeled motor vehicle in traffic accident

X● **V42.9**   Unspecified car occupant injured in collision with two- or three-wheeled motor vehicle in traffic accident

● **V43**   Car occupant injured in collision with car, pick-up truck or van

The appropriate 7th character is to be added to each code from category V43

> A   initial encounter
> D   subsequent encounter
> S   sequela

● **V43.0**   Car driver injured in collision with car, pick-up truck or van in nontraffic accident

X● **V43.01**   Car driver injured in collision with sport utility vehicle in nontraffic accident

X● **V43.02**   Car driver injured in collision with other type car in nontraffic accident

X● **V43.03**   Car driver injured in collision with pick-up truck in nontraffic accident

X● **V43.04**   Car driver injured in collision with van in nontraffic accident

● **V43.1**   Car passenger injured in collision with car, pick-up truck or van in nontraffic accident

X● **V43.11**   Car passenger injured in collision with sport utility vehicle in nontraffic accident

X● **V43.12**   Car passenger injured in collision with other type car in nontraffic accident

X● **V43.13**   Car passenger injured in collision with pick-up truck in nontraffic accident

X● **V43.14**   Car passenger injured in collision with van in nontraffic accident

● **V43.2**   Person on outside of car injured in collision with car, pick-up truck or van in nontraffic accident

X● **V43.21**   Person on outside of car injured in collision with sport utility vehicle in nontraffic accident

X● **V43.22**   Person on outside of car injured in collision with other type car in nontraffic accident

X● **V43.23**   Person on outside of car injured in collision with pick-up truck in nontraffic accident

X● **V43.24**   Person on outside of car injured in collision with van in nontraffic accident

▶ New   ⇒ Revised   ~~deleted~~ Deleted   Excludes 1   Excludes 2   Includes   Use additional   Code first   Code also   Key words

OGCR Official Guidelines   X Assign placeholder X   ● Use Additional Character(s)   ▌ Manifestation Code   🦠 Hierarchical Condition Category   **Coding Clinic**

● **V43.3** Unspecified car occupant injured in collision with car, pick-up truck or van in nontraffic accident

   X ● **V43.31** Unspecified car occupant injured in collision with sport utility vehicle in nontraffic accident

   X ● **V43.32** Unspecified car occupant injured in collision with other type car in nontraffic accident

   X ● **V43.33** Unspecified car occupant injured in collision with pick-up truck in nontraffic accident

   X ● **V43.34** Unspecified car occupant injured in collision with van in nontraffic accident

● **V43.4** Person boarding or alighting a car injured in collision with car, pick-up truck or van

   X ● **V43.41** Person boarding or alighting a car injured in collision with sport utility vehicle

   X ● **V43.42** Person boarding or alighting a car injured in collision with other type car

   X ● **V43.43** Person boarding or alighting a car injured in collision with pick-up truck

   X ● **V43.44** Person boarding or alighting a car injured in collision with van

● **V43.5** Car driver injured in collision with car, pick-up truck or van in traffic accident

   X ● **V43.51** Car driver injured in collision with sport utility vehicle in traffic accident

   X ● **V43.52** Car driver injured in collision with other type car in traffic accident

   X ● **V43.53** Car driver injured in collision with pick-up truck in traffic accident

   X ● **V43.54** Car driver injured in collision with van in traffic accident

● **V43.6** Car passenger injured in collision with car, pick-up truck or van in traffic accident

   X ● **V43.61** Car passenger injured in collision with sport utility vehicle in traffic accident
       Coding Clinic: 2015, Q1, P5-7

   X ● **V43.62** Car passenger injured in collision with other type car in traffic accident

   X ● **V43.63** Car passenger injured in collision with pick-up truck in traffic accident

   X ● **V43.64** Car passenger injured in collision with van in traffic accident

● **V43.7** Person on outside of car injured in collision with car, pick-up truck or van in traffic accident

   X ● **V43.71** Person on outside of car injured in collision with sport utility vehicle in traffic accident

   X ● **V43.72** Person on outside of car injured in collision with other type car in traffic accident

   X ● **V43.73** Person on outside of car injured in collision with pick-up truck in traffic accident

   X ● **V43.74** Person on outside of car injured in collision with van in traffic accident

● **V43.9** Unspecified car occupant injured in collision with car, pick-up truck or van in traffic accident

   X ● **V43.91** Unspecified car occupant injured in collision with sport utility vehicle in traffic accident

   X ● **V43.92** Unspecified car occupant injured in collision with other type car in traffic accident

   X ● **V43.93** Unspecified car occupant injured in collision with pick-up truck in traffic accident

   X ● **V43.94** Unspecified car occupant injured in collision with van in traffic accident

● **V44** Car occupant injured in collision with heavy transport vehicle or bus

   Excludes1 car occupant injured in collision with military vehicle (V49.81)

   The appropriate 7th character is to be added to each code from category V44

A	initial encounter
D	subsequent encounter
S	sequela

   X ● **V44.0** Car driver injured in collision with heavy transport vehicle or bus in nontraffic accident

   X ● **V44.1** Car passenger injured in collision with heavy transport vehicle or bus in nontraffic accident

   X ● **V44.2** Person on outside of car injured in collision with heavy transport vehicle or bus in nontraffic accident

   X ● **V44.3** Unspecified car occupant injured in collision with heavy transport vehicle or bus in nontraffic accident

   X ● **V44.4** Person boarding or alighting a car injured in collision with heavy transport vehicle or bus

   X ● **V44.5** Car driver injured in collision with heavy transport vehicle or bus in traffic accident

   X ● **V44.6** Car passenger injured in collision with heavy transport vehicle or bus in traffic accident

   X ● **V44.7** Person on outside of car injured in collision with heavy transport vehicle or bus in traffic accident

   X ● **V44.9** Unspecified car occupant injured in collision with heavy transport vehicle or bus in traffic accident

● **V45** Car occupant injured in collision with railway train or railway vehicle

   The appropriate 7th character is to be added to each code from category V45

A	initial encounter
D	subsequent encounter
S	sequela

   X ● **V45.0** Car driver injured in collision with railway train or railway vehicle in nontraffic accident

   X ● **V45.1** Car passenger injured in collision with railway train or railway vehicle in nontraffic accident

   X ● **V45.2** Person on outside of car injured in collision with railway train or railway vehicle in nontraffic accident

   X ● **V45.3** Unspecified car occupant injured in collision with railway train or railway vehicle in nontraffic accident

   X ● **V45.4** Person boarding or alighting a car injured in collision with railway train or railway vehicle

   X ● **V45.5** Car driver injured in collision with railway train or railway vehicle in traffic accident

   X ● **V45.6** Car passenger injured in collision with railway train or railway vehicle in traffic accident

   X ● **V45.7** Person on outside of car injured in collision with railway train or railway vehicle in traffic accident

   X ● **V45.9** Unspecified car occupant injured in collision with railway train or railway vehicle in traffic accident

● **V46** Car occupant injured in collision with other nonmotor vehicle

   Includes collision with animal-drawn vehicle, animal being ridden, streetcar

   The appropriate 7th character is to be added to each code from category V46

A	initial encounter
D	subsequent encounter
S	sequela

   X ● **V46.0** Car driver injured in collision with other nonmotor vehicle in nontraffic accident

   X ● **V46.1** Car passenger injured in collision with other nonmotor vehicle in nontraffic accident

X ● **V46.2**   **Person** on outside of car injured in collision with other nonmotor vehicle in **nontraffic accident**

X ● **V46.3**   **Unspecified** car occupant injured in collision with other nonmotor vehicle in **nontraffic accident**

X ● **V46.4**   **Person** boarding or alighting a car injured in collision with other nonmotor vehicle

X ● **V46.5**   Car **driver** injured in collision with other nonmotor vehicle in **traffic accident**

X ● **V46.6**   Car **passenger** injured in collision with other nonmotor vehicle in **traffic accident**

X ● **V46.7**   **Person** on outside of car injured in collision with other nonmotor vehicle in **traffic accident**

X ● **V46.9**   **Unspecified** car occupant injured in collision with other nonmotor vehicle in **traffic accident**

● **V47**   **Car occupant injured in collision with fixed or stationary object**

The appropriate 7th character is to be added to each code from category V47

> A   initial encounter
> D   subsequent encounter
> S   sequela

Coding Clinic: 2016, Q4, P73

X ● **V47.0**   Car **driver** injured in collision with fixed or stationary object in **nontraffic accident**

X ● **V47.1**   Car **passenger** injured in collision with fixed or stationary object in **nontraffic accident**

X ● **V47.2**   **Person** on outside of car injured in collision with fixed or stationary object in **nontraffic accident**

X ● **V47.3**   **Unspecified** car occupant injured in collision with fixed or stationary object in **nontraffic accident**

X ● **V47.4**   **Person** boarding or alighting a car injured in collision with fixed or stationary object

X ● **V47.5**   Car **driver** injured in collision with fixed or stationary object in **traffic accident**

X ● **V47.6**   Car **passenger** injured in collision with fixed or stationary object in **traffic accident**

X ● **V47.7**   **Person** on outside of car injured in collision with fixed or stationary object in **traffic accident**

X ● **V47.9**   **Unspecified** car occupant injured in collision with fixed or stationary object in **traffic accident**

● **V48**   **Car occupant injured in noncollision transport accident**

> **Includes**   overturning car NOS
> overturning car without collision

The appropriate 7th character is to be added to each code from category V48

> A   initial encounter
> D   subsequent encounter
> S   sequela

X ● **V48.0**   Car **driver** injured in noncollision transport accident in **nontraffic accident**

X ● **V48.1**   Car **passenger** injured in noncollision transport accident in **nontraffic accident**

X ● **V48.2**   **Person** on outside of car injured in noncollision transport accident in **nontraffic accident**

X ● **V48.3**   **Unspecified** car occupant injured in noncollision transport accident in **nontraffic accident**

X ● **V48.4**   **Person** boarding or alighting a car injured in noncollision transport accident

X ● **V48.5**   Car **driver** injured in noncollision transport accident in **traffic accident**

X ● **V48.6**   Car **passenger** injured in noncollision transport accident in **traffic accident**

X ● **V48.7**   **Person** on outside of car injured in noncollision transport accident in **traffic accident**

X ● **V48.9**   **Unspecified** car occupant injured in noncollision transport accident in **traffic accident**

● **V49**   **Car occupant injured in other and unspecified transport accidents**

The appropriate 7th character is to be added to each code from category V49

> A   initial encounter
> D   subsequent encounter
> S   sequela

● **V49.0**   **Driver** injured in collision with other and unspecified motor vehicles in **nontraffic accident**

X ● **V49.00**   **Driver** injured in collision with **unspecified** motor vehicles in nontraffic accident

X ● **V49.09**   **Driver** injured in collision with **other** motor vehicles in nontraffic accident

● **V49.1**   **Passenger** injured in collision with other and unspecified motor vehicles in **nontraffic accident**

X ● **V49.10**   **Passenger** injured in collision with **unspecified** motor vehicles in nontraffic accident

X ● **V49.19**   **Passenger** injured in collision with **other** motor vehicles in nontraffic accident

● **V49.2**   **Unspecified** car occupant injured in collision with other and unspecified motor vehicles in **nontraffic accident**

X ● **V49.20**   **Unspecified** car occupant injured in collision with **unspecified** motor vehicles in nontraffic accident

Car collision NOS, nontraffic

X ● **V49.29**   **Unspecified** car occupant injured in collision with **other** motor vehicles in nontraffic accident

X ● **V49.3**   Car occupant (driver) (passenger) injured in **unspecified** **nontraffic accident**

Car accident NOS, nontraffic
Car occupant injured in nontraffic accident NOS

● **V49.4**   **Driver** injured in collision with other and unspecified motor vehicles in **traffic accident**

X ● **V49.40**   **Driver** injured in collision with **unspecified** motor vehicles in traffic accident

X ● **V49.49**   **Driver** injured in collision with **other** motor vehicles in traffic accident

● **V49.5**   **Passenger** injured in collision with other and unspecified motor vehicles in **traffic accident**

X ● **V49.50**   **Passenger** injured in collision with **unspecified** motor vehicles in traffic accident

X ● **V49.59**   **Passenger** injured in collision with **other** motor vehicles in traffic accident

● **V49.6**   **Unspecified** car occupant injured in collision with other and unspecified motor vehicles in **traffic accident**

X ● **V49.60**   **Unspecified** car occupant injured in collision with **unspecified** motor vehicles in traffic accident

Car collision NOS (traffic)

X ● **V49.69**   **Unspecified** car occupant injured in collision with **other** motor vehicles in traffic accident

● **V49.8**   **Car occupant (driver) (passenger) injured in other specified transport accidents**

X ● **V49.81**   Car occupant (driver) (passenger) injured in transport accident with **military** vehicle

X ● **V49.88**   Car occupant (driver) (passenger) injured in other specified transport accidents

X ● **V49.9**   Car occupant (driver) (passenger) injured in **unspecified** traffic accident

Car accident NOS
Coding Clinic: 2015, Q1, P11

OCCUPANT OF PICK-UP TRUCK OR VAN INJURED IN TRANSPORT ACCIDENT (V50-V59)

Includes	a four- or six-wheel motor vehicle designed primarily for carrying passengers and property but weighing less than the local limit for classification as a heavy goods vehicle
	minibus
	minivan
	sport utility vehicle (SUV)
	truck
	van
Excludes1	heavy transport vehicle (V60-V69)

● **V50** Occupant of pick-up truck or van injured in collision with pedestrian or animal

> **Excludes1**   pick-up truck or van collision with animal-drawn vehicle or animal being ridden (V56.-)

> The appropriate 7th character is to be added to each code from category V50

A	initial encounter
D	subsequent encounter
S	sequela

X● **V50.0** Driver of pick-up truck or van injured in collision with pedestrian or animal in nontraffic accident

X● **V50.1** Passenger in pick-up truck or van injured in collision with pedestrian or animal in nontraffic accident

X● **V50.2** Person on outside of pick-up truck or van injured in collision with pedestrian or animal in nontraffic accident

X● **V50.3** Unspecified occupant of pick-up truck or van injured in collision with pedestrian or animal in nontraffic accident

X● **V50.4** Person boarding or alighting a pick-up truck or van injured in collision with pedestrian or animal

X● **V50.5** Driver of pick-up truck or van injured in collision with pedestrian or animal in traffic accident

X● **V50.6** Passenger in pick-up truck or van injured in collision with pedestrian or animal in traffic accident

X● **V50.7** Person on outside of pick-up truck or van injured in collision with pedestrian or animal in traffic accident

X● **V50.9** Unspecified occupant of pick-up truck or van injured in collision with pedestrian or animal in traffic accident

● **V51** Occupant of pick-up truck or van injured in collision with pedal cycle

> The appropriate 7th character is to be added to each code from category V51

A	initial encounter
D	subsequent encounter
S	sequela

X● **V51.0** Driver of pick-up truck or van injured in collision with pedal cycle in nontraffic accident

X● **V51.1** Passenger in pick-up truck or van injured in collision with pedal cycle in nontraffic accident

X● **V51.2** Person on outside of pick-up truck or van injured in collision with pedal cycle in nontraffic accident

X● **V51.3** Unspecified occupant of pick-up truck or van injured in collision with pedal cycle in nontraffic accident

X● **V51.4** Person boarding or alighting a pick-up truck or van injured in collision with pedal cycle

X● **V51.5** Driver of pick-up truck or van injured in collision with pedal cycle in traffic accident

X● **V51.6** Passenger in pick-up truck or van injured in collision with pedal cycle in traffic accident

X● **V51.7** Person on outside of pick-up truck or van injured in collision with pedal cycle in traffic accident

X● **V51.9** Unspecified occupant of pick-up truck or van injured in collision with pedal cycle in traffic accident

● **V52** Occupant of pick-up truck or van injured in collision with two- or three-wheeled motor vehicle

> The appropriate 7th character is to be added to each code from category V52

A	initial encounter
D	subsequent encounter
S	sequela

X● **V52.0** Driver of pick-up truck or van injured in collision with two- or three-wheeled motor vehicle in nontraffic accident

X● **V52.1** Passenger in pick-up truck or van injured in collision with two- or three-wheeled motor vehicle in nontraffic accident

X● **V52.2** Person on outside of pick-up truck or van injured in collision with two- or three-wheeled motor vehicle in nontraffic accident

X● **V52.3** Unspecified occupant of pick-up truck or van injured in collision with two- or three-wheeled motor vehicle in nontraffic accident

X● **V52.4** Person boarding or alighting a pick-up truck or van injured in collision with two- or three-wheeled motor vehicle

X● **V52.5** Driver of pick-up truck or van injured in collision with two- or three-wheeled motor vehicle in traffic accident

X● **V52.6** Passenger in pick-up truck or van injured in collision with two- or three-wheeled motor vehicle in traffic accident

X● **V52.7** Person on outside of pick-up truck or van injured in collision with two- or three-wheeled motor vehicle in traffic accident

X● **V52.9** Unspecified occupant of pick-up truck or van injured in collision with two- or three-wheeled motor vehicle in traffic accident

● **V53** Occupant of pick-up truck or van injured in collision with car, pick-up truck or van

> The appropriate 7th character is to be added to each code from category V53

A	initial encounter
D	subsequent encounter
S	sequela

X● **V53.0** Driver of pick-up truck or van injured in collision with car, pick-up truck or van in nontraffic accident

X● **V53.1** Passenger in pick-up truck or van injured in collision with car, pick-up truck or van in nontraffic accident

X● **V53.2** Person on outside of pick-up truck or van injured in collision with car, pick-up truck or van in nontraffic accident

X● **V53.3** Unspecified occupant of pick-up truck or van injured in collision with car, pick-up truck or van in nontraffic accident

X● **V53.4** Person boarding or alighting a pick-up truck or van injured in collision with car, pick-up truck or van

X● **V53.5** Driver of pick-up truck or van injured in collision with car, pick-up truck or van in traffic accident

X● **V53.6** Passenger in pick-up truck or van injured in collision with car, pick-up truck or van in traffic accident

X● **V53.7** Person on outside of pick-up truck or van injured in collision with car, pick-up truck or van in traffic accident

X● **V53.9** Unspecified occupant of pick-up truck or van injured in collision with car, pick-up truck or van in traffic accident

CHAPTER 20 (V00-Y99)

● **V54** Occupant of pick-up truck or van injured in collision with heavy transport vehicle or bus

  Excludes1 occupant of pick-up truck or van injured in collision with military vehicle (V59.81)

  The appropriate 7th character is to be added to each code from category V54

  A initial encounter
  D subsequent encounter
  S sequela

X● **V54.0** Driver of pick-up truck or van injured in collision with heavy transport vehicle or bus in nontraffic accident

X● **V54.1** Passenger in pick-up truck or van injured in collision with heavy transport vehicle or bus in nontraffic accident

X● **V54.2** Person on outside of pick-up truck or van injured in collision with heavy transport vehicle or bus in nontraffic accident

X● **V54.3** Unspecified occupant of pick-up truck or van injured in collision with heavy transport vehicle or bus in nontraffic accident

X● **V54.4** Person boarding or alighting a pick-up truck or van injured in collision with heavy transport vehicle or bus

X● **V54.5** Driver of pick-up truck or van injured in collision with heavy transport vehicle or bus in traffic accident

X● **V54.6** Passenger in pick-up truck or van injured in collision with heavy transport vehicle or bus in traffic accident

X● **V54.7** Person on outside of pick-up truck or van injured in collision with heavy transport vehicle or bus in traffic accident

X● **V54.9** Unspecified occupant of pick-up truck or van injured in collision with heavy transport vehicle or bus in traffic accident

● **V55** Occupant of pick-up truck or van injured in collision with railway train or railway vehicle

  The appropriate 7th character is to be added to each code from category V55

  A initial encounter
  D subsequent encounter
  S sequela

X● **V55.0** Driver of pick-up truck or van injured in collision with railway train or railway vehicle in nontraffic accident

X● **V55.1** Passenger in pick-up truck or van injured in collision with railway train or railway vehicle in nontraffic accident

X● **V55.2** Person on outside of pick-up truck or van injured in collision with railway train or railway vehicle in nontraffic accident

X● **V55.3** Unspecified occupant of pick-up truck or van injured in collision with railway train or railway vehicle in nontraffic accident

X● **V55.4** Person boarding or alighting a pick-up truck or van injured in collision with railway train or railway vehicle

X● **V55.5** Driver of pick-up truck or van injured in collision with railway train or railway vehicle in traffic accident

X● **V55.6** Passenger in pick-up truck or van injured in collision with railway train or railway vehicle in traffic accident

X● **V55.7** Person on outside of pick-up truck or van injured in collision with railway train or railway vehicle in traffic accident

X● **V55.9** Unspecified occupant of pick-up truck or van injured in collision with railway train or railway vehicle in traffic accident

● **V56** Occupant of pick-up truck or van injured in collision with other nonmotor vehicle

  Includes collision with animal-drawn vehicle, animal being ridden, streetcar

  The appropriate 7th character is to be added to each code from category V56

  A initial encounter
  D subsequent encounter
  S sequela

X● **V56.0** Driver of pick-up truck or van injured in collision with other nonmotor vehicle in nontraffic accident

X● **V56.1** Passenger in pick-up truck or van injured in collision with other nonmotor vehicle in nontraffic accident

X● **V56.2** Person on outside of pick-up truck or van injured in collision with other nonmotor vehicle in nontraffic accident

X● **V56.3** Unspecified occupant of pick-up truck or van injured in collision with other nonmotor vehicle in nontraffic accident

X● **V56.4** Person boarding or alighting a pick-up truck or van injured in collision with other nonmotor vehicle

X● **V56.5** Driver of pick-up truck or van injured in collision with other nonmotor vehicle in traffic accident

X● **V56.6** Passenger in pick-up truck or van injured in collision with other nonmotor vehicle in traffic accident

X● **V56.7** Person on outside of pick-up truck or van injured in collision with other nonmotor vehicle in traffic accident

X● **V56.9** Unspecified occupant of pick-up truck or van injured in collision with other nonmotor vehicle in traffic accident

● **V57** Occupant of pick-up truck or van injured in collision with fixed or stationary object

  The appropriate 7th character is to be added to each code from category V57

  A initial encounter
  D subsequent encounter
  S sequela

X● **V57.0** Driver of pick-up truck or van injured in collision with fixed or stationary object in nontraffic accident

X● **V57.1** Passenger in pick-up truck or van injured in collision with fixed or stationary object in nontraffic accident

X● **V57.2** Person on outside of pick-up truck or van injured in collision with fixed or stationary object in nontraffic accident

X● **V57.3** Unspecified occupant of pick-up truck or van injured in collision with fixed or stationary object in nontraffic accident

X● **V57.4** Person boarding or alighting a pick-up truck or van injured in collision with fixed or stationary object

X● **V57.5** Driver of pick-up truck or van injured in collision with fixed or stationary object in traffic accident

X● **V57.6** Passenger in pick-up truck or van injured in collision with fixed or stationary object in traffic accident

X● **V57.7** Person on outside of pick-up truck or van injured in collision with fixed or stationary object in traffic accident

X● **V57.9** Unspecified occupant of pick-up truck or van injured in collision with fixed or stationary object in traffic accident

● **V58** **Occupant of pick-up truck or van injured in noncollision transport accident**

> **Includes**   overturning pick-up truck or van NOS
> overturning pick-up truck or van without collision

The appropriate 7th character is to be added to each code from category V58

> A   initial encounter
> D   subsequent encounter
> S   sequela

X ● **V58.0** **Driver of pick-up truck or van injured in noncollision transport accident in nontraffic accident**

X ● **V58.1** **Passenger in pick-up truck or van injured in noncollision transport accident in nontraffic accident**

X ● **V58.2** **Person on outside of pick-up truck or van injured in noncollision transport accident in nontraffic accident**

X ● **V58.3** **Unspecified occupant of pick-up truck or van injured in noncollision transport accident in nontraffic accident**

X ● **V58.4** **Person boarding or alighting a pick-up truck or van injured in noncollision transport accident**

X ● **V58.5** **Driver of pick-up truck or van injured in noncollision transport accident in traffic accident**

X ● **V58.6** **Passenger in pick-up truck or van injured in noncollision transport accident in traffic accident**

X ● **V58.7** **Person on outside of pick-up truck or van injured in noncollision transport accident in traffic accident**

X ● **V58.9** **Unspecified occupant of pick-up truck or van injured in noncollision transport accident in traffic accident**

● **V59** **Occupant of pick-up truck or van injured in other and unspecified transport accidents**

The appropriate 7th character is to be added to each code from category V59

> A   initial encounter
> D   subsequent encounter
> S   sequela

● **V59.0** **Driver of pick-up truck or van injured in collision with other and unspecified motor vehicles in nontraffic accident**

    X ● **V59.00** **Driver of pick-up truck or van injured in collision with unspecified motor vehicles in nontraffic accident**

    X ● **V59.09** **Driver of pick-up truck or van injured in collision with other motor vehicles in nontraffic accident**

● **V59.1** **Passenger in pick-up truck or van injured in collision with other and unspecified motor vehicles in nontraffic accident**

    X ● **V59.10** **Passenger in pick-up truck or van injured in collision with unspecified motor vehicles in nontraffic accident**

    X ● **V59.19** **Passenger in pick-up truck or van injured in collision with other motor vehicles in nontraffic accident**

● **V59.2** **Unspecified occupant of pick-up truck or van injured in collision with other and unspecified motor vehicles in nontraffic accident**

    X ● **V59.20** **Unspecified occupant of pick-up truck or van injured in collision with unspecified motor vehicles in nontraffic accident**
> Collision NOS involving pick-up truck or van, nontraffic

    X ● **V59.29** **Unspecified occupant of pick-up truck or van injured in collision with other motor vehicles in nontraffic accident**

X ● **V59.3** **Occupant (driver) (passenger) of pick-up truck or van injured in unspecified nontraffic accident**
> Accident NOS involving pick-up truck or van, nontraffic
> Occupant of pick-up truck or van injured in nontraffic accident NOS

● **V59.4** **Driver of pick-up truck or van injured in collision with other and unspecified motor vehicles in traffic accident**

    X ● **V59.40** **Driver of pick-up truck or van injured in collision with unspecified motor vehicles in traffic accident**

    X ● **V59.49** **Driver of pick-up truck or van injured in collision with other motor vehicles in traffic accident**

● **V59.5** **Passenger in pick-up truck or van injured in collision with other and unspecified motor vehicles in traffic accident**

    X ● **V59.50** **Passenger in pick-up truck or van injured in collision with unspecified motor vehicles in traffic accident**

    X ● **V59.59** **Passenger in pick-up truck or van injured in collision with other motor vehicles in traffic accident**

● **V59.6** **Unspecified occupant of pick-up truck or van injured in collision with other and unspecified motor vehicles in traffic accident**

    X ● **V59.60** **Unspecified occupant of pick-up truck or van injured in collision with unspecified motor vehicles in traffic accident**
> Collision NOS involving pick-up truck or van (traffic)

    X ● **V59.69** **Unspecified occupant of pick-up truck or van injured in collision with other motor vehicles in traffic accident**

● **V59.8** **Occupant (driver) (passenger) of pick-up truck or van injured in other specified transport accidents**

    X ● **V59.81** **Occupant (driver) (passenger) of pick-up truck or van injured in transport accident with military vehicle**

    X ● **V59.88** **Occupant (driver) (passenger) of pick-up truck or van injured in other specified transport accidents**

X ● **V59.9** **Occupant (driver) (passenger) of pick-up truck or van injured in unspecified traffic accident**
> Accident NOS involving pick-up truck or van

OCCUPANT OF HEAVY TRANSPORT VEHICLE INJURED IN TRANSPORT ACCIDENT (V60-V69)

> **Includes**   18 wheeler
> armored car
> panel truck

> **Excludes1**   bus
> motorcoach

● **V60** **Occupant of heavy transport vehicle injured in collision with pedestrian or animal**

> **Excludes1**   heavy transport vehicle collision with animal-drawn vehicle or animal being ridden (V66.-)

The appropriate 7th character is to be added to each code from category V60

> A   initial encounter
> D   subsequent encounter
> S   sequela

X ● **V60.0** **Driver of heavy transport vehicle injured in collision with pedestrian or animal in nontraffic accident**

X ● **V60.1** **Passenger in heavy transport vehicle injured in collision with pedestrian or animal in nontraffic accident**

X ● **V60.2** **Person on outside of heavy transport vehicle injured in collision with pedestrian or animal in nontraffic accident**

X ● **V60.3** **Unspecified occupant of heavy transport vehicle injured in collision with pedestrian or animal in nontraffic accident**

X ● **V60.4** **Person boarding or alighting a heavy transport vehicle injured in collision with pedestrian or animal**

X ● **V60.5** **Driver of heavy transport vehicle injured in collision with pedestrian or animal in traffic accident**

X ⬤ **V60.6**   **Passenger in heavy transport vehicle injured in collision with pedestrian or animal in** traffic accident

X ⬤ **V60.7**   **Person on outside of heavy transport vehicle injured in collision with pedestrian or animal in** traffic accident

X ⬤ **V60.9**   **Unspecified occupant of heavy transport vehicle injured in collision with pedestrian or animal in** traffic accident

⬤ **V61**   **Occupant of heavy transport vehicle injured in collision with pedal cycle**

The appropriate 7th character is to be added to each code from category V61

A	initial encounter
D	subsequent encounter
S	sequela

X ⬤ **V61.0**   **Driver of heavy transport vehicle injured in collision with pedal cycle in** nontraffic accident

X ⬤ **V61.1**   **Passenger in heavy transport vehicle injured in collision with pedal cycle in** nontraffic accident

X ⬤ **V61.2**   **Person on outside of heavy transport vehicle injured in collision with pedal cycle in** nontraffic accident

X ⬤ **V61.3**   **Unspecified occupant of heavy transport vehicle injured in collision with pedal cycle in** nontraffic accident

X ⬤ **V61.4**   **Person boarding or alighting a heavy transport vehicle injured in collision with pedal cycle while boarding or alighting**

X ⬤ **V61.5**   **Driver of heavy transport vehicle injured in collision with pedal cycle in** traffic accident

X ⬤ **V61.6**   **Passenger in heavy transport vehicle injured in collision with pedal cycle in** traffic accident

X ⬤ **V61.7**   **Person on outside of heavy transport vehicle injured in collision with pedal cycle in** traffic accident

X ⬤ **V61.9**   **Unspecified occupant of heavy transport vehicle injured in collision with pedal cycle in** traffic accident

⬤ **V62**   **Occupant of heavy transport vehicle injured in collision with two- or three-wheeled motor vehicle**

The appropriate 7th character is to be added to each code from category V62

A	initial encounter
D	subsequent encounter
S	sequela

X ⬤ **V62.0**   **Driver of heavy transport vehicle injured in collision with two- or three-wheeled motor vehicle in** nontraffic accident

X ⬤ **V62.1**   **Passenger in heavy transport vehicle injured in collision with two- or three-wheeled motor vehicle in** nontraffic accident

X ⬤ **V62.2**   **Person on outside of heavy transport vehicle injured in collision with two- or three-wheeled motor vehicle in** nontraffic accident

X ⬤ **V62.3**   **Unspecified occupant of heavy transport vehicle injured in collision with two- or three-wheeled motor vehicle in** nontraffic accident

X ⬤ **V62.4**   **Person boarding or alighting a heavy transport vehicle injured in collision with two- or three-wheeled motor vehicle**

X ⬤ **V62.5**   **Driver of heavy transport vehicle injured in collision with two- or three-wheeled motor vehicle in** traffic accident

X ⬤ **V62.6**   **Passenger in heavy transport vehicle injured in collision with two- or three-wheeled motor vehicle in** traffic accident

X ⬤ **V62.7**   **Person on outside of heavy transport vehicle injured in collision with two- or three-wheeled motor vehicle in** traffic accident

X ⬤ **V62.9**   **Unspecified occupant of heavy transport vehicle injured in collision with two- or three-wheeled motor vehicle in** traffic accident

⬤ **V63**   **Occupant of heavy transport vehicle injured in collision with car, pick-up truck or van**

The appropriate 7th character is to be added to each code from category V63

A	initial encounter
D	subsequent encounter
S	sequela

X ⬤ **V63.0**   **Driver of heavy transport vehicle injured in collision with car, pick-up truck or van in** nontraffic accident

X ⬤ **V63.1**   **Passenger in heavy transport vehicle injured in collision with car, pick-up truck or van in** nontraffic accident

X ⬤ **V63.2**   **Person on outside of heavy transport vehicle injured in collision with car, pick-up truck or van in** nontraffic accident

X ⬤ **V63.3**   **Unspecified occupant of heavy transport vehicle injured in collision with car, pick-up truck or van in** nontraffic accident

X ⬤ **V63.4**   **Person boarding or alighting a heavy transport vehicle injured in collision with car, pick-up truck or van**

X ⬤ **V63.5**   **Driver of heavy transport vehicle injured in collision with car, pick-up truck or van in** traffic accident

X ⬤ **V63.6**   **Passenger in heavy transport vehicle injured in collision with car, pick-up truck or van in** traffic accident

X ⬤ **V63.7**   **Person on outside of heavy transport vehicle injured in collision with car, pick-up truck or van in** traffic accident

X ⬤ **V63.9**   **Unspecified occupant of heavy transport vehicle injured in collision with car, pick-up truck or van in** traffic accident

⬤ **V64**   **Occupant of heavy transport vehicle injured in collision with heavy transport vehicle or bus**

> **Excludes 1**   occupant of heavy transport vehicle injured in collision with military vehicle (V69.81)

The appropriate 7th character is to be added to each code from category V64

A	initial encounter
D	subsequent encounter
S	sequela

X ⬤ **V64.0**   **Driver of heavy transport vehicle injured in collision with heavy transport vehicle or bus in** nontraffic accident

X ⬤ **V64.1**   **Passenger in heavy transport vehicle injured in collision with heavy transport vehicle or bus in** nontraffic accident

X ⬤ **V64.2**   **Person on outside of heavy transport vehicle injured in collision with heavy transport vehicle or bus in** nontraffic accident

X ⬤ **V64.3**   **Unspecified occupant of heavy transport vehicle injured in collision with heavy transport vehicle or bus in** nontraffic accident

X ⬤ **V64.4**   **Person boarding or alighting a heavy transport vehicle injured in collision with heavy transport vehicle or bus while boarding or alighting**

X ⬤ **V64.5**   **Driver of heavy transport vehicle injured in collision with heavy transport vehicle or bus in** traffic accident

X ⬤ **V64.6**   **Passenger in heavy transport vehicle injured in collision with heavy transport vehicle or bus in** traffic accident

X ⬤ **V64.7**   **Person on outside of heavy transport vehicle injured in collision with heavy transport vehicle or bus in** traffic accident

X ⬤ **V64.9**   **Unspecified occupant of heavy transport vehicle injured in collision with heavy transport vehicle or bus in** traffic accident

▶ New   ⟹ Revised   ~~deleted~~ Deleted   Excludes 1   Excludes 2   Includes   Use additional   Code first   Code also   Key words

OGCR Official Guidelines   X Assign placeholder X   ⬤ Use Additional Character(s)   ▶ Manifestation Code   🏷 Hierarchical Condition Category   Coding Clinic

● **V65 Occupant of heavy transport vehicle injured in collision with railway train or railway vehicle**

The appropriate 7th character is to be added to each code from category V65

A	initial encounter
D	subsequent encounter
S	sequela

X ● **V65.0 Driver of heavy transport vehicle injured in collision with railway train or railway vehicle in nontraffic accident**

X ● **V65.1 Passenger in heavy transport vehicle injured in collision with railway train or railway vehicle in nontraffic accident**

X ● **V65.2 Person on outside of heavy transport vehicle injured in collision with railway train or railway vehicle in nontraffic accident**

X ● **V65.3 Unspecified occupant of heavy transport vehicle injured in collision with railway train or railway vehicle in nontraffic accident**

X ● **V65.4 Person boarding or alighting a heavy transport vehicle injured in collision with railway train or railway vehicle**

X ● **V65.5 Driver of heavy transport vehicle injured in collision with railway train or railway vehicle in traffic accident**

X ● **V65.6 Passenger in heavy transport vehicle injured in collision with railway train or railway vehicle in traffic accident**

X ● **V65.7 Person on outside of heavy transport vehicle injured in collision with railway train or railway vehicle in traffic accident**

X ● **V65.9 Unspecified occupant of heavy transport vehicle injured in collision with railway train or railway vehicle in traffic accident**

● **V66 Occupant of heavy transport vehicle injured in collision with other nonmotor vehicle**

Includes	collision with animal-drawn vehicle, animal being ridden, streetcar

The appropriate 7th character is to be added to each code from category V66

A	initial encounter
D	subsequent encounter
S	sequela

X ● **V66.0 Driver of heavy transport vehicle injured in collision with other nonmotor vehicle in nontraffic accident**

X ● **V66.1 Passenger in heavy transport vehicle injured in collision with other nonmotor vehicle in nontraffic accident**

X ● **V66.2 Person on outside of heavy transport vehicle injured in collision with other nonmotor vehicle in nontraffic accident**

X ● **V66.3 Unspecified occupant of heavy transport vehicle injured in collision with other nonmotor vehicle in nontraffic accident**

X ● **V66.4 Person boarding or alighting a heavy transport vehicle injured in collision with other nonmotor vehicle**

X ● **V66.5 Driver of heavy transport vehicle injured in collision with other nonmotor vehicle in traffic accident**

X ● **V66.6 Passenger in heavy transport vehicle injured in collision with other nonmotor vehicle in traffic accident**

X ● **V66.7 Person on outside of heavy transport vehicle injured in collision with other nonmotor vehicle in traffic accident**

X ● **V66.9 Unspecified occupant of heavy transport vehicle injured in collision with other nonmotor vehicle in traffic accident**

● **V67 Occupant of heavy transport vehicle injured in collision with fixed or stationary object**

The appropriate 7th character is to be added to each code from category V67

A	initial encounter
D	subsequent encounter
S	sequela

X ● **V67.0 Driver of heavy transport vehicle injured in collision with fixed or stationary object in nontraffic accident**

X ● **V67.1 Passenger in heavy transport vehicle injured in collision with fixed or stationary object in nontraffic accident**

X ● **V67.2 Person on outside of heavy transport vehicle injured in collision with fixed or stationary object in nontraffic accident**

X ● **V67.3 Unspecified occupant of heavy transport vehicle injured in collision with fixed or stationary object in nontraffic accident**

X ● **V67.4 Person boarding or alighting a heavy transport vehicle injured in collision with fixed or stationary object**

X ● **V67.5 Driver of heavy transport vehicle injured in collision with fixed or stationary object in traffic accident**

X ● **V67.6 Passenger in heavy transport vehicle injured in collision with fixed or stationary object in traffic accident**

X ● **V67.7 Person on outside of heavy transport vehicle injured in collision with fixed or stationary object in traffic accident**

X ● **V67.9 Unspecified occupant of heavy transport vehicle injured in collision with fixed or stationary object in traffic accident**

● **V68 Occupant of heavy transport vehicle injured in noncollision transport accident**

Includes	overturning heavy transport vehicle NOS overturning heavy transport vehicle without collision

The appropriate 7th character is to be added to each code from category V68

A	initial encounter
D	subsequent encounter
S	sequela

X ● **V68.0 Driver of heavy transport vehicle injured in noncollision transport accident in nontraffic accident**

X ● **V68.1 Passenger in heavy transport vehicle injured in noncollision transport accident in nontraffic accident**

X ● **V68.2 Person on outside of heavy transport vehicle injured in noncollision transport accident in nontraffic accident**

X ● **V68.3 Unspecified occupant of heavy transport vehicle injured in noncollision transport accident in nontraffic accident**

X ● **V68.4 Person boarding or alighting a heavy transport vehicle injured in noncollision transport accident**

X ● **V68.5 Driver of heavy transport vehicle injured in noncollision transport accident in traffic accident**

X ● **V68.6 Passenger in heavy transport vehicle injured in noncollision transport accident in traffic accident**

X ● **V68.7 Person on outside of heavy transport vehicle injured in noncollision transport accident in traffic accident**

X ● **V68.9 Unspecified occupant of heavy transport vehicle injured in noncollision transport accident in traffic accident**

CHAPTER 20 (V00-Y99)

● **V69** **Occupant of heavy transport vehicle injured in other and unspecified transport accidents**

The appropriate 7th character is to be added to each code from category V69

A	initial encounter
D	subsequent encounter
S	sequela

● **V69.0** **Driver of heavy transport vehicle injured in collision with other and unspecified motor vehicles in nontraffic accident**

  X ● **V69.00** Driver of heavy transport vehicle injured in collision with unspecified motor vehicles in nontraffic accident

  X ● **V69.09** Driver of heavy transport vehicle injured in collision with other motor vehicles in nontraffic accident

● **V69.1** **Passenger in heavy transport vehicle injured in collision with other and unspecified motor vehicles in nontraffic accident**

  X ● **V69.10** Passenger in heavy transport vehicle injured in collision with unspecified motor vehicles in nontraffic accident

  X ● **V69.19** Passenger in heavy transport vehicle injured in collision with other motor vehicles in nontraffic accident

● **V69.2** **Unspecified occupant of heavy transport vehicle injured in collision with other and unspecified motor vehicles in nontraffic accident**

  X ● **V69.20** Unspecified occupant of heavy transport vehicle injured in collision with unspecified motor vehicles in nontraffic accident

       Collision NOS involving heavy transport vehicle, nontraffic

  X ● **V69.29** Unspecified occupant of heavy transport vehicle injured in collision with other motor vehicles in nontraffic accident

X ● **V69.3** **Occupant (driver) (passenger) of heavy transport vehicle injured in unspecified nontraffic accident**

       Accident NOS involving heavy transport vehicle, nontraffic

       Occupant of heavy transport vehicle injured in nontraffic accident NOS

● **V69.4** **Driver of heavy transport vehicle injured in collision with other and unspecified motor vehicles in traffic accident**

  X ● **V69.40** Driver of heavy transport vehicle injured in collision with unspecified motor vehicles in traffic accident

  X ● **V69.49** Driver of heavy transport vehicle injured in collision with other motor vehicles in traffic accident

● **V69.5** **Passenger in heavy transport vehicle injured in collision with other and unspecified motor vehicles in traffic accident**

  X ● **V69.50** Passenger in heavy transport vehicle injured in collision with unspecified motor vehicles in traffic accident

  X ● **V69.59** Passenger in heavy transport vehicle injured in collision with other motor vehicles in traffic accident

● **V69.6** **Unspecified occupant of heavy transport vehicle injured in collision with other and unspecified motor vehicles in traffic accident**

  X ● **V69.60** Unspecified occupant of heavy transport vehicle injured in collision with unspecified motor vehicles in traffic accident

       Collision NOS involving heavy transport vehicle (traffic)

  X ● **V69.69** Unspecified occupant of heavy transport vehicle injured in collision with other motor vehicles in traffic accident

● **V69.8** **Occupant (driver) (passenger) of heavy transport vehicle injured in other specified transport accidents**

  X ● **V69.81** Occupant (driver) (passenger) of heavy transport vehicle injured in transport accidents with military vehicle

  X ● **V69.88** Occupant (driver) (passenger) of heavy transport vehicle injured in other specified transport accidents

X ● **V69.9** **Occupant (driver) (passenger) of heavy transport vehicle injured in unspecified traffic accident**

       Accident NOS involving heavy transport vehicle

BUS OCCUPANT INJURED IN TRANSPORT ACCIDENT (V70-V79)

Includes	motorcoach
Excludes1	minibus (V50-V59)

● **V70** **Bus occupant injured in collision with pedestrian or animal**

  Excludes1   bus collision with animal-drawn vehicle or animal being ridden (V76.-)

The appropriate 7th character is to be added to each code from category V70

A	initial encounter
D	subsequent encounter
S	sequela

  X ● **V70.0** Driver of bus injured in collision with pedestrian or animal in nontraffic accident

  X ● **V70.1** Passenger on bus injured in collision with pedestrian or animal in nontraffic accident

  X ● **V70.2** Person on outside of bus injured in collision with pedestrian or animal in nontraffic accident

  X ● **V70.3** Unspecified occupant of bus injured in collision with pedestrian or animal in nontraffic accident

  X ● **V70.4** Person boarding or alighting from bus injured in collision with pedestrian or animal

  X ● **V70.5** Driver of bus injured in collision with pedestrian or animal in traffic accident

  X ● **V70.6** Passenger on bus injured in collision with pedestrian or animal in traffic accident

  X ● **V70.7** Person on outside of bus injured in collision with pedestrian or animal in traffic accident

  X ● **V70.9** Unspecified occupant of bus injured in collision with pedestrian or animal in traffic accident

● **V71** **Bus occupant injured in collision with pedal cycle**

The appropriate 7th character is to be added to each code from category V71

A	initial encounter
D	subsequent encounter
S	sequela

  X ● **V71.0** Driver of bus injured in collision with pedal cycle in nontraffic accident

  X ● **V71.1** Passenger on bus injured in collision with pedal cycle in nontraffic accident

  X ● **V71.2** Person on outside of bus injured in collision with pedal cycle in nontraffic accident

  X ● **V71.3** Unspecified occupant of bus injured in collision with pedal cycle in nontraffic accident

  X ● **V71.4** Person boarding or alighting from bus injured in collision with pedal cycle

  X ● **V71.5** Driver of bus injured in collision with pedal cycle in traffic accident

  X ● **V71.6** Passenger on bus injured in collision with pedal cycle in traffic accident

  X ● **V71.7** Person on outside of bus injured in collision with pedal cycle in traffic accident

  X ● **V71.9** Unspecified occupant of bus injured in collision with pedal cycle in traffic accident

▶ New   ⇒ Revised   ~~deleted~~ Deleted   Excludes 1   Excludes 2   Includes   Use additional   Code first   Code also   Key words

OGCR Official Guidelines   X Assign placeholder X   ● Use Additional Character(s)   ▶ Manifestation Code   🏥 Hierarchical Condition Category   Coding Clinic

● **V72** **Bus occupant injured in collision with two- or three-wheeled motor vehicle**

> The appropriate 7th character is to be added to each code from category V72

> | | |
> |---|---|
> | A | initial encounter |
> | D | subsequent encounter |
> | S | sequela |

X● **V72.0** **Driver** of bus injured in collision with two- or three-wheeled motor vehicle in nontraffic accident

X● **V72.1** **Passenger** on bus injured in collision with two- or three-wheeled motor vehicle in nontraffic accident

X● **V72.2** **Person on outside** of bus injured in collision with two- or three-wheeled motor vehicle in nontraffic accident

X● **V72.3** **Unspecified** occupant of bus injured in collision with two- or three-wheeled motor vehicle in nontraffic accident

X● **V72.4** **Person boarding or alighting** from bus injured in collision with two- or three-wheeled motor vehicle

X● **V72.5** **Driver** of bus injured in collision with two- or three-wheeled motor vehicle in traffic accident

X● **V72.6** **Passenger** on bus injured in collision with two- or three-wheeled motor vehicle in traffic accident

X● **V72.7** **Person on outside** of bus injured in collision with two- or three-wheeled motor vehicle in traffic accident

X● **V72.9** **Unspecified** occupant of bus injured in collision with two- or three-wheeled motor vehicle in traffic accident

● **V73** **Bus occupant injured in collision with car, pick-up truck or van**

> The appropriate 7th character is to be added to each code from category V73

> | | |
> |---|---|
> | A | initial encounter |
> | D | subsequent encounter |
> | S | sequela |

X● **V73.0** **Driver** of bus injured in collision with car, pick-up truck or van in nontraffic accident

X● **V73.1** **Passenger** on bus injured in collision with car, pick-up truck or van in nontraffic accident

X● **V73.2** **Person on outside** of bus injured in collision with car, pick-up truck or van in nontraffic accident

X● **V73.3** **Unspecified** occupant of bus injured in collision with car, pick-up truck or van in nontraffic accident

X● **V73.4** **Person boarding or alighting** from bus injured in collision with car, pick-up truck or van

X● **V73.5** **Driver** of bus injured in collision with car, pick-up truck or van in traffic accident

X● **V73.6** **Passenger** on bus injured in collision with car, pick-up truck or van in traffic accident

X● **V73.7** **Person on outside** of bus injured in collision with car, pick-up truck or van in traffic accident

X● **V73.9** **Unspecified** occupant of bus injured in collision with car, pick-up truck or van in traffic accident

● **V74** **Bus occupant injured in collision with heavy transport vehicle or bus**

> **Excludes1** bus occupant injured in collision with military vehicle (V79.81)

> The appropriate 7th character is to be added to each code from category V74

> | | |
> |---|---|
> | A | initial encounter |
> | D | subsequent encounter |
> | S | sequela |

X● **V74.0** **Driver** of bus injured in collision with heavy transport vehicle or bus in nontraffic accident

X● **V74.1** **Passenger** on bus injured in collision with heavy transport vehicle or bus in nontraffic accident

X● **V74.2** **Person on outside** of bus injured in collision with heavy transport vehicle or bus in nontraffic accident

X● **V74.3** **Unspecified** occupant of bus injured in collision with heavy transport vehicle or bus in nontraffic accident

X● **V74.4** **Person boarding or alighting** from bus injured in collision with heavy transport vehicle or bus

X● **V74.5** **Driver** of bus injured in collision with heavy transport vehicle or bus in traffic accident

X● **V74.6** **Passenger** on bus injured in collision with heavy transport vehicle or bus in traffic accident

X● **V74.7** **Person on outside** of bus injured in collision with heavy transport vehicle or bus in traffic accident

X● **V74.9** **Unspecified** occupant of bus injured in collision with heavy transport vehicle or bus in traffic accident

● **V75** **Bus occupant injured in collision with railway train or railway vehicle**

> The appropriate 7th character is to be added to each code from category V75

> | | |
> |---|---|
> | A | initial encounter |
> | D | subsequent encounter |
> | S | sequela |

X● **V75.0** **Driver** of bus injured in collision with railway train or railway vehicle in nontraffic accident

X● **V75.1** **Passenger** on bus injured in collision with railway train or railway vehicle in nontraffic accident

X● **V75.2** **Person on outside** of bus injured in collision with railway train or railway vehicle in nontraffic accident

X● **V75.3** **Unspecified** occupant of bus injured in collision with railway train or railway vehicle in nontraffic accident

X● **V75.4** **Person boarding or alighting** from bus injured in collision with railway train or railway vehicle

X● **V75.5** **Driver** of bus injured in collision with railway train or railway vehicle in traffic accident

X● **V75.6** **Passenger** on bus injured in collision with railway train or railway vehicle in traffic accident

X● **V75.7** **Person on outside** of bus injured in collision with railway train or railway vehicle in traffic accident

X● **V75.9** **Unspecified** occupant of bus injured in collision with railway train or railway vehicle in traffic accident

● **V76** **Bus occupant injured in collision with other nonmotor vehicle**

> **Includes** collision with animal-drawn vehicle, animal being ridden, streetcar

> The appropriate 7th character is to be added to each code from category V76

> | | |
> |---|---|
> | A | initial encounter |
> | D | subsequent encounter |
> | S | sequela |

X● **V76.0** **Driver** of bus injured in collision with other nonmotor vehicle in nontraffic accident

X● **V76.1** **Passenger** on bus injured in collision with other nonmotor vehicle in nontraffic accident

X● **V76.2** **Person on outside** of bus injured in collision with other nonmotor vehicle in nontraffic accident

X● **V76.3** **Unspecified** occupant of bus injured in collision with other nonmotor vehicle in nontraffic accident

X● **V76.4** **Person boarding or alighting** from bus injured in collision with other nonmotor vehicle

X● **V76.5** **Driver** of bus injured in collision with other nonmotor vehicle in traffic accident

X● **V76.6** **Passenger** on bus injured in collision with other nonmotor vehicle in traffic accident

X● **V76.7** **Person on outside** of bus injured in collision with other nonmotor vehicle in traffic accident

X● **V76.9** **Unspecified** occupant of bus injured in collision with other nonmotor vehicle in traffic accident

CHAPTER 20 (V00-Y99)

● V77 **Bus occupant injured in collision with fixed or stationary object**

The appropriate 7th character is to be added to each code from category V77

A	initial encounter
D	subsequent encounter
S	sequela

X ● **V77.0** Driver of bus injured in collision with fixed or stationary object in nontraffic accident

X ● **V77.1** Passenger on bus injured in collision with fixed or stationary object in nontraffic accident

X ● **V77.2** Person on outside of bus injured in collision with fixed or stationary object in nontraffic accident

X ● **V77.3** Unspecified occupant of bus injured in collision with fixed or stationary object in nontraffic accident

X ● **V77.4** Person boarding or alighting from bus injured in collision with fixed or stationary object

X ● **V77.5** Driver of bus injured in collision with fixed or stationary object in traffic accident

X ● **V77.6** Passenger on bus injured in collision with fixed or stationary object in traffic accident

X ● **V77.7** Person on outside of bus injured in collision with fixed or stationary object in traffic accident

X ● **V77.9** Unspecified occupant of bus injured in collision with fixed or stationary object in traffic accident

● V78 **Bus occupant injured in noncollision transport accident**

Includes overturning bus NOS
overturning bus without collision

The appropriate 7th character is to be added to each code from category V78

A	initial encounter
D	subsequent encounter
S	sequela

X ● **V78.0** Driver of bus injured in noncollision transport accident in nontraffic accident

X ● **V78.1** Passenger on bus injured in noncollision transport accident in nontraffic accident

X ● **V78.2** Person on outside of bus injured in noncollision transport accident in nontraffic accident

X ● **V78.3** Unspecified occupant of bus injured in noncollision transport accident in nontraffic accident

X ● **V78.4** Person boarding or alighting from bus injured in noncollision transport accident

X ● **V78.5** Driver of bus injured in noncollision transport accident in traffic accident

X ● **V78.6** Passenger on bus injured in noncollision transport accident in traffic accident

X ● **V78.7** Person on outside of bus injured in noncollision transport accident in traffic accident

X ● **V78.9** Unspecified occupant of bus injured in noncollision transport accident in traffic accident

● V79 **Bus occupant injured in other and unspecified transport accidents**

The appropriate 7th character is to be added to each code from category V79

A	initial encounter
D	subsequent encounter
S	sequela

● **V79.0** Driver of bus injured in collision with other and unspecified motor vehicles in nontraffic accident

X ● **V79.00** Driver of bus injured in collision with unspecified motor vehicles in nontraffic accident

X ● **V79.09** Driver of bus injured in collision with other motor vehicles in nontraffic accident

● **V79.1** Passenger on bus injured in collision with other and unspecified motor vehicles in nontraffic accident

X ● **V79.10** Passenger on bus injured in collision with unspecified motor vehicles in nontraffic accident

X ● **V79.19** Passenger on bus injured in collision with other motor vehicles in nontraffic accident

● **V79.2** Unspecified bus occupant injured in collision with other and unspecified motor vehicles in nontraffic accident

X ● **V79.20** Unspecified bus occupant injured in collision with unspecified motor vehicles in nontraffic accident
Bus collision NOS, nontraffic

X ● **V79.29** Unspecified bus occupant injured in collision with other motor vehicles in nontraffic accident

X ● **V79.3** Bus occupant (driver) (passenger) injured in unspecified nontraffic accident
Bus accident NOS, nontraffic
Bus occupant injured in nontraffic accident NOS

● **V79.4** Driver of bus injured in collision with other and unspecified motor vehicles in traffic accident

X ● **V79.40** Driver of bus injured in collision with unspecified motor vehicles in traffic accident

X ● **V79.49** Driver of bus injured in collision with other motor vehicles in traffic accident

● **V79.5** Passenger on bus injured in collision with other and unspecified motor vehicles in traffic accident

X ● **V79.50** Passenger on bus injured in collision with unspecified motor vehicles in traffic accident

X ● **V79.59** Passenger on bus injured in collision with other motor vehicles in traffic accident

● **V79.6** Unspecified bus occupant injured in collision with other and unspecified motor vehicles in traffic accident

X ● **V79.60** Unspecified bus occupant injured in collision with unspecified motor vehicles in traffic accident
Bus collision NOS (traffic)

X ● **V79.69** Unspecified bus occupant injured in collision with other motor vehicles in traffic accident

● **V79.8** Bus occupant (driver) (passenger) injured in other specified transport accidents

X ● **V79.81** Bus occupant (driver) (passenger) injured in transport accidents with military vehicle

X ● **V79.88** Bus occupant (driver) (passenger) injured in other specified transport accidents

X ● **V79.9** Bus occupant (driver) (passenger) injured in unspecified traffic accident
Bus accident NOS

OTHER LAND TRANSPORT ACCIDENTS (V80-V89)

● V80 **Animal-rider or occupant of animal-drawn vehicle injured in transport accident**

The appropriate 7th character is to be added to each code from category V80

A	initial encounter
D	subsequent encounter
S	sequela

● **V80.0** Animal-rider or occupant of animal drawn vehicle injured by fall from or being thrown from animal or animal-drawn vehicle in noncollision accident

● **V80.01** Animal-rider injured by fall from or being thrown from animal in noncollision accident

● **V80.010** Animal-rider injured by fall from or being thrown from horse in noncollision accident

● **V80.018** Animal-rider injured by fall from or being thrown from other animal in noncollision accident

▶ New   ⟹ Revised   ~~deleted~~ Deleted   Excludes 1   Excludes 2   Includes   Use additional   Code first   Code also   Key words

OGCR Official Guidelines   X Assign placeholder X   ● Use Additional Character(s)   ▸ Manifestation Code   🦠 Hierarchical Condition Category   Coding Clinic

X ● **V80.02** Occupant of animal-drawn vehicle injured by fall from or being thrown from animal-drawn vehicle in noncollision accident
Overturning animal-drawn vehicle NOS
Overturning animal-drawn vehicle without collision

● **V80.1** Animal-rider or occupant of animal-drawn vehicle injured in collision with pedestrian or animal

Excludes1 animal-rider or animal-drawn vehicle collision with animal-drawn vehicle or animal being ridden (V80.7)

X ● **V80.11** Animal-rider injured in collision with pedestrian or animal

X ● **V80.12** Occupant of animal-drawn vehicle injured in collision with pedestrian or animal

● **V80.2** Animal-rider or occupant of animal-drawn vehicle injured in collision with pedal cycle

X ● **V80.21** Animal-rider injured in collision with pedal cycle

X ● **V80.22** Occupant of animal-drawn vehicle injured in collision with pedal cycle

● **V80.3** Animal-rider or occupant of animal-drawn vehicle injured in collision with two- or three-wheeled motor vehicle

X ● **V80.31** Animal-rider injured in collision with two- or three-wheeled motor vehicle

X ● **V80.32** Occupant of animal-drawn vehicle injured in collision with two- or three-wheeled motor vehicle

● **V80.4** Animal-rider or occupant of animal-drawn vehicle injured in collision with car, pick-up truck, van, heavy transport vehicle or bus

Excludes1 animal-rider injured in collision with military vehicle (V80.910)
occupant of animal-drawn vehicle injured in collision with military vehicle (V80.920)

X ● **V80.41** Animal-rider injured in collision with car, pick-up truck, van, heavy transport vehicle or bus

X ● **V80.42** Occupant of animal-drawn vehicle injured in collision with car, pick-up truck, van, heavy transport vehicle or bus

● **V80.5** Animal-rider or occupant of animal-drawn vehicle injured in collision with other specified motor vehicle

X ● **V80.51** Animal-rider injured in collision with other specified motor vehicle

X ● **V80.52** Occupant of animal-drawn vehicle injured in collision with other specified motor vehicle

● **V80.6** Animal-rider or occupant of animal-drawn vehicle injured in collision with railway train or railway vehicle

X ● **V80.61** Animal-rider injured in collision with railway train or railway vehicle

X ● **V80.62** Occupant of animal-drawn vehicle injured in collision with railway train or railway vehicle

● **V80.7** Animal-rider or occupant of animal-drawn vehicle injured in collision with other nonmotor vehicles

● **V80.71** Animal-rider or occupant of animal-drawn vehicle injured in collision with animal being ridden

● **V80.710** Animal-rider injured in collision with other animal being ridden

● **V80.711** Occupant of animal-drawn vehicle injured in collision with animal being ridden

● **V80.72** Animal-rider or occupant of animal-drawn vehicle injured in collision with other animal-drawn vehicle

● **V80.720** Animal-rider injured in collision with animal-drawn vehicle

● **V80.721** Occupant of animal-drawn vehicle injured in collision with other animal-drawn vehicle

● **V80.73** Animal-rider or occupant of animal-drawn vehicle injured in collision with streetcar

● **V80.730** Animal-rider injured in collision with streetcar

● **V80.731** Occupant of animal-drawn vehicle injured in collision with streetcar

● **V80.79** Animal-rider or occupant of animal-drawn vehicle injured in collision with other nonmotor vehicles

● **V80.790** Animal-rider injured in collision with other nonmotor vehicles

● **V80.791** Occupant of animal-drawn vehicle injured in collision with other nonmotor vehicles

● **V80.8** Animal-rider or occupant of animal-drawn vehicle injured in collision with fixed or stationary object

X ● **V80.81** Animal-rider injured in collision with fixed or stationary object

X ● **V80.82** Occupant of animal-drawn vehicle injured in collision with fixed or stationary object

● **V80.9** Animal-rider or occupant of animal-drawn vehicle injured in other and unspecified transport accidents

● **V80.91** Animal-rider injured in other and unspecified transport accidents

● **V80.910** Animal-rider injured in transport accident with military vehicle

● **V80.918** Animal-rider injured in other transport accident

● **V80.919** Animal-rider injured in unspecified transport accident
Animal rider accident NOS

● **V80.92** Occupant of animal-drawn vehicle injured in other and unspecified transport accidents

● **V80.920** Occupant of animal-drawn vehicle injured in transport accident with military vehicle

● **V80.928** Occupant of animal-drawn vehicle injured in other transport accident

● **V80.929** Occupant of animal-drawn vehicle injured in unspecified transport accident
Animal-drawn vehicle accident NOS

● **V81** Occupant of railway train or railway vehicle injured in transport accident

Includes derailment of railway train or railway vehicle
person on outside of train

Excludes1 streetcar (V82.-)

The appropriate 7th character is to be added to each code from category V81

A	initial encounter
D	subsequent encounter
S	sequela

X ● **V81.0** Occupant of railway train or railway vehicle injured in collision with motor vehicle in nontraffic accident

Excludes1 occupant of railway train or railway vehicle injured due to collision with military vehicle (V81.83)

X ● **V81.1** Occupant of railway train or railway vehicle injured in collision with motor vehicle in traffic accident

Excludes1 occupant of railway train or railway vehicle injured due to collision with military vehicle (V81.83)

X ● **V81.2** Occupant of railway train or railway vehicle injured in collision with or hit by rolling stock

X ● **V81.3** Occupant of railway train or railway vehicle injured in collision with other object
Railway collision NOS

X ● **V81.4** Person injured while boarding or alighting from railway train or railway vehicle

CHAPTER 20 (V00-Y99)

X ● **V81.5**   **Occupant of railway train or railway vehicle injured by fall in railway train or railway vehicle**

X ● **V81.6**   **Occupant of railway train or railway vehicle injured by fall from railway train or railway vehicle**

X ● **V81.7**   **Occupant of railway train or railway vehicle injured in derailment without antecedent collision**

● **V81.8**   **Occupant of railway train or railway vehicle injured in other specified railway accidents**

     X ● **V81.81**   **Occupant of railway train or railway vehicle injured due to explosion or fire on train**

     X ● **V81.82**   **Occupant of railway train or railway vehicle injured due to object falling onto train**

         Occupant of railway train or railway vehicle injured due to falling earth onto train

         Occupant of railway train or railway vehicle injured due to falling rocks onto train

         Occupant of railway train or railway vehicle injured due to falling snow onto train

         Occupant of railway train or railway vehicle injured due to falling trees onto train

     X ● **V81.83**   **Occupant of railway train or railway vehicle injured due to collision with military vehicle**

     X ● **V81.89**   **Occupant of railway train or railway vehicle injured due to other specified railway accident**

X ● **V81.9**   **Occupant of railway train or railway vehicle injured in unspecified railway accident**

     Railway accident NOS

● **V82**   **Occupant of powered streetcar injured in transport accident**

Includes	interurban electric car
	person on outside of streetcar
	tram (car)
	trolley (car)

Excludes1	bus (V70-V79)
	motorcoach (V70-V79)
	nonpowered streetcar (V76.-)
	train (V81.-)

The appropriate 7th character is to be added to each code from category V82

A	initial encounter
D	subsequent encounter
S	sequela

X ● **V82.0**   **Occupant of streetcar injured in collision with motor vehicle in nontraffic accident**

X ● **V82.1**   **Occupant of streetcar injured in collision with motor vehicle in traffic accident**

X ● **V82.2**   **Occupant of streetcar injured in collision with or hit by rolling stock**

X ● **V82.3**   **Occupant of streetcar injured in collision with other object**

Excludes1	collision with animal-drawn vehicle or animal being ridden (V82.8)

X ● **V82.4**   **Person injured while boarding or alighting from streetcar**

X ● **V82.5**   **Occupant of streetcar injured by fall in streetcar**

Excludes1	fall in streetcar:
	while boarding or alighting (V82.4)
	with antecedent collision (V82.0-V82.3)

X ● **V82.6**   **Occupant of streetcar injured by fall from streetcar**

Excludes1	fall from streetcar:
	while boarding or alighting (V82.4)
	with antecedent collision (V82.0-V82.3)

X ● **V82.7**   **Occupant of streetcar injured in derailment without antecedent collision**

Excludes1	occupant of streetcar injured in derailment with antecedent collision (V82.0-V82.3)

X ● **V82.8**   **Occupant of streetcar injured in other specified transport accidents**

     Streetcar collision with military vehicle

     Streetcar collision with train or nonmotor vehicles

X ● **V82.9**   **Occupant of streetcar injured in unspecified traffic accident**

     Streetcar accident NOS

● **V83**   **Occupant of special vehicle mainly used on industrial premises injured in transport accident**

Includes	battery-powered airport passenger vehicle
	battery-powered truck (baggage) (mail)
	coal-car in mine
	forklift (truck)
	logging car
	self-propelled industrial truck
	station baggage truck (powered)
	tram, truck, or tub (powered) in mine or quarry

Excludes1	special construction vehicles (V85.-)
	special industrial vehicle in stationary use or maintenance (W31.-)

The appropriate 7th character is to be added to each code from category V83

A	initial encounter
D	subsequent encounter
S	sequela

X ● **V83.0**   **Driver of special industrial vehicle injured in traffic accident**

X ● **V83.1**   **Passenger of special industrial vehicle injured in traffic accident**

X ● **V83.2**   **Person on outside of special industrial vehicle injured in traffic accident**

X ● **V83.3**   **Unspecified occupant of special industrial vehicle injured in traffic accident**

X ● **V83.4**   **Person injured while boarding or alighting from special industrial vehicle**

X ● **V83.5**   **Driver of special industrial vehicle injured in nontraffic accident**

X ● **V83.6**   **Passenger of special industrial vehicle injured in nontraffic accident**

X ● **V83.7**   **Person on outside of special industrial vehicle injured in nontraffic accident**

X ● **V83.9**   **Unspecified occupant of special industrial vehicle injured in nontraffic accident**

     Special-industrial-vehicle accident NOS

● **V84**   **Occupant of special vehicle mainly used in agriculture injured in transport accident**

Includes	self-propelled farm machinery
	tractor (and trailer)

Excludes1	animal-powered farm machinery accident (W30.8-)
	contact with combine harvester (W30.0)
	special agricultural vehicle in stationary use or maintenance (W30.-)

The appropriate 7th character is to be added to each code from category V84

A	initial encounter
D	subsequent encounter
S	sequela

X ● **V84.0**   **Driver of special agricultural vehicle injured in traffic accident**

X ● **V84.1**   **Passenger of special agricultural vehicle injured in traffic accident**

X ● **V84.2**   **Person on outside of special agricultural vehicle injured in traffic accident**

X ● **V84.3**   **Unspecified occupant of special agricultural vehicle injured in traffic accident**

X ● **V84.4**   **Person injured while boarding or alighting from special agricultural vehicle**

X ● **V84.5**   **Driver of special agricultural vehicle injured in nontraffic accident**

X ● **V84.6**   **Passenger of special agricultural vehicle injured in nontraffic accident**

X● **V84.7 Person on outside of special agricultural vehicle injured in nontraffic accident**

X● **V84.9 Unspecified occupant of special agricultural vehicle injured in nontraffic accident**
Special-agricultural vehicle accident NOS

● **V85 Occupant of special construction vehicle injured in transport accident**

Includes	bulldozer
	digger
	dump truck
	earth-leveller
	mechanical shovel
	road-roller

Excludes1	special industrial vehicle (V83.-)
	special construction vehicle in stationary use or maintenance (W31.-)

The appropriate 7th character is to be added to each code from category V85

A	initial encounter
D	subsequent encounter
S	sequela

X● **V85.0 Driver of special construction vehicle injured in traffic accident**

X● **V85.1 Passenger of special construction vehicle injured in traffic accident**

X● **V85.2 Person on outside of special construction vehicle injured in traffic accident**

X● **V85.3 Unspecified occupant of special construction vehicle injured in traffic accident**

X● **V85.4 Person injured while boarding or alighting from special construction vehicle**

X● **V85.5 Driver of special construction vehicle injured in nontraffic accident**

X● **V85.6 Passenger of special construction vehicle injured in nontraffic accident**

X● **V85.7 Person on outside of special construction vehicle injured in nontraffic accident**

X● **V85.9 Unspecified occupant of special construction vehicle injured in nontraffic accident**
Special-construction-vehicle accident NOS

● **V86 Occupant of special all-terrain or other off-road motor vehicle, injured in transport accident**

Excludes1	special all-terrain vehicle in stationary use or maintenance (W31.-)
	sport-utility vehicle (V50-V59)
	three-wheeled motor vehicle designed for on-road use (V30-V39)

The appropriate 7th character is to be added to each code from category V86

A	initial encounter
D	subsequent encounter
S	sequela

● **V86.0 Driver of special all-terrain or other off-road motor vehicle injured in traffic accident**

X● **V86.01 Driver of ambulance or fire engine injured in traffic accident**

X● **V86.02 Driver of snowmobile injured in traffic accident**

X● **V86.03 Driver of dune buggy injured in traffic accident**

X● **V86.04 Driver of military vehicle injured in traffic accident**

X● **V86.05 Driver of 3- or 4-wheeled all-terrain vehicle (ATV) injured in traffic accident**

X● **V86.06 Driver of dirt bike or motor/cross bike injured in traffic accident**

X● **V86.09 Driver of other off-road special all-terrain or other off-road vehicle injured in traffic accident**
Driver of go cart injured in traffic accident
Driver of golf cart injured in traffic accident

● **V86.1 Passenger of special all-terrain or other off-road motor vehicle injured in traffic accident**

X● **V86.11 Passenger of ambulance or fire engine injured in traffic accident**

X● **V86.12 Passenger of snowmobile injured in traffic accident**

X● **V86.13 Passenger of dune buggy injured in traffic accident**

X● **V86.14 Passenger of military vehicle injured in traffic accident**

X● **V86.15 Passenger of 3- or 4-wheeled all-terrain vehicle (ATV) injured in traffic accident**

X● **V86.16 Passenger of dirt bike or motor/cross bike injured in traffic accident**

X● **V86.19 Passenger of other off-road special all-terrain or other off-road off-road motor vehicle injured in traffic accident**
Passenger of go cart injured in traffic accident
Passenger of golf cart injured in traffic accident

● **V86.2 Person on outside of special all-terrain or other off-road motor vehicle injured in traffic accident**

X● **V86.21 Person on outside of ambulance or fire engine injured in traffic accident**

X● **V86.22 Person on outside of snowmobile injured in traffic accident**

X● **V86.23 Person on outside of dune buggy injured in traffic accident**

X● **V86.24 Person on outside of military vehicle injured in traffic accident**

X● **V86.25 Person on outside of 3- or 4-wheeled all-terrain vehicle (ATV) injured in traffic accident**

X● **V86.26 Person on outside of dirt bike or motor/cross bike injured in traffic accident**

X● **V86.29 Person on outside of other special all-terrain or other off-road motor vehicle injured in traffic accident**
Person on outside of go cart in traffic accident
Person on outside of golf cart injured in traffic accident

● **V86.3 Unspecified occupant of special all-terrain or other off-road motor vehicle injured in traffic accident**

X● **V86.31 Unspecified occupant of ambulance or fire engine injured in traffic accident**

X● **V86.32 Unspecified occupant of snowmobile injured in traffic accident**

X● **V86.33 Unspecified occupant of dune buggy injured in traffic accident**

X● **V86.34 Unspecified occupant of military vehicle injured in traffic accident**

X● **V86.35 Unspecified occupant of 3- or 4-wheeled all-terrain vehicle (ATV) injured in traffic accident**

X● **V86.36 Unspecified occupant of dirt bike or motor/cross bike injured in traffic accident**

X● **V86.39 Unspecified occupant of other special all-terrain or other off-road motor vehicle injured in traffic accident**
Unspecified occupant of go cart injured in traffic accident
Unspecified occupant of golf cart injured in traffic accident

● **V86.4 Person injured while boarding or alighting from special all-terrain or other off-road motor vehicle**

X● **V86.41 Person injured while boarding or alighting from ambulance or fire engine**

X● **V86.42 Person injured while boarding or alighting from snowmobile**

X● **V86.43 Person injured while boarding or alighting from dune buggy**

X● **V86.44 Person injured while boarding or alighting from military vehicle**

X● **V86.45 Person injured while boarding or alighting from a 3- or 4-wheeled all-terrain vehicle (ATV)**

CHAPTER 20 (V00-Y99)

X ● **V86.46**   **Person injured while boarding or alighting from a dirt bike or motor/cross bike**

X ● **V86.49**   **Person injured while boarding or alighting from other special all-terrain or other off-road motor vehicle**

Person injured while boarding or alighting from go cart

Person injured while boarding or alighting from golf cart

● **V86.5**   **Driver of special all-terrain or other off-road motor vehicle injured in nontraffic accident**

X ● **V86.51**   **Driver of ambulance or fire engine injured in nontraffic accident**

X ● **V86.52**   **Driver of snowmobile injured in nontraffic accident**

X ● **V86.53**   **Driver of dune buggy injured in nontraffic accident**

X ● **V86.54**   **Driver of military vehicle injured in nontraffic accident**

X ● **V86.55**   **Driver of 3- or 4-wheeled all-terrain vehicle (ATV) injured in nontraffic accident**

X ● **V86.56**   **Driver of dirt bike or motor/cross bike injured in nontraffic accident**

X ● **V86.59**   **Driver of other off-road special all-terrain or other off-road motor vehicle injured in nontraffic accident**

Driver of go cart injured in nontraffic accident

Driver of golf cart injured in nontraffic accident

● **V86.6**   **Passenger of special all-terrain or other off-road motor vehicle injured in nontraffic accident**

X ● **V86.61**   **Passenger of ambulance or fire engine injured in nontraffic accident**

X ● **V86.62**   **Passenger of snowmobile injured in nontraffic accident**

X ● **V86.63**   **Passenger of dune buggy injured in nontraffic accident**

X ● **V86.64**   **Passenger of military vehicle injured in nontraffic accident**

X ● **V86.65**   **Passenger of 3- or 4-wheeled all-terrain vehicle (ATV) injured in nontraffic accident**

X ● **V86.66**   **Passenger of dirt bike or motor/cross bike injured in nontraffic accident**

X ● **V86.69**   **Passenger of other special all-terrain or other off-road vehicle injured in nontraffic accident**

Passenger of go cart injured in nontraffic accident

Passenger of golf cart injured in nontraffic accident

● **V86.7**   **Person on outside of special all-terrain or other off-road motor vehicle injured in nontraffic accident**

X ● **V86.71**   **Person on outside of ambulance or fire engine injured in nontraffic accident**

X ● **V86.72**   **Person on outside of snowmobile injured in nontraffic accident**

X ● **V86.73**   **Person on outside of dune buggy injured in nontraffic accident**

X ● **V86.74**   **Person on outside of military vehicle injured in nontraffic accident**

X ● **V86.75**   **Person on outside of 3- or 4-wheeled all-terrain vehicle (ATV) injured in nontraffic accident**

X ● **V86.76**   **Person on outside of dirt bike or motor/cross bike injured in nontraffic accident**

X ● **V86.79**   **Person on outside of other special all-terrain or other off-road motor vehicles injured in nontraffic accident**

Person on outside of go cart injured in nontraffic accident

Person on outside of golf cart injured in nontraffic accident

● **V86.9**   **Unspecified occupant of special all-terrain or other off-road motor vehicle injured in nontraffic accident**

X ● **V86.91**   **Unspecified occupant of ambulance or fire engine injured in nontraffic accident**

X ● **V86.92**   **Unspecified occupant of snowmobile injured in nontraffic accident**

X ● **V86.93**   **Unspecified occupant of dune buggy injured in nontraffic accident**

X ● **V86.94**   **Unspecified occupant of military vehicle injured in nontraffic accident**

X ● **V86.95**   **Unspecified occupant of 3- or 4-wheeled all-terrain vehicle (ATV) injured in nontraffic accident**

X ● **V86.96**   **Unspecified occupant of dirt bike or motor/cross bike injured in nontraffic accident**

X ● **V86.99**   **Unspecified occupant of other special all-terrain or other off-road motor vehicle injured in nontraffic accident**

Off-road motor-vehicle accident NOS

Other motor-vehicle accident NOS

Unspecified occupant of go cart injured in nontraffic accident

Unspecified occupant of golf cart injured in nontraffic accident

Unspecified occupant of race car injured in nontraffic accident

● **V87**   **Traffic accident of specified type but victim's mode of transport unknown**

> **Excludes1**   collision involving:
> pedal cycle (V10-V19)
> pedestrian (V01-V09)

The appropriate 7th character is to be added to each code from category V87

> A   initial encounter
> D   subsequent encounter
> S   sequela

X ● **V87.0**   **Person injured in collision between car and two- or three-wheeled powered vehicle (traffic)**

X ● **V87.1**   **Person injured in collision between other motor vehicle and two- or three-wheeled motor vehicle (traffic)**

X ● **V87.2**   **Person injured in collision between car and pick-up truck or van (traffic)**

X ● **V87.3**   **Person injured in collision between car and bus (traffic)**

X ● **V87.4**   **Person injured in collision between car and heavy transport vehicle (traffic)**

X ● **V87.5**   **Person injured in collision between heavy transport vehicle and bus (traffic)**

X ● **V87.6**   **Person injured in collision between railway train or railway vehicle and car (traffic)**

X ● **V87.7**   **Person injured in collision between other specified motor vehicles (traffic)**

X ● **V87.8**   **Person injured in other specified noncollision transport accidents involving motor vehicle (traffic)**

X ● **V87.9**   **Person injured in other specified (collision) (noncollision) transport accidents involving nonmotor vehicle (traffic)**

● **V88**   **Nontraffic accident of specified type but victim's mode of transport unknown**

> **Excludes1**   collision involving:
> pedal cycle (V10-V19)
> pedestrian (V01-V09)

The appropriate 7th character is to be added to each code from category V88

> A   initial encounter
> D   subsequent encounter
> S   sequela

X ● **V88.0**   **Person injured in collision between car and two- or three-wheeled motor vehicle, nontraffic**

X ● **V88.1**   **Person injured in collision between other motor vehicle and two- or three-wheeled motor vehicle, nontraffic**

X ● **V88.2**   **Person injured in collision between car and pick-up truck or van, nontraffic**

X● **V88.3**   Person injured in collision between car and bus, nontraffic

X● **V88.4**   Person injured in collision between car and heavy transport vehicle, nontraffic

X● **V88.5**   Person injured in collision between heavy transport vehicle and bus, nontraffic

X● **V88.6**   Person injured in collision between railway train or railway vehicle and car, nontraffic

X● **V88.7**   Person injured in collision between other specified motor vehicle, nontraffic

X● **V88.8**   Person injured in other specified noncollision transport accidents involving motor vehicle, nontraffic

X● **V88.9**   Person injured in other specified (collision) (noncollision) transport accidents involving nonmotor vehicle, nontraffic

●**V89**   Motor- or nonmotor-vehicle accident, type of vehicle unspecified

> The appropriate 7th character is to be added to each code from category V89

> | | |
> |---|---|
> | A | initial encounter |
> | D | subsequent encounter |
> | S | sequela |

X● **V89.0**   Person injured in unspecified motor-vehicle accident, nontraffic
> Motor-vehicle accident NOS, nontraffic

X● **V89.1**   Person injured in unspecified nonmotor-vehicle accident, nontraffic
> Nonmotor-vehicle accident NOS (nontraffic)

X● **V89.2**   Person injured in unspecified motor-vehicle accident, traffic
> Motor-vehicle accident [MVA] NOS
> Road (traffic) accident [RTA] NOS

X● **V89.3**   Person injured in unspecified nonmotor-vehicle accident, traffic
> Nonmotor-vehicle traffic accident NOS

X● **V89.9**   Person injured in unspecified vehicle accident
> Collision NOS

WATER TRANSPORT ACCIDENTS (V90-V94)

●**V90**   Drowning and submersion due to accident to watercraft

> Excludes1   civilian water transport accident involving military watercraft (V94.81-)
> fall into water not from watercraft (W16.-)
> military watercraft accident in military or war operations (Y36.0-, Y37.0-)
> water-transport–related drowning or submersion without accident to watercraft (V92.-)

> The appropriate 7th character is to be added to each code from category V90

> | | |
> |---|---|
> | A | initial encounter |
> | D | subsequent encounter |
> | S | sequela |

●**V90.0**   Drowning and submersion due to watercraft overturning

X● **V90.00**   Drowning and submersion due to merchant ship overturning

X● **V90.01**   Drowning and submersion due to passenger ship overturning
> Drowning and submersion due to ferry-boat overturning
> Drowning and submersion due to liner overturning

X● **V90.02**   Drowning and submersion due to fishing boat overturning

X● **V90.03**   Drowning and submersion due to other powered watercraft overturning
> Drowning and submersion due to hovercraft (on open water) overturning
> Drowning and submersion due to jet ski overturning

X● **V90.04**   Drowning and submersion due to sailboat overturning

X● **V90.05**   Drowning and submersion due to canoe or kayak overturning

X● **V90.06**   Drowning and submersion due to (nonpowered) inflatable craft overturning

X● **V90.08**   Drowning and submersion due to other unpowered watercraft overturning
> Drowning and submersion due to windsurfer overturning

X● **V90.09**   Drowning and submersion due to unspecified watercraft overturning
> Drowning and submersion due to boat NOS overturning
> Drowning and submersion due to ship NOS overturning
> Drowning and submersion due to watercraft NOS overturning

●**V90.1**   Drowning and submersion due to watercraft sinking

X● **V90.10**   Drowning and submersion due to merchant ship sinking

X● **V90.11**   Drowning and submersion due to passenger ship sinking
> Drowning and submersion due to ferry-boat sinking
> Drowning and submersion due to liner sinking

X● **V90.12**   Drowning and submersion due to fishing boat sinking

X● **V90.13**   Drowning and submersion due to other powered watercraft sinking
> Drowning and submersion due to hovercraft (on open water) sinking
> Drowning and submersion due to jet ski sinking

X● **V90.14**   Drowning and submersion due to sailboat sinking

X● **V90.15**   Drowning and submersion due to canoe or kayak sinking

X● **V90.16**   Drowning and submersion due to (nonpowered) inflatable craft sinking

X● **V90.18**   Drowning and submersion due to other unpowered watercraft sinking

X● **V90.19**   Drowning and submersion due to unspecified watercraft sinking
> Drowning and submersion due to boat NOS sinking
> Drowning and submersion due to ship NOS sinking
> Drowning and submersion due to watercraft NOS sinking

●**V90.2**   Drowning and submersion due to falling or jumping from burning watercraft

X● **V90.20**   Drowning and submersion due to falling or jumping from burning merchant ship

X● **V90.21**   Drowning and submersion due to falling or jumping from burning passenger ship
> Drowning and submersion due to falling or jumping from burning ferry-boat
> Drowning and submersion due to falling or jumping from burning liner

X● **V90.22**   Drowning and submersion due to falling or jumping from burning fishing boat

X● **V90.23**   Drowning and submersion due to falling or jumping from other burning powered watercraft
> Drowning and submersion due to falling and jumping from burning hovercraft (on open water)
> Drowning and submersion due to falling and jumping from burning jet ski

X● **V90.24**   Drowning and submersion due to falling or jumping from burning sailboat

X● **V90.25**   Drowning and submersion due to falling or jumping from burning canoe or kayak

X ● **V90.26** **Drowning and submersion due to falling or jumping from burning (nonpowered) inflatable craft**

X ● **V90.27** **Drowning and submersion due to falling or jumping from burning water-skis**

X ● **V90.28** **Drowning and submersion due to falling or jumping from other burning unpowered watercraft**
Drowning and submersion due to falling and jumping from burning surf-board
Drowning and submersion due to falling and jumping from burning windsurfer

X ● **V90.29** **Drowning and submersion due to falling or jumping from unspecified burning watercraft**
Drowning and submersion due to falling or jumping from burning boat NOS
Drowning and submersion due to falling or jumping from burning ship NOS
Drowning and submersion due to falling or jumping from burning watercraft NOS

● **V90.3** **Drowning and submersion due to falling or jumping from crushed watercraft**

X ● **V90.30** **Drowning and submersion due to falling or jumping from crushed merchant ship**

X ● **V90.31** **Drowning and submersion due to falling or jumping from crushed passenger ship**
Drowning and submersion due to falling and jumping from crushed ferry-boat
Drowning and submersion due to falling and jumping from crushed liner

X ● **V90.32** **Drowning and submersion due to falling or jumping from crushed fishing boat**

X ● **V90.33** **Drowning and submersion due to falling or jumping from other crushed powered watercraft**
Drowning and submersion due to falling and jumping from crushed hovercraft
Drowning and submersion due to falling and jumping from crushed jet ski

X ● **V90.34** **Drowning and submersion due to falling or jumping from crushed sailboat**

X ● **V90.35** **Drowning and submersion due to falling or jumping from crushed canoe or kayak**

X ● **V90.36** **Drowning and submersion due to falling or jumping from crushed (nonpowered) inflatable craft**

X ● **V90.37** **Drowning and submersion due to falling or jumping from crushed water-skis**

X ● **V90.38** **Drowning and submersion due to falling or jumping from other crushed unpowered watercraft**
Drowning and submersion due to falling and jumping from crushed surf-board
Drowning and submersion due to falling and jumping from crushed windsurfer

X ● **V90.39** **Drowning and submersion due to falling or jumping from crushed unspecified watercraft**
Drowning and submersion due to falling and jumping from crushed boat NOS
Drowning and submersion due to falling and jumping from crushed ship NOS
Drowning and submersion due to falling and jumping from crushed watercraft NOS

● **V90.8** **Drowning and submersion due to other accident to watercraft**

X ● **V90.80** **Drowning and submersion due to other accident to merchant ship**

X ● **V90.81** **Drowning and submersion due to other accident to passenger ship**
Drowning and submersion due to other accident to ferry-boat
Drowning and submersion due to other accident to liner

X ● **V90.82** **Drowning and submersion due to other accident to fishing boat**

X ● **V90.83** **Drowning and submersion due to other accident to other powered watercraft**
Drowning and submersion due to other accident to hovercraft (on open water)
Drowning and submersion due to other accident to jet ski

X ● **V90.84** **Drowning and submersion due to other accident to sailboat**

X ● **V90.85** **Drowning and submersion due to other accident to canoe or kayak**

X ● **V90.86** **Drowning and submersion due to other accident to (nonpowered) inflatable craft**

X ● **V90.87** **Drowning and submersion due to other accident to water-skis**

X ● **V90.88** **Drowning and submersion due to other accident to other unpowered watercraft**
Drowning and submersion due to other accident to surf-board
Drowning and submersion due to other accident to windsurfer

X ● **V90.89** **Drowning and submersion due to other accident to unspecified watercraft**
Drowning and submersion due to other accident to boat NOS
Drowning and submersion due to other accident to ship NOS
Drowning and submersion due to other accident to watercraft NOS

● **V91** **Other injury due to accident to watercraft**

> **Includes**   any injury except drowning and submersion as a result of an accident to watercraft

> **Excludes1**   civilian water transport accident involving military watercraft (V94.81-)
military watercraft accident in military or war operations (Y36, Y37.-)

> **Excludes2**   drowning and submersion due to accident to watercraft (V90.-)

The appropriate 7th character is to be added to each code from category V91

A	initial encounter
D	subsequent encounter
S	sequela

● **V91.0** **Burn due to watercraft on fire**

> **Excludes1**   burn from localized fire or explosion on board ship without accident to watercraft (V93.-)

X ● **V91.00** **Burn due to merchant ship on fire**

X ● **V91.01** **Burn due to passenger ship on fire**
Burn due to ferry-boat on fire
Burn due to liner on fire

X ● **V91.02** **Burn due to fishing boat on fire**

X ● **V91.03** **Burn due to other powered watercraft on fire**
Burn due to hovercraft (on open water) on fire
Burn due to jet ski on fire

X ● **V91.04** **Burn due to sailboat on fire**

X ● **V91.05** **Burn due to canoe or kayak on fire**

X ● **V91.06** **Burn due to (nonpowered) inflatable craft on fire**

X ● **V91.07** **Burn due to water-skis on fire**

X ● **V91.08** **Burn due to other unpowered watercraft on fire**

X ● **V91.09** **Burn due to unspecified watercraft on fire**
Burn due to boat NOS on fire
Burn due to ship NOS on fire
Burn due to watercraft NOS on fire

▶ New   ⇒ Revised   ~~deleted~~ Deleted   Excludes 1   Excludes 2   Includes   Use additional   Code first   Code also   Key words
OGCR Official Guidelines   X Assign placeholder X   ● Use Additional Character(s)   ▶ Manifestation Code   🗣 Hierarchical Condition Category   Coding Clinic

● **V91.1 Crushed between watercraft and other watercraft or other object due to collision**

Crushed by lifeboat after abandoning ship in a collision

Note: Select the specified type of watercraft that the victim was on at the time of the collision.

X● **V91.10 Crushed between merchant ship and other watercraft or other object due to collision**

X● **V91.11 Crushed between passenger ship and other watercraft or other object due to collision**

Crushed between ferry-boat and other watercraft or other object due to collision

Crushed between liner and other watercraft or other object due to collision

X● **V91.12 Crushed between fishing boat and other watercraft or other object due to collision**

X● **V91.13 Crushed between other powered watercraft and other watercraft or other object due to collision**

Crushed between hovercraft (on open water) and other watercraft or other object due to collision

Crushed between jet ski and other watercraft or other object due to collision

X● **V91.14 Crushed between sailboat and other watercraft or other object due to collision**

X● **V91.15 Crushed between canoe or kayak and other watercraft or other object due to collision**

X● **V91.16 Crushed between (nonpowered) inflatable craft and other watercraft or other object due to collision**

X● **V91.18 Crushed between other unpowered watercraft and other watercraft or other object due to collision**

Crushed between surfboard and other watercraft or other object due to collision

Crushed between windsurfer and other watercraft or other object due to collision

X● **V91.19 Crushed between unspecified watercraft and other watercraft or other object due to collision**

Crushed between boat NOS and other watercraft or other object due to collision

Crushed between ship NOS and other watercraft or other object due to collision

Crushed between watercraft NOS and other watercraft or other object due to collision

● **V91.2 Fall due to collision between watercraft and other watercraft or other object**

Fall while remaining on watercraft after collision

Note: Select the specified type of watercraft that the victim was on at the time of the collision.

Excludes1 crushed between watercraft and other watercraft and other object due to collision (V91.1-)

drowning and submersion due to falling from crushed watercraft (V90.3-)

X● **V91.20 Fall due to collision between merchant ship and other watercraft or other object**

X● **V91.21 Fall due to collision between passenger ship and other watercraft or other object**

Fall due to collision between ferry-boat and other watercraft or other object

Fall due to collision between liner and other watercraft or other object

X● **V91.22 Fall due to collision between fishing boat and other watercraft or other object**

X● **V91.23 Fall due to collision between other powered watercraft and other watercraft or other object**

Fall due to collision between hovercraft (on open water) and other watercraft or other object

Fall due to collision between jet ski and other watercraft or other object

X● **V91.24 Fall due to collision between sailboat and other watercraft or other object**

X● **V91.25 Fall due to collision between canoe or kayak and other watercraft or other object**

X● **V91.26 Fall due to collision between (nonpowered) inflatable craft and other watercraft or other object**

X● **V91.29 Fall due to collision between unspecified watercraft and other watercraft or other object**

Fall due to collision between boat NOS and other watercraft or other object

Fall due to collision between ship NOS and other watercraft or other object

Fall due to collision between watercraft NOS and other watercraft or other object

● **V91.3 Hit or struck by falling object due to accident to watercraft**

Hit or struck by falling object (part of damaged watercraft or other object) after falling or jumping from damaged watercraft

Excludes2 drowning or submersion due to fall or jumping from damaged watercraft (V90.2-, V90.3-)

X● **V91.30 Hit or struck by falling object due to accident to merchant ship**

X● **V91.31 Hit or struck by falling object due to accident to passenger ship**

Hit or struck by falling object due to accident to ferry-boat

Hit or struck by falling object due to accident to liner

X● **V91.32 Hit or struck by falling object due to accident to fishing boat**

X● **V91.33 Hit or struck by falling object due to accident to other powered watercraft**

Hit or struck by falling object due to accident to hovercraft (on open water)

Hit or struck by falling object due to accident to jet ski

X● **V91.34 Hit or struck by falling object due to accident to sailboat**

X● **V91.35 Hit or struck by falling object due to accident to canoe or kayak**

X● **V91.36 Hit or struck by falling object due to accident to (nonpowered) inflatable craft**

X● **V91.37 Hit or struck by falling object due to accident to water-skis**

Hit by water-skis after jumping off of waterskis

X● **V91.38 Hit or struck by falling object due to accident to other unpowered watercraft**

Hit or struck by surf-board after falling off damaged surf-board

Hit or struck by object after falling off damaged windsurfer

X● **V91.39 Hit or struck by falling object due to accident to unspecified watercraft**

Hit or struck by falling object due to accident to boat NOS

Hit or struck by falling object due to accident to ship NOS

Hit or struck by falling object due to accident to watercraft NOS

● **V91.8 Other injury due to other accident to watercraft**

X● **V91.80 Other injury due to other accident to merchant ship**

X● **V91.81 Other injury due to other accident to passenger ship**

Other injury due to other accident to ferry-boat

Other injury due to other accident to liner

X● **V91.82 Other injury due to other accident to fishing boat**

X● **V91.83 Other injury due to other accident to other powered watercraft**

Other injury due to other accident to hovercraft (on open water)

Other injury due to other accident to jet ski

CHAPTER 20 (V00-Y99)

X● **V91.84 Other injury due to other accident to sailboat**

X● **V91.85 Other injury due to other accident to canoe or kayak**

X● **V91.86 Other injury due to other accident to (nonpowered) inflatable craft**

X● **V91.87 Other injury due to other accident to water-skis**

X● **V91.88 Other injury due to other accident to other unpowered watercraft**
   Other injury due to other accident to surf-board
   Other injury due to other accident to windsurfer

X● **V91.89 Other injury due to other accident to unspecified watercraft**
   Other injury due to other accident to boat NOS
   Other injury due to other accident to ship NOS
   Other injury due to other accident to watercraft NOS

● **V92 Drowning and submersion due to accident on board watercraft, without accident to watercraft**

   Excludes1   civilian water transport accident involving military watercraft (V94.81-)
    drowning or submersion due to accident to watercraft (V90-V91)
    drowning or submersion of diver who voluntarily jumps from boat not involved in an accident (W16.711, W16.721)
    fall into water without watercraft (W16.-)
    military watercraft accident in military or war operations (Y36, Y37)

   The appropriate 7th character is to be added to each code from category V92

> A   initial encounter
> D   subsequent encounter
> S   sequela

● **V92.0 Drowning and submersion due to fall off watercraft**
   Drowning and submersion due to fall from gangplank of watercraft
   Drowning and submersion due to fall overboard watercraft

   Excludes2   hitting head on object or bottom of body of water due to fall from watercraft (V94.0-)

X● **V92.00 Drowning and submersion due to fall off merchant ship**

X● **V92.01 Drowning and submersion due to fall off passenger ship**
   Drowning and submersion due to fall off ferry-boat
   Drowning and submersion due to fall off liner

X● **V92.02 Drowning and submersion due to fall off fishing boat**

X● **V92.03 Drowning and submersion due to fall off other powered watercraft**
   Drowning and submersion due to fall off hovercraft (on open water)
   Drowning and submersion due to fall off jet ski

X● **V92.04 Drowning and submersion due to fall off sailboat**

X● **V92.05 Drowning and submersion due to fall off canoe or kayak**

X● **V92.06 Drowning and submersion due to fall off (nonpowered) inflatable craft**

X● **V92.07 Drowning and submersion due to fall off water-skis**

   Excludes1   drowning and submersion due to falling off burning water-skis (V90.27)
    drowning and submersion due to falling off crushed water-skis (V90.37)
    hit by boat while water-skiing NOS (V94.X)

X● **V92.08 Drowning and submersion due to fall off other unpowered watercraft**
   Drowning and submersion due to fall off surf-board
   Drowning and submersion due to fall off windsurfer

   Excludes1   drowning and submersion due to fall off burning unpowered watercraft (V90.28)
    drowning and submersion due to fall off crushed unpowered watercraft (V90.38)
    drowning and submersion due to fall off damaged unpowered watercraft (V90.88)
    drowning and submersion due to rider of nonpowered watercraft being hit by other watercraft (V94.-)
    other injury due to rider of nonpowered watercraft being hit by other watercraft (V94.-)

X● **V92.09 Drowning and submersion due to fall off unspecified watercraft**
   Drowning and submersion due to fall off boat NOS
   Drowning and submersion due to fall off ship
   Drowning and submersion due to fall off watercraft NOS

● **V92.1 Drowning and submersion due to being thrown overboard by motion of watercraft**

   Excludes1   drowning and submersion due to fall off surf-board (V92.08)
    drowning and submersion due to fall off water-skis (V92.07)
    drowning and submersion due to fall off windsurfer (V92.08)

X● **V92.10 Drowning and submersion due to being thrown overboard by motion of merchant ship**

X● **V92.11 Drowning and submersion due to being thrown overboard by motion of passenger ship**
   Drowning and submersion due to being thrown overboard by motion of ferry-boat
   Drowning and submersion due to being thrown overboard by motion of liner

X● **V92.12 Drowning and submersion due to being thrown overboard by motion of fishing boat**

X● **V92.13 Drowning and submersion due to being thrown overboard by motion of other powered watercraft**
   Drowning and submersion due to being thrown overboard by motion of hovercraft

X● **V92.14 Drowning and submersion due to being thrown overboard by motion of sailboat**

X● **V92.15 Drowning and submersion due to being thrown overboard by motion of canoe or kayak**

X● **V92.16 Drowning and submersion due to being thrown overboard by motion of (nonpowered) inflatable craft**

X● **V92.19 Drowning and submersion due to being thrown overboard by motion of unspecified watercraft**
   Drowning and submersion due to being thrown overboard by motion of boat NOS
   Drowning and submersion due to being thrown overboard by motion of ship NOS
   Drowning and submersion due to being thrown overboard by motion of watercraft NOS

▶ New   ⇒ Revised   ~~deleted~~ Deleted   Excludes 1   Excludes 2   Includes   Use additional   Code first   Code also   Key words
OGCR Official Guidelines   X Assign placeholder X   ● Use Additional Character(s)   ▶ Manifestation Code   🝢 Hierarchical Condition Category   **Coding Clinic**

● **V92.2** **Drowning and submersion due to being** washed overboard from watercraft
  Code first any associated cataclysm (X37.0-)

X● **V92.20** Drowning and submersion due to being washed overboard from merchant ship

X● **V92.21** Drowning and submersion due to being washed overboard from passenger ship
  Drowning and submersion due to being washed overboard from ferry-boat
  Drowning and submersion due to being washed overboard from liner

X● **V92.22** Drowning and submersion due to being washed overboard from fishing boat

X● **V92.23** Drowning and submersion due to being washed overboard from other powered watercraft
  Drowning and submersion due to being washed overboard from hovercraft (on open water)
  Drowning and submersion due to being washed overboard from jet ski

X● **V92.24** Drowning and submersion due to being washed overboard from sailboat

X● **V92.25** Drowning and submersion due to being washed overboard from canoe or kayak

X● **V92.26** Drowning and submersion due to being washed overboard from (nonpowered) inflatable craft

X● **V92.27** Drowning and submersion due to being washed overboard from water-skis
  Excludes1 drowning and submersion due to fall off water-skis (V92.07)

X● **V92.28** Drowning and submersion due to being washed overboard from other unpowered watercraft
  Drowning and submersion due to being washed overboard from surf-board
  Drowning and submersion due to being washed overboard from windsurfer

X● **V92.29** Drowning and submersion due to being washed overboard from unspecified watercraft
  Drowning and submersion due to being washed overboard from boat NOS
  Drowning and submersion due to being washed overboard from ship NOS
  Drowning and submersion due to being washed overboard from watercraft NOS

● **V93** **Other injury due to accident on board watercraft, without accident to watercraft**
  Excludes1 civilian water transport accident involving military watercraft (V94.81-)
    other injury due to accident to watercraft (V91.-)
    military watercraft accident in military or war operations (Y36, Y37.-)
  Excludes2 drowning and submersion due to accident on board watercraft, without accident to watercraft (V92.-)
  The appropriate 7th character is to be added to each code from category V93

A	initial encounter
D	subsequent encounter
S	sequela

● **V93.0** **Burn due to** localized fire on board **watercraft**
  Excludes1 burn due to watercraft on fire (V91.0-)

X● **V93.00** Burn due to localized fire on board merchant vessel

X● **V93.01** Burn due to localized fire on board passenger vessel
  Burn due to localized fire on board ferry-boat
  Burn due to localized fire on board liner

X● **V93.02** Burn due to localized fire on board fishing boat

X● **V93.03** Burn due to localized fire on board other powered watercraft
  Burn due to localized fire on board hovercraft
  Burn due to localized fire on board jet ski

X● **V93.04** Burn due to localized fire on board sailboat

X● **V93.09** Burn due to localized fire on board unspecified watercraft
  Burn due to localized fire on board boat NOS
  Burn due to localized fire on board ship NOS
  Burn due to localized fire on board watercraft NOS

● **V93.1** **Other burn on board watercraft**
  Burn due to source other than fire on board watercraft
  Excludes1 burn due to watercraft on fire (V91.0-)

X● **V93.10** Other burn on board merchant vessel

X● **V93.11** Other burn on board passenger vessel
  Other burn on board ferry-boat
  Other burn on board liner

X● **V93.12** Other burn on board fishing boat

X● **V93.13** Other burn on board other powered watercraft
  Other burn on board hovercraft
  Other burn on board jet ski

X● **V93.14** Other burn on board sailboat

X● **V93.19** Other burn on board unspecified watercraft
  Other burn on board boat NOS
  Other burn on board ship NOS
  Other burn on board watercraft NOS

● **V93.2** **Heat exposure on board watercraft**
  Excludes1 exposure to man-made heat not aboard watercraft (W92)
    exposure to natural heat while on board watercraft (X30)
    exposure to sunlight while on board watercraft (X32)
  Excludes2 burn due to fire on board watercraft (V93.0-)

X● **V93.20** Heat exposure on board merchant ship

X● **V93.21** Heat exposure on board passenger ship
  Heat exposure on board ferry-boat
  Heat exposure on board liner

X● **V93.22** Heat exposure on board fishing boat

X● **V93.23** Heat exposure on board other powered watercraft
  Heat exposure on board hovercraft

X● **V93.24** Heat exposure on board sailboat

X● **V93.29** Heat exposure on board unspecified watercraft
  Heat exposure on board boat NOS
  Heat exposure on board ship NOS
  Heat exposure on board watercraft NOS

● **V93.3** **Fall on board watercraft**
  Excludes1 fall due to collision of watercraft (V91.2-)

X● **V93.30** Fall on board merchant ship

X● **V93.31** Fall on board passenger ship
  Fall on board ferry-boat
  Fall on board liner

X● **V93.32** Fall on board fishing boat

X● **V93.33** Fall on board other powered watercraft
  Fall on board hovercraft (on open water)
  Fall on board jet ski

X● **V93.34** Fall on board sailboat

X● **V93.35** Fall on board canoe or kayak

X● **V93.36** Fall on board (nonpowered) inflatable craft

X● **V93.38** Fall on board other unpowered watercraft

X● **V93.39** Fall on board unspecified watercraft
  Fall on board boat NOS
  Fall on board ship NOS
  Fall on board watercraft NOS

CHAPTER 20 (V00-Y99)

- **V93.4   Struck by falling object on board watercraft**
  Hit by falling object on board watercraft
  > **Excludes1**   struck by falling object due to accident to watercraft (V91.3)
  - X● **V93.40   Struck by falling object on merchant ship**
  - X● **V93.41   Struck by falling object on passenger ship**
    Struck by falling object on ferry-boat
    Struck by falling object on liner
  - X● **V93.42   Struck by falling object on fishing boat**
  - X● **V93.43   Struck by falling object on other powered watercraft**
    Struck by falling object on hovercraft
  - X● **V93.44   Struck by falling object on sailboat**
  - X● **V93.48   Struck by falling object on other unpowered watercraft**
  - X● **V93.49   Struck by falling object on unspecified watercraft**
- **V93.5   Explosion on board watercraft**
  Boiler explosion on steamship
  > **Excludes2**   fire on board watercraft (V93.0-)
  - X● **V93.50   Explosion on board merchant ship**
  - X● **V93.51   Explosion on board passenger ship**
    Explosion on board ferry-boat
    Explosion on board liner
  - X● **V93.52   Explosion on board fishing boat**
  - X● **V93.53   Explosion on board other powered watercraft**
    Explosion on board hovercraft
    Explosion on board jet ski
  - X● **V93.54   Explosion on board sailboat**
  - X● **V93.59   Explosion on board unspecified watercraft**
    Explosion on board boat NOS
    Explosion on board ship NOS
    Explosion on board watercraft NOS
- **V93.6   Machinery accident on board watercraft**
  > **Excludes1**   machinery explosion on board watercraft (V93.4-)
  > machinery fire on board watercraft (V93.0-)
  - X● **V93.60   Machinery accident on board merchant ship**
  - X● **V93.61   Machinery accident on board passenger ship**
    Machinery accident on board ferry-boat
    Machinery accident on board liner
  - X● **V93.62   Machinery accident on board fishing boat**
  - X● **V93.63   Machinery accident on board other powered watercraft**
    Machinery accident on board hovercraft
  - X● **V93.64   Machinery accident on board sailboat**
  - X● **V93.69   Machinery accident on board unspecified watercraft**
    Machinery accident on board boat NOS
    Machinery accident on board ship NOS
    Machinery accident on board watercraft NOS
- **V93.8   Other injury due to other accident on board watercraft**
  Accidental poisoning by gases or fumes on watercraft
  - X● **V93.80   Other injury due to other accident on board merchant ship**
  - X● **V93.81   Other injury due to other accident on board passenger ship**
    Other injury due to other accident on board ferry-boat
    Other injury due to other accident on board liner
  - X● **V93.82   Other injury due to other accident on board fishing boat**
  - X● **V93.83   Other injury due to other accident on board other powered watercraft**
    Other injury due to other accident on board hovercraft
    Other injury due to other accident on board jet ski
  - X● **V93.84   Other injury due to other accident on board sailboat**

- X● **V93.85   Other injury due to other accident on board canoe or kayak**
- X● **V93.86   Other injury due to other accident on board (nonpowered) inflatable craft**
- X● **V93.87   Other injury due to other accident on board water-skis**
  Hit or struck by object while waterskiing
- X● **V93.88   Other injury due to other accident on board other unpowered watercraft**
  Hit or struck by object while surfing
  Hit or struck by object while on board windsurfer
- X● **V93.89   Other injury due to other accident on board unspecified watercraft**
  Other injury due to other accident on board boat NOS
  Other injury due to other accident on board ship NOS
  Other injury due to other accident on board watercraft NOS

- ● **V94   Other and unspecified water transport accidents**
  > **Excludes1**   military watercraft accidents in military or war operations (Y36, Y37)

  The appropriate 7th character is to be added to each code from category V94

A	initial encounter
D	subsequent encounter
S	sequela

  - X● **V94.0   Hitting object or bottom of body of water due to fall from watercraft**
    > **Excludes2**   drowning and submersion due to fall from watercraft (V92.0-)
  - **V94.1   Bather struck by watercraft**
    Swimmer hit by watercraft
    - X● **V94.11   Bather struck by powered watercraft**
    - X● **V94.12   Bather struck by nonpowered watercraft**
  - **V94.2   Rider of nonpowered watercraft struck by other watercraft**
    - X● **V94.21   Rider of nonpowered watercraft struck by other nonpowered watercraft**
      Canoer hit by other nonpowered watercraft
      Surfer hit by other nonpowered watercraft
      Windsurfer hit by other nonpowered watercraft
    - X● **V94.22   Rider of nonpowered watercraft struck by powered watercraft**
      Canoer hit by motorboat
      Surfer hit by motorboat
      Windsurfer hit by motorboat
  - **V94.3   Injury to rider of (inflatable) watercraft being pulled behind other watercraft**
    - X● **V94.31   Injury to rider of (inflatable) recreational watercraft being pulled behind other watercraft**
      Injury to rider of inner-tube pulled behind motor boat
    - X● **V94.32   Injury to rider of non-recreational watercraft being pulled behind other watercraft**
      Injury to occupant of dingy being pulled behind boat or ship
      Injury to occupant of life-raft being pulled behind boat or ship
  - X● **V94.4   Injury to barefoot water-skier**
    Injury to person being pulled behind boat or ship
  - **V94.8   Other water transport accident**
    - ● **V94.81   Water transport accident involving military watercraft**
      - ● **V94.810   Civilian watercraft involved in water transport accident with military watercraft**
        Passenger on civilian watercraft injured due to accident with military watercraft

X ● **V94.811** Civilian in water injured by military watercraft

X ● **V94.818** Other water transport accident involving military watercraft

X ● **V94.89** Other water transport accident

X ● **V94.9** Unspecified water transport accident
Water transport accident NOS

AIR AND SPACE TRANSPORT ACCIDENTS (V95-V97)

Excludes1   military aircraft accidents in military or war operations (Y36, Y37)

● **V95** Accident to powered aircraft causing injury to occupant

The appropriate 7th character is to be added to each code from category V95

A	initial encounter
D	subsequent encounter
S	sequela

● **V95.0** Helicopter accident injuring occupant

X ● **V95.00** Unspecified helicopter accident injuring occupant

X ● **V95.01** Helicopter crash injuring occupant

X ● **V95.02** Forced landing of helicopter injuring occupant

X ● **V95.03** Helicopter collision injuring occupant
Helicopter collision with any object, fixed, movable or moving

X ● **V95.04** Helicopter fire injuring occupant

X ● **V95.05** Helicopter explosion injuring occupant

X ● **V95.09** Other helicopter accident injuring occupant

● **V95.1** Ultralight, microlight or powered-glider accident injuring occupant

X ● **V95.10** Unspecified ultralight, microlight or powered-glider accident injuring occupant

X ● **V95.11** Ultralight, microlight or powered-glider crash injuring occupant

X ● **V95.12** Forced landing of ultralight, microlight or powered-glider injuring occupant

X ● **V95.13** Ultralight, microlight or powered-glider collision injuring occupant
Ultralight, microlight or powered-glider collision with any object, fixed, movable or moving

X ● **V95.14** Ultralight, microlight or powered-glider fire injuring occupant

X ● **V95.15** Ultralight, microlight or powered-glider explosion injuring occupant

X ● **V95.19** Other ultralight, microlight or powered-glider accident injuring occupant

● **V95.2** Other private fixed-wing aircraft accident injuring occupant

X ● **V95.20** Unspecified accident to other private fixed-wing aircraft, injuring occupant

X ● **V95.21** Other private fixed-wing aircraft crash injuring occupant

X ● **V95.22** Forced landing of other private fixed-wing aircraft injuring occupant

X ● **V95.23** Other private fixed-wing aircraft collision injuring occupant
Other private fixed-wing aircraft collision with any object, fixed, movable or moving

X ● **V95.24** Other private fixed-wing aircraft fire injuring occupant

X ● **V95.25** Other private fixed-wing aircraft explosion injuring occupant

X ● **V95.29** Other accident to other private fixed-wing aircraft injuring occupant

● **V95.3** Commercial fixed-wing aircraft accident injuring occupant

X ● **V95.30** Unspecified accident to commercial fixed-wing aircraft injuring occupant

X ● **V95.31** Commercial fixed-wing aircraft crash injuring occupant

X ● **V95.32** Forced landing of commercial fixed-wing aircraft injuring occupant

X ● **V95.33** Commercial fixed-wing aircraft collision injuring occupant
Commercial fixed-wing aircraft collision with any object, fixed, movable or moving

X ● **V95.34** Commercial fixed-wing aircraft fire injuring occupant

X ● **V95.35** Commercial fixed-wing aircraft explosion injuring occupant

X ● **V95.39** Other accident to commercial fixed-wing aircraft injuring occupant

● **V95.4** Spacecraft accident injuring occupant

X ● **V95.40** Unspecified spacecraft accident injuring occupant

X ● **V95.41** Spacecraft crash injuring occupant

X ● **V95.42** Forced landing of spacecraft injuring occupant

X ● **V95.43** Spacecraft collision injuring occupant
Spacecraft collision with any object, fixed, moveable or moving

X ● **V95.44** Spacecraft fire injuring occupant

X ● **V95.45** Spacecraft explosion injuring occupant

X ● **V95.49** Other spacecraft accident injuring occupant

X ● **V95.8** Other powered aircraft accidents injuring occupant

X ● **V95.9** Unspecified aircraft accident injuring occupant
Aircraft accident NOS
Air transport accident NOS

● **V96** Accident to nonpowered aircraft causing injury to occupant

The appropriate 7th character is to be added to each code from category V96

A	initial encounter
D	subsequent encounter
S	sequela

● **V96.0** Balloon accident injuring occupant

X ● **V96.00** Unspecified balloon accident injuring occupant

X ● **V96.01** Balloon crash injuring occupant

X ● **V96.02** Forced landing of balloon injuring occupant

X ● **V96.03** Balloon collision injuring occupant
Balloon collision with any object, fixed, moveable or moving

X ● **V96.04** Balloon fire injuring occupant

X ● **V96.05** Balloon explosion injuring occupant

X ● **V96.09** Other balloon accident injuring occupant

● **V96.1** Hang-glider accident injuring occupant

X ● **V96.10** Unspecified hang-glider accident injuring occupant

X ● **V96.11** Hang-glider crash injuring occupant

X ● **V96.12** Forced landing of hang-glider injuring occupant

X ● **V96.13** Hang-glider collision injuring occupant
Hang-glider collision with any object, fixed, moveable or moving

X ● **V96.14** Hang-glider fire injuring occupant

X ● **V96.15** Hang-glider explosion injuring occupant

X ● **V96.19** Other hang-glider accident injuring occupant

● **V96.2** Glider (nonpowered) accident injuring occupant

X ● **V96.20** Unspecified glider (nonpowered) accident injuring occupant

X ● **V96.21** Glider (nonpowered) crash injuring occupant

X ● **V96.22** Forced landing of glider (nonpowered) injuring occupant

X ● **V96.23**   Glider (nonpowered) **collision** injuring occupant
> Glider (nonpowered) collision with any object, fixed, moveable or moving

X ● **V96.24**   Glider (nonpowered) **fire** injuring occupant

X ● **V96.25**   Glider (nonpowered) **explosion** injuring occupant

X ● **V96.29**   **Other glider (nonpowered) accident** injuring occupant

X ● **V96.8**   Other nonpowered-aircraft accidents injuring occupant
> Kite carrying a person accident injuring occupant

X ● **V96.9**   **Unspecified** nonpowered-aircraft accident injuring occupant
> Nonpowered-aircraft accident NOS

● **V97**   Other specified air transport accidents
> The appropriate 7th character is to be added to each code from category V97

A	initial encounter
D	subsequent encounter
S	sequela

X ● **V97.0**   Occupant of aircraft injured in other specified air transport accidents
> Fall in, on or from aircraft in air transport accident
>
> **Excludes1**   accident while boarding or alighting aircraft (V97.1)

X ● **V97.1**   Person injured while boarding or alighting from aircraft

● **V97.2**   Parachutist accident

    X ● **V97.21**   Parachutist **entangled in object**
> Parachutist landing in tree

    X ● **V97.22**   Parachutist **injured on landing**

    X ● **V97.29**   **Other parachutist accident**

● **V97.3**   Person on ground injured in air transport accident

    X ● **V97.31**   Hit by object falling from aircraft
> Hit by crashing aircraft
> Injured by aircraft hitting house
> Injured by aircraft hitting car

    X ● **V97.32**   Injured by rotating propeller

    X ● **V97.33**   Sucked into jet engine

    X ● **V97.39**   Other injury to person on ground due to air transport accident

● **V97.8**   Other air transport accidents, not elsewhere classified
> **Excludes1**   aircraft accident NOS (V95.9)
>   exposure to changes in air pressure during ascent or descent (W94.-)

    ● **V97.81**   Air transport accident involving military aircraft

       ● **V97.810**   Civilian aircraft involved in air transport accident with military aircraft
> Passenger in civilian aircraft injured due to accident with military aircraft

       ● **V97.811**   Civilian injured by military aircraft

       ● **V97.818**   Other air transport accident involving military aircraft

    X ● **V97.89**   Other air transport accidents, not elsewhere classified
> Injury from machinery on aircraft

OTHER AND UNSPECIFIED TRANSPORT ACCIDENTS (V98-V99)

> **Excludes1**   vehicle accident, type of vehicle unspecified (V89.-)

● **V98**   Other specified transport accidents
> The appropriate 7th character is to be added to each code from category V98

A	initial encounter
D	subsequent encounter
S	sequela

X ● **V98.0**   Accident to, on or involving **cable-car, not on rails**
> Caught or dragged by cable-car, not on rails
> Fall or jump from cable-car, not on rails
> Object thrown from or in cable-car, not on rails

X ● **V98.1**   Accident to, on or involving **land-yacht**

X ● **V98.2**   Accident to, on or involving **ice yacht**

X ● **V98.3**   Accident to, on or involving **ski lift**
> Accident to, on or involving ski chair-lift
> Accident to, on or involving ski-lift with gondola

X ● **V98.8**   **Other specified transport accidents**

X ● **V99**   Unspecified transport accident
> The appropriate 7th character is to be added to code V99

A	initial encounter
D	subsequent encounter
S	sequela

OTHER EXTERNAL CAUSES OF ACCIDENTAL INJURY (W00-X58)

SLIPPING, TRIPPING, STUMBLING AND FALLS (W00-W19)

> **Excludes1**   assault involving a fall (Y01-Y02)
>   fall from animal (V80.-)
>   fall (in) (from) machinery (in operation) (W28-W31)
>   fall (in) (from) transport vehicle (V01-V99)
>   intentional self-harm involving a fall (X80-X81)
>
> **Excludes2**   at risk for fall (history of fall) Z91.81
>   fall (in) (from) burning building (X00.-)
>   fall into fire (X00-X04, X08)

● **W00**   Fall due to ice and snow
> **Includes**   pedestrian on foot falling (slipping) on ice and snow
>
> **Excludes1**   fall on (from) ice and snow involving pedestrian conveyance (V00.-)
>   fall from stairs and steps not due to ice and snow (W10.-)

> The appropriate 7th character is to be added to each code from category W00

A	initial encounter
D	subsequent encounter
S	sequela

X ● **W00.0**   Fall on **same level due to ice and snow**
> **Coding Clinic: 2016, Q2, P5**

X ● **W00.1**   Fall **from stairs and steps due to ice and snow**

X ● **W00.2**   **Other fall from one level to another due to ice and snow**

X ● **W00.9**   **Unspecified fall due to ice and snow**

● **W01**   Fall on same level from slipping, tripping and stumbling
> **Includes**   fall on moving sidewalk
>
> **Excludes1**   fall due to bumping (striking) against object (W18.0-)
>   fall in shower or bathtub (W18.2-)
>   fall on same level NOS (W18.30)
>   fall on same level from slipping, tripping and stumbling due to ice or snow (W00.0)
>   fall off or from toilet (W18.1-)
>   slipping, tripping and stumbling NOS (W18.40)
>   slipping, tripping and stumbling without falling (W18.4-)

> The appropriate 7th character is to be added to each code from category W01

A	initial encounter
D	subsequent encounter
S	sequela

X ● **W01.0**   Fall on same level from slipping, tripping and stumbling **without subsequent striking against object**
> Falling over animal

    ● **W01.1**   Fall on same level from slipping, tripping and stumbling **with subsequent striking against object**

X ● **W01.10** Fall on same level from slipping, tripping and stumbling with subsequent striking against unspecified object

● **W01.11** Fall on same level from slipping, tripping and stumbling with subsequent striking against sharp object

　　● **W01.110** Fall on same level from slipping, tripping and stumbling with subsequent striking against sharp glass

　　● **W01.111** Fall on same level from slipping, tripping and stumbling with subsequent striking against power tool or machine

　　● **W01.118** Fall on same level from slipping, tripping and stumbling with subsequent striking against other sharp object

　　● **W01.119** Fall on same level from slipping, tripping and stumbling with subsequent striking against unspecified sharp object

● **W01.19** Fall on same level from slipping, tripping and stumbling with subsequent striking against other object

　　● **W01.190** Fall on same level from slipping, tripping and stumbling with subsequent striking against furniture
　　　　Coding Clinic: 2021, Q1, P5

　　● **W01.198** Fall on same level from slipping, tripping and stumbling with subsequent striking against other object

X ● **W03** Other fall on same level due to collision with another person
Fall due to non-transport collision with other person

Excludes1　collision with another person without fall (W51)
crushed or pushed by a crowd or human stampede (W52)
fall involving pedestrian conveyance (V00-V09)
fall due to ice or snow (W00)
fall on same level NOS (W18.30)

The appropriate 7th character is to be added to code W03

A	initial encounter
D	subsequent encounter
S	sequela

Coding Clinic: 2015, Q1, P9-10; 2012, Q4, P108

X ● **W04** Fall while being carried or supported by other persons
Accidentally dropped while being carried

The appropriate 7th character is to be added to code W04

A	initial encounter
D	subsequent encounter
S	sequel

● **W05** Fall from non-moving wheelchair, nonmotorized scooter and motorized mobility scooter

Excludes1　fall from moving wheelchair (powered) (V00.811)
fall from moving motorized mobility scooter (V00.831)
fall from nonmotorized scooter (V00.141)

The appropriate 7th character is to be added to each code from category W05

A	initial encounter
D	subsequent encounter
S	sequela

X ● **W05.0** Fall from non-moving wheelchair
Coding Clinic: 2019, Q2, P27

X ● **W05.1** Fall from non-moving nonmotorized scooter

X ● **W05.2** Fall from non-moving motorized mobility scooter

X ● **W06** Fall from bed
The appropriate 7th character is to be added to code W06

A	initial encounter
D	subsequent encounter
S	sequela

X ● **W07** Fall from chair
The appropriate 7th character is to be added to code W07

A	initial encounter
D	subsequent encounter
S	sequela

X ● **W08** Fall from other furniture
The appropriate 7th character is to be added to code W08

A	initial encounter
D	subsequent encounter
S	sequela

● **W09** Fall on and from playground equipment
Excludes1　fall involving recreational machinery (W31)
The appropriate 7th character is to be added to each code from category W09

A	initial encounter
D	subsequent encounter
S	sequela

X ● **W09.0** Fall on or from playground slide
X ● **W09.1** Fall from playground swing
X ● **W09.2** Fall on or from jungle gym
X ● **W09.8** Fall on or from other playground equipment

● **W10** Fall on and from stairs and steps
Excludes1　fall from stairs and steps due to ice and snow (W00.1)
The appropriate 7th character is to be added to each code from category W10

A	initial encounter
D	subsequent encounter
S	sequela

X ● **W10.0** Fall (on) (from) escalator
X ● **W10.1** Fall (on) (from) sidewalk curb
X ● **W10.2** Fall (on) (from) incline
Fall (on) (from) ramp
X ● **W10.8** Fall (on) (from) other stairs and steps
X ● **W10.9** Fall (on) (from) unspecified stairs and steps

X ● **W11** Fall on and from ladder
The appropriate 7th character is to be added to code W11

A	initial encounter
D	subsequent encounter
S	sequela

X ● **W12** Fall on and from scaffolding
The appropriate 7th character is to be added to code W12

A	initial encounter
D	subsequent encounter
S	sequela

● **W13** Fall from, out of or through building or structure
The appropriate 7th character is to be added to each code from category W13

A	initial encounter
D	subsequent encounter
S	sequela

CHAPTER 20 (V00-Y99)

X ● **W13.0** **Fall from, out of or through balcony**
Fall from, out of or through railing

X ● **W13.1** **Fall from, out of or through bridge**

X ● **W13.2** **Fall from, out of or through roof**

X ● **W13.3** **Fall through floor**

X ● **W13.4** **Fall from, out of or through window**

Excludes2   fall with subsequent striking against sharp glass (W01.110-)

X ● **W13.8** **Fall from, out of or through other building or structure**
Fall from, out of or through viaduct
Fall from, out of or through wall
Fall from, out of or through flag-pole

X ● **W13.9** **Fall from, out of or through building, not otherwise specified**

Excludes1   collapse of a building or structure (W20.-)
fall or jump from burning building or structure (X00.-)

X ● **W14** **Fall from tree**

The appropriate 7th character is to be added to code W14

A	initial encounter
D	subsequent encounter
S	sequela

X ● **W15** **Fall from cliff**

The appropriate 7th character is to be added to code W15

A	initial encounter
D	subsequent encounter
S	sequela

● **W16** **Fall, jump or diving into water**

Excludes1   accidental non-watercraft drowning and submersion not involving fall (W65-W74)
effects of air pressure from diving (W94.-)
fall into water from watercraft (V90-V94)
hitting an object or against bottom when falling from watercraft (V94.0)

Excludes2   striking or hitting diving board (W21.4)

The appropriate 7th character is to be added to each code from category W16

A	initial encounter
D	subsequent encounter
S	sequela

● **W16.0** **Fall into swimming pool**
Fall into swimming pool NOS

Excludes1   fall into empty swimming pool (W17.3)

● **W16.01** **Fall into swimming pool striking water surface**

● **W16.011** **Fall into swimming pool striking water surface causing drowning and submersion**

Excludes1   drowning and submersion while in swimming pool without fall (W67)

● **W16.012** **Fall into swimming pool striking water surface causing other injury**

● **W16.02** **Fall into swimming pool striking bottom**

● **W16.021** **Fall into swimming pool striking bottom causing drowning and submersion**

Excludes1   drowning and submersion while in swimming pool without fall (W67)

● **W16.022** **Fall into swimming pool striking bottom causing other injury**

● **W16.03** **Fall into swimming pool striking wall**

● **W16.031** **Fall into swimming pool striking wall causing drowning and submersion**

Excludes1   drowning and submersion while in swimming pool without fall (W67)

● **W16.032** **Fall into swimming pool striking wall causing other injury**

● **W16.1** **Fall into natural body of water**
Fall into lake
Fall into open sea
Fall into river
Fall into stream

● **W16.11** **Fall into natural body of water striking water surface**

● **W16.111** **Fall into natural body of water striking water surface causing drowning and submersion**

Excludes1   drowning and submersion while in natural body of water without fall (W69)

● **W16.112** **Fall into natural body of water striking water surface causing other injury**

● **W16.12** **Fall into natural body of water striking bottom**

● **W16.121** **Fall into natural body of water striking bottom causing drowning and submersion**

Excludes1   drowning and submersion while in natural body of water without fall (W69)

● **W16.122** **Fall into natural body of water striking bottom causing other injury**

● **W16.13** **Fall into natural body of water striking side**

● **W16.131** **Fall into natural body of water striking side causing drowning and submersion**

Excludes1   drowning and submersion while in natural body of water without fall (W69)

● **W16.132** **Fall into natural body of water striking side causing other injury**

● **W16.2** **Fall in (into) filled bathtub or bucket of water**

● **W16.21** **Fall in (into) filled bathtub**

Excludes1   fall into empty bathtub (W18.2)

● **W16.211** **Fall in (into) filled bathtub causing drowning and submersion**

Excludes1   drowning and submersion while in filled bathtub without fall (W65)

● **W16.212** **Fall in (into) filled bathtub causing other injury**

● **W16.22** **Fall in (into) bucket of water**

● **W16.221** **Fall in (into) bucket of water causing drowning and submersion**

● **W16.222** **Fall in (into) bucket of water causing other injury**

▶ New   ⇒ Revised   ~~deleted~~ Deleted   Excludes 1   Excludes 2   Includes   Use additional   Code first   Code also   Key words

OGCR Official Guidelines   X Assign placeholder X   ● Use Additional Character(s)   ▶ Manifestation Code   🏥 Hierarchical Condition Category   **Coding Clinic**

● **W16.3   Fall into other water**
     Fall into fountain
     Fall into reservoir

   ● **W16.31   Fall into other water striking water surface**

     ● **W16.311   Fall into other water striking water surface causing drowning and submersion**

       Excludes1   drowning and submersion while in other water without fall (W73)

     ● **W16.312   Fall into other water striking water surface causing other injury**

   ● **W16.32   Fall into other water striking bottom**

     ● **W16.321   Fall into other water striking bottom causing drowning and submersion**

       Excludes1   drowning and submersion while in other water without fall (W73)

     ● **W16.322   Fall into other water striking bottom causing other injury**

   ● **W16.33   Fall into other water striking wall**

     ● **W16.331   Fall into other water striking wall causing drowning and submersion**

       Excludes1   drowning and submersion while in other water without fall (W73)

     ● **W16.332   Fall into other water striking wall causing other injury**

● **W16.4   Fall into unspecified water**

   X ● **W16.41   Fall into unspecified water causing drowning and submersion**

   X ● **W16.42   Fall into unspecified water causing other injury**

● **W16.5   Jumping or diving into swimming pool**

   ● **W16.51   Jumping or diving into swimming pool striking water surface**

     ● **W16.511   Jumping or diving into swimming pool striking water surface causing drowning and submersion**

       Excludes1   drowning and submersion while in swimming pool without jumping or diving (W67)

     ● **W16.512   Jumping or diving into swimming pool striking water surface causing other injury**

   ● **W16.52   Jumping or diving into swimming pool striking bottom**

     ● **W16.521   Jumping or diving into swimming pool striking bottom causing drowning and submersion**

       Excludes1   drowning and submersion while in swimming pool without jumping or diving (W67)

     ● **W16.522   Jumping or diving into swimming pool striking bottom causing other injury**

● **W16.53   Jumping or diving into swimming pool striking wall**

   ● **W16.531   Jumping or diving into swimming pool striking wall causing drowning and submersion**

     Excludes1   drowning and submersion while in swimming pool without jumping or diving (W67)

   ● **W16.532   Jumping or diving into swimming pool striking wall causing other injury**

● **W16.6   Jumping or diving into natural body of water**
     Jumping or diving into lake
     Jumping or diving into open sea
     Jumping or diving into river
     Jumping or diving into stream

   ● **W16.61   Jumping or diving into natural body of water striking water surface**

     ● **W16.611   Jumping or diving into natural body of water striking water surface causing drowning and submersion**

       Excludes1   drowning and submersion while in natural body of water without jumping or diving (W69)

     ● **W16.612   Jumping or diving into natural body of water striking water surface causing other injury**

   ● **W16.62   Jumping or diving into natural body of water striking bottom**

     ● **W16.621   Jumping or diving into natural body of water striking bottom causing drowning and submersion**

       Excludes1   drowning and submersion while in natural body of water without jumping or diving (W69)

     ● **W16.622   Jumping or diving into natural body of water striking bottom causing other injury**

● **W16.7   Jumping or diving from boat**

   Excludes1   fall from boat into water - see watercraft accident (V90-V94)

   ● **W16.71   Jumping or diving from boat striking water surface**

     ● **W16.711   Jumping or diving from boat striking water surface causing drowning and submersion**

     ● **W16.712   Jumping or diving from boat striking water surface causing other injury**

   ● **W16.72   Jumping or diving from boat striking bottom**

     ● **W16.721   Jumping or diving from boat striking bottom causing drowning and submersion**

     ● **W16.722   Jumping or diving from boat striking bottom causing other injury**

CHAPTER 20 (V00-Y99)

● **W16.8** **Jumping or diving into other water**
Jumping or diving into fountain
Jumping or diving into reservoir

● **W16.81** **Jumping or diving into other water striking water surface**

● **W16.811** **Jumping or diving into other water striking water surface causing drowning and submersion**

Excludes1   drowning and submersion while in other water without jumping or diving (W73)

● **W16.812** **Jumping or diving into other water striking water surface causing other injury**

● **W16.82** **Jumping or diving into other water striking bottom**

● **W16.821** **Jumping or diving into other water striking bottom causing drowning and submersion**

Excludes1   drowning and submersion while in other water without jumping or diving (W73)

● **W16.822** **Jumping or diving into other water striking bottom causing other injury**

● **W16.83** **Jumping or diving into other water striking wall**

● **W16.831** **Jumping or diving into other water striking wall causing drowning and submersion**

Excludes1   drowning and submersion while in other water without jumping or diving (W73)

● **W16.832** **Jumping or diving into other water striking wall causing other injury**

● **W16.9** **Jumping or diving into unspecified water**

X ● **W16.91** **Jumping or diving into unspecified water causing drowning and submersion**

X ● **W16.92** **Jumping or diving into unspecified water causing other injury**

● **W17** **Other fall from one level to another**

The appropriate 7th character is to be added to each code from category W17

A	initial encounter
D	subsequent encounter
S	sequela

X ● **W17.0** **Fall into well**

X ● **W17.1** **Fall into storm drain or manhole**

X ● **W17.2** **Fall into hole**
Fall into pit

X ● **W17.3** **Fall into empty swimming pool**

Excludes1   fall into filled swimming pool (W16.0-)

X ● **W17.4** **Fall from dock**

● **W17.8** **Other fall from one level to another**

X ● **W17.81** **Fall down embankment (hill)**

X ● **W17.82** **Fall from (out of) grocery cart**
Fall due to grocery cart tipping over

X ● **W17.89** **Other fall from one level to another**
Fall from cherry picker
Fall from lifting device
Fall from mobile elevated work platform [MEWP]
Fall from sky lift
Coding Clinic: 2015, Q2, P6

● **W18** **Other slipping, tripping and stumbling and falls**

The appropriate 7th character is to be added to each code from category W18

A	initial encounter
D	subsequent encounter
S	sequela

● **W18.0** **Fall due to bumping against object**
Striking against object with subsequent fall

Excludes1   fall on same level due to slipping, tripping, or stumbling with subsequent striking against object (W01.1-)

X ● **W18.00** **Striking against unspecified object with subsequent fall**

X ● **W18.01** **Striking against sports equipment with subsequent fall**

X ● **W18.02** **Striking against glass with subsequent fall**

X ● **W18.09** **Striking against other object with subsequent fall**

● **W18.1** **Fall from or off toilet**

X ● **W18.11** **Fall from or off toilet without subsequent striking against object**
Fall from (off) toilet NOS

X ● **W18.12** **Fall from or off toilet with subsequent striking against object**

X ● **W18.2** **Fall in (into) shower or empty bathtub**

Excludes1   fall in full bathtub causing drowning or submersion (W16.21-)

● **W18.3** **Other and unspecified fall on same level**

X ● **W18.30** **Fall on same level, unspecified**

X ● **W18.31** **Fall on same level due to stepping on an object**
Fall on same level due to stepping on an animal

Excludes1   slipping, tripping and stumbling without fall due to stepping on animal (W18.41)

X ● **W18.39** **Other fall on same level**

● **W18.4** **Slipping, tripping and stumbling without falling**

Excludes1   collision with another person without fall (W51)

X ● **W18.40** **Slipping, tripping and stumbling without falling, unspecified**

X ● **W18.41** **Slipping, tripping and stumbling without falling due to stepping on object**
Slipping, tripping and stumbling without falling due to stepping on animal

Excludes1   slipping, tripping and stumbling with fall due to stepping on animal (W18.31)

X ● **W18.42** **Slipping, tripping and stumbling without falling due to stepping into hole or opening**

X ● **W18.43** **Slipping, tripping and stumbling without falling due to stepping from one level to another**

X ● **W18.49** **Other slipping, tripping and stumbling without falling**

X ● **W19** **Unspecified fall**
Accidental fall NOS

The appropriate 7th character is to be added to code W19

A	initial encounter
D	subsequent encounter
S	sequela

Coding Clinic: 2021, Q2, P5; 2012, Q4, P95

▶ New   ⇒ Revised   ~~deleted~~ Deleted   Excludes 1   Excludes 2   Includes   Use additional   Code first   Code also   Key words

   OGCR Official Guidelines   X Assign placeholder X   ● Use Additional Character(s)   ▶ Manifestation Code   🔲 Hierarchical Condition Category   **Coding Clinic**

EXPOSURE TO INANIMATE MECHANICAL FORCES (W20-W49)

Excludes1   assault (X92-Y09)
contact or collision with animals or persons
(W50-W64)
exposure to inanimate mechanical forces
involving military or war operations (Y36.-,
Y37.-)
intentional self-harm (X71-X83)

Coding Clinic: 2016, Q4, P129

● **W20   Struck by thrown, projected or falling object**

Code first any associated:
cataclysm (X34-X39)
lightning strike (T75.00)

Excludes1   falling object in machinery accident (W24,
W28-W31)
falling object in transport accident (V01-V99)
object set in motion by explosion (W35-W40)
object set in motion by firearm (W32-W34)
struck by thrown sports equipment (W21.-)

The appropriate 7th character is to be added to each code from
category W20

A	initial encounter
D	subsequent encounter
S	sequela

X● **W20.0   Struck by falling object in cave-in**
Excludes2   asphyxiation due to cave-in (T71.21)

X● **W20.1   Struck by object due to collapse of building**
Excludes1   struck by object due to collapse of
burning building (X00.2, X02.2)

X● **W20.8   Other cause of strike by thrown, projected or falling
object**
Excludes1   struck by thrown sports equipment
(W21.-)

● **W21   Striking against or struck by sports equipment**

Excludes1   assault with sports equipment (Y08.0-)
striking against or struck by sports equipment
with subsequent fall (W18.01)

The appropriate 7th character is to be added to each code from
category W21

A	initial encounter
D	subsequent encounter
S	sequela

● **W21.0   Struck by hit or thrown ball**
X● **W21.00   Struck by hit or thrown ball, unspecified type**
X● **W21.01   Struck by football**
X● **W21.02   Struck by soccer ball**
X● **W21.03   Struck by baseball**
X● **W21.04   Struck by golf ball**
X● **W21.05   Struck by basketball**
X● **W21.06   Struck by volleyball**
X● **W21.07   Struck by softball**
X● **W21.09   Struck by other hit or thrown ball**
● **W21.1   Struck by bat, racquet or club**
X● **W21.11   Struck by baseball bat**
X● **W21.12   Struck by tennis racquet**
X● **W21.13   Struck by golf club**
X● **W21.19   Struck by other bat, racquet or club**
● **W21.2   Struck by hockey stick or puck**
● **W21.21   Struck by hockey stick**
● **W21.210   Struck by ice hockey stick**
● **W21.211   Struck by field hockey stick**

● **W21.22   Struck by hockey puck**
● **W21.220   Struck by ice hockey puck**
● **W21.221   Struck by field hockey puck**
● **W21.3   Struck by sports foot wear**
X● **W21.31   Struck by shoe cleats**
Stepped on by shoe cleats
X● **W21.32   Struck by skate blades**
Skated over by skate blades
X● **W21.39   Struck by other sports foot wear**
X● **W21.4   Striking against diving board**
Use additional code for subsequent falling into water, if
applicable (W16.-)
● **W21.8   Striking against or struck by other sports equipment**
X● **W21.81   Striking against or struck by football helmet**
X● **W21.89   Striking against or struck by other sports
equipment**
X● **W21.9   Striking against or struck by unspecified sports
equipment**

● **W22   Striking against or struck by other objects**

Excludes1   striking against or struck by object with
subsequent fall (W18.09)

The appropriate 7th character is to be added to each code from
category W22

A	initial encounter
D	subsequent encounter
S	sequela

● **W22.0   Striking against stationary object**
Excludes1   striking against stationary sports
equipment (W21.8)
X● **W22.01   Walked into wall**
X● **W22.02   Walked into lamppost**
X● **W22.03   Walked into furniture**
● **W22.04   Striking against wall of swimming pool**
● **W22.041   Striking against wall of swimming
pool causing drowning and
submersion**
Excludes1   drowning and
submersion
while swimming
without striking
against wall
(W67)

● **W22.042   Striking against wall of swimming
pool causing other injury**
X● **W22.09   Striking against other stationary object**
● **W22.1   Striking against or struck by automobile airbag**
X● **W22.10   Striking against or struck by unspecified
automobile airbag**
X● **W22.11   Striking against or struck by driver side
automobile airbag**
X● **W22.12   Striking against or struck by front passenger
side automobile airbag**
X● **W22.19   Striking against or struck by other automobile
airbag**
X● **W22.8   Striking against or struck by other objects**
Striking against or struck by object NOS
Excludes1   struck by thrown, projected or falling
object (W20.-)

CHAPTER 20 (V00-Y99)

CHAPTER 20 (V00-Y99)

● **W23 Caught, crushed, jammed or pinched in or between objects**

> **Excludes1**   injury caused by cutting or piercing instruments (W25-W27)
> injury caused by firearms malfunction (W32.1, W33.1-, W34.1-)
> injury caused by lifting and transmission devices (W24.-)
> injury caused by machinery (W28-W31)
> injury caused by nonpowered hand tools (W27.-)
> injury caused by transport vehicle being used as a means of transportation (V01-V99)
> injury caused by struck by thrown, projected or falling object (W20.-)

The appropriate 7th character is to be added to each code from category W23

A	initial encounter
D	subsequent encounter
S	sequela

X● **W23.0 Caught, crushed, jammed, or pinched between moving objects**

X● **W23.1 Caught, crushed, jammed, or pinched between stationary objects**

▶X● **W23.2 Caught, crushed, jammed or pinched between a moving and stationary object**

● **W24 Contact with lifting and transmission devices, not elsewhere classified**

> **Excludes1**   transport accidents (V01-V99)

The appropriate 7th character is to be added to each code from category W24

A	initial encounter
D	subsequent encounter
S	sequela

X● **W24.0 Contact with lifting devices, not elsewhere classified**
> Contact with chain hoist
> Contact with drive belt
> Contact with pulley (block)

X● **W24.1 Contact with transmission devices, not elsewhere classified**
> Contact with transmission belt or cable

X● **W25 Contact with sharp glass**

> *Code first any associated:*
> injury due to flying glass from explosion or firearm discharge (W32-W40)
> transport accident (V00-V99)

> **Excludes1**   fall on same level due to slipping, tripping and stumbling with subsequent striking against sharp glass (W01.110-)
> striking against sharp glass with subsequent fall (W18.02-)

> **Excludes2**   glass embedded in skin (W45.-)

The appropriate 7th character is to be added to code W25

A	initial encounter
D	subsequent encounter
S	sequela

● **W26 Contact with other sharp objects**

> **Excludes2**   sharp object(s) embedded in skin (W45.-)

The appropriate 7th character is to be added to each code from category W26

A	initial encounter
D	subsequent encounter
S	sequela

Coding Clinic: 2016, Q4, P73

X● **W26.0 Contact with knife**
> **Excludes1**   contact with electric knife (W29.1)

X● **W26.1 Contact with sword or dagger**

X● **W26.2 Contact with edge of stiff paper**
> Paper cut
> **Coding Clinic: 2016, Q4, P73**

X● **W26.8 Contact with other sharp object(s), not elsewhere classified**
> Contact with tin can lid
> **Coding Clinic: 2016, Q4, P73**

X● **W26.9 Contact with unspecified sharp object(s)**
> **Coding Clinic: 2016, Q4, P73**

● **W27 Contact with nonpowered hand tool**

The appropriate 7th character is to be added to each code from category W27

A	initial encounter
D	subsequent encounter
S	sequela

X● **W27.0 Contact with workbench tool**
> Contact with auger
> Contact with axe
> Contact with chisel
> Contact with handsaw
> Contact with screwdriver

X● **W27.1 Contact with garden tool**
> Contact with hoe
> Contact with nonpowered lawn mower
> Contact with pitchfork
> Contact with rake

X● **W27.2 Contact with scissors**

X● **W27.3 Contact with needle (sewing)**
> **Excludes1**   contact with hypodermic needle (W46.-)

X● **W27.4 Contact with kitchen utensil**
> Contact with fork
> Contact with ice-pick
> Contact with can-opener NOS

X● **W27.5 Contact with paper-cutter**

X● **W27.8 Contact with other nonpowered hand tool**
> Contact with nonpowered sewing machine
> Contact with shovel

X● **W28 Contact with powered lawn mower**
> Powered lawn mower (commercial) (residential)
> **Excludes1**   contact with nonpowered lawn mower (W27.1)
> **Excludes2**   exposure to electric current (W86.-)

The appropriate 7th character is to be added to code W28

A	initial encounter
D	subsequent encounter
S	sequela

● **W29 Contact with other powered hand tools and household machinery**
> **Excludes1**   contact with commercial machinery (W31.82)
> contact with hot household appliance (X15)
> contact with nonpowered hand tool (W27.-)
> exposure to electric current (W86)

The appropriate 7th character is to be added to each code from category W29

A	initial encounter
D	subsequent encounter
S	sequela

X● **W29.0 Contact with powered kitchen appliance**
> Contact with blender
> Contact with can-opener
> Contact with garbage disposal
> Contact with mixer

X● **W29.1 Contact with electric knife**

X● **W29.2 Contact with other powered household machinery**
> Contact with electric fan
> Contact with powered dryer (clothes) (powered) (spin)
> Contact with washing-machine
> Contact with sewing machine

▶ New   ⇒ Revised   ~~deleted~~ Deleted   Excludes 1   Excludes 2   Includes   Use additional   Code first   Code also   Key words

OGCR Official Guidelines   X Assign placeholder X   ● Use Additional Character(s)   ▶ Manifestation Code   🐾 Hierarchical Condition Category   Coding Clinic

X● **W29.3 Contact with powered garden and outdoor hand tools and machinery**
    Contact with chainsaw
    Contact with edger
    Contact with garden cultivator (tiller)
    Contact with hedge trimmer
    Contact with other powered garden tool
       Excludes1   contact with powered lawn mower (W28)

X● **W29.4 Contact with nail gun**

X● **W29.8 Contact with other powered hand tools and household machinery**
    Contact with do-it-yourself tool NOS

● **W30 Contact with agricultural machinery**
    Includes   animal-powered farm machine
    Excludes1   agricultural transport vehicle accident (V01-V99)
                explosion of grain store (W40.8)
                exposure to electric current (W86.-)

The appropriate 7th character is to be added to each code from category W30

A	initial encounter
D	subsequent encounter
S	sequela

X● **W30.0 Contact with combine harvester**
    Contact with reaper
    Contact with thresher

X● **W30.1 Contact with power take-off devices (PTO)**

X● **W30.2 Contact with hay derrick**

X● **W30.3 Contact with grain storage elevator**
       Excludes1   explosion of grain store (W40.8)

● **W30.8 Contact with other specified agricultural machinery**
   X● **W30.81 Contact with agricultural transport vehicle in stationary use**
       Contact with agricultural transport vehicle under repair, not on public roadway
          Excludes1   agricultural transport vehicle accident (V01-V99)

   X● **W30.89 Contact with other specified agricultural machinery**

X● **W30.9 Contact with unspecified agricultural machinery**
    Contact with farm machinery NOS

● **W31 Contact with other and unspecified machinery**
    Excludes1   contact with agricultural machinery (W30.-)
                contact with machinery in transport under own power or being towed by a vehicle (V01-V99)
                exposure to electric current (W86)

The appropriate 7th character is to be added to each code from category W31

A	initial encounter
D	subsequent encounter
S	sequela

X● **W31.0 Contact with mining and earth-drilling machinery**
    Contact with bore or drill (land) (seabed)
    Contact with shaft hoist
    Contact with shaft lift
    Contact with undercutter

X● **W31.1 Contact with metalworking machines**
    Contact with abrasive wheel
    Contact with forging machine
    Contact with lathe
    Contact with mechanical shears
    Contact with metal drilling machine
    Contact with milling machine
    Contact with power press
    Contact with rolling-mill
    Contact with metal sawing machine

X● **W31.2 Contact with powered woodworking and forming machines**
    Contact with band saw
    Contact with bench saw
    Contact with circular saw
    Contact with molding machine
    Contact with overhead plane
    Contact with powered saw
    Contact with radial saw
    Contact with sander
       Excludes1   nonpowered woodworking tools (W27.0)

X● **W31.3 Contact with prime movers**
    Contact with gas turbine
    Contact with internal combustion engine
    Contact with steam engine
    Contact with water driven turbine

● **W31.8 Contact with other specified machinery**
   X● **W31.81 Contact with recreational machinery**
       Contact with roller-coaster

   X● **W31.82 Contact with other commercial machinery**
       Contact with commercial electric fan
       Contact with commercial kitchen appliances
       Contact with commercial powered dryer (clothes) (powered) (spin)
       Contact with commercial washing-machine
       Contact with commercial sewing machine
          Excludes1   contact with household machinery (W29.-)
                     contact with powered lawn mower (W28)

   X● **W31.83 Contact with special construction vehicle in stationary use**
       Contact with special construction vehicle under repair, not on public roadway
          Excludes1   special construction vehicle accident (V01-V99)

   X● **W31.89 Contact with other specified machinery**

X● **W31.9 Contact with unspecified machinery**
    Contact with machinery NOS

● **W32 Accidental handgun discharge and malfunction**
    Includes   accidental discharge and malfunction of gun for single hand use
            accidental discharge and malfunction of pistol
            accidental discharge and malfunction of revolver
            handgun discharge and malfunction NOS
    Excludes1   accidental airgun discharge and malfunction (W34.010, W34.110)
            accidental BB gun discharge and malfunction (W34.010, W34.110)
            accidental pellet gun discharge and malfunction (W34.010, W34.110)
            accidental shotgun discharge and malfunction (W33.01, W33.11)
            assault by handgun discharge (X93)
            handgun discharge involving legal intervention (Y35.0-)
            handgun discharge involving military or war operations (Y36.4-)
            intentional self-harm by handgun discharge (X72)
            Very pistol discharge and malfunction (W34.09, W34.19)

The appropriate 7th character is to be added to each code from category W32

A	initial encounter
D	subsequent encounter
S	sequela

X● **W32.0 Accidental handgun discharge**

X● **W32.1 Accidental handgun malfunction**
    Injury due to explosion of handgun (parts)
    Injury due to malfunction of mechanism or component of handgun
    Injury due to recoil of handgun
    Powder burn from handgun

● **W33 Accidental rifle, shotgun and larger firearm discharge and malfunction**

> **Includes**   rifle, shotgun and larger firearm discharge and malfunction NOS

> **Excludes1**   accidental airgun discharge and malfunction (W34.010, W34.110)
> accidental BB gun discharge and malfunction (W34.010, W34.110)
> accidental handgun discharge and malfunction (W32.-)
> accidental pellet gun discharge and malfunction (W34.010, W34.110)
> assault by rifle, shotgun and larger firearm discharge (X94)
> firearm discharge involving legal intervention (Y35.0-)
> firearm discharge involving military or war operations (Y36.4-)
> intentional self-harm by rifle, shotgun and larger firearm discharge (X73)

> The appropriate 7th character is to be added to each code from category W33

> | A | initial encounter |
> | D | subsequent encounter |
> | S | sequela |

● **W33.0 Accidental rifle, shotgun and larger firearm discharge**

X● **W33.00 Accidental discharge of unspecified larger firearm**
Discharge of unspecified larger firearm NOS

X● **W33.01 Accidental discharge of shotgun**
Discharge of shotgun NOS

X● **W33.02 Accidental discharge of hunting rifle**
Discharge of hunting rifle NOS

X● **W33.03 Accidental discharge of machine gun**
Discharge of machine gun NOS

X● **W33.09 Accidental discharge of other larger firearm**
Discharge of other larger firearm NOS

● **W33.1 Accidental rifle, shotgun and larger firearm malfunction**
Injury due to explosion of rifle, shotgun and larger firearm (parts)
Injury due to malfunction of mechanism or component of rifle, shotgun and larger firearm
Injury due to piercing, cutting, crushing or pinching due to (by) slide trigger mechanism, scope or other gun part
Injury due to recoil of rifle, shotgun and larger firearm
Powder burn from rifle, shotgun and larger firearm

X● **W33.10 Accidental malfunction of unspecified larger firearm**
Malfunction of unspecified larger firearm NOS

X● **W33.11 Accidental malfunction of shotgun**
Malfunction of shotgun NOS

X● **W33.12 Accidental malfunction of hunting rifle**
Malfunction of hunting rifle NOS

X● **W33.13 Accidental malfunction of machine gun**
Malfunction of machine gun NOS

X● **W33.19 Accidental malfunction of other larger firearm**
Malfunction of other larger firearm NOS

● **W34 Accidental discharge and malfunction from other and unspecified firearms and guns**

> The appropriate 7th character is to be added to each code from category W34

> | A | initial encounter |
> | D | subsequent encounter |
> | S | sequela |

● **W34.0 Accidental discharge from other and unspecified firearms and guns**

X● **W34.00 Accidental discharge from unspecified firearms or gun**
Discharge from firearm NOS
Gunshot wound NOS
Shot NOS
Coding Clinic: 2015, Q1, P17

● **W34.01 Accidental discharge of gas, air or spring-operated guns**

● **W34.010 Accidental discharge of airgun**
Accidental discharge of BB gun
Accidental discharge of pellet gun

● **W34.011 Accidental discharge of paintball gun**
Accidental injury due to paintball discharge

● **W34.018 Accidental discharge of other gas, air or spring-operated gun**

X● **W34.09 Accidental discharge from other specified firearms**
Accidental discharge from Very pistol [flare]

● **W34.1 Accidental malfunction from other and unspecified firearms and guns**

X● **W34.10 Accidental malfunction from unspecified firearms or gun**
Firearm malfunction NOS

● **W34.11 Accidental malfunction of gas, air or spring-operated guns**

● **W34.110 Accidental malfunction of airgun**
Accidental malfunction of BB gun
Accidental malfunction of pellet gun

● **W34.111 Accidental malfunction of paintball gun**
Accidental injury due to paintball gun malfunction

● **W34.118 Accidental malfunction of other gas, air or spring-operated gun**

X● **W34.19 Accidental malfunction from other specified firearms**
Accidental malfunction from Very pistol [flare]

X● **W35 Explosion and rupture of boiler**

> **Excludes1**   explosion and rupture of boiler on watercraft (V93.4)

> The appropriate 7th character is to be added to code W35

> | A | initial encounter |
> | D | subsequent encounter |
> | S | sequela |

● **W36 Explosion and rupture of gas cylinder**

> The appropriate 7th character is to be added to each code from category W36

> | A | initial encounter |
> | D | subsequent encounter |
> | S | sequela |

X● **W36.1 Explosion and rupture of aerosol can**
X● **W36.2 Explosion and rupture of air tank**
X● **W36.3 Explosion and rupture of pressurized-gas tank**
X● **W36.8 Explosion and rupture of other gas cylinder**
X● **W36.9 Explosion and rupture of unspecified gas cylinder**

▶ New   ⇒ Revised   ~~deleted~~ Deleted   Excludes 1   Excludes 2   Includes   Use additional   Code first   Code also   Key words
OGCR Official Guidelines   X Assign placeholder X   ● Use Additional Character(s)   ▶ Manifestation Code   🏷 Hierarchical Condition Category   **Coding Clinic**

● **W37   Explosion and rupture of** pressurized tire, pipe or hose

> The appropriate 7th character is to be added to each code from category W37

> | A | initial encounter |
> |---|---|
> | D | subsequent encounter |
> | S | sequela |

X ● **W37.0   Explosion of** bicycle tire

X ● **W37.8   Explosion and rupture of** other pressurized tire, pipe or hose

X ● **W38   Explosion and rupture of** other specified pressurized devices

> The appropriate 7th character is to be added to code W38

> | A | initial encounter |
> |---|---|
> | D | subsequent encounter |
> | S | sequela |

X ● **W39   Discharge of** firework

> The appropriate 7th character is to be added to code W39

> | A | initial encounter |
> |---|---|
> | D | subsequent encounter |
> | S | sequela |

● **W40   Explosion of other materials**

> **Excludes1**   assault by explosive material (X96)
> explosion involving legal intervention (Y35.1-)
> explosion involving military or war operations (Y36.0-, Y36.2-)
> intentional self-harm by explosive material (X75)

> The appropriate 7th character is to be added to each code from category W40

> | A | initial encounter |
> |---|---|
> | D | subsequent encounter |
> | S | sequela |

X ● **W40.0   Explosion of blasting material**
> Explosion of blasting cap
> Explosion of detonator
> Explosion of dynamite
> Explosion of explosive (any) used in blasting operations

X ● **W40.1   Explosion of** explosive gases
> Explosion of acetylene
> Explosion of butane
> Explosion of coal gas
> Explosion in mine NOS
> Explosion of explosive gas
> Explosion of fire damp
> Explosion of gasoline fumes
> Explosion of methane
> Explosion of propane

X ● **W40.8   Explosion of** other specified explosive materials
> Explosion in dump NOS
> Explosion in factory NOS
> Explosion in grain store
> Explosion in munitions

> > **Excludes1**   explosion involving legal intervention (Y35.1-)
> > explosion involving military or war operations (Y36.0-, Y36.2-)

X ● **W40.9   Explosion of** unspecified explosive materials
> Explosion NOS

● **W42   Exposure to noise**

> The appropriate 7th character is to be added to each code from category W42

> | A | initial encounter |
> |---|---|
> | D | subsequent encounter |
> | S | sequela |

X ● **W42.0   Exposure to** supersonic waves

X ● **W42.9   Exposure to other noise**
> Exposure to sound waves NOS

● **W45   Foreign body or object entering through skin**

> **Includes**   foreign body or object embedded in skin
> nail embedded in skin

> **Excludes2**   contact with hand tools (nonpowered) (powered) (W27-W29)
> contact with other sharp object(s) (W26.-)
> contact with sharp glass (W25.-)
> struck by objects (W20-W22)

> The appropriate 7th character is to be added to each code from category W45

> | A | initial encounter |
> |---|---|
> | D | subsequent encounter |
> | S | sequela |

X ● **W45.0   Nail entering through skin**

X ● **W45.8   Other foreign body or object entering through skin**
> Splinter in skin NOS

● **W46   Contact with hypodermic needle**

> The appropriate 7th character is to be added to each code from category W46

> | A | initial encounter |
> |---|---|
> | D | subsequent encounter |
> | S | sequela |

X ● **W46.0   Contact with hypodermic needle**
> Hypodermic needle stick NOS

X ● **W46.1   Contact with** contaminated **hypodermic needle**

● **W49   Exposure to other inanimate mechanical forces**

> **Includes**   exposure to abnormal gravitational [G] forces
> exposure to inanimate mechanical forces NEC

> **Excludes1**   exposure to inanimate mechanical forces involving military or war operations (Y36.-, Y37.-)

> The appropriate 7th character is to be added to each code from category W49

> | A | initial encounter |
> |---|---|
> | D | subsequent encounter |
> | S | sequela |

● **W49.0   Item causing external constriction**

> X ● **W49.01   Hair causing external constriction**
> X ● **W49.02   String or thread causing external constriction**
> X ● **W49.03   Rubber band causing external constriction**
> X ● **W49.04   Ring or other jewelry causing external constriction**
> X ● **W49.09   Other item causing external constriction**

X ● **W49.9   Exposure to other** inanimate mechanical forces

---

EXPOSURE TO ANIMATE MECHANICAL FORCES (W50-W64)

> **Excludes1**   toxic effect of contact with venomous animals and plants (T63.-)

● **W50   Accidental hit, strike, kick, twist, bite or scratch by another person**

> **Includes**   hit, strike, kick, twist, bite, or scratch by another person NOS

> **Excludes1**   assault by bodily force (Y04)
> struck by objects (W20-W22)

> The appropriate 7th character is to be added to each code from category W50

> | A | initial encounter |
> |---|---|
> | D | subsequent encounter |
> | S | sequela |

X ● **W50.0   Accidental hit or strike by another person**
> Hit or strike by another person NOS

X ● **W50.1   Accidental kick by another person**
> Kick by another person NOS

X ● **W50.2 Accidental twist by another person**
Twist by another person NOS
Coding Clinic: 2015, Q1, P8

X ● **W50.3 Accidental bite by another person**
Human bite
Bite by another person NOS

X ● **W50.4 Accidental scratch by another person**
Scratch by another person NOS

X ●**W51 Accidental striking against or bumped into by another person**
Excludes1 assault by striking against or bumping into by another person (Y04.2)
fall due to collision with another person (W03)
The appropriate 7th character is to be added to code W51

A initial encounter
D subsequent encounter
S sequela

X ●**W52 Crushed, pushed or stepped on by crowd or human stampede**
Crushed, pushed or stepped on by crowd or human stampede with or without fall
The appropriate 7th character is to be added to code W52

A initial encounter
D subsequent encounter
S sequela

●**W53 Contact with rodent**
Includes contact with saliva, feces or urine of rodent
The appropriate 7th character is to be added to each code from category W53

A initial encounter
D subsequent encounter
S sequela

● **W53.0 Contact with mouse**
X ● **W53.01 Bitten by mouse**
X ● **W53.09 Other contact with mouse**
● **W53.1 Contact with rat**
X ● **W53.11 Bitten by rat**
X ● **W53.19 Other contact with rat**
● **W53.2 Contact with squirrel**
X ● **W53.21 Bitten by squirrel**
X ● **W53.29 Other contact with squirrel**
● **W53.8 Contact with other rodent**
X ● **W53.81 Bitten by other rodent**
X ● **W53.89 Other contact with other rodent**

●**W54 Contact with dog**
Includes contact with saliva, feces or urine of dog
The appropriate 7th character is to be added to each code from category W54

A initial encounter
D subsequent encounter
S sequela

X ● **W54.0 Bitten by dog**
X ● **W54.1 Struck by dog**
Knocked over by dog
X ● **W54.8 Other contact with dog**

●**W55 Contact with other mammals**
Includes contact with saliva, feces or urine of mammal
Excludes1 animal being ridden - see transport accidents
bitten or struck by dog (W54)
bitten or struck by rodent (W53.-)
contact with marine mammals (W56.X-)
The appropriate 7th character is to be added to each code from category W55

A initial encounter
D subsequent encounter
S sequela

● **W55.0 Contact with cat**
X ● **W55.01 Bitten by cat**
X ● **W55.03 Scratched by cat**
X ● **W55.09 Other contact with cat**
● **W55.1 Contact with horse**
X ● **W55.11 Bitten by horse**
X ● **W55.12 Struck by horse**
X ● **W55.19 Other contact with horse**
● **W55.2 Contact with cow**
Contact with bull
X ● **W55.21 Bitten by cow**
X ● **W55.22 Struck by cow**
Gored by bull
X ● **W55.29 Other contact with cow**
● **W55.3 Contact with other hoof stock**
Contact with goats
Contact with sheep
X ● **W55.31 Bitten by other hoof stock**
X ● **W55.32 Struck by other hoof stock**
Gored by goat
Gored by ram
X ● **W55.39 Other contact with other hoof stock**
● **W55.4 Contact with pig**
X ● **W55.41 Bitten by pig**
X ● **W55.42 Struck by pig**
X ● **W55.49 Other contact with pig**
● **W55.5 Contact with raccoon**
X ● **W55.51 Bitten by raccoon**
X ● **W55.52 Struck by raccoon**
X ● **W55.59 Other contact with raccoon**
● **W55.8 Contact with other mammals**
X ● **W55.81 Bitten by other mammals**
X ● **W55.82 Struck by other mammals**
X ● **W55.89 Other contact with other mammals**

●**W56 Contact with nonvenomous marine animal**
Excludes1 contact with venomous marine animal (T63.-)
The appropriate 7th character is to be added to each code from category W56

A initial encounter
D subsequent encounter
S sequela

● **W56.0 Contact with dolphin**
X ● **W56.01 Bitten by dolphin**
X ● **W56.02 Struck by dolphin**
X ● **W56.09 Other contact with dolphin**
● **W56.1 Contact with sea lion**
X ● **W56.11 Bitten by sea lion**
X ● **W56.12 Struck by sea lion**
X ● **W56.19 Other contact with sea lion**

● W56.2 Contact with orca
      Contact with killer whale
  X ● W56.21 Bitten by orca
  X ● W56.22 Struck by orca
  X ● W56.29 Other contact with orca
● W56.3 Contact with other marine mammals
  X ● W56.31 Bitten by other marine mammals
  X ● W56.32 Struck by other marine mammals
  X ● W56.39 Other contact with other marine mammals
● W56.4 Contact with shark
  X ● W56.41 Bitten by shark
  X ● W56.42 Struck by shark
  X ● W56.49 Other contact with shark
● W56.5 Contact with other fish
  X ● W56.51 Bitten by other fish
  X ● W56.52 Struck by other fish
  X ● W56.59 Other contact with other fish
● W56.8 Contact with other nonvenomous marine animals
  X ● W56.81 Bitten by other nonvenomous marine animals
  X ● W56.82 Struck by other nonvenomous marine animals
  X ● W56.89 Other contact with other nonvenomous marine animals

X ● W57 Bitten or stung by nonvenomous insect and other nonvenomous arthropods
  Excludes1   contact with venomous insects and arthropods (T63.2-, T63.3-, T63.4-)
  The appropriate 7th character is to be added to code W57

A	initial encounter
D	subsequent encounter
S	sequela

● W58 Contact with crocodile or alligator
  The appropriate 7th character is to be added to each code from category W58

A	initial encounter
D	subsequent encounter
S	sequela

● W58.0 Contact with alligator
  X ● W58.01 Bitten by alligator
  X ● W58.02 Struck by alligator
  X ● W58.03 Crushed by alligator
  X ● W58.09 Other contact with alligator
● W58.1 Contact with crocodile
  X ● W58.11 Bitten by crocodile
  X ● W58.12 Struck by crocodile
  X ● W58.13 Crushed by crocodile
  X ● W58.19 Other contact with crocodile

● W59 Contact with other nonvenomous reptiles
  Excludes1   contact with venomous reptile (T63.0-, T63.1-)
  The appropriate 7th character is to be added to each code from category W59

A	initial encounter
D	subsequent encounter
S	sequela

● W59.0 Contact with nonvenomous lizards
  X ● W59.01 Bitten by nonvenomous lizards
  X ● W59.02 Struck by nonvenomous lizards
  X ● W59.09 Other contact with nonvenomous lizards
      Exposure to nonvenomous lizards

● W59.1 Contact with nonvenomous snakes
  X ● W59.11 Bitten by nonvenomous snake
  X ● W59.12 Struck by nonvenomous snake
  X ● W59.13 Crushed by nonvenomous snake
  X ● W59.19 Other contact with nonvenomous snake
● W59.2 Contact with turtles
  Excludes1   contact with tortoises (W59.8-)
  X ● W59.21 Bitten by turtle
  X ● W59.22 Struck by turtle
  X ● W59.29 Other contact with turtle
      Exposure to turtles
● W59.8 Contact with other nonvenomous reptiles
  X ● W59.81 Bitten by other nonvenomous reptiles
  X ● W59.82 Struck by other nonvenomous reptiles
  X ● W59.83 Crushed by other nonvenomous reptiles
  X ● W59.89 Other contact with other nonvenomous reptiles

X ● W60 Contact with nonvenomous plant thorns and spines and sharp leaves
  Excludes1   contact with venomous plants (T63.X7-)
  The appropriate 7th character is to be added to code W60

A	initial encounter
D	subsequent encounter
S	sequela

● W61 Contact with birds (domestic) (wild)
  Includes   contact with excreta of birds
  The appropriate 7th character is to be added to each code from category W61

A	initial encounter
D	subsequent encounter
S	sequela

● W61.0 Contact with parrot
  X ● W61.01 Bitten by parrot
  X ● W61.02 Struck by parrot
  X ● W61.09 Other contact with parrot
      Exposure to parrots
● W61.1 Contact with macaw
  X ● W61.11 Bitten by macaw
  X ● W61.12 Struck by macaw
  X ● W61.19 Other contact with macaw
      Exposure to macaws
● W61.2 Contact with other psittacines
  X ● W61.21 Bitten by other psittacines
  X ● W61.22 Struck by other psittacines
  X ● W61.29 Other contact with other psittacines
      Exposure to other psittacines
● W61.3 Contact with chicken
  X ● W61.32 Struck by chicken
  X ● W61.33 Pecked by chicken
  X ● W61.39 Other contact with chicken
      Exposure to chickens
● W61.4 Contact with turkey
  X ● W61.42 Struck by turkey
  X ● W61.43 Pecked by turkey
  X ● W61.49 Other contact with turkey
● W61.5 Contact with goose
  X ● W61.51 Bitten by goose
  X ● W61.52 Struck by goose
  X ● W61.59 Other contact with goose

- ● W61.6 **Contact with duck**
  - X ● W61.61 **Bitten by duck**
  - X ● W61.62 **Struck by duck**
  - X ● W61.69 **Other contact with duck**
- ● W61.9 **Contact with other birds**
  - X ● W61.91 **Bitten by other birds**
  - X ● W61.92 **Struck by other birds**
  - X ● W61.99 **Other contact with other birds**
    Contact with bird NOS

● W62 **Contact with nonvenomous amphibians**

> **Excludes1** contact with venomous amphibians (T63.81-R63.83)

The appropriate 7th character is to be added to each code from category W62

A	initial encounter
D	subsequent encounter
S	sequela

- X ● W62.0 **Contact with nonvenomous frogs**
- X ● W62.1 **Contact with nonvenomous toads**
- X ● W62.9 **Contact with other nonvenomous amphibians**

X ● W64 **Exposure to other animate mechanical forces**

> **Includes** exposure to nonvenomous animal NOS
>
> **Excludes1** contact with venomous animal (T63.-)

The appropriate 7th character is to be added to code W64

A	initial encounter
D	subsequent encounter
S	sequela

ACCIDENTAL NON-TRANSPORT DROWNING AND SUBMERSION (W65-W74)

> **Excludes1** accidental drowning and submersion due to fall into water (W16.-)
> accidental drowning and submersion due to water transport accident (V90.-, V92.-)
>
> **Excludes2** accidental drowning and submersion due to cataclysm (X34-X39)

X ● W65 **Accidental drowning and submersion while in bathtub**

> **Excludes1** accidental drowning and submersion due to fall in (into) bathtub (W16.211)

The appropriate 7th character is to be added to code W65

A	initial encounter
D	subsequent encounter
S	sequela

X ● W67 **Accidental drowning and submersion while in swimming pool**

> **Excludes1** accidental drowning and submersion due to fall into swimming pool (W16.011, W16.021, W16.031)
> accidental drowning and submersion due to striking into wall of swimming pool (W22.041)

The appropriate 7th character is to be added to code W67

A	initial encounter
D	subsequent encounter
S	sequela

X ● W69 **Accidental drowning and submersion while in natural water**
  Accidental drowning and submersion while in lake
  Accidental drowning and submersion while in open sea
  Accidental drowning and submersion while in river
  Accidental drowning and submersion while in stream

> **Excludes1** accidental drowning and submersion due to fall into natural body of water (W16.111, W16.121, W16.131)

The appropriate 7th character is to be added to code W69

A	initial encounter
D	subsequent encounter
S	sequela

X ● W73 **Other specified cause of accidental non-transport drowning and submersion**
  Accidental drowning and submersion while in quenching tank
  Accidental drowning and submersion while in reservoir

> **Excludes1** accidental drowning and submersion due to fall into other water (W16.311, W16.321, W16.331)

The appropriate 7th character is to be added to code W73

A	initial encounter
D	subsequent encounter
S	sequela

X ● W74 **Unspecified cause of accidental drowning and submersion**
  Drowning NOS

The appropriate 7th character is to be added to code W74

A	initial encounter
D	subsequent encounter
S	sequela

EXPOSURE TO ELECTRIC CURRENT, RADIATION AND EXTREME AMBIENT AIR TEMPERATURE AND PRESSURE (W85-W99)

> **Excludes1** exposure to:
> failure in dosage of radiation or temperature during surgical and medical care (Y63.2-Y63.5)
> lightning (T75.0-)
> natural cold (X31)
> natural heat (X30)
> natural radiation NOS (X39)
> radiological procedure and radiotherapy (Y84.2)
> sunlight (X32)

X ● W85 **Exposure to electric transmission lines**
  Broken power line

The appropriate 7th character is to be added to code W85

A	initial encounter
D	subsequent encounter
S	sequela

● W86 **Exposure to other specified electric current**

The appropriate 7th character is to be added to each code from category W86

A	initial encounter
D	subsequent encounter
S	sequela

- X ● W86.0 **Exposure to domestic wiring and appliances**
- X ● W86.1 **Exposure to industrial wiring, appliances and electrical machinery**
  Exposure to conductors
  Exposure to control apparatus
  Exposure to electrical equipment and machinery
  Exposure to transformers

X● **W86.8 Exposure to other electric current**
     Exposure to wiring and appliances in or on farm (not farmhouse)
     Exposure to wiring and appliances outdoors
     Exposure to wiring and appliances in or on public building
     Exposure to wiring and appliances in or on residential institutions
     Exposure to wiring and appliances in or on schools

● **W88 Exposure to ionizing radiation**

     Excludes1   exposure to sunlight (X32)

     The appropriate 7th character is to be added to each code from category W88

A	initial encounter
D	subsequent encounter
S	sequela

X● **W88.0 Exposure to X-rays**
X● **W88.1 Exposure to radioactive isotopes**
X● **W88.8 Exposure to other ionizing radiation**

● **W89 Exposure to man-made visible and ultraviolet light**

     Includes   exposure to welding light (arc)
     Excludes2   exposure to sunlight (X32)

     The appropriate 7th character is to be added to each code from category W89

A	initial encounter
D	subsequent encounter
S	sequela

X● **W89.0 Exposure to welding light (arc)**
X● **W89.1 Exposure to tanning bed**
X● **W89.8 Exposure to other man-made visible and ultraviolet light**
X● **W89.9 Exposure to unspecified man-made visible and ultraviolet light**

● **W90 Exposure to other nonionizing radiation**

     Excludes2   exposure to sunlight (X32)

     The appropriate 7th character is to be added to each code from category W90

A	initial encounter
D	subsequent encounter
S	sequela

X● **W90.0 Exposure to radiofrequency**
X● **W90.1 Exposure to infrared radiation**
X● **W90.2 Exposure to laser radiation**
X● **W90.8 Exposure to other nonionizing radiation**

X● **W92 Exposure to excessive heat of man-made origin**

     The appropriate 7th character is to be added to code W92

A	initial encounter
D	subsequent encounter
S	sequela

● **W93 Exposure to excessive cold of man-made origin**

     The appropriate 7th character is to be added to each code from category W93

A	initial encounter
D	subsequent encounter
S	sequela

● **W93.0 Contact with or inhalation of dry ice**
   X● **W93.01 Contact with dry ice**
   X● **W93.02 Inhalation of dry ice**

● **W93.1 Contact with or inhalation of liquid air**
   X● **W93.11 Contact with liquid air**
     Contact with liquid hydrogen
     Contact with liquid nitrogen
   X● **W93.12 Inhalation of liquid air**
     Inhalation of liquid hydrogen
     Inhalation of liquid nitrogen

X● **W93.2 Prolonged exposure in deep freeze unit or refrigerator**
X● **W93.8 Exposure to other excessive cold of man-made origin**

● **W94 Exposure to high and low air pressure and changes in air pressure**

     The appropriate 7th character is to be added to each code from category W94

A	initial encounter
D	subsequent encounter
S	sequela

X● **W94.0 Exposure to prolonged high air pressure**
● **W94.1 Exposure to prolonged low air pressure**
   X● **W94.11 Exposure to residence or prolonged visit at high altitude**
   X● **W94.12 Exposure to other prolonged low air pressure**
● **W94.2 Exposure to rapid changes in air pressure during ascent**
   X● **W94.21 Exposure to reduction in atmospheric pressure while surfacing from deep-water diving**
   X● **W94.22 Exposure to reduction in atmospheric pressure while surfacing from underground**
   X● **W94.23 Exposure to sudden change in air pressure in aircraft during ascent**
   X● **W94.29 Exposure to other rapid changes in air pressure during ascent**
● **W94.3 Exposure to rapid changes in air pressure during descent**
   X● **W94.31 Exposure to sudden change in air pressure in aircraft during descent**
   X● **W94.32 Exposure to high air pressure from rapid descent in water**
   X● **W94.39 Exposure to other rapid changes in air pressure during descent**

X●**W99 Exposure to other man-made environmental factors**

     The appropriate 7th character is to be added to code W99

A	initial encounter
D	subsequent encounter
S	sequela

EXPOSURE TO SMOKE, FIRE AND FLAMES (X00-X08)

Excludes1   arson (X97)
Excludes2   explosions (W35-W40)
     lightning (T75.0-)
     transport accident (V01-V99)

● **X00 Exposure to uncontrolled fire in building or structure**

     Includes   conflagration in building or structure

     Code first any associated cataclysm

     Excludes2   exposure to ignition or melting of nightwear (X05)
     exposure to ignition or melting of other clothing and apparel (X06.-)
     exposure to other specified smoke, fire and flames (X08.-)

     The appropriate 7th character is to be added to each code from category X00

A	initial encounter
D	subsequent encounter
S	sequela

X● **X00.0 Exposure to flames in uncontrolled fire in building or structure**
     Coding Clinic: 2016, Q2, P5-6; 2015, Q1, P19

X● **X00.1 Exposure to smoke in uncontrolled fire in building or structure**

X ● **X00.2** **Injury due to collapse** of burning building or structure in uncontrolled fire

> **Excludes1**   injury due to collapse of building not on fire (W20.1)

X ● **X00.3** **Fall from** burning building or structure in uncontrolled fire

X ● **X00.4** **Hit by object** from burning building or structure in uncontrolled fire

X ● **X00.5** **Jump from** burning building or structure in uncontrolled fire

X ● **X00.8** **Other** exposure to uncontrolled fire in building or structure

● **X01** **Exposure to uncontrolled fire, not in building or structure**

> **Includes**   exposure to forest fire

The appropriate 7th character is to be added to each code from category X01

> A   initial encounter
> D   subsequent encounter
> S   sequela

X ● **X01.0** **Exposure to flames** in uncontrolled fire, not in building or structure

X ● **X01.1** **Exposure to smoke** in uncontrolled fire, not in building or structure

X ● **X01.3** **Fall due to** uncontrolled fire, not in building or structure

X ● **X01.4** **Hit by object** due to uncontrolled fire, not in building or structure

X ● **X01.8** **Other** exposure to uncontrolled fire, not in building or structure

● **X02** **Exposure to controlled fire in building or structure**

> **Includes**   exposure to fire in fireplace exposure to fire in stove

The appropriate 7th character is to be added to each code from category X02

> A   initial encounter
> D   subsequent encounter
> S   sequela

X ● **X02.0** **Exposure to flames** in controlled fire in building or structure

X ● **X02.1** **Exposure to smoke** in controlled fire in building or structure

X ● **X02.2** **Injury due to collapse** of burning building or structure in controlled fire

> **Excludes1**   injury due to collapse of building not on fire (W20.1)

X ● **X02.3** **Fall from** burning building or structure in controlled fire

X ● **X02.4** **Hit by object** from burning building or structure in controlled fire

X ● **X02.5** **Jump from** burning building or structure in controlled fire

X ● **X02.8** **Other** exposure to controlled fire in building or structure

● **X03** **Exposure to controlled fire, not in building or structure**

> **Includes**   exposure to bon fire exposure to camp fire exposure to trash fire

The appropriate 7th character is to be added to each code from category X03

> A   initial encounter
> D   subsequent encounter
> S   sequela

X ● **X03.0** **Exposure to flames** in controlled fire, not in building or structure
> **Coding Clinic: 2015, Q1, P19**

X ● **X03.1** **Exposure to smoke** in controlled fire, not in building or structure

X ● **X03.3** **Fall due to** controlled fire, not in building or structure

X ● **X03.4** **Hit by object** due to controlled fire, not in building or structure

X ● **X03.8** **Other** exposure to controlled fire, not in building or structure

● **X04** **Exposure to ignition of highly flammable material**

> Exposure to ignition of gasoline
> Exposure to ignition of kerosene
> Exposure to ignition of petrol

> **Excludes2**   exposure to ignition or melting of nightwear (X05)
> exposure to ignition or melting of other clothing and apparel (X06)

The appropriate 7th character is to be added to code X04

> A   initial encounter
> D   subsequent encounter
> S   sequela

Coding Clinic: 2016, Q2, P4

X ● **X05** **Exposure to ignition or melting of nightwear**

> **Excludes2**   exposure to uncontrolled fire in building or structure (X00.-)
> exposure to uncontrolled fire, not in building or structure (X01.-)
> exposure to controlled fire in building or structure (X02.-)
> exposure to controlled fire, not in building or structure (X03.-)
> exposure to ignition of highly flammable materials (X04.-)

The appropriate 7th character is to be added to code X05

> A   initial encounter
> D   subsequent encounter
> S   sequela

● **X06** **Exposure to ignition or melting of other clothing and apparel**

> **Excludes2**   exposure to uncontrolled fire in building or structure (X00.-)
> exposure to uncontrolled fire, not in building or structure (X01.-)
> exposure to controlled fire in building or structure (X02.-)
> exposure to controlled fire, not in building or structure (X03.-)
> exposure to ignition of highly flammable materials (X04.-)

The appropriate 7th character is to be added to each code from category X06

> A   initial encounter
> D   subsequent encounter
> S   sequela

X ● **X06.0** **Exposure to ignition of** plastic jewelry

X ● **X06.1** **Exposure to melting of** plastic jewelry

X ● **X06.2** **Exposure to ignition of** other clothing and apparel

X ● **X06.3** **Exposure to melting of** other clothing and apparel

● **X08** **Exposure to other specified smoke, fire and flames**

The appropriate 7th character is to be added to each code from category X08

> A   initial encounter
> D   subsequent encounter
> S   sequela

● **X08.0** **Exposure to bed fire**
> Exposure to mattress fire

X ● **X08.00** **Exposure to bed fire due to unspecified** burning material

X ● **X08.01** **Exposure to bed fire due to burning cigarette**
> **Coding Clinic: 2015, Q1, P19**

X ● **X08.09** **Exposure to bed fire due to other** burning material

▶ New   ⇒ Revised   ~~deleted~~ Deleted   Excludes 1   Excludes 2   Includes   Use additional   Code first   Code also   Key words

OGCR Official Guidelines   X Assign placeholder X   ● Use Additional Character(s)   ) Manifestation Code   🕭 Hierarchical Condition Category   **Coding Clinic**

● **X08.1**   **Exposure to sofa fire**
   X ● **X08.10**   Exposure to sofa fire due to unspecified burning material
   X ● **X08.11**   Exposure to sofa fire due to burning cigarette
   X ● **X08.19**   Exposure to sofa fire due to other burning material

● **X08.2**   **Exposure to other furniture fire**
   X ● **X08.20**   Exposure to other furniture fire due to unspecified burning material
   X ● **X08.21**   Exposure to other furniture fire due to burning cigarette
   X ● **X08.29**   Exposure to other furniture fire due to other burning material

X ● **X08.8**   **Exposure to other specified smoke, fire and flames**

CONTACT WITH HEAT AND HOT SUBSTANCES (X10-X19)

Excludes1   exposure to excessive natural heat (X30)
               exposure to fire and flames (X00-X08)

● **X10**   **Contact with hot drinks, food, fats and cooking oils**
The appropriate 7th character is to be added to each code from category X10

A	initial encounter
D	subsequent encounter
S	sequela

X ● **X10.0**   **Contact with hot drinks**
X ● **X10.1**   **Contact with hot food**
X ● **X10.2**   **Contact with fats and cooking oils**

● **X11**   **Contact with hot tap-water**
Includes   contact with boiling tap-water
            contact with boiling water NOS
Excludes1   contact with water heated on stove (X12)
The appropriate 7th character is to be added to each code from category X11

A	initial encounter
D	subsequent encounter
S	sequela

X ● **X11.0**   **Contact with hot water in bath or tub**
     Excludes1   contact with running hot water in bath or tub (X11.1)
X ● **X11.1**   **Contact with running hot water**
     Contact with hot water running out of hose
     Contact with hot water running out of tap
X ● **X11.8**   **Contact with other hot tap-water**
     Contact with hot water in bucket
     Contact with hot tap-water NOS

X ● **X12**   **Contact with other hot fluids**
     Contact with water heated on stove
Excludes1   hot (liquid) metals (X18)
The appropriate 7th character is to be added to code X12

A	initial encounter
D	subsequent encounter
S	sequela

● **X13**   **Contact with steam and other hot vapors**
The appropriate 7th character is to be added to each code from category X13

A	initial encounter
D	subsequent encounter
S	sequela

X ● **X13.0**   **Inhalation of steam and other hot vapors**
X ● **X13.1**   **Other contact with steam and other hot vapors**

● **X14**   **Contact with hot air and other hot gases**
The appropriate 7th character is to be added to each code from category X14

A	initial encounter
D	subsequent encounter
S	sequela

X ● **X14.0**   **Inhalation of hot air and gases**
X ● **X14.1**   **Other contact with hot air and other hot gases**

● **X15**   **Contact with hot household appliances**
     Excludes1   contact with heating appliances (X16)
               contact with powered household appliances (W29.-)
               exposure to controlled fire in building or structure due to household appliance (X02.8)
               exposure to household appliances electrical current (W86.0)
The appropriate 7th character is to be added to each code from category X15

A	initial encounter
D	subsequent encounter
S	sequela

X ● **X15.0**   **Contact with hot stove (kitchen)**
X ● **X15.1**   **Contact with hot toaster**
X ● **X15.2**   **Contact with hotplate**
X ● **X15.3**   **Contact with hot saucepan or skillet**
     ▶Contact with hot cooking pan
     ▶Contact with hot cooking pot
X ● **X15.8**   **Contact with other hot household appliances**
     Contact with cooker
     Contact with kettle
     Contact with light bulbs

X ● **X16**   **Contact with hot heating appliances, radiators and pipes**
     Excludes1   contact with powered appliances (W29.-)
               exposure to controlled fire in building or structure due to appliance (X02.8)
               exposure to industrial appliances electrical current (W86.1)
The appropriate 7th character is to be added to code X16

A	initial encounter
D	subsequent encounter
S	sequela

X ● **X17**   **Contact with hot engines, machinery and tools**
     Excludes1   contact with hot heating appliances, radiators and pipes (X16)
               contact with hot household appliances (X15)
The appropriate 7th character is to be added to code X17

A	initial encounter
D	subsequent encounter
S	sequela

X ● **X18**   **Contact with other hot metals**
     Contact with liquid metal
The appropriate 7th character is to be added to code X18

A	initial encounter
D	subsequent encounter
S	sequela

X ● **X19**   **Contact with other heat and hot substances**
     Excludes1   objects that are not normally hot, e.g., an object made hot by a house fire (X00-X08)
The appropriate 7th character is to be added to code X19

A	initial encounter
D	subsequent encounter
S	sequela

CHAPTER 20 (V00-Y99)

EXPOSURE TO FORCES OF NATURE (X30-X39)

X ● **X30   Exposure to excessive natural heat**
Exposure to excessive heat as the cause of sunstroke
Exposure to heat NOS

Excludes1   excessive heat of man-made origin (W92)
exposure to man-made radiation (W89)
exposure to sunlight (X32)
exposure to tanning bed (W89)

The appropriate 7th character is to be added to code X30

A	initial encounter
D	subsequent encounter
S	sequela

X ● **X31   Exposure to excessive natural cold**
Excessive cold as the cause of chilblains NOS
Excessive cold as the cause of immersion foot or hand
Exposure to cold NOS
Exposure to weather conditions

Excludes1   cold of man-made origin (W93.-)
contact with or inhalation of dry ice (W93.-)
contact with or inhalation of liquefied gas (W93.-)

The appropriate 7th character is to be added to code X31

A	initial encounter
D	subsequent encounter
S	sequela

X ● **X32   Exposure to sunlight**

Excludes1   man-made radiation (tanning bed) (W89)

Excludes2   radiation-related disorders of the skin and
subcutaneous tissue (L55-L59)

The appropriate 7th character is to be added to code X32

A	initial encounter
D	subsequent encounter
S	sequela

X ● **X34   Earthquake**

Excludes2   tidal wave (tsunami) due to earthquake (X37.41)

The appropriate 7th character is to be added to code X34

A	initial encounter
D	subsequent encounter
S	sequela

X ● **X35   Volcanic eruption**

Excludes2   tidal wave (tsunami) due to volcanic eruption
(X37.41)

The appropriate 7th character is to be added to code X35

A	initial encounter
D	subsequent encounter
S	sequela

● **X36   Avalanche, landslide and other earth movements**

Includes   victim of mudslide of cataclysmic nature

Excludes1   earthquake (X34)

Excludes2   transport accident involving collision with
avalanche or landslide not in motion
(V01-V99)

The appropriate 7th character is to be added to each code from
category X36

A	initial encounter
D	subsequent encounter
S	sequela

X ● **X36.0   Collapse of dam or man-made structure causing earth
movement**

X ● **X36.1   Avalanche, landslide, or mudslide**

● **X37   Cataclysmic storm**

The appropriate 7th character is to be added to each code from
category X37

A	initial encounter
D	subsequent encounter
S	sequela

X ● **X37.0   Hurricane**
Storm surge   Typhoon

X ● **X37.1   Tornado**
Cyclone   Twister

X ● **X37.2   Blizzard (snow) (ice)**

X ● **X37.3   Dust storm**

● **X37.4   Tidalwave**

X ● **X37.41   Tidal wave due to earthquake or volcanic
eruption**
Tidal wave NOS
Tsunami

X ● **X37.42   Tidal wave due to storm**

X ● **X37.43   Tidal wave due to landslide**

X ● **X37.8   Other cataclysmic storms**
Cloudburst
Torrential rain

Excludes2   flood (X38)

X ● **X37.9   Unspecified cataclysmic storm**
Storm NOS

Excludes1   collapse of dam or man-made structure
causing earth movement (X36.0)

X ● **X38   Flood**
Flood arising from remote storm
Flood of cataclysmic nature arising from melting snow
Flood resulting directly from storm

Excludes1   collapse of dam or man-made structure causing
earth movement (X36.0)
tidal wave NOS (X37.41)
tidal wave caused by storm (X37.42)

The appropriate 7th character is to be added to code X38

A	initial encounter
D	subsequent encounter
S	sequela

● **X39   Exposure to other forces of nature**

The appropriate 7th character is to be added to each code from
category X39

A	initial encounter
D	subsequent encounter
S	sequela

● **X39.0   Exposure to natural radiation**

Excludes1   contact with and (suspected) exposure to
radon and other naturally occurring
radiation (Z77.123)
exposure to man-made radiation
(W88-W90)
exposure to sunlight (X32)

X ● **X39.01   Exposure to radon**

X ● **X39.08   Exposure to other natural radiation**

X ● **X39.8   Other exposure to forces of nature**

▶ New   ⇒ Revised   deleted Deleted   Excludes 1   Excludes 2   Includes   Use additional   Code first   Code also   Key words

OGCR Official Guidelines   X Assign placeholder X   ● Use Additional Character(s)   ▌ Manifestation Code   🦥 Hierarchical Condition Category   **Coding Clinic**

OVEREXERTION AND STRENUOUS OR REPETITIVE MOVEMENTS (X50)

● **X50   Overexertion and strenuous or repetitive movements**

The appropriate 7th character is to be added to each code from category X50

A	initial encounter
D	subsequent encounter
S	sequela

Coding Clinic: 2016, Q4, P73-74

X ● **X50.0   Overexertion from strenuous movement or load**
Lifting heavy objects
Lifting weights
Coding Clinic: 2016, Q4, P74

X ● **X50.1   Overexertion from prolonged static or awkward postures**
Prolonged bending
Prolonged kneeling
Prolonged reaching
Prolonged sitting
Prolonged standing
Prolonged twisting
Static bending
Static kneeling
Static reaching
Static sitting
Static standing
Static twisting

X ● **X50.3   Overexertion from repetitive movements**
Use of hand as hammer

Excludes2   Overuse from prolonged static or awkward postures (X50.1)
Coding Clinic: 2016, Q4, P74

X ● **X50.9   Other and unspecified overexertion or strenuous movements or postures**
Contact pressure
Contact stress

ACCIDENTAL EXPOSURE TO OTHER SPECIFIED FACTORS (X52, X58)

X ● **X52   Prolonged stay in weightless environment**
Weightlessness in spacecraft (simulator)

The appropriate 7th character is to be added to code X52

A	initial encounter
D	subsequent encounter
S	sequela

X ● **X58   Exposure to other specified factors**
Accident NOS
Exposure NOS

The appropriate 7th character is to be added to code X58

A	initial encounter
D	subsequent encounter
S	sequela

INTENTIONAL SELF-HARM (X71-X83)

Purposely self-inflicted injury
Suicide (attempted)

● **X71   Intentional self-harm by drowning and submersion**

The appropriate 7th character is to be added to each code from category X71

A	initial encounter
D	subsequent encounter
S	sequela

X ● **X71.0   Intentional self-harm by drowning and submersion while in bathtub** A, D, S 🐾

X ● **X71.1   Intentional self-harm by drowning and submersion while in swimming pool** A, D, S 🐾

X ● **X71.2   Intentional self-harm by drowning and submersion after jump into swimming pool** A, D, S 🐾

X ● **X71.3   Intentional self-harm by drowning and submersion in natural water** A, D, S 🐾

X ● **X71.8   Other intentional self-harm by drowning and submersion** A, D, S 🐾

X ● **X71.9   Intentional self-harm by drowning and submersion, unspecified** A, D, S 🐾

X ● **X72   Intentional self-harm by handgun discharge** A, D, S 🐾
Intentional self-harm by gun for single hand use
Intentional self-harm by pistol
Intentional self-harm by revolver

Excludes1   Very pistol (X74.8)

The appropriate 7th character is to be added to code X72

A	initial encounter
D	subsequent encounter
S	sequela

● **X73   Intentional self-harm by rifle, shotgun and larger firearm discharge**

Excludes1   airgun (X74.01)

The appropriate 7th character is to be added to each code from category X73

A	initial encounter
D	subsequent encounter
S	sequela

X ● **X73.0   Intentional self-harm by shotgun discharge** A, D, S 🐾

X ● **X73.1   Intentional self-harm by hunting rifle discharge** A, D, S 🐾

X ● **X73.2   Intentional self-harm by machine gun discharge** A, D, S 🐾

X ● **X73.8   Intentional self-harm by other larger firearm discharge** A, D, S 🐾

X ● **X73.9   Intentional self-harm by unspecified larger firearm discharge** A, D, S 🐾

● **X74   Intentional self-harm by other and unspecified firearm and gun discharge**

The appropriate 7th character is to be added to each code from category X74

A	initial encounter
D	subsequent encounter
S	sequela

● **X74.0   Intentional self-harm by gas, air or spring-operated guns**

X ● **X74.01   Intentional self-harm by airgun** A, D, S 🐾
Intentional self-harm by BB gun discharge
Intentional self-harm by pellet gun discharge

X ● **X74.02   Intentional self-harm by paintball gun** A, D, S 🐾

X ● **X74.09   Intentional self-harm by other gas, air or spring-operated gun** A, D, S 🐾

X ● **X74.8   Intentional self-harm by other firearm discharge** A, D, S 🐾
Intentional self-harm by Very pistol [flare] discharge

X ● **X74.9   Intentional self-harm by unspecified firearm discharge** A, D, S 🐾

X ● **X75   Intentional self-harm by explosive material** A, D, S 🐾

The appropriate 7th character is to be added to code X75

A	initial encounter
D	subsequent encounter
S	sequela

X ● **X76   Intentional self-harm by smoke, fire and flames** A, D, S 🐾

The appropriate 7th character is to be added to code X76

A	initial encounter
D	subsequent encounter
S	sequela

CHAPTER 20 (V00-Y99)

CHAPTER 20 (V00-Y99)

● **X77**   **Intentional self-harm by steam, hot vapors and hot objects**

The appropriate 7th character is to be added to each code from category X77

A	initial encounter
D	subsequent encounter
S	sequela

X● **X77.0**   Intentional self-harm by steam or hot vapors A, D, S 🐾
X● **X77.1**   Intentional self-harm by hot tap water A, D, S 🐾
X● **X77.2**   Intentional self-harm by other hot fluids A, D, S 🐾
X● **X77.3**   Intentional self-harm by hot household appliances A, D, S 🐾
X● **X77.8**   Intentional self-harm by other hot objects A, D, S 🐾
X● **X77.9**   Intentional self-harm by unspecified hot objects A, D, S 🐾

● **X78**   **Intentional self-harm by sharp object**

The appropriate 7th character is to be added to each code from category X78

A	initial encounter
D	subsequent encounter
S	sequela

X● **X78.0**   Intentional self-harm by sharp glass A, D, S 🐾
X● **X78.1**   Intentional self-harm by knife A, D, S 🐾
X● **X78.2**   Intentional self-harm by sword or dagger A, D, S 🐾
X● **X78.8**   Intentional self-harm by other sharp object A, D, S 🐾
      Coding Clinic: 2022, Q1, P27
X● **X78.9**   Intentional self-harm by unspecified sharp object A, D, S 🐾

X● **X79**   **Intentional self-harm by blunt object A, D, S 🐾**

The appropriate 7th character is to be added to code X79

A	initial encounter
D	subsequent encounter
S	sequela

X● **X80**   **Intentional self-harm by jumping from a high place A, D, S 🐾**
      Intentional fall from one level to another

The appropriate 7th character is to be added to code X80

A	initial encounter
D	subsequent encounter
S	sequela

● **X81**   **Intentional self-harm by jumping or lying in front of moving object**

The appropriate 7th character is to be added to each code from category X81

A	initial encounter
D	subsequent encounter
S	sequela

X● **X81.0**   Intentional self-harm by jumping or lying in front of motor vehicle A, D, S 🐾
X● **X81.1**   Intentional self-harm by jumping or lying in front of (subway) train A, D, S 🐾
X● **X81.8**   Intentional self-harm by jumping or lying in front of other moving object A, D, S 🐾

● **X82**   **Intentional self-harm by crashing of motor vehicle**

The appropriate 7th character is to be added to each code from category X82

A	initial encounter
D	subsequent encounter
S	sequela

X● **X82.0**   Intentional collision of motor vehicle with other motor vehicle A, D, S 🐾
X● **X82.1**   Intentional collision of motor vehicle with train A, D, S 🐾

X● **X82.2**   Intentional collision of motor vehicle with tree A, D, S 🐾
X● **X82.8**   Other intentional self-harm by crashing of motor vehicle A, D, S 🐾

● **X83**   **Intentional self-harm by other specified means**

> **Excludes1**   intentional self-harm by poisoning or contact with toxic substance - see Table of Drugs and Chemicals

The appropriate 7th character is to be added to each code from category X83

A	initial encounter
D	subsequent encounter
S	sequela

X● **X83.0**   Intentional self-harm by crashing of aircraft A, D, S 🐾
X● **X83.1**   Intentional self-harm by electrocution A, D, S 🐾
X● **X83.2**   Intentional self-harm by exposure to extremes of cold A, D, S 🐾
X● **X83.8**   Intentional self-harm by other specified means A, D, S 🐾

ASSAULT (X92-Y09)

> **Includes**   homicide injuries inflicted by another person with intent to injure or kill, by any means

> **Excludes1**   injuries due to legal intervention (Y35.-)
> injuries due to operations of war (Y36.-)
> injuries due to terrorism (Y38.-)

● **X92**   **Assault by drowning and submersion**

The appropriate 7th character is to be added to each code from category X92

A	initial encounter
D	subsequent encounter
S	sequela

X● **X92.0**   Assault by drowning and submersion while in bathtub
X● **X92.1**   Assault by drowning and submersion while in swimming pool
X● **X92.2**   Assault by drowning and submersion after push into swimming pool
X● **X92.3**   Assault by drowning and submersion in natural water
X● **X92.8**   Other assault by drowning and submersion
X● **X92.9**   Assault by drowning and submersion, unspecified

X● **X93**   **Assault by handgun discharge**
      Assault by discharge of gun for single hand use
      Assault by discharge of pistol
      Assault by discharge of revolver

> **Excludes1**   Very pistol (X95.8)

The appropriate 7th character is to be added to code X93

A	initial encounter
D	subsequent encounter
S	sequela

● **X94**   **Assault by rifle, shotgun and larger firearm discharge**

> **Excludes1**   airgun (X95.01)

The appropriate 7th character is to be added to each code from category X94

A	initial encounter
D	subsequent encounter
S	sequela

X● **X94.0**   Assault by shotgun
X● **X94.1**   Assault by hunting rifle
X● **X94.2**   Assault by machine gun
X● **X94.8**   Assault by other larger firearm discharge
X● **X94.9**   Assault by unspecified larger firearm discharge

---

▶ New   ⇒ Revised   ~~deleted~~ Deleted   Excludes 1   Excludes 2   Includes   Use additional   Code first   Code also   Key words

OGCR Official Guidelines   X Assign placeholder X   ● Use Additional Character(s)   ▷ Manifestation Code   🐾 Hierarchical Condition Category   **Coding Clinic**

● **X95 Assault by other and unspecified firearm and gun discharge**

The appropriate 7th character is to be added to each code from category X95

A	initial encounter
D	subsequent encounter
S	sequela

● **X95.0 Assault by gas, air or spring-operated guns**

X● **X95.01 Assault by airgun discharge**
Assault by BB gun discharge
Assault by pellet gun discharge

X● **X95.02 Assault by paintball gun discharge**

X● **X95.09 Assault by other gas, air or spring-operated gun**

X● **X95.8 Assault by other firearm discharge**
Assault by very pistol [flare] discharge

X● **X95.9 Assault by unspecified firearm discharge**
Coding Clinic: 2016, Q3, P24

● **X96 Assault by explosive material**

Excludes1   incendiary device (X97)
terrorism involving explosive material (Y38.2-)

The appropriate 7th character is to be added to each code from category X96

A	initial encounter
D	subsequent encounter
S	sequela

X● **X96.0 Assault by antipersonnel bomb**

Excludes1   antipersonnel bomb use in military or war (Y36.2-)

X● **X96.1 Assault by gasoline bomb**

X● **X96.2 Assault by letter bomb**

X● **X96.3 Assault by fertilizer bomb**

X● **X96.4 Assault by pipe bomb**

X● **X96.8 Assault by other specified explosive**

X● **X96.9 Assault by unspecified explosive**

X● **X97 Assault by smoke, fire and flames**
Assault by arson
Assault by cigarettes
Assault by incendiary device

The appropriate 7th character is to be added to code X97

A	initial encounter
D	subsequent encounter
S	sequela

● **X98 Assault by steam, hot vapors and hot objects**

The appropriate 7th character is to be added to each code from category X98

A	initial encounter
D	subsequent encounter
S	sequela

X● **X98.0 Assault by steam or hot vapors**

X● **X98.1 Assault by hot tap water**

X● **X98.2 Assault by hot fluids**

X● **X98.3 Assault by hot household appliances**

X● **X98.8 Assault by other hot objects**

X● **X98.9 Assault by unspecified hot objects**

● **X99 Assault by sharp object**

Excludes1   assault by strike by sports equipment (Y08.0-)

The appropriate 7th character is to be added to each code from category X99

A	initial encounter
D	subsequent encounter
S	sequela

X● **X99.0 Assault by sharp glass**

X● **X99.1 Assault by knife**

X● **X99.2 Assault by sword or dagger**

X● **X99.8 Assault by other sharp object**

X● **X99.9 Assault by unspecified sharp object**
Assault by stabbing NOS

X● **Y00 Assault by blunt object**

Excludes1   assault by strike by sports equipment (Y08.0)

The appropriate 7th character is to be added to code Y00

A	initial encounter
D	subsequent encounter
S	sequela

X● **Y01 Assault by pushing from high place**

The appropriate 7th character is to be added to code Y01

A	initial encounter
D	subsequent encounter
S	sequela

● **Y02 Assault by pushing or placing victim in front of moving object**

The appropriate 7th character is to be added to each code from category Y02

A	initial encounter
D	subsequent encounter
S	sequela

X● **Y02.0 Assault by pushing or placing victim in front of motor vehicle**

X● **Y02.1 Assault by pushing or placing victim in front of (subway) train**

X● **Y02.8 Assault by pushing or placing victim in front of other moving object**

● **Y03 Assault by crashing of motor vehicle**

The appropriate 7th character is to be added to each code from category Y03

A	initial encounter
D	subsequent encounter
S	sequela

X● **Y03.0 Assault by being hit or run over by motor vehicle**

X● **Y03.8 Other assault by crashing of motor vehicle**

● **Y04 Assault by bodily force**

Excludes1   assault by:
submersion (X92.-)
use of weapon (X93-X95, X99, Y00)

The appropriate 7th character is to be added to each code from category Y04

A	initial encounter
D	subsequent encounter
S	sequela

X● **Y04.0 Assault by unarmed brawl or fight**

X● **Y04.1 Assault by human bite**

X● **Y04.2 Assault by strike against or bumped into by another person**

X● **Y04.8 Assault by other bodily force**
Assault by bodily force NOS

CHAPTER 20 (V00-Y99)

OGCR Section I.C.19.f.

Adult and child abuse, neglect and other maltreatment

Sequence first the appropriate code from categories T74 or T76 for abuse, neglect and other maltreatment, followed by any accompanying mental health or injury code(s).

If the documentation in the medical record states abuse or neglect it is coded as confirmed (T74.-). It is coded as suspected if it is documented as suspected (T76.-).

For cases of confirmed abuse or neglect an external cause code from the assault section (X92-Y09) should be added to identify the cause of any physical injuries. A perpetrator code (Y07) should be added when the perpetrator of the abuse is known. For suspected cases of abuse or neglect, do not report external cause or perpetrator code.

If a suspected case of abuse, neglect or mistreatment is ruled out during an encounter code Z04.71, Encounter for examination and observation following alleged physical adult abuse, ruled out, or code Z04.72, Encounter for examination and observation following alleged adult rape, should be used, not a code from T76.

If a suspected case of alleged rape or sexual abuse is ruled out during an encounter code Z04.41, Encounter for examination and observation following alleged adult rape or code Z04.42, Encounter for examination and observation following alleged child rape should be used, not a code from T76.

● **Y07**   **Perpetrator of assault, maltreatment and neglect**

     Note: Codes from this category are for use only in cases of confirmed abuse (T74.-)

        Selection of the correct perpetrator code is based on the relationship between the perpetrator and the victim

        Includes   perpetrator of abandonment
                        perpetrator of emotional neglect
                        perpetrator of mental cruelty
                        perpetrator of physical abuse
                        perpetrator of physical neglect
                        perpetrator of sexual abuse
                        perpetrator of torture

     Coding Clinic: 2016, Q4, P129

● **Y07.0**   **Spouse or partner, perpetrator of maltreatment and neglect**
        Spouse or partner, perpetrator of maltreatment and neglect against spouse or partner

     Y07.01   **Husband, perpetrator of maltreatment and neglect**

     Y07.02   **Wife, perpetrator of maltreatment and neglect**

     Y07.03   **Male partner, perpetrator of maltreatment and neglect**

     Y07.04   **Female partner, perpetrator of maltreatment and neglect**

● **Y07.1**   **Parent (adoptive) (biological), perpetrator of maltreatment and neglect**

     Y07.11   **Biological father, perpetrator of maltreatment and neglect**

     Y07.12   **Biological mother, perpetrator of maltreatment and neglect**

     Y07.13   **Adoptive father, perpetrator of maltreatment and neglect**

     Y07.14   **Adoptive mother, perpetrator of maltreatment and neglect**

● **Y07.4**   **Other family member, perpetrator of maltreatment and neglect**

  ● **Y07.41**   **Sibling, perpetrator of maltreatment and neglect**

       Excludes1   stepsibling, perpetrator of maltreatment and neglect (Y07.435, Y07.436)

     Y07.410   **Brother, perpetrator of maltreatment and neglect**

     Y07.411   **Sister, perpetrator of maltreatment and neglect**

● **Y07.42**   **Foster parent, perpetrator of maltreatment and neglect**

     Y07.420   **Foster father, perpetrator of maltreatment and neglect**

     Y07.421   **Foster mother, perpetrator of maltreatment and neglect**

● **Y07.43**   **Stepparent or stepsibling, perpetrator of maltreatment and neglect**

     Y07.430   **Stepfather, perpetrator of maltreatment and neglect**

     Y07.432   **Male friend of parent (co-residing in household), perpetrator of maltreatment and neglect**

     Y07.433   **Stepmother, perpetrator of maltreatment and neglect**

     Y07.434   **Female friend of parent (co-residing in household), perpetrator of maltreatment and neglect**

     Y07.435   **Stepbrother, perpetrator or maltreatment and neglect**

     Y07.436   **Stepsister, perpetrator of maltreatment and neglect**

● **Y07.49**   **Other family member, perpetrator of maltreatment and neglect**

     Y07.490   **Male cousin, perpetrator of maltreatment and neglect**

     Y07.491   **Female cousin, perpetrator of maltreatment and neglect**

     Y07.499   **Other family member, perpetrator of maltreatment and neglect**

● **Y07.5**   **Non-family member, perpetrator of maltreatment and neglect**

     Y07.50   **Unspecified non-family member, perpetrator of maltreatment and neglect**

● **Y07.51**   **Daycare provider, perpetrator of maltreatment and neglect**

     Y07.510   **At-home childcare provider, perpetrator of maltreatment and neglect**

     Y07.511   **Daycare center childcare provider, perpetrator of maltreatment and neglect**

     Y07.512   **At-home adultcare provider, perpetrator of maltreatment and neglect**

     Y07.513   **Adultcare center provider, perpetrator of maltreatment and neglect**

     Y07.519   **Unspecified daycare provider, perpetrator of maltreatment and neglect**

● **Y07.52**   **Healthcare provider, perpetrator of maltreatment and neglect**

     Y07.521   **Mental health provider, perpetrator of maltreatment and neglect**

     Y07.528   **Other therapist or healthcare provider, perpetrator of maltreatment and neglect**
        Nurse perpetrator of maltreatment and neglect
        Occupational therapist perpetrator of maltreatment and neglect
        Physical therapist perpetrator of maltreatment and neglect
        Speech therapist perpetrator of maltreatment and neglect

     Y07.529   **Unspecified healthcare provider, perpetrator of maltreatment and neglect**

▶ New   ➡ Revised   ~~deleted~~ Deleted   Excludes 1   Excludes 2   Includes   Use additional   Code first   Code also   Key words

OGCR Official Guidelines   X Assign placeholder X   ● Use Additional Character(s)   ▌Manifestation Code   🏷 Hierarchical Condition Category   **Coding Clinic**

Y07.53   **Teacher or instructor, perpetrator of maltreatment and neglect**
     Coach, perpetrator of maltreatment and neglect

Y07.59   **Other non-family member, perpetrator of maltreatment and neglect**

Y07.6   **Multiple perpetrators of maltreatment and neglect**

Y07.9   **Unspecified perpetrator of maltreatment and neglect**

● **Y08   Assault by other specified means**

The appropriate 7th character is to be added to each code from category Y08

A	initial encounter
D	subsequent encounter
S	sequela

● **Y08.0   Assault by strike by sport equipment**

X● **Y08.01   Assault by strike by hockey stick**

X● **Y08.02   Assault by strike by baseball bat**

X● **Y08.09   Assault by strike by other specified type of sport equipment**

● **Y08.8   Assault by other specified means**

X● **Y08.81   Assault by crashing of aircraft**

X● **Y08.89   Assault by other specified means**

● **Y09   Assault by unspecified means**
Assassination (attempted) NOS
Homicide (attempted) NOS
Manslaughter (attempted) NOS
Murder (attempted) NOS

EVENT OF UNDETERMINED INTENT (Y21-Y33)

Undetermined intent is only for use when there is specific documentation in the record that the intent of the injury cannot be determined. If no such documentation is present, code to accidental (unintentional)

● **Y21   Drowning and submersion, undetermined intent**

The appropriate 7th character is to be added to each code from category Y21

A	initial encounter
D	subsequent encounter
S	sequela

X● **Y21.0   Drowning and submersion while in bathtub, undetermined intent**

X● **Y21.1   Drowning and submersion after fall into bathtub, undetermined intent**

X● **Y21.2   Drowning and submersion while in swimming pool, undetermined intent**

X● **Y21.3   Drowning and submersion after fall into swimming pool, undetermined intent**

X● **Y21.4   Drowning and submersion in natural water, undetermined intent**

X● **Y21.8   Other drowning and submersion, undetermined intent**

X● **Y21.9   Unspecified drowning and submersion, undetermined intent**

X● **Y22   Handgun discharge, undetermined intent**
Discharge of gun for single hand use, undetermined intent
Discharge of pistol, undetermined intent
Discharge of revolver, undetermined intent

Excludes2   very pistol (Y24.8)

The appropriate 7th character is to be added to code Y22

A	initial encounter
D	subsequent encounter
S	sequela

● **Y23   Rifle, shotgun and larger firearm discharge, undetermined intent**

Excludes2   airgun (Y24.0)

The appropriate 7th character is to be added to each code from category Y23

A	initial encounter
D	subsequent encounter
S	sequela

X● **Y23.0   Shotgun discharge, undetermined intent**

X● **Y23.1   Hunting rifle discharge, undetermined intent**

X● **Y23.2   Military firearm discharge, undetermined intent**

X● **Y23.3   Machine gun discharge, undetermined intent**

X● **Y23.8   Other larger firearm discharge, undetermined intent**

X● **Y23.9   Unspecified larger firearm discharge, undetermined intent**

● **Y24   Other and unspecified firearm discharge, undetermined intent**

The appropriate 7th character is to be added to each code from category Y24

A	initial encounter
D	subsequent encounter
S	sequela

X● **Y24.0   Airgun discharge, undetermined intent**
BB gun discharge, undetermined intent
Pellet gun discharge, undetermined intent

X● **Y24.8   Other firearm discharge, undetermined intent**
Paintball gun discharge, undetermined intent
Very pistol [flare] discharge, undetermined intent

X● **Y24.9   Unspecified firearm discharge, undetermined intent**

X● **Y25   Contact with explosive material, undetermined intent**

The appropriate 7th character is to be added to code Y25

A	initial encounter
D	subsequent encounter
S	sequela

X● **Y26   Exposure to smoke, fire and flames, undetermined intent**

The appropriate 7th character is to be added to code Y26

A	initial encounter
D	subsequent encounter
S	sequela

● **Y27   Contact with steam, hot vapors and hot objects, undetermined intent**

The appropriate 7th character is to be added to each code from category Y27

A	initial encounter
D	subsequent encounter
S	sequela

X● **Y27.0   Contact with steam and hot vapors, undetermined intent**

X● **Y27.1   Contact with hot tap water, undetermined intent**

X● **Y27.2   Contact with hot fluids, undetermined intent**

X● **Y27.3   Contact with hot household appliance, undetermined intent**

X● **Y27.8   Contact with other hot objects, undetermined intent**

X● **Y27.9   Contact with unspecified hot objects, undetermined intent**

● **Y28   Contact with sharp object, undetermined intent**

The appropriate 7th character is to be added to each code from category Y28

A	initial encounter
D	subsequent encounter
S	sequela

X● **Y28.0   Contact with sharp glass, undetermined intent**

X● **Y28.1   Contact with knife, undetermined intent**

X ⬤ **Y28.2**   Contact with sword or dagger, undetermined intent

X ⬤ **Y28.8**   Contact with other sharp object, undetermined intent

X ⬤ **Y28.9**   Contact with unspecified sharp object, undetermined intent

X ⬤ **Y29**   Contact with blunt object, undetermined intent

The appropriate 7th character is to be added to code Y29

A	initial encounter
D	subsequent encounter
S	sequela

X ⬤ **Y30**   Falling, jumping or pushed from a high place, undetermined intent

Victim falling from one level to another, undetermined intent

The appropriate 7th character is to be added to code Y30

A	initial encounter
D	subsequent encounter
S	sequela

X ⬤ **Y31**   Falling, lying or running before or into moving object, undetermined intent

The appropriate 7th character is to be added to code Y31

A	initial encounter
D	subsequent encounter
S	sequela

X ⬤ **Y32**   Crashing of motor vehicle, undetermined intent

The appropriate 7th character is to be added to code Y32

A	initial encounter
D	subsequent encounter
S	sequela

X ⬤ **Y33**   Other specified events, undetermined intent

The appropriate 7th character is to be added to code Y33

A	initial encounter
D	subsequent encounter
S	sequela

LEGAL INTERVENTION, OPERATIONS OF WAR, MILITARY OPERATIONS, AND TERRORISM (Y35-Y38)

⬤ **Y35**   Legal intervention

Includes   any injury sustained as a result of an encounter with any law enforcement official, serving in any capacity at the time of the encounter, whether on-duty or off-duty. Includes: injury to law enforcement official, suspect and bystander

The appropriate 7th character is to be added to each code from category Y35

A	initial encounter
D	subsequent encounter
S	sequela

⬤ **Y35.0**   Legal intervention involving firearm discharge

⬤ **Y35.00**   Legal intervention involving unspecified firearm discharge

Legal intervention involving gunshot wound

Legal intervention involving shot NOS

⬤ **Y35.001**   Legal intervention involving unspecified firearm discharge, law enforcement official injured

⬤ **Y35.002**   Legal intervention involving unspecified firearm discharge, bystander injured

⬤ **Y35.003**   Legal intervention involving unspecified firearm discharge, suspect injured

⬤ **Y35.009**   Legal intervention involving unspecified firearm discharge, unspecified person injured

⬤ **Y35.01**   Legal intervention involving injury by machine gun

⬤ **Y35.011**   Legal intervention involving injury by machine gun, law enforcement official injured

⬤ **Y35.012**   Legal intervention involving injury by machine gun, bystander injured

⬤ **Y35.013**   Legal intervention involving injury by machine gun, suspect injured

⬤ **Y35.019**   Legal intervention involving injury by machine gun, unspecified person injured

⬤ **Y35.02**   Legal intervention involving injury by handgun

⬤ **Y35.021**   Legal intervention involving injury by handgun, law enforcement official injured

⬤ **Y35.022**   Legal intervention involving injury by handgun, bystander injured

⬤ **Y35.023**   Legal intervention involving injury by handgun, suspect injured

⬤ **Y35.029**   Legal intervention involving injury by handgun, unspecified person injured

⬤ **Y35.03**   Legal intervention involving injury by rifle pellet

⬤ **Y35.031**   Legal intervention involving injury by rifle pellet, law enforcement official injured

⬤ **Y35.032**   Legal intervention involving injury by rifle pellet, bystander injured

⬤ **Y35.033**   Legal intervention involving injury by rifle pellet, suspect injured

⬤ **Y35.039**   Legal intervention involving injury by rifle pellet, unspecified person injured

⬤ **Y35.04**   Legal intervention involving injury by rubber bullet

⬤ **Y35.041**   Legal intervention involving injury by rubber bullet, law enforcement official injured

⬤ **Y35.042**   Legal intervention involving injury by rubber bullet, bystander injured

⬤ **Y35.043**   Legal intervention involving injury by rubber bullet, suspect injured

⬤ **Y35.049**   Legal intervention involving injury by rubber bullet, unspecified person injured

⬤ **Y35.09**   Legal intervention involving other firearm discharge

⬤ **Y35.091**   Legal intervention involving other firearm discharge, law enforcement official injured

⬤ **Y35.092**   Legal intervention involving other firearm discharge, bystander injured

⬤ **Y35.093**   Legal intervention involving other firearm discharge, suspect injured

⬤ **Y35.099**   Legal intervention involving other firearm discharge, unspecified person injured

● **Y35.1** Legal intervention involving explosives
  ● **Y35.10** Legal intervention involving unspecified explosives
    ● **Y35.101** Legal intervention involving unspecified explosives, law enforcement official injured
    ● **Y35.102** Legal intervention involving unspecified explosives, bystander injured
    ● **Y35.103** Legal intervention involving unspecified explosives, suspect injured
    ● **Y35.109** Legal intervention involving unspecified explosives, unspecified person injured
  ● **Y35.11** Legal intervention involving injury by dynamite
    ● **Y35.111** Legal intervention involving injury by dynamite, law enforcement official injured
    ● **Y35.112** Legal intervention involving injury by dynamite, bystander injured
    ● **Y35.113** Legal intervention involving injury by dynamite, suspect injured
    ● **Y35.119** Legal intervention involving injury by dynamite, unspecified person injured
  ● **Y35.12** Legal intervention involving injury by explosive shell
    ● **Y35.121** Legal intervention involving injury by explosive shell, law enforcement official injured
    ● **Y35.122** Legal intervention involving injury by explosive shell, bystander injured
    ● **Y35.123** Legal intervention involving injury by explosive shell, suspect injured
    ● **Y35.129** Legal intervention involving other explosives, unspecified person injured
  ● **Y35.19** Legal intervention involving other explosives
    Legal intervention involving injury by grenade
    Legal intervention involving injury by mortar bomb
    ● **Y35.191** Legal intervention involving other explosives, law enforcement official injured
    ● **Y35.192** Legal intervention involving other explosives, bystander injured
    ● **Y35.193** Legal intervention involving other explosives, suspect injured
    ● **Y35.199** Legal intervention involving other explosives, unspecified person injured
● **Y35.2** Legal intervention involving gas
    Legal intervention involving asphyxiation by gas
    Legal intervention involving poisoning by gas
  ● **Y35.20** Legal intervention involving unspecified gas
    ● **Y35.201** Legal intervention involving unspecified gas, law enforcement official injured
    ● **Y35.202** Legal intervention involving unspecified gas, bystander injured
    ● **Y35.203** Legal intervention involving unspecified gas, suspect injured
    ● **Y35.209** Legal intervention involving unspecified gas, unspecified person injured

● **Y35.21** Legal intervention involving injury by tear gas
    ● **Y35.211** Legal intervention involving injury by tear gas, law enforcement official injured
    ● **Y35.212** Legal intervention involving injury by tear gas, bystander injured
    ● **Y35.213** Legal intervention involving injury by tear gas, suspect injured
    ● **Y35.219** Legal intervention involving injury by tear gas, unspecified person injured
  ● **Y35.29** Legal intervention involving other gas
    ● **Y35.291** Legal intervention involving other gas, law enforcement official injured
    ● **Y35.292** Legal intervention involving other gas, bystander injured
    ● **Y35.293** Legal intervention involving other gas, suspect injured
    ● **Y35.299** Legal intervention involving other gas, unspecified person injured
● **Y35.3** Legal intervention involving blunt objects
    Legal intervention involving being hit or struck by blunt object
  ● **Y35.30** Legal intervention involving unspecified blunt objects
    ● **Y35.301** Legal intervention involving unspecified blunt objects, law enforcement official injured
    ● **Y35.302** Legal intervention involving unspecified blunt objects, bystander injured
    ● **Y35.303** Legal intervention involving unspecified blunt objects, suspect injured
    ● **Y35.309** Legal intervention involving unspecified blunt objects, unspecified person injured
  ● **Y35.31** Legal intervention involving baton
    ● **Y35.311** Legal intervention involving baton, law enforcement official injured
    ● **Y35.312** Legal intervention involving baton, bystander injured
    ● **Y35.313** Legal intervention involving baton, suspect injured
    ● **Y35.319** Legal intervention involving baton, unspecified person injured
  ● **Y35.39** Legal intervention involving other blunt objects
    ● **Y35.391** Legal intervention involving other blunt objects, law enforcement official injured
    ● **Y35.392** Legal intervention involving other blunt objects, bystander injured
    ● **Y35.393** Legal intervention involving other blunt objects, suspect injured
    ● **Y35.399** Legal intervention involving other blunt objects, unspecified person injured
● **Y35.4** Legal intervention involving sharp objects
    Legal intervention involving being cut by sharp objects
    Legal intervention involving being stabbed by sharp objects
  ● **Y35.40** Legal intervention involving unspecified sharp objects
    ● **Y35.401** Legal intervention involving unspecified sharp objects, law enforcement official injured
    ● **Y35.402** Legal intervention involving unspecified sharp objects, bystander injured

● Y35.403   Legal intervention involving unspecified sharp objects, suspect injured

● Y35.409   Legal intervention involving unspecified sharp objects, unspecified person injured

● Y35.41   Legal intervention involving bayonet

  ● Y35.411   Legal intervention involving bayonet, law enforcement official injured

  ● Y35.412   Legal intervention involving bayonet, bystander injured

  ● Y35.413   Legal intervention involving bayonet, suspect injured

  ● Y35.419   Legal intervention involving bayonet, unspecified person injured

● Y35.49   Legal intervention involving other sharp objects

  ● Y35.491   Legal intervention involving other sharp objects, law enforcement official injured

  ● Y35.492   Legal intervention involving other sharp objects, bystander injured

  ● Y35.493   Legal intervention involving other sharp objects, suspect injured

  ● Y35.499   Legal intervention involving other sharp objects, unspecified person injured

● Y35.8   Legal intervention involving other specified means

● Y35.81   Legal intervention involving manhandling

  ● Y35.811   Legal intervention involving manhandling, law enforcement official injured

  ● Y35.812   Legal intervention involving manhandling, bystander injured

  ● Y35.813   Legal intervention involving manhandling, suspect injured

  ● Y35.819   Legal intervention involving manhandling, unspecified person injured

● Y35.83   Legal intervention involving a conducted energy device
     Electroshock device (taser)
     Stun gun

  ● Y35.831   Legal intervention involving a conducted energy device, law enforcement official injured

  ● Y35.832   Legal intervention involving a conducted energy device, bystander injured

  ● Y35.833   Legal intervention involving a conducted energy device, suspect injured

  ● Y35.839   Legal intervention involving a conducted energy device, unspecified person injured

● Y35.89   Legal intervention involving other specified means

  ● Y35.891   Legal intervention involving other specified means, law enforcement official injured

  ● Y35.892   Legal intervention involving other specified means, bystander injured

  ● Y35.893   Legal intervention involving other specified means, suspect injured
     Coding Clinic: 2018, Q1, P5

  ● Y35.899   Legal intervention involving other specified means, unspecified person injured

● Y35.9   Legal intervention, means unspecified

  X ● Y35.91   Legal intervention, means unspecified, law enforcement official injured

  X ● Y35.92   Legal intervention, means unspecified, bystander injured

  X ● Y35.93   Legal intervention, means unspecified, suspect injured

  X ● Y35.99   Legal intervention, means unspecified, unspecified person injured

● Y36   Operations of war

Includes   injuries to military personnel and civilians caused by war, civil insurrection, and peacekeeping missions

Excludes1   injury to military personnel occurring during peacetime military operations (Y37.-)

➠ military vehicles involved in transport accidents with non-military vehicle during peacetime (V09.01, V09.21, V19.81, V29.818, V39.81, V49.81, V59.81, V69.81, V79.81)

The appropriate 7th character is to be added to each code from category Y36

A	initial encounter
D	subsequent encounter
S	sequela

● Y36.0   War operations involving explosion of marine weapons
     Weapons and military watercraft

  ● Y36.00   War operations involving explosion of unspecified marine weapon
     War operations involving underwater blast NOS

    ● Y36.000   War operations involving explosion of unspecified marine weapon, military personnel

    ● Y36.001   War operations involving explosion of unspecified marine weapon, civilian

  ● Y36.01   War operations involving explosion of depth-charge

    ● Y36.010   War operations involving explosion of depth-charge, military personnel

    ● Y36.011   War operations involving explosion of depth-charge, civilian

  ● Y36.02   War operations involving explosion of marine mine
     War operations involving explosion of marine mine, at sea or in harbor

    ● Y36.020   War operations involving explosion of marine mine, military personnel

    ● Y36.021   War operations involving explosion of marine mine, civilian

  ● Y36.03   War operations involving explosion of sea-based artillery shell

    ● Y36.030   War operations involving explosion of sea-based artillery shell, military personnel

    ● Y36.031   War operations involving explosion of sea-based artillery shell, civilian

  ● Y36.04   War operations involving explosion of torpedo

    ● Y36.040   War operations involving explosion of torpedo, military personnel

    ● Y36.041   War operations involving explosion of torpedo, civilian

● **Y36.05** War operations involving accidental detonation of onboard marine weapons

　　● **Y36.050** War operations involving accidental detonation of onboard marine weapons, military personnel

　　● **Y36.051** War operations involving accidental detonation of onboard marine weapons, civilian

● **Y36.09** War operations involving explosion of other marine weapons

　　● **Y36.090** War operations involving explosion of other marine weapons, military personnel

　　● **Y36.091** War operations involving explosion of other marine weapons, civilian

● **Y36.1** War operations involving destruction of aircraft

　　● **Y36.10** War operations involving unspecified destruction of aircraft

　　　　● **Y36.100** War operations involving unspecified destruction of aircraft, military personnel

　　　　● **Y36.101** War operations involving unspecified destruction of aircraft, civilian

　　● **Y36.11** War operations involving destruction of aircraft due to enemy fire or explosives

　　　　War operations involving destruction of aircraft due to air to air missile
　　　　War operations involving destruction of aircraft due to explosive placed on aircraft
　　　　War operations involving destruction of aircraft due to rocket propelled grenade [RPG]
　　　　War operations involving destruction of aircraft due to small arms fire
　　　　War operations involving destruction of aircraft due to surface to air missile

　　　　● **Y36.110** War operations involving destruction of aircraft due to enemy fire or explosives, military personnel

　　　　● **Y36.111** War operations involving destruction of aircraft due to enemy fire or explosives, civilian

　　● **Y36.12** War operations involving destruction of aircraft due to collision with other aircraft

　　　　● **Y36.120** War operations involving destruction of aircraft due to collision with other aircraft, military personnel

　　　　● **Y36.121** War operations involving destruction of aircraft due to collision with other aircraft, civilian

　　● **Y36.13** War operations involving destruction of aircraft due to onboard fire

　　　　● **Y36.130** War operations involving destruction of aircraft due to onboard fire, military personnel

　　　　● **Y36.131** War operations involving destruction of aircraft due to onboard fire, civilian

　　● **Y36.14** War operations involving destruction of aircraft due to accidental detonation of onboard munitions and explosives

　　　　● **Y36.140** War operations involving destruction of aircraft due to accidental detonation of onboard munitions and explosives, military personnel

　　　　● **Y36.141** War operations involving destruction of aircraft due to accidental detonation of onboard munitions and explosives, civilian

● **Y36.19** War operations involving other destruction of aircraft

　　● **Y36.190** War operations involving other destruction of aircraft, military personnel

　　● **Y36.191** War operations involving other destruction of aircraft, civilian

● **Y36.2** War operations involving other explosions and fragments

　　Excludes1 war operations involving explosion of aircraft (Y36.1-)
　　　　　　war operations involving explosion of marine weapons (Y36.0-)
　　　　　　war operations involving explosion of nuclear weapons (Y36.5-)
　　　　　　war operations involving explosion occurring after cessation of hostilities (Y36.8-)

　　● **Y36.20** War operations involving unspecified explosion and fragments

　　　　War operations involving air blast NOS
　　　　War operations involving blast NOS
　　　　War operations involving blast fragments NOS
　　　　War operations involving blast wave NOS
　　　　War operations involving blast wind NOS
　　　　War operations involving explosion NOS
　　　　War operations involving explosion of bomb NOS

　　　　● **Y36.200** War operations involving unspecified explosion and fragments, military personnel

　　　　● **Y36.201** War operations involving unspecified explosion and fragments, civilian

　　● **Y36.21** War operations involving explosion of aerial bomb

　　　　● **Y36.210** War operations involving explosion of aerial bomb, military personnel

　　　　● **Y36.211** War operations involving explosion of aerial bomb, civilian

　　● **Y36.22** War operations involving explosion of guided missile

　　　　● **Y36.220** War operations involving explosion of guided missile, military personnel

　　　　● **Y36.221** War operations involving explosion of guided missile, civilian

　　● **Y36.23** War operations involving explosion of improvised explosive device [IED]

　　　　War operations involving explosion of person-borne improvised explosive device [IED]
　　　　War operations involving explosion of vehicle-borne improvised explosive device [IED]
　　　　War operations involving explosion of roadside improvised explosive device [IED]

　　　　● **Y36.230** War operations involving explosion of improvised explosive device [IED], military personnel

　　　　● **Y36.231** War operations involving explosion of improvised explosive device [IED], civilian

　　● **Y36.24** War operations involving explosion due to accidental detonation and discharge of own munitions or munitions launch device

　　　　● **Y36.240** War operations involving explosion due to accidental detonation and discharge of own munitions or munitions launch device, military personnel

　　　　● **Y36.241** War operations involving explosion due to accidental detonation and discharge of own munitions or munitions launch device, civilian

CHAPTER 2Ø (VØØ-Y99)

● Y36.25　War operations involving fragments from munitions
- ● Y36.250　War operations involving fragments from munitions, military personnel
- ● Y36.251　War operations involving fragments from munitions, civilian

● Y36.26　War operations involving fragments of improvised explosive device [IED]
War operations involving fragments of person-borne improvised explosive device [IED]
War operations involving fragments of vehicle-borne improvised explosive device [IED]
War operations involving fragments of roadside improvised explosive device [IED]
- ● Y36.260　War operations involving fragments of improvised explosive device [IED], military personnel
- ● Y36.261　War operations involving fragments of improvised explosive device [IED], civilian

● Y36.27　War operations involving fragments from weapons
- ● Y36.270　War operations involving fragments from weapons, military personnel
- ● Y36.271　War operations involving fragments from weapons, civilian

● Y36.29　War operations involving other explosions and fragments
War operations involving explosion of grenade
War operations involving explosions of land mine
War operations involving shrapnel NOS
- ● Y36.290　War operations involving other explosions and fragments, military personnel
- ● Y36.291　War operations involving other explosions and fragments, civilian

● Y36.3　War operations involving fires, conflagrations and hot substances
War operations involving smoke, fumes, and heat from fires, conflagrations and hot substances

Excludes 1　war operations involving fires and conflagrations aboard military aircraft (Y36.1-)
war operations involving fires and conflagrations aboard military watercraft (Y36.0-)
war operations involving fires and conflagrations caused indirectly by conventional weapons (Y36.2-)
war operations involving fires and thermal effects of nuclear weapons (Y36.53-)

- ● Y36.30　War operations involving unspecified fire, conflagration and hot substance
- ● Y36.300　War operations involving unspecified fire, conflagration and hot substance, military personnel
- ● Y36.301　War operations involving unspecified fire, conflagration and hot substance, civilian

● Y36.31　War operations involving gasoline bomb
War operations involving incendiary bomb
War operations involving petrol bomb
- ● Y36.310　War operations involving gasoline bomb, military personnel
- ● Y36.311　War operations involving gasoline bomb, civilian

● Y36.32　War operations involving incendiary bullet
- ● Y36.320　War operations involving incendiary bullet, military personnel
- ● Y36.321　War operations involving incendiary bullet, civilian

● Y36.33　War operations involving flamethrower
- ● Y36.330　War operations involving flamethrower, military personnel
- ● Y36.331　War operations involving flamethrower, civilian

● Y36.39　War operations involving other fires, conflagrations and hot substances
- ● Y36.390　War operations involving other fires, conflagrations and hot substances, military personnel
- ● Y36.391　War operations involving other fires, conflagrations and hot substances, civilian

● Y36.4　War operations involving firearm discharge and other forms of conventional warfare

● Y36.41　War operations involving rubber bullets
- ● Y36.410　War operations involving rubber bullets, military personnel
- ● Y36.411　War operations involving rubber bullets, civilian

● Y36.42　War operations involving firearms pellets
- ● Y36.420　War operations involving firearms pellets, military personnel
- ● Y36.421　War operations involving firearms pellets, civilian

● Y36.43　War operations involving other firearms discharge
War operations involving bullets NOS

Excludes 1　war operations involving munitions fragments (Y36.25-)
war operations involving incendiary bullets (Y36.32-)

- ● Y36.430　War operations involving other firearms discharge, military personnel
- ● Y36.431　War operations involving other firearms discharge, civilian

● Y36.44　War operations involving unarmed hand to hand combat

Excludes 1　war operations involving combat using blunt or piercing object (Y36.45-)
war operations involving intentional restriction of air and airway (Y36.46-)
war operations involving unintentional restriction of air and airway (Y36.47-)

- ● Y36.440　War operations involving unarmed hand to hand combat, military personnel
- ● Y36.441　War operations involving unarmed hand to hand combat, civilian

● Y36.45　War operations involving combat using blunt or piercing object
- ● Y36.450　War operations involving combat using blunt or piercing object, military personnel
- ● Y36.451　War operations involving combat using blunt or piercing object, civilian

● Y36.46   War operations involving intentional restriction of air and airway
    ● Y36.460   War operations involving intentional restriction of air and airway, military personnel
    ● Y36.461   War operations involving intentional restriction of air and airway, civilian
● Y36.47   War operations involving unintentional restriction of air and airway
    ● Y36.470   War operations involving unintentional restriction of air and airway, military personnel
    ● Y36.471   War operations involving unintentional restriction of air and airway, civilian
● Y36.49   War operations involving other forms of conventional warfare
    ● Y36.490   War operations involving other forms of conventional warfare, military personnel
    ● Y36.491   War operations involving other forms of conventional warfare, civilian
● Y36.5   War operations involving nuclear weapons
    War operations involving dirty bomb NOS
● Y36.50   War operations involving unspecified effect of nuclear weapon
    ● Y36.500   War operations involving unspecified effect of nuclear weapon, military personnel
    ● Y36.501   War operations involving unspecified effect of nuclear weapon, civilian
● Y36.51   War operations involving direct blast effect of nuclear weapon
    War operations involving blast pressure of nuclear weapon
    ● Y36.510   War operations involving direct blast effect of nuclear weapon, military personnel
    ● Y36.511   War operations involving direct blast effect of nuclear weapon, civilian
● Y36.52   War operations involving indirect blast effect of nuclear weapon
    War operations involving being thrown by blast of nuclear weapon
    War operations involving being struck or crushed by blast debris of nuclear weapon
    ● Y36.520   War operations involving indirect blast effect of nuclear weapon, military personnel
    ● Y36.521   War operations involving indirect blast effect of nuclear weapon, civilian
● Y36.53   War operations involving thermal radiation effect of nuclear weapon
    War operations involving direct heat from nuclear weapon
    War operation involving fireball effects from nuclear weapon
    ● Y36.530   War operations involving thermal radiation effect of nuclear weapon, military personnel
    ● Y36.531   War operations involving thermal radiation effect of nuclear weapon, civilian

● Y36.54   War operation involving nuclear radiation effects of nuclear weapon
    War operation involving acute radiation exposure from nuclear weapon
    War operation involving exposure to immediate ionizing radiation from nuclear weapon
    War operation involving fallout exposure from nuclear weapon
    War operation involving secondary effects of nuclear weapons
    ● Y36.540   War operation involving nuclear radiation effects of nuclear weapon, military personnel
    ● Y36.541   War operation involving nuclear radiation effects of nuclear weapon, civilian
● Y36.59   War operation involving other effects of nuclear weapons
    ● Y36.590   War operation involving other effects of nuclear weapons, military personnel
    ● Y36.591   War operation involving other effects of nuclear weapons, civilian
● Y36.6   War operations involving biological weapons
    ● Y36.6X   War operations involving biological weapons
        ● Y36.6X0   War operations involving biological weapons, military personnel
        ● Y36.6X1   War operations involving biological weapons, civilian
● Y36.7   War operations involving chemical weapons and other forms of unconventional warfare
    Excludes1   war operations involving incendiary devices (Y36.3-, Y36.5-)
    ● Y36.7X   War operations involving chemical weapons and other forms of unconventional warfare
        ● Y36.7X0   War operations involving chemical weapons and other forms of unconventional warfare, military personnel
        ● Y36.7X1   War operations involving chemical weapons and other forms of unconventional warfare, civilian
● Y36.8   War operations occurring after cessation of hostilities
    War operations classifiable to categories Y36.0-Y36.8 but occurring after cessation of hostilities
    ● Y36.81   Explosion of mine placed during war operations but exploding after cessation of hostilities
        ● Y36.810   Explosion of mine placed during war operations but exploding after cessation of hostilities, military personnel
        ● Y36.811   Explosion of mine placed during war operations but exploding after cessation of hostilities, civilian
    ● Y36.82   Explosion of bomb placed during war operations but exploding after cessation of hostilities
        ● Y36.820   Explosion of bomb placed during war operations but exploding after cessation of hostilities, military personnel
        ● Y36.821   Explosion of bomb placed during war operations but exploding after cessation of hostilities, civilian

CHAPTER 20 (V00-Y99)

● **Y36.88** Other war operations occurring after cessation of hostilities

● **Y36.880** Other war operations occurring after cessation of hostilities, military personnel

● **Y36.881** Other war operations occurring after cessation of hostilities, civilian

● **Y36.89** Unspecified war operations occurring after cessation of hostilities

● **Y36.890** Unspecified war operations occurring after cessation of hostilities, military personnel

● **Y36.891** Unspecified war operations occurring after cessation of hostilities, civilian

● **Y36.9** Other and unspecified war operations

X ● **Y36.90** War operations, unspecified

X ● **Y36.91** War operations involving unspecified weapon of mass destruction [WMD]

X ● **Y36.92** War operations involving friendly fire

● **Y37** **Military operations**

Includes Injuries to military personnel and civilians occurring during peacetime on military property and during routine military exercises and operations

Excludes1 military aircraft involved in aircraft accident with civilian aircraft (V97.81-)
➡ military vehicles involved in transport accident with civilian vehicle (V09.01, V09.21, V19.81, V29.818, V39.81, V49.81, V59.81, V69.81, V79.81)
military watercraft involved in water transport accident with civilian watercraft (V94.81-)
war operations (Y36.-)

The appropriate 7th character is to be added to each code from category Y37

A	initial encounter
D	subsequent encounter
S	sequela

● **Y37.0** Military operations involving explosion of marine weapons

● **Y37.00** Military operations involving explosion of unspecified marine weapon
Military operations involving underwater blast NOS

● **Y37.000** Military operations involving explosion of unspecified marine weapon, military personnel

● **Y37.001** Military operations involving explosion of unspecified marine weapon, civilian

● **Y37.01** Military operations involving explosion of depth-charge

● **Y37.010** Military operations involving explosion of depth-charge, military personnel

● **Y37.011** Military operations involving explosion of depth-charge, civilian

● **Y37.02** Military operations involving explosion of marine mine
Military operations involving explosion of marine mine, at sea or in harbor

● **Y37.020** Military operations involving explosion of marine mine, military personnel

● **Y37.021** Military operations involving explosion of marine mine, civilian

● **Y37.03** Military operations involving explosion of sea-based artillery shell

● **Y37.030** Military operations involving explosion of sea-based artillery shell, military personnel

● **Y37.031** Military operations involving explosion of sea-based artillery shell, civilian

● **Y37.04** Military operations involving explosion of torpedo

● **Y37.040** Military operations involving explosion of torpedo, military personnel

● **Y37.041** Military operations involving explosion of torpedo, civilian

● **Y37.05** Military operations involving accidental detonation of onboard marine weapons

● **Y37.050** Military operations involving accidental detonation of onboard marine weapons, military personnel

● **Y37.051** Military operations involving accidental detonation of onboard marine weapons, civilian

● **Y37.09** Military operations involving explosion of other marine weapons

● **Y37.090** Military operations involving explosion of other marine weapons, military personnel

● **Y37.091** Military operations involving explosion of other marine weapons, civilian

● **Y37.1** Military operations involving destruction of aircraft

● **Y37.10** Military operations involving unspecified destruction of aircraft

● **Y37.100** Military operations involving unspecified destruction of aircraft, military personnel

● **Y37.101** Military operations involving unspecified destruction of aircraft, civilian

● **Y37.11** Military operations involving destruction of aircraft due to enemy fire or explosives
Military operations involving destruction of aircraft due to air to air missile
Military operations involving destruction of aircraft due to explosive placed on aircraft
Military operations involving destruction of aircraft due to rocket propelled grenade [RPG]
Military operations involving destruction of aircraft due to small arms fire
Military operations involving destruction of aircraft due to surface to air missile

● **Y37.110** Military operations involving destruction of aircraft due to enemy fire or explosives, military personnel

● **Y37.111** Military operations involving destruction of aircraft due to enemy fire or explosives, civilian

● **Y37.12** Military operations involving destruction of aircraft due to collision with other aircraft

● **Y37.120** Military operations involving destruction of aircraft due to collision with other aircraft, military personnel

● **Y37.121** Military operations involving destruction of aircraft due to collision with other aircraft, civilian

● Y37.13   Military operations involving destruction of aircraft due to onboard fire
   ● Y37.130   Military operations involving destruction of aircraft due to onboard fire, military personnel
   ● Y37.131   Military operations involving destruction of aircraft due to onboard fire, civilian

● Y37.14   Military operations involving destruction of aircraft due to accidental detonation of onboard munitions and explosives
   ● Y37.140   Military operations involving destruction of aircraft due to accidental detonation of onboard munitions and explosives, military personnel
   ● Y37.141   Military operations involving destruction of aircraft due to accidental detonation of onboard munitions and explosives, civilian

● Y37.19   Military operations involving other destruction of aircraft
   ● Y37.190   Military operations involving other destruction of aircraft, military personnel
   ● Y37.191   Military operations involving other destruction of aircraft, civilian

● Y37.2   Military operations involving other explosions and fragments

   Excludes1   military operations involving explosion of aircraft (Y37.1-)
               military operations involving explosion of marine weapons (Y37.0-)
               military operations involving explosion of nuclear weapons (Y37.5-)

● Y37.20   Military operations involving unspecified explosion and fragments
   Military operations involving air blast NOS
   Military operations involving blast NOS
   Military operations involving blast fragments NOS
   Military operations involving blast wave NOS
   Military operations involving blast wind NOS
   Military operations involving explosion NOS
   Military operations involving explosion of bomb NOS
   ● Y37.200   Military operations involving unspecified explosion and fragments, military personnel
   ● Y37.201   Military operations involving unspecified explosion and fragments, civilian

● Y37.21   Military operations involving explosion of aerial bomb
   ● Y37.210   Military operations involving explosion of aerial bomb, military personnel
   ● Y37.211   Military operations involving explosion of aerial bomb, civilian

● Y37.22   Military operations involving explosion of guided missile
   ● Y37.220   Military operations involving explosion of guided missile, military personnel
   ● Y37.221   Military operations involving explosion of guided missile, civilian

● Y37.23   Military operations involving explosion of improvised explosive device [IED]
   Military operations involving explosion of person-borne improvised explosive device [IED]
   Military operations involving explosion of vehicle-borne improvised explosive device [IED]
   Military operations involving explosion of roadside improvised explosive device [IED]
   ● Y37.230   Military operations involving explosion of improvised explosive device [IED], military personnel
   ● Y37.231   Military operations involving explosion of improvised explosive device [IED], civilian

● Y37.24   Military operations involving explosion due to accidental detonation and discharge of own munitions or munitions launch device
   ● Y37.240   Military operations involving explosion due to accidental detonation and discharge of own munitions or munitions launch device, military personnel
   ● Y37.241   Military operations involving explosion due to accidental detonation and discharge of own munitions or munitions launch device, civilian

● Y37.25   Military operations involving fragments from munitions
   ● Y37.250   Military operations involving fragments from munitions, military personnel
   ● Y37.251   Military operations involving fragments from munitions, civilian

● Y37.26   Military operations involving fragments of improvised explosive device [IED]
   Military operations involving fragments of person-borne improvised explosive device [IED]
   Military operations involving fragments of vehicle-borne improvised explosive device [IED]
   Military operations involving fragments of roadside improvised explosive device [IED]
   ● Y37.260   Military operations involving fragments of improvised explosive device [IED], military personnel
   ● Y37.261   Military operations involving fragments of improvised explosive device [IED], civilian

● Y37.27   Military operations involving fragments from weapons
   ● Y37.270   Military operations involving fragments from weapons, military personnel
   ● Y37.271   Military operations involving fragments from weapons, civilian

● Y37.29   Military operations involving other explosions and fragments
   Military operations involving explosion of grenade
   Military operations involving explosions of land mine
   Military operations involving shrapnel NOS
   ● Y37.290   Military operations involving other explosions and fragments, military personnel
   ● Y37.291   Military operations involving other explosions and fragments, civilian

CHAPTER 20 (V00-Y99)

Y37.3 Military operations involving fires, conflagrations and hot substances
Military operations involving smoke, fumes, and heat from fires, conflagrations and hot substances

Excludes1 military operations involving fires and conflagrations aboard military aircraft (Y37.1-)
military operations involving fires and conflagrations aboard military watercraft (Y37.0-)
military operations involving fires and conflagrations caused indirectly by conventional weapons (Y37.2-)
military operations involving fires and thermal effects of nuclear weapons (Y36.53-)

Y37.30 Military operations involving unspecified fire, conflagration and hot substance

Y37.300 Military operations involving unspecified fire, conflagration and hot substance, military personnel

Y37.301 Military operations involving unspecified fire, conflagration and hot substance, civilian

Y37.31 Military operations involving gasoline bomb
Military operations involving incendiary bomb
Military operations involving petrol bomb

Y37.310 Military operations involving gasoline bomb, military personnel

Y37.311 Military operations involving gasoline bomb, civilian

Y37.32 Military operations involving incendiary bullet

Y37.320 Military operations involving incendiary bullet, military personnel

Y37.321 Military operations involving incendiary bullet, civilian

Y37.33 Military operations involving flamethrower

Y37.330 Military operations involving flamethrower, military personnel

Y37.331 Military operations involving flamethrower, civilian

Y37.39 Military operations involving other fires, conflagrations and hot substances

Y37.390 Military operations involving other fires, conflagrations and hot substances, military personnel

Y37.391 Military operations involving other fires, conflagrations and hot substances, civilian

Y37.4 Military operations involving firearm discharge and other forms of conventional warfare

Y37.41 Military operations involving rubber bullets

Y37.410 Military operations involving rubber bullets, military personnel

Y37.411 Military operations involving rubber bullets, civilian

Y37.42 Military operations involving firearms pellets

Y37.420 Military operations involving firearms pellets, military personnel

Y37.421 Military operations involving firearms pellets, civilian

Y37.43 Military operations involving other firearms discharge
Military operations involving bullets NOS

Excludes1 military operations involving munitions fragments (Y37.25-)
military operations involving incendiary bullets (Y37.32-)

Y37.430 Military operations involving other firearms discharge, military personnel

Y37.431 Military operations involving other firearms discharge, civilian

Y37.44 Military operations involving unarmed hand to hand combat

Excludes1 military operations involving combat using blunt or piercing object (Y37.45-)
military operations involving intentional restriction of air and airway (Y37.46-)
military operations involving unintentional restriction of air and airway (Y37.47-)

Y37.440 Military operations involving unarmed hand to hand combat, military personnel

Y37.441 Military operations involving unarmed hand to hand combat, civilian

Y37.45 Military operations involving combat using blunt or piercing object

Y37.450 Military operations involving combat using blunt or piercing object, military personnel

Y37.451 Military operations involving combat using blunt or piercing object, civilian

Y37.46 Military operations involving intentional restriction of air and airway

Y37.460 Military operations involving intentional restriction of air and airway, military personnel

Y37.461 Military operations involving intentional restriction of air and airway, civilian

Y37.47 Military operations involving unintentional restriction of air and airway

Y37.470 Military operations involving unintentional restriction of air and airway, military personnel

Y37.471 Military operations involving unintentional restriction of air and airway, civilian

Y37.49 Military operations involving other forms of conventional warfare

Y37.490 Military operations involving other forms of conventional warfare, military personnel

Y37.491 Military operations involving other forms of conventional warfare, civilian

Y37.5 Military operations involving nuclear weapons
Military operation involving dirty bomb NOS

Y37.50 Military operations involving unspecified effect of nuclear weapon

Y37.500 Military operations involving unspecified effect of nuclear weapon, military personnel

Y37.501 Military operations involving unspecified effect of nuclear weapon, civilian

Y37.51 Military operations involving direct blast effect of nuclear weapon
Military operations involving blast pressure of nuclear weapon

Y37.510 Military operations involving direct blast effect of nuclear weapon, military personnel

Y37.511 Military operations involving direct blast effect of nuclear weapon, civilian

▶ New   ⇒ Revised   ~~deleted~~ Deleted   Excludes 1   Excludes 2   Includes   Use additional   Code first   Code also   Key words

OGCR Official Guidelines   X Assign placeholder X   ● Use Additional Character(s)   ▮ Manifestation Code   ⦿ Hierarchical Condition Category   Coding Clinic

● **Y37.52** Military operations involving indirect blast effect of nuclear weapon
  Military operations involving being thrown by blast of nuclear weapon
  Military operations involving being struck or crushed by blast debris of nuclear weapon

 ● **Y37.520** Military operations involving indirect blast effect of nuclear weapon, military personnel

 ● **Y37.521** Military operations involving indirect blast effect of nuclear weapon, civilian

● **Y37.53** Military operations involving thermal radiation effect of nuclear weapon
  Military operations involving direct heat from nuclear weapon
  Military operation involving fireball effects from nuclear weapon

 ● **Y37.530** Military operations involving thermal radiation effect of nuclear weapon, military personnel

 ● **Y37.531** Military operations involving thermal radiation effect of nuclear weapon, civilian

● **Y37.54** Military operation involving nuclear radiation effects of nuclear weapon
  Military operation involving acute radiation exposure from nuclear weapon
  Military operation involving exposure to immediate ionizing radiation from nuclear weapon
  Military operation involving fallout exposure from nuclear weapon
  Military operation involving secondary effects of nuclear weapons

 ● **Y37.540** Military operation involving nuclear radiation effects of nuclear weapon, military personnel

 ● **Y37.541** Military operation involving nuclear radiation effects of nuclear weapon, civilian

● **Y37.59** Military operation involving other effects of nuclear weapons

 ● **Y37.590** Military operation involving other effects of nuclear weapons, military personnel

 ● **Y37.591** Military operation involving other effects of nuclear weapons, civilian

● **Y37.6** Military operations involving biological weapons

 ● **Y37.6X** Military operations involving biological weapons

  ● **Y37.6X0** Military operations involving biological weapons, military personnel

  ● **Y37.6X1** Military operations involving biological weapons, civilian

● **Y37.7** Military operations involving chemical weapons and other forms of unconventional warfare

   Excludes1 military operations involving incendiary devices (Y36.3-, Y36.5-)

 ● **Y37.7X** Military operations involving chemical weapons and other forms of unconventional warfare

  ● **Y37.7X0** Military operations involving chemical weapons and other forms of unconventional warfare, military personnel

  ● **Y37.7X1** Military operations involving chemical weapons and other forms of unconventional warfare, civilian

● **Y37.9** Other and unspecified military operations

 X ● **Y37.90** Military operations, unspecified

 X ● **Y37.91** Military operations involving unspecified weapon of mass destruction [WMD]

 X ● **Y37.92** Military operations involving friendly fire

● **Y38** Terrorism
  These codes are for use to identify injuries resulting from the unlawful use of force or violence against persons or property to intimidate or coerce a government, the civilian population, or any segment thereof, in furtherance of political or social objective
  Use additional code for place of occurrence (Y92.-)
  The appropriate 7th character is to be added to each code from category Y38

A	initial encounter
D	subsequent encounter
S	sequela

● **Y38.0** Terrorism involving explosion of marine weapons
  Terrorism involving depth-charge
  Terrorism involving marine mine
  Terrorism involving mine NOS, at sea or in harbor
  Terrorism involving sea-based artillery shell
  Terrorism involving torpedo
  Terrorism involving underwater blast

 ● **Y38.0X** Terrorism involving explosion of marine weapons

  ● **Y38.0X1** Terrorism involving explosion of marine weapons, public safety official injured

  ● **Y38.0X2** Terrorism involving explosion of marine weapons, civilian injured

  ● **Y38.0X3** Terrorism involving explosion of marine weapons, terrorist injured

● **Y38.1** Terrorism involving destruction of aircraft
  Terrorism involving aircraft burned
  Terrorism involving aircraft exploded
  Terrorism involving aircraft being shot down
  Terrorism involving aircraft used as a weapon

 ● **Y38.1X** Terrorism involving destruction of aircraft

  ● **Y38.1X1** Terrorism involving destruction of aircraft, public safety official injured

  ● **Y38.1X2** Terrorism involving destruction of aircraft, civilian injured

  ● **Y38.1X3** Terrorism involving destruction of aircraft, terrorist injured

● **Y38.2** Terrorism involving other explosions and fragments
  Terrorism involving antipersonnel (fragments) bomb
  Terrorism involving blast NOS
  Terrorism involving explosion NOS
  Terrorism involving explosion of breech block
  Terrorism involving explosion of cannon block
  Terrorism involving explosion (fragments) of artillery shell
  Terrorism involving explosion (fragments) of bomb
  Terrorism involving explosion (fragments) of grenade
  Terrorism involving explosion (fragments) of guided missile
  Terrorism involving explosion (fragments) of land mine
  Terrorism involving explosion of mortar bomb
  Terrorism involving explosion of munitions
  Terrorism involving explosion (fragments) of rocket
  Terrorism involving explosion (fragments) of shell
  Terrorism involving shrapnel
  Terrorism involving mine NOS, on land

   Excludes1 terrorism involving explosion of nuclear weapon (Y38.5)
     terrorism involving suicide bomber (Y38.81)

 ● **Y38.2X** Terrorism involving other explosions and fragments

  ● **Y38.2X1** Terrorism involving other explosions and fragments, public safety official injured

  ● **Y38.2X2** Terrorism involving other explosions and fragments, civilian injured

  ● **Y38.2X3** Terrorism involving other explosions and fragments, terrorist injured

CHAPTER 20 (V00-Y99)

● **Y38.3** **Terrorism involving fires, conflagration and hot substances**
    Terrorism involving conflagration NOS
    Terrorism involving fire NOS
    Terrorism involving petrol bomb
    Excludes1   terrorism involving fire or heat of nuclear weapon (Y38.5)

  ● **Y38.3X** **Terrorism involving fires, conflagration and hot substances**
    ● **Y38.3X1** **Terrorism involving fires, conflagration and hot substances, public safety official injured**
    ● **Y38.3X2** **Terrorism involving fires, conflagration and hot substances, civilian injured**
    ● **Y38.3X3** **Terrorism involving fires, conflagration and hot substances, terrorist injured**

● **Y38.4** **Terrorism involving firearms**
    Terrorism involving carbine bullet
    Terrorism involving machine gun bullet
    Terrorism involving pellets (shotgun)
    Terrorism involving pistol bullet
    Terrorism involving rifle bullet
    Terrorism involving rubber (rifle) bullet
  ● **Y38.4X** **Terrorism involving firearms**
    ● **Y38.4X1** **Terrorism involving firearms, public safety official injured**
    ● **Y38.4X2** **Terrorism involving firearms, civilian injured**
    ● **Y38.4X3** **Terrorism involving firearms, terrorist injured**

● **Y38.5** **Terrorism involving nuclear weapons**
    Terrorism involving blast effects of nuclear weapon
    Terrorism involving exposure to ionizing radiation from nuclear weapon
    Terrorism involving fireball effect of nuclear weapon
    Terrorism involving heat from nuclear weapon
  ● **Y38.5X** **Terrorism involving nuclear weapons**
    ● **Y38.5X1** **Terrorism involving nuclear weapons, public safety official injured**
    ● **Y38.5X2** **Terrorism involving nuclear weapons, civilian injured**
    ● **Y38.5X3** **Terrorism involving nuclear weapons, terrorist injured**

● **Y38.6** **Terrorism involving biological weapons**
    Terrorism involving anthrax
    Terrorism involving cholera
    A serious, often deadly, infectious disease of the small intestine
    Terrorism involving smallpox
  ● **Y38.6X** **Terrorism involving biological weapons**
    ● **Y38.6X1** **Terrorism involving biological weapons, public safety official injured**
    ● **Y38.6X2** **Terrorism involving biological weapons, civilian injured**
    ● **Y38.6X3** **Terrorism involving biological weapons, terrorist injured**

● **Y38.7** **Terrorism involving chemical weapons**
    Terrorism involving gases, fumes, chemicals
    Terrorism involving hydrogen cyanide
    Terrorism involving phosgene
    Terrorism involving sarin
  ● **Y38.7X** **Terrorism involving chemical weapons**
    ● **Y38.7X1** **Terrorism involving chemical weapons, public safety official injured**
    ● **Y38.7X2** **Terrorism involving chemical weapons, civilian injured**
    ● **Y38.7X3** **Terrorism involving chemical weapons, terrorist injured**

● **Y38.8** **Terrorism involving other and unspecified means**
  ● **Y38.80** **Terrorism involving unspecified means**
    Terrorism NOS
  ● **Y38.81** **Terrorism involving suicide bomber**
    ● **Y38.811** **Terrorism involving suicide bomber, public safety official injured**
    ● **Y38.812** **Terrorism involving suicide bomber, civilian injured**
  ● **Y38.89** **Terrorism involving other means**
    Terrorism involving drowning and submersion
    Terrorism involving lasers
    Terrorism involving piercing or stabbing instruments
    ● **Y38.891** **Terrorism involving other means, public safety official injured**
    ● **Y38.892** **Terrorism involving other means, civilian injured**
    ● **Y38.893** **Terrorism involving other means, terrorist injured**

● **Y38.9** **Terrorism, secondary effects**
    Note: This code is for use to identify conditions occurring subsequent to a terrorist attack not those that are due to the initial terrorist attack.
  ● **Y38.9X** **Terrorism, secondary effects**
    ● **Y38.9X1** **Terrorism, secondary effects, public safety official injured**
    ● **Y38.9X2** **Terrorism, secondary effects, civilian injured categories**

COMPLICATIONS OF MEDICAL AND SURGICAL CARE (Y62-Y84)

Includes complications of medical devices surgical and medical procedures as the cause of abnormal reaction of the patient, or of later complication, without mention of misadventure at the time of the procedure

MISADVENTURES TO PATIENTS DURING SURGICAL AND MEDICAL CARE (Y62-Y69)

Excludes1 surgical and medical procedures as the cause of abnormal reaction of the patient, without mention of misadventure at the time of the procedure (Y83-Y84)

● **Y62** **Failure of sterile precautions during surgical and medical care**
  Y62.0 **Failure of sterile precautions during surgical operation**
  Y62.1 **Failure of sterile precautions during infusion or transfusion**
  Y62.2 **Failure of sterile precautions during kidney dialysis and other perfusion**
  Y62.3 **Failure of sterile precautions during injection or immunization**
  Y62.4 **Failure of sterile precautions during endoscopic examination**
  Y62.5 **Failure of sterile precautions during heart catheterization**
  Y62.6 **Failure of sterile precautions during aspiration, puncture and other catheterization**
  Y62.8 **Failure of sterile precautions during other surgical and medical care**
  Y62.9 **Failure of sterile precautions during unspecified surgical and medical care**

● **Y63** **Failure in dosage during surgical and medical care**
  Excludes2 accidental overdose of drug or wrong drug given in error (T36-T50)
  Y63.0 **Excessive amount of blood or other fluid given during transfusion or infusion**
  Y63.1 **Incorrect dilution of fluid used during infusion**
  Y63.2 **Overdose of radiation given during therapy**

Y63.3 Inadvertent exposure of patient to radiation during medical care

Y63.4 Failure in dosage in electroshock or insulin-shock therapy

Y63.5 Inappropriate temperature in local application and packing

Y63.6 Underdosing and nonadministration of necessary drug, medicament or biological substance

Y63.8 Failure in dosage during other surgical and medical care

Y63.9 Failure in dosage during unspecified surgical and medical care

● Y64 Contaminated medical or biological substances

Y64.0 Contaminated medical or biological substance, transfused or infused

Y64.1 Contaminated medical or biological substance, injected or used for immunization

Y64.8 Contaminated medical or biological substance administered by other means

Y64.9 Contaminated medical or biological substance administered by unspecified means
Administered contaminated medical or biological substance NOS

● Y65 Other misadventures during surgical and medical care

Y65.0 Mismatched blood in transfusion

Y65.1 Wrong fluid used in infusion

Y65.2 Failure in suture or ligature during surgical operation

Y65.3 Endotracheal tube wrongly placed during anesthetic procedure

Y65.4 Failure to introduce or to remove other tube or instrument

● Y65.5 Performance of wrong procedure (operation)

● Y65.51 Performance of wrong procedure (operation) on correct patient
Wrong device implanted into correct surgical site

Excludes1 performance of correct procedure (operation) on wrong side or body part (Y65.53)

● Y65.52 Performance of procedure (operation) on patient not scheduled for surgery
Performance of procedure (operation) intended for another patient
Performance of procedure (operation) on wrong patient

● Y65.53 Performance of correct procedure (operation) on wrong side or body part
Performance of correct procedure (operation) on wrong side
Performance of correct procedure (operation) on wrong site

Y65.8 Other specified misadventures during surgical and medical care
Coding Clinic: 2019, Q2, P24

Y66 Nonadministration of surgical and medical care
Premature cessation of surgical and medical care

Excludes1 DNR status (Z66)
palliative care (Z51.5)

Y69 Unspecified misadventure during surgical and medical care

MEDICAL DEVICES ASSOCIATED WITH ADVERSE INCIDENTS IN DIAGNOSTIC AND THERAPEUTIC USE (Y70-Y82)

Includes breakdown or malfunction of medical devices (during use) (after implantation) (ongoing use)

Excludes2 later complications following use of medical devices without breakdown or malfunctioning of device (Y83-Y84)
misadventure to patients during surgical and medical care, classifiable to (Y62-Y69)
surgical and other medical procedures as the cause of abnormal reaction of the patient, or of later complication, without mention of misadventure at the time of the procedure (Y83-Y84)

● Y70 Anesthesiology devices associated with adverse incidents

Y70.0 Diagnostic and monitoring anesthesiology devices associated with adverse incidents

Y70.1 Therapeutic (nonsurgical) and rehabilitative anesthesiology devices associated with adverse incidents

Y70.2 Prosthetic and other implants, materials and accessory anesthesiology devices associated with adverse incidents

Y70.3 Surgical instruments, materials and anesthesiology devices (including sutures) associated with adverse incidents

Y70.8 Miscellaneous anesthesiology devices associated with adverse incidents, not elsewhere classified

● Y71 Cardiovascular devices associated with adverse incidents

Y71.0 Diagnostic and monitoring cardiovascular devices associated with adverse incidents

Y71.1 Therapeutic (nonsurgical) and rehabilitative cardiovascular devices associated with adverse incidents

Y71.2 Prosthetic and other implants, materials and accessory cardiovascular devices associated with adverse incidents

Y71.3 Surgical instruments, materials and cardiovascular devices (including sutures) associated with adverse incidents

Y71.8 Miscellaneous cardiovascular devices associated with adverse incidents, not elsewhere classified

● Y72 Otorhinolaryngological devices associated with adverse incidents

Y72.0 Diagnostic and monitoring otorhinolaryngological devices associated with adverse incidents

Y72.1 Therapeutic (nonsurgical) and rehabilitative otorhinolaryngological devices associated with adverse incidents

Y72.2 Prosthetic and other implants, materials and accessory otorhinolaryngological devices associated with adverse incidents

Y72.3 Surgical instruments, materials and otorhinolaryngological devices (including sutures) associated with adverse incidents

Y72.8 Miscellaneous otorhinolaryngological devices associated with adverse incidents, not elsewhere classified

● Y73 Gastroenterology and urology devices associated with adverse incidents

Y73.0 Diagnostic and monitoring gastroenterology and urology devices associated with adverse incidents

Y73.1 Therapeutic (nonsurgical) and rehabilitative gastroenterology and urology devices associated with adverse incidents

Y73.2 Prosthetic and other implants, materials and accessory gastroenterology and urology devices associated with adverse incidents

Y73.3   Surgical instruments, materials and gastroenterology and urology devices (including sutures) associated with adverse incidents

Y73.8   Miscellaneous gastroenterology and urology devices associated with adverse incidents, not elsewhere classified

● Y74   General hospital and personal-use devices associated with adverse incidents

Y74.0   Diagnostic and monitoring general hospital and personal-use devices associated with adverse incidents

Y74.1   Therapeutic (nonsurgical) and rehabilitative general hospital and personal-use devices associated with adverse incidents

Y74.2   Prosthetic and other implants, materials and accessory general hospital and personal-use devices associated with adverse incidents

Y74.3   Surgical instruments, materials and general hospital and personal-use devices (including sutures) associated with adverse incidents

Y74.8   Miscellaneous general hospital and personal-use devices associated with adverse incidents, not elsewhere classified

● Y75   Neurological devices associated with adverse incidents

Y75.0   Diagnostic and monitoring neurological devices associated with adverse incidents

Y75.1   Therapeutic (nonsurgical) and rehabilitative neurological devices associated with adverse incidents

Y75.2   Prosthetic and other implants, materials and neurological devices associated with adverse incidents

Y75.3   Surgical instruments, materials and neurological devices (including sutures) associated with adverse incidents

Y75.8   Miscellaneous neurological devices associated with adverse incidents, not elsewhere classified

● Y76   Obstetric and gynecological devices associated with adverse incidents

Y76.0   Diagnostic and monitoring obstetric and gynecological devices associated with adverse incidents ♀

Y76.1   Therapeutic (nonsurgical) and rehabilitative obstetric and gynecological devices associated with adverse incidents ♀

Y76.2   Prosthetic and other implants, materials and accessory obstetric and gynecological devices associated with adverse incidents ♀

Y76.3   Surgical instruments, materials and obstetric and gynecological devices (including sutures) associated with adverse incidents ♀

Y76.8   Miscellaneous obstetric and gynecological devices associated with adverse incidents, not elsewhere classified ♀

● Y77   Ophthalmic devices associated with adverse incidents

Y77.0   Diagnostic and monitoring ophthalmic devices associated with adverse incidents

● Y77.1   Therapeutic (nonsurgical) and rehabilitative ophthalmic devices associated with adverse incidents

Y77.11   Contact lens associated with adverse incidents
Rigid gas permeable contact lens associated with adverse incidents
Soft (hydrophilic) contact lens associated with adverse incidents

Y77.19   Other therapeutic (nonsurgical) and rehabilitative ophthalmic devices associated with adverse incidents

Y77.2   Prosthetic and other implants, materials and accessory ophthalmic devices associated with adverse incidents

Y77.3   Surgical instruments, materials and ophthalmic devices (including sutures) associated with adverse incidents

Y77.8   Miscellaneous ophthalmic devices associated with adverse incidents, not elsewhere classified

● Y78   Radiological devices associated with adverse incidents

Y78.0   Diagnostic and monitoring radiological devices associated with adverse incidents

Y78.1   Therapeutic (nonsurgical) and rehabilitative radiological devices associated with adverse incidents

Y78.2   Prosthetic and other implants, materials and accessory radiological devices associated with adverse incidents

Y78.3   Surgical instruments, materials and radiological devices (including sutures) associated with adverse incidents

Y78.8   Miscellaneous radiological devices associated with adverse incidents, not elsewhere classified

● Y79   Orthopedic devices associated with adverse incidents

Y79.0   Diagnostic and monitoring orthopedic devices associated with adverse incidents

Y79.1   Therapeutic (nonsurgical) and rehabilitative orthopedic devices associated with adverse incidents

Y79.2   Prosthetic and other implants, materials and accessory orthopedic devices associated with adverse incidents

Y79.3   Surgical instruments, materials and orthopedic devices (including sutures) associated with adverse incidents

Y79.8   Miscellaneous orthopedic devices associated with adverse incidents, not elsewhere classified

● Y80   Physical medicine devices associated with adverse incidents

Y80.0   Diagnostic and monitoring physical medicine devices associated with adverse incidents

Y80.1   Therapeutic (nonsurgical) and rehabilitative physical medicine devices associated with adverse incidents

Y80.2   Prosthetic and other implants, materials and accessory physical medicine devices associated with adverse incidents

Y80.3   Surgical instruments, materials and physical medicine devices (including sutures) associated with adverse incidents

Y80.8   Miscellaneous physical medicine devices associated with adverse incidents, not elsewhere classified

● Y81   General- and plastic-surgery devices associated with adverse incidents

Y81.0   Diagnostic and monitoring general- and plastic-surgery devices associated with adverse incidents

Y81.1   Therapeutic (nonsurgical) and rehabilitative general- and plastic-surgery devices associated with adverse incidents

Y81.2   Prosthetic and other implants, materials and accessory general- and plastic-surgery devices associated with adverse incidents

Y81.3   Surgical instruments, materials and general- and plastic-surgery devices (including sutures) associated with adverse incidents

Y81.8   Miscellaneous general- and plastic-surgery devices associated with adverse incidents, not elsewhere classified

● Y82   Other and unspecified medical devices associated with adverse incidents

Y82.8   Other medical devices associated with adverse incidents

Y82.9   Unspecified medical devices associated with adverse incidents

▶ New   ⇒ Revised   ~~deleted~~ Deleted   Excludes 1   Excludes 2   Includes   Use additional   Code first   Code also   Key words

OGCR Official Guidelines   X Assign placeholder X   ● Use Additional Character(s)   ▌ Manifestation Code   ⍟ Hierarchical Condition Category   Coding Clinic

SURGICAL AND OTHER MEDICAL PROCEDURES AS THE CAUSE OF ABNORMAL REACTION OF THE PATIENT, OR OF LATER COMPLICATION, WITHOUT MENTION OF MISADVENTURE AT THE TIME OF THE PROCEDURE (Y83-Y84)

> **Excludes1** misadventures to patients during surgical and medical care, classifiable to (Y62-Y69)
>
> **Excludes2** breakdown or malfunctioning of medical device (after implantation) (during procedure) (ongoing use) (Y70-Y82)

● **Y83 Surgical operation and other surgical procedures as the cause of abnormal reaction of the patient, or of later complication, without mention of misadventure at the time of the procedure**

Y83.0 Surgical operation with transplant of whole organ as the cause of abnormal reaction of the patient, or of later complication, without mention of misadventure at the time of the procedure

Y83.1 Surgical operation with implant of artificial internal device as the cause of abnormal reaction of the patient, or of later complication, without mention of misadventure at the time of the procedure

Y83.2 Surgical operation with anastomosis, bypass or graft as the cause of abnormal reaction of the patient, or of later complication, without mention of misadventure at the time of the procedure

Y83.3 Surgical operation with formation of external stoma as the cause of abnormal reaction of the patient, or of later complication, without mention of misadventure at the time of the procedure

Y83.4 Other reconstructive surgery as the cause of abnormal reaction of the patient, or of later complication, without mention of misadventure at the time of the procedure

Y83.5 Amputation of limb(s) as the cause of abnormal reaction of the patient, or of later complication, without mention of misadventure at the time of the procedure

Y83.6 Removal of other organ (partial) (total) as the cause of abnormal reaction of the patient, or of later complication, without mention of misadventure at the time of the procedure

Y83.8 Other surgical procedures as the cause of abnormal reaction of the patient, or of later complication, without mention of misadventure at the time of the procedure

Y83.9 Surgical procedure, unspecified as the cause of abnormal reaction of the patient, or of later complication, without mention of misadventure at the time of the procedure

● **Y84 Other medical procedures as the cause of abnormal reaction of the patient, or of later complication, without mention of misadventure at the time of the procedure**

Y84.0 Cardiac catheterization as the cause of abnormal reaction of the patient, or of later complication, without mention of misadventure at the time of the procedure

Y84.1 Kidney dialysis as the cause of abnormal reaction of the patient, or of later complication, without mention of misadventure at the time of the procedure

Y84.2 Radiological procedure and radiotherapy as the cause of abnormal reaction of the patient, or of later complication, without mention of misadventure at the time of the procedure
Coding Clinic: 2019, Q1, P21; 2017, Q1, P34

Y84.3 Shock therapy as the cause of abnormal reaction of the patient, or of later complication, without mention of misadventure at the time of the procedure

Y84.4 Aspiration of fluid as the cause of abnormal reaction of the patient, or of later complication, without mention of misadventure at the time of the procedure

Y84.5 Insertion of gastric or duodenal sound as the cause of abnormal reaction of the patient, or of later complication, without mention of misadventure at the time of the procedure

Y84.6 Urinary catheterization as the cause of abnormal reaction of the patient, or of later complication, without mention of misadventure at the time of the procedure

Y84.7 Blood-sampling as the cause of abnormal reaction of the patient, or of later complication, without mention of misadventure at the time of the procedure

Y84.8 Other medical procedures as the cause of abnormal reaction of the patient, or of later complication, without mention of misadventure at the time of the procedure
Coding Clinic: 2021, Q1, P5

Y84.9 Medical procedure, unspecified as the cause of abnormal reaction of the patient, or of later complication, without mention of misadventure at the time of the procedure

SUPPLEMENTARY FACTORS RELATED TO CAUSES OF MORBIDITY CLASSIFIED ELSEWHERE (Y90-Y99)

Note: These categories may be used to provide supplementary information concerning causes of morbidity. They are not to be used for single-condition coding.

● **Y90 Evidence of alcohol involvement determined by blood alcohol level**
Code first any associated alcohol related disorders (F10)

Y90.0 Blood alcohol level of less than 20 mg/100 ml

Y90.1 Blood alcohol level of 20-39 mg/100 ml

Y90.2 Blood alcohol level of 40-59 mg/100 ml

Y90.3 Blood alcohol level of 60-79 mg/100 ml

Y90.4 Blood alcohol level of 80-99 mg/100 ml

Y90.5 Blood alcohol level of 100-119 mg/100 ml

Y90.6 Blood alcohol level of 120-199 mg/100 ml

Y90.7 Blood alcohol level of 200-239 mg/100 ml

Y90.8 Blood alcohol level of 240 mg/100 ml or more

Y90.9 Presence of alcohol in blood, level not specified

OGCR Section I.C.20.b.

> Place of Occurrence Guideline
>
> Codes from category Y92, Place of occurrence of the external cause, are secondary codes for use after other external cause codes to identify the location of the patient at the time of injury or other condition.
>
> Generally, a place of occurrence code is assigned only once, at the initial encounter for treatment. However, in the rare instance that a new injury occurs during hospitalization, an additional place of occurrence code may be assigned. No 7th characters are used for Y92. Only one code from Y92 should be recorded on a medical record.
>
> Do not use place of occurrence code Y92.9 if the place is not stated or is not applicable.

● **Y92 Place of occurrence of the external cause**
The following category is for use, when relevant, to identify the place of occurrence of the external cause. Use in conjunction with an activity code.
Place of occurrence should be recorded only at the initial encounter for treatment

● **Y92.0 Non-institutional (private) residence as the place of occurrence of the external cause**

> **Excludes1** abandoned or derelict house (Y92.89)
> home under construction but not yet occupied (Y92.6-)
> institutional place of residence (Y92.1-)

● **Y92.00** Unspecified non-institutional (private) residence as the place of occurrence of the external cause

Y92.000 Kitchen of unspecified non-institutional (private) residence as the place of occurrence of the external cause

Y92.001 Dining room of unspecified non-institutional (private) residence as the place of occurrence of the external cause

Y92.002 Bathroom of unspecified non-institutional (private) residence as the place of occurrence of the external cause

Y92.003 Bedroom of unspecified non-institutional (private) residence as the place of occurrence of the external cause

Y92.007 Garden or yard of unspecified non-institutional (private) residence as the place of occurrence of the external cause

Y92.008 Other place in unspecified non-institutional (private) residence as the place of occurrence of the external cause

Y92.009 Unspecified place in unspecified non-institutional (private) residence as the place of occurrence of the external cause

Home (NOS) as the place of occurrence of the external cause
Coding Clinic: 2021, Q2, P5

● **Y92.01** Single-family non-institutional (private) house as the place of occurrence of the external cause
Farmhouse as the place of occurrence of the external cause

Excludes1   barn (Y92.71)
chicken coop or hen house (Y92.72)
farm field (Y92.73)
orchard (Y92.74)
single family mobile home or trailer (Y92.02-)
slaughter house (Y92.86)

Y92.010 Kitchen of single-family (private) house as the place of occurrence of the external cause

Y92.011 Dining room of single-family (private) house as the place of occurrence of the external cause

Y92.012 Bathroom of single-family (private) house as the place of occurrence of the external cause

Y92.013 Bedroom of single-family (private) house as the place of occurrence of the external cause

Y92.014 Private driveway to single-family (private) house as the place of occurrence of the external cause

Y92.015 Private garage of single-family (private) house as the place of occurrence of the external cause

Y92.016 Swimming pool in single-family (private) house or garden as the place of occurrence of the external cause

Y92.017 Garden or yard in single-family (private) house as the place of occurrence of the external cause

Y92.018 Other place in single-family (private) house as the place of occurrence of the external cause

Y92.019 Unspecified place in single-family (private) house as the place of occurrence of the external cause

● **Y92.02** Mobile home as the place of occurrence of the external cause

Y92.020 Kitchen in mobile home as the place of occurrence of the external cause

Y92.021 Dining room in mobile home as the place of occurrence of the external cause

Y92.022 Bathroom in mobile home as the place of occurrence of the external cause

Y92.023 Bedroom in mobile home as the place of occurrence of the external cause

Y92.024 Driveway of mobile home as the place of occurrence of the external cause

Y92.025 Garage of mobile home as the place of occurrence of the external cause

Y92.026 Swimming pool of mobile home as the place of occurrence of the external cause

Y92.027 Garden or yard of mobile home as the place of occurrence of the external cause

Y92.028 Other place in mobile home as the place of occurrence of the external cause

Y92.029 Unspecified place in mobile home as the place of occurrence of the external cause

● **Y92.03** Apartment as the place of occurrence of the external cause
Condominium as the place of occurrence of the external cause
Co-op apartment as the place of occurrence of the external cause

Y92.030 Kitchen in apartment as the place of occurrence of the external cause

Y92.031 Bathroom in apartment as the place of occurrence of the external cause

Y92.032 Bedroom in apartment as the place of occurrence of the external cause

Y92.038 Other place in apartment as the place of occurrence of the external cause

Y92.039 Unspecified place in apartment as the place of occurrence of the external cause

● **Y92.04** Boarding-house as the place of occurrence of the external cause

Y92.040 Kitchen in boarding-house as the place of occurrence of the external cause

Y92.041 Bathroom in boarding-house as the place of occurrence of the external cause

Y92.042 Bedroom in boarding-house as the place of occurrence of the external cause

Y92.043 Driveway of boarding-house as the place of occurrence of the external cause

Y92.044 Garage of boarding-house as the place of occurrence of the external cause

Y92.045 Swimming pool of boarding-house as the place of occurrence of the external cause

Y92.046 Garden or yard of boarding-house as the place of occurrence of the external cause

Y92.048　Other place in boarding-house as the place of occurrence of the external cause

Y92.049　Unspecified place in boarding-house as the place of occurrence of the external cause

● Y92.09　Other non-institutional residence as the place of occurrence of the external cause

Y92.090　Kitchen in other non-institutional residence as the place of occurrence of the external cause

Y92.091　Bathroom in other non-institutional residence as the place of occurrence of the external cause

Y92.092　Bedroom in other non-institutional residence as the place of occurrence of the external cause

Y92.093　Driveway of other non-institutional residence as the place of occurrence of the external cause

Y92.094　Garage of other non-institutional residence as the place of occurrence of the external cause

Y92.095　Swimming pool of other non-institutional residence as the place of occurrence of the external cause

Y92.096　Garden or yard of other non-institutional residence as the place of occurrence of the external cause

Y92.098　Other place in other non-institutional residence as the place of occurrence of the external cause

Y92.099　Unspecified place in other non-institutional residence as the place of occurrence of the external cause
　　　　　Coding Clinic: 2017, Q2, P10

● Y92.1　Institutional (nonprivate) residence as the place of occurrence of the external cause

Y92.10　Unspecified residential institution as the place of occurrence of the external cause

● Y92.11　Children's home and orphanage as the place of occurrence of the external cause

Y92.110　Kitchen in children's home and orphanage as the place of occurrence of the external cause

Y92.111　Bathroom in children's home and orphanage as the place of occurrence of the external cause

Y92.112　Bedroom in children's home and orphanage as the place of occurrence of the external cause

Y92.113　Driveway of children's home and orphanage as the place of occurrence of the external cause

Y92.114　Garage of children's home and orphanage as the place of occurrence of the external cause

Y92.115　Swimming pool of children's home and orphanage as the place of occurrence of the external cause

Y92.116　Garden or yard of children's home and orphanage as the place of occurrence of the external cause

Y92.118　Other place in children's home and orphanage as the place of occurrence of the external cause

Y92.119　Unspecified place in children's home and orphanage as the place of occurrence of the external cause

● Y92.12　Nursing home as the place of occurrence of the external cause
　　　　Home for the sick as the place of occurrence of the external cause
　　　　Hospice as the place of occurrence of the external cause

Y92.120　Kitchen in nursing home as the place of occurrence of the external cause

Y92.121　Bathroom in nursing home as the place of occurrence of the external cause

Y92.122　Bedroom in nursing home as the place of occurrence of the external cause

Y92.123　Driveway of nursing home as the place of occurrence of the external cause

Y92.124　Garage of nursing home as the place of occurrence of the external cause

Y92.125　Swimming pool of nursing home as the place of occurrence of the external cause

Y92.126　Garden or yard of nursing home as the place of occurrence of the external cause

Y92.128　Other place in nursing home as the place of occurrence of the external cause

Y92.129　Unspecified place in nursing home as the place of occurrence of the external cause
　　　　　Coding Clinic: 2017, Q2, P10

● Y92.13　Military base as the place of occurrence of the external cause

Excludes1　military training grounds (Y92.83)

Y92.130　Kitchen on military base as the place of occurrence of the external cause

Y92.131　Mess hall on military base as the place of occurrence of the external cause

Y92.133　Barracks on military base as the place of occurrence of the external cause

Y92.135　Garage on military base as the place of occurrence of the external cause

Y92.136　Swimming pool on military base as the place of occurrence of the external cause

Y92.137　Garden or yard on military base as the place of occurrence of the external cause

Y92.138　Other place on military base as the place of occurrence of the external cause

Y92.139　Unspecified place military base as the place of occurrence of the external cause

● Y92.14　Prison as the place of occurrence of the external cause

Y92.140　Kitchen in prison as the place of occurrence of the external cause

Y92.141　Dining room in prison as the place of occurrence of the external cause

Y92.142　Bathroom in prison as the place of occurrence of the external cause

Y92.143　Cell of prison as the place of occurrence of the external cause

Y92.146   Swimming pool of prison as the place of occurrence of the external cause

Y92.147   Courtyard of prison as the place of occurrence of the external cause

Y92.148   Other place in prison as the place of occurrence of the external cause

Y92.149   Unspecified place in prison as the place of occurrence of the external cause

● Y92.15   Reform school as the place of occurrence of the external cause

Y92.150   Kitchen in reform school as the place of occurrence of the external cause

Y92.151   Dining room in reform school as the place of occurrence of the external cause

Y92.152   Bathroom in reform school as the place of occurrence of the external cause

Y92.153   Bedroom in reform school as the place of occurrence of the external cause

Y92.154   Driveway of reform school as the place of occurrence of the external cause

Y92.155   Garage of reform school as the place of occurrence of the external cause

Y92.156   Swimming pool of reform school as the place of occurrence of the external cause

Y92.157   Garden or yard of reform school as the place of occurrence of the external cause

Y92.158   Other place in reform school as the place of occurrence of the external cause

Y92.159   Unspecified place in reform school as the place of occurrence of the external cause

● Y92.16   School dormitory as the place of occurrence of the external cause

Excludes1   reform school as the place of occurrence of the external cause (Y92.15-)
school buildings and grounds as the place of occurrence of the external cause (Y92.2-)
school sports and athletic areas as the place of occurrence of the external cause (Y92.3-)

Y92.160   Kitchen in school dormitory as the place of occurrence of the external cause

Y92.161   Dining room in school dormitory as the place of occurrence of the external cause

Y92.162   Bathroom in school dormitory as the place of occurrence of the external cause

Y92.163   Bedroom in school dormitory as the place of occurrence of the external cause

Y92.168   Other place in school dormitory as the place of occurrence of the external cause

Y92.169   Unspecified place in school dormitory as the place of occurrence of the external cause

● Y92.19   Other specified residential institution as the place of occurrence of the external cause

Y92.190   Kitchen in other specified residential institution as the place of occurrence of the external cause

Y92.191   Dining room in other specified residential institution as the place of occurrence of the external cause

Y92.192   Bathroom in other specified residential institution as the place of occurrence of the external cause

Y92.193   Bedroom in other specified residential institution as the place of occurrence of the external cause

Y92.194   Driveway of other specified residential institution as the place of occurrence of the external cause

Y92.195   Garage of other specified residential institution as the place of occurrence of the external cause

Y92.196   Pool of other specified residential institution as the place of occurrence of the external cause

Y92.197   Garden or yard of other specified residential institution as the place of occurrence of the external cause

Y92.198   Other place in other specified residential institution as the place of occurrence of the external cause
Coding Clinic: 2017, Q2, P11

Y92.199   Unspecified place in other specified residential institution as the place of occurrence of the external cause
Coding Clinic: 2017, Q2, P10

● Y92.2   School, other institution and public administrative area as the place of occurrence of the external cause
Building and adjacent grounds used by the general public or by a particular group of the public

Excludes1   building under construction as the place of occurrence of the external cause (Y92.6)
residential institution as the place of occurrence of the external cause (Y92.1)
school dormitory as the place of occurrence of the external cause (Y92.16-)
sports and athletics area of schools as the place of occurrence of the external cause (Y92.3-)

● Y92.21   School (private) (public) (state) as the place of occurrence of the external cause

Y92.210   Daycare center as the place of occurrence of the external cause

Y92.211   Elementary school as the place of occurrence of the external cause
Kindergarten as the place of occurrence of the external cause

Y92.212   Middle school as the place of occurrence of the external cause

Y92.213   High school as the place of occurrence of the external cause
Coding Clinic: 2012, Q4, P108

Y92.214   College as the place of occurrence of the external cause
University as the place of occurrence of the external cause

Y92.215   Trade school as the place of occurrence of the external cause

Y92.218   Other school as the place of occurrence of the external cause

Y92.219   Unspecified school as the place of occurrence of the external cause

Y92.22 Religious institution as the place of occurrence of the external cause
  Church as the place of occurrence of the external cause
  Mosque as the place of occurrence of the external cause
  Synagogue as the place of occurrence of the external cause

● **Y92.23 Hospital** as the place of occurrence of the external cause

  Excludes1 ambulatory (outpatient) health services establishments (Y92.53-)
  home for the sick as the place of occurrence of the external cause (Y92.12-)
  hospice as the place of occurrence of the external cause (Y92.12-)
  nursing home as the place of occurrence of the external cause (Y92.12-)

  Y92.230 **Patient room** in hospital as the place of occurrence of the external cause
  Y92.231 **Patient bathroom** in hospital as the place of occurrence of the external cause
  Y92.232 **Corridor** of hospital as the place of occurrence of the external cause
  Y92.233 **Cafeteria** of hospital as the place of occurrence of the external cause
  Y92.234 **Operating room** of hospital as the place of occurrence of the external cause
  Y92.238 **Other place** in hospital as the place of occurrence of the external cause
  Y92.239 **Unspecified** place in hospital as the place of occurrence of the external cause

● **Y92.24 Public administrative building** as the place of occurrence of the external cause
  Y92.240 **Courthouse** as the place of occurrence of the external cause
  Y92.241 **Library** as the place of occurrence of the external cause
  Y92.242 **Post office** as the place of occurrence of the external cause
  Y92.243 **City hall** as the place of occurrence of the external cause
  Y92.248 **Other** public administrative building as the place of occurrence of the external cause

● **Y92.25 Cultural building** as the place of occurrence of the external cause
  Y92.250 **Art gallery** as the place of occurrence of the external cause
  Y92.251 **Museum** as the place of occurrence of the external cause
  Y92.252 **Music hall** as the place of occurrence of the external cause
  Y92.253 **Opera house** as the place of occurrence of the external cause
  Y92.254 **Theater (live)** as the place of occurrence of the external cause
  Y92.258 **Other cultural public building** as the place of occurrence of the external cause

  Y92.26 Movie house or cinema as the place of occurrence of the external cause

  Y92.29 Other specified public building as the place of occurrence of the external cause
  Assembly hall as the place of occurrence of the external cause
  Clubhouse as the place of occurrence of the external cause

● **Y92.3 Sports and athletics area** as the place of occurrence of the external cause

● **Y92.31 Athletic court** as the place of occurrence of the external cause

  Excludes1 tennis court in private home or garden (Y92.09)

  Y92.310 **Basketball court** as the place of occurrence of the external cause
  Y92.311 **Squash court** as the place of occurrence of the external cause
  Y92.312 **Tennis court** as the place of occurrence of the external cause
  Y92.318 **Other athletic court** as the place of occurrence of the external cause

● **Y92.32 Athletic field** as the place of occurrence of the external cause
  Y92.320 **Baseball field** as the place of occurrence of the external cause
  Y92.321 **Football field** as the place of occurrence of the external cause
  Y92.322 **Soccer field** as the place of occurrence of the external cause
  Y92.328 **Other athletic field** as the place of occurrence of the external cause
    Cricket field as the place of occurrence of the external cause
    Hockey field as the place of occurrence of the external cause

● **Y92.33 Skating rink** as the place of occurrence of the external cause
  Y92.330 **Ice skating rink (indoor) (outdoor)** as the place of occurrence of the external cause
  Y92.331 **Roller skating rink** as the place of occurrence of the external cause

  Y92.34 Swimming pool (public) as the place of occurrence of the external cause

  Excludes1 swimming pool in private home or garden (Y92.016)

  Y92.39 Other specified sports and athletic area as the place of occurrence of the external cause
    Golf-course as the place of occurrence of the external cause
    Gymnasium as the place of occurrence of the external cause
    Riding-school as the place of occurrence of the external cause
    Stadium as the place of occurrence of the external cause

● **Y92.4 Street, highway and other paved roadways** as the place of occurrence of the external cause

  Excludes1 private driveway of residence (Y92.014, Y92.024, Y92.043, Y92.093, Y92.113, Y92.123, Y92.154, Y92.194)

● **Y92.41 Street and highway** as the place of occurrence of the external cause
  Y92.410 **Unspecified** street and highway as the place of occurrence of the external cause
    Road NOS as the place of occurrence of the external cause
  Y92.411 **Interstate highway** as the place of occurrence of the external cause
    Freeway as the place of occurrence of the external cause
    Motorway as the place of occurrence of the external cause
  Y92.412 **Parkway** as the place of occurrence of the external cause
  Y92.413 **State road** as the place of occurrence of the external cause

Y92.414   Local residential or business street as the place of occurrence of the external cause

Y92.415   Exit ramp or entrance ramp of street or highway as the place of occurrence of the external cause

● **Y92.48**   Other paved roadways as the place of occurrence of the external cause

Y92.480   Sidewalk as the place of occurrence of the external cause

Y92.481   Parking lot as the place of occurrence of the external cause

Y92.482   Bike path as the place of occurrence of the external cause

Y92.488   Other paved roadways as the place of occurrence of the external cause

● **Y92.5**   Trade and service area as the place of occurrence of the external cause

> **Excludes1**   garage in private home (Y92.015)
> schools and other public administration buildings (Y92.2-)

● **Y92.51**   Private commercial establishments as the place of occurrence of the external cause

Y92.510   Bank as the place of occurrence of the external cause

Y92.511   Restaurant or café as the place of occurrence of the external cause

Y92.512   Supermarket, store or market as the place of occurrence of the external cause

Y92.513   Shop (commercial) as the place of occurrence of the external cause

● **Y92.52**   Service areas as the place of occurrence of the external cause

Y92.520   Airport as the place of occurrence of the external cause

Y92.521   Bus station as the place of occurrence of the external cause

Y92.522   Railway station as the place of occurrence of the external cause

Y92.523   Highway rest stop as the place of occurrence of the external cause

Y92.524   Gas station as the place of occurrence of the external cause
> Petroleum station as the place of occurrence of the external cause
> Service station as the place of occurrence of the external cause

● **Y92.53**   Ambulatory health services establishments as the place of occurrence of the external cause

Y92.530   Ambulatory surgery center as the place of occurrence of the external cause
> Outpatient surgery center, including that connected with a hospital as the place of occurrence of the external cause
> Same day surgery center, including that connected with a hospital as the place of occurrence of the external cause

Y92.531   Health care provider office as the place of occurrence of the external cause
> Physician office as the place of occurrence of the external cause

Y92.532   Urgent care center as the place of occurrence of the external cause

Y92.538   Other ambulatory health services establishments as the place of occurrence of the external cause
> **Coding Clinic: 2019, Q1, P21**

Y92.59   Other trade areas as the place of occurrence of the external cause
> Office building as the place of occurrence of the external cause
> Casino as the place of occurrence of the external cause
> Garage (commercial) as the place of occurrence of the external cause
> Hotel as the place of occurrence of the external cause
> Radio or television station as the place of occurrence of the external cause
> Shopping mall as the place of occurrence of the external cause
> Warehouse as the place of occurrence of the external cause

● **Y92.6**   Industrial and construction area as the place of occurrence of the external cause

Y92.61   Building [any] under construction as the place of occurrence of the external cause

Y92.62   Dock or shipyard as the place of occurrence of the external cause
> Dockyard as the place of occurrence of the external cause
> Dry dock as the place of occurrence of the external cause
> Shipyard as the place of occurrence of the external cause

Y92.63   Factory as the place of occurrence of the external cause
> Factory building as the place of occurrence of the external cause
> Factory premises as the place of occurrence of the external cause
> Industrial yard as the place of occurrence of the external cause

Y92.64   Mine or pit as the place of occurrence of the external cause
> Mine as the place of occurrence of the external cause

Y92.65   Oil rig as the place of occurrence of the external cause
> Pit (coal) (gravel) (sand) as the place of occurrence of the external cause

Y92.69   Other specified industrial and construction area as the place of occurrence of the external cause
> Gasworks as the place of occurrence of the external cause
> Power-station (coal) (nuclear) (oil) as the place of occurrence of the external cause
> Tunnel under construction as the place of occurrence of the external cause
> Workshop as the place of occurrence of the external cause

● **Y92.7**   Farm as the place of occurrence of the external cause
> Ranch as the place of occurrence of the external cause
> **Excludes1**   farmhouse and home premises of farm (Y92.01-)

Y92.71   Barn as the place of occurrence of the external cause

Y92.72   Chicken coop as the place of occurrence of the external cause
> Hen house as the place of occurrence of the external cause

Y92.73   Farm field as the place of occurrence of the external cause

Y92.74   Orchard as the place of occurrence of the external cause

Y92.79   Other farm location as the place of occurrence of the external cause

▶ New   ⇒ Revised   ~~deleted~~ Deleted   Excludes 1   Excludes 2   Includes   Use additional   Code first   Code also   Key words

OGCR Official Guidelines   **X** Assign placeholder X   ● Use Additional Character(s)   ▶ Manifestation Code   🍄 Hierarchical Condition Category   **Coding Clinic**

● **Y92.8** **Other places** as the place of occurrence of the external cause

　● **Y92.81** **Transport vehicle** as the place of occurrence of the external cause

　　　Excludes1　transport accidents (V00-V99)

　　　Y92.810　**Car** as the place of occurrence of the external cause

　　　Y92.811　**Bus** as the place of occurrence of the external cause

　　　Y92.812　**Truck** as the place of occurrence of the external cause

　　　Y92.813　**Airplane** as the place of occurrence of the external cause

　　　Y92.814　**Boat** as the place of occurrence of the external cause

　　　Y92.815　**Train** as the place of occurrence of the external cause

　　　Y92.816　**Subway car** as the place of occurrence of the external cause

　　　Y92.818　**Other transport vehicle** as the place of occurrence of the external cause

　● **Y92.82** **Wilderness area**

　　　Y92.820　**Desert** as the place of occurrence of the external cause

　　　Y92.821　**Forest** as the place of occurrence of the external cause

　　　Y92.828　**Other wilderness area** as the place of occurrence of the external cause

　　　　　　Swamp as the place of occurrence of the external cause

　　　　　　Mountain as the place of occurrence of the external cause

　　　　　　Marsh as the place of occurrence of the external cause

　　　　　　Prairie as the place of occurrence of the external cause

　● **Y92.83** **Recreation area** as the place of occurrence of the external cause

　　　Y92.830　**Public park** as the place of occurrence of the external cause

　　　Y92.831　**Amusement park** as the place of occurrence of the external cause

　　　Y92.832　**Beach** as the place of occurrence of the external cause

　　　　　　Seashore as the place of occurrence of the external cause

　　　Y92.833　**Campsite** as the place of occurrence of the external cause

　　　Y92.834　**Zoological garden (zoo)** as the place of occurrence of the external cause

　　　Y92.838　**Other recreation area** as the place of occurrence of the external cause

　　Y92.84 **Military training ground** as the place of occurrence of the external cause

　　Y92.85 **Railroad track** as the place of occurrence of the external cause

　　Y92.86 **Slaughter house** as the place of occurrence of the external cause

　　Y92.89 **Other specified places** as the place of occurrence of the external cause

　　　　　Derelict house as the place of occurrence of the external cause

OGCR Section I.C.20.b.

Do not use place of occurrence code Y92.9 if the place is not stated or is not applicable.

Y92.9 **Unspecified place** or not applicable

OGCR　See Section I.C.20.c.

Activity Code

Assign a code from category Y93, Activity code, to describe the activity of the patient at the time the injury or other health condition occurred.

An activity code is used only once, at the initial encounter for treatment. Only one code from Y93 should be recorded on a medical record.

The activity codes are not applicable to poisonings, adverse effects, misadventures or sequela.

Do not assign Y93.9, Unspecified activity, if the activity is not stated.

A code from category Y93 is appropriate for use with external cause and intent codes if identifying the activity provides additional information about the event.

● **Y93** **Activity codes**

　Note: Category Y93 is provided for use to indicate the activity of the person seeking healthcare for an injury or health condition, such as a heart attack while shoveling snow, which resulted from, or was contributed to, by the activity. These codes are appropriate for use for both acute injuries, such as those from Chapter 19, and conditions that are due to the long-term, cumulative effects of an activity, such as those from Chapter 13. They are also appropriate for use with external cause codes for cause and intent if identifying the activity provides additional information on the event. These codes should be used in conjunction with codes for external cause status (Y99) and place of occurrence (Y92).

　This section contains the following broad activity categories:

　　Y93.0　Activities involving walking and running

　　Y93.1　Activities involving water and water craft

　　Y93.2　Activities involving ice and snow

　　Y93.3　Activities involving climbing, rappelling, and jumping off

　　Y93.4　Activities involving dancing and other rhythmic movement

　　Y93.5　Activities involving other sports and athletics played individually

　　Y93.6　Activities involving other sports and athletics played as a team or group

　　Y93.7　Activities involving other specified sports and athletics

　　Y93.A　Activities involving other cardiorespiratory exercise

　　Y93.B　Activities involving other muscle strengthening exercises

　　Y93.C　Activities involving computer technology and electronic devices

　　Y93.D　Activities involving arts and handcrafts

　　Y93.E　Activities involving personal hygiene and interior property and clothing maintenance

　　Y93.F　Activities involving caregiving

　　Y93.G　Activities involving food preparation, cooking and grilling

　　Y93.H　Activities involving exterior property and land maintenance, building and construction

　　Y93.I　Activities involving roller coasters and other types of external motion

　　Y93.J　Activities involving playing musical instrument

　　Y93.K　Activities involving animal care

　　Y93.8　Activities, other specified

　　Y93.9　Activity, unspecified

● **Y93.0** **Activities involving walking and running**

　　Excludes1　Activity, walking an animal (Y93.K1)

　　　　　Activity, walking or running on a treadmill (Y93.A1)

　　Y93.01　**Activity, walking, marching and hiking**

　　　　Activity, walking, marching and hiking on level or elevated terrain

　　　　Excludes1　activity, mountain climbing (Y93.31)

　　Y93.02　**Activity, running**

CHAPTER 20 (V00-Y99)

● **Y93.1   Activities involving water and water craft**
        Excludes1   activities involving ice (Y93.2-)

    Y93.11   **Activity, swimming**

    Y93.12   **Activity, springboard and platform diving**

    Y93.13   **Activity, water polo**

    Y93.14   **Activity, water aerobics and water exercise**

    Y93.15   **Activity, underwater diving and snorkeling**
            Activity, SCUBA diving

    Y93.16   **Activity, rowing, canoeing, kayaking, rafting and tubing**
            Activity, canoeing, kayaking, rafting and
                tubing in calm and turbulent water

    Y93.17   **Activity, water skiing and wake boarding**

    Y93.18   **Activity, surfing, windsurfing and boogie boarding**
            Activity, water sliding

    Y93.19   **Activity, other involving water and watercraft**
            Activity involving water NOS
            Activity, parasailing
            Activity, water survival training and testing

● **Y93.2   Activities involving ice and snow**
        Excludes1   activity, shoveling ice and snow (Y93.H1)

    Y93.21   **Activity, ice skating**
            Activity, figure skating (singles) (pairs)
            Activity, ice dancing
            Excludes1   activity, ice hockey (Y93.22)

    Y93.22   **Activity, ice hockey**

    Y93.23   **Activity, snow (alpine) (downhill) skiing, snowboarding, sledding, tobogganing and snow tubing**
            Excludes1   activity, cross country skiing
                        (Y93.24)

    Y93.24   **Activity, cross country skiing**
            Activity, nordic skiing

    Y93.29   **Activity, other activity involving ice and snow**
            Activity, activity involving ice and snow NOS

● **Y93.3   Activities involving climbing, rappelling and jumping off**
        Excludes1   activity, hiking on level or elevated
                        terrain (Y93.01)
                     activity, jumping rope (Y93.56)
                     activity, trampoline jumping (Y93.44)

    Y93.31   **Activity, mountain climbing, rock climbing and wall climbing**

    Y93.32   **Activity, rappelling**

    Y93.33   **Activity, BASE jumping**
            Activity, building, Antenna, Span, Earth
                jumping

    Y93.34   **Activity, bungee jumping**

    Y93.35   **Activity, hang gliding**

    Y93.39   **Activity, other activity involving climbing, rappelling and jumping off**

● **Y93.4   Activities involving dancing and other rhythmic movement**
        Excludes1   activity, martial arts (Y93.75)

    Y93.41   **Activity, dancing**
            Coding Clinic: 2012, Q4, P108

    Y93.42   **Activity, yoga**

    Y93.43   **Activity, gymnastics**
            Activity, rhythmic gymnastics
            Excludes1   activity, trampolining (Y93.44)

    Y93.44   **Activity, trampolining**

    Y93.45   **Activity, cheerleading**

    Y93.49   **Activity, other involving dancing and other rhythmic movements**

● **Y93.5   Activities involving other sports and athletics played individually**
        Excludes1   activity, dancing (Y93.41)
                     activity, gymnastic (Y93.43)
                     activity, trampolining (Y93.44)
                     activity, yoga (Y93.42)

    Y93.51   **Activity, roller skating (inline) and skateboarding**

    Y93.52   **Activity, horseback riding**

    Y93.53   **Activity, golf**

    Y93.54   **Activity, bowling**

    Y93.55   **Activity, bike riding**

    Y93.56   **Activity, jumping rope**

    Y93.57   **Activity, non-running track and field events**
            Excludes1   activity, running (any form)
                        (Y93.02)

    Y93.59   **Activity, other involving other sports and athletics played individually**
            Excludes1   activities involving climbing,
                        rappelling, and jumping
                        (Y93.3-)
                     activities involving ice and snow
                        (Y93.2-)
                     activities involving walking and
                        running (Y93.0-)
                     activities involving water and
                        watercraft (Y93.1-)

● **Y93.6   Activities involving other sports and athletics played as a team or group**
        Excludes1   activity, ice hockey (Y93.22)
                     activity, water polo (Y93.13)

    Y93.61   **Activity, American tackle football**
            Activity, football NOS

    Y93.62   **Activity, American flag or touch football**

    Y93.63   **Activity, rugby**

    Y93.64   **Activity, baseball**
            Activity, softball

    Y93.65   **Activity, lacrosse and field hockey**
            Coding Clinic: 2015, Q1, P9

    Y93.66   **Activity, soccer**

    Y93.67   **Activity, basketball**
            Coding Clinic: 2019, Q4, P18

    Y93.68   **Activity, volleyball (beach) (court)**

    Y93.6A   **Activity, physical games generally associated with school recess, summer camp and children**
            Activity, capture the flag
            Activity, dodge ball
            Activity, four square
            Activity, kickball

    Y93.69   **Activity, other involving other sports and athletics played as a team or group**
            Cricket

● **Y93.7   Activities involving other specified sports and athletics**

    Y93.71   **Activity, boxing**

    Y93.72   **Activity, wrestling**

    Y93.73   **Activity, racquet and hand sports**
            Activity, handball
            Activity, racquetball
            Activity, squash
            Activity, tennis

    Y93.74   **Activity, frisbee**
            Activity, ultimate frisbee

    Y93.75   **Activity, martial arts**
            Activity, combatives

    Y93.79   **Activity, other specified sports and athletics**
            Excludes1   sports and athletics activities
                        specified in categories
                        Y93.0-Y93.6

CHAPTER 20 (V00-Y99)

● **Y93.A** **Activities involving other cardiorespiratory exercise**
　　　Activities involving physical training

　　Y93.A1 **Activity, exercise machines primarily for cardiorespiratory conditioning**
　　　　Activity, elliptical and stepper machines
　　　　Activity, stationary bike
　　　　Activity, treadmill

　　Y93.A2 **Activity, calisthenics**
　　　　Activity, jumping jacks
　　　　Activity, warm up and cool down

　　Y93.A3 **Activity, aerobic and step exercise**

　　Y93.A4 **Activity, circuit training**

　　Y93.A5 **Activity, obstacle course**
　　　　Activity, challenge course
　　　　Activity, confidence course

　　Y93.A6 **Activity, grass drills**
　　　　Activity, guerilla drills

　　Y93.A9 **Activity, other involving other cardiorespiratory exercise**

　　　　Excludes1　activities involving cardiorespiratory exercise specified in categories Y93.0-Y93.7

● **Y93.B** **Activity involving other muscle strengthening exercises**

　　Y93.B1 **Activity, exercise machines primarily for muscle strengthening**

　　Y93.B2 **Activity, push-ups, pull-ups, sit-ups**

　　Y93.B3 **Activity, free weights**
　　　　Activity, barbells
　　　　Activity, dumbbells

　　Y93.B4 **Activity, pilates**

　　Y93.B9 **Activity, other involving other muscle strengthening exercises**

　　　　Excludes1　activities involving muscle strengthening specified in categories Y93.0-Y93.A

● **Y93.C** **Activities involving computer technology and electronic devices**

　　　　Excludes1　activity, electronic musical keyboard or instruments (Y93.J-)

　　Y93.C1 **Activity, computer keyboarding**
　　　　Activity, electronic game playing using keyboard or other stationary device

　　Y93.C2 **Activity, hand held interactive electronic device**
　　　　Activity, cellular telephone and communication device
　　　　Activity, electronic game playing using interactive device

　　　　Excludes1　activity, electronic game playing using keyboard or other stationary device (Y93.C1)

　　Y93.C9 **Activity, other involving computer technology and electronic devices**

● **Y93.D** **Activities involving arts and handcrafts**

　　　　Excludes1　activities involving playing musical instrument (Y93.J-)

　　Y93.D1 **Knitting and crocheting**

　　Y93.D2 **Sewing**

　　Y93.D3 **Furniture building and finishing**
　　　　Furniture repair

　　Y93.D9 **Activity, other involving arts and handcrafts**

● **Y93.E** **Activities involving personal hygiene and interior property and clothing maintenance**

　　　　Excludes1　activities involving cooking and grilling (Y93.G-)
　　　　　　activities involving exterior property and land maintenance, building and construction (Y93.H-)
　　　　　　activity involving caregiving (Y93.F-)
　　　　　　activity, dishwashing (Y93.G1)
　　　　　　activity, food preparation (Y93.G1)
　　　　　　activity, gardening (Y93.H2)

　　Y93.E1 **Activity, personal bathing and showering**

　　Y93.E2 **Activity, laundry**

　　Y93.E3 **Activity, vacuuming**

　　Y93.E4 **Activity, ironing**

　　Y93.E5 **Activity, floor mopping and cleaning**

　　Y93.E6 **Activity, residential relocation**
　　　　Activity, packing up and unpacking involved in moving to a new residence

　　Y93.E8 **Activity, other personal hygiene activity**

　　Y93.E9 **Activity, other household maintenance**

● **Y93.F** **Activities involving person providing caregiving**
　　　Activity involving the provider of caregiving

　　Y93.F1 **Activity, caregiving involving bathing**

　　Y93.F2 **Activity, caregiving involving lifting**
　　　　Coding Clinic: 2016, Q4, P74

　　Y93.F9 **Activity, other caregiving**

● **Y93.G** **Activities involving food preparation, cooking and grilling**

　　Y93.G1 **Activity, food preparation and clean up**
　　　　Activity, dishwashing

　　Y93.G2 **Activity, grilling and smoking food**

　　Y93.G3 **Activity, cooking and baking**
　　　　Activity, use of stove, oven and microwave oven

　　Y93.G9 **Activity, other activity involving cooking and grilling**

● **Y93.H** **Activities involving property and land maintenance, building and construction**

　　Y93.H1 **Activity, digging, shoveling and raking**
　　　　Activity, dirt digging
　　　　Activity, raking leaves
　　　　Activity, snow shoveling

　　Y93.H2 **Activity, gardening and landscaping**
　　　　Activity, pruning, trimming shrubs, weeding

　　Y93.H3 **Activity, building and construction**

　　Y93.H9 **Activity, other activity involving property and land maintenance, building and construction**

● **Y93.I** **Activities involving roller coasters and other types of external motion**

　　Y93.I1 **Activity, rollercoaster riding**

　　Y93.I9 **Activity, other involving external motion**

● **Y93.J** **Activities involving playing musical instrument**
　　　Activity involving playing electric musical instrument

　　Y93.J1 **Activity, piano playing**
　　　　Activity, musical keyboard (electronic) playing

　　Y93.J2 **Activity, drum and other percussion instrument playing**

　　Y93.J3 **Activity, string instrument playing**

　　Y93.J4 **Activity, winds and brass instrument playing**

● Y93.K **Activities involving animal care**
  Excludes1 activity, horseback riding (Y93.52)
  Y93.K1 **Activity, walking an animal**
  Y93.K2 **Activity, milking an animal**
  Y93.K3 **Activity, grooming and shearing an animal**
  Y93.K9 **Activity, other activity involving animal care**

● Y93.8 **Other activity**
  Coding Clinic: 2016, Q4, P74
  Y93.81 **Activity, refereeing a sports activity**
  Y93.82 **Activity, spectator at an event**
  Y93.83 **Activity, rough housing and horseplay**
      Coding Clinic: 2015, Q1, P8
  Y93.84 **Activity, sleeping**
  Y93.85 **Activity, choking game**
      Activity, blackout game
      Activity, fainting game
      Activity, pass out game
      Coding Clinic: 2016, Q4, P74-76
  Y93.89 **Activity, other specified**

  OGCR See Section I.C.20.c.

  Do not assign Y93.9, Unspecified activity, if the activity is not stated.

● Y93.9 **Activity, unspecified**

Y95 **Nosocomial condition**

● Y99 **External cause status**
  Note: A single code from category Y99 should be used in conjunction with the external cause code(s) assigned to a record to indicate the status of the person at the time the event occurred.
  Coding Clinic: 2016, Q4, P74

Y99.0 **Civilian activity done for income or pay**
    Civilian activity done for financial or other compensation
    Excludes1 military activity (Y99.1)
        volunteer activity (Y99.2)

Y99.1 **Military activity**
    Excludes1 activity of off duty military personnel (Y99.8)

Y99.2 **Volunteer activity**
    Excludes1 activity of child or other family member assisting in compensated work of other family member (Y99.8)

Y99.8 **Other external cause status**
    Activity NEC
    Activity of child or other family member assisting in compensated work of other family member
    Hobby not done for income
    Leisure activity
    Off-duty activity of military personnel
    Recreation or sport not for income or while a student
    Student activity
    Excludes1 civilian activity done for income or compensation (Y99.0)
        military activity (Y99.1)
    Coding Clinic: 2012, Q4, P108

Y99.9 **Unspecified external cause status**

CHAPTER 21

FACTORS INFLUENCING HEALTH STATUS AND CONTACT WITH HEALTH SERVICES (Z00-Z99)

OGCR Chapter-Specific Coding Guidelines

21. **Chapter 21: Factors influencing health status and contact with health services (Z00-Z99)**
Note: The chapter specific guidelines provide additional information about the use of Z codes for specified encounters.

a. Use of Z codes in any healthcare setting
Z codes are for use in any healthcare setting. Z codes may be used as either a first-listed (principal diagnosis code in the inpatient setting) or secondary code, depending on the circumstances of the encounter. Certain Z codes may only be used as first-listed or principal diagnosis.

b. Z Codes indicate a reason for an encounter
Z codes are not procedure codes. A corresponding procedure code must accompany a Z code to describe any procedure performed.

c. Categories of Z Codes

1) Contact/Exposure
Category Z20 indicates contact with, and suspected exposure to, communicable diseases. These codes are for patients who do not show any sign or symptom of a disease but are suspected to have been exposed to it by close personal contact with an infected individual or are in an area where a disease is epidemic.

Category Z77, Other contact with and (suspected) exposures hazardous to health, indicates contact with and suspected exposures hazardous to health.

Contact/exposure codes may be used as a first-listed code to explain an encounter for testing, or, more commonly, as a secondary code to identify a potential risk.

2) Inoculations and vaccinations
Code Z23 is for encounters for inoculations and vaccinations. It indicates that a patient is being seen to receive a prophylactic inoculation against a disease. Procedure codes are required to identify the actual administration of the injection and the type(s) of immunizations given. Code Z23 may be used as a secondary code if the inoculation is given as a routine part of preventive health care, such as a well-baby visit.

3) Status
Status codes indicate that a patient is either a carrier of a disease or has the sequelae or residual of a past disease or condition. This includes such things as the presence of prosthetic or mechanical devices resulting from past treatment. A status code is informative, because the status may affect the course of treatment and its outcome. A status code is distinct from a history code. The history code indicates that the patient no longer has the condition.

A status code should not be used with a diagnosis code from one of the body system chapters, if the diagnosis code includes the information provided by the status code. For example, code Z94.1, Heart transplant status, should not be used with a code from subcategory T86.2, Complications of heart transplant. The status code does not provide additional information. The complication code indicates that the patient is a heart transplant patient.

For encounters for weaning from a mechanical ventilator, assign a code from subcategory J96.1, Chronic respiratory failure, followed by code Z99.11, Dependence on respirator [ventilator] status.

The status Z codes/categories are:

Z14   Genetic carrier
Genetic carrier status indicates that a person carries a gene, associated with a particular disease, which may be passed to offspring who may develop that disease. The person does not have the disease and is not at risk of developing the disease.

Z15   Genetic susceptibility to disease Genetic susceptibility indicates that a person has a gene that increases the risk of that person developing the disease.

Codes from category Z15 should not be used as principal or first-listed codes. If the patient has the condition to which he/she is susceptible, and that condition is the reason for the encounter, the code for the current condition should be sequenced first. If the patient is being seen for follow-up after completed treatment for this condition, and the condition no longer exists, a follow-up

code should be sequenced first, followed by the appropriate personal history and genetic susceptibility codes. If the purpose of the encounter is genetic counseling associated with procreative management, code Z31.5, Encounter for genetic counseling, should be assigned as the first-listed code, followed by a code from category Z15. Additional codes should be assigned for any applicable family or personal history.

Z16   Resistance to antimicrobial drugs
This code indicates that a patient has a condition that is resistant to antimicrobial drug treatment. Sequence the infection code first.

Z17   Estrogen receptor status

Z18   Retained foreign body fragments

Z19   Hormone sensitivity malignancy status

Z21   Asymptomatic HIV infection status This code indicates that a patient has tested positive for HIV but has manifested no signs or symptoms of the disease.

Z22   Carrier of infectious disease Carrier status indicates that a person harbors the specific organisms of a disease without manifest symptoms and is capable of transmitting the infection.

Z28.3   Underimmunization status

Z33.1   Pregnant state, incidental This code is a secondary code only for use when the pregnancy is in no way complicating the reason for visit. Otherwise, a code from the obstetric chapter is required.

Z66   Do not resuscitate
This code may be used when it is documented by the provider that a patient is on do not resuscitate status at any time during the stay.

Z67   Blood type

Z68   Body mass index (BMI)
BMI codes should only be assigned when the associated diagnosis (such as overweight or obesity) meets the definition of a reportable diagnosis (see Section III, Reporting Additional Diagnoses). Do not assign BMI codes during pregnancy. See Section I.B.14 for BMI documentation by clinicians other than the patient's provider.

Z74.01   Bed confinement status

Z76.82   Awaiting organ transplant status

Z78   Other specified health status
Code Z78.1, Physical restraint status, may be used when it is documented by the provider that a patient has been put in restraints during the current encounter. Please note that this code should not be reported when it is documented by the provider that a patient is temporarily restrained during a procedure.

Z79   Long-term (current) drug therapy
Codes from this category indicate a patient's continuous use of a prescribed drug (including such things as aspirin therapy) for the long-term treatment of a condition or for prophylactic use. It is not for use for patients who have addictions to drugs. This subcategory is not for use of medications for detoxification or maintenance programs to prevent withdrawal symptoms in patients with drug dependence (e.g., methadone maintenance for opiate dependence). Assign the appropriate code for the drug dependence instead.

Assign a code from Z79 if the patient is receiving a medication for an extended period as a prophylactic measure (such as for the prevention of deep vein thrombosis) or as treatment of a chronic condition (such as arthritis) or a disease requiring a lengthy course of treatment (such as cancer). Do not assign a code from category Z79 for medication being administered for a brief period of time to treat an acute illness or injury (such as a course of antibiotics to treat acute bronchitis).

Z88   Allergy status to drugs, medicaments and biological substances Except: Z88.9, Allergy status to unspecified drugs, medicaments and biological substances status

Z89   Acquired absence of limb

Z90   Acquired absence of organs, not elsewhere classified

Z91.0-   Allergy status, other than to drugs and biological substances

Z92.82   Status post administration of tPA (rtPA) in a different facility within the last 24 hours prior to admission to a current facility Assign code Z92.82, Status post administration of tPA (rtPA) in a different facility within the last 24 hours prior to admission to current facility, as a secondary diagnosis when a patient is received by transfer into a facility and documentation indicates they were administered tissue plasminogen activator (tPA) within the last 24 hours prior to admission to the current facility. This guideline applies even if the patient is still receiving the tPA at the time they are received into the current facility. The appropriate code for the condition for which the tPA was administered (such as cerebrovascular disease or myocardial infarction) should be assigned first. Code Z92.82 is only applicable to the receiving facility record and not to the transferring facility record.

Z93	Artificial opening status
Z94	Transplanted organ and tissue status
Z95	Presence of cardiac and vascular implants and grafts
Z96	Presence of other functional implants
Z97	Presence of other devices
Z98	Other postprocedural states

Assign code Z98.85, Transplanted organ removal status, to indicate that a transplanted organ has been previously removed. This code should not be assigned for the encounter in which the transplanted organ is removed. The complication necessitating removal of the transplant organ should be assigned for that encounter.

See Section I.C.19. for information on the coding of organ transplant complications.

| Z99 | Dependence on enabling machines and devices, not elsewhere classified |

Note: Categories Z89-Z90 and Z93-Z99 are for use only if there are no complications or malfunctions of the organ or tissue replaced, the amputation site or the equipment on which the patient is dependent.

4) History (of)

There are two types of history Z codes, personal and family. Personal history codes explain a patient's past medical condition that no longer exists and is not receiving any treatment, but that has the potential for recurrence, and therefore may require continued monitoring.

Family history codes are for use when a patient has a family member(s) who has had a particular disease that causes the patient to be at higher risk of also contracting the disease.

Personal history codes may be used in conjunction with follow-up codes and family history codes may be used in conjunction with screening codes to explain the need for a test or procedure. History codes are also acceptable on any medical record regardless of the reason for visit. A history of an illness, even if no longer present, is important information that may alter the type of treatment ordered.

The history Z code categories are:

Z80	Family history of primary malignant neoplasm
Z81	Family history of mental and behavioral disorders
Z82	Family history of certain disabilities and chronic diseases (leading to disablement)
Z83	Family history of other specific disorders
Z84	Family history of other conditions
Z85	Personal history of malignant neoplasm
Z86	Personal history of certain other diseases
Z87	Personal history of other diseases and conditions
Z91.4-	Personal history of psychological trauma, not elsewhere classified
Z91.5	Personal history of self-harm
Z91.81	History of falling
Z91.82	Personal history of military deployment
Z92	Personal history of medical treatment Except: Z92.0, Personal history of contraception Except: Z92.82, Status post administration of tPA (rtPA) in a different facility within the last 24 hours prior to admission to a current facility

5) Screening

Screening is the testing for disease or disease precursors in seemingly well individuals so that early detection and treatment can be provided for those who test positive for the disease (e.g., screening mammogram).

The testing of a person to rule out or confirm a suspected diagnosis because the patient has some sign or symptom is a diagnostic examination, not a screening. In these cases, the sign or symptom is used to explain the reason for the test.

A screening code may be a first-listed code if the reason for the visit is specifically the screening exam. It may also be used as an additional code if the screening is done during an office visit for other health problems. A screening code is not necessary if the screening is inherent to a routine examination, such as a pap smear done during a routine pelvic examination.

Should a condition be discovered during the screening then the code for the condition may be assigned as an additional diagnosis.

The Z code indicates that a screening exam is planned. A procedure code is required to confirm that the screening was performed.

The screening Z codes/categories:

Z11	Encounter for screening for infectious and parasitic diseases
Z12	Encounter for screening for malignant neoplasms
Z13	Encounter for screening for other diseases and disorders Except: Z13.9, Encounter for screening, unspecified
Z36	Encounter for antenatal screening for mother

6) Observation

There are three observation Z code categories. They are for use in very limited circumstances when a person is being observed for a suspected condition that is ruled out. The observation codes are not for use if an injury or illness or any signs or symptoms related to the suspected condition are present. In such cases the diagnosis/symptom code is used with the corresponding external cause code.

The observation codes are to be used as principal diagnosis only. The only exception to this is when the principal diagnosis is required to be a code from category Z38, Liveborn infants according to place of birth and type of delivery. Then a code from category Z05, Encounter for observation and evaluation of newborn for suspected diseases and conditions ruled out, is sequenced after the Z38 code. Additional codes may be used in addition to the observation code but only if they are unrelated to the suspected condition being observed.

Codes from subcategory Z03.7 Encounter for suspected maternal and fetal conditions ruled out, may either be used as a first-listed or as an additional code assignment depending on the case. They are for use in very limited circumstances on a maternal record when an encounter is for a suspected maternal or fetal condition that is ruled out during that encounter (for example, a maternal or fetal condition may be suspected due to an abnormal test result). These codes should not be used when the condition is confirmed. In those cases, the confirmed condition should be coded. In addition, these codes are not for use if an illness or any signs or symptoms related to the suspected condition or problem are present. In such cases the diagnosis/symptom code is used.

Additional codes may be used in addition to the code from subcategory Z03.7, but only if they are unrelated to the suspected condition being evaluated.

Codes from subcategory Z03.7 may not be used for encounters for antenatal screening of mother. *See Section I.C.21. Screening.*

For encounters for suspected fetal condition that are inconclusive following testing and evaluation, assign the appropriate code from category O35, O36, O40 or O41.

The observation Z code categories:

Z03	Encounter for medical observation for suspected diseases and conditions ruled out
Z04	Encounter for examination and observation for other reasons Except: Z04.9, Encounter for examination and observation for unspecified reason
Z05	Encounter for observation and evaluation of newborn for suspected diseases and conditions ruled out

7) Aftercare

Aftercare visit codes cover situations when the initial treatment of a disease has been performed and the patient requires continued care during the healing or recovery phase, or for the long-term consequences of the disease. The aftercare Z code should not be used if treatment is directed at a current, acute disease. The diagnosis code is to be used in these cases.

Exceptions to this rule are codes Z51.0, Encounter for antineoplastic radiation therapy, and codes from subcategory Z51.1, Encounter for antineoplastic chemotherapy and immunotherapy. These codes are to be first-listed, followed by the diagnosis code when a patient's encounter is solely to receive radiation therapy, chemotherapy, or immunotherapy for the treatment of a neoplasm. If the reason for the encounter is more than one type of antineoplastic therapy, code Z51.0 and a code from subcategory Z51.1 may be assigned together, in which case one of these codes would be reported as a secondary diagnosis.

The aftercare Z codes should also not be used for aftercare for injuries. For aftercare of an injury, assign the acute injury code with the appropriate 7th character (for subsequent encounter).

The aftercare codes are generally first-listed to explain the specific reason for the encounter. An aftercare code may be used as an additional code when some type of aftercare is provided in addition to the reason for admission and no diagnosis code is applicable. An example of this would be the closure of a colostomy during an encounter for treatment of another condition.

Aftercare codes should be used in conjunction with other aftercare codes or diagnosis codes to provide better detail on the specifics of an aftercare encounter visit, unless otherwise directed by the classification. Should a patient receive multiple types of antineoplastic therapy during the same encounter, code Z51.0, Encounter for antineoplastic radiation therapy, and codes from subcategory Z51.1, Encounter for antineoplastic chemotherapy and immunotherapy, may be used together on a record. The sequencing of multiple aftercare codes depends on the circumstances of the encounter.

Certain aftercare Z code categories need a secondary diagnosis code to describe the resolving condition or sequelae. For others, the condition is included in the code title.

Additional Z code aftercare category terms include fitting and adjustment, and attention to artificial openings.

Status Z codes may be used with aftercare Z codes to indicate the nature of the aftercare. For example code Z95.1, Presence of aortocoronary bypass graft, may be used with code Z48.812, Encounter for surgical aftercare following surgery on the circulatory system, to indicate the surgery for which the aftercare is being performed. A status code should not be used when the aftercare code indicates the type of status, such as using Z43.0, Encounter for attention to tracheostomy, with Z93.0, Tracheostomy status.

The aftercare Z category/codes:

Z42	Encounter for plastic and reconstructive surgery following medical procedure or healed injury
Z43	Encounter for attention to artificial openings
Z44	Encounter for fitting and adjustment of external prosthetic device
Z45	Encounter for adjustment and management of implanted device
Z46	Encounter for fitting and adjustment of other devices
Z47	Orthopedic aftercare
Z48	Encounter for other postprocedural aftercare
Z49	Encounter for care involving renal dialysis
Z51	Encounter for other aftercare and medical care

8) Follow-up

The follow-up codes are used to explain continuing surveillance following completed treatment of a disease, condition, or injury. They imply that the condition has been fully treated and no longer exists. They should not be confused with aftercare codes, or injury codes with a 7th character for subsequent encounter, that explain ongoing care of a healing condition or its sequelae. Follow-up codes may be used in conjunction with history codes to provide the full picture of the healed condition and its treatment. The follow-up code is sequenced first, followed by the history code.

A follow-up code may be used to explain multiple visits. Should a condition be found to have recurred on the follow-up visit, then the diagnosis code for the condition should be assigned in place of the follow-up code.

The follow-up Z code categories:

Z08	Encounter for follow-up examination after completed treatment for malignant neoplasm
Z09	Encounter for follow-up examination after completed treatment for conditions other than malignant neoplasm
Z39	Encounter for maternal postpartum care and examination

9) Donor

Codes in category Z52, Donors of organs and tissues, are used for living individuals who are donating blood or other body tissue.

These codes are only for individuals donating for others, not for self-donations. They are not used to identify cadaveric donations.

10) Counseling

Counseling Z codes are used when a patient or family member receives assistance in the aftermath of an illness or injury, or when support is required in coping with family or social problems.

The counseling Z codes/categories:

Z30.0-	Encounter for general counseling and advice on contraception
Z31.5	Encounter for procreative genetic counseling
Z31.6-	Encounter for general counseling and advice on procreation
Z32.2	Encounter for childbirth instruction
Z32.3	Encounter for childcare instruction
Z69	Encounter for mental health services for victim and perpetrator of abuse
Z70	Counseling related to sexual attitude, behavior and orientation
Z71	Persons encountering health services for other counseling and medical advice, not elsewhere classified
Z76.81	Expectant mother prebirth pediatrician visit

11) Encounters for Obstetrical and Reproductive Services

See Section I.C.15. Pregnancy, Childbirth, and the Puerperium, for further instruction on the use of these codes.

Z codes for pregnancy are for use in those circumstances when none of the problems or complications included in the codes from the Obstetrics chapter exist (a routine prenatal visit or postpartum care). Codes in category Z34, Encounter for supervision of normal pregnancy, are always first listed and are not to be used with any other code from the OB chapter.

Codes in category Z3A, Weeks of gestation, may be assigned to provide additional information about the pregnancy. Category Z3A codes should not be assigned for pregnancies with abortive outcomes (categories O00-O08), elective termination of pregnancy (code Z33.2), nor for postpartum conditions, as category Z3A is not applicable to these conditions. The date of the admission should be used to determine weeks of gestation for inpatient admissions that encompass more than one gestational week.

The outcome of delivery, category Z37, should be included on all maternal delivery records. It is always a secondary code. Codes in category Z37 should not be used on the newborn record.

Z codes for family planning (contraceptive) or procreative management and counseling should be included on an obstetric record either during the pregnancy or the postpartum stage, if applicable.

Z codes/categories for obstetrical and reproductive services:

Z30	Encounter for contraceptive management
Z31	Encounter for procreative management
Z32.2	Encounter for childbirth instruction
Z32.3	Encounter for childcare instruction
Z33	Pregnant state
Z34	Encounter for supervision of normal pregnancy
Z36	Encounter for antenatal screening of mother
Z3A	Weeks of gestation
Z37	Outcome of delivery
Z39	Encounter for maternal postpartum care and examination
Z76.81	Expectant mother prebirth pediatrician visit

12) Newborns and Infants

See Section I.C.16. Newborn (Perinatal) Guidelines, for further instruction on the use of these codes.

Newborn Z codes/categories:

Z76.1	Encounter for health supervision and care of foundling
Z00.1-	Encounter for routine child health examination
Z38	Liveborn infants according to place of birth and type of delivery

13) Routine and administrative examinations

The Z codes allow for the description of encounters for routine examinations, such as, a general check-up, or, examinations for administrative purposes, such as, a pre-employment physical. The codes are not to be used if the examination is for diagnosis of a suspected condition or for treatment purposes. In such cases the diagnosis code is used. During a routine exam, should a diagnosis or condition be discovered, it should be coded as an additional code. Pre-existing and chronic conditions and history codes may also be included as additional codes as long as the examination is for administrative purposes and not focused on any particular condition.

Some of the codes for routine health examinations distinguish between "with" and "without" abnormal findings. Code assignment depends on the information that is known at the time the encounter is being coded. For example, if no abnormal findings were found during the examination, but the encounter is being coded before test results are back, it is acceptable to assign the code for "without abnormal findings." When assigning a code for "with abnormal findings," additional code(s) should be assigned to identify the specific abnormal finding(s).

Pre-operative examination and pre-procedural laboratory examination Z codes are for use only in those situations when a patient is being cleared for a procedure or surgery and no treatment is given.

The Z codes/categories for routine and administrative examinations:

Z00	Encounter for general examination without complaint, suspected or reported diagnosis
Z01	Encounter for other special examination without complaint, suspected or reported diagnosis
Z02	Encounter for administrative examination Except: Z02.9, Encounter for administrative examinations, unspecified
Z32.0-	Encounter for pregnancy test

14) Miscellaneous Z codes

The miscellaneous Z codes capture a number of other health care encounters that do not fall into one of the other categories. Certain of these codes identify the reason for the encounter; others are for use as additional codes that provide useful information on circumstances that may affect a patient's care and treatment.

Prophylactic Organ Removal

For encounters specifically for prophylactic removal of an organ (such as prophylactic removal of breasts due to a genetic susceptibility to cancer or a family history of cancer), the principal or first-listed code should be a code from category Z40, Encounter for prophylactic surgery, followed by the appropriate codes to identify the associated risk factor (such as genetic susceptibility or family history).

If the patient has a malignancy of one site and is having prophylactic removal at another site to prevent either a new primary malignancy or metastatic disease, a code for the malignancy should also be assigned in addition to a code from subcategory Z40.0, Encounter for prophylactic surgery for risk factors related to malignant neoplasms. A Z40.0 code should not be assigned if the patient is having organ removal for treatment of a malignancy, such as the removal of the testes for the treatment of prostate cancer.

Miscellaneous Z codes/categories:

Z28	Immunization not carried out Except: Z28.3, Underimmunization status
Z29	Encounter for other prophylactic measures
Z40	Encounter for prophylactic surgery
Z41	Encounter for procedures for purposes other than remedying health state Except: Z41.9, Encounter for procedure for purposes other than remedying health state, unspecified
Z53	Persons encountering health services for specific procedures and treatment, not carried out
Z55	Problems related to education and literacy
Z56	Problems related to employment and unemployment
Z57	Occupational exposure to risk factors
Z58	Problems related to physical environment
Z59	Problems related to housing and economic circumstances
Z60	Problems related to social environment
Z62	Problems related to upbringing
Z63	Other problems related to primary support group, including family circumstances
Z64	Problems related to certain psychosocial circumstances
Z65	Problems related to other psychosocial circumstances
Z72	Problems related to lifestyle Note: These codes should be assigned only when the documentation specifies that the patient has an associated problem
Z73	Problems related to life management difficulty

Z74	Problems related to care provider dependency Except: Z74.01, Bed confinement status
Z75	Problems related to medical facilities and other health care
Z76.0	Encounter for issue of repeat prescription
Z76.3	Healthy person accompanying sick person
Z76.4	Other boarder to healthcare facility
Z76.5	Malingerer [conscious simulation]
Z91.1-	Patient's noncompliance with medical treatment and regimen
Z91.83	Wandering in diseases classified elsewhere
Z91.84-	Oral health risk factors
Z91.89	Other specified personal risk factors, not elsewhere classified

See Section I.B.14 for Z55-Z65 Persons with potential health hazards related to socioeconomic and psychosocial circumstances, documentation by clinicians other than the patient's provider.

15) Nonspecific Z codes

Certain Z codes are so non-specific, or potentially redundant with other codes in the classification, that there can be little justification for their use in the inpatient setting. Their use in the outpatient setting should be limited to those instances when there is no further documentation to permit more precise coding. Otherwise, any sign or symptom or any other reason for visit that is captured in another code should be used.

Nonspecific Z codes/categories:

Z02.9	Encounter for administrative examinations, unspecified
Z04.9	Encounter for examination and observation for unspecified reason
Z13.9	Encounter for screening, unspecified
Z41.9	Encounter for procedure for purposes other than remedying health state, unspecified
Z52.9	Donor of unspecified organ or tissue
Z86.59	Personal history of other mental and behavioral disorders
Z88.9	Allergy status to unspecified drugs, medicaments and biological substances status
Z92.0	Personal history of contraception

16) Z Codes That May Only Be Principal/First-Listed Diagnosis

The following Z codes/categories may only be reported as the principal/first-listed diagnosis, except when there are multiple encounters on the same day and the medical records for the encounters are combined:

Z00	Encounter for general examination without complaint, suspected or reported diagnosis Except: Z00.6
Z01	Encounter for other special examination without complaint, suspected or reported diagnosis
Z02	Encounter for administrative examination
Z03	Encounter for medical observation for suspected diseases and conditions ruled out
Z04	Encounter for examination and observation for other reasons
Z33.2	Encounter for elective termination of pregnancy
Z31.81	Encounter for male factor infertility in female patient
Z31.83	Encounter for assisted reproductive fertility procedure cycle
Z31.84	Encounter for fertility preservation procedure
Z34	Encounter for supervision of normal pregnancy
Z39	Encounter for maternal postpartum care and examination
Z38	Liveborn infants according to place of birth and type of delivery
Z40	Encounter for prophylactic surgery
Z42	Encounter for plastic and reconstructive surgery following medical procedure or healed injury
Z51.0	Encounter for antineoplastic radiation therapy
Z51.1-	Encounter for antineoplastic chemotherapy and immunotherapy
Z52	Donors of organs and tissues Except: Z52.9, Donor of unspecified organ or tissue
Z76.1	Encounter for health supervision and care of foundling
Z76.2	Encounter for health supervision and care of other healthy infant and child
Z99.12	Encounter for respirator [ventilator] dependence during power failure

CHAPTER 21

FACTORS INFLUENCING HEALTH STATUS AND CONTACT WITH HEALTH SERVICES (Z00-Z99)

Note: Z codes represent reasons for encounters. A corresponding procedure code must accompany a Z code if a procedure is performed. Categories Z00-Z99 are provided for occasions when circumstances other than a disease, injury or external cause classifiable to categories A00-Y89 are recorded as "diagnoses" or "problems." This can arise in two main ways:

(a) When a person who may or may not be sick encounters the health services for some specific purpose, such as to receive limited care or service for a current condition, to donate an organ or tissue, to receive prophylactic vaccination (immunization), or to discuss a problem which is in itself not a disease or injury.

(b) When some circumstance or problem is present which influences the person's health status but is not in itself a current illness or injury.

This chapter contains the following blocks:

Z00-Z13	Persons encountering health services for examination
Z14-Z15	Genetic carrier and genetic susceptibility to disease
Z16	Resistance to antimicrobial drugs
Z17	Estrogen receptor status
Z18	Retained foreign body fragments
Z19	Hormone sensitivity malignancy status
Z20-Z29	Persons with potential health hazards related to communicable diseases
Z30-Z39	Persons encountering health services in circumstances related to reproduction
Z40-Z53	Encounters for other specific health care
Z55-Z65	Persons with potential health hazards related to socioeconomic and psychosocial circumstances
Z66	Do not resuscitate status
Z67	Blood type
Z68	Body mass index (BMI)
Z69-Z76	Persons encountering health services in other circumstances
Z77-Z99	Persons with potential health hazards related to family and personal history and certain conditions influencing health status

PERSONS ENCOUNTERING HEALTH SERVICES FOR EXAMINATIONS (Z00-Z13)

Note: Nonspecific abnormal findings disclosed at the time of these examinations are classified to categories R70-R94.

> **Excludes1**   examinations related to pregnancy and reproduction (Z30-Z36, Z39.-)

● **Z00**   **Encounter for general examination without complaint, suspected or reported diagnosis**

> **Excludes1**   encounter for examination for administrative purposes (Z02.-)
>
> **Excludes2**   encounter for pre-procedural examinations (Z01.81-)
> special screening examinations (Z11-Z13)

● **Z00.0**   **Encounter for general adult medical examination**
Encounter for adult periodic examination (annual) (physical) and any associated laboratory and radiologic examinations

> **Excludes1**   encounter for examination of sign or symptom - code to sign or symptom
> general health check-up of infant or child (Z00.12.-)

Coding Clinic: 2016, Q4, P131

    Z00.00   **Encounter for general adult medical examination without abnormal findings**   A
Encounter for adult health check-up NOS
Coding Clinic: 2017, Q4, P95; 2016, Q1, P37

    Z00.01   **Encounter for general adult medical examination with abnormal findings**   A
Use additional code to identify abnormal findings
Coding Clinic: 2016, Q1, P36

● **Z00.1**   **Encounter for newborn, infant and child health examinations**

● **Z00.11**   **Newborn health examination**
Health check for child under 29 days old
Use additional code to identify any abnormal findings

> **Excludes1**   health check for child over 28 days old (Z00.12-)

    Z00.110   **Health examination for newborn under 8 days old**   N
Health check for newborn under 8 days old

    Z00.111   **Health examination for newborn 8 to 28 days old**   N
Health check for newborn 8 to 28 days old
Newborn weight check

● **Z00.12**   **Encounter for routine child health examination**
Immunizations appropriate for age
Health check (routine) for child over 28 days old
Routine developmental screening of infant or child
Routine vision and hearing testing

> **Excludes1**   health check for child under 29 days old (Z00.11-)
> health supervision of foundling or other healthy infant or child (Z76.1-Z76.2)
> newborn health examination (Z00.11-)

    Z00.121   **Encounter for routine child health examination with abnormal findings**   P
Use additional code to identify abnormal findings
Coding Clinic: 2017, Q4, P95; 2016, Q1, P34-35

    Z00.129   **Encounter for routine child health examination without abnormal findings**   P
Encounter for routine child health examination NOS
Coding Clinic: 2016, Q1, P34

Z00.2   **Encounter for examination for period of rapid growth in childhood**   P

Z00.3   **Encounter for examination for adolescent development state**   P
Encounter for puberty development state

Z00.5   **Encounter for examination of potential donor of organ and tissue**

Z00.6   **Encounter for examination for normal comparison and control in clinical research program**
Examination of participant or control in clinical research program

● **Z00.7**   **Encounter for examination for period of delayed growth in childhood**

    Z00.70   **Encounter for examination for period of delayed growth in childhood without abnormal findings**   P

    Z00.71   **Encounter for examination for period of delayed growth in childhood with abnormal findings**   P
Use additional code to identify abnormal findings

Z00.8   **Encounter for other general examination**
Encounter for health examination in population surveys

● **Z01**   **Encounter for other special examination without complaint, suspected or reported diagnosis**

     Includes   routine examination of specific system

     Note: Codes from category Z01 represent the reason for the encounter. A separate procedure code is required to identify any examinations or procedures performed.

     Excludes1   encounter for examination for administrative purposes (Z02.-)

                encounter for examination for suspected conditions, proven not to exist (Z03.-)

                encounter for laboratory and radiologic examinations as a component of general medical examinations (Z00.0-)

                encounter for laboratory, radiologic and imaging examinations for sign(s) and symptom(s) - code to the sign(s) or symptom(s)

     Excludes2   screening examinations (Z11-Z13)

● **Z01.0**   **Encounter for examination of eyes and vision**

     Excludes1   examination for driving license (Z02.4)

   Z01.00   **Encounter for examination of eyes and vision without abnormal findings**

       Encounter for examination of eyes and vision NOS

   Z01.01   **Encounter for examination of eyes and vision with abnormal findings**

       Use additional code to identify abnormal findings

       Coding Clinic: 2016, Q4, P21

●   **Z01.02**   **Encounter for examination of eyes and vision following failed vision screening**

     Excludes1   encounter for examination of eyes and vision with abnormal findings (Z01.01)

            encounter for examination of eyes and vision without abnormal findings (Z01.00)

     ● **Z01.020**   **Encounter for examination of eyes and vision following failed vision screening without abnormal findings**

     ● **Z01.021**   **Encounter for examination of eyes and vision following failed vision screening with abnormal findings**

       Use additional code to identify abnormal findings

● **Z01.1**   **Encounter for examination of ears and hearing**

   Z01.10   **Encounter for examination of ears and hearing without abnormal findings**

       Encounter for examination of ears and hearing NOS

       Coding Clinic: 2016, Q4, P25

●   **Z01.11**   **Encounter for examination of ears and hearing with abnormal findings**

       Coding Clinic: 2016, Q3, P18

     Z01.110   **Encounter for hearing examination following failed hearing screening**

       Coding Clinic: 2016, Q3, P18-19

     Z01.118   **Encounter for examination of ears and hearing with other abnormal findings**

       Use additional code to identify abnormal findings

       Coding Clinic: 2016, Q3, P17

   Z01.12   **Encounter for hearing conservation and treatment**

● **Z01.2**   **Encounter for dental examination and cleaning**

   Z01.20   **Encounter for dental examination and cleaning without abnormal findings**

       Encounter for dental examination and cleaning NOS

   Z01.21   **Encounter for dental examination and cleaning with abnormal findings**

       Use additional code to identify abnormal findings

● **Z01.3**   **Encounter for examination of blood pressure**

   Z01.30   **Encounter for examination of blood pressure without abnormal findings**

       Encounter for examination of blood pressure NOS

   Z01.31   **Encounter for examination of blood pressure with abnormal findings**

       Use additional code to identify abnormal findings

● **Z01.4**   **Encounter for gynecological examination**

     Excludes2   pregnancy examination or test (Z32.0-)

            routine examination for contraceptive maintenance (Z30.4-)

●   **Z01.41**   **Encounter for routine gynecological examination**

       Encounter for general gynecological examination with or without cervical smear

       Encounter for gynecological examination (general) (routine) NOS

       Encounter for pelvic examination (annual) (periodic)

       Use additional code:

         for screening for human papillomavirus, if applicable (Z11.51)

         for screening vaginal pap smear, if applicable (Z12.72)

         to identify acquired absence of uterus, if applicable (Z90.71-)

     Excludes1   gynecologic examination status-post hysterectomy for malignant condition (Z08)

            screening cervical pap smear not a part of a routine gynecological examination (Z12.4)

     Z01.411   **Encounter for gynecological examination (general) (routine) with abnormal findings** ♀

       Use additional code to identify any abnormal findings

     Z01.419   **Encounter for gynecological examination (general) (routine) without abnormal findings** ♀

   Z01.42   **Encounter for cervical smear to confirm findings of recent normal smear following initial abnormal smear** ♀

● **Z01.8**   **Encounter for other specified special examinations**

●   **Z01.81**   **Encounter for preprocedural examinations**

       Encounter for preoperative examinations

       Encounter for radiological and imaging examinations as part of preprocedural examination

     Z01.810   **Encounter for preprocedural cardiovascular examination**

     Z01.811   **Encounter for preprocedural respiratory examination**

     Z01.812   **Encounter for preprocedural laboratory examination**

       Blood and urine tests prior to treatment or procedure

       Coding Clinic: 2021, Q1, P38

     Z01.818   **Encounter for other preprocedural examination**

       Encounter for preprocedural examination NOS

       Encounter for examinations prior to antineoplastic chemotherapy

   Z01.82   **Encounter for allergy testing**

     Excludes1   encounter for antibody response examination (Z01.84)

   Z01.83   **Encounter for blood typing**

       Encounter for Rh typing

Z01.84   Encounter for antibody response examination
Encounter for immunity status testing

> **Excludes1**   encounter for allergy testing (Z01.82)

Z01.89   Encounter for other specified special examinations

● **Z02**   **Encounter for administrative examination**

Z02.0   **Encounter for examination for admission to educational institution**
Encounter for examination for admission to preschool (education)
Encounter for examination for re-admission to school following illness or medical treatment

Z02.1   **Encounter for pre-employment examination**

Z02.2   **Encounter for examination for admission to residential institution**

> **Excludes1**   examination for admission to prison (Z02.89)

Z02.3   **Encounter for examination for recruitment to armed forces**

Z02.4   **Encounter for examination for driving license**

Z02.5   **Encounter for examination for participation in sport**

> **Excludes1**   blood-alcohol and blood-drug test (Z02.83)

Z02.6   **Encounter for examination for insurance purposes**

● **Z02.7**   **Encounter for issue of medical certificate**

> **Excludes1**   encounter for general medical examination (Z00-Z01, Z02.0-Z02.6, Z02.8-Z02.9)

Z02.71   Encounter for disability determination
Encounter for issue of medical certificate of incapacity
Encounter for issue of medical certificate of invalidity

Z02.79   Encounter for issue of other medical certificate

● **Z02.8**   **Encounter for other administrative examinations**

Z02.81   Encounter for paternity testing

Z02.82   Encounter for adoption services

Z02.83   Encounter for blood-alcohol and blood-drug test
Use additional code for findings of alcohol or drugs in blood (R78.-)

Z02.89   Encounter for other administrative examinations
Encounter for examination for admission to prison
Encounter for examination for admission to summer camp
Encounter for immigration examination
Encounter for naturalization examination
Encounter for premarital examination

> **Excludes1**   health supervision of foundling or other healthy infant or child (Z76.1-Z76.2)

Z02.9   **Encounter for administrative examinations, unspecified**

OGCR Section II.C.21.c.6.

Observation

There are three observation Z code categories. They are for use in very limited circumstances when a person is being observed for a suspected condition that is ruled out. The observation codes are not for use if an injury or illnesses or any signs or symptoms related to the suspected condition are present. In such cases the diagnosis/symptom code is used with the corresponding external cause code.

The observation codes are to be used as principal diagnosis only. The only exception to this is when the principal diagnosis is required to be a code from category Z38, Liveborn infants according to place of birth and type of delivery. Then a code from category Z05, Encounter for observation and evaluation of newborn for suspected diseases and conditions ruled out, is sequenced after the Z38 code. Additional codes may be used in addition to the observation code but only if they are unrelated to the suspected condition being observed.

Codes from subcategory Z03.7 Encounter for suspected maternal and fetal conditions ruled out, may either be used as a first listed or as an additional code assignment depending on the case. They are for use in very limited circumstances on a maternal record when an encounter is for a suspected maternal or fetal condition that is ruled out during that encounter (for example, a maternal or fetal condition may be suspected due to an abnormal test result). These codes should not be used when the condition is confirmed. In those cases, the confirmed condition should be coded. In addition, these codes are not for use if an illness or any signs or symptoms related to the suspected condition or problem are present. In such cases the diagnosis/symptom code is used.

Additional codes may be used in addition to the code from subcategory Z03.7, but only if they are unrelated to the suspected condition being evaluated.

Codes from subcategory Z03.7 may not be used for encounters for antenatal screening of mother. *See Section I.C.21. Screening.*

For encounters for suspected fetal condition that are inconclusive following testing and evaluation, assign the appropriate code from category O35, O36, O40 or O41.

The observation Z code categories:

Z03   Encounter for medical observation for suspected diseases and conditions ruled out

Z04   Encounter for examination and observation for other reasons Except: Z04.9, Encounter for examination and observation for unspecified reason

Z05   Encounter for observation and evaluation of newborn for suspected diseases and conditions ruled out

● **Z03**   **Encounter for medical observation for suspected diseases and conditions ruled out**
This category is to be used when a person without a diagnosis is suspected of having an abnormal condition, without signs or symptoms, which requires study, but after examination and observation, is ruled out. This category is also for use for administrative and legal observation status.

> **Excludes1**   contact with and (suspected) exposures hazardous to health (Z77.-)
> encounter for observation and evaluation of newborn for suspected diseases and conditions ruled out (Z05.-)
> person with feared complaint in whom no diagnosis is made (Z71.1)
> signs or symptoms under study - code to signs or symptoms

Z03.6   **Encounter for observation for suspected toxic effect from ingested substance ruled out**
Encounter for observation for suspected adverse effect from drug
Encounter for observation for suspected poisoning

● **Z03.7** **Encounter for suspected maternal and fetal conditions ruled out**

Encounter for suspected maternal and fetal conditions not found

> **Excludes1**   known or suspected fetal anomalies affecting management of mother, not ruled out (O26.-, O35.-, O36.-, O40.-, O41.-)

Z03.71 **Encounter for suspected problem with amniotic cavity and membrane ruled out** ♀   M

Encounter for suspected oligohydramnios ruled out

Encounter for suspected polyhydramnios ruled out

Z03.72 **Encounter for suspected placental problem ruled out** ♀   M

Z03.73 **Encounter for suspected fetal anomaly ruled out** ♀   M

Coding Clinic: 2016, Q4, P6

Z03.74 **Encounter for suspected problem with fetal growth ruled out** ♀   M

Z03.75 **Encounter for suspected cervical shortening ruled out** ♀   M

Z03.79 **Encounter for other suspected maternal and fetal conditions ruled out** ♀   M

Coding Clinic: 2016, Q4, P7

● **Z03.8** **Encounter for observation for other suspected diseases and conditions ruled out**

● **Z03.81** **Encounter for observation for suspected exposure to biological agents ruled out**

Z03.810 **Encounter for observation for suspected exposure to anthrax ruled out**

Z03.818 **Encounter for observation for suspected exposure to other biological agents ruled out**

● **Z03.82** **Encounter for observation for suspected foreign body ruled out**

> **Excludes1**   retained foreign body (Z18.-)
> retained foreign body in eyelid (H02.81)
> residual foreign body in soft tissue (M79.5)
>
> **Excludes2**   confirmed foreign body ingestion or aspiration including:
> foreign body in alimentary tract (T18)
> foreign body in ear (T16)
> foreign body on external eye (T15)
> foreign body in respiratory tract (T17)

Z03.821 **Encounter for observation for suspected ingested foreign body ruled out**

Z03.822 **Encounter for observation for suspected aspirated (inhaled) foreign body ruled out**

Z03.823 **Encounter for observation for suspected inserted (injected) foreign body ruled out**

Encounter for observation for suspected inserted (injected) foreign body in eye ruled out

Encounter for observation for suspected inserted (injected) foreign body in orifice ruled out

Encounter for observation for suspected inserted (injected) foreign body in skin ruled out

▶ **Z03.83** **Encounter for observation for suspected conditions related to home physiologic monitoring device ruled out**

> ▶ Encounter for observation for apnea alarm without findings
> ▶ Encounter for observation for bradycardia alarm without findings
> ▶ Encounter for observation for malfunction of home cardiorespiratory monitor
> ▶ Encounter for observation for non-specific findings home physiologic monitoring device
> ▶ Encounter for observation for pulse oximeter alarm without findings

> ▶ **Excludes1**   apnea NOS (R06.81)
>   ▶ neonatal bradycardia (P29.12)
>   ▶ newborn apnea (P28.4-)
>   ▶ primary sleep apnea of newborn (P28.3-)
>   ▶ sleep apnea (G47.3-)

Z03.89 **Encounter for observation for other suspected diseases and conditions ruled out**

● **Z04** **Encounter for examination and observation for other reasons**

> **Includes**   encounter for examination for medicolegal reasons
> This category is to be used when a person without a diagnosis is suspected of having an abnormal condition, without signs or symptoms, which requires study, but after examination and observation, is ruled-out. This category is also for use for administrative and legal observation status.

Z04.1 **Encounter for examination and observation following transport accident**

> **Excludes1**   encounter for examination and observation following work accident (Z04.2)

Coding Clinic: 2019, Q2, P11

Z04.2 **Encounter for examination and observation following work accident**

Z04.3 **Encounter for examination and observation following other accident**

● **Z04.4** **Encounter for examination and observation following alleged rape**

Encounter for examination and observation of victim following alleged rape

Encounter for examination and observation of victim following alleged sexual abuse

Coding Clinic: 2016, Q4, P129

Z04.41 **Encounter for examination and observation following alleged adult rape**   A

Suspected adult rape, ruled out

Suspected adult sexual abuse, ruled out

Z04.42 **Encounter for examination and observation following alleged child rape**   P

Suspected child rape, ruled out

Suspected child sexual abuse, ruled out

Z04.6 **Encounter for general psychiatric examination, requested by authority**

● **Z04.7** **Encounter for examination and observation following alleged physical abuse**

Z04.71 **Encounter for examination and observation following alleged adult physical abuse**   A

Suspected adult physical abuse, ruled out

> **Excludes1**   confirmed case of adult physical abuse (T74.-)
> encounter for examination and observation following alleged adult sexual abuse (Z04.41)
> suspected case of adult physical abuse, not ruled out (T76.-)

CHAPTER 21 (Z00-Z99)

▶ New   ⟹ Revised   ~~deleted~~ Deleted   Excludes 1   Excludes 2   Includes   Use additional   Code first   Code also   Key words

OGCR Official Guidelines   X Assign placeholder X   ● Use Additional Character(s)   ▶ Manifestation Code   🔖 Hierarchical Condition Category   **Coding Clinic**

Z04.72   **Encounter for examination and observation following alleged child physical abuse**   P

Suspected child physical abuse, ruled out

Excludes1   confirmed case of child physical abuse (T74.-)

encounter for examination and observation following alleged child sexual abuse (Z04.42)

suspected case of child physical abuse, not ruled out (T76.-)

● **Z04.8**   **Encounter for examination and observation for other specified reasons**

Encounter for examination and observation for request for expert evidence

Z04.81   **Encounter for examination and observation of victim following forced sexual exploitation**

Z04.82   **Encounter for examination and observation of victim following forced labor exploitation**

Z04.89   **Encounter for examination and observation for other specified reasons**

Z04.9   **Encounter for examination and observation for unspecified reason**

Encounter for observation NOS

● **Z05**   **Encounter for observation and evaluation of newborn for suspected diseases and conditions ruled out**

This category is to be used for newborns, within the neonatal period (the first 28 days of life), who are suspected of having an abnormal condition, but without signs or symptoms, and which, after examination and observation, is ruled out.

Coding Clinic: 2022, Q1, P17-18; 2019, Q2, P11; 2016, Q4, P54, 77, 126-127, 130

Z05.0   **Observation and evaluation of newborn for suspected cardiac condition ruled out**   N

Z05.1   **Observation and evaluation of newborn for suspected infectious condition ruled out**   N

Coding Clinic: 2019, Q2, P11

Z05.2   **Observation and evaluation of newborn for suspected neurological condition ruled out**   N

Z05.3   **Observation and evaluation of newborn for suspected respiratory condition ruled out**   N

● **Z05.4**   **Observation and evaluation of newborn for suspected genetic, metabolic or immunologic condition ruled out**

Z05.41   **Observation and evaluation of newborn for suspected genetic condition ruled out**   N

Coding Clinic: 2016, Q4, P55

Z05.42   **Observation and evaluation of newborn for suspected metabolic condition ruled out**   N

Z05.43   **Observation and evaluation of newborn for suspected immunologic condition ruled out**   N

Z05.5   **Observation and evaluation of newborn for suspected gastrointestinal condition ruled out**   N

Z05.6   **Observation and evaluation of newborn for suspected genitourinary condition ruled out**   N

● **Z05.7**   **Observation and evaluation of newborn for suspected skin, subcutaneous, musculoskeletal and connective tissue condition ruled out**

Z05.71   **Observation and evaluation of newborn for suspected skin and subcutaneous tissue condition ruled out**   N

Z05.72   **Observation and evaluation of newborn for suspected musculoskeletal condition ruled out**   N

Z05.73   **Observation and evaluation of newborn for suspected connective tissue condition ruled out**   N

Z05.8   **Observation and evaluation of newborn for other specified suspected condition ruled out**   N

Coding Clinic: 2022, Q1, P17-18

Z05.9   **Observation and evaluation of newborn for unspecified suspected condition ruled out**   N

OGCR See Section II.C.21.c.8.

The follow-up codes are used to explain continuing surveillance following completed treatment of a disease, condition, or injury. They imply that the condition has been fully treated and no longer exists. They should not be confused with aftercare codes, or injury codes with 7th character "D," that explain ongoing care of a healing condition or its sequelae. Follow-up codes may be used in conjunction with history codes to provide the full picture of the healed condition and its treatment. The follow-up code is sequenced first, followed by the history code.

A follow-up code may be used to explain multiple visits. Should a condition be found to have recurred on the follow-up visit, then the diagnosis code for the condition should be assigned in place of the follow-up code.

The follow-up Z code categories:

Z08   Encounter for follow-up examination after completed treatment for malignant neoplasm

Z09   Encounter for follow-up examination after completed treatment for conditions other than malignant neoplasm

Z39   Encounter for maternal postpartum care and examination

Z08   **Encounter for follow-up examination after completed treatment for malignant neoplasm**

Medical surveillance following completed treatment

Use additional code to identify any acquired absence of organs (Z90.-)

Use additional code to identify the personal history of malignant neoplasm (Z85.-)

Excludes1   aftercare following medical care (Z43-Z49, Z51)

Z09   **Encounter for follow-up examination after completed treatment for conditions other than malignant neoplasm**

Medical surveillance following completed treatment

Use additional code to identify any applicable history of disease code (Z86.-, Z87.-)

Excludes1   aftercare following medical care (Z43-Z49, Z51)

surveillance of contraception (Z30.4-)

surveillance of prosthetic and other medical devices (Z44-Z46)

Coding Clinic: 2021, Q1, P33; 2017, Q1, P9; 2015, Q1, P8

OGCR Section II.C.21.c.5.

Screening

Screening is the testing for disease or disease precursors in seemingly well individuals so that early detection and treatment can be provided for those who test positive for the disease (e.g., screening mammogram).

The testing of a person to rule out or confirm a suspected diagnosis because the patient has some sign or symptom is a diagnostic examination, not a screening. In these cases, the sign or symptom is used to explain the reason for the test.

A screening code may be a first listed code if the reason for the visit is specifically the screening exam. It may also be used as an additional code if the screening is done during an office visit for other health problems. A screening code is not necessary if the screening is inherent to a routine examination, such as a pap smear done during a routine pelvic examination.

Should a condition be discovered during the screening then the code for the condition may be assigned as an additional diagnosis.

The Z code indicates that a screening exam is planned. A procedure code is required to confirm that the screening was performed.

The screening Z codes/categories:

Z11   Encounter for screening for infectious and parasitic diseases

Z12   Encounter for screening for malignant neoplasms

Z13   Encounter for screening for other diseases and disorders

     Except: Z13.9, Encounter for screening, unspecified

Z36   Encounter for antenatal screening for mother

CHAPTER 21 (Z00-Z99)

CHAPTER 21 (Z00-Z99)

● **Z11**   Encounter for screening for infectious and parasitic diseases
Screening is the testing for disease or disease precursors in asymptomatic individuals so that early detection and treatment can be provided for those who test positive for the disease.

> **Excludes1**   encounter for diagnostic examination - code to sign or symptom

Z11.0   Encounter for screening for intestinal infectious diseases
Encounter for screening for active tuberculosis disease

Z11.1   Encounter for screening for respiratory tuberculosis

Z11.2   Encounter for screening for other bacterial diseases

Z11.3   Encounter for screening for infections with a predominantly sexual mode of transmission

> **Excludes2**   encounter for screening for human immunodeficiency virus [HIV] (Z11.4)
> encounter for screening for human papillomavirus (Z11.51)

Z11.4   Encounter for screening for human immunodeficiency virus [HIV]

● **Z11.5**   Encounter for screening for other viral diseases

> **Excludes2**   encounter for screening for viral intestinal disease (Z11.0)

Z11.51   Encounter for screening for human papillomavirus (HPV)

Z11.52   Encounter for screening for COVID-19
Coding Clinic: 2021, Q1, P37, 42

Z11.59   Encounter for screening for other viral diseases
Coding Clinic: 2021, Q1, P37

Z11.6   Encounter for screening for other protozoal diseases and helminthiases
Diseases or infestations caused by parasitic worms

> **Excludes2**   encounter for screening for protozoal intestinal disease (Z11.0)

Z11.7   Encounter for testing for latent tuberculosis infection

Z11.8   Encounter for screening for other infectious and parasitic diseases
Encounter for screening for chlamydia
Encounter for screening for rickettsial
Encounter for screening for spirochetal
Encounter for screening for mycoses

Z11.9   Encounter for screening for infectious and parasitic diseases, unspecified

● **Z12**   Encounter for screening for malignant neoplasms
Screening is the testing for disease or disease precursors in asymptomatic individuals so that early detection and treatment can be provided for those who test positive for the disease.

Use additional code to identify any family history of malignant neoplasm (Z80.-)

> **Excludes1**   encounter for diagnostic examination - code to sign or symptom

Z12.0   Encounter for screening for malignant neoplasm of stomach

● **Z12.1**   Encounter for screening for malignant neoplasm of intestinal tract

Z12.10   Encounter for screening for malignant neoplasm of intestinal tract, unspecified

Z12.11   Encounter for screening for malignant neoplasm of colon
Encounter for screening colonoscopy NOS
Coding Clinic: 2018, Q1, P7; 2017, Q1, P8-9

Z12.12   Encounter for screening for malignant neoplasm of rectum

Z12.13   Encounter for screening for malignant neoplasm of small intestine

Z12.2   Encounter for screening for malignant neoplasm of respiratory organs

● **Z12.3**   Encounter for screening for malignant neoplasm of breast

Z12.31   Encounter for screening mammogram for malignant neoplasm of breast

> **Excludes1**   inconclusive mammogram (R92.2)
> Coding Clinic: 2015, Q1, P24

Z12.39   Encounter for other screening for malignant neoplasm of breast

Z12.4   Encounter for screening for malignant neoplasm of cervix ♀
Encounter for screening pap smear for malignant neoplasm of cervix

> **Excludes1**   when screening is part of general gynecological examination (Z01.4-)

> **Excludes2**   encounter for screening for human papillomavirus (Z11.51)

Z12.5   Encounter for screening for malignant neoplasm of prostate ♂

Z12.6   Encounter for screening for malignant neoplasm of bladder

● **Z12.7**   Encounter for screening for malignant neoplasm of other genitourinary organs

Z12.71   Encounter for screening for malignant neoplasm of testis ♂

Z12.72   Encounter for screening for malignant neoplasm of vagina ♀
Vaginal pap smear status - post hysterectomy for non-malignant condition
Use additional code to identify acquired absence of uterus (Z90.71-)

> **Excludes1**   vaginal pap smear status - post hysterectomy for malignant conditions (Z08)

Z12.73   Encounter for screening for malignant neoplasm of ovary ♀

Z12.79   Encounter for screening for malignant neoplasm of other genitourinary organs

● **Z12.8**   Encounter for screening for malignant neoplasm of other sites

Z12.81   Encounter for screening for malignant neoplasm of oral cavity

Z12.82   Encounter for screening for malignant neoplasm of nervous system

Z12.83   Encounter for screening for malignant neoplasm of skin

Z12.89   Encounter for screening for malignant neoplasm of other sites
Coding Clinic: 2021, Q1, P15

Z12.9   Encounter for screening for malignant neoplasm, site unspecified

● **Z13**   Encounter for screening for other diseases and disorders
Screening is the testing for disease or disease precursors in asymptomatic individuals so that early detection and treatment can be provided for those who test positive for the disease.

> **Excludes1**   encounter for diagnostic examination - code to sign or symptom

Z13.0   Encounter for screening for diseases of the blood and blood-forming organs and certain disorders involving the immune mechanism

Z13.1   Encounter for screening for diabetes mellitus

● **Z13.2** Encounter for screening for nutritional, metabolic and other endocrine disorders

    Z13.21 Encounter for screening for nutritional disorder

    ● **Z13.22** Encounter for screening for metabolic disorder

        Z13.220 Encounter for screening for lipoid disorders

            Encounter for screening for cholesterol level

            Encounter for screening for hypercholesterolemia

            Encounter for screening for hyperlipidemia

        Z13.228 Encounter for screening for other metabolic disorders

    Z13.29 Encounter for screening for other suspected endocrine disorder

        Excludes2 encounter for screening for diabetes mellitus (Z13.1)

● **Z13.3** Encounter for screening examination for mental health and behavioral disorders

    Z13.30 Encounter for screening examination for mental health and behavioral disorders, unspecified

    Z13.31 Encounter for screening for depression

        Encounter for screening for depression, adult

        Encounter for screening for depression for child or adolescent

    Z13.32 Encounter for screening for maternal depression ♀

        Encounter for screening for perinatal depression

    Z13.39 Encounter for screening examination for other mental health and behavioral disorders

        Encounter for screening for alcoholism

        Encounter for screening for intellectual disabilities

● **Z13.4** Encounter for screening for certain developmental disorders in childhood   P

    Encounter for development testing of infant or child

    Encounter for screening for developmental handicaps in early childhood

    Excludes2 encounter for routine child health examination (Z00.12-)

    Z13.40 Encounter for screening for unspecified developmental delays

    Z13.41 Encounter for autism screening

    Z13.42 Encounter for screening for global developmental delays (milestones)

        Encounter for screening for developmental handicaps in early childhood

    Z13.49 Encounter for screening for other developmental delays

● **Z13.5** Encounter for screening for eye and ear disorders

    Excludes2 encounter for general hearing examination (Z01.1-)

        encounter for general vision examination (Z01.0-)

    Coding Clinic: 2016, Q3, P17

Z13.6 Encounter for screening for cardiovascular disorders

● **Z13.7** Encounter for screening for genetic and chromosomal anomalies

    Excludes1 genetic testing for procreative management (Z31.4-)

    Z13.71 Encounter for nonprocreative screening for genetic disease carrier status

    Z13.79 Encounter for other screening for genetic and chromosomal anomalies

● **Z13.8** Encounter for screening for other specified diseases and disorders

    Excludes2 screening for malignant neoplasms (Z12.-)

● **Z13.81** Encounter for screening for digestive system disorders

    Z13.810 Encounter for screening for upper gastrointestinal disorder

    Z13.811 Encounter for screening for lower gastrointestinal disorder

        Excludes1 encounter for screening for intestinal infectious disease (Z11.0)

    Z13.818 Encounter for screening for other digestive system disorders

● **Z13.82** Encounter for screening for musculoskeletal disorder

    Z13.820 Encounter for screening for osteoporosis

    Z13.828 Encounter for screening for other musculoskeletal disorder

    Z13.83 Encounter for screening for respiratory disorder NEC

        Excludes1 encounter for screening for respiratory tuberculosis (Z11.1)

    Z13.84 Encounter for screening for dental disorders

● **Z13.85** Encounter for screening for nervous system disorders

    Z13.850 Encounter for screening for traumatic brain injury

    Z13.858 Encounter for screening for other nervous system disorders

    Z13.88 Encounter for screening for disorder due to exposure to contaminants

        Excludes1 those exposed to contaminants without suspected disorders (Z57-Z77.-)

    Z13.89 Encounter for screening for other disorder

        Encounter for screening for genitourinary disorders

Z13.9 Encounter for screening, unspecified

GENETIC CARRIER AND GENETIC SUSCEPTIBILITY TO DISEASE (Z14-Z15)

● **Z14** Genetic carrier

  ● **Z14.0** Hemophilia A carrier

    Z14.01 Asymptomatic hemophilia A carrier

    Z14.02 Symptomatic hemophilia A carrier

  Z14.1 Cystic fibrosis carrier

  Z14.8 Genetic carrier of other disease

● **Z15** Genetic susceptibility to disease

    Excludes1 chromosomal anomalies (Q90-Q99)

    Includes confirmed abnormal gene

    Use additional code, if applicable, for any associated family history of the disease (Z80-Z84)

  ● **Z15.0** Genetic susceptibility to malignant neoplasm

    Code first if applicable, any current malignant neoplasm (C00-C75, C81-C96)

    Use additional code, if applicable, for any personal history of malignant neoplasm (Z85.-)

    Z15.01 Genetic susceptibility to malignant neoplasm of breast

    Z15.02 Genetic susceptibility to malignant neoplasm of ovary ♀

    Z15.03 Genetic susceptibility to malignant neoplasm of prostate ♂

    Z15.04 Genetic susceptibility to malignant neoplasm of endometrium ♀

    Z15.09 Genetic susceptibility to other malignant neoplasm

        Coding Clinic: 2021, Q1, P15

CHAPTER 21 (Z00-Z99)

● **Z15.8   Genetic susceptibility to other disease**

    Z15.81   Genetic susceptibility to multiple endocrine neoplasia [MEN]

        Excludes1   multiple endocrine neoplasia [MEN] syndromes (E31.2-)

    Z15.89   Genetic susceptibility to other disease

RESISTANCE TO ANTIMICROBIAL DRUGS (Z16)

● **Z16   Resistance to antimicrobial drugs**

    Note: The codes in this category are provided for use as additional codes to identify the resistance and non-responsiveness of a condition to antimicrobial drugs.

    Code first the infection

    Excludes1   Methicillin resistant Staphylococcus aureus infection (A49.02)
        Methicillin resistant Staphylococcus aureus pneumonia (J15.212)
        Sepsis due to Methicillin resistant Staphylococcus aureus (A41.02)

● **Z16.1   Resistance to beta lactam antibiotics**

    Z16.10   Resistance to unspecified beta lactam antibiotics

    Z16.11   Resistance to penicillins
        Resistance to amoxicillin
        Resistance to ampicillin

    Z16.12   Extended spectrum beta lactamase (ESBL) resistance

        Excludes2   Methicillin resistant Staphylococcus aureus infection in diseases classified elsewhere (B95.62)

    Z16.19   Resistance to other specified beta lactam antibiotics
        Resistance to cephalosporins

● **Z16.2   Resistance to other antibiotics**

    Z16.20   Resistance to unspecified antibiotic
        Resistance to antibiotics NOS

    Z16.21   Resistance to vancomycin

    Z16.22   Resistance to vancomycin related antibiotics

    Z16.23   Resistance to quinolones and fluoroquinolones

    Z16.24   Resistance to multiple antibiotics

    Z16.29   Resistance to other single specified antibiotic
        Resistance to aminoglycosides
        Resistance to macrolides
        Resistance to sulfonamides
        Resistance to tetracyclines

● **Z16.3   Resistance to other antimicrobial drugs**

    Excludes1   resistance to antibiotics (Z16.1-, Z16.2-)

    Z16.30   Resistance to unspecified antimicrobial drugs
        Drug resistance NOS

    Z16.31   Resistance to antiparasitic drug(s)
        Resistance to quinine and related compounds

    Z16.32   Resistance to antifungal drug(s)

    Z16.33   Resistance to antiviral drug(s)

● **Z16.34   Resistance to antimycobacterial drug(s)**
        Resistance to tuberculostatics

    Z16.341   Resistance to single antimycobacterial drug
        Resistance to antimycobacterial drug NOS

    Z16.342   Resistance to multiple antimycobacterial drugs

    Z16.35   Resistance to multiple antimicrobial drugs
        Excludes1   Resistance to multiple antibiotics only (Z16.24)

    Z16.39   Resistance to other specified antimicrobial drug

ESTROGEN RECEPTOR STATUS (Z17)

● **Z17   Estrogen receptor status**

    Code first malignant neoplasm of breast (C50.-)

    Z17.0   Estrogen receptor positive status [ER+]

    Z17.1   Estrogen receptor negative status [ER-]

RETAINED FOREIGN BODY FRAGMENTS (Z18)

● **Z18   Retained foreign body fragments**

    Includes   embedded fragment (status)
        embedded splinter (status)
        retained foreign body status

    Excludes1   artificial joint prosthesis status (Z96.6-)
        foreign body accidentally left during a procedure (T81.5-)
        foreign body entering through orifice (T15-T19)
        in situ cardiac device (Z95.-)
        organ or tissue replaced by means other than transplant (Z96.-, Z97.-)
        organ or tissue replaced by transplant (Z94.-)
        personal history of retained foreign body fully removed Z87.821
        superficial foreign body (non-embedded splinter) - code to superficial foreign body, by site

● **Z18.0   Retained radioactive fragments**

    Z18.01   Retained depleted uranium fragments

    Z18.09   Other retained radioactive fragments
        Other retained depleted isotope fragments
        Retained nontherapeutic radioactive fragments

● **Z18.1   Retained metal fragments**

    Excludes1   retained radioactive metal fragments (Z18.01-Z18.09)

    Z18.10   Retained metal fragments, unspecified
        Retained metal fragment NOS

    Z18.11   Retained magnetic metal fragments

    Z18.12   Retained nonmagnetic metal fragments

    Z18.2   Retained plastic fragments
        Acrylics fragments
        Diethylhexylphthalates fragments
        Isocyanate fragments

● **Z18.3   Retained organic fragments**

    Z18.31   Retained animal quills or spines

    Z18.32   Retained tooth

    Z18.33   Retained wood fragments

    Z18.39   Other retained organic fragments

● **Z18.8   Other specified retained foreign body**

    Z18.81   Retained glass fragments

    Z18.83   Retained stone or crystalline fragments
        Retained concrete or cement fragments

    Z18.89   Other specified retained foreign body fragments
        Coding Clinic: 2016, Q3, P24

    Z18.9   Retained foreign body fragments, unspecified material

HORMONE SENSITIVITY MALIGNANCY STATUS (Z19)

● **Z19   Hormone sensitivity malignancy status**

    Code first malignant neoplasm —see Table of Neoplasms, by site, malignant
    Coding Clinic: 2016, Q4, P129

    Z19.1   Hormone sensitive malignancy status
        Coding Clinic: 2016, Q4, P76

    Z19.2   Hormone resistant malignancy status
        Castrate resistant prostate malignancy status
        Coding Clinic: 2016, Q4, P76

▶ New   ▦ Revised   ~~deleted~~ Deleted   Excludes 1   Excludes 2   Includes   Use additional   Code first   Code also   Key words

OGCR Official Guidelines   **X** Assign placeholder X   ● Use Additional Character(s)   ▌ Manifestation Code   🔾 Hierarchical Condition Category   **Coding Clinic**

PERSONS WITH POTENTIAL HEALTH HAZARDS RELATED TO COMMUNICABLE DISEASES (Z20-Z29)

● **Z20** **Contact with and (suspected) exposure to communicable diseases**

    Excludes1   carrier of infectious disease (Z22.-)
           diagnosed current infectious or parasitic disease - see Alphabetic Index

    Excludes2   personal history of infectious and parasitic diseases (Z86.1-)

    Coding Clinic: 2021, Q1, P37

● **Z20.0** **Contact with and (suspected) exposure to intestinal infectious diseases**

    Z20.01 Contact with and (suspected) exposure to intestinal infectious diseases due to Escherichia coli (E. coli)

    Z20.09 Contact with and (suspected) exposure to other intestinal infectious diseases

 Z20.1 Contact with and (suspected) exposure to tuberculosis

 Z20.2 Contact with and (suspected) exposure to infections with a predominantly sexual mode of transmission

 Z20.3 Contact with and (suspected) exposure to rabies

 Z20.4 Contact with and (suspected) exposure to rubella

 Z20.5 Contact with and (suspected) exposure to viral hepatitis

 Z20.6 Contact with and (suspected) exposure to human immunodeficiency virus [HIV]

    Excludes1 asymptomatic human immunodeficiency virus [HIV]
       HIV infection status (Z21)

 Z20.7 Contact with and (suspected) exposure to pediculosis, acariasis and other infestations

● **Z20.8** **Contact with and (suspected) exposure to other communicable diseases**

●   **Z20.81** **Contact with and (suspected) exposure to other bacterial communicable diseases**

        Z20.810 Contact with and (suspected) exposure to anthrax

        Z20.811 Contact with and (suspected) exposure to meningococcus

        Z20.818 Contact with and (suspected) exposure to other bacterial communicable diseases

●   **Z20.82** **Contact with and (suspected) exposure to other viral communicable diseases**

        Z20.820 Contact with and (suspected) exposure to varicella

        Z20.821 Contact with and (suspected) exposure to Zika virus

        Z20.822 Contact with and (suspected) exposure to COVID-19
           Contact with and (suspected) exposure to SARS-CoV-2
           Coding Clinic: 2022, Q2, P28,29; 2021, Q4, P109; 2021, Q1, P37-39, 42

        Z20.828 Contact with and (suspected) exposure to other viral communicable diseases
           Coding Clinic: 2021, Q1, P37-39; 2016, Q4, P6-7, 121

    Z20.89 Contact with and (suspected) exposure to other communicable diseases

 Z20.9 Contact with and (suspected) exposure to unspecified communicable disease

● **Z21** **Asymptomatic human immunodeficiency virus [HIV] infection status** 🔒
    HIV positive NOS

    Code first Human immunodeficiency virus [HIV] disease complicating pregnancy, childbirth and the puerperium, if applicable (O98.7-)

    Excludes1 acquired immunodeficiency syndrome (B20)
       contact with human immunodeficiency virus [HIV] (Z20.6)
       exposure to human immunodeficiency virus [HIV] (Z20.6)
       human immunodeficiency virus [HIV] disease (B20)
       inconclusive laboratory evidence of human immunodeficiency virus [HIV] (R75)

    Coding Clinic: 2022, Q1, P37; 2019, Q1, P10-11

● **Z22** **Carrier of infectious disease**

    Includes   colonization status
           suspected carrier

    Excludes2 carrier of viral hepatitis (B18.-)

 Z22.0 Carrier of typhoid

 Z22.1 Carrier of other intestinal infectious diseases

 Z22.2 Carrier of diphtheria

● **Z22.3** **Carrier of other specified bacterial diseases**

    Z22.31 Carrier of bacterial disease due to meningococci

●   **Z22.32** Carrier of bacterial disease due to staphylococci

        Z22.321 Carrier or suspected carrier of Methicillin susceptible Staphylococcus aureus
           MSSA colonization

        Z22.322 Carrier or suspected carrier of Methicillin resistant Staphylococcus aureus
           MRSA colonization

●   **Z22.33** Carrier of bacterial disease due to streptococci

        Z22.330 Carrier of Group B streptococcus

          Excludes1 Carrier of streptococcus group B (GBS) complicating pregnancy, childbirth and the puerperium (O99.82-)

        Z22.338 Carrier of other streptococcus

    Z22.39 Carrier of other specified bacterial diseases

 Z22.4 Carrier of infections with a predominantly sexual mode of transmission

 Z22.6 Carrier of human T-lymphotropic virus type-1 [HTLV-1] infection

 Z22.7 Latent tuberculosis
    Latent tuberculosis infection (LTBI)

    Excludes1 nonspecific reaction to cell mediated immunity measurement of gamma interferon antigen response without active tuberculosis (R76.12)
       nonspecific reaction to tuberculin skin test without active tuberculosis (R76.11)

 Z22.8 Carrier of other infectious diseases

 Z22.9 Carrier of infectious disease, unspecified

Z23 **Encounter for immunization**

    Code first any routine childhood examination

    Note: Procedure codes are required to identify the types of immunizations given.

    Code also, if applicable, encounter for immunization safety counseling (Z71.85)

CHAPTER 21 (Z00-Z99)

● **Z28   Immunization not carried out and underimmunization status**

     Includes   vaccination not carried out

     Code also, if applicable, encounter for immunization safety counseling (Z71.85)

    ● **Z28.0   Immunization not carried out because of contraindication**

       Z28.01   Immunization not carried out because of acute illness of patient

       Z28.02   Immunization not carried out because of chronic illness or condition of patient

       Z28.03   Immunization not carried out because of immune compromised state of patient

       Z28.04   Immunization not carried out because of patient allergy to vaccine or component

       Z28.09   Immunization not carried out because of other contraindication

     Z28.1   Immunization not carried out because of patient decision for reasons of belief or group pressure

       Immunization not carried out because of religious belief

    ● **Z28.2   Immunization not carried out because of patient decision for other and unspecified reason**

       Z28.20   Immunization not carried out because of patient decision for unspecified reason

       Z28.21   Immunization not carried out because of patient refusal

       Z28.29   Immunization not carried out because of patient decision for other reason

     Z28.3   Underimmunization status

       Coding Clinic: 2021, Q4, P110

       Use additional code, if applicable, to identify:

       immunization not carried out because of contraindication (Z28.0-)

       immunization not carried out because of patient decision for other and unspecified reason (Z28.2-)

       immunization not carried out because of patient decision for reasons of belief or group pressure (Z28.1)

       immunization not carried out for other reason (Z28.8-)

       Z28.31   Underimmunization for COVID-19 status

         Note: These codes should not be used for individuals who are not eligible for the COVID-19 vaccines, as determined by the healthcare provider.

         Z28.310   Unvaccinated for COVID-19

         Z28.311   Partially vaccinated for COVID-19

       Z28.39   Other underimmunization status

         Delinquent immunization status

         Lapsed immunization schedule status

    ● **Z28.8   Immunization not carried out for other reason**

       Z28.81   Immunization not carried out due to patient having had the disease

       Z28.82   Immunization not carried out because of caregiver refusal

         Immunization not carried out because of guardian refusal

         Immunization not carried out because of parent refusal

         Excludes1   immunization not carried out because of caregiver refusal because of religious belief (Z28.1)

       Z28.83   Immunization not carried out due to unavailability of vaccine

         Delay in delivery of vaccine

         Lack of availability of vaccine

         Manufacturer delay of vaccine

       Z28.89   Immunization not carried out for other reason

     Z28.9   Immunization not carried out for unspecified reason

● **Z29   Encounter for other prophylactic measures**

     Excludes1   desensitization to allergens (Z51.6)

                 prophylactic surgery (Z40.-)

     Coding Clinic: 2016, Q4, P130

    ● **Z29.1   Encounter for prophylactic immunotherapy**

       Encounter for administration of immunoglobulin

       Coding Clinic: 2016, Q4, P78-79

       Z29.11   Encounter for prophylactic immunotherapy for respiratory syncytial virus (RSV)

       Z29.12   Encounter for prophylactic antivenin

       Z29.13   Encounter for prophylactic Rho(D) immune globulin

         Coding Clinic: 2019, Q3, P5

       Z29.14   Encounter for prophylactic rabies immune globin

     Z29.3   Encounter for prophylactic fluoride administration

       Coding Clinic: 2016, Q4, P79

     Z29.8   Encounter for other specified prophylactic measures

       Coding Clinic: 2022, Q2, P27; 2016, Q4, P79

     Z29.9   Encounter for prophylactic measures, unspecified

       Coding Clinic: 2016, Q4, P79

PERSONS ENCOUNTERING HEALTH SERVICES IN CIRCUMSTANCES RELATED TO REPRODUCTION (Z30-Z39)

● **Z30   Encounter for contraceptive management**

    ● **Z30.0   Encounter for general counseling and advice on contraception**

      ● **Z30.01   Encounter for initial prescription of contraceptives**

         Excludes1   encounter for surveillance of contraceptives (Z30.4-)

         Z30.011   Encounter for initial prescription of contraceptive pills ♀

         Z30.012   Encounter for prescription of emergency contraception ♀

           Encounter for postcoital contraception

         Z30.013   Encounter for initial prescription of injectable contraceptive ♀

         Z30.014   Encounter for initial prescription of intrauterine contraceptive device ♀

           Excludes1   encounter for insertion of intrauterine contraceptive device (Z30.430, Z30.432)

         Z30.015   Encounter for initial prescription of vaginal ring hormonal contraceptive ♀

           Coding Clinic: 2016, Q4, P78

         Z30.016   Encounter for initial prescription of transdermal patch hormonal contraceptive device

           Coding Clinic: 2016, Q4, P78

         Z30.017   Encounter for initial prescription of implantable subdermal contraceptive

           Coding Clinic: 2016, Q4, P78

         Z30.018   Encounter for initial prescription of other contraceptives ♀

           Encounter for initial prescription of barrier contraception

           Encounter for initial prescription of diaphragm

         Z30.019   Encounter for initial prescription of contraceptives, unspecified ♀

      Z30.02   Counseling and instruction in natural family planning to avoid pregnancy

      Z30.09   Encounter for other general counseling and advice on contraception

        Encounter for family planning advice NOS

     Z30.2   Encounter for sterilization

       Coding Clinic: 2021, Q3, P13

▶ New   ⇒ Revised   ~~deleted~~ Deleted   Excludes 1   Excludes 2   Includes   Use additional   Code first   Code also   Key words

OGCR Official Guidelines   X Assign placeholder X   ● Use Additional Character(s)   ▶ Manifestation Code   🏷 Hierarchical Condition Category   **Coding Clinic**

● **Z30.4** **Encounter for surveillance of contraceptives**
    Z30.40 Encounter for surveillance of contraceptives, **unspecified**
    Z30.41 Encounter for surveillance of contraceptive pills ♀
        Encounter for repeat prescription for contraceptive pill
    Z30.42 Encounter for surveillance of injectable contraceptive ♀
●   **Z30.43** Encounter for surveillance of intrauterine contraceptive device
        Z30.430 Encounter for insertion of intrauterine contraceptive device ♀
        Z30.431 Encounter for routine checking of intrauterine contraceptive device ♀
        Z30.432 Encounter for removal of intrauterine contraceptive device ♀
        Z30.433 Encounter for removal and reinsertion of intrauterine contraceptive device ♀
            Encounter for replacement of intrauterine contraceptive device
    Z30.44 Encounter for surveillance of vaginal ring hormonal contraceptive device ♀
        Coding Clinic: 2016, Q4, P78
    Z30.45 Encounter for surveillance of transdermal patch hormonal contraceptive device ♀
        Coding Clinic: 2016, Q4, P78
    Z30.46 Encounter for surveillance of implantable subdermal contraceptive ♀
        Encounter for checking, reinsertion or removal of implantable subdermal contraceptive
        Coding Clinic: 2016, Q4, P78
    Z30.49 Encounter for surveillance of other contraceptives ♀
        Encounter for surveillance of barrier contraception
        Encounter for surveillance of diaphragm

Z30.8 **Encounter for other contraceptive management**
    Encounter for postvasectomy sperm count
    Encounter for routine examination for contraceptive maintenance
    Excludes1 sperm count following sterilization reversal (Z31.42)
            sperm count for fertility testing (Z31.41)

Z30.9 **Encounter for contraceptive management, unspecified**

● **Z31** **Encounter for procreative management**
    Excludes2 complications associated with artificial fertilization (N98.-)
            female infertility (N97.-)
            male infertility (N46.-)

Z31.0 **Encounter for reversal of previous sterilization**

● **Z31.4** **Encounter for procreative investigation and testing**
    Excludes1 postvasectomy sperm count (Z30.8)
    Z31.41 Encounter for fertility testing
        Encounter for fallopian tube patency testing
        Encounter for sperm count for fertility testing
    Z31.42 Aftercare following sterilization reversal
        Sperm count following sterilization reversal
●   **Z31.43** Encounter for genetic testing of female for procreative management
        Use additional code for recurrent pregnancy loss, if applicable (N96, O26.2-)
        Excludes1 nonprocreative genetic testing (Z13.7-)
        Z31.430 Encounter of female for testing for genetic disease carrier status for procreative management ♀
        Z31.438 Encounter for other genetic testing of female for procreative management ♀

●   **Z31.44** Encounter for genetic testing of male for procreative management
        Excludes1 nonprocreative genetic testing (Z13.7-)
        Z31.440 Encounter of male for testing for genetic disease carrier status for procreative management ♂
        Z31.441 Encounter for testing of male partner of patient with recurrent pregnancy loss ♂   A
        Z31.448 Encounter for other genetic testing of male for procreative management ♂ A
    Z31.49 Encounter for other procreative investigation and testing

Z31.5 **Encounter for procreative genetic counseling**

● **Z31.6** **Encounter for general counseling and advice on procreation**
    Z31.61 Procreative counseling and advice using natural family planning
    Z31.62 Encounter for fertility preservation counseling
        Encounter for fertility preservation counseling prior to cancer therapy
        Encounter for fertility preservation counseling prior to surgical removal of gonads
    Z31.69 Encounter for other general counseling and advice on procreation

Z31.7 **Encounter for procreative management and counseling for gestational carrier** ♀
    Excludes1 pregnant state, gestational carrier (Z33.3)
    Coding Clinic: 2016, Q4, P78

● **Z31.8** **Encounter for other procreative management**
    Z31.81 Encounter for male factor infertility in female patient ♀
    Z31.82 Encounter for Rh incompatibility status ♀
        Coding Clinic: 2015, Q3, P40
    Z31.83 Encounter for assisted reproductive fertility procedure cycle ♀
        Patient undergoing in vitro fertilization cycle
        Use additional code to identify the type of infertility
        Excludes1 pre-cycle diagnosis and testing - code to reason for encounter
        Coding Clinic: 2022, Q2, P15,16
    Z31.84 Encounter for fertility preservation procedure
        Encounter for fertility preservation procedure prior to cancer therapy
        Encounter for fertility preservation procedure prior to surgical removal of gonads
    Z31.89 Encounter for other procreative management

Z31.9 **Encounter for procreative management, unspecified**

● **Z32** **Encounter for pregnancy test and childbirth and childcare instruction**
●   **Z32.0** **Encounter for pregnancy test**
    Z32.00 Encounter for pregnancy test, result unknown ♀
        Encounter for pregnancy test NOS
    Z32.01 Encounter for pregnancy test, result positive ♀ M
    Z32.02 Encounter for pregnancy test, result negative ♀

Z32.2 **Encounter for childbirth instruction**

Z32.3 **Encounter for childcare instruction**
    Encounter for prenatal or postpartum childcare instruction

● **Z33** **Pregnant state**
    Z33.1 **Pregnant state, incidental** ♀   M
        Pregnancy NOS
        Pregnant state NOS
        Excludes1 complications of pregnancy (O00-O9A)
            pregnant state, gestational carrier (Z33.3)
    Z33.2 **Encounter for elective termination of pregnancy** ♀   M
        Excludes1 early fetal death with retention of dead fetus (O02.1)
            late fetal death (O36.4)
            spontaneous abortion (O03)
        Coding Clinic: 2016, Q4, P130

CHAPTER 21 (Z00-Z99)

Figure 21-1 Trimesters. (From Shiland, Betsy J. Medical Terminology & Anatomy for ICD-10 Coding, ed 2, Mosby, 2015)

First trimester (0 to 14 weeks)
Second trimester (14 to 28 weeks)
Third trimester (28 weeks to delivery)

Z33.3 Pregnant state, gestational carrier ♀
   Excludes1 encounter for procreative management and counseling for gestational carrier (Z31.7)
   Coding Clinic: 2016, Q4, P78

Z34 Encounter for supervision of normal pregnancy
   Excludes1 any complication of pregnancy (O00-O9A)
   encounter for pregnancy test (Z32.0-)
   encounter for supervision of high risk pregnancy (O09.-)
   Coding Clinic: 2016, Q4, P6

Z34.0 Encounter for supervision of normal first pregnancy
  Z34.00 Encounter for supervision of normal first pregnancy, unspecified trimester ♀ M
  Z34.01 Encounter for supervision of normal first pregnancy, first trimester ♀ M
  Z34.02 Encounter for supervision of normal first pregnancy, second trimester ♀ M
  Z34.03 Encounter for supervision of normal first pregnancy, third trimester ♀ M

Z34.8 Encounter for supervision of other normal pregnancy
  Z34.80 Encounter for supervision of other normal pregnancy, unspecified trimester ♀ M
  Z34.81 Encounter for supervision of other normal pregnancy, first trimester ♀ M
  Z34.82 Encounter for supervision of other normal pregnancy, second trimester ♀ M
  Z34.83 Encounter for supervision of other normal pregnancy, third trimester ♀ M

Z34.9 Encounter for supervision of normal pregnancy, unspecified
  Z34.90 Encounter for supervision of normal pregnancy, unspecified, unspecified trimester ♀ M
  Z34.91 Encounter for supervision of normal pregnancy, unspecified, first trimester ♀ M
  Z34.92 Encounter for supervision of normal pregnancy, unspecified, second trimester ♀ M
  Z34.93 Encounter for supervision of normal pregnancy, unspecified, third trimester ♀ M

Z36 Encounter for antenatal screening of mother ♀
  Includes Encounter for placental sample (taken vaginally)
  Screening is the testing for disease or disease precursors in asymptomatic individuals so that early detection and treatment can be provided for those who test positive for the disease.
  Excludes1 diagnostic examination - code to sign or symptom
  encounter for suspected maternal and fetal conditions ruled out (Z03.7-)
  suspected fetal condition affecting management of pregnancy - code to condition in Chapter 15
  Excludes2 abnormal findings on antenatal screening of mother (O28.-)
  genetic counseling and testing (Z31.43-, Z31.5)
  routine prenatal care (Z34)

Z36.0 Encounter for antenatal screening for chromosomal anomalies ♀ M
Z36.1 Encounter for antenatal screening for raised alphafetoprotein level ♀ M
  Encounter for antenatal screening for elevated maternal serum alphafetoprotein level
Z36.2 Encounter for other antenatal screening follow-up ♀ M
  Non-visualized anatomy on a previous scan
Z36.3 Encounter for antenatal screening for malformations ♀ M
  Screening for a suspected anomaly
Z36.4 Encounter for antenatal screening for fetal growth retardation ♀ M
  Intrauterine growth restriction (IUGR)/small-for-dates
Z36.5 Encounter for antenatal screening for isoimmunization ♀ M
Z36.8 Encounter for other antenatal screening
  Z36.81 Encounter for antenatal screening for hydrops fetalis ♀ M
  Z36.82 Encounter for antenatal screening for nuchal translucency ♀ M
  Z36.83 Encounter for fetal screening for congenital cardiac abnormalities ♀ M
  Z36.84 Encounter for antenatal screening for fetal lung maturity ♀ M
  Z36.85 Encounter for antenatal screening for Streptococcus B ♀ M
  Z36.86 Encounter for antenatal screening for cervical length ♀ M
   Screening for risk of pre-term labor
  Z36.87 Encounter for antenatal screening for uncertain dates ♀ M
  Z36.88 Encounter for antenatal screening for fetal macrosomia ♀ M
   Screening for large-for-dates
  Z36.89 Encounter for other specified antenatal screening ♀ M
  Z36.8A Encounter for antenatal screening for other genetic defects ♀ M
Z36.9 Encounter for antenatal screening, unspecified ♀ M

Z3A Weeks of gestation
  Note: Codes from category Z3A are for use, only on the maternal record, to indicate the weeks of gestation of the pregnancy, if known.
  Code first obstetric condition or encounter for delivery (O09-O60, O80-O82)
  Coding Clinic: 2022, Q2, P3-4; 2016, Q4, P130; 2013, Q2, P33

Z3A.0 Weeks of gestation of pregnancy, unspecified or less than 10 weeks
  Z3A.00 Weeks of gestation of pregnancy not specified ♀ M
  Z3A.01 Less than 8 weeks gestation of pregnancy ♀ M
  Z3A.08 8 weeks gestation of pregnancy ♀ M
  Z3A.09 9 weeks gestation of pregnancy ♀ M
Z3A.1 Weeks of gestation of pregnancy, weeks 10-19
  Z3A.10 10 weeks gestation of pregnancy ♀ M
  Z3A.11 11 weeks gestation of pregnancy ♀ M
  Z3A.12 12 weeks gestation of pregnancy ♀ M
  Z3A.13 13 weeks gestation of pregnancy ♀ M
  Z3A.14 14 weeks gestation of pregnancy ♀ M
  Z3A.15 15 weeks gestation of pregnancy ♀ M
  Z3A.16 16 weeks gestation of pregnancy ♀ M
   Coding Clinic: 2016, Q4, P5
  Z3A.17 17 weeks gestation of pregnancy ♀ M
  Z3A.18 18 weeks gestation of pregnancy ♀ M
   Coding Clinic: 2019, Q2, P11
  Z3A.19 19 weeks gestation of pregnancy ♀ M
Z3A.2 Weeks of gestation of pregnancy, weeks 20-29
  Z3A.20 20 weeks gestation of pregnancy M
   Coding Clinic: 2016, Q4, P6
  Z3A.21 21 weeks gestation of pregnancy ♀ M

Z3A.22   22 weeks gestation of pregnancy ♀   M
Coding Clinic: 2016, Q4, P6

Z3A.23   23 weeks gestation of pregnancy ♀   M

Z3A.24   24 weeks gestation of pregnancy ♀   M

Z3A.25   25 weeks gestation of pregnancy ♀   M

Z3A.26   26 weeks gestation of pregnancy ♀   M

Z3A.27   27 weeks gestation of pregnancy ♀   M

Z3A.28   28 weeks gestation of pregnancy ♀   M

Z3A.29   29 weeks gestation of pregnancy ♀   M

● Z3A.3   Weeks of gestation of pregnancy, weeks 30-39

Z3A.30   30 weeks gestation of pregnancy ♀   M

Z3A.31   31 weeks gestation of pregnancy ♀   M

Z3A.32   32 weeks gestation of pregnancy ♀   M
Coding Clinic: 2016, Q4, P6

Z3A.33   33 weeks gestation of pregnancy ♀   M

Z3A.34   34 weeks gestation of pregnancy ♀   M

Z3A.35   35 weeks gestation of pregnancy ♀   M

Z3A.36   36 weeks gestation of pregnancy ♀   M

Z3A.37   37 weeks gestation of pregnancy ♀   M

Z3A.38   38 weeks gestation of pregnancy ♀   M
Coding Clinic: 2016, Q2, P34

Z3A.39   39 weeks gestation of pregnancy ♀   M

● Z3A.4   Weeks of gestation of pregnancy, weeks 40 or greater

Z3A.40   40 weeks gestation of pregnancy ♀   M

Z3A.41   41 weeks gestation of pregnancy ♀   M

Z3A.42   42 weeks gestation of pregnancy ♀   M

Z3A.49   Greater than 42 weeks gestation of pregnancy ♀   M

● Z37   **Outcome of delivery**
This category is intended for use as an additional code to identify the outcome of delivery on the mother's record. It is not for use on the newborn record.

   Excludes1   stillbirth (P95)

Z37.0   Single live birth ♀   M
Coding Clinic: 2016, Q2, P34

Z37.1   Single stillbirth ♀   M

Z37.2   Twins, both liveborn ♀   M

Z37.3   Twins, one liveborn and one stillborn ♀   M

Z37.4   Twins, both stillborn ♀   M

● Z37.5   Other multiple births, all liveborn

Z37.50   Multiple births, unspecified, all liveborn ♀   M

Z37.51   Triplets, all liveborn ♀   M

Z37.52   Quadruplets, all liveborn ♀   M

Z37.53   Quintuplets, all liveborn ♀   M

Z37.54   Sextuplets, all liveborn ♀   M

Z37.59   Other multiple births, all liveborn ♀   M

● Z37.6   Other multiple births, some liveborn

Z37.60   Multiple births, unspecified, some liveborn ♀ M

Z37.61   Triplets, some liveborn ♀   M

Z37.62   Quadruplets, some liveborn ♀   M

Z37.63   Quintuplets, some liveborn ♀   M

Z37.64   Sextuplets, some liveborn ♀   M

Z37.69   Other multiple births, some liveborn ♀   M

Z37.7   Other multiple births, all stillborn ♀   M

Z37.9   Outcome of delivery, unspecified ♀   M
Multiple birth NOS
Single birth NOS

● Z38   **Liveborn infants according to place of birth and type of delivery**
This category is for use as the principal code on the initial record of a newborn baby. It is to be used for the initial birth record only. It is not to be used on the mother's record.
Coding Clinic: 2017, Q2, P6-7; 2016, Q4, P126-127, 130; 2015, Q2, P15

● Z38.0   Single liveborn infant, born in hospital
Single liveborn infant, born in birthing center or other health care facility
Coding Clinic: 2017, Q2, P5-7

Z38.00   Single liveborn infant, delivered vaginally   N
Coding Clinic: 2021, Q4, P23; 2018, Q4, P26; 2016, Q4, P7, 55

Z38.01   Single liveborn infant, delivered by cesarean   N
Coding Clinic: 2017, Q2, P7; 2016, Q3, P18

Z38.1   Single liveborn infant, born outside hospital   N

Z38.2   Single liveborn infant, unspecified as to place of birth   N
Single liveborn infant NOS

● Z38.3   Twin liveborn infant, born in hospital

Z38.30   Twin liveborn infant, delivered vaginally   N

Z38.31   Twin liveborn infant, delivered by cesarean   N

Z38.4   Twin liveborn infant, born outside hospital   N

Z38.5   Twin liveborn infant, unspecified as to place of birth   N

● Z38.6   Other multiple liveborn infant, born in hospital

Z38.61   Triplet liveborn infant, delivered vaginally   N

Z38.62   Triplet liveborn infant, delivered by cesarean   N

Z38.63   Quadruplet liveborn infant, delivered vaginally   N

Z38.64   Quadruplet liveborn infant, delivered by cesarean   N

Z38.65   Quintuplet liveborn infant, delivered vaginally   N

Z38.66   Quintuplet liveborn infant, delivered by cesarean   N

Z38.68   Other multiple liveborn infant, delivered vaginally   N

Z38.69   Other multiple liveborn infant, delivered by cesarean   N

Z38.7   Other multiple liveborn infant, born outside hospital   N

Z38.8   Other multiple liveborn infant, unspecified as to place of birth   N

● Z39   **Encounter for maternal postpartum care and examination**

Z39.0   Encounter for care and examination of mother immediately after delivery ♀   M
Care and observation in uncomplicated cases when the delivery occurs outside a healthcare facility

   Excludes1   care for postpartum complication - see Alphabetic index

Coding Clinic: 2021, Q3, P13

Z39.1   Encounter for care and examination of lactating mother ♀   M
Encounter for supervision of lactation

   Excludes1   disorders of lactation (O92.-)

Z39.2   Encounter for routine postpartum follow-up ♀   M

ENCOUNTERS FOR OTHER SPECIFIC HEALTH CARE (Z40-Z53)

Categories Z40-Z53 are intended for use to indicate a reason for care. They may be used for patients who have already been treated for a disease or injury, but who are receiving aftercare or prophylactic care, or care to consolidate the treatment, or to deal with a residual state

   Excludes2   follow-up examination for medical surveillance after treatment (Z08-Z09)

● Z40   **Encounter for prophylactic surgery**

   Excludes1   organ donations (Z52.-)
therapeutic organ removal - code to condition

Coding Clinic: 2016, Q4, P79

● Z40.0   Encounter for prophylactic surgery for risk factors related to malignant neoplasms
Admission for prophylactic organ removal
Use additional code to identify risk factor

Z40.00   Encounter for prophylactic removal of unspecified organ

Z40.01   Encounter for prophylactic removal of breast

Z40.02   Encounter for prophylactic removal of ovary(s) ♀
Encounter for prophylactic removal of ovary(s) and fallopian tube(s)

CHAPTER 21 (Z00-Z99)

CHAPTER 21 (Z00–Z99)

Z40.03   Encounter for prophylactic removal of fallopian tube(s) ♀

Z40.09   Encounter for prophylactic removal of other organ

Z40.8   Encounter for other prophylactic surgery

Z40.9   Encounter for prophylactic surgery, unspecified

● Z41   Encounter for procedures for purposes other than remedying health state

   Z41.1   Encounter for cosmetic surgery
      Encounter for cosmetic breast implant
      Encounter for cosmetic procedure

      Excludes1   encounter for plastic and reconstructive surgery following medical procedure or healed injury (Z42.-)
          encounter for post-mastectomy breast implantation (Z42.1)

   Z41.2   Encounter for routine and ritual male circumcision ♂

   Z41.3   Encounter for ear piercing

   Z41.8   Encounter for other procedures for purposes other than remedying health state

   Z41.9   Encounter for procedure for purposes other than remedying health state, unspecified

● Z42   Encounter for plastic and reconstructive surgery following medical procedure or healed injury

      Excludes1   encounter for cosmetic plastic surgery (Z41.1)
          encounter for plastic surgery for treatment of current injury - code to relevent injury

   Z42.1   Encounter for breast reconstruction following mastectomy

      Excludes1   deformity and disproportion of reconstructed breast (N65.1-)

   Z42.8   Encounter for other plastic and reconstructive surgery following medical procedure or healed injury
      Coding Clinic: 2017, Q1, P42

● Z43   Encounter for attention to artificial openings

      Includes   closure of artificial openings
          passage of sounds or bougies through artificial openings
          reforming artificial openings
          removal of catheter from artificial openings
          toilet or cleansing of artificial openings

      Excludes1   complications of external stoma (J95.0-, K94.-, N99.5-)

      Excludes2   fitting and adjustment of prosthetic and other devices (Z44-Z46)

   Z43.0   Encounter for attention to tracheostomy 🐾

   Z43.1   Encounter for attention to gastrostomy 🐾

      Excludes2   artificial opening status only, without need for care (Z93.-)

   Z43.2   Encounter for attention to ileostomy 🐾
      Coding Clinic: 2016, Q3, P5

   Z43.3   Encounter for attention to colostomy 🐾

   Z43.4   Encounter for attention to other artificial openings of digestive tract 🐾

   Z43.5   Encounter for attention to cystostomy 🐾

   Z43.6   Encounter for attention to other artificial openings of urinary tract 🐾
      Encounter for attention to nephrostomy
      Encounter for attention to ureterostomy
      Encounter for attention to urethrostomy

   Z43.7   Encounter for attention to artificial vagina

   Z43.8   Encounter for attention to other artificial openings 🐾

   Z43.9   Encounter for attention to unspecified artificial opening 🐾

● Z44   Encounter for fitting and adjustment of external prosthetic device

      Includes   removal or replacement of external prosthetic device

      Excludes1   malfunction or other complications of device - see Alphabetical Index presence of prosthetic device (Z97.-)

● Z44.0   Encounter for fitting and adjustment of artificial arm

   ● Z44.00   Encounter for fitting and adjustment of unspecified artificial arm

      Z44.001   Encounter for fitting and adjustment of unspecified right artificial arm

      Z44.002   Encounter for fitting and adjustment of unspecified left artificial arm

      Z44.009   Encounter for fitting and adjustment of unspecified artificial arm, unspecified arm

   ● Z44.01   Encounter for fitting and adjustment of complete artificial arm

      Z44.011   Encounter for fitting and adjustment of complete right artificial arm

      Z44.012   Encounter for fitting and adjustment of complete left artificial arm

      Z44.019   Encounter for fitting and adjustment of complete artificial arm, unspecified arm

   ● Z44.02   Encounter for fitting and adjustment of partial artificial arm

      Z44.021   Encounter for fitting and adjustment of partial artificial right arm

      Z44.022   Encounter for fitting and adjustment of partial artificial left arm

      Z44.029   Encounter for fitting and adjustment of partial artificial arm, unspecified arm

● Z44.1   Encounter for fitting and adjustment of artificial leg

   ● Z44.10   Encounter for fitting and adjustment of unspecified artificial leg

      Z44.101   Encounter for fitting and adjustment of unspecified right artificial leg 🐾

      Z44.102   Encounter for fitting and adjustment of unspecified left artificial leg 🐾

      Z44.109   Encounter for fitting and adjustment of unspecified artificial leg, unspecified leg 🐾

   ● Z44.11   Encounter for fitting and adjustment of complete artificial leg

      Z44.111   Encounter for fitting and adjustment of complete right artificial leg 🐾

      Z44.112   Encounter for fitting and adjustment of complete left artificial leg 🐾

      Z44.119   Encounter for fitting and adjustment of complete artificial leg, unspecified leg 🐾

   ● Z44.12   Encounter for fitting and adjustment of partial artificial leg

      Z44.121   Encounter for fitting and adjustment of partial artificial right leg 🐾

      Z44.122   Encounter for fitting and adjustment of partial artificial left leg 🐾

      Z44.129   Encounter for fitting and adjustment of partial artificial leg, unspecified leg 🐾

● Z44.2   Encounter for fitting and adjustment of artificial eye

      Excludes1   mechanical complication of ocular prosthesis (T85.3)

   Z44.20   Encounter for fitting and adjustment of artificial eye, unspecified

   Z44.21   Encounter for fitting and adjustment of artificial right eye

   Z44.22   Encounter for fitting and adjustment of artificial left eye

▶ New   ⇒ Revised   ~~deleted~~ Deleted   Excludes 1   Excludes 2   Includes   Use additional   Code first   Code also   Key words
OGCR Official Guidelines   X Assign placeholder X   ● Use Additional Character(s)   ❙ Manifestation Code   🐾 Hierarchical Condition Category   **Coding Clinic**

● **Z44.3**   **Encounter for fitting and adjustment of external breast prosthesis**

     Excludes1   complications of breast implant (T85.4-)
                         encounter for adjustment or removal of breast implant (Z45.81-)
                         encounter for initial breast implant insertion for cosmetic breast augmentation (Z41.1)
                         encounter for breast reconstruction following mastectomy (Z42.1)

     Z44.30   Encounter for fitting and adjustment of external breast prosthesis, **unspecified** breast

     Z44.31   Encounter for fitting and adjustment of external **right** breast prosthesis

     Z44.32   Encounter for fitting and adjustment of external **left** breast prosthesis

   Z44.8   Encounter for fitting and adjustment of **other external** prosthetic devices

   Z44.9   Encounter for fitting and adjustment of **unspecified** external prosthetic device

● **Z45**   **Encounter for adjustment and management of implanted device**

     Includes   removal or replacement of implanted device

     Excludes1   malfunction or other complications of device - see Alphabetical Index

     Excludes2   encounter for fitting and adjustment of non-implanted device (Z46.-)

   ● **Z45.0**   **Encounter for adjustment and management of cardiac device**

     ● **Z45.01**   **Encounter for adjustment and management of cardiac pacemaker**
          Encounter for adjustment and management of cardiac resynchronization therapy pacemaker (CRT-P)

         Excludes1   encounter for adjustment and management of automatic implantable cardiac defibrillator with synchronous cardiac pacemaker (Z45.02)

        Z45.010   **Encounter for checking and testing of cardiac pacemaker pulse generator [battery]**
            Encounter for replacing cardiac pacemaker pulse generator [battery]

        Z45.018   **Encounter for adjustment and management of other part of cardiac pacemaker**

          Excludes1   presence of other part of cardiac pacemaker (Z95.0)

          Excludes2   presence of prosthetic and other devices (Z95.1-Z95.5, Z95.811-Z97)

     Z45.02   **Encounter for adjustment and management of automatic implantable cardiac defibrillator**
         Encounter for adjustment and management of automatic implantable cardiac defibrillator with synchronous cardiac pacemaker
         Encounter for adjustment and management of cardiac resynchronization therapy defibrillator (CRT-D)

     Z45.09   **Encounter for adjustment and management of other cardiac device**

   Z45.1   **Encounter for adjustment and management of infusion pump**

● **Z45.2**   **Encounter for adjustment and management of vascular access device**
     Encounter for adjustment and management of vascular catheters

     Excludes1   encounter for adjustment and management of renal dialysis catheter (Z49.01)

● **Z45.3**   **Encounter for adjustment and management of implanted devices of the special senses**

   Z45.31   **Encounter for adjustment and management of implanted visual substitution device**

   ● **Z45.32**   **Encounter for adjustment and management of implanted hearing device**

     Excludes1   encounter for fitting and adjustment of hearing aide (Z46.1)

     Z45.320   **Encounter for adjustment and management of bone conduction device**

     Z45.321   **Encounter for adjustment and management of cochlear device**

     Z45.328   **Encounter for adjustment and management of other implanted hearing device**

● **Z45.4**   **Encounter for adjustment and management of implanted nervous system device**

   Z45.41   **Encounter for adjustment and management of cerebrospinal fluid drainage device**
     Encounter for adjustment and management of cerebral ventricular (communicating) shunt

   Z45.42   **Encounter for adjustment and management of neuropacemaker**
     Encounter for adjustment and management of brain neurostimulator
     Encounter for adjustment and management of gastric neurostimulator
     Encounter for adjustment and management of peripheral nerve neurostimulator
     Encounter for adjustment and management of sacral nerve neurostimulator
     Encounter for adjustment and management of spinal cord neurostimulator
     Encounter for adjustment and management of vagus nerve neurostimulator

   Z45.49   **Encounter for adjustment and management of other implanted nervous system device**

● **Z45.8**   **Encounter for adjustment and management of other implanted devices**

   ● **Z45.81**   **Encounter for adjustment or removal of breast implant**
     Encounter for elective implant exchange (different material) (different size)
     Encounter for removal of tissue expander with or without synchronous insertion of permanent implant

     Excludes1   complications of breast implant (T85.4-)
                     encounter for initial breast implant insertion for cosmetic breast augmentation (Z41.1)
                     encounter for breast reconstruction following mastectomy (Z42.1)

     Z45.811   **Encounter for adjustment or removal of right breast implant**

     Z45.812   **Encounter for adjustment or removal of left breast implant**

     Z45.819   **Encounter for adjustment or removal of unspecified breast implant**

   Z45.82   **Encounter for adjustment or removal of myringotomy device (stent) (tube)**

   Z45.89   **Encounter for adjustment and management of other implanted devices**

   Z45.9   **Encounter for adjustment and management of unspecified implanted device**

● **Z46 Encounter for fitting and adjustment of other devices**

Includes removal or replacement of other device

Excludes1 malfunction or other complications of device - see Alphabetical Index

Excludes2 encounter for fitting and management of implanted devices (Z45.-)
issue of repeat prescription only (Z76.0)
presence of prosthetic and other devices (Z95-Z97)

Z46.0 Encounter for fitting and adjustment of spectacles and contact lenses

Z46.1 Encounter for fitting and adjustment of hearing aid

Excludes1 encounter for adjustment and management of implanted hearing device (Z45.32-)

Z46.2 Encounter for fitting and adjustment of other devices related to nervous system and special senses

Excludes2 encounter for adjustment and management of implanted nervous system device (Z45.4-)
encounter for adjustment and management of implanted visual substitution device (Z45.31)

Z46.3 Encounter for fitting and adjustment of dental prosthetic device

Encounter for fitting and adjustment of dentures

Z46.4 Encounter for fitting and adjustment of orthodontic device

● **Z46.5 Encounter for fitting and adjustment of other gastrointestinal appliance and device**

Excludes1 encounter for attention to artificial openings of digestive tract (Z43.1-Z43.4)

Z46.51 Encounter for fitting and adjustment of gastric lap band

Z46.59 Encounter for fitting and adjustment of other gastrointestinal appliance and device

Z46.6 Encounter for fitting and adjustment of urinary device

Excludes2 attention to artificial openings of urinary tract (Z43.5, Z43.6)

● **Z46.8 Encounter for fitting and adjustment of other specified devices**

Z46.81 Encounter for fitting and adjustment of insulin pump

Encounter for insulin pump instruction and training
Encounter for insulin pump titration

Z46.82 Encounter for fitting and adjustment of non-vascular catheter

Z46.89 Encounter for fitting and adjustment of other specified devices

Encounter for fitting and adjustment of wheelchair

Z46.9 Encounter for fitting and adjustment of unspecified device

● **Z47 Orthopedic aftercare**

Excludes1 aftercare for healing fracture - code to fracture with 7th character D

Z47.1 Aftercare following joint replacement surgery

Use additional code to identify the joint (Z96.6-)
Coding Clinic: 2020, Q1, P23-24

Z47.2 Encounter for removal of internal fixation device

Excludes1 encounter for adjustment of internal fixation device for fracture treatment - code to fracture with appropriate 7th character
encounter for removal of external fixation device - code to fracture with 7th character D
infection or inflammatory reaction to internal fixation device (T84.6-)
mechanical complication of internal fixation device (T84.1-)

● **Z47.3 Aftercare following explantation of joint prosthesis**

Aftercare following explantation of joint prosthesis, staged procedure
Encounter for joint prosthesis insertion following prior explantation of joint prosthesis
Coding Clinic: 2020, Q1, P23; 2015, Q1, P17

Z47.31 Aftercare following explantation of shoulder joint prosthesis

Excludes1 acquired absence of shoulder joint following prior explantation of shoulder joint prosthesis (Z89.23-)
shoulder joint prosthesis explantation status (Z89.23-)

Z47.32 Aftercare following explantation of hip joint prosthesis

Excludes1 acquired absence of hip joint following prior explantation of hip joint prosthesis (Z89.62-)
hip joint prosthesis explantation status (Z89.62-)
Coding Clinic: 2015, Q1, P17

Z47.33 Aftercare following explantation of knee joint prosthesis

Excludes1 acquired absence of knee joint following prior explantation of knee prosthesis (Z89.52-)
knee joint prosthesis explantation status (Z89.52-)

● **Z47.8 Encounter for other orthopedic aftercare**

Z47.81 Encounter for orthopedic aftercare following surgical amputation

Use additional code to identify the limb amputated (Z89.-)

Z47.82 Encounter for orthopedic aftercare following scoliosis surgery

Z47.89 Encounter for other orthopedic aftercare
Coding Clinic: 2015, Q1, P8

● **Z48 Encounter for other postprocedural aftercare**

Excludes1 encounter for aftercare following injury - code to Injury, by site, with appropriate 7th character for subsequent encounter
encounter for follow-up examination after completed treatment (Z08-Z09)

Excludes2 encounter for attention to artificial openings (Z43.-)
encounter for fitting and adjustment of prosthetic and other devices (Z44-Z46)

● **Z48.0 Encounter for attention to dressings, sutures and drains**

Excludes1 encounter for planned postprocedural wound closure (Z48.1)

Z48.00 Encounter for change or removal of nonsurgical wound dressing

Encounter for change or removal of wound dressing NOS

Z48.01 Encounter for change or removal of surgical wound dressing
Coding Clinic: 2019, Q2, P33; 2015, Q4, P38

Z48.02 Encounter for removal of sutures

Encounter for removal of staples
Coding Clinic: 2015, Q1, P6

Z48.03 Encounter for change or removal of drains

Z48.1 Encounter for planned postprocedural wound closure

Excludes1 encounter for attention to dressings and sutures (Z48.0-)

▶ New ⇒ Revised ~~deleted~~ Deleted | Excludes 1 | Excludes 2 | Includes | Use additional | Code first | Code also | Key words

OGCR Official Guidelines X Assign placeholder X ● Use Additional Character(s)) Manifestation Code 🦠 Hierarchical Condition Category **Coding Clinic**

● **Z48.2**   Encounter for aftercare following organ transplant
    Z48.21   Encounter for aftercare following heart transplant 🔧
    Z48.22   Encounter for aftercare following kidney transplant
    Z48.23   Encounter for aftercare following liver transplant 🔧
    Z48.24   Encounter for aftercare following lung transplant 🔧
  ● **Z48.28**   Encounter for aftercare following multiple organ transplant
      Z48.280   Encounter for aftercare following heart-lung transplant 🔧
      Z48.288   Encounter for aftercare following multiple organ transplant
  ● **Z48.29**   Encounter for aftercare following other organ transplant
      Z48.290   Encounter for aftercare following bone marrow transplant 🔧
      Z48.298   Encounter for aftercare following other organ transplant

Z48.3   Aftercare following surgery for neoplasm
    Use additional code to identify the neoplasm

● **Z48.8**   Encounter for other specified postprocedural aftercare
  ● **Z48.81**   Encounter for surgical aftercare following surgery on specified body systems
      These codes identify the body system requiring aftercare. They are for use in conjunction with other aftercare codes to fully explain the aftercare encounter. The condition treated should also be coded if still present.
      Excludes1   aftercare for injury - code the injury with 7th character D
              aftercare following surgery for neoplasm (Z48.3)
      Excludes2   aftercare following organ transplant (Z48.2-)
              orthopedic aftercare (Z47.-)
      Z48.810   Encounter for surgical aftercare following surgery on the sense organs
      Z48.811   Encounter for surgical aftercare following surgery on the nervous system
        Excludes2   encounter for surgical aftercare following surgery on the sense organs (Z48.810)
      Z48.812   Encounter for surgical aftercare following surgery on the circulatory system
        Coding Clinic: 2012, Q4, P96
      Z48.813   Encounter for surgical aftercare following surgery on the respiratory system
        Coding Clinic: 2019, Q2, P33
      Z48.814   Encounter for surgical aftercare following surgery on the teeth or oral cavity
      Z48.815   Encounter for surgical aftercare following surgery on the digestive system
        Coding Clinic: 2015, Q4, P38
      Z48.816   Encounter for surgical aftercare following surgery on the genitourinary system
        Excludes1   encounter for aftercare following sterilization reversal (Z31.42)

      Z48.817   Encounter for surgical aftercare following surgery on the skin and subcutaneous tissue
        Coding Clinic: 2015, Q1, P6
     Z48.89   Encounter for other specified surgical aftercare

● **Z49**   Encounter for care involving renal dialysis
    Code also associated end stage renal disease (N18.6)
  ● **Z49.0**   Preparatory care for renal dialysis
      Encounter for dialysis instruction and training
     Z49.01   Encounter for fitting and adjustment of extracorporeal dialysis catheter 🔧
       Removal or replacement of renal dialysis catheter
       Toilet or cleansing of renal dialysis catheter
     Z49.02   Encounter for fitting and adjustment of peritoneal dialysis catheter 🔧
  ● **Z49.3**   Encounter for adequacy testing for dialysis
     Z49.31   Encounter for adequacy testing for hemodialysis 🔧
     Z49.32   Encounter for adequacy testing for peritoneal dialysis 🔧
       Encounter for peritoneal equilibration test

● **Z51**   Encounter for other aftercare and medical care
    Code also condition requiring care
    Excludes1   follow-up examination after treatment (Z08-Z09)
    Coding Clinic: 2017, Q1, P49; 2016, Q4, P130
    Z51.0   Encounter for antineoplastic radiation therapy
      Coding Clinic: 2017, Q4, P103
  ● **Z51.1**   Encounter for antineoplastic chemotherapy and immunotherapy
     Excludes2   encounter for chemotherapy and immunotherapy for nonneoplastic condition-code to condition
     Z51.11   Encounter for antineoplastic chemotherapy
       Coding Clinic: 2022, Q1, P16; 2015, Q3, P19
     Z51.12   Encounter for antineoplastic immunotherapy
    Z51.5   Encounter for palliative care
      Coding Clinic: 2022, Q1, P19; 2017, Q1, P48-49
    Z51.6   Encounter for desensitization to allergens
      Coding Clinic: 2016, Q4, P77-79
  ● **Z51.8**   Encounter for other specified aftercare
     Excludes1   holiday relief care (Z75.5)
     Z51.81   Encounter for therapeutic drug level monitoring
       Code also any long-term (current) drug therapy (Z79.-)
       Excludes1   encounter for blood-drug test for administrative or medicolegal reasons (Z02.83)
     Z51.89   Encounter for other specified aftercare
       Coding Clinic: 2012, Q4, P96-97

● **Z52**   Donors of organs and tissues
    Includes   autologous and other living donors
    Excludes1   cadaveric donor - omit code
              examination of potential donor (Z00.5)
    Coding Clinic: 2012, Q4, P100
  ● **Z52.0**   Blood donor
    ● **Z52.00**   Unspecified blood donor
       Z52.000   Unspecified donor, whole blood
       Z52.001   Unspecified donor, stem cells
       Z52.008   Unspecified donor, other blood
    ● **Z52.01**   Autologous blood donor
       Z52.010   Autologous donor, whole blood
       Z52.011   Autologous donor, stem cells
       Z52.018   Autologous donor, other blood

CHAPTER 21 (Z00-Z99)

● **Z52.09**   **Other blood donor**
Volunteer donor
  Z52.090   Other blood donor, whole blood
  Z52.091   Other blood donor, stem cells
  Z52.098   Other blood donor, other blood
● **Z52.1**   **Skin donor**
  Z52.10   Skin donor, unspecified
  Z52.11   Skin donor, autologous
  Z52.19   Skin donor, other
● **Z52.2**   **Bone donor**
  Z52.20   Bone donor, unspecified
  Z52.21   Bone donor, autologous
  Z52.29   Bone donor, other
  Z52.3   **Bone marrow donor**
  Z52.4   **Kidney donor**
  Z52.5   **Cornea donor**
  Z52.6   **Liver donor**
      Coding Clinic: 2012, Q4, P100
● **Z52.8**   **Donor of other specified organs or tissues**
  ● **Z52.81**   **Egg (Oocyte) donor**
    Z52.810   Egg (Oocyte) donor under age 35, anonymous recipient ♀
        Egg donor under age 35 NOS
    Z52.811   Egg (Oocyte) donor under age 35, designated recipient ♀
    Z52.812   Egg (Oocyte) donor age 35 and over, anonymous recipient ♀
        Egg donor age 35 and over NOS
    Z52.813   Egg (Oocyte) donor age 35 and over, designated recipient ♀
    Z52.819   Egg (Oocyte) donor, unspecified ♀
  Z52.89   Donor of other specified organs or tissues
  Z52.9   **Donor of unspecified organ or tissue**
      Donor NOS
● **Z53**   **Persons encountering health services for specific procedures and treatment, not carried out**
● **Z53.0**   **Procedure and treatment not carried out because of contraindication**
  Z53.01   Procedure and treatment not carried out due to patient smoking
  Z53.09   Procedure and treatment not carried out because of other contraindication
  Z53.1   **Procedure and treatment not carried out because of patient's decision for reasons of belief and group pressure**
● **Z53.2**   **Procedure and treatment not carried out because of patient's decision for other and unspecified reasons**
  Z53.20   Procedure and treatment not carried out because of patient's decision for unspecified reasons
  Z53.21   Procedure and treatment not carried out due to patient leaving prior to being seen by health care provider
  Z53.29   Procedure and treatment not carried out because of patient's decision for other reasons
● **Z53.3**   **Procedure converted to open procedure**
      Coding Clinic: 2016, Q4, P79
  Z53.31   Laparoscopic surgical procedure converted to open procedure
      Coding Clinic: 2016, Q4, P100
  Z53.32   Thoracoscopic surgical procedure converted to open procedure
  Z53.33   Arthroscopic surgical procedure converted to open procedure
  Z53.39   Other specified procedure converted to open procedure
  Z53.8   **Procedure and treatment not carried out for other reasons**
  Z53.9   **Procedure and treatment not carried out, unspecified reason**

PERSONS WITH POTENTIAL HEALTH HAZARDS RELATED TO SOCIOECONOMIC AND PSYCHOSOCIAL CIRCUMSTANCES (Z55-Z65)

● **Z55**   **Problems related to education and literacy**
      Excludes1   disorders of psychological development (F80-F89)
  Z55.0   Illiteracy and low-level literacy
  Z55.1   Schooling unavailable and unattainable
  Z55.2   Failed school examinations
  Z55.3   Underachievement in school
  Z55.4   Educational maladjustment and discord with teachers and classmates
  Z55.5   Less than a high school diploma
        No general equivalence degree (GED)
  Z55.8   Other problems related to education and literacy
        Problems related to inadequate teaching
  Z55.9   Problems related to education and literacy, unspecified
        Academic problems NOS
● **Z56**   **Problems related to employment and unemployment**
      Excludes2   occupational exposure to risk factors (Z57.-)
            problems related to housing and economic circumstances (Z59.-)
  Z56.0   Unemployment, unspecified
  Z56.1   Change of job
  Z56.2   Threat of job loss
  Z56.3   Stressful work schedule
  Z56.4   Discord with boss and workmates
  Z56.5   Uncongenial work environment
        Difficult conditions at work
  Z56.6   Other physical and mental strain related to work
● **Z56.8**   **Other problems related to employment**
  Z56.81   Sexual harassment on the job
  Z56.82   Military deployment status
        Individual (civilian or military) currently deployed in theater or in support of military war, peacekeeping and humanitarian operations
  Z56.89   Other problems related to employment
  Z56.9   Unspecified problems related to employment
        Occupational problems NOS
● **Z57**   **Occupational exposure to risk factors**
  Z57.0   Occupational exposure to noise
  Z57.1   Occupational exposure to radiation
  Z57.2   Occupational exposure to dust
● **Z57.3**   **Occupational exposure to other air contaminants**
  Z57.31   Occupational exposure to environmental tobacco smoke
        Excludes2   exposure to environmental tobacco smoke (Z77.22)
  Z57.39   Occupational exposure to other air contaminants
  Z57.4   Occupational exposure to toxic agents in agriculture
        Occupational exposure to solids, liquids, gases or vapors in agriculture
  Z57.5   Occupational exposure to toxic agents in other industries
        Occupational exposure to solids, liquids, gases or vapors in other industries
  Z57.6   Occupational exposure to extreme temperature
  Z57.7   Occupational exposure to vibration
  Z57.8   Occupational exposure to other risk factors
  Z57.9   Occupational exposure to unspecified risk factor
● **Z58**   **Problems related to physical environment**
      Excludes2   occupational exposure (Z57.-)
  Z58.6   Inadequate drinking-water supply
        Lack of safe drinking water
        Excludes2   deprivation of water (T73.1)
● **Z59**   **Problems related to housing and economic circumstances**
      Excludes2   problems related to upbringing (Z62.-)

- **Z59.0 Homelessness**
    - Z59.00 **Homelessness unspecified**
    - Z59.01 **Sheltered homelessness**
        - Doubled up
        - Living in a shelter such as: motel, scattered site housing, temporary or transitional living situation
    - Z59.02 **Unsheltered homelessness**
        - Residing in place not meant for human habitation such as: abandoned buildings, cars, parks, sidewalk
        - Residing on the street
- **Z59.1 Inadequate housing**
    - Lack of heating
    - Restriction of space
    - Technical defects in home preventing adequate care
    - Unsatisfactory surroundings
    - **Excludes1** problems related to the natural and physical environment (Z77.1-)
- Z59.2 **Discord with neighbors, lodgers and landlord**
- Z59.3 **Problems related to living in residential institution**
    - Boarding-school resident
    - **Excludes1** institutional upbringing (Z62.2)
- **Z59.4 Lack of adequate food**
    - **Excludes2** deprivation of food (T73.0)
        - effects of hunger (T73.0)
        - inappropriate diet or eating habits (Z72.4)
        - malnutrition (E40-E46)
    - Z59.41 **Food insecurity**
    - Z59.48 **Other specified lack of adequate food**
        - Inadequate food
        - Lack of food
- Z59.5 **Extreme poverty**
- Z59.6 **Low income**
- Z59.7 **Insufficient social insurance and welfare support**
- **Z59.8 Other problems related to housing and economic circumstances**
    - **Z59.81 Housing instability, housed**
        - Foreclosure on home loan
        - Past due on rent or mortgage
        - Unwanted multiple moves in the last 12 months
        - Z59.811 **Housing instability, housed, with risk of homelessness**
            - Imminent risk of homelessness
        - Z59.812 **Housing instability, housed, homelessness in past 12 months**
        - Z59.819 **Housing instability, housed unspecified**
    - Z59.82 **Transportation insecurity**
        - Excessive transportation time
        - Inaccessible transportation
        - Inadequate transportation
        - Lack of transportation
        - Unaffordable transportation
        - Unreliable transportation
        - Unsafe transportation
    - Z59.86 **Financial insecurity**
        - Bankruptcy
        - Burdensome debt
        - Economic strain
        - Financial strain
        - Money problems
        - Running out of money
        - Unable to make ends meet
        - **Excludes2** extreme poverty (Z59.5)
            - low income (Z59.6)
            - material hardship, not elsewhere classified (Z59.87)

- Z59.87 **Material hardship**
    - Material deprivation
    - Unable to obtain adequate childcare
    - Unable to obtain adequate clothing
    - Unable to obtain adequate utilities
    - Unable to obtain basic needs
    - **Excludes2** extreme poverty (Z59.5)
        - financial insecurity, not elsewhere classified (Z59.86)
        - low income (Z59.6)
    - Z59.89 **Other problems related to housing and economic circumstances**
        - Foreclosure on loan
        - Isolated dwelling
        - Problems with creditors
- Z59.9 **Problem related to housing and economic circumstances, unspecified**
- **Z60 Problems related to social environment**
    - Z60.0 **Problems of adjustment to life-cycle transitions**
        - Empty nest syndrome
        - Phase of life problem
        - Problem with adjustment to retirement [pension]
    - Z60.2 **Problems related to living alone**
    - Z60.3 **Acculturation difficulty**
        - Problem with migration
        - Problem with social transplantation
    - Z60.4 **Social exclusion and rejection**
        - Exclusion and rejection on the basis of personal characteristics, such as unusual physical appearance, illness or behavior.
        - **Excludes1** target of adverse discrimination such as for racial or religious reasons (Z60.5)
    - Z60.5 **Target of (perceived) adverse discrimination and persecution**
        - **Excludes1** social exclusion and rejection (Z60.4)
    - Z60.8 **Other problems related to social environment**
    - Z60.9 **Problem related to social environment, unspecified**
- **Z62 Problems related to upbringing**
    - **Includes** current and past negative life events in childhood
        - current and past problems of a child related to upbringing
    - **Excludes2** maltreatment syndrome (T74.-)
        - problems related to housing and economic circumstances (Z59.-)
    - Z62.0 **Inadequate parental supervision and control**
    - Z62.1 **Parental overprotection**
    - **Z62.2 Upbringing away from parents**
        - **Excludes1** problems with boarding school (Z59.3)
        - Z62.21 **Child in welfare custody**   P
            - Child in care of non-parental family member
            - Child in foster care
            - **Excludes2** problem for parent due to child in welfare custody (Z63.5)
        - Z62.22 **Institutional upbringing**
            - Child living in orphanage or group home
        - Z62.29 **Other upbringing away from parents**
    - Z62.3 **Hostility towards and scapegoating of child**   P
    - Z62.6 **Inappropriate (excessive) parental pressure**
    - **Z62.8 Other specified problems related to upbringing**
        - **Z62.81 Personal history of abuse in childhood**
            - Z62.810 **Personal history of physical and sexual abuse in childhood**
                - **Excludes1** current child physical abuse (T74.12, T76.12)
                    - current child sexual abuse (T74.22, T76.22)

CHAPTER 21 (Z00-Z99)

CHAPTER 21 (Z00-Z99)

Z62.811   Personal history of psychological abuse in childhood

> **Excludes1**   current child psychological abuse (T74.32, T76.32)

Z62.812   Personal history of neglect in childhood

> **Excludes1**   current child neglect (T74.02, T76.02)

Z62.813   Personal history of forced labor or sexual exploitation in childhood

Z62.819   Personal history of unspecified abuse in childhood

> **Excludes1**   current child abuse NOS (T74.92, T76.92)

● **Z62.82   Parent-child conflict**

Z62.820   Parent-biological child conflict
Parent-child problem NOS

Z62.821   Parent-adopted child conflict

Z62.822   Parent-foster child conflict

● **Z62.89   Other specified problems related to upbringing**

Z62.890   Parent-child estrangement NEC

Z62.891   Sibling rivalry

Z62.898   Other specified problems related to upbringing

Z62.9   Problem related to upbringing, unspecified

● **Z63   Other problems related to primary support group, including family circumstances**

> **Excludes2**   maltreatment syndrome (T74.-, T76)
> parent-child problems (Z62.-)
> problems related to negative life events in childhood (Z62.-)
> problems related to upbringing (Z62.-)

Z63.0   Problems in relationship with spouse or partner
Relationship distress with spouse or intimate partner

> **Excludes1**   counseling for spousal or partner abuse problems (Z69.1)
> counseling related to sexual attitude, behavior, and orientation (Z70.-)

Z63.1   Problems in relationship with in-laws

● **Z63.3   Absence of family member**

> **Excludes1**   absence of family member due to disappearance and death (Z63.4)
> absence of family member due to separation and divorce (Z63.5)

Z63.31   Absence of family member due to military deployment
Individual or family affected by other family member being on military deployment

> **Excludes1**   family disruption due to return of family member from military deployment (Z63.71)

Z63.32   Other absence of family member

Z63.4   Disappearance and death of family member
Assumed death of family member
Bereavement

Z63.5   Disruption of family by separation and divorce
Marital estrangement

Z63.6   Dependent relative needing care at home

● **Z63.7   Other stressful life events affecting family and household**

Z63.71   Stress on family due to return of family member from military deployment
Individual or family affected by family member having returned from military deployment (current or past conflict)

Z63.72   Alcoholism and drug addiction in family

Z63.79   Other stressful life events affecting family and household
Anxiety (normal) about sick person in family
Health problems within family
Ill or disturbed family member
Isolated family

Z63.8   Other specified problems related to primary support group
Family discord NOS
Family estrangement NOS
High expressed emotional level within family
Inadequate family support NOS
Inadequate or distorted communication within family

Z63.9   Problem related to primary support group, unspecified
Relationship disorder NOS

● **Z64   Problems related to certain psychosocial circumstances**

Z64.0   Problems related to unwanted pregnancy ♀

Z64.1   Problems related to multiparity ♀

Z64.4   Discord with counselors
Discord with probation officer
Discord with social worker

● **Z65   Problems related to other psychosocial circumstances**

Z65.0   Conviction in civil and criminal proceedings without imprisonment

Z65.1   Imprisonment and other incarceration

Z65.2   Problems related to release from prison

Z65.3   Problems related to other legal circumstances
Arrest
Child custody or support proceedings
Litigation
Prosecution

Z65.4   Victim of crime and terrorism
Victim of torture

Z65.5   Exposure to disaster, war and other hostilities

> **Excludes1**   target of perceived discrimination or persecution (Z60.5)

Z65.8   Other specified problems related to psychosocial circumstances
Religious or spiritual problem

Z65.9   Problem related to unspecified psychosocial circumstances

---

DO NOT RESUSCITATE STATUS (Z66)

Z66   Do not resuscitate
DNR status

BLOOD TYPE (Z67)

● **Z67   Blood type**
Coding Clinic: 2015, Q3, P40

● **Z67.1   Type A blood**

Z67.10   Type A blood, Rh positive

Z67.11   Type A blood, Rh negative

● **Z67.2   Type B blood**

Z67.20   Type B blood, Rh positive

Z67.21   Type B blood, Rh negative

● **Z67.3   Type AB blood**

Z67.30   Type AB blood, Rh positive

Z67.31   Type AB blood, Rh negative

● **Z67.4   Type O blood**

Z67.40   Type O blood, Rh positive

Z67.41   Type O blood, Rh negative

● **Z67.9   Unspecified blood type**

Z67.90   Unspecified blood type, Rh positive

Z67.91   Unspecified blood type, Rh negative
Coding Clinic: 2015, Q3, P40

▶ New   ⇒ Revised   ~~deleted~~ Deleted   Excludes 1   Excludes 2   Includes   Use additional   Code first   Code also   Key words

OGCR Official Guidelines   X Assign placeholder X   ● Use Additional Character(s)   ▶ Manifestation Code   🏷 Hierarchical Condition Category   Coding Clinic

BODY MASS INDEX [BMI] (Z68)

OGCR Section I.B.14.

General Coding Guidelines

14. Documentation for BMI, Depth of Non-pressure ulcers, Pressure Ulcer Stages, Coma Scale, and NIH Stroke Scale

For the Body Mass Index (BMI), depth of non-pressure chronic ulcers, pressure ulcer stage, coma scale, and NIH stroke scale (NIHSS) codes, code assignment may be based on medical record documentation from clinicians who are not the patient's provider (i.e., physician or other qualified healthcare practitioner legally accountable for establishing the patient's diagnosis), since this information is typically documented by other clinicians involved in the care of the patient (e.g., a dietitian often documents the BMI, a nurse often documents the pressure ulcer stages, and an emergency medical technician often documents the coma scale). However, the associated diagnosis (such as overweight, obesity, acute stroke, or pressure ulcer) must be documented by the patient's provider. If there is conflicting medical record documentation, either from the same clinician or different clinicians, the patient's attending provider should be queried for clarification.

The BMI, coma scale, and NIHSS codes should only be reported as secondary diagnoses.

- **Z68**   **Body mass index [BMI]**
  Kilograms per meters squared
  Note: BMI adult codes are for use for persons 20 years of age or older.
  BMI pediatric codes are for use for persons 2-19 years of age.
  These percentiles are based on the growth charts published by the Centers for Disease Control and Prevention (CDC)
  Coding Clinic: 2018, Q4, P81; 2016, Q4, P129

     Z68.1   Body mass index [BMI] **19.9 or less, adult**   A
            Coding Clinic: 2017, Q1, P39

-    **Z68.2**   Body mass index [BMI] **20-29, adult**
       Z68.20   Body mass index [BMI] 20.0-20.9, adult   A
       Z68.21   Body mass index [BMI] 21.0-21.9, adult   A
       Z68.22   Body mass index [BMI] 22.0-22.9, adult   A
       Z68.23   Body mass index [BMI] 23.0-23.9, adult   A
       Z68.24   Body mass index [BMI] 24.0-24.9, adult   A
       Z68.25   Body mass index [BMI] 25.0-25.9, adult   A
       Z68.26   Body mass index [BMI] 26.0-26.9, adult   A
       Z68.27   Body mass index [BMI] 27.0-27.9, adult   A
       Z68.28   Body mass index [BMI] 28.0-28.9, adult   A
       Z68.29   Body mass index [BMI] 29.0-29.9, adult   A

-    **Z68.3**   Body mass index [BMI] **30-39, adult**
       Z68.30   Body mass index [BMI] 30.0-30.9, adult   A
       Z68.31   Body mass index [BMI] 31.0-31.9, adult   A
       Z68.32   Body mass index [BMI] 32.0-32.9, adult   A
       Z68.33   Body mass index [BMI] 33.0-33.9, adult   A
       Z68.34   Body mass index [BMI] 34.0-34.9, adult   A
       Z68.35   Body mass index [BMI] 35.0-35.9, adult   A
       Z68.36   Body mass index [BMI] 36.0-36.9, adult   A
       Z68.37   Body mass index [BMI] 37.0-37.9, adult   A
       Z68.38   Body mass index [BMI] 38.0-38.9, adult   A
       Z68.39   Body mass index [BMI] 39.0-39.9, adult   A

-    **Z68.4**   Body mass index [BMI] **40 or greater, adult**
       Z68.41   Body mass index [BMI] 40.0-44.9, adult   A
       Z68.42   Body mass index [BMI] 45.0-49.9, adult   A
       Z68.43   Body mass index [BMI] 50.0-59.9, adult   A
       Z68.44   Body mass index [BMI] 60.0-69.9, adult   A
       Z68.45   Body mass index [BMI] 70 or greater, adult   A

-    **Z68.5**   Body mass index [BMI] **pediatric**
           Coding Clinic: 2018, Q4, P81
       Z68.51   Body mass index [BMI] pediatric, **less than 5th percentile for age**
              Coding Clinic: 2018, Q4, P82

     Z68.52   Body mass index [BMI] pediatric, **5th percentile to less than 85th percentile for age**
     Z68.53   Body mass index [BMI] pediatric, **85th percentile to less than 95th percentile for age**
     Z68.54   Body mass index [BMI] pediatric, **greater than or equal to 95th percentile for age**

PERSONS ENCOUNTERING HEALTH SERVICES IN OTHER CIRCUMSTANCES (Z69-Z76)

- **Z69**   **Encounter for mental health services for victim and perpetrator of abuse**
       Includes   counseling for victims and perpetrators of abuse

-    **Z69.0**   **Encounter for mental health services for child abuse problems**

  -    **Z69.01**   **Encounter for mental health services for parental child abuse**

         Z69.010   **Encounter for mental health services for victim of parental child abuse**   P
              Encounter for mental health services for victim of child abuse by parent
              Encounter for mental health services for victim of child neglect by parent
              Encounter for mental health services for victim of child psychological abuse by parent
              Encounter for mental health services for victim of child sexual abuse by parent

         Z69.011   **Encounter for mental health services for perpetrator of parental child abuse**
              Encounter for mental health services for perpetrator of parental child neglect
              Encounter for mental health services for perpetrator of parental child psychological abuse
              Encounter for mental health services for perpetrator of parental child sexual abuse

         Excludes1   encounter for mental health services for non-parental child abuse (Z69.02-)

  -    **Z69.02**   **Encounter for mental health services for non-parental child abuse**

         Z69.020   **Encounter for mental health services for victim of non-parental child abuse**   P
              Encounter for mental health services for victim of non-parental child neglect
              Encounter for mental health services for victim of non-parental child psychological abuse
              Encounter for mental health services for victim of non-parental child sexual abuse

         Z69.021   **Encounter for mental health services for perpetrator of non- parental child abuse**
              Encounter for mental health services for perpetrator of non-parental child neglect
              Encounter for mental health services for perpetrator of non-parental child psychological abuse
              Encounter for mental health services for perpetrator of non-parental child sexual abuse

CHAPTER 21 (Z00-Z99)

● **Z69.1** **Encounter for mental health services for spousal or partner abuse problems**

    Z69.11 **Encounter for mental health services for victim of spousal or partner abuse**
        Encounter for mental health services for victim of spouse or partner neglect
        Encounter for mental health services for victim of spouse or partner psychological abuse
        Encounter for mental health services for victim of spouse or partner violence, physical

    Z69.12 **Encounter for mental health services for perpetrator of spousal or partner abuse**
        Encounter for mental health services for perpetrator of spouse or partner neglect
        Encounter for mental health services for perpetrator of spouse or partner psychological abuse
        Encounter for mental health services for perpetrator of spouse or partner violence, physical
        Encounter for mental health services for perpetrator of spouse or partner violence, sexual

● **Z69.8** **Encounter for mental health services for victim or perpetrator of other abuse**

    Z69.81 **Encounter for mental health services for victim of other abuse**
        Encounter for mental health services for victim of non-spousal adult abuse
        Encounter for mental health services for victim of spouse or partner violence, sexual
        Encounter for rape victim counseling

    Z69.82 **Encounter for mental health services for perpetrator of other abuse**
        Encounter for mental health services for perpetrator of non-spousal adult abuse

● **Z70** **Counseling related to sexual attitude, behavior and orientation**
    Includes   encounter for mental health services for sexual attitude, behavior and orientation
    Excludes2   contraceptive or procreative counseling (Z30-Z31)

    Z70.0 **Counseling related to sexual attitude**

    Z70.1 **Counseling related to patient's sexual behavior and orientation**
        Patient concerned regarding impotence
        Patient concerned regarding non-responsiveness
        Patient concerned regarding promiscuity
        Patient concerned regarding sexual orientation

    Z70.2 **Counseling related to sexual behavior and orientation of third party**
        Advice sought regarding sexual behavior and orientation of child
        Advice sought regarding sexual behavior and orientation of partner
        Advice sought regarding sexual behavior and orientation of spouse

    Z70.3 **Counseling related to combined concerns regarding sexual attitude, behavior and orientation**

    Z70.8 **Other sex counseling**
        Encounter for sex education

    Z70.9 **Sex counseling, unspecified**

● **Z71** **Persons encountering health services for other counseling and medical advice, not elsewhere classified**
    Excludes2   contraceptive or procreation counseling (Z30-Z31)
                 sex counseling (Z70.-)

    Z71.0 **Person encountering health services to consult on behalf of another person**
        Person encountering health services to seek advice or treatment for non-attending third party
    Excludes2   anxiety (normal) about sick person in family (Z63.7)
                 expectant (adoptive) parent(s) pre-birth pediatrician visit (Z76.81)

Z71.1 **Person with feared health complaint in whom no diagnosis is made**
    Person encountering health services with feared condition which was not demonstrated
    Person encountering health services in which problem was normal state
    "Worried well"
    Excludes1   medical observation for suspected diseases and conditions proven not to exist (Z03.-)

    Coding Clinic: 2016, Q4, P7

Z71.2 **Person consulting for explanation of examination or test findings**

Z71.3 **Dietary counseling and surveillance**
    Use additional code for any associated underlying medical condition
    Use additional code to identify body mass index (BMI), if known (Z68.-)

● **Z71.4** **Alcohol abuse counseling and surveillance**
    Use additional code for alcohol abuse or dependence (F10.-)

    Z71.41 **Alcohol abuse counseling and surveillance of alcoholic**

    Z71.42 **Counseling for family member of alcoholic**
        Counseling for significant other, partner, or friend of alcoholic

● **Z71.5** **Drug abuse counseling and surveillance**
    Use additional code for drug abuse or dependence (F11-F16, F18-F19)

    Z71.51 **Drug abuse counseling and surveillance of drug abuser**

    Z71.52 **Counseling for family member of drug abuser**
        Counseling for significant other, partner, or friend of drug abuser

Z71.6 **Tobacco abuse counseling**
    Use additional code for nicotine dependence (F17.-)

Z71.7 **Human immunodeficiency virus [HIV] counseling**

● **Z71.8** **Other specified counseling**
    Excludes2   counseling for contraception (Z30.0-)

    Z71.81 **Spiritual or religious counseling**

    Z71.82 **Exercise counseling**

    Z71.83 **Encounter for nonprocreative genetic counseling**
        Excludes1   counseling for procreative genetics (Z31.5)
                  counseling for procreative management (Z31.6)

    Z71.84 **Encounter for health counseling related to travel**
        Encounter for health risk and safety counseling for (international) travel
        Code also, if applicable, encounter for immunization (Z23)
        Excludes2   encounter for administrative examination (Z02.-)
                  encounter for other special examination without complaint, suspected or reported diagnosis (Z01.-)

    Z71.85 **Encounter for immunization safety counseling**
        Encounter for vaccine product safety counseling
        Code also, if applicable, encounter for immunization (Z23)
        Code also, if applicable, immunization not carried out (Z28.-)
        Excludes1   encounter for health counseling related to travel (Z71.84)

CHAPTER 21 (Z00-Z99)

▶ New   ⇒ Revised   ~~deleted~~ Deleted   Excludes 1   Excludes 2   Includes   Use additional   Code first   Code also   Key words

OGCR Official Guidelines   X Assign placeholder X   ● Use Additional Character(s)   ▶ Manifestation Code   🔁 Hierarchical Condition Category   Coding Clinic

▶**Z71.87**   **Encounter for pediatric-to-adult transition counseling**
- ▶Code also chronic condition, if applicable, such as:
  - ▶autism spectrum disorder (F84.0)
  - ▶congenital malformations of the circulatory system (Q20-Q28)
  - ▶cystic fibrosis (E84.-)
  - ▶sickle-cell disorder (D57.-)

▶**Z71.88**   **Encounter for counseling for socioeconomic factors**

Z71.89   **Other specified counseling**

Z71.9   **Counseling, unspecified**
Encounter for medical advice NOS

●**Z72**   **Problems related to lifestyle**
> **Excludes2**   problems related to life-management difficulty (Z73.-)
> problems related to socioeconomic and psychosocial circumstances (Z55-Z65)

Coding Clinic: 2016, Q4, P130

Z72.0   **Tobacco use**
Tobacco use NOS
> **Excludes1**   history of tobacco dependence (Z87.891)
> nicotine dependence (F17.2-)
> tobacco dependence (F17.2-)
> tobacco use during pregnancy (O99.33-)

Z72.3   **Lack of physical exercise**

Z72.4   **Inappropriate diet and eating habits**
> **Excludes1**   behavioral eating disorders of infancy or childhood (F98.2.-F98.3)
> eating disorders (F50.-)
> lack of adequate food (Z59.48)
> malnutrition and other nutritional deficiencies (E40-E64)

●**Z72.5**   **High risk sexual behavior**
Promiscuity
> **Excludes1**   paraphilias (F65)

Z72.51   **High risk heterosexual behavior**

Z72.52   **High risk homosexual behavior**

Z72.53   **High risk bisexual behavior**

Z72.6   **Gambling and betting**
> **Excludes1**   compulsive or pathological gambling (F63.0)

●**Z72.8**   **Other problems related to lifestyle**

●**Z72.81**   **Antisocial behavior**
> **Excludes1**   conduct disorders (F91.-)

Z72.810   **Child and adolescent antisocial behavior**   P
Antisocial behavior (child) (adolescent) without manifest psychiatric disorder
Delinquency NOS
Group delinquency
Offenses in the context of gang membership
Stealing in company with others
Truancy from school

Z72.811   **Adult antisocial behavior**   A
Adult antisocial behavior without manifest psychiatric disorder

●**Z72.82**   **Problems related to sleep**

Z72.820   **Sleep deprivation**
Lack of adequate sleep
> **Excludes1**   insomnia (G47.0-)

Z72.821   **Inadequate sleep hygiene**
Bad sleep habits
Irregular sleep habits
Unhealthy sleep wake schedule
> **Excludes1**   insomnia (F51.0-, G47.0-)

▶**Z72.823**   **Risk of suffocation (smothering) under another while sleeping**
- ▶Child-caregiver co-sleeping
- ▶Infant bed-sharing

Z72.89   **Other problems related to lifestyle**
Self-damaging behavior

Z72.9   **Problem related to lifestyle, unspecified**

●**Z73**   **Problems related to life management difficulty**
> **Excludes2**   problems related to socioeconomic and psychosocial circumstances (Z55-Z65)

Z73.0   **Burn-out**

Z73.1   **Type A behavior pattern**

Z73.2   **Lack of relaxation and leisure**

Z73.3   **Stress, not elsewhere classified**
Physical and mental strain NOS
> **Excludes1**   stress related to employment or unemployment (Z56.-)

Z73.4   **Inadequate social skills, not elsewhere classified**

Z73.5   **Social role conflict, not elsewhere classified**

Z73.6   **Limitation of activities due to disability**
> **Excludes1**   care-provider dependency (Z74.-)

●**Z73.8**   **Other problems related to life management difficulty**

●**Z73.81**   **Behavioral insomnia of childhood**

Z73.810   **Behavioral insomnia of childhood, sleep-onset association type**   P

Z73.811   **Behavioral insomnia of childhood, limit setting type**   P

Z73.812   **Behavioral insomnia of childhood, combined type**   P

Z73.819   **Behavioral insomnia of childhood, unspecified type**   P

Z73.82   **Dual sensory impairment**

Z73.89   **Other problems related to life management difficulty**

Z73.9   **Problem related to life management difficulty, unspecified**

●**Z74**   **Problems related to care provider dependency**
> **Excludes2**   dependence on enabling machines or devices NEC (Z99.-)

●**Z74.0**   **Reduced mobility**

Z74.01   **Bed confinement status**
Bedridden

Z74.09   **Other reduced mobility**
Chairridden
Reduced mobility NOS
> **Excludes2**   wheelchair dependence (Z99.3)

Z74.1   **Need for assistance with personal care**

Z74.2   **Need for assistance at home and no other household member able to render care**

Z74.3   **Need for continuous supervision**

Z74.8   **Other problems related to care provider dependency**

Z74.9   **Problem related to care provider dependency, unspecified**

●**Z75**   **Problems related to medical facilities and other health care**

Z75.0   **Medical services not available in home**
> **Excludes1**   no other household member able to render care (Z74.2)

Z75.1   **Person awaiting admission to adequate facility elsewhere**

Z75.2   **Other waiting period for investigation and treatment**

Z75.3   **Unavailability and inaccessibility of health care facilities**
> **Excludes1**   bed unavailable (Z75.1)

Z75.4   **Unavailability and inaccessibility of other helping agencies**

Z75.5   **Holiday relief care**

CHAPTER 21 (Z00-Z99)

Z75.8   Other problems related to medical facilities and other health care

Z75.9   Unspecified problem related to medical facilities and other health care

● **Z76**   Persons encountering health services in other circumstances

Z76.0   Encounter for issue of repeat prescription
Encounter for issue of repeat prescription for appliance
Encounter for issue of repeat prescription for medicaments
Encounter for issue of repeat prescription for spectacles

    Excludes2   issue of medical certificate (Z02.7)
repeat prescription for contraceptive (Z30.4-)

Z76.1   Encounter for health supervision and care of foundling

Z76.2   Encounter for health supervision and care of other healthy infant and child   P
Encounter for medical or nursing care or supervision of healthy infant under circumstances such as adverse socioeconomic conditions at home
Encounter for medical or nursing care or supervision of healthy infant under circumstances such as awaiting foster or adoptive placement
Encounter for medical or nursing care or supervision of healthy infant under circumstances such as maternal illness
Encounter for medical or nursing care or supervision of healthy infant under circumstances such as number of children at home preventing or interfering with normal care

Z76.3   Healthy person accompanying sick person

Z76.4   Other boarder to healthcare facility

    Excludes1   homelessness (Z59.0-)

Z76.5   Malingerer [conscious simulation]
Person feigning illness (with obvious motivation)

    Excludes1   factitious disorder (F68.1-, F68.A)
peregrinating patient (F68.1-)

● **Z76.8**   Persons encountering health services in other specified circumstances

Z76.81   Expectant parent(s) prebirth pediatrician visit
Pre-adoption pediatrician visit for adoptive parent(s)

Z76.82   Awaiting organ transplant status
Patient waiting for organ availability

Z76.89   Persons encountering health services in other specified circumstances
Persons encountering health services NOS

PERSONS WITH POTENTIAL HEALTH HAZARDS RELATED TO FAMILY AND PERSONAL HISTORY AND CERTAIN CONDITIONS INFLUENCING HEALTH STATUS (Z77-Z99)

    Code also any follow-up examination (Z08-Z09)

● **Z77**   Other contact with and (suspected) exposures hazardous to health

    Includes   contact with and (suspected) exposures to potential hazards to health

    Excludes2   contact with and (suspected) exposure to communicable diseases (Z20.-)
exposure to (parental) (environmental) tobacco smoke in the perinatal period (P96.81)
newborn affected by noxious substances transmitted via placenta or breast milk (P04.-)
occupational exposure to risk factors (Z57.-)
retained foreign body (Z18.-)
retained foreign body fully removed (Z87.821)
toxic effects of substances chiefly nonmedicinal as to source (T51-T65)

● **Z77.0**   Contact with and (suspected) exposure to hazardous, chiefly nonmedicinal, chemicals

   ● **Z77.01**   Contact with and (suspected) exposure to hazardous metals

      Z77.010   Contact with and (suspected) exposure to arsenic

Z77.011   Contact with and (suspected) exposure to lead

Z77.012   Contact with and (suspected) exposure to uranium

    Excludes1   retained depleted uranium fragments (Z18.01)

Z77.018   Contact with and (suspected) exposure to other hazardous metals
Contact with and (suspected) exposure to chromium compounds
Contact with and (suspected) exposure to nickel dust

● **Z77.02**   Contact with and (suspected) exposure to hazardous aromatic compounds

Z77.020   Contact with and (suspected) exposure to aromatic amines

Z77.021   Contact with and (suspected) exposure to benzene

Z77.028   Contact with and (suspected) exposure to other hazardous aromatic compounds
Aromatic dyes NOS
Polycyclic aromatic hydrocarbons

● **Z77.09**   Contact with and (suspected) exposure to other hazardous, chiefly nonmedicinal, chemicals

Z77.090   Contact with and (suspected) exposure to asbestos

Z77.098   Contact with and (suspected) exposure to other hazardous, chiefly nonmedicinal, chemicals
Dyes NOS

● **Z77.1**   Contact with and (suspected) exposure to environmental pollution and hazards in the physical environment

● **Z77.11**   Contact with and (suspected) exposure to environmental pollution

Z77.110   Contact with and (suspected) exposure to air pollution

Z77.111   Contact with and (suspected) exposure to water pollution

Z77.112   Contact with and (suspected) exposure to soil pollution

Z77.118   Contact with and (suspected) exposure to other environmental pollution

● **Z77.12**   Contact with and (suspected) exposure to hazards in the physical environment

Z77.120   Contact with and (suspected) exposure to mold (toxic)

Z77.121   Contact with and (suspected) exposure to harmful algae and algae toxins
Contact with and (suspected) exposure to (harmful) algae bloom NOS
Contact with and (suspected) exposure to blue-green algae bloom
Contact with and (suspected) exposure to brown tide
Contact with and (suspected) exposure to cyanobacteria bloom
Contact with and (suspected) exposure to Florida red tide
Contact with and (suspected) exposure to pfiesteria piscicida
Contact with and (suspected) exposure to red tide

Z77.122   Contact with and (suspected) exposure to noise

▶ New   ⮕ Revised   ~~deleted~~ Deleted   Excludes 1   Excludes 2   Includes   Use additional   Code first   Code also   Key words

OGCR Official Guidelines   X Assign placeholder X   ● Use Additional Character(s)   ▸ Manifestation Code   ◕ Hierarchical Condition Category   **Coding Clinic**

Z77.123 **Contact with and (suspected) exposure to radon and other naturally occurring radiation**

Excludes2 radiation exposure as the cause of a confirmed condition (W88-W90, X39.0-)

radiation sickness NOS (T66)

Z77.128 **Contact with and (suspected) exposure to other hazards in the physical environment**

● Z77.2 **Contact with and (suspected) exposure to other hazardous substances**

Z77.21 **Contact with and (suspected) exposure to potentially hazardous body fluids**

Z77.22 **Contact with and (suspected) exposure to environmental tobacco smoke (acute) (chronic)**

Exposure to second hand tobacco smoke (acute) (chronic)

Passive smoking (acute) (chronic)

Excludes1 nicotine dependence (F17.-) tobacco use (Z72.0)

Excludes2 occupational exposure to environmental tobacco smoke (Z57.31)

Z77.29 **Contact with and (suspected) exposure to other hazardous substances**

Coding Clinic: 2016, Q2, P34

Z77.9 **Other contact with and (suspected) exposures hazardous to health**

● Z78 **Other specified health status**

Excludes2 asymptomatic human immunodeficiency virus [HIV] infection status (Z21)

postprocedural status (Z93-Z99)

sex reassignment status (Z87.890)

Z78.0 **Asymptomatic menopausal state** ♀ A

Menopausal state NOS

Postmenopausal status NOS

Excludes2 symptomatic menopausal state (N95.1)

Z78.1 **Physical restraint status**

Excludes1 physical restraint due to a procedure - omit code

Z78.9 **Other specified health status**

● Z79 **Long term (current) drug therapy**

Includes long term (current) drug use for prophylactic purposes

Code also any therapeutic drug level monitoring (Z51.81)

Excludes2 drug abuse and dependence (F11-F19)

drug use complicating pregnancy, childbirth, and the puerperium (O99.32-)

● Z79.0 **Long term (current) use of anticoagulants and antithrombotics/antiplatelets**

Excludes2 long term (current) use of aspirin (Z79.82)

Coding Clinic: 2021, Q1, P12-13

Z79.01 **Long term (current) use of anticoagulants**

Coding Clinic: 2022, Q2, P17; 2021, Q1, P5

Z79.02 **Long term (current) use of antithrombotics/ antiplatelets**

Z79.1 **Long term (current) use of non-steroidal anti-inflammatories (NSAID)**

Excludes2 long term (current) use of aspirin (Z79.82)

Z79.2 **Long term (current) use of antibiotics**

Z79.3 **Long term (current) use of hormonal contraceptives**

Long term (current) use of birth control pill or patch

Z79.4 **Long term (current) use of insulin** 🔁

▶ **Excludes2** long-term (current) use of injectable non-insulin antidiabetic drugs (Z79.85)

long term (current) use of oral hypoglycemic drugs (Z79.84)

long term (current) use of oral antidiabetic drugs (Z79.84)

● Z79.5 **Long term (current) use of steroids**

Z79.51 **Long term (current) use of inhaled steroids**

Z79.52 **Long term (current) use of systemic steroids**

▶ ● Z79.6 **Long term (current) use of immunomodulators and immunosuppressants**

▶ **Excludes2** long term (current) use of steroids (Z79.5-)

▶ long term (current) use of agents affecting estrogen receptors and estrogen levels (Z79.81-)

▶ Z79.60 **Long term (current) use of unspecified immunomodulators and immunosuppressants**

▶ Z79.61 **Long term (current) use of immunomodulator**

▶ Long term (current) use of apremilast

▶ Long term (current) use of immunomodulatory imide drug

▶ Long term (current) use of lenalidomide

▶ Long term (current) use of pomalidomide

▶ ● Z79.62 **Long term (current) use of immunosuppressant**

▶ Z79.620 **Long term (current) use of immunosuppressive biologic**

▶ Long term (current) use of adalimumab

▶ Long term (current) use of etanercept

▶ Long term (current) use of infliximab

▶ Long term (current) use of monoclonal antibodies

▶ Z79.621 **Long term (current) use of calcineurin inhibitor**

▶ Long term (current) use of cyclosporine

▶ Long term (current) use of tacrolimus

▶ Z79.622 **Long term (current) use of Janus kinase inhibitor**

▶ Long term (current) use of tofacitinib

▶ Z79.623 **Long term (current) use of mammalian target of rapamycin (mTOR) inhibitor**

▶ Long term (current) use of sirolimus

▶ Z79.624 **Long term (current) use of inhibitors of nucleotide synthesis**

▶ Long term (current) use of azathioprine

▶ Long term (current) use omycophenolate

▶ Long term (current) use of purine synthesis (IMDH) inhibitors

▶ ● Z79.63 **Long term (current) use of chemotherapeutic agent**

▶ Z79.630 **Long term (current) use of alkylating agent**

▶ Long term (current) use of chlorambucil

▶ Long term (current) use of cisplatin

▶ Long term (current) use of cyclophosphamide

▶ Z79.631 **Long term (current) use of antimetabolite agent**

▶ Long term (current) use of 5-fluorouracil

▶ Long term (current) use of 6-mercaptopurine

▶ Long term (current) use of cytarabine

▶ Long term (current) use of methotrexate

CHAPTER 21 (Z00-Z99)

▶Z79.632 **Long term (current) use of antitumor antibiotic**
▶Long term (current) use of bleomycin
▶Long term (current) use of doxorubicin
▶Long term (current) use of mitomycin C

▶Z79.633 **Long term (current) use of mitotic inhibitor**
▶Long term (current) use of paclitaxel
▶Long term (current) use of plant alkaloids
▶Long term (current) use of vinblastine
▶Long term (current) use of vincristine

▶Z79.634 **Long term (current) use of topoisomerase inhibitor**
▶Long term (current) use of etoposide
▶Long term (current) use of irinotecan
▶Long term (current) use of topotecan

▶Z79.64 **Long term (current) use of myelosuppressive agent**
▶Long term (current) use of hydroxyurea

▶Z79.69 **Long term (current) use of other immunomodulators and immunosuppressants**

● Z79.8 **Other long term (current) drug therapy**

● Z79.81 **Long term (current) use of agents affecting estrogen receptors and estrogen levels**
Code first, if applicable:
malignant neoplasm of breast (C50.-)
malignant neoplasm of prostate (C61)

Use additional code, if applicable, to identify:
estrogen receptor positive status (Z17.0)
family history of breast cancer (Z80.3)
genetic susceptibility to malignant neoplasm (cancer) (Z15.0-)
personal history of breast cancer (Z85.3)
personal history of prostate cancer (Z85.46)
postmenopausal status (Z78.0)

Excludes1 hormone replacement therapy (Z79.890)

Z79.810 **Long term (current) use of selective estrogen receptor modulators (SERMs)**
Long term (current) use of raloxifene (Evista)
Long term (current) use of tamoxifen (Nolvadex)
Long term (current) use of toremifene (Fareston)

Z79.811 **Long term (current) use of aromatase inhibitors**
Long term (current) use of anastrozole (Arimidex)
Long term (current) use of exemestane (Aromasin)
Long term (current) use of letrozole (Femara)

Z79.818 **Long term (current) use of other agents affecting estrogen receptors and estrogen levels**
Long term (current) use of estrogen receptor downregulators
Long term (current) use of fulvestrant (Faslodex)
Long term (current) use of gonadotropin-releasing hormone (GnRH) agonist
Long term (current) use of goserelin acetate (Zoladex)
Long term (current) use of leuprolide acetate (leuprorelin) (Lupron)
Long term (current) use of megestrol acetate (Megace)

Z79.82 **Long term (current) use of aspirin**

Z79.83 **Long term (current) use of bisphosphonates**
Coding Clinic: 2016, Q4, P42

Z79.84 **Long term (current) use of oral hypoglycemic drugs**
Long term (current) use of oral antidiabetic drugs
▶ **Excludes2** long-term (current) use of injectable non-insulin antidiabetic drugs (Z79.85)
long term (current) use of insulin (Z79.4)
Coding Clinic: 2016, Q4, P76, 121-122, 126

▶Z79.85 **Long-term (current) use of injectable non-insulin antidiabetic drugs**
▶ **Excludes2** long term (current) use of insulin (Z79.4)
▶long term (current) use of oral hypoglycemic drugs (Z79.84)

● Z79.89 **Other long term (current) drug therapy**
Z79.890 **Hormone replacement therapy**
Z79.891 **Long term (current) use of opiate analgesic**
Long term (current) use of methadone for pain management
Excludes1 methadone use NOS (F11.9-)
use of methadone for treatment of heroin addiction (F11.2-)

Z79.899 **Other long term (current) drug therapy**
Coding Clinic: 2015, Q4, P34, Q3, P21

● Z80 **Family history of primary malignant neoplasm**

Z80.0 **Family history of malignant neoplasm of digestive organs**
Conditions classifiable to C15-C26
Coding Clinic: 2018, Q1, P7

Z80.1 **Family history of malignant neoplasm of trachea, bronchus and lung**
Conditions classifiable to C33-C34

Z80.2 **Family history of malignant neoplasm of other respiratory and intrathoracic organs**
Conditions classifiable to C30-C32, C37-C39

Z80.3 **Family history of malignant neoplasm of breast**
Conditions classifiable to C50.-

● Z80.4 **Family history of malignant neoplasm of genital organs**
Conditions classifiable to C51-C63

Z80.41 **Family history of malignant neoplasm of ovary**

Z80.42 **Family history of malignant neoplasm of prostate**

Z80.43 **Family history of malignant neoplasm of testis**

Z80.49 **Family history of malignant neoplasm of other genital organs**

● Z80.5 **Family history of malignant neoplasm of urinary tract**
Conditions classifiable to C64-C68

Z80.51 **Family history of malignant neoplasm of kidney**

Z80.52 **Family history of malignant neoplasm of bladder**

Z80.59 **Family history of malignant neoplasm of other urinary tract organ**

Z80.6 **Family history of leukemia**
Conditions classifiable to C91-C95

Z80.7 **Family history of other malignant neoplasms of lymphoid, hematopoietic and related tissues**
Conditions classifiable to C81-C90, C96.-

▶ New   ⇒ Revised   ~~deleted~~ Deleted   Excludes 1   Excludes 2   Includes   Use additional   Code first   Code also   Key words

OGCR Official Guidelines   X Assign placeholder X   ● Use Additional Character(s)   ▷ Manifestation Code   🔖 Hierarchical Condition Category   Coding Clinic

Z80.8   Family history of malignant neoplasm of other organs or systems
Conditions classifiable to C00-C14, C40-C49, C69-C79

Z80.9   Family history of malignant neoplasm, unspecified
Conditions classifiable to C80.1

● Z81   Family history of mental and behavioral disorders

Z81.0   Family history of intellectual disabilities
Conditions classifiable to F70-F79

Z81.1   Family history of alcohol abuse and dependence
Conditions classifiable to F10.-

Z81.2   Family history of tobacco abuse and dependence
Conditions classifiable to F17.-

Z81.3   Family history of other psychoactive substance abuse and dependence
Conditions classifiable to F11-F16, F18-F19

Z81.4   Family history of other substance abuse and dependence
Conditions classifiable to F55

Z81.8   Family history of other mental and behavioral disorders
Conditions classifiable elsewhere in F01-F99

● Z82   Family history of certain disabilities and chronic diseases (leading to disablement)

Z82.0   Family history of epilepsy and other diseases of the nervous system
Conditions classifiable to G00-G99

Z82.1   Family history of blindness and visual loss
Conditions classifiable to H54.-

Z82.2   Family history of deafness and hearing loss
Conditions classifiable to H90-H91

Z82.3   Family history of stroke
Conditions classifiable to I60-I64

● Z82.4   Family history of ischemic heart disease and other diseases of the circulatory system
Conditions classifiable to I00-I5A, I65-I99

Z82.41   Family history of sudden cardiac death

Z82.49   Family history of ischemic heart disease and other diseases of the circulatory system

Z82.5   Family history of asthma and other chronic lower respiratory diseases
Conditions classifiable to J40-J47

Excludes2   family history of other diseases of the respiratory system (Z83.6)

● Z82.6   Family history of arthritis and other diseases of the musculoskeletal system and connective tissue
Conditions classifiable to M00-M99

Z82.61   Family history of arthritis

Z82.62   Family history of osteoporosis

Z82.69   Family history of other diseases of the musculoskeletal system and connective tissue

● Z82.7   Family history of congenital malformations, deformations and chromosomal abnormalities
Conditions classifiable to Q00-Q99

Z82.71   Family history of polycystic kidney

Z82.79   Family history of other congenital malformations, deformations and chromosomal abnormalities

Z82.8   Family history of other disabilities and chronic diseases leading to disablement, not elsewhere classified

● Z83   Family history of other specific disorders

Excludes2   contact with and (suspected) exposure to communicable disease in the family (Z20.-)

Z83.0   Family history of human immunodeficiency virus [HIV] disease
Conditions classifiable to B20

Z83.1   Family history of other infectious and parasitic diseases
Conditions classifiable to A00-B19, B25-B94, B99

Z83.2   Family history of diseases of the blood and blood-forming organs and certain disorders involving the immune mechanism
Conditions classifiable to D50-D89

Z83.3   Family history of diabetes mellitus
Conditions classifiable to E08-E13

● Z83.4   Family history of other endocrine, nutritional and metabolic diseases
Conditions classifiable to E00-E07, E15-E88

Z83.41   Family history of multiple endocrine neoplasia [MEN] syndrome

Z83.42   Family history of familial hypercholesterolemia
Coding Clinic: 2016, Q4, P77

● Z83.43   Family history of other disorder of lipoprotein metabolism and other lipidemias

Z83.430   Family history of elevated lipoprotein(a)
Family history of elevated Lp(a)

Z83.438   Family history of other disorder of lipoprotein metabolism and other lipidemia
Family history of familial combined hyperlipidemia

Z83.49   Family history of other endocrine, nutritional and metabolic diseases

● Z83.5   Family history of eye and ear disorders

● Z83.51   Family history of eye disorders
Conditions classifiable to H00-H53, H55-H59

Excludes2   family history of blindness and visual loss (Z82.1)

Z83.511   Family history of glaucoma

Z83.518   Family history of other specified eye disorder

Z83.52   Family history of ear disorders
Conditions classifiable to H60-H83, H92-H95

Excludes2   family history of deafness and hearing loss (Z82.2)

Z83.6   Family history of other diseases of the respiratory system
Conditions classifiable to J00-J39, J60-J99

Excludes2   family history of asthma and other chronic lower respiratory diseases (Z82.5)

● Z83.7   Family history of diseases of the digestive system
Conditions classifiable to K00-K93

Z83.71   Family history of colonic polyps

Excludes2   family history of malignant neoplasm of digestive organs (Z80.0)

Coding Clinic: 2021, Q1, P15

Z83.79   Family history of other diseases of the digestive system

● Z84   Family history of other conditions

Z84.0   Family history of diseases of the skin and subcutaneous tissue
Conditions classifiable to L00-L99

Z84.1   Family history of disorders of kidney and ureter
Conditions classifiable to N00-N29

Z84.2   Family history of other diseases of the genitourinary system
Conditions classifiable to N30-N99
Coding Clinic: 2016, Q4, P77

Z84.3   Family history of consanguinity

● Z84.8   Family history of other specified conditions

Z84.81   Family history of carrier of genetic disease
Coding Clinic: 2021, Q1, P15

Z84.82   Family history of sudden infant death syndrome
Family history of SIDS

Z84.89   Family history of other specified conditions

● **Z85   Personal history of malignant neoplasm**

Code first any follow-up examination after treatment of malignant neoplasm (Z08)

Use additional code to identify:

alcohol use and dependence (F10.-)

exposure to environmental tobacco smoke (Z77.22)

history of tobacco dependence (Z87.891)

occupational exposure to environmental tobacco smoke (Z57.31)

tobacco dependence (F17.-)

tobacco use (Z72.0)

Excludes2   personal history of benign neoplasm (Z86.01-)
personal history of carcinoma-in-situ (Z86.00-)

● **Z85.0   Personal history of malignant neoplasm of digestive organs**

     Z85.00   Personal history of malignant neoplasm of unspecified digestive organ

     Z85.01   Personal history of malignant neoplasm of esophagus
           Conditions classifiable to C15

●   **Z85.02   Personal history of malignant neoplasm of stomach**

         Z85.020   Personal history of malignant carcinoid tumor of stomach
              Conditions classifiable to C7A.092

         Z85.028   Personal history of other malignant neoplasm of stomach
              Conditions classifiable to C16

●   **Z85.03   Personal history of malignant neoplasm of large intestine**

         Z85.030   Personal history of malignant carcinoid tumor of large intestine
              Conditions classifiable to C7A.022-C7A.025, C7A.029

         Z85.038   Personal history of other malignant neoplasm of large intestine
              Conditions classifiable to C18

●   **Z85.04   Personal history of malignant neoplasm of rectum, rectosigmoid junction, and anus**

         Z85.040   Personal history of malignant carcinoid tumor of rectum
              Conditions classifiable to C7A.026

         Z85.048   Personal history of other malignant neoplasm of rectum, rectosigmoid junction, and anus
              Conditions classifiable to C19-C21

     Z85.05   Personal history of malignant neoplasm of liver
           Conditions classifiable to C22

●   **Z85.06   Personal history of malignant neoplasm of small intestine**

         Z85.060   Personal history of malignant carcinoid tumor of small intestine
              Conditions classifiable to C7A.01-

         Z85.068   Personal history of other malignant neoplasm of small intestine
              Conditions classifiable to C17

     Z85.07   Personal history of malignant neoplasm of pancreas
           Conditions classifiable to C25

     Z85.09   Personal history of malignant neoplasm of other digestive organs

● **Z85.1   Personal history of malignant neoplasm of trachea, bronchus and lung**

●   **Z85.11   Personal history of malignant neoplasm of bronchus and lung**

         Z85.110   Personal history of malignant carcinoid tumor of bronchus and lung
              Conditions classifiable to C7A.090

         Z85.118   Personal history of other malignant neoplasm of bronchus and lung
              Conditions classifiable to C34

     Z85.12   Personal history of malignant neoplasm of trachea
           Conditions classifiable to C33

● **Z85.2   Personal history of malignant neoplasm of other respiratory and intrathoracic organs**

     Z85.20   Personal history of malignant neoplasm of unspecified respiratory organ

     Z85.21   Personal history of malignant neoplasm of larynx
           Conditions classifiable to C32

     Z85.22   Personal history of malignant neoplasm of nasal cavities, middle ear, and accessory sinuses
           Conditions classifiable to C30-C31

●   **Z85.23   Personal history of malignant neoplasm of thymus**

         Z85.230   Personal history of malignant carcinoid tumor of thymus
              Conditions classifiable to C7A.091

         Z85.238   Personal history of other malignant neoplasm of thymus
              Conditions classifiable to C37

     Z85.29   Personal history of malignant neoplasm of other respiratory and intrathoracic organs

Z85.3   Personal history of malignant neoplasm of breast
      Conditions classifiable to C50.-

● **Z85.4   Personal history of malignant neoplasm of genital organs**
      Conditions classifiable to C51-C63

     Z85.40   Personal history of malignant neoplasm of unspecified female genital organ ♀

     Z85.41   Personal history of malignant neoplasm of cervix uteri ♀

     Z85.42   Personal history of malignant neoplasm of other parts of uterus ♀

     Z85.43   Personal history of malignant neoplasm of ovary ♀

     Z85.44   Personal history of malignant neoplasm of other female genital organs ♀

     Z85.45   Personal history of malignant neoplasm of unspecified male genital organ ♂

     Z85.46   Personal history of malignant neoplasm of prostate ♂

     Z85.47   Personal history of malignant neoplasm of testis ♂

     Z85.48   Personal history of malignant neoplasm of epididymis ♂

     Z85.49   Personal history of malignant neoplasm of other male genital organs ♂

● **Z85.5   Personal history of malignant neoplasm of urinary tract**
      Conditions classifiable to C64-C68

     Z85.50   Personal history of malignant neoplasm of unspecified urinary tract organ

     Z85.51   Personal history of malignant neoplasm of bladder

●   **Z85.52   Personal history of malignant neoplasm of kidney**

         Excludes1   personal history of malignant neoplasm of renal pelvis (Z85.53)

         Z85.520   Personal history of malignant carcinoid tumor of kidney
              Conditions classifiable to C7A.093

         Z85.528   Personal history of other malignant neoplasm of kidney
              Conditions classifiable to C64

     Z85.53   Personal history of malignant neoplasm of renal pelvis

     Z85.54   Personal history of malignant neoplasm of ureter

     Z85.59   Personal history of malignant neoplasm of other urinary tract organ

▶ New   ⇒ Revised   ~~deleted~~ Deleted   Excludes 1   Excludes 2   Includes   Use additional   Code first   Code also   Key words

OGCR Official Guidelines   X Assign placeholder X   ● Use Additional Character(s)   ⟩ Manifestation Code   🔖 Hierarchical Condition Category   **Coding Clinic**

Z85.6   Personal history of leukemia
Conditions classifiable to C91-C95

     Excludes1   leukemia in remission C91.0-C95.9 with
5th character 1

● **Z85.7**   Personal history of other malignant neoplasms of
lymphoid, hematopoietic and related tissues

     Z85.71   Personal history of Hodgkin lymphoma
Conditions classifiable to C81

     Z85.72   Personal history of non-Hodgkin lymphomas
Conditions classifiable to C82-C85

     Z85.79   Personal history of other malignant neoplasms
of lymphoid, hematopoietic and related tissues
Conditions classifiable to C88-C90, C96

       Excludes1   multiple myeloma in remission
(C90.01)
plasma cell leukemia in
remission (C90.11)
plasmacytoma in remission
(C90.21)

● **Z85.8**   Personal history of malignant neoplasms of other organs
and systems
Conditions classifiable to C00-C14, C40-C49, C69-C75,
C7A.098, C76-C79

   ● **Z85.81**   Personal history of malignant neoplasm of lip,
oral cavity, and pharynx
Conditions classifiable to C00-C14

     Z85.810   Personal history of malignant
neoplasm of tongue

     Z85.818   Personal history of malignant
neoplasm of other sites of lip, oral
cavity, and pharynx

     Z85.819   Personal history of malignant
neoplasm of unspecified site of lip,
oral cavity, and pharynx

   ● **Z85.82**   Personal history of malignant neoplasm of skin

     Z85.820   Personal history of malignant
melanoma of skin
Conditions classifiable to C43

     Z85.821   Personal history of Merkel cell
carcinoma
Conditions classifiable to C4A

     Z85.828   Personal history of other malignant
neoplasm of skin
Conditions classifiable to C44

   ● **Z85.83**   Personal history of malignant neoplasm of
bone and soft tissue
Conditions classifiable to C40-C41; C45-C49

     Z85.830   Personal history of malignant
neoplasm of bone

     Z85.831   Personal history of malignant
neoplasm of soft tissue

       Excludes2   personal history
of malignant
neoplasm of skin
(Z85.82-)

   ● **Z85.84**   Personal history of malignant neoplasm of eye
and nervous tissue
Conditions classifiable to C69-C72

     Z85.840   Personal history of malignant
neoplasm of eye

     Z85.841   Personal history of malignant
neoplasm of brain

     Z85.848   Personal history of malignant
neoplasm of other parts of nervous
tissue

   ● **Z85.85**   Personal history of malignant neoplasm of
endocrine glands
Conditions classifiable to C73-C75

     Z85.850   Personal history of malignant
neoplasm of thyroid

     Z85.858   Personal history of malignant
neoplasm of other endocrine glands

   Z85.89   Personal history of malignant neoplasm of
other organs and systems
Conditions classifiable to C7A.098, C76,
C77-C79

Z85.9   Personal history of malignant neoplasm, unspecified
Conditions classifiable to C7A.00, C80.1

● **Z86**   Personal history of certain other diseases

Code first any follow-up examination after treatment (Z09)

   ● **Z86.0**   Personal history of in-situ and benign neoplasms and
neoplasms of uncertain behavior

     Excludes2   personal history of malignant neoplasms
(Z85.-)

   ● **Z86.00**   Personal history of in-situ neoplasm
Conditions classifiable to D00-D09

     Z86.000   Personal history of in-situ neoplasm
of breast
Conditions classifiable to D05

     Z86.001   Personal history of in-situ neoplasm
of cervix uteri ♀
Conditions classifiable to D06
Personal history of cervical
intraepithelial neoplasia III
[CIN III]

     Z86.002   Personal history of in-situ neoplasm of
other and unspecified genital organs
Conditions classifiable to D07
Personal history of high-grade
prostatic intraepithelial
neoplasia III [HGPIN III]
Personal history of vaginal
intraepithelial neoplasia III
[VAIN III]
Personal history of vulvar
intraepithelial neoplasia III
[VIN III]

     Z86.003   Personal history of in-situ neoplasm
of oral cavity, esophagus and stomach
Conditions classifiable to D00

     Z86.004   Personal history of in-situ neoplasm
of other and unspecified digestive
organs
Conditions classifiable to D01
Personal history of anal intraepithelial
neoplasia (AIN III)

     Z86.005   Personal history of in-situ neoplasm
of middle ear and respiratory system
Conditions classifiable to D02

     Z86.006   Personal history of melanoma in-situ
Conditions classifiable to D03

       Excludes2   sites other than skin -
code to personal
history of in-situ
neoplasm of the
site

     Z86.007   Personal history of in-situ neoplasm
of skin
Conditions classifiable to D04
Personal history of carcinoma in situ
of skin

     Z86.008   Personal history of in-situ neoplasm
of other site
Conditions classifiable to D09

   ● **Z86.01**   Personal history of benign neoplasm
Coding Clinic: 2017, Q1, P14

     Z86.010   Personal history of colonic polyps
Coding Clinic: 2021, Q1, P15; 2017, Q1, P9,
P14

     Z86.011   Personal history of benign neoplasm
of the brain

Z86.012   **Personal history of benign carcinoid tumor**

Z86.018   **Personal history of other benign neoplasm**
Coding Clinic: 2017, Q1, P14

Z86.03   **Personal history of neoplasm of uncertain behavior**

● Z86.1   **Personal history of infectious and parasitic diseases**
Conditions classifiable to A00-B89, B99

Excludes1   personal history of infectious diseases specific to a body system sequelae of infectious and parasitic diseases (B90-B94)
Coding Clinic: 2016, Q4, P5

Z86.11   **Personal history of tuberculosis**

Z86.12   **Personal history of poliomyelitis**

Z86.13   **Personal history of malaria**

Z86.14   **Personal history of Methicillin resistant Staphylococcus aureus infection**
Personal history of MRSA infection

Z86.15   **Personal history of latent tuberculosis infection**

Z86.16   **Personal history of COVID-19**
Excludes1   post COVID-19 condition (U09.9)
Coding Clinic: 2021, Q4, P103-105, 107-108; 2021, Q1, P34-35, 40-42, 44, 46

Z86.19   **Personal history of other infectious and parasitic diseases**
Coding Clinic: 2021, Q1, P34-35, 40-41

Z86.2   **Personal history of diseases of the blood and blood-forming organs and certain disorders involving the immune mechanism**
Conditions classifiable to D50-D89

● Z86.3   **Personal history of endocrine, nutritional and metabolic diseases**
Conditions classifiable to E00-E88

Z86.31   **Personal history of diabetic foot ulcer**
Excludes2   current diabetic foot ulcer (E08.621, E09.621, E10.621, E11.621, E13.621)

Z86.32   **Personal history of gestational diabetes** ♀
Personal history of conditions classifiable to O24.4-
Excludes1   gestational diabetes mellitus in current pregnancy (O24.4-)

Z86.39   **Personal history of other endocrine, nutritional and metabolic disease**
Coding Clinic: 2020, Q1, P13

● Z86.5   **Personal history of mental and behavioral disorders**
Conditions classifiable to F40-F59

Z86.51   **Personal history of combat and operational stress reaction**   A

Z86.59   **Personal history of other mental and behavioral disorders**

● Z86.6   **Personal history of diseases of the nervous system and sense organs**
Conditions classifiable to G00-G99, H00-H95

Z86.61   **Personal history of infections of the central nervous system**
Personal history of encephalitis
Personal history of meningitis

Z86.69   **Personal history of other diseases of the nervous system and sense organs**
Coding Clinic: 2016, Q4, P25

● Z86.7   **Personal history of diseases of the circulatory system**
Conditions classifiable to I00-I99
Excludes2   old myocardial infarction (I25.2)
personal history of anaphylactic shock (Z87.892)
postmyocardial infarction syndrome (I24.1)

● Z86.71   **Personal history of venous thrombosis and embolism**

Z86.711   **Personal history of pulmonary embolism**

Z86.718   **Personal history of other venous thrombosis and embolism**

Z86.72   **Personal history of thrombophlebitis**

Z86.73   **Personal history of transient ischemic attack (TIA), and cerebral infarction without residual deficits**
Personal history of prolonged reversible ischemic neurological deficit (PRIND)
Personal history of stroke NOS without residual deficits
Excludes1   personal history of traumatic brain injury (Z87.820)
sequelae of cerebrovascular disease (I69.-)
Coding Clinic: 2012, Q4, P3

Z86.74   **Personal history of sudden cardiac arrest**
Personal history of sudden cardiac death successfully resuscitated

Z86.79   **Personal history of other diseases of the circulatory system**
Coding Clinic: 2022, Q2, P15; 2020, Q1, P13

● Z87   **Personal history of other diseases and conditions**
Code first any follow-up examination after treatment (Z09)

● Z87.0   **Personal history of diseases of the respiratory system**
Conditions classifiable to J00-J99

Z87.01   **Personal history of pneumonia (recurrent)**

Z87.09   **Personal history of other diseases of the respiratory system**

● Z87.1   **Personal history of diseases of the digestive system**
Conditions classifiable to K00-K93

Z87.11   **Personal history of peptic ulcer disease**

Z87.19   **Personal history of other diseases of the digestive system**
Coding Clinic: 2017, Q1, P14

Z87.2   **Personal history of diseases of the skin and subcutaneous tissue**
Conditions classifiable to L00-L99
Excludes2   personal history of diabetic foot ulcer (Z86.31)

● Z87.3   **Personal history of diseases of the musculoskeletal system and connective tissue**
Conditions classifiable to M00-M99
Excludes2   personal history of (healed) traumatic fracture (Z87.81)

● Z87.31   **Personal history of (healed) nontraumatic fracture**

Z87.310   **Personal history of (healed) osteoporosis fracture**
Personal history of (healed) fragility fracture
Personal history of (healed) collapsed vertebra due to osteoporosis

Z87.311   **Personal history of (healed) other pathological fracture**
Personal history of (healed) collapsed vertebra NOS
Excludes2   personal history of osteoporosis fracture (Z87.310)

Z87.312   **Personal history of (healed) stress fracture**
Personal history of (healed) fatigue fracture

Z87.39   **Personal history of other diseases of the musculoskeletal system and connective tissue**

CHAPTER 21 (Z00-Z99)

▶ New   ⇏ Revised   ~~deleted~~ Deleted   Excludes 1   Excludes 2   Includes   Use additional   Code first   Code also   Key words
OGCR Official Guidelines   X Assign placeholder X   ● Use Additional Character(s)   ▌ Manifestation Code   ✎ Hierarchical Condition Category   Coding Clinic

● **Z87.4** **Personal history of diseases of genitourinary system**
Conditions classifiable to N00-N99

● **Z87.41** **Personal history of dysplasia of the female genital tract**

> **Excludes1** personal history of intraepithelial neoplasia III of female genital tract (Z86.001, Z86.008)
> personal history of malignant neoplasm of female genital tract (Z85.40-Z85.44)

Z87.410 **Personal history of cervical dysplasia** ♀

Z87.411 **Personal history of vaginal dysplasia** ♀

Z87.412 **Personal history of vulvar dysplasia** ♀

Z87.42 **Personal history of other diseases of the female genital tract** ♀

● **Z87.43** **Personal history of diseases of male genital organs**

Z87.430 **Personal history of prostatic dysplasia** ♂

> **Excludes1** personal history of malignant neoplasm of prostate (Z85.46)

Z87.438 **Personal history of other diseases of male genital organs** ♂

● **Z87.44** **Personal history of diseases of urinary system**

> **Excludes1** personal history of malignant neoplasm of cervix uteri (Z85.41)

Z87.440 **Personal history of urinary (tract) infections**

Z87.441 **Personal history of nephrotic syndrome**

Z87.442 **Personal history of urinary calculi**
Personal history of kidney stones

Z87.448 **Personal history of other diseases of urinary system**

● **Z87.5** **Personal history of complications of pregnancy, childbirth and the puerperium**
Conditions classifiable to O00-O9A

> **Excludes2** recurrent pregnancy loss (N96)

Z87.51 **Personal history of pre-term labor** ♀

> **Excludes1** current pregnancy with history of pre-term labor (O09.21-)

Z87.59 **Personal history of other complications of pregnancy, childbirth and the puerperium** ♀
Personal history of trophoblastic disease

▶ ● **Z87.6** **Personal history of certain (corrected) conditions arising in the perinatal period**
▶ Conditions classifiable to P00-P96

> ▶ **Excludes1** personal history of (corrected) congenital malformations (Z87.7-)

▶ Z87.61 **Personal history of (corrected) necrotizing enterocolitis of newborn**

▶ Z87.68 **Personal history of other (corrected) conditions arising in the perinatal period**

● **Z87.7** **Personal history of (corrected) congenital malformations**
Conditions classifiable to Q00-Q89 that have been repaired or corrected

> **Excludes1** congenital malformations that have been partially corrected or repair but which still require medical treatment - code to condition

> **Excludes2** other postprocedural states (Z98.-)
> personal history of medical treatment (Z92.-)
> presence of cardiac and vascular implants and grafts (Z95.-)
> presence of other devices (Z97.-)
> presence of other functional implants (Z96.-)
> transplanted organ and tissue status (Z94.-)

● **Z87.71** **Personal history of (corrected) congenital malformations of genitourinary system**

Z87.710 **Personal history of (corrected) hypospadias** ♂

Z87.718 **Personal history of other specified (corrected) congenital malformations of genitourinary system**

● **Z87.72** **Personal history of (corrected) congenital malformations of nervous system and sense organs**

Z87.720 **Personal history of (corrected) congenital malformations of eye**

Z87.721 **Personal history of (corrected) congenital malformations of ear**

Z87.728 **Personal history of other specified (corrected) congenital malformations of nervous system and sense organs**

● **Z87.73** **Personal history of (corrected) congenital malformations of digestive system**

Z87.730 **Personal history of (corrected) cleft lip and palate**

▶ Z87.731 **Personal history of (corrected) tracheoesophageal fistula or atresia**

▶ Z87.732 **Personal history of (corrected) persistent cloaca or cloacal malformations**

Z87.738 **Personal history of other specified (corrected) congenital malformations of digestive system**

Z87.74 **Personal history of (corrected) congenital malformations of heart and circulatory system**

Z87.75 **Personal history of (corrected) congenital malformations of respiratory system**

● **Z87.76** **Personal history of (corrected) congenital malformations of integument, limbs and musculoskeletal system**

▶ Z87.760 **Personal history of (corrected) congenital diaphragmatic hernia or other congenital diaphragm malformations**

▶ Z87.761 **Personal history of (corrected) gastroschisis**

▶ Z87.762 **Personal history of (corrected) prune belly malformation**

▶ Z87.763 **Personal history of other (corrected) congenital abdominal wall malformations**

▶ Z87.768 **Personal history of other specified (corrected) congenital malformations of integument, limbs and musculoskeletal system**

● **Z87.79** **Personal history of other (corrected) congenital malformations**

Z87.790 **Personal history of (corrected) congenital malformations of face and neck**

Z87.798 **Personal history of other (corrected) congenital malformations**

● **Z87.8** **Personal history of other specified conditions**

> **Excludes2** personal history of self harm (Z91.5-)

Z87.81 **Personal history of (healed) traumatic fracture**

> **Excludes2** personal history of (healed) nontraumatic fracture (Z87.31-)

CHAPTER 21 (Z00-Z99)

CHAPTER 21 (Z00-Z99)

● **Z87.82** **Personal history of other (healed) physical injury and trauma**
Conditions classifiable to S00-T88, except traumatic fractures

Z87.820 **Personal history of traumatic brain injury**
Excludes1 personal history of transient ischemic attack (TIA), and cerebral infarction without residual deficits (Z86.73)

Z87.821 **Personal history of retained foreign body fully removed**

Z87.828 **Personal history of other (healed) physical injury and trauma**

● **Z87.89** **Personal history of other specified conditions**

Z87.890 **Personal history of sex reassignment**

Z87.891 **Personal history of nicotine dependence**
Excludes1 current nicotine dependence (F17.2-)
Coding Clinic: 2017, Q2, P27

Z87.892 **Personal history of anaphylaxis**
Code also allergy status such as:
allergy status to drugs, medicaments and biological substances (Z88.-)
allergy status, other than to drugs and biological substances (Z91.0-)

Z87.898 **Personal history of other specified conditions**
Coding Clinic: 2013, Q1, P21

● **Z88** **Allergy status to drugs, medicaments and biological substances**
Excludes2 allergy status, other than to drugs and biological substances (Z91.0-)

Z88.0 **Allergy status to penicillin**

Z88.1 **Allergy status to other antibiotic agents**

Z88.2 **Allergy status to sulfonamides**
Coding Clinic: 2015, Q3, P23

Z88.3 **Allergy status to other anti-infective agents**

Z88.4 **Allergy status to anesthetic agent**

Z88.5 **Allergy status to narcotic agent**

Z88.6 **Allergy status to analgesic agent**

Z88.7 **Allergy status to serum and vaccine**

Z88.8 **Allergy status to other drugs, medicaments and biological substances**

Z88.9 **Allergy status to unspecified drugs, medicaments and biological substances**

● **Z89** **Acquired absence of limb**
Includes amputation status
postprocedural loss of limb
post-traumatic loss of limb
Excludes1 acquired deformities of limbs (M20-M21)
congenital absence of limbs (Q71-Q73)

● **Z89.0** **Acquired absence of thumb and other finger(s)**

● **Z89.01** **Acquired absence of thumb**
Z89.011 **Acquired absence of right thumb**
Z89.012 **Acquired absence of left thumb**
Z89.019 **Acquired absence of unspecified thumb**

● **Z89.02** **Acquired absence of other finger(s)**
Excludes2 acquired absence of thumb (Z89.01-)
Z89.021 **Acquired absence of right finger(s)**

Z89.022 **Acquired absence of left finger(s)**
Z89.029 **Acquired absence of unspecified finger(s)**

● **Z89.1** **Acquired absence of hand and wrist**
● **Z89.11** **Acquired absence of hand**
Z89.111 **Acquired absence of right hand**
Z89.112 **Acquired absence of left hand**
Z89.119 **Acquired absence of unspecified hand**

● **Z89.12** **Acquired absence of wrist**
Disarticulation at wrist
Z89.121 **Acquired absence of right wrist**
Z89.122 **Acquired absence of left wrist**
Z89.129 **Acquired absence of unspecified wrist**

● **Z89.2** **Acquired absence of upper limb above wrist**
● **Z89.20** **Acquired absence of upper limb, unspecified level**
Z89.201 **Acquired absence of right upper limb, unspecified level**
Z89.202 **Acquired absence of left upper limb, unspecified level**
Z89.209 **Acquired absence of unspecified upper limb, unspecified level**
Acquired absence of arm NOS

● **Z89.21** **Acquired absence of upper limb below elbow**
Z89.211 **Acquired absence of right upper limb below elbow**
Z89.212 **Acquired absence of left upper limb below elbow**
Z89.219 **Acquired absence of unspecified upper limb below elbow**

● **Z89.22** **Acquired absence of upper limb above elbow**
Disarticulation at elbow
Z89.221 **Acquired absence of right upper limb above elbow**
Z89.222 **Acquired absence of left upper limb above elbow**
Z89.229 **Acquired absence of unspecified upper limb above elbow**

● **Z89.23** **Acquired absence of shoulder**
Acquired absence of shoulder joint following explantation of shoulder joint prosthesis, with or without presence of antibiotic-impregnated cement spacer
Z89.231 **Acquired absence of right shoulder**
Z89.232 **Acquired absence of left shoulder**
Z89.239 **Acquired absence of unspecified shoulder**

● **Z89.4** **Acquired absence of toe(s), foot, and ankle**
● **Z89.41** **Acquired absence of great toe**
Z89.411 **Acquired absence of right great toe** 🏷
Z89.412 **Acquired absence of left great toe** 🏷
Z89.419 **Acquired absence of unspecified great toe** 🏷

● **Z89.42** **Acquired absence of other toe(s)**
Excludes2 acquired absence of great toe (Z89.41-)
Z89.421 **Acquired absence of other right toe(s)** 🏷
Z89.422 **Acquired absence of other left toe(s)** 🏷
Z89.429 **Acquired absence of other toe(s), unspecified side** 🏷

● **Z89.43** **Acquired absence of foot**
Z89.431 **Acquired absence of right foot** 🏷
Z89.432 **Acquired absence of left foot** 🏷
Z89.439 **Acquired absence of unspecified foot** 🏷

▶ New   ⇒ Revised   ~~deleted~~ Deleted   Excludes 1   Excludes 2   Includes   Use additional   Code first   Code also   Key words
OGCR Official Guidelines   X Assign placeholder X   ● Use Additional Character(s)   ▶ Manifestation Code   🏷 Hierarchical Condition Category   Coding Clinic

● **Z89.44   Acquired absence of** ankle
Disarticulation of ankle

Z89.441   **Acquired absence of** right ankle 🔖

Z89.442   **Acquired absence of** left ankle 🔖

Z89.449   **Acquired absence of** unspecified
ankle 🔖

● **Z89.5   Acquired absence of** leg below knee

● **Z89.51   Acquired absence of** leg below knee

Z89.511   **Acquired absence of** right leg below
knee 🔖

Z89.512   **Acquired absence of** left leg below
knee 🔖

Z89.519   **Acquired absence of** unspecified leg
below knee 🔖

● **Z89.52   Acquired absence of** knee
Acquired absence of knee joint following
explantation of knee joint prosthesis,
with or without presence of antibiotic-
impregnated cement spacer

Z89.521   **Acquired absence of** right knee

Z89.522   **Acquired absence of** left knee

Z89.529   **Acquired absence of** unspecified knee

● **Z89.6   Acquired absence of** leg above knee

● **Z89.61   Acquired absence of** leg above knee
Acquired absence of leg NOS
Disarticulation at knee

Z89.611   **Acquired absence of** right leg above
knee 🔖

Z89.612   **Acquired absence of** left leg above
knee 🔖

Z89.619   **Acquired absence of** unspecified leg
above knee 🔖

● **Z89.62   Acquired absence of** hip
Acquired absence of hip joint following
explantation of hip joint prosthesis,
with or without presence of antibiotic-
impregnated cement spacer
Disarticulation at hip

Z89.621   **Acquired absence of** right hip joint

Z89.622   **Acquired absence of** left hip joint

Z89.629   **Acquired absence of** unspecified hip
joint

● **Z89.9   Acquired absence of limb, unspecified**

● **Z90   Acquired absence of organs, not elsewhere classified**

Includes   postprocedural or post-traumatic loss of body
part NEC

Excludes1   congenital absence - see Alphabetical Index

Excludes2   postprocedural absence of endocrine glands
(E89.-)

● **Z90.0   Acquired absence of** part of head and neck

Z90.01   **Acquired absence of** eye

Z90.02   **Acquired absence of** larynx

Z90.09   **Acquired absence of** other part of head and
neck
Acquired absence of nose

Excludes2   teeth (K08.1)

● **Z90.1   Acquired absence of** breast and nipple

Z90.10   **Acquired absence of** unspecified breast and
nipple

Z90.11   **Acquired absence of** right breast and nipple

Z90.12   **Acquired absence of** left breast and nipple

Z90.13   **Acquired absence of** bilateral breasts and
nipples

Z90.2   **Acquired absence of** lung [part of]

Z90.3   **Acquired absence of** stomach [part of]

● **Z90.4   Acquired absence of** other specified parts of digestive
tract

● **Z90.41   Acquired absence of** pancreas
Code also exocrine pancreatic insufficiency
(K86.81)
Use additional code to identify any associated:
diabetes mellitus, postpancreatectomy
(E13.-)
insulin use (Z79.4)

Z90.410   **Acquired total absence of pancreas**
Acquired absence of pancreas NOS

Z90.411   **Acquired partial absence of pancreas**

Z90.49   **Acquired absence of** other specified parts of
digestive tract

Z90.5   **Acquired absence of** kidney

Z90.6   **Acquired absence of** other parts of urinary tract
Acquired absence of bladder

● **Z90.7   Acquired absence of** genital organ(s)

Excludes1   personal history of sex reassignment
(Z87.890)

Excludes2   female genital mutilation status (N90.81-)

● **Z90.71   Acquired absence of** cervix and uterus

Z90.710   **Acquired absence of** both cervix and
uterus ♀
Acquired absence of uterus NOS
Status post total hysterectomy

Z90.711   **Acquired absence of** uterus with
remaining cervical stump ♀
Status post partial hysterectomy
with remaining cervical stump

Z90.712   **Acquired absence of** cervix with
remaining uterus ♀

● **Z90.72   Acquired absence of** ovaries

Z90.721   **Acquired absence of** ovaries,
unilateral ♀

Z90.722   **Acquired absence of** ovaries,
bilateral ♀

Z90.79   **Acquired absence of** other genital organ(s)

● **Z90.8   Acquired absence of other organs**

Z90.81   **Acquired absence of** spleen

Z90.89   **Acquired absence of** other organs

● **Z91   Personal risk factors, not elsewhere classified**

Excludes2   contact with and (suspected) exposures
hazardous to health (Z77.-)
exposure to pollution and other problems related
to physical environment (Z77.1-)
female genital mutilation status (N90.81-)
occupational exposure to risk factors (Z57.-)
personal history of physical injury and trauma
(Z87.81, Z87.82-)

● **Z91.0   Allergy status, other than to drugs and biological
substances**

Excludes2   allergy status to drugs, medicaments, and
biological substances (Z88.-)

● **Z91.01   Food allergy status**

Excludes2   food additives allergy status
(Z91.02)

Z91.010   **Allergy to** peanuts

Z91.011   **Allergy to** milk products

Excludes1   lactose intolerance
(E73.-)

Z91.012   **Allergy to** eggs

Z91.013   **Allergy to** seafood
Allergy to shellfish
Allergy to octopus or squid ink

Z91.014   **Allergy to** mammalian meats
Allergy to beef
Allergy to lamb
Allergy to pork
Allergy to red meats

Z91.018   **Allergy to other foods**
Allergy to nuts other than peanuts

Z91.02   **Food additives allergy status**

● **Z91.03**   **Insect allergy status**

Z91.030   **Bee allergy status**

Z91.038   **Other insect allergy status**

● **Z91.04**   **Nonmedicinal substance allergy status**

Z91.040   **Latex allergy status**
Latex sensitivity status

Z91.041   **Radiographic dye allergy status**
Allergy status to contrast media used for diagnostic X-ray procedure

Z91.048   **Other nonmedicinal substance allergy status**

Z91.09   **Other allergy status, other than to drugs and biological substances**

● **Z91.1**   **Patient's noncompliance with medical treatment and regimen**

▶ **Excludes 2**   caregiver noncompliance with patient's medical treatment and regimen (Z91.A-)

● **Z91.11**   **Patient's noncompliance with dietary regimen**
▶Code also, if applicable, food insecurity (Z59.4-)

▶ **Z91.110**   **Patient's noncompliance with dietary regimen due to financial hardship**

▶ **Z91.118**   **Patient's noncompliance with dietary regimen for other reason**
▶Inability to comply with dietary regimen

▶ **Z91.119**   **Patient's noncompliance with dietary regimen due to unspecified reason**

● **Z91.12**   **Patient's intentional underdosing of medication regimen**
Code first underdosing of medication (T36-T50) with fifth or sixth character 6

Excludes1   adverse effect of prescribed drug taken as directed - code to adverse effect
poisoning (overdose) - code to poisoning

Z91.120   **Patient's intentional underdosing of medication regimen due to financial hardship**

Z91.128   **Patient's intentional underdosing of medication regimen for other reason**

● **Z91.13**   **Patient's unintentional underdosing of medication regimen**
Code first underdosing of medication (T36-T50) with fifth or sixth character 6

Excludes1   adverse effect of prescribed drug taken as directed - code to adverse effect
poisoning (overdose) - code to poisoning

Z91.130   **Patient's unintentional underdosing of medication regimen due to age-related debility**

Z91.138   **Patient's unintentional underdosing of medication regimen for other reason**

Z91.14   **Patient's other noncompliance with medication regimen**
Patient's underdosing of medication NOS
Coding Clinic: 2022, Q1, P36

● **Z91.15**   **Patient's noncompliance with renal dialysis** 🝖

● **Z91.19**   **Patient's noncompliance with other medical treatment and regimen**
⇒Patient's nonadherence to medical treatment

▶ **Z91.190**   **Patient's noncompliance with other medical treatment and regimen due to financial hardship**

▶ **Z91.198**   **Patient's noncompliance with other medical treatment and regimen for other reason**

▶ **Z91.199**   **Patient's noncompliance with other medical treatment and regimen due to unspecified reason**

● **Z91.4**   **Personal history of psychological trauma, not elsewhere classified**

● **Z91.41**   **Personal history of adult abuse**
Excludes2   personal history of abuse in childhood (Z62.81-)

Z91.410   **Personal history of adult physical and sexual abuse**   A
Excludes1   current adult physical abuse (T74.11, T76.11)
current adult sexual abuse (T74.21, T76.11)

Z91.411   **Personal history of adult psychological abuse**   A

Z91.412   **Personal history of adult neglect**   A
Excludes1   current adult neglect (T74.01, T76.01)

Z91.419   **Personal history of unspecified adult abuse**   A

Z91.42   **Personal history of forced labor or sexual exploitation**

Z91.49   **Other personal history of psychological trauma, not elsewhere classified**

● **Z91.5**   **Personal history of self-harm**
Code also mental health disorder, if known

Z91.51   **Personal history of suicidal behavior**
Personal history of parasuicide
Personal history of self-poisoning
Personal history of suicide attempt

Z91.52   **Personal history of nonsuicidal self-harm**
Personal history of nonsuicidal self-injury
Personal history of self-inflicted injury without suicidal intent
Personal history of self-mutilation

● **Z91.8**   **Other specified personal risk factors, not elsewhere classified**

Z91.81   **History of falling**
At risk for falling

Z91.82   **Personal history of military deployment**   A
Individual (civilian or military) with past history of military war, peacekeeping and humanitarian deployment (current or past conflict)
Returned from military deployment

▷ **Z91.83**   *Wandering in diseases classified elsewhere*
Code first underlying disorder such as:
Alzheimer's disease (G30.-)
autism or pervasive developmental disorder (F84.-)
intellectual disabilities (F70-F79)
⇒unspecified dementia with behavioral disturbance (F03.9-, F03.A-, F03.B-, F03.C-)

● **Z91.84**   **Oral health risk factors**
    Z91.841   **Risk for dental caries, low**
    Z91.842   **Risk for dental caries, moderate**
    Z91.843   **Risk for dental caries, high**
    Z91.849   **Unspecified risk for dental caries**
   Z91.89   **Other specified personal risk factors, not elsewhere classified**
       Coding Clinic: 2017, Q1, P46

● **Z92**   **Personal history of medical treatment**
   Excludes2   postprocedural states (Z98.-)
  Z92.0   **Personal history of contraception**
    Excludes1   counseling or management of current contraceptive practices (Z30.-)
        long term (current) use of contraception (Z79.3)
        presence of (intrauterine) contraceptive device (Z97.5)
● **Z92.2**   **Personal history of drug therapy**
    Excludes2   long term (current) drug therapy (Z79.-)
   Z92.21   **Personal history of antineoplastic chemotherapy**
   Z92.22   **Personal history of monoclonal drug therapy**
   Z92.23   **Personal history of estrogen therapy**
● **Z92.24**   **Personal history of steroid therapy**
    Z92.240   **Personal history of inhaled steroid therapy**
    Z92.241   **Personal history of systemic steroid therapy**
        Personal history of steroid therapy NOS
   Z92.25   **Personal history of immunosuppression therapy**
     Excludes2   personal history of steroid therapy (Z92.24)
   Z92.29   **Personal history of other drug therapy**
  Z92.3   **Personal history of irradiation**
     Personal history of exposure to therapeutic radiation
    Excludes1   exposure to radiation in the physical environment (Z77.12)
        occupational exposure to radiation (Z57.1)
● **Z92.8**   **Personal history of other medical treatment**
     Coding Clinic: 2016, Q4, P72
   Z92.81   **Personal history of extracorporeal membrane oxygenation (ECMO)**
   Z92.82   **Status post administration of tPA (rtPA) in a different facility within the last 24 hours prior to admission to current facility**
     Code first condition requiring tPA administration, such as:
       acute cerebral infarction (I63.-)
       acute myocardial infarction (I21.-, I22.-)
   Z92.83   **Personal history of failed moderate sedation**
     Personal history of failed conscious sedation
     Excludes2   failed moderate sedation during procedure (T88.52)
   Z92.84   **Personal history of unintended awareness under general anesthesia**
     Excludes2   unintended awareness under general anesthesia during procedure (T88.53)
       Coding Clinic: 2016, Q4, P72, 77

● **Z92.85**   **Personal history of cellular therapy**
   Z92.850   **Personal history of Chimeric Antigen Receptor T-cell therapy**
      Personal history of CAR T-cell therapy
   Z92.858   **Personal history of other cellular therapy**
   Z92.859   **Personal history of cellular therapy, unspecified**
  Z92.86   **Personal history of gene therapy**
  Z92.89   **Personal history of other medical treatment**
     Coding Clinic: 2020, Q1, P18
▶● **Z91.A**   **Caregiver's noncompliance with patient's medical treatment and regimen**
 ▶● **Z91.A1**   **Caregiver's noncompliance with patient's dietary regimen**
   ▶ Caregiver's inability to comply with patient's dietary regimen
   ▶ Code also, if applicable, food insecurity (Z59.4-)
  ▶ **Z91.A10**   **Caregiver's noncompliance with patient's dietary regimen due to financial hardship**
  ▶ **Z91.A18**   **Caregiver's noncompliance with patient's dietary regimen for other reason**
 ▶● **Z91.A2**   **Caregiver's intentional underdosing of patient's medication regimen**
   ▶ *Code first underdosing of medication (T36-T50) with fifth or sixth character 6*
  ▶ **Z91.A20**   **Caregiver's intentional underdosing of patient's medication regimen due to financial hardship**
  ▶ **Z91.A28**   **Caregiver's intentional underdosing of medication regimen for other reason**
 ▶ **Z91.A3**   **Caregiver's unintentional underdosing of patient's medication regimen**
   ▶ *Code first underdosing of medication (T36-T50) with fifth or sixth character 6*
 ▶ **Z91.A4**   **Caregiver's other noncompliance with patient's medication regimen**
   ▶ Caregiver's underdosing of patient's medication NOS
 ▶ **Z91.A5**   **Caregiver's noncompliance with patient's renal dialysis**
 ▶ **Z91.A9**   **Caregiver's noncompliance with patient's other medical treatment and regimen**
   ▶ Caregiver's nonadherence to patient's medical treatment

● **Z93**   **Artificial opening status**
   Excludes1   artificial openings requiring attention or management (Z43.-)
       complications of external stoma (J95.0-, K94.-, N99.5-)
   Z93.0   **Tracheostomy status** 🐾
   Z93.1   **Gastrostomy status** 🐾
   Z93.2   **Ileostomy status** 🐾
   Z93.3   **Colostomy status** 🐾
   Z93.4   **Other artificial openings of gastrointestinal tract status** 🐾
● **Z93.5**   **Cystostomy status**
   Z93.50   **Unspecified cystostomy status** 🐾
   Z93.51   **Cutaneous-vesicostomy status** 🐾
   Z93.52   **Appendico-vesicostomy status** 🐾
   Z93.59   **Other cystostomy status** 🐾

CHAPTER 21 (Z00-Z99)

Z93.6   Other artificial openings of urinary tract status 🗝
        Nephrostomy status
        Ureterostomy status
        Urethrostomy status

Z93.8   Other artificial opening status 🗝

Z93.9   Artificial opening status, unspecified 🗝

● **Z94**   Transplanted organ and tissue status

     Includes   organ or tissue replaced by heterogenous or homogenous transplant

     Excludes1   complications of transplanted organ or tissue - see Alphabetical Index

     Excludes2   presence of vascular grafts (Z95.-)

Z94.0   Kidney transplant status

Z94.1   Heart transplant status 🗝

     Excludes1   artificial heart status (Z95.812)
                 heart-valve replacement status (Z95.2-Z95.4)

Z94.2   Lung transplant status 🗝

Z94.3   Heart and lungs transplant status 🗝

Z94.4   Liver transplant status 🗝

Z94.5   Skin transplant status
        Autogenous skin transplant status

Z94.6   Bone transplant status

Z94.7   Corneal transplant status

● **Z94.8**   Other transplanted organ and tissue status

     Z94.81   Bone marrow transplant status 🗝

     Z94.82   Intestine transplant status 🗝

     Z94.83   Pancreas transplant status 🗝

     Z94.84   Stem cells transplant status 🗝

     Z94.89   Other transplanted organ and tissue status

Z94.9   Transplanted organ and tissue status, unspecified

● **Z95**   Presence of cardiac and vascular implants and grafts

     Excludes2   complications of cardiac and vascular devices, implants and grafts (T82.-)

Z95.0   Presence of cardiac pacemaker
        Presence of cardiac resynchronization therapy (CRT-P) pacemaker

     Excludes1   adjustment or management of cardiac device (Z45.0-)
                 adjustment or management of cardiac pacemaker (Z45.0)
                 presence of automatic (implantable) cardiac defibrillator with synchronous cardiac pacemaker (Z95.810)

      Coding Clinic: 2019, Q1, P33

Z95.1   Presence of aortocoronary bypass graft
        Presence of coronary artery bypass graft

Z95.2   Presence of prosthetic heart valve
        Presence of heart valve NOS

Z95.3   Presence of xenogenic heart valve

Z95.4   Presence of other heart-valve replacement

Z95.5   Presence of coronary angioplasty implant and graft

     Excludes1   coronary angioplasty status without implant and graft (Z98.61)

● **Z95.8**   Presence of other cardiac and vascular implants and grafts

    ● **Z95.81**   Presence of other cardiac implants and grafts

         Z95.810   Presence of automatic (implantable) cardiac defibrillator
                Presence of automatic (implantable) cardiac defibrillator with synchronous cardiac pacemaker
                Presence of cardiac resynchronization therapy defibrillator (CRT-D)
                Presence of cardioverter-defibrillator (ICD)

          Coding Clinic: 2022, Q2, P15

     Z95.811   Presence of heart assist device 🗝

     Z95.812   Presence of fully implantable artificial heart 🗝

     Z95.818   Presence of other cardiac implants and grafts

    ● **Z95.82**   Presence of other vascular implants and grafts

         Z95.820   Peripheral vascular angioplasty status with implants and grafts

           Excludes1   peripheral vascular angioplasty without implant and graft (Z98.62)

         Z95.828   Presence of other vascular implants and grafts
             Presence of intravascular prosthesis NEC

Z95.9   Presence of cardiac and vascular implant and graft, unspecified

● **Z96**   Presence of other functional implants

     Excludes2   complications of internal prosthetic devices, implants and grafts (T82-T85)
                 fitting and adjustment of prosthetic and other devices (Z44-Z46)

Z96.0   Presence of urogenital implants

Z96.1   Presence of intraocular lens
        Presence of pseudophakia

● **Z96.2**   Presence of otological and audiological implants

     Z96.20   Presence of otological and audiological implant, unspecified

     Z96.21   Cochlear implant status

     Z96.22   Myringotomy tube(s) status

     Z96.29   Presence of other otological and audiological implants
            Presence of bone-conduction hearing device
            Presence of eustachian tube stent
            Stapes replacement

Z96.3   Presence of artificial larynx

● **Z96.4**   Presence of endocrine implants

     Z96.41   Presence of insulin pump (external) (internal)

     Z96.49   Presence of other endocrine implants

Z96.5   Presence of tooth-root and mandibular implants

● **Z96.6**   Presence of orthopedic joint implants

     Z96.60   Presence of unspecified orthopedic joint implant

    ● **Z96.61**   Presence of artificial shoulder joint

         Z96.611   Presence of right artificial shoulder joint

         Z96.612   Presence of left artificial shoulder joint

         Z96.619   Presence of unspecified artificial shoulder joint

    ● **Z96.62**   Presence of artificial elbow joint

         Z96.621   Presence of right artificial elbow joint

         Z96.622   Presence of left artificial elbow joint

         Z96.629   Presence of unspecified artificial elbow joint

    ● **Z96.63**   Presence of artificial wrist joint

         Z96.631   Presence of right artificial wrist joint

         Z96.632   Presence of left artificial wrist joint

         Z96.639   Presence of unspecified artificial wrist joint

    ● **Z96.64**   Presence of artificial hip joint
        Hip-joint replacement (partial) (total)

         Z96.641   Presence of right artificial hip joint
            Coding Clinic: 2016, Q3, P17

         Z96.642   Presence of left artificial hip joint
            Coding Clinic: 2015, Q1, P16

▶ New   ⇒ Revised   ~~deleted~~ Deleted   Excludes 1   Excludes 2   Includes   Use additional   Code first   Code also   Key words

OGCR Official Guidelines   X Assign placeholder X   ● Use Additional Character(s)   ▌ Manifestation Code   🗝 Hierarchical Condition Category   **Coding Clinic**

Z96.643   Presence of artificial hip joint, bilateral

Z96.649   Presence of unspecified artificial hip joint

● Z96.65   Presence of artificial knee joint

Z96.651   Presence of right artificial knee joint

Z96.652   Presence of left artificial knee joint
       Coding Clinic: 2019, Q3, P16

Z96.653   Presence of artificial knee joint, bilateral

Z96.659   Presence of unspecified artificial knee joint

● Z96.66   Presence of artificial ankle joint

Z96.661   Presence of right artificial ankle joint

Z96.662   Presence of left artificial ankle joint

Z96.669   Presence of unspecified artificial ankle joint

● Z96.69   Presence of other orthopedic joint implants

Z96.691   Finger-joint replacement of right hand

Z96.692   Finger-joint replacement of left hand

Z96.693   Finger-joint replacement, bilateral

Z96.698   Presence of other orthopedic joint implants

Z96.7   Presence of other bone and tendon implants
     Presence of skull plate

● Z96.8   Presence of other specified functional implants

Z96.81   Presence of artificial skin

Z96.82   Presence of neurostimulator
     Presence of brain neurostimulator
     Presence of gastric neurostimulator
     Presence of peripheral nerve neurostimulator
     Presence of sacral nerve neurostimulator
     Presence of spinal cord neurostimulator
     Presence of vagus nerve neurostimulator

Z96.89   Presence of other specified functional implants

Z96.9   Presence of functional implant, unspecified

● Z97   **Presence of other devices**

Excludes2   fitting and adjustment of prosthetic and other devices (Z44-Z46)
     presence of cerebrospinal fluid drainage device (Z98.2)

Z97.0   Presence of artificial eye

● Z97.1   Presence of artificial limb (complete) (partial)

Z97.10   Presence of artificial limb (complete) (partial), unspecified

Z97.11   Presence of artificial right arm (complete) (partial)

Z97.12   Presence of artificial left arm (complete) (partial)

Z97.13   Presence of artificial right leg (complete) (partial)

Z97.14   Presence of artificial left leg (complete) (partial)

Z97.15   Presence of artificial arms, bilateral (complete) (partial)

Z97.16   Presence of artificial legs, bilateral (complete) (partial)

Z97.2   Presence of dental prosthetic device (complete) (partial)
     Presence of dentures (complete) (partial)

Z97.3   Presence of spectacles and contact lenses

Z97.4   Presence of external hearing-aid

Z97.5   Presence of (intrauterine) contraceptive device ♀

Excludes1   checking, reinsertion or removal of implantable subdermal contraceptive (Z30.46)
     checking, reinsertion or removal of intrauterine contraceptive device (Z30.43-)

Z97.8   Presence of other specified devices

● Z98   **Other postprocedural states**

Excludes2   aftercare (Z43-Z49, Z51)
     follow-up medical care (Z08-Z09)
     postprocedural complication - see Alphabetical Index

Z98.0   Intestinal bypass and anastomosis status

Excludes2   bariatric surgery status (Z98.84)
     gastric bypass status (Z98.84)
     obesity surgery status (Z98.84)

Z98.1   Arthrodesis status

Z98.2   Presence of cerebrospinal fluid drainage device
     Presence of CSF shunt

Z98.3   Post therapeutic collapse of lung status
     Code first underlying disease

● Z98.4   Cataract extraction status
     Use additional code to identify intraocular lens implant status (Z96.1)

Excludes1   aphakia (H27.0)

Z98.41   Cataract extraction status, right eye

Z98.42   Cataract extraction status, left eye

Z98.49   Cataract extraction status, unspecified eye

● Z98.5   Sterilization status

Excludes1   female infertility (N97.-)
     male infertility (N46.-)

Z98.51   Tubal ligation status ♀

Z98.52   Vasectomy status ♂   A

● Z98.6   Angioplasty status

Z98.61   Coronary angioplasty status

Excludes1   coronary angioplasty status with implant and graft (Z95.5)

Z98.62   Peripheral vascular angioplasty status

Excludes1   peripheral vascular angioplasty status with implant and graft (Z95.820)

● Z98.8   Other specified postprocedural states
     Coding Clinic: 2016, Q4, P76

● Z98.81   Dental procedure status

Z98.810   Dental sealant status

Z98.811   Dental restoration status
     Dental crown status
     Dental fillings status

Z98.818   Other dental procedure status

Z98.82   Breast implant status

Excludes1   breast implant removal status (Z98.86)

Z98.83   Filtering (vitreous) bleb after glaucoma surgery status

Excludes1   inflammation (infection) of postprocedural bleb (H59.4-)

Z98.84   Bariatric surgery status
     Gastric banding status
     Gastric bypass status for obesity
     Obesity surgery status

Excludes1   bariatric surgery status complicating pregnancy, childbirth, or the puerperium (O99.84)

Excludes2   intestinal bypass and anastomosis status (Z98.0)

     Coding Clinic: 2020, Q1, P12

Z98.85   **Transplanted organ removal status**
Transplanted organ previously removed due to complication, failure, rejection or infection
> **Excludes1**   encounter for removal of transplanted organ - code to complication of transplanted organ (T86.-)

Z98.86   **Personal history of breast implant removal**

● **Z98.87**   **Personal history of in utero procedure**

Z98.870   **Personal history of in utero procedure during pregnancy** ♀
> **Excludes2**   complications from in utero procedure for current pregnancy (O35.7)
> supervision of current pregnancy with history of in utero procedure during previous pregnancy (O09.82-)

Z98.871   **Personal history of in utero procedure while a fetus**

● **Z98.89**   **Other specified postprocedural states**
Coding Clinic: 2016, Q4, P76

Z98.890   **Other specified postprocedural states**
Personal history of surgery, not elsewhere classified

Z98.891   **History of uterine scar from previous surgery** ♀
> **Excludes1**   Maternal care due to uterine scar from previous surgery (O34.2-)
Coding Clinic: 2016, Q4, P52, P76

● **Z99**   **Dependence on enabling machines and devices, not elsewhere classified**
Coding Clinic: 2020, Q1, P11

Z99.0   **Dependence on aspirator**

● **Z99.1**   **Dependence on respirator**
Dependence on ventilator

Z99.11   **Dependence on respirator [ventilator] status** 🦠
Coding Clinic: 2018, Q1, P14; 2015, Q1, P21

Z99.12   **Encounter for respirator [ventilator] dependence during power failure** 🦠
> **Excludes1**   mechanical complication of respirator [ventilator] (J95.850)

Z99.2   **Dependence on renal dialysis** 🦠
Hemodialysis status
Peritoneal dialysis status
Presence of arteriovenous shunt for dialysis
Renal dialysis status NOS
> **Excludes1**   encounter for fitting and adjustment of dialysis catheter (Z49.0-)
> **Excludes2**   noncompliance with renal dialysis (Z91.15)
Coding Clinic: 2016, Q1, P13

Z99.3   **Dependence on wheelchair**
Wheelchair confinement status
Code first cause of dependence, such as:
muscular dystrophy (G71.0-)
obesity (E66.-)

● **Z99.8**   **Dependence on other enabling machines and devices**

Z99.81   **Dependence on supplemental oxygen**
Dependence on long-term oxygen

Z99.89   **Dependence on other enabling machines and devices**
Dependence on machine or device NOS
Coding Clinic: 2020, Q1, P11

CHAPTER 22

CODES FOR SPECIAL PURPOSES (U00-U85)

Note: Codes from this chapter are for use on newborn records only, never on maternal records.

This chapter contains the following blocks:

U00-U49	Provisional assignment of new diseases of uncertain etiology or emergency use

---

PROVISIONAL ASSIGNMENT OF NEW DISEASES OF UNCERTAIN ETIOLOGY OR EMERGENCY USE (U00-U49)

U07　Emergency use of U07

　U07.0　Vaping-related disorder

　　　Dabbing related lung damage
　　　Dabbing related lung injury
　　　E-cigarette, or vaping, product use associated lung injury [EVALI]
　　　Electronic cigarette related lung damage
　　　Electronic cigarette related lung injury
　　　Use additional code to identify manifestations, such as:
　　　　abdominal pain (R10.84)
　　　　acute respiratory distress syndrome (J80)
　　　　diarrhea (R19.7)
　　　　drug-induced interstitial lung disorder (J70.4)
　　　　lipoid pneumonia (J69.1)
　　　　weight loss (R63.4)

U07.1　COVID-19

　Use additional code to identify pneumonia or other manifestations

　Excludes1　coronavirus infection, unspecified (B34.2)
　　　　　　coronavirus as the cause of diseases classified elsewhere (B97.2-)
　　　　　　pneumonia due to SARS-associated coronavirus (J12.81)

　Coding Clinic: 2022, Q2, P29; 2021, Q4, P109; 2021, Q1, P31-33, 36, 39-40, 47, 49

● **U09 Post COVID-19 condition**

　U09.9 Post COVID-19 condition, unspecified

　　Note: This code enables establishment of a link with COVID-19.

　　　This code is not to be used in cases that are still presenting with active COVID-19. However, an exception is made in cases of re-infection with COVID-19, occurring with a condition related to prior COVID-19.

　　Post-acute sequela of COVID-19

　　Code first the specific condition related to COVID-19 if known, such as:
　　　　chronic respiratory failure (J96.1-)
　　　　loss of smell (R43.8)
　　　　loss of taste (R43.8)
　　　　multisystem inflammatory syndrome (M35.81)
　　　　pulmonary embolism (I26.-)
　　　　pulmonary fibrosis (J84.10)

　　Coding Clinic: 2021, Q4, P102-104,106

ELSEVIER

Trust Elsevier to support ~~you~~ every step of your coding career!

From beginning to advanced, from the classroom to the workplace, from application to certiÿcation, Elsevier coding solutions are your guide to greater opportunities and successful career advancement.

 ## Step One: Lear

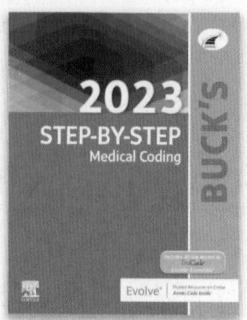

Buck's Step-by-Step Medical Coding, 2023 Editio
ISBN: 978-0-323-87412-0

Also available:

Buck's Workbook for Step-by-Step Medical Coding, 2023 Edition
ISBN: 978-0-323-87406-9

Buck's Medical Coding Online for Step-by-Step Medical Coding, 2023 Edition
ISBN: 978-0-323-87420-5

 ## Step Two: Practic

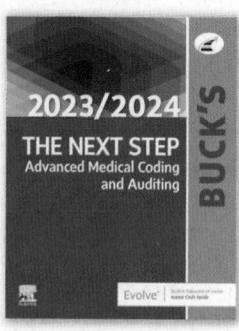

Buck's The Next Step: Advanced Medical Coding and Auditing, 2023/2024 Edition
ISBN: 978-0-323-87411-3

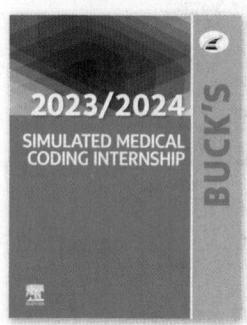

Buck's Simulated Medical Coding Internship, 2023/2024 Edition
ISBN: 978-0-323-87419-9

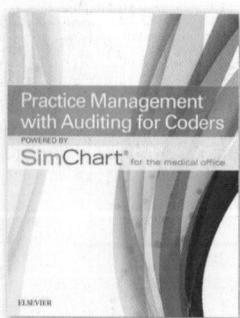

Practice Management with Auditing for Coders Powered by SimChart for the Medical Office
ISBN: 978-0-323-43011-1

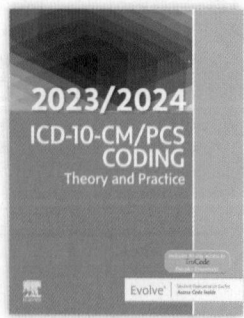

ICD-10-CM/PCS Coding: Theory and Practice, 2023/2024 Edition
ISBN: 978-0-323-87405-2